Veterinary Anesthesia and Analgesia

The Fifth Edition of Lumb and Jones

Edited by

Kurt A. Grimm

Leigh A. Lamont

William J. Tranquilli

Stephen A. Greene

and

Sheilah A. Robertson

WILEY Blackwell

Editorial Offices
1606 Golden Aspen Drive, Suites 103 and 104, Ames, Iowa 50010, USA
The Atrium, Southern Gate, Chichester, West Sussex, PO19 8SQ, UK
9600 Garsington Road, Oxford, OX4 2DQ, UK

For details of our global editorial offices, for customer services and for information about how to apply for permission to reuse the copyright material in this book please see our website at www.wiley.com/wiley-blackwell.

Library of Congress Cataloging-in-Publication Data

Veterinary anesthesia and analgesia (Grimm)
Veterinary anesthesia and analgesia / edited by Dr. Kurt A. Grimm, Dr. Leigh A. Lamont, William J. Tranquilli, Stephen A. Greene, and Sheilah A. Robertson. – Fifth edition.
p. ; cm.
Preceded by: Lumb & Jones' veterinary anesthesia and analgesia / edited by William J. Tranquilli, John C. Thurmon, and Kurt A. Grimm. 4th ed. Ames, Iowa : Blackwell Pub., c2007.
Includes bibliographical references and index.
ISBN 978-1-118-52623-1 (cloth)
1. Veterinary anesthesia. I. Grimm, Kurt A., editor. II. Lamont, Leigh A., editor. III. Tranquilli, William J., editor. IV. Greene, Stephen A., editor. V. Robertson, Sheilah A., editor. VI. Lumb & Jones' veterinary anesthesia and analgesia. Preceded by work: VII. Title.
[DNLM: 1. Anesthesia–veterinary. 2. Analgesia–veterinary. SF 914]
SF914.L82 2015
636.089'796–dc23

2014048480

A catalogue record for this book is available from the British Library.

Wiley also publishes its books in a variety of electronic formats. Some content that appears in print may not be available in electronic books.

Cover images (from left to right): Cat: Photo from iStock.com. iStock #16988839. © SondraP 6-26-11; Horse: Photo from iStock.com. iStock #14701119. © Groomes Photography 10-30-10; Goat: Photo from iStock.com. iStock #17108939. © LazingBee 7-10-11; Mouse: Photo from iStock.com. iStock #16390014. © lculig 4-26-11; Dog: Photo from iStock.com. iStock #16146668. © CountryStyle Photography 3-29-11.
Cover design by Andy Meaden

Set in 9/11pt Minion by SPi Publisher Services, Pondicherry, India

Veterinary Anesthesia and Analgesia

The Fifth Edition of Lumb and Jones

Edited by

Kurt A. Grimm

Leigh A. Lamont

William J. Tranquilli

Stephen A. Greene

and

Sheilah A. Robertson

WILEY Blackwell

Editorial Offices
1606 Golden Aspen Drive, Suites 103 and 104, Ames, Iowa 50010, USA
The Atrium, Southern Gate, Chichester, West Sussex, PO19 8SQ, UK
9600 Garsington Road, Oxford, OX4 2DQ, UK

For details of our global editorial offices, for customer services and for information about how to apply for permission to reuse the copyright material in this book please see our website at www.wiley.com/wiley-blackwell.

Library of Congress Cataloging-in-Publication Data

Veterinary anesthesia and analgesia (Grimm)
Veterinary anesthesia and analgesia / edited by Dr. Kurt A. Grimm, Dr. Leigh A. Lamont, William J. Tranquilli, Stephen A. Greene, and Sheilah A. Robertson. – Fifth edition.
p. ; cm.
Preceded by: Lumb & Jones' veterinary anesthesia and analgesia / edited by William J. Tranquilli, John C. Thurmon, and Kurt A. Grimm. 4th ed. Ames, Iowa : Blackwell Pub., c2007.
Includes bibliographical references and index.
ISBN 978-1-118-52623-1 (cloth)
1. Veterinary anesthesia. I. Grimm, Kurt A., editor. II. Lamont, Leigh A., editor. III. Tranquilli, William J., editor. IV. Greene, Stephen A., editor. V. Robertson, Sheilah A., editor. VI. Lumb & Jones' veterinary anesthesia and analgesia. Preceded by work: VII. Title.
[DNLM: 1. Anesthesia–veterinary. 2. Analgesia–veterinary. SF 914]
SF914.L82 2015
636.089'796–dc23

2014048480

A catalogue record for this book is available from the British Library.

Wiley also publishes its books in a variety of electronic formats. Some content that appears in print may not be available in electronic books.

Cover images (from left to right): Cat: Photo from iStock.com. iStock #16988839. © SondraP 6-26-11; Horse: Photo from iStock.com. iStock #14701119. © Groomes Photography 10-30-10; Goat: Photo from iStock.com. iStock #17108939. © LazingBee 7-10-11; Mouse: Photo from iStock.com. iStock #16390014. © lculig 4-26-11; Dog: Photo from iStock.com. iStock #16146668. © CountryStyle Photography 3-29-11.
Cover design by Andy Meaden

Set in 9/11pt Minion by SPi Publisher Services, Pondicherry, India

Contents

Dedication

The fifth edition of this text is dedicated to the many people who support and make up the specialty of veterinary anesthesia and analgesia including all animal care providers, veterinarians, and scientists striving to advance humane veterinary care.

The editors wish to dedicate our efforts in bringing the fifth edition of *Veterinary Anesthesia and Analgesia* to publication to our parents for imparting the values of hard work, loyalty, and patience; to our teachers and colleagues for the belief that scientific knowledge gives us the best chance to know what is real; to the animals in our care who have taught us so much; to our significant others for their support; and to those who learn from this text for making everything joyful and worthwhile.

Foreword

The extensively referenced content, important additions, and timely revisions of the fifth edition of *Veterinary Anesthesia and Analgesia* provide an impressive documentation of the basic and applied clinical science essential to the safe delivery of animal anesthesia and pain management. As such, this text continues to be the most complete source of information on this subject matter for students, practitioners, and specialists alike. The fifth edition once again sets a high standard as the most comprehensive textbook on veterinary anesthesia and analgesia within veterinary literature.

As previous editors of *Lumb and Jones' Veterinary Anesthesia*, we wish to acknowledge the efforts of the contributors, 85 in all, with special thanks to Drs. Grimm, Lamont, Tranquilli, Greene, and Robertson for assuming the editorship of such a large endeavor. As we enter the 21st century, the publication of *Veterinary Anesthesia and Analgesia: The Fifth Edition of Lumb and Jones* in 2015 serves to highlight the importance, significance, and necessity of continually improving animal anesthesia and analgesia. With their combined efforts, the contributing authors and editors have admirably upheld this text's long-standing reputation as an indispensable resource in advancing and improving animal welfare.

William Lumb
Wynn Jones
John Thurmon

Preface

The first edition of *Veterinary Anesthesia* was published in 1973; the second edition followed in 1984. The third edition, entitled *Lumb and Jones' Veterinary Anesthesia*, was published in 1996. The fourth edition was renamed *Lumb and Jones' Veterinary Anesthesia and Analgesia* and was published in 2007. Now in its 42nd year, a fifth edition of this text is available to the veterinary profession and scientific community.

Many improvements have occurred in veterinary anesthesia and analgesia in parallel with the evolution of veterinary medicine, as each succeeding edition of this text updates and documents these advances. This effort has continued within the chapters and pages of the fifth edition. As the specialty of veterinary anesthesia and analgesia has become recognized and established throughout the world, the knowledge and clinical practice of sophisticated anesthesia and analgesia is no longer defined by its initial academic beginnings. This revision, entitled *Veterinary Anesthesia and Analgesia: The Fifth Edition of Lumb and Jones*, reflects the current editors' collective view that the specialty of veterinary anesthesia and analgesia has secured a well-deserved and respected place among recognized specialties within the greater global veterinary community. This accomplishment is evidenced by the international makeup of the contributing authorship of the fifth edition and is supported by the worldwide practice of more advanced anesthesia and pain management care.

As editors, we have endeavored to provide information on multiple species and the important physiology and pharmacology for safe delivery of anesthetics and analgesics in a variety of patients and clinical conditions. The volume of space required in presenting newer knowledge and evolving issues pertinent to veterinary anesthesia and analgesia in 2015 makes the retention of much of the previous editions' text impossible. Fortunately, this information, much of which is of historical interest, remains available to interested individuals within earlier editions. As such, we wish to acknowledge the valuable contributions made by all previous authors and editors of this landmark text.

This edition has over 80 contributing authors, offering a wide range of scientific training and clinical experience. Many contributors are anesthesiologists, but a number of authors are specialists in other areas, including clinical pharmacology, surgery, medicine, critical care, cardiology, urology, and laboratory animal medicine. It is hoped that this diversity in author expertise will help provide a more comprehensive perspective when managing patients suffering from a variety of clinical conditions and diseases.

The editors of the fifth edition are indebted to the contributing authors for the many hours each devoted to the preparation of their chapters. Many of these authors have dedicated their careers to the advancement of veterinary anesthesiology, pain management, and the humane treatment of animals. In so doing, they have made numerous contributions to the advancement of veterinary medicine during their lives. Among these is Dr. Steve C. Haskins, whose unexpected passing saddened the veterinary community worldwide. His chapter contributions on anesthetic monitoring in the third, fourth, and fifth editions may be regarded as one of the most comprehensive discussions of the fundamental principles of anesthetic monitoring. Dr. Haskin's dedication to the discovery of new knowledge and his love of teaching were driven by his joy of seeing students learn. Our loss, with his passing, as with all great teachers, is immeasurable.

As the current editors, it is our hope that this revision will be viewed both as a textbook and as a comprehensive source of scientific knowledge relevant to the clinical management of anesthesia and provision of analgesic therapy. Information on the immobilization and anesthesia of wild, zoo, and laboratory animals will be found in chapters devoted to the comparative aspects of anesthesia in these species. In addition to chapters on cardiovascular, respiratory, nervous system, and acid–base physiology, the pharmacology of various classes of drugs employed in the delivery of anesthesia and analgesia has been updated. Chapters on anesthetic equipment, monitoring, and regional analgesic techniques are provided. Chapters covering anesthetic and analgesic considerations for patients undergoing renal replacement therapy, cardiac pacemaker implantation, and cardiopulmonary bypass have been added. Chapters continue to be devoted to the anesthesia of specific species and classes of animals including dogs, cats, horses, swine, ruminants, laboratory animals, zoo animals, free ranging terrestrial and aquatic mammals, birds, reptiles, amphibians, and fish. Anesthetic considerations for patients with conditions affecting specific body systems have been consolidated into single-system chapters.

We would like to personally thank the many contributing authors for their generous sharing of knowledge and our families and co-workers for allowing us the time necessary to complete this work. Finally, we thank the staff at Wiley Blackwell for their support and encouragement.

Kurt A. Grimm
Leigh A. Lamont
William J. Tranquilli
Stephen A. Greene
Sheilah A. Robertson

Contributors List

Jennifer G. Adams, DVM, DACVIM (LA), DACVAA
Hull, Georgia, USA

Jon M. Arnemo, DVM, PhD, DECZM
Hedmark University College
Campus Evenstad, Norway
Swedish University of Agricultural Sciences
Umeå, Sweden

Sébastien H. Bauquier, DMV, MANZCVS, DACVAA
Faculty of Veterinary and Agricultural Sciences, University of Melbourne
Werribee, Victoria, Australia

Richard M. Bednarski, DVM, MS, DACVAA
College of Veterinary Medicine, The Ohio State University
Columbus, Ohio, USA

Stephanie H. Berry, DVM, MS, DACVAA
Atlantic Veterinary College
University of Prince Edward Island
Charlottetown, Prince Edward Island, Canada

Thierry Beths, DVM, Cert VA, MRCVS, PhD
Faculty of Veterinary and Agricultural Sciences, University of Melbourne,
Werribee, Victoria, Australia

Regula Bettschart-Wolfensberger, Prof.Dr.med.vet., PhD, DECVAA
Vetsuisse Faculty, Section Anaesthesiology
University of Zurich
Zurich, Switzerland

Lori A. Bidwell, DVM, DACVAA
College of Veterinary Medicine
Michigan State University
East Lansing, Michigan, USA

Benjamin M. Brainard, VMD, DACVAA, DACVECC
Department of Small Animal Medicine and Surgery
College of Veterinary Medicine
University of Georgia
Athens, Georgia, USA

Dave C. Brodbelt, MA, VetMB, PhD, DVA, DECVAA, FHEA, MRCVS
Veterinary Epidemiology, Economics and Public Health Group
Royal Veterinary College
North Mymms, Hertfordshire, UK

Robert J. Brosnan, DVM, PhD, DACVAA
Department of Surgical and Radiological Sciences, School of Veterinary Medicine
University of California
Davis, California, USA

David B. Brunson, DVM, MS, DACVAA
Zoetis, LLC
Florham Park, New Jersey, USA

Steven C. Budsberg, DVM, MS, DACVS
College of Veterinary Medicine
University of Georgia
Athens, Georgia, USA

Barret J. Bulmer, DVM, MS, DACVIM-Cardiology
Tufts Veterinary Emergency Treatment and Specialties
Walpole, Massachusetts, USA

Christopher R. Byron, DVM, MS, DACVS
Virginia-Maryland College of Veterinary Medicine
Virginia Tech
Blacksburg, Virginia, USA

Luis Campoy, LV, CertVA, DECVAA, MRCVS
Department of Clinical Sciences
College of Veterinary Medicine
Cornell University
Ithaca, New York, USA

Rachael E. Carpenter, DVM
Virginia-Maryland Regional College of Veterinary Medicine
Blacksburg, Virginia, USA

Nigel Anthony Caulkett, DVM, MVetSc, DACVAA
Department of Veterinary Clinical and Diagnostic Science
University of Calgary
Calgary, Alberta, Canada

Amandeep S. Chohan, BVSc & AH, MVSc, MS, DACVAA
Veterinary Teaching Hospital
Washington State University
Pullman, Washington, USA

Stuart C. Clark-Price, DVM, MS, DACVIM(LA), DACVAA
Department of Veterinary Clinical Medicine
College of Veterinary Medicine
University of Illinois
Urbana, Illinois, USA

Elizabeth B. Davidow, DVM, DACVECC
ACCES BluePearl
Seattle, Washington, USA

Helio A. de Morais, DVM, MS, PhD, DACVIM(SA), DACVIM-Cardiology
College of Veterinary Medicine
Oregon State University
Corvallis, Oregon, USA

Timothy M. Fan, DVM, PhD, DACVIM-Oncology
Department of Veterinary Clinical Medicine
College of Veterinary Medicine
University of Illinois at Urbana-Champaign
Urbana, Illinois, USA

Juliana Peboni Figueiredo, MV, MS, DACVAA
Small Animal Medicine and Surgery Academic Program
St. George's University – School of Veterinary Medicine
Grenada, West Indies

Derek Flaherty, BVMS, DVA, DECVAA, MRCA, MRCVS
School of Veterinary Medicine
University of Glasgow
Glasgow, Scotland, UK

Paul A. Flecknell, VetMB, PhD, DECVAA, DECLAM
Institute of Neuroscience
Newcastle University
Newcastle upon Tyne, UK

Fernando Garcia-Pereira, DVM, MS, DACVAA
Large Animal Clinical Sciences
College of Veterinary Medicine
University of Florida
Gainesville, Florida, USA

Gregory F. Grauer, DVM, MS, DACVIM(SA)
Department of Clinical Sciences
College of Veterinary Medicine
Kansas State University
Manhattan, Kansas, USA

Thomas K. Graves, DVM, MS, PhD, DACVIM(SA)
College of Veterinary Medicine
Midwestern University
Glendale, Arizona, USA

Stephen A. Greene, DVM, MS, DACVAA
Washington State University, Pullman, Washington, USA

Kurt A. Grimm, DVM, MS, PhD, DACVAA, DACVCP
Veterinary Specialist Services, PC
Conifer, Colorado, USA

Marjorie E. Gross, DVM, MS, DACVAA
Oklahoma State University
Center for Veterinary Health Sciences
Stillwater, Oklahoma, USA

Tamara L. Grubb, DVM, PhD, DACVAA
Veterinary Clinical Sciences, Washington State University
Pullman, Washington, USA

Sandee M. Hartsfield, DVM, MS, DACVAA
Department of Small Animal Clinical Sciences
College of Veterinary Medicine and Biomedical Sciences
Texas A&M University
College Station, Texas, USA

Steve C. Haskins, DVM, MS, DACVAA, DACVECC
School of Veterinary Medicine, University of California
Davis, California, USA

Rebecca A. Johnson, DVM, MS, PhD, DACVAA
School of Veterinary Medicine
University of Wisconsin
Madison, Wisconsin, USA

Robert D. Keegan, DVM, DACVAA
Department of Veterinary Clinical Sciences
College of Veterinary Medicine
Washington State University
Pullman, Washington, USA

Carolyn L. Kerr, DVM, DVSc, PhD, DACVAA
Department of Clinical Studies
Ontario Veterinary College
University of Guelph
Guelph, Ontario, Canada

Butch KuKanich, DVM, PhD, DACVCP
Department of Anatomy and Physiology
College of Veterinary Medicine
Kansas State University
Manhattan, Kansas, USA

Leigh A. Lamont, DVM, MS, DACVAA
Atlantic Veterinary College, University of Prince Edward Island, Canada

Phillip Lerche, BVSc, PhD, DACVAA
Veterinary Clinical Sciences, The Ohio State University
Columbus, Ohio, USA

HuiChu Lin, DVM, MS, DACVAA
College of Veterinary Medicine, Auburn University
Auburn, Alabama, USA

Andrea L. Looney, DVM, DACVAA, DACVSMR
Massachusetts Veterinary Referral Hospital, IVG Hospitals
Woburn, Massachusetts, USA

John W. Ludders, DVM, DACVAA
College of Veterinary Medicine
Cornell University
Ithaca, New York, USA

Lais M. Malavasi, DVM, MS, PhD
Department of Veterinary Clinical Sciences
College of Veterinary Medicine
Washington State University
Pullman, Washington, USA

Khursheed R. Mama, DVM, DACVAA
Department of Clinical Sciences
Colorado State University
Fort Collins, Colorado, USA

Elizabeth A. Martinez, DVM, DACVAA
College of Veterinary Medicine
Texas A&M University
College Station, Texas, USA

Wayne N. McDonell, DVM, MSc, PhD, DACVAA
University Professor Emeritus
Department of Clinical Studies, Ontario Veterinary College
University of Guelph
Guelph, Ontario, Canada

Carolyn M. McKune, DVM, DACVAA
Mythos Veterinary, LLC
Gainesville, Florida, USA

Kristin Messenger, DVM, PhD, DACVAA, DACVCP
Department of Molecular Biomedical Sciences
College of Veterinary Medicine
North Carolina State University
Raleigh, North Carolina, USA

Robert E. Meyer, DVM, DACVAA
College of Veterinary Medicine
Mississippi State University
Mississippi, USA

Cornelia I. Mosley, Dr.med.vet, DACVAA
Ontario Veterinary College
University of Guelph, Canada

Craig A. Mosley, DVM, MSc, DACVAA
Mosley Veterinary Anesthesia Services
Rockwood, Ontario, Canada

William W. Muir, DVM, PhD, DACVAA, DACVECC
VCPCS
Columbus, Ohio, USA

Joanna C. Murrell, BVSc. (Hons), PhD, DECVAA, MRCVS
School of Veterinary Sciences
University of Bristol
Langford, North Somerset, UK

Andrea M. Nolan, MVB, MRCVS, DVA, PhD, DECVAA, DECVPT
Edinburgh Napier University
Edinburgh, Scotland, UK

Klaus A. Otto, Dr.med.vet., PD, DACVAA, DECVAA, DECLAM
Institut für Versuchstierkunde und Zentrales Tierlaboratorium
Medizinische Hochschule Hannover
Hannover, Germany

Mark A. Oyama, DVM, DACVIM-Cardiology
Department of Clinical Studies-Philadelphia
University of Pennsylvania
Philadelphia, Pennsylvania, USA

Luisito S. Pablo, DVM, MS, DACVAA
College of Veterinary Medicine
Auburn University
Auburn, Alabama, USA

Daniel S. J. Pang, BVSc, MSc, PhD, DACVAA, DECVAA, MRCVS
Faculty of Veterinary Medicine and Hotchkiss Brain Institute
University of Calgary
Calgary, Alberta, Canada

Mark G. Papich, DVM, MS, DACVCP
Department of Molecular Biomedical Sciences
College of Veterinary Medicine
North Carolina State University
Raleigh, North Carolina, USA

Peter J. Pascoe, BVSc, DVA, DACVAA, DECVAA
Department of Surgical and Radiological Sciences
School of Veterinary Medicine
University of California
Davis, California, USA

Santiago Peralta, DVM, DAVDC
Department of Clinical Sciences
College of Veterinary Medicine
Cornell University
Ithaca, New York, USA

Tania E. Perez Jimenez, DVM, MS
College of Veterinary Medicine
Washington State University
Pullman, Washington, USA

Sandra Z. Perkowski, VMD, PhD, DACVAA
Department of Clinical Studies-Philadelphia
School of Veterinary Medicine
University of Pennsylvania
Philadelphia, Pennsylvania, USA

Glenn R. Pettifer, BA(Hons), BSc, DVM, DVSc, DACVAA
College of Veterinarians of Ontario
Guelph, Ontario, Canada

Bruno H. Pypendop, DrVetMed, DrVetSci, DACVAA
Department of Surgical and Radiological Sciences
School of Veterinary Medicine
University of California
Davis, California, USA

Marc R. Raffe, DVM, MS, DACVAA, DACVECC
Veterinary Anesthesia and Critical Care Associates LLC
St. Paul, Minnesota, USA

David C. Rankin, DVM, MS, DACVAA
Department of Clinical Sciences
Kansas State University
Manhattan, Kansas, USA

Matt Read, DVM, MVSc, DACVAA
Faculty of Veterinary Medicine
University of Calgary
Calgary, Alberta, Canada

Thomas W. Riebold, DVM, DACVAA
Veterinary Teaching Hospital
College of Veterinary Medicine
Oregon State University
Corvallis, Oregon, USA

Eva Rioja Garcia, DVM, DVSc, PhD, DACVAA
School of Veterinary Science
University of Liverpool
Leahurst Campus, UK

Sheilah A. Robertson, BVMS (Hons), PhD, DACVAA, DECVAA, DACAW, DECAWBM (WSEL)
Michigan State University, East Lansing
Michigan, USA

Molly K. Shepard, DVM, DACVAA
University of Georgia
Athens, Georgia, USA

André C. Shih, DVM, DACVAA
University of Florida College of Veterinary Medicine
Gainesville, Florida, USA

Melissa Sinclair, DVM, DVSc, DACVAA
Department of Clinical Studies
Ontario Veterinary College
University of Guelph
Guelph, Ontario, Canada

Julie A. Smith, DVM, DACVAA
MedVet Medical and Cancer Centers for Pets
Worthington, Ohio, USA

Eugene P. Steffey, VMD, PhD DACVAA, DECVAA, MRCVSHonAssoc, Dr.h.c.(Univ of Berne)
Emeritus Professor
Department of Surgical and Radiological Sciences
School of Veterinary Medicine
University of California
Davis, California, USA

Aurelie A. Thomas, DVM, MSc, MRCVS
Comparative Biology Centre
Newcastle University, Medical School
Newcastle upon Tyne, UK

William J. Tranquilli, DVM, MS, DACVAA
College of Veterinary Medicine
University of Illinois at Urbana-Champaign
Champaign, Illinois, USA

Cynthia M. Trim, BVSc, DVA, DACVAA, DECVAA
Department of Large Animal Medicine
College of Veterinary Medicine
University of Georgia
Athens, Georgia, USA

Alexander Valverde, DVM, DVSc, DACVAA
Department of Clinical Studies
Ontario Veterinary College
University of Guelph
Guelph, Ontario, Canada

Alessio Vigani, DVM, PhD, DACVAA, DACVECC
Department of Clinical Sciences
College of Veterinary Medicine
North Carolina State University
Raleigh, North Carolina, USA

Kate L. White, MA, Vet MB, DVA, DECVAA, MRCVS
School of Veterinary Medicine and Science
University of Nottingham
Nottingham, UK

Ted Whittem, BVSc, PhD, DACVCP, FANZCVS
Faculty of Veterinary and Agricultural Sciences
University of Melbourne
Werribee, Victoria, Australia

Ashley J. Wiese, DVM, MS, DACVAA
Department of Anesthesia
MedVet Medical and Cancer Center for Pets
Cincinnati, Ohio, USA

Deborah V. Wilson, BVSc(Hons), MS, DACVAA
Department of Large Animal Clinical Sciences
College of Veterinary Medicine
Michigan State University
East Lansing, Michigan, USA

Bonnie D. Wright, DVM, DACVAA
Fort Collins Veterinary Emergency and Rehabilitation Hospital
Fort Collins, Colorado, USA

SECTION 1

General Topics

1 Introduction: Use, Definitions, History, Concepts, Classification, and Considerations for Anesthesia and Analgesia

William J. Tranquilli[1] and Kurt A. Grimm[2]
[1]College of Veterinary Medicine, University of Illinois at Urbana-Champaign, Urbana, Illinois, USA
[2]Veterinary Specialist Services, PC, Conifer, Colorado, USA

Chapter contents

Introduction

Veterinary anesthesia continues to evolve as a science and specialty within the veterinary profession. The major drivers of change are advances in medical technology and pharmaceutical development for domesticated animals or those adapted from human anesthesiology; research in physiology, pharmacology, and clinical trials for human and veterinary patients that provide better evidence-based guidance for patient care; and socioeconomic and demographic changes in countries where animals serve evolving roles. Veterinary anesthesiologists will continue to be advocates for patient safety, humane care through education about pain management and quality of life, and educators of the profession and society at large about the current best practices in anesthesia, analgesia, and pain management.

Use of anesthesia, sedation, and analgesia

Proper use of anesthetics, sedatives, and analgesics can alleviate pain, create amnesia, and produce muscle relaxation essential for safe and humane patient care [1]. Important uses include facilitation of immobilization for various diagnostic, surgical, and therapeutic procedures; safe transportation of wild and exotic animals; and euthanasia and the humane slaughter of food animals. Anesthesia, sedation, and analgesic drug administration are not without significant patient risk and are not recommended for trivial reasons. The continued development of better techniques and drugs along with the concerted and continuing effort to educate veterinary care providers has minimized the overall risk of anesthesia and pain alleviation in an ever-increasing and more sophisticated patient care environment. Any discussion with the animal-owning public, such as that occurring with owners when obtaining informed consent, requires use of proper terminology to convey the issues central to the safe delivery of veterinary anesthesia and pain therapy.

Definitions

The term *anesthesia*, derived from the Greek term *anaisthaesia*, meaning 'insensibility,' is used to describe the loss of sensation to the entire or any part of the body. Anesthesia is induced by drugs that depress the activity of nervous tissue locally, regionally, or within the central nervous system (CNS). From a pharmacological viewpoint, there has been a significant redefining of the term general anesthesia [2]. Both central nervous stimulants and depressants can be useful general anesthetics [3].

Management of pain in patients involves the use of drugs which are often called *analgesics*. The term is derived from *an*, which is the negative or without, and *alges(is)*, meaning pain [4]. Clinical management of pain often results in varying degrees of effectiveness that represent states of *hypoalgesia*, or decreased sensation of pain. It is important to understand that the administration of an analgesic drug does not necessarily create the state of analgesia.

Several terms are commonly used in describing the effects of anesthetic and pain-inhibiting drugs:

1 *Analgesia* is the absence of pain in response to stimulation which would normally be painful. The term is generally reserved for describing a state in a conscious patient [5].
2 *Nociception* is the neural process of encoding noxious stimuli [5]. Nociception is the physiologic process that underlies the conscious perception of pain. Nociception does not require consciousness and can continue unabated during

Veterinary Anesthesia and Analgesia: The Fifth Edition of Lumb and Jones.
Edited by Kurt A. Grimm, Leigh A. Lamont, William J. Tranquilli, Stephen A. Greene and Sheilah A. Robertson.

general anesthesia if techniques that interrupt or inhibit the transduction, transmission, and modulation of nociceptive stimuli are not included.

3 *Pain* is an unpleasant sensory and emotional experience associated with actual or potential tissue damage, or described in terms of such damage [5].
4 *Tranquilization* results in behavioral change wherein anxiety is relieved and the patient becomes relaxed but remains aware of its surroundings. Tranquilizers are drugs that result in tranquilization when administered; however, many prefer to use the term anxiolytic or anti-anxiety drug when describing drugs that result in both reduced anxiety and relaxation.
5 *Sedation* is a state characterized by central depression accompanied by drowsiness and some degree of centrally induced relaxation. The patient is generally unaware of its surroundings but can become aroused and is responsive to noxious stimulation. Sedatives are not recommended by themselves to immobilize a patient during times which painful stimuli are likely to occur.
6 *Narcosis* is a drug-induced state of deep sleep from which the patient cannot be easily aroused. Narcosis may or may not be accompanied by antinociception, depending on the techniques and drugs used.
7 *Hypnosis* is a condition of artificially induced sleep, or a trance resembling sleep, resulting from moderate depression of the CNS from which the patient is readily aroused.
8 *Local analgesia* (*anesthesia*) is a loss of pain sensation in a circumscribed body area.
9 *Regional analgesia* (*anesthesia*) is insensibility to pain in a larger, though limited, body area usually defined by the pattern of innervation of the effected nerve(s) (e.g., paralumbar nerve blockade and anesthesia).
10 *General anesthesia* is drug-induced unconsciousness that is characterized by controlled but reversible depression of the CNS and perception. In this state, the patient is not arousable by noxious stimulation. Sensory, motor, and autonomic reflex functions are attenuated to varying degrees, depending upon the specific drug(s) and technique(s) used.
11 *Surgical general anesthesia* is the state/plane of anesthesia that provides unconsciousness, amnesia, muscular relaxation, and hypoalgesia sufficient for painless surgery.
12 *Balanced anesthesia* is achieved by the simultaneous use of multiple drugs and techniques. Drugs are targeted to attenuate specifically individual components of the anesthetic state, that is, amnesia, antinociception, muscle relaxation, and alteration of autonomic reflexes.
13 *Dissociative anesthesia* is induced by drugs (e.g., ketamine) that dissociate the thalamocortic and limbic systems. This form of anesthesia is characterized by a cataleptoid state in which eyes remain open and swallowing reflexes remain intact. Skeletal muscle hypertonus persists unless a strong sedative or peripheral or central muscle relaxant is co-administered.

Brief history of animal anesthesia

In 1800, Sir Humphrey Davy suggested that nitrous oxide might have anesthetic properties. Twenty four years later, H. H. Hickman demonstrated that pain associated with surgery in dogs could be alleviated by inhalation of a mixture of nitrous oxide and carbon dioxide. He reasoned that the latter increased the rate and depth of breathing, thus enhancing the effects of nitrous oxide. More recent studies have shown that unconsciousness can be induced in 30–40 s in piglets breathing carbon dioxide (50%) in oxygen (50%) [6].

It was not until 1842 that diethyl ether was used for human anesthesia. Two years later, a dentist, Horace Wells, rediscovered the anesthetic properties of nitrous oxide. Although this finding was neglected for several years, nitrous oxide was introduced to human anesthesia in 1862. C. T. Jackson, a Boston physician, was the first to employ diethyl ether extensively in animals [7].

Chloroform was discovered by Liebig in 1831, but it was not until 1847 that it was first used to induce anesthesia in animals by Flourens and in people by J. Y. Simpson of Edinburgh, Scotland. With the introduction of chloroform, reports began to appear in the veterinary literature of its use in animals. Dadd routinely used general anesthesia in animals and was one of the first in the United States to advocate humane treatment of animals and the application of scientific principles (i.e., anesthesia) in veterinary surgery [8].

In 1875, Ore published the first monograph on intravenous anesthesia using chloral hydrate; 3 years later, Humbert described its use in horses. Pirogoff was the first to attempt rectal anesthesia with chloral hydrate in 1847. Intraperitoneal injection was first used in 1892 in France. Thus, various routes of administration of general anesthetics to animals had been identified and minimally investigated by the end of the 19th century.

After the initial isolation of cocaine by Albert Niemann of Germany in 1860, Anrep, in 1878, suggested the possibility of using cocaine as a local anesthetic. In 1884, Kohler used cocaine for local anesthesia of the eye, and Halsted described cocaine regional anesthesia a year later. Its use was popularized by Sir Frederick Hobday, an English veterinarian. Thereafter, G. L. Corning was credited for using cocaine for spinal anesthesia in dogs in 1885. From his description, however, it would appear that he induced epidural anesthesia. In 1898, August Bier of Germany induced true spinal anesthesia in animals and then in himself and an assistant [9].

While local infiltration was popularized by Reclus (1890) and Schleich (1892), conduction regional anesthesia had been earlier introduced by Halsted and Hall in New York in 1884. These techniques increased in popularity with the discovery of local anesthetics less toxic than cocaine. These developments enabled Cuille and Sendrail (1901) in France to induce subarachnoid anesthesia in horses, cattle, and dogs. Cathelin (1901) reported epidural anesthesia in dogs, but it remained for Retzgen, Benesch, and Brook to utilize this technique in larger species during the 1920s. Although paralumbar anesthesia was employed in humans by Sellheim in 1909, it was not until the 1940s that Farquharson and Formston applied this technique in cattle. Despite these promising advancements in local analgesic techniques in the latter half of the 19th century, likely owing to the many unfavorable results, general anesthesia and humane surgery were not readily adopted by the veterinary profession until well into the 20th century. It is sad to say, but a 'heavy hand,' without analgesia/anesthesia or even sedation, was the stock in trade of many 'large animal' practicing veterinarians well into the latter half of the 20th century.

In smaller domestic animals, diethyl ether and chloroform were commonly administered in the early part of the 20th century. However, general anesthesia became more widely accepted after the discovery of barbiturates in the late 1920s and, in particular, with the development of pentobarbital in 1930. Barbiturate anesthesia received an additional boost with the introduction of the thiobarbiturates and particularly thiopental in 1934. Because of rough, prolonged recovery, the acceptance of barbiturate general anesthesia in larger species of animals was delayed until phenothiazine derivatives were also introduced by Charpentier in France in 1950.

General anesthesia of large farm animals was further advanced by the discovery of fluorinated hydrocarbons and the development of 'large animal' inhalant anesthetic equipment for safe administration. The discovery of newer classes of drugs together with their safe co-administration (e.g., tranquilizers, opioids, α_2-adrenergic receptor agonists, dissociatives, muscle relaxants, and inhalant anesthetics) has further advanced the safety and utility of veterinary anesthesia for both large and small animal species [10].

The modern era of veterinary anesthesia was initiated during the last three decades of the 20th century facilitated by the establishment of anesthesia specialty colleges within North America and Europe. Stated organizational missions were the improvement of patient safety and the development of new techniques and knowledge paralleling the advances made in human anesthesia. New drugs and techniques are continually being evaluated for clinical usefulness in a variety of species and individual patient pathologies. In addition, an appreciation of patient monitoring for improved safety has led to the adaptation of technologies such as pulse oximetry, capnography, and blood pressure measurement. The veterinary anesthesiologist's value as a member of the patient care team has led to an ever-increasing presence in private veterinary practice. A more sophisticated approach to anesthesia care has become evident with an increasing patient age demographic. This demand will continue to expand the anesthesiologist's importance to our profession beyond the traditional roles of university instructors and pharmaceutical researchers. Demand has also been bolstered by the veterinary profession's quest to improve patient quality of life through better pain management. Many anesthesiologists have been leaders in this area through continued research and the creation of evidence-based species-specific pain-assessment scales and therapeutic guidelines.

History of North American organizations

During the late 1960s and early 1970s, a small group of physician anesthesiologists made it possible for a number of future diplomates of the American College of Veterinary Anesthesiologists (ACVA), now the American College of Veterinary Anesthesia and Analgesia (ACVAA), to participate in their training programs and to learn about the development of new anesthetic drugs and techniques. Among these physicians were Robert Dripps, University of Pennsylvania; Arthur Keats, Baylor University; Mort Shulman and Max Sadolv, University of Illinois; and Edmond I. Eger, University of California Medical College. During this same period, E. W. Jones (Oklahoma State University) and William Lumb (Colorado State University) were making significant contributions to the field of veterinary anesthesiology. Jerry Gillespie had made significant contributions through his work on the respiratory function of anesthetized horses and William Muir was reporting on the cardiopulmonary effects of various anesthetic drugs in various species.

Even though there were many dedicated faculty within North American veterinary colleges and research laboratories, it was not until 1970 that a major effort was made at organizing veterinarians interested in anesthesiology as a stand-alone specialty. Initially, the American Society of Veterinary Anesthesia (ASVA) was established. Membership of the ASVA was open to all individuals working in the veterinary profession who had an interest in veterinary anesthesiology. In 1970, the first organizational meeting was held in conjunction with the American Veterinary Medical Association (AVMA) to coordinate the efforts/interest of all those wishing to develop the specialty of veterinary anesthesiology. Their primary goal was to improve anesthetic techniques and to disseminate knowledge whenever and wherever possible. Charles Short was elected the first President of the new society. The ASVA was designed expressly to promote dissemination of information irrespective of individual training or background. Of major emphasis was the selection of individuals to speak at the ASVA and other scientific and educational meetings. As the ASVA developed, publication of original research and review articles seemed in order. Bruce Heath accepted editorial responsibilities for manuscripts submitted for the ASVA journal. In 1971, John Thurmon chaired the Ad Hoc Committee to establish the American College of Veterinary Anesthesiologists (ACVA). The AVMA had established guidelines for the selection of founding-charter diplomat of specialty organizations. The Ad Hoc Committee requirements for charter diplomat status in a specialty included 10 years of active service in the specialty, significant publication, intensive training, and either being a recognized head of an anesthesiology program or spending a major portion of one's professional time in anesthesia or a closely related subject area. Seven members of the ASVA were found to meet these qualifications becoming the founding diplomats of the ACVA.

Between 1970 and 1975, the constitution and bylaws were drafted and formalized. In 1975, the AVMA Council on Education recommended preliminary approval of the ACVA and it was confirmed by the AVMA House of Delegates in that same year. Thus, the ACVA was officially established in North America. Of importance throughout this process were the insight and efforts of William Lumb and E. Wynn Jones. They greatly assisted in the establishment of the ACVA because of their sincere interest in the sound principles of veterinary anesthesiology. During this same period, several didactic texts had been published further establishing anesthesia as a stand-alone discipline and specialty within veterinary medicine. The first edition of this text, *Lumb and Jones' Veterinary Anesthesia*, was published in 1973, *Clinical Veterinary Anesthesia*, edited by Charles Short, was published in 1974, and the *Textbook of Veterinary Anesthesia*, edited by Larry Soma, was published in 1971.

During the late 1970s, many of the founding diplomats established residency training programs in their respective veterinary colleges. From 1975 to 1980, the ACVA developed continuing education programs, programs in self-improvement, and programs for testing and certification of new diplomats. Along with residency training programs, anesthesiology faculty positions were being created in a number of universities across North America. In 1980, an effort headed by then president Eugene Steffey sought and achieved the full accreditation of the ACVA by the AVMA.

During the past four decades, a number of additional organizations have promoted and contributed greatly to the advancement of veterinary anesthesia. They include the Association of

Veterinary Anaesthetists of Great Britain and Ireland (AVA) and the Veterinary Anesthesia and Surgery Association in Japan. These associations along with the ACVA were instrumental in organizing the first International Congress of Veterinary Anesthesiology with its stated objective of globally advancing the field of veterinary anesthesiology. The first International Congress was held in Cambridge, England, in 1982, and has been held continually triannually ever since at various locations around the world on nearly every continent.

Concurrently, during the latter decades of the 20th century, organized veterinary anesthesiology was being advanced in Western Europe. Veterinary anesthesiologists in the United Kingdom had established the Association of Veterinary Anaesthetists and awarded the Diploma of Veterinary Anaesthesia to those with advanced specialty training. Later, interest in board specialization became increasingly evident in the United Kingdom and many European countries, resulting in the establishment of the European College of Veterinary Anesthesiologists (ECVA). In order to better recognize the central role anesthesiologists have in providing and advancing pain management, both the ECVA and ACVA subsequently sought and were granted approval to incorporate the word 'analgesia' into their names. Thus, the colleges were renamed the European College of Veterinary Anesthesia and Analgesia (ECVAA) and the American College of Veterinary Anesthesia and Analgesia (ACVAA). Currently, a number of veterinary anesthesiologists are boarded by both the ACVAA and ECVAA with both organizations recognizing the legitimacy of either credential, allowing residency training programs supervised by ACVAA diplomats to qualify candidates to sit the ECVAA Board Exam and vice versa. For further information concerning the early history of veterinary anesthesia, the reader is referred to additional sources [11–14].

The establishment of the ACVAA and the ECVAA has helped to advance veterinary anesthesia and pain management on a global scale through their efforts to promote research, create knowledge and enhance its dissemination via annual scientific meetings and publications. The ACVAA and ECVAA have as their official scientific publication the *Journal of Veterinary Anaesthesia and Analgesia*, which also serves as the official publication of the International Veterinary Academy of Pain Management (IVAPM).

During the early 2000s, in an effort to improve out-reach to practitioners interested in humane care and to increase pain management awareness and continuing education programs for practicing veterinarians, the IVAPM was initially conceived of at the annual Veterinary Midwest Anesthesia and Analgesia Conference (VMAAC) Scientific Meeting. The organization's stated mission was to advance the multidisciplinary approach to pain management within the wider veterinary community and was supported by an ongoing academic–pharmaceutical industry partnership, the Companion Animal Pain Management Consortium, led by ACVAA diplomats Charles Short (president of the original ASVA), William Tranquilli, and James Gaynor. Appropriately, the first President-Elect of the IVAPM was the then current President of the ACVA, Peter Hellyer. Interestingly, at the time of this writing (early 2014), the current IVAPM President-Elect, Bonnie Wright, continues to represent the legacy of ACVAA leadership in the field of veterinary analgesia and pain management.

Indeed, alleviating animal pain and suffering is an increasingly important and defining issue for 21st century veterinary medicine. Today, academic and private practice anesthesiologists, practitioners, veterinary technicians, research and industry veterinarians, and animal scientists alike are increasingly working together through organizations such as the ACVAA, ECVAA, IVAPM, AVA, AVTA, and others, toward the common goals of creating new knowledge, coordinating educational programs, and advancing veterinary anesthesia, analgesia, and pain management.

Anesthesiologist defined

A boarded *anesthesiologist* is a person with a doctoral degree who has been certified by either the ACVAA or ECVAA and legally qualified to administer anesthetics and related techniques [15]. The term *anesthetist* has more variable meaning because in some European countries an anesthetist is equivalent to an anesthesiologist, but in North America and many other countries anesthetist refers to a person who administers anesthetics who is not board certified or possibly not a physician or veterinarian. Perhaps the most appropriate way to define a *veterinary anesthesiologist* is by recognizing that the veterinarian has been extensively trained and supervised by either ACVAA or ECVAA diplomats and credentialed by a veterinary certifying anesthesia and analgesia specialty examination (i.e., either the ACVAA or ECVAA Certifying Board Exam) whose expertise consists of anesthetic and analgesic delivery and risk management across a wide array of species and medical circumstances.

Early conceptual stages of anesthesia

Throughout the early years of anesthetic administration (diethyl ether) to human and veterinary patients alike, the assessment of anesthetic depth was a learned skill, appreciated most fully by individuals with much experience and the courage to learn from trial and error. John Snow was the first physician to attempt to classify the depth of anesthesia based on observation of the patient [16]. Teaching new anesthetists how much anesthetic to administer required close oversight by an experienced person. This system became strained during periods of high demand for anesthetists such as was encountered during the First World War.

Dr Arthur Guedel was a physician from Indianapolis, Indiana, who served in the First World War. One of his tasks was to train orderlies and nurses to administer diethyl ether to wounded solders. Guedel thus developed guidelines through the use of a wall chart that could be used by anesthetists to gauge the depth of anesthesia (Table 1.1) [17].

While Guedel's original observations were made in human patients anesthetized with diethyl ether, they were subsequently adapted for use with other inhalant anesthetics such as halothane. Four progressive stages of anesthesia beginning at its initial administration and ending at near death were characterized. Within stage 3 there are three or four sub-classifications listed (Box 1.1). These planes of anesthesia represent the progressive central nervous system depression that can be observed while a patient is within a surgical depth of anesthesia.

Modern anesthetic techniques seldom utilize only inhalant anesthesia, which has led to less reliance on Guedel's classification. Incorporation of other drugs into balanced anesthetic techniques (e.g., antimuscarinics and dissociative anesthetics)

Table 1.1 Characteristics of the stages of general anesthesia.

Stage of Anesthesia		I	II	III				IV
				Plane				
				1	2	3	4	
System Affected	Characteristic Observed			Light	Medium		Deep	
Cardiovascular	Pulse[a]	Tachycardia		Progressive bradycardia				Weak or imperceptible
	Blood pressure[a]	Hypertension		Normal	Increasing hypotension			Shock level
	Capillary refill	1 s or less			Progressive delay			3 s or longer
	Dysrhythmia probability	+++	+++	++	+		++	++++
Respiratory	Respiratory rate[a]	Irregular or increased		Progressive decrease			Slow irregular	Ceased; may gasp terminally
	Respiratory depth[a]	Irregular or increased		Progressive decrease			Irregular	Ceased
	Mucous membrane, skin color	Normal					Cyanosis	Pale to white
	Respiratory action	May be breatholding		Thoracoabdominal, abdominal			Diaphragmatic	Ceased
	Cough reflex	++++	+++	+	Lost			
	Laryngeal reflex	++++	May vocalize	Lost				
	Intubation possible	No	Yes					
Gastrointestinal	Salivation	++++	+++	+	Diminished absent, except in ruminants			Absent
	Oropharyngeal reflex	++++	+++	+	Lost			
	Vomition probability	+++	+++	+	Very slight			
	Reflux (regurgitation) potential	None		Increases with relaxation				++++
	Tympany (rumen, cecum)	None		Potential increases with duration of anesthesia				
Ocular	Pupils	Dilated		Normal or constricted, progressive dilation				Acutely dilated
	Corneal reflex	Normal	+++	Diminishes, lost (horses may persist)				Absent
	Lacrimation	Normal	+++	+	Diminishes, absent			Absent
	Photomotor reflex	Normal	+++	+	Diminishes, absent			Absent
	Palpebral reflex	Normal	+++	+	Diminishes, absent			Absent
	Eyeball position	Normal	Variable	Ventromedial in dogs and cats or central				
	Nystagmus	++++	Especially horses and cows				+	None
Musculoskeletal	Jaw tone	++++	++++	Decreased, minimal			Lost	
	Limb muscle tone	++++	++++	Decreased, minimal			Lost	
	Abdominal muscle tone	++++	++++	++	Decreased, minimal			Lost
	Sphincters (anus, bladder)	May void		Progressive relaxation			Control lost	
Nervous	Sensorium	+++	+	Lost				
	Pedal reflex	++++	++++	Decreased	Absent			
	Reaction to surgical manipulation	++++	++++	+	None			

[a]Surgical stimulation causes increased heart rate, blood pressure and respiratory rate via autonomic responses that persist in plane 2. Vagal reflexes due to visceral traction persist in plane 3.
+ to ++++ = degree present.

greatly influence the reflexive and autonomic responses of the patient. In light of this, a greater reliance on monitoring patient physiologic parameters such as blood pressure, respiration, and neuromuscular tone has become common. Use of electroencephalographic monitoring of CNS activity (e.g., bispectral index monitoring) is currently of great interest and increasing in clinical application to insure adequate anesthetic depth for surgical procedures. Interestingly, a comparison of bispectral index monitoring with Guedel's classic signs for anesthetic depth in humans anesthetized with diethyl ether has a relatively good correlation (Fig. 1.1) [18]. Nevertheless, and despite the incorporation of many new monitoring modalities in daily practice, the anesthetist should continue to have some understanding of the correlation of changing physical signs with anesthetic depth progression. Thus, Guedel's early observational classification will likely continue to have relevancy.

Box 1.1 Stages of anesthesia observed during inhalant anesthesia.

Stage I. The stage of voluntary movement is defined as lasting from initial administration to loss of consciousness. Some analgesia may be present in the deeper phases of this stage. Excited, apprehensive animals may struggle violently and voluntarily hold their breath for short periods. Epinephrine release causes a strong, rapid heartbeat and pupillary dilation. Salivation is frequent in some species, as are urination and defecation. With the approach of stage II, animals become progressively ataxic, lose their ability to stand, and assume lateral recumbency.

Stage II. The stage of delirium or involuntary movement. As the CNS becomes depressed, patients lose all voluntary control. By definition, this stage lasts from loss of consciousness to the onset of a regular pattern of breathing. As a result of anesthetic depression of the CNS, reflexes become more primitive and exaggerated. Patients react to external stimuli by violent reflex struggling, breath holding, tachypnea, and hyperventilation. Continued catecholamine release causes a fast, strong heartbeat, cardiac arrhythmias may occur, and the pupils may be widely dilated. Eyelash and palpebral reflexes are prominent. Nystagmus commonly occurs in horses. During this stage, animals may whine, cry, bellow, or neigh, depending on the species concerned. In some species, especially ruminants and cats, salivation may be excessive; in dogs, cats, and goats, vomiting may be evoked. The larynx of cats and pigs is very sensitive at this stage, and stimulation may cause laryngeal spasms.

Stage III. The stage of surgical anesthesia is characterized by unconsciousness with progressive depression of the reflexes. Muscular relaxation develops, and ventilation becomes slow and regular. Vomiting and swallowing reflexes are lost.

In humans, this stage has been further divided into planes 1–4 for finer differentiation. Others have suggested the simpler classification of light, medium, and deep. Light anesthesia persists until eyeball movement ceases. Medium anesthesia is characterized by progressive intercostal paralysis, and deep anesthesia by diaphragmatic respiration. A medium depth of unconsciousness or anesthesia has traditionally been considered a light plane of surgical anesthesia (stage III, plane 2) characterized by stable respiration and pulse rate, abolished laryngeal reflexes, a sluggish palpebral reflex, a strong corneal reflex, and adequate muscle relaxation and analgesia for most surgical procedures. Deep surgical anesthesia (stage III, plane 3) is characterized by decreased intercostal muscle function and tidal volume, increased respiration rate, profound muscle relaxation, diaphragmatic breathing, a weak corneal reflex, and a centered and dilated pupil.

Stage IV. Extreme CNS depression. Respirations cease and the heart continues to beat for only a short time. Blood pressure is at the shock level, capillary refill of visible mucous membranes is markedly delayed, and the pupils are widely dilated. Death quickly intervenes unless immediate resuscitative steps are taken. If the anesthetic is withdrawn and artificial respiration is initiated before myocardial collapse, these effects may be overcome and patients will go through the various stages in reverse.

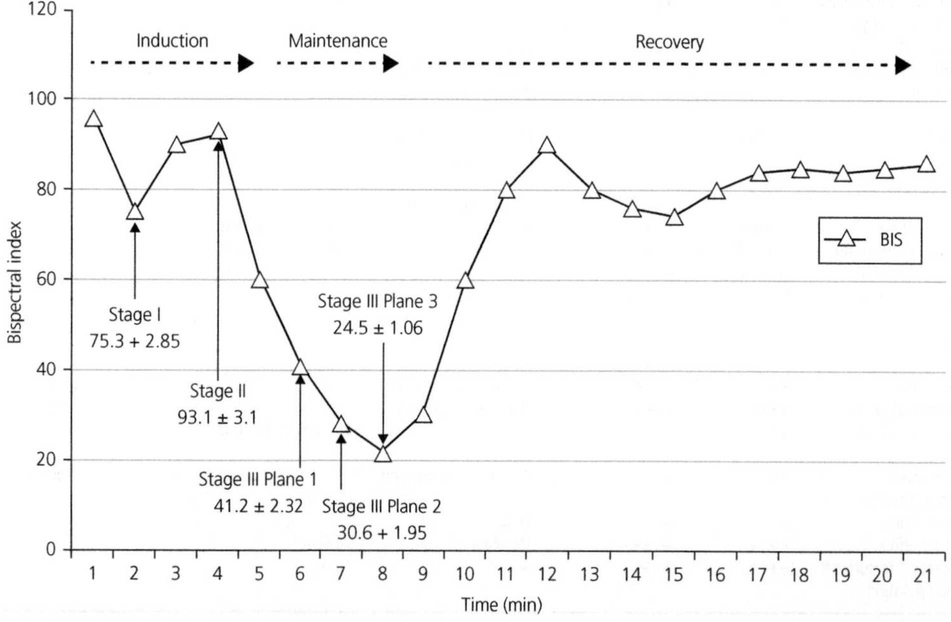

Figure 1.1 Bispectral index (BIS) values under various stages of ether anesthesia (mean ± SD). Source: [18]. Reproduced with permission of Lippincott Williams & Wilkins.

Classification of anesthesia

The diverse uses for anesthesia (as it relates to immobilization, muscle relaxation, and antinociception) and the requirements peculiar to species, age, and disease state necessitate the use of a variety of drugs, drug combinations, and methods. Anesthetic technique is often classified according to the type of drug and/or method/route of drug administration:

1 *Inhalation*: Anesthetic gases or vapors are inhaled in combination with oxygen.
2 *Injectable*: Anesthetic solutions are injected intravenously, intramuscularly, and subcutaneously. Other injectable routes include intrathoracic and intraperitoneal. These last two routes are not generally recommended.
3 *Total intravenous anesthesia (TIVA), partial intravenous anesthesia (PIVA) and targeted controlled infusion (TCI)*: Anesthetic techniques that utilize intravenous infusion of one or more drugs to produce a suitable anesthetic state. Some automated infusion systems are available that allow input of patient parameters and

pharmacokinetic information for specific drugs and allow the anesthesiologist to target a predetermined plasma drug concentration (TCI).

4 *Oral or rectal*: These routes are ordinarily used for liquid anesthetics, analgesics, or suppositories. There is often a greater degree of inter-species and inter-individual variability in the dose–response relationship of orally administered drugs due to differences in absorption and first-pass hepatic metabolism.
5 *Local and conduction*: Anesthetic drug is applied topically, injected locally into or around the surgical site (field block), or injected around a large nerve trunk supplying a specific region (conduction or regional nerve block). In the last instance, the injection may be perineural (nerve block) or into the epidural or subarachnoid space.
6 *Electronarcosis, electroanesthesia, or electrosleep*: Electrical currents are passed through the cerebrum to induce deep narcosis. Even though there have been successful studies, this form of anesthesia has never gained popularity and is rarely used in veterinary practice. Electronarcosis should not be confused with the inhumane practice of electroimmobilization.
7 *Transcutaneous electrical nerve stimulation (TENS, TNS, or TES)*: Local analgesia is induced by low-intensity, high-frequency electric stimulation of the skin through surface electrodes. TENS has many similarities to electroacupuncture.
8 *Hypnosis*: A non-drug-induced trance-like state sometimes employed in rabbits and birds.
9 *Twilight anesthesia*: A state of heavy sedation where the patient is still conscious, but cooperative, and has limited or no recall (amnesia). This technique is popular for outpatient anesthesia in human medicine for diagnostic procedures and for minor surgical procedures when combined with local anesthetics and additional analgesic drugs. *Twilight anesthesia* is a term in common use by laypeople to connote heavy sedation and does not refer to a specific anesthetic procedure or technique.
10 *Acupuncture*: A system of therapy using long, fine needles to induce analgesia. Additional modalities of acupuncture point stimulation have been utilized, including mechanical and electrical stimulation.
11 *Hypothermia*: Body temperature is decreased, either locally or generally, to supplement insensitivity and decrease anesthetic drug requirement, and reduce metabolic needs. It is primarily used in neonates or in patients undergoing cardiovascular surgery.

Environmental considerations

Concerns about potential adverse effects associated with the use of anesthetic drugs fall into three general categories. The first is patient-experienced adverse drug reactions, which can be classified into seven types: dose-related (Augmented or type A), non-dose-related (Bizarre or type B), dose-related and time-related (Chronic or type C), time-related (Delayed or type D), withdrawal (End of use or type E), failure of therapy (Failure or type F), and genetic reactions (type G) [19]. Specific patient-experienced adverse drug reactions are reviewed in other areas of this text.

A second type of adverse effect is experienced by health and veterinary care providers exposed to anesthetic drugs and gases during the performance of their daily tasks. Acute exposure through accidental needle penetration or through accidental spillage of drugs will always be a risk. Many employers have standard operating procedures in place, instructing employees how to limit their exposure and how to proceed if exposure occurs. Chronic workplace exposure to low levels of inhalant anesthetic agents has been a concern since their use began and, although studied repeatedly, questions still exist about the relative risk of toxicity such as infertility, miscarriage, cancer, and other chronic health problems. Part of the difficulty in determining safe levels of exposure is related to the apparently low incidence of adverse effects and the potentially long lag period between exposure and expression of toxicity. Usually the question is approached through large epidemiological studies of healthcare providers that are administering anesthetics. This introduces many confounders such as provider age, agents in use, coexisting health problems, and measurement of actual provider exposure, which may make interpretation and generalization of results problematic. Occupational exposure to inhalant anesthetics is addressed in Chapter 16, Inhalant Anesthetics.

The third type of anesthetic adverse effect is environmental. Historically, drug development and clinical use of anesthetic agents did not consider the resources consumed to produce drugs, or their ultimate fate once eliminated by the patient. Of the inhalant anesthetics in clinical use, desflurane is responsible for the largest greenhouse gas emission (both carbon dioxide and halogenated compounds) during its lifecycle. It is approximately 15 times that of isoflurane and 20 times that of sevoflurane on a per MAC-hour basis. The concurrent use of nitrous oxide to facilitate delivery of inhalant anesthetics further increases emissions. The impact of the contemporary inhalant anesthetics on ozone depletion has also been studied [20]. Although these agents do have some potential for ozone depletion, their relative contribution is low and the impact on global warming through this mechanism is minor. For all of the inhalation anesthetics, their eventual release as waste anesthetic gases into the atmosphere is the largest contributor to their greenhouse gas footprint and global warming potential.

Propofol's impact on greenhouse gas emission is much smaller, by nearly four orders of magnitude, than that of desflurane or nitrous oxide. The greenhouse gas emission associated with propofol and many other injectable anesthetic drugs is primarily related to their production and consumption of fossil fuels needed to manufacture and deliver the drugs [21,22].

References

1 Short CE. The management of animal pain: where have we been, where are we now, and where are we going? *Vet J* 2003; **165**: 101–103.
2 Heavner JE. Veterinary anesthesia update. *J Am Vet Med Assoc* 1983; **182**: 30.
3 Winters WD, Ferrer AT, Guzman-Flores C. The cataleptic state induced by ketamine: a review of the neuropharmacology of anesthesia. *Neuropharmacology* 1972; **11**: 303–315.
4 Askitopoulou H, Ramoutsaki IA, Konsolaki E. Analgesia and anesthesia: etymology and literary history of related Greek words. *Anesth Analg* 2000; **91**(2): 486–491.
5 International Association for the Study of Pain. *IASP Taxonomy*. http://www.iasp-pain.org/Education/Content.aspx?ItemNumber=1698 (accessed 15 September 2014).
6 Thurmon JC, Benson GJ. Anesthesia in ruminants and swine. In: Howard JL, ed. *Current Veterinary Therapy*, vol. 3. Philadelphia: WB Saunders, 1993; 58–76.
7 Jackson CT. Etherization of Animals. *Report of the Commissioner of Patients for the Year of 1853*. Washington, DC: Beverly Tucker, Senate Printer, 1853, **59**.
8 Dadd GH. *The Modern Horse Doctor*. Boston: JP Jewett, 1854.
9 Keys TE. The development of anesthesia. *Anesthesiology* 1942; **3**: 11–23.
10 Stevenson DE. The evolution of veterinary anesthesia. *Br Vet J* 1963; **119**: 477.
11 Clark AJ. Aspects of the history of anesthetics. *Br Med J* 1938; **ii**: 1029.
12 Smithcors JE. The early use of anesthesia in veterinary practice. *Br Vet J* 1957; **113**: 284.
13 Lee JA. *A Synopsis of Anesthesia*, 4th edn. Baltimore: Williams & Wilkins, 1959.
14 Miller RD. *Anesthesia*, 2nd edn. New York: Churchill Livingstone, 1986.
15 Medical Dictionary. *Medical Dictionary, Medical Terminology*. http://www.medilexicon.com/medicaldictionary.php (accessed 1 December 2012).

16 Snow J. *On the Inhalation of the Vapor of Ether in Surgical Operations.* London: Churchill, 1847.
17 California Pacific Medical Center. http://www.cpmc.org/professionals/hslibrary/collections/guedel/ (accessed 15 September 2014).
18 Bhargava AK, Setlur R, Sreevastava D. Correlation of bispectral index and Guedel's stages of ether anesthesia. *Anesth Analg* 2004; **98**(1): 132–134.
19 Edwards IR, Aronson JK. Adverse drug reactions: definitions, diagnosis, and management. *Lancet* 2000; **356**(9237): 1255–1259.
20 Langbein T, Sonntag H, Trapp D, *et al.* Volatile anaesthetics and the atmosphere: atmospheric lifetimes and atmospheric effects of halothane, enflurane, isoflurane, desflurane and sevoflurane. *Br J Anaesth* 1999; **82**(1): 66–73.
21 Sherman J, Le C, Lamers V, Eckelman M. Life cycle greenhouse gas emissions of anesthetic drugs. *Anesth Analg* 2012; **114**(5): 1086–1090.
22 Ryan SM, Nielsen CJ. Global warming potential of inhaled anesthetics: application to clinical use. *Anesth Analg* 2010; **111**(1): 92–98.

2 Anesthetic Risk and Informed Consent

Dave C. Brodbelt[1], Derek Flaherty[2] and Glenn R. Pettifer[3]

[1] Veterinary Epidemiology, Economics and Public Health Group, Royal Veterinary College, North Mymms, Hertfordshire, UK
[2] School of Veterinary Medicine, University of Glasgow, Glasgow, Scotland, UK
[3] College of Veterinarians of Ontario, Guelph, Ontario, Canada

Chapter contents

Anesthetic risk assessment

Perioperative assessment of anesthetic risk is a valuable exercise in order to minimize complications and optimize anesthetic safety. A number of studies have been published in relation to anesthetic morbidity and mortality in both small and large animals, and based on this evidence improved recognition of the risks of anesthesia and those patients that require greatest care and preoperative management could help improve standards of veterinary anesthesia and patient outcome.

General overview – preoperative patient risk assessment

Patient health assessment

The preoperative assessment of an animal's health status is valuable to acknowledge preanesthetic risks, to identify management priorities and to advise clients appropriately prior to anesthesia and surgery. Health status has been consistently reported to be associated with anesthetic death in humans and in the spectrum of species commonly seen in veterinary anesthesia. Increased American Society of Anesthesiologists(ASA) grade [1,2] (see Table 2.1) has been associated with an increased risk of death in a number of small animal anesthetic studies [3–12], in horses [13,14], and in human anesthesia [15–34].

Anesthetic agents cause cardiopulmonary depression and the presence of pre-existing pathology is likely to predispose to greater anesthetic-induced physiologic disturbance [35]. Disturbances of major body systems will make the patient less tolerant of physiologic depression induced by anesthesia. Pre-existing cardiopulmonary pathology is particularly relevant in the immediate preoperative period, as anesthetic-related mortality is likely to involve respiratory or cardiovascular compromise, and most anesthetics depress one or both systems at clinical levels of anesthesia [35].

Hematologic and biochemical abnormalities may also be a significant consideration. In particular, anemia will reduce oxygen-carrying capacity and predispose to hypoxia, and hypoproteinemia has been theorized to increase the response of the patient to highly protein-bound drugs and result in relative overdose [35]. Renal disease is also important, particularly if dehydration or uremia is present, as under these conditions the renal system will have a lower tolerance to anesthesia and the patient may be more sensitive to some anesthetics and perioperative drugs such as non-steroidal anti-inflammatory agents. Neurologic disease may be relevant with respect to the occurrence of postoperative seizures, increased sensitivity to anesthetics, and when cardiopulmonary function is affected, e.g., medullary pathology can depress ventilation and cardiovascular function. Additionally, liver and endocrine disease may influence the response to anesthesia, with diabetes mellitus and potential intraoperative cellular changes in glucose concentrations being particularly relevant [36].

Hence some form of physical health status assessment is an important preanesthetic consideration. Most frequently, ASA grade [1,2] has been described. However, the repeatability and agreement between observers of such scoring systems have been questioned and evidence suggests that inter-observer agreement in ASA health status classification is poor in veterinary anesthesia [37]. Other assessment systems exist in human medicine, including the Acute Physiology and Chronic Health Evaluation (APACHE), and the Physiological and Operative Severity Score for the enUmeration of Mortality and morbidity (POSSUM) and in pediatric practice the Neurological, Airway, Respiratory, Cardiovascular and Other (NARCO) score, and all were observed to predict perioperative risk [38–40]. However, these systems are complex, require more time to complete, and have yet to be evaluated for agreement between observers in a veterinary context. Hence, at present, there appears

Veterinary Anesthesia and Analgesia: The Fifth Edition of Lumb and Jones.
Edited by Kurt A. Grimm, Leigh A. Lamont, William J. Tranquilli, Stephen A. Greene and Sheilah A. Robertson.

Table 2.1 Classification of physical status[a].

Category	Physical Status	Possible Examples of This Category
1	Normal healthy patients	No discernible disease; animals entered for ovariohysterectomy, ear trim, caudectomy, or castration
2	Patients with mild systemic disease	Skin tumor, fracture without shock, uncomplicated hernia, cryptorchidectomy, localized infection, or compensated cardiac disease
3	Patients with severe systemic disease	Fever, dehydration, anemia, cachexia, or moderate hypovolemia
4	Patients with severe systemic disease that is a constant threat to life	Uremia, toxemia, severe dehydration and hypovolemia, anemia, cardiac decompensation, emaciation, or high fever
5	Moribund patients not expected to survive 1 day with or without operation	Extreme shock and dehydration, terminal malignancy or infection, or severe trauma

[a]This classification is the same as that adopted by the American Society of Anesthesiologists.

to be little consensus as to the optimal method of patient health status assessment for consistent and efficient classification across observers and caution should be exercised in over-interpreting individual health status assessments. Nonetheless, there is a body of evidence that highlights that sicker patients are more likely to die perioperatively and therefore some form of preoperative patient assessment would be advisable to distinguish sick from healthy patients, to identify those at greater risk, and to manage patients appropriately in order to try to minimize risk prior to, during, and after anesthesia.

Preanesthetic blood testing

Given the fact that organ dysfunction and various pathologic conditions such as anemia or hypoproteinemia may contribute to increased anesthetic morbidity or mortality, it would seem sensible to make every effort to detect these prior to general anesthesia. For this reason, routine preanesthetic blood screening is commonly recommended by many veterinary practitioners and, indeed, some anesthesia specialists. However, although there is no doubt that prior biochemical and hematologic analyses are of definite value in certain patient groups, the question remains as to whether their use can be justified for every patient, in particular healthy animals undergoing elective procedures.

An internet search for 'Preanesthetic blood screening in animals' (https://www.google.com, accessed August 2013) returned over six million 'hits,' of which a substantial proportion appeared to be veterinary practices each detailing their reasons and prices for carrying out such a procedure; interestingly, the search term returned virtually no scientific papers relating to the practice. In addition, as with much information to be found on the internet, many of the relevant web pages providing advice on the subject were written by people with no apparent scientific background or credentials for discussing such a topic, with the majority of these being pet owner discussion forums. Although there may be no genuine scientific or clinical background behind these types of discussion groups, they almost certainly help perpetuate the 'need' for ubiquitous preanesthetic blood testing, but given that many veterinary professionals also recommend its routine use, it obviously cannot all be dependent on owner perceptions. So, is there actually a sound rationale upon which the need for preanesthetic biochemical and hematologic sampling is based?

There are numerous studies in human anesthesia now questioning the necessity for preanesthetic laboratory testing in healthy patients [41–43], with each of these demonstrating that – for subjects with no demonstrable abnormalities on the basis of history and clinical examination – there appears to be no reduction in perianesthetic complications if prior blood sampling has been carried out. The UK National Institute for Health and Care Excellence (NICE) gathers evidence from a variety of sources and then produces recommendations for human clinicians for various medical and surgical interventions. In terms of preanesthetic blood testing, NICE subdivides its recommendations based on both the age of the patient and the 'grade' of surgery the subject is undergoing, with a grading system (from least to most invasive) of 1–4 (separate grading systems are used for those undergoing neurologic or cardiovascular surgery). There is a huge number of different surgeries allocated to each grade. Examples of grade 1 procedures include surgery on the external nose or nasal septum, or on the prepuce; grade 2 procedures include tonsillectomy or inguinal hernia repair; grade 3 total mastectomy or hysterectomy and grade 4 total hip replacement or renal transplantation [44]. Based on this system, NICE recommends a full blood count only in those humans over 60 years old when undergoing moderate to major surgical procedures (surgical severity grading of ≥2), in all adults undergoing major surgery (surgical severity grade ≥3), or in those with severe renal disease [44]. Similarly, recommended biochemical testing (urea, creatinine, and electrolytes) is only advocated in patients older than 60 years of age and undergoing a procedure of surgical severity ≥3, for all adults having surgery of severity grade 4 (the maximum grade), or in the presence of any renal disease or severe cardiovascular disease [44].

The recommendations for preanesthetic blood screening are even more restrictive in human pediatric patients (<less than 16 years old). If the individual is ASA 1, no routine preanesthetic testing is advised regardless of the grade of surgery being undertaken, the only exceptions being if the child is undergoing either neurologic or cardiovascular procedures [44]. Surprisingly, standard guidelines do not appear to have been published for children who are ≥ ASA 2. The discrepancy between the sampling recommendations for human pediatric patients and adults probably relates to the increased incidence of comorbidities in the latter. As a result of the NICE recommendations, the guidelines of the Association of Anaesthetists of Great Britain and Ireland (AAGBI) [45] for human anesthesia conclude: 'Routine pre-operative investigations are expensive, labour intensive and of questionable value, especially as they may contribute to morbidity or cause additional delays due to spurious results.'

Aside from the issue of erroneous results impacting on the efficiency of case throughput, it is also important to remember that the reference ranges established for most laboratory tests incorporate only approximately 80% of the population, i.e., around one in five animals that are perfectly healthy will return laboratory results that are outside the 'normal' range, which may then lead to further unnecessary investigations being carried out, in addition to delaying the planned procedure. Hence it is important to interpret carefully test results obtained and to view them as part of the overall assessment of the patient.

The AAGBI also takes the view that history and examination performed by appropriately trained and competent personnel remain the most efficient and accurate way of initially detecting significant morbidity: 'Thus, it is important that, where preanaesthetic blood screening is carried out, it is seen as an adjunct to a full clinical examination, rather than an alternative.' While this is undoubtedly the case in both veterinary and human anesthesia, the results from human studies relating to preanesthetic blood screening of healthy patients may not be directly applicable to animals. This is because the majority of humans are both cognitive and verbal, and are able to self-report health issues. Veterinary clinicians, on the other hand, obtain the relevant health information by proxy (the owner), which may mean that important details are not identified. Thus, it is possible that a higher incidence of abnormalities may be detected on preanesthetic screening of animals than has been reported for humans.

Given that the consensus opinion from human anesthesia seems to be that preanesthetic blood sampling appears to be justifiable only in 'sicker' patients, and that healthy individuals undergoing elective procedures do not benefit from this practice, what recommendations should be put in place for veterinary anesthesia? There appear to be at least three studies relating to the validity of routine preanesthetic blood screening in animals. Toews and Campbell [46] performed a complete blood count in 102 horses undergoing cryptorchidectomy and then determined whether any abnormalities detected impacted on the risk of surgical complications. They found that 55 animals had results outside the reference range for at least one hematologic parameter, but there was no correlation between those demonstrating abnormal values and the likelihood of either intra- or postoperative surgical complications, nor did these abnormalities dictate alterations in patient management. Alef and colleagues [47] analyzed results from over 1500 dogs undergoing anesthesia at the University of Leipzig, and reported that if no potential issues were identified in either the animal's history or clinical examination, 'the changes revealed by preoperative screening were usually of little clinical relevance and did not prompt major changes to the anesthetic technique.' They concluded that preanesthetic blood screening is, therefore, unlikely to yield additional important information in most cases. However, the same study also documented that of those dogs where the history and clinical examination would not normally have resulted in preanesthetic laboratory testing being performed at their institution (equivalent to 84% of the dogs recruited), 8% demonstrated biochemical or hematologic abnormalities that would have reclassified them as a higher ASA status, even if this may not necessarily have altered the anesthetic protocol. In addition, they also identified that surgery would have been postponed due to the laboratory findings in 0.8% of these dogs where preanesthetic blood screening would not usually have been performed, while 1.5% would have received additional preanesthetic therapy. Although the authors concluded that only 0.2% of dogs in the study would have required an alteration to their proposed anesthetic protocol based on the biochemical or hematologic results, the implication that undiagnosed pathology may be detected prior to anesthesia using 'routine' screening may have implications for whether the owner decides to proceed with anesthesia/surgery, and may also alter the expected prognosis for the animal. Thus, despite the fact that preanesthetic biochemical and hematologic testing may not alter how the subsequent anesthetic is actually performed in most animals, it may in reality be the deciding factor as to whether the procedure goes ahead.

Given that advancing age is one component impacting on the NICE recommendations regarding preanesthetic blood screening in humans, it would be useful to know whether abnormal results are more likely to be detected in this same patient group in veterinary anesthesia, and any potential impact that this may have. In this regard, Joubert [48] assessed whether hematologic and biochemical analyses were of value in geriatric dogs (>7 years of age) presented for anesthesia. Of the 101 dogs recruited to the study, 30 new diagnoses (e.g., neoplasia, hyperadrenocorticism) were made on the basis of the blood sample, with 13 animals not undergoing general anesthesia as a result of the new diagnosis. However, similarly to the conclusions of the study by Alef and colleagues [47], Joubert [48]suggested that although preanesthetic screening had revealed the presence of subclinical disease in almost 30% of the dogs in the study, and that screening of geriatric patients is important, 'the value of screening before anesthesia is perhaps more questionable in terms of anesthetic practice but it is an appropriate time to perform such an evaluation.' In other words, although preanesthetic blood testing may be of value in uncovering undiagnosed pathology in geriatric patients, there was little evidence that what was detected would actually impact on either how the subsequent anesthetic was managed, or the overall outcome from it. However, this study did identify that over 10% of the dogs had their anesthesia cancelled due solely to the findings of the preanesthetic blood screening, which is obviously of significance.

Interestingly, and somewhat in contrast to the previous studies, work within the Confidential Enquiry into Perioperative Small Animal Fatalities (CEPSAF) highlighted a reduction in risk when preoperative bloods were taken in higher ASA grade patients. CEPSAF was a multicenter study undertaken in the UK between 2002 and 2004 and involved over 100 practices and data from approximately 200 000 dogs and cats [49]. When analyzing risk factors for anesthetic death in sick dogs (ASA 3–5), having a preoperative blood test was associated with reduced odds of death, particularly in ASA grade 4–5 dogs [50]. This association was not detected in the overall analyses where ASA grade 1–5 dogs were considered together or in cats, but does suggest that preoperative biochemistry and hematology are most likely to be merited in the sicker animals that are anesthetized.

Thus, based on the evidence from human anesthesia, and from a smaller number of published veterinary studies, there would appear to be negligible benefit to apparently healthy animals (ASA 1) of biochemical or hematologic screening prior to anesthesia in terms of either anesthetic risk reduction or alteration of the anesthetic protocol; however, given that a significant percentage of animals may have the procedure cancelled based on the results of these tests (due either to a worsened prognosis or the need for further treatment prior to anesthesia), this may counterbalance the preceding argument. Overall, the requirement for preanesthetic blood screening in ASA 1 animals is likely to remain a contentious issue, with valid arguments both for and against.

The situation in animals that are ASA 2 or greater, however, is probably more clear cut, with the published veterinary studies providing some justification that preanesthetic screening may be of value in terms of potentially altering anesthetic management and outcome.

Aside from the impact (or lack thereof) that preanesthetic screening may have on the subsequent conduct of anesthesia and ultimate outcome for veterinary patients, there is perhaps another factor that may require consideration, namely that of potential litigation. It seems that an increasing number of clients are willing (sometimes overly so) to 'point the finger of blame' at the veterinarian when things go wrong in relation to anesthesia, even when in many cases this may be completely unjustified. Hence the genuine reason why many veterinary practices carry out routine preanesthetic screening may be more to do with 'covering one's back' rather than providing the ability to alter anesthetic management suitably if abnormalities are actually detected. It is impossible to say what the legal system may make of a healthy animal undergoing an elective procedure that dies during anesthesia where no preoperative blood sampling had been performed, but based on the recommendations from human anesthesia and the lack of evidence of any benefit in the few veterinary studies that have been carried out, it would appear difficult for them to state that preanesthetic biochemical or hematologic screening is a basic standard of care. Given that there is a more limited evidence base for 'sicker' animals, it may be considered wise to perform preanesthetic screening in patients of ASA 2 or above, from both standard of care and litigation points of view.

Morbidity and mortality

Nonfatal complications tend to occur more frequently than mortal events, although they have been less often documented in the veterinary literature. Reported small animal morbidity risks range from 2–10% [4,5,10,51]. Work in small and large animal anesthesia has acknowledged the difficulty of ensuring consistent detection and recording of morbid events in the practice setting [3,4,52,53]. Small animal practice standards of monitoring of anesthesia are often superficial [54–56] and, unless a given complication results in obvious patient disturbance, it may go unnoticed. Hence, in considering morbid complications, only major events, most likely to be consistently observed, that could contribute substantial physiologic disturbance and that could have the greatest impact on a patient (other than death) will be discussed here.

Small animal anesthesia morbidity

Small animal anesthesia morbidity studies have most frequently been veterinary teaching hospital based, with a few primary practice-based studies also reporting major non-fatal complications [3–5,10,51,56,57]. Conditions consistently described include respiratory, cardiovascular, renal, gastrointestinal, thermoregulatory, and neurologic complications.

Respiratory complications were observed in 0.54% of dog and 0.34% of cat anesthetics in a study of practitioners in Ontario, Canada, and included respiratory depression or apnea, respiratory distress, and difficulty with intubation (although the definitions of these were not stated) [4]. In a veterinary teaching hospital setting, similar respiratory complications were observed, but more often. Hypoventilation and hypercapnia (defined as partial pressure of arterial carbon dioxide or end-tidal carbon dioxide >55 mmHg) were reported in 1.3% and in 1 of 683 dogs and cats undergoing anesthesia, respectively, and hypoxemia (partial pressure of arterial oxygen <60 mmHg or hemoglobin arterial oxygen saturation <90%) was reported in 0.5% of dogs and occasionally airway compromise was also noted [51]. More recently in a Spanish veterinary school hospital, hypoventilation (defined as minute ventilation <100 mL/kg/min) was observed in over 60% and hypoxemia (defined as an SpO_2 < 90%) in 16% of anesthetized dogs [57].

Cardiovascular compromise in small animals included the development of cardiac arrhythmias, notably bradycardia in 0.62% and 0.14% of dog and cat anesthetics in a primary practice setting, although the latter was classified as <60 beats/min and irregular or <50 beats/min and regular for both dogs and cats [4]. In contrast, in a teaching hospital setting, the most frequently recorded cardiovascular complications were hypotension (defined as systolic arterial pressure <80 mmHg or mean arterial pressure <60 mmHg and observed in 7% and 8.5% of dogs and cats, respectively), and cardiac arrhythmias (2.5% and 1.8% of dog and cats, respectively) [51]. Hosgood and Scholl [5,10] reported similar levels of arrhythmias in a teaching hospital environment, with 4% of dogs and 3.6% of cats exhibiting cardiac arrhythmias. The arrhythmias recorded included premature ventricular contractions, sick sinus syndrome, second-degree heart block, and ventricular tachycardia. Bradycardia (heart rate <50 bpm) was reported in approximately 36% and hypotension (mean arterial blood pressure <60 mmHg, or systolic arterial blood pressure <90 mmHg) in nearly 38% of dogs anesthetized at a veterinary school hospital in Spain [57].

Regurgitation was the most frequently documented perioperative gastrointestinal complication. The risk of regurgitation in dogs without pre-existing predisposing disease has been reported in some studies to be between 0.42 and 0.74% [58–60], whereas another report documented a substantially greater risk of regurgitation (5.5%) [61]. The variation in frequency across these studies likely reflects differences in procedures performed, premedication and anesthetic drugs and doses used, and the dog populations studied. The risk of gastroesophageal reflux, which may result in substantial esophageal mucosa injury, has been previously reported at a much higher level of 16–17% and even up to 27–60%, again depending on the animals studied and anesthetic drugs administered, suggesting that the risk of mucosal injury may be much greater than the proportion of patients where reflux is observed [58,59,61,62].

Hypothermia, where monitored, was a particularly common complication. In a veterinary teaching hospital study, 85% of dogs had a temperature recorded perioperatively of less than 37.3 °C and 51% of cats had a body temperature less than 35.0 °C during or after anesthesia [5,10]. Recent work in a veterinary university hospital in Spain highlighted perioperative hypothermia in over 70% of cats and 32% of dogs (body temperature <36.5 °C) [63,64].

Poor recoveries have also been documented, often recorded as prolonged return to consciousness, and these were seen in 0.14–0.18% of dog and cat anesthetics in one study [4]. A smaller number of dogs and cats exhibited complications including excitement in recovery, collapse, prolonged hypothermia, reduced consciousness after an apparently normal recovery, and renal failure [4]. Further, occasional case reports of perioperative blindness have been published, but there are limited data on the frequency of this complication relative to the number of animals anesthetized [65,66]. Interestingly, the use of a mouth gag was reported in 16 of 20 cats observed with postanesthetic cortical blindness, although data relating to denominator use of a mouth gag in general were not available, limiting the ability to conclude an association between the use of a gag or a procedure and the development of blindness [65].

Large animal anesthesia morbidity

A range of non-fatal complications have been reported, although information on their frequency in general equine populations is limited. Cardiovascular compromise, as reported in small animal anesthesia, is a major consideration in equine anesthesia. Hypotension and brady- and tachyarrhythmias have been described. In particular, second-degree atrioventricular block, atrial fibrillation, and ventricular premature contractions have all been reported [67]. Respiratory morbid complications have centered on hypoventilation and hypercapnia and hypoxemia, and these have frequently been reported as potential complications of equine anesthesia [67,68].

In contrast to small animal anesthesia, horses appear to demonstrate a wider range of postoperative complications, including fractures and soft tissue injury, myopathy, neuropathy, and myelopathy, and many result in death or euthanasia [67]. There are limited data on the frequency of these events when non-fatal, although evidence of these complications resulting in mortality highlights their importance. Fractures have been reported intermittently and have often resulted in euthanasia. In the Confidential Enquiry into Perioperative Equine Fatalities (CEPEF), a multicenter prospective study of complications in equine anesthesia, fractures were estimated to be the cause of 25% of anesthetic deaths, myopathy 7%, and CNS complications 5.5% [53]. Similarly, in a single-center study in Kentucky (USA), fractures were the cause of 19% of deaths or euthanasias and neuropathy and myopathy 7% [69]. Other complications reported included postanesthetic colic, which in a multicenter study in the United Kingdom was estimated at approximately 5% of all anesthetized horses [70].

Mortality studies

Small animal anesthetic fatalities

Risks of anesthetic death

Mortality, in contrast to morbidity, has been more consistently observed and has been reported extensively in the veterinary literature. In small animal anesthesia, the risk of death has been documented over the last 50 years [71], and trends to reduction in risk over time have been reported (see Table 2.2). Referral center- and university-based studies generally have reported higher death risks due to the nature of their patients and procedures, whereas practice-based studies tended to reflect healthier populations and simpler procedures. Direct comparison of risks of death between studies has been limited by a number of factors, including variations in study case definitions, study populations, and procedures performed.

Initial institution-based studies from the United States documented a wide range of relatively high risks of mortality. An early study at the Angell Memorial Animal Hospital in Boston published risks of anesthetic death of 0.26% in dogs, 0.36% in cats, and 5% in other species [72]. Colorado State University reported higher risks

Table 2.2 Summary risks of anesthetic death in dogs and cats published in primary practice and institutional studies.

Location [Ref.]	Year	Institution of Practice	Risk of Anesthetic Death (%)	
			Dog	Cat
Angell Memorial AH, Boston [72]	1946–50	Institution	0.26	0.36
CSU, Colorado [73]	1955–57	Institution	1.08	1.79
Wheatridge AH, Colorado [73]	1960–69	Institution	0.23	0.40
Univ. Missouri, VH [73]	1968–69	Institution	0.8	0.53
CSU, Colorado [74]	1979–81	Institution	0.43	0.26
CSU, Colorado [51]	1993–94	Institution	0.43	0.35
Louisiana State [5, 10]	1995–96	Institution	1.49	5.80
RVC, London [6]	1999–2002	Institution	0.58	–
Scotland [75]	1975	Practice	–	0.31
Vermont [76]	1989	Practice	0.11	0.06
UK [3]	1984–86	Practice	0.23	0.29
Ontario, Canada [4]	1993	Practice	0.11	0.10
Finland [77]	1993	Practice	0.13 in small animals	
South Africa [56]	1999	Practice	0.08 in dogs and cats	
UK [7]	2002–04	Practice	0.17	0.24
Spain [11]	2007–08	Practice	1.39 in dogs and cats	
France [12]	2008–10	Practice	1.35 in dogs and cats	

CSU = Colorado State University, AH = Animal Hospital, VH = Veterinary Hospital, RVC = Royal Veterinary College.

of 1.08% in dogs and 1.79% in cats between 1955 and 1957 [73], and the Wheatridge Animal Hospital (Colorado) reported anesthetic death risks of 0.23% in dogs and 0.40% in cats between 1960 and 1969 [73]. At a similar time, the University of Missouri Veterinary Hospital reported mortality risks of 0.8% in dogs and 0.53% in cats [73]. More recent referral center studies have reported lower risks of mortality, suggesting that outcomes have improved. Further work at Colorado State University documented risks of 0.43% in dogs and 0.26% in cats between 1979 and 1981 and 0.43% in dogs and 0.35% in cats between 1993 and 1994 [51,74]. Louisiana State University reported higher risks of perioperative death of 1.49% of dogs and 5.80% of cats at their institution between 1995 and 1996, although this related to all deaths, not just anesthetic-related mortality [5,10]. Work at the Royal Veterinary College in the United Kingdom reported an anesthetic-related mortality risk of 0.58% in dogs between 1999 and 2002 [6]. Based on the more recent work described above, the risk of anesthetic-related death in the referral setting would appear to be of the order of 0.25–0.60% in dogs and cats.

Work undertaken in small animal primary practice has generally documented lower risks of mortality than referral-based studies. An early practice-based study evaluated feline mortality in Scotland (United Kingdom) and published a risk of death of 0.31% in cats [75]. This was followed by a further survey of small animal anesthetic practice, undertaken in Vermont (United States), which reported the risk of death to be 0.11% and 0.06% in dogs and cats, respectively [76]. A similar study was undertaken in Finland in 1993 and reported a risk of death of 0.13% in small animals in general [77]. A more recent retrospective study evaluated mortality in a South African practice population in 1999 and estimated a mortality risk of 0.08% in dogs and cats [56], and a private veterinary clinic in France reported a risk of anesthetic death of 1.35% overall and 0.12% for healthy patients (ASA 1–2) [12]. The health status of the patients anesthetized in these studies was not always recorded, although it was likely to reflect relatively healthy animals and partly explains the generally lower risks reported.

The first prospective multicenter cohort study of small animal practice complications was undertaken between 1984 and 1986 in the United Kingdom [3]. Fifty-three practices were recruited, 41 881 anesthetics were recorded and anesthetic risks of death of 0.23% in dogs and 0.29% in cats were reported. For healthy patients (ASA grades 1–2, see Table 2.1), the death risks were 0.12% in dogs and 0.18% in cats, whereas in ill patients (ASA grades 3–5, see Table 2.1), over 3% of dogs and cats died perioperatively. Perioperative deaths in healthy patients (ASA 1–2), occurring during or shortly after surgery, were considered 'primarily due to anesthesia' unless an obvious surgical cause was present, whereas in sick patients (ASA 3–5), all deaths independent of cause were reported. This was followed by a further prospective multicenter cohort study of anesthetic mortality in small animal veterinary practice in Ontario, Canada [4]. During the 6 month study period, 8087 dogs and 8702 cats were anesthetized and 0.11% of dogs and 0.10% of cats had cardiac arrests and died. For healthy animals (ASA 1–2), the risks were 0.067% in dogs and 0.048% in cats, whereas for sick patients (ASA 3–5), 0.46% of dogs and 0.92% of cats died of a cardiac arrest. Only perioperative deaths within an unspecified follow-up period resulting from cardiac arrest were included.

The largest recent multicenter small animal practice-based study, the Confidential Enquiry into Perioperative Small Animal Fatalities (CEPSAF), was undertaken in the United Kingdom between 2002 and 2004 and 98 036 anesthetics and sedations were recorded in dogs and 79 178 in cats, across 117 participating centers [49]. Anesthetic- and sedation-related death was defined as perioperative death within 48 h of termination of the procedure, except where death was due solely to inoperable surgical or pre-existing medical conditions (i.e., anesthesia and sedation could not be reasonably excluded from contributing to the death). The risk of anesthetic- and sedation-related death was approximately 0.17% in dogs and 0.24% in cats (Tables 2.2 and 2.3). In healthy patients (ASA 1–2), the risks were 0.05% and 0.11% in dogs and cats, respectively, whereas in sick patients (ASA 3–5) over 1% of dogs and cats died (Table 2.4). Rabbits were the third most commonly anesthetized species in practice but the risks of anesthetic-related death were substantially higher, with 0.73% of healthy rabbits and 7.37% of sick rabbits dying. The risks in other small animal species were also high, between 1 and 4% (Table 2.3).

Subsequent to CEPSAF, a further prospective study was undertaken with 39 Spanish veterinary clinics and recorded data from 2012 anesthetics. Anesthetic death was defined as perioperative death within 24 h of the procedure end and a risk of death of 1.29% overall was reported, with risks in healthy dogs and cats of 0.33% and in sick animals 4.06% [11].

In summary, recent estimates of anesthetic-related death risks in small animal practice appeared to be of the order of 0.1–0.3%, although in some circumstances this may be higher, with the risk in healthy dogs and cats being approximately 0.05–0.30% and in sick dogs and cats 1–4% [3,4,11,12,49,56,76]. Cats appeared to be at greater risk of death than dogs in some work [3,49], and rabbits and other companion animal species appeared to be at even higher risk where studied [7]. In referral institutions, mortality ranged from 0.30 to 0.60% in dogs and cats [5,6,10,49,51].

Table 2.3 Anesthetic- and sedation-related risk of death in small animals in CEPSAF [7].

Species	No. of Anesthetic- and Sedation-related Deaths	No. Anesthetized and Sedated	Risk of Anesthetic-related Death (%) (95% Confidence Interval, %)
Dog	163	98036	0.17 (0.14–0.19)
Cat	189	79178	0.24 (0.20–0.27)
Rabbit	114	8209	1.39 (1.14–1.64)
Guinea Pig	49	1288	3.80 (2.76–4.85)
Hamsters	9	246	3.66 (1.69–6.83)
Chinchilla	11	334	3.29 (1.38–5.21)
Rat	8	398	2.01 (0.87–3.92)

Source: [7]. Reproduced with permission of Wiley.

Table 2.4 Risk of anesthetic- and sedation-related death in healthy and sick dogs, cats, and rabbits in CEPSAF [7].

Species	Health Status[a]	No. of Deaths[b]	Estimated No. of Anesthetics and Sedations	Risk of Anesthetic-related death (%) (95% Confidence Interval, %)
Dog	Healthy(ASA 1–2)	49	90618	0.05 (0.04–0.07)
	Sick(ASA 3–5)	99	7418	1.33 (1.07–1.60)
Cat	Healthy(ASA 1–2)	81	72473	0.11 (0.09–0.14)
	Sick(ASA 3–5)	94	6705	1.40 (1.12–1.68)
Rabbit	Healthy(ASA 1–2)	56	7652	0.73 (0.54–0.93)
	Sick(ASA 3–5)	41	557	7.37 (5.20–9.54)

[a] ASA 1–2, no/mild preoperative disease; ASA 3–5, severe preoperative disease.
[b] Only deaths where detailed information was available were included here.
Source: [7]. Reproduced with permission of Wiley.

Causes of anesthetic death

The physiologic cause of many anesthetic deaths may be multifactorial, although cardiovascular and respiratory complications represent the primary causes of many perioperative deaths reported. Other causes reported include gastrointestinal-, neurologic-, and hepatic- or renal-related deaths. Cardiac arrest has been reported to result from cardiac arrhythmias associated with increased circulating catecholamines, myocardial hypoxia, specific anesthetic agents, pre-existing pathology, specific procedures (e.g., vagal traction and enucleation), and myocardial depression due to relative anesthetic overdose [35,78] Between 30 and 70% of deaths resulted from relative anesthetic overdose and myocardial depression, cardiac arrhythmias or circulatory failure, and hypovolemia in a number of studies [3–5,56,74]. Halothane, ether, and thiobarbiturate anesthesia were frequently associated with anesthetic overdose in earlier work [3,76]. Dogs more frequently had cardiovascular complications than cats in one study and high-risk patients were the most likely patients to die from circulatory failure, often when hypovolemic [3].

Respiratory complications represented the other main cause of anesthetic-related death. Respiratory complications were an underlying cause of death in 30–40% of dogs and about 40–50% of cats [3,4,74]. Problems related to endotracheal intubation and respiratory obstruction represented the majority of feline respiratory causes of death [3,4]. In dogs, complications with endotracheal intubation and respiratory failure were equally reported, although in brachycephalic dogs respiratory obstruction was the principal cause of respiratory complications [3,4,76].

In small animal anesthesia, causes other than respiratory and cardiovascular complications have infrequently been reported, although have included postoperative renal failure, iliac thrombosis in cats, aspiration of gastric contents, anaphylactic reactions, failure to regain consciousness, and unknown causes [3,4,56,76]. The last causes, often arising when patients were not being closely watched, represented approximately 5–20% of patients.

Timing of death

The timing of anesthetic deaths has varied, with more recent studies increasingly highlighting the postoperative period. Albrecht and Blakely [72] reported in an early study only one death during induction and one during recovery, with the remainder of the deaths occurring during maintenance of anesthesia. In contrast, work at Colorado State University in the 1950s reported that of 36 dog and cat deaths, 17% occurred during induction, 22% during maintenance, and interestingly the majority (61%) during recovery [73]. However, later work at Colorado (1979–1981) reported mostly intraoperative deaths [74] and work there in the 1990s reported that only approximately 25% of dogs and cats died during recovery, with the rest dying during anesthesia [51]. Other referral institutions reported differing high-risk periods; Hosgood and Scholl [5,10] documented that 9 of 14 (61%) deaths in dogs and 4 of 7 (57%) in cats occurred postoperatively, although the number of deaths recorded was small and included all causes of death.

In the primary practice setting, only the larger studies quantified the timing of fatalities. Clarke and Hall [3] reported deaths occurring principally during anesthesia. In dogs, 22% died on induction of anesthesia, 55% during maintenance, and 18% in recovery, whereas in cats, 30% died during induction, 39% during anesthesia, and 31% during recovery. Similarly, in the study in Ontario, Canada [4], most dogs and cats died during anesthesia (6/9 dogs and 7/8 cats) and only 33% and 13% of dogs and cats, respectively, died postoperatively (3/9 dogs and 1/8 cats). More recently, CEPSAF

Table 2.5 Timing of death in dogs, cats, and rabbits in CEPSAF [7].

Timing of Death	Dogs	Cats	Rabbits
After premedication	1 (1%)	2 (1%)	0
Induction of anesthesia	9 (6%)	14 (8%)	6 (6%)
Maintenance of anesthesia	68 (46%)	53 (30%)	29 (30%)
Postoperative death[a]:	70 (47%)	106 (61%)	62 (64%)
0–3 h PO	31	66	26
3–6 h PO	11	9	7
6–12 h PO	12	7	13
12–24 h PO	13	12	9
24–48 h PO	3	10	3
Unknown time	0	2	4
Total[b]	148 (100%)	175 (100%)	97 (100%)

[a]Postoperative (PO) deaths were additionally categorized by time after anesthesia.
[b]Only deaths where detailed information was available were included here.
Source: [7]. Reproduced with permission of Wiley.

highlighted the postoperative period as the most common time for dogs, cats. and rabbits to die [49]. Over 60% of cats and rabbits and nearly 50% of dogs died during this time period (see Table 2.5). Notably, most of these postoperative deaths occurred within 3 h of termination of the procedure, suggesting that increased vigilance, particularly in the early postoperative period, could reduce the risk of death. Subsequent to this study, work in Spain further highlighted the postoperative period, with over 75% of dogs dying in this multiclinic practice study after anesthesia [11]. Hence, increasingly, the postoperative period represented a high-risk time and close monitoring and management until full recovery is observed are to be recommended.

Risk factors for anesthetic death

Early institution-based studies suggested contributory factors without providing in-depth analysis of risk factors [72,73]. The use of specific drugs was associated with higher mortality in dogs and cats, and trauma patients, neutering procedures, certain breeds including brachycephalic, terrier, and spaniel breeds in dogs were frequently represented amongst the fatalities [72–74]. Old age and poor health status were associated with increased odds of mortality in dogs and poor health status only in cats in a subsequent referral-based study [5,10]. Work at the Royal Veterinary College also reported poor health status as increasing odds and additionally premedication with acepromazine being associated with reduced odds of death in dogs [6]. Although they identified important risk factors, all of these studies were single-center referral studies with small sample sizes and limited abilities to detect more than a small number of major risk factors.

Early practice-based work was also limited in its ability to evaluate risk factors. Dodman [75] identified a trend to reduced risk with thiopental (thiopentone)/halothane anesthesia relative to other drugs in feline anesthetic practice. In a later study, Dodman and Lamb [76] identified high risk with xylazine administration and in brachycephalic breeds, although in both of these studies quantification of risk factors was limited. Clarke and Hall identified a number of risk factors for anesthetic death in healthy dogs and cats [3]. Higher risks were seen with administration of the α_2-adrenergic receptor agonist xylazine and reduced risk with premedication with atropine or acepromazine. In cats, endotracheal intubation, induction of anesthesia with a volatile agent, thiopental, methohexital (methohexitone), ketamine, halothane, ether, and nitrous oxide use were also associated with higher risks of death and administration of alphadolone/alphaxalone (Saffan®) with lower risks, although statistical comparisons were not made. In dogs, Pekingese were the most commonly reported breed to die. Administration of xylazine was associated with higher risk of death whereas halothane and thiopental use was associated with lower death risks. The Ontario study identified similar risk factors with xylazine administration and sick patients (ASA 3–5) being at increased odds of cardiac arrest in dogs, whereas in cats, sick patients (ASA 3–5) were at greater risk while the presence of a technician monitoring anesthesia reduced the risk [4] A study at a single center in France also highlighted increased risk with poor health status [12], and this was supported by a multicenter study in Spain [11].

More recently in CEPSAF, within larger study populations a number of risk factors were evaluated within multivariable logistic regression models for cats and dogs [9,79]. In cats, increasing ASA grade, procedural urgency, major versus minor intended procedures, increasing age, extremes of weight, endotracheal intubation, and the use of fluid therapy were associated with increased odds of anesthetic and sedation-related death (Table 2.6) [79]. Pulse and pulse oximetry monitoring were associated with a reduction in odds. In dogs, poorer health status (based on ASA grade), greater procedural urgency, major versus minor intended procedures, old age, and low weight were associated with anesthetic-related death. Additionally, increasing duration of the procedure and the anesthetic induction and maintenance combination used were associated with increased odds of anesthetic-related death. Maintenance with halothane after induction of anesthesia with an injectable anesthetic agent and dogs undergoing total inhalational anesthesia were both associated with an approximately sixfold increase in odds compared with isoflurane maintenance after induction of anesthesia with an injectable anesthetic agent [9].

The association between patient health status (ASA grade) and anesthetic-related death was repeatedly documented in many of the studies described and has been discussed above [3–6,11,12,50,79]. Pre-existing pathology may reduce the therapeutic index of administered anesthetics, predispose to cardiopulmonary depression, and depress other physiologic functions significantly. Additionally, in CEPSAF, procedural urgency was associated with increased odds of death [9,79]. Hence greater attention to preoperative assessment and stabilization of the patient prior to the procedure could substantially reduce fatalities.

Increased risk with increasing age, independent of patient physical status (ASA grade), was also identified as an important risk factor; however, only some of the more recent work in small animals has reported this [5,9,79]. Old patients may be more susceptible to the depressant effects of anesthetics, to hypothermia via impaired thermoregulatory mechanisms, and to prolonged recovery due to tendencies to reduced metabolic function and hypothermia [80–82].

Increased odds of death reported for small dogs and cats in CEPSAF [9,79] were consistent with work in pediatric anesthesia [83]. Smaller patients could be more prone to drug overdose, to hypothermia, and to perioperative management difficulties (e.g., intravenous catheter placement, endotracheal intubation). Increased risk with increasing weight seen in cats likely reflected, at least in part, risks associated with obesity [79]. Interestingly, although there was a tendency to a breed association in dogs in CEPSAF, after adjusting for weight this association dropped out. This suggested that a major aspect of the risk associated with breed could be related to animal size [9]. Nonetheless, other work has reported increased complications with brachycephalics and terrier breeds [3,4,73], and caution with the anesthesia of these breeds may be advisable.

Table 2.6 Multivariable model of risk factors for anesthetic- and sedation-related death in cats in CEPSAF [8].

Risk Factor	Categories	Odds Ratio[a]	95% Confidence Interval (%)	P value
Health status (ASA grade[b])	ASA 4–5 vs ASA 3 vs ASA 1–2 (trend[c])	3.2	2.0–5.0	<0.001
Urgency of procedure	Emergency vs urgent vs scheduled (trend[c])	1.6	1.0–2.5	0.050
Intended procedure	Minor procedure	1		
	Major procedure	2.7	1.4–5.4	0.005
Age	0–0.5 years	0.4	0.1–2.4	0.058
	0.5–5 years	1		
	5–12 years	1.7	0.9–3.0	
	12 years–max.	2.1	1.1–3.9	
Weight	0–2 kg	15.7	2.9–83.6	
	2–6 kg	1		
	6 kg–max.	2.8	1.1–7.4	
	Unknown	1.1	0.2–5.5	0.002
Endotracheal (ET) intubation	No ET tube	1		
	ET tube	1.9	1.0–3.7	0.042
Pulse and pulse oximeter used	None	1		
	Pulse assessed only	0.3	0.2–0.6	
	Pulse oximeter used only	0.2	0.1–0.5	
	Pulse and pulse oximeter	0.2	0.1–0.4	<0.001
Perioperative intravenous (IV) fluids	No fluids given	1		
	IV catheter used only	0.7	0.2–2.5	
	IV fluids given	3.9	2.2–7.1	<0.001

[a]Odds ratios greater than 1.0 indicate increased odds whereas odds ratios less than 1.0 indicate reduced odds of anesthetic-related death.
[b]ASA 1–2, healthy/moderate disease only; ASA 3, severe disease, limiting activity; ASA 4–5, life-threatening disease.
[c]Trend represents the odds ratio for a one-category increase in the risk factor.
Source: [8]. Reproduced with permission of Oxford University Press.

Increasing risk for patients presenting for major procedures, as documented in CEPSAF [79], was consistent with work in equine anesthesia [14,53]. More complex and invasive procedures were likely to impose greater stress on patient physiology, and when assessing patient risk prior to anesthesia, assessment of the procedure's complexity should be considered. Increasing duration, in addition to type of procedure, was associated with increased risk in dogs in CEPSAF [9]. Longer procedures could expose the patient to extended periods of physiologic compromise, increased hypothermia and fluid loss and could be expected to predispose to greater risk [35]. The previously unreported association of increased risk of death associated with fluid therapy administration in cats in CEPSAF was surprising [79]. Although this may have reflected in part residual confounding, a component of the increased odds may have been related to excessive administration of fluids and fluid overload. Careful fluid administration and monitoring are recommended in cats, although further work is needed to confirm this observation.

The reduction in odds of anesthetic-related death with pulse and pulse oximetry monitoring in cats in CEPSAF has not been reported previously in small animals [79]. Theoretical analyses in human anesthesia support these findings and have suggested that pulse oximetry would have detected 40–82% of reported perioperative incidents, and when combined with capnography 88–93% [84–86]. These associations suggest that some form of assessment of cardiovascular function (pulse quality and rate) and respiratory function (oxygen saturation and end-tidal CO_2) may be important in minimizing mortality.

The role of specific anesthetic drugs in anesthetic death has been evaluated in a number of small animal studies. The premedication administered was a risk factor in a number of studies in dogs and cats [3,4,6,53]. Early work had identified acepromazine as being associated with reduced odds of death [3,6] and major morbid complications [4], compared with no premedication, whereas the α_2-adrenergic receptor agonist xylazine was associated with increased odds of death [3,4]. In CEPSAF, although there were trends to reduced odds with the administration of acepromazine, after adjustment for major confounders this was not a major factor in dogs or cats. Further, when evaluating premedication with the α_2-adrenergic receptor agonist medetomidine, no increased odds of death was detected [9,79]. Xylazine has been found to reduce the threshold to catecholamine-induced arrhythmias under halothane anesthesia [87,88], whereas medetomidine did not [89]. This difference, combined with a greater awareness of the physiologic effects and a better understanding of the optimal method of administration of α_2-adrenergic receptor agonists, may be the basis of a lack of increased risk with medetomidine compared with acepromazine observed in CEPSAF.

The specific induction agent used did not appear important in CEPSAF, in contrast to the tendency for increased risk with the use of thiopental and ketamine in cats and lower risk with alphadolone/alphaxalone (Saffan®) in cats and thiopental in dogs in the last United Kingdom study [3,9,79]. The lack of a consistent difference in risks with different induction agents likely reflects that the effect of induction agent was small. The maintenance agent used, however, was relevant to dogs in CEPSAF, and isoflurane appeared to be associated with reduced odds compared with halothane after induction of anesthesia with an injectable anesthetic agent. This is supported by clinical studies indicating that although isoflurane induces greater respiratory depression and vasodilation than halothane, it causes less direct myocardial depression and sensitizes the heart less to catecholamine-induced arrhythmias, and on balance would appear to cause less overall cardiovascular depression [90–99].

In summary, only the more recent studies have critically evaluated risk factors for death [3–6,9–12,50,79]. Commonly reported risk factors for death include poor health status, old age, poor monitoring, endotracheal intubation in cats, and possible breed associations in dogs [3–6,9,10,79]. Additionally, CEPSAF identified a number of previously unreported risk factors, including the use of pulse oximetry and pulse monitoring reducing odds and fluid therapy increasing odds of death in cats and isoflurane maintenance being associated with reduced odds compared with halothane after an induction of anesthesia with an injectable anesthetic agent in dogs [9,79]. Awareness of these risk factors can aid veterinarians in identifying preoperatively those patients at greatest risk of mortality and in perioperatively managing patients appropriately to reduce mortality.

Large animal anesthetic mortality

Risk of anesthetic death

Work in large animals has concentrated on equine anesthetic complications. Earlier studies focused principally on referral institution populations and death risks were most frequently divided into elective and emergency populations, with the latter principally representing acute abdominal or 'colic' surgery. Mitchell [100] conducted a retrospective study at the Royal (Dick) Vet School (United Kingdom) between 1962 and 1968; 473 horses were anesthetized and seven deaths occurred (1.47%). Short, at the University of Missouri, reported a smaller retrospective study of 125 horses anesthetized, with no deaths [73]. Heath reported an overall single-clinic perioperative equine mortality risk, between 1968 and 1970, at Colorado State University of 4.35% (13 deaths out of 295 anesthetics) [73]. The anesthetic death risk decreased to 1.69% when only anesthetic-related deaths were considered. In a follow-up study at Colorado State University, a reduced overall death risk of 1.18% was reported [74]. Many of these fatalities were due to horses undergoing emergency gastrointestinal surgery that were high-risk patients, and all of these studies were limited by their small sample size, and could only reflect approximate estimates of the frequency of death.

Tevick [101] retrospectively identified a single-clinic equine perioperative mortality risk of 2.70% over a 17-year period, but this was reduced to 0.8% when due to 'anesthesia alone.' The majority of these deaths occurred within 24 h of anesthesia. Gastrointestinal surgery represented the major operation type in those that died and the majority of these patients were deemed high-risk cases. Further single-center reports concentrated on specific hospital populations. Evaluating horses undergoing colic surgery, Trim and colleagues [102] conducted a single-clinic retrospective survey and found a perioperative death risk of 12.5% within 3 days of anesthesia and 20% within 16 days. In contrast, Young and Taylor excluded gastrointestinal surgery and reported a lower single-clinic death risk over a 7-year period of 0.68% [103,104]. Subsequently, Liverpool Veterinary School (United Kingdom) reported mortality risks for both elective and emergency procedures in a retrospective single-clinic study [105,106]. Of 2276 anesthetics, 1279 were classified elective and 995 emergency procedures. Horses were followed until discharged. Of the elective cases, eight died and anesthesia and surgery contributed to the death (0.63%) and one (0.078%) died solely due to anesthesia [106]. For non-colic emergencies, the surgical/anesthetic death risk was 2% and for colic surgeries it was 4.35% [105]. The overall surgical/anesthetic death risk for elective and emergency procedures was 2%. Subsequent to this, Bidwell and colleagues [69] reported reduced risks at a another single center in Kentucky (United States). Of 17 961 horses anesthetized at the clinic between 1997 and 2001, 0.12% died with deaths classified as directly related to anesthesia and 0.24% died or were euthanized within 7 days. These estimates were lower than in previous work and likely reflected, at least in part, differences in populations studied and duration of procedures (most procedures were less than 1 h). All of these reports were single-center studies, the precision of some of their estimates was likely to be limited by their sample sizes, and the risks were highly specific to the populations anesthetized.

The first prospective multicenter perioperative cohort study of equine anesthesia, the Confidential Enquiry into Perioperative Equine Fatalities (CEPEF), was undertaken in the United Kingdom between 1991 and 1997 [52,53]. Of a total of 41 824 horses anesthetized, 39 025 were alive and 785 were dead 7 days postoperatively, giving a death risk of 1.89% [53]. When emergency abdominal surgery and delivery of foals were excluded, the death risk decreased to 0.90% [53]. This was followed by CEPEF 3, a randomized controlled trial of 8242 horses comparing isoflurane with halothane anesthesia [13]. Although representing maintenance of anesthesia with inhalation agents only, they reported similar risks to their previous work. An overall death risk of 1.61% was reported in horses, but when colic and other emergency surgery were excluded a risk of approximately 0.9% was reported. In both of these studies, perioperative death was defined as unexpected death or euthanasia for perioperative complications within 7 days of anesthesia.

In summary, overall anesthetic death risks of approximately 2.0%, decreasing amongst non-emergency horses to approximately 1.0% and in some populations even further, have been reported [13,52,53,69,103,104,106]. Where anesthesia was considered the sole cause of death, a risk of 0.1% was estimated [106]. Emergency anesthetics had a death risk of nearer 1 in 10–30 [52,53,102,105].

Causes of anesthetic death

In equine anesthesia, cardiac arrest and cardiovascular collapse were major causes of death, resulting in 20–50% of all reported deaths [52,53,101,103–106]. Respiratory complications, in contrast, were infrequently reported. Although Tevik [101] did not distinguish respiratory from cardiovascular causes, which when combined accounted for all ten anesthetic deaths described, other studies have reported less than 25% of all deaths as resulting from respiratory compromise [52,53,103–106]. Johnston and colleagues [52,53] documented that only 4% of deaths resulted from respiratory problems.

Non-cardiopulmonary causes have been reported as the cause of death or euthanasia in up to 77% of all equine fatalities [13,52,53, 101,103–106]. Johnston and colleagues [52,53] attributed death in 55% of all cases to fractures on recovery, postoperative myopathy, and abdominal complications such as sepsis and colitis. Young and Taylor [103] reported deaths due to postoperative myopathy and fractures in seven of nine deaths, whereas Bidwell and colleagues [69] reported fractures and myopathy were the basis of over 50% of anesthetic deaths at their center. Rarely have horses been reported 'found dead' or dying of unknown cause, perhaps because horses are more closely observed on recovery than many small animal patients. Johnston and colleagues classified only 5% of equine fatalities as 'found dead' [53].

Timing of anesthetic death

Consistent with work in small animals, recent work in equine anesthesia has also highlighted the postoperative period as a major period of risk. Johnston and colleagues [52,53] reported over 44% of deaths as postoperative events. Young and Taylor [103] reported postoperative fatalities in seven of nine deaths. In the most recent single-clinic study, over 50% of 22 deaths classified as related to anesthesia occurred postoperatively [69]. Hence, although intraoperative concerns remain important, close attention to the postoperative period is also merited in equine anesthesia.

Risk factors for anesthetic death

A number of single-center retrospective studies identified risk factors associated with perioperative complications in horses. In studies undertaken at Colorado State University, anesthetic overdose was considered a major cause of death or euthanasia, and many fatalities were associated with emergency gastrointestinal surgery and high-risk status [73,74]. Tevick [101] identified gastrointestinal surgery as the principal operation type in those horses that died and the majority of these were deemed high-risk cases. Amongst horses undergoing acute emergency abdominal surgery, long duration of anesthesia and intraoperative hypotension were associated with increased risk of death in a further single-center retrospective study [102]. When factors were evaluated in non-colic horses, similar risk factors were identified [103,104].

Intraoperative fluids and inotropic support were associated with reduced risk of fatal myopathy, whereas long procedures and old age were associated with increased risk of death or myopathy. Subsequent work evaluated both elective and emergency procedures in a further retrospective single-clinic study [105,106]. High ASA grade in the elective cases, e.g., elective exploratory laparotomy for 'colic,' was associated with increased risk of death, and amongst emergency patients acute abdominal surgery ('colic' surgery) increased risk.

The prospective multicenter cohort undertaken by Johnston and colleagues [52,53] evaluated risk factors more thoroughly in a large population of anesthetized horses. They identified anesthesia of pregnant mares, foals, horses undergoing abdominal surgery, orthopedic cases requiring internal fixation, long operation time, positioning in dorsal recumbency, lack of sedation, and the use of xylazine as a premedicant with increased risk. Acepromazine premedication and total intravenous anesthesia were associated with reduced risk. The subsequent phase of the work, a randomized clinical trial of isoflurane and halothane for maintenance of anesthesia, reported similar findings [13]. In general, no difference in outcome between the two inhalant anesthetics was found, but in horses aged 2–5 years, isoflurane was associated with reduced odds. In both treatment groups, increased risk was seen with orthopedic and emergency abdominal surgery whereas reduced risk occurred with monitoring of blood pressure, and with ear, nose, and throat and urogenital surgery.

This multicenter work has been uniquely able to quantify specific risk factors and drug associations [13,52,53], but the patterns are similar to those reported in the other equine studies. The work in equine anesthesia indicates risk factors similar to those published in other species. In particular, emergency, abdominal, and orthopedic surgery, long operations, poor health status, and extremes of age were commonly reported factors associated with death. In addition, risks associated with specific anesthetic agents have been addressed, and lack of sedation and xylazine administration were associated with increased risk whereas acepromazine premedication, total intravenous anesthesia, isoflurane in 2–5-year-old horses,. and blood pressure monitoring were associated with reduced risk.

Informed consent

In addition to furnishing the anesthesia provider with information that could inform risk management strategies, an assessment of peri-anesthetic risk is an essential component in the process of informed owner consent. With the assistance of the anesthesia provider, an owner presented with an assessment of the significant risks associated with a proposed procedure for their animal is led to a point of decision-making where they can consent to accept the risk, or refuse consent because of perceived unmitigatable risk. This process of obtaining informed owner consent or refusal involves a conversation between the owner and the anesthesia provider centering on a discussion of relevant and significant risks. At a time where information is readily available (rightly or wrongly) to the public, animal owners can seek out anesthesia care with existing conceptions about anesthesia-related risk. The possibility of such preconceptions mandates the need for a discussion of risk even further.

Included in an informed consent discussion will be an acknowledgment of the extra-label use of drugs, if any. The process of veterinary anesthesia frequently involves the extra-label use of drugs of which the client should be informed. In many cases, the extra-label use of a drug is associated with low-level risk and consent for such use of each drug is impractical. Rather, a blanket acknowledgment and brief discussion of the well-documented, low-level risk of extra-label use of these drugs should be made. In instances where extra-label use is not associated with significant precedence and the risk may be greater, informed consent for the specific use of this particular drug should be obtained.

Clients and animal owners operate under varied perceptions regarding the role of the veterinary anesthesiologist in the delivery of anesthesia care. Hence an informed consent discussion should include an outline of the roles of the various individuals who will be involved in the delivery of anesthesia during a particular procedure. It may be that a certified anesthesia specialist [Diploma in Veterinary Anaesthesia (DVA), Diplomate of the European College of Veterinary Anaesthesia and Analgesia (DECVAA), or Diplomate of the American College of Veterinary Anesthesia and Analgesia (DACVAA)] is involved in the prescribing of a suitable anesthesia protocol and supervises the subsequent delivery of anesthesia care. Specific delivery of that care may be delegated to a non-veterinarian who may be a certified technician or nurse specialist or generalist.

Models for the delivery of anesthesia care are numerous. Proper informed client consent will include a discussion that leads to client understanding and acceptance of the model employed. The documentation of informed consent can be as simple as the notation in the case record of the elements of the process that were discussed with the client. In cases where the associated risks of the procedure are more substantial, a prepared consent form may assist in structuring the informed consent conversation in a systematic way that affords consideration of all of the attendant, significant risks. Although the use of a signed consent form may serve to underscore the existence of real and substantial risk, a frank and informed discussion with an owner remains central to the process of informed consent.

In summary, much improvement in small and large animal anesthesia has occurred over the last 50 years. Risks have reduced and standards of care have improved substantially, and a clearer understanding of factors associated with these complications has aided further improvements. Additionally, the successful communication of these risks to owners and clients is central to the provision of safe anesthesia and the maintenance of realistic owner expectations. Ongoing evaluation of risks and risk factors is merited to sustain and further improve veterinary anesthesia.

References

1 Anon. New classification of physical status. *Anesthesiology* 1963; **24**: 111.

2 American Society of Anesthesiologists. *ASA Physical Status Classification*. Park Ridge, IL: American Society of Anesthesiologists, 2010.

3 Clarke KW, Hall LW. A survey of anaesthesia in small animal practice: AVA/BSAVA report. *J Vet Anaesth* 1990; **17**: 4–10.

4 Dyson DH, Maxie MG, Schnurr D. Morbidity and mortality associated with anesthetic management in small animal veterinary practice in Ontario. *J Am Anim Hosp Assoc* 1998; **34**(4): 325–335.

5 Hosgood G, Scholl DT. Evaluation of age as a risk factor for perianesthetic morbidity and mortality in the dog. *J Vet Emerg Crit Care* 1998; **8**(3): 222–236.

6 Brodbelt DC, Hammond RA, Tuminaro D, *et al.* Risk factors for anaesthetic-related death in referred dogs. *Vet Rec* 2006; **158**: 563–564.

7 Brodbelt DC, Blissitt KJ, Hammond RA, *et al.* The Risk of Death: The Confidential Enquiry into Perioperative Small Animal Fatalities (CEPSAF). *Vet Anaesth Analg* 2008; **35**(5): 365–373.

8 Brodbelt DC, Pfeiffer DU, Young LE, Wood JL. Risk factors for anaesthetic-related death in cats: results from the Confidential Enquiry into Perioperative Small Animal Fatalities (CEPSAF). *Br J Anaesth* 2007; **99**(5): 617–623.

9 Brodbelt DC, Pfeifer DU, Young L, Wood JLN. Risk factors for anesthetic-related death in dogs: results from the Confidential Enquiry into Perioperative Small Animal Fatalities (CEPSAF). *J Am Vet Med Assoc* 2008; **233**(7): 1096–1104.

10 Hosgood G, Scholl DT. Evaluation of age and American Society of Anesthesiologists (ASA) physical status as risk factors for perianesthetic morbidity and mortality in the cat. *J Vet Emerg Crit Care* 2002; **12**(1): 9–15.

11 Gil L, Redondo JI. Canine anaesthetic death in Spain: a multicenter prospective cohort study of 2012 cases. *Vet Anaesth Analg* 2013; **40**(6): e57–e67.

12 Bille C, Auvigne V, Libermann S, *et al.* Risk of anaesthetic mortality in dogs and cats: an observational cohort study of 3546 cases. *Vet Anaesth Analg* 2012; **39**(1): 59–68.

13 Eastment JK, Johnston GM, Taylor PM, *et al.* Is isoflurane safer than halothane in equine anesthesia: results from a multicenter randomised controlled trial. Proceedings of a Meeting of the Society of Veterinary Epidemiology and Preventative Medicine, Cambridge, UK, 4 April 2002.

14 Johnston GM, Eastment JK, Taylor PM, Wood JLN. Is isoflurane safer than halothane in equine anaesthesia? Results from a prospective multicenter randomised controlled trial. *Equine Vet J* 2004; **36**(1): 64–71.

15 NCEPOD. NCEPOD and perioperative deaths of children. *Lancet* 1990; **335**(8704): 1498–1500.

16 Marx GF, Mateo CV, Orkin LR. Computer analysis of postanesthetic deaths. *Anesthesiology* 1973; **39**(1): 54–58.

17 Wolters U, Wolf T, Stutzer H, Schroder T. ASA classification and perioperative variables as predictors of postoperative outcome. *Br J Anaesth* 1996; **77**: 217–222.

18 Cohen MM, Duncan PG, Tate RB. Does anesthesia contribute to operative mortality? *JAMA* 1988; **260**: 2859–2863.

19 Donati A, Ruzzi M, Adrario E, *et al.* A new and feasible model for predicting operative risk. *Br J Anaesth* 2004; **93**(3): 393–399.

20 Morita K, Kawashima Y, Irita K, *et al.* Perioperative mortality and morbidity in 1999 with a special reference to age in 466 certified training hospitals of Japanese Society of Anesthesiologists – Report of Committee on Operating Room Safety of Japanese Society of Anesthesiologists. *Masui* 2001; **50**(8): 909–921.

21 Biboulet P, Aubus P, Dubourdieu J, *et al.* Fatal and non fatal cardiac arrest related to anesthesia. *Can J Anaesth* 2001; **48**(4): 326–332.

22 Buck N, Devlin HB, Lunn JN. *The Report of a Confidential Enquiry into Perioperative Deaths 1987*. London: Nuffield Provincial Hospitals Trust, The King's Fund, 1988.

23 Forrest JB, Cahalan MK, Rehder K, *et al.* Multicenter study of general anesthesia. II. *Results. Anesthesiology* 1990; **72**(2): 262–268.

24 Forrest JB, Rehder K, Cahalan MK, Goldsmith CH. Multicenter study of general anesthesia. III. Predictors of severe perioperative adverse outcomes. *Anesthesiology* 1992; **76**(1): 3–15.

25 Hovi-Viander M. Death associated with anaesthesia in Finland. *Br J Anaesth* 1980; **52**(5): 483–489.

26 Lunn JN, Mushin WW. Mortality associated with anaesthesia. *Anaesthesia* 1982; **37**: 856.

27 McKenzie AG. Mortality associated with anaesthesia at Zimbabwean teaching hospitals. *S Afr Med J* 1996; **86**(4): 338–342.

28 Pedersen T. Complications and death following anaesthesia. A prospective study with special reference to the influence of patient-, anaesthesia-, and surgery-related risk factors. *Dan Med Bull* 1994; **41**(3): 319–331.

29 Pedersen T, Eliasen K, Henriksen E. A prospective study of mortality associated with anaesthesia and surgery: risk indicators of mortality in hospital. *Acta Anaesthesiol Scand* 1990; **34**(3): 176–182.

30 Pottecher T, Tiret L, Desmonts JM, *et al.* Cardiac arrest related to anaesthesia: a prospective survey in France (1978–1982). *Eur J Anaesthesiol* 1984; **1**(4): 305–318.

31 Tikkanen J, Hovi-Viander M. Death associated with anaesthesia and surgery in Finland in 1986 compared to 1975. *Acta Anaesthesiol Scand* 1995; **39**(2): 262–267.

32 Tiret L, Desmonts JM, Hatton F, Vourc'h G. Complications associated with anaesthesia – a prospective survey in France. *Can Anaesth Soc J* 1986; **33**(3 Pt 1): 336–344.

33 Warden JC, Borton CL, Horan BF. Mortality associated with anaesthesia in New South Wales, 1984–1990. *Med J Aust* 1994; **161**(10): 585–593.

34 Warden JC, Horan BF. Deaths attributed to anaesthesia in New South Wales, 1984–1990. *Anaesth Intensive Care* 1996; **24**(1): 66–73.

35 Hall LW, Clarke KW, Trim CM. *Veterinary Anaesthesia*, 10th edn. London: WB Saunders, 2001.

36 Johnson CB. Endocrine disease. In: Seymour C, Gleed RD, eds. *Manual of Small Animal Anaesthesia and Analgesia*. Cheltenham: BSAVA, 1999; 223–230.

37 McMillan M, Brearley J. Assessment of the variation in American Society of Anaesthesiologists Physical Status Classification assignment in small animal anaesthesia. *Vet Anaesth Analg* 2013; **40**(3): 229–236.

38 Knaus W, Draper E, Wagner D, Zimmerman J. APACHE II: a severity of disease classification system. *Crit Care Med* 1985; **13**(10): 818–829.

39 Malviya S, Voepel-Lewis T, Chiravuri S, *et al.* Does an objective system-based approach improve assessment of perioperative risk in children? A preliminary evaluation of the 'NARCO'. *Br J Anaesth* 2011; **106**(3): 352–358.

40 Neary W, Heather B, Earnshaw J. The Physiological and Operative Severity Score for the enUmeration of Mortality and morbidity (POSSUM). *Br J Surg* 2003; **90**(2): 157–165.

41 Schein O, Katz J, Bass E, *et al.* The value of routine preoperative medical testing before cataract surgery. Study of Medical Testing for Cataract Surgery. *N Engl J Med* 2000; **342**(3): 168–175.

42 Chung F, Yuan H, Yin L, *et al.* Elimination of preoperative testing in ambulatory surgery. *Anesth Analg* 2009; **108**(2): 467–475.

43 Benarroch-Gampel J, Sheffield K, Duncan C, *et al.* Preoperative laboratory testing in patients undergoing elective, low-risk ambulatory surgery. *Ann Surg* 2012; **256**(3): 518–528.

44 NICE. Preoperative Tests. The Use of Routine Preoperative Tests for Elective Surgery. Evidence, Methods and Guidance. London: National Institute for Clinical Excellence, 2003.

45 AAGBI. AAGBI Safety Guideline 2. Pre-operative Assessment and Patient Preparation: the Role of the Anaesthetist. London: The Association of Anaesthetists of Great Britain and Ireland, 2010; 22–23.

46 Toews A, Campbell J. Influence of preoperative complete blood cell counts on surgical outcomes in healthy horses: 102 cases (1986–1996). *J Am Vet Med Assoc* 1997; **211**(7): 887–888.

47 Alef M, von Praun F, Oechtering G. Is routine pre-anaesthetic haematological and biochemical screening justified in dogs? *Vet Anaesth Analg* 2008; **35**(2): 132–140.

48 Joubert KE. Pre-anaesthetic screening of geriatric dogs. *J S Afr Vet Assoc* 2007; **78**(1): 31–35.

49 Brodbelt DC, Blissitt KJ, Hammond RA, *et al.* The risk of death: The Confidential Enquiry into Perioperative Small Animal Fatalities. *Vet Anaesth Analg* 2008; **35**(5): 365–373.

50 Brodbelt DC. The Confidential Enquiry into Perioperative Small Animal Fatalities. London: London University, 2006.

51 Gaynor JS, Dunlop CI, Wagner AE, *et al.* Complications and mortality associated with anesthesia in dogs and cats. *J Am Anim Hosp Assoc* 1999; **35**: 13–17.

52 Johnston GM, Taylor PM, Holmes MA, Wood JLN. Confidential Enquiry of Perioperative Equine Fatalities (CEPEF-1): preliminary results. *Equine Vet J* 1995; **27**(3): 193–200.

53 Johnston GM, Eastment JK, Wood JLN, Taylor PM. Confidential Enquiry of Perioperative Equine Fatalities (CEPEF): mortality results of Phases 1 and 2. *Vet Anaesth Analg* 2002; **29**: 159–170.

54 Wagner AE, Hellyer PW. Survey of anesthesia techniques and concerns in private veterinary practice. *J Am Vet Med Assoc* 2000; **217**(11): 1652–1657.

55 Nicholson A, Watson ADJ. Survey on small animal anaesthesia. *Aust Vet J* 2001; **79**(9): 613–619.

56 Joubert KE. Routine veterinary anaesthetic management practice in South Africa. *J S Afr Vet Assoc* 2000; **71**(3): 166–172.

57 Redondo J, Rubio M, Soler G, *et al.* Normal values and incidence of cardiorespiratory complications in dogs during general anaesthesia. A review of 1281 cases. *J Vet Med A Physiol Pathol Clin Med* 2007; **54**(9): 470–477.

58 Galatos AD, Raptopoulos D. Gastro-oesophageal reflux during anaesthesia in the dog: the effect of age, positioning and type of surgical procedure. *Vet Rec* 1995; **137**(20): 513–516.

59 Galatos AD, Raptopoulos D. Gastro-oesophageal reflux during anaesthesia in the dog: the effect of preoperative fasting and premedication. *Vet Rec* 1995; **137**(19): 479–483.

60 Lamata C, Loughton V, Jones M, *et al.* Risk of peri-operative regurgitation in a referral hospital population of dogs. *Vet Anaesth Analg* 2012; **39**(3): 266–274.

61 Wilson DV, Evans AT, Miller R. Effects of preanesthetic administration of morphine on gastroesophageal reflux and regurgitation during anesthesia in dogs. *Am J Vet Res* 2005; **66**(3): 386–390.

62 Wilson DV, Boruta DT, Evans AT. Influence of halothane, isoflurane, and sevoflurane on gastroesophageal reflux during anesthesia in dogs. *Am J Vet Res* 2006; **67**(11): 1821–1825.

63 Redondo J, Suesta P, Gil L, *et al.* Retrospective study of the prevalence of postanaesthetic hypothermia in cats. *Vet Rec* 2012; **170**(8): 206.

64 Redondo J, Suesta P, Serra I, *et al.* Retrospective study of the prevalence of postanaesthetic hypothermia in dogs. *Vet Rec* 2012; **171**(15): 374.

65 Stiles J, Weil A, Packer R, Lantz G. Post-anesthetic cortical blindness in cats: twenty cases. *Vet J* 2012; **193**(2): 367–373.

66 Jurk I, Thibodeau M, Whitney K, *et al.* Acute vision loss after general anesthesia in a cat. *Vet Ophthalmol* 2001; **4**: 155–158.

67 Wagner AE. Complications in equine anesthesia. *Vet Clin North Am Equine Pract* 2008; **24**(3): 735–752.

68 Taylor PM, Clarke KW. *Handbook of Equine Anaesthesia*. Edinburgh: WB Saunders, 1999.

69 Bidwell LA, Bramlage LR, Rood WA. Equine perioperative fatalities associated with general anaesthesia at a private practice – a retrospective case series. *Vet Anaesth Analg* 2007; **34**(1): 23–30.

70 Senior J, Pinchbeck G, Allister R, *et al.* Post anaesthetic colic in horses: a preventable complication? *Equine Vet J* 2006; **38**(5): 479–484.

71 Jones RS. Comparative mortality in anaesthesia. *Br J Anaesth* 2001; **87**(6): 813–815.

72 Albrecht DT, Blakely CL. Anesthetic mortality: a five-year survey of the records of the Angell Memorial Animal Hospital. *J Am Vet Med Assoc* 1951; **119**: 429.

73 Lumb WV, Jones EW. *Veterinary Anesthesia*. Philadelphia: Lea and Febiger, 1973.

74 Lumb WV, Jones EW. *Veterinary Anesthesia*, 2nd edn. Philadelphia: Lea and Febiger, 1984.

75 Dodman NH. Feline anaesthesia survey. *J Small Anim Pract* 1977; **18**: 653–658.

76 Dodman NH, Lamb LA. Survey of small animal anesthetic practice in Vermont. *J Am Anim Hosp Assoc* 1992; **28**: 439–444.

77 Rintasalo J, Vainio O. A survey on anaesthetic practice in Finnish veterinary clinics. *Suom Elainlaakaril* 1995; **101**(9): 541–544.

78 Hall LW, Taylor PM. *Anaesthesia of the Cat*, 1st edn. London: Baillière Tindall, 1994.

79 Brodbelt DC, Pfeifer DU, Young L, Wood JL. Risk factors for anaesthetic-related death in cats: results from the Confidential Enquiry into Perioperative Small Animal Fatalities (CEPSAF). *Br J Anaesth* 2007; **99**: 617–623.

80 Meyer RE. Geriatric patients. In: Seymour C, Gleed RD, eds. *Manual of Small Animal Anaesthesia and Analgesia*, 2nd edn. Cheltenham: BSAVA, 1999; 253–256.

81 Waterman AE. Maintenance of body temperature during anaesthesia. *J Vet Anaesth* 1981; **9**: 73–85.

82 Dhupa N. Hypothermia in dogs and cats. *Compend Contin Educ Pract Vet* 1995; **17**(1): 61–68.

83 Campling EA, Devlin HB, Lunn JN. *The Report of the National Confidential Enquiry into Perioperative Deaths 1989*. London: Nuffield Provincial Hospitals Trust, The King's Fund, 1990.

84 Webb RK, Van der Walt JH, Runciman WB, *et al.* The Australian Incident Monitoring Study. Which monitor? An analysis of 2000 incident reports. *Anaesth Intensive Care* 1993; **21**: 529–542.

85 Tinker JH, Dull DL, Caplan RA, *et al.* Role of monitoring devices in prevention of anesthetic mishaps: a closed claims analysis. *Anesthesiology* 1989; **71**(4): 541–546.

86 Eichhorn JH, Cooper JB, Cullen DJ, *et al.* Standards for patient monitoring during anesthesia at Harvard Medical School. *JAMA* 1986; **256**: 1017–1020.

87 Tranquilli WJ, Thurmon JC, Benson GJ, Davis LE. Alterations in the arrhythmogenic dose of epinephrine (ADE) following xylazine administration to halothane-anesthetised dogs. *J Vet Pharmacol Ther* 1986; **9**: 198–203.

88 Muir WW, Werner LL, Hamlin RL. Effects of xylazine and acetylpromazine upon induced ventricular fibrillation in dogs anesthetised with thiamylal and halothane. *Am J Vet Res* 1975; **36**: 1299–1303.

89 Pettifer GR, Dyson DH, McDonnell WN. An evaluation of the influence of medetomidine hydrochloride and atipamizole hydrochloride on the arrhythmogenic dose of epinephrine in dogs during halothane anaesthesia. *Can J Vet Res* 1996; **60**: 1–6.

90 Tranquilli WJ, Thurmon JC, Benson GJ. Alterations in epinephrine-induced arrhythmias after xylazine and subsequent yohimbine administration in isoflurane-anesthetised dogs. *Am J Vet Res* 1988; **49**(7): 1072–1075.

91 Hellebrekers LJ. Comparison of isoflurane and halothane as inhalation anaesthetics in the dog. *Vet Q* 1986; **8**(3): 183–188.

92 Lemke KA, Tranquilli WJ, Thurmon JC, *et al.* Alterations in the arrhythmogenic dose of epinephrine following xylazine or medetomidine administration to isoflurane-anesthetised dogs. *Am J Vet Res* 1993; **54**(12): 2139–2145.

93 Hikasa Y, Okabe C, Takase K, Ogasawara S. Ventricular arrhythmogenic dose of adrenaline during sevoflurane, isoflurane and halothane anaesthesia either with or without ketamine or thiopentone in cats. *Res Vet Sci* 1996; **60**: 134–137.

94 Hikasa Y, Ohe N, Takase K, Ogasawara S. Cardiopulmonary effects of sevoflurane in cats: comparison with isoflurane, halothane and enflurane. *Res Vet Sci* 1997; **63**: 205–210.

95 Steffey EP, Howland MA. Isoflurane potency in the dog and cat. *Am J Vet Res* 1977; **38**(11): 1833–1836.

96 Steffey EP, Gillespie JR, Berry JD, *et al.* Circulatory effects of halothane and halothane–nitrous oxide anesthesia in the dog: spontaneous ventilation. *Am J Vet Res* 1975; **36**: 197–200.

97 Joas TA, Stevens WC. Comparison of the arrhythmic dose of epinephrine during forane, halothane and fluroxene anesthesia in dogs. *Anesthesiology* 1971; **35**: 48–53.

98 Hodgson DS, Dunlop CI, Chapman PL, Grandy JL. Cardiopulmonary effects of anesthesia induced and maintained with isoflurane in cats. *Am J Vet Res* 1998; **59**(2): 182–185.

99 Grandy JL, Hodgson DS, Dunlop CI, *et al.* Cardiopulmonary effects of halothane anesthesia in cats. *Am J Vet Res* 1989; **50**(10): 1729–1732.

100 Mitchell B. Equine anaesthesia: an assessment of techniques used in clinical practice. *Equine Vet J* 1970; **1**(6):261–274.

101 Tevik A. The role of anesthesia in surgical mortality. *Nord Vetinarmed* 1983; **35**: 175–179.

102 Trim CM, Adams JG, Cowgill LM, Ward SL. A retrospective survey of anaesthesia in horses with colic. *Equine Vet J Suppl* 1989; **7**: 84–90.

103 Young SS, Taylor PM. Factors influencing the outcome of equine anaesthesia: a review of 1,314 cases. *Equine Vet J* 1993; **25**(2): 147–151.

104 Young SS, Taylor PM. Factors leading to serious anaesthetic-related problems in equine anaesthesia. *J Vet Anaesth* 1990; **17**: 59.

105 Mee AM, Cripps PJ, Jones RS. A retrospective study of mortality associated with general anaesthesia in horses: emergency procedures. *Vet Rec* 1998; **142**(12): 307–309.

106 Mee AM, Cripps PJ, Jones RS. A retrospective study of mortality associated with general anaesthesia in horses: elective procedures. *Vet Rec* 1998; **142**(11): 275–276.

3 Anesthesia Equipment

Craig A. Mosley
Mosley Veterinary Anesthesia Services, Rockwood, Ontario, Canada

Chapter contents

Introduction

The delivery and maintenance of safe anesthesia have become increasingly dependent upon mechanical and electrical equipment. It is necessary for the anesthetist to have a thorough understanding of equipment function and potential patient and personnel risks before adaptation for routine patient care. Anesthesia equipment includes various airway support products, oxygen delivery devices, anesthetic machines, scavenging systems, ventilators, and many configurations of patient monitors and other support products. The products available to the veterinary anesthetist include nearly any human-patient product that can be adapted for use in veterinary anesthesia, regularly produced items specifically for the veterinary market, and many limited-production and/or custom products that may only be occasionally available. There are several excellent textbooks devoted to describing in great detail the anesthetic equipment available for use in human anesthesia [1–4] and, although not entirely applicable to veterinary anesthesia, much of the equipment used is the same (i.e., vaporizers, laryngoscopes, endotracheal tubes, some anesthetic machines) or can be adapted from human products. As such, it would be impossible to discuss all of the anesthetic related equipment and products available today in a single chapter. This chapter provides the reader with the operating principles and a practical working overview of common anesthetic-related products (i.e., endotracheal tubes, intubating aids, etc.), the

Veterinary Anesthesia and Analgesia: The Fifth Edition of Lumb and Jones.
Edited by Kurt A. Grimm, Leigh A. Lamont, William J. Tranquilli, Stephen A. Greene and Sheilah A. Robertson.

anesthetic machine, vaporizers, breathing circuits, and ventilators. In addition, there are products that have been designed specifically for veterinary use which are described in more detail here.

Safety and design

Since 1989 and 2000, respectively, human anesthetic breathing circuits (i.e., circle system) and anesthesia machines sold in North America must meet minimum design and safety standards established by organizations such as the American Society for Testing and Materials (ASTM) and the Canadian Standards Association (CSA). The standards were most recently updated in 2005, ASTM F1850 (Standard Specification for Particular Requirements for Anesthesia Workstations and Their Components). Anesthetic machines designed for veterinary use are not required to meet any specific design or safety standards beyond those associated with basic hazards to the operator (i.e., electrical safety requirements). Safety features are often added on an *ad hoc* basis and there are no requirements for demonstrating equipment efficacy. Ideally, some safety features, such as airway pressure alarms, should be integral to the design of the anesthetic machine. The inclusion of some of these safety systems on anesthetic machines may help eliminate preventable anesthetic accidents. However, until safety and design standards are adopted by the manufacturers of veterinary anesthetic equipment, there will remain equipment options of varying quality, efficacy, and safety available for delivering inhalant anesthetics to veterinary patients. Ancillary and support equipment for veterinary patients, including patient monitors and ventilators, are similarly devoid of required efficacy and safety testing. Fortunately, most reputable manufacturers and distributors readily provide the specifications, accuracy, and any testing for efficacy of their designs. Regardless of the presence of standards, it will always be incumbent upon the veterinary anesthetist to understand thoroughly the function, principles of operation, and use of all anesthetic-related pieces of equipment and to ensure that the machine or piece of equipment is designed suitably well to accomplish their functions safely.

Introduction to airway management and support equipment

Airway management and support are vital for the safe delivery of anesthesia. Most, if not all, anesthetics cause respiratory depression at doses suitable for anesthesia. In addition, relaxation and/or loss of airway reflexes make the patient more prone to upper airway obstruction. Both of these factors put the anesthetized patient at higher risk for the development of hypoxia. Additionally, the inhalant anesthetics require delivery to the lungs while minimizing environmental and personnel exposure to waste anesthetic gases. For these reasons, airway management and support are critical aspects of properly performed inhalant general anesthesia.

Endotracheal tubes, lung isolation devices, supraglottic airway devices, laryngoscopes, intubation aids and techniques

Endotracheal tubes

Endotracheal tubes are commonly used to maintain an airway in anesthetized patients. Supraglottic airway devices (SGADs) have also been evaluated in a number of domestic species and may be suitable alternatives in some instances [5–9]. A properly placed endotracheal tube or supraglottic airway device with a properly inflated cuff provides a patent airway, facilitates positive pressure ventilation, protects the lungs from aspiration of fluids, and prevents contamination of the work environment with waste anesthetic gases. Occasionally it is desirable to limit airway management to one lung field (i.e., thoracoscopy), and specially designed equipment is available to accomplish this task in dogs.

There are many styles and types of endotracheal tubes available that can be used in veterinary medicine. Most are manufactured for humans but can also be used in most small animal patients. There are some veterinary-specific products available for patients requiring tube sizes larger and smaller than those available for human use. Endotracheal tubes manufactured for human patients must have various markings and abbreviations directly on the tube that describes each tube's characteristics and also depth of insertion. The markings may include the manufacturer, internal (I.D.) and outer (O.D.) tube diameter and length, and codes indicating tissue toxicity or implantation testing (e.g., F29) (Fig. 3.1). There is no requirement for similar markings on tubes manufactured solely for veterinary use, but it is common for them to minimally list tube diameters and length. Endotracheal tubes are often sized according to their internal diameters. For example, a size 6.0 endotracheal tube refers to a tube with an internal diameter of 6 mm. Some tubes manufactured specifically for the veterinary market have their sizes indicated using the French gauge/catheter scale, and this should, but may not always, reflect the internal size of the tube. The outer diameter for any given tube size may vary depending upon the construction of the tube. Endotracheal tubes having thicker walls will have greater differences between the internal and outer diameters. This can become important when selecting tubes for very small patients. Very thick-walled tubes will effectively reduce the internal airway diameter compared with a thin-walled tube as ultimately the size of endotracheal tube that can be placed in a patient is limited by the outer diameter of the tube and not the inner diameter. However, very thin-walled soft tubes are susceptible to obstruction by external compression or kinking (Fig. 3.2).

Common endotracheal tube materials include polyvinyl chloride, silicone, or red rubber. Clear endotracheal tubes are generally preferred so that they can be inspected visually for the presence of mucus or blood intraoperatively, or debris within the tube lumen after cleaning. Generally, the largest size of endotracheal tube that will fit without causing trauma in the patient's trachea should be used. Although various 'rules-of-thumb' for selecting tube size exist, it is probably easiest to estimate the most appropriate tube size by palpating the individual patient's cervical trachea. The tube should not extend distally beyond the thoracic inlet and ideally should not extend rostrally beyond the patient's incisors, as any additional tube length extending beyond the patient's incisors will increase mechanical deadspace. If the endotracheal tube is too long, and further insertion would lead to the possibility of endobronchial intubation, the machine end can be cut and the endotracheal tube connector reinserted.

The most commonly used type of endotracheal tube in both large and small animals is the cuffed Murphy-type tube shown in Fig. 3.1. Cole-type and guarded (spiral embedded, armored) tubes are also occasionally used in veterinary medicine. Cole tubes are an uncuffed tube that has a smaller diameter at the patient (distal) end relative to the machine (proximal) end. The distal smaller diameter portion of the tube is inserted into the trachea to a point where the shoulder contacts the larynx, forming a seal. However, Cole tubes will not produce the same degree of airway security as a standard cuffed tube and are normally used only in very small patients for

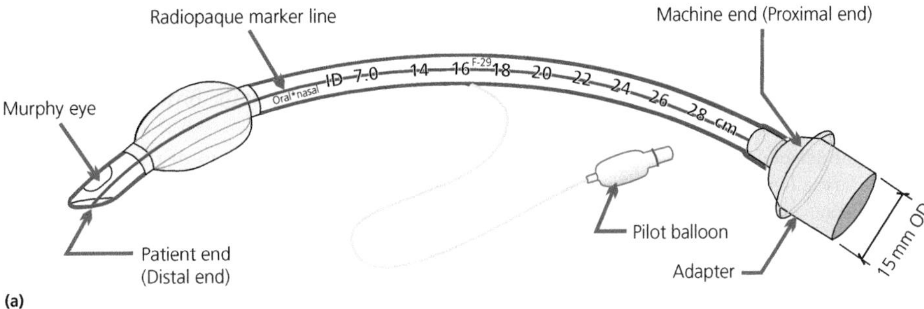

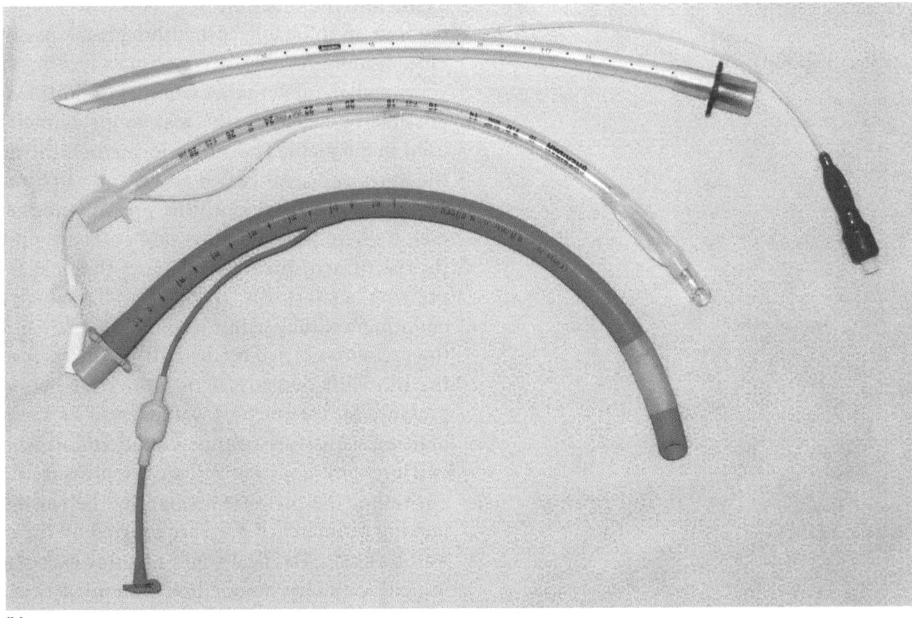

Figure 3.1 Most endotracheal tubes have common design features (a). However, the specific design and materials can vary among the various manufacturers. Tubes can be made of silicone, polyvinyl chloride and red rubber (b, top to bottom). Source: part b, Craig Mosley, Mosley Veterinary Anesthesia Services, Rockwood, ON, Canada.

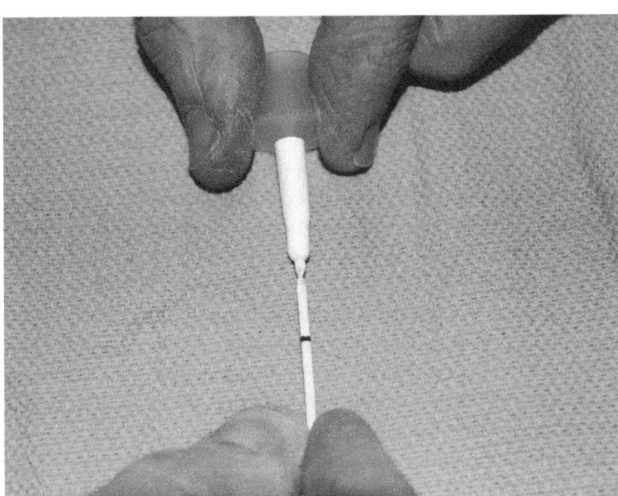

Figure 3.2 Very thin-walled endotracheal tubes are prone to occlusion from external compression or twisting. Continual evaluation of the endotracheal tube for patency is required when thin pliable walled endotracheal tubes are used. Source: Craig Mosley, Mosley Veterinary Anesthesia Services, Rockwood, ON, Canada.

short-term intubation (see Fig. 3.3). Guarded tubes incorporate a metal or nylon spiral-wound reinforcing wire into the endotracheal tube wall that helps prevent tube collapse and occlusion (Fig. 3.4). Guarded tubes are useful in situations where the tube is likely to be compressed or kinked, such as procedures requiring extreme flexion of the head and neck (e.g., cervical cerebrospinal fluid collection and ophthalmic procedures) or those that involve compression of the trachea (e.g., tracheal retraction during ventral approach to the cervical spinal cord).

The machine end of the tube contains the endotracheal tube connector. The most proximal portion of the connector used for small animals and human patients is a uniform size (15 mm O.D.) facilitating universal connection to all standard anesthetic circuits. Tubes designed for use in large animals typically have larger connectors which include metal-type and funnel-type connectors. The distal (patient) end of the connector varies in size according to the diameter of the endotracheal tube. Endotracheal tube adapters may also incorporate gas sampling ports (Fig. 3.5). These are particularly useful in small patients where minimizing equipment deadspace may be important and may improve the accuracy of gas sampling in smaller patients where non-rebreathing systems are often used.

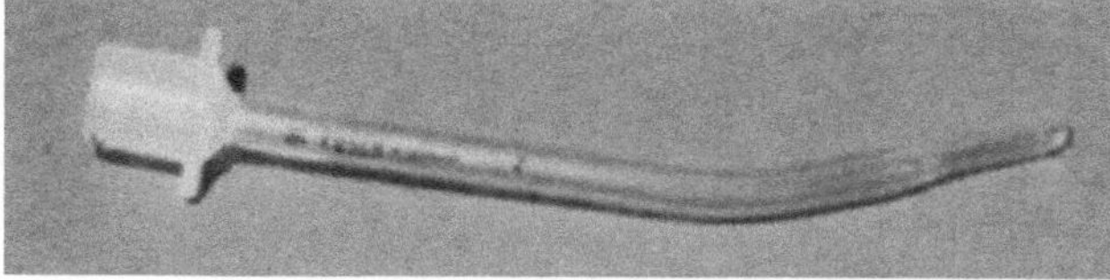

Figure 3.3 Cole endotracheal tube demonstrating the tapered shoulder used to position the tube in the larynx forming a seal. Note that the tube does not have a cuff or pilot balloon.

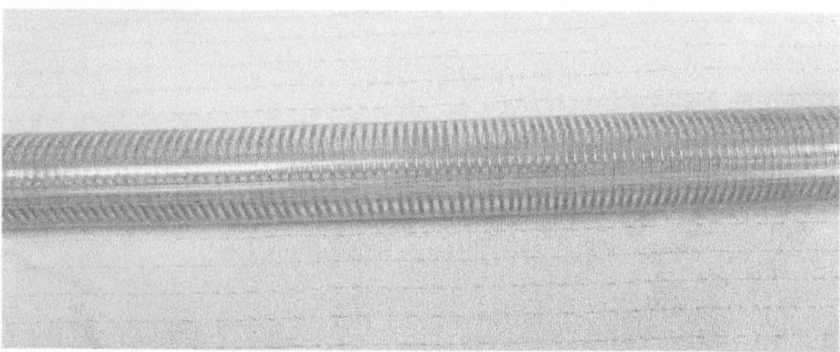

(a)

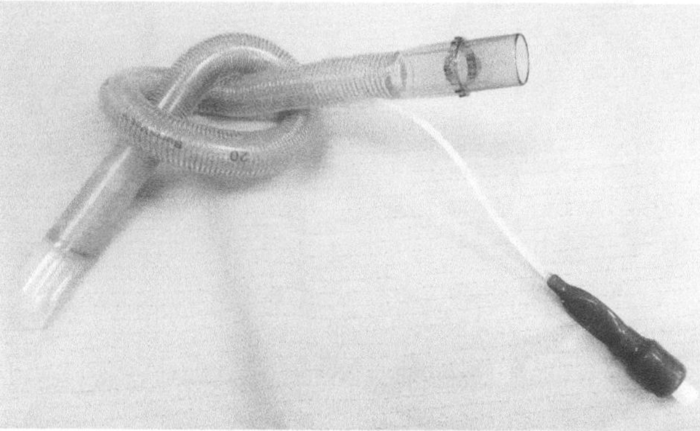

(b)

Figure 3.4 Guarded tubes contain a metal or nylon spiral wire (a) that prevents collapse if the tubes are bent or folded (b). Source: Craig Mosley, Mosley Veterinary Anesthesia Services, Rockwood, ON, Canada.

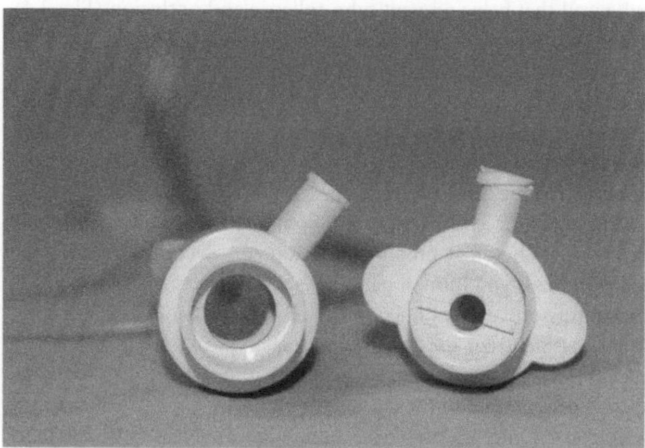

Figure 3.5 Two endotracheal tube adapters that incorporate a gas sampling port. Note the internal diameter (volume) of the pediatric design on the right. This type of design can help improve the accuracy of side stream end tidal gas sampling in smaller patients. Source: Craig Mosley, Mosley Veterinary Anesthesia Services, Rockwood, ON, Canada.

Endotracheal tubes designed for large animals are normally manufactured with a silicone funnel adapter attached (Fig. 3.6) that is designed to fit over the large animal Y-piece (54 mm O.D.). There are also stainless-steel endotracheal tube adapters (22 O.D.) that are designed to fit the Bivona insert sometimes found on large animal Y-pieces.

The patient (distal) end of the endotracheal tube is normally beveled. Murphy-type tubes have a hole in the endotracheal tube wall opposite the bevel, referred to as a Murphy eye or hole (see Fig. 3.1a). The purpose of the hole is to provide an alternative route for gas flow should the beveled opening becoming occluded. Those endotracheal tubes without a Murphy eye are referred to as Magill-type tubes. Most endotracheal tube sizes can be found without an inflatable cuff, although the use of cuffed tubes provides a more reliable airway. Tubes lacking cuffs tend to be the very small diameter tubes where the addition of a cuff may not be possible or will limit the maximum diameter tube that can be used in a patient. The cuff is located on the machine-end side of the Murphy eye for cuffed tubes, and can be a low-volume, high-pressure or high-volume, low-pressure design (Fig. 3.7). In general, high-volume, low-pressure cuffs are preferred to minimize the risk of ischemic tracheal injury that may result from excessive pressure against the tracheal wall. When a properly fitting endotracheal tube with a high-volume, low-pressure cuff is used, the pressure exerted by the cuff on the tracheal wall is similar to the intracuff pressure. This allows for better estimation of the pressure on the tracheal wall exerted by the cuff. When using a high-pressure, low-volume cuffed endotracheal tube, the intracuff pressure does not reflect the pressure on the tracheal wall but rather the pressure created by the elastic recoil of the cuff, making estimates of pressure exerted by the cuff on the tracheal wall difficult. Tracheal wall pressures exceeding 48 cmH_2O may impede capillary blood flow, potentially causing ischemic tracheal damage, and pressure below 18 mmHg may increase the risk of aspiration [10]. There are also several cases of tracheal rupture or disruption reported in veterinary medicine leading to pneumothorax, pneumomediastinum, and/or subcutaneous emphysema [11].

A reliable method for ensuring that cuff pressures are within the recommended range is to use a cuff monitor to inflate high volume, low pressure cuffs. A cuff monitor is essentially a low-pressure manometer similar to those used for Doppler blood pressure measurement that is attached to the pilot balloon of the cuff and provides a measure of intracuff pressure. Other commercially available cuff inflation guides are available for the human market and can be adapted to veterinary use (Fig. 3.8). Alternatively, it is more common to use a leak test, performed by inflating the cuff until a leak is no longer audible while maintaining airway pressures of 20–30 cmH_2O. The pilot balloon used for inflating the endotracheal tube cuff is connected to the cuff via a channel incorporated into the endotracheal tube and normally includes a syringe activated self-sealing valve system. However, there are also valveless pilot balloons that do not self-seal and require occlusion using either a clamp or plug.

Recently, an uncuffed self-sealing endotracheal tube (Safe-Seal™, Innovative Animal Products, Rochester, MN, USA, 55901) has been introduced into the veterinary market. The tube is designed with a series of flexible ringed flanges at the patient end of the endotracheal tube that deform to the contours of the trachea, forming a seal against the tracheal wall eliminating the need to inflate a cuff (Fig. 3.9). There are currently no independent research studies

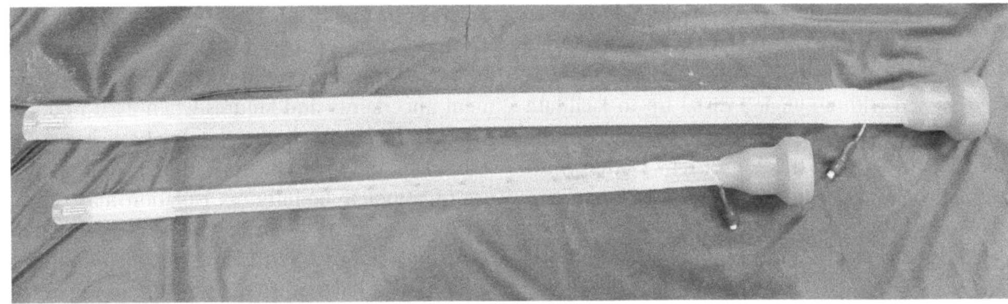

Figure 3.6 Two endotracheal tubes used for large animal anesthesia. These tubes are typically silicone and are commonly manufactured with a silicone funnel adapter that is compatible with the Y-piece of most large animal anesthetic breathing circuits. Source: Craig Mosley, Mosley Veterinary Anesthesia Services, Rockwood, ON, Canada.

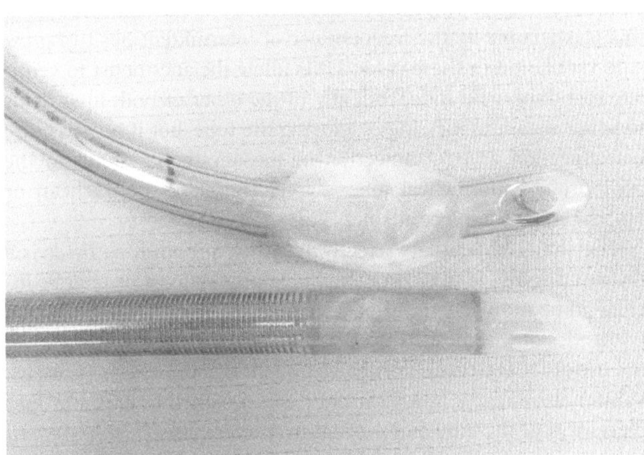

Figure 3.7 The upper endotracheal tube has a high-volume, low-pressure cuff whereas the lower endotracheal tube shows an example of a high-pressure, low-volume cuff. Note the bulkiness that can be associated with the high-volume, low-pressure cuff compared with the low-volume, high-pressure cuff. The bulkiness associated with some cuffs can limit the endotracheal tube size, which can be problematic in very small patients. However, high-volume, low-pressure cuffs may help reduce tracheal damage resulting from cuff over-inflation. Source: Craig Mosley, Mosley Veterinary Anesthesia Services, Rockwood, ON, Canada.

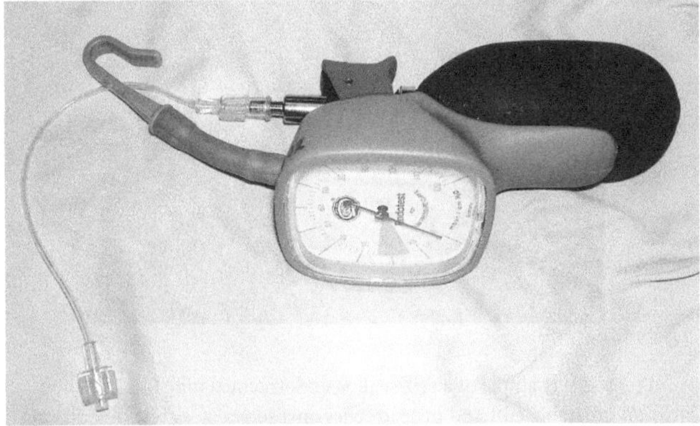

(a)

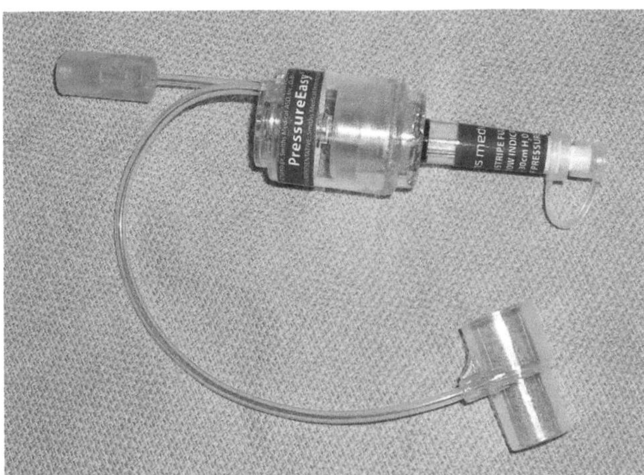

(b)

Figure 3.8 An endotracheal tube inflation guide or monitor can be used to evaluate the intracuff pressures of the endotracheal tube and may help avoid tracheal injury secondary to excessive tracheal wall pressures. Several styles are available. Source: Craig Mosley, Mosley Veterinary Anesthesia Services, Rockwood, ON, Canada.

evaluating the effectiveness of this tube for use in veterinary anesthesia. It is available with only a limited number of internal tube diameters and differs from a conventional endotracheal tube in that it has no Murphy's eye or inflatable cuff.

Endotracheal tubes for isolating one lung

In addition to the endotracheal tubes described above, there are tubes specially designed for isolating or ventilating one lung. Indications for the use of these tubes include improving surgical conditions for various thoracic procedures (i.e., thoracoscopy), the control of contamination or hemorrhage, and use in circumstances where unilateral pathology exists. There are generally three methods of isolating or ventilating a single lung; a double-lumen tube (DLT), a bronchial blocker, or by using a long, standard endotracheal tube as an endobronchial tube.

Endobronchial intubation for single lung ventilation or isolation is probably the least desirable as it provides less direct control for making changes in the non-intubated lung. However, it does not require specialized equipment, apart from a sufficiently long endotracheal tube, and is relatively easy to perform. Endobronchial intubation has been used in dogs successfully and may be an alternative when DLTs and bronchial blockers are not available [12,13].

DLTs tend to be the preferred option in human medicine. All commercially available DLTs have been designed specifically for human patients and have been adapted for use in dogs. There have been several types evaluated in a range of dog sizes and breeds

[14–17]. DLTs consist of two single-lumen tubes bonded together and are available as right- or left-sided tubes (Fig. 3.10), where right and left designate which mainstem bronchus the tube is designed to fit. Most DLTs are designed with an angled distal tip to facilitate placement into either the right or left bronchus. The three most commonly available styles of DLTs are the Robertshaw, Carlens, and White. The tubes have two elliptical cuffs: one occludes the trachea and the other occludes the bronchus (Fig. 3.11). The bronchial cuff and pilot balloon are normally colored blue for differentiation from the tracheal cuff.

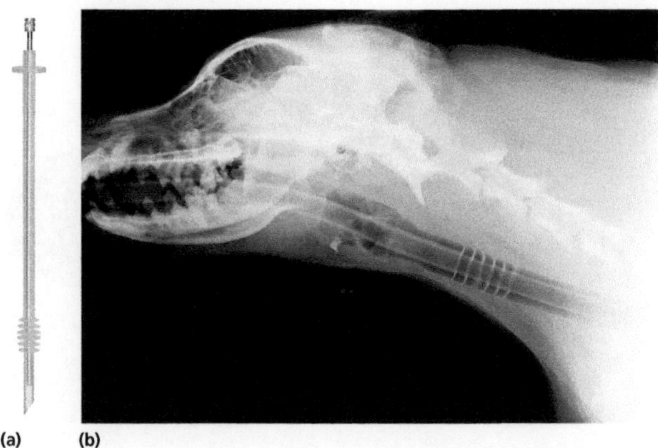

Figure 3.9 An example of a self-sealing endotracheal tube (a). The tube lacks an inflatable cuff and instead relies on a series of soft flexible flanges to provide airway security (b). Source: Craig Mosley, Mosley Veterinary Anesthesia Services, Rockwood, ON, Canada.

The bronchial cuffs of right-sided tubes vary in shape and design in order to facilitate ventilation of the upper right lung lobe in humans. The use of right-sided tubes can introduce greater placement uncertainty and failures when used in dogs, as the right cranial lung lobe bronchus of the dog branches more proximally than in humans and the bronchial cuff may occlude the bronchus or failure of complete hemithorax isolation may occur. In general, left-sided tubes are most often used and can be used effectively for both right- and left-sided procedures. Even if proximal clamping or transection of the left mainstem bronchus is required, the left-sided tube can simply be withdrawn into the trachea so the distal bronchial portion of the tube does not interfere with clamping. The internal lumen of the tracheal portion of the tube is oval or D-shaped and the sizes are designated using the French scale, ranging from 26 to 41 Fr. The reduced lumen size will increase resistance to breathing compared to an appropriately sized standard single lumen tube, but this is overcome by the frequent use of intermittent positive pressure ventilation in these cases. DLTs allow the anesthetist to ventilate each lung field independently of the other or both lung fields together without replacing or moving the tube, but it does require disconnection and reconnection of the anesthetic circuit to the appropriate endotracheal tube adapter (bronchial or tracheal) or both by using a Y-piece adapter (Fig. 3.12).

The ability to ventilate selectively either or both lung fields is a distinct advantage over bronchial blocking systems or endobronchial intubation when surgical conditions require operating on both sides of the chest. However, the available sizes typically limit the use of DLTs to dogs between 5 and 20 kg. Some DLTs (Carlens, White) also incorporate a carinal hook designed to aid in proper placement of the tube and prevent movement after positioning. In veterinary patients, this modification may actually hinder rather than contribute to correct tube placement [14]. Additional care should also be taken when placing DLTs with a carinal hook to

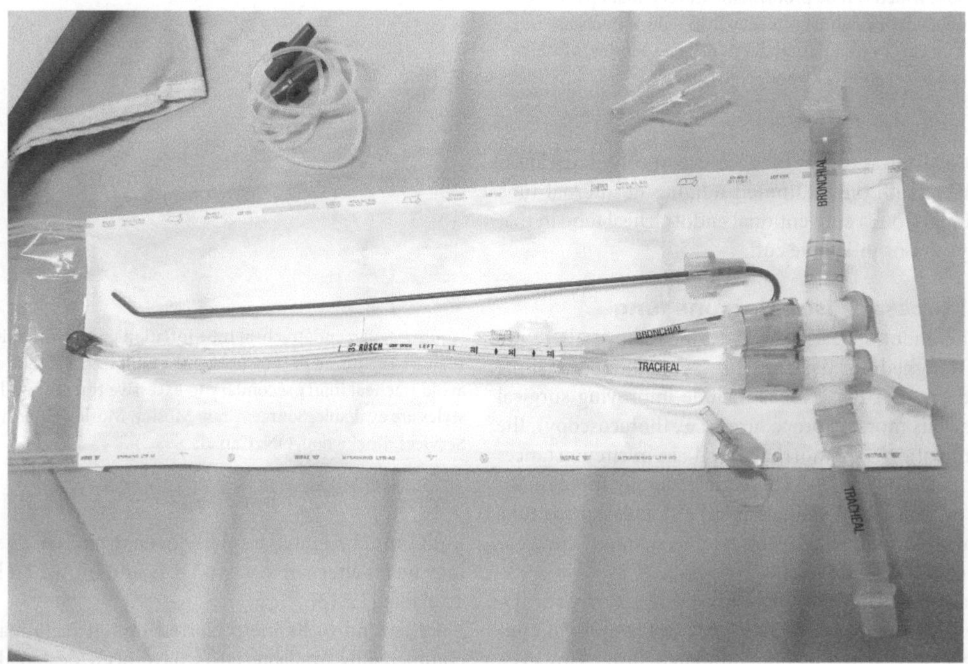

Figure 3.10 An example of a left-sided Robertshaw double-lumen endotracheal tube. DLTs can be used to ventilate selectively one or both lung fields in appropriately sized dogs. Source: Craig Mosley, Mosley Veterinary Anesthesia Services, Rockwood, ON, Canada.

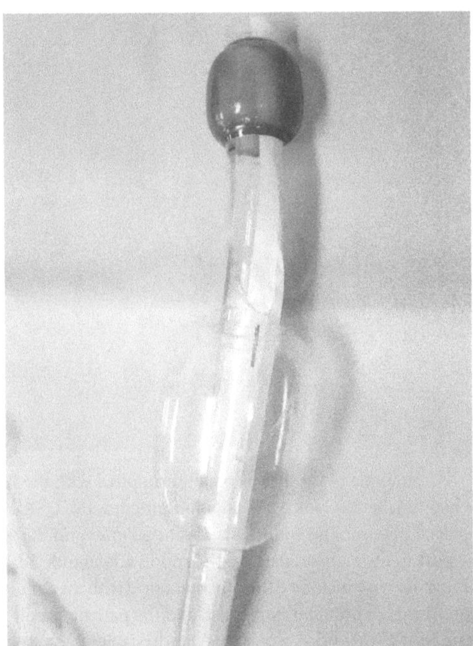

Figure 3.11 A closer image demonstrating the distal end of a left-sided Robertshaw double-lumen endotracheal tube. Note the angle of the distal end of the tube and the two cuffs. The more distal blue cuff is the bronchial cuff. This tube is designed to facilitate placement into the left mainstem bronchus. Source: Craig Mosley, Mosley Veterinary Anesthesia Services, Rockwood, ON, Canada.

ensure that it does not catch on any tissues or structures when introducing the tube into the trachea. For this reason, the Robertshaw left-sided DLT is probably the most versatile type for use in dogs. In veterinary patients, correct placement of a DLT is generally confirmed by direct visualization using a small-diameter bronchoscope. Recently, a thoracoscopic assisted technique has also been described [14]. Correct and complete placement is further confirmed by ventilating both the right and left lung fields while auscultating for lung sounds. Correct and complete placement should ventilate all intended lung fields (i.e., right or left) without ventilating any lung fields on the contralateral side. Although blind placement is possible using some tubes, it is associated with a relatively high failure to achieve correct and complete tube placement [14]. Small movements of the tube and/or patient may disrupt correct and complete placement and occasionally bronchial cuffs will prolapse into the trachea, leading to complete airway obstruction. Vigilance is required by the anesthetist to recognize and correct any positional problems should they occur (e.g., deflation of bronchial cuff).

Bronchial blockers represent another system for facilitating one-lung isolation or ventilation in dogs (Fig. 3.13) [13,15,18,19]. In human anesthesia they are often used when patient size precludes the use of a DLT or when anatomic abnormalities or differences are present that may preclude optimal tube fit. That they are very adaptable for use over a wider range of patient sizes and are not as anatomically specific as DLTs are distinct advantages of using bronchial blockers in veterinary anesthesia. However, independent lung ventilation is not possible without withdrawing and replacing the bronchial blocker in the contralateral bronchus.

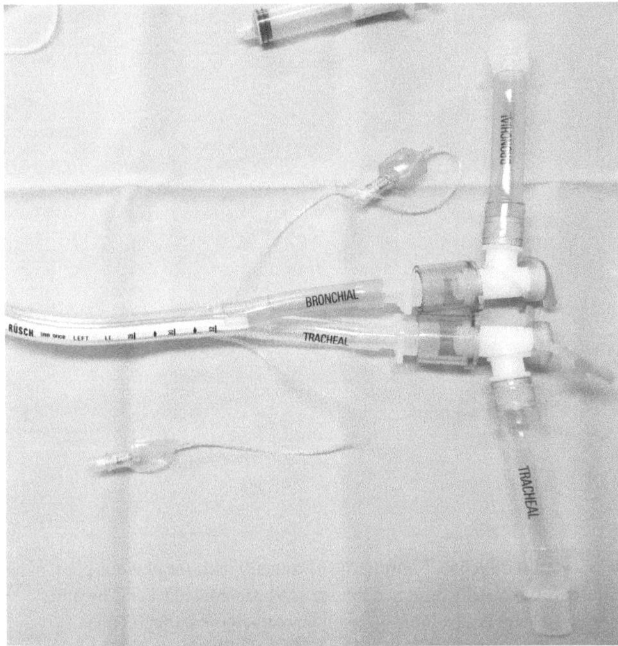

(a)

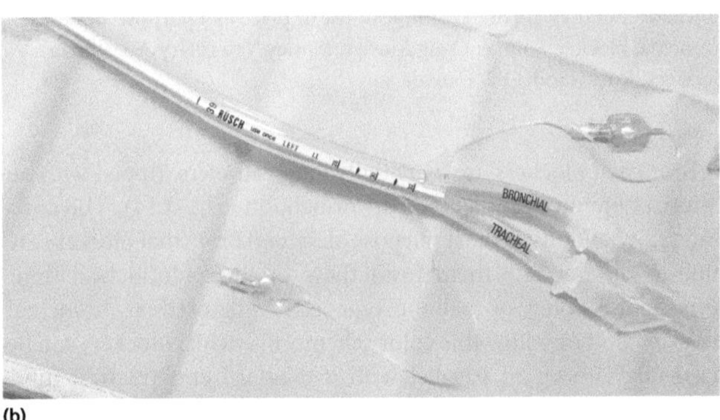

(b)

Figure 3.12 DLTs can be used to ventilate (or collapse) each lung field independently or can ventilate both lung fields simultaneously. (a) The adapter configuration required for independent lung field ventilation (or collapse) and (b) the use of a Y-adapter to facilitate simultaneous ventilation of both lung fields. Note the blue pilot balloon cuff and the blue tubing corresponding to the bronchial portion of the tube. Source: Craig Mosley, Mosley Veterinary Anesthesia Services, Rockwood, ON, Canada.

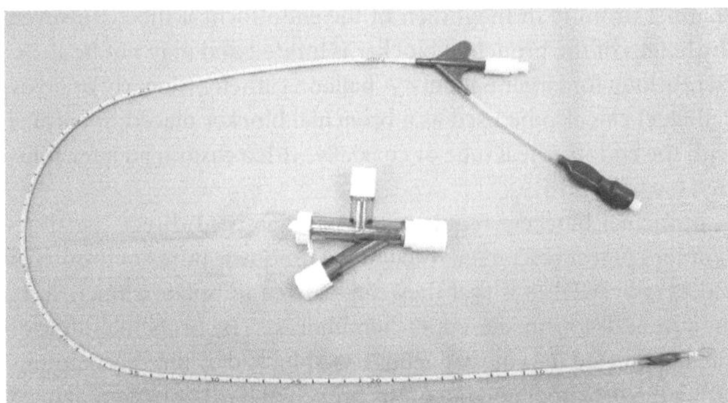

Figure 3.13 An example of a bronchial blocking system commonly used in veterinary medicine. The system consists of a bronchial blocker (balloon-tipped catheter) and a swivel adapter allowing for coaxial placement of the blocker. Source: Craig Mosley, Mosley Veterinary Anesthesia Services, Rockwood, ON, Canada.

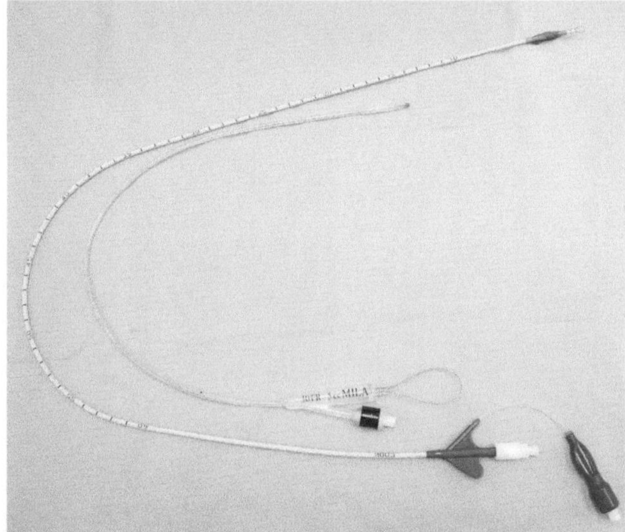

Figure 3.14 The yellow (or outermost) catheter with the obvious pilot balloon is specifically designed for use as a bronchial blocker. The inner shorter catheter is a balloon-tipped Foley catheter. Although Foley catheters are not designed for use as bronchial blockers, they have been placed alongside endotracheal tubes and used successfully for bronchial blockade, but they are not as simple to use or place as a purpose-designed bronchial blocker. Source: Craig Mosley, Mosley Veterinary Anesthesia Services, Rockwood, ON, Canada.

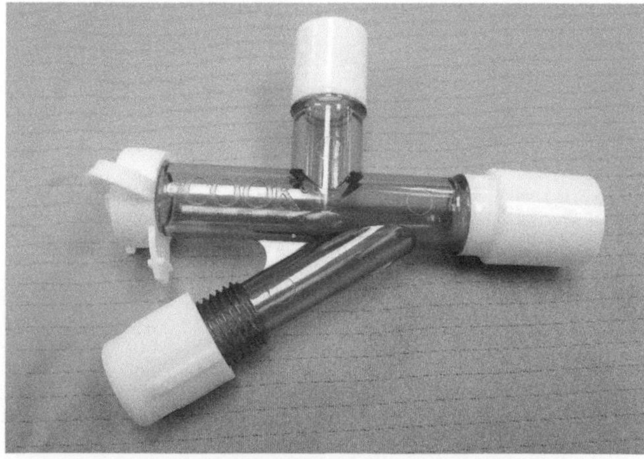

Figure 3.15 An example of the airway adapter supplied with the Arndt Endobronchial Blocker™ (Cook Medical, Bloomington, IN, USA). The adapter is placed between the endotracheal tube adapter and the breathing circuit. The port to the right attaches to the endotracheal tube adapter; the ports moving clockwise include the bronchial port (with an annular compression fitting), a bronchoscope port, and the patient circuit port. Source: Craig Mosley, Mosley Veterinary Anesthesia Services, Rockwood, ON, Canada.

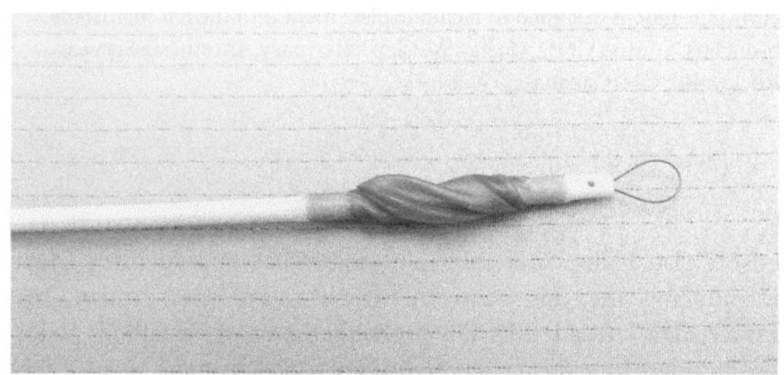

Figure 3.16 The distal end of an Arndt Endobronchial Blocker™ (Cook Medical, Bloomington, IN, USA) showing the wire loop used to facilitate proper placement using a bronchoscope. Source: Craig Mosley, Mosley Veterinary Anesthesia Services, Rockwood, ON, Canada.

Bronchial blockers are essentially long catheters, tipped with an elliptical or round inflatable cuff or balloon (Fig. 3.14). The cuffs and pilot balloons of most purpose-designed bronchial blockers are blue to differentiate them from those of the endotracheal tube. Expectedly, Foley or balloon-type catheters used as bronchial blockers do not follow this color scheme. Bronchial blockers can be used coaxially or in parallel with a standard endotracheal tube. Various swivel adapters are supplied with commercially available bronchial blockers to facilitate coaxial use. The swivel adapters connect to the endotracheal tube adapter and have ports for passing the bronchial blocker, a bronchoscope, and a connector for the anesthetic circuit (Fig. 3.15).

The ports are designed in a way to prevent leakage and to secure the bronchial blocker once it is in place. There is also a commercially available human coaxial product (Univent® tube, Teleflex Inc., Limerick, PA, USA) that incorporates the bronchial blocker in a channel running in the lumen of the endotracheal tube. However, the length of the bronchial blocker is limited and may not be sufficiently long for larger patients. A balloon catheter (Fogarty or Foley catheter) can also be used as a bronchial blocker placed in parallel with the endotracheal tube or coaxially with a custom adapter solution (see Fig. 3.14).

Bronchial blockers require fiber-optic-assisted direct visualization for correct placement. One of the unique features of bronchial blockers over DLTs is that they can be used to isolate a single lung lobe in addition to the entire hemithorax. The bronchial blocker can be directed into the bronchus to be blocked by directly manipulating the proximal portion of the bronchial blocker or by placing a guide wire into the bronchus to be blocked and sliding the bronchial blocker over the guide wire. One bronchial blocker (Ardnt Endobronchial Blocker™, Cook Medical, Bloomington, IN, USA) has a small wire loop exiting the distal end of the blocker (Fig. 3.16). The loop can be used to facilitate placement by sliding the loop over the end of the bronchoscope. Once correct placement has been achieved, the balloon or cuff can be inflated, precluding ventilation of that lung region. The lung is then allowed to collapse by opening the bronchial blocker catheter channel. The open channel can be used for continuous positive airway pressure (CPAP) application, oxygen insufflation, and/or suctioning. Placement of the bronchial blocker in the right bronchus can be challenging owing to the proximal branching of the cranial lung lobe. Prolapse of a bronchial blocker into the trachea can lead to complete airway obstruction; this is most likely to occur when placed proximally in the bronchus and/or if the tube and bronchial blocker assembly are withdrawn inadvertently when moving or manipulating the patient.

Supraglottic airway devices

Supraglottic airway devices (SGADs), also commonly referred to as laryngeal mask airways (LMAs), are becoming increasingly popular for veterinary use. There are a large number of products available that were designed for humans that have been adapted for veterinary use. However, these products have been optimized specifically

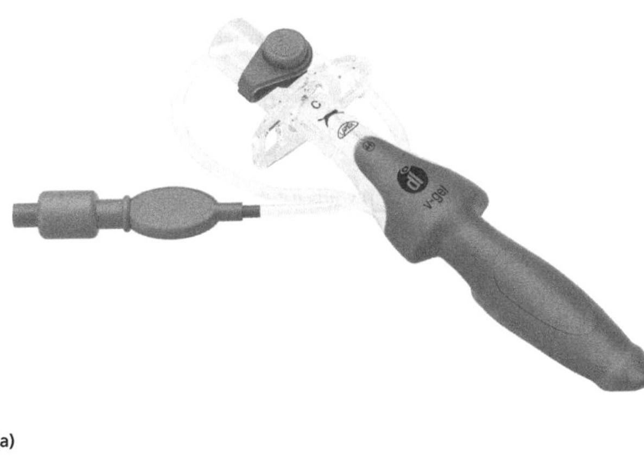

(a)

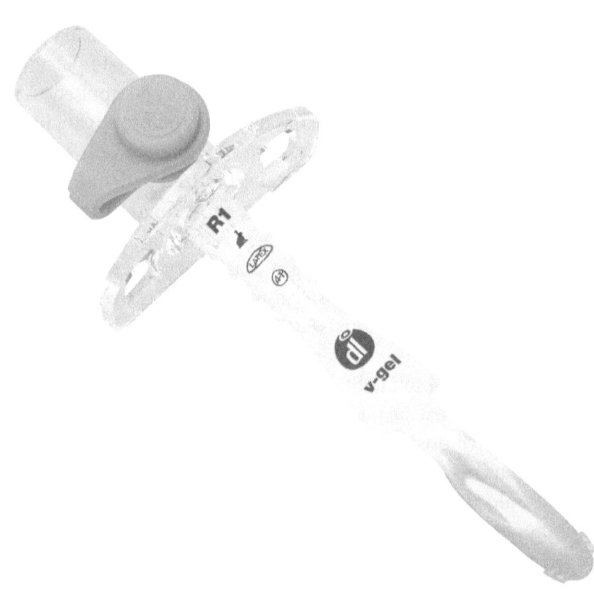

(b)

Figure 3.17 Veterinary-specific laryngeal masks (v-gel®) designed for use in cats (a) and rabbits (b). These masks can be used as alternatives to tracheal intubation and may be easier to place than endotracheal tubes in some species. Source: Docsinnovent Ltd, London, UK. Reproduced with permission of Docsinnovent Ltd.

for the orolaryngeal/pharyngeal anatomy of humans and may not conform well to the varied anatomy, patient size, species, and breeds commonly encountered in veterinary medicine. Appropriate use of these products is important as inappropriate SGAD and/or patient selection may lead to placement difficulties/failures, damage to tissues of the oropharyngeal region, and/or improper protection and patency of the airway. Recently, a veterinary-specific SGAD has been introduced (cat and rabbit v-gel®, Docsinnovent Ltd, London, UK) designed for use in cats and rabbits (Fig. 3.17).

SGADs represent an alternative to endotracheal intubation for maintenance of a patent airway and there is some evidence that they may be simpler and faster to place than endotracheal tubes in some species [20–22]. There is also some evidence that less anesthetic is required for placement of an SGAD compared with an endotracheal tube [7]. SGADs do not require the use of a laryngoscope for placement and do not enter the larynx or trachea. A typical device consists of a tube, similar to an endotracheal tube, connected to an elliptical mask that has an inflatable outer edge. When placed and inflated correctly, they form a seal around the glottis. The criteria for correct SGAD placement have been described for various species and should be reviewed prior to using these devices [20,22,23]. Properly placed and inflated SGADs are not associated with greater leakage of anesthetic gases compared with endotracheal tubes and positive pressure ventilation using an SGAD has been successfully performed and evaluated in several veterinary species [6,8,20, 24–26]. The use of SGADs is still relatively uncommon in veterinary medicine but as their use increases and further large prospective studies are completed, additional advantages and disadvantages related to relatively rare events (e.g., gastroesophageal reflux and subsequent aspiration, significant post extubation airway irritation) may be detected.

Laryngoscopes

Laryngoscopes consist of a handle and lighted blade; and are used to aid tracheal intubation and oropharyngeal evaluation during intubation. Unfortunately, laryngoscopes are often considered an optional piece of anesthetic-related equipment but their proper use can be vital for successful intubation in some patients (e.g., brachycephalics and patients with laryngeal/oral trauma). Regardless of the absolute need for laryngoscope-assisted intubation, its use is recommended for all intubations to ensure that the anesthetist maintains the motor skills and coordination to use a laryngoscope properly and so that a cursory oropharyngeal evaluation can be performed.

There are several styles and types of laryngoscopes and blades available. Some laryngoscopes have a fixed blade (i.e., one blade type and size) and may be made of plastic whereas others are designed for use with multiple blade sizes and styles of blades and are made of stainless steel. Because there is such a range of patient sizes, with different oral cavity configurations, found in veterinary medicine the option to use multiple blades is a significant advantage when selecting a laryngoscope. The handle may also vary in size and, although this rarely impacts the functional use of the laryngoscope, a smaller handle may be more comfortable and easier to manipulate for some anesthetists, particularly when used for intubating very small patients. The handles are usually specific for either fiber-optic or bulb-in-blade illumination, although there are some handles that can accept either type of blade illumination system. There is no clear advantage of one lighting system over the other.

There are two main types of blades that are used in veterinary medicine, the MacIntosh and the Miller blade. Both come in a wide range of sizes (000–5). The MacIntosh is a curved blade with a prominent vertical flange whereas the Miller is a straight blade with a less prominent vertical flange; both are suitable for intubation of most patients and the decision to use one over the other is often determined by personal preference (Fig. 3.18). However, the prominent flange of the MacIntosh blade can potentially interfere with laryngeal visualization when used for intubating veterinary patients (see below). In addition to the standard sized blades available in human medicine, extremely long (~300 mm) Miller-style blades (useful for intubating swine, camelids, sheep. and goats) are also available.

Interestingly, the majority of human-designed laryngoscope blades and endotracheal tubes are designed for anesthetist's using their right hand to pass the endotracheal tube while their left hand holds the laryngoscope. The endotracheal tube bevel faces the left when viewing the tube from the concave aspect and the laryngoscope blade flange is normally on the right side of the blade when

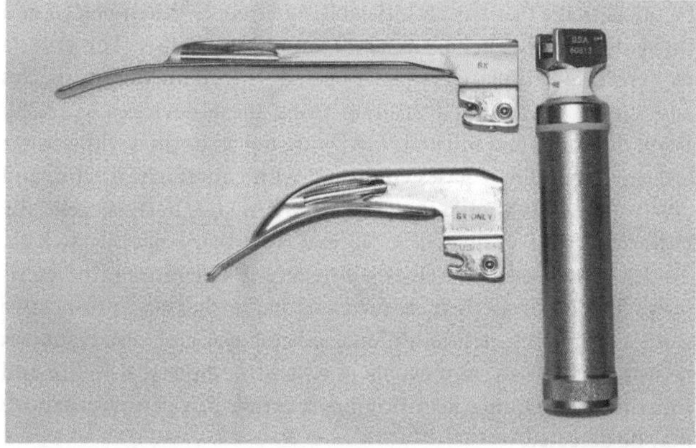

Figure 3.18 Laryngoscope handle with Miller (upper) and Macintosh (lower) blades. Note the more prominent vertical flange on the Macintosh blade. This flange may impair visualization of the larynx when intubating a patient in sternal recumbency using the right hand. Source: Craig Mosley, Mosley Veterinary Anesthesia Services, Rockwood, ON, Canada.

viewing the blade from the top. This configuration provides optimal visualization of the larynx when intubating a patient in the supine position (dorsal recumbency) where the laryngoscope is held with the blade in a downward position (inverted) and the endotracheal tube is held with the concave surface directed upwards. However, most veterinary patients are intubated in sternal recumbency where the flange of the laryngoscope when held in the left hand can obscure visualization and the bevel of the endotracheal tube will do little to improve visualization when held in the right hand. There are left-handed MacIntosh blades available that may be more appropriate for routine intubation in veterinary species as these blades place the flange on the left side of the blade, improving visualization of the laryngeal area when the laryngoscope is held in the left hand in an upright position. Since the Miller blade's flange is far less prominent, there is no real need for a left-handed design.

Intubation aids and techniques

Orotracheal intubation of most veterinary patients does not require any special equipment beyond the use of a laryngoscope and a familiarity with normal patient anatomy. However, there are circumstances and situations resulting from anatomic features, pathology, or trauma that make oral endotracheal intubation difficult or impossible. It is important that the veterinary anesthetist be familiar with and prepared to use alternative techniques to obtain a patent airway. The following sections present some of the options available, the associated equipment and describes the techniques in general terms. For more specific details, the reader should consult species-specific chapters in this book or other species-specific veterinary anesthesia references [27].

Nasotracheal intubation

Nasotracheal intubation is a useful technique for procedures involving the oral cavity where a standard orotracheal tube may preclude or limit optimal surgical or diagnostic access or it can be used for procedures in sedated conscious animals that will not tolerate an orotracheal tube but require oxygen supplementation and support. Nasotracheal intubation can also be safely used for the administration of inhalant anesthetics for inducing anesthesia in some animals (foals and calves) [28,29]. The technique for nasotracheal intubation has been described in foals, calves, horses, camelids, rabbits, and a kangaroo but has certainly been performed and not reported in many other animal species [28–32].

The characteristics of an ideal nasotracheal tube include a tube with minimal curvature and a suitable length to pass distal of the larynx. The tube should be made of inert material (e.g., silicone rubber) and have relatively thin walls for maximum internal diameter, although this may increase the risk of tube compression or kinking. Low-volume, high-pressure cuffs are typically less bulky and may be less traumatic during placement, but high-volume, low-pressure cuffs may be best for longer periods of anesthesia. Tube size will be dependent upon species and patient size but will often be smaller than an appropriately sized orotracheal tube. The smaller internal diameter can increase resistance to gas flow and may be a problem for some spontaneously breathing patients.

Nasotracheal intubation involves passage of a properly sized endotracheal tube through the nostril, nasal meatus, and larynx and into the trachea. Lidocaine-containing gel can facilitate placement and provides lubrication for the tube. It should be applied to the nostril and rostral portion of the nasal passage before advancing the tube in awake or sedated animals. A sterile water-soluble lubricant without lidocaine is appropriate for anesthetized patients. The tube should be passed gently and may require some rotation and redirection in order to facilitate passage between nasal conchae. Nasal hemorrhage or other tissue damage occasionally occurs during this procedure, particularly if excessive force or an excessively large tube is used relative to the nasal passages, or the tube is passed into the incorrect nasal meatus. In general, the patient's head and neck should be extended to facilitate passage of the tube from the nasopharynx into the trachea. However, species differences may necessitate alternative positioning or further manipulation of the head, neck, and laryngeal positions.

Air should move freely through a correctly placed tube during spontaneous ventilation. Confirmation of correct tube placement can be readily, and initially, assessed by using a bulb syringe adapted to the end of the nasotracheal tube. Once the tube is in place, the bulb can be squeezed and attached to the tube; if it readily expands, this suggests the tube is an airway, and if the bulb fails to expand, it is likely that the tube has entered the esophagus (Fig. 3.19). Further confirmation of correct tube placement using auscultation of lung sounds during manual ventilation and/or capnography waveform appearance should be used for definitive confirmation.

Extubation following nasotracheal intubation should be done carefully. After deflation of the cuff, the tube should be withdrawn slowly and deliberately, with the patient's head restrained to avoid any sudden, jerky motions. Rapid, rough extubation may cause nasal hemorrhage.

Wire- or tube-guided techniques

Wire- or tube-guided techniques are sometimes used when direct visualization of the laryngeal opening is not possible or obscured. This is commonly a result of species-specific anatomic features (e.g., rabbits, brachycephalic breeds) and patient size relative to available equipment. For example, the laryngoscope may be too small to be effective in a cow and manual palpation and guide tube placement using a small-diameter tube is frequently used to facilitate passage of the desired endotracheal tube; in very small patients the presence of both the laryngoscope and the endotracheal tube may obscure visualization and a thin wire can be initially placed to facilitate intubation [33].

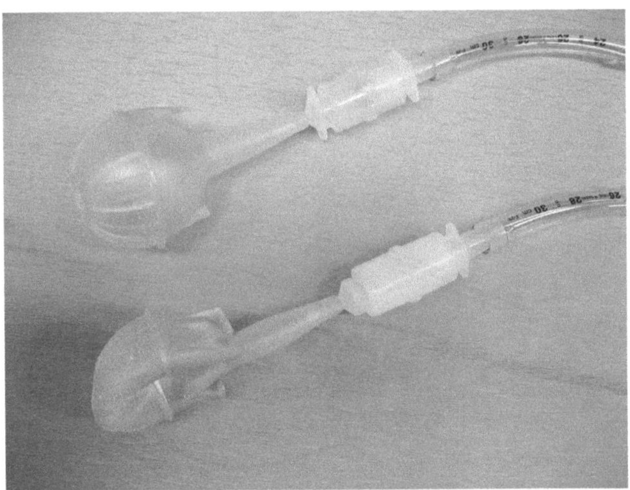

Figure 3.19 A suction bulb adapted to the end of an endotracheal tube can be used for the rapid assessment of correct endotracheal intubation. The bulb is deflated and attached to the tube using an appropriately sized adapter. If the endotracheal tube is in the trachea, the bulb should immediately reinflate. If the endotracheal tube is in the esophagus, the bulb will not generally reinflate. This technique provides a rapid assessment of proper intubation when direct visualization is not possible (i.e. nasotracheal intubation) but should always be used in conjunction with additional methods of confirming proper endotracheal intubation (i.e., observation of capnography waveform or auscultation of lung sounds during manual ventilation). Source: Thomas Riebold, College of Veterinary Medicine, Oregon State University, Corvallis, OR, USA. Reproduced with permission of Thomas Riebold.

In some patients, trauma or other pathological conditions (nasopharyngeal polyp or mass) may obscure the laryngeal opening with only a small portion visible. In these circumstances, the placement of a small-diameter tube or wire can be used as a guide for placement of a properly sized endotracheal tube (Fig. 3.20). The technique involves using a guide (wire or tube) with a smaller outer diameter than the internal diameter of the intended endotracheal tube. It should also be sufficiently long to allow complete intubation (about half the distance from the cricoid cartilage to the thoracic inlet) while still allowing the tube to be placed over the guide leaving a portion of the guide available for the operator to hold while advancing the tube (Fig. 3.21). The tube or wire should be blunt-ended so as not to damage the trachea or associated structures. The wire guides associated with some intravenous catheters (e.g., multiple-lumen jugular catheters) are blunt-ended and make excellent wire guides for some small patients. The guide is first appropriately placed and then the endotracheal tube is fed over the guide and through the laryngeal opening blindly; occasionally, slight rotation of the tube is required and passing the tube through the larynx during inspiration when the arytenoids are fully abducted helps facilitate smooth passage. The guide is then removed and the tube secured into place.

Endoscope-guided technique

Laryngoscopy with a flexible or rigid endoscope can be useful for assisting intubation in patients with abnormal anatomy or disease processes involving the pharynx, head, or neck. It is also often used in patients that can be challenging to intubate using direct visualization (e.g., pygmy rabbits and other small mammals). Depending

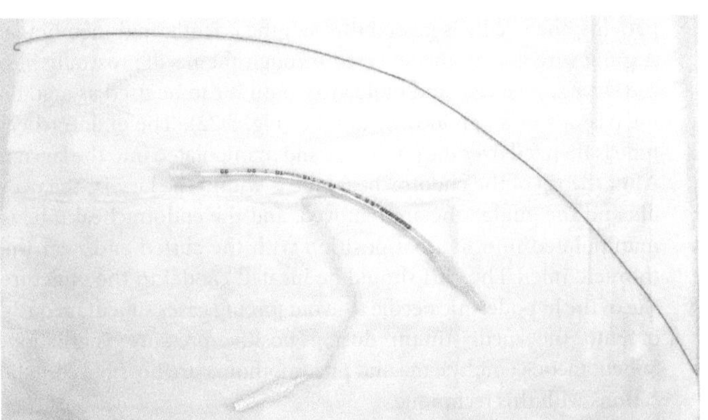

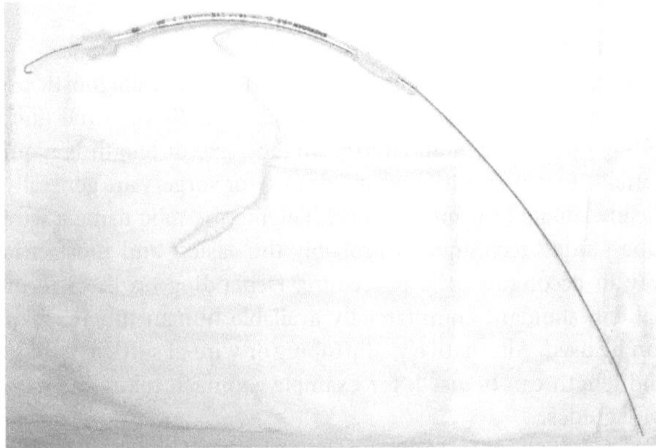

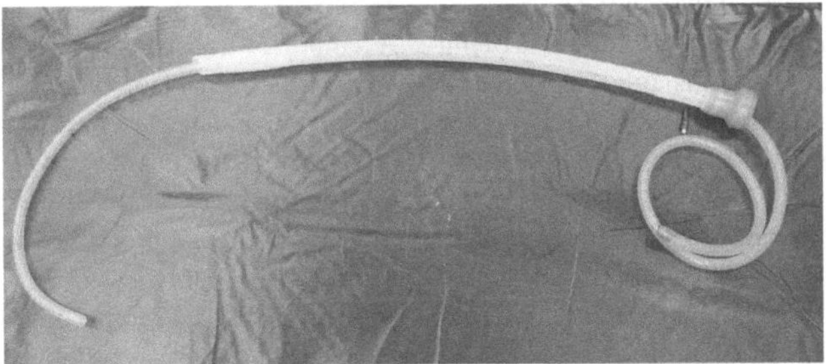

Figure 3.20 Examples of various guide wires and tube combinations used for guided endotracheal intubation. A wire or tube guide smaller, and typically easier to place, than the appropriately sized endotracheal tube is first placed in the trachea. The endotracheal tube is then fed over the guide, normally without further visualization. Once endotracheal intubation has been achieved, the guide is removed. Source: Craig Mosley, Mosley Veterinary Anesthesia Services, Rockwood, ON, Canada.

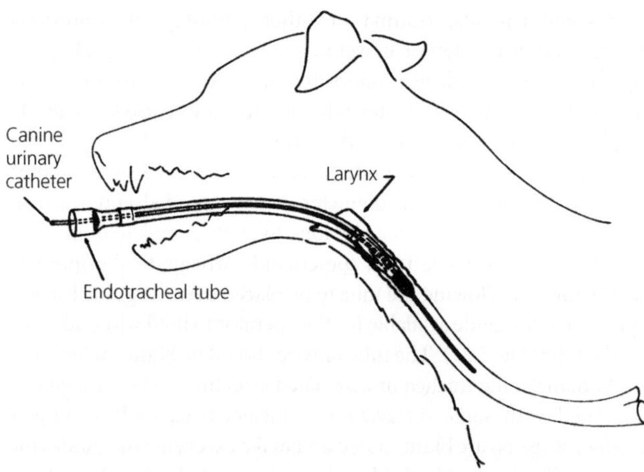

Figure 3.21 Diagram illustrating the passage of an endotracheal tube into the trachea of a dog using a guide device (urinary catheter). Source: Hartsfield SM. Alternate methods of endotracheal intubation in small animals with emphasis on patients with oropharyngeal pathology. *Tex Vet Med J* 1985; **47**: 25. Reproduced with permission of TVMA.

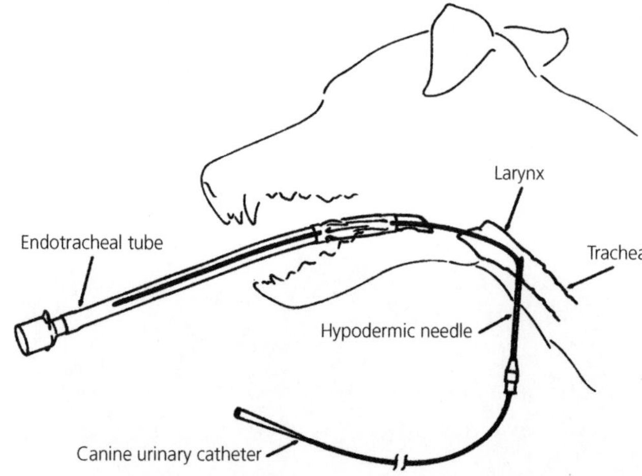

Figure 3.22 Illustration of intubation using a retrograde guide device in a dog. Catheter guide wires or other blunt-ended wires are optimal for this procedure owing to their small diameter. This technique should be reserved for cases that cannot be intubated by other methods. Source: Hartsfield SM. Alternate methods of endotracheal intubation in small animals with emphasis on patients with oropharyngeal pathology. *Tex Vet Med J* 1985; **47**: 25. Reproduced with permission of TVMA.

on the species and the specific conditions, the endoscope can be placed inside the endotracheal tube to guide intubation directly or passed orally beside the endotracheal tube to guide correct placement visually. Rabbits and other small mammals are frequently intubated using this technique [34]. When appropriate, endoscopes can also be used to facilitate nasotracheal intubation. This technique can be particularly advantageous in horses (and other large animals) with abnormal oropharyngeal, laryngeal, and/or nasal anatomy where direct visualization using a laryngoscope is virtually impossible without specialized custom equipment.

Endotracheal tube exchangers

Changing endotracheal tubes during a surgical or diagnostic procedure in an anesthetized animal is occasionally required due to a failing cuff or when an alternative tube size or length is required. Patients that are positioned and draped for surgery are generally not ideally situated for intubation. Changing the tube using a wire- or tube-guided technique is probably the easiest and most efficient way to accomplish the procedure. Depending on the size of the patient, standard commercially available human tube exchangers can be used. Alternatively, any tubing or wire of sufficient diameter and length can be used, for example, stomach tubes and catheter wire guides.

To change endotracheal tubes, the guide (tube or wire) is inserted through the original endotracheal tube to the area of the midcervical trachea. It should be noted that if the patient is being maintained under anesthesia using an inhalant anesthetic, it should be discontinued during tube exchange. Depending on the duration required to exchange the tube, the patient's anesthetic depth may become very light and additional intravenous anesthetic and a means to administer it should be readily available. Next, the endotracheal tube cuff is deflated, and the endotracheal tube is pulled over the guide without removing the guide from the trachea. Then, the new endotracheal tube is maneuvered through the larynx and into the trachea by using the guide to direct its passage. The cuff of the new tube is inflated to protect the airway, and the new tube is secured in the manner appropriate for the specific species.

Retrograde intubation

If direct visualization of at least a portion of the glottis is impossible, retrograde intubation may be performed. Retrograde intubation has been evaluated as an alternative technique for endotracheal intubation in South America camelids and mice [35,36] and a cadaveric study has been performed in rabbits [37]. The technique essentially involves passing a needle through the skin of the ventral neck and into the trachea between upper tracheal rings. In human patients, the needle is passed through the cricothyroid membrane. A guidewire is then maneuvered through the needle rostrally into the larynx, pharynx, and oral cavity until it can be used as a guide for passage of an endotracheal tube (Fig. 3.22). The endotracheal tube is then fed over the guidewire and manipulated into the larynx. After the tip of the endotracheal tube is within the larynx, the needle and the guide tube are removed, and the endotracheal tube is manipulated into its final position with the cuffed end near the thoracic inlet. The cuff should be located caudal to the puncture site of the hypodermic needle to avoid forcing gases subcutaneously or into the mediastinum during positive-pressure ventilation. Subcutaneous emphysema and pneumothorax are possible complications with this technique.

Tracheostomy

A temporary tracheostomy can be performed for airway management during anesthesia. However, as it is invasive it is typically reserved for those patients where even with guided assistance, oro- or nasotracheal intubation is not possible owing to anatomy, pathology, or surgical procedures. Occasionally a tracheostomy may be recommended to facilitate a surgical procedure involving the oropharynx, although if appropriate a pharyngostomy tube may represent a more desirable alternative. Tracheostomy tube placement may also be used when there is a reasonable expectation that the patient will require an ongoing tracheostomy following the anesthetic procedure (e.g., incomplete resection of laryngeal tumor). Occasionally patients may present to anesthesia with an emergency tracheostomy already present as the result of acute upper airway obstruction.

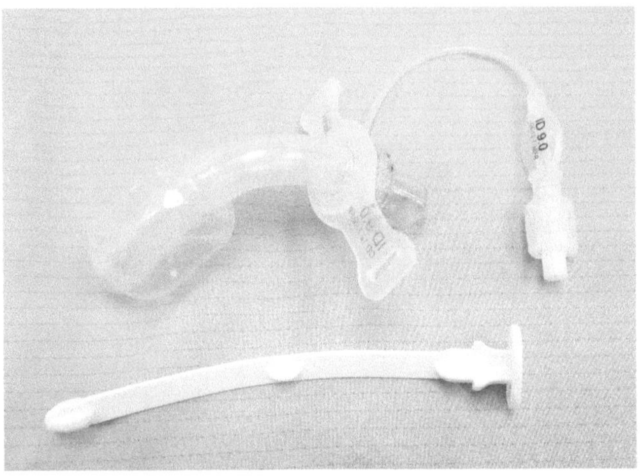

Figure 3.23 An example of a cuffed tracheostomy tube with an inner stylet to ease placement. Some tubes are also designed with a removal inner tube to facilitate cleaning of the tube. Source: Craig Mosley, Mosley Veterinary Anesthesia Services, Rockwood, ON, Canada.

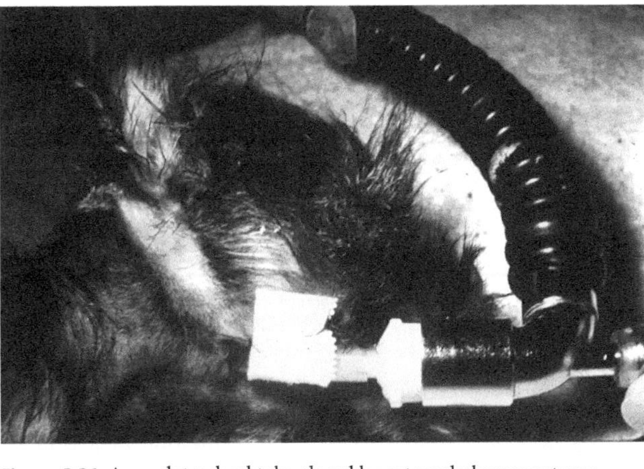

Figure 3.24 An endotracheal tube placed by external pharyngostomy in a small dog to facilitate oropharyngeal surgery. Source: Hartsfield SM. Alternate methods of endotracheal intubation in small animals with emphasis on patients with oropharyngeal pathology. *Tex Vet Med J* 1985; **47**: 25. Reproduced with permission of TVMA.

Intubation via a tracheostomy is relatively simply to perform but may be complicated in patients with very small-diameter tracheas or those with very thickened and calcified tracheal rings (e.g., some brachycephalics). A standard endotracheal tube or tracheostomy tube can be used for intubation; however, care should be taken when using a standard length endotracheal tube as endobronchial intubation can easily result. Tracheostomy tubes are generally short with a pronounced curvature in the tube and an inner stylet to ease placement (Fig. 3.23). The curvature also allow the tube to be secured flatly to the patient's neck and tubes are normally fitted with a standard 15 mm endotracheal tube adapter, inflatable cuffs, and pilot balloons, although many of the smaller sized tubes will be uncuffed. Some tracheostomy tubes also have an inner removable cannula to facilitate cleaning and longer term maintenance of tracheostomy tubes in patients. Care of the tube is very important. Neglected tubes that are not cleaned regularly can be obstructed by mucus that dries within the lumen of the tube.

Tracheostomy has been associated with infection, granulomas, tracheal stricture, cartilage damage, hemorrhage, pneumothorax, subcutaneous emphysema, tracheocutaneous or tracheoesophageal fistula, aspiration, dysphagia, and tracheal malacia; hence tracheostomy should not be considered an innocuous procedure. The specific techniques, indications, and outcomes have been reviewed in cattle, horses, dogs, and cats [38–42].

Lateral pharyngotomy

A lateral pharyngotomy is an alternative to a tracheostomy and suitable for facilitating surgical procedures of the mandible, maxilla, or oral cavity. The use of a pharyngotomy provides improved visualization within the operative field during oropharyngeal surgery and normal dental occlusion to aid in the proper reduction of mandibular or maxillary fractures. It is also a potentially less invasive alternative to a tracheostomy when oral or nasal airway management is undesirable or unfeasible for facilitating a surgical procedure.

This technique has been described in detail elsewhere (Fig. 3.24) [43]. The basics of tube placement involve passage of a correctly sized, cuffed endotracheal tube and making a routine skin incision near the angle of the mandible. Then, hemostats are bluntly passed through the skin incision into the caudal part of the pharynx. After the endotracheal tube adapter has been removed, the adapter end of the tube is grasped and pulled from the pharynx, through the subcutaneous tissue, and through the skin incision. The endotracheal tube adapter is replaced, and the tube is reconnected to the breathing system for maintenance. A correctly placed tube should be secured to the skin with tape and several sutures.

Techniques of oxygen administration

Supplemental oxygen is used in anesthetized and critically ill patients to increase the partial pressure of oxygen in arterial blood (PaO_2) and to promote the delivery of oxygen to the tissues. When a patient is breathing room air, values for PaO_2 that are less than 80 mmHg indicate the potential for hypoxemia. Any patient in respiratory distress or those likely to experience hypoxia in the perianesthetic period (e.g., brachycephalic breeds) should be provided with supplemental oxygen. If the PaO_2 decreases to less than 60 mmHg, the need for supplemental oxygen is indicated. It is also important to recall that both hemoglobin and tissue perfusion play fundamental roles in ensuring sufficient delivery of oxygen to tissues and when indicated red blood cell transfusions and/or cardiovascular support may be required in addition to providing supplemental oxygen to prevent cellular hypoxia.

The fraction of oxygen in inspired gases (F_IO_2) plays a significant role in establishing the PaO_2. As a rule, the PaO_2 value should be approximately five times the F_IO_2 value if there are no major abnormalities in the matching of pulmonary ventilation and perfusion. Supplemental oxygen can be an effective way of correcting hypoxemia in animals with diffusion abnormalities, ventilation–perfusion mismatching, and/or hypoventilation. In addition to oxygen supplementation, the specific underlying condition(s) contributing to hypoxemia should be addressed when possible. Supplemental oxygen may not significantly improve PaO_2 in patients with substantial right to left vascular shunts (pulmonary or cardiac shunts).

Several techniques can be used to administer oxygen to anesthetized and ill patients. The effectiveness of oxygen supplementation is assessed by evaluation of the patient's clinical responses (e.g., improvement in mucous membrane color and character of

Table 3.1 Approximate F_IO_2 values obtained from various oxygen supplementation techniques for dogs and cats[a].

Technique	Approximate F_IO_2 Obtainable (%)	Flow Rate
Flow by oxygen	25–40	0.5–5 L/min
Face mask	35–60	2–8 L/min
Nasal insufflation	30–70	100–150 mL/kg/min
Tracheal insufflation	40–60	50 mL/kg/min
Oxygen cages	25–50	Variable

[a] These values are not applicable for all veterinary species during all circumstances and will be flow rate and respiratory character (rate and depth) dependent.

ventilation), by measuring the F_IO_2, and by monitoring of PaO_2, arterial oxygen saturation (SaO_2), and saturation of peripheral oxygen (SpO_2). Although PaO_2 and SaO_2 data are reliable, they require periodic arterial blood sampling and the use of a blood gas analyzer. The SpO_2 can be conveniently measured by pulse oximetry. Pulse oximetry is a practical method for non-invasive, moment-to-moment estimation of the saturation of hemoglobin with oxygen in anesthetized, recovering, and ill patients [44–51]. Various techniques for supplementing oxygen to patients are outlined below and Table 3.1 summarizes the approximate F_IO_2 obtained using each of the commonly available techniques in dogs and cats.

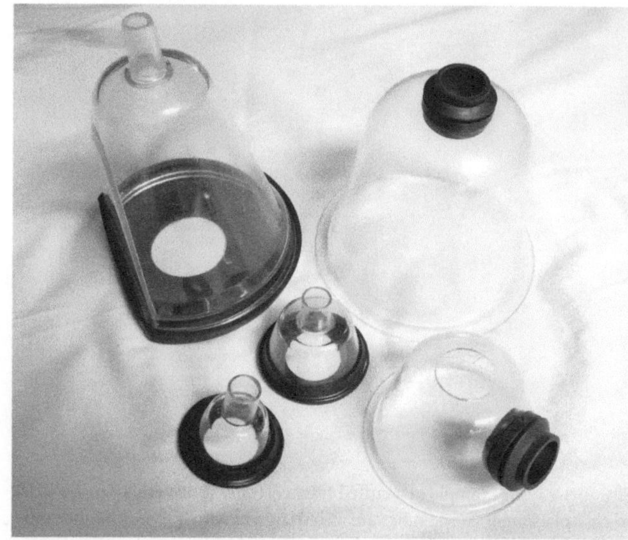

Figure 3.25 Commercial face masks are available in many styles and sizes. A face mask should be chosen to minimize the potential for rebreathing of exhaled gases (i.e., snug fitting), especially when used with the rubber diaphragm in place. Source: Craig Mosley, Mosley Veterinary Anesthesia Services, Rockwood, ON, Canada.

Mask delivery

Masks for delivery of oxygen to veterinary patients are useful for preoxygenation immediately before induction of anesthesia and for conscious patients experiencing respiratory distress. The use of masks for oxygenation requires constant attention, and some patients will not accept a mask unless they are sedated. Both factors limit the effectiveness of masks in conscious patients. Indeed, some patients object to a mask so vigorously that the increase in oxygen consumption associated with restraint may nullify the benefits of a greater F_IO_2. If the oxygen mask is attached to an anesthetic breathing circuit, the circuit should be flushed in order to reduce anesthetic odors and potentially improve compliance, but this is variably useful.

The flow rates generally recommended for increasing F_IO_2 when using masks are variable among species. For example, flow rates of 10–15 L/min of supplemental oxygen have been recommended to increase the inspired-oxygen concentration to approximately 35–60% in adult horses, although supporting studies are lacking and nasal and tracheal insufflation represent better, more practical options in larger patients. Flow rates for smaller patients, including dogs and cats, usually range from 2 to 8 L/min to produce 30–60% inspired oxygen concentration [52], although specific supporting studies are lacking. With a tight-fitting mask, higher flow rates of oxygen tend to produce greater F_IO_2 values and less rebreathing of expired carbon dioxide.

Tight-fitting masks should be used with a breathing system (anesthetic circuit or manual resuscitation bag) with a reservoir that can meet the patient's tidal volume demands or with a vented or valved mask allowing entrainment of air from outside the mask. As an example, a dog with a tidal volume of 300 mL and an inspiratory time of 1 s has a peak inspiratory gas flow of approximately 18 L/min, which exceeds the practical flow rate for oxygen during masking. High inspiratory flow rates can be accommodated if the mask is attached to an anesthetic breathing system with a reservoir bag or a mask fitted to a manual resuscitation bag. In addition, an appropriate breathing system has an overflow that prevents the buildup of excessive pressure with a tight-fitting mask. Alternatively, a loose-fitting mask that allows room air to be entrained can be used, but entrained room air will reduce inspired F_IO_2 associated with supplemental oxygen delivery.

Face masks for oxygen supplementation in veterinary patients are readily available (Fig. 3.25). Most consist of a clear plastic cone fitted with a black rubber diaphragm that can improve fit and sealing around a patient's face. Unless they are sedated or otherwise minimally responsive, most conscious patients rarely accept snug-fitting face masks. Although face masks designed specifically for very small patients are available (Fig. 3.26), it is common to use a plastic syringe case, latex glove and endotracheal tube adapter to 'custom' design a face mask (Fig. 3.27). Traffic cones have been adapted and fitted to pigs for delivery of inhalant anesthetics.

Nasal insufflation

Insufflation involves delivery of oxygen into the patient's airway at relatively high flow rates; the patient inspires oxygen and room air, the relative proportions of each being determined primarily by the oxygen flow rate and the rate of gas flow during inspiration. Insufflation can be accomplished by a variety of methods. For horses recovering from anesthesia, oxygen may be delivered from a flowmeter through a delivery tube and into an appropriately sized insufflation tube in the horse's nasal cavity or trachea. Appropriately sized endotracheal tubes or large animal stomach tubes are often used as nasal tubes. Intact stomach tubes are sufficiently long that they may also be used for tracheal insufflation if advanced through the nasal cavity and into the trachea. For most conscious patients, oxygen is insufflated through a nasal catheter, the tip of which is positioned in the nasopharynx. The catheter is usually made of soft rubber, and the tube should have several fenestrations to minimize jetting lesions from developing in the nasopharyngeal mucosa. For awake patients, instilling 2% lidocaine (or lidocaine gel) or 0.5% proparacaine into the nasal passage with the patient's head and neck extended and held upward may facilitate passage of the tube.

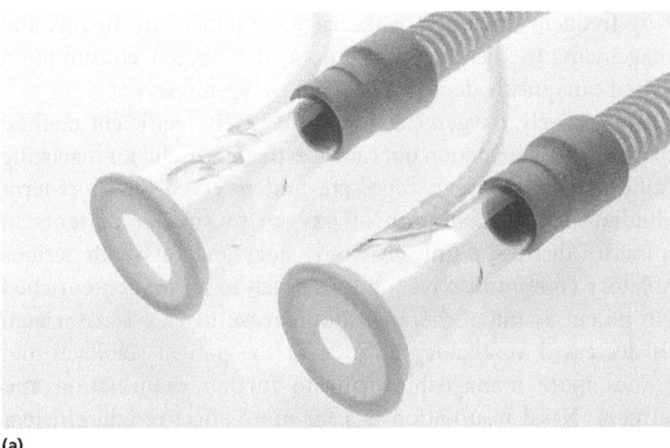
(a)

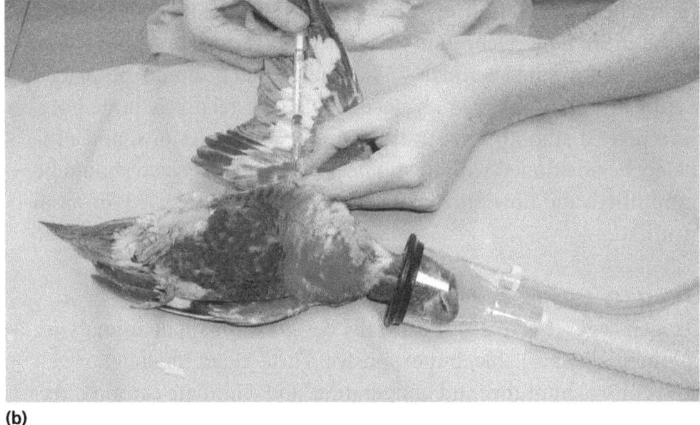
(b)

Figure 3.26 Commercial facemasks designed specifically for use with very small patients. The masks are used with two sizes of interchangeable diaphragms. Source: Advanced Anesthesia Specialists, Phoenix, AZ, USA. Reproduced with permission of Advanced Anesthesia Specialists.

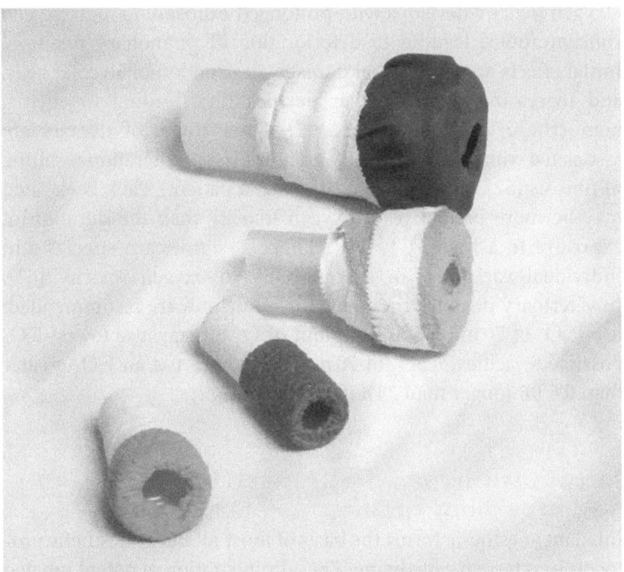

Figure 3.27 Face masks can be fashioned from syringe cases and rubber gloves are often made for use in very small patients. Source: Craig Mosley, Mosley Veterinary Anesthesia Services, Rockwood, ON, Canada.

Placement involves insertion of a suitable sized insufflation catheter into the nasal passage and the nasopharynx, the distance being approximately the same as from the tip of the nose to the medial canthus of the eye. Specifically designed nasal insufflation catheters (with multiple fenestrations) are available or they can be made from feeding tubes or other soft non-reactive tubing and adapted to the oxygen delivery line. The external portion of the catheter is secured to the patient's head with tissue adhesive, tape, and/or sutures or staples. A flexible length of tubing supplies oxygen from a flowmeter and allows the patient some freedom for movement in a cage or stall. Changing the catheter to the opposite nasal passage every 1–2 days has been recommended to prevent pressure necrosis, jet lesions, and accumulation of mucus [53]. Humidification of the oxygen is also advisable if the need for insufflation will be for more than a short period of time.

The flow-rate requirements for oxygen during insufflation are variable, the patient's ventilation character and the desired F_IO_2 being two important factors impacting suitable flow rates. Following anesthesia, adult horses require a minimum of 15 L/min of oxygen flow to improve the PaO_2 in arterial blood, and proportionally lower flows (e.g., 5 L/min) are suitable for smaller horses, foals, and calves [54–57]. In small animals, flow rates of 1–7 L/min are typically used for the administration of nasal oxygen. Approximate flow rates for dogs and cats to achieve rather specific ranges of F_IO_2 have been suggested, but monitoring of SpO_2 or PaO_2 should ultimately guide flow rate adjustment [58]. In dogs, various flow rates of 100% oxygen administered intranasally were studied, and flow rates of 50, 100, 150, and 200 mL/kg/min produced inspired-oxygen concentrations measured at the tracheal bifurcation of 28, 37, 40, and 47, respectively [53]. To prevent mucosal drying with prolonged insufflation, oxygen should be flowed through a bubble-type humidifier. Frequently, bilateral nasal insufflation catheters are placed and can be expected to improve the maximum achievable F_IO_2, achieving up to 80% at 200 mL/kg/min [59].

Tracheal insufflation

Tracheal insufflation can be achieved via nasotracheal or transtracheal oxygen administration. These techniques are useful for patients suffering from conditions causing upper airway obstruction.

Nasotracheal insufflation is achieved by passing a catheter through the nares into the trachea. In conscious animals, this process is normally performed after instilling a topical local anesthetic (lidocaine, proparacaine) into the nose and using a lubricant containing a local anesthetic (lidocaine gel). To facilitate tube placement into the trachea rather than the esophagus, the neck should be extended. Conscious patients will frequently cough as the catheter enters the larynx; coughing can be reduced by instilling a small amount of topical lidocaine through the nasotracheal tube on to the laryngeal area. Proper nasotracheal tube placement can be assessed by demonstrating a lack of negative pressure when air is evacuated from the tube/catheter. Air can be evacuated by attaching an appropriately sized syringe or compressed suction bulb to the catheter. If negative pressure is detected while evacuating air from the tube, this suggests that the tube is not in the trachea and may have been swallowed by the patient and is in the esophagus.

A transtracheal catheter can be placed percutaneously into the trachea through the cricothyroid membrane or between tracheal rings near the larynx and can be used to insufflate oxygen to a compromised patient. Intratracheal administration of 100% oxygen has been evaluated in dogs, and flow rates of 10, 25, 50, 100, 150, 200, and 250 mL/kg/min produced inspired-oxygen concentrations at the tracheal bifurcation of 25, 32, 47, 67, 70, 78, and 86%, respectively [58]. The technique for tracheal insufflation has been described for small animals [58]. The catheter should be placed aseptically, be of the over-the-needle type, be relatively large bore, have several smooth fenestrations to prevent jet lesions, and ultimately be positioned with the tip near the carina. Oxygen should be humidified, and flow rates should approximate those used for nasal insufflation.

Oxygen cages

Oxygen cages (Fig. 3.28) specifically designed for small animals are commercially available, but expensive. These cages regulate oxygen flow, control humidity and temperature, and eliminate carbon dioxide from exhaled gases. Most oxygen cages are capable of producing oxygen concentrations between 30 and 60% but the flow rates required can be as high as 15 L/min [60]. However, there is considerable variability in design and efficacy among many commercially available products. There is also considerable variation for the time required to obtain desired oxygen concentration, 30–45 min [60]. Factors that will influence this include internal volume of the cage, air tightness of the cage, and how often the cage is opened. For small animals, flow rates of oxygen, cage temperature, and cage humidity have been recommended to be less than 10 L/min (but this will depend greatly on overall efficiency of the cage), approximately 22 °C, and 40–50%, respectively [61]. Oxygen concentrations of 30–40% generally are adequate for patients with moderate pulmonary disease [62]. Oxygen cages are not practical for horses or larger animals and, even in smaller animals, the effectiveness of an oxygen cage diminishes as body size increases. Smaller patients can be managed easily in oxygen cages, but temperature and humidity are more difficult to control with larger dogs. A major disadvantage of an oxygen cage is that the animal must be removed from the cage (or the doors opened) for examination and treatment, requiring the patient to breath room air or oxygen by mask during this period.

Prior to purchasing an oxygen cage, it is important to understand fully its operation and oxygen requirements. Significant amounts of oxygen can be consumed by oxygen cages that are poorly sealed and during frequent openings of the cage for patient treatments and management. In these circumstances, the oxygen consumption required can quickly deplete a hospital's oxygen reserves.

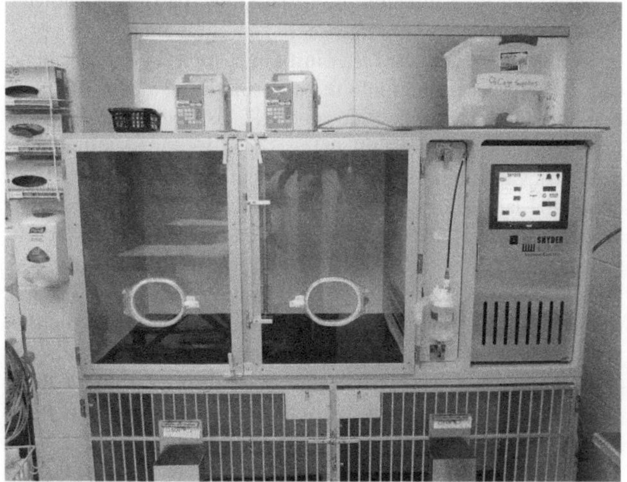

Figure 3.28 Commercial oxygen cages are available that can precisely control the oxygen concentration within in the cage and remove exhaled CO_2. Many frequently also incorporate humidity and temperature control (heating and cooling). Source: Craig Mosley, Mosley Veterinary Anesthesia Services, Rockwood, ON, Canada.

Comparatively, oxygen cages are a relatively inefficient method of oxygen supplementation but can be extremely useful for managing specific patients. Oxygen cages are best reserved for short-term immediate supplementation of oxygen to smaller patients in respiratory distress. Clinically, some dogs and cats with serious ventilatory compromise respond very well to an oxygen-enriched environment as initial therapy; the increase in F_IO_2 is associated with decreased ventilatory effort, and the patient stabilizes and becomes more manageable prior to further examination and treatment. Nasal insufflation is a far more effective and efficient method of oxygen supplementation in most circumstances, particularly those requiring longer term supplementation, even for smaller dogs and cats.

Oxygen toxicity

Oxygen toxicity develops with prolonged exposure to high oxygen concentrations, leading to deterioration of pulmonary function. Initial effects are endothelial damage, destruction of alveolar cells, and increasing microvascular permeability, leading to edema, hemorrhage, and congestion [52]. Later stages of toxicity are associated with alveolar type II and fibroblast proliferation resulting in fibrosis [52]. The length of time that a patient's PaO_2 is elevated may be more predictive of oxygen toxicity than the duration of exposure to a high F_IO_2 [63]. There is significant species and individual variability in susceptibility to oxygen toxicity [63]. In veterinary patients, the following guidelines are recommended: use PaO_2 of 70 mmHg as endpoint of O_2 therapy, use lowest F_IO_2 possible to achieve PaO_2 of 70 mmHg, do not use an F_IO_2 greater than 0.6 for longer than 24 h if possible [52].

Introduction anesthetic machine and breathing circuits

Inhalant anesthesia forms the basis of most modern anesthetic protocols in veterinary medicine. The administration of potent inhaled anesthetics requires specific delivery techniques. The anesthetic machine permits the delivery of a precise yet variable combination of inhalant anesthetic and oxygen. The basic components and functions of all anesthetic machines are similar but significant design differences exist among them. Machines can be very simple, for example those used for mobile applications, to very complex anesthetic workstations with built-in ventilators, monitors, and safety systems (Fig. 3.29). Regardless of the complexity of the design, all anesthetic machines share common components: a source of oxygen, a regulator for oxygen (this may be part of the gas supply system), a flowmeter for oxygen, and a vaporizer. If additional gases are used (e.g., nitrous oxide), there will also be a source, regulator, and flowmeter for each gas that generally parallels the path of oxygen with some exceptions (e.g., oxygen flush valve). The basic anesthetic machine is then used in conjunction with a breathing circuit and anesthetic waste gas scavenging system for delivery of anesthetic to the patient.

Medical gas supply

Anesthetic machines ideally have two gas supplies, one from small, high-pressure tanks attached directly to the machine and a second source often originating from a hospital's central pipeline supply.

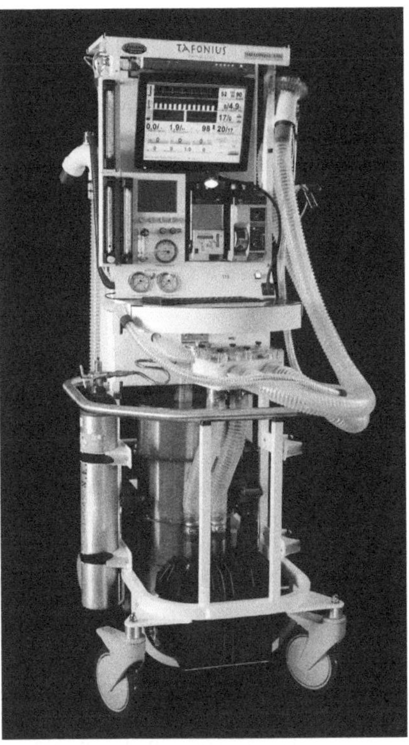

(a)

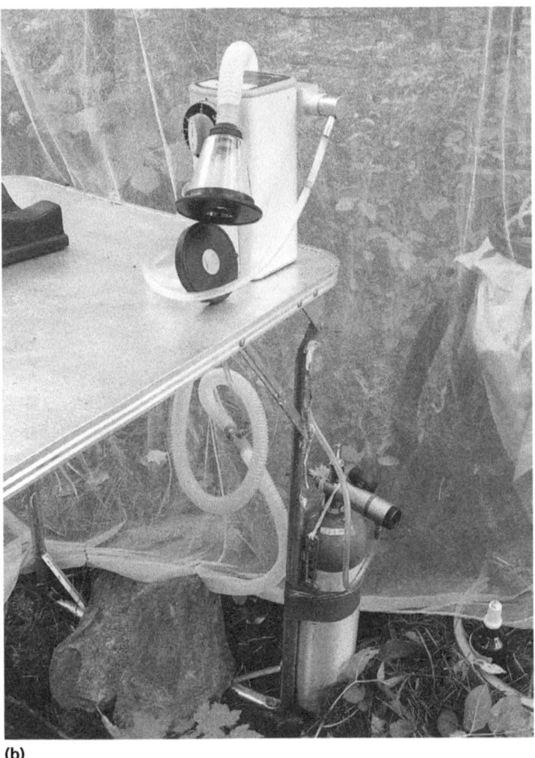

(b)

Figure 3.29 Anesthetic machines for veterinary use can vary considerably in their complexity and sophistication. (a) A complete veterinary anesthetic workstation for large animal use and (b) a portable anesthetic system for field use. Both systems provide all the components necessary for the controlled delivery of inhalant anesthetics. Source: part a, Hallowell EMC, Pittsfield, MA, USA. Reproduced with permission of Hallowell EMC. Source: part b, Craig Mosley, Mosley Veterinary Anesthesia Services, Rockwood, ON, Canada.

The small tanks mounted directly to the anesthesia machine are normally intended to be used as back-up or reserve gas sources should the pipeline malfunction or for working in an area without access to the pipeline. Oxygen is by far the most commonly used medical gas during veterinary anesthesia, with nitrous oxide being used in conjunction with oxygen as an adjunct carrier gas for the inhalants much less frequently. Most medical gases are normally stored under high pressure in gas cylinders of various sizes or in low-pressure insulated cryogenic liquid bulk tanks. The characteristics (e.g., working pressure) and capacity of the gas cylinders vary with the type of gas they contain (see Table 3.2). Alternatively, oxygen concentrators can be used to supply a hospital with its oxygen requirements in circumstances where obtaining and storing tanks are inconvenient, impossible, or prohibitively expensive (e.g., remote communities). Most oxygen concentrators use a system of absorbing nitrogen from air to produce gas with an oxygen concentration between 90 and 96%. Recently, small, integrated, single-machine oxygen-concentrating units have been made available in the veterinary market (Pureline™, Supera Anesthesia Innovations, Clackamas, OR, USA) (Fig. 3.30).

Most modern veterinary facilities will have some form of central gas supply and pipeline distribution system delivering medical gases to various work sites. The complexity of these systems can vary significantly, from a small bank of large (G or H) cylinders and a regulator to more complex systems consisting of multiple large liquid oxygen tanks, automatic manifolds, regulators, alarms, and banks of large high-pressure cylinders for back up (Fig. 3.31). The size and complexity of the gas distribution system will depend upon the gas needs, area of required gas distribution, and the number of work sites required. Proper installation of large gas distribution systems is essential for safety and efficacy. All gas installations should be installed and properly evaluated by those with expertise in this area prior to using them to deliver gas to patients.

Table 3.2 Characteristics of medical gas cylinders [2].

Size	Gas	Gas Symbol	Color Code (U.S.)	Capacity and Pressure (at 70°F)	Empty Cylinder Weight (pounds)
E	Oxygen	O_2	Green	660 L 1900 psi	14
E	Nitrous oxide	N_2O	Blue	1590 L 745 psi	14
G	Nitrous oxide	N_2O	Blue	13,800 L 745 psi	97
H	Oxygen	O_2	Green	6900 L 2200 psi	119
H	Nitrous oxide	N_2O	Blue	15,800 L 745 psi	119

psi, pounds per square inch.

Medical gas safety

There are several international (ASTM), national, and local documents related to the safe use, transport, and storage of pressurized gases. There are also standards surrounding the installation of medical gas piping systems and some of these provisions have been incorporated into hospital accreditation requirements in veterinary medicine. However, the specific guidelines can vary significantly among jurisdictions and regions. There have been several well-documented medical accidents related to the inappropriate use of

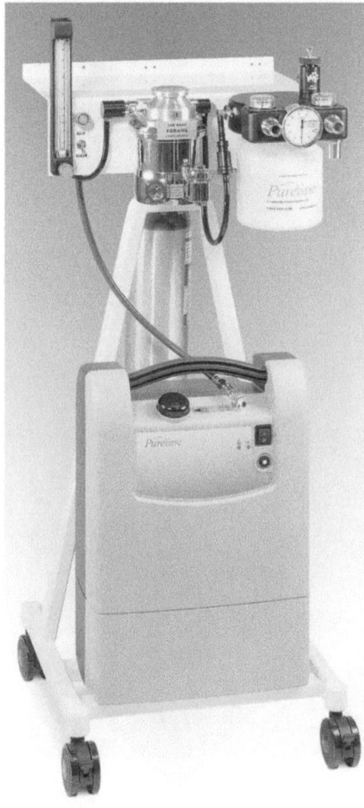

Figure 3.30 Small, quiet, portable oxygen concentrators are becoming increasingly available as an alternative to using refillable compressed gas tanks. This figure depicts an anesthesia machine with a built-in oxygen concentrator. The oxygen concentrator is located in the case on the bottom of the machine. Source: Supera Anesthesia Innovations, Clackamas, OR, USA. Reproduced with permission of Supera Anesthesia Innovations.

medical gases in humans, but the incidence of such accidents seems to be decreasing [64,65]. The reduction of such accidents is likely due in large part to better monitoring and maintenance of gas delivery systems. Consequently, there are several safety systems that have been developed to help reduce and eliminate these problems. For example, all anesthetic equipment has a gas-specific non-interchangeable connector that is part of the base unit (anesthetic machine, ventilator). These connectors, diameter index safety system, pin index safety system, and quick connector are described below.

Color coding

Gas cylinders and gas lines are commonly color coded to avoid improper use, but color coding systems can vary among countries. For example, oxygen is colored white in Canada and green in the United States. In addition to color coding, all tanks have a labeling scheme consisting of various shaped labels, key words, and colors that are all used to identify hazards associated with the gas they contain. Most tanks originating from gas supply facilities normally have perforated tags (full, in use, empty) to track the cylinder's use status.

Diameter index safety system

The diameter index safety system (DISS) is a non-interchangeable gas-specific threaded connection system (Fig. 3.32). DISS is the gas connection used almost universally by all equipment and cylinder manufactures for the connection of medical gases.

Quick connectors

There are many proprietary (manufacturer-specific) quick connect systems that have been developed. These are standardized within a manufacturer but are not generally compatible with the quick connect systems of another manufacturer (Fig. 3.33). These systems

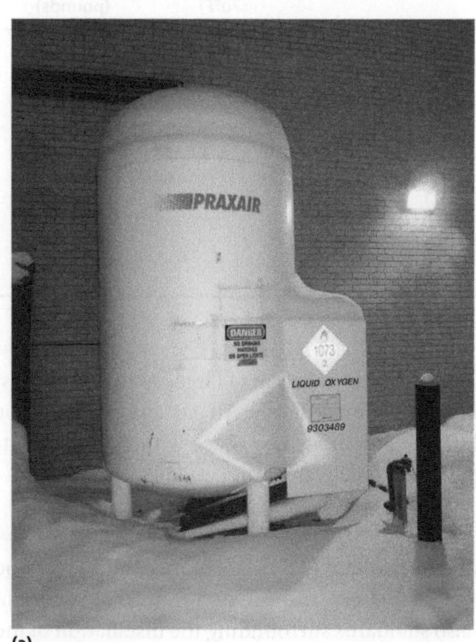

(a)

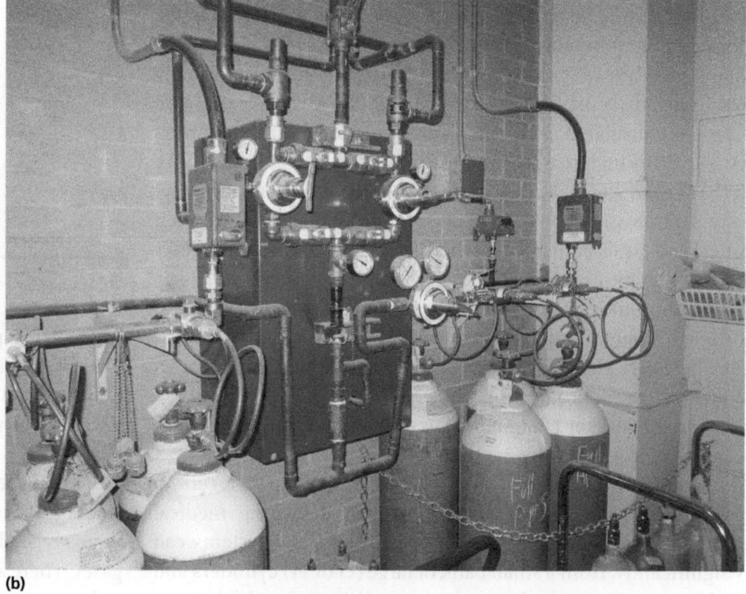

(b)

Figure 3.31 Bulk oxygen requirements for larger hospitals are frequently met using large liquid oxygen tanks (a) or banks of compressed gas tanks (b). Both of these systems are normally designed with a backup supply should the main supply fail or become depleted. Source: Craig Mosley, Mosley Veterinary Anesthesia Services, Rockwood, ON, Canada.

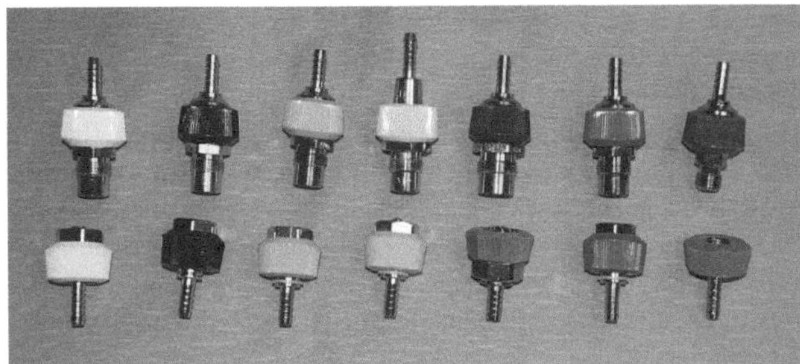

Figure 3.32 The diameter index safety system (DISS) uses a gas-specific non-interchangeable thread pattern to avoid incorrect gas delivery. Gases are also color coded as apparent in the figure. Source: Thomas Riebold, College of Veterinary Medicine, Oregon State University, Corvallis, OR, USA. Reproduced with permission of Thomas Riebold.

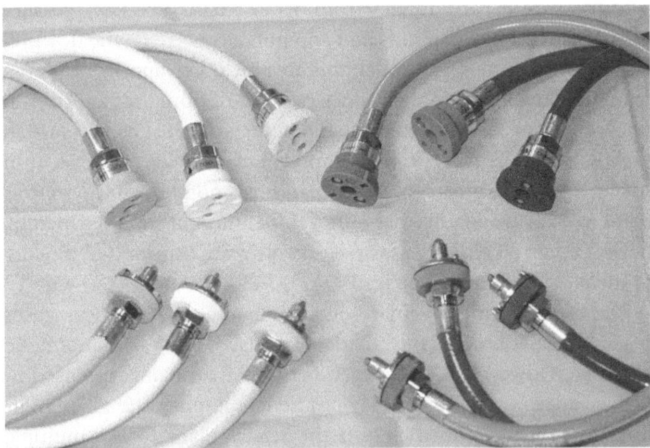

Figure 3.33 Proprietary quick-connect gas couplings are available to ease frequent connecting and disconnecting of gas lines. These systems, such as the Ohmeda system pictured here, are manufacturer specific and are incompatible among various manufacturers. Source: Thomas Riebold, College of Veterinary Medicine, Oregon State University, Corvallis, OR, USA. Reproduced with permission of Thomas Riebold.

facilitate rapid connecting and disconnecting of gas hoses and may be useful in situations where frequent connects and disconnects are required (e.g., multipurpose work areas).

Pin index safety system

The pin index safety system (PISS) uses gas-specific pin patterns that only allow connections between the appropriate cylinder yokes and small gas cylinders (E size). The PISS is commonly found on the yokes mounted on anesthesia machines and some cylinder-specific regulators/flowmeters (Fig. 3.34).

Pressure-reducing valve (regulator)

The pressure-reducing valve (regulator) is a key component required to bring the high pressures of gas cylinders down to a more reasonable and safe working pressure (i.e., 40–55 psi). Regulators also reduce or prevent fluctuations in pressure as the tank empties. Regulators are normally found wherever a high-pressure gas cylinder is in use (e.g., gas pipelines, cylinder connected directly to machine) (see Fig. 3.35). The regulators used for pipelines are normally adjustable whereas those on most anesthesia machines are set by the manufacturer. The ASTM standard requires that regulators on anesthesia machines be set to use preferentially pipeline gases before using gas from the backup cylinder on the anesthesia machine. However, since neither pipeline systems nor veterinary anesthesia machines are required to meet ASTM standards, it is not uncommon for machines to draw from the reserve or backup tank preferentially rather than the pipeline. This problem can be avoided by ensuring that the pipeline pressure is set approximately 5 psi higher than the anesthesia machine's regulator for the reserve oxygen cylinder.

Pressure gauges

Pressure gauges are commonly used to measure cylinder pressures, pipeline pressures, anesthetic machine working pressures, and pressures within the breathing system. Cylinder, pipeline, and anesthetic machine working pressures are normally expressed in pounds per square inch (psi) or kilopascals (kPa), whereas the pressures within the breathing system of the anesthetic machine are normally

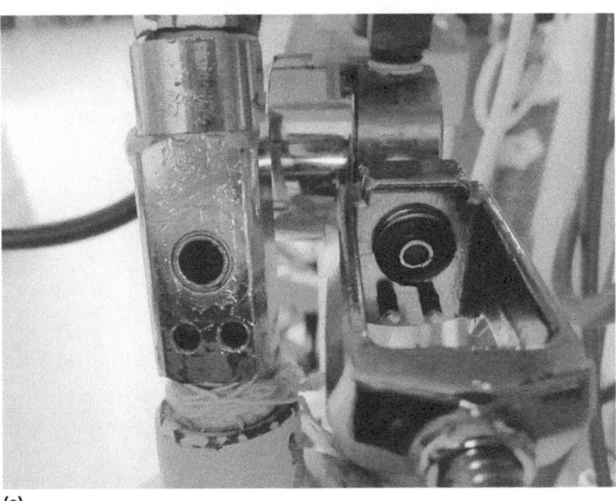

(a)

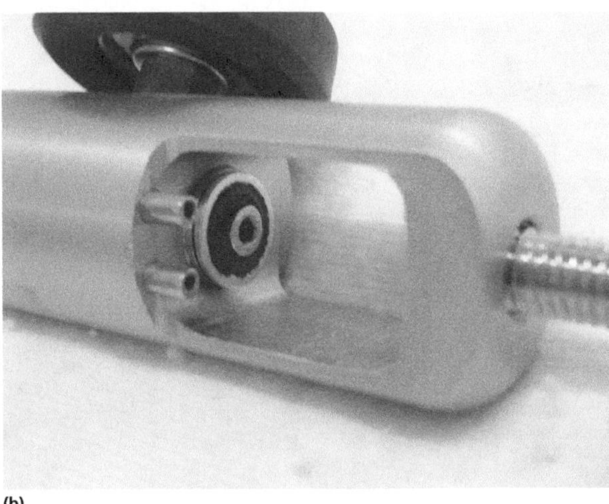

(b)

Figure 3.34 The pin index safety system (PISS) uses a series of gas-specific pin positions on the yolk that correspond to similarly positioned pin receiver ports on the tank. (a) The PISS typical of the cylinder yolk of an anesthesia machine. (b) The PISS being used on a combination regulator/flowmeter for the delivery of oxygen. Source: Craig Mosley, Mosley Veterinary Anesthesia Services, Rockwood, ON, Canada.

expressed in centimeters of water (cmH_2O) (Fig. 3.36). The gauge measuring the pressure of the breathing system is often also referred to as a pressure manometer. The information provided by these gauges is vital for safe operation of anesthesia equipment.

The modern anesthetic machine

Gas flow within the anesthetic machine

The basic anesthesia delivery apparatus is made up from a series of parts that work collectively to deliver inhalant anesthetics safely and support breathing. These components include: the gas delivery system, the vaporizer, the breathing circuit, and the waste gas scavenge system. Perhaps the simplest way to describe an anesthetic machine is to describe the components in order of the flow of gas through the machine, from source to patient. However, prior to describing these components, it is important to recognize that the pressures of gas vary at different locations in an anesthesia machine and knowledge of these pressures facilitates the evaluation and safe operation of these machines. There are high-, intermediate-, and low-pressure areas. The high-pressure area accepts gases at cylinder pressure and reduces and regulates the pressure; this area includes gas cylinders, hanger yokes, yoke blocks, high-pressure hoses, pressure gauges, and regulators, and the pressure may be as high as 2200 psi. The intermediate-pressure area accepts gases from the central pipeline or from the regulators on the anesthesia machine and conducts them to the flush valve and flowmeters; this area includes pipeline inlets, power outlets for ventilators, conduits from pipeline inlets to flowmeters, and conduits from regulators to flowmeters, the flowmeter assembly, and the oxygen-flush apparatus. The pressure usually ranges from 40 to 55 psi. The low-pressure area consists of the conduits and components between the flowmeter and the common gas outlet; this area includes vaporizers, piping from the flowmeters to the vaporizer, conduit from the vaporizer to the common gas outlet, and the breathing system. The pressure in the low-pressure area is close to ambient pressure. Pressures within the low-pressure area can vary depending upon how the system is being used (e.g., positive pressure ventilation) but should generally never exceed 30 cmH_2O as these pressures are transmitted directly to the patient's lungs (see Fig. 3.37).

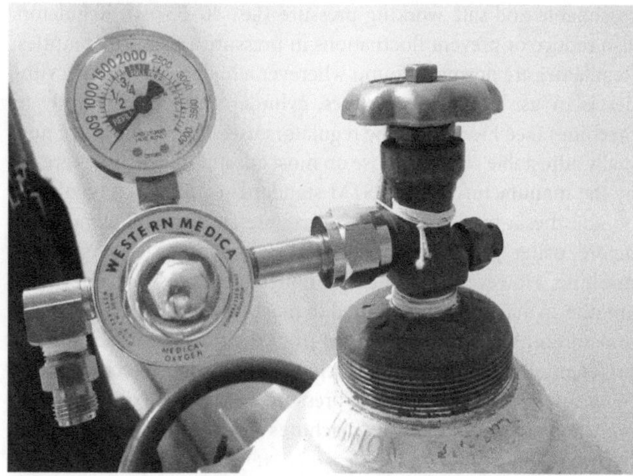

Figure 3.35 Pressure-reducing valves/regulators are used to decrease the pressure of the gas in a compressed gas cylinder down to a lower pressure, sometimes referred to as the working pressure, normally 45–55 psi. These valves maintain a constant pressure delivery from the gas supply and help prevent fluctuations associated with gas depletion and use. Source: Craig Mosley, Mosley Veterinary Anesthesia Services, Rockwood, ON, Canada.

Occasionally in veterinary medicine, multiple medical gases (e.g., oxygen, air, nitrous oxide) are used with the anesthetic machine. However, 100% oxygen is normally the only gas used to deliver anesthesia and power anesthetic equipment (e.g., ventilators) in veterinary medicine. If the reader plans to use multiple gases for delivering anesthesia, it is their responsibility to understand fully the implications of the usage (indications and contraindications) and to ensure that the anesthetic equipment is properly designed and monitored to prevent the possibility of

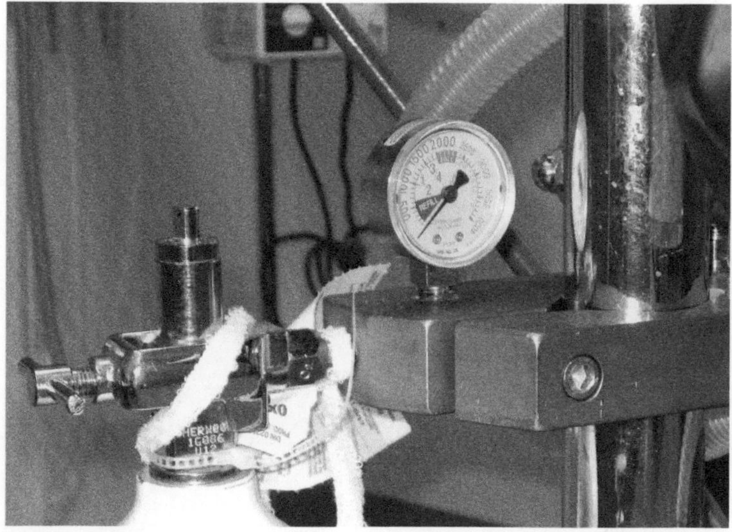

(a)

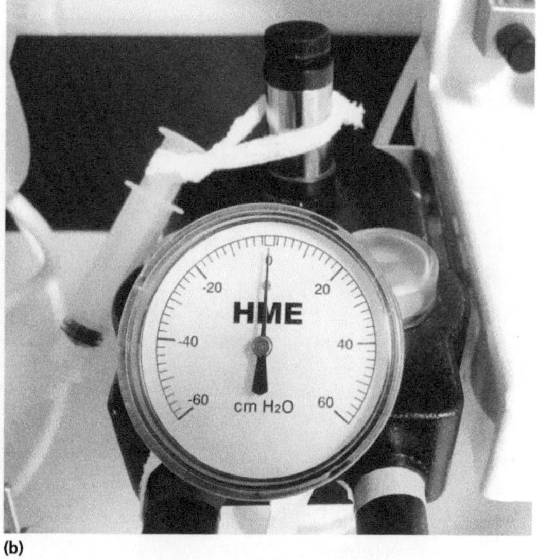

(b)

Figure 3.36 Pressure gauges are used to measure pressure in gas cylinders, anesthetic machines and breathing systems. (a) A pressure gauge associated with a compressed gas tank, measured in pounds per square inch (psi). (b) The pressure gauge found commonly on most anesthetic breathing circuits. Note that the pressure in the breathing circuit is measured in cmH_2O. Source: Craig Mosley, Mosley Veterinary Anesthesia Services, Rockwood, ON, Canada.

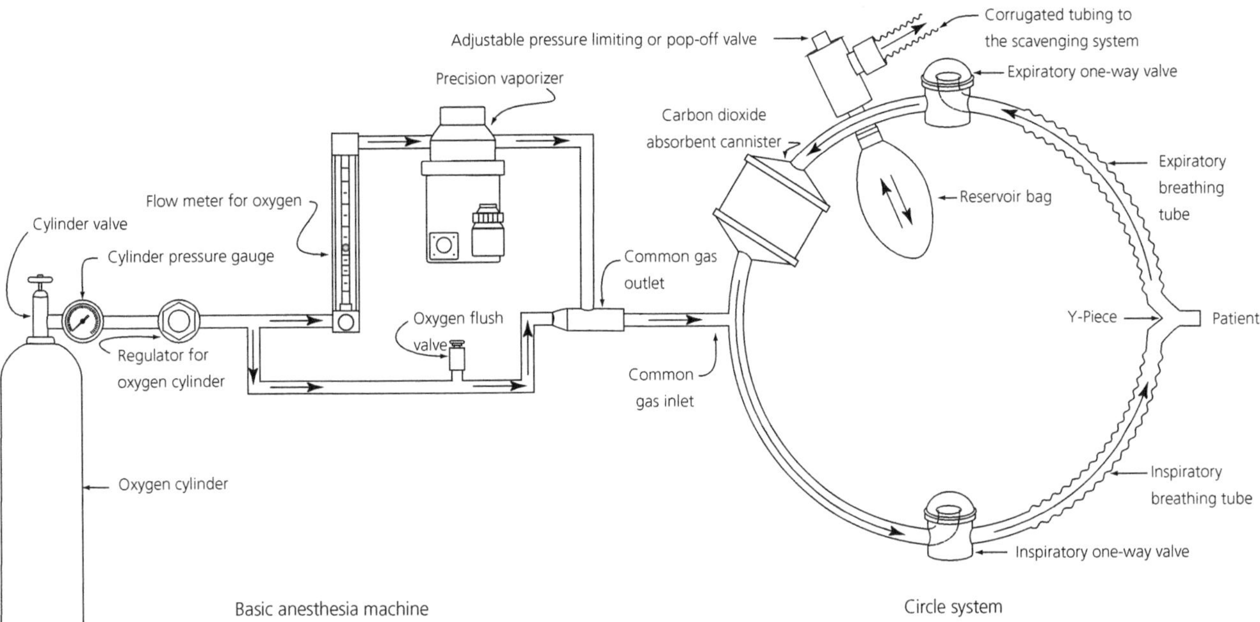

Figure 3.37 Diagram of the basic anesthetic machine and circle breathing system. The exact positions of the various components and specific features can vary markedly among manufacturers. Source: Kath Klassen, Vancouver Animal Emergency Clinic, Vancouver, Canada. Reproduced with permission of Kath Klassen.

delivering a hypoxic gas mixture to the patient. All human machines must have a proportioning system associated with the oxygen flow and oxygen concentration monitors to ensure that a hypoxic gas mixture cannot be delivered; this is not generally the case with veterinary anesthesia machines.

The flow of gas within an anesthetic machine may take multiple routes once it enters the intermediate pressure areas of the machine. Minimally, gas must be delivered to the flowmeter, where it is then directed to the vaporizer and subsequently to the patient. However, in addition to this route of movement, there may be several more routes available for gas distribution in the anesthesia machine. Normally on most anesthesia machines intermediate pressure gas is also diverted to a fresh gas flush valve that bypasses the flowmeter and vaporizer and delivers fresh gas directly to the breathing circuit. There are circumstances where flush valves may not be present or are unavailable on veterinary anesthesia machines. Additionally, gas from the intermediate pressure area may be diverted to one or more auxiliary oxygen outlets that may be used as the driving gas for a built-in or external ventilator or an external oxygen flowmeter.

Flowmeters

Flowmeters control the rate of gas delivery to the low-pressure area of the anesthetic machine and determine the fresh gas flow (FGF) to the anesthetic circuit. There must be a separate flowmeter for each gas type used with the anesthetic machine (Fig. 3.38). The type of breathing system used, the volume of the breathing circuit and the size of the patient are all factors that influence the rate of FGF.

There are several flowmeter designs available, but most are based on a tapered gas tube with a moveable float. The gas normally flows into the bottom of the tube and out at the top. The tube is narrower at the bottom and wider at the top, so as the float moves up the tube more gas can flow around the float, producing higher flow rates (Fig. 3.39) The amount of gas entering the tube is controlled by a

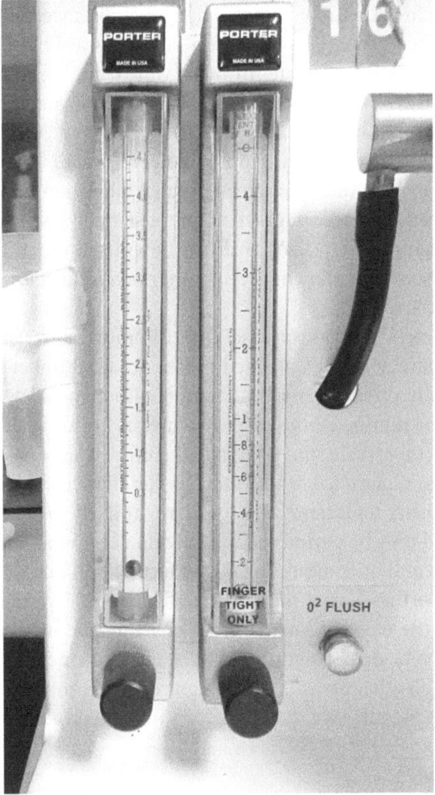

Figure 3.38 Two flowmeters arranged in parallel on an anesthetic machine with nitrous oxide (blue) on the left and oxygen (green) on the right. Flowmeters on human anesthesia machines must conform to specific positioning (i.e. oxygen right-most flowmeter) and control-knob dimension (i.e. oxygen is furled and protrudes out furthest); this is not the case for flowmeters on anesthestic machines designed solely for veterinary use. Source: Craig Mosley, Mosley Veterinary Anesthesia Services, Rockwood, ON, Canada.

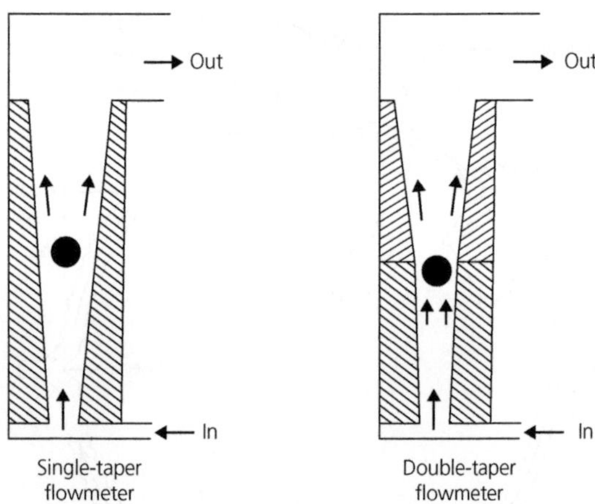

Figure 3.39 Diagram of a flowmeter illustrating gas flow from bottom to top with single and double tapers. As the flow indicator (bobbin, ball, or spindle) rises, flow increases because the orifice size increases. The double taper allows increased accuracy at the lower end of the tube while accurately metering higher flows from the top. Source: Hartsfield SM. Machines and breathing systems for administration of inhalation anesthetics. In: Short CE, ed. *Principles and Practices of Veterinary Anesthesia*. Baltimore: Williams & Wilkins, 1987; 395. Reproduced with permission of Lippincott Williams & Wilkins.

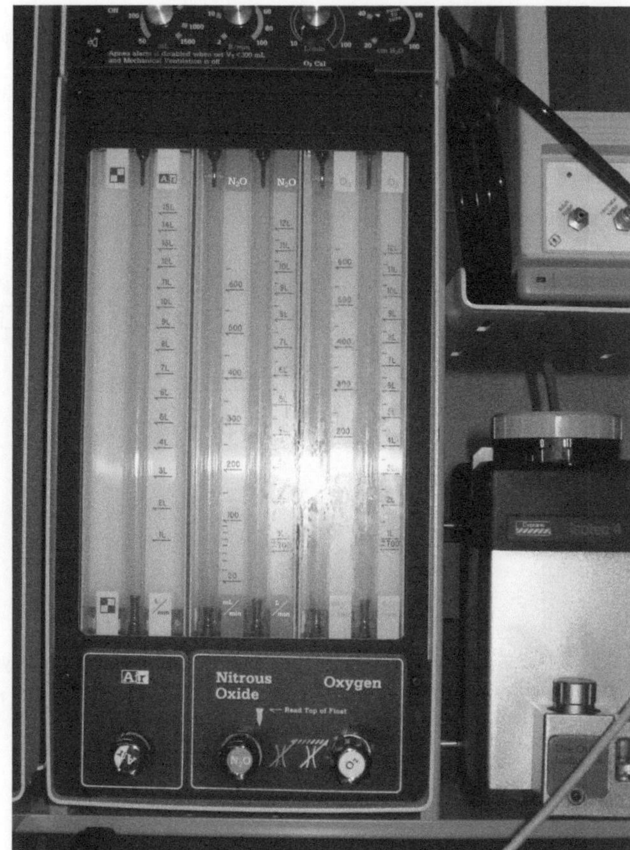

Figure 3.40 An example of multiple flowmeters being used on a single anesthetic machine designed for human use. Note the positioning of the flowmeters and shape of the control knobs. Also note that the nitrous oxide and oxygen flowmeters are dual-stage flowmeters in series allowing for increased precision of gas delivery. Source: Craig Mosley, Mosley Veterinary Anesthesia Services, Rockwood, ON, Canada.

flow-control knob that adjusts a needle valve. A float indicates the gas flow on a calibrated scale. The gas flow rates are normally expressed in mL/min or L/min. The spatial distance between vertical markings on the flowmeter do not necessarily correspond to equal changes in flow rate. In other words, the distance between 0 and 1000 mL as measured vertically on the flowmeter may not be the same as the vertical distance between 1000 and 2000 mL. This is similar to the spatial separation of the percentages found on many vaporizers where there is a greater spatial allocation on the dial for normal working percentages than for those rarely used. Some anesthetic machines may also have two flowmeters for the same gas placed in series for allowing even greater precision at lower gas flow rates (Fig. 3.40).

Flowmeters are gas specific and calibrated at 760 mmHg and 20 °C; accuracy may be affected if they are used under conditions significantly different from calibration, although this is rarely significant for routine clinical use. Flowmeters are also calibrated as a unit (flow tube, scale, and float) and therefore if any one of these fail it is best to replace the whole unit. Gasket, flow-control dial/knob, and/or washer replacement or repair are unlikely to affect accuracy but should only be performed by individuals familiar with flowmeter design and operation. The flow-control knob on contemporary human anesthesia machines must conform to ASTM standards. For example, the oxygen flow-control knob must be uniquely shaped and it must be on the right-most side of the flowmeter bank downstream of all other gases. These design considerations are important for minimizing the accidental delivery of hypoxic gas mixtures.

Vaporizers

Vaporizers change liquid anesthetic into vapor and meter the amount of vapor leaving the vaporizer. Most modern vaporizers are agent-specific, concentration-calibrated, variable-bypass, flow-over the wick, out of the circle, and high-resistance (or plenum) vaporizers that are compensated for temperature, flow, and back-pressure. Non-precision, low-resistance, in the circle vaporizers continue to be found in veterinary medicine owing to their lower cost, but without proper inspired inhalant gas monitoring these vaporizers would seem to pose unnecessary risk during anesthesia and their use should probably be discouraged unless used in conjunction with anesthetic agent monitors. Vaporizers work by splitting the carrier gas to flow into the vaporizing chamber (where it picks up anesthetic vapor) or to the bypass channel where it does not (Fig. 3.41). The ratio of the amount of gas that picks up inhalant to the gas that bypasses the inhalant, along with the vapor pressure of the volatile anesthetic, will determine the final concentration of the gas leaving the vaporizer. The output from the vaporizer is expressed as a concentration (e.g., volume percent) of vapor in the gas leaving the vaporizer.

Temperature, flow, and pressure are all factors that can potentially alter vaporizer output. The mechanisms for temperature, flow, and pressure compensation vary among vaporizer manufacturers and models. In general, most modern precision compensated vaporizers will maintain consistent output at flows between 0.5 and 10 L/min, temperatures between 15 and 35 °C, and pressure changes associated with positive pressure ventilation and the use of the flush valve.

Temperature compensation

Temperature compensation is achieved through using materials for vaporizer construction that supply and conduct heat efficiently, promoting greater thermostability. In addition, most vaporizers

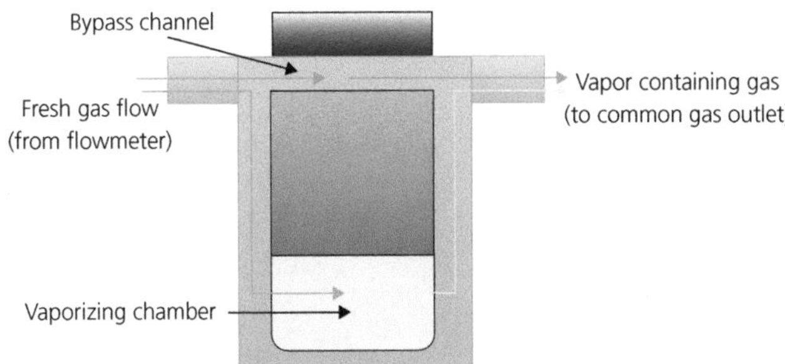

Figure 3.41 Schematic of a generic variable-bypass vaporizer demonstrating the splitting of the fresh gas flow to the vaporizing chamber and bypass channel. The splitting ratio and vapor pressure of the volatile anesthetic will determine the final percent output from the vaporizer. Source: Craig Mosley, Mosley Veterinary Anesthesia Services, Rockwood, ON, Canada.

have mechanical and a few have electrical circuit driven thermocompensation systems. These vaporizers compensate for temperature changes by altering the splitting ratio so that a greater or lesser amount of gas is conducted through the vaporizing chamber as the temperature changes during use. In mechanical systems, as the vaporizer cools, the thermal element restricts gas flow to the bypass chamber, causing more carrier gas to enter the vaporizing chamber. The opposite will occur if the vaporizer becomes too warm. The exact thermocompensation systems vary among manufacturers but the thermal element is normally a heat-sensitive metal(s) that will reliably expand and contract when subjected to temperature changes.

Flow rate

Changes in gas flow rate through the vaporizer can potentially lead to changes in output. For example, if the flow is excessively high, complete saturation of the gas moving through the vaporizing chamber may not occur, leading to a reduction in output. Flow rate compensation is achieved by ensuring reliable and consistent saturation of all gas flowing through the vaporization chamber by using a series of wicks, baffles, and spiral tracks to facilitate liquid gas vaporization. These techniques are used to increase the surface area of the carrier gas–liquid interface, ensuring that all the gas exiting the vaporization chamber is fully saturated. All properly functioning modern vaporizers have very predictable outputs within a clinically useful range of gas flow rates (500–2000 mL/min).

Back-pressure

Back-pressure on the vaporizer can occur during intermittent positive pressure ventilation or with the use of the flush valve, and this effect can increase vaporizer output if compensation mechanisms are not in place. There are a number of ways in which the effects of back-pressure are minimized in modern vaporizers. One is to reduce the size of the vaporizing chamber relative to the bypass chamber. Another option is to use a long, spiral, or small-diameter tube connecting the vaporizer chamber to the bypass channel. Both will reduce the amount of pressurized gas reaching the vaporizing chamber. The use of one-way check valves immediately upstream from the vaporizer can also prevent the effects of back-pressure and they are incorporated into some machines. One-way check valves are also sometimes used downstream of the flush valve (upstream of the vaporizer) to prevent back-pressure associated with use of the flush valve.

There are many vaporizers available for use in veterinary anesthesia but most are based on three main styles of vaporizers: the Ohmeda Tec, Dräger Vapor, and Penlon Sigma series. The primary differences among vaporizer series include capacity of the vaporization chamber (larger chambers allow longer times between fillings, particularly useful for large animal applications), susceptibility to alterations in output due to tipping (rarely a consideration under normal circumstances), and mounting options. All are very accurate and well designed; the use of one over another is often more about personal preference and availability than performance differences.

Most vaporizers are mechanical devices requiring no external power to function normally. However, as a result of the unique vapor properties of desflurane, specially designed heated vaporizers are required to ensure consistent output. Despite the need for external power, most desflurane vaporizers function very similarly to standard variable bypass vaporizers, although technically they are classified as measured flow vaporizers; see the description of the Tec 6 vaporizer below. There are also electronic vaporizers available for use in both human (Aladin cassette vaporizer, GE Healthcare) and veterinary anesthesia (Vetland EX3000 Electronic Vaporization System). These vaporizers function as variable bypass vaporizers but the splitting ratio of the carrier gas is determined electronically rather than mechanically. Since the system is electronic, various manufacturer and user alarm settings can be incorporated. For example, the vaporizer may alert the user if unusually high concentrations of anesthetic are being delivered from the vaporizer or if the vaporizer setting has not been altered within a specified time period, potentially avoiding inadvertent anesthetic overdoses (e.g., the vaporizer output is momentarily increased and the user forgets to reduce the setting). Although electronic systems arguably provide additional information that may be valuable to the anesthetist, they may also be more prone to problems and damage related to the fact they rely on properly operating electronics to function.

Vaporizers can be filled using a standard screw-capped filler port or an agent-specific keyed filler port. Keyed filler ports are intended to prevent inadvertent filling of a vaporizer with the wrong anesthetic agent (Fig. 3.42). Most modern vaporizers are extremely dependable and durable, requiring very little routine maintenance and care. However, maintenance and care should be performed according to the manufacturer's recommendations and only by a qualified technician.

Vaporizers are generally mounted on what is referred to as the 'back bar,' which simply refers to the rail or mounting system used to hold vaporizers on the machine. Most veterinary vaporizers use cagemount systems for securing the vaporizer to the back bar; this system uses 23 mm taper push fittings (inlet and outlet, female and male) to attach the vaporizer to the gas delivery system and the vaporizer is bolted directly to the back bar (Fig. 3.43). The tapered fittings are often referred to as vaporizer caps, adapters, or elbows.

There are also several proprietary mounting bracket systems that allow vaporizers to be easily removed, for example, the GE Healthcare Ohmeda Selectatec and the Dräger Interlock, with the former being significantly more popular. The Selectatec mount consist of two vertically situated male valve ports, between the inlet and outlet ports is an accessory pin and locking recess (Fig. 3.44). Selectatec compatible vaporizers have two female ports with a recessed assembly to receive the accessory pin. The vaporizer is lowered on to the male valve ports and then locked into place using the locking knob located on the vaporizer. The O-rings on the male valve ports ensure a gas-tight seal between the vaporizer and the Selectatec mount. Loss or deformation of these rings can lead to leaks between the vaporizer and mount. The vaporizer cannot be turned on unless it is locked in place on the mount. When the vaporizer is turned on (Tec 4, 5, 6, 7),

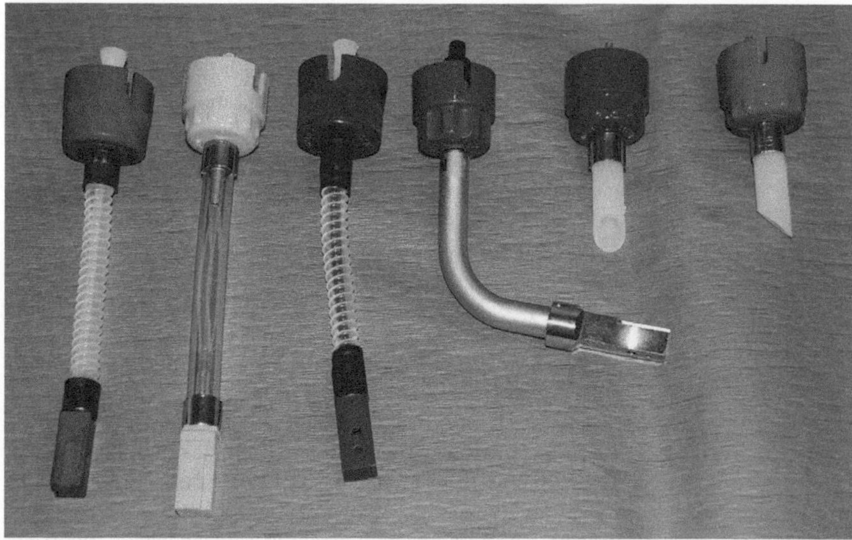

(a)

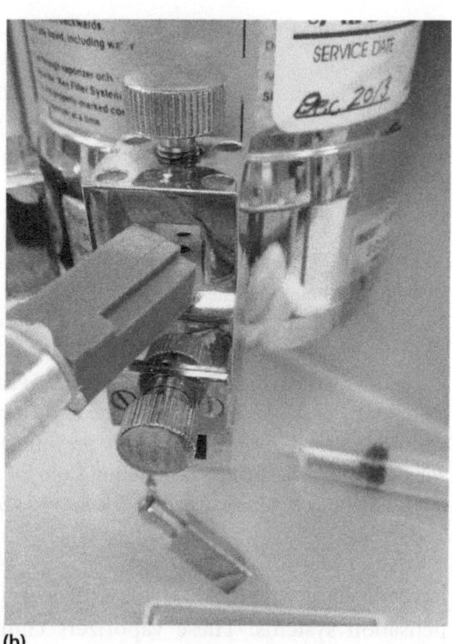

(b)

Figure 3.42 Many vaporizers are filled using agent-specific filler keys represented by the four fillers located on the left in a. The keys are indexed to both the bottle and vaporizer (b) and prevent inadvertent filling of a vaporizer with the wrong anesthetic agent. There are also many vaporizers that are not equipped with a keyed filler port and instead use a standard screw-topped filler port. Filling of these vaporizers is best performed using an inhalant-specific filler spout (second right-most in a). These are indexed to a specific agent bottle but not the vaporizer. Source: part a, Thomas Riebold, College of Veterinary Medicine, Oregon State University, Corvallis, OR, USA. Reproduced with permission of Thomas Riebold. Source: part b, Craig Mosley, Mosley Veterinary Anesthesia Services, Rockwood, ON, Canada.

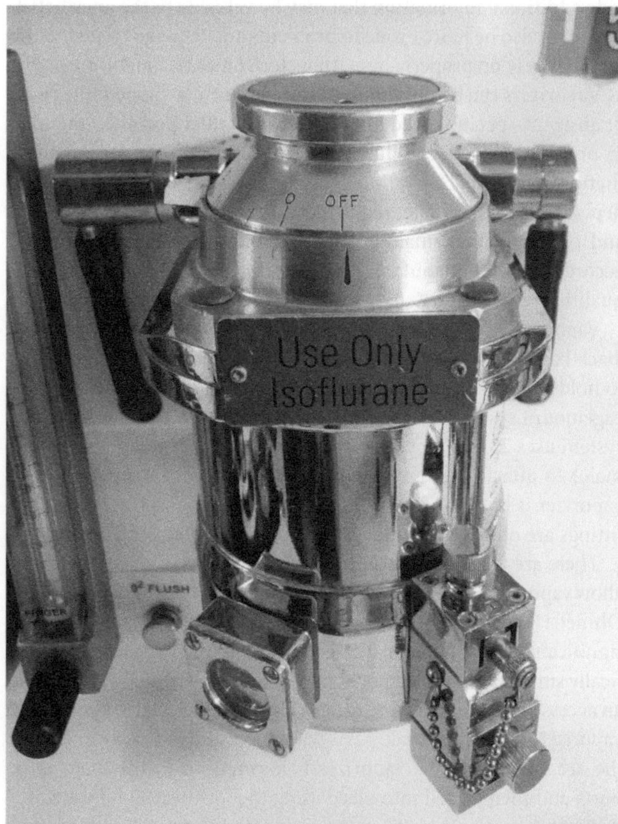

Figure 3.43 An example of a typical cagemount vaporizer with tapered push fittings for delivery of gas to and from the vaporizer. Source: Craig Mosley, Mosley Veterinary Anesthesia Services, Rockwood, ON, Canada.

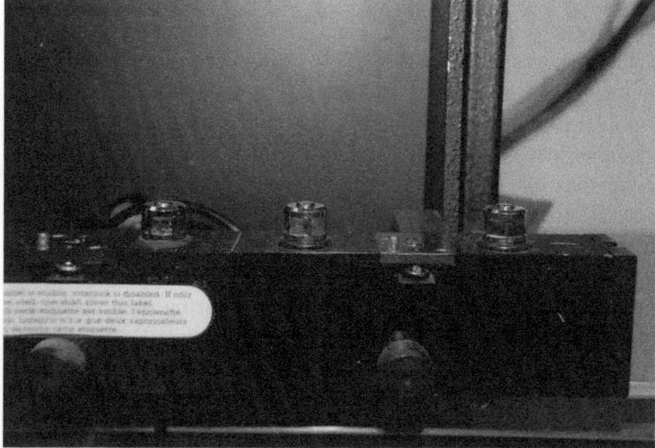

Figure 3.44 A Selectatec mounting bar for Tec style vaporizers. This mounting system is convenient for quick placement and removal of vaporizers. The vertical male ports deliver gas to and from the vaporizer; the pin between the two ports is the locking system used to mount the vaporizer The vaporizer must be locked in place before the control dial can be turned on. Source: Thomas Riebold, College of Veterinary Medicine, Oregon State University, Corvallis, OR, USA. Reproduced with permission of Thomas Riebold.

a retractable spindle depresses the ball valve in the male valve ports, allowing gas to flow from the vaporizer to the anesthetic machine. Tec 4 and above vaporizer models also incorporate a safety interlock system (vaporizer exclusion/isolation) that uses a horizontal push rod system that ensures that only one vaporizer can be used at a time when multiple vaporizers are mounted in series on a Selectatec mount. The Dräger Interlock mount system is very similar to the Selectatec mount and also includes a safety interlink system;

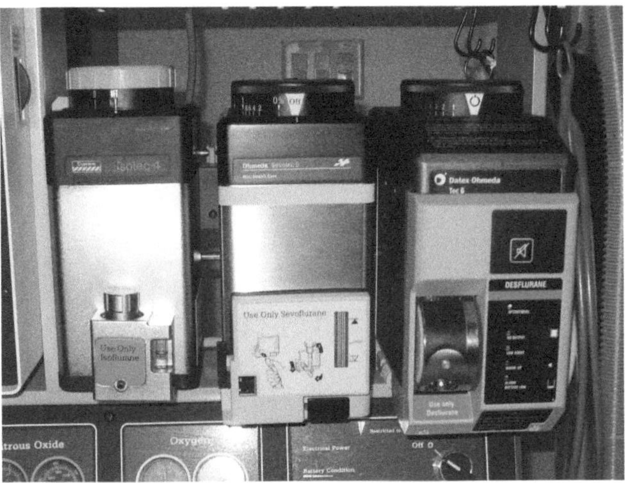

Figure 3.45 A machine mounted with several of the Ohmeda/Datex-Ohmeda Tec series of vaporizers. From the left: the Tec 4, Tec 5, and Tec 6 vaporizers. Source: Craig Mosley, Mosley Veterinary Anesthesia Services, Rockwood, ON, Canada.

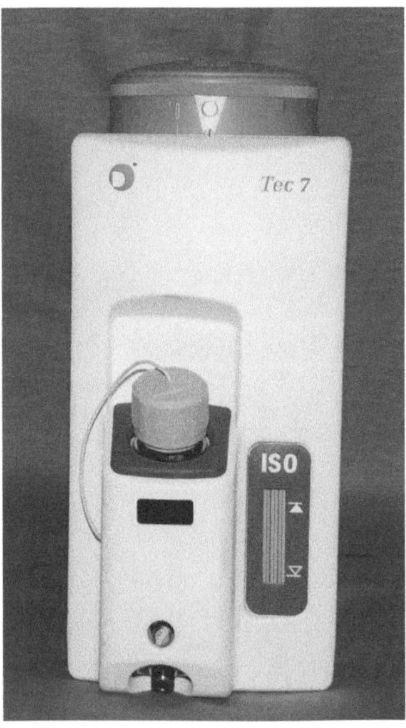

Figure 3.46 A Datex-Ohmeda/GE Healthcare Tec 7 isoflurane-specific vaporizer. The Tec 7 series is the latest variable-bypass plenum vaporizer series offered by Datex-Ohmeda/GE Healthcare. Source: Thomas Riebold, College of Veterinary Medicine, Oregon State University, Corvallis, OR, USA. Reproduced with permission of Thomas Riebold.

however, the dimensions are unique, meaning that each system can only be used with a vaporizer compatible with the individual mounting system. Most vaporizers are available in models compatible with the Selectatec mounting system.

Descriptions of vaporizers common in veterinary medicine

The vaporizers described here are some of those most commonly being used in veterinary anesthesia. Earlier vaporizers no longer being manufactured may still be in use and some have been described in earlier editions of this book and elsewhere [66].

Ohmeda/Datex-Ohmeda/GE Healthcare Tec vaporizers

Tec vaporizers specifically designed for halothane or isoflurane vaporization, particularly the Fluotec Mark 3 and Isotec 3, are commonly used in veterinary anesthesia and are described in more detail below. They are considered reliable and are temperature, flow, and back-pressure compensated under normal operating conditions. The Fluotec Mark 3 predecessor, the Fluotec Mark 2, is no longer being manufactured, but may still be available as used equipment and still found in some veterinary practices [66]. It was associated with relatively poor performance characteristics and replacement with more accurate and reliable units should be considered. Tec 4, 5, 6, and 7 vaporizers have superseded the Tec 3 vaporizers for use with contemporary human anesthesia machines [2]. The Tec 4 was only available for the delivery of isoflurane and the Tec 6 is a desflurane-specific model (Fig. 3.45). The Tec 5 series is available for delivery of enflurane, halothane, isoflurane, and sevoflurane and has been replaced by the more recent Tec 7 series of vaporizers (Fig. 3.46). These vaporizers are becoming increasingly common for use in veterinary anesthesia and various publications and the specific operating manuals offer information about their use and performance [1].

Tec 3 vaporizers

These vaporizers are classified as variable bypass, flow-over with wick, automatic thermocompensation, agent specific, high resistance and back-pressure compensated [67]. The Tec 3 model includes the Fluotec Mark 3, the Pentec Mark 2, and the Isotec 3 vaporizers (Fig. 3.47). The Tec 3 vaporizer is temperature compensated with a bimetallic, temperature-sensitive element associated with the vaporization chamber. Output from the Tec 3 vaporizer is nearly linear over the range of concentrations and flow rates that would typically be selected for veterinary patients (250 mL/min–6 L/min). Back-pressure compensation is accomplished in the internal design of the vaporizer with a long tube leading to the vaporization chamber, an expansion area in the tube, and exclusion of wicks from the area of the vaporization chamber near the inlet [67].

Tec 4 and 5 vaporizers

These vaporizers are classified as variable bypass, flow-over with wick, automatic thermocompensation, agent specific, high resistance and back-pressure compensated [67]. The vaporizer's main design features over earlier models are associated with its obligatory use with a Selectatec mounting system. The Tec 4 was the earliest version of these vaporizers and was only available for isoflurane delivery (Fig. 3.48). The Tec 5 is available for the delivery of enflurane, halothane, isoflurane, and sevoflurane and can be found in either a key or funnel filled configuration (Fig. 3.49). When the dial is turned to '0' and the flowmeter is activated, all of the gas bypasses the vaporizer through the Selectatec mount rather than the passing through the vaporizers bypass channel. Only when the vaporizer is turned from '0' will the gas enter the vaporizer. Temperature compensation is accomplished through a bimetallic strip located in the bypass channel; as the temperature decreases, less gas is allowed through the bypass channel so that relatively more gas passes through the vaporizing chamber. Tec 5 vaporizers also feature a safety interlock system (vaporizer isolation/exclusion system), activated when multiple vaporizers are mounted in series.

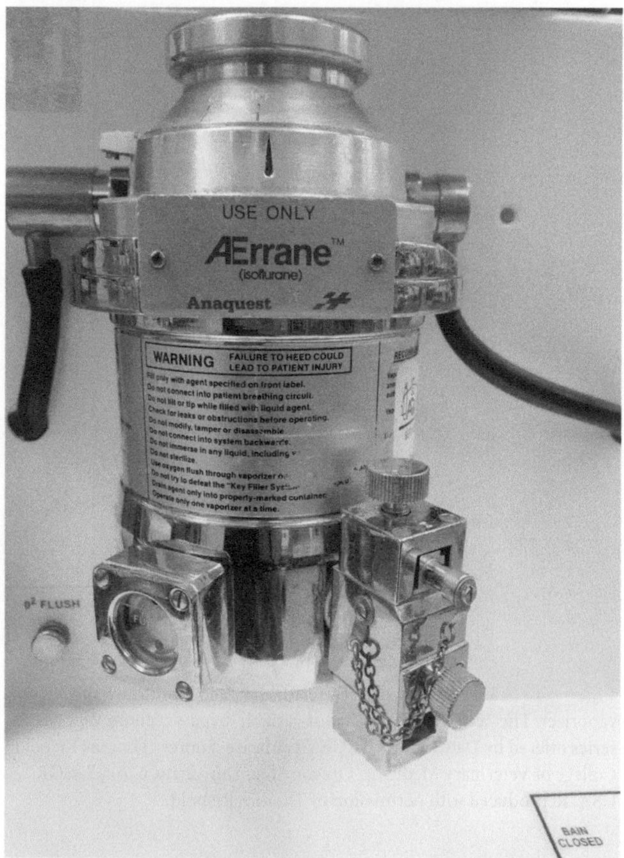

Figure 3.47 An example of a Tec 3 style isoflurane-specific vaporizer. This style of vaporizer is very common in many veterinary practices. Source: Craig Mosley, Mosley Veterinary Anesthesia Services, Rockwood, ON, Canada.

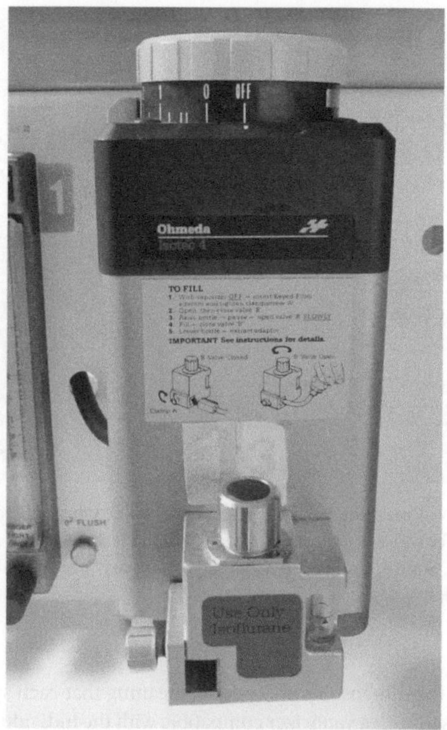

Figure 3.48 The Ohmeda Tec 4 (IsoTec) was the first vaporizer designed for use with the Selectatec mounting system and was only available for the delivery of isoflurane. Source: Craig Mosley, Mosley Veterinary Anesthesia Services, Rockwood, ON, Canada.

Tec 6

The Tec 6 vaporizer is designed for use only with desflurane (Fig. 3.50). Owing to its relatively low potency and low boiling point (near room temperature), desflurane liquid requires heating to ensure complete and stable vaporization of the liquid and accurate vaporizer output. The vaporizer is classified as a measured-flow vaporizer, automatic thermocompensation, agent specific, high resistance (see below) and back-pressure compensated. The vaporizer uses electronics to indicate its operational status, the level of agent, to control the pressure balance (between the diluent/bypass gas and the vaporized inhalant), to heat the liquid desflurane, and to charge the backup battery. The vaporizer can only be turned on once the electronics determine it to be operable. The heaters in the agent sump heat the desflurane to 39 °C, producing saturated desflurane at a vapor pressure of approximately 1500 mmHg in the reservoir.

When the vaporizer is turned on, the valve is opened and the pressurized vapor moves to a pressure regulator that reduces the pressure to that normally found in a high-resistance (plenum) vaporizer (10–20 cmH_2O). The desflurane vapor then moves to a variable restrictor controlled by the concentration selection dial, where it is added to the carrier gas leaving the vaporizer. The fresh gas (carrier gas) flow into the vaporizer passes through a fixed restrictor that increases its pressure to that normally found in a high-resistance (plenum) vaporizer. Two independent pressure

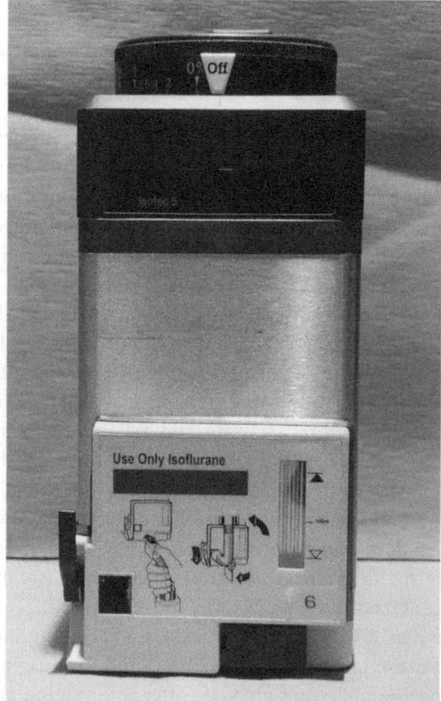

Figure 3.49 The Tec 5 series of vaporizers included enflurane-, halothane-, isoflurane-, and sevoflurane-specific models. The Tec 5 model also incorporated an interlock safety system that prevents multiple vaporizers from being turned on when mounted in series. Source: Thomas Riebold, College of Veterinary Medicine, Oregon State University, Corvallis, OR, USA. Reproduced with permission of Thomas Riebold.

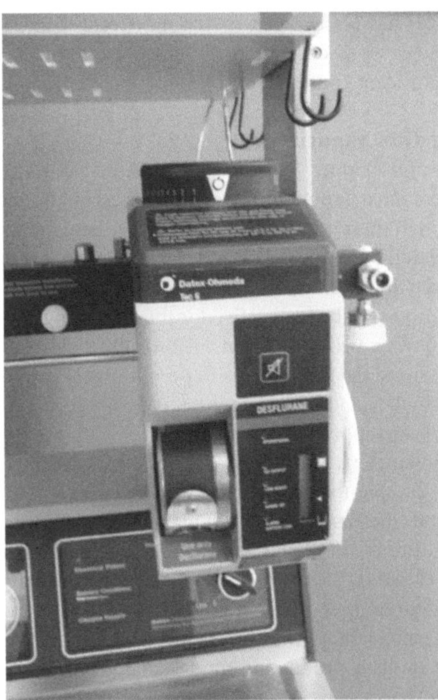

Figure 3.50 The Datex-Ohmeda Tec 6 vaporizer is a desflurane-specific model incorporating a heated vaporizing chamber. The Tec 6 Plus from Datex-Ohmeda/GE Healthcare is the latest available in this vaporizer series. Source: Craig Mosley, Mosley Veterinary Anesthesia Services, Rockwood, ON, Canada.

sensors in the pathway detect pressure changes and instruct the pressure regulator to change the desflurane pressure (and flow) proportionately so as to maintain the set vapor concentration. For example, if the fresh gas flow rate is increased, the pressure created by the carrier gas moving through the fixed restrictor will increase. This will then instruct the desflurane pressure (and flow) to increase proportionately, maintaining the vaporizer output despite changes in carrier gas flow. If the readings from the two sensors are not similar, the vaporizer will shut off the vaporizing chamber, initiating an alarm. The filler port accepts only the specific filler nozzle associated with the desflurane bottle.

Dräger vapor vaporizers: Vapor 19.1

Dräger Vapor 19.1 series vaporizers are commonly found in veterinary medicine. An interlock compatible model is also available, the Vapor 19.3 series. The Vapor 19.1 probably first became popular in veterinary anesthesia for large animal applications (Fig. 3.51). The Vapor 19.1 had a significantly larger inhalant reservoir capacity relative to the standard Tec 3 and 4 vaporizers commonly used at the time (although extended capacity Tec 3 models were also produced). The larger inhalant reservoir is well suited to the increased inhalant demands associated with large animal inhalant anesthesia and reduced the likelihood of needing to refill the vaporizer in the middle of a case. The Vapor 19.1 series vaporizers are classified as variable bypass, flow-over with wick, automatic thermocompensation, high resistance, agent specific and pressure compensated [67]. Specific vaporizers are available for sevoflurane, isoflurane, enflurane and halothane, administration. Temperature compensation is

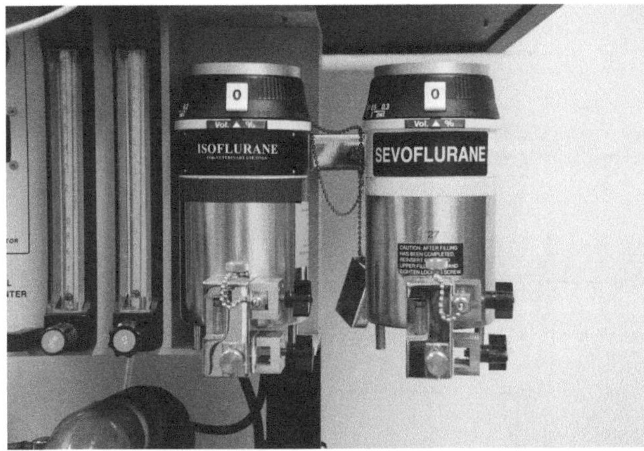

Figure 3.51 Isoflurane and sevoflurane Dräger Vapor 19.1 vaporizers mounted on a large animal anesthesia machine. These vaporizers probably first became popular for use in veterinary medicine for providing large animal anesthesia owing to their relatively large inhalant reservoir, requiring less filling during a case. Source: Thomas Riebold, College of Veterinary Medicine, Oregon State University, Corvallis, OR, USA. Reproduced with permission of Thomas Riebold.

automatic with a temperature compensator. The temperature compensator makes use of the thermal characteristics of two different materials to expand or contract the bypass channel, decreasing or increasing the amount of gas passing through the vaporization chamber. Pressure compensation is accomplished by the presence of a long spiral inlet tube to the vaporization chamber [2]. This vaporizer is accurate from 0.3 to 15 L/min of fresh gas flow at the lower settings on the control dial, but complete saturation may not occur at higher settings with higher flows. The vaporizer is designed for operation (temperature compensation) in the range 10–40 °C [2]. Dräger also produces desflurane-specific vaporizers, the D Vapor and the DIVA, which are additional examples of measure flow vaporizers, similar to the Tec 6.

Penlon Sigma Delta vaporizers

Penlon Sigma Delta vaporizers are another type of vaporizer occasionally used in veterinary medicine. The Sigma Delta vaporizer (Fig. 3.52) is classified as variable bypass, flow-over with wick, temperature compensated, high resistance, agent specific, and VOC [67]. Specific vaporizers are available for sevoflurane, isoflurane, enflurane, and halothane administration. Penlon also produces a desflurane vaporizer, the Sigma Alpha. Temperature compensation is through a thermostat in the bypass channel. The operating temperature is between 15 and 35 °C and the temperature-compensating mechanism reacts slowly, requiring 1–2 h to compensate for changes in room temperature. This vaporizer is accurate from 0.2 to 15 L/min of fresh gas flow at all dial settings, with only slightly decreased output at lower settings and slightly increased output at higher settings when using very low flow rates.

Ohio calibrated vaporizer

This vaporizer (Fig. 3.53) has been available for veterinary use and was commonly employed on human anesthesia machines for many years. It is classified as variable bypass, flow-over with wick, automatically temperature compensated, agent specific, VOC, and high resistance [67]. Specific units are manufactured for isoflurane, halothane, and sevoflurane administration. These vaporizers were

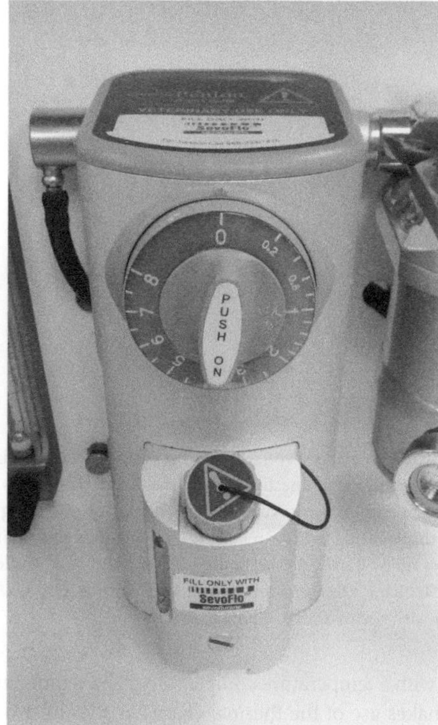

Figure 3.52 A sevoflurane-specific Penlon Sigma Delta vaporizer. The Sigma Delta is also available for the delivery of enflurane, halothane, and isoflurane. Source: Craig Mosley, Mosley Veterinary Anesthesia Services, Rockwood, ON, Canada.

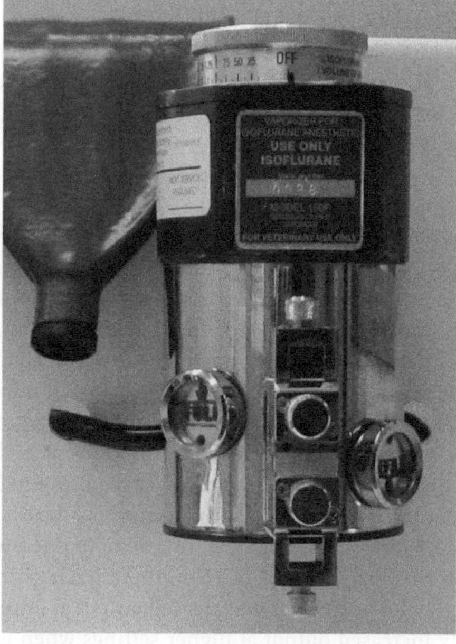

Figure 3.53 An isoflurane-specific Ohio vaporizer. It has also been manufactured for the delivery of halothane and sevoflurane. Source: Craig Mosley, Mosley Veterinary Anesthesia Services, Rockwood, ON, Canada.

designed for accuracy at fresh gas flows between 0.3 and 10 L/min, and temperature compensation occurs between 16 and 32 °C. Tilting these vaporizers up to 20° while in use or up to 45° when not in use does not cause problems. Greater tipping of the vaporizer may cause delivery of high concentrations. Between paper wicks, the vaporizer has plastic spacers that may react with enflurane or isoflurane to cause discoloration of the liquid anesthetic, apparently without significant consequences [67].

Measured-flow vaporizers

Verni-Trol and Copper Kettles are flowmeter-controlled vaporizers that were once popular for use in anesthesia of human patients [67]. Although these vaporizers are no longer being manufactured, are not covered by the ASTM standards for anesthesia equipment, and are rarely found in clinical use (or otherwise), a description of their operation may be instructive for those wanting an alternative explanation of vaporizer function. Historically they are also important as they were the first devices to permit precise vaporization of liquid anesthetics and served as the precursors to today's modern variable-bypass vaporizers.

These flowmeter-controlled vaporizers are classified as measured flow, bubble-through, high resistance, VOC, temperature compensated (thermally stable with manual flow adjustments based on temperature of the liquid anesthetic), and multipurpose. They have been classified as saturation vaporizers. These vaporizers are constructed of copper (Copper Kettle) or silicon bronze (Verni-Trol) for thermostability. Back-pressure compensation mechanisms are present on later production models and can be fitted on older models (e.g., check valves). Since these vaporizers are multipurpose or universal, they can accurately vaporize halothane, isoflurane, sevoflurane, or methoxyflurane, and should be clearly labeled for the agent in use.

With measured-flow vaporizers, manual adjustments of flow rates are required to account for variations in total gas flow, day-to-day changes in temperature, and changes in liquid temperature during use, especially with high fresh gas flow rates. In most cases, a calculator is supplied with each vaporizer for determining proper flow rates. Anesthesia machines with measured-flow vaporizers have two oxygen flowmeters: One flowmeter routes all of its oxygen through the vaporization chamber, where it is fully saturated with anesthetic; the other flowmeter supplies oxygen that bypasses the vaporizer and supplies oxygen to meet the patient's requirements. By manually altering the ratio of gas going to the vaporizer to that bypassing the vaporizer, precise concentrations of anesthetic could be delivered to the patient. Both gas sources combine at a mixing valve to achieve the proper anesthetic concentration before gases enter the breathing system. Modern agent-specific variable-bypass vaporizers simply eliminated the need to determine and adjust these ratios manually. Further details concerning the use of measured-flow vaporizers can be found in earlier editions of this book [66].

Maintenance of vaporizers

Vaporizers require maintenance. In general, the best policy is to follow the manufacturer's guidelines for care and servicing. Recommendations vary but, regardless of the maintenance schedule, servicing should be performed on a vaporizer if, based on the responses of patients, the dialed anesthetic concentration is suspected to be erroneous, or if any of the components of the vaporizer function improperly (e.g., the control dial is difficult to adjust). Servicing as recommended by the manufacturer often includes an evaluation of operation, cleaning, changing of filters, replacement of worn parts, and recalibration. Halothane and methoxyflurane contain preservatives (thymol and butylated hydroxytoluene, respectively) that are not highly volatile and therefore collect in the vaporization chambers and on the wicks,

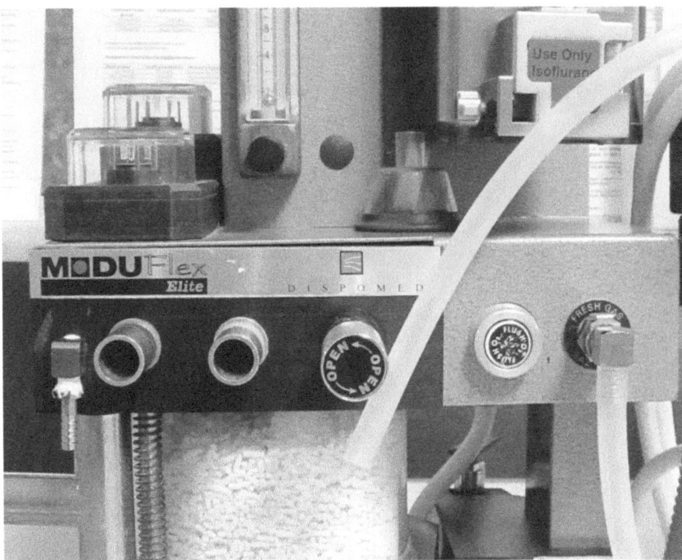

(a)

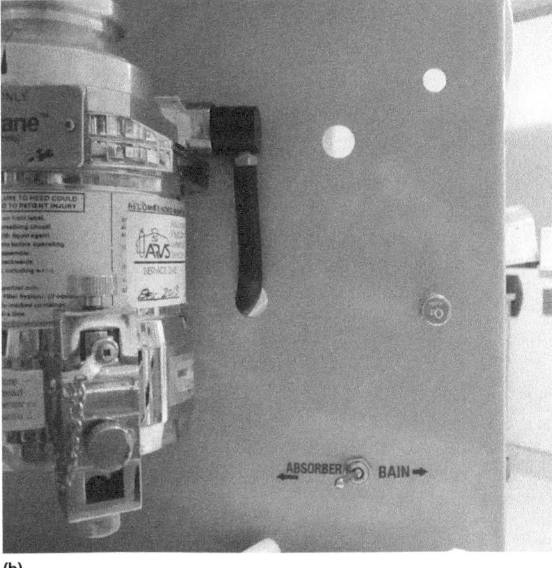

(b)

Figure 3.54 Examples of various flush valve buttons on anesthetic machines. (a) The oxygen flush button is recessed in a protective collar to prevent inadvertent activation if bumped. Many flush buttons are relatively small and are unprotected from accidental activation. (b). Source: Craig Mosley, Mosley Veterinary Anesthesia Services, Rockwood, ON, Canada.

potentially affecting anesthetic output. These vaporizers should be periodically drained to remove most of these preservatives. Vaporizers should not be overfilled or tipped significantly once filled. They should also be drained before removal from the anesthesia machine for service. In the past, flushing a vaporizer with diethyl ether to dissolve preservatives that collect within it has been recommended. Owing to the flammability and explosiveness of diethyl ether, and the common use of 100% oxygen as a carrier gas, this is no longer recommended. Flushing the vaporizer does not eliminate the need for regular service by a certified vaporizer technician.

Use of the wrong anesthetic in an agent-specific vaporizer

Using an agent-specific vaporizer for an anesthetic for which the vaporizer is not calibrated is problematic, especially if the introduction of an anesthetic is unintentional (i.e., the operator does not realize the mistake). Lower than indicated anesthetic output is expected if an anesthetic with a lower vapor pressure is placed in a vaporizer designed for a drug with a higher vapor pressure (e.g., sevoflurane used in an isoflurane vaporizer). Conversely, a highly volatile anesthetic in an agent-specific vaporizer designed for a drug with a lower vapor pressure is likely to produce a high, potentially lethal concentration. The differential potencies of the drugs in question would be expected to affect the depth of anesthesia in either situation.

During the introduction of isoflurane into veterinary anesthesia, it was commonly administered with agent-specific halothane vaporizers that were relabeled, but not recalibrated for isoflurane. Because the vapor pressures of halothane and isoflurane are similar (e.g., 243 and 240 mmHg at 20 °C, respectively), the output was not expected to differ greatly from the control-dial setting. Indeed, halothane vaporizers produce concentrations of isoflurane that are reasonably close to the dial setting for halothane [68]. Nevertheless, current manufacturer recommendations are against the use of isoflurane in halothane-specific vaporizers and vice versa [69]. Depending on the vaporizer and conditions of operation, isoflurane in a halothane vaporizer may produce 25–50% more vapor than expected, and halothane in an isoflurane-specific vaporizer usually delivers a concentration that is lower than expected [69]. If isoflurane is to be used in an agent-specific halothane vaporizer, the vaporizer should be serviced and completely recalibrated for isoflurane. Complete calibration implies that the vaporizer has been tested for accuracy with an anesthetic-gas analyzer at various carrier gas flow rates and various temperatures to assure reliable function.

Oxygen flush valve

Oxygen flush valves are found on most, but not all, veterinary anesthetic machines. There is no convention regarding location, size, or design of the flush valve in veterinary medicine and they vary dramatically (e.g., button, toggle, or switch) (Fig. 3.54). Flush valves on human anesthetic machines must be a recessed button type and easily accessible on the front of the machine. Flush valves are designed to rapidly deliver large volumes of non-anesthetic-containing gas to the patient breathing circuit in emergency situations. The flow originates downstream of the regulator within the intermediate pressure area of the anesthetic machine (~50 psi) and bypasses the flowmeter and vaporizer, delivering gas at rates ranging between 35 and 75 L/min to the patient circuit. To avoid overpressuring the patient circuit, the flush valve should not be used, or be used very cautiously with non-rebreathing circuits, circuits attached to mechanical ventilators, and circuits with very low volumes (e.g., pediatric circle systems) as pressures within the breathing circuit may temporarily rise, creating dangerously high pressures to the patient's lungs. The adjustable pressure-limiting (APL) valves should be fully open at all times to help prevent overpressurizing the breathing circuit.

Common gas outlet

The common gas outlet leads from the anesthetic machine to the breathing circuit (Fig. 3.55). Gas reaching the common gas outlet has traveled from the gas supply (cylinder or pipeline), through the regulator, flowmeter, and vaporizer. The gas flowing from the common

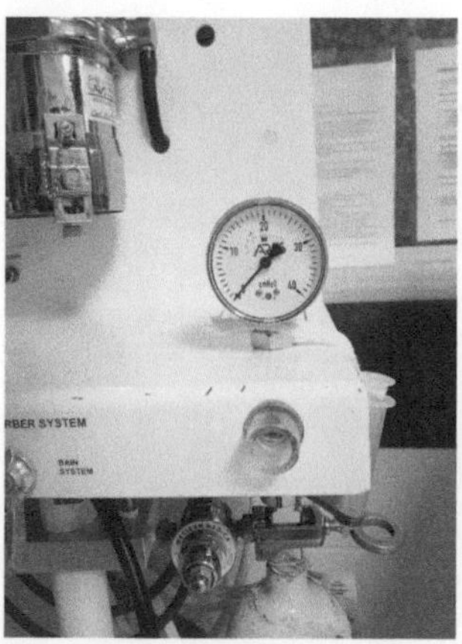

(a)

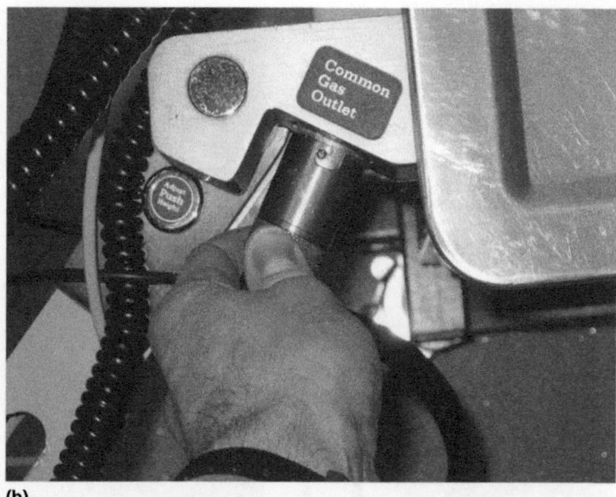

(b)

Figure 3.55 Common gas outlets deliver gas from the anesthetic machine to the patient breathing circuit. Push-type taper connections are common in veterinary medicine (a). Locking common gas outlets are standard on human anesthesia machines (b). Locking systems will help prevent inadvertent disconnection from the gas supply from the machine to the breathing circuit. Source: Craig Mosley, Mosley Veterinary Anesthesia Services, Rockwood, ON, Canada.

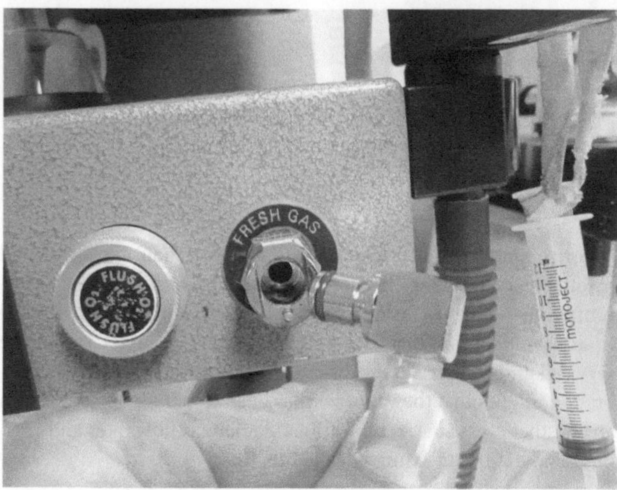

Figure 3.56 A quick-connect/disconnect system used for the common gas outlet on a machine designed solely for veterinary use can be a safety feature preventing inadvertent disconnections between the patient circuit and anesthesia machine. Source: Craig Mosley, Mosley Veterinary Anesthesia Services, Rockwood, ON, Canada.

gas outlet normally delivers the anesthetic and carrier gas(es) to the patient circuit at the concentration and flow rate determined by the vaporizer setting and flowmeter flow rate. However, the concentration of inhalant gas from the common gas outlet is not usually equivalent to the gas concentration inhaled by the patient when using rebreathing circuits, particularly when using low flow rates, due to dilution of incoming gases with those already in the patient circuit. The exact configuration of the common gas outlet varies among manufacturers but it is normally a taper 15 mm I.D. port. Human anesthesia machines must have a locking mechanism in place to prevent inadvertent disconnection from the machine (Fig. 3.55), but this is not a requirement in veterinary medicine. However, at least one company designs their fresh gas outlet with a quick-connect system to prevent inadvertent disconnections (Fig. 3.56).

Breathing systems

Although some parts of the breathing system are built into anesthesia machines (e.g., the circle system carbon dioxide absorbent canister), breathing systems are considered separately from the actual anesthesia machine (i.e., components upstream of the fresh gas outlet). This is a convenient way to discuss breathing systems in veterinary medicine as on any single anesthetic machine the breathing system may be frequently changed depending upon the needs of the patient or the circumstances in which anesthetic is delivered (Fig. 3.57). The primary purposes of the breathing system are to direct oxygen to the patient, deliver anesthetic gas to the patient, remove carbon dioxide from inhaled breaths (or prevent significant rebreathing of carbon dioxide), and provide a means of controlling ventilation.

Breathing systems have been classified using numerous schemes with little uniformity or consensus of nomenclature (i.e., open, semi-open, and semi-closed). For this reason, it is suggested that these terms be abandoned and rather a description of the flow rates and breathing system (e.g., circle system, Mapleson D system) are all that is needed. For clarity, it is easiest to classify the breathing circuits into one of two groups: those designed for rebreathing of exhaled gases (rebreathing or partial rebreathing system) and those designed to be used under circumstances of minimal to no rebreathing (non-rebreathing systems). Some have argued that this classification is somewhat of a misnomer since, depending upon the specific system used and the fresh gas flow rates used, a rebreathing system may have minimal rebreathing occurring (i.e., excessively high fresh gas flows) or a non-rebreathing system may not completely prevent rebreathing (i.e., inadequate/low fresh gas flow). To help circumvent this debate, it has been suggested that in addition to describing the design of the breathing circuit, the fresh gas flow rate should be provided to describe fully how the system is being used [70]. The fresh gas flow rate should be expressed in mL/kg/min in veterinary medicine owing to the vast range of patient sizes encountered. Additionally, the degree of rebreathing with breathing circuits can be affected by other factors such as the equipment deadspace and the patient's respiratory pattern. Breathing systems have been designed to function as rebreathing or non-rebreathing systems and should be used in the manner for which they were originally intended.

Rebreathing (circle system)

The circle system is the most commonly used rebreathing system and will be the only one described here, although other types of rebreathing systems have been used (e.g., to-and-fro). Descriptions of these rarely used systems can be found in earlier editions of this book [66]. The circle system is designed to produce a unidirectional flow of gas through the system and has a means of absorbing carbon dioxide from exhaled gases. The components of the circle system include a fresh gas inlet, inspiratory one-way valve, breathing tubes,

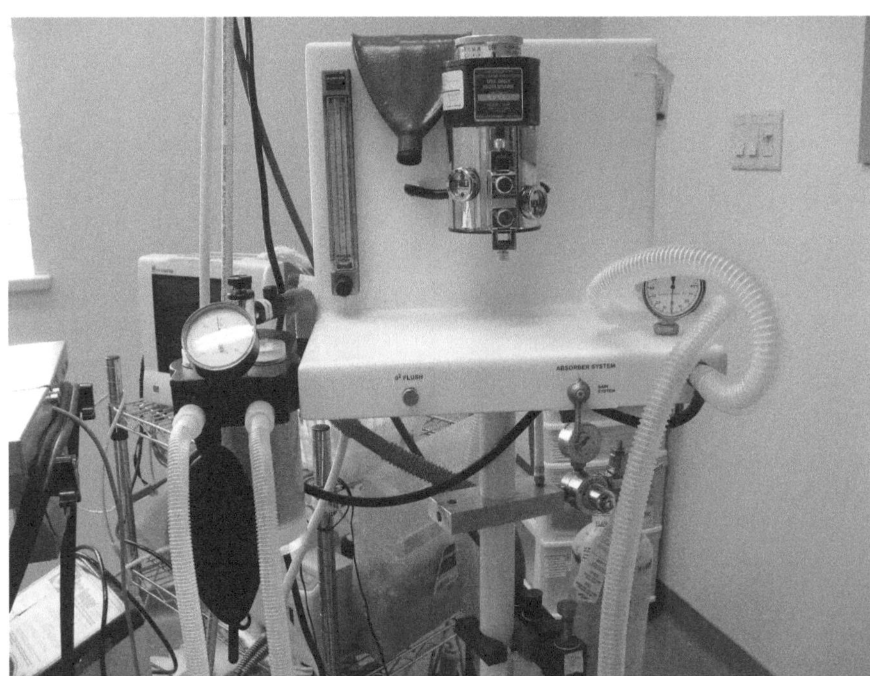

Figure 3.57 An example of an anesthetic machine mounted with both a circle (left) and Bain breathing (right) circuit. Changing gas flow to the circuits is achieved through the use of switch handle located on the lower right front of the machine. There is no obvious common gas outlet on this machine as it is integrated into the breathing circuit toggle switch. Source: Craig Mosley, Mosley Veterinary Anesthesia Services, Rockwood, ON, Canada.

expiratory one-way valve, APL valve, reservoir bag. and carbon dioxide absorber (see Fig. 3.37).

The fresh gas flows used with a circle system determine the amount of rebreathing; full rebreathing (closed), partial rebreathing (semi-closed or low flow) and minimal rebreathing. Historically, many terms have been applied to describe the amount of rebreathing, but there is no universally accepted standard or description of these terms. However, it has been suggested by several authors that the use of the terms open, semi-open and semi-closed should be dropped to avoid confusion [71].

Full (complete) rebreathing

This describes a circle system using flow rates equal to, or nearing, the metabolic oxygen consumption of the patient, between 3 and 14 mL/kg/min. This is sometimes also described as a closed system, but it may be best to avoid using such terms to avoid confusion. Note that in a 'closed system' the APL is not normally closed since that could create a potentially dangerous situation should fresh gas flow rates exceed metabolic oxygen requirements.

Partial rebreathing

This generally describes a circle system using a flow rate greater than metabolic oxygen consumption (e.g., 20 mL/kg/min) but less than that required to prevent rebreathing. Since this is a very large range, it is often divided arbitrarily into low flow (20–50 mL/kg/min), mid ('so-so') flow (50–100 mL/kg/min) and high flow (100–200 mL/kg/min), although this is not a universally accepted description.

Non- (minimal) rebreathing circle system

This describes a circle system using flow rates greater than 200 mL/kg/min (flow rates that would normally not be used in most circumstances). Such unusually high flow rates may result when circle systems are used for maintenance of anesthesia in very small patients (<5 kg) with flow rates of 1000 mL/min or greater. Frequently in veterinary medicine, it is suggested that flow rates below 1000 mL/min should not be used. Although this recommendation may be clinically useful for preventing some anesthetic delivery errors, most modern anesthetic systems (i.e., vaporizers) continue to function optimally down to flow rates of 200–500 mL/min. With the availability of low-volume, low-deadspace pediatric and neonatal circle systems coupled with improved patient monitoring (pulse oximetry and end tidal carbon dioxide), it is common to use circle systems with partial rebreathing flow rates (i.e., <1000 mL/min) in small patients (<5 kg).

It is most economical in terms of both oxygen and inhalant anesthetic use to employ low flow rates when possible. Lower flow rates are also associated with less environmental contamination by halogenated hydrocarbons (all commonly available inhaled anesthetics) and marginally improved maintenance of body temperature. However, lower flow rates are also associated with decreased anesthetic gas delivery (unless higher vaporizer settings are utilized). Additionally, when low carrier gas flows are used (relative to the volume of the circuit), the time required to change the anesthetic concentration within the circuit significantly increases.

Most inhalant anesthetics are delivered initially using relatively high fresh gas flow rates (e.g., 50–100 mL/kg/min for dogs) to facilitate rapid inspired concentration increases within the system and to replace the anesthetic vapor that is dissolving into patient tissues during the initial uptake period of inhalant anesthesia delivery. The flow rates are then decreased (e.g., to 20–50 mL/kg/min for dogs) after the initial uptake period (e.g., the first 10–20 min.) to economize on gas use and waste. The initial and maintenance recommended flow rates (mL/kg/min) often used clinically tend to be much higher in smaller patients (e.g., cats) relative to larger patients (e.g., horses). This ensures that the patient's inspired gas concentration is more reflective of the concentration of anesthetic gas delivered from the vaporizer. This is in contrast to using low fresh gas flow rates where the inspired patient anesthetic concentration will not necessarily reflect the vaporizer concentration of gas until nearing equilibration. Use of anesthetic agent analyzers to monitor inspired and expired anesthetic partial pressures greatly facilitates

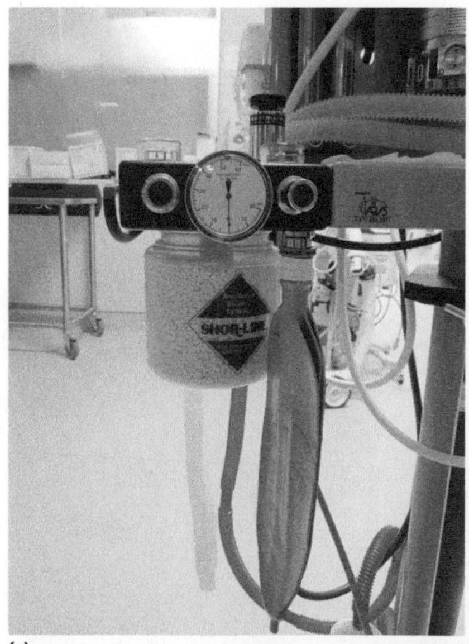

(a)

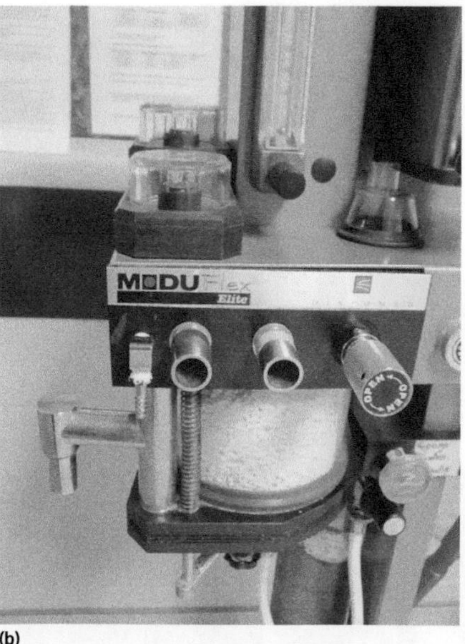

(b)

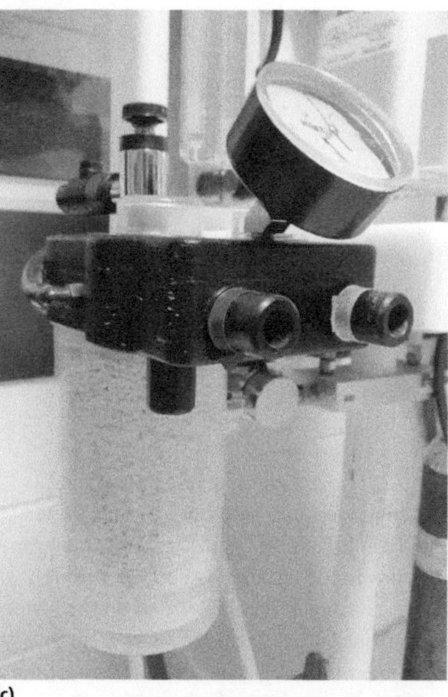
(c)

Figure 3.58 Examples of various circle rebreathing circuits used in veterinary medicine. The degree of integration into the anesthetic machine and added details vary markedly among manufacturers but the essential features and function are similar. Source: Craig Mosley, Mosley Veterinary Anesthesia Services, Rockwood, ON, Canada.

decision-making with respect to vaporizer settings and timing changes in gas flows when using lower carrier gas flows. The interaction between the vaporizer output, circuit volume, patient size, and flow rate is often an unfamiliar and difficult concept to grasp. Equating anesthetic delivery to a constant-rate infusion of an intravenous drug is perhaps a more familiar comparison for understanding inhalant anesthetic delivery.

The configuration and features of available circle systems vary somewhat depending upon the manufacturer, but in general a common pattern of gas flow is followed through the fresh gas inlet, the inspiratory one-way valve, the inspiratory and expiratory breathing tubes (into and out of patient), the expiratory one-way valve, the adjustable pressure-limiting (APL) valve, the reservoir bag, and the carbon dioxide absorbing canister back to the fresh gas inlet (Fig. 3.58). Some circle systems may also have additional incorporated features such as a switch to automatically engage the mechanical ventilator and oxygen sensor ports (Fig. 3.59).

Fresh gas inlet

The fresh gas inlet is the site of gas delivery to the circle system from the common gas outlet of the anesthetic machine. The fresh gas inlet is normally found after the carbon dioxide absorber and before the inspiratory one-way valve.

Inspiratory one-way valve

During inspiration, the inspiratory one-way valve opens, allowing gas to move from the fresh gas inlet and reservoir bag to the valve into the inspiratory limb of the breathing circuit. These valves normally consist of a clear dome (for direct visualization of valve function), a light-weight valve, and a valve housing (valve seat and valve guides). The valves are normally accessible for cleaning and repair through a removable cover. During expiration, the inspiratory valve is closed, preventing exhaled gas from entering the inspiratory limb of the breathing circuit, forcing it into the expiratory limb of the breathing circuit. At least one system (Matrx circle system, Midmark Animal Health, Versailles, OH, USA) also incorporates a negative pressure relief valve, providing an alternative path of gas flow (room air) to the patient should the inspiratory valve become stuck in the closed position (Fig. 3.60).

Breathing circuit tubing

The most basic breathing circuit is made up of a corrugated plastic or rubber inspiratory and expiratory limbs. The corrugated tubing helps prevent kinking and allows for some expansion if the breathing circuit is subjected to compression or traction. The two breathing limbs are connected via a Y-piece that connects to the endotracheal tube or facemask. There are also various coaxial designs that place the inspiratory limb within the expiratory limb of the breathing circuit. Coaxial systems reduce the bulk associated with the breathing system and (at least theoretically) facilitate warming the inspired gases by the expired gases. The Universal F-circuit (a coaxial breathing system) is designed to function with standard circle systems (e.g., 22 mm O.D. connectors of the circle system). Most breathing circuits are adapted for use with all circle systems as the fitting diameters are standardized. However, there is a proprietary coaxial circuit available that utilizes non-standard-sized circle system connectors requiring the use of a proprietary circle system (Moduflex Coaxial Breathing Circuit, Dispomed, Joliette, QC, Canada). There are also several sizes of breathing circuits available that vary in length, volume, and the amount of deadspace to meet various anesthetic requirements. Pediatric and neonatal rebreathing circuits are normally low-volume and low-deadspace systems, allowing them to function optimally in small patients (i.e., those with small tidal volumes) (Figure 3.61).

Expiratory one-way valve

The expiratory one-way valve functions together with the inspiratory one-way valve, closing upon inspiration and opening during expiration. This valve helps direct gas into the expiratory limb of the breathing system, through the expiratory valve and into the reservoir bag.

Reservoir bag

The reservoir bag is also referred to as a breathing or rebreathing bag. The purpose of the reservoir bag is to provide a compliant reservoir of gas that changes volume with the patient's expiration and inspiration. It is commonly recommended that the reservoir bag have a volume that is approximately 5–10 times the patient's normal tidal volume (10–20 mL/kg) or roughly equivalent to the patient's minute volume. Ultimately, the reservoir bag should be large enough to provide a reasonably sized reservoir of gas but not so large that it becomes difficult to observe movements of the bag associated with breathing. In addition, a very large reservoir bag will contribute to the overall functional volume of the rebreathing system (i.e., circle system), contributing to slower rates of change in anesthetic concentration within the breathing system when the

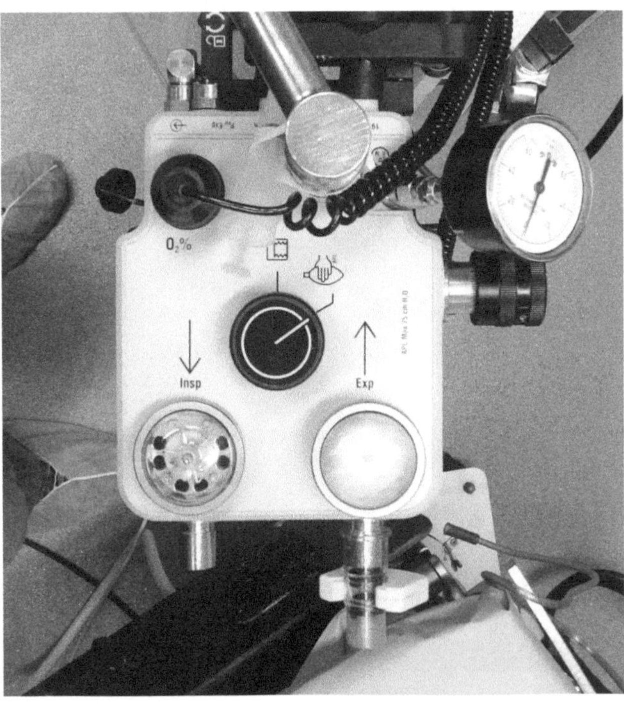

Figure 3.59 An example of a circle breathing system on an anesthetic machine with a built-in ventilator that uses a switch to engage the ventilator circuit. This can minimize the potential for misconnections, disconnections, or kinked hoses during ventilator set up. Source: Craig Mosley, Mosley Veterinary Anesthesia Services, Rockwood, ON, Canada.

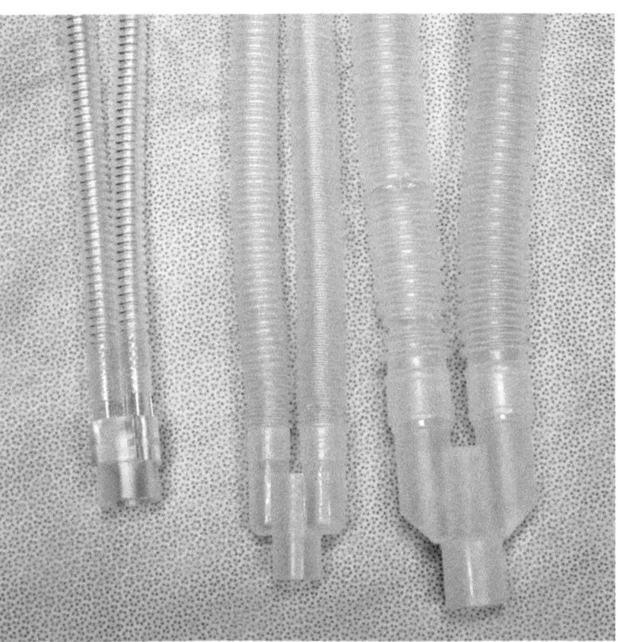

Figure 3.61 The Y-piece of three different-sized circle system circuits demonstrating the difference in deadspace. Circle system circuits are commonly available in neonatal/pediatric and adult configurations (middle and right, respectively). The system on the left is a veterinary-specific circuit designed specifically for very small patients and has minimal deadspace associated with its use. Source: Craig Mosley, Mosley Veterinary Anesthesia Services, Rockwood, ON, Canada.

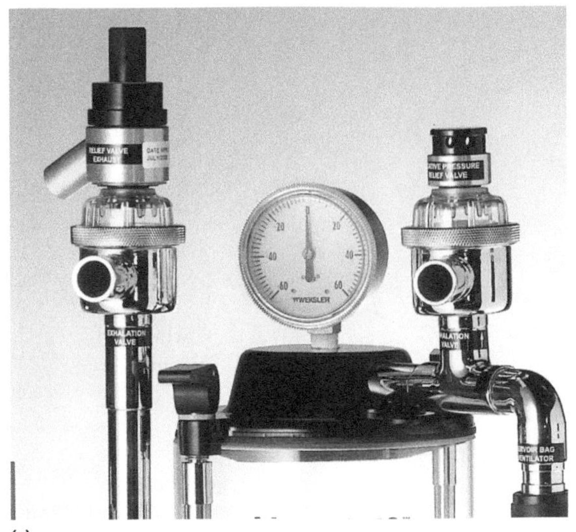

(a)

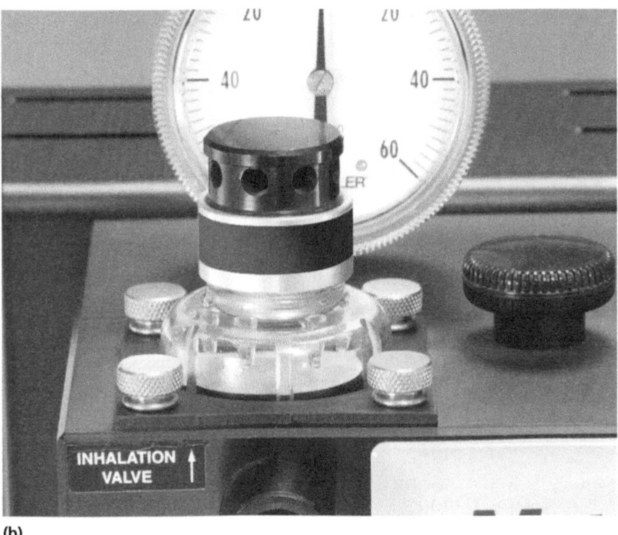

(b)

Figure 3.60 Negative pressure relief valves are incorporated into some circle systems and will be activated (allowing the patient to inhale air from the room) should the inspiratory valve become occluded or stuck.

vaporizer output is altered. This would not be the case when using a non-rebreathing system.

Adjustable pressure-limiting valve

The adjustable pressure-limiting (APL) valve is also commonly referred to as the overflow, pop-off, or pressure relief valve. The APL is a safety valve allowing excess gas to escape from the patient circuit. If the valve is functioning properly, gas should escape if system pressures exceed 1–3 cmH_2O. Normally it should be left fully open at all times unless positive pressure ventilation is being used, and then it should be immediately reopened when ventilation ceases to prevent excessive pressure from building in the patient circuit. The APL is partially closed in some instances to prevent collapse of the reservoir bag due the negative pressure/vacuum from the scavenging system. Although this can remedy the situation, it is discouraged because it can lead to closure of the valve, leading to excessive pressure building up in the patient circuit. If the reservoir bag continually collapses under normal use, this indicates the need to adjust the central vacuum/scavenge system and or the need to incorporate a properly functioning scavenging interface to offset this effect.

Several manufacturers market products that allow intermittent closure of the APL system. These devices allow temporary closure of outflow to the scavenge system when a button is depressed. These momentary closure systems are built directly into some APL valves or can be added to currently used APL valves (Fig. 3.62). These are

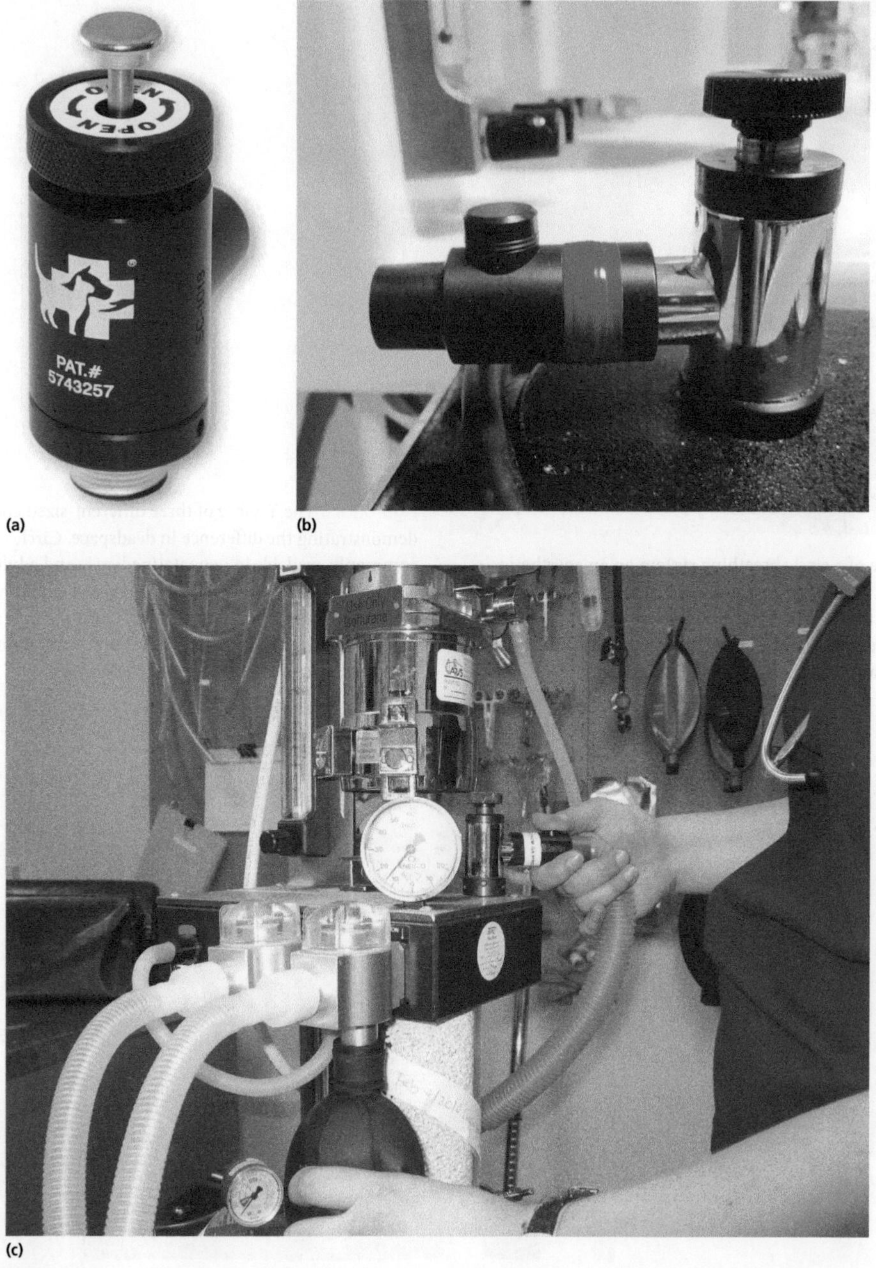

Figure 3.62 An example of a momentary closure valve built into the adjustable pressure-limiting (APL) valve (a) and a momentary closure valve that can be added to any standard APL valve (b). (c) Demonstration of the use of a momentary occlusion valve to deliver a breath to a patient. Source: part a, Supera Anesthesia Innovations, Clackamas, OR, USA. Reproduced with permission of Supera Anesthesia Innovations. Source: parts B and C, Craig Mosley, Mosley Veterinary Anesthesia Services, Rockwood, ON, Canada.

valuable additions to the APL valve system and help to prevent excessive pressure associated with an inadvertently closed APL valve that can lead to patient barotrauma or death. They also greatly facilitate the ease and safety of manual intermittent positive pressure ventilation.

Carbon dioxide absorber

The carbon dioxide absorber contains the chemical absorbent for removing carbon dioxide from exhaled gases. There are many types (dual canister, disposable, etc.) and sizes of carbon dioxide absorbers available (Fig. 3.63). All contain some type of screen to prevent absorbent granules from entering the breathing circuit and most contain a baffling system to prevent channeling of gases within the absorber canister. However, despite the screens, the absorbent granules and/or dust will occasionally enter the breathing circuit. This is probably most commonly encountered in large animal systems where relatively high peak flows of gas (associated with inspiration and expiration) are more common. Gas flow patterns within canisters vary considerably, but canister design normally attempts to ensure optimal and efficient absorbent use.

It is often suggested in veterinary medicine that the absorber canister must be twice the patient's tidal volume to ensure complete absorption of carbon dioxide, but there seems to be little evidence to support this statement. Most large animal machine canisters rarely have a volume equal to twice the patient's tidal volume and may in fact have a volume less than the patient's tidal volume. Moreover, many carbon dioxide absorbers used in human anesthetic machines have volumes less than the patient's tidal volume. Smaller canisters are often preferred to ensure more frequent changing of the absorbent, lessening the likelihood that toxic products will be produced by desiccated absorbent. However, the relative efficiency of absorption (i.e., the carbon dioxide load absorbed when an absorbent appears exhausted) may improve with larger carbon dioxide absorbers [4]. Smaller carbon dioxide absorbers will reduce the internal volume of the breathing circuit, leading to vaporizer concentration changes being reflected more rapidly in the inspired gas concentration, but will require more frequent absorbent changes.

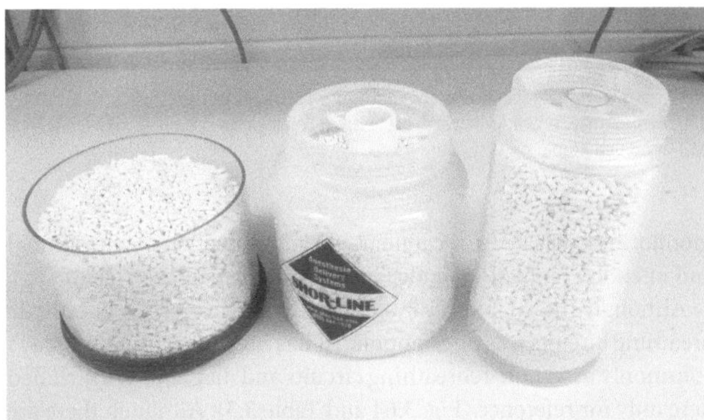

Figure 3.63 Three different absorber canisters. The canister on the far left is a bulk flow-through type canister where the exhaled gas from the patient circuit enters one side (i.e., top) of the canister and exits the other (i.e., bottom) upon inspiration. The two canisters on the right utilize a conducting tube to direct the exhaled or inhaled gases in a predictable pattern through the canister. Gas must enter and exit the canister from the same opening (i.e., the top) through different paths. Source: Craig Mosley, Mosley Veterinary Anesthesia Services, Rockwood, ON, Canada.

Carbon dioxide absorbents

The general principle of carbon dioxide absorption involves a base (absorbent) neutralizing an acid (CO_2). The end products of the reaction are water, a carbonate (e.g., calcium carbonate) and heat production. The principal component of most commonly used absorbents is calcium hydroxide [$Ca(OH)_2$]. There are currently three absorbents available in North America: soda lime, Baralyme (barium lime), and Amsorb (calcium hydroxide lime), with soda lime being the most commonly used. Soda lime is approximately 80% calcium hydroxide, 15% water, and 4% sodium hydroxide (NaOH). Baralyme is a mixture of approximately 20% barium hydroxide and 80% calcium hydroxide, and may also contain some potassium hydroxide. Amsorb, marketed as Amsorb® Plus, consists of approximately 80% calcium hydroxide, 1% calcium sulfate hemihydrate, 3% calcium chloride, and 15% water. Amsorb is the newest absorbent and is associated with minimal (if any) carbon monoxide production, minimal Compound A production and the least amount of sevoflurane degradation compared with soda lime and Baralyme [72]. The absorptive capacities of soda lime and Baralyme are approximately 25 and 27 L of carbon dioxide per 100 g, respectively, with Amsorb absorption being about 50% that of soda lime [73].

The absorption of CO_2 in soda lime occurs through a series of chemical reactions. CO_2 first combines with water to form carbonic acid, which then reacts with the hydroxides to form sodium (or potassium) carbonate, water, and heat. The calcium hydroxide then accepts the carbonate to form calcium carbonate and regenerate sodium (or potassium) hydroxide.

1 $CO_2 + H_2O \rightleftharpoons H_2CO_3$
2 $H_2CO_3 + 2NaOH\ (KOH) \rightarrow Na_2CO_3\ (K_2CO_3) + 2H_2O + \text{heat}$
3 $Na_2CO_3\ (K_2CO_3) + Ca(OH)_2 \rightarrow CaCO_3 + 2NaOH\ (KOH)$

Some CO_2 may react directly with the calcium hydroxide, but the reaction is relatively slow compared with the process utilizing sodium or potassium hydroxide.

$$H_2CO_3 + Ca(OH)_2 \rightarrow CaCO_3 + 2H_2O + \text{heat}$$

The reaction of Baralyme differs in that more water is liberated by the direct reaction of CO_2 with the barium hydroxide.

1 $Ba(OH)_2 + 8H_2O + CO_2 \rightarrow BaCO_3 + 9H_2O + \text{heat}$
2 $9H_2O + 9CO_2 \rightarrow 9H_2CO_3$

then by direct reactions (below) and by KOH and NaOH (as above)

3 $9H_2CO_3 + 9Ca(OH)_2 \rightarrow 9CaCO_3 + 18H_2O + \text{heat}$

The reaction of Amsorb is simpler, with the CO_2 reacting with water to form carbonic acid and the carbonic acid reacting directly with the calcium hydroxide to form calcium carbonate.

1 $CO_2 + H_2O \rightleftharpoons H_2CO_3$
2 $H_2CO_3 + Ca(OH)_2 \rightarrow CaCO_3 + 2H_2O + \text{heat}$

When in continuous use, the absorbents may appear exhausted (i.e., indicator color change) before the absorption capacity of the granules is exceeded. Granules normally turn from white to purple or pink as they become exhausted depending upon the indicator used. Ethyl Violet (purple) and phenolphthalein (red) are pH-sensitive indicators commonly added to the granules to help identify absorbent exhaustion. The color change should not be used as the only indicator of absorbent exhaustion. It is common for absorbent that has changed color to turn back to white if allowed to stand unused for several hours. Fresh absorbent is normally easily crumbled under pressure whereas used absorbent becomes hard (calcium carbonate). Additionally, since the reaction of carbon dioxide absorption produces heat and moisture, the activity of the absorbent may be evaluated by looking for evidence of both heat and moisture development within the canister. Also, where available, capnography can be used to detect absorbent exhaustion. The rate of absorbent exhaustion will be determined by the size of the patient (CO_2 production) and the rate of fresh gas flow (mL/kg/min). Absorbent exhaustion will occur faster in larger patients and when low fresh gas flow rates are used. The absorbent canister should be filled carefully to avoid overfilling, packing granules in the canister, and spilling granules into the breathing system.

Some degradation of inhalant anesthetics occurs with their exposure to carbon dioxide absorbents. Normally this degradation is insignificant. However, sevoflurane can decompose to a potentially nephrotoxic compound, Compound A. Factors associated with increasing production of Compound A include a high concentration of sevoflurane, low fresh gas flow rates, dry absorbent, high temperature and use of barium lime. The significance of Compound A production for human and other animal health effects has been widely debated, but its clinical significance appears to be of little concern in dogs and cats. Carbon monoxide can also be produced when desflurane, enflurane, or isoflurane is passed through dry absorbents containing a strong alkali (potassium or sodium hydroxide). Most human cases of carbon monoxide poisoning have been reported to occur during the first general anesthetic administered from a little-used anesthetic machine. In human anesthesia, it is recommended to use only non-desiccated absorbents containing no potassium hydroxide and little or no sodium hydroxide. Although carbon monoxide poisoning associated with anesthetic use in veterinary medicine seems to be a very rare occurrence (or it is simply not recognized), similar recommendations are probably applicable.

Non-rebreathing systems

Non-rebreathing systems are characterized by the absence of unidirectional valves and a carbon dioxide absorber. Rather than relying on carbon dioxide absorption for removal of CO_2, these systems depend on high fresh gas flow rates to flush CO_2 from the circuit. Non-rebreathing systems are normally not used for patients exceeding 10 kg as they become far less economical owing to the use of high fresh gas flow rates required to prevent rebreathing of CO_2. Recommended flow rates to minimize the rebreathing of expired CO_2 range from 130 to 300 mL/kg/min, although values as high as 600 mL/kg/min have been recommended. The wide range of recommended flow rates likely has something to do with fact that in addition to the fresh gas flow rate, the patient's intrinsic respiratory pattern will influence if rebreathing occurs (discussed later).

Non-rebreathing systems have historically been recommended, somewhat arbitrarily, for use in all patients less than 5 kg, citing lower resistance during breathing, less equipment deadspace, and smaller total circuit volume. However, by using newer pediatric, neonatal, and small patient-specific rebreathing circuits, many of the advantages normally associated with non-rebreathing systems are negated and it is possible to maintain patients less than 5 kg safely using rebreathing systems provided that the patient's tidal volume is adequate to actuate the unidirectional valves. Small patient-specific circuits generally have no more, and in some case less, deadspace and total volume than standard non-rebreathing systems (Fig. 3.61).

There is no minimum patient size for using a rebreathing system generally accepted among anesthesiologists. The minimum patient size generally ranges between 3 and 7 kg, although individual anesthetists may choose patient sizes outside this range depending upon monitoring available (e.g., capnography for evaluation of rebreathing) and intended ventilation mode (spontaneous versus controlled).

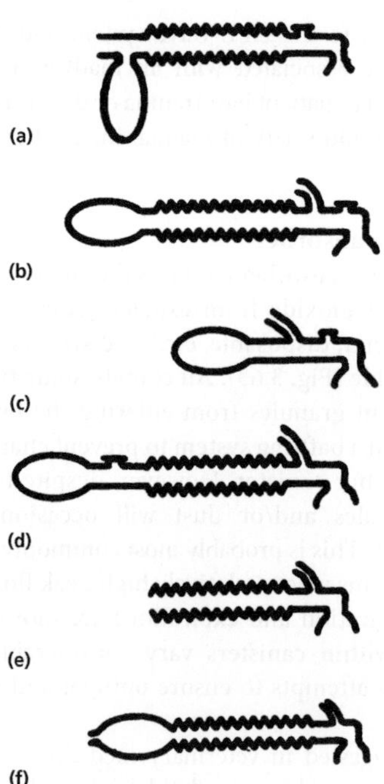

Figure 3.64 Diagrams of each of the historically described Mapleson breathing systems (a–f). Source: Rayburn RL. Pediatric anesthesia circuits. Annual Refresher Course Lecture 117, Washington, DC, 1981. Reprinted with permission of the American Society of Anesthesiologists.

Table 3.3 Characteristics of the Mapleson breathing systems.

Class	Fresh Gas Inlet	Overflow Location	Presence of a Reservoir	Corrugated Tubing	Example System
A	Near the reservoir	Near the patient	Yes	Yes	Magill
B	Near the patient	Near the patient	Yes	Yes	[a]
C	Near the patient	Near the patient	Yes	No	[a]
D	Near the patient	Away from the patient[b]	Yes	Yes	[a]
MD[c]	Near the patient	Away from the patient	Yes	Yes	Bain
E	Near the patient	Away from the patient	No	Yes	T-piece
F	Near the patient	Away from the patient[b]	Yes	Yes	Jackson-Rees

[a] No system in this classification is commonly used in veterinary anesthesia.
[b] The overflow may be located between the reservoir and the corrugated tubing of the system.
[c] MD, modified Mapleson D system.

Although the Mapleson system for classification of anesthetic breathing circuits was once popular, it has little relevance for today's commonly used non-rebreathing circuits and diagrams are included here only for reference (Fig. 3.64 and Table 3.3). Although there are often three or more non-rebreathing systems commonly described for use in veterinary medicine in North America, all are nearly functionally identical and based on two of the six historically described Mapleson systems: D and F (see Fig. 3.65).

The non-rebreathing system include a fresh gas-conducting hose, patient connection, exhalation conducting tubing (normally corrugated), excess gas venting system, and a reservoir bag. All

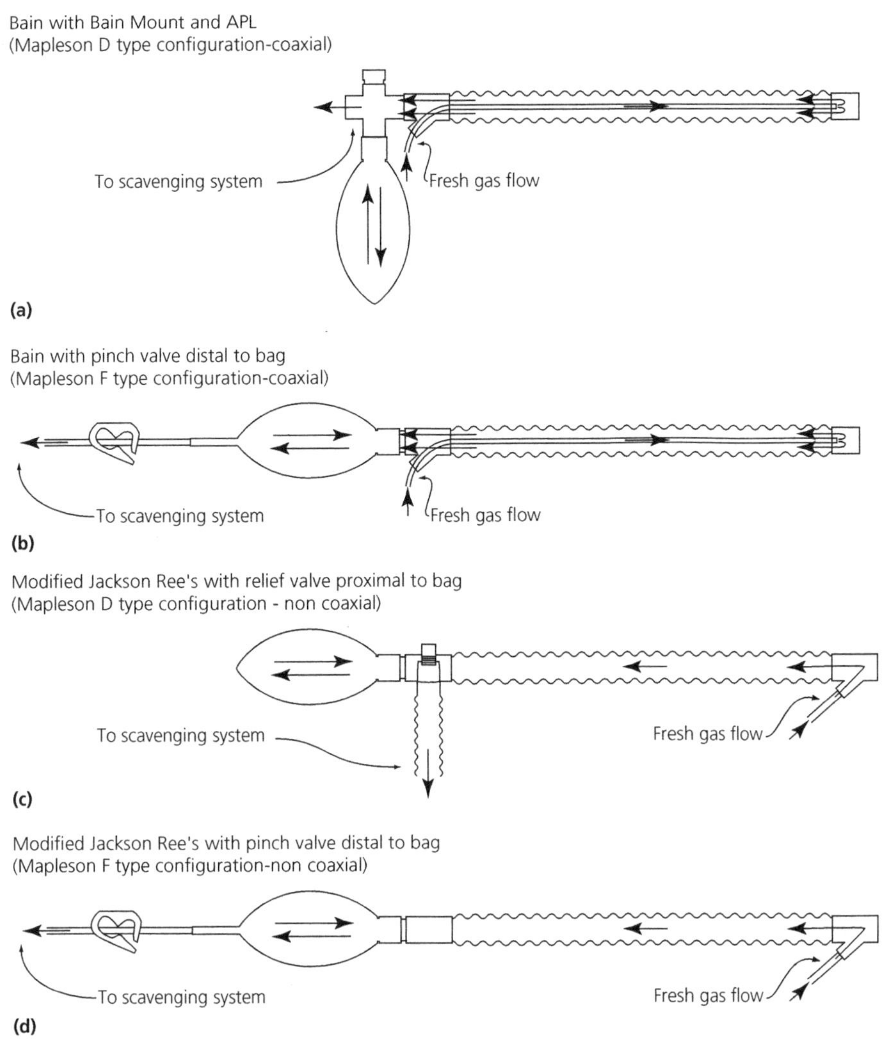

Figure 3.65 Diagrams of the Mapleson systems (D and F) used most commonly as the foundation for modern non-rebreathing systems. Most modern non-rebreathing systems are modifications of the Mapleson classification and can no longer be strictly classified as one type or the other. For example, a Bain system is a coaxial system like the Mapleson D system and can be configured with the exhaust gas exiting prior to the rebreathing bag – Mapleson D (a) – or after the rebreathing bag – Mapleson F (b). The Jackson Rees system is a non-coaxial system that can be configured similarly with the exhaust gas exiting either before – Mapleson D (c) – or after the rebreathing bag – Mapleson F (d). Source: Kath Klassen, Vancouver Animal Emergency Clinic, Vancouver, Canada. Reproduced with permission of Kath Klassen.

commonly used systems have the fresh gas flow entering near the patient connection and rely on the fresh gas inflow to displace the CO_2-containing expired breath down a variable length of conducting tubing towards the reservoir bag and ultimately into the scavenge system. High fresh gas flows are necessary to help minimize the rebreathing of expired gases.

During the expiratory pause, the high fresh gas flow from the fresh gas-conducting tube pushes the exhaled gas from the previous expiration down the exhalation conducting tube away from the patient towards the reservoir bag. When the patient inspires, it inspires gas coming from both the fresh gas-conducting tube and the exhalation conducting tube. Under normal circumstances (i.e., patient with a normal respiratory pattern and inspiratory flow rate), the majority of the inspired breath comes from the exhalation conducting tube. In some circumstance (i.e., patients with unusual respiratory patterns), a patient may rebreath exhaled gases despite seemingly sufficient fresh gas flows. For example, a patient with rapid breathing may not have an expiratory pause of sufficient duration for CO_2 to be washed distal enough from the patient end of the tube to prevent rebreathing, particularly if a sufficiently large breath is taken. End-tidal carbon dioxide monitoring can be useful in determining if adequate fresh gas flows are being used to minimize rebreathing.

The Bain and the Modified Jackson Rees systems are probably the names most commonly applied to non-rebreathing systems, but they do not adequately describe the systems as they are frequently used in veterinary medicine. Neither system is a specifically defined system in that they are not always reliably configured in the same manner. Based on the historical descriptions of these circuits the Bain circuit (based on a Mapleson D system) would have an APL valve proximal to the rebreathing bag whereas the Modified Jackson Rees (based on a Mapleson F system) would have a pinch or stopcock valve located distal to the rebreathing bag. However, both breathing systems can be adapted for use with a mounting block and various reservoir bag and venting system combinations, making strict classification

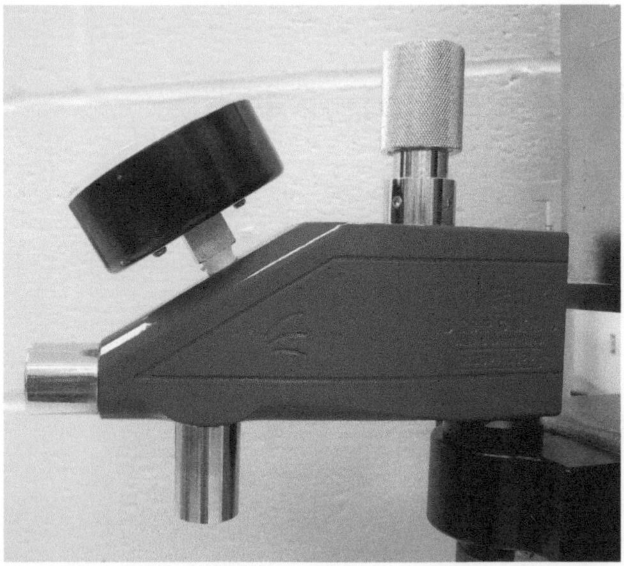

Figure 3.66 A mounting block (sometimes also referred to as a Bain mount, although they are not exclusive for use with Bain circuits only) provides fixed connection points for the non-rebreathing circuit, the reservoir bag, and scavenge tubing. Most also incorporate an adjustable pressure-limiting (APL) valve and pressure gauge. Source: Craig Mosley, Mosley Veterinary Anesthesia Services, Rockwood, ON, Canada.

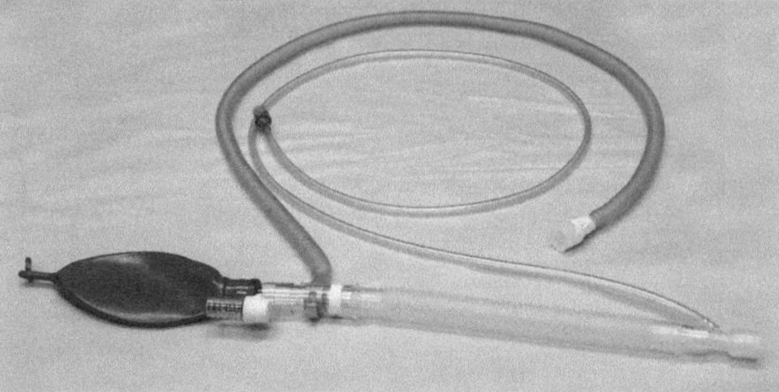

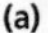

(a)

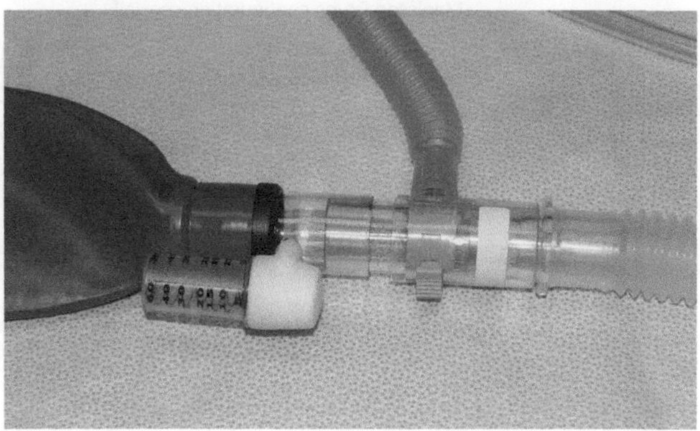

(b)

Figure 3.67 An example of a disposable resuscitation bag manometer that can be adapted for use with most non-rebreathing systems. The presence of the manometer will allow the anesthetist to evaluate better the airway pressures within the breathing system. Source: Craig Mosley, Mosley Veterinary Anesthesia Services, Rockwood, ON, Canada.

nearly impossible. Essentially the main difference between how the two systems function clinically is that one is a coaxial design (Bain) and the other is not (Modified Jackson Rees). Perhaps a less confusing and consistent way to classify the commonly used non-rebreathing circuits in veterinary medicine would be based on the configuration of the conducting tubing (i.e., coaxial or non-coaxial), location of scavenging system (i.e., proximal or distal to the reservoir bag), and method of scavenging (APL valve, pinch valve, or stopcock type valve).

The coaxial design of the Bain system reduces the overall bulk and provides a method for potentially warming the cold inspired gases. Mounting blocks are convenient methods for arranging non-rebreathing systems by providing fixed connection points for the breathing circuit, reservoir bag, and scavenge tubing (Fig. 3.66). Use of a mounting block minimizes the potential for misconnections, disconnections, or kinked hoses. The fixed positioning relative to the anesthetic machine also allows the anesthetist to assess readily the integrity of all connections.

Non-rebreathing systems used without a mounting block can be placed anywhere in the anesthetic work area and run the risk of being covered by drapes hanging off surgical tables or being pulled or caught by moving legs or equipment in the operating room, all increasing the possibility of anesthetic complications. Most mounting blocks also have a pressure manometer built into the system, which is an invaluable addition enabling the user to monitor and assess changes in airway pressure. Most non-rebreathing systems sold to veterinarians are not configured with a pressure manometer as part of the standard system, which, along with high fresh gas flows and relatively small circuit volumes, exposes patients to the potential for accidental barotrauma. One solution to overcome this problem if a mounting block with manometer is not available is to purchase disposable pressure manometers designed for use with a resuscitation bag. These can be easily placed within all non-rebreathing systems, used many times over, and are an inexpensive method of evaluating airway pressures (Fig. 3.67). Alternatively, high patient pressure alarms are available that can be inserted into the system between the patient and the valve used to isolate the system from the scavenging.

Waste gas scavenge system

The scavenge system directs waste gases from the anesthetic breathing circuit out of the immediate workspace and into the atmosphere. Ideally, the scavenging system includes the APL valve, an interface, and a waste gas elimination system (Fig. 3.68), although it is important to note that these components may not be found as part of all scavenge systems. Many systems in use consist of a hose connected to the APL (or other breathing circuit outlet) to a vent leading outside the immediate work area. The waste gas elimination system may be either an active or a passive system. A passive system does not use negative pressure (e.g., it opens to atmospheric pressure) whereas an active system uses a slight vacuum. The type of waste gas elimination system will determine the need and type of waste gas interface required. Passive waste gas systems may use an activated charcoal canister to inactivate halogenated anesthetics or they may divert the waste anesthetic gases through a short conduit outside the work environment directly to the atmosphere.

Negative pressure scavenge (vacuum) systems are increasingly being used in veterinary medicine. They may be part of a surgical vacuum (suction) system, stand-alone vacuum, fan/blower system, or other design since there are no specific standards regarding

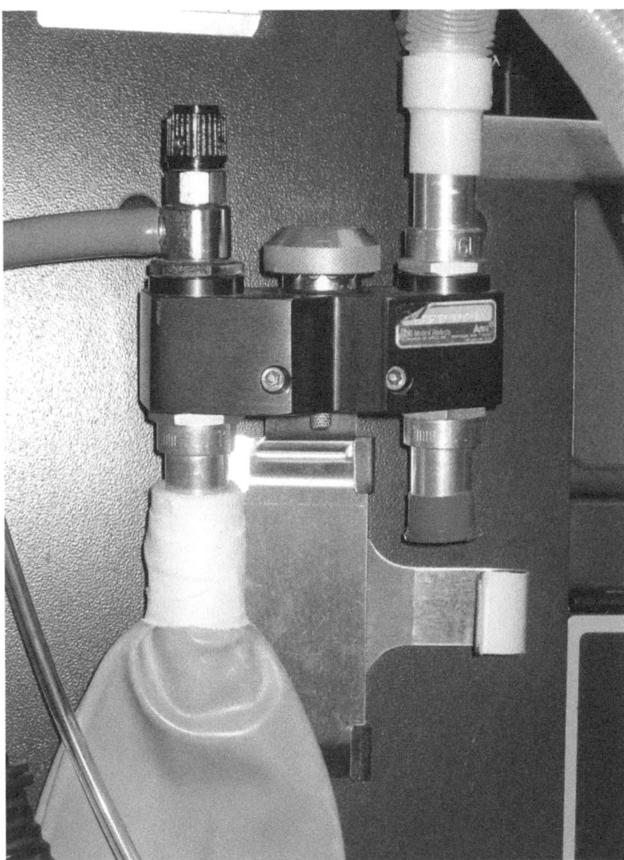

Figure 3.68 An adjustable scavenge interface with both positive and negative pressure relief functions. These types of interfaces work well with active scavenging systems. Source: Craig Mosley, Mosley Veterinary Anesthesia Services, Rockwood, ON, Canada.

these systems. All negative pressure scavenge systems require some type of scavenge interface to operate properly and prevent the patient airway from experiencing a vacuum. Ideally, waste gas scavenge interfaces should have means of managing both excessive positive and negative pressure, a reservoir system to accommodate changes in waste gas delivery to the scavenge system, and a means of inactivating any halogenated gas that escapes the scavenging system (Fig. 3.69). Most scavenge interfaces fail to meet all these specifications under all the variable circumstances encountered during use (e.g., high negative pressure scavenge systems, pressure alterations within the vacuum system, marked alterations in the rate of waste gases exhausted to the scavenge system), but most perform adequately under normal operating conditions.

Low negative pressure scavenging systems (blower or fan systems) work well with most scavenge interfaces. These systems are often dedicated for waste gas scavenge and may be centrally located or located at the machine itself. These are often blower- or fan-driven systems that do not maintain a steady evacuation rate (negative pressure) at all times and in all locations. Several factors, such as the number of sites they serve, distance from the blower or fan, and the number of sites being used, can affect evacuation rates at any given location. Higher negative pressure scavenge systems are most commonly found in larger facilities with centrally located medical vacuum systems and the active scavenge system works off the same negative pressure system as used for medical suction. Although it is often seen as more convenient and cost-effective to use the same vacuum system for all functions in the hospital, there are some unique challenges associated with this type of installation. Since these systems are under a significant amount of negative pressure relative to that needed for scavenging, they require adjustable scavenge interfaces to regulate the level of suction at the scavenge interface and frequent minor adjustments to prevent collapse of the reservoir bag of the breathing system. Regardless of the type of scavenging system used, canisters of activated charcoal should be available for situations where other modes of waste anesthetic gas scavenge are not available (e.g., when moving patients attached to the anesthetic machine, or when working in areas without scavenging facilities).

Routine anesthesia machine checkout procedure

Routine evaluation of the anesthetic machine and associated systems prior to and throughout the anesthetic period should be part of every anesthetist's standard operating procedures (SOP). Historically, equipment failures appear to have been a relatively common cause of anesthetic-related morbidity and mortality [2]. However, with improvements in technology and monitoring and the adoption of universal safety standards for human anesthetic equipment, complications related to equipment malfunctions have been reduced. Preanesthetic equipment checkout recommendations for human anesthetic equipment have been developed in conjunction with regulatory, industry and anesthesia personnel and published in many countries. Unfortunately, there is no generally recognized standard for preanesthetic checkout recommendations in veterinary medicine. However, an excellent checklist for veterinary anesthetists developed by Hartsfield has been proposed that is based on the US Food and Drug Administration's Center for Devices and Radiological Health 'Anesthesia Apparatus Checkout Recommendations' [66,74]. Table 3.4 presents a modified summary of the checklist proposed by Hartsfield.

Anesthesia ventilators

The anesthesia ventilator is designed to provide patient ventilation in the perianesthetic period. Most anesthesia ventilators lack the sophistication of control and function found in intensive care unit (ICU) ventilators and work best when used to ventilate patients with relatively normal lung function and simple ventilation needs. However, some human- and veterinary-specific anesthesia ventilators now offer features and performance rivaling those of a basic ICU ventilator. In North America, anesthesia ventilators designed for use in humans are subject to a series of international and national standards, whereas ventilators designed for the veterinary market are under no obligations to meet any similar design standards. Once again this makes it imperative that the veterinary anesthetist not only fully understands the physiological and practical implications of ventilator use but is also intimately familiar with the design, function, and troubleshooting of any ventilator used.

Classification

Ventilators are variably classified by a number of different criteria describing their design and control. Unfortunately, there are several inconsistencies in the use of the terminology and their definitions. There is also no generally accepted consensus as to how to classify anesthesia ventilators and some ventilators simply cannot be adequately described using current classification schemes. For example, some modern human anesthesia ventilators are sophisticated processor-controlled machines capable of multiple ventilation modes and deliver similar performance to ICU ventilators, hence

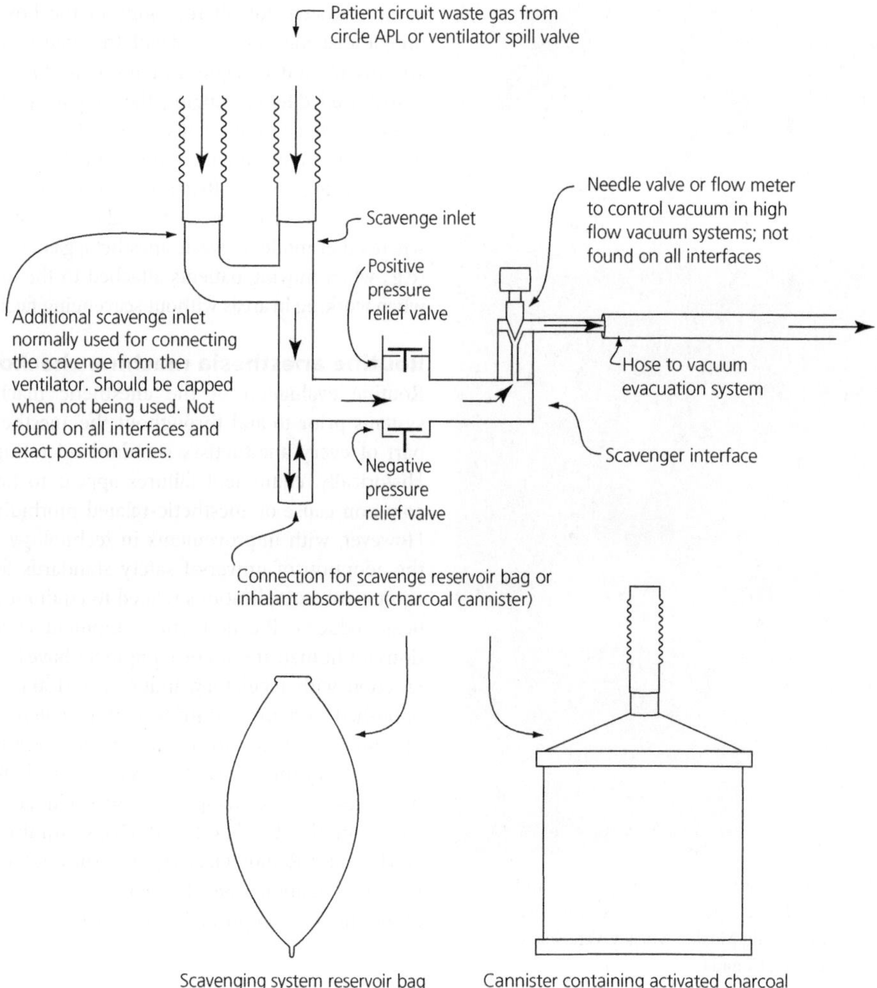

Figure 3.69 Diagram of a scavenge interface. The exact configurations of commercially available scavenge interfaces vary considerably and may not contain all the components shown. Source: Kath Klassen, Vancouver Animal Emergency Clinic, Vancouver, Canada. Reproduced with permission of Kath Klassen.

they are not easily classified using current criteria. The most commonly used criteria used to describe or classify ventilators include the major control variable, the type of power source, the drive mechanism, the cycling mechanism, and the type of bellows.

Major control variable

Most ventilators are described as pressure- or volume-controlled ventilators. This refers to the target, preset, or limiting variable used to determine the tidal volume delivered by the ventilator. In a volume-limited ventilator, the tidal volume is predetermined and will be delivered regardless of the associated pressures required to do so. This is not a precisely accurate statement as many ventilators (anesthetic machines/circuits) have built-in pressure relief or alarm systems that will activate and limit the volume delivered if excessively high airway pressures are reached. Additionally, changes in circuit and patient compliance will alter the actual tidal volume delivered to the patient compared with the apparent tidal volume set on the ventilator (see the later section Factors That Affect Delivered Tidal Volume). This effect is normally negligible as sustained significant changes in system or patient respiratory compliance are unlikely during a routine case. With a pressure-limited ventilator, a peak inspiratory pressure preset is used to limit the tidal volume delivered to the patient. The delivered volume can be affected by changes in patient respiratory or circuit compliance/resistance, inspiratory flow rates, leaks, inspiratory time, and the location of the pressure sensor.

Power source

The power source typically refers to what is required to operate a mechanical ventilator. It may be compressed gas, electricity, or both. Although not generally accepted, it may be more useful to classify ventilators based on what actually powers positive pressure ventilation: compressed gas or an electronically controlled piston. Although historically many ventilators did not contain sophisticated microprocessors requiring electricity and required only compressed gas to function, most modern ventilators have some electrical components regardless of what actually produces positive pressure ventilation. The drive mechanism normally refers more specifically to how positive pressure ventilation is actually produced.

Drive mechanism/circuit

Either compressed gas or an electronically driven mechanical device, such as a piston, can drive ventilators. Ventilators using compressed gas for power are normally referred to as dual-circuit ventilators as they have two gas circuits, one containing gas to power the ventilator and the other containing gas being delivered to the patient. Ventilators that do not use gas to power ventilation are referred to as single-circuit ventilators. However, there is at least

Table 3.4 Ensuring that all equipment is properly functioning is a crucial step that should be performed prior to initiating anesthesia. The proposed equipment checkout recommendations are based on the Food and Drug Administration's Center for Devices and Radiological Health "Anesthesia Apparatus Checkout Recommendations."

Veterinary Anesthesia Apparatus Checkout Recommendations*

This anesthesia checkout list does not replace the experience of a knowledgeable operator continuously monitoring the anesthetic equipment. All parts of the anesthesia machine and breathing system should be present, properly functioning, free of defects, and correctly connected. This checklist includes the assessment of automated ventilators and patient monitors if they are present.

High pressure system

Central gas supplies (oxygen, nitrous oxide, air) should be adequate in quantity and pressure. The central pipeline pressure should not fluctuate and should remain at its preset level (normally about 50 psi) when flowmeters on the anesthesia machine are adjusted to a 3–5 L/min flow rate.

Portable gas supplies (oxygen cylinders on the anesthesia machine) should be adequate in quantity and pressure. These cylinders should be evaluated for leaks. With the flowmeter off and the cylinder valve open, there should be no audible leaks or decrease in cylinder pressure over time (i.e., 10 min).

Low pressure system

Test the flowmeters of each gas. With the flow control off the float should rest on the bottom of the glass tube. Adjust the flowmeter throughout its full range, the float should move smoothly with no sticking or erratic movements.

Vaporizers should be filled, filler caps tightened and the control dial in the off position. The inlet and outlet connections should be in place and secure.

Leak test the low pressure system.

a. Attach a "suction bulb" to the common gas outlet.
b. Squeeze the bulb until fully collapsed.
c. Verify the bulb stays fully collapsed for at least 10 seconds.
d. Open each vaporizer one at a time, if more than two vaporizers, and repeat steps (b) and (c) with each vaporizer.

Scavenging system

Ensure proper connection between the scavenging system and the APL valve.

Adjust the waste gas vacuum flow, if possible, to meet the needs of the individual case.

With the APL fully open and the wye piece occluded.

a. Allow the scavenge reservoir back to fully collapse and verify that the circuit pressure gauge reads about zero.
b. With the oxygen flush valve activated, allow the scavenge reservoir bag to distend fully and then verify that the circuit pressure gauge reads less than 10 cmH_2O.

If the scavenging system involves a charcoal canister, the quality of the charcoal absorbent should be ensured.

Breathing system

Rebreathing (circle) system

Ensure the selected circuit and reservoir bag size are appropriate for the patient.

Check the breathing system is complete, undamaged, and unobstructed.

Verify that the carbon dioxide absorbent is adequate.

Perform a leak test of the breathing system.

a. Set all gas flows to zero (or minimum).
b. Close the APL valve and occlude the wye piece.
c. Pressurize the breathing system using the flush valve to a pressure of about 30 cmH_2O.
d. Ensure the pressure remains fixed for at least 10 seconds. Alternatively, the leak rate required to maintain at 30 cmH_2O should be less than 300 mL/min.
e. Open the APL and ensure the pressure decreases appropriately.

Non-rebreathing system

Ensure the selected circuit and reservoir bag size are appropriate for the patient.

Check the breathing system is complete, undamaged, and unobstructed.

Perform a leak test of the breathing system.

a. Set all gas flows to zero (or minimum).
b. Close the APL valve and occlude the patient port.
c. Pressurize the breathing system using the flush valve to a pressure of about 30 cmH_2O. If there is no pressure gauge associated with the breathing system the reservoir bag should remain fully distended with no loss of pressure.
d. For Bain systems (coaxial Mapleson D) the integrity of the inner tube should be evaluated. With the flowmeter set to 1 L/min, the inner tube should be briefly occluded and the float of the flowmeter should fall to near zero.
e. Open the APL and ensure the pressure decreases appropriately.

Ventilator

Place a second reservoir bag on the patient circuit, appropriate for the size of the patient.

Set the appropriate ventilator parameters for the patient.

Connect the ventilator as directed by the manufacturer and fill the bellows and reservoir bag using the flush valve.

Turn the ventilator on and ensure adequate tidal volumes are delivered and that during expiration the bellows fill completely.

Check for the proper action of the unidirectional valves of the circle, if applicable.

Manipulate ventilation parameters to ensure all are functioning normally.

Turn off the ventilator and disconnect as directed by the manufacturer.

Monitors

Ensure all cables and connectors are present.

Ensure all alarms are appropriately set.

*Owing to the significant variability and lack of standards among veterinary anesthesia equipment not all checkout procedures will apply to all anesthetic machines.

one commercially available ventilator design that uses compressed gas as its power source but contains neither a bellows nor a piston and is technically a single-circuit ventilator, the Penlon Nuffield 200 (Penlon Ltd, Abingdon, UK). However, this ventilator can also be combined with a bellows canister system (bag in a box), creating a dual-circuit ventilator. The lack of physical barrier in this design can potentially allow mixing of gas from the circuit used to power the ventilator with gas from the patient circuit. However, the clinical significance of mixing is minimal provided that fresh gas flow rates are suitable to ensure non-rebreathing. Any mixing between ventilator driving gas and patient circuit gas should only involve the exhaled patient gas being moved through the breathing circuit destined for evacuation and collection into the scavenging system.

Cycling mechanism

The cycling mechanism is a term that is used to describe how a ventilator cycles from inspiration to expiration and back. It is probably also the term used most inconsistently. The cycling in most ventilators is determined by a timing mechanism, although in at least one commonly used ventilator (Bird Mark series ventilators), pressure rather than time can be used to cycle the ventilator. An electronic microprocessor or a fluid logic unit can control the timing mechanism. Electronic timing mechanisms dominate current ventilators, although some fluid logic control systems are still produced. Before the advent of readily available microprocessors and electronics, fluid logic control was popular and can be found on many older ventilators still in use today (e.g. Air-Shields, Ohio V5A, and Metomatic). Electronic microprocessor units essentially open and close valves allowing gas to drive the ventilator or, in the case of a piston design, they activate movement of the piston. Fluid logic units work through use of compressed gas, normally at a constant pressure, to activate timing valves for inspiration and expiration. The amount of gas needed to activate these timing valves and hence inspiratory and expiratory times can be altered by increasing or decreasing the flow of gas into the timing valve, producing shorter or longer activation times. Ultimately, these valves are opened and closed by changes in gas pressure within the timing valves and it is likely this fact that has led to some confusion and misuse of terminology. Although pressure changes are used to activate the inspiratory and expiratory timers, these ventilators are strictly still time cycled with pressure being used to produce predictable fluid timers. The term pressure-cycled ventilators should be reserved for those ventilators where pressure within the patient circuit is responsible for cycling the ventilator. The Bird Mark series of ventilators can be pressure cycled. The timing for inspiration in these ventilators is a function of the duration of time required to attain a specific pressure within the patient circuit during positive pressure ventilation. The cycling duration can be modified by gas flow rates driving the ventilator and changes in patient lung compliance. When using these ventilators, the inspiration will continue until a specific pressure threshold is achieved regardless of the time required to achieve the pressure. The term volume cycled has been applied to anesthesia ventilators; however, timing mechanisms are generally the foundation of these ventilators and the term volume cycled should be reserved for describing a specific mode of ventilation normally possible only using an ICU-type ventilator and some advanced anesthesia ventilators equipped with spirometry and microprocessors capable of compensating for tidal volume changes caused by changes in lung and circuit compliance. The use of the terms pressure and volume cycled should not be confused with the terms pressure and volume limited, which are used to describe the principle factors that limit the tidal volume delivered to a patient. In essence, all time-cycled ventilators are volume limited and only pressure-cycled ventilators are pressure limited.

Bellows

If a ventilator has a bellows, they can be classified as ascending or descending. This terminology refers to the direction of the bellows during expiration and often creates confusion. The terms 'standing' and 'hanging' are perhaps more intuitive and are used to describe the ascending and descending bellows configuration, respectively. This then refers to the position of the bellows during the expiratory pause or prior to the initiation of ventilation.

Introduction to single- and dual-circuit ventilators

Most anesthesia ventilators used in veterinary medicine are electronically time-cycled ventilators and can be classified as either a dual-circuit gas-driven ventilator or single-circuit piston-driven ventilator. However, there are at least two compressed gas-powered ventilators that can be used as both dual- and single-circuit ventilators, depending upon how they are configured. They will be discussed separately later (see Single-Circuit Compressed Gas-Powered Ventilators). It is important to note that the use of the term single-circuit ventilator by itself can be misleading. Historically, it has been used to describe ventilators using two gases (ventilator driving gas and patient circuit gas) that operate within a single circuit (i.e., there is no physical barrier between the gases). In this situation, there is the possibility of ventilator driving gas mixing with gas in the patient circuit. It is therefore more descriptive to include the terms 'piston-driven' or 'compressed gas-driven' when using the term 'single-circuit' to describe veterinary ventilators.

The anesthesia ventilator normally replaces the reservoir bag and APL valve of the anesthesia machine with a bellows (or piston chamber) and spill valve (i.e., dump or relief valve), respectively, but even here there are exceptions in ventilator design and use. One manufacturer's design does not replace the reservoir bag and APL valve of the anesthetic machine but instead it is simply added to the patient circuit (Merlin, Vetronic Services, Abbotskerswell, Devon, UK).

Single-circuit piston-driven ventilators

Piston-driven ventilators use electronically controlled pistons to compress gas in the breathing circuit. The use of an electronically controlled piston eliminates the need for a second circuit (i.e., the driving gas), and this typically enables the ventilator to deliver tidal volumes more precisely since it will not be influenced by the presence of a compressible driving gas. Piston-driven ventilators are also more efficient in terms of gas use since additional gas is not required to drive the ventilator and they are normally controlled by sophisticated electronics that can provide more advanced modes of ventilation and cycling options. Electrical power is used to raise and lower the piston using a servomotor and ball screw assembly (linear actuator). Piston-driven ventilators can offer the user a very wide range of sophisticated ventilation options typically unavailable using common dual-circuit ventilators.

Each piston-driven ventilator is unique in its specific design but most will share some of the following features: a cylinder, piston, linear actuator, rolling diaphragms, and positive/negative pressure relief valves. The exact configuration of each component and mechanism for facilitating expiration and spontaneous breathing will vary among manufacturers. The Tafonius large animal anesthetic workstation ventilator (Hallowell EMC, Pittsfield, MA, USA) is a veterinary-specific piston-driven ventilator and will be used as an example for describing the operation of a piston-driven anesthetic ventilator. Descriptions of other piston-driven ventilators designed for human use such as the Dräger Apollo, Divan, or Fabius GS ventilator are available elsewhere [75].

There are two rolling diaphragms that seal the piston of the Tafonius ventilator to prevent mixing of ambient and patient circuit gas (Fig. 3.70). The lower diaphragm seals the breathing gas below the piston in the breathing system. The upper diaphragm seals the upper side of the lower diaphragm from ambient air, creating a space between the two diaphragms. A vacuum is applied to this space that holds the two diaphragms tightly against the piston and cylinder walls. As the piston is actuated it moves downward and the space below the lower diaphragm decreases, forcing gas into the patient's lungs; at the end of inspiration the patient exhales and the piston rises. During controlled ventilation, the piston drives the inspiration according to the ventilator settings. When the patient expires, the piston moves in response to the measured airway pressure, measured at the patient Y-piece. When the airway pressure increases by 0.5 cmH_2O the piston is moved up enough to bring the airway pressure back to zero. This correction is made every 5 ms (200 times per second). This ensures that unless

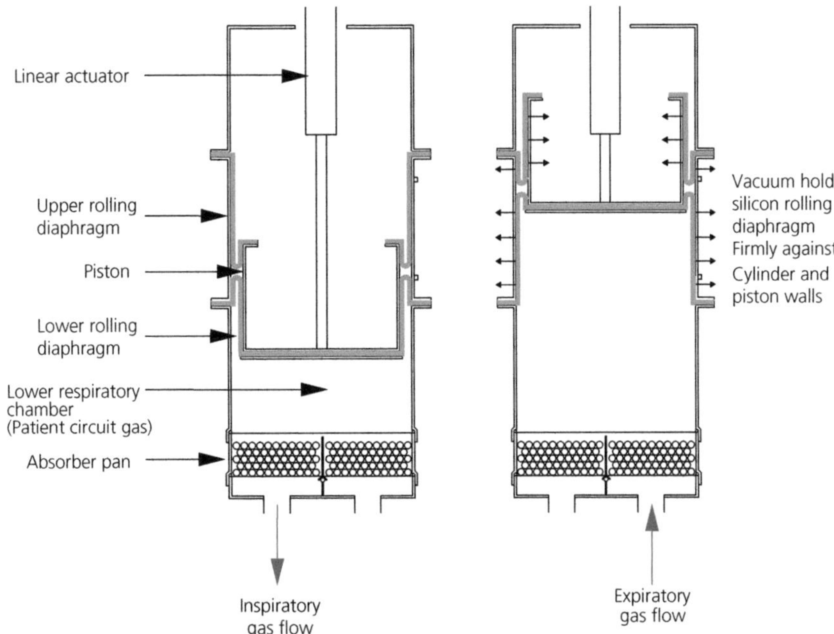

Figure 3.70 Configuration of a piston-driven ventilator (Tafonius rolling diaphragm system) during inspiration (left) and expiration (right), demonstrating various features and general principles of operation. Source: Hallowell EMC, Pittsfield, MA, USA. Modified diagram reproduced with permission of Hallowell EMC.

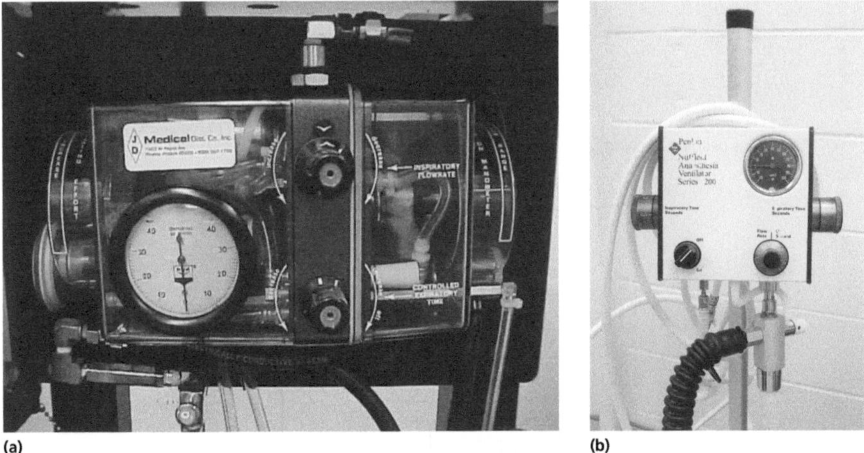

Figure 3.71 The Bird respirator (a) and Penlon Nuffield 200 ventilator (b) are examples of compressed gas powered ventilators. They can be used as single and dual circuit ventilators although the latter configuration is by far the most commonly used and most intuitive configuration. The patient valve, located on the bottom of the Penlon Nuffield ventilator, acts as a connection point for the ventilator drive gas controlled by the control unit, the conducting hose to the patient circuit (black corrugated tube) and the spill valve to the scavenge. Drive gas is delivered to this valve during inspiration pushing gas towards the patient. During expiration the valve opens allowing excess gas to spill into the scavenge system. Source: Craig Mosley, Mosley Veterinary Anesthesia Services, Rockwood, ON, Canada.

desired there is no resistance to exhalation (i.e., positive end expiratory pressure or PEEP).

Most standard standing bellows will have mandatory PEEP (2–4 cmH_2O) due to the design of the ventilator spill valve that is required to compensate for the weight of the bellows. During spontaneous breathing, the piston moves both upwards (expiration) and downwards (inspiration) in response to changes in measured airway pressure, ensuring that the airway pressure is maintained near zero. Expiration will occur as noted above, while conversely during inspiration when the airway pressure decreases by 0.5 cmH_2O the piston will move down enough to bring the airway pressure back to zero. Electronic positive and negative relief valves are located at the scavenging manifold to protect against excessive positive or negative pressure within the patient circuit.

Single-circuit compressed gas-powered ventilators

There are at least two compressed gas-powered ventilators available in veterinary anesthesia that can be configured as single-circuit ventilators: Bird Mark series ventilators and Penlon Nuffield 200 ventilators (Fig. 3.71). When used as a single-circuit ventilator there is no physical barrier between the gas that drives ventilation and the gas in the patient circuit. However, these ventilators do have two separate gas 'circuits,' the ventilator driving gas and the patient circuit gas, hence the use of the term 'single-circuit' is slightly misleading. The patient gas and the ventilator driving gas simply move within (or share) the same continuous circuit, with no physical barrier between the ventilator drive gas and the patient gas. Hence they operate within a single physically uninterrupted gas circuit. It is important to note that the Bird Mark respirators and Penlon Nuffield 200 are commonly used as dual-circuit ventilators by combining them with bellows in a canister ('bag in a box'), as described later. A gas-powered single-circuit ventilator should only be used with non-rebreathing flow rates (non-rebreathing breathing circuits – Mapleson D or F) to prevent contamination of the patient circuit with ventilator drive gas. As non-rebreathing flow rates are required, these types of ventilator configurations are best suited for use in smaller patients, although it is possible to ventilate larger patients requiring tidal volumes of approximately 1000 mL, but the efficiency of gas (oxygen and inhalant) consumption required is markedly reduced.

The Penlon Nuffield 200 ventilator is marketed and described as a single-circuit ventilator (see Fig. 3.71b). The ventilator is connected to the bag mount of the circuit by a long corrugated tube that acts as a 'reservoir,' replacing the reservoir bag. The ventilator drive gas moves 'to and from' the patient through this tube. The patient's exhaled gases will also move through this tube and will be scavenged from a so-called 'patient' valve. The patient valve acts as a spill valve, allowing all excess gas – the drive gas from the ventilator, exhaled gas from the patient, and any excess fresh gas flow – to leave the system. The ventilator drive gas and the patient gas move within the same circuit without any physical separation, hence the term 'single-circuit.' During inspiration, the patient valve closes, forcing the ventilator driving gas into the 'reservoir' tube, compressing the circuit gas back towards the patient, leading to inspiration. During the expiratory pause, the patient valve opens, allowing the ventilator driving gas to exit the system immediately as the pressure within the circuit drops back to zero. This gas is followed by the exhaled gas of the patient being pushed away from the patient as a result of the non-rebreathing fresh gas flow being delivered to the patient circuit. The fresh gas flow rate must be sufficiently high to prevent rebreathing of expired gases (i.e., a volume of fresh gas greater than or matching the patient's tidal volume must be delivered to the circuit during each respiratory cycle in order to minimize rebreathing of CO_2). The tidal volume is created by the combined effect of the volume of drive gas delivered by the ventilator and the volume of fresh gas flow entering the circuit during inspiration.

Dual-circuit ventilators

Dual-circuit ventilators have a physical separation between the ventilator driving gas and the patient circuit gas. Dual-circuit ventilators are comprised of the bellows assembly and the control mechanism for the drive gas. The control mechanism is normally

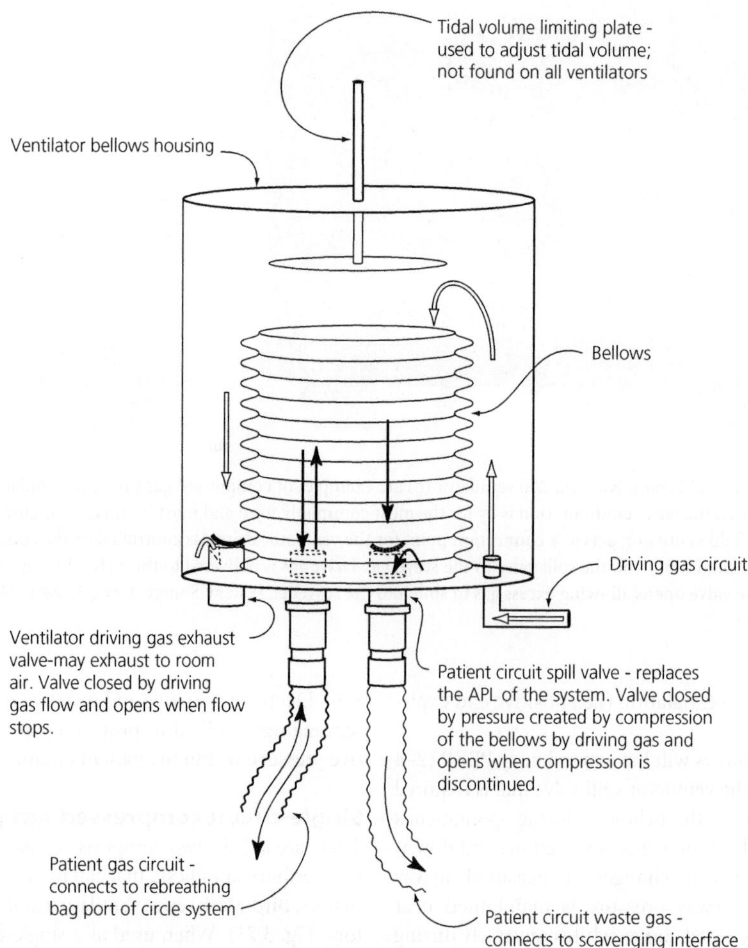

Figure 3.72 Schematic diagram of a generic dual-circuit ventilator demonstrating the gas flows within the ventilator during inspiration and expiration. Note that the exact position and design of the various components vary among manufacturers. Source: Kath Klassen, Vancouver Animal Emergency Clinic, Vancouver, Canada. Reproduced with permission of Kath Klassen.

an electronic microprocessor in most modern ventilators, but some older ventilators used fluid logic units to control the drive gas. The bellows assembly replaces the reservoir bag and APL valve and is comprised of the following components: bellows, housing, housing exhaust valve, spill valve, and ventilator hose connection (Fig. 3.72).

The primary circuit is continuous with the patient circuit and consists of the bellows and the spill valve. The second circuit contains the driving gas used to compress the bellows. The breathing circuit and the driving gas circuit are not connected; the bellows acts as a compliant barrier between these two circuits. Drive gas is allowed into the bellows housing for a specific period of time and delivered at a specified rate; during this time, the housing exhaust valve is closed, causing compression of the bellows and closing the spill valve. This forces gas inside the bellows to move towards the patient's lungs, expanding the chest. During expiration, the driving gas is discontinued (the housing pressure and consequently the patient circuit pressure drop) and the gas in the bellows housing is allowed to escape from an exhaust valve, allowing the patient to exhale passively into the bellows. The spill valve reopens, allowing excess fresh gas flow from the patient circuit to escape, preventing pressure from building up within the patient circuit. Although there are specific design differences in the way these functions are accomplished among dual-circuit ventilators, the general principles are similar.

Bellows (configuration)

The bellows is an accordion-like device attached to either the top or bottom of the bellows assembly. Anesthesia ventilators can be configured with ascending (standing) or descending (hanging) bellows (Fig. 3.73). The terms ascending and descending refer to the direction in which the bellows moves during exhalation and have been used historically to describe the orientation of the bellows. However, it is becoming increasingly common to replace these terms with standing (ascending) or hanging (descending) to describe the position of the bellows during the expiratory pause; this is often considered a more intuitive description of the configuration of the bellows. The majority of modern ventilators use a standing (ascending) bellows configuration where the bellows moves towards the base of the ventilator during inspiration and upon exhalation they expand upwards. The tidal volume may be set by adjusting the inspiratory time and/or flow rate, or by a plate or other limiting device that limits the excursion of the bellows (see Fig. 3.72).

The spill valves on ventilators with standing bellows normally pose slight resistance (2–4 cmH_2O) to opening, thus creating slight PEEP in the system. This is to counteract the tendency of the bellows to collapse due to their weight and elastic nature. In the case of very large and heavy bellows, this may have the effect of producing a clinically relevant amount of PEEP. In some cases this may be considered desirable, but at least one manufacturer has developed a method to overcome this PEEP effect by providing the option of applying a slight vacuum to the interior of the bellows housing. A desirable feature of the standing bellows configuration is that should a leak occur in the breathing system, the bellows will fail to expand fully and progressively collapse during the expiratory pause. A leak can be readily detected by an observant anesthetist.

The hanging (descending) bellows is attached to the top of the ventilator assembly and is compressed upwards during inspiration. During exhalation, the bellows descends passively, facilitated by a

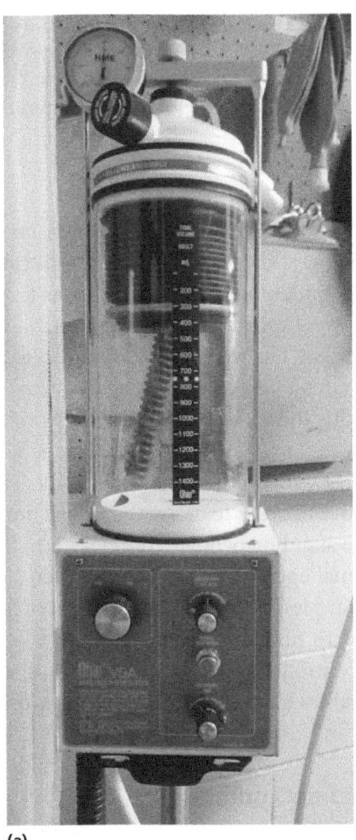
(a)

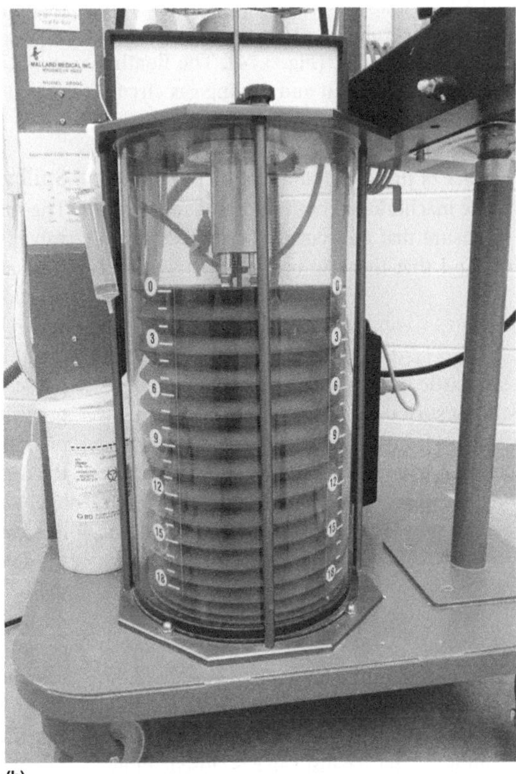
(b)

Figure 3.73 The Ohio V5A anesthesia ventilator is an example of a descending or hanging bellows configuration (a). A weight is used in the most dependent portion of the bellows to facilitate descent of the bellows during exhalation; this may also lead to a failure to recognize a disconnection or leak as the bellows will appear to move appropriately regardless of whether it is connected to a patient. The bellows of the Mallard 2800 large animal anesthesia ventilator (b) is an example of an ascending or standing bellows configuration. Standing or ascending bellows normally produce slight positive pressure during the expiratory pause. Source: Craig Mosley, Mosley Veterinary Anesthesia Services, Rockwood, ON, Canada.

weight placed in the dependent portion of the bellows. As the bellows descends, it can cause a slight negative pressure in the bellows and breathing system. If a leak or disconnection develops in the breathing system, the weight of the bellows will cause the bellow to expand normally, drawing extraneous gases into the breathing system through the leak or a negative pressure relief valve. During the subsequent inspiration, not only will the gas in the breathing circuit be diluted by the non-anesthetic-containing gases, but all or some of the inspiration will be lost through the leak. Leaks (particularly large leaks) in the breathing system are not as readily identified by visually assessing the bellows using this type of ventilator configuration compared with the standing configuration. However, it is possible to detect small leaks that are made more significant by high pressure. For example, a small leak between the ETT cuff and the trachea of the patient will become much more significant as the airway pressures associated with IPPV rise; this will direct some of the tidal volume intended for the patient into the room. Upon exhalation, a volume of gas inadequate to replace the volume lost from the bellows during inspiration will be expelled from the animal's lungs. The bellows will then attempt to fall but will do so more slowly if the rate of aspiration of room air through a small leak (and volume contributed to the system via the fresh gas flow) is less than that required for the bellows to fall normally. The result will be a bellows that falls very slowly or does not fall completely before the next inspiration occurs. This effect is most commonly recognized during ventilation of large patients where the leak is often relatively small (and is increased with positive pressure), the tidal volume is relatively large, and the fresh gas flows are low relative to the patient's tidal volume.

There is at least one unique dual-circuit ventilator (Anesthesia WorkStation, Hallowell EMC, Pittsfield, MA, USA) designed specifically for patients requiring tidal volumes of less than 100 mL that replaces the bellows with a floating disc (Fig. 3.74). The floating disc separates the patient breathing circuit and driving gas circuit. In this configuration, the driving gas and patient circuit do not come into contact with one another but they do move back and forth across the same surface of the ventilation tube. This configuration requires very precise machining of both the ventilation tube and the floating disc to ensure that gas remains separated within their respective circuits and that the disc moves freely without significant resistance.

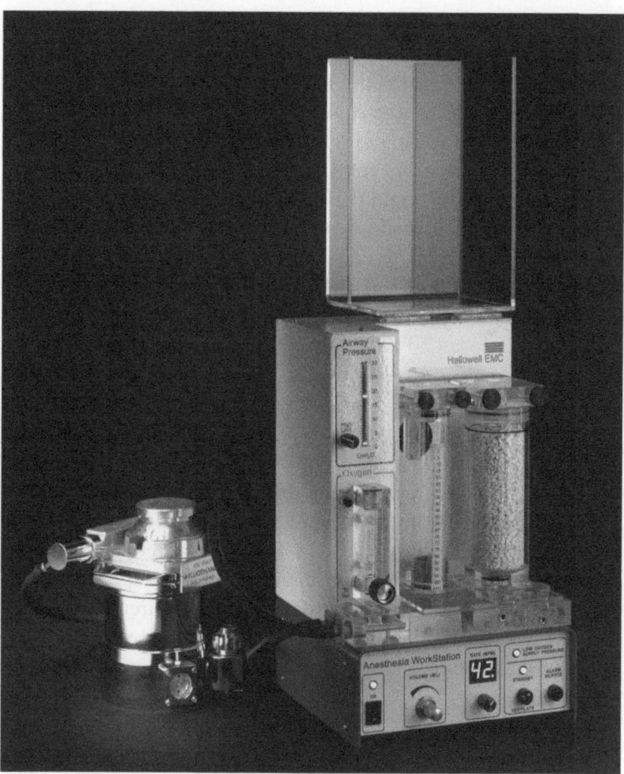

Figure 3.74 The Hallowell Anesthesia WorkStation (AWS) is a ventilator and circle breathing system designed specifically for very small animal patients (those between 150 g and 7 kg). The system features a unique ventilator that utilizes a floating puck, rather than a bellows, to separate the ventilator drive gas from the patient breathing circuit. The circle system is also optimized for very small patients with a low volume (circuit and absorbent canister) and a nearly zero deadspace Y-piece. Source: Hallowell EMC, Pittsfield, MA, USA. Reproduced with permission of Hallowell EMC.

Bellows housing

A housing made of clear plastic that allows observation of bellows movement by the anesthetist surrounds the bellows. The housing is sealed and can be pressurized during ventilator cycling, causing compression of the bellows. A scale is normally present on the side of the bellows indicating the approximate tidal volume delivered. However, this volume is usually not precisely equivalent to the actual tidal volume received by the patient (see Factors Affecting Tidal Volume below).

Exhaust valve

The exhaust valve allows communication between the inside of the bellows housing and the external atmosphere on pneumatically driven ventilators (i.e., those that use compressed gases to squeeze the bellows). During inspiration, the exhaust valve is closed, allowing the driving gas to build pressure within the housing. During exhalation, the exhaust valve opens (and driving gas delivery stops), allowing the pressure to drop and the bellows to re-expand. Piston-driven ventilators have no need for an exhaust valve.

Spill valve

The spill valve replaces the function of the anesthetic machine's APL valve (which is still present, but closed during mechanical ventilation) and is sometimes also referred to as a vent valve, dump valve, overflow valve, expired gas outlet, pop-off valve, relief valve, or pressure relief valve. The valve is used to direct excess fresh gas from the breathing circuit into the scavenge system during the expiratory pause. During the ventilator's inspiratory cycle, the valve is closed to prevent escape of gas into the scavenge system and allow positive pressure to develop in the breathing circuit. This is similar to closing the APL valve in order to deliver a manual breath using the reservoir bag. With a standing bellows configuration, the spill valve normally has a minimal opening pressure of between 2 and 4 cmH_2O to offset the downward force created by the weight of the bellows. This allows the bellows to fill completely during exhalation. The spill valve is normally controlled pneumatically in ventilators using gas to compress the bellows, but in the case of piston-driven ventilators it may be opened and closed electronically.

Ventilator hose connection

The ventilator hose connection is a standard sized outlet (22 mm male conical fitting) normally found on the back of the ventilator bellows assembly. A length of standard sized corrugated tubing is used between the ventilator hose connection and the machine's fitting that normally holds the reservoir bag. On anesthetic machines with built-in ventilators, this connection is often accomplished through the use of a switch or dial minimizing the potential for misconnections, disconnections, or kinked hoses.

Control of ventilator driving gas

The driving gas supplied to the ventilator is normally under intermediate pressure (35–55 psi) and is delivered at a specified flow rate for a specific period of time to produce a volume of gas sufficient to compress the bellows and ventilate the patient's lungs. The driving gas is typically 100% oxygen and is used because it is usually readily available and to minimize the potential for reducing the oxygen concentration of the breathing circuit should a leak develop between the two ventilator circuits (breathing and driving gas circuit).

The driving gas flow to the ventilator is normally controlled electronically with dials labeled to adjust three essential variables: the duration of time driving gas is allowed into the bellows housing (inspiratory time), the rate at which the driving gas flows into the bellows housing (inspiratory flow rate), and the pause between inhalations (expiratory time). By manipulating these three variables, the more commonly described variables respiratory frequency (*f*), tidal volume (V_t) and the inspiratory-to-expiratory ratio (I:E) can be controlled. Fluid logic-controlled ventilators are slightly less intuitive to operate but essentially through manipulations related to pressure thresholds, flow rates, and time the same variables can be controlled.

Factors that affect delivered tidal volume

Unless mechanisms for compensation are built into the anesthesia ventilator, various factors can affect the actual tidal volume delivered to the patient. Under most circumstances, and by using proper monitoring and setup procedures, these factors are insignificant.

Fresh gas flow

Although many modern human anesthesia ventilators compensate for changes in fresh gas flow, most veterinary ventilators do not. The electronics of most veterinary anesthesia ventilators are designed to deliver a set amount of driving gas regardless of the actual compression of the bellows. During inspiration, the fresh gas flow will continue into the patient circuit, contributing to the patient's actual tidal volume. Increasing the fresh gas flow or prolonging the inspiratory time will lead to larger tidal volumes. Although this effect may be insignificant in most patients, it can become significant in very small patients where a fresh gas flow of 1000 mL/min will contribute roughly 17 mL/s of gas to the patients tidal volume during inspiration.

Compliance and compression volumes

Changes in compliance of the breathing system can be accompanied by changes in the tidal volume of gas delivered to the patient. Increases in the compliance of a breathing system can be accompanied by decreases in the patient tidal volume as more of the delivered gas volume is expended expanding the breathing components. In addition, changes in airway pressures associated with ventilation and/or changes in lung compliance may alter the actual tidal volume of gas that the patient receives as gas volume is compressible when subjected to increasing pressures.

Leaks

Leaks within the system (e.g., around the endotracheal tube) will impact the delivered tidal volume as some gas will escape through these leaks, leading to a reduction in the delivered tidal volume. Although side-stream airway gas monitors are not considered leaks, they do aspirate a small volume of gas from the breathing system (50–250 mL/min or 0.8–4 mL/s) that may marginally reduce tidal volume unless the gas is reintroduced as it leaves the monitor. This effect is normally negligible but may be significant in patients requiring extremely small tidal volumes (i.e., <50 mL).

Alarms

There are no standard alarm configurations for veterinary anesthesia ventilators. Some of the more commonly found alarms are described below.

Low driving gas pressure alarm

This alarm is sometimes also referred to as the low-pressure alarm and will detect when the driving gas pressure falls below a preset value (i.e., 35 psi). A drop in driving gas pressure below a certain level may lead to a decrease in delivered tidal volume.

Airway pressure alarms

Both high and low airway pressure alarms are available on some ventilators. These are important to help protect a patient from barotrauma (high airway pressure) and help detect leaks or disconnects. The alarm settings may be preset by the manufacturer or adjusted by the user. Occasionally preset alarms are not compatible with the ventilation requirements in some patients. For example, a minimum airway pressure alarm set at 6 cmH_2O may exceed the maximum airway pressures used when ventilating very small patients with extremely compliant chests (e.g., kittens, puppies, reptiles, and birds).

Determinants of tidal volume

One of the principal risks associated with mechanical ventilation is inadvertent volutrauma or barotrauma to the patient's lungs if ventilator settings are improperly set. Fortunately, most of these errors are unlikely to be catastrophic as the vigilant anesthetist should immediately notice these errors. The tidal volume on most pneumatically driven ventilators is limited (or determined) by the flow rate of gas entering the bellows housing and the duration of time that this gas is allowed to enter the bellows. Some ventilators will also use mechanical limiting devices to restrict movement of the bellows, thus effectively limiting the tidal volume that can be delivered regardless of changes in inspiratory flow rate and times (Mallard 2400V, Mallard Medical, Redding, CA, USA, and Dräger Large Animal Ventilator). One common recommendation when initiating mechanical ventilation in a patient is to start with low tidal volume settings and increase these based on monitored parameters once the ventilation is initiated. This is an especially important consideration if no mechanical volume-limiting device is present on the ventilator.

Tidal volume on most ventilators is controlled by dials variously labeled inspiratory flow rate, tidal volume, or minute volume and will be impacted by inspiratory time, I:E ratio and respiratory rate. It is important to review the settings prior to the initiation of ventilation and to be fully aware of how changes in any one parameter may affect others. For example, if the respiratory rate is reduced on some ventilators, the inspiratory time will automatically be increased to reflect the new respiratory rate, leading to an increase in tidal volume (i.e., the inspiratory flow rate remains the same but the duration of inspiration increases).

Proper ventilator setup and monitoring

Prior to using an anesthesia ventilator it is important for the anesthetist to determine clearly the desired ventilator settings. Typical settings used for small and large animal patients are listed in Table 3.5. The anesthetist should have a solid understanding of the

Table 3.5 Guideline parameters for initiating intermittent positive pressure ventilation in small animal patients and horses[a].

Patient	Respiratory Rate (breaths/min)	Tidal Volume (mL/kg)	Inspiratory Pressure (cmH_2O)	I:E Ratio
Small animal	10–15	10–20	10–15	1:2
Equine	6–8	10–20	10–25	1:3–1:4

[a]It is important to recognize that these are only guidelines and that specific settings can vary significantly among patients depending upon patient factors such as breed, body condition, and disease. Additionally, ventilator limitations may influence the specific parameters attainable (e.g., minimum inspiratory flow limits). Ultimately, the adequacy of ventilation is best evaluated individually in each patient using capnography and/or blood gas analysis.

indications, contraindications, and physiology of IPPV prior to initiating ventilation. In addition, the anesthetist should ensure that they are familiar with all the features and proper operation of the ventilator they are using by reviewing the manufacturer's instructions. Improper use of positive pressure ventilation equipment can lead to unnecessary morbidity and mortality. The following steps are intended as a general overview to ventilator setup and may not be applicable for all ventilators, patients, and circumstances.

- Ensure power is available to the ventilator; most ventilators will require a source of compressed gas and an electrical supply.
- Connect the scavenge hose from the ventilator to a scavenge system. Many scavenge interfaces have two scavenging ports, one for the anesthetic machine and the other for a ventilator.
- Empty the reservoir bag into the scavenge system, remove the reservoir bag, and connect the ventilator breathing hose to the reservoir bag mount. Close the APL valve. Some machines with built-in ventilators do not require removal of the reservoir bag and closure of the APL; instead, a switch or dial is used to isolate the reservoir bag and APL from the ventilator.
- Allow the bellows to fill. This can be facilitated by momentarily increasing the fresh gas flow rate. The flush valve should not be used for this purpose unless the fresh gas flow cannot be suitably increased to fill the bellows in a relatively rapid fashion (e.g., large animal ventilator).
- Initiate ventilation based on the predetermined ventilation parameters. It is generally best to start with tidal volumes at the lower end of the typical range to avoid barotrauma or volutrauma. Under all circumstances it is vital immediately and then routinely to evaluate the peak airway pressures and other monitored parameters (e.g., end tidal CO_2, arterial blood gas analysis, and arterial blood pressure) to assess the adequacy of ventilator settings.

Selected ventilator models

Although not all-inclusive, the following discussion describes ventilators that are appropriate for veterinary patients. Some of these ventilators were designed specifically to support anesthetized veterinary patients, whereas others were designed for human use but are applicable to veterinary patients or can be modified for veterinary use. The classification, principles of operation, and other points about the general function of each ventilator are included. Before operating a ventilator, the user should consult the operating manuals and follow all pre-use evaluation procedures recommended by the manufacturer.

Dräger Small Animal Ventilator (SAV)

This ventilator was marketed as an optional component for the Dräger Narkovet 2 Anesthesia Machine and was available on a mobile stand (universal pole) specifically designed for the ventilator. Currently the ventilator is not being manufactured, but these ventilators remain in use for veterinary anesthesia. The SAV is classified as double-circuit, time-cycled, with an ascending (standing) bellows; it is pneumatically powered and has fluidic circuitry. The pressure of the driving gas should be between 40 and 60 psi. The controls include a power ('on–off') switch, a tidal volume adjustment rod to set the attached plate within the bellows housing to the selected tidal volume (200–1600 mL), a frequency control knob (10–30 breaths/min), and an inspiratory flow knob to control the rate of flow into the bellows housing to deliver the breath. The inspiratory flow knob is normally set so that the bellows is fully compressed at the end of the inspiratory phase; however, the bellows should not be deformed at the end of inspiration. Deformation of the bellows at the end of inspiration may indicate an increase in tidal volume by as much as 100 mL. The inspiratory flow control setting affects the peak inspiratory pressure that is achieved and the inspiratory time. Higher inspiratory flows produce shorter inspiratory times and tend to produce higher peak inspiratory pressures. The ratio of inspiratory to expiratory time phase is preset to 1:2. The ventilator spill valve behind the bellows chamber compensates for the continuous entry of fresh gases into the breathing system. Because the ventilator uses an ascending bellows, the effect of gravity on the bellows maintains a PEEP of approximately 2 cmH_2O.

Before using the ventilator, the proper connections to the gas supply and scavenger system should be made, and the appropriate pre-use checkout procedures should be preformed for all equipment. Assuming that the anesthesia machine, breathing system, and ventilator are functional, the following is a reasonable step-by-step approach to the operation of this ventilator with a circle breathing system:

1. The tidal volume adjustment rod is set appropriately for the patient.
2. Corrugated tubing from the ventilator's breathing-hose terminal is connected to the circle system's reservoir-bag mount.
3. The circle system's APL valve (adjustable pressure-limiting or pop-off valve) is closed.
4. The frequency of ventilation is adjusted to approximate the desired number of breaths per minute.
5. The ventilator's power switch is turned on.
6. The inspiratory flow control knob is adjusted to produce the desired inspiratory time to deliver the preset tidal volume.
7. The frequency of ventilation and inspiratory flow may need to be readjusted to achieve the desired rate of breathing and inspiratory time.

Engler ADS 1000 and 2000 veterinary Anesthesia Delivery System and critical care ventilator

This microprocessor-controlled ventilator is marketed for use with a vaporizer or for patients not requiring an inhalant anesthetic (e.g., critical care patients). The ventilator–anesthesia system functions as a non-rebreathing circuit (unidirectional circuit), does not incorporate a bellows assembly or piston canister, and does not include a canister for chemical absorbent to eliminate carbon dioxide. It is not intended for connection to another breathing system.

This ventilator fits into the single-circuit class and is powered electrically and pneumatically. However, it is different in its function from both piston- and pneumatically driven single-circuit ventilators. The ventilator only delivers gas intermittently to the patient (i.e., during inspiration) and, if used with a vaporizer, the ventilation drive gas moves through the vaporizer. In most other ventilation systems, gas flow to the vaporizer is independent of drive gas flow delivered by the ventilator and continuous. There is no possibility for rebreathing and the gas flow is unidirectional.

According to the operating manual, the ventilator must be supplied with oxygen at a pressure of 50 (normal mode) or 5 psi (laboratory/low-flow mode) for the display to report the minute volume per kilogram of body weight accurately. When in laboratory mode, only tidal volume is reported. When used in normal mode, the ventilator's microprocessor will determine (estimate) the values for the various ventilatory parameters to be provided based on the patient's body weight. However, it is important to note that the preselected values may not optimally ventilate all patients and manual adjustments of ventilator parameters based on blood gas analysis and/or end-tidal CO_2 values should be used to ensure proper patient ventilation. The manufacturer's specifications suggest the ADS 2000 is capable of ventilating patients less than 1 and up to 68 kg. The ventilator is also capable of operating in an assist ventilation mode, delivering a breath each time the patient attempts to inspire spontaneously. The sensitivity of this feature is manually controlled by the user. The Engler ADS 2000 features updated electronics and microprocessor but is functionally the same as the Engler ADS 1000.

This ventilator acts as a non-rebreathing circuit leading to excessive oxygen and inhalant anesthetic consumption when used in larger patients, particularly those over 10 kg. It is also important to note that the gas flow rates required to produce the tidal volumes required for larger patients may fall outside the recommended flow rates (200–15000 mL/min) for most vaporizers. For example, to produce a tidal volume of 600 mL using a 2 s inspiratory time will require the ventilator to deliver gas at a rate of 300 mL/s or 18 L/min to achieve the desired tidal volume. There is also some concern about the accuracy of vaporizer output resulting from the intermittent nature of carrier gas delivery to the vaporizer. When using this ventilator with a vaporizer, it is probably best to ensure that ventilator flow rates fall within those recommended by the vaporizer manufacturer to ensure accurate output.

The front panel of the ventilator has the following controls and components: power switch, mask-mode switch, set–run switch, weight-selection buttons, fill–hold button, breath button, display for various ventilatory parameters with adjustments for these parameters below the display, two ports for attachment of corrugated breathing tubes, and a gas sampling input port (this port was absent on earlier ADS 1000 models).

Before attempting to use the ventilator, the operator should read the manual supplied by the manufacturer and be very familiar with how ventilatory parameters can be modified manually as the preset values may not be optimal for individual patients. The following is a summary of the manufacturer's guidelines for operating the ventilator, but is not intended to replace or supplant the manual supplied for the ventilator:

1 Connect the green oxygen hose on the back of the ventilator to an oxygen source (50 or 5 psi).
2 Attach the circle system tubes to the breathing-circuit ports on the front of the ventilator.
3 Connect the scavenger out port on the back of the ventilator to the hospital scavenger system.
4 Connect the electric cord to an electric outlet.
5 Attach the vaporizer connectors to the appropriate ports on the back of the ventilator.
6 Attach the gas sampling line to the appropriate circuit adapter and gas sampling port on the ventilator.
7 Allow the ventilator to complete the self-diagnostic test described in the operator's manual. The test will help to determine failure of the safety pop-off valve, inadequate oxygen supply, and the presence of leaks.
8 After diagnostics are complete, the mask function should be off and the set–run switch should be in the set position. The display will then show settings for a 20 kg patient (flow rate of 24 L/min, 9 breaths/min, peak inspiratory pressure of 15 cmH_2O, and the assist mode in the off position).
9 Using the weight-up or weight-down button, enter the correct weight of the patient in kilograms into the display, and the ventilator will automatically set the ventilatory parameters based on the patient's weight. Ventilation will be completely controlled (the default setting for assist is off).

Once these steps have been completed, the patient should be anesthetized and intubated with a cuffed endotracheal tube. The Y-piece connecting the breathing tubes should be attached to the endotracheal tube connector and the vaporizer should be set appropriately. The ventilator's set–run switch should be set to run. Controlled ventilation should begin.

Hallowell EMC 2000 and 2002, and Matrx 3000 anesthesia ventilators

These ventilators (Fig. 3.75) were designed for use with standard small animal anesthesia machines and breathing systems (circle and non-rebreathing circuits). The connections to the breathing system, scavenger, and driving gas are located on the back of the unit. The Matrx 3000 model is the Hallowell EMC 2000 model ventilator produced for Matrx/Midmark. The 2002 model has essentially replaced the 2000 model, but many 2000 models are still in use. The primary difference between the two models is the fine inspiratory flow adjustment dial that was added to the 2002 model.

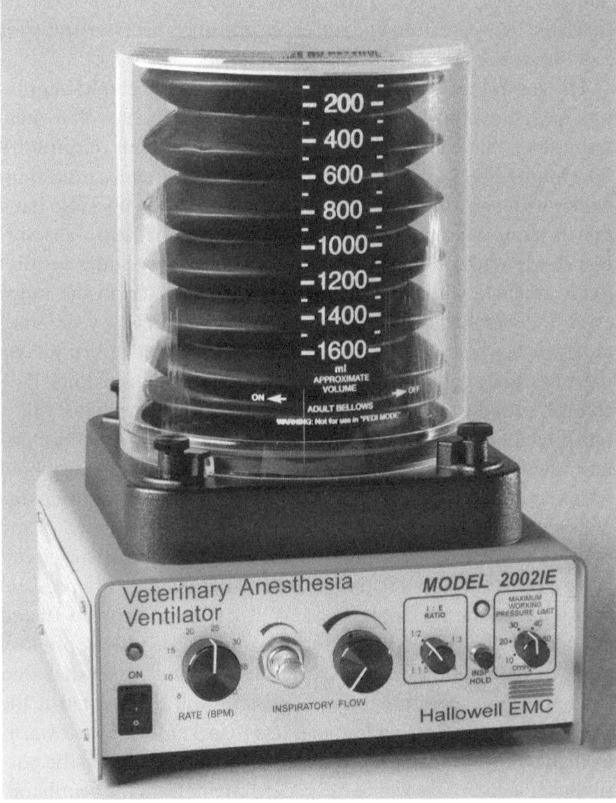

Figure 3.75 The Hallowell 2002 ventilator features a fine inspiratory flow dial, improving its ability to deliver more precise tidal volumes. It is also available with or without an adjustable I:E ratio. Source: Hallowell EMC, Pittsfield, MA, USA. Reproduced with permission of Hallowell EMC.

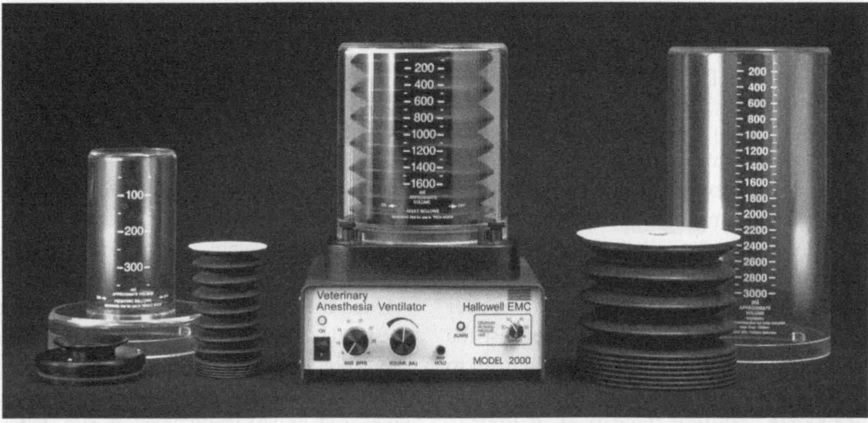

Figure 3.76 Many ventilators are available with different sizes of interchangeable bellows. This feature is convenient when ventilating patients requiring markedly different tidal volumes, but the bellows does not generally change the overall function of the ventilator (i.e. a small bellows does not mean that smaller tidal volumes can be achieved with the ventilator, it simply provides more precision in estimating tidal volume from movement of the bellows; the minimum tidal volume will be determined by the inspiratory flow rate and inspiratory time). Source: Hallowell EMC, Pittsfield, MA, USA. Reproduced with permission of Hallowell EMC.

This addition allows for more precise tidal volume control, particularly when small tidal volumes are required. This ventilator is classified as double-circuit and time-cycled with an ascending (standing) bellows and is electrically powered. The ventilator is pneumatically driven and electronically controlled by an electrically activated solenoid valve that allows gas pressure to be supplied to the volume control during the inspiratory phase of the ventilatory cycle. The ventilator's power switch is incorporated into the respiratory-rate control. The pressure of the driving-gas supply (either oxygen, nitrogen, or compressed conditioned air) should be regulated between 30 and 60 psi. High pressure is necessary only for high inspiratory flow rates in larger patients.

The control modules of the EMC 2000 and 2002 model ventilators have the following adjustable components: the on–off switch, respiratory-rate control knob, a volume control knob (inspiratory flow Model 2002), an inspiratory hold push button, and a maximum working pressure limit (MWPL) selector. The 2002 model also has a fine inspiratory flow adjustment (see Fig. 3.75). The ratio of inspiratory to expiratory time phase is preset at 1:2. However, this ventilator is available with an optional adjustable I:E ratio in the range 1:1.5–1:4, enabling users greater flexibility in selecting ventilatory parameters. The inspiratory flow control is a variable orifice-metering valve that regulates the driving-gas flow. The inspiratory flow control is used to set tidal volume. It regulates the inspiratory flow rate directly, and a higher inspiratory flow rate at any given respiratory rate will produce a greater tidal volume. The inspiratory hold push button interrupts the ventilatory cycle and prevents discharge of gas from the bellows housing until the button is released or the MWPL is reached. The MWPL is measured in the patient circuit using a coupling placed in the patient circuit extending to a pressure transducer in the ventilator. The MWPL can be set between 10 and 60 cmH_2O. If the MWPL is reached at any time, the inspiratory phase of ventilation is terminated, an alarm sounds, and exhalation is allowed. Low breathing-system pressure will be detected if the pressure at the end of inspiration is less than 5 cmH_2O; a red warning light will illuminate and an alarm will sound, indicating the possibility of a disconnection of the patient circuit from the ventilator.

Three sizes of interchangeable bellows and bellows housings are available to enable various sizes of patients to be ventilated effectively (Fig. 3.76). With the proper bellows, the manufacturer indicates that tidal volumes as small as 20 mL and as large as 3 L can be delivered and that the patient can effectively breathe spontaneously from the bellows when the ventilator is not in operation. The ventilator spill valve compensates for the continuous entry of fresh gas into the breathing system, and the resistance of the spill valve creates a PEEP of 2–3 cmH_2O.

Before using the ventilator, connections to the gas supply and scavenger system should be made and the appropriate pre-use checkout procedures followed. Assuming proper functioning of the anesthesia machine, breathing system, and ventilator, the following is a reasonable operational approach for this ventilator with a circle breathing system:

1 The MWPL selector is set to the desired maximum pressure (safety limit), and the pressure coupler is connected to the breathing system according to the manufacturer's recommendations.
2 Corrugated tubing from the ventilator's breathing system connector is attached to the circle system's reservoir-bag mount, and the ventilator is attached to the scavenger system.
3 The circle system's pop-off (APL) valve is closed.
4 The ventilator's volume control is adjusted to the minimum setting.
5 The ventilator's power-rate switch is turned on and the desired frequency of ventilation is set.
6 The volume control knob (inspiratory flow on Model 2002) is adjusted to produce a flow of gas during inspiration that produces the desired tidal volume and/or peak inspiratory pressure.

Mallard Medical Model 2400V anesthesia ventilator

This ventilator was originally designed to allow continuous mechanical ventilation of anesthetized pediatric and adult human patients. It is sold to veterinarians as a stand-alone unit for use with a breathing system and anesthesia machine (Fig. 3.77). Classified as a double-circuit ventilator, it has electric power and is pneumatically driven. The ventilator is controlled by a microprocessor, and the manufacturer describes the ventilator as electronically time cycled and volume limited. The tidal volume is selected by limiting the upward expansion of the bellows by use of a bellows expansion limiting device. Tidal volume is adjusted by moving a cylinder and plate within the bellows housing to coincide with the desired setting in milliliters. The cylinder within the bellows housing is secured by

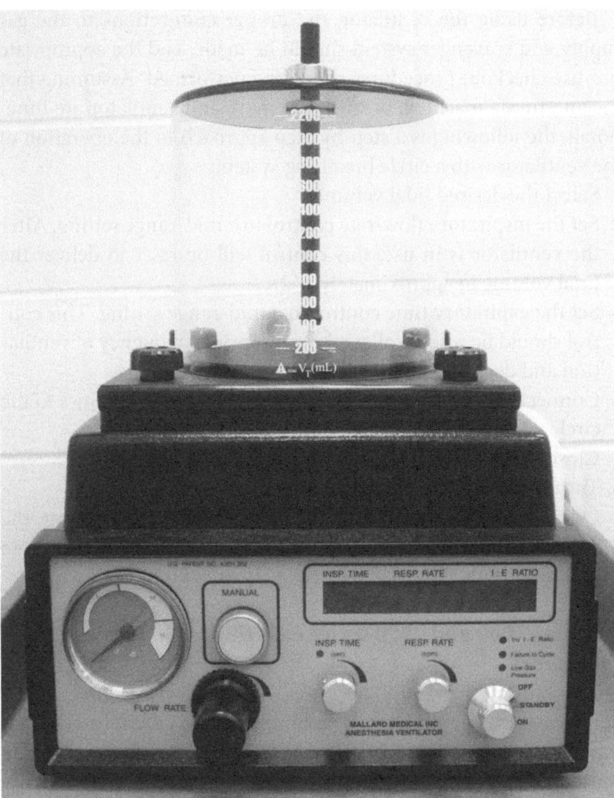

Figure 3.77 The Mallard 2400V anesthesia ventilator. The ventilator can be volume limited through the use of an adjustable bellows limiting device, or alternatively the volume can be limited through changes in the driving gas flow rate. Source: Craig Mosley, Mosley Veterinary Anesthesia Services, Rockwood, ON, Canada.

a control knob (nut) located on the top center of the housing. This ventilator employs an ascending (standing) bellows. The bellows is pneumatically driven, and the ventilator operates at a driving gas pressure of 50 ± 10 psi.

The controls are positioned on a console, which is located below the bellows housing. A master on–standby–off switch is present in the right lower corner of the console's front panel; the standby mode allows preselection of respiratory rate and inspiratory time (see Fig. 3.77). The I:E ratio is computed from these settings and displayed digitally on light-emitting diode (LED) displays before mechanical ventilation is initiated. Respiratory rate and inspiratory time are controlled by ten-turn potentiometers to allow selection of 2–80 breaths/min (respiratory rate) and 0.1–3.0 s (inspiratory time), respectively. The I:E ratio display shows the relationship of inspiratory time to expiratory time, giving inspiratory time a value of 1. A black control knob located in the lower left portion of the front panel allows adjustment of inspiratory flow rate (10–100 L/min), and a display gauge near the control knob indicates whether the flow being used is low, medium, or high. The flow rate is normally adjusted to ensure complete compression of the bellows at the end of inspiration. If the flow rate is set higher than needed, it will produce a rapid time to peak inspiration volume and an inspiratory hold. A green push button is located in the front center portion of the control console; this button activates inspiration as long as the button is pushed in. This button can be used to maintain mechanical ventilation in the event of a power failure and can be used to sigh the patient.

Two sizes of bellows are available: the adult bellows provides tidal volumes ranging from 200 to 2200 mL and the pediatric bellows from 50 to 300 mL. An exhalation valve assembly is located on the back of the control console. This valve is closed pneumatically during the inspiratory phase of ventilation and opens automatically during the expiratory phase. Excess gas from the patient circuit also exits through this valve to prevent the buildup of pressure. The post (19 mm) of this valve should be attached to a scavenger system for elimination of waste gases from the working environment. With an ascending bellows, PEEP (usually 2–3 cmH_2O) will be present. In addition, PEEP of up to 20 cmH_2O can be added to the system with the control knob of the optional PEEP valve. Also, an adjustable overpressure spill valve within the console is preset to 80 cmH_2O, and this limits the maximum pressure that can be developed in the patient breathing circuit. Externally, this pressure can be adjusted from 20 to 100 cmH_2O. This ventilator has audible alarms if the ventilator fails to cycle or if an electric power failure occurs. In addition, the LED displays will indicate selection of an inverse I:E ratio, failure of the ventilator to cycle, and low supply-gas pressure (<30 psi).

Before using the ventilator, the proper connections to the gas supply and scavenger system should be made, and the appropriate pre-use checkout procedures should be performed. Assuming proper functioning of the anesthesia machine, breathing system, and ventilator, the following is a reasonable operational approach for this ventilator with a circle breathing system:

1 Prior to clinical applications, refer to the operating manual for instructions and conduct performance verification procedures.
2 Select the appropriate control settings for the tidal volume by limiting the upward expansion of the bellows.
3 Place the master switch in the standby mode and dial the desired settings for the respiratory rate and the inspiratory time, based on the patient's needs.
4 Set the inspiratory flow control to the desired rate of flow, low, medium, or high, depending on the needs of the patient.
5 Connect the corrugated tubing from the ventilator's bellows to the circle system's reservoir-bag mount and attach the ventilator to the scavenger system.
6 Close the circle system's pop-off (APL) valve.
7 Set the master switch to the on position.
8 The ventilator should cycle according to the selected settings, and only minor adjustments should be necessary (e.g., slight alterations of inspiratory time).

Ohio V5A ventilator

This ventilator is shown in Fig. 3.73a. This unit was produced for human use and is capable of delivering tidal volumes in the range 20–1400 mL. This ventilator is no longer produced but is still available. The Metomatic, a small animal-specific model, produced by Ohio Medical Products, is also no longer produced although it may still be found in some veterinary practices and has been described elsewhere [66]. The Metomatic and the V5A are very similar in overall design, although the Metomatic offered an assist mode for ventilation and could be set to limit the tidal volume based on pressure. Arguably the Metomatic offered more features for precisely controlling ventilation but is perhaps less intuitive for those unfamiliar with IPPV. The V5A is classified as a double-circuit and time-cycled ventilator with fluidic circuitry and a descending (hanging) bellows. The ventilator is powered and driven pneumatically and will function properly with an oxygen-supply pressure to 40–75 psi.

Controls for this ventilator are as follows: power (on–off) switch, inspiratory flow-rate control, expiratory time control, and a manual inspiration button. There is also a dial on the side of the ventilator canister used to control tidal volume by limiting descent of the bellows (Fig. 3.78). The power switch controls a valve that supplies pneumatic power to the ventilator. The tidal volume control dial adjusts the bellows from 0 to 1400 mL (20–300 mL pediatric bellows). The inspiratory flow-rate control regulates the rate of delivery of gas to the ventilator canister compressing the bellows during inspiration and is adjustable from 6 to 100 L/min. It should be set to deliver the complete tidal volume from the bellows over a reasonable period of time, normally 1–2 s. The expiratory time control adjusts the time between the end of one inspiratory phase of respiration and the beginning of the next and can be varied from 1 to 10 s; essentially, it is a setting for respiratory rate, although rate is influenced to some extent by other controls (e.g., inspiratory time). The manual inspiration push button allows the initiation of inspiration at any point during the respiratory cycle by depressing and immediately releasing the button. If the push button is depressed and held, inspiration will be initiated, and the bellows will remain at the end-inspiratory position until the button is released. The ventilator is also equipped with a low airway pressure alarm. This is a useful feature as a leak is not easily detected through observation of the ventilator bellows in a descending/hanging configuration. The ventilator provides a spill valve (pop-off valve) to allow the escape of excess gases that are delivered to the patient circuit. Generally, the pressure in the patient circuit returns to zero at end of expiration, since a descending bellows is employed.

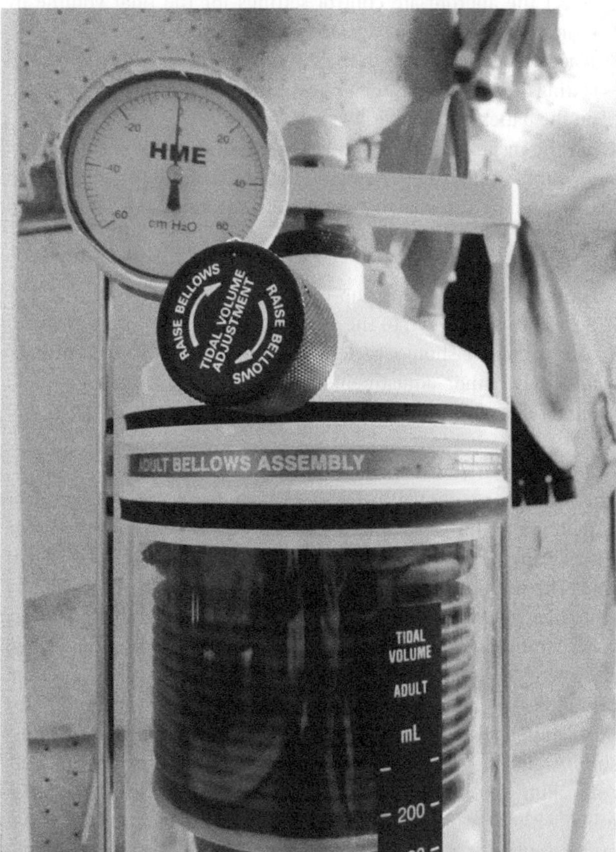

Figure 3.78 The tidal volume delivered to a patient using a 'hanging' bellows ventilator is often controlled by using an adjustable dial that limits the descent of the bellows. Source: Craig Mosley, Mosley Veterinary Anesthesia Services, Rockwood, ON, Canada.

Before using the ventilator, the proper connections to the gas supply and scavenger system should be made, and the appropriate pre-use checkout procedures should be performed. Assuming that the anesthesia machine, breathing system, and ventilator are functional, the following is a step-by-step approach to the operation of the ventilator with a circle breathing system:

1 Select the desired tidal volume.
2 Set the inspiratory flow-rate control to a mid-range setting. After the ventilator is in use, this control will be reset to deliver the tidal volume in approximately 1–2 s.
3 Set the expiratory time control to a mid-range setting. This control should be reset to allow the appropriate frequency of ventilation and desired I:E ratio after the ventilator is in use.
4 Connect the corrugated tube from the ventilator's bellows to the circle system's reservoir-bag port.
5 Close the pop-off (APL) valve of the breathing system.
6 Turn the power switch on.
7 Observe the character and rate of ventilation, and refine the adjustments of the various controls. Usually, inspiratory flow rate is adjusted first, followed by frequency or expiratory time.

Ohmeda 7000 and 7800 series electronic anesthesia ventilators

The Ohmeda 7000 and 7800 series ventilators are double-circuit human anesthesia ventilators with a pneumatically driven ascending/standing bellows (Fig. 3.79). The 7000 ventilator is electronically controlled with a preset minute volume, whereas the 7800 is electronically controlled with a preset tidal volume, which may be a specific advantage (as discussed below).

Both ventilators can be fitted with either an adult or a pediatric bellows, and they have been used extensively in human anesthesia [1, 75]. These ventilators are available used and are readily applicable to small animal anesthesia. The scale on the bellows housing ranges from 100 to 1600 mL on the adult bellows and from 0 to 300 mL on the pediatric bellows. The bellows assembly exhaust port is 19 mm O.D., the connection to the anesthesia machine is 22 mm, and there is a high-pressure (50 psi) diameter index safety system (DISS) fitting for an oxygen line for the driving-gas circuit. The driving-gas supply is oxygen at 50 psi, which is reduced to 38 psi by a precision regulator within the ventilator. During the expiratory phase, gas from the patient circuit (flow from the anesthesia machine) enters the bellows. The ventilator spill opens when the bellows is fully distended and a pressure of 2.5 cmH_2O has been exceeded; excess gas from the patient circuit is vented into the scavenger system. The controls and specific details of each model series are discussed separately below.

The 7000 series control module (see Fig. 3.79a) has six controls, namely the minute volume dial (2–30 L/min with the adult bellows and 2–12 L/min with the pediatric bellows), the respiratory-rate dial (6–40 breaths/min), the I:E ratio dial (1:1–1:3), power (on–off) switch, the sigh switch (to provide a 'sigh' equal to 150% of the tidal volume once every 64 breaths), and a manual cycle button (used to initiate inspiration manually only during the expiratory phase). The controls for ventilation (minute volume, respiratory rate and I:E ratio) are not interactive. If minute volume is increased and the rate held constant, the tidal volume will increase. Hence changing the minute volume is normally used to change the patient's tidal volume, although it is important to recognize that changing the respiratory rate can also change the tidal volume. If the respiratory rate is decreased while the minute volume is held constant, the tidal volume will increase. Inappropriate use of any ventilator without

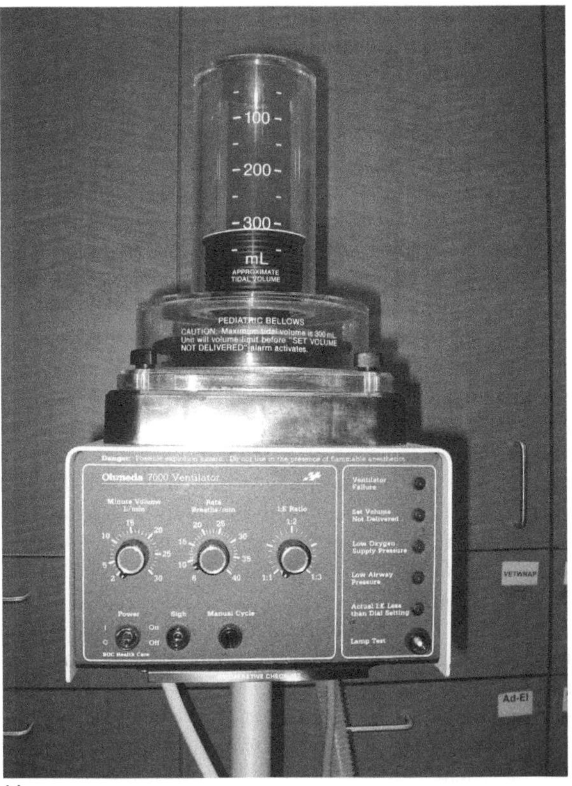

(a)

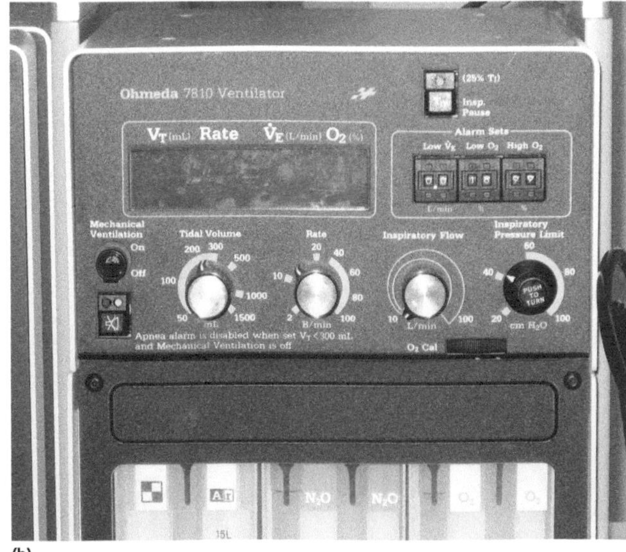

(b)

Figure 3.79 An Ohmeda 7000 series stand-alone ventilator (a) and a built-in Ohmeda 7800 series (Model 7810 shown) (b) showing the control panel. The Ohmeda 7800 provides greater functionality with built-in adjustable alarm parameters. Both of these ventilators are designed for use in humans but work well for most veterinary patients. Source: Craig Mosley, Mosley Veterinary Anesthesia Services, Rockwood, ON, Canada.

proper regard for how changes in one parameter may affect ancillary variables can be potentially dangerous (i.e., volutrauma or barotrauma) for the patient.

The 7800 series represents an evolution of the 7000 series providing additional functionality, built-in alarms and more intuitive control (see Fig. 3.79b). The respiratory parameters and the inspired oxygen concentration are displayed on a liquid crystal screen. There is a ventilation (on–off) toggle switch, alarm silence button (silences alarms for 30 s), tidal volume dial (50–1500 mL), respiratory rate dial (2–100 breaths/min), an inspiratory flow dial (10–100 L/min), an inspiratory pressure limit dial (20–100 cmH_2O; sustained alarm is 50% of set limit), an inspiratory pause switch (25% of inspiratory time), and a main power (on–off) toggle switch. There are also input plugins for an oxygen sensor (measuring percent inspired oxygen) and spirometer (measuring actual volume exhaled). There are three sets of toggle wheels for alarm settings: low minute ventilation, low oxygen concentration, and high oxygen concentration. The controls for ventilation (tidal volume, respiratory rate, and inspiratory flow rate) are not interactive. However, unlike the 7000 series, only changes to the tidal volume dial will result in changes in the tidal volume being delivered to the patient, which makes it less likely that an inadvertently large tidal volume will be delivered. Changing each of the ventilation controls (tidal volume, respiratory rate, and inspiratory flow rate) will alter its associated ventilator variable but will only lead to ancillary changes in the I:E ratio rather than delivered tidal volume. Normally the ventilator is set by selecting the desired tidal volume and respiratory rate, with the inspiratory flow rate being used to select an appropriate I:E ratio.

The manufacturer recommends a bellows assembly-leak test. With the ventilator attached to a circle breathing system with the breathing system's pop-off valve closed, the Y-piece occluded, all fresh gas flow off, and the bellows filled from the anesthesia machine's oxygen-flush valve, the bellows should drop no more than 100 mL/min. If a significant leak is present, the ventilator should not be used until the leak has been sealed. If the anesthesia machine, breathing system, and ventilator are all in proper working order, as indicated by pre-use checkout procedures, the following guidelines are appropriate for use of the ventilator:

1 Properly connect the electric and pneumatic power sources for the ventilator.
2 7000 series ventilators set the desired values for minute volume, respiratory rate (frequency), and I:E ratio. 7800 series ventilators set the desired values for tidal volume, respiratory rate, and I:E ratio (normally done by adjusting inspiratory flow rate). The alarm settings should be appropriately set.
3 Make the appropriate connections from the ventilator bellows to the circle system's reservoir bag port and to the scavenger system.
4 Close the pop-off (APL) valve of the circle system.
5 Make sure that the bellows is completely filled with oxygen–anesthetic mixture.
6 Switch the power control to on.
7 Make final adjustments to minute volume and respiratory rate to meet the needs of the patient.

Surgivet SAV 2500

This ventilator (Fig. 3.80) was designed for use with standard small animal anesthesia machines and breathing systems (circle

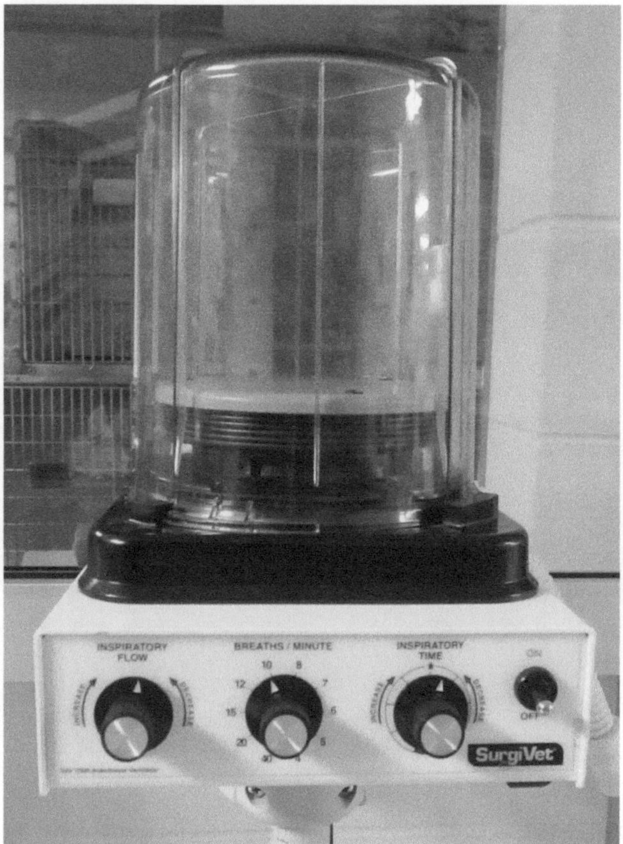

Figure 3.80 The Surgivet SAV 2500 showing the various control dials used to set respiratory parameters. Source: Craig Mosley, Mosley Veterinary Anesthesia Services, Rockwood, ON, Canada.

and non-rebreathing circuits). This ventilator is classified as double circuit and time cycled with an ascending (standing) bellows; it is pneumatically driven and electrically controlled. The pressure of the driving-gas supply (oxygen, nitrogen, or compressed conditioned air) should be regulated between 50 and 55 psi.

The control module for the SAV 2500 ventilator has the following adjustable components located on the front of the ventilator control unit: the on–off switch, inspiratory time dial, breaths per minute, and inspiratory flow. A transport breath button (pneumatic manual) and an adjustable pressure relief valve are located on the back of the base or control unit. The on–off switch initiates IPPV, the inspiratory time dial adjusts the time allowed for inspiration, and the breaths per minute is used to set the number of respiratory cycles that the ventilator will deliver over time. An appropriate I:E ratio is obtained by adjusting the inspiratory time relative to the number of breaths per minute. The inspiratory flow determines the rate at which gas is delivered to the bellows housing during the inspiratory time and hence the compression of the bellows; it is essentially used to set the tidal volume. However, like many other ventilators, these dials are independent of one another and changes in one will independently affect various respiratory parameters. For example, increasing inspiratory time or inspiratory flow rate will both increase tidal volume. Adjusting the breaths per minute will not alter tidal volume but will affect the I:E ratio. Changes should be made carefully with all ventilators and an immediate reassessment of ventilator parameters (tidal volume, peak airway pressures, I:E ratio) should be made following all adjustments.

The transport button is pneumatically operated and can be used to ventilate a patient should electrical power be interrupted or temporarily unavailable. When the button is depressed it delivers gas into the bellows housing, compressing the bellows until the button is released or when it exceeds the pressure relief valve limits. This button can be activated at any point during the ventilator cycle, making it possible to deliver 'stacked' breaths (potentially leading to the delivery of an excessively large breath). The adjustable pressure relief valve adapted between the driving gas port of the control unit and the bellows housing limits the maximum pressure that can be generated by the driving gas helping to eliminate the possibility of patient barotrauma. The valve when closed will open at 60 cmH_2O (±5 cmH_2O) but can be adjusted to open at incrementally lower pressures down to almost 0 cmH_2O. Three sizes of interchangeable bellows (300, 1500, 3000 mL) are available to facilitate ventilation in various sizes of patients. The ventilator spill valve compensates for the continuous entry of fresh gas into the breathing system, and the resistance of the spill valve creates a PEEP of 2–3 cmH_2O. An MRI-compatible ventilator model (SAV 2550) is also available but it differs considerably from the SAV 2500 and is not discussed here.

Before using the ventilator, connections to the gas supply and scavenger system should be made, and the appropriate pre-use checkout procedures followed. Assuming proper functioning of the anesthesia machine, breathing system, and ventilator, the following is a reasonable operational approach for this ventilator with a circle breathing system:

1 The adjustable pressure relief valve can be set to open at the desired level. Although this is not absolutely necessary, setting it to a reasonable opening pressure (30–40 cmH_2O) can help minimize the risk of accidental ventilator-induced barotrauma.
2 Corrugated tubing from the ventilator's breathing system connector is attached to the circle system's reservoir-bag mount, and the ventilator is attached to the scavenger system.
3 The circle system's pop-off (APL) valve is closed.
4 The ventilator's breaths per minute is set to the desired frequency.
5 The ventilator's inspiratory time is set. When the dial is turned to the 12 o'clock position (marked by an asterisk), the inspiratory time will be approximately 1 s.
6 The inspiratory flow dial should be set to a low setting initially to avoid delivering an inadvertently large tidal volume to the patient and the ventilator should be switched on. The inspiratory flow control dial is adjusted to produce a flow of gas during inspiration that produces the desired tidal volume and/or peak inspiratory pressure.
7 Make final adjustments to inspiratory flow rate, inspiratory time, and breaths per minute to meet the needs of the patient.

Vetronics Merlin small animal ventilator

The Merlin is a computer-controlled small animal ventilator designed specifically for small animal practice (Fig. 3.81). It is capable of delivering tidal volumes from 1 to 800 mL. The Merlin differs from most other commonly used veterinary ventilators in that it is piston driven and can be computer controlled. The ventilator is classified as single-circuit and electronically time-, pressure-, or volume-cycled with a piston drive mechanism using a ventilator chamber; it is electrically powered and driven and computer controlled. The actual ventilation delivery system works similarly to a large syringe controlled precisely by a computer or microprocessor. The ventilator is capable of providing both controlled and assist modes of ventilation. The ventilator can be configured for use with

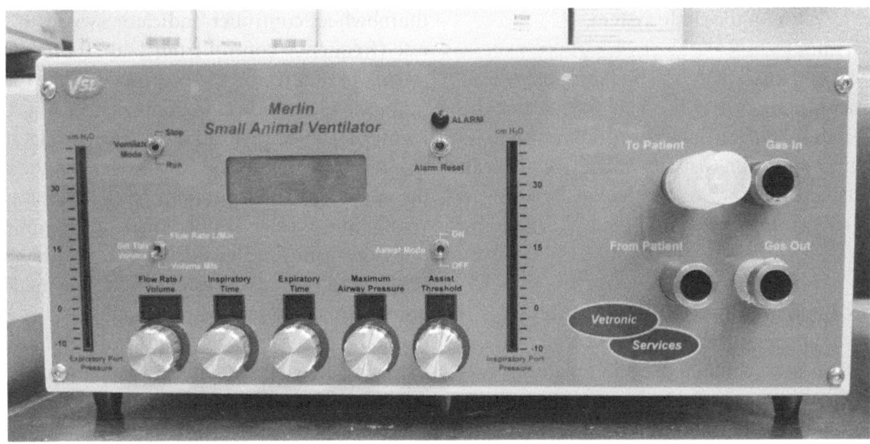

Figure 3.81 The front of the Merlin small animal ventilator showing its various control dials and connection points to the breathing circuit. It is important to note that for proper operation a one-way valve must always be in place on the 'To Patient' port. Source: Craig Mosley, Mosley Veterinary Anesthesia Services, Rockwood, ON, Canada.

both rebreathing and non-rebreathing systems and does not require a separate gas supply, it only uses gas from the patient circuit and the electronically controlled piston to produce ventilation. In order to function properly when used with a non-rebreathing circuit, it is necessary to ensure that anesthetic machine fresh gas flow rates slightly exceed the minute ventilation delivered by the ventilator.

The ventilator control panel includes (see Fig. 3.81) flow rate/volume control (0.1–25 L/min or 1–800 mL), inspiratory time control (0.1–9.1 s), expiratory time control (0.1–9.1 s), maximum airway pressure (1–60 cmH_2O), assist threshold (−1 to −10 cmH_2O), ventilate mode switch (run–stop), and tidal volume set switch (volume or flow rate). Through the use of the various controls, the ventilator can be set to deliver a tidal volume limited by volume, time, or pressure variables. The volume-limited control mode is generally the easiest and most intuitive to use for most anesthetists. However, the ability to use it as a pressure-limited ventilator and in assist mode may be useful under specific circumstances. The front panel also contains a liquid crystal display screen that shows the following: tidal volume, minute volume, I:E ratio, respiratory rate, measure airway pressure, measure system compliance, and causes of alarm conditions. There are also two pressure monitors that show airway pressures in the inspiratory and expiratory limbs of the anesthetic circuit. There are four standard 22 mm stainless-steel tapered fittings to connect the breathing system to the ventilator labeled gas-in, gas-out, patient gas delivery and patient gas exhaust. A non-return one-way valve must also be placed in the inspiratory limb to ensure unidirectional gas flow.

It is important to be completely familiar with the operation and limitations of any piece of anesthetic equipment prior to using it with a patient. If the anesthesia machine, breathing system, and ventilator are all in proper working order as indicated by pre-use checkout procedures and the ventilator is being used in volume-limited control mode, the following guidelines are appropriate for use of the ventilator:

1 Properly connect the electric power sources for the ventilator.
2 Ensure the ventilator is in stop mode, tidal volume is in volume mode and the assist setting is off.
3 Set the desired tidal volume (10–20 mL/kg), inspiratory time (1–2 s), expiratory time (1–4 s), and maximum airway pressure (20–30 cmH_2O). It is not necessary to set the assist threshold unless this mode is being used.
4 Make the appropriate connections from the ventilator to the anesthetic machine and patient as described by the manufacturer. This includes placement of the one-way non-return valve on the patient inspiratory limb. The reservoir bag should remain in place and the adjustable pressure-limiting valve (pop-off valve) should NOT be closed.
5 Switch the ventilator to run mode.
6 Make final adjustments to tidal volume, inspiratory time, and expiratory time to meet the needs of the patient.

Dräger Large Animal Anesthesia Ventilator

This ventilator is included as a part of the Narkovet-E Large Animal Anesthesia Machine; the entire system is called the Narkovet-E Large Animal Anesthesia Control Center. The ventilator was not marketed as a stand-alone unit for large animal anesthesia. Although they are no longer being manufactured, some of these ventilator–anesthesia machine combinations remain in use in veterinary hospitals. The ventilator is powered pneumatically, generally at a pressure of 50 psi. It is classed as double-circuit, tidal volume preset, time-cycled, and pneumatically driven with a descending/hanging bellows, and it uses fluidic circuitry. The controls include an on–off switch, a tidal volume control with a scale of 4–15 L on the bellows housing, a frequency control (6–18 breaths/min), and a flow control knob that determines inspiratory flow (a combination of flow and maximum pressure being delivered to the bellows compartment); the manufacturer recommends that the flow setting be adjusted so that the bellows always reaches the upper stop. The I:E ratio of 1:2 is preset.

Before using the ventilator, the proper connections to the gas supply and scavenger system should be made, and the appropriate pre-use checkout procedures should be performed. The instruction manual for ventilators includes a standard pre-use check for the ventilator. The following is a logical approach to the operation of the ventilator with a circle breathing system:

1 Connect the compressed gas supply hose to the ventilator.
2 Adjust the tidal volume control to the appropriate setting for the patient and ensure that the self-locking mechanism is engaged to prevent inadvertent movement of the bellows stop plate during use.
3 Attach the corrugated breathing hose from the bellows to the reservoir-bag port of the circle system.

4 Close the pop-off (APL) valve on the circle system.
5 Turn the power switch on.
6 Adjust the frequency control knob to the desired respiratory rate.
7 Adjust the flow control knob so that the bellows reaches the upper stop at end inspiration. If the bellows does not return to its original position during expiration (usually indicative of a leak in the patient circuit), the bellows can be filled by using a higher flow from the oxygen flowmeter, and the leak should be corrected.

Narkovet- E Electronic Large Animal Control Center

This is a combination of Dräger's Narkovet E-2 Large Animal Anesthesia System (anesthesia machine and circle breathing system) with a Dräger AV-E ventilator (Fig. 3.82). The ventilator is not available as a stand-alone unit for large animals and is no longer being manufactured, but machines are still in use. The ventilator is classified as double-circuit, tidal volume preset, and time-cycled, with a descending bellows. The ventilator is electronically controlled and pneumatically driven. It is powered electrically and pneumatically (40–60 psi with oxygen, but air is an option). The controls include an on–off switch, a self-locking knob located below the bellows assembly to control the tidal volume (4–15 L), a

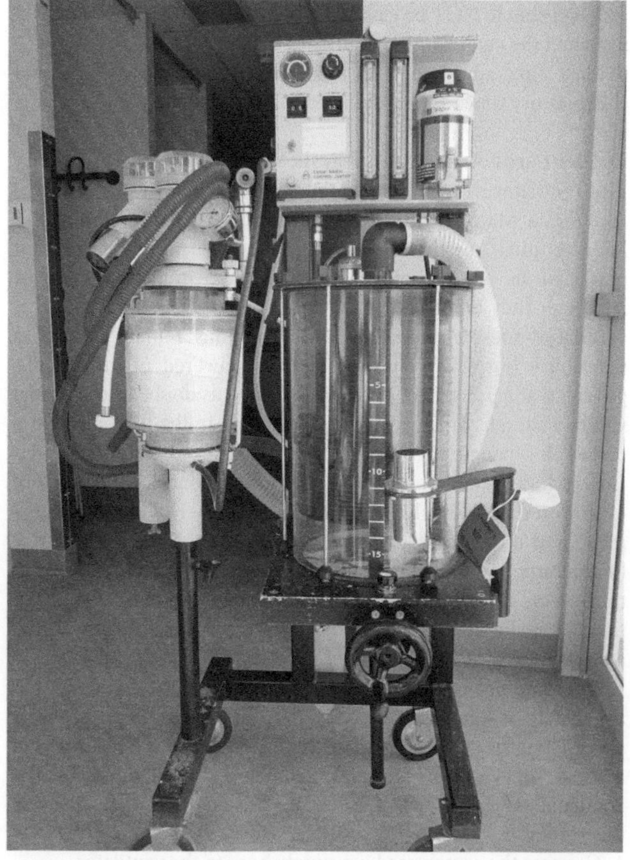

Figure 3.82 The Dräger Narkovet-E Electronic Large Animal Control Center: the bellows and bellows housing with markings for tidal volume (4–15 L), the corrugated breathing hose from the bellows to the circle system (behind the bellows housing), and the self-locking knob or wheel (bottom center) for selection of tidal volume. The controls are located above the bellows on the left. Source: Craig Mosley, Mosley Veterinary Anesthesia Services, Rockwood, ON, Canada.

thumbwheel controller–indicator switch to adjust the respiratory rate (frequency control from 1 to 30 breaths/min), a flow control setting to determine the inspiratory flow rate, and the I:E control (a thumbwheel indicator–controller to adjust the I:E ratio in increments of 0.5 from 1:1 to 1:4.5). The manufacturer recommends that the flow control knob be adjusted so that the bellows always reaches the upper stop of inspiration. The ventilator provides for controlled ventilation; assisted ventilation is not an option.

Before using the ventilator, the proper connections to the gas supply and scavenger system should be made, and the appropriate pre-use checkout procedures should be performed. The instruction manual for the ventilator includes a standard pre-use checklist. The following is a step-by-step approach to the operation of the ventilator with a circle breathing system:

1 Connect the gas supply (oxygen hose) to the anesthesia machine and ventilator.
2 Adjust the tidal volume control to the appropriate setting for the patient and ensure that the self-locking mechanism is engaged to prevent inadvertent movement of the bellows stop plate.
3 Select the desired frequency of ventilation.
4 Select the desired I:E ratio.
5 Attach the corrugated breathing hose from the bellows to the reservoir bag port of the circle system.
6 Close the pop-off (APL) valve on the circle system.
7 Turn the power supply switch on.
8 Adjust the flow control knob so that the bellows reaches the upper stop at end inspiration. If the bellows does not return to its original location during expiration, it can be filled by increasing the flow from the oxygen flowmeter.

Mallard Medical Rachel Model 2800 series anesthesia ventilator

This ventilator (Fig. 3.83) is a microprocessor-based, electronic control system used to control ventilation in large animals being maintained on circle breathing systems. The 2800 series has been upgraded since its initial introduction. The earlier Models 2800A and 2800B of the series are still widely used in veterinary practice; the most recent Model 2800C features updated electronics and display and an optional air flowmeter for controlling F_IO_2, and the bellows is reduced from 21 to 18 L, but it retains all the performance of the earlier models and is functionally very similar. The ventilator is currently available as part of a complete large animal anesthetic machine and circle system breathing circuit. The stand for the ventilator and the bellows is designed for the attachment of a circle breathing system and two vaporizers for inhalant anesthetics, and it has shelves to accommodate physiological monitoring devices. The ventilator is classified as dual-circuit and time-cycled and it is pneumatically driven and electronically controlled with an ascending (standing) bellows configuration.

Most of the functional considerations for the Model 2800C are similar to those for the Model 2400V used for small animal applications. The control console for the 2800C is located above the bellows housing instead of below the housing as it is in the 2400V, and LED displays are employed as they are in the 2400V. The ventilator is controlled by a microprocessor, but the pneumatics have been modified for generation of greater inspiratory flow rates, which are adjustable from 10 to 600 L/min. The control dials include flow rate dial (10–660 L/min), inspiratory time, respiratory rate (2–15 breaths per minute), a power switch (off–on–standby), and a manual ventilation button. The tidal volume is controlled by adjusting the flow rate dial until the desired tidal volume is obtained (read from the

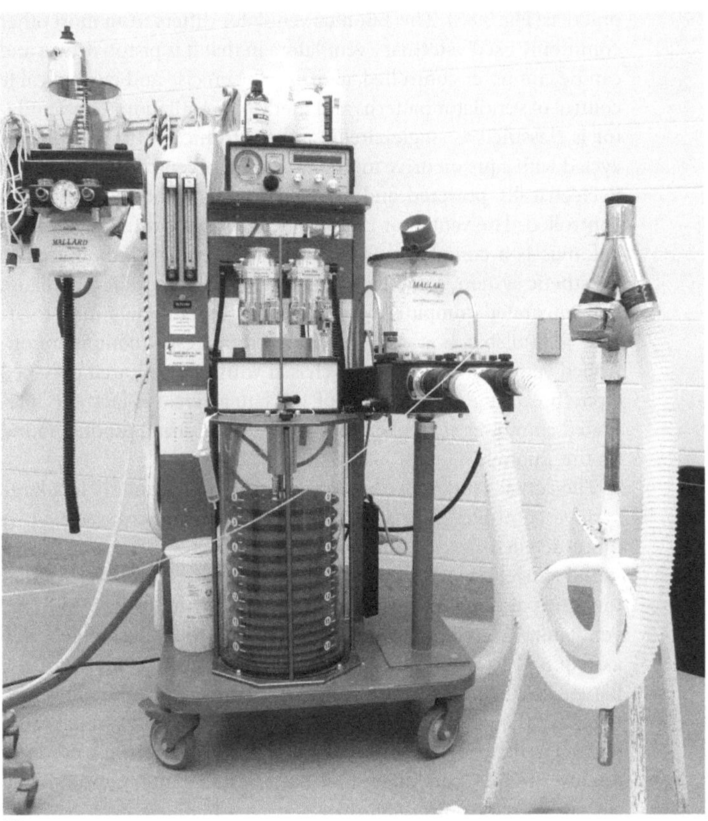
(a)

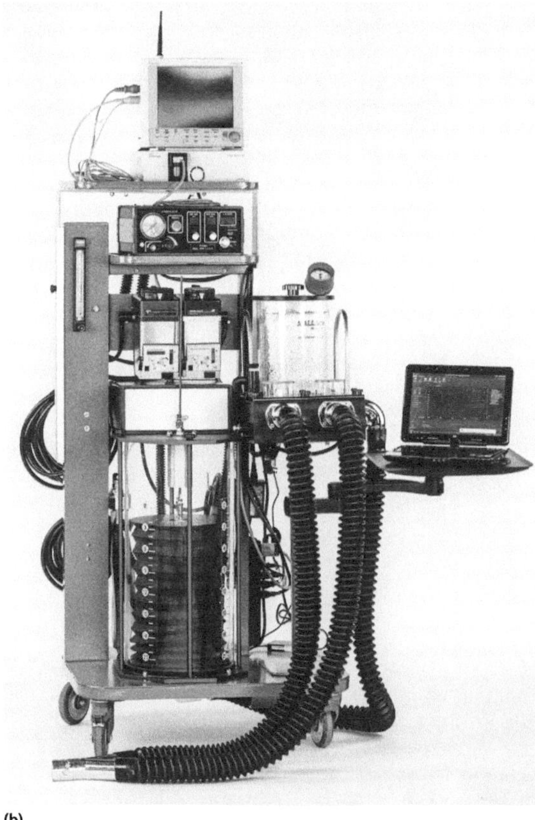
(b)

Figure 3.83 The Mallard 2800 large animal anesthetic machine and ventilator is available with an optional small animal circuit and ventilator, mounted on the top left of the machine in (a). The ventilator uses the same control system as the large animal ventilator. The Mallard 2800 is also available in many custom configurations as shown in (b). Source: part a, Craig Mosley, Mosley Veterinary Anesthesia Services, Rockwood, ON, Canada. Source, part b: Ron E. Mandsager, College of Veterinary Medicine, Oregon State University, Veterinary Teaching Hospital, Corvallis, OR, USA. Reproduced with permission of Ron E. Mandsager.

bellows canister) and the I:E ratio is calculated based on the selected inspiratory time and respiratory rate. The manual ventilation button will deliver the selected flow rate to compress the bellows as long as it is depressed and will operate even in circumstances where power is unavailable. The bellows (18 or 21 L) is standing and ascends during expiration. Like other ventilators with standing bellows, the Model 2800C produces PEEP. This is a result of the above atmospheric pressure required to activate (open) the spill valve(s) in order to offset the effect of gravity due to the weight of the bellows. The spill valves of the 2800C are unique in that they are a pair of spring-activated valves located on the top of the bellows and are activated to open only once the bellows reaches maximum ascension and the pin in the top of the spill valves is depressed, opening the valves (Fig. 3.84). The gas exiting the spill valves is then exhausted into a hollow cylinder located at the top of the bellows housing and removed. The pressure to activate the spill valves, resulting in PEEP, is between 4 and 6 cmH_2O. The amount of PEEP can also be controlled by a pneumatic vacuum pump on the 2800C: the pump creates negative pressure between the bellows and the bellows housing during the expiratory phase of ventilation and functions to reduce the level of PEEP according to the adjustments made by the operator. An ambient end-expiratory pressure may be achieved, although activation of this function is rarely needed and indeed the PEEP provided by the ventilator may even be beneficial. The patient is often allowed to breathe spontaneously through the bellows even if the ventilator is off or in standby mode as the work of breathing is not significantly increased; this avoids the need to use a reservoir bag and disconnect and reconnect should ventilation be required. The hosing from the bellows to the circle system can be removed, facilitating drainage of moisture from the machine. There is also a 'holding' assembly located on the top of the bellows that can be used to hold the bellows fully inflated when not in use to facilitate drying of the bellows. An MRI-compatible model is also available.

Before using the ventilator, the proper connections to the gas and electric power supplies and the scavenger system should be made, and the appropriate pre-use checkout procedures should be performed for all equipment. The following is a reasonable operational approach for the Model 2800C ventilator with a circle breathing system:

1 Place the master switch in the standby mode and dial the desired settings for respiratory rate and inspiratory time, according to the patient's needs.
2 Set the inspiratory flow control to the desired rate of flow – low, medium, or high – depending on the patient's needs; it is generally best to start at the low or medium rate to ensure excessive tidal volumes are not inadvertently administered.
3 Connect the corrugated tubing from the ventilator's bellows to the circle system's reservoir-bag mount and the ventilator exhalation port to the scavenger system. Close the circle system's

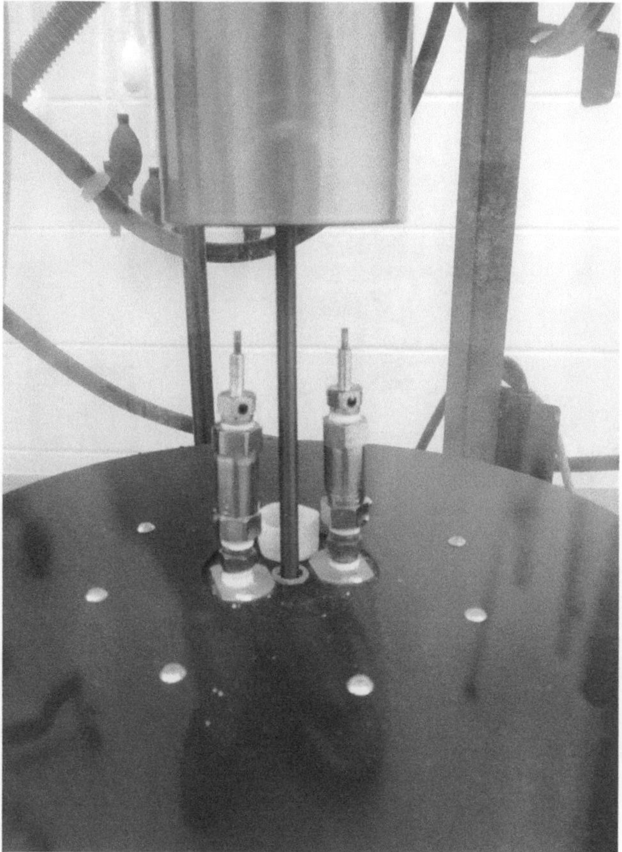

Figure 3.84 The ventilator spill valves of the Mallard Model 2800 are situated on the top of the bellows (spindle-shaped stainless-steel fixtures on top of the bellows) within the ventilator canister. When the bellows reaches full ascent, a pin in the top of the spill valve is depressed, allowing excess gas flow to escape. Note the stainless-steel cylinder (above the spill valves) in the top of the bellows housing into which the excess gas is evacuated. Source: Craig Mosley, Mosley Veterinary Anesthesia Services, Rockwood, ON, Canada.

pop-off (APL) valve and release the ventilator's bellows. Ensure that the bellows is fully inflated and positioned at zero. Under normal use circumstances, the ventilator often remains continuously connected to the breathing circuit for convenience during a case as the patient can breathe through the bellows in this configuration standing (ascending) without any additional effort.

4 Turn the master switch on, and inspiration should begin.
5 If the bellows does not return to zero, this may suggest a leak in the system; the bellows can be filled by turning up the flowmeter or alternatively by using the flush valve, and the leak should be identified and corrected. If the flush valve is used to fill the bellows, the anesthetic concentration in the breathing circuit will be reduced.
6 The flow rate, inspiratory time, and respiratory rate can then be further adjusted to produce the appropriate ventilator parameters for the patient.
7 Finally, if desired, the PEEP control can be adjusted to set the desired end-expiratory pressure.

Hallowell Tafonius and Tafonius Junior

The Tafonius ventilator is a microprocessor/computer-controlled large animal ventilator designed specifically for large animal practice (Fig. 3.85). The Tafonius ventilator differs from most other commonly used veterinary ventilators in that it is piston driven and can be computer controlled, allowing for precise and customizable control of ventilator patterns and modes of ventilation. The ventilator is classified as single-circuit and electronically timed, volume-cycled with a piston drive mechanism using a ventilator chamber; it is electrically powered and driven and microprocessor/computer controlled. The ventilator is available in several configurations; the Tafonius is a complete anesthetic workstation (including a circle anesthetic system, complete patient monitoring module, ventilator, and integrated computer controller) and the Tafonius Junior version is available as a stand-alone microprocessor/computer-controlled ventilator or can be purchased with the Hallowell designed circle breathing system; both of the latter versions lack the integrated computer controller and patient monitoring module found on the Tafonius.

The actual ventilation delivery system works similarly to a large syringe controlled precisely by a computer or microprocessor. A more detailed description of the piston drive mechanism can be found above. It is important to note that similarly to other ventilators, the patient can breathe spontaneously while connected to the ventilator. The piston in the ventilator will move instantaneously as required to maintain an airway pressure near 0 cmH_2O at the patient circuit Y-piece. Although a reservoir-bag attachment is provided, it is not necessary to use it if spontaneous ventilation is desired in the patient. As the ventilator requires electronic power to operate, there is an integrated battery and battery monitoring system should a power failure occur.

The ventilator is capable of providing both controlled and assist modes of ventilation. Control of the ventilator is accomplished via the ventilator's auxiliary computer/microprocessor (Tafonius and Tafonius Junior) or via the integrated computer running the Tafonius system software found on the standard (complete) Tafonius anesthetic workstation. With appropriate programming, the integrated computer and Tafonius software could be used to customize ventilator control to produce nearly limitless breathing patterns. Primary ventilator control is achieved by altering the following parameters: tidal volume (0.1–20 L), respiratory rate (1–20 breaths/min), inspiratory time (0.5–4.0 s), and maximum work pressure limit (10–80 cmH_2O). The microprocessor will automatically determine expiratory time and inspiratory flow rate based on these preset parameters within the limits of the equipment (maximum inspiratory flow rate 900 L/min and minimum expiratory time 0.5 s). Other ventilation controls include user-defined assist mode and CPAP/PEEP. There is also a dump valve button that functions as an electronic pop-off or spill valve found on conventional ventilators and a buffer volume button used to determine the size of the 'virtual' reservoir bag. A detailed operational description of this ventilator is beyond the scope of this discussion as it will depend on the specific ventilator configuration being used (Tafonius or Tafonius Junior) and whether the ventilator is being controlled using the auxiliary ventilator control panel or the integrated computer system running the Tafonius software. However, ease of use of the ventilator is very comparable to that of other ventilators.

Before using the ventilator, the proper connections to the gas and electric power supplies and the scavenger system should be made. It is necessary for the Tafonius ventilators to perform an automatic start-up checkout procedure that calibrates the pressure transducers, initializes the piston, and leak tests the machine. The results of this self-test will display on the auxiliary control screen and/or the integrated computer.

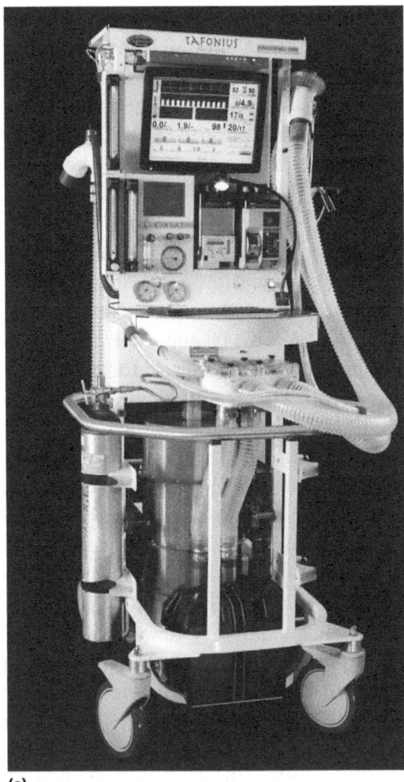

(a)

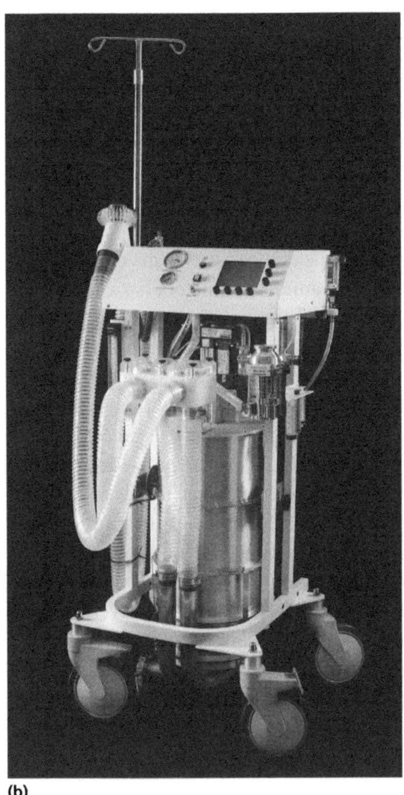

(b)

Figure 3.85 The Tafonius (a) and Tafonuis Junior (b) are microprocessor/computer-controlled piston large animal ventilators. The ventilator is available in a stand-alone configuration (Tafonius Junior) or with an integrated large animal anesthetic machine and patient monitoring system (Tafonius). Source: Hallowell EMC, Pittsfield, MA, USA. Reproduced with permission of Hallowell EMC.

Surgivet DHV1000 large animal ventilator

This large animal specific ventilator can be purchased as a stand-alone ventilator compatible for use with any standard large animal anesthesia machine or purchased as part of a complete anesthesia workstation (LDS 3000 Large animal anesthesia Machine) (Fig. 3.86). The ventilator is classified as dual-circuit, tidal volume preset/limited, and time-cycled and is pneumatically driven and electronically controlled with a descending/hanging bellows configuration.

The controls on the control module include power switch (on–off), respiratory rate dial, inspiratory time dial, flow dial (inspiratory gas flow), and a manual ventilation button. There is also a turn wheel located on the side of the control module used to adjust the maximum descent of the bellows.

Before using the ventilator, the proper connections to the gas supply and scavenger system should be made, and the appropriate pre-use checkout procedures should be performed. The instruction manual for the ventilator includes a standard pre-use checklist. The following is a step-by-step approach to the operation of the ventilator with a circle breathing system:

1 Connect the gas supply (oxygen hose) to the anesthesia machine and ventilator.
2 Adjust the tidal volume control wheel to the appropriate setting for the patient.
3 Select the desired respiratory rate.
4 Select the desired inspiratory time.
5 Attach the corrugated breathing hose from the bellows to the reservoir-bag port of the circle system.
6 Close the pop-off (APL) valve on the circle system.

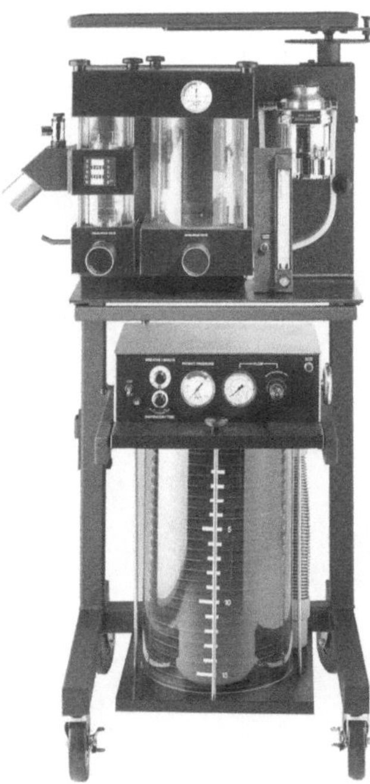

Figure 3.86 The Surgivet DHV large animal ventilator can be purchased alone or as part of a complete large animal workstation as shown here. In this configuration, the ventilator unit is mounted on the machine cart below the large animal circle. Source: Smith Medical, Norwell, MA, USA. Reproduced with permission of Smith Medical.

7 Turn the power supply switch on.
8 Adjust the flow control knob so that the bellows reaches the upper stop at end inspiration.
9 The flow rate, inspiratory time, and respiratory rate can then be further adjusted to produce the appropriate ventilator parameters for the patient.

Bird Mark respirator-driven ventilators

The Bird Mark 7 respirator was one of the first systems used to drive and control both small and large animal ventilators (so-called 'bag-in-a-barrel' ventilators) and are still being used today (Fig. 3.87). The Bird Mark 7 was originally developed as a single-circuit respirator for humans and was not designed principally as an anesthetic ventilator; however, by applying the respirator function to a bag or bellows in a 'box or barrel,' a dual-circuit ventilator is created.

Uniquely, Bird respirator-driven ventilators can be used in control, assist, or assist-control modes and have the capability of limiting tidal volume based on airway pressure. This differs from most contemporary ventilators that only offer control modes of ventilation and tend to limit tidal volume based on the volume of gas delivered. Bird Mark 7 respirators are used to control and drive both JD Medical's LAV-2000 and -3000 series large animal ventilators. Although other Bird respirator-driven ventilators are not discussed here, the general principles of operation are similar although the design details may vary significantly.

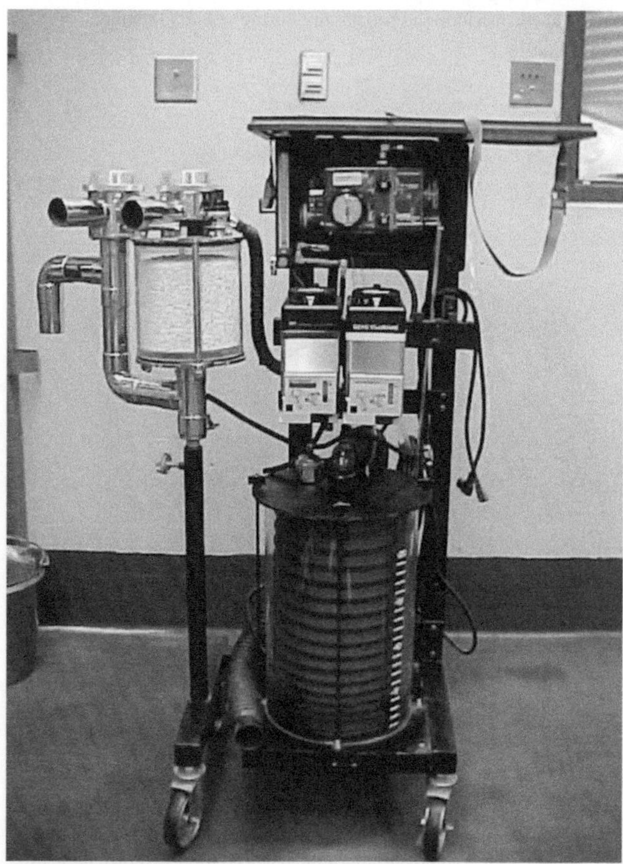

Figure 3.87 An example of a Bird Mark 7 respirator being used as the controller of a large animal anesthesia ventilator. Source: Thomas Riebold, College of Veterinary Medicine, Oregon State University, Corvallis, OR, USA. Reproduced with permission of Thomas Riebold.

The JD Medical LAV-3000 is a stand-alone ventilator that can be used with any LA anesthetic machine and the LAV-2000 is an integrated ventilator and anesthesia machine available in several predesigned and custom configurations. The LAVC-2000 and -3000 systems can be converted to a 5 L system for use in foals by adding a 5000 mL bellows and a canister (bellows housing) insert. A modified Mark 7 respirator drives the bellows in the ventilator system. When the system is operating, the Bird ventilator supplies gas to pressurize the space between the bellows and the bellows housing (canister) to force the bellows in an upward motion delivering gases from the bellows, through the interface hose, to the breathing system. The LAVC-2000 and -3000 are classified as dual-circuit, pressure-limited, and time-cycled and are pneumatically controlled and driven with a descending/hanging bellows configuration.

The controls on a Bird Mark 7 (Fig 3.88) inspiratory pressure, inspiratory flow rate, expiratory time (apnea control), and inspiratory sensitivity. In addition, a manometer, a hand timer (push-pull mechanism) used to manually initiate/end respiration, and a DISS connector for the source of pneumatic power are features of the ventilator. With the modified Bird Mark 7, inspiratory pressure can be varied from 5 to 65 cm H_2O, inspiratory sensitivity from −0.5 to −5 cm H_2O, expiratory time from 5 to 15 s, and inspiratory flow from 0 to over 450 L/min. The pneumatic power source should be delivered to the inlet of the ventilator at 50 psi. The bellows can deliver a tidal volume of up to 20 L. Inspiration can be started or stopped by use of a hand timer. The Bird Mark 7 is a pressure-cycled ventilator unless the push-pull manual cycling rod is pulled out, which causes the ventilator to be time cycled.

Before using the Model LAV-3000 ventilator for controlling ventilation during anesthesia, the power-supply and scavenger system should be connected, and the appropriate pre-use checkout procedures should be performed for all equipment. The following is a reasonable operational approach for the ventilator with a circle breathing system in the control mode:

1 Set the inspiratory sensitivity control to a high setting to minimize the possibility of patient-initiated ventilation.
2 Set the inspiratory pressure control to the range 20–30 cmH_2O and readjust the setting to achieve the desired tidal volume after steps 5 and 6 have been completed.

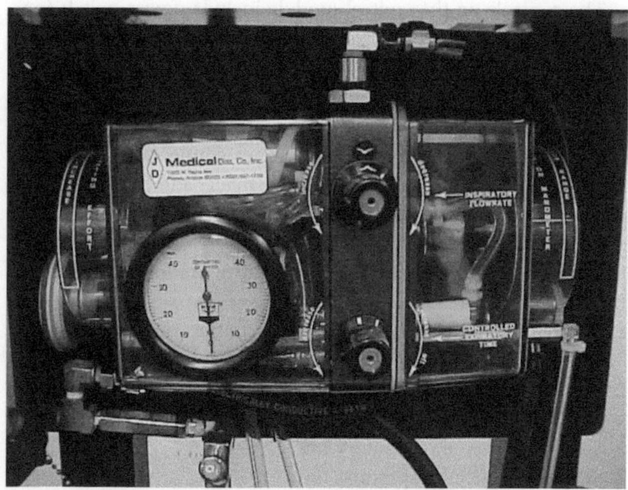

Figure 3.88 A Bird Mark 7 respirator showing the various controls used to control a ventilator. Source: Thomas Riebold, College of Veterinary Medicine, Oregon State University, Corvallis, OR, USA. Reproduced with permission of Thomas Riebold.

3 Connect the corrugated hose (interface hose) from the bellows to the reservoir-bag port of the circle system.
4 Close the pop-off (APL) valve of the circle system. Then, the bellows may need to be filled by increasing the flow of oxygen to the patient circuit (oxygen flowmeter on the anesthesia machine).
5 Turn the inspiratory flow control on to start the ventilator and set the flow control to deliver a tidal volume in approximately 1.5–3.0 s.
6 Set the expiratory time control to establish a respiratory rate appropriate for the patient, often 7–10 breaths/min.
7 For final settings, the operator should understand that there are interactions between the controls on a Bird ventilator (e.g., changing inspiratory flow may affect respiratory rate and vice versa).

Respiratory assist devices

Several types and brands of respiratory assist devices are available. Some are completely manual in operation (resuscitation bags with one-way valves) and some use compressed gas (oxygen) to assist ventilation (demand valves). The mechanics of these devices have been reviewed [2].

Manual resuscitators

A manual resuscitator is appropriate for application of IPPV to small veterinary patients. Several brands of resuscitators are available. The basic components of a manual resuscitator are a compressible self-expanding bag, a bag-refill valve, and a non-rebreathing valve. Some resuscitators can be attached to a source of oxygen to enrich the oxygen content of inspired gases (Fig. 3.89). Manual resuscitators can be fitted with a reservoir to serve as a source of oxygen when the oxygen flow to the resuscitator does not meet the filling demands of the resuscitator.

Demand valves

A demand valve can be used to deliver intermittent positive pressure ventilation (Fig. 3.90). The demand valve is set to deliver oxygen when the patient begins to inspire (creating slight negative pressure activating gas delivery) until exhalation starts or until a certain preset pressure is reached. Expiration is passive through the valve outlet. The outlet may be restrictive to expiration in large patients. The device can be disconnected from the endotracheal tube after inspiration to decrease the resistance to exhalation. A demand valve can be triggered manually to deliver oxygen to the patient as long as the activation button is held down or until the preset pressure limit is reached. Alternately compressing and releasing the control button allows application of IPPV. A demand valve with the capacity for a high inspiratory flow rate is most desirable for use in large animals; demand valves generating low inspiratory flows will cause an excessively long inspiratory time in patients requiring a large tidal volume.

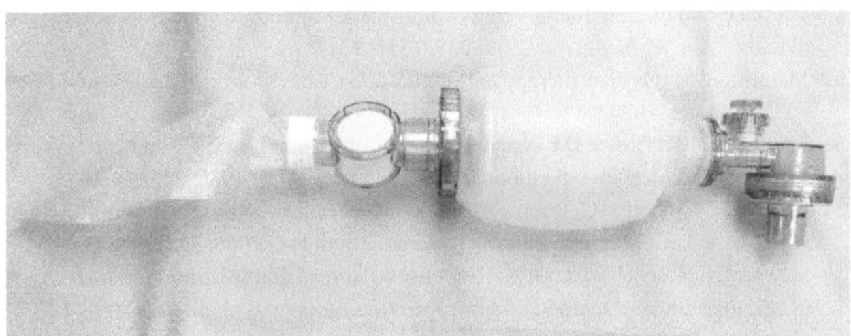

Figure 3.89 An example of a resuscitation bag suitable for use in veterinary medicine. This bag also has an expandable reservoir (left of image) to serve as a reservoir of enriched gas if being used with supplemental oxygen. However, it is important to note that resuscitation bags do not require supplemental gas delivery for use. Source: Craig Mosley, Mosley Veterinary Anesthesia Services, Rockwood, ON, Canada.

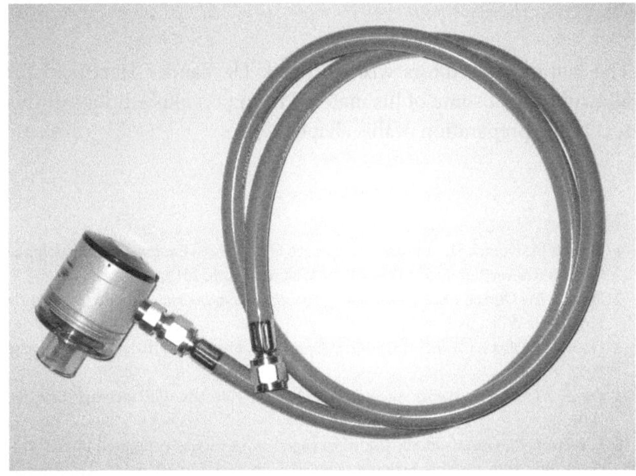

Figure 3.90 A demand valve is an oxygen delivery system that can be used to perform manual intermittent positive pressure ventilation. Sourc: Craig Mosley, Mosley Veterinary Anesthesia Services, Rockwood, ON, Canada.

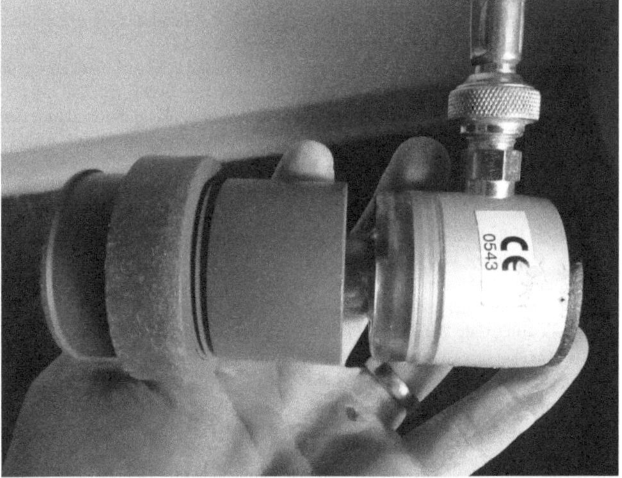

Figure 3.91 Demand valves are normally designed to fit standard endotracheal tube adapters. Large animal-specific adapters are normally required for use with the funnel-type (shown) or 22 mm O.D. stainless-steel adapters normally associated with large animal endotracheal tubes. Source: Craig Mosley, Mosley Veterinary Anesthesia Services, Rockwood, ON, Canada.

Demand valves are available from various manufacturers. Most will deliver a maximum flow rate of approximately 160 L/min at 50 psi and are frequently available as a low-flow model (40 L/min). The high-flow models are most suitable for large animal veterinary applications. The Hudson demand valve has been described for use in horses but is no longer readily available [76]. It delivers approximately 200 L/min if the oxygen-supply pressure is 50 psi and more than 275 L/min if the supply pressure is 80 psi. Demand valves are normally designed to accept a standard endotracheal tube connector (15 mm O.D.) and a standard face mask (22 mm O.D.), although various adapters are available in veterinary medicine for large animal endotracheal tube adapters (funnel-type and stainless-steel 22 mm O.D. adapters) (Fig. 3.91).

Acknowledgement

The author and editors wish to thank Dr. Sandee Hartsfield for allowing use of some of his material from previous editions of this text in the preparation of this chapter.

References

1 Dorsch JA, Dorsch SE. *A Practical Approach to Anesthesia Equipment*. Philadelphia: Wolters Kluwer/Lippincott Williams & Wilkins Health, 2010.

2 Dorsch JA, Dorsch SE. *Understanding Anesthesia Equipment*, 5th edn. New York: Lippincott Williams & Wilkins, 2008.

3 Davey AJ, Diba A. *Ward's Anaesthetic Equipment*, 6th edn. Philadelphia: Saunders, 2012.

4 Davey AJ, Diba A. *Ward's Anaesthetic Equipment*, 5th edn. Philadelphia: Elsevier, 2005.

5 Fulkerson PJ, Gustafson SB. Use of laryngeal mask airway compared to endotracheal tube with positive-pressure ventilation in anesthetized swine. *Vet Anaesth Analg* 2007; **34**: 284–288.

6 Cassu RN, Luna SP, Teixeira Neto FJ, *et al*. Evaluation of laryngeal mask as an alternative to endotracheal intubation in cats anesthetized under spontaneous or controlled ventilation. *Vet Anaesth Analg* 2004; **31**: 213–221.

7 Wiederstein I, Auer U, Moens Y. Laryngeal mask airway insertion requires less propofol than endotracheal intubation in dogs. *Vet Anaesth Analg* 2006; **33**: 201–206.

8 Wiederstein I, Moens YP. Guidelines and criteria for the placement of laryngeal mask airways in dogs. *Vet Anaesth Analg* 2008; **35**: 374–382.

9 Kazakos GM, Anagnostou T, Savvas I, *et al*. Use of the laryngeal mask airway in rabbits: placement and efficacy. *Lab Anim (NY)* 2007; **36**: 29–34.

10 Stewart SL, Secrest JA, Norwood BR, *et al*. A comparison of endotracheal tube cuff pressures using estimation techniques and direct intracuff measurement. *AANA J* 2003; **71**: 443–447.

11 Mitchell SL, McCarthy R, Rudloff E, *et al*. Tracheal rupture associated with intubation in cats: 20 cases (1996–1998). *J Am Vet Med Assoc* 2000; **216**: 1592–1595.

12 Jackson J, Richter KP, Launer DP. Thoracoscopic partial pericardiectomy in 13 dogs. *J Vet Intern Med* 1999; **13**: 529–533.

13 Radlinsky MG, Mason DE, Biller DS, *et al*. Thoracoscopic visualization and ligation of the thoracic duct in dogs. *Vet Surg* 2002; **31**: 138–146.

14 Mayhew PD, Culp WT, Pascoe PJ, *et al*. Evaluation of blind thoracoscopic-assisted placement of three double-lumen endobronchial tube designs for one-lung ventilation in dogs. *Vet Surg* 2012; **41**: 664–670.

15 Cantwell SL, Duke T, Walsh PJ, *et al*. One-lung versus two-lung ventilation in the closed-chest anesthetized dog: a comparison of cardiopulmonary parameters. *Vet Surg* 2000; **29**: 365–373.

16 Adami C, Axiak S, Rytz U, *et al*. Alternating one lung ventilation using a double lumen endobronchial tube and providing CPAP to the non-ventilated lung in a dog. *Vet Anaesth Analg* 2011; **38**: 70–76.

17 Mayhew KN, Mayhew PD, Sorrell-Raschi L, *et al*. Thoracoscopic subphrenic pericardectomy using double-lumen endobronchial intubation for alternating one-lung ventilation. *Vet Surg* 2009; **38**: 961–966.

18 Bauquier SH, Culp WT, Lin RC, *et al*. One-lung ventilation using a wire-guided endobronchial blocker for thoracoscopic pericardial fenestration in a dog. *Can Vet J* 2010; **51**: 1135–1138.

19 Lansdowne JL, Monnet E, Twedt DC, *et al*. Thoracoscopic lung lobectomy for treatment of lung tumors in dogs. *Vet Surg* 2005; **34**: 530–535.

20 Fulkerson PJ, Gustafson SB. Use of laryngeal mask airway compared to endotracheal tube with positive-pressure ventilation in anesthetized swine. *Vet Anaesth Analg* 2007; **34**: 284–288.

21 Smith JC, Robertson LD, Auhll A, *et al*. Endotracheal tubes versus laryngeal mask airways in rabbit inhalation anesthesia: ease of use and waste gas emissions. *Contemp Top Lab Anim Sci* 2004; **43**: 22–25.

22 van Oostrom H, Krauss MW, Sap R. A comparison between the v-gel supraglottic airway device and the cuffed endotracheal tube for airway management in spontaneously breathing cats during isoflurane anaesthesia. *Vet Anaesth Analg* 2013; **40**: 265–271.

23 Wiederstein I, Moens YP. Guidelines and criteria for the placement of laryngeal mask airways in dogs. *Vet Anaesth Analg* 2008; **35**: 374–382.

24 Bateman L, Ludders JW, Gleed RD, *et al*. Comparison between facemask and laryngeal mask airway in rabbits during isoflurane anesthesia. *Vet Anaesth Analg* 2005; **32**: 280–288.

25 Johnson JA, Atkins AL, Heard DJ. Application of the laryngeal mask airway for anesthesia in three chimpanzees and one gibbon. *J Zoo Wildl Med* 2010; **41**: 535–537.

26 Cerveny SN, D'Agostino JJ, Davis MR, *et al*. Comparison of laryngeal mask airway use with endotracheal intubation during anesthesia of western lowland gorillas (*Gorilla gorilla gorilla*). *J Zoo Wildl Med* 2012; **43**: 759–767.

27 West G, Heard DJ, Caulkett N. *Zoo Animal and Wildlife Immobilization and Anesthesia*. Ames, IA: Blackwell Publishing, 2007; 718.

28 Read MR, Read EK, Duke T, *et al*. Cardiopulmonary effects and induction and recovery characteristics of isoflurane and sevoflurane in foals. *J Am Vet Med Assoc* 2002; **221**: 393–398.

29 Quandt JE, Robinson EP. Nasotracheal intubation in calves. *J Am Vet Med Assoc* 1996; **209**: 967–968.

30 Bauquier SH, Golder FJ. Extended anaesthesia and nasotracheal intubation of a red kangaroo (*Macropus rufus*). *Aust Vet J* 2010; **88**: 449–450.

31 Riebold TW, Engel HN, Grubb TL, *et al*. Orotracheal and nasotracheal intubation in llamas. *J Am Vet Med Assoc* 1994; **204**: 779–783.

32 Stephens Devalle JM. Successful management of rabbit anesthesia through the use of nasotracheal intubation. *J Am Assoc Lab Anim Sci* 2009; **48**: 166–170.

33 Hamacher J, Arras M, Bootz F, *et al*. Microscopic wire guide-based orotracheal mouse intubation: description, evaluation and comparison with transillumination. *Lab Anim* 2008; **42**: 222–230.

34 Johnson DH. Endoscopic intubation of exotic companion mammals. *Vet Clin North Am Exot Anim Pract* 2010; **13**: 273–289.

35 Byers SR, Cary JA, Farnsworth KD. Comparison of endotracheal intubation techniques in llamas. *Can Vet J* 2009; **50**: 745–749.

36 Zhao X, Wu N, Zhou J, *et al*. A technique for retrograde intubation in mice. *Lab Anim* 2006; **35**: 39–42.

37 Corleta O, Habazettl H, Kreimeier U, *et al*. Modified retrograde orotracheal intubation techniques for airway access in rabbits. *Eur Surg Res* 1992; **24**: 129–132.

38 Chesen AB, Rakestraw PC. Indications for and short- and long-term outcome of permanent tracheostomy performed in standing horses: 82 cases (1995–2005). *J Am Vet Med Assoc* 2008; **232**: 1352–1356.

39 Hedlund CS. Tracheostomy. *Probl Vet Med* 1991; **3**: 198–209.

40 McClure SR, Taylor TS, Honnas CM, *et al*. Permanent tracheostomy in standing horses: technique and results. *Vet Surg* 1995; **24**: 231–234.

41 Nichols S. Tracheotomy and tracheostomy tube placement in cattle. *Vet Clin North Am Food Anim Pract* 2008; **24**: 307–317.

42 Nicholson I, Baines S. Complications associated with temporary tracheostomy tubes in 42 dogs (1998 to 2007). *J Small Anim Pract* 2012; **53**: 108–114.

43 Hartsfield SM, Gendreau CL, Smith CW, *et al*. Endotracheal intubation by pharyngotomy. *J Am Anim Hosp Assoc* 1977; **13**: 71–74.

44 Huss BT, Anderson MA, Branson KR, *et al*. Evaluation of pulse oximeter probes and probe placement in healthy dogs. *J Am Anim Hosp Assoc* 1995; **31**: 9–14.

45 Jacobson JD, Miller MW, Matthews NS, *et al*. Evaluation of accuracy of pulse oximetry in dogs. *Am J Vet Res* 1992; **53**: 537–540.

46 Chaffin MK, Matthews NS, Cohen ND, *et al*. Evaluation of pulse oximetry in anaesthetised foals using multiple combinations of transducer type and transducer attachment site. *Equine Vet J* 1996; **28**: 437–445.

47 Koenig J, McDonell W, Valverde A. Accuracy of pulse oximetry and capnography in healthy and compromised horses during spontaneous and controlled ventilation. *Can J Vet Res* 2003; **67**: 169–174.

48 Matthews NS, Hartsfield SM, Sanders EA, *et al*. Evaluation of pulse oximetry in horses surgically treated for colic. *Equine Vet J* 1994; **26**: 114–116.

49 Nishimura R, Kim H, Matsunaga S, *et al*. Evaluation of pulse oximetry in anesthetized dogs. *J Vet Med Sci* 1991; **53**: 1117–1118.

50 Quinn CT, Raisis AL, Musk GC. Evaluation of Masimo signal extraction technology pulse oximetry in anaesthetized pregnant sheep. *Vet Anaesth Analg* 2013; **40**: 149–156.

51 Wong DM, Alcott CJ, Wang C, *et al*. Agreement between arterial partial pressure of carbon dioxide and saturation of hemoglobin with oxygen values obtained by direct arterial blood measurements versus noninvasive methods in conscious healthy and ill foals. *J Am Vet Med Assoc* 2011; **239**: 1341–1347.

52 Manning AM. Oxygen therapy and toxicity. *Vet Clin North Am Small Anim Pract* 2002; **32**: 1005–1020.

53 Fitzpatrick RK, Crowe DT. Nasal oxygen administration in dogs and cats: experimental and clinical investigations. *J Am Anim Hosp Assoc* 1986; **22**: 293–300.

54 Wilson DV, Schott HC, Robinson NE, *et al*. Response to nasopharyngeal oxygen administration in horses with lung disease. *Equine Vet J* 2006; **38**: 219–223.

55 Stewart JH, Rose RJ, Barko AM. Response to oxygen administration in foals: effect of age, duration and method of administration on arterial blood gas values. *Equine Vet J* 1984; **16**: 329–331.

56 Rose RJ, Hodgson DR, Leadon DP, *et al*. Effect of intranasal oxygen administration on arterial blood gas and acid base parameters in spontaneously delivered, term induced and induced premature foals. *Res Vet Sci* 1983; **34**: 159–162.

57 Bleul UT, Bircher BM, Kahn WK. Effect of intranasal oxygen administration on blood gas variables and outcome in neonatal calves with respiratory distress syndrome: 20 cases (2004–2006). *J Am Vet Med Assoc* 2008; **233**: 289–293.

58 Mann FA, Wagner-Mann C, Allert JA, *et al.* Comparison of intranasal and intratracheal oxygen administration in healthy awake dogs. *Am J Vet Res* 1992; **53**: 856–860.

59 Dunphy ED, Mann FA, Dodam JR, *et al.* Comparison of unilateral versus bilateral nasal catheters for oxygen administration in dogs. *J Vet Emerg Crit Care* 2002; **12**: 213–294.

60 Crowe DT. Oxygen therapy. In: Bonagura JD, Twedt DC, Hawkins EC, eds. *Kirk's Current Veterinary Therapy XIV*. St Louis, MO: Saunders Elsevier, 2009; 596–602.

61 Court MH. Respiratory support of the critically ill small animal patient. In: Murtaugh RJ, Kaplan PM, eds. *Veterinary Emergency and Critical Care Medicine.* St. Louis, MO: Mosby, 1992; 575.

62 Fairman NB. Evaluation of pulse oximetry as a continuous monitoring technique in critically ill dogs in the small animal intensive care unit. *J Vet Emerg Crit Care* 1992; **2**: 50–56.

63 Lumb AB. Hyperoxia and oxygen toxicity. *Nunn's Applied Respiratory Physiology*, 7th edn. Edinburgh: Churchill Livingstone Elsevier, 2010; 377–390.

64 Caplan RA, Vistica MF, Posner KL, *et al.* Adverse anesthetic outcomes arising from gas delivery equipment: a closed claims analysis. *Anesthesiology* 1997; **87**: 741–748.

65 Mehta SP, Eisenkraft JB, Posner KL, *et al.* Patient injuries from anesthesia gas delivery equipment: a closed claims update. *Anesthesiology* 2013; **119**: 788–795.

66 Hartsfield SM. Anesthetic machines and breathing systems. In: Tranquilli WJ, Thurmon JC, Grimm KA, eds. *Lumb and Jones' Veterinary Anesthesia and Analgesia*, 4th edn. Ames, IA: Blackwell Publishing, 2007; 453–494.

67 Dorsch JA, Dorsch SE. *Understanding Anesthesia Equipment*, 4th edn. Baltimore: Lippincott Williams & Wilkins, 1999.

68 Steffey EP, Woliner MJ, Howland D. Accuracy of isoflurane delivery by halothane-specific vaporizers. *Am J Vet Res* 1983; **44**: 1072–1078.

69 Dorsch JA, Dorsch SE. *Understanding Anesthesia Equipment: Construction, Care, and Complications*, 3rd edn. Baltimore: Williams & Wilkins, 1994.

70 Hamilton WK. Nomenclature of inhalation anesthetic systems. *Anesthesiology* 1964; **25**: 3–5.

71 Dorsch JA, Dorsch SE. The breathing sytem: general principles, common components, and classifications. *Understanding Anesthesia Equipment.* New York: Lippincott Williams & Wilkins, 2008; 191–208.

72 Kharasch ED, Powers KM, Artru AA. Comparison of Amsorb, sodalime, and Baralyme degradation of volatile anesthetics and formation of carbon monoxide and compound a in swine *in vivo*. *Anesthesiology* 2002; **96**: 173–182.

73 Higuchi H, Adachi Y, Arimura S, *et al.* The carbon dioxide absorption capacity of Amsorb is half that of soda lime. *Anesth Analg* 2001; **93**: 221–225.

74 Hartsfield SM. Anesthesia euipment. In: Carroll GL, ed. *Small Animal Anesthesia and Analgesia*. Ames, IA: Blackwell Publishing, 2008; 3–24.

75 Dorsch JA, Dorsch SE. Anesthesia ventilators. In: *Understanding Anesthetic Equipment*, 5th edn. New York: Lippincott Williams & Wilkins, 2008; 310–372.

76 Riebold TW, Evans AT, Robinson NE. Evaluation of the demand valve for resuscitation of horses. *J Am Vet Med Assoc* 1980; **176**: 623–626.

4 Monitoring Anesthetized Patients

Steve C. Haskins
School of Veterinary Medicine, University of California, Davis, California, USA

Chapter contents

Introduction

The primary focus of monitoring anesthetized patients is the assessment of (1) depth of anesthesia, (2) cardiovascular and pulmonary consequences of the anesthetized state, and (3) temperature. Too light a level of anesthesia fails to achieve all of the basic goals of anesthesia. Animals that are too deeply anesthetized may suffer adverse cardiopulmonary consequences and death. General anesthesia predisposes to hypothermia, which, in turn, predisposes to excess anesthetic depth and a number of cardiopulmonary problems. Hyperthermia is not common but, if severe, can cause widespread tissue damage.

There are many aspects of cardiovascular and pulmonary function that can be monitored. Any single measure defines only itself and cannot be used to define the overall status of the system. It is important to assess all of the available individual parameters of cardiovascular and pulmonary function, and then to form a composite estimate of overall function (Fig. 4.1). The cardiovascular system is subdivided into preload parameters ('is the pump being sufficiently primed?'), heart parameters ('is the pump pumping?'), and forward flow parameters ('are the tissues being perfused?'). Is the heart rate and rhythm satisfactory; is contractility sufficient? Of the 'forward flow' parameters, are stroke volume and cardiac output, blood pressure, vasomotor tone, and tissue perfusion adequate? How is the animal ventilating? How is it oxygenating?

Monitoring anesthetic depth

The purpose of assuring an appropriate level of anesthesia is to assure lack of patient awareness, recall, pain, and movement while avoiding excessive levels of anesthesia and its attendant problems (hypoventilation and hypoxemia; reduced cardiac output, hypotension, inadequate tissue perfusion, and prolonged recovery). Anesthetic depth is determined by: (1) the amount of anesthetic drug(s) in the brain, (2) the magnitude of surgical (or environmental) stimulation, and (3) underlying conditions that have synergistic CNS depressant effects (i.e., hypothermia, hypotension). Anesthetic depth can be fairly volatile if there are abrupt changes in any of the determinants. The specific anesthetic drugs used are important; some are good CNS depressants but poor analgesics whereas others are good analgesics but poor CNS depressants. Although anesthetic infusion rates for intravenous drugs and end-tidal concentrations for gaseous drugs are two of the factors used to help estimate anesthetic depth, they do not define anesthetic depth.

Physical signs of anesthetic depth

Anesthetic depth has traditionally been divided into stages and planes. Stage I is the awake state of awareness, including all of the levels of obtundation down to loss of consciousness, which marks the beginning of stage II. Stage II is the excitement stage heralded by spontaneous muscular movement; the cessation of spontaneous muscle movement and onset of a regular pattern of breathing marks

Veterinary Anesthesia and Analgesia: The Fifth Edition of Lumb and Jones.
Edited by Kurt A. Grimm, Leigh A. Lamont, William J. Tranquilli, Stephen A. Greene and Sheilah A. Robertson.

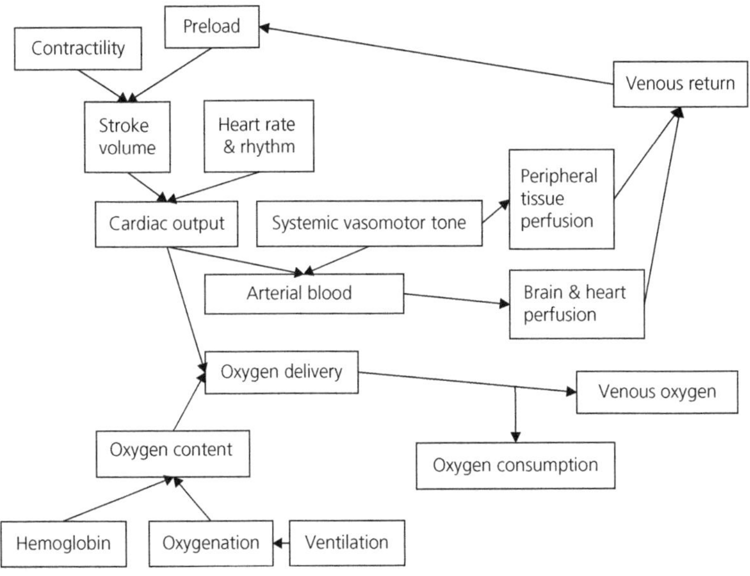

Figure 4.1 Overview of cardiopulmonary function. Preload and myocardial contractility generate a stroke volume. Heart rate (which may be negatively impacted by arrhythmias) and stroke volume determine cardiac output. Afterload impedance to cardiac output is not pictured because it is seldom a problem in anesthesia. Cardiac output and peripheral vasomotor tone determine blood pressure. Peripheral vasomotor tone is the important determinant of peripheral tissue perfusion. Arterial blood pressure is the important determinant of brain and heart perfusion. Veins conduct blood back to the heart (preload). Hemoglobin concentration and oxygenation determine blood oxygen content. Oxygen content and cardiac output determine oxygen delivery. The amount of oxygen taken out of the blood by the tissues (or carbon dioxide produced by the tissues) determines venous oxygen (or carbon dioxide).

Table 4.1 Physical signs of anesthetic depth within Stage III.

Plane	Eyeball Position	Palpebral Reflex	Pupil Size	PLR[a]	Corneal Moistness	Eyelid Muscle Tone	Mandibular Muscle Tone	Reflex Movement Response to Nociception	Physiologic Response to Nociception[b]
1. Light	Central	+	Medium to large	+	Moist	Lots	Lots	Maybe	Yes
2. Light–medium	Rotated med-vent	0	Small to medium	+	Moist	Some	Some	No	Maybe
3. Deep–medium	Rotated med-vent	0	Medium to large	0	Intermediate	Little	Little	No	No
4. Deep	Central	0	Large	0	Dry	None	None	No	No

[a] PLR = pupillary light response.
[b] Physiologic responses to nociception include increases in heart rate, blood pressure, or respiratory rate.

the end of stage II and the beginning of stage III (the surgical stage of anesthesia). Stage III is divided into four planes, which can be characterized by changes in readily available physical signs and progressive loss of reflexes (Table 4.1). Stage IV is characterized by extreme CNS depression and respiratory arrest. Cardiac arrest and death will result if the CNS depression is not reversed. Unfortunately, animals seldom behave according to the books and may simultaneously exhibit signs consistent with two or more planes. The anesthetist assesses each sign and then interprets them to estimate anesthetic depth. When the signs of anesthetic depth are unclear or contradictory, anesthetic drug administration should be gently decreased until it is clear that the animal is at an appropriate level. The intra-anesthetic depth goal is plane 2. Plane 1 might be too responsive and plane 4 is too close to death. Plane 3 is acceptable, but it is deeper than is often needed, particularly towards the end of the operative procedure.

A physiologic response to surgical stimulation defines a patient as being light but does not necessarily define a patient as being too light (Table 4.1). Animals lose consciousness (i.e., awareness) long before they lose spontaneous movement and physiologic responses. MACawake [minimum alveolar concentration (MAC) to prevent response to verbal command in 50% of patients] for halothane is about 0.4% [1]. MACincision (MAC to prevent muscular movement in response to a strong surgical stimulus) is about 0.9% and MAC_{BAR} (MAC to block the autonomic response to skin incision) is about 1.1%. The MACawake and the MACincision for isoflurane and sevoflurane were reported to be 0.39 and 1.3% and 0.61 and 2.0%, respectively [2]. If an animal exhibits a physiologic change or even moves slightly in response to surgical stimulation (provided that it does not move enough to interfere with the surgical procedure), it can be a good sign: it proves that the anesthesia level is light and not deep and that awareness is highly unlikely.

The recent history of anesthetic dosing is an important component of depth of anesthesia assessment; large dosages should be associated with a deep level of anesthesia and vice versa. Typical anesthetic drug dose administration does not guarantee that the animal is not over-anesthetized or at a typical anesthetic plane. Also, there is no obligatory correlation between level of anesthesia and physiologic consequence of anesthesia; animals can be lightly anesthetized and still be apneic, hypoxemic, or hypotensive.

Spontaneous movement is a reliable sign of a light level of anesthesia with most anesthetics. Focal facial or neck muscle twitching is a characteristic of some drugs (e.g., etomidate and propofol) and should not be interpreted, *per se*, to indicate a light level of anesthesia. Reflex movement in response to surgical stimulation is a more reliable sign of a light level of anesthesia.

An abrupt increase in heart rate, blood pressure, or breathing rate in response to surgical stimulation is a reliable sign of a light or light–medium level of anesthesia. In general, physiologic parameters such as heart rate, arterial blood pressure, breathing rate, and minute ventilation should trend downwards when an animal becomes more deeply anesthetized and vice versa. Breathing becomes shallower and the abdominal (diaphragm) component becomes more predominant at deeper levels of anesthesia. However, increases in these parameters should not be considered reliable premonitory guides to depth of anesthesia; it often happens that these parameters do not change until after the animal's anesthesia level suddenly becomes too light. Physiologic parameters are more importantly used to characterize the physiologic status of the patient. With increasing or decreasing trends of any physiologic parameter, other signs of anesthetic depth should be assessed before making any changes in the rate of drug administration.

Masticatory and eyelid muscle tone gradually decrease as anesthetic depth deepens. Masticatory muscle tone must be indexed to the species and size of the patient. Young animals such as puppies never exhibit much muscle tone whereas large animals always exhibit a lot. Ruminants and swine may exhibit spontaneous chewing when they are lightly anesthetized [3].

In small animals, with traditional anesthetics, the eyeball position is central at light and deep levels of anesthesia and (usually) ventro-medially rotated in planes 2 and 3. The eyeball does not rotate with ketamine. In horses, the eyeball can rotate, but not reliably so, and spontaneous nystagmus can occur. A very slow ('roving') eyeball might represent a medium level of anesthesia whereas a fast nystagmus represents a light level of anesthesia. Nystagmus may also occur in light levels of anesthesia in ruminants and swine, but disappears at deeper levels as the eyeball rotates ventrally. Nystagmus does not normally occur in surgically anesthetized small animals.

The presence of a palpebral reflex is a reliable indicator of a light level of anesthesia; the absence of it suggests a medium or deep level. Some individuals never exhibit a palpebral reflex or it has become fatigued with repeated testing. With ketamine, the palpebral reflex is always present and the eyelids remain open. The pupillary light reflex (PLR) (pupillary constriction in response to a bright light) and a dazzle reflex (a blink in response to a bright light) are reliable indicators of a light to light–medium level of anesthesia. The PLR may be minimized by the administration of parasympatholytics.

Lacrimation (tear production) decreases and stops at deeper levels of anesthesia. Lacrimation in horses is a sign of a light level of anesthesia. The presence of gag and swallow reflexes indicates a light level of anesthesia in nearly all species.

Electroencephalographic monitoring of anesthetic depth

Most of the physical signs of anesthetic depth are facial signs that depend upon muscle function, which is problematic when anesthetist access to the patient's head is limited or if neuromuscular blocking agents are used. In addition, because the physical signs of anesthetic depth are notoriously inaccurate, there is great interest in 'seeing what's happening on the inside.' The encephalogram (EEG) and its derived indices of brain activity offer just such an opportunity. The EEG changes from a low-amplitude, high-frequency wave pattern during the awake state to a high-amplitude, low-frequency pattern during anesthesia to burst suppression (intermittent periods of electrical silence), and finally persistent electrical silence with deep levels of anesthesia. The raw EEG requires a considerable volume of recording and also specialized training and expertise for interpretation. Computer analysis and processing of the raw EEG facilitate interpretation of EEG signals. Electroencephalograph voltage (power) changes as a function of time (time domain) generate indices such as total EEG power (TOTPOW), median power frequency, and burst suppression. Interpretational algorithms (by fast Fourier transformation) also examine signal activity as a function of frequency (frequency domain) and generate indices such as spectral edge frequency (SEF95) (the frequency below which 95% of the total EEG power resides), median frequency (MF) (the median EEG power frequency), and the relative power of the delta (0.5–3.5 Hz), theta (3.5–7.0 Hz), alpha (7–13 Hz), and beta (13–30 Hz) frequency ranges compared with total EEG power [4]. Such indices have been used to characterize anesthetic depth in people [5–8] and animals [9–12]. Bispectral Index™, cerebral state index, and Narcotrend™ may represent a more integrated and user-friendly approach to EEG analysis compared with the classic indices.

The Bispectral Index™ (BIS™) (Aspect Medical Systems) is a processed electroencephalogram that quantifies the degree of anesthetic induced cortical depression. The BIS index represents a variably weighted value derived from four subparameters: (1) burst suppression ratio (time domain); (2) a QUAZI value (time domain); (3) $beta_2$ power ratio in the 30–47 Hz range compared with that in the 11–20 Hz range (frequency domain); and (4) the bispectral biocoherence ratio of peaks in the 0.5–47 Hz range compared with the 40–47 Hz range (frequency domain) [13]. The BIS monitor does not require calibration and displays a bar graph denoting signal quality and amount of muscle artifact. Excessive muscle movement can interfere with the BIS computation [14]. BIS has been used to help assure that patients are well anesthetized, pain free, and unaware [13,15]. The monitor displays a number between 0 and 100: values >90 in patients are compatible with awake and alert, 80–90 with anxiolysis, 60–80 with moderate obtundation, <60 with loss of recall, <50 with unresponsiveness to verbal stimuli, <40 with the loss of muscular movement in response to a noxious stimulus, <20 with burst suppression (deep anesthesia), and 0 with isoelectric activity. In dogs, a BIS index of 60–70 was reported to be compatible with completion of the surgical procedure [16]. BIS has been extensively studied in humans, primarily as an index of sedation [17,18] or depth of anesthesia [8,12,19–23]. It has also been used as an index of brain function in neurologic patients [24,25]. MAC_{BAR} and MAC_{BIS} (the MAC at which a nociceptive stimulus causes an increase in BIS to 60) has been reported for cats [19]. One canine study using the BIS monitoring system, with electrodes placed either longitudinally or laterally, on the top of the head reported that the BIS index was highly variable and did not track end-tidal isoflurane concentrations very well [26]. Not all anesthetics affect BIS in the same way; propofol, midazolam, and thiopental strongly depress it, inhalational anesthetics have an intermediate effect, opioids have little effect, and nitrous oxide and ketamine tend to increase it [13].

A cerebral state index (CSI) using a cerebral state monitor (CSM) (Danmeter, Odense, Denmark) has been reported [27]. There are three clip electrode attachments: forehead (+), occipital (–), and parietal (reference). The CSI index is calculated from an algorithm which considers two energy bands (β and α), the β:α ratio, and burst suppression (BS), a quotient that considers the amount of time of zero EEG activity. The monitor displays EEG, CSI, BS, EMG, and signal quality index (SQI). CSI values >90 represent awake, 80–90 sedation, and <80 unconscious. CSI progressively decreased with increasing propofol infusion but was not well correlated with the physical signs of anesthetic depth evaluated in this study [28]. In a final study, the authors concluded that while CSI could predict deep levels of anesthesia, it was not too discriminative with regard to differentiating anesthetic levels used clinically [29].

The Narcotrend™ monitor (Monitor Technik, Bad Bramstedt, Germany) analyzes the raw EEG and then categorizes the levels of sedation as awake (A0), subvigilant (A1/A2), sedation (B0/B1/B2), anesthesia (C0/C1/C2), moderate anesthesia (D0/D1/D2), deep anesthesia/burst suppression (E), and coma/electrical silence (F) [30]. Auditory evoked EEG responses (AEP) have been used primarily to assess neurologic function in CNS disease but have also been used to assess anesthetic depth and awareness/recall [31]. Many studies have used sensory (to a noxious stimulus) evoked EEG or BIS, hemodynamic changes, and movement responses to evaluate nociception.

All EEG indices are subject to large and anesthetic drug variations. Depending upon the magnitude of the stimulation and the depth of anesthesia, stimulus-induced EEG changes could represent either an arousal pattern or a pattern that suggests a deeper level of anesthesia (the paradoxical response) [9,32]. The EEG does not reflect analgesic properties of an anesthetic drug, only its hypnotic properties. EEG indices may aide in the evaluation of anesthetic depth, but none have taken the place of, and indeed, may not be any more accurate than, physical evaluation of anesthetic depth.

Cardiovascular system

Heart rate and rhythm

Heart rate is an important determinant of cardiac output. Heart rates (bpm) in normal animals are highly variable: 60–120 for large dogs, 80–160 for small dogs, 120–220 for cats, 35–45 for horses, and 70–90 for small ruminants. A change in heart rate is a sensitive index of a change in the physiologic status of the patient. Excessive bradycardia diminishes cardiac output even though stroke volume may increase due to longer diastolic filling times. Excessive tachycardia can diminish cardiac output due to shortened diastolic filling time and reduced stroke volume. Causes of bradycardia and tachycardia are listed in Tables 4.2 and 4.3, respectively. There is no consensus as to when bradycardia should be treated, but a conservative treatment trigger guideline might be something like (estimated as about 20–30% below low normal) <50 for large dogs, <60 for small dogs, <90 for cats, <25 for horses, and <55 for small ruminants. Certainly bradycardia should be treated when it is associated with any evidence of poor cardiac output, blood pressure, or tissue perfusion. In dogs, heart rates of 51 ± 5 and 54 ± 8 were associated with cardiac indexes of 130 ± 19 mL/min/kg (about 79% of normal) [33] and 2.24 ± 0.64 L/min/m^2 (about 50% of normal) [34], respectively. Mean blood pressure was maintained by enhanced systemic vascular resistance. In both reports, there was evidence of increased tissue oxygen extraction, but in neither report was there evidence of tissue hypoxia. Common causes of bradycardia which are not responsive to pharmacological treatment are severe hypothermia, cardiac conduction abnormalities, and severe myocardial hypoxemia. In most cases, treatment involves the administration of an anticholinergic and/or a sympathomimetic, although an underlying cause should be sought.

In people, because of coronary artery disease, sinus tachycardia is much feared because the increased myocardial oxygen consumption may exceed a limited oxygen delivery capability. In animals, the main concern is how tachycardia impacts diastolic filling and whether it is associated with ventricular arrhythmias. Similarly to bradycardia, it is not known exactly when tachycardia should be treated. In dogs, a pacing rate of approximately 240 (for 2–3 weeks) has been used as a model for inducing heart failure, but this hardly serves as a guideline for acute tachycardia during anesthesia. Conservative intervention trigger levels might be something like (estimated as about 20% above high normal) >150 for large dogs, >190 for small dogs, >260 for cats, >55 for horses, and >110 for small ruminants. Certainly tachycardia should be addressed when it is associated with any evidence of poor cardiac output, blood pressure, or tissue perfusion. Care should be exercised to determine whether tachycardia is the primary cause of hemodynamic problems, or compensation for another, underlying problem (e.g., elevation of heart rate to compensate for acute blood loss). Treating tachycardia for the sake of normalizing heart rate may cause rapid cardiovascular decompensation if tachycardia is, in fact, compensatory. Treatment must involve identification and correction of the underlying disorder; beta-blockers are rarely indicated.

Causes of supraventricular or ventricular tachycardia are listed in Table 4.4. The concerns and treatment trigger levels for supraventricular tachycardia are similar to those for sinus tachycardia. Ventricular arrhythmias are different in that treatment triggers fall into two categories: (1) if there is any evidence of impaired forward blood flow (cardiac output, blood pressure, or tissue perfusion); or (2) if there is any concern that the ventricular rhythm may proceed to ventricular fibrillation. The criteria for the latter include: (1) an instantaneous rate >180–200 bpm (If there are periods of paroxysmal tachycardia, the instantaneous heart rate is calculated as if the paroxysm lasted for an entire minute); (2) a worsening arrhythmia (an increasing number or an increasing multiformity); or (3) R-on-T (the ectopic complex overlies the T-wave of the preceding depolarization; a vulnerable time to stimulate ventricular fibrillation). If there is an observable isoelectric period between the two QRST complexes, there is no R-on-T; if the last waveform runs into the next waveform without an isoelectric period (even once), there may be R-on-T and the condition is worthy of treatment.

Table 4.2 Potential causes of bradycardia.

Anesthetic agents	α_2-Adrenergic receptor agonists, opioid agonists, overdose of any anesthetic
Increased vagal tone	Endotracheal tube, abdominal nociception, traction on ocular muscles, high blood pressure
Metabolic	Hypothermia, end-stage hypoxemia, hyperkalemia
Heart disease	Sick sinus syndrome, A–V conduction disturbance

Table 4.3 Potential causes of tachycardia.

Light level of anesthesia	Nociceptive response during surgery; arousal to sensory input
Drugs	Ketamine, parasympatholytics, sympathomimetics
Metabolic	Hypovolemia, hypoxemia, hypercapnia, hyperthermia, postoperative pain
Disease	Pheochromocytoma, hyperthyroidism
Heart disease	Supraventricular tachycardia, ventricular tachycardia

Table 4.4 Potential causes of arrhythmias.

Supraventricular	See tachycardia	
	Heart disease	Atrial dilation, myocarditis
Ventricular	See tachycardia	
	Heart disease	DCM[a], HCM[a], myocarditis
	Iatrogenic	Intracardiac catheters, chest tubes
	Metabolic	Thoracic and non-thoracic trauma, visceral disease (GDV[a]), hyperkalemia, hypokalemia
	Anesthetics	Thiopental, halothane, α_2-adrenergic receptor agonists
	Miscellaneous	Increased intracranial pressure, cerebral hypoxia, digitalis toxicity

[a] DCM = dilative cardiomyopathy; HCM = hypertrophic cardiomyopathy; GDV = gastric dilation/volvulus.

Table 4.5 Potential causes of hypotension.

Low venous return	Hypovolemia secondary to pre-existing dehydration, blood loss, plasma exudation at surgical site, PPV[a], abdominal compartment syndrome
Poor diastolic function	HCM[a], pericardial tamponade, fibrosis (endo-, epi-, myocardial), excess tachycardia
Poor systolic function	DCM[a], negative inotropic effect of anesthetics, β-receptor blockers, calcium-channel blockers, antiarrhythmics
Impaired systolic efficiency	Ventricular arrhythmias, atrioventricular valve insufficiency, outflow tract obstruction
Bradycardia	See Table 4.2
Low SVR[a]	Vasodilation secondary to anesthetic drugs, patent ductus arteriosus, sepsis

[a] PPV = positive pressure ventilation; HCM = hypertrophic cardiomyopathy; DCM = dilative cardiomyopathy; SVR = systemic vascular resistance.

Table 4.6 Potential causes of hypertension.

Vasoconstriction	Light level of anesthesia, sympathomimetic drugs, renal failure, Cushing's disease, hyperthyroidism, pheochromocytoma
	Elevated intracranial pressure

Arterial blood pressure

Arterial blood pressure is arterial hydrostatic pressure compared with atmospheric pressure. Arterial blood pressure is determined by the arterial compartment blood volume and the arterial compartment wall tone. The intra-arterial blood volume is the balance between inflow (cardiac output) and outflow (diastolic run-off). Cardiac output is the product of stroke volume and heart rate, and diastolic run-off is determined by vasomotor tone. Systolic pressure is the highest intra-arterial pressure of each cardiac cycle; and is primarily determined by stroke volume and arterial system compliance. Diastolic pressure is the lowest pressure prior to the next heart beat and is primarily determined by the rate of diastolic run-off (vasomotor tone) and heart rate. Mean pressure is the average of the area under the pulse pressure waveform, not the arithmetic mean of the measured systolic and diastolic pressure. Systolic, diastolic, and mean blood pressure measurements in normal dogs and cats are variable depending on the level of stress, body position, and measurement technique, but are approximately 100–160, 60–100, and 80–120 mmHg, respectively [35–39]. Horses, goats, and sheep have slightly lower values: 90–130, 60–90, and 70–110 mmHg, respectively.

When the blood pressure becomes too low, cerebral and coronary perfusion will be compromised. In general, one becomes concerned about excessive hypotension when the mean blood pressure decreases below about 60 mmHg or the systolic blood pressure decreases below about 80 mmHg, in any species. In ideal situations, the mean blood pressure should be maintained above 80 mmHg and the systolic blood pressure above 100 mmHg. Hypotension may be caused by hypovolemia, poor cardiac output, or vasodilation (Table 4.5).

Severe acute hypertension, even though it may be transient, may cause edema and hemorrhage anywhere, but the brain and the lungs are the primary organs of concern. Sustained hypertension may generate issues with high cardiac afterload, ocular retinopathy or choroidopathy, and retinal detachment, encephalopathy, and eventually renal disease. In general, one becomes concerned about acute, persistent hypertension when mean blood pressure exceeds 140 mmHg or the systolic blood pressure exceeds 180 mmHg, or with chronic hypertension when the mean blood pressure exceeds 120 mmHg and the systolic 160 mmHg [39]. These values are just suggestions; decisions about treatment are based on a variety of factors: (1) reliability and repeatability of the measurement, (2) stage of operative procedure (patients are often transiently hypotensive immediately after anesthesia induction and it typically resolves itself without specific treatment; hypotension at the end of the procedure corrects itself as inhalant anesthetic effects wane), (3) the persistent nature and magnitude of hypotension, and (4) the potential adverse consequences of the proposed treatment. One must guard against the use of treatment trigger values without regard to concomitant disease (pathophysiologic) processes. Hypertension is generally attributed to vasoconstriction (Table 4.6).

Arterial blood pressure can be measured indirectly by sphygmomanometry or directly via an arterial catheter. Some methodologies measure/report all three blood pressures (systolic, diastolic, and mean) whereas others measure only systolic. Of the three pressures, mean arterial blood pressure is physiologically the most important to the anesthetist; it represents the average upstream pressure for tissue perfusion and the average afterload to the heart. When a measuring device measures all three pressures, the clinician should focus primarily on the mean pressure. Sometimes, for example, especially during direct blood pressure measurement, systolic pressures will measure high whereas mean pressure measures within the normal range (see frequency response discussion under Direct blood pressure measurement). This patient should be defined as normotensive because of the mean pressure, in spite of the high systolic pressure reading.

Indirect blood pressure measurement

Arterial blood pressure can be measured indirectly by sphygmomanometry, which involves the application of an occlusive cuff over an artery in a cylindrical appendage. The forelimb, hindlimb, and tail are commonly used in animals. The width of the cuff should be about 30–40% of the circumference of the appendage. This provides some consistency in how the cuff applies pressure to the underlying tissue. Cuffs that are too narrow tend to overestimate blood pressure whereas cuffs that are too wide tend to underestimate it [40]. The cuff should be placed snugly around the leg. If it is applied too tightly, the pressure measurements will be erroneously low since the cuff itself, acting as a tourniquet, will partially occlude the underlying artery. If the cuff is too loose, the pressure measurements will be erroneously high since excessive cuff pressure will be required to occlude the underlying artery. The subtleties of cuff width to appendage size, cuff application, how the cuff applies pressure to the underlying tissues, and location of the arteries inevitably lead to variation and inaccuracy of measurements with sphygmomanometry.

During measurement, inflation of the cuff applies pressure to the underlying tissues and will totally occlude blood flow when the cuff pressure exceeds systolic blood pressure. As the cuff pressure is gradually decreased, blood will begin to flow intermittently when the cuff pressure falls below the systolic pressure. The cuff pressure should be reduced slowly, especially when heart rates are slow, so as not to miss the highest systolic event. As the cuff is deflated, small, positive deflections of the cuff pressure may be observed each time the pulse wave hits the cuff. The manometer pressure at which this positive oscillation begins to occur corresponds approximately to systolic blood pressure. The oscillations will be maximal at mean arterial pressure and will suddenly diminute at approximately diastolic pressure.

As the cuff pressure is decreased below the systolic pressure, blood will begin to flow intermittently past the cuff. Flow distal to the cuff can be digitally palpated or, if the vessel is large enough, auscultated (Korotkoff sounds). The cuff pressure at which the first palpable pulse, or auscultated tapping sound, occurs approximates systolic blood pressure. The sudden diminution of sounds approximates diastolic pressure. Amplifying stethoscopes could be used in the smaller arteries of animals.

Doppler ultrasound instrumentation involves the application of a pair of small piezoelectric ultrasound crystals over an artery distal to the cuff. One of the piezoelectric crystals transmits ultrasound energy into the tissue. The ultrasound signal is phase shifted by movement of the underlying tissues (Doppler shift) and transmitted back to the receiving crystal. The change in frequency between the transmitted and the received signal is detected and electronically transduced into an audible signal. The cuff pressure at which the first audible flow sounds are heard approximates systolic blood pressure. This instrument cannot measure diastolic pressure. Sometimes a secondary sound will follow closely the primary sound as the cuff pressure is further decreased (a double blood flow sound associated with each heart beat). This occurs when the cuff pressure is in the dicrotic notch of the pulse pressure waveform; the subsequent transient rise in blood pressure exceeds cuff pressure and flow transiently recurs. The cuff pressure at which this occurs is not diastolic pressure and should not be recorded as such. Other Doppler instruments generate signals from the movement of the arterial wall and can be used to measure both systolic and diastolic blood pressures.

Oscillometry is a popular method of indirect blood pressure measurement because it is easy to use, requiring just the application of the occlusion cuff. The instruments automatically inflate and deflate the cuff (the timing of measurements is set by the operator). The oscillometer analyzes the fluctuations of pressure within the cuff as it is slowly deflated. Systolic and diastolic pressures are measured at the first and last pulse-associated fluctuations in cuff pressure, and mean pressure is taken as the cuff pressure at which maximal pressure oscillations occur. Systolic, diastolic, and mean blood pressure and heart rate are then displayed. Small vessel size (due either to small vessel size or to vasoconstriction) and motion can interfere with measurements.

There are multiple guidelines for validating the accuracy and repeatability (precision) of blood pressure instrumentation [41]; the latest is the European Society for Hypertension International Protocol Version 2 (ESH-IP2) [42]. Protocols, in their entirety, contain a fair number of testing and analysis requirements but at their core they require a certain level of accuracy compared with some gold standard (generally direct blood pressure measurements). The ESH-IP2 protocol, in the phase 1 portion, requires that the test instrument measures within 5 mmHg 73% of the time, within 10 mmHg 87% of the time, and within 15 mmHg 96% of the time (any two of the three) or within 5 mmHg 65% of the time, within 10 mmHg 81% of the time, and within 15 mmHg 93% of the time (all three) with a cross spectrum of normotensive, hypertensive, and hypotensive subjects. Published veterinary standards suggest that the test instrument should measure within 10 mmHg of the reference instrument >50% of the time and within 20 mmHg >80% of the time [39].

Indirect blood pressure measurement techniques exhibit variable precision and accuracy, but provide a reasonable surrogate marker of direct mean pressure measurements in humans [43–45], dogs [38,46–50], cats [51–53], rabbits [54], and foals [55]. Noninvasive techniques tend to underestimate systolic pressure [43,45–48,52, 56,57], to overestimate blood pressure in hypotensive patients,[43, 45,48,49,57], and to exhibit wider variability compared with direct arterial blood pressure [48,52,53,58–61]. Some studies report a poor correlation between indirect and direct blood pressure measurements [48,50,52,59]. Comparative trials test both the instruments and the technical aspects associated with the use of that measuring system. When the results do not agree (or when they do), it is not possible to know if the fault lies with the test instrument or the reference instrument, with methodological issues such as cuff placement for non-invasive methods [55], frequency/damping with invasive methods, or the specific pressure compared (systolic, diastolic, or mean).

Direct blood pressure measurement

Direct measurement of arterial blood pressure, via an arterial catheter, is more continuous and less variable than using indirect methods. The dorsal metatarsal, radial/carpal, coccygeal, lingual, femoral, and auricular arteries are commonly used in dogs and cats, the facial and metatarsal arteries in horses, and auricular arteries in ruminants and swine. The subcutaneous tissues around peripheral arteries are relatively tight and hematoma formation at the time of catheter removal is rarely a problem (compared with the femoral, lingual or carotid artery sites). Cats have a few unique problems: (1) their arteries are small for percutaneous catheterization and some expertise is required; (2) arteries soon constrict with cut-down manipulation; and (3) collateral circulation is sparse; placement of femoral or metatarsal catheters may be associated with foot ischemia if adequate collateral circulation is not available (remove the catheter at the earliest sign of coolness). Catheter patency is preserved either by intermittent, frequent flushing or by continuous flushing with low-flow, high-pressure heparinized saline (1000 U per 500 mL). Blood pressure normally oscillates and, during the relatively higher phase, blood will push into the tip of the catheter and clot if care is not taken to prevent it.

There are improvised devices that could be used to measure mean arterial blood pressure, but most people gravitate to disposable commercial transducers because they are easier to use. The measuring device could simply be a long fluid administration set suspended from some high point [a mean blood pressure of 140 mmHg is equivalent to a 186 cm (75 in) column of water] (Fig. 4.2). The measuring device could also be an aneroid manometer system (Fig. 4.3). The arterial catheter can also be attached to a commercial transducer and physiograph.

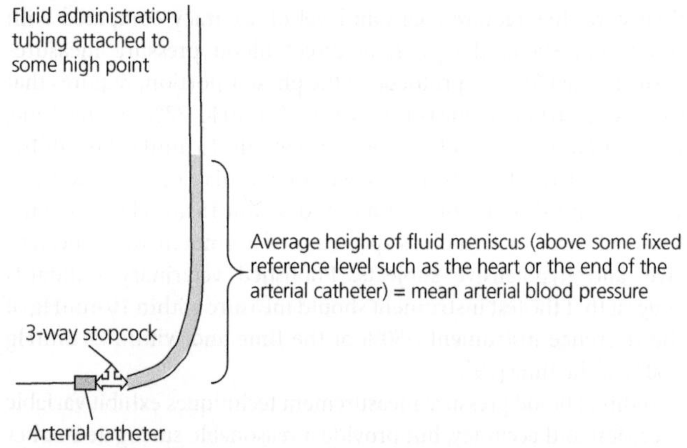

Figure 4.2 Column manometer for measuring central venous or arterial blood pressure. Pressure measurement procedure: (1) turn the three-way stopcock off to the patient; (2) inject fluid into the tubing to a level well above that of the patient; (3) open the three-way stopcock between the patient and the column of fluid, allowing fluid to gravitate into the patient (never allow the patient's blood pressure to fill the fluid column – it will clot in the catheter); (4) measure the average equilibrated height of the fluid column; (5) adjust the units to mmHg ($mmHg = 0.736 \times cmH_2O$). Blood pressure oscillations will clot the catheter between measurements. Either close the stopcock to the patient between measurements or flush the catheter frequently or attach a continuous low-volume infusion device.

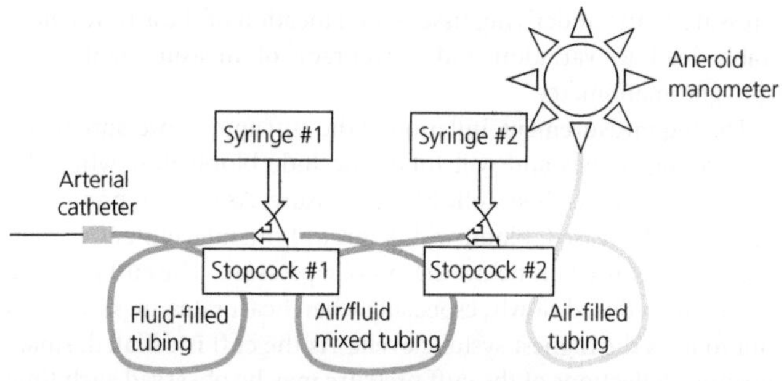

Figure 4.3 Aneroid manometer system for measuring arterial blood pressure. The fluid-filled tubing is always charged with sterile fluid. The air-fill tubing never contains fluid (aneroid manometers do not tolerate wetting very well; if fluid appears in this tubing, replace it). The air/fluid middle tubing will intermittently contain air or fluid. To make a measurement: (1) close stopcock #1 to the patient and stopcock #2 to the aneroid manometer; (2) expel all the fluid in the air/fluid mixed, middle tubing, left over from the previous measurement, by injecting air from syringe #2 out through stopcock #1 (do not inject air into the patient); (3) close stopcock #2 to the syringe and inject sterile saline from syringe #1 into the tubing towards the aneroid manometer until the registered pressure is well above mean arterial blood pressure of the patient; (4) close stopcock #1 to the syringe, allowing saline to flow from the high pressure within the tubing into the patient; (5) the equilibrated pressure represents mean arterial blood pressure. The aneroid manometer can be at any level with reference to the patient provided that the fluid meniscus in the tubing is at a fixed reference level (such as the heart). The needle may oscillate with each heart beat; this does not represent systolic or diastolic pressure because there is too much inertia in the system. The needle may oscillate with ventilation; take the measurement between breaths. All maneuvers must be accomplished in a sterile manner.

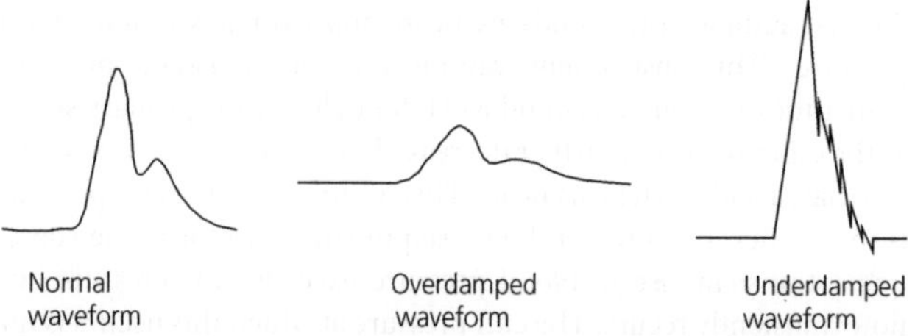

Figure 4.4 Normal, overdamped, and underdamped arterial pulse pressure waveforms.

The transducer should be periodically zeroed to atmospheric pressure. A stopcock (usually the one closest to the transducer) is closed to the patient, and opened between the transducer and the atmosphere while pressing the 'zero' option on the monitor. The stopcock that is opened for the zeroing process must be at the reference level of the heart for accuracy to be maintained. Although it is common practice to position the transducer also at heart level, with modern patient monitors this is not absolutely necessary if the stopcock is located away from the transducer. Monitors internally compensate for vertical differences between the patient and the transducer with an 'offset pressure.' Once zeroed, the relative height of the transducer cannot be changed without re-zeroing. With older patient monitors without this offset feature, the transducer and the zeroing stopcock must be placed at the level of the heart. Although not normally necessary with systems used for clinical monitoring, the accuracy of the transducer can be checked with a mercury manometer.

The extension tubing between the catheter and the transducer should be as short as practical and should be constructed of non-expansible (low-compliance) plastic tubing (as opposed to regular intravenous fluid extension sets) to minimize damped signals. The fidelity of the reproduction of the pulse pressure waveform by a fluid-filled measuring system is the result of a complex interaction between the frequency response of the catheter and measuring system, and patient factors such as heart rate and systolic vigor. The frequency response of the measuring system is determined by two important parameters: its resonant frequency (the rate of system oscillation in response to a change in pressure) and its damping coefficient (the rate at which the oscillations come to rest after the change in pressure) [43,62]. Generally, smaller catheters, longer and more compliant tubing, and blood clots or air bubbles overdamp a signal. An overdamped signal results in a flattened tracing (systolic pressures are lower than they really are and diastolic pressures are higher) (Fig. 4.4). If this occurs, check the measuring system for leaks, kinks, clots, or air bubbles. If this does not fix the overdamping, switch to shorter or less compliant tubing. A larger catheter would lessen overdamping, but frequently catheter size is limited by the size of the patient. Underdamping occurs when the frequency response of the measuring system is similar to that of the source pulse pressure waveform. The recorded waveform will be exaggerated – the systolic pressure will be higher than reality and exhibit a 'spiked' appearance (Fig. 4.4). The displayed systolic pressure may appear unreasonably higher than the mean pressure. The diastolic pressure will also be erroneously low and sharp pressure oscillations may over-ride the normally smooth descent of the pulse pressure waveform (Fig. 4.4). If underdamping occurs, change something in the measuring system: remove kinks, clots, or air bubbles, add an air bubble, change to longer or shorter tubing, change to more or less compliant tubing. Most commercial transducer and monitoring systems underdamp. One can alter systolic pressure at will by changing the characteristics of the measuring system. For clinical purposes, this is usually not much of a concern since monitoring and therapeutic decisions emphasize mean pressure. This may be problematic in studies which compare indirect blood pressure measuring techniques with direct arterial blood pressure measurements (which are usually considered to be a gold standard).

The frequency response of the measurement system can be assessed by the dynamic pressure response test (Fig. 4.5). This involves the sudden release of pressure on the measurement system, such as is done by flushing the catheter with the continuous flush device, and observing the oscillation pattern as the pressure returns to baseline. During the flush procedure, the registered pressure equals that of the pressure bag (usually >300 mmHg). When the flushing procedure is abruptly terminated, the pressure should return to baseline after about 1–2 negative and 1–2 positive oscillations (Fig. 4.5) [43,62]. The appropriateness of the frequency response of the measuring system for a particular patient is determined by a combination of the resonant frequency and the damping (Fig. 4.6).

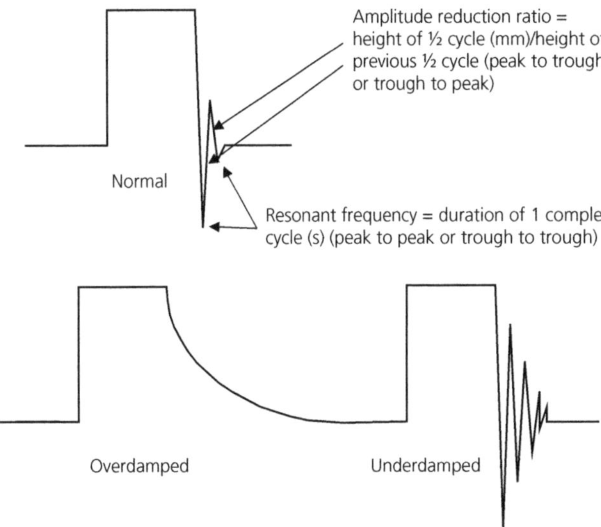

Figure 4.5 Dynamic pressure response test to determine resonant frequency and amplitude reduction ratio of a measuring system. A high pressure is applied to the measuring system while it is attached to the patient (usually with the flush device). The pressure is suddenly released and the oscillations in pressure as it returns to baseline are observed. With an optimally damped system, the waveform should oscillate 1–2 negative and 1–2 positive deflections before returning to baseline. With an overdamped system, the waveform returns smoothly, but slowly, to baseline. With an underdamped system, the waveform oscillates more than two full cycles before it returns to baseline. Resonant frequency is calculated as the duration of one complete cycle (peak to peak or trough to trough). Typical resonant frequencies of common measuring systems are between 10 and 25 Hz (one complete cycle in 0.04–0.1 s) [43, 62]. The optimal resonant frequency of a measuring system is dependent upon heart rate and systolic vigor. It is recommended that the resonant frequency be 6–10 times that of the heart rate (6–10 Hz for a heart rate of 60 bpm, 12–20 Hz for a heart rate of 120 bpm, 18–30 Hz for a heart rate of 180 bpm, and 24–40 Hz for a heart rate of 240 bpm) [43]. Amplitude reduction ratio is the height of any half complete cycle (peak to trough or trough to peak) divided by the height of the previous half cycle. Typical values are 0.2–0.6 [43, 62]. Ideally, a measuring system would have a high resonant frequency and a low amplitude reduction ratio (0.1–0.4).

Cardiac preload

Preload is defined *in vitro* as muscle stretch prior to muscle contraction. *In vivo*, it is defined by the formula: stress = (ventricular pressure × ventricular wall thickness)/ventricular diameter. These parameters can be measured clinically (see discussion below regarding Doppler ultrasound-based methods of assessing contractility), but usually they are not. It is assumed that preload would be proportional to end-diastolic ventricular volume (another parameter that is not usually measured clinically). Hence the first approximation of preload that is routinely measured in clinical patients is end-diastolic diameter by echocardiography. End-diastolic diameter in normal dogs is reported to be $1.44 \times kg^{0.32}$ in the dog and 1.5 ± 0.2 cm in the cat [63]. If a chest radiograph is available, the diameter of the posterior vena cava (normally about 2.5 × width of the adjacent ribs) may provide some insight into the central venous blood volume. Clinically, the ease of jugular vein distention may be informative; a jugular vein that cannot be raised much by applying digital pressure into the thoracic inlet is likely to be associated with low venous volume, venous pressure, and hypovolemia; and vice versa for hypervolemia or heart failure [64]. A distant, and often inaccurate, surrogate marker of left ventricular preload is central venous pressure.

Central venous pressure

Central venous pressure (CVP) is the luminal pressure of the intrathoracic vena cava. Peripheral venous pressure is variably higher than CVP, is subject to unpredictable extraneous influences, and is not a reliable indicator of CVP [65,66]. CVP is determined by the relationship between central blood volume and venous tone. Central blood volume is determined by venous return and cardiac output. Verification of a well-placed, unobstructed catheter can be ascertained by observing small fluctuations in the fluid meniscus within the column manometer (Fig. 4.2) or displayed on the physiograph, synchronous with the heart beat, and larger excursions synchronous with ventilation. Large fluctuations synchronous with each heart beat may indicate that the end of the catheter is positioned within the right ventricle. Direct observation of the CVP waveform may help identify that the catheter tip is in the proper location (Fig. 4.7). Measurements should be made during the expiratory pause phase of the breathing cycle (during either spontaneous or positive pressure ventilation), since changes in pleural pressure affect the luminal pressure within the anterior vena cava. Erroneously high CVP measurements will occur if the tip of the catheter is positioned in the right ventricle or if there is significant tricuspid insufficiency.

The normal CVP in dogs and cats is approximately 0–10 cmH_2O. In laterally recumbent horses, CVP has been reported to be 15–25 cmH_2O [67,68], and in dorsally recumbent or standing horses 5–10 cmH_2O [67,69]. In horses, when a central venous catheter is not available, jugular venous pressures may be used as a surrogate marker of CVP [68]. CVP is often used as a marker of circulating blood volume even though it is not, *per se*, a measure of preload volume (it is a measure of preload pressure). Below-range pressure values suggest absolute or relative hypovolemia and that the patient may benefit from a rapid bolus of fluids. Above-range pressure values indicate absolute or relative hypervolemia and that fluid therapy should perhaps be stopped. Central venous pressure is used as a measure of the relationship between blood volume and blood volume capacity and is often used to help determine the endpoint for acute, large fluid volume resuscitation. Central venous pressure measurements can also

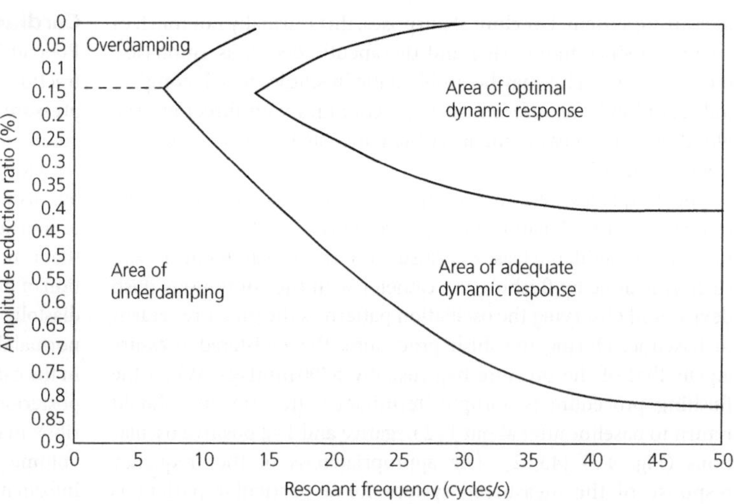

Figure 4.6 Resonant frequency:amplitude reduction ratio of monitoring systems. Resonant frequency rates and amplitude reduction ratio combinations below the 'acceptable' (dashed) line in the lower left quadrant of the table represent underdamping, while combinations above the 'acceptable' (dashed) line in the upper left corner of the table represent overdamping. Most monitoring systems are underdamped. Redrawn from published resonant frequency and amplitude reduction ratio:damping coefficient plots [43, 62].

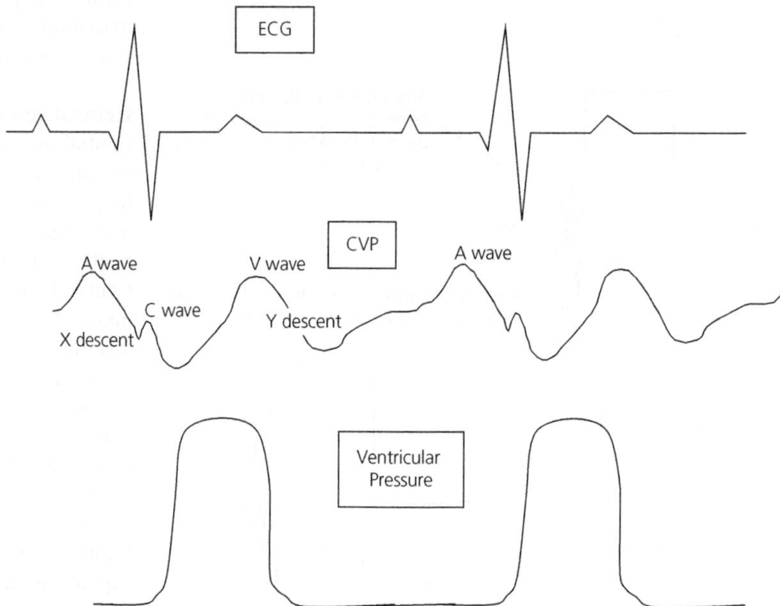

Figure 4.7 Central venous pressure tracing. The A wave represents atrial contraction and occurs after the ECG P wave and before the beginning of the QRS wave. The X descent is the pressure drop associated with atrial relaxation. The C wave, which may or may not be observed, is the reflected wave and bulging of the A–V valve upwards into the atrium associated with ventricular contraction. The upswing in pressure after the X descent and prior to the V wave is the increase in atrial pressure associated with venous return during the time of ventricular contraction (the A–V valve is closed). The V wave is not a cardiac event, but the plateau of the atrial filling. The Y descent marks ventricular relaxation and the drop in atrial pressure as the A–V valves open and blood rushes into the ventricle. The increasing pressure between the Y descent and the next A wave is atrial and ventricular filling prior to the next atrial contraction. Mitral regurgitation will obliterate the X descent – the C wave to the V wave will become one positive wave. If the catheter has inadvertently been placed in the ventricle, the tracing will be that typical of a ventricular pressure tracing.

track acute volume unloading as in the case of acute blood loss or anesthetic-induced vasodilation. Central venous pressure is not a good monitor of day-to-day fluid balance; it is a measure of the central blood volume:venous tone relationship and cannot 'see' whether the interstitial fluid compartment is under- or overloaded. Overall, CVP is a poor predictor of stroke volume or cardiac output [70].

Initial CVP measurements are often neither profoundly low nor high, and are difficult to interpret in isolation of history and other cardiovascular variables [71]. However, response to therapy can often be very informative. A decreasing CVP measurement in response to fluid therapy suggests venodilation and is the cardiovascular system's way of saying 'thanks for the fluids and could I have some more please'; one then continues with fluid administration until the CVP works its way all the way down and back up again to a mid to high normal value. A rapidly increasing CVP in response to fluid therapy suggests cardiac intolerance to the fluid load and that further fluid loading should stop. Central venous pressure is a measure of the ability of the heart to pump venous return volume and should be measured whenever heart failure is a concern.

Mean systemic filling pressure

Because central venous pressure is heavily influenced by venomotor tone and pleural pressure, it is a notoriously poor predictor of volume status [72]. Since, however, venous return is critical to cardiac output [73], there is continuing effort to find ways to characterize the functional circulating volume, the relationship between blood volume and blood volume capacity, to help with fluid therapy decisions. The measurement of blood volume would provide some information; however, it would be insufficient to characterize the functional status of the relationship since vascular tone and volume capacity can be considerably variable. Mean systemic filling pressure (Pmsf), literally, is the system-wide equilibrated pressure after a cardiac arrest (usually about 10–15 mmHg) and it is also very similar to postcapillary venous pressure in an animal with a beating heart [73]. It is P_1 in the equation

$$\text{flow} = (P_1 - P_2)/R$$

where R is resistance to flow, which can be rewritten as

$$\text{venous return} = (\text{Pmsf} - \text{CVP})/\text{venous resistance}$$

A venoconstrictor such as norepinephrine or phenylephrine, for instance, may increase venous return by increasing Pmsf or may diminish venous return by increasing venous resistance. Studies have reported both an increased [74–77] and a decreased [77,78] cardiac output with norepinephrine administration.

Short of a cardiac arrest, Pmsf determination in critical or anesthetized patients can be complicated. One method involves a series of inspiratory hold maneuvers at airway pressures of 5, 15, 25, and 35 cmH_2O, coupled with simultaneous CVP and cardiac output measurements [79,80]. The CVP and cardiac output data points are plotted and extrapolated back to a cardiac output of zero to extrapolate Pmsf. A second method involves mathematical modeling and human-derived data [80]. The third, which would be easy to accomplish in routine veterinary settings, is based on the assumption that the appendage venous system behaves similarly to the systemic venous system [80]. With this technique, a rapidly inflating tourniquet (to provide a stop-flow event) is applied to an appendage with a preplaced arterial or venous catheter, which is attached to a pressure-measuring device. After about 20–30 s, arterial and venous blood pressures will be equilibrated and this pressure is taken to represent Pmsf [80–82]. Initial reports suggest that Pmsf estimations by this approach generate values that are not different from those generated by the first, more complicated procedure [80].

Mean systemic filling pressure has been used to characterize the functional status of the circulating blood volume and to identify hypovolemic patients that would benefit from fluid therapy [79]. It could also be used to predict which patients are likely to experience an increase in cardiac output with the administration of norepinephrine (subjects with higher Pmsf) [77]. From a research perspective, venous return (which is assumed to equal cardiac output), Pmsf, and CVP measurements can be used to calculate venous resistance; total systemic compliance can be calculated from a known volume load and pre/post-Pmsf measurements.

Assessing thoracic blood flow impairment

A functional estimation of Pmsf and circulating blood volume can be derived from the fact that positive pressure ventilation impedes intrathoracic venous return, diastolic filling of the heart, and stroke volume. The magnitude of the decrement in stroke volume caused by positive pressure inflation of the lungs can be used as an index of central blood volume [83–90]. The magnitude of decrement in stroke volume can be assessed by the decrease in (1) systolic blood pressure, (2) mean blood pressure, (3) pulse pressure (systolic – diastolic pressure), (4) digital evaluation of pulse quality (the area under the pulse pressure waveform), or (5) plethysmographic monitoring of the area under the pulse pressure waveform, caused by inflating the lung. Stroke volume variation as measured by the Vigileo™/FloTrac™ system (Edwards Lifesciences, Irvine, CA, USA) reliably predicted hypovolemia and fluid responsiveness [91] whereas the PRAM/MostCare™ device (Vytech Health, Padova, Italy) did not [92]. The magnitude of thoracic blood flow impairment is, of course, also dependent upon peak airway pressure, inspiratory time, and cycle rate [93], and this would have to be consistent and standardized in order for this maneuver to have any meaning with reference to circulating blood volume. This procedure is also only intended for use in patients with normal lungs and a closed chest. Diffuse lung disease decreases pulmonary compliance, which diminishes the transfer of pressure from the airways to the pleural space, which diminishes the magnitude of thoracic blood flow impairment to a given ventilator pressure setting. Area under the pulse pressure waveform decrements of >10–13% (with 'reasonable' ventilator settings in subjects with normal lungs) were reported to predict hypovolemia and fluid bolus responsiveness [92,94].

Stroke volume

Stroke volume can be estimated by Doppler ultrasonography by several methods [95–98]. (1) Ventricular end-diastolic diameter (EDD) and ventricular end-systolic diameter (ESD) are measured, then end-diastolic volume (EDV) and end-systolic volume (ESV) are calculated. Stroke volume is calculated as the difference between EDV and ESV. (2) Stroke volume can be calculated by measuring the flow velocity through a structure (often the aortic valve) of known diameter [99]. (3) Stroke volume can be determined by computed tomography (CT) [98] and magnetic resonance imaging (MRI), but these are primarily research tools in anesthetized patients.

The area under the pulse pressure waveform bears some correlation with stroke volume [94,100]. The pulse pressure waveform can be qualitatively characterized by digital palpation of an artery (compared with normal); a tall, wide ('bounding') pulse is likely associated with a large stroke volume whereas a short, narrow ('thready') pulse is likely associated with a small stroke volume. The pulse pressure waveform can also be real-time digitally integrated [101]. At a given arterial compliance, there is an association between the change in the area under the pulse pressure waveform and the stroke volume, and this is the basis of several commercial cardiac output measuring devices (see pulse contour methods in the following section Cardiac Output). When compliance or impedance changes, the quantitative relationship between pulse pressure waveform and stroke volume also changes. Commercial devices that continuously measure and assess the pulse pressure waveform, and then compute cardiac output, usually require intermittent resetting of the computation constant (via input of independent cardiac output measurements) in order to account for changes in compliance and flow impedance (due to retrograde reflected pressure waves) over time.

Cardiac output

Many monitored parameters, such as arterial blood pressure, although important in their own right, may have little to do with forward flow and tissue perfusion. It has been recognized for some time that minimally invasive cardiac output would be a useful addition to anesthetic monitoring. It is worth noting that one of the weaknesses of global indicators of perfusion, including cardiac output and superficial indicators (MM color and CRT), is they do not necessarily reflect the reality of critical organ blood flow. There are normal and necessary changes in regional blood flow distribution along with local oxygen utilization during anesthesia and sedation. An example is with the administration of α_2-adrenergic receptor agonist administration where cardiac output may drop by more than 50%, but regional blood flow decreases much more in skeletal muscle and adipose tissue than in kidney and brain. The clinical significance of changes in cardiac output should always be interpreted within context (e.g., awake patient with normal vasomotor control versus sedated or anesthetized dog with pharmacologically modified vasodilation or constriction). There are many ways to estimate cardiac output, including indicator dilution techniques (thermodilution and lithium dilution), Fick principle-based techniques, pulse contour analysis techniques, transthoracic bioimpedance, and echocardiographic techniques.

Oxygen content, delivery, and consumption

Cardiac output is important but is only one half of the determinants of global oxygen delivery (DO_2); the other half is oxygen content. Oxygen content can be measured, but it is usually calculated as

$$(1.34 \times Hb \times SO_2) + (0.003 \times PO_2)$$

where Hb = hemoglobin concentration (g/dL), SO_2 = oxyhemoglobin saturation, and PO_2 = partial pressure of oxygen in blood (content can be calculated for arterial or venous blood). DO_2 is calculated as cardiac output × oxygen content. DO_2 is important in that it meets tissue oxygen demand. Values for cardiac output, DO_2, and oxygen consumption (VO_2) in normal dogs have been reported [102]. Representative values for other domestic species are included in Table 23.1 in Chapter 23. Anesthesia typically (but not always) decreases cardiac output and DO_2 [103–107]. Anesthesia also typically (but not always) reduces metabolic oxygen consumption [103–105,107,108] by direct and indirect (via hypothermia) depression of metabolic rate, and this partially offsets the problem of decreased DO_2. In addition, when DO_2 starts to decrease, oxygen extraction increases and tissue oxygen requirements continue to be met (delivery-independent oxygen consumption). Oxygen extraction typically increases during general anesthesia [103–105]. Eventually, a point is reached where further decreases in DO_2 are associated with decreases in VO_2 and the onset of tissue hypoxia (delivery-dependent oxygen consumption). The point at which oxygen consumption transitions from delivery independent to delivery dependent is termed the point of critical oxygen delivery. One might think that critical oxygen delivery should decrease during general anesthesia as a direct result of the decrease in metabolic oxygen consumption, but critical oxygen delivery is increased with all anesthetics, in a dose-related manner, and occurs at a lower oxygen extraction ratio, suggesting impaired tissue oxygen extraction [104,105]. This effect on critical oxygen delivery has been attributed to the manner in which anesthetics disturb peripheral blood flow. DO_2 in normal awake dogs has been reported to be 29.5 ± 8.8 mL/min/kg (790 ± 259 mL/min/m^2) [102]. Critical oxygen delivery was reported to be 6.9 mL/min/kg under light pentobarbital anesthesia, increasing to 9–14 mL/min/kg with enflurane, isoflurane, halothane, alfentanil, propofol, etomidate, and higher dosages of pentobarbital [104,105]. Ketamine was the exception in that it did not increase critical oxygen delivery significantly.

From the above oxygen content equation, it is apparent that hemoglobin concentration plays a major role in determining oxygen content. Whether or not animals are anemic prior to induction of general anesthesia, hemoglobin concentrations invariably decrease intraoperatively from anesthetic induced vaso- and splenic dilation, the administration of non-hemoglobin-containing fluids, and intraoperative blood loss. Historically, in humans, the trigger for a hemoglobin transfusion has been a hemoglobin concentration of about 10 g/dL [a packed cell volume (PCV) of 30%] [109]. Subsequent studies in humans have suggested that a more relaxed trigger of 7 g/dL (PCV = 21%) is associated with at least as good, and perhaps better, morbidity and mortality statistics [109]. In veterinary medicine, anesthesiologists have historically used hemoglobin values of 7–8 g/dL (PCV 20–25%) as a trigger for blood transfusion. In animals with immune-mediated hemolytic anemia, it is well accepted to withhold blood transfusions until the hemoglobin concentration has dropped to very low levels of about 5 g/dL (PCV = 15%). This idea is reinforced by the very real chance and negative consequences of a transfusion reaction. In human medicine, in individuals reluctant to participate in blood transfusions, mortality rate does not statistically increase until the hemoglobin concentration decreases below about 5 g/dL (PCV = 15%) [109]. There are many examples of human and veterinary patients surviving much greater levels of anemia, especially if anemia is chronic. Hemoglobin concentration and oxygen content are only one half of the determinants of DO_2 and variations in the subject's ability to increase cardiac output to compensate for anemia may account for much of the patient-to-patient variation in critical oxygen delivery. Animals with anemia diseases but without cardiac impairment (e.g., immune-mediated anemia) may be able to tolerate lower hemoglobin levels by increasing cardiac output, and animals with impaired cardiac function (e.g., sepsis) or under general anesthesia [110,111] likely benefit from higher transfusion trigger levels (Hb 8–9 g/dL; PCV 24–27%). Critical hemoglobin levels in anesthetized dogs have been reported to be in the range 3–4 g/dL [111],; however, this is not a guideline, it is a figure to stay far away from.

Myocardial contractility

Anesthesiologists, intensivists, and physiologists are concerned about the effects of drugs and diseases on the inherent contractility of the myocardium. Contractility is usually not measured but poor contractility is suspected when preload parameters (history of recent fluid loading, ease of jugular vein distention, central venous pressure, posterior vena cava diameter, end-diastolic ventricular volume) suggest high preload and the forward flow parameters [blood pressure, pulse quality, parameters of vasomotor tone (capillary refill time), and parameters of tissue perfusion (appendage temperature, metabolic acidosis, lactate, central venous PO_2)] suggest poor cardiac output in animals without known heart disease (cardiomyopathies, mitral insufficiency, aortic stenosis, pericardial tamponade, or fibrosis). Contractility is the intrinsic rate and force of muscle fiber shortening in a no-load situation. In a living animal, the heart is never unloaded, so myocardial contractility, in addition to its inherent force of contraction, is influenced by preload augmentation and afterload impedance. Augmentation of preload by fluid therapy or venoconstriction increases presystolic muscle stretch and contractility measured by most indices of contractility. Afterload is the impedance to muscle contraction and the generation of a stroke volume. Afterload *in vitro* is the weight that the muscle must lift and afterload *in vivo* is systolic wall stress: (ventricular pressure × radius)/muscle thickness. Inherent contractility is also heart rate dependent [112,113]; an increase in heart rate augments myocardial sarcoplasmic calcium transients and contractility.

Pressure-based methods of assessing contractility

Contractility can be characterized by the rate of pressure development in a ventricle during the contractile process. A pressure transducer-tipped catheter inserted into the ventricle (the left ventricle is usually the ventricle of concern) measures the change in pressures throughout the cardiac cycle. The maximum rate of change of ventricular pressure during the isovolumic contraction phase (Fig. 4.8a) is termed peak dP/dt [114,115]. The clinical disadvantage of this technique is the requirement for a ventricular catheter.

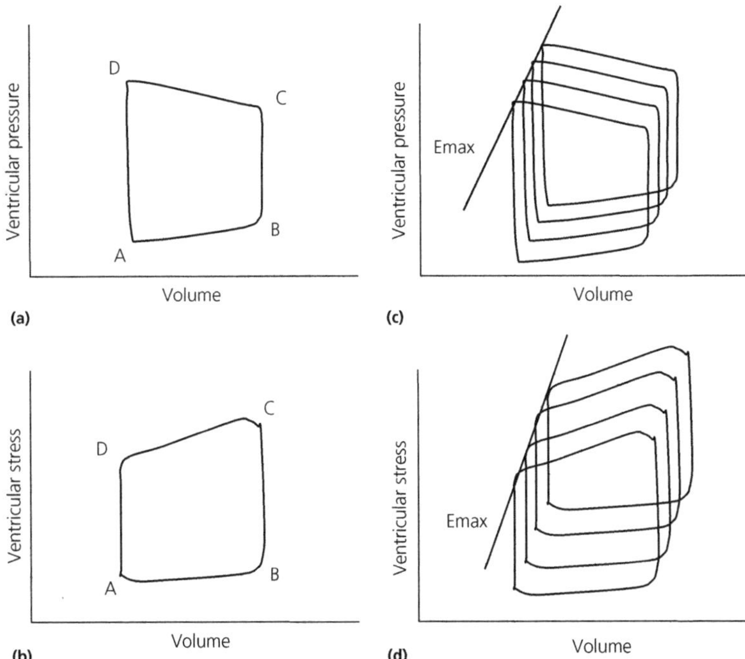

Figure 4.8 Ventricular pressure–volume (a) and stress–volume (b) loops. A to B = ventricular filling; B to C = isovolumic contraction; C to D = ventricular ejection; D to A = isovolumic relaxation. A series of pressure–volume loops (c) and stress–volume loops (d) following vasoconstrictor or fluid administration. A line drawn through the end-systolic points of the loops is Emax and the slope of this line is a preload- and afterload-independent marker of myocardial contractility.

Combining ventricular pressure measurements with serial assessment of changes in ventricular volume (usually Doppler ultrasound derived) allows the construction of a ventricular pressure:volume loop (Fig. 4.8a). Acute changes in preload (fluid administration) or afterload (vasoconstrictor administration) changes the end-systolic pressure–volume point in an upward direction (Fig. 4.8c). The slope of the line drawn through several end-systolic pressure–volume points (Emax) characterizes myocardial contractility independent of preload and afterload [116]. Generating several pressure–volume curves or end-systolic pressure–volume points is, however, technically time consuming. Definition of the entire loop requires ventricular catheterization; however, the end-systolic pressure (defined as systolic arterial blood pressure)–volume [defined by calculating end systolic volume (ESV) from Doppler-derived end systolic diameter (ESD)] points is a non-invasive method of estimating Emax [117].

The d*P*/d*t* of the ventricle determines the d*P*/d*t* of the upsweep of the pulse pressure waveform. The pulse waveform provides an indirect way of estimating ventricular contractility without using a ventricular catheter. Some commercial pulse pressure waveform analyzers (PiCCO$_2$™ and Most Care™) have the ability to generate a measure of contractility based upon the rate of change of the pulse pressure waveform [118].

Doppler ultrasound-based methods of assessing contractility

Doppler ultrasound technology has revolutionized the ability to assess non-invasively indices of myocardial contractility in clinical situations. Accurate and repeatable cardiac ultrasound assessments require training and practice. Anesthesiologists and intensivists who may not have developed the expertise to make such measurements reliably [119,120] should still be familiar with how to interpret them. A qualitative assessment of myocardial function can be obtained by visual inspection of the echocardiogram; a heart with poor contractility will be seen to contract slowly and incompletely compared with normal. Standard cardiac ultrasound examinations commonly report some indices that correlate with contractility. Minor axis end-diastolic diameter (EDD) and end-systolic diameter (ESD) are measured (Table 4.7). Fractional shortening (FS) is calculated as (EDD - ESD/EDD). Typical values for FS are 25–45% in dogs and 30–55% in cats [63]; a decrease in contractility would be associated with a decrease in fractional shortening. A note of caution in interpreting FS is that the compensatory increase in EDD that occurs in animals with congestive heart failure can restore FS to normal numbers even though contractility, *per se*, is decreased. End-diastolic volume (EDV) and end-systolic volume (ESV) can be calculated from EDD and ESD, respectively [95–97]. Stroke volume (SV) is calculated from the difference between EDV and ESV and ejection fraction (EF) is calculated as SV/EDV. EF typically exceeds 50%. When a heart contracts less vigorously, ESV, SV, and EF are decreased. FS, SV, and EF are preload, afterload, and heart rate dependent.

Mitral regurgitation presents a special problem with these parameters because a variable portion of the reduction in ESD, FS, ESV, and EF that occurs during systole constitutes retrograde blood flow into the left atrium. In these situations, the subjective shape of the regurgitant jet may, however, be informative; a low peak velocity and a slow rate of change in velocity may suggest poor contractility [97, 121]. In the presence of mitral regurgitaiton, a Doppler-derived d*P*/d*t* can be derived from initial rate of change of the regurgitant jet [97,121,122]; d*P*/d*t* in normal dogs generally exceed 1800 mmHg/s [121] and can be as high 3000–4000 mmHg/s [112].

The velocity of circumferential fractional shortening (Vcf) is calculated as FS/ET, where ET = ejection time. ET is the time from initial opening of the aortic valve until its closure. A surrogate marker of ET might be from the initial upstroke of the arterial pulse pressure waveform to the depth of the dicrotic notch. Vcf is relatively preload independent but is heart rate and afterload dependent. A heart rate-corrected Vcf can be calculated as [123,124]

$$\mathrm{FS}/\left\{\mathrm{ET}\times[\mathrm{R}-\mathrm{R\ interval(ms)}]^{1/2}\right\}$$

Table 4.7 Doppler-derived variables and systolic time intervals for normal dogs and cats [63,96,121,125].

Parameter[a]	Dog	Cat
LVEDD (cm)	$1.44 \times kg^{0.32}$; 2.0–5.5 (small to large)	1.2–1.8
LVESD (cm)	$0.69 \times kg^{0.41}$; 1.0–4.0 (small to large)	0.5–1.0
LVEDV (mL/kg)	2.4–4.8 (large to small)	1.5–2.0
LVESV (mL/kg)	0.81–0.97 (small to large)	0.14–0.43
SV (mL/kg)	1.4–4.0 (large to small)	1.4–1.6
EF (%)	60–80	70–90
FS (%)	25–50	25–60
Vcf (circumferences/s)	2.0–3.5	2.8–4.8
PEP (ms)	50–75	40–50
LVET (ms)	150–270	110–160
LVETi (ms)	210–310	200–220
PEP + LVET (ms)	200–330	140–180
PEP/LVET	0.15–0.40	0.35–0.45

[a] LVEDD = left ventricular end-diastolic diameter; LVESD = left ventricular end-systolic diameter; LVEDV = left ventricular end-diastolic volume (calculated by the Teichholz formula: $(7 \times D^3)/(2.4 + D)$; LVESV = left ventricular end-systolic volume (calculated by the Teichholz formula as above; SV = stroke volume; EF = ejection fraction; FS = fractional shortening; Vcf = velocity of circumferential fractional shortening; PEP = pre-ejection period; LVET = left ventricular ejection time; LVETi = LVET indexed to heart rate.

Myocardial strain is the idea that afterload is more than just pressure; it is myocardial stress (ventricular pressure × radius/wall thickness). The shape of the stress–volume loop is different from that of the pressure–volume loop in that the top of the stress–volume loop is angled downwards (Fig. 4.8b); myocardial stress decreases over the course of systole. Doppler imaging is capable of defining ventricular radius and wall thickness. Ventricular pressure can be measured directly or indirectly from arterial blood pressure (systolic pressure ≈ end-systolic ventricular pressure), and then ventricular wall stress can be calculated. Emax can be determined from a set of end-systolic wall stress points (Fig. 4.8d) and the slope of line characterizes contractility in a load-independent manner. End-systolic wall stress, *per se*, has been reported to be a non-load-dependent marker of contractility [124]. Myocardial strain and rate of strain development are relatively preload- and afterload-independent indices of contractility [97,115,123,125].

Three-dimensional Doppler imaging is currently the best technique for measuring ventricular volumes [97]. Measurements, calculated volumes, and EF can be accomplished in real time and correlate well with CT and MRI [126]. Tissue Doppler imaging uses high-velocity filters to isolate myocardial wall acceleration (from that of blood) during systole and can be used to calculate d*P*/d*t* [97]. Radial and longitudinal endocardial ventricular velocities have been reported during systole, and early and late diastole, for unanesthetized and anesthetized dogs [127,128], awake normal cats [129,130], and cats with cardiomyopathy [131]. Decreased contraction velocities during systole suggest poor contractility; decreased relaxation velocities during diastole reflect diastolic dysfunction [97]. A myocardial performance index (MPI or Tei) is calculated as (isovolumic contraction time + isovolumic relaxation time)/ejection time and provides an overall assessment of ventricular function. Contractility augmentation decreases both values in the numerator more than the denominator and MPI decreases, whereas contractility inhibition does the opposite [132]. Dobutamine augmentation of contractility increased all measurements of contractility (increased systolic pressure, +d*P*/d*t*, and decreased isovolemic contraction time) and relaxation (–d*P*/d*t*, decreased isovolemic relaxation time); esmolol inhibition of myocardial β_1 receptors decreased all measurements of contractility and relaxation [132].

Systolic time intervals

Systolic time intervals are also a measure of myocardial contractility and can be determined with or without the aid of Doppler ultrasound [133–135]. The pre-ejection period (PEP) is the time from the beginning of the QRS wave on the ECG to the opening of the aortic valve. The opening of the aortic valve can be determined by visual observation of the aortic valve with Doppler ultrasound or it can be taken as the beginning of the upstroke of the aortic pressure waveform. Left ventricular ejection time (LVET) is the time from the opening to the closure of the aortic valve. Closure of the aortic valve can be determined by visual observation of the valve with Doppler ultrasound, the depth of the dicrotic notch of the pulse pressure waveform, or the beginning of the second heart sound on a phonocardiogram. Total electromechanical systole = PEP + LVET. PEP (pre) and LVET (after) indices are load and heart rate dependent. The PEP/LVET index minimizes the effects of preload and afterload. A decrease in contractility prolongs PEP and LVET and increases the PEP/LVET index.

Systemic vascular resistance and tissue perfusion

Physical signs

Peripheral and visceral perfusion are primarily regulated by vasomotor tone; at the microvascular level vasoconstriction impairs it whereas vasodilation improves it. Vasoconstriction increases blood pressure whereas vasodilation decreases it. Vasomotor tone can be assessed by mucous membrane color (paler than normal = vasoconstriction; redder than normal = vasodilation), capillary refill time (<1 s = vasodilation; >2 s = vasoconstriction); toe-web/core temperature gradient (>4 °C = vasoconstriction; <2 °C = vasodilation) [136,137]. Vasoconstriction may be caused by hypovolemia, heart failure, hypothermia, or the administration of vasoconstrictor drugs. Vasodilation may be caused by the systemic inflammatory response, hyperthermia, or the administration of vasodilator drugs.

Calculation of systemic vascular resistance

Systemic vascular resistance (SVR) is calculated as: mean arterial blood pressure (ABPm – CVP) (in mmHg)/cardiac output indexed to body weight (mL/min/kg) or surface area (L/min/m²). SVR is commonly reported as $dyn \cdot s \cdot cm^{-5}/m^2$:

$$[ABPm - CVP(mmHg) \times 79.92]/CI(L/min/m^2)$$

Systemic vascular resistance in normal dogs has been reported to be between about 1800 and 2100 $dyn\,s\,cm^{-5}/m^2$ [102] increasing to 2500–3000 $dyn\,s\,cm^{-5}/m^2$ with moderate hypovolemia [138]. The effect of anesthetics on SVR varies with drug, drug dosage, and baseline SVR.

Metabolic markers of tissue perfusion

Arterial–venous oxygen differences

As mentioned previously, one way to measure cardiac output is the Fick equation:

$$CO = \text{oxygen consumption}/(CaO_2 - CmvO_2)$$

where CaO_2 = oxygen content of arterial blood and $CmvO_2$ = oxygen content of mixed venous blood. Oxygen consumption, however, is not usually measured. If one assumes that it does not change too much, at least over the course of a short procedure, it can be dropped from the Fick equation, leaving cardiac output inversely proportional to CaO_2 – $CmvO_2$. In two canine studies, CaO_2 – $CmvO_2$ was reported to increase from 3.8 ± 1.2 to 7.1 ± 1.9 mL/dL with moderate hypovolemia [138] and from 4.0 ± 0.8 to 8.9 ± 2.1 mL/dL at critical oxygen delivery during severe hypovolemia, and ultimately to 13.1 ± 2.0 mL/dL just prior to the collapse of arterial blood pressure [139]. The CaO_2 – $CmvO_2$ gradient can be used as a global marker of the increased oxygen extraction that occurs when oxygen delivery decreases for any reason. Oxygen extraction expressed as a percentage [(CaO_2 – $CmvO_2$)/CaO_2] is a similar global marker. In two canine studies, oxygen extraction was reported to increase from 20.9 ± 6.2 to 42.3 ± 9.6% with moderate hypovolemia [138] and from 22.4 ± 4.5 to 53.5 ± 10.4% at critical oxygen delivery in severe hypovolemia, and ultimately to 84.2 ± 9.5% just prior to the collapse of arterial blood pressure [139].

A further abbreviation of the oxygen Fick equation is to drop CaO_2 and simply add it to the list of abnormalities that can cause a decreased $CmvO_2$ (oxygen delivery ≈ venous oxygen). Since blood oxygen content, hemoglobin saturation, and PO_2 are directionally related, any expression of the amount of oxygen in mixed venous blood will suffice for this purpose; PO_2 is the easiest to obtain. However, peripheral venous blood will not suffice [140] because it only represents local tissue extraction; blood must be obtained from a location as close to the pulmonary artery as possible for a global measurement. Mixed venous PO_2, saturation, and oxygen content reportedly decrease from 49 ± 6 mmHg, 78 ± 6%, and 13.8 ± 2.2 mL/dL to 35 ± 5 mmHg, 56 ± 9%, and 9.6 ± 2.5 mL/dL, respectively, in moderate hypovolemia [138]. In another canine acute hemorrhage model, SvO_2 decreased from 73 ± 4 to 42 ± 9% at critical oxygen delivery in severe hypovolemia and ultimately to 17 ± 9% just prior to the collapse of arterial blood pressure [139]. Venous oxygen can also be used to mark improved oxygen delivery with therapy. In a cohort of critically ill humans, dobutamine augmentation of cardiac output decreased oxygen extraction from 48 to 36% and increased mixed venous oxygen saturation from 49 to 61% [141]. Other studies have reported weak correlations between venous oxygen saturation and cardiac output in human ICU patients [142] and in piglets of hemorrhagic, anemic, and hypoxemic models [143].

Venous–arterial PCO_2 gradient

Cardiac output can also be determined by the carbon dioxide Fick equation:

$$CO = \text{carbon dioxide production}/(CmvCO_2 - CaCO_2)$$

where $CmvCO_2$ = carbon dioxide content of mixed venous blood and $CaCO_2$ = carbon dioxide content of arterial blood. One of the methods of measuring cardiac output ($PiCCO_2$) uses this principle. Carbon dioxide production, however, is not usually measured and, assuming that it has not change too much, it can be dropped from the above equation:

$$\text{cardiac output} \approx CmvCO_2 - CaCO_2$$

Carbon dioxide content can be calculated, but since carbon dioxide is so soluble (the PCO_2–CO_2 content curve is nearly linear within the broad range of PCO_2 values seen clinically) [144], measured $PmvCO_2$ and $PaCO_2$ can be used directly without converting to content. When cardiac output and tissue perfusion decrease, and carbon dioxide production continues at its previous level, there will be an increase in venous carbon dioxide. In three canine acute hemorrhage models, venous – arterial PCO_2 was reported to increase from 4.2 ± 1.5 to 10.7 ± 3.9 mmHg [138], from 5.2 to 12.9 mmHg in moderate hypovolemia, and from 4.3 ± 1.3 to 12.9 ± 5.2 mmHg at critical oxygen delivery in severe hypovolemia, and ultimately to 32.9 ± 10.0 mmHg just prior to the collapse of arterial blood pressure [139]. In a pig model of severe hypovolemic shock, $CmvCO_2$ – $CaCO_2$ increased from 2 ± 6 to 26 ± 5 mmHg after blood pressure had been maintained at 50 mmHg for 2 h [145]. $CmvCO_2$ – $CaCO_2$ can also be used to track response to therapy; it decreased from 9 to 5 mmHg with dobutamine augmentation of cardiac output in people [141].

Lactate and metabolic acidosis

Lactate is a measure of poor tissue oxygenation and is commonly measured in clinical patients. However, blood lactate is a global measure that disproportionately overweights large tissue masses, and may not be a sensitive acute measure of oxygen deficiency in tissues that have low mass but high oxygen demand (e.g., brain or kidney). Therefore, it may not accurately represent vital organ status during anesthesia, but may be better used for predicting mortality in ICU patients that can survive long enough for significant accumulation to occur, and which have higher metabolic demand of muscle and other large tissue masses than anesthetized, hypothermic patients. In a pig model of severe hypovolemic shock, lactate increased from about 1.5 to about 14 mmol/L after blood pressure had been maintained at 50 mmHg for 2 h [145]. In a canine acute hemorrhage model, lactate increased from 2.4 ± 0.9 to 3.5 ± 1.4 mmol/L at critical oxygen delivery with severe hypovolemia, and ultimately to 8.9 ± 3.8 mmol/L just prior to the collapse of arterial blood pressure [139].

Base deficit worsened from −2.2 ± 2.4 to −6.3 ± 2.9 mEq/L in moderate hypovolemia [138] and from −2.4 ± 4.0 to −16.1 ± 3.9 mEq/L in severe hypovolemia in dogs [146]. In three canine hypovolemia models, the arterial – venous pH gradient increased from 0.02 ± 0.01 to 0.06 ± 0.03 units [138] and from 0.03 ± 0.05 to 0.09 ± 0.11 units [146] during moderate hypovolemia, from 0.03 ± 0.01 to 0.06 ± 0.03 units at critical oxygen delivery with severe hypovolemia, and ultimately to 0.14 ± 0.04 units just prior to the collapse of arterial blood pressure [139].

Tissue PO_2, PCO_2, and pH

Poor tissue perfusion results in decreased tissue PO_2 and pH and increased PCO_2. Such measurements might provide earlier and more organ-specific warning of poor tissue perfusion than do measures from the venous blood flowing from those tissues. There are a variety of ways to measure tissue PO_2, PCO_2, and pH: PO_2 catheter-tip electrodes, PCO_2 catheter-tip electrodes, pH catheter-tip electrodes, gastric capnometry, and sublingual capnometry.

Tissue PO_2 (PtO_2) can be measured either with catheter-tipped PO_2 electrodes [146–148] or with transcutaneous sensors [149,150]. The measurement of decreased PtO_2 is a sensitive index of poor peripheral perfusion [146,147] and decreased PtO_2 significantly increases mortality risk in critically ill patients [150].

Transcutaneous catheter-tipped pH electrodes can be used to measure tissue pH [146,148]. Tissue pH is a sensitive marker of poor tissue perfusion [146,147]. A fiber-optic multiparameter (PO_2, PCO_2, and pH) catheter (Diametrics Medical) that could be placed in any tissue has been investigated [146–148], but is not available at the time of this writing.

Gastric tonometry is a technique based on the fact that as tissue PCO_2 increases in malperfusion states, the carbon dioxide diffuses into the lumen of the stomach in direct proportion to its accumulation in the gastric tissues. Gastric lumen PCO_2 ($PgCO_2$) can be measured via either a PCO_2 sensor-tipped catheter [151,152] or a balloon-tipped catheter [153–155]. Carbon dioxide diffuses into the lumen of the balloon, which, after a suitable equilibration time, is aspirated and the PCO_2 is measured. Systems are available that automatically inflate the balloon, then withdraw and analyze the gas sample after a 10 min dwell time (Tonometrics). Gastric PCO_2 should be below 50 mmHg or less than 10 mmHg above $PaCO_2$; values of >60 mmHg or of >20 mmHg higher than $PaCO_2$ suggest gastric malperfusion [154–156]. In a pig model of severe hypovolemia, $PgCO_2$ increased from about 60 to about 110 mmHg after blood pressure had been maintained at 50 mmHg for 2 h [145]. The $PgCO_2$–$PaCO_2$ gradient increases with anything that impairs tissue oxygenation: ischemia [146,153,157], hypoxemia [157], and severe anemia (PCV 15%) [155]. Both $PgCO_2$ and $PgCO_2$–$PaCO_2$ gradient should be assessed [158]. Raw $PgCO_2$ values may be increased with systemic hypercapnia without visceral malperfusion (the $PgCO_2$–$PaCO_2$ gradient would be normal). In transition states, the $PgCO_2$–$PaCO_2$ gradient may be misleading because it takes about 20 min for tissue PCO_2 to equilibrate with $PaCO_2$. A persistently elevated $PgCO_2$ following therapy is associated with increased mortality [151,154].

Sublingual capnometry ($PslCO_2$) (Optical Sensors) compares very well with $PgCO_2$ as a measure of peripheral tissue perfusion [145]. The sensor is not as invasive as the gastric catheter but, owing to its location, is more prone to technical errors. In pig models of severe hypovolemia, $PslCO_2$ increased from about 60 to about 120 mmHg after blood pressure had been maintained at 50–55 mmHg for 2 h [145,159]. Sublingual capnometry (both raw $PslCO_2$ and $PaCO_2$–$PslCO_2$ gradient) was reported to be a sensitive index of poor tissue perfusion; non-survivors had persistently higher values [160,161].

Microvascular Imaging

There are many ways to visualize the microcirculation in clinical patients [161–168]: laser-Doppler flowmetry (PeriFlux™, Perimed), laser speckle contrast imaging, polarized spectroscopy, orthogonal polarization spectral imaging (OPS) (Cytoscan™, Cytometrics), sidestream darkfield imaging (Microscan™, Microvision Medical), light videomicroscopy, fluorescence videomicroscopy, wide-field microscopy, and Doppler ultrasound. Capillary size and shape, density and heterogeneity, and blood flow and blood flow velocity can be determined. Many systems employ a hand-held videomicroscope for bed-side application. Microvascular imaging has been used to evaluate peripheral/regional blood flow [75] and vascular reactivity [169] in various disease states.

Pulmonary system

Breathing rate, rhythm, and effort

The breathing rate can vary widely and, except for extreme values, is of limited value as a respiratory parameter. A change in breathing rate, however, is a sensitive indicator of a change in the underlying status of the patient. Bradypnea may be a sign of deep anesthesia or hypothermia. Apnea is common following induction of anesthesia and can occur even in animals that are very lightly anesthetized. Arrhythmic breathing patterns are indicative of a problem with the central pattern generator in the medulla. A Cheyne–Stokes breathing pattern (cycling between hyperventilation and hypoventilation) may be seen in otherwise healthy anesthetized horses and an apneustic breathing pattern (inspiratory hold) may be seen in otherwise healthy dogs and cats anesthetized with ketamine. There are many causes of tachypnea and exaggerated breathing effort during anesthesia (Box 4.1).

Box 4.1 Causes of tachypnea and exaggerated breathing effort.

- Light level of anesthesia
- Deep level of anesthesia
- Hypoxemia, hypercapnia, hyperthermia
- Hypotension
- Atelectasis
- Airway obstruction, pleural space filling disorder, pulmonary parenchymal disease
- Excitement stage of recovery
- Postoperative pain
- Postoperative delirium (any drug but particularly following opioids and benzodiazepines)
- Postoperative distended urinary bladder

Ventilometry, deadspace, and compliance

Ventilation volume can be estimated by visual observation of the chest or rebreathing bag or measured by ventilometry. Normal tidal volume ranges between about 6 and 15 mL/kg. A small tidal volume may be acceptable if the breathing rate is sufficiently rapid to accomplish normal alveolar minute ventilation. Normal total minute ventilation ranges between 150 and 250 mL/kg/min in awake patients. Ventilometry can measure total ventilation but it cannot measure the proportion that is distributed to deadspace versus to functional alveoli. Physiologic deadspace (anatomic and alveolar) ranges between 30 and 50% of tidal volume and minute ventilation in a normal patient breathing a normal tidal volume; the remaining balance is termed functional alveolar ventilation [170–174]. Physiologic deadspace (%) will be higher with rapid, shallow breathing and lower with slow, deep breathing. Physiologic deadspace is calculated as

$$Vd/Vt = (PaCO_2 - PmeCO_2)/(PaCO_2 - P_ICO_2)$$

where Vd = deadspace volume, Vt = tidal volume, Vd/Vt = ratio of deadspace to total tidal volume, $PaCO_2$ = arterial partial pressure of carbon dioxide, $PmeCO_2$ = mixed-expired PCO_2, and P_ICO_2 = inspired PCO_2. Deadspace (%) × measured tidal volume or minute ventilation calculates absolute values (mL/kg) for deadspace. Vt − Vd = Valv, where Valv = alveolar ventilation. Effective alveolar minute ventilation is typically defined by $PaCO_2$. A high measured total minute ventilation in combination with a normal $PaCO_2$ is indicative of increased deadspace ventilation.

Compliance is calculated as expired tidal volume divided by the change in pressure that it took to generate the tidal volume. The change in airway pressure during positive pressure ventilation is calculated as peak or pause pressure minus end-expiratory pressure. During spontaneous ventilation, the change in transpulmonary pressure requires the measurement of pleural pressure (which is usually done via a balloon-tipped catheter placed in the lower esophagus). If, for instance, 10 cmH_2O of pressure generated a tidal volume of 10 mL/kg, the compliance would be calculated to be 1 $mL/kg/cmH_2O$. If the measurements are made during the cyclic breathing process (using peak pressure), the calculated value is termed dynamic compliance. If the measurements are made after a short (or a long) inspiratory pause (pause pressure), the value is termed static compliance.

With positive pressure ventilation, during airway pressurization, some of the volume that left the ventilator is taken up by compression of gases within the anesthetic circuit and by breathing circuit expansion. This volume never reaches the patient but will be measured as part of the expired tidal volume. Many anesthesia ventilators do not compensate for this effect and higher measured tidal volume will result in erroneous assumptions about the patient and incorrect compliance calculations. This may be particularly important in very small animals where the volume of circuit compression and expansion represents a larger percentage of the total measured tidal volume. The volume of compression and expansion for a given anesthetic circuit and ventilation technique can be determined by disconnecting the patient and recording the measured tidal volume (at the same peak inspiratory pressure observed while ventilating the patient) while the patient port of the Y-piece is plugged. This volume of compression and expansion should then be subtracted from the measured tidal volume prior to calculating compliance. Compliance is decreased by restrictive pulmonary, pleural, or thoracic wall disease.

Partial pressure of carbon dioxide (PCO_2)

The PCO_2 measuring electrode of a blood gas analyzer consists of a hydrogen ion-sensitive, silver–silver chloride measuring half-cell and a reference half-cell. Carbon dioxide diffuses from the test solution, in proportion to its partial pressure, across a semipermeable silicone membrane. Carbon dioxide combines with water and increases the hydrogen ion concentration (carbonic acid equilibration) of the inside solution. The hydrogen ion causes an electrical potential difference between the half-cells that is proportional to the change in hydrogen ion concentration, which is proportional to the change in PCO_2.

The arterial PCO_2 ($PaCO_2$) is a measure of the effective alveolar minute ventilation and normally ranges between 35 and 45 mmHg. Acceptable $PaCO_2$ values may be higher in anesthetized small animals and is considerably higher (60–80 mmHg) in anesthetized horses [175] and cattle [3]. A $PaCO_2$ in excess of 60 mmHg may be associated with excessive respiratory acidosis and is usually considered to represent sufficient hypoventilation to warrant positive pressure ventilation in small animals. $PaCO_2$ values below 20 mmHg are associated with respiratory alkalosis and a decreased cerebral blood flow, which may impair cerebral oxygenation. Acceptable values should be maintained closer to awake values for patients with central nervous system disease, pre-existing metabolic acid–base abnormalities, or significant hyperkalemia. The causes of hypercapnia and hypocapnia are listed in Table 4.8.

Venous PCO_2 is usually 3–6 mmHg higher than arterial PCO_2 in stable states [102] and can generally be used as a surrogate marker of $PaCO_2$. $PvCO_2$ is variably higher in transition states and during hypovolemia [138], poor cardiac output, or anemia. An increased arterial–venous PCO_2 gradient suggests decreased tissue perfusion. The PCO_2 in a sample of gas taken at the end of an exhalation ($PetCO_2$) can also be used as a surrogate marker of $PaCO_2$. $PetCO_2$ is usually 3–6 mmHg lower than $PaCO_2$ in dogs and 10–15 mmHg lower in horses [176].

Capnometry is the measure of carbon dioxide in the respiratory gases. The most common method of measuring gaseous carbon dioxide is by infrared light absorption, with absorption being proportional to the partial pressure of the gas. Carbon dioxide can also be measured by Raman spectroscopy, where a monochromatic argon light beam is passed through the gas sample. The light is absorbed and then re-emitted at a different wavelength that is specific to the gas molecule that absorbed it. Mass spectrometry, based upon separation of the various gas species by an electron beam in a magnetic field, can also be used to measure carbon dioxide, but these analyzers are expensive, bulky, and not commonly used in clinical medicine.

Table 4.8 Potential causes of hypocapnia and hypercapnia.

Hypocapnia – hyperventilation	Light level of anesthesia, hypoxemia, hyperthermia, hypotension, inappropriate ventilator settings, early pulmonary parenchymal disease
	Postoperation: excitement stage of recovery, delirium, pain, distended urinary bladder, sepsis
Hypercapnia – hypoventilation	Excessive depth of anesthesia, neuromuscular disease, airway obstruction, pleural space-filling disorder, late pulmonary parenchymal disease, inappropriate ventilator settings, malfunctioning anesthetic machine (unidirectional valves stuck, soda lime exhaustion), low fresh gas flow with non-rebreathing circuits

With mainstream capnometers, the patient breathes through a cell or cuvette surrounded by an infrared transmitter and photosensor system. The cuvette is heated to help minimize condensation on its windows. The CO_2 signal is transmitted immediately to a display device so displayed waveforms are near-real time. Cuvettes are somewhat bulky and add deadspace and resistance to the breathing circuit. Sidestream capnometers aspirate a gas sample from the airway (usually at a flow rate between 50 and 200 mL/min) and the CO_2 measurement occurs away from the airway in the analyzer. There is a delay of about 3 s between the time when the sample is aspirated and the time when they are measured and displayed on the device (the time delay is determined by length and diameter of the aspiration tube and the aspiration flow rate). Sidestream sample ports should be placed dorsally in the airway to minimize occlusion with respiratory secretions. The aspirated sample should be returned to the anesthetic circuit to minimize depletion of circuit volume with low-flow techniques or to the scavenging system to minimize environmental pollution. Aspiration tubing of sidestream capnometers can also be placed nasally or can be attached to a tracheal catheter for CO_2 monitoring [177].

There are two types of capnography: time:PCO_2 and volume:PCO_2. Time capnography is represented by the familiar analyzer used in clinical practice [178]; PCO_2 is expressed as a function of time during the entire respiratory cycle (Fig. 4.9). The presence of a typical signal can be used to verify that the endotracheal tube is properly placed in the trachea at the beginning of the procedure. A sudden cessation of the capnogram such that it appears 'stuck' in the plateau phase represents severe bradypnea/apnea or an obstructed aspiration tube. A sudden disappearance of the capnogram (such that it appears to be 'stuck' at zero) could be caused by apnea, accidental extubation, or disconnection/obstruction of the breathing system or aspiration tube. If the animal is being ventilated, a 'stuck at zero' capnogram could also represent cardiac arrest. Other aberrations in the capnogram are illustrated in Fig. 4.10.

Volume capnography plots expired CO_2 against expired volume (Fig. 4.11) [179]. Tidal volume, anatomic and alveolar deadspace, physiologic deadspace, effective alveolar tidal volume, end-tidal

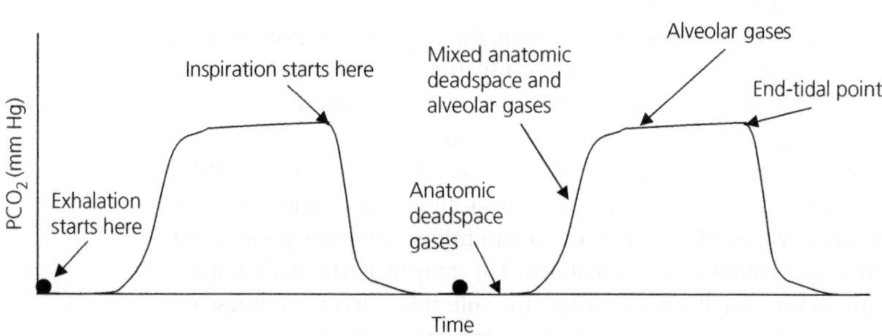

Figure 4.9 Time capnography. Exhalation starts at the black dots; the first gas exhaled is anatomic deadspace and is CO_2 free. The PCO_2 line then slopes upwards and this represents a mixture of deadspace and alveolar gases. A shallow slope to this line coupled with a steeper slope to the plateau portion suggests impaired alveolar emptying such as would occur with lower airway narrowing. The plateau, which represents alveolar gases, may (or may not) slope upwards slightly due to the continued delivery of venous carbon dioxide to the alveoli during exhalation. End-tidal CO_2 is the highest PCO_2 before the next inspiration. Inspired gases should contain no carbon dioxide; the capnogram should go to zero during inspiration.

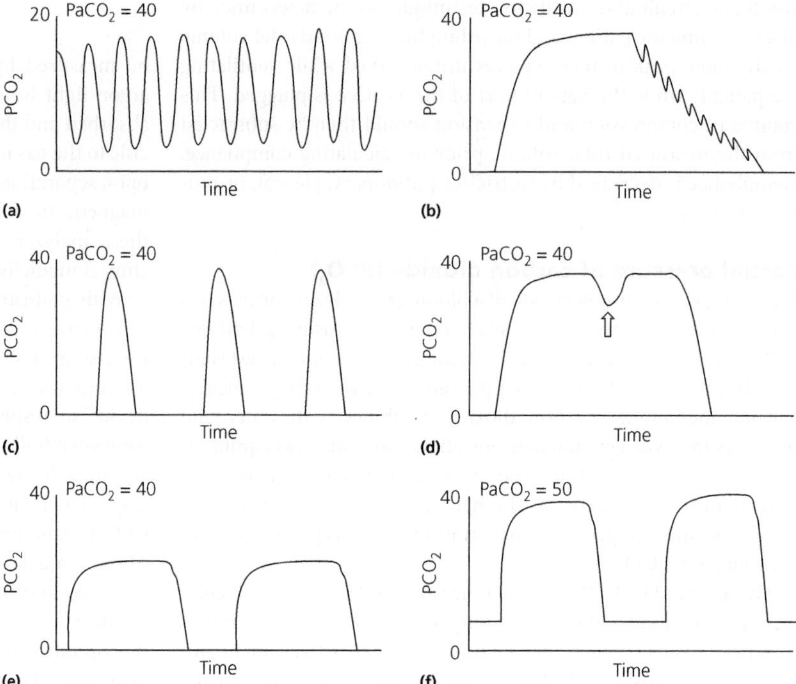

Figure 4.10 Abnormal capnograms. (a) Capnogram oscillates with ventilation but does not return to zero with inspiration and does not approach $PaCO_2$. Tachynpnea without good separation of anatomic deadspace and alveolar gases. Displayed end-tidal PCO_2 values are not representative of $PaCO_2$. (b) Cardiac oscillations of airway pressure. (c) Capnogram rises with exhalation but does not plateau and returns to baseline before the animal inspires. Sample port too close to fresh gas inflow. (d) A small negative divot in the capnogram represents a spontaneous inspiratory effort prior to a proper inspiration. (e) Capnogram shape is not abnormal but the plateau is very low compared with $PaCO_2$. Excessive alveolar deadspace (hypovolemia; thromboembolism). (f) Capnogram shape is not abnormal but the baseline does not return to zero with inspiration. Deadspace rebreathing.

PCO_2, alveolar PCO_2, eliminated CO_2 volume, and mixed-expired CO_2 can be determined. A flattening of the curve (less steep phase II coupled with a less 'plateaued' phase III) suggests increased physiologic deadspace, due either to lower airway obstructive disease [179,180] or to increased alveolar deadspace ventilation due to hypovolemia or pulmonary thromboembolism [181]. As with time capnography, accidental extubation and cardiac arrest will cause the volumetric capnogram to flatten to zero. Positive pressure ventilation may either flatten the slope (due to increased alveolar deadspace ventilation) or normalize the slope (due to recruitment of collapsed lung units).

Oxygen

Partial pressure of oxygen in arterial blood (PaO_2)

The PaO_2 is the partial pressure (the vapor pressure) of oxygen dissolved in solution in the plasma of arterial blood and is measured with a blood gas analyzer. The oxygen electrode is usually a silver anode/platinum cathode system in an electrolyte solution separated from the unknown solution by a semipermeable membrane. The chemical reaction of the binding of oxygen at the cathode drives the oxidation (electron release) from the adjacent silver anode, which changes the current between the two electrodes in direct proportion to the PO_2.

Atmospheric oxygen is normally ventilated into the alveoli and then diffuses across the respiratory membrane along partial pressure gradients into the plasma. The PaO_2 is a measure of the ability of the lungs to move oxygen from the atmosphere to the blood. Anything which interferes with these processes will decrease plasma PO_2. The normal PaO_2 at sea level (breathing 21% oxygen) ranges between 80 and 110 mmHg. Hypoxemia is generally defined as a $PaO_2 < 80$ mmHg, and potentially life-threatening hypoxemia as a $PaO_2 < 60$ mmHg. Hyperoxemia is defined as a $PaO_2 > 110$ mmHg and is the norm when breathing oxygen-enriched gas mixtures during anesthesia.

Blood oxygen can also be expressed as a concentration or content (mL/dL whole blood), but this parameter is primarily determined by hemoglobin concentration and is not considered, *per se*, a marker of hypoxemia or hyperoxemia. Oxygen content has a great deal to do with oxygen delivery and is discussed under that heading.

Arterial blood samples must be used for the assessment of pulmonary function. Venous blood comes from the tissues and is more

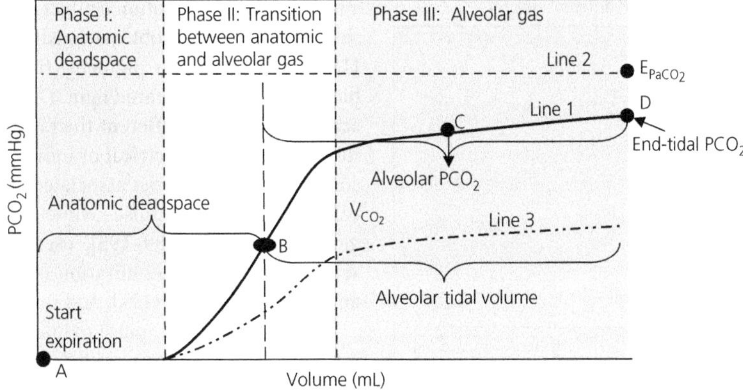

Figure 4.11 Volumetric capnography. The capnogram displays only the expired CO_2 as a function of volume; the analyzer resets itself after each inspiration; inspiratory PCO_2 is not visible. Expiration begins at the black dot in the lower left-hand corner of the figure (A) and the first gas exhaled is that of airway deadspace (phase I). The sloping line of phase II (Line 1) represents a mixture of airway deadspace and alveolar gases. The phase III plateau (Line 1) represents alveolar gases and often continues to escalate until the end of the breath. End-tidal PCO_2 is the highest PCO_2 at the end of the breath (D). $PaCO_2$ (measured separately) is usually 3–6 mmHg higher than end-tidal PCO_2. The horizontal dashed line (Line 2) at the level of $PaCO_2$ is the theoretical expired PCO_2 (E) if there were no airway or alveolar deadspace. Airway deadspace can be estimated as the expired volume at which the PCO_2 is half-way between zero (at the beginning of phase II) and the shoulder of the plateau (at the end of phase II) (B). The area under the curve of Line 1 represents the volume of carbon dioxide expelled during that breath (V_{CO2}). The total volume of exhaled CO_2 (V_{CO2}) is derived from integrating volume and CO_2 over time. The area above the curve of Line 1, to the left of the mid-phase II vertical line (B), and below Line 2 is airway deadspace inefficiency. The area above the curve and to the right of the mid-phase II vertical line (B), and below Line 2 is alveolar deadspace (high V/Q) and atelectasis (0 V/Q) inefficiency. Mixed-expired PCO_2 ($PmeCO_2$) is calculated as V_{CO_2}/tidal volume. Average alveolar PCO_2 ($PavealveCO_2$) is the PCO_2 on the horizontal axis of Line 1, mid-way between the phase II vertical line and the endpoint of the breath (C). Physiologic deadspace (%) is calculated by the Bohr equation, ($PaCO_2$ – $PmeCO_2$)/($PaCO_2$ – P_ICO_2), where P_ICO_2 = inspired PCO_2. Airway deadspace (%) can be calculated as either ($PavealveCO_2$ – $PmeCO_2$)/($PavealvCO_2$ – P_ICO_2) or ($PetCO_2$ – $PmeCO_2$)/($PetCO_2$ – P_ICO_2). Alveolar deadspace (%) is calculated as physiologic deadspace – airway deadspace. Physiologic, airway, and alveolar deadspace (mL) are calculated as physiologic, airway, or alveolar deadspace (%) × tidal volume. A flattening of the curve (less steep phase II coupled with a less 'plateaued' phase III) (Line 3) is compatible with lower airway narrowing or increased alveolar deadspace ventilation. Phase I of exhalation is the inspired gas of that breath and an above-zero PCO_2 represents an increased inspired PCO_2 (excessive apparatus deadspace or exhausted soda lime).

a reflection of tissue function than lung function and is discussed under the heading of tissue perfusion. The details of blood sampling and storage prior to analysis have been detailed elsewhere [65, 182,183]. The blood sample must be taken as anaerobically as possible (exposure to air will change the partial pressures of both oxygen and carbon dioxide) and analyzed as soon as possible (*in vitro* metabolism and diffusion of gases into and through the plastic of the syringe will change the partial pressures of both oxygen and carbon dioxide) [184]. Excessive dilution with anticoagulant should be avoided [185].

Blood gases are measured at the temperature of the blood gas analyzer water bath (usually 37 °C). Ideally, the animal's body temperature would be identical with that of the water bath, but this seldom occurs with veterinary species. When the animal's body temperature is different from that of the water bath, there will be *in vitro* changes in the measured pH and blood gases associated with the change in temperature. Normal ranges for a hypothermic or hyperthermic patient are different than those for the normothermic patient, but these reference values have not been established. There is some debate about whether or not to correct for measured values to the temperature of the patient. If one wants to know what is actually happening in the patient and wants to compare measurements across a span of body temperatures, the temperature-corrected values should be used (alpha-stat). If the clinician is contemplating therapy to correct an abnormality, using normothermic reference points, then the uncorrected values should be used (pH-stat). A recent meta-analysis reviewed the controversy regarding which approach resulted in better neurological outcome following deep hypothermia and concluded that the alpha-stat approach was better for adults and pH-stat was better for pediatrics. Several referenced publications reported no difference [186].

Hemoglobin saturation with oxygen (SO_2)

Oxygen diffuses from the plasma into the red blood cell and binds to hemoglobin. There is a directional correlation between PO_2 and SO_2 but the association is not linear (Fig. 4.12). The same pulmonary processes that determine PaO_2, also determine SaO_2, and SaO_2 is often used as a surrogate marker of PaO_2; SpO_2 is a surrogate marker of SaO_2. Hemoglobin saturation is measured by red to infrared light absorption in either a bench-top oximeter (using arterial blood) (SaO_2) or non-invasively with a pulse oximeter (SpO_2). The normal range for SaO_2 or SpO_2 is about 98–99%. Hypoxemia is defined as an SaO_2 or SpO_2 of less than about 95% and serious hypoxemia is defined as an SaO_2 or SpO_2 of less than about 90% in people; these values are somewhat higher in horses and lower in dogs and cats (Fig. 4.12).

Hemoglobin saturation with oxygen can be measured with a bench-top co-oximeter (SaO_2) using many wavelengths of red to infrared light. The different hemoglobin species (reduced hemoglobin, oxyhemoglobin, methemoglobin, and carboxyhemoglobin) absorb light differently. The co-oximeter then calculates the relative concentration of each of these hemoglobin species from the pattern of light absorption. Pulse oximeters use only two wavelengths of light (660 and 940 nm) and are designed to measure only oxygenated hemoglobin. Pulse oximeters may operate on the principle either of absorbed light (where the light signal is transmitted through a tissue bed to a photodetector on the opposite side of the light-emitting diode) or of reflected light (where the light signal is

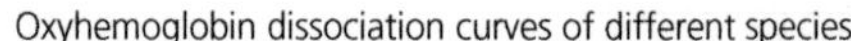

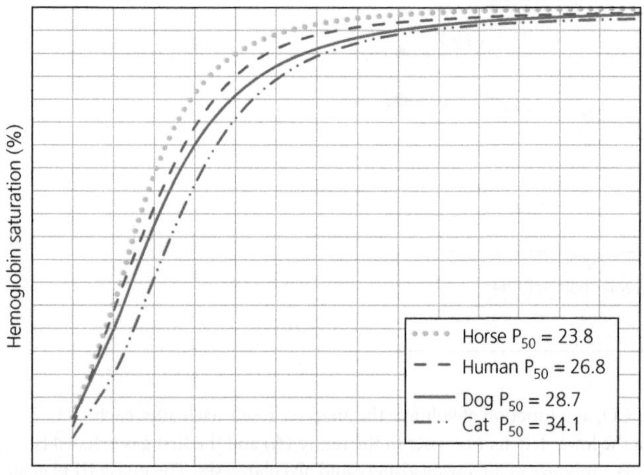

Figure 4.12 Oxyhemoglobin dissociation curves for the horse[260], humans [261], dog, [205], and cat [262]. Cattle were reported to have a P_{50} of about 25 mmHg [263], and an oxyhemoglobin curve between that of horses and people. Goats were reported to have a P_{50} of 29 mmHg [264], and a curve that would overlie that of dogs.

reflected off tissues back to an optical sensor on the same side as the light-emitting diode). Unfortunately, skin, tissue, and venous blood also absorb red to infrared light and the pulse oximeter must have some way to subtract this background light absorption from that of the tissue of interest – arterial blood; this is the 'pulse' part of the pulse oximeter. Pulse oximeters generally will not display an oxyhemoglobin value, much less an accurate one, if they cannot detect a pulse. In this regard, pulse oximeters also function as a monitor of peripheral pulse quality. SpO_2 is then calculated from the ratio of the pulse-added light absorbance at the 660 nm wavelength to that at the 940 nm wavelength [187].

The SO_2–PO_2 relationship is fairly linear and steep below a PO_2 of about 40 mmHg and fairly linear and flat above a PO_2 of about 80 mmHg (Fig. 4.12). There are several important clinical implications of this SO_2–PO_2 relationship. Most importantly, the difference between normoxemia and hypoxemia is only a few saturation percentage points, and severe hypoxemia is only a few saturation percentage points further down the curve.. Small changes in SpO_2 represent large changes in PaO_2 in this region of the oxyhemoglobin dissociation curve. Second, severe hypoxemia is defined at a level when the hemoglobin is still 90% saturated. It is the partial pressure of oxygen in the plasma, not hemoglobin saturation, which drives diffusion of oxygen into the tissues. PO_2 is the driving force; SO_2 (more specifically oxygen content) is the reservoir that prevents the rapid decrease in capillary PO_2 that would otherwise occur when oxygen diffuses out of the blood. Third, saturation measurements cannot detect the difference between a PaO_2 of 100 and 500 mmHg. This difference is important when monitoring and tracking the progress of animals breathing an enriched oxygen mixture. With these, and a few additional caveats, pulse oximeters monitor hypoxemia non-invasively, continuously, and automatically.

Under ideal laboratory conditions, pulse oximeters accurately estimate *in vitro* SaO_2 measurements. The accuracy of a pulse oximeter is greatest within the range 80–95%, and is determined by the accuracy of the empirical algorithm programmed into the instrument. Under clinical conditions, pulse oximeter measurements can vary widely [188]. Motion artifact and low signal-to-noise ratio are the most frequent problems causing inaccuracy in pulse oximetry [187]. Skin and skin pigment, tissue, and venous and capillary blood also absorb infrared light. Differences in tissue absorption or scattering of light, different thicknesses of tissue, smaller pulsatile flow patterns and electrical or optical interference may account for some of the inaccuracies associated with pulse oximeters. For clinical purposes, most pulse oximeters sufficiently estimate hemoglobin saturation [189–195], except in severe situations such as severe hemoglobin desaturation (<70%) [189,193,195,196], severe anemia (PCV <10%) [197], and severe vasoconstriction [187].

In clinical practice, pulse oximeter readings can either be accurate or they can be erroneously low (they almost never read erroneously high). So how does one decide if a low measurement is real? [198]. The measurement is more likely to be accurate if the displayed pulse rate is the same as that of the patient and if the displayed number increases towards normal with oxygen supplementation and decreases again with room air breathing. One of the common reasons for poor instrument performance is its inability to detect a peripheral pulse either because the animal is hypovolemic or vasoconstricted, or because the probe has been left in one place for too long, causing compression of the underlying tissues. If the probe is moved to several different locations; the highest reading is likely to be the most accurate estimate of SaO_2. Suspected hypoxemia should be corroborated with other clinical signs and an arterial blood gas analysis if necessary.

Pulse oximeters use only two wavelengths (660 and 940 nm) and are designed to measure only oxygenated hemoglobin. If methemoglobin or carboxyhemoglobin is present, it will simply confuse the analyzer. owing to the biphasic absorption of methemoglobin at both the 660 and 940 nm wavelengths, abnormal accumulations of this hemoglobin species tend to push the pulse oximeter reading toward 85% [199,200]. Carboxyhemoglobin absorbs light like oxyhemoglobin at 660 nm but hardly at all at 940 nm, which a pulse oximeter interprets as oxyhemoglobin; increasing the apparent oxyhemoglobin value [201]. Fetal hemoglobin and hemoglobin-based blood substitutes have very little effect on measured hemoglobin saturation [187,202]. Indocyanine green dye and methylene blue dye absorb light and will generate false low saturation measurements [187].

Many blood gas analyzers list oxyhemoglobin saturation on their printout. This is usually a calculated rather than a measured value. The calculation is usually based upon the normal human oxyhemoglobin dissociation curve. Oxyhemoglobin curves vary from species to species [203,204] (Fig. 4.12), but the curve can also vary between breeds within a species and between age and individuals within a breed [205–211]. P_{50} is the PO_2 at which the hemoglobin is 50% saturated. It is commonly used to define the position of the oxyhemoglobin curve, with a higher number indicating a right-shifted curve and a lower number a left-shifted curve [212]. P_{50} values for canine breeds vary between 25.8 and 35.8 mmHg [205] and for cats between 31 [211] and 36 mmHg [213, 214], depending on their relative concentration of hemoblogin A versus hemoglobin B [209]. Bovine P_{50} reportedly varies between 25 and 31 mmHg [205,215,216], and ovine P_{50} between 30 and 40 mmHg [204,215,217]. The curve also changes with different disease conditions (anemia) and with changes in pH, CO_2, and temperature. The important point is that using the human oxyhemoglobin relationship to analyze blood from various canine breeds is probably acceptable since it is within the range of the spectrum of dog oxyhemoglobin relationships. The use of dog curves for dog blood is not more accurate. The oxyhemoglobin relationships for horses and cats are shifted more to the left and right, respectively, and SO_2 calculations using the human oxyhemoglobin relationship from PO_2 measurements will be less accurate. If great accuracy is required, oxyhemoglobin itself must be measured [218,219]. The absorbance spectra of dog, cat, horse, cow, and pig oxyhemoglobin are sufficiently similar to that of human hemoglobin that analyzers based upon human algorithms of light absorbance are satisfactorily accurate for animals [220,221].

Cyanosis

Grayish to bluish discoloration of mucous membranes signals the presence of unoxygenated hemoglobin in the observed tissues. The observation of cyanosis is dependent upon the concentration of deoxygenated hemoglobin present, the visual acuity of the observer (some individuals can see it earlier than others), lighting (it is more readily detected in a well-lit room than in the shadows of a cage), and the type of lighting used (it is more readily detectable with incandescent as opposed to fluorescent lighting) [222]. In general, it requires an absolute concentration of unoxygenated hemoglobin of 5 g/dL to manifest sufficient cyanosis to be observed visually [223]. This is important for two reasons. First, if an animal had a hemoglobin concentration of 15 g/dL, cyanosis would manifest when the arterial blood saturation decreased to 67% (equivalent to a PaO_2 of about 37 mmHg) (Fig. 4.12). When cyanosis is manifested as a sign of hypoxemia (central cyanosis as with pneumonia), it is always a late sign of severe hypoxemia. Second, cyanosis is not a reliable sign of hypoxemia in an anemic patient because PO_2 driving pressures will have fallen to lethal levels long before hemoglobin is sufficiently desaturated to manifest cyanosis.

Methemoglobin is oxidized hemoglobin and cannot reversibly bind oxygen. Methemoglobinemia imparts a brownish to bluish discoloration to the mucous membranes and it proportionately reduces the concentration of oxyhemoglobin. PaO_2 is normal because pulmonary function is normal. The problem is the inability of the hemoglobin to bind the oxygen. Pulse oximeters are likely to display a value towards 85%. Another cause of cyanosis is stagnant peripheral blood flow, the extreme example being α_2-adrenergic receptor agonist-mediated peripheral vasoconstriction (peripheral cyanosis). When peripheral blood flow is slow, there is more time for more oxygen to diffuse into the tissues, which creates more unoxygenated hemoglobin in the capillaries. Peripheral cyanosis may not signal a lack of oxygen delivery to other tissues such as brain, kidney, or heart. Vasoconstriction diminishes capillary blood flow, membranes appear pale or white because there is very little blood in these capillary beds, and cyanosis may not be manifested even if the animal is hypoxemic. Vasodilation (lots of blood in the capillary beds), coupled with hypoxemia, or sluggish blood flow (lots of unoxygenated blood), generates the 'purple' discoloration common to late-stage septic shock.

Hypoxemia

There are three categorical causes of hypoxemia: low inspired oxygen concentration, hypoventilation, or venous admixture (Table 4.9). A fourth cause of hypoxemia can be a reduced venous oxygen content [224–227] secondary to low cardiac output or sluggish peripheral blood flow (shock) or high oxygen extraction by the tissues (seizures). Normally, venous blood is fully arterialized (reoxygenated) in about one-third of the normal pulmonary transit time [144]. When the venous oxygen content is very low, it takes more oxygen and more time for the capillary blood to be arterialized. This lowers alveolar PO_2 (P_AO_2) and therefore PaO_2. PaO_2 will be further reduced if the equilibration time exceeds the transit time. In practice, the impact of low venous oxygen and blood flow is often offset by a decrease in shunt fraction, which diminishes the decrease in PaO_2 [144,227]. Low venous oxygen is verified by measuring central venous oxygen.

Table 4.9 Categorical causes of hypoxemia.

Cause	Examples
Low inspired oxygen	Improper functioning apparatus to which the animal is attached; depleted oxygen supply; altitude
Hypoventilation	Neuromuscular impairment (intracranial disease or general anesthesia, cervical spinal cord disease, or a peripheral neuromuscular disorder), upper or lower airway obstruction, abdominal distention causing anterior displacement of the diaphragm, large chest wall 'flail' segments or open pneumothorax, or pleural space filling disorders
Venous admixture	Diffuse lung disease
Low V/Q regions[a]	Moderate to severe diffuse lung disease
Atelectasis	Severe to very severe diffuse lung disease
Diffusion defects	Moderate to severe, diffuse lung disease
Right-to-left shunts	Right-to-left PDA[b] and VSD[b]; intrapulmonary A–V anatomic shunts

[a] V = ventilation; Q = perfusion; low V/Q ratio = low ventilation compared with blood flow due to either low regional ventilation or high regional perfusion.
[b] PDA = patent ductus arteriosus; VSD = ventricular septal defect.

Low inspired oxygen secondary to mechanical failure or accidental delivery of a hypoxic gas mixture should be considered any time an animal is attached to mechanical apparatus such as a face mask, anesthetic circuit, or ventilator, or is in an enclosed environment such as an oxygen cage. Inspired or ambient oxygen concentration can be measured with a variety of commercially available oxygen meters. The effect of altitude on inspired PO_2 is only a concern for individuals practicing at altitude (Table 4.10).

Hypoventilation can be caused by a variety of neuromuscular or respiratory disorders (Tables 4.9 and 4.11). Hypoventilation is defined by an elevated $PaCO_2$ or one of its surrogate markers ($PetCO_2$ or $PvCO_2$). A decrease in alveolar minute ventilation decreases the delivery of oxygen to the alveoli. Increasing the inspired oxygen concentration is very effective in preventing/treating hypoxemia secondary to hypoventilation.

Venous admixture is all of the ways in which venous blood can get from the right side to the left side of the circulation without being properly oxygenated. There are four causes of venous admixture (Table 4.9): (a) low ventilation/perfusion ratio (V/Q); (b) small airway and alveolar collapse [atelectasis; lung units with zero ventilation but with perfusion (0 V/Q)]; (c) diffusion defects; and (d) anatomic right-to-left shunts. A high V/Q ratio does not cause hypoxemia. Most diffuse lung disease will have a variable combination of several of the above mechanisms, but one often predominates. Venous blood that flows through the lung without being oxygenated (right-to-left anatomic shunts and atelectasis) admixes with optimally arterialized blood from the more normally functioning regions of the lung, reducing the net oxygen content and PaO_2. Venous blood that is partially arterialized (low V/Q and diffusion impairment) admixes with arterialized blood, reducing the net oxygen content and PaO_2. There is usually a small amount of venous admixture in the normal lung (<5%) [102]. An increased venous admixture represents a reduced blood oxygenating efficiency and pulmonary parenchymal disease.

Table 4.10 Effect of altitude on barometric pressure, inspired oxygen, and PaO_2.

Altitude (ft/m)	P_B (mmHg/mbar)[a]	P_IO_2 (mmHg)[b]	PaO_2 @ $PaCO_2$ 40[c] (mmHg)	PaO_2 @ (compensated $PaCO_2$)[d]	Added Value Rule[e]
Sea level	760/1013	149	95	95 @ 40	120
1000/305	733/976	143	89	90 @ 39	115
2000/610	707/942	138	84	86 @ 38	110
3000/915	682/909	133	79	82 @ 37	106
4000/1220	659/878	128	74	78 @ 36	101
5000/1525	634/844	123	69	75 @ 35	98
6000/1830	609/811	118	64	71 @ 34	93
7000/2135	586/781	113	59	67 @ 33	89
8000/2440	564/751	108	54	63 @ 32	84
9000/2745	543/723	104	50	60 @ 31	81
10000/3050	523/697	99	45	56 @ 30	76
12000/3355	483/643	91	37	50 @ 28	69
15000/4575	429/571	80	26	44 @ 24	60

[a] P_B = barometric pressure.
[b] P_IO_2 = inspired partial pressure of oxygen. Atmospheric oxygen concentration is 21% at any altitude, but as altitude increases the barometric pressure decreases and the $PatmO_2$ represented by 21% decreases.
[c] Assumes an $P_{A\text{-}a}O_2$ gradient of 10 mmHg and an RQ of 0.9.
[d] Individuals at altitude tend to hyperventilate to compensate for the low atmospheric PO_2.
[e] See discussion for $PaCO_2 + PaO_2$ added value rule.

Table 4.11 P/% O_2 ratio, $P_{A\text{-}a}O_2/PaO_2$ ratio, arterial/(calculated) alveolar PO_2 ratio, and $P_{A\text{-}a}O_2$/% inspired oxygen of normal lungs at different inspired oxygen concentrations.

Inspired oxygen (%)	Minimum expected PaO_2	PaO_2/% inspired O_2	$P_{A\text{-}a}O_2/PaO_2$	a/A gradient	$P_{A\text{-}a}O_2$/% inspired
21	80	4	0.31	0.76	1.20
40	200	5	0.20	0.83	1.00
60	300	5	0.27	0.79	1.37
80	400	5	0.31	0.76	1.55
100	500	5	0.33	0.75	1.66

Low V/Q occurs secondary to small airway narrowing (bronchospasm, fluid accumulation along the walls of the lower airways, or epithelial edema), which impairs ventilation (V) to the associated alveoli. Low V/Q may also occur with increased blood flow (Q) (pulmonary thromboembolism). The low V/Q mechanism of hypoxemia is common and, like global hypoventilation, is very responsive to oxygen therapy. Small airway and alveolar collapse occurs when the accumulation of airway fluids (transudate, exudates, or blood) reaches a critical surface tension, at which time the airway and alveolus collapse. Small airway and alveolar collapse in lower regions of the lung is also commonly caused by positional atelectasis (e.g., general anesthesia or coma). Small airway and alveolar collapse is a common mechanism of hypoxemia and is not responsive to oxygen but is very responsive to increases in the airway or transpulmonary pressure. Diffusion impairment, due to a thickened respiratory membrane, is an uncommon cause of hypoxemia. Transcapillary fluid leaks do not accumulate within the interstitial space at the level of the respiratory membrane [228]. In order for a diffusion defect to occur, the flat type I pneumocytes have to be damaged by inhalation or inflammatory injury. In the healing process, the thick, cuboidal type II pneumocytes proliferate across the surface of the respiratory membrane [229]. This represents a substantial diffusion defect until such time as the type II pneumocytes mature into type I pneumocytes. Diffusion defects are partially responsive to oxygen therapy. Right-to-left anatomic shunts (e.g., patent ductus arteriosis or ventricular septal defect with pulmonary hypertension or tetralogy of Fallot) are not common and are not responsive to either oxygen or positive pressure ventilation; some are amenable to surgical intervention.

Estimating the magnitude of the venous admixture

In pulmonary parenchymal disease, lungs often fail in their ability to oxygenate the blood prior to failing in their ability to remove carbon dioxide (hypoxemia and hypocapnia are common presentations in animals with lung disease). Although this is commonly ascribed to the fact that carbon dioxide is more soluble than oxygen, oxygen diffusion defects play a minor role in the hypoxemia of acute lung disease. Rather, alveolar–capillary units that are working relatively well can easily compensate for those that are working relatively poorly with respect to carbon dioxide elimination, but not for oxygen intake, because of the location on their respective dissociation curves where the action occurs. The PCO_2:CO_2 content relationship is fairly linear over a wide range of clinically relevant PCO_2 values [144]. Alveoli that are working more normally can very effectively lower capillary CO_2 content and thereby compensate and, indeed, overcompensate for poorly functioning alveoli. The portion of the PO_2:O_2 content relationship above a PO_2 of about 80 mmHg is, however, fairly flat (Fig. 4.12). Alveoli that are working normally can hyperventilate and increase P_AO_2, but they cannot increase blood oxygen content enough to compensate for poorly functioning alveoli in any significant way. Thus, $PaCO_2$ can be used to define alveolar minute ventilation whereas PaO_2 cannot. PaO_2 simply defines blood oxygenation whereas some combination of $PaCO_2$ and PaO_2 defines venous admixture.

There are many ways to quantitate venous admixture. In general, it is recommended to estimate venous admixture with the prevailing conditions of treatment rather than under some arbitrary condition (such as 'always while breathing room air' or 'always while breathing 100% oxygen' or 'always off ventilator support' or 'always at certain ventilator settings'). While the latter approach may provide a more consistent evaluation of the underlying pathophysiology, the former approach better indexes therapeutic effectiveness and guides the withdrawal of such support. Increasing inspired oxygen (F_IO_2) will almost always increase PaO_2, but it may also simultaneously improve (by improving oxygenation of low V/Q regions) or worsen (by increasing the regions of 0 V/Q via absorption atelectasis) indices of venous admixture [230–232].

Increasing mean airway pressure with positive pressure ventilation (including PEEP and CPAP) will reopen collapsed small airways and thereby improve indices of lung function when 0 V/Q is a predominant mechanism of the baseline hypoxemia [233].

When breathing 21% oxygen, the $PaCO_2$:PaO_2 reciprocal calculation will give the clinician some idea about lung function. In the alveoli, water vapor is fixed at about 50 mmHg by virtue of alveolar gases being 100% saturated at body temperature and nitrogen is fixed at about 560 mmHg by virtue of being in equilibrium with the Earth's atmosphere. Oxygen and carbon dioxide are reciprocally related. Ventilation delivers oxygen and removes carbon dioxide to the alveoli, whereas venous blood delivers carbon dioxide and removes oxygen from the alveoli. The O_2:CO_2 'trade' occurs at almost a 1:1 ratio [determined by metabolism; there is slightly less CO_2 produced than oxygen consumed (respiratory quotient)]. Normal $PaCO_2$ is 40 mmHg and the minimum PaO_2 compatible with 'normoxemia' is 80 mmHg. If the $PaCO_2$ decreases by 20 mmHg by hyperventilation, the PaO_2 should increase by about 20 mmHg. A PaO_2 value less than 100 mmHg, when the $PaCO_2$ is 20 mmHg, suggests venous admixture, and vice versa, if the $PaCO_2$ increases by 20 mmHg, the PaO_2 should decrease by about the same amount.

Another version of the $PaCO_2$:PaO_2 reciprocal relationship is the $PaCO_2 + PaO_2$ added value. When breathing 21% oxygen, at sea level, the $PaCO_2 + PaO_2$ normally adds to a least 120 mmHg. An added value of less than 120 mmHg suggests the presence of venous admixture and, the greater the discrepancy, the worse is the lung function. With oxygen breathing, or at altitude, this added value rule or '120 rule' cannot be used. At altitude, atmospheric and alveolar and arterial PO_2 are decreased and the 'added value rule' is proportionately decreased (Table 4.10).

The alveolar–arterial PO_2 gradient ($P_{A-a}O_2$) is a common index of pulmonary oxygenating efficiency. Alveolar PO_2 (P_AO_2) is calculated by the alveolar air equation:

$$P_AO_2 = \left[\left(P_B - P_{H_2O}\right) \times \%\ \text{inspired oxygen}\right] - PaCO_2\left(1/RQ\right)$$

where P_B = barometric pressure, P_{H_2O} = saturated water vapor pressure at body temperature, and RQ = respiratory quotient. Barometric pressure can be measured or can be obtained from the local weather station. For simplicity, it can be assumed to be an average value for the altitude of the area (Table 4.10), 760 mmHg at sea level. Saturated water vapor pressure at 38.1 °C (100.6 °F) is 50 mmHg. At sea level, breathing 21% oxygen, inspired oxygen (P_IO_2) is calculated as (760 – 50) × 0.21 = 149 mmHg (which for simplicity can be rounded up to 150 mmHg in the short formula): P_AO_2 = 150 – $PaCO_2$(1.1); RQ is assumed to be 0.9 (1/0.9 = 1.1). Respiratory quotient in critically ill people and dogs varies considerably, depending upon the metabolic circumstances. In critically ill people, RQ was reported to vary between 0.85 and 0.95[234,235]. In dogs with a variety of diseases, RQ varies between a narrow range of 0.8–0.9 [236–239] and a broad range of 0.7–1.0 [240, 241]. The average of all 54 reported RQ values from the references cited is 0.86 ± 0.06. The value was rounded to 0.9 for the proposed calculations herein because it represents an RQ value close to the mean of that reported and because it allows easy calculation at the cage side (1/0.9 = 1.1). When using a spreadsheet, 0.86 may be a more representative average, realizing that individual RQ values vary widely. $P_{A-a}O_2$ is calculated as the difference between the calculated P_AO_2 and the measured PaO_2. The $P_{A-a}O_2$ gradient has been reported to be less than 10 mmHg in normal dogs [102]; values above 20 mmHg are considered to represent decreased oxygenating efficiency (some venous admixture).

The full alveolar air equation can be used at any altitude [with the appropriate change in barometric pressure (Table 4.10)]. The full alveolar air equation can be used at any inspired oxygen concentration. Unfortunately, the normal $P_{A-a}O_2$ gradient increases at higher inspired oxygen concentrations and may be as high as 100–150 mmHg at an inspired oxygen concentration of 100%. Interim values have not been determined, but one idea is that the $P_{A-a}O_2$ gradient should be between a value equal to the inspired oxygen concentration and a value equal to 1.5 × the inspired oxygen concentration (i.e., at 80% inspired, the $P_{A-a}O_2$ should be 80–120 mmHg; values greater than 120 mmHg would indicate venous admixture). Many approaches have been used to compensate for the variation in $P_{A-a}O_2$ associated with variations in inspired oxygen (Table 4.11): (1) PaO_2/inspired oxygen (P/F ratio)(see discussion below) [values <5 (or 500) suggest venous admixture); (2) the respiratory index (RI): RI = $P_{A-a}O_2/PaO_2$ (normal calculated values range between 0.2 and 0.33; values >0.4 suggest venous admixture); (3) arterial/alveolar PO_2 index [230,240] (normal calculated values range between 0.75 to 0.83; values <0.70 suggest venous admixture); and (4) $P_{A-a}O_2$/% inspired oxygen (normal calculated values range between 1.0 and 1.7; values >1.8 suggest venous admixture). Of the four, PaO_2/inspired oxygen (P/F ratio) is the easiest to calculate and the others, for all of their extra math, do not increase the accuracy of the assessment.

When breathing 21% oxygen, changes in P_ACO_2 have an important impact on P_AO_2 and, therefore, on PaO_2. When breathing 21% oxygen, $PaCO_2$ must be taken into account as it has been done in the approaches discussed above. With progressively higher inspired oxygen concentrations, changes in $PaCO_2$ have quantitatively less important effects on P_AO_2 and have, for convenience, been ignored in this method of estimating venous admixture. When an animal is breathing a known high oxygen concentration, as is common during anesthesia, simply divide the measured PaO_2 by the inspired oxygen concentration, which can be expressed as either 21–100% (PaO_2/% ratio) or 0.21–1.0 (PaO_2/F_IO_2 ratio). The lower this dividend, the worse is the lung function (Table 4.12). The advantages of this P/F approach are its simplicity and that it allows cage-side comparisons regarding lung performance at different inspired oxygen concentrations. The P/F ratio, unfortunately, is not as linear as one would hope for [230,231]. Although fairly linear between inspired oxygen concentrations of 40 and 80% with true shunts of less than 30% and between 40 and 100% with true shunts >30% [230] the actual shape of the curve can vary substantially, in a biphasic manner at different inspired oxygen concentrations and with different magnitudes of shunt and different arterial–venous oxygen content differences [231]. Upward trends in P/F ratio in response to therapy provide the clinician with a guide to therapeutic effectiveness and downward trends can be used to guide the withdrawal of such support. The P/F ratio index provides a functional assessment of lung

Table 4.12 PaO_2/% inspired oxygen and PaO_2/F_IO_2 ratios associated with worsening venous admixture.

	PaO_2/inspired O_2 concentration (21–100%) (P/% ratio)	**PaO_2/F_IO_2 (0.21–1.0) (P/F ratio)**
Normal	>5	>500
Mild venous admixture	3–5	300–500
Moderate venous admixture	2–3	200–300
Severe venous admixture	<2	<200

oxygenating efficiency at the current inspired oxygen and ventilator settings, in the face of the current lung pathophysiology. The oxygenation index [(mean airway pressure × % inspired oxygen)/PaO_2] has been suggested as a means of better characterizing underlying lung pathophysiology and minimizing variations in the P/F ratio index due to variations in F_IO_2 and mean airway pressure [242, 243]. $PaCO_2$ values have been ignored in this calculation, but this does not mean that $PaCO_2$ has no influence. If $PaCO_2$ values vary widely between two comparisons, one can accept that comparable P/F values probably have to vary by more than 20% in order to represent a true change in oxygenating efficiency. Consistency between measurements may be enhanced by adding the measured $PaCO_2$ to the calculated P/F ratio (or $PaCO_2 \times 0.01$ to the P/% ratio) (two calculations need vary by only about 10% to represent a true difference when $PaCO_2$ is incorporated in the calculation). The P/F calculation should not be used when the animal is breathing (21% oxygen). When breathing ambient air, calculations can be misleading, particularly when $PaCO_2$ values are elevated.

If a mixed venous blood sample (pulmonary artery, right atrium) can be obtained, the venous admixture can be calculated:

$$Q_S/Q_T = (CcO_2 - CaO_2)/(CcO_2 - CmvO_2)$$

where Q_S = shunt fraction, Q_T = cardiac output, Q_S/Q_T = venous admixture expressed as a percent of cardiac output, CcO_2 = oxygen content of end-capillary blood, CaO_2 = oxygen content of arterial blood, and $CmvO_2$ = oxygen content of mixed venous blood. Jugular venous blood is sometimes used as a surrogate for pulmonary arterial blood. Arterial and mixed venous PO_2 is measured and oxygen content (mL/dL) is calculated as

$$(1.34 \times Hb \times SO_2) + (0.003 \times PO_2)$$

where SO_2 is percentage hemoglobin saturation with oxygen. Capillary PO_2 is assumed to be equal to calculated P_AO_2, which is used to calculate capillary oxygen content. PO_2 is measured and SO_2 is either measured or extrapolated from a standard oxyhemoglobin dissociation curve [which is the value reported on the printout from the blood gas analyzers, or can be derived manually from an oxyhemoglobin dissociation curve (Fig. 4.12)]. Venous admixture is normally less than 5% [102]. Values over 10% are considered to be increased, and may increase to over 50% in severe, diffuse lung disease. Although the venous admixture equation seems like a lot of math, it is considered the most accurate method of estimating venous admixture [244]. Spreadsheets make it easy. If blood samples are taken while the patient is breathing room air, all of the categorical mechanisms of venous admixture are assessed. If blood samples are taken while the patient is breathing 100% oxygen, the low V/Q mechanism of hypoxemia is eliminated from the assessment and diffusion defects are minimized. In this usage, the formula is referred to as the 'shunt' formula because it assesses the magnitude of the remaining two causes of venous admixture: physiologic shunts secondary to atelectasis and true anatomic shunts. Like all of the previously discussed venous admixture indices, values calculated by this formula are also affected by changes in inspired oxygen concentration [230,232,244,245] and by changes in mean airway pressure [245].

Obtaining a mixed-venous blood sample is sometimes difficult. One approach calculates venous oxygen content from arterial oxygen content and assumed oxygen consumption. This approach has been reported to generate acceptable results for the calculation of venous admixture in people [246] and sheep[247]: $CmvO_2 = CaO_2 - 3.5$ mL/dL, where 3.5 mL/dL is a representative oxygen consumption in people. $CmvO_2$ was reported to be 3.6 in a large series of dogs[102], so this formula will probably work also in dogs, provided that the animal's metabolic rate doesn't vary too much. This calculated $CmvO_2$ is then plugged into the venous admixture formula to calculate Qs/Qt.

Temperature

Hypothermia

Hypothermia during anesthesia may be associated with anesthetic drug depression of muscular activity, metabolism, and hypothalamic thermostatic mechanisms. Heat loss may be augmented by evaporation of surgical scrub solutions from the skin surface, by the infusion of room temperature fluids, by contact with cold, uninsulated surfaces, and by evaporation of surface fluid from an exposed body cavity. Core temperature can be measured with either esophageal or rectal thermistors attached to a continuously displayed thermometer. Core body temperatures down to 36 °C (96 °F) are often not associated with detrimental effects [248,249], although immune function impairment may lead to increased risk of infection and altered enzyme kinetics may predispose to coagulation and hemostatic abnormalities. Non-shivering thermogenesis will increase and there may be some shivering thermogenesis during recovery. Recovery should not be prolonged in any noticeable way. Body temperatures of 32–34 °C (90–94 °F) are associated with reduced anesthetic requirements (normothermic amounts of anesthetic will over-anesthetize these patients), and recovery will be prolonged. Shivering will occur in most animals but some animals will not shiver and will have to be artificially rewarmed. Body temperatures of 28–30 °C (82–86 °F) have a marked CNS depressant effect (little if any anesthetic agent is required). Shivering thermogenesis will not occur and these animals will have to be artificially rewarmed. Atrial arrhythmias may occur. Oxygen consumption is reduced to about 50% of normal, heart rate and cardiac output to about 35–40% of normal, and arterial blood pressure to about 60% of normal [248]. Cerebral metabolism is about 25% of normal. Body temperatures of 25–26 °C (77–80 °F) are associated with prolongation of the PR interval and widened QRS complexes, increased myocardial automaticity, decreased tissue oxygen delivery out of proportion to decreases in oxygen requirement resulting in anaerobic metabolism, lactic acidosis, and rewarming acidemia. Blood viscosity is about 200% of normal. Body temperatures of 22–23 °C (72–74 °F) are usually associated with ventricular fibrillation. Intraoperative hypothermia is usually mild to moderate and, provided that appropriate safeguards are exercised, is seldom detrimental to the patient in the long term. The greatest problem with intraoperative hypothermia is the non-recognition of it. The continued administration of normothermic amounts of anesthetic to a hypothermic patient results in anesthetic overdose.

Hyperthermia

Fever is a reset thermostat caused by the release of endogenous pyrogens (interleukin-I) from monocytes [250] in response to infections, tissue damage, and/or antigen–antibody reactions. Hyperthermia, without a reset thermostat, is pathologic. It can occur in large dogs that are cocooned on the operating table with many layers of drapes or overzealous use of supplemental heat sources. Hyperthermia may be potentiated by surface vasoconstriction, thick coats (e.g., Newfoundland dogs), light levels of anesthesia, and some drugs (e.g., ketamine and opioids, especially in cats). Mild degrees of hyperthermia are not harmful to the patient and may represent an appropriate fever. Mild hyperthermia (less than 40 °C or 104 °F) does not normally require symptomatic treatment. Cell damage starts to occur at body temperatures above 42 °C (108 °F), when oxygen delivery can no longer keep pace with increased metabolism and oxygen consumption. Severe hyperthermia causes multiple organ dysfunction and failure: renal, hepatic, gastrointestinal failure, myocardial and skeletal muscle, cerebral edema, disseminated intravascular coagulation, hypoxemia, metabolic acidosis, and hyperkalemia [251]. Malignant hyperthermia is a rapidly and relentlessly progressive increase in body temperature associated with metabolic heat production of disturbed intracellular calcium cycling [252,253]. Muscle hypertonicity may or may not occur, depending on the cellular calcium concentration. The defect has been identified in families of people and pigs, and a malignant hyperthermia-like syndrome has been reported in dogs [254,255], cats [256,257], and horses [258, 259]. Aggressive cooling of the animal, by any and all means possible, is indicated.

References

1 Stanski DR. Monitoring depth of anesthesia. In: Miller RD, ed. *Anesthesia*. New York: Churchill Livingstone, 1990; 1001–1029.

2 Katoh T, Suguro Y, Nakajima R, *et al.* Blood concentration of sevoflurane and isoflurane on recovery from anaesthesia. *Br J Anaesth* 1992; **69**: 259–262.

3 Tranquilli WJ. Techniques of inhalation anesthesia in ruminants and swine. In: *Veterinary Clinics of North America; Food Animal Practice*. Philadephia: WB Saunders, 1986; 593–619.

4 Rampil IJ. A primer for EEG signal processing in anesthesia. *Anesthesiology* 1998; **89**: 980–1002.

5 Mi WD, Sakai T, Singh H, *et al.* Hypnotic endpoints vs the bispectral index, 95% spectral edge frequency and median frequency during propofol infusion with or without fentanyl. *Eur J Anaesth* 1999; **16**: 47–54.

6 Schwender D, Daunderer M, Mulzer S, *et al.* Spectral edge frequency of the electroencephalogram to monitor 'depth' of anaesthesia with isoflurane or propofol. *Br J Anaesth* 1996; **77**: 179–184.

7 Drummond JC, Brann CA, Perkins DE, Wolfe DE. A comparison of median frequency, spectral edge frequency, a frequency band power ratio, total power, and dominance shift in the determination of depth of anesthesia. *Acta Anaesth Scand* 1991; **35**: 693–699.

8 Schmidt GN, Bischoff P, Standl T, *et al.* Comparative evaluation of Narcotrend™, Bispectral Index™, and classical electroencephalographic variables during induction, maintenance, and emergence of a propofol/remifentanil anesthesia. *Anesth Analg* 2004; **98**: 1346–1353.

9 Otto KA, Mally P. Noxious stimulation during orthopaedic surgery results in EEG 'arousal' or 'paradoxical arousal' reaction in isoflurane-anaesthetised sheep. *Res Vet Sci* 2003; **75**: 103–112.

10 Otto KA, Short CE. Electroencephalographic power spectrum analysis as a monitor of anesthetic depth in horses. *Vet Surg* 2004; **20**: 362–371.

11 Miller SM, Short CE, Ekstrom PM. Quantitative electroencephalographic evaluation to determine the quality of analgesia during anesthesia of horses for arthroscopic surgery. *Am J Vet Res* 2004; **56**: 374–379.

12 Martin-Cancho MF, Lima JR, Luis L, *et al.* Bispectral index, spectral edge frequency 95%, and median frequency recorded for various concentrations of isoflurane and sevoflurane in pigs. *Am J Vet Res* 2003; **64**: 866–873.

13 Vuyk J, Mertens M. Bispectral index scale (BIS) monitoring and intravenous anaesthesia. In: Vuyk J, Schraag S, eds. *Advances in Modeling and Clinical Applications of Intravenous Anaesthesia*. New York: Kluwer Academic/Plenum Publishers, 2003; 95–104.

14 Nasraway SA, Wu EC, Kelleher RM, *et al.* How reliable is the Bispectral Index in critically ill patients? A prospective, comparative, single-blinded observer study. *Crit Care Med* 2002; **30**: 1483–1487.

15 Mashour GA, Shanks A, Tremper KK, *et al.* Prevention of intraoperative awareness with explicit recall in an unselected surgical population: a randomized comparative effectiveness trial. *Anesthesiology* 2012; **117**: 717–725.

16 de Mattos-Junior E, Ito KC, Conti-Patara A, *et al.* Bispectral monitoring in dogs subjected to ovariohysterectomy and anesthetized with halothane, isoflurane or sevoflurane. *Vet Anaesth Analg* 2011; **38**: 475–483.

17 Simmons LE, Riker RR, Prato BS, Fraser GL. Assessing sedation during intensive care unit mechanical ventilation with the Bispectral Index and the Sedation–Agitation Scale. *Crit Care Med* 1999; **27**: 1499–1504.

18 DeDeyne C, Struys M, Decruyenaere J, *et al.* Use of continuous bispectral EEG monitoring to assess depth of sedation in ICU patients. *Intens Care Med* 1998; **24**: 1294–1298.

19 March PA, Muir WW. Minimum alveolar concentration measures of central nervous system activation in cats anesthetized with isoflurane. *Am J Vet Res* 2003; **64**: 1528–1533.

20 Greene SA, Benson GJ, Tranquilli WJ, Grimm KA. Relationship of canine bispectral index to multiples of sevoflurane minimal alveolar concentration, using patch or subdermal electrodes. *Comp Med* 2002; **52**: 424–428.

21 Muthuswamy J, Sharma A. A study of electroencephalographic descriptors and end-tidal concentration in estimating depth of anesthesia. *J Clin Monit* 1996; **12**: 353–364.

22 March PA, Muir WW. Use of the bispectral index as a monitor of anesthetic depth in cats anesthetized with isoflurane. *Am J Vet Res* 2003; **64**: 1534–1541.

23 Rosow C, Manberg PJ. Bispectral index monitoring. *Anesth Clin North Am* 2001; **19**: 947–966.

24 Gilbert TT, Wagner MR, Halukurike V, *et al.* Use of bispectral electroencephalogram monitoring to assess neurologic status in unsedated, critically ill patients. *Crit Care Med* 2001; **29**: 1996–2000.

25 Fabregas N, Gambus PL, Valero R, *et al.* Can bispectral index monitoring predict recovery of consciousness in patients with severe brain injury? *Anesthesiology* 2004; **101**: 43–51.

26 Campagnol D, Teixeira Neto FJ, Monteiro ER, *et al.* Use of bispectral index to monitor depth of anesthesia in isoflurane-anesthetized dogs. *Am J Vet Res* 2007; **68**: 1300–1307.

27 Ribeiro LM, Ferreira DA, Bressan NM, *et al.* Brain monitoring in dogs using the cerebral state index during the induction of anaesthesia via target-controlled infusion of propofol. *Res Vet Sci* 2008; **85**: 227–232.

28 Ribeiro LM, Ferreira DA, Brás S, *et al.* Correlation between clinical signs of depth of anaesthesia and cerebral state index responses in dogs during induction of anaesthesia with propofol. *Res Vet Sci* 2009; **87**: 287–291.

29 Ribeiro LM, Ferreira DA, Brás S, *et al.* Correlation between clinical signs of depth of anaesthesia and cerebral state index responses in dogs with different target controlled infusions of propofol. *Vet Anaesth Analg* 2012; **39**: 21–28.

30 Bauerle K, Greim CA, Schroth M, *et al.* Prediction of depth of sedation and anaesthesia by the Narcotrend™ EEG monitor. *Br J Anaesth* 2004; **92**: 841–845.

31 Schraag S, Kenny GNC. Auditory evoked potentials; a clinical or a research tool? In: Vuyk J, Schraag S, eds. *Advances in Modeling and Clinical Applications of Intravenous Anaesthesia*. New York: Kluwer Academic/Plenum Publishers, 2003; 105–113.

32 Kiyama S,Tsuzaki K. Processed electroencephalogram during combined extradural and general anaesthesia. *Br J Anaesth* 1997; **78**: 751–753.

33 Copland VS, Haskins SC, Patz JD. Cardiovascular and pulmonary effects of atropine reversal of oxymorphone-induced bradycardia in dogs. *Vet Surg* 1992; **21**: 414–417.

34 Ilkiw JE, Pascoe PJ, Haskins SC, *et al.* The cardiovascular sparing effect of fentanyl and atropine, administered to enflurane anesthetized dogs. *Can J Vet Res* 1994; **58**: 248–253.

35 Remillard RL, Ross JN, Eddy J. Variance of indirect blood pressure measurements and prevalence of hypertension in clinically normal dogs. *Am J Vet Res* 1991; **52**: 561–565.

36 Kallet AJ, Cowgill LD, Kass PH. Comparison of blood pressure measurements obtained in dogs by use of indirect oscillometry in a veterinary clinic versus at home. *J Am Vet Med Assoc* 1997; **210**: 651–654.

37 Sansom J, Rogers K, Wood JLN, Blood pressure assessment in healthy cats and cats with hypertensive retinopathy. *Am J Vet Res* 2004; **65**: 245–252.

38 Stephen RL, Rapoport GS. Clinical comparison of three methods to measure blood pressure in nonsedated dogs. *J Am Vet Med Assoc* 1999; **215**: 1623–1628.

39 Brown S, Atkins C, Bagley R. Guidelines for the identification, evaluation, and management of systemic hypertension in dogs and cats. *J Vet Intern Med* 2007; **21**: 542–558.

40 Valtonen MH, Eriksson LM. The effect of cuff width on accuracy of indirect measurement of blood pressure in dogs. *Res Vet Sci* 1970; **11**: 358–362.

41 Hodgkinson JA, Sheppard JP, Heneghan C, *et al.* Accuracy of ambulatory blood pressure monitors: a systemic review of validation studies. *J Hypertension* 2013; **31**: 239–250.

42 O'Brien E, Atkins N, Stergiou GS, *et al.* European Society of Hypertension International protocol revision 2012 for the validation of blood pressure measuring devices in adults. *Blood Press Monit* 2010; **15**: 23–38.

43 Mark JB. *Atlas of Cardiovascular Monitoring*. New York: Churchill Livingstone, 1998.

44 Thien T, Adiyaman A, Staessen JA, Deinum J. Blood pressure measurement in the year 2008: revival of oscillometry? *Neth J Med* 2008; **66**: 453–456.

45 Lehman LH, Saeed M, Talmor D, *et al.* Methods of blood pressure measurement in the ICU. *Crit Care Med* 2013; **41**: 34–40.
46 McMurphy RM, Stoll MR, McCubrey R. Accuracy of an oscillometric blood pressure monitor during phenylephrine-induced hypertension in dogs. *Am J Vet Res* 2006; **67**: 1541–1545.
47 Deflandre CJA, Hellebrekers LJ. Clinical evaluation of the Surgivet V60046, a non-invasive blood pressure monitor in anaesthetized dogs. *Vet Anaesth Analg* 2008; **35**: 13–21.
48 Bosiack AP, Mann FA, Dodman JR, *et al.* Comparison of ultrasonic Doppler flow monitor, oscillometric, and direct arterial blood pressure measurements in ill dogs. *J Vet Emerg Crit Care* 2010; **20**: 207–215.
49 Garafolo N, Neto TFJ, Alvaides RK, *et al.* Agreement between direct, oscillometric and Doppler ultrasound blood pressures using three different cuff positions in anesthetized dogs. *Vet Anaesth Analg* 2012; **39**: 324–334.
50 Acierno MJ, Fauth E, Mitchell MA, daCunha A. Measuring the level of agreement between directly measured blood pressure and pressure readings obtained with a veterinary-specific oscillometric unit in anesthetized dogs. *J Vet Emerg Crit Care* 2013; **23**: 37–40.
51 Pedersen KM, Butler MA, Ersboll AK, Pedersen HD. Evaluation of an oscillometric blood pressure monitor for use in anesthetized cats. *J Am Vet Med Assoc* 2002; **221**: 646–650.
52 Acierno MJ, Seaton D, Mitchell MA, daCunha A. Agreement between directly measured blood pressure and pressures obtained with three veterinary-specific oscillometric units in cats. *J Am Vet Med Assoc* 2010; **237**: 402–406.
53 Zwijnenberg RJ, del Rio CL, Cobb RM, *et al.* Evaluation of oscillometric and vascular access port arterial blood pressure measurement techniques versus implanted telemetry in anesthetized cats. *Am J Vet Res* 2011; **72**: 1015–1021.
54 Harvey L, Knowles T, Murison PJ. Comparison of direct and Doppler arterial blood pressure measurements in rabbits during isoflurane anaesthesia. *Vet Anaesth Analg* 2012; **39**: 174–184.
55 Giguère S, Knowles HA Jr, Valverde A, *et al.* Accuracy of indirect measurement of blood pressure in neonatal foals. *J Vet Intern Med* 2005; **19**: 571–576.
56 Grandy JL, Dunlop CI, Hodgson DS, *et al.* Evaluation of the Doppler ultrasonic method of measuring systolic arterial blood pressure in cats. *Am J Vet Res* 1992; **53**: 1166–1169.
57 Gourdeau M, Martin R, Lamarche Y, Tetreault L. Oscillometry and direct blood pressure: a comparative clinical study during deliberate hypotension. *Can Anaesth Soc J* 1986; **33**: 300–307.
58 Bur A, Hirschi MM, Herkner H, *et al.* Accuracy of oscillometric blood pressure measurement according to the relation between cuff size and upper-arm circumference in critically ill patients. *Crit Care Med* 2000; **28**: 371–376.
59 Shih A, Robertson S, Vigania A, *et al.* Evaluation of an indirect oscillometric blood pressure monitor in normotensive and hypotensive anesthetized dogs. *J Vet Emerg Crit Care* 2010; **20**: 313–318.
60 Chetboul V, Tissier R, Gouni V, *et al.* Comparison of Doppler ultrasonography and high-definition oscillometry for blood pressure measurements in healthy awake dogs. *Am J Vet Res* 2010; **71**: 766–772.
61 Wernick MB, Hopfner R, Francey T, Howard J. Comparison of arterial blood pressure measurements and hypertension scores obtained by use of three indirect measurement devices in hospitalized dogs. *J Am Vet Med Assoc* 2012; **240**: 962–968.
62 Gardner RM. Direct blood pressure measurement – dynamic response requirements. *Anesthesiology* 1981; **54**: 227–236.
63 Kittleson MD, Kienle RD. *Small Animal Cardiovascular Medicine.* St Louis, MO: Mosby, 1998.
64 Jennings PB, Coppinger TS. Use of external jugular venous distention in the dog to estimate central venous pressure. *J Am Anim Hosp Assoc* 1975; **11**: 668–672.
65 Haskins SC. Standards and techniques of equipment utilization. In: Sattler FP, Knowles RP, Whittick WG, eds. *Veterinary Critical Care.* Philadelphia: Lea and Febiger, 1981; 73.
66 Chow RS, Kass PH, Haskins SC. Evaluation of peripheral and central venous pressure in awake dogs and cats. *Am J Vet Res* 2006; **67**: 1987–1991.
67 Riebold TW. Monitoring equine anesthesia. In: Turner AS, ed. *Veterinary Clinics of North America; Equine Practice.* Philadelphia: WB Saunders, 1990; 607–624.
68 Tam K, Rezende M, Boscan P. Correlation between jugular and central venous pressure in laterally recumbent horses. *Vet Anaesth Analg* 2011; **38**: 580–583.
69 Wilsterman S, Hackett ES, Rao S, Hackett TB. A technique for central venous pressure measurement in normal horses. *J Vet Emerg Crit Care* 2009; **19**: 241–246.
70 Kumar A, Anel R, Bunnel E, *et al.* Pulmonary artery occlusion pressure and central venous pressure fail to predict ventricular filling volume, cardiac performance, or the response to volume infusion in normal subjects. *Crit Care Med* 2004; **32**: 691–699.
71 Magder S. Central venous pressure: a useful but not so simple measurement. *Crit Care Med* 2006; **34**: 2224–2227.
72 Osman D, Ridel C, Ray P, *et al.* Cardiac filling pressures are not appropriate to predict hemodynamic response to volume challenge. *Crit Care Med* 2007; **35**: 64–68.
73 Funk DJ, Jacosohn E, Kumar A. The role of venous return in critical illness and shock – Part I: physiology. *Crit Care Med* 2013; **41**: 255–262.
74 Valverde A, Giguère S, Sanchez C, *et al.* Effects of dobutamine, norepinephrine, and vasopressin on cardiovascular function in anesthetized neonatal foals with induced hypotension. *Am J Vet Res* 2006; **67**: 1730–1737.
75 Jhanji S, Stirling S, Patel N, *et al.* The effect of increasing doses of norepinephrine on tissue oxygenation and microvascular flow in patients with septic shock. *Crit Care Med* 2009; **37**: 1961–1966.
76 Persichini R, Silva S, Teboul JL, *et al.* Effects of norepinephrine on mean systemic pressure and venous return in human septic shock. *Crit Care Med* 2012; **40**: 3146–3153.
77 Maas JJ, Pinsky MR, de Wilde RB, *et al.* Cardiac output responses to norepinephrine in postoperative cardiac surgery patients: interpretation with venous return and cardiac function curves. *Crit Care Med* 2013; **41**: 143–150.
78 Craig CA, Haskins SC, Hildebrand SV. The cardiopulmonary effects of dobutamine and norepinephrine in isoflurane-anesthetized foals. *Vet Anesth Analg* 2007; **14**: 177–187.
79 Maas JJ, Geerts BF, van den Berg PCM, *et al.* Assessment of venous return curve and mean systemic filling pressure in postoperative cardiac surgery patients. *Crit Care Med* 2009; **37**: 912–918.
80 Maas JJ, Pinsky MR, Geerts BF, *et al.* Estimation of mean systemic filling pressure in postoperative cardiac surgery patients with three methods. *Intensive Care Med* 2012; **38**: 1452–1460.
81 Sheldon CA, Balik E, Dhanalal K, *et al.* Peripheral postcapillary venous pressure – a new hemodynamic monitoring parameter. *Surgery* 1982; **92**: 663–668.
82 Sheldon CA, Cerra FB, Bohnhoff N, *et al.* Peripheral venous pressure: a new, more sensitive monitor of effective blood volume during hemorrhagic shock and resuscitation. *Surgery* 1983; **94**: 399–406.
83 Perel A, Pizov R, Cotev S. Systolic blood pressure variation is a sensitive indicator of hypovolemia in ventilated dogs subjected to graded hemorrhage. *Anesthesiology* 1987; **67**: 498–502.
84 Szold A, Pizov R, Segal E, Perel A. The effect of tidal volume and intravascular volume state on systolic pressure variation in ventilated dogs. *Intensive Care Med* 1989; **15**: 368–371.
85 Tavernier B, Makhotine O, Lebuffe G, *et al.* Systolic pressure variation as a guide to fluid therapy in patients with sepsis-induced hypotension. *Anesthesiology* 1998; **89**: 1313–1321.
86 Reuter DA, Kirchner A, Felbinger TW, *et al.* Usefulness of left ventricular stroke volume variation to assess fluid responsiveness in patients with reduced cardiac function. *Crit Care Med* 2003; **31**: 1399–1404.
87 Huang CC, Fu JY, Hu HC, *et al.* Prediction of fluid responsiveness in acute respiratory distress syndrome patients ventilated with low tidal volume and high positive end-expiratory pressure. *Crit Care Med* 2008; **36**: 2810–2816.
88 Marik PE, Cavallazzi R, Vasu T, Hirani A. Dynamic changes in arterial waveform derived variables and fluid responsiveness in mechanically ventilated patients: a systematic review of the literature. *Crit Care Med* 2009; **37**: 2642–2647.
89 Loupec T, Nanadoumgar H, Frasca D, *et al.* Pleth variability index predicts fluid responsiveness in critically ill patients. *Crit Care Med* 2011; **39**: 294–299.
90 Fielding CL, Stolba DN. Pulse pressure variation and systolic pressure variation in horses undergoing general anesthesia, *J Vet Emerg Crit Care* 2012; **22**: 372–375.
91 Biais M, Nouette-Gaulain K, Roullet S, *et al.* Evaluation of stroke volume variation measured by Vigileo™/FloTrac™ system and aortic Doppler echocardiography. *Anesth Analg* 2009; **109**: 466–469.
92 Biais M, Cottenceau V, Stecken L, *et al.* Evaluation of stroke volume variations obtained with the pressure recording analytic method. *Crit Care Med* 2012; **40**: 1186–1191.
93 Kim HK, Pinsky MR. Effect of tidal volume, sampling duration, and cardiac contractility on pulse pressure and stroke volume variation during positive-pressure ventilation. *Crit Care Med* 2008; **36**: 2858–2862.
94 Michard F, Teboul JL. Predicting fluid responsiveness in ICU patients: a critical analysis of the evidence. *Chest* 2002; **121**: 2000–2008.
95 Lee M, Park N, Lee S, *et al.* Comparison of echocardiography with dual-source computed tomography for assessment of left ventricular volume in healthy Beagles. *Am J Vet Res* 2013; **74**: 62–69.
96 Moise NS, Fox PR. Echocardiography and Doppler imaging. In: Fox PR, Sisson D, Moise NS, eds. *Textbook of Canine and Feline Cardiology*, 2nd edn. Philadelphia: WB Saunders, 1999; 130–171.
97 Dittoe N, Stultz D, Schwartz BP, Hahn HS. Quantitative left ventricular systolic function: from chamber to myocardium. *Crit Care Med* 2007; **35**: S330–S339.
98 Henjes CR, Hungerbühler S, Bojarski IB, *et al.* Comparison of multi-detector row computed tomography with echocardiography for assessment of left ventricular function in healthy dogs. *Am J Vet Res* 2012; **73**: 393–403.
99 Brown DJ, Knight DH, King RR, Use of pulsed-wave Doppler echocardiography to determine aortic and pulmonary velocity and flow variables in clinically normal dogs. *Am J Vet Res* 1991; **52**: 543–550.

100 Monnet X, Letierce A, Hamzaoui O, *et al.* Arterial pressure allows monitoring the changes in cardiac output induced by volume expansion but not by norepinephrine. *Crit Care Med* 2011; **39**: 1394–1399.
101 Sun JX, Reisner AT, Saeed M, *et al.* The cardiac output from blood pressure algorithms trial. *Crit Care Med* 2009; **37**: 72–80.
102 Haskins SC, Pascoe PJ, Ilkiw JE, *et al.* Reference cardiopulmonary values in normal dogs. *Comp Med* 2005; **55**: 158–163.
103 Rock P, Beattie C, Kimball AW, *et al.* Halothane alters the oxygen consumption-oxygen delivery relationship compared with conscious state. *Anesthesiology* 1990; **73**: 1186–1197.
104 Van der Linden P, Gilbart E, Engelman E, *et al.* Effects of anesthetic agents on systemic critical O_2 delivery. *J Appl Physiol* 1991; **71**: 83–93.
105 Van der Linden P, Schmartz D, Gilbart E, *et al.* Effects of propofol, etomidate, and pentobarbital on critical oxygen delivery. *Crit Care Med* 2000; **28**: 2492–2499.
106 Pypendop BH, Ilkiw JE. Hemodynamic effects of sevoflurane in cats. *Am J Vet Res* 2004; **65**: 20–25.
107 Haskins SC. Comparative cardiovascular and pulmonary effects of sedatives and anesthetic agents and anesthetic drug selection for the trauma patient. *J Vet Emerg Crit Care* 2006; **16**: 300–328.
108 Mikat M, Peters J, Zindler M, Arndt JO. Whole body oxygen consumption in awake, sleeping, and anesthetized dogs. *Anesthesiology* 1984; **60**: 220–227.
109 McLellan SA, McClelland DBL,Walsh TS. Anaemia and red blood cell transfusion in the critically ill patient. *Blood Rev* 2003; **17**: 195–208.
110 Ickx BE, Rigolet M, Van der Linden J. Cardiovascular and metabolic response to acute normovolemic anemia. *Anesthesiology* 2000; **93**: 1011–1016.
111 Van der Linden J, De Hert S, Mathieu N, *et al.* Tolerance to acute isovolemic hemodilution. Effect of anesthetic depth. *Anesthesiology* 2003; **99**: 97–104.
112 Higgins CB, Vatner SF, Franklin D, Braunwald E. Extent of regulation of the heart's contractile state in the conscious dog. *J Clin Invest* 1973; **52**: 1187–1194.
113 Bombardini T. Myocardial contractility in the echo lab: molecular, cellular and pathophysiogical base. *Cardiovasc Ultrasound* 2005; **3**: 27.
114 Rhodes J, Udelson JE, Marx GR, *et al.* A new noninvasive method for the estimation of peak dP/dt. *Circulation* 1993; **88**: 2693–2699.
115 Culwell NM, Bonagura JD, Schober KE. Comparison of echocardiographic indices of myocardial strain with invasive measurements of left ventricular systolic function in anesthetized healthy dogs. *Am J Vet Res* 2011; **72**: 650–660.
116 Suga H, Sagawa K, Shoukas AA. Load independence of the instantaneous pressure–volume ratio of the canine left ventricle and effects of epinephrine and heart rate on the ratio. *Circ Res* 1973; **32**: 314–322.
117 Opie LH. *Heart Physiology*, 4th edn. Philadelphia: Lippincott Williams & Wilkins, 2004.
118 Scolletta S, Bodson L, Donadello K, *et al.* Assessment of left ventricular function by pulse wave analysis in critically ill patients. *Intensive Care Med* 2013; **39**: 1025–1033.
119 Lawrence JP. Physics and instrumentation of ultrasound. *Crit Care Med* 2007; **35**: S314–S322.
120 Mazraeshahi RM, Farmer JC, Porembka DT. A suggested curriculum in echocardiography for critical care physicians. *Crit Care Med* 2007; **35**: S431–S433.
121 Bonagura JD, Schober KE. Can ventricular function be assessed by echocardiography in chronic canine mitral valve disease? *J Small Anim Pract* 2009; **50**: 12–24.
122 Asano K, Masui Y, Masuda K, Fujinaga T. Noninvasive estimation of cardiac systolic function using continuous-wave Doppler echocardiography in dogs with experimental mitral regurgitation. *Aust Vet J* 2002; **80**: 25–28.
123 Colan SD, Borow KM, Neumann A. Left ventricular end-systolic wall stress-velocity of fiber shortening relation: a load-independent index of myocardial contractility. *J Am Coll Cardiol* 1984; **4**: 715–724.
124 Courand JA, Marshall J, Chang Y, King ME. Clinical applications of wall-stress analysis in the pediatric intensive care unit. *Crit Care Med* 2001; **29**: 526–533.
125 Takano H, Fujii Y, Ishikawa R, *et al.* Comparison of left ventricular contraction profiles among small, medium, and large dogs by use of two-dimensional speckle-tracking echocardiography. *Am J Vet Res* 2010; **71**: 421–427.
126 Sugeng L, Mor-Avi V, Weinert L, *et al.* Quantitative assessment of left ventricular size and function: side-by-side comparison of real-time three-dimensional echocardiography and computed tomography with magnetic resonance reference. *Circulation* 2006; **114**: 654–661
127 McEntee K, Clercx C, Amory H, *et al.* Doppler echocardiographic study of left and right ventricular function during dobutamine stress testing in conscious healthy dogs. *Am J Vet Res* 1999; **60**: 865–867.
128 Chetboul V, Athanassiadis N, Carlos C, *et al.* Assessment of repeatability, reproducibility, and effect of anesthesia on determination of radial and longitudinal left ventricular velocities via tissue Doppler imaging in dogs. *Am J Vet Res* 2004; **65**: 909–915.
129 Koffas H, Dukes-McEwan J, Corcoran BM, *et al.* Peak mean myocardial velocities and velocity gradients measured by color M-mode tissue Doppler imaging in healthy cats. *J Vet Intern Med* 2003; **17**: 510–524.
130 Chetboul V, Athanassiadis N, Carlos C, *et al.* Quantification, repeatability, and reproducibility of feline radial and longitudinal left ventricular velocities by tissue Doppler imaging. *Am J Vet Res* 2004; **65**: 566–572.
131 Gavaghan BJ, Kittleson MD, Fisher KJ, *et al.* Quantification of left ventricular diastolic wall motion by Doppler tissue imaging in healthy cats and cats with cardiomyopathy. *Am J Vet Res* 1999; **60**: 1478–1486.
132 Hori Y, Sato S, Hoshi F, Higuchi S. Assessment of longitudinal tissue Doppler imaging of the left ventricular septum and free wall as an indicator of left ventricular systolic function in dogs. *Am J Vet Res* 2007; **68**: 1051–1057.
133 Piper FS, Andrysco RM, Hamlin RL. A totally noninvasive method for obtaining systolic time intervals in the dog. *Am J Vet Res* 1978; **39**: 1822–1826.
134 Lewis RP, Rittger SE, Forester WF, Boudoulas H. A critical review of the systolic time intervals. *Circulation* 1977; **56**: 146–158.
135 Paival RP, Carvalho P, Couceiro R, *et al.* Beat-to-beat systolic time-interval measurement from heart sounds and ECG. *Physiol Meas* 2012; **33**: 177–194.
136 Kolata RJ. The significance of changes in toe web temperature in dogs in circulatory shock. *Proc Gaines Vet Symp* 1978; **28**: 21–26.
137 Lima A, Jansen TC, van Bommel J, *et al.* The prognostic value of the subjective assessment of peripheral perfusion in critically ill patients. *Crit Care Med* 2009; **37**: 934–938.
138 Haskins SC, Pascoe PJ, Ilkiw JE, *et al.* The effect of moderate hypovolemia on cardiopulmonary function in dogs. *J Vet Emerg Crit Care* 2005; **15**: 100–109.
139 Van der Linden P, Rausin I, Deltell A, *et al.* Detection of tissue hypoxia by arterio-venous gradient for PCO_2 and pH in anesthetized dogs during progressive hemorrhage. *Anesth Analg* 1995; **80**: 269–275.
140 van Beest PA, van der Schors A, Liefers H, *et al.* Femoral venous oxygen saturation is no surrogate for central venous oxygen saturation. *Crit Care Med* 2012; **40**: 3196–3201.
141 Teboul JL, Mercat A, Lenique F, *et al.* Value of the venous-arterial PCO_2 gradient to reflect the oxygen supply to demand in humans: effects of dobutamine. *Crit Care Med* 1998; **26**: 979–980.
142 Mahutte CK, Jaffe MB, Sasse SA, *et al.* Relationship of thermodilution cardiac output to metabolic measurements and mixed venous oxygen saturation. *Chest* 1993; **104**: 1236–1242.
143 van der Hoeven MA, Maertzdorf WJ, Blanco CE. Relationship between mixed venous oxygen saturation and markers of tissue oxygenation in progressive hypoxic hypoxia and in isovolemic anemic hypoxia in 8- to 12-day-old piglets. *Crit Care Med* 1999; 27: 1885–1892.
144 Lumb AB. *Nunn's Applied Respiratory Physiology*, 6th edn. Oxford: Butterworth Heinemann, 2005.
145 Povoas HP, Weil MH, Tang W, *et al.* Comparisons between sublingual and gastric tonometry during hemorrhagic shock. *Chest* 2000; **118**: 1127–1132.
146 McKinley BA, Butler BD. Comparison of skeletal muscle PO_2, PCO_2, and pH with gastric tonometric PCO_2 and pH in hemorrhagic shock. *Crit Care Med* 1999; **27**: 1869–1877.
147 Clavijo-Alvarez JA, Sims CA, Pinsky MR, Puyana JC. Monitoring skeletal muscle and subcutaneous tissue acid–base status and oxygenation during hemorrhagic shock and resuscitation. *Shock* 2005; **24**: 270–275.
148 Soller BR, Heard SO, Cingo NA, *et al.* Application of fiberoptic sensors for the study of hepatic dysoxia in swine hemorrhagic shock. *Crit Care Med* 2001; **29**: 1438–1444.
149 Shoemaker WC, Thangathurai D, Wo CC, *et al.* Intraoperative evaluation of tissue perfusion in high-risk patients by invasive and noninvasive hemodynamic monitoring. *Crit Care Med* 1999; **27**: 2147–2152.
150 Tatevossian RG, Wo CC, Velmahos GC, *et al.* Transcutaneous oxygen and CO_2 as early warning of tissue hypoxia and hemodynamic shock in critically ill emergency patients. *Crit Care Med* 2000; **28**: 2248–2253.
151 Fries M, Weil MH, Sun S, *et al.* Increases in tissue PCO_2 during circulatory shock reflect selective decreases in capillary blood flow. *Crit Care Med* 2006; **34**: 446–452.
152 Imai T, Sekiguchi T, Nagai Y, *et al.* Continuous monitoring of gastric intraluminal carbon dioxide pressure, cardiac output, and end-tidal carbon dioxide pressure in the perioperative period in patients receiving cardiovascular surgery using cardiopulmonary bypass. *Crit Care Med* 2002; **30**: 44–51.
153 Nezu Y, Sakaue Y, Hara Y, *et al.* Evaluation of intestinal intramucosal pH, arterial and portal venous blood gas values, and intestinal blood flow during small intestinal ischemia and reperfusion in dogs. *Am J Vet Res* 2002; **63**: 804–810.
154 Jakob SM, Parviainen I, Ruokonen E, *et al.* Tonometry revisited: perfusion-related, metabolic, and respiratory components of gastric mucosal acidosis in acute cardiorespiratory failure. *Shock* 2008; **29**: 543–548.
155 Perin D, Cruz RJ Jr, Silva E, Poli-de-Figueiredo LF. Low hematocrit impairs gastric mucosal CO_2 removal during experimental severe normovolemic hemodilution. *Clinics (Sao Paulo)* 2006; **61**: 445–452.
156 Ruffolo DC, Headley JM. Regional carbon dioxide monitoring: a different look at tissue perfusion. *AACN Clin Issues* 2003; **14**: 168–175.

157 Nevière R, Chagnon JL, Teboul JL, *et al.* Small intestine intramucosal PCO_2 and microvascular blood flow during hypoxic and ischemic hypoxia. *Crit Care Med* 2002; **30**: 379–384.
158 Guzman JA, Kruse JA. Gut mucosal-arterial PCO_2 gradient as an indicator of splanchnic perfusion during systemic hypo- and hypercapnia. *Crit Care Med* 1999; **27**: 2760–2765.
159 Pellis T, Weil MH, Tang W, *et al.* Increases in both buccal and sublingual partial pressure of carbon dioxide reflect decreases of tissue blood flows in a porcine model during hemorrhagic shock. *Trauma* 2005; **58**: 817–824.
160 Awan ZA, Wester T, Kvernebo K. Human microvascular imaging: a review of skin and tongue videomicroscopy techniques and analysing variables. *Clin Physiol Funct Imaging* 2010; **30**: 79–88.
161 Marik PE, Bankov A. Sublingual capnometry versus traditional markers of tissue oxygenation in critically ill patients. *Crit Care Med* 2003; **31**: 818–822.
162 Daly SM, Leahy MJ. 'Go with the flow': a review of methods and advancements in blood flow imaging. *J Biophotonics* 2013; **6**: 217–255.
163 Manning TO, Monteiro-Riviere NA, Bristol DG, Riviere JE. Cutaneous laser-Doppler velocimetry in nine animal species. *Am J Vet Res* 1991; **52**: 1960–1964.
164 De Backer D, Creteur J, Preiser JC, *et al.* Microvascular blood flow is altered in patients with sepsis. *Am J Respir Crit Care Med* 2002; **166**: 98–104.
165 Trzeciak S, Dellinger RP, Parrillo JE, *et al.* Early microcirculatory perfusion derangements in patients with severe sepsis and septic shock: relationship to hemodynamics, oxygen transport, and survival. *Ann Emerg Med* 2007; **49**: 88–98.
166 Jhanji S, Vivian-Smith A, Lecena-Arnaro S, *et al.* Haemodynamic optimisation improves tissue microvascular flow and oxygenation after major surgery: a randomized controlled trial. *Crit Care* 2010; **14**: R151.
167 Choi JY, Lee WH, Yoo TK, *et al.* A new severity predicting index for hemorrhagic shock using lactate concentration and peripheral perfusion in a rat model. *Shock* 2012; **38**: 635–641.
168 Fang X, Tang W, Sun S, *et al.* Comparison of buccal microcirculation between septic and hemorrhagic shock. *Crit Care Med* 2006; **34**: S447–S453.
169 Puissant C, Abraham P, Durand S, *et al.* Reproducibility of non-invasive assessment of skin endothelial function using laser Doppler flowmetry and laser speckle contrast imaging. *PLoS One* 2013; **8**(4): e61320.
170 Haskins SC, Patz JD. Effects of small and large face masks and translaryngeal and tracheostomy intubation on ventilation, upper-airway deadspace, and arterial blood gases. *Am J Vet Res* 1986; **47**: 945–948.
171 Mauderly JL, Pickrell JA. Pulmonary function testing of unanesthetized beagle dogs. In: Harmison LT, ed. *Research Animals in Medicine.* Washington, DC: US Department of Health, Education, and Welfare, 1973; 665–679.
172 Beck KC, Vettermann J, Rehder K. Gas exchange in dogs in the prone and supine positions. *J Appl Physiol* 1992; **72**: 2292–2297.
173 Collier CR, Mead J. Pulmonary exchange as related to altered pulmonary mechanics in anesthetized dogs. *J Appl Physiol* 1964; **19**: 659–664.
174 Bennet RA, Orton EC, Tucker A, Heiller CL. Cardiopulmonary changes in conscious dogs with induced progressive pneumothorax. *Am J Vet Res* 1989; **50**: 284.
175 Riebold TW. Monitoring equine anesthesia. In: Turner AS, ed. *Veterinary Clinics of North America; Equine Practice.* Philadelphia: WB Saunders, 1990; 607–624.
176 Hubbell JAE. Monitoring. In: Muir WW, Hubbell JAE, eds. *Equine Anesthesia Monitoring and Emergency Therapy.* St Louis, MO: Mosby Year Book, 1991; 153–178.
177 Pang D, Hethey J, Caulkett NA, Duke T. Partial pressure of end-tidal CO_2 sampled via an intranasal catheter as a substitute for partial pressure of arterial CO_2 in dogs. *J Vet Emerg Crit Care* 2007; **17**: 143–148.
178 Barter LS. Capnography. In: Burkitt-Creedon JM, Davis H, eds. *Advanced Monitoring and Procedures for Small Animal Emergency and Critical Care.* Chichester: John Wiley & Sons, Ltd, 2012; 340–348.
179 Tusman G, Gogniat E, Bohm SH, *et al.* Reference values for volumetric capnography-derived non-invasive parameters in healthy individuals. *J Clin Monit Comput* 2013; **27**: 281–288.
180 Herholz CP, Gerber V, Tschudi P, *et al.* Use of volumetric capnography to identify pulmonary dysfunction in horses with and without clinically apparent recurrent airway obstruction. *Am J Vet Res* 2003; **64**: 338–345.
181 Tusman G, Suarez-Sipmann F, Paez G, *et al.* States of low pulmonary blood flow can be detected non-invasively at the bedside measuring alveolar deadspace. *J Clin Monit Comput* 2012; **26**: 183–190.
182 Gray S, Powell LL. Blood gas analysis. In: Burkitt-Creedon JM, Davis H, eds. *Advanced Monitoring and Procedures for Small Animal Emergency and Critical Care.* Chichester: John Wiley & Sons, Ltd, 2012; 286–292.
183 Kennedy SA, Constable PD, Sen I, Couetil L. Effects of syringe type and storage conditions on results of equine blood gas and acid-base analysis. *Am J Vet Res* 2012; **73**: 979–987.
184 Rezende ML, Haskins SC, Hopper K. The effects of ice-water storage on blood gas and acid–base measurements. *J Vet Emerg Crit Care* 2006; **17**: 67–71.
185 Hopper K, Rezende ML, Haskins SC. Assessment of the effect of dilution of blood samples with sodium heparin on blood gas, electrolyte, and lactate measurements in dogs. *Am J Vet Res* 2005; **65**: 656–660.
186 Anuar K, Aziz A, Meduoye A. Is pH-stat or alpha-stat the best technique to follow in patients undergoing deep hypothermic circulatory arrest? *Interact Cardiovasc Thorac Surg* 2010; **10**: 271–282.
187 Tremper KK, Barker SJ. Pulse oximetry. *Anesthesiology* 1989; **70**: 98–108.
188 Hendricks JC, King LG. Practicality, usefulness, and limits of pulse oximetry in critical small animal patients. *J Vet Emerg Crit Care* 1993; **2**: 5–12.
189 Barton LJ, Devey JJ, Gorski S, *et al.* Evaluation of transmittance and reflectance pulse oximetry in a canine model of hypotension and desaturation. *J Vet Emerg Crit Care* 1997; **6**: 21–28.
190 White GA, Matthews NS, Hartsfield SM, *et al.* Pulse oximetry for estimation of oxygenation in dogs with experimental pneumothorax. *J Vet Emerg Crit Care* 1995; **4**: 69–76.
191 Fairman NB. Evaluation of pulse oximetry as a continuous monitoring technique in critically ill dogs in a small animal intensive care unit. *J Vet Emerg Crit Care* 1993; **2**: 50–56.
192 Sendak MJ, Harris AP, Donham RT. Accuracy of pulse oximetry during arterial oxyhemoglobin desaturation in dogs. *Anesthesiology* 1988; **68**: 111–114.
193 Jacobson JD, Miller MW, Matthews NS, *et al.* Evaluation of accuracy of pulse oximetry in dogs. *Am J Vet Res* 1992; **53**: 537–540.
194 Huss BT, Anderson MA, Branson RR, *et al.* Evaluation of pulse oximeter probes and probe placement in healthy dogs. *J Am Anim Hosp Assoc* 1995; **31**: 9–14.
195 Grosenbaugh DA, Alben JO, Muir WW. Absorbance spectra of inter-species hemoglobins in the visible and near infrared regions. *J Vet Emerg Crit Care* 1998; **7**: 36–42.
196 Sidi A, Rush W, Gravenstein N, *et al.* Pulse oximetry fails to accurately detect low levels of arterial hemoglobin oxygen saturation in dogs. *J Clin Monit* 1987; **3**: 257–262.
197 Lee S, Tremper KK, Barker SJ. Effects of anemia on pulse oximetry and continuous mixed venous hemoglobin saturation monitoring in dogs. *Anesthesiology* 1991; **75**: 118–122.
198 Ayres DA. Pulse oximetry and CO-oximetry. In: Burkitt-Creedon JM, Davis H, eds. *Advanced Monitoring and Procedures for Small Animal Emergency and Critical Care.* Chichester: John Wiley & Sons, Ltd, 2012; 274–285.
199 Barker SJ, Tremper KK, Hyatt J. Effects of methemoglobinemia on pulse oximetry and mixed venous oximetry. *Anesthesiology* 1989; **70**: 112–117.
200 Anderson ST, Hajduczek J, Barker SJ. Benzocaine-induced methemoglobinemia in an adult: accuracy of pulse oximetry with methemoglobinemia. *Anesth Analg* 1988; **67**: 1099–1101.
201 Barker SJ, Tremper KK. The effect of carbon monoxide inhalation on pulse oximetry and transcutaneous PO_2. *Anesthesiology* 1987; **66**: 677–679.
202 Aaron AA, Genevieve SA, Steinke JM, Shepherd AP. Co-oximetry interference by hemoglobin-based blood substitutes. *Anesth Analg* 2001; **92**: 863–869.
203 Bunn HF. The role of 2,3-diphosphoglycerate in mediating hemoglobin function of mammalian red cells. *Ann N Y Acad Sci* 1974; **241**: 498–512.
204 Scott AF, Bunn HF, Brush AH. The phylogenetic distribution of red cell 2,3-diphosphoglycerate and its interaction with mammalian hemoglobins. *J Exp Zool* 1977; **201**: 269–288.
205 Clerbaux T, Gustin P, Detry B, *et al.* Comparative study of the oxyhaemoglobin dissociation curve of four mammals: man, dog, horse, and cattle. *Comp Biochem Physiol* 1993; **106**: 687–694.
206 Samaja M, Gattinoni L. Oxygen affinity in the blood of sheep. *Resp Physiol* 1978; **34**: 385–392.
207 Chiodi H. Comparative study of the blood gas transport in high altitude and sea level camelidae and goats. *Resp Physiol* 1970; **11**: 84–93.
208 Dawson TJ, Evans JV. Effect of hypoxia on oxygen transport in sheep with different hemoglobin types. *J Appl Physiol* 1966; **210**: 1021–1025.
209 Bauman R, Haller EA. Cat haemoglobins A and B: differences in the interaction with Cl–, phosphate, and CO_2. *Biochem Biophys Res Commun* 1975; **65**: 220–227.
210 Mauk AG, Huang YP, Skogen W, *et al.* The effect of hemoglobin phenotype on whole blood oxygen saturation and erythrocyte organic phosphate concentration in the domestic cat (Felis catus). *Comp Biochem Physiol* 1975; **51**: 487–489.
211 Gustin P, Detry B, Robert A, *et al.* Influence of age and breed on the binding of oxygen to red blood cells of bovine calves. *J Appl Physiol* 1997; **82**: 784–790.
212 Oneglia C, Fabris C, Modica A, *et al.* The oxygen affinity of normal human whole blood measured by double tonometry. I. P50 and n factor. *Boll Soc Ital Biol Sper* 1984; **60**: 421–427.
213 Herbert DA, Mitchell RA. Blood gas tensions and acid–base balance in awake cats. *J Appl Physiol* 1971; **30**: 434–436.
214 Herrmann K, Haskins S. Determination of P50 for feline hemoglobin. *J Vet Emerg Crit Care* 2005; **13**: 26–31.

215 Nakashima M, Noda H, Hasegaera M, Ikai A. The oxygen affinity of mammalian hemoglobins in the absence of 2,3-diphosphoglycerate in relation to body weight. *Comp Biochem Physiol* 1985; **82A**: 583–589.

216 Smith RC, Garbutt GJ, Isaacks RE, Harkness DR. Oxgen binding of fetal and adult bovine hemoglobin in the presence of organic phosphates and uric acid riboside. *Hemoglobin* 1979; **3**: 47–55.

217 Meshia G. Properties of fetal and adult hemoglobin in sheep at altitude. *Q J Exp Physiol* 1961; **46**: 156–160.

218 Johnson PA, Bihari DJ, Raper RF, *et al.* A comparison between direct and calculated oxygen saturation in intensive care. *Anaesth Intensive Care* 1993; **21**: 72–75.

219 Scott NE, Haskins SC, Aldrich J, *et al.* Comparison of measured oxyhemoglobin saturation and oxygen content with analyze-calculated values and hand-calculated values obtained in unsedated healthy dogs. *Am J Vet Res* 2005; **66**: 1273–1277.

220 Grosenbaugh DA, Muir WW. Accuracy of noninvasive oxyhemoglobin saturation, end-tidal carbon dioxide concentration, and blood pressure monitoring during experimentally induced hypoxemia, hypotension, or hypertension in anesthetized dogs. *Am J Vet Res* 1998; **59**: 205–212.

221 Zijlstra WG, Burrsma A. Spectrophotometry of hemoglobin: a comparison of dog and man. *Comp Biochem Physiol* 1987; **88**: 251–255.

222 Kelman GR, Nunn JF. Clinical recognition of hypoxaemia under fluorescent lamps. *Lancet* 1966; **i**: 1400–1403.

223 Martin L, Khalil H. How much reduced hemoglobin is necessary to generate central cyanosis? *Chest* 1990; **87**: 182–185.

224 Huttemeier PC, Ringsted C, Eliasen K, Mogensen T. Ventilation-perfusion inequality during endotoxin-induced pulmonary vasoconstriction in conscious sheep: mechanisms of hypoxia. *Clin Physiol* 1988; **8**: 351–358.

225 Santolicandro A, Prediletto R, Formai E, *et al.* Mechanisms of hypoxemia and hypocapnia in pulmonary embolism. *Am J Respir Crit Care Med* 1995; **152**: 336–347.

226 Cooper CB, Celli B. Venous admixture in COPD: pathophysiology and therapeutic approaches. *J Chron Obstruct Pulmon Dis* 2008; **5**: 376–381.

227 Bishop MJ, Cheney FW. Effects of pulmonary blood flow and mixed venous O_2 tension on gas exchange in dogs. *Anesthesiology* 1983; **58**: 130–135.

228 Staub NC. The pathogenesis of pulmonary edema. *Prog Cardiovasc Dis* 1980; **23**: 53–80.

229 Ware LB, Matthay MA. The acute respiratory distress syndrome. *N Engl J Med* 2000; **342**: 1334–1349.

230 Gowda MS, Klocke RA. Variability of indices of hypoxemia in adult respiratory distress syndrome. *Crit Care Med* 1997; **25**: 41–45.

231 Aboab J, Louis B, Jonson B, Brochard L. Relationship between PaO_2/FIO_2 ratio and FIO_2: a mathematical description. *Intensive Care Med* 2006; **32**: 1494–1497.

232 Whiteley JP, Gavaghan DJ, Hahn DEW. Variation of venous admixture, SF6 shunt, PaO_2, and the PaO2/FIO_2 ratio with FIO_2. *Br J Anaesth* 2002; **88**: 771–778.

233 Ferguson ND, Kacmarek RM, Chiche JD, *et al.* Screening of ARDS patients using standardized ventilator settings: influence on enrollment in a clinical trial. *Intensive Care Med* 2004; **30**: 1111–1116.

234 Mann S, Westenskow DR, Houtchens BA. Measured and predicted caloric expenditure in the acutely ill. *Crit Care Med* 1985; **13**: 173–176.

235 Vernon DD, Witte MK. Effect of neuromuscular blockade on oxygen consumption and energy expenditure in sedated, mechanically ventilated children. *Crit Care Med* 2000; **28**: 1569–1571.

236 Ogilvie GK, Salman MD, Kesel ML, Fettman MJ. Effect of anesthesia and surgery on energy expenditure determined by indirect calorimetry in dogs with malignant and nonmalignant conditions. *Am J Vet Res* 1996; **57**: 1321–1326.

237 Ogilvie GK, Walters LM, Salman MD, Fettman MJ. Resting energy expenditure in dogs with nonhematopoietic malignancies before and after excision of tumors. *Am J Vet Res* 1996; **57**: 1463–1467.

238 Walton RS, Wingfield WE, Ogilvie GK, *et al.* Energy expenditure in 104 postoperative and traumatically injured dogs with indirect calorimetry. *J Vet Emerg Crit Care* 1997; **6**: 71–79.

239 Mazzaferro EM, Hackett TB, Stein TP, *et al.* Metabolic alterations in dogs with osteosarcoma. *Am J Vet Res* 2001; **62**: 1234–1239.

240 Walters LM, Ogilvie GK, Salman MD, *et al.* Repeatability of energy expenditure measurements in clinically normal dogs by use of indirect calorimetry. *Am J Vet Res* 1993; **54**: 1881–1885.

241 O'Toole E, Miller CW, Wilson BA, *et al.* Comparison of the standard predictive equation for calculation of resting energy expenditure with indirect calorimetry in hospitalized and healthy dogs. *J Am Vet Med Assoc* 2004; **225**: 58–64.

242 Covelli HD, Nessan VJ, Tuttle WK. Oxygen derived variables in acute respiratory failure. *Crit Care Med* 1983; **1**: 646–649.

243 Phua J, Stewart TE, Ferguson ND. Acute respiratory distress syndrome 40 year later: time to revisit its definition. *Crit Care Med* 2008; **36**: 2912–2921.

244 Wandrup JH. Quanifying pulmonary oxygen transfer deficits in critically ill patients. *Acta Anaesth Scand* 1996; **107**: 37–44.

245 Oliven A, Abinader E, Bursztein S. Influence of varying inspired oxygen tensions on the pulmonary venous admixture (shunt) of mechanically ventilated patients. *Crit Care Med* 1980; **8**: 99–101.

246 El-Khatib MF, Jamaleddine GW. A new oxygenation index for reflecting intrapulmonary shunting in patients undergoing open-heart surgery. *Chest* 2004; **125**: 592–596.

247 Araos JD, Larenza MP, Boston RC, *et al.* Use of the oxygen content-based index, Fshunt, as an indicator of pulmonary venous admixture at various inspired oxygen fractions in anesthetized sheep. *Am J Vet Res* 2012; **73**: 2013–2020.

248 Blair E. *Clinical Hypothermia.* New York: McGraw-Hill, 1964.

249 Danzl DF. Accidental hypothermia. In: Rosen P, Baker FJ, Barkin RM, *et al.*, eds. *Emergency Medicine.* St Louis, MO: Mosby, 1988; 663–692.

250 Thomas H. Fever. In: Rosen P, Baker FJ, Barkin RM, *et al.*, eds. *Emergency Medicine.* St Louis, MO: Mosby, 1988; 309–320.

251 Callaham M. Heat Illness. In: Rosen P, Baker FJ, Barkin RM, *et al.*, eds. *Emergency Medicine.* St Louis, MO: Mosby, 1988; 693–717.

252 Gronert GA. Malignant hyperthermia. *Anesthesiology* 1980; **53**: 395–423.

253 Ayres SM, Keenan RL. The hyperthermic syndromes. In: Ayres SM, Grenvik A, Holbrook PR, Shoemaker WC, eds. *Textbook of Critical Care.* Philadelphia: WB Saunders, 1995; 1520–1523.

254 Short CE, Paddleford RR. Malignant hyperpyrexia in the dog. *Anesthesiology* 1973; **39**: 462–463.

255 Bagshaw RJ, Cox RH, Knight DH, Detweiler DK. Malignant hyperthemia in a greyhound. *J Am Vet Med Assoc* 1978; **172**: 61–62.

256 de Jong RH, Heavner JE, Amory DW. Malignant hyperpyrexia in the cat. *Anesthesiology* 1974; **41**: 608–609.

257 Bellah JR. Suspected malignant hyperthermia after halothane anesthesia in a cat. *Vet Surg* 1989; **18**: 483–486.

258 McClure JJ. Malignant hyperthermia in the horse: case report. *Minn Vet* 1975; **15**: 12–15.

259 Klein LV. Case report: a hot horse. *Vet Anesth* 1975; **2**: 41–44.

260 Smale K, Anderson LS, Butler PJ, An algorithm to describe the oxygen equilibrium curve for the thoroughbred racehorse. *Equine Vet J* 1994; **26**: 500–502.

261 Kelman GR, Digital computer subroutine for the conversion of oxygen tension into saturation. *J Appl Physiol* 1966; **21**: 1375–1376.

262 Cambier C, Wierinckx M, Clerbaux T, *et al.* Haemoglobin oxygen affinity and regulating factors of the blood oxygen transport in canine and feline blood. *Res Vet Sci* 2004; **77**: 83–88.

263 Gustin P, Clerbaux T, Willems E, *et al.* Oxygen transport properties of blood in two different bovine breeds. *Comp Biochem Physiol* 1988; **89A**: 553–558.

264 Haskins SC, Rezende ML, The caprine oxyhemoglobin dissociation curve. *Res Vet Sci* 2006; **80**: 103–108.

5 Anesthetic Emergencies and Resuscitation

Deborah V. Wilson[1] and André C. Shih[2]

[1]Department of Large Animal Clinical Sciences, College of Veterinary Medicine, Michigan State University, East Lansing, Michigan, USA
[2]University of Florida College of Veterinary Medicine, Gainesville, Florida, USA

Chapter contents

Introduction

Anesthesia is a very complex, dynamic domain that is labor intensive, can be equipment intensive, and requires accuracy and attention to detail for a good outcome. Errors and unforeseen events occur with low frequency, catastrophic events usually cannot be predicted, and mistakes are not always reversible. Human factors are integral to the anesthesia domain. Even for elective surgery in the healthy patient there is a small but ever-present risk of injury, brain damage, and death [1–5]. The most recent measure of anesthesia-associated mortality was 0.17% in canine anesthetics, 0.24% in cats and 1.39% in rabbits [3]. Assessment and management of perioperative risk are discussed in Chapter 2.

It has been shown that the majority (70%) of anesthetic complications occurring in people involved human error [6–8]. Anesthetic complications associated with other causes are reported with variable frequency in other species. Hypotension, apnea, dysrhythmias, hypoxemia, and airway problems were reported in 12% of dogs and 10.5% of cats in one study from a busy University Veterinary Teaching Hospital [1]. Eight years later, in a group of 1281 well-monitored dogs, the most commonly reported anesthesia-associated complications were hypoventilation (63%), hypothermia (53%), and hypotension (38%), with an anesthesia-associated mortality rate of 0.9% [9].

Cardiovascular

Derangements of cardiovascular function occur commonly in most species under anesthesia.

Hypotension

Defined as a mean arterial pressure less than 60 mmHg (and systolic pressure ≤80 mmHg), hypotension occurs in up to 38% of dogs under anesthesia [9,10]. Patients with more severe disease (ASA physical status III and IV) generally have lower blood pressure under anesthesia than those with less severe disease [9]. Hypotension jeopardizes perfusion of all organs, has been shown to triple the risk of intra- and postanesthetic death for mares with dystocia, and is associated with increased risk of perianesthetic death in horses with large colon torsion [11,12].

Many factors are associated with the development of hypotension, including effects of most anesthetic agents, hypovolemia, hemorrhage, myocardial damage, humoral mediators, and peripheral vasodilation.

Treatment of hypotension should be aimed at the probable cause, but generally should start with a reduction in anesthetic depth and a fluid bolus (assuming no cardiovascular disease which would be adversely affected by a fluid bolus). Infusion of dopamine or dobutamine, or a bolus dose of ephedrine, would be next in the

Veterinary Anesthesia and Analgesia: The Fifth Edition of Lumb and Jones.
Edited by Kurt A. Grimm, Leigh A. Lamont, William J. Tranquilli, Stephen A. Greene and Sheilah A. Robertson.

treatment algorithm. Vasopressors such as phenylephrine, norepinephrine, and vasopressin are only occasionally required and may result in decreased tissue perfusion if not carefully titrated.

Hemorrhage

Acute hemorrhage results in hypovolemia and a reduction in blood oxygen-carrying capacity. A significant decrease in circulating blood volume is not well tolerated in the anesthetized patient. A blood volume loss of 10–20% is clinically detectable, and life-threatening circulatory failure occurs with an uncorrected blood volume loss of 30–40% [13]. Life-threatening hemorrhage is a relatively rare event during surgery, occurring in about 2% of canine major surgeries [1].

Blood loss during surgery may be insidious or obvious, and quantifying blood loss can be difficult [14]. Most often the severity of hemorrhage is assessed by its impact on the patient. Severe blood loss in most domestic species causes tachycardia, reduced arterial pressure, a decrease in pulse pressure, decreased area under the arterial pulse waveform, and peripheral vasoconstriction leading to pale mucus membranes [15,16]. Some of theses signs (e.g., tachycardia) may be masked by anesthetic or adjunctive drugs, making early detection of significant hemorrhage challenging. The base deficit, increased lactate, and changes in bicarbonate, arterial oxygenation and venous pH correlate with volume of blood lost [17–19], but usually lag other physiological signs of blood loss or tissue hypoxemia. The anesthetized horse manifests most of the above changes, but heart rate is remarkably steady and usually stays at pre-hemorrhage levels [17].

Minimizing ischemia and tissue hypoperfusion are the goals of blood volume replacement. Treatment usually begins with the administration of a balanced polyionic crystalloid solution, with a rough guideline that acutely, the volume administered is three times the volume of shed blood (due to rapid extravasation of this fluid). Dilution of the remaining red blood cells is inevitable, which further reduces hematocrit, the concentration of clotting factors and platelets, although improved cardiac output may balance the decreased oxygen-carrying capacity. In cases of severe hemorrhage, more specific therapy should be administered. Transfusion of whole blood, hemoglobin solution, or blood component products would follow if oxygen-carrying capacity or coagulation is compromised. The rate at which lactate levels normalize with treatment is correlated strongly with outcome [19,20].

Cardiac dysrhythmias

Cardiac dysrhythmias occur in >60% of human patients undergoing anesthesia and surgery, and seem as prevalent in animal patients [21,22]. Holter monitoring of 50 young, healthy dogs before, during, and after routine ovariohysterectomy or orchidectomy detected second-degree atrioventricular block (AVB) in 26 dogs and ventricular premature complexes (VPCs) in 22 (44%), and showed that atrial premature complexes were also common (32%) [10].

Cardiac dysrhythmias can occur as a result of pre-existing medical conditions and as a response to surgery and anesthesia. Some conditions, such as gastric dilation/volvulus, trauma and splenic disease, are well known to be associated with cardiac dysrhythmias [23–25]. Anesthesia for cervical spinal decompression is also associated with a high incidence of dysrhythmias and VPCs, but not thoracic or lumbar spinal surgery [26].

Several drugs used during anesthesia predispose the patient to conduction abnormalities and potentiate the development of arrhythmias [27]. Phenothiazine tranquilizers have been associated with sinus bradycardia, sinus arrest, and occasional first- and second-degree heart block. Xylazine administration produces a 30% reduction in the arrhythmogenic dose of epinephrine in dogs, although the clinical relevance of this experimental design remains debated [28]. In dogs, administration of dexmedetomidine was associated with low heart rate but no VPCs [29]. Atropine and glycopyrrolate can cause sinus tachycardia and increased myocardial work. Muscarinic blockade increases the arrhythmogenic dose of epinephrine in dogs, but reduces the arrhythmogenic dose of dobutamine by 66% in horses [30,31]. Most opioids have been associated with bradyarrhythmias.

Administration of thiopental and ketamine increases the likelihood of epinephrine-induced dysrhythmias during halothane and isoflurane anesthesia [27,32,33] whereas Telazol® [34]. does not. Halothane potentiates the arrhythmogenic effect of epinephrine much more than isoflurane [35]. Two studies have shown that where VPCs occur in healthy dogs during inhalant anesthesia, either changing to a different inhalant or increasing the depth of inhalant anesthesia may eliminate the VPCs [36,37].

Most perioperative dysrhythmias have little clinical significance, and are monitored but not treated. However, perioperative ventricular arrhythmias detected in cats may be associated with occult myocardial disease and usually warrant further evaluation. A bradyarrhythmia requires treatment if there is evidence that perfusion is inadequate (discolored mucous membranes, low blood pressure), asystole appears imminent, or the arterial blood pressure becomes heart rate dependent. When blood pressure monitoring is not utilized, some anesthetists choose to treat bradycardia when the heart rate is less than some threshold (many veterinarians use 60 bpm in dogs and 20 bpm in horses for this limit). Although the usual treatment for bradycardia is administration of an antimuscarinic, treatment of an α_2-adrenergic receptor agonist-induced bradyarrhythmia observed with concurrent normo- or hypertension may be better resolved with an α_2-adrenergic receptor antagonist (e.g., atipamezole) [38].

A tachyarrhythmia will require treatment if pulse deficits and/or hypotension occur, or when runs of VPCs, an increasing frequency of VPCs, or multi-focal VPCs are present. Treatment involves correcting any obvious physiologic abnormalities (low pH, hypercarbia, hypoxia, electrolyte derangements such as low K^+) and administering antiarrhythmic drugs (e.g., lidocaine or procainamide). Esmolol infusion is a very effective treatment for epinephrine-induced ventricular tachyarrhythmias but may result in decreased myocardial contractility [39]. In the patient with traumatic myocarditis, arrhythmias and myocardial dysfunction peak about 24–48 h after the injury, and it may be prudent to delay surgery beyond this time if possible [24].

Anaphylaxis

Allergic (antigen–immune complex mediated) reactions involving anesthetics are relatively uncommon, and require previous exposure to the agent, or one like it. However, anaphylactoid reactions cause severe systemic histamine release, and prior exposure to the drug is not required. Severe cardiovascular collapse with hypotension, tachycardia with arrhythmias, pulmonary hypertension, portal hypertension, and cutaneous changes such as wheals or edema occur during an anaphylactic reaction. This type of reaction can be life threatening and usually requires aggressive treatment.

Allergic reactions during anesthesia in people are most commonly reported to follow administration of antibiotics and neuromuscular blocking agents [40]. Other agents have been implicated in animals, but caution should be used when recording or communicating an adverse event as 'allergic' in origin (in the absence of supporting documentation), since this may create future medicolegal difficulties. Anaphylactic reactions have been reported following thiopental administration in dogs [41,42], manifesting as obvious straining with passage of mucoid, bloody diarrhea within minutes of injection. Meperidine administration is associated with significant cutaneous histamine release with swelling and wheal formation in 10% of dogs [43]. Propofol administration carries the potential to induce anaphylaxis (most likely associated with drug carrier components), although this has yet to be reported in animals.

Other agents associated with severe reactions are the intravenous contrast agents used during imaging, including iodinated agents and gadolinium. Two dogs administered iodinated agents developed hypotension, heart rate changes, diarrhea and periorbital edema. A series of three dogs receiving IV gadolinium developed severe facial, periorbital, and sublingual edema, and one of the three developed a severe systemic reaction including profound hypotension [44,45].

When tachycardia, arrhythmias, and hypotension are present, oxygen, IV fluids, IV antihistamines (diphenhydramine), and corticosteroids are indicated for treatment and occasionally epinephrine and cardiopulmonary resuscitation (CPR) will be necessary.

Cardiopulmonary arrest

Introduction

Cardiopulmonary arrest (CPA) is a dynamic, time-dependent process occurring secondary to failed cardiac contractility, which results in either ventricular asystole, pulseless electrical activity (PEA), pulseless ventricular tachycardia (VT), or ventricular fibrillation (VF) [46]. The aims of CPR are to provide blood flow to the heart and brain until restoration of spontaneous circulation [47]. Successful CPR combines basic life support (BLS) and advanced life support (ALS) techniques, in addition to postresuscitation care [48].

The use of *cardiopulmonary resuscitation* as a medical term was not adopted until 1958, when treatment of cardiopulmonary arrest shifted from open chest cardiac massage to closed chest compression and defibrillation [46]. Cardiopulmonary resuscitation has overwhelmingly poor outcomes in both human and veterinary medicine. Initial CPR success or *return of spontaneous circulation* (ROSC) in dogs and cats is 28–35 and 42–44% respectively [49,50]. Unfortunately, after CPR, the survival-to-discharge rates drop to 4.1–6.0% in dogs and 7–9% in cats [49]. Every minute spent performing CPR adds significant morbidity risk and the success rate decreases rapidly [46].

The outcome of CPR is strongly influenced by timely initiation of effective interventions. To ensure the highest chance of success, hospital staff should be prepared and trained to respond to the crisis quickly and efficiently. During treatment of an arrest, the veterinarian in charge will usually take a central role coordinating the resuscitation procedures (e.g., running the code). It is important that the anesthesia team is well trained in current CPR procedures. Regardless of initial training, there is always time-related decay of skills. Refresher training and mock CPR simulation every 6 months are recommended [51]. The necessary emergency drugs and equipment should be organized in one place (e.g., crash cart) and should be adequately stocked, regularly audited, and placed in a readily accessible area. It should include supplies for venous access, airway management, and initial pharmacological therapy. It is wise also to have a surgical kit for emergency thoracotomy, tracheostomy, and venous dissection.

Box 5.1 Summary of current CPR guidelines: key CPR points [53]. Be prepared: maintain a well-stocked, centrally located crash cart and train staff members in advance

- Perform chest compression at rate of at least 100/minute, compressing the chest by one-third to one-half of its width
- Maintain continuous chest compression with complete chest recoil
- Perform 2 minute CPR cycles with minimal interruption between rescuers
- Provide asynchronous ventilation with rate of 10 breaths/ per minute and full breath in approximately 1 second with 10 ml/kg tidal volume
- For ventricular fibrillation or pulseless ventricular tachycardia, administer electrical conversion (defibrillation, preferably using a biphasic defibrillator) promptly, followed by chest compression

Guidelines for performing CPR have been implemented in human medicine for some time. In 1992, the International Liaison Committee on Resuscitation (ILCOR) was created in order to develop an internationally accepted CPR protocol. The ILCOR is composed of the American Heart Association (AHA), the European Resuscitation Council, and the Heart and Stroke Foundation of Canada, among others. Protocols were based on research discussed at the International Consensus Conference for Cardiopulmonary Resuscitation and Emergency Cardiovascular Science and Treatment. The ILCOR produced the first international CPR Guidelines in 2000 and revised the protocol in 2005 and 2010 [46].

Until recently, veterinary CPR recommendations were largely based on a combination of clinician preference and the ILCOR guidelines [52]. In 2012, the Reassessment Campaign on Veterinary Resuscitation (RECOVER) was organized in order to provide comprehensive, evidence-based CPR guidelines for veterinary medicine. Most RECOVER initiative participants were Diplomates of the American College of Veterinary Anesthesia and Analgesia (ACVAA) or the American College of Veterinary Emergency and Critical Care (ACVECC) [52]. This was a collaborative initiative that systematically evaluated the published evidence regarding 75 topics relevant to small animal CPR, and generated CPR guidelines (Box 5.1) [52]. If continually updated, the RECOVER initiative should be able to bridge some of the knowledge gaps in veterinary CPR [51]. All hospital staff involved in CPR, particularly the anesthesia and emergency staff, should be aware of these guidelines; they should also be aware of the reasons for any guideline changes and of the current knowledge gaps in veterinary medicine.

Basic life support

Basic life support (BLS) is the foundation for all modern CPR. It consists of recognition of CPA, initiation of chest compressions, and airway management, combined with assisted ventilation [53]. Studies have shown that the quality of BLS performed is directly related to ROSC and survival rate [53]. In 2010, ILCOR human CPR guidelines changed the order of intervention for all age groups (except newborns) from the classical airway (A), breathing (B) and chest compression (C) – ABC – to chest compression (C) first, followed by airway (A) and then breathing (B) (i.e., CAB). This change was made in part because securing an airway in humans is fairly challenging and the prolonged intubation time causes a delay in initiation of chest compression, which negatively impacts ROSC. Furthermore, a large percentage of CPA in humans is due to primary cardiac disease (myocardial ischemia) [53].

In veterinary medicine, there is no evidence supporting benefits of CAB resuscitation over standard ABC resuscitation [53]. There are few data in veterinary medicine regarding the epidemiology of CPA, but it is fair to assume that many veterinary CPA cases are due to ventilatory/pulmonary failure and not myocardial ischemia. Furthermore, in most small animals it is fairly easy to intubate and secure an airway. When multiple trained rescuers are available, chest compression, securing an airway, and ventilation can be initiated almost simultaneously. Current small animal CPR guidelines therefore dictate that in unwitnessed CPA or CPA **not** due to primary cardiac disease, traditional ventilation first or ABC resuscitation is acceptable. In witnessed CPA due to primary cardiac disease, the compression first (or CAB resuscitation) is recommended [53].

Chest compression

In order to maximize blood flow to the myocardium and brain, it is essential to start chest compression early, and to provide the highest quality compressions while paying attention to complete and effective chest recoil [53]. Rescuers should be trained to minimize any interruption to chest compression. Both the 2010 ILCOR human CPR guidelines and the 2012 RECOVER veterinary CPR guidelines recommend a compression rate of *at least* 100 per minute. This is different from the 2005 guidelines, which suggested *approximately* 100 per minute. Although this is a subtle change, the implication is that the more frequent the compressions the better. In animal studies, chest compression rates as high as 120–150 per minute have been associated with good cardiac output and improved coronary blood flow [53].

Myocardial blood flow is determined by the coronary perfusion pressure (C_oPP), defined as the difference between aortic diastolic and right atrial diastolic pressures:

$$C_oPP = DAP - RAP$$

where DAP is diastolic aortic pressure and RAP is right atrial pressure (diastolic). Cerebral blood flow correlates with cerebral perfusion pressure (C_EPP):

$$C_EPP = MAP - ICP$$

where MAP is mean arterial pressure and ICP is intracranial pressure.

A healthy animal can maintain a fairly constant cerebral blood flow within a wide range of cerebral perfusion pressures (50–150 mmHg); during cardiac arrest, however, the autoregulatory mechanism is disrupted and the relationship between cerebral blood flow and cerebral perfusion pressure becomes linear. Hemodynamic optimization during CPR is therefore important in order to minimize adverse cardiac and neurological sequelae [54]. Veterinary CPR guidelines recommend compressing the chest by one-third to one-half of its width to maximize vital organ blood flow [53]. Depth of chest compression has been positively correlated with improved aortic pressure [53]. Institution of effective cardiac compression restores the pressure gradient between the aorta and right atrium, with return of coronary perfusion and a corresponding marked increase in the likelihood of ROSC [55].

Chest compression provides forward blood flow by one or a combination of two mechanisms. The thoracic pump theory states that blood moves out of the thoracic cavity due to an increase in intrathoracic pressure (IttP). This mechanism is thought to occur primarily in animals with a body weight greater than 15–20 kg [56]. The cardiac pump theory explains the development of forward blood flow in smaller animals and refers to actual mechanical compression of the heart by the thoracic wall during the compression cycle [56]. The decompression phase of the CPR cycle (also known as chest recoil) is as important as the compression phase for successful resuscitation. Incomplete chest recoil leaves residual positive IttP that in turn decreases venous return and stroke volume [57–59]. By not allowing full recoil of the chest, IttP remains positive during the decompression phase of CPR, decreasing the pressure gradient between extra- and intrathoracic vessels and diminishing the rate of blood return to the thorax [57,59].

Both human and veterinary CPR guidelines emphasize the importance of continuous chest compression with minimal interruption [53,54]. Even short pauses during CPR acutely decrease the aortic pressure for a significant time and decrease the likelihood of ROSC. Compressions should be performed in approximately 2 min cycles with compressors alternating between cycles. Performance of high-quality chest compression is a strenuous exercise that can rapidly lead to fatigue. Rescuer fatigue decreases the number of adequate compressions and causes the rescuer to rest their hands on the patient's thorax (leaning into the chest), decreasing the effectiveness of chest recoil [60–62]. Longer CPR cycles (5 min) have resulted in a lower number of correct chest compressions compared with shorter cycles (2 min), 18 and 67%, respectively [53].

If multiple rescuers are present, intermittent abdominal compression (IAC) and chest compression can be performed. Abdominal compression has been shown to improve venous return and hemodynamic values in animal CPR models, with little risk to the patient [53]. With this technique, the abdomen is compressed during the relaxation phase of chest compression.

During normal closed chest compression, the cardiac output generated is only 20–30% of normal. Open-chest CPR is more effective in optimizing hemodynamic values and achieving ROSC. In cases of elevated IttP such as tension pneumothorax, pleural fluid, pericardial effusion, severe abdominal distension (gastric dilatation volvulus), or the presence of flail chest, prompt open-chest CPR should be advocated. Open-chest CPR also allows for temporary occlusion (cross-clamping) of the descending aorta, maximizing cerebral and myocardial perfusion. Cross-clamping can be performed by encircling the descending aorta using either a Penrose drain or a red rubber catheter. Open-chest CPR requires significant resources, carries some risk to the rescuer, and demands an intensive care unit postoperatively [63].

Breathing

A high percentage of CPA in veterinary medicine is due to hypoxia and hypoventilation; therefore, securing the airway and adequate ventilation are essential during CPR. During CPR, an airway should be rapidly established by orotracheal intubation. After the airway has been secured, the patient should be ventilated manually with the maximal available inspired oxygen mixture (e.g., $F_IO_2 \approx 1.0$). No studies have yet evaluated the optimal tidal volume and inspiratory time for dogs and cats during CPR. Current guidelines include a ventilation rate of 10 breaths/min without interruption of chest compression [53]. A full breath should be given in approximately 1 s and with a 10 mL/kg tidal volume. A slower inspiratory time would subject the patient to a high IttP for a longer period, decreasing venous return (VR), increasing right ventricular afterload and decreasing left ventricular dispensability [53]. The reduction in VR correlates with peak inspiratory pressure, plateau pressure, and inspiratory:expiratory (I:E) ratio. Excessive ventilation has been associated with an increased mortality rate [64]. In an animal CPR model, the survival rate was 85.7% with ventilation at 12 breaths/min, compared with 14.3% at 30 breaths/min [64]. If there is only one rescuer and chest compression needs to cease for ventilation to occur, the ideal compression:ventilation (C:V) ratio in dogs and cats is currently undetermined, but a C:V ratio of 30:2 is reasonable [64].

Advanced life support

Advanced life support (ALS) includes pharmacological therapy and correction of electrolyte disturbances and volume deficits, along with prompt defibrillation when appropriate [63].

Pharmacological therapy

Few advances have been made recently in pharmacotherapy for CPR (Table 5.1). Many clinicians erroneously focus on drug therapy during resuscitation. In fact, the 2010 ILCOR guidelines de-emphasize the use of drugs, devices, and other distracters, and instead emphasize high-quality BLS.

Vasopressors increase systemic vascular resistance, increasing aortic pressure and directing more of the intravascular volume from the peripheral circulation to the central compartment [63]. Both epinephrine and vasopressin are reasonable choices for all types of cardiac arrest. At the correct dosage, epinephrine acts on both α- (vasoconstrictor) and β-adrenergic receptors (inotropic and chronotropic). An appropriate epinephrine dosage regimen is 0.01 mg/kg IV every 3–5 min. Although a higher dose (0.1 mg/kg) of epinephrine initially increases ROSC, this does not improve hospital discharge rate (survival) and is no longer recommended for CPR.

Table 5.1 Pharmacotherapy during CPR.

Drug	Dose Regimen	Comments
Epinephrine	0.01 mg/kg IV every 3–5 min	Use acceptable in most cases of CPA; causes peripheral vasoconstriction and increased aortic pressure
Vasopressin	0.8 IU/kg IV every 5 min	Use acceptable in most cases of CPA; causes peripheral vasoconstriction and increased aortic pressure
Atropine	0.05 mg/kg IV every 5 min	Routine use is not recommended but may be used in animal CPA after high vagal tone (e.g., vomiting, diarrhea)
Lidocaine	2 mg/kg IV	Routine use is not recommended but may be used in shock-resistant VT or VF
Amiodarone	5 mg/kg	Routine use is not recommended but may be used in shock-resistant VT or VF
Corticosteroid	NA	Routine use is not recommended
Sodium bicarbonate	1 mEq/kg	Routine use is not recommended but may be used in prolonged CPA or CPA due to severe hyperkalemia or severe metabolic acidosis
Calcium gluconate	50 mg/kg	Routine use is not recommended but may be used in CPA due to calcium channel blocker overdose, severe hypocalcemia, or severe hyperkalemia

Vasopressin is a non-catecholamine vasopressor that acts on peripheral vessels (V_1 receptors) while decreasing cellular hyperpolarization and increasing intracellular calcium concentration. In comparison with epinephrine, vasopressin has a longer half-life and seems to be more efficacious in a hypoxic, acidotic environment. An appropriate vasopressin dosage regimen is 0.8 IU/kg IV every 5 min. Vasopressin may be superior to epinephrine in certain conditions, such as prolonged CPA or CPA due to hypovolemia [63]. In the majority of cases, however, vasopressin and epinephrine can be used interchangeably as first-line vasopressors during CPR. Large-scale human studies have not shown a difference in patient outcome for use of vasopressin versus epinephrine during CPR [63].

The 2010 ILCOR guidelines do not recommend the routine use of atropine during CPR. A human CPR study revealed that the use of atropine with epinephrine produced a worse outcome than epinephrine alone. However, for animal CPA after a high vagal tone event (e.g., vomiting, diarrhea), use of atropine is reasonable [63].

The 2010 ILCOR guidelines do not recommend the routine use of antiarrhythmic drugs during CPR. Use of lidocaine can cause vasodilation and a decrease in cardiac output. In pulseless VT and VF, early and rapid defibrillation is advised. In dogs with shock-resistant VT or VF, amiodarone is a choice, although hypotension and anaphylactic reaction have been reported in this species following amiodarone administration. Lidocaine or β-adrenergic receptor blockers (e.g., esmolol) can be an alternative for resistant VT or VF when amiodarone is not available.

The 2010 ILCOR guidelines do not recommend the routine use of steroids during CPR. The use of corticosteroids can cause coagulopathy, hyperglycemia, and immunosuppression, all of which are deleterious post-arrest [63].

The 2010 ILCOR guidelines do not recommend the routine use of sodium bicarbonate during CPR. Bicarbonate administration may cause paradoxical cerebral acidosis, hyperosmolarity, and decreased catecholamine effectiveness. Bicarbonate use may be considered in prolonged CPA or for CPA due to severe hyperkalemia or severe metabolic acidosis. An appropriate dose of sodium bicarbonate dose is 1–2 mEq/kg IV [63].

The 2010 ILCOR guidelines do not recommend the routine use of calcium during CPR. Calcium administration may cause cellular apoptosis with impaired neurological outcome and myocardial damage. The use of calcium may be considered for CPA due to calcium channel blocker overdose, severe hypocalcemia or severe hyperkalemia [63]. An appropriate calcium gluconate dose is 50–100 mg/kg IV.

The use of fluid therapy was not evaluated by the 2012 RECOVER initiative. Fluid therapy is essential if CPA was caused by hypovolemia or hemorrhage. Aggressive fluid therapy can be detrimental to euvolemic patients. Fluid boluses increase central venous pressure (CVP) and right atrial pressure (RAP), which decreases cerebral and coronary perfusion pressures. The 2010 ILCOR guidelines do not recommend aggressive fluid therapy during routine CPR of a euvolemic patient.

Defibrillation

In the event of ventricular fibrillation (VF) or pulseless ventricular tachycardia (VT), the recommendation is to start chest compression and then immediately perform electrical conversion (defibrillation). Implementation of chest compression before defibrillation is beneficial when there is a delayed response time (>4 min) to CPA. It is important for the rescuer to understand that BLS compression should resume *immediately* after shock defibrillation, with no interruption until after a full CPR cycle has been completed.

When choosing a defibrillator, preference should be given to biphasic waveform defibrillators. Biphasic defibrillators have been found to be as effective as or more effective than monophasic defibrillators. Biphasic defibrillators require less energy for successful defibrillation and produce less tissue trauma and less cardiac damage [65]. Electrical defibrillation should start at 2–5 J/kg with a 50% increase in energy for each subsequent attempt.

CPR and anesthesia

Few studies have looked at the incidence of CPA in veterinary practice. A recent study reported 204 CPA events (161 dogs and 43 cats) in a teaching hospital over a 5 year period. Of these, only 19 (0.1%) occurred in patients under anesthesia [49,53]. Despite the rare occurrence of CPA during anesthesia, these cases deserve special attention. Animals that experience CPA during anesthesia have a significantly higher chance of successful resuscitation than animals that are not under anesthesia when they arrest [63]. Anesthetized patients usually have venous access established and are intubated, breathing oxygen. Additionally, CPA should be recognized more quickly because the patient is being monitored adequately.

If anesthesia-related CPA is due to drug overdose, reversal agents should be administered if appropriate. Agents such as naloxone, flumazenil and atipamezole should be administered in the case of opioid, benzodiazepine or α_2-adrenergic receptor agonist overdose, respectively. All inhalant anesthetics cause myocardial depression and their use should be terminated during CPR. Lipid rescue (discussed later in this chapter) may be considered in animals with CPA due to local anesthetic overdose.

If CPA occurs during an abdominal surgery, open-chest CPR performed by reaching the heart through the diaphragm should be considered. During the approach, care must be taken to avoid lacerating the vena cava and aorta.

Postresuscitation care

Postcardiac arrest syndrome (coined by ILCOR in 2008) refers to the pathophysiologic events following ROSC. This syndrome includes brain injury, acute kidney disease, myocardial damage, severe vasodilation and coagulopathy, secondary to low blood flow and subsequent ischemia–reperfusion injury [65]. Systemic inflammatory response syndrome (SIRS) and acute respiratory distress syndrome (ARDS) can follow. Mortality (second arrest) is very common in the first 24 h after resuscitation. Postcardiac arrest care should be aggressive and the patient monitored intensively. Goals for treatment are listed in Table 5.2. Therapeutic protocols are based on goal-directed hemodynamic optimization, cerebral protection, and therapeutic hypothermia [65].

Hemodynamic optimization

To avoid further morbidity, adequate organ perfusion should be re-established during the postcardiac arrest phase. Respiratory goals are to maintain a PaO_2 of 80–100 mmHg or a saturation of 94–98%. Hyperoxemia (PaO_2 > 100 mmHg) can cause an increase in free radical and neurological injury. Hypoventilation is common after CPR. It is important to ensure spontaneous or mechanical ventilation that maintains a $PaCO_2$ of ~32–43 mmHg. The major cardiovascular goal is to maintain systolic blood pressure at 100–200 mmHg (mean blood pressure at 80–100 mmHg). Hypotension can be indicative of hypovolemia or decreased vascular resistance. In these cases, the use of fluid therapy, inotropes, and vasopressors is indicated.

Table 5.2 Post-CPR goals.

Goal	Possible Intervention
Optimize pulmonary function: Maintain saturation 94–98% Maintain PaO_2 80–100 mmHg Maintain $PaCO_2$ ~ 32–43 mmHg	Oxygen supplementation Positive pressure ventilation (IPPV)
Optimize vital organ perfusion: Systolic blood pressure 100–200 mmHg Mean blood pressure 80–100 mmHg Lactate <2.5 mmol/L	Inotropes Fluid therapy Vasopressors
Cerebral protection	Therapeutic hypothermia Hypertonic saline Avoid seizures Total intravenous anesthesia (TIVA)
Prevent recurrent arrest: Recheck electrolytes Monitor ECG and invasive blood pressure	Blood transfusion

Therapeutic hypothermia

There is little information about therapeutic hypothermia (TH) for postcardiac arrest syndrome in veterinary medicine. Advantages of TH include reductions in cerebral oxygen requirement, brain metabolic demand, excitatory neurotransmitters, inflammatory cytokines, and free radicals, together with inhibition of neuronal cell apoptosis [65]. Mild hypothermia (97 °F) seems to be a safe target, although the ideal target temperature and the speed of rewarming have not yet been established in veterinary medicine. In humans, postarrest hypothermia reduced hospital mortality by 20% after cardiac arrest resulting from VF, but this benefit was not observed in patients suffering from PEA or asystole [65]. Therapeutic hypothermia might therefore be beneficial in only a specific subgroup of patients, such as after ventricular fibrillation. Complications from TH include discomfort, increased tissue healing time, and coagulopathy.

Adjunct CPR Devices

An impedance threshold device (ITD) is a device connected to the endotracheal tube, which controls air entry to the lungs. The ITD contains pressure-sensitive valves that require a certain inspiratory threshold (or 'cracking pressure') to be reached prior to inflow of inspiratory gas. The cracking pressure is set at the time of manufacture. During the decompression phase of CPR, the pressure in the patient's upper airway decreases and causes closure of the valve. By enhancing negative IttP during recoil of the chest, the ITD can augment venous return and increase cardiac output [54].

The ITD has been shown to be beneficial in improving C_oPP and aortic pressure. A porcine cardiac arrest model has been used to investigate the effects of an ITD on vital organ perfusion during CPR [66]. A fully functional ITD was used for the experimental group and a sham ITD, which did not occlude the airway during the decompression phase of CPR, was used for the control group. Intrathoracic pressures were lower in the functional ITD group (−5.2 ± 0.5 mmHg) compared with the non-functional group (−1.1 ± 0.2 mmHg). In the functional ITD group, vital organ blood flow was increased with a doubling of C_oPP. In comparison with the control group, the ITD group showed improvements in IttP, CPP, mean arterial pressure, and survival rate (54.5% versus 18.1% in controls) [66]. The Resuscitation Outcomes Consortium (ROC) PRIMED (Prehospital Resuscitation using an IMpedance valve and Early versus Delayed analysis) was the largest human multicenter double-blinded clinical study designed to investigate the effect of the ITD in out-of-hospital cardiac arrest survival-to-discharge [67].

This study found that the use of an ITD improved short-term but not long-term survival [67].

Owing to its effects on intrathoracic cardiovascular dynamics, there is concern that the ITD can possibly cause pulmonary pathology. Development of pulmonary edema may occur because the increased transthoracic pressure differences (between intrathoracic and alveolar pressures) may favor capillary leakage. However, no evidence of pulmonary edema or organ damage was found in pigs after use of an ITD [59]. On a microscopic level, there was no evidence of atelectasis, pulmonary hemorrhage, or edema in this study [59]. An ITD should not be recommended for small dogs (<5 kg) or cats. Contraindications for the ResQPod® ITD (Advanced Circulatory, Roseville, MN, USA). include congestive heart failure, dilated cardiomyopathy, pulmonary hypertension, aortic stenosis, flail chest, chest pain, and shortness of breath. Clinical ITD use in veterinary patients is still being evaluated.

Respiratory system

Respiratory problems are implicated in up to 50% of canine and 66% of feline anesthetic-related deaths [1,2,5]. Severe hypoventilation occurs in up to two-thirds of dogs under anesthesia and has few associated clinical signs [9], and therefore will be missed unless tidal volume or carbon dioxide levels are specifically measured. Support of respiration is of vital importance for a good outcome from anesthesia.

Respiratory depression

Respiratory depression is defined as a condition where insufficient carbon dioxide is cleared from the lungs, detected as an increase in arterial or end-tidal carbon dioxide rather than a decrease in respiratory rate. Anesthetic agents all cause some degree of respiratory depression. Hypercapnia will not be detected unless carbon dioxide is being measured. While a slight elevation above normal can be beneficial for most patients (permissive hypercapnia), if a significant lowering of end-tidal carbon dioxide concentration is desired, either the anesthetic level should be decreased or it may be necessary to commit to either manual or mechanically controlled ventilation of that patient.

Apnea is an extreme manifestation of respiratory depression, which should be treated immediately by endotracheal intubation and ventilation with oxygen. Untreated apnea will lead rapidly to hypoxia, resulting in severe respiratory acidosis and cardiac arrest. Apnea occurs commonly during anesthesia and some of the causes of apnea include rapid injection of anesthetic induction drugs or opioid analgesics, and excessive depth under inhalant anesthesia. Although rare, apnea is one of the first signs of brainstem herniation and of cardiac arrest.

Hypoxia

Hypoxia ($PaO_2 < 60$ mmHg) is reported to occur in 0.5% of dogs under anesthesia while breathing enriched oxygen mixtures, most commonly in cases undergoing thoracotomy, endoscopy, and bronchoscopy [1]. Hypoxia usually occurs without cyanosis, and will only be detected when mild by pulse oximetry or arterial blood gas analysis. This is a solid endorsement of the routine use of pulse oximetry in every patient during anesthesia and recovery. Hypoxemia is associated with lactic acidosis, malignant arrhythmias, and cardiac, muscular, renal, and neurological damage, ultimately terminating in cardiac arrest.

While there are some conditions and procedures commonly associated with hypoxia, it is most threatening to a patient when it is severe and undetected. Some conditions encountered during routine clinical practice, and associated with unexpected hypoxemia, include endobronchial intubation (iatrogenic), a mucus-occluded endotracheal tube, kinking or cuff-induced occlusion of an inserted endotracheal tube, and the presence of undiagnosed pleural fluid (Fig. 5.1) or undiagnosed pneumothorax.

Another cause of hypoxemia is airway obstruction secondary to laryngospasm, occurring most commonly in the cat and especially after administration of thiobarbiturates, or in response to direct stimulation of the glottic area. If laryngospasm occurs, 2% lidocaine either IV or (more commonly) applied directly to the arytenoid cartilages will usually relax the spasm and permit the passage of the endotracheal tube through the larynx. Prophylactic application of lidocaine to the arytenoid cartilages is standard procedure for some anesthetists when intubating cats and swine.

Brachycephalic breeds are particularly prone to airway obstruction during the perianesthetic period. They are prone to obstruct and die if left unattended after having been given sedatives or anesthetic drugs. Short-acting agents that leave little residual drug effect should allow these dogs to wake up rapidly and get back airway control. These cases are high risk and should be labor intensive to ensure a good outcome.

Pulmonary edema associated with hypoxia is reported to occur occasionally in horses during recovery from anesthesia and is probably associated with upper airway obstruction. These cases manifest with tachypnea, struggling, and foamy nasal discharge [68]. Treatment is supportive: airway patency should be ensured and oxygen and furosemide administered.

Treatment of hypoxia should progress as needed from oxygen administration (either nasally, mask, or chamber) to endotracheal intubation and controlled ventilation incorporating increased peak airway pressure and appropriate levels of positive end-expiratory pressure. Monitoring arterial oxygenation through arterial blood gas analysis or pulse oximetry will be useful in guiding therapy.

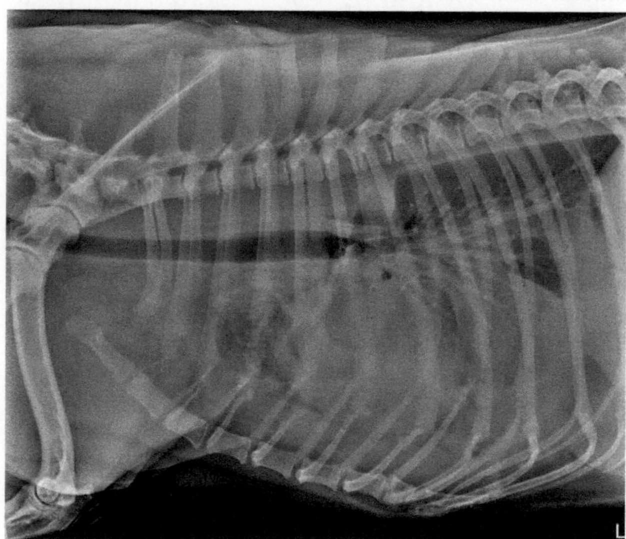

Figure 5.1 Lateral thoracic radiograph of a dog with clinically undetected pleural fluid, which developed hemoglobin desaturation and arterial hypoxemia during anesthesia for CT of a neck mass.

Acute pneumothorax

Pneumothorax can be categorized by etiology as spontaneous, traumatic, or iatrogenic [69]. Pneumothorax complicating anesthesia is a very rare occurrence. Pneumothorax has been observed to occur as a complication of surgeries including laparoscopic liver biopsy, cranial abdominal surgery, and repair of diaphragmatic hernia. Bronchial lavage using a rigid catheter has also been observed by one of the authors (D.V.W.) to produce fatal pneumothorax. In patients with pulmonary contusions or pulmonary bullae, the development of pneumothorax is an anticipated risk. Tracheal lacerations secondary to intubation of cats may manifest as pneumothorax soon after intubation, although subcutaneous crepitation is often noticed first.

In dogs with pneumothorax, the thorax expands progressively, allowing the patient to tolerate a volume of pleural air that is 2.5–3.5 times the functional residual capacity (FRC approximately 45 mL/kg) [70,71]. At maximal expansion of the chest, the inspiratory muscles (including the diaphragm) cannot work and respiration becomes severely compromised and may cease [72,73]. If tension pneumothorax exists, not only do the lungs collapse, but as intra-thoracic air accumulates and IttP increases, collapse of the vena cava and even aorta leads rapidly to cardiovascular collapse and death.

The clinical appearance of pneumothorax may mimic that of severe bronchospasm. Other potential rule-outs for the clinical signs include airway obstruction and endobronchial intubation. A rapid and shallow respiratory pattern will be manifested, with activation of the accessory muscles of respiration as hypoxemia progresses, leading to an abnormal, gasping type of inspiration. This can look like, and is, a preterminal (agonal) respiratory pattern. The thoracic wall can be hyper-resonant on percussion and may be acutely tympanic if a tension pneumothorax is present [69]. Diminished breath sounds, tachycardia, and hypotension will all be observed. Increasing airway pressure (during mechanical ventilation) and reduced thoracic compliance are observed. Eventual cyanosis and cardiac arrest will follow if no intervention occurs. Monitoring pulse oximetry, chest wall compliance during intermittent manual ventilation, end-tidal carbon dioxide, and arterial blood pressure will often give a relatively early indication that something has changed within the thoracic cavity and a tension pneumothorax should be suspected.

In the case where a chest wall defect is present (open pneumothorax), or during repair of diaphragmatic hernia, initiating positive pressure ventilation will stabilize the patient until the defect can be located and repaired. In the case of a closed pneumothorax, where air cannot escape and accumulates in the chest, initiating positive pressure ventilation may cause rapid progression to tension pneumothorax. When compressing the rebreathing bag, it can feel like trying to ventilate a brick – no air moves in or out.

Pneumothorax may rapidly progress to cardiac arrest, so diagnosis and treatment are time critical and a definitive response to the situation can be life saving. Treatment begins with attention to ABC, as in all collapsed patients. Thoracic radiography will easily reveal the condition, but with the typical acute onset and rapid progression of this problem, diagnostic thoracocentesis should usually be the initial intervention [69]. Confirmation of the problem and definitive treatment involve drainage of the pleural air. Tube thoracostomy may be required if ongoing air leakage is present, evidenced by symptom recurrence and the need for repeated chest drainage.

Bronchospasm

Any patient could develop fulminant bronchospasm under anesthesia, the result of a drug reaction or physical intervention of the airway. In species with particularly reactive airways, such as the cat and sheep, endotracheal intubation may occasionally precipitate profound bronchospasm. Fluid instillation during broncho-alveolar lavage can initiate bronchospasm and is often associated with an oxygen-responsive hypoxia [74]. Bronchospasm will also occur as a response to aspiration of rumen or gastric contents. Fortunately, this is a rare event.

History, clinical signs, timeline of events, and response to treatment should allow diagnosis. Clinical signs encountered in a patient with bronchospasm will include difficulty maintaining acceptable hemoglobin saturation, tachypnea, tachycardia, and increasing airway pressures if being ventilated, a characteristic waveform is observed on the capnograph, and wheezing may be auscultated. In extreme cases, air may not move into the chest, and no respiratory sounds will be heard.

Patients with inflamed or reactive airways generally do well under inhalant anesthesia since halothane, isoflurane, and sevoflurane, but not desflurane, cause bronchial relaxation [75]. Ketamine also produces bronchial relaxation [76].

Bronchospasm can occur as a new event during recovery from anesthesia. Manifesting as wheezing and tachypnea, this has been observed in three horses recovering from inhalant anesthesia (D.V. Wilson, unpublished observation). It was postulated that those horses were experiencing a rebound bronchoconstriction. A rapid response to IV atropine (two horses) or inhaled albuterol (one horse), and a subsequent normal recovery from anesthesia, were observed in all three. Bronchospasm and laryngospasm have also been shown to occur in children following isoflurane anesthesia [77].

Treatment of bronchospasm is usually initiated with a bronchodilator such as albuterol, either by mask or into the breathing circle near the endotracheal tube. When ventilation of the lungs is not possible; or nebulizer use impractical, administration of terbutaline SQ or IV, or atropine, should result in rapid and effective bronchodilation. If cardiac arrest is imminent, then epinephrine and CPR may be required.

If aspiration of ruminal or stomach contents is suspected or witnessed, pulmonary lavage should be considered. In non-ruminants such lavage is more controversial.

Volutrauma and barotrauma

Even brief periods of lung overinflation can lead to air leak and extra-alveolar air accumulation [78,79]. Barotrauma and pneumothorax following a closed adjustable pressure-limiting (APL) valve have been reported in a cat [80]. More importantly, even brief periods of lung overexpansion cause increases in endothelial and epithelial permeability leading to edema, and severe ultrastructural damage [78,79]. This can lead to fulminant pulmonary edema with tracheal flooding, severe hypoxemia, and death [81]. Although lung overinflation usually follows inadvertent prolonged closure or malfunction of the APL valve, upper airway obstruction has also been implicated in the development of fulminant pulmonary edema in horses recovering from anesthesia [68]. Use of an airway pressure monitor allows early detection of most cases of accidental APL valve closure.

Tracheal tears

Iatrogenic tracheal tears occur following approximately 1 in 20 000 intubations in people, with women more affected [82]. The small airway of the domestic cat also places them at risk [83]. Tracheal tears associated with endotracheal intubation are localized, iatrogenic tears of the dorsal, longitudinal trachealis muscle, most commonly reported in the cat (Fig. 5.2), and occasionally in small dogs [84]. Two retrospective studies reported data from 36 cats with tracheal tears [85,86]. The tears were from 2 to 5 cm in length and occurred most commonly at the level of the thoracic inlet, less often in the thoracic portion of the trachea or extending to the carina [83,85,86]. The interval between anesthesia and diagnosis of the tear varied from 4 h to 14 days. Risk factors include dental procedures (83% of cases), the use of a stylet, and multiple position changes, although no one factor was associated with all cases. It is possible that cuff overinflation is the cause of some tracheal tears. It was found that in 19 cats it took an average of 1.6 mL of air in the cuff of the endotracheal tube to obtain an air-tight seal [85]. However, forcing up to 10 mL of air into both a high-pressure, low-volume cuff and a low-pressure, high-volume cuff was shown to cause tracheal rupture in the majority of cats in each group (3/5 and 4/5 cats, respectively) [85].

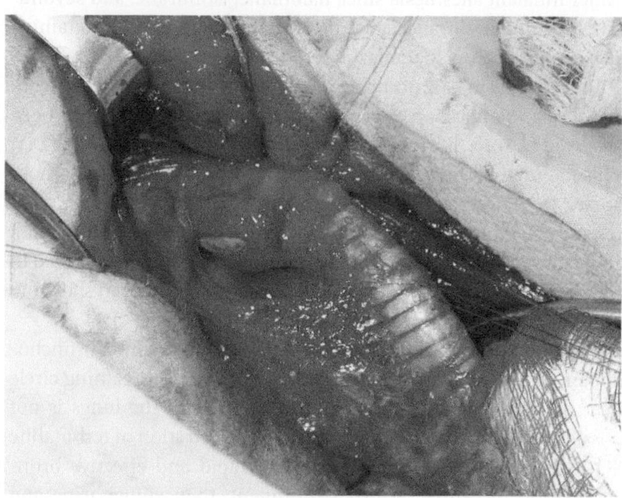

Figure 5.2 Tracheal tear in a cat, exposed during surgical repair of the lesion. Source: Dr Bryden J. Stanley, Department of Small Animal Clinical Sciences, Michigan State University, East Lansing, MI, USA. Reproduced with permission of Dr Bryden J. Stanley.

The predominant clinical sign associated with tracheal tears is impressive subcutaneous emphysema of the cervical region, which spreads rapidly, and subsequent respiratory distress (Fig 5.3). Radiographed patients usually have pneumomediastinum, with spread to pneumothorax and to the retroperitoneal space also having been reported [85–87]. Bronchoscopy will not always reveal the tear [86], and CT has been used to identify the site of the rupture in some cases [88].

Approximately half of the cats presenting with postintubation tracheal tears will improve with conservative treatment, oxygen therapy, and cage rest [85,86]. Progressive dyspnea is an indication for surgical intervention [85,87]. The anesthetic plan for surgical repair of a tracheal tear should begin with smooth IV induction and endotracheal intubation with a smaller tube than anticipated, which is long enough to pass to the carina, hopefully below the tear. Cats

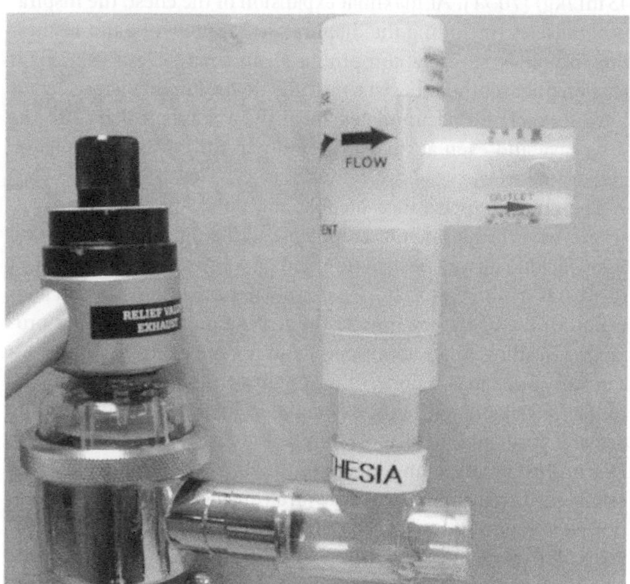

Figure 5.4 Modification of the breathing circle, with a PEEP valve inserted to act as a pressure relief valve. Source: Dr Tom Evans, Veterinary Clinical Center, Michigan State University, East Lansing, MI, USA. Reproduced with permission of Dr Tom Evans.

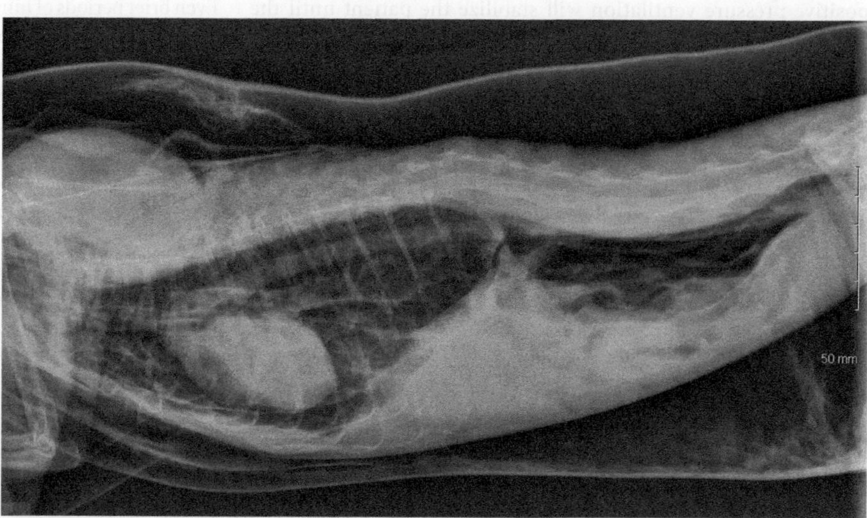

Figure 5.3 Lateral thoracic radiograph of a cat with a tracheal tear, showing extensive subcutaneous emphysema, and extensive air tracking in the mediastinum and retroperitoneal space.

with a tear extending to the carina will present the greatest anesthetic challenge and mortality during surgery is high [85,89].

Pulmonary aspiration

Aspiration pneumonia (AP) has become a well-recognized sequel to anesthesia in dogs, with reports that anesthesia precedes 13–16% of all AP cases [90–92]. Based upon a large, multicenter, retrospective study, the estimated prevalence of postanesthetic AP in dogs is 0.17%, or 1.7 out of every 1000 anesthetic events [93]. In most dogs, the aspiration event is not witnessed, so developing protective strategies for patients at risk is an important goal [93].

Procedures associated with high risk of subsequent AP include upper airway surgery, neurosurgery, laparotomy, thoracotomy, and endoscopy [93]. Interestingly, dogs undergoing orthopedic surgery were unlikely to develop AP. Factors significantly associated with the development of postanesthetic AP include regurgitation during anesthesia or recovery, and administration of opioids (specifically hydromorphone) at induction. Combining risk factors, such as a dog regurgitating during a high-risk procedure, significantly increased the likelihood of AP [93].

Aspirated acidic material induces severe alveolar damage and airway hyper-responsiveness [94], which manifests as bronchospasm and hypoxia. The diagnosis of AP in dogs has been based on a combination of history, clinical signs, arterial hemoglobin desaturation, thoracic radiographs, transtracheal wash with bacterial cultures, or necropsy [90–92,95,97].

Prevention would be ideal and proton pump inhibitors and prokinetics have been shown to reduce the likelihood of gastroesophageal reflux (GER) and should help patients at risk [98,99]. Other antiemetic classes may also offer protection during recovery. Once AP has occurred, treatment should be symptomatic, to include antibiotics, oxygen, and perhaps bronchodilators if wheezing is noted.

Drug factors

Anecdotally, drug handling errors are common in veterinary anesthesia, although published data on their prevalence are lacking. Drug swaps, whether the syringe was labeled or not, seem most common, and many of these may cause a brief flurry of action, but not significant consequences (a 'near miss'). Potassium chloride can cause a lethal accident when inadvertently given IV, although a more commonly encountered problem is local anesthetics, especially bupivacaine, being inadvertently given IV. Clearly, labeling syringes and paying attention to the drug label are both important habits to acquire.

Some measure has been made of these drug handling errors in human anesthesia. One study of 8000 anesthetics in two New Zealand hospitals used an anonymous and self-reporting system (survey completion) to determine that the anesthetic-related drug administration error rate was 0.75%, with a 'near miss' rate of 0.37%. This study determined that the most frequent errors were dose errors (20%), and drug substitutions (20%). Most errors (63%) involved IV boluses, 20% involved infusions, and 15% inhalational agents [100,101].

Strategies shown to reduce the chance of these errors include always reading the label carefully, the legibility and contents of ampule and syringe labels should be optimized to agreed standards, syringes should be labeled, and labels should be checked with another person or device before drugs are given [102].

Drug overdosage is cited as a cause of anesthesia-related mortality [2]. In veterinary medicine, there is no measure of the frequency of this type of event. Recognition of a drug overdose can be difficult, but this event may manifest as hypotension, cardiovascular collapse, cardiac arrhythmias, or prolonged recovery from anesthesia. One report described a dog receiving a 10-fold overdose of meperidine, with good outcome [103]. Another dog received a 26-fold overdose of intrathecal morphine and required intensive care for 60 h, with eventual recovery [104].

Treatment of an overdose begins with supportive care, and administration of the antagonist if the agent is reversible, such as with the opioid receptor agonists, the benzodiazepines and the α_2-adrenergic receptor agonists.

Intravenous lipid emulsion (ILE) is an emerging therapy for overdosage of lipophilic agents, dubbed LipidRescue™ [105]. ILE is considered to create a lipid 'sink' removing active drug from the circulation [106]. Although derived specifically to treat local anesthetic toxicity, lipid rescue should be considered for any overdosage of a drug with lipid affinity, particularly bupivacaine, ropivacaine, lidocaine, carprofen, chlorpromazine, diazepam, ketoprofen, propofol, thiopentone, or trazodone [107–112].

Equipment

Adjustable pressure-limiting valve closure

The pop-off or adjustable pressure-limiting (APL) valve is a component of every anesthesia circuit and some non-rebreathing systems. This valve performs an essential function in preventing excessive pressure from accumulating in the breathing circle while allowing intermittent closure for ventilation. It should remain open in all situations except when the patient is on a mechanical ventilator with an integral and automatic APL.

Inadvertent and persistent closure of the APL occurs frequently during anesthesia. Although there is no published frequency of this event, one report of 148 canine fatalities included two from a closed APL [4]. Based upon observations in clinical practice, there is a much higher 'near miss' rate. With a closed APL valve and oxygen flowing, pressure in the breathing circle climbs rapidly, and plateaus at around the elastic limit of the rebreathing bag. Volutrauma, pneumothorax, or failure of venous return and subsequent cardiac arrest, or all of these, can occur [80].

Deriving a pattern of behaviors to prevent this event is important. First, it is critical that the normal functioning of the APL valve is assessed during each machine check-out, prior to every use. Commercial high patient pressure alarms (Smiths Medical PM, Waukesha, WI, USA) can be purchased that allow variable alarm limits to be set (Fig. 5.5a). A cheaper method is to place a commercially available 20 cmH_2O PEEP valve in the breathing circuit, to act as a pressure-relief valve (Fig. 5.4). This approach has the disadvantage of having a fixed relief pressure, which can be problematic during intermittent positive pressure ventilation, and the overflow gases are not scavenged. Numerous models of commercially available spring-loaded waste gas occlusion valves can be placed downstream of the primary APL to allow intermittent closure of the waste gas pathway without permanently closing the APL (Fig. 5.5b).

Tipped vaporizer

Many anesthesia machines are top-heavy and have a narrow base, and when moving the machine accidental inversion becomes possible. If a precision vaporizer tips over, or even if it moves beyond 45° from the vertical plane, it should be immediately removed from service and evaluated for proper function. A dangerous situation may occur where the vaporizer output can be

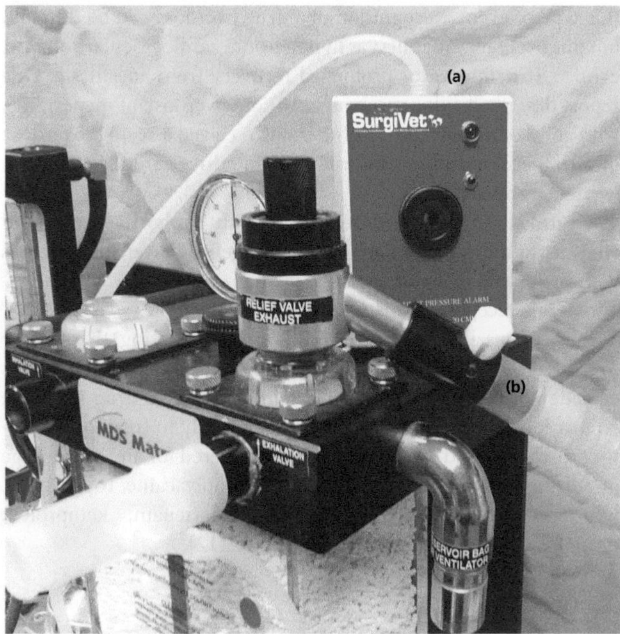

Figure 5.5 (a) Adjustable high patient pressure alarm inserted into the breathing circuit and (b) pop-off occlusion valve. Source: Kurt Grimm, Veterinary Specialist Services, Conifer, CO, USA. Reproduced with permission of Kurt Grimm.

much higher than the vaporizer setting, a situation that can rapidly be lethal. If the vaporizer is dropped from a significant height, it may be prudent to seek professional servicing to verify proper functioning.

Regional anesthesia

Peripheral nerve blocks and regional blocks are becoming common in practice. These techniques can provide very effective analgesia for patients with pain from many causes.

Toxicity

Local anesthetic-induced cardiovascular collapse and cardiac arrest are a rare but catastrophic sequel to regional anesthesia. Careful attention to dosing, and to injection technique, helps prevent this problem. In anesthetized dogs, toxicity may manifest as hypotension and cardiovascular collapse. Seizures and wide-complex ventricular tachycardia may be seen in some animals [113]. Resuscitation from severe bupivacaine intoxication using inotropes, epinephrine, and/or CPR will be successful in about half of cases and recoveries can be rapid (80% will be normotensive 20 min after resuscitation) [113]. A relatively new therapeutic strategy is intravenous lipid emulsion (ILE), which has been shown to be effective in the treatment of some cases of local anesthetic-induced collapse and cardiac arrest [106,109–112,114–117]. Use of ILE is considered off-label, with appropriate dosing relatively free of side-effects [108,109]. Clinical guidelines have been published for its use in people, and guidelines for animal use are extrapolated from those [108].

While in people ILE for treatment of local anesthetic toxicosis is recommended only after treatment of cardiac arrest has failed to establish ROSC (after at least 20 min), the accumulating evidence supports the early use of lipid infusion once signs of local anesthetic toxicity are manifest, to attenuate progression of the local anesthetic toxic syndrome [105,108].

The published guidelines recommend treating local anesthetic toxicity with ILE with a bolus 1.5 mL/kg (lean body mass) IV over 1 min, followed by continuous infusion of 0.25 mL/kg/min, continuing the infusion for at least 10 min after attaining circulatory stability. Bolus administration can be repeated once or twice for persistent cardiovascular collapse, and doubling the lipid infusion rate may be beneficial if blood pressure remains low [105,108]. The recommended upper dose of lipid is 10–12 mL/kg/24 h.

Complications

Reports of complications following regional nerve block include prolonged nerve dysfunction and bilateral spread following unilateral nerve blockade (probable epidural migration) [118]. Where the block persists unexpectedly it is likely that intraneural injection has occurred, although the use of electrostimulation and ultrasound guidance has not eliminated these problems. High-pressure intraneural injections have been shown to cause persistent nerve damage, whereas the effects of low-pressure intraneural injections resolve rapidly [109].

Complications of epidural injection are more commonly encountered. Up to 50% of dogs receiving an epidural opioid will experience urine retention [120]. If unattended to, urine retention may lead to acute urinary bladder rupture, or chronic urinary bladder dysfunction. Occasionally myoclonus, neuritis, and pruritis may follow epidural or intrathecal morphine injection (the preservative-free solution), which requires management with prolonged sedation or anesthesia until the signs abate [121]. Delayed hair regrowth is a relatively common postepidural complication with no effective treatment to date.

Other factors

Many other derangements in homeostasis are associated with anesthesia. Some commonly occurring ones will be discussed here.

Regurgitation

Regurgitation is a passive process, which occurs where a sufficient volume of gastric contents moves up the esophagus and passes the upper esophageal sphincter to be observed exiting the mouth or nose. Sometimes the regurgitated material is clear fluid, often it is brown or yellow, and usually acidic. Regurgitation is a marker for gastroesophageal reflux, and occurs in approximately 12% of cases of GER, meaning that most cases of GER are clinically silent [122,123]. Regurgitated material can cause problems for patients in three ways. First, regurgitation is associated with aspiration pneumonia [92,93,97]; second, ulcerative esophagitis and stricture formation may follow, in an estimated 1 in 1000 anesthetics [124]; and third, the gastric contents induce nasal and pharyngeal irritation, which can contribute to patient discomfort following anesthesia.

Regurgitation is better prevented than treated. Antacids, in particular esomeprazole, do not prevent GER under anesthesia, but make the refluxate less acidic [98]. Administration of cisapride and metoclopramide both reduce the risk but do not prevent all cases of GER [98,99]. Careful local treatment of the esophagus with lavage and instillation of dilute bicarbonate will normalize the luminal pH, but has not been evaluated for prevention of esophagitis [125].

Hypothermia

Hypothermia occurs in association with anesthesia due to a combination of the cold hospital environment and altered patient thermoregulation. With normal handling, dogs have been shown to experience an average decrease in rectal temperature of 1.9 °C in the first hour of anesthesia, although this appears to vary considerably with patient size and the type of surgical procedure [126]. Despite increasing attempts to preserve body heat, and warm patients, hypothermia is very common, with half the dogs in one recent study being moderately or severely hypothermic during anesthesia and surgery [9]. Many anesthetic drugs contribute to prolonged postoperative hypothermia, including opioids, inhalant anesthetics, and α_2-adrenergic receptor agonists, although α_2-adrenergic receptor agonists may initially slow loss of body heat through peripheral vasoconstriction [127–129].

While hypothermia causes substantial protection against ischemia and hypoxia [130], a reduction of core body temperature is associated with some potentially deleterious effects. Peripheral vasoconstriction, reduced cutaneous perfusion, lactic acidosis, reduced drug metabolism, slowed coagulation [130], suppressed activity of polymorphonuclear cells, reduced bacterial killing, and suppression of immune reactivity all occur in the perioperative period as core temperature falls [131–133].

Hypothermia can be limited by increasing the ambient temperature, but this is seldom feasible. Circulating warm water pads, especially applied to the legs, have been shown to help preserve body heat in dogs [134]. Forced-air warming systems are the most efficient and effective means of preserving and increasing body heat in the anesthetized patient. This warming technique has been shown to delay or reduce the rate of heat loss in horses, people, dogs, and parrots [135–137]. Efficacy of the method is well established, and forced-air heating is both inexpensive and remarkably safe [136,137].

Another warming system currently available is the Hot Dog® (Augustine Temperature Management, Eden Prairie, MN, USA) resistive warming blanket, especially effective for smaller patients. There are few comparisons of the two warming systems, but in people undergoing major facial surgery, although the forced-air warming system and the Hot Dog resistive warming blanket were both effective, the forced-air warming system rewarmed twice as fast as the Hot Dog [137]. No matter which supplemental heat source is used, increasing body surface contact and minimizing exposure to the environment will limit heat loss.

Humidification and warming of inhaled gas have been shown to be ineffective as a sole means of maintaining core temperature in dogs or cats [126,138–140]. Supplemental heat sources not specifically designed for anesthetized patients should not be used in anesthetized or sedated patients. These patients cannot sense the impending thermal injury and, coupled with altered peripheral blood flow distribution, are at risk of thermal burns. The use of uncovered electric heating pads or hot water bottles is discouraged because of potential thermal injury [141,142].

Hyperthermia

Although hypothermia is the most common temperature derangement associated with anesthesia, occasionally an animal will hyperthermic. Hyperthermia results from excessive heating (iatrogenic) or as a possible response to several drugs. Accidental hyperthermia is more likely with a warm ambient temperature, in animals with thick hair coats, and with the use of active heating. To avoid overheating patients, it is important to monitor body temperature perioperatively.

Two specific drug-induced causes of hyperthermia occur in the domestic species, namely opioid-induced hyperthermia in cats and malignant hyperthermia (MH). All opioids used in cats are implicated in causing hyperthermia [143–145]. Hydromorphone is associated with most reports of temperature elevations in cats, but administration of full and partial μ-agonists, and κ-agonists, have been shown to produce mild to moderate increases in body temperature. Opioid-associated hyperthermia will occur in about 50% of cats, and is clearly associated with altered central thermoregulation [143,144]. Temperature increases usually occur in the first 5 h following drug administration [143,145–147]. Ketamine has also been reported to produce a mild increase in core temperature for 1 h [145], and may also have a weak additive effect with hydromorphone [143,148].

Most cases of opioid-induced hyperthermia are self-limiting, but temperatures over 104 °F (40 °C) warrant attention such as removal of the heat source, provision of a cooler environment, or simply the use of a fan. Where extreme temperature elevation persists following opioid administration in a cat, IV naloxone should rapidly reduce temperature to normal, although analgesia will also be lost [143].

Malignant hyperthermia (MH) is an inherited membrane-linked abnormality (ryanodine receptor gene mutation, RYR1) that has been described in many species, including pigs, dogs, cats, and horses [149–152]. The prevalence of MH is very low, occurring in people 9.6 times per million inpatient anesthetics, and often associated with succinylcholine administration [153]. Known triggering agents include all potent inhalation anesthetics, succinylcholine, and stress [154].

Affected patients are usually panting, tachypneic, tachycardic, hypercarbic, and vasodilated, with a progressive metabolic acidosis. The temperature elevation comes late in the syndrome, and can rise rapidly (1 °C/5 min). Treatment should include removal of any triggering agent, ventilation with 100% oxygen, administration of dantrolene (2.5 mg/kg IV or 10 mg/kg by stomach tube), and aggressive cooling. Mortality rates from MH were approximately 80% in human patients until implementation of programs emphasizing early recognition, MH-safe anesthetics and dantrolene, which reduced it to approximately 5%.

Electrolyte abnormalities

Of the serum electrolyte derangements that can occur under anesthesia, hyperkalemia is the most immediately life threatening [155,156]. Arrhythmias resulting from hyperkalemia may not respond to conventional antiarrhythmic therapies, can lead to cardiac arrest, and may not respond to treatment of hyperkalemia [155–161]. The common causes of hyperkalemia include transfusion of old stored blood, chronic heparin therapy (dogs), uroperitoneum (especially foals and cats), iatrogenic (potassium penicillin or KCl), hyperkalemic periodic paralysis, and acute hypoadrenocorticism crisis (Addison's disease) [156–161].

Horses that carry the gene for hyperkalemic periodic paralysis (HYPP) are at greater anesthetic risk and should be closely monitored [156,161]. They are also often large and heavily muscled, making them prone to postanesthetic myopathy. Diet change, the stress of fasting, anesthesia, and pain may lead to a crisis in the perianesthetic period. Signs of a crisis of HYPP are apparent even in the anesthetized horse, including muscle tremors, sweating, and characteristic ECG changes [156,157,161]. If a horse has an episode of HYPP during anesthesia, provided that the condition is recognized and treated appropriately, the horse can make an uneventful recovery [161]. Aggressive lowering of serum potassium using dextrose with or without insulin, sodium bicarbonate, and calcium can lead to resolution of an episode of HYPP under anesthesia [157–161].

Injuries

Various non-lethal events contribute to anesthesia-associated morbidity. There is no current measure of the prevalence of these injuries. Included would be corneal ulcers, soft tissue trauma, burns from heating devices, drug-induced tissue necrosis, blindness, facial neuropathy, myoneuropathy, and long bone fractures. The last three conditions are relevant to the equine species, and will be discussed in other parts of this text.

Thermal injury has been reported following anesthesia and can be devastating. There are a number of heating systems now available that are very effective and designed specifically for anesthetized patients. The use of gloves containing hot water or most electric heating pads are not recommended [141,142].

Postanesthetic blindness in cats has been reported. A recent collection of 20 cases determined that 13 followed dental procedures (12 with spring-held mouth gag), four followed endoscopy (all with mouth gag), and three followed cardiac arrest [162]. Most (17/20) of these cats had other neurologic abnormalities beyond blindness, such as circling, ataxia, head tilt, weakness, opisthotonus, decreased conscious proprioception, and abnormal mentation. Fourteen of the 20 cats regained vision, with the time from insult until return of vision ranging from 1 day to 6 weeks. Signs of cortical ischemia were found where cats with postanesthetic blindness underwent necropsy [162–165].

While hypotension and hypoxia have been variously attributed as primary causative factors in this catastrophic event, the role of the spring-held mouth gag is emerging. The blood supply to the feline brain is almost entirely from the maxillary artery, and a widely deployed mouth gag has been demonstrated to induce maxillary artery hypoperfusion in cats [165].

Prolonged recovery

Prolonged recovery from anesthesia is reported to occur in 0.15% of dogs (12 of 8087) and in 0.18% of cats (16 of 8702) [3]. The period after anesthesia is discontinued and, while the patient is recovering from the effects of anesthesia and surgery, is just as critical for the patient as the anesthetic period. Over 60% of anesthesia-associated mortality in cats and rabbits, and nearly 50% in dogs, occurs after anesthesia has ended [4].

There are several common causes of delayed recovery, including hypothermia, and profound drug effect (over-narcotization secondary to aggressive pain management) is increasingly common). Metabolic derangements such as hypothyroidism, adrenal insufficiency, and hypoglycemia may not be recognized before surgery, and have been associated with delayed recovery from anesthesia [166]. Potential causes of hypoglycemia are prolonged starvation, patients with a low body condition score (cachectic), sepsis, hepatic insufficiency, hypoadrenocorticism, insulinoma, non-islet cell neoplasia, glycogen storage disease, and hypoadrenocorticism. Hypoglycemia can be clinically silent in the anesthetized patient, and signs of sympathetic overactivity or ventricular arrhythmias may be the only detectable evidence of a life-threatening hypoglycemia [166,167].

Occasionally a patient with undiagnosed elevated intracranial pressure (from a brain tumor or hydrocephalus) has their condition further compromised by anesthesia, and this only becomes apparent when they either stop breathing or fail to recover from anesthesia. Careful monitoring of end-tidal carbon dioxide, arterial blood pressure, and anesthetic depth may help with intraoperative management of these cases and prevent decompensation.

Critical event debriefing

The term *risk management* was developed by the insurance industry and adopted by the healthcare industry to describe processes used to prevent injury, litigation, and financial loss [168,169]. The overarching goal of this process is to use analysis of adverse events to prevent similar injuries from occurring in subsequent patients, and this is discussed at greater length in other chapters.

Analysis of adverse events should start with an unbiased and non-judgmental review of all events leading up to the accident. Once a clear picture has been formed of what happened, the next step should be the formation or modification of operating procedures that make replication of the adverse event less likely. There will always be things that could have been done differently, but time and effort should be focused on those which would have made a difference in the outcome. An adverse outcome is devastating for all involved, but is better borne where it is perceived that something has been learned and thus the level of care will be improved.

There are significant similarities between aviation and anesthesia; most notably, both are equipment intensive, and a critical event or malfunction may prove rapidly fatal. In aviation there are well-defined processes for investigation and evaluation of the events leading up to an accident. An independent board, the National Transportation Safety Board (NTSB), with analysis and publication of the findings, leads the process of accident investigation. There is also an anonymous reporting system, the Aviation Safety Reporting System (ASRS), that allows the collection, analysis, and publication of events that were considered hazardous by the participants, and may have caused a near miss but did not lead to an accident. We would like to propose a similar approach in veterinary anesthesia.

References

1 Gaynor JS, Dunlop CI, Wagner AE, *et al.* Complications and mortality associated with anesthesia in dogs and cats. *J Am Anim Hosp Assoc* 1999; **35**: 13–17.

2 Dyson DH, Maxie MG, Schnurr D. Morbidity and mortality associated with anesthetic management in small animal veterinary practice in Ontario. *J Am Anim Hosp Assoc* 1998; **34**: 325–335.

3 Brodbelt DC, Blisset KJ, Hammond RA, *et al.* The risk of death: the Confidential Enquiry into Perioperative Small Animal Fatalities. *Vet Anaesth Analg* 2008; **35**: 365–373.

4 Brodbelt DC, Pfeiffer DU, Young LE, *et al.* Results of the Confidential Enquiry into Perioperative Small Animal Fatalities regarding risk factors for anesthetic-related death in dogs. *J Am Vet Med Assoc* 2008; **233**: 1096–1104.

5 Cooper JB, Newbower RS, Kitz RJ. An analysis of major errors and equipment failures in anesthesia management: considerations for prevention and detection. *Anesthesiology* 1984; **60**: 34–42.

6 Cooper JB, Newbower RS, Long CE, *et al.* Preventable anesthesia mishaps: a study of human factors. *Anesthesiology* 1978; **49**: 399–406.

7 Cooper JB, Cullen DJ, Nemeskal R, *et al.* Effects of information feedback and pulse oximetry on the incidence of anesthesia complications. *Anesthesiology* 1987; **67**: 686–694.

8 Cooper JB, Gaba D. No myth: anesthesia is a model for addressing patient safety. *Anesthesiology* 2002; **97**: 1335–1337.

9 Redondo JL, Rubio M, Soler G, *et al.* Normal values and incidence of cardiorespiratory complications in dogs during general anesthesia. A review of 1281 cases. *J Vet Med A Physiol Pathol Clin Med* 2007; **54**: 470–477.

10 Duerr FM, Carr AP, Duke T, *et al.* Prevalence of perioperative arrhythmias in 50 young, healthy dogs. *Can Vet J* 2007; **48**: 169–177.

11 Kelleher ME, Brosnan RJ, Kass PH, *et al.* Use of physiologic and arterial blood gas variables to predict short-term survival in horses with large colon volvulus. *Vet Surg* 2013; **42**: 107–113.
12 Rioja E, Costa MC, Valverde A. Perioperative risk factors for mortality and length of hospitalization in mares with dystocia undergoing general anesthesia: a retrospective study. *Can Vet J* 2012; **53**: 502–510.
13 Magdesian KG, Fielding CL, Rhodes DM. Changes in central venous pressure and blood lactate concentration in response to acute blood loss in horses. *J Am Vet Med Assoc* 2006; **229**: 1458–1462.
14 Trim CM, Eaton SA, Parks AH. Severe nasal hemorrhage in an anesthetized horse. *J Am Vet Med Assoc* 1997; **210**: 1324–1327.
15 Schmall LM, Muir WW, Robertson JT. Haemodynamic effects of small volume hypertonic saline in experimentally induced haemorrhagic shock. *Equine Vet J* 1990; **22**: 273–277.
16 Skillman JJ, Olson JE, Lyons JH, *et al.* The hemodynamic effect of acute blood loss in normal man, with observations on the effect of the Valsalva maneuver and breath holding. *Ann Surg* 1967; **166**: 713–738.
17 Wilson DV, Shance PU, Rondenay Y. The cardiopulmonary effects of severe blood loss in anesthetized horses. *Vet Anaesth Analg* 2003; **30**: 80–86.
18 Waisman Y, Eichacker PQ, Banks SM, *et al.* Acute hemorrhage in dogs: construction and validation of models to quantify blood loss. *J Appl Physiol* 1993; **74**: 510–519.
19 Dutton RP. Current concepts in hemorrhagic shock. *Anesth Clin* 2007; **25**: 23–34.
20 Abramson D, Scalea TM, Hitchcock R, *et al.* Lactate clearance and survival following injury. *J Trauma* 1993; **35**: 584–588.
21 Katz RL, Bigger JT. Cardiac arrhythmias during anesthesia and operation. *Anesthesiology* 1970; **33**: 193–213.
22 Bertrand CA, Steiner NV, Jameson AG. Disturbances of cardiac rhythm during anesthesia and surgery. *J Am Med Assoc* 1971; **216**: 1615–1617.
23 Muir WW III, Lipowitz AJ. Cardiac dysrhythmias associated with gastric dilatation-volvulus in the dog. *J Am Vet Med Assoc* 1978; **172**: 683–689.
24 Macintire DK, Snider TG III. Cardiac arrhythmias associated with multiple trauma in dogs. *J Am Vet Med Assoc* 1984; **184**: 541–545.
25 Marino DJ, Matthiessen DT, Fox PR, *et al.* Ventricular arrhythmias n dogs undergoing splenectomy: a prospective study. *Vet Surg* 1994; **23**: 101–106.
26 Stauffer JL, Gleed RD, Short CE, *et al.* Cardiac dysrhythmias during anesthesia for cervical decompression in the dog. *Am J Vet Res* 1988; **49**: 1143–1146.
27 Atlee JL, Bosnjak ZJ. Mechanisms for cardiac dysrhythmias during anesthesia. *Anesthesiology* 1990; **72**: 347–374.
28 Tranquilli WJ, Thurmon JC, Benson GJ, *et al.* Alteration in the arrhythmogenic dose of epinephrine (ADE) following xylazine administration to halothane-anesthetized dogs. *J Vet Pharmacol Ther* 1986; **9**: 198–203.
29 Kuusela E, Raekallio M, Hietanen H, *et al.* 24-hour holter-monitoring in the perianesthetic period in dogs premedicated with dexmedetomidine. *Vet J* 2002; **164**: 235–239.
30 Lemke KA, Tranquilli WJ. Anesthetics, arrhythmias, and myocardial sensitization to epinephrine. *J Am Vet Med Assoc* 1994; **205**: 1679–1684.
31 Light GS, Hellyer PW. Effects of atropine on the arrhythmogenic dose of dobutamine in xylazine-thiamylal-halothane anesthetized horses. *Am J Vet Res* 1993; **54**: 2099–2103.
32 Atlee JL, Roberts JL. Thiopental and epinephrine-induced dysrhythmias in dogs anesthetized with enflurane or isoflurane. *Anesth Analg* 1986; **65**: 437–443.
33 Hikasa Y, Okabe C, Takase K, *et al.* Ventricular arrhythmogenic dose of adrenaline during sevoflurane, isoflurane, and halothane anaesthesia either with or without ketamine or thiopentone in cats. *Res Vet Sci* 1996; **60**: 134–137.
34 Bednarski RM, Muir WW. Ventricular arrhythmogenic dose of epinephrine in dogs and cats anesthetized with tiletamine/zolazepam and halothane. *Am J Vet Res* 1990; **51**: 1468–1470.
35 Pettifer G, Dyson D, McDonnell W. The arrhythmogenic dose of epinephrine in halothane and isoflurane anesthetized dogs: an assessment of repeatability. *Can J Vet Res* 1997; **61**: 221–226.
36 Muir WW, Hubbell JAE, Flaherty S. Increasing halothane concentration abolishes anesthesia-associated arrhythmias in cats and dogs. *J Am Vet Med Assoc* 1988; **192**: 1730–1735.
37 Hubbell JAE, Muir WW, Bednarski RM, Bednarski LS. Change of inhalation anesthetic agents for management of ventricular premature depolarizations in anesthetized cats and dogs. *J Am Vet Med Assoc* 1984; **185**:643–646.
38 Alibhai HI, Clarke KW, Lee YH, *et al.* Cardiopulmonary effects of combinations of medetomidine hydrochloride and atropine sulphate in dogs. *Vet Rec* 1996; **138**: 11–13.
39 Dimich I, Lingham R, Narang J, *et al.* Esmolol prevents and suppresses arrhythmias during halothane anaesthesia in dogs. *Can J Anaesth* 1992; **39**: 83–86.
40 Dewachter P, Mouton-Faivre C, Castells MC, *et al.* Anesthesia in the patient with multiple drug allergies: are all allergies the same? *Curr Opin Anaesthesiol* 2011; **24**: 320–325.
41 Burren VS, Mason KV. Supected anaphylaxis to thiopentone in a dog. *Aust Vet J* 1986; **63**: 384–385.
42 Mason TA. Anaphylactic response to thiopentone in a dog. *Vet Rec* 1976; **98**: 136.
43 Wilson DV, Evans AT, Mauer W. The effect of preanesthetic meperidine on gastroesophageal reflux during anesthesia in dogs. *Vet Anaesth Analg* 2007; **34**: 15–22.
44 Pollard RE, Pascoe PJ. Severe reaction to intravenous administration of an ionic iodinated contrast agent in two anesthetized dogs. *J Am Vet Med Assoc* 2008; **233**: 274–278.
45 Girad NM, Leece EA. Suspected anaphylactoid reaction following intravenous administration of a gadolinium-based contrast agent in three dogs undergoing magnetic resonance imaging. *Vet Anaesth Analg* 2010; **37**: 352–356.
46 Carabini L, Tamul P, Afifi S. Cardiopulmonary to cardiocerebral resuscitation: current challenges and future directions. *Int Anesthesiol Clin* 2009; **47**: 1–13.
47 Plunkett SJ, McMichael M. Cardiopulmonary resuscitation in small animal medicine: an update. *J Vet Intern Med* 2008; **22**: 9–25.
48 Cole SG, Otto CM, Hughes D. Cardiopulmonary cerebral resuscitation in small animals – a clinical practice review (Part III). *J Vet Emerg Crit Care* 2003; **13**: 13–23.
49 Hofmeister EH, Brainard BM, Egger CM, *et al.* Prognostic factors for dogs and cats with cardiopulmonary arrest treated by cardiopulmonary cerebral resuscitation at a university teaching hospital. *J Am Vet Med Assoc* 2009; **235**: 50–57.
50 Kass PH, Haskins SC. Survival following cardiopulmonary resuscitation in dogs and cats. *J Vet Emerg Crit Care* 1992; **2**: 23–25.
51 Fletcher DJ, Boller M, Brainard BM, *et al.* RECOVER evidence and knowledge gap analysis on veterinary CPR. Part 7. Clinical guidelines. *J Vet Emerg Crit Care* 2012; **22**: S102–S131.
52 Boller M, Fletcher DJ. RECOVER evidence and knowledge gap analysis on veterinary CPR. Part 1. Evidence analysis and consensus process: collaborative path toward small animal CPR guidelines. *J Vet Emerg Crit Care* 2012; **22**: S4–S12.
53 Hopper K, Epstein ES, Fletcher DJ, *et al.* RECOVER evidence and knowledge gap analysis on veterinary CPR. Part 3. Basic life support. *J Vet Emerg Crit Care* 2012; **22**: S26–S43.
54 Buckley GJ. Shih A, Garcia Pereira FL, Band C. The effect of using an impedance threshold device on hemodynamic parameters during cardiopulmonary resuscitation in dogs. *J Vet Emerg Crit Care* 2012; **22**: 435–440.
55 Andreka P, Frenneaux M. Haemodynamics of cardiac arrest and resuscitation *Curr Opin Crit Care* 2006; **12**: 198–203.
56 Evans T, Wilson D. Anesthetic emergencies and procedures. In: Tranquilli WJ, Thurmon JC, Grimm KA, eds. *Lumb and Jones' Veterinary Anesthesia and Analgesia*, 4th edn. Ames, IA: Blackwell Publishing, 2007; 1033–1048.
57 Frascone RJ, Bitz D, Lurie K. Combination of active compression decompression cardiopulmonary resuscitation and the inspiratory impedance threshold device: state of the art. *Curr Opin Crit Care* 2004; **10**: 193–201.
58 Chandra NC, Beyar R, Halperin HR, *et al.* Vital organ perfusion during assisted circulation by manipulation of intrathoracic pressure. *Circulation* 1991; **84**: 279–286.
59 Yannopoulos D, McKnite S, Aufderheide TP, *et al.* Effects of incomplete chest wall decompression during cardiopulmonary resuscitation on coronary and cerebral perfusion pressures in a porcine model of cardiac arrest. *Resuscitation* 2005; **64**: 363–372.
60 Sugerman NT, Edelson DP, Leary M, *et al.* Rescuer fatigue during actual in-hospital cardiopulmonary resuscitation with audiovisual feedback: a prospective multicenter study. *Resuscitation* 2009; **80**: 981–984.
61 Haque IU, Udassi JP, Udassi S, *et al.* Chest compression quality and rescuer fatigue with increased compression to ventilation ratio during single rescuer pediatric CPR. *Resuscitation* 2008; **79**: 82–89.
62 Heidenreich JW, Berg RA, Higdon TA, *et al.* Rescuer fatigue: standard versus continuous chest-compression cardiopulmonary resuscitation. *Acad Emerg Med* 2006; **13**: 1020–1026.
63 Rozaski EA, Rush JE, Buckley GJ, *et al.* RECOVER evidence and knowledge gap analysis on veterinary CPR. Part 4. Advanced life support. *J Vet Emerg Crit Care* 2012; **22**: S44–S64.
64 Cournand A, Motley H, Werko L. Physiological studies of the effects of intermittent positive pressure breathing on cardiac output in man. *Am J Physiol* 1948; **152**: 162–174.
65 Mottram A, Page R Advances in resuscitation. *Circulation* 2012; **126**: 991–1002.
66 Laurie K, Zielinski T, McKnit S, *et al.* Improving the efficacy of cardiopulmonary rescuscitation with an inspiratory threshold valve. *Crit Care Med* 2000; **28**(11 Suppl): 207–209.
67 Aufderheide T, Kudenchuk P, Hedges JR, *et al.* Resuscitation Outcomes Consortium (ROC) PRIMED cardiac arrest trial methods. Part 1: rationale and methodology for the impedance threshold device (ITD) protocol. *Resuscitation* 2008; **78**: 179–185.
68 Senior M. Post-anaesthetic pulmonary oedema in horses: a review. *Vet Anaesth Analg* 2005; **32**: 193–200.
69 Pawloski DR, Broaddus KD. Pneumothorax: a review. *J Am Anim Hosp Assoc* 2010; **46**: 385–397.

70 Kramek BA, Caywood DD. Pneumothorax. *Vet Clin North Am Small Anim Pract* 1987; **17**: 285–300.

71 Bennett RA, Orton EC, Tucker A, *et al.* Cardiopulmonary changes in conscious dogs with induced progressive pneumothorax. *Am J Vet Res* 1989; **50**: 280–284.

72 Boscan P, Watson Z, Spangler T, *et al.* Adverse effect of complete thoracic evacuation during chronic pneumothorax in a dog. *Vet Anaesth Analg* 2007; **34**: 143–148.

73 Hemingway A, Simmons DH. Respiratory response to acute progressive pneumothorax. *J Appl Physiol* 1958; **13**: 165–170.

74 Hawkins EC, DeNicola DB, Kuehn NF. Bronchoalveolar lavage in the evaluation of pulmonary disease in the dog and cat. State of the art. *J Vet Intern Med* 1999; **4**: 267–274.

75 Jat KR, Chawla D. Ketamine for management of acute exacerbations of asthma in children. *Cochrane Database Syst Rev* 2012; (**11**): CD009293.

76 Goff MJ, Arain SR, Ficke DJ, *et al.* Absence of bronchodilation during desflurane anesthesia. *Anesthesiology* 2000; **93**: 404–408.

77 Pappas AL, Sukhani R, Lurie J, *et al.* Severity of airway hyperreactivity associated with laryngeal mask airway removal: correlation with volatile anesthetic choice and depth of anesthesia. *J Clin Anesth* 2001; **13**: 498–503.

78 Dreyfuss D, Saumon G. Barotrauma is volutrauma, but which volume is responsible? *Intensive Care Med* 1992; **18**: 139–141.

79 Dreyfuss D, Soler P, Basset G, *et al.* High inflation pressure pulmonary edema. Respective effects of high airway pressure, high tidal volume and positive end-expiratory pressure. *Am Rev Respir Dis* 1988; **137**: 1159–1164.

80 Manning MM, Brunson DB. Barotrauma in a cat. *J Am Vet Med Assoc* 1994; **205**: 62–64.

81 Webb HH, Tierney DF. Experimental pulmonary edema due to intermittent positive pressure ventilation with high inflation pressures. Protection by positive end expiratory pressure. *Am Rev Respir Dis* 1974; **110**: 556–565.

82 Lampi L. Tracheal tears: conservative treatment. *Interact Cardiovasc Thorac Surg* 2004; **3**: 401–405.

83 Wong WT, Brock KA. Tracheal laceration from endotracheal intubation in a cat. *Vet Rec* 1994; **134**: 622–624.

84 Alderson B, Senior JM, Dugdale AH. Tracheal necrosis following tracheal intubation in a dog. *J Small Anim Pract* 2006; **47**: 754–756.

85 Hardie EM, Spodnick GJ, Gilson SD, *et al.* Tracheal rupture in cats: 16 cases (1983–1998). *J Am Vet Med Assoc* 1999; **214**: 508–512.

86 Mitchell SL, McCarthy R, Rudloff E, *et al.* Tracheal rupture associated with intubation in cats: 20 cases (1996–1998). *J Am Vet Med Assoc* 2000; **216**: 1592–1595.

87 Gabor S, Renner H, Pinter H, *et al.* Indications for surgery in tracheobronchial ruptures. *Eur J Cardiothorac Surg* 2001; **20**: 399–404.

88 Bhandal J, Kuzma A. Tracheal rupture in a cat: diagnosis by computed tomography. *Can Vet J* 2008; **49**: 595–597.

89 Kastner SBR, Grundmann S, Bettschart-Wolfensberger R. Unstable endobronchial intubation in a cat undergoing tracheal laceration repair. *Vet Anaesth Analg* 2004; **31**: 227–230.

90 Kogan DA, Johnson LR, Sturges BK, *et al.* Etiology and clinical outcome in dogs with aspiration pneumonia: 88 cases (2004–2006). *J Am Vet Med Assoc* 2008; **233**: 1748–1755.

91 Kogan, DA, Johnson LR, Jandrey KE, *et al.* Clinical, clinicopathologic, and radiographic findings in dogs with aspiration pneumonia: 88 cases (2004–2006). *J Am Vet Med Assoc* 2008; **233**: 1742–1747.

92 Tart KM, Babski DM, Lee JA. Potential risk, prognostic indicators, and diagnostic and treatment modalities affecting survival in dogs with presumptive aspiration pneumonia: 125 cases (2005–2008). *J Vet Emerg Crit Care* 2010; **20**: 319–329.

93 Ovbey DH, Wilson DV, Bednarski RM, *et al.* Incidence and risk factors for canine post-anesthetic aspiration pneumonia (1999–2009) : a multicenter study. *Vet Anaesth Analg* 2014; **41**: 127–136.

94 Allen GB, Leclair TR, von Reyn J, *et al.* Acid aspiration-induced airways hyperresponsiveness in mice. *J Appl Physiol* 2009; **107**: 1763–1770.

95 Alwood AJ, Brainard BM, LaFond E, *et al.* Post-operative pulmonary complications in dogs undergoing laparotomy: frequency, characterization, and disease-related risk factors. *J Vet Emerg Crit Care* 2006; **16**: 176–183.

96 Brainard BM, Alwood AJ, Kushner LI, *et al.* Post-operative pulmonary complications in dogs undergoing laparotomy: anesthetic and perioperative factors. *J Vet Emerg Crit Care* 2006; **16**: 184–191.

97 Fransson BA, Bagley RS, Gay JM, *et al.* Pneumonia after intracranial surgery in dogs. *Vet Surg* 2001; **30**: 432–439.

98 Zacuto AC, Marks SL, Osborn KL, *et al.* The influence of esomeprazole and cisapride on gastroesophageal reflux during anesthesia in dogs. *J Vet Intern Med* 2012; **26**: 518–525.

99 Wilson DV, Evans AT, Mauer W. Influence of metoclopramide on gastroesophageal reflux during anesthesia. *Am J Vet Res* 2006; **67**: 26–31.

100 Wheeler SJ, Wheeler DW. Mediation errors in anaesthesia and critical care. *Anaesthesia* 2005; **60**: 257–273.

101 Webster CS, Merry AF, Larsson L, *et al.* The frequency and nature of drug administration error during anaesthesia. *Anaesth Intensive Care* 2001; **29**: 494–500.

102 Jensen LS, Merry AF, Webster CS, *et al.* Evidence-based strategies for preventing drug administration errors during anaesthesia. *Anaesthesia* 2004; **59**: 493–504.

103 Golder FJ, Wilson J, Larenza MP, Fink OT. Suspected acute meperidine toxicity in a dog. *Vet Anaesth Analg* 2010; **37**: 471–477.

104 De Cunha AE, Carter JE, Grafinger M, *et al.* Intrathecal morphine overdose in a dog. *J Am Vet Med Assoc* 2007; **230**: 1665–1668.

105 Weinberg G. *LipidRescue™ Resuscitation for Drug Toxicity*. http://www.lipidrescue.org (accessed 19 January 2012).

106 O'Brien TQ, Clark-Price SC, Evans EE, *et al.* Infusion of a lipid emulsion to treat lidocaine intoxication in a cat. *J Am Vet Med Assoc* 2010; **237**: 1455–1458.

107 Weinberg GL. Lipid infusion therapy: translation to clinical practice. *Anaesthes Analg* 2008; **106**: 1340–1342.

108 Fernandez AL, Lee JA, Rahilly L, *et al.* The use of intravenous lipid emulsion as an antidote in veterinary toxicology. *J Vet Emerg Crit Care* 2011; **21**: 309–320.

109 Kaplan A, Whelan M. The use of IV lipid emulsion for lipophilic drug toxicities. *J Am Anim Hosp Assoc* 2012; **48**: 221–227.

110 Litz RJ, Popp M, Stehr SN, *et al.* Successful resuscitation of a patient with ropivacaine-induced asystole after axillary plexus block using lipid infusion. *Anaesthesia* 2006; **61**: 800–801.

111 Levine M, Brooks DE, Franken A, *et al.* Delayed-onset seizure and cardiac arrest after amitryptalline overdose, treated with intravenous lipid emulsion therapy. *Pediatrics* 2012; **130**: 432–438.

112 Litz RJ, Roessel T, Heller AR, *et al.* Reversal of central nervous system and cardiac toxicity after local anesthetic intoxication by lipid emulsion injection. *Anesth Analg* 2008; **106**: 1575–1577.

113 Groban L, Deal DD, Vernon, JC, *et al.* Cardiac resuscitation after incremental overdosage with lidocaine, bupivacaine, levo-bupivacaine and ropivacaine in anesthetized dogs. *Anaesth Analg* 2001; **92**: 37–43.

114 Rosenblatt MA, Abel M, Fischer GW, *et al.* Successful use of a 20% lipid emulsion to resuscitate a patient after a presumed bupivacaine related cardiac arrest. *Anesthesiology* 2006; **105**: 217–218.

115 Picard J, Ward SC, Zumpe R, *et al.* Guidelines and the adoption of 'lipid rescue' therapy for local anaesthetic toxicity. *Anaesthesia* 2009; **64**: 122–125.

116 Weinberg G, Ripper R, Feinstein DL, Hoffman W. Lipid emulsion infusion rescues dogs from bupivacaine-induced cardiac toxicity. *Reg Anesth Pain Med* 2003; **28**: 198–202.

117 Ludot H, Tharin JY, Belouadah M, *et al.* Successful resuscitation after ropivacaine and lidocaine-induced ventricular arrhythmia following posterior lumbar plexus block in a child. *Anesth Analg* 2008; **106**: 1572–1574.

118 Vettorato E, Bradbrook M, Gurney M, *et al.* Peripheral nerve blocks of the pelvic limb in dogs: a retrospective clinical study. *Vet Comp Orthop Traumatol* 2012; **25**: 314–320.

119 Kapur E, Vuckovic L, Dilberovic F, *et al.* Neurologic and histologic outcome after intraneural injections of lidocaine in canine sciatic nerves. *Acta Anaesthiol Scand* 2007; **51**: 101–107.

120 Campoy L, Martin-Flores M, Ludders JW, *et al.* Comparison of bupivacaine femoral and sciatic nerve block versus bupivacaine and morphine epidural for stifle surgery in dogs. *Vet Anaesth Analg* 2012; **39**: 91–98.

121 Kona-Boun JJ, Silim A, Troncy E. Evaluation of epidural administration of morphine or morphine and bupivacaine for postoperative analgesia after premedication with an opioid analgesic and orthopedic surgery in dogs. *J Am Vet Med Assoc* 2006; **229**: 1103–1112.

122 Wilson DV, Evans AT, Millar R. The effect of preanesthetic morphine on gastroesophageal reflux and regurgitation during anesthesia in dogs. *Am J Vet Res* 2005; **66**: 386–390.

123 Wilson DV, Evans AT, Mauer W. The effect of preanesthetic meperidine on gastroesophageal reflux during anesthesia in dogs. *Vet Anaesth Analg* 2007; **34**: 15–22.

124 Wilson DV, Walshaw R. Post-anesthetic esophageal dysfunction in 13 dogs. *J Am Anim Hosp Assoc* 2004; **40**: 455–460.

125 Wilson DV, Evans AT. Effect of topical treatment on esophageal pH during acid reflux in dogs. *Vet Anaesth Analg* 2007; **34**: 339–343.

126 Tan C, Govendir M, Zaki S, *et al.* Evaluation of four warming procedures to minimize heat loss induced by anaesthesia and surgery in dogs. *Aust Vet J* 2004; **82**: 65–68.

127 Sessler DI, Olofsson CI, Rubinstein EH, *et al.* The thermoregulatory threshold in humans during halothane anesthesia. *Anesthesiology* 1988; **68**: 836–842.

128 Vainio O. Introduction to the clinical pharmacology of medetomidine. *Acta Vet Scand Suppl* 1989; **85**: 85–88.

129 Barnhart MD, Hubbell JAE, Muir WW, *et al.* Pharmacokinetics, pharmacodynamics, and analgesic effects of morphine after rectal, intramuscular, and intravenous administration in dogs. *Am J Vet Res* 2000; **61**: 24–28.

130 Georgiou AP, Manara AR. Role of therapeutic hypothermia in improving outcome after traumatic brain injury: a systematic review. *Br J Anaesth* 2013; **110**: 357–367.
131 Pottie RG, Dart CM, Perkins NR, *et al.* Effect of hypothermia on recovery from general anaesthesia in the dog. *Aust Vet J* 2007; **85**: 158–162.
132 Putzu M, Casati A, Berti M, *et al.* Clinical complications, monitoring and management of perioperative mild hypothermia: anesthesiological failures. *Acta Biomed* 2007; **78**: 163–169.
133 Beilin B, Shavit Y, Razumovsky J, *et al.* Effects of mild hypothermia on cellular immune responses. *Anesthesiology* 1998; **89**: 1133–1140.
134 Cabell LW, Perkowski SZ, Gregor T, *et al.* The effects of active peripheral skin warming on perioperative hypothermia in dogs. *Vet Surg* 1997; **26**: 79–85.
135 Tomasic M. Temporal changes in core body temperature in anesthetized adult horses. *Am J Vet Res* 1999; **60**: 556–562.
136 Rembert FS, Smith JA, Hosgood G. *et al.* Comparison of traditional thermal support devices with the forced-air warmer system in anesthetized Hispaniolan Amazon parrots (*Amazona ventralis*). *J Avian Med Surg* 2001; **15**: 187–193.
137 Roder G, Sessler DI, Roth G, *et al.* Intra-operative rewarming with Hot Dog resistive heating and forced-air heating: a trial of lower-body warming. *Anaesthesia* 2011; **66**: 667–674.
138 Haskins SC, Patz JD. Effect of inspired-air warming and humidification in the prevention of hypothermia during general anesthesia in cats. *Am J Vet Res* 1980; **41**: 1669–1673.
139 Raffe MR, Martin FB. Effect of inspired air heat and humidification on anesthetic-induced hypothermia in dogs. *Am J Vet Res* 1983; **44**: 455–458.
140 Hofmeister EH, Brainard BM, Braun C, *et al.* Effect of a heat and moisture exchanger on heat loss in isoflurane-anesthetized dogs undergoing single-limb orthopedic surgeries. *J Am Vet Med Assoc* 2011; **239**: 1561–1565.
141 Swaim SF, Lee AH, Hughes KS. Heating pads and thermal burns in small animals. *J Am Anim Hosp Assoc* 1989; **25**: 156–162.
142 Dunlop CI, Daunt DA, Haskins SC. Thermal burns in four dogs during anesthesia. *Vet Surg* 1989; **18**: 242–246.
143 Niedfeldt RL, Robertson SA. Postanesthetic hyperthermia in cats: a retrospective comparison between hydromorphone and buprenorphine. *Vet Anaesth Analg* 2006; **33**: 381–389.
144 Posner LP, Gleed RD, Erb HN, *et al.* Post-anesthetic hyperthermia in cats. *Vet Anaesth Analg* 2007; **34**: 40–47.
145 Posner LP, Pavuk A, Rokshar JL, *et al.* Effects of opioids and anesthetic drugs on body temperature in cats. *Vet Anaesth Analg* 2010; **37**: 35–43.
146 Clark WG, Cumby HR. Hyperthermic responses to central and peripheral injections of morphine sulfate in the cat. *Br J Pharmacol* 1978; **63**: 65–71.
147 Gellasch KL, Kruse-Elliott KT, Osmond CS *et al.* Comparison of transdermal administration of fentanyl versus intramuscular administration of butorphanol for analgesia after onychectomy in cats. *J Am Vet Med Assoc* 2002; **220**: 1020–1024.
148 Kilos MB, Graham LF, Lee J. Comparison of two anesthetic protocols for feline blood donation. *Vet Anaesth Analg* 2010; **37**: 230–239.
149 Bellah JR, Robertson SR, Buergelt CD, *et al.* Suspected malignant hyperthermia after halothane anesthesia in a cat. *Vet Surg* 1989; **18**: 483–488.
150 Bagshaw RJ, Cox RH, Knight DH, *et al.* Malignant hyperthermia in a greyhound. *J Am Vet Med Assoc* 1978; **172**: 61–62.
151 Waldron-Mease EW, Klein LV, Rosenberg H, *et al.* Malignant hyperthermia in a halothane-anesthetized horse. *J Am Vet Med Assoc* 1981; **179**: 896–898.
152 Gronert GA. Malignant hyperthermia. *Anesthesiology* 1980; **53**: 395–423.
153 Dexter F, Epstein RH, Wachtel RE, *et al.* Estimate of the relative risk of succinylcholine for malignant hyperthermia. *Anesth Analg* 2013; **116**: 118–122.
154 Migita T, Mukaida K, Kosayashi M, *et al.* The severity of sevoflurane-induced malignant hyperthermia. *Acta Anaesthesiol Scand* 2012; **56**: 351–356.
155 Richardson DW, Kohn CW. Uroperitoneum in the foal. *J Am Vet Med Assoc* 1983; **182**: 267–271.
156 Waldridge BM, Lin HC, Purohit RC. Anesthetic management of horses with hyperkalemic periodic paralysis. *Comp Cont Educ Pract Vet* 1996; **18**: 1030–1039.
157 Bailey JE, Pablo L, Hubbell JAE. Hyperkalemic periodic paralysis episode during halothane anesthesia in a horse. *J Am Vet Med Assoc* 1996; **208**: 1859–1865.
158 Cornick JL, Seahorn TL, Hartsfield SM. Hyperthermia during isoflurane anesthesia in a horse with suspected hyperkalemic periodic paralysis. *Equine Vet J* 1994; **26**: 511–514.
159 Robertson SA, Green SL, Carter SW, *et al.* Postanesthetic recumbency associated with hyperkalemic periodic paralysis in a quarter horse. *J Am Vet Med Assoc* 1992; **201**: 1209–1212.
160 Baetge CL. Anesthesia case of the month. Hyperkalemic periodic paralysis. *J Am Vet Med Assoc* 2007; **230**: 33–36.
161 Pang DS, Panizzi L, Paterson JM. Successful treatment of hyperkalemic periodic paralysis in a horse during isoflurane anesthesia. *Vet Anaesth Analg* 2011; **38**: 113–120.
162 Stiles J, Weil AB, Packer RA, *et al.* Post-anesthetic cortical blindness in cats: twenty cases. *Vet J* 2012; **193**: 367–373.
163 Jurk IR, Thibodeau MS, Whitney K, *et al.* Acute vision loss after general anesthesia in a cat. *Vet Ophthalmol* 2001; **4**: 155–158.
164 Son WG, Jung BY, Kwon TE, *et al.* Acute temporary visual loss after general anesthesia in a cat. *J Vet Clin* 2009; **26**: 480–482.
165 Barton-Lamb AL, Martin-Flores M, Scrivani PV, *et al.* Evaluation of maxillary arterial blood flow in anesthetized cats with the mouth closed and open. *Vet J.* 2013; **196**: 325–331.
166 Lane IF, Matwichuk CL, Carpenter LG, Behrend EN. Profound postanesthetic hypoglycemia attributable to glucocorticoid deficiency in 2 dogs. *Can Vet J* 1999; **40**: 497–500.
167 Chelliah YR. Ventricular arrhythmias associated with hypoglycaemia. *Anaesth Intensive Care* 2000; **28**: 698–700.
168 Davies JM. On-site risk management. *Can J Anaesth* 1991; **38**: 1029–1030.
169 Armstrong JN, Davies JM. A systematic method for the investigation of anaesthetic incidents. *Can J Anaesth* 1991; **38**: 1033–1035.

6 Euthanasia and Humane Killing

Robert E. Meyer
College of Veterinary Medicine, Mississippi State University, Mississippi, USA

Chapter contents

Introduction

Anesthesiology and the intentional killing of animals at first glance seem to have diametrically opposing goals. The former is concerned with maintaining life whereas the latter takes it; indeed, the act of performing euthanasia can be both physically and emotionally difficult for animal workers, caretakers, and veterinarians because of this perceived conflict [1,2]. However, the humane treatment of animals has increasingly become a subject for public debate and discussion, and a conservative and humane approach to the intentional killing of any creature is warranted, justifiable, and expected by society. As veterinarians, we take an oath on entry to the profession '... to use my scientific knowledge and skills for the benefit of society through the protection of animal health and welfare, the prevention and relief of animal suffering, the conservation of livestock resources ...' [3]; further, we are reminded that our moral duty is to the welfare of animals under our care [4,5]. Therefore, whether for welfare concerns, food and fiber production, or in response to natural or human disasters, our duty as compassionate veterinarians is to minimize or eliminate animal pain, anxiety, and distress. Viewed in this context, veterinary anesthetists and anesthesiologists are uniquely positioned to contribute meaningfully to matters pertaining to the humane taking of animal life.

Determining the humaneness of euthanasia, slaughter, or depopulation methods can be difficult because as humans we can never fully know or understand the subjective experiences of animals during loss of consciousness. This problem has vexed veterinary medicine since 1847 when, after administering the then newly described ether anesthetic to dogs and cats, the eminent British veterinarian Edward Mayhew concluded [6]:

> The results of these trials are not calculated to inspire any very sanguine hopes. We cannot tell whether the cries emitted are evidence of pain or not; but they are suggestive of agony to the listener, and, without testimony to the contrary, must be regarded as evidence of suffering. The process, therefore, is not calculated to attain the object for which in veterinary practice it would be most generally employed, namely, to relieve the owner from the impression that his animal was subjected to torture. In another light, it is not likely to be of much practical utility.

One of the defining characteristics in humans undergoing anesthesia is feeling as if one is having an 'out-of-body experience,' suggesting a disconnection between one's sense of self and one's awareness of time and space [7]. Although we cannot know for certain the subjective experiences of animals, one can speculate that similar feelings of disorientation may contribute to apparent signs of animal distress observed during anesthesia. Fortunately, the development of anesthesia methods for animals continued despite Dr Mayhew's initial misgivings.

Determining the humaneness of killing methods depends on our ability to assess pain and consciousness within the contexts of method and application. Events such as vocalization, paddling, or convulsions are often interpreted as unequivocal evidence of animal suffering. Although unpleasant to observe, such events have much less effect on animal welfare when they occur after loss of consciousness.

This purpose of this chapter is to review the mechanisms and methods used for the intentional taking of animal life, including during the fetal stage, within the contexts of pain perception and consciousness. Recently described novel methods of low atmospheric pressure stunning and foam depopulation for poultry are described, in addition to

Veterinary Anesthesia and Analgesia: The Fifth Edition of Lumb and Jones.
Edited by Kurt A. Grimm, Leigh A. Lamont, William J. Tranquilli, Stephen A. Greene and Sheilah A. Robertson.

considerations on agent purity requirements for humane killing. For a more detailed overview of euthanasia, including recommendations and procedures for specific species, readers are strongly encouraged to consult the most recent guidelines issued by the American Veterinary Medical Association (AVMA) [8], the Canadian Council on Animal Care (CCAC) [9], and the World Organisation for Animal Health (OIE) [10].

Terminology

Euthanasia (derived from the Greek *eu + thanatos*, or 'good death') generally refers to the goal of ending the life of an individual animal in a way that minimizes or eliminates pain and distress. Currently, the term is applied to situations where death is induced in a manner that is (a) in accord with an animal's interests and/or because it is a matter of welfare (humane disposition) and (b) where humane techniques are applied to induce the most rapid, painless, and distress-free death possible. Hence, for an act of intentional killing to be considered euthanasia, both humane disposition and humane techniques must be considered together [8]. Euthanasia is not a substitute for poor veterinary care, and should never be considered as the 'easy way out' or as a means to justify questionable management decisions. Rather, euthanasia provides a humane and responsible solution to improve animal welfare by alleviating animal suffering.

There is debate as to whether the term *euthanasia* appropriately describes the killing of some animals at the end of biological experiments and of unwanted shelter animals; extensive discussion regarding these issues can be found in papers by McMillan [11] and Pavlovik and co-workers [12]. For a more extensive review of the moral and ethical considerations of euthanasia, including the decision processes, the reader is directed to the 2013 AVMA Guidelines on Euthanasia [8].

Humane slaughter refers to processes and methods employed to intentionally kill animals raised for food, fur, or fiber production. The term applies both to individual animals killed on-farm and to commercial production processes. From a welfare perspective, the term is inclusive of the transport and handling of an animal, the methods employed to induce unconsciousness, the period until unconsciousness is verified, and the time of death when the animal is ready for entry into the food chain. This means that efforts must be made to minimize and, where possible, eliminate distress, pain, suffering, or anxiety associated with the entire process of bringing that animal to slaughter. Although some humane slaughter methods may employ euthanasia techniques, not all humane slaughter methods meet the criteria required to be considered euthanasia.

In addition to animal welfare concerns, important considerations with regard to humane slaughter processes include public health and safety, food safety and quality, environmental and economic sustainability, production adequacy and sustainability, occupational health and impact on the labor force, international animal welfare and trade standards, and religious and cultural aspects. In the United States, methods for humane slaughter are federally codified for cattle, calves, horses, mules, sheep, and swine by the 1958 Humane Slaughter (HS) Act and the 1978 Humane Methods of Livestock Slaughter Act (Pub. L. 85-765; 7 USC 1901 *et seq.*) (Pub. L. 85-765, Sec. 1, Aug. 27, 1958, 72 Stat. 862; Pub. L. 85-765, §2, Aug. 27, 1958, 72 Stat. 862; Pub. L. 95-445, §5(a), Oct. 10, 1978, 92 Stat. 1069) [13]. Although methods for the humane slaughter of poultry, fish, and rabbits are not specifically included in the 1958 and 1978 Acts, similar considerations should be applied to these species.

Depopulation is defined as the rapid destruction of large numbers of animals in response to emergencies, such as the control of catastrophic infectious diseases, or exigent situations caused by natural or human disasters. As defined by the AVMA, the term applies to methods by which large numbers of animals must be destroyed quickly and efficiently with as much consideration given to the welfare of the animals as practicable, but where the circumstances and tasks facing those performing the depopulation are understood to be extenuating [14].

Depopulation is especially problematic from a welfare standpoint owing to several factors, including the sheer number of animals potentially involved, the need for rapid and decisive responses to limit disease spread or economic damage, and the potential for extenuating circumstances limiting availability or deployment of supplies, equipment, and personnel. This combination of factors can lead to consideration of expedient, rather than humane, solutions. For example, in large confinement production facilities, loss of system ventilation, whether by intentional or accidental means, will eventually result in animal death. Although application of mass depopulation methods may result in the same ultimate outcome, it is our duty as compassionate veterinarians to develop and employ methods that minimize animal suffering under these adverse circumstances. As with humane slaughter methods, depopulation may employ euthanasia techniques, but not all depopulation methods may meet the criteria to be considered euthanasia.

Within the 2013 AVMA Euthanasia Guidelines, methods are classified as *Acceptable*, *Acceptable with Conditions*, and *Unacceptable*; similar terminology is applied throughout this chapter:

- *Acceptable* methods are those that consistently produce a humane death when used alone or as the sole means of producing death.
- *Acceptable with Conditions* methods are those techniques that may require certain conditions to be met to produce humane death consistently, may have greater potential for operator error or to be a safety hazard, are not well documented in the scientific literature, or may require a secondary method to ensure death. Methods 'acceptable with conditions' are equivalent to 'acceptable methods' when all criteria for application of a method can be met.
- *Unacceptable* methods and techniques are those deemed inhumane under any conditions or pose a substantial risk to the human applying the technique. Examples include, but are not necessarily limited to:
  - Certain anesthetic agents and adjuncts, such as chloral hydrate, chloroform, diethyl ether, neuromuscular blocking agents in conscious vertebrate animals (includes nicotine; also $MgSO_4$, KCl, and all depolarizing and non-depolarizing curariform agents).
  - Certain chemicals, such as cyanide, formaldehyde, household products and solvents, cleaning products and disinfectants, pesticides, and strychnine.
  - Certain physical methods, such as air embolism, burning, rapid decompression, drowning, exsanguination, hypothermia, manually applied blunt force trauma to the head (exceptions apply), non-penetrating captive bolts (exceptions apply), rapid freezing (exceptions apply), smothering, and thoracic compression.
- Adjunctive methods are procedures and practices that should not be used as a sole or primary method, but which can be used in conjunction with acceptable methods to bring about humane

death following initial loss of consciousness. Examples include, but are not necessarily limited to:
- Exsanguination, pithing, intravenous or intracardiac $MgSO_4$ or KCl, or creating a pneumothorax.

The following criteria were used in the 2013 AVMA Guidelines on Euthanasia to evaluate methods used to take the life of animals intentionally:
- Ability to induce loss of consciousness and death with a minimum of pain and distress.
- Time required to induce loss of consciousness.
- Reliability.
- Safety of personnel.
- Irreversibility.
- Compatibility with intended animal use and purpose.
- Documented emotional effect on observers or operators.
- Compatibility with subsequent evaluation, examination, or use of tissue.
- Drug availability and human abuse potential.
- Compatibility with species, age, and health status.
- Ability to maintain equipment in proper working order.
- Safety for predators or scavengers should the carcass be consumed.
- Legal requirements.
- Environmental impacts of the method or carcass disposition.

Further, application of humane killing methods must be performed in accord with applicable national, regional, or local laws governing drug acquisition and storage, occupational safety, and methods used for euthanasia and disposal of animals, with special attention to individual species requirements where possible. If drugs have been used, careful consideration must be given to appropriate carcass disposal and steps should be taken to avoid environmental contamination or harm to other animals [8].

Selection of the most appropriate killing method for a particular situation will depend on several factors, including the species and number of animals involved, available means for animal handling and restraint, the skill and proficiency of personnel, and the methods and equipment available. Information in the scientific literature and available from practical experience focuses primarily on domesticated animals, but the same general considerations can be applied to all species. There will be less-than-perfect situations in which methods listed as 'acceptable' or 'acceptable with conditions' may not be possible, such that a method or agent that is the best under the circumstances will be applied. It should be noted that any useful and potentially humane killing method can become inhumane through poor technique, improper application, or lack of strict adherence to specified conditions and contingencies.

Pain and consciousness

Euthanasia, humane slaughter, and depopulation methods initially produce unconsciousness through three basic mechanisms: (1) direct depression of neurons necessary for life functions; (2) hypoxia; and (3) physical disruption of brain activity. Death follows as the circulatory and respiratory centers fail, or as hypoxia or reduced pH renders intracellular processes non-functional. However, loss of consciousness occurs at substantially different rates, such that the suitability of any particular agent or method depends on whether an animal experiences pain or distress prior to loss of consciousness.

Pain is defined as a conscious perception. Pain is subjective in the sense that individuals can differ in their perceptions of intensity and also in their physical and behavioral responses. The International Association for the Study of Pain (IASP) describes pain as [15]:

> An unpleasant sensory and emotional experience associated with actual or potential tissue damage, or described in terms of such damage. Activity induced in the nociceptor and nociceptive pathways by a noxious stimulus is not pain, which is always a psychological state, even though we may well appreciate that pain most often has a proximate physical cause.

Based on mammalian models, the perception of pain requires nerve impulses from peripheral nociceptors to reach an awake, functioning cerebral cortex and associated subcortical brain structures. Impulses from peripheral nociceptors are conducted by primary afferent fibers to either the spinal cord or the brainstem and two general sets of neural networks. Reflex withdrawal and flexion in response to nociceptive input are mediated at the spinal level, while ascending nociceptive pathways carry impulses to the reticular formation, hypothalamus, thalamus, and cerebral cortex (somatosensory cortex and limbic system) for conscious sensory processing and spatial localization. This distinction is important, in that movements observed in response to nociception can be due to spinally mediated reflex activity (unconscious), cerebral cortical and subcortical processing (conscious), or a combination of the two. Consequently, the choice of specific killing agent or method is less critical if it is to be used on an animal that is already anesthetized or rendered unconscious, provided that the animal does not regain consciousness prior to death.

Although the perception of pain requires a conscious experience, defining consciousness, and therefore the ability to perceive pain, across many species is difficult. Amnesia, defined as loss of memory function in which old memories cannot be remembered or new memories cannot be formed, is a defining characteristic of anesthesia, in that with sufficient quantities, all anesthetics are capable of producing a state of amnesia where new memories cannot be formed [7]. Unconsciousness, defined as loss of individual awareness, occurs when the brain's ability to integrate information is blocked or disrupted. Anesthetics produce unconsciousness either by preventing integration (blocking interactions among specialized brain regions) or by reducing information (shrinking the number of activity patterns available to cortical networks) received by the cerebral cortex or equivalent structure or structures. Further, the abrupt loss of consciousness that occurs at a critical concentration of anesthetic implies that the integrated workings of the interconnected neural states underlying consciousness may collapse nonlinearly [16,17].

In humans, onset of anesthetic-induced unconsciousness has been functionally defined by loss of appropriate response to verbal command; in animals, loss of consciousness is functionally defined by loss of the righting reflex (LORR), also called loss of position (LOP) [18–20]. This definition, introduced with the discovery of general anesthesia over 160 years ago, is still useful because it is an easily observable, integrated whole-animal response that is applicable to a wide variety of species. Although surrogate measures of brain activity such as an electroencephalogram or functional MRI are often applied in this context, these methods cannot yet provide definitive answers as to onset of either human or animal unconsciousness; limitations of these methods for this purpose are reviewed later in the section Evaluating Animal Distress. The usefulness of LOP/LORR as an easily observable proxy for loss of animal consciousness was recently reinforced when a reduction in alpha:delta brain wave ratios was found to coincide with LOP in chickens [21,22].

Vocalization or physical movement observed during application of humane killing methods is often interpreted as unequivocal evidence of consciousness. While purposeful escape behaviors should not be observed during the transition to unconsciousness, human and animal studies confirm that amnesia is produced and conscious awareness is blocked at less than half the anesthetic concentration required to abolish physical movement [19]. Once consciousness is lost, subsequent activities, such as seizures, vocalization, reflex struggling, breath holding, and tachypnea, can be attributed to the 'excitement' phase or anesthesia stage 2, which by definition lasts from loss of consciousness to the onset of a regular breathing pattern [23,24]. Hence vocalization and non-purposeful movements observed following LORR/LOP are not necessarily signs of conscious perception by an animal.

Previously, it was thought that finfish, amphibians, reptiles, and invertebrates lacked the anatomic structures necessary to perceive pain as we understand it in birds and mammals. However, most invertebrates respond to noxious stimuli and many have endogenous opioids [25], and there is increasing taxa-specific evidence of the efficacy of analgesics to minimize the impact of noxious stimuli on amphibians and reptiles [26,27]. Suggestions that fish responses to pain merely represent simple reflexes [28] have been refuted by studies demonstrating differing forebrain and midbrain electrical activity in response to nociceptor stimulation [29,30]; further, finfish exhibit learning and memory consolidation when taught to avoid noxious stimuli [31]. Based on the above considerations, killing methods that 'result in rapid loss of consciousness' and 'minimize pain and distress' should be strived for, even in those species where it is difficult to determine that these criteria have been met.

Mechanisms of action

Physical methods (e.g., gunshot, captive bolt, cerebral electrocution, blunt force trauma, maceration) produce instantaneous unconsciousness by destroying, or rendering non-functional, brain regions responsible for cortical integration; death quickly follows when the midbrain centers controlling respiration and cardiac activity fail. Signs of effective stun and onset of unconsciousness in cattle include immediate collapse (LORR/LOP) and a several-second period of tetanic spasm, followed by slow hind limb movements of increasing frequency [32–34]; however, there is species variability in this response. The corneal reflex will be absent [35]. Signs of effective electrocution are loss of righting reflex, loss of eye blink and moving object tracking, extension of the limbs, opisthotonos, downward rotation of the eyeballs, and tonic (rigid) spasm changing to clonic (paddling) spasm, with eventual muscle flaccidity [33,36,37]. The corneal reflex will be absent [35]. Although generalized seizures may be observed following effective application of physical methods, these most often follow loss of consciousness. Physical methods are inexpensive, humane, and painless if performed properly, and leave no drug residues in the carcass. Furthermore, animals presumably experience less fear and anxiety with methods that require little preparatory handling. However, as noted in the section Choice of Killing Method Relative to Onset of Unconsciousness, physical methods usually require more direct physical proximity with the animals to be euthanized, which can be both offensive and upsetting for the operator. Physical disruption methods are often followed by adjunctive methods such as exsanguination or pithing to ensure death.

Decapitation and cervical dislocation as physical methods of humane killing require separate comment. Electrical activity in the brain can persist for up to 30 s following these methods [38–41]; interpretation of the significance of this activity is controversial [42]. As discussed in the section Evaluating Animal Distress, brain electrical activity cannot yet provide definitive answers as to the precise onset of unconsciousness. Other studies [43–47] indicate such activity does not imply the ability to perceive pain and conclude that loss of consciousness develops rapidly.

Anesthetics and carbon dioxide (CO_2) inhalation initially produce loss of consciousness through direct depression of the cortical neural system; death subsequently occurs due to respiratory or cardiovascular failure associated with agent overdose. Acute hypercapnea (defined as >5% atmospheric CO_2) rapidly reduces intracellular pH, producing unconsciousness and a reversible anesthetic state characterized by reduction of both basal and evoked neural activities [48–51] and inhibits central *N*-methyl-D-aspartate (NMDA) receptors [52]. In contrast to inert gas killing methods, exposure to CO_2 does not rely on the induction of hypoxia to cause unconsciousness and death and can kill over a wide range of concentrations [53].

Hypoxia is commonly achieved by displacing oxygen; this can be achieved through exposure to high concentrations of inert gases, such as nitrogen or argon. To be effective, O_2 levels of <2% must be achieved and maintained, as re-establishment of a concentration of O_2 of 6% or greater prior to death will allow immediate recovery [53–56]. Carbon monoxide binds avidly to hemoglobin and produces hypoxemia by blocking uptake of oxygen within red blood cells. Exsanguination is another method of inducing hypoxemia, albeit indirectly, to ensure death in already unconscious or moribund animals. Low atmospheric pressure stunning of poultry (LAPS) represents a recent refinement in producing hypoxia (see the section Low Atmospheric Pressure Stunning). Whether a hypoxia-based method is classified as stunning or killing depends on the amount of time the animal remains in the modified atmosphere; killing methods eliminate the concern that animals may regain consciousness. Hypoxia-based methods are not appropriate for those species or stages of development that are tolerant to prolonged periods of hypoxemia.

Nitrous oxide (N_2O) is not a potent anesthetic in animals. The effective dose for N_2O is above 100 vol.%; therefore, it cannot be used alone in any species at normal atmospheric pressure without producing hypoxia prior to respiratory or cardiac arrest. In humans, the minimum alveolar concentration (MAC) (defined as the median effective dose preventing purposeful movement; see Chapter 16) for N_2O is 104 vol.%; its potency in other species is less than half that in humans (i.e., approximately 200 vol.%). By comparison, the MAC for isoflurane is approximately 1.4 vol.%. Up to 70 vol.% N_2O can be added to an inhaled fluorocarbon anesthetic–oxygen vapor to speed the onset of unconsciousness through the 'second gas effect.' However, owing to its reduced potency in animals, N_2O will only reduce the fluorocarbon anesthetic MAC by 20–30%, or about half that expected in humans [57]. The combination of CO_2 with N_2O, administered at a displacement rate of 20 and 60% of the chamber volume per minute, produced LORR in C57Bl/6 and CD1 mice 10.3% faster than CO_2 alone (N_2O–CO_2, 96.7 ± 7.9 s; CO_2, 108.7 ± 9.4 s), and may represent a refinement over the use of CO_2 alone [58].

A gradual displacement rate between 10 and 30% of the container volume per minute is currently recommended for administration of CO_2 for euthanasia [8]. The build-up, or wash-in, of gases within enclosed spaces is an exponential process dependent on chamber volume and gas displacement rate, such that time to loss of consciousness, and eventually death, will be a function of the time constant for that container [59]. The time constant can be calculated as the chamber volume divided by the gas displacement rate [59]. When starting from a gas concentration near zero, one time constant is required to reach a washed-in gas concentration of 63 vol.% such that a gas volume displacement rate of 20%/min represents a time constant of 5 min (1 divided by 0.2). Thus, applying any vapor or gas at a displacement rate of 20% of the container volume per minute will result in an exponential rise to 63 vol.% of the wash-in gas concentration within 5 min for a container of any size [59,60].

The application of inhaled gases into enclosed spaces can be further refined to meet specific inflow rates, delivery points, and optimal gas concentration profiles through use of computational fluid dynamic (CFD) modeling. Gas distribution and temperature within containers can be modeled in three dimensions using CFD software running inside desktop computer-aided design (CAD) systems. CFD simulation has proved to be a very powerful tool for modeling transient gas concentrations during gas wash-in and wash-out. It has further reduced the need for time- and labor-intensive experimental testing of many design alternatives for on-farm depopulation methods without the need for extensive experimental testing [61].

Loss of consciousness, as LORR/LOP, should always precede loss of muscle movement. However, as with the physical killing methods, some animals may exhibit motor activity or convulsions following loss of consciousness with anesthetics or with hypoxia-based methods. Indeed, anesthesia, coma, and generalized seizures all represent a loss of consciousness where both arousal and awareness in humans is low or absent [62]. Characteristic signs of effective neural depression are similar to those observed with physical methods or with deep levels of anesthesia, including LORR/LOP, loss of eye blink and corneal reflexes, and muscle flaccidity. Inhaled and hypoxia-based methods require a number of conditions and contingencies for their proper and appropriate use, such that they are currently classified as 'acceptable with conditions' in the 2013 AVMA Guidelines [8].

Agents and methods that prevent movement through muscle paralysis without inhibiting or disrupting the cerebral cortex or equivalent structures (e.g., succinylcholine, strychnine, curare, nicotine, and potassium or magnesium salts) are not acceptable as sole agents for humane killing of vertebrates because they result in conscious perception of distress and pain prior to death. In contrast, magnesium salts are considered to be acceptable as the sole agent for euthanasia in many invertebrates owing to the absence of evidence for cerebral activity in some members of these taxa [63,64]; further, there is evidence that the magnesium ion acts centrally to suppress neural activity of cephalopods [65].

In summary, the cerebral cortex or equivalent structure(s) and associated subcortical structures must be functional for conscious perception of pain to occur. If the cerebral cortex is non-functional because of neuronal depression, hypoxia, or physical disruption, pain is not experienced. Although distressing to observers, reflex motor activity or physical signs occurring following loss of consciousness, as LORR/LOP, is not perceived by the animal as pain or distress. Given that we are limited to applying humane killing methods based on these three basic mechanisms, efforts should be directed towards education of involved personnel and towards achieving technical proficiency and refinement in the application of currently approved methods [66].

Evaluating animal distress

Stress and the resulting responses have been divided into three phases [67]. Eustress results when harmless stimuli initiate adaptive responses that are beneficial to the animal. Neutral stress results when the animal's response to stimuli causes neither harmful nor beneficial effects to the animal. Distress results when an animal's response to stimuli interferes with its well-being and comfort [68]. Distress may be created by the conditions prior to application of stunning or killing methods (e.g., transport conditions, environment, or restraint), or by the conditions under which methods are applied (e.g., gradual gas/vapor displacement or immersion [69]). Simply placing Sprague–Dawley rats into an unfamiliar exposure chamber containing room air produces arousal, if not distress [70]. Pigs are social animals and prefer not to be isolated from one another; consequently, moving them to the CO_2 stunning box in groups, rather than lining them up single-file as needed for electric stunning, improves voluntary forward movement, reduces handling stress, and reduces electric prod use [71]. Gradual-fill inhaled methods may be less stressful than more rapid displacements [72]. Distress may manifest behaviorally [e.g., overt escape behaviors, approach–avoidance preferences (aversion)] or physiologically [e.g., changes in heart rate, sympathetic nervous system (SNS) activity, hypothalamic–pituitary axis (HPA) activity], such that a 'one size fits all' approach cannot be easily applied to evaluate killing methods or determine specific species applications.

Both sympathetic nervous system (SNS) and hypothalamic–pituitary–adrenal axis (HPAA) activation are well accepted as stress response markers. However, it has been suggested that responses to systemic stressors associated with immediate survival, such as hypoxia and hypercapnia, are likely directly relayed from brainstem nuclei and are not associated with higher order CNS processing and conscious experiences [73]. Marked increases in circulating catecholamines, glucagon, insulin, lactate, and free fatty acids have been reported in porcine experimental models where brain death is induced following induction of general anesthesia [74–76]. Forslid and Augustinsson reported that concentrations of norepinephrine and lactate increased 1 min after exposure of pigs to CO_2 [77]. Borovsky and co-workers found an increase in norepinephrine in rats following 30 s of exposure to 100% CO_2 [78]. Similarly, Reed and co-workers exposed rats to 20–25 s of CO_2, which was sufficient to render them recumbent, unconscious, and unresponsive, and observed tenfold increases in vasopressin and oxytocin concentrations [79]. Hypothalamic vasopressin-containing neurons are similarly activated in response to CO_2 exposure in both awake and anesthetized rats [80]. In pigs undergoing euthanasia with physical methods resulting in immediate unconsciousness (e.g., captive bolt; two-point electrocution) or inhaled methods where onset of unconsciousness is delayed (CO_2; 70% N_2–30% CO_2), cortisol levels were observed to be similar, whereas plasma norepinephrine and lactate were similarly increased in all groups [81]; although all gases and mixtures induced open-mouthed breathing prior to loss of righting reflex, the mean latency to onset of open-mouth breathing and subsequent loss of righting reflex was substantially longer with 70% N_2–30% CO_2 than with CO_2 [82]. The fact that levels of stress hormones observed were similar with both physical and inhaled methods illustrates the difficulty in differentiating conscious from unconscious distress where interpretation is complicated by continued exposure during the period between loss of consciousness and death.

Behavioral assessment (e.g., purposeful escape behaviors; open-mouth breathing) and aversion testing have been used to evaluate subjectively, inhaled killing methods in several species; these methods have recently been reviewed [8]. Aversion, defined as a desire to avoid or retreat from a stimulus, is usually determined using approach–avoidance studies, where the strength of avoidance to a particular situation or condition is determined by the animal's choice to forego a desirable reward. This quantitative feature makes aversion a powerful tool for behavior studies. However, it is important to note that although aversion is a measure of preference and may imply unpleasantness, aversion itself does not necessarily indicate pain or distress; further, approach–avoidance tests fail to distinguish adequately between aversion and distress, which is the inability to respond appropriately (either behaviorally or physiologically) to a stressor [69]. In addition, agents identified as being less aversive (e.g., Ar or N_2 gas mixtures) can still produce overt and extended signs of behavioral distress (e.g., open-mouth breathing) prior to loss of consciousness under certain conditions of administration (e.g., gradual displacement application) [82,83].

Measurements of brain electrical function, such as electroencephalogram (EEG), bispectral analysis (BIS), and visual and auditory evoked potentials (VEP, AEP), have been used to quantify the unconscious state. In humans, the issue is intraoperative awareness under anesthesia; in animals, the problem is procedural humaneness relative to onset of unconsciousness. The problem is even more complex in animals where we cannot question them directly and must infer from their actions and responses.

Brain electrical activity is acknowledged to be limited for this purpose, especially when trying to conflate electrical activity with a complex process such as consciousness. EEG is not a direct measure of consciousness – it measures brain electrical activity, and while that activity changes with levels of consciousness, EEG cannot provide definitive answers as to onset of unconsciousness using the current state of the art. Although consciousness must vanish at some level between behavioral unresponsiveness and the induction of a flat EEG (indicating the cessation of the brain's electrical activity and brain death), current EEG-based brain function monitors are limited in their ability to indicate directly the presence or absence of unconsciousness, especially around the transition point [16,84]; also, it is not always clear which EEG patterns are indicators of activation by stress or pain [85].

A recent editorial neatly sums up the issues [86]:

> The electroencephalogram has been the Holy Grail of anesthetic depth monitoring for more than half a century but has fallen on hard times lately, largely because the focus of the dialog changed from electroencephalogram as a monitor of 'depth' to one of intraoperative awareness ... consciousness and intraoperative awareness are neurobiologically exceedingly complex phenomena. This makes these states difficult to capture or evaluate with electroencephalography, no matter the parameter or sophistication of the processing algorithm. Recent studies examining the efficacy of the electroencephalogram bispectral index for minimizing the risk of intraoperative awareness confirm as much.

Although loss of visual evoked potentials (VEPs) is associated with brain death, visual cortex neurons remain responsive to flash stimulation under desflurane anesthesia [87], and reduction in flash-induced gamma oscillations in rat visual cortex is not a unitary correlate of anesthetic-induced unconsciousness [88]. Large inter-individual variations in auditory evoked potential (AEP) and BIS analysis make it impossible to discriminate subtle changes of clinical state of consciousness in real time during propofol anesthesia [89].

Similarly, blood oxygen level-dependent (BOLD) MRI is a multifactorial surrogate for cerebral blood flow or cerebral blood volume, both of which are actual measures of neural activity. Although a BOLD MRI response is generally a good surrogate measure of neuronal activity, it is based on hemodynamic changes which may not reflect actual neural activity patterns, especially during anesthesia or under pharmacological challenge; rather, observed effects may be directly due to drug effects, or indirectly through changes in autonomic activity, blood pressure, cardiac output, or respiration [90,91]. In contrast, imaging of cerebral blood flow using positron emission tomography (PET) has been used in human volunteers during manipulation of consciousness with anesthetics combined with response to verbal command [17]; application of this method to explore the transition between the conscious and unconsciousness state in animals will be difficult.

Choice of killing method relative to onset of unconsciousness

The suitability of any particular agent or method for humane killing depends largely on whether distress and/or pain are experienced prior to loss of consciousness. While a 'gentle' death that takes longer is generally preferable to a rapid but more distressing death [85], in some species and under some circumstances, the most humane and pragmatic option may require the use of less than ideal agents or conditions resulting in rapid unconsciousness with few or no outward signs of distress [8]. Any perceived distress or discomfort associated with a specific killing method occurring prior to loss of consciousness must therefore be weighed against adverse welfare that may occur due to handling or restraining procedures [53].

People are disturbed less by the euthanasia process when they feel distanced from the physical act of euthanasia or when animals exhibit little or no movement. As noted previously, reflex and convulsive motor activities can be particularly unsettling, such that choice of stunning or killing method is substantially influenced by the perceptions and preferences of those individuals to whom the task has been charged. For example, laboratory technicians reported they felt more comfortable using inhaled methods, where they were more dissociated from the animals' death, than directly killing the animal with cervical dislocation [92]. Focus groups of North Carolina swine farm managers preferred methods 'where you give a shot and the animal goes to sleep,' even when those methods prolonged time to death, over captive bolt and blunt force cranial trauma [93]. Injectable and inhaled killing methods can provide that distance, which may partially explain their widespread usage for this purpose.

Killing methods where unconsciousness is delayed have the potential to affect animal welfare adversely. With inhalational methods, onset of unconsciousness relies on a critical concentration of gases or vapors within the alveoli and blood for effect; similarly, onset of unconsciousness following administration of injectable agents is dependent on achieving an effective concentration at the site of action. This depends on the properties of the agent and route of administration; loss of consciousness can be relatively quick following direct injection into the circulatory system whereas injectable agent administration by non-intravenous routes can delay the process. Accordingly, both inhaled methods and non-intravenous administration of barbiturate acid derivatives are currently classified as 'acceptable with conditions' [8].

Interestingly, more than 40% of human children aged 2–10 years display distress behaviors during sevoflurane induction, with 17%

displaying significant distress and more than 30% physically resisting during induction [94]. Fear in children undergoing anesthesia may be due to odor, feel of the mask, or a true phobia of the mask [95]. That anesthetic agents can produce distress and aversion in humans raises concerns for their use in animals, in that the US Government Principles for the Utilization and Care of Vertebrate Animals Used in Testing, Research, and Training state: 'Unless the contrary is established, investigators should consider that procedures that cause pain or distress in human beings may cause pain or distress in other animals' [96]. Despite evidence of distress and aversion, anesthesia continues to be clinically administered to both humans and animals because the benefits associated with use greatly outweigh any distress and/or aversion the agents themselves may cause.

An intravenous (IV) overdose of a barbiturate acid derivative, such as pentobarbital or secobarbital, is currently recommended for euthanasia of companion animals [8]. These agents are no longer commonly used veterinary anesthetics, and few veterinarians today have had clinical experience of using them outside the context of euthanasia. Onset of unconsciousness with IV administration of pentobarbital or secobarbital usually occurs within 30–60 s [97]; however, maximal depth of anesthesia may not be attained for 1 min or longer [98]. It is important to understand that overdoses of these agents are utilized to ensure death and do not result in faster induction times. Pentobarbital inductions are quiet in most cases; however, struggling, excitement, and/or vocalization are occasionally observed, with the recommendation to hold the animal firmly as the head begins to fall to help avoid provoking an excitement phase during induction [99].

Non-intravenous administration of barbiturates is currently categorized as 'acceptable with conditions' when IV access would be distressful, dangerous, or impractical due to animal size or behavioral considerations [8]. Administration by the intraperitoneal (IP) route is noted to produce a slow induction of anesthesia with excitement and vocalization, unpredictable levels of anesthesia, and damage to viscera in both dogs and cats [99]. In adult male Crl:CD(BR) rats, IP administration of 40 and 50 mg/kg pentobarbital produced loss of righting in 4.7 ± 1.4 and 3.5 ± 1.4 min, respectively [100]; similar findings were reported in male and female Wistar U:WU(Cpb) rats [101]. Cats from an animal shelter administered 346.6 mg/kg pentobarbital and 17.7 mg/kg lidocaine intrahepatically while conscious showed incoordination in 0.45 min (27 s) and recumbency in 1.11 min (67 s) [102]. Although time to loss of consciousness in cats receiving IP pentobarbital was not reported, incoordination and recumbency were stated to be 'significantly prolonged,' with 25% of cats in the IP group and 9% of cats in the intrahepatic group showing at least 30 s of what was characterized as anesthesia Stage 1 and 2 excitement [102]. As both pentobarbital and secobarbital are highly alkaline, with a pH of ~10, IP administration is associated with significant peritoneal irritation and pain, evidenced as upregulation in spinal c-fos expression following administration of pentobarbital, even with the addition of the local anesthetic lidocaine [103].

When a gas or vapor is first introduced into a large air-filled confined space using gradual displacement methods, animals are not immediately exposed to conditions known to be aversive or painful. Time between onset of signs of distress and LOP with inhaled methods depends on the agent and displacement rate. Generally, loss of consciousness will be more rapid if animals are initially exposed to a high concentration of an inhaled agent. For example, the induction time for neonatal pigs is 90 s when exposed to 5 vol.% isoflurane [104] and 120 s for 5 vol.% halothane [105]. For many agents and species, however, forced exposure to high inhalant concentrations can be aversive and distressing, such that gradual exposure may be the most pragmatic and humane option.

Flecknell and co-workers reported violent struggling accompanied by apnea and bradycardia in rabbits administered isoflurane, halothane, and sevoflurane by mask or induction chamber, and concluded that these agents were aversive and should be avoided whenever possible [106]. Leach and co-workers found inhaled anesthetic vapors to be associated with some degree of aversion in laboratory rodents, with increasing aversion noted as concentration increased; halothane was least aversive for rats, and halothane and enflurane were least aversive for mice [107–109]. Makowska and Weary also reported halothane and isoflurane to be aversive to male Wistar rats, but less so than CO_2 [110].

Carbon monoxide is reported to be aversive to laboratory rats, but not as aversive as CO_2 [111]. Carbon monoxide produces LOP at approximately 5 vol.% concentration in male Wistar rats; however, time to LOP varies with CO displacement rate (104 s at 3% volume displacement rate; 64 s at 6% volume displacement rate; 53 s at 7% volume displacement rate) [111]; for comparison, a 10% CO atmosphere could be achieved within 30 s with administration of 100% CO at a volume displacement rate equivalent to 20% of the chamber volume per minute.

Aversion to the inert gases argon (Ar) and nitrogen (N_2) depends largely on species and conditions of administration [8]. Hypoxia resulting from exposure to these gases is aversive to rats, mice, and mink. In contrast, these gases appear not to be directly aversive to poultry, and the resulting hypoxia appears to be non-aversive or only mildly aversive. Similarly, Ar or N_2 gas mixtures do not appear to be directly aversive to pigs and seem to reduce, but not eliminate, behavioral responses to hypoxia [56]. However, based on the wash-in and wash-out exponential functions, gradual displacement administration of inert gases results in prolonged exposure to hypoxic conditions and can produce overt signs of behavioral distress, such as open-mouth breathing, for an extended period prior to loss of consciousness in laboratory rodents [70,72], pigs [82], and poultry [83].

Distress during CO_2 exposure has been examined using behavioral assessment and aversion testing [8]. Variability in behavioral responses to CO_2 has been reported for rats and mice [69,72, 112–118], pigs [54, 56, 119–122], and poultry [123–132]. Although signs of distress have been reported in animals in some studies, other researchers have not consistently observed these effects. This may be due to variations in gas administration and exposure methods, types of behaviors assessed, and animal strains tested.

Using preference and approach–avoidance testing, rats and mice show aversion to CO_2 concentrations sufficient to induce unconsciousness [108,109], and are willing to forgo a palatable food reward to avoid exposure to CO_2 concentrations of approximately 15% and higher [110,133] after up to 24 h of food deprivation [134]. Mink will avoid a chamber containing a desirable novel object when it contains 100% CO_2 [135]. In contrast to other species, a large proportion of chickens and turkeys will enter a chamber containing moderate concentrations of CO_2 (60%) to gain access to food or social contact [128,130,132]. Following incapacitation and prior to loss of consciousness, birds in these studies show behaviors such as open-beak breathing and head shaking; these behaviors, however, may not be associated with distress because birds do not withdraw from CO_2 when these behaviors occur [126]. Exposure to CO_2 levels up to 30 vol.% do not appear to be aversive to pigs, as

Duroc and Large White pigs, when given a choice, will tolerate 30 vol.% CO_2 to gain access to a food reward [54,120]. Hence it appears that birds and pigs are more willing than rodents and mink to tolerate CO_2 at concentrations sufficient to induce LORR/LOP.

Carbon dioxide exposure using gradual fill methods is less likely to cause pain due to nociceptor activation by carbonic acid prior to onset of unconsciousness, such that a CO_2 displacement rate between 10 and 30% of the chamber volume per minute is currently recommended for euthanasia [8,9]. When administered at these rates, unconsciousness occurs prior to exposure to CO_2 levels known to produce nociceptor stimulation [69,72]. In humans, rats, and cats, nociceptors begin to respond at CO_2 concentrations of approximately 40 vol.% [136–139]. Humans report that discomfort begins between 30 and 50 vol.% CO_2, and intensifies to overt pain with higher concentrations [140–142]. In rodents, distress begins at approximately 15 vol.% CO_2 concentration and lasts to onset of unconsciousness approximately 30 s later. Unconsciousness occurs within 106 s at a CO_2 concentration of approximately 30 vol.% with a CO_2 displacement rate equivalent to 17–20% of the chamber volume [118,133,142,143]. A slower 10%/min displacement increases time to onset of unconsciousness to 156 s at a CO_2 concentration of 21% [72]. When CO_2 is administered to neonatal pigs at 20% of the chamber volume per minute, unconsciousness (loss of righting reflex) occurs within 80 ± 15 s at a CO_2 concentration of approximately 22 vol.% [82]. The CO_2 concentrations required to produce LOP for broilers, layers, turkeys, and ducks are 19.0, 19.9, 19.3, and 23.8 vol.%, respectively [124].

Genetics may play a role in CO_2 response variability. Panic disorder in humans is genetically linked to enhanced sensitivity to CO_2 [144]. The fear network, comprising the hippocampus, the medial prefrontal cortex, and the amygdala and its brainstem projections, appears to be abnormally sensitive to CO_2 in these patients [145]. The genetic background of some pigs, especially excitable lines such as the Hampshire and German Landrace, has been associated with animals that react poorly to CO_2 stunning, whereas calmer genetic lines combining the Yorkshire or Dutch Landrace conformations show much milder reactions [146]. Given a choice, Duroc and Large White pigs will tolerate 30% CO_2 to gain access to a food reward, but will forego the reward to avoid exposure to 90% CO_2, even after a 24 h period of food deprivation [54,120]. A shock with an electric prod, however, is more aversive to Landrace × Large White pigs than inhaling 60 or 90% CO_2, with pigs inhaling 60% CO_2 willing to re-enter the crate containing CO_2 [119]. Until further research is conducted, one can conclude that exposure to high levels of CO_2 may be humane for certain genetic lines of pigs and stressful for others [146].

Recent studies involving mice have found regions of the amygdala associated with fear behavior to contain acid-sensing ion channels (ASIC) sensitive to elevated CO_2 [147]. Fear behaviors and aversion in response to CO_2 exposure were reduced in mice in which the ASIC receptors were eliminated or inhibited, suggesting that aversive responses to CO_2 in rodents, and potentially other species, are mediated in part by an innate fear response. Further studies defining the presence of ASIC and their role in CO_2-induced fear in other rodent strains, and also other animal species, are warranted.

The practice of immersion in a container prefilled with 100% CO_2 is now considered 'unacceptable' for euthanasia [8,9]. However, a distinction must be made between immersion, where conscious animals are placed directly into a high concentration of a gas or vapor within a container, and commercial controlled atmosphere stunning (CAS) processes as employed for the stunning of poultry and hogs. Unlike immersion, animals experience their introduction into CAS atmospheres gradually; this can be through physical transport at a controlled rate into a contained stunning atmosphere gradient, through controlled introduction of stunning gases into an enclosed space, or by controlled reduction of atmospheric pressure to produce hypoxia. Sequential combinations (so-called 'two-step' or 'multi-phase' processes) may utilize one gas or gas mixture to induce unconsciousness prior to exposure to a different gas mixture or higher gas concentration. Animal transport or introduction rate may be slow or relatively quick, depending on the process, gases utilized, and the specific species. Further, denser than air gases such as CO_2 layer into defined gradients within an enclosed space [148]. Thus, animals are not immediately exposed to conditions known to be aversive or painful with CAS. The design of commercial CAS systems has been reviewed by Grandin [146].

Uncertainty exists as to the usefulness and feasibility of substituting inhaled anesthetic agents for CO_2 with respect to animal welfare and human health and safety [8,85]. Inhaled halocarbon anesthetics have been proposed as alternatives to CO_2 for rodent euthanasia [85,110,111,149] and the Canadian Council on Animal Care (CCAC) recently adopted this position when feasible [9]. However, inhaled anesthetics are known to produce varying degrees of aversion in rodents [107–110,149], and produce aversion, distress, and escape behaviors during anesthetic induction in other animal species [106] and humans [94,95]. Isoflurane anesthesia administered prior to CO_2 euthanasia increased adverse behavioral signs of distress and c-fos expression in the brains of female CD1 mice [69]. Consistent with the principles governing wash-in and wash-out of gases within closed containers, five of ten isoflurane-anesthetized mice showed signs of recovery of consciousness when CO_2 was added to the container [69]. Premedication with acepromazine or midazolam prior to exposure to CO_2 administered at a 20%/min displacement rate did not significantly alter observed behaviors but did induce significantly higher c-fos expression [69]. Large amounts of inhaled anesthetics are absorbed and significant amounts remain in the body for days, even after apparent recovery [150], making these agents unsuitable for euthanasia of food-producing animals.

Fetal sentience and euthanasia

Fetal sentience during euthanasia of pregnant animals and ovariohysterectomy of pregnant dogs and cats has been extensively reviewed by Mellor and co-workers [151–154] and White [155]. Concerns about fetal suffering during humane slaughter of pregnant animals or ovariohysterectomy of pregnant dogs and cats may arise, at least in part, because of observation of fetal body and respiratory movements. However, these movements are a part of normal fetal physiology *in utero* and should not, in and of themselves, be a cause for welfare concerns. Although the term 'fetal distress' has been used in the past, it is not meant to indicate or imply conscious emotional distress, awareness, or conscious suffering and is currently considered to be imprecise and non-specific in this context [155].

In an extensive review of fetal physiology and pain perception, Mellor and Diesch [151] asserted that 'an animal must be both sentient and conscious for suffering to occur'; in other words, the animal must have adequate neural development for sensory perception or sentience and must also be in an awake conscious state. All mammalian embryos or fetuses studied to date remain in an unconscious state throughout pregnancy and birth [152]. This occurs in some species due to exceptional neurological immaturity (e.g., certain marsupials) or moderate neurological immaturity (e.g., cats, dogs, rabbits, rats, and mice). In those species which are neurologically mature at birth (e.g., cattle, deer, goats, sheep, horses, and guinea pigs), initial neurological immaturity is combined with *in utero* neuro-inhibitors. These neuro-inhibitors are unique to prenatal life and include adenosine (a potent promoter of sleep and/or unconsciousness), allopregnanolone and pregnanolone (neuroactive steroids with well-established anesthetic, sedative/hypnotic, and analgesic effects, synthesized by the fetal brain), and prostaglandin D_2 (a potent sleep-inducing agent, synthesized by the fetal brain). Consciousness occurs within minutes or hours following birth in these species largely due to the combined effect of decreasing neuro-inhibition and the onset of strong neuro-activation. Further, an isoelectric EEG, which is incompatible with consciousness, rapidly appears after cessation of placental oxygen supply. Thus, embryos and fetuses cannot consciously experience sensations or feeling such as breathlessness or pain, and cannot suffer while dying *in utero* after the death of the dam, whatever the cause of her death. A rather similar, but qualified, conclusion has been drawn regarding the possibility that consciousness may not occur until after hatching in domestic chickens [156].

Low atmospheric pressure stunning

Low atmospheric pressure stunning (LAPS) is a recently described method for stunning poultry prior to humane slaughter. Unconsciousness occurs following a controlled and gradual reduction of barometric pressure due to hypoxia [157,158]. A significant advantage of LAPS over electrical stunning and 'live-dump' controlled atmosphere stunning (CAS) using gas is elimination of welfare issues associated with dumping live birds onto the conveyor line, and eliminating the need to handle live birds manually. The European Union allows the use of a vacuum chamber for slaughter of the farmed quail, partridge, and pheasant [159] and the method is currently undergoing commercial testing for broiler stunning in the United States under a USDA Office of New Technology Testing Approval.

Rapid decompression is currently deemed 'unacceptable' for euthanasia [8]. LAPS is not rapid decompression, but rather negative atmospheric pressure applied gradually over time, typically over 1 min in broilers, which results in an acute hypoxic state not unlike being in an unpressurized airplane at altitude. Maximum observed negative pressure during commercial broiler LAPS corresponds to an estimated atmospheric pressure of 156 mmHg and inspired PO_2 of 33 mmHg (R.E. Meyer, personal observation at OK Foods, Fort Smith, AR, USA, 8 March 2012). Thus, LAPS PO_2 at maximum negative pressure is equivalent to a 4% oxygen atmosphere at sea level (33 mmHg/760 mmHg). For comparison, the atmospheric pressure (P_B) on top of Mount Everest (elevation approximately 29 000 ft) is 225 mmHg and the PO_2 is 47 mmHg; at 40 000 ft, P_B is 141 mmHg and PO_2 is 30 mmHg.

Rapid decompression can cause both pain and distress through expansion of gases present in enclosed spaces [160]. In the case of birds, however, gases are unlikely to be trapped in the lungs or abdomen during LAPS, and are therefore unlikely to become a source of abdominal distention, due to the unique anatomic structure of the avian respiratory system. Avian lungs are open at both ends, rigid, attached to the ribs, and do not change size during ventilation. Attached to the lungs are nine air sacs that fill all spaces within the thoracic and abdominal cavities. Because birds lack a diaphragm, they move air in and out during sternal movement using the intercostal and abdominal muscles; air movement is simultaneous and continuous with no passive or relaxed period. Hence it is unlikely that significant amounts of gas can be trapped within the avian lungs or abdomen unless the trachea was blocked for some reason [161]. In contrast to reports of hemorrhagic lesions in the lungs, brain, and heart of animals undergoing rapid decompression [162], no such lesions were observed in birds undergoing LAPS [158]. Corticosterone concentrations in LAPS-stunned broilers were nearly half the levels observed in electrically stunned birds [158].

During commercial operation, birds undergoing LAPS remain within palletized shipping cages. Following the LAPS cycle, the palletized cages containing unconscious birds are moved to the dumping station and moved by conveyor belt to the shackling area prior to entry to the processing line. LAPS target pressures for broilers are achieved within 1 min from the start of the LAPS cycle and maintained for 4 min 40 s to assure that recovery to consciousness does not occur prior to exsanguination [158]. Time to first coordinated animal movement was 58.7 ± 3.0 s, with 'light-headedness' (defined as time from first head movement to first wing flap) noted within 69.3 ± 6.4 s; LOP occurred within 64.9 ± 6.1 s. Wing and leg paddling was infrequent, lasting 15.1 ± 1.1 s following LOP. Neither mandibulation (movements of the beak as if the bird was responding to sensations in the mouth) nor deep open-bill breathing was observed in LAPS birds; bill breathing and mandibulation are commonly reported during controlled atmosphere stunning with various gas mixtures [163]. Based on EEG studies, increasing slow (delta) wave activity consistent with a gradual loss of consciousness occurs within 10 s of the start of the LAPS cycle, peaking between 30 and 40 s and coincident with LOP and first brief movements [164]. The same group also determined that heart rate decreases over time during LAPS, implying minimal additional sympathetic nervous system stimulation, and concluded that LAPS is a humane approach that can potentially improve the welfare of poultry at slaughter by inducing unconsciousness without distress, eliminating live shackling, and ensuring that every bird is adequately stunned before exsanguination [164].

Foam depopulation

Foam depopulation methods were initially developed as an alternative to modified atmosphere depopulation methods for floor-raised poultry [165]. Advantages of foam over other depopulation methods include reduced overall time required to depopulate farms, reduced number of workers required and their potential exposure to zoonotic diseases, less physical activity while wearing personal protective equipment, suppression of airborne particulates, enhancement of carcass disposal using in-house composting, and greater flexibility of use in various style poultry houses, including those structurally damaged [166].

Foam depopulation uses medium- or high-expansion foam-generating equipment to create a blanket of water-based foam to cover the animals. Most current foam depopulation equipment uses compressed or ambient air to create the bubbles. Immersion in the foam produces rapid airway blockage and occlusion, resulting in death by suffocation. Water-based foam requires less time to death than CO_2 gas, with similar pretreatment and post-mortem corticosterone levels [165]. Based on cessation of EEG activity, water-based foam was as consistent as CO_2 gas, and more consistent than a 70% Ar–30% CO_2 gas mix [167]; EEG cessation time with ambient air-foam was not statistically different from that for CO_2-filled foam [165]. Foam is also an effective depopulation tool for chukar partridges, quail, ducks, and turkeys [168].

Water-based foam depopulation for poultry was conditionally approved in 2006 by the United States Department of Agriculture Animal and Plant Health Service (USDA APHIS). The use of foam is not an AVMA-approved method of euthanasia [8], but the AVMA has issued policy statements indicating that it 'supports the use of water-based foam as a method of mass depopulation in accord with the conditions and performance standards outlined by the USDA APHIS' [14]. The use of foam is conditionally approved for situations in which animals are (1) infected with a potentially zoonotic disease, (2) experiencing an outbreak of a rapidly spreading infectious disease that cannot be easily contained, or (3) housed in structurally unsound buildings.

Raj and co-workers [169] raised animal welfare concerns because water-based foam filled with ambient air produces airway occlusion, a form of suffocation; they proposed increasing bubble size as a means to reduce airway occlusion in addition to incorporating an inert gas in the foam to produce unconsciousness prior to death. Gerritzen and co-workers evaluated responses of broilers, ducks, and turkeys to CO_2-filled foam and N_2-filled foam [170]. Exposure of poultry to CO_2-filled foam resulted in an earlier induction of a transitional state of the EEG than when exposed to N_2-filled foam; the effect of CO_2 on consciousness started before the birds were submerged. After submersion, there was no difference in reduction of conscious state between CO_2- and N_2-filled foam, and it was concluded that the anoxic effects of both gas-filled foams were comparable and acceptable, with the warning that birds submerged under the leading edge of the foam with a height less than 80 cm are likely to be at risk of compromised welfare in the event of technical failure of the foam system. High-expansion nitrogen-filled foam is currently being investigated within the European Union as a means to perform pig welfare culls under European Council Regulation No. 1099/2009 [171].

Agent purity and euthanasia

The Office for Laboratory Animal Welfare (OLAW) and the USDA provide guidance on the use of non-pharmaceutical-grade substances. Both OLAW and USDA agree that pharmaceutical-grade chemicals and other substances, when available, must be used to avoid toxicity or side-effects that may threaten the health and welfare of vertebrate animals or interfere with the interpretation of research results. However, the decision to use non-pharmaceutical-grade substances rests with the Institutional Animal Care Committee [172]. OLAW, together with USDA and the International Association for the Assessment and Accreditation of Laboratory Animal Care (AAALAC), offers guidance on this issue [173]. Basically, the highest grade equivalent chemical reagent should be used if no equivalent veterinary or human drug is available for experimental use.

In the case of inhaled gases, industrial or food grades may be of similar or higher purity than medical grades. The federal government technical and USP specifications for CO_2 are detailed in BB-C-101D [174]. Grade A CO_2 is defined by BB-C-101D as conforming to the requirements of the US Pharmacopeia/National Formulary (USP/NF), whereas Grade B CO_2 is defined as having purity of no less than 99.5 vol.%. Grade A gases are manufactured under certified Good Manufacturing Practices (cGMP) as defined by federal statute 21 CFR 211.84 and meet the applicable specifications of the USP/NF, which include a certificate of analysis, validated analytical procedures, lot number assignment, traceability, and recall procedures [175]. Industrial grade gases generally do not have these cGMP attributes. Users wishing to substitute Grade B or industrial-grade gases will need to confirm with their gas supplier that product purity is equivalent to or greater than the corresponding medical or Grade A product.

Euthanasia in the clinical setting

Barbiturates and barbituric acid derivatives (e.g., sodium pentobarbital, secobarbital, pentobarbital combination products), administered IV, are acceptable for euthanasia of conscious animals [8]. These agents can be administered as the sole agent, or as a second step following sedation or general anesthesia. With the exception of IM delivery of select injectable anesthetics (e.g., an α_2-agonist combined with ketamine), the subcutaneous, intramuscular, intrapulmonary, and intrathecal routes of administration are unacceptable for administration of injectable euthanasia agents because of the limited information available regarding their effectiveness and the high probability of pain associated with injection in awake animals [8].

When IV access would be distressful, dangerous, or impractical (e.g., small patient size such as puppies, kittens, small dogs and cats, rodents, non-domestic species, or behavioral considerations for some small exotic mammals and feral domestic animals), barbiturates may be conditionally administered intraperitoneal (e.g., sodium pentobarbital, secobarbital; not pentobarbital combination products as these have only been approved for IV and intracardiac administration). Administration by the IP route has potential for peritoneal irritation and pain and, as noted previously, results in delayed loss of consciousness; hence this route is considered 'acceptable with conditions' by the AVMA [8]. In unconscious or anesthetized animals, intra-organ injections (e.g., intraosseous, intracardiac, intrahepatic, intrasplenic, intrarenal) may be used as an alternative. Intra-organ injections may speed the rate of barbiturate uptake over standard IP injections and, when an owner is present, this approach may be preferred over the IP route [8].

Proper carcass disposal is important, as animals euthanized with barbiturates create risks for scavengers and other animals that may consume portions of the animal's remains; further, renderers may not accept animal remains contaminated with barbiturate residues.

Injectable anesthetic overdose (e.g., combination of ketamine and an α_2-agonist given IV, IP, or IM or propofol given IV) is acceptable for euthanasia when animal size, restraint requirements, or other circumstances indicate that these drugs are the best option. Assurance of death is paramount and may require a second step (e.g., a barbiturate, or additional doses of the anesthetic), or use of an acceptable adjunctive method (e.g., potassium chloride, 1–2 mmol/kg, 75–150 mg/kg, or 1–2 mEq K^+/kg, administered IV or IC) [8]. Potassium chloride or a saturated magnesium sulfate solution can only be used adjunctively to euthanize unconscious animals (defined as unresponsive to noxious stimuli) or under general anesthesia [8].

Alternatives to barbiturates for euthanasia include T-61 and Tributame™. T-61 is acceptable as an agent of euthanasia, provided that it is administered appropriately by trained individuals. Slow IV injection is necessary to avoid muscular paralysis prior to unconsciousness. Administration of T-61 by routes other than IV is unacceptable [8]. T-61 is not currently being manufactured in the United States but is obtainable from Canada. Tributame, although not currently in production in the United States, is also an acceptable euthanasia drug for dogs provided that it is administered IV by an appropriately trained individual at recommended dosages and at proper injection rates. If barbiturates are not available, its extra-label use in cats may be considered; however, adverse reactions, such as agonal breathing, have been reported and the current FDA-approved Tributame label recommends against its use in cats. Routes of Tributame administration other than IV injection are not acceptable [8].

References

1 Arluke, A. Trapped in a guilt cage. *New Sci Publ* 1992; **134**: 33–35.

2 Whiting TL, Marion CR. Perpetration-induced traumatic stress – a risk for veterinarians involved in the destruction of healthy animals. *Can Vet J* 2011; **52**: 794–796.

3 American Veterinary Medical Association. *Veterinarian's Oath*, 2013. https://www.avma.org/KB/Policies/Pages/veterinarians-oath.aspx (accessed 30 April 2013).

4 Rollin BE. The use and abuse of Aesculapian authority in veterinary medicine. *J Am Vet Med Assoc* 2002; **220**: 1144–1149.

5 Rollin BE. Euthanasia and the quality of life. *J Am Vet Med Assoc* 2006; **228**: 1014–1016.

6 Carter HE. Historical cases. *J Small Anim Pract* 1984; **25**: 31–35.

7 Alkire MT. General anesthesia. In: Banks WP, ed. *Encyclopedia of Consciousness*. Oxford: Elsevier/Academic Press, 2009; 296–313.

8 American Veterinary Medical Association. *AVMA Guidelines for the Euthanasia of Animals*, 2013. https://www.avma.org/KB/Policies/Pages/Euthanasia-Guidelines.aspx (accessed 30 April 2013).

9 Canadian Council on Animal Care. *CCAC Guidelines on: Euthanasia of Animals Used in Science*, 2010. http://www.ccac.ca/Documents/Standards/Guidelines/Euthanasia.pdf (accessed 30 April 2013).

10 OIE – World Organisation for Animal Health. *OIE's Achievements in Animal Welfare*, 2013 http://www.oie.int/animal-welfare/animal-welfare-key-themes/ (accessed 30 April 2013).

11 McMillan FD. Rethinking euthanasia: death as an unintentional outcome. *J Am Vet Med Assoc* 2001; **219**: 1204–1206.

12 Pavlovic D, Spassov A, Lehmann C. Euthanasia: in defense of a good, ancient word. *J Clin Res Bioeth* 2011; **2**: 105.

13 United States Code. 7 USC Chapter 48 – *Humane Methods of Livestock Slaughter*. http://uscode.house.gov/view.xhtml?req=granuleid%3AUSC-prelim-title7-chapter48&edition=prelim (accessed 20 November 2014).

14 American Veterinary Medical Association. *Poultry Depopulation*, 2013. https://www.avma.org/KB/Policies/Pages/Poultry-Depopulation.aspx (accessed 30 April 2013).

15 International Association for the Study of Pain. *IASP Terms*. http://www.iasp-pain.org/Education/Content.aspx?ItemNumber=1698&navItemNumber=576#Pain (accessed 20 November 2014).

16 Alkire MT, Hudetz AG, Tononi G. Consciousness and anesthesia. *Science* 2008; **322**:876–880.

17 Långsjö JW, Alkire MT, Kaskinoro K, *et al*. Returning from oblivion: imaging the neural core of consciousness. *J Neurosci* 2012; **32**: 4935–4943.

18 Hendrickx JF, Eger EI II, Sonner JM, *et al*. Is synergy the rule? A review of anesthetic interactions producing hypnosis and immobility. *Anesth Analg* 2008; **107**: 494–506.

19 Antognini JF, Barter L, Carstens E. Overview: movement as an index of anesthetic depth in humans and experimental animals. *Comp Med* 2005; **55**: 413–418.

20 Zeller, W, Mettler D, Schatzmann U. Untersuchungen zur Betäubung des Schlachtgeflügels mit Kohlendioxid. *Fleischwirtschaft* 1988; **68**: 1308–1312 (as cited in Raj ABM, Gregory NG. Effect of rate of induction of carbon dioxide anaesthesia on the time of onset of unconsciousness and convulsions. *Res Vet Sci*. 1990; **49**: 360–363).

21 McKeegan DEF, Sparks NHC, Sandilands V, *et al*. Physiological responses of laying hens during whole-house killing with carbon dioxide. *Br Poult Sci* 2011; **52**: 645–657.

22 Benson ER, Alphin RL, Rankin MK, *et al*. Evaluation of EEG based determination of unconsciousness vs. loss of posture in broilers. *Res Vet Sci* 2012; **93**: 960–964.

23 Muir WW. Considerations for general anesthesia. In: Tranquilli WJ, Thurmon JC, Grimm KA, eds. *Lumb and Jones' Veterinary Anesthesia and Analgesia*, 4th edn. Ames, IA: Blackwell Publishing, 2007; 7–30.

24 Erhardt W, Ring C, Kraft H, *et al*. CO_2 stunning of swine for slaughter from the anesthesiological viewpoint. *Dtsch Tierarztl Wochenschr* 1989; **96**: 92–99.

25 Dyakonova VE. Role of opioid peptides in behavior of invertebrates. *J Evol Biochem Physiol* 2001; **37**: 335–347.

26 Sladky KK, Kinney ME, Johnson SM. Analgesic efficacy of butorphanol and morphine in bearded dragons and corn snakes. *J Am Vet Med Assoc* 2008; **233**: 267–273.

27 Baker BB, Sladky KK, Johnson SM. Evaluation of the analgesic effects of oral and subcutaneous tramadol administration in red eared slider turtles. *J Am Vet Med Assoc* 2011; **238**: 220–227.

28 Rose JD. The neurobehavioral nature of fishes and the question of awareness and pain. *Rev Fish Sci* 2002; **10**: 1–38.

29 Nordgreen J, Horsberg TE, Ranheim B, *et al*. Somatosensory evoked potentials in the telencephalon of Atlantic salmon (*Salmo salar*) following galvanic stimulation of the tail. *J Comp Physiol A Neuroethol Sens Neural Behav Physiol* 2007; **193**: 1235–1242.

30 Dunlop R, Laming P. Mechanoreceptive and nociceptive responses in the central nervous system of goldfish (*Carassius auratus*) and trout (*Oncorhynchus mykiss*). *J Pain* 2005; **6**: 561–568.

31 Braithwaite VA. Cognition in fish. *Behav Physiol Fish* 2006; **24**: 1–37.

32 Finnie JW. Neuropathologic changes produced by non-penetrating percussive captive bolt stunning of cattle. *N Z Vet J* 1995; **43**: 183–185.

33 Blackmore DK, Newhook JC. The assessment of insensibility in sheep, calves and pigs during slaughter. In: Eikelenboom G. ed. *Stunning of Animals for Slaughter*. Boston: Martinus Nijhoff Publishers, 1983: 13–25.

34 Gregory NG. Animal welfare at markets and during transport and slaughter. *Meat Sci* 2008; **80**: 2–11.

35 Gregory NG, Lee JL, Widdicombe JP. Depth of concussion in cattle shot by penetrating captive bolt. *Meat Sci* 2007; **77**: 499–503.

36 Vogel KD, Badtram G, Claus JR, *et al*. Head-only followed by cardiac arrest electrical stunning is an effective alternative to head-only electrical stunning in pigs. *J Anim Sci* 2011; **89**: 1412–1418.

37 Blackmore DK, Newhook JC. Electroencephalographic studies of stunning and slaughter of sheep and calves. 3. The duration of insensibility induced by electrical stunning in sheep and calves. *Meat Sci* 1982; **7**: 19–28.

38 Cartner SC, Barlow SC, Ness TJ. Loss of cortical function in mice after decapitation, cervical dislocation, potassium chloride injection, and CO_2 inhalation. *Comp Med* 2007; **57**: 570–573.

39 Close B, Banister K, Baumans V, *et al*. Recommendations for euthanasia of experimental animals: Part 2. DGXI of the European Commission. *Lab Anim* 1997; **31**: 1–32.

40 Close B, Banister K, Baumans V, *et al*. Recommendations for euthanasia of experimental animals: Part 1. DGXI of the European Commission. *Lab Anim* 1996; **30**: 293–316.

41 Gregory NG, Wotton SB. Effect of slaughter on the spontaneous and evoked activity of the brain. *Br Poult Sci* 1986; **27**: 195–205.

42 Bates G. Humane issues surrounding decapitation reconsidered. *J Am Vet Med Assoc* 2010; **237**: 1024–1026.

43 Holson RR. Euthanasia by decapitation: evidence that this technique produces prompt, painless unconsciousness in laboratory rodents. *Neurotoxicol Teratol* 1992; **14**: 253–257.

44 Derr RF. Pain perception in decapitated rat brain. *Life Sci* 1991; **49**: 1399–1402.

45 Vanderwolf CH, Buzak DP, Cain RK, *et al*. Neocortical and hippocampal electrical activity following decapitation in the rat. *Brain Res* 1988; **451**: 340–344.

46 Mikeska JA, Klemm WR. EEG evaluation of humaneness of asphyxia and decapitation euthanasia of the laboratory rat. *Lab Anim Sci* 1975; **25**: 175–179.

47 van Rijn CM, Krijnen H, Menting-Hermeling S, Coenen AM. Decapitation in rats: latency to unconsciousness and the 'wave of death'. *PLoS ONE* 2011; **6**: e16514

48 Martoft L, Lomholt L, Kolthoff C, *et al*. Effects of CO_2 anaesthesia on central nervous system activity in swine. *Lab Anim* 2002; **36**: 115–126.

49 Raj ABM, Johnson SP, Wotton SB, *et al*. Welfare implications of gas stunning pigs. 3. The time to loss of somatosensory evoked potentials and spontaneous electrocorticogram of pigs during exposure to gases. *Vet J* 1997; **153**: 329–339.

50 Ring C, Erhardt W, Kraft H, *et al*. CO_2 anaesthesia of slaughter pigs. *Fleischwirtschaft* 1988; **68**: 1304–1307.

51 Forslid A. Transient neocortical, hippocampal, and amygdaloid EEG silence induced by one minute inhalation of high CO_2 concentration in swine. *Acta Physiol Scand* 1987; **130**: 1–10.

52 Brosnan RJ, Pham TL. Carbon dioxide negatively modulates *N*-methyl-D-aspartate receptors. *Br J Anaesth* 2008; **101**: 673–679.

53 Raj M. Humane killing of nonhuman animals for disease control purposes. *J Appl Anim Welf Sci* 2008; **11**: 112–124.

54 Raj ABM, Gregory NG. Welfare implications of the gas stunning of pigs: 1. Determination of aversion to the initial inhalation of carbon dioxide or argon. *Anim Welf* 1995; **4**: 273–280.

55 Raj ABM. Behaviour of pigs exposed to mixtures of gases and the time required to stun and kill them: welfare implications. *Vet Rec* 1999; **144**: 165–168.

56 Dalmau A, Rodriguez P, Llonch P, *et al*. Stunning pigs with different gas mixtures: aversion in pigs. *Anim Welf* 2010; **19**: 325–333.

57 Steffey EP, Mama KR. Inhalation anesthetics. In: Tranquilli WJ, Thurmon JC, Grimm KA, eds. *Lumb and Jones' Veterinary Anesthesia and Analgesia*, 4th edn. Ames, IA: Blackwell Publishing, 2007; 355–393.
58 Thomas AA, Flecknell PA, Golledge HD. Combining nitrous oxide with carbon dioxide decreases the time to loss of consciousness during euthanasia in mice – refinement of animal welfare? *PLoS One* 2012; **7**: e32290.
59 Meyer RE, Morrow WEM. Carbon dioxide for emergency on-farm euthanasia of swine. *J Swine Health Prod* 2005; **13**: 210–217.
60 Meyer R.E. Principles of carbon dioxide displacement. *Lab Anim* 2008; **37**: 241–242.
61 Stikeleather LF, Morrow WEM, Meyer RE, *et al.* CFD Simulation of gas mixing for evaluation of design alternatives for on-farm mass-depopulation of swine in a disease emergency. Technical Presentation 121338237, American Society of Agricultural and Biological Engineers, Dallas, TX, 29 July–1 August 2012. http://elibrary.asabe.org/azdez.asp?JID=5&AID=41889&CID=dall2012&T=1 (accessed 2 May 2013).
62 Cavanna AE, Shah, S, Eddy CM, *et al.* Consciousness: a neurological perspective. *Behav Neurol* 2011; **24**: 107–116.
63 Reilly JS. ed. *Euthanasia of Animals Used for Scientific Purposes*. Adelaide, SA: Australia and New Zealand Council for the Care of Animals in Research and Teaching, Department of Environmental Biology, Adelaide University, 2001.
64 Murray MJ. Euthanasia. In: Lewbart GA, ed. *Invertebrate Medicine*. Ames, IA: Blackwell Publishing, 2006; 303–304.
65 Messenger JB, Nixon M, Ryan KP. Magnesium chloride as an anaesthetic for cephalopods. *Comp Biochem Physiol C* 1985; **82**: 203–205.
66 Meyer RE, Morrow WEM. Euthanasia. In: Rollin BE, Benson GJ, eds. *Improving the Well-being of Farm Animals: Maximizing Welfare and Minimizing Pain and Suffering*. Ames, IA: Blackwell Publishing, 2004; 351–362.
67 Breazile JE, Kitchell RL. Euthanasia for laboratory animals. *Fed Proc* 1969; **28**: 1577–1579.
68 McMillan FD. Comfort as the primary goal in veterinary medical practice. *J Am Vet Med Assoc* 1998; **212**: 1370–1374.
69 Valentine H, Williams WO, Maurer KJ. Sedation or inhalant anesthesia before euthanasia with CO_2 does not reduce behavioral or physiologic signs of pain and stress in mice. *J Am Assoc Lab Anim Sci* 2012; **51**: 50–57.
70 Sharp J, Azar T, Lawson D. Comparison of carbon dioxide, argon, and nitrogen for inducing unconsciousness or euthanasia of rats. *J Am Assoc Lab Anim Sci* 2006; **45**: 21–25.
71 Barton Gade P, Christensen L. *Transportation and Pre-stun Handling: CO_2 Systems*. Danish Meat Research Institute, 2002. www.butina.eu/fileadmin/user_upload/images/articles/transport.pdf (accessed 30 April 2013).
72 Burkholder TH, Niel L, Weed JL, *et al.* Comparison of carbon dioxide and argon euthanasia: effects on behavior, heart rate, and respiratory lesions in rats. *J Am Assoc Lab Anim Sci.* 2010; **49**: 448–453.
73 Herman JP, Cullinan WE. Neurocircuitry of stress: central control of the hypothalamo-pituitary-adrenocortical axis. *Trends Neurosci* 1997; **20**: 78–84.
74 Barklin A, Larsson A, Vestergaard C, *et al.* Does brain death induce a pro-inflammatory response at the organ level in a porcine model? *Acta Anaesthesiol Scand* 2008; **52**: 621–627.
75 Chiari P, Hadour G, Michel P, *et al.* Biphasic response after brain death induction: prominent part of catecholamines release in this phenomenon. *J Heart Lung Transplant* 2000; **19**: 675–682.
76 Licker M, Schweizer A, Hohn L, Morel DR. Haemodynamic and metabolic changes induced by repeated episodes of hypoxia in pigs. *Acta Anaesthesiol Scand* 1998; **42**: 957–965.
77 Forslid A, Augustinsson O. Acidosis, hypoxia and stress hormone release in response to one minute inhalation of 80% CO_2 in swine. *Acta Physiol Scand* 1988; **132**: 222–231.
78 Borovsky V, Herman M, Dunphy G, *et al.* CO_2 asphyxia increases plasma norepinephrine in rats via sympathetic nerves. *Am J Physiol* 1998; **274**: R19–R22.
79 Reed B, Varon J, Chait BT, *et al.* Carbon dioxide-induced anesthesia results in a rapid increase in plasma levels of vasopressin. *Endocrinology* 2009; **150**: 2934–2939.
80 Kc P, Haxhiu MA, Trouth CO, *et al.* CO_2-induced c-Fos expression in hypothalamic vasopressin containing neurons. *Resp Physiol* 2002; **129**: 289–296.
81 Morrow WEM, Meyer R, Whitley J, *et al.* Pre- and post-euthanasia concentrations of cortisol, norepinephrine and lactate in pigs. In: *Proceedings, American Association of Swine Veterinarians 2013 Annual Meeting, 2-5 March 2013, San Diego, CA*: **399**.
82 Meyer RE, Morrow WEM, Stikeleather LF, *et al.* Time to loss of consciousness using CO_2 or 70% N_2/30% CO_2 for pig euthanasia. In: *Proceedings, American Association of Swine Veterinarians 2013 Annual Meeting, 2-5 March 2013, San Diego, CA*: **47**.
83 Webster AB, Collett SR. A mobile modified-atmosphere killing system for small-flock depopulation. *J Appl Poult Res* 2012; **21**: 131–144.
84 Mashour GA, Orser BA, Avidan MS. Intraoperative awareness – from neurobiology to clinical practice. *Anesthesiology* 2011; **114**: 1218–1233.
85 Hawkins P, Playle L, Golledge H, *et al.* *Newcastle Consensus Meeting on Carbon Dioxide Euthanasia of Laboratory Animals*. Available at: http://www.academia.edu/3320424/Newcastle_concensus_meeting_on_carbon_dioxide_euthanasia_of_laboratory_animals (accessed 20 November 2014).
86 Crosby G, Culley D. Processed electroencephalogram and depth of anesthesia: window to nowhere or into the brain? *Anesthesiology* 2012; **116**: 235–237.
87 Hudetz AG, Vizuete JA, Imas OA. Desflurane selectively suppresses long-latency cortical neuronal response to flash in the rat. *Anesthesiology* 2009; **111**: 231–239.
88 Imas OA, Ropella KM, Ward BD, *et al.* Volatile anesthetics enhance flash-induced gamma oscillations in rat visual cortex. *Anesthesiology* 2005; **102**: 937–947.
89 Barr G, Anderson RE, Jakobsson JG. A study of bispectral analysis and auditory evoked potential indices during propofol-induced hypnosis in volunteers: the effect of an episode of wakefulness on explicit and implicit memory. *Anaesthesia* 2001; **56**: 888–893.
90 Baudelet C, Gallez B. Effect of anesthesia on the signal intensity in tumors using BOLD-MRI: comparison with flow measurements by laser Doppler flowmetry and oxygen measurements by luminescence-based probes. *Magn Reson Imaging* 2004; **22**: 905–912.
91 Steward CA, Marsden CA, Prior MJW, *et al.* Methodological considerations in rat brain BOLD contrast pharmacological MRI. *Psychopharmacology* 2005; **180**: 687–704.
92 Arluke A. Uneasiness among laboratory technicians. *Occup Med* 1999; **14**: 305–316.
93 Matthis JS. *Selected Employee Attributes and Perceptions Regarding Methods and Animal Welfare Concerns Associated with Swine Euthanasia*. Dissertation submitted to the Graduate Faculty of North Carolina State University in partial fulfillment of the requirements for the degree of Doctor of Education, Occupational Education, Raleigh, NC, 2004.
94 Chorney JM, Kain ZN. Behavioral analysis of children's response to induction of anesthesia. *Anesth Analg* 2009; **109**: 1434–1440.
95 Przybylo HJ, Tarbell SE, Stevenson GW. Mask fear in children presenting for anesthesia: aversion, phobia, or both? *Paediatr Anaesth* 2005; **15**: 366–370.
96 Interagency Research Animal Committee. *U.S. Government Principles for the Utilization and Care of Vertebrate Animals Used in Testing, Research and Training*, 2002. http://grants.nih.gov/grants/olaw/references/phspol.htm#USGovPrinciples. (accessed 30 April 2013).
97 Branson KR. Injectable and alternative anesthetic techniques. In: Tranquilli WJ, Thurmon JC, Grimm KA, eds. *Lumb and Jones' Veterinary Anesthesia and Analgesia*, 4th edn. Ames, IA: Blackwell Publishing, 2007; 273–299.
98 Price HL. The pharmacodynamics of thiobarbiturates. In: Soma LR, ed. *Textbook of Veterinary Anesthesiology*. Baltimore: Williams & Wilkins, 1971; 105–110.
99 Hall LW, Clarke KW. Anaesthesia of the dog. In: Hall LW, Clarke KW, eds. *Veterinary Anaesthesia*, 8th edn. London: Baillière Tindall, 1983; 305–340.
100 Field KJ, While WJ, Lang CM. Anaesthetic effects of chloral hydrate, pentobarbitone and urethane in adult male rats *Lab Anim* 1993; **27**: 258–269.
101 Haberham ZL, van den Brom WE, Venker-van Haagen AJ, *et al.* EEG evaluation of reflex testing as assessment of depth of pentobarbital anaesthesia in the rat. *Lab Anim* 1999; **33**: 47–57.
102 Grier RL, Schaffer CB. Evaluation of intraperitoneal and intrahepatic administration of a euthanasia agent in animal shelter cats. *J Am Vet Med Assoc* 1990; **197**: 1611–1615.
103 Svendsen O, Kok L, Lauritzen B. Nociception after intraperitoneal injection of a sodium pentobarbitone formulation with and without lidocaine in rats quantified by expression of neuronal c-fos in the spinal cord – a preliminary study. *Lab Anim* 2007; **41**: 197–203.
104 Walker B, Jäggin N, Doherr M, *et al.* Inhalation anaesthesia for castration of newborn piglets: experiences with isoflurane and isoflurane/NO. *J Vet Med A Physiol Pathol Clin Med* 2004; **51**: 150–154.
105 Jäggin N., Kohler I, Blum J, *et al.* Die Kastration von neugeborenen Ferkeln unter Halothananästhesie. *Prakt Tierarzt* 2001; **12**: 1054–1061.
106 Flecknell PA, Roughan JV, Hedenqvist P. Induction of anaesthesia with sevoflurane and isoflurane in the rabbit. *Lab Anim* 1999; **33**: 41–46.
107 Leach MC, Bowell VA, Allan TF, *et al.* Measurement of aversion to determine humane methods of anaesthesia and euthanasia. *Anim Welf* 2004; **13**: S77–S86.
108 Leach MC, Bowell VA, Allan TF, *et al.* Aversion to gaseous euthanasia agents in rats and mice. *Comp Med* 2002; **52**: 249–257.
109 Leach MC, Bowell VA, Allan TF, *et al.* Degrees of aversion shown by rats and mice to different concentrations of inhalational anaesthetics. *Vet Rec* 2002; **150**: 808–815.
110 Makowska LJ, Weary DM. Rat aversion to induction with inhaled anaesthetics. *Appl Anim Behav Sci* 2009; **119**: 229–235.
111 Makowska IJ, Weary DM. Rat aversion to carbon monoxide. *Appl Anim Behav Sci* 2009, **121**: 148–151.

112 Niel L, Weary DM. Behavioural responses of rats to gradual-fill carbon dioxide euthanasia and reduced oxygen concentrations. *Appl Anim Behav Sci* 2006; **100**: 295–308.
113 Hackbarth H, Kuppers N, Bohnet W. Euthanasia of rats with carbon dioxide – animal welfare aspects. *Lab Anim* 2000; **34**: 91–96.
114 Smith W, Harrap SB. Behavioural and cardiovascular responses of rats to euthanasia using carbon dioxide gas. *Lab Anim* 1997; **31**: 337–346.
115 Coenen AML, Drinkenburg W, Hoenderken R, *et al.* Carbon dioxide euthanasia in rats: oxygen supplementation minimizes signs of agitation and asphyxia. *Lab Anim* 1995; **29**: 262–268.
116 Blackshaw JK, Fenwick DC, Beattie AW, *et al.* The behavior of chickens, mice and rats during euthanasia with chloroform, carbon dioxide and ether. *Lab Anim* 1988; **22**: 67–75.
117 Britt DP. The humaneness of carbon dioxide as an agent of euthanasia for laboratory rodents. In: *Euthanasia of Unwanted, Injured or Diseased Animals or for Educational or Scientific Purposes. Proceedings of a Symposium Organized by Universities Federation for Animal Welfare in Association with Humane Slaughter Association, Zoological Society of London, 19th September 1986.* Potters Bar: Universities Federation for Animal Welfare, 1987; 19–31.
118 Hornett TD, Haynes AR Comparison of carbon dioxide/air mixture and nitrogen/air mixture for the euthanasia of rodents. Design of a system for inhalation euthanasia. *Anim Technol* 1984; **35**: 93–99.
119 Jongman EC, Barnett JL, Hemsworth PH. The aversiveness of carbon dioxide stunning in pigs and a comparison of the CO_2 stunner crate vs. the V-restrainer. *Appl Anim Behav Sci* 2000; **67**: 67–76
120 Raj ABM, Gregory NG. Welfare implications of the gas stunning of pigs 2. Stress of induction of anaesthesia. *Anim Welf* 1996; **5**: 71–78.
121 Troeger K, Woltersdorf W. Gas anesthesia of slaughter pigs. 1. Stunning experiments under laboratory conditions with fat pigs of known halothane reaction type – meat quality, animal protection. *Fleischwirtschaft* 1991; **71**: 1063–1068.
122 Dodman NH. Observations on use of Wernberg dip-lift carbon dioxide apparatus for pre-slaughter anesthesia of pigs. *Br Vet J* 1977; **133**: 71–80.
123 Gerritzen M, Lambooij B, Reimert H, *et al.* A note on behaviour of poultry exposed to increasing carbon dioxide concentrations. *Appl Anim Behav Sci* 2007; **108**: 179–185.
124 Gerritzen MS, Lambooij E, Reimert HG, *et al.* Susceptibility of duck and turkey to severe hypercapnic hypoxia. *Poult Sci* 2006; **85**: 1055–1061.
125 McKeegan DEF, McIntyre JA, Demmers TGM, *et al.* Physiological and behavioural responses of broilers to controlled atmosphere stunning: implications for welfare. *Anim Welf* 2007; **16**: 409–426.
126 McKeegan DEF, McIntyre J, Demmers TGM, *et al.* Behavioural responses of broiler chickens during acute exposure to gaseous stimulation. *Appl Anim Behav Sci* 2006; **99**: 271–286.
127 Webster AB, Fletcher DL. Reaction of laying hens and broilers to different gases used for stunning poultry. *Poult Sci* 2001; **80**: 1371–1377.
128 Webster AB, Fletcher DL. Assessment of the aversion of hens to different gas atmospheres using an approach-avoidance test. *Appl Anim Behav Sci* 2004; **88**: 275–287.
129 Abeyesinghe SM, McKeegan DEF, McLeman MA, *et al.* Controlled atmosphere stunning of broiler chickens. I. Effects on behaviour, physiology and meat quality in a pilot scale system at a processing plant. *Br Poult Sci* 2007; **48**: 406–423.
130 Gerritzen MA, Lambooij E, Hillebrand SJW, *et al.* Behavioral responses of broilers to different gaseous atmospheres. *Poult Sci* 2000; **79**: 928–933.
131 Lambooij E, Gerritzen MA, Engel B, *et al.* Behavioural responses during exposure of broiler chickens to different gas mixtures. *Appl Anim Behav Sci* 1999; **62**: 255–265.
132 Raj ABM. Aversive reactions of turkeys to argon, carbon dioxide and a mixture of carbon dioxide and argon. *Vet Rec* 1996; **138**: 592–593.
133 Niel L, Weary DM. Rats avoid exposure to carbon dioxide and argon. *Appl Anim Behav Sci* 2007; **107**: 100–109.
134 Kirkden RD, Niel L, Stewart SA, *et al.* Gas killing of rats: the effect of supplemental oxygen on aversion to carbon dioxide. *Anim Welf* 2008; **17**: 79–87.
135 Cooper J, Mason G, Raj M. Determination of the aversion of farmed mink (*Mustela vison*) to carbon dioxide. *Vet Rec* 1998; **143**: 359–361.
136 Chen XJ, Gallar J, Pozo MA, *et al.* CO_2 stimulation of the cornea – a comparison between human sensation and nerve activity in polymodal nociceptive afferents of the cat. *Eur J Neurosci* 1995; **7**: 1154–1163.
137 Peppel P, Anton F. Responses of rat medullary dorsal horn neurons following intranasal noxious chemical stimulation – effects of stimulus intensity, duration and interstimulus interval. *J Neurophysiol* 1993; **70**: 2260–2275.
138 Thurauf N, Hummel T, Kettenmann B, *et al.* Nociceptive and reflexive responses recorded from the human nasal mucosa. *Brain Res* 1993; **629**: 293–299.
139 Anton F, Peppel P, Euchner I, *et al.* Noxious chemical stimulation – responses of rat trigeminal brain stem neurons to CO_2 pulses applied to the nasal mucosa. *Neurosci Lett* 1991; **123**: 208–211.
140 Feng YW, Simpson TL. Nociceptive sensation and sensitivity evoked from human cornea and conjunctiva stimulated by CO_2. *Invest Ophthalmol Vis Sci* 2003; **44**: 529–532.
141 Thurauf N, Gunther M, Pauli E, *et al.* Sensitivity of the negative mucosal potential to the trigeminal target stimulus CO_2. *Brain Res* 2002; **942**: 79–86.
142 Danneman PJ, Stein S, Walshaw SO. Humane and practical implications of using carbon dioxide mixed with oxygen for anesthesia or euthanasia of rats. *Lab Anim Sci* 1997; **47**: 376–385.
143 Hewett TA, Kovacs MS, Artwohl JE, *et al.* A comparison of euthanasia methods in rats, using carbon dioxide in prefilled and fixed flow-rate filled chambers. *Lab Anim Sci* 1993; **43**: 579–582.
144 Battaglia M, Ogliari A, Harris J, *et al.* A genetic study of the acute anxious response to carbon dioxide stimulation in man. *J Psychiatr Res* 2007; **41**: 906–917.
145 Nardi AE, Freire RC, Zin WA. Panic disorder and control of breathing. *Respir Physiol Neurobiol* 2009; **167**: 133–143.
146 Grandin T. Improving livestock, poultry, and fish welfare in slaughter plants with auditing programmes. In: Grandin T, ed. *Improving Animal Welfare: a Practical Approach.* Wallingford: CAB International, 2010; 160–185.
147 Ziemann AE, Allen JE, Dahdaleh NS, *et al.* The amygdala is a chemosensor that detects carbon dioxide and acidosis to elicit fear behavior. *Cell* 2009; **139**: 1012–1021.
148 Dalmau A, Llonch P, Rodriguez P, *et al.* Stunning pigs with different gas mixtures: gas stability. *Anim Welf* 2010; **19**: 315–323.
149 Wong D, Makowska IJ, Weary DM. Rat aversion to isoflurane versus carbon dioxide. *Biol Lett* 2013; **9**(1): 20121000.
150 Lockwood G. Theoretical context-sensitive elimination times for inhalational anaesthetics. *Br J Anaesth* 2010; **104**: 648–655.
151 Mellor DJ, Diesch TJ. Onset of sentience: the potential for suffering in fetal and newborn farm animals. *Appl Anim Behav Sci* 2006; **100**: 48–57.
152 Mellor DJ. Galloping colts, fetal feelings, and reassuring regulations: putting animal-welfare science into practice. *J Vet Med Educ* 2010; **37**: 94–100.
153 Mellor DJ, Diesch TJ, Johnson CB. Should mammalian fetuses be excluded from regulations protecting animals during experiments? Proceedings of the 7th World Congress on Alternatives and Animal Use in the Life Sciences 2010. *ALTEX* 2010; **27**(Special Issue): 199–202.
154 Mellor D J, Diesch T J, Johnson CB. When do mammalian young become sentient? Proceedings of the 7th World Congress on Alternatives and Animal Use in the Life Sciences 2010. *ALTEX* 2010; **27**(Special Issue): 275–280.
155 White SC. Prevention of fetal suffering during ovariohysterectomy of pregnant animals. *J Am Vet Med Assoc* 2012; **240**: 1160–1163.
156 Mellor DJ, Diesch TJ. Birth and hatching: key events in the onset of awareness in the lamb and chick. *N Z Vet.* 2007; **55**: 51–60.
157 Purswell JL, Thaxton JP, Branton SL. Identifying process variables for a low atmospheric pressure stunning–killing system. *J Appl Poult Res* 2007; **16**: 509–513.
158 Vizzier-Thaxton Y, Christensen KD, Schilling MW, *et al.* A new humane method of stunning broilers using low atmospheric pressure. *J Appl Poult Res* 2010; **19**: 341–348.
159 Directorate General, Health and Consumer Protection, European Commission. Council Directive 93/119/EC. *Protection of Animals at the Time of Slaughter or Killing.* Brussels: European Commission, 2003.
160 Booth NH. Effect of rapid decompression and associated hypoxic phenomena in euthanasia of animals: a review. *J Am Vet Med Assoc* 1978; **173**: 308–314.
161 Fedde MR. Relationship of structure and function of the avian respiratory system to disease susceptibility. *Poult Sci* 1998; **77**: 1130–1138.
162 Van Liere EJ. *Anoxia: Its Effect on the Body.* Chicago:University of Chicago Press, 1943.
163 Coenen AML, Lankhaar J, Lowe JC, *et al.* Remote monitoring of electroencephalogram, electrocardiogram, and behavior during controlled atmosphere stunning in broilers: implications for welfare. *Poult Sci* 2009; **88**: 10–19.
164 McKeegan DE, Sandercock DA, Gerritzen MA. Physiological responses to low atmospheric pressure stunning and the implications for welfare. *Poult Sci.* 2013; **92**: 858–868.
165 Benson E, Malone GW, Alphin RL, *et al.* Foam-based mass emergency depopulation of floor-reared meat-type poultry operations. *Poult Sci* 2007; **86**: 219–224.
166 Malone B, Benson E, Alphin B, *et al.* Methods of mass depopulation for poultry flocks with highly infectious disease. In: *Proceedings to ANECA Symposium on Emerging Diseases*, Queretaro, Mexico, November 2007.
167 Alphin RL, Rankin MK, Johnson KJ, *et al.* Comparison of water-based foam and inert-gas mass emergency depopulation methods. *Avian Dis* 2010; **54**(s1):757–762.
168 Benson ER, Alphin RL, Dawson MD, *et al.* Use of water-based foam to depopulate ducks and other species. *Poult Sci* 2009; **88**: 904–910.
169 Raj ABM, Smith C, Hickman G. Novel method for killing poultry in houses with dry foam created using nitrogen. *Vet Rec* 2008; **162**: 722–723.

170 Gerritzen MA, Reimert HGM, Hindle VA, *et al. Welfare Assessment of Gas-filled Foam as an Agent for Killing Poultry*, Wageningen UR Livestock Research Report 399, 2010. http://library.wur.nl/WebQuery/wurpubs/403154 (accessed 29 June 2012).

171 Pig Progress. *Nitrogen Gas Foam for Humane Culling of Pigs*, 2013. http://www.pigprogress.net/Pork-Processing/Slaughtering--Processing/2013/4/Nitrogen-gas-foam-for-humane-culling-of-pigs-1222270W/, 2013 (accessed 1 May 2013).

172 Office of Laboratory Animal Welfare. *Position Statement 3) Non-Pharmaceutical-Grade Substances*, 2012 http://grants.nih.gov/grants/olaw/positionstatement_guide.htm#nonpharma (accessed 1 May 2013).

173 Office of Laboratory Animal Welfare. *OLAW Online Seminars – Seminar Recordings and Reference Materials*, 2014. http://grants.nih.gov/grants/olaw/educational_resources.htm (accessed 1 May 2013).

174 General Services Administration. *Metric BB-C-101D, Federal Specification Carbon Dioxide (CO_2): Technical and USP.* everyspec.com/FED_SPECS/B/download.php?spec=BB-C-101D.031791.PDF (accessed 20 November 2014).

175 Linde. *VERISEQ® Pharmaceutical Grade Gases. Carbon Dioxide*, 2013. http://www.lindeus.com/internet.lg.lg.usa/en/images/VERISEQ_CarbonDioxide138_7034.pdf (accessed 1 May 2013).

SECTION 2

Pharmacology

7 General Pharmacology of Anesthetic and Analgesic Drugs

Ted Whittem, Thierry Beths and Sébastien H. Bauquier
Faculty of Veterinary and Agricultural Sciences, University of Melbourne, Werribee, Victoria, Australia

Chapter contents

Introduction

Anesthesia and pain management are two branches of veterinary clinical medicine that inarguably are inextricably intertwined with clinical pharmacology. A thorough, deep, and workable understanding of the principles of clinical pharmacology is fundamental to successful clinical practice in these disciplines. The primary objective of this chapter is to introduce these fundamental pharmacological concepts as they relate to the practice of anesthesia, and to do so in sufficient detail to provide the basis for which sound clinical decisions can be made, even when specific evidence to support the decision is unavailable or unknown. This chapter also strives to provide the nascent anesthetic scientist with an elementary understanding of some of the commonly used research methods and tools for pharmacokinetic research in veterinary clinical pharmacology.

Classical receptor theory

To allow communication between organs and between cells, the body uses messengers or signals. The role of the biological receptors is to convert signals into different forms of stimuli that will induce a reaction from the cell or organ. The French scientist Claude Bernard (1813–1878) was the first to demonstrate the existence of circulating messengers allowing communication between different parts of the body [1]. This discovery was the prelude to the receptor theory.

A receptor is a component of a cell, usually a protein or glycoprotein, which interacts with the signaling messenger substance. Classically, the signaling messenger substance is called a ligand. Ligands can be, for example, hormones or drugs. The combination of a drug-ligand with its receptor induces pharmacological effects; the initial effect is called the 'action' of the drug whereas succeeding

Veterinary Anesthesia and Analgesia: The Fifth Edition of Lumb and Jones.
Edited by Kurt A. Grimm, Leigh A. Lamont, William J. Tranquilli, Stephen A. Greene and Sheilah A. Robertson.

effects are called drug 'effects' [2]. The relationship between a ligand and its receptor follows the law of mass action:

$$[\mathrm{L}]+[\mathrm{R}] \underset{K_d}{\overset{K_a}{\rightleftharpoons}} [\mathrm{LR}] \tag{7.1}$$

where

$$K_a = \frac{1}{K_d} = \frac{[\mathrm{LR}]}{[\mathrm{L}][\mathrm{R}]}$$

where K_a is the rate constant of association of the ligand with the receptor, K_d is the rate constant of dissociation of the ligand with the receptor, [L] is the concentration of unbound ligand, [R] is the concentration of unbound receptor, and [LR] is the concentration of bound receptors.

Affinity and activity of a ligand

The affinity describes the relationship between a particular receptor and its ligand: from eqn (7.1), if the amount of ligand administered is just enough to occupy 50% of the receptors, then

$$[\mathrm{LR}]=[\mathrm{R}] \xrightarrow{\text{yields}} K_a = \frac{[\mathrm{R}]}{[\mathrm{L}][\mathrm{R}]} \xrightarrow{\text{yields}} K_a = \frac{1}{[\mathrm{L}]} \tag{7.2}$$

A high K_a (and a low K_d) implies that at equilibrium the number of unbound ligand molecules is low, showing a high affinity of the ligand for the receptor. Conversely, a low K_a (and a high K_d) indicates a poor affinity of the ligand for the receptor. However, a ligand can have a strong affinity to a receptor without producing an effect. The activity will describe the ability of a ligand to induce an action. For example, the mu (μ) and kappa (κ) opioid receptors are the main opioid receptors involved in opioid modulation of pain. Buprenorphine is classified as a partial μ-opioid agonist. It has a high affinity for the μ-opioid receptor and as a consequence its effects, although moderate, are difficult to antagonize [3]. Butorphanol is classified as an agonist–antagonist opioid [2]. It produces its effect by activating the κ-opioid receptors and also binds to μ-opioid receptors. However, even though butorphanol has a strong affinity for the μ-opioid receptors, it is unable to activate them and will cause no action from the association with those receptors.

Selectivity and specificity of a ligand

The selectivity of a ligand determines its capacity to produce a particular effect. A highly selective drug will only produce one effect through activity at only one class or subclass of receptor. Dopamine is a catecholamine that produces different cardiovascular effects at different doses; when given at a relatively low dose, it will increase myocardial contractility (β-adrenergic receptor mediated); however, when the dose is increased, dopamine will induce some peripheral vasoconstriction (α-adrenergic receptor mediated). This lack of selectivity occurs because dopamine acts as a ligand at different subclasses of adrenergic receptors with varying affinity. In contrast, dobutamine is a more selective catecholamine (β-adrenergic receptor mediated only) and its main effect will be to increase myocardial contractility without inducing major peripheral vasoconstriction [4].

The specificity of a ligand describes its capacity to associate with only one specific type of receptor. The effects of a highly specific ligand can be numerous but are due to only one type of receptor–ligand interaction. For example, atropine associates with one specific type of receptor even though these receptors are present in different tissues and the effects are diverse [5]. In comparison, inhalant anesthetics will interact with several different receptors to induce their broad effect, unconsciousness [6].

Assessment of the ligand–receptor interaction

It can be difficult to assess directly the interaction of a receptor with its ligand by observing the number of bound or unbound receptors or even by looking at drug action. As a consequence, investigators often measure the effects of the drugs to try to quantify the receptor occupancy. The effect of the drug is proportional to the concentration of ligand molecules available to bind, which is a function of the dose and method of administration of the ligand, physicochemical and pharmacokinetic properties of the ligand, and location of the receptor. Delays from dosing to onset of pharmacological effects are common and are often referred to as the lag time. The delays can be due to the relative difficulty of a ligand reaching the receptor (pharmacokinetics) or can be due to post-transduction delay (pharmacodynamics). For example, glucocorticoid receptors are nuclear receptors which, when not bound to a ligand such as cortisol or another glucocorticoid, are located in the cytosol. Once activated by ligand binding, the glucocorticoid receptor drug complex is actively transported into the nucleus, where it induces the transcription of genes coding for anti-inflammatory proteins and inhibits the transcription of genes usually upregulated by inflammatory mediators [7]. In this case, the onset of activity is post-transduction and the long lag time explains why glucocorticoids fail to show good results as emergency drugs.

Receptor agonists and antagonists: Definition and examples

The term agonist comes from the Greek *agōnistēs*, meaning contestant or champion. An agonist ligand is a ligand that binds to the receptor and usually activates it the same way that endogenous molecules would. An agonist ligand can be a full agonist, fully activating the receptor, or a partial agonist that does not fully activate the receptor and therefore produces a less intense maximum effect (see below). It is unknown why some molecules work as full agonists and others as partial agonists; however, the beginning of the explanation involves the receptor state concept (see below). For example, morphine and buprenorphine are a full μ-opioid agonist and partial μ-opioid agonist, respectively. Accordingly, morphine can provide better analgesic effects than buprenorphine, even though buprenorphine's affinity for the μ-opioid receptors is higher than that of morphine.

A ligand can also be classified as a neutral antagonist. In this case, the ligand will bind to the receptor but will be unable to activate it. No action following the association of the ligand with the receptor will be seen. This association is usually competitive but can also be non-competitive. The competitive inhibition of the receptor can be overcome by administering a large enough amount of an agonist ligand whereas the same action will have no effect if the inhibition is non-competitive.

Reverse agonists are ligands that will activate the receptor but will induce opposite effects to the agonist ligands. Another way to see it is to consider that a receptor has a baseline agonist effect that is not nil, and the administration of the reverse agonist will decrease the baseline effect. The explanation of this phenomenon is based on the receptor state theory discussed below. If the agonist effect is to provide analgesia, the reverse agonist effect will be to increase the sensation of pain.

Flumazenil and Ro 19-4603 are examples of competitive neutral antagonist and reverse agonist, respectively. Mandema *et al.* studied the averaged concentration–EEG effect relationships of all individual rats that had received an intravenous bolus administration of midazolam, flumazenil, or Ro 19-4603. Midazolam was followed by a positive effect whereas flumazenil and Ro 19-4603 were followed by neutral and negative effects, respectively [8].

Confusion between neutral antagonist and reverse agonist can occur when the baseline agonist effect is minimal. Also, the classification of agonist, partial agonist, neutral antagonist, and reverse agonist applies for a ligand in relation to a particular receptor and the overall effect of a drug may be different from the effect expected from its action on a particular receptor. Although naloxone is a well-known opioid antagonist, low doses can induce analgesic effects. The mechanism by which an opioid antagonist can enhance the opioid agonist effect is unknown, although it could be explained by its effects on: increasing the release of endogenous ligands, upregulation of postsynaptic receptors, inhibiting counteraction by Gs proteins, uncoupling of filament A, and attenuating the increase in expression of GFAP [9].

Receptor state theory

The classic receptor theory implies that the receptor is by default in a non-activated form and needs an agonist ligand in order to be activated. Although the non-activated receptor form represents most of the receptors, experiments have shown that without the presence of an agonist ligand some receptors can exist in their activated form. The role of the ligand would then be not to activate the receptor but to stabilize the receptor's activated form. The two major implications of this theory are the existence of a baseline agonist effect for the receptor and the differentiation between antagonist drugs and inverse agonist drugs.

Receptor structure

Receptors are mainly multiprotein entities and so have four levels of structure. The primary structure is a linear sequence of amino acids, the secondary structure is a regular local sub-structure (α-helix or β-sheets), the tertiary structure is the three-dimensional structure of a single peptide molecule, and the quaternary structure is the combination of the multiple tertiary structures of different proteins linked together. All these levels of structure are of particular importance, as a ligand will have to fit with these four levels of structure to be able to associate with and activate the receptor.

The aim of this section is to illustrate the study of receptor structures using a few examples only of receptors that have a particular importance in the field of anesthesia. The discussion will be limited to some membrane receptors, ion channels, and G-protein receptors.

Sodium ion channel

One key role of the sodium channel is to allow the genesis of action potentials [10]. Indeed, sodium channels are voltage-gated ion channels that conduct the sodium cation into the cell, generating an action potential. When the membrane potential equals the resting potential of the cell, the channels are closed. However, as the membrane potential increases, the conformation of the central pore of the channel changes, increasing sodium permeability and allowing influx of sodium ions, and consequently initiating or propagating an action potential. This change of conformation is made possible by the presence of particular transmembrane-spanning segments (α-helices) called voltage sensors.

The sodium channel is constituted from three peptide subunits: one α glycoprotein subunit and two accessory β subunits [10] (Fig. 7.1). The α subunit is composed of four homologous domains and each domain contains six transmembrane-spanning segments. The primary structure of one of these segments includes a high number of positively charged amino acids, and when the membrane potential increases, the positively charged segments move towards the extracellular side of the membrane, changing the conformation of the channel. Although their mechanism of action is not completely understood, the local anesthetics work by blocking these channels, thus preventing the formation of action potentials.

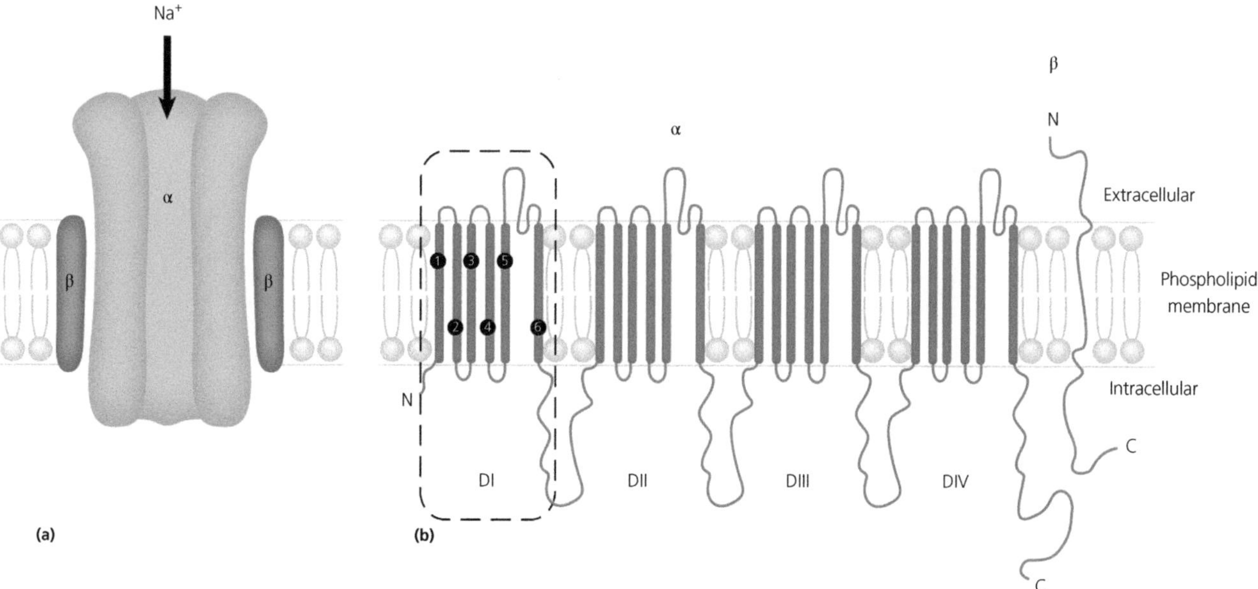

Figure 7.1 Structure of the sodium channel. (a) Schematic of a sodium channel composed of one α subunit and two accessory β subunits. (b) Schematic of the α glycoprotein subunit showing the four homologous domains (DI–DIV) containing six membrane-spanning segments numbered 1–6. The primary structure of segment 4 includes positively charged amino acids placed at every fourth position. When the membrane potential increases, the positively charged segments move towards the extracellular side of the membrane, changing the conformation of the channel and allowing more sodium cations to enter the cell.

GABA Receptors

Activated by the neurotransmitter ligand γ-aminobutyric acid (GABA), the neuroinhibitory GABA receptors ($GABA_A$ and $GABA_B$) are mainly present in the central nervous system in mammals. The $GABA_A$ (fast response) receptors are anion channels whereas the $GABA_B$ (slow response) receptors are G-protein-coupled receptors. Of this ligand's receptor types, only the $GABA_A$ receptor will be addressed here.

$GABA_A$ Receptors

The $GABA_A$ receptors are ligand-gated anion channels that allow the passage of chloride anions into the cell. The hyperpolarization of the neuron following activation of the receptor inhibits subsequent depolarization of the neuron, reducing central nervous system activity. γ-Aminobutyric acid is the main agonist of this receptor. Most of the drugs used in anesthesia that bind to the $GABA_A$ receptor do not directly activate the receptor but induce an allosteric change (i.e., change of the quaternary structure) of the conformation of the receptor and are called allosteric modulators. Barbiturates, benzodiazepines, propofol, etomidate, alfaxalone, inhalant anesthetics, and ethanol are examples of ligands that increase the efficiency of the receptor, allowing greater hyperpolarization of the neuron, and are therefore called positive allosteric modulators [11]. The benzodiazepine reversal agent flumazenil decreases the efficiency of the receptor and is therefore a negative allosteric modulator.

The $GABA_A$ receptor is a heteropentamer (five subunits) comprising α, β, and γ subunits, with many combinations of those subunits being possible [11]. Agonist and antagonist ligands and allosteric modulators bind to specific sites of these subunits as illustrated in Fig. 7.2a. Also, each subunit has four transmembrane-spanning (α-helix) segments creating the chloride channel (Fig. 7.2b).

AMPA and NMDA Receptors

The α-aminohydroxymethylisoxazolepropionic acid (AMPA) and *N*-methyl-D-aspartate (NMDA) receptors are both cation channels. Their endogenous agonist is glutamate [12] and they usually coexist on the same postsynaptic membranes. Their interaction is thought to be one key element of central sensitization.

AMPA Receptor

The AMPA receptor is a ligand-gated ionotropic receptor. This cation channel allows the entry of Na^+ into the cell and the exit of K^+ from the cell. The AMPA receptor is composed of four subunits, with each subunit having four membrane-spanning segments which create the cation channel [12]. Similarly to the $GABA_A$ receptor, the association with an agonist ligand induces a conformation change allowing the channel to open. The amount of glutamate being released in the synapse will dictate the amount of cation transfer, and consequently the degree of depolarization of the postsynaptic neuron induced by the AMPA receptor–ligand interaction.

NMDA Receptor

The NMDA receptor is both a ligand-gated and voltage-gated ionotropic receptor [12] (Fig. 7.3). This cation channel allows the entry of Na^+ and Ca^{2+} into the cell and the exit of K^+ out of the cell. In contrast to the AMPA receptor, a molecule of Mg^{2+} keeps the channel closed until a strong enough depolarization of the postsynaptic membrane occurs. Although weak activation of the AMPA receptor is not sufficient to activate the NMDA receptor, multiple or stronger activation of the AMPA receptor will induce a strong enough depolarization of the postsynaptic membrane to release the Mg^{2+} from inside the channel of the NMDA receptor.

Glutamate and aspartate are the main endogenous agonists for the NMDA receptor and glycine is a co-agonist required to open the channel efficiently. NMDA is a partial agonist and amantidine, gabapentin, ketamine, and phencyclidine derivatives, ethanol, xenon, nitrous oxide, and some opioids (methadone and tramadol) are NMDA receptor antagonists. Magnesium, sodium, calcium, potassium, zinc, and copper are modulators of the NMDA receptor.

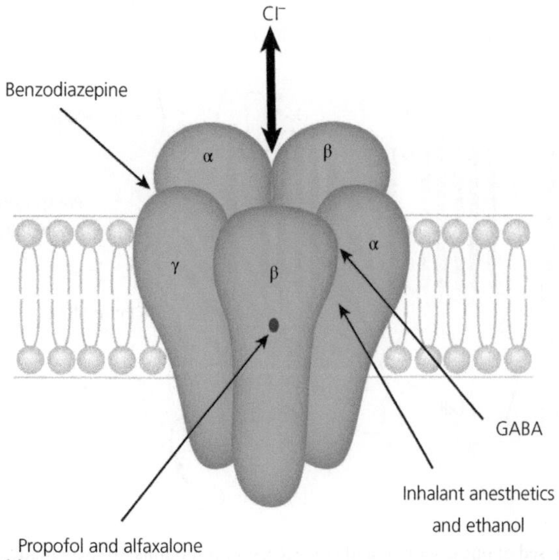

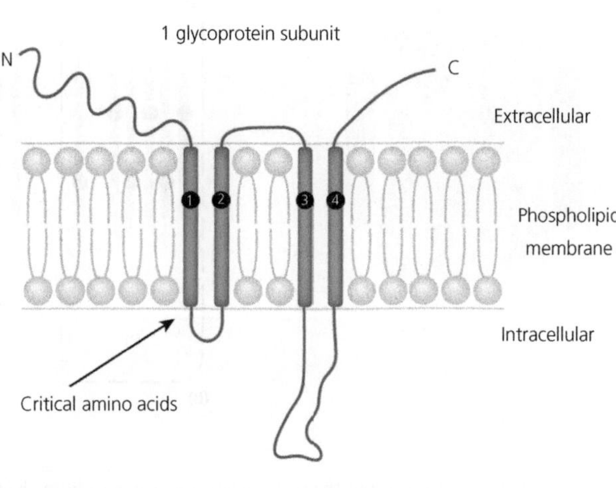

Figure 7.2 Structure of the $GABA_A$ receptors. (a) Schematic of a $GABA_A$ receptor composed of two α, two β, and one γ subunits showing the binding site of the agonist GABA and of the allosteric modulators benzodiazepines, inhalant anesthetics, ethanol, propofol, and alfaxalone. (b) Schematic of one glycoprotein subunit showing the four membrane-spanning segments numbered 1–4.

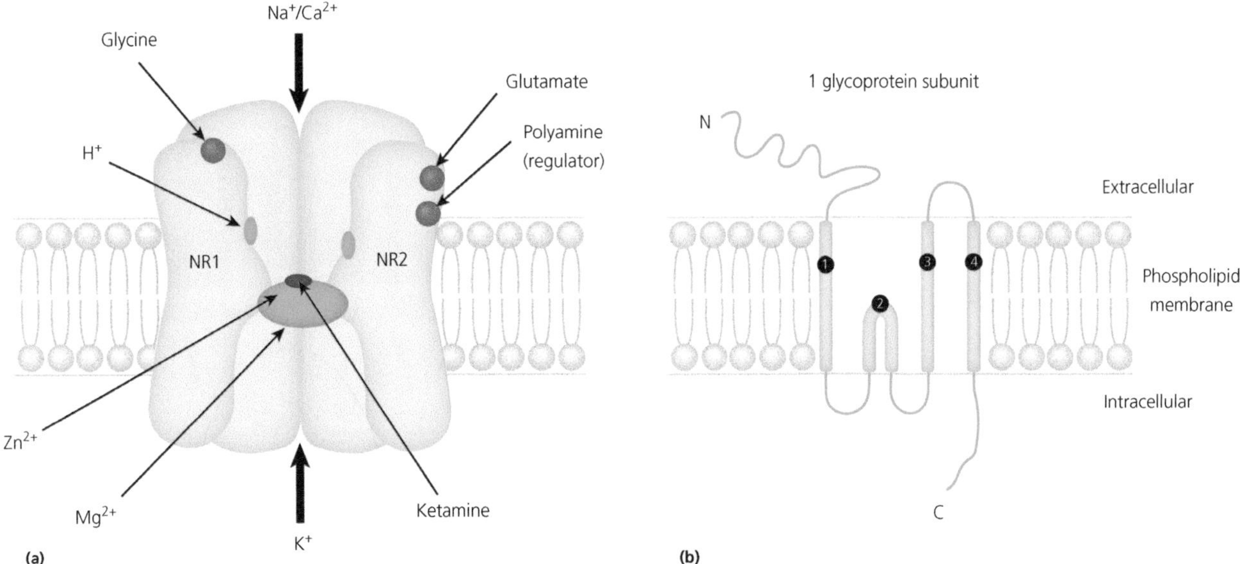

Figure 7.3 Structure of the NMDA receptors. (a) Schematic of an NMDA receptor composed of four subunits (two NR1 subunits and two NR2 subunits) showing the binding site of the agonists glutamate, the co-agonist glycine, the antagonist ketamine, and the modulators zinc and copper. Other axillary subunits have also been described. (b) Schematic of one glycoprotein subunit showing the four membrane-spanning segments numbered 1–4. It should be noted that segment numbered 2 does not cross the membrane but kinks back on itself towards the intracellular side of the membrane.

G-Protein receptors – second messengers

To transduce extracellular signals, some transmembrane receptors use intermediaries such as guanine nucleotide-binding proteins (G-proteins). A series of intracellular biochemical events (or second messengers) are initiated by the receptor–ligand interaction and ultimately lead to the observation of the clinical effect. Guanosine triphosphate (GTP) supplies the energy required by such complex G-protein receptors. These receptors are some of the most common and important receptors. The β-adrenergic receptor will be discussed as an example of a G-protein coupled receptor.

β-Adrenergic receptors

There are three types of β-adrenergic receptors: β_1 found in the cardiac sarcolemma, β_2 found in the bronchial and vasculature smooth muscle, and β_3 found in adipose tissue. The β-adrenergic receptors are linked to the adenylyl cyclase (AC) enzyme system through the G-proteins and are activated by the endogenous β-adrenergic agonists epinephrine and norepinephrine. The stimulatory G-protein (G_s or $G\alpha_s$), linked to the β-adrenergic receptor, is composed of α, β, and γ subunits and is located on the intracellular side of the cellular membrane. By default, the α subunit is associated with guanosine diphosphate (GDP) and the protein is considered switched off. However, interaction of the β-adrenergic receptor with norepinephrine or epinephrine changes its conformation, allowing guanosine triphosphate (GTP) to replace the GDP on the α subunit, and the protein is switched on. The associated AC is stimulated, inducing the production of cyclic AMP (cAMP), which in turn activates protein kinase A (PKA) and numerous downstream enzymes (Fig. 7.4). The AC can also be inhibited by the inhibitory G-proteins (G_i or $G\alpha_i$), which have a similar mechanism of activation to G_s. Indeed, G_i is linked to a β_2-adrenergic receptor and is a likely mechanism of modulation.

Clinical evaluation of drug effects

To study pharmacodynamics, or the effects of a drug on the whole body, one can evaluate the efficacy, potency, concentration–response relationship, effective dose, lethal dose, and the therapeutic index. Although one general pharmacological principle remains – the more drug, the more effects (the effects being measured either within an individual or within a population) – the occurrences of U-shaped (or inverted U-shaped) dose–response curves are widely and independently observed phenomena [13]. 'Hormesis' defines dose–response relationships characterized by stimulatory effects at low dose and inhibitory effects at higher dose, resulting in an inverted U-shaped dose–response curve. With naloxone as one example of this hormetic response (see the above paragraph on receptor agonist and antagonist), all receptors assessed to date display dose–response relationships with identifiable mechanisms regulated by agonist concentration gradient [13].

Efficacy, potency, and concentration–response relationship

Earlier in the chapter, it was described how the association of a ligand with a receptor follows the laws of mass action [eqn (7.1)]. The total concentration of receptors, $[R_T]$, is equal to the sum of [LR] plus [R], and if [R] is replaced by [RT] – [LR] in eqn (7.1), the relationship becomes

$$\frac{1}{K_d} = \frac{[LR]}{[L]([R_T]-[R])} \tag{7.3}$$

which rearranges to

$$\frac{[LR]}{[R_T]} = \frac{[L]}{[L]+K_d} \tag{7.4}$$

Also, knowing that the maximum efficacy (E_{max}) represents the maximal pharmacological effect of a drug or a ligand, and that the

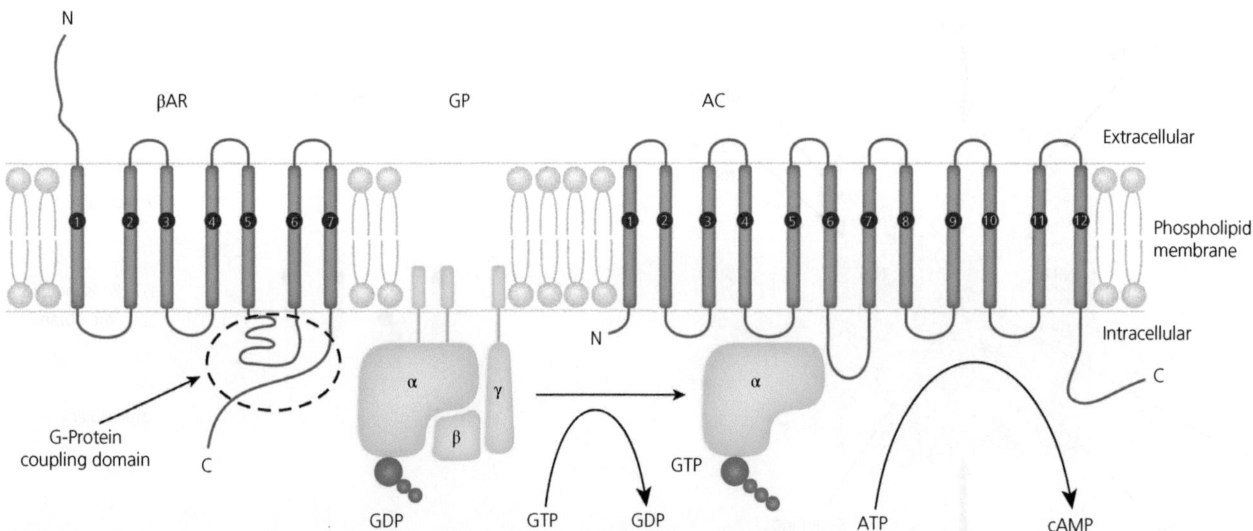

Figure 7.4 Illustration of the association between the β-adrenergic receptor (βAR), G-proteins (GP) and adenylate cyclase (AC). The βAR and AC glycoproteins are showing 7 and 12 membrane-spanning segments respectively. The GP is composed of α, β, and γ subunits and is located on the intracellular side of the cellular membrane. The conformation of the βAR and the GP are closely linked together. When an agonist ligand binds to the βAR and changes its conformation, the α subunit of the GP also changes conformation, allowing a GTP (guanosine triphosphate) to bind instead of a GDP (guanosine diphosphate). The α subunit of the GP is switched on and will stimulate the AC, inducing the production of cAMP (cyclic AMP) from ATP (adenosine triphosphate).

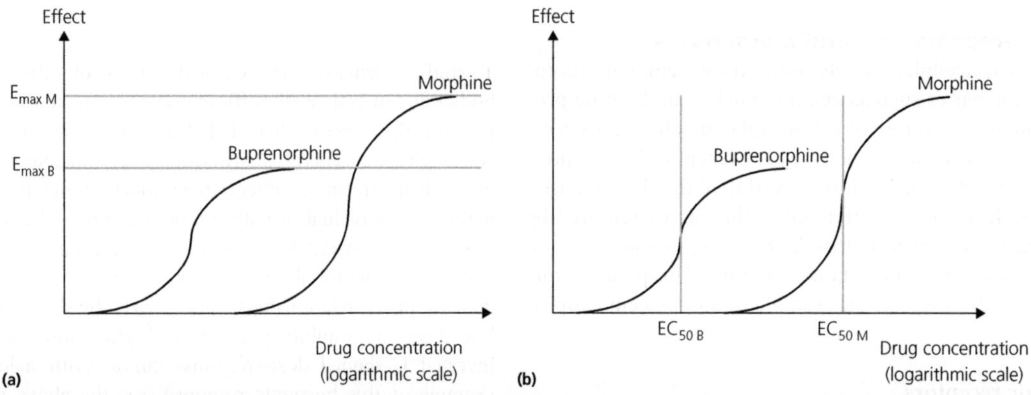

Figure 7.5 Illustration of the concentration–response relationships of the two opioids morphine and buprenorphine, the considered measured effect being analgesia. (a) The maximal analgesic effect of buprenorphine ($E_{max\,B}$) is lower than that of morphine ($E_{max\,M}$). Indeed, morphine is a full opioid μ agonist whereas buprenorphine is a partial μ opioid agonist. (b) The concentration of drug needed to obtain a pharmacological effect equal to 50% of the maximal effect is lower for buprenorphine ($EC_{50\,B}$) than for morphine ($EC_{50\,M}$). Consequently, buprenorphine is considered to be more potent than morphine.

pharmacological effect (E) of the drug is directly proportional to the percentage of activated receptors [14], then eqn 7.4 becomes

$$\frac{E}{E_{max}} = \frac{[L]}{[L]+K_d} \xrightarrow{\text{yields}} E = \frac{E_{max}[L]}{K_d+[L]} \tag{7.5}$$

This equation indicates a sigmoid relationship between the logarithm of the concentration of ligand and the effect (concentration–response relationship) and that in the absence of ligand the effect approaches nil. However, the receptor state theory implies the existence of a baseline agonist effect (E_0) of the receptor and this baseline effect is taken into consideration in Hill's equation:

$$E = \frac{(E_{max} - E_0)[L]}{K_d + [L]} \tag{7.6}$$

The concentration–response relationship is usually illustrated showing the effect as a function of the ligand's concentration (or other measure of exposure). The term potency characterizes the concentration of drug needed to obtain a pharmacological effect equal to 50% of E_{max}, i.e., the EC_{50}. The lower the EC_{50}, the less drug is needed to achieve the required effect and the higher the potency of the drug (Fig. 7.5).

Effective dose, lethal dose, toxic dose, and therapeutic index

The effective dose (ED_{50}) corresponds to the dose of drug necessary to induce the desired effect in 50% of the animals to which it is administered. Similarly, the lethal dose (LD_{50}) corresponds to the dose of drug necessary to induce death in 50% of the animals to which the drug is administered. In most human trials, the

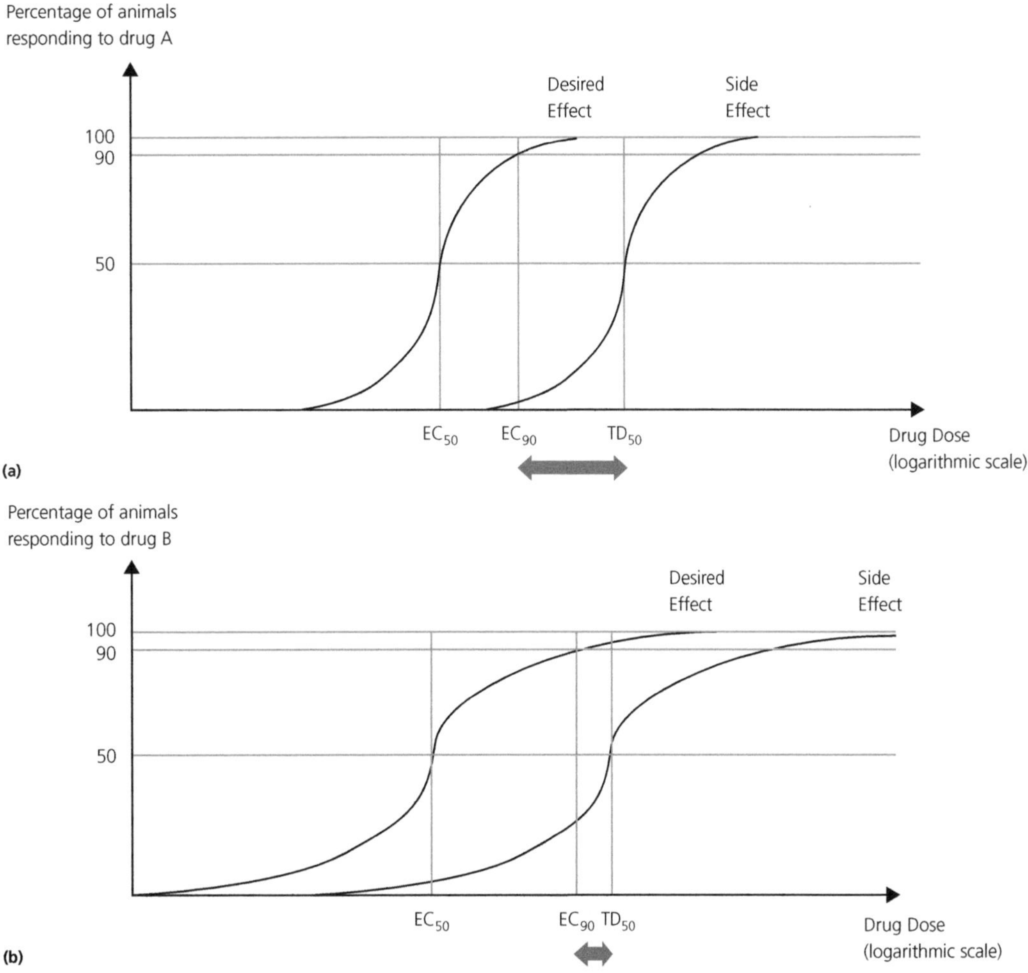

Figure 7.6 Illustration of the limitation of the therapeutic index to establish the safety profile of a drug. Drugs A and B have the same therapeutic index (ED_{50}/TD_{50}, the ratio of the effective dose in 50% of the population to the toxic dose in 50% of the population) but different dose–response curve slopes. (a) The EC_{90} (effective dose in 90% of the population) of drug A is significantly different from the TD_{50}, implying that most of the population will benefit from drug A without encountering side effects. (b) The EC_{90} of drug B is similar to the TD_{50}, implying that a large part of the population that benefit from drug B will encounter toxic effects.

lethal dose is not established, and is replaced by the toxic dose (TD_{50}). The TD_{50} corresponds to the dose of drug necessary to induce toxic effects in 50% of the patients to whom it is administered. The therapeutic index is the ratio LD_{50}:ED_{50} or TD_{50}:ED_{50}. The higher the therapeutic index, the safer the drug is considered to be. However, the therapeutic index does not take into consideration the slope of the concentration–response curve. Two drugs, A and B, with the same therapeutic index and given at ED_{90} (the effective dose in 90% of the population) can induce a significantly different prevalence of side effects and therefore the therapeutic index is not useful as a measure of a drug's clinical safety (Fig. 7.6).

It is fundamental to recognize that variability between the sensitivity of individuals to drug effects results in a range of doses that may be effective or toxic in some individuals and not in others. It is less self-evident, but equally important, to recognize that between-occasion variability in response to a fixed dose exists within an individual. The sum of between-individual and between-occasion variability causes uncertainty in the dose–response correlation, necessitating attention to the individual response on each occasion of drug administration.

Pharmacokinetics and pharmacodynamics

When drugs are administered to animals, two interactions are initiated. First, the animal's body initiates its actions on the drug; absorption, distribution, metabolism, and elimination (ADME). These processes are described by the discipline called pharmacokinetics. At the same time, the drug initiates its actions on the body and this process is described by the discipline called pharmacodynamics.

Fundamentals of pharmacodynamics

As discussed above, the interaction of free drug with its receptor stimulates the effect response by the organism. The association between receptor-drug concentration and response can differ between drugs, receptor systems, and occasions. As discussed above, the effect response is regarded as directly proportional to ratio of the receptor drug concentration to the total receptor concentration [14]. Experimental description of the effect response helps us to illustrate and understand the nature and extent of drug responses.

One of the purposes of drug effect response modeling is to allow one to make predictions of the outcome from clinical use of the drug. Consequently, a good pharmacodynamic model is one that closely describes the data and allows the development and evaluation of hypotheses about the drug's effect response at doses not directly tested. Several routine approaches are made to describe pharmacodynamic effect response data mathematically.

Where the effect response being measured is induced by a drug–receptor complex between 20 and 80% of maximal binding capacity at a single receptor class, then the effect response is often approximately log–linear in relation to drug concentration. Therefore, in the absence of a maximal effect being achieved, where E is the effect response measure, C is the drug concentration and E_0 is a constant that represents baseline activity, the effect response measure can be approximated by a straight line:

$$E = m\ln C + E_0 \tag{7.7}$$

In single receptor systems but where a maximal response is measured so that the effect response measure approaches an asymptote, the shape of the response curve may be described in the same form as for receptor binding [eqn 7.5]. If E_{max} is the maximum achievable response and EC_{50} is the concentration at which a response is achieved equal to 50% of the E_{max}, the effect response can sometimes be described as

$$E = \frac{E_{max}C}{EC_{50} + C} \tag{7.8}$$

Sometimes, the relationship between drug concentration and effect response reflects changes in the sensitivity of the signaling pathway to the presence of the drug. This may be a function of biological processes such as receptor tachyphylaxis or may be unrelated to known processes. These cases are not well approximated by the E_{max} model shown above, but can often be better described by the following related equation, where h (the Hill coefficient) modifies the steepness of the effect response curve:

$$E = \frac{(E_{max}C)^h}{EC_{50}{}^h + C^h} \tag{7.9}$$

when $h = 1$, this equation reduces to the standard E_{max} model of eqn 7.8. For example, the dose–response curves illustrated in Fig. 7.6a versus Fig. 7.6b are examples of curves with the same E_{max} and EC_{50} but with different slopes, hence they would have differing values for h.

More complex models are needed for drugs that achieve the measured effect response through multiple signaling pathways, and for effect responses that are not objectively measured on continuous distributions. During the 1950s, Robins and Rall formulated the 'free hormone hypothesis,' which is now generally accepted to be true both for hormones and for drugs [15]. Robins and Rall presented a convincing argument that, where a hormone (or drug) is present in protein-bound and unbound (or free) forms in equilibrium, the activity of the drug or hormone at its site of action is proportional to the concentration of the free drug or free hormone in the plasma, irrespective of the total drug or hormone concentration. Based on the assumption that free drugs can diffuse readily to their sites of action, or that there are alternative facilitated or active processes that assist drugs to reach their site of action, the free hormone hypothesis allows the linkage of the plasma concentration to the drug's effect response. Consequently, the plasma pharmacokinetics of a drug are usually associated with the degree, extent, and duration of drug effect.

Fundamentals of pharmacokinetics

Most pharmacokinetic processes within mammalian bodies occur as saturable processes (Michaelis–Menten kinetics): the speed at which a process occurs has an upper limit that can be reached, at least in theory. However, we can simplify the mathematics for pharmacokinetics by assuming that processes occur either at constant rates (zero order) or rates constant in proportion to the concentration of administered drug (first order). This simplification is usually acceptable because usually the concentration range of drugs used is narrow.

Zero-order processes are those in which the change of drug concentration in a body fluid such as plasma or urine occurs at a constant rate, irrespective of the concentration of the drug present in that body fluid. Since this process is constant, the equation for a straight line can be used. Consequently, the equation for a zero-order elimination has the following form:

$$C(t) = C(0) - k_0 t \tag{7.10}$$

where $C(t)$ is the concentration of the drug in the sample at any time t and the zero-order elimination rate (k_0) is the slope of the curve when concentration is plotted as a function of time, and is called the 'zero-order rate equation.' This is the equation for a straight line, i.e., $y = b + mx$, where y is the concentration in the sample, $C(0)$ is the y-intercept when $x = 0$, and x is time.

Sometimes, drug delivery devices or formulations are designed purposefully to achieve zero-order delivery (constant rate delivery) to maintain a constant effect of the drug for a prolonged period. Constant rate delivery is discussed later in this chapter.

In contrast to zero-order processes, a first-order process is one where the rate of change in concentration of drug in a body fluid is proportional to the concentration of the drug in that fluid at that time. This is an exponential function conforming to a straight line on a semi-logarithmic plot:

$$\ln C(t) = \ln C(0) - k_{el} t \tag{7.11}$$

where $\ln C(t)$ is the natural logarithm of the concentration of drug in the sample at any time t and the first-order elimination rate constant (k_{el}) is the slope. This reduces to

$$C(t) = C(0)e^{-k_{el}t} \tag{7.12}$$

which is called the 'first-order rate equation.' Many drugs used in anesthesia and analgesia adhere to first-order pharmacokinetics with respect to their elimination from the body and there are several drugs that are absorbed and eliminated by zero-order processes (Fig. 7.7).

Half-life of elimination

The elimination half-life of a drug is the time interval needed for the plasma concentration to be reduced to 50% (half) of its initial value [16]. Drugs eliminated by zero-order kinetics have half-lives that are a function of the plasma concentration of the drug at the beginning of the time interval. This parameter therefore is not constant for these drugs. In contrast, drugs eliminated by first-order kinetics have elimination half-lives that are fixed at a constant rate

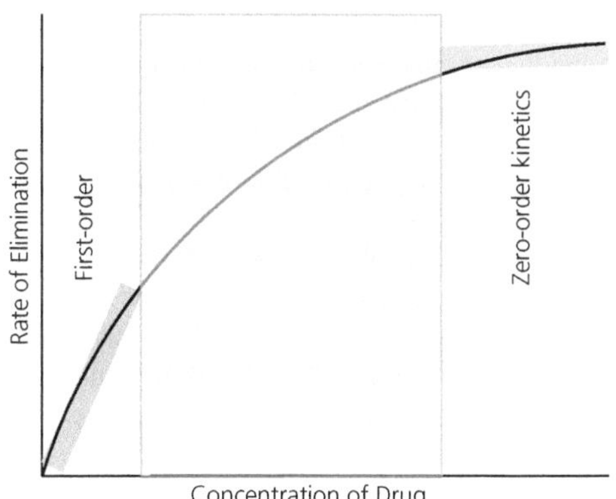

Figure 7.7 For most drugs, the elimination processes obey saturable kinetics, but at the concentrations used clinically most drugs approximate linear 'first-order' pharmacokinetics because the elimination processes are not approaching saturation.

per unit time. The half-life is inversely proportional to the rate of elimination (k_{el}):

$$C(t) = C(0)e^{-k_{el}t} \tag{7.13}$$

$$\frac{1}{2}C(0) = C(0)e^{-k_{el}t_{1/2}} \tag{7.14}$$

$$\frac{1}{2} = e^{-k_{el}t_{1/2}} \tag{7.15}$$

$$\ln\left(\frac{1}{2}\right) = -k_{el}t_{1/2} \tag{7.16}$$

$$0.693 = -k_{el}t_{1/2} \tag{7.17}$$

$$t_{1/2} = \frac{0.693}{k_{el}} \tag{7.18}$$

Superficially, the concept of elimination half-life appears easy to understand. However, this is a hybrid parameter and is influenced by many factors. Both metabolism and elimination commonly affect the elimination half-life of a drug. Some factors that affect the rate of metabolism of a drug include the species, the age, the gender, the bodyweight, disease states (especially renal and hepatic diseases), and drug interactions.

The time one must wait after administering a drug or changing a drug dose rate before attaining a new steady-state plasma concentration, or before attaining complete elimination of a drug, is a function solely of the half-life of that drug. If the fraction of drug that is eliminated is F_E, from the first-order rate equation we can derive:

$$F_E = 1 - e^{-k_{el}t} \tag{7.19}$$

For practical purposes in clinical veterinary practice, approximately 4–5 half-lives must pass before a change in dose achieves a new steady-state plasma concentration (at about 97% of total). Similarly, approximately 4–5 half-lives must pass after cessation of administration before effectively all of the drug is eliminated.

Apparent volume of distribution

The mass of drug in the body at any time is proportional to the concentration measured in the sample space (often the plasma) at any time and can be expressed as the following equality:

$$X_B = CV_d \tag{7.20}$$

where X_B is the mass of drug in the body and V_d is a proportionality constant. This proportionality constant V_d is known as the apparent volume of distribution [17]. The reason why the word 'apparent' is used to describe the parameter is that although it has units of volume it does not actually represent any particular physiological or anatomic space and cannot be attributed to any such space from any simple physiological or pharmacokinetic analysis.

It is clear that each sample space will have its own volume parameter, so in complex models each 'compartment' will have an individual volume; for example, the volume of the circulation is often referred to as the volume of the 'central compartment'(V_c). The sum of all volumes, central and peripheral, is often referred to as the 'volume of distribution at steady state' (V_{dss}). Understanding and having an estimate for volume parameters facilitate dose calculations; for example:

$$\text{loading dose} = C_{(\text{desired})}V_c \tag{7.21}$$

Just as there are several different volume parameters, there are also different methods to calculate them. It is important to understand that estimates of a volume parameter might be differently derived and therefore have different absolute values.

Particular volume parameters are better suited to particular uses; for example, the apparent volume of the central compartment (V_c) is usually used for calculating loading doses for rapidly acting or toxic drugs such as an induction doses of anesthetic, whereas the apparent volume of distribution at steady state (V_{dss}) is often used for calculating constant rate infusions or repeated analgesic drug dosing regimens (see the discussion below in the section Constant Rate Therapy).

Within a species, the apparent volume of distribution varies from individual to individual. Individual factors that affect the volume of distribution include the state of hydration, the age and gender of the animal, the body weight, and the body composition (fat, muscle, water ratios), the protein content of serum especially for protein bound drugs, the presence of plasma expanders such as lipids after a meal, and drug interactions (especially due to competition for binding sites).

Total body clearance

Total body clearance (Cl) is defined as the volume of blood from which drug is completely removed per unit of time. Total body clearance is often referred to simply as "clearance" and the units for clearance are volume per unit time (e.g., mL/min or L/h), often normalized by body weight (e.g., mL/min/kg). Clearance is a measure of the efficiency of drug elimination and is often directly compared or contrasted with cardiac output in the species under examination.

Total body clearance describes the relationship between the rate of excretion of a drug and the plasma concentration. If X_E is the mass of drug eliminated from the body and equals $-X_B$ if no further dose is administered, total body clearance can be described algebraically as follows:

$$Cl = \frac{-\frac{dX_B}{dt}}{C} \tag{7.22}$$

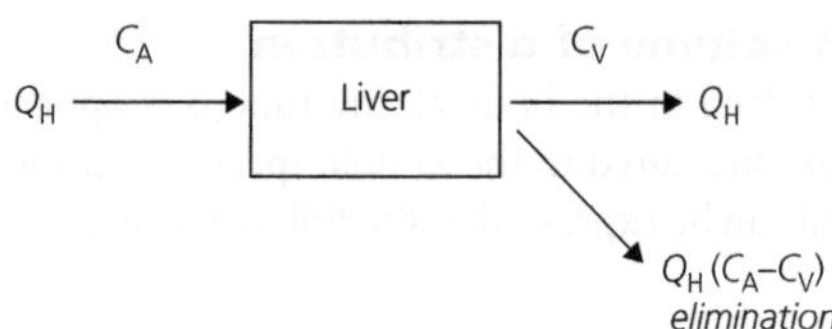

Figure 7.8 Hepatic clearance of drugs is estimated from hepatic blood flow (Q_H) and the concentration difference between the drug in the hepatic blood inflow (C_A) and outflow (C_V).

$$Cl = \frac{X_B k_{el}}{C} \tag{7.23}$$

However, we have already seen that $X_B = CV_d$ [(eqn 7.20]. Therefore, in this simplified example:

$$Cl = k_{el} V_d \tag{7.24}$$

Clearance can thereby be understood as a function of both volume of distribution and the concentration of drug present in the sample space. Although this is demonstrated to be true for total body clearance, it is useful to foresee that it can be extrapolated to clearance from individual compartments in complicated multi-compartment systems.

Total body clearance is a sum of the clearance achieved by all mechanisms. Although some anesthetic drugs are cleared by the lungs, the two most important components are usually attributed to hepatic and renal clearance. Total body clearance can be defined as follows:

$$Cl_T = Cl_H + Cl_R + Cl_{other} \tag{7.25}$$

where Cl_H and Cl_R are the clearance due to hepatic and renal mechanisms, respectively. Total body clearance (Cl_T) is a very important pharmacokinetic parameter and must be comprehensively understood [18].

Hepatic clearance

Consider the flow diagram in Fig. 7.8, where Q_H is the rate of organ blood flow through the liver, C_A is the concentration of drug in the arterial blood, C_V is the concentration of drug in the venous blood and $Q_H(C_A - C_V)$ is the rate of elimination by the liver.

Then, since

$$Cl = \frac{\frac{dX_E}{dt}}{C} \tag{7.26}$$

$$Cl_H = \frac{\text{rate of elimination}}{C_A} \tag{7.27}$$

$$Cl_H = \frac{Q_H(C_A - C_V)}{C_A} \tag{7.28}$$

Now, since the fraction of drug removed from the blood on each pass of the blood through the liver is the extraction ratio (*ER*), it can be seen that

$$ER = \frac{C_A - C_V}{C_A} \tag{7.29}$$

and hence by substitution

$$Cl_H = Q_H ER \tag{7.30}$$

Because most body systems and processes are saturable, the liver in each individual animal has a maximum capacity for removing a drug from the blood when there are no blood flow constrictions. This capacity for drug elimination by the combination of biotransformation and by excretion in the bile is a function of liver mass and of the amount and activity of the enzymes of drug metabolism that are present in that individual's hepatocytes. This maximum capacity for drug removal from the blood is the intrinsic ability of the liver to remove drug; the innate capacity of the liver to clear drug is known as its intrinsic clearance (Cl_I). An understanding of the concept of intrinsic clearance allows us to redefine the extraction ratio in terms of intrinsic clearance:

$$ER = \frac{Cl_I}{Q_H + Cl_I} \tag{7.31}$$

Therefore, by substitution:

$$Cl_H = \frac{Q_H Cl_I}{Q_H + Cl_I} \tag{7.32}$$

A corollary to the free hormone hypothesis is that the availability of a hormone or drug for binding to receptors or to enzymes of biotransformation is proportional to the free concentration. If *fu* is the fraction of drug not bound to plasma proteins (i.e., the free fraction) and $Cl_I{}'$ is the intrinsic clearance for free drug only, it can be seen that

$$Cl_I = fuCl_I' \tag{7.33}$$

For each drug in each individual, a relationship will exist between the intrinsic hepatic clearance and that animal's particular hepatic blood flow. This relationship between drugs is likely to be a continuum from one extreme, where intrinsic clearance is very much less than hepatic blood flow, to the other extreme, where hepatic intrinsic clearance is very much greater than hepatic blood flow.

If intrinsic clearance is very much less than hepatic blood flow, then intrinsic clearance is not a significant contributor to the denominator in the following equation:

$$Cl_H = \frac{Q_H Cl_I}{Q_H + Cl_I} \tag{7.34}$$

and therefore in this special case where intrinsic clearance is much less than hepatic blood flow, by cancellation it can be seen that

$$Cl_H = Cl_I \tag{7.35}$$

Since intrinsic hepatic clearance is the product of the fraction unbound and the intrinsic clearance for free drug only, it is clear that in this special case hepatic clearance is proportional to the fraction of drug unbound [19]. It is with drugs for which this special set of conditions is valid that alterations to plasma protein binding of the drug can significantly affect the rate of that drug's excretion. Similarly, for these drugs, induction of hepatic enzymes for biotransformation can have a large effect on their elimination rate, as discussed further below.

Now let us consider the alternative case where the intrinsic hepatic clearance is very much greater than hepatic blood flow. In this case, it is the contribution of hepatic blood flow to the denominator of eqn 7.34 that is insignificant. Consequently, in this alternative special case:

$$Cl_H = Q_H \tag{7.36}$$

Box 7.1 Example 1: high hepatic clearance drugs.

This example illustrates what the effect would be of doubling the intrinsic hepatic clearance rate of a drug where hepatic clearance is very much greater than hepatic blood flow.

$Cl_I >> Q_H$, e.g., propranolol
$Cl_I = 7.0$ L/min
$Q_H = 1.5$ L/min
$ER = 7/(7+1.5)$
$= 0.82$

$Cl_H = Q_H \times ER$
$= 1.5 \times 0.82$
$= 1.23$ L/min

After enzyme induction:
$Cl_I = 14.0$ L/min
$Q_H = 1.5$ L/min
$ER = 14/(14+1.5)$
$= 0.9$

$Cl_H = Q_H \times ER$
$= 1.5 \times 0.9$
$= 1.35$ L/min

Box 7.2 Example 2: low hepatic clearance drugs.

This example illustrates what the effect would be of doubling the intrinsic hepatic clearance rate of a drug where hepatic clearance is very much less than hepatic blood flow.

$Cl_I << Q_H$, e.g., theophylline
$Cl_I = 0.1$ L/min
$Q_H = 1.5$ L/min
$ER = 0.1/(0.1+1.5)$
$= 0.06$

$Cl_H = Q_H \times ER$
$= 1.5 \times 0.06$
$= 0.094$ L/min

After enzyme induction:
$Cl_I = 0.2$ L/min
$Q_H = 1.5$ L/min
$ER = 0.2/(0.2+1.5)$
$= 0.12$

$Cl_H = Q_H \times ER$
$= 1.5 \times 0.12$
$= 0.18$ L/min

For drugs that conform to this set of special conditions, it is clear that alterations in hepatic blood flow will profoundly influence the rate of hepatic clearance. The elimination of such drugs will be dependent upon factors such as cardiac output and normal structure and function of hepatic blood vessels. Anesthesiologists understand that many of the drugs that are used markedly affect cardiac output and regional blood flow and that surgical procedures and pathology can also lead to marked changes in hepatic blood flow. Therefore, the rate of elimination of many common anesthetic drugs can be markedly different from expectation as either the animal's pathophysiology or the procedure cause a departure from normal hepatic blood flow.

It can be seen in Example 1 in Box 7.1 that doubling the intrinsic hepatic clearance for a high intrinsic clearance drug resulted in an increase in the rate of hepatic clearance by a factor of only 1.09, whereas in Example 2 in Box 7.2 the doubling of the intrinsic hepatic clearance rate for a low intrinsic hepatic clearance drug resulted in a doubling of its hepatic clearance.

Since the intrinsic clearance (Cl_I) is the product of the fraction unbound (*fu*) and the intrinsic clearance for the unbound fraction (Cl_I'), an increase in Cl_I' can be caused either by increasing the displacement of the drug from binding sites and hence increasing *fu*, or by inducing the activity or expression of enzymes of metabolism through enzyme induction. In the former case, changing the plasma protein binding would result in a change of the volume of distribution of the drug, whereas in the latter case, a change in the expression of enzymes on metabolism would result in a change in the excretion rate constant for the drug.

It is also notable that drugs with a high intrinsic hepatic clearance consequently have high extraction ratios and therefore they have a low bioavailability (*F*) when administered by the oral route:

$$F = 1 - ER \tag{7.37}$$

This is known as the first pass effect and is clinically a very real effect with some drugs. The first pass effect is the explanation on occasions for markedly different dose rates for some drugs when administered by oral versus parenteral routes (e.g., opioids).

In clinical anesthesiology, drug interactions are thought to cause alterations in hepatic clearance. Although there is little published evidence that such interactions are clinical realities, the clinician should be aware of which drugs have intrinsically high and which have intrinsically low hepatic clearance in order to anticipate correctly the need to adjust dose rates in cases where multiple drug protocols are being used. An additional point to consider is that many drugs have multiple mechanisms involved in the establishment of their plasma concentrations (e.g., hepatic biotransformation and redistribution as with propofol), hence the clinical impact of changes in hepatic clearance may not be as great as predicted.

Renal clearance

Renal clearance defines the relationship between the rate of change of the amount of drug in the urine and the plasma drug concentration. Algebraically, this can be expressed as follows:

$$Cl_R = \frac{\frac{dX_u}{dt}}{C} \tag{7.38}$$

where Cl_R is the renal clearance, X_u is the amount of drug in the urine, and *C* is the plasma concentration. It is important to note that the clearance of drug from the plasma by the kidneys is achieved by the summation of renal filtration and active renal tubular secretion of drug into the urinary ultrafiltrate. Renal clearance is diminished from this sum by any tubular resorption of drug that might occur. If *RF* is the rate of renal filtration, *RS* is the rate of renal secretion, and *RR* is the rate of renal resorption:

$$Cl_R = \frac{RF}{C} + \frac{RS}{C} + \frac{RR}{C} \tag{7.39}$$

It should be noted that drug bound to plasma proteins cannot be filtered because of the size-exclusion capability of the glomerulus. Therefore, the rate of renal filtration is a function of the glomerular filtration rate (*GFR*) and the plasma concentration of unbound drug. If C_u is the concentration of unbound drug in the plasma:

$$RF = GFR \times C_u \tag{7.40}$$

Since

$$fu = \frac{C_u}{C} \tag{7.41}$$

$$RF = GFR \times fu \times C \tag{7.42}$$

Therefore, in the absence of renal secretion or resorption:

$$Cl_R = \frac{GFR \times fu \times C}{C} \tag{7.43}$$

$$Cl_R = GFR \times fu \tag{7.44}$$

It is obvious that if the fraction unbound is $fu = 1$ (i.e., if no drug is bound to plasma proteins) then the renal clearance of the drug equals the glomerular filtration rate. For practical purposes, this is accepted as true for the endogenous metabolite of muscle creatinine, for the inert carbohydrate xenobiotic inulin, and for the radiographic contrast agent iohexol, which allows their use for measuring renal filtration rate.

If renal clearance is greater than the product of the fraction unbound and glomerular filtration rate, then renal secretion must be occurring. If renal clearance is less than the product of fraction unbound and glomerular filtration rate, then renal resorption must be occurring.

Absorption

It is usually accepted that drugs formulated for standard delivery methods are absorbed by concentration-dependent processes that are linear (i.e., first-order processes). When drugs are administered by routes other than intravenously, the rate of absorption across membranes which are barriers to entry is proportional to the difference in concentration across the membrane, the area of the membrane, and its permeability to the drug. Surface area can be manipulated, for example, by giving a dose in aliquots to multiple sites. The concentration of drug in the formulation will partially determine the steepness of the diffusion gradient for drug absorption (e.g., transdermal fentanyl solution). The concentration of the drug in the formulation may be altered by dilution prior to administration or after injection due to water movement as a function of an osmotic gradient. The rates of lymph and blood flow, cardiac output, and factors controlling local blood flow can alter the concentration gradient. The proximity of an administration to impermeable boundaries such as fascial plains and fat is an important determinant of the rate of drug absorption and is to some extent controllable by appropriate choice of injection site. These factors can result in unexpected inefficacy or toxicity with high-potency drugs because of changes in the rate and extent of drug absorption.

A special case is that of constant rate intravenous infusions and some transdermal patch delivery devices. In these cases, the administration of drug is achieved at a constant rate per unit time (i.e., it is zero order). For zero-order delivery when elimination is first order, the following equation approximates the predicted plasma concentration:

$$C(t) = \frac{k_0}{(V_d k_{el})(1 - e^{-k_{el}t})} \tag{7.45}$$

Now, since as time approaches infinity $e^{-k_{el}t}$ approaches zero, under this assumption the concentration at steady state (C_{ss}) is

$$C_{ss} \cong \frac{k_0}{V_d k_{el}} \tag{7.46}$$

However, we have seen earlier that

$$Cl = k_{el} V_d \tag{7.47}$$

Hence by substitution and rearrangement, we can determine that for a drug of known total body clearance, to maintain a target steady-state plasma concentration the zero-order infusion rate (k_0) must equal the elimination rate and can be calculated as

$$k_0 = C_{ss} Cl = \text{elimination rate} \tag{7.48}$$

Bioavailability

The bioavailability (F) of a drug is the fraction of the dose given that finds its way into the systemic circulation [20]. It should be noted that this is not necessarily equal to the fraction of the dose that is absorbed, since a drug might be absorbed (e.g., across the gastrointestinal lumen) but removed by metabolism from the portal blood by the liver or from the pulmonary blood by the lungs, before reaching the systemic circulation. Similarly, for topically applied drugs, the skin is an organ of drug metabolism and might biotransform a drug already absorbed before it reaches the circulation.

The bioavailability for a drug by a given route is calculated by comparing the total drug exposure of the dose with that achieved when the same dose is delivered intravenously. However, drugs administered by any route may be incompletely delivered to the systemic circulation. Even for simple intravenous injection, a drug may have bioavailability less than 100% if it is metabolized or excreted by the lungs.

Pharmacokinetics of inhalant anesthetic agents

The absorption, disposition, and fate of inhalant agents, like any agent administered to an animal, adhere to the principles of pharmacokinetics. However, both absorption and elimination of inhalational agents are mostly through the lungs and are is therefore influenced by all the factors acting on their alveolar partial pressure (P_A). The role of the lungs causes inhalant agents to behave differently from injectable agents, seemingly counterintuitive for the clinician who is more familiar with IV pharmacokinetics. Whereas the speed of induction will be proportional to the cardiac output (CO) for the intravenous hypnotic agents, it will be inversely proportional for the inhalant due to the negative effect of the high CO on P_A. Similarly, an increase in blood solubility of the inhalant agent will drive more drug from the alveoli into the blood, resulting in a decrease in P_A and consequently in a decrease in the speed of induction. These factors are discussed in detail in Chapter 16.

Linear and non-linear pharmacokinetics

When the behavior of a drug in the body obeys the principle of superposition, the pharmacokinetics are said to conform to a linear pharmacokinetic model. The principle of superposition states that the response to any combination of inputs must equal the sum of the responses when input separately. For pharmacokinetics, the input is the dose and the response is the sample's drug concentration. The clinical effect of linear pharmacokinetics is that plasma drug concentrations achieved after changes of drug dose are predictable because, for example, doubling of the dose would achieve twice the plasma concentration [21]. In contrast to drugs with zero-order pharmacokinetics, drugs that display first-order pharmacokinetics are usually approximated well by linear pharmacokinetic models.

Generally, having linear pharmacokinetics indicates that a drug behaves predictably; for example, in a stochastic system, each molecule of the drug introduced to the body moves through the system independently of all other molecules of the same drug introduced to the system, in addition to any daughter molecules produced through metabolism [22]. Exceptions do occur and warrant careful clinical use, such as for the analgesic non-steroidal anti-inflammatory drug (NSAID) phenylbutazone in both the dog and the horse, which appears to have linear pharmacokinetics because it shows a log–linear plasma drug concentration decay after any chosen dose. However, the primary metabolite oxphenbutazone interferes with its parent moiety's metabolism, hence this is a non-stochastic system. The result is that the elimination half-life is dose dependent and therefore the pharmacokinetics of phenylbutazone in these species are non-linear [23–25].

A typical use of clinical pharmacokinetics depends on the assumptions of linearity and superposition, assumptions that are violated for many drugs used in anesthesia and pain management. Non-linearity may be due to changes wrought by the drug on its own absorption, distribution, metabolism, or elimination. Changes can be either immediate or delayed. It is no great challenge to identify examples of drugs used in the practice of anesthesia and analgesia that create non-stochastic pharmacokinetics.

Experiments in pharmacokinetics

Background knowledge of the pharmacokinetics of a drug is necessary to permit the proper use of that drug in clinical cases. Therefore, with new drugs, or older drugs for new applications, it is important to describe adequately their pharmacokinetics in the target population. There are several important steps in the design and conduct of pharmacokinetic experiments that ensure the yield of informative results (Box 7.3).

Preparation for the study

In order to plan the study properly, it is necessary to have a reasonable prediction of its outcome. Therefore, the conduct of a pilot study is the foundation of a well-planned pharmacokinetic experiment. Predictions are needed of the approximate target plasma concentration, the likely elimination rate constant, the probability of linear pharmacokinetics, and the likelihood that the formulation might markedly affect the pharmacokinetics.

The approximate target plasma concentration needs to be known so that the analytical assay can be planned, developed, and validated. The assay must be capable of accurately measuring concentrations at least tenfold lower than the minimum effective concentration. It is important to have a validated assay prior to initiation of sample collection. Assay validation parameters that are minimally required include the inter- and intra-day coefficients of variation at the lowest and highest concentrations of the standard curve, measures of linearity of the standard curve (or statistical evaluation of non-linear standard curves), robustness of the assay, especially between laboratory technicians and equipment (if different technicians and equipment are likely to be used), the stability of stock and standard solutions at storage temperatures, the stability of samples at −20 and possibly −80 °C, the extent of analyte recovery through the sample preparation process, and the lower limit of quantification (LLOQ) [26]. The minimum acceptable sample volume must be known, derived from the intersection of the LLOQ and the expected minimum target concentration.

The likely elimination rate constant, or elimination half-life, informs the experimental design. An accepted rule of thumb is that it is not possible to predict the half-life of a drug accurately unless several samples are collected over at least 2–3 half-lives. If sample collection is not sufficiently frequent and prolonged, or if the assay used is not sufficiently sensitive, then the experiment can be compromised by this lack of planning. Where pilot data in the target species are unavailable, it is reasonable to use allometric scaling from data in other species in order to obtain suitable estimates for experimental design. Methods that can be used for this allometry are available [27], and there are examples of the use of such methods for pharmacokinetic studies in veterinary medicine [28].

Many drugs for anesthesia are rather lipophilic. Their lack of water solubility increases the need for biotransformation. Biotransformation processes are often saturable. Furthermore, most anesthetic drugs have been demonstrated to affect cardiac output and regional tissue blood flow. Therefore, it is common that anesthetic drugs have non-linear pharmacokinetics. The external validity of the planned experiment, i.e., the ability to extrapolate its results to novel clinical situations, requires the experiment to demonstrate whether the drug behaves with linear pharmacokinetics. The simplest way to address this question in the first instance is to perform the experiment at multiple doses [29].

Whereas the pharmacokinetics of an active moiety can be markedly influenced by the formulation excipients, this is generally not true for intravenous preparations. If the study is planned to evaluate a formulation that is to be administered by a route other than intravenous, then attention to the effect of formulation is needed. In order to describe completely the new formulation's pharmacokinetics, it is necessary to have access to the pharmacokinetics of the active moiety after intravenous administration. If these data are not available, then the study should be planned to include both the intravenous and the intended routes of administration.

Experimental design and conduct

The background understanding gained from the preparation for the study will determine the optimum study design. Study types that are commonly used include the naive pooled data set, the standard two-stage approach, a pharmacokinetic–pharmacodynamic (PK–PD)

Box 7.3 Example 3: steps for planning and conduct of pharmacokinetic experiments.

1. Conduct a pilot study OR choose a suitable PK model and determine parameter estimates from the literature with or without the use of inter-species allometry.
2. Determine the target plasma concentration.
3. Develop and validate the analytical assay.
4. Choose the dosing strategy; doses, frequency, formulation, routes of administration.
5. Choose the sampling strategy; sample space, sample frequency and volume, sample processing and storage.
6. Choose the study design; consult a statistician if needed.
7. Conduct the study.
8. Analyze the results.
9. Review the results for plausibility and repeat steps 8 and 9 as many times as needed, changing methodology as needed to establish robustness of estimates.
10. Return to step 4 and repeat if your assumptions for step 1 were not realistic.

study, or a population pharmacokinetic (POP-PK) approach [30]. The study type will influence the chosen experimental design. The naive pooled study type is the least desirable. In this study type, all the data from all the animals are pooled together for data analysis. Taking this approach loses the opportunity to develop an understanding of differences between animals within the population or of the variance within a population. Although suboptimal, naive pooled studies are sometimes necessary when each individual animal is only able to be sampled on one or two occasions. This restriction occurs when the sample volume is large relative to the circulating blood volume, where the act of sampling is likely to alter the pharmacokinetics at subsequent time points, or where the species to be evaluated is difficult to capture, handle, or restrain. Before planning a study of this type, the researcher should consider whether a population approach is possible, since if it is possible then it is likely to result in more useful outcomes.

The most frequently used study type is the standard two-stage approach. Usually a cohort is enrolled of similar individuals from the target population. After dosing, each individual is sampled at the same time points and on multiple occasions. After a suitable washout period, generally accepted to be longer than five half-lives of the drug, the cohort can be dosed again and similarly sampled so as to evaluate either the dose proportionality or the effect of a chosen manipulation on the drug's pharmacokinetics. Typical manipulations include changes in dose, presence or absence of concomitant medications, or modeled disease states. The data from each individual are analyzed independently and the resulting predicted variables are used to generate estimates for the mean variables in the population. Routine statistical comparisons can be made between the results before and after the manipulation. These statistical comparisons are enhanced by careful choice of experimental design, paying attention to randomization, balance, bias elimination, masking, and *a priori* decisions for statistical evaluation of the resulting data. Typically, these study designs lend themselves to evaluation using general linear models with factors for dose, sequence, animal, period, sequence plus animal interactions, and other manipulations.

The PK–PD type of study is an embellishment of the standard two-stage approach. In PK–PD studies, data are collected to measure the drug concentration, and usually at the same time points samples or measurements are also taken to assess one or more effects of the drug. Ideally, the targeted effect outcome can be evaluated using a rigorous and objective measure. Alternatively, a surrogate variable can be used. Surrogate variables used for evaluation of efficacy include biological markers such as intermediate enzyme activities or second messenger concentrations. Once again, the data from each animal are analyzed independently and then combined to generate estimates for the population variables, but the nature of the data analysis differs in complexity from PK-only studies. Typically, PK–PD studies are used to evaluate the correlation between dose and effect, to predict ideal doses better, and to gain better understandings of the drug effect on pathophysiologic processes. The data need to support the determination of the pharmacokinetic and statistical models as in a standard two-stage analysis, plus the superimposition of a model for the relationship between drug concentration and efficacy. Therefore, it is necessary to have 'rich' data (i.e., a large number of sample time points per animal) in order to estimate a larger number of variables accurately.

The POP-PK approach is an excellent type of study to evaluate the pharmacokinetics of a drug in clinical cases. For this study type, a small number of samples, usually 2–5, is taken from each case at times convenient for that case; preferably animals are sampled at different times from one individual to another. In addition, data are collected from each case which describe covariates that are hypothesized to have potential to affect the pharmacokinetics of the drug. Generally, it is expected that 30–50 cases will be needed to describe adequately the effect of each covariate. It is necessary to have access to a previous study that adequately describes a suitable structural model for the pharmacokinetics of the drug. Alternatively, a small number of individual cases should be sampled sufficiently frequently to describe the drug's pharmacokinetic adequately. Usually, the population modeling is performed on a subset of the available data and the resulting model is validated using the data that were excluded from model development. The POP-PK approach allows the identification of those factors within the clinical population that might markedly alter the pharmacokinetics and hence also alter the efficacy or toxicity of the drug. Such knowledge allows for an appropriate evidence-based adaptation of clinical dosing regimens based on individual animal characteristics.

Data analysis – compartmental models

The availability of off-the-shelf pharmacokinetic analysis software, including purpose-written programs and spreadsheet plug-ins, has all but eliminated the potential barrier (or energy of activation) needed to initiate pharmacokinetic data analysis. These programs allow the researcher to enter time and concentration data and, without further intellectual input, to obtain tables of estimates of pharmacokinetic variables. The temptation to take this approach can result in the rejection of manuscripts submitted to peer-reviewed publications. A skilled and systematic approach to the review, evaluation, and then analysis of pharmacokinetic data is necessary, since within this mathematical discipline it is necessary to make subjective decisions and evaluate the legitimacy of assumptions. Evaluation of pharmacokinetic data requires the researcher to determine both the ideal pharmacokinetic structural model and the ideal statistical model needed to describe the data adequately.

Classical pharmacokinetic models include the one-, two-, and three-compartment mammillary models with first-order elimination only from the central compartment and administration only to the central compartment. Alternatively, non-compartmental modeling (sometimes erroneously referred to as model-independent analysis) is often used. The purpose of any of these modeling approaches is to evaluate the data so as to derive estimates of pharmacokinetic variables. These estimates may then be used to make predictions of outcome. The accuracy of the predictions will depend on external validity of the modeling approach taken.

For one-, two-, and three-compartmental models, when plotted on semi-logarithmic axes, the data appear to draw one, two, or three straight lines, respectively. Referring to the first-order rate equation discussed earlier [eqn 7.12], a common representation of these models is as follows, with i as the number of compartments and k_i the slopes of the ith straight portion of the plasma concentration versus time curve. At this time, it is useful to begin to consider that all experiments include some imprecision, or variability, represented by ε:

$$C(t) = \sum_i \left(A_i e^{-k_i t} \right) + \varepsilon \tag{7.49}$$

For compartmental analysis of data, a typical first step is to plot the time and concentration data on semi-logarithmic axes. Working with the example of intravenous administration of alfaxalone to a greyhound dog [31], the first step is to check that the data can be

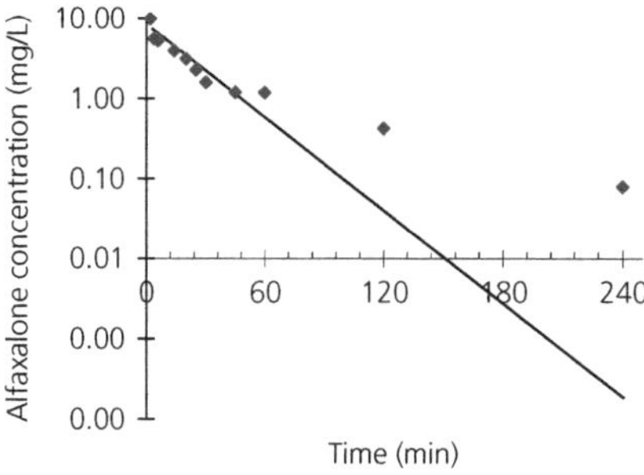

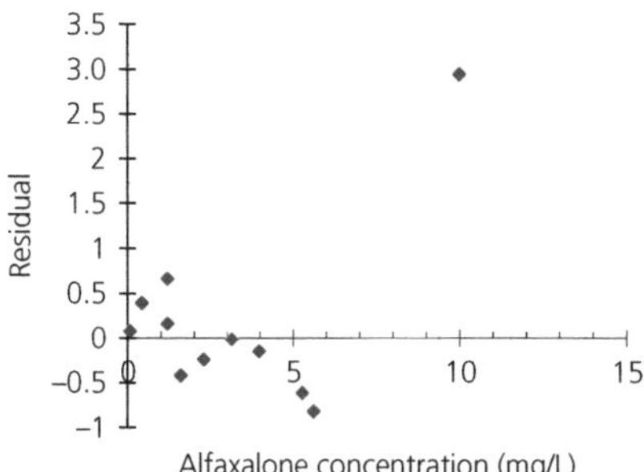

Figure 7.9 Plasma concentration versus time on semi-logarithmic axes and residuals versus concentration, after intravenous administration of 2 mg/kg alfaxalone to a greyhound dog [31], showing failure to be approximated by a single straight line.

described by a single straight line. If so, it suggests that a one-compartment model is appropriate. In this case (Fig. 7.9), it is clear that a single straight line does not adequately describe these data. The line does not 'fit to' the data and the residuals; in other words, the differences between the measured concentration $C(t)$ and the concentration predicted $\hat{C}(t)$ for each time point are not randomly distributed around zero. Accordingly, for these data we would choose to evaluate them next in a two-compartment model. This example shows that it is necessary to review each animal's data graphically in order to direct the modeling software towards an acceptable solution. Whether a correct choice has been made is subsequently confirmed by statistically comparing the output of the model parameters for a one- versus a two- (or more) compartment model, often using Akaike's Information Criterion (AIC) as the test statistic [32]. The process of fitting the best model to the data is iterative. We choose an objective criterion, such as the sum of the squares of the errors (SSE), and iterate in search for the solution that minimizes this criterion.

Having chosen the pharmacokinetic model for this example as

$$C(t) = A_1 e^{-k_1 t} + A_2 e^{-k_2 t} \tag{7.50}$$

we now must estimate the model's variables A_i and k_i. It should be noted that it is possible to parameterize compartmental models for intercepts and rates as described above using the first-order rate equation, or using the inter-compartmental rate micro-constants, or in terms of clearance and volume. Some authorities prefer the latter approach [33].

Some computer software requires manual input of initial estimates for model variables and some packages derive their own initial estimates. The choice of initial estimates can markedly affect the outcome of the model fitting. It is good practice to test one's model for robustness to variation in the initial estimates. If different initial estimates yield different results, then the pharmacokinetic model or the statistical model may be unsuited to the data.

It is still premature to make the statistical comparison between models, because first a statistical model must be chosen for this process. The statistical model needs to describe the relationship between the dependent variable (usually the plasma concentration) and the distribution of its estimates around the mean value (i.e., variance). A variety of variance models are used in pharmacokinetic analyses. Frequently the SSE is not weighted if the distribution of the residuals is homoscedastic. If, however, an examination of residuals has a pattern or a non-random distribution and there is confidence that the pharmacokinetic model is sound, then the model for variance should be changed. The variance model can markedly impact the resulting parameter estimates. For example, the same alfaxalone data can be compared with the residuals unweighted or weighted.

For these data the residuals are evenly scattered with the weighted SSE model, derived in this case by summing the products of each squared error and the reciprocal of its corresponding measured drug concentration (i.e., $1/y$) (Fig. 7.10). Having chosen the pharmacokinetic model and the model for variance, then next step in data analysis is to repeat the pharmacokinetic modeling for all animals, using the same chosen statistical model, and then to compare the fits statistically using a test such as AIC. Note that the variance model must be unchanged in order to evaluate the best-fitting pharmacokinetic structural model. Finally, one must review the model and evaluate its deficiencies. If necessary, the process must be repeated from the beginning to correct errors in experimental design, data collection, analysis, or interpretation [34].

Software for pharmacokinetic model fitting usually offers options to choose the mathematical approach, the 'size' of the steps, and the number of iterations. Making the wrong decisions can result in inaccurate or imprecise parameter estimates. The three main mathematical approaches are those which directly compare the minimizing criterion either using random iterations to vary the parameter estimates (e.g., Monte Carlo) or using a simple stepwise approach (e.g., simplex), or 'gradient' methods that use either first- or second-order derivatives of the minimizing criterion (e.g., Gauss–Newton and Marquardt) [35]. Monte Carlo and simplex methods are robust to poor initial parameter estimates but tend to be slow and computer intensive. With Monte Carlo approaches, care should be taken not to restrict the number of iterations greatly. For simplex methods, one should start with large step sizes and gradually reduce the step size through several runs of the minimization process, to avoid finding false solutions. The gradient methods tend to require good initial estimates in order to proceed, but they have high reliability of quickly finding the best solution, if they have had a good starting point. Often data are analyzed first with a simplex method, then the results of that analysis can be used as the initial estimates for a gradient method.

Data analysis – non-compartmental models

After planning and conducting a pharmacokinetic experiment for a compartmental modeling approach as described above, it is possible to analyze the data using a non-compartmental approach. This approach has the advantage of being applicable to both stochastic and non-stochastic pharmacokinetics and results in the calculation of volumes of distribution, clearance, and mean time parameters.

Generally, mean time parameters describe the average total time spent by molecules in a kinetic space after introduction to that space. The kinetic space is defined by the experimental design, where the samples are derived from the sample space and may represent homogeneous or heterogeneous kinetic spaces. A homogeneous kinetic

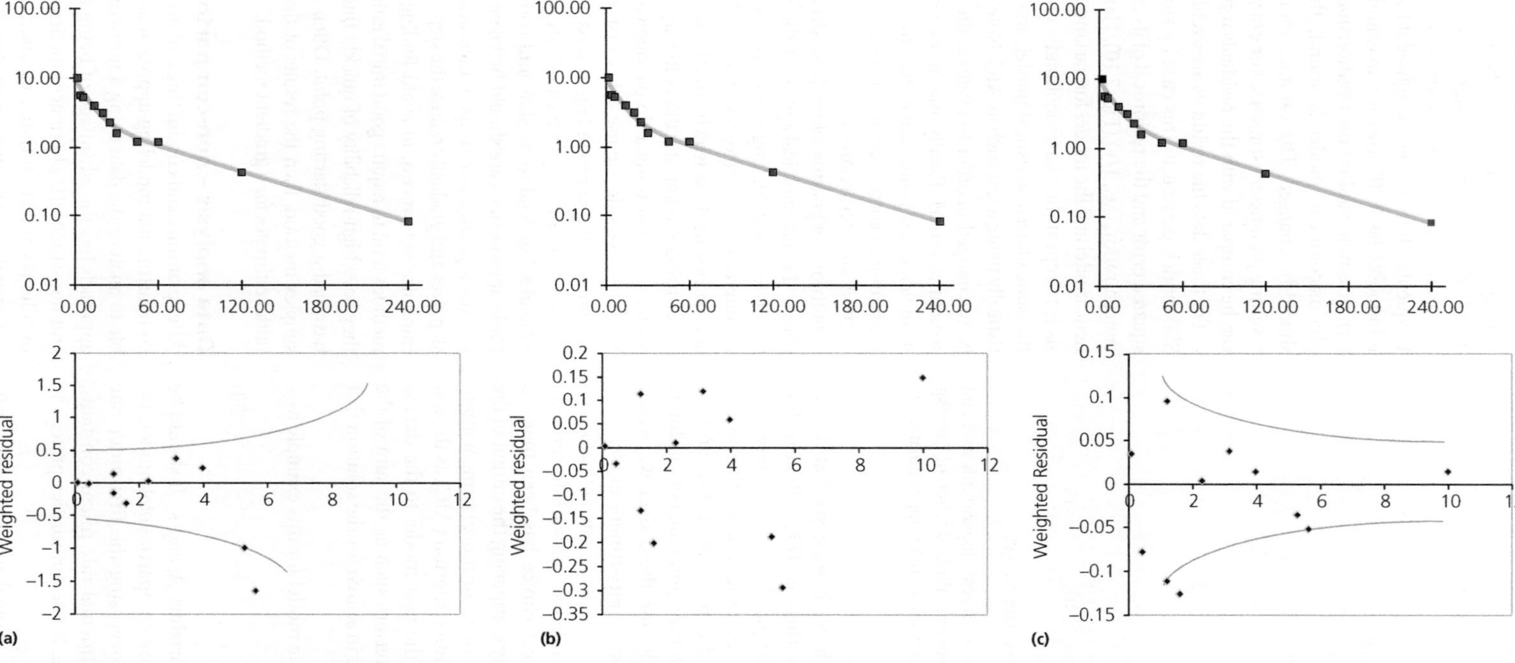

Figure 7.10 Plasma concentration versus time on semi-logarithmic axes and residuals versus concentration, after intravenous administration of 2 mg/kg alfaxalone to a greyhound dog [31], fitted using a two-compartment model, showing the effect of changing the variance models on the distribution of residuals: weight[var(y)]. = $1/y^z$, where (a) $z = 0$, (b) $z = 1$, and (c) $z = 2$.

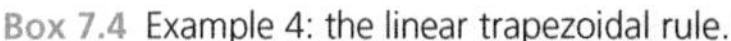

Box 7.4 Example 4: the linear trapezoidal rule.

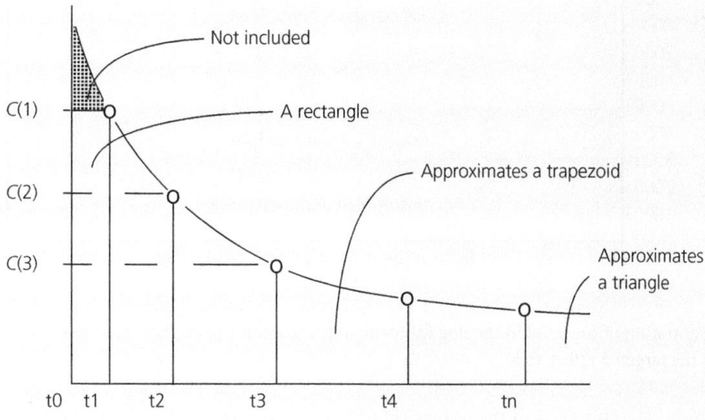

The linear trapezoidal rule

The area under the plasma concentration versus time curve can be estimated using the linear trapezoidal rule using the equation

$$AUC_{(0-\infty)} = \sum_{t=1}^{n}\left(\left\{\left[\frac{C(t)+C(t-1)}{2}\right]\left[t-(t-1)\right]\right\}+\frac{C(n)}{k_{el}}\right)$$

The accuracy of this estimate depends upon the frequency and choice of sample time points, the lower limit of quantification of the assay, the terminal slope of the elimination curve (k_{el}), and the dimension of the excluded initial and estimated final triangles. Subtle changes to the equation are needed for non-intravenous data [36].

space is analogous to a single compartment in a compartmental model whereas a heterogeneous kinetic space is likened to a grouping of multiple independent compartments of a complex compartmental model. This is an important concept to understand when interpreting the meaning of mean time parameters [22].

The mathematics routinely used for the non-compartmental approach [36] are simpler than for compartmental modeling, although their derivation and hence ease of understanding are more opaque. It is important to note that many of the frequently used equations rely on the same underlying assumption of linear pharmacokinetics [22]. The two most important calculated variables used for parameter estimation in non-compartmental analyses are the area under the concentration versus time curve from the time of introduction of the dose ($t=0$) until infinity [$AUC_{(0-\infty)}$], and the area under the first moment of the concentration versus time curve from the time of dosing ($t=0$) until infinity [$AUMC_{(0-\infty)}$]. These are usually calculated from the data using the linear or log-linear trapezoidal methods (Box 7.4) [37].

Errors in estimation of these variables result in misleading pharmacokinetic parameter estimates. The most common error in estimating AUC and AUMC is failing to define the pharmacokinetic curve for an adequate time period, resulting in a large portion of the total area being under the portion of the curve that is after the last quantified time point, i.e., the portion of the curve that is extrapolated. As a rule of thumb, if the proportion of the total area that was extrapolated is greater than 20%, then the experimental design is inadequate for this approach to data analysis. Parts of the experimental design that need to be re-evaluated in this case are the duration and frequency of sampling and the lower limit of quantification of the assay.

Non-compartmental modeling can provide the same useful pharmacokinetic parameters that are used for dose calculation and for understanding the need for alterations to pharmacokinetics in diseased animals. There are differences of opinion as to whether the added complexity in data analysis for compartmental modeling provides great benefit over the simpler arithmetic of non-compartmental approaches for generation of pharmacokinetic variable estimates.

Data analysis in more complex models

The examples discussed above are conveniently simple. However, there are many variations from these simple modeling approaches that can become necessary to describe data adequately. The compartmental models introduced above are used with an implicit understanding of their many assumptions. The implications of these assumptions are especially troubling to anesthesiologists. The most problematic of these assumptions is that there is assumed to be instantaneous mixing of the drug after introduction to a large, homogeneous central compartment. Pharmacokinetic studies rarely include sample collection at less than 2 min after an intravenous dose because it has been demonstrated that complete mixing of a rapid intravenous bolus dose in the dog is delayed for approximately 1 min [38]. For intravenous general anesthesia, many of the important pharmacodynamic events are well under way or completed within 2 min, but the simple compartmental and non-compartmental models do not assist us to understand the rapid pharmacokinetic changes that drive these events. Physiologically based pharmacokinetic (PBPK) models make allowance for individual organ and tissue blood flow as a proportion of cardiac output. Appropriate PBPK study designs allow the determination of the extraction ratio for each organ of interest and the drug clearance achieved by that organ and estimation of organ or tissue drug concentration. For example, the evaluation of propofol administration using PBPK models led to a better understanding of the effect of slow intravenous administration on the duration of anesthesia, markedly altering anesthetic practice and ultimately improving quality of transition to volatile anesthetic [39,40]. Finally, PBPK models allow understanding of the effect of drug recirculation on

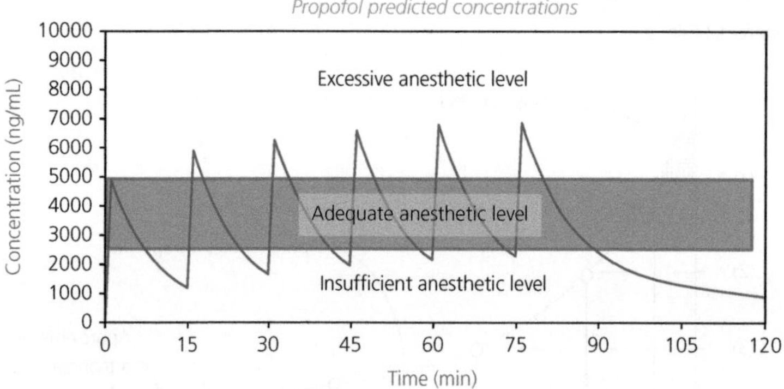

Figure 7.11 Simulated plasma concentration of propofol in the dog following repeated bolus (4 mg/kg) injections over time. Propofol is injected every 15 min. The shaded area represents the targeted effect area.

the arterial and venous drug concentrations, an understanding that is fundamental to modern intravenous anesthesia [38,41].

For drugs where there are multiple points of drug input, such as complex formulations with non-linear absorption, data analysis that uses a deconvolution approach may be needed: the intravenous pharmacokinetics can be defined independently in each individual, then progressing to modeling of the absorption phases.

Delayed absorption or distribution can result in a lag between dosing and changes in concentration, or between the appearance of drug in the sample space and its distribution to the site of action. This is frequently exemplified by NSAIDs. Modeling NSAIDs in PK–PD models can require inclusion of lag-times in the models [42].

Using mixed effects hierarchical modeling, known as population pharmacokinetics (POP-PK), allows the estimation of large numbers of model parameters and more careful characterization of the sources of variance. Purpose-written software with capabilities such as convolution and deconvolution and parametric and non-parametric nonlinear mixed effects modeling in data analysis is necessary, as are targeted training and deep expertise in understanding and implementing such data analyses.

Constant rate therapy

Constant rate therapy is used when maintenance of a specific plasma concentration and its consequent effect is desired. Constant rate therapy is usually achieved intravenously, although constant rate release devices and systems are also available such as patches and slow-release injectable agents [43]. To produce a sustained drug plasma concentration, a constant rate of absorption is required. For simplicity, we will consider that such devices behave similarly to a constant rate IV infusion. To provide constant rate therapy and maintain constant plasma concentration using IV administration, two techniques are usually described [44]: intermittent bolus injection and continuous infusion. The aim with both of these techniques is to administer drug at a rate equal to its clearance.

Intermittent boluses

Intermittent IV bolus administration is a very simple technique. The only equipment needed consists of an IV catheter and a syringe containing the agents (anesthetic, analgesic, etc.). After injection of the loading dose, the effect can be maintained by repeated injections. After each injection, the plasma drug concentration reaches a peak and then starts to decrease as a function of distribution and clearance. This decrease in plasma drug concentration will cause a decrease in drug concentration at the effect site that will reach a point where the effect will not be adequate (e.g., patient waking up, breakthrough pain), and a new bolus will be necessary for the desired effect to be re-established. With intermittent IV bolus administration, the drug plasma concentration tends to oscillate between peaks of relative excess and troughs of ineffective amount (Fig. 7.11). In addition to the very poor consistency in the targeted effect, this technique can result in the administration of a large total drug dose and consequently can cause a slower and longer recovery from the effect [44,45].

Continuous rate infusion

By eliminating the peaks and troughs in plasma concentration that occur with the intermittent bolus technique, continuous infusion results in a better quality of effect and a decrease in the total drug dose delivered [44,45]. The cheapest and least accurate way to maintain a continuous infusion is to use a bag containing the chosen agent(s) and an administration set [44,46]. The flow rate can be adjusted by varying the radius of the infusion tubing using a 'regulating' clamp (Fig. 7.12). The infusion rate can be calculated

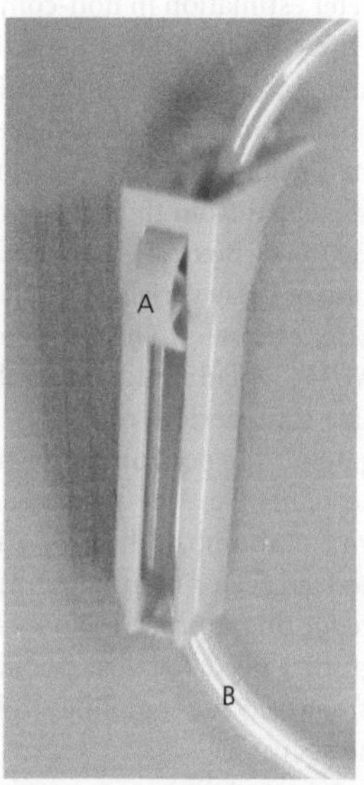

Figure 7.12 'Regulating' clamp used to modify the radius of the infusion tubing. The wheel (A) allows modification of the radius of the infusion tubing (B), allowing the speed of the infusion to be varied.

knowing the volume of each drop (e.g., 20 versus 60 drops/mL) and counting the drip rate. In this system, the speed of infusion is gravity dependent and depends also on the diameter and length of the connecting tube, the size of the drops, the size of the cannula, the viscosity of the agent, the height of the fluid, and the venous pressure of the patient. As the fluid decreases in the bag, the infusion rate decreases and needs readjusting.

Infusion pumps and syringe drivers allow a more controlled continuous, accurate, and safer infusion [44,46]. Larger volume infusions will be administered accurately using an infusion pump whereas a syringe driver is more appropriate for smaller volumes at slower rates.

Potential hazards with infusion pumps and syringe drivers include a too rapid rate of infusion (administration set not properly clamped), failure of power (main and battery), infusion of air, and continued infusion although the cannula has become extravascular. Modern infusion devices are able to detect some of these faults, such as air in the system and line blockage. In addition, with syringe drivers the clinician should also be aware that the position of the device is important: if positioned higher than the patient's heart, siphoning may occur due to the weight of the liquid [44], which will result in a larger volume of drug being administered than was programmed. To avoid this, the device must have protection against the syringe plunger moving faster than its motor drive. Conversely, a position of the syringe driver that is lower than the vascular access port can result in less agent being infused than programmed, owing both to the back-pressure from the venous bed and to the weight of the liquid. To avoid these hazards, infusion sets should incorporate a one-way valve system. Further, if the syringe driver is positioned vertically, the outlet should be placed downwards so as to avoid infusing bubbles formed by gas coming out of solution.

When choosing an infusion pump or a syringe driver, the clinician should consider the following: versatility (choice of bolus or infusion mode), internal calculator for choice of dosing scheme, choice of infusion rates, possibility of using different-sized syringes (even from different manufacturers), light weight, clear display of drug administered and infusion rate, simple protocol for initiation or change of infusion rates, digital interface for record keeping, and external automated control and alarms for tubing disconnection, high pressure, and presence of bubbles in the tubing [44,47].

Continuous rate infusion can be classified as being either non-pharmacokinetic or pharmacokinetic dependent.

Non-pharmacokinetic-dependent infusion systems – constant rate infusion (CRI) and rate-controlled infusion (RCI)

When using a constant rate infusion (CRI), the clinician decides empirically on an infusion rate and maintains that rate for the whole procedure. Unfortunately, with such a system, the plasma drug concentration that is achieved is not controlled. Choice of CRI is not appropriate for drugs with relatively long elimination half-lives: at the beginning of the procedure the plasma drug concentration will be low and might not provide an adequate effect. With time, the concentration will climb as the mass of drug accumulates in the animal and the effect of the agent will become more adequate. If the procedure is prolonged, the plasma drug concentration may reach the point at which undesired side-effects occur (Fig. 7.13). To avoid the initial lack of effect, a loading dose may be administered immediately prior to beginning the CRI (Fig. 7.14). Unfortunately, in prolonged CRI therapy, monitoring for undesired clinical effects is the only practical approach available to alert the clinician to drug accumulation. Despite these shortcomings, CRI is a useful technique in some clinical settings, for example, the administration of morphine to dogs for analgesia or of ketamine in the triple drip anesthesia technique in the horse.

To minimize drug accumulation and the consequent side-effects, the clinician can change the drug infusion rate according to the observed needs of the patient. This technique [rate-controlled infusion (RCI)] can provide a much smoother anesthesia with less total drug used, but frequent adjustments might sometimes be necessary to fine tune the infusion to the patient's needs.

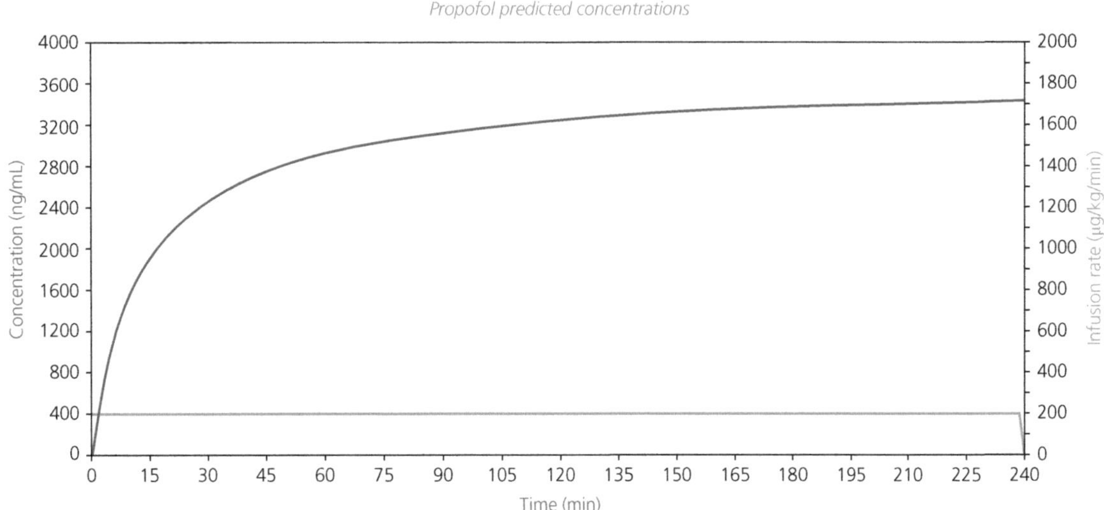

Figure 7.13 Simulated plasma concentration of propofol in the dog during a constant rate infusion over time, derived using the PK simulator PK-SIM (Specialised Data Systems, Jenkintown, PA, USA) and PK parameters of propofol [46]. The blue line represents the predicted plasma concentration. The green line represents the infusion rate (200 µg/kg/min). The infusion rate can be based on empirical data or, as in this case, on pharmacokinetic data.

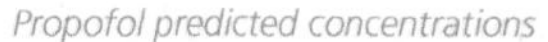

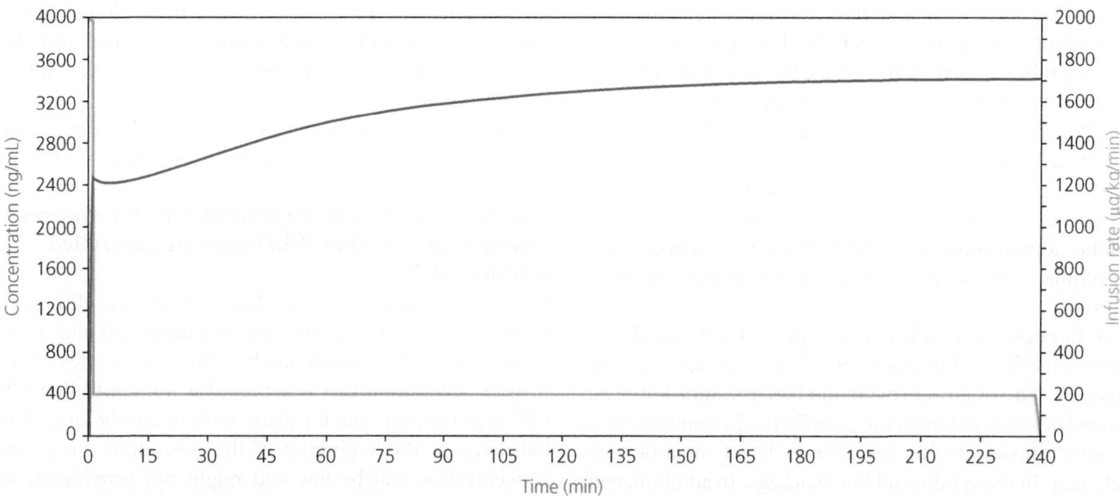

Figure 7.14 Simulated plasma concentration of propofol in the dog after a bolus injection followed by a constant rate infusion over time, derived using the PK simulator PK-SIM (Specialised Data Systems, Jenkintown, PA, USA) and PK parameters of propofol [46]. The blue line represents the predicted plasma concentration. The green line represents the loading dose (2 mg/kg) and the following infusion rate (200 µg/kg/min). The bolus or loading dose and the infusion rate can be based on empirical data or, as in this case, on pharmacokinetic data.

Pharmacokinetic-dependent infusion systems

Knowing a specific agent's pharmacokinetics and its effective plasma concentration allows the development of an infusion scheme that targets the desired plasma drug concentration. The techniques for PK-dependent infusion can be either manually controlled using an RCI or a stepped infusion, or electronically controlled with the help of a computer adjusting the speed of infusion, i.e., target controlled infusion (TCI). The more reliant the technique is on pre-existing PK data, the more the achieved plasma drug concentration will depend on the quality and relevance of the PK model used and the similarities of the patient and the experimental subjects used for initial data collection. Therefore, deviations from the conditions under which the PK data were obtained may result in unexpected plasma dug concentrations. Deviations that should be considered include different species, breed, gender, age, disease state, and concurrent medications.

To maintain a constant targeted plasma drug concentration, i.e., a steady-state plasma drug concentration (C_{ss}), the amount of drug infused must equal the amount of drug being eliminated. This can be expressed by the following equation

$$\text{maintenance rate} = \text{elimination rate} \tag{7.51}$$

Assuming first-order elimination, the mass of drug eliminated per unit time (the elimination rate) will depend on the plasma drug concentration at steady state (C_{ss}) of the agent and the clearance (Cl) [see eqn 7.48]. Therefore, the necessary maintenance infusion rate (k_0) will depend on both the targeted drug plasma concentration at steady state (C_{ss}) and the drug's total body clearance. As observed with the non-PK-dependent CRI (Fig. 7.13), it will take about 4–5 times the elimination half-life for the plasma drug concentration to approach its accumulation plateau. Of course, if an estimate of the V_c is available, a loading dose can also be calculated and administered before the start of the CRI to reach an effective plasma concentration more rapidly (Fig. 7.14). The clinician must realize that although an effective targeted plasma concentration has been reached, it will still take 4–5 half-lives before C_{ss} is reached (Fig. 7.15).

To calculate the loading dose, there are two possible methods: either calculating the dose to fill the central compartment (V_c) or calculating the dose to fill the total distribution volume at steady state (V_{ss}). With the first method using V_c only, the plasma drug concentration obtained will be low whereas with the second method (V_{ss}), there will be an overshoot and an initial increased risk of side-effects.

These simple approaches of applied PK are not always suitable for anesthesia or analgesia and more complex infusion strategies can better achieve the desired initial blood concentration. Ideal infusion schemes can be predicted using known PK parameters and a computer simulation program. Stepped infusion [48–50] consists of a series of CRIs aimed at reaching the targeted plasma drug concentration as rapidly as possible while neither under- nor overshooting (Fig. 7.16). Usually, using a small number of infusion steps help to ensure a practical series.

With a stepped infusion, a fast initial infusion is administered to fill the V_c, followed by a maintenance infusion that will be determined by the desired target or central compartment drug concentration and the drug's rate of clearance [49]. Unfortunately, like the CRI system, the stepped infusion system is very rigid and difficult to adapt to the clinical situation [44,51]. A low target will result in inadequate anesthesia and a high target will result in increased side-effects (hypotension, apnea, delayed recovery).

In 1968, Kruger-Thiemer described an infusion scheme known as BET, standing for Bolus (loading dose), Elimination (steady-state rate of infusion according to drug's elimination) and Transfer (exponentially decreasing rate to match the redistribution of drug from the central compartment to peripheral sites) [48]. In 1981, by interfacing a computer to an infusion pump, Schwilden demonstrated the clinical application of the BET infusion scheme [52]. The first drugs to be administered by this system were etomidate and alfentanil in 1983 [53]. The development of new pumps, computer systems, and infusion rate control algorithms to enable the anesthetist to vary the target plasma drug concentration followed [54]. The first target-controlled infusion (TCI) system was described by Schuttler and colleagues in 1988 [55]. It was only 8

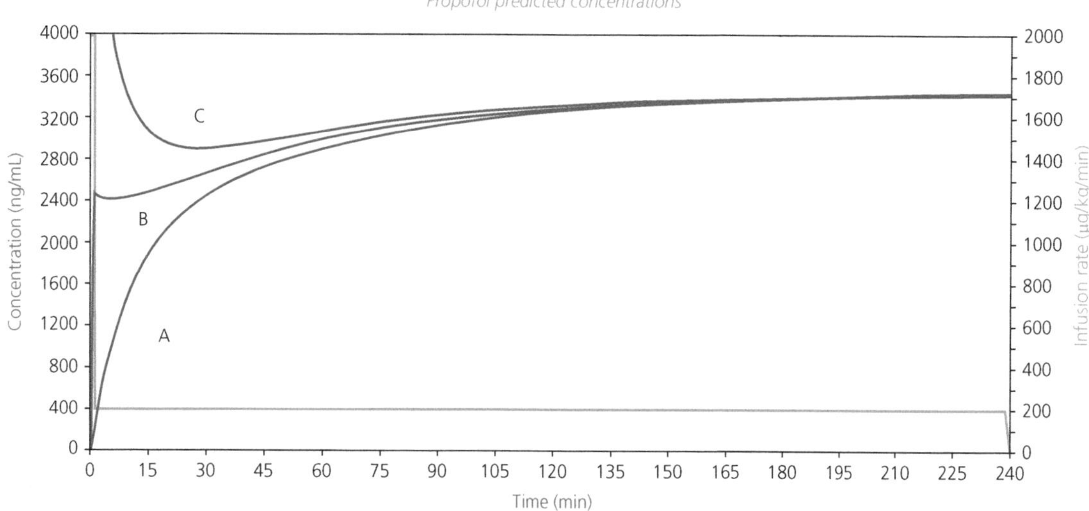

Figure 7.15 Simulated plasma concentration of propofol in the dog during a constant rate infusion over time (a) or preceded by a bolus of 2 mg/kg (b) and 4 mg/kg (c), derived using the PK simulator PK-SIM (Specialised Data Systems, Jenkintown, PA, USA) and PK parameters of propofol [46]. The blue line represents the predicted plasma concentration. The green line represents the loading doses (2 and 4 mg/kg) and the following infusion rate (200 µg/kg/min). This graph shows that 3–4 half-lives are still necessary to reach the steady-state concentration (C_{ss}), without a loading dose preceding the CRI. The bolus or loading dose and the infusion rate can be based on empirical data or, as in this case, on pharmacokinetic data.

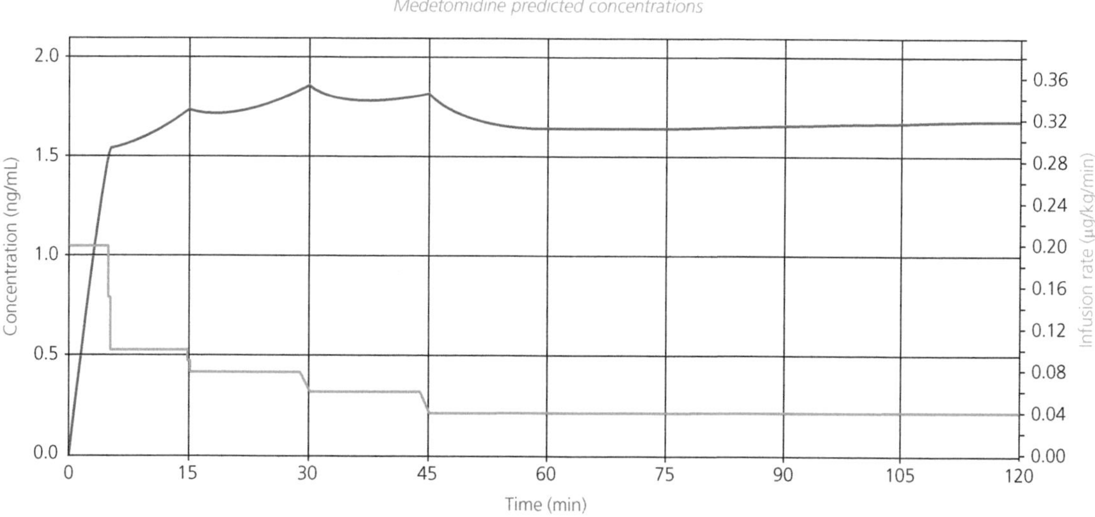

Figure 7.16 Five-step infusion (green line) of medetomidine in the dog with a target blood concentration of 1.7 ng/mL and the predicted plasma concentration of medetomidine (blue line), derived using the PK simulator PK-SIM (Specialised Data Systems, Jenkintown, PA, USA).

years later, in 1996, that the first commercial TCI system for use with propofol in humans was launched [56,57].

The fundamental principles and development of the TCI system were described by Gray and Kenny [58] and Glen [57]. Succinctly, a TCI system is a computer programmed with a set of PK parameters (specific for a species and a drug) and coupled with a syringe driver. The computer pump control algorithm calculates the infusion rate that is necessary to achieve a blood target concentration. Once the target blood concentration has been achieved, the computer will control the pump to maintain the blood target concentration.

The speed of infusion is calculated as follows:

$$\text{infusion rate} = C_t V_c \left(k_{12} e^{k_{21} t} + k_{13} e^{k_{31} t}\right) \tag{7.52}$$

where C_t is the targeted concentration, V_c is the volume of the central compartment, t is time, and k_{12}, k_{21}, k_{13}, k_{31} are the microconstants describing the movement of the agent between the different compartments of the three-compartment model [59].

To begin, a bolus is calculated ($C_t \times V_c$) and administered. As illustrated by the equation, if the target is kept constant, the infusion rate will decrease exponentially over time to match the cumulative characteristic of the agent [60]. At any point the clinician can choose to modify the target. An increase in target concentration will result in injection of a calculated bolus dose using the same formula as above ($C_t \times V_c$), but where C_t is the difference between the current C and the new C_t. It will then be followed by an exponentially decreasing infusion rate that will be higher than the

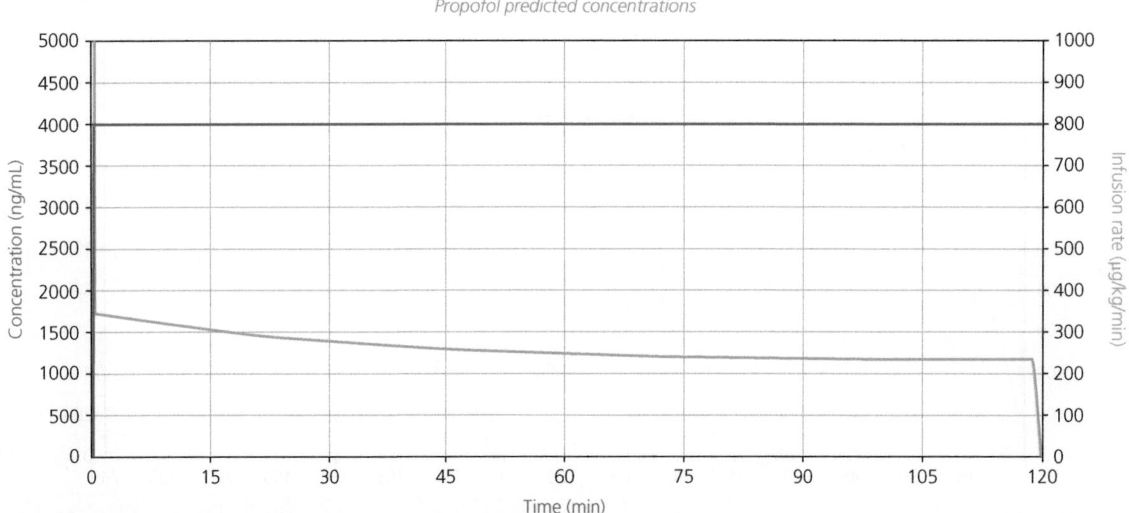

Figure 7.17 Simulated plasma concentration of propofol in the dog during a target-controlled infusion (TCI) over time, derived using the PK simulator PK-SIM (Specialised Data Systems, Jenkintown, PA, USA) and PK parameters of propofol [46]. The blue line represents the plasma concentration with a propofol target of 4000 ng/mL. The green line represents the exponentially decreasing infusion rate.

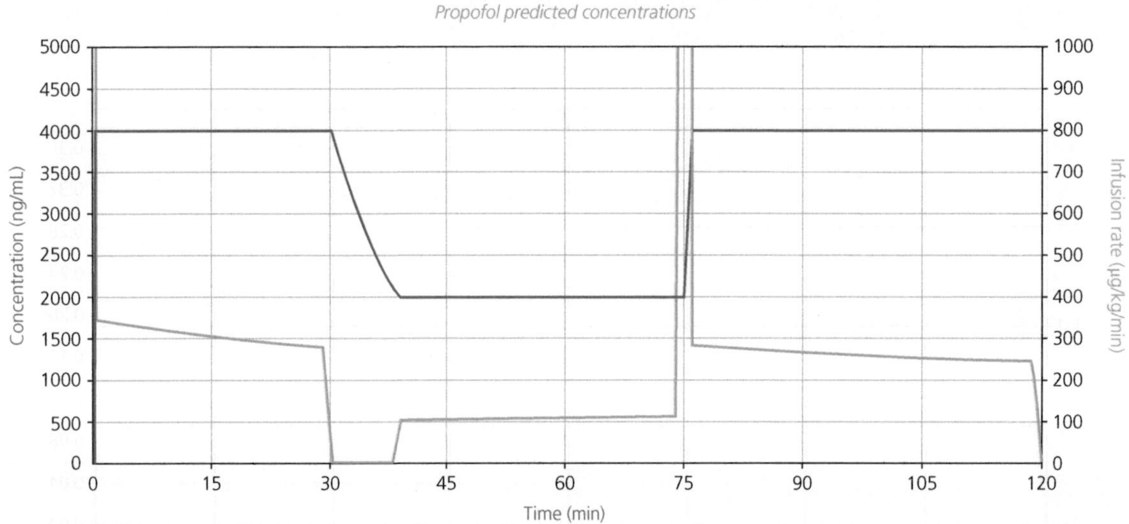

Figure 7.18 Simulated plasma concentration of propofol in the dog during a target-controlled infusion (TCI) over time, derived using the PK simulator PK-SIM (Specialised Data Systems, Jenkintown, PA, USA) and PK parameters of propofol [46]. This graph simulates an anesthesia where the clinician, 30 min after targeting a propofol plasma concentration (blue line) of 4000 ng/mL, decided to decrease the level anesthesia with a new propofol plasma concentration of 2000 ng/mL. Then 45 min later, the anesthesia is deepened by the change to a new propofol plasma concentration (4000 ng/mL). The green line represents the exponentially decreasing infusion rate for the different plasma concentration. Note that the infusion stopped at time 30 min, allowing the propofol plasma concentration to decrease from 4000 to 2000 ng/mL. Note the bolus injection given time 75 min when the propofol plasma concentration was once again changed to 4000 ng/mL.

original infusion rate. Following a decrease in target concentration, the infusion will cease until the new target, as predicted by the computer, is reached. Thereafter, an exponentially decreasing infusion rate will resume, at a lower rate than previously [60]. Examples of these schemes are illustrated in Figs 7.17 and 7.18.

The accuracy of a TCI system is dependent on the PK variables that have been used to program the device. Consequently, the system must be validated before general use in clinical practice. The evaluation of the predictive performance of a TCI system is carried out by comparing the drug concentrations predicted by the system with the measured drug concentrations in either venous or arterial blood samples taken at various time points during anesthesia, over a range of target concentrations, according to a methodology that has been used by many authors [61–71]. This methodology is based on the calculation of the percentage prediction error (*PE*%) as the difference between measured and predicted values expressed as a percentage of the predicted value [65]:

$$PE\% = \frac{\text{measured concentration} - \text{predicted concentration}}{\text{predicted concentration}} \times 100 \quad (7.53)$$

Using values of *PE*% derived at each measurement point, a number of indices of performance in an individual subject are calculated.

The median prediction error (*MDPE*%), provides a measure of bias to indicate whether measured concentrations are systematically above or below targeted values. The median absolute prediction error (*MDAPE*%) measures inaccuracy and gives information on the typical size of the difference between measured and targeted concentrations [69,72].

$$MDPE\% = \text{median}\left\{PE_{ij}, j = 1, \ldots, N_i\right\} \quad (7.54)$$

where N_i is the number of $|PE|$ values obtained for the ith subject, and

$$MDAPE\% = \left\{\left|PE_{ij}\right|, j = 1, \ldots, N_i\right\} \quad (7.55)$$

Two other indices are wobble and divergence, both of which reflect time-related changes. Wobble measures the total intra-individual variability in performance error, and divergence describes any systematic time-related changes in measured concentrations away from or towards the targeted concentration. A positive value indicates a widening of the gap between the predicted and measured concentrations over time, while a negative value indicates that the measured concentrations converge on the predicted values. Information regarding how those can be calculated can be found elsewhere [64,69,72].

Although no reference values have been reported for divergence or wobble, it has been suggested that the performance of a TCI system is clinically acceptable if the bias (*MDPE*%) is not greater than ±10–0% and the inaccuracy (*MDAPE*%) falls between 15 and 40% [60,64,67,73]. In veterinary medicine, such systems have been developed and validated for propofol in the dog [62], for alfentanil in the cat [74–76], and for lidocaine, alfentanil and detomidine in the horse [76–78].

Context-sensitive half-life

Knowledge of the PK of an agent combined with a computer-driven infusion pump allows for a more precise infusion and an easier titration to effect, which could result in quicker recovery. In fact, after cessation of the infusion, the duration of drug effect is more dependent on the PK of the agent than the method of administration [79]. Moreover, for most of the agents, the time to recovery increases with the duration of the infusion. This dependence comprises the concept of context-sensitive half-life (CSHL), wherein the context is the variation of the duration of the infusion [80, 81]. The CSHL is the time from the end of the infusion necessary for the plasma's drug concentration to decrease by 50%. For most anesthetic agents, after a bolus injection the duration of their clinical effect is mostly dependent on redistribution of the drug from the brain to other tissues. After infusion, however, the explanation of the mechanism for recovery from anesthesia varies [81]. Because most anesthetic drugs behave according to multiple compartmental pharmacokinetics, different explanations are needed for different durations of infusion. For short-term infusions, the CSHL will be dependent on redistribution (e.g., a short period of thiopental administration). For moderate infusion times, the CSHL will depend on both the drug's distribution and elimination. For long infusions where the peripheral compartments (tissues) are saturated, the CSHL will approach the true elimination half-life of the drug ($t_{½}$) [81].

The CSHLs for some drugs in cats have recently been described (Fig. 7.19). Drugs vary in their sensitivity to context; fentanyl is very context sensitive whereas remifentanil is context insensitive [82].

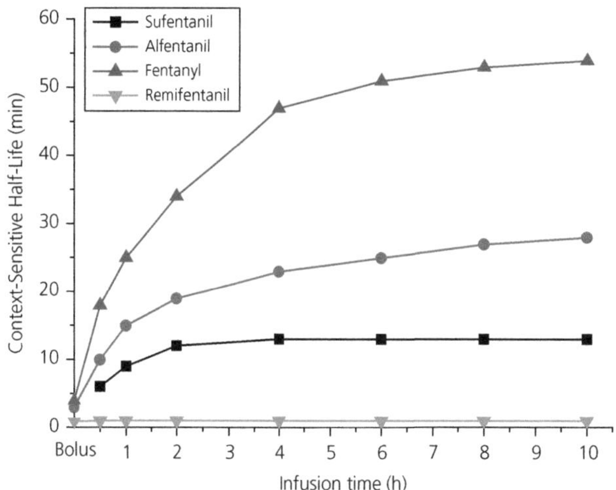

Figure 7.19 Context-sensitive half-lives for four opioids after a bolus and infusion of different duration (0.5–10 h) in isoflurane-anesthetized cats. Source: adapted from [82].

The CSHL is interesting in the clinical setting mostly if it corresponds to the dissipation of a specific observable drug effect (i.e., recovery of spontaneous breathing, recovery of the swallowing reflex, etc.). As this desired clinical effect can occur earlier or later than the 50% decrease of the drug, investigators often provide the times needed for 20%, 50% (CSHL) and 80% decrements in drug concentration. The clinician is usually more interested in the drug concentration at the effect site than in the plasma [83].

A more general term, which was first described in humans for the recovery from opioids, is the context-sensitive effect-site 'decrement' time in which the decrease in concentration is modeled specifically for the compartment of the effect site [59,84]. This parameter allows the clinician to determine better when to stop an infusion (to allow awakening at the end of a surgery). To achieve this, the clinician needs to remember the decrease in concentration necessary for the recovery (percentage), the duration of the infusion (context), and the context-sensitive effect-site decrement time required for the necessary decrease [59].

In 2000, Struys and colleagues [85] compared a TCI system targeting plasma concentration with a TCI system targeting the effect-site concentration. They concluded that targeting the effect-site compartment resulted in less variability and greater predictability in the time to loss of consciousness. They also observed that when targeting the effect site, the onset of drug effect was quicker and without adverse hemodynamic consequences. An effect-site PK parameter (k_{e0}) has been incorporated into human TCI systems to reflect the passage of the drug from the blood to the effect site [86]. The k_{e0} value can be determined during an integrated PK–PD study [87]. Unfortunately, with this method, the k_{e0} value will be specific for this set of PK parameters and will result in poor predictions of the time course of drug effect if one wanted to use it with a different set of PK parameters [86,88]. To be able to link the k_{e0} from an integrated PK–PD study to PK parameters determined in another study, Minto and colleagues in 2003 introduced the time of maximum effect-site concentration (t_{peak}) [87]. Knowing the t_{peak} for a specific agent, the investigator can calculate the value of k_{e0} that accurately predicts t_{peak} when using the set of parameters of interest. With simulations for thiopentone, remifentanil, and propofol, Minto and colleagues showed that the k_{e0} value determined through the t_{peak} method better approximated the time course of drug effect than the simple transfer of a k_{e0} value from one set of PK parameters to another. The usefulness of integrated PK–PD incorporating effect-site rate constants and time of maximum effect site concentration has not yet been explored extensively in veterinary anesthesiology.

Drug interactions

Combinations of drugs may occasionally result in drug–drug interactions, which can be synergistic, antagonistic, or additive [89]. These interactions can be explained by three mechanisms: physicochemical, PK, and PD.

Physicochemical Interactions

Physicochemical interactions usually occur when two incompatible drugs are mixed together *in vitro* (e.g., pH difference). The interaction can take several forms, including changes in physical stability of complex formulations, changes in solubility with precipitation, changes in chemical stability of active or excipient ingredients, adsorption onto delivery device surfaces, and chelation or chemical reactions such as reduction or oxidation. These *in vitro* interactions may be inconsistent between different formulations of the same active ingredients, so clinicians should not assume that a combination which is proven acceptable with particular brands of products will necessarily be equally acceptable with alternative product brands. Unless specific data are available as evidence that a particular combination is without interaction, *in vitro* mixtures should be avoided. Commonly known incompatibilities are tabulated in previous editions of this book and are listed in most common formularies [90].

Pharmacokinetic interactions

Interactions during the different PK phases of absorption, distribution, elimination, or biotransformation are each possible. Some such interactions are used as a deliberate mechanism to alter drug action or duration, e.g., the inclusion of epinephrine in formulations of lidocaine delays the systemic absorption of the lidocaine, prolonging its local action. Although drug interactions in distribution can occur as a function of their interaction at cell membrane transporters in peripheral tissues, these interactions are not described as having clinical relevance in anesthesia and analgesia. Alterations to plasma protein binding by competition between drugs for the same binding site were thought to be of clinical importance [91], but a more thorough understanding of clearance, as discussed above, has led to an understanding that displacement of drugs from protein binding does not markedly alter the unbound fraction in circulation, and therefore affects elimination rate more than efficacy [19]. Consequently, there is a need for many clinicians to 'unlearn' the dogma that has been taught of the potential for clinical toxicity from drug interactions through displacement from plasma protein-binding sites by competition between concomitantly administered drugs.

Drug–drug interactions during biotransformation are generally more frequent [89], and can be of clinical significance depending on the hepatic intrinsic clearance for each drug, as discussed earlier in this chapter. Hepatic drug metabolism can be studied *in vitro* or *in vivo*. *In vitro* studies on PK interactions are both time- and cost-effective. They offer the opportunity to investigate specific biotransformation pathways under strictly controlled conditions and to investigate the ability of a drug to alter the metabolism of other drugs. For these reasons, *in vitro* studies form part of the screening processes used by pharmaceutical companies in the selection of new drugs [92–94]. However, both *in vitro* and *in vivo* evidence for drug–drug interactions in metabolism should be interpreted with care, as there is a growing understanding of the extent of genetic polymorphism among individuals or breeds of the same species (e.g., reduced hepatic metabolism of butorphanol in certain dog breeds)and its impact on drug metabolism and toxicity [95,96]. The well-described sensitivity of the rough collies to ivermectin has been attributed to a frame-shift mutation within the multidrug resistance (*MDR1*) gene, which has now been discovered within several other related breed of dogs [97–99]. However, the clinical relevance of this mutation in canine anesthesia has not been demonstrated. Further, it is not possible to extrapolate drug metabolism evidence between species as major differences exist in metabolic pathways and enzyme activities [100,101].

Elimination or clearance of a drug is also subject to drug–drug interactions. Whereas inhibition of the clearance would result in an increase in the drug concentration, possibly to toxic levels, increases in clearance would result in a decrease in the drug blood concentration and possibly lack of efficacy and/or therapeutic failure. Both the inhibition and the induction of drug clearance can affect either the CYPs (see Phase I metabolism) or the transporters (see Phase III metabolism). Clinically important interactions affecting elimination or clearance are rare.

In addition to those two types of clearance alteration, other causes have been described. Pharmacokinetic interaction can be mediated physiologically. For example, it has been well documented that during CRI or TCI with drugs of high intrinsic hepatic clearance, increases in cardiac output will result in decreases in plasma drug concentration and consequent changes to efficacy, and vice versa. This alteration in hepatic clearance related to change in cardiac output has been demonstrated with propofol in humans, sheep, and pigs and likely occurs with many anesthetics and analgesics [39,102–106].

Pharmacodynamic interactions

Pharmacodynamic interactions result in the modification of the response of the body to one or more concomitantly administered drugs. These modifications can be due to mechanisms such as the alteration of the receptor sensitivity or affinity to one agent by the other. Alternatively, the production of additive or inhibitory effects can occur either through action at different effect sites or by actions through alternative receptor mechanisms. Interactions through PD mechanisms are common clinical realities, such as the sparing effect of opioids or α_2-adrenergic receptor agonists on the MAC values of an inhalant agents or propofol infusion. However, when considering clinically important drug–drug inter-relationships, it is worth noting that inter-individual PD variability frequently ranges between 300 and 400% and inter-individual variance of PK can be in the order of 70–80% [107,108]. This inter-individual PK and PD variability makes it difficult to identify an unexpected clinical occurrence as an unwanted drug interaction rather than simply a function of inter-individual variability.

There are two major types of studies developed to assess PD interactions, either isobolographic analyses or response surface modeling techniques. Knowledge from studies using these methods permits dosing decisions designed to maximize or minimize an interaction. Interactions are often deleterious to clinical case management, but can also be beneficial (e.g., optimizing speed of induction of anesthesia, increasing hemodynamic stability at induction and during maintenance of anesthesia, decreasing time to awakening, optimizing spontaneous respiration, and minimizing the level of postoperative pain) [107,109,110].

Isobolographic analyses

Isobolographic studies evaluate the effects of different concentrations of two agents on a specific effect, such as loss of consciousness. Different dosing pair combinations resulting in the same effect are evaluated. An isobole can be constructed by drawing a line through those 'iso-effective' combinations. A straight line called the 'line of additivity' or 'additive interaction' is drawn between the two concentrations for each single agent associated with the same effect (Fig. 7.20). Synergism is usually associated with a concave-up shaped isobole whereas infra-additivity is associated with a concave-down shaped isobole. One of the main problems with this system is that the information is only in two dimensions and only gives the information for a specific effect level (i.e., EC_{50} or EC_{95}) [109].

Response surface analyses

To describe a more complete set of effect levels (EC_{01}–EC_{99}), a response surface is constructed using three-dimensional graphs that incorporate all the available isoboles for different levels of the effect (Fig. 7.21). In such a system, each single combination of the two drugs is a point on a surface, the height of which is the drug effect of interest [111]. Different mathematical approaches have

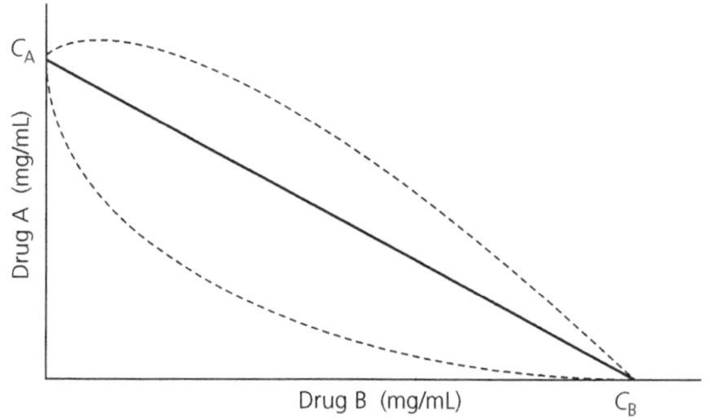

Figure 7.20 Example of an isobole for two agents, A and B, when given alone (C_A and C_B) and when given in combination to induce an effect such as endotracheal intubation. The isobole can take different shapes depending of the nature of the interaction between the two agents.

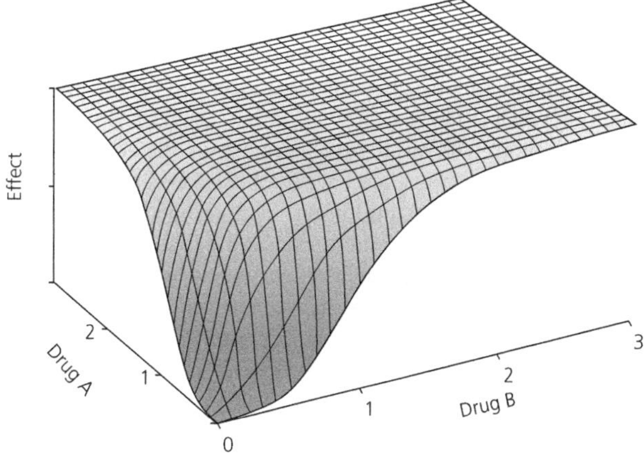

Figure 7.21 Modeling of a response (effect) surface between two hypothetical agents, A and B. Source: adapted from [109].

been described to produce the response surface [112,113]. It has been proposed that while the mathematical approach of Minto *et al.* [112] is appropriate for the analysis of unimodal endpoints (loss of consciousness, return of consciousness), Bol *et al.*'s approach [113] was better suited to analyze multimodal endpoints (adequacy of anesthesia which includes hypnotic and analgesic components) [114]. If one is studying the interaction of drugs which on their own do not produce the studied effect, other models have been proposed, such as the Reduced Greco, Fixed C50O Hierarchical, and Scaled C50O Hierarchical models [115]. To determine the optimal response, these models can be used in combinations with PK data [116]. In humans, PK–PD modeling of propofol and different opioids has been used to maximize the use of both agents [110]. The PK–PD modeling determines the various optimal propofol–opioid concentrations associated with intra-operative adequacy of anesthesia and the most rapid return to consciousness thereafter. As expected, the optimal propofol concentration changes with both the opioid used and the length of infusion [107,110].

Adverse drug reactions

Adverse drug reactions (ADRs) and adverse drug events (ADEs) are collective terms that are each used to describe events that include both undesired effects and inefficacy, relative to the expected effects after drug administration [117,118]. Evaluation of ADEs divides them into several categories, although the categories are not exclusive: dose-related, non-dose-related, dose- and time-related, time-related, withdrawal, and unexpected inefficacy.

Population variability in drug-response blurs the boundary between ADEs that are non-dose-related (unexpected events) and dose-related (inefficacy, toxicity). Toxic events can occur at unexpectedly low doses in sensitive individuals. Apparent inefficacy can occur at labeled doses, when the labeled dose is established using population parameters such as the effective dose for a proportion of the population. For example, in some regulatory territories the labeled dose of alfaxalone is its ED_{90} [119].

Drugs that induce physiological adaptation, receptor downregulation or tachyphylaxis, and enzyme induction or inhibition can result in time-related undesired effects. These effects can be either direct or be caused by drug interactions, as discussed previously. Developing tolerance can result in the onset of inefficacy, or upon their withdrawal unexpected ADEs can occur because of the unmasking of the adapted physiological changes. Although such ADEs are rarely recognized in veterinary medicine, some drugs frequently used possess characteristics that lead to these time-related ADEs (e.g., adrenergic agonists such as clenbuterol [120] and opiate analgesics) [121].

Voluntary reports of ADEs submitted through voluntary reporting schemes are likely to underestimate the true number of ADEs that occur. Despite this likely under-reporting, large numbers of ADEs are reported each year. Within the drug classes of relevance to the practice of anesthesia and analgesia, the NSAIDs are the category of drugs about which ADEs are most numerously reported [118]. Relative to the number of doses used, voluntary reports of ADEs for anesthetic induction agents such as propofol, ketamine, and alfaxalone are relatively rare [122].

Regulatory agencies and drug manufacturers endeavor to assess each ADE and assign a causal probability classification. A commonly used causality classification is a categorical system that is subjectively based: certain, probable, possible, unlikely, unassessable [117]. Some regulatory jurisdictions use a flow chart scoring system [123]. Drug products that receive a high number of 'certain' or 'probable' assessments are occasionally subject to regulatory review. For example, a high number of ADEs to an injectable propofol in Australia in 2004 [124] resulted in a regulatory review with subsequent mandatory label changes warning of ADEs to one of its excipients.

Drug metabolism

Metabolism of administered xenobiotics can result in their activation from ineffective prodrugs, transformation or modification of the extent or nature of their activity, or detoxification and facilitation of their excretion. Metabolism of drugs, or biotransformation, is classically described as occurring in two phases. A xenobiotic may be metabolized by either or both of these phases depending on the physicochemical properties of the drug and the species of animal. Phase I biotransformations aim to convert fat-soluble (lipophilic) compounds into water-soluble (hydrophilic) compounds ready for immediate renal clearance, or to add chemically reactive sites to a relatively chemically inert molecule so as to allow further biotransformation. Secondary biotransformation processes can be either further Phase I reactions or may be conjugation reactions. In general, conjugation reactions attach the exogenous compound covalently to a substrate, which increases both the molecular weight and the water solubility of the complex. Conjugation reactions collectively are called Phase II reactions. The chemical reactions associated with Phases I and II are reported in Table 7.1 [125–144].

The water-soluble compounds formed during Phase I and II metabolism need to be transported out of the cells prior to excretion. Some excretion processes are also transcellular, requiring further transport across biological membranes. These transcellular transport processes have recently been labeled as a 'third phase' or Phase III of the drug metabolism process [145]. Factors described as affecting drug metabolism include species, gender, genetics, age, hormone and disease status, drug–drug interactions, diet, and environment (i.e., nearly everything!) [146,147].

Phase I biotransformation

The bulk of the Phase I biotransformation reactions are performed by a family of enzymes called the cytochrome P450 isoenzymes (CYPs), which are found mostly in the liver, but also in the gastrointestinal tract, skin, brain, lung, kidney, and other tissues [148]. The CYPs are principally located on the endoplasmic reticulum of the metabolically active cells and are mainly responsible for oxidation, reduction, hydrolysis, and hydration reactions, which prepare xenobiotics for Phase II conjugation reactions.

Table 7.1 Chemical reactions usually associated with Phase I and Phase II metabolism.

Phase I	Phase II
Oxidation – involving CYP[a]	Glucuronidation
Oxidation – others	Glycosidation
Reduction	Sulfation
Hydrolysis	Methylation
Hydration	Acetylation
Others:	Amino acid conjugation
Isomerization	Glutathione conjugation
Ring cyclization	Condensation
Dimerization	Fatty acid conjugation
Transamidation	
Decarboxylation	
Dethioacetylation	
N-Carboylation	

[a] Cytochrome P450.

Source: adapted from Gibson GG, Skett P, eds. *Introduction to Drug Metabolism. An Introduction*, 3rd edn. Andover: Cengage Learning EMEA, 2001.

The CYPs are hemoproteins that exhibit a spectral absorbance maximum at 450 nm when reduced and complexed with carbon monoxide. The general reaction catalyzed by the CYPs can be written as follows:

$$\mathrm{NADPH + H^+ + O_2 + RH \xrightarrow{CYT\,P450} CYT\,P\,450 \rightarrow NADP^+ + H_2O + ROH}$$

where RH represents an oxidizable drug substrate and ROH its hydroxylated metabolite.

The CYP isoenzymes are a superfamily with a modern classification and nomenclature derived from gene cloning and sequencing [149]. The superfamily is divided into families that are themselves divided into subfamilies, depending on the percentage of their genome that the CYPs have in common. The enzyme families are described by an Arabic number, the subfamilies by a capital letter, and a final Arabic number denotes individual enzymes. Although some CYPs have been screened and identified in human, mouse, rats, and monkeys (only a handful are known in dogs so far, including CYP 1A1, 1A2, 2B11, 2E, 2C21, 2C41, 2D15, 3A12, and 3A26 [150,151]. In dogs, CYP 2B11 has been recognized as being responsible for propofol hydroxylation and also for the breed differences seen in propofol metabolism [152,153]. whereas CYP3A seems to be the main contributor to medetomidine metabolism [137].

Induction and inhibition of drug metabolism can lead to drug–drug interactions. The CYP enzymes are most commonly responsible for the metabolism-based interactions [89], the pharmacokinetics of which have been discussed above under Hepatic Clearance. Induction of enzyme activity results from several factors: increased synthesis, decreased degradation, activation of pre-existing components, or a combination of these three processes [92]. In dogs, phenobarbital increases the activity of CYP 2B11, 2C21, and 3A26, rifampin induces CYP 3A26, and omeprazole induces CYP 1A2 [150]. Further, in the rat, ketamine has been shown to induce propofol metabolism [154]. Four facts are of importance for the clinician to remember regarding enzyme induction: (1) induction is usually a slow process (days to weeks), (2) the effect on drug concentration can alter treatment outcomes, (3) clinical relevance is mostly confined to drugs with low intrinsic hepatic clearance, and (4) the process is usually reversible [155].

An inhibitor will result in a decrease in metabolic enzyme activity. Four main processes have been described that cause CYP inhibition: competitive inhibition, non-competitive inhibition, uncompetitive inhibition, and mechanism-based inhibition [156]. Inhibition of an biotransformation enzyme is mostly reversible in nature, but occasionally can be irreversible and lead to permanent loss of enzyme activity until new enzymes are synthesized [92]. Unlike induction, CYP inhibition is usually an immediate response. The clinical consequences of enzyme inhibition are usually a higher plasma drug concentrations and/or prolonged elimination half-life, increasing the risk of accumulation and toxic effects. Table 7.2 provides a non-exhaustive list of veterinary anesthesia-related agents that can inhibit CYP isoenzymes.

Table 7.2 Non-exhaustive list of anesthesia-related agents with CYP inhibitory activity in different species.

Drug	Species	Ref.
Propofol	Human	125–134
	Rat	135
	Hamster	125, 128
	Pig	
Medetomidine	Dog	136–138
	Rat	136, 138
	Fish	139, 140
Dexmedetomidine	Human	141–143
	Dog	136
	Rat	136, 144
Levmedetomidine	Human	142
	Dog	136
	Rat	136, 144
Atipamezole	Dogs	138

Phase II biotransformation or conjugation

During this phase, endogenous and xenobiotic metabolites will be conjugated, resulting in products of higher molecular weight and usually less activity than their substrates. The products of conjugation are excreted either by the bile, if they are have high molecular weight, or in the urine, if they have both lower molecular weight and high water solubility [149]. Although this phase is generally seen as enhancing the detoxification effect, in some cases the conjugation may result in activated metabolites and increase toxicity [148].

Different mechanisms are involved in conjugations: glucuronidation, sulfation, methylation, acetylation, amino acid conjugation, glutathione conjugation, and fatty acid conjugation. Glucuronidation is quantitatively the most important form of conjugation for drugs in most species and endogenous compounds and can occur with alcohols, phenols, hydroxylamines, carboxylic acids, and so on. Glutathione is regarded as a protective compound in the body for the removal of potentially toxic electrophilic compounds such as epoxides, haloalkanes, nitroalkanes, alkenes, and aromatic halo and nitro compounds. Sulfation is a major metabolic pathway for phenols [157]. The enzymes that facilitate conjugation reactions belong to a superfamily of enzymes and include sulfotransferases (SULT), UDP-glucuronosyltransferases (UGT) and glutathione *S*-transferases (GST) [148].

Transport of metabolites (Phase III biotransformation)

Drug transporters can be found in numerous tissues (intestine, liver, kidney, and brain) and are involved in absorption, distribution, and excretion. They are usually transmembrane transporters which may aid drug and drug–metabolite movement and they include P-glycoprotein (P-gp), organic anion-transporting polypeptide 2 (OATP2) and multidrug resistance-associated protein (MRP). The MRP and the P-gp are called ATP-binding cassette (ABC) transporters as they utilize the energy from ATP to transport substrate across the cell membrane [148]. In the liver, these transporters are found on the canicular membrane where they are involved in the biliary excretion of both parent drugs and their metabolites, and the transporters are also found on the sinusoidal membrane where they are responsible for the uptake of drugs from the blood into the hepatocytes [158]. In the kidneys, the organic anion and cation transport systems are found on brush border and basolateral membranes of the tubular epithelial cells and are responsible for the secretion of drugs into the urine [148,158].

Just as for the CYPs, transporter activity can be increased or decreased and can play a role in both drug absorption and drug elimination. For example, in humans, fruit juices are well-known inhibitors of organic anion transporters and result in reduced oral drug bioavailability. Also in humans, the hepatic and/or renal excretion of digoxin is altered by verapamil and quinidine, which are potent inhibitors of P-gp. The inhibition of P-gp results in increased plasma concentration of the cardiac glycosides [158–160].

Isomers and stereoisomers

Although labeled simply with the active drug's pharmacopeial name, many of the drug products commonly used contain more than one form of the active molecule. Drug molecules often are carbon-based entities, the majority of which have multiple structural molecular forms, called isomers. Isomers can be either constitutional isomers or stereoisomers. Constitutional isomers are those with the same number and type of atoms, but where the connectivity between the atoms differs (e.g., propane versus cyclopropane). Stereoisomers occur either because of the inflexibility of carbon–carbon double bonds (*cis–trans* isomers), or because a carbon molecule may have four different covalently bonded moieties, thus creating one or more chirally active centers (enantiomers and diastereomers).

Constitutional isomers pose little practical clinical problem, as drug products rarely contain mixtures of such isomers. Similarly, because *cis–trans* isomers usually have major differences in affinity for drug receptors or metabolizing enzymes, products rarely have more than a minor contamination of the less active isomer. In contrast to non-chiral isomers, chirally active stereoisomers pose a major consideration for clinical pharmacology, pharmacokinetics, and anesthesia. There are two types of chiral stereoisomers, enantiomers and diastereomers. Enantiomers are chirally active stereoisomers that have planar symmetry, i.e., one form is the mirror image of the other. Where a molecule has two chirally active centers, there is a possibility of four isomers. Two of the possible pairings result in symmetry and are stereoisomers, but the other four pairing permutations do not have planar symmetry, and are called diastereomers. Products that contain a mixture of enantiomers are called a racemic mixture.

For stereoisomers there are two naming conventions that do not necessarily align. The *R–S* system of naming involves a deliberate orientation of the molecule in space, then reading the direction of descending atomic mass; clockwise is *R*, where *R* is from the Latin *rectus* = straight, and anticlockwise is *S*, where *S* is from the Latin *sinister* = left. Alternatively, if polarized light rotates to the right when passed through a solution of an enantiomer, then the enantiomer is designated the dextrorotatory (+) isomer and the image is the levorotatory (−) isomer. Many of the drugs used in anesthesia have chiral isomers and are marketed as racemic mixtures, e.g., thiopental, ketamine, carprofen, and ketoprofen. The mammalian body is a very chiral environment and enantiomers can have markedly different efficacy, potency, safety, and pharmacokinetics [161–165]. Sometimes these differences are exemplified or altered by unequal binding to albumin [166,167]. Further, for some drugs, the mammalian isomerase enzymes can convert isomers between forms, but for other enantiomers such enzyme isomerization is not achieved [168].

As techniques for the manufacture of purified enantiomers become cheaper, products are likely to be marketed that comprise pure enantiomers or non-racemic mixtures. These products may have different efficacy and toxicity profiles from their racemic look-alikes, and may require attention to different dosing regimens, (e.g., medetomidine versus dexmedetomidine).

Effect of formulation

Most of the drug products that we commonly use are not labeled with information about their contents, other than the name and concentration of the active molecule. The drug products usually contain a far greater mass of other 'ingredients' called excipients. The excipients can have marked effects on drug efficacy and safety.

An example of formulation effects is illustrative of the need for clinical attention to formulation. The white-colored propofol is formulated as a stabilized emulsion using oil and emulsifiers to provide a useful formulation that maintains its physical stability for a suitable shelf life. However, aqueous solutions are preferred for intravenous use and therefore efforts have been made recently to formulate an aqueous solution of propofol. Several successful approaches have resulted in formulations that appear initially to have similar properties to the pioneer milky emulsion [169,170]. However, aqueous microemulsion formulations have been marketed in several countries in which the solubilization was achieved using various polyethoxylated detergents. These aqueous preparations have resulted in reported adverse drug reactions such as anaphylaxis and increased pain on injection [171,172].

Just as isomerization can result in more than one form of the active drug's molecule, other variations of form for the active ingredient can markedly alter a drug's pharmacokinetics. Many oral drugs are dosed as compressed tablets. The active drug in the tablet may be the drug's free base or may be an ionic or organic salt. The drug may be in a dry, amorphous form, or may be crystals. Different salts and different crystal shapes can have markedly different solubilities, causing large changes in bioavailability.

The preparation of a consistently performing, effective, and stable formulation is a high-level pharmaceutical skill. In most major global territories, the manufacturers of products are regulated by governing authorities, providing users with assurance that the product will perform as labeled. In contrast, the recent adoption of products sourced from unlicensed manufacturers, such as compounding pharmacies, may be problematic. Unlicensed manufacturers are of unknown skill and their processes and products are not evaluated, reviewed, or approved. In human and veterinary medicine, there are numerous examples of morbidity and mortality that are directly attributable to poor knowledge, lack of skill, or unsatisfactory processes of and by compounding pharmacies [173–175].

References

1 Bernard C. Analyse physiologique des propriétés des systèmes musculaire et nerveux au moyen du curare. *C R Acad Sci* 1856; **43**: 825–829.

2 Adams HR. *Veterinary Pharmacology and Therapeutics*, 8th edn.Ames, IA: Iowa State University Press, 2001.

3 Heit HA, Gourlay DL. Buprenorphine: new tricks with an old molecule for pain management. *Clin J Pain* 2008; **24**(2): 93–97.

4 Povoa P, Carneiro AH. Adrenergic support in septic shock: a critical review. *Hosp Pract* 2010; **38**(1): 62–63.

5 Goodman LS, Gilman A, Brunton LL. *Goodman & Gilman's Manual of Pharmacology and Therapeutics*. New York: McGraw-Hill Medical, 2008.

6 Sonner JM, Antognini JF, Dutton RC, *et al.* Inhaled anesthetics and immobility: mechanisms, mysteries, and minimum alveolar anesthetic concentration. *Anesth Analg* 2003; **97**(3): 718–740.

7 Barnes PJ. Glucocorticosteroids: current and future directions. *Br J Pharmacol* 2011; **163**(1): 29–33.

8 Mandema JW, Kuck MT, Danhof M. Differences in intrinsic efficacy of benzodiazepines are reflected in their concentration–EEG effect relationship. *Br J Pharmacol* 1992; **105**(1): 164–170.

9 Taylor R Jr, Pergolizzi JV Jr, Porreca F, Raffa RB. Opioid antagonists for pain. *Expert Opin Investig Drugs* 2013; **22**(4): 517–525.

10 Yu FH, Catterall WA. Overview of the voltage-gated sodium channel family. *Genome Biol* 2003; **4**(3): 207.

11 Johnston GA. GABAA receptor pharmacology. *Pharmacol Ther* 1996; **69**(3): 173–198.

12 Traynelis SF, Wollmuth LP, McBain CJ, *et al.* Glutamate receptor ion channels: structure, regulation, and function. *Pharmacol Rev* 2010; **62**(3): 405–496.

13 Calabrese EJ, Baldwin LA. U-shaped dose-responses in biology, toxicology, and public health. *Annu Rev Public Health* 2001; **22**: 15–33.

14 Ariens EJ. Affinity and intrinsic activity in the theory of competitive inhibition. I. Problems and theory. *Arch Int Pharmacodyn Ther* 1954; **99**(1): 32–39.

15 Robbins J, Rall JE. The interaction of thyroid hormones and protein in biological fluids. *Recent Prog Hormone Res* 1957; **13**: 161–202; discussion, 202–208.

16 Toutain PL, Bousquet-Melou A. Plasma terminal half-life. *J Vet Pharmacol Ther* 2004; **27**(6): 427–439.

17 Toutain PL, Bousquet-Melou A. Volumes of distribution. *J Vet Pharmacol Ther* 2004; **27**(6): 441–453.

18 Toutain PL, Bousquet-Melou A. Plasma clearance. *J Vet Pharmacol Ther* 2004; **27**(6): 415–425.

19 Toutain PL, Bousquet-Melou A. Free drug fraction vs free drug concentration: a matter of frequent confusion. *J Vet Pharmacol Ther* 2002; **25**(6): 460–463.

20 Toutain PL, Bousquet-Melou A. Bioavailability and its assessment. *J Vet Pharmacol Ther* 2004; **27**(6): 455–466.

21 Thron CD. Linearity and superposition in pharmacokinetics. *Pharmacol Rev* 1974; **26**(1): 3–31.

22 Veng-Pedersen P. Mean time parameters in pharmacokinetics. Definition, computation and clinical implications (Part 1). *Clin Pharmacokinet* 1989; **17**(5): 345–366.

23 Dayton PG, Cucinell SA, Weiss M, Perel JM. Dose-dependence of drug plasma level decline in dogs. *J Pharmacol Exp Ther* 1967; **158**(2): 305–316.

24 Maylin GA. Disposition of phenylbutazone in the horse. In: *Proceedings of the 20th Convention of the Association of American Equine Practitioners*. Lexington, KY: Association of American Equine Practitioners, 1974; 243–248.

25 Lees P, Taylor JBO, Higgins AJ, Sharma SC. Phenylbutazone and oxyphenbutazone distribution into tissue fluids in the horse. *J Vet Pharmacol Ther* 1986; **9**: 204–212.

26 Ng LL. *Reviewer Guidance: Validation of Chromatographic Methods*. Washington DC: Food and Drug Administration: Center for Drug Evaluation and Research, 1994. http://www.fda.gov/downloads/Drugs/Guidances/UCM134409.pdf (accessed 10 September 2014).

27 Mordenti J. Man versus beast: pharmacokinetic scaling in mammals. *J Pharm Sci* 1986; **75**(11): 1028–1040.

28 Fiakpui NN, Hogan DF, Whittem T, *et al.* Dose determination of fondaparinux in healthy cats. *Am J Vet Res* 2012; **73**(4): 556–561.

29 Committee for Veterinary Medicinal Products. *Guidelines for the Conduct of Pharmacokinetic Studies in Target Animal Species*. London: European Agency for the Evaluation of Medicinal Products, 2000.

30 Sheiner LB. The population approach to pharmacokinetic data analysis: rationale and standard data analysis methods. *Drug Metab Rev* 1984; **15**(1–2): 153–171.

31 Pasloske K, Sauer B, Perkins N, Whittem T. Plasma pharmacokinetics of alfaxalone in both premedicated and unpremedicated Greyhound dogs after single, intravenous administration of Alfaxan at a clinical dose. *J Vet Pharmacol Ther* 2009; **32**(5): 510–513.

32 Yamaoka K, Nakagawa T, Uno T. Application of Akaike's Information Criterion (AIC) in the evaluation of linear pharmacokinetic equations. *J Pharmacokinet Biopharm* 1978; **6**(2): 165–175.

33 Sheiner LB, Beal SL. Evaluation of methods for estimating population pharmacokinetic parameters. III. Monoexponential model: routine clinical pharmacokinetic data. *J Pharmacokinet Biopharm* 1983; **11**(3): 303–319.

34 Sheiner LB. Analysis of pharmacokinetic data using parametric models: regression models. *J Pharmacokinet Biopharm* 1984; **12**(1): 93–117.

35 Sheiner LB. Analysis of pharmacokinetic data using parametric models. II. Point estimates of an individual's parameters. *J Pharmacokinet Biopharm* 1985; **13**(5): 515–540.

36 Gibaldi M, Perrier D. Noncompartmental analysis based on statistical moment theory. In: Swarbrick J, ed. *Pharmacokinetics*, 2nd edn. New York: Marcel Dekker, 1982; 409–417.

37 Purves RD. Optimum numerical integration methods for estimating area-under-the-curve (AUC) and area-under-the-moment-curve (AUMC). *J Pharmacokinet Biopharm* 1992; **20**(3): 211–226.

38 Avram MJ, Krejcie TC, Niemann CU, *et al.* Isoflurane alters the recirculatory pharmacokinetics of physiologic markers. *Anesthesiology* 2000; **92**(6): 1757–1768.

39 Upton RN, Ludbrook GL. A model of the kinetics and dynamics of induction of anaesthesia in sheep: variable estimation for thiopental and comparison with propofol. *Br J Anaesth* 1999; **82**(6): 890–899.
40 Upton RN, Ludbrook GL. A physiological model of induction of anaesthesia with propofol in sheep. 1. Structure and estimation of variables. *Br J Anaesth* 1997; **79**(4): 497–504.
41 Krejcie TC, Avram MJ. Recirculatory pharmacokinetic modeling: what goes around, comes around. *Anesth Analg* 2012; **115**(2): 223–226.
42 Giraudel JM, Diquelou A, Laroute V, *et al.* Pharmacokinetic/pharmacodynamic modelling of NSAIDs in a model of reversible inflammation in the cat. *Br J Pharmacol* 2005; **146**(5): 642–653.
43 Rowland M, Tozer TN. Constant-rate Therapy. In: Troy DB, ed.. *Clinical Pharmacokinetics and Pharmacodynamics: Concepts and Applications*, 4th edn. Baltimore: Lippincott Williams & Wilkins, 2011; 259–292.
44 Smith I, White PF. Intravenous anaesthesia delivery and monitoring systems. In: Hahn CEW, Adams AP, eds. *Total Intravenous Anaesthesia*. London: BMJ Books, 1998; 98–127.
45 Padfield NL. Administration of intravenous anaesthesia/total intravenous anaesthesia. In: Tait M, ed. *Total Intravenous Anaesthesia*. London: Butterworth Heinemann, 2000; 66–76.
46 Beths T. Total intravenous techniques for anaesthesia. *In Practice* 2007; **29**(7): 410–414.
47 Glass PS, Jacobs JR, Quill TJ. Intravenous drug delivery systems. In: Fragen RJ, ed. *Drug Infusions in Anesthesiology*. New York: Raven Press, 1991; 23–61.
48 Kruger-Thiemer E. Continuous intravenous infusion and multicompartment accumulation. *Eur J Pharmacol* 1968; **4**(3): 317–324.
49 Wagner JG. A safe method for rapidly achieving plasma concentration plateaus. *Clin Pharmacol Ther* 1974; **16**(4): 691–700.
50 Miller DR. Intravenous infusion anaesthesia and delivery devices. *Can J Anaesth* 1994; **41**(7): 639–651.
51 Gepts E. Pharmacokinetic concepts for TCI anaesthesia. *Anaesthesia* 1998; **53**(Suppl 1): 4–12.
52 Schwilden H. A general method for calculating the dosage scheme in linear pharmacokinetics. *Eur J Clin Pharmacol* 1981; **20**(5): 379–386.
53 Schuttler J, Schwilden H, Stoekel H. Pharmacokinetics as applied to total intravenous anaesthesia. Practical implications. *Anaesthesia* 1983; **38**(Suppl): 53–56.
54 Alvis JM, Reves JG, Govier AV, *et al.* Computer-assisted continuous infusions of fentanyl during cardiac anesthesia: comparison with a manual method. *Anesthesiology* 1985; **63**(1): 41–49.
55 Schuttler J, Kloos S, Schwilden H, Stoeckel H. Total intravenous anaesthesia with propofol and alfentanil by computer-assisted infusion. *Anaesthesia* 1988; **43**(Suppl): 2–7.
56 Milne SE, Kenny GN. Target controlled infusions. *Curr Anaesth Crit Care* 1998; **9**: 174–179.
57 Glen JB. The development and future of target controlled infusion. *Adv Exp Med Biol* 2003; **523**: 123–133.
58 Gray JM, Kenny GN. Development of the technology for 'Diprifusor' TCI systems. *Anaesthesia* 1998; **53**(Suppl 1): 22–27.
59 Glass SA, Shafer SL, Reves JG. Intravenous drug delivery systems. In: Krehling E, ed. *Miller's Anesthesia*. Philadelphia: Churchill Livingstone Elsevier, 2009; 825.
60 Egan TD. Target-controlled drug delivery: progress toward an intravenous 'vaporizer' and automated anesthetic administration. *Anesthesiology* 2003; **99**(5): 1214–1219.
61 Short TG, Lim TA, Tam YH. Prospective evaluation of pharmacokinetic model-controlled infusion of propofol in adult patients. *Br J Anaesth* 1996; **76**(2): 313–315.
62 Beths T, Glen JB, Reid J, *et al.* Evaluation and optimisation of a target-controlled infusion system for administering propofol to dogs as part of a total intravenous anaesthetic technique during dental surgery. *Vet Rec* 2001; **148**(7): 198–203.
63 Oei-Lim VL, White M, Kalkman CJ, *et al.* Pharmacokinetics of propofol during conscious sedation using target-controlled infusion in anxious patients undergoing dental treatment. *Br J Anaesth* 1998; **80**(3): 324–331.
64 Swinhoe CF, Peacock JE, Glen JB, Reilly CS. Evaluation of the predictive performance of a 'Diprifusor' TCI system. *Anaesthesia* 1998; **53**(Suppl 1): 61–67.
65 Varvel JR. Measuring the predictive performance of computer-controlled infusion pumps. *J Pharmacokinet Biopharm* 2002; **20**(1): 63–94.
66 Slepchenko G, Simon N, Goubaux B, *et al.* Performance of target-controlled sufentanil infusion in obese patients. *Anesthesiology* 2003; **98**(1): 65–73.
67 Li YH, Xu JH, Yang JJ, *et al.* Predictive performance of 'Diprifusor' TCI system in patients during upper abdominal surgery under propofol/fentanyl anesthesia. *J Zhejiang Univ Sci B* 2005; **6**(1): 43–48.
68 Ko YP, Hsu YW, Hsu K, *et al.* Simulation analysis of the performance of target-controlled infusion of propofol in Chinese patients. *Acta Anaesthesiol Taiwan* 2007; **45**(3): 141–147.
69 Coetzee JF, Glen JB, Wium CA, Boshoff L. Pharmacokinetic model selection for target controlled infusions of propofol. Assessment of three parameter sets. *Anesthesiology* 1995; **82**(6): 1328–1345.
70 Vuyk J, Engbers FH, Burm AG, *et al.* Performance of computer-controlled infusion of propofol: an evaluation of five pharmacokinetic parameter sets. *Anesth Analg* 1995; **81**(6): 1275–1282.
71 Glen JB. The development of 'Diprifusor': a TCI system for propofol. *Anaesthesia* 1998; **53**(Suppl 1): 13–21.
72 Varvel JR, Donoho DL, Shafer SL. Measuring the predictive performance of computer-controlled infusion pumps. *J Pharmacokinet Biopharm* 1992; **20**(1): 63–64.
73 Glass PS. Pharmacokinetic basis of intravenous drug delivery. *Baillière's Clin Anaesth* 1991; **5**(3): 735–775.
74 Ilkiw JE, Pascoe PJ, Fisher LD. Effect of alfentanil on the minimum alveolar concentration of isoflurane in cats. *Am J Vet Res* 1997; **58**(11): 1274–1279.
75 Pypendop BH, Ilkiw JE. Assessment of the hemodynamic effects of lidocaine administered IV in isoflurane-anesthetized cats. *Am J Vet Res* 2005; **66**(4): 661–668.
76 Pypendop BH, Ilkiw JE, Robertson SA. Effects of intravenous administration of lidocaine on the thermal threshold in cats. *Am J Vet Res* 2006; **67**(1): 16–20.
77 Pascoe PJ, Steffey EP, Black WD, *et al.* Evaluation of the effect of alfentanil on the minimum alveolar concentration of halothane in horses. *Am J Vet Res* 1993; **54**(8): 1327–1332.
78 Daunt DA, Dunlop CI, Chapman PL, *et al.* Cardiopulmonary and behavioral responses to computer-driven infusion of detomidine in standing horses. *Am J Vet Res* 1993; **54**(12): 2075–2082.
79 Shafer SL, Varvel JR. Pharmacokinetics, pharmacodynamics, and rational opioid selection. *Anesthesiology* 1991; **74**(1): 53–63.
80 Lagneau F, Tod M, Marty J. Clinical applications of intravenous anaesthetics pharmacology: the example of hypnotics and opioids. *Ann Fr Anesth Reanim* 2004; **23**(10): 986–997.
81 Bailey JM. Context-sensitive half-times: what are they and how valuable are they in anaesthesiology? *Clin Pharmacokinet* 2002; **41**(11): 793–799.
82 Pypendop BH. Context-sensitive half-times of fentanyl, alfentanil, sufentanil, and remifentanil in cats anesthetized with isoflurane obtained by pharmacokinetic simulation. Presented at the 11th World Congress of Veterinary Anaesthesiology, Cape Town, 2013.
83 Engbers F. Basic pharmacokinetic principles for intravenous anaesthesia. In: Vuyk J, Schraag S, eds. *Advances in Modelling and Clinical Applications of Intravenous Anaesthesia*. New York: Kluwer Academic/Plenum Publishers, 2003; 3–8.
84 Youngs EJ, Shafer SL. Pharmacokinetic parameters relevant to recovery from opioids. *Anesthesiology* 1994; **81**(4): 833–842.
85 Struys MM, De Smet T, Depoorter B, *et al.* Comparison of plasma compartment versus two methods for effect compartment-controlled target-controlled infusion for propofol. *Anesthesiology* 2000; **92**(2): 399–406.
86 Wakeling HG, Zimmerman JB, Howell S, Glass PS. Targeting effect compartment or central compartment concentration of propofol: what predicts loss of consciousness? *Anesthesiology* 1999; **90**(1): 92–97.
87 Minto CF, Schnider TW, Gregg KM, *et al.* Using the time of maximum effect site concentration to combine pharmacokinetics and pharmacodynamics. *Anesthesiology* 2003; **99**(2): 324–333.
88 Gentry WB, Krejcie TC, Henthorn TK, *et al.* Effect of infusion rate on thiopental dose–response relationships. Assessment of a pharmacokinetic–pharmacodynamic model. *Anesthesiology* 1994; **81**(2): 316–324.
89 Benet LZ, Kroetz DL, Sheiner LB. Pharmacokinetics. In: Molinoff PB, Ruddon RW, eds. *Goodman and Gilman's The Pharmacological Basis of Therapeutics*, 9th edn. New York: McGraw-Hill, 1996; 3–8.
90 Plumb DC. *Plumb's Veterinary Drug Handbook*, 5th edn. Ames, IA: Blackwell Publishing Professional, 2005.
91 Aarons L. Kinetics of drug–drug interactions. *Pharmacol Ther* 1981; **14**(3): 321–344.
92 Gibson GG, Skett P. Induction and Inhibition of Drug Metabolism. In: Gibson GG, Skett P, eds. *Introduction to Drug Metabolism*, 3rd edn. Andover: Cengage Learning EMEA, 2001; 87–118.
93 Lin JH, Lu AY. Inhibition and induction of cytochrome P450 and the clinical implications. *Clin Pharmacokinet* 1998; **35**(5): 361–390.
94 Venkatakrishnan K, von Moltke LL, Obach RS, Greenblatt DJ. Drug metabolism and drug interactions: application and clinical value of *in vitro* models. *Curr Drug Metab* 2003; **4**(5): 423–459.
95 Funk-Keenan J, Sacco J, Wong YY, *et al.* Evaluation of polymorphisms in the sulfonamide detoxification genes CYB5A and CYB5R3 in dogs with sulfonamide hypersensitivity. *J Vet Intern Med* 2012; **26**(5): 1126–1133.
96 Paulson SK, Engel L, Reitz B, *et al.* Evidence for polymorphism in the canine metabolism of the cyclooxygenase 2 inhibitor, celecoxib. *Drug Metab Dispos* 1999; **27**(10): 1133–1142.

97 Gramer I, Leidolf R, Doring B, *et al.* Breed distribution of the nt230(del4) MDR1 mutation in dogs. *Vet J* 2011; **189**(1): 67–71.

98 Geyer J, Doring B, Godoy JR, *et al.* Frequency of the nt230 (del4) MDR1 mutation in collies and related dog breeds in Germany. *J Vet Pharmacol Ther* 2005; **28**(6): 545–551.

99 Mealey KL, Bentjen SA, Gay JM, Cantor GH. Ivermectin sensitivity in collies is associated with a deletion mutation of the mdr1 gene. *Pharmacogenetics* 2001; **11**(8): 727–733.

100 Fink-Gremmels J. Implications of hepatic cytochrome P450-related biotransformation processes in veterinary sciences. *Eur J Pharmacol* 2008; **585**(2–3): 502–509.

101 Sharer JE, Shipley LA, Vandenbranden MR, *et al.* Comparisons of phase I and phase II in vitro hepatic enzyme activities of human, dog, rhesus monkey, and cynomolgus monkey. *Drug Metab Dispos* 1995; **23**(11): 1231–1241.

102 Takizawa D, Hiraoka H, Nakamura K, *et al.* Influence of the prone position on propofol pharmacokinetics. *Anaesthesia* 2004; **59**(12): 1250–1251.

103 Takizawa D, Nishikawa K, Sato E, *et al.* A dopamine infusion decreases propofol concentration during epidural blockade under general anesthesia. *Can J Anaesth* 2005; **52**(5): 463–466.

104 Takizawa E, Ito N, Ishizeki J, *et al.* The effect of positive end-expiratory pressure ventilation on propofol concentrations during general anesthesia in humans. *Fundam Clin Pharmacol* 2006; **20**(5): 489–492.

105 Myburgh JA, Upton RN, Grant C, Martinez A. Epinephrine, norepinephrine and dopamine infusions decrease propofol concentrations during continuous propofol infusion in an ovine model. *Intensive Care Med* 2001; **27**(1): 276–282.

106 Kurita T, Morita K, Kazama T, Sato S. Influence of cardiac output on plasma propofol concentrations during constant infusion in swine. *Anesthesiology* 2002; **96**(6): 1498–1503.

107 Lichtenbelt BJ, Mertens M, Vuyk J. Strategies to optimise propofol–opioid anaesthesia. *Clin Pharmacokinet* 2004; **43**(9): 577–593.

108 Vuyk J. TCI: supplementation and drug interactions. *Anaesthesia* 1998; **53**(Suppl 1): 35–41.

109 Minto C, Vuyk J. Response surface modelling of drug interactions. *Adv Exp Med Biol* 2003; **523**: 35–43.

110 Vuyk J. Clinical interpretation of pharmacokinetic and pharmacodynamic propofol–opioid interactions. *Acta Anaesthesiol Belg* 2001; **52**(4): 445–451.

111 Short TG, Ho TY, Minto CF, *et al.* Efficient trial design for eliciting a pharmacokinetic–pharmacodynamic model-based response surface describing the interaction between two intravenous anesthetic drugs. *Anesthesiology* 2002; **96**(2): 400–408.

112 Minto CF, Schnider TW, Short TG, *et al.* Response surface model for anesthetic drug interactions. *Anesthesiology* 2000; **92**(6): 1603–1616.

113 Bol CJ, Vogelaar JP, Tang JP, Mandema JW. Quantification of pharmacodynamic interactions between dexmedetomidine and midazolam in the rat. *J Pharmacol Exp Ther* 2000; **294**(1): 347–355.

114 Mertens MJ, Olofsen E, Engbers FH, *et al.* Propofol reduces perioperative remifentanil requirements in a synergistic manner: response surface modeling of perioperative remifentanil–propofol interactions. *Anesthesiology* 2003; **99**(2): 347–359.

115 Heyse B, Proost JH, Schumacher PM, *et al.* Sevoflurane remifentanil interaction: comparison of different response surface models. *Anesthesiology* 2012; **116**(2): 311–323.

116 Manyam SC, Gupta DK, Johnson KB, *et al.* Opioid–volatile anesthetic synergy: a response surface model with remifentanil and sevoflurane as prototypes. *Anesthesiology* 2006; **105**(2): 267–278.

117 Edwards IR, Aronson JK. Adverse drug reactions: definitions, diagnosis, and management. *Lancet* 2000; **356**(9237): 1255–1259.

118 Hampshire VA, Doddy FM, Post LO, *et al.* Adverse drug event reports at the United States Food And Drug Administration Center for Veterinary Medicine. *J Am Vet Med Assoc* 2004; **225**(4): 533–536.

119 Emmerich I, Ungemach F. Neue Arzneimittel für Kleintiere 2008. *Tierärztliche Praxis Kleintiere* 2009; **37**(6): 399–409.

120 Thompson JA, Eades SC, Chapman AM, *et al.* Effects of clenbuterol administration on serum biochemical, histologic, and echocardiographic measurements of muscle injury in exercising horses. *Am J Vet Res* 2012; **73**(6): 875–883.

121 Stanton-Hicks MdA, Wüst HJ, Koch U, *et al.* Experimental tachyphylaxis: development of a continuous epidural dog model. In: Wüst H, Stanton-Hicks MdA, eds. *New Aspects in Regional Anesthesia 4*. Berlin: Springer, 1986; 32–38.

122 APVMA. *Report of Adverse Experiences for Veterinary Medicines and Agricultural Chemicals; Calendar Year 2009*. Canberra: Australian Pesticides and Veterinary Medicines Authority, 2010.

123 Kramer MS, Leventhal JM, Hutchinson TA, Feinstein AR. An algorithm for the operational assessment of adverse drug reactions: I. Background, description, and instructions for use. *J Am Med Assoc* 1979; **242**(7): 623–632.

124 APVMA. *Report of Adverse Experiences 2009 Calendar Year; Veterinary Medicines*. Canberra: Australian Pesticides and Veterinary Medicines Authority, 2010.

125 Janicki PK, James MF, Erskine WA. Propofol inhibits enzymatic degradation of alfentanil and sufentanil by isolated liver microsomes *in vitro*. *Br J Anaesth* 1992; **68**(3): 311–312.

126 Chen TL, Ueng TH, Chen SH, *et al.* Human cytochrome P450 mono-oxygenase system is suppressed by propofol. *Br J Anaesth* 1995; **74**(5): 558–562.

127 McKillop D, Wild MJ, Butters CJ, Simcock C. Effects of propofol on human hepatic microsomal cytochrome P450 activities. *Xenobiotica* 1998; **28**(9): 845–853.

128 Lejus C, Fautrel A, Malledant Y, Guillouzo A. Inhibition of cytochrome P450 2E1 by propofol in human and porcine liver microsomes. *Biochem Pharmacol* 2002; **64**(7): 1151–1156.

129 Inomata S, Nagashima A, Osaka Y, *et al.* Propofol inhibits lidocaine metabolism in human and rat liver microsomes. *J Anesth* 2003; **17**(4): 246–250.

130 Yang LQ, Yu WF, Cao YF, *et al. Potential inhibition of cytochrome P450 3A4 by propofol in human primary hepatocytes*. 2003; **9**(9): 1959–1962.

131 Osaka Y, Inomata S, Tanaka E, *et al.* Effect of propofol on ropivacaine metabolism in human liver microsomes. *J Anesth* 2006; **20**(1): 60–63.

132 Baker MT, Chadam MV, Ronnenberg WC. Inhibitory effects of propofol on cytochrome P450 activities in rat hepatic microsomes. *Anesth Analg* 1993; **76**(4): 817–821.

133 Gemayel J, Geloen A, Mion F. Propofol-induced cytochrome P450 inhibition: an *in vitro* and *in vivo* study in rats. *Life Sci* 2001; **68**(26): 2957–2965.

134 Yamazaki H, Shimizu M, Nagashima T, *et al.* Rat cytochrome P450 2C11 in liver microsomes involved in oxidation of anesthetic agent propofol and deactivated by prior treatment with propofol. *Drug Metab Dispos* 2006; **34**(11): 1803–1805.

135 Chen TL, Wang MJ, Huang CH, *et al.* Difference between *in vivo* and *in vitro* effects of propofol on defluorination and metabolic activities of hamster hepatic cytochrome P450-dependent mono-oxygenases. *Br J Anaesth* 1995; **75**(4): 462–466.

136 Beths T, Glen JB, Reid J, Nolan AM. The inhibitory effect of medetomidine and its enantiomers on canine and rat liver microsomal propofol metabolism in vitro. Presented at the World Congress of Veterinary Anaesthesiology, University of Tennessee, September 2003.

137 Duhamel MC, Troncy E, Beaudry F. Metabolic stability and determination of cytochrome P450 isoenzymes' contribution to the metabolism of medetomidine in dog liver microsomes. *Biomed Chromatogr* 2010; **24**(8): 868–877.

138 Baratta MT, Zaya MJ, White JA, Locuson CW. Canine CYP2B11 metabolizes and is inhibited by anesthetic agents often co-administered in dogs. *J Vet Pharmacol Ther* 2010; **33**(1): 50–55.

139 Lennquist A, Celander M C, Forlin L. Effects of medetomidine on hepatic EROD activity in three species of fish. *Ecotoxicol Environ Saf* 2008; **69**(1): 74–79.

140 Lennquist A, Hilvarsson A, Forlin L. Responses in fish exposed to medetomidine, a new antifouling agent. *Mar Environ Res* 2010; **69**(Suppl); S43–S45.

141 Kharasch ED, Hill HF, Eddy AC. Influence of dexmedetomidine and clonidine on human liver microsomal alfentanil metabolism. *Anesthesiology* 1991; **75**(3): 520–524.

142 Kharasch ED, Herrmann S, Labroo R. Ketamine as a probe for medetomidine stereoisomer inhibition of human liver microsomal drug metabolism. *Anesthesiology* 1992; **77**(6): 1208–1214.

143 Rodrigues AD, Roberts EM. The *in vitro* interaction of dexmedetomidine with human liver microsomal cytochrome P4502D6 (CYP2D6). *Drug Metab Dispos* 1997; **25**(5): 651–655.

144 Pelkonen O, Puurunen J, Arvela P, Lammintausta R. Comparative effects of medetomidine enantiomers on *in vitro* and *in vivo* microsomal drug metabolism. *Pharmacol Toxicol* 1991; **69**(3): 189–194.

145 Coleman MD. Drug biotransformational systems – origins and aims. *Human Drug Metabolism. An Introduction*, 2nd edn. Chichester: Wiley-Blackwell, 2010; 13–22.

146 Gibson GG, Skett P. Factors affecting drug metabolism: internal factors. In: Gibson GG, Skett P, eds. *Introduction to Drug Metabolism*, 3rd edn. Andover: Cengage Learning EMEA, 2001; 119–145.

147 Gibson GG, Skett P. Factors affecting Drug Metabolism: External Factors. In: Gibson GG, Skett P, eds. *Introduction to Drug Metabolism*, 3rd edn. Andover: Cengage Learning EMEA, 2001; 146–170.

148 Xu C, Li CY, Kong AN. Induction of phase I, II and III drug metabolism/transport by xenobiotics. *Arch Pharm Res* 2005; **28**(3): 249–268.

149 Chang GW, Kam PC. The physiological and pharmacological roles of cytochrome P450 isoenzymes. *Anaesthesia* 1999; **54**(1): 42–50.

150 Trepanier LA. Cytochrome P450 and its role in veterinary drug interactions. *Vet Clin North Am Small Anim Pract*. 2006; **36**(5): 975–985.

151 Martignoni M, Groothuis GM, de Kanter R. Species differences between mouse, rat, dog, monkey and human CYP-mediated drug metabolism, inhibition and induction. *Expert Opin Drug Metab Toxicol* 2006; **2**(6): 875–894.

152 Court MH, Hay-Kraus BL, Hill DW, *et al.* Propofol hydroxylation by dog liver microsomes: assay development and dog breed differences. *Drug Metab Dispos* 1999; **27**(11): 1293–1299.

153 Hay Kraus BL, Greenblatt DJ, Venkatakrishnan K, Court MH. Evidence for propofol hydroxylation by cytochrome P4502B11 in canine liver microsomes: breed and gender differences. *Xenobiotica* 2000; **30**(6): 575–588.

154 Chan WH, Chen TL, Chen RM, *et al.* Propofol metabolism is enhanced after repetitive ketamine administration in rats: the role of cytochrome P-50 2B induction. *Br J Anaesth* 2006; **97**(3): 351–58.

155 Coleman MD. Induction of cytochrome P450 systems. *Human Drug Metabolism. An Introduction*, 2nd edn. Chichester: Wiley-Blackwell, 2010; 65–92.

156 Coleman MD. Cytochrome P450 inhibition. *Human Drug Metabolism. An Introduction*, 2nd edn. Chichester: Wiley-Blackwell, 2010; 93–124.

157 Gibson GG, Skett P. Pathways of drug metabolism In: Giaccone G, Skett P, eds. *Introduction to Drug Metabolism*, 3rd edn. Andover: Cengage Learning EMEA, 2001; 1–6.

158 Mizuno N, Niwa T, Yotsumoto Y, Sugiyama Y. Impact of drug transporter studies on drug discovery and development. *Pharmacol Rev* 2003; **55**(3): 425–461.

159 Hedman A, Angelin B, Arvidsson A, *et al.* Interactions in the renal and biliary elimination of digoxin: stereoselective difference between quinine and quinidine. *Clin Pharmacol Ther* 1990; **47**(1): 20–26.

160 Hedman A, Angelin B, Arvidsson A, *et al.* Digoxin–verapamil interaction: reduction of biliary but not renal digoxin clearance in humans. *Clin Pharmacol Ther* 1991; **49**(3): 256–262.

161 Mather LE, Duke CC, Ladd LA, *et al.* Direct cardiac effects of coronary site-directed thiopental and its enantiomers: a comparison to propofol in conscious sheep. *Anesthesiology* 2004; **101**(2): 354–364.

162 Larenza MP, Knobloch M, Landoni MF, *et al.* Stereoselective pharmacokinetics of ketamine and norketamine after racemic ketamine or S-ketamine administration in Shetland ponies sedated with xylazine. *Vet J* 2008; **177**(3): 432–435.

163 Larenza MP, Ringer SK, Kutter AP, *et al.* Evaluation of anesthesia recovery quality after low-dose racemic or S-ketamine infusions during anesthesia with isoflurane in horses. *Am J Vet Res* 2009; **70**(6): 710–718.

164 Lipscomb VJ, AliAbadi FS, Lees P, *et al.* Clinical efficacy and pharmacokinetics of carprofen in the treatment of dogs with osteoarthritis. *Vet Rec* 2002; **150**(22): 684–689.

165 Arifah AK, Landoni MF, Frean SP, Lees P. Pharmacodynamics and pharmacokinetics of ketoprofen enantiomers in sheep. *Am J Vet Res* 2001; **62**(1): 77–86.

166 Lapicque F, Muller N, Payan E, *et al.* Protein binding and stereoselectivity of nonsteroidal anti-inflammatory drugs. *Clin Pharmacokinet* 1993; **25**(2): 115–123.

167 Rahman MH, Maruyama T, Okada T, *et al.* Study of interaction of carprofen and its enantiomers with human serum albumin. II. Stereoselective site-to-site displacement of carprofen by ibuprofen. *Biochem Pharmacol* 1993; **46**(10): 1733–1740.

168 Jamali F, Lovlin R, Aberg G. Bi-directional chiral inversion of ketoprofen in CD-1mice. *Chirality* 1997; **9**(1): 29–31.

169 McIntosh MP, Rajewski RA. Comparative canine pharmacokinetics–pharmacodynamics of fospropofol disodium injection, propofol emulsion, and cyclodextrin-enabled propofol solution following bolus parenteral administration. *J Pharm Sci* 2012; **101**(9): 3547–3552.

170 Trapani G, Latrofa A, Franco M, *et al.* Inclusion complexation of propofol with 2-hydroxypropyl-beta-cyclodextrin. Physicochemical, nuclear magnetic resonance spectroscopic studies, and anesthetic properties in rat. *J Pharm Sci* 1998; **87**(4): 514–518.

171 Lee SJ, Kim SI, Jung BI, *et al.* Suspected anaphylactic reaction associated with microemulsion propofol during anesthesia induction. *J Korean Med Sci* 2012; **27**(7): 827–829.

172 Jung JA, Choi BM, Cho SH, *et al.* Effectiveness, safety, and pharmacokinetic and pharmacodynamic characteristics of microemulsion propofol in patients undergoing elective surgery under total intravenous anaesthesia. *Br J Anaesth* 2010; **104**(5): 563–576.

173 Desta B, Maldonado G, Reid H, *et al.* Acute selenium toxicosis in polo ponies. *J Vet Diagn Invest* 2011; **23**(3): 623–628.

174 Kairuz TE, Gargiulo D, Bunt C, Garg S. Quality, safety and efficacy in the 'off-label' use of medicines. *Curr Drug Saf* 2007; **2**(1): 89–95.

175 Gershman MD, Kennedy DJ, Noble-Wang J, *et al.* Multistate outbreak of *Pseudomonas fluorescens* bloodstream infection after exposure to contaminated heparinized saline flush prepared by a compounding pharmacy. *Clin Infect Dis* 2008; **47**(11): 1372–1379.

8 Anticholinergics

Phillip Lerche
Veterinary Clinical Sciences, The Ohio State University, Columbus, Ohio, USA

Chapter contents

Introduction

Anticholinergic drugs are commonly used in veterinary anesthesia to treat and/or prevent anesthetic and preanesthetic bradycardia, decrease airway and salivary secretions, dilate the pupil, block vagally mediated reflexes (viscerovagal, oculocardiac, Branham), and block the effects of parasympathomimetic drugs. Historically, inhalant anesthetics such as diethyl ether produced profound parasympathetic effects that resulted in hypersalivation and bradycardia. As such, anticholinergics were consistently used preoperatively to counteract these unwanted adverse effects. Modern inhalant anesthetics have lesser effects on the autonomic nervous system, making the indiscriminate use of anticholinergic drugs less popular. The administration of an anticholinergic drug as part of a patient's premedication should be based on a thorough knowledge of the drug's benefits and risks, taking into account the drugs to be co-administered, species, age and disease status of the patient, and the procedure being performed.

History

Plants such as deadly nightshade (*Atropa belladonna*) (Fig. 8.1), henbane (*Hyoscyamus niger*), mandrake (*Mandragora officilanis*), and *Datura* species contain naturally occurring tropane alkaloids (atropine, hyoscyamine, and scopolamine) in concentrations that are potentially toxic to most species. Ingesting 3–5 nightshade berries may prove lethal to a person, for example. Despite this risk, extracts from these plants have been used since ancient times for their anesthetic, mydriatic, antidiarrheal, and analgesic properties. In the 1830s, atropine was isolated from deadly nightshade and in the 1880s hyoscine from henbane, paving the way for a clearer understanding of how the autonomic nervous system functions and the eventual discovery of the neurotransmitter acetylcholine [1,2]. The anticholinergic preparations used in modern veterinary anesthesia have a relatively high margin of safety by comparison.

General pharmacology

Modern anticholinergics exert their effects by competitively antagonizing acetylcholine at postganglionic muscarinic cholinergic receptors in the parasympathetic nervous system. This has led some to prefer the use of the term *antimuscarinics* to differentiate the drugs that only act as antagonists at muscarinic receptors from some naturally occurring compounds that can non-specifically antagonize both muscarinic and nicotinic acetylcholine receptors. Muscarinic receptors have five subtypes, classified as M1–M5, based on the order in which they were cloned [3]. Intracellular signaling by activation of the different subtypes occurs via coupling to multiple G proteins, with single receptor subtypes being capable of activating more than one G protein in the same cell [4]. The muscarinic receptors can be placed into two groups based on the primary G protein to which they couple: M1, M3, and M5 couple with $G_{q/11}$-type proteins, and M2 and M4 couple with $G_{i/o}$-type proteins. There is also evidence that M1, M2, and M3 receptors can cause actions via non-G-protein mechanisms, such as protein kinase [5]. In addition to being able to activate different G-proteins, the muscarinic receptor subtypes show a tissue-specific anatomic distribution, and physiologic response (Table 8.1).

Atropine and glycopyrrolate, the anticholinergics most commonly used in veterinary anesthesia, are relatively unselective in their binding to muscarinic receptor subtypes. Different tissue types, however, appear to have different responses to clinically administered doses of these drugs (Table 8.2) [6]. Receptors in salivary, cardiac, and bronchial tissues are more sensitive than those in the urinary and gastrointestinal tracts.

Veterinary Anesthesia and Analgesia: The Fifth Edition of Lumb and Jones.
Edited by Kurt A. Grimm, Leigh A. Lamont, William J. Tranquilli, Stephen A. Greene and Sheilah A. Robertson.

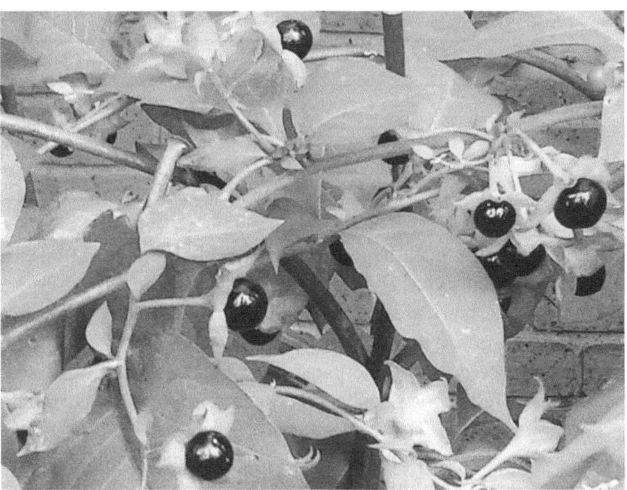

Figure 8.1 Deadly nightshade (*Atropa belladonna*) plant with berries.

Table 8.1 Muscarinic receptor subtypes, cellular response, tissue location, and physiologic responses in mammals.

Receptor	Cellular Response	Tissue Location	Physiologic Response
M_1	PLC activated ↑ IP_3, DAG, Ca^{2+}, PKC, cAMP	CNS Stomach	Neuron depolarization H^+ secretion
M_2	PLC activated ↑ or ↓ AC	Lungs Heart (SA and AV nodes, atrial myocardium)	Bronchoconstriction Bradycardia, AV block ↓ Inotropy
M_3	PLC activated ↑ IP_3, DAG, Ca^{2+} ↑ NO	CNS Salivary glands Airway smooth muscle Vascular endothelium	 Salivation Bronchoconstriction, ↑ secretions Vasodilation
M_4	↓ AC	CNS Heart	?
M_5	PLC activated ↑ IP_3, DAG, Ca^{2+} ↓ PKA, cAMP	CNS	?

AC, adenylate cyclase; AV, atrioventricular; cAMP, cyclic adenosine monophosphate; CNS, central nervous system; DAG, diacylglycerol; IP_3, inositol triphosphate; NO, nitric oxide; PLC, phospholipase C; PKA, protein kinase A; PKC, protein kinase C; SA, sinoatrial;?, specific action unclear or undefined.

Table 8.2 Comparison of clinical effects of systemically administered atropine and glycopyrrolate.

Drug	Antisialagogue Effects	Heart Rate Increase	Smooth Muscle Relaxation	Ocular Effects
Atropine	+	+++	++	++
Glycopyrrolate	++	+	++	0

Anticholinergic effects in the heart are mediated by pre- and postsynaptic M2 receptors located in the sinoatrial and atrioventricular nodes and also in the atrial myocardium. Systemic anticholinergic drug administration typically leads to an increase in sinus rate, acceleration of atrioventricular nodal conduction, and increased atrial contractility. The increase in heart rate may result in tachycardia and tachydysrhythmias, which may be unwanted, particularly if these changes result in decreased cardiac output or significantly increased myocardial oxygen consumption. Routine use of anticholinergics should be avoided in patients with hypertrophic or restrictive forms of cardiomyopathy.

Sometimes, worsening of bradycardia may occur immediately following anticholinergic administration. This paradoxical effect has been postulated to be due to more rapid blockade of presynaptic M1 receptors that inhibits the negative feedback mechanism, resulting in a transient increase in acetylcholine release and further slowing of the heart rate [7]. In this scenario, waiting a few minutes or repeating the dose of anticholinergic administered will typically induce blockade of postsynaptic M2 receptors, resulting in the desired increase in heart rate.

Bronchodilation and reduced airway secretions via M2 and M3 receptor antagonism can decrease airway resistance and the likelihood of airway obstruction, but can contribute to hypoventilation and, theoretically, decreased arterial oxygen tension as a result of increased anatomic deadspace. Additionally, in many species the viscosity of the airway secretions increases as the volume is decreased following an anticholinergic administration, potentially offsetting any benefit with respect to reducing airway secretions.

In the eye, cholinergic fibers originating from cranial nerve III innervate the circular muscles (sphincter pupillae) of the iris that control pupil diameter, and also the ciliary muscle that controls the shape of the lens, facilitating accommodation. Topical application of anticholinergic drugs to the cornea blocks the action of acetylcholine at both of these sites and results in mydriasis and cyclopegia. This has been well documented for atropine in numerous species, including sheep, goats, cats, and horses [8–12], and for glycopyrrolate in rabbits [13]. Topical application of anticholinergic drugs has also been shown to acutely increase intraocular pressure (IOP) caused by drainage angle closure in cats [10], but not in sheep and horses [8,12]. These mixed findings have led some to suggest that this route of administration should be avoided in patients with pre-existing elevations of IOP or those predisposed to developing angle-closure glaucoma.

The potential to induce mydriatic and cyclopegic effects with systemic (i.e., either intravenous or intramuscular) administration of anticholinergics is lower than with topical administration, and is probably drug and dose dependent. Scopolamine, a drug rarely used in veterinary medicine, appears to have the most potent ocular effects when administered systemically, followed by atropine and finally glycopyrrolate. There are few data for any species to suggest that systemic administration of atropine or glycopyrrolate at clinically relevant doses for treatment of reflex or drug-induced bradycardia would cause adverse effects in patients with glaucoma. Both drugs can, however, decrease tear production, resulting in corneal drying [14,15].

Anticholinergics that cross the blood–brain barrier, such as scopolamine and atropine, also have the potential to induce sedation and prolong anesthetic recovery when administered systemically via M1 receptor antagonism. In the case of atropine, however, its sedative potential when clinically relevant doses are administered is negligible.

Anticholinergics (M3) are effective antisialogogues in monogastrics. In ruminants, however, salivation is not inhibited completely; rather, the saliva becomes more viscous to the point where the thickened, ropy saliva may pose a risk of causing airway obstruction. Routine anticholinergic use is therefore not recommended in ruminants, with the exception of treating intraoperative bradycardia.

Although the dose of an anticholinergic required to decrease gastrointestinal motility via blockade of M3 receptors is higher than that required to treat bradycardia, there is some risk of gastrointestinal ileus following administration. This may lead to symptoms of colic in horses, hence the routine use of anticholinergics is generally avoided in this species [16]. As with ruminants, anticholinergic use in horses should be reserved for treating intraoperative bradycardia. In monogastrics, anticholinergics have been shown to decrease lower esophageal sphincter function, which may lead to an increased risk of gastroesophageal reflux and associated complications such as aspiration pneumonia, esophagitis, and esophageal stricture [17].

Specific anticholinergic drugs

Atropine

Pharmacology

Atropine is a racemic mixture of L- and D-hyoscyamine, with the L-isomer being responsible for the majority of the drug's activity. The atropine molecule has a lipid-soluble tertiary amine structure consisting of a tropic acid ester linked to an organic base (see Fig. 8.2), and it easily crosses the blood–brain and blood–placenta barriers [18].

Onset of action after intravenous (IV) and intramuscular (IM) atropine administration is approximately 1 and 5 min, respectively, in dogs, with an increase in heart rate lasting for about 30 min [19]. Other body systems are generally affected for one to several hours, although mydriasis after topical administration can persist for up to 3 days.

The metabolism of atropine varies between species. Atropine is rapidly cleared from the central compartment via hydrolysis to inactive metabolites, with some being excreted unchanged by the kidneys in dogs and people. Rabbits, on the other hand, eat the leaves of the usually toxic deadly nightshade with impunity because they have the ability to metabolize atropine-like compounds rapidly via a plasma esterase, atropinase, which may render typical clinical doses ineffective. Not all rabbits possess large amounts of this enzyme, hence the full picture of how this species metabolizes atropine is yet to be elucidated [20]. In cats, hepatic and renal esterases contribute to atropine's clearance from the plasma.

Clinical use

Atropine is mostly used to prevent or treat bradycardia associated with anesthesia. Intramuscular and IV dosing is preferred over the subcutaneous route by most anesthesiologists in order to maximize absorption and minimize onset time.

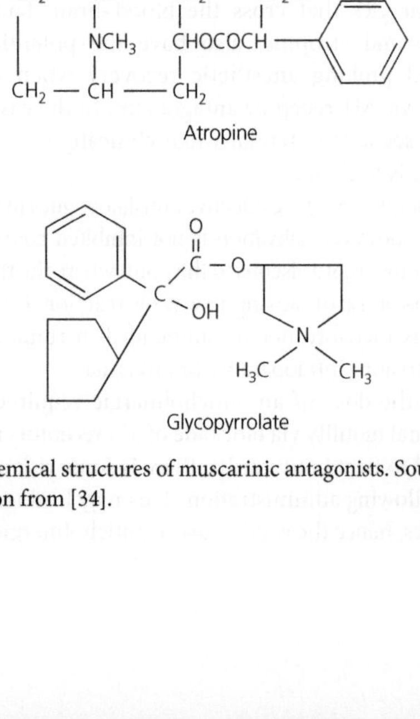

Atropine

Glycopyrrolate

Figure 8.2 Chemical structures of muscarinic antagonists. Source: adapted with permission from [34].

Table 8.3 Dose ranges for atropine and glycopyrrolate (mg/kg).

Animal	Atropine	Glycopyrrolate
Cats and dogs	0.02–0.04	0.005–0.01
Horses	0.02–0.04	0.0025–0.005
Ruminants	0.04–0.08	0.0025–0.005
Pigs	0.04–0.08	0.0025–0.005

Cardiac rhythm disturbances associated with atropine administration can be pronounced [21]. Transient bradycardia and second-degree atrioventricular block are common parasympathomimetic effects that tend to occur more frequently with administration of lower doses [22]. Evidence suggests that these paradoxical effects result from initial blockade of presynaptic peripheral M1 receptors that normally inhibit acetylcholine release. This causes a transient increase in acetylcholine prior to the onset of atropine-induced postsynaptic M2 receptor blockade [7]. The resulting bradycardia (with or without atrioventricular block) typically resolves spontaneously with establishment of postsynaptic blockade, or upon administration of a supplemental dose of drug. In sheep, unexpected bradycardia has been reported after administration of a higher dose (0.08 mg/kg IV) of atropine [23]. It surprisingly resolved after administration of edrophonium, the reasons for which are not clear (see Table 8.3 for dose ranges).

Dose-dependent tachycardia is frequently observed following atropine administration [19]. The mean dose required to increase heart rate by 50% in conscious dogs was reported to be approximately 0.04 mg/kg IV [19]. Greater increases in heart rate may be observed in patients with high pre-existing vagal tone, a phenomenon called 'excess tachycardia.' In addition, occasional premature ventricular contractions have also been reported in dogs but are not necessarily proportional to the magnitude of tachycardia [22]. Although transient tachycardia is generally well tolerated in normal healthy veterinary patients, atropine should be used with caution in those who may be adversely impacted by tachycardia, such as patients with hypertrophic or restrictive forms of cardiomyopathy.

Atropine is commonly used prior to administration of cholinergic drugs such as neostigmine and edrophonium when reversing neuromuscular blockade (see Chapter 14). Additionally, atropine has historically been recommended during cardiopulmonary–cerebral resuscitation (CPR). It can be delivered via the endotracheal tube at two to three times the usual IV dose if venous access has not been established prior to cardiopulmonary collapse.

Glycopyrrolate

Pharmacology

Glycopyrrolate is a synthetic quaternary ammonium compound that is poorly lipid soluble, making it difficult for the molecule to cross the blood–brain or blood–placenta barriers [18]. The molecule consists of a mandelic acid ester linked to an organic base (see Fig. 8.2). Glycopyrrolate has four times the potency of atropine.

The onset of action of glycopyrrolate is slightly slower than that of atropine, usually occurring within a few minutes. In people, the duration of action is similar to that of atropine, but in conscious dogs cardiovascular effects lasted for approximately 1 h, which was longer than those for atropine [24]. Glycopyrrolate is cleared from the plasma relatively rapidly, with most of it being excreted unchanged in the urine.

Whereas topical glycopyrrolate has been shown readily to induce persistent mydriasis and cycloplegia in rabbits [13], systemic administration of clinically relevant doses is reported to have minimal effects on ocular parameters in dogs [25,26].

In people, the purported benefit of glycopyrrolate over atropine is its improved cardiovascular parameters with less risk of tachycardia. This is not the case in dogs, where drug effects on the cardiovascular system are similar between the two anticholinergics [22].

The effect of glycopyrrolate on gastrointestinal motility has been evaluated in anesthetized dogs and horses. Motility was decreased for up to 30 min in dogs and the duration of decreased motility in horses was dose dependent, lasting for over 6 h after a 0.005 mg/kg IV dose [27,28]. Development of colic postoperatively in horses is multifactorial and antimuscarinic drug administration may be a contributing factor. Of 17 horses that received glycopyrrolate intraoperatively, one subsequently showed signs of colic [29,30].

Clinical use

Glycopyrrolate is mostly used to treat or prevent bradycardia in the perioperative period. It can also be used to counteract the cholinergic effects when reversing neuromuscular blockade with a cholinergic drug such as neostigmine, and in some countries the two drugs are combined in a single preparation for this purpose. It is not used as an emergency drug in CPR when atropine is available owing to its longer onset time. See Table 8.3 for dose ranges.

Drug combinations

Anticholinergics are water soluble and have historically been used in premixed combinations of preanesthetic medications in small animal anesthesia such as 'BAG' (butorphanol, acepromazine, glycopyrrolate) and 'superBAG' (buprenorphine, acepromazine, glycopyrrolate). Anticholinergics are often selected to counteract the bradycardia associated with the use of α_2-adrenergic receptor agonists. Clinically, it is important to determine whether the bradycardia is a baroreceptor response to an increase in arterial blood pressure secondary to peripheral vasoconstriction, or is due to centrally mediated suppression of sympathetic output with accompanying low blood pressure. Increasing the heart rate in the face of arterial vasoconstriction has the potential to decrease cardiac output further while significantly increasing myocardial oxygen consumption [31]. Cardiac output is usually not significantly improved when dogs are sedated with dexmedetomidine compared with dexmedetomidine and atropine. The routine use of atropine was not recommended by the authors owing to the detection of cardiac arrhythmias when atropine was co-administered and lack of any clear benefit [32]. Similarly, Monteiro *et al.* found no benefit in sedating cats with dexmedetomidine and atropine versus dexmedetomidine alone, although cardiac output was not measured [33]. The rationale for use of an anticholinergic with an α_2-adrenergic receptor agonist when preceding general anesthesia (versus sedation) has yet to be critically evaluated.

Following the use of α_2-adrenergic receptor agonists, if the arterial blood pressure is low, administration of an anticholinergic may be considered to counter bradycardia and improve blood pressure. However, if bradycardia is secondary to decreased sympathetic nervous system activity, antagonism of parasympathetic influence on the sinus node may not cause improvement in heart rate. In those cases, administration of a sympathomimetic agent (e.g., ephedrine), or reversal of the α_2-adrenergic receptor agonist, may be beneficial.

It is important to consider that adverse effects of combinations of drugs may be additive. For example, anticholinergics, opioids, and α_2-adrenergic agonists can all decrease gastrointestinal activity. Although this does not preclude the use of anticholinergics as part of a preanesthetic medication, their use should not be indiscriminate and instead should be based on a risk–benefit analysis for the individual patient.

References

1 Lee MR. *Solanaceae* III: henbane, hags and Hawley Harvey Crippen. *J R Coll Physicians Edinb* 2006; **36**: 366–373.

2 Lee MR. *Solanaceae* IV: *Atropa belladonna*, deadly nightshade. *J R Coll Physicians Edinb* 2007; **37**: 77–84.

3 Caulfield MP, Birdsall NJM. International Union of Pharmacology. XVII. Classification of muscarinic acetylcholine receptors. *Pharmacol Rev* 1998; **50**: 279–290.

4 Karakiulakis G, Roth M. Muscarinic receptors and their antagonists in COPD: anti-inflammatory and antiremodeling effects. *Mediators Inflamm* 2012; **409580.**

5 Rosenblum K, Futter M, Jones M, *et al.* ERKI/II regulation by the muscarinic acetylcholine receptors in neurons. *J Neurosci* 2000; **20**: 977–985.

6 Stoelting RK, Hillier SC. Anticholinergic drugs. *Pharmacology and Physiology in Anesthetic Practice*, 4 edn. Philadelphia: Lippinott Williams & Wilkins, 2006; 266–275.

7 Wellstein A, Pitschner HF. Complex dose–response curves of atropine in man explained by different functions of M1- and M2-cholinoceptors. *Naunyn Schmiedeberg's Arch Pharmacol* 1988; **338**: 19–27.

8 Ribeiro AP, Crivelaro RM, Teixeira PP, *et al.* Effects of different mydriatics on intraocular pressure, pupil diameter, and ruminal and intestinal motility in healthy sheep. *Vet Ophthalmol* 2013; doi: 10.1111/vop.12121 (epub ahead of print).

9 Whelan NC, Castillo-Alcala FC, Lizarraga I. Efficacy of tropicamide, homatropine, cyclopentolate, atropine and hyoscine as mydriatics in Angora goats. *N Z Vet J* 2011; **59**: 328–331.

10 Stadtbäumer K, Frommlet F, Nell B. Effects of mydriatics on intracoluar pressure and pupil size in the normal feline eye. *Vet Ophthalmol* 2006; **9**: 233–237.

11 Davis JL, Stewart T, Brazik E, *et al.* The effect of topical administration of atropine sulfate on the normal equine pupil: influence of age, breed and gender. *Vet Ophthalmol* 2003; **6**: 329–332.

12 Mughannam AJ, Buyukmihci NC, Kass PH. Effect of topical atropine on intraocular pressure and pupil diameter in the normal horse eye. *Vet Ophthalmol* 1999; **2**: 213–215.

13 Varsanno D, Rothamn S, Haas K, *et al.* The mydriatic effect of topical glycopyrrolate. *Graefes Arch Clin Exp Ophthalmol* 1996; **234**: 205–207.

14 Ludders JW, Heavner JE. Effect of atropine on tear formation in anesthetized dogs. *J Am Vet Med Assoc* 1979; **175**: 585–586.

15 Arnett BD, Brightman AH, Mussleman EE. Effect of atropine sulfate on tear production in the cat when used with ketamine hydrochloride and acetylpromazine maleate. *J Am Vet Med Assoc* 1984; **185**: 214–215.

16 Ducharme NG, Fubini SL. Gastrointestinal complications associated with the use of atropine in horses. *J Am Vet Med Assoc* 1983; **167**: 200–202.

17 Roush JK, Keene BW, Eicker SW, *et al.* Effects of atropine and glycopyrrolate on esophageal, gastric and tracheal pH in anesthetized dogs. *Vet Surg* 1990; **19**: 88–92.

18 Proakis AG, Harris GB. Comparative penetration of glycopyrrolate and atropine across the blood–brain and placental barriers in anesthetized dogs. *Anesthesiology* 1978; **48**: 339–344.

19 Hendrix PK, Robinson EP. Effects of a selective and a nonselective muscarinic cholinergic antagonist on heart rate and intestinal motility in dogs. *J Vet Pharmacol Ther* 1997; **20**: 387–395.

20 Harrison PK, Tattersall JE, Gosden E. The presence of atropinesterase activity in animal plasma. *Naunyn Schmiedebergs Arch Pharmacol* 2000; **373**: 230–236.

21 Muir WW. Effects of atropine on cardiac rate and rhythm in dogs. *J Am Vet Med Assoc* 1978; **172**: 917–921.

22 Richards DL, Clutton RE, Boyd C. Electrocardiographic findings following intravenous glycopyrrolate to sedated dogs: a comparison with atropine. *J Assoc Vet Anaesth* 1989; **16**: 46–50.

23 Clutton RE, Glasby MA. Cardiovascular and autonomic nervous effects of edrophonium and atropine combinations during neuromuscular blockade antagonism in sheep. *Vet Anaesth Analg* 2008; **35**: 191–200.

24 Lemke, KA. Electrocardiographic and cardiopulmonary effects of intramuscular administration of glycopyrrolate and romifidine in conscious Beagle dogs. *Vet Anaesth Analg* 2001; **28**: 75–86.

25 Frischmeyer KJ, Miller PE, Bellay Y, *et al.* Parenteral anticholinergics in dogs with normal and elevated intraocular pressure. *Vet Surg* 1993; **22**: 230–234.

26 Hall, LW, Clarke, KW, Trim CM. Principles of sedation, analgesia and premedication. *Veterinary Anaesthesia*, 10th edn. Philadelphia: Saunders, 2000; 75–112.

27 Short CE, Paddleford RR, Cloyd GD. Glycopyrrolate for prevention of pulmonary complications during anesthesia. *Mod Vet Pract* 1974; **55**: 194–196.

28 Singh S, McDonell WN, Young SS, *et al.* The effect of glycopyrrolate on heart rate and intestinal motility in conscious horses. *J Vet Anaesth* 1997; **24**: 14–19.

29 Gonçalves S, Julliand V, Leblond A. Risk factors associated with colic in horses. *Vet Res* 2002; **33**: 641–652.

30 Dyson DH, Pascoe PJ, McDonell WN. Effects of intravenously administered glycopyrrolate in anesthetized horses. *Can Vet J* 1999; **40**: 29–32.

31 Lemke KA, Tranquilli WJ, Thurmon JC, *et al.* Hemodynamic effects of atropine and glycopyrrolate in isoflurane–xylazine-anesthetized dogs. *Vet Surg* 1993; **22**: 163–169.

32 Congdon JM, Marquez M, Niyom S, Boscan P. Evaluation of the sedative and cardiovascular effects of intramuscular administration of dexmedetomidine with and without concurrent atropine administration in dogs. *J Am Vet Med Assoc* 2011; **239**: 81–89.

33 Monteiro ER, Campagnol D, Parrilha LR, Furlan LZ. Evaluation of cardiorespiratory effects of combinations of dexmedetomidine and atropine in cats. *J Feline Med Surg* 2009; **11**: 783–792.

34 Stoelting RK. Anticholinergic drugs. *Pharmacology and Physiology in Anesthetic Practice*, 3rd edn. Philadelphia: Lippincott-Raven, 1999; 238–246.

9 Adrenergic Agents

Joanna C. Murrell
School of Veterinary Sciences, University of Bristol, Langford, North Somerset, UK

Chapter contents

Introduction

Adrenergic agents are drugs that act on the sympathetic nervous system (SNS) and as such are widely used in veterinary anesthesia for the management of cardiorespiratory function. In order to understand the mechanism of action of the different drugs, it is important to have a thorough knowledge of the physiology of adrenergic receptors and the autonomic nervous system (see Chapter 28). Table 9.1 provides a brief overview of the distributions, effects, and mechanisms of action of adrenergic and dopaminergic receptors. This is useful to help predict the physiologic effects of the different drugs acting at these receptors types.

There are a number of different systems that can be used to classify adrenergic agents, for example, the receptor at which the drug exerts an effect, whether the drug is an agonist or antagonist at the receptor, or whether the drug is a naturally occurring or synthetic agent. Classification of adrenergic agents can also be confusing because some agents act at more than one type of receptor (e.g., ephedrine is an agonist at both α- and β-adrenergic receptors) whereas others may act differentially at receptors depending on dose (e.g., dopamine is a β_1-adrenergic agonist when administered at low doses, but at higher doses α_1-agonist effects tend to predominate).

Adrenergic agents that are agonists at α_1-, β_1- and β_2-receptors are also classified as sympathomimetics because they cause stimulation or activation of the SNS. Drugs acting at dopamine receptors are also sympathomimetics and therefore are included in this chapter. Sympathomimetics can also be classified according to whether they have a direct effect at adrenergic receptors or whether they act indirectly by causing the release of norepinephrine. In contrast, antagonists at α- and β-receptors are classified as sympatholytics because they reduce the level of activation of the SNS.

Catecholamines and other adrenergic agonists

The structure of sympathomimetics is based on a benzene ring with various amine side-chains attached at the C1 position. Where a hydroxyl group is present at the C3 and C4 positions, the agent is known as a catecholamine (because 3,4-dihydroxybenzene is otherwise known as catechol). In this chapter, the naturally occurring catecholamines are discussed first, followed by synthetic catecholamines and then other non-catecholamine synthetic adrenergic agents. The synthetic adrenergic agents are classified according to receptor type and whether they act as agonists or antagonists.

Naturally occurring catecholamines

Epinephrine

Epinephrine acts non-selectively and directly as an agonist at all of the adrenergic receptors (i.e., α_1, α_2, β_1, and β_2) (see Table 9.1). In veterinary anesthesia, epinephrine is principally used to support cardiovascular function during cardiopulmonary resuscitation.

Epinephrine for systemic administration is available in vials and prefilled syringes at concentrations of 0.1 mg/mL (1:10 000) and 1 mg/mL (1:1000). It must be protected from light and therefore is presented in colored glass vials or prefilled syringes stored inside protective packaging. In animals, it is administered systemically by intravenous injection or via the airway during resuscitation (intratracheal administration), although for humans, epinephrine is also available in a metered aerosol preparation to treat swelling associated with upper airway obstruction due to its vasoconstrictive effects. Epinephrine is also formulated with local anesthetic solutions for infiltration at concentrations ranging from 1:200 000 to

Veterinary Anesthesia and Analgesia: The Fifth Edition of Lumb and Jones.
Edited by Kurt A. Grimm, Leigh A. Lamont, William J. Tranquilli, Stephen A. Greene and Sheilah A. Robertson.

Table 9.1 Adrenergic and dopaminergic receptor distributions, effects, and mechanisms of action.

Receptor	Subtype	Location	Effects When Stimulated	Mechanism of Action
Alpha (α)	1	Smooth muscle (blood vessels, bronchi, GI system, uterus, urinary system)	Contraction of smooth muscle, vasoconstriction	Excitatory G-protein coupled receptor linked to PLC; receptor binding activates PLC, which increases intracellular IP_3 and leads to an increase in intracellular [Ca^{2+}]
	2	Throughout the CNS Platelets	Sedation, analgesia, attenuation of sympathetically mediated responses Platelet aggregation	Inhibitory G-protein coupled receptor linked to AC; receptor binding reduces AC activity which leads to a decrease in intracellular [cAMP]
Beta (β)	1	Heart	Positive inotropic and chronotropic effects	Excitatory G-protein coupled receptor linked to AC; receptor binding activates AC and leads to an increase in intracellular [cAMP]
	2	Smooth muscle (blood vessels, bronchi, GI system, uterus, urinary system) Heart	Relaxation of smooth muscle, vasodilation Positive inotropic and chronotropic effects (minor)	Excitatory G-protein coupled receptor linked to AC; receptor binding activates AC and leads to an increase in intracellular [cAMP]; cAMP activates PKA and also increases activity of Na^+/K^+ ATPase activity, causing hyperpolarization
	3	Adipose tissue	Lipolysis	Excitatory G-protein coupled receptor linked to AC; receptor binding activates AC and leads to an increase in intracellular [cAMP]
Dopamine	1	Throughout the CNS Vascular smooth muscle, kidney, sympathetic ganglia, etc.	Modulates extrapyramidal activity Vasodilation of renal and mesenteric vasculature	Excitatory G-protein coupled receptor linked to AC; receptor binding activates AC and leads to an increase in intracellular [cAMP]
	2	Throughout the CNS Vascular smooth muscle, kidney, sympathetic ganglia, etc.	Reduced pituitary hormone output Inhibit further noradrenaline release	Inhibitory G-protein coupled receptor linked to AC; receptor binding reduces AC activity, which leads to a decrease in intracellular [cAMP]

GI, gastrointestinal; PLC, phospholipase C; IP_3, inositol triphosphate; AC, adenylyl cyclase; cAMP, cyclic adenosine monophosphate; PKA, protein kinase A; CNS, central nervous system.

1:80 000. Most formulations contain racemic epinephrine, although the L-isomer is the active form.

Cardiovascular system effects

The cardiovascular effects of epinephrine are dose dependent. Low doses of epinephrine administered by bolus (0.01 mg/kg IV) cause β_1- and β_2-adrenergic agonist effects to predominate. The cardiac effects of β_1-adrenergic receptor agonism result in increased cardiac output, myocardial oxygen consumption, coronary artery dilation, and a reduced threshold for arrhythmias. In low doses, peripheral β_2-adrenergic agonist effects result in a decrease in diastolic blood pressure and peripheral vascular resistance. At high doses (0.1 mg/kg IV), α_1-adrenergic effects predominate, causing a marked rise in systemic vascular resistance.

Data describing the detailed cardiovascular effects of epinephrine in different species are sparse. However, in cats anesthetized with isoflurane, the cardiovascular effects of epinephrine infusion at dose rates of 0.125–2 μg/kg/min were dose dependent [1]. All infusion rates caused increases in packed cell volume (PCV) due to α_1-adrenergic-induced splenic contraction [2], arterial oxygen content, heart rate, cardiac index, and stroke volume index (SVI) [1]. Increases in SVI were greatest with infusion rates of 1 and 2 μg/kg/min. Mean arterial blood pressure increased at infusion rates of 0.5 μg/kg/min and higher. At the infusion rates tested, epinephrine was not associated with an increase in systemic vascular resistance, reflecting the predominant β-adrenergic effects at these lower dose rates. However, the increases in blood pressure and cardiac index were also associated with increased lactate concentrations and progressive metabolic acidosis. The cardiovascular effects of epinephrine waned after the end of the infusion and the majority of the parameters returned to preinfusion values 30 min later. Extravasation of epinephrine can cause tissue necrosis due to localized vasoconstriction, hence care must be taken during intravenous administration.

Epinephrine, along with other catecholamines, is recognized to be proarrhythmogenic, causing a decrease in threshold for ventricular fibrillation and increased incidence of premature ventricular contractions and missed beats [3]. The precise mechanisms underlying the proarrhythmogenic effects of epinephrine are complex and are likely multifactorial [4]. Agonist effects at postsynaptic α_1- and β_1-adrenergic receptors on myocardial cells are implicated, in addition to activation of cardiac cholinergic reflexes [3].

Importantly, some anesthetic agents, notably halothane, are recognized to sensitize the myocardium to catecholamine-induced arrhythmias [5]. The proarrhythmogenic effects of epinephrine during halothane anesthesia have been documented in a wide range of species, including dogs [4], cats [6], horses [7], and swine [8]. Similarly to the proarrhythmogenic effects of catecholamines in awake animals, the mechanisms are multiple and complex and are considered to involve α_1-adrenergic, β_1-adrenergic, and cholinergic receptors in the heart [3, 4]. In comparison with halothane, isoflurane and sevoflurane do not sensitize the myocardium to epinephrine to any great extent [9, 10].

The effects of other anesthetic agents, in combination with halothane, on the arrhythmogenic dose of epinephrine have also been investigated in a variety of species. Xylazine does not alter the arrhythmogenic dose of epinephrine in horses induced with thiopental and maintained with halothane [11]. Ketamine decreases the arrhythmogenic dose of epinephrine in halothane-anesthetized cats [12,13] and dogs [14].

Other effects

Epinephrine will produce a small increase in minute volume through its bronchodilator effects, which are β_2-adrenergic receptor mediated. Pulmonary vascular resistance is increased at higher dose rates reflecting agonism at pulmonary vascular α_1-adrenergic receptors [15].

Epinephrine has wide-ranging effects on metabolism that are dose dependent. Basal metabolic rate is increased, resulting in a slight increase in body temperature following administration [1]. Plasma glucose concentration is increased via multiple mechanisms, including inhibition of insulin secretion (an α_2- and β_2-adrenergic effect), glycogenolysis in liver and muscle (an α_1- and β_2-adrenergic effect), lipolysis (a β_2- and β_3-adrenergic effect), and gluconeogenesis (an

α_1- and β_2-adrenergic effect). Serum potassium concentration will increase initially following epinephrine administration, followed by hypokalemia caused by increased uptake of potassium into cells (a β_2-effect).

Anesthetic requirement is related to the release of CNS catecholamines [16]; therefore, it would be predicted that epinephrine will increase the minimum alveolar concentration (MAC) of volatile agents. However, no effect of low-dose epinephrine on the MAC of halothane was reported in dogs [17].

Epinephrine causes the release of renin from the kidney through multiple mechanisms, including stimulation of intrarenal β_1- and β_2-adrenergic receptors in addition to extrarenal adrenergic receptors [18,19]. Renal blood flow is moderately decreased due to regional vasoconstriction.

Pharmacokinetics

Epinephrine has a very short half-life due to rapid metabolism, necessitating frequent redosing or administration by infusion for a prolonged effect. Following intravenous administration, epinephrine is rapidly metabolized by mitochondrial monoamine oxidase and catechol-*O*-methyltransferase within the liver, kidney, and circulation to inactive metabolites (3-methoxy-4-hydroxymandelic acid and metanephrine). The metabolites are conjugated with glucuronic acid or sulfates and excreted in the urine.

Norepinephrine

Norepinephrine acts as an agonist at α_1-, α_2- and β_1-adrenergic receptors, with effects at α-adrenergic receptors predominating at clinically used dose rates (see Table 9.1). Norepinephrine is predominantly used during anesthesia to manage hypotension, particularly when caused by a reduction in systemic vascular resistance (i.e., vasodilation) due to sepsis or administration of volatile anesthetic agents.

Norepinephrine differs from epinephrine in the absence of a methyl group on the nitrogen atom. It is generally supplied as a 1 mg/mL solution in the form of the bitartrate salt with the preservative sodium metabisulfite.

Cardiovascular system effects

At very low dose rates (0.025 µg/kg/min), norepinephrine's β_1-adrenergic receptor-mediated effects predominate and are manifested as increases in heart rate and cardiac output and decreases in systemic vascular resistance [20]. At higher dose rates (greater than 0.5–1.5 µg/kg/min), norepinephrine causes dose-dependent increases in systolic, diastolic, and mean arterial blood pressures, cardiac output, and systemic and pulmonary vascular resistance [21–23]. Norepinephrine will also cause coronary vasodilation to promote increased coronary blood flow. Tachycardia is less likely when compared with administration of epinephrine.

Norepinephrine (0.3 and 1.0 µg/kg/min) was effective at improving cardiovascular function and maintaining splanchnic function in foals [22] and alpacas [23] with isoflurane-induced hypotension. At high doses, the increased systemic vascular resistance will ultimately reduce cardiac output and increase myocardial oxygen consumption due to the increase in afterload [24]. Extravasation of norepinephrine can cause tissue necrosis due to localized vasoconstriction, hence care must be taken during intravenous administration. The arrhythmogenic effects of norepinephrine are similar to those of epinephrine.

Pharmacokinetics

Exogenously administered norepinephrine is metabolized similarly to epinephrine and has a short half-life. Unlike epinephrine, approximately 25% of administered norepinephrine is extracted from the circulation as it passes through the lung, where it is deactivated by monoamine oxidase and catechol-*O*-methyltransferase in the endothelial cells of the pulmonary microvasculature [25].

Dopamine

The receptor effects of dopamine are dose dependent. At low doses (1–2 µg/kg/min), effects on dopamine (DA)-1 and DA-2 receptors predominate. As dose rates increase further, β_1- and β_2-adrenergic receptor effects predominate. Finally, α_1-adrenergic receptor effects are noted at infusion rates greater than 10 µg/kg/min (see Table 9.1). Dopamine will also stimulate the release of endogenous norepinephrine from presynaptic storage sites at adrenergic receptors to cause an endogenous sympathomimetic effect. Dopamine is predominantly used by continuous rate infusion to improve hemodynamic parameters.

Dopamine is available as an injectable preparation, typically as a 40 mg/mL dopamine hydrochloride solution. It contains the preservative sodium metabisulfite. Dopamine hydrochloride in 100 mL dextrose 5% is also commercially available in a range of concentrations from 0.8 to 6.4 mg/mL.

Cardiovascular system effects

At dose rates less than 10 µg/kg/min, the β_1-adrenergic effects of dopamine predominate, leading to increases in myocardial contractility, heart rate, cardiac output, and coronary blood flow. At dose rates greater than 10 µg/kg/min, α_1-adrenergic agonist effects dominate, leading to increased systemic and pulmonary vascular resistance, venous return, and PCV due to splenic contraction. Tachycardia can occur at higher dose rates. A reduction in mean arterial blood pressure and cardiac output generally occurs after cessation of dopamine infusions, with return to preinfusion values within 30 min, leading to the recommendation that administration of dopamine be stopped in a stepwise manner [1].

The cardiovascular effects of dopamine given by continuous rate infusion have been studied in dogs, cats, and horses during volatile agent anesthesia. In dogs anesthetized with isoflurane, increasing infusion rates of dopamine from 3 to 20 µg/kg/min caused a dose-dependent increase in cardiac index and blood pressure, with increases in heart rate and systemic vascular resistance noted at dose rates greater than 7 µg/kg/min [26]. Doses less than 7 µg/kg/min were insufficient to support hemodynamic variables using the defined criteria (e.g., mean arterial blood pressure greater than 70 mmHg). At a dopamine infusion rate of 10 µg/kg/min and greater, there was a marked increase in systemic vascular resistance and a reduction in stroke volume, reflecting increased myocardial work associated with the increased afterload. This dose recommendation is supported by other studies investigating the dose-dependent effects of dopamine in dogs [27–30].

Similar dose-dependent effects have been reported in cats [1], with infusion rates around 10 µg/kg/min necessary to maintain mean arterial blood pressure above 70 mmHg in cats anesthetized with isoflurane. Wiese *et al.* [31] investigated the effects of a dopamine infusion on cardiovascular variables in cats with hypertrophic cardiomyopathy anesthetized with isoflurane. Dopamine infusion rates between 2.5 and 10 µg/kg/min increased heart rate, blood pressure, cardiac output, and oxygen delivery; while global oxygen consumption was reduced. However, all six cats in the study developed premature ventricular complexes and the authors suggested that dopamine may have negatively impacted myocardial oxygen consumption, which was not measured, despite the observed increase in global oxygen delivery.

In horses, the effect of dopamine infusion for management of hypotension during volatile agent anesthesia has been widely investigated. A dopamine infusion rate of 5 μg/kg/min increases myocardial contractility and cardiac output with little effect on blood pressure [32–36]. This is attributed to a reduction in systemic vascular resistance caused by a decrease in smooth muscle vascular tone elicited by stimulation of DA-1 and DA-2 receptors [37] in the absence of α_1-adrenergic receptor agonist effects, which are only activated at higher doses.

Extravasation of dopamine can cause tissue necrosis due to localized vasoconstriction; therefore, care must be taken during intravenous administration. Dopamine has the potential to be proarrhythmogenic at higher doses (10 μg/kg/min or greater).

Other effects

Infusions of dopamine attenuate the response of the carotid body to hypoxemia [38]. Early studies suggested that at very low doses (less than 2 μg/kg/min), dopamine infusions had a renal specific action, preferentially increasing renal blood flow and causing renal artery dilation, leading to a concomitant increase in urine output [39,40]. This was attributed to an effect of dopamine at renal DA-1 and DA-2 receptors. Consequentially, in human patients, there was significant use of low-dose dopamine for the management of acute renal failure in the intensive care unit [41]. However, it is now recognized that increased urine output associated with dopamine administration is caused by improved hemodynamic function [42,43] in combination with inhibition of proximal tubular Na^+ reabsorption [44]. Dopamine will produce vasodilation in mesenteric vascular beds [45] mediated by DA-1 receptor activation [46].

Pharmacokinetics

Dopamine has a short half-life of approximately 3 min, and therefore is given by continuous rate infusion. Onset of action after the start of an infusion can be up to 5 min. Dopamine is metabolized via monoamine oxidase and catechol-*O*-methyltransferase in the liver, kidney, and plasma to inactive compounds that are excreted in the urine as sulfate and glucuronide conjugates. About 25% is converted to norepinephrine in sympathetic nerve terminals.

Synthetic catecholamines

Dobutamine

Dobutamine primarily stimulates β_1-adrenergic receptors, but at higher dose rates (5–10 μg/kg/min) will also stimulate β_2- and α_1-adrenergic receptors. It does not exert an effect at α_2-adrenergic receptors. Dobutamine is principally used to augment low cardiac output states associated with reduced myocardial function. It is very commonly used in equine inhalant anesthesia to manage hypotension.

Dobutamine is a direct-acting synthetic catecholamine that is a derivative of isoproterenol. It is available in a range of concentrations from 12.5 to 50 mg/mL; the solution usually contains sodium metabisulfite preservative.

Cardiovascular system effects

The effects on the cardiovascular system are dose dependent and have been well described in cats, dogs, and horses. In halothane-anesthetized normotensive horses, a very low-dose infusion of dobutamine for 30 min (0.5 μg/kg/min) increased systolic, diastolic, and mean arterial blood pressure but did not increase myocardial contractility or cardiac output; PCV was also increased [47]. Infusion rates of 4–5 μg/kg/min to halothane-anesthetized horses increased arterial blood pressure and cardiac output with minimal effects on heart rate and systemic vascular resistance [32,35,48]. Dobutamine at 10 μg/kg/min tends to increase systemic vascular resistance and heart rate, with increases in cardiac output at high doses attributed to both inotropic and chronotropic effects of the drug [32,36]. In comparison with dopamine, dopexamine, and phenylephrine, dobutamine has been shown to have a more consistent effect in increasing intramuscular blood flow in ponies anesthetized with halothane [36].

In isoflurane-anesthetized dogs, dobutamine at doses up to 10 μg/kg/min had more limited effects on blood pressure, but caused increases in cardiac output, heart rate, and systemic vascular resistance [26,29]. The authors noted that owing to the limited effect of dobutamine on blood pressure, assessment of the effectiveness of dobutamine to improve hemodynamic function was challenging in the absence of cardiac output measurements.

In cats, dobutamine at similar dose rates to those studied in dogs also had limited effects on blood pressure and increased heart rate [1]. Systemic vascular resistance decreased, reflecting the β_2-adrenergic receptor agonist effects of the drug causing peripheral vasodilation in skeletal muscle.

Like other catecholamines, dobutamine has the potential to be proarrhythmogenic at high doses (10 μg/kg/min or greater).

Pharmacokinetics

Dobutamine has a short half-life and is therefore administered by continuous-rate infusion. It is predominantly metabolized via catechol-*O*-methyltransferase in the liver to inactive metabolites that are conjugated and excreted in the urine.

Dopexamine

Dopexamine is a potent stimulator of β_2-adrenergic receptors with weak agonist effects at β_1, DA-1 and DA-2 receptors. It has no effect on α_1-adrenergic receptors. Dopexamine inhibits the neuronal uptake of endogenous catecholamines. In human medicine, dopexamine is primarily used to improve cardiac output and mesenteric perfusion. The potential ability of dopexamine to protect hepatosplanchnic and renal blood flow has resulted in the recommendation of dopexamine over other positive inotropes such as dopamine and dobutamine for use in patients particularly at risk of poor splanchnic blood flow, although evidence to support this contention is lacking [49]. Dopexamine is available as a 10 mg/mL solution in 5 mL vials.

Cardiovascular system effects

Dopexamine has a positive inotropic effect via cardiac β_2-adrenergic receptors, although systemic blood pressure may fall due to β_2-receptor-mediated vasodilation of peripheral blood vessels, particularly in skeletal muscle. The reduction in systemic vascular resistance helps to promote an increase in cardiac output. The cardiovascular effects of dopexamine infusion at dose rates varying from 1 to 10 μg/kg/min have been investigated in horses anesthetized with halothane [36,50–52]. Low doses (1–2.5 μg/kg/min) increased blood pressure and cardiac output, but higher dose rates (at or above 5 μg/kg/min) were associated with tachycardia, cardiac arrhythmias, muscle twitching, and poor recoveries from anesthesia. Therefore, despite the positive hemodynamic effects of dopexamine, administration to support hemodynamic function during anesthesia in horses is not recommended.

There are a few reports on the investigation of the effects of dopexamine infusions in dogs; dopexamine increased cardiac output and heart rate in a dose-dependent manner [53,54], with one study indicating that the arrhythmogenic potential of dopexamine is lower than that of dopamine [55]. These studies evaluated infusion rates between 0.25 and 3.5 μg/kg/min. Despite the potential advantages of increased cardiac output with reduced systemic vascular resistance, and therefore a more limited effect on myocardial oxygen consumption compared with other inotropes, dopexamine is not commonly used clinically in dogs.

Other effects

Dopexamine causes bronchodilation via β_2-adrenergic receptors. Blood flow to the gastrointestinal system and kidneys is increased due to increased cardiac output and reduced regional vascular resistance; there is a concomitant increase in urine output. The clinical benefit of selecting dopexamine over other inotropes in human patients where increased splanchnic perfusion is desirable has been debated [56].

Pharmacokinetics

Dopexamine has a short half-life and is rapidly metabolized by *O*-methylation and sulfation in the liver [57].

Isoproterenol (isoprenaline)

Isoproterenol is a very potent synthetic catecholamine that is an agonist at β_1- and β_2-adrenergic receptors. It has no α-adrenergic receptor effects. Isoproterenol is used to increase heart rate and myocardial contractility during anesthesia. In human medicine, isoproterenol may also be used to promote abnormal electrical activity of the heart during electrophysiological studies. Low doses of isoproterenol are used as a 'test dose' to detect intravascular needle placement during epidural anesthesia in children. This is to prevent inadvertent intravascular injection of local anesthetics that may be associated with adverse effects [58]. There are very limited data on the clinical use of isoproterenol in animals.

Isoproterenol is typically available as a 0.2 mg/mL solution that contains sodium metabisulfite as a preservative. It should be protected from light.

Cardiovascular system effects

Stimulation of β_1-adrenergic receptors causes an increase in heart rate, myocardial contractility, and cardiac output [59]. Agonist effects at β_2-adrenergic receptors generally reduce systemic vascular resistance such that the mean arterial blood pressure falls. At higher infusion rates (2.5 μg/kg/min), myocardial oxygen delivery is likely to be compromised owing to the combined effects of increased heart rate reducing coronary filling time, while decreased systemic blood pressure reduces coronary perfusion [60]. However, a very low-dose infusion (0.1 μg/kg/min) of isoproterenol in dogs anesthetized with isoflurane increased cardiac output and heart rate while increasing myocardial blood flow such that adequate myocardial oxygenation was maintained [59]. This was attributed to metabolically driven vasodilation of coronary blood vessels rather than direct stimulation of coronary vasculature β_2-adrenergic receptors. Given these actions, the administration of a potent β_1/β_2-agonist such as isoproterenol to a low blood volume patient (e.g., hemorrhagic shock or severe dehydration) dependent upon intense compensatory vasoconstriction for coronary perfusion pressure is problematic and discouraged, unless and until blood and stroke volume can be restored.

Isoproterenol has well-characterized proarrhythmogenic effects through its effects on ion channel kinetics and promotion of intracellular calcium accumulation and tachycardia [61].

Other Effects

Isoproterenol is a potent bronchodilator, increasing anatomic deadspace and thus ventilation perfusion mismatching; which has the potential to causes systemic hypoxemia. It causes stimulation of the central nervous system and therefore can increase the level of arousal during general anesthesia [62]. Isoproterenol increases splanchnic and renal blood flow via selective vasodilation mediated by stimulation of β-adrenergic receptors [63].

Typical metabolic effects of β-adrenergic receptor stimulation are seen following isoproterenol administration, including increases in blood glucose and free fatty acid concentrations, and a decrease in serum potassium concentration caused by a shift of potassium into cells.

Pharmacokinetics

Isoproterenol has a short half-life. It is rapidly metabolized by catechol-*O*-methyltransferase in the liver, in addition to being excreted in the urine unchanged [64]. In addition, both isoproterenol and its metabolites may be excreted as conjugated sulfates in the urine.

α_1-adrenergic receptor agonists

Phenylephrine

Phenylephrine is a direct-acting sympathomimetic amine with potent α_1-adrenergic receptor agonist effects and therefore it is often referred to as 'vasopressor'. It has no effect on β-adrenergic receptors. Phenylephrine is used systemically during anesthesia to increase systemic vascular resistance and therefore increase blood pressure. Phenylephrine can also be administered topically to mucosal surfaces to produce localized vasoconstriction and reduce edema or hemorrhage. In the horse, phenylephrine may be used in the medical management of nephrosplenic entrapment prior to rolling or laparoscopic surgical correction of the condition. The aim of phenylephrine administration is to reduce splenic size and therefore facilitate medical or surgical correction of the entrapment.

Phenylephrine is typically available for injection as a 10 mg/mL solution as the hydrochloride salt. However, phenylephrine is also present in some topical eye preparations and is a common ingredient in decongestants for use in people.

Cardiovascular system effects

Administered systemically, phenylephrine causes a dose-dependent increase in systemic vascular resistance and mean arterial blood pressure and a reflex reduction in heart rate. Cardiac output is usually minimally altered or may fall as a result of increased afterload combined with bradycardia. In horses, phenylephrine is typically infused intravenously at a rate of 1 μg/kg/min preceded by a 2 μg/kg loading dose [47,65] until the blood pressure is increased. The hemodynamic effects wane rapidly once the infusion is terminated. Systemic and pulmonary vascular resistances are increased, and there is a limited effect on cardiac output. Phenylephrine at dose rates between 0.25 and 2 μg/kg/min did not improve skeletal muscle blood flow in horses anesthetized with halothane [36,47]. Frederick *et al.* [66] reported five cases of severe phenylephrine-associated hemorrhage in aged horses. The phenylephrine was administered to facilitate management of nephrosplenic entrapment and the hemorrhage was attributed to secondary hypertension caused by increased systemic vascular resistance. The negative effects of phenylephrine on cardiac output and skeletal muscle blood flow suggest that phenylephrine should not be used to manage hypotension primarily caused by myocardial depression in anesthetized horses.

There are limited clinical data on the use of phenylephrine in dogs, but a few experimental studies have investigated the cardiovascular effects of infusion. A dose of at least 0.4 µg/kg/min was necessary to increase mean arterial blood pressure significantly in conscious dogs [67], followed by linear increases in blood pressure up to the maximum infusion rate evaluated of 4 µg/kg/min. A reduction in heart rate occurred at the lowest infusion rate tested (0.008 µg/kg/min), which was attributed to a vagally mediated reflex bradycardia [67]. Phenylephrine at 0.14 mg/kg was necessary to manage hypotension caused by acepromazine in halothane-anesthetized dogs [68].

The cardiovascular effects of phenylephrine have been studied in healthy cats anesthetized with isoflurane [1] and in cats with hypertrophic cardiomyopathy [31]. In healthy cats, infusion rates of 0.125–2 µg/kg/min were studied. Mean arterial blood pressure was significantly increased at infusion rates at and above 1 µg/kg/min, which was associated with increased systemic vascular resistance. Heart rate did not change as isoflurane likely obtunded baroreflex-mediated reflex activity. In contrast to horses, these infusion rates were associated with an increase in cardiac output; oxygen delivery was also increased, which was attributed to an increase in PCV and cardiac output. Phenylephrine infusion rates of 0.25–1 µg/kg/min were studied in cats with hypertrophic myopathy anesthetized with isoflurane [31]. Similar changes in heart rate and blood pressure to those observed in healthy cats were reported; there was no change in cardiac output, but oxygen delivery increased with no change in global oxygen consumption.

There is little evidence to suggest that phenylephrine is proarrhythmogenic when used clinically.

Other effects

Phenylephrine has no stimulatory effects on the central nervous system. Hepatic and renal blood flow are reduced, mediated by α_1-adrenergic receptor-induced vasoconstriction [69,70]. Phenylephrine will reduce uterine blood flow and it is generally recommended to avoid administration during pregnancy due to potential adverse effects on fetal oxygen delivery [71].

Intranasal administration of phenylephrine to anesthetized horses prior to recovery from anesthesia is used to reduce nasal edema and the potential for upper airway obstruction [72]. Administration of 5 mL of 0.15% phenylephrine solution into each nostril approximately 50 min before extubation was sufficient to reduce nasal edema and significantly reduced the requirement for placement of a nasal tube during recovery in the majority of horses studied (20 horses) compared with a control group (20 horses). No adverse cardiovascular effects following administration were noted.

Topical eye drops containing 10% phenylephrine hydrochloride caused increased blood pressure in both anesthetized and conscious dogs [73,74].

Pharmacokinetics

Phenylephrine has a short half-life when administered intravenously. It is metabolized in the liver by monoamine oxidase.

Methoxamine

Methoxamine is a direct-acting sympathomimetic amine with specific α_1-adrenergic receptor agonist effects and is also classified as a vasopressor. The clinical effects of methoxamine are similar to those of phenylephrine; however, methoxamine is purported to have a longer duration of action, despite limited pharmacological data on systemically administered methoxamine in animals. Methoxamine is reported to predominantly cause vasoconstriction of arterioles, with little effect at capacitance vessels. In horses, a dose of 0.04 mg/kg IV approximately 5–10 min before induction of anesthesia did not modulate halothane-induced hypotension during the maintenance phase of anesthesia, with no effect on mean arterial blood pressure, heart rate, cardiac output, or central venous pressure [75]. However, experimental studies have demonstrated the cardiovascular effects of methoxamine in other species. Doses of methoxamine from 0.4 to 6.0 mg/kg in lambs caused an increase in cardiac output, attributed to stimulation of α_1-adrenergic receptors in the lamb myocardium [76]. In contrast, no positive inotropic action was reported in dogs [77,78], suggesting species-specific effects of methoxamine on the myocardium.

Methoxamine is available as a 20 mg/mL solution as the hydrochloride salt for intravenous injection.

α_2-Adrenergic receptor agonists

Dexmedetomidine, medetomidine, detomidine, xylazine, romifidine

These agents are not classified as sympathomimetics but they are used extensively in veterinary medicine for their excellent sedative and analgesic properties. Their other α_2-adrenergic receptor-mediated effects are considered, in most instances, to be adverse side-effects. For a complete discussion of α_2-adrenergic receptor agonist pharmacology, see Chapter 10.

β_2-Adrenergic receptor agonists

Clenbuterol, albuterol (salbutamol), terbutaline

Clenbuterol, albuterol, and terbutaline are predominantly used for the management of bronchospasm in people with asthma. In veterinary medicine, they are used to treat bronchospasm in both awake and anesthetized animals. In addition, clenbuterol has been used illegally to increase the muscle mass and reduce the fat composition of carcasses of food-producing animals.

Clenbuterol has Marketing Authorization for administration to horses for the management of chronic obstructive pulmonary disease and is available as an injectable solution for administration intravenously, and also as syrup and granule preparations for oral administration. An injectable preparation is also licensed for administration to cattle to delay the onset of parturition by causing uterine relaxation. Albuterol and terbutaline are not licensed for administration to animals but are available as aerosol and oral preparations for the management of asthma in people.

Cardiovascular system effects

At high doses, this class of agents can also exert agonist effects at β_1-adrenergic receptors causing tachycardia, whereas at lower doses decreases in blood pressure are noted due to β_2-adrenergic receptor-mediated vasodilation.

These agents are noted to be proarrythmogenic as they shorten the refractory period of the atrioventricular node, slow ventricular conduction, and shorten the refractory period of the ventricular myocardium [79]. The arrythmogenic effects are likely to be more pronounced during concurrent hypoxemia (e.g., caused by an increase in shunt fraction) or during hypokalemia.

Other effects

These agents stimulate Na^+/K^+ ATPase, leading to increased intracellular uptake of K^+ and hypokalemia. The blood glucose concentration typically increases. In the respiratory system, they cause relaxation of bronchial smooth muscle and reversal of hypoxic pulmonary vasoconstriction (see below).

Clenbuterol and albuterol have been evaluated in anesthetized horses for the management of hypoxemia. Data pertaining to the clinical effects of clenbuterol (IV) are conflicting. Early studies investigating clenbuterol at 0.8 and 2.4 mg/kg IV reported improved arterial oxygenation in horses anesthetized with halothane [80,81], with a prolonged duration of effect of up to 90 min. However, more recent studies have found no effect of clenbuterol on arterial oxygen concentrations at similar doses rates, or a potentiation of hypoxemia [36,82]. Potentiation of hypoxemia [82] was attributed to an increased shunt fraction associated with bronchodilation and a reduction in hypoxic pulmonary vasoconstriction. At these dose rates clenbuterol caused hemodynamic effects consistent with β_2-adrenergic receptor stimulation; causing a small increase in heart rate and cardiac output that persisted for up to 30 min after administration and that was associated with a transient increase in muscle perfusion. Adverse effects of clenbuterol include profuse sweating and increased oxygen consumption associated with the sympathomimetic effects on cardiovascular function. Consequently, clenbuterol administered intravenously is not recommended as a treatment for hypoxemia in anesthetized horses.

Albuterol, administered via inhalation through the endotracheal tube, has been shown to improve arterial oxygenation in anesthetized horses, predominantly through a sympathomimetic effect on hemodynamic function. Robertson and Bailey [83] administered 2 μg/kg albuterol using a human metered dose inhaler, with the dose delivered over a number of consecutive breaths at the start of each inspiration. This treatment was administered to 81 horses during volatile agent anesthesia when PaO_2 decreased below 70 mmHg. The authors reported an almost twofold increase in PaO_2 within 20 min of administration, with no concurrent effects on heart rate or mean arterial blood pressure. Patschova *et al.* [84] investigated the effects of the same dose (2 μg/kg) administered via the endotracheal tube on arterial oxygen concentrations and hemodynamics in isoflurane-anesthetized horses. There was a significant increase in cardiac output 15 min after albuterol administration, persisting for the duration of the monitored period (60 min). There was a transient increase in heart rate while mean arterial blood pressure was unchanged, which was attributed to a reduction in systemic vascular resistance mediated by β_2-adrenergic receptors. The PaO_2:F_IO_2 ratio improved, but to a lesser extent than reported by Robertson and Bailey [83], and coincided with the peak effect of albuterol on cardiac output. These data suggest that improvements in oxygenation following albuterol administration arise predominantly from the positive hemodynamic effects of the drug. Collectively, these studies support the use of inhaled albuterol to manage hypoxemia in anesthetized horses.

There are no clinical reports of administration of this class of drugs to dogs during anesthesia; however, a number of studies have investigated the efficacy of inhaled albuterol in the management of bronchospasm in cats [85–87]. Albuterol at 100 μg/kg, delivered via a face mask immediately prior to induction of anesthesia, was effective at reducing bronchoconstriction in response to bronchoalveolar lavage in both normal cats and cats with experimentally induced asthma [85]. This investigation did not monitor for concurrent cardiovascular effects of drug administration. Terbutaline is also used in cats for the management of bronchospasm during bronchoscopy and bronchoalveolar lavage, particularly in cats with asthma. A dose of 0.01 mg/kg IM or SC has a duration of action of about 4 h, with peak effects occurring approximately 15 min after administration [88].

Mixed α- and β-adrenergic receptor agonists

Ephedrine

Ephedrine has both direct and indirect sympathomimetic actions, acting as an agonist at α_1-, α_2-, β_1-, and β_2-adrenergic receptors. It also inhibits the action of monoamine oxidase on norepinephrine. Tachyphylaxis occurs with repeated dosing due to depletion of norepinephrine stores and therefore a reduction in the magnitude of indirect sympathomimetic effects [89].

Ephedrine is used in the management of hypotension during anesthesia. Its longer duration of action compared with many other vasopressors and inotropes allows the administration of an intravenous bolus to produce clinical effects, removing the necessity for administration of drugs by continuous-rate infusion. Infusions can be more time consuming to prepare and therefore delay the initiation of vasopressor or inotropic therapy.

Ephedrine is available in a variety of formulations for human use as a decongestant. For use during anesthesia, a 30 or 50 mg/mL solution is typically used. There are at least four isomers of ephedrine, all of which show some activity in dogs and cats [90], although this may vary between species [91]; two of the isomers are termed pseudoephedrine and the other two ephedrine. The commercially available medical preparation is L-ephedrine.

Cardiovascular system effects

Ephedrine increases cardiac output, heart rate, blood pressure, coronary blood flow, and myocardial oxygen consumption. In horses anesthetized with halothane, administration of ephedrine (0.06 mg/kg IV) caused an increase in cardiac output and mean arterial blood pressure, with minimal effect on systemic vascular resistance [92]. The increase in cardiac output was attributed to increased stroke volume rather than a chronotropic effect. The effect of ephedrine was detected at 10 min (the first measured time point) after administration and persisted for 45–60 min. In this study, there was a concurrent increase in PaO_2, attributed to the effect of increased cardiac output on pulmonary perfusion. A similar dose of ephedrine administered to halothane-anesthetized horses with blood pressures below 65 mmHg also caused an increase in mean arterial blood pressure, detected 5 min after administration [48]; heart rate was unchanged and there was no significant increase in PCV.

In dogs, single doses of ephedrine have been evaluated for the management of isoflurane-induced hypotension during anesthesia [30,93]. Chen *et al.* [30] administered ephedrine at 0.2 mg/kg IV to dogs with a mean arterial blood pressure lower than 70 mmHg and documented increased cardiac output, stroke volume, blood pressure, and global oxygen delivery; however, these effects were very transient, with a duration of effect of approximately 5 min. A repeat dose of ephedrine given 10 min later was ineffective at improving any cardiovascular parameters, which was attributed to tachyphylaxis. These findings were similar to those in an earlier study by Wagner *et al.* [93], although they investigated three different doses of ephedrine and found a more sustained increase in hemodynamic parameters following a 0.25 mg/kg dose, persisting for up to 30 min after administration. In contrast to the effect of ephedrine in horses, PCV increased at the higher dose in dogs, and this was attributed to α-adrenergic-induced splenic contraction [94].

There are limited clinical data on the administration of ephedrine to cats. Egger *et al.* [95] reported the cardiovascular effects of ephedrine at 0.1 mg/kg IM in cats anesthetized with acepromazine, ketamine, and isoflurane. The ephedrine was given 10 min before induction of anesthesia and was noted to delay the onset of hypotension (defined as a systolic arterial blood pressure of less than 80 mmHg) until 25 min after induction of anesthesia, compared with cats administered saline. No other cardiovascular changes occurred; however, cardiovascular monitoring was less rigorous in this study compared with studies in dogs and horses.

As with other sympathomimetics, administration of ephedrine may promote cardiac arrhythmias.

Other effects

Ephedrine causes stimulation of the respiratory system and bronchodilation similar to other drugs with β_2-adrenergic receptor agonist activity [see clenbuterol in the section Clenbuterol, Albuterol (Salbutamol), Terbutaline for details].

Ephedrine reduces renal blood flow with an associated reduction in glomerular filtration rate, attributed to regional vasoconstriction following stimulation of α_1-adrenergic receptors [96].

Pharmacokinetics

The pharmacokinetics of ephedrine have been described in the dog [97]. It undergoes rapid *N*-demethylation to norephedrine, which also has vasopressor effects and is likely to contribute to the hemodynamic effects of ephedrine seen in this species. There are limited data available on the metabolism of ephedrine in cats or horses, but data in ponies suggests that ephedrine is also metabolized to norephedrine [98].

Metaraminol

Similarly to ephedrine, metaraminol is a synthetic amine with both direct and indirect sympathomimetic effects that acts predominantly on α-adrenergic receptors with some β-adrenergic receptor activity. In contrast to ephedrine, owing to relatively greater effects at α_1-adrenergic receptors, its major cardiovascular action is to increase blood pressure through an increase in systemic vascular resistance; consequently, cardiac output often falls. Metaraminol is not commonly used in veterinary anesthesia.

Adrenergic receptor antagonists

Adrenergic receptor antagonists prevent the actions of sympathomimetic amines on adrenergic receptors and are therefore called sympatholytics. This class of drug can be subdivided depending on whether a drug is an antagonist at α- or β-adrenergic receptors, and then further subdivided according to whether it is selective for the α_1, α_2, β_1, or β_2-subtype.

α_1-Adrenergic receptor antagonists

Prazosin

Prazosin, a quinazoline derivative, is a highly selective α_1-adrenergic receptor antagonist. It is used predominantly for the management of functional urethral obstruction in cats and dogs. Stimulation of α_1-adrenergic receptors in the bladder neck and proximal urethra narrow the bladder outlet maintaining continence. Inappropriate contraction of the bladder neck or urethra during voiding prevents normal urine flow and is termed functional urethral obstruction. Although prazosin is not used during the management of anesthesia, it is important to understand the physiological effects of the drug and their relevance to anesthesia because of the requirement to anesthetize dogs and cats that are receiving prazosin therapy. Prazosin is available in an oral preparation (0.5–2 mg tablets) and an injectable form. The oral preparation is used most commonly in animals.

Cardiovascular system effects

Prazosin produces vasodilation of arteries and veins and reduces systemic vascular resistance; this is associated with a reduction in blood pressure, with diastolic blood pressure being impacted most significantly. There is little or no reflex tachycardia, which is attributed to a reduction in central thoracic sympathetic outflow [99]. There are limited clinical data on the cardiovascular effects of oral prazosin in cats or dogs. In a small study of three dogs, prazosin 0.025 mg/kg administered intravenously caused a maximal reduction in blood pressure that occurred 10 min after administration, but did not cause clinical hypotension (i.e., mean arterial blood pressure less than 70 mmHg). However, anecdotally, clinical signs attributable to hypotension have been reported in cats receiving prazosin for functional urethral obstruction. Prazosin is recommended for administration every 8–12 h in cats and dogs for the management of functional urethral obstruction. Therefore, in order to reduce the likelihood of hypotension during anesthesia of animals receiving prazosin for this purpose, it is reasonable to recommend cessation of administration 12–24 h before induction of anesthesia. Prazosin may also be used in the management of hemodynamic function in patients with pheochromocytoma, although phenoxybenzamine is more commonly used for this purpose (see below).

Pharmacokinetics

The pharmacokinetics of oral and intravenous prazosin have been described in awake dogs and dogs anesthetized with sodium pentobarbital [100]. Orally, although well absorbed from the gastrointestinal tract, prazosin has a relatively low bioavailability (approximately 38%), with hepatic extraction contributing to a major proportion of the presystemic metabolism of the drug. Following intravenous administration, initial plasma concentrations decrease rapidly due to extensive tissue distribution. The major liver hepatic pathways were demethylation, amide hydrolysis and *O*-glucuronidation [100, 101]. Anesthesia had a minimal effect on the pharmacokinetics of prazosin; however, it is predicted that drug metabolism would be significantly slowed in animals with liver dysfunction. The pharmacokinetics of prazosin in cats have not been described.

α_2-Adrenergic receptor antagonists

Atipamezole, yohimbine, tolazoline

In veterinary anesthesia, these agents are used for the reversal of sedation produced by α_2-adrenergic receptor agonists such as medetomidine and dexmedetomidine. See Chapter 10 for a description of the pharmacology of this class of drugs.

Non-selective α-adrenergic receptor antagonists

Phentolamine

Phentolamine is a competitive non-selective α-adrenergic receptor blocker, with three times greater affinity for α_1- than α_2-adrenergic receptors. During anesthesia, phentolamine is used in the management of hypertensive crises due to excessive administration of sympathomimetics and pheochromocytoma, especially during tumor manipulation. In human dentistry, a preparation of phentolamine is available to reverse the effects of local anesthetic administration [102]. Vasodilation produced by α-adrenergic receptor blockade increases the systemic absorption of local anesthetics and therefore shortens the duration of sensory blockade. Phentolamine is also used in the management of pain associated with complex regional pain syndrome in people, although there are limited clinical data to support use in this context [103]. There are very limited published clinical data on the administration of phentolamine to companion animals. Phentolamine is available as a 10 mg/mL injectable preparation.

Blockade of postjunctional vascular α_1- and α_2-adrenergic receptors causes vasodilation and hypotension. Blockade of presynaptic α_2-adrenergic receptors facilitates norepinephrine release, leading to tachycardia and an increase in cardiac output. Pulmonary artery pressure is also reduced.

Phentolamine can cause an increase in insulin secretion, precipitating hypoglycemia; it is advisable to monitor blood glucose following administration. The drug is metabolized in the liver, with a short half-life following intravenous administration (approximately 20 min in people). There are no published data on the specific metabolic pathways of phentolamine in companion animals.

Phenoxybenzamine

Phenoxybenzamine is a long-acting, non-selective α-adrenergic receptor blocker, with greater affinity for α_1- than α_2-adrenergic receptors. Its effects are mediated by a reactive intermediate that forms a covalent bond and alkylates the α-adrenergic receptor, resulting in irreversible blockade. In addition to receptor blockade, phenoxybenzamine also inhibits neuronal and extraneuronal uptake of catecholamines.

In veterinary patients, phenoxybenzamine is most commonly used for the preoperative management of pheochromocytoma, administered orally. The aims of administration are to reverse chronic vasoconstriction due to increased circulating concentrations of epinephrine and norepinephrine that are produced by the tumor, and thereby facilitate expansion of intravascular volume. The long duration of action of oral phenoxybenzamine allows twice daily dosing.

In people, preoperative stabilization of patients with pheochromocytoma with oral phenoxybenzamine significantly decreases mortality rates in the perioperative period [104]. Phenoxybenzamine is also used to control changes in heart rate and blood pressure during surgical tumor manipulation, where the irreversible nature of the adrenergic blockade results in greater efficacy compared with shorter acting competitive blockers such as phentolamine.

A retrospective study in dogs with pheochromocytoma [105] also found preoperative administration of phenoxybenzamine for a median period of 20 days before adrenalectomy also decreased mortality compared with untreated controls. The long duration of action can result in persistent hypotension following tumor removal, however; therefore, some anesthetists elect to stop administration of phenoxybenzamine 48 h prior to surgery. Phenoxybenzamine may also be used in the management of functional urethral obstruction in dogs and cats, where more limited effects on blood pressure are advantageous compared with treatment with prazosin [106]. Phenoxybenzamine is available as an oral and injectable preparation.

The cardiovascular effects of phenoxybenzamine are similar to those of phentolamine. Phenoxybenzamine does not prevent arrhythmias from occurring during adrenalectomy for pheochromocytoma removal as a result of tumor manipulation. In people, concurrent β-adrenergic blockade is sometimes instituted to control arrhythmias and reduce tachycardias resulting from β-adrenergic receptor stimulation [107]. The requirement for concurrent β-blockade depends on the tumor type and associated hormone secretion. In dogs with pheochromocytoma, oral doses of approximately 0.6 mg/kg every 12 h reduced mortality in the perioperative period [105]. Doses of 0.5 mg/kg twice daily have been recommended in cats.

A reduction in central nervous system sympathetic outflow as a result of adrenergic blockade can cause mild sedation in treated animals, although this is not normally of sufficient magnitude to cause clinically relevant effects.

Phenoxybenzamine is incompletely and variably absorbed from the gut of people, with an oral bioavailability of about 25%. It is reasonable to assume that this is also the case in monogastric animals. The drug is extensively metabolized in the liver and excreted in urine and bile. Although the plasma half-life is 24 h in people, the duration of action can be up to 3 days, reflecting the biologic requirement of new α-adrenergic receptor synthesis for effects to wane and eventually terminate.

β_1-Adrenergic receptor antagonists

General properties of β-adrenergic receptor antagonists are presented in Table 9.2. β-Adrenergic receptor antagonists (commonly termed 'beta-blockers') are all competitive antagonists with varying degrees of selectivity for β_1- and β_2-adrenergic receptors. Some beta-blockers have intrinsic sympathomimetic activity (ISA), resulting in a partial agonist effect at β_1, β_2, or both types of adrenergic receptors. [108]. Membrane-stabilizing activity, similar to that of local anesthetics on the cardiac action potential, is also a feature of some β-adrenergic receptor antagonists, although concentrations greater than those achieved by therapeutic doses are usually required to elicit this effect.

The therapeutic usefulness of β-adrenergic receptor antagonists is mediated through their effect at β_1-adrenergic receptors, while concurrent effects at β_2-receptors are deemed undesirable. Atenolol and esmolol demonstrate β_1-adrenergic receptor selectivity, although at high doses antagonist effects at β_2-receptors also occur.

β-Adrenergic receptor antagonists that have ISA are able to stimulate these receptors and oppose the stimulating effects of catecholamines in a competitive way. Therefore, the balance between agonism and antagonism depends on the circulating level of catecholamines. Beta-blockers with ISA are partial agonists at β-adrenergic receptors and elicit a submaximal response at full receptor occupancy. The presence of ISA results in less resting bradycardia and a smaller reduction in cardiac output than are observed with beta-blockers without ISA [109]. In the long term, they may produce arterial vasodilation and increase arterial compliance,

Table 9.2 Comparison of receptor selectivity, intrinsic sympathomimetic activity, and membrane stabilizing activity of beta adrenergic receptor antagonists used in veterinary medicine.

Drug	β_1-Receptor Selectivity	Intrinsic Sympathomimetic Activity	Membrane-Stabilizing Activity
Atenolol	+	+	–
Esmolol	++	–	–
Metoprolol	++	–	+
Pindolol	–	++	+
Propranolol	–	–	++
Sotalol	–	–	–

which is postulated to be beneficial in the management of hypertension in humans [109].

In human medicine, β-adrenergic receptor antagonists are predominantly used in the treatment of hypertension, angina, and myocardial infarction. These drugs are also widely used in veterinary medicine, predominantly for the management of the hemodynamic and neuroendocrine consequences of cardiac disease, including the management of cardiac arrhythmias. Therefore, it is important to have a good understanding of the clinical pharmacology of β-adrenergic receptor antagonists in order to determine potential effects during anesthesia in animals receiving therapy. During anesthesia, beta-blockers are predominantly used in the management of inappropriate tachycardia, where the increased heart rate is having a negative effect on hemodynamic function. They are also used in the perioperative management of pheochromocytomas to prevent reflex tachycardia associated with α-adrenergic blockade therapy, and to control arrhythmias and tachycardias associated with β-adrenergic receptor stimulation due to hormone secretion from the tumor.

β-Adrenergic receptor antagonists decrease the heart rate by reducing automaticity in the sinoatrial node and prolonging the conduction time in the atrioventricular node. A reduction in heart rate lengthens diastole and therefore can improve coronary perfusion and increase regional myocardial oxygen delivery. They are class II antiarrhythmic agents and are mainly used to treat arrhythmias associated with high circulating levels of catecholamines. At the same time, they have a negative inotropic effect, which decreases oxygen demand, thereby collectively improving the balance between myocardial oxygen supply and demand. Potential negative effects on cardiovascular function are a prolonged systolic ejection time, dilation of ventricles, and an increase in coronary vascular resistance due to the antagonism of coronary vasodilatory β_2-adrenergic receptors. In human patients with poor left ventricular function, β-blockade is recognized to be a risk factor for the development of cardiac failure [110].

Beta-blockers control blood pressure [111] predominantly through a reduction in heart rate and cardiac output and also via inhibition of the renin–angiotensin system due to blockade of β_1-adrenergic receptors at the juxtaglomerular apparatus. A reduction in circulating angiotensin II will ameliorate vasoconstriction that also drives the secretion of aldosterone. However, when β-adrenergic blockers are administered acutely during anesthesia, the reductions in cardiac output and heart rate are the primary mechanisms responsible for decreased blood pressure.

High doses of all beta-blockers, irrespective of selectivity for β_1-adrenergic receptors at clinical dose rates, will precipitate bronchospasm via blockade of β_2-adrenergic receptors in bronchioles, opposing tonic sympathetically mediated bronchodilation [112].

The metabolic effects of beta-blockers are complex owing to the multiple pathways and organs involved in the regulation of blood glucose concentration. However, beta-blockers can lead both to an increase in blood glucose concentration (through peripheral insulin resistance and decreased insulin secretion from pancreatic cells) and to a decrease in blood glucose concentration (by mitigating the normal increase that occurs during exercise). They can also have complex effects on lipid metabolism, resulting in increased plasma triglycerides [113].

Atenolol

Atenolol is a relatively cardioselective (i.e., β_1) adrenergic receptor antagonist that is available as tablet and syrup formulations for oral administration, and as an injectable preparation (0.5 mg/mL) for intravenous use. Although it is not widely administered during anesthesia, atenolol is prescribed to delay the onset of adverse sequelae in cats with hypertrophic cardiomyopathy and for the management of ventricular arrhythmias in cats and dogs; therefore, knowledge of atenolol pharmacology is important. It is worth noting that in human medicine, continuation of β-adrenergic blocker therapy is generally recommended in the perioperative period for patients with cardiac disease [114,115].

In cats, atenolol is well absorbed orally, with recommended clinical doses producing plasma concentrations that are within the therapeutic range within 1 h of oral administration, with effects that persist for up to 12 h, allowing twice daily dosing [116]. Twice daily dosing with atenolol, orally, is also recommended in dogs [117]. In people, atenolol is excreted unchanged in the urine, and effects are therefore more prolonged in patients with renal impairment; whether this is also the case in small animals is unknown.

Esmolol

Esmolol is highly selective for the β_1-adrenergic receptor and is very lipophilic, with a rapid onset and offset of action when given intravenously; therefore, it is the beta-blocker of choice for use during anesthesia to control tachycardia, hypertension, and acute supraventricular tachycardia associated with inappropriate sympathetic nervous system activity. It is commonly given by infusion, using a controlled infusion apparatus in order to prevent overdose. In dogs and cats, a bolus dose of 2 μg/kg followed by an infusion of 50 μg/kg/min is generally recommended to decrease heart rate and systolic function [118,119]. Esmolol is rapidly metabolized by red blood cell esterases to an essentially inactive metabolite with a long half-life and methanol. It has no intrinsic sympathomimetic activity or membrane-stabilizing properties.

Metoprolol

Metoprolol is also relatively selective for the β_1-adrenergic receptor and has no intrinsic sympathomimetic activity. It is available as an oral tablet preparation and has been evaluated in the management of dogs with acquired cardiac disease [120]. Metoprolol is rapidly absorbed from the gut but undergoes very high first-pass metabolism, giving an oral bioavailability of approximately 50% across species [121,122]. The half-life of metoprolol is approximately 2 h in dogs [123], with twice daily dosing generally recommended. In humans, rats, dogs, and horses, metabolism is via oxidative pathways, with metoprolol and its metabolites excreted mainly in urine in an unconjugated form [122].

Non-selective β-adrenergic receptor antagonists

Pindolol

Pindolol is a non-selective β-adrenergic antagonist with intrinsic sympathomimetic and membrane-stabilizing properties that is also a serotonin receptor (5-HT1A/1B) antagonist [124]. In addition to the typical cardiovascular effects of the drug, pindolol may potentiate analgesia provided by tramadol in dogs [125], presumably due to augmentation of serotonergic effects of tramadol by activation of the serotonergic modulatory system.

Propranolol

Propranolol is a non-selective β-adrenergic antagonist without intrinsic sympathomimetic activity. It is available as a racemic mixture, although the *S*-isomer confers most of the therapeutic cardiac effects of the drug. The *R*-isomer prevents the peripheral conversion of thyroxine (T4) to triiodothyronine (T3) in people, although whether this effect is also present in animal species has not yet been determined. Propranolol is available as injectable and oral preparations; in animals it is most commonly administered orally for the control of heart rate and hypertension prior to thyroidectomy in cats with hyperthyroidism, or as part of the presurgical management of animals with pheochromocytoma. Use of propranolol during anesthesia has been largely superseded by the availability of esmolol, which has greater selectivity for the β_1-adrenergic receptor. Propranolol is well absorbed through the gut, but has a very high first-pass hepatic metabolism in humans, dogs, rats, and cats [126,127]. The major metabolic pathways for propranolol also occur in the liver [127]. It is noteworthy that the metabolism of oral propranolol is prolonged in hyperthyroid compared with euthyroid cats [128], necessitating dosing adjustments.

Sotalol

Sotalol, in addition to being a non-selective β-adrenergic antagonist without intrinsic sympathomimetic activity, is a class III antiarrhythmic and has potassium channel-blocking effects. It is most commonly used orally to treat ventricular tachyarrhythmias and has been shown to reduce the number of ventricular premature contractions in Boxer dogs with familial ventricular arrhythmias [117]. It is well absorbed from the gut when administered orally and is excreted largely unchanged in the urine; therefore, renal impairment will significantly reduce clearance. In dogs, the plasma half-life is approximately 4 h [129].

References

1 Pascoe PJ, Ilkiw JE, Pypendop BH. Effects of increasing infusion rates of dopamine, dobutamine, epinephrine, and phenylephrine in healthy anesthetized cats. *Am J Vet Res* 2006; **67**: 1491–1499.

2 Grassi-Kassisse DM, Faro R, Withrington PG, *et al.* Characterisation of functional endothelin receptors in the canine isolated perfused spleen. *Eur J Pharmacol* 1995; **282**: 57–63.

3 Igić R. Mechanism of epinephrine-induced dysrhythmias in rat involves local cholinergic activation. *Can J Physiol Pharmacol* 1996; **74**: 85–88.

4 Maze M, Smith CM. Identification of receptor mechanism mediating epinephrine-induced arrhythmias during halothane anesthesia in the dog. *Anesthesiology* 1983; **59**: 322–326.

5 Katz RL, Bigger JT Jr. Cardiac arrhythmias during anesthesia and operation. *Anesthesiology* 1970; **33**: 193–213.

6 Black GW, Clarke RS, Howard PJ, McCullough H. The cardiovascular effects of teflurane in the cat. *Br J Anaesth* 1969; **41**: 288–296.

7 Lees P, Tavernor WD. Influence of halothane and catecholamines on heart rate and rhythm in the horse. *Br J Pharmacol* 1970; **39**: 149–159.

8 Tranquilli WJ, Thurmon JC, Benson GJ. Halothane-catecholamine arrhythmias in swine (*Sus scrofa*). *Am J Vet Res* 1986; **47**: 2134–2137.

9 Hikasa Y, Okabe C, Takase K, Ogasawara S. Ventricular arrhythmogenic dose of adrenaline during sevoflurane, isoflurane, and halothane anaesthesia either with or without ketamine or thiopentone in cats. *Res Vet Sci* 1996; **60**: 134–137.

10 Pettifer G, Dyson D, McDonell W. The arrhythmogenic dose of epinephrine in halothane and isoflurane anesthetized dogs: an assessment of repeatability. *Can J Vet Res* 1997; **61**: 221–226.

11 Gaynor JS, Bednarski RM, Muir WW III. Effect of xylazine on the arrhythmogenic dose of epinephrine in thiamylal/halothane-anesthetized horses. *Am J Vet Res* 1992; **53**: 2350–2354.

12 Bednarski RM, Majors LJ. Ketamine and the arrhythmogenic dose of epinephrine in cats anesthetized with halothane and isoflurane. *Am J Vet Res* 1986; **47**: 2122–2125.

13 Bednarski RM, Sams RA, Majors LJ, Ashcraft S. Reduction of the ventricular arrhythmogenic dose of epinephrine by ketamine administration in halothane-anesthetized cats. *Am J Vet Res* 1988; **49**: 350–354.

14 Niiya S. The effect of ketamine on epinephrine-induced arrhythmias in dogs anesthetized with halothane-nitrous oxide, *Masui* 1990; **39**: 1652–1659.

15 Kaye AD, Hoover JM, Baber SR, *et al.* Effects of norepinephrine on alpha-subtype receptors in the feline pulmonary vascular bed. *Crit Care Med* 2004; **32**: 2300–2303.

16 Miller RD, Way WL, Eger EI II. The effects of alpha-methyldopa, reserpine, guanethidine, and iproniazid on minimum alveolar anesthetic requirement (MAC). *Anesthesiology* 1968; **29**: 1153–1158.

17 Steffey EP, Eger EI. The effect of seven vasopressors of halothane MAC in dogs. *Br J Anaesth* 1975; **47**: 435–438.

18 Johnson MD. Circulating epinephrine stimulates renin secretion in anesthetized dogs by activation of extrarenal adrenoceptors. *Am J Physiol* 1984; **246**: F676–F684.

19 Johnson MD, Whitener CJ, Sears TS. Epinephrine-induced renin secretion is not initiated by cardiac adrenoceptors. *Am J Physiol* 1988; **254**: E265–E271.

20 Laks M, Callis G, Swan HJ. Hemodynamic effects of low doses of norepinephrine in the conscious dog. *Am J Physiol* 1971; **220**: 171–173.

21 Melchior JC, Pinaud M, Blanloeil Y, *et al.* Hemodynamic effects of continuous norepinephrine infusion in dogs with and without hyperkinetic endotoxic shock. *Crit Care Med* 1987; **15**: 687–691.

22 Valverde A, Giguère S, Sanchez LC, *et al.* Effects of dobutamine, norepinephrine, and vasopressin on cardiovascular function in anesthetized neonatal foals with induced hypotension. *Am J Vet Res* 2006; **67**: 1730–1737.

23 Vincent CJ, Hawley AT, Rozanski EA, *et al.* Cardiopulmonary effects of dobutamine and norepinephrine infusion in healthy anesthetized alpacas. *Am J Vet Res* 2009; **70**: 1236–1242.

24 Bakker J, Vincent JL. Effects of norepinephrine and dobutamine on oxygen transport and consumption in a dog model of endotoxic shock. *Crit Care Med* 1993; **21**: 425–432.

25 Gillis CN, Pitt BR. The fate of circulating amines within the pulmonary circulation. *Annu Rev Physiol* 1982; **44**: 269–281.

26 Rosati M, Dyson DH, Sinclair MD, Sears WC. Response of hypotensive dogs to dopamine hydrochloride and dobutamine hydrochloride during deep isoflurane anesthesia. *Am J Vet Res* 2007; **68**: 483–494.

27 Brooks HL, Stein PD, Matson JL, Hyland JW. Dopamine-induced alterations in coronary hemodynamics in dogs. *Circ Res* 1969; **24**: 699–704.

28 Scott A, Chakrabarti MK, Hall GM. Oxygen transport during dopamine infusion in dogs. *Br J Anaesth* 1979; **51**: 1011–1019.

29 Dyson DH, Sinclair MD. Impact of dopamine or dobutamine infusions on cardiovascular variables after rapid blood loss and volume replacement during isoflurane-induced anesthesia in dogs. *Am J Vet Res* 2006; **67**: 1121–1130.

30 Chen HC, Sinclair MD, Dyson DH. Use of ephedrine and dopamine in dogs for the management of hypotension in routine clinical cases under isoflurane anesthesia. *Vet Anaesth Analg* 2007; **34**: 301–311.

31 Wiese AJ, Barter LS, Ilkiw JE, *et al.* Cardiovascular and respiratory effects of incremental doses of dopamine and phenylephrine in the management of isoflurane-induced hypotension in cats with hypertrophic cardiomyopathy. *Am J Vet Res* 2012; **73**: 908–916.

32 Swanson CR, Muir WW III, Bednarski RM, *et al.* Hemodynamic responses in halothane-anesthetized horses given infusions of dopamine or dobutamine. *Am J Vet Res* 1985; **46**: 365–370.

33 Trim CM, Moore JN, White NA. Cardiopulmonary effects of dopamine hydrochloride in anaesthetised horses. *Equine Vet J* 1985; **17**: 41–44.

34 Robertson SA, Malark JA, Steele CJ, Chen CL. Metabolic, hormonal, and hemodynamic changes during dopamine infusions in halothane anesthetized horses. *Vet Surg* 1996; **25**: 88–97.

35 Young LE, Blissitt KJ, Clutton RE, Molony V. Haemodynamic effects of a sixty minute infusion of dopamine hydrochloride in horses anaesthetised with halothane. *Equine Vet J* 1998; **30**: 310–316.

36 Lee YH, Clarke KW, Alibhai HI, Song D. Effects of dopamine, dobutamine, dopexamine, phenylephrine, and saline solution on intramuscular blood flow and other cardiopulmonary variables in halothane-anesthetized ponies. *Am J Vet Res* 1998; **59**: 1463–1472.

37 Lokhandwala MF, Jandhyala BS. The role of sympathetic nervous system in the vascular actions of dopamine. *J Pharmacol Exp Ther* 1979; **210**: 120–126.

38 Tatsumi K, Pickett CK, Weil JV. Decreased carotid body hypoxic sensitivity in chronic hypoxia: role of dopamine. *Respir Physiol* 1995; **101**: 47–57.

39 McNay JL, Mcdonald RH Jr, Goldberg LI. Direct renal vasodilatation produced by dopamine in the dog. *Circ Res* 1965; **16**: 510–517.

40 MacCannell KL, McNay JL, Meyer MB, Goldberg LL. Dopamine in the treatment of hypotension and shock. *N Engl J Med* 1966; **275**: 1389–1398.

41 Karthik S, Lisbon A. Low-dose dopamine in the intensive care unit. *Semin Dial* 2006; **19**: 465–471.

42 Clark KL, Robertson MJ, Drew GM. Do renal tubular dopamine receptors mediate dopamine-induced diuresis in the anesthetized cat? *J Cardiovasc Pharmacol* 1991; **17**: 267–276.

43 Furukawa S, Nagashima Y, Hoshi K, *et al.* Effects of dopamine infusion on cardiac and renal blood flows in dogs. *J Vet Med Sci* 2002; **64**: 41–44.

44 Takemoto F, Cohen HT, Satoh T, Katz AI. Dopamine inhibits Na/K-ATPase in single tubules and cultured cells from distal nephron. *Pflugers Arch* 1992; **421**: 302–306.

45 Clark BJ, Menninger K. Peripheral dopamine receptors. *Circ Res* 1980; **46**: I59–I63.

46 Voelckel WG, Lindner KH, Wenzel V, Bonatti JO, *et al.*. Effect of small-dose dopamine on mesenteric blood flow and renal function in a pig model of cardiopulmonary resuscitation with vasopressin. *Anesth Analg* 1999; **89**: 1430–1436.

47 Raisis AL, Young LE, Blissitt KJ, *et al.* Effect of a 30-minute infusion of dobutamine hydrochloride on hind limb blood flow and hemodynamics in halothane-anesthetized horses. *Am J Vet Res* 2000; **61**: 1282–1288.

48 Hellyer PW, Wagner AE, Mama KR, Gaynor JS. The effects of dobutamine and ephedrine on packed cell volume, total protein, heart rate, and blood pressure in anaesthetized horses. *J Vet Pharmacol Ther* 1998; **21**: 497–499.

49 Renton MC, Snowden CP. Dopexamine and its role in the protection of hepatosplanchnic and renal perfusion in high-risk surgical and critically ill patients. *Br J Anaesth* 2005; **94**: 459–467.

50 Muir WW III. Inotropic mechanisms of dopexamine hydrochloride in horses. *Am J Vet Res* 1992; **53**: 1343–1346.

51 Muir WW III. Cardiovascular effects of dopexamine HCl in conscious and halothane-anaesthetised horses. *Equine Vet J Suppl* 1992; **(11)**: 24–29.

52 Young LE, Blissitt KJ, Clutton RE, Molony V. Temporal effects of an infusion of dopexamine hydrochloride in horses anesthetized with halothane. *Am J Vet Res* 1997; **58**: 516–523.

53 Einstein R, Abdul-Hussein N, Wong TW, *et al.* Cardiovascular actions of dopexamine in anaesthetized and conscious dogs. *Br J Pharmacol* 1994; **111**: 199–204.

54 Scheeren TW, Arndt JO. Different response of oxygen consumption and cardiac output to various endogenous and synthetic catecholamines in awake dogs. *Crit Care Med* 2008; **28**: 3861–3868.

55 Neustein SM, Dimich I, Sampson I, *et al.* Arrhythmogenic potential of dopexamine hydrochloride during halothane anaesthesia in dogs. *Can J Anaesth* 1994; **41**: 542–546.

56 Asfar P, De Backer D, Meier-Hellmann A, *et al.* Clinical review: influence of vasoactive and other therapies on intestinal and hepatic circulations in patients with septic shock. *Crit Care* 2004; **8**: 170–179.

57 Gray PA, Jones T, Park GR. Blood concentrations of dopexamine in patients during and after orthotopic liver transplantation. *Br J Clin Pharmacol* 1994; **37**: 89–92.

58 Tobias JD. Caudal epidural block: a review of test dosing and recognition of systemic injection in children. *Anesth Analg* 2001; **93**: 1156–1161.

59 Crystal GJ, Salem MR. Beta-adrenergic stimulation restores oxygen extraction reserve during acute normovolemic hemodilution. *Anesth Analg* 2002; **95**: 851–857.

60 Sandusky GE, Means JR, Todd GC. Comparative cardiovascular toxicity in dogs given inotropic agents by continuous intravenous infusion. *Toxicol Pathol* 1990; **18**: 268–278.

61 Volders PG, Kulcśar A, Vos MA, *et al.* Similarities between early and delayed afterdepolarizations induced by isoproterenol in canine ventricular myocytes. *Cardiovasc Res* 1997; **34**: 348–359.

62 O'Neill DK, Aizer A, Linton P, *et al.* Isoproterenol infusion increases level of consciousness during catheter ablation of atrial fibrillation. *J Interv Card Electrophysiol* 2012; **34**: 137–142.

63 Zhang H, De Jongh R, De Backer D, *et al.* Effects of alpha - and beta-adrenergic stimulation on hepatosplanchnic perfusion and oxygen extraction in endotoxic shock. *Crit Care Med* 2001; **29**: 581–588.

64 Szefler SJ, Acara M. Isoproterenol excretion and metabolism in the isolated perfused rat kidney. *J Pharmacol Exp Ther* 1979; **210**: 295–300.

65 Linton RA, Young LE, Marlin DJ, *et al.* Cardiac output measured by lithium dilution, thermodilution, and transesophageal Doppler echocardiography in anesthetized horses. *Am J Vet Res* 2000; **61**: 731–737.

66 Frederick J, Giguère S, Butterworth K, *et al.* Severe phenylephrine-associated hemorrhage in five aged horses. *J Am Vet Med Assoc* 2010; **237**: 830–834.

67 Robinson JL. Effect of vasopressin and phenylephrine on arterial pressure and heart rate in conscious dogs. *Am J Physiol* 1986; **251**: H253–H260.

68 Ludders JW, Reitan JA, Martucci R, *et al.* Blood pressure response to phenylephrine infusion in halothane-anesthetized dogs given acetylpromazine maleate. *Am J Vet Res* 1983; **44**: 996–999.

69 Richardson PD, Withrington PG. The role of beta-adrenoceptors in the responses of the hepatic arterial vascular bed of the dog to phenylephrine, isoproterenol, noradrenaline and adrenaline. *Br J Pharmacol* 1977; **60**: 239–249.

70 Strandhoy JW, Wolff DW, Buckalew VM Jr. Renal alpha 1- and alpha 2-adrenoceptor mediated vasoconstriction in dogs. *J Hypertens Suppl* 1984; **2**: S151–S153.

71 Erkinaro T, Mäkikallio K, Kavasmaa T, *et al.* Effects of ephedrine and phenylephrine on uterine and placental circulations and fetal outcome following fetal hypoxaemia and epidural-induced hypotension in a sheep model. *Br J Anaesth* 2004; **93**: 825–832.

72 Lukasik VM, Gleed RD, Scarlett JM, *et al.* Intranasal phenylephrine reduces post anesthetic upper airway obstruction in horses. *Equine Vet J* 1997; **29**: 236–238.

73 Herring IP, Jacobson JD, Pickett JP. Cardiovascular effects of topical ophthalmic 10% phenylephrine in dogs. *Vet Ophthalmol* 2004; **7**: 41–46.

74 Martin-Flores M, Mercure-McKenzie TM, Campoy L, *et al.* Controlled retrospective study of the effects of eyedrops containing phenylephrine hydrochloride and scopolamine hydrobromide on mean arterial blood pressure in anesthetized dogs. *Am J Vet Res* 2010; **71**: 1407–1412.

75 Dyson DH, Pascoe PJ. Influence of preinduction methoxamine, lactated Ringer solution, or hypertonic saline solution infusion or postinduction dobutamine infusion on anesthetic-induced hypotension in horses. *Am J Vet Res* 1990; **51**: 17–21.

76 Lee JC, Fripp RR, Downing SE. Myocardial responses to alpha-adrenoceptor stimulation with methoxamine hydrochloride in lambs. *Am J Physiol* 1982; **242**: H405–H410.

77 Brewster WR, Osgood PF, Isaacs JP, *et al.* Haemodynamic effects of a pressor amine (methoxamine) with predominant vasoconstrictor activity. *Circ Res* 1960; **8**: 980–988.

78 Imai S, Shigei T, Hashimoto K. Cardiac actions of methoxamine with special reference to its antagonistic action to epinephrine. *Circ Res* 1961; **9**: 552–560.

79 Canepa-Anson R, Dawson JR, Frankl WS, *et al.*. Beta 2 adrenoceptor agonists. Pharmacology, metabolic effects and arrhythmias. *Eur Heart J* 1982; (Suppl D): 129–134.

80 Gleed RD, Dobson A. Effect of clenbuterol on arterial oxygen tension in the anaesthetised horse. *Res Vet Sci* 1990; **48**: 331–337.

81 Keegan RD, Gleed RD, Sanders EA, *et al.* Treatment of low arterial oxygen tension in anesthetized horses with clenbuterol. *Vet Surg* 1991; **20**: 148–152.

82 Dodam JR, Moon RE, Olson NC, *et al.* Effects of clenbuterol hydrochloride on pulmonary gas exchange and hemodynamics in anesthetized horses. *Am J Vet Res* 1993; **54**: 776–782.

83 Robertson SA, Bailey JE. Aerosolized salbutamol (albuterol) improves PaO_2 in hypoxaemic anaesthetized horses - a prospective clinical trial in 81 horses. *Vet Anaesth Analg* 2002; **29**: 212–218.

84 Patschova M, Kabes R, Krisova S. The effects of inhalation salbutamol administration on systemic and pulmonary hemodynamic, pulmonary mechanics and oxygen balance during general anaesthesia in the horse. *Vet Med (Czech)* 2010; **55**: 445–456.

85 Kirschvink N, Leemans J, Delvaux F, *et al.* Bronchodilators in bronchoscopy-induced airflow limitation in allergen-sensitized cats. *J Vet Intern Med* 2005; **19**: 161–167.

86 Leemans J, Kirschvink N, Clercx C, *et al.* Functional response to inhaled salbutamol and/or ipratropium bromide in Ascaris suum-sensitised cats with allergen-induced bronchospasms. *Vet J* 2010; **186**: 76–83.

87 Leemans J, Kirschvink N, Bernaerts F, *et al.* Salmeterol or doxycycline do not inhibit acute bronchospasm and airway inflammation in cats with experimentally-induced asthma. *Vet J* 2012; **192**: 49–56.

88 Padrid P, Church DB. Drugs used in the management of respiratory diseases. In: Maddison J, Page SW, Church D, eds. *Small Animal Clinical Pharmacology*, 2nd edn. Edinburgh: Saunders Elsevier, 2008: 458–468.

89 Takasaki K, Urabe M, Yamamoto R. Tachyphylaxis of indirectly acting sympathomimetic amines. II. Recovery of tyramine tachyphylaxis and crossed tachyphylaxis between tyramine and other indirectly acting sympathomimetic amines in dogs. *Kurume Med J* 1972; **19**: 11–22.

90 Patil PN, Tye A, Lapidus JB. A pharmacological study of the ephedrine isomers. *J Pharmacol Exp Ther* 1965; **148**: 158–168.

91 Young R, Glennon RA. Discriminative stimulus properties of (–)-ephedrine. *Pharmacol Biochem Behav* 1998; **60**: 771–775.

92 Grandy JL, Hodgson DS, Dunlop CI, *et al.* Cardiopulmonary effects of ephedrine in halothane-anesthetized horses. *J Vet Pharmacol Ther* 1989; **12**: 389–396.

93 Wagner AE, Dunlop CI, Chapman PL. Effects of ephedrine on cardiovascular function and oxygen delivery in isoflurane-anesthetized dogs. *Am J Vet Res* 1993; **54**: 1917–1922.

94 Davies BN, Withrington PG. The actions of drugs on the smooth muscle of the capsule and blood vessels of the spleen. *Pharmacol Rev* 1973; **25**: 373–413.

95 Egger C, McCrackin MA, Hofmeister E, *et al.* Efficacy of preanesthetic intramuscular administration of ephedrine for prevention of anesthesia-induced hypotension in cats and dogs. *Can Vet J* 2009; **50**: 179–184.

96 Amorin RB, Braz JR, Castiglia YM, *et al.* Effects of ephedrine on cardiovascular and renal function of dogs anesthetized with sodium pentobarbital. *Rev Bras Anestesiol* 2002; **52**: 434–445.

97 Axelrod J. Studies on sympathomimetic amines I. The biotransformation and physiological disposition of *l*-ephedrine and *l*-norephedrine. *J Pharm Exp Ther* 1953; **109**: 62–73.

98 Nicholson JD. The metabolism of *l*-ephedrine in ponies. *Arch Int Pharmacodyn Ther* 1970; **188**: 375–386.

99 Ramage AG. The effect of prazosin, indoramin and phentolamine on sympathetic nerve activity. *Eur J Pharmacol* 1984; **106**: 507–513.

100 Rubin P, Yee YG, Anderson M, Blaschke T. Prazosin first-pass metabolism and hepatic extraction in the dog. *J Cardiovasc Pharmacol* 1979; **1**: 641–647.

101 Erve JC, Vashishtha SC, DeMaio W, Talaat RE. Metabolism of prazosin in rat, dog, and human liver microsomes and cryopreserved rat and human hepatocytes and characterization of metabolites by liquid chromatography/tandem mass spectrometry. *Drug Metab Dispos* 2007; **35**: 908–916.
102 Becker DE, Reed KL. Local anesthetics: review of pharmacological considerations. *Anesth Prog* 2012; **59**: 90–101.
103 Rowbotham MC. Pharmacologic management of complex regional pain syndrome. *Clin J Pain* 2006; **22**: 425–429.
104 Russell WJ, Metcalfe IR, Tonkin AL, Frewin DB. The preoperative management of phaeochromocytoma. *Anaesth Intensive Care* 1998; **26**: 196–200.
105 Herrera MA, Mehl ML, Kass PH, *et al.* Predictive factors and the effect of phenoxybenzamine on outcome in dogs undergoing adrenalectomy for pheochromocytoma. *J Vet Intern Med* 2008; **22**: 1333–1339.
106 Fischer JR, Lane IF, Cribb AE. Urethral pressure profile and hemodynamic effects of phenoxybenzamine and prazosin in non-sedated male beagle dogs. *Can J Vet Res* 2003; **67**: 30–38.
107 Myklejord DJ. Undiagnosed pheochromocytoma: the anesthesiologist nightmare. *Clin Med Res* 2004; **2**: 59–62.
108 Frishman WH, Saunders E. β-Adrenergic blockers. *J Clin Hypertens* 2011; **13**: 649–653.
109 Jaillon P. Relevance of intrinsic sympathomimetic activity for beta blockers. *Am J Cardiol* 1990; **66**: 21C–23C.
110 Ventura HO, Kalapura T. Beta-blocker therapy and severe heart failure: myth or reality? *Congest Heart Fail* 2003; **9**: 197–202.
111 Wiysonge CS, Bradley HA, Volmink J, *et al.* Beta-blockers for hypertension. *Cochrane Database Syst Rev* 2012; (**11**): CD002003.
112 Foresi A, Cavigioli G, Signorelli G, *et al.* Is the use of beta-blockers in COPD still an unresolved dilemma? *Respiration* 2010; **80**: 177–187.
113 Fonseca VA. Effects of beta-blockers on glucose and lipid metabolism. *Curr Med Res Opin* 2010; **26**: 615–629.
114 Flynn BC, Vernick WJ, Ellis JE. β-Blockade in the perioperative management of the patient with cardiac disease undergoing non-cardiac surgery. *Br J Anaesth* 2011; **107**: 13–15.
115 Flier S, Buhre WF, van Klei WA. Cardioprotective effects of perioperative β-blockade in vascular surgery patients: fact or fiction? *Curr Opin Anaesthesiol* 2011; **24**: 104–110.
116 Khor KH, Campbell FE, Charles BG, *et al.* Comparative pharmacokinetics and pharmacodynamics of tablet, suspension and paste formulations of atenolol in cats. *J Vet Pharmacol Ther* 2012; **35**: 437–445.
117 Meurs KM, Spier AW, Wright NA, *et al.* Comparison of the effects of four antiarrhythmic treatments for familial ventricular arrhythmias in Boxers. *J Am Vet Med Assoc* 2002; **221**: 522–527.
118 Quon CY, Gorczynski RJ. Pharmacodynamics and onset of action of esmolol in anesthetized dogs. *J Pharmacol Exp Ther* 1986; **237**: 912–918.
119 Schober KE, Fuentes VL, Bonagura JD. Comparison between invasive hemodynamic measurements and noninvasive assessment of left ventricular diastolic function by use of Doppler echocardiography in healthy anesthetized cats. *Am J Vet Res* 2003; **64**: 93–103.
120 Rush JE, Freeman LM, Hiler C, Brown DJ. Use of metoprolol in dogs with acquired cardiac disease. *J Vet Cardiol* 2002; **4**: 23–28.
121 Fang J, Semple HA, Song J. Determination of metoprolol and its four metabolites in dog plasma. *J Chromatogr B* 2004; **809**: 9–14.
122 Dumasia MC. In vivo biotransformation of metoprolol in the horse and on-column esterification of the aminocarboxylic acid metabolite by alcohols during solid phase extraction using mixed mode columns. *J Pharm Biomed Anal* 2006; **40**: 75–81.
123 Regårdh CG, Ek L, Hoffmann KJ. Plasma levels and beta-blocking effect of alpha-hydroxymetoprolol – metabolite of metoprolol – in the dog. *J Pharmacokinet Biopharm* 1979; **7**: 471–479.
124 Romero L, Bel N, Artigas F, *et al.* Effect of pindolol on the function of pre- and postsynaptic 5-HT1A receptors: in vivo microdialysis and electrophysiological studies in the rat brain. *Neuropsychopharmacology* 1996; **15**: 349–360.
125 Kongara K, Chambers P, Johnson CB. Glomerular filtration rate after tramadol, parecoxib and pindolol following anaesthesia and analgesia in comparison with morphine in dogs. *Vet Anaesth Analg* 2009; **36**: 86–94.
126 Mills PC, Siebert GA, Roberts MS. A model to study intestinal and hepatic metabolism of propranolol in the dog. *J Vet Pharmacol Ther* 2004; **27**: 45–48.
127 Baughman TM, Talarico CL, Soglia JR. Evaluation of the metabolism of propranolol by linear ion trap technology in mouse, rat, dog, monkey, and human cryopreserved hepatocytes. *Rapid Commun Mass Spectrom* 2009; **23**: 2146–2150.
128 Jacobs G, Whittem T, Sams R, *et al.* Pharmacokinetics of propranolol in healthy cats during euthyroid and hyperthyroid states. *Am J Vet Res* 1997; **58**: 398–403.
129 Ishizaki T, Tawara K. Relationship between pharmacokinetics and pharmacodynamics of the beta adrenergic blocking drug sotalol in dogs. *J Pharmacol Exp Ther* 1979; **211**: 331–337.

10 Sedatives and Tranquilizers

David C. Rankin
Department of Clinical Sciences, Kansas State University, Manhattan, Kansas, USA

Chapter contents

Introduction

Sedatives and tranquilizers play an important role in day-to-day veterinary practice. The use of these medications as part of an anesthetic regimen has many advantages, including, but not limited to, calming the patient, facilitating intravenous catheterization, analgesia, reduced sympathetic responses to surgical stimulation, reduced anesthetic requirements, and promoting smooth induction and recovery. The selection of drugs should be individualized to the patient. Age, patient temperament, pathologic processes, blood volume status, and so on should be considered when selecting drugs and doses.

The distinction between a tranquilizer and sedative is often nebulous due to species and dosing differences. For example, α_2-adrenergic receptor agonists are effective in both horses and cattle, but cattle may require one-tenth the horse dose to achieve the same level of sedation. Phenothiazines are efficacious in dogs and horses but not so in swine. These distinctions are discussed in this chapter and in chapters pertaining to techniques in different species.

In general, a tranquilizer induces a feeling of calm (anxiolysis). Sedatives, while reducing anxiety, also reduce overall response to external stimuli. Analgesia is a feature of some sedatives but certainly not all. Clinical practice demonstrates that different species can vary widely in their response to a class of medication. Individuals within a species may also display varying effects of a medication. Terminology will vary in different sources; in this chapter, all the medications are termed sedatives, knowing that effects will vary with species and dose.

There are a variety of classes of sedatives currently used in veterinary medicine. Phenothiazines, benzodiazepines, α_2-adrenergic receptor agonists, butyrophenones, and opioids are frequently used to produce a state of calming, sedation, and possibly analgesia depending on the medications used.

Phenothiazines

Background

Phenothiazines are commonly used by themselves as sedatives, or in combinations as premedication prior to anesthesia. In humans, drugs of this class are used for antipsychotic and antiemetic effects. At clinically relevant doses, they inhibit conditioned avoidance behaviors with a reduction in spontaneous motor activity [1]. Extrapyramidal side-effects have been noted, typically with long-term use in humans or overdose in veterinary patients (tremor, coma/catalepsy, and rigidity). They exhibit activity at a wide variety of receptors, including adrenergic, muscarinic, dopaminergic, serotonergic, and histamine receptors.

The sedative effects of the phenothiazines are mediated primarily by blockade of dopamine receptors, specifically D2 receptors. This pre- and postsynaptic G-protein coupled receptor blockade leads to a decrease in cAMP and adenylate cyclase activity, calcium conductance, and alterations in postsynaptic potassium conductance. Blockade of α_1-adrenergic, muscarinic, and histamine (H1) receptors may also play a role in sedation. α_1-Adrenergic receptor antagonism mediates the decrease in blood pressure noted with this group of medications, and may play a role in the decrease in thermoregulatory control (tendency towards poikilothermia) along with serotonin blockade.

Veterinary Anesthesia and Analgesia: The Fifth Edition of Lumb and Jones.
Edited by Kurt A. Grimm, Leigh A. Lamont, William J. Tranquilli, Stephen A. Greene and Sheilah A. Robertson.

Acepromazine

Acepromazine is one of the most widely used sedatives in veterinary practice. It is labeled for use in small and large animals in many countries. It is generally reliable as a sedative when given parentally, and often at doses lower than the label dose. Muscle relaxation is a hallmark of this sedation. Acepromazine has no analgesic properties by itself, and it is frequently given in combination with opioids to produce neuroleptanalgesia, a state characterized by sedation and analgesia. Decreased systemic vascular resistance and blood pressure are the main adverse effects of acepromazine usage.

The hemodynamic impact of acepromazine is highly variable, but can be significant in some individuals. Stroke volume, cardiac output, and arterial blood pressure has been shown to decrease by 20–30% in conscious dogs administered 0.1 mg/kg IV [2,3]. Conscious horses administered 0.1 mg/kg IV showed a 20–30% decrease in mean aortic pressure and a 10–15% decrease in cardiac output [4]. Mean arterial pressure measured at the tail (not corrected for height) was significantly reduced in standing horses receiving 0.1 mg/kg acepromazine [5]. Standing horses receiving 0.04 mg/kg acepromazine IV had lower facial artery pressures but no real change in digital palmar arterial flow compared with saline-treated horses [6].

Blood pressure can also be reduced in anesthetized dogs and horses. Dogs anesthetized with halothane receiving acepromazine at 0.05, 0.125, and 0.25 mg/kg IV displayed reductions in mean arterial pressure of 2.3, 9.4, and 16.8%, respectively [7]. Anesthetized horses receiving IV acepromazine at 0.03 mg/kg showed a decrease in mean arterial blood pressure of up to 25% [8]. Clearly, once anesthetized, dogs and horses (and likely other mammals) receiving acepromazine can have significant changes in hemodynamics. Clinical experience suggests that mammals premedicated with low, clinically applicable doses of acepromazine rarely display such dramatic decreases in blood pressure. That said, it is important that monitoring blood pressure be part of the clinical delivery of anesthesia. Heart rate is typically not affected, and when it is it may rise to compensate for decreased systemic vascular resistance and blood pressure [2,4]. Premedication with acepromazine will increase the dose of epinephrine required to induce a ventricular arrhythmia, likely due to α-adrenergic receptor blockade [9–11].

Acepromazine administration has little effect on pulmonary function. Respiratory rates often decrease but blood gases and pH are not typically affected because tidal volume is increased to maintain adequate minute ventilation [4,12]. Acepromazine has been shown to have no impact on respiratory rate and blood gases in halothane-anesthetized horses [8].

Acepromazine administration has a significant dose-dependent impact on inhalant anesthetic requirements. In dogs, acepromazine at 0.2 mg/kg reduced halothane requirement by 28% and isoflurane requirement by 48% [13]. In another study of dogs anesthetized with halothane, IM administration of acepromazine at 0.02 and 0.2 mg/kg reduced the minimum alveolar concentration (MAC) by 34 and 44%, respectively [14]. Ponies receiving 0.05 mg/kg acepromazine IV reduced halothane MAC by 37% [15]. This across-species MAC reduction of 28–48% dictates that patients receiving acepromazine be closely monitored during anesthetic events, with anesthetic administration appropriately adjusted.

Hematologic effects of acepromazine administration include decreased packed cell volume (PCV) and a reduction of platelet aggregation. Hematocrit is reduced in some dogs and horses by 20–30% shortly after acepromazine administration as a result of splenic engorgement after α_1-adrenergic receptor blockade [6,16–18]. This effect can last several hours. Platelet aggregation was shown by Barr *et al.* [19] to be affected transiently, but recent work by Conner *et al.* [20] demonstrated no impact on clot formation.

> **Box 10.1** Acepromazine and seizures?
>
> Acepromazine has long been associated with seizures. The association grew from a study looking at high-dose chlorpromazine altering EEG activity in epileptic dogs. Recent retrospective studies seem to indicate that acepromazine used in dogs with seizure disorders does not lead to a higher incidence of issues.

Acepromazine has antiemetic properties. Administration of acepromazine 15 min prior to a variety of opioids reduced the incidence of vomiting from 45 to 18%. Lower esophageal tone and gastric emptying are reduced with acepromazine in dogs [21–23]. Despite the changes, acepromazine with low-dose butorphanol was considered acceptable for restraint when performing upper gastrointestinal contrast studies in healthy dogs [23]. In horses, acepromazine administration is associated with similar effects on gastrointestinal motility [24,25].

Penile prolapse (priapism) in stallions has been associated with acepromazine administration [26,27]. A 2011 retrospective study by Driessen *et al.* showed that 2.4% of male horses developed penile prolapse lasting 1–4 h [27]. One stallion in the review (0.02%) developed a prolapse lasting more than 12 h but less than 18 h. The incidence of permanent penile paralysis is apparently low but may be of catastrophic consequence in valuable breeding males. Glomerular filtration is maintained in dogs premedicated with acepromazine [28,29]. Acepromazine reduces urethral pressure in male cats anesthetized with halothane [30].

Clinical Application

Acepromazine is a reliable sedative in most dogs, cats, horses, and cattle. Dogs given 0.05 mg/kg acepromazine IV display mild to moderate sedation within 10 min [31]. Sedation scores in dogs receiving 0.02 mg/kg acepromazine IV are elevated out to 80 min compared with baseline [32]. Acepromazine is frequently used in horses as a tranquilizer prior to further sedation and induction of anesthesia for surgical or diagnostic procedures [17,27]. The duration of effect can be long, and no specific reversal agent exists for acepromazine.

Box 10.1 summarizes the association between acepromazine administration and seizures.

Benzodiazepines

Background

γ-Aminobutyric acid (GABA) is the primary inhibitory neurotransmitter in the central nervous system (CNS) [33]. Benzodiazepines exert their influence on the CNS by enhancing the $GABA_A$ receptor's affinity for GABA, resulting in increased chloride conductance and hyperpolarization of postsynaptic cell membranes [34]. The $GABA_A$ receptor is a pentameric combination of homologous subunits with a central pore, spanning the cell membrane. The receptor is frequently described in terms of its α subunit expression. The benzodiazepine binding site is usually located on the α_1, α_2, and γ subunits [35]. Barbiturates, ethanol, etomidate, and propofol also all have activity on $GABA_A$ receptors, and synergistic effects can result in significant CNS depression. Benzodiazepines enhance endogenous GABA binding to the receptor. The lack of direct agonist activity leads to a wide safety margin as far as CNS depression is concerned.

The response to benzodiazepines is multifactorial. The location of α_1 and α_2 subunits on the receptors, the location of the receptor in the CNS, the specific drug's affinity for the variety of subreceptors on the GABA receptor, lipid solubility, and overall pharmacokinetics all play a role in the clinical effect of a particular drug and dose.

All benzodiazepines share a common chemical structure, in which a benzene ring is linked to a seven-membered diazepine ring. They are classed as agonists, antagonists, and inverse agonists.

Agonists facilitate the activity of GABA. This results in sedation, anxiolysis, muscle relaxation, and anticonvulsant effects typically associated with these medications. Effects vary as discussed above. Diazepam and midazolam are the most commonly used parenterally administered benzodiazepines during veterinary anesthesia. Endogenous benzodiazepines ('endozepines') exist, but their synthetic pathways remain unelucidated [36–38]. Inverse agonists, when bound to the receptor site, produce an effect opposite to that of agonists. In the case of benzodiazepine receptor physiology, this results in seizures and anxiety (e.g., β-carboline alkaloids) [1]. Antagonists at benzodiazepine receptors have affinity for the receptor but little or no intrinsic activity. They block the effects of both agonists and inverse agonists. There is no antagonistic effect on other GABA agonists, like propofol, ethanol, or barbiturates. Flumazenil is currently the only commercially available benzodiazepine antagonist available in the United States.

Diazepam

Diazepam is currently one of the most common benzodiazepines given to veterinary patients. Diazepam is poorly water soluble and is therefore supplied for injection in a solution of an organic solvent, including propylene glycol and ethanol. It has a pH of 6.6–6.9 and is viscid, causing potential pain with IV or IM injection. Diazepam is light sensitive (photodegradation) and will bind to plastics if exposed to light for long periods [39,40]. It is frequently used as an anticonvulsant, as a mild sedative in small animal species, and as an adjunct to ketamine anesthesia in dogs, cats, and horses. Diazepam is rapidly absorbed from the gastrointestinal tract, with very high bioavailability via this route. It is metabolized by hepatic microsomal enzymes utilizing an oxidative pathway [41–43].

In dogs, the elimination half-life of diazepam following IV administration is approximately 3.2 h [44]. Active metabolites (nordiazepam and oxazepam) appear within 2 h and eventually exceed diazepam concentrations, with half-lives of 3.6 and 5.7 h, respectively. Greyhounds given 0.5 mg/kg diazepam IV resulted in an estimated 1.0 h terminal half-life of the parent drug. The oxazepam metabolite had a mean terminal half-life of 6.2 h, indicating that breed differences do exist [41].

Cats receiving very high doses of diazepam (5, 10, and 20 mg/kg) IV show a half-life of diazepam of 5.5 h. About 50% of the diazepam is converted quickly to nordiazepam, which has a half-life of 21 h [45].

Horses receiving 0.05–0.4 mg/kg diazepam IV demonstrated a half-life of the parent drug of 2.5–21.6 h. Nordiazepam and oxazepam were not detected in plasma but were present in urine, suggesting rapid excretion in this species [46]. The terminal half-life of diazepam is unchanged during the first 21 days of life and repeated doses of diazepam should be given with caution [47].

Clinical doses of parenterally administered diazepam result in minimal depression of ventilation, cardiac output, and oxygen delivery. Heart rate, myocardial contractility, cardiac output, and arterial blood pressure are effectively unchanged in dogs after IV administration of diazepam at doses of 0.5, 1.0, and 2.5 mg/kg [48]. Blood gas values were unchanged in horses given doses of diazepam from 0.05 to 0.4 mg/kg [46].

Clinical application

In general terms, diazepam is an unreliable sedative but is useful for providing central muscle relaxation and as an anticonvulsant. It is frequently given to many species prior to or in conjunction with ketamine to ameliorate the central excitatory effects associated with cyclohexamines. The necessity for this practice is not absolute if premedication with other drugs (e.g., opioids or α_2-adrenergic receptor agonists) provides appropriate preinduction sedation. Diazepam has been used with propofol in a similar manner, to reduce the dose of propofol and minimize hemodynamic changes associated with propofol use [49,50]. The MAC is modestly reduced with diazepam administration [51,52].

When used as an anticonvulsant, higher doses than those used for premedication are frequently given. Dogs and cats are routinely given 0.5–1.0 mg/kg IV or rectally to control seizures, whereas 0.1–0.2 mg/kg IV is usually given to horses. Care should be taken with repeat dosing, as metabolites (which have sedative effects but minimal anticonvulsant effects) are cleared slowly.

Midazolam

Midazolam is the other main benzodiazepine used perianesthetically by veterinarians. At a pH of less than 4.0 the drug is highly water soluble owing to an open diazepine ring. At physiologic pH, its diazepine ring closes, rendering the drug lipid soluble and able to cross the blood–brain barrier rapidly to cause its central effects [53]. In addition to frequent intravenous administration, it is rapidly absorbed after IM administration, so it is given by this route for convenience in0020animals that are uncooperative or which do not have intravenous catheters. It is used in a wide variety of species (e.g., swine, ferrets, dogs, cats, horses, and birds). Like diazepam, midazolam is sensitive to light and undergoes photodegradation.

In dogs, bioavailability following IM injection is greater than 90% and peak plasma concentrations occur within 15 min [54]. Enteral bioavailability is high and affected by pH within the gastrointestinal tract where absorption is occurring [55]. An intranasal gel formulation is also available and showed bioavailability of 70.4% in dogs. Nasal drops and spray have also been studied [56–58]. Midazolam given to dogs at 0.5 mg/kg IV had an elimination half-life of 77 min [54]. The median terminal half-life in horses is approximately 216 and 408 min at 0.05 and 0.1 mg/kg IV, respectively, demonstrating dose-dependent kinetics [59]. Similarly to diazepam, midazolam is metabolized by hepatic microsomal enzymes [60].

The cardiovascular effects of midazolam are minor in most cases. Heart rate and cardiac output decrease by 10–20% in dogs given between 0.25 and 1.0 mg/kg [48]. Heart rate decreased in cats given midazolam–butorphanol as a preanesthetic sedative combination. Cardiac output decreased by 23% compared with a saline control; however, the impact of butorphanol on heart rate and therefore cardiac output needs to be taken into consideration [61]. Blood pressure may decrease as a result of central effects on vasomotor centers [1]. Blood gas values are minimally changed in most animals, as was shown in swine [62,63]. It is presumed that the effects of midazolam on ventilation in dogs and cats are similar to those of diazepam.

Clinical Application

Like diazepam, midazolam is unpredictable as a sedative. Dogs administered midazolam IV at 0.5 mg/kg display mild sedation and muscle relaxation but also occasionally agitation [54]. Cats tend to be less sedate, with excitement or agitation evident as doses increase (from 0.05 mg/kg to a non-clinical dose of 5.0 mg/kg) [64–66]. Horses do not typically display sedation but show muscle relaxation and ataxia at doses of 0.05 and 0.1 mg/kg IV [59]. Ferrets and rabbits sedate reasonably well with midazolam, and nasal administration has been studied in rabbits [67]. Midazolam use in a wide variety of bird species has been evaluated and mild to moderate sedation is usually noted.

Like diazepam, midazolam is frequently given to reduce the central excitatory effects of ketamine [66,68,69]. It is also co-administered during induction to reduce the dose of other injectable anesthetics (e.g., propofol or alphaxalone) [47,70–75]. A reduction in MAC is also noted with midazolam use [76,77]. It can be used for its anticonvulsant effects in veterinary species [78].

α_2-Adrenergic receptor agonists

Frequently used in both large and small animal patients, α_2-adrenergic receptor agonists provide sedation, analgesia, and muscle relaxation. Commonly used drugs include xylazine, detomidine, romifidine, medetomidine, and dexmedetomidine. They can be reliably reversed with administration of selective antagonists.

α_2-Adrenergic receptors are scattered throughout the body, in neural tissue, most organs, and extra-synaptically in vascular tissue and platelets. This wide distribution results in a variety of undesired effects when giving an α_2-adrenergic receptor agonist for sedation and/or analgesia. A variety of α_2-adrenergic receptor subtypes have been identified using molecular techniques. Currently, four subtypes are commonly described: α_{2a} receptors are located in the cerebral cortex and brainstem and are the primary source of sedation and supraspinal analgesia in addition to centrally mediated bradycardia and hypotension; α_{2b} receptors are located in the spinal cord and vascular endothelium with stimulation resulting in spinal analgesia, vasoconstriction, and peripherally mediated bradycardia; α_{2c} receptors are also located in the spinal cord, modulating spinal analgesia and possibly thermoregulation; and α_{2d} receptors have been cloned and are thought to be similar to α_{2a} in function and distribution [1].

Current α_2-adrenergic receptor agonists in clinical use also have some impact on α_1-adrenergic receptors (Box 10.2). α_1-Adrenergic receptor agonist action typically results in excitation and increased motor activity in animals. The less selective for α_2-adrenergic receptor a drug is, the more likely in theory rigidity and/or paradoxical excitement may be noted. Arterial injection may also result in these signs and should be avoided. Xylazine is the least specific of currently used drugs.

Box 10.2 α_2:α_1 adrenergic receptor selectivity for selected α_2-adrenergic receptor agonists.

Xylazine 160:1
Detomidine 260:1
Romifidine 340:1
Medetomidine 1620:1
Dexmedetomidine 1620:1

α_2-Adrenergic receptors are G-coupled proteins. In general, when stimulated they inhibit adenyl cyclase activity, leading to a decrease in cAMP concentrations within the cell. Some effects of α_2-adrenergic receptor stimulation do not require G-protein coupling, such as their inhibition of platelet aggregation.

In the CNS, α_2-adrenergic receptor agonist binding leads to sedation, analgesia, muscle relaxation, and centrally mediated effects on heart rate and afterload (through decreased sympathetic nervous system activity). Peripherally, increased systemic vascular resistance (afterload) is noted, which will be discussed shortly.

Effects of α_2-adrenergic receptor agonists

It was noted previously that the broad distribution of α_2-receptors leads to a wide variety of physiologic effects when administered.

Central Nervous System

Fundamentally, the occupancy of α_2-adrenergic receptors in the CNS by one of the α_2-agonists reduces norepinephrine release and may prevent occupancy of receptors. In the brainstem, binding of agonists to α_2-adrenergic receptors in the locus coeruleus and rostroventral lateral medulla (the primary areas for sympathetic outflow from the CNS) cause sedation as the discharge frequency of tracts into the cortex slows.

Rigidity, seizures, and/or excitement have been noted following accidental intracarotid injection of xylazine in horses. Failure to sedate, or paradoxical excitement, can result when animals are excited, fearful, in pain, or otherwise stressed (Box 10.3). These conditions result in high circulating catecholamine levels and can be difficult to overcome with medication [79].

Analgesia results from agonist binding to α_2-adrenergic receptors at various points in the nociceptive pathways. Receptors have been isolated in the dorsal horn of the spinal cord and in the brainstem. Afferent input into the dorsal horn from nociceptors in the periphery continues but is modulated and dampened by the decrease in norepinephrine release (presynaptic inhibition) and occupancy of those receptors (postsynaptic inhibition).

Intracranial pressure (ICP), at least in dogs, appears to be unaffected with the use of medetomidine, with a modest increase in cerebral perfusion pressure [80]. Other studies [81,82] have demonstrated a decrease in cerebral blood flow with dexmedetomidine in dogs and rabbits (which would tend to decrease ICP but also decrease oxygen delivery); therefore, care must be taken when considering the use of α_2-adrenergic receptor agonists in patients with altered intracranial hemodynamics. Mice administered dexmedetomidine displayed attenuated neuronal injury and preserved neurologic function following experimental interruptions in cord blood flow, which supports the clinical observation that this class of drugs can be used carefully in patients with neurological disease [83].

Respiratory

Normal blood gas parameters are generally maintained when using α_2-adrenergic receptor agonists alone [84–87]. When used in conjunction with other sedatives, opioids, or anesthetics, blood gas

Box 10.3 Sedation.

Despite profound sedation, it is important to realize that animals sedated with these medications can be very touch and sound sensitive. Care should be taken regarding rapid arousal from loud noises or movement.

values can be variable, but often are indicative of respiratory depression. Mucous membrane color frequently becomes 'muddy' or pale blue/gray when these medications are administered, as peripheral vasoconstriction slows blood flow in the periphery. The prolonged capillary transit time allows more oxygen extraction, resulting in a greater amount of deoxygenated hemoglobin being present at the end of the capillary. This often exceeds the 5 mg/dL threshold of deoxygenated hemoglobin associated with the observation of cyanosis. It should be appreciated that the arterial oxygen partial pressure is often normal or near normal and therefore cyanosis in this context has a different implication than when it is present in arterial blood and is due to respiratory disease or severe hypoventilation.

Ventilatory drive can be affected, and care should be taken when administering α_2-adrenergic receptor agonists to patients with borderline respiratory function or CNS depression [87,88]. Sheep are prone to hypoxemia following the use of α_2-adrenergic receptor agonists, likely a result of pulmonary edema secondary to pulmonary parenchymal damage. Care should be used when using this class of drug in sheep, or it should be avoided altogether [89–92].

Cardiovascular

The cardiovascular effects of α_2-adrenergic receptor agonists are likely to cause the greatest concern with their use in veterinary patients. The species-dependent distribution of α_1- and α_2-adrenergic receptors in the periphery can lead to wide variability in systemic vascular resistance, blood pressure, heart rate and rhythm, and blood flow with their clinical use. In general, bradycardia is noted. Initially it is primarily a baroreceptor (vagal)-mediated reflex due to increased systemic vascular resistance. As vascular resistance returns to normal, persistent bradycardia is often the result of decreased central sympathetic outflow. Antimuscarinic drugs are often effective at increasing heart rate initially (also causing severe hypertension), but they are often less effective in the later phases. In those patients, sympathomimetic drugs (e.g., ephedrine) may be more effective at increasing heart rate. The decision about which approach is most rational requires concurrent information about arterial blood pressure.

Cardiac output is usually decreased with α_2-adrenergic agonist administration. This is usually secondary to the reduction in heart rate in an attempt to maintain physiological blood pressure in the face of increased systemic vascular resistance. Tissue blood flow is decreased as a result, but it should be appreciated that the reduction is not uniform across all tissue beds and skeletal muscle, adipose tissue, and other non-vital tissues usually are reduced to the greatest extent. Indiscriminately using antimuscarinics to increase heart rate does not increase cardiac output proportionally. In fact, this practice may result in hypertension, increased myocardial oxygen consumption, and arrhythmias while only marginally increasing cardiac output.

Gastrointestinal

Gastrointestinal motility is typically decreased and gastric emptying time may be delayed.

Specific drugs

Xylazine

Xylazine has been used in clinical practice by veterinarians since the late 1960s. Initially used in cattle, its application spread rapidly to other species. Currently, the Food Animal Residue Avoidance Databank does not list xylazine as approved for use in food animal species in the United States, although its use is common [93].

Pharmacokinetics

The elimination half-life of xylazine after IV administration is generally similar across studied species. Cattle and dogs demonstrated xylazine elimination half-lives of about 30 min after 0.2 and 1.4 mg/kg doses, respectively. The elimination half-life in horses was slightly longer at 50 min following a 0.6 mg/kg dose. After IM administration of these doses, cattle and dog plasma levels peaked around 15 min and with similar elimination half-lives as with IV administration [94].

Pharmacodynamics

Onset of sedation and analgesia is rapid following IV and IM administration. Subcutaneous administration usually results in poor sedation owing to the reduced systemic absorption following local vasoconstriction. Clinically applicable doses produce sedation and analgesia in horses within 5–10 min, and persist for 30–60 min. The analgesic and sedative effects are comparable in duration. Few data exist regarding onset of sedation in dogs, but clinical experience would support a rapid onset in dogs and cats also.

Cardiovascular

Administration of xylazine produces a reflex bradycardia that is persistent, as central effects of α_2-adrenergic receptor agonist action outweigh the peripheral effects [84]. Initial hypertension is relatively brief and subsequent hypotension frequently follows. Cardiac output is reduced by up to 50% in dogs and horses, and blood pressure can decrease by 20–30% in the hypotensive phase, especially if arousal from sedation is delayed [4,84,95]. Stroke volume tends to be preserved as the heart rate slows, and the decrease in cardiac output is linked primarily to decreases in heart rate. IM administration of xylazine tends to have less of an impact on cardiac output and rate, although in most individuals it is still significant [84,96]. Sinus bradycardia and second-degree atrioventricular block are the most commonly noted arrhythmia with xylazine administration, although other abnormal rhythms may be observed [84,97].

Respiratory

The respiratory rate usually decreases, but PaO_2, $PaCO_2$, and pH are typically unchanged with clinically used doses of xylazine. This is because the tidal volume increases as the rate falls, resulting in a consistent minute ventilation [97,98]. Higher doses of xylazine in dogs (1.0 mg/kg) can result in a decreased minute ventilation, physiologic deadspace, and oxygen delivery to tissues [97]. Horses anesthetized with halothane showed decreases in PaO_2 when administered xylazine at doses of 0.5–1.0 mg/kg) [99]. These decreases are likely the result of ventilation/perfusion mismatch as a result of alterations in cardiac output and pulmonary vascular tone. PaO_2 frequently decreases after xylazine administration to sheep, which is likely the result of pulmonary inflammation and edema due to the specific intravascular macrophages in this species [89,90].

Gastrointestinal

Xylazine administration can produce salivation, emesis, and reflux. Emesis (in those species that vomit) is likely a result of central α_2-adrenergic receptor stimulation, as pretreatment with yohimbine (α_2-adrenergic receptor antagonist) limits this effect [100]. Gastrointestinal motility, including rumen contractions, is reduced with xylazine administration. This effect is reversible with antagonist administration, provided that excessive gas accumulation (ileus) is not present [101]. Motility of the cecum and colon of horses is also reduced [102]. The analgesic effect and smooth muscle relaxation mediated by α_2-adrenergic receptors may be part of the analgesic impact of xylazine when used as an adjunct for the treatment of colic in horses. The resulting sedation and analgesia can help prevent self-trauma. Intestinal blood flow is reduced, to an extent inconsistent with the decrease in cardiac output, highlighting the impact that α_2-receptors have in the gastrointestinal vasculature [103].

Genitourinary

Urine production reliably increases following xylazine administration, accompanied by a decrease in the specific gravity and osmolality of the urine [104–106]. Normal micturition reflexes are maintained, although urethral pressures can be lowered with xylazine use [107, 108]. Myometrial tone and intrauterine pressure increase in cattle after xylazine administration [109,110]. Intrauterine pressure is also increased in horses, regardless of the α_2-adrenergic receptor agonist used (at equipotent doses) [111]. Xylazine also reduces uterine oxygen delivery [112]. No current data exist on the incidence of negative sequelae to xylazine use in pregnant animals, but caution seems prudent owing to the impact on uterine blood flow and tone, and also the reduction in cardiac output and potential reduction in oxygen delivery to tissues. In many cases, the inclusion of an α_2-adrenergic agonist in the anesthetic protocol is based on a risk–benefit evaluation of the risk to the mother from a poor induction and recovery, and the potential benefit to both from a smooth anesthetic with some degree of fetal oxygen deficit. This is often species dependent and also is based on the availability of other suitable sedatives.

Clinical application

Xylazine is used in dogs and cats for short-term sedation and analgesia for diagnostic or minor surgical procedures. Neuroleptanalgesia is achieved when α_2-adrenergic receptor agonists are combined with opioids. Xylazine is also given with ketamine for restraint or for brief surgical procedures when injectable anesthesia is preferred. It is useful as a premedication, providing good sedation for IV catheter placement and reduced doses of induction agent. Bradycardia and bradyarrythmia are common and should be treated with anticholinergics when appropriate (blood pressure and ECG monitoring is helpful in determining the need for anticholinergic administration).

In horses, xylazine is used for standing restraint/sedation and analgesia. It is frequently used as a premedication for induction of general anesthesia. It can be used as part of an injectable anesthetic technique, either in combination with ketamine or as part of an infusion containing guaifenesin and ketamine, frequently referred to as 'Triple Drip' or 'GKX'. Cattle require a much lower dose (on the order of one-tenth of an equine dose) to provide equipotent sedation. Bovine breeds sensitive to xylazine (e.g., Brahman cattle), sick or debilitated animals, and animals having received prior α_2-adrenergic receptor agonists (e.g., horses with colic presenting for general anesthesia) should receive lower initial doses of xylazine [113]. Accidental intracarotid injections should be avoided as they will usually lead to convulsions. Seizures should be treated appropriately, with intubation and support as necessary.

Detomidine

Detomidine is primarily used in horses, but is occasionally used in other species. It is more potent than xylazine, requiring lower milligram amounts to achieve similar sedation.

Pharmacokinetics

In resting horses, detomidine given at 40 μg/kg IV had a median half-life of 26 min and a median clearance time of 37 min. After supramaximal exercise, the median half-life was 46 min and the median clearance time was 20 min. The volume of distribution increased from 585 to 1296 mL/kg following exercise [114]. Another study demonstrated, at an IV dose of 30.0 μg/kg, a mean elimination half-life of 26 min. Horses given the same dose IM had a mean elimination half-life of 53 min [115]. Cattle receiving 80 μg/kg IV or IM showed a rapid absorption and distribution, with an elimination half-life of 1.3 h following the IV dose and 2.6 h following the IM dose [116].

Detomidine is available in some countries as a gel for sublingual use in horses. The mean bioavailability was 22% after sublingual dosing of 40 μg/kg, compared with 38.2% following the same dose IM [117].

Pharmacodynamics

Peak sedation in horses is rapid, approximately 5 min following appropriate IV dosing, and lasts about 1 h [118,119]. Analgesia and sedation with detomidine administered at 20 μg/kg IV to horses appear equipotent with xylazine administered at 1.0 mg/kg but last longer (up to 46 min) [118,120].

Cardiovascular

Detomidine produces dose-dependent changes in cardiovascular function that wane with clearance of the drug. Detomidine at 10 μg/kg IV reduces heart rate within 2 min, and may induce sinoatrial block or second-degree atrioventricular block. Systolic function is impaired with increases in left ventricular internal diameter noted via echocardiography [121,122]. Cardiac output is decreased by up to 50%, with significant increases in mean blood pressure and systemic vascular resistance at doses ranging from 10 to 40 μg/kg IV. Constant-rate infusion (CRI) administration of detomidine to anesthetized horses results in similar cardiovascular changes that persist with the duration of the CRI [123].

Respiratory

Detomidine administration (when given alone) does not have a great impact on respiratory rate. $PaCO_2$ increases slightly, with clinically negligible changes in PaO_2. Oxygen delivery is reduced as cardiac output decreases. The pulmonary shunt fraction is relatively unchanged but modest increases in V/Q were noted following IV administration of detomidine [124].

Gastrointestinal

Detomidine is a potent analgesic for gastrointestinal pain in horses. The effect and duration are dose dependent and can last several hours with doses greater than 20 μg/kg. Myoelectric activity and motility are reduced. Gastrointestinal blood flow can be impacted negatively [125–127].

Genitourinary

Urine flow is increased with detomidine administration [128,129]. Intrauterine pressure is increased, as with xylazine [111]. Uterine myoelectric activity was increased in normal non-gravid mares receiving detomidine [130], but mares in the last trimester showed no effect or decreased myoelectric activity [131]. Caution in pregnant animals seems warranted.

Clinical application

Detomidine is frequently used to facilitate standing sedation/restraint for a variety of procedures (e.g., ophthalmic, dental) where the practitioner needs more time than xylazine will provide. It is effective as an analgesic, but its duration and associated cardiovascular effects make it less appealing as a premedication for surgery with some practitioners.

Romifidine

Romifidine is another α_2-adrenergic receptor agonist labeled for use in horses in many countries. It is not intended for use in horses intended for human consumption. Its use in dogs and cats is off-label, but has been reported.

Pharmacokinetics

Romifidine administered at 80 μg/kg IV over 2 min to thoroughbred horses fitted a two-compartment model. The elimination half-life was estimated at 138 min with a C_{max} of 51 ng/mL measured at 4 min after injection. Clearance from plasma was 32 mL/min/kg [132].

Pharmacodynamics

Romifidine produces profound sedation in the horse, with peak sedation occurring at approximately 15 min following IV administration. Sedative effects were noted up to 2 h after administration [132]. Sedative effects of romifidine were longer lasting than those of xylazine and detomidine in standing horses [133].

Beagle dogs receiving 20–120 μg/kg romifidine IV demonstrated profound sedation, particularly at higher doses [134]. The IV and SC routes both provided quick uptake and sedation [135]. In most species, ataxia is considered to be less with romifidine compared to other α_2-adrenergic receptor agonists.

Cardiorespiratory

The cardiovascular effects of romifidine are similar to those of other α_2-adrenergic receptor agonists. Bradycardia was noted in horses receiving 80 μg/kg, and the presence of second-degree AV block was detected. Mean arterial blood pressure was elevated by 15% at 5 min, declining to values below baseline by 60 min. The cardiac index was significantly reduced in the same time period [132]. This effect is similar to that in previous studies of other α_2-adrenergic receptor agonists [136,137].

Dogs demonstrate similar dose-dependent effects following romifidine administration. Beagle dogs receiving doses of 5, 10, 25, 50, or 100 μg/kg all had significant decreases in heart rate (up to 70%) and cardiac index (35–50%). Stroke index was unchanged. Blood pressure initially rose, but eventually decreased to below baseline. Systemic vascular resistance exhibited a profound increase at all doses (184–443% increase) [138].

Effects on the respiratory system seem similar to those of other α_2-adrenergic receptor agonists.

Other side effects

Romifidine was similar to xylazine and detomidine with respect to changes in intrauterine pressure [111]. It is presumed that uterine blood flow is affected in the same manner. Romifidine appears to increase urine production [138] and blood glucose concentrations [138–140].

Clinical application

Romifidine produces reliable sedation and analgesia in horses. It is used in a variety of combinations in horses for standing procedures and as a premedication prior to general anesthesia. Its duration should be taken into account when planning general anesthesia.

Dexmedetomidine/medetomidine

Dexmedetomidine is primarily used in dogs and cats, but is also used in other species. It is the dextrorotatory isomer of medetomidine, which is currently no longer available except as formulations prepared for wildlife capture/restraint. Both medetomidine and dexmedetomidine are potent sedatives/analgesics.

Pharmacokinetics

The pharmacokinetics of dexmedetomidine and racemic medetomidine are very similar in dogs. All of the pharmacologic actions of medetomidine are due to the dextrorotatory isomer which is isolated in dexmedetomidine. Administration of medetomidine at 40 μg/kg IV and dexmedetomidine at 20 and 10 μg/kg IV produced peak sedation at 10–20 min at plasma concentrations of 18.5, 14, and 5.5 ng/mL, respectively, in dogs. Terminal half-lives of 0.96, 0.78, and 0.66 h were reported [141]. Administration of levomedetomidine produced no apparent sedation or analgesia. Clearance of levomedetomidine was faster [141]. In cats anesthetized with isoflurane, receiving 10 μg/kg dexmedetomidine IV over 5 min, a terminal half-life of 198 min (range 129–295 min) was estimated [142]. Ponies receiving dexmedetomidine at 3.5 μg/kg IV (deemed comparable to 7 μg/kg medetomidine, or 1.0 mg/kg xylazine) demonstrated a rapid decline in plasma levels, falling below the detection limit within 60–90 min. Plasma half-lives of 19 min in young ponies and of 28 min in more mature ponies have been reported [143]. Medetomidine administration in horses at 10 μg/kg IV produced peak plasma concentrations at 6.4 min, with an elimination half-life of 29 min [144]. Oral transmucosal administration of medetomidine to cats produced similar sedation to IM injection but took longer to achieve peak plasma concentrations (43 versus 21 min, respectively). Individual variation was suspected to be secondary to salivation and drug loss [145]. Dexmedetomidine has been used in a similar fashion, sometimes combined with buprenorphine in cats [146–148].

Pharmacodynamics

Dexmedetomidine produces sedation and analgesia in dogs and cats. Peak sedation in dogs following a dose of 20 or 40 μg/kg IV was achieved in 10 min. Peak analgesia occurred at about 20 min. Moderate sedation was still noted at 40 min and several dogs remained recumbent at 90 min. Dogs receiving dexmedetomidine at 10 μg/kg followed a similar clinical picture. Medetomidine and dexmedetomidine can have a significant impact on anesthetic requirements. Medetomidine infused at 3.5 μg/kg/h in horses decreased the MAC of desflurane by 28% [149]. CRI of dexmedetomidine in dogs at 0.5 and 3.0 μg/kg/h, after 0.5 and 3.0 μg/kg IV given as loading doses, reduced the MAC of isoflurane by 18 and 59%, respectively [150]. Dogs receiving 20 μg/kg IV dexmedetomidine showed a MAC reduction of 88% at 30 min [151].

Cats receiving a targeted infusion of dexmedetomidine showed a dose-dependent decrease in the MAC of isoflurane [152]. Cats receiving a CRI of dexmedetomidine or epidural dexmedetomidine, concurrently with a lidocaine epidural, also displayed a decrease in MAC [153]. Analgesia seems to correlate with sedation in terms of onset, peak, and duration [144,154].

Cardiopulmonary

The cardiopulmonary effects of dexmedetomidine and medetomidine seem to be similar to those of other α_2-adrenergic receptor agonists. Heart rate decreases, cardiac output decreases, and systemic vascular resistance increases [141,143,145,148,153–155]. Systemic arterial blood pressure increases initially followed by hypotension once sympatholytic effects predominate. Changes can also be seen in left ventricular work and pulmonary vascular resistance [155]. Dexmedetomidine at 10 and 20 μg/kg reduced the heart rate in dogs by 60 and 66%, respectively, within 5 min of IV injection. Systolic and diastolic blood pressure increased in a stepwise fashion, with peak effects (20 and 26% changes) at 5 min [141]. Cardiac output decreased by approximately 66% in isoflurane-anesthetized dogs, and increased slowly to half of baseline over 3.5 h. Systemic vascular resistance was increased and corresponded to the change in cardiac output. Contractility was not significantly affected in the dogs [151]. Cardiac output was reduced significantly in horses but returned to baseline levels after 30 min [143]. Blood flow appeared to be directed to vital organs, preserving flow to the brain, heart, kidneys, and liver [156]. This study used radiolabeled microspheres injected into the arterial system, so hepatic portal flow was not studied directly. Global oxygen requirements were reduced and blood flow to vital organs was maintained above a level associated with hypoperfusion and oxygen debt. Coronary vasoconstriction seems to be balanced with oxygen demand by local metabolic control in anesthetized dogs. Arterial blood gas analysis showed little central alteration with dexmedetomidine or medetomidine administration.

Other adverse effects

As with all α_2-adrenergic agonists, the plasma glucose concentration is generally increased with dexmedetomidine or medetomidine administration [144,155,157–159]. Medetomidine at 20, 40, and 60 μg/kg IV in pregnant dogs affected uterine motor activity, with a decrease at 20 μg/kg and an increase in activity at 40 and 60 μg/kg [160]. Urine production is increased in dogs [161–163] and cats [164].

Clinical application

Dexmedetomidine produces reliable sedation and analgesia of varying duration depending on the species in question. It is frequently used in conjunction with opioids to augment analgesia. It is useful as a premedication for general anesthesia, presuming that the patient has no comorbidities that preclude its use. It is frequently used as a sole sedative agent for radiography or with a local anesthetic for minor surgical procedures. Like other α_2-adrenergic receptor agonists, it is reversible; atipamezole is the most commonly used α_2-adrenergic receptor antagonist for medetomidine and dexmedetomidine reversal.

α_2-Adrenergic receptor antagonists

The ability to antagonize pharmacologically the cardiovascular, sedative, and analgesic actions of α_2-adrenergic receptor agonists is a major reason why this class of sedative analgesic drugs are used in veterinary practice. The three antagonist drugs of current clinical interest are yohimbine, tolazoline, and atipamezole. Atipamezole has replaced the others in small and exotic animal practice primarily because of the increasing use of highly specific agonists such as medetomidine and dexmedetomidine; however, yohimbine can still be useful if xylazine is used in small animal patients. In food animal practice, yohimbine and tolazoline are used since the primary α_2-adrenergic agonist in use is xylazine. Equine practitioners generally do not reverse the sedation from α_2-adrenergic agonists owing to concern abut excitation during emergence, but many practices have tolazoline for emergency use.

Reversal of α_2-adrenergic agonists should not be done without consideration of the potential for patient excitation, loss of analgesia, and adverse cardiovascular effects, including tachycardia and hypotension. Intravenous administration often results in rapid vasodilation if animals still have high systemic vascular resistance from agonist action on vascular smooth muscle α_2-adrenergic receptors. If vasodilation occurs without an accompanying increase in heart rate and cardiac output, severe hypotension often results. Although usually transient, this degree of hypotension may not be tolerated by some patients, hence intramuscular administration is often preferred unless the reversal is for emergency purposes. Intramuscular administration usually is effective; however, some animals may have prolonged sedation or incomplete reversal despite an adequate dose. In those patients, it is likely that vasoconstriction in the muscle tissue significantly slows the absorption of the antagonist, resulting in slow reversal. Administration of an additional partial dose of the antagonist intravenously may rapidly result in complete recovery since it bypasses tissue absorption, but it may be prudent to wait until the heart rate begins to increase before intravenous administration is performed to minimize hypotension.

References

1 Katzung BG, ed. *Basic and Clinical Pharmacology*, 9th edn. New York: McGraw Hill, 2004.
2 Coulter DB, Whelan SC, Wilson RC, *et al.* Determination of blood pressure by indirect methods in dogs given acetylpromazine maleate. *Cornell Vet* 1981; **71**: 75–84.
3 Stepien RL, Bonagura JD, Bednarski RM, *et al.* Cardiorespiratory effects of acepromazine maleate and buprenorphine hydrochloride in clinically normal dogs. *Am J Vet Res* 1983; **44**: 996–999.
4 Muir WW, Skarda RT, Sheehan W. Hemodynamic and respiratory effects of a xylazine–acetylpromazine drug combination in horses. *Am J Vet Res* 1979; **40**: 1518–1522.
5 Pequito M, Amory H, Serteyn D, *et al.* Comparison of the sedative and hemodynamic effects of acepromazine and promethazine in the standing horse. *J Equine Vet Sci* 2012; **32**: 799–804.
6 Leise BS, Fugler LA, Stokes AM, *et al.* Effects of intramuscular administration of acepromazine on palmar digital blood flow, palmar digital arterial pressure, transverse facial arterial pressure, and packed cell volume in clinically healthy, conscious horses. *Vet Surg* 2007; **36**: 717–723.
7 Ludders JW, Reitan JA, Martucci R, *et al.* Blood pressure response to phenylephrine infusion in halothane anesthetized dogs given acetylpromazine maleate. *Am J Vet Res* 1983; **44**: 996–999.
8 Steffey EP, Kelly AB, Farver TB, *et al.* Cardiovascular and respiratory effects of acetylpromazine and xylazine on halothane anesthetized horses. *J Vet Pharmacol Ther* 1985; **8**: 290–302.
9 Muir WW, Werner LL, Hamlin RL. Effects of xylazine and acetylpromazine upon induced ventricular fibrillation in dogs anesthetized with thiamylal and halothane. *Am J Vet Res* 1975; **36**: 1299–1303.
10 Dyson D, Pettifer G. Evaluation of the arrhythmogenicity of a low dose of acepromazine: comparison with xylazine. *Can J Vet Res* 1997; **61**: 241–245.
11 Lemke KA, Tranquilli WJ. Anesthetics, arrhythmias, and myocardial sensitization to epinephrine. *J Am Vet Med Assoc* 1994; **205**: 1679–1684.
12 Popovic NA, Mullane JF, Yhap EO. Effects of acetylpromazine maleate on certain cardiorespiratory responses in dogs. *Am J Vet Res* 1972; **33**: 1819–1824.
13 Webb AI, O'Brien JM. The effect of acepromazine maleate on the anesthetic potency of halothane and isoflurane. *J Am Anim Hosp Assoc* 1988; **24**: 609–613.
14 Heard DJ, Webb AI, Daniels RT. Effect of acepromazine on the anesthetic requirement of halothane in the dog. *Am J Vet Res* 1986; **47**: 2113–2115.
15 Doherty TJ, Geiser DR, Rohrback BW. Effect of acepromazine and butorphanol on halothane minimum alveolar concentration in ponies. *Equine Vet J* 1997; **29**: 374–376.
16 Ballard S, Shults T, Kownacki AA, *et al.* The pharmacokinetics, pharmacological responses and behavioral effects of acepromazine in the horse. *J Vet Pharmacol Ther* 1982; **5**: 21–31.
17 Marroum PJ, Webb AI, Aeschbacher G, *et al.* Pharmacokinetics and pharmacodynamics of acepromazine in horses. *Am J Vet Res* 1994; **55**: 1428–1433.
18 Lang SM, Eglen RM, Henry AC. Acetylpromazine administration: its effect on canine haematology. *Vet Rec* 1979; **105**: 397–398.

19 Barr SC, Ludders JW, Looney AL, *et al.* Platelet aggregation in dogs after sedation with acepromazine and atropine and during subsequent general anesthesia and surgery. *Am J Vet Res* 1992; **53**: 2067–2070.

20 Conner BJ, Hanel RM, Hansen BD, *et al.* Effects of acepromazine maleate on platelet function assessed by use of adenosine diphosphate activated- and arachidonic acid- activated modified thromboelastography in healthy dogs. *Am J Vet Res* 2012; **73**: 595–601.

21 Strombeck DR, Harrold D. Effects of atropine, acepromazine, meperidine, and xylazine on gastroesophageal sphincter pressure in the dog. *Am J Vet Res* 1985; **46**: 963–965.

22 Hall JA, Magne ML, Twedt DC. Effect of acepromazine, diazepam, fentanyl-droperidol, and oxymorphone on gastroesophageal sphincter pressure in healthy dogs. *Am J Vet Res* 1987; **48**: 556–557.

23 Scrivani PV, Bednarski RM, Myer CW. Effects of acepromazine and butorphanol on positive-contrast upper gastrointestinal tract examination in dogs. *Am J Vet Res* 1998; **59**: 1227–1233.

24 Davies JV, Gerring EL. Effect of spasmolytic analgesic drugs on the motility patterns of the equine small intestine. *Res Vet Sci* 1983; **34**: 334–339.

25 Doherty TJ, Andrews FM, Provenza MK, *et al.* The effect of sedation on gastric emptying of a liquid marker in ponies. *Vet Surg* 1999; **28**: 375–379.

26 Pearson H, Weaver BM. Priapism after sedation, neuroleptanalgesia, and anaesthesia in the horse. *Equine Vet J* 1979; **11**: 33–35.

27 Driessen B, Zarucco L, Kalir B, Bertolotti L. Contemporary use of acepromazine in the anaesthetic management of male horses and ponies: a retrospective study and opinion poll. *Equine Vet J* 2011; **43**: 88–98.

28 Bostrom I, Nyman G, Kampa N, *et al.* Effects of acepromazine on renal function in anesthetized dogs. *Am J Vet Res* 2003; **64**: 590–598.

29 Newell SM, Ko JC, Ginn PE, *et al.* Effects of three sedative protocols on glomerular filtration rate in clinically normal dogs. *Am J Vet Res* 1997; **58**: 446–450.

30 Marks SL, Straeter-Knowlen IM, Moore M, *et al.* Effects of acepromazine maleate and phenoxybenzamine on urethral pressure profiles of anesthetized, healthy, sexually intact male cats. *Am J Vet Res* 1996; **57**: 1497–1500.

31 Alvaides RK, Teixeira Neto FJ, Aguiar AJA, *et al.* Sedative and cardiorespiratory effects of acepromazine or atropine given before dexmedetomidine in dogs. *Vet Rec* 2008; **162**: 852–856.

32 Saponaro V, Crovace A, De Marzo L, *et al.* Echocardiographic evaluation of the cardiovascular effects of medetomidine, acepromazine and their combination in healthy dogs. *Res Vet Sci* 2013; **95**: 687–692.

33 Holliday TA, Cunningham JG, Gutnick MJ. Comparative clinical and electroencephalographic studies of canine epilepsy. *Epilepsia* 1970; **11**: 281–292.

34 Tobias KM, Marioni-Henry K, Wagner R. A retrospective study on the use of acepromazine maleate in dogs with seizures. *J Am Anim Hosp Assoc* 2006; **42**: 283–289.

35 McConnell J, Kirby R, Rudloff E. Administration of acepromazine maleate to 31 dogs with a history of seizures. *J Vet Emerg Crit Care* 2007; 17: 262–267.

36 Goodchild CS. GABA receptors and benzodiazepines. *Br J Anaesth* 1993; **71**: 127–133.

37 Engin E, Liu J, Uwe R. α2-Containing GABAA receptors: a target for the development of novel treatment strategies for CNS disorders. *Pharmacol Ther* 2012; **136**: 142–152.

38 Mohler H, Richards JG. The benzodiazepine receptor: a pharmacological control element of brain function. *Eur J Anaesthesiol Suppl* 1988; **2**: 15–24.

39 Baraldi M, Avallone R, Corsi L, *et al.* Endogenous benzodiazepines. *Therapie* 2000; **55**: 143–146.

40 Cortelli P, Avallone R, Baraldi M, *et al.* Endozepines in recurrent stupor. *Sleep Med Rev* 2005; 9: 477–487.

41 Ahboucha S, Gamrani H, Baker G. GABAergic neurosteroids: the 'endogenous benzodiazepines' of acute liver failure. *Neurochem Int* 2012; **60**: 707–714.

42 Treleano A, Wolz G, Brandsch R, Welle F. Investigation into the adsorption of nitroglycerine and diazepam into PVC tubes and alternative tube materials during application. *Int J Pharm* 2009; **369**(1–2): 30–37.

43 Winsnes M, Jeffsson R, Sjoberg B. Diazepam absorption to infusion sets and plastic syringes. *Acta Anaesthesiol Scand* 1981; **25**: 93–96.

44 KuKanich B, Nauss JL. Pharmacokinetics of the cytochrome P-450 substrates phenytoin, theophylline, and diazepam in healthy Greyhound dogs. *Vet Pharm Ther* 2011; **35**: 275–281.

45 Stoelting RK, Hillier SC, eds. *Pharmacology and Physiology in Anesthetic Practice*, 4th edn. Philadelphia: Lippincott Williams & Wilkins, 2006.

46 Shou M, Norcross R, Sandig G, *et al.* Substrate specificity and kinetic properties of seven heterologously expressed dog cytochromes p450. *Drug Metab Dispos* 2003; **31**: 1161–1169.

47 Loscher W, Frey HH. Pharmacokinetics of diazepam in the dog. *Arch Int Pharmacodyn Ther* 1981; **254**: 180–195.

48 Cotler S, Gustafson JH, Colburn WA. Pharmacokinetics of diazepam and nordiazepam in the cat. *J Pharm Sci* 1984; 73: 348–351.

49 Muir WW, Sams RA, Huffman RH, *et al.* Pharmacodynamic and pharmacokinetic properties of diazepam in horses. *Am J Vet Res* 1982; **43**: 1756–1762.

50 Robinson R, Borer-Weir K. A dose titration study into the effects of diazepam or midazolam on the propofol dose requirements for induction of general anaesthesia in client owned dogs, premedicated with methadone and acepromazine. *Vet Anesth Analg* 2013; **40**: 455–463.

51 Jones DJ, Stehling LC, Zauder HL. Cardiovascular responses to diazepam and midazolam maleate in the dog. *Anesthesiology* 1979; **51**: 430–434.

52 Fayyaz S, Kerr CL, Dyson DH, *et al.* The cardiopulmonary effects of anesthetic induction with isoflurane, ketamine–diazepam or propofol–diazepam in the hypovolemic dog. *Vet Anesth Analg* 2009; **36**: 110–120.

53 Ko JC, Payton ME, White AG, *et al.* Effects of intravenous diazepam or microdose medetomidine on propofol induced sedation in dogs. *J Am Anim Hosp Assoc* 2006; **42**: 18–27.

54 Matthews NS, Dollar NS, Shawley RV. Halothane sparing effect of benzodiazepines in ponies. *Cornell Vet* 1990; **80**: 259–265.

55 Hellyer PW, Mama KR, Shafford HL, *et al.* Effects of diazepam and flumazenil on minimum alveolar concentrations for dogs anesthetized with isoflurane or a combination of isoflurane and fentanyl. *Am J Vet Res* 2001; **62**: 555–560.

56 Kanto JH. Midazolam: the first water-soluble benzodiazepine. Pharmacology, pharmacokinetics and efficacy in insomnia and anesthesia. *Pharmacotherapy* 1985; **5**: 138–155.

57 Court MH, Greenblatt DJ. Pharmacokinetics and preliminary observations of behavioral changes following administration of midazolam to dogs. *J Vet Pharm Ther* 1992; **15**: 343–350.

58 Zhang J, Niu S, Zhang H, Streisand JB. Oral mucosal absorption of midazolam in dogs is strongly pH dependent. *J Pharm Sci* 2002; **91**: 980–982.

59 Eagleson JS, Platt SR, Strong DL, *et al.* Bioavailability of a novel midazolam gel after intranasal administration in dogs. *Am J Vet Res* 2012; **73**: 539–545.

60 Henry RJ, Ruano N, Casto D, Wolf RH. A pharmacokinetic study of midazolam in dogs: nasal drop vs. atomizer administration. *Pediatr Dent* 1998; **20**: 321–326.

61 Lui CY, Amidon GL, Goldberg A. Intranasal absorption of flurazepam, midazolam, and triazolam in dogs. *J Pharm Sci* 1991; **80**: 1125–1129.

62 Hubbell JAE, Kelly EM, Aarnes TK, *et al.* Pharmacokinetics of midazolam after intravenous administration to horses. *Equine Vet J* 2013; **45**: 721–725.

63 KuKanich B, Hubin M. The pharmacokinetics of ketoconazole and its effects on the pharmacokinetics of midazolam and fentanyl in dogs. *J Vet Pharmacol Ther* 2010; **33**: 42–49.

64 Biermann K, Hungerbuhler S, Mischke R, *et al.* Sedative, cardiovascular, haematologic and biochemical effects of four different drug combinations administered intramuscularly in cats. *Vet Anesth Analg* 2012; **39**: 137–150.

65 Cassu RN, Crociolli GC, Diniz MS, *et al.* Continuous infusion rate of midazolam alone or in combination with fentanyl for endoscopy in swine. *Cienc Rural* 2012; **42**: 2206–2212.

66 Smith AC, Zellner JL, Spinale FG, *et al.* Sedative and cardiovascular effects of midazolam in swine. *Lab Anim Sci* 1991; **41**: 157–161.

67 Ilkiw JE, Suter CM, Farver TB, *et al.* The behavior of healthy awake cats following intravenous and intramuscular administration of midazolam. *J Vet Pharmacol Ther* 1996; **19**: 205–216.

68 Ilkiw JE, Suter CM, McNeal D, *et al.* The effect of intravenous administration of variable dose midazolam after fixed dose ketamine in healthy awake cats. *J Vet Pharmacol Ther* 1996; **19**: 217–224.

69 Ilkiw JE, Suter CM, McNeal D, *et al.* The optimal intravenous dose of midazolam after intravenous ketamine in healthy awake cats. *J Vet Pharmacol Ther* 1998; **21**: 54–61.

70 Robertson SA, Eberhart S. Efficacy of the intranasal route for administration of anesthetic agents to adult rabbits. *Lab Anim Sci* 1994; **44**: 159–165.

71 Gangl M, Grulke S, Detilleux J, *et al.* Comparison of thiopentone/guaifenesin, ketamine/guaifenesin and ketamine/midazolam for the induction of horses to be anesthetized with isoflurane. *Vet Rec* 2001; **149**: 147–151.

72 Hellyer PW, Freeman LC, Hubbell JA. Induction of anesthesia with diazepam–ketamine and midazolam–ketamine in greyhounds. *Vet Surg* 1991; **20**: 143–147.

73 Greene SA, Benson GJ, Hartsfield SM. Thiamylal sparing effect of midazolam for canine endotracheal intubation: a clinical study of 118 dogs. *Vet Surg* 1993; **22**: 69–72.

74 Hopkins A, Giuffrida M, Larenza MP. Midazolam, as a co-induction agent, has propofol sparing effects but also decreases systolic blood pressure in healthy dogs. *Vet Anesth Analg* 2014; **41**: 64–72.

75 Sanchez A, Belda E, Escobar M, *et al.* Effects of altering the sequence of midazolam and propofol during co-induction of anesthesia. *Vet Anesth Analg* 2013; **40**: 359–366.

76 Hall RI, Szlam F, Hug CC Jr. Pharmacokinetics and pharmacodynamics of midazolam in the enflurane-anesthetized dog. *J Pharmacokinet Biopharm* 1988; **16**: 251–262.

77 Seddighi R, Egger CM, Rohrbach BW, *et al.* The effect of midazolam on the end-tidal concentration of isoflurane necessary to prevent movement in dogs. *Vet Anesth Analg* 2011; **38**: 195–202.
78 Schwartz M, Munana KR, Nettifee-Osborne JA, *et al.* The pharmacokinetics of midazolam after intravenous, intramuscular, and rectal administration in healthy dogs. *J Vet Pharm Ther* 2013; **36**: 471–477.
79 Clarke KW, England GCW. Medetomidine, a new sedative-analgesic for use in the dog and its reversal with atipamezole. *J Small Anim Pract* 1989; **30**: 343–348.
80 Keegan RD, Greene SA, Bagley RS, *et al.* Effects of medetomidine administration on intracranial pressure and cardiovascular variables of isoflurane anesthetized dogs. *Am J Vet Res* 1995; **56**: 193–198.
81 Ishiyama T, Dohi I, Iida H, *et al.* Mechanisms of dexmedetomidine induced cerebrovascular effects in canine in vivo experiments. *Anesth Analg* 1995; **81**: 1208–1215.
82 Zornow MH, Fleischer JE, Scheller MS, *et al.* Dexmedetomidine, an alpha 2-adrenergic agonist, decreases cerebral blood flow in the isoflurane-anesthetized dog. *Anesth Analg* 1990; **70**: 624–630.
83 Bell MT, Puskas F, Bennett DT, *et al.* Dexmedetomidine, an alpha-2a adrenergic agonist, promotes ischemic tolerance in a murine model of spinal cord ischemia-reperfusion. *J Thorac Cardiovasc Surg* 2014; **147**: 500–506.
84 Klide AM, Calderwood HW, Soma LR. Cardiopulmonary effects of xylazine in dogs. *Am J Vet Res* 1975; **36**: 931–935.
85 Selmi AL, Barbudo-Selmi GR, Moreira CF, *et al.* Evaluation of sedative and cardiorespiratory effects of romifidine and romifidine-butorphanol in cats. *J Am Vet Med Assoc* 2002; **221**: 506–510.
86 Lamont LA, Bulmer BJ, Grimm KA, *et al.* Cardiopulmonary evaluation of the use of medetomidine hydrochloride in cats. *Am J Vet Res* 2001; **62**: 1745–1749.
87 Bloor BC, Abdul-Rasool I, Temp J, *et al.* The effects of medetomidine, an α2-adrenergic agonist, on ventilatory drive in the dog. *Acta Vet Scand* 1989; (Suppl 85): 65–70.
88 Lerche P, Muir WW. Effect of medetomidine on breathing and inspiratory neuromuscular drive in conscious dogs. *Am J Vet Res* 2004; **65**: 720–724.
89 Celly CS, Atwal OS, McDonell WN, Black WD. Histopathologic alterations induced in the lungs of sheep by use of alpha2-adrenergic receptor agonists. *Am J Vet Res* 1999; **60**: 154–161.
90 Celly CS, McDonell WN, Black WD. Cardiopulmonary effects of the alpha2-adrenoceptor agonists medetomidine and ST-91 in anesthetized sheep. *J Pharmacol Exp Ther* 1999; **289**: 712–720.
91 Kästner SB. Alpha2-agonists in sheep: a review. *Vet Anaesth Analg* 2006; **33**: 79–96.
92 Kästner SB, Ohlerth S, Pospischil A, *et al.* Dexmedetomidine-induced pulmonary alterations in sheep. *Res Vet Sci* 2007; **83**: 217–226.
93 Haskell SR, Gehring R, Payne MA, *et al.* Update on FARAD food animal drug withholding recommendations. *J Am Vet Med Assoc* 2003; **223**: 1277–1278.
94 Garcia-Villar R, Toutain PL, Alvinerie M, Ruckebusch Y. The pharmacokinetics of xylazine hydrochloride: an interspecific study. *J Vet Pharmacol Ther* 1981; **4**: 87–92.
95 Kerr DD, Jones EW, Holbert D, *et al.* Sedative and other effects of xylazine given to horses. *Am J Vet Res* 1972; **33**: 525–532.
96 McCashin FB, Gabel AA. Evaluation of xylazine as a sedative and preanesthetic agent in horses. *Am J Vet Res* 1975; **36**: 1421–1429.
97 Haskins SC, Patz JD, Farver TB. Xylazine and xylazine-ketamine in dogs. *Am J Vet Res* 1986; **47**: 636–641.
98 Lavoie JP, Pasco JR, Kurpershoek CJ. Effects of xylazine on ventilation in in horses. *Am J Vet Res* 1992; **53**: 916–920.
99 Steffey EP, Kelly AB, Farver TB, *et al.* Cardiovascular and respiratory effects of acetylpromazine and xylazine on halothane-anesthetized horses. *J Vet Pharmacol Ther* 1985; **8**: 290–302.
100 Hikasa Y, Ogasawara S, Takase K. Alpha adrenoceptor subtypes involved in the emetic action of dogs. *J Pharmacol Exp Ther* 1992; **261**: 746–754.
101 Ruckebusch Y, Allal C. Depression of reticulo-ruminal motor functions through the stimulation of α_2-adrenoceptors. *J Vet Pharmacol Ther* 1987; **10**: 1–10.
102 Rutkowski JA, Ross MW, Cullen K. Effects of xylazine and/or butorphanol or neostigmine on myoelectric activity of the cecum and right ventral colon in female ponies. *Am J Vet Res* 1989; **50**: 1096–1101.
103 Evades SC, Moore JN. Blockage of endotoxin-induced cecal hypo-perfusion and ileus with an α_2-antagonist in horses. *Am J Vet Res* 1993; **54**: 586–590.
104 Thurmon JC, Nelson DR, Hartsfield SM, *et al.* Effects of xylazine hydrochloride on urine in cattle. *Aust Vet J* 1978; **54**: 178–180.
105 Thurmon JC, Steffey EP, Zinkl JG, *et al.* Xylazine causes transient dose related hyperglycemia and increased urine volumes in mares. *Am J Vet Res* 1984; **45**: 224–227.
106 Trim CM, Hanson RR. Effects of xylazine on renal function and plasma glucose in ponies. *Vet Rec* 1986; **118**: 65–67.
107 Moreau PM, Lees GE, Gross DR. Simultaneous cystometry and uroflowmetry (micturition study) for evaluation of the caudal part of the urinary tract in dogs: reference values for healthy animals sedated with xylazine. *Am J Vet Res* 1983; **44**: 1774–1781.
108 Richter KP, Ling GV. Effects of xylazine on the urethral pressure profile of healthy dogs. *Am J Vet Res* 1985; **46**: 1881–1886.
109 LeBlanc MM, Hubbell JA, Smith HC. The effects of xylazine hydrochloride on intrauterine pressure in the cow. *Theriogenology* 1984; **21**: 681–690.
110 Jansen CA, Lowe KC, Nathanielsz PW. The effects of xylazine on uterine activity, fetal, and maternal oxygenation, cardiovascular function and fetal breathing. *Am J Obstet Gynecol* 1984; **148**: 386–390.
111 Schatzmann U, Jossfck H, Starffer JL, *et al.* Effects of alpha 2-agonists on intrauterine pressure and sedation in horses: comparison between detomidine, romifidine, and xylazine. *Zentralbl Veterinarmed A* 1994; **41**: 523–529.
112 Hodgson DS, Dunlop CI, Chapman PL, *et al.* Cardiopulmonary effects of xylazine and acepromazine in pregnant cows in late gestation. *Am J Vet Res* 2002; **63**: 1695–1699.
113 Greene SA, Thurmon JC. Xylazine: a review of its pharmacology and use in veterinary medicine. *J Vet Pharm Ther* 1988; **11**: 295–313.
114 Hubbell JAE, Sams RA, Schmall LM, *et al.* Pharmacokinetics of detomidine administered to horses at rest and after maximal exercise. *Equine Vet J* 2009; **5**: 419–422.
115 Grimsrud KN, Mama KR, Thomasy SM, *et al.* Pharmacokinetics of detomidine and its metabolites following intravenous and intramuscular administration in horses. *Equine Vet J* 2009; **4**: 361–365.
116 Salonen JS, Vaha-Vahe T, Vainio O, *et al.* Single dose pharmacokinetics of detomidine the horse and cow. *J Vet Pharm Ther* 1989; **12**: 65–72.
117 Kaukinen H, Aspegren J, Hyyppa S, *et al.* Bioavailability of detomidine administered sublingually to horses as an oromucosal gel. *J Vet Pharm Ther* 2011; **34**: 76–81.
118 Lowe JE, Hilfiger J. Analgesic and sedative effects of detomidine compared to xylazine in a colic model using IV and IM routes of administration. *Acta Vet Scand Suppl* 1986; **82**: 85–95.
119 Hubbell JAE, Muir WW. Use of the α_2-adrenergic receptor agonists xylazine and detomidine in the perianesthetic period in the horse. *Equine Vet Educ* 2004; **16**: 326–332.
120 England GC, Clarke KW, Goossens L. A comparison of the sedative effects of three α2-adrenoceptor agonists (romifidine, detomidine, and xylazine) in the horse. *J Vet Pharm Ther* 1992; **15**: 194–201.
121 Buhl R, Ersboll AK, Larsen NH, *et al.* The effects of detomidine, romifidine or acepromazine on echocardiographic measurement and cardiac function in normal horses. *Vet Anesth Analg* 2006; **34**: 1–8.
122 Yamashita K, Tsubakishita S, Futaoka S, *et al.* Cardiovascular effects of medetomidine, detomidine, and xylazine in horses. *J Vet Med Sci* 2000; **62**: 1025–1032.
123 Schauvliege S, Marcilla MG, Verryken K, *et al.* Effects of a constant rate infusion of detomidine on cardiovascular function, isoflurane requirements, and recovery quality in horses. *Vet Anesth Analg* 2011; **38**: 544–554.
124 Nyman G, Marntell S, Edner A, *et al.* Effect of sedation with detomidine and butorphanol on pulmonary gas exchange in the horse. *Acta Vet Scand* 2009; **51**: 22.
125 Merritt AM, Burrow JA, Hartless CS, *et al.* Effect of xylazine, detomidine, and a combination of xylazine and butorphanol on equine duodenal motility. *Am J Vet Res* 1998; **59**: 619–623.
126 Koenig J, Cote N. Equine gastrointestinal motility – ileus and pharmacological modification. *Can Vet J* 2006; **47**: 551–559.
127 Malone E, Graham L. Management of gastrointestinal pain. *Vet Clin Equine* 2002; **18**: 133–158.
128 Nunez E, Steffey EP, Ocampo L, *et al.* Effects of alpha2 adrenergic receptor agonists on urine production in horses deprived of food and water. *Am J Vet Res* 2004; **65**: 1342–1346.
129 Steffey EP, Pascoe PJ. Detomidine reduces isoflurane anesthetic requirement (MAC) in horses. *Vet Anesth Analg* 2002; **29**: 223–227.
130 Von Reitzenstein M, Callahan MA, Hansen PJ, LeBlanc MM. Aberration in uterine contractile patterns in mares with delayed uterine clearance after administration of detomidine and oxytocin. *Theriogenology* 2002; **58**: 887–898.
131 Jedruch J, Gajewski Z, Kuussaari J. The effect of detomidine hydrochloride on the electrical activity of uterus in pregnant mares. *Acta Vet Scan* 1989; **30**: 307–311.
132 Wojtasiak-Wypart M, Soma LR, Rudy JA, *et al.* Pharmacokinetic profile and pharmacodynamic effects of romifidine hydrochloride in the horse. *J Vet Pharmacol Ther* 2012; **35**: 478–488.
133 England GCW, Clarke KW, Goossens L. A comparison of the sedative effects of three alpha 2-adrenoceptor agonists (romifidine, detomidine and xylazine) in the horse. *J Vet Pharmacol Ther* 1992; **15**: 194–201.
134 England GCW, Flack TE, Hollingworth E, *et al.* Sedative effects of romifidine in the dog. *J Small Anim Pract* 1996; **37**: 19–25.

135 England GCW, Thompson S. The influence of route of administration upon the sedative effect of romifidine in dogs. *J Vet Anaesth* 1997; **24**: 21–23.

136 Freeman SL, Bowe IM, Bettschart-Wolfensberger R, *et al.* Cardiovascular effects of romifidine in the standing horse. *Res Vet Sci* 2002; **72**: 123–129.

137 Clarke KW, England GC, Goossens L. Sedative and cardiovascular effects of romifidine, alone and in combination with butorphanol in the horse. *J Vet Anaesth* 1991; **18**: 25–29.

138 Gasthuys F, Martens A, Goossens L, *et al.* A quantitative study of the diuretic effects of romifidine in the horse. *J Vet Anaesth* 1996; **23**: 6–10.

139 Ringer SK, Schwarzwald CC, Portier K, *et al.* Blood glucose, acid–base and electrolyte changes during loading doses of α_2-adrenergic agonists followed by constant rate infusions in horses. *Vet J* 2013; **198**: 684–689.

140 Pypendop BH, Verstegen JP. Cardiovascular effects of romifidine in dogs. *Am J Vet Res* 2001; **62**: 490–495.

141 Kuusela E, Raekallio M, Anttila M, *et al.* Clinical effects and pharmacokinetics of medetomidine and its enantiomers in dogs. *J Vet Pharmcol Ther* 2000; **23**: 15–20.

142 Escobar A, Pypendop BH, Siao KT, *et al.* Pharmacokinetics of dexmedetomidine administered intravenously in isoflurane anesthetized cats. *Am J Vet Res* 2012; **73**: 285–289.

143 Bettschart-Wolfensberger R, Freeman SL, Bowen IM, *et al.* Cardiopulmonary effects and pharmacokinetics of IV dexmedetomidine in ponies. *Equine Vet J* 2005; **37**: 60–64.

144 Grimsrud KN, Mama KR, Steffey EP, Stanley SD. Pharmacokinetics and pharmacodynamics of intravenous medetomidine in the horse. *Vet Anaesth Analg* 2012; **39**: 38–48.

145 Ansah OB, Raekallio M, Vainio O. Comparing oral and intramuscular administration of medetomidine in cats. *J Vet Anaesth* 1998; **25**: 41–46.

146 Slingsby LS, Taylor OM, Monroe T. Thermal antinociception after dexmedetomidine administration in cats: a comparison between intramuscular and oral transmucosal administration. *J Feline Med Surg* 2009; **11**: 829–834.

147 Santos LCP, Ludders JW, Erb HN, *et al.* Sedative and cardiorespiratory effects of dexmedetomidine and buprenorphine administered to cats via oral transmucosal or intramuscular routes. *Vet Anesth Analg* 2010; **37**: 417–424.

148 Porters N, Bosmans T, Debille M, *et al.* Sedative and antinociceptive effects of dexmedetomidine and buprenorphine after oral transmucosal or intramuscular administration in cats. *Vet Anaesth Analg* 2014; **41**: 90–96.

149 Bettschart-Wolfensberger R, Jäggin-Schmucker N, Lendl C, *et al.* Minimal alveolar concentration of desflurane in combination with an infusion of medetomidine for the anaesthesia of ponies. *Vet Rec* 2001; **148**: 264–267.

150 Pascoe PJ, Raekallio M, Kuusela E, *et al.* Changes in the minimum alveolar concentration of isoflurane and some cardiopulmonary measurements during three continuous infusion rates of dexmedetomidine in dogs. *Vet Anesth Analg* 2005; **33**: 97–103.

151 Bloor BC, Frankland M, Alper G, *et al.* Hemodynamic and sedative effects of dexmedetomidine in dog. *J Pharm Exp Ther* 1992; **263**: 690–697.

152 Escobar A, Pypendop BH, Siao KT, *et al.* Effect of dexmedetomidine on the minimum alveolar concentration of isoflurane in cats. *J Vet Pharmacol Ther* 2011; **35**: 163–168.

153 Souza SS, Intelisano TR, de Biaggi CP, *et al.* Cardiopulmonary and isoflurane sparing effects of epidural or intravenous infusion of dexmedetomidine in cats undergoing surgery with epidural lidocaine. *Vet Anaesth Analg* 2010; **37**: 106–115.

154 Murrell JC, Hellebrekers LJ. Medetomidine and dexmedetomidine: a review of cardiovascular effects and antinociceptive properties in the dog. *Vet Anaesth Analg* 2005; **32**: 117–127.

155 Pypendop BH, Barter LS, Stanley SD, *et al.* Hemodynamic effects of dexmedetomidine in isoflurane-anesthetized cats. *Vet Anaesth Analg* 2011; **38**: 555–567.

156 Lawrence CJ, Prinzen FW, de Lange S. The effect of dexmedetomidine on nutrient organ blood flow. *Anesth Analg* 1996; **83**: 1160–1165.

157 Roekaerts P, Prinzen F, de Lange S. Coronary vascular effects of dexmedetomidine during reactive hyperemia in the anaesthetized dog. *J Cardiothorac Vasc Anesth* 1996; **10**: 619–626.

158 Sharma R, Kumar A, Kumar A, *et al.* Comparison of xylazine and dexmedetomidine as a premedicant for general anesthesia in dogs. *Indian J Anim Sci* 2014; **84**: 8–12.

159 Restitutti F, Raekallio M, Vainionpaa M, *et al.* Plasma glucose, insulin, free fatty acids, lactate and cortisol concentration in dexmedetomidine sedated dogs with or without MK-467: a peripheral alpha 2 adrenoceptor antagonist. *Vet J* 2012; **193**: 481–485.

160 Jedruch J, Gajewski Z, Ratajska-Michalczak R. Uterine motor responses to an alpha 2 adrenergic agonist medetomidine hydrochloride in the bitches during the end of gestation and the post-partum period. *Acta Vet Scand Suppl* 1989; **85**: 129–134.

161 Burton S, Lemke KA, Ihle SL, Mackenzie AL. Effects of medetomidine on serum osmolality; urine volume, osmolality and pH; free water clearance; and fractional clearance of sodium, chloride, potassium, and glucose in dogs. *Am J Vet Res* 1998; **59**: 756–761.

162 Saleh N, Aoki M, Shimada T, *et al.* Renal effects of medetomidine in isoflurane anesthetized dogs with special reference to its diuretic action. *J Vet Med Sci* 2005; **67**: 461–465.

163 Talukder MH, Hikasa Y. Diuretic effects of medetomidine compared with xylazine in healthy dogs. *Can J Vet Res* 2009; **73**: 224–236.

164 Murahata Y, Hikasa Y. Comparison of the diuretic effects of medetomidine hydrochloride and xylazine hydrochloride in healthy cats. *Am J Vet Res* 2012; **73**: 1871–1880.

11 Opioids

Butch KuKanich[1] **and Ashley J. Wiese**[2]

[1]Department of Anatomy and Physiology, College of Veterinary Medicine, Kansas State University, Manhattan, Kansas, USA

[2]Department of Anesthesia, MedVet Medical and Cancer Center for Pets, Cincinnati, Ohio, USA

Chapter contents

Introduction

An opiate is a drug derived from opium (a mixture of compounds prepared from a species of poppy, *Papaver somniferum*) and an opioid is a drug which is not derived from opium but interacts at the opioid receptor. For the context of this chapter, opioid will refer to any drug that interacts at an opioid receptor. Opioids are the prototypical analgesics, antitussives, and antidiarrheal drug class. The opioid receptor system or opioid effects have been identified in numerous animal species including ascarids [1], scallops [2], fish [3], reptiles [4], birds [5], and mammals.

Opioid receptors

Three opioid receptor types have been definitively identified: mu (μ), kappa (κ), and delta (δ). Opioid receptor nomenclature has evolved over the years as shown in Table 11.1 [6,7]. There are variants of the μ opioid receptor which may explain the relative species sensitivity to opioid adverse effects, including dysphoria, or the relative insensitivity to opioid adverse effects. Alternative splicing may produce differences in the structure and function of the receptor despite the receptors being produced from the same gene [8]. A specific strain of mice (CXBX) are 5–10-fold less sensitive to morphine, but are similarly sensitive as 'standard' mice (CD1) to methadone, heroin, and fentanyl, suggesting different opioid receptor subtypes [8]. Additionally, single nucleotide polymorphisms (SNP) have been identified in dogs which may also increase the diversity in receptor structure and function, resulting in altered drug effects. For example, a SNP has been identified with high prevalence in dogs experiencing dysphoria in association with opioid administration [9]. Therefore different sensitivities to μ opioids (pharmacodynamic variability) may be due in part to individual differences in the types of μ opioid receptor subtypes. The original Greek nomenclature, the most widely accepted system in the medical literature, is one of the nomenclature systems currently

Veterinary Anesthesia and Analgesia: The Fifth Edition of Lumb and Jones.
Edited by Kurt A. Grimm, Leigh A. Lamont, William J. Tranquilli, Stephen A. Greene and Sheilah A. Robertson.

Table 11.1 Opioid receptor nomenclature.

Anatomic and pharmacologic classification using Greek nomenclature 1977	IUPHAR 1996	IUPHAR 2013
Vas deferens (*d*elta)	OP1	δ, delta, DOP
*K*etocyclazocine (*k*appa)	OP2	κ, kappa, KOP
*M*orphine (*mu*)	OP3	μ, mu, MOP
	OP4	NOP

IUPHAR = International Union of Pharmacology.

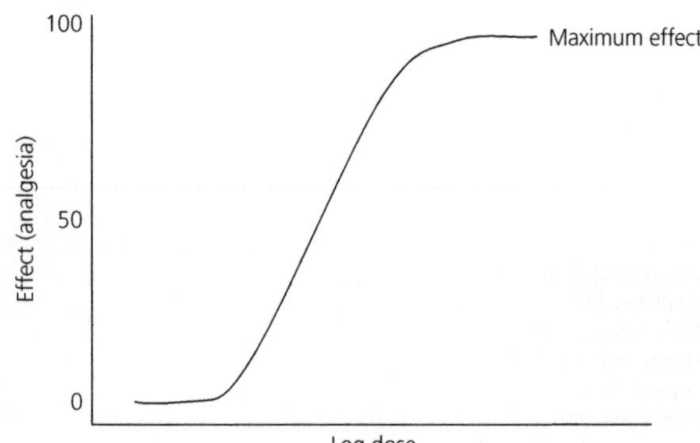

Figure 11.1 A typical dose–response curve for an opioid. The effect increases as the dose (or plasma concentration) increases until it plateaus at a maximum effect. This dose–response curve could represent fentanyl.

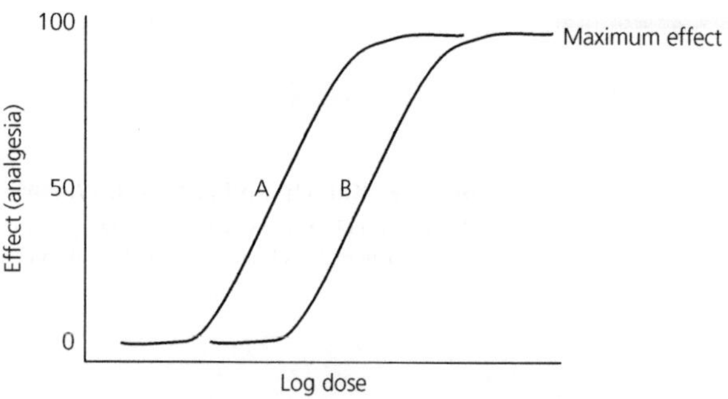

Figure 11.2 Dose–response curves for two opioids with equal efficacy but different potencies. This example could represent morphine (*line B*) and fentanyl (*line A*). The dose of fentanyl needed to achieve a desired analgesic effect is lower, but the analgesic effects of fentanyl and morphine will be similar.

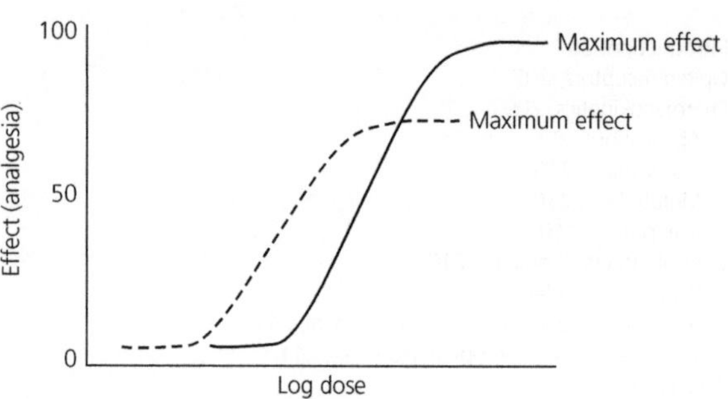

Figure 11.3 Dose–response curves for two opioids with different efficacies and potencies. This example could represent morphine (*solid line*) and buprenorphine (*dashed line*). Despite buprenorphine being a more potent drug, the maximum analgesic effect of morphine is greater.

supported by the International Union of Pharmacology (IUPHAR), and will be the nomenclature system used in this chapter.

The nociception/orphanin FQ receptor, so named for its endogenous ligand, is often referred to as the N/OFQ [NOP] receptor in the medical literature [10,11]. This receptor possesses significant homology to other opioid receptors although naloxone hydrochloride does not have significant antagonistic action at this receptor. The N/OFQ [NOP] receptor has been investigated but details of the interactions of the endogenous ligand(s) with the receptor and the clinical implications of the N/OFQ [NOP] receptor are not well described. Interestingly, antagonists of the N/OFQ [NOP] receptor produce analgesia and may be a target for future development of analgesics or analgesic adjuncts. β-Endorphin is the primary endogenous ligand for the μ opioid receptor; leucine- and methionine-enkephalin are the primary endogenous ligands for the κ opioid receptor; and dynorphin A is the primary endogenous ligand for the δ opioid receptor.

Opioid-class drugs can be further classified by the receptor or receptors they interact with as well as the effect elicited (e.g., concentration- or dose–response relationship). A full agonist will produce a dose-dependent increase in effect until maximum stimulation of the receptor is achieved (Figs 11.1 and 11.2). A partial agonist produces a dose-dependent increase in effect, but plateaus at a maximum effect less than the maximum effect of a full agonist (Fig. 11.3).

An antagonist binds to a receptor with high affinity; however, it produces no effect and inhibits the binding of agonists (both endogenous and exogenous). Administration of an antagonist will therefore 'reverse' the receptor-mediated effects of an agonist by inhibiting binding of the agonist and displacing previously bound agonists due to the greater receptor affinity of the antagonist. Most opioid receptor antagonists are considered competitive antagonists based on their lack of intrinsic activity and the ability for high concentrations of agonists to overcome their effect to produce a maximal effect (the dose–response curve is shifted to the right). Administration of a partial agonist can act as an antagonist by partially reversing the effects of a full agonist (shifting the dose–response curve to the right) and may be preferred over an antagonist such as naloxone if some analgesia is still desired.

The potency of an opioid simply describes the relative dose needed to elicit a response, most commonly analgesia (measured as a change in latency of withdrawal or increased threshold to a noxious stimulus) for opioids. For example, fentanyl is more potent than morphine, which means the dose of fentanyl (0.01 mg/kg) needed to produce an equivalent analgesic response to morphine (1 mg/kg) is lower (see Fig. 11.2). Note that potency does not describe duration of effect or efficacy. In the example of fentanyl (0.01 mg/kg) and morphine (1 mg/kg), both opioids produce equivalent maximal analgesic effects. The duration of fentanyl analgesia is expected to be approximately 1 h or less depending on the dose, but morphine may last as long as 4–6 h depending on the dose [12]. While fentanyl and morphine can be equally efficacious analgesics since both are μ opioid agonists, the typical dose of morphine is 100-fold greater than that of fentanyl since morphine is less potent than fentanyl.

Opioid receptors are located throughout the body, including the brain, spinal cord, chemoreceptor trigger zone, gastrointestinal tract, synovium, urinary tract, leukocytes, and uterus, among other tissues. Therefore it is not surprising to observe widespread effects of systemically administered opioids (see section on pharmacodynamics). Opioid receptors are Gi-protein coupled receptors with proposed molecular effects that include inhibition of adenylyl cyclase, decreased formation of cyclic adenosine monophosphate (cAMP), inhibition of Ca^{2+} channels in presynaptic neurons resulting in decreased release of excitatory neurotransmitters (e.g., glutamate and substance P), and enhancement of cellular potassium (K^+) outflow in postsynaptic neurons resulting in hyperpolarization of nociceptive neurons and nociceptors and increased activation thresholds.

Pharmacokinetics

Pharmacokinetics describes what the animal's body does to a drug. The absorption, distribution, metabolism (biotransformation), and elimination (ADME) are typical processes described with pharmacokinetics. Pharmacokinetic studies are useful in estimating the rate and extent of drug absorption, the plasma concentrations achieved with a given dose in a given species or patient population, the persistence of drug after a given dose, and sometimes the potential for drug interactions. Some pharmacokinetic parameter estimates of commonly used opioids in healthy dogs and cats are presented in Table 11.2.

Absorption

Opioids are lipophilic compounds so they are typically well absorbed when administered intramuscularly (IM), subcutaneously (SC) or *per os* (PO). However, PO administration usually results in substantial first-pass metabolism for many opioid drugs and as a result, opioids generally have low oral bioavailability and may be ineffective when administered by this route at standard doses. An exception is that some drugs can produce active metabolites (e.g., codeine in humans).

First-pass metabolism occurs when drugs are absorbed from the gastrointestinal system (usually following oral administration). As drugs pass through the mucosa, intestinal metabolizing enzymes (both Phase I metabolic reactions and Phase II conjugation reactions) can biotransform the drug before it enters the intestinal capillary system. If the drug enters the intestinal capillaries intact, it then enters the portal vein and liver where further metabolism occurs. Any drug that makes it through the liver intact can enter the systemic circulation and be distributed to elicit an effect. Therefore, despite a large fraction of the opioid being absorbed, a relatively small amount enters the systemic circulation in an active form where interactions with opioid receptors can elicit an effect. Opioids administered by IM and SC routes tend to be absorbed rapidly and with a high bioavailability. Unless sustained-release (SR) formulations are used (e.g., buprenorphine SR intended for SC administration), a prolonged effect (compared to IV) is not typically expected from IM or SC administration.

Transdermal administration bypasses the gastrointestinal tract and does not lead to first-pass metabolism. However, the stratum corneum presents a substantial barrier to drug absorption for some drugs. Fentanyl has chemical characteristics which suggest that transdermal absorption can result in useful drug concentrations and a transdermal fentanyl solution is approved for use in dogs and transdermal fentanyl patches designed for human skin are occasionally used off-label in some veterinary species. However, not all fentanyl preparations are absorbed well transdermally which is demonstrated by some pluronic lecithin organogel (PLO) formulations of fentanyl [13–15]. Other opioids will usually be poorly absorbed by the transdermal route unless a specially designed vehicle or formulation is used which facilitates movement across the dermal layers. Therefore transdermal products should only be recommended for veterinary patients if data exist to support the use of that specific product, and compounding of products should be limited to cases where sufficient pharmacokinetics studies have been performed.

Transmucosal drug administration is another route of administration that bypasses first-pass metabolism. The mucosal barrier is thinner and more vascular than the stratum corneum and is therefore less of a barrier. The oral transmucosal uptake of buprenorphine has been assessed in several species including the cat, dog, and horse [16–21]. Buprenorphine is lipophilic and can be absorbed by this route; however, it is only effective if the drug is not swallowed. Some data suggest transmucosal buprenorphine may be a viable route in cats, but it is still somewhat variable due to conditions (e.g., pH) that can alter its chemical properties [19,20]. The extent of transmucosal buprenorphine absorption in dogs is relatively small and may not be a practical route of delivery in this species due to volume and cost limitations, although preclinical pain models have demonstrated some efficacy [16,22]. A more complete discussion of buprenorphine is included later in this chapter.

Table 11.2 Selected pharmacokinetic parameters of some opioids in dogs and cats.

	T½ (h)		Cl (mL/min/kg)		Vd (L/kg)		Oral %F	
	Dogs	Cats	Dogs	Cats	Dogs	Cats	Dogs	Cats
Morphine	1.2	1.3	60	24	4	2.6	5–20%	
Oxymorphone	0.8	1.6	52	26	3.7	2.5		
Hydromorphone	1.0	1.6	68	28	4.5	3.1		
Fentanyl	3–6	~2.5	35	20	10	2.6		
Meperidine (Pethidine)	0.8	1.8	43	40	1.9	4.0	11%	
Methadone	2–4		30		3.5		<5%	
Oxycodone (PO data only)	1.9						low	
Hydrocodone	1.7		41		5.0		40–84%	
Codeine	1.5		36		3.2		4%	
Buprenorphine	5	6.9	16	16	17.5	7.1	3–6%	
Butorphanol (IM data only)	1.6	6.6	57	12.7	8.0	7.7	<20%	
Nalbuphine	1.2		46		4.6		5.6%	
Tramadol	0.8	2.2	55	20.8	3.0	3.0	<10%	93

T½ = terminal half-life; Cl = plasma clearance; Vd = volume of distribution; %F = fraction of the dose absorbed (bioavailability); PO = per os; IM = intramuscular. For IM data Cl and Vd are calculated per fraction of the dose absorbed.

Distribution

Opioids are lipophilic compounds; therefore they are capable of diffusing throughout the body. The primary effect site of opioids is the central nervous system (CNS) for analgesia, antitussive effects, and sedation. Therefore the drug must penetrate into the CNS to elicit these effects. Most clinically useful opioids do penetrate the CNS well, but the P-glycoprotein efflux pump (an active transporter) can efflux absorbed drug from the CNS back into the vasculature, in part limiting central effects. For example, loperamide is a μ opioid agonist used clinically as an antidiarrheal that initially diffuses well throughout the body, including into the CNS. However, once loperamide diffuses across the capillary membrane into the CNS, the P-glycoprotein efflux pumps transport it back into the vasculature, limiting its ability to elicit a central effect in most animals. An exception is in animals deficient in functional P-glycoprotein efflux pumps, such as dogs with homozygous mutations in the gene (MDR1) expressing P-glycoprotein efflux pumps (e.g., 'ivermectin sensitive' Collies) [23]. These dogs exhibit significant central effects of loperamide including heavy sedation which can be reversed by administration of the opioid antagonist naloxone. Morphine, methadone, fentanyl, buprenorphine, and oxycodone have been shown in humans or rodents to be substrates for P-glycoprotein but the extent of their transport by the canine P-glycoprotein is not reported [25–27]. When using known MDR1 substrates in heterozygote or homozygote MDR1 gene mutation carriers, increased duration and intensity of effect may be recognized, although many factors can contribute to the individual variability in patient response to opioids.

Distribution is also affected by relative regional blood flow of tissues and organs. Intravenous bolus administration of a drug results in the highest plasma concentrations at the end of the bolus dose and then plasma drug concentrations decrease over time due to drug metabolism and elimination and movement of drug from the plasma into the tissues. Some tissues have a high ratio of blood flow to organ mass (e.g., brain, liver, kidney, lungs, heart, endocrine glands) and are often referred to as well-perfused or vessel-rich tissues. Since these tissues receive the greatest blood flow per tissue mass, equilibrium between plasma concentrations and tissue concentrations occurs the most rapidly (assuming the drug is highly lipophilic and rapidly crosses the lipid tissue barriers). Since equilibrium occurs the most rapidly, equilibrium occurs at relatively higher plasma concentrations than in tissue less well perfused and as a result the peak effect in the tissues occurs rapidly after IV drug administration (Fig. 11.4). After equilibrium is reached between the well-perfused tissue plasma, tissue concentrations drop due to metabolism and distribution to less well-perfused tissues. Clinically, the phenomenon results in a loss of effect (due to drug movement out of the CNS) more rapidly than predicted by the elimination half-life. As an example, fentanyl has a short duration of effect after intravenous administration, typically less than an hour depending on the dose and duration of administration, despite a terminal half-life in the range of 3–4 h (see Fentanyl).

Morphine is not nearly as lipophilic as fentanyl and as such, peak effects may not occur until about 45 min after IV injection due to slower movement into the CNS limited by the drug's lipophilicity. However, clinically relevant effects can occur within 5–15 min so use as a perioperative analgesic is reasonable (see Morphine). The slower distribution into and out of the CNS can be advantageous as epidural injection of morphine can produce a longer duration of effect due to the much higher concentrations of morphine achieved at the spinal opioid receptors and the slower distribution out of the CNS.

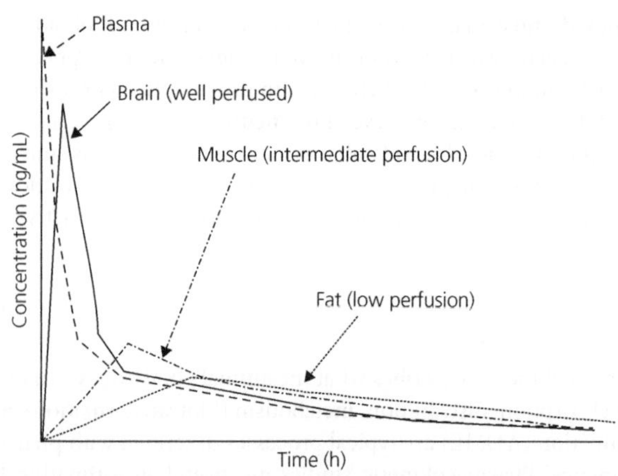

Figure 11.4 Distribution is affected by the relative regional blood flow of tissues and organs. Intravenous bolus administration of a drug results in the highest plasma concentrations at the end of the bolus administration. The plasma concentrations then decrease rapidly due to drug metabolism and excretion, and movement of drug from the plasma into the tissues (redistribution). Some tissues have a high ratio of blood flow to organ mass (well perfused) and equilibrium between the plasma and tissue occurs rapidly. Other tissues with less blood flow per unit mass, but which comprise a large amount of total body mass (e.g. skeletal muscle) or which have a high capacity for lipophilic compounds (adipose tissue), can play a significant role in termination of CNS action by absorbing drug that leaves the CNS. This redistribution of the drug may play a greater role than metabolism in termination of CNS effects for some anesthetic and analgesic drugs.

Metabolism

Most opioids undergo extensive metabolism in mammalian species. Opioids can undergo Phase I and/or Phase II metabolism depending on the specific drug and species. For example, most species metabolize morphine by Phase II glucuronide conjugation to morphine-3-glucuronide but the cat, which is relatively deficient in some types of glucuronidase action, still rapidly and efficiently eliminates morphine by sulfate conjugation [28,29]. Remifentanil is different compared to the other opioids as it is hydrolyzed by plasma esterases, independent of hepatic metabolism (see Remifentanil). Opioid metabolites in general are less potent (or there may be complete loss of activity) than the parent drug. Although morphine-6-glucuronide is often cited as an active metabolite of morphine, it must be given by intracerebroventricular injection to elicit an effect as it is not lipophilic enough to effectively penetrate the CNS to produce a central effect. There are few reported drug–drug metabolism interactions in veterinary patients, but chloramphenicol can significantly decrease the metabolism of methadone in dogs [30].

Elimination

Opioids are typically metabolized prior to elimination in mammalian species, although some excretion of parent drug can occur via the urine or feces. Opioid metabolites are usually more water soluble and are often eliminated in the urine but they can be eliminated in the feces by biliary secretion as well.

Clinical effects of opioids

Variability of effects

Although the effects and common doses of opioids are routinely referenced, it is important to recognize the large variability in their effects in a patient population. This variability can be due to individual pharmacodynamic and pharmacokinetic differences, as well as any number of other potential environmental, behavioral, genetic, sex, and breed differences which can alter the patient's response. Therefore variability should be expected in patients of different breeds, with different degrees and causes of pain, different concurrent diseases and administered a variety of concurrent medications. The dosage of an opioid should be titrated for each specific patient with recommended dosages used only as a guideline or starting point. For example, a commonly published dose of morphine in dogs is 0.5 mg/kg IV q 6 h. However, if the patient is still painful after administration, the dose may need to be increased or the dosing interval may need to be reduced. Likewise, if adverse effects occur (e.g., profound sedation) but analgesia is adequate, either the dose can be lowered or the dosing interval extended. Use of variable rate intravenous infusions can facilitate dose titration in patients which are likely to have variable requirements or are at risk of significant adverse effects (e.g., following severe trauma). Pharmacogenetic differences may also be responsible for individual animal and species variability in response to opioid therapy, for example opioid-induced dysphoria in dogs [9].

Tolerance, dependence, and withdrawal

Tolerance is the loss of *in vivo* potency (i.e., shifting of the dose–response curve to the right) of a drug or therapy over time. As a result of tolerance, higher doses of opioids may be needed in order to achieve a similar effect. Although tolerance is a well-recognized phenomenon of opioid administration in humans, it is not as well recognized clinically in veterinary patients. However, experimentally, tolerance and withdrawal can be observed in animals [31,32]. Drug dependence in humans can be physical or psychological. While psychological dependence in veterinary species appears rare or non-existent, physical dependence may occur although it would appear to be less common than in people. Signs of withdrawal include lethargy, anorexia, nausea, vomiting, aggression, muscle twitching, and muscle weakness. Dogs administered μ opioid agonists for periods of 7 days or more could display signs of opioid withdrawal if they are given a drug that can reverse the μ opioid effects (i.e., partial μ agonists, μ antagonist/κ agonist combinations or μ antagonists) (BK, personal observation).

The effect of pain on opioid response

Many preclinical studies of opioids are conducted in healthy animals without naturally occurring pain, although the effect opioids elicit in a clinical patient with naturally occurring pain may be different. The presence of pain may blunt some of the undesired effects of opioids in animals. For example, morphine routinely may cause vomiting and dysphoria (which is dose and route dependent) when administered to healthy dogs. However, vomiting and dysphoria are less frequently observed in painful dogs. Similarly, in painful feline patients, sedation or euphoria is the common effect of morphine and dysphoria is rarely observed under these circumstances.

Analgesia

The most common indication for opioid administration is pain management (i.e., hypoalgesia or analgesia). Morphine is considered the prototypical opioid analgesic (Table 11.3). Opioids (μ, κ, and δ) decrease the release of excitatory neurotransmitters and hypopolarize nociceptors, resulting in decreased transmission within the spinal cord. Supraspinal effects of opioids (e.g., analgesia, sedation, altered thermoregulation, and respiratory depression) have been described with microinjection of morphine into various brain sites [33]. Perhaps the best described supraspinal area contributing to analgesia is the periaqueductal gray (PAG) region [34]. Binding of opioid agonists to receptors within the PAG results in inhibition of γ-amino butyric acid (GABA) interneurons leading to activation of medullary pathways that selectively inhibit dorsal horn nociceptive neurons. In the bulbospinal pathways, this results in release of norepinephrine and serotonin in the dorsal horn of the spinal cord. Spinally mediated analgesic effects of opioids, as discussed previously, are mediated by inhibition of presynaptic neurotransmitter release and postsynaptic hyperpolarization of neuronal membranes leading to decreased excitability. Analgesic effects related to peripheral opioid administration (e.g., intra-articular morphine) are mediated through more localized peripheral opioid receptors, an effect that is naloxone reversible [35]. Peripheral opioid receptors appear to be activated and upregulated by trauma or inflammation and can be targeted by local administration of opioids to produce an analgesic effect [36,37]. Intra-articular opioids reduce nerve terminal excitability of primary afferents with enhanced spontaneous activity, as observed in inflamed joints, and provide some mild anti-inflammatory effects [38]. Thus, peripherally opioids act as antihyperalgesics.

Systemic analgesic doses of opioids are more effective at decreasing pain transmitted by C-fiber nociceptors (the slow-conducting, unmyelinated nerves associated with dull aching pain) than by A-δ fibers (fast-conducting, myelinated nerves associated with sharp, discrete pain). This is the reason why analgesic doses of opioids used alone may not produce effective analgesia (anesthesia) for surgical stimulation. High intravenous doses or epidural administration

Table 11.3 Opioid receptors and their associated effects when activated by an appropriate opioid agonist.

μ Opioid receptor	κ Opioid receptor	δ Opioid receptor
• Analgesia (spinal & supraspinal) • Antidiuresis • Decreased biliary secretions • Decreased gastrointestinal propulsive motility • Decreased gastrointestinal secretions • Decreased urine voiding reflex • Decreased uterine contractions • Emesis/antiemesis (drug specific) • Euphoria • Immunomodulation • Increased appetite • Miosis/mydriasis (species specific) • Respiratory depression • Sedation	• Analgesia (spinal & supraspinal) • Decreased gastrointestinal propulsive motility • Decreased gastrointestinal secretions • Diuresis (inhibits antidiuretic hormone release) • Increased appetite • Miosis/mydriasis (species specific) • Sedation	• Analgesia (spinal & supraspinal) • Immunomodulation • Increased appetite

(which saturate spinal opioid receptors at the site of administration) result in effects on both C-fiber and A-δ fiber nociceptors. High doses of opioids such as fentanyl are capable of producing anesthesia (unconsciousness) in humans, but are accompanied by significant adverse effects such as profound respiratory depression. Use of very high doses of opioids by themselves is usually unsatisfactory for producing surgical anesthesia in dogs and cats, although clinically recommended dosages can result in significant anesthetic-sparing effects in most situations. Despite saturable effects at spinal opioid receptors, epidural opioids will not prevent transmission of all tactile and nociceptive input (an effect that can be produced by appropriate doses of local anesthetics) and thus will blunt the nociceptive response to surgery, but not block all surgical stimulation.

Full μ agonists (e.g., morphine, hydromorphone, fentanyl, remifentanil, alfentanil, oxymorphone, and methadone) produce the most profound analgesic effects. The partial μ agonist buprenorphine produces a clinically useful analgesic effect that is generally less profound than a full μ agonist and as such is only expected to be useful for mild to moderate pain. However, clinical studies suggest that buprenorphine may be as effective as full opioid agonists (e.g., morphine) for some types of pain in cats and horses with fewer adverse effects [39–43]. Butorphanol is generally considered to be a μ antagonist and κ agonist with relatively modest analgesic effects. However, some reports show that butorphanol may produce more profound analgesic effects than buprenorphine in certain species such as some birds[44], although studies are conflicting in cats, horses, and rodents [42,45,46]. Generally butorphanol has less of an effect than a full μ agonist opioid [47]. It has a 'reputation' of being a less effective drug in dogs but the lack of efficacy is often due to an inappropriately low dose being administered (0.4 mg/kg has been recommended as an appropriate dose)[48,49] or due to its short duration of action (dose dependent) which is typically less than 2 h.

Sedation and excitation

Opioids typically produce dose-dependent sedation when administered alone, but can produce more profound sedation when combined with other sedatives such as phenothiazines and α_2-adrenergic receptor agonists. However, higher doses of opioids or rapid IV administration (producing high plasma concentrations quickly) may produce excitation. Some species, for example the cat and horse [50–53], appear more likely to exhibit excitatory and dysphoric effects with opioids than others (e.g., dog, pig). Breed may also influence how a patient responds (e.g., northern breed dogs such as Huskies often vocalize). The issue of CNS excitation and behavioral effects of opioids in horses has been complicated by reports and investigational studies where clinically irrelevant doses of opioids were administered. The reader is referred to articles addressing the use of opioid analgesics in horses with consideration of dose and behavioral effects [54,55].

Rapid IV administration of opioids produces high concentrations initially, even at clinically appropriate doses, and can produce a transient excitement in any species. Excitation usually occurs within a few minutes but is often short-lived. In contrast, dysphoria may last for hours and can include hypersensitivity, thrashing, ataxia, and vocalization. Confounding factors such as other drugs (e.g., anesthetics and sedatives), uncontrolled or poorly recognized pain, and underlying behavioral differences may contribute to dysphoria in individual dogs. Recently, a single nucleotide polymorphism in the μ opioid receptor has been identified and has been reported to occur with a greater prevalence in dogs displaying opioid-associated dysphoria [9]. Although dysphoria is often recognized clinically in dogs, comprehensive studies or comparisons between opioids are not available in peer-reviewed literature.

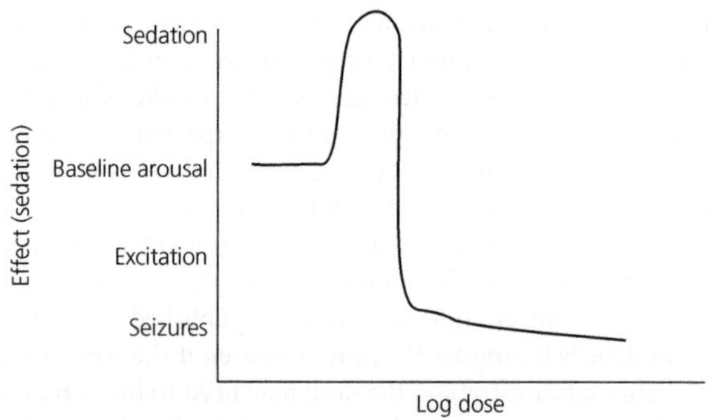

Figure 11.5 The expected dose–response curve for the sedative effects of opioids. Although initial increases in opioid doses produce increasing sedation, some species will respond to ever increasing doses with excitation and finally seizures with massive overdosages. Cats and horses are two species that are more likely to manifest the excitatory effects of opioids.

High (supratherapeutic) doses of opioids in cats and horses can also produce excitement similar to that seen in dogs and may last for hours (Fig. 11.5).

Although cats and horses are often noted as being species in which opioids routinely produce CNS stimulation, this is not necessarily the case. Due to pharmacokinetic differences in cats (a smaller volume of distribution), a dose of 0.2 mg/kg morphine produces similar plasma concentrations as 0.5 mg/kg in the dog and as such, lower doses of morphine (compared to dogs) are often well tolerated in cats and rarely produce CNS excitation (especially in the presence of pain) [56,57]. Additionally, in one study 'morphine mania' was consistently produced in cats with IV doses of 20 mg/kg which is 100 times the clinically recommended dose. However, doses less than 5 mg/kg IV failed to produce excitatory responses in cats [50] and doses up to 2 mg/kg IV (ten times the clinically recommended dose) have been reported to be well tolerated in cats with no excitation noted [58]. Clinically relevant doses of 0.2 mg/kg IV did not produce dysphoria or excitement but rather signs of euphoria (increased affection, purring, kneading) in non-painful cats assessed with thermal and mechanical threshold [59]. Similarly in horses, the clinically recommended dose of morphine is 0.1–0.2 mg/kg, which produces plasma concentrations similar to 0.5 mg/kg in dogs. It is generally well tolerated and excitation is not routinely observed. Higher doses of opioids in horses reliably produce excitation or stimulation. Morphine at doses of 0.6–0.66 mg/kg, almost 2.5 times the recommended dose, has been shown to produce excitement [53,60].

Another manifestation of opioid-induced neuroexcitation in horses is increased locomotor activity. Horses administered μ opioid agonists show characteristic pacing and weaving patterns. Opioid agonist-antagonists also produce increased locomotor activity which is often accompanied by ataxia [61,62]. Increased dopamine release in the brain has been suggested as a possible mechanism for increased locomotor activity. Drugs that decrease dopamine release show some efficacy at reducing step counts; however, administration of specific DA1 and DA2 receptor antagonists was not successful in significantly reducing activity [63,64].

Respiratory depression

Opioids cause a dose-dependent respiratory depression in most veterinary species, but in conscious animals it typically plateaus at a level that does not warrant intervention. During anesthesia, opioids contribute to respiratory depression associated with other drugs (e.g., inhalant anesthetics). Adequate patient monitoring allows early detection of significant respiratory depression and allows better patient management during the anesthetic period. Respiratory depression is characterized by increased $PaCO_2$ and is primarily mediated by supraspinal μ opioid receptors. It is important to differentiate a drop in respiratory rate (breaths per minute) versus true respiratory depression (decreased alveolar minute ventilation). Respiratory rate can be depressed but not result in respiratory depression if tidal volume increases to maintain alveolar minute ventilation. Clinically relevant doses of opioids usually produce minor effects in veterinary species and rarely result in adverse events in healthy animals [65–68]. However, animals administered concurrent potent respiratory depressants such as anesthetics, animals with underlying moderate to severe respiratory disease, and animals with increased intracranial pressure (e.g., head trauma or intracranial neoplasia) would be at increased risk for respiratory depression. However, even in these high-risk patients, the respiratory depressant effects of opioids are less than that reported in humans and are not an absolute contraindication for opioid use provided monitoring is appropriate. Opioid-related respiratory depression can be fatal in humans, but fatalities are rare in animals unless patient monitoring is inadequate or serious neurological disease is present.

Increased chest wall rigidity, or so-called 'wooden chest' syndrome, has been described in human pediatric and adult patients administered large doses of μ opioid agonists [69,70]. While not commonly reported in the veterinary literature, clinically similar syndromes have been observed by the authors in dogs. Experimentally, supratherapeutic doses of fentanyl (20–60 μg/kg IV) decrease inspiratory, and increase and prolong expiratory neuron activity (tonic discharges), resulting in increased excitatory drive to intercostal interneurons and abdominal motor neurons that control chest wall compliance. The increase in intercostal and abdominal muscle tension leads to an increase in chest wall rigidity and decreased thoracic wall compliance. Similar effects are produced on pharyngeal constrictor and motor neurons and result in tonic vocal fold closure and pharyngeal obstruction of airflow, consequently increasing airflow resistance and resting abdominal musculature wall tension [71].

Opioids readily cross the placental barrier and effects on the fetus are expected if opioids are administered prior to a cesarean section. Therefore, monitoring of neonates for opioid effects is recommended and naloxone (an opioid antagonist) can be administered if needed.

Antitussive effects

Opioids produce their antitussive effects directly at the cough center in the medulla oblongata by actions at both μ and κ opioid receptors. Opioids are considered the prototypical antitussives and many are highly effective. Clinically, the antitussive effects of opioids are notable, for example, increased endotracheal tube tolerance. Opioid and benzodiazepine combinations may be used as an anesthetic induction technique to allow endotracheal intubation in certain species and clinical settings (e.g., sick or debilitated dogs) and to increase tolerance to the endotracheal tube in the postanesthetic and intensive care setting. Opioid receptor agonists (often in combination with phenothiazines or α_2-adrenergic receptor agonists) can also be used to facilitate standing procedures (e.g., laryngoscopy or transtracheal lavage) in large animals [72–74]. The antitussive effects are independent of respiratory depressant effects and can occur with no detectable depression in respiration. Antitussive effects are also independent of analgesic effects. Butorphanol tablets (Torbutrol®, Food and Drug Administration approved for dogs) and hydrocodone are some of the most commonly used oral opioid antitussives in veterinary practice. Co-phenotrope (Lomotil®), a combination of the opioid diphenoxylate and atropine, has gained popularity in the medical management of tracheal collapse in dogs. Other options include codeine and dihydrocodeine which have variable efficacy.

Cardiovascular effects

In animals, clinically relevant doses of opioids have minor direct effects on the cardiovascular system [65,75]. Bradycardia commonly occurs in dogs as a result of centrally mediated enhanced parasympathetic activity in neurons innervating the heart, but administration of antimuscarinics (e.g., atropine or glycopyrrolate) can block or reverse this effect. During mild bradycardia, cardiac output is usually maintained by an increased stroke volume. This typically results in a beneficial or protective effect on the heart due to less work and oxygen consumption. Caution is advised in allowing heart rate to markedly decrease as a result of opioid administration, particularly in young animals (where cardiac output is more heart rate dependent) and during general anesthesia since cardiac output may decrease as heart rate decreases. Treatment with an antimuscarinic to increase heart rate will restore and may even increase cardiac output [76]. Awake horses and cats may show no change, or an increase in heart rate when given opioids. However, when administered during general anesthesia, a decrease in heart rate may occur in cats whereas the heart rate in horses tends not to change. The vascular effects of opioids are usually minimal, with minor increases or decreases in systemic vascular resistance and blood pressure occurring. High doses of morphine (3 mg/kg IV; six times the clinically recommended dose) in pentobarbital anesthetized dogs produced more profound effects resulting in a marked decrease in blood pressure, but this was not associated with mortality in healthy dogs [77].

Part of the observed effect seen with high doses of morphine in dogs is thought to be mediated by histamine release from mast cells. Circulating histamine levels can be increased 800-fold following 3 mg/kg of morphine given IV. Mast cell degranulation and histamine release with associated hemodynamic and anaphylactic responses (hypotension, tachycardia, bronchospasm) are dependent on the opioid administered, dose, and route of administration, with rapid intravenous injection being the most provocative method for triggering histamine release [75,78–81]. Histamine release has also been linked to the development of arachnoid membrane granulomas following intrathecal morphine administration in dogs [82,83]. Histamine release and granuloma formation is not opioid receptor mediated (it is not reversible with opioid antagonists) but can be managed with mast cell stabilizers (e.g., cromolyn) [83]. Clinically relevant doses of morphine (0.5 mg/kg IV or less) in healthy dogs usually produce no detrimental effect on mean arterial blood pressure [75,78,79]. Administration of 1 mg/kg IV morphine has been shown to result in significant release of histamine, but hypotension did not occur. Therefore morphine can be safely administered as a slow IV bolus (0.25–0.5 mg/kg) in healthy dogs. The effects of IV morphine on histamine release in dogs with mast cell tumors have not been reported and until such data are available, it may be wise to either administer morphine by IM or SC routes or use another opioid.

The cardiovascular effects of opioids are more pronounced when administered concurrently with drugs that affect cardiac output (anesthetics) and vascular resistance (phenothiazines, α_2-adrenergic receptor agonists). However, the overall effects are still minor and profound changes in cardiac output, systemic vascular resistance, and blood pressure are more likely due to the other drugs administered and not the opioid itself.

Nausea, emetic, and antiemetic effects

Opioids can produce either emetic or antiemetic effects depending on the opioid, dose, and route of administration. Emetic effects of opioids occur when dopamine receptors within the chemoreceptor trigger zone are stimulated. The δ receptor appears to be involved in the emetic effect whereas the μ and/or κ receptors may be involved in antiemetic effects [84]. Ileus can occur with opioids which can result in nausea and vomiting independent of direct stimulation of the emetic pathway; in these cases a prokinetic drug (e.g., metoclopramide, cisapride) may be useful for controlling emesis. Maropitant, a neurokinin 1 receptor antagonist, administered 1 h prior to opioid administration can reduce the incidence of emesis, retching, and clinical signs of nausea in dogs by preventing binding of substance P to neurokinin 1 receptors in the emetic center in the brain [85].

Low doses of morphine tend to produce an emetic effect through stimulation of dopamine receptors in the chemoreceptor trigger zone. Higher doses or multiple doses of morphine tend to produce an antiemetic effect (e.g., emesis can occur with the first morphine dose, but subsequently an antiemetic effect is more prominent). Fentanyl, butorphanol, and methadone tend to produce a more prominent antiemetic effect which may be related to faster penetration into the CNS and inhibition of the emetic center [86–88]. The route of administration also appears to influence the likelihood of emesis, with subcutaneous or intramuscular administration of opioids more likely to result in emesis than the intravenous route [89]. Prior administration of acepromazine significantly reduces the likelihood of opioid-induced emesis in dogs [90].

Pupil diameter

The effects of opioids on pupil diameter vary between individuals and species. In general, dogs, rabbits, and rats tend to exhibit miosis caused by increased outflow in parasympathetic neurons leaving the Edinger-Westphal nucleus. These parasympathetic neurons innervate the sphincter pupillae (constrictor) muscle, leading to contraction of the iris [91]. Cats, horses, and ruminants tend to exhibit mydriasis, an effect that is incompletely understood but likely due to both a peripherally driven, sympathetically mediated response generated by the release of catecholamines from the adrenal glands acting on the pupil and a central component, possibly at the Edinger-Westphal nucleus [92,93]. The effect on the pupil may be masked by concurrent drug administration (e.g., anticholinergic agents) or by endogenous catecholamine release (e.g., stress response or pain). Therefore pupillary effects of opioids are not specific and are quite variable.

Gastrointestinal motility

Gastrointestinal (GI) motility is controlled by the myenteric plexus and is dependent upon neurotransmitters released from enteric neurons. The major neurotransmitters include acetylcholine (ACh), serotonin (5-HT), vasoactive intestinal peptide (VIP), and nitric oxide (NO). ACh activates the cholinergic excitatory motor neurons while NO and VIP control the non-cholinergic inhibitory motor neurons. Together, the balance between ACh and NO plus VIP release coordinates contractile and propulsive gut motility. Opioids inhibit the release of these motility-modifying neurotransmitters, thereby impairing coordination of motility and inhibition of colonic (morphine) and jejunal (butorphanol) motility [94]. Opioids can produce effects on gastrointestinal motility by both peripheral (μ receptor) and central (μ and κ receptor) mechanisms. The primary effects of opioids on the intestinal tract include decreased propulsive contractions, increased non-propulsive contractions (enhancing fluid absorption), and decreased GI fluid secretions. These effects are thought to be mediated by a decrease in the release of acetylcholine and substance P. The net effect of these actions is either a constipating or antidiarrheal effect depending on the condition of the GI tract. Opioids can also increase the tone of the stomach antrum and duodenum and as such can make passage of an endoscope more difficult for some clinicians. The effect of μ opioid receptors on the bile duct is dose dependent, with increased bile duct tone and increased bile duct sphincter tone observed with low doses and decreased tone at high dose [95,96]. While sphincter of Oddi spasm and increased gall bladder pressure are documented side-effects of μ opioid agonists, the clinical relevance of this in biliary surgery remains uncertain.

Although dogs and cats tend to tolerate the short-term effects of opioids on the GI tract well, horses may be more profoundly affected and monitoring GI output and motility is recommended whenever opioids are administered in more than a single dose. Constipation, ileus, and obstruction are potential adverse effects of opioids in horses and can be clinically substantial. A few reviews have explored this topic specifically in horses [97,98]. Morphine decreases propulsive intestinal motility and moisture of gastrointestinal contents and in one study was associated with a four-fold greater risk of colic compared with the use of butorphanol or no opioid administration [99,100]. The correlation of reduced gastrointestinal tract motility, lower fecal production, and increased incidence of colic often leads to conservative use of opioids in horses. The data are conflicting, however, as other studies have failed to identify an increased risk for colic following opioid administration, suggesting that differences in the duration of opioid administration (single dose as a preanesthetic versus multi-day dosing) and concurrent medications may contribute to these reported adverse effects [99,101]. The gastrointestinal inhibitory effects are more profound when opioids are combined with α_2-adrenergic receptor agonists. For example, both xylazine and detomidine caused a marked reduction in intestinal motility for up to 1 h after treatment when given alone [102]. The peripherally acting opioid antagonist *N*-methylnaltrexone administered to horses partially prevented the adverse gastrointestinal effects while preserving central analgesic effects [103].

The peripherally acting opioid loperamide is an effective antidiarrheal drug despite the lack of central effects in most animals. Due to lack of central effects, loperamide is not a controlled substance and is available over the counter in the United States.

Urinary tract effects

The specific effect an opioid has on urinary tract function depends on the drug and the receptors it binds to. Urinary tract effects of systemically administered opioids are not frequently recognized in veterinary species, but can occur. Opioid agonists administered epidurally or intrathecally may cause urine retention to varying degrees due to a spinal opioid receptor-mediated decrease in detrusor muscle contraction, increased tone of urinary sphincters, and inhibition of micturition [104–106]. Morphine is associated with a longer duration of urine retention following epidural or intrathecal administration due to its longer residence time in the epidural or subarachnoid space allowing for continued spinal inhibition of micturition [104]. The incidence of urine retention following epidural administration of opioids to dogs is reported to vary from 0% to 44% [107–109] and intrathecally from 5% to 8% [110,111] and varies based on the opioid, concomitant administration of other drugs that may contribute to urine retention, and the definition of urine retention. Fewer data are available for cats but one study identified urine retention in 9% of cats that received epidural morphine in combination with bupivacaine [107]. The urodynamic effects of epidural opioids are reversible with systemically administered naloxone [112]. While these effects are thought to be more dependent on spinal than local effects, urinary retention has occurred with the peripherally acting opioid loperamide.

Mu opioid agonists decrease urine production [113]. Although the mechanism is not well defined, stimulation of arginine vasopressin (AVP, also known as antidiuretic hormone) release was demonstrated in anesthetized dogs administered large doses of fentanyl [114] whereas this effect was not apparent in anesthetized dogs given morphine [115]. The influence of opioid, dose, and anesthetic (injectable vs inhalant) may contribute to these conflicting results. In contrast, κ opioid agonists enhance urine production resulting in a diuretic response due to decreased release of AVP [116,117].

Thermoregulation

The effects of opioids on thermoregulation are species specific. Opioids tend to interfere with normal thermoregulation (e.g., produce a hypothermic response) in dogs, rabbits, and birds which can be profound with high doses or when combined with other drugs (e.g., phenothiazines and inhalant anesthetics) that have an effect on thermoregulation. Opioids appear to directly interact with neurons in the preoptic anterior hypothalamus to alter the thermoregulatory set point and compensatory responses [118]. Dogs commonly start to pant within a few minutes of opioid administration, which decreases body temperature. Body temperatures can decrease to values below 37.2–37.8°C (99–100°F) when opioids are administered at clinically appropriate dosages to conscious dogs [119,120]. There have been no reported long-term adverse effects attributed to a mild decrease in body temperature. However, much larger changes can be seen when opioids are administered at high dosages or combined with other drugs (e.g., phenothiazines, inhalant anesthetics) and temperatures can easily drop below 35°C (95°F) if thermal support and patient monitoring are inadequate. Hypothermia is associated with prolonged recovery from anesthesia which may be detrimental in specific situations [121].

Hyperthermia has also been observed after administration of opioids in cats, horses, swine, goats, and cattle. Body temperature in cats can become substantially increased with temperatures as high as 41.6 °C (107 °F) being reported [122,123]. In cats undergoing general anesthesia, hyperthermia has been noted following administration of hydromorphone, morphine, buprenorphine, and butorphanol for up to 5 h after extubation, and anesthesia combined with surgery may increase the magnitude of the hyperthermic response [123]. Therefore body temperature should be monitored in cats receiving opioids for at least 5 h following the end of anesthesia. Successful reduction in temperature following naloxone administration and lack of reduction in temperature following non-steroidal anti-inflammatory drugs support an opioid receptor-mediated mechanism for the hyperthermia [124]. Active cooling measures (removing blankets from the animal's cage, use of a fan, and/or wetting the paw pads with alcohol) may be effective for halting temperature rises and/or reducing temperature in hyperthermic animals.

Biphasic temperature changes following morphine administration are observed in mice and rats and appear to be dose related [125,126]. Immobilization of zoo and wild animals with potent opioids (e.g., etorphine, carfentanil, thiafentanil) is often associated with increases in body temperature. While it is likely that these opioids may exert an effect on the preoptic anterior hypothalamus to change the thermoregulatory set point as in domestic species, the stress response generated by capture appears to be the predominant underlying cause for the observed hyperthermia [127]. Additionally, the relative doses of opioids used for immobilization are much larger than the doses administered for analgesia so this may be a dose-dependent effect.

Immune system effects

The effects of opioids on the immune system appear to be drug, dose, and duration dependent. A complex interaction between the immune, endocrine, and autonomic nervous system is thought to be involved. Morphine suppresses natural killer cell activity, inflammatory cytokines, and mitogen-induced lymphocyte proliferation through supraspinal mechanisms [128,129]. Pain and tissue injury related to surgery produce similar immunosuppressive actions so, especially in the acute setting, administration of opioids to relieve pain likely protects against the pathologic immune effects of pain and surgery [130]. Fentanyl, remifentanil, and tramadol have protective effects on natural killer cell function by preserving and even increasing their function at some doses [131–133]. Additionally, opioid receptors are present on leukocytes and direct effects are expected. However, it is well established that pain produces immunosuppressant effects and withholding opioids worsens immune system function in a painful patient [130].

Opioids have been associated with both immunostimulatory and immunosuppressive effects. In cats acute administration of morphine (two 2 mg/kg SC doses per week) delayed the effects of experimentally induced feline immunodeficiency virus (FIV) infection [31]. A separate study assessing chronic administration of morphine with escalating doses (starting at 0.5 mg/kg SC bid increasing to a final dose of 1 mg/kg SC bid) over 21 weeks also demonstrated no negative effects on experimental FIV infection in cats and displayed some protective effects compared to untreated control animals [58].

In human patients who are chronic opioid abusers, immunosuppressive effects of opioids are routinely observed. However, it is unclear how this applies to veterinary medicine as there is no corresponding group of animals that are chronically receiving therapeutic (high) doses of opioids.

Minimum alveolar concentration (MAC) reducing effects

Opioids are capable of inhalant anesthetic MAC reduction, a phenomenon that is species, dose, and opioid receptor dependent. Opioids that act as full agonists primarily at the μ opioid receptor (e.g., morphine, fentanyl) in general produce the greatest magnitude of inhalant anesthetic-sparing effects compared to partial

Table 11.4 Morphine dosages in selected species.

	IV	IV infusion	IM/SC	PO
Dog	0.25–0.5 mg/kg q 2–4 h	0.1–0.2 mg/kg/h	0.25–1 mg/kg q 2–4 h	NR
Cat	0.1–0.25 mg/kg q 2–4 h	0.05–0.1 mg/kg/h	0.1–0.25 mg/kg q 2–4 h	NR
Horse	0.1–0.2 mg/kg q 8 h*		0.1–0.2 mg/kg q 8 h	NR
Cattle				NR
Sheep			≤10 mg total dose	NR
Goat			≤10 mg total dose	NR
Swine			0.2–0.5 mg/kg	NR
Rat/mouse			2–5 mg/kg q 4 h	NR
Guinea pig/hamster			2–5 mg/kg q 4 h	NR
Rabbit			2–5 mg/kg q 4 h	NR
Primate			0.5–2 mg/kg q 4–6 h	NR
Ferret			0.5 mg/kg q 4–6 h	NR

IV = intravenous; IM = intramuscular; SC = subcutaneous; PO = per os; NR = not recommended. * Clinically, an adult horse (450 kg) is often given 45–60 mg IV.

agonists (buprenorphine) or agonist-antagonists (butorphanol) [134]. Full opioid agonists produce dose-dependent MAC reduction in dogs although a ceiling effect is observed [135–138]. Anesthetic-sparing effects are generally accomplished with single intravenous doses of longer acting opioids (e.g., morphine, hydromorphone, oxymorphone) or continuous intravenous infusions of short-acting opioids (e.g., fentanyl, remifentanil) although non-intravenous methods of administration, including the epidural route, also produce anesthetic-sparing effects [139].

Horses and cats given systemic opioids exhibit comparatively less inhalant anesthetic-sparing effect compared to dogs,[134,140–143], with one study failing to demonstrate any anesthetic-sparing effect in cats administered remifentanil infusions up to 75 times the analgesic effective concentration (EC_{50}) [144]. Others have even demonstrated increased anesthetic requirements when fentanyl and morphine were administered to horses at high doses [51,145]. Goats, pigs, sheep, and cattle exhibit more MAC-sparing effects with opioids than horses and cats, but less than that observed in dogs [146]. Opioids produce dose-dependent inhalant-sparing effects in rodents, but partial agonists demonstrate an equal sparing effect to full agonists [147–149].

Varying densities of μ, δ, and κ opioid receptors have been identified in the brain and spinal cord of multiple avian species [5,150–152]. Forebrain opioid receptor distribution in avian species likely differs the most from mammals whereas spinal cord and brainstem receptor distribution appears to be well preserved across species. Full μ opioid agonists and mixed agonist-antagonists have demonstrated similar MAC reduction in multiple avian species [153,154]. Inhalant sparing effects of tramadol appear to be a result of its action at opioid receptors as opposed to its effect on serotonin and norepinephrine reuptake inhibition or at α-adrenergic receptors [155].

Opioid agonists

Morphine

Morphine is still widely used in veterinary medicine due to its safety, efficacy, tolerability, and cost-effectiveness. Morphine elicits its effects primarily as a full μ opioid agonist, but higher doses can also result in κ receptor agonist effects. Morphine is effective for mild to severe pain in veterinary mammalian species with increasing doses producing increasing analgesic effects. For example, 0.25 mg/kg IM as a single dose may be effective for postoperative pain following removal of a subcutaneous lipoma in a dog, but 1 mg/kg IM q 2 h may be needed to control postoperative pain immediately following a total ear canal ablation. Individual animal pain assessment is essential. Dose recommendations are included in Table 11.4.

Morphine is less lipophilic (octanol/water partition coefficient of approximately 1.2), making it an ideal opioid for administration as a single epidural injection, providing sustained analgesia for up to 24 h [107,156–160].

Dogs

Histamine release has been documented after IV (0.5 and 1 mg/kg) administration of morphine in dogs, but substantial cardiovascular effects were not observed in awake dogs at either dose [75]. In contrast, a 3 mg/kg IV bolus produced profound hypotension in dogs anesthetized with pentobarbital [77] but in conscious dogs, 3 mg/kg IV over 5 min did not produce detrimental cardiovascular effects [161]. It is unclear how pentobarbital affected the response to the higher dose of morphine, but intravenous doses exceeding 1 mg/kg are discouraged and 0.5 mg/kg IV in dogs may be a better maximum dose to administer as a bolus (over 1–2 min).

There is a 5–15 min lag time from IV administration to onset of clinical effects in dogs with a maximum effect noted around 30–45 min after administration [162,163]. The half-life of morphine is short, approximately 1 h, requiring frequent administration or a constant rate infusion to maintain the desired effects. A constant rate infusion of 0.1–1.0 mg/kg/h following a 0.3–0.5 mg/kg IM or IV dose is generally effective for moderate to severe pain in dogs [164]. Oral and rectal morphine is poorly and erratically absorbed in dogs and is not recommended. Transdermal (pluronic lecithin organogel) formulations of morphine are not absorbed systemically and are not recommended [13]. Due to rapid and near complete absorption of morphine administered IM or SC, dosing is the same for these routes as for IV administration.

Morphine is primarily metabolized to morphine-3-glucuronide in dogs which is inactive and very low concentrations of the active metabolite morphine-6-glucuronide are formed [165]. There is no accumulation of morphine-6-glucuronide after 7 days of infusion [165]. Morphine undergoes about 50% hepatic metabolism and 50% extrahepatic metabolism in dogs, compared to near complete hepatic metabolism of most other opioids, therefore it may be a suitable opioid in dogs with hepatic dysfunction, although dose adjustments would be needed [166].

Adverse effects of morphine in dogs include nausea, vomiting, defecation immediately after administration, constipation with long-term administration, sedation, panting, hypothermia, bradycardia (but no effects on cardiac output in healthy dogs), decreased urine voiding and production. Morphine can produce mild respiratory depression but at clinically relevant dosages, this is not a major concern in healthy animals. Morphine should be avoided in animals with pre-existing head trauma or increased intracranial pressure due to the risk for emesis. Morphine is not contraindicated in animals with respiratory depression, severe respiratory disease or receiving other drugs causing respiratory depression, but these animals should be monitored closely. Administration of morphine as a constant rate infusion can minimize respiratory depressive effects by avoiding high initial concentrations. Morphine can be administered to neonates as young as 2 days old with minimal effects on respiration even though compared to adults, puppies are more sensitive to its respiratory depressive actions [167].

Intra-articular administration of morphine is an effective means of providing analgesia following arthroscopy in canine subjects. A dose of 0.1 mg/kg of morphine diluted in normal saline or appropriate local anesthetic to 1 mL/10 kg body weight may be injected into the joint before surgery and/or after joint closure [168].

Cats

Morphine is an effective analgesic and well tolerated in cats when administered at appropriate dosages. Although studies have reliably produced CNS excitation in cats, the doses used were much higher (5–20 mg/kg) than those currently recommended clinically (0.1–0.25 mg/kg) [50]. Morphine doses of 2–3 mg/kg have been well tolerated in cats despite being higher than clinically recommended [58]. Unwanted effects in cats are similar to those in dogs and additional behaviors, which are not usually considered undesirable, including purring, kneading, rubbing, euphoria, mydriasis, and marked affection may be observed [59].

The metabolism of morphine in cats is primarily through sulfate conjugation which is rapid. Morphine's terminal half-life is approximately 1 h which is similar to dogs [57]. The volume of distribution for morphine is smaller in cats and this appears to be the reason the clinically recommended dose in cats is lower than that of dogs (see Table 11.2).

Horses

Morphine is well tolerated in horses when administered at clinically appropriate doses. Although morphine is reported to cause excitation and other adverse CNS effects in horses, the doses administered were higher (exceeding 0.5 mg/kg) than the clinically recommended dose of 0.1–0.2 mg/kg [51–53]. Morphine may increase the risk of colic in postoperative orthopedic patients [100] but other studies have not reported that morphine increases adverse GI effects in surgical patients. It should be noted that orthopedic patients did not represent a large percentage of the patient population in these studies [169,170]. Morphine can be administered as the sole drug in horses, but is often combined with sedatives or tranquilizers. Systemic side-effects of morphine can be avoided when regional techniques are employed [171,172]. Intra-articular morphine provides analgesia and anti-inflammatory effects in experimentally induced lipopolysaccharide synovitis models for up to 24 h [173]. Morphine doses of approximately 0.05 mg/kg are routinely used for intra-articular administration in horses.

Ruminants and swine

The use of morphine in ruminants and swine is limited and few data are available although both species tolerate opioids at dosages frequently prescribed for dogs. The lack of residue depletion studies makes it problematic to develop slaughter withdrawal times. A reliable resource such as the Food Animal Residue Avoidance Databank (FARAD) (in the United States) should be consulted prior to administering morphine to a food-producing species.

Oxymorphone

Oxymorphone is a synthetic opioid that elicits its effect as a full μ opioid agonist. Oxymorphone is more potent than morphine. The effects of oxymorphone are similar to those of morphine but it tends to produce less nausea and vomiting when administered at equianalgesic doses and does not commonly produce histamine release when administered IV. The duration of effect of oxymorphone approximates that of morphine. Oxymorphone may be administered IV as a bolus (over 1 min) or infusion, SC or IM to dogs with a reported dose range of 0.05–0.2 mg/kg [174,175]. The bioavailability of oxymorphone PO is poor and as such this is not an effective route of administration in veterinary species. Oxymorphone is primarily metabolized by conjugate formation, but small amounts are excreted as other metabolites and intact drug in dogs. Doses used in cats tend to be lower than in dogs, with 0.03–0.05 mg/kg IM, SC, or IV being the dose range routinely suggested. Oxymorphone produces similar effects in horses as morphine, but due to its higher cost it is rarely used. There are minimal data on oxymorphone use in food-producing animals and as such limited data on withdrawal times. Specific dose regimens are included in Table 11.5.

Hydromorphone

Hydromorphone is a full μ opioid agonist which produces effects very similar to morphine when administered in equianalgesic doses. It is more potent than morphine and its duration of effect is similar. Hydromorphone produces minimal histamine release when administered IV in dogs [175]. It may be more likely to cause postoperative hyperthermia in cats compared to other opioids,[124] but hyperthermia has also been noted following morphine, buprenorphine, and butorphanol administration in this species [123]. Subcutaneous administration of hydromorphone in cats may result in slow absorption and long lag time [89]. Hydromorphone can be administered IV as a bolus (over 1 min) or infusion or IM, but is not expected to be

Table 11.5 Oxymorphone dosages in selected species.

	IV	IV infusion	IM/SC	PO
Dog	0.05–0.1 mg/kg q 2–4 h	0.005–0.01 mg/kg/h	0.05–0.1 mg/kg q 2–4 h	NR
Cat	0.025–0.05 mg/kg q 2–3 h	0.0025–0.005 mg/kg/h	0.02–-0.05 mg/kg q 2–4 h	NR
Horse	0.01–0.02 mg/kg q 8 h	NR	0.01–0.02 mg/kg q 8 h	NR
Rat/mouse			0.2–0.5 mg/kg q 4 h	NR
Guinea pig/hamster			0.2–0.5 mg/kg q 4 h	NR
Rabbit			0.2–0.5 mg/kg q 4 h	NR
Primate			0.05–0.2 mg/kg q 4–6 h	NR
Ferret			0.05 mg/kg q 4–6 h	NR

IV = intravenous; IM = intramuscular; SC = subcutaneous; PO = per os; NR = not recommended.

Table 11.6 Hydromorphone dosages in selected species.

	IV	IV infusion	IM/SC	PO
Dog	0.05–0.1 mg/kg q 2–4 h	0.02–0.04 mg/kg/h	0.1 mg/kg q 2–4 h	NR
Cat	0.05–0.1 mg/kg q 2–4 h	0.02–0.03 mg/kg/h	0.05–0.1 mg/kg q 2–4 h	NR
Horse	0.01–0.02 mg/kg once	NR	0.01–0.02 mg/kg once	NR
Rat/mouse			0.3–0.7 mg/kg q 4 h	NR
Guinea pig/hamster			0.3–0.7 mg/kg q 4 h	NR
Rabbit			0.3–0.7 mg/kg q 4 h	NR
Primate			0.1–0.3 mg/kg q 4–6 h	NR
Ferret			0.05–0.1 mg/kg q 4–6 h	NR

IV = intravenous; IM = intramuscular; SC = subcutaneous; PO = per os; NR = not recommended.

Table 11.7 Fentanyl dosages in selected species.

	IV	IV infusion	IM/SC	Transdermal solution
Dog	0.005–0.010 mg/kg q 0.5–2 h	0.002–0.005 mg/kg/h	0.005–0.015 mg/kg q 1–3 h	2.7 mg/kg once
Cat	0.005–0.010 mg/kg q 0.5–2 h	0.002–0.005 mg/kg/h	0.005–0.015 mg/kg q 1–3 h	
Horse	0.002–0.004 mg/kg q 3–4 h	0.0003–0.0005 mg/kg/h	0.002–0.004 mg/kg q 3–4 h	

1000 μg = 1 mg.
Intravenous doses may be higher when used as an adjunct to general anesthesia provided appropriate monitoring is available.
IV = intravenous; IM = intramuscular; SC = subcutaneous.

effective PO due to poor bioavailability. Based on results using a thermal threshold model and administration of 0.1 mg/kg, it is less effective in cats when administered SC as opposed to IM or IV [89]. Specific dose regimens are included in Table 11.6.

Fentanyl

Fentanyl is a full μ opioid agonist which is much more potent than morphine with a short duration of effect when administered IV (bolus), IM, or SC. Fentanyl results in less nausea and vomiting than morphine and produces a predominant antiemetic effect. However, if fentanyl administration results in ileus, then nausea and vomiting may occur. The pharmacokinetics of IV and SC fentanyl have been reported. Fentanyl can be administered IV as a bolus or infusion, SC or IM, but is not expected to be effective PO due to poor bioavailability. Fentanyl produces mild pain on SC administration, but mixing with 8.4% sodium bicarbonate (1 mL sodium bicarbonate:20 mL fentanyl) eliminates pain on injection [176]. Its use by routes other than IV is usually limited by the large volume of injection needed for all but the smallest of patients. The duration of effect of fentanyl administered IV, SC, or IM is short with an expected duration of 30 min to 2 h depending on the dose and route. Therefore fentanyl is often administered by an IV infusion. It is also available as a veterinary approved transdermal solution and as human approved transdermal patches. Specific dose regimens are included in Table 11.7.

The pharmacokinetics [177], efficacy [119], and margin of safety [178] of the transdermal fentanyl solution (TFS) in dogs have been published. The TFS appears effective if applied 4 h prior to surgery with a duration of effect of at least 4 days after administration in postoperative orthopedic patients. The TFS is recommended only as a single dose. The variability in absorption and duration of effect can be profound; therefore patients should be monitored throughout the postoperative period for adequate analgesia and also for adverse effects, as with other opioid regimens. Due to the great variability, the extra-label use at a reduced dose may be beneficial in animals at risk of the effects of limited or slow metabolism (e.g., mild pain conditions, hypothermic, aged, severely sick animals). Naloxone can effectively reverse adverse effects of TFS and typically requires a single administration to improve patient responsiveness. A risk minimization and action plan (RiskMAP) has been developed for TFS and educational training for veterinarians, veterinary staff, and clients is required prior to its use. People administering the drug should wear latex or nitrile gloves, protective glasses, and a laboratory coat to minimize the potential for accidental exposure. Dogs should be restrained for approximately 2 min after application and the site should not be disturbed for at least 5 min following application to allow for drying. Hospital staff who handle these dogs after administration should wear gloves. Clients should be instructed not to have contact with the application site for at least 72 h and the animal must be isolated from children for 72 h. TFS absorption in cats is not the same as in dogs and the product is not approved for use in cats.

Transdermal fentanyl patches are available as human approved products and have been used in veterinary patients [179,180]. In dogs, up to 24 h may be required until effective drug concentrations are reached which is longer than the 4 h lag for TFS. The duration of effect of the fentanyl patch ranges from 24 to 72 h after patch application (approximately 48 h of efficacy). The lag time to reach effective plasma concentrations is shorter in cats, approximately 12 h, with a duration of effect until approximately 100 h (~4 days) after application. The variability in absorption and effect of transdermal fentanyl patches is substantial, so some animals may have their pain poorly controlled with the patch and others may experience adverse effects. It is also important to instruct the clients on safe handling and disposal of used patches. The patch is easily removed, depending on site of application, and can be consumed by the animal, so close monitoring by the staff or client is advised [181]. Removal by the client or anyone else with access to the animal, including children, is possible and abuse and liability potential [182] are high.

Methadone

Methadone is a μ opioid agonist with similar effects and potency to morphine. It also has effects as an *N*-methyl D-aspartate (NMDA) antagonist which may make it a more effective analgesic for chronic

Table 11.8 Methadone (racemic) dosages in selected species. The dose of levo-methadone would be half the dose of racemic methadone.

	IV	IV infusion	IM/SC	PO
Dog	0.25–0.5 mg/kg q 3–4 h	0.05–0.2 mg/kg/h	0.25–0.5 mg/kg q 3–4 h	NR
Cat	0.1–0.25 mg/kg q 3–4 h	0.05–0.1 mg/kg/h	0.1–0.25 mg/kg q 3–4 h	NR
Horse	0.15–0.25 mg/kg q 4–8 h	NR	0.15–0.25 mg/kg q 4–8 h	NR

IV = intravenous; IM = intramuscular; SC = subcutaneous; PO = per os; NR = not recommended.

and refractory pain than morphine and also decrease the development of tolerance. There are two optical isomers of methadone (D- and L- forms), both of which bind to and antagonize the NMDA receptor [183]. The pharmacokinetics of methadone are similar to morphine. Methadone may be administered IV as a bolus (over 1 min) or infusion, SC or IM, but repeated SC or IM administration may result in tissue irritation or damage. In contrast to humans, methadone has a low oral bioavailability in most veterinary species and as such is not expected to be effective when administered PO [30]. Methadone is metabolized by metabolic pathways inhibited by chloramphenicol (and possibly other hepatic enzyme inhibitors) in dogs (and potentially other species) and therefore markedly prolonged effects can occur in animals treated concurrently with both drugs [30]. Methadone exhibits synergistic effects when combined with some μ opioid agonists such as morphine [184]. It has been administered by the oral transmucosal route to horses and cats and appears to be well tolerated [185,186]. Specific dose regimens are included in Table 11.8.

Meperidine (Pethidine)

Meperidine is a μ opioid agonist. Meperidine and its metabolite normeperidine (in humans) may produce serotonergic effects so it is not recommended to administer meperidine with other serotonergic drugs or monoamine oxidase inhibitors. Normeperidine appears to be a minor metabolite in dogs. Meperidine, in contrast to other opioids, has negative inotropic effects and also possesses antimuscarinic effects [187,188]. Local anesthetic effects have also been demonstrated with meperidine and it has been used alone for intravenous regional anesthesia [189]. Meperidine may be administered IV as a bolus (over 2–3 min) SC or IM, but oral bioavailability is poor. The typical doses of meperidine are 5–10 mg/kg IM q 2–3 h for dogs and 3–5 mg/kg IM q 2–4 h in cats. The duration of effect is short with clinical effects ranging from 0.5 to 2 h in dogs but slightly longer in cats (up to 3 h) [57,190]. Meperidine causes more histamine release than equipotent doses of morphine and rapid IV bolus administration can produce adverse cardiovascular effects [191] in addition to severe, species-specific adverse effects. In horses, hyperesthesia, muscle fasciculations, and sweating in addition to adverse cardiovascular effects are reported [192]. Meperidine rarely causes panting, unlike other μ opioid agonists, and is effective at reducing shivering, possibly through its agonist effects at the α_2B-adrenergic receptor subtypes [193].

Hydrocodone

Hydrocodone is a μ opioid agonist available in oral dosage forms. Although the oral bioavailability of hydrocodone in dogs is relatively poor, it is variably metabolized to hydromorphone which may produce opioid effects [194]. Hydrocodone has long been used as an effective antitussive in dogs, but clinical studies evaluating its analgesic efficacy are not reported. Hydrocodone may prove to be a useful analgesic in dogs. A dose of 0.25–0.5 mg/kg of hydrocodone PO q 8–12 h is anticipated to produce plasma drug concentrations consistent with analgesia, but analgesic efficacy studies are not reported [194]. Studies assessing hydrocodone in cats have also not been reported. Most hydrocodone formulations are combination products with non-steroidal anti-inflammatory drugs, acetaminophen (paracetamol) or homatropine. Hydrocodone formulations with acetaminophen are contraindicated in cats due to concerns of acetaminophen toxicity.

Codeine

Codeine is a naturally occurring alkaloid structurally similar to morphine. It is classified as a μ opioid agonist. Codeine can be administered IV as a bolus (over 1 min) or infusion, SC or IM. Codeine has a 60% oral bioavailability in humans with approximately 10% of the dose metabolized to morphine. In contrast, in dogs codeine only has a 4% oral bioavailability and negligible amounts of morphine were detected as a metabolite in dogs and cats [195–197]. Large amounts of codeine-6-glucuronide were formed in dogs which may provide some opioid effects and norcodeine was the primary metabolite recovered in the urine in cats. The efficacy of IV codeine (2.5–5 mg/kg) in experimental models in dogs indicated that it produced a much shorter duration of antinociception compared to morphine administered at 0.25 mg/kg IV [198]. The efficacy of PO codeine in dogs is expected to be low at best. There are no reports of codeine plasma pharmacokinetics or analgesic efficacy in cats. Current recommended dosages of codeine in dogs are 1.1–2.2 mg/kg codeine PO q 8–12 h, most often administered in combination with acetaminophen. There are formulations that do not contain acetaminophen which can be administered to dogs and cats, but formulations with acetaminophen should never be administered to cats.

Oxycodone

Oxycodone is a μ opioid agonist available in oral dosage forms. It is not commonly used in veterinary medicine. Limited studies suggest it has a low oral bioavailability in dogs and is rapidly eliminated and as such the data suggest it is not an effective PO drug in dogs [199]. No data or evidence for oxycodone use in cats are available.

Sufentanil, alfentanil, remifentanil

Sufentanil and alfentanil are fentanyl derivatives of differing potencies that produce effects very similar to fentanyl. They are typically administered by IV infusion. Remifentanil is also a fentanyl derivative that is metabolized primarily by extrahepatic metabolism by plasma esterases which results in a very short elimination half-life (approximately 6 min); therefore animals with impaired hepatic function should still have a consistent and predictable elimination of the drug [200]. Constant rate infusions of remifentanil are necessary to provide continued pain relief because of its very short half-life. Clinical analgesic effects subside quickly after discontinuation of a constant rate infusion and provision of additional opioids with a more sustained duration of action are recommended to ensure adequate ongoing pain control. Remifentanil is as efficacious as fentanyl and similar doses are used for producing MAC reduction in dogs and cats although a ceiling effect is appreciated in both species [135,141].

Etorphine, carfentanil, and thiafentanil

Etorphine and carfentanil are highly potent opioid agonists used for capture and restraint of wildlife and exotic animals. Special caution is advised when using these highly potent drugs because very small volumes (0.01 mL) can be lethal to humans. These drugs should only be handled with at least two people present and with adequate opioid antagonists (e.g., naltrexone, diprenorphine) immediately available. These drugs are often combined with other drugs such as α_2-adrenergic receptor agonists to produce reliable sedation.

Partial opioid agonists and agonist/antagonists

Buprenorphine

Buprenorphine is a μ opioid receptor partial agonist, approximately 25 times more potent than morphine. Buprenorphine can be administered IV as a bolus (over 1 min) or infusion, SC, IM, or specifically to cats by oral transmucosal administration. The subcutaneous and oral transmucosal route of administration for buprenorphine in cats is less effective than IV or IM routes in the perioperative setting [19]. Specific dose regimens are included in Table 11.9.

Its effects are similar to morphine but it has a lower maximal efficacy in many models. However, buprenorphine may be more effective than morphine for chronic pain. The safety profile of buprenorphine is very large and even supratherapeutic doses produce minor adverse effects on the cardiovascular and respiratory systems. In contrast to morphine, buprenorphine seems to produce less nausea and vomiting, but these may still occur. Buprenorphine may produce fewer adverse effects in cats compared to morphine. In horses the adverse effects of buprenorphine are similar to those reported for morphine. The peak effects appear to occur approximately 45–90 min after IV administration, similar to morphine, but clinically relevant effects appear within 20 min of IV dosing [201]. Buprenorphine may antagonize the effects of full μ agonists, but the degree of antagonism may not be complete [202]. Prior administration of buprenorphine is believed to render subsequent administration of full μ agonists less effective or ineffective due to its much greater affinity at the μ opioid receptor [202]. The degree of this interference is likely determined by the relative doses, the timing between doses, the species, and the type of nociceptive environment. This receptor interference persists for the duration of buprenorphine's effect. The duration of analgesic effect is expected to be longer than morphine, 4–8 h and up to 12 h depending on the dose, route, species, pain intensity, and individual response to the drug. The oral bioavailability (swallowed) of buprenorphine is poor and so this is not a viable route of administration [203,204]. However, oral transmucosal (OTM) administration to cats can be a clinically relevant route of administration [20]. The oral pH of cats (8.0–9.0) closely approximates buprenorphine's pKa (8.4), allowing good absorption of OTM buprenorphine whereas acidifying the formulation may limit absorption and thus clinical efficacy [18,19]. OTM administration of buprenorphine in dogs results in reasonable uptake and produces antinociceptive effects but larger volumes may be cost-prohibitive in large dogs [17,22]. OTM buprenorphine is not an effective route of administration in horses [205]. Transdermal buprenorphine patches are available in some countries, but initial studies in dogs indicated a slow absorption (T_{max} range 48–60 h) and the mean plasma concentrations were low for the first 36 h with a total duration of 72 h [201]. Buprenorphine was absorbed better from transdermal patches in cats with a 12–24 h lag to target concentrations which persisted until about 96 h even when the patch was removed at 72 h [206]. Further studies assessing the efficacy and adverse effects of the buprenorphine transdermal patch in cats are needed.

Table 11.9 Buprenorphine dosages in selected species.

	IV/IM/SC	Oral transmucosal	PO
Dog	0.01–0.04 mg/kg q 4–8 h	NR	NR
Cat	0.01–0.02 mg/kg q 4–8 h 0.24 mg/kg SC*	0.01–0.02 mg/kg q 4–12 h	NR
Horse	0.005–0.01 mg/kg	NR	NR
Rat/mouse	0.05–0.1 mg/kg q 4–12 h	NR	NR
Guinea pig/hamster	0.05–0.1 mg/kg 4–12 h	NR	NR
Rabbit	0.01–0.05 mg/kg q 4–12 h	NR	NR
Primate	0.005–0.01 mg/kg q 4–12 h	NR	NR
Ferret	0.01–0.03 mg/kg q 4–12 h	NR	NR

IV = intravenous; IM = intramuscular; SC = subcutaneous; PO = per os; NR = not recommended.
* Simbadol™, 1.8 mg/ml.

A new formulation of buprenorphine has been approved by the FDA, Simbadol®, for once daily SC administration for up to 3 days to cats for the control of postoperative pain. Safety (up to 5x label dose) and efficacy (ovariohysterectomy, castration, and onychectomy) studies were completed for the drug approval process; however at the time of publication no peer-reviewed studies incorporating a control group had been published. Recommended dosing for cats is 0.24 mg/kg SC once daily for up to three days.

Sustained-release (SR) buprenorphine, a compounded, unapproved drug formulation delivered in a biodegradable matrix allowing controlled release over 72 h, and administered SC, has been demonstrated to provide analgesic effects for up to 72 h in postsurgical models (cats and rats) and in thermal threshold models (mice and rats) [207–209]. There are no data available for the use of this compounded drug in dogs. Recommended doses for SR buprenorphine (3 mg/mL) in cats and dogs range from 0.12 mg/kg SC to 0.12–0.27 mg/kg SC, respectively. However, this is a compounded formulation and as such does not have the safety and efficacy data an FDA approved formulation requires, nor the same requirements for consistent manufacturing or evidence of dose proportional pharmacokinetics in different species. It is also unclear if this SR compounded formula results in dose-dependent release when the surface area changes with the volume injected. A formulation of buprenorphine extended release (1 mg/mL) is marketed as an indexed, unapproved drug in the USA for use in rats only. Recommended doses of SR buprenorphine in laboratory rats and mice range from 1.0–1.5 mg/kg SC to 0.5–1.0 mg/kg SC, respectively, and provide pain control for 72 h. Due to the high affinity of buprenorphine for μ opioid receptors, complete antagonism with opioid antagonists may be difficult.

Butorphanol

Butorphanol is a μ antagonist to partial μ agonist and κ opioid agonist approved for use in some veterinary species such as the dog (oral only), cat and horse, but approval varies among countries. Butorphanol may be administered as an IV bolus (over 1 min), constant rate infusion, and by the SC and IM routes. Specific dose regimens are included in Table 11.10.

Table 11.10 Butorphanol dosages for analgesia.

	IV/IM/SC	IV infusion	PO
Dog	0.2–0.4 mg/kg q 1–4 h	0.1–0.2 mg/kg/h	NR
Cat	0.2–0.4 mg/kg q 1–4 h	0.1–0.2 mg/kg/h	NR
Horse	0.005–0.1 mg/kg q 2–6 hours	0.01–0.025 mg/kg/h	NR
Ruminant	0.05–0.2 mg/kg q 4–12 h		NR
Rabbit	0.1–0.5 mg/kg 4–6 h		NR

IV = intravenous; IM = intramuscular; SC = subcutaneous; PO = per os; NR = not recommended.
Typical clinical doses are 5–10 mg/horse IV repeated as necessary. Doses can range considerably due to breed, sex, temperament, body size, age, concurrently administered sedatives, and pain intensity.

The oral bioavailability of butorphanol is low and will not reliably produce effective analgesia by this route in dogs and cats, despite its ability to produce antitussive and some sedative effects when administered PO. Similar to buprenorphine, an effect plateau (ceiling effect) occurs with butorphanol where increasing doses do not produce increasing analgesic effects. The efficacy of butorphanol is dose dependent with higher doses producing clinically relevant analgesia, but the effect is less than with morphine. Dose–response studies demonstrate that duration of effect is also dose dependent with higher doses, up to a peak effective dose, producing a more prolonged effect in horses and dogs, although this was not found to be true in cats [48,60,210,211]. Therefore butorphanol can be used clinically to control mild to moderate pain if appropriate dosages are administered and the relatively short duration of action is considered. However, for severe pain (e.g., trauma, postoperative total ear canal ablation, etc.) butorphanol is not expected to be completely effective.

Butorphanol is a more efficacious antitussive than morphine or codeine [74,212]. Butorphanol tablets (Torbutrol®) are FDA approved in the USA as an antitussive in dogs. In contrast to morphine, butorphanol is an antiemetic and has been used to prevent chemotherapy-induced emesis [87]. The adverse effects of butorphanol are similar to morphine, but occur with less severity. While butorphanol in general may cause less dysphoria at clinical doses and may be less likely to cause CNS excitement than full μ agonists in horses and cats, large doses, as with other opioids, are likely to induce ataxia, excitement or dysphoria [211].

Administration of butorphanol (0.1 mg/kg IV) to non-painful horses produces increased locomotor activity and reduction in GI motility; thus the total dose administered and presence or absence of pain likely contributes to the development of adverse effects in horses [61]. Particularly in horses, adverse CNS effects are likely due to large peak plasma concentrations as constant rate infusions were associated with fewer adverse CNS effects [213]. Butorphanol may decrease GI motility and can result in ileus and colic in horses, but the gastrointestinal effects are variable depending on the intestinal segments studied [214–216]. Despite the potential adverse GI effects, it is an effective analgesic in both visceral pain models and for colic surgery, particularly when combined with α_2-adrenergic receptor agonists [217–219].

Butorphanol is a substrate of P-glycoprotein and has been speculated to cause sedation that is more profound and prolonged in dogs with the MDR1 gene mutation [220]. Although no well-designed studies have been performed, it is conservatively recommended that dogs heterozygous for the MDR1 mutation should be given a reduced dose (25% less) whereas dogs homozygous for the MDR1 mutation should be administered doses 30–50% lower than recommended doses for normal dogs.

Nalbuphine

Nalbuphine is a μ antagonist and κ agonist opioid (similar to butorphanol) occasionally used in veterinary species. It is not currently a Drug Enforcement Agency (USA) scheduled drug. The potency, pharmacokinetics, and duration of effect of nalbuphine are similar to morphine, but the analgesic effects are expected to be less. The efficacy of nalbuphine is likely to be sufficient for mild and maybe moderate pain, but extensive analgesic studies in veterinary species are lacking [221]. Adverse effects of nalbuphine are generally mild but can include panting, nausea, vomiting, and CNS stimulation if administered rapidly IV or in higher doses to horses. Doses of 0.25–1 mg/kg IM, SC, or IV are commonly used in dogs and cats. According to the human approved label, nalbuphine has greater antagonist activity at equianalgesic doses compared to pentazocine and butorphanol and antagonist activity approximately one-quarter that of nalorphine. Fewer sedative effects are produced with nalbuphine compared to pentazocine, butorphanol, and nalorphine. Based on the human approval, nalbuphine appears to produce adverse gastrointestinal effects less frequently than other agonist-antagonists or full agonists.

Pentazocine

Pentazocine is a μ antagonist and κ agonist opioid rarely used in veterinary species. Its efficacy is thought to be limited to mild to moderate pain and the duration of effect is 1–3 h although one study demonstrated analgesic effects as long as those reported for morphine (4 h) [218]. Following orthopedic surgery in dogs, morphine, buprenorphine, and pentazocine were all assessed as providing adequate analgesia [222].

Tramadol

Tramadol is a centrally acting analgesic that elicits its effects through several different mechanisms. The primary analgesic effect in humans is due to metabolism of tramadol to O-desmethyltramadol (M1) which acts as a full μ opioid agonist. Additional effects can occur due to activity of both tramadol and M1 as serotonin and norepinephrine reuptake inhibitors. However, studies in humans have demonstrated that without formation of O-desmethyltramadol, tramadol has little analgesic effect [223].

The metabolism of tramadol has been examined in dogs [224], cats [225], and horses [226]. Dogs and horses do not make substantial amounts of O-desmethyltramadol and as a consequence analgesic effects are predicted to be weak at best. Plasma concentrations of tramadol following 7 days of continuous PO administration were reduced to only 33% of those reached on day 1, further suggesting that tramadol may be a poor analgesic choice in dogs for chronic administration without patient monitoring and dose adjustments [227]. In contrast, cats produce substantial amounts of O-desmethyltramadol and it is likely an effective analgesic, although the bitter taste makes routine oral administration difficult. Doses of tramadol in dogs and horses in the range of 5–10 mg/kg PO q 8 h would provide tramadol concentrations within ranges achieved in humans. In cats, a dose of 1–2 mg/kg PO q 8–12 h is expected to produce O-desmethyltramadol plasma concentrations considered clinically effective in humans. However, results of controlled clinical trials have not been published for cats. Tramadol is also available as a solution for injection in some countries. Since the bioavailability of injectable tramadol is higher than oral tramadol, the dose of the injectable solution is lower with a recommended range of 2–4 mg/kg.

Tramadol can have some clinically relevant drug interactions with other drugs that affect serotonin receptor activation. It is recommended that tramadol not be combined with meperidine, tricyclic antidepressants (amitriptyline, clomipramine), or selective serotonin reuptake inhibitors (fluoxetine, paroxetine) due to the risk of serotonin syndrome. When severe, serotonin syndrome can present as fever, seizures, muscle tremors/fasciculations, hyperthermia, salivation, and rarely death [228].

The toxicology of tramadol has been studied in dogs [227]. Single oral administration of tramadol at a dose of 450 mg/kg was not lethal, but adverse effects included restlessness, unsteady gait, reduced spontaneous activity, mydriasis, salivation, vomiting, tremors, convulsions, cyanosis, and dyspnea. Dogs administered tramadol at 5, 12, and 20 mg/kg PO q 12 h for one year had minimal adverse effects with the only observed adverse effects being mydriasis and weight loss. Dogs administered tramadol 25 mg/kg and 60 mg/kg PO q 24 h for six months had adverse effects including vomiting and convulsions. Convulsions can be effectively managed with an anticonvulsant such as diazepam and anecdotally many dogs respond to a single dose.

Opioid antagonists

The primary indications for administering an opioid antagonist is for the reversal of severe opioid-related adverse effects or reversing sedation after a non-painful procedure. As previously stated, the safety margin of opioids is very large and life-threatening adverse effects, even with substantial overdoses, are rare in most animals if supportive measures are instituted. The duration of effect of opioid antagonists is often shorter than the opioid agonist and as such multiple doses may need to be administered. Administration of an opioid antagonist to a painful animal may result in adverse cardiovascular sequelae which are presumably due to unmitigated pain from reversal of both exogenous and endogenous opioids and therefore opioid antagonists should be administered to effect in these patients rather than giving a single predetermined dose. The administration of nalbuphine or butorphanol will also reverse μ opioid effects but maintain some analgesia due to their effect as κ agonists and this may be a more reasonable choice for a painful animal.

Naloxone

Naloxone is a commonly administered opioid antagonist. It acts primarily as a μ opioid antagonist, but antagonist effects can also occur at κ and δ opioid receptors. Naloxone can elicit convulsions due to some GABA antagonist actions although this is usually not a clinical consideration. High doses of naloxone will antagonize the central effects of opioid agonists that may cause the animal to experience acute pain and associated sympathetic stimulation with serious consequences including tachycardia, hypertension, pulmonary edema, and cardiac arrhythmias. It is best to administer naloxone to effect by careful titration and multiple doses may be needed to maintain antagonistic effects due to its short duration of action [229,230]. A typical dose range of naloxone is 0.001–0.04 mg/kg IV. It is advisable to start at the low end of the dose range and repeat administration every 1–2 min until the desired effect is achieved (e.g., cessation of dysphoria or increase in respiratory rate).

Naloxone also has effects as a Toll-like 4 (TLR4) receptor antagonist. The TLR4 receptor appears to be stimulated by morphine administration, resulting in allodynia at some doses. Administration of low-dose naloxone can block TLR4 allodynia associated with morphine administration in rodent models of peripheral nerve injury [231]. Reviews of the use of opioid antagonists for the management of pain in humans have been published [232,233]. A study in research cats using thermal and mechanical nociceptive models failed to show a benefit of naloxone in combination with buprenorphine compared to buprenorphine alone, but it is unclear how the research model applies to clinical pain in cats [234].

Naltrexone

Naltrexone is an opioid antagonist at the μ, κ, and δ receptors. Naltrexone is often administered to reverse the sedative effects of carfentanil in wildlife and zoo animals, but would be effective in reversing other opioids as well. The longer duration of action, at least twice that of naloxone, makes it desirable in wildlife and zoo animals where repeat dosing may not be possible. The dose of naltrexone is 100 mg per 1 mg of carfentanil administered with typically one-quarter of the dose administered IV and the remainder administered SC. Limited information is available on naltrexone administration to companion animals with doses being described only recently in cats [235]. Low dosages of naloxone and naltrexone have been administered to humans prior to or after surgery to reduce the potential for side-effects (constipation and urine retention) without interfering with analgesia, but these adverse effects are not as common in dogs and cats [234,236].

Methylnaltrexone

Methylnaltrexone is a quaternary derivative of naltrexone that, due to its greater polarity and lower lipid solubility, only acts peripherally as it is excluded from the CNS. The primary indication is for controlling GI adverse effects, including ileus, without affecting central analgesic effects. Preliminary studies in horses indicate that methylnaltrexone may have some beneficial effects in preventing GI motility problems associated with opioid use, but it is costly and further studies are needed [103,237].

References

1 Goumon Y, Casares F, Pryor S, *et al.* Ascaris suum, an intestinal parasite, produces morphine. *J Immunol* 2000; **165**: 339–343.

2 Liu D, Sun H. Immunohistological detection of mu, delta and kappa opioid-like receptors in the gill, gonad, and hemocytes of the scallop Chlamys farreri. *Connect Tissue Res* 2010; **51**: 67–70.

3 Chadzinska M, Hermsen T, Savelkoul HF, *et al.* Cloning of opioid receptors in common carp (Cyprinus carpio L.) and their involvement in regulation of stress and immune response. *Brain, Behav Immun* 2009; **23**: 257–266.

4 Xia Y, Haddad GG. Major difference in the expression of delta- and mu-opioid receptors between turtle and rat brain. *J Compar Neurol* 2001; **436**: 202–210.

5 Kawate T, Sakamoto H, Yang C, *et al.* Immunohistochemical study of delta and mu opioid receptors on synaptic glomeruli with substance P-positive central terminals in chicken dorsal horn. *Neurosci Res* 2005; **53**: 279–287.

6 Lord JAH, Waterfield AA, Hughes J, *et al.* Endogenous opioid peptides: multiple agonists and receptors. *Nature* 1977; **267**: 495–499.

7 Dhawan BN, Cesselin F, Raghubir R, *et al.* International Union of Pharmacology. XII. Classification for opioid receptors. *Pharmacol Rev* 1996; **48**: 567–592.

8 Pasternak GW, Pan YX. Mu opioids and their receptors: evolution of a concept. *Pharmacol Rev* 2013; **65**: 1257–1317.

9 Hawley AT, Wetmore LA. Identification of single nucleotide polymorphisms within exon 1 of the canine mu-opioid receptor gene. *Vet Anaesth Analg* 2010; **37**: 79–82.

10 Reinscheid RK, Nothacker HP, Bourson A, *et al.* Orphanin-FQ: a neuropeptide that activates an opioid-like G protein-coupled receptor. *Science* 1995; **270**: 792–794.

11 Meunier JC, Mollereau C, Toll L, *et al.* Isolation and structure of the endogenous agonist of opioid receptor-like ORL-1 receptor. *Nature* 1995; **377**: 532–535.

12 Wegner K, Horais KA, Tozier NA, *et al.* Development of a canine nociceptive thermal escape model. *J Neurosci Methods* 2008; **168**: 88–97.

13 Krotscheck U, Boothe DM, Boothe HW. Evaluation of transdermal morphine and fentanyl pluronic lecithin organogel administration in dogs. *Vet Ther* 2004; **5**: 202–211.

14 Robertson SA, Taylor PM, Sear JW, *et al.* Relationship between plasma concentrations and analgesia after intravenous fentanyl and disposition after other routes of administration in cats. *J Vet Pharmacol Ther* 2005; **28**: 87–93.
15 Hofmeister EH, Egger, CM. Transdermal fentanyl patches in small animals. *J Am Anim Hosp Assoc* 2004; **40**: 468–478.
16 Ko JC, Freeman LJ, Barletta M, *et al.* Efficacy of oral transmucosal and intravenous administration of buprenorphine before surgery for postoperative analgesia in dogs undergoing ovariohysterectomy. *J Am Vet Med Assoc* 2011; **238**: 318–328.
17 Abbo LA, Ko JC, Maxwell LK, *et al.* Pharmacokinetics of buprenorphine following intravenous and oral transmucosal administration in dogs. *Vet Ther* 2008; **9**: 83–93.
18 Robertson SA, Taylor PM, Sear JW. Systemic uptake of buprenorphine by cats after oral mucosal administration. *Vet Rec* 2003; **152**:675–678.
19 Giordano T, Steagall PV, Ferriera TH, *et al.* Postoperative analgesic effects of intravenous, intramuscular, subcutaneous or oral transmucosal buprenorphine administered to cats undergoing ovariohysterectomy. *Vet Anaesth Anal* 2010; **37**: 357–366.
20 Robertson SA, Lascelles BDX, Taylor PM, *et al.* PK-PD modeling of buprenorphine in cats: intravenous and oral transmucosal administration. *J Vet Pharmacol Ther* 2005; **28**: 453–460.
21 Walker AF. Sublingual administration of buprenorphine for long-term analgesia in the horse. *Vet Rec* 2007 9; **160**: 808–809.
22 Niyom S, Mama KR, de Rezende ML. Comparison of the analgesic efficacy of oral ABT-116 administration with that of transmucosal buprenorphine administration in dogs. *Am J Vet Res* 2012; **73**: 476–481.
23 Edwards G. Ivermectin: does P-glycoprotein play a role in neurotoxicity? *Filaria J* 2003; **24**(2 Suppl 1): S8.
24 Mercer SL, Coop A. Opioid analgesics and P-glycoprotein efflux transporters: a potential systems-level contribution to analgesic tolerance. *Curr Top Med Chem* 2011; **11**: 1157–1164.
25 Wandel C, Kim R, Wood M, *et al.* Interaction of morphine, fentanyl, sufentanil, alfentanil, and loperamide with the efflux drug transporter P-glycoprotein. *Anesthesiology* 2002; **96**: 913–920.
26 Henthorn TK, Liu Y, Mahapatro M, *et al.* Active transport of fentanyl by the blood–brain barrier. *J Pharmacol Exp Ther* 1999; **289**: 1084–1089.
27 Brown SM, Campbell SD, Crafford A, *et al.* P-Glycoprotein is a major determinant of norbuprenorphine brain exposure and antinociception. *J Pharm Exp Ther* 2012; **343**: 53–61.
28 Court MH, Greenblatt DJ. Molecular basis for deficient acetaminophen glucuronidation in cats. An interspecies comparison of enzyme kinetics in liver microsomes. *Biochem Pharmacol* 1997; **53**: 1041–1047.
29 Yeh SY, Chernov HI, Woods LA. Metabolism of morphine by cats. *J Pharm Sci* 1971; **60**: 469–471.
30 KuKanich B, KuKanich KS, Rodriguez J. The effects of cytochrome P450 inhibitors on oral methadone on Greyhound dogs. *J Vet Intern Med* 2011; **25**: 741.
31 Barr MC, Huitron-Resendiz S, Sanchez-Alavez M, *et al.* Escalating morphine exposures followed by withdrawal in feline immunodeficiency virus-infected cats: a model for HIV infection in chronic opiate abusers. *Drug Alcohol Depend* 2003; **72**: 141–149.
32 Martin WR, Eades CG, Thompson WO, *et al.* Morphine physical dependence in the dog. *J Pharmacol Exp Ther* 1974; **189**: 759–771.
33 Yaksh TL, Rudy TA. Narcotic analgestics: CSN sites and mechanisms of action as revealed by intracerebral injection techniques. *Pain* 1978; **4**: 299–359.
34 Yaksh TL, Rudy TA. Microinjection of morphine into the periaqueductal gray evokes the release of serotonin from spinal cord. *Brain Res* 1979; **171**: 176–181.
35 Stein C, Comisel K, Haimerl E, *et al.* Analgesic effect of intraarticular morphine after arthroscopic knee surgery. *N Engl J Med* 1991; **325**: 1123–1126.
36 Stein C. Peripheral mechanisms of opioid analgesia. *Anesth Analg* 1993; **76**: 182–191.
37 Keates HL, Cramond T, Smith MT. Intraarticular and periarticular opioid binding in inflamed tissue in experimental canine arthritis. *Anesth Analg* 1999; **89**: 409–415.
38 van Loon JP, de Grauw JC, van Dierendonck M, *et al.* Intra-articular opioid analgesia is effective in reducing pain and inflammation in an equine LPS induced synovitis model. *Equine Vet J* 2010; **42**: 412–419.
39 Robertson SA, Taylor PM, Lascelles BD, *et al.* Changes in thermal threshold response in eight cats after administration of buprenorphine, butorphanol and morphine. *Vet Rec* 2003; **153**: 462–465.
40 Polson S, Taylor PM, Yates D. Analgesia after feline ovariohysterectomy under midazolam-medetomidine-ketamine anaesthesia with buprenorphine or butorphanol, and carprofen or meloxicam: a prospective, randomised clinical trial. *J Feline Med Surg* 2012; **14**: 553–559.
41 Johnson JA, Robertson SA, Pypendop BH. Antinociceptive effects of butorphanol, buprenorphine, or both, administered intramuscularly in cats. *Am J Vet Res* 2007; **68**: 699–703.
42 Love EJ, Taylor PM, Murrell J, *et al.* Effects of acepromazine, butorphanol and buprenorphine on thermal and mechanical nociceptive thresholds in horses. *Equine Vet J* 2012; **44**: 221–225.
43 Fischer BL, Ludders JW, Asakawa M, *et al.* A comparison of epidural buprenorphine plus detomidine with morphine plus detomidine in horses undergoing bilateral stifle arthroscopy. *Vet Anaesth Analg* 2009; **36**: 67–76.
44 Paul-Murphy JR, Brunson DB, Miletic V. Analgesic effects of butorphanol and buprenorphine in conscious African grey parrots (Psittacus erithacus erithacus and Psittacus erithacus timneh). *Am J Vet Res* 1999; **60**: 1218–1221.
45 Taylor PM, Kirby JJ, Robinson C, *et al.* A prospective multi-centre clinical trial to compare buprenorphine and butorphanol for postoperative analgesia in cats. *J Feline Med Surg* 2010; **12**: 247–255.
46 Gades NM, Danneman PJ, Wixson SK, *et al.* The magnitude and duration of the analgesic effect of morphine, butorphanol, and buprenorphine in rats and mice. *Contemp Top Lab Anim Sci* 2000; **39**: 8–13.
47 Morgan D, Cook CD, Smith MA, *et al.* An examination of the interactions between the antinociceptive effects of morphine and various mu-opioids: the role of intrinsic efficacy and stimulus intensity. *Anesth Analg* 1999; **88**: 407–413.
48 Houghton KJ, Rech RH, Sawyer DC, *et al.* Dose–response of intravenous butorphanol to increase visceral nociceptive threshold in dogs. *Proc Soc Exp Biol Med* 1991; **197**: 290–296.
49 Sawyer DC, Rech RH, Durham RA, *et al.* Dose response to butorphanol administered subcutaneously to increase visceral nociceptive threshold in dogs. *Am J Vet Res* 1991; **52**: 1826–1830.
50 Sturtevant FM, Drill VA. Tranquilizing drugs and morphine-mania in cats. *Nature* 1957; **179**: 1253.
51 Steffey EP, Eisele JH, Baggot JD. Interactions of morphine and isoflurane in horses. *Am J Vet Res* 2003; **64**: 166–175.
52 Pascoe PJ, Black WD, Claxton JM, *et al.* The pharmacokinetics and locomotor activity of alfentanil in the horse. *J Vet Pharmacol Ther* 1991; **14**: 317–325.
53 Combie J, Dougherty J, Nugent E, *et al.* The pharmacology of narcotic analgesics in the horse. IV. Dose- and time-response relationships for behavioral responses to morphine, meperidine, pentazocine, anileridine, methadone, and hydromorphone. *J Equine Med Surg* 1979; **3**: 377–385.
54 Kamerling S, Wood T, DeQuick D, *et al.* Narcotic analgesics, their detection and pain measurement in the horse: a review. *Equine Vet J* 1989; **21**: 4–12.
55 Clutton RE. Opioid analgesia in horses. *Vet Clin Eq* 2010; **26**: 493–514.
56 KuKanich B, Lascelles BD, Papich MG. Pharmacokinetics of morphine and plasma concentrations of morphine-6-glucuronide following morphine administration to dogs. *J Vet Pharmacol Ther* 2005; **28**: 371–376.
57 Taylor PM, Robertson SA, Dixon MJ, *et al.* Morphine, pethidine and buprenorphine disposition in the cat. *J Pharmacol Exp Ther* 2001; **24**: 391–398.
58 Barr MC, Billaud JN, Selway DR, *et al.* Effects of multiple acute morphine exposures on feline immunodeficiency virus disease progression. *J Infect Dis* 2000; **182**: 725–732.
59 Steagall PV, Carnicelli P, Taylor PM, *et al.* Effects of subcutaneous methadone, morphine, buprenorphine or saline on thermal and pressure thresholds in cats. *J Vet Pharmacol Ther* 2006; **29**: 531–537.
60 Kalpravidh M, Lumb WV, Wright M, *et al.* Effects of butorphanol, flunixin, levorphanol, morphine, and xylazine in ponies. *Am J Vet Res* 1984; **45**: 217–223.
61 Knych HK, Casbeer HC, McKemie DS, *et al.* Pharmacokinetics and pharmacodynamics of butorphanol following intravenous administration to the horse. *J Vet Pharmacol Ther* 2013; **36**: 21–30.
62 Carregaro AB, Luna SP, Mataqueiro MI, *et al.* Effects of buprenorphine on nociception and spontaneous locomotor activity in horses. *Am J Vet Res* 2007; **68**: 246–250.
63 Combie J, Shults T, Nugent EC, *et al.* Pharmacology of narcotic analgesics in the horse: selective blockade of narcotic-induced locomotor activity. *Am J Vet Res* 1981; **42**: 716–721.
64 Pascoe PJ, Taylor PM. Effects of dopamine antagonists on alfentanil-induced locomotor activity in horses. *Vet Anaesth Analg* 2003; **30**: 165–171.
65 Grimm KA, Tranquilli WJ, Gross DR, *et al.* Cardiopulmonary effects of fentanyl in conscious dogs and dogs sedated with a continuous rate infusion of medetomidine. *Am J Vet Res* 2005; **66**: 1222–1226.
66 Wunsch LA, Schmidt BK, Krugner-Higby LA, *et al.* A comparison of the effects of hydromorphone HCl and a novel extended release hydromorphone on arterial blood gas values in conscious healthy dogs. *Res Vet Sci* 2010; **88**: 154–158.
67 Maiante AA, Teixeira Neto FJ, Beier SL, *et al.* Comparison of the cardio-respiratory effects of methadone and morphine in conscious dogs. *J Pharmacol Exp Ther* 2009; **32**: 317–328.
68 Campbell VL, Drobatz KJ, Perkowski SZ. Postoperative hypoxemia and hypercarbia in healthy dogs undergoing routine ovariohysterectomy or castration and receiving butorphanol or hydromorphone for analgesia. *J Am Vet Med Assoc* 2003; **222**: 330–336.
69 Coruh B, Tonelli MR, Park DR. Fentanyl-induced chest wall rigidity. *Chest* 2013; **143**: 1145–1146.
70 Vaughn RL, Bennett CR. Fentanyl chest wall rigidity syndrome – a case report. *Anesth Prog* 1981; **28**: 50–51.

71 Lalley PM. μ-opioid receptor agonists effects on medullary respiratory neurons in the cat: evidence for involvement in certain types of ventilatory disturbances. *Am J Physiol Regul Integr Comp Physiol* 2003; **285**: R1287–R1304.

72 Boudreau AE, Bersenas AM, Kerr CL, *et al.* A comparison of 3 anesthetic protocols for 24 hours of mechanical ventilation in cats. *J Vet Emerg Crit Care* 2012; **22**: 239–252.

73 Ethier MR, Mathews KA, Valverde A, *et al.* Evaluation of the efficacy and safety for use of two sedation and analgesia protocols to facilitate assisted ventilation of healthy dogs. *Am J Vet Res* 2008; **69**: 1351–1359.

74 Westermann CM, Laan TT, van Nieuwstadt RA, *et al.* Effects of antitussive agents administered before bronchoalveolar lavage in horses. *Am J Vet Res* 2005; **66**: 1420–1424.

75 Guedes AG, Papich MG, Rude EP, *et al.* Comparison of plasma histamine levels after intravenous administration of hydromorphone and morphine in dogs. *J Pharmacol Exp Ther* 2007; **30**: 516–522.

76 Ilkiw JE, Pascoe PJ, Haskins SC, *et al.* The cardiovascular sparing effect of fentanyl and atropine, administered to enflurane anesthetized dogs. *Can J Vet Res* 1994; **58**: 248–253.

77 Muldoon SM, Freas W, Mahla ME, *et al.* Plasma histamine and catecholamine levels during hypotension induced by morphine and compound 48/80. *J Cardiovasc Pharmacol* 1987; **9**: 578–583.

78 Robinson EP, Faggella AM, Henry DP, *et al.* Comparison of histamine release induced by morphine and oxymorphone administration in dogs. *Am J Vet Res* 1988; **49**: 1699–1701.

79 Muldoon SM, Donlon MA, Todd R, *et al.* Plasma histamine and hemodynamic responses following administration of nalbuphine and morphine. *Agents Actions* 1984; **15**: 229–234.

80 Schurig JE, Cavanagh RL, Buyniski JP. Effect of butorphanol and morphine on pulmonary mechanics, arterial blood pressure and venous plasma histamine in the anesthetized dog. *Arch Int Pharmacodyn Ther* 1978; **233**: 296–304.

81 Akcasu A, Yillar DO, Akkan AG, *et al.* The role of mast cells in the genesis of acute manifestations following the intravenous injection of meperidine in dogs. *J Basic Clin Physiol Pharmacol* 2009; **20**: 67–72.

82 Allen JW, Horais KA, Tozier NA, *et al.* Time course and role of morphine dose and concentration in intrathecal granuloma formation in dogs: a combined magnetic resonance imaging and histopathology investigation. *Anesthesiology* 2006; **105**: 581–589.

83 Yaksh TL, Allen JW, Veesart SL, *et al.* Role of meningeal mast cells in intrathecal morphine-evoked granuloma formation. *Anesthesiology* 2013; **118**: 664–678.

84 Blancquaert JP, Lefebvre RA, Willems JL. Emetic and antiemetic effects of opioids in the dog. *Eur J Pharmacol* 1986; **128**: 143–150.

85 Hay-Kraus BL. Efficacy of maropitant in preventing vomiting in dogs premedicated with hydromorphone. *Vet Anaesth Analg* 2013; **40**: 28–34.

86 Monteiro ER, Junior AR, Assis HM, *et al.* Comparative study on the sedative effects of morphine, methadone, butorphanol or tramadol, in combination with acepromazine, in dogs. *Vet Anaesth Analg* 2009; **36**: 25–33.

87 Moore AS, Rand WM, Berg J, *et al.* Evaluation of butorphanol and cyproheptadine for prevention of cisplatin-induced vomiting in dogs. *J Am Vet Med Assoc* 1994; **205**: 441–443.

88 Schurig JE, Florczyk AP, Rose WC, *et al.* Antiemetic activity of butorphanol against cisplatin-induced emesis in ferrets and dogs. *Cancer Treat Rep* 1982; **66**: 1831–1835.

89 Robertson SA, Wegner K, Lascelles BD. Antinociceptive and side-effects of hydromorphone after subcutaneous administration in cats. *J Feline Med Surg* 2009; **11**: 76–81.

90 Valverde A, Cantwell S, Hernandez J, *et al.* Effects of acepromazine on the incidence of vomiting associated with opioid administration in dogs. *Vet Anaesth Analg* 2004; **31**: 40–45.

91 Lee HK, Wang SC. Mechanism of morphine-induced miosis in the dog. *J Pharmacol Exp Ther* 1975; **192**: 415–431.

92 Wallenstein MC, Wang SC. Mechanism of morphine-induced mydriasis in the cat. *Am J Physiol* 1979; **236**: R292–296.

93 Sharpe LG, Pickworth WB. Opposite pupillary size effects in the cat and dog after microinjections of morphine, normorphine and clonidine in the Edinger-Wesphal nucleus. *Brain Res Bull* 1985; **15**: 329–333.

94 Brock C, Olesen SS, Olesen AE, *et al.* Opioid-induced bowel dysfunction: pathophysiology and management. *Drugs* 2012; **72**: 1847–1865.

95 Vatashsky E, Haskel Y, Nissan S, *et al.* Effect of morphine on the mechanical activity of common bile duct isolated from the guinea pig. *Anesth Analg* 1987; **66**: 245–248.

96 Johnson EE. Morphine: a dual effect at the canine choledochoduodenal junction. *J Pharmacol Exp Ther* 1981; **219**: 274–280.

97 Kohn CW, Muir WW. Selected aspects of the clinical pharmacology of visceral analgesics and gut motility modifying drugs in the horse. *J Vet Intern Med* 1988; **2**: 85–91.

98 Koenig J, Cote N. Equine gastrointestinal motility – ileus and pharmacological modification. *Can Vet J* 2006; **47**: 551–559.

99 Boscan P, van Hoogmoed LM, Farver TB, *et al.* Evaluation of the effects of the opioid agonist morphine on gastrointestinal tract function in horses. *Am J Vet Res* 2006; **67**: 992–997.

100 Senior JM, Pinchbeck GL, Dugdale AH, *et al.* Retrospective study of the risk factors and prevalence of colic in horses after orthopaedic surgery. *Vet Rec* 2004; **155**: 321–325.

101 Andersen MS, Clark L, Dyson SJ, *et al.* Risk factors for colic in horses after general anaesthesia for MRI or nonabdominal surgery: absence of evidence of effect from perianaesthetic morphine. *Equine Vet J* 2006; **38**: 368–374.

102 Merritt AM, Burrow JA, Hartless CS. Effect of xylazine, detomidine, and a combination of xylazine and butorphanol on equine duodenal motility. *Am J Vet Res* 1998; **59**: 619–623.

103 Boscan P, van Hoogmoed LM, Pypendop BH, *et al.* Pharmacokinetics of the opioid antagonist N-methylnaltrexone and evaluation of its effects on gastrointestinal tract function in horses treated or not treated with morphine. *Am J Vet Res* 2006; **67**: 998–1004.

104 Baldini G, Bagry H, Aprikian A, *et al.* Postoperative urinary retention: anesthetic and perioperative considerations. *Anesthesiology* 2009; **110**: 1139–1157.

105 Drenger B, Magora F. Urodynamic studies after intrathecal fentanyl and buprenorphine in the dog. *Anesth Analg* 1989; **69**: 348–353.

106 Malinovsky JM, Le Normand L, Lepage JY, *et al.* The urodynamic effects of intravenous opioids and ketoprofen in humans. *Anesth Analg* 1998; **87**: 456–461.

107 Troncy E, Junot S, Keroack S, *et al.* Results of preemptive epidural administration of morphine with or without bupivacaine in dogs and cats undergoing surgery: 265 cases (1997–1999). *J Am Vet Med Assoc* 2002; **221**: 666–672.

108 Campoy L, Martin-Flores M, Ludders JW, *et al.* Comparison of bupivacaine femoral and sciatic nerve block versus bupivacaine and morphine epidural for stifle surgery in dogs. *Vet Anaesth Analag* 2012; **39**: 91–98.

109 Pekcan Z, Koc B. The post-operative analgesic effects of epidurally administered morphine and transdermal fentanyl patch after ovariohysterectomy in dogs. *Vet Anaesth Analg* 2010; **37**: 557–565.

110 Sarotti D, Rabozzi R, Franci P. A retrospective study of efficacy and side effects of intrathecal administration of hyperbaric bupivacaine and morphine solution in 39 dogs undergoing hind limb orthopaedic surgery. *Vet Anaesth Analag* 2013; **40**: 220–224.

111 Sarotti D, Rabozzi R, Corletto F. Efficacy and side effects of intraoperative analgesia with intrathecal bupivacaine and levobupivacaine: a retrospective study in 82 dogs. *Vet Anaesth Analg* 2011; **38**: 240–251.

112 Rawal N, Mollefors K, Axelsson K, *et al.* An experimental study of urodynamic effects of epidural morphine and of naloxone reversal. *Anesth Analg* 1983; **62**: 641–647.

113 Anderson MK, Day TK. Effects of morphine and fentanyl constant rate infusion on urine output in healthy and traumatized dogs. *Vet Anaesth Analg* 2008; **35**: 528–536.

114 Biswai AV, Liu WS, Stanley TH, *et al.* The effects of large doses of fentanyl and fentanyl with nitrous oxide on renal function in the dog. *Can Anaesth Soc J* 1976; **23**: 296–302.

115 Robertson SA, Hauptman JG, Nachreiner RF, *et al.* Effects of acetylpromazine or morphine on urine production in halothane-anesthetized dogs. *Am J Vet Res* 2001; **62**: 1922–1927.

116 Leander JD, Hart JC, Zerbe RL. Kappa agonist-induced diuresis: evidence for stereoselectivity, strain differences, independence of hydration variables and a result of decreased plasma vasopressin levels. *J Pharmacol Exp Ther* 1987; **242**: 33–39.

117 Craft RM, Ulibarri CM, Raub DJ. Kappa opioid-induced diuresis in female vs. male rats. *Pharmacol Biochem Behav* 2000; **65**: 53–59.

118 Adler MW, Geller ED, Rosow CE, *et al.* The opioid system and temperature regulation. *Annu Rev Pharmacol Toxicol* 1988; **28**: 429–449.

119 Linton DD, Wilson MG, Newbound GC, *et al.* The effectiveness of a long-acting transdermal fentanyl solution compared to buprenorphine for the control of postoperative pain in dogs in a randomized, multicentered clinical study. *J Pharmacol Exp Ther* 2012; **35**(Suppl 2): 53–64.

120 Guedes AG, Papich MG, Rude EP, *et al.* Pharmacokinetics and physiological effects of intravenous hydromorphone in conscious dogs. *J Pharmacol Exp Ther* 2008; **31**: 334–343.

121 Pottie RG, Dart CM, Perkins NR, *et al.* Effect of hypothermia on recovery from general anaesthesia in the dog. *Austral Vet J* 2007; **85**: 158–162.

122 Posner LP, Gleed RD, Erb HN, *et al.* Post-anesthetic hyperthermia in cats. *Vet Anaesth Analg* 2007; **34**: 40–47.

123 Posner LP, Pavuk AA, Rokshar JL, *et al.* Effects of opioids and anesthetic drugs on body temperature in cats. *Vet Anaesth Analg* 2010; **37**: 35–43.

124 Niedfeldt RL, Robertson SA. Postanesthetic hyperthermia in cats: a retrospective comparison between hydromorphone and buprenorphine. *Vet Anaesth Analg* 2006; **33**: 381–389.

125 Geller EB, Hawk C, Keinath SH, *et al.* Subclasses of opioids based on body temperature change in rats: acute subcutaneous administration. *J Pharmacol Exp Ther* 1983; **225**: 391–398.
126 Rosow CE, Miller JM, Pelikan EW, *et al.* Opiates and thermoregulation in mice. I. Agonists. *J Pharmacol Exp Ther* 1980; **213**: 273–283.
127 Meyer LC, Fick L, Matthee A, *et al.* Hyperthermia in captured impala (Aepyceros melampus): a fright not flight response. *J Wildl Dis* 2008; **44**: 404–416.
128 Page GG. Immunologic effects of opioids in the presence or absence of pain. *J Pain Symptom Manage* 2005; **29**: S25–31.
129 Mellon RD, Bayer BM. Evidence for central opioid receptors in the immunomodulatory effects of morphine: review of potential mechanism(s) of action. *J Neuroimmunol* 1998; **83**: 19–28.
130 Page GG. The immune-suppressive effects of pain. In: Machelska H, Stein C, eds. *Immune Mechanisms of Pain and Analgesia*. Dordrecht: Kluwer Academic, 2003; 117–125.
131 Cronin AJ, Aucutt-Walter NM, Budinetz T, *et al.* Low-dose remifentanil infusion does not impair natural killer cell function in healthy volunteers. *Br J Anaesth* 2003; **91**: 805–809.
132 Yeager MP, Procopio MA, DeLeo JA, *et al.* Intravenous fentanyl increases natural killer cell cytotoxicity and circulating CD16(+) lymphocytes in humans. *Anesth Analg* 2002; **94**: 94–99.
133 Gaspani L, Bianchi M, Limiroli E, *et al.* The analgesic drug tramadol prevents the effect of surgery on natural killer cell activity and metastatic colonization in rats. *J Neuroimmunol* 2002; **129**: 18–24.
134 Ilkiw JE, Pascoe PJ, Tripp LD. Effects of morphine, butorphanol, buprenorphine, and U50488H on the minimum alveolar concentration of isoflurane in cats. *Am J Vet Res* 2002; **63**: 1198–1202.
135 Monteiro ER, Teixeira-Neto FJ, Campagnol D, *et al.* Effects of remifentanil on the minimum alveolar concentration of isoflurane in dogs. *Am J Vet Res* 2010; **71**: 150–156.
136 Glass PS, Gan TJ, Howell S, *et al.* Drug interactions: volatile anesthetics and opioids. *J Clin Anesth* 1997; **9**(6 Suppl): 18S–22S.
137 Michelsen LG, Salmenperä M, Hug CC Jr, *et al.* Anesthetic potency of remifentanil in dogs. *Anesthesiology* 1996; **84**: 865–872.
138 Machado CE, Dyson DH, Grant MM. Effects of oxymorphone and hydromorphone on the minimum alveolar concentration of isoflurane in dogs. *Vet Anaesth Analg* 2006; **33**: 70–77.
139 Valverde A, Dyson DH, McDonell WN. Epidural morphine reduces halothane MAC in the dog. *Can J Anaesth* 1989; **36**: 629–632.
140 Villalba M, Santiago I, Gomez de Segura IA. Effects of constant rate infusion of lidocaine and ketamine, with or without morphine, on isoflurane MAC in horses. *Equine Vet J* 2011; **43**: 721–726.
141 Ferreira TH, Aguiar AJ, Valverde A, *et al.* Effect of remifentanil hydrochloride administered via constant rate infusion on the minimum alveolar concentration of isoflurane in cats. *Am J Vet Res* 2009; **70**: 581–588.
142 Ferreira TH, Steffey EP, Mama KR, *et al.* Determination of the sevoflurane sparing effect of methadone in cats. *Vet Anaesth Analg* 2011; **38**: 310–319.
143 Ilkiw JE, Pascoe PJ, Fisher LD. Effect of alfentanil on the minimum alveolar concentration of isoflurane in cats. *Am J Vet Res* 1997; **58**: 1274–1279.
144 Brosnan RJ, Pypendop BH, Siao KT, *et al.* Effects of remifentanil on measures of anesthetic immobility and analgesia in cats. *Am J Vet Res* 2009; **70**: 1065–1071.
145 Knych HK, Steffey EP, Mama KR, *et al.* Effects of high plasma fentanyl concentrations on minimum alveolar concentration of isoflurane in horses. *Am J Vet Res* 2009; **70**: 1193–1200.
146 Doherty TJ, Will WA, Rohrbach BW, *et al.* Effect of morphine and flunixin meglumine on isoflurane minimum alveolar concentration in goats. *Vet Anaesth Analg* 2004; **31**: 97–101.
147 Criado AB, Gómez de Segura IA, Tendillo FJ, *et al.* Reduction of isoflurane MAC with buprenorphine and morphine in rats. *Lab Anim* 2000; **34**: 252–259.
148 Criado AB, Gómez e Segura IA. Reduction of isoflurane MAC by fentanyl or remifentanil in rats. *Vet Anaesth Analg* 2003; **30**: 250–256.
149 Abreu M, Aguado D, Benito J, *et al.* Reduction of the sevoflurane minimum alveolar concentration induced by methadone, tramadol, butorphanol and morphine in rats. *Lab Anim* 2012; **46**: 200–206.
150 Khurshid N, Agarwal V, Iyengar S. Expression of mu- and delta-opioid receptors in song control regions of adult male zebra finches (Taenopygia guttata). *J Chem Neuroanat* 2009; **37**: 158–169.
151 Csillag A, Bourne RC, Stewart MG. Distribution of mu, delta, and kappa opioid receptor binding sites in the brain of the one-day-old domestic chick (Gallus domesticus): an in vitro quantitative autoradiographic study. *J Comp Neurol* 1990; **302**: 543–551.
152 Reiner A, Brauth SE, Kitt CA, *et al.* Distribution of mu, delta, and kappa opiate receptor types in the forebrain and midbrain of pigeons. *J Comp Neurol* 1989; **280**: 359–382.
153 Escobar A, Valadao CA, Brosnan RJ, *et al.* Effects of butorphanol on the minimum anesthetic concentration for sevoflurane in guineafowl (Numida meleagris). *Am J Vet Res* 2012; **73**: 183–188.
154 Concannon KT, Dodam JR, Hellyer PW. Influence of a mu- and kappa-opioid agonist on isoflurane minimal anesthetic concentration in chickens. *Am J Vet Res* 1995; **56**: 806–811.
155 de Wolff MH, Leather HA, Wouters PF. Effects of tramadol on minimum alveolar concentration (MAC) of isoflurane in rats. *Br J Anaesth* 1999; **83**: 780–783.
156 Levin VA. Relationship of octanol/water partition coefficient and molecular weight to rat brain capillary permeability. *J Med Chem* 1980; **23**: 682–684.
157 Pacharinsak C, Greene SA, Keegan RD, *et al.* Postoperative analgesia in dogs receiving epidural morphine plus medetomidine. *J Vet Pharmacol Ther* 2003; **26**: 71–77.
158 Torske KE, Dyson DH. Epidural analgesia and anesthesia. *Vet Clin North Am Small Anim Pract* 2000; **30**: 859–874.
159 Dobromylskyj P, Flecknell PA, Lascelles BD, *et al.* Management of postoperative and other acute pain. In: Flecknell P, Waterman-Pearson A, eds. *Pain Management in Animals*. London: WB Saunders, 2000; 102.
160 Cousins MJ, Mather LE. Intrathecal and epidural administration of opioids. *Anesthesiology* 1984; **61**: 276–310.
161 Priano LL, Vatner SF. Morphine effects on cardiac output and regional blood flow distribution in conscious dogs. *Anesthesiology* 1981; **55**: 236–243.
162 KuKanich B, Lascelles BD, Papich MG. Use of a von Frey device for evaluation of pharmacokinetics and pharmacodynamics of morphine after intravenous administration as an infusion or multiple doses in dogs. *Am J Vet Res* 2005; **66**: 1968–1974.
163 KuKanich B, Lascelles BDX, Riviere JE, *et al.* Pharmacokinetic-pharmacodynamics modeling of morphine in dogs. *J Vet Intern Med* 2007; **21**: 617.
164 Lucas AN, Firth AM, Anderson GA, *et al.* Comparison of the effects of morphine administered by constant-rate intravenous infusion or intermittent intramuscular injection in dogs. *J Am Vet Med Assoc* 2001; **218**: 884–891.
165 Yoshimura K, Horiuchi M, Konishi M, *et al.* Physical dependence on morphine induced in dogs via the use of miniosmotic pumps. *J Pharmacol Toxicol Methods* 1993; **30**: 85–95.
166 Jacqz E, Ward S, Johnson R, *et al.* Extrahepatic glucuronidation of morphine in the dog. *Drug Metab Dispos* 1986; **14**: 627–630.
167 Bragg P, Zwass MS, Lau M, *et al.* Opioid pharmacodynamics in neonatal dogs: differences between morphine and fentanyl. *J Appl Physiol* 1995; **79**: 1519–1524.
168 Day TK, Pepper WT, Tobias TA, *et al.* Comparison of intra-articular and epidural morphine for analgesia following stifle arthrotomy in dogs. *Vet Surg* 1995; **24**: 522–530.
169 Devine EP, KuKanich B, Beard WL. Pharmacokinetics of intramuscularly administered morphine in horses. *J Am Vet Med Assoc* 2013; **243**: 105–112.
170 Mircica E, Clutton RE, Kyles KW, *et al.* Problems associated with perioperative morphine in horses: a retrospective case analysis. *Vet Anaesth Analg* 2003; **30**: 147–155.
171 Santos LC, de Moraes AN, Saito ME. Effects of intraarticular ropivacaine and morphine on lipopolysaccharide-induced synovitis in horses. *Vet Anaesth Analg* 2009; **36**: 280–286.
172 Lindegaard C, Thomsen MH, Larsen S, *et al.* Analgesic efficacy of intra-articular morphine in experimentally induced radiocarpal synovitis in horses. *Vet Anaesth Analg* 2010; **37**: 171–185.
173 Lindegaard C, Gleerup KB, Thomsen MH, *et al.* Anti-inflammatory effects of intra-articular administration of morphine in horses with experimentally induced synovitis. *Am J Vet Res* 2010; **71**: 69–75.
174 Mathews KA, Paley DM, Foster RA, *et al.* A comparison of ketorolac with flunixin, butorphanol, and oxymorphone in controlling postoperative pain in dogs. *Can Vet J* 1996; **37**: 557–567.
175 Smith LJ, Yu JK, Bjorling DE, *et al.* Effects of hydromorphone or oxymorphone, with or without acepromazine, on preanesthetic sedation, physiologic values, and histamine release in dogs. *J Am Vet Med Assoc* 2001; **218**: 1101–1105.
176 KuKanich B. Pharmacokinetics of subcutaneous fentanyl in Greyhounds. *Vet J* 2011; **190**: e140–142.
177 Freise KJ, Linton DD, Newbound GC, *et al.* Population pharmacokinetics of transdermal fentanyl solution following a single dose administered prior to soft tissue and orthopedic surgery in dogs. *J Vet Pharmacol Ther* 2012; **35**(Suppl 2): 65–72.
178 Savides MC, Pohland RC, Wilkie DA, *et al.* The margin of safety of a single application of transdermal fentanyl solution when administered at multiples of the therapeutic dose to laboratory dogs. *J Vet Pharmacol Ther* 2012; **35**(Suppl 2): 35–43.
179 Kyles AE, Papich MG, Hardie EM. Disposition of transdermally administered fentanyl in dogs. *Am J Vet Res* 1996; **57**: 715–719.
180 Lee DD. Papich MG, Hardie EM. Comparison of pharmacokinetics of fentanyl after intravenous and transdermal administration in cats. *Am J Vet Res* 2000; **61**: 672–677.
181 Schmiedt CW, Bjorling DE. Accidental prehension and suspected transmucosal or oral absorption of fentanyl from a transdermal patch in a dog. *Vet Anaesth Analg* 2007; **34**: 70–73.

182 Teske J, Weller JP, Larsch K, *et al.* Fatal outcome in a child after ingestion of a transdermal fentanyl patch. *Int J Legal Med* 2007; **121**: 147–151.
183 Gorman AL, Elliott KJ, Inturrisi CE. The d- and l-isomers of methadone bind to the non-competitive site on the N-methyl-D-aspartate (NMDA) receptor in rat forebrain and spinal cord. *Neurosci Lett* 1997; **223**: 5–8.
184 Bolan EA, Tallarida RJ, Pasternak GW. Synergy between mu opioid ligands: evidence for functional interactions among mu opioid receptor subtypes. *J Vet Pharmacol Ther* 2002; **303**: 557–562.
185 Linardi RL, Stokes AM, Barker SA, *et al.* Pharmacokinetics of the injectable formulation of methadone hydrochloride administered orally in horses. *J Vet Pharmacol Ther* 2009; **32**: 492–497.
186 Pypendop B, Ilkiw JE, Shilo-Benjamini Y. Bioavailability of morphine, methadone, hydromorphone, and oxymorphone following buccal administration in cats. *J Vet Pharmacol Ther* 2014; **37**: 295–300.
187 Priano LL, Vatner SF. Generalized cardiovascular and regional hemodynamic effects of meperidine in conscious dogs. *Anesth Analg* 1981; **60**: 649–654.
188 Huang YF, Upton RN, Rutten AJ, *et al.* The hemodynamic effects of intravenous bolus doses of meperidine in conscious sheep. *Anesth Analg* 1994; **78**: 442–449.
189 Reuben SS, Steinberg RB, Lurie SD, *et al.* A dose–response study of intravenous regional anesthesia with meperidine. *Anesth Analg* 1999; **88**: 831–835.
190 Waterman AE, Kalthum W. Use of opioids in providing postoperative analgesia in the dog: a double-blind trial of pethidine, pentazocine, buprenorphine, and butorphanol In: Short CE, van Poznack A, eds. *Animal Pain*. New York: Churchill Livingstone, 1992; 466–479.
191 Flacke JW, Flacke WE, Bloor BC, *et al.* Histamine release by four narcotics: a double-blind study in humans. *Anesth Analg* 1987; **66**: 723–730.
192 Clutton RE. Unexpected responses following intravenous pethidine injection in two horses. *Equine Vet J* 1987; **19**: 72–73.
193 Takada K, Clark DJ, Davies MF, *et al.* Meperidine exerts agonist activity at the alpha(2B)-adrenoceptor subtype. *Anesthesiology* 2002; **96(6)**: 1420–1426.
194 KuKanich B, Spade J. Pharmacokinetics of hydrocodone and hydromorphone after oral hydrocodone in healthy Greyhound dogs. *Vet J* 2013; **196**: 266–268.
195 Yeh SY, Woods LA. Excretion of codeine and its metabolites by dogs, rabbits and cats. *Arch Int Pharmacodyn Ther* 1971; **191**: 231–242.
196 Findlay JW, Jones EC, Welch RM. Radioimmunoassay determination of the absolute oral bioavailabilities and O-demethylation of codeine and hydrocodone in the dog. *Drug Metab Dispos* 1979; **7**: 310–314.
197 KuKanich B. Pharmacokinetics of acetaminophen, codeine, and the codeine metabolites morphine and codeine-6-glucuronide in healthy Greyhound dogs. *J Vet Pharmacol Ther* 2010; **33**: 15–21.
198 Martin WR, Eades CG, Fraser HF, *et al.* Use of hindlimb reflexes of the chronic spinal dog for comparing analgesics. *J Vet Pharmacol Ther* 1964; **144**: 8–11.
199 Weinstein SH, Gaylord JC. Determination of oxycodone in plasma and identification of a major metabolite. *J Pharmaceut Sci* 1979; **68**: 527–528.
200 Hoke JF, Cunningham F, James MK, *et al.* Comparative pharmacokinetics and pharmacodynamics of remifentanil, its principal metabolite (GR90291) and alfentanil in dogs. *J Pharmacol Exp Ther* 1997; **281**: 226–232.
201 Pieper K, Schuster T, Levionnois O, *et al.* Antinociceptive efficacy and plasma concentrations of transdermal buprenorphine in dogs. *Vet J* 2011; **187**: 335–341.
202 Goyenechea Jaramillo LA, Murrell JC, Hellebrekers LJ. Investigation of the interaction between buprenorphine and sufentanil during anaesthesia for ovariectomy in dogs. *Vet Anaesth Analg* 2006; **33**: 399–407.
203 Martin LB, Thompson AC, Martin T, Kristal MB. Analgesic efficacy of orally administered buprenorphine in rats. *Comp Med* 2001; **51(1)**: 43–48.
204 Thompson AC, Kristal MB, Sallaj A, *et al.* Analgesic efficacy of orally administered buprenorphine in rats: methodologic considerations. *Comp Med* 2004; **54(3)**: 293–300.
205 Messenger KM, Davis JL, LaFevers DH, *et al.* Intravenous and sublingual buprenorphine in horses: pharmacokinetics and influence of sampling site. *Vet Anaesth Analg* 2011; **38**: 374–384.
206 Murrell JC, Robertson SA, Taylor PM, *et al.* Use of a transdermal matrix patch of buprenorphine in cats: preliminary pharmacokinetic and pharmacodynamic data. *Vet Rec* 2007; **160**: 578–583.
207 Catbagan DL, Quimby JM, Mama KR, *et al.* Comparison of the efficacy and adverse effects of sustained-release buprenorphine hydrochloride following subcutaneous administration and buprenorphine hydrochloride following oral transmucosal administration in cats undergoing ovariohysterectomy. *Am J Vet Res* 2011; **72**: 461–466.
208 Foley PL, Liang H, Crichlow AR. Evaluation of a sustained release formulation of buprenorphine for analgesia in rats. *J Am Assoc Lab Anim Sci* 2011; **50**: 198–204.
209 Carbone ET, Lindstrom KE, Diep S, *et al.* Duration of action of sustained-release buprenorphine in 2 strains of mice. *J Am Assoc Lab Anim Sci* 2012; **51**: 815–819.
210 Sawyer DC, Rech RH, Durham RA, *et al.* Dose response to butorphanol administered subcutaneously to increase visceral nociceptive threshold in dogs. *Am J Vet Res* 1991; **52**: 1826–1830.
211 Lascelles BD, Robertson SA. Use of thermal threshold response to evaluate the antinociceptive effects of butorphanol in cats. *Am J Vet Res* 2004; **65**: 1085–1089.
212 Cavanagh RL, Gylys JA, Bierwagen ME. Antitussive properties of butorphanol. *Arch Int Pharmacodyn Ther* 1976; **220**: 258–268.
213 Sellon DC, Monroe VL, Roberts MC, *et al.* Pharmacokinetics and adverse effects of butorphanol administered by single intravenous injection or continuous intravenous infusion in horses. *Am J Vet Res* 2001; **62**: 183–189.
214 Sanchez LC, Elfenbein JR, Robertson SA. Effect of acepromazine, butorphanol, or N-butylscopolammonium bromide on visceral and somatic nociception and duodenal motility in conscious horses. *Am J Vet Res* 2008; **69**: 579–585.
215 Merritt AM, Campbell-Thompson ML, Lowrey S. Effect of butorphanol on equine antroduodenal motility. *Equine Vet J* 1989; 7(Suppl): 21–23.
216 Sojka JE, Adams SB, Lamar CH, *et al.* Effect of butorphanol, pentazocine, meperidine, or metoclopramide on intestinal motility in female ponies. *Am J Vet Res* 1988; **49**: 527–529.
217 Sellon DC, Roberts MC, Blikslager AT, *et al.* Effects of continuous rate intravenous infusion of butorphanol on physiologic and outcome variables in horses after celiotomy. *J Vet Intern Med* 2004; **18**: 555–563.
218 Muir WW, Robertson JT. Visceral analgesia: effects of xylazine, butorphanol, meperidine, and pentazocine in horses. *Am J Vet Res* 1985; **46**: 2081–2084.
219 Kohn CW, Muir WW. Selected aspects of the clinical pharmacology of visceral analgesic and gut motility modifying drugs in the horse. *J Vet Intern Med* 1988; **2**: 85–91.
220 Mealey KL. Adverse drug reactions in herding breed dogs: the role of p-glycoprotein. *Compendium* 2006; **28**: 23–33.
221 Frazillo Fde, DeRossi R, Jardim PH, *et al.* Effects of epidural nalbuphine on intraoperative isoflurane and postoperative analgesic requirements in dogs. *Acta Cir Bras* 2014; **29**: 38–46.
222 Taylor PM, Houlton JEF. Post-operative analgesia in the dog: a comparison of morphine, buprenorphine and pentazocine. *J Small Anim Pract* 1984; **25**: 437–451.
223 Stamer UM, Musshoff F, Kobilay M, *et al.* Concentrations of tramadol and O-desmethyltramadol enantiomers in different CYP2D6 genotypes. *Clin Pharmacol Ther* 2007; **82**: 41–47.
224 Kukanich B, Papich MG. Pharmacokinetics and antinociceptive effects of oral tramadol hydrochloride administration in Greyhounds. *Am J Vet Res* 2011; **72**: 256–262.
225 Pypendop BH, Siao KT, Ilkiw JE. Effects of tramadol hydrochloride on the thermal threshold in cats. *Am J Vet Res* 2009; **70**: 1465–1470.
226 Knych HK, Corado CR, McKemie DS, *et al.* Pharmacokinetics and pharmacodynamics of tramadol in horses following oral administration. *J Vet Pharmacol Ther* 2013; **36**: 389–398.
227 Matthiesen T, Wöhrmann T, Coogan TP, *et al.* The experimental toxicology of tramadol: an overview. *Toxicol Lett* 1998; **95**: 63–71.
228 Mohammad-Zadeh LF, Moses L, Gwaltney-Brant SM. Serotonin: a review. *Vet Pharmacol Ther* 2008; **31**: 187–199.
229 Veng-Pedersen P, Wilhelm JA, Zakszewski TB, *et al.* Duration of opioid antagonism by nalmefene and naloxone in the dog: an integrated pharmacokinetic/pharmacodynamic comparison. *J Pharm Sci* 1995; **84**: 1101–1106.
230 Wilhelm JA, Veng-Pedersen P, Zakszewski TB, *et al.* Duration of opioid antagonism by nalmefene and naloxone in the dog. A nonparametric pharmacodynamic comparison based on generalized cross-validated spline estimation. *Int J Clin Pharmacol Ther* 1995; **33**: 540–545.
231 Grace PM, Greene LI, Strand KA, *et al.* Repeated morphine enhances peripheral nerve injury-induced allodynia via TLR4 and P2X7 activation in the lumbar spinal cord. Presented at the Society for Neuroscience Annual Meeting, San Diego, CA, USA, 2013.
232 Taylor R Jr, Pergolizzi JV Jr, Porreca F, *et al.* Opioid antagonists for pain. *Expert Opin Invest Drugs* 2013; **22**: 517–525.
233 Leavitt SD. Opioid antagonists, naloxone & naltrexone – aids for pain management. *Pain Treatment Topics*, 2009. http://pain-topics.org/pdf/OpioidAntagonistsForPain.pdf (accessed 23 January 2014).
234 Slingsby LS, Murrell JC, Taylor PM. Buprenorphine in combination with naloxone at a ratio of 15:1 does not enhance antinociception from buprenorphine in healthy cats. *Vet J* 2012; **192**: 523–524.
235 Pypendop BH, Brosnan RJ, Ilkiw JE. Use of naltrexone to antagonize high doses of remifentanil in cats: a dose-finding study. *Vet Anaesth Analg* 2011; **38**: 594–597.
236 Movafegh A, Shoeibi G, Ansari M, *et al.* Naloxone infusion and post-hysterectomy morphine consumption: a double-blind, placebo-controlled study. *Acta Anaesthesiol Scand* 2012; **56**: 1241–1249.
237 van Hoogmoed LM, Boscan PL. In vitro evaluation of the effect of the opioid antagonist N-methylnaltrexone on motility of the equine jejunum and pelvic flexure. *Equine Vet J* 2005; **37**: 325–328.

12 Non-Steroidal Anti-Inflammatory Drugs

Mark G. Papich and Kristin Messenger
Department of Molecular Biomedical Sciences, College of Veterinary Medicine, North Carolina State University, Raleigh, North Carolina, USA

Chapter contents

Introduction

Non-steroidal anti-inflammatory drugs (NSAIDs) are among the most important drugs used in all species of animals. They possess both analgesic and anti-inflammatory properties. Because they are not controlled or scheduled drugs they can be easily prescribed and dispensed. There are a variety of formulations and routes of administration to choose from that include oral tablets, oral caplets, oral liquids, chewable tablets, paste (for horses), oral transmucosal mist, transdermal, and injectable solutions for intravenous or subcutaneous administration. There are many NSAIDs to choose from (Table 12.1, Box 12.1).

This chapter will focus primarily on the drugs used in many countries, but the reader should consider that availability, registration, licensing, and approvals by regulatory authorities vary greatly. There are older drugs that may be used (e.g., aspirin and dipyrone) but for which the pharmacology has not been re-examined for animals in many years. These older drugs will not be covered in this chapter but details of their pharmacology may be found in previous editions of this text (book) and other older textbooks. Although this chapter focuses primarily on the major veterinary species of dogs, cats, horses, and cattle, the use of NSAIDs in other animals should not be overlooked. There has been extensive work in zoo and exotic species. Surprising differences and some similarities exist in the pharmacokinetics and pharmacodynamics in these other species. It is beyond the scope of this chapter to address all the other animal species in which NSAIDs are administered; therefore, the reader is encouraged to consult species-specific publications for more guidance.

Information on the pharmacology of these agents has been provided by Lees [1] as well as many other authors. Complete monographs of these drugs were published in 2004 and are available at no charge on-line at www.aavpt.org (search words: "veterinary drug monographs"). A review of NSAID pharmacology and use in small animals has been provided by KuKanich *et al.* [2] and an analysis of adverse reactions in dogs by Monteiro-Steagall *et al.* [3]. The pharmacokinetic and pharmacodynamic actions of many NSAIDs have been reviewed extensively by Lees *et al.* [4,5]. Guidelines for clinical use in dogs [2,6], cats [7,8], and food animals [9] are available in species-specific reviews. A description of the chemistry, mechanism of action, and clinical use of the COXIB-class of NSAIDs is also available [10–12].

Mechanism of action

Metabolism of arachidonic acid

As shown in Fig. 12.1, arachidonic acid, a fatty acid consisting of 20 carbons, is released from cell membranes by the enzyme phospholipase A_2 (PLA_2). Arachidonic acid is the predominant fatty acid in animal cell membranes. The products of arachidonic

Veterinary Anesthesia and Analgesia: The Fifth Edition of Lumb and Jones.
Edited by Kurt A. Grimm, Leigh A. Lamont, William J. Tranquilli, Stephen A. Greene and Sheilah A. Robertson.

Table 12.1 Structures and pharmacologic parameters for selected nonsteroidal anti-inflammatory drugs (NSAIDS) commonly used in animals.

Drug	Chemical group and structure	COX-1 or COX-2 inhibitory	Half-life	V_D	F%*	Protein binding*
Carprofen	Propionic acid 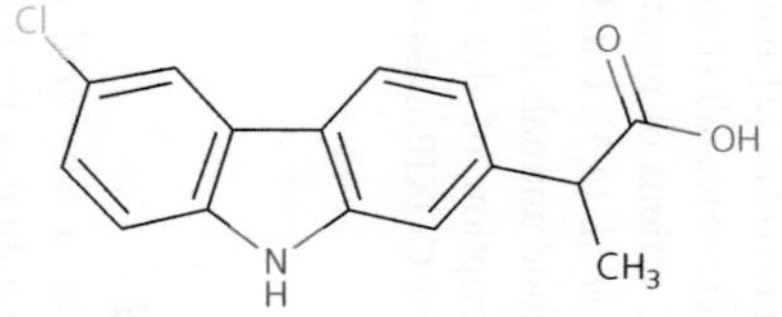	Preferential for COX-2	Dogs: 11.7 h (after 100 mg single IV bolus) and ~8 h (range 4.5–9.8 h) (oral) Horses: (S+) 7.95 +/– 2.18h, and 9.68 +/– 1.29h Cats: 20 +/– 16.6 h (range 9–49); and 10.7 +/– 5.17 h (S+) Calves: 37 +/–2.4 h (S+) Cows: 30.7 +/– 2.3 h (43 +/– 2.3 h with mastitis)	Dogs: 0.14 +/– 0.02 L/kg Cats: 0.14 +/– 0.05 L/kg; and 0.25 L/kg Horses: 0.307 +/– 0.036 L/kg Cows: 0.091 +/– 0.003 L/kg Calves: 0.163 +/– 0.002 L/kg	Dogs: >90% (oral)	>99%
Deracoxib	Coxib (diaryl substituted pyrazole) 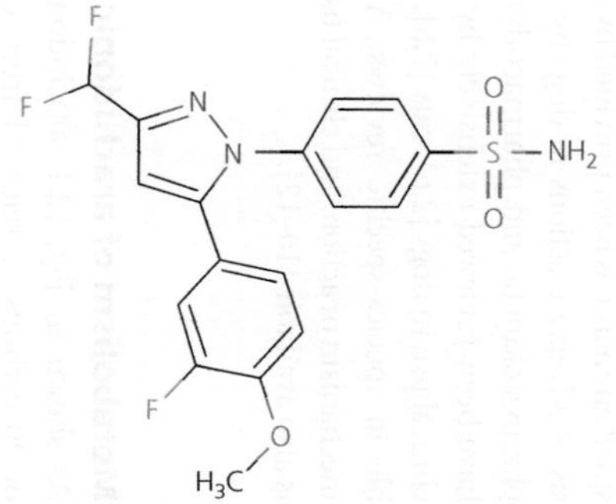	Selective for COX-2	Dogs: following IV administration: 3 h at 2–3 mg/kg Cats: 7.9 h	Dogs: ~1.5 L/kg	Dogs: >90% at 2 mg/kg (oral)	>90%
Robenacoxib	Coxib 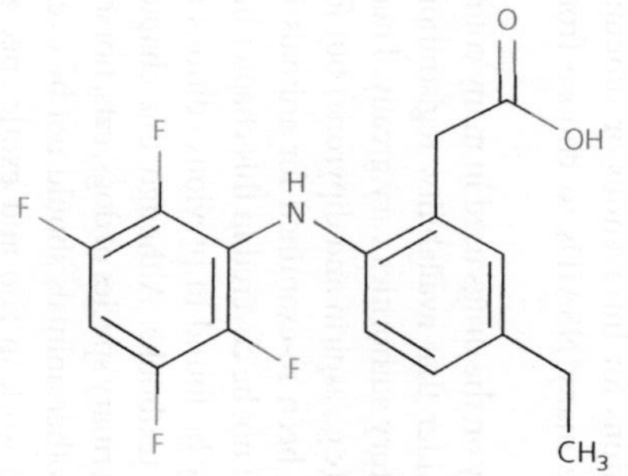	Selective for COX-2	Dogs: 0.63 and 1.1 h Cats: 1.49, 1.87, 0.84, and 0.78 h (depending on the study)	Dogs: 0.24 L/kg Cats:0.13 and 0.19 L/kg, depending on the study	Dogs: 84% non-fed; 62% fed Cats: 49% non-fed, 10% fed	Dogs: 98% Cats: 99.9%
Etodolac	Pyranocarboxylic acid 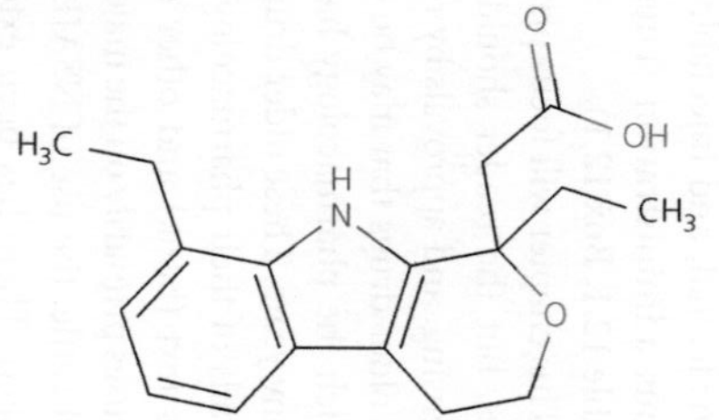	Non-selective for COX-2 or preferential for COX-2, depending on the study	Dogs: fasted: 7.66 ± 2.05 h (oral), non-fasted: 11.98 ± 5.52 h (oral), 9.7 +/– 0.97 h (IV) Horses: 2.85 h (mean)	Dogs: 1.14 L/kg Horses: 0.29 +/- 0.09 L/kg	Dogs: ~100% Horses: 77% (range 43–100%)	>95%

Firocoxib	Coxib 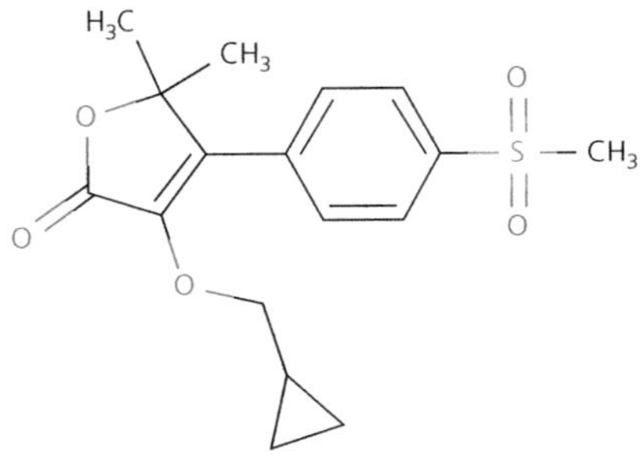	Selective for COX-2. The most highly selective of all the veterinary NSAIDs	Dogs: 7.8 h (CV ± 30%) Horses: 33.8 +/−11.2 h IV, 29.6 +/−7.5 h oral (longer after multiple doses, 36.5 +/− 9.5 h)	Dogs: ~4.6 L/kg Horses: 1.7 +/− 0.4 L/kg	Dogs: ~38% (oral) Horses: 79% +/− 31	Dogs: 96% Horses >97%
Ketoprofen	Propionic acid 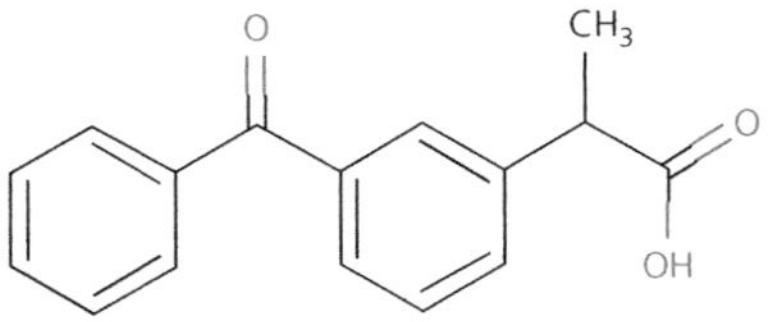	Non-selective for COX-2	*S*-(+)-enantiomer Dogs: 1.65 ± 0.48 h (oral) Cats: 1.5 h Horses: 0.37–1.51 h (depending on the study) Calves: 0.42–2.19 h (depending on study and age)	*S*-(+)-enantiomer. Dogs: 0.39 +/− 0.07 L/kg Horses: 0.14 +/− 0.02 L/kg and 0.22 +/− 0.08 L/kg Calves: 0.26 +/− 0.06 L/kg	Dogs, Cats: almost 100% Horses: 52%	Horses: 93%
Mavacoxib	Coxib 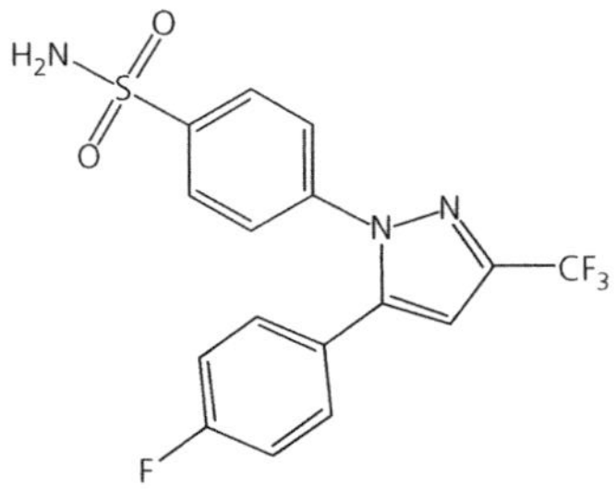	COX-2 selective	Median 17 days (8–39 days) in Beagle dogs, and 39 days in field trial dogs, with some dogs >80 days	1.6 L/kg	Fasted: 46.1%; fed 87.4% (dose is based on fed dogs)	98%
Meloxicam	Enolic acid derivative (oxicam) 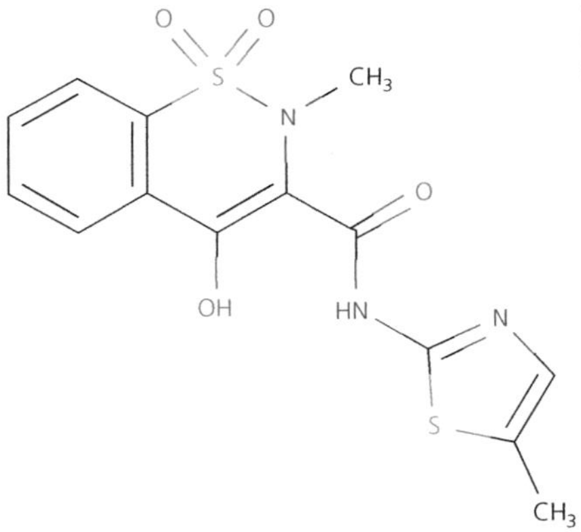	Meloxicam is considered to be COX-2 preferential because at high doses its COX-2 specificity diminishes	Dogs: 24.0 ± 26.2% h (IV), 23.7 ± 30.0% h (oral) Cats: 26–37 h (depending on study) Horse: 8.54 +/− 3.02 h, 5.15 h (average of range of doses) and 10.2 +/− 3.0 h in fed horses Cattle: 20–30 h depending on the study (cows 14.6 h)	Dogs: ~0.32 +/− 20% L/kg (VD_{AREA}) Horses: 0.23 and 0.12 L/kg (depending on study) Cats: 0.245 L/kg (VD/F) Cattle: 0.194 L/kg	Dogs: 100% Horses: 85.3 +/− 19.4% (non-fed), 95.9 +/− 13.2 % (fed) Cattle: 100%	Dogs: 97% Horses: 98.5%

(Continued)

Table 12.1 (*Continued*)

Drug	Chemical group and structure	COX-1 or COX-2 inhibitory	Half-life	V_D	F%*	Protein binding*
Phenylbutazone	Pyrazolone (pyrazolidinedione) 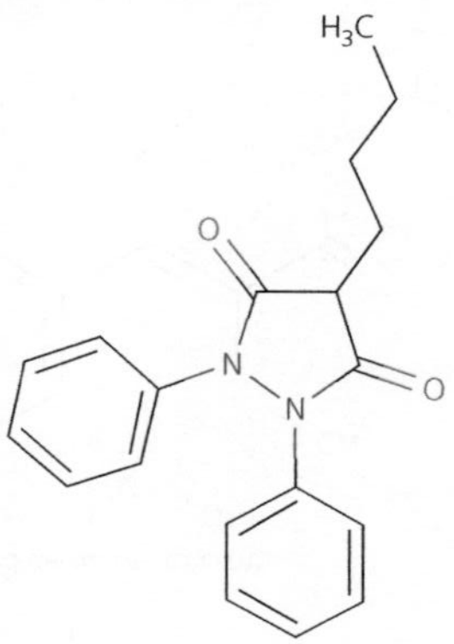 H_3C O N N O	Non-selective for COX-2	Horses: 5.4 +/– 0.5 h Calves: 53.4 +/– 5.1 h Bulls: 62 h Cows: 36–55 h (depending on study) Dogs: 4–6 h	Cattle: 0.13–0.14 L/kg Horses: 0.14 L/kg	Cattle: 54–69% and 69–89% (depen-ding on study) Horses: 70% (delayed with feeding)	Horses: 99% Cattle: 93–98%
Flunixin	Anthranilic adic (pyridinecarboxylic acid) 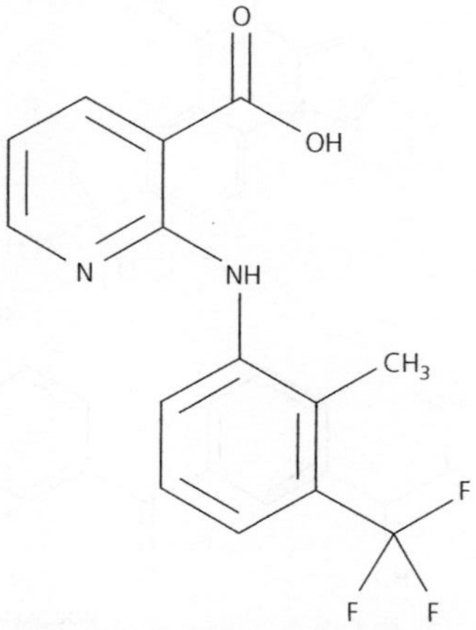 O OH N NH CH_3 F F F	Non-selective for COX-2	Horses: 1.7–3.4 h (depending on study) Cows: 3–8 h (depending on study) Dogs: 3.7 h Cats: 6.6 h	Horses: 0.15 +/– 0.04 L/kg Dogs: 0.18 +/– 0.08 L/kg Cats: 0.75 L/kg Cows: 0.42, 0.78, and 0.50 L/kg in different studies	Dogs: approx-imately 100% Horses: 72%	>90%

*Data for dogs, unless otherwise stated. VD, apparent volume of distribution (for most drugs, at steady state); F%, fraction of oral dose absorbed.
T½, half-life; V_D, apparent volume of distribution; CL, systemic clearance; F%, percent bioavailability after oral administration. Colored portions of the structure represent the reactive groups.
Pharmacokinetics from references: 26,27,29,30,41–43,45,48–50,57,67,105,115, and 145–155.

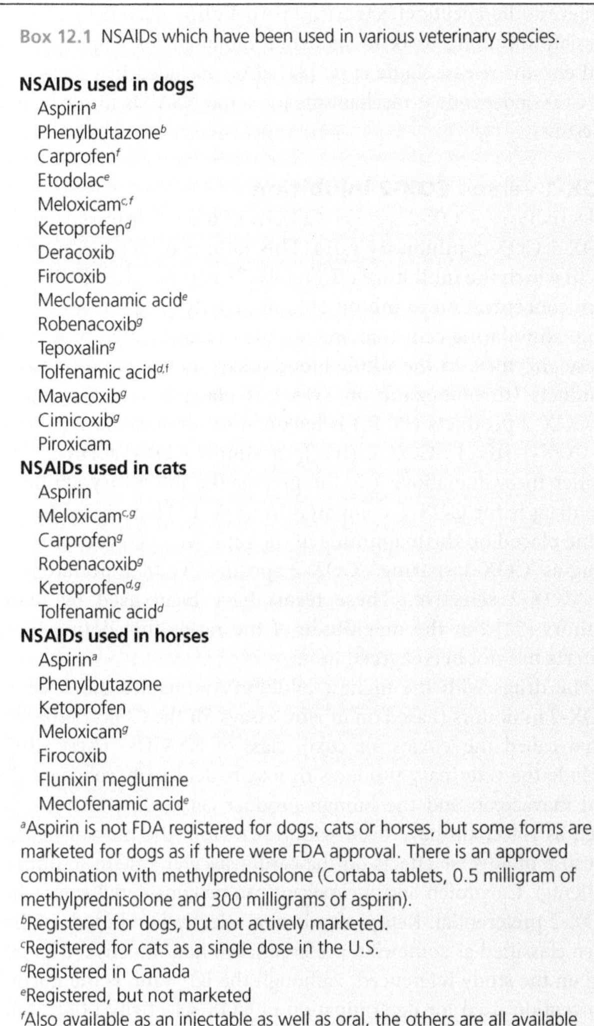

Box 12.1 NSAIDs which have been used in various veterinary species.

NSAIDs used in dogs

- Aspirin[a]
- Phenylbutazone[b]
- Carprofen[f]
- Etodolac[e]
- Meloxicam[c,f]
- Ketoprofen[d]
- Deracoxib
- Firocoxib
- Meclofenamic acid[e]
- Robenacoxib[g]
- Tepoxalin[g]
- Tolfenamic acid[d,f]
- Mavacoxib[g]
- Cimicoxib[g]
- Piroxicam

NSAIDs used in cats

- Aspirin
- Meloxicam[c,g]
- Carprofen[g]
- Robenacoxib[g]
- Ketoprofen[d,g]
- Tolfenamic acid[d]

NSAIDs used in horses

- Aspirin[a]
- Phenylbutazone
- Ketoprofen
- Meloxicam[g]
- Firocoxib
- Flunixin meglumine
- Meclofenamic acid[e]

[a]Aspirin is not FDA registered for dogs, cats or horses, but some forms are marketed for dogs as if there were FDA approval. There is an approved combination with methylprednisolone (Cortaba tablets, 0.5 milligram of methylprednisolone and 300 milligrams of aspirin).
[b]Registered for dogs, but not actively marketed.
[c]Registered for cats as a single dose in the U.S.
[d]Registered in Canada
[e]Registered, but not marketed
[f]Also available as an injectable as well as oral, the others are all available in oral forms.
[g]Registered in other countries, but not the U.S. (Robenacoxib approved in U.S. for cats)

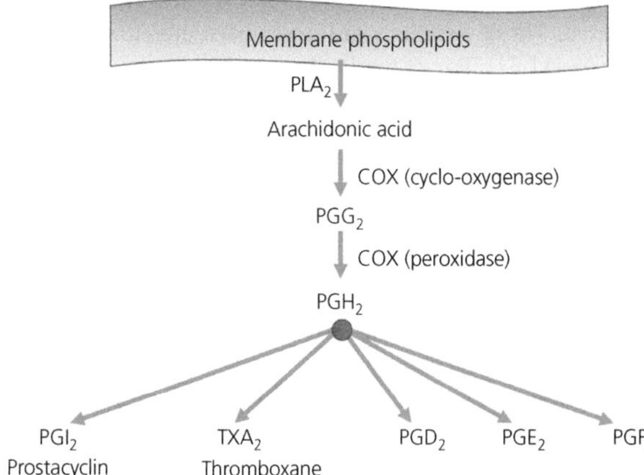

Figure 12.1 Membrane phospholipids are the source of arachidonic acid, the major eicosanoid in animals. Arachidonic acid is further metabolized by cyclo-oxygenase enzymes (COX) to the various prostaglandins (PGs), prostacyclin, and thromboxane to produce clinical, immunologic, and physiologic functions. The COX enzymes are the targets for non-steroidal anti-inflammatory drugs (NSAIDs).

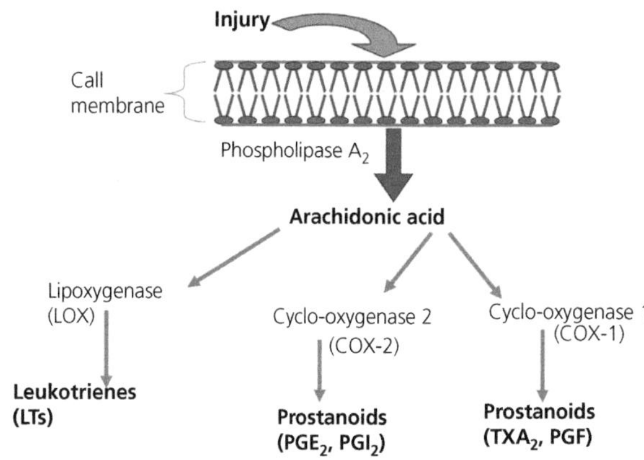

Figure 12.2 Metabolism of arachidonic acid products. The cell membrane generates arachidonic acid via de-esterification by the enzyme phospholipase A_2. Arachidonic acid is further metabolized by cyclo-oxygenase enzymes (COX-1 and COX-2) to the various prostaglandins (PGs), prostacyclin, and thromboxane to produce clinical, immunologic, and physiologic functions. An alternative pathway is via the lipoxygenase enzyme (LOX) which produces the inflammatory leukotrienes (LOX). The COX enzymes are the targets for non-steroidal anti-inflammatory drugs (NSAIDs), but do not ordinarily affect the LOX enzymes.

acid biotransformation are referred to as eicosanoids because of their structure of 20 carbons (Greek *eikosi* = 20). Most arachidonic acid is recycled back to the cell membranes, but in the face of various stimuli, arachidonic acid may be acted upon by cyclo-oxygenase (COX) or lipoxygenase (LOX) enzymes to form various eicosanoids which have a role in homeostasis and disease (Fig. 12.2). Prostanoids are specific eicosanoids that are further metabolized into the various prostaglandins (PGD_2, $PGF_2\alpha$, and PGE_2), prostacyclin (PGI_2), and thromboxane (TXA_2). These products act locally via G-protein coupled receptors to generate inflammatory and immunological responses and are also responsible for important physiological functions. A group of lipoxygenase (LOX) products, the leukotrienes (LT), are also responsible for inflammation, but are not inhibited by the traditional drugs covered in this chapter and will not be further discussed.

There are drugs which inhibit lipoxygenase and leukotriene formation, although their use is mainly as a therapy for bronchoconstrictive disease and investigations into their use as analgesics have been disappointing. It is worth noting that when COX-inhibiting NSAIDs are administered to animals, there is evidence that some shunting of substrate toward the LOX pathway may occur which is why a warning to patients with asthma is usually included for NSAIDs approved for use in human patients [13,14].

The action of NSAIDs is to inhibit COX enzymes and alter the formation of the prostanoids [15]. The significant development that improved the understanding of NSAIDs' mechanism of action occurred in the early 1990s when new details about the targets of these drugs emerged [16,17]. It was elucidated that there are two isoenzymes (isoforms) of cyclo-oxygenase (also known as prostaglandin synthase) that are responsible for synthesis of prostaglandins. Prostaglandin synthase-1 (COX-1) is usually simplistically described as a constitutive enzyme expressed in tissues [16,17]. Prostaglandins, prostacyclin, and thromboxane synthesized by this enzyme are responsible for normal physiologic functions. Prostaglandin synthase-2 (COX-2), on the other hand, is inducible (upregulated) and synthesized by macrophages and inflammatory cells after stimulation by cytokines and other mediators of inflammation. In 2002, a third isozyme of COX was described [18,19]. The COX-3 enzyme is a splice variant from the COX-1 gene, which to date has only been identified in the canine brain, human brain, and heart [19]. It is hypothesized that the mechanism of action of acetaminophen (paracetamol) is by inhibition of COX-3 although this hypothesis predated the discovery of the COX-3 splicing varient [18,19].

This explanation of cyclo-oxygenase function is overly simplistic. Both enzymes can participate in regulatory and homeostatic function, and both can produce pain and inflammation. The predominant enzyme is a reflection of the tissue or cell type in which it is produced. For example, COX-1 is the dominant enzyme in platelets and COX-2 is the dominant enzyme in inflammatory cells. In bone, COX-1 is expressed under normal conditions, but COX-2 is expressed during mechanical stress. Some COX-2 products are important for homeostatic function, and COX-1 products are involved in pain and inflammation. Prostaglandin synthesis is inherently higher in canine gastric mucosa than duodenal mucosa [20,21] but COX-2 production of prostaglandins can be upregulated in these tissues, responding to inflammatory stimuli to produce a protective and healing role [22]. COX-2 products are also important in normal renal function. COX-2 may be upregulated under conditions that may be stressful to the kidney, such as hypovolemia or severe hypotension [23].

Therefore, the perception that COX-2 is a 'bad' enzyme, and COX-1 is a 'good' enzyme is too simplistic because we now understand that there is some overlap in the functions of these isoforms on organs [24]. Drugs that inhibit these enzymes (e.g., the NSAIDs) can be effective and/or harmful regardless of whether or not they are selective or non-selective in their action on these enzymes. Nevertheless, some of the most recently developed NSAIDs have targeted COX-2 inhibition, so that COX-1 is spared as much as possible with the goal of producing analgesia and suppressing inflammation without inhibiting physiologically important prostanoids in various organs and tissues.

Other possible mechanisms of action

Although it is assumed that prostaglandin inhibition in both peripheral and nervous system (spinal and brain) tissues is the most important mechanism of action for most NSAIDs, there may be other mechanisms to explain some of their effects. These properties have not been accepted as a mechanism as universally as prostaglandin inhibition, but deserve some consideration. Some NSAIDs, including salicylates, may inhibit nuclear factor kappa-B (NF-κB) which promotes synthesis of other inflammatory mediators. There is not universal agreement on the mechanism of action of carprofen, which is one of the most commonly used NSAIDs in dogs. Some evidence indicates that it inhibits prostaglandins *in vitro* [25] but carprofen did not show an *in vivo* antiprostaglandin effect in dogs [26,27]. In another study, the investigators were unable to show that carprofen inhibited either COX-1 or COX-2 [28], suggesting either a central mechanism of action or activity on other pathways. More recent data by the authors (unpublished data) show that carprofen significantly inhibits PGE_2 (a biomarker for COX-2) directly at sites of inflammation in dogs, providing evidence that carprofen does indeed act on COX-2.

In horses, similar questions have been raised. Lees *et al.* [29] concluded that the anti-inflammatory effects of carprofen in horses were not caused by cyclo-oxygenase inhibition. In another study in the same laboratory [30], they concluded that recommended doses of carprofen produce minimal inhibition of COX and it is likely to achieve its therapeutic effects at least partially through other pathways, possibly including weak to moderate inhibition of 5-lipoxygenase and enzyme release. Little *et al.* [31] also concluded that there may be COX-independent mechanisms for some NSAIDs in the equine intestine.

COX-1 versus COX-2 inhibition

Selectivity of COX-2 versus COX-1 is often expressed as the COX-1:COX-2 inhibitory ratio. This ratio is derived from studies in which the inhibitory effect, usually expressed as the inhibitory concentration to inhibit 50% of activity (IC_{50}), is measured from stimulating cells that are capable of expressing products of these enzymes. In the whole blood assay, the source for COX-1 products (thromboxane or TXA_2) is platelets and the source of COX-2 products (PGE_2) is leukocytes. The ratio is expressed as COX-1 [IC_{50}] : COX-2 [IC_{50}], or simply COX-1:COX-2. The higher the value above 1.0, the greater the inhibitory action of the drug is for COX-2 compared to COX-1. There is subjective value placed on the magnitude of the ratio when considering the drug as 'COX-1 sparing,' 'COX-2 specific,' 'COX-2 preferential' or 'COX-2 selective.' These terms have been used by many authors [32] but the magnitude of the ratios that define these criteria has not been agreed upon.

The drugs with the highest inhibitory ratios are the selective COX-2 inhibitors (based on *in vitro* assays for the COX-2 enzyme) often called the 'coxibs' or coxib class of NSAIDs. These drugs include the veterinary products firocoxib, deracoxib, robenacoxib, and mavacoxib and the human product celecoxib (other coxibs such as rofecoxib have been withdrawn from the human market because of adverse effects on the cardiovascular system in human patients). Carprofen and meloxicam can be considered somewhat COX-2 preferential. Ketoprofen is non-selective, and etodolac has been classified as somewhat preferential to non-selective, depending on the study referenced. Although the IC_{50} ratio is the normal convention used for determination of COX selectivity [4,5], some investigators have proposed that a higher inhibitory concentration ratio (e.g., IC_{80}) may be better for predicting clinical efficacy, because such a high degree of inhibition may be necessary for analgesia or anti-inflammatory effects [33].

Comparisons of COX-1 versus COX-2 inhibition of veterinary NSAIDs varies among the drugs, animal species, and study technique used. These variations in the reported literature were listed previously [11,34]. For example, deracoxib is considered a highly selective COX-2 inhibitor based on an assay performed in purified enzymes [35]. In this study, the COX-1:COX-2 ratio was 1275, much higher than other drugs tested. But when tested in canine whole blood and compared to other NSAIDs, deracoxib had a ratio of only 12. In the same study, carprofen had a ratio of 6–7 and firocoxib had a ratio of 384–427 [36]. The ratio for etodolac has been reported as 8.1 in humans but 0.52–0.53 in dogs. Another study with etodolac showed that the selectivity for COX-2 was ten times greater in people than dogs [35,37].

In a study using canine enzyme systems, carprofen had a COX-1:COX-2 ratio of 129 [25] but in another study, using cell lines of another species (sheep and rodent), the ratio was 1.0 [15] and in a study using canine macrophages, the ratio was 1.75 [38]. Yet another study on carprofen showed a ratio of 5.3, which was 1000 times less potent in whole blood than in cell culture [39]. Lees *et al.* [5,30] pointed out the differences among species and concluded that for human cells carprofen is relatively selective for COX-1; for canine and feline cells carprofen shows preferential activity against COX-2; and for equine cells it is non-selective or slightly preferential for COX-2.

In view of the discrepancies among studies and techniques, it is now generally accepted that the whole blood assay should be the gold standard for determining COX-1/COX-2 specificity because it most closely simulates the appropriate physiologic conditions [4,5,32,33]. The first use of this technique was in 1992 [40] and it is now used in most veterinary drug studies. The advantage of the whole blood assay is that it incorporates the components into the assay that normally occur in circulating blood: proteins, cells, platelets, and enzymes. These components are not present in isolated cells or enzyme systems used for some earlier assays. Because the NSAIDs are highly protein bound, this is particularly important as only a small fraction, the unbound fraction, is biologically active in blood. The whole blood assay measures COX-2 products (PGE_2) from stimulated leukocytes and COX-1 products (TXA_2) from stimulated platelets.

Pharmacokinetic properties

Pharmacokinetic parameter estimates for NSAIDs can be examined using the available data from research reports and the drug package inserts. Some selected values are shown in Table 12.1 and are derived from a variety of sources. There are some common features possessed by the NSAIDs used in animals. All have high protein binding (>90%). Generally, all are well absorbed after oral administration and are weak acids that have high lipophilicity at physiologic tissue pH. The lipid/water partition coefficients, reported as the logarithm of the partition coefficient, or LogP, for these drugs is greater than or near 2.0. If the LogP for a medication is close to or above 2.0, diffusion across biologic membranes is favored (unless restricted by protein binding) and oral absorption is favored by high lipophilicity. Being weak acids, the lipophilicity (LogD) is highest at the low pH of the stomach and is lower, but still above 0.0, at the physiologic pH of 7.0. Meloxicam is an exception because the LogD is -0.75 at a pH of 7.0. Mavacoxib is another exception, because it is a weak base.

Both lipophilicity and protein binding affect a drug's volume of distribution. The volume of distribution varies considerably among the NSAIDs (see Table 12.1). For many drugs, high protein binding is associated with a small volume of distribution because protein binding decreases diffusion out of the extracellular compartment (e.g., plasma and extracellular fluid), but this is not a consistent feature of the NSAIDs. Carprofen and phenylbutazone have the lowest volume of distribution at 0.14 L/kg (lower than extracellular water volume), and most NSAIDs have volumes of distribution less than 1.0 L/kg. However, firocoxib, deracoxib, and etodolac all have volumes of distribution greater than 1.0 L/kg. Firocoxib has the highest volume of distribution (approximately 4.6 L/kg in dogs) [41] while it has the lowest lipophilicity (LogP 1.96). Interestingly, carprofen has one of the highest lipophilicity values among the NSAIDS (LogP of 3.79), but also has the lowest volume of distribution.

The estimated plasma half-life varies considerably among the NSAIDs, and among species (see Table 12.1). For example, in dogs, it is <1 h for robenacoxib, 1.6 h for ketoprofen, 3 h for deracoxib, and up to 24 h for meloxicam. Phenylbutazone ranges from 5–6 h in dogs and horses to over 50 h in cattle. Firocoxib has a half-life of 7.8 h in dogs, but 30 h or more in horses. Mavacoxib, an NSAID approved for dogs in Europe but not the United States, is unusual in that it has very low systemic clearance, resulting in a half-life in laboratory Beagles of 15.5–19.3 days. However, in osteoarthritic dogs of other breeds the half-life was highly variable with an average of 44 days, but exceeding 80 days in some dogs [42,43].

Despite these differences, the half-life does not appear to influence dosing intervals. In other words, the canine-approved labels for these drugs generally state once-daily oral administration for osteoarthritis or soft tissue inflammation despite the disparate half-lives. Mavacoxib is a notable exception with initial dosing at a 14-day interval with subsequent doses given every 30 days [43].

One of the reasons why plasma drug pharmacokinetic parameters (e.g., half-life) may not predict the dose interval is because of a lag-time between the tissue concentrations and blood concentrations. Even the drugs with short half-lives can be administered once daily because the tissue concentrations and inhibitory effects persist much longer. Protein binding has historically been used to explain the long persistence in tissues, but more recent data challenge this assumption. The high lipophilicity of these drugs also may explain the long tissue half-lives because high lipophilicity favors intracellular distribution, which can serve as a reservoir for prolonged tissue levels.

The NSAIDs are biotransformed by hepatic mechanisms, which is characteristic of lipophilic, poorly water-soluble compounds, and they have relatively low systemic clearance. Clearance values are not listed in Table 12.1, but all NSAIDs have clearance values of approximately 0.4 L/kg/h (6.67 mL/kg/min) or less. With liver blood flow being approximately 30 mL/kg/min in dogs [44], such a low value for these NSAIDs would qualify them as low clearance compounds. Mavacoxib is an extreme example with systemic clearance of only 0.0027 L/kg/h in Beagle dogs [42]. Similar properties are observed for the NSAIDs in other species in which the systemic clearance is much lower than liver blood flow. There are a few exceptions: systemic clearance of meloxicam in horses is approximately 3–5 times higher than in humans and three times higher than in dogs [45,46]. One of the newest NSAIDs used in dogs and cats in Europe is robenacoxib (approved for cats only in the US). It has a clearance of approximately 9–12 mL/kg/min in cats [47] and 13 mL/kg/min in dogs [48], which is much higher than the other NSAIDs. It also has a correspondingly short half-life in each of these species.

Gastrointestinal absorption is generally high for the formulations approved for animals (close to 100%), but there are exceptions. Firocoxib and mavacoxib are unusual with only 38% and 46% oral bioavailability in dogs, respectively. Robenacoxib has unusually low bioavailability in cats that is significantly affected by feeding (see below). There are also lower values for oral absorption of some drugs in horses and cattle (see Table 12.1).

Feeding may increase, inhibit, or delay absorption of concurrently administered NSAIDs. For example, feeding horses at the same time as oral phenylbutazone administration does not decrease absorption but it is delayed significantly, presumably because of binding to materials in feed and release in the distal intestine [49]. Robenacoxib is highly affected by feeding with oral absorption of 10% in fed cats versus 49% in fasted cats [50] and 62% in fed dogs versus 84% in fasted dogs [48]. Mavacoxib (unique because it is a weak base instead of a weak acid) is affected in the opposite direction, with feeding increasing the oral absorption from 46% to 87% [42]. Meloxicam oral absorption is only slightly affected by feeding in horses (see Table 12.1).

Stereoisomerism

The propionic acid derivatives (carprofen and ketoprofen) exist as *R*-(−) and *S*-(+) chiral enantiomers. Chirality is important because each isomer may show different pharmacokinetic and pharmacodynamic behavior. For example, the *S*-(+)-enantiomer (eutomer) is most active (lowest IC_{50}) for prostaglandin inhibition for these two NSAIDs. Etodolac also exists as a chiral enantiomer, with the *S*-(+)-isomer being more active. None of the other drugs listed in Table 12.1 have chiral enantiomers.

Pharmacokinetic-pharmacodynamic (PK-PD) properties

There has been tremendous interest in comparing the pharmacodynamic studies that measure COX-1 and COX-2 inhibitory concentrations, or observations of clinical response, with the estimated pharmacokinetic parameters of the drug to derive optimal and safe dosing for animals. These approaches were described in a review by Lees and colleagues [4,5] and demonstrated for specific drugs in studies by Giraudel *et al.* [51–53]. This approach was used to characterize the dose for the newest NSAID in dogs and cats, robenacoxib [47,51–55], and was used to evaluate NSAIDs for horses [45,46].

The approach by these investigators was to use a blood concentration corresponding to 80% inhibition of COX-2 (IC_{80}) to produce a therapeutic effect, and a 20% inhibition of COX-1 (IC_{20}) to avoid adverse effects. As reviewed by Hinz and Brune [56] and Warner *et al.* [33], using 80% COX-2 inhibition to predict clinical effects was selected because a drug concentration that inhibits the enzyme by only 50% may not be enough to produce a therapeutic effect. Using these inhibitory concentration values as targets, PK-PD modeling can be used to derive doses to attain optimal blood concentrations. The doses derived are intended to be starting points from which other studies investigating the clinical safety and effectiveness can be planned. For example, using the PK-PD modeling approach, investigators determined a dose of meloxicam of 0.17 mg/kg every 24 h in cats [52]. This dose of meloxicam deviates from doses derived from clinical studies because it is below the US Food and Drug Administration-registered single dose (0.3 mg/kg) for cats [57] but higher than the chronic dose registered in other countries, including Europe [58]. On the other hand, this approach correctly identified the optimum dose of 2 mg/kg of robenacoxib in cats [47,53,55,59] and dogs [60].

In Vivo assessment of PK-PD models

Rather than using an *in vitro* assay such as the whole blood assay to measure cyclo-oxygenase inhibition as the pharmacodynamic (PD) surrogate marker for efficacy, another approach is to use an *in vivo* measure. An *in vivo* measure is more likely to reflect physiologic and pathologic conditions and predict clinical outcome. Several *in vivo* models have been used to test NSAIDs in animals which are described in more detail by Lees *et al.* [4]. A typical *in vivo* model involves inducing inflammation in a tissue cage and measuring the inhibition of the inflammatory response in relation to the drug concentration. Alternatively, the model may use an injection of an irritant into a joint followed by an observation of the response by measuring the degree of lameness produced, heat, and/or pain [47]. Values such as 50% inhibitory concentration (IC_{50}) can be estimated from the *in vivo* model as it was for the *in vitro* model and used to derive an effective dose. One example of this approach was used to derive a dose for meloxicam in cats. Inflammation was induced in experimental cats and the response was matched to pharmacokinetic parameters for PK-PD modeling [51]. These investigators calculated a single dose of 0.25–0.3 mg/kg of meloxicam to produce optimum analgesic, anti-inflammatory, and antipyretic effects. This dose agrees with the dose derived from clinical trials that led to the current FDA-registered dose for cats in the United States [57] but is higher than the dose used clinically by many practitioners.

Adverse effects of NSAIDs

Gastrointestinal injury

Among the adverse reactions caused by NSAIDs, gastrointestinal problems are the most frequent reason to discontinue NSAID therapy or consider alternative treatment. Gastrointestinal adverse events, including vomiting, diarrhea, inappetance, and ulceration, have been documented in the veterinary literature, primarily in dogs and horses but also for other species.

Gastrointestinal toxicity is likely caused by at least two mechanisms: direct irritation of the drug on the gastrointestinal mucosa and the result of prostaglandin inhibition [22,51–64]. Direct mucosal irritation occurs because acidic NSAIDs become more lipophilic in the acid milieu of the stomach and diffuse into the gastric mucosa cells, where they cause injury. Direct effects also occur in the intestine where NSAIDs within the lumen can directly injure the intestinal villi. Diagnostic techniques have previously focused on stomach injury, but it is now apparent that the intestine is also an important site of direct injury [63,64]. Drugs that enter the lumen via the bile perhaps pose a higher risk for injury, which presents a greater problem for the NSAIDs that undergo enterohepatic recycling and produce high biliary concentrations. These effects may not result in perforation but may be an important cause of the nausea, vomiting, and diarrhea observed in animals following administration of NSAIDs.

Prostaglandins (along with other eicosanoid products such as lipoxins) have a cytoprotective effect on the gastrointestinal mucosa. Inhibition of prostaglandins by NSAIDs results in decreased cytoprotection, diminished blood flow, decreased synthesis of protective mucus, and inhibition of mucosal cell turnover and repair. This can lead to gastritis, enteritis, erosions, ulcers, and perforation. Because NSAIDs also can inhibit platelet function, injury to the gastrointestinal tract that causes bleeding can be exacerbated and result in significant blood loss. Serious complications have been observed with NSAID use in practically all animal species and are discussed with specific examples provided below.

Canine examples of gastrointestinal injury

The gastrointestinal effects of any NSAID can range from mild gastritis and vomiting, to severe gastrointestinal ulceration, bleeding, and death. Vomiting, anorexia, nausea, and diarrhea are by far the most common events documented [34]. Gastrointestinal ulceration and perforation are rare, but can be catastrophic. An examination of published reports of gastrointestinal injury related to administration of NSAID in animals indicates that the most (but not all) serious problems are caused by doses that are higher than recommended [65,66]. This is usually a result of accidental ingestion, administration of incorrect dose, or using inaccurate body weight. Overdosage is studied prior to regulatory approval by administration of exaggerated doses (e.g., 5× or 10×) in target animal safety studies performed by pharmaceutical sponsors and results are available in Freedom of Information (FOI) documents. Some drugs may lose their COX-2 selectivity at high doses [62]. Dose-dependent toxicity was shown for etodolac; at the label dose it was safe, but at higher doses (2.7× dose) it produced gastrointestinal lesions, and at the highest dose (5.3× dose), it caused death [67]. At high doses, meloxicam also produced gastrointestinal injury in dogs [66,68,69].

As with most NSAIDs, individual patients can have adverse effects at lower doses and according to one report, the sponsors of meloxicam in Europe recommended reducing the original approved dose from 0.2 mg/kg to 0.1 mg/kg because of some initial gastrointestinal problems [70].

Factors that may increase the risk of gastrointestinal injury include concurrent corticosteroid administration and/or concurrent gastrointestinal disease or injury. In people, there is now evidence that genetic variation may determine one's susceptibility to NSAIDs. Whether or not this is a factor in animals is undetermined but is presumed to be likely due to genetic diversity [71].

In the gastrointestinal tract of healthy dogs, COX-1 is the primary enzyme that produces prostaglandins (primarily PGE_2) [39]. COX-2 is normally present, but is upregulated after exposure to an irritant [20]. In the canine stomach there is a relatively high level of COX-1-synthesized prostaglandins because of the requirement to protect the stomach from high shear forces and gastric acid, and produce mucosal bicarbonate. Therefore, it is logical that inhibition of COX-1 in the stomach would increase the risk of gastric erosions and ulcers. In the duodenum, on the other hand, the prostaglandin requirement is lower because there is less acid, less requirement for mucosal bicarbonate (bicarbonate is secreted by the pancreas), and less shear force because of the trituration of food that has already occurred in the stomach. However, clinical observation would suggest that the proximal duodenum is the site of many catastrophic NSAID-associated perforating ulcers in dogs. Injury or insult to the duodenum induces COX-2 to produce protective and healing prostaglandins. If the COX-2-mediated prostaglandins are inhibited by NSAIDs, it may increase the risk of duodenal ulceration. This particular adverse event has been observed following treatment with deracoxib, one of the most selective COX-2 inhibitors in dogs [65]. Although most dogs in this report were predisposed to injury because of other factors, it appeared to be the administration of this selective COX-2 inhibitor that was the trigger for the duodenal injury.

Although there are several drugs available for use in dogs (see Box 12.1), there is no evidence in the published literature of controlled clinical trials to show that one NSAID is noticeably safer for the gastrointestinal tract than another [34]. For example, in a study in which carprofen, meloxicam, and ketoprofen were compared in dogs using endoscopic evaluation after 7 and 28 days of administration, there was no statistical difference among the drugs with respect to development of gastroduodenal lesions [70]. In another study that compared the gastrointestinal effects of recommended doses of carprofen, etodolac, and aspirin on the canine stomach and duodenum for 28 days, etodolac and carprofen produced significantly fewer lesions than aspirin [72]. Lesion scores in the carprofen and etodolac groups were no different from administration of placebo.

Equine examples of gastrointestinal injury

The NSAIDs are the drugs most commonly used to treat pain and inflammation in horses. As in other animals, gastric ulceration and intestinal injury have posed important limitations to their use. Gastric ulcers and related syndromes are a major health problem in horses, especially in performance horses and foals with stressful clinical illness. Gastric and intestinal injury in horses is a multifactorial problem and NSAIDs are just one of the factors contributing to the problem [73]. Phenylbutazone-induced injury to the gastrointestinal tract of horses has been documented in the literature for at least 30 years, and details of these findings can be found in other publications [1,74]. As described earlier, the pathophysiology is related to inhibition of protective prostaglandins in the stomach, coupled with high stress, exercise, and diet. The most severe ulcers in horses occur in the glandular mucosa because this is the region where prostaglandin inhibition plays the most important role.

Effects on the equine intestine also have been extensively studied. These have been reviewed by Marshall and Blikslager [75] and Tomlinson and Blikslager [76], and specific agents have been examined [31,77]. Although NSAIDs are commonly used in the management of pain and endotoxemia associated with colic in the horse [78], the effects must be balanced against the association with adverse gastrointestinal effects, including right dorsal colitis, and inhibition of mucosal barrier healing. Flunixin meglumine, one of the agents most commonly administered for this indication, decreases small intestine barrier function. When the equine intestine is exposed to flunixin, it inhibits recovery after intestinal ischemia and increases permeability to lipopolysaccharide (LPS). By contrast, experimental evidence suggests that those NSAIDs with anti-inflammatory effects either independent of cyclo-oxygenase inhibition or a COX-2-selective mode of action may offer significant advantages over traditional NSAIDs [31,77].

Non-steroidal anti-inflammatory agents, particularly phenylbutazone, can also affect the equine colon, producing the syndrome of right dorsal colitis [79]. The pathophysiology is not completely understood, but it is known that phenylbutazone administration to horses can cause hypoalbuminemia, neutropenia, changes in blood flow to the right dorsal colon, and alterations in luminal concentrations of volatile fatty acids (VFA) [79].

Gastrointestinal adaptation and chronic NSAID administration

One of the features consistent in clinical and basic research studies of NSAIDs is that animals may exhibit an initial adverse reaction to these agents, but tolerance often develops with continued administration. Indeed, there are accounts of dogs, cats, horses, and people that have survived on daily administration of NSAIDs for a majority of their lives. What accounts for this tolerance? The process of gastrointestinal adaptation involves many factors. Studies by Brzozowski *et al.* [80] showed attenuation of gastric mucosal injury after repeated exposure to aspirin. Gastric adaptation may be attributed to enhanced production of growth factors, increased cell proliferation, and mucosal regeneration. These authors also argued that gastric adaptation was a long-lasting effect that produces increased resistance of the adapted mucosa to subsequent damage by ulcerogenic agents.

Most information and review papers on this topic deal primarily with laboratory rodents, but studies in dogs from many years ago [81–88] demonstrated adaptation to administration of aspirin. These reports showed that gastric lesions were observed initially following aspirin treatment, but after 1–2 weeks of aspirin treatment the lesions resolved in the face of continued administration. The adaptation to aspirin in the dogs was accompanied by a rise in gastric blood flow, reduction in inflammatory cell infiltration, and an increase in mucosal cell regeneration and mucosal content of epidermal growth factor [83–88]. These observations are consistent with stimulation of a protective factor known as aspirin-triggered lipoxin (ATL) [86–88]. This factor is produced by acetylated COX-2 and inhibited by COX-2 inhibitors. Additional evidence for upregulation of COX-2 after mucosal injury was demonstrated by Wooten *et al.* [20]. COX-2 was increased in the duodenum of dogs after 3 days of administration of aspirin [20]. The phenomenon of adaptation related to chronic administration is not without controversy as other studies have failed to demonstrate gastric adaptation after aspirin administration to dogs. When dogs received aspirin at a unusually high dose of 25 mg/kg every 8 h, there was no evidence of adaptation, and lesions were as severe or worse on day 28 compared to earlier in the study [89].

Kidney injury related to NSAID administration

In the kidney, prostaglandins play an important role in modulating the tone of blood vessels and regulating salt and water balance. Renal injury caused by NSAIDs has been described in people, and horses, but is not as well documented in small animals, although clinical experience indicates it happens frequently enough to be of concern to the practitioner. Reported cases of toxicity often occurred when high doses were used or when there were other risk factors [90]. Renal injury occurs as a result of inhibition of renal prostaglandin synthesis. Animals with decreased renal perfusion caused by dehydration, anesthesia, shock, or pre-existing renal disease are at greater risk for NSAID-induced renal ischemia [90–92].

In healthy animals the kidneys are usually able to compensate for NSAID-associated effects. Because these agents are not inherently nephrotoxic, renal damage is usually associated with coexisting clinical or occult renal compromise [93]. In the face of factors that produce renal compromise (e.g., dehydration, tubular dysfunction, electrolyte depletion, and hemodynamic changes associated with anesthesia), the kidney is dependent on COX-1 and COX-2 for prostaglandin synthesis to regulate water homeostasis, tubular function, and renal blood flow [94].

Acute kidney injury associated with NSAIDs is characterized by decreased renal perfusion, sodium and fluid retention, decreased tubular function, and azotemia. In people, pain in the kidney area has been reported. One should not assume that NSAIDs that are more specific for the COX-2 enzyme are safer for the kidneys. Both COX-1 and COX-2 enzymes are involved in renal blood flow regulation and tubular function. Some of the prostaglandins that play an important role in salt and water regulation and hemodynamics in the kidney are synthesized by COX-2 enzymes [23,95]. Administration of a specific COX-2 inhibitor to salt-depleted people decreased renal blood flow, glomerular filtration rate, and electrolyte excretion [95]. Corticosteroids may also increase the risk of injury because it was shown that administration of prednisolone to dogs in combination with either meloxicam or ketoprofen has a potential for serious adverse effects on the kidneys as well as the gastrointestinal tract [96].

There is another form of analgesic nephritis, usually caused by chronic use of acetaminophen (paracetamol) in people [97]. This syndrome has not been described in domestic animals.

Examples in dogs

Of the currently available NSAIDs used in dogs, the effects of carprofen and meloxicam on renal function have been most extensively studied. Because these drugs are used perioperatively, investigations were performed to determine if there was any evidence of acute kidney injury, particularly in association with anesthesia. Based on these studies, the risk of kidney injury from these medications appears to be low. In one study, carprofen, ketorolac, and ketoprofen were examined in healthy dogs undergoing surgery, but without IV fluid administration. There were minor increases in renal tubular epithelial cells in urine sediment, but carprofen had no adverse effects on renal function [93]. Some ketorolac and ketoprofen-treated dogs had transient azotemia. In other studies, administration of carprofen to anesthetized healthy dogs had no adverse effects on renal function [98–102].

Meloxicam did not produce adverse renal effects in healthy dogs after short-term administration, with and without the inodilator pimobendan [103]. In healthy dogs anesthetized and given acepromazine to produce hypotension, preanesthetic administration of meloxicam did not produce any alteration of kidney function, although generalization of the results from this model to other anesthetic protocols is difficult [104]. Healthy dogs administered meloxicam prior to anesthesia and an electrical nociceptive stimulus did not have decreased renal function associated with treatment [102].

Renal effects following deracoxib administration to dogs were reported by the manufacturer [105]. At high doses, there is a dose-dependent effect on renal tubules. It is well tolerated in most healthy dogs at up to 10 mg/kg for 6 months, but there is a potential for a dose-dependent renal tubular degeneration/regeneration at doses of 6 mg/kg or higher (clinically approved dose for long-term treatment is 1–2 mg/kg per day). Long-term administration of carprofen, etodolac, flunixin, ketoprofen, or meloxicam to dogs did not induce any evidence of renal injury as measured by urinalysis and serum biochemistry [106].

The common theme in many of the studies cited above was that dogs were healthy, generally young, and NSAIDs were dosed once daily within the recommended range. Deviations from this study design, use of higher doses, longer duration of treatment, or administration to clinical patients with comorbidities could produce different results.

Examples in cats

Because it is often older cats that are treated with NSAIDs for degenerative joint disease (DJD) and surgery, veterinarians and pet owners are concerned about the effects these drugs may have on renal function. The effects of both short- and long-term use have attracted attention. One of the reasons for concern is a so-called black box warning issued by the United States Food and Drug Administration in 2010 which stated that 'Repeated use of meloxicam in cats has been associated with acute renal failure and death. Do not administer additional injectable or oral meloxicam to cats.' This prompted several studies because overt and subclinical chronic kidney disease (CKD) is common in the population of cats most often treated with NSAIDs long term. Follow-up studies have helped to mitigate this concern. The study by Surdyk *et al.* [107]. showed that in cats with reduced renal function, but euvolemic, NSAIDs did not alter kidney function. In their study, neither meloxicam nor acetylsalicylic acid had a measurable effect on urinary clearance of exogenously administered creatinine, serum creatinine concentration, or the protein to creatinine ratio. They concluded that kidney function of euvolemic cats with normal or reduced renal function is not dependent on cyclo-oxygenase function and therefore not likely impacted by NSAID administration.

Meloxicam is licensed for chronic use in cats in several countries (not in the United States), and is the drug recommended for long-term administration, by consensus, from a group of feline medicine experts [8]. Three important studies have concluded that chronic administration of meloxicam to cats can be both safe and effective. Oral meloxicam was safe and palatable for long-term treatment of DJD in cats when given with food at a dose of 0.01–0.03 mg/kg/day

[108]. Gowan *et al.* [109] concluded in a study with aged cats with CKD that long-term therapy with meloxicam (0.02 mg/kg daily) can be administered safely. These cats tolerated meloxicam with daily administration despite their kidney disease. And finally, in a follow-up study, the same investigators [110] concluded that long-term management with oral meloxicam in cats did not reduce the lifespan of cats with pre-existent stable CKD. Many cats actually had a better outcome associated with meloxicam treatment. These studies have resolved some concerns about the use of NSAIDs, at least meloxicam, when administered to aged cats and to cats with CKD. It should be noted that the doses prescribed in these studies are lower than the approved label dose [57,58], and in fact lower than the dose recommended in the review by Sparkes *et al.* [8].

Studies have also been completed on the newest NSAID approved for cats, robenacoxib. In safety studies using healthy cats, the data show that robenacoxib was well tolerated even when treatment was for longer, and at higher doses than approved [111]. When prescribing NSAIDs for long-term use in any animal, client education and informed consent are important. Regularly scheduled patient follow-up evaluations are helpful to assess the benefit of therapy and to recognize any adverse effects.

Hepatic safety

Any NSAID has the potential for causing liver injury [112]. As pointed out earlier, these are lipophilic drugs that undergo extensive hepatic metabolism. The liver is exposed to high concentrations of the parent drug and metabolites. Injury caused by NSAID can be idiosyncratic (unpredictable, non-dose related) or intrinsic (predictable and dose related) [113,114]. Toxicity resulting from high doses of acetaminophen and aspirin is intrinsic; reactions to other drugs tend to be idiosyncratic and unpredictable.

Prescribing NSAIDs for animals with hepatic disease has been questioned because of the role of the liver in metabolizing these drugs, but there is no evidence that prior hepatic disease predisposes a patient to NSAID-induced liver injury when properly dosed. Drug enzyme systems are remarkably preserved in hepatic disease and pre-existing hepatic disease is not necessarily a contraindication for administration of an NSAID. Patients with liver disease may be more prone to gastrointestinal ulceration, and there is concern that administration of NSAIDs could increase the risk of this complication.

Carprofen has received the most attention related to drug-induced liver injury in small animal medicine but the potential exists for all NSAIDs. Carprofen was approved by United States Food and Drug Administration in October 1996 for relief of pain and inflammation in dogs [115]. Before this approval, it was registered for treatment of dogs in Europe and was evaluated in clinical trials [116]. In studies in dogs with arthritis, it was effective and had a low incidence of adverse effects [116]. In longer term studies, in which carprofen was administered from 2 weeks to 5 years, the incidence of adverse reactions was only 1.3% [115]. Vomiting, diarrhea, anorexia, and lethargy were the most common adverse reactions documented. Attention was focused on the hepatic toxicity of carprofen because of a published report documenting liver injury in a series of dogs presented to a referral hospital [117]. In the report cited [117], 21 dogs were described in which carprofen was associated with acute, idiosyncratic hepatotoxicosis. Affected dogs had diminished appetites, vomited, and were icteric with elevations in hepatic enzymes and bilirubin. Dogs received the recommended dose and developed signs an average of 19 days after therapy was initiated. No predisposing conditions were identified and most dogs recovered without further consequences following cessation of drug administration and supportive medical care. Many of the dogs in that report were Labrador Retrievers, but there is no additional evidence to show that this breed has an increased risk of carprofen hepatotoxicity [118]. Among other drugs, firocoxib caused fatty liver changes in young dogs when administered at high doses (Merial manufacturer's data) [41]. Signs of hepatic injury are among the most common adverse events reported for carprofen to the Food and Drug Administration's Center for Veterinary Medicine adverse events reporting site (www.fda.gov).

Despite common recommendation by veterinarians, there is no evidence that dietary supplements such as silymarin (milk thistle, silybin, Marin®), S-adenosyl-methionine (SAMe, Denosyl®), or combinations of both (Denamarin®, NutraMax®) have any benefit in preventing liver injury from NSAIDs. Idiosyncratic reactions are rare (1 in 1000 to 1 in 10 000 patients). Nevertheless, any unexplained increase in hepatic enzymes or bilirubin 7–90 days after initiating NSAID administration should be investigated. Fortunately, liver injury is generally reversible with supportive care and avoidance of additional inciting causes.

Injury to cartilage

With chronic use some NSAIDs have been shown to accelerate articular cartilage lesions in arthritic joints. This has been demonstrated experimentally when NSAIDs were administered at high doses in canine arthritis models; however, the clinical significance is uncertain. Most of the currently used drugs have not been shown to accelerate degradation of articular cartilage *in vivo* [119].

Blood coagulation effects: Platelet inhibition and thrombotic abnormalities

Non-steroidal anti-inflammatory drugs which inhibit COX-1 can reduce thromboxane (TXA_2) synthesis in platelets and decrease platelet function. In some instances this may lead to clinical episodes of increased perioperative bleeding. Aspirin, at low doses, is the most specific COX-1 inhibitor because the acetyl group (aspirin = acetylsalicylic acid) inhibits the cyclo-oxygenase in platelets irreversibly. Non-acetylated NSAIDs inhibit platelets only when their concentrations in blood are maintained at inhibitory levels. Therefore, the effects from non-aspirin NSAIDs are brief and rarely lead to clinical complications. Ketoprofen is a non-selective COX inhibitor that has been reported to alter hemostasis [120]. A clinical trial by Lemke *et al.* [121] in dogs undergoing ovariohysterectomy found that preoperative ketoprofen administration resulted in an inhibition of platelet aggregation but there were no effects on buccal mucosal bleeding time. The authors concluded that as long as dogs were otherwise healthy, with no other known bleeding problems, ketoprofen could be used safely as a preoperative analgesic and anti-inflammatory drug [121]. Drugs that are specific COX-2 inhibitors, or that spare COX-1, have little clinical effect on platelets although *in vitro* testing may demonstrate effects.

Risks in people compared to animals

In the human literature, there has been a concern that COX-2-specific inhibitors may increase the risk of cardiovascular events, particularly myocardial infarction, thrombosis, strokes, and sudden death [122,123]. Similar problems have not been identified in animals. Cardiovascular safety is a concern in people using COX-2-selective drugs because these drugs preserve COX-1 which may promote platelet aggregation and vasoconstriction [122]. This is the reason that the once popular drug rofecoxib was voluntarily taken off the market by the manufacturer [123], and this was soon followed by the withdrawal of valdecoxib. Some experts believe that the high COX-2 selectivity of this drug led to this increased risk [124–126].

Drug selection

There are several NSAID choices available to veterinarians (see Box 12.1). Over the past several years the profession has learned some important information about these drugs that should help guide treatment. One of the most significant lessons is that *we really do not know which NSAID drug is most efficacious and safest in a given individual.* Each has advantages and disadvantages. There are different dosage forms including injectable, oral solutions, oral transmucosal, conventional tablets, chewable tablets, equine pastes, and transdermal formulations. Initial dosing for healthy patients is well established (Table 12.2). Choice of product will depend on the clinical situation, owner preference, prior observed efficacy, and compliance. There are veterinary generic formulations of popular drugs and there are some human-labeled drugs that are used off-label (e.g., aspirin, naproxen, and piroxicam).

COX-2 inhibition as selection criterion

After the discovery of the two isoenzymes COX-1 and -2, there was a focus in drug development on highly selective COX-2 inhibitors. Drugs that emerged from this work were celecoxib, valdecoxib (now discontinued), and rofecoxib (now discontinued) [127]. At one time, these coxibs were among the top-selling prescription drugs of any category in human medicine.

Deracoxib was the first veterinary drug in this group followed by firocoxib and robenacoxib. Mavacoxib and cimicoxib have been licensed for use in dogs in Europe. Although these drugs have a higher COX-1/COX-2 inhibitory ratio than older NSAIDs, clinical superiority has not been demonstrated in large patient populations. In fact, one of the veterinary drugs with selective COX-2 inhibitory action, deracoxib, was shown to be safe in studies performed by Bergh and Budsberg [10] but as discussed earlier, gastrointestinal perforation and bleeding have been reported in association with deracoxib use in dogs [65]. In canine efficacy studies, firocoxib was compared to etodolac and carprofen and was shown in some measurements to have better improvement in lameness scores. Studies that have assessed safety among drugs have been scarce and of low statistical power. The results available indicate that firocoxib, carprofen, and etodolac all are similar with respect to incidence of vomiting and anorexia in dogs. But with respect to diarrhea there was a lower incidence with firocoxib compared to carprofen and etodolac and less melena compared to etodolac [41]. The studies with robenacoxib in cats have shown good safety and efficacy. It was superior to meloxicam in a clinical study [128] but was non-inferior to older NSAIDs such as ketoprofen in terms of safety and efficacy [54,129].

Evaluations of the coxibs in people show that they are not necessarily more effective than older drugs, but they may be safer for the gastrointestinal tract [130] during short-term evaluations. There is no evidence that selective COX-2 inhibitors are superior for long-term therapy than older established drugs, which included drugs with mixed COX-1/COX-2 inhibition in terms of gastrointestinal safety and efficacy [131,132]. With an exception for intestinal injury in horses, which is discussed elsewhere in this chapter, there is little evidence in other studies in veterinary species that drugs with higher COX-1/COX-2 ratios produce fewer gastrointestinal or renal adverse effects than drugs with low ratios.

Table 12.2 Reported or regulatory agency approved dosages for NSAIDs in animals[a] [41,57,67,105,115,156].

Drug	Cats	Dogs	Horses	Cattle
Aspirin	10 mg/kg q48h oral	10–20 mg/kg q8–12 h, oral	25–50 mg/kg q8h, oral	100 mg/kg q12h, oral
Carprofen	1–4 mg/kg given once by injection	4.4 mg/kg q24h, or 2.2 mg/kg q12h, oral	0.7 mg/kg q24h, oral or IV	1.4 mg/kg, once, SC or IV
Deracoxib	1 mg/kg oral, once	3–4 mg/kg q24h, oral for up to 7 days, then 1–2 mg/kg q24h oral	No dose established	No dose established
Etodolac	No dose established	10–15 mg/kg q24h, oral	23 mg/kg oral q24h	No dose established
Firocoxib	1.5 mg/kg, oral, once	5 mg/kg q24h, oral	0.1 mg/kg q24h, oral, for up to 14 days, or 0.09 mg/kg q24h, IV, for up to 5 days	Not recommended
Flunixin	1 mg/kg once, IV, SC, or IM	1 mg/kg, oral, IV or IM, once	1 mg/kg q24h, for up to 5 days IM or IV, or 1 mg/kg oral q24h	1–2 mg/kg, q24h, IV, for up to 3 days
Meloxicam	0.1 mg/kg initially, then 0.05 mg/kg per day, then reduce dose to every other day, or 0.02 mg/kg per day	0.2 mg/kg initial dose oral, SC, or IV, then 0.1 mg/kg q24h, oral	0.6 mg/kg, q24h, IV or oral	0.5 mg/kg, q24h, IM, IV, or SC
Naproxen	Not recommended	5 mg/kg initial, then 2 mg/kg q48h, oral	10 mg/kg q12h, oral	Not recommended
Phenylbutazone	6–8 mg/kg q12h, oral	15–22 mg/kg q12h, oral	4.4–8.8 mg/kg per day, oral (limit highest dose to 2–4 days). 2.2–4.4 mg/kg IV per day for 2–4 days	17–25 m/kg initial dose, then 2.5–5 mg/kg q24h or 10–14 mg/kg q48h PO
Piroxicam	0.3 mg/kg q24h, oral, or 1 mg per cat, q24h, oral	0.3 mg/kg, q24h, or q48h, oral	No dose established	Not recommended
Robenacoxib	1–2.4 mg/kg oral per day	1–2 mg/kg q24h, oral	No dose established	Not recommended
Mavacoxib	Not recommended	2 mg/kg orally once, repeat in 14 days, then repeat every 30 days up to 6.5 months	Not recommended	Not recommended

[a]Dosing information and label information including species, indicated uses, and precautionary warnings vary by regulatory jurisdiction. Appropriateness of use within the local regulatory environment should be verified by the prescribing veterinarian.
IV = intravenous; IM = intramuscular; PO = per os; SC = subcutaneous.

Selection of NSAIDs for dogs

For acute pain (e.g., postoperative pain) there is good evidence of efficacy from oral and injectable formulations and this has been published in previous reports and reviews. Drugs discussed previously and listed in Tables 12.1 and 12.2 have been used in these instances. These drugs have been used in the short term to decrease fever and decrease pain from surgery or trauma. Preoperative injections of carprofen in dogs were shown to be beneficial for decreasing postoperative pain after ovariohysterectomy [133]. Meloxicam has been reported to be effective in dogs for perioperative use [134,135] and was shown to be superior to butorphanol in some pain assessments.

Oral NSAIDs may be used for acute treatment of myositis, arthritis, and postoperative pain, or they may be administered chronically for relief of osteoarthritis-related pain. Drugs that have been administered in the United States to small animals are listed in Box 12.1, and some veterinarians have also used human-label drugs such as aspirin, piroxicam, and naproxen. If human-label drugs are considered, consult appropriate references for accurate dosing because it may differ from the human dose schedule (see Table 12.2). The approved veterinary drugs used most often in dogs are carprofen, etodolac, meloxicam, firocoxib, and deracoxib. Tepoxalin has been removed from the market by the sponsor. In countries outside the US, other NSAIDs approved for dogs include ketoprofen, mavacoxib, cimicoxib ,and tolfenamic acid.

For long-term use there are no controlled studies that indicate which drug is the most effective and likely there is individual variation in response to treatment. When drugs are compared to one another, it is difficult, using subjective measurements, to demonstrate differences between these drugs for reducing pain in animals. Robust and validated objective measures of pain are lacking in veterinary medicine. Clinical trials used for regulatory approval sometimes use 'non-inferior' criteria for comparison to another approved drug. Without a very large number of patients, achieving the statistical power to detect differences among drugs in clinical veterinary studies is difficult.

With several choices of NSAIDs for treating dogs with osteoarthritis, selection can be frustrating for veterinary clinicians. Like people, there may be greater differences among individuals in their response than there are differences among the drugs. Response to treatment may also vary over time and with disease progression, further complicating pharmacologic management of this disease. Historically, veterinarians often selected aspirin or phenylbutazone as an initial drug, and then progressed to off-label human drugs (e.g., piroxicam) or other agents as an alternative. With availability of several veterinary-approved NSAIDs for which there are excellent published studies and FDA or foreign approval to guide clinical use and safe dosages, it is difficult to justify using non-approved drugs for which safety and efficacy data are unavailable. Among the drugs available (see Box 12.1), there may be variations among animals with respect to tolerance of adverse effects and clinical response. It is a rational approach to consider keeping at least two or more NSAIDs in clinical inventory so that clinicians have an opportunity to discover the NSAID that is best tolerated, most effective, and easiest to administer in each patient.

Selection of NSAIDs for cats

Excellent in-depth reviews are available for guidance on the use of NSAIDs in cats. Readers are encouraged to consult publications by Lascelles *et al.* [7], Sparkes *et al.* [8], and Bennett and Johnston [136]. Treatment of degenerative joint disease and other sources of long-term pain in cats has not been addressed adequately in the past and these papers help raise awareness of these conditions.

Veterinarians have been reluctant to prescribe NSAIDs to cats because of a fear of adverse effects. The adverse effects of salicylates (aspirin) in cats are well documented. Cats are susceptible because of slow clearance and dose-dependent elimination. Affected cats may have hyperthermia, respiratory alkalosis, metabolic acidosis, methemoglobinemia, hemorrhagic gastritis, and kidney and liver injury. Cats also are prone to acetaminophen toxicosis because of their deficiency in the drug-metabolizing enzyme UDP-glucuronosyltransferase [137]. Despite the apparent sensitivity of cats to some adverse effects of NSAIDs, aspirin has been used at doses of 10 mg/kg every other day. There are also reports of the safe use of ketoprofen (registered in Canada and European countries for use in cats) at a dose of 1 mg/kg/day × 4 days and flunixin meglumine (1 mg/kg once) in cats for short-term treatment.

In the United States injectable meloxicam is approved by the FDA only for a single dose in cats at 0.3 mg/kg. Meloxicam (oral formulation) is licensed for long-term use in cats in Europe, Australia, and New Zealand and, by consensus, was the drug recommended by a group of feline medicine experts for repeated administration [8]. Extra-label drug use (ELDU) in non-food animals is legal in the United States. After the ISFM and AAFP consensus guidelines were published [8], robenacoxib became available for cats in the US and Europe. Robenacoxib has favorable pharmacokinetic and safety properties that would make this an acceptable choice for repeated dosing. When cats were administered high doses (5× dose) of meloxicam, vomiting and other gastrointestinal problems were reported. With repeated doses (9 days) of 0.3 mg/kg per day to cats, inflamed gastrointestinal mucosa and ulceration were observed [57]. Nevertheless, many veterinarians have administered meloxicam to cats multiple times at much lower doses. As discussed under the section on renal adverse effects, meloxicam has been administered safely and long term at a dose of 0.01–0.03 mg/kg [108] and in aged cats with kidney disease at a dose of 0.02 mg/kg daily [109,110]. Some regimens recommend meloxicam in cats at 0.1 mg/kg initially, followed by decreasing doses. One such regimen recommends that if a favorable response is seen in the first few days, increase the dose interval to once every 48–72 h, and then lower the dose to 0.05 mg/kg or less (0.025 mg/kg) as long as efficacy persists. In Europe and other countries, the approved dose for cats is 0.05 mg/kg per day for chronic use with safety data from the sponsor to support this claim.

The newest approved NSAID for use in cats (but not dogs) in the United States is robenacoxib. The recommended dose has been optimized through PK-PD and safety studies [47,51–54,111]. The FDA-approved dose in the US is 1 mg/kg orally per day with a range of 1–2.4 mg/kg/day for a maximum of 3 days, while in some European countries the approved cat dose is 1 mg/kg body weight per day for up to 6 days. Availability of drug formulations differs between countries. In the US there is a 6 mg unscored tablet for use in cats only. In Europe and other countries it is also available as 5, 10, 20, and 40 mg tablets for dogs, and a 20 mg/mL injectable solution.

Carprofen (injectable solution) is approved for single-dose administration to cats in Europe. Repeated dosing of carprofen in cats has been discouraged because of reports of gastroduodenal toxicosis and high individual variation in half-life when administered at canine dose rates. There is one report of firocoxib administration in cats [138]. Firocoxib was effective for attenuating experimentally induced fever in cats at doses of 0.75–3 mg/kg (single dose).

Selection of NSAIDs for horses

For horses, phenylbutazone has been used more often than any other NSAID, and many experts still believe that it is the most cost-effective treatment, especially for oral treatment of musculoskeletal inflammation and pain. Flunixin meglumine is the most commonly utilized injectable NSAID for acute soft tissue injury, endotoxemia, and abdominal pain [139]. Additional NSAIDs are listed in the articles by Valverde and Gunkel [140] and Marshall and Blikslager [75]. These include injectable ketoprofen and the equine oral paste or injectable formulation of firocoxib. Oral treatment with meloxicam is approved in some countries, and occasionally meclofenamic acid has been used. In some countries (not US), carprofen is licensed for use in horses at an intravenous dose of 0.7 mg/kg, which can be repeated once after 24 h.

Flunixin has a long history in the treatment of acute pain and inflammation associated with colic in horses. The rationale for this treatment has focused on the inhibition of prostanoids that are responsible for hemodynamic changes during endotoxemia [78,139]. However, recent work [31,75–77,141] has indicated that non-selective NSAIDs such as flunixin may increase the risk of intestinal injury. These studies indicate that selective NSAIDs such as firocoxib may have a safety advantage.

NSAID selection for food animals

In the US, flunixin meglumine is FDA approved for the treatment of inflammation and fever in food animals. All other NSAIDs are considered off-label and withdrawal times should be determined from a reliable source such as the Food Animal Residue Avoidance Databank (FARAD) [142]. NSAIDs used off-label in food animals include aspirin, phenylbutazone (prohibited from use in dairy cattle), dipyrone (prohibited by the FDA), carprofen, ketoprofen, and meloxicam (approved for use in Europe in cattle and pigs). Doses used in food animals are listed in the article by Valverde and Gunkel [140] and in Table 12.2.

There is some evidence that NSAIDs provide analgesia and reduce stress in food animals following surgery. Meloxicam, which is approved in Europe for use in cattle and pigs, has been used in sows to treat mastitis-metritis-agalactia (MMA) syndrome [143,144] at a dose of 0.4 mg/kg IM.

Summary

In summary, the pharmacokinetics of NSAIDs in common domesticated species are included in specific tables as are their clinical dosages. For NSAID use in specific clinical situations and pathologies, the reader is referred to other species- and pain syndrome-specific chapters in this fifth edition of *Veterinary Anesthesia and Analgesia.*

References

1 Lees P. Analgesic, anti-inflammatory, antipyretic drugs. In: Riviere JE, Papich MG, eds. *Veterinary Pharmacology and Therapeutics*, 9th edn. Chichester: Wiley, 2009; 457–492.

2 KuKanich B, Bidgood T, Knesl O. Clinical pharmacology of nonsteroidal anti-inflammatory drugs in dogs. *Vet Anaesth Analg* 2012; **39**(1): 69–90.

3 Monteiro-Steagall BP, Steagall PVM, Lascelles BDX. Systematic review of nonsteroidal anti-inflammatory drug-induced adverse effects in dogs. *J Vet Intern Med* 2012; **27**(5): 1011–1019.

4 Lees P, Giraudel J, Landoni MF, Toutain PL. PK-PD integration and PK-PD modelling of nonsteroidal anti-inflammatory drugs: principles and applications in veterinary pharmacology. *J Vet Pharmacol Ther* 2004; **27**(6): 491–502.

5 Lees P, Landoni MF, Giraudel J, Toutain PL. Pharmacodynamics and pharmacokinetics of nonsteroidal anti-inflammatory drugs in species of veterinary interest. *J Vet Pharmacol Ther* 2004; **27**(6): 479–490.

6 Lascelles BDX, McFarland JM, Swann H. Guidelines for safe and effective use of NSAIDs in dogs. *Vet Ther* 2005; **6**(3): 237–250.

7 Lascelles BDX, Court MH, Hardie EM, Robertson SA. Nonsteroidal anti-inflammatory drugs in cats: a review. *Vet Anesth Analg* 2007; **34**: 228–250.

8 Sparkes AH, Heiene R, Lascelles BDX, *et al*. ISFM and AAFP consensus guidelines: long-term use of NSAIDs in cats. *J Feline Med Surg* 2010; **12**(7): 521–538.

9 Coetzee JF. A review of analgesic compounds used in food animals in the United States. *Vet Clin North Am Food Anim Pract* 2013; **29**(1): 11–28.

10 Bergh MS, Budsberg SC. The Coxib NSAIDs: potential clinical and pharmacologic importance in veterinary medicine. *J Vet Intern Med* 2005; **19**: 633–643.

11 Papich MG. An update on nonsteroidal anti-inflammatory drugs (NSAIDs) in small animals. *Vet Clin North Am Food Anim Pract* 2008; **38**(6): 1243–1266.

12 Papich MG. Pharmacologic considerations for opiate analgesic and nonsteroidal anti-inflammatory drugs. *Vet Clin North Am Food Anim Pract* 2000; **30**: 815–837.

13 Charlier C, Michaux C. Dual inhibition of cyclooxygenase-2 (COX-2) and 5-lipoxygenase (5-LOX) as a new strategy to provide safer non-steroidal anti-inflammatory drugs. *Eur J Med Chem* 2003; **38**(7-8): 645–659.

14 Park S, Heo D, Sung M. The shunting of arachidonic acid metabolism to 5-lipoxygenase and cytochrome P450 epoxygenase antagonizes the anti-cancer effect of cyclooxygenase-2 inhibition in head and neck cancer cells. *Cell Oncol* 2012; **35**: 1–8.

15 Vane JR, Botting RM. New insights into the mode of action of anti-inflammatory drugs. *Inflamm Res* 1995; **44**: 1–10.

16 Meade EA, Smith WL, DeWitt DL. Pharmacology of prostaglandin endoperoxide synthase isozymes-1 and -2. *Ann NY Acad Sci* 1994; **714**: 136–142.

17 Laneuville O, Breuer DK, DeWitt DL, *et al*. Differential inhibition of human prostaglandin endoperoxide synthases-1 and -2 by nonsteroidal anti-inflammatory drugs. *J Pharm Exp Ther* 1994; **271**: 927–934.

18 Chandrasekharan NV, Dai H, Roos KL, *et al*. COX-3, a cyclooxygenase-1 variant inhibited by acetaminophen and other analgesic/antipyretic drugs: cloning, structure, and expression. *Proc Natl Acad Sci USA* 2002; **99**(21): 13926–13931.

19 Davies NM, Good RL, Roupe KA, Yáñez JA. Cyclooxygenase-3: axiom, dogma, anaomaly, enigma or splice error? – not as easy as 1, 2, 3. *J Pharm Pharmaceut Sci* 2004; **7**(2): 217–226.

20 Wooten JG, Blikslager AT, Ryan KA, *et al*. Cyclooxygenase expression and prostanoid production in pyloric and duodenal mucosae in dogs after administration of nonsteroidal anti-inflammatory drugs. *Am J Vet Res* 2008; **69**(4): 457–464.

21 Punke JP, Speas AL, Reynolds LR, Budsberg SC. Effects of firocoxib, meloxicam, and tepoxalin on prostanoid and leukotriene production by duodenal mucosa and other tissues of osteoarthritic dogs. *Am J Vet Res* 2008; **69**(9): 1203–1209.

22 Konturek SJ, Konturek PC, Brzozowski T. Prostaglandins and ulcer healing. *J Physiol Pharmacol* 2005; **56**(Suppl 5): 5–31.

23 Brater DC. Effects of nonsteroidal anti-inflammatory drugs on renal function: focus on cyclooxygenase-20selective inhibition. *Am J Med* 1999; **107**(6): 65–70.

24 Bertolini A, Ottani A, Sandrini M. Dual acting anti-inflammatory drugs: a reappraisal. *Pharmacol Res* 2001; **44**: 437–450.

25 Ricketts AP, Lundy KM, Seibel SB. Evaluation of selective inhibition of canine cyclooxygenase 1 and 2 by carprofen and other nonsteroidal anti-inflammatory drugs. *Am J Vet Res* 1998; **59**: 1441–1446.

26 McKellar QA, Pearson T, Bogan JA, *et al*. Pharmacokinetics, tolerance and serum thromboxane inhibition of carprofen in the dog. *J Small Anim Pract* 1990; **31**(9): 443–448.

27 McKellar QA, Delatour P, Lees P. Stereospecific pharmacodynamics and pharmacokinetics of carprofen in the dog. *J Vet Pharmacol Ther* 1994; **17**: 447–454.

28 Bryant CE, Farnfield BA, Janicke HJ. Evaluation of the ability of carprofen and flunixin meglumine to inhibit activation of nuclear factor kappa B. *Am J Vet Res* 2003; **64**: 211–215.

29 Lees P, McKellar Q, May SA, Ludwig B. Pharmacodynamics and pharmacokinetics of carprofen in the horse. *Equine Vet J* 1994; **26**(3): 203–208.

30 Lees P, Aliabadi FS, Landoni MF. Pharmacodynamics and enantioselective pharmacokinetics of racemic carprofen in the horse. *J Vet Pharmacol Ther* 2002; **25**(6): 433–448.

31 Little D, Brown SA, Campbell NB, *et al*. Effects of the cyclooxygenase inhibitor meloxicam on recovery of ischemia-injured equine jejunum. *Am J Vet Res* 2007; **68**(6): 614–624.

32 Pairet M, van Ryn J. Experimental models used to investigate the differential inhibition of cyclooxygenase-1 and cyclooxygenase-2 by Nonsteroidal anti-inflammatory drugs. *Inflamm Res* 1998; **47**(Suppl 2): S93–S101.

33 Warner TD, Giuliano F, Vojnovic I, *et al*. Nonsteroid drug selectivities for cyclo-oxygenase-1 rather than cyclo-oxygenase-2 are associated with human gastrointestinal toxicity: a full in vitro analysis. *Proc Natl Acad Sci USA* 1999; **96**: 7563–7568.

34 Fox SM. Nonsteroidal anti-inflammatory drugs. In: Carroll GL, ed. *Small Animal Anesthesia and Analgesia*. Ames, IA: Blackwell Publishing, 2008; 143–157.

35 Gierse JK, Staten NR, Casperson GF, *et al.* Cloning, expression, and selective inhibition of canine cyclooxygenase-1 and cyclooxygenase-2. *Vet Ther* 2002; **3**: 270–280.

36 McCann ME, Andersen DR, Zhang D, *et al.* In vitro effects and in vivo efficacy of a novel cyclo-oxygenase-2 inhibitor in dogs with experimentally induced synovitis. *Am J Vet Res* 2004; **65**: 503–512.

37 Glaser KB. Cyclooxygenase selectivity and NSAIDs: cyclooxygenase-2 selectivity of etodolac (Lodine). *Inflammopharmacology* 1995; **3**: 335–345.

38 Kay-Mugford P, Benn SJ, LaMarre J, Conlon P. In vitro effects of nonsteroidal anti-inflammatory drugs on cyclooxygenase activity in dogs. *Am J Vet Res* 2000; **61**: 802–810.

39 Wilson JE, Chandrasekharan NV, Westover KD, *et al.* Determination of expression of cyclooxygenase-1 and -2 isozymes in canine tissues and their differential sensitivity to nonsteroidal anti-inflammatory drugs. *Am J Vet Res* 2004; **65**: 810–818.

40 Patrignani P, Panara MR, Greco A, *et al.* Biochemical and pharmacological characterization of the cyclooxygenase activity of human blood prostaglandin endoperoxide synthases. *J Pharmacol Exp Ther* 1994; **271(3)**: 1705–1712.

41 US Food and Drug Administration. Freedom of information summary: Previcox chewable tablets (NADA 141-230). Approval Date: July 21, 2004. www.fda.gov/Downloads/Animalveterinary/Products/Approvedanimaldrugproducts/Foiadrugsummaries/Ucm118041.Pdf (accessed 15 September 2014).

42 Cox SR, Lesman SP, Boucher JF, *et al.* The pharmacokinetics of mavacoxib, a long-acting COX-2 inhibitor, in young adult laboratory dogs. *J Vet Pharmacol Ther* 2010; **33(5)**: 461–470.

43 Cox SR, Liao S, Payne-Johnson M, *et al.* Population pharmacokinetics of mavacoxib in osteoarthritic dogs. *J Vet Pharmacol Ther* 2011; **34(1)**: 1–11.

44 Gabrielsson J, Weiner D. *Pharmacokinetic and Pharmacodynamic Data Analysis: Concepts and Applications*, 4th edn. Stockholm, Sweden: Swedish Pharmaceutical Press, 2007.

45 Toutain PL, Reymond N, Laroute V, *et al.* Pharmacokinetics of meloxicam in plasma and urine of horses. *Am J Vet Res* 2004; **65(11)**: 1542–1547.

46 Toutain PL, Cester CC. Pharmacokinetic-pharmacodynamic relationships and dose response to meloxicam in horses with induced arthritis in the right carpal joint.*Am J Vet Res* 2004; **65(11)**: 1533–1541.

47 Pelligand L, King JN, Toutain PL, *et al.* Pharmacokinetic/pharmacodynamic modelling of robenacoxib in a feline tissue cage model of inflammation. *J Vet Pharmacol Ther* 2012; **35(1)**: 19–32.

48 Jung M, Lees P, Seewald W, King JN. Analytical determination and pharmacokinetics of robenacoxib in the dog. *J Vet Pharmacol Ther* 2009; **32(1)**: 41–48.

49 Maitho TE, Lees P, Taylor JB. Absorption and pharmacokinetics of phenylbutazone in Welsh Mountain ponies. *J Vet Pharmacol Ther* 1986; **9**: 26–39.

50 King JN, Jung M, Maurer MP, *et al.* Effects of route of administration and feeding schedule on pharmacokinetics of robenacoxib in cats. *Am J Vet Res* 2013; **74(3)**: 465–472.

51 Giraudel JM, Diquelou A, Laroute V, *et al.* Pharmacokinetic/pharmacodynamic modelling of NSAIDs in a model of reversible inflammation in the cat. *Br J Pharmacol* 2005; **146(5)**: 642–653.

52 Giraudel JM, Diquelou A, Lees P, Toutain PL. Development and validation of a new model of inflammation in the cat and selection of surrogate endpoints for testing anti-inflammatory drugs. *J Vet Pharmacol Ther* 2005; **28(3)**: 275–285.

53 Giraudel JM, King JN, Jeunesse EC, *et al.* Use of a pharmacokinetic/pharmacodynamics approach in the cat to determine a dosage regimen for the COX-2 selective drug robenacoxib. *J Vet Pharmacol Ther* 2009; **32**: 18–30.

54 Giraudel JM, Gruet P, Alexander DG, *et al.* Evaluation of orally administered robenacoxib versus ketoprofen for treatment of acute pain and inflammation associated with musculoskeletal disorders in cats. *Am J Vet Res* 2010; **71(7)**: 710–719.

55 King JN, Rudaz C, Borer L, *et al.* *In vitro* and *ex vivo* inhibition of canine cyclooxygenase isoforms by robenacoxib: a comparative study. *Res Vet Sci* 2010; **88(3)**: 497–506.

56 Hinz B, Brune K. Can drug removals involving cyclooxygenase-2 inhibitors be avoided? A plea for human pharmacology. *Trends Pharmacol Sci* 2008; **29(8)**: 391–397.

57 US Food and Drug Administration. Freedom of information summary: Metacam oral suspension (NADA 141-213). Approval Date: April 15, 2003. www.fda.gov/downloads/animalveterinary/products/approvedanimaldrugproducts/foiadrugsummaries/ucm118006.pdf (accessed 15 September 2014).

58 European Agency for the Evaluation of Medicinal Products. Meloxicam summary report. June 1997. EMEA/MRL/236/97.

59 Giraudel JM, Toutain PL, King JN, Lees P. Differential inhibition of cyclooxygenase isoenzymes in the cat by the NSAID robenacoxib. *J Vet Pharmacol Ther* 2009; **32**: 31–40.

60 Schmid VB, Spreng DE, Seewald W, *et al.* Analgesic and anti-inflammatory actions of robenacoxib in acute joint inflammation in the dogs. *J Vet Pharmacol Ther* 2009; **33**: 118–131.

61 Whittle BJ. Mechanisms underlying intestinal injury induced by anti-inflammatory COX inhibitors. *Eur J Pharmacol* 2004; **500(1-3)**: 427–439.

62 Wolfe MM, Lichtenstein DR, Singh G. Gastrointestinal toxicity of nonsteroidal antiinflammatory drugs. *N Engl J Med* 1999; **340**: 1888–1899.

63 Fortun PJ, Hawkey CJ. Nonsteroidal antiinflammatory drugs and the small intestine. *Curr Opin Gastroenterol* 2005; **21(2)**: 169–175.

64 Treinen-Moslen M, Kanz MF. Intestinal tract injury by drugs: importance of metabolite delivery by yellow bile road. *Pharmacol Ther* 2006; **112(3)**: 649–667.

65 Lascelles BDX, Blikslager AT, Fox SM, Reece D. Gastrointestinal tract perforation in dogs treated with a selective cyclooxygenase-2 inhibitor: 29 cases (2002–2003). *J Am Vet Med Assoc* 2005; **227**: 1112–1117.

66 Enberg TB, Braun LD, Kuzma AB. Gastrointestinal perforation in five dogs associated with the administration of meloxicam. *J Vet Emerg Crit Care* 2006; **16**: 34–43.

67 US Food and Drug Administration. Freedom of information summary: EtoGesic tablets (NADA 141-108). Approval Date: July 22, 1998. www.fda.gov/ohrms/dockets/98fr/NADA141-108-FOIS082703.pdf.pdf (accessed 15 September 2014).

68 Doig PA, Purbrick KA, Hare JE, McKeown DB. Clinical efficacy and tolerance of meloxicam in dogs with chronic osteoarthritis. *Can Vet J* 2000; **41(4)**: 296–300.

69 Jones CJ, Streppa HK, Harmon BG, Budsberg SC. In vivo effects of meloxicam and aspirin on blood, gastric mucosal, and synovial fluid prostanoid synthesis in dogs. *Am J Vet Res* 2002; **63**: 1527–1531.

70 Forsyth SF, Guilford WG, Haslett SJ, Godfrey J. Endoscopy of the gastroduodenal mucosa after carprofen, meloxicam and ketoprofen administration in dogs. *J Small Anim Pract* 1998; **39**: 421–424.

71 Lee YS, Kim H, Wu TX, *et al.* Genetically mediated interindividual variation in analgesic responses to cyclooxygenase inhibitory drugs. *Clin Pharmacol Ther* 2006 **79(5)**: 407–418.

72 Reimer ME, Johnston SA, Leib MS, *et al.* The gastrointestinal effects of buffered aspirin, carprofen, and etodolac in healthy dogs. *J Vet Intern Med* 1999; **13**: 472–477.

73 Nadeau JA, Andrews FM. Equine gastric ulcer syndrome: the continuing conundrum. *Equine Vet J* 2009; **41(7)**: 611–615.

74 Tobin T, Chay S, Kamerling S, *et al.* Phenylbutazone in the horse: a review. *J Vet Pharmacol Ther* 1986; **9(1)**: 1–25.

75 Marshall JF, Blikslager AT. The effect of nonsteroidal anti-inflammatory drugs on the equine intestine. *Equine Vet J* 2011; **43(s39)**: 140–144.

76 Tomlinson J, Blikslager A. Role of nonsteroidal anti-inflammatory drugs in gastrointestinal tract injury and repair. *J Am Vet Med Assoc* 2003; **222(7)**: 946–951.

77 Tomlinson JE, Blikslager AT. Effects of cyclooxygenase inhibitors flunixin and deracoxib on permeability of ischaemic-injured equine jejunum. *Equine Vet J* 2005; **37(1)**: 75–80.

78 Moore JN. Nonsteroidal anti-inflammatory drug therapy for endotoxemia: we're doing the right thing, aren't we? *Compendium Cont Educat* 1989; **11**: 741–744.

79 McConnico RS, Morgan TW, Williams CC, *et al.* Pathophysiologic effects of phenylbutazone on the right dorsal colon in horses. *Am J Vet Res* 2008; **69**: 1496–1505.

80 Brzozowski T, Konturek PC, Konturek SJ, *et al.* Role of prostaglandins in gastroprotection and gastric adaptation. *J Physiol Pharmacol* 2005; **56(Suppl 5)**: 33–55.

81 Hurley JW, Crandal LA. The effects of salicylates upon the stomach of dogs. *Gasteroenterology* 1964; **46**: 36–43.

82 Phillips BM. Aspirin-induced gastrointestinal microbleeding in dogs. *Toxicol Appl Pharmacol* 1973; **24**: 182–189.

83 Konturek JW, Dembinski A, Stoll R, *et al.* Mucosal adaptation to aspirin induced gastric damage in humans. Studies on blood flow, gastric mucosal growth, and neutrophil activation. *Gut* 1994; **35**: 1197–1204.

84 Taylor LA, Crawford LM. Aspirin-induced gastrointestinal lesions in dogs. *J Am Vet Med Assoc* 1968; **152(6)**: 617–619.

85 Souza MH, de Lima OM Jr, Zamuner SR, *et al.* Gastritis increases resistance to aspirin-induced mucosal injury via COX-2-mediated lipoxin synthesis. *Am J Physiol Gastrointest Liver Physiol* 2003; **285(1)**: G54–61.

86 Wallace JL, Fiorucci S. A magic bullet for mucosal protection and aspirin is the trigger! *Trends Pharmacol Sci* 2003; **24(7)**: 323–236.

87 Wallace JL, Zamuner SR, McKnight W, *et al.* Aspirin, but not NO-releasing aspirin (NCX-4016), interacts with selective COX-2 inhibitors to aggravate gastric damage and inflammation. *Am J Physiol Gastrointest Liver Physiol* 2004; **286(1)**: G76–81.

88 Fiorucci S, de Lima OM Jr, Mencarelli A, *et al.* Cyclooxygenase-2-derived lipoxin A4 increases gastric resistance to aspirin-induced damage. *Gastroenterology* 2002; **123(5)**:1598–1606.

89 Sennello KA, Leib MS. Effects of deracoxib or buffered aspirin on the gastric mucosa of healthy dogs. *J Vet Intern Med* 2006; **20**: 1291–1296.

90 Mathews KA, Doherty T, Dyson DH, *et al.* Nephrotoxicity in dogs associated with methoxyflurane anesthesia and flunixin meglumine analgesia. *Can Vet J* 1990; **31**: 766–771.

91 Mathews KA. Nonsteroidal anti-inflammatory analgesics in pain management in dogs and cats. *Can Vet J* 1996; **37**: 539–545.

92 Gunson DE, Soma LR. Renal papillary necrosis in horses after phenylbutazone and water deprivation. *Vet Pathol* 1983; **20(5)**: 603–610.

93 Lobetti RG, Joubert KE. Effect of administration of nonsteroidal anti-inflammatory drugs before surgery on renal function in clinically normal dogs. *Am J Vet Res* 2000; **61**: 1501–1506.

94 Gambaro G, Perazella MA. Adverse renal effects of anti-inflammatory agents: evaluation of selective and nonselective cyclooxygenase inhibitors. *J Intern Med* 2003; **253**: 643–652.

95 Rossat J, Maillard M, Nussberger JU, *et al.* Renal effects of selective cyclooxygenase-2 inhibition in normotensive salt-depleted subjects. *Clin Pharmacol Ther* 1999; **66**: 76–84.

96 Narita T, Sato R, Motoishi K, *et al.* The interaction between orally administered non-steroidal anti-inflammatory drugs and prednisolone in healthy dogs. *J Vet Med Sci* 2007; **69(4)**: 353–363.

97 de Broe ME, Elseviers MM. Analgesic nephropathy. *N Engl J Med* 1998; **338**: 446–452.

98 Frendin JH, Boström IM, Kampa N, *et al.* Effects of carprofen on renal function during medetomidine-propofol-isoflurane anesthesia in dogs. *Am J Vet Res* 2006; **67(12)**: 1967–1973.

99 Ko JCH, Miyabiyashi T, Mandsager RE, *et al.* Renal effects of carprofen administered to healthy dogs anesthetized with propofol and isoflurane. *Am J Vet Med Assoc* 2000; **217**: 346–349.

100 Bergmann HML, Nolte IJA, Kramer S. Effects of preoperative administration of carprofen on renal function and hemostasis in dogs undergoing surgery for fracture repair. *Am J Vet Res* 2005; **66**: 1356–1363.

101 Boström IM, Nyman GC, Lord PF, *et al.* Effects of carprofen on renal function and results of serum biochemical and hematologic analyses in anesthetized dogs that had low blood pressure during anesthesia. *Am J Vet Res* 2002; **63**: 712–721.

102 Crandell DE, Mathews KA, Dyson DH. Effect of meloxicam and carprofen on renal function when administered to healthy dogs prior to anesthesia and painful stimulation. *Am J Vet Res* 2004; **65(10)**: 1384–1390.

103 Fusellier M, Desfontis JC, LeRoux A, *et al.* Effect of short-term treatment with meloxicam and pimobendan on the renal function in healthy beagle dogs. *J Vet Pharmacol Ther* 2008; **31**: 150–155.

104 Boström IM, Nyman G, Hoppe A, Lord P. Effects of meloxicam on renal function in dogs with hypotension during anaesthesia. *Vet Anaesth Analg* 2006; **33(1)**: 62–69.

105 US Food and Drug Administration. Freedom of information summary: Deramaxx chewable tablets (NADA 141-203). Approval Date: August 21, 2002. www.fda.gov/downloads/AnimalVeterinary/Products/ApprovedAnimalDrugProducts/FOIADrugSummaries/ucm117640.pdf (accessed 15 September 2014).

106 Luna SP, Basílio AC, Steagall PV, *et al.* Evaluation of adverse effects of long-term oral administration of carprofen, etodolac, flunixin meglumine, ketoprofen, and meloxicam in dogs. *Am J Vet Res* 2007; **68(3)**: 258–264.

107 Surdyk KK, Brown CA, Brown SA. Evaluation of glomerular filtration rate in cats with reduced renal mass and administered meloxicam and acetylsalicylic acid. *Am J Vet Res* 2013; **74(4)**: 648–651.

108 Gunew MN, Menrath VH, Marshall RD. Long-term safety, efficacy and palatability of oral meloxicam at 0.01–0.03 mg/kg for treatment of osteoarthritic pain in cats. *J Feline Med Surg* 2008; **10(3)**: 235–241.

109 Gowan RA, Lingard AE, Johnston L, *et al.* Retrospective case–control study of the effects of long-term dosing with meloxicam on renal function in aged cats with degenerative joint disease. *J Feline Med Surg* 2011; **13(10)**: 752–761.

110 Gowan RA, Baral RM, Lingard AE, *et al.* A retrospective analysis of the effects of meloxicam on the longevity of aged cats with and without overt chronic kidney disease. *J Feline Med Surg* 2012; **14(12)**: 876–881.

111 King JN, Hotz R, Reagan EL, *et al.* Safety of oral robenacoxib in the cat. *J Vet Pharmacol Ther* 2012; **35(3)**: 290–300.

112 Lee WM. Drug induced hepatotoxicity. *N Engl J Med* 2003; **349**: 474–485.

113 Bjorkman D. Nonsteroidal anti-inflammatory drug-associated toxicity of the liver, lower gastrointestinal tract, and esophagus. *Am J Med* 1998; **105(Suppl 5A)**: 17S–21S.

114 Tolman KG. Hepatotoxicity of non-narcotic analgesics. *Am J Med* 1998; **105(Suppl 1B)**: 13S–17S.

115 US Food and Drug Administration. Freedom of information summary: Rimadyl tablets (NADA 141-053). Approval Date: October 25, 1996.

116 Vasseur PB, Johnson AL, Budsberg SC, *et al.* Randomized, controlled trial of the efficacy of carprofen, a nonsteroidal antiinflammatory drug, in the treatment of osteoarthritis in dogs. *J Am Vet Med Assoc* 1995; **206**: 807–811.

117 MacPhail CM, Lappin MR, Meyer DJ, *et al.* Hepatocellular toxicosis associated with administration of carprofen in 21 dogs. *J Am Vet Med Assoc* 1998; **212**: 1895–1901.

118 Hickford FH, Barr SC, Erb HN. Effect of carprofen on hemostatic variables in dogs. *Am J Vet Res* 2001; **62(10)**: 1642–1646.

119 Budsberg SC, Stoker AM, Johnston SA, *et al.* In vitro effects of meloxicam on metabolism in articular chondrocytes from dogs with naturally occurring osteoarthritis. *Am J Vet Res* 2013; **74(9)**: 1198–1205.

120 Niemi TT, Taxell C, Rosenberg PH. Comparison of the effect of intravenous ketoprofen, ketorolac and diclofenac on platelet function in volunteers. *Acta Anaesthesiol Scand* 1997; **41(10)**: 1353–1358.

121 Lemke KA, Runyon CL, Horney BS. Effects of preoperative administration of ketoprofen on whole blood platelet aggregation, buccal mucosal bleeding time, and hematologic indices in dogs undergoing elective ovariohysterectomy. *J Am Vet Med Assoc* 2002; **220(12)**: 1818–1822.

122 Mukherjee D, Nissen SE, Topol EJ. Risk of cardiovascular events associated with selective COX-2 inhibitors. *JAMA* 2001; **286**: 954–959.

123 Eisenberg RS. Learning the value of drugs – is rofecoxib a regulatory success story? *N Engl J Med* 2005; **352**: 1285–1287.

124 Fitzgerald GA. Coxibs and cardiovascular disease. *N Engl J Med* 2004; **351**: 1709–1711.

125 Topol EJ. Failing the public health - rofecoxib, Merck and the FDA. *N Engl J Med* 2004; **351**: 1707–1709.

126 Drazen JM. COX-2 inhibitors – a lesson in unexpected problems. *N Engl J Med* 2005; **352**: 1131–1132.

127 Fitzgerald GA, Patrono C. The coxibs, selective inhibitors of cyclooxygenase-2. *N Engl J Med* 2001; **345**: 433–442.

128 Kamata M, King JN, Seewald W, *et al.* Comparison of injectable robenacoxib versus meloxicam for peri-operative use in cats: results of a randomised clinical trial. *Vet J* 2012; **193(1)**: 114–118.

129 Sano T, King JN, Seewald W, *et al.* Comparison of oral robenacoxib and ketoprofen for the treatment of acute pain and inflammation associated with musculoskeletal disorders in cats: a randomised clinical trial. *Vet J* 2012; **193(2)**: 397–403.

130 Peterson WL, Cryer B. COX-1-sparing NSAIDs – is the enthusiasm justified? *JAMA* 1999; **282**: 1961–1963.

131 Jüni P, Rutjes AWS, Dieppe PA. Are selective COX 2 inhibitors superior to traditional nonsteroidal anti-inflammatory drugs? *BMJ* 2002; **324**: 1287–1288.

132 Rainsford KD. The ever-emerging anti-inflammatories. Have there been any real advances? *J Physiol* 2001; **95**: 11–19.

133 Lascelles BDX, Cripps PJ, Jones A, Waterman-Pearson AE. Efficacy and kinetics of carprofen, administered preoperatively or postoperatively, for the prevention of pain in dogs undergoing ovariohysterectomy. *Vet Surg* 1998; **27**: 568–582.

134 Mathews KA, Pettifer G, Foster R, McDonell W. Safety and efficacy of preoperative administration of meloxicam, compared with that of ketoprofen and butorphanol in dogs undergoing abdominal surgery. *Am J Vet Res* 2001; **62(6)**: 882–888.

135 Budsberg SC, Cross AR, Quandt JE, *et al.* Evaluation of intravenous administration of meloxicam for perioperative pain management following stifle joint surgery in dogs. *Am J Vet Res* 2002; **63(11)**: 1557–1563.

136 Bennett D, Johnston P. Osteoarthritis in the cat. How should it be managed and treated? *J Feline Med Surg* 2012; **14(1)**: 76–84.

137 Hjelle JJ, Grauer GF. Acetaminophen-induced toxicosis in dogs and cats. *J Am Vet Med Assoc* 1986; **188**: 742–746.

138 McCann ME, Rickes EL, Hora DF, *et al.* In vitro effects and in vivo efficacy of a novel cyclooxygenase-2 inhibitor in cats with lipopolysaccharide-induced pyrexia. *Am J Vet Res* 2005; **66**: 1278–1284.

139 Morresey PR. Therapeutic intervention strategies in endotoxemia. *Compend Contin Educ Vet* 2001; **23**: 925–931.

140 Valverde A, Gunkel CI. Pain management in horses and farm animals. *J Vet Emerg Crit Care* 2005; **15(4)**: 295–307.

141 Cook VL, Meyer CT, Campbell NB, Blikslager AT. Effect of firocoxib or flunixin meglumine on recovery of ischemic-injured equine jejunum. *Am J Vet Res* 2009; **70(8)**: 992–1000.

142 Smith GW, Davis JL, Tell LA, *et al.* FARAD Digest: Extralabel use of nonsteroidal anti-inflammatory drugs in cattle. *J Am Vet Med Assoc* 2008; **232**: 697–701.

143 Coetzee JF, Mosher RA, KuKanich B, *et al.* Pharmacokinetics and effect of intravenous meloxicam in weaned Holstein calves following scoop dehorning without local anesthesia. *BMC Vet Res* 2012; **8(1)**: 1–15.

144 Hirsch AC, Philipp H, Kleemann R. Investigation on the efficacy of meloxicam in sows with mastitis–metritis–agalactia syndrome. *J Vet Pharmacol Ther* 2003; **26(5)**: 355–360.

145 Delatour P, Foot R, Foster AP, *et al.* Pharmacodynamics and chiralpharmacokinetics of carprofen in calves. *Br Vet J* 1996; **152(2)**: 183–198.

146 Letendre LT, Tessman RK, McClure SR, *et al.* Pharmacokinetics of firocoxib after administration of multiple consecutive daily doses to horses. *Am J Vet Res* 2008; **69(11)**: 1399–1405.

147 Lohuis JACM, Werven TV, Brand A, *et al.* Pharmacodynamics and pharmacokinetics of carprofen, a non-steroidal anti-inflammatory drug, in healthy cows and

cows with Escherichia coli endotoxin-induced mastitis. *J Vet Pharmacol Ther* 1991; **14**(3): 219–229.

148 Malreddy PR, Coetzee JF, KuKanich B, Gehring R. Pharmacokinetics and milk secretion of gabapentin and meloxicam co-administered orally in Holstein-Friesian cows. *J Vet Pharmacol Ther* 2013; **36**(1): 14–20.

149 Montoya L, Ambros L, Kreil V, *et al.* A pharmacokinetic comparison of meloxicam and ketoprofen following oral administration to healthy dogs. *Vet Res Commun* 2004; **28**(5): 415–428.

150 Mosher RA, Coetzee JF, Cull CA, *et al.* Pharmacokinetics of oral meloxicam in ruminant and preruminant calves. *J Vet Pharmacol Ther* 2012; **35**(4): 373–381.

151 Noble G, Edwards S, Lievaart J, *et al.* Pharmacokinetics and safety of single and multiple oral doses of meloxicam in adult horses. *J Vet Intern Med* 2012; **26**(5): 1192–1201.

152 Parton K, Balmer TV, Boyle J, *et al.* The pharmacokinetics and effects of intravenously administered carprofen and salicylate on gastrointestinal mucosa and selected biochemical measurements in healthy cats. *J Vet Pharmacol Ther* 2000; **23**(2): 73–80.

153 Silber HE, Burgener C, Letellier IM, *et al.* Population pharmacokinetic analysis of blood and joint synovial fluid concentrations of robenacoxib from healthy dogs and dogs with osteoarthritis. *Pharmaceut Res* 2010; **27**(12): 2633–2645.

154 Sinclair MD, Mealey KL, Matthews NS, *et al.* Comparative pharmacokinetics of meloxicam in clinically normal horses and donkeys. *Am J Vet Res* 2006; **67**(6): 1082–1085.

155 Busch U, Schmid J, Heinzel G, *et al.* Pharmacokinetics of meloxicam in animals and the relevance to humans. *Drug Metab Dispos* 1998; **26**(6): 576–584.

156 Papich MG. *Saunders Handbook of Veterinary Drugs*, 3rd edn. St Louis, MO: Elsevier, 2011.

13 Anesthetic and Analgesic Adjunctive Drugs

Daniel S. J. Pang
Faculty of Veterinary Medicine and Hotchkiss Brain Institute, University of Calgary, Calgary, Alberta, Canada

Chapter contents

Introduction

Adjunctive drugs can be broadly described as drugs which fall outside common clinical use but may provide a benefit beyond that of more commonly used drugs or are less readily characterized because they play a supportive role in the provision of anesthesia and analgesia. Some of the drugs described in this chapter may enter the mainstream as evidence supporting their use grows, while others may remain unconventional, restricted to second- or third-line therapy, or fall out of use as alternatives are identified. This chapter is divided into non-analgesic and analgesic adjuncts.

Non-analgesic adjuncts

Dantrolene

Dantrolene is a peripherally acting muscle relaxant, producing skeletal muscle relaxation through ryanodine receptor antagonism [1,2]. There are three isoforms of ryanodine receptors with RYR1 believed to be predominant in skeletal muscle. Receptors are located in organelle (i.e., mitochondrial, endoplasmic and sarcoplasmic reticular, and nuclear) membranes. The mechanism of dantrolene's action is not fully understood but its primary effect is to reduce calcium release from the sarcoplasmic reticulum into the cytoplasm, thereby dissociating excitation-contraction coupling. Its muscle-relaxing properties are limited to skeletal muscle though cardiac depression has been reported in dogs when administered at high doses (greater than 5 mg/kg) or in combination with verapamil [3]. At therapeutic intravenous (IV) doses (1–5 mg/kg) in dogs and cats, minute ventilation during general anesthesia is reduced through depression of both respiratory rate and tidal volume [4,5].

Dantrolene is primarily indicated for the treatment and prevention of malignant hyperthermia (MH) [6–12], and rhabdomyolysis [13–17], with recent interest in a potential role in cytoprotection [1,2].

Shortly after MH was first reported in humans [18,19] and pigs [20,21], the successful use of dantrolene for prevention and treatment of MH was published with the experiments performed in pigs [12]. It has since been used to treat MH in dogs [7] and horses [10].

Dantrolene is used in the prevention and treatment of exertional rhabdomyolyis in horses [14,16], though use in rhabdomyolysis in a dog [13] and tetanus in cats [17] have also been reported. In horses, approximately 2–4 mg/kg orally (PO) given 60–90 min prior to exercise has been effective in preventing exertional rhabdomyolysis in horses prone to the condition [14,16].

Dantrolene undergoes hepatic metabolism, primarily hydroxylation, in the dog and horse. Metabolites and up to 1% of unchanged dantrolene are excreted in urine and bile [22–24].

Dosages in horses are as follows: 1.9 mg/kg IV loading dose followed by oral dosing at 2.5 mg/kg every 60 min [23], or 4 mg/kg PO [10,24].

Dosages in dogs and cats are as follows: 1–3 mg/kg IV (low end of dose range for muscle relaxation and high end for treatment of malignant hyperthermia); 5–6 mg/kg PO once daily as prophylaxis.

Veterinary Anesthesia and Analgesia: The Fifth Edition of Lumb and Jones.
Edited by Kurt A. Grimm, Leigh A. Lamont, William J. Tranquilli, Stephen A. Greene and Sheilah A. Robertson.

Dosages in pigs are as follows: 1–3 mg/kg IV for treatment of malignant hyperthermia; 5 mg/kg PO for prophylaxis.

Dantrolene is available as a 0.33 mg/mL solution for injection and as 100 mg capsules. Solutions of reconstituted dantrolene are light sensitive and stable for 6 h [2].

Doxapram

The analeptic (central nervous system stimulant) agent doxapram has a long history of use in veterinary medicine and has been applied in a wide variety of situations including arousal from sedation/anesthesia [25–27], cardiopulmonay resuscitation [28–30], stimulation of respiration in neonates and following drug-induced respiratory depression [31–39], and assessment of laryngeal function [40–42].

The mechanism of action leading to respiratory stimulation is likely a combination of central and peripheral effects [43–45]. Electrophysiological studies in cats and dogs showed increased activity of the respiratory nuclei of the medulla when given therapeutic doses of doxapram [43]. As the dose was increased, cortical stimulation occurred followed by convulsions. A safety margin of 20–60:1 was cited before onset of central stimulation and convulsions. Experimental evidence suggests that stimulation of respiration is dose dependent, with activation of peripheral aortic and carotid receptors occurring at doses (0.05–0.25 mg/kg IV) below those typically used clinically [44]. As the dose is increased (0.5–5 mg/kg IV), stimulation of respiratory and non-respiratory brainstem neurons occurs [44]. There is limited evidence for interspecies variability in the doxapram dose effective for respiratory stimulation versus CNS arousal. Low doses of doxapram are successful in eliciting respiratory stimulation in cats before cardiovascular or CNS stimulation occurs [43–45], but higher doses may be necessary in other species. It is unclear to what extent this dose dependency occurs in dogs and horses, with evidence of CNS arousal occurring at doses effective for respiratory stimulation [31,32,46,47].

The molecular mechanisms underlying peripheral and central control of respiration are an active research area. Recent evidence suggests involvement of two-pore domain potassium channels and these channels may also be involved in the mechanism of inhalational anesthesia [48–50]. See Yost (2006) for a complete review [51].

Doxapram has the ability to significantly increase minute ventilation through an increase in both respiratory rate and tidal volume, leading to the term 'pharmacologic ventilator' [52]. However, its effects are short-lived, reflecting a rapid decline in plasma levels following an intravenous bolus [53]. Doxapram undergoes hepatic metabolism in dogs with renal excretion of metabolites. A similar pharmacokinetic profile is observed in horses with a rapid decline in plasma levels following IV bolus administration, extensive hepatic metabolism, and renal excretion of metabolites [54].

Doxapram administration also results in modest increases in arterial blood pressure and heart rate in humans [52]. While cardiovascular changes are short-lived in healthy animals (i.e., several minutes), one report of its use in dogs rendered hypovolemic from controlled hemorrhage showed sustained increases in cardiac output and arterial blood pressure for up to 1 h [47]. Doxapram does not induce cardiac arrhythmias in dogs anesthetized with halothane or cycloproprane even in the presence of epinephrine and hypercapnia [55].

In healthy adult horses and those with experimentally induced respiratory disease, a dose of 0.3 mg/kg (IV) resulted in an approximately 50% increase in respiratory rate and tidal volume [56]. The duration of action was not described. During halothane anesthesia, preceded with acepromazine and thiopental in ponies, the addition of doxapram (0.05 mg/kg/min) resulted in a return of arterial carbon dioxide tension ($PaCO_2$) and pH to near normal levels, with an increase in respiratory rate (tidal volume was not measured) [31]. An increase in mean arterial blood pressure of approximately 20% without an accompanying increase in heart rate was observed during doxapram infusion. Interestingly, the infusion of doxapram was associated with a reduction in plane of anesthesia, necessitating an increase in halothane vaporizer setting.

In cats anesthetized with a preparation of alfaxalone/alfadolone (i.e., Saffan®), administration of doxapram (7.5 mg/kg IV) resulted in a 181% increase in minute ventilation which lasted for several minutes [33]. A similar pattern was seen in cats anesthetized with thiopental [33]. At this dose, heart rates increased for several minutes during both thiopental and Saffan® anesthesia to approximately 15–20% above the pre-doxapram period. Recovery was faster in the Saffan® group with the addition of doxapram, and no change was observed in the thiopental group.

The use of doxapram in patients with a history of seizures is controversial [51]. While it is clear that cortical activity increases in a dose-dependent fashion, it is unclear if this constitutes proconvulsant activity. Care should be exercised when administering doxapram in patients with a history of seizures. As always, the use of appropriate dosing (i.e., to effect) is critical.

Two areas of active doxapram usage are in foal and calf neonatal medicine and assessment of laryngeal function in dogs. Retrospective data from a cohort of foals with hypoxic-ischemic encephalopathy (neonatal maladjustment syndrome) revealed doxapram (0.02–0.05 mg/kg/min IV) to be more effective than caffeine (loading dose of 7.5–12 mg/kg followed by 2.5–5 mg/kg/day PO via nasogastric tube) at reducing $PaCO_2$ for at least 12 h [35]. However, foals remained acidemic with no significant increase in pH. The reduction in $PaCO_2$ was achieved with an increase in tidal volume as respiratory rate did not increase. No effects on heart rate were observed and there was no difference in mortality rates. These data agreed with an earlier retrospective study in healthy foals showing no advantage of caffeine over saline in correcting respiratory acidosis created with isoflurane anesthesia [34]. Furthermore, a doxapram dosing regimen of 0.5 mg/kg followed by 0.03 mg/kg/min IV was as effective as 0.5 mg/kg followed by 0.08 mg/kg/min. Giguere *et al.* also reported an improvement in arterial oxygen tension (PaO_2) following doxapram administration, compared with saline control or caffeine [34]. In contrast to adult horses, the effects of doxapram on cardiovascular function differed, with a small but significant increase in heart rate observed in healthy foals regardless of doxapram dose. The mechanism of increased ventilation also differed; minute ventilation was increased in healthy foals as a result of increased respiratory rate and not tidal volume. Doxapram also resulted in a modest increase in mean arterial blood pressure of approximately 10 mmHg.

In calves, a comparison of doxapram (2 mg/kg IV) and theophylline (7 mg/kg IV) showed a marked increase in respiratory rate with doxapram but not theophylline, resulting in a doubling of respiratory rate 10 min after drug administration followed by a steady decline over the next 2 h (which was the end of the recording period). The effect on $PaCO_2$ (maximal decrease of approximate 20 mmHg) and PaO_2 (maximal increase of approximate 15 mmHg) peaked 30 s following administration, followed by a steady return towards baseline over the recording period. Small increases in heart rate (120 to 155 beats per minute) and systemic systolic arterial blood pressure (105 to 112 mmHg) were also observed without a significant change in cardiac output. A greater change (20 mmHg increase) was observed in systolic pulmonary arterial blood pressures. The authors concluded that the transient respiratory stimulation following doxapram administration could be beneficial in newborn calves when positive pressure ventilation was not possible. Interestingly, a systematic review of doxapram use in human infants did not identify a clear advantage associated with doxapram use over saline [57] and there is evidence that doxapram may cause cortical damage due to a reduction in cerebral blood flow [58–60].

A comparison of the effects of doxapram on laryngeal function in normal dogs and those with laryngeal paralysis found that doxapram was useful in differentiating the two populations [41]. Following premedication with acepromazine (0.022 mg/kg IM in diseased dogs and 0.2 mg/kg IM in normal dogs) with butorphanol (0.44 mg/kg IM), animals were preoxygenated for 5 min and general anesthesia induced with isoflurane delivered by mask. Doxapram was administered at 1.1 mg/kg IV following induction and recording of baseline video. At baseline, the normalized glottal gap area was significantly larger in dogs with laryngeal paralysis during both inspiration and expiration. Following doxapram administration, the normalized glottal gap area at inspiration was significantly reduced in dogs with laryngeal paralysis compared to normal dogs, and the area during expiration was significantly greater in dogs with laryngeal paralysis. These results reflect the paradoxical movement of the arytenoid cartilages in diseased dogs, with inward collapse of the arytenoid cartilages as subatmospheric thoracic pressure is generated. The dramatic changes observed allowed for diagnosis but also led the authors to warn of the need to potentially intubate the airway to provide oxygen.

Another group of investigators used a different anesthetic protocol consisting of the following premedication: butorphanol 0.22 mg/kg IV, acepromazine 0.05 mg/kg SC, and glycopyrrolate 0.005 mg/kg SC. Anesthesia was induced with propofol to effect and doxapram was administered at 2.2 mg/kg IV. Their results differed in that doxapram administration resulted in significant arytenoid cartilage movement which was not observed by Tobias *et al.* [41]. Unfortunately, as no diseased group was used as a comparison in the Miller *et al.* (2002) study [40], it is not possible to determine potential differences between diseased and healthy populations.

In horses, laryngeal function has been evaluated by comparison of the following techniques compared to animals standing at rest with a twitch: rest without twitch, manual occlusion of nostrils, post exercise (lunging at canter), swallowing, doxapram (40 mg/kg IV), and xylazine (0.5 mg/kg IV) [42]. Subjectively, doxapram resulted in an increased respiratory rate in approximately half of the horses examined (total $n = 7$), but the most successful technique for stimulating deep breaths was manual nostril occlusion.

An internet survey of 600 veterinarians in small animal practice, with or without board certification in critical care and emergency medicine or anesthesia, showed that while doxapram was as frequently available to both specialists and practitioners (74% and 81%, respectively), a significantly higher percentage of general practitioners had used it during cerebral-cardiopulmonary resuscitation (CPR) (29% and 70%, respectively) [30]. This contrasts starkly with the current evidence-based CPR guidelines in which doxapram is not mentioned [28]. Experimental animal and human infant evidence indicates that doxapram may reduce cerebral oxygen flow, compromising cortical oxygen delivery, and may result in long-term brain damage [58–61].

The use of doxapram at 0.1–0.2 mg/kg IV has also been suggested to facilitate recovery from general anesthesia in horses, when appropriate, by increasing the level of arousal and stimulating respiration, thereby speeding reduction in alveolar concentrations of inhalational agents [62].

Other species in which doxapram use has been recorded are cattle (1 mg/kg IV was effective in speeding recovery from xylazine), camels (0.05–0.13 mg/kg IV was effective at speeding recovery from xylazine in Bactrian camels), llamas (2.2 mg/kg IV was not effective in reversing xylazine), and southern elephant seals (appeared to cause CNS stimulation at 5 mg/kg when used to aid recovery from a range of drug combinations; therefore authors recommended 2 mg/kg) [63–66].

Famotidine and omeprazole

Acid secretion in the stomach is initiated at the level of parietal cells by gastrin, histamine type 2 (H_2), and muscarinic (M_3) receptors. Receptor activation results in increased proton pump activity on the luminal side of the cell via calcium- or cAMP-dependent pathways. Several H_2 receptor antagonists (famotidine, ranitidine, and cimetidine) have been used clinically. Famotidine and ranitidine are 20–50 and 4–10 times more potent than cimetidine, respectively. Perioperative use is usually to offset risk of gastrointestinal ulceration, with common indications including stress- or NSAID-related abomasal and gastric ulcers in calves, foals, and horses, and following regurgitation during anesthesia in dogs.

In a small cross-over study involving five healthy horses, a comparison of famotidine and ranitidine found a high degree of individual variation in measured gastric fluid pH following administration of either drug at a range of dosages [67]. Each horse received famotidine (0.5 mg/kg, 1 mg/kg, and 2 mg/kg) and ranidi-tine (4.4 mg/kg and 6.6 mg/kg) via nasogastric tube. For famotidine, gastric fluid pH increased above 6 in three of five horses receiving 0.5 mg/kg, five of five horses receiving 1 mg/kg, and three of five horses receiving 2 mg/kg. For ranitidine, gastric fluid pH increased above 6 in four of five horses receiving 4.4 mg/kg and five of five horses receiving 6.6 mg/kg. Ranitidine demonstrated a tendency to result in a longer elevation of gastric fluid pH (166 ± 106 min versus 98 ± 110 min; mean ± SD). The drug response varied considerably between horses, leading the authors to suggest a dose of 6.6 mg/kg ranitidine. Similar studies in 2–6-day old foals and milk-fed calves resulted in recommended dosages of ranitidine of 6.6 mg/kg PO three times daily and 50 mg/kg PO three times daily, respectively [68,69]. However, more recent evidence highlights the risk of extrapolating the need for H_2 antagonists in critically ill foals without measurement of gastric pH [70]. This study found that almost 50% of hospitalized foals had a baseline gastric pH which was alkaline. Data supporting the use of famotidine in calves and foals are not available.

Omeprazole is a proton pump inhibitor which acts on the proton pump located at the luminal surface of gastric parietal cells. Clinical evidence (described below) suggests that it is more effective at raising gastric pH above 3, a level correlated with healing gastric and duodenal ulcers in humans [71]. The dose in dogs and cats is 1–2.5 mg/kg PO once daily [72,73], and 1–4 mg/kg PO once daily in horses and foals, with the low end of dose range for ulcer prevention and the higher end for treatment [74–76].

The perioperative use of famotidine in dogs and cats is commonly performed in cases with suspected gastrointestinal ulceration or in patients at risk of ulceration. Recommended doses of famotidine in dogs and cats vary widely due to limited clinical data. In dogs,

0.1–0.5 mg/kg twice daily or 1 mg/kg once daily (PO, IV, SC, IM) has been advocated. In cats, 0.2–0.25 mg/kg once or twice daily (IM, SC, PO, IV) has been suggested. Slow IV administration in cats is recommended based on anecdotal evidence that fast injection (i.e., less than 5 min) is associated with hemolysis as a result of the benzyl alcohol component of the injectable formulation. However, a retrospective study in which hospital policy was that famotidine be administered over 5 min IV did not identify an effect on packed cell volume (PCV) [77]. The same study showed no change in PCV when cats received famotidine SC. There are limited clinical data demonstrating efficacy of famotidine in dogs, and omeprazole may be superior at raising gastric pH for a useful period of time [72,78]. A recent study in dogs with exercise-induced gastritis and clinically relevant gastric ulcers showed famotidine (approximately 1 mg/kg PO once daily) to be superior to no treatment in preventing gastric ulcers but inferior to omeprazole (approximately 0.85 mg/kg PO once daily) [78]. In healthy adult dogs, famotidine (0.5 mg/kg IV twice daily) resulted in a significant elevation of gastric pH above saline control and ranitidine, but did not raise pH as high, or for as long, as omeprazole (1 mg/kg PO once daily). Increasing the dosing frequency of famotidine to three times daily did not result in any improvement [72].

The preoperative use of omeprazole (or its *S*-enantiomer, esomeprazole) has demonstrated variable results [79,80]. In one study, the administration of esomeprazole (two doses 12 h apart at 1 mg/kg IV prior to induction of general anesthesia) resulted in a less acidic reflux but did not reduce the incidence of reflux [79]. In contrast, another study reporting the use of preoperative omeprazole (single dose, 1 mg/kg PO at least 4 h prior to induction of general anesthesia) showed a reduction in the number of gastroesophageal reflux and regurgitation episodes [80]. A direct comparison between findings is difficult due to differences in study design. Zacuto *et al.* also had another treatment group, esomeprazole (1 mg/kg IV) with cisapride (1 mg/kg IV), which resulted in less acidic reflux but also a significant reduction in the number of reflux events compared to the control and omeprazole groups [79]. Consequently, there is no clear answer regarding the best choice of preventive therapy but it is important to recognize that, while the incidence of gastroesophageal reflux is relatively high (up to approximately 50%) [81,82], the incidence of complications such as esophageal stricture formation is extremely low [83].

There is a theoretical concern with chronic omeprazole therapy resulting in a change in gastric fauna and bacterial overgrowth, potentially increasing the risk of pneumonia in patients predisposed to regurgitation, such as those with megaesophagus. Another potential concern is the effect of omeprazole to inhibit the cytochrome (CYP) P450 system, specifically CYP2C19, responsible for diazepam metabolism [84,85]. There is currently no evidence that this is of clinical significance in veterinary medicine, and the large therapeutic margin of diazepam may reduce the risk of adverse events.

Famotidine is available as 10 mg tablets (other strengths may be available), an 8 mg/mL suspension, and a 10 mg/mL solution for injection.

Omeprazole is available as 20 and 40 mg capsules and is licensed as an oral paste in horses (370 mg/g of paste).

Guaifenesin (GG, glyceryl guaiacolate ether)

Guaifenesin, originally derived from the *Guaiacum* genus of trees, is a centrally acting skeletal muscle relaxant with sedative properties primarily co-administered IV with injectable anesthetic agents for the induction and maintenance of general anesthesia in horses and ruminants. Historically, it was used for this indication in humans along with a role in the management of tetanus. It has been in use in veterinary anesthesia since the 1960s [86,87]. In humans, it is currently used exclusively as an expectorant [88]. The mechanism(s) of action of guaifenesin are largely unknown, but evidence from the 1950s suggests sites of action in both the brain (brainstem and subcortical regions) and spinal cord (polysynaptic reflex inhibition) affected by interneuron depression, resulting in sedation and muscle relaxation [87,89]. There is extremely limited evidence to suggest it has any analgesic properties and none are typically attributed [87]. It has a wide therapeutic margin, with doses resulting in cardiopulmonary side-effects such as hypotension, respiratory depression, and apneustic breathing pattern, being approximately 70–80% greater than that required to induce recumbency in horses (75–150 mg/kg) [86–90].

Cardiovascular effects are mild when guaifenesin is administered on its own at therapeutic doses, with no change in heart rate, cardiac output, central venous pressure or respiratory rate, and approximately a 20% decrease in mean arterial blood pressure [91,92]. Similarly, respiratory effects are minimal and the physiologic changes associated with recumbency appear to have a greater effect than any respiratory depression from guaifenesin [93]. Minute ventilation is maintained as a result of increased respiratory rate offsetting a decrease in tidal volume, indicating a sparing effect on the respiratory muscles [91]. An elegant study by Schatzmann *et al.* demonstrated minimal changes in PaO_2 when horses were administered guaifenesin (100 mg/kg, IV) but remained standing [93].

Overdose in horses results in a period of transient muscle spasm and mydriasis as the dose approaches 180 mg/kg (IV), followed by loss of palpebral reflex, with death following respiratory or cardiac arrest at approximately 460 mg/kg [86]. Guaifenesin undergoes hepatic metabolism with glucuronidation followed by renal excretion. A sex difference in elimination has been identified in ponies with more rapid elimination in females [94].

Guaifenesin is commonly prepared as a 5–15% solution with 0.9% saline or 5% dextrose solution, though it can also be solubilized in sterile water. There is a concentration-dependent risk of hemolysis which appears unrelated to the speed of administration [87,93,95]. Hemolysis has been documented in horses when the concentration exceeds a 15% solution, and in cattle when it exceeds 5% [87,93,96]. Intravascular thrombus formation is also dose related and concentrations of greater than 7% are associated with increased risk of thrombosis [93,97,98]. This effect is related to solution concentration rather than speed of administration, with reported histologic changes including endothelial loss with formation of a fibrin clot [97]. With a 10% solution the thrombus is not occlusive [97].

The drug is prone to precipitate out of solution when stored below room temperature (22 °C) but this is reversible with gentle heating such as immersion in a warm water bath [86]. Perivascular injection has been associated with tissue necrosis [86] and administration via an IV catheter is recommended. Urticaria attributed to guaifenesin has also been reported [99]. In the reported case, the horse also received xylazine, ketamine, butorphanol, bupivacaine, and isoflurane, but the timing of the appearance of urticaria and failure of recurrence during two subsequent anesthetic episodes without guaifenesin raised the index of suspicion.

Maropitant

Maropitant is a neurokinin (NK1) receptor antagonist licensed as an antiemetic in dogs and cats. It is highly protein bound and undergoes extensive hepatic metabolism by CYP3A enzymes [100]. Oral bioavailability is approximately 20% in dogs and 50% in cats [101].

Neurokinin receptor antagonism by maropitant reduces binding of the neuropeptide neurotransmitter substance P. Substance P is intimately involved in the brainstem nuclei (area postrema, nucleus tractus solitarius, and vagal dorsal motor nucleus) facilitating emesis [102].

The most frequently encountered and reported adverse event is pain on injection [103]. The commercial preparation of maropitant is formulated with β-cyclodextrin to increase solubility and the binding relationship is temperature dependent. As the free, unbound maropitant is suspected to cause pain on injection, refrigerating the solution was investigated as a means to reduce this reaction. An injectate temperature of 4 °C was associated with a mild response ('twitching of the skin, licking of the fur, or digging at the injection site') in one out of 17 dogs; the remaining 16 dogs did not react to injection. In contrast, injections at 25 °C were associated with a painful response in nine out of 17 dogs, four of which were moderate-severe ('short-term vocalization, jumping, wincing, prolonged yelping or aggression') [103]. This pattern of responses was reflected with a concurrent visual analogue scale (VAS) score, showing that a 25 °C injectate temperature resulted in a significantly greater VAS than maropitant at 4 °C (or saline at both 4 °C and 25 °C) [103].

As an antiemetic, maropitant has been shown to be effective in cats and dogs in a variety of situations, including motion sickness, chemotherapy, and non-specific gastritis [101,104–109]. Its efficacy has compared favorably to metoclopramide, chlorpromazine, and ondansetron with a range of emetogens and clinical conditions [104,110].

Specific to anesthesia and analgesia, maropitant has been investigated for potential analgesic properties [111–113] and efficacy in reducing emesis following premedication with hydromorphone [114].

A MAC-sparing effect ranging from 16% to 30% has been shown in two nociceptive models: tail clamp and ovary and ovarian ligament stimulation [111–113]. The range in MAC-sparing effect may reflect the different study models or doses used in each study, or both. A loading dose of 5 mg/kg IV followed by 150 μg/kg/h resulted in a MAC reduction of 16% after a tail clamp stimulus during sevoflurane anesthesia compared to control [111]. Administration of maropitant via the epidural route did not reduce MAC in the same model and the authors suggested that inappropriate dose, failure to cross dural membranes or a restricted site of action may have contributed [111]. In contrast, in an ovary and ovarian ligament stimulation model, a lower IV dose of maropitant (1 mg/kg IV followed by 30 μg/kg/h) resulted in a 24% decrease in the MAC of sevoflurane [112]. Increasing the maropitant dose to 5 mg/kg IV followed by infusion at 150 μg/kg/h resulted in a small (non-significant) further reduction in MAC of 30% [112]. A similar study in cats (same nociceptive model and anesthetic agent) but with a single IV bolus of maropitant (1 mg/kg) resulted in a MAC reduction of 15% [113]. Increasing the dose of maropitant did not lead to a further decrease in MAC.

The putative sites of antinociceptive action of maropitant are NK1 receptors of the central and peripheral nervous systems, where NK1 receptors have been identified on sensory afferent nerves [115], in spinal cord [116], and in brain and viscera [117]. Current experimental evidence with visceral and somatic nociceptive models suggests a potential role as an analgesic agent.

Maropitant's antiemetic effect has been documented in dogs and cats receiving hydromorphone [114] or xylazine [101]. In cats, 1 mg/kg of maropitant administered 2 h prior to xylazine (0.44 mg/kg IM) significantly reduced emesis by 76%, 90%, and 100% for the SC, PO, and IV routes of administration, respectively [101]. Additionally, administration of 1 mg/kg maropitant orally 24 h prior to xylazine administration resulted in a 66% reduction in emetic events [111–113]. When 1 mg/kg of maropitant was administered SC 1 h prior to hydromorphone (0.1 mg/kg IM) in healthy dogs, emesis, retching, and nausea did not occur [114]. This compared to incidences of emesis, retching, and nausea of 66%, 11%, and 22%, respectively, in the saline control group. Compared to the use of acepromazine as a strategy for reducing emesis following hydromorphone administration [118], maropitant appears to be more effective.

The antiemetic efficacy of maropitant in the face of a wide range of emetogenic insults likely reflects its central site of action at the common pathway governing emesis.

The injectable formulation (10 mg/mL) is effective at 1 mg/kg SC in dogs and cats.

Methocarbamol

Methocarbamol is a centrally acting muscle relaxant that selectively inhibits spinal and supraspinal polysynaptic reflexes through its action on interneurons, without direct effects on skeletal muscle [119,120]. It is commonly used in human medicine for back pain with a muscular component [121]. Use in veterinary medicine has historically been associated with tetanus [122–124], metaldehyde and pyrethrin/permethrin toxicity [125–127], and exertional rhabdomyolysis [128,129]. More recently, it has been successfully used for the management of acute muscle strain in combination with rest, physical therapy and non-steroidal anti-inflammatory drugs (NSAIDs) [130]. Higher doses may result in sedation and this should be accounted for when used in combination with sedative and anesthetic agents.

Pharmacokinetics have been studied in dogs [131] and horses [128,129,132]. Therapeutic serum concentrations are achieved rapidly by an oral route of administration in dogs and horses [131,132]. Extensive hepatic metabolism (dealkylation and hydroxylation followed by conjugation) is followed by primarily urinary excretion of metabolites [131]. Guaifenesin is a metabolite of methocarbamol produced in low concentrations in horses [128,129].

The recommended dose of methocarbamol in cats and dogs is 40–60 mg/kg (PO, IV) three times daily for one day followed by 20–40 mg/kg (PO, IV) three times daily until symptoms resolve [130]. Higher doses may result in toxicity and potential effects of co-administration of drugs with CNS depressant effects should be taken into account [122,124,133]. One case series reported doses of 55–100 mg/kg IV every 30–60 min in dogs with tetanus, though its efficacy was questioned when compared to other muscle relaxants/sedatives employed [124]. Per rectum administration (55–200 mg/kg, up to 330 mg/kg/day per rectum every 6–8 h) has been reported when an IV formulation was not available [133]. Its use is associated with few side-effects, with a human study finding the incidence of adverse events similar to that of placebo [121]. Administration of methocarbamol at therapeutic doses does not result in cardiopulmonay changes.

Overdose may result in sedation and excessive muscle weakness with any effects being short-lived.

Methocarbamol is available as 500 and 750 mg tablets, and as a 100 mg/mL solution for injection.

Metoclopramide

Metoclopramide is primarily indicated as an antiemetic in small animals. It is less effective than maropitant which works to block the final pathway controlling emesis [110]. It has also been investigated for use in promotion of gastric emptying and reduction of gastroesophageal reflux [134,135]. Metoclopramide increases gastroesophageal sphincter tone [136,137] and promotes peristalsis of the duodenum along with an improvement in antropyloroduodenal co-ordination; together these effects promote gastric emptying in healthy dogs [138]. Supporting evidence for its use in promoting gastric emptying in clinical cases is limited [134]. Following a dose of 0.3 mg/kg in dogs 1 week after gastropexy for correction of gastric dilatation-volvulus, metoclopramide did not promote gastric emptying [134].

In a comparison of two doses of metoclopramide (loading dose of 1 mg/kg then 1 mg/kg/h IV, or 0.4 mg/kg then 0.3 mg/kg/h IV) in dogs undergoing orthopedic surgery, the low and high doses of metoclopramide resulted in a reduction of the risk of gastroesophageal reflux by 34% and 54%, respectively [135]. Given the low risk of clinical sequelae following gastroesophageal reflux, the case for pre-emptive therapy is unclear.

The drug has multiple sites of action, including serotonin receptor antagonism in the CNS and dopamine (D_2) receptor antagonism in the CNS and gastrointestinal tract [102]. Metabolism is primarily hepatic with a high first-pass effect [139]. The recommended doses in dogs and cats are 0.25–0.5 mg/kg IV, IM, or PO every 8–12 h (higher doses may be required in refractory cases). For continuous rate infusion (CRI) a loading dose of 0.4 mg/kg then 0.3–1 mg/kg/h is recommended.

The administration of metoclopramide in horses and ponies has demonstrated limited efficacy [140]. Doses of 0.06–0.25 mg/kg caused restlessness, sedation, and occasionally colic. Lack of supporting evidence for beneficial large intestinal effects does not indicate its use in colic [141].

Use in cattle is limited as the dose effective at increasing reticular motility (0.3 mg/kg IM) in healthy animals was associated with neurological signs (restlessness then depression) [142]. The effects of the reported effective dose were short-lived, lasting no more than 20 min. Similarly, in calves, metoclopramide (0.1 mg/kg IM) was no better than saline at increasing abomasal motility or emptying rate [143].

Available formulations include 5 and 10 mg tablets, 1 mg/mL oral solution, and 5 mg/mL injectable solution.

Ondansetron and dolasetron

Ondansetron and dolasetron are serotonin (5-HT_3) receptor antagonists often administered as antiemetics prior to chemotherapy [144]. Ondansetron has been shown to be highly effective in cisplatin-induced emesis in dogs and doxorubicin-induced emesis in ferrets [145]. Cisplatin induces emesis through peripheral activity on the gastric mucosa to activate 5-HT_3 receptors in vagal and sympathetic afferents to the emetic center of the brainstem [146,147], and ondansetron and dolasetron block this pathway at the level of the emetic center. Anecdotal evidence suggests success in treating nausea and vomiting associated with renal and hepatic disease as well as gastroenteritis [148].

Unlike maropitant which acts at the final common pathway controlling emesis, ondansetron is less effective against a broad range of emetogens. For example, it has been shown to be less effective than maropitant in preventing emesis resulting from apomorphine administration in dogs [110].

Evidence from clinical human literature does not suggest a difference in efficacy between dolasetron and ondansetron [149]. A similar comparison has not been studied in a clinical veterinary setting.

While adverse effects have not been reported in dogs and cats, in 2010 the United States Food and Drug Administration released a drug safety communication contraindicating the use of injectable dolasetron for the prevention of nausea and vomiting associated with chemotherapy in humans [150]. This resulted from evidence of electrocardiographic QT prolongation and torsade de pointes associated with IV administration. The warning did not extend to oral therapy.

In the dog, dolasetron undergoes hepatic metabolism, producing the active metabolite reduced-dolasetron. This metabolite and the unchanged drug are both excreted in urine and feces [151]. Ondansetron metabolism is mediated by CYP3A4 in the liver with excretion of metabolites in urine and feces [152]. Ondansetron dose in cats and dogs is 0.5–1 mg/kg twice daily (IV or PO) or 30 min prior to chemotherapy. A lower dose may be effective in reducing emesis associated with other emetogens. For example, 0.22 mg/kg IV reduced the incidence of emesis when co-administered with dexmedetomidine in cats [153]. The dose of dolasetron in dogs and cats is 0.6–1 mg/kg once daily (IV or PO).

Available formulations of ondansetron include 4 and 8 mg tablets, 4 mg/5 mL oral solution, and 2 mg/mL injectable solution. Dolasetron is available as 50 and 100 mg tablets and a 20 mg/mL solution.

Procainamide

Procainamide is a Class 1a (Singh-Vaughan Williams and Keefe classifications) antiarrhythmic agent with efficacy for the treatment of supraventricular and ventricular tachyarrhythmias (VT). It is a derivative of the local anesthetic procaine (ester linkage replaced with amide). Through sodium channel blockade it reduces the rate of rise of phase 0 of the cardiac action potential, raises the threshold potential and prolongs the refractory period. It also has some anticholinergic effects. It is often used as a second-line therapy for VT resistant to lidocaine.

A comparison between procainamide and lidocaine for the management of postoperative ventricular arrhythmias (i.e., ventricular premature contractions (VPCs), ventricular tachycardia, R-on-T phenomenon, and multiform VPCs) in a mixed population of medium-large breed dogs showed each drug to be equally effective in restoring sinus rhythm [154]. Procainamide was administered as a loading dose, 10 mg/kg IV over 5 min, then an infusion of 20 μg/kg/min IV. No side-effects were associated with procainamide administration.

Efficacy in the treatment of atrial fibrillation is mainly from experimental models of induced arrhythmia studies in dogs, with one recent case report [155,156]. The clinical case report describes the successful use of procainamide (14.3 mg/kg IV over 15 min) to treat atrial fibrillation associated with pericardiocentesis and unresponsive to a single dose of lidocaine (1.2 mg/kg IV). Procainamide administration resulted in cardioversion to a sinus rhythm [155]. In Boxers, two studies have reported the efficacy of antiarrhythmic agents in terms of median survival time [157] and response of ventricular arrhythmias [158]. Caro-Vadillo *et al.* did not find a significant effect on median survival time (age and the presence of syncope were better predictors) between the following treatments: sotalol, mexiletine-atenolol, or procainamide (20–26 mg/kg PO every 8 h) [157]. Meurs *et al.*, in a comparison between procainamide (20–26 mg/kg PO every 8 h), atenolol, sotalol or mexiletine-atenolol, found that only sotalol or mexiletine-atenolol were effective at reducing the number and severity of VPCs and heart rate [158]. However, none of the treatments resulted in an improvement in the incidence of syncope, though it is possible the study was underpowered for this outcome.

There is limited evidence of its use in horses or other species, with one report of failed therapy for ventricular extrasystoles and VT at a total dose of 20 mg/kg over two administrations given at a 2 h interval [159]. The pharmacokinetics of procainamide have been reported in horses where, unlike dogs [160], the active metabolite NAPA (*N*-acetylprocainamide) is produced which has class III antiarrhythmic activity (i.e., it prolongs the cardiac action potential) [161].

An effective dose in dogs is 10 mg/kg IV over 10 min followed by an infusion of 20 μg/kg/min [154]. Single or repeated bolus injection of 1–2 mg/kg IV may be effective in dogs for the management of short-duration ventricular ectopic activity associated with surgical manipulation or catecholamine release. The recommended dose in cats is a loading dose of 1–2 mg/kg slowly IV followed by an infusion of 10–20 μg/kg/min.

Toxicity manifests as a widening of the QRS complex, additional arrhythmias and hypotension [158].

It is available as 250, 375, and 500 mg tablets and a 100 mg/mL solution for injection.

Sodium nitroprusside (SNP)

Sodium nitroprusside elicits arterial and venous dilation through the liberation of the potent endogenous vasodilator nitric oxide (NO). Cyanide ions are also produced as a by-product. For an in-depth review of nitric oxide physiology, the reader is referred to Forstermann and Sessa [162]. Following administration of SNP, its vascular effects are mediated locally in the vascular endothelium and underlying smooth muscle. SNP produces NO (from reaction with oxyhemoglobin, also generating methemoglobin) which in turn activates soluble guanylyl cyclase, increasing levels of cyclic GMP in the vascular musculature. Cyclic GMP inhibits entry of calcium into smooth muscle cells and increases uptake of intracellular calcium by smooth endoplasmic reticulum, with the resultant effect of vasodilation.

When delivered by IV infusion, SNP has a rapid onset and offset, allowing titration to effect. Dose rates of 1–5 μg/kg/min have been reported in dogs and cats [163]. Close monitoring of systemic arterial blood pressure and heart rate and rhythm is essential due to the risk of inadvertent hypotension or reflex tachycardia. The rapid offset of SNP is due to the short half-life of NO which is rapidly oxidized to nitrite [164]. Cyanide ions, produced with NO from SNP, are metabolized by the liver to thiocyanate which is then excreted by the kidneys [165]. In cases of overdose or hepatic or renal insufficiency, there is a risk of cyanide and thiocyanate toxicity. Toxicity manifests as tachycardia, hyperventilation, metabolic acidosis (as cyanide binds cytochrome oxidase, thereby inhibiting aerobic metabolism), and seizures. Toxicity can be treated with thiosulfate (6 mg/kg/h IV in dogs) [166–168]. Solutions of SNP are light sensitive, turning from a light orange/straw-colored solution when fresh (reconstituted with 5% dextrose) to dark brown/blue upon exposure to light. The solution should be discarded if this occurs.

Nitroprusside is available in 10 and 25 mg/mL solutions for injection following dilution.

Vasopressin (Antidiuretic Hormone, Arginine Vasopressin, AVP) and desmopressin (DDAVP)

The primary perioperative indication for vasopressin is in cardiopulmonary resuscitation and refractory hypotension [28,169–175]. It is a potent vasoconstrictor, acting on V_{1a} receptors of vascular smooth muscle, though it also displays activity at V_{1b} (anterior pituitary) and V_2 (renal collecting duct) receptors [176]. Its analogue, desmopressin (DDAVP), is used in the treatment of central diabetes insipidus [177–179] and management of coagulopathy [180–182].

Vasopressin is an alternative vasopressor to epinephrine for use during CPR, though there is no clear evidence supporting its role as a replacement for epinephrine. Recent veterinary [28,173] and human [171] CPR guidelines suggest its use (0.8 U/kg IV) on alternating rounds of CPR instead of epinephrine. Due to lack of β_1-adrenergic receptor activity, it may reduce the risk of myocardial ischemia compared with epinephrine, though it will still cause coronary vasoconstriction. An additional potential advantage over epinephrine is that V_1 receptors, unlike α_1-adrenergic receptors, remain responsive in an acidic environment [183]. Reports of clinical use in the veterinary literature are mixed [170,174], with vasopressin showing no benefit over epinephrine in a randomized comparison using a standardized CPR technique [174], but associated with an improved rate of return to spontaneous circulation in a hospital-wide study [170]. A meta-analysis demonstrated a potential improvement in return of spontaneous circulation associated with its use, though contributing studies were predominantly in porcine models of ventricular fibrillation [175]. A systematic review of three human trials did not show a clear benefit of vasopressin over epinephrine [169].

Vasopressin can be administered via the endotracheal route if necessary, with one animal study suggesting that the same dose as that recommended for IV use is effective [184].

What has become clear from the Reassessment Campaign on Veterinary Resuscitation (RECOVER) initiative [185] is that there is wide variability in study design and reporting of animal models of CPR, making it difficult to draw firm conclusions from currently available experimental evidence. Anecdotal reports suggest use of vasopressin in cases of refractory hypotension, though the available veterinary literature is sparse and human studies are contradictory [172,186–188]. This is likely a reflection of the heterogeneity of clinical and experimental studies [188]. Infusion rates of 1–4 mU/kg/min and 0.1–2.5 mU/kg/min have been suggested in dogs and foals, respectively [172,186]. Users should be aware of the potential for detrimental hypoperfusion of vascular beds resulting from the resultant vasoconstriction [189]. Desmopressin acetate, a synthetic analogue of vasopressin with reduced vascular effects, is used for perioperative management of patients with von Willebrand disease [181,190] and management of central diabetes insipidus [177–179].

Von Willebrand disease, the most common canine hereditary defect of hemostasis, is classified according to one of three subtypes, with type 1 being the least severe and most common, especially in Doberman Pinschers [191]. Management consists of both non-transfusion and transfusion therapy, based on disease severity and clinical presentation. Non-transfusion therapy includes appropriate patient management (i.e., good surgical technique, minimizing use of drugs with antiplatelet activity, careful handling) and DDAVP. Administration of 1 µg/kg SC or IV [190] 30 min prior to surgery may support hemostasis but the response is more variable in dogs than humans [181,190]. Administration of DDAVP intranasally or into the conjunctival sac is commonly performed but there is limited supporting evidence of its efficacy via this route in von Willebrand disease.

Other reported uses for DDAVP include support of hemostasis following administration of aspirin prior to surgery [192,193] and as a prophylactic measure to manage postoperative diabetes insipidus following hypophysectomy [182].

Injectable vasopressin is available as a 20 U/mL solution. DDAVP is available as a 4 µg/mL injectable solution, 0.1 and 0.2 mg tablets, 100 µg/mL spray, and a 0.01% solution for intranasal administration.

Analgesic adjuncts

Amantadine and memantine

The dopamine agonist and *N*-methyl-D-aspartate (NMDA) receptor antagonist amantadine was originally used as an antiviral agent [194,195] but has entered clinical use in human medicine for diseases and presentations as varied as Parkinson's disease [196], traumatic brain injury, and pain. Its continued use in the management of Parkinson's disease arose serendipitously from a patient with Parkinson's disease noticing an improvement in motor function while taking amantadine for influenza [197]. Recent meta-analysis and systematic reviews have indicated a potential role for amantadine in traumatic brain injury (TBI) though further studies are required to confirm promising earlier findings [198,199]. Human studies have demonstrated improved arousal when amantadine was administered between 3 days and 4 weeks following TBI, and purported mechanisms are through CNS stimulation mediated by amantadine's dopaminergic activity and reduced neurotoxicity through its NMDA receptor antagonism [200,201]. Its use in animals is currently limited to an experimental model of TBI in rats where learning and hippocampal neuron survival were improved with amantadine administration 1 h following TBI [202].

Amantadine and memantine have also been studied for their potential analgesic properties mediated through NMDA receptor antagonism [203]. Amantadine's analgesic efficacy appears to be limited to cases of chronic pain, particularly where central sensitization may play a role, such as in chronic arthritis [204] and limb amputation [205–207]. In a population of dogs with pelvic limb lameness and pain refractory to NSAID use, Lascelles *et al.* showed that activity increased after 3 weeks of combination therapy with meloxicam (0.1 mg/kg PO once daily) and amantadine (3–5 mg/kg PO once daily) [204]. An alternative dosing regimen of 2–10 mg/kg PO 2–3 times daily has been suggested, though it would be sensible to monitor for CNS excitation at the higher end of the dose range [208].

More work is required to clarify the potential role of amantadine and memantine in chronic pain, with a recent meta-analysis identifying a lack of strong evidence for its use in people with a range of neuropathic pain etiologies [207].

Its use has been suggested in cats at a dose of 3–5 mg/kg PO once or twice daily for the management of chronic arthritic pain though published evidence of its efficacy is sparse [203,208].

There are limited pharmacokinetic data available for its use in companion animals. It undergoes primarily renal excretion in dogs [209] and there are limited dose–response data from rats [210]. As a result of its dopaminergic properties, CNS stimulation is a predicted side-effect from overdose, and caution should be exercised in patients receiving other dopamine agonists (e.g., the monoamine oxidase inhibitor selegiline), or agents inhibiting the reuptake of serotonin (e.g., the tricyclic antidepressants such as amitriptyline, and the selective serotonin reuptake inhibitors such as fluoxetine). Such combinations risk the occurrence of serotonin syndrome, a potentially fatal syndrome characterized by signs of CNS stimulation, muscular tremors and autonomic stimulation including tachycardia, tachypnea, and hypertension [211,212]. The risk is likely increased in the presence of hepatic insufficiency as monoamine oxidase inhibitors and selective serotonin reuptake inhibitors are metabolized by the CYP 450 pathway. Specific to anesthesia, there is evidence from human medicine that the phenylpiperidine opioids (meperidine, fentanyl, and fentanyl's congeners, tramadol and methadone) all increase the CNS concentration of serotonin to varying degrees and in some instances have contributed to serotonin syndrome although the risk to veterinary patients remains unknown [213,214].

A less studied use of amantadine, and its derivative memantine, is as a local anesthetic. Local anesthesia appears to be mediated through sodium channel-blocking properties in addition to NMDA receptor antagonism [210,215]. It remains to be seen if there are significant advantages over traditional local anesthetics such as lidocaine and bupivacaine.

Amantadine is available as 100 mg tablets and capsules, and as a 10 mg/mL syrup. Memantine is available as 5 and 10 mg tablets, and as a 2 mg/mL oral formulation.

Amitriptyline and nortriptyline

The tricyclic antidepressant amitriptyline is indicated for behavioral disorders (e.g., obsessive-compulsive disorder) [216], idiopathic feline lower urinary tract disease (IFLUTD) [217,218], and more recently neuropathic pain states [219]. Tricyclic antidepressants are selective serotonin reuptake inhibitors, increasing synaptic levels of serotonin and norepinephrine. This appears to be the primary mechanism mediating their useful behavioral modification effects. However, other less well-understood mechanisms of action may also contribute to their clinical potential as analgesics [219]. These include sodium channel blockade [220], NMDA receptor antagonism [221], and antihistamine activity [222], but not opioid receptor activity [223].

Amitriptyline, 1–2 mg/kg/day, is commonly prescribed for management of IFLUTD, though the mechanism of action leading to resolution of clinical signs is still subject to speculation, including serotonin reuptake inhibition, antihistamine, and anticholinergic activity [217]. Prospective studies indicate that treatment periods greater than 7 days are necessary to observe improvements of clinical signs [217,218,224].

Its use for the treatment of neuropathic pain in clinical cases is largely anecdotal with few reported cases [219,225]. The case series reported by Cashmore *et al.* describes three cases of neuropathic pain in dogs, two of which responded successfully to amitriptyline (1.1–1.3 mg/kg PO twice daily) [219]. One case exhibited mechanical allodynia and dysesthesia over the facial dermatome innervated by the infraorbital branch of the right trigeminal nerve. The dog did not respond to gabapentin (12.5 mg/kg PO twice daily) but responded rapidly to amitriptyline (1.3 mg/kg PO twice daily) with resolution of clinical signs over 6 weeks. Owner-initiated discontinuation of therapy resulted in a return of clinical signs within 3 days and the dog was maintained on long-term amitriptyline therapy thereafter. The second successful case was of intermittent lumbar pain with diffuse mechanical allodynia. Amitriptyline (1.1 mg/kg PO twice daily) resulted in an improvement of clinical signs within 1 week and resolution of clinical signs by 1 month. Discontinuation of therapy resulted in a return of pain within 2 days, and the dog was then maintained on long-term amitriptyline therapy. The final reported case involved mechanical allodynia associated with ulnar and median nerve lesions which was non-responsive to amitriptyline (1.4 mg/kg PO twice daily) but responded to gabapentin (14.3 mg/kg PO twice daily). A commonly reported adverse effect of amitriptyline, sedation, was also reported by the owners. All of these cases were non-responsive to initial trials with NSAIDs, steroids, and opioids.

A feline case of neuropathic pain following femoral fracture repair, iatrogenic sciatic nerve trauma, and subsequent amputation exhibited suspected neuropathic pain (phantom limb pain) approximately 1 month following amputation [225]. The cat was frequently shaking the amputation stump though there was no response to palpation of the area. Following an IV infusion of morphine, ketamine, and lidocaine for 37 h followed by transmucosal buprenorphine (approximately 0.03 mg/kg twice daily) and oral amitriptyline (approximately 2 mg/kg twice daily), the cat was ambulating normally at discharge. At follow-up 10 months later, ambulation was normal without observed shaking of the amputation stump. Neuropathic pain has also been implicated in syringomyelia [226] and some cases of head shaking in horses [227].

Hepatic metabolism of amitriptyline results in production of the active metabolite nortriptyline in dogs and humans [228]. Both amitriptyline and nortriptyline are also excreted unchanged in urine, and caution should therefore be exercised in animals with renal insufficiency. Nortriptyline is used clinically as a treatment for neuropathic pain in humans [229], though its use in animals has not been reported.

The recommended route of administration is oral [230]; transdermal application is not effective at raising plasma drug levels and intrathecal administration resulted in marked spinal cord pathology [221].

Adverse effects on the heart include tachycardia mediated via an anticholinergic effect and potential fatal ventricular tachyarrhythmias from overdose (exceeding approximately 15 mg/kg IV) [231,232]. Ventricular tachyarrhythmias are preceded by prolongation of the QRS complex. No ECG abnormalities were detected in dogs receiving appropriate doses of amitriptyline (0.74–2.5 mg/kg PO every 12 h) for behavioral disorders [233]. Other signs of toxicity in conscious dogs include hypersalivation and vomiting. Common side-effects at therapeutic doses are weight gain and sedation [234]. While there is a theoretical risk of triggering serotonin syndrome with the concurrent use of tricyclic antidepressants and monoamine oxidase inhibitors, this risk (at least in humans) is believed to be low with amitriptyline [214].

Available formulations of amitriptyline include 10, 25, 50, 75, 100, and 150 mg tablets. Available formulations of nortriptyline include 10, 25, 50, and 75 mg tablets and 10 mg/5 mL oral solution.

Gabapentin and pregabalin

Gabapentin and pregabalin are structural analogues of γ-aminobutyric acid (GABA), but do not interact with GABA receptors to produce analgesia. Historically gabapentin has been prescribed as an anticonvulsant in humans and veterinary species, but is being used increasingly for neuropathic and perioperative pain in humans. Recent systematic reviews and meta-analyses have identified some promising results but more work is required to confirm its efficacy and roles [235–238]. There is a growing body of veterinary literature describing its use in dogs [219,239–243], cats [244–247], horses [248–251], and cattle [252–254], though questions remain regarding its efficacy and appropriate dosing regimens.

The mechanism of action of gabapentin and pregabalin is not fully understood. They do not appear to interact with GABA, NMDA or dopamine receptors, with evidence suggesting inhibition of N-type voltage-dependent neuronal calcium channels, a previously unidentified pharmacological target for analgesics [255,256]. Inhibition leads to a reduction of calcium influx into neurons, in turn reducing the release of a range of excitatory and inhibitory neurotransmitters, altering channel trafficking and stimulating the movement of channels away from neuronal cell membranes [255].

Pharmacokinetic data are available for dogs [243,257], cats [244], horses [248,249], and cattle [252,254]. In dogs, a short terminal half-life suggests the need for frequent dosing; this is supported by limited clinical evidence indicating that the therapeutic dose is in the range of 10–20 mg/kg PO 2–3 times daily [219,239,241,242].

Gabapentin has been used to successfully improve clinical signs in a case series of Cavalier King Charles Spaniels with Chiari malformation and syringomyelia [241]. A prospective clinical trial comparing gabapentin to a gelatin capsule placebo in dogs undergoing thoracic limb amputation did not identify an advantage of gabapentin in the management of postoperative pain [242]. However, the authors conceded that the study may have been underpowered and it is possible that the dose used (10 mg/kg total daily dose) was subtherapeutic. Similarly, a prospective clinical trial using gabapentin (10 mg/kg PO twice daily) as an adjunctive analgesic agent resulted in a non-significant reduction in pain scores compared to placebo for hemilaminectomy surgery [239]. In addition to potential limitations from insufficient power, the potent analgesia provided by concurrent opioid administration and the complexity of the pain model led the authors to suggest that the dosage of gabapentin be tailored to an individual animal's response, as is performed in humans, rather than adhering to rigid dosing regimens. A series of three cases of neuropathic pain (partial avulsion of ulnar and median spinal nerve roots, sensory trigeminal neuropathy, and presumed spinal cord neuropathy) reported successful pain management with gabapentin (14 mg/kg PO twice daily) or amitriptyline [219]. Interestingly, when one drug failed to improve clinical symptoms, switching to the other was often successful.

Pharmacokinetic data in cats suggest a dosing regimen of 8 mg/kg PO every 8 h, or 3 mg/kg PO every 6 h, in order to achieve plasma concentrations associated with analgesia in humans [244]. However, an increase in thermal threshold did not occur when gabapentin was administered orally at 5, 10 or 30 mg/kg [245]. These doses resulted in plasma drug concentrations in excess of those associated with analgesia in humans, leaving the authors to question the utility of gabapentin in healthy cats and the adequacy of the pain model. Sedation was not associated with gabapentin in this study at any dose, though it is a common adverse effect in dogs [258]. The same investigators were not able to show a MAC-sparing effect of gabapentin on isoflurane despite achieving plasma drug concentrations almost double those reported to be effective in humans, though this does not rule out an analgesic effect [246]. A report of two cases of polytrauma from road traffic accidents describes the successful use of gabapentin in response to clinical signs indicative of mechanical allodynia [247]. In both cases, gabapentin (10 mg/kg PO every 8 h) was administered following development of mechanical allodynia 24–48h after a surgical procedure. In each case, clinical signs resolved 24h later, allowing a stepping down of all analgesics. While promising, these cases reflect multimodal management (i.e., cats also received opioids, NSAIDs, and locoregional analgesia) of polytrauma, making it difficult to interpret gabapentin's contribution in isolation.

In a study reporting pharmacokinetic and behavioral data in horses, following 20 mg/kg PO or IV, no significant changes in heart rate or mean arterial blood pressure were recorded [249]. Sedation, scored as mild to moderate, occurred in all horses for 1h following IV gabapentin. The frequency of drinking and standing at rest increased and decreased, respectively, over the 11-h observation period. Oral dosing of gabapentin had a lower bioavailability in horses (16%) compared to dogs (80%), which is likely to influence dosing requirements. No metabolites were detected in equine plasma, indicating that metabolism may be similar to that reported in humans, with the majority of drug excreted unchanged in urine. These pharmacokinetic data were in broad agreement with those previously reported in this species [248].

Reports of the clinical use of gabapentin in horses are scarce [250,251]. Following debridement of subsolar seromas, subsequent infection and ongoing chronic laminitis and tendonitis, gabapentin (2–3.3 mg/kg PO every 8–12h) was included in a complex multimodal analgesic plan which also included opioids, NSAIDs, locoregional analgesia, α_2-adrenergic receptor agonists and ketamine at various times [250]. Though it is impossible to assess the contribution of gabapentin in this case, no adverse effects were noted and an improvement in pain score coincided with initiation of gabapentin (along with concurrent perineural administration of bupivacaine). In a horse displaying signs of pain attributed to femoral neuropathy and associated left pelvic limb paresis following surgery for colic, gabapentin administration was initiated (2.5 mg/kg PO every 8h for 24h, then every 12h) following a lack of response to xylazine, butorphanol, flunixin and a lidocaine CRI, and adverse effects (marked sedation) from a detomidine CRI. Two hours after administration of gabapentin, during which time detomidine CRI (3µg/kg/h IV) and acepromazine (0.03 mg/kg IV every 6h) were continued, the mare became less agitated and clinical signs (i.e., circling and pawing with the affected hoof) improved further over the following 36h.

Pharmacokinetic and some pharmacodynamic data are available in adult cows [254] and calves [252,254]. A comparison of gabapentin (15 mg/kg PO once 1h prior to dehorning) with flunixin, meloxicam, and meloxicam with gabapentin did not result in significant differences between groups or compared with placebo in plasma cortisol concentrations or eye temperature. The results for mechanical nociceptive threshold were equivocal. Weight gain was the only parameter to show a difference between analgesic treatments and placebo. Average daily weight gain was greater in calves treated with meloxicam and gabapentin than placebo, gabapentin alone or meloxicam alone. A combination of gabapentin (15 mg/kg PO) and meloxicam (0.5 mg/kg PO) resulted in plasma levels of gabapentin greater than 2µg/mL (which is the threshold associated with analgesia in humans) for 15h [252]. Compared with horses and dogs where maximal plasma concentrations were achieved within 2h, peak concentrations in calves were not reached until 7h post administration. In adult Holstein-Friesian cows, the time to achieve maximal plasma concentrations of gabapentin (10–20 mg/kg PO co-administered with meloxicam 1 mg/kg PO) was also slow, taking over 8h [254]. Both gabapentin and meloxicam concentrations in milk took 3 days to drop below the level of detection.

In dogs, approximately 30–35% of an administered dose of gabapentin undergoes hepatic metabolism while unchanged drug is excreted by the kidneys [257]. The metabolism of gabapentin has not been reported in the cat.

Sedation has been reported as an adverse effect in dogs and horses receiving gabapentin [249,258] but not cats or cattle.

While pharmacokinetic data for the use of pregabalin for analgesia in dogs suggest that plasma concentrations associated with analgesia in humans are achieved with 4 mg/kg PO [259], its clinical use as an analgesic in this species remains anecdotal. Potential adverse effects include sedation and ataxia at higher doses. Similarly in horses, a dose of 4 mg/kg PO every 8h has been suggested based on pharmacokinetic data. Pharmacodynamic and/or clinical studies are required to validate these data.

Gabapentin is available as tablets and capsules (100, 300, 400, 600, 800 mg) and as a 50 mg/mL oral formulation. Pregabalin is available as capsules (25, 50, 75, 100, 150, 200, 225, 300 mg) and an oral solution (20 mg/mL).

Tramadol

Tramadol is a racemic mixture and has been described as an 'atypical' opioid due to the potential provision of analgesia via opioid and non-opioid (i.e., monoamine uptake inhibition) mechanisms [260]. Interestingly, both enantiomers of the parent compound and the M_1 metabolite (*O*-desmethyltramadol) contribute to analgesia. Norepinephrine reuptake inhibition results from activity of the (-)-enantiomer of tramadol, serotonin (5-HT) reuptake inhibition results from activity of the (+)-enantiomer of tramadol, and µ opioid receptor agonism results from activity of the (+)-enantiomer of the M_1 metabolite and the (+)-enantiomer of tramadol [260–262]. It is therefore clear that the potential for interindividual as well as inter- and intraspecies variation in analgesic potency may occur as a result of variations in metabolism.

The metabolic pathways of tramadol have been described in the dog [263–266], cat [267], horse [268–270], alpaca [271], and llama [272].

In humans, metabolism of tramadol to the active M_1 metabolite is mediated by CYP2D6. In veterinary species, the CYP P450 enzyme responsible for tramadol has not been identified. In the dog, there appears to be limited production of the M_1 metabolite, indicating that analgesia is largely dependent on activity of the parent compound [262–266]. While the therapeutic plasma concentration of M_1 is unknown in the dog, measured levels are substantially below those associated with analgesia in humans. This may explain the variability in efficacy observed clinically, with a similar pattern observed in a subsection of humans who are 'poor metabolizers' (i.e., those lacking the CYP2D6 isozyme) and consequently experience substantially lower analgesia from tramadol [273]. As tramadol is excreted largely unchanged in urine, hepatic dysfunction would not be expected to result in complications with therapeutic dosing.

In cats, metabolism of tramadol is significant, resulting in M_1 metabolite concentrations associated with analgesia in humans [274]. Clearance was lower than reported in dogs, indicating that less frequent dosing may be effective. Excretion of parent drug and metabolites is suspected to be renal.

In horses, the majority of studies show that tramadol is metabolized to the M_1 metabolite at concentrations which may contribute to analgesia [268–270]. However, low bioavailability (less than 10%)

and rapid clearance may limit the utility of oral administration. Clearance, as in dogs and cats, is via renal excretion. Tramadol may prove more effective in llamas as significant concentrations of the M_1 metabolite were detected following IV and IM administration, but clearance was similar to that reported in horses, which could make frequent dosing necessary [272]. In alpacas, a study of six adult animals discovered wide interindividual variation in oral absorption (ranging from 6% to 20%) and rapid clearance, with variable detection of the M_1 metabolite [271]. At doses of 3.4–4 mg/kg IV, the following adverse effects were observed: head tremor, ataxia, and star gazing. A lower rate of infusion (i.e., the same dose but administered over 10 min) or oral dosing were not associated with side-effects. Further work is needed to identify an effective dose in alpacas.

Tramadol's pharmacokinetic profile in dogs may explain its variable performance in clinical studies [275–278]. A 26–36% sevoflurane MAC reduction effect has been shown [279]. In a population of dogs with osteoarthritis, oral tramadol (4 mg/kg every 8 h) resulted in effective analgesia as assessed by owner questionnaire (the canine brief pain inventory), but not activity monitoring, gait analysis and requirement for rescue medication [280]. A combination of small sample sizes and treatment effects reduced study power substantially, contributing to the lack of observed significance. Additionally, plasma tramadol levels were below the threshold associated with analgesia as early as 3 h after dosing. Two studies in dogs comparing extradural and IV (2 mg/kg) or extradural and IM (2 mg/kg) tramadol in dogs for either a tibial plateau leveling osteotomy procedure (TPLO) or ovariohysterectomy failed to show an advantage of extradural administration; both routes of administration provided adequate analgesia [276,277].

Clinical data in horses are limited, with large variability in tramadol dosing regimens impeding interpretation of data. Further work, preferably combined pharmacokinetic and pharmacodynamic studies, is required though the dose-dependent incidence of adverse effects and rapid clearance may limit the drug's use in this species [281,282]. Extradural administration (0.5–1 mg/kg) shows promise and may be a useful alternative route, providing analgesia and limiting CNS stimulation [283,284]. The extradural administration of tramadol has also been reported in cattle and lambs [285,286].

Sedation was observed with tramadol doses greater than 2 mg/kg IV in dogs [266,287]. In cats 1 mg/kg SC had variable behavioral effects with six of eight cats exhibiting signs of euphoria and two cats appearing dysphoric [288]. Reliance on renal excretion of parent drug and the active M_1 metabolite implies that renal dysfunction might result in adverse effects [289], though none have been reported in veterinary species. Doses of tramadol greater than 3.1 mg/kg IV in horses were associated with a significant (i.e., approximately 100%) increase in respiratory rate, 50% reduction in borborygmus, and trembling [290]. At lower doses (0.3 mg/kg IV), signs associated with CNS stimulation (i.e., head nodding) were observed.

In dogs, oral administration at 10 mg/kg was associated with analgesia using a pressure pain model at 5–6 h post administration, and doses of 5–10 mg/kg every 6–8 h have been recommended [264]. Oral administration of tramadol beyond 1 week may result in a reduction in plasma drug concentrations through an unknown mechanism [291]. Preoperative IV and IM administration at 2 mg/kg has been effective for ovariohysterectomy and TPLO surgery [276–278].

In cats, oral administration at 8.6–11.6 mg/kg was effective at reducing the MAC of sevoflurane [292]. A 2 mg/kg SC dose was no more effective than placebo following ovariohysterectomy when assessed with an interactive VAS and composite pain score, though there was a lower requirement for rescue analgesia compared with placebo [293]. Similarly, 1 mg/kg SC did not substantially increase either pressure or thermal threshold responses in cats [288]. Doses between 2 and 4 mg/kg PO were effective in increasing the thermal threshold in cats and the authors calculated that a dose of 4 mg/kg PO every 6 h may provide appropriate analgesia [274]. Extradural administration of tramadol at 1 mg/kg in cats receiving a mechanical stimulation resulted in effective analgesia compared to saline control but did not last as long as extradural morphine [294]. In horses, a dose of 2 mg/kg IV did not result in significant reductions in skin twitch latency or hoof withdrawal reflex during exposure to thermal stimulation [290]. While higher doses may have resulted in analgesia, the 2 mg/kg dose was selected as adverse effects were observed with higher doses.

Tapentadol

The analgesic agent tapentadol was designed with the aims of combining μ opioid receptor agonism and norepinephrine reuptake inhibition without dependency on generating active metabolites, as is the case with tramadol [295,296]. Tapentadol has a higher affinity (approximately 50-fold) for the μ opioid receptor compared to tramadol, but lower affinity compared to the M_1 metabolite of tramadol. Compared to tramadol, it has similar potency for inhibition of norepinephrine reuptake, and lesser potency (approximately five-fold) at inhibiting serotonin reuptake inhibition [295]. These activities, without a reliance on metabolism to an active metabolite, make tapentadol an attractive analgesic option though evidence of its use in veterinary species is limited. The pharmacokinetics have been described in dogs [297] and the drug appears to holds promise, particularly in those species that do not produce significant quantities of the active M_1 metabolite. In dogs, it has a low oral bioavailability and is expected, as in humans, to undergo extensive hepatic metabolism (glucuronidation) to generate an inactive metabolite [297]. A recommended dose is not currently available.

References

1 Boys JA, Toledo AH, Anaya-Prado R, *et al.* Effects of dantrolene on ischemia-reperfusion injury in animal models: a review of outcomes in heart, brain, liver, and kidney. *J Invest Med* 2010; **58**: 875–882.

2 Inan S, Wei H. The cytoprotective effects of dantrolene: a ryanodine receptor antagonist. *Anesth Analg* 2010; **111**: 1400–1410.

3 Lynch Cr, Durbin CGJ, Fisher NA, *et al.* Effects of dantrolene and verapamil on atrioventricular conduction and cardiovascular performance in dogs. *Anesth Analg* 1986; **65**: 252–258.

4 Oliven A, Deal ECJ, Kelsen SG. Effect of dantrolene on ventilation and respiratory muscle activity in anaesthetized dogs. *Br J Anaesth* 1990; **64**: 207–213.

5 Bowman WC, Houston J, Khan HH, *et al.* Effects of dantrolene sodium on respiratory and other muscles and on respiratory parameters in the anaesthetised cat. *Eur J Pharmacol* 1979; **55**: 293–303.

6 Bagshaw RJ, Cox RH, Rosenberg H. Dantrolene treatment of malignant hyperthermia. *J Am Vet Med Assoc* 1981; **178**: 1129.

7 Kirmayer AH, Klide AM, Purvance JE. Malignant hyperthermia in a dog: case report and review of the syndrome. *J Am Vet Med Assoc* 1984; **185**: 978–982.

8 Nelson TE. Malignant hyperthermia in dogs. *J Am Vet Med Assoc* 1991; **198**: 989–994.

9 Rand JS, O'Brien PJ. Exercise-induced malignant hyperthermia in an English springer spaniel. *J Am Vet Med Assoc* 1987; **190**: 1013–1014.

10 Klein L, Ailes N, Fackelman GE, *et al.* Postanesthetic equine myopathy suggestive of malignant hyperthermia. A case report. *Vet Surg* 1989; **18**: 479–482.

11 Waldron-Mease E, Klein LV, Rosenberg H, *et al.* Malignant hyperthermia in a halothane-anesthetized horse. *J Am Vet Med Assoc* 1981; **179**: 896–898.

12 Harrison GG. Control of the malignant hyperpyrexic syndrome in MHS swine by dantrolene sodium. *Br J Anaesth* 1975; **47**: 62–65.

13 Wells RJ, Sedacca CD, Aman AM, *et al.* Successful management of a dog that had severe rhabdomyolysis with myocardial and respiratory failure. *J Am Vet Med Assoc* 2009; **234**: 1049–1054.
14 McKenzie EC, Valberg SJ, Godden SM, *et al.* Effect of oral administration of dantrolene sodium on serum creatine kinase activity after exercise in horses with recurrent exertional rhabdomyolysis. *Am J Vet Res* 2004; **65**: 74–79.
15 McKenzie EC, Garrett RL, Payton ME, *et al.* Effect of feed restriction on plasma dantrolene concentrations in horses. *Equine Vet J Suppl* 2010; 613–617.
16 Edwards JG, Newtont JR, Ramzan PH, *et al.* The efficacy of dantrolene sodium in controlling exertional rhabdomyolysis in the Thoroughbred racehorse. *Equine Vet J* 2003; **35**: 707–711.
17 Takano K. Effect of dantrolene sodium upon the activity of the hind leg muscle of the cat with local tetanus. *Naunyn Schmiedebergs Arch Pharmacol* 1976; **293**: 195–196.
18 Denborough MA, Lovell RRH. Anaesthetic deaths in a family. *Lancet* 1960; **276**: 45.
19 Denborough MA, Forster JFA, Lovell RRH, *et al.* Anesthetic deaths in a family. *Br J Anaesth* 1962; **34**: 395–396.
20 Jones EW, Nelson TE, Anderson IL, *et al.* Malignant hyperthermia of swine. *Anesthesiology* 1972; **36**: 42–51.
21 Hall LW, Woolf N, Bradley JW, *et al.* Unusual reaction to suxamethonium chloride. *BMJ* 1966; **2**: 1305.
22 Wuis EW, Janssen MG, Vree TB, *et al.* Determination of a dantrolene metabolite, 5-(p-nitrophenyl)-2-furoic acid, in plasma and urine by high-performance liquid chromatography. *J Chromatogr* 1990; **526**: 575–580.
23 Court MH, Engelking LR, Dodman NH, *et al.* Pharmacokinetics of dantrolene sodium in horses. *J Vet Pharmacol Ther* 1987; **10**: 218–226.
24 DiMaio Knych HK, Arthur RM, Taylor A, *et al.* Pharmacokinetics and metabolism of dantrolene in horses. *J Vet Pharmacol Ther* 2011; **34**: 238–246.
25 Hatch RC, Jernigan AD, Wilson RC, *et al.* Prompt arousal from fentanyl-droperidol-pentobarbital anesthesia in dogs: a preliminary study. *Can J Vet Res* 1986; **50**: 251–258.
26 Short CE. Doxapram for reversing xylazine sedation [letter]. *J Am Vet Med Assoc* 1984; **184(3)**: 237, 258.
27 Zapata M, Hofmeister EH. Refinement of the dose of doxapram to counteract the sedative effects of acepromazine in dogs. *J Small Anim Pract* 2013; **54**: 405–408.
28 Fletcher DJ, Boller M, Brainard BM, *et al.* RECOVER evidence and knowledge gap analysis on veterinary CPR. Part 7: Clinical guidelines. *J Vet Emerg Crit Care* 2012; **22(Suppl 1)**: S102–131.
29 Nicholson A, Watson A. Survey on small animal anaesthesia. *Aust Vet J* 2001; **79**: 613–619.
30 Boller M, Kellett-Gregory L, Shofer FS, *et al.* The clinical practice of CPCR in small animals: an internet-based survey. *J Vet Emerg Crit Care* 2010; **20**: 558–570.
31 Taylor PM. Doxapram infusion during halothane anaesthesia in ponies. *Equine Vet J* 1990; **22**: 329–332.
32 Roy RC, Stullken EH. Electroencephalographic evidence of arousal in dogs from halothane after doxapram, physostigmine, or naloxone. *Anesthesiology* 1981; **55**: 392–397.
33 Curtis R, Evans JM. The effect of doxapram hydrochloride on cats anaesthetized with either Saffan or thiopentone sodium. *J Small Anim Pract* 1981; **22**: 77–83.
34 Giguere S, Sanchez LC, Shih A, *et al.* Comparison of the effects of caffeine and doxapram on respiratory and cardiovascular function in foals with induced respiratory acidosis. *Am J Vet Res* 2007; **68**: 1407–1416.
35 Giguere S, Slade JK, Sanchez LC. Retrospective comparison of caffeine and doxapram for the treatment of hypercapnia in foals with hypoxic-ischemic encephalopathy. *J Vet Intern Med* 2008; **22**: 401–405.
36 Bleul U, Bircher B, Jud RS, *et al.* Respiratory and cardiovascular effects of doxapram and theophylline for the treatment of asphyxia in neonatal calves. *Theriogenology* 2010; **73**: 612–619.
37 Short CE, Cloyd GD, Ward JW. An evaluation of doxapram hydrochloride to control respiration in dogs during and after inhalation anesthesia. *Vet Med Small Anim Clin* 1970; **65**: 787–790.
38 Short CE, Cloyd GD. The use of doxapram hydrochloride with inhalation anesthetics in horses. II. *Vet Med Small Anim Clin* 1970; **65**: 260–261.
39 Short CE, Cloyd GD, Ward JW. The use of doxapram hydrochloride with intravenous anesthetics in horses. I. *Vet Med Small Anim Clin* 1970; **65**: 157–160.
40 Miller CJ, McKiernan BC, Pace J, *et al.* The effects of doxapram hydrochloride (dopram-V) on laryngeal function in healthy dogs. *J Vet Intern Med* 2002; **16**: 524–528.
41 Tobias KM, Jackson AM, Harvey RC. Effects of doxapram HCl on laryngeal function of normal dogs and dogs with naturally occurring laryngeal paralysis. *Vet Anaesth Analg* 2004; **31**: 258–263.
42 Archer RM, Lindsay WA, Duncan ID. A comparison of techniques to enhance the evaluation of equine laryngeal function. *Equine Vet J* 1991; **23**: 104–107.
43 Funderburk WH, Oliver KL, Ward JW. Electrophysiologic analysis of the site of action of doxapram hydrochloride. *J Pharmacol Exp Ther* 1966; **151**: 360–368.
44 Hirsh K, Wang SC. Selective respiratory stimulating action of doxapram compared to pentylenetetrazaol. *J Pharmacol Exp Ther* 1974; **189**: 1–11.
45 Kato H, Buckley JP. Possible sites of action of the respiratory stimulant effect of doxapram hydrochloride. *J Pharmacol Exp Ther* 1964; **144**: 260–264.
46 Soma LR, Kenny R. Respiratory, cardiovascular, metabolic and electroencephalographic effects of doxapram hydrochloride in the dog. *Am J Vet Res* 1967; **28**: 191–198.
47 Kim SI, Winnie AP, Collins VJ, *et al.* Hemodynamic responses to doxapram in normovolemic and hypovolemic dogs. *Anesth Analg* 1971; **50**: 705–710.
48 Pang DS, Robledo CJ, Carr DR, *et al.* An unexpected role for TASK-3 potassium channels in network oscillations with implications for sleep mechanisms and anesthetic action. *Proc Natl Acad Sci USA* 2009; **106**: 17546–17551.
49 Cotten JF. TASK-1 (KCNK3) and TASK-3 (KCNK9) tandem pore potassium channel antagonists stimulate breathing in isoflurane-anesthetized rats. *Anesth Analg* 2013; **116**: 810–816.
50 Trapp S, Aller MI, Wisden W, *et al.* A role for TASK-1 (KCNK3) channels in the chemosensory control of breathing. *J Neurosci* 2008; **28**: 8844–8850.
51 Yost CS. A new look at the respiratory stimulant doxapram. *CNS Drug Rev* 2006; **12**: 236–249.
52 Winnie AP, Collins VJ. The search for a pharmacologic ventilator. *Acta Anaesthesiol Scand* 1966; **23(Suppl)**: 63–71.
53 Bruce RB, Pitts JE, Pinchbeck F, *et al.* Excretion, distribution, and metabolism of doxapram hydrochloride. *J Med Chem* 1965; **8**: 157–164.
54 Sams RA, Detra RL, Muir WW. Pharmacokinetics and metabolism of intravenous doxapram in horses. *Equine Vet J Suppl* 1992; 45–51.
55 Huffington P, Craythorne NW. Effect of doxapram on heart rhythm during anesthesia in dog and man. *Anesth Analg* 1966; **45**: 558–563.
56 Aguilera-Tejero E, Pascoe JR, Smith BL, *et al* The effect of doxapram-induced hyperventilation on respiratory mechanics in horses. *Res Vet Sci* 1997; **62**: 143–146.
57 Henderson-Smart DJ, Steer PA. Doxapram treatment for apnea in preterm infants. *Cochrane Database Syst Rev* 2004; **4**: CD000074.
58 Uehara H, Yoshioka H, Nagai H, *et al.* Doxapram accentuates white matter injury in neonatal rats following bilateral carotid artery occlusion. *Neurosci Lett* 2000; **281**: 191–194.
59 Roll C, Horsch S. Effect of doxapram on cerebral blood flow velocity in preterm infants. *Neuropediatrics* 2004; **35**: 126–129.
60 Dani C, Bertini G, Pezzati M, *et al.* Brain hemodynamic effects of doxapram in preterm infants. *Biol Neonate* 2006; **89**: 69–74.
61 Sreenan C, Etches PC, Demianczuk N, *et al.* Isolated mental developmental delay in very low birth weight infants: association with prolonged doxapram therapy for apnea. *J Pediatr* 2001; **139**: 832–837.
62 Hubbell JAE, Muir WW. Considerations for induction, maintenance and recovery. In: Hubbell JAE, Muir WW, eds. *Equine Anesthesia: Monitoring and Emergency Therapy*. Philadelphia: Elsevier Saunders, 2009; 381–396.
63 Zahner JM, Hatch RC, Wilson RC, *et al.* Antagonism of xylazine sedation in steers by doxapram and 4-aminopyridine. *Am J Vet Res* 1984; **45**: 2546–2551.
64 Riebold TW, Kaneps AJ, Schmotzer WB. Reversal of xylazine-induced sedation in llamas, using doxapram or 4-aminopyridine and yohimbine. *J Am Vet Med Assoc* 1986; **189**: 1059–1061.
65 Said AH. Some aspects of anaesthesia in the camel. *Vet Rec* 1964; **76**: 550.
66 Woods R, McLean S, Nicol S, *et al.* Antagonism of some cyclohexamine-based drug combinations used for chemical restraint of southern elephant seals (Mirounga leonina). *Aust Vet J* 1995; **72**: 165–171.
67 Murray MJ, Grodinsky C. The effects of famotidine, ranitidine and magnesium hydroxide/aluminium hydroxide on gastric fluid pH in adult horses. *Equine Vet J Suppl* 1992; 52–55.
68 Ahmed AF, Constable PD, Misk NA. Effect of orally administered cimetidine and ranitidine on abomasal luminal pH in clinically normal milk-fed calves. *Am J Vet Res* 2001; **62**: 1531–1538.
69 Sanchez LC, Lester GD, Merritt AM. Effect of ranitidine on intragastric pH in clinically normal neonatal foals. *J Am Vet Med Assoc* 1998; **212**: 1407–1412.
70 Sanchez LC, Lester GD, Merritt AM. Intragastric pH in critically ill neonatal foals and the effect of ranitidine. *J Am Vet Med Assoc* 2001; **218**: 907–911.
71 Huang JQ, Hunt RH. Pharmacological and pharmacodynamic essentials of H(2)-receptor antagonists and proton pump inhibitors for the practising physician. *Best Pract Res Clin Gastroenterol* 2001; **15**: 355–370.
72 Bersenas AM, Mathews KA, Allen DG, *et al.* Effects of ranitidine, famotidine, pantoprazole, and omeprazole on intragastric pH in dogs. *Am J Vet Res* 2005; **66**: 425–431.
73 Tolbert K, Bissett S, King A, *et al.* Efficacy of oral famotidine and 2 omeprazole formulations for the control of intragastric pH in dogs. *J Vet Intern Med* 2011; **25**: 47–54.
74 Andrews FM, Doherty TJ, Blackford JT, *et al.* Effects of orally administered enteric-coated omeprazole on gastric acid secretion in horses. *Am J Vet Res* 1999; **60**: 929–931.

75 Murray MJ. Suppression of gastric acidity in horses. *J Am Vet Med Assoc* 1997; **211**: 37–40.

76 Sanchez LC, Murray MJ, Merritt AM. Effect of omeprazole paste on intragastric pH in clinically normal neonatal foals. *Am J Vet Res* 2004; **65**: 1039–1041.

77 de Brito Galvao JF, Trepanier LA. Risk of hemolytic anemia with intravenous administration of famotidine to hospitalized cats. *J Vet Intern Med* 2008; **22**: 325–329.

78 Williamson KK, Willard MD, Payton ME, *et al.* Efficacy of omeprazole versus high-dose famotidine for prevention of exercise-induced gastritis in racing Alaskan sled dogs. *J Vet Intern Med* 2010; **24**: 285–288.

79 Zacuto AC, Marks SL, Osborn J, *et al.* The influence of esomeprazole and cisapride on gastroesophageal reflux during anesthesia in dogs. *J Vet Intern Med* 2012; **26**: 518–525.

80 Panti A, Bennett RC, Corletto F, *et al.* The effect of omeprazole on oesophageal pH in dogs during anaesthesia. *J Small Anim Pract* 2009; **50**: 540–544.

81 Adamama-Moraitou KK, Rallis TS, Prassinos NN, *et al.* Benign esophageal stricture in the dog and cat: a retrospective study of 20 cases. *Can J Vet Res* 2002; **66**: 55–59.

82 Wilson DV, Walshaw R. Postanesthetic esophageal dysfunction in 13 dogs. *J Am Anim Hosp Assoc* 2004; **40**: 455–460.

83 Pearson H, Darke PG, Gibbs C, *et al.* Reflux oesophagitis and stricture formation after anaesthesia: a review of seven cases in dogs and cats. *J Small Anim Pract* 1978; **19**: 507–519.

84 Andersson T, Cederberg C, Edvardsson G, *et al.* Effect of omeprazole treatment on diazepam plasma levels in slow versus normal rapid metabolizers of omeprazole. *Clin Pharmacol Ther* 1990; **47**: 79–85.

85 Hassan-Alin M, Andersson T, Niazi M, *et al.* A pharmacokinetic study comparing single and repeated oral doses of 20 mg and 40 mg omeprazole and its two optical isomers, S-omeprazole (esomeprazole) and R-omeprazole, in healthy subjects. *Eur J Clin Pharmacol* 2005; **60**: 779–784.

86 Funk KA. Glyceryl guaiacolate: some effects and indications in horses. *Equine Vet J* 1973; **5**: 15–19.

87 Funk KA. Glyceryl guaiacolate: a centrally acting muscle relaxant. *Equine Vet J* 1970; **2**: 173–178.

88 Seagrave J, Albrecht H, Park YS, *et al.* Effect of guaifenesin on mucin production, rheology, and mucociliary transport in differentiated human airway epithelial cells. *Exp Lung Res* 2011; **37**: 606–614.

89 Posner LP, Burns P. Injectable anesthetic agents. In: Riviere JE, Papich MG, eds. *Veterinary Pharmacology and Therapeutics*. Chichester: Wiley-Blackwell, 2009; 265–289.

90 Muir WW. Intravenous anesthetic drugs. In: Muir WW, Hubbell JAE, eds. *Equine Anesthesia: Monitoring and Emergency Therapy*. Philadelphia: Elsevier Saunders, 2009; 243–259.

91 Hubbell JA, Muir WW, Sams RA. Guaifenesin: cardiopulmonary effects and plasma concentrations in horses. *Am J Vet Res* 1980; **41**: 1751–1755.

92 Tavernor WD. The influence of guaiacol glycerol ether on cardiovascular and respiratory function in the horse. *Res Vet Sci* 1970; **11**: 91–93.

93 Schatzmann U, Tschudi P, Held JP, *et al.* An investigation of the action and haemolytic effect of glyceryl guaiacolate in the horse. *Equine Vet J* 1978; **10**: 224–228.

94 Davis LE, Wolff WA. Pharmacokinetics and metabolism of glyceryl guaiacolate in ponies. *Am J Vet Res* 1970; **31**: 469–473.

95 Mostert JW, Metz J. Observations on the haemolytic activity of guaiacol glycerol ether. *Br J Anaesth* 1963; **35**: 461–464.

96 Wall R, Muir WW. Hemolytic potential of guaifenesin in cattle. *Cornell Vet* 1990; **80**: 209–216.

97 Herschl MA, Trim CM, Mahaffey EA. Effects of 5% and 10% guaifenesin infusion on equine vascular endothelium. *Vet Surg* 1992; **21**: 494–497.

98 Dickson LR, Badcoe LM, Burbidge H, *et al.* Jugular thrombophlebitis resulting from an anaesthetic induction technique in the horse. *Equine Vet J* 1990; **22**: 177–179.

99 Matthews NS, Light GS, Sanders EA, *et al.* Urticarial response during anesthesia in a horse. *Equine Vet J* 1993; **25**: 555–556.

100 Benchaoui HA, Cox SR, Schneider RP, *et al.* The pharmacokinetics of maropitant, a novel neurokinin type-1 receptor antagonist, in dogs. *J Vet Pharmacol Ther* 2007; **30**: 336–344.

101 Hickman MA, Cox SR, Mahabir S, *et al.* Safety, pharmacokinetics and use of the novel NK-1 receptor antagonist maropitant (Cerenia) for the prevention of emesis and motion sickness in cats. *J Vet Pharmacol Ther* 2008; **31**: 220–229.

102 Diemunsch P, Grelot L. Potential of substance P antagonists as antiemetics. *Drugs* 2000; **60**: 533–546.

103 Narishetty ST, Galvan B, Coscarelli E, *et al.* Effect of refrigeration of the antiemetic Cerenia (maropitant) on pain on injection. *Vet Ther* 2009; **10**: 93–102.

104 de la Puente-Redondo VA, Siedek EM, Benchaoui HA, *et al.* The antiemetic efficacy of maropitant (Cerenia) in the treatment of ongoing emesis caused by a wide range of underlying clinical aetiologies in canine patients in Europe. *J Small Anim Pract* 2007; **48**: 93–98.

105 de la Puente-Redondo VA, Tilt N, Rowan TG, *et al.* Efficacy of maropitant for treatment and prevention of emesis caused by intravenous infusion of cisplatin in dogs. *Am J Vet Res* 2007; **68**: 48–56.

106 Vail DM, Rodabaugh HS, Conder GA, *et al.* Efficacy of injectable maropitant (Cerenia) in a randomized clinical trial for prevention and treatment of cisplatin-induced emesis in dogs presented as veterinary patients. *Vet Comp Oncol* 2007; **5**: 38–46.

107 Rau SE, Barber LG, Burgess KE. Efficacy of maropitant in the prevention of delayed vomiting associated with administration of doxorubicin to dogs. *J Vet Intern Med* 2010; **24**: 1452–1457.

108 Ramsey DS, Kincaid K, Watkins JA, *et al.* Safety and efficacy of injectable and oral maropitant, a selective neurokinin 1 receptor antagonist, in a randomized clinical trial for treatment of vomiting in dogs. *J Vet Pharmacol Ther* 2008; **31**: 538–543.

109 Conder GA, Sedlacek HS, Boucher JF, *et al.* Efficacy and safety of maropitant, a selective neurokinin 1 receptor antagonist, in two randomized clinical trials for prevention of vomiting due to motion sickness in dogs. *J Vet Pharmacol Ther* 2008; **31**: 528–532.

110 Sedlacek HS, Ramsey DS, Boucher JF, *et al.* Comparative efficacy of maropitant and selected drugs in preventing emesis induced by centrally or peripherally acting emetogens in dogs. *J Vet Pharmacol Ther* 2008; **31**: 533–537.

111 Alvillar BM, Boscan P, Mama KR, *et al.* Effect of epidural and intravenous use of the neurokinin-1 (NK-1) receptor antagonist maropitant on the sevoflurane minimum alveolar concentration (MAC) in dogs. *Vet Anaesth Analg* 2012; **39**: 201–205.

112 Boscan P, Monnet E, Mama K, *et al.* Effect of maropitant, a neurokinin 1 receptor antagonist, on anesthetic requirements during noxious visceral stimulation of the ovary in dogs. *Am J Vet Res* 2011; **72**: 1576–1579.

113 Niyom S, Boscan P, Twedt DC, *et al.* Effect of maropitant, a neurokinin-1 receptor antagonist, on the minimum alveolar concentration of sevoflurane during stimulation of the ovarian ligament in cats. *Vet Anaesth Analg* 2013; **40**: 425–431.

114 Hay Kraus BL. Efficacy of maropitant in preventing vomiting in dogs premedicated with hydromorphone. *Vet Anaesth Analg* 2013; **40**: 28–34.

115 Inoue M, Kobayashi M, Kozaki S, *et al.* Nociceptin/orphanin FQ-induced nociceptive responses through substance P release from peripheral nerve endings in mice. *Proc Natl Acad Sci USA* 1998; **95**: 10949–10953.

116 Morris R, Cheunsuang O, Stewart A, *et al.* Spinal dorsal horn neurone targets for nociceptive primary afferents: do single neurone morphological characteristics suggest how nociceptive information is processed at the spinal level. *Brain Res Brain Res Rev* 2004; **46**: 173-190.

117 Mantyh PW, Gates T, Mantyh CR, *et al.* Autoradiographic localization and characterization of tachykinin receptor binding sites in the rat brain and peripheral tissues. *J Neurosci* 1989; **9**: 258–279.

118 Valverde A, Cantwell S, Hernandez J, *et al.* Effects of acepromazine on the incidence of vomiting associated with opioid administration in dogs. *Vet Anaesth Analg* 2004; **31**: 40–45.

119 Roszkowski AP. A pharmacological comparison of therapeutically useful centrally acting skeletal muscle relaxants. *J Pharmacol Exp Ther* 1960; **129**: 75–81.

120 Witkin LB, Spitaletta P, Galdi F, *et al.* Some neuropharmacologic effects of four mephenesin-like agents in mice. *Toxicol Appl Pharmacol* 1960; **2**: 264–269.

121 Valtonen EJ. A double-blind trial of methocarbamol versus placebo in painful muscle spasm. *Curr Med Res Opin* 1975; **3**: 382–385.

122 Simmonds EE, Alwood AJ, Costello MF. Magnesium sulfate as an adjunct therapy in the management of severe generalized tetanus in a dog. *J Vet Emerg Crit Care* 2011; **21**: 542–546.

123 Burkitt JM, Sturges BK, Jandrey KE, *et al.* Risk factors associated with outcome in dogs with tetanus: 38 cases (1987–2005). *J Am Vet Med Assoc* 2007; **230**: 76–83.

124 Bandt C, Rozanski EA, Steinberg T, *et al.* Retrospective study of tetanus in 20 dogs: 1988–2004. *J Am Anim Hosp Assoc* 2007; **43**: 143–148.

125 Boland LA, Angles JM. Feline permethrin toxicity: retrospective study of 42 cases. *J Feline Med Surg* 2010; **12**: 61–71.

126 Bates NS, Sutton NM, Campbell A. Suspected metaldehyde slug bait poisoning in dogs: a retrospective analysis of cases reported to the Veterinary Poisons Information Service. *Vet Rec* 2012; **171**: 324.

127 Richardson JA. Permethrin spot-on toxicosis in cats. *J Vet Emerg Crit Care* 2000; **10**: 103–106.

128 Muir WW, Sams RA, Ashcraft S. Pharmacologic and pharmacokinetic properties of methocarbamol in the horse. *Am J Vet Res* 1984; **45**: 2256–2260.

129 Muir WW, Sams RA, Ashcraft S. The pharmacology and pharmacokinetics of high-dose methocarbamol in horses. *Equine Vet J Suppl* 1992; 41–44.

130 Nielsen C, Pluhar GE. Diagnosis and treatment of hind limb muscle strain injuries in 22 dogs. *Vet Comp Orthop Traumatol* 2005; **18**: 247–253.

131 Bruce RB, Turnbull LB, Newman JH. Metabolism of methocarbamol in the rat, dog, and human. *J Pharm Sci* 1971; **60**: 104–106.

132 Cunningham FE, Fisher JH, Bevelle C, *et al.* The pharmacokinetics of methocarbamol in the thoroughbred race horse. *J Vet Pharmacol Ther* 1992; **15**: 96–100.
133 Dymond NL, Swift IM. Permethrin toxicity in cats: a retrospective study of 20 cases. *Aust Vet J* 2008; **86**: 219–223.
134 Hall JA, Solie TN, Seim HB, *et al.* Effect of metoclopramide on fed-state gastric myoelectric and motor activity in dogs. *Am J Vet Res* 1996; **57**: 1616–1622.
135 Wilson DV, Evans AT, Mauer WA. Influence of metoclopramide on gastroesophageal reflux in anesthetized dogs. *Am J Vet Res* 2006; **67**: 26–31.
136 Strombeck DR, Harrold D. Effect of gastrin, histamine, serotonin, and adrenergic amines on gastroesophageal sphincter pressure in the dog. *Am J Vet Res* 1985; **46**: 1684–1690.
137 Punto L, Mokka RE, Kairaluoma MI, *et al.* Effect of metoclopramide on the lower oesophageal sphincter. An experimental study in dogs. *Med Biol* 1977; **55**: 66–68.
138 Orihata M, Sarna SK. Contractile mechanisms of action of gastroprokinetic agents: cisapride, metoclopramide, and domperidone. *Am J Physiol* 1994; **266**: G665–676.
139 Bakke OM, Segura J. The absorption and elimination of metoclopramide in three animal species. *J Pharm Pharmacol* 1976; **28**: 32–39.
140 Kohn CW, Muir WW. Selected aspects of the clinical pharmacology of visceral analgesics and gut motility modifying drugs in the horse. *J Vet Intern Med* 1988; **2**: 85–91.
141 Sojka JE, Adams SB, Lamar CH, *et al.* Effect of butorphanol, pentazocine, meperidine, or metoclopramide on intestinal motility in female ponies. *Am J Vet Res* 1988; **49**: 527–529.
142 El-Khodery SA, Sato M. Ultrasonographic assessment of the reticular motility in cows after administration of different doses of metoclopramide and neostigmine. *Vet Res Commun* 2008; **32**: 473–480.
143 Wittek T, Constable PD. Assessment of the effects of erythromycin, neostigmine, and metoclopramide on abomasal motility and emptying rate in calves. *Am J Vet Res* 2005; **66**: 545–552.
144 Butler A, Hill JM, Ireland SJ, *et al.* Pharmacological properties of GR38032F, a novel antagonist at 5-HT3 receptors. *Br J Pharmacol* 1988; **94**: 397–412.
145 Sagrada A, Turconi M, Bonali P, *et al.* Antiemetic activity of the new 5-HT3 antagonist DAU 6215 in animal models of cancer chemotherapy and radiation. *Cancer Chemother Pharmacol* 1991; **28**: 470–474.
146 Fukui H, Yamamoto M, Sato S. Vagal afferent fibers and peripheral 5-HT3 receptors mediate cisplatin-induced emesis in dogs. *Jpn J Pharmacol* 1992; **59**: 221–226.
147 Miller AD, Nonaka S. Mechanisms of vomiting induced by serotonin-3 receptor agonists in the cat: effect of vagotomy, splanchnicectomy or area postrema lesion. *J Pharmacol Exp Ther* 1992; **260**: 509–517.
148 Ogilvie GK. Dolasetron: a new option for nausea and vomiting. *J Am Anim Hosp Assoc* 2000; **36**: 481–483.
149 Zarate E, Watcha MF, White PF, *et al.* A comparison of the costs and efficacy of ondansetron versus dolasetron for antiemetic prophylaxis. *Anesth Analg* 2000; **90**: 1352–1358.
150 FDA. FDA Drug Safety Communication: Abnormal heart rhythms associated with use of Anzemet (dolasetron mesylate). www.fda.gov/drugs/drugsafety/ucm237081.htm (accessed 16 September 2014).
151 Dow J, Francesco GF, Berg C. Comparison of the pharmacokinetics of dolasetron and its major active metabolite, reduced dolasetron, in dog. *J Pharm Sci* 1996; **85**: 685–689.
152 Somers GI, Harris AJ, Bayliss MK, *et al.* The metabolism of the 5HT3 antagonists ondansetron, alosetron and GR87442 I: a comparison of in vitro and in vivo metabolism and in vitro enzyme kinetics in rat, dog and human hepatocytes, microsomes and recombinant human enzymes. *Xenobiotica* 2007; **37**: 832–854.
153 Santos LC, Ludders JW, Erb HN, *et al.* A randomized, blinded, controlled trial of the antiemetic effect of ondansetron on dexmedetomidine-induced emesis in cats. *Vet Anaesth Analg* 2011; **38**: 320–327.
154 Chandler JC, Monnet E, Staatz AJ. Comparison of acute hemodynamic effects of lidocaine and procainamide for postoperative ventricular arrhythmias in dogs. *J Am Anim Hosp Assoc* 2006; **42**: 262–268.
155 Fries R, Saunders AB. Use of procainamide for conversion of acute onset AF following pericardiocentesis in a dog. *J Am Anim Hosp Assoc* 2012; **48**: 429–433.
156 Chou CC, Zhou S, Miyauchi Y, *et al.* Effects of procainamide on electrical activity in thoracic veins and atria in canine model of sustained atrial fibrillation. *Am J Physiol Heart Circ Physiol* 2004; **286**: H1936–1945.
157 Caro-Vadillo A, Garcia-Guasch L, Carreton E, *et al.* Arrhythmogenic right ventricular cardiomyopathy in boxer dogs: a retrospective study of survival. *Vet Rec* 2013; **172**: 268.
158 Meurs KM, Spier AW, Wright NA, *et al.* Comparison of the effects of four antiarrhythmic treatments for familial ventricular arrhythmias in Boxers. *J Am Vet Med Assoc* 2002; **221**: 522–527.
159 Wijnberg ID, Ververs FF. Phenytoin sodium as a treatment for ventricular dysrhythmia in horses. *J Vet Intern Med* 2004; **18**: 350–353.
160 Papich MG, Davis LE, Davis CA. Procainamide in the dog: antiarrhythmic plasma concentrations after intravenous administration. *J Vet Pharmacol Ther* 1986; **9**: 359–369.
161 Ellis EJ, Ravis WR, Malloy M, *et al.* The pharmacokinetics and pharmacodynamics of procainamide in horses after intravenous administration. *J Vet Pharmacol Ther* 1994; **17**: 265–270.
162 Forstermann U, Sessa WC. Nitric oxide synthases: regulation and function. *Eur Heart J* 2012; **33**: 829–837, 837a–837d.
163 Ginn JA, Bentley E, Stepien RL. Systemic hypertension and hypertensive retinopathy following PPA overdose in a dog. *J Am Anim Hosp Assoc* 2013; **49**: 46–53.
164 Kelm M. Nitric oxide metabolism and breakdown. *Biochim Biophys Acta* 1999; **1411**: 273–289.
165 Thomas C, Svehla L, Moffett BS. Sodium-nitroprusside-induced cyanide toxicity in pediatric patients. *Expert Opin Drug Saf* 2009; **8**: 599–602.
166 Michenfelder JD, Tinker JH. Cyanide toxicity and thiosulfate protection during chronic administration of sodium nitroprusside in the dog: correlation with a human case. *Anesthesiology* 1977; **47**: 441–448.
167 Ivankovich AD, Braverman B, Shulman M, *et al.* Prevention of nitroprusside toxicity with thiosulfate in dogs. *Anesth Analg* 1982; **61**: 120–126.
168 Michenfelder JD. Cyanide release from sodium nitroprusside in the dog. *Anesthesiology* 1977; **46**: 196–201.
169 Sillberg VA, Perry JJ, Stiell IG, *et al.* Is the combination of vasopressin and epinephrine superior to repeated doses of epinephrine alone in the treatment of cardiac arrest – a systematic review. *Resuscitation* 2008; **79**: 380–386.
170 Hofmeister EH, Brainard BM, Egger CM, *et al.* Prognostic indicators for dogs and cats with cardiopulmonary arrest treated by cardiopulmonary cerebral resuscitation at a university teaching hospital. *J Am Vet Med Assoc* 2009; **235**: 50–57.
171 Neumar RW, Otto CW, Link MS, *et al.* Part 8: adult advanced cardiovascular life support: 2010 American Heart Association Guidelines for Cardiopulmonary Resuscitation and Emergency Cardiovascular Care. *Circulation* 2010; **122**: S729–767.
172 Dickey EJ, McKenzie Hr, Johnson A, *et al.* Use of pressor therapy in 34 hypotensive critically ill neonatal foals. *Aust Vet J* 2010; **88**: 472–477.
173 Fletcher DJ, Boller M. Updates in small animal cardiopulmonary resuscitation. *Vet Clin North Am Small Anim Pract* 2013; **43**: 971–987.
174 Buckley GJ, Rozanski EA, Rush JE. Randomized, blinded comparison of epinephrine and vasopressin for treatment of naturally occurring cardiopulmonary arrest in dogs. *J Vet Intern Med* 2011; **25**: 1334–1340.
175 Biondi-Zoccai GG, Abbate A, Parisi Q, *et al.* Is vasopressin superior to adrenaline or placebo in the management of cardiac arrest? A meta-analysis. *Resuscitation* 2003; **59**: 221–224.
176 Koshimizu TA, Nakamura K, Egashira N, *et al.* Vasopressin V1a and V1b receptors: from molecules to physiological systems. *Physiol Rev* 2012; **92**: 1813–1864.
177 Schott HC. Water homeostasis and diabetes insipidus in horses. *Vet Clin North Am Equine Pract* 2011; **27**: 175–195.
178 Kranenburg LC, Thelen MH, Westermann CM, *et al.* Use of desmopressin eye drops in the treatment of equine congenital central diabetes insipidus. *Vet Rec* 2010; **167**: 790–791.
179 Simpson CJ, Mansfield CS, Milne ME, *et al.* Central diabetes insipidus in a cat with central nervous system B cell lymphoma. *J Feline Med Surg* 2011; **13**: 787–792.
180 Mansell PD, Parry BW. Changes in factor VIII: coagulant activity and von Willebrand factor antigen concentration after subcutaneous injection of desmopressin in dogs with mild hemophilia A. *J Vet Intern Med* 1991; **5**: 191–194.
181 Callan MB, Giger U. Effect of desmopressin acetate administration on primary hemostasis in Doberman Pinschers with type-1 von Willebrand disease as assessed by a point-of-care instrument. *Am J Vet Res* 2002; **63**: 1700–1706.
182 Hara Y, Masuda H, Taoda T, *et al.* Prophylactic efficacy of desmopressin acetate for diabetes insipidus after hypophysectomy in the dog. *J Vet Med Sci* 2003; **65**: 17–22.
183 Fox AW, May RE, Mitch WE. Comparison of peptide and nonpeptide receptor-mediated responses in rat tail artery. *J Cardiovasc Pharmacol* 1992; **20**: 282–289.
184 Wenzel V, Lindner KH, Prengel AW, *et al.* Endobronchial vasopressin improves survival during cardiopulmonary resuscitation in pigs. *Anesthesiology* 1997; **86**: 1375–1381.
185 Reassessment Campaign on Veterinary Resuscitation(RECOVER). www.acvecc-recover.org (accessed 16 September 2014).
186 Morales D, Madigan J, Cullinane S, *et al.* Reversal by vasopressin of intractable hypotension in the late phase of hemorrhagic shock. *Circulation* 1999; **100**: 226–229.
187 Cohn SM. Potential benefit of vasopressin in resuscitation of hemorrhagic shock. *J Trauma* 2007; **62**: S56–57.
188 Russell JA. Bench-to-bedside review: vasopressin in the management of septic shock. *Crit Care* 2011; **15**: 226.

189 Valverde A, Giguere S, Sanchez LC, *et al.* Effects of dobutamine, norepinephrine, and vasopressin on cardiovascular function in anesthetized neonatal foals with induced hypotension. *Am J Vet Res* 2006; **67**: 1730–1737.

190 Kraus KH, Turrentine MA, Jergens AE, *et al.* Effect of desmopressin acetate on bleeding times and plasma von Willebrand factor in Doberman pinscher dogs with von Willebrand's disease. *Vet Surg* 1989; **18**: 103–109.

191 Brooks MB, Catafalmo JL. Platelet disorders and von Willebrand disease. In: Ettinger SJ, Feldman EC, eds. *Textbook of Veterinary Internal Medicine*. Philadelphia: Elsevier Saunders, 2005; 1918–1929.

192 Di Mauro FM, Holowaychuk MK. Intravenous administration of desmopressin acetate to reverse acetylsalicylic acid-induced coagulopathy in three dogs. *J Vet Emerg Crit Care* 2013; **23**(4): 455–458.

193 Sakai M, Watari T, Miura T, *et al.* Effects of DDAVP administrated subcutaneously in dogs with aspirin-induced platelet dysfunction and hemostatic impairment due to chronic liver diseases. *J Vet Med Sci* 2003; **65**: 83–86.

194 Grunert RR, McGahen JW, Davies WL. The *in vivo* antiviral activity of 1-adamantanamine (amantadine). I. Prophylactic and therapeutic activity against influenza viruses. *Virology* 1965; **26**: 262–269.

195 Lee SM, Yen HL. Targeting the host or the virus: current and novel concepts for antiviral approaches against influenza virus infection. *Antiviral Res* 2012; **96**: 391–404.

196 Hubsher G, Haider M, Okun MS. Amantadine: the journey from fighting flu to treating Parkinson disease. *Neurology* 2012; **78**: 1096–1099.

197 Schwab RS, England AC, Poskanzer DC, *et al.* Amantadine in the treament of Parkinson's disease. *JAMA* 1969; **208**: 1168–1170.

198 Wheaton P, Mathias JL, Vink R. Impact of early pharmacological treatment on cognitive and behavioral outcome after traumatic brain injury in adults: a meta-analysis. *J Clin Psychopharmacol* 2009; **29**: 468–477.

199 Frenette AJ, Kanji S, Rees L, *et al.* Efficacy and safety of dopamine agonists in traumatic brain injury: a systematic review of randomized controlled trials. *J Neurotrauma* 2012; **29**: 1–18.

200 Saniova B, Drobny M, Kneslova L, *et al.* The outcome of patients with severe head injuries treated with amantadine sulphate. *J Neural Transm* 2004; **111**: 511–514.

201 Giacino JT, Whyte J, Bagiella E, *et al.* Placebo-controlled trial of amantadine for severe traumatic brain injury. *N Engl J Med* 2012; **366**: 819–826.

202 Wang T, Huang XJ, Van KC, *et al.* Amantadine improves cognitive outcome and increases neuronal survival after fluid percussion TBI in rats. *J Neurotrauma* 2014; **31**(4): 470–477.

203 Robertson SA. Managing pain in feline patients. *Vet Clin North Am Small Anim Pract* 2008; **38**: 1267–1290.

204 Lascelles BD, Gaynor JS, Smith ES, *et al.* Amantadine in a multimodal analgesic regimen for alleviation of refractory osteoarthritis pain in dogs. *J Vet Intern Med* 2008; **22**: 53–59.

205 Suzuki M. Role of N-methyl-D-aspartate receptor antagonists in postoperative pain management. *Curr Opin Anaesthesiol* 2009; **22**: 618–622.

206 Eisenberg E, Pud D. Can patients with chronic neuropathic pain be cured by acute administration of the NMDA receptor antagonist amantadine? *Pain* 1998; **74**: 337–339.

207 Collins S, Sigtermans MJ, Dahan A, *et al.* NMDA receptor antagonists for the treatment of neuropathic pain. *Pain Med* 2010; **11**: 1726–1742.

208 Pozzi A, Muir WW, Traverso F. Prevention of central sensitization and pain by N-methyl-D-aspartate receptor antagonists. *J Am Vet Med Assoc* 2006; **228**: 53–60.

209 Bleidner WE, Harmon JB, Hewes WE, *et al.* Absorption, distribution and excretion of amantadine hydrochloride. *J Pharmacol Exp Ther* 1965; **150**: 484–490.

210 Chen YW, Chu CC, Chen YC, *et al.* The local anesthetic effect of memantine on infiltrative cutaneous analgesia in the rat. *Anesth Analg* 2011; **113**: 191–195.

211 Crowell-Davis SL, Poggiagliolmi S. Understanding behavior: serotonin syndrome. *Compend Contin Educ Vet* 2008; **30**: 490–493.

212 Mohammad-Zadeh LF, Moses L, Gwaltney-Brant SM. Serotonin: a review. *J Vet Pharmacol Ther* 2008; **31**: 187–199.

213 Kitson R, Carr B. Tramadol and severe serotonin syndrome. *Anaesthesia* 2005; **60**: 934–935.

214 Gillman PK. Monoamine oxidase inhibitors, opioid analgesics and serotonin toxicity. *Br J Anaesth* 2005; **95**: 434–441.

215 Chen YW, Shieh JP, Chen YC, *et al.* Cutaneous analgesia after subcutaneous injection of memantine and amantadine and their systemic toxicity in rats. *Eur J Pharmacol* 2012; **693**: 25–30.

216 Overall KL, Dunham AE. Clinical features and outcome in dogs and cats with obsessive-compulsive disorder: 126 cases (1989–2000). *J Am Vet Med Assoc* 2002; **221**: 1445–1452.

217 Kraijer M, Fink-Gremmels J, Nickel RF. The short-term clinical efficacy of amitriptyline in the management of idiopathic feline lower urinary tract disease: a controlled clinical study. *J Feline Med Surg* 2003; **5**: 191–196.

218 Kruger JM, Conway TS, Kaneene JB, *et al.* Randomized controlled trial of the efficacy of short-term amitriptyline administration for treatment of acute, nonobstructive, idiopathic lower urinary tract disease in cats. *J Am Vet Med Assoc* 2003; **222**: 749–758.

219 Cashmore RG, Harcourt-Brown TR, Freeman PM, *et al.* Clinical diagnosis and treatment of suspected neuropathic pain in three dogs. *Aust Vet J* 2009; **87**: 45–50.

220 Wang GK, Russell C, Wang SY. State-dependent block of voltage-gated Na+ channels by amitriptyline via the local anesthetic receptor and its implication for neuropathic pain. *Pain* 2004; **110**: 166–174.

221 Yaksh TL, Tozier N, Horais KA, *et al.* Toxicology profile of N-methyl-D-aspartate antagonists delivered by intrathecal infusion in the canine model. *Anesthesiology* 2008; **108**: 938–949.

222 Irman-Florjanc T, Stanovnik L. Tricyclic antidepressants change plasma histamine kinetics after its secretion induced by compound 48/80 in the rat. *Inflamm Res* 1998; **47**(Suppl 1): S26–27.

223 Bohren Y, Karavelic D, Tessier LH, *et al.* Mu-opioid receptors are not necessary for nortriptyline treatment of neuropathic allodynia. *Eur J Pain* 2010; **14**: 700–704.

224 Chew DJ, Buffington CA, Kendall MS, *et al.* Amitriptyline treatment for severe recurrent idiopathic cystitis in cats. *J Am Vet Med Assoc* 1998; **213**: 1282–1286.

225 O'Hagan BJ. Neuropathic pain in a cat post-amputation. *Aust Vet J* 2006; **84**: 83–86.

226 Rusbridge C, Jeffery ND. Pathophysiology and treatment of neuropathic pain associated with syringomyelia. *Vet J* 2008; **175**: 164–172.

227 Newton SA, Knottenbelt DC, Eldridge PR. Headshaking in horses: possible aetiopathogenesis suggested by the results of diagnostic tests and several treatment regimes used in 20 cases. *Equine Vet J* 2000; **32**: 208–216.

228 Hucker HB, Balletto AJ, Demetriades J, *et al.* Urinary metabolites of amitriptyline in the dog. *Drug Metab Dispos* 1977; **5**: 132–142.

229 Dworkin RH, O'Connor AB, Backonja M, *et al.* Pharmacologic management of neuropathic pain: evidence-based recommendations. *Pain* 2007; **132**: 237–251.

230 Mealey KL, Peck KE, Bennett BS, *et al.* Systemic absorption of amitriptyline and buspirone after oral and transdermal administration to healthy cats. *J Vet Intern Med* 2004; **18**: 43–46.

231 Nattel S, Keable H, Sasyniuk BI. Experimental amitriptyline intoxication: electrophysiologic manifestations and management. *J Cardiovasc Pharmacol* 1984; **6**: 83–89.

232 Kwok YH, Mitchelson F. Comparison of the antimuscarinic activity of mianserin and amitriptyline in the cat superior cervical ganglion. *Naunyn Schmiedebergs Arch Pharmacol* 1981; **316**: 161–164.

233 Reich MR, Ohad DG, Overall KL, *et al.* Electrocardiographic assessment of antianxiety medication in dogs and correlation with serum drug concentration. *J Am Vet Med Assoc* 2000; **216**: 1571–1575.

234 Chew DJ, Buffington CA, Kendall MS, *et al.* Amitriptyline treatment for severe recurrent idiopathic cystitis in cats. *J Am Vet Med Assoc* 1998; **213**: 1282–1286.

235 Abbass K. Efficacy of gabapentin for treatment of adults with phantom limb pain. *Ann Pharmacother* 2012; **46**: 1707–1711.

236 Chaparro LE, Smith SA, Moore RA, *et al.* Pharmacotherapy for the prevention of chronic pain after surgery in adults. *Cochrane Database Syst Rev* 2013; **7**: CD008307.

237 Snedecor SJ, Sudharshan L, Cappelleri JC, *et al.* Systematic review and comparison of pharmacologic therapies for neuropathic pain associated with spinal cord injury. *J Pain Res* 2013; **6**: 539–547.

238 Zakkar M, Frazer S, Hunt I. Is there a role for gabapentin in preventing or treating pain following thoracic surgery? *Interact Cardiovasc Thorac Surg* 2013; **17**(4): 716–719.

239 Aghighi SA, Tipold A, Piechotta M, *et al.* Assessment of the effects of adjunctive gabapentin on postoperative pain after intervertebral disc surgery in dogs. *Vet Anaesth Analg* 2012; **39**: 636–646.

240 Plessas IN, Rusbridge C, Driver CJ, *et al.* Long-term outcome of Cavalier King Charles spaniel dogs with clinical signs associated with Chiari-like malformation and syringomyelia. *Vet Rec* 2012; **171**: 501.

241 Wolfe KC, Poma R. Syringomyelia in the Cavalier King Charles spaniel (CKCS) dog. *Can Vet J* 2010; **51**: 95–102.

242 Wagner AE, Mich PM, Uhrig SR, *et al.* Clinical evaluation of perioperative administration of gabapentin as an adjunct for postoperative analgesia in dogs undergoing amputation of a forelimb. *J Am Vet Med Assoc* 2010; **236**: 751–756.

243 Kukanich B, Cohen RL. Pharmacokinetics of oral gabapentin in greyhound dogs. *Vet J* 2011; **187**: 133–135.

244 Siao KT, Pypendop BH, Ilkiw JE. Pharmacokinetics of gabapentin in cats. *Am J Vet Res* 2010; **71**: 817–821.

245 Pypendop BH, Siao KT, Ilkiw JE. Thermal antinociceptive effect of orally administered gabapentin in healthy cats. *Am J Vet Res* 2010; **71**: 1027–1032.

246 Reid P, Pypendop BH, Ilkiw JE. The effects of intravenous gabapentin administration on the minimum alveolar concentration of isoflurane in cats. *Anesth Analg* 2010; **111**: 633–637.

247 Vettorato E, Corletto F. Gabapentin as part of multi-modal analgesia in two cats suffering multiple injuries. *Vet Anaesth Analg* 2011; **38**: 518–520.
248 Dirikolu L, Dafalla A, Ely KJ, *et al.* Pharmacokinetics of gabapentin in horses. *J Vet Pharmacol Ther* 2008; **31**: 175–177.
249 Terry RL, McDonnell SM, van Eps AW, *et al.* Pharmacokinetic profile and behavioral effects of gabapentin in the horse. *J Vet Pharmacol Ther* 2010; **33**: 485–494.
250 Dutton DW, Lasnhnits KJ, Wegner K. Managing severe hoof pain in a horse using multimodal analgesia and a modified composite pain score. *Equine Vet Educ* 2009; **21**: 37–43.
251 Davis JL, Posner LP, Elce Y. Gabapentin for the treatment of neuropathic pain in a pregnant horse. *J Am Vet Med Assoc* 2007; **231**: 755–758.
252 Coetzee JF, Mosher RA, Kohake LE, *et al.* Pharmacokinetics of oral gabapentin alone or co-administered with meloxicam in ruminant beef calves. *Vet J* 2011; **190**: 98–102.
253 Glynn HD, Coetzee JF, Edwards-Callaway LN, *et al.* The pharmacokinetics and effects of meloxicam, gabapentin, and flunixin in postweaning dairy calves following dehorning with local anesthesia. *J Vet Pharmacol Ther* 2013; **36**(6): 550–561.
254 Malreddy PR, Coetzee JF, Kukanich B, *et al.* Pharmacokinetics and milk secretion of gabapentin and meloxicam co-administered orally in Holstein-Friesian cows. *J Vet Pharmacol Ther* 2013; **36**: 14–20.
255 Taylor CP. Mechanisms of analgesia by gabapentin and pregabalin – calcium channel alpha2-delta [Cavalpha2-delta] ligands. *Pain* 2009; **142**: 13–16.
256 Field MJ, Cox PJ, Stott E, *et al.* Identification of the alpha2-delta-1 subunit of voltage-dependent calcium channels as a molecular target for pain mediating the analgesic actions of pregabalin. *Proc Natl Acad Sci USA* 2006; **103**: 17537–17542.
257 Radulovic LL, Turck D, von Hodenberg A, *et al.* Disposition of gabapentin (neurontin) in mice, rats, dogs, and monkeys. *Drug Metab Dispos* 1995; **23**: 441–448.
258 Platt SR, Adams V, Garosi LS, *et al.* Treatment with gabapentin of 11 dogs with refractory idiopathic epilepsy. *Vet Rec* 2006; **159**: 881–884.
259 Salazar V, Dewey CW, Schwark W, *et al.* Pharmacokinetics of single-dose oral pregabalin administration in normal dogs. *Vet Anaesth Analg* 2009; **36**: 574–580.
260 Raffa RB, Friderichs E, Reimann W, *et al.* Opioid and nonopioid components independently contribute to the mechanism of action of tramadol, an 'atypical' opioid analgesic. *J Pharmacol Exp Ther* 1992; **260**: 275–285.
261 Frink MC, Hennies HH, Englberger W, *et al.* Influence of tramadol on neurotransmitter systems of the rat brain. *Arzneimittelforschung* 1996; **46**: 1029–1036.
262 Raffa RB, Friderichs E, Reimann W, *et al.* Complementary and synergistic antinociceptive interaction between the enantiomers of tramadol. *J Pharmacol Exp Ther* 1993; **267**: 331–340.
263 KuKanich B, Papich MG. Pharmacokinetics of tramadol and the metabolite O-desmethyltramadol in dogs. *J Vet Pharmacol Ther* 2004; **27**: 239–246.
264 Kukanich B, Papich MG. Pharmacokinetics and antinociceptive effects of oral tramadol hydrochloride administration in Greyhounds. *Am J Vet Res* 2011; **72**: 256–262.
265 Giorgi M, del Carlo S, Saccomanni G, *et al.* Pharmacokinetics of tramadol and its major metabolites following rectal and intravenous administration in dogs. *N Z Vet J* 2009; **57**: 146–152.
266 McMillan CJ, Livingston A, Clark CR, *et al.* Pharmacokinetics of intravenous tramadol in dogs. *Can J Vet Res* 2008; **72**: 325–331.
267 Pypendop BH, Ilkiw JE. Pharmacokinetics of tramadol, and its metabolite O-desmethyl-tramadol, in cats. *J Vet Pharmacol Ther* 2008; **31**: 52–59.
268 Cox S, Villarino N, Doherty T. Determination of oral tramadol pharmacokinetics in horses. *Res Vet Sci* 2010; **89**: 236–241.
269 Shilo Y, Britzi M, Eytan B, *et al.* Pharmacokinetics of tramadol in horses after intravenous, intramuscular and oral administration. *J Vet Pharmacol Ther* 2008; **31**: 60–65.
270 Stewart AJ, Boothe DM, Cruz-Espindola C, *et al.* Pharmacokinetics of tramadol and metabolites O-desmethyltramadol and N-desmethyltramadol in adult horses. *Am J Vet Res* 2011; **72**: 967–974.
271 Edmondson MA, Duran SH, Boothe DM, *et al.* Pharmacokinetics of tramadol and its major metabolites in alpacas following intravenous and oral administration. *J Vet Pharmacol Ther* 2012; **35**: 389–396.
272 Cox S, Martin-Jimenez T, van Amstel S, *et al.* Pharmacokinetics of intravenous and intramuscular tramadol in llamas. *J Vet Pharmacol Ther* 2011; **34**: 259–264.
273 Poulsen L, Arendt-Nielsen L, Brosen K, *et al.* The hypoalgesic effect of tramadol in relation to CYP2D6. *Clin Pharmacol Ther* 1996; **60**: 636–644.
274 Pypendop BH, Siao KT, Ilkiw JE. Effects of tramadol hydrochloride on the thermal threshold in cats. *Am J Vet Res* 2009; **70**: 1465–1470.
275 Davila D, Keeshen TP, Evans RB, *et al.* Comparison of the analgesic efficacy of perioperative firocoxib and tramadol administration in dogs undergoing tibial plateau leveling osteotomy. *J Am Vet Med Assoc* 2013; **243**: 225–231.
276 Vettorato E, Zonca A, Isola M, *et al.* Pharmacokinetics and efficacy of intravenous and extradural tramadol in dogs. *Vet J* 2010; **183**: 310–315.
277 Mastrocinque S, Almeida TF, Tatarunas AC, *et al.* Comparison of epidural and systemic tramadol for analgesia following ovariohysterectomy. *J Am Anim Hosp Assoc* 2012; **48**: 310–319.
278 Mastrocinque S, Fantoni DT. A comparison of preoperative tramadol and morphine for the control of early postoperative pain in canine ovariohysterectomy. *Vet Anaesth Analg* 2003; **30**: 220–228.
279 Seddighi MR, Egger CM, Rohrbach BW, *et al.* Effects of tramadol on the minimum alveolar concentration of sevoflurane in dogs. *Vet Anaesth Analg* 2009; **36**: 334–340.
280 Malek S, Sample SJ, Schwartz Z, *et al.* Effect of analgesic therapy on clinical outcome measures in a randomized controlled trial using client-owned dogs with hip osteoarthritis. *BMC Vet Res* 2012; **8**: 185.
281 Knych HK, Corado CR, McKemie DS, *et al.* Pharmacokinetics and pharmacodynamics of tramadol in horses following oral administration. *J Vet Pharmacol Ther* 2013; **36**: 389–398.
282 Knych HK, Corado CR, McKemie DS, *et al.* Pharmacokinetics and selected pharmacodynamic effects of tramadol following intravenous administration to the horse. *Equine Vet J* 2013; **45**: 490–496.
283 Natalini CC, Robinson EP. Evaluation of the analgesic effects of epidurally administered morphine, alfentanil, butorphanol, tramadol, and U50488H in horses. *Am J Vet Res* 2000; **61**: 1579–1586.
284 DeRossi R, Modolo TJ, Maciel FB, *et al.* Efficacy of epidural lidocaine combined with tramadol or neostigmine on perineal analgesia in the horse. *Equine Vet J* 2013; **45**: 497–502.
285 Bigham AS, Habibian S, Ghasemian F, *et al.* Caudal epidural injection of lidocaine, tramadol, and lidocaine-tramadol for epidural anesthesia in cattle. *J Vet Pharmacol Ther* 2010; **33**: 439–443.
286 Habibian S, Bigham AS, Aali E. Comparison of lidocaine, tramadol, and lidocaine-tramadol for epidural analgesia in lambs. *Res Vet Sci* 2011; **91**: 434–438.
287 Monteiro ER, Junior AR, Assis HM, *et al.* Comparative study on the sedative effects of morphine, methadone, butorphanol or tramadol, in combination with acepromazine, in dogs. *Vet Anaesth Analg* 2009; **36**: 25–33.
288 Steagall PV, Taylor PM, Brondani JT, *et al.* Antinociceptive effects of tramadol and acepromazine in cats. *J Feline Med Surg* 2008; **10**: 24–31.
289 Barnung SK, Treschow M, Borgbjerg FM. Respiratory depression following oral tramadol in a patient with impaired renal function. *Pain* 1997; **71**: 111–112.
290 Dhanjal JK, Wilson DV, Robinson E, *et al.* Intravenous tramadol: effects, nociceptive properties, and pharmacokinetics in horses. *Vet Anaesth Analg* 2009; **36**: 581–590.
291 Matthiesen T, Wohrmann T, Coogan TP, *et al.* The experimental toxicology of tramadol: an overview. *Toxicol Lett* 1998; **95**: 63–71.
292 Ko JC, Abbo LA, Weil AB, *et al.* Effect of orally administered tramadol alone or with an intravenously administered opioid on minimum alveolar concentration of sevoflurane in cats. *J Am Vet Med Assoc* 2008; **232**: 1834–1840.
293 Brondani JT, Luna SP, Marcello GC, *et al.* Perioperative administration of vedaprofen, tramadol or their combination does not interfere with platelet aggregation, bleeding time and biochemical variables in cats. *J Feline Med Surg* 2009; **11**: 503–509.
294 Castro DS, Silva MF, Shih AC, *et al.* Comparison between the analgesic effects of morphine and tramadol delivered epidurally in cats receiving a standardized noxious stimulation. *J Feline Med Surg* 2009; **11**: 948–953.
295 Raffa RB, Buschmann H, Christoph T, *et al.* Mechanistic and functional differentiation of tapentadol and tramadol. *Expert Opin Pharmacother* 2012; **13**: 1437–1449.
296 Tzschentke TM, Christoph T, Kogel B, *et al.* (-)-(1R,2R)-3-(3-dimethylamino-1-ethyl-2-methyl-propyl)-phenol hydrochloride (tapentadol HCl): a novel mu-opioid receptor agonist/norepinephrine reuptake inhibitor with broad-spectrum analgesic properties. *J Pharmacol Exp Ther* 2007; **323**: 265–276.
297 Giorgi M, Meizler A, Mills PC. Pharmacokinetics of the novel atypical opioid tapentadol following oral and intravenous administration in dogs. *Vet J* 2012; **194**: 309–313.

14 Muscle Relaxants and Neuromuscular Blockade

Robert D. Keegan
Department of Veterinary Clinical Sciences, College of Veterinary Medicine, Washington State University, Pullman, Washington, USA

Chapter contents

History of muscle relaxants

Muscle relaxants are a group of anesthetic adjuncts administered to improve relaxation of skeletal muscles during surgical or diagnostic procedures. The term neuromuscular blocking agents (NMBAs) is a cumbersome but descriptive name that refers to the fact that this class of drugs produce their effects by action at the neuromuscular junction. The more general term muscle relaxant refers to any drug having relaxant properties and would include centrally acting agents such as benzodiazepines, α_2-adrenergic receptor agonists, and guaifenesin. Beneficial effects of NMBA administration during general anesthesia include facilitation of tracheal intubation, reduction of skeletal muscle tone at light planes of inhalant or injectable anesthesia, and prevention of patient movement during delicate ocular, neurologic, or cardiothoracic surgery. While used frequently in human anesthesia and in some veterinary specialty practices such as ophthalmology, the use of NMBAs in general veterinary practice is limited. Inhalant anesthetics such as isoflurane are complete anesthetics in that they fulfill the 'triad of anesthesia'; that is, they provide unconsciousness, analgesia, and muscle relaxation. All three of these properties are required to permit most invasive surgical procedures. Of the three properties of the triad, inhalant anesthetics are very good at producing loss of consciousness at comparatively light planes of anesthesia while substantially deeper planes are required to provide analgesia and muscle relaxation. Indeed, these last two properties are provided by potent inhalant anesthetics only by virtue of general CNS depression. Unfortunately, deeper planes of inhalant anesthetics are associated with a decrease in cardiovascular function, thus the properties of muscle relaxation and analgesia are accompanied by the adverse effect of reduced cardiovascular performance. In young, healthy animals having good cardiovascular reserve this may be tolerated, but in patients with poor cardiovascular function, significant morbidity and mortality may result.

Veterinary Anesthesia and Analgesia: The Fifth Edition of Lumb and Jones.
Edited by Kurt A. Grimm, Leigh A. Lamont, William J. Tranquilli, Stephen A. Greene and Sheilah A. Robertson.

Rather than using an inhalant anesthetic to provide all three components of the triad, a safer, smoother anesthetic technique, particularly in patients with cardiovascular compromise, may be one that uses low concentrations of inhalant anesthetic to provide unconsciousness, opioids to provide analgesia, and a NMBA to provide muscle relaxation. Techniques such as this may be termed *balanced anesthesia* in that a mixture of agents at smaller doses is chosen based upon what they do reasonably well. Balanced anesthesia techniques are frequently chosen because they provide optimal conditions for both the surgeon and the patient.

The introduction of NMBAs into anesthesiology is a relatively recent event in medical practice, occurring in 1942. South Americans had for centuries been using a poison, derived from the tropical plant *Chondodendron tomentosum,* on the heads of their hunting arrows which had the property of causing paralysis and death to quarry. Such a poison was an obvious advantage in that animals suffering even a minor wound would succumb and be harvested by the hunter. The existence of this poison, known as curare, was recognized outside South America, but what possible use would an arrow poison have in medicine? The link was made when the explorer Richard Gill returned from the jungles of Ecuador and was diagnosed with multiple sclerosis. The suggestion that the spastic paralysis might be relieved by administration of the arrow poison led Gill to overcome his disability and return to the South American jungle. He returned to the United States in the late 1930s having obtained a quantity of curare which he sold to a pharmaceutical company who purified the raw mixture and marketed it under the trade name of Intocostrin. Initially Intocostrin was used only in psychiatric medicine to control seizures that were associated with treatments of psychotic states. A physician in the company realized the potential the drug might have in the field of anesthesiology and convinced an anesthesiologist to undertake studies in humans. This was to be a monumental undertaking as the anesthesia community of the day was understandably not receptive to administration of a paralytic arrow poison to surgical patients. Indeed, the mere suggestion that one would administer a drug which would intentionally cause respiratory arrest was unthinkable to a generation of physicians who had grown up with the motto 'where there is breath, there is hope.' Studies which suggested that d-tubocurarine, a quaternary alkaloid having a benzylisoquinolinium structure, isolated from raw curare, was safe and useful for producing abdominal muscle relaxation during general anesthesia began to emerge and use of the drug spread to Britain by 1945 [1].

Another drug with paralytic properties similar to d-tubocurarine but having the advantage of rapid onset and offset, succinylcholine, was introduced into human practice in the early 1950s [1]. Reports of veterinary use of NMBAs in dogs began to appear also in the early 1950s [2] and administration of succinylcholine to horses was described in the 1960s [3].

Both d-tubocurarine [4] and succinylcholine have a number of undesirable cardiovascular effects. Both agents can affect autonomic ganglia and cardiac muscarinic receptors, and cause release of histamine. Although succinlycholine has the advantage of rapid onset and offset compared with d-tubocurarine, additional disadvantages of possible hyperkalemia, arrhythmias, postanesthetic myalgia, and the changing nature of its block dictated that other NMBAs would be developed.

Synthetic relaxants developed during the ensuing years included gallamine, decamethonium, alcuronium and finally the steroid-based pancuronium. Most are now only of historical interest, although alcuronium is still frequently used in many parts of the world and the steroid molecule of pancuronium serves as a parent molecule of several contemporary NMBAs. Atracurium and vecuronium, introduced in the 1980s, have the advantage of minimal to no cardiovascular effects, minimal histamine release, and a controllable and predictable duration of action. Both are widely used in human anesthesia practice. Recently developed NMBAs include doxacurium, pipecuronium, and cisatracurium. All of these drugs represent continuing efforts to develop neuromuscular blockade with fewer cardiovascular and hemodynamic side-effects.

A prime indication for the use of NMBAs in human practice is tracheal intubation during induction of anesthesia. Despite its undesirable effects, succinylcholine remains the gold standard for facilitating tracheal intubation in humans primarily due to rapid onset and short duration of action. A search for a non-depolarizing alternative to succinylcholine has resulted in the development of mivacurium, an analogue of atracurium, and rocuronium, a steroidal drug derived from pancuronium. Despite improvements in speed of onset, neither mivacurium nor rocuronicum is able to facilitate human tracheal intubation as rapidly as succinylcholine. The latest NMBA to be developed, gantacurium, has an ultra-short duration of action and an onset time approaching that of succinylcholine. Structurally distinct from any previously released NMBA, gantacurium is currently undergoing human clinical trials and may eventually replace succinylcholine as an adjunct to human tracheal intubation.

Physiology of the neuromuscular junction

All NMBAs exert their effects at the neuromuscular junction or motor endplate. The neuromuscular junction forms the interface between the large myelinated motor nerve and the muscle that is supplied by that nerve. The neuromuscular junction itself may be divided into the prejunctional motor nerve ending, the synaptic cleft, and the postjunctional membrane of the skeletal muscle fiber. Present on the pre- and postjunctional areas of the neuromuscular junction are nicotinic receptors which bind and respond to acetylcholine (ACh) or another suitable ligand. The prejunctional receptor is thought to be important in the synthesis and mobilization of ACh stores but not for its release [5]. There appear to be two types of postjunctional receptors, junctional and extrajunctional [6]. The junctional receptor is found on the motor endplates of normal adult animals and is responsible for binding with the released ACh and effecting a muscle contraction. Junctional receptors are therefore responsible for the relaxant effect seen when a NMBA is administered. The extrajunctional receptors are not normally present in the muscles of typical adults but they have importance because they are synthesized by muscles that are receiving a less than normal degree of motor nerve stimulation [7]. Thus they are produced by muscles following a spinal cord or peripheral nerve injury or after a period of disuse as when a limb is casted. They are also present in neonates. The location of extrajunctional receptors is not restricted to the motor endplate and they may be located over the entire muscle cell surface [8,9].

Extrajunctional receptors appear to be more sensitive to depolarizing NMBAa such as succinylcholine and less sensitive to non-depolarizing NMBAs such as atracurium [10]. If the degree of neural deficit is severe, extrajunctional receptors may be numerous and widely distributed over the muscle membrane. Such patients may have very different responses to the actions of depolarizing NMBA and thus profound release of intracellular K^+ with concomitant adverse cardiac effects may result if succinylcholine is administered to these patients [11].

The prejunctional nerve ending synthesizes and stores a quantity of ACh in synaptic vesicles and this ACh acts as a neurotransmitter, thus coupling the nerve impulse with a resultant muscular contraction. During the course of normal neuromuscular transmission, an action potential arrives at the prejunctional motor nerve ending causing depolarization of the nerve terminal which results in release of ACh. The release of packets or quanta of ACh in response to membrane depolarization is a Ca^{++}-dependent process. The depolarization of the nerve membrane results in activation of adenylate cyclase which converts adenosine triphosphate to cyclic adenosine monophosphate. The resultant conversion results in Ca^{++} entry into the nerve terminal and subsequent release of ACh into the synaptic cleft. As mentioned previously, ACh is the neurotransmitter that effectively couples the nerve action potential into a muscular contraction. This coupling is accomplished by interaction of ACh with the postjunctional nicotinic receptor.

The interaction of ACh with the nicotinic receptor is associated with the development of an endplate potential (a muscle cell action potential) and ultimately muscular contraction. The ACh released from the prejunctional nerve cell is short-lived in that it is rapidly hydrolyzed into choline and acetate via the enzyme acetylcholinesterase. Thus the postjunctional muscle cell is depolarized by the endplate potential created by the binding of ACh to the receptor and then is repolarized as the ACh is removed from the receptor and is hydrolyzed.

The postjunctional receptors are concentrated on the endplate immediately opposite the ACh release sites on the prejunctional membrane [12]. Electron microscopy of these receptors shows them to have a central pit surrounded by a raised circular area [13,14] and thus they look similar to a spool of thread that is viewed end on. The raised circular area is the mouth of a cylinder of a receptor protein that protrudes through the membrane and contains the binding sites where ACh and other ligands attach. The pit is the opening of an ion channel that is contained within the cylinder and runs throughout its length. The receptor protein is composed of five subunits composed of two α, and one each of β, γ, and δ subunits. They are arranged into a cylinder having a potential space, the ion channel, contained within [15]. The opening of the channel is controlled by the ACh binding sites present in the two α subunits. When molecules of ACh are bound to the binding sites on each of the two α subunits, the protein rotates into a new configuration and in so doing opens the ion channel and permits ion flow [16]. The channel permits the flow of small cations but not large cations or anions. Thus during normal neuromuscular transmission, binding of two molecules of ACh to the α subunits opens the channel and permits Na^+ and Ca^{++} to flow in and K^+ to flow out of the channel. Electrical current flow thus occurs with resultant depolarization of the postjunctional membrane [17]. As the ACh molecules leave the receptor and are hydrolyzed by acetylcholinesterase, the ion channel closes, current flow stops and repolarization of the membrane occurs.

Binding of ligands to the receptor is a competitive process. Whichever suitable ligand is present in highest concentration in the vicinity of the receptor will win the competition and affect the outcome. Since two molecules of ACh are required to bind to each of the α subunits on the receptor [18], antagonists have a distinct advantage in that they need only bind to one of the subunits to prevent normal neuromuscular transmission. Contraction of the muscle does not occur in response to motor nerve depolarization and paralysis results.

The interaction of ACh and NMBA at the postjunctional receptors is a dynamic process of binding and release and, coupled with the sheer number of receptors present (10–20,000/μm^2), the success or failure of neuromuscular transmission in the presence of a NMBA is determined by the concentration of the NMBA versus the concentration of ACh. A high percentage of receptors binding ACh favors muscular contraction while a high percentage of receptors binding NMBA favors paralysis. This suggests a method for reversing paralysis induced by a NMBA. Increasing the concentration of ACh compared with the concentration of NMBA will increase the probability that ACh will win the competition for the receptor and restore normal neuromuscular transmission. Clinically this is accomplished by administration of acetylcholinesterase inhibitors. When an anticholinesterase drug such as neostigmine is administered, the available ACh is not degraded immediately, but persists within the synapse and is able to repeatedly interact with receptors. This tips the competitive balance in favor of ACh; more receptors participate in current flow and global muscle strength increases. Such interaction is also seen as the activity of a NMBA wanes due to elimination of the drug.

Pharmacology

Ligand–receptor interactions

The classic interaction of a NMBA such as d-tubocurarine or atracurium and the cholinergic receptor involves a competitive binding of the drug to the receptor, thus inhibiting the coupling of nerve action potential transmission with muscular contraction. There are at least two other less understood mechanisms, desensitization and channel blockade, where drugs may interact with the ACh receptors and disrupt neuromuscular transmission. Earlier it was stated that the cholinergic receptor is in an inactive state with its potential ion channel collapsed when two molecules of ACh are not attached to the α subunits' binding sites. Binding of ACh to each of the two α subunits of the receptor causes conformational change and allows the ion channel to open to the active state, depolarization occurs and muscle contraction ensues. A third possibility exists and is called the desensitized state. Receptors existing in the desensitized state bind ACh to the α subunits but conformational change and channel opening do not occur, so the receptor is said to be desensitized. A number of drugs including agonists, antagonists, and inhalant anesthetics appear to be able to switch the cholinergic receptor to the desensitized state.

The desensitized state hypothesis explains the synergistic action that inhalant anesthetics have with NMBAs since it is known clinically that low doses of NMBA achieve an acceptable degree of relaxation when the patient is anesthetized with a volatile anesthetic. A large number of drugs may cause or promote desensitization such as succinylcholine, thiopental, Ca^{++} channel blockers, local anesthetics, phenothiazines, cyclohexamines, inhalant anesthetics, and some antibiotics [19–22]. Channel blockade can occur when the cholinergic receptor binds an agonist to each of the α subunits, the ion channel opens, and a molecule becomes stuck within the channel. This is possible because the mouth of the ion channel is much wider than the transmembrane spanning region, thus permitting molecules to enter the channel but not to cross it. Entrapped molecules act like plugs in a funnel and interfere with the normal passage of ions in response to the binding of ACh. Channel blockade therefore blocks normal neuromuscular transmission not by competing for binding sites on the nicotinic receptor, but by interfering with the depolarization process in response to binding of an agonist [23,24]. This is an important distinction because the paralysis induced by channel blockade may not be antagonized by administration of an anticholinesterase. In fact, inhibition of cholinesterase enzyme may make the block more intense since the opening of more ion channels in response to a greater concentration of ACh may provide a greater opportunity for the offending molecules to become trapped within the channel.

It is known that many drugs can cause channel blockade but the fact that NMBAs themselves can cause blockage of the neuromuscular receptor channels may provide a partial explanation as to why administration of an anticholinesterase drug in an effort to antagonize a profound neuromuscular blockade may actually intensify rather than lessen the paralysis [25,26].

Depolarizing and non-depolarizing drugs

Earlier a distinction was made between two main categories of NMBA: non-depolarizing represented by drugs such as d-tubocurarine and atracurium and depolarizing represented by succinylcholine. Both groups have affinity for the ACh receptor and therefore act as competitors of ACh. However, their intrinsic activity once bound to the receptor site is very different. Non-depolarizing drugs bind to the receptor but do not activate it. That is, the ion channel is not opened in response to their binding. These non-depolarizing drugs may be thought of as competing for the receptor, thus preventing the endogenous ligand, ACh, from binding and causing current flow. The onset of action of these drugs is characterized by a progressive weakening of muscle contraction and ultimately flaccid paralysis.

Depolarizing drugs also bind to the receptor and, similar to the actions of ACh, the receptor is stimulated, undergoes conformational change and results in current flow and depolarization of the postjunctional membrane. Unlike ACh, however, succinylcholine and other depolarizing NMBAs are not susceptible to breakdown by acetylcholinesterase and thus the ion channel remains open and repolarization does not occur. The persistent state of depolarization associated with administration of a depolarizing NMBA results in inexcitability of the motor endplate and, as with a non-depolarizing NMBA, a flaccid paralysis.

In addition to the differing mechanism of action of the depolarizing drugs, several other differences are clinically apparent when comparing depolarizing and non-depolarizing NMBA. The initial depolarization of the motor endplate associated with succinylcholine binding to and activating the postjunctional ACh receptors leads to the initial, unco-ordinated contractions seen clinically as fasciculations. Large doses of succinylcholine, repeated administration, or administration of the drug as an infusion result in a change in the character of the block from the classic depolarizing action described above to a block known as Phase II block which resembles that of non-depolarizing drugs such as d-tubocurarine. Despite years of investigation into the genesis of Phase II block, its mechanism is still not clearly understood. Prolonged exposure of the cholinergic receptors to the agonist succinylcholine likely results in receptor desensitization, channel blockade or a combination of both. Both receptor desensitization and channel blockade have properties that would mimic those of the non-depolarizing NMBAs and thus would change the nature of the succinylcholine-induced block.

Individual neuromuscular blocking drugs

The NMBAs are quaternary ammonium compounds designed to mimic the quaternary nitrogen atom of ACh. They bind to the cholinergic receptors at the motor endplate as well as to cholinergic receptors located in autonomic ganglia. Most NMBAs are positively charged, water-soluble compounds that have a limited volume of distribution and, in many cases, limited hepatic metabolism. The water-soluble nature of these compounds dictates that their pharmacokinetics differ markedly from most anesthetic drugs clinicians are familiar with such as thiopental, propofol, and ketamine. A hallmark of these lipid-soluble anesthetic agents is their rapid onset of action and their rapid termination of effect after IV administration (see Table 14.1). The lipid solubility of these agents dictates that the induction drugs will gain entrance to the site of action in the brain by rapidly crossing cellular membranes such as the blood–brain barrier. Termination of anesthetic effect is achieved by rapid metabolism and by redistribution to the skeletal muscles and ultimately the adipose tissue.

Table 14.1 Approximate doses and duration of action of muscle relaxants given intravenously to dogs.

Muscle relaxant	Approximate dose (μg/kg)	Approximate duration (min)	Twitch recovery signifying end point of duration (% of baseline twitch)	References
Atracurium	200–400	17–28.9	50%	38
Doxacurium	3.5	108	75%	56
Gantacurium	60	3–6	95%	63
Mivacurium	10	35.1	100%	58
Pancuronium	22–100	31–108	50–100%	68
Pipecuronium	3.7–50	16–80.7	50%	55
Rocuronium	122	6.7	90%	50, 51
Succinylcholine	300–400	22–29	10–50%	33
d-Tubocurarine	130	100	50%	4
Vecuronium	14–200	15–42	50%	4, 47

Note: Twitch recovery applies to those experimental studies where evoked muscle contractions following nerve stimulation were measured.

The poor lipid solubility of the NMBAs is primarily due to the positive charges present at the quaternary ammonium moieties of the molecules [27]. The low lipid solubility exhibited by the NMBAs dictates the pharmacokinetics and pharmacodynamics of these drugs. Transfer across membrane structures including the placenta and blood–brain barrier is poor, resulting in decreased distribution compared with the lipid-soluble anesthetic drugs. Hepatic metabolism and redistribution to sites other than the skeletal muscles are usually not major mechanisms whereby the action of the NMBA is terminated. Exceptions include vecuronium where biliary excretion is important in the elimination of vecuronium from the body [28]. Due to their water solubility, most NMBAs are easily excreted by glomerular filtration into the urine and are generally not reabsorbed by the renal tubules. The water-soluble nature of these drugs may also contribute to the observation that neonates require higher relative doses of NMBA since neonates have a higher percentage of body water, and thus a higher volume for water-soluble drugs to distribute into, than do adults. Some reported doses for NMBAs in dogs, cats, and horses are included in Table 14.2.

Succinylcholine

Succinylcholine is currently the only depolarizing NMBA used clinically in veterinary medicine. Structurally, the succinylcholine molecule is two acetylcholine molecules joined together, or diacetylcholine. The drug is so rapidly hydrolyzed in plasma by the enzyme pseudocholinesterase (plasma cholinesterase) that only a small fraction of the original injected dose survives degradation in plasma to reach the site of action at the neuromuscular junction. Very little pseudocholinesterase is present in the synaptic cleft so

Table 14.2 Intravenous doses of selected neuromuscular junction blocking agents used in the dog, cat, and horse.

Drug (mg/kg)	Dog	Cat	Horse
Succinylcholine	0.3–0.4	0.2	0.12–0.15
Pancuronium	0.07–0.1	0.06–0.1	0.12
Atracurium	0.1–0.2	0.1–0.25	0.07–0.15
Vecuronium	0.1	0.025–0.1	0.1
Pipecuronium	0.05	0.003	
Cisatracurium	0.075–0.3	0.05–0.3	
Mivacurium	0.01–0.05	0.08	
Gantacurium (GW280430A)	0.06	0.06	
Rocuronium	0.1–0.6	0.1–0.6	0.3–0.6
Doxacurium	0.002–0.005		

Equipotent doses for neuromuscular junction blocking agents are often reported at the ED_{95}. Clinical paralysis may require more or less drug depending on the concurrent anesthetic agents used, the speed of onset required, the duration of block desired, and the area of the body where muscle relaxation is needed. Repeated doses are usually administered at approximately half of the original dose required to cause paralysis.

termination of succinylcholine-induced paralysis is due to diffusion of the drug away from the neuromuscular junction and into the extracellular fluid. Paradoxically, the rapid degradation of succinylcholine in the plasma is responsible for the rapid onset of effect achieved by the drug. Because of the rapid degradation by plasma pseudocholinesterase, comparatively large doses of succinylcholine may be administered without fear of an increased duration of effect. The higher the initial dose of a NMBA, the more rapid the onset of paralysis but also, in the case of all currently available NMBAs except succinylcholine and perhaps gantacurium, a significant increase in the duration of action results. Because of the rapid onset of effect and short duration of action, succinylcholine is often referred to as the relaxant of choice to facilitate human endotracheal intubation. Use of NMBAs to facilitate endotracheal tube placement is not common in veterinary practice since, with the arguable exception of the cat and pig, laryngeal activity is rarely an impediment to tracheal intubation.

Pseudocholinesterase is synthesized in the liver and production is decreased by liver disease, chronic anemia, malnutrition, burns, pregnancy, cytotoxic drugs, metoclopramide, and cholinesterase inhibitor drugs [29–32]. A reduction in plasma cholinesterase activity may be expected to result in a prolonged duration of action of succinylcholine [33]. Administration of organophosphate insecticides such as diclorovos and trichlorfon to horses has been shown to reduce pseudocholinesterase activity and prolong the duration of succinylcholine-induced neuromuscular blockade [34]. Conversely, cats wearing a dichlorvos flea collar had no increased duration of effect from succinylcholine [35].

Pancuronium

Pancuronium was the first in a series of non-depolarizing NMBAs having a steroid molecule base structure. The drug has a dose-dependent onset of approximately 5 min and a duration of action ranging from 40 to 60 min in dogs [36]. Repeated doses have a cumulative effect so administration via infusion is not common. A large fraction of the drug is excreted by the kidney, the remainder is metabolized by the liver. As may be expected, the duration of action is increased in patients presenting with renal insufficiency. In addition to having affinity for the cholinergic receptors at the neuromuscular junction, pancuronium also appears to block cardiac muscarinic receptors, resulting in an increase in heart rate. This effect appears to vary among species and usually is not a clinical concern. The muscaranic blocking effect and associated tachycardia appear to be due to the presence of a second positive charge attached to the steroid ring. Removal of a single methyl group and thus of the positive charge creates vecuronium, a NMBA essentially devoid of cardiovascular effects.

Atracurium

Atracurium is a short-acting non-depolarizing NMBA having a benzylisoquinoline structure similar to that of d-tubocurarine. The drug has a dose-dependent onset of approximately 5 minu and dependent duration of action of approximately 30 min in dogs [37]. Repeated doses do not tend to be cumulative so longer term maintenance of neuromuscular blockade via infusion is viable. Atracurium is unique in that almost half of the drug is degraded by Hofmann elimination and non-specific ester hydrolysis. The remaining fraction of the drug is degraded by as yet undefined routes although evidence exists that duration of action is not prolonged in humans with hepatic or renal failure [38,39]. Hepatic metabolism and renal excretion are thus not strictly necessary for termination of the paralytic effect and consequently atracurium may be administered to patients with hepatic or renal insufficiency without an increase in the duration of action. The drug should be refrigerated and is supplied at a pH of 3.25–3.65 to slow degradation. Hofmann elimination is not a biologic process and does not require enzymatic activity. When injected IV at physiologic pH and temperature, atracurium spontaneously decomposes into laudanosine and a quaternary monoacrylate. Laudanosine is a known CNS stimulant and has the potential to induce seizures. Unlike atracurium, laudanosine is dependent upon hepatic clearance so laudanosine plasma concentrations may be elevated in patients with hepatic insufficiency. Despite the theoretical concerns, laudanosine-induced CNS stimulation and resultant seizures are unlikely in clinical patients unless the drug is used for prolonged periods of time as might occur in intensive care settings.

Since Hofmann elimination is a pH- and temperature-dependent process, hypothermia will increase the duration of atracurium neuromuscular blockade and will decrease the infusion rate necessary to maintain neuromuscular blockade [40]. Ester hydrolysis of atracurium is accomplished by several plasma esterases not related to plasma cholinesterase. In contrast to the depolarizing relaxant succinylcholine, duration of action is not prolonged in the presence of cholinesterase inhibitors.

Many NMBAs with the benzylisoquinolone structure are associated with histamine release and a varying degree of resultant hypotension. d-Tubocurarine, the prototypical benzylisoquinolone NMBA, is among the most potent histamine-releasing NMBAs but newer drugs having the benzylisoquinolone structure such as atracurium and mivacurium require several times the ED_{95} dose required for neuromuscular blockade before appreciable amounts of histamine are released [41,42]. Although atracurium has the potential to result in histamine release, problems such as hypotension and tachycardia are not usually observed in clinical cases.

Cisatracurium

Atracurium is a racemic mixture of ten optical isomers. The 1R-*cis*, 1R′-*cis* isomer, or cisatracurium, comprises approximately 15% of racemic atracurium and has approximately four times the potency and a reduced potential for histamine release. Indeed, in a study of cats, plasma histamine concentrations were unchanged when up to 60 times the ED_{95} of cisatracurium was administered [43]. Cisatracurium has a similar onset and duration of action as atracurium. Hofmann elimination is responsible for greater than half of the administered dose of cisatracurium but unlike atracurium, ester hydrolysis does not occur. As with atracurium, the Hofmann elimination process results in laudanosine production. Since cisatracurium is approximately four times as potent as atracurium, the administered dose is correspondingly less as is the resultant production of laudanosine [44].

Vecuronium

Introduced in the 1980s, vecuronium was one of the first NMBAs devoid of cardiovascular effects. The discovery that the vagolytic properties seen with administration of pancuronium were due to the presence of two positive charges within the steroid molecule led investigators to remove a single methyl group from the parent pancuronium molecule. Vecuronium, the resultant drug, does not induce tachycardia or promote histamine release [45]. Indeed, in dogs vecuronium does not alter arterial blood pressure [46]. This drug has a dose-dependent onset of action of approximately 5 min and an intermediate 30-min duration of action similar to that of atracurium. As with atracurium, a cumulative effect with subsequent doses is not a prominent feature of this drug. Vecuronium is unstable when prepared in solution and thus it is supplied as a lyophilized powder that is reconstituted with sterile water prior to injection. The powder does not need refrigeration and once reconstituted, the solution is stable for 24 h. Slightly more than half of the drug is metabolized by hepatic microsomes and excreted in the bile while a significant fraction undergoes renal elimination [47]. In humans the duration of action of vecuronium is either slightly prolonged or unchanged in patients exhibiting renal insufficiency. In patients with hepatic failure the duration of action is prolonged only if increased doses are administered [48].

Rocuronium

Rocuronium is a derivative of vecuronium, having approximately one-eighth the potency of the parent compound. Since vecuronium and rocuronium have similar molecular weights and rocuronium has lower potency, a larger injected dose of rocuronium places a greater number of molecules near the neuromuscular junction, translating into a more rapid onset of neuromuscular blockade. Despite a more rapid onset compared with atracurium and vecuronium, rocuronium cannot provide optimal conditions for human tracheal intubation as quickly as succinylcholine. Duration of action in the dog is similar to that of vecuronium and atracurium [49,50]. Similar to vecuronium, rocuronium seems to be virtually without cardiovascular adverse effects and does not cause histamine release [51]. The primary route of elimination is via the hepatic system while a small fraction is eliminated via the kidney [42]. The neuromuscular blocking effects of rocuronium and vecuronium can be reversed by the administration of suggammadex, a chelating agent that preferentially binds to and physically removes the NMBA from the motor endplate [52–54].

Pipecuronium

Pipecuronium is another steroid relaxant derived from pancuronium. Manipulation of the steroid structure has resulted in a relaxant that has greatly reduced antimuscarinic effects so pipecuronium is free of tachycardic effects while retaining a long duration of action. It has resulted in hypotension in dogs [55]. Similar to pancuronium, pipecuronium is eliminated primarily via the renal route with a smaller fraction undergoing biliary excretion.

Doxacurium

Doxacurium is a very potent benzylisoquinilone NMBA having a long duration of action [56]. Similar to other benzylisoquinilone NMBAs such as atracurium, the drug does not have vagolytic properties or result in ganglion blockade. Similar to cisatracurium, administration of clinically useful doses of doxacurium does not result in appreciable histamine release. Doxacurium appears to be minimally metabolized and is excreted unchanged into the bile and urine.

Mivacurium

Mivacurium is a rapid-acting, short-duration NMBA marketed for use in human tracheal intubation. Similar to the related benzylisoquinolone drug atracurium, mivacurium has the potential to induce histamine release, particularly if high doses are administered as often occurs when a rapid onset of effect is desirable. Mivacurium is degraded by plasma pseudocholinesterase and metabolites do not have appreciable neuromuscular blocking activity. Typical administered doses in humans have a duration of action of approximately 25 min, thus being one-half to one-third shorter than atracurium. Mivacurium shows marked differences in potency and in duration of action among species, being much more potent in dogs than in humans. Indeed, in dogs one-third of the typical human dose is associated with a duration of blockade that is five times longer than in humans [57]. The differences in duration of action between species may in part reflect the circulating quantity of pseudocholinesterase present since normal plasma cholinesterase values for dogs are from 19% to 76% of human values [58]. In addition, it is possible that canine pseudocholinesterase enzyme has differing affinity for the three primary isomers of mivacurium found in the proprietary formulation [49]. Clinical observations in cats indicate that mivacurium has a much shorter duration of action in this species compared with dogs (RDK personal observation).

Gantacurium

Gantacurium is a rapid-acting, ultra-short duration non-depolarizing NMBA currently undergoing human clinical trials. It is structurally distinct from the traditional steroidal and benzylisoquinolinium compounds and is classified as an asymmetric mixed-onium cholorfumerate. Gantacurium is not stable in aqueous solution and, similar to vecuronium, the drug is provided as a lyophilized powder that is reconstituted prior to administration. The dose in humans required to produce a 95% block (ED_{95}) is 0.19 mg/kg [59]. Following IV bolus administration of 0.45–0.54 mg/kg (2.5–3× ED_{95}), optimal conditions for intubation were achieved in 90 s [57,60]. In addition to having a rapid onset in humans, gantacurium has a short duration of action of approximately 14 min for a dose of 0.4 mg/kg and, similar to succinylcholine, increasing the administered dose in an effort to increase onset does not markedly increase duration of action [61]. In dogs anesthetized with thiopental, nitrous oxide, and isoflurane, the ED_{95} was 0.06 mg/kg, onset time was 107 s, and duration of action was 5.2 min [62].

In humans, gantacurium has the potential to release histamine at doses exceeding 2.5× ED_{95}. The histamine release was accompanied by clinically significant decreases in blood pressure, increases in heart rate, and facial redness [57]. Conversely, clinically significant histamine release was not observed in dogs at IV bolus doses up to 25× ED_{95} [60].

Gantacurium has two degradation pathways that account for its predictably ultra-short duration of action. The first pathway is a pH-sensitive hydrolysis in plasma while the second involves the binding of the non-essential amino acid cysteine to the gantacurium ring structure. Endogenous or exogenously administered cysteine replaces a chlorine atom and saturates the double bond of the fumerate moiety [63]. The gantacurium is thus rendered inactive and neuromuscular transmission resumes.

Non-neuromuscular effects of NMBAs

The NMBAs have a primary action at the nicotinic cholinergic receptors at the motor nerve plate but may also have effects at other cholinergic receptors throughout the body. Cholinergic receptors that may be affected by NMBA include cardiac muscarinic receptors and autonomic nervous system ganglia. Many of these undesirable effects involve either a blocking of the receptor or a mimicking of the action of ACh. In addition, many NMBAs promote the release of histamine and other vasoactive substances from mast cells. Still other undesirable effects may result from the initial muscle fasciculation associated with administration of depolarizing NMBAs such as succinylcholine.

Cardiovascular effects

Acetylcholine is the primary neurotransmitter at not only the nicotinic receptors at the motor endplate of skeletal muscles but at muscarinic receptors of the parasympathetic nervous system and at sympathetic ganglia as well. ACh is the primary neurotransmitter of pre- and postganglionic neurons within the parasympathetic nervous system while the sympathetic nervous system employs ACh as a preganglionic neurotransmitter. The ubiquitous presence of ACh and the structural similarities between ACh and the NMBAs provide opportunity for the NMBAs to have effects in addition to their paralytic actions. Stimulation or blocking of cardiac muscarinic receptors or of sympathetic ganglia may result in either increases or decreases in heart rate and the development of cardiac dysrhythmias. Succinylcholine can mimic the effect of ACh at cardiac muscarinic receptors, resulting in sinus bradycardia, junctional rhythms and even sinus arrest [64,65]. In contrast, by virtue of its ACh-like effects at sympathetic ganglia, administration of succinylcholine may result in increases in heart rate and blood pressure [66].

Non-depolarizing drugs, particularly the older agents, may also influence a patient's cardiovascular status. The rapid IV injection of a paralyzing dose of d-tubocurarine can result in a significant decrease in blood pressure. One possible mechanism is that the injected d-tubocurarine blocks the action of ACh at sympathetic ganglia, thus resulting in an effective decrease in sympathetic tone with resultant hypotension. Alternatively, histamine release associated with the rapid IV administration of d-tubocurarine is probably responsible for the majority of the hypotension seen since slow IV administration or prior administration of an antihistamine drug attenuates the decrease in blood pressure that is observed following administration [67]. Rapid IV administration of pancuronium is associated with an increase in heart rate and corresponding increases in arterial pressure and cardiac output [68,69]. This tachycardic effect has been shown to be due to blockade of cardiac muscarinic receptors and resultant decreased parasympathetic nervous system activity [70]. In addition there is evidence that pancuronium may stimulate the release of norepinephrine from sympathetic nerves [71].

The modest increase in heart rate is not always disadvantageous, particularly when drugs having bradycardic effects such as the opioids are co-administered to a patient receiving pancuronium. The ability of pancuronium to induce an increase in heart rate is inconsistent between species. In dogs, pancuronium increases heart rate, blood pressure, and cardiac output [55,56]. The heart rates of horses anesthetized with halothane and administered pancuronium did not change [72] but ponies had an increase in both heart rate and blood pressure [73]. Similar to the effect on horses, pancuronium did not change heart rate or blood pressure in anesthetized calves [74] but did result in increases in heart rate and blood pressure in pigs [75].

The newer, intermediate duration agents such as atracurium and vecuronium are virtually devoid of cardiovascular effects. Atracurium and mivacurium do have the potential to result in histamine release, but decreases in blood pressure are rarely seen clinically if the drugs are not administered as a rapid IV bolus. The newest drugs, pipecuronium, doxacurium, and rocuronium, were designed with cardiovascular stability in mind and are unlikely to be associated with profound changes in cardiovascular function.

Histamine release

The quaternary ammonium structure inherent in the NMBAs is responsible for the propensity of many of these compounds to result in histamine release following IV injection. Release of histamine in animals results in vasodilation, a decrease in blood pressure and possibly a compensatory increase in heart rate. Histamine release is usually associated with administration of the benzylisoquinoline class of NMBA but has been reported with steroid relaxants having low potency [76]. The relaxant d-tubocurarine is a potent releaser of histamine at doses required to produce neuromuscular block and thus histamine release, vasodilation and increased heart rate are commonly encountered [54]. For the newer NMBAs, the dose necessary to evoke clinically significant histamine release is much higher than the dose necessary to produce relaxation. For example, in humans approximately 2.5 times the ED_{95} dose of atracurium is required to cause clinically significant histamine release [77]. Pretreatment of patients with H_1 and H_2 receptor antagonists is effective in preventing the effects associated with histamine release [78]. In clinical patients, worries about histamine release with use of the newer NMBAs may be avoided simply by administering relaxants via slow IV injection and refraining from administration of greater than recommended doses.

Placental transfer

All clinically used NMBAs are large, hydrophilic polar molecules and as a consequence their transfer across cell membranes, including the placenta, is limited. At doses used clinically, placental transfer of relaxants is minimal and effects on the neonate are unlikely. There is current widespread use of NMBAs in human cesarean operations and atracurium and succinylcholine have been used clinically in small and large domestic animals without detection of effects on the neonate. Administration of NMBAs such as pancuronium, succinylcholine, gallamine, and d-tubocurarine to pregnant ferrets and cats does not impair muscle twitch strength in the neonate [79].

Central nervous system effects

Being large, polar, hydrophilic molecules, the NMBAs do not cross cell membranes readily. However, evidence exists that most of these drugs do gain entrance into the CSF and may be associated with resultant CNS effects. In one study, pancuronium was reported to reduce the MAC of halothane in humans [80]. However, a subsequent study found that pancuronium, atracurium or vecuronium had no effect on the MAC of halothane in humans [81]. Accidental administration of NMBA into the CSF has resulted in myotonia, autonomic effects, and seizures [82,83]. Laudanosine is a product of atracurium degradation that easily crosses the blood–brain barrier in dogs [84] and, in large doses, may result in CNS stimulation. Clinically used dosages of atracurium, however, are extremely unlikely to result in the formation of sufficient quantity of laudanosine to cause CNS stimulation.

Protein binding

All non-depolarizing NMBAs are protein bound, but the clinical significance of such binding is unclear. Presumably only the unbound fraction of drug is available to interact at ACh receptors and induce paralysis. In addition, protein binding would be expected to reduce renal elimination since only free unbound drug is filtered at the glomerulus. In human studies of patients with hepatic cirrhosis with decreased plasma protein concentrations, the proportion of d-tubocurarine, pancuronium, and vecuronium bound to plasma protein was not different compared with healthy patients having normal plasma protein concentrations [85,86]. Thus, despite the theoretical concerns of low plasma protein increasing the proportion of free, active drug, the amount of NMBA that is protein bound in hypoproteinemic states seems to remain unchanged.

Non-neuromuscular effects of succinylcholine

Several undesirable non-neuromuscular side-effects are associated with the administration of clinically useful doses of the non-depolarizing NMBA succinylcholine. These effects include hyperkalemia, increased intraocular, intracranial and intragastric pressure, and muscle soreness.

Hyperkalemia

Administration of succinylcholine is associated with a transient increase in serum potassium levels. Succinylcholine binds to and activates the nicotinic motor endplate receptors but unlike Ach, succinylcholine is not immediately degraded by acetylcholinesterase enzyme. Thus, a state of depolarization characterized by open ion channels persists. When the ion channels are open, potassium ions are able to exit from the muscle fiber into the extracellular fluid space. As a result, serum potassium concentrations rise transiently following administration of succinylcholine. However, in healthy patients this transient increase is without adverse effects provided that cardiovascular disease is not present and preadministration potassium levels are normal. In patients presenting with burns, severe muscle trauma, muscular denervation, nerve damage or neuromuscular disease, extrajunctional ACh receptors proliferate over the surface of the muscle fiber membrane. This increase in receptor density is associated with an increase in sensitivity to the depolarizing muscle relaxants and an increase in the amount of intracellular potassium released in response to administration of succinylcholine. The increase in ACh receptor density does not occur before about 2 days following the injury and seems to persist for 2–3 months [87]. Similar to the effect seen with burns or denervation injuries, prolonged immobilization of a limb is also associated with an increase in ACh receptor density. As with burn patients, increases in serum potassium levels may be expected if succinylcholine is administered to these patients.

Intraocular pressure

Administration of succinylcholine is associated with an increase in intraocular pressure. In humans, the intraocular pressure peaks at 2–4 min and remains increased for at least 6 min following administration [88]. The mechanism responsible for the increase in intraocular pressure is presently unknown but likely involves the circulation to the eye since administration of the calcium channel blocker nifedipine attenuates the increase [89]. Administration of succinylcholine to patients presenting with penetrating eye injuries has the potential to result in loss of global contents. In humans, controversy exists as to whether administration of a non-depolarizing NMBA prior to succinylcholine prevents the increase in intraocular pressure. However, since most domestic animals are easily intubated without the aid of a NMBA, it is probably prudent to avoid succinylcholine in veterinary patients presenting with penetrating eye injuries. It is important to realize that any induction technique which provokes gagging or forceful coughing will also raise intraocular and intracranial pressure and thus must be avoided in patients presenting with an open globe. Thus induction with a rapid and smooth-acting injectable anesthetic agent is crucial, making certain that adequate anesthetic depth has been achieved prior to attempting tracheal intubation.

Intragastric pressure

The administration of succinylcholine causes an initial depolarization of the motor endplate that is manifest clinically as fasciculations of the skeletal muscles. The muscle fasciculations cause abdominal compression and a resultant increase in intragastric pressure. The increase in intragastric pressure could theoretically increase the incidence of regurgitation and may worsen outcome in dogs presenting with gastric dilation volvulus.

Intracranial pressure

The transient muscle fasciculation induced by succinylcholine may be responsible for the increase in intracranial pressure seen following its administration. In humans the increase in intracranial pressure may be prevented by prior administration of the non-depolarizing NMBA d-tubocurarine. Again, since most domestic animals are usually readily intubated without use of a rapid-acting NMBA, it is recommended that succinylcholine be avoided in patients presenting with raised intracranial pressure. As with penetrating eye injuries, a rapid smooth induction of anesthesia free of coughing and struggling is desirable to prevent unnecessary increases in intracranial pressure.

Muscle responses

Administration of succinylcholine is often associated with postanesthetic muscle soreness. It has been suggested that this postanesthetic myalgia results from muscle fasciculation that occurs during the initial depolarization of the motor endplate [90]. Further, there appears to be good correlation between the intensity of the fasciculation and the intensity of the muscle pain [91]. Although skeletal muscle enzymes such as creatine kinase increase in both humans [92,93] and animals[94] following administration of succinylcholine, it is presently unknown if animals experience muscle pain similar to that of humans.

Muscle relaxants in anesthetized animals

Most animals can be intubated relatively easily without paralysis, and muscle relaxation caused by inhalant anesthetic agents is adequate for most procedures. While human patients are frequently given muscle relaxants to facilitate endotracheal intubation and surgical access, the use of muscle relaxants in veterinary practice is not as common. When considering use of NMBAs, veterinarians should first become familiar with their pharmacology and the clinical implementation of mechanical ventilation in addition to developing skills at monitoring depth of anesthesia in paralyzed patients.

Indications

Muscle relaxants may be administered for numerous reasons. They are typically given with hypnotic drugs to eliminate laryngeal spasm and facilitate rapid control of the airway. The need for a motionless, centrally positioned eye during intraocular or corneal surgery often requires the use of a muscle relaxant. Other indications include prevention of unconscious spontaneous movement, reduced resistance to controlled ventilation, and facilitation of surgical access during surgery.

Precautions

Because the muscles of respiration are paralyzed, ventilation must be controlled, either by a mechanical ventilator or by a staff member who can manually ventilate the patient until muscle strength is restored. Muscle relaxants have no sedative, anesthetic, or analgesic properties, so it is critical that the animal be adequately anesthetized to render it completely unconscious. Assessing the level of anesthesia in a paralyzed patient is more difficult than in a non-paralyzed patient because some indicators of depth (e.g. purposeful movement in response to a noxious stimulus, palpebral response, and jaw tone) are abolished. When including an NMBA in an anesthetic protocol, anesthetists must be certain they can reliably maintain an adequate plane of surgical anesthesia and level of ventilation.

Historically, muscle relaxants have been given alone to animals for capture or restraint, including use as the sole agent for brief surgical procedures (e.g. equine castration). At this time, the use of such inhumane practices is not justified because of the widespread availability of safe and effective anesthetics. The administration of an NMBA alone to an awake patient for immobilization purposes is also considered inhumane.

Selection

When choosing a muscle relaxant, one must consider many factors including the species, the reason for paralysis, the duration, the health status of the patient, and concurrent drug administration. Relaxants will differ in the onset and duration of action, cardiovascular effects, and route of elimination. If a rapid onset and brief action are needed, the choice might be rocuronium or mivacurium, whereas doxacurium may be selected for longer action without significant cardiovascular effects. Atracurium is metabolized via Hofmann elimination and may be a good choice when hepatic or renal disease is present [38,39].

Because many factors will affect the intensity and duration of muscle paralysis, monitoring of neuromuscular blockade is useful for titrating the dose needed for the desired effect. It is important to remember that individual muscle groups respond differently to muscle relaxants. The diaphragm is less sensitive to the effects of muscle relaxants compared with the muscles of the limbs [95]. Therefore, a higher dose may be required to abolish spontaneous ventilation compared with the dose for facilitation of fracture reduction. In horses, when a dose of muscle relaxant required to abolish the hoof twitch is administered, the facial twitch will often remain, though at reduced strength [96, 97]. When not monitoring hoof twitch tension, it should be appreciated that the facial twitch may be present even when adequate relaxation has been achieved in the limb for performing the surgical procedure.

Factors affecting neuromuscular blockade

A number of factors can influence the duration of action, intensity, and recovery from neuromuscular blockade. Whenever a muscle relaxant is administered, neuromuscular function can be monitored during the anesthetic and recovery periods to minimize overdosing and residual paralysis.

Impaired metabolism and excretion

Hepatic insufficiency may alter the initial effect of non-depolarizing muscle relaxants because of an increase in the volume of distribution. However, their effect may be increased due to decreased elimination, especially when drugs dependent on hepatic biotransformation (e.g. vecuronium) are administered [98–100]. Impaired liver function may also prolong or cause residual neuromuscular blockade [101]. In general, muscle relaxants are not highly protein bound to albumin, typically less than 50% [102–105]. Thus, the net effect of low albumin may not be clinically significant. Decreased esterase activity may slow the biotransformation of mivacurium and atracurium. Patients with biliary obstruction may have reduced hepatic clearance of muscle relaxants [106]. The clinical impact of hepatic failure depends on the specific NMBA and dose administered.

In patients with renal insufficiency, paralysis may be prolonged when muscle relaxants that rely predominantly on renal elimination (gallamine, pancuronium, or doxacurium) are given [107–110]. Recovery from mivacurium administration may also be prolonged, possibly because of decreased pseudocholinesterase activity [111]. Atracurium pharmacokinetics are generally unaffected, but if a constant-rate infusion is given to a patient with renal failure, laudanosine levels may be increased [112]. It is best to avoid the use of high doses, repeated doses, or continuous infusions of muscle relaxants that primarily depend on renal elimination in patients with significant renal disease.

Anesthetic drugs

Inhalant anesthetic agents cause a time- and dose-dependent enhancement of the intensity and duration of block produced by muscle relaxants [113]. The explanation for this interaction is complex, with inhalational agents suppressing motor-evoked potentials in response to spinal cord and transcranial stimulation. Muscle contractility is altered, and variation in regional muscle blood flow causes a greater fraction of the relaxant to reach the site of action [114]. The effects are greatest after administration of a long-acting relaxant or during a continuous infusion. The order of potency of some of the inhalational anesthetics in enhancing muscle relaxant effects is as follows: diethyl ether > enflurane > isoflurane > desflurane > halothane [114]. Also, antagonism of the block may be delayed, especially if inhalant anesthesia is continued after administration of the reversal agent. Monitoring of neuromuscular function helps to facilitate the appropriate dosing of muscle relaxants during inhalational anesthesia. Most injectable anesthetic agents have only minor effects on the neuromuscular blocking properties of muscle relaxants. Induction agents, such as thiopental, ketamine and propofol, may minimally enhance neuromuscular blockade [114].

Acid–base disturbances

Generally, respiratory acidosis increases the intensity of muscle blockade, whereas respiratory alkalosis decreases the effect [115–118]. Both metabolic acidosis and alkalosis may potentiate the effects of muscle relaxants and make it more difficult to antagonize relaxant-induced muscle paralysis [115,116,118,119].

Electrolyte disturbances

Alterations in serum concentration of potassium, magnesium, and calcium influence neuromuscular blockade. Decreases in extracellular potassium result in hyperpolarization of the endplate and resistance to ACh-induced depolarization [120]. A relative increase in extracellular potassium lowers the resting membrane potential, opposing the effect of the muscle relaxant [120]. Increased serum magnesium concentrations compete with ionized calcium, decreasing ACh release. Accordingly, in patients given magnesium sulfate, the duration of action of muscle relaxants may increase [121]. Hypocalcemia decreases ACh release, muscle action potential, and muscle contraction strength, thus increasing the effect of the neuromuscular block [120,122]. Typically, hypercalcemia decreases the effect of d-tubocurarine, pancuronium, and possibly other NMBAs, resulting in a higher dose requirement to achieve paralysis [120].

Hypothermia

This generally slows drug elimination and decreases nerve conduction and muscle contraction. The overall clinical effect will vary with the degree of hypothermia and the NMBA administered.

Age

Youth is associated with altered dose requirements of muscle relaxants. Receptor immaturity and decreased clearance appear to increase the potency of muscle relaxants in the young [123–125]. On the other hand, very young animals may require higher doses of muscle relaxants because of increased extracellular fluid and a larger volume of distribution when compared with adults. In addition, younger animals experience a faster onset of drug action while neuromuscular function recovers more quickly, so a lower dose of antagonist is usually required at the termination of the procedure [126].

Although the data from published studies are not always clear-cut, old age may be associated with an increase in the effect of muscle relaxants, perhaps because of a lower volume of distribution and decreased rate of clearance. In elderly human patients, a delay in reversal and the need for higher doses of reversal agents are common, and likely attributable to slower spontaneous recovery [127,128].

Neuromuscular disorders

Animals with neuromuscular disorders may exhibit unpredictable responses to both depolarizing and non-depolarizing muscle relaxants. Care should be taken when administering muscle relaxants to patients with neuromuscular disorders or a history of muscle weakness or wasting. Peripheral neuropathies may be classified as idiopathic, familial, metabolic, or immune mediated. In human patients, peripheral neuropathy may increase the effect of non-depolarizing muscle relaxants because of neural damage and the possibility of denervation-induced upregulation [129]. These patients may also be predisposed to succinylcholine-induced hyperkalemia [130]. Diseases such as tick paralysis and botulism impair presynaptic release of ACh. Patients with presynaptic neuromuscular disorders show an increased sensitivity to non-depolarizing muscle relaxants. Myasthenia gravis is an autoimmune disease that causes generalized muscle weakness from a decrease in the number of ACh receptors on the motor endplate muscle membrane. ACh is released normally, but its effect on the postsynaptic membrane is reduced. Patients with myasthenia gravis may be resistant to succinylcholine-induced paralysis, but are extremely sensitive to non-depolarizing relaxants and have an increased sensitivity to succinylcholine-induced Phase II block [131,132]. These patients do not appear to be more sensitive to succinylcholine-induced hyperkalemia or malignant hyperthermia [133]. From published reports of dogs with myasthenia gravis, the initial dose recommendations of atracurium and vecuronium are 0.1 mg/kg and 0.02 mg/kg, respectively [134,135].

Antimicrobial and other drug interactions

The most notable effects on neuromuscular blockade occur with the administration of polymyxin and aminoglycoside antimicrobials, but can also occur with tetracycline, lincomycin, and clindamycin. Polymyxins may depress postsynaptic sensitivity to ACh and enhance channel block [136,137]. Antagonism with either neostigmine or calcium may be difficult and unreliable [137]. Aminoglycosides, such as gentamicin, kanamycin, neomycin, streptomycin, and tobramycin, have a presynaptic site of action, as evidenced by depressed ACh release. The ability to antagonize blockade with calcium supports this mechanism and site of action [137]. Studies in anesthetized cats and horses given atracurium have shown a significant decrease in twitch tension after administration of gentamicin (2 mg/kg IV), but recovery times were not significantly changed [138,139]. Cats given gentamicin (10 mg/kg IV) during neuromuscular blockade have shown a significant decrease in tibialis cranialis twitch response [140]. Furthermore, dogs given a single daily dose of gentamicin (6 mg/kg IV as a bolus) had significantly decreased twitch tension, while recovery time did not differ from that for controls [141].

Tetracycline administration presumably depresses ACh release through calcium chelation. The enhanced blockade is usually reversible with calcium, but not neostigmine administration [137]. The primary site of the inhibitory action of lincomycin may be directly on the muscle. It may also have slight presynaptic and postsynaptic activity. This effect is poorly reversed with neostigmine or calcium but partially reversed with 4-aminopyridine [137]. Clindamycin has a greater neuromuscular blocking effect than lincomycin. The mechanism is direct inhibition of the muscle, and reversal is difficult with either calcium or neostigmine administration [137]. Penicillins and cephalosporins appear to have a negligible effect on overall neuromuscular function [137]. Nevertheless, whenever an antibiotic is administered to a patient also given a muscle relaxant, the possibility of an enhanced block and/or residual paralysis should be considered. Close patient monitoring is recommended well into the recovery period.

Lithium administration may also increase or prolong neuromuscular blockade by competing with sodium and decreasing ACh release. The effects of muscle relaxants have been potentiated by numerous classes of drugs, including β-blockers, doxapram, anticonvulsants, steroids, and H_2 receptor antagonists [114].

Monitoring neuromuscular blockade

Neuromuscular function may be monitored whenever a muscle relaxant is administered. Appropriate monitoring will facilitate proper dosing of both the muscle relaxant and its antagonist. To prevent residual paralysis and muscle weakness in the recovery period, it is important that monitoring be continued until the function is fully restored. Evoked motor responses to peripheral nerve stimulation are used to evaluate the degree of neuromuscular blockade. Many handheld peripheral nerve stimulators are available (Fig. 14.1).

Sites of stimulation

Sites for stimulation of peripheral motor nerves in dogs and cats include the peroneal and ulnar nerves (Figs 14.2, 14.3). In horses,

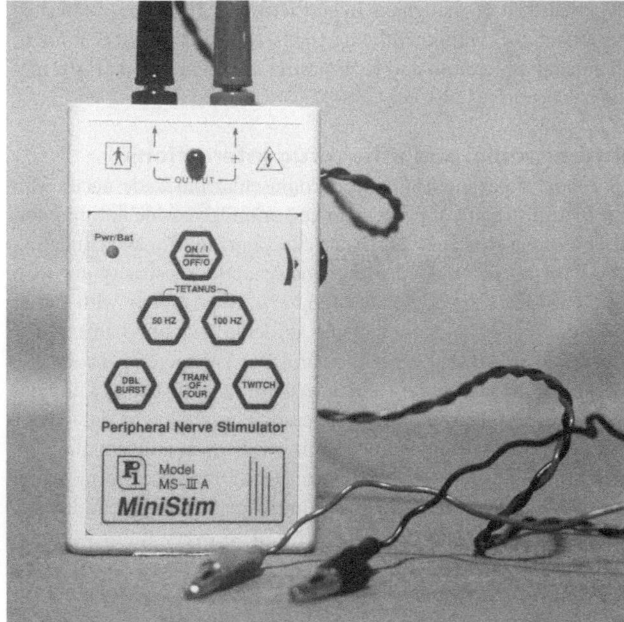

Figure 14.1 Peripheral nerve stimulator.

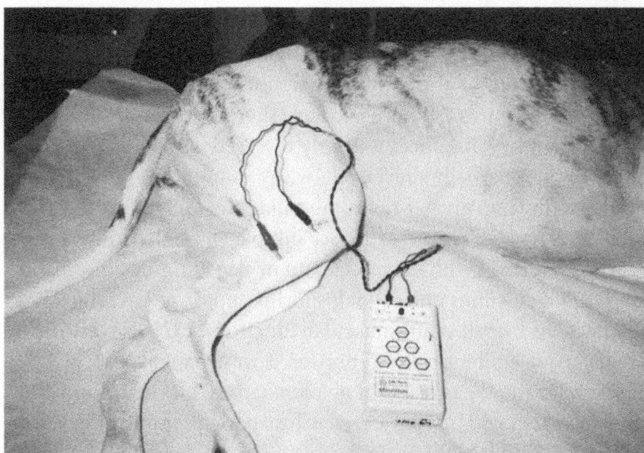

Figure 14.2 Superficial peroneal nerve stimulation in a dog.

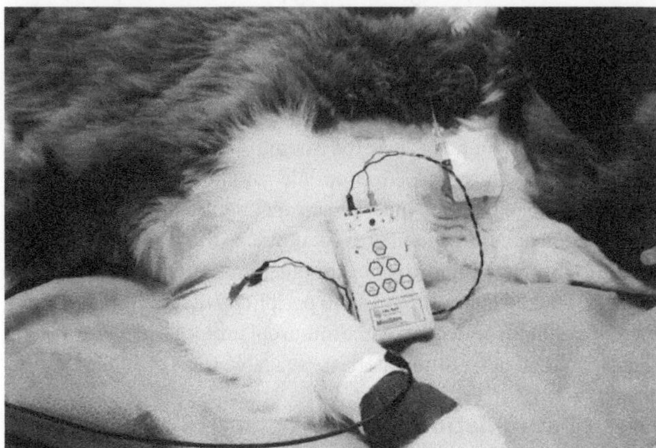

Figure 14.3 Ulnar nerve stimulation in a dog.

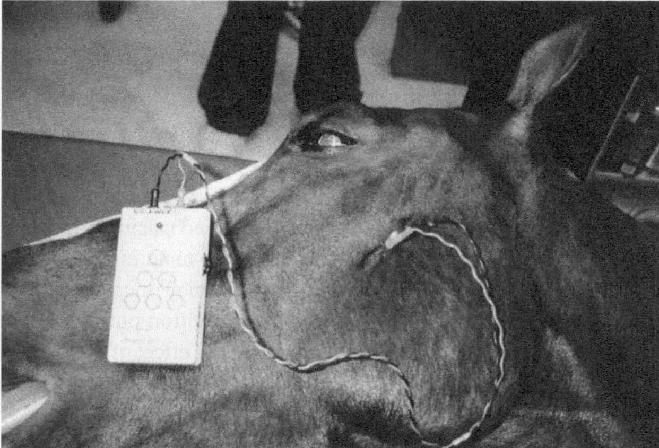

Figure 14.4 Facial nerve stimulation in a horse.

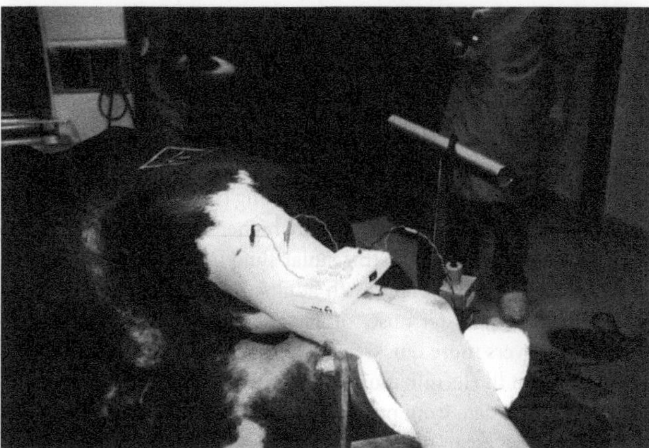

Figure 14.5 Peroneal nerve stimulation in a horse.

the facial nerve and superficial peroneal nerve are most commonly used (Figs 14.4, 14.5). Contact electrodes are placed over the nerve to be stimulated, and the resultant motor response is compared with the prerelaxant response.

Electrical stimulation characteristics

When monitoring neuromuscular function in veterinary patients, there are standard methods for stimulating peripheral nerves. The output from the peripheral nerve stimulator should be a square-wave stimulus lasting 0.2–0.3 ms. Ideally, the output current of the nerve stimulator should be adjustable, enabling a supramaximal impulse (i.e. a current slightly greater than that required to elicit the maximum motor response) to be applied to the nerve. A supramaximal stimulus ensures that all fibers in the nerve bundle are depolarized. Since muscle fibers contract in an all-or-none fashion, any subsequent changes in the evoked motor response during supramaximal stimulation of the peripheral nerve are caused by changes at the neuromuscular junction or muscle level, not by loss of nerve fiber input.

Pattern of stimulation

Ideally, the peripheral nerve stimulator should have a variable output and be capable of providing single-twitch, train-of-four, tetanic, and double-burst patterns of stimulation. Examples of the evoked muscle response to supramaximal stimulation before and after

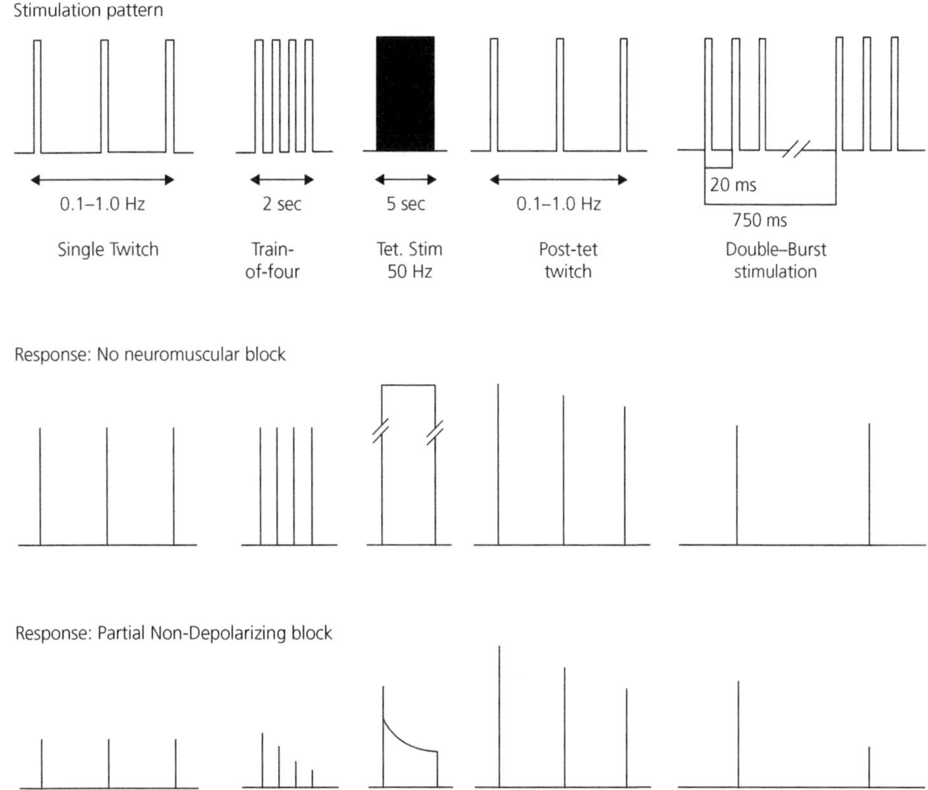

Figure 14.6 Different peripheral nerve stimulation patterns for monitoring neuromuscular function (*top panel*). Under each pattern is shown the characteristics of the evoked muscle responses measured mechanically before (*center panel*) and during (*bottom panel*) partial block.

administration of a muscle relaxant are presented in Fig. 14.6. Partial neuromuscular block with depolarizing and non-depolarizing relaxants modifies the recorded responses to these stimulation patterns. These modified responses are summarized in Table 14.3.

Single twitch

When using the single twitch, the simplest form of nerve stimulation, the degree of relaxation is assessed by dividing the elicited response by the prerelaxant response. The prerelaxant response is the twitch response measured immediately prior to the administration of the muscle relaxant. Since ACh release is decreased by the prejunctional effects of the relaxant, the frequency of single-twitch stimulation should be no greater than approximately one twitch every 7–10s [142]. If the stimulus is applied too frequently, the resultant twitch response will be artificially low, causing inaccuracy in determination of the degree of relaxation. Twitch response is not depressed until 75–80% of receptors are blocked and will be abolished when approximately 90–95% of receptors are blocked [143].

Train of four

The train-of-four (TOF) pattern of stimulation is the delivery of four supramaximal impulses over 2s (2Hz). The TOF can be repeated every 10–20s without significant temporal effects. The relaxation level is determined by comparing the ratio of the intensity of the fourth twitch to the first twitch (T_4:T_1 ratio). Since the TOF serves as its own control, it is not necessary to determine baseline values prior to relaxant administration, although proper stimulator function should be verified before paralysis. In the absence of neuromuscular blockade, the T_4:T_1 ratio will be 1.0. After a non-depolarizing muscle relaxant is administered, when approximately

Table 14.3 Responses during partial neuromuscular block.[a]

Criteria	Depolarizing Block	Nondepolarizing Block	Phase II Block
Fasciculation before onset of block	Yes	No	–
Time for onset	Short	Longer	–
Single twitch	Depressed	Depressed	Depressed
Tetanic height	Depressed	Depressed	Depressed
Tetanic fade	Minimal or absent	Present and marked	Present and marked
Train-of-four fade	Minimal or absent	Present and marked	Present and marked
Posttetanic facilitation	Minimal or absent	Present	Present
Response to anticholinesterases	Block is prolonged	Block is antagonized	Block is antagonized

[a]Distinguishing features of depolarizing, nondepolarizing, and succinylcholine–induced phase **II** block. The left column lists the different patterns of nerve stimulation or other characteristic, and the second, third, and fourth columns list the respective responses in the presence of partial neuromuscular block.

70% of receptors are occupied the twitches will fade, beginning with the fourth, followed by the third, second, and first twitches [144]. The dose of relaxant given will determine the degree of fade, the strength of any remaining twitches, and how long the twitches are absent. During recovery, the twitches will reappear in reverse order. A T_4:T_1 ratio of 0.7 or greater is associated with adequate clinical signs of recovery from the muscle relaxant [145].

During the Phase I block from a depolarizing relaxant, the TOF fade will be absent. However, repeat administration or continuous infusion of the depolarizing drug can cause a Phase II block. When this occurs, fade will be seen following a TOF stimulus (see Table 14.3) [146].

Tetanic stimulation

Sustained muscle contraction is achieved by continuously delivering a high-frequency (50 Hz) supramaximal stimulus for 5 s [146]. Partial neuromuscular blockade from non-depolarizing relaxant administration will reduce tetanic height and cause fade [147]. Although this pattern of stimulation is helpful for detecting residual neuromuscular blockade during the anesthetic recovery period, it is important to remember that tetanic stimulation can be painful for lightly anesthetized or conscious patients [148].

Post-tetanic facilitation

Post-tetanic facilitation is an increase in an evoked response from a stimulus delivered shortly after tetanic stimulation. This is thought to be caused by increased ACh release from the nerve terminal, but other theories exist [143]. It is characterized by either an increase in twitch strength or a decrease in the degree of fade in response to a single-twitch, TOF, or double-burst pattern of stimulation. Post-tetanic facilitation is often the first clinical indicator of recovery from neuromuscular blockade [149,150].

Double-burst stimulation

Double-burst stimulation (DBS) is the delivery of two minitetanic bursts, two to four impulses each, delivered at a rate of 50 Hz and 750 ms apart. When DBS is used, a ratio of the response to the second burst compared with the response to the first burst (D_2:D_1) is calculated. DBS may be superior to TOF because not only does DBS correlate highly to TOF when assessed via mechanomyography, but fade is more readily seen with DBS using both visual and tactile means [143]. An additional advantage of DBS is that D_1 is detectable at a deeper level of neuromuscular blockade than is T_1 [151].

Quantifying evoked responses

Whenever a muscle relaxant is administered, patients should be monitored until normal neuromuscular function is restored. Residual blockade during the recovery period can cause serious complications. Proper monitoring provides information about the degree and duration of neuromuscular blockade, and assures the observer that no residual blockade is present prior to recovery from anesthesia. In veterinary patients, the most common method used for assessing the degree of neuromuscular blockade is visual observation of the evoked response from peripheral nerve stimulation. With experienced observers, visual observation is adequate in most clinical situations. However, more accurate evaluation of the depth and duration of block is best achieved when the muscle response is recorded and measured. The two methods for accurately quantifying the evoked response are mechanically recorded, where the twitch tension by the muscle is measured using a force displacement transducer, and electromyographically recorded, where the muscle action potential is measured.

Mechanomyography

Mechanomyography (MMG) measures the evoked response of the stimulated muscle by force translation. The use of this method has been described in cats, dogs, horses, ponies, cows, and llamas [49,138,139,152–154]. With the limb immobilized, stimulating electrodes are placed over a peripheral nerve (peroneal or ulnar). The force transducer is attached to a paw or hoof at a right angle to the direction of muscle contraction. For maximum evoked muscle-twitch tension, a resting tension of 100–300 g should be applied. A supramaximal stimulus is applied to the nerve by using a single-twitch, TOF, or double-burst stimulation pattern. The resultant twitch tension can then be quantified. By using MMG, the depth and duration of neuromuscular blockade can be determined accurately. However, limitations make its use in many clinical situations impractical. To prevent changes in resting tension and twitch angle, the limb must be immobilized and no movement should occur during the recording period [155].

Electromyography

Electromyography (EMG) measures the compound action potential of muscle fibers contracting during a supramaximal stimulus of a peripheral motor nerve. With the stimulating electrodes placed over a peripheral nerve, the recording electrode is placed over the innervation zone of the muscle, midway between its origin and insertion. Also required are a reference electrode, placed over the insertion site, and a ground electrode, placed between the other two electrodes. EMG has the advantage of requiring less (or no) limb immobilization and no resting tension, and there are more choices as to which muscles may be used [155]. In a study in dogs given atracurium, there was no statistical difference between MMG and EMG during TOF stimulation for either T_1 or T_4:T_1 [156]. The disadvantage of EMG is that it may be difficult to obtain proper electrode placement for accurate results, particularly in smaller patients. Until a standard method is developed and validated for various species and sites of monitoring, MMG will remain the gold standard for quantifying evoked responses.

Reversal of neuromuscular blockade

Non-depolarizing blockade

As previously reviewed, acetylcholinesterase is present in high concentrations at the neuromuscular junction. It hydrolyzes ACh into choline and acetic acid, terminating the effects of ACh. The effects of non-depolarizing muscle relaxants are antagonized by administering an anticholinesterase (also known as an acetylcholinesterase inhibitor). This class of drug inhibits the enzyme acetylcholinesterase, increasing the concentration of ACh molecules at the neuromuscular junction. Since non-depolarizing muscle relaxants and ACh compete for the same postsynaptic binding sites, the ACh increase can tip the balance of competition in favor of ACh, and neuromuscular transmission is restored.

The anticholinesterase drugs used to antagonize neuromuscular blockade include edrophonium, neostigmine, and pyridostigmine. They differ in how they inhibit acetylcholinesterase activity. Edrophonium produces a reversible inhibition by electrostatic attachment to the anionic site and by hydrogen bonding at the esteratic site on acetylcholinesterase. The action of edrophonium is relatively brief because a covalent bond is not formed and ACh can easily compete with edrophonium for access to the enzyme. Neostigmine and pyridostigmine inhibit acetylcholinesterase by forming a carbamyl-ester complex at the esteratic site of acetylcholinesterase. This bond lasts longer when compared with the bond of the enzyme with ACh, thereby preventing acetylcholinesterase from accessing ACh.

The reversal agents vary in their onset of action. In order from the shortest to the longest onset is edrophonium < neostigmine < pyridostigmine. In human patients, neostigmine is 4.4 times more potent than pyridostigmine and 5.7 times more potent than edrophonium for reversal of non-depolarizing neuromuscular blockade [157]. The duration of action is similar for both neostigmine and edrophonium, whereas that of pyridostigmine is approximately 40% longer [157,158]. In cats, neostigmine is 12 times more potent than edrophonium [159].

Antiacetylcholinesterase agents are primarily metabolized by the liver, with hepatic biotransformation eliminating 50% of a neostigmine dose, 30% of an edrophonium dose, and 25% of a pyridostigmine dose. Renal excretion eliminates the remainder of the drug. Patients with renal failure will have prolonged elimination of an anticholinesterase drug.

The ACh accumulation following the administration of an anticholinesterase drug is not specific to the neuromuscular junction. While nicotinic effects occur at the neuromuscular junction and autonomic ganglia, muscarinic cholinergic effects occur because of inhibition of acetylcholinesterase at the sinus node, smooth muscle, and glands. Clinical effects of increased ACh concentrations at these sites include bradycardia, sinus arrest, bronchospasm, miosis, intestinal hyperperistalsis, and salivation. For this reason, it is advised that an anticholinergic drug, either atropine or glycopyrrolate, be administered immediately prior to reversal of neuromuscular blockade with an anticholinesterase. When choosing between atropine and glycopyrrolate, one must consider that atropine has a faster onset of action, which is more likely to cause an initial tachycardia, and will cross the blood–brain and blood–placenta barriers. Compared with neostigmine and pyridostigmine, the muscarinic effects of edrophonium are mild, so it may be chosen for reversal when one wants to avoid the use of an anticholinergic. For example, edrophonium is frequently chosen in equine patients because anticholinergic drug administration has been associated with the development of ileus and colic.

Depolarizing blockade

Recovery from succinylcholine (Phase I block) is rapid and spontaneous because of succinylcholine hydrolysis by plasma cholinesterases. Recovery may be delayed in patients with decreases in plasma cholinesterase activity. The administration of an anticholinesterase would actually prolong the depolarizing block [160]. On the other hand, a Phase II block from succinylcholine can be antagonized similarly to the non-depolarizing muscle relaxants, emphasizing the need for determining the type (Phase I or Phase II) of block present when using succinylcholine (see Table 14.3) [161,162].

Centrally acting muscle relaxants

Guaifenesin

Guaifenesin is used routinely as a muscle relaxant in large animal species. Its mechanism of action is to disrupt nerve impulse transmission at the level of the internuncial neurons of the spinal cord, brainstem, and subcortical areas of the brain. At therapeutic doses, skeletal muscle relaxes, but there is little effect on the respiratory muscles or diaphragm. Guaifenesin does not provide analgesia or produce unconsciousness. Therefore, it should not be used alone for any painful surgical or diagnostic procedure. No antagonist is available to reverse the muscle relaxant effects of guaifenesin.

Guaifenesin is commercially available as either a powder, which is reconstituted to the desired concentration with sterile water, or as a ready-made solution. Concentrations of 5%, 10%, and 15% have been used, with a 5% solution in 5% dextrose being the most common. Guaifenesin administered intravenously in high concentrations (>10%) can cause hemolysis, hemoglobinuria, and venous thrombosis [163]. Tissue can be damaged if guaifenesin is inadvertently administered perivascularly [163].

The cardiopulmonary effects of guaifenesin, alone or in combination with xylazine, ketamine, or thiobarbiturates, have been studied in horses. When guaifenesin is given alone, heart rate, respiratory rate, right atrial pressure, pulmonary arterial pressure, and cardiac output are unchanged. Systolic, diastolic, and mean arterial pressures are decreased. Xylazine (1.1 mg/kg IV), given prior to guaifenesin administration, reduced the dose necessary to achieve lateral recumbency (88 ± 10 mg/kg) compared with guaifenesin alone (134 ± 34 mg/kg). The addition of xylazine typically decreases heart rate, respiratory rate, cardiac output, and arterial oxygen partial pressure (PaO_2). Central venous pressure increases, whereas systolic, diastolic, and mean arterial blood pressures commonly decrease [164,165].

Guaifenesin can be combined with thiopental for both induction and maintenance of anesthesia in horses. Following premedication with either xylazine or acepromazine, a combination of guaifenesin and thiopental (2–3 g of thiopental in 1 L of 5% guaifenesin) is given for induction or, alternatively, guaifenesin is given until the horse is wobbly and buckling at the knees, and then a bolus of thiopental (4 mg/kg) is administered. Short periods of anesthesia (<1 h) can be maintained by a continuous infusion of the guaifenesin-thiopental combination.

A significant amount of guaifenesin crosses the placental barrier in pregnant mares [165]. Stallions may have up to 1.5 times longer action compared with mares. The longer recovery time in male horses is attributed to slower drug elimination from the plasma [166].

Guaifenesin has also been combined with thiobarbiturates or ketamine for use in cattle, small ruminants, and swine [167,168]. Although guaifenesin has been used in dogs, the large volume requirement makes it impractical for routine use in this species [169]. However, when combined with a thiobarbiturate or ketamine combined with xylazine, guaifenesin has proven an effective component when immobilizing dogs [170].

Dantrolene

Dantrolene is a hydantoin derivative that interferes with excitation-contraction coupling, thus relaxing skeletal muscle through a decrease in the amount of calcium released from the sarcoplasmic reticulum. Therapeutic doses do not adversely affect cardiac or smooth muscle and do not depress respiration [171]. Dantrolene is the drug of choice for the treatment of malignant hyperthermia. In swine, the recommended dose is 1–3 mg/kg IV when treating a malignant hyperthermia crisis and 5 mg/kg orally for prophylaxis [172]. Dantrolene is supplied in 20 mg vials in powder form with 3 g of mannitol to improve solubility. It is reconstituted using 60 mL of sterile water to achieve a concentration of 0.33 mg/mL. The oral preparation comes in various sized capsules.

The prophylactic use of dantrolene in animal patients prone to malignant hyperthermia is no longer routinely recommended. Pretreatment with dantrolene prior to anesthesia does not guarantee effective blood levels and, in equine patients, may produce unwanted skeletal muscle weakness during the recovery period. In susceptible patients, an anesthetic regimen using non-triggering anesthetics should be used, and dantrolene should be immediately available. However, the intravenous preparation of dantrolene may be cost prohibitive and not economically justifiable for many veterinary clinics to keep in stock. Most human hospital pharmacies have the intravenous formulation and may sell the needed amount to the veterinary clinic when required. Compounding the oral preparation for intravenous use has been described. The process is complex and time consuming, but dantrolene powder can be stored for rapid reconstitution during a malignant hyperthermia crisis [173,174].

Metabolism of dantrolene is via the liver through oxidative and reductive pathways. Metabolites and the unchanged drug are excreted in the urine. Dantrolene can cause muscle weakness, nausea, and diarrhea. Fatal hepatitis has occurred in human patients after chronic treatment with dantrolene [175]. Severe myocardial depression has been reported when dantrolene is administered concurrently with verapamil or other calcium channel blockers [176,177]. Synergism, resulting in a delayed recovery of neuromuscular function, has been observed with dantrolene and vecuronium co-administration [178].

References

1 Foldes FF, McNall PG, Borrego-Hinojosa JM. Succinyl-choline, a new approach to muscular relaxation in anaesthesiology. *N Engl J Med* 1952; **247**: 596–600.
2 Pickett D. Curare in canine surgery. *J Am Vet Med Assoc* 1951; **119**: 346–353.
3 Miller RM. Psychological effects of succinylcholine chloride immobilization in the horse. *Vet Med Small Anim Clin* 1966; **61**: 941–943.
4 Booij LH, Edwards RP, Sohn YJ, Miller RD. Cardiovascular and neuromuscular effects of Org NC 45, pancuronium, metocurine, and d-tubocurarine in dogs. *Anesth Analg* 1980; **59**: 26–30.
5 Bowman WC. Prejunctional and postjunctional cholinoceptors at the neuromuscular junction. *Anes Analg* 1980; **59**: 935–943.
6 Edwards C. The effects of innervation on the properties of acetylcholine receptors in muscle. *Neuroscience* 1979; **4**: 565–584.
7 Steinbach JH. Neuromuscular junctions and alpha-bungarotoxin-binding sites in denervated and contralateral cat skeletal muscles. *J Physiol* 1981; **313**: 513–528.
8 Fambrough DM. Control of acetylcholine receptors in skeletal muscle. *Physiol Rev* 1979; **59**: 165–227.
9 Stya M, Axelrod D. Mobility of extrajunctional acetylcholine receptors on denervated adult muscle fibers. *J Neurosci* 1984; **4**: 70–74.
10 Azar I. The response of patients with neuromuscular disorders to muscle relaxants: a review. *Anesthesiology* 1984; **61**: 173–187.
11 Gronert GA, Theye RA. Pathophysiology of hyperkalemia induced by succinylcholine. *Anesthesiology* 1975; **43**: 89–99.
12 Hirokawa N, Heuser JE. Internal and external differentiations of the postsynaptic membrane at the neuromuscular junction. *J Neurocytol* 1982; **11**: 487–510.
13 Changeux JP, Bon F, Cartaud J, *et al.* Allosteric properties of the acetylcholine receptor protein from Torpedo marmorata. *Cold Spring Harb Symp Quant Biol* 1983; **48**: 35–52.
14 Stroud RM. Acetycholine receptor structure, function, and evolution. *Annu Rev Cell Biol* 1982; **1**: 317–351.
15 Fairclough RH, Finer-Moore J, Love RA, *et al.* Subunit organization and structure of an acetylcholine receptor. *Cold Spring Harb Symp Quant Biol* 1983; **48**: 9–20.
16 Guy HR. A structural model of the acetylcholine receptor channel based on partition energy and helix packing calculations. *Biophys J* 1984; **45**: 249–261.
17 Neubig RR, Boyd ND, Cohen JB. Conformations of Torpedo acetylcholine receptor associated with ion transport and desensitization. *Biochemistry* 1982; **21**: 3460–3467.
18 Sheridan RE, Lester HA. Functional stoichiometry at the nicotinic receptor. *J Gen Physiol* 1982; **80**: 499–515.
19 Brown RD, Taylor P. The influence of antibiotics on agonist occupation and functional states of the nicotinic acetylcholine receptor. *Mol Pharmacol* 1983; **23**: 8–16.
20 Madsen BW, Albuquerque EX. The narcotic antagonist naltrexone has a biphasic effect on the nicotinic acetylcholine receptor. *FEBS Lett* 1985; **182**: 20–24.
21 Albuquerque EX, Akiake A, Shaw DP, Rickett DL. The interaction of anticholinesterase agents with the acetylcholine receptor-ionic channel complex. *Fundam Appl Toxicol* 1984; **4**: S27–S33.
22 Cohen JB, Boyd ND, Shera NS. Interactions of anesthetics with nicotinic postsynaptic membranes isolated from Torpedo electric tissue. *Progr Anesth* 1980; **2**:165–174.
23 Dreyer F. Acetylcholine receptor. *Br J Anaesth* 1982; **54**: 115–130.
24 Lambert JJ, Durant NN, Henderson EG. Drug-induced modification of ionic conductance at the neuromuscular junction. *Annu Rev Pharmacol Toxicol* 1983; **23**: 505–539.
25 Colquhoun D, Sheridan RE. The modes of action of gallamine. *Proc R Soc Lond B Biol Sci* 1981; **211**: 181–203.
26 Ogden DC, Colquhoun D. Ion channel block by acetylcholine, carbachol, and suberyldicholine at the frog neuromuscular junction. *Proc R Soc Lond B Biol Sci* 1985; **225**: 329–355.
27 Shanks CA. Pharmacokinetics of the nondepolarizing neuromuscular relaxants applied to calculation of bolus and infusion dosage regimens. *Anesthesiology* 1986; **64**: 72–86.
28 Upton RA, Nguyen TL, Miller RD, Castagnoli N Jr. Renal and biliary elimination of vecuronium (ORG NC 45) and pancuronium in rats. *Anesth Analg* 1982; **61**: 313–316.
29 Birch JH, Foldes FF, Rendell-Baker L. Causes and prevention of prolonged apnea with succinylcholine. *Curr Res Anesth Analg* 1956; **35**: 609–633.
30 Pantuck EJ. Ecothiopate iodide eye drops and prolonged response to suxamethonium. *Br J Anaesth* 1966; **38**: 406–407.
31 Kopman AF, Strachovsky G, Lichtenstein L. Prolonged response to succinylcholine following physostigmine. *Anesthesiology* 1978; **49**: 142–143.
32 Bentz EW, Stoelting RK. Prolonged response to succinylcholine following pancuronium reversal with pyridostigmine. *Anesthesiology* 1976; **44**: 258–260.
33 Jones RS, Heckmann R, Wuersch W. Observations on the duration of action of suxamethonium in the dog. *Br Vet J* 1978; **134**: 521–523.
34 Short CE, Cuneio J, Cupp D. Organophosphate-induced complications during anesthetic management in the horse. *J Am Vet Med Assoc* 1971; **159**: 1319–1327.
35 Reynolds WT. Use of suxamethonium in cats fitted with dichlorvos flea collars. *Aust Vet J* 1985; **62**: 106–107.
36 Gleed RD, Jones RS. Observations on the neuromuscular blocking action of gallamine and pancuronium and their reversal by neostigmine. *Res Vet Sci* 1982; **32**: 324–326.
37 Jones RS, Hunter JM, Utting JE. Neuromuscular blocking action of atracurium in the dog and its reversal by neostigmine. *Res Vet Sci* 1983; **34**: 173–176.
38 Fisher DM, Canfell PC, Fahey MR, *et al.* Elimination of atracurium in humans: contribution of Hofmann elimination and ester hydrolysis versus organ-based elimination. *Anesthesiology* 1986; **65**: 6–12.
39 Fahey MR, Rupp SM, Fisher DM, *et al.* The pharmacokinetics and pharmacodynamics of atracurium in patients with and without renal failure. *Anesthesiology* 1984; **61**: 699–702.
40 Playfor SD, Thomas DA, Choonara I. The effect of induced hypothermia on the duration of action of atracurium when given by infusion to critically ill children. *Paediatr Anaesth* 2000; **10**: 83–88.
41 Scott RP, Savarese JJ, Basta SJ, *et al.* Clinical pharmacology of atracurium given in high dose. *Br J Anaesth* 1986; **58**: 834–838.
42 Stoops CM, Curtis CA, Kovach DA, *et al.* Hemodynamic effects of mivacurium chloride administered to patients during oxygen-sufentanil anesthesia for coronary artery bypass grafting or valve replacement. *Anesth Analg* 1989; **68**: 333–339.
43 Wastila WB, Maehr RB, Turner GL, *et al.* Comparative pharmacology of cisatracurium (51W89), atracurium, and five isomers in cats. *Anesthesiology* 1996; **85**: 169–177.
44 Sparr HJ, Beaufort TM, Fuchs-Buder T. Newer neuromuscular blocking agents: how do they compare with established agents? *Drugs* 2001; **61**: 919–942.
45 Morris RB, Cahalan MK, Miller RD, *et al.* The cardiovascular effects of vecuronium (ORG NC45) and pancuronium in patients undergoing coronary artery bypass grafting. *Anesthesiology* 1983; **58**: 438–440.
46 Jones RS. Neuromuscular blocking action of vecuronium in the dog and its reversal by neostigmine. *Res Vet Sci* 1985; **38**: 193–196.
47 Caldwell JE, Szenohradszky J, Segredo V, *et al.* The pharmacodynamics and pharmacokinetics of the metabolite 3-desacetylvecuronium (ORG 7268) and its parent compound, vecuronium, in human volunteers. *J Pharmacol Exp Ther* 1994; **270**: 1216–1222.
48 Lebrault C, Berger JL, D'Hollander AA, *et al.* Pharmacokinetics and pharmacodynamics of vecuronium (ORG NC 45) in patients with cirrhosis. *Anesthesiology* 1985; **62**: 601–605.
49 Cason B, Baker DG, Hickey RF, *et al.* Cardiovascular and neuromuscular effects of three steroidal neuromuscular blocking drugs in dogs (ORG 9616, ORG 9426, ORG 9991). *Anesth Analg* 1990; **70**: 382–388.
50 Gyermek L, Chingmuh L, Cho YM, Nguyen N. Neuromuscular pharmacology of TAAC3, a new nondepolarizing muscle relaxant with rapid onset and ultrashort duration of action. *Anesth Analg* 2002; **94**: 879–885.
51 Hudson ME, Rothfield KP, Tullock WC, Firestone LL. Haemodynamic effects of rocuronium bromide in adult cardiac surgical patients. *Can J Anaesth* 1998; **45**: 139–143.
52 Adam JM, Bennet DJ, Bom A, *et al.* Cyclodextrin host molecules as reversal agents for the neuromuscular blocker rocuronium bromide: synthesis and structure-activity relationships. *J Med Chem* 2002; **45**: 555–562.
53 Naguib M. Sugammadex: another milestone in clinical neuromuscular pharmacology. *Anesth Analg* 2007; **104**: 575–581.
54 Puhringer FK, Rox C, Sielenkamper AW, *et al.* Reversal of profound, high-dose rocuronium-induced neuromuscular blockade by sugammadex at two different time points. *Anesthesiology* 2008; **109**: 188–197.
55 Jones RS. Observations on the neuromuscular blocking action of pipecuronium in the dog. *Res Vet Sci* 1987; **43**: 101–103.
56 Martinez EA, Wooldridge AA, Hartsfield SM, Mealey KL. Neuromuscular effects of doxacurium chloride in isoflurane-anesthetized dogs. *Vet Surg* 1998; **27**: 2792–2783.
57 Smith LJ, Moon PF, Lukasik VM, Erb HN. Duration of action and hemodynamic properties of mivacurium chloride in dogs anesthetized with halothane. *Am J Vet Res* 1999; **60**: 1047–1050.

58 Smith LJ, Schwark WS, Cook DR, *et al.* Pharmacokinetic variables of mivacurium chloride after intravenous administration in dogs. *Am J Vet Res* 1999; **60**: 1051–1054.

59 Belmont MR, Lien CA, Tjan J, *et al.* Clinical pharmacology of GW280430A in humans. *Anesthesiology* 2004; **100**: 768–763.

60 Caldwell JE. The continuing search for a succinylcholine replacement. *Anesthesiology* 2004; **100**: 763–764.

61 Lien CA. Development and potential clinical impact of ultra-short acting neuromuscular blocking agents. *Br J Anaesth* 2011; **107(S1)**: I60–I71.

62 Heerdt PM, Kang R, The' A, *et al.* Cardiopulmonary effects of the novel neuromuscular blocking drug GW280430A (AV430A) in dogs. *Anesthesiology* 2004; **100**: 846–851.

63 Lein CA. The pharmacology of GW280430A: a new nondepolarizing neuromuscular blocking agent. *Semin Anesth Perioperat Med Pain* 2002; **21**: 86–91.

64 Leigh MD, McCoy DD, Belton MK, Lewis GB Jr. Bradycardia following intravenous administration of succinylcholine chloride to infants and children. *Anesthesiology* 1957; **18**: 698–702.

65 Schoenstadt DA, Whitcher CE. Observations on the mechanism of succinyldicholine-induced cardiac arrhythmias. *Anesthesiology* 1963; **24**: 358–362.

66 Galindo AH, Davis TB. Succinylcholine and cardiac excitability. *Anesthesiology* 1962; **23**: 32–40.

67 Moss J, Rosow CE, Savarese JJ, *et al.* Role of histamine in the hypotensive action of d-tubocurarine in humans. *Anesthesiology* 1981; **55**: 19–25.

68 Booij LH, Edwards RP, Sohn YJ, Miller RD. Cardiovascular and neuromuscular effects of Org NC 45, pancuronium, metocurine, and d-tubocurarine in dogs. *Anesth Analg* 1980; **59**: 26–30.

69 Reitan JA, Warpinski MA. Cardiovascular effects of pancuronium bromide in mongrel dogs. *Am J Vet Res* 1975; **36**: 1309–1311.

70 Durant NN, Marshall IG, Savage DS, *et al.* The neuromuscular and autonomic blocking activities of pancuronium, Org NC 45, and other pancuronium analogues, in the cat. *J Pharm Pharmacol* 1979; **31**: 831–836.

71 Domenech JS, Garcia RC, Sastain JM, *et al.* Pancuronium bromide: an indirect sympathomimetic agent. *Br J Anaesth* 1976; **48**: 1143–1148.

72 Klein L, Hopkins J, Beck E, Burton B. Cumulative dose responses to gallamine, pancuronium, and neostigmine in halothane-anesthetized horses: neuromuscular and cardiovascular effects. *Am J Vet Res* 1983; **44**: 786–792.

73 Manley SV, Steffey EP, Howitt GA, Woliner M. Cardiovascular and neuromuscular effects of pancuronium bromide in the pony. *Am J Vet Res* 1983; **44**: 1349–1353.

74 Hildebrand SV, Howitt GA. Neuromuscular and cardiovascular effects of pancuronium bromide in calves anesthetized with halothane. *Am J Vet Res* 1984; **45**: 1549–1552.

75 Muir AW, Marshall RJ. Comparative neuromuscular blocking effects of vecuronium, pancuronium, Org 6368 and suxamethonium in the anaesthetized domestic pig. *Br J Anaesth* 1987; **59**: 622–629.

76 Savarese JJ, Caldwell JE, Lien CA, Miller RD. Pharmacology of muscle relaxants and their antagonists. In: Miller RD, ed. *Anesthesia*, 5th edn. Philadelphia: Churchill Livingstone, 2000: 412–490.

77 Basta SJ, Savarese JJ, Ali HH, *et al.* Histamine-releasing potencies of atracurium, dimethyl tubocurarine and tubocurarine. *Br J Anaesth* 1983; **55(Suppl 1)**: 105S–106S.

78 Scott RP, Savarese JJ, Basta SJ, *et al.* Atracurium: clinical strategies for preventing histamine release and attenuating the haemodynamic response. *Br J Anaesth* 1985; **57**: 550–553.

79 Evans CA, Waud DR. Do maternally administered neuromuscular blocking agents interfere with fetal neuromuscular transmission? *Anesth Analg* 1973; **52**: 548–552.

80 Forbes AR, Cohen NH, Eger EI II. Pancuronium reduces halothane requirement in man. *Anesth Analg* 1979; **58**: 497–499.

81 Fahey MR, Sessler DI, Cannon JE, *et al.* Atracurium, vecuronium, and pancuronium do not alter the minimum alveolar concentration of halothane in humans. *Anesthesiology* 1989; **71**: 53–56.

82 Peduto VA, Gungui P, di Martino MR, Napoleone M. Accidental subarachnoid injection of pancuronium. *Anesth Analg* 1989; **69**: 516–517.

83 Goonewardene TW, Sentheshanmuganathan S, Kamalanathan S, Kanagasunderam R. Accidental subarachnoid injection of gallamine. A case report. *Br J Anaesth* 1975; **47**: 889–893.

84 Hennis PJ, Fahey MR, Canfell PC, *et al.* Pharmacology of laudanosine in dogs. *Anesthesiology* 1986; **65**: 56–60.

85 Ghoneim MM, Kramer E, Bannow R, *et al.* Binding of d-tubocurarine to plasma proteins in normal man and in patients with hepatic or renal disease. *Anesthesiology* 1973; **39**: 410–415.

86 Duvaldestin P, Henzel D. Binding of tubocurarine, fazadinium, pancuronium and Org NC 45 to serum proteins in normal man and in patients with cirrhosis. *Br J Anaesth* 1982; **54**: 513–516.

87 Carter JG, Sokoll MD, Gergis SD. Effect of spinal cord transection on neuromuscular function in the rat. *Anesthesiology* 1981; **55**: 542–546.

88 Pandey K, Badola RP, Kumar S. Time course of intraocular hypertension produced by suxamethonium. *Br J Anaesth* 1972; **44**: 191–196.

89 Indu B, Batra YK, Puri GD, Singh H. Nifedipine attenuates the intraocular pressure response to intubation following succinylcholine. *Can J Anaesth* 1989; **36**: 269–272.

90 Waters DJ, Mapleson WW. Suxamethonium pains: hypothesis and observation. *Anaesthesia* 1971; **26**: 127–141.

91 Magee DA, Robinson RJ. Effect of stretch exercises on suxamethonium induced fasciculations and myalgia. *Br J Anaesth* 1987; **59**: 596–601.

92 Maddineni VR, Mirakhur RK, Cooper AR. Myalgia and biochemical changes following suxamethonium after induction of anaesthesia with thiopentone or propofol. *Anaesthesia* 1993; **48**: 626–628.

93 McLoughlin C, Leslie K, Caldwell JE. Influence of dose on suxamethonium-induced muscle damage. *Br J Anaesth* 1994; **73**: 194–198.

94 Benson GJ, Hartsfield SM, Manning JP, Thurmon JC. Biochemical effects of succinylcholine chloride in mechanically ventilated horses anesthetized with halothane in oxygen. *Am J Vet Res* 1980; **41**: 754–756.

95 Silverman DG, Brull SJ. Features of neurostimulation. In: Silverman DG, ed. *Neuromuscular Block in Perioperative and Intensive Care.* Philadelphia: JB Lippincott, 1994; 23–36.

96 Klein LV. Neuromuscular blocking agents in equine anesthesia. *Vet Clin North Am Large Anim Pract* 1981; **3**: 135–161.

97 Hildebrand SV, Holland M, Copland VS, *et al.* Clinical use of the neuromuscular blocking agents atracurium and pancuronium for equine anesthesia. *J Am Vet Med Assoc* 1989; **195**: 212–219.

98 Duvaldstein P, Agoston S, Henzel D, *et al.* Pancuronium pharmacokinetics in patients with liver cirrhosis. *Br J Anaesth* 1978; **50**: 1131–1136.

99 Duvaldstein P, Berger JL, Videcoq M, Desmonts JM. Pharmacokinetics and pharmacodynamics of Org NC 45 in patients with cirrhosis. *Anesthesiology* 1982; **57**: A238.

100 Bencine AF, Houwertjes MC, Agoston S. Effects of hepatic uptake of vecuronium bromide and its putative metabolites on their neuromuscular blocking actions in the cat. *Br J Anaesth* 1985; **57**: 789–795.

101 Silverman DG, Mirakhur RK. Reversal of nondepolarizing block. In: Silverman DG, ed. *Neuromuscular Block in Perioperative and Intensive Care.* Philadelphia: JB Lippincott, 1994; 217–238.

102 Wood M. Plasma binding and limitation of drug access to site of action. *Anesthesiology* 1991; **75**: 721–723.

103 Wood M. Plasma drug binding: implications for anesthesiologists. *Anesth Analg* 1986; **65**: 786–804.

104 Wood M, Stone WJ, Wood AJ. Plasma binding of pancuronium: effects of age, sex, and disease. *Anesth Analg* 1983; **62**: 29–32.

105 Skivington MA. Protein binding of three titrated muscle relaxants. *Br J Anaesth* 1972; **44**: 1030–1034.

106 Lebrault C, Duvaldestin P, Henzel D, *et al.* Pharmacokinetics and pharmacodynamics of vecuronium in patients with cholestasis. *Br J Anaesth* 1986; **58**: 983–987.

107 Agoston S, Vermeer GA, Kersten UW, Meijer DKF. The fate of pancuronium bromide in man. *Acta Anaesthesiol Scand* 1973; **17**: 267–275.

108 Cook DR, Freeman JA, Lai AA, *et al.* Pharmacokinetics and pharmacodynamics of doxacurium in normal patients and in those with hepatic or renal failure. *Anesth Analg* 1991; **72**: 145–150.

109 Miller RD, Stevens WC, Way WL. The effect of renal failure and hyperkalemia on the duration of pancuronium neuromuscular blockade in man. *Anesth Analg* 1972: **52**; 661–666.

110 Cooper R, Maddineni VR, Mirakhur RK, *et al.* Time course of neuromuscular effect and pharmacokinetics of rocuronium bromide (ORG 9426) during isoflurane anesthesia in patients with and without renal failure. *Br J Anaesth* 1993; **71**: 222–226.

111 Phillips BJ, Hunter JM. The use of mivacurium chloride by constant infusion in the anephric patient. *Br J Anaesth* 1992; **68**: 492–498.

112 Ward S, Boheimer N, Weatherly BC, *et al.* Pharmacokinetics of atracurium and its metabolites in patients with normal renal function, and in patients with renal failure. *Br J Anaesth* 1987; **59**: 697–706.

113 Withington DE, Donati F, Bevan DR, Varin F. Potentiation of atracurium neuromuscular blockade by enflurane: time-course of effect. *Anesth Analg* 1991; **72**: 469–473.

114 Silverman DG, Mirakhur RK. Effect of other agents on nondepolarizing relaxants. In: Silverman DG, ed. *Neuromuscular Block in Perioperative and Intensive Care.* Philadelphia: JB Lippincott, 1994; 104–122.

115 Crul-Sluijter EJ, Crul JF. Acidosis and neuromuscular blockade. *Acta Anaesthesiol Scand* 1974; **18**: 224–236.

116 Funk DI, Crul JF, Pol FM. Effects of changes in acid-base balance on neuromuscular blockade produced by ORG-NC 45. *Acta Anaesthesiol Scand* 1980; **24**: 119–124.

117 Gencarelli PJ, Swen J, Koot HWJ, Miller RD. The effects of hypercarbia and hypocarbia on pancuronium and vecuronium neuromuscular blockades in anesthetized humans. *Anesthesiology* 1983; **59**: 376–380.
118 Hughes R, Chapple DJ. The pharmacology of atracurium: a new competitive neuromuscular blocking agent. *Br J Anaesth* 1981; **53**: 31–44.
119 Miller RD, Roderick LL. The influence of acid-base changes on neostigmine antagonism of pancuronium neuromuscular blockade. *Br J Anaesth* 1978; **50**: 317–324.
120 Waud BE, Waud DR. Interaction of calcium and potassium with neuromuscular blocking agents. *Br J Anaesth* 1980; **52**: 863–866.
121 Ghoneim MM, Long JP. The interaction between magnesium and other neuromuscular blocking agents. *Anesthesiology* 1970; **32**: 23–27.
122 Gramstad L, Hysing ES. Effect of ionized calcium on the neuromuscular blocking actions of atracurium and vecuronium in the cat. *Br J Anaesth* 1990; **64**: 199–206.
123 Meakin G, Morton RH, Wareham AC. Age-dependent variations in response to tubocurarine in the isolated rat diaphragm. *Br J Anaesth* 1992; **68**: 161–163.
124 Meretoja OA. Is vecuronium a long-acting neuromuscular blocking agent in neonates and infants? *Br J Anaesth* 1989; **62**: 184–187.
125 Meakin G, Shaw EA, Baker RD, Morris P. Comparison of atracurium-induced neuromuscular blockade in neonates, infants, and children. *Br J Anaesth* 1988; **60**: 171–175.
126 Debaene B, Meistelman C, d'Hollander A. Recovery from vecuronium neuromuscular blockade following neostigmine administration in infants, children, and adults during halothane anesthesia. *Anesthesiology* 1989; **71**: 840–844.
127 Marsh RHK, Chjmielewski AT, Goat VA. Recovery from pancuronium: a comparison between old and young patients. *Anaesthesia* 1980; **35**: 1193–1196.
128 Young WI, Matteo RS, Ornstein E. Duration of action of neostigmine and pyridostigmine in the elderly. *Anesth Analg* 1988; **67**: 775–778.
129 Fikes LL, Dodman NH, Court MH. Anaesthesia for small animal patients with neuromuscular disease. *Br Vet J* 1990; **146**: 487–499.
130 Fergusson RJ, Wright DJ, Willey RF, *et al.* Suxamethonium is dangerous in polyneuropathy. *BMJ (Clin Res Ed)* 1981; **282**: 298–299.
131 Nilsson E, Meretoja OA. Vecuronium dose-response and maintenance requirements in patients with myasthenia gravis. *Anesthesiology* 1990; **73**: 28–32.
132 Eisenkraft JB, Book WJ, Mann SM, Papatestas AE. Resistance to succinylcholine in myasthenia gravis: a dose-response study. *Anesthesiology* 1988; **69**: 760–763.
133 Silverman DG. Myasthenia gravis and myasthenic syndrome. In: Silverman DG, ed. *Neuromuscular Block in Perioperative and Intensive Care*. Philadelphia: JB Lippincott, 1994; 324–331.
134 Jones RS, Sharp NJH. Use of the muscle relaxant atracurium in a myasthenic dog. *Vet Rec* 1985; **117**: 500–501.
135 Jones RS, Brown A, Watkins PE. Use of the muscle relaxant atracurium in a myasthenic dog. *Vet Rec* 1988; **122**: 611.
136 Singh TN, Marshall IG, Harvey AC. Pre- and postjunctional blocking effects of aminoglycoside, polymyxin, tetracycline, and lincosamide antibiotics. *Br J Anaesth* 1982; **54**: 1295–1305.
137 Sucoll MD, Gergis SD. Antibiotics and neuromuscular function. *Anesthesiology* 1981; **55**: 148–159.
138 Hildebrand SV, Hill T. Interaction of gentamycin and atracurium in anaesthetized horses. *Equine Vet J* 1994; **26**: 209–211.
139 Forsyth SF, Ilkiw JE, Hildebrand SV. Effect of gentamicin administration on the neuromuscular blockade induced by atracurium in cats. *Am J Vet Res* 1990; **51**: 1675–1678.
140 Potter JM, Edeson RG, Campbell RJ, Forbes AM. Potentiation by gentamicin of non-depolarizing neuromuscular block in the cat. *Anaesth Intensive Care* 1980; **8**: 20–25.
141 Martinez EA, Mealey KL, Wooldridge AA, *et al.* Pharmacokinetics, effects on renal function, and potentiation of atracurium-induced neuromuscular blockade after administration of a high dose of gentamicin in isoflurane-anesthetized dogs. *Am J Vet Res* 1996; **57**: 1623–1626.
142 Ali HH, Savarese JJ. Stimulus frequency and dose-response curve to d-tubocurarine in man. *Anesthesiology* 1980; **52**: 36–39.
143 Silverman DG, Brull SJ. Patterns of stimulation. In: Silverman DG, ed. *Neuromuscular Block in Perioperative and Intensive Care*. Philadelphia: JB Lippincott, 1994; 37–50.
144 Waud BE, Waud DR. The relationship between the response to 'train-of-four' stimulation and receptor occlusion during competitive neuromuscular block. *Anesthesiology* 1972; **37**: 413–416.
145 Brand JB, Cullen DJ, Wilson NE, Ali HH. Spontaneous recovery from nondepolarizing neuromuscular blockade: correlation between clinical and evoked response. *Anesth Analg* 1977; **56**: 55–58.
146 Klein LV. Neuromuscular blocking agents. In: Short CE, ed. *Principles and Practice of Veterinary Anesthesia*. Baltimore, MD: Williams and Wilkins, 1987; 134–153.
147 Hildebrand SV. Neuromuscular blocking agents in equine anesthesia. *Vet Clin North Am Equine Pract* 1990; **6**: 587–606.
148 Hildebrand SV. Neuromuscular blocking agents. *Vet Clin North Am Small Anim Pract* 1992; **22**: 341–346.
149 Torda TA, Graham GG, Tsui D. Neuromuscular sensitivity to atracurium in humans. *Anaesth Intensive Care* 1990; **18**: 62–68.
150 Viby-Morgenson J, Howardy-Hansen P, Chraemmer-Jorgensen B, *et al.* Posttetanic count (PTC): a new method of evaluating an intense nondepolarizing neuromuscular blockade. *Anesthesiology* 1981; **55**: 458–461.
151 Braude N, Vyvyan HAL, Jordan MJ. Intraoperative assessment of atracurium-induced neuromuscular block using double burst stimulation. *Br J Anaesth* 1991; **67**: 574–578.
152 Hildebrand SV, Howitt GA. Dosage requirement of pancuronium in halothane-anesthetized ponies: a comparison of cumulative and single-dose administration. *Am J Vet Res* 1984; **45**: 2441–2444.
153 Bowen JM. Monitoring neuromuscular function in intact animals. *Am J Vet Res* 1969; **30**: 857–859.
154 Hildebrand SV, Hill T. Neuromuscular blockade by atracurium in llamas. *Vet Surg* 1991; **20**: 153–154.
155 Law SC, Cook DR. Monitoring the neuromuscular junction. In: Lake CL, ed. *Clinical Monitoring*. Philadelphia: WB Saunders, 1990; 719–755.
156 Martinez EA, Hartsfield SM, Carroll GL. Comparison of two methods to assess neuromuscular blockade in anesthetized dogs. *Vet Surg* 1998; **28**: 127.
157 Cronnelly R, Morris RB, Miller RD. Edrophonium: duration of action and atropine requirement in humans during halothane anesthesia. *Anesthesiology* 1982; **57**: 261–265.
158 Morris RB, Cronnelly R, Miller RD, *et al.* Pharmacokinetics of edrophonium and neostigmine when antagonizing d-tubocurarine neuromuscular blockade in man. *Anesthesiology* 1981; **54**: 399–402.
159 Baird WLM, Bowman WC, Kerr WJ. Some actions of NC 45 and of edrophonium in the anesthetized cat and man. *Br J Anaesth* 1982; **54**: 375–385.
160 Jones RS, Heckmann R, Wuersch W. The effect of neostigmine on the duration of action of suxamethonium in the dog. *Br Vet J* 1980; **136**: 71–73.
161 Lee C. Train-of-four fade and edrophonium antagonism of neuromuscular block by succinylcholine in man. *Anesth Analg* 1976; **55**: 663–667.
162 Cullen LK, Jones RS. The effect of neostigmine on suxamethonium neuromuscular block in the dog. *Res Vet Sci* 1980; **29**: 266–268.
163 Hall LW, Clarke KW, Trim CM. *Veterinary Anaesthesia*, 10th edn. London: WB Saunders, 2001; 149–178.
164 Hubbell JAE, Muir WW, Sams RA. Guaifenesin: cardiopulmonary effects and plasma concentrations in horses. *Am J Vet Res* 1980; **41**: 1751–1755.
165 Greene SA, Thurmon JC, Tranquilli WJ, Benson GJ. Cardiopulmonary effects of continuous intravenous infusion of guaifenesin, ketamine, and xylazine in ponies. *Am J Vet Res* 1986; **47**: 2364–2367.
166 Davis LE, Wolff WA. Pharmacokinetics and metabolism of glyceryl guaiacolate in ponies. *Am J Vet Res* 1970; **31**: 469–473.
167 Carroll GL, Hartsfield SM. General anesthetic techniques in ruminants. *Vet Clin North Am Food Anim Pract* 1996; **12**: 627–661.
168 Moon PF, Smith LJ. General anesthetic techniques in swine. *Vet Clin North Am Food Anim Pract* 1996; **12**: 663–691.
169 Tavernor WD, Jones EW. Observations on the cardiovascular and respiratory effects of guaiacol glycerol ether in conscious and anaesthetized dogs. *J Small Anim Pract* 1970; **11**: 177–184.
170 Benson GJ, Thurmon JC, Tranquilli WJ, Smith CW. Cardiopulmonary effects of an intravenous infusion of guaifenesin, ketamine, and xylazine in dogs. *Am J Vet Res* 1985; **46**: 1896–1898.
171 Pinder RM, Brogden RN, Speight TM, Avery GS. Dantrolene sodium: a review of its pharmacological properties and therapeutic efficacy in spasticity. *Drugs* 1977; **13**: 3–23.
172 Gronert GA, Milde JH, Theye RA. Dantrolene in porcine malignant hyperthermia. *Anesthesiology* 1976; **41**: 488–495.
173 Gronert GA, Mansfield E, Theye RA. Rapidly soluble dantrolene for intravenous use. In: Aldrete JA, Britt BA, eds. *Malignant Hyperthermia*. New York: Grune and Stratton, 1978; 535–536.
174 O'Brien PJ, Forsyth GW. Preparation of injectable dantrolene for emergency treatment of malignant hyperthermia-like syndromes. *Can Vet J* 1983; **24**: 200–204.
175 Stoelting RK. *Pharmacology and Physiology in Anesthetic Practice*, 2nd edn. Philadelphia: JB Lippincott, 1991; 541–548.
176 Roewer N, Rumberger E, Bode H, *et al.* Electrophysiological and mechanical interactions of verapamil and dantrolene on isolated heart muscle. *Anesthesiology* 1985; **63**: A274.
177 Bezer G. Dantrolene sodium intravenous – verapamil. *Anesth Intensive Care* 1985; **13**: 108–110.
178 Dreissen JJ, Wuis EW, Gieden JM. Prolonged vecuronium neuromuscular blockade in a patient receiving oral dantrolene. *Anesthesiology* 1985; **62**: 523–524.

15 Injectable Anesthetics

Stephanie H. Berry
Atlantic Veterinary College, University of Prince Edward Island, Charlottetown, Prince Edward Island, Canada

Chapter contents

Introduction

Injectable anesthetic drugs produce reliable sedation and anesthesia in veterinary patients. Most commonly, these agents are administered intravenously to induce an unconscious state suitable for intubation and transition to an inhalant anesthetic. However, when administered by constant rate infusion, intermittent bolus or intramuscularly, injectable anesthetics can also be used to maintain anesthesia for short periods of time.

Ideally, injectable anesthetics would be water soluble, have a long shelf-life, and be stable when exposed to heat and light. Only a small volume of drug would be needed to produce anesthesia, and these agents would have a large safety margin. Their duration of action would be short, with no cumulative effects, and they would be readily metabolized into non-toxic metabolites and/or excreted from the body. Their half-lives would be well characterized, as would their maximum residual limits so that withdrawal times could be established for animals destined for human consumption. Analgesia adequate for the procedure and some degree of muscle relaxation would also be produced by ideal injectable anesthetics. Most importantly perhaps, the ideal injectable anesthetic would not create unpredictable life-threatening changes in cardiovascular and respiratory function.

An injectable anesthetic that possesses all of these characteristics has not yet been produced. When selecting an injectable anesthetic, the practitioner should consider the pharmacokinetics and pharmacodynamics of the agent as well as the patient's physical status in order to select the most appropriate agent and dose for that individual patient.

Barbiturates

Chemical structure

Barbiturates have been used in veterinary medicine for decades as both injectable anesthetics and anticonvulsants. All of the drugs in this category are derivatives of barbituric acid, a combination of urea and malonic acid (Fig. 15.1). While barbituric acid does not have sedative or hypnotic properties, side-chains added at position

Veterinary Anesthesia and Analgesia: The Fifth Edition of Lumb and Jones.
Edited by Kurt A. Grimm, Leigh A. Lamont, William J. Tranquilli, Stephen A. Greene and Sheilah A. Robertson.

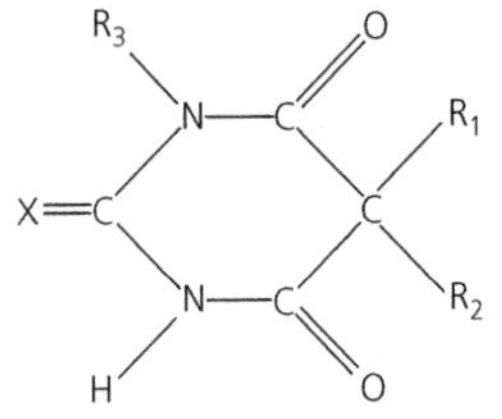

Figure 15.1 General formula of barbiturates.

5 in the pyrimidine nucleus impart hypnotic activity. The length of the side-chain at position 5 influences the potency and duration of action of these drugs, with longer side-chains increasing potency. If a sulfur atom replaces the oxygen atom at position 2, an active barbiturate with a faster onset of action and a shorter duration is produced. In general, any modification of the barbiturate that increases the lipophilicity of the molecule will increase its potency while shortening the onset time and duration of action. Many barbiturates (thiopental, thiamylal, methohexital) have asymmetric carbon atoms in one of the side-chains attached to the barbiturate ring at position 5, which results in stereoisomers. Despite differences in potency of the stereoisomers (L-isomers are nearly twice as potent as D-isomers), barbiturates are supplied as racemic mixtures.

Commonly, barbiturates are classified by their duration of action (long, intermediate, short, and ultra-short) or their chemical structure. Thiobarbiturates (thiopental and thiamylal) are those with a sulfur atom at position 2, while oxybarbiturates (pentobarbital, phenobarbital, and methohexital) have an oxygen atom at position 2.

Ultra-short acting thiobarbiturates are commonly used for anesthetic induction. Historically, thiopental was the most commonly used ultra-short acting barbiturate in veterinary medicine. It is a yellow crystalline powder buffered with sodium bicarbonate which is usually reconstituted with sterile water or saline to produce 2.5%, 5%, or 10% solutions. The resulting solution is alkaline (pH 10–11) and can cause tissue necrosis if injected perivascularly. The reconstituted solution is stable at room temperature for up to 1 week [1]. As the solution ages, crystals precipitate which results in a progressive loss of potency; therefore, higher doses may be needed to induce anesthesia.

Thiamylal is an ultra-short acting thiobarbiturate that differs from thiopental in that the ethyl radical in thiopental has been replaced with an allyl radical. While thiamylal was commonly used in veterinary medicine for some time, it is no longer commercially available.

Methohexital is an ultra-short acting oxybarbiturate that possesses a methyl group at the N-1 position. This results in a drug that is twice as potent as thiopental, but also has an increased incidence of excitatory side-effects. Methohexital sodium is supplied as a powder and is reconstituted with sterile water or saline to produce a 2.5% solution that is stable for up to 6 weeks if refrigerated [2].

Pentobarbital is classified as a short-acting oxybarbiturate that is identical to methohexital but lacks a methyl group at the N-1 position. It undergoes extensive hepatic metabolism and is totally dependent on the liver for biotransformation and elimination. The duration of action of pentobarbital is typically 4–8 times longer than that of thiopental in most species. Sheep and goats, however, are rapid metabolizers of the drug and require supplemental doses if anesthesia is to be maintained beyond 20–30 min. The longer duration of action, combined with a low therapeutic index, has resulted in pentobarbital being replaced as a general anesthetic in most domestic species. It is still used as an injectable anesthetic in laboratory rodents, particularly for non-recovery procedures, and remains the primary ingredient in most commercially available euthanasia solutions.

Mechanism of action

Barbiturates produce central nervous system (CNS) depression by activating the ionotropic subtype of the γ-aminobutyric acid (GABA) receptor known as $GABA_A$ [3]. Activation of the $GABA_A$ receptor increases transmembrane chloride conduction, resulting in hyperpolarization of the postsynaptic cell membrane. It appears that the barbiturates reduce the rate of dissociation of GABA from its receptor, which increases the duration of chloride channel opening. At increasing drug concentrations, barbiturates can mimic the action of GABA and activate the chloride channels directly [3,4]. Ultimately, inhibition of the postsynaptic neuron results in central nervous system depression and loss of consciousness.

Pharmacokinetics

After intravenous administration of thiopental, the drug mixes within the blood and is delivered to body tissues in accordance with the rate of perfusion, the tissue affinity for the drug, and the relative concentration of thiopental in the blood and tissues. Well-perfused, small-volume tissues such as the brain equilibrate rapidly with the thiopental concentrations in the blood, inducing anesthesia. The concentration of thiopental in the blood and brain falls rapidly as the drug redistributes to less perfused muscular tissues, allowing the animal to regain consciousness. The principal factor limiting anesthetic duration after a single dose of thiopental is redistribution from the brain to other tissues [5]. Therefore, when thiopental is administered in large doses, as repeated doses or as a constant rate infusion, recovery from anesthesia may be prolonged as tissues (e.g., muscle) approach equilibrium with the concentration of thiopental in the blood. This equilibrium progressively decreases the capacity of the tissues to remove the drug from the blood [6,7]. Additionally, obesity increases the mean disposition residence time of thiopental and this is associated with a prolongation of terminal half-life although the increased adipose mass will serve to remove more drug from the blood and speed clinical recovery from a single bolus [8].

Distribution of the barbiturates within the body is determined by factors such as time, protein binding, degree of ionization, and lipid solubility. Lipid solubility increases with the substitution of a sulfur molecule at carbon position 2 in the barbiturate ring. As previously stated, an increase in lipid solubility increases potency and shortens onset and duration of action. Protein binding correlates with lipid solubility, with those barbiturates that are highly lipophilic (thiopental) also being highly bound to protein. Decreased protein binding due to displacement from binding sites by other drugs (aspirin, phenylbutazone) or hypoproteinemia may lead to increased drug effects.

The acid dissociation constant (pKa) and pH of the environment can be used to predict the proportion of ionization of the barbiturates for any given condition. The pKa is the pH at which the barbiturate exists 50% in the ionized and 50% in non-ionized form. For a barbiturate to penetrate the lipid layer of a cell, it needs to be in the non-ionized form. Therefore, as blood becomes more acidic, more non-ionized drug exists. This leads to an increase in the barbiturate's CNS penetration and clinical effectiveness. The reverse is also true: with more alkaline blood the ionized form is favored and the anesthetic effect is reduced.

Pharmacokinetic parameters of thiopental have been described in the dog, sheep, and rabbit [9]. The initial volume of distribution was 38.1 ± 18.4, 44.5 ± 9.1, and 38.6 ± 10.0 mL/kg respectively [9]. The elimination half-life was shown to be shortest in the rabbit (43.1 ± 3.4 min) and longest in the sheep (251.9 ± 107.8 min) [9]. Elimination half-life in the dog was 182.4 ± 57.9 min [9].

Metabolism of the barbiturates occurs in the liver followed by excretion by the kidneys. Biotransformation in the liver occurs primarily in the endoplasmic reticulum of hepatocytes and can result in hepatic enzyme induction (P450 system) [5]. The reserve capacity of the liver is quite large so significant hepatic dysfunction must be present before there is a prolongation of the duration of action of barbiturates [10].

Pharmacodynamics

Central nervous system

As noted previously, administration of barbiturates results in CNS depression and anesthesia. The electroencephalogram (EEG) is depressed in a dose-dependent fashion with the administration of thiopental, with the awake α pattern progressing to δ and θ waves until there is burst suppression and a flat EEG [11]. The barbiturates appear to possess cerebroprotectant properties. Cerebral metabolism of oxygen ($CMRO_2$) is reduced by up to 55% in a dose-dependent fashion [12]. Cerebral blood flow and intracranial pressure (ICP) are also decreased in parallel with the reduction in $CMRO_2$ [12]. Cerebral perfusion pressure is usually not adversely affected, however, because the ICP decreases more than the mean arterial pressure. Several studies have been performed evaluating thiopental as a cerebroprotectant and have shown that it may be of some clinical value. In dogs pretreated with thiopental and subjected to isolated brainstem ischemia, auditory evoked potentials were increased compared to those dogs that were not pretreated with thiopental [13]. Additionally, it was demonstrated that the mitigating effect of immediate postarrest hypothermia in dogs with postischemic encephalopathy might be enhanced by thiopental [14]. These properties make thiopental an appropriate choice for patients with intracranial disease or a history of seizures. Methohexital has been associated with CNS excitation and epileptiform seizures, making it a poor choice for patients with seizures. Intraocular pressure (IOP) is reduced slightly by thiopental administration [15].

Cardiovascular system

Administration of lower doses of thiopental results in a decrease in stroke volume and myocardial contractility [16]. A mild decrease in arterial blood pressure can be seen, but it is often offset by a compensatory increase in heart rate. Venodilation after thiopental administration can lead to sequestration of red blood cells in the spleen, an increase in splenic size, and a decrease in packed cell volume. Vasodilation of cutaneous and skeletal blood vessels may also predispose the patient to hypothermia. Ventricular arrhythmias, particularly ventricular bigeminy, have also been demonstrated [17]. The incidence of these arrhythmias may be reduced with adequate ventilation and oxygenation prior to thiopental administration. Thiopental sensitizes the myocardium to epinephrine-induced arrhythmias in many species studied [18].

Respiratory system

Barbiturate administration for the induction of anesthesia causes dose-dependent depression of ventilatory centers along with decreased responsiveness to hypoxemia and hypercarbia [19]. There is also a decrease in respiratory rate and minute ventilation [20]. Transient periods of apnea are commonly reported after large, rapidly administered doses of thiopental. Thiopental has also been shown to cause bronchoconstriction in the dog [21]. However, laryngeal reflexes may be less affected with thiopental administration compared to other induction agents so it may be a good choice for evaluation of laryngeal function [22]. Thiopental has also been shown to reduce mucociliary clearance in the dog [23].

Hepatic, renal, and gastrointestinal systems

Healthy patients have little change in hepatic or gastrointestinal function after induction of anesthesia with thiopental and only modest decreases in hepatic blood flow may be seen. Barbiturates stimulate an increase in microsomal enzymes, but only after 2–7 days of sustained drug administration [24].

While gastrointestinal effects such as diarrhea or intestinal stasis have not been reported with barbiturate administration, thiopental has been shown to decrease the tone of the lower esophageal sphincter in cats [25].

Renal blood flow may be decreased slightly by thiopental administration, most likely due to decreases in systemic blood pressure and cardiac output. A 15 mg/kg dose of thiopental in the dog resulted in a mean glomerular filtration rate of 2.04 ± 0.36 mL/min/kg, which did not differ significantly from other induction agents [26].

Fetal/neonatal effects

Intravenous barbiturates cross the placenta and establish a dynamic equilibrium between maternal and fetal circulation. However, it should be remembered that the placental circulation passes through the liver before reaching the fetal CNS, thereby reducing overall drug exposure for most highly metabolized drugs. In a study performed in dogs, thiopental more profoundly depressed neurological reflexes in puppies born by cesarean section compared to propofol or epidural anesthesia [27]. Additionally, uterine blood flow transiently decreased in pregnant ewes induced with thiopental [28].

Analgesic effects

It should be noted that barbiturates do not produce antinociception (and analgesia only during unconsciousness); therefore additional analgesics should be administered to patients undergoing painful procedures. In fact, at subanesthetic doses, the barbiturates may actually be hyperalgesic. However, this effect is controversial, and likely not clinically significant [29].

Species-specific effects

Canine

Documented breed-associated differences in anesthetic pharmacokinetics and pharmacodynamics are uncommon. However, among canine breeds, Greyhounds are relatively deficient in the hepatic microsomal enzymes that are needed to metabolize the thiobarbiturates. This deficiency, along with lean bodies and low fat stores, potentially result in prolonged recoveries from thiopental anesthesia when larger doses are administered [24]. Barbiturate anesthetics are often not recommended for sighthound breeds (e.g., Greyhound, Irish Wolfhound, Afghan Hound) but use of anesthetic-sparing premedications and minimal thiobarbiturate doses has allowed safe anesthetic induction in these breeds with minimal delay in recovery.

Equine

The pharmacokinetics of a single dose of thiopental at 11 mg/kg has been studied following administration to horses [30]. In that study a three compartment open model best described the pharmacokinetics of thiopental. In plasma, thiopental has a very rapid initial distribution phase, with a half-life of 1.4 ± 1.2 min and 1.3 ± 0.7 min in horses and ponies, respectively. While horses had a somewhat shorter elimination half-life (147 ± 21 min) than ponies (222 ± 44 min), no obvious difference in clearance of the drug between horses (3.5 ± 0.5 mL/kg/min) and ponies (3.6 ± 0.8 mL/kg/min) was noted [30].

Thiopental should not be administered to horses without prior sedation with an α_2-adrenergic receptor agonist, as significant excitement and incoordination may result. Additionally, anesthesia induction with guaifenesin and thiopental in horses that have just undergone maximal exercise is not recommended [31].

Ruminant

The pharmacokinetics of thiopental in sheep has also been described using a three compartment open model [32]. The volume of distribution was 1005 ± 196 mL/kg, total body clearance was 3.5 ± 0.8 mL/kg/min and half-life was 196 ± 64 min in that study. Time of awaking was 36.6 ± 6.36 min [32]. The authors suggest that the relatively short duration of action of thiopental should be attributed mainly to elimination of the drug by hepatic metabolism and uptake by body fat [32]. This theory differs from the widely held belief that redistribution of thiopental terminates its anesthetic action. Toutain *et al.* proposed that this is perhaps due to differences in regional blood flow between sheep and monogastric species, although this remains unestablished [32].

Swine

Barbiturates are effective anesthetic agents in swine limited only by the difficulty of intravenous access in these species [33,34], although care should be used when administering thiopental to hypovolemic pigs as the anesthetic requirement for thiopental is reduced by approximately 35% in these animals [35]. Barbiturates do not trigger malignant hyperthermia in swine.

Clinical use

The induction doses of thiopental used in veterinary species are listed in Table 15.1. It should be noted that the dose required to induce anesthesia and facilitate endotracheal intubation is altered by premedications and the patient's physical status. Patients that are premedicated with other CNS depressants, are hypovolemic, hypoproteinemic, acidotic and/or uremic will require less thiopental to induce anesthesia. Thiopental should be administered intravenously, preferably through an intravenous catheter, and the dose should be titrated to effect. Induction of anesthesia is rapid, occurring in approximately 20–30 s after administration. Because periods of apnea are often reported after induction of anesthesia with thiopental, equipment to facilitate intubation with a cuffed endotracheal tube and to assist ventilation should be immediately available. The duration of action of thiopental is quite short with the distribution/redistribution phase lasting 14.9 ± 3.3 min in dogs [10].

Table 15.1 Barbiturate dosages in various species.

	Thiopental mg/kg IV	Pentobarbital mg/kg IV
Dog	8–22	2–30
Cat	8–22	2–15
Horse	4–15	
Cow	4–22	
Sheep	8–15	20–30
Llama	6–15	
Pig	5–12	

IV = intravenous.

Perivascular administration of thiopental is associated with tissue necrosis, especially at higher concentrations (e.g., 5%). If inadvertent perivascular injection occurs, dilution of the drug should be attempted. This is best accomplished by injection of saline through the needle or catheter that still remains in place. At the same time, lidocaine can be injected to produce vasodilation and local anesthesia.

In order to reduce the incidence of ventricular arrhythmias, intravenous lidocaine has been investigated as a co-induction agent with thiobarbiturates. Thiopental administered to dogs at a dose of 11 mg/kg and lidocaine at a dose of 8.8 mg/kg produced a smooth induction with no arrhythmias and less cardiovascular depression as compared to thiopental alone [36]. This technique may not be suitable for all species since the intravenous administration of a relatively large dose of lidocaine may cause toxicity. Mixtures of thiopental and propofol (1:1) have also been used in the dog [37]. The dose of each drug required for induction was reduced and induction quality was similar to that of thiopental or propofol alone. Recovery times and quality of recovery were similar to those of propofol and superior to those of thiopental alone [37]. It should be noted that the mixture should inhibit bacterial growth and is bactericidal after 48 h against *Staphylococcus aureus, Escherichia coli, Pseudomonas aeruginosa,* and *Candida albicans* [38]. Mixtures of thiopental and propofol at a ratio of less than 1:1 do not maintain bactericidal properties [38]. Proper evaluation of drug stability in these mixtures is lacking, but they appear to maintain relatively normal potency.

Propofol

Propofol is chemically distinct from all other intravenous drugs used to induce or maintain anesthesia. Awakening from anesthesia has been found to be more rapid with propofol than with other induction agents. It is this rapid return to consciousness with minimal residual effects that has made propofol such a popular induction agent in both human and veterinary anesthesia. Its first use as an anesthetic in people was reported in 1977 [39].

Chemical structure

Propofol is a substituted isopropylphenol (2,6-diisopropylphenol) that can be used to produce sedation, as well as to induce and maintain anesthesia. It is formulated as proprietary variations of a oil in water emulsion containing 1% propofol, 10% soybean oil, 2.25% glycerol, and 1.2% purified egg phosphatide. Propofol is relatively insoluble in aqueous solutions, but is highly lipid soluble. It is a slightly viscous, milky white substance with a pH of 6.5–8.5. This formulation of propofol is stable at room temperature and not light sensitive. Most formulations do not contain preservatives and therefore will support bacterial or fungal growth; therefore strict aseptic technique should be used when using multidose vials of propofol [40]. According to most labels, opened vials should be used or discarded before 6 h. When using propofol as a constant rate infusion, it would be prudent to discard intravenous tubing and administration sets every 12 h or if gross bacterial contamination occurs.

A lipid-free microemulsion formulation of propofol has been developed to increase vial shelf-life when broached, reduce infection risk by the addition of antimicrobial agents, reduce inherent emulsion instability, and reduce pain on injection [41]. Additionally, a propofol formulation for the veterinary market containing benzyl alcohol has also been developed for use in dogs which has an increased shelf-life of 28 days once the vial is opened [42].

In addition, other formulation approaches have been developed in attempts to reduce or eliminate the problem of injection-related pain, including prodrug approaches [43]. Of these, fospropofol is the most successful prodrug investigated to date. It is a water-soluble aqueous solution and reportedly causes less pain at injection in human patients than emulsion formulations. Fospropofol has been administered to dogs in a small prospective pharmacokinetic-pharmacodynamic study which demonstrated that onset time and duration were significantly longer for fospropofol compared to the emulsion formulation [44].

Mechanism of action

Like the barbiturates, propofol appears to exert its anesthetic effects through an interaction with $GABA_A$ receptors [45]. Propofol also inhibits the *N*-methyl-D-aspartate (NMDA) receptor through modulation of channel gating which may also contribute to its central nervous system effects [46].

Pharmacokinetics

Propofol pharmacokinetics can be described by a two compartment open model, with a rapid distribution phase followed by a slower clearance phase [47]. Following intravenous injection of propofol, it rapidly moves into the CNS, resulting in induction of anesthesia. It then is rapidly redistributed from the brain to other tissues in the body, terminating its anesthetic action. In most species (cats are an exception), propofol undergoes rapid and extensive hepatic metabolism resulting in production of inactive water-soluble sulfide and glucuronide metabolites. These are then excreted by the kidneys [48]. Clearance of propofol from the plasma exceeds hepatic blood flow, which emphasizes the importance of tissue uptake and suggests that extrahepatic metabolism or extrarenal excretion may occur [49]. In humans, there is no evidence of impaired elimination of propofol in patients with cirrhosis of the liver and extrahepatic metabolism has been confirmed in the anhepatic phase of liver transplant patients [49,50]. In cats, extrahepatic metabolism of propofol has been demonstrated in the pulmonary tissue [51]. In cats with hepatic lipidosis, anesthetic induction with propofol for placement of a feeding tube did not increase morbidity or mortality despite the anticipated alteration of drug action [52].

The pharmacokinetics of propofol have been thoroughly studied in the dog [47,53,54]. Propofol's lipophilic nature results in a large apparent volume of distribution (17.9 L/kg) as well as steady-state volume of distribution (9.7 ml/kg) [47]. Due to rapid redistribution of the drug into other tissues as well as rapid and extensive metabolism, the initial distribution half-life is short as is the rate of disappearance from plasma. Greyhounds appear to have a smaller apparent volume of distribution and steady-state volume of distribution, which suggests that recovery from propofol anesthesia in Greyhounds will be slower [54]. Dogs greater than 8.5 years of age also have been shown to have a slower clearance rate compared to younger dogs [53]. The rapid distribution and clearance of propofol make it a suitable choice for maintenance of anesthesia by constant rate infusion of the drug in many species. In most species (except cats), propofol does not accumulate after repeated doses and/or prolonged infusion of the drug, so recovery from anesthesia remains rapid and of good quality [55,56].

Pharmacodynamics

Central nervous system

Intravenous injection of propofol results in rapid CNS depression and induction of anesthesia. Much like the barbiturates, propofol reduces ICP and $CMRO_2$ [57]. Cerebral perfusion pressure is reduced slightly in patients with normal ICP, but in patients with elevated ICP, the drop in cerebral perfusion pressure is significant and may not be beneficial [58]. Brain responsiveness to carbon dioxide and cerebral metabolic autoregulation is maintained during propofol administration [57]; however, this response may be modified by concurrent administration of other drugs such as opioids. Propofol produces cortical EEG changes similar to the barbiturates, including the incidence of burst suppression with administration of high doses [57]. Propofol possesses anticonvulsant effects and can be used in the treatment of refractory seizures [59,60].

Cardiovascular system

The most prominent cardiovascular effect of propofol administration is a decrease in arterial blood pressure. Decreases in systemic vascular resistance and cardiac output are also seen [61, 62]. The myocardial depression and vasodilation appear to be dose (and plasma concentration) dependent [61]. These cardiovascular effects may be more profound in patients that are hypovolemic [63], geriatric, or have compromised left ventricular function [64]. Unlike thiopental, however, administration of propofol does not usually result in a compensatory increase in heart rate. Propofol does appear to sensitize the myocardium to epinephrine-induced arrhythmias, but does not appear to be arrhythmogenic [65].

Respiratory system

Much like thiopental, propofol causes dose-dependent depression of ventilation and postinduction apnea with transient cyanosis occurring regularly [66]. The incidence of apnea appears to be related to dose and rate of administration, with rapid injection rates making apnea more likely to occur [66]. The ventilatory response to hypoxemia [67] and carbon dioxide [68] is reduced by propofol [69], and the administration of opioids may enhance propofol's effect on ventilation [70]. Respiratory effects are also seen when propofol is administered as a constant rate infusion, with propofol decreasing tidal volume and respiratory rate [68].

Hepatic, renal, and gastrointestinal systems

Propofol does not adversely affect hepatic blood flow [71] or glomerular filtration rate in dogs [26]. In humans, propofol has been shown to be a very effective antiemetic. In fact, subanesthetic doses of propofol may be used post anesthesia to treat nausea and vomiting [72]; however, this effect has not been demonstrated in domestic animals.

Muscle

Like thiopental, propofol produces muscle relaxation. Occasionally, however, myoclonic movements have been reported in both humans and dogs [73,74]. These movements resolve spontaneously.

Fetal/neonatal effects

Propofol readily crosses the placenta but it is rapidly cleared from the neonatal circulation [75]. It is considered an acceptable choice for dogs undergoing cesarean section, as effects on healthy puppies are minimal [76].

Analgesic effects

Propofol produces neither antinociception nor hyperalgesia [29]. Animals undergoing painful procedures should therefore receive appropriate analgesics as part of the anesthetic plan.

Species-specific effects

Canine

Propofol can be administered intravenously for sedation and induction of anesthesia. It is also well suited to use as a constant rate infusion for the maintenance of anesthesia. Propofol is often recommended for use in Greyhounds. The dose required for induction of anesthesia in Greyhounds is the same as mixed breed dogs, but the recovery time is longer in Greyhounds [47].

As mentioned previously, the lipid-based emulsion formulation of propofol is capable of supporting microbial growth. In a retrospective study of clean wounds in dogs and cats, animals receiving propofol were 3.8 times more likely to develop wound infections compared to animals that did not receive propofol [77]. Causal mechanisms have not been established and the numerous confounding factors of wound infection rates would caution against overemphasizing the results of this study. However, strict aseptic techniques should be followed when using propofol as an anesthetic and prompt disposal of unused drug should reduce the potential for drug contamination and any impact that would have on infection rates.

The lipid-free microemulsion formulation of propofol has been evaluated in the dog [78] and appears to be pharmacokinetically and pharmacodynamically similar to the lipid formulation. However, it has been reported that intravenous injection of the microemulsion formulation resulted in severe pain and complications in dogs [79].

Feline

Repeated daily administration of propofol can induce oxidative injuries to feline red blood cells [80]. Heinz body formation, facial edema, generalized malaise, anorexia, and diarrhea were all reported in one study in which cats received propofol on consecutive days. Heinz body formation was significantly increased by the third day of propofol administration and recovery times were significantly increased after the second consecutive day [80]. However, in another study repeated propofol anesthesia was evaluated and no relevant hematologic changes were reported [81].

The formulation of propofol containing benzyl alcohol (Propoflo 28®) has been evaluated in cats [42]. While there has been concern regarding this formulation due to potential adverse effects of benzyl alcohol on feline blood and nervous systems, it has been shown that administration to healthy cats of normal to high clinical doses of the formulation did not cause organ toxicity [42]. The lipid-free microemulsion formulation has also been evaluated in cats [41,82] and, when compared to the lipid emulsion formulation, produces comparable pharmacokinetic, pharmacodynamic, and physiologic responses [41].

Equine

The clinical effects of propofol in the horse are similar to those seen in other species. Intravenous administration of propofol following sedation produces rapid induction of anesthesia, a short duration of action, and a rapid, smooth recovery [83,84]. However, propofol can produce unpredictable behavioral responses and excitation at the time of induction, thereby limiting its use as a routine induction agent in adult horses [85]. These adverse effects at the time of induction appear to be prevented, however, by the intravenous administration of guaifenesin for 3 min prior to propofol administration [86].

Propofol, either solely or in combination with other drugs, has been used effectively as a constant rate infusion in horses to maintain anesthesia [87–89]. While adverse events at induction were noted with propofol administration, horses appeared calm and coordinated in recovery [85]. This prompted the investigation of propofol, in combination with xylazine, as a potential modulator of recovery [90,91]. In these reports, it was noted that a combination of xylazine and propofol might be of some benefit as the quality of recovery was significantly improved [90,91].

The non-lipid microemulsion formulation of propofol has also been evaluated in the horse [92,93]. A 3 h continuous rate infusion produced similar cardiopulmonary and biochemical results to those reported when the lipid formulation was used [93]. However, in a different study of the pharmacokinetics, investigators urged caution when using propofol to maintain anesthesia due to variable kinetics, poor analgesia, and myoclonal activity [92].

Ruminant

Propofol has been satisfactorily used as an induction agent in sheep [94], goats [95], cows [96], and camelids [97]. Reported characteristics of propofol anesthesia in these species are similar to those reported in other veterinary species. Induction is rapid and smooth, duration of action is short, and recovery is of good quality. Cardiopulmonary effects are similar to those reported in other species.

The pharmacokinetics of propofol have been described in the goat. The mean elimination half-life was short (15.5 min), the volume of distribution at steady state was large (2.56 L/kg) and the clearance rate was rapid (275 mL/kg/min) [95]. These values differ from those obtained in sheep where the mean elimination half-life was 56.6 ± 13.1 min, volume of distribution was 1.037 ± 0.48 L/kg, and clearance was 85.4 ± 28.0 mL/kg/min [98].

Swine

Propofol does not induce malignant hyperthermia in susceptible swine [99]. As with other species, respiratory depression and apnea have been reported with propofol administration [100].

Clinical use

Propofol doses commonly used to induce anesthesia in veterinary patients are given in Table 15.2. It should be noted that the dose required to achieve endotracheal intubation is altered by premedications and

Table 15.2 Propofol dosages in various species.

	Induction dose (mg/kg) IV	Constant rate infusion mg/kg/min
Dog	3[a]–10	0.2–0.6
Cat	5–10	0.2–1.0
Horse	2–3[a], 6–8	0.2–0.4
Foal	2	0.33
Donkey	2	0.21
Pig	2–3	0.1–0.2
Llama	2	0.4
Ferret	2–4	
Rabbit	2–10	
Sheep	2–6	0.3–0.4
Goat	3–6	0.3

[a]Premedicated.
IV = intravenous.

the physical status of the patient. Patients that are debilitated and/or have received CNS depressants will often require less propofol for induction.

Propofol should be administered intravenously, preferably through an intravenous catheter, and the dose should be titrated to effect. Once administered, anesthetic effects usually occur within 20–30 s, although in states of low cardiac output the lag period may be prolonged. The quality of induction with propofol is good with a smooth transition to unconsciousness. To reduce the incidence of postinduction apnea, it is often recommended that the titrated dose of propofol should be administered slowly (over 60–90 s). However, apnea may still occur. Transient apnea is seldom a problem (except when airway establishment is difficult or impossible such as with some oropharyngeal conditions) as long as the anesthetist is prepared to intubate with an endotracheal tube and assist or control ventilation until spontaneous respiration begins. Duration of unconsciousness ranges from 2 to 8 min and the quality of recovery is often good.

While perivascular injection of propofol will not produce anesthesia, it is not associated with tissue necrosis. Pain on intravenous injection has been reported, and appears to be associated with injection of propofol into smaller vessels, not necessarily perivascular administration. To decrease the incidence of injection pain, clinicians may choose to inject propofol into larger vessels, administer a small dose of lidocaine intravenously prior to propofol injection, or dilute the dose by administering propofol into a running intravenous fluid line.

Dissociative anesthetics

The dissociatives are phencyclidine derivatives that produce a so-called state of 'dissociative anesthesia' characterized by dissociation of the thalamocortical and limbic systems causing a change in awareness [101]. Ketamine hydrochloride and tiletamine hydrochloride are the dissociative anesthetics most commonly used in veterinary medicine.

Chemical structure

Ketamine is 2-(o-chlorophenol)-2-(methylamino)-cyclohexanone hydrochloride. Two optical isomers of ketamine exist due to an asymmetric carbon. Most formulations contain the racemic mixture, but a purified *S*-ketamine formulation is available in some countries. The positive (*S*) isomer produces more intense analgesia, is metabolized more rapidly, and has a lower incidence of emergence reactions than the negative (*R*) isomer [102]. Racemic ketamine is available as a 10% aqueous solution. It has a pH of 3.5–5.5 and is preserved by benzethonium chloride.

Tiletamine is 2-(ethylamino)-2-(2-thienyl)-cyclohexanone hydrochloride. It is only available in combination with the benzodiazepine zolazepam, and is marketed under the names Telazol® and Zoletil®. Tiletamine/zolazepam combinations are available as a white powder that is reconstituted with 5 mL of diluent. The final concentrations of tiletamine and zolazepam depend on the product being used.

Mechanism of action

The dissociative anesthetics act on NMDA, opioid, monoaminergic, and muscarinic receptors. Additionally, they interact with voltage-gated calcium channels [103,104]. Interestingly, the dissociatives do not appear to interact with GABA receptors as the other injectable anesthetics do.

Ketamine and tiletamine are non-competitive antagonists at the NMDA receptor. They bind to the phencyclidine-binding site, which prevents glutamate, an excitatory neurotransmitter, from binding. Prevention of glutamate binding results in depression of the thalamocortical, limbic, and reticular activating systems.

Dissociatives have also been reported to have action at μ, δ, and κ opioid receptors [105]. Activity at the opioid receptors imparts analgesic properties unlike other injectable anesthetics, although the clinical significance of this action at clinically relevant doses is debatable. Additionally, the dissociatives' interaction at monoaminergic receptors may also contribute to antinociception [104]. Because dissociative anesthesia is associated with anticholinergic symptoms (emergence delirium, bronchodilation, and sympathomimetic actions), it is thought that these drugs have antagonist activity at muscarinic receptors [104]. However, many of these effects may also be related to the sympathetic nervous system-stimulating effects of ketamine and tiletamine.

Pharmacokinetics

The dissociatives are similar to other injectable anesthetics in that they have a relatively rapid onset of action (especially when administered intravenously), short duration, and are highly lipophilic. Unlike other injectable anesthetics, the dissociatives are also effective when administered intramuscularly (IM). Peak plasma concentrations occur within 1 min of IV administration and within 10 min following IM injection. The high lipid solubility of the dissociatives ensures that the blood–brain barrier is crossed quickly, which establishes effective brain concentrations of the drugs [106].

In most species, metabolism of the dissociatives occurs in the liver. Ketamine is demethylated by hepatic microsomal enzymes, producing the active metabolite norketamine. Eventually, norketamine is hydroxylated and then conjugated to form water-soluble and inactive glucuronide metabolites that are excreted by the kidney [107]. This process differs in the cat, where ketamine is biotransformed to norketamine, which is excreted unchanged in the urine [108]. Dissociatives should be used with care in animals with significant hepatic and/or renal dysfunction as prolonged anesthetic times may result.

Tiletamine also undergoes hepatic metabolism and renal excretion. Since tiletamine is only supplied with zolazepam, the action of the benzodiazepine should also be discussed. In cats, the duration of action of zolazepam is longer than that of tiletamine. This means that the CNS effects of the benzodiazepine (sedation) are present longer than those of tiletamine. In the dog, the reverse is true; the duration of action of tiletamine is longer than zolazepam. This means that the effects of the dissociative are observed, including muscle rigidity, sympathetic stimulation, and emergence delirium. Pigs appear to have a slow, calm recovery from tiletamine/zolazepam combinations, while in horses an agitated recovery may be seen if additional sedation is not provided. If significant plasma levels of tiletamine are present, reversal of the benzodiazepine with flumazenil may result in an anxious recovery.

Pharmacodynamics

Central nervous system

Dissociative anesthesia resembles a cataleptic state in which the patient does not appear to be asleep, but does not respond to external stimuli. As mentioned previously, antagonism of the NMDA receptor leads to a dissociation of the limbic and thalamocortical systems [101]. Unlike other injectable anesthetics, the dissociatives increase cerebral blood flow and $CMRO_2$ [109]. Cerebral vasodilation and an increase in blood pressure result in an increase in ICP [110]. It appears that this increase can be attenuated if ventilation is controlled and animals remain eucapnic [111]. Administration of thiopental or a benzodiazepine has also been shown to reduce ketamine-induced increases in ICP [106]. Clinicians should still exercise caution, however, when using dissociatives in patients that have or are suspected of having increased ICP.

Epileptiform EEG patterns are seen after ketamine administration [112], resulting in the recommendation that dissociatives be avoided in patients with seizure disorders. However, it has been shown that ketamine does not alter the seizure threshold in epileptic patients [113]. Additionally, there is evidence that ketamine possesses anticonvulsant as well as neuroprotective activity [114].

Abnormal behavior that may progress to emergence delirium may occur during recovery from dissociative anesthesia. Misrepresentation of visual and auditory stimuli may be responsible for this reaction [107]. A patient experiencing an emergence reaction may be ataxic, hyper-reflexive, sensitive to touch, have increased motor activity, and may have a violent recovery. These reactions are usually temporary and resolve within a few hours. Administration of CNS depressants such as benzodiazepines, acepromazine, or α_2-adrenergic receptor agonists may decrease the incidence and/or the severity of these reactions [107].

Cardiovascular system

Ketamine has a direct negative cardiac inotropic effect [115], but it is usually overcome by central sympathetic stimulation. Intravenous administration of ketamine increases systemic and pulmonary arterial pressure, heart rate, cardiac output, myocardial oxygen requirements, and cardiac work [116]. It is likely that these changes are the result of direct stimulation of the CNS leading to increased sympathetic nervous system outflow [117]. Ketamine also inhibits norepinephrine reuptake into postganglionic sympathetic nerve endings, leading to an increased concentration of plasma catecholamines [118]. Critically ill patients may respond to induction of anesthesia with ketamine with a decrease in systemic blood pressure and cardiac output. The catecholamine stores and the sympathetic nervous system's compensatory mechanism may be exhausted, unveiling ketamine's negative inotropic effects [119]. While healthy animals are usually tolerant of increased cardiac work, myocardial oxygen requirements, and heart rate, ketamine should be used with caution in those animals that have severe cardiovascular disease (e.g., uncontrolled hypertension, cardiomyopathy, or heart failure), and those that are already tachycardic and/or dysrhythmic. Stimulation of the cardiovascular system in these patients may not be desirable.

Respiratory system

Unlike other injectable anesthetics, ketamine does not cause significant respiratory depression. Ventilatory responses to hypoxia and carbon dioxide are maintained in animals receiving ketamine as the sole anesthetic agent [120]. When ketamine is administered with other CNS depressants, significant respiratory depression can occur. Ketamine administration has been associated with an 'apneustic' respiratory pattern, characterized by a prolonged inspiratory duration and relatively short expiratory time [121]. Despite this altered respiratory pattern, carbon dioxide levels and minute ventilation usually remain within normal limits.

Ketamine is a bronchial smooth muscle relaxant and causes bronchodilation and a decrease in airway resistance [122]. This makes it an attractive choice when anesthetizing animals with asthma or obstructive airway diseases such as chronic obstructive pulmonary disease. Pharyngeal and laryngeal reflexes remain intact when ketamine is used as the sole anesthetic agent [123]. It should be noted, however, that these reflexes are often uncoordinated and not protective. An endotracheal tube should always be placed to prevent aspiration. Maintaining a secure airway is especially important because ketamine increases salivation and respiratory tract secretions [106]. These can be reduced with the administration of an anticholinergic.

Hepatic, renal, gastrointestinal systems

Laboratory tests that indicate hepatic or renal function are not altered by the administration of dissociatives. Gastrointestinal motility is unchanged after the administration of ketamine in the dog [124].

Analgesic effects

As previously discussed, the action of the dissociatives at NMDA and opioid receptors imparts analgesic properties. In fact, it has been demonstrated that subanesthetic doses of ketamine produce profound analgesia especially in situations of somatic pain [103]. Additionally, blockade of the excitatory neurotransmitter glutamate at the NMDA receptor by the dissociatives is thought to play a role in preventing or minimizing central sensitization or wind-up pain. Therefore, pre-emptive administration of ketamine prior to painful stimuli may play a role in attenuating central sensitization [125].

Muscle

Unlike the previously discussed injectable anesthetic agents, the dissociatives produce little muscle relaxation. In fact, the dissociatives may cause muscle rigidity and often spontaneous movement of the limbs, trunk, and/or head. Substantial increases in IOP are seen after ketamine administration which may be a result of increased tone of the extraocular muscles [126]. Muscle relaxation can be improved with the co-administration of benzodiazepines or α_2-adrenergic receptor agonists.

Fetal/Neonatal Effects

Ketamine crosses the placenta and enters fetal circulation. In a study evaluating neurologic reflexes in puppies born via cesarean section, anesthetic induction of the dam with ketamine and midazolam resulted in the most depression of neurologic reflexes when compared with other injectable induction drugs [27].

Species-specific effects

Canine

The dissociatives can be administered either intravenously or intramuscularly to produce a range of effects from sedation to anesthesia. Induction of anesthesia with ketamine alone can lead to muscle rigidity, spontaneous movement, and undesirable recoveries. Therefore, it is usually administered with a co-induction agent such as a benzodiazepine. Because tiletamine is supplied as a combination with zolazepam, there is no need for additional benzodiazepine for intravenous administration.

Intramuscular ketamine or tiletamine/zolazepam combinations are frequently combined with an α_2-adrenergic receptor agonist and an opioid to produce excellent immobilization with muscle relaxation and analgesia. Table 15.3 shows dosages of ketamine alone or in combination with other anesthetics commonly used in the dog. Table 15.4 shows common doses and usage of Telazol® in dogs.

Table 15.3 Ketamine dosages when used alone or in combination in dogs.

Agent	Dose (mg/kg)	Route	Duration (minutes)	Effect
Ketamine alone	10	IV	7–23	Short duration, anesthesia inadequate for surgery
Acepromazine Ketamine	0.2 10	IV	31–47	Clinical anesthesia, less muscle rigidity
Acepromazine Ketamine	0.22 11–18	IM		Restraint, spastic movements, prolonged recovery
Xylazine Ketamine	0.55–1.1 IM 22 IV to effect	IM/IV	28–36	Surgical anesthesia, muscle relaxation, analgesia for abdominal surgery
Atropine Xylazine Ketamine	0.04 1.1 11	IV	17–35	Increased risk with dogs with cardiopulmonary compromise
Atropine Xylazine Ketamine	0.04 1.1 22	IM	17–35	Increased risk with dogs with cardiopulmonary compromise
Metomidine Ketamine	0.04 5	IM	25–35	Longer muscle relaxation and recovery than xylazine/ketamine
Diazapam Ketamine	0.28 5.5	IV		Suitable induction for sighthounds
Midazolam Ketamine	0.5 10	IV	10–16	Increased heart rate, mild respiratory depression, good muscle relaxation

Modified from Tranquilli WJ, Thurmon JC, Grimm KA, eds. *Lumb and Jones' Veterinary Anesthesia and Analgesia*, 4th edn. Ames, IA: Blackwell Publishing, 2007; Figure 12.1, 304.
IM = intramuscular; IV = intravenous.

Table 15.4 Telazol® dosages alone or in combination in dogs.

Agent	Dose (mg/kg)	Route	Duration (minutes)	Effect
Telazol	9.9	IM	10–30	Rough recovery
Telazol	6.6	IV	7–27	
Telazol Xylazine Butorphanol	8.8 1.1 0.22	IM	100	Clinical anesthesia, good muscle relaxation, good analgesia
Butorphanol Telazol	0.7 9.3–11.9	IM		Unsatisfactory sedation in vicious dogs
Acepromazine Telazol	0.6–3.0 17.5–21.1	IM		Adequate sedation in vicious dogs

Modified from Tranquilli WJ, Thurmon JC, Grimm KA, eds. *Lumb and Jones' Veterinary Anesthesia and Analgesia*, 4th edn. Ames, IA: Blackwell Publishing, 2007; Figure 12.2, p.305.
IM = intramuscular; IV = intravenous.

Feline

The dissociatives have been used to produce a range of effects from sedation to anesthesia in cats. These drugs can be administered intravenously or intramuscularly. Ketamine is also absorbed through the oral mucosa. In particularly fractious cats, ketamine can be sprayed into the mouth to effectively induce sedation and facilitate the induction of anesthesia [127]. Copious salivation usually results due to the bitter taste and/or low pH of ketamine.

α_2-Adrenergic receptor agonists, benzodiazepines, and/or acepromazine are commonly administered in combination with intramuscular ketamine. The combination of dexmedetomidine, ketamine, and an opioid produces excellent chemical restraint/anesthesia, muscle relaxation, and analgesia [128].

Table 15.5 Telazol® dosages alone or in combination in cats.

Agent	Dose (mg/kg)	Route	Duration (minutes)	Effect
Telazol alone	6–40 (average 12.8)	IM	40–70	Salivation, apneustic breathing
Telazol alone	12.8	IV	35–70	Salivation, apneustic breathing
Acepromazine Telazol	0.1 3.4 ± 1.09	IM		Adequate anesthesia for castration
Telazol Ketamine Xylazine	3.3 2.64 0.66	IM	34–52	Smooth induction and recovery, excellent muscle relaxation, good analgesia

Modified from Tranquilli WJ, Thurmon JC, Grimm KA, eds. *Lumb and Jones' Veterinary Anesthesia and Analgesia*, 4th edn. Ames, IA: Blackwell Publishing, 2007; Figure 12.4, p.308.
IM = intramuscular; IV = intravenous.

Tiletamine/zolazepam powder (500 mg) has been reconstituted with xylazine (100 mg) and ketamine (400 mg) to form a potent chemical restraint/anesthesia cocktail that can be administered intramuscularly [129,130]. Care must be exercised when administering the drug combination since the overall volume is very small and accurate measurement important. Additionally, careful patient monitoring to prevent profound hypothermia is required since prolonged recovery may result due to low metabolism. Flumazenil and/or an α_2-adrenergic receptor antagonist have been used to speed recovery from this combination. Table 15.5 shows common combinations and dosages of Telazol® in cats.

The use of tiletamine/zolazepam combinations in large felids, especially tigers, is not recommended. Adverse reactions including delayed recovery, hind limb paresis, hyper-reflexia, seizures, and death have been reported [131].

Equine

The dissociatives, particularly ketamine, are used extensively in equine anesthesia. Intravenous administration of the dissociatives rapidly and smoothly induces anesthesia provided that adequate sedation has been achieved prior to their administration. If the dissociatives are administered before adequate sedation has been provided, excitement will occur. Some muscle rigidity and involuntary movement may still occur when ketamine is used; therefore it is frequently combined with a co-induction agent such as a benzodiazepine, α_2-adrenergic receptor agonist or guaifenesin.

Anesthesia can be maintained by administering additional intravenous doses of ketamine. These doses may be administered as intermittent boluses or as a constant rate infusion. When used as a constant rate infusion, ketamine is frequently combined with sedatives and analgesic agents (e.g., α_2-adrenergic receptor agonists, guaifenesin, and opioids) in a combination commonly referred to as 'triple drip.' Commonly used doses for ketamine in combination with other anesthetic agents can be found in Table 15.6.

Tiletamine/zolazepam combinations can be administered IV to induce anesthesia in the horse after adequate sedation has been achieved. It should be noted, however, that recovery from tiletamine/zolazepam anesthesia is sometimes associated with excitement and incoordination if additional sedatives such as α_2-adrenergic receptor agonists are not administered or anesthesia is not prolonged with inhalants [132]. Table 15.7 shows dosages for tiletamine in horses.

Table 15.6 Ketamine dosages alone or in combination in horses.

Agent	Dose (mg/kg)	Route	Duration (minutes)	Effect
Xylazine Ketamine	1.1 2.2	IV	12–35	Smooth induction and recovery, inadequate muscle relaxation
Xylazine Butorphanol Ketamine	1.1 0.1–0.2 2.2	IV	18–56 depending on breed	Behavioral changes, muscle relaxation, good analgesia
Xylazine Ketamine Methadone	1.1 2.2 0.1	IV		Satisfactory anesthesia
Methadone Acepromazine Xylazine Ketamine	0.1 0.15 1.1 2.2	IV		Inadequate anesthesia
Acepromazine Methadone Ketamine	0.04 0.04 2.0–2.5	IV	3–18	Muscle tremors
Guiafenesin Xylazine Ketamine	50 0.5 1.0	IV	120	Low blood pressure and hypoventilation
Guiafenesin Ketamine	50 1.5–2.2			Less cardiovascular depression than barbiturate/guiafenesin
Xylazine Diazepam Ketamine	1.1 0.1 2.0	IV		Supplement with 200–750 mg ketamine, maintain with halothane, good muscle relaxation
Xylazine Temazepam Ketamine	1.1 0.044 2.2	IV		Longer recumbency
Romifidine Ketamine	0.1 2.0–2.2	IV	10–25	Initial limb rigidity, mild tremor
Romifidine Midazolam Ketamine	0.08 0.06 2.2	IV	25–40	May require additional dose of M and K Smooth recovery
Methotrimeprazine Midazolam Guaifenesin Ketamine	0.5 0.1 100 1.6	IV		Induction of anesthesia, smooth recovery
Detomidine Ketamine	0.02 2.2	IV	10–43	Required more time than xylazine-ketamine to assume recumbency, occasional poor recovery, longer hypertension
Guaifenesin Detomidine Ketamine	50 0.04 4	IV	140	Surgical anesthesia but may require additional ketamine during surgery, good recovery
Detomidine Butorphanol Ketamine	0.02 0.04 2.2	IV	18–67	Smooth induction Smoother recovery Muscle relaxation

Modified from Tranquilli WJ, Thurmon JC, Grimm KA, eds. *Lumb and Jones' Veterinary Anesthesia and Analgesia*, 4th edn. Ames, IA: Blackwell Publishing, 2007; Figure 12.5, p.309.
IM = intramuscular; IV = intravenous.

Table 15.7 Ketamine and tiletamine dosages in various species.

Species	Dose of ketamine (mg/kg)	Dose of tiletamine/ zolazepam (mg/kg)
Dog	5–10 IV	1 IV 3–6 IM
Cat	5–10 IV 5–15 IM	4–7 IM
Horse	2–2.2 IV (after adequate sedation)	1–3 IV (after adequate sedation)
Cattle	2–4 IV	2–4 IV
Pig	10 IM	6 IM

IM = intramuscular; IV = intravenous.

Ruminant

The dissociatives can be used in ruminants to induce anesthesia. Sedation and muscle relaxation are usually improved by the administration of an α_2-adrenergic receptor agonist or benzodiazepine prior to the administration of ketamine. Anesthesia can be maintained with a constant rate infusion of ketamine or by a combination of ketamine, guaifenesin, and xylazine.

Subanesthetic doses of ketamine (in combination with xylazine) have been administered to calves to produce sedation prior to castration [133]. This so-called 'ketamine stun' technique may be an efficacious and cost-effective alternative or adjunct to local anesthesia for castration [133]. See Table 15.7 for dosages of the dissociatives in ruminants.

Swine

The dissociatives have been used extensively in swine for chemical restraint and anesthesia. Ketamine does not induce malignant hyperthermia in susceptible pigs, although its use in these animals has been controversial [134]. Similar to other species, ketamine as a sole anesthetic agent produces poor muscle relaxation so it is commonly combined with azaperone, benzodiazepines and/or α_2-adrenergic receptor agonists for sedation and anesthesia. Tiletamine/zolazepam combinations are commonly reconstituted with 250 mg of xylazine and 250 mg of ketamine and used as an injectable anesthetic in swine [135]. See Table 15.7 for dosages of dissociative anesthetics in swine.

Clinical use

The tables mentioned previously list the commonly used doses of ketamine and tiletamine/zolazepam combinations. Both intravenous and intramuscular routes of administration are listed. The total dose required to induce anesthesia will be affected by premedications, the patient's physical status, and route of administration. Clinicians should evaluate patients carefully to determine if the dosage needs to be altered.

Depending on the dose administered, intramuscular injection of dissociatives produces effects ranging from rapid and reliable chemical immobilization to general anesthesia. Onset of action occurs within 10 min of intramuscular injection. Duration of anesthesia is dependent on the dose administered, but usually longer following intramuscular injection due to the higher overall dose. Reversal of the sedative/tranquilizer used in combination with the dissociative should not occur until the effects of the dissociative have waned. Early reversal of sedatives may lead to emergence delirium and a rough recovery.

Intravenous administration of ketamine plus a benzodiazepine or tiletamine/zolazepam combinations results in anesthetic induction in approximately 45–90 s. The quality of induction is good, but clinicians should remember that ocular, laryngeal, and pharyngeal reflexes may remain intact. The eyes stay open, but the patient is anesthetized. Anesthetic duration of a single induction dose of ketamine/diazepam or tiletamine/zolazepam combinations is approximately 20 min. Recovery from intravenous dissociative administration is usually of good quality, especially if other drugs (e.g., α_2-adrenergic receptor agonists) are co-administered or anesthesia prolonged with inhalants.

Etomidate

Synthesized in 1964 and introduced into human medical practice in 1972, etomidate has been used as an induction and maintenance agent due to its minimal cardiopulmonary and cerebral protective effects [136,137]. Recent interest in etomidate derivatives such as methoxycarbonyl etomidate (MOC-etomidate) has resulted in an improved understanding of etomidate pharmacology and adverse effects.

Chemical structure

Etomidate is an imidazole derivative, *R*-(+)-pentylethyl-1H-imidazole-5 carboxylate sulfate, which exists in two isomers, with only the (+) isomer producing hypnosis. Etomidate is unstable in neutral solutions and is insoluble in water. It is supplied as a 0.2% solution in 35% propylene glycol with a pH of 6.9. Commercially available etomidate preparations have a high osmolality which may result in some of its adverse effects including the potential for erythrocyte damage.

Mechanism of action

Similar to other injectable anesthetics, etomidate has agonist activity at the GABA receptor [3]. Etomidate enhances the action of the inhibitory neurotransmitter GABA, which increases chloride conduction into the cell, resulting in hyperpolarization of the postsynaptic neuron. The hyperpolarization of the postsynaptic neuron results in CNS depression and hypnosis.

Pharmacokinetics

The pharmacokinetics of etomidate have been described in cats and people as an open three compartment model [138,139]. Etomidate is redistributed rapidly in the cat (0.05 h) and its elimination half-life is 2.89 h [139]. The volume of distribution at steady state is large (4.88 ± 2.25 L/kg in cats) and total clearance occurs over 2.47 ± 0.78 L/kg/h [139]. Etomidate penetrates the brain quickly, resulting in a rapid induction of anesthesia. Recovery from a single intravenous injection of etomidate is also rapid due to redistribution of the drug from the brain to inactive tissue sites. Approximately 75% of etomidate is bound to albumin, therefore conditions where albumin concentrations are decreased result in increases in the pharmacologically active drug [140]. The therapeutic index (LD_{50}/ED_{50}) of etomidate in rats is quite large (26.0) compared to thiopental (4.6) [141].

Etomidate undergoes hydrolysis of its ethyl ester side-chain that forms a water-soluble, pharmacologically inactive metabolite that is excreted in the urine, bile, and feces. Hepatic enzymes and plasma esterases carry out the hydrolysis. The hydrolysis of the drug is nearly complete as less than 3% of etomidate is excreted unchanged in the urine [142,143].

Pharmacodynamics

Central nervous system

The primary CNS effect of etomidate is hypnosis that is accomplished through GABA agonist activity. In cats, etomidate decreases the spontaneous firing of cortical neurons as well as the firing rate of neurons in the thalamus and reticular formation. This depression of neuronal activity likely contributes to anesthetic-induced unconsciousness [144].

Etomidate causes vasoconstriction of the cerebral vasculature and reduces cerebral blood flow and $CMRO_2$ [145,146]. Because mean arterial blood pressure is unchanged after etomidate administration, cerebral perfusion pressure is maintained [146]. As a result, previously elevated intracranial pressure is reduced after etomidate administration much like it is after thiopental administration [147,148]. In a canine model of cerebral hypoperfusion, cerebral oxygen extraction fraction did not change during hypotension when etomidate was administered. Therefore it was concluded that etomidate may preserve the cerebral metabolic state [149]. Reducing the cerebral metabolic rate of oxygen consumption while lowering the rate of rise of intracranial pressure and producing immobilization may reduce the effects of a hypoxic insult to the brain of animals [150]. Etomidate produces changes in the EEG similar to the barbiturates [148], but it has also been associated with grand mal seizures [151]. For this reason, some anesthetists argue against etomidate's use in patients with a history of seizures.

Cardiovascular system

Intravenous administration of etomidate in healthy animals is characterized by cardiovascular stability. A single induction dose of etomidate results in minimal to no changes in heart rate, stroke volume, cardiac output, mean arterial blood pressure, central venous pressure, or cardiac index [152,153]. In a canine isolated papillary muscle preparation, etomidate produced less myocardial depression than an equally potent dose of thiopental [154]. Baroreceptor function and sympathetic nervous system responses appear to remain intact after etomidate administration, further contributing to hemodynamic stability [155]. When administered to hypovolemic dogs, etomidate produced minimal changes in cardiopulmonary variables [156]. In dogs with dilated cardiomyopathy, however, arterial blood pressure remains stable during etomidate anesthesia due to increases in arterial resistance and aortic impedance along with decreases in aortic compliance [157]. This indicates that arterial pressure is maintained due to an increase in left ventricular afterload, which adversely affects left ventricular systolic and diastolic performance in patients with impaired left ventricular function [157]. It should be emphasized that etomidate is usually only suitable for induction of anesthesia and that the greatest cardiovascular effects the patient is likely to experience will be due to the drugs used to maintain anesthesia (usually inhalant anesthetics) which may negate or alter any potential benefits from using etomidate.

Respiratory system

Etomidate has minimal effects on the respiratory system. Postinduction apnea has been reported after rapid intravenous administration [158]. In most patients, any reduction in tidal volume that is seen after etomidate administration is usually offset by an increase in respiratory rate [136].

Hepatic, renal, and gastrointestinal systems

Etomidate does not decrease renal blood flow or glomerular filtration rate.[26]. Hepatic and renal function tests are not affected by etomidate administration [138].

Endocrine system

Adrenocortical suppression has been documented after etomidate administration. Etomidate causes a dose-dependent inhibition of the conversion of cholesterol to cortisol [159]. This suppression of the adrenocortical system persists for at least 6 h in the dog [160] and 5 h in the cat [161]. This has been a proposed mechanism for the increased mortality in human patients observed in some studies following etomidate anesthesia. Care should be exercised when anesthetizing patients with existing adrenocortical disease (e.g., Addison's disease), highly stressed patients or when etomidate is being used as a constant rate infusion to maintain anesthesia. Infusion of etomidate for long durations is not recommended.

Analgesic effects

Etomidate does not produce antinociception; therefore patients undergoing painful procedures should have appropriate analgesics administered during the perioperative period.

Muscle

Myoclonus, dystonia, and tremor can occur with etomidate administration [162]. It is thought that this is the result of disinhibition of subcortical structures that normally suppress extrapyramidal motor activity [163]. Myoclonic activity can be decreased with adequate premedication and/or the intravenous administration of a benzodiazepine immediately prior to etomidate administration [162].

Pain on injection

Intravenous administration of etomidate frequently results in pain. It is thought that this is due to the propylene glycol vehicle or the hyperosmolar nature of the commercial product. The incidence of pain can be lessened by administration of etomidate into a large vein, through a running intravenous line, or intravenous administration of an opioid immediately prior to etomidate administration [162].

Other considerations

The current formulation of etomidate in propylene glycol results in a solution with an osmolality of 4640 mOsm/L. This is hyperosmotic when compared to plasma (osmolality approximately 300 mOsm/L) and has been associated with intravascular hemolysis. In dogs, clinically significant hemolysis has been reported following prolonged administration of etomidate [164].

Species-specific effects

Canine

Despite side-effects of administration such as vomiting, myoclonus, excitement, and hemolysis, etomidate still should be considered as an intravenous induction agent in patients with cardiovascular instability, increased intracranial pressure, and/or cirrhosis [165].

Feline

The pharmacokinetics of etomidate have been described in the cat and are detailed above. When used as an induction agent in normal cats, etomidate has been demonstrated to be an acceptable induction agent producing minimal cardiopulmonary effects [166]. Additionally, when investigated as an intravenous induction agent for cats with decreased cardiovascular reserve, etomidate administered at a dose of 1–2 mg/kg titrated to effect was determined to be effective. Excessive salivation was noted in all cats, however [166]. It should be noted that due to the fragility of feline red blood cells, cats may be more likely to have intravascular hemolysis when etomidate is administered.

Equine

Etomidate is not used clinically in horses.

Ruminant

Etomidate has been studied in pregnant ewes. Fresno *et al.* studied the cardiovascular and acid–base effects of etomidate in the pregnant ewe and fetus [167]. It was determined that an intravenous bolus of 1 mg/kg of etomidate did not depress cardiovascular function in the ewe or fetus. When etomidate was administered as a constant rate infusion for 1 h, the maternal heart rate and blood pressure increased during the second half of the infusion and in the initial stages of recovery. Acid–base alterations led to transient but slight respiratory depression of the mother and fetus, which may have been due to a combination of etomidate and positioning of the animal [167]. Placental transfer of etomidate was also examined in pregnant ewes. It was determined that etomidate crosses the placenta rapidly and reaches the fetus in high amounts. However, cumulative effects of etomidate in the fetus were not demonstrated because fetal elimination occurred just as quickly as it did in the dam [168].

The inhibitory effects of etomidate on basal and ACTH-stimulated cortisol synthesis by isolated bovine adrenocortical cells have also been investigated. In concentrations likely to be achieved

Table 15.8 Etomidate dosages in various species.

Species	Dose (mg/kg) IV
Dog	0.5–4.0
Cat	0.5–4.0
Pig	2–4

IV = intravenous.

during anesthesia, etomidate blocks cortisol output by these isolated bovine cells [169].

Swine

Etomidate has been used as an intravenous induction agent in swine [170]. As in other species, it provides cardiovascular stability, decreases cerebral blood flow, and renal blood flow remains essentially unchanged [171]. Additionally, it does not trigger malignant hyperthermia in susceptible pigs [172].

Clinical use

Doses of etomidate commonly used in domestic species are given in Table 15.8. Clinicians should note that the dose needed to achieve endotracheal intubation is affected by the patient's physical status and prior administration of other CNS depressants (e.g., sedatives, tranquilizers, opioids). Etomidate may be a reasonable anesthetic induction agent for those patients with some types of myocardial disease, cardiovascular instability, and/or intracranial lesions [165].

Induction of anesthesia with etomidate is rapid and endotracheal intubation is usually possible within 30 s of administration. As noted previously, pain on intravenous injection has been described. The incidence of injection pain may be reduced by intravenous administration of an opioid analgesic prior to etomidate injection, administration of etomidate through an intravenous catheter placed in a large vein, and/or administration of etomidate via a running intravenous line. Myoclonus following intravenous etomidate administration has also been described. Adequate premedication with sedatives such as benzodiazepines may reduce the incidence of myoclonic activity.

The duration of anesthesia after intravenous administration of etomidate is dose dependent, but awaking from a single dose of etomidate is more rapid than after barbiturate administration [136]. Anesthesia can be maintained by administering etomidate as a constant rate infusion as there is little evidence of cumulative drug effect. However, maintenance of anesthesia with etomidate is not recommended due to the previously discussed adrenocortical suppression and erythrocyte damage.

Alfaxalone

Alfaxalone has been used in veterinary medicine since its anesthetic properties were described in 1971 [173]. Because alfaxalone is poorly water soluble, it was originally combined with a weak anesthetic, alphadolone, and formulated in a 20% polyoxyethylated castor oil vehicle. Althesin® was formulated for human use while Saffan® was marketed for veterinary use. This combination of two neurosteroids was used to induce and/or maintain anesthesia in a variety of domestic species including cats, horses, pigs, and sheep [174]. However, the castor oil formulation, Cremophor EL®, was associated with hyperemia in cats [175] and histamine release with resultant anaphylactic reactions in dogs [173]. More recently, a solution containing alfaxalone in a non-cremophor (cyclodextran) vehicle (Alfaxan-CD®) has been approved for dogs and cats in several countries. This formulation is not associated with histamine release [176]. The following discussion centers on this newer formulation of alfaxalone.

Chemical structure

Alfaxalone (3-α-hydroxy-5-α-pregnane-11,20-dione) is a neuroactive steroid molecule capable of inducing anesthesia. It is supplied as a 1% solution in 2-hydroxypropyl-β-cyclodextrin. The solution does not contain an antimicrobial preservative so any solution remaining in the vial following withdrawal of the required dose should be discarded.

Mechanism of action

As with many of the other injectable anesthetic agents, alfaxalone produces CNS depression by activity at GABA receptors [177]. Binding of alfaxalone to GABA receptors increases chloride conduction into the cell, resulting in hyperpolarization of the postsynaptic membrane. This, in turn, inhibits the pathways responsible for arousal and awareness. When present in lower concentrations, alfaxalone will modulate ion currents through the GABA receptor. At higher concentrations, however, alfaxalone acts as a GABA agonist, similar to the barbiturates [177].

Pharmacokinetics

The pharmacokinetics of alfaxalone have been determined in dogs, cats, and horses. The volume of distribution after doses of 2 and 5 mg/kg is 2.4 L/kg in dogs and 1.8 L/kg in cats. In cats, the mean terminal plasma elimination half-life (t½) is approximately 45 min for a 5 mg/kg dose, while mean plasma clearance is 25.1 ± 7.6 mL/kg/min [178]. In dogs, the t½ is approximately 25 min for a 2 mg/kg dose. Plasma clearance for a 2 mg/kg dose is 59.4 ± 12.9 mL/kg/min [176]. The duration of anesthesia, t½, and plasma clearance for alfaxalone in non-premedicated Greyhounds are similar to those reported in Beagles [179]. In the horse, the volume of distribution after a 1 mg/kg dose is 1.6 ± 0.4 L/kg. The t½ of a 1 mg/kg dose is 33.4 min and the plasma clearance of a 1 mg/kg dose of alfaxalone is 37.1 ± 11.1 mL/kg/min [180]. In foals premedicated with butorphanol, 3 mg/kg of alfaxalone had a mean plasma elimination half-life of 22.8 ± 5.2 min, and an observed plasma clearance and volume of distribution of 19.9 ± 5.9 mL/kg/min and 0.6 ± 0.2 L/kg, respectively [181].

It appears alfaxalone undergoes both cytochrome P450-dependent (Phase I) and conjugation-dependent (Phase II) hepatic metabolism. Cats and dogs seem to form the same five Phase I metabolites of alfaxalone. While cats produce alfaxalone sulfate and alfaxalone glucuronide in Phase II, dogs are observed to produce alfaxalone glucuronide. These metabolites are then eliminated by the hepatic/fecal and renal routes (Jurox summary of product characteristics).

Pharmacodynamics

Central nervous system

Alfaxalone administration produces unconsciousness and a dose-dependent reduction in EEG activity [182]. Cerebral blood flow, intracranial pressure, and cerebral metabolic oxygen demands are all decreased [183]. The duration of anesthesia and unresponsiveness to noxious stimuli increases with increasing dosages of alfaxalone in cats and dogs. In dogs anesthetized with halothane, alfaxalone administration resulted in changes in the electroencephalogram.

These changes included a shift in the dominant frequency band to δ from β, occasional burst suppression, and decreases in median and spectral edge frequency [182].

Cardiovascular system

Intravenous administration of alfaxalone produces dose-dependent cardiovascular depression in dogs and cats. Arterial blood pressure, cardiac output, and heart rate decreased in cats that were given 15 mg/kg and 50 mg/kg of intravenous alfaxalone. In those animals that received the 50 mg/kg dose, the decrease in systolic blood pressure was marked, and did not return to a clinically acceptable value for approximately 15–30 min. In dogs that received 6 and 20 mg/kg of alfaxalone intravenously, heart rate increased while arterial blood pressure and mean pulmonary arterial pressure decreased in a dose-dependent fashion. It should be noted, however, that when alfaxalone was administered to dogs and cats at clinically relevant doses (5 mg/kg in cats and 2 mg/kg in dogs), cardiovascular parameters remained quite stable. Studies utilizing clinical doses of alfaxalone in horses, sheep, and swine have also demonstrated stable cardiovascular parameters.

Respiratory system

In dogs and cats, the administration of alfaxalone produces dose-dependent respiratory depression, with apnea being the most common side-effect [184,185]. In dogs, the duration of apnea was related to the dose of alfaxalone administered [184]. Dose-dependent decreases in respiratory rate, minute volume, and arterial partial pressure of oxygen were noted in both dogs and cats [184,185]. The arterial partial pressure of carbon dioxide ($PaCO_2$) increased in cats receiving 50 mg/kg and dogs receiving 6 and 20 mg/kg [184,185]. Neither apnea nor increases in $PaCO_2$ occurred in dogs that received 2 mg/kg of alfaxalone [183]. As with the cardiovascular parameters, the respiratory effects of alfaxalone are manageable when administered at clinically relevant doses.

Hepatic, renal, and gastrointestinal systems

To the author's knowledge, no controlled studies examining the effect of alfaxalone alone on hepatic or renal blood flow have been published. Studies involving alfaxalone-alphadolone have demonstrated that renal function in rats is only transiently altered, if changed at all [186,187], while a study in dogs showed that renal blood flow remained unchanged [188]. Administration of alfaxalone-alphadolone in Greyhounds decreased hepatic blood flow and hepatic oxygen supply [189]. As discussed previously, alfaxalone undergoes cytochrome P450 hepatic metabolism. Induction of the cytochrome P450 enzyme leads to an increase in the rate of alfaxalone degradation, which may decrease the duration of anesthesia [190].

Other effects

Alfaxalone is a steroid compound derived from progesterone; therefore it is possible that sex-specific metabolism could produce pharmacokinetic differences between male and female animals. However, in studies describing the pharmacokinetics of alfaxalone, sex does not appear to have an effect on any of the key variables. Therefore, alfaxalone can be administered at the same dose to either sex [177].

Species-specific effects

Canine

In a multicenter clinical trial involving 231 dogs, alfaxalone was found to be a safe and effective agent for the induction and maintenance of anesthesia [191]. In this study, the average induction dose for alfaxalone was 2.2 mg/kg in non-premedicated dogs and 1.6 mg/kg in dogs that received premedications [191]. This reduction in the dose of alfaxalone needed for induction after premedication has been demonstrated in other studies [192,193].

As described previously, cardiovascular and respiratory parameters remain quite stable in dogs that are administered alfaxalone at clinically relevant doses, with postinduction apnea being the most commonly reported side-effect [184]. When compared to etomidate, induction of anesthesia with alfaxalone resulted in tachycardia and an increase in cardiac index. Additionally, arterial blood pressure and systemic vascular resistance index were decreased, although both remained at clinically acceptable values [152]. When used in a clinical study involving dogs of poor anesthetic risk, alfaxalone did not produce significant changes in systolic blood pressure and was determined to be a clinically acceptable induction agent [194].

Alfaxalone has been delivered as a constant rate infusion to maintain anesthesia in dogs, and has been shown to be an effective anesthetic producing clinically acceptable hemodynamic values [195]. Constant rate infusions of alfaxalone produce effective anesthesia for surgical procedures [196,197]. Doses of 0.07 mg/kg/min adjusted to maintain adequate anesthetic depth [196] and 0.11 ± 0.01 mg/kg/min [197] produced satisfactory anesthesia in dogs undergoing ovariohysterectomy. In both studies, significant respiratory depression was observed, therefore ventilatory monitoring is recommended [196,197].

Alfaxalone has also been evaluated in dogs less than 12 weeks of age and has been determined to be a suitable induction agent [198]. Additionally, it has been used to induce anesthesia in dogs prior to cesarean section [199]. Seventy-four bitches were included in the study, 26 of which received alfaxalone to induce anesthesia. Puppy vigor scores were higher in those dogs receiving alfaxalone when compared to those receiving propofol, but survival rates 24 h after birth were similar between groups (97% for alfaxalone and 98% for propofol) [199].

Other studies of alfaxalone in the dog show that intravenous administration for induction of anesthesia will increase intraocular pressure [200]. And unlike some formulations of propofol and etomidate, intravenous injection of alfaxalone does not cause pain on injection [79].

Recovery from alfaxalone anesthesia is longer compared to propofol and has been associated with adverse events such as paddling, rigidity, myoclonus, and vocalization [191,201]. However, these events lasted less than 2 min and did not result in injury or require treatment [201].

Feline

Alfaxalone has been used for sedation as well as induction and maintenance of anesthesia in the cat. Subcutaneous administration of alfaxalone and butorphanol in hyperthyroid cats resulted in adequate sedation for oral administration of iodine-131 [202]. However, in another study, intramuscular alfaxalone in combination with dexmedetomidine and hydromorphone resulted in prolonged recoveries with excitement, ataxia and hyper-reactivity in all cats and therefore this route of administration for alfaxalone was not recommended [203].

When used intravenously at clinically relevant doses to induce anesthesia, alfaxalone produces dose-dependent anesthesia and unresponsiveness to noxious stimuli [185]. As noted previously, cardiopulmonary parameters remain relatively stable with hypoventilation and hypoxia being the most frequent side-effects of the administration of high doses of alfaxalone [185]. When compared to propofol, intravenous administration of alfaxalone resulted in similar and clinically acceptable inductions, cardiorespiratory variables, and recoveries [204]. In cats 3–12 months of age, intravenous administration of alfaxalone produced a smooth induction of anesthesia with a rapid recovery [205]. Alfaxalone has also been demonstrated to be a suitable induction and maintenance agent in cats less than 12 weeks of age [206].

Administration of intermittent intravenous bolus doses of alfaxalone does not appear to result in plasma accumulation in cats or increase recovery times, so it can be used as a constant rate infusion to maintain anesthesia [178]. In cats premedicated with morphine and dexmedetomidine undergoing neutering procedures, alfaxalone induction and constant rate infusion (1.7 mg/kg and 0.18 mg/kg/min, respectively) were effective for surgical anesthesia [207].

Similar to the dog, minor adverse events have been noted during recovery in animals that have received alfaxalone. When compared to propofol, cats receiving alfaxalone were more likely to have episodes of paddling and trembling during recovery [208]. However, most recoveries were assessed as smooth overall and were similar to those in cats receiving propofol [208].

Equine

Alfaxalone has been used to induce and maintain anesthesia in horses [209–211]. When administered intravenously to horses following xylazine and guaifenesin, 1 mg/kg of alfaxalone satisfactorily induced anesthesia, although tremors/shaking were reported [210]. When compared with ketamine, 1 mg/kg of alfaxalone with 0.02 mg/kg diazepam IV produced shorter induction times (18 ± 4 s) with similar anesthesia times [211]. Recovery scores, however, were significantly worse in horses receiving alfaxalone [211]. Alfaxalone has also been administered as a constant rate infusion to maintain general anesthesia in horses undergoing field castration. In this study, alfaxalone at a dose of 2 mg/kg/h and medetomidine at a dose of 5 μg/kg/h were determined to be suitable for short-term field anesthesia in the horse [209].

Ruminant

Alfaxalone has been shown to produce acceptable anesthesia while maintaining cardiovascular and respiratory function in sheep [212,213]. It has been demonstrated that a constant rate infusion of alfaxalone in desflurane-anesthetized sheep reduced inhalant requirements while cardiorespiratory parameters remained similar to sheep anesthetized with desflurane alone [212]. In another study, a 2 mg/kg intravenous dose of alfaxalone produced minimal changes in cardiopulmonary and acid–base variables [213]. Alfaxalone has also been shown to have no effect on intraocular pressure in sheep; however, marked myosis was observed [214].

Swine

Alfaxalone has been used to induce sedation and anesthesia in pigs. Alfaxalone alone or in combination with diazepam has been injected intramuscularly in pigs. This rapidly produced recumbency, deep sedation, and minimal side-effects. It was noted that this combination may be useful for premedication in pigs, but that the volume of injectate would limit its use to small pigs [215]. Induction of anesthesia with intravenous alfaxalone has also been described in swine. In pigs premedicated with intramuscular azaperone, intravenous alfaxalone resulted in satisfactory conditions for intubation with minimal side-effects [216].

Table 15.9 Alfaxalone dosages in various species.

Species	Intravenous induction of anesthesia (mg/kg)	Constant rate infusion (mg/kg/min)	Sedation dose (mg/kg)
Dog	0.5–2.2	0.07–0.12	
Cat	0.5–5.0	0.18	3.0 SC
Horse	1–3	0.033[14]	
Foal	3		
Sheep	1.2–2.6		
Pig	0.6–1.1		5.0 IM

Administered with 5 μg/kg/h medetomidine
IM = intramuscular; SC = subcutaneous.

Clinical use

Table 15.9 lists commonly used doses for alfaxalone. As with all injectable induction agents, the dose should be tailored according to concurrent drug administration and physical status.

As discussed previously, alfaxalone can be effective when administered intravenously or intramuscularly. However, due to volume of injection, the intramuscular route of administration should be limited to small patients.

While recovering from alfaxalone anesthesia, it is recommended that animals be left in a quiet, dark area where they are not handled or disturbed except for necessary monitoring. Paddling of the limbs, muscle twitching, hyper-reactivity, and ataxia have been reported in animals that are recovering from alfaxalone anesthesia. These reactions may be obtunded by the use of sedative agents.

Other drugs

The following injectable anesthetic agents are no longer routinely used in clinical practice but do have historical significance in the study of veterinary anesthesia or are occasionally of interest to laboratory investigators.

Metomidate

Metomidate is the first compound of the imidazole class of anesthetics that was designed as a non-barbiturate intravenous hypnotic drug. It is freely soluble in water but aqueous solutions are unstable and should be used within 24 h. It was introduced initially as a hypnotic for pigs, horses [217], and a variety of avian species. When given by intravenous injection, metomidate produces loss of consciousness quickly. It has a short duration of action of less than 25 min; however animals will sleep for several hours. Recovery in horses may be extremely violent [218].

Metomidate anesthesia is characterized by cardiovascular stability. Mild hypotension results initially, along with a decrease in heart rate and a slight decrease in cardiac output. Minute ventilation also remains stable with a slightly decreased respiratory rate, but increased tidal volume. Metomidate produces profound muscle relaxation but little analgesia, so it must be combined with analgesics for surgical procedures [218]. Further development of the imidazole compounds created the superior substance etomidate, which has gained use in human and veterinary medicine.

Chloral hydrate

Chloral hydrate, 1,1,1-trichloro-2,2-dihydroxyethane, is a hypnotic that was first introduced in 1869. It is a crystalline substance that has a distinct odor and volatizes slowly at room temperature. It is readily soluble in water and aqueous solutions remain generally stable. Chloral hydrate is metabolized after administration to trichloroethanol which is responsible for most of the observed effects.

Although the mechanism of action is unknown, it is likely that trichloroethanol interacts with the GABA receptor in a similar fashion as the other injectable anesthetics. When administered, chloral hydrate produces dose-dependent sedation. The dose required to produce anesthesia approaches the minimum lethal dose, so its margin of safety is quite narrow. The effects of an intravenous injection are slow to occur which makes it difficult to assess the degree of sedation or depression. Even after slow administration, sedation continues to deepen for a few minutes after the injection is stopped, likely due to the lag time created by the metabolism to trichloroethanol.

Myocardial contractility is reduced, resulting in hypotension. The respiratory system is mildly affected by chloral hydrate administration but at doses needed to produce anesthesia, respiratory depression can be severe. Ventricular fibrillation and sudden death in the recovery period have been reported. To mitigate the risk of death, the addition of either magnesium sulfate, pentobarbital, or both has been used.

Historically, chloral hydrate has been used for sedation in horses and cattle either intravenously or orally. Chloral hydrate is irritating to both stomach and mucous membranes; its irritating nature means that perivascular injection results in necrosis and sloughing of the vessel wall and the surrounding tissues. If intravenous injection is continued until a surgical plane of anesthesia is reached, recovery will be prolonged.

Magnesium sulfate

Magnesium sulfate is probably better thought of as a muscle relaxant and CNS depressant rather than an injectable anesthetic. When combined with chloral hydrate, it hastens the onset of anesthesia, increases its depth, and reduces the toxicity associated with chloral hydrate. The recommended mixture is two parts chloral hydrate to one part magnesium sulfate.

Dilute solutions of magnesium sulfate have been used to induce anesthesia in small animal patients. However, magnesium sulfate administration results in global depression of the CNS, and respiratory arrest occurs frequently. Magnesium sulfate has been used for euthanasia, but it should only be administered after the animal is rendered unconscious with another anesthetic agent.

Chloralose

Chloralose is a solution prepared by heating glucose and chloral hydrate. Its use as an anesthetic is limited to laboratory animals being used in non-survival surgical experiments. Anesthesia produced with chloralose is similar to chloral hydrate but the effects last 8–10 h. Compared to chloral hydrate, blood pressure is elevated, as is the heart rate and respiratory rate [218]. Chloralose is transformed to chloraldehyde and glucose and the safety margin is relatively large. Recovery from chloralose anesthesia is slow and marked by paddling and muscle fasciculations. Consequently, there is little indication for its use in veterinary medicine.

References

1 Haws JL, Herman N, Clark Y, *et al.* The chemical stability and sterility of sodium thiopental after preparation. *Anesth Analg* 1998; **86(1)**: 208–213.

2 Beeman CS, Dembo J, Bogardus A. Stability of reconstituted methohexital sodium. *J Oral Maxillofac Surg* 1994; **52(4)**: 393–396.

3 Olsen RW, Li GD. GABA(A) receptors as molecular targets of general anesthetics: identification of binding sites provides clues to allosteric modulation. *Can J Anaesth* 2011; **58(2)**: 206–215.

4 Tanelian DL, Kosek P, Mody I *et al.* The role of the GABAA receptor/chloride channel complex in anesthesia. *Anesthesiology* 1993; **78(4)**: 757–776.

5 Saidman LJ. Uptake, distribution, and elimination of barbiturates. In: Eger EI, ed. *Anesthetic Uptake and Action*, 2nd edn. Baltimore, MD: Williams & Wilkins, 1974.

6 Russo H, Bressolle F. Pharmacodynamics and pharmacokinetics of thiopental. *Clin Pharmacokinet* 1998; **35(2)**: 95–134.

7 Price HL. A dynamic concept of the distribution of thiopental in the human body. *Anesthesiology* 1960; **21**: 40–45.

8 Weiss M. How does obesity affect residence time dispersion and the shape of drug disposition curves? Thiopental as an example. *J Pharmacokinet Pharmacodynam* 2008; **35(3)**: 325–336.

9 Ilkiw JE, Benthuysen JA, Ebling WF, *et al.* A comparative study of the pharmacokinetics of thiopental in the rabbit, sheep and dog. *J Vet Pharmacol Ther* 1991; **14(2)**: 134–140.

10 Brandon RA, Baggot JD. The pharmacokinetics of thiopentone. *J Vet Pharmacol Ther* 1981; **4(2)**: 79–85.

11 Kiersey DK, Bickford RG, Faulconer A. Electro-encephalographic patterns produced by thiopental sodium during surgical operations; description and classification. *Br J Anaesth* 1951; **23(3)**: 141–152.

12 Albrecht RF, Miletich DJ, Rosenberg R, *et al.* Cerebral blood flow and metabolic changes from induction to onset of anesthesia with halothane or pentobarbital. *Anesthesiology* 1977; **47(3)**: 252–256.

13 Guo J, White JA, Batjer HH. The protective effects of thiopental on brain stem ischemia. *Neurosurgery* 1995; **37(3)**: 490–495.

14 Ebmeyer U, Safar P, Radovsky A, *et al.* Thiopental combination treatments for cerebral resuscitation after prolonged cardiac arrest in dogs. Exploratory outcome study. *Resuscitation* 2000; **45(2)**: 119–131.

15 Hofmeister EH, Williams CO, Braun C, *et al.* Propofol versus thiopental: effects on peri-induction intraocular pressures in normal dogs. *Vet Anaesth Analg* 2008; **35(4)**: 275–281.

16 Turner DM, Ilkiw JE. Cardiovascular and respiratory effects of three rapidly acting barbiturates in dogs. *Am J Vet Res* 1990; **51(4)**: 598–604.

17 Muir WW. Thiobarbiturate-induced dysrhythmias: the role of heart rate and autonomic imbalance. *Am J Vet Res* 1977; **38(9)**: 1377–1381.

18 Hayashi Y, Sumikawa K, Yamatodani A, *et al.* Myocardial sensitization by thiopental to arrhythmogenic action of epinephrine in dogs. *Anesthesiology* 1989; **71(6)**: 929–935.

19 Hirshman CA, McCullough RE, Cohen PJ, *et al.* Hypoxic ventilatory drive in dogs during thiopental, ketamine, or pentobarbital anesthesia. *Anesthesiology* 1975; **43(6)**: 628–634.

20 Quandt JE, Robinson EP, Rivers WJ, *et al.* Cardiorespiratory and anesthetic effects of propofol and thiopental in dogs. *Am J Vet Res* 1998; **59(9)**: 1137–1143.

21 Hirota K, Ohtomo N, Hashimoto Y, *et al.* Effects of thiopental on airway calibre in dogs: direct visualization method using a superfine fibreoptic bronchoscope. *Br J Anaesth* 1998; **81(2)**: 203–207.

22 Jackson AM, Tobias K, Long C, *et al.* Effects of various anesthetic agents on laryngeal motion during laryngoscopy in normal dogs. *Vet Surg* 2004; **33(2)**: 102–106.

23 Forbes AR, Gamsu G. Depression of lung mucociliary clearance by thiopental and halothane. *Anesth Analg* 1979; **58(5)**: 387–389.

24 Sams RA, Muir WW. Effects of phenobarbital on thiopental pharmacokinetics in greyhounds. *Am J Vet Res* 1988; **49(2)**: 245–249.

25 Hashim MA, Waterman AE. Effects of thiopentone, propofol, alphaxalone-alphadolone, ketamine and xylazine-ketamine on lower oesophageal sphincter pressure and barrier pressure in cats. *Vet Rec* 1991; **129(7)**: 137–139.

26 Chang J, Kim S, Jung J, *et al.* Evaluation of the effects of thiopental, propofol, and etomidate on glomerular filtration rate measured by the use of dynamic computed tomography in dogs. *Am J Vet Res* 2011; **72(1)**: 146–151.

27 Luna SP, Cassu RN, Castro GB, *et al.* Effects of four anaesthetic protocols on the neurological and cardiorespiratory variables of puppies born by Caesarean section. *Vet Rec* 2004; **154(13)**: 387–389.

28 Alon E, Ball RH, Gillie MH, *et al.* Effects of propofol and thiopental on maternal and fetal cardiovascular and acid-base variables in the pregnant ewe. *Anesthesiology* 1993; **78(3)**: 562–576.

29 Wilder-Smith OH, Kolletzki M, Wilder-Smith CH. Sedation with intravenous infusions of propofol or thiopentone. Effects on pain perception. *Anaesthesia* 1995; **50(3)**: 218–222.

30 Abass BT, Weaver BM, Staddon GE, *et al.* Pharmacokinetics of thiopentone in the horse. *J Vet Pharmacol Ther* 1994; **17(5)**: 331–338.

31 Hubbell JA, Hinchcliff KW, Schmall LM, *et al.* Anesthetic, cardiorespiratory, and metabolic effects of four intravenous anesthetic regimens induced in horses immediately after maximal exercise. *Am J Vet Res* 2000; **61(12)**: 1545–1552.

32 Toutain PL, Brandon RA, Alvinerie M, *et al.* Thiopentone pharmacokinetics and electrocorticogram pattern in sheep. *J Vet Pharmacol Ther* 1983; **6(3)**: 201–209.

33 Softeland E, Framstad T, Thorsen T, *et al.* Evaluation of thiopentone-midazolam-fentanyl anaesthesia in pigs. *Lab Anim* 1995; **29(3):** 269–275.

34 Dyess DL, Tacchi E, Powell RQ, *et al.* Development of a protocol to provide prolonged general anesthesia to pregnant sows. *J Invest Surg* 1994; **7(3):** 235–242.

35 Weiskopf RB, Bogetz MS. Haemorrhage decreases the anaesthetic requirement for ketamine and thiopentone in the pig. *Br J Anaesth* 1985; **57(10):** 1022–1025.

36 Rawlings CA, Kolata RJ. Cardiopulmonary effects of thiopental/lidocaine combination during anesthetic induction in the dog. *Am J Vet Res* 1983; **44(1):** 144–149.

37 Ko JC, Golder FJ, Mandsager RE, *et al.* Anesthetic and cardiorespiratory effects of a 1:1 mixture of propofol and thiopental sodium in dogs. *J Am Vet Med Assoc*1999; **215(9):** 1292–1296.

38 Joubert KE, Picard J, Sethusa M. Inhibition of bacterial growth by different mixtures of propofol and thiopentone. *J S Afr Vet Assoc* 2005; **76(2):** 85–89.

39 Kay B, Rolly G. I.C.I. 35868, a new intravenous induction agent. *Acta Anaesth Belg* 1977; **28(4):** 303–316.

40 Wachowski I, Jolly DT, Hrazdil J, *et al.* The growth of microorganisms in propofol and mixtures of propofol and lidocaine. *Anesth Analg* 1999; **88(1):** 209–212.

41 Cleale RM, Muir WW, Waselau AC, *et al.* Pharmacokinetic and pharmacodynamic evaluation of propofol administered to cats in a novel, aqueous, nano-droplet formulation or as an oil-in-water macroemulsion. *J Vet Pharmacol Ther* 2009; **32(5):** 436–445.

42 Taylor PM, Chengelis CP, Miller WR, *et al.* Evaluation of propofol containing 2% benzyl alcohol preservative in cats. *J Feline Med Surg* 2012; **14(8):** 516–526.

43 Altomare C1, Trapani G, Latrofa A, *et al.* Highly water-soluble derivatives of the anesthetic agent propofol: in vitro and in vivo evaluation of cyclic amino acid esters. *Eur J Pharmaceut Sci* 2003; **20(1):** 17–26.

44 McIntosh MP1, Rajewski RA. Comparative canine pharmacokinetics-pharmacodynamics of fospropofol disodium injection, propofol emulsion, and cyclodextrin-enabled propofol solution following bolus parenteral administration. *J Pharmaceut Sci* 2012; **101(9):** 3547–3552.

45 Ying SW, Goldstein PA. Propofol suppresses synaptic responsiveness of somatosensory relay neurons to excitatory input by potentiating GABA(A) receptor chloride channels. *Molec Pain* 2005; **1:** 2.

46 Orser BA, Bertlik M, Wang LY, *et al.* Inhibition by propofol (2,6 di-isopropylphenol) of the N-methyl-D-aspartate subtype of glutamate receptor in cultured hippocampal neurones. *Br J Pharmacol* 1995; **116(2):** 1761–1768.

47 Zoran DL, Riedesel DH, Dyer DC. Pharmacokinetics of propofol in mixed-breed dogs and greyhounds. *Am J Vet Res* 1993; **54(5):** 755–760.

48 Hay-Kraus BL, Greenblatt DJ, Venkatakrishnan K, *et al.* Evidence for propofol hydroxylation by cytochrome P4502B11 in canine liver microsomes: breed and gender differences. *Xenobiotica* 2000; **30(6):** 575–588.

49 Veroli P, O'Kelly B, Bertrand F, *et al.* Extrahepatic metabolism of propofol in man during the anhepatic phase of orthotopic liver transplantation. *Br J Anaesth* 1992; **68(2):** 183–186.

50 Servin F, Cockshott ID, Farinotti R, *et al.* Pharmacokinetics of propofol infusions in patients with cirrhosis. *Br J Anaesth* 1990; **65(2):** 177–183.

51 Matot I, Neely CF, Katz RY, *et al.* Pulmonary uptake of propofol in cats. Effect of fentanyl and halothane. *Anesthesiology* 1993; **78(6):** 1157–1165.

52 Posner LP, Asakawa M, Erb HN. Use of propofol for anesthesia in cats with primary hepatic lipidosis: 44 cases (1995–2004). *J Am Vet Med Assoc*2008; **232(12):** 1841–1843.

53 Reid J, Nolan AM. Pharmacokinetics of propofol as an induction agent in geriatric dogs. *Res Vet Sci* 1996; **61(2):** 169–171.

54 Court MH, Hay-Kraus BL, Hill DW, *et al.* Propofol hydroxylation by dog liver microsomes: assay development and dog breed differences. *Drug Metab Dispos*1999; **27(11):** 1293–1299.

55 Adam HK, Glen JB, Hoyle PA. Pharmacokinetics in laboratory animals of ICI 35 868, a new i.v. anaesthetic agent. *Br J Anaesth* 1980; **52(8):** 743–746.

56 Mandsager RE, Clarke CR, Shawley RV, *et al.* Effects of chloramphenicol on infusion pharmacokinetics of propofol in greyhounds. *Am J Vet Res* 1995; **56(1):** 95–99.

57 Artru AA, Shapira Y, Bowdle TA. Electroencephalogram, cerebral metabolic, and vascular responses to propofol anesthesia in dogs. *J Neurosurg Anesthesiol* 1992; **4(2):** 99–109.

58 Herregods L, Verbeke J, Rolly G, *et al.* Effect of propofol on elevated intracranial pressure. Preliminary results *Anaesthesia* 1988; **43(Suppl):** 107–109.

59 Cheng MA, Tempelhoff R, Silbergeld DL, *et al.* Large-dose propofol alone in adult epileptic patients: electrocorticographic results. *Anesth Analg* 1996; **83(1):** 169–174.

60 Steffen F, Grasmueck S. Propofol for treatment of refractory seizures in dogs and a cat with intracranial disorders. *J Small Anim Pract* 2000; **41(11):** 496–499.

61 Goodchild CS, Serrao JM. Cardiovascular effects of propofol in the anaesthetized dog. *Br J Anaesth* 1989; **63(1):** 87–92.

62 Brussel T, Theissen JL, Vigfusson G, *et al.* Hemodynamic and cardiodynamic effects of propofol and etomidate: negative inotropic properties of propofol. *Anesth Analg* 1989; **69(1):** 35–40.

63 Ilkiw JE, Haskins SC, Patz JD. Cardiovascular and respiratory effects of thiopental administration in hypovolemic dogs. *Am J Vet Res* 1991; **52(4):** 576–580.

64 Pagel PS, Hettrick DA, Kersten JR, *et al.* Cardiovascular effects of propofol in dogs with dilated cardiomyopathy. *Anesthesiology* 1998; **88(1):** 180–189.

65 Kamibayashi T, Hayashi Y, Sumikawa K, *et al.* Enhancement by propofol of epinephrine-induced arrhythmias in dogs. *Anesthesiology* 1991; **75(6):** 1035–1040.

66 Muir WW, Gadawski JE. Respiratory depression and apnea induced by propofol in dogs. *Am J Vet Res* 1998; **59(2):** 157–161.

67 Blouin RT, Seifert HA, Babenco HD, *et al.* Propofol depresses the hypoxic ventilatory response during conscious sedation and isohypercapnia. *Anesthesiology* 1993; **79(6):** 1177–1182.

68 Goodman NW, Black AM, Carter JA. Some ventilatory effects of propofol as sole anaesthetic agent. *Br J Anaesth* 1987; **59(12):** 1497–1503.

69 Ponte J, Sadler CL. Effect of thiopentone, etomidate and propofol on carotid body chemoreceptor activity in the rabbit and the cat. *Br J Anaesth* 1989; **62(1):** 41–45.

70 Taylor MB, Grounds RM, Mulrooney PD, *et al.* Ventilatory effects of propofol during induction of anaesthesia. Comparison with thiopentone. *Anaesthesia* 1986; **41(8):** 816–820.

71 Haberer JP, Audibert G, Saunier CG, *et al.* Effect of propofol and thiopentone on regional blood flow in brain and peripheral tissues during normoxia and hypoxia in the dog. *Clin Physiol* 1993; **13(2):** 197–207.

72 Apfel CC, Korttila K, Abdalla M, *et al.* A factorial trial of six interventions for the prevention of postoperative nausea and vomiting. *N Engl J Med* 2004; **350(24):** 2441–2451.

73 Smedile LE, Duke T, Taylor SM. Excitatory movements in a dog following propofol anesthesia. *J Am Anim Hosp Assoc*1996; **32(4):** 365–368.

74 Nimmaanrat S. Myoclonic movements following induction of anesthesia with propofol: a case report. *J Med Assoc Thailand* 2005; **88(12):** 1955–1957.

75 Andaluz A, Tusell J, Trasserres O, *et al.* Transplacental transfer of propofol in pregnant ewes. *Vet J* 2003; **166(2):** 198–204.

76 Doebeli A, Michel E, Bettschart R, *et al.* Apgar score after induction of anesthesia for canine cesarean section with alfaxalone versus propofol. *Theriogenology* 2013; **80(8):** 850–854.

77 Heldmann E, Brown DC, Shofer F. The association of propofol usage with postoperative wound infection rate in clean wounds: a retrospective study. *Vet Surg* 1999; **28(4):** 256–259.

78 Lee SH, Ghim JL, Song MH, *et al.* Pharmacokinetics and pharmacodynamics of a new reformulated microemulsion and the long-chain triglyceride emulsion of propofol in beagle dogs. *Br J Pharmacol* 2009; **158(8):** 1982–1995.

79 Michou JN, Leece EA, Brearley JC. Comparison of pain on injection during induction of anaesthesia with alfaxalone and two formulations of propofol in dogs. *Vet Anaesth Analg* 2012; **39(3):** 275–281.

80 Andress JL, Day TK, Day D. The effects of consecutive day propofol anesthesia on feline red blood cells. *Vet Surg* 1995; **24(3):** 277–282.

81 Bley CR, Roos M, Price J, *et al.* Clinical assessment of repeated propofol-associated anesthesia in cats. *J Am Vet Med Assoc*2007; **231(9):** 1347–1353.

82 Wiese AJ, Lerche P, Cleale RM, *et al.* Investigation of escalating and large bolus doses of a novel, nano-droplet, aqueous 1% propofol formulation in cats. *Vet Anaesth Analg* 2010; **37(3):** 250–257.

83 Nolan AM, Hall LW. Total intravenous anaesthesia in the horse with propofol. *Equine Vet J* 1985; **17(5):** 394–398.

84 Mama KR, Steffey EP, Pascoe PJ. Evaluation of propofol as a general anesthetic for horses. *Vet Surg* 1995; **24(2):** 188–194.

85 Mama KR, Steffey EP, Pascoe PJ. Evaluation of propofol for general anesthesia in premedicated horses. *Am J Vet Res* 1996; **57(4):** 512–516.

86 Brosnan RJ, Steffey EP, Escobar A, *et al.* Anesthetic induction with guaifenesin and propofol in adult horses. *Am J Vet Res* 2011; **72(12):** 1569–1575.

87 Oku K, Ohta M, Katoh T, *et al.* Cardiovascular effects of continuous propofol infusion in horses. *J Vet Med Sci* 2006; **68(8):** 773–778.

88 Umar MA, Yamashita K, Kushiro T, *et al.* Evaluation of total intravenous anesthesia with propofol or ketamine-medetomidine-propofol combination in horses. *J Am Vet Med Assoc* 2006; **228(8):** 1221–1227.

89 Ishizuka T, Itami T, Tamura J, *et al.* Anesthetic and cardiorespiratory effects of propofol, medetomidine, lidocaine and butorphanol total intravenous anesthesia in horses. *J Vet Med Sci* 2013; **75(2):** 165–172.

90 Wagner AE, Mama KR, Steffey EP, *et al.* Evaluation of infusions of xylazine with ketamine or propofol to modulate recovery following sevoflurane anesthesia in horses. *Am J Vet Res* 2012; **73(3):** 346–352.

91 Steffey EP, Mama KR, Brosnan RJ, *et al.* Effect of administration of propofol and xylazine hydrochloride on recovery of horses after four hours of anesthesia with desflurane. *Am J Vet Res* 2009; **70(8):** 956–963.

92 Boscan P, Rezende ML, Grimsrud K, *et al.* Pharmacokinetic profile in relation to anaesthesia characteristics after a 5% micellar microemulsion of propofol in the horse. *Br J Anaesth* 2010; **104(3):** 330–337.
93 Rezende ML, Boscan P, Stanley SD, *et al.* Evaluation of cardiovascular, respiratory and biochemical effects, and anesthetic induction and recovery behavior in horses anesthetized with a 5% micellar microemulsion propofol formulation. *Vet Anaesth Analg* 2010; **37(5):** 440–450.
94 Lin HC, Purohit RC, Powe TA. Anesthesia in sheep with propofol or with xylazine-ketamine followed by halothane. *Vet Surg* 1997; **26(3):** 247–252.
95 Reid J, Nolan AM, Welsh E. Propofol as an induction agent in the goat: a pharmacokinetic study. *J Vet Pharmacol Ther* 1993; **16(4):** 488–493.
96 Cagnardi P, Zonca A, Gallo M, *et al.* Pharmacokinetics of propofol in calves undergoing abdominal surgery. *Vet Res Commun* 2009; **Suppl 1:** 177–179.
97 Duke T, Egger CM, Ferguson JG, *et al.* Cardiopulmonary effects of propofol infusion in llamas. *Am J Vet Res* 1997; **58(2):** 153–156.
98 Correia D, Nolan AM, Reid J. Pharmacokinetics of propofol infusions, either alone or with ketamine, in sheep premedicated with acepromazine and papaveretum. *Res Vet Sci* 1996; **60(3):** 213–217.
99 Foster PS, Hopkinson KC, Denborough MA. Propofol anaesthesia in malignant hyperpyrexia susceptible swine. *Clin Exper Pharmacol Physiol* 1992; **19(3):** 183–186.
100 Kaiser GM, Breuckmann F, Aker S, *et al.* Anesthesia for cardiovascular interventions and magnetic resonance imaging in pigs. *J Am Assoc Lab Anim Sci* 2007; **46(2):** 30–33.
101 Reich DL, Silvay G. Ketamine: an update on the first twenty-five years of clinical experience. *Can J Anaesth* 1989; **36(2):** 186–197.
102 White PF, Ham J, Way WL, *et al.* Pharmacology of ketamine isomers in surgical patients. *Anesthesiology* 1980; **52(3):** 231–239.
103 Annetta MG, Iemma D, Garisto C, *et al.* Ketamine: new indications for an old drug. *Curr Drug Targ* 2005; **6(7):** 789–794.
104 Hirota K, Lambert DG. Ketamine: its mechanism(s) of action and unusual clinical uses. *Br J Anaesth* 1996; **77(4):** 441–444.
105 Hustveit O, Maurset A, Oye I. Interaction of the chiral forms of ketamine with opioid, phencyclidine, sigma and muscarinic receptors. *Pharmacol Toxicol* 1995; **77(6):** 355–359.
106 Stoelting RK. Nonbarbiturate induction drugs. In: Stoelting RK, ed. *Pharmacology and Physiology in Anesthetic Practice*, 3rd edn. Philadelphia: Lippincott, Williams & Wilkins, **1999**, 140–157.
107 White PF, Way WL, Trevor AJ. Ketamine – its pharmacology and therapeutic uses. *Anesthesiology* 1982; **56(2):** 119–136.
108 Hanna RM, Borchard RE, Schmidt SL. Pharmacokinetics of ketamine HCl and metabolite I in the cat: a comparison of i.v., i.m., and rectal administration. *J Vet Pharmacol Ther* 1988; **11(1):** 84–93.
109 Dawson B, Michenfelder JD, Theye RA. Effects of ketamine on canine cerebral blood flow and metabolism: modification by prior administration of thiopental. *Anesth Analg* 1971; **50(3):** 443–447.
110 Takeshita H, Okuda Y, Sari A. The effects of ketamine on cerebral circulation and metabolism in man. *Anesthesiology* 1972; **36(1):** 69–75.
111 Pfenninger E, Dick W, Ahnefeld FW. The influence of ketamine on both normal and raised intracranial pressure of artificially ventilated animals. *Eur J Anaesthesiol* 1985; **2(3):** 297–307.
112 Kayama Y. Ketamine and EEG seizure waves: interaction with anti-epileptic drugs. *Br J Anaesth* 1982; **54(8):** 879–883.
113 Celesia GG, Chen RC, Bamforth BJ. Effects of ketamine in epilepsy. *Neurology* 1975; **25(2):** 169–172.
114 Reder BS, Trapp LD, Troutman KC. Ketamine suppression of chemically induced convulsions in the two-day-old white leghorn cockerel. *Anesth Analg* 1980; **59(6):** 406–409.
115 Diaz FA, Bianco JA, Bello A, *et al.* Effects of ketamine on canine cardiovascular function. *Br J Anaesth* 1976; **48(10):** 941–946.
116 Haskins SC, Farver TB, Patz JD. Ketamine in dogs. *Am J Vet Res* 1985; **46(9):** 1855–1860.
117 Wong DH, Jenkins LC. An experimental study of the mechanism of action of ketamine on the central nervous system. *Can Anaesth Soc J* 1974; **21(1):** 57–67.
118 Baraka A, Harrison T, Kachachi T. Catecholamine levels after ketamine anesthesia in man. *Anesth Analg* 1973; **52(2):** 198–200.
119 Waxman K, Shoemaker WC, Lippmann M. Cardiovascular effects of anesthetic induction with ketamine. *Anesth Analg* 1980; **59(5):** 355–358.
120 Soliman MG, Brindle GF, Kuster G. Response to hypercapnia under ketamine anaesthesia. *Can Anaesth Soc J* 1975; **22(4):** 486-494.
121 Jaspar N, Mazzarelli M, Tessier C, *et al.* Effect of ketamine on control of breathing in cats. *J Appl Physiol* 1983; **55(3):** 851–859.
122 Hirshman CA, Downes H, Farbood A, *et al.* Ketamine block of bronchospasm in experimental canine asthma. *Br J Anaesth* 1979; **51(8):** 713–718.
123 Taylor PA, Towey RM. Ketamine anaesthesia. *BMJ* 1971; **3(5771):** 432.
124 Fass J, Bares R, Hermsdorf V, *et al.* Effects of intravenous ketamine on gastrointestinal motility in the dog. *Intensive Care Med* 1995; **21(7):** 584–589.
125 Aida S, Yamakura T, Baba H, *et al.* Preemptive analgesia by intravenous low-dose ketamine and epidural morphine in gastrectomy: a randomized double-blind study. *Anesthesiology* 2000; **92(6):** 1624–1630.
126 Kovalcuka L, Birgele E, Bandere D, *et al.* The effects of ketamine hydrochloride and diazepam on the intraocular pressure and pupil diameter of the dog's eye. *Vet Ophthalmol* 2013; **16(1):** 29–34.
127 Wetzel RW, Ramsay EC. Comparison of four regimens for intraoral administration of medication to induce sedation in cats prior to euthanasia. *J Am Vet Med Assoc*1998; **213(2):** 243–245.
128 Harrison KA, Robertson SA, Levy JK, *et al.* Evaluation of medetomidine, ketamine and buprenorphine for neutering feral cats. *J Feline Med Surg* 2011; **13(12):** 896–902.
129 Cistola AM, Golder FJ, Centonze LA, *et al.* Anesthetic and physiologic effects of tiletamine, zolazepam, ketamine, and xylazine combination (TKX) in feral cats undergoing surgical sterilization. *J Feline Med Surg* 2004; **6(5):** 297–303.
130 Cruz ML, Luna SP, de Castro GB, *et al.* A preliminary trial comparison of several anesthetic techniques in cats. *Can Vet J* 2000; **41(6):** 481–485.
131 Gunkel C, Lafortune M. Felids. In: West G, Heard D, Caulkett N, eds. *Zoo Animal and Wildlife Immobilization and Anesthesia*. Ames, IA: Blackwell Publishing, 2007; 443–458.
132 Muir WW, Lerche P, Robertson JT, *et al.* Comparison of four drug combinations for total intravenous anesthesia of horses undergoing surgical removal of an abdominal testis. *J Am Vet Med Assoc* 2000; **217(6):** 869–873.
133 Coetzee JF, Gehring R, Tarus-Sang J, *et al.* Effect of sub-anesthetic xylazine and ketamine ('ketamine stun') administered to calves immediately prior to castration. *Vet Anaesth Analg* 2010; **37(6):** 566–578.
134 Dershwitz M, Sreter FA, Ryan JF. Ketamine does not trigger malignant hyperthermia in susceptible swine. *Anesth Analg* 1989; **69(4):** 501–503.
135 Ko JC, Williams BL, Smith VL, *et al.* Comparison of Telazol, Telazol-ketamine, Telazol-xylazine, and Telazol-ketamine-xylazine as chemical restraint and anesthetic induction combination in swine. *Lab Anim Sci* 1993; **43(5):** 476–480.
136 Nagel ML, Muir WW, Nguyen K. Comparison of the cardiopulmonary effects of etomidate and thiamylal in dogs. *Am J Vet Res* 1979; **40(2):** 193–196.
137 Tulleken CA, van Dieren A, Jonkman J, *et al.* Clinical and experimental experience with etomidate as a brain protective agent. *J Cerebr Blood Flow Metab* 1982; **2**(Suppl 1): S92–97.
138 Van Hamme MJ, Ghoneim MM, Ambre JJ. Pharmacokinetics of etomidate, a new intravenous anesthetic. *Anesthesiology* 1978; **49(4):** 274–277.
139 Wertz EM, Benson GJ, Thurmon JC, *et al.* Pharmacokinetics of etomidate in cats. *Am J Vet Res* 1990; **51(2):** 281–285.
140 Meuldermans WE, Heykants JJ. The plasma protein binding and distribution of etomidate in dog, rat and human blood. *Arch Int Pharmacodyn Ther* 1976; **221(1):** 150–162.
141 Janssen PA, Niemegeers CJ, Marsboom RP. Etomidate, a potent non-barbiturate hypnotic. Intravenous etomidate in mice, rats, guinea-pigs, rabbits and dogs. *Arch Int Pharmacodyn Ther* 1975; **214(1):** 92–132.
142 Gooding JM, Corssen G. Etomidate: an ultrashort-acting nonbarbiturate agent for anesthesia induction. *Anesth Analg* 1976; **55(2):** 286–289.
143 Heykants JJ, Meuldermans WE, Michiels LJ, *et al.* Distribution, metabolism and excretion of etomidate, a short-acting hypnotic drug, in the rat. Comparative study of (R)-(+)-(–)-etomidate. *Arch Int Pharmacodyn Ther* 1975; **216(1):** 113–129.
144 Andrada J, Livingston P, Lee BJ, *et al.* Propofol and etomidate depress cortical, thalamic, and reticular formation neurons during anesthetic-induced unconsciousness. *Anesth Analg* 2012 **114(3):** 661–669.
145 Milde LN, Milde JH, Michenfelder JD. Cerebral functional, metabolic, and hemodynamic effects of etomidate in dogs. *Anesthesiology* 1985; **63(4):** 371–377.
146 Cold GE, Eskesen V, Eriksen H, *et al.* CBF and CMRO2 during continuous etomidate infusion supplemented with N2O and fentanyl in patients with supratentorial cerebral tumour. A dose-response study. *Acta Anaesthesiol Scand* 1985; **29(5):** 490–494.
147 Dearden NM, McDowall DG. Comparison of etomidate and althesin in the reduction of increased intracranial pressure after head injury. *Br J Anaesth* 1985; **57(4):** 361–368.
148 Ghoneim MM, Yamada T. Etomidate: a clinical and electroencephalographic comparison with thiopental. *Anesth Analg* 1977; **56(4):** 479–485.
149 Frizzell RT, Meyer YJ, Borchers DJ, *et al.* The effects of etomidate on cerebral metabolism and blood flow in a canine model for hypoperfusion. *J Neurosurg* 1991; **74(2):** 263–269.
150 Wauquier A. Profile of etomidate. A hypnotic, anticonvulsant and brain protective compound. *Anaesthesia* 1983; **38(Suppl):** 26–33.

151 Ebrahim ZY, DeBoer GE, Luders H, *et al.* Effect of etomidate on the electroencephalogram of patients with epilepsy. *Anesth Analg* 1986; **65(10):** 1004–1006.
152 Rodriguez JM, Munoz-Rascon P, Navarrete-Calvo R, *et al.* Comparison of the cardiopulmonary parameters after induction of anaesthesia with alphaxalone or etomidate in dogs. *Vet Anaesth Analg* 2012; **39(4):** 357–365.
153 Sams L, Braun C, Allman D, *et al.* A comparison of the effects of propofol and etomidate on the induction of anesthesia and on cardiopulmonary parameters in dogs. *Vet Anaesth Analg* 2008; **35(6):** 488–494.
154 Kissin I, Motomura S, Aultman DF, *et al.* Inotropic and anesthetic potencies of etomidate and thiopental in dogs. *Anesth Analg* 1983; **62(11):** 961–965.
155 Priano LL, Bernards C, Marrone B. Effect of anesthetic induction agents on cardiovascular neuroregulation in dogs. *Anesth Analg* 1989; **68(3):** 344–349.
156 Pascoe PJ, Ilkiw JE, Haskins SC, *et al.* Cardiopulmonary effects of etomidate in hypovolemic dogs. *Am J Vet Res* 1992; **53(11):** 2178–2182.
157 Pagel PS, Hettrick DA, Kersten JR, *et al.* Etomidate adversely alters determinants of left ventricular afterload in dogs with dilated cardiomyopathy. *Anesth Analg* 1998; **86(5):** 932–938.
158 Choi SD, Spaulding BC, Gross JB, *et al.* Comparison of the ventilatory effects of etomidate and methohexital. *Anesthesiology* 1985; **62(4):** 442–447.
159 Fraser R, Watt I, Gray CE, *et al.* The effect of etomidate on adrenocortical function in dogs before and during hemorrhagic shock. *Endocrinology* 1984; **115(6):** 2266–2270.
160 Dodam JR, Kruse-Elliott KT, Aucoin DP, *et al.* Duration of etomidate-induced adrenocortical suppression during surgery in dogs. *Am J Vet Res* 1990; **51(5):** 786–788.
161 Moon PF. Cortisol suppression in cats after induction of anesthesia with etomidate, compared with ketamine-diazepam combination. *Am J Vet Res* 1997; **58(8):** 868–871.
162 Muir WW, Mason DE. Side effects of etomidate in dogs. *J Am Vet Med Assoc* 1989; **194(10):** 1430–1434.
163 Reddy RV, Moorthy SS, Dierdorf SF, *et al.* Excitatory effects and electroencephalographic correlation of etomidate, thiopental, methohexital, and propofol. *Anesth Analg* 1993; **77(5):** 1008–1011.
164 Moon PF. Acute toxicosis in two dogs associated with etomidate-propylene glycol infusion. *Lab Anim Sci* 1994; **44(6):** 590–594.
165 Robertson S. Advantages of etomidate use as an anesthetic agent. *Vet Clin North Am Small Anim Pract* 1992; **22(2):** 277–280.
166 Akkerdaas LC, Sap R, Hellebreker LJ. An alternative premedication and induction regime for cats with a decreased cardio-vascular reserve. *Vet Quart* 1998; **20(Suppl 1):** S108.
167 Fresno L, Andaluz A, Moll X, *et al.* The effects on maternal and fetal cardiovascular and acid-base variables after the administration of etomidate in the pregnant ewe. *Vet J* 2008; **177(1):** 94–103.
168 Fresno L, Andaluz A, Moll X, *et al.* Placental transfer of etomidate in pregnant ewes after an intravenous bolus dose and continuous infusion. *Vet J* 2008; **175(3):** 395–402.
169 Kenyon CJ, McNeil LM, Fraser R. Comparison of the effects of etomidate, thiopentone and propofol on cortisol synthesis. *Br J Anaesth* 1985; **57(5):** 509–511.
170 Clutton RE, Blissitt KJ, Bradley AA, *et al.* Comparison of three injectable anaesthetic techniques in pigs. *Vet Rec* 1997; **141(6):** 140–146.
171 Prakash O, Dhasmana KM, Verdouw PD, *et al.* Cardiovascular effects of etomidate with emphasis on regional myocardial blood flow and performance. *Br J Anaesth* 1981; **53(6):** 591–599.
172 Suresh MS, Nelson TE. Malignant hyperthermia: is etomidate safe? *Anesth Analg* 1985; **64(4):** 420–424.
173 Child KJ, Currie JP, Dis B, *et al.* The pharmacological properties in animals of CT1341 – a new steroid anaesthetic agent. *Br J Anaesth* 1971; **43(1):** 2–13.
174 Hall LW. Althesin in the larger animal. *Postgrad Med J* 1972; **48(Suppl 2):** 55–58.
175 Dodman NH. Complications of saffan anaesthesia in cats. *Vet Rec* 1980; **107(21):** 481–483.
176 Ferre PJ, Pasloske K, Whittem T, *et al.* Plasma pharmacokinetics of alfaxalone in dogs after an intravenous bolus of Alfaxan-CD RTU. *Vet Anaesth Analg* 2006; **33(4):** 229–236.
177 Cottrell GA, Lambert JJ, Peters JA. Modulation of GABAA receptor activity by alphaxalone. *Br J Pharmacol* 1987; **90(3):** 491–500.
178 Whittem T, Pasloske KS, Heit MC, *et al.* The pharmacokinetics and pharmacodynamics of alfaxalone in cats after single and multiple intravenous administration of Alfaxan at clinical and supraclinical doses. *J Vet Pharmacol Ther* 2008; **31(6):** 571–579.
179 Pasloske K, Sauer B, Perkins N, *et al.* Plasma pharmacokinetics of alfaxalone in both premedicated and unpremedicated Greyhound dogs after single, intravenous administration of Alfaxan at a clinical dose. *J Vet Pharmacol Ther* 2009; **32(5):** 510–513.
180 Goodwin WA, Keates HL, Pasloske K, *et al.* The pharmacokinetics and pharmacodynamics of the injectable anaesthetic alfaxalone in the horse. *Vet Anaesth Analg* 2011; **38(5):** 431–438.
181 Goodwin W, Keates H, Pasloske K, *et al.* Plasma pharmacokinetics and pharmacodynamics of alfaxalone in neonatal foals after an intravenous bolus of alfaxalone following premedication with butorphanol tartrate. *Vet Anaesth Analg* 2012; **39(5):** 503–510.
182 Ambrisko TD, Johnson CB, Chambers P. Effect of alfaxalone infusion on the electroencephalogram of dogs anaesthetized with halothane. *Vet Anaesth Analg* 2011; **38(6):** 529–535.
183 Rasmussen NJ, Rosendal T, Overgaard J. Althesin in neurosurgical patients: effects on cerebral hemodynamics and metabolism. *Acta Anaesthesiol Scand* 1978; **22(3):** 257–269.
184 Muir W, Lerche P, Wiese A, *et al.* Cardiorespiratory and anesthetic effects of clinical and supraclinical doses of alfaxalone in dogs. *Vet Anaesth Analg* 2008; **35(6):** 451–462.
185 Muir W, Lerche P, Wiese A, *et al.* The cardiorespiratory and anesthetic effects of clinical and supraclinical doses of alfaxalone in cats. *Vet Anaesth Analg* 2009; **36(1):** 42–54.
186 Petersen JS, Shalmi M, Christensen S, *et al.* Comparison of the renal effects of six sedating agents in rats. *Physiol Behav* 1996; **60(3):** 759–765.
187 Chen CF, Chapman BJ, Munday KA. The effect of althesin, ketamine or pentothal on renal function in saline loaded rats. *Clin Exper Pharmacol Physiol* 1985; **12(2):** 99–105.
188 Patschke D, Passian J, Tarnow J, *et al.* Effect of althesin on renal perfusion in anaesthetized dogs. *Can Anaesth Soc J* 1975; **22(2):** 138–143.
189 Thomson IA, Fitch W, Hughes RL, *et al.* Effects of certain i.v. anaesthetics on liver blood flow and hepatic oxygen consumption in the greyhound. *Br J Anaesth* 1986; **58(1):** 69–80.
190 Sear JW, McGivan JD. Metabolism of alphaxalone in the rat: evidence for the limitation of the anaesthetic effect by the rate of degradation through the hepatic mixed function oxygenase system. *Br J Anaesth* 1981; **53(4):** 417–424.
191 Pasloske K, Gazzard B, Perkins N, *et al.* A multicentre clinical trial evaluating the efficacy and safety of Alfaxan-CD RTU administered to dogs for induction and maintenance of anesthesia. Presented at the British Small Animal Veterinary Association Congress, 2005; Birmingham, UK.
192 Pinelas R, Alibhai HI, Mathis A, *et al.* Effects of different doses of dexmedetomidine on anaesthetic induction with alfaxalone – a clinical trial. *Vet Anaesth Analg* 2014; **41(4):** 378–385.
193 Maddern K, Adams VJ, Hill NA, *et al.* Alfaxalone induction dose following administration of medetomidine and butorphanol in the dog. *Vet Anaesth Analg* 2010; **37(1):** 7–13.
194 Psatha E, Alibhai HI, Jimenez-Lozano A, *et al.* Clinical efficacy and cardiorespiratory effects of alfaxalone, or diazepam/fentanyl for induction of anaesthesia in dogs that are a poor anaesthetic risk. *Vet Anaesth Analg* 2011; **38(1):** 24–36.
195 Ambros B, Duke-Novakovski T, Pasloske KS. Comparison of the anesthetic efficacy and cardiopulmonary effects of continuous rate infusions of alfaxalone-2-hydroxypropyl-beta-cyclodextrin and propofol in dogs. *Am J Vet Res* 2008; **69(11):** 1391–1398.
196 Herbert GL, Bowlt KL, Ford-Fennah V, *et al.* Alfaxalone for total intravenous anaesthesia in dogs undergoing ovariohysterectomy: a comparison of premedication with acepromazine or dexmedetomidine. *Vet Anaesth Analg* 2013; **40(2):** 124–133.
197 Suarez MA, Dzikiti BT, Stegmann FG, *et al.* Comparison of alfaxalone and propofol administered as total intravenous anaesthesia for ovariohysterectomy in dogs. *Vet Anaesth Analg* 2012; **39(3):** 236–244.
198 O'Hagan B, Pasloske K, McKinnon C, *et al.* Clinical evaluation of alfaxalone as an anaesthetic induction agent in dogs less than 12 weeks of age. *Aust Vet J* 2012; **90(9):** 346–350.
199 Metcalfe S, Hulands-Nave A, Bell M, *et al.* A multi-centre clinical trial evaluating the efficacy and safety of Alfaxan administered to bitches for induction of anesthesia prior to caesarean section. Presented at the World Small Animal Veterinary Congress, 2008; Dublin, Ireland.
200 Hasiuk MM, Forde N, Cooke A, *et al.* A comparison of alfaxalone and propofol on intraocular pressure in healthy dogs. *Vet Ophthalmol* 2013; Nov 18 (epub ahead of print).
201 Maney JK, Shepard MK, Braun C, *et al.* A comparison of cardiopulmonary and anesthetic effects of an induction dose of alfaxalone or propofol in dogs. *Vet Anaesth Analg* 2013; **40(3):** 237–244.
202 Ramoo S, Bradbury LA, Anderson GA, *et al.* Sedation of hyperthyroid cats with subcutaneous administration of a combination of alfaxalone and butorphanol. *Aust Vet J* 2013; **91(4):** 131–136.

203 Grubb TL, Greene SA, Perez TE. Cardiovascular and respiratory effects, and quality of anesthesia produced by alfaxalone administered intramuscularly to cats sedated with dexmedetomidine and hydromorphone. *J Feline Med Surg* 2013; **15**(**10**): 858–865.
204 Taboada FM, Murison PJ. Induction of anaesthesia with alfaxalone or propofol before isoflurane maintenance in cats. *Vet Rec* 2010; **167**(**3**): 85–89.
205 Zaki S, Ticehurst K, Miyaki Y. Clinical evaluation of Alfaxan-CD(R) as an intravenous anaesthetic in young cats. *Aust Vet J* 2009; **87**(**3**): 82–87.
206 O'Hagan BJ, Pasloske K, McKinnon C, *et al.* Clinical evaluation of alfaxalone as an anaesthetic induction agent in cats less than 12 weeks of age. *Aust Vet J* 2012; **90**(**10**): 395–401.
207 Beths T, Touzot-Jourde G, Musk G, *et al.* Clinical evaluation of alfaxalone to induce and maintain anaesthesia in cats undergoing neutering procedures. *J Feline Med Surg* 2013; **16**(**8**): 609–615.
208 Mathis A, Pinelas R, Brodbelt DC, *et al.* Comparison of quality of recovery from anaesthesia in cats induced with propofol or alfaxalone. *Vet Anaesth Analg* 2012; **39**(**3**): 282–290.
209 Goodwin WA, Keates HL, Pearson M, *et al.* Alfaxalone and medetomidine intravenous infusion to maintain anaesthesia in colts undergoing field castration. *Equine Vet J* 2013; **45**(**3**): 315–319.
210 Keates HL, van Eps AW, Pearson MR. Alfaxalone compared with ketamine for induction of anaesthesia in horses following xylazine and guaifenesin. *Vet Anaesth Analg* 2012; **39**(**6**): 591–598.
211 Kloppel H, Leece EA. Comparison of ketamine and alfaxalone for induction and maintenance of anaesthesia in ponies undergoing castration. *Vet Anaesth Analg* 2011; **38**(**1**): 37–43.
212 Granados MM, Dominguez JM, Fernandez-Sarmiento A, *et al.* Anaesthetic and cardiorespiratory effects of a constant-rate infusion of alfaxalone in desflurane-anaesthetised sheep. *Vet Rec* 2012; **171**(**5**): 125.
213 Andaluz A, Felez-Ocana N, Santos L, *et al.* The effects on cardio-respiratory and acid-base variables of the anaesthetic alfaxalone in a 2-hydroxypropyl-beta-cyclodextrin (HPCD) formulation in sheep. *Vet J* 2012; **191**(**3**): 389–392.
214 Torres MD, Andaluz A, Garcia F, *et al.* Effects of an intravenous bolus of alfaxalone versus propofol on intraocular pressure in sheep. *Vet Rec* 2012; **170**(**9**): 226.
215 Santos Gonzalez M, Bertran de Lis BT, Tendillo Cortijo FJ. Effects of intramuscular alfaxalone alone or in combination with diazepam in swine. *Vet Anaesth Analg* 2013; **40**(**4**): 399–402.
216 Keates H. Induction of anaesthesia in pigs using a new alphaxalone formulation. *Vet Rec* 2003; **153**(**20**): 627–628.
217 Hillidge CJ, Lees P, Serrano L. Investigations of azaperone-metomidate anaesthesia in the horse. *Vet Rec* 1973; **93**(**11**): 307–311.
218 Hall LW, Clarke KW. General pharmacology of the intravenous anesthetics. In: Hall LW, Clarke KW, eds. *Veterinary Anesthesia*. Chichester: Baillière Tindall, 1983; 74–93.

16 Inhalation Anesthetics

Eugene P. Steffey[1], Khursheed R. Mama[2] and Robert J. Brosnan[1]

[1]Department of Surgical and Radiological Sciences, School of Veterinary Medicine, University of California, Davis, California, USA
[2]Department of Clinical Sciences, Colorado State University, Fort Collins, Colorado, USA

Chapter contents

Introduction

Inhalation anesthetics are used widely for the anesthetic management of animals. They are unique among the anesthetic drugs because they are administered, and in large part removed from the body, via the lungs. Their popularity arises in part because their pharmacokinetic characteristics favor predictable and rapid adjustment of anesthetic depth. In addition, a special apparatus is usually used to deliver the inhaled agents. This apparatus includes a source of oxygen (O_2) and a patient breathing circuit, which in turn usually includes an endotracheal tube or face mask, a means of eliminating carbon dioxide (CO_2), and a compliant gas reservoir. These components help minimize patient morbidity or mortality because they facilitate lung ventilation and improved arterial oxygenation. In addition, inhalation anesthetics in gas samples can be readily measured continuously. Measurement of inhalation anesthetic concentration enhances the precision and safety of anesthetic management beyond the extent commonly possible with injectable anesthetic agents.

Over the nearly 150 years that inhalation anesthesia has been used in clinical practice, less than 20 agents have actually been introduced and approved for general use with patients (Fig. 16.1) [1]. Less than ten of these have a history of widespread clinical use in veterinary medicine, and only four are of current veterinary importance in North America. It is this group of anesthetics that are the focus of this chapter. Isoflurane is currently considered the most widely used veterinary inhalation anesthetic in North America, with sevoflurane a close second. Other inhalation anesthetics include desflurane and the gaseous agent nitrous oxide (N_2O), which are used much less for veterinary patients. Halothane, once the most popular volatile anesthetic throughout the world, is no longer commercially distributed in North America. However, it remains available elsewhere (at least on a limited basis) and considering the agent's widespread international distribution, we will continue to include information here on some actions of clinical importance to veterinary anesthesia.

Two additional volatile agents continue to receive brief attention for different reasons. Methoxyflurane, an agent popular during the period of about 1960 to 1990, has not been commercially available in North America for many years. However, because of some of its physicochemical characteristics, mention here has value especially to students of our clinical discipline and pharmacologists and permits easy comparison to agents of more current interest. Enflurane, introduced for use in human patients in 1972 and still commercially available, has little or no use in veterinary practice in North America. Information on this volatile anesthetic was included in previous editions of this text. However, because enflurane is only in very limited and focused veterinary use elsewhere, we have deleted most information about this agent in the present chapter and refer interested readers to the fourth edition of this text for coverage. Although of investigational and very limited human patient interest, a review of xenon is again not included in this animal patient-focused chapter.

Veterinary Anesthesia and Analgesia: The Fifth Edition of Lumb and Jones.
Edited by Kurt A. Grimm, Leigh A. Lamont, William J. Tranquilli, Stephen A. Greene and Sheilah A. Robertson.

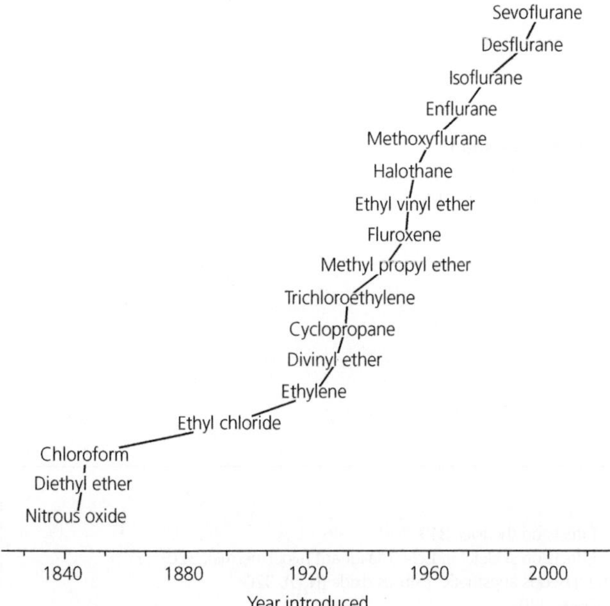

Figure 16.1 Inhalation anesthetics introduced for widespread clinical use. Source: Adapted from Karzai W, Haberstroh J, Muller W, Priebe H-J. Rapid increase in inspired desflurane concentration does not elicit a hyperdynamic circulatory response in the pig. *Lab Anim* 1997; **31**: 279–282.

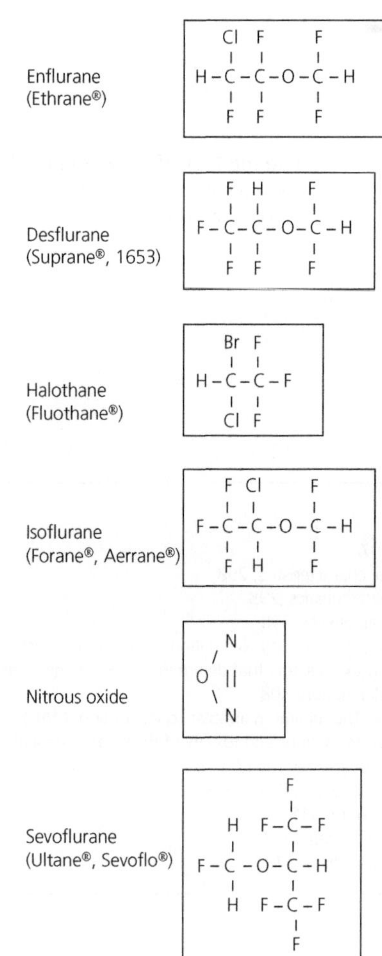

Figure 16.2 Chemical structure of inhalation anesthetics in current use for animals. Trade names are given in parentheses.

In this edition, information on agents of largely historical interest again has not been included. Readers interested in aspects of these formerly used agents are referred to the earlier editions of this and other textbooks [2–6]. Examples of such agents are diethyl ether and chloroform. A more complete listing is noted in Fig. 16.1.

Physicochemical characteristics

The chemical structure of inhalation anesthetics and their physical properties determine their actions and safety of administration. An in-depth analysis of the impact of agent chemical structure and physical properties is beyond the scope of this chapter. However, brief discussion of aspects of Fig. 16.2 and Table 16.1 is appropriate because the physicochemical characteristics summarized determine and/or influence practical considerations of their clinical use. For example, they determine the form in which the agents are supplied by the manufacturer (e.g., as a gas or liquid) and account for the resistance of the anesthetic molecule to degradation by physical factors (e.g., heat, light) and substances it contacts during use (e.g., metal components of the anesthetic delivery apparatus and the CO_2 absorbents such as soda lime). The equipment necessary to safely deliver the agent to the patient (e.g., vaporizer, breathing circuit) is influenced by some of these properties, as are the agent's uptake, distribution within, and elimination (including potential for metabolic breakdown) from the patient. In summary, a knowledge and understanding of fundamental properties permits intelligent use of contemporary anesthetics.

Chemical characteristics

Most contemporary inhalation anesthetics are organic compounds, except N_2O (Fig. 16.2) (cyclopropane and xenon are other notable inorganic anesthetics). Agents of current interest are further classified as either aliphatic (i.e., straight or branch chained) hydrocarbons or ethers (i.e., two organic radicals attached to an atom of oxygen; the general structure is ROR'). In the continued search for a less reactive, more potent, nonflammable inhalation anesthetic, focus on halogenation (i.e., addition of fluorine, chlorine, or bromine) of these compounds has predominated. Chlorine and bromine especially convert many compounds of low anesthetic potency into more potent drugs. Historically, interest in fluorinated derivatives was delayed until the 1940s because of difficulties in synthesis, and thus quantities available for study were limited. Methods of synthesis, although difficult, improved considerably and facilitated new agent discovery (see Fig. 16.2). It is interesting that organic fluorinated compounds are a group of extreme contrasts – some are toxic, others are not; some are inert, others are highly reactive. In some anesthetics, fluorine is substituted for chlorine or bromine to improve stability, but at the expense of reduced anesthetic potency and solubility.

Halothane (see Fig. 16.2) is a halogenated, aliphatic saturated hydrocarbon (ethane). Predictions that halogenated structure would provide non-flammability and molecular stability encouraged the development of halothane in the early 1950s. However, soon after clinical introduction it was observed that the concurrent presence of halothane and catecholamines increased the incidence of cardiac arrhythmias, especially in human patients. An ether linkage in the

Table 16.1 Some physical and chemical properties of inhalation anesthetics in current clinical use for animals.

Property	Desflurane	Enflurane	Halothane	Isoflurane	Methoxyflurane[a]	N_2O	Sevoflurane
Molecular weight (g)	168	185	197	185	165	44	200
Liquid specific gravity (20°C)(g/mL)	1.47	1.52	1.86	1.49	1.42	1.42	1.52
Boiling point (°C)	23.5	57	50	49	105	-89	59
Vapor pressure (mmHg)							
20°C	700(413)	172	243	240	23	–	160
24°C	804	207	288	286	28	–	183
mL vapor/mL liquid at 20°C	209.7	197.5	227	194.7	206.9	–	182.7
Preservative	None	None	Yes	None	Not available	None	Yes
Stability in:							
Soda lime	Yes	Yes	No	Yes	No	Yes	No
UV light	Yes	Yes	No	Yes	No	Yes	??

[a]Methoxyflurane is no longer available.
UV = ultraviolet.

molecule reduces the incidence of cardiac arrhythmias. Consequently, this chemical structure is a predominant characteristic of all agents which have been developed or entered clinical use since the introduction of halothane (see Fig. 16.2).

Despite many favorable characteristics and improvements over earlier anesthetics (see Fig. 16.1) that included improved chemical stability, halothane is susceptible to decomposition. Accordingly, it is stored in dark bottles and a very small amount of a preservative, thymol, is added to slow decomposition. Thymol is much less volatile than halothane and over time concentrates within the devices used to control delivery of the volatile anesthetic (i.e., vaporizers) and causes them to malfunction. To achieve greater molecular stability, fluorine is substituted for chlorine or bromine in the anesthetic molecule. This chemical manipulation added shelf-life to the substance and negated the need for additives such as thymol. Unfortunately, the fluorine ion is also toxic to some tissues (e.g., kidneys), which is of clinical concern if the parent compound (e.g., historically, most notably methoxyflurane) is not resistant to metabolism (see Fig. 16.2).

Physical characteristics

Life is supported via a constant interchange of respiratory gases (O_2 and CO_2) between cells and the external environment and blood transport. Inhalation anesthetics similarly gain entrance and exit the body via the respiratory system and their movement from a container to sites of action in the central nervous system involves similar considerations as respiratory gases. Early in the process of controlled transfer, the agent is diluted to an appropriate amount (partial pressure or concentration) and directed to the respiratory system in a gas mixture that contains enough O_2 to support life. The chain of events that ensues is influenced by many physical and chemical characteristics that can be quantitatively described (Tables 16.1–16.4). The practical clinical applications of these quantitative descriptions are reviewed here. Limited space does not permit in-depth review of all underlying principles, and readers interested in further background information are referred elsewhere [7,8].

The physical characteristics of importance to our understanding of the action of inhalation anesthetics can be conveniently divided into two general categories: those that determine the means by which the agents are administered and those that help determine their kinetics in the body. This information is applied in the clinical manipulation of anesthetic induction and recovery and in facilitating changes in anesthetic-induced CNS depression in a timely fashion.

Properties determining methods of administration

A variety of physical/chemical properties determine the means by which inhalation anesthetics are administered. These include characteristics such as boiling point, liquid density (specific gravity), and vapor pressure.

General principles: A brief review

Molecules are in a constant state of motion and exhibit a force of mutual attraction. The degree of attraction is evident by the state in which the substance exists (i.e., solid, liquid, or gas). Molecular motion increases as energy (e.g., in the form of heat) is added to the molecular aggregate and decreases as energy is removed. With increased motion, there is a reduction in the intermolecular forces; if conditions are extreme enough, a change in physical state may ensue. All substances exist naturally in a particular state but can be made to exist (at least in theory) in any or all phases by altering conditions. Water, as an example, exists as ice (mutual molecular attraction is great), liquid water, or water vapor (attraction considerably reduced) depending upon conditions.

Gas versus vapor

Inhalation anesthetics are either gases or vapors. In relation to inhalation anesthetics, the term *gas* refers to an agent, such as N_2O, that exists in its gaseous form at room temperature and sea level pressure. The term *vapor* indicates the gaseous state of a substance that at ambient temperature and pressure is a liquid. With the exception of N_2O, all the contemporary anesthetics fall into this category. Desflurane (see Table 16.1) is one volatile liquid that comes close to the transition stage and offers some unique (among the inhalation anesthetics) considerations to be discussed later in this chapter.

Whether inhalation agents are supplied as a gas or volatile liquid under ambient conditions, the same physical principles apply to each agent when it is in the gaseous state. Molecules move about in haphazard fashion at high speeds and collide with each other or the walls of the containing vessel. The force per unit area of the bombardment is measurable and referred to as pressure. In the case of gases, if the space or volume in which the gas is enclosed is increased, the number of bombardments decreases (i.e., a smaller number of molecular collisions per unit time) and then the pressure decreases. The behavior of gases is predictably described by various gas laws. Relationships such as those described by Boyle's law (volume vs pressure), Charles's law (volume vs temperature), Gay-Lussac's law (temperature vs pressure), Dalton's law of partial pressure (the total pressure of a mixture of gases is equal to the sum of the partial pressures of all the gaseous substances present), and

Table 16.2 Partition coefficients (solvent/gas) of some inhalation anesthetics at 37°C.

Solvent	Desflurane	Enflurane	Halothane	Isoflurane	Methoxyflurane	N_2O	Sevoflurane
Water	–	0.78	0.82	0.62	4.50	0.47	0.60
Blood	0.42	2.00	2.54	1.46	15.00	0.47	0.68
Olive oil	18.70	96.00	224.00	91.00	970.00	1.40	47.00
Brain	1.30	2.70	1.90	1.60	20.00	0.50	1.70
Liver	1.30	3.70	2.10	1.80	29.00	0.38	1.80
Kidney	1.00	1.90	1.00	1.20	11.00	0.40	1.20
Muscle	2.00	2.20	3.40	2.90	16.00	0.54	3.10
Fat	27.00	83.00	51.00	45.00	902.00	1.08	48.00

Tissue samples are derived from human sources. Data are from sources referenced in the previous edition of this text.

Table 16.3 Blood/gas partition coefficients for desflurane, halothane, isoflurane, methoxyflurane, and sevoflurane in species of common clinical and/or research interest in veterinary medicine, including for comparison similarly derived values for humans.

	Desflurane	Halothane	Isoflurane	Methoxyflurane	Sevoflurane	Nitrous oxide
Cat	0.58	–	1.40	26.4	0.59	–
Cow	0.44	2.40 [415]	1.22	11.3	0.52	–
Dog	0.63	3.51 [415]	1.40	26.1	0.66	0.43 [416]
Goat	0.52	–	1.37	13.0	0.56	–
Horse	0.54	1.77 [415]	1.13	13.0	0.65	–
Pig	0.50	–	1.07	11.1	0.52	–
Rat	0.61	6.56 [417]	1.41	17.7	0.74	–
Rabbit	0.72	4.36 [418]	1.37	25.0	0.70	–
Sheep	0.50	–	1.24	13.2	0.56	–
Human	0.50	2.54 [417]	1.32	14.3	0.64	0.41 [416]

Values are taken mostly from the 2012 reported work of Soares *et al.* [419] except where indicated. Values are reported for 37°C. A dash indicates the value was not found.

Table 16.4 Rubber or plastic/gas partition coefficients at room temperature.

Solvent	Desflurane	Enflurane	Halothane	Isoflurane	Methoxyflurane	Nitrous oxide	Sevoflurane	Reference
Rubber	–	74	120	62	630	1.2	–	[1]
	19	–	190	49	–	–	29	[420]
Poly(vinyl chloride)	–	120	190	110	–	–	–	[1]
	35	–	233	114	–	–	69	[420]
Poly(ethylene)	–	~2	26	~2	118	–	–	[1]
	16	–	128	58	–	–	31	[420]

These data are summarized from multiple sources as reported in Eger [1], with some differences in methods of determination. The data from Targ *et al.* [420] indicate more recently derived data which unlike earlier data were recorded following complete equilibration with these materials. Where there is overlap, the ranking of partition coefficients is consistent with halothane > isoflurane > sevoflurane > desflurane. Combining both groupings yields methoxyflurane > halothane > enflurane > isoflurane > sevoflurane > desflurane > N_2O.

others are important to our overall understanding of aspects of respiratory and anesthetic gases and vapors. However, in-depth descriptions of these principles are beyond the scope of this chapter and readers are referred elsewhere for this information [8].

Methods of description

Quantities of inhalation anesthetic agent are usually characterized by one of three methods: pressure (e.g., in mmHg), concentration (in vol %) or mass (in mg or g). The form most familiar to clinicians is that of concentration (e.g., X% of agent A in relation to the whole gas mixture). Agent analysis monitoring equipment samples inspired and expired gases and provides readings for inhalation anesthetics. Precision vaporizers used to control delivery of inhalation anesthetics are calibrated in percentage of agent, and effective doses are almost always reported in percentages.

Pressure is also an important way of describing inhalation anesthetics and is further discussed under the heading of anesthetic potency. A mixture of gases in a closed container will exert a pressure on the walls of the container. The individual pressure of each gas in a mixture of gases is referred to as its *partial pressure.* As noted earlier, this expression of the behavior of a mixture of gases is known as Dalton's law, and its use in understanding inhalation anesthesia is inescapable. Use of the concept of partial pressure is important in understanding inhalation anesthetic action in a multiphase biologic system because, unlike concentration, the partial pressure of an agent is the same in different compartments that are in equilibrium with each other. That is, in contradistinction to concentration or volume percent, an expression of the relative ratio of gas molecules in a mixture, partial pressure is an expression of the absolute value.

Molecular weight and agent density are used in many calculations to convert from liquid to vapor volumes and mass. Briefly (and in simplified fashion), Avogadro's principle is that equal volume of all gases under the same conditions of temperature and pressure contain the same number of molecules (6.0226×10^{23} [Avogadro's number] per gram molecular weight). Furthermore, under standard conditions the number of gas molecules in a gram molecular weight of a substance occupies 22.4 liters. In order to compare properties of different substances of similar state, it is necessary to do so under comparable conditions; with respect to gases

a Isoflurane specific gravity = 1.49 g/mL, therefore:
1mL liquid isoflurane = 1 mL × 1.49 g/mL = 1.49 g

b Since molecular weight of isoflurane = 185 g (from Table 13-1, then:
1.49 g ÷ 185 g = 0.0081 mol of liquid

c Since 1 mol of gas = 22.4 L, then:
0.0081 mol × 22,400 mL/mol = 181.4 mL of isoflurane vapor at 0C, 1 atm

d But vapor is at 20C not 0C (i.e., 273 K),
So, 181.4 × 293/273 = 194.7 mL vapor/mL liquid isoflurane at 20C and at sea level pressure

For substantial variation in ambient pressure, the final figure noted above would have to be further "corrected" by a factor of: 760/ambient barometric pressure

Figure 16.3 Example of calculations to determine the volume of isoflurane vapor at 20°C from 1 mL of isoflurane liquid.

a Total isoflurane vapor delivered over 2 hours (120 min) estimated at:
3%/100 × 6 LPM = 0.18 LPM × 120 min = 21.60 L/120 min = 21,600 mL/120min

vs

3%/100 × 4 LPM = 0.12 LPM × 120 min = 14.4 L/120 min = 14,400 mL/120min

b Total vapor volume saved:

21,600 mL/120 min – 14,400 mL/120 min = 7,200 mL vapor/120 min saved

c Total liquid isoflurane volume saved/2 hours

7,200 mL vapor ÷ 194.7 mL vapor/mL liquid = 36.98 mL of isoflurane liquid

(194.7 mL vapor/mL liquid can be calculated as in Fig. 13.4 or taken from Table 13-1)

The economic value of reducing isoflurane consumption can then be determined by calculating the product of the liquid volume saved and the purchase cost/mL of isoflurane liquid

Figure 16.4 Problem: Determine the savings in isoflurane liquid afforded by reducing the fresh gas (e.g., O_2) inflow rate from 6 Lpm (liters per minute) to 4 Lpm, given that the average delivered (vaporizer setting) concentration for 2 h is 3%.

and liquids, this usually means with reference to pressure and temperature. Unless otherwise indicated, physical scientists have arbitrarily selected *standard conditions* as 0°C (273°K in absolute scale) and 760 mmHg pressure (1 atmosphere at sea level). If conditions differ, appropriate temperature and/or pressure corrections must be applied to resultant data.

The weight of a given volume of liquid, gas, or vapor may be expressed in terms of its density or specific gravity. The density is an absolute value of mass (usually grams) per unit volume (for liquids, volume = 1 mL; for gases, 1 liter at standard conditions). The specific gravity is a relative value; that is, the ratio of the weight of a unit volume of one substance to a similar volume of water in the case of liquids or air in the case of gases (or vapors) under similar conditions. The value of both air and water is one. At least for clinical purposes, the value for density and specific gravity for an inhalation anesthetic is the same. Thus, for example, we can determine the volume of isoflurane gas (vapor) at 20°C from 1 mL of isoflurane liquid according to the scheme given in Fig. 16.3. This type of calculation has practical applications. For example, to determine the savings in isoflurane liquid afforded by reducing the fresh gas (e.g., O_2) inflow rate, a series of calculations as presented in Fig. 16.4 can be made.

Vapor pressure Molecules of liquids are in constant random motion. Some of those in the surface layer gain sufficient velocity to overcome the attractive forces of neighboring molecules and in escaping from the surface, enter the vapor phase. The change in state from a liquid to a gas phase is known as *vaporization* or *evaporation.* This process is dynamic and in a closed container that is kept at a constant temperature, eventually reaches an equilibrium whereby there is no further net loss of molecules to the gas phase (i.e., the numbers of molecules leaving and returning to the liquid phase are equal). The gas phase at this point is saturated.

Molecules of a vapor exert a force per unit area or pressure in exactly the same manner as do molecules of a gas. The pressure (units of measure are mmHg) that the vapor molecules exert when the liquid and vapor phases are in equilibrium is known as the *vapor pressure.* Thus, the vapor pressure of an anesthetic is a measure of its ability to evaporate; that is, it is a measure of the tendency for molecules in the liquid state to enter the gaseous (vapor) phase. The vapor pressure of a volatile anesthetic must be at least sufficient to provide enough molecules of anesthetic in the vapor state to produce anesthesia at ambient conditions. The *saturated vapor pressure* represents a maximum concentration of molecules in the vapor state that exists for a given liquid at each temperature. Herein lies a practical difference between substances classified as a gas or vapor; a gas can be administered over a range of concentrations from 0% to 100%, whereas the vapor has a ceiling that is dictated by its vapor pressure. The *saturated vapor concentration* can be easily determined by relating the vapor pressure to the ambient pressure. For example, in the case of isoflurane (see Table 16.1), a maximal concentration of 32% isoflurane is possible under usual conditions and 20°C (i.e [240/760] × 100 = 32%, where 760 mmHg is the barometric pressure at sea level). With other variables considered constant, the greater the vapor pressure, the greater the concentration of the drug deliverable to the patient. Therefore, again from Table 16.1, isoflurane, for example, is more volatile than methoxyflurane under similar conditions. The barometric pressure also influences the final concentration of an agent. For example, in locations such as Denver, Colorado, where the altitude is about 5000 feet above sea level and the barometric pressure is only about 635 mmHg, the saturated vapor concentration of isoflurane at 20°C is now (240/635) × 100 = 37.8%.

It is important to recognize that the saturated vapor pressure at 1 atmosphere is unique for each volatile anesthetic agent and depends only on its temperature. In this case the effect of barometric pressure can be neglected over ranges normally encountered in the practice of anesthesia. Thus, for a given agent, the graph of the saturated vapor pressure versus temperature is a curve as shown in Fig. 16.5. From this graph it can be seen that if the temperature of the liquid is increased, more molecules escape the liquid phase and enter the gaseous phase. The greater number of molecules in the vapor phase results in a greater vapor pressure and vapor concentration. Conversely, if the liquid is cooled, the reverse occurs and vapor concentration decreases. Liquid cooling may occur not only as a result of ambient conditions but also as a natural consequence of the vaporization process. For example, during vaporization the 'fastest' molecules at the surface escape first. With depletion of these 'high-energy' molecules, the average kinetic energy of those left behind is reduced and there is a tendency for the temperature of the remaining liquid to fall if this process is not compensated for externally. As the temperature decreases, the vapor pressure, and thus the vapor concentration, also decreases.

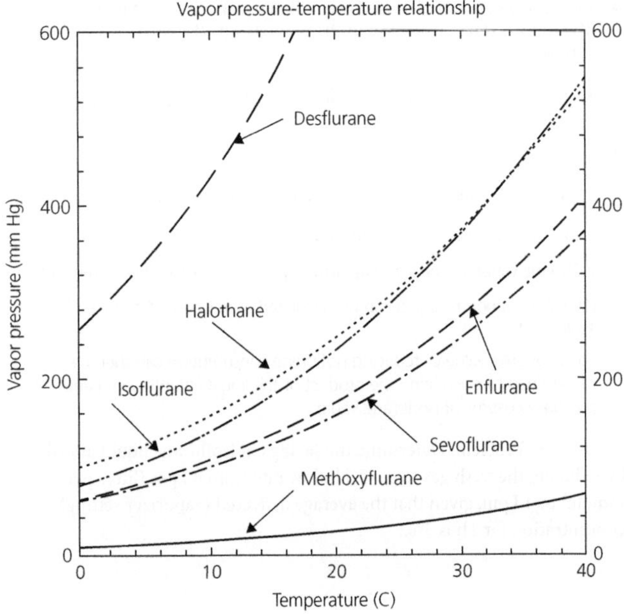

Figure 16.5 Vapor pressure as a function of temperature for six volatile anesthetics. Curves are generated from Antoine equations.

Boiling point The boiling point of a liquid is defined as the temperature at which the vapor pressure of the liquid is equal to the atmospheric pressure. Customarily, the boiling temperature is stated at the standard atmospheric pressure of 760 mmHg. The boiling point decreases with increasing altitude because the vapor pressure does not change but the barometric pressure decreases. The boiling point of N_2O is −89°C (see Table 16.1) at 1 atmosphere pressure at sea level. It is thus a gas under operating room conditions. Because of this, it is distributed for clinical purposes in steel tanks compressed to the liquid state at about 750 psi (pounds per square inch; 750 psi/14.9 psi [1 atmosphere] = 50 atmospheres pressure). As the N_2O gas is drawn from the tank, liquid N_2O is vaporized and the over-riding gas pressure remains constant until no further liquid remains in the tank. At that point, only N_2O gas remains, and the gas pressure decreases from this point as remaining gas is vented from the tank. Consequently, the weight of the N_2O minus the weight of the tank rather than the gas pressure within the tank is a more accurate guide to the remaining amount of N_2O in the tank [9].

Desflurane also possesses an interesting consideration because its boiling point (see Table 16.1) is near room temperature. This characteristic accounted for an interesting engineering challenge in developing an administration device (i.e., a vaporizer) for routine use in the relatively constant environment of the operating room and limits further consideration of its use in all but a narrow range of circumstances commonly encountered in veterinary medical applications. For example, because of its low boiling point, even evaporative cooling has large influences on vapor pressure and thus the vapor concentration of gas mixtures delivered to the patient.

Calculation of Anesthetic Concentration Delivered by a Vaporizer

The saturated vapor pressure of most volatile anesthetics is of such magnitude that the maximal concentration of anesthetic attainable at usual operating room conditions is above the range of concentrations that are commonly necessary for safe clinical anesthetic management. Therefore, some control of the delivered concentration is necessary and usually provided by a device known as a *vaporizer.* The purpose of the vaporizer is to dilute the vapor generated from the liquid anesthetic with O_2 (or O_2 plus N_2O, or O_2 plus air mixtures) to produce a more satisfactory inspired anesthetic concentration. This anesthetic dilution is usually accomplished as indicated in the model shown in Fig. 16.6 by diverting the gas entering the vaporizer into two streams: one that enters the vaporizing chamber (anesthetic chamber volume: V_{anes}) and the other that bypasses the vaporizing chamber (dilution volume or $V_{dilution}$). If the vaporizer is efficient, the carrier gas passing through the vaporizing chamber becomes completely saturated to an anesthetic concentration (%) reflected by (anesthetic agent vapor pressure/atmospheric pressure) × 100, at the vaporizer chamber temperature. The resultant anesthetic concentration then is decreased (diluted) downstream by the second gas stream to a 'working' concentration. In modern, precision, agent-specific vaporizers no mental effort is required – just set the dial, as the manufacturers have precalibrated the vaporizer for accurate delivery of the dialed concentration (within some variability, say 10% of delivered concentration, allowance). Nevertheless, it is helpful to our overall understanding to know the principles underlying this convenience and how to apply these principles in the use of older, non-compensated measured flow vaporizers.

To calculate the anesthetic concentration from the vaporizer, one must know the vapor pressure of the agent (at the temperature of use), the atmospheric pressure, the fresh gas flow entering the vaporizing chamber, and the diluent gas flow. Then,

$$\% \text{ anesthetic} = \text{flow of anesthetic from the vaporizing chamber/totalgas flow.}$$

More detail for interested readers is given in Fig. 16.6.

Properties influencing drug ginetics: Solubility

Anesthetic gases and vapors dissolve in liquids and solids. The solubility of an anesthetic is a major characteristic of the agent and has important clinical ramifications. For example, anesthetic solubility in blood and body tissues is a primary factor in the rate of uptake and its distribution within the body. It is therefore a primary determinant of the speed of anesthetic induction and recovery. Solubility in lipid bears a strong relationship to anesthetic potency, and its tendency to dissolve in anesthetic delivery components such as rubber goods influences equipment selection and other aspects of anesthetic management.

Solubility of gases

As previously mentioned, molecules of a gas that overlie a liquid surface are in random motion and some penetrate the liquid surface. After entering the liquid, they intermingle with the molecules of the liquid (i.e., the gas dissolves in the liquid). There is a net movement of the gas into the liquid until equilibrium is established between the dissolved gas in the liquid and the undissolved portion above the liquid. At this time, there is no further net gain of gas molecules by the liquid, and the number of gas molecules entering the liquid equals the number leaving. The gas molecules within the liquid exert the same pressure or tension that they exert in the gas phase. If the pressure (i.e., the number of gas molecules overlying the liquid) is increased, more molecules pass into the liquid and the pressure within the liquid is increased. This net inward movement of gas molecules continues until a new equilibrium is established between the pressure of the gas in the liquid and that overlying the liquid. Alternatively, if the pressure of gas overlying the liquid is

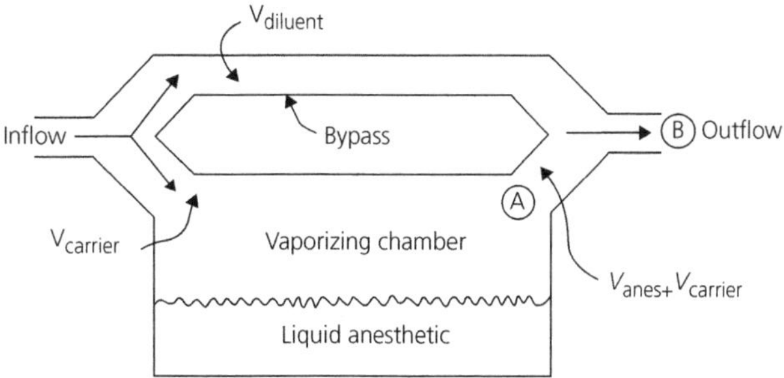

Steps:

1 The saturated *concentration* of anesthetic in the anesthetic vaporizing chamber and leaving it (ideally at A above) is calculated knowing the saturated vapor pressure (P_{VP}) (from Table 2) and barometric pressure (P_B).
For example:

$$\text{Halothane\%} = \frac{243}{760} \times 100 = 32.0\% \qquad \textbf{a}$$

2 The *volume* of anesthetic leaving the vaporizing chamber is the original volume of the carrier gas (O_2) entering the anesthetic vaporizing chamber ($V_{carrier}$) and the volume of anesthetic (V_{halo}) added to it.

$$\text{Halothane\%} - \frac{V_{halo}}{V_{carrier} + V_{halo}} \times 100 \qquad \textbf{b}$$

Halothane% is known from (a) above and $V_{carrier}$ is known from control of a flowmeter (e.g., a measured flow vaporizer) or via the design characteristics of a commercial, agent-specific, vaporizer that automatically "splits" the fresh gas flow from a single flow meter. In the first case, two gas flow controls are necessary, one for $V_{carrier}$ and one for a automatic fresh gas flow alteration, the equation is then solved for V_{halo} (expressed in ml of halothane vapor).
For example, if $V_{carrier}$ = 100mL O_2, then

$$32\% = \frac{V_{halo}}{100 + V_{halo}} \times 100$$

$$3200 + 32V_{halo} = 100V_{halo}$$

$$3200 = 68V_{halo}$$

$$V_{halo} = 47.1 \text{ mL halothane vapor}$$

3 V_{halo} is then contained in a total gas volume at B of

$$V_{total\ gas} = V_{halo} + V_{carrier} + V_{diluent} \qquad \textbf{c}$$

Where $V_{diluent}$ is set by the anesthetist using a second gas control (i.e., flowmeter; units here of mL/min) or by the vaporizer design and dial setting.
Then in our example for a $V_{diluent}$ of 1000 mL (in 1 minute)

$$V_{total} = 47.1 + 100 + 1000$$
$$= 1147 \text{ ml (rounded off)}$$

4 So the final halothane vapor concentration is determined by

$$\text{halothane\%} = \frac{V_{halo}}{V_{Total}} \times 100$$

Again, in our example,

$$\text{halothane\%} = \frac{47.1}{1147} = 4.1\%$$

Alternatively, with some basic algebraic work with equations given above, the same numbers can be applied to the resultant formula given below to arrive at the anesthetic concentration. The condensed formula is :

$$\text{Anesthetic concentration (\%)} = \frac{V_{carrier} \cdot P_{VP} \cdot 100}{V_{diluent} \cdot (P_B - P_{VP}) + (V_{carrier} \cdot P_B)}$$

Figure 16.6 An anesthetic vaporizer model to assist in illustrating the principles associated with the calculation of the vapor concentration of an inhalation anesthetic emerging from a vaporizer. Conditions associated with halothane delivery in San Francisco (i.e., at sea level; barometric pressure = 760 mm Hg) at 20°C are used as an example of general principles.

somehow decreased below that in the liquid, gas molecules escape from the liquid. This net outward movement of gas molecules from the liquid phase continues until equilibrium between the two phases is re-established.

The amount, that is, the total number of molecules of a given gas dissolving in a solvent, depends on the chemical nature of the gas itself, the partial pressure of the gas, the nature of the solvent, and the temperature. This relationship is described by Henry's law:

$$V = S \times P$$

where V is the volume of gas, P is the partial pressure of the gas, and S is the solubility coefficient for the gas in the solvent at a given temperature. Henry's law applies to gases that do not combine chemically with the solvent to form compounds.

Before leaving this basic information, a brief focus on a number of variations may be helpful. First, it is important to recognize that if the atmosphere that overlies the solvent is made up of a mixture of gases, then each gas dissolves in the solvent in proportion to the partial pressure of the individual gases. The total pressure exerted by the molecules of all gases within the solvent equals the total gas pressure lying above the solvent.

Within the body there is a partition of anesthetic gases between blood and body tissues in accordance with Henry's law. This process can perhaps be better understood by visualizing a system composed of three compartments (e.g., gas, water, and oil) contained in a closed container (Fig. 16.7). In such a system the gas overlies the oil, which in turn overlies the water. Because there is a passive gradient from the gas phase to the oil, gas molecules move into the oil compartment. This movement in turn develops a gradient for the gas molecules in oil relative to water. If gas is continually added above the oil, there will be a continual net movement of the gas molecules from the gas phase into both the oil and, in turn, the water. At a given temperature, when no more gas dissolves in the solvent, the solvent is said to be *fully saturated.* At this point the pressure of the gas molecules within the three compartments will be equal but the amount (i.e., the number of molecules or volume of gas) partitioned between the two liquids will vary with the nature of the liquid and gas. Finally, it is important to understand that the amount of gas that goes into solution depends upon the temperature

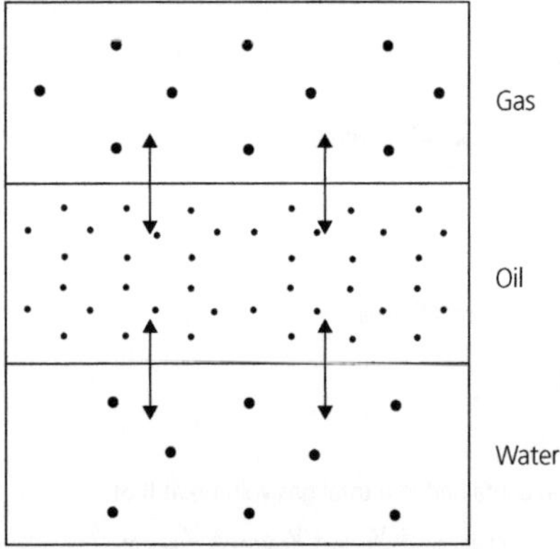

Figure 16.7 Diagrammatic representation of an anesthetic gas distributing itself among three compartments (gas, oil, water). At equilibrium, the number of anesthetic molecules in the three compartments differs but the pressure exerted by the anesthetic molecules is the same in each compartment.

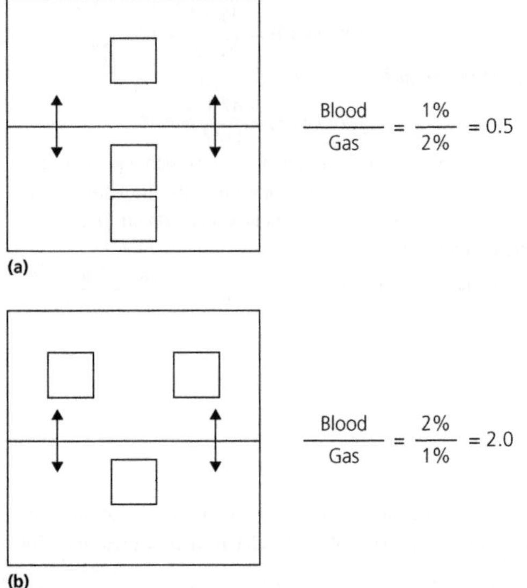

Figure 16.8 Blood gas partition coefficient illustration. Source: Adapted from Eger EI II. *Anesthetic Uptake and Action*. Baltimore, MD: Williams & Wilkins. 1974.

of the solvent. Less gas dissolves in a solvent as temperature increases, and more gas is taken up as solvent temperature decreases. For example, as water is heated air bubbles appear inside the container as a result of the decreasing solubility of the air in water. Conversely, as blood is cooled from a normal body temperature (e.g., hypothermia), gases become more soluble in blood.

The extent to which a gas will dissolve in a given solvent is usually expressed in terms of its solubility coefficient (see Table 16.2). With inhalation anesthetics, solubility is most commonly measured and expressed as a partition coefficient (PC). Other measurements of solubility include the Bunson and Ostwald solubility coefficients [8,10].

The PC is the concentration ratio of an anesthetic in the solvent and gas phases (e.g., blood and gas; Fig. 16.8) or between two tissue solvents (e.g., brain and blood; see Table 16.2). It thus describes the capacity of a given solvent to dissolve the anesthetic gas. That is, how the anesthetic will *partition* itself between the gas and the liquid solvent phases after equilibrium has been reached. Remember, anesthetic gas movement occurs because of a partial pressure difference in the gas and liquid solvent phases, so when there is no longer any anesthetic partial pressure difference, there is no longer any net movement of anesthetic and equilibrium has been achieved. Solvent/gas PCs are summarized in Table 16.2. Values noted in this table are for human tissues because they are most widely available in the anesthesia literature. Comparative data for blood solubility of desflurane, isoflurane, and sevoflurane in a variety of species of clinical interest in veterinary medicine are listed in Table 16.3. Regardless of the species, it is important to emphasize that many factors can alter anesthetic agent solubility [10–13]. Perhaps the most notable after the nature of the solvent is that of temperature.

Of all the PCs that have been described or are of interest, two are of particular importance in the practical understanding of anesthetic action. They are the blood/gas and the oil/gas solubility coefficients.

Blood/gas partition coefficient Blood/gas solubility coefficients (see Tables 16.2 and 16.3) provide a means for predicting the speed of anesthetic induction, recovery, and change of anesthetic depth. Assume, for example, that anesthetic A has a blood/gas PC value of 15. This means that the concentration of the anesthetic in blood will be 15 times greater at equilibrium than that in alveolar gas. Expressed differently, the same volume of blood, say 1 mL, will hold 15 times more of anesthetic A than 1 mL of alveolar gas despite an equal partial pressure. Alternatively, consider anesthetic B with a PC of 1.4. This PC indicates that at equilibrium, the amount of anesthetic B is only 1.4 times greater in blood than it is in alveolar air. Comparing the PC of anesthetic A with that of anesthetic B indicates that anesthetic A is much more soluble in blood than B (nearly 11 times more soluble: 15/1.4). From this, and assuming other conditions are equal, anesthetic A will require a longer time of administration to attain a partial pressure in the body for a particular endpoint (say, anesthetic induction) than will anesthetic B. Also, since there is more of anesthetic A contained in blood and other body tissues under similar conditions, elimination (and therefore anesthetic recovery) will be prolonged when compared to anesthetic B.

Oil/gas partition coefficient The oil/gas PC is another solubility characteristic of clinical importance (see Tables 16.2 and 16.3). This PC describes the ratio of the concentration of an anesthetic in oil (olive oil is the standard) and gas phases at equilibrium. The oil/gas PC correlates directly with anesthetic potency (see Anesthetic Dose: The Minimum Alveolar Concentration (MAC) and Mechanism of Action both later in this chapter) and describes the capacity of lipids for anesthetic.

Other partition coefficients Solubility characteristics for various tissues (see Tables 16.2 and 16.3) and other media, such as rubber and plastic (see Table 16.4), are also important. For example, the solubility of a tissue determines in part the quantity of anesthetic removed from the blood to which it is exposed. The higher the tissue solubility, the longer it will take to saturate the tissue with anesthetic agent. Thus, other things considered equal, anesthetics that are very soluble in tissues will require a longer period for induction and recovery. If the amount of rubber goods in the apparatus used to deliver the anesthetic to the patient is substantial and the anesthetic agent solubility in rubber is large (as for example was common with equipment in use prior to the the 21st century), the amount of uptake of anesthetic agent by the rubber may also be of clinical significance.

Pharmacokinetics: Uptake and elimination of inhalation anesthetics

The aim in administering an inhalation anesthetic to a patient is to achieve an adequate partial pressure or tension of anesthetic (P_{anes}) in the central nervous system (CNS, e.g., brain; for purposes of this discussion considerations of anesthetic delivery to spinal cord sites of action are considered similar to those of the brain) to cause a desired level of CNS depression commensurate with the definition of general anesthesia. Anesthetic depth varies directly with P_{anes} in brain tissue. The rate of change of anesthetic depth is of obvious clinical importance and is directly dependent upon the rate of change in anesthetic tensions in the various media in which it is contained before reaching the brain. Thus, knowledge of the factors that govern these relationships is of fundamental importance to skillful control of general inhalation anesthesia.

Inhalation anesthetics are unique among the classes of drugs that are used to produce general anesthesia because they are administered via the lungs. The pharmacokinetics of the inhaled anesthetics describe the rate of their uptake by blood from the lungs, distribution in the body, and eventual elimination by the lungs and other routes. Readers seeking more in-depth coverage are directed to reviews by Eger [10,14,15] and Mapleson [16].

Inhalation anesthetics, similar to the gases of respiration (i.e., O_2 and CO_2), move down a series of partial pressure gradients from regions of higher tension to those of lower tension until equilibrium (i.e., equal pressure throughout the apparatus and body tissues) is established. Thus, on induction, the P_{anes} at its source in the vaporizer is high, as is dictated by the vapor pressure, and progressively decreases as anesthetic travels from vaporizer to patient breathing circuit, from circuit to lungs, from lungs to arterial blood, and finally, from arterial blood to body tissues (e.g., the brain; Fig. 16.9).

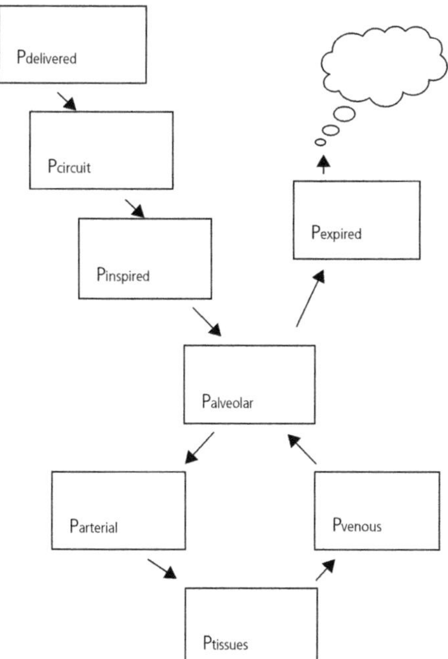

Figure 16.9 The flow pattern of inhalation anesthetic agents during anesthetic induction and recovery. Inhalation anesthesia may be viewed as the development of a series of partial pressure (tension) gradients. During induction there is a high anesthetic tension in the vaporizer that decreases progressively as the flow of anesthetic gas moves from its source to the brain. Some of these gradients are easily manipulated by the anesthetist; others are not, or are difficult to achieve.

Of these, the alveolar partial pressure (P_A) of anesthetic is pivotal. The brain has a rich blood supply and the anesthetic in arterial blood (P_aAnes) rapidly equilibrates with brain tissue (P_{brain}Anes). Usually gas exchange at the alveolar level is sufficiently efficient that the P_aAnes is close to P_AAnes. Thus, the P_{brain}Anes closely follows P_AAnes, and by controlling the P_AAnes there is a reliable indirect way for controlling P_{brain}Anes and anesthetic depth.

At this point it may also be helpful to recall that although the partial pressure of anesthetic is of primary importance, we frequently define clinical dose of an inhaled anesthetic in terms of concentration (*C*, i.e., vol %). As previously noted, this is because it is common practice for the clinician to regulate and/or measure respiratory and anesthetic gases in volume percent. In addition, in the gaseous phase, the relationship between the P_{anes} and the C_{anes} is a simple one:

$$P_{anes} = \text{fractional anesthetic concentration} \times \text{total ambient pressure.}$$

The fractional anesthetic concentration is of course $C_{anes}/100$. However, as reviewed in the preceding section, in blood or tissues the actual *quantity* of anesthetic depends on both the P_{anes} and the anesthetic solubility (as measured by partition coefficient) within the solvent (e.g., blood or oil). Consequently, at equilibrium, the *partial pressure* of the gas in the alveoli and among tissue compartments will be equal although *concentrations* will vary within these tissues.

Anesthetic uptake: Factors that determine the P_A of anesthetic

The P_A of anesthetic is a balance between anesthetic input (i.e., delivery to the alveoli) and loss (uptake by blood and body tissues) from the lungs. A rapid rise in the P_A of anesthetic is associated with a rapid anesthetic induction or change in anesthetic depth. Factors that contribute to a rapid change in the P_A of anesthetic are summarized in Fig. 16.10.

Delivery to the alveoli

Delivery of anesthetic to the alveoli and therefore the rate of rise of the alveolar concentration or fraction (F_A) toward the inspired concentration or fraction (F_I) depends on the inspired anesthetic concentration itself and the magnitude of alveolar ventilation. Increasing either one of these or both increases the rate of rise of the P_A of anesthetic; that is, with other things considered equal, there is an increase in speed of anesthetic induction or change in anesthetic level.

A Increased alveolar delivery
- **1** Increased inspired anesthetic concentration
  - **a** Increased vaporization of agent
  - **b** Increased vaporizer dial setting
  - **c** Increased fresh gas inflow
  - **d** Decreased gas volume of patient breathing circuit
- **2** Increased alveolar ventilation
  - **a** Increased minute ventilation
  - **b** Decreased dead space ventilation

B Decreased removal from the alveoli
- **1** Decreased blood solubility of anesthetic
- **2** Decreased cardiac output
- **3** Decreased alveolar–venous anesthetic gradient

Figure 16.10 Factors related to a rapid change in alveolar anesthetic tension (P_A).

Inspired concentration

The inspired concentration has a number of variables controlling it. First of all, the upper limit of inspired concentration is dictated by the agent vapor pressure, which in turn is dependent on temperature. This may be especially important considering the breadth of veterinary medical application of inhaled anesthesia and methods of vaporizing volatile anesthetics under widely diverse conditions (some environmental conditions are quite hostile).

Characteristics of the patient breathing system can also be a major factor in generating a suitable inspired concentration under usual operating room conditions. Characteristics of special importance include the volume of the system, the amount of rubber or plastic components of the system, the position of the vaporizer relative to the breathing circuit (i.e., within or outside the circuit), and the fresh gas inflow to the patient breathing circuit. The patient breathing circuit contains a gas volume that must be replaced with gas containing the desired anesthetic concentration. Thus, the volume of the breathing circuit serves as a buffer to delay the rise of anesthetic concentration. In the management of small animals (i.e., less than 10 kg), a non-rebreathing patient circuit and/or a relatively high fresh gas inflow into the patient breathing circuit is usually used, so there should *not* be a clinically important difference between the delivered (e.g., vaporizer dial setting) and the inspired concentration. That is, when the vaporizer dial setting is adjusted to the desired concentration setting, the fresh gas plus anesthetic flowing from the vaporizer almost immediately contains the dialed anesthetic vapor concentration. In addition, the total gas flow is high relative to the volume of the delivery circuit, so the anesthetic concentration in the inspired breath is rapidly increased. However, with larger animals (i.e., greater than 10 kg), a circle, CO_2 absorber (i.e., rebreathing), patient breathing circuit is most commonly used for inhalation anesthesia. The volume of this breathing circuit may be very large compared to fresh gas inflow. This volume markedly delays the rate of rise of inspired anesthetic concentration because the residual gas volume must be 'washed out' and replaced by anesthetic containing fresh gas in order for the inspired concentration to increase to that delivered from the vaporizer (Fig. 16.11). In addition, rebreathing of exhaled gas (minus CO_2) occurs to varying degrees with these circuits. The inspired gas is composed of exhaled and fresh gases. Because the expired gas contains less anesthetic than the fresh gas, the inspired anesthetic gas concentration will be less than that of the fresh gas leaving the vaporizer.

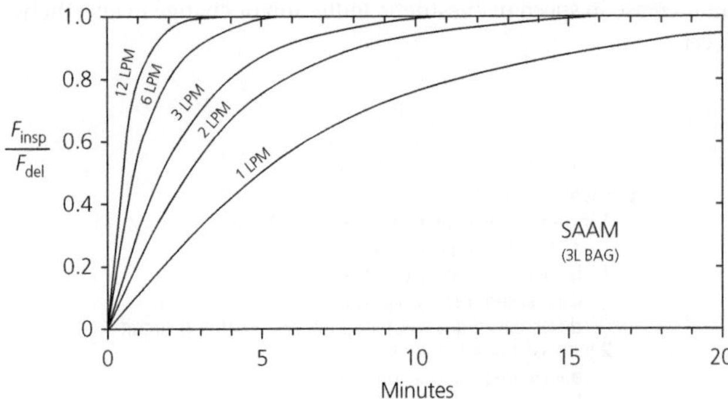

Figure 16.11 A comparison of the rate of increase of inspired halothane concentration toward a constant delivered concentration F_{insp}/F_{del} in a 7 L small animal anesthetic breathing circuit (SAAM) at fresh gas flow rates of 1, 3, 6, and 12 Lpm. Source: Steffey EP, Howland D Jr. Rate of change of halothane concentration in a large animal circle anesthetic system. *Am J Vet Res* 1977; **38**(12): 1993–1996.

In veterinary applications, the delaying influence of the circle circuit is most notable with anesthetic management of very large animals such as horses [17] and cattle and/or when using a closed circuit fresh gas flow rate (i.e., where O_2 is the fresh gas and its inflow [plus anesthetic] to the circuit just meets the metabolic needs of the patient). With closed circuit delivery, the fresh gas inflow is very low relative to the circuit volume [7,10,17].

The high solubility of some anesthetics (e.g., methoxyflurane; see Table 16.4) in rubber and plastic delays development of an appropriate inspired anesthetic concentration. The loss of anesthetic to these equipment 'sinks' increases the apparent volume of the anesthetic circuitry and may, in some cases, be clinically important (e.g., the use of rubber hoses and a large rubber rebreathing bag on circuits designed for anesthetic management of horses). With the newest inhalation anesthetics and more modern anesthetic delivery equipment, this issue is of minor or no clinical importance.

Positioning the vaporizer in relation to the patient breathing circuit will influence inspired anesthetic concentration [16,18]. For example, with the vaporizer positioned within a circle rebreathing circuit, a decrease in inspired concentration will follow an increase in fresh gas inflow to the circuit, whereas an increase in inspired concentration will result if the vaporizer is positioned outside the circuit (Table 16.5). With the loss of methoxyflurane to clinical practice, nearly all, if not all, vaporizers in use in North America are agent-specific, precision vaporizers. This style of vaporizer is always placed upstream and outside the patient breathing circuit.

Alveolar ventilation

An increase in alveolar ventilation increases the rate of delivery of inhalation anesthetic to the alveolus (Fig. 16.12). If unopposed by blood and tissue uptake of anesthetic, alveolar ventilation would rapidly increase the alveolar concentration of anesthetic so that within minutes the alveolar concentration would equal the inspired concentration. However, in reality, the input created by alveolar ventilation is countered by absorption of anesthetic into blood. Predictably, hypoventilation decreases the rate at which the alveolar concentration increases over time compared to the inspired concentration (i.e., anesthetic induction is slowed). Alveolar ventilation is altered by changes in anesthetic depth (increased depth usually means decreased ventilation), mechanical ventilation (usually increased ventilation), and deadspace ventilation (i.e., for constant minute ventilation a decrease in deadspace ventilation results in an increase in alveolar ventilation).

Alveolar ventilation and thus the alveolar anesthetic concentration can also be influenced by administering a potent inhalation anesthetic like halothane in conjunction with N_2O. Very early in the administration of N_2O (during the period of large volume uptake; the first 5–10 min of delivery), the rate of rise of the alveolar concentration of the concurrently administered inhalation anesthetic is increased. This is commonly referred to as the *second gas effect*, and this phenomenon can be applied clinically to speed anesthetic induction [10,14,19].

Table 16.5 Vaporizer positioning within or outside a circle patient rebreathing circuit influences inspired anesthetic concentration.

Factor	Vaporizer positioning	
	Out of circuit	In circuit
Increase ventilation	Decrease	Increase
Increase fresh gas (O_2) inflow to circuit	Increase	Decrease

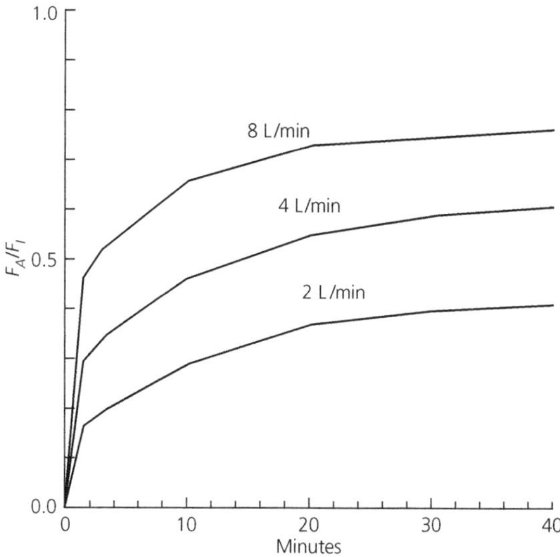

Figure 16.12 The effect of ventilation on the rise of the alveolar (F_A) concentration of halothane toward the inspired (F_I) concentration. As noted, the F_A:F_I ratio increases more rapidly as ventilation is increased from 2 to 8 L/min. Source: Redrawn with permission from from Eger EI II. *Anesthetic Uptake and Action*. Baltimore, MD: Williams & Wilkins. 1974.

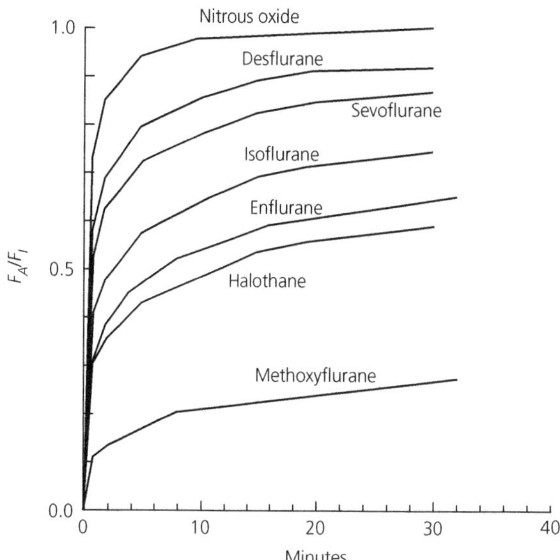

Figure 16.13 The rise in the alveolar (F_A) anesthetic concentration toward the inspired (F_I) concentration. Note the rise is most rapid with the least soluble anesthetic, N_2O, and slowest with the most soluble anesthetic, methoxyflurane. All data are from studies of humans. The curves are redrawn from Eger [1,414].

Removal from alveoli: Uptake by blood

As noted by Eger [10], anesthetic uptake is the product of three factors: solubility (S, the blood/gas solubility; see Table 16.4), cardiac output (CO), and the difference in the anesthetic partial pressure between the alveolus and venous blood returning to the lungs $\left(P_A - P_{\bar{V}}/P_{bar}\right)$ expressed in mmHg: that is:

$$\text{Uptake} = S \times CO\left(P_A - P_{\bar{V}}/P_{bar}\right)$$

where P_{bar} = barometric pressure in mmHg. Note that if any of these three factors equals zero there is no further uptake of anesthetic by blood.

Solubility

As previously discussed, the solubility of an inhalation anesthetic in blood and tissues is characterized by its partition coefficient (PC; see Tables 16.2 and 16.3). Remember that a PC describes how an inhalation anesthetic distributes itself between two phases or two solvents (e.g., the quantity of agent in blood and alveoli [gas] or blood and muscle, respectively) once equilibrium is established (i.e., when the anesthetic partial pressure is equal). Based on blood/gas PCs, inhalation anesthetics range from highly soluble (methoxyflurane) to poorly soluble (N_2O, desflurane, and sevoflurane). Agents such as halothane and isoflurane are intermediate.

Compared to an anesthetic with high blood solubility (PC), an agent with low blood solubility is associated with a more rapid equilibration because a smaller amount of anesthetic must be dissolved in the blood before equilibrium is reached with the gas phase. In the case of the agent with a high blood/gas PC, the blood acts like a large 'sink' into which the anesthetic is poured and accordingly blood is 'reluctant' to give up the agent to other tissues (such as the brain). The blood serves as a conduit for drug delivery to the brain and as such can be visualized as a pharmacologically inactive reservoir that is interposed between the lungs and the agent's site of desired pharmacologic activity (i.e., brain). Therefore, an anesthetic agent with a low blood/gas PC is usually more desirable than a highly soluble agent, because it is associated with (a) a more rapid anesthetic induction (i.e., more rapid rate of rise in alveolar concentration during induction; Fig. 16.13); (b) more precise control of anesthetic depth (i.e., alveolar concentration during the anesthetic maintenance); and (c) a more rapid elimination of anesthetic and recovery (i.e., a rapid decrease in alveolar concentration during recovery).

Cardiac output

The amount of blood flowing through the lungs and on to body tissues also influences anesthetic uptake from the lungs. The greater the CO, the more blood passing through the lungs carrying away anesthetic from the alveoli. Thus a large CO, like increased anesthetic agent blood solubility, delays the alveolar rise of P_{anes} (Fig. 16.14). Patient excitement is an example in which a relatively large CO is anticipated. Conversely, a reduced CO should be anticipated with a patient with poor myocardial function or severe bradycardia. Such a situation would be associated with an increase in the rate of rise of the P_A of the anesthetic and this, along with other factors, makes the anesthetic induction more rapid and risky.

Alveolar to venous anesthetic partial pressure difference

The magnitude of difference in anesthetic partial pressure between the alveoli and mixed venous blood returning to the lungs is related to the amount of uptake of anesthetic by tissues. It is not surprising that the largest gradient occurs during induction. Once the tissues no longer absorb anesthetic (i.e., equilibrium is reached), there is no longer any uptake of anesthetic from the lungs because $P_{\bar{V}} = P_A$ (i.e., the mixed venous blood returning to the lungs contains as much anesthetic as when it left the lungs). The changes in gradient between the initiation of induction and equilibration result in part from the relative distribution of CO. In this regard it is important to recognize that roughly 70–80% of the CO is normally directed to only a small volume of body tissues in a lean individual [20,21].

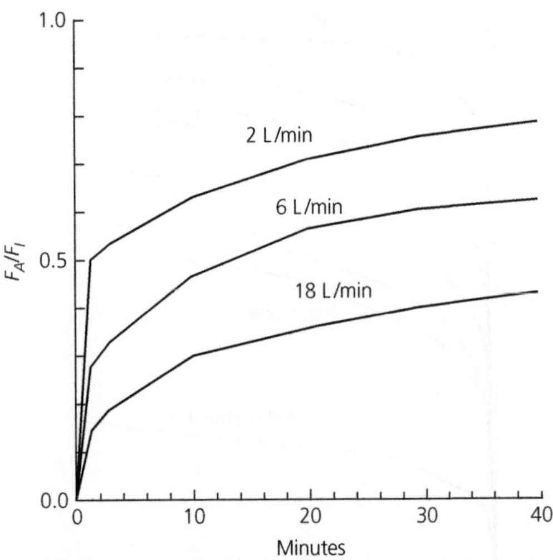

Figure 16.14 The effect of cardiac output on the rise of the alveolar (F_A) concentration of halothane toward the inspired (F_I) concentration. As noted, the F_A:F_I ratio increases more rapidly as cardiac output is decreased from 18 to 2 L/min. Source: Redrawn with permission from Eger EI II. *Anesthetic Uptake and Action*. Baltimore, MD: Williams & Wilkins. 1974.

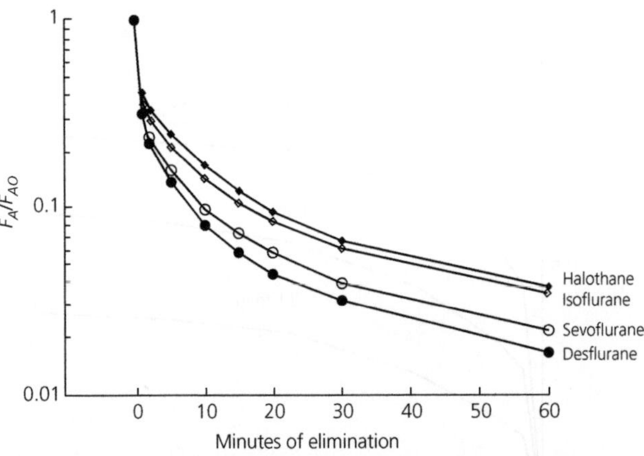

Figure 16.15 The fall in alveolar (F_A) concentration relative to the alveolar concentration at the end of anesthesia (F_{AO}). Note that the newest, most insoluble, volatile anesthetic, desflurane, is eliminated in humans more rapidly than the other contemporary potent anesthetics. Not shown is information for methoxyflurane. If present, the curve for methoxyflurane would appear above that for halothane. Source: Reproduced with permission from Eger EI II. Desflurane animal and human pharmacology: aspects of kinetics, safety, and MAC. *Anesth Analg* 1992; **75**: S3–S9.

Tissues such as the brain, heart, hepatoportal system, and kidneys represent only about 10% of the body mass but normally receive about 75% of the total blood flow each minute. As a result, these highly perfused tissues equilibrate rapidly with arterial anesthetic partial pressure when compared to other body tissues (actual timing is influenced by agent solubility). Since the venous anesthetic pressure or tension equals that in the tissue within 10 or 15 min, about 75% of the blood returning to the lungs is the same as the alveolar tension. This presumes there has been no change in arterial anesthetic partial pressure during this time and thus uptake is reduced. Skin and muscle comprise the major bulk of the body (about 50% in humans) but at rest receive only about 15–20% of the CO, so saturation of these tissues takes hours to accomplish. Fat is a variable component of body bulk and receives only a small proportion of blood flow. Consequently, anesthetic saturation of this tissue is very slow because all anesthetics are considerably more soluble in fat than other tissue groups (see Tables 16.2 and 16.3).

Other factors can influence the magnitude of the alveolar to arterial anesthetic partial pressure gradient. For example, abnormalities of ventilation/perfusion result in an alveolar-arterial gradient proportional to the degree of abnormality [10,22,23]. Others include loss of anesthetic via the skin [24–26] and into closed gas spaces [10,14,19], and metabolism [10,14].

Overview

The rate at which the alveolar anesthetic concentration increases relative to the inspired concentration (i.e., the rate of change in anesthetic level) is often summarized as a plot of the ratio of F_A:F_I versus time. The position of individual curves representing different anesthetics on a plot is related to the solubility characteristics of the anesthetics (see Fig. 16.13). The shape of the graph of F_A:F_I versus time is similar for all anesthetics (see Fig. 16.13). There is a rapid rise initially that results from the effect of alveolar ventilation bringing anesthetic into the lung. There is then a decrease in the rate of rise of the curve as uptake by the blood occurs. With time, the highly perfused tissues of the body equilibrate with incoming blood so that eventually about three-quarters of the total blood flow returning to the heart has the same anesthetic partial pressure as it had when it left the lungs. Thus, further uptake from the lung is decreased and the rate of approach of the F_A to F_I over time is further decreased.

Anesthetic elimination

Recovery from inhalation anesthesia results from the elimination of anesthetic from the CNS. This requires a decrease in alveolar anesthetic partial pressure (concentration), which in turn fosters a decrease in arterial and then CNS anesthetic partial pressure (see Fig. 16.10). Prominent factors accounting for recovery are the same as those for anesthetic induction. The percent clearance of an inhaled anesthetic can be expressed as:

$$\%\text{clearance} = 100 \times V_A \div \left(\text{agent blood/gas PC} \times \text{CO} + V_A\right) \quad [27]$$

Therefore, factors such as alveolar ventilation, cardiac output, and especially agent solubility greatly influence recovery from inhalation anesthesia. Indeed, the graphic curves representing the wash-out of anesthetic from alveoli versus time (Fig. 16.15) are essentially inverses of the wash-in curves. That is, the wash-out of the less soluble anesthetics is high at first (i.e., rapid wash-out by ventilation of the lung functional residual capacity), then rapidly declines to a lower output level that continues to decrease but at a slower rate. The wash-out of more soluble agents is also high at first, but the magnitude of decrease in alveolar anesthetic concentration is less and decreases more gradually with time (see Fig. 16.15).

An important factor during the wash-out period is the duration of anesthesia. This effect and a comparison of this effect between three agents spanning a range of blood solubilities are summarized in Fig. 16.16 [28]. Times to recovery from anesthesia in, for example, rats correlate with values for blood solubility of anesthetics (Fig. 16.17) [29]. If a patient rebreathing anesthetic circuit (e.g., circle system) is in use and the patient is not disconnected from the circuit at the end of anesthesia, the circuit itself may also reduce the rate of recovery, just as the circuit was shown to decrease the rate of rise of anesthetic during induction. This influence of rebreathing

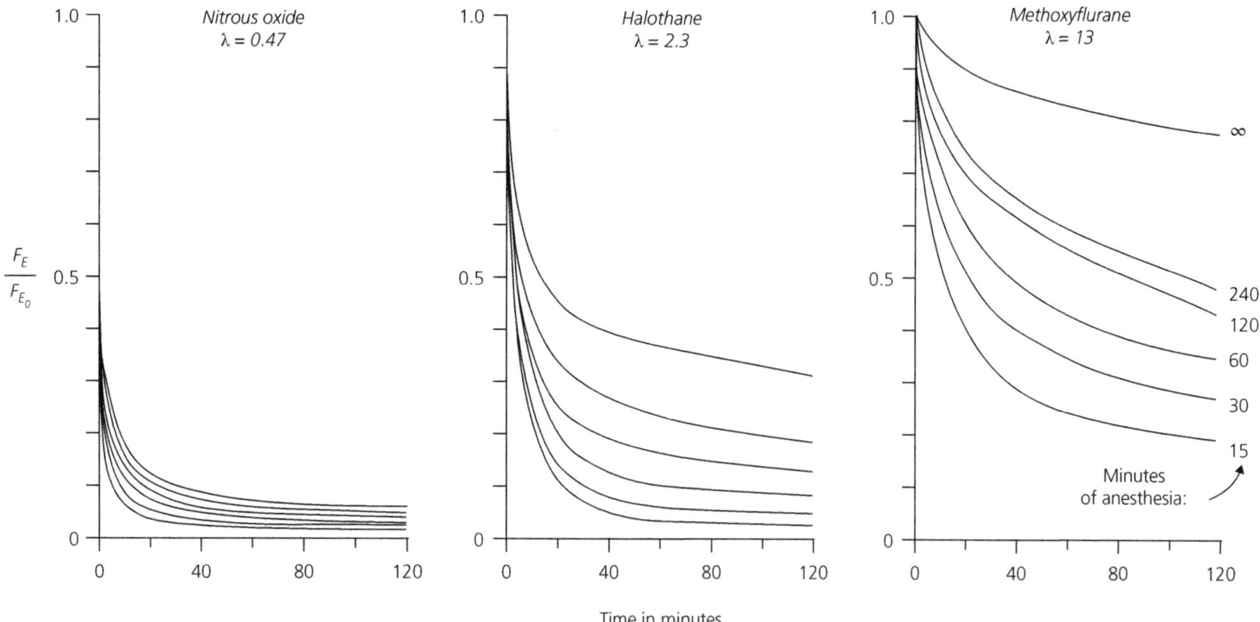

Figure 16.16 The decrease in the alveolar (F_E) anesthetic concentration from the concentration at the time of breathing circuit disconnect (i.e., the beginning of recovery from anesthesia; F_{EO}) is influenced by both the solubility (λ) of anesthetic and the duration of anesthesia. Source: Redrawn with permission from Stoelting RK, Eger EI II. The effects of ventilation and anesthetic solubility on recovery from anesthesia: an in vivo and analog analysis before and after equilibration. *Anesthesiology* 1969; **30**(3): 290–296.

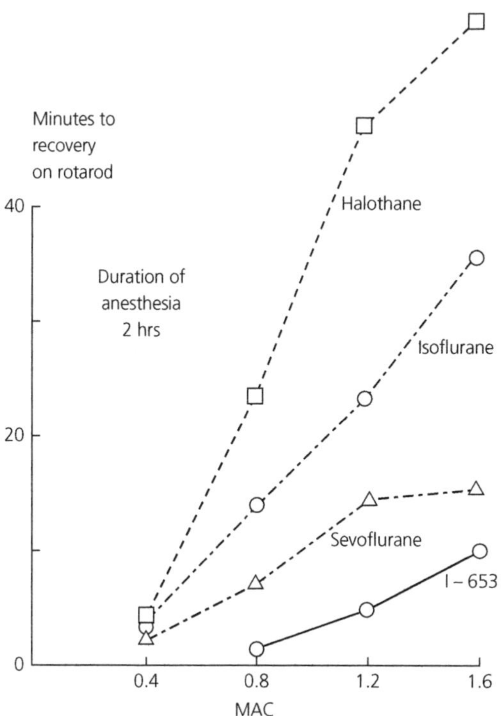

Figure 16.17 Increasing the delivered concentration of inhalation anesthetic increased the time to recovery of the motor co-ordination necessary to remain atop a 6 cm rod rotating at 8 rpm. The duration of anesthesia was constant for all trials. Source: Redrawn with permission from Eger EI II, Johnson BH. Rates of awakening from anesthesia with I-653, halothane, isoflurane, and sevoflurane – a test of the effect of anesthetic concentration and duration in rats. *Anesth Analg* 1987; **66**: 977–983.

circuits can be reduced by directing high flow rates of anesthetic-free O_2 into the anesthetic circuit (i.e., applying principles of a non-rebreathing circuit).

Other factors that are important to varying degrees to inhalation anesthetic elimination from the body include percutaneous loss, intertissue diffusion of agents, and metabolism. Transcutaneous movement of inhalation agent occurs, but the amount under consideration is small [24–27,30]. Intertissue diffusion is of theoretical interest, but its clinical importance is limited [27,31,32]. In this regard, the impact of obesity on recovery from anesthesia may be important to consider clinically [27]. Metabolism may also play a small role with some inhalation anesthetics (e.g., methoxyflurane and perhaps even halothane), especially when associated with prolonged anesthesia [31,33–35].

A special consideration associated with recovery following use of N_2O deserves comment. *Diffusion hypoxia* is a possibility at the end of N_2O administration when the patient breathes air immediately rather than O_2 for at least a brief transition period (i.e., 5–10 min) [36–38]. In this case a large volume of N_2O returns to the lung from the blood. This early rapid inflow of N_2O to the lung displaces other gases within the lung. If at this time the patient is breathing air (only about 21% O_2) rather than 100% O_2, N_2O dilutes alveolar O_2, further reducing O_2 partial pressure from levels found in ambient air. This may cause life-threatening reductions in arterial oxygenation. Since the major effect is in the first few minutes after discontinuing N_2O, the condition can be prevented by administering high inspired fractions of O_2 at the conclusion of N_2O administration rather than allowing the patient to immediately breathe ambient air.

Biotransformation

Most inhalation anesthetics are not chemically inert [39]. They undergo varying degrees of metabolism, primarily in the liver but also to lesser degrees in the lung, kidney, and intestinal tract

Table 16.6 Biotransformation of inhalation anesthetics in humans.

Anesthetic	% of Anesthetic metabolized	
Methoxyflurane	50–75	[35,42]
Halothane	20–46	[35,41,421]
Sevoflurane	2–5	[54,422]
Enflurane	2–8	[35,423]
Isoflurane	0.2	[424]
Desflurane	0.02	[57]
Nitrous oxide	0.004	[361,362]

[33],[40–43]. The importance of this is two-fold. First, in a very limited way, metabolism may facilitate anesthetic recovery. Second and more important is the potential for acute and chronic toxicities by intermediate or end- metabolites of inhalation agents, especially on kidneys, liver, and reproductive organs [33,43].

The magnitude of metabolism of inhalation anesthetic agents varies greatly and is determined by a variety of factors including the chemical structure, hepatic enzyme activity (cytochrome P_{450} enzymes located in the endoplasmic reticulum of the hepatocyte), the blood concentration of the anesthetic [44], disease states, and genetic factors (i.e., some species and individuals are more active metabolizers of these drugs than others, e.g., humans versus rats).

An indication of the extent of biotransformation of contemporary inhalation anesthetics is given in Table 16.6. The degradation of sevoflurane occurs *in vivo* to about the same extent as isoflurane, perhaps a bit more depending on circumstances, and as indicated by transient postanesthetic increases in blood and urinary fluoride levels in rats [45–49], dogs [48]. horses [50–52], swine [53], and humans [54]. The peak serum fluoride concentrations observed in humans during and following sevoflurane anesthesia are low, and nephrotoxicity is not expected [54,55]. Desflurane resists degradation *in vivo* [53,56,57]. The increase in serum inorganic fluoride is much smaller than that found with isoflurane [53,56,57].

For further information on the biotransformation of inhalation anesthetics in general and for specific details regarding individual anesthetic agents, readers are referred to reviews by Baden and Rice [33], Mazze and Fujinaga [43], and Njoku et al. [58].

Anesthetic dose: The minimum alveolar concentration (MAC)

In 1963 Merkel and Eger described what has become the standard index of anesthetic potency for inhalation anesthetics, *MAC* [59]. MAC is defined as the minimum alveolar concentration of an anesthetic at 1 atmosphere that produces immobility in 50% of subjects exposed to a supramaximal noxious stimulus. Thus MAC corresponds to the effective $dose_{50}$ or ED_{50}; half of the subjects are anesthetized and half have not yet reached that 'level.' The dose that corresponds to the ED_{95} (95% of the individuals are anesthetized), at least in humans, is 20–40% greater than MAC [60]. Anesthetic potency of an inhaled anesthetic is inversely related to MAC (i.e., potency = 1/MAC). From information presented earlier, it also follows that MAC is inversely related to the oil/gas PC. Thus, a very potent anesthetic like methoxyflurane which has a high oil/gas PC has a low MAC, whereas an agent with a low oil/gas PC has a high MAC.

A number of characteristics of MAC deserve emphasis [10]. First, the A in MAC represents *alveolar* concentration, not inspired or delivered (as, for example, from a vaporizer). This is important because the alveolar concentration is easily monitored with contemporary technology. Also, as we reviewed earlier, after sufficient time for equilibration (minutes), alveolar partial pressure will closely approximate arterial and brain (CNS) anesthetic partial pressures.

Second, MAC is defined in terms of volumes percent of 1 atmosphere and therefore represents an anesthetic partial pressure (P) at the anesthetic site of action (i.e., remember $P_x = (C/100)\ P_{bar}$, where P_x stands for the partial pressure of the anesthetic in the gas mixture, C is the anesthetic concentration in vol % and P_{bar} is the barometric or total pressure of the gas mixture). Thus, although the concentration at MAC for a given agent may vary depending on ambient pressure conditions (e.g., sea level vs high altitude), the anesthetic partial pressure always remains the same. For example, MAC for isoflurane in healthy dogs is reported as 1.63 volumes %. The study reporting this value was conducted at near sea level conditions at Davis, CA (i.e., P_{bar} of 760 mmHg). Based on discussion above, MAC of 1.63% represents an alveolar isoflurane partial pressure (P_{iso}) of 11.6 mmHg. In comparison, for the same dog at Mexico City (elevation 2240 M above sea level; P_{bar} = 584 mmHg), the alveolar P_{iso} at MAC is expected to be the same as determined at Davis, CA (i.e., 11.6 mmHg); however, MAC (i.e., the alveolar concentration) would be about 2.17%.

Finally, it is important to note that MAC is determined in healthy animals under laboratory conditions in the *absence* of other drugs and circumstances common to clinical use that may modify the requirements for anesthesia. General techniques for determining MAC in animals are given elsewhere [10,61–64]. In determining MAC in humans, the initial surgical skin incision has been the standard noxious stimulus used [10]. For the determination of MAC in smaller animals (mice to dogs and pigs) [10,65,66], the standard stimulus has been application of a forceps or other surgical clamp to the base of the tail or the base of the dewclaw of the limb (e.g., pigs [64]), while electrical stimulus applied beneath the oral mucus membranes is most commonly used in larger species such as horses [62].

The MAC values for contemporary inhalation anesthetics for a variety of mammals commonly encountered in veterinary medicine are summarized in Table 16.7A, while the ED_{50} values for non-mammalian species are given in Table 16.7B. Values for humans are also given for comparison. For values of agents of historical interest such as methoxyflurane, enflurane or diethyl ether, readers are referred to the review in an earlier edition of this book or elsewhere [10,66].

Since its original introduction, the MAC concept has been extended to other stimulus endpoints in an effort to better define and understand the anesthetic state. For example, Stoelting and coworkers [67] determined the value for MAC of an anesthetic at which humans opened their eyes on verbal command during emergence from anesthesia; this has been termed 'MAC-awake.' The verbal stimulus is of course less intense than the surgical incision in humans and thus the response occurs at a lower concentration of anesthetic than movement following incision. The end-tidal concentration preventing movement in response to tracheal intubation (MAC for intubation) is more stimulating to humans than surgical incision and was described by Yakaitis and colleagues [68,69]. Roizen and colleagues [70] reported an even greater alveolar concentration necessary to prevent adrenergic response (rise in endogenous catecholamines) to skin incision (also in human patients) compared to the concentration necessary to just prevent movement; this is known as MAC-BAR. Similarly, Boscan and colleagues showed that ovarian/ovarian ligament traction increased

Table 16.7A MAC values (%) for a variety of mammals at sea level or near sea level conditions.

	Desflurane	Halothane	Isoflurane	Sevoflurane	Nitrous oxide
Cat	9.79 [425]	0.99 [427,428]	1.28 [431]	2.58 [433]	255 [429]
	10.27 [426]	1.14 [429]	1.50 [428]	3.07 [428]	
		1.19 [430]	1.61 [430]	3.41 [426]	
			1.63 [244]		
			1.90 [426]		
			2.21 [432]		
Cow		0.76 [434](calf)	1.14 [435]		223 [434] [(calf)
Dog	7.2 [436]	0.86 [90]	1.28 [244]	2.10 [127]	188 [439]
	7.68–8.19 [437]	0.87 [429,439,440]	1.30 [198]	2.36 [441]	222 [429]
	10.3 [438]	0.89 [243,441]	1.31 [444]		297 [446]
		0.92 [442]	1.39 [244]		
		0.93 [443]	1.39-1.50 [445]		
Ferret		1.01 [447]	1.52 [447]		267 [447]
			1.74 [448]		
Goat		1.29 [449]	1.2 [100]	2.33 [449]	
		1.3 [450]	1.23 [451]		
			1.29 [449]		
			1.31 [452]		
			1.43 [453]		
			1.5 [450]		
Horse	7.02 [454]	0.88 [62]	1.31 [62]	2.31 [459]	205 [280]
	8.06 [209]	0.95 [455]	1.43 [199]	2.84 [52]	
		1.02 [456]	1.44 [457]		
		1.05 [200]	1.64 [458]		
Monkey		0.89 [429]	1.28 [460]		200 [429]
		1.15 [460]	1.46 [198]		
Mouse	6.6–9.1[a] [461]	0.95 [462]	1.31–1.77[a] [461]	2.7 [465]	150 [466]
		1.00 [463]	1.35 [462]		275 [463]
		1.19–1.37[a] [461]	1.41 [463]		
		1.59 [464]			
Pig	10.00 [64]	0.90 [467]	1.45 [470]	1.97 [473]	162 [471]
		0.91 [468]	1.48 [467]	2.12 [467]	195 [472]
		1.25 [469]	1.51 [198]	2.53 [474]	277 [469]
			1.55 [471]	2.66 [135]	
			1.75 [472]		
			2.04 [64]		
Rabbit	8.90 [436]	0.80 [475]	2.05 [478]	3.70 [482]	
		0.82 [476]	2.07 [479]		
		1.05 [477]	2.12 [480]		
		1.39 [478]			
		1.42 [479]			
		1.44 [480]			
		1.56 [481]			
Rat	5.72 [483]	0.81 [487]	1.17 [487]	2.99 [489]	136 [497]
	6.48 [484]	0.95 [488]	1.28 [495]	2.40 [490]	155 [498]
	6.85 [485]	1.02 [489]	1.30 [496]	2.50 [45]	204 [250]
	7.10 [486]	1.03 [462]	1.38 [491]		221 [499]
		1.10 [490]	1.46 [462]		235 [499]
		1.11 [491]	1.46 [485]		
		1.13 [492,493]	1.58 [448,488]		
		1.17 [494]			
		1.23 [485]			
Sheep		0.97 [500]	1.58 [500]		
Human	6.00 [501]	0.73 [502]	1.15 [506]	1.58 [507]	104 [513]
(30–60 years)		0.74 [503,504]		1.71 [508]	
		0.77 [505]		1.83 [509]	
				1.84 [510]	
				1.85 [511]	
				1.9 [512]	
				2.05 [482]	

[a] Absolute value related to strain.

sevoflurane MAC compared to tail clamp in dogs [71]. Thus a group of response curves is possible and dependent upon the strength of the stimulus applied.

In a single species the variability in MAC (response to a noxious stimulus) is generally small and is not substantially influenced by gender, duration of anesthesia, variation of $PaCO_2$ (from 10 to 90 mmHg), metabolic alkalosis or acidosis, variation in PaO_2 (from 40 to 500 mmHg), moderate anemia, or moderate hypotension (see Table 16.7A) [10,66,72]. Even between species, the variability in MAC for a given agent is usually not large. However, there is at least one notable exception (see Table 16.7A). In humans, the MAC for N_2O is 104%, making it the least potent of the inhalation anesthetics currently used in this species. Its potency in other species is less than half that in humans (i.e., around 200%). Because the N_2O MAC is above 100% it cannot be used by itself at 1 atmosphere pressure in any species and still provide adequate amounts of O_2.

Table 16.7B ED_{50} values for a variety of non-mammals at sea level or near sea level conditions.

	Desflurane	Halothane	Isoflurane	Sevoflurane	Nitrous oxide
Birds:					
Chicken		0.85 [63]	1.15 [514]		
Cockatoo			1.44 [515]		
Crane			1.34 [516]		
Duck		1.04 [517]	1.30 [517]		
Guinea			1.45 [518]	2.9 [520]	220 [518]
fowl			2.05 [519]		
Hawk					
Parrot,			1.47 [515]		
Amazon					
Parrot,			1.91 [515]		
African Grey			1.07 [521]		
Parrot,					
thick-billed					
Pigeon			1.51 [518]		154 [518]
			1.45 [522]		
Other:					
Goldfish		0.76 [523]			
Toad		0.67 [524]			82.2 [524]

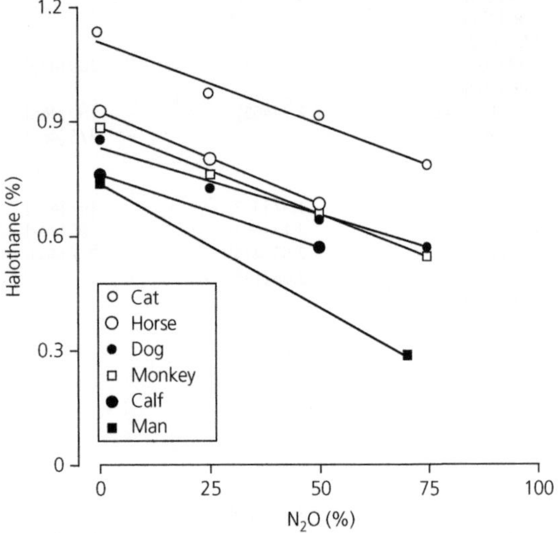

Figure 16.18 When N_2O is combined with halothane the alveolar concentration of halothane at MAC is decreased. However, the halothane sparing imposed by N_2O is less in animals compared to humans. Source: Reproduced with permission from Steffey EP, Eger EI II. Nitrous oxide in veterinary practice and animal research. In: Eger EI II, ed. *Nitrous Oxide/N_2O*. New York: Elsiever, 1984; 305–312.

Consequently, and assuming that MAC values for combinations of inhaled anesthetics are additive, N_2O is usually administered with another more potent agent to thereby reduce the concentration of the second agent necessary for anesthesia (see Fig. 16.18). However, because of the potency difference between animals and humans, the amount of reduction differs in an important way. For example, administration of 60% N_2O with halothane reduces the amount of halothane needed to produce MAC by about 55% in healthy humans (see Fig. 16.18) but reduces it only by about 20–30% in dogs. As noted in Fig. 16.18, the response of other animals most closely resembles the dog. Some factors that are known to influence MAC are given in Table 16.8.

Equipotent doses (i.e., equivalent concentrations of different anesthetics at MAC) are useful for comparing effects of inhalation anesthetics on vital organs. In this regard, anesthetic dose is commonly defined in terms of multiples of MAC (i.e., 1.5 or 2.0 times MAC, or simply 1.5 MAC or 2.0 MAC). From the preceding discussion, therefore, the ED_{50} equals MAC or 1.0 MAC and represents a light level of anesthesia (clearly inadequate in 50% of otherwise unmedicated, healthy animals). The ED_{95} is 1.2 to 1.4 MAC, and 2.0 MAC represents a deep level of anesthesia, in some cases even an anesthetic overdose. The authors will use the concept of MAC multiples later to compare drug effects and contrast pharmacodynamics of multiple doses of a specific drug.

Pharmacodynamics: Actions and toxicity of the volatile inhalation anesthetics on body systems

All contemporary inhalation anesthetic agents in one way or another influence vital organ function. Some actions are inevitable and accompany the use of all agents, whereas other actions are a special or prominent feature of one or a number of the agents. In addition, dose–response relationships of inhalation anesthetics are not necessarily parallel. Differences in action, and especially undesirable action, of specific anesthetic agents form the basis for selecting one agent over another for a particular patient and/or procedure. Undesirable actions also provide primary impetus for development of new agents and/or anesthetic techniques.

Data from healthy animals exposed to equipotent alveolar concentrations of these drugs under controlled circumstances provide foundation information for this review. In other cases, results of studies of human volunteers form the basis of our understanding of some drug actions because actions in animals of common clinical focus in veterinary medicine have not been described. Because animals are commonly allowed to breathe spontaneously during clinical management of general anesthesia (vs controlled mechanical ventilation), investigational results obtained from spontaneously breathing test animals are often considered baseline by veterinarians. However, in the broader anesthesiology and pharmacology literature, results of studies from human volunteers or animals administered precise amounts of inhalation anesthetics during controlled ventilation (and normocapnia) most commonly form the basis of comparison of pharmacodynamic differences. It is important to stress that many variables other than mode of ventilation commonly accompany anesthetic management of animals in both clinical and laboratory settings. These variables influence drug pharmacokinetics and pharmacodynamics and may cause individuals to respond differently from test subjects that were studied

Table 16.8 Some factors that influence the value of MAC (anesthetic requirement).

No change	Increase	Decrease
Arterial blood pressure	Drugs causing CNS stimulation:	Drugs causing CNS depression[a]:
	– Amphetamine	– Other inhaled anesthetic N_2O [19]
>50 mmHg [525]	– Ephedrine	–Injectable anesthetics:
	– Morphine (horse) [200]	ketamine [309]
Atropine, glycopyrrolate, scopolamine [427]	– Laudanosine [481]	lidocaine [432, 443]
	– Physostigmine [526]	thiopental [527]
Duration of anesthesia	Hyperthermia (to 42°C)	– Preanesthetic medication: acepromazine [528–530]
		diazepam [531–533]
Gender		detomidine [457]
		fentanyl [534]
Hyperkalemia, hypokalemia		medetomidine [535, 536]
		meperidine [307]
Metabolic acid–base change		midazolam [537]
		morphine [538]
PaO_2 >40 mmHg		xylazine [458]
		– Other:
$PaCO_2$ 15–95 mmHg		adenosine
		central anticholinergic [526]
		5-HT antagonist [539]
		Arterial blood pressure <50 mmHg
		Hyponatremia
		Hypothermia
		Increasing adult age
		PaO_2 <40 mmHg
		$PaCO_2$ >95 mmHg
		Pregnancy

[a] The list of example drugs is intended to be representative, not exhaustive. The list is summarized from previous reviews [10,61,66] except where indicated by reference numbers.

under standardized conditions. Such confounding variables include species, duration of anesthesia, noxious (painful) stimulation, coexisting disease, concurrent medications, variation in body temperature, and extremes of age as examples.

Central nervous system (CNS)

Inhalation anesthetics affect the CNS in many ways. Mostly these agents are selected because they induce a reversible, dose-related state of CNS (somatic, motor), but also hemodynamic and endocrine unresponsiveness to noxious stimulation, i.e., a state of general anesthesia. Interestingly, although clinical anesthesia was introduced more than 150 years ago, the mechanisms and sites by which general anesthetics (including the inhalation anesthetics) cause unresponsiveness to surgical or other forms of noxious stimulation remain unknown [73]. Inhalation anesthetics influence electrical activity of the brain, cerebral metabolism, cerebral perfusion, intracranial pressure, and analgesia – issues of critical importance to the anesthetic management of animals. Our systematic review will start with a focus on mechanisms of action of inhalation anesthetics within the CNS.

Mechanism of action

Molecular mechanisms of action

Background As a class, inhaled anesthetics exhibit unusual actions that set them apart from most other pharmacologic agents. Most drugs rely on a unique molecular size, shape, volume, charge, polarity, functional group, or other structural motif in order to bind with a specific target molecule and induce a functional change, as set forth by Fisher's Schloss und Schlüssel (lock and key) description of specific enzyme–substrate or protein–drug interactions [74]. Yet inhaled anesthetics share no chemical or structural commonalities; they range in composition from single atoms (xenon) and diatomic elements (nitrogen) to inorganic molecules (nitrous oxide) and hydrocarbons of varying lengths containing any number of halogens and organic functional groups, including alkanes (chloroform, halothane), alkenes (trichloroethylene), alcohols (ethanol), ethers (isoflurane, sevoflurane, desflurane), and combinations thereof (ethyl vinyl ether, fluroxene). Even endogenous by-products of metabolism such as CO_2 [75], ammonia [76], and ketones [77] exert anesthetic effects. Such chemical diversity among drug 'keys' is incongruent with classical notions of drug–ligand interactions.

Inhaled anesthetic efficacy is not limited to humans and domestic mammals. Rather, they reversibly immobilize all vertebrate and invertebrate animals in which they have been studied, including worms, fish, amphibians, reptiles, and birds. In fact, efficacy is not limited to the animal kingdom, as inhaled anesthetics can even prevent movement in protozoa [78] and plants (those with touch-sensitive contractile leaves) [79]. It is unknown why these pharmacologic effects should be conserved across such diverse phyla, especially since most anesthetics are not found in nature and there is no obvious selective pressure underlying anesthetic sensitivity. It suggests, perhaps, that the molecular mechanism underlying inhaled anesthetic action involves interactions with cellular components that are essential to all life.

Molecular sites: Lipid and aqueous theories Meyer [80] and Overton [81] noted that narcotic potency correlated with anesthetic solubility in oil from which they concluded that the cell lipid membrane served as the site of anesthetic action. However, non-specific lipid theories do not adequately explain effect differences between anesthetic sterioisomers [82] or the existence of the anesthetic cut-off effect and non-immobilizers, compounds that lack an immobilizing effect at concentrations predicted by the Meyer–Overton hypothesis to produce general anesthesia [83]. More recently, Cantor [84] hypothesized that anesthetics may alter molecular composition and forces within a bilayer plane and cause a change in the lateral pressure profile exerted upon proteins within the lipid membrane. Since non-immobilizers may not access interfacial regions of the membrane critical to modulation of embedded protein receptors [85] and since ion channels and membrane lipids themselves have chiral centers that may interact differently with anesthetic stereoisomers, this theory could address inconsistencies presented by the older Meyer–Overton lipid theory of action.

Miller [86] and Pauling [87] each proposed an aqueous site of action whereby the ordering of water into gas hydrates or clathrates alters electrical conductance across the cell membrane to produce unconsciousness. However, anesthetic MAC correlates better with lipid solubility than with hydrate dissociation pressure [88,89]. In addition, enthalpy for anesthetic hydrate formation is much greater than calculated for *in vivo* hypothermia MAC studies [90] and the extreme transience of anesthetic clathrate formation with reduced water concentration at anesthetic binding sites [91] makes a bulk aqueous phase site of action unlikely.

Molecular sites: Protein theories Inhaled anesthetics also bind proteins and can modulate function even in the absence of a lipid environment [92]. In general, agents potentiate inhibitory cell targets such as γ-aminobutyric acid type A ($GABA_A$) receptors, glycine receptors, and two-pore domain potassium channels; these same agents inhibit excitatory cell targets such as *N*-methyl-d-aspartate (NMDA) receptors, α-amino-3-hydroxy-5-methyl-4-isoxazole-propionic acid (AMPA) receptors, nicotinic receptors, and voltage-gated sodium channels [73,82]. In many of these proteins, specific mutations at putative anesthetic binding sites alter anesthetic effects on receptor kinetics or ion conductance, and can sometimes render the receptor insensitive to one or more anesthetics altogether. And yet this evidence for specific protein–receptor ligand interactions is inconsistent with the ability for so many chemically unrelated substances to modulate so many phylogenetically unrelated proteins. It is also unclear why the type of pharmacologic effect on a receptor or channel – either potentiation or inhibition – should vary depending on whether the receptor or channel itself is inhibitory or excitatory. How does the anesthetic 'know' whether the receptor is inhibitory or excitatory? Finally, the creation of several mutant anesthetic-resistant receptor knock-in or knock-out mice models has so far failed to produce animals with any substantial resistance to the immobilizing effects of anesthetics.

Inability to identify *the* receptor critical to anesthetic action may in fact suggest that immobility is the product of multiple cell receptor and ion channel target modulations [93] acting in a combination of in-parallel and in-series cell pathways and neuronal circuits to decrease cell excitability [94]. Such a model, in which the anesthetic MAC greatly exceeds the dissociation constant between the anesthetic and its relevant protein targets, also predicts steep dose responses (large Hill coefficients) and additive combinatorial effects that are hallmarks of most inhaled anesthetic actions both *in vivo* [95] and *in vitro* [96]. Multiple relevant sites of action would also explain why loss of anesthetic efficacy at one cellular target consequently produces greater anesthetic modulation of other putative cellular targets at MAC [97,98].

Anatomic sites of action

Traditionally, this summary state we refer to as general anesthesia was assumed to result from a focus in the brain. However, mounting evidence is causing a shift in thinking such that this state we know as general anesthesia is likely the collection of a number of endpoints that are distinct and site specific, and include supraspinal and spinal events. For example, actions focused in the brain (especially the cerebral cortex, amygdala, and hippocampus) mediate such centrally recognized components of general anesthesia as hypnosis (sleep) and amnesia (at least in humans) while the spinal cord appears to be a critical site of anesthetic action that suppresses noxious-evoked movement [99–101].

In an experimental goat model in which the cerebral circulation was isolated from the rest of the body, selective brain isoflurane administration more than doubled the anesthetic requirement for immobility compared to whole-body isoflurane administration. This demonstrated that the spinal cord, and not the brain, is principally responsible for preventing movement during surgery with inhaled anesthetics [100]. Within the spinal cord, immobility is most likely produced by depression of locomotor neuronal networks located in the ventral horn.

In contrast, amnestic effects of inhaled anesthetics are produced by actions within the brain, most probably within the amygdala and hippocampus [102]. Lesions created within the amygdala of rats can block amnestic actions of sevoflurane [103]. On electroencephalography, hippocampal-dependent θ-rhythm frequency slows in proportion to the amnestic effects observed with subanesthetic concentrations of isoflurane in rats [104]. Furthermore, mutant mice lacking the gene encoding either the α_4 or β_3 subunits of $GABA_A$ receptors are resistant to isoflurane depression of hippocampus-dependent learning and memory [105,106] and antagonism of α_5 subunit-containing $GABA_A$ receptors restores hippocampal-dependent memory during sevoflurane administration [107]. Clearly, the mechanisms of inhaled anesthetic action responsible for amnesia are different from those responsible for immobility.

At concentrations above MAC, it is presumed that inhaled anesthetics sufficiently depress cortical function to prevent animals from experiencing motivational-affective dimensions of pain [108]. Additionally, concentrations of modern volatile agents (halothane, enflurane, isoflurane, sevoflurane, desflurane) between 0.8 to 1.0 times MAC decrease, but do not ablate, wind-up and central sensitization and so may help prevent heightened postoperative pain sensitivity; however, higher concentrations of contemporary drugs offer no further benefit in this regard [109,110]. Volatile anesthetic concentrations between 0.4 to 0.8 times MAC decrease withdrawal responses to noxious stimuli, but lower concentrations can actually cause hyperalgesia with a peak effect at 0.1 times MAC [111,112] due to potent nicotinic cholinergic receptor inhibition [113]. In contrast, the gaseous anesthetics xenon and nitrous oxide produce analgesia via glutamatergic receptor inhibition [114] and in the case of nitrous oxide, through additional modulation of noradrenergic-opioid receptor pathways [115]. Anatomically, analgesic actions occur both supraspinally and within the dorsal horn of the spinal cord, and are likely responsible for greater blunting of autonomic responses associated with these gases compared to the modern volatile agents.

Electroencephalographic (EEG) effects

The EEG is used to help identify pathologic brain disorders and predict outcome of brain insults. Studies have shown that general anesthesia alters EEG parameters; however, all anesthetics do not produce exactly the same changes in EEG pattern as dose (anesthetic depth) increases, therefore the generic correlation of the raw EEG with anesthetic dose is not precise. Indeed, despite some weak correlations and its usefulness as an indication of changing anesthetic depth, no parameter has had sensitivity and specificity sufficient to justify use of the EEG alone as a reliable index of anesthetic depth [116]. With technological advances in recent years, research has focused on use of processed EEG parameters (e.g., the bispectral index) as improved descriptions of anesthetic states. However, this subject is beyond the scope of this chapter and therefore is explored elsewhere in this text.

In general, as the depth of anesthesia increases from awake states, the electric activity of the cerebral cortex becomes desynchronized. Using isoflurane as an example of the general EEG response to volatile anesthetics [1], there is initially an increased frequency of the EEG activity (alveolar concentrations less than 0.4 MAC). With further increases in anesthetic concentration, a decrease in frequency and increased amplitude of the EEG waves occur. The wave amplitude increases to a peak (about 1 MAC) and then with further dose increase it progressively declines (burst suppression occurs at about 1.5 MAC, i.e., bursts of slow high-voltage activity separated by electrical silence) and eventually becomes flat line. With isoflurane an isoelectric pattern occurs at about 2.0 MAC while at the other extreme, it is not seen with halothane until >3.5 MAC. Electrical silence does not occur with enflurane. The two newest volatile anesthetics, sevoflurane and desflurane, cause dose-related changes similar to those of isoflurane [117–119]. Systematic studies of EEG activity in humans [120] and dogs [121] showed that enflurane was associated with spontaneous or noise-initiated intensified seizures. In addition, enflurane induces seizure activity that is associated with substantial increases in cerebral blood flow and cerebral metabolic use of O_2. The EEG responses to the two newest anesthetics, desflurane and sevoflurane, are reportedly similar to those of isoflurane [117–119] and all three can suppress drug-induced convulsive behavior [122–126]. However, there are reports of seizure activity in animals [127,128] and human patients [129,130] during sevoflurane anesthesia.

Cerebral metabolism

All volatile anesthetics decrease cerebral metabolic rate (CMR; cerebral oxygen consumption). The magnitude of decrease is least with halothane but similar with isoflurane, sevoflurane, and desflurane [117,122,127,131,132].

Cerebral blood flow (CBF), cerebral perfusion pressure (CPP)

The volatile anesthetics cause either no change or more often an increase in CBF [117,122,127,132–135]. The effect on CBF is likely the sum of a tendency to decrease as a result of both anesthesia reducing cerebral oxygen consumption and increase due to vasodilation caused by direct anesthetic action on intracranial vascular smooth muscle [136]. This can be summarized by saying the ratio of CBF relative to CMR is increased by the potent inhalation anesthetics and such action increases brain blood volume and, in turn, intracranial pressure. The effect is anesthetic dose related and influenced by agent. The rank order of CBF increase is generally regarded as greatest with halothane, less with enflurane, isoflurane and desflurane, and least with sevoflurane [72,137,138]. Interestingly, nitrous oxide reportedly causes more cerebral vasodilation than equipotent doses of isoflurane [139].

Cerebral perfusion pressure (CPP) is defined as the difference between mean arterial blood pressure (MAP) and intracranial pressure (ICP); it represents the driving pressure for blood flow to the brain. The potent volatile agents depress cardiovascular function and decrease MAP, and thus decrease CPP [140]. Nonetheless, as previously noted, CBF typically increases due to dose-dependent cerebral vasodilation that reduces vascular resistance [141], despite dose-dependent reduction in EEG activity and CMR. Through possible actions on nitric oxide synthase [142–145], cyclo-oxygenase [142] and adenylate cylase [146], vasodilation caused by potent volatile anesthetics leads to a loss of cerebrovascular autoregulation, reflected by an uncoupling of cerebral perfusion from cerebral oxygen demand.

In addition to specific agent effects, anesthetic modulation of cerebral hemodynamics depends upon agent dose, anesthetic time, animal species studied, and hyper- or hypoventilation. For example, at 0.5 times MAC, cerebrovascular autoregulation during anesthesia with potent inhaled agents is slowed or obtunded; however, at concentrations greater than MAC, cerebrovascular autoregulation is significantly and progressively diminished as cerebral blood flow becomes simply a function of CPP [147,148]. Effects on CBF have been shown to be anesthetic duration dependent in animals [149–152] but not in humans [153]. The blood flow increase is presumably due to time-dependent increases in nitric oxide synthase inhibition [152]. Carbon dioxide tension further affects autoregulation. Autoregulation is lost and CBF is increased at lower inhaled anesthetic doses when animals are allowed to hypoventilate [154] although this interaction between CO_2 and agent is greater with isoflurane than for sevoflurane [155].

Intracranial pressure (ICP)

The inhalation anesthetics produce an increase in ICP and this change parallels the increase in CBF [117,137]. Thus, regardless of the species, cerebrovascular autoregulation, CBF and ICP can be better preserved at a given MAC-multiple of a haloether anesthetic when hyperventilation is maintained concurrently and $PaCO_2$ is reduced [156,157].

Although most anesthetic effects on cerebral hemodynamics are similar among humans and small animal research models, the same does not hold true for horses, and perhaps other very large animal species. Intracranial pressure in awake horses remains constant irrespective of head position [158] but cerebral vasodilation during inhalant anesthesia causes large increases in intracranial pressure, sometimes similar in magnitude to values seen in human severe head trauma patients – that is, exacerbated by dorsal recumbency, head-down positioning, hypercapnia during spontaneous ventilation, and anesthetic time during controlled ventilation [159–162]. Surprisingly, over a wide range of perfusion pressures, isoflurane-anesthetized horses maintain regional cerebral blood flow relatively constant, albeit at a low flow that may still place animals at risk for tissue hypoxia [163]. Blood flow to the thoracolumbar spinal cord is particularly low, and further reduction may predispose to postanesthetic myelomalacia in horses.

Respiratory system

Inhalation anesthetics depress respiratory system function. The volatile agents in particular decrease ventilation in a drug-specific and species-specific manner. Depending on conditions, including species of interest, some of the most commonly considered measures of breathing effectiveness, i.e., breathing rate and depth (tidal volume), may not be revealing or may even be misleading. In general, spontaneous ventilation progressively decreases as inhalation anesthetic dose is increased because at low doses tidal volume decreases more than frequency increases. As anesthetic dose is further increased, respiratory frequency also decreases. In otherwise unmedicated animals (including humans) anesthetized with volatile agents, respiratory arrest occurs at 1.5–3 MAC (Table 16.9). The overall decrease in minute ventilation and the likely variable increase in deadspace ventilation (resulting in an increase in the deadspace to tidal volume ratio, $V_D{:}V_t$, from a normal of about 0.3 to 0.5 or more) result in a reduction in alveolar ventilation. Decreases in alveolar ventilation are out of proportion to decreases in CO_2 production (O_2 utilization is decreased by general anesthesia), such that $PaCO_2$ increases (Fig. 16.19). In addition, the normal

Table 16.9 Apneic Index (AI) in various species.

	Desflurane		Halothane		Isoflurane	
	MAC	AI	MAC	AI	MAC	AI
Cat					1.63	2.4 [244]
Dog	7.2	2.4 [177]	0.87	2.9 [440]	1.28	2.5 [244]
Horse			0.88	2.6 [62]	1.31	2.3 [62]
Pig	9.8	1.6 [177, 540]				
Rat			1.11	2.3 [251]	1.38	3.1 [250]
Human	7.25	1.8 [179]	0.77	2.3 [179]	1.15	1.7 [179]

Minimum alveolar concentration (MAC) is given in volumes % and the AI is a ratio of the end-tidal anesthetic concentration at apnea and MAC. Similar data are not currently available for sevoflurane.

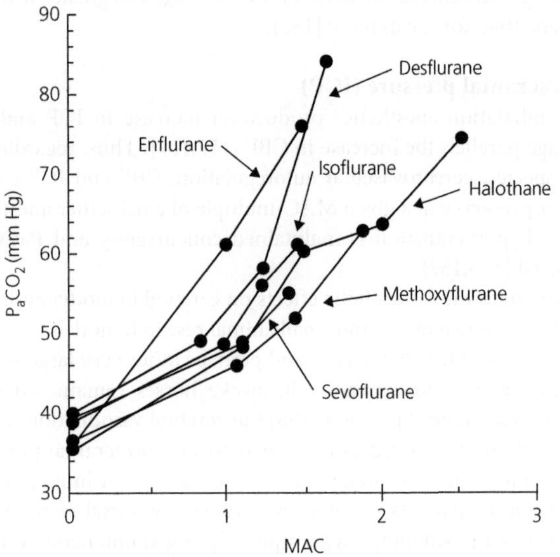

Figure 16.19 Respiratory response to an increase in the alveolar concentration (expressed as a multiple of MAC) of inhalation anesthetics in humans. Data are taken from multiple sources [165, 179–183].

stimulation of ventilation caused by increased $PaCO_2$ (or decreased PaO_2) is depressed by the inhalation anesthetics, presumably via the action of these agents directly on the medullary and peripheral (aortic and carotid body) chemoreceptors [164–167].

Bronchospasm is associated with some conditions that contribute to increased airway resistance. A variety of early studies indicated that among anesthetics available at the time, halothane was the most effective bronchodilator [168,169]. That effect is believed to result, at least partially, from decreased cholinergic neurotransmission [170,171]. Therefore, it was often recommended for patients at risk of bronchospasm. The work of Hirshman and colleagues suggests that isoflurane and perhaps enflurane were as effective in decreasing experimentally produced airway resistance and therefore were good alternatives to halothane [172,173]. Recent work with isoflurane, sevoflurane, and desflurane indicate that relaxation of constricted bronchial muscles by these agents is at least equal to or exceeds that caused by halothane [171,174,175].

Avoiding airway irritation during administration of inhalation anesthetics is important, especially during induction of anesthesia because it may cause breath holding, coughing, and laryngospasm (particularly in some species such as primates, human and nonhuman) that in turn result in arterial oxyhemoglobin desaturation. At least in humans, none of the potent inhalation anesthetics seem to have irritant properties at subanesthetic concentrations. However, patient objection and airway irritation are evident with desflurane (and to a lesser degree with isoflurane [176]) at concentrations of 7% or greater [177,178] and as a result desflurane is not commonly used for anesthetic induction of human patients.

Arterial carbon dioxide tension ($PaCO_2$)

The $PaCO_2$ is the most frequently used measure of respiratory system response to general anesthetics. All contemporary inhalation anesthetics depress alveolar ventilation and increase $PaCO_2$ in dose-related fashion. Fig. 16.19 summarizes the effects of inhalation anesthetics in humans, the species for which data are most complete [165,179–183]. Because appropriate data in the species of interest to veterinary anesthetists are incomplete, rank order of the magnitude of hypoventilation caused by the four contemporary volatile anesthetics at a common alveolar dose cannot be expressed with authority. Indeed, species variability is an important confounder (see below).

Factors influencing respiratory effects

Mode of ventilation

Ventilation is often assisted or controlled during inhalation anesthesia to compensate for the anesthetic-induced respiratory depression. Controlled mechanical ventilation is used to predictably maintain a normal or some other specific $PaCO_2$, during anesthesia. Assisted ventilation (i.e., the anesthetist augments tidal volume but the animal determines its own breathing frequency) is used to attempt to improve the efficiency of oxygenating arterial blood and reduce the work of breathing but is usually not effective in substantially lowering $PaCO_2$ compared to circumstances associated with spontaneous ventilation (i.e., the animal controls both the rate and depth of breathing) [184,185].

Duration of anesthesia

Respiratory function, including $PaCO_2$, is little changed for as long as up to 10 h of constant, low-dose halothane (or methoxyflurane) in dogs [186,187]. This is also supported by studies of humans [188] anesthetized with constant low-dose halothane. However, in horses anesthetized for 5 h with a constant dose of 1.2 MAC isoflurane, a substantial temporal increase in $PaCO_2$ was noted [189]. A similar but more modest trend was noted in horses when halothane was used for anesthesia [190,191]. At least in some species, if alveolar dose of halothane is increased above about 1–1.3 MAC and maintained constant at a heightened level, the magnitude of change in hypoventilation also worsens with time [187]. Conversely, there is evidence for recovery from the ventilatory depressant effects of volatile anesthetics in humans [183].

Surgery and other noxious stimulation

Noxious stimulation may result in sufficient central nervous stimulation to lessen the ventilatory depression of the inhalation anesthetic [192–195]. This effect is diminished with increasing anesthetic depth.

Concurrent drugs

In humans, the substitution of N_2O for an equivalent amount of a concurrently administered volatile agent such as isoflurane results in a lower $PaCO_2$ than that seen with the volatile agent alone [19]. However, in dogs and monkeys anesthetized with halothane, ventilation was at least as, and sometimes more, depressed when N_2O was substituted for a portion of the halothane [196,197]. The addition of opioid drugs like morphine may increase the respiratory depression produced by an inhalation anesthetic [194,198–200].

Cardiovascular system

All volatile inhalation anesthetics cause dose-dependent and drug-specific changes in cardiovascular performance. The magnitude and sometimes direction of change may be influenced by other variables that often accompany general anesthesia (Box 16.1). The mechanisms of cardiovascular effects are diverse but often include direct myocardial depression and a decrease in sympathoadrenal activity.

Cardiac output (CO)

All of the volatile anesthetics can decrease CO. The magnitude of change is dose related and dependent upon agent. In general, among the contemporary agents in use with animals, halothane is most depressing to CO [1,201–203]. Desflurane in many ways is similar in cardiovascular action to isoflurane while sevoflurane has characteristics resembling both halothane and isoflurane. All of the newer volatile anesthetics tend to preserve CO at clinically useful concentrations, facilitated by reductions in systemic vascular resistance [177,204–212]. However, the direct effect of volatile agents on CO (if vascular resistence is maintained) is often a decrease in stroke volume as a result of dose-related depression in myocardial contractility [1,177,208,213–215].

The effect of inhalation anesthetics on heart rate (HR) is variable and depends on agent and species. For example, in humans HR is not substantially altered with halothane anesthesia but is usually increased by isoflurane, desflurane, and sevoflurane [211,216,217]. Compared to conditions in awake, calm dogs, HR is increased with all four of the anesthetics listed [207,212]. There is evidence to suggest that differences between agents in the degree of increase in HR in dogs are explained by differences in their vagolytic activity [210]. In the dog the HR usually remains constant over a range of clinically useful alveolar concentrations in the absence of other modifying factors (e.g., noxious stimulation) [201,202,207,212,218,219].

Cardiac rhythm and catecholamines

Inhalation anesthetics may increase the automaticity of the myocardium and the likelihood of propagated impulses from ectopic sites, especially from within the ventricle [220]. While spontaneous dysrhythmias were most notable with earlier inhalation anesthetics (e.g., halothane), it appears that none of the three most recently introduced ether-derivative agents predispose the heart to extrasystoles. However, adrenergic agonist-associated dysrhythmias may be exaggerated by the presence of inhalant anesthetics [221]. The association of cardiac dysrhythmias with adrenergic drugs and anesthetic agents has received extensive study.

Halothane markedly reduces the amount of epinephrine necessary to cause ventricular premature contractions [222]. There is some evidence that deeper levels of halothane decrease this incidence [223–225], but this is not a consistent finding [226]. Enflurane and methoxyflurane are less likely to sensitize the heart to arrhythmogenic effects of epinephrine, and isoflurane, desflurane, and sevoflurane are least arrhythmogenic [1,225,227–232]. The potential for dysrhythmias follows administration of most catecholamine-type drugs although the magnitude of such potential varies with the drug co-administered [232–237] and other associated conditions [238].

Box 16.1 Factors that influence cardiovascular effects of inhalation anesthetics.

- Anesthetic dose
- Duration of anesthesia
- Concurrent drug therapy
- Intravenous fluid therapy
- Magnitude of $PaCO_2$
- Mechanical ventilation
- Noxious stimulation

Regional blood flow

A fundamental principle of circulatory function is that blood flow is sufficient to deliver adequate amounts of O_2 and nutrients to tissues and to remove metabolic waste. However, tissues have very different requirements for blood flow per unit volume of tissue and these tissue-specific blood flow requirements change with conditions (e.g., basal vs exercise or 'flight or fight'). In general, blood flow to each tissue is usually maintained at a level only slightly more than that required for metabolic activity by the tissue. Unfortunately, inhalation anesthetics not only reduce total blood flow (i.e., cardiac output) but they also impact the distribution of blood flow to tissues. In most patients the changes are qualitatively similar for all the contemporary agents, but in others agents have clear differences. Dose of anesthetic and species differences add further impact to their ultimate effect. Detailed information on the many permutations of anesthetic effects on regional blood flow is not available for all species and is beyond the scope of this chapter. However, references are included here as an introduction to this much broader topic [205,239–242].

Arterial blood pressure

Volatile anesthetics cause a dose-dependent decrease in arterial blood pressure (Fig. 16.20) [52,201,205,209,212,242–247]. In general, the dose-related decrease in arterial blood pressure is similar regardless of the species studied [62,201,203,206,243,245–248]. The

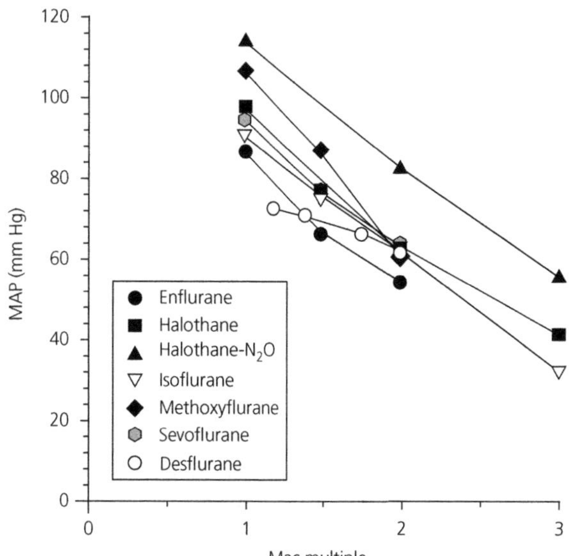

Figure 16.20 Inhalation anesthetics cause a dose (expressed as multiples of MAC)-dependent decrease in mean arterial blood pressure (MAP) in dogs whose ventilation is mechanically controlled to produce eucapnia. Data are from multiple sources [202,205,212,243, 245].

Table 16.10 Anesthetic-induced cardiovascular depression as expressed by cardiovascular anesthetic indices.

	Desflurane	Halothane	Isoflurane
Dog[a]	2.84		2.69
Pig[b]	2.45		3.02
Rat[c]		3.0	5.7

[a] The anesthetic concentration causing death in ventilated dogs related to MAC [177].
[b] Mean fatal dose related to MAC [540].
[c] Heart concentration of anesthetic at cardiovascular failure related to heart concentration of anesthetic at establishment of anesthesia [250, 251].

dose-related decrease in blood pressure with all four of the contemporary agents is usually related to a decrease in stroke volume but in some cases (agent and/or species), a decrease in peripheral vascular resistance may play an important role. This common scenario in animals differs from results generally reported from studies with humans anesthetized with isoflurane, sevoflurane and desflurane, where pressure decreases primarily from a decrease in systemic vascular resistance [15,249]. Indices of anesthetic influence on cardiovascular collapse are given in Table 16.10 [201,250,251].

Factors tnfluencing circulatory effects

A variety of circumstances associated with the anesthetic management of veterinary patients may add to or oppose the primary effects of the anesthetic. The most profound modifications of drug action are usually on cardiovascular function. They may include mechanical ventilation and alterations in $PaCO_2$, noxious (surgical) stimulation, duration of anesthesia, and coexisting drugs.

Mode of ventilation and $PaCO_2$

There may be considerable difference in the cardiovascular effects of inhalation anesthetics in animals breathing spontaneously compared to when their breathing is mechanically controlled (e.g., intermittent positive pressure ventilation or IPPV) to produce and maintain a normal $PaCO_2$. In general, cardiovascular function is usually depressed during IPPV relative to spontaneous ventilation. This results from either the direct mechanical actions (i.e., intermittent elevation of intrathoracic pressure and resultant decrease in venous return to the heart) or lessening of the indirect pharmacologic action of $PaCO_2$ [252], or both. Carbon dioxide has pharmacologic actions important to these considerations. For example, an increased $PaCO_2$ has direct depressant actions on the heart and smooth muscle of the peripheral blood vessels (i.e., vessel dilation) but indirect (via sympathetic nervous system) stimulation of circulatory function. In generally healthy, sympathetically intact animals, the stimulatory actions of hypercapnia usually predominate, so increased CO and arterial blood pressure usually accompany an increase in $PaCO_2$, becoming lower when $PaCO_2$ is normalized [52,184,203,246,248,253–258].

Noxious stimulation

Noxious stimulation during anesthesia modifies the circulatory effect of inhalation anesthetics via stimulation of the sympathetic nervous system. An increase in arterial blood pressure and heart rate (cardiac output) commonly accompanies noxious stimulation [70,194,195,259,260]. The response is anesthetic dose related. For example, Roizen *et al.* [70] and Yasuda *et al.* [259] showed that deeper levels of halothane and enflurane decreased or prevented surgically induced increases in serum norepinephrine levels in human patients. Anesthetic doses that block the response are in the range of 1.5–2.0 MAC [70,259]. Similar responses have been reported for animals as well [261–266].

Duration of anesthesia

Some cardiovascular effects of inhalation anesthetics may change with duration of anesthesia. For example, in humans halothane anesthesia lasting 5–6 h is associated with an increase in values of some measures of cardiovascular function such as CO and heart rate [254,267]. Similarly, varying degrees of time-related changes have been reported with enflurane [183], desflurane [217,268,269], and others [216,268–272]. Temporal changes in cardiovascular function have also been reported in a variety of animals with halothane [187,190,273,274], isoflurane [189,273,275], and sevoflurane [275]. Dose of anesthetic [187,216,276] and body posture during anesthesia [191,277] apparently also play a temporal role in some species.

The causes of these changes remain unclear. *In vitro*, depression of the cat papillary muscle exposed to a constant concentration of halothane does not vary over a 3-h period [278]. This observation suggests that temporal effects associated with inhalation anesthetics are not the result of improved intrinsic cardiac function. Studies of human volunteers have shown that temporal responses to halothane can be prevented if the subjects are given propranolol before anesthesia, suggesting the mechanism is related to increasing sympathetic nervous system activity [279].

Usually the temporal changes associated with inhalation anesthetics are of only minor or no concern to the clinician. However, such changes must be considered in interpreting results of laboratory studies in which these agents are used for anesthetic management.

Concurrent drugs

Drugs administered immediately before or in conjunction with inhalation anesthetics (preanesthetic medication, injectable anesthetic induction drugs, vasoactive and cardiotonic drugs, etc.) may influence cardiovascular function by altering the anesthetic requirement (i.e., MAC and thereby increased or decreased anesthetic level) or by their own direct action on cardiovascular performance or sympathetic nervous system function.

For example, N_2O is used on occasion to substitute for a portion of a potent inhalation anesthetic. Because of its own anesthetic potency (albeit low; remember the MAC for N_2O in animals is in the range of 2 atmospheres; see Table 16.7A), its use may facilitate delivery of a reduced amount of the potent volatile agent, and thereby contribute to some cardiovascular sparing. Nitrous oxide may depress the myocardium directly, but these effects are usually counterbalanced by its sympathomimetic effect, resulting in a net improvement in cardiovascular function compared to conditions without N_2O. In animal patients, the magnitude of N_2O effect is limited and species dependent [196,197,245,280–283].

Injectable drugs such as acepromazine, α_2-adrenergic receptor agonists, thiobarbiturates, dissociatives (e.g., ketamine), and others are frequently administered to animals as part of their anesthetic management. They confound the primary effects of the inhalation anesthetics and may accentuate cardiovascular depression. On the other hand, sympathomimetic drugs such as ephedrine [284], dopamine, and dobutamine [285,286] are frequently given to counteract unwanted cardiovascular depressions of the anesthetic.

Effects on the kidneys

It is generally regarded that clinically used volatile inhalation anesthetics produce similar mild, reversible, dose-related decreases in renal blood flow and glomerular filtration rate and that such changes largely reflect an anesthetic-induced decrease in cardiac output [249]. However, some studies show little or no change in these kidney-related parameters [45,240,287,288].

As a consequence of the anesthetic-induced decrease in glomerular filtration, healthy anesthetized animals commonly produce a smaller volume of concentrated urine compared to when awake. An increase in serum urea nitrogen, creatinine, and inorganic phosphate may accompany prolonged anesthesia [289–292]. The reduction in renal function is highly influenced by the animal's state of hydration and hemodynamics during anesthesia [293]. Intravenous fluid therapy and prevention of a marked reduction in renal blood flow will lessen or counteract the tendency for reduced renal function. In most cases, especially in healthy animals, effects of inhalation anesthesia on renal function are rapidly reversed after anesthesia.

Among the inhalation anesthetics, methoxyflurane was the most nephrotoxic. Although it is no longer available in North America for use in human or animal patients, it is of pathophysiologic interest and therefore will be briefly reviewed. In humans and some strains of rats, methoxyflurane caused renal failure that was characterized not by oliguria but by a large urine volume (polyuric) unresponsive to vasopressin [33]. This was caused by the biotransformation of methoxyflurane and the large release of free fluoride ion (both in peak levels and in the prolonged exposure due to high adipose accumulation of methoxyflurane during anesthesia) that in turn caused direct damage to the renal tubules. Although renal injury in animals is rare, it has been reported in dogs when methoxyflurane was used in combination with tetracycline antibiotics [294] and flunixin [294].

With the possible exception of enflurane and sevoflurane, the breakdown of other inhalation anesthetics does not pose a risk of fluoride-induced nephrotoxicity. Biotransformation of enflurane and sevoflurane by humans following moderate duration of anesthesia causes serum inorganic fluoride concentrations to increase even beyond the 50 μmol/L level, which is normally considered the nephrotoxic threshold in humans [33,249,295,296]. However, clinical, histological or biochemical evidence of injury related to increases in fluoride has only rarely been reported in human patients. The over-riding consensus is that sevoflurane has little potential for nephrotoxicity as a result of defluorination [33,249].

Two factors may explain the general lack of injury despite the body's ability to degrade sevoflurane. In 1977, Mazze *et al.* proposed that the area under the serum fluoride concentration versus time curve may be a more important determinant of nephrotoxicity than peak serum fluoride concentration [297]. Because sevoflurane is poorly soluble and is rapidly eliminated via the lungs, the duration of its availability for biotransformation is notably limited. More recently, Kharasch and co-workers proposed another consideration [298]. Sevoflurane is primarily metabolized by the liver while hepatic and renal sites were important for methoxyflurane breakdown. The relative lack of intrarenal anesthetic defluorination may markedly reduce its nephrotoxic potential. Studies have confirmed the increase in serum fluoride in horses anesthetized with sevoflurane [50–52]. In these reports, the magnitude and time course of fluoride increase were similar to those reported for humans. As with humans, there has been no evidence of untoward renal effects associated with the increase in fluoride in horses.

Early reports of sevoflurane noted its degradation by CO_2 absorbents such as soda lime and Baralyme [46,54]. A nephrotoxic breakdown product, Compound A, is produced [46]. Compound A can cause renal injury and death in rats [299] and the concentration threshold for nephrotoxicity in rats [300–302] is within the range of concentrations that may be found associated with the anesthetic management of human patients [303]. However, reports of nephrotoxicity in humans are rare and point to alternative mechanisms of toxicity such as species-dependent metabolic degradation of Compound A to directly nephrotoxic compounds. Not surprisingly, Compound A is formed in the breathing circuits used for animals (except non-rebreathing circuits which do not use CO_2 absorbent) [304]. The ultimate importance of *in vitro* sevoflurane degradation to the well-being of veterinary patients like dogs, cats, and horses [51] remains to be established. Regardless, because of concerns associated with anesthetic management of human patients, most commercially available absorbents now used in the US no longer contain KOH or NaOH.

Effects on the liver

Depression of hepatic function and hepatocellular damage may be caused by the action of volatile anesthetics. Effects may be mild and transient or permanent, and injury may be by direct or indirect action. Studies by Reilly *et al.* [305] suggested that halothane (but likely also other potent inhalation anesthetics) substantially inhibits drug-metabolizing capacity in the liver. A reduction in intrinsic hepatic clearance of drugs, along with anesthetic-induced alteration of other pharmacokinetically important variables (e.g., reduced hepatic blood flow), delays drug removal or an increase in plasma drug concentration during anesthesia. Examples of such circumstances have been reported [305–309]. Prolonged or increased (relative to conditions in the unanesthetized animal) plasma concentrations of some drugs have important toxic implications, especially in physiologically compromised patients.

All of the potent inhalation anesthetics are capable of causing hepatocellular injury by reducing liver blood flow and oxygen delivery. However, available data suggest that of the four contemporary volatile anesthetics, isoflurane is most likely to better maintain liver O_2 delivery and thus is the agent least likely to produce haptocyte injury. Sevoflurane and desflurane are similar to isoflurane, whereas halothane produces the most striking adverse changes [33,205,239,240,242,310–315]. Results of studies indicate that confounding factors including N_2O [316], concurrent hypoxia [314,317–319], prior induction of hepatic drug-metabolizing enzymes [320,321], mode of ventilation [322], and positive end-expired pressure [323] may worsen conditions and increase the likelihood of hepatocellular damage.

It now appears that halothane produces two types of hepatotoxicity in susceptible individuals. One is a mild, self-limiting postanesthetic form of hepatocellular damage and associated increase in serum concentrations of liver enzymes. Signs of hepatotoxicity occur shortly after anesthetic exposure. The other is a rare, severe, often fatal hepatotoxicity with delayed onset. The fulminant hepatopathy appears limited to human patients (i.e., 'halothane hepatitis') and is thought to be an immune-mediated toxicity [324,325]. The mechanism of halothane hepatitis may also be genetic associated [326]. The increased incidence of hepatic injury associated with halothane is the principal factor leading to the decrease in use of halothane for human patients nearly three decades ago.

Effects on skeletal muscle: Malignant hyperthermia

Malignant hyperthermia (MH) is a potentially life-threatening pharmacogenetic myopathy that is most commonly reported in susceptible human patients [327,328] and swine [329]. However, reports of its occurrence in other species exist [330–336]. Its clinicopathological, histopathological, and genetic basis has recently been further described for the horse [337–339]. All of the four contemporary volatile anesthetics can initiate MH, but halothane is the most potent triggering agent (relative to other inhalation anesthetics) [328]. The syndrome is characterized by a rapid rise in cellular metabolic activity that, if not treated quickly, causes death. Monitoring of temperature, CO_2 production, and other signs of metabolic imbalance (arterial blood gases) is warranted in susceptible/suspected patients. Patients known to be susceptible to MH can be anesthetized safely. Avoidance of triggering agents and prophylactic dantrolene given before anesthesia are effective in blocking the onset of MH [328].

The gaseous anesthetic: Nitrous oxide (N_2O)

Nitrous oxide was introduced into clinical practice more than 150 years ago. Since then its use has formed the basis for more general anesthetic techniques of human patients than any other single inhalation agent [19]. Its widespread use resulted from many desirable properties, including low blood solubility (see Table 16.2), limited cardiovascular and respiratory system depression, and minimal toxicity [19]. Its use in the anesthetic management of animals became a natural extension of its use for humans.

Dose

Nitrous oxide is not the ideal anesthetic for humans or animals. As discussed earlier in this chapter, N_2O is not a potent anesthetic (see Table 16.7A) and will not anesthetize a fit, healthy individual when given alone. To maximize the benefits of N_2O, it is usually used in high inspired concentrations. However, as the concentration of N_2O is increased, there is a change in the proportion and partial pressure of the various other constituents of the inspired breath, notably O_2. Consequently, to avoid hypoxemia, 75% of the inspired breath is the highest fraction that can be safely administered under conditions at sea level. Use of N_2O at locations above sea level requires a lower N_2O concentration to ensure an adequate P_IO_2.

Nitrous oxide has less value in the anesthetic management of animals than in that of humans because the anesthetic potency of N_2O in most animals studied is only about half (or less) that found for humans (for example, MAC for the dog is about 200% vs about 100% for humans; see Table 16.7A) [10,283]. Thus, the value of N_2O in veterinary clinical practice is as an anesthetic adjuvant, that is, accompanying other inhaled or injectable drugs. Since the effects of N_2O on vital organ function (including cardiovascular and respiratory) in the absence of hypoxemia are small in most veterinary patients, benefit is afforded by allowing a certain reduction in the amount of the primary, more potent, inhaled or injectable anesthetic agents.

Pharmacokinetics

Nitrous oxide's low blood solubility (see Table 16.2) is responsible for its rapid onset of action. Although it does not have the potency to produce anesthesia by itself, it may be used to speed induction of inhalation anesthesia as a result of its own (albeit limited) central nervous system effects and, as mentioned earlier, also by augmenting the uptake of a concurrently administered, more potent volatile anesthetic such as halothane, the 'second gas effect' [10,19,340,341]. When a high concentration of N_2O is given concurrently in a mixture with an inhalation agent (e.g., N_2O plus halothane), the alveolar concentration of the simultaneously administered anesthetic (halothane) increases more rapidly than when the 'second' gas had been administered without N_2O. The second gas effect is the result of an increased inspiratory volume secondary to the large volume of N_2O taken up [340] and a concentrating effect on the second gas in a smaller volume (and thus increased gradient for transfer to blood) as a result of the uptake of the large volume of N_2O [10,341]. Results of a more recent study with desflurane confirm previous findings for the second gas effect [342].

Pharmacodynamics

As noted previously, N_2O's effects on cardiovascular and respiratory function (other than reducing the inspired O_2 concentration) are small compared to other inhalation anesthetics. It does depress myocardial function directly, but its sympathetic stimulation properties counteract some of the direct depression (its own as well as that from accompanying volatile anesthetics) [283,343]. As a result of its sympathetic nervous system activation, it may contribute to a desirable increased arterial blood pressure [280,344] or an undesirable increased incidence of cardiac arrhythmias [345,346]. There is evidence to suggest that its use contributes to myocardial ischemia in some circumstances [347–350]. Overall, a conservative outlook regarding N_2O use relative to respiration and circulation is that significant concern is warranted only in patients with initially compromised function [351,352]. As with any agent, its advantages and disadvantages should be considered on an individual patient basis.

Nitrous oxide has little or no effect on liver and kidney function [353–355]. Although there is evidence of N_2O-induced interference with production of red and white blood cells by bone marrow, the risk of adverse outcomes to a subject exposed under most clinical veterinary circumstances is little or none [354,356]. However, prolonged exposure to N_2O causes megaloblastic hematopoiesis and polyneuropathy. Seriously ill patients may have increased sensitivity to these toxicities. Problems result from N_2O-induced inactivation of the vitamin B_{12}-dependent enzyme methionine synthase, an enzyme that controls inter-relations between vitamin B_{12} and folic acid metabolism [357]. Although an occasional patient may develop signs suggestive of vitamin B_{12} and folic acid deficiency after an anesthetic technique that included N_2O, this is a rare event in human and animal patients [354,358]. Prolonged occupational or abusive exposure to N_2O may be equally harmful and should be considered in management plans of veterinary practices [33,354,359,360]. Nitrous oxide is rapidly and mainly eliminated in the exhaled breath. The extent of biotransformation (to molecular N_2) is very small and mainly by intestinal flora (see Table 16.6) [33,361,362].

Transfer of N_2O to closed gas spaces

Gas spaces exist or may exist in the body under a variety of conditions. For example, gas is normally found in the stomach and intestines. The gut is a dynamic reservoir; the gas it contains is freely movable into and out of it according to the laws of diffusion. The gas in the gut originates from air swallowing, normal production from bacterial processes, chemical reactions, and diffusion from the blood. There is marked variability in both composition and volume of stomach and bowel gas (e.g., herbivore vs carnivore). There are other natural air cavities, such as the air sinuses and the middle ear, and then there are circumstances in which air may be electively or inadvertently introduced as part of diagnostic or therapeutic actions (e.g., pneumoencephalogram, pneumocystogram, endoscopy, vascular air emboli, etc.).

Potential problems associated with gas spaces arise when an animal breathing air is given a gas mixture containing a high partial pressure of N_2O [10,19]. Nitrogen (N_2) is the major component of air (80%) and of most gas spaces within the body (methane, CO_2, and hydrogen are also found in variable quantities in the gut). When N_2O is introduced into the inspired breath, a re-equilibration of gases in the gas space begins with N_2O quickly entering and N_2 slowly leaving. That is, because of its greater blood solubility the volume of N_2O that can be transported to a closed gas space is many times the volume of N_2 that can be carried away [10]. For example, the blood/gas partition coefficient for N_2O is 0.47 (see Table 16.2), whereas that for N_2 is about 0.015 [363]. Thus, N_2O is more than 30 times more soluble in blood than N_2 (0.47/0.015). The result of the net transfer of gas to the gas space can be manifested as an increase in volume, as with the gut [364,365], pneumothorax [365], or blood embolus [366,367], an increase in pressure (e.g., middle ear [368,369], pneumoencephalogram [370]), or both (as the distending limits of the compliant container are reached). Usually air is used to inflate the cuff of an endotracheal tube. This cuff is another relatively compliant, enclosed air space. Nitrous oxide will similarly expand this gas space and may increase the pressure exerted on the tracheal wall [371–373].

Diffusion hypoxia

A further consideration for the differential movement of N_2O and N_2 occurs at the end of anesthesia when N_2O is discontinued. Because of the large volume of N_2O stored in the body during anesthesia and the unequal change of N_2O for N_2, a deficiency in blood oxygenation may occur at the end of anesthesia if air is abruptly substituted for N_2O. As discussed earlier in this chapter, this condition is referred to as *diffusion hypoxia* [36,37]. The rapid outpouring of N_2O from the blood into the lung results in a transient but marked decrease in alveolar PO_2 with a resultant decrease in PaO_2.

Interaction with respiratory gas monitoring

Routine monitoring of expired CO_2 is increasingly important in the operating room of veterinary hospitals. Nitrous oxide interferes with the accurate detection of CO_2 with some monitoring devices. This interaction must be considered in decisions regarding the purchasing of equipment and overall anesthetic management plan. A more complete summary of the advantages and disadvantages of N_2O use is available elsewhere [19]. A brief summary of practical consideration of N_2O use in veterinary practice is also available [374,375].

Waste inhalation anesthetics

Occupational exposure: Trace concentrations of inhalation anesthetics

Operating room personnel are often exposed to low concentrations of inhalation anesthetics. Contamination of ambient air occurs via vaporizer filling, known and unknown leaks in the patient breathing circuit, and careless spillage of liquid agent. Another source of anesthetic gas exposure is disconnection of a patient from an anesthetic machine at the end of a procedure without first flushing the system with anesthetic-free gas, and allowing the patient to expire into the machine for several minutes. Measurable amounts of anesthetic gases and vapors are present in operating room air under a variety of conditions [376–383]. Personnel inhale and, as shown by studies, retain these agents for some time [384,385]. The slow rate of elimination of some vapors (especially the more blood-soluble agents like halothane) allows accumulation of retained trace anesthetic quantities from one day to the next.

Concern is raised because epidemiologic studies of humans and laboratory studies of animals have suggested that chronic exposure to trace levels of anesthetics may constitute a health hazard. The possibility that chronic exposure to low levels of anesthetic agents constitutes a hazard to health science personnel has attracted and maintained worldwide interest since the early 1970s. Of particular concern are reports that inhaled anesthetics possess mutagenic, carcinogenic, or teratogenic potential. Depending on the point in life at which exposure occurs, there is concern that these underlying mechanisms in turn may result in an increased incidence in fetal death, spontaneous abortion, birth defects or cancer in exposed workers [386–388]. However, to date, no genotoxic effect of long-term or short-term exposure to inhaled anesthetics has been demonstrated in humans and '...the conclusion from both animal and human studies is that there is no carcinogenic risk either from exposure to the currently used inhaled anesthetics' [33].

Although the data to date, especially regarding effects on human reproduction, remain equivocal, a firm cause-and-effect relationship between chronic exposure to trace levels of anesthetics and human health problems does not exist. Although the risk of long-term exposure to trace concentrations of anesthetics for those in operating room conditions appears minimal, current evidence is suggestive enough to cause concern and to encourage practices to reduce the contamination by anesthetics of operating room personnel. Indeed, within the United States, there are three federal agencies concerned with possible hazards associated with exposure to waste anesthetic gases: the National Institute for Occupational Safety and Health (NIOSH), an agency of the Department of Health, Education and Welfare, the Occupational Safety and Health Administration (OSHA), an agency of the Department of Labor, and the Food and Drug Administration (FDA). Levels of exposure have been recommended and published by NIOSH as 2.0 parts per million (ppm) for volatile agents and 25 ppm for N_2O [386]. In this regard, inexpensive methods to reduce and control anesthetic exposure by operating room personnel are available and should be used (Box 16.2). Indeed, the spillage of inhalation anesthetic agents into the operating room environment has been reduced significantly since the 1970s by the widespread introduction of anesthetic delivery equipment scavenging systems. However, with the exception of anesthetic adsorbent systems, most systems used deposit the waste gases directly and unchanged into the atmosphere.

Frequent monitoring of actual levels of anesthetic gas/vapor is of obvious value and is encouraged in specialized circumstances

Box 16.2 Methods to reduce occupational exposure to inhalation anesthetics in the operating room.

1 Educate personnel.
2 Use waste gas *scavenger* to collect gas from the pressure relief (pop-off) valve of the patient breathing circuit and ventilator.
3 Conduct *regular inspection* and *maintenance* to detect and repair leaks in anesthetic machines and patient breathing circuits, piped gas supplies (N_2O), etc.
4 *Alter work practices* (e.g., minimize leaks around face mask, turn off vaporizer/fresh gas flow when patient breathing circuit not attached to patient).
5 Adequately ventilate operating rooms and recovery rooms/areas.
6 Monitor room trace anesthetic gas levels.

and/or environments of high use. Likely the greatest impact results from educating personnel about the potential problem of waste anesthetic gases and methods for controlling exposure levels [386–389]. For further information on this subject readers are directed to a more complete report of current knowledge and conclusions from available data that have been developed by the American Society of Anesthesiologists (ASA) Task Force on Trace Anesthetic Gases of the ASA Committee on Occupational Health of Operating Room Personnel [390]. Commentary and recommendations on control of waste anesthetic gases in the veterinary medical workplace have also been articulated by the American College of Veterinary Anesthesiology and Analgesia (www.acvaa.org/docs/2013_ACVAA_Waste_Anesthetic_Gas_Recommendations.pdf) [391].

While exposure by personnel during anesthetic delivery equipment preparation and clean-up, inhalation anesthetic induction procedures and when working with anesthetic equipment that is not leak free is most notable, the postanesthetic recovery period is not without concern. Postanesthetic care personel in the environment of hospital care of humans are also exposed to gases eliminated from patients. Studies of human postanesthetic care circumstances have reported quantities of volatile anesthetic concentrations that in some cases approach NIOSH recommended maximum exposure limits [392,393]. Similar circumstances are undoubtly also present in veterinary medicine, particularly the veterinary hospitals (small and large animal patients) with large daily inhalation anesthesia requirements. For example, horses recovering from inhalation anesthesia in a relatively small room with limited fresh air changes per unit time can likely raise the concentration of exhaled inhalation anesthetic considerably and in such cases likewise approach or perhaps exceed OSHA recommended maximum amounts.

Environmental implications of inhalation anesthetics

Research and commentary regarding the impact (or lack of impact) of contemporary general anesthetic gases and vapors on the global environment have been ongoing in the medical literature since early concerns were publicly voiced about stratospheric ozone destruction by man-made halogenated organic compounds [394,395] and biomedical contributions to the global atmosphere of exponentially increasing concentrations of N_2O, and other 'greenhouse gases' [396].

Before proceeding to focus on anesthetic gases, a brief review of selected aspects of atmospheric science seems appropriate. Earth is surrounded by an atmosphere that gradually changes its composition (via molecular diffusion) with altitude. The inner two layers of our atmosphere important to life are the innermost (closest to earth) troposphere (upper limit at about 5–10 miles above the earth's surface) and the outer of these two layers, the stratosphere (reaching up to 30 miles above earth). Circumstances associated with the uppermost layers of our environment, the mesosphere, thermosphere and exosphere, are not important to the present discussion. Life on earth depends on solar energy. Of the sunlight that ultimately reaches the earth's surface, some is reflected upward again as infrared radiation. Emission of infrared radiation into space is an important mechanism by which the earth's temperature is regulated, i.e., the heat caused by infrared radiation is absorbed by 'greenhouse gases' such as water vapor, carbon dioxide, ozone, methane, and others which in turn slows the energy's escape from the troposphere and thus regulates climatic conditions by trapping the heat. Therefore, the greenhouse effect is an essential environmental prerequisite for life on earth as without it conditions on earth would be far too cold to sustain the ecosystem as we know it. Additions (quantitative and qualitative) to greenhouse gases distort and accelerate the natural process and result in more such gases in the atmosphere than are necessary to regulate and maintain an ideal temperature on earth; global warming is a consequence. The other layer associated with this discussion, the stratospheric ozone layer, shields the earth's surface from the sun's harmful ultraviolet (UV) radiation.

The major atmospheric effects that result from emission of inhalation anesthetics are their contributions to ozone depletion in the stratosphere and to greenhouse warming in the troposphere. The stratospheric ozone layer is known to be damaged by the rapid, widespread global usage, and subsequent atmospheric presence, of volatile, synthetic, long-lived organochlorine- and bromine-containing compounds (chlorofluorocarbons; CFCs). Indeed, knowledge of ozone depletion by CFCs was one of the major environmental issues of the 20th century and is sure to continue in a major way well into the 21st century. The CFCs causing most of the original worldwide concern regarding destruction of the ozone layer were those used as refrigerants, aerosol propellants, cleaning solutions, and foaming agents [397,398].

As halogenated compounds, all of the contemporary volatile anesthetics are in theory potentially destructive to the ozone layer [399–401]. However, in effect only chlorine-containing halothane and, much less so, isoflurane are of concern in this regard (substances that contain only fluorine do not harm the ozone layer). In addition, the relative contribution of these two volatile agents has been estimated to be at most only 0.01% of the annual global release of CFCs [399] and thus their resulting impact on ozone depletion is comparatively small [401,402]. Historically, CFCs have been considered the dominant ozone-depleting substances but N_2O shares many similarities with the CFCs and N_2O emission has been highlighted as '... the single most important ozone-depleting emission and is expected to remain the largest throughout the 21st century ...' [403]. The inhalation anesthetics including N_2O are not regulated by the 1987 Montreal Protocol on Substances That Deplete the Ozone Layer (the Montreal Protocol to the Vienna Convention for the Protection of the Ozone Layer is an international agreement designed to protect the ozone layer, ratified by 197 states) [404]. Although the magnitude of stratospheric impact of halothane and isoflurane is controversial, there is increasing concern that as a result of the effectiveness of the Montreal Protocol and associated efforts to decrease CFCs globally, the influence of the volatile anesthetics on ozone depletion is becoming proportionally more important [401].

As noted previously, both N_2O and the volatile agents affect global warming. The impact of the volatile agents is small relative to the much larger players such as CO_2, methane, etc., so present debate relates more to their potential status [401,402,405–408]. For example, in their recently published assessment of the impact on global climate of general anesthetic gases, Sulbaek Andersen *et al.* [402] estimated that 'the inhaled anesthetics released during the approximately 200 million anesthetic procedures performed globally each year, globally have a climate impact that is approximately 0.01% ... of that of the CO_2 released from global fossil fuel combustion.' Regardless, the majority of impacts of inhalation anesthetics are due to desflurane which has the highest heat trapping effect of the inhalation anesthetics [405,406,409,410], and N_2O which is released to the atmosphere in the greatest quantity [397,399,400,402,405,410]. In an attempt to provide contemporary comparative relevance, Ryan and Nielsen [405] note that, on an hourly basis and given the US average of 398 g of CO_2 emissions/mile of auto driving, '... using desflurane equates with driving 235–470 miles per hour of anesthetic use, whereas sevoflurane and isoflurane equate with driving 18 and 20–40 miles per hour of anesthetic use, respectively.'

References

1 Eger EI II. *Isoflurane (Forane): A Compendium and Reference*, 2nd edn. Madison, WI: Anaquest, 1985.
2 Soma LR. *Textbook of Veterinary Anesthesia*. Baltimore, MD: Williams & Wilkins, 1971.
3 Hall LW. *Wright's Veterinary Anaesthesia and Analgesia*, 7th edn. London: Baillière Tindall, 1971.
4 Lumb WV, Jones EW. *Veterinary Anesthesia*. Philadelphia: Lea & Febiger, 1973.
5 Short CE. Inhalant anesthetics. In: Short CE, ed. *Principles & Practice of Veterinary Anesthesia*. Baltimore, MD: Williams & Wilkins, 1987; 70–90.
6 Steffey EP, Mama KR. Inhalation anesthetics. In: Tranquilli WJ, Thurmon JC, Grimm KA, eds. *Lumb and Jones' Veterinary Anesthesia and Analgesia*, 4th edn. Ames, IA: Blackwell Publishing, 2007; 355–393.
7 Lowe HJ, Ernst EA. *The Quantitative Practice of Anesthesia: Use of Closed Circuit*. Baltimore, MD: Williams & Wilkins, 1981.
8 Hill DW. *Physics Applied to Anaesthesia*, 4th edn. London: Butterworth, 1980.
9 Haskins S, Sansome AL. A time-table for exhaustion of nitrous oxide cylinders using cylinder pressure. *Vet Anesth* 1979; **6**: 6–8.
10 Eger EI II. *Anesthetic Uptake and Action*. Baltimore, MD: Williams & Wilkins, 1974.
11 Mapleson WW, Allott PR, Steward A. The variability of partition coefficients for halothane in the rabbit. *Br J Anaesth* 1972; **44**: 650.
12 Eger RR, Eger EI II. Effect of temperature and age on the solubility of enflurane, halothane, isoflurane, and methoxyflurane in human blood. *Anesth Analg* 1985; **64**: 640–642.
13 Lerman J, Schmitt-Bantel BI, Gregory GA, *et al.* Effect of age on the solubility of volatile anesthetics in human tissues. *Anesthesiology* 1986; **65**(3): 307–312.
14 Eger EI II. Uptake and distribution. In: Miller RD, ed. *Anesthesia*, 5th edn. Philadelphia: Churchill Livingstone, 2000; 74–95.
15 Eger EI II, Eisenkraft JB, Weiskopf RB. *The Pharmacology of Inhaled Anesthetics*, 2nd edn. San Francisco, CA: Dannemiller Memorial Educational Foundation, 2003.
16 Mapleson WW. Pharmacokinetics of inhalational anaesthetics. In: Nunn JF, Utting JE, Brown BR Jr, eds. *General Anaesthesia*, 5th edn. London: Butterworths, 1989; 44–59.
17 Steffey EP, Howland D Jr. Rate of change of halothane concentration in a large animal circle anesthetic system. *Am J Vet Res* 1977; **38**(12): 1993–1996.
18 Mapleson WW. The concentration of anaesthetics in closed circuits, with special reference to halothane. I. Theoretical studies. *Br J Anaesth* 1960; **32**: 298–309.
19 Eger EI II. *Nitrous Oxide/ N2O*. New York: Elsevier, 1985.
20 Webb AI. The effect of species differences in the uptake and distribution of inhalant anesthetic agents. In: Grandy J, Hildebrand S, McDonell W, *et al.*, eds. In: *Proceedings of the Second International Congress of Veterinary Anesthesia*. Santa Barbara, CA: Veterinary Practice Publishing Co., 1985; 27–32.
21 Staddon GE, Weaver BMQ, Webb AI. Distribution of cardiac output in anaesthetized horses. *Res Vet Sci* 1979; **27**: 38–45.
22 Eger EI II, Severinghaus JW. Effect of uneven pulmonary distribution of blood and gas on induction with inhalation anesthetics. *Anesthesiology* 1964; **25**: 620–626.
23 Stoelting RK. The effect of right to left shunt on the rate of increase of arterial anesthetic concentration. *Anesthesiology* 1972; **36**: 352–356.
24 Stoelting RK, Eger EI II. Percutaneous loss of nitrous oxide, cyclopropane, ether and halothane in man. *Anesthesiology* 1969; **30**(3): 278–283.
25 Fassoulaki A, Lockhart SH, Freire BA, *et al.* Percutaneous loss of desflurane, isoflurane, and halothane in humans. *Anesthesiology* 1991; **74**: 479–483.
26 Lockhart SH, Yasuda N, Peterson N, *et al.* Comparison of percutaneous losses of sevoflurane and isoflurane in humans. *Anesth Analg* 1991; **72**: 212–215.
27 Eger EI II, Saidman LJ. Illustrations of inhaled anesthetic uptake, including intertissue diffusion to and from fat. *Anesth Analg* 2005; **100**: 1020–1033.
28 Stoelting RK, Eger EI II. The effects of ventilation and anesthetic solubility on recovery from anesthesia: an in vivo and analog analysis before and after equilibration. *Anesthesiology* 1969; **30**(3): 290–296.
29 Eger EI II, Johnson BH. Rates of awakening from anesthesia with I-653, halothane, isoflurane, and sevoflurane – a test of the effect of anesthetic concentration and duration in rats. *Anesth Analg* 1987; **66**: 977–983.
30 Cullen BF, Eger EI II. Diffusion of nitrous oxide, cyclopropane, and halothane through human skin and amniotic membrane. *Anesthesiology* 1972; **36**: 168–173.
31 Carpenter RL, Eger EI II, Johnson BH, *et al.* Does the duration of anesthetic administration affect the pharmacokinetics or metabolism of inhaled anesthetics in humans? *Anesth Analg* 1987; **66**: 1–8.
32 Laster MJ, Taheri S, Eger EI, *et al.* Visceral losses of desflurane, isoflurane, and halothane in swine. *Anesth Analg* 1991; **73**: 209–212.
33 Baden JM, Rice SA. Metabolism and toxicity of inhaled anesthetics. In: Miller RD, ed. *Anesthesia*, 5th edn. New York: Churchill Livingstone, 2000; 147–173.
34 Cahalan MK, Johnson BH, Eger EI II. Relationship of concentrations of halothane and enflurane to their metabolism and elimination in man. *Anesthesiology* 1981; **54**: 3–8.
35 Carpenter RL, Eger EI II, Johnson BH, *et al.* The extent of metabolism of inhaled anesthetics in humans. *Anesthesiology* 1986; **65**: 201–206.
36 Fink BR. Diffusion anoxia. *Anesthesiology* 1955; **16**: 511–519.
37 Rackow H, Salanitre E, Frumin MH. Dilution of alveolar gases during nitrous oxide excretion in man. *J Appl Physiol* 1961; **16**(4): 723–728.
38 Sheffer L, Steffenson JL, Birch AA. Nitrous oxide-induced diffusion hypoxia in patients breathing spontaneously. *Anesthesiology* 1972; **37**: 436–439.
39 Van Dyke RA, Chenoweth MB, van Poznak A. Metabolism of volatile anesthetics. I. Conversion in vivo of several anesthetics to 14-CO_2 and chloride. *Biochem Pharmacol* 1964; **13**: 1239–1247.
40 Stier A, Alter H, Hessler O, Rehder K. Urinary excretion of bromide in halothane anesthesia. *Anesth Analg* 1964; **43**: 723–728.
41 Rehder K, Forbes J, Alter H, *et al.* Halothane biotransformation in man: a quantitative study. *Anesthesiology* 1967; **28**: 711–715.
42 Holaday DA, Rudofsky S, Treuhaft PS. The metabolic degradation of methoxyflurane in man. *Anesthesiology* 1970; **33**(6): 579–593.
43 Mazze RI, Fujinaga M. Biotransformation of inhalational anaesthetics. In: Nunn JF, Utting JE, Brown BR, eds. *General Anaesthesia*, 5th edn. London: Butterworths, 1989; 73–85.
44 Sawyer DC, Eger EI II, Bahlman SH, *et al.* Concentration dependence of hepatic halothane metabolism. *Anesthesiology* 1971; **34**: 230–235.
45 Cook TL, Beppu WJ, Hitt BA, *et al.* Renal effects and metabolism of sevoflurane in Fischer 344 rats: an in-vivo and in-vitro comparison with methoxyflurane. *Anesthesiology* 1975; **43**: 70–77.
46 Wallin RF, Regan BM, Napoli MD, Stern IJ. Sevoflurane: a new inhalational anesthetic agent. *Anesth Analg* 1975; **54**: 758–766.
47 Cook TL, Beppu WJ, Hitt BA, *et al.* A comparison of renal effects and metabolism of sevoflurane and methoxyflurane in enzyme-induced rats. *Anesth Analg* 1975; **54**: 829–835.
48 Martis L, Lynch S, Napoli MD, Woods EF. Biotransformation of sevoflurane in dogs and rats. *Anesth Analg* 1981; **60**: 186–191.
49 Rice SA, Dooley JR, Mazze RI. Metabolism by rat hepatic microsomes of fluorinated ether anesthetics following ethanol consumption. *Anesthesiology* 1983; **58**: 237–241.
50 Aida H, Mizuno Y, Hobo S, *et al.* Cardiovascular and pulmonary effects of sevoflurane anesthesia in horses. *Vet Surg* 1996; **25**: 164–170.
51 Driessen B, Zarucco L, Steffey EP, *et al.* Serum fluoride concentrations, biochemical and histopathological changes associated with prolonged sevoflurane anaesthesia in horses. *J Vet Med A Physiol Pathol Clin Med* 2002; **49**: 337–347.
52 Steffey EP, Mama KR, Galey F, *et al.* Effects of sevoflurane dose and mode of ventilation on cardiopulmonary function and blood biochemical variables in horses. *Am J Vet Res* 2005; **66**(4): 606–614.
53 Koblin DD, Weiskopf RB, Holmes MA, *et al.* Metabolism of I-653 and isoflurane in swine. *Anesth Analg* 1989; **68**: 147–149.
54 Holaday DA, Smith FR. Clinical characteristics and biotransformation of sevoflurane in healthy human volunteers. *Anesthesiology* 1981; **54**: 100–106.
55 Frink EJ Jr, Malan TP Jr, Brown EA, *et al.* Plasma inorganic fluoride levels with sevoflurane anesthesia in morbidly obese and nonobese patients. *Anesth Analg* 1993; **76**: 1333–1337.
56 Koblin DD, Eger EI II, Johnson BH, *et al.* I-653 resists degradation in rats. *Anesth Analg* 1988; **67**: 534–539.
57 Sutton TS, Koblin DD, Gruenke LD, *et al.* Fluoride metabolites after prolonged exposure of volunteers and patients to desflurane. *Anesth Analg* 1991; **73**: 180–185.
58 Njoku D, Laster MJ, Gong DH, *et al.* Biotransformation of halothane, enflurane, isoflurane, and desflurane to trifluoroacetylated liver proteins: association between protein acylation and hepatic injury. *Anesth Analg* 1997; **84**(1): 173–178.
59 Merkel G, Eger EI II. A comparative study of halothane and halopropane anesthesia: including method for determining equipotency. *Anesthesiology* 1963; **24**(3): 346–357.
60 deJong RH, Eger EI II. MAC expanded: AD50 and AD95 values of common inhalation anesthetics in man. *Anesthesiology* 1975; **42**: 408–419.
61 Stanski DR. Monitoring depth of anesthesia. In: Miller RD, ed. *Anesthesia*, 5th edn. Philadelphia: Churchill Livingstone, 2000; 1087–116.
62 Steffey EP, Howland D Jr, Giri S, Eger EI II. Enflurane, halothane and isoflurane potency in horses. *Am J Vet Res* 1977; **38**: 1037–1039.
63 Ludders JW, Mitchell GS, Schaefer SI. Minimum anesthetic dose and cardiopulmonary response for halothane in chickens. *Am J Vet Res* 1988; **49**: 929–933.
64 Eger EI II, Johnson BH, Weiskopf RB, *et al.* Minimum alveolar concentration of I-653 and isoflurane in pigs: definition of a supramaximal stimulus. *Anesth Analg* 1988; **67**: 1174–1177.
65 Eger EI II, Saidman LJ, Brandstater B. Minimal alveolar anesthetic concentration: a standard of anesthetic potency. *Anesthesiology* 1965; **26**: 756–763.
66 Quasha AL, Eger EI II, Tinker JH. Determination and applications of MAC. *Anesthesiology* 1980; **53**(4): 315–334.

67 Stoelting RK, Longnecker DE, Eger EI II. Minimum alveolar concentrations in man on awakening from methoxyflurane, halothane, ether and fluroxene anesthesia: MAC awake. *Anesthesiology* 1970; **33**: 5–9.

68 Yakaitis RW, Blitt CD, Angiulo JP. End-tidal halothane concentration for endotracheal intubation. *Anesthesiology* 1977; **47**: 386–388.

69 Yakaitis RW, Blitt CD, Angiulo JP. End-tidal enflurane concentration for endotracheal intubation. *Anesthesiology* 1979; **50**: 59–61.

70 Roizen MF, Horrigan RW, Frazer BM. Anesthetic doses blocking adrenergic (stress) and cardiovascular responses to incision – MAC BAR. *Anesthesiology* 1981; **54**: 390–398.

71 Boscan P, Monnet E, Mama K, *et al.* A dog model to study ovary, ovarian ligament and visceral pain. *Vet Anaesth Analg* 2011; **38**(3): 260–266.

72 Drummond JC, Patel PM. Cerebral physiolgy and the effects of anesthetics and techniques. In: Miller RD, ed. *Anesthesia*, 5th edn. Philadelphia: Churchill Livingstone, 2000; 695–733.

73 Sonner JM, Antognini JF, Dutton RC, *et al.* Inhaled anesthetics and immobility: mechanisms, mysteries, and minimum alveolar anesthetic concentration. *Anesth Analg* 2003; **97**(3): 718–740.

74 Fischer E. Einfluss der configuration auf die wirkung der enzyme. *Der Dtsch Chem Ges* 1894; **27**: 2985–2993.

75 Brosnan RJ, Eger EI II, Laster MJ, Sonner JM. Anesthetic properties of carbon dioxide in the rat. *Anesth Analg* 2007; **105**(1): 103–106.

76 Brosnan RJ, Yang L, Milutinovic PS, *et al.* Ammonia has anesthteic properties. *Anesth Analg* 2007; **104**(6): 1430–1433.

77 Won A, Oh I, Liao M, Sonner JM, *et al.* The minimum alveolar anesthetic concentration of 2-, 3-, and 4- alcohols and ketones in rats: relevance to anesthetic mechanisms. *Anesth Analg* 2006; **102**(5): 1419–1426.

78 Nunn JF, Sturrock JE, Willis EJ, *et al.* The effect of inhalational anaesthetics on the swimming velocity of Tetrahymena pyriformis. *J Cell Sci* 1974; **15**: 537–554.

79 Livingston JS. On the anaesthetic effects of chloroform, ether, and amylene on sensitive plants. *Trans Bot Soc Edinburgh* 1860; **6**: 323–325.

80 Meyer H. Zur theorie der alkoholnarkose. *Naunyn-Schmiedeberg Arch Pharmacol* 1899; **42**: 109–118.

81 Overton CE. *Studies of Narcosis.* London: Chapman and Hall, 1991.

82 Brosnan R, Gong D, Cotten J, *et al.* Chirality in anesthesia II: stereoselective modulation of ion channel function by secondary alcohol enantiomers. *Anesth Analg* 2006; **103**(1): 86–91.

83 Koblin DD, Chortkoff BS, Laster MJ, *et al.* Polyhalogenated and perfluorinated compounds that disobey the Meyer–Overton hypothesis. *Anesth Analg* 1994; **79**: 1043–1048.

84 Cantor RS. Breaking the Meyer–Overton rule: predicted effects of varying stiffness and interfacial activity on the intrinsic potency of anesthetics. *Biophys J* 2001; **80**(5): 2284–2297.

85 Phorille A, Wilson MA, New MH, Chipot C. Concentrations of anesthetics across the water–membrane interface; the Meyer–Overton hypothesis revisited. *Toxicol Lett* 1998; **100–101**: 421–430.

86 Miller SL. A theory of gaseous anesthetics. *Proc Natl Acad Sci USA* 1961; **47**: 1515–1524.

87 Pauling L. A molecular theory of general anesthesia. *Science* 1961; **134**: 15–21.

88 Miller KW, Paton WD, Smith EB. Site of action of general aneaesthetics. *Nature* 1965; **206**: 574–547.

89 Eger EI II, Lundgren C, Miller SL, Stevens WC. Anesthetic potencies of sulfur hexafluoride, carbon tetrafluoride, chloroform and ethrane in dogs: correlation with the hydrate and lipid theories of anesthetic action. *Anesthesiology* 1969; **30**(2): 129–135.

90 Eger EI II, Saidman LJ, Brandstater B. Temperature dependence of halothane and cylcopropane anesthesia in dogs: correlation with some theories of anesthetic action. *Anesthesiology* 1965; **26**(6): 764–770.

91 Willenbring D, Xu Y, Tang P. The role of structured water in mediating general anesthetic action on alpha4beta2 nAChR. *Phys Chem Chem Phys* 2010; **12**: 10263–10269.

92 Franks NP, Lieb WR. Do general anaesthetics act by competitive binding to specific receptors? *Nature* 1984; **310**: 599–602.

93 Eckenhoff RG, Johansson JS. On the relevance of 'clinically relevant concentrations' of inhaled anesthetics in in vitro experiments. *Anesthesiology* 1999; **91**: 856–860.

94 Shafer SL, Hendrickx JFA, Flood P, *et al.* Additivity versus synergy: a theoretical analysis of implications for anestheteic mechanisms. *Anesth Analg* 2008; **107**(2): 507–524.

95 Eger EI II, Tang M, Liao M, *et al.* Inhaled anesthetics do not combine to produce synergistic effects regarding minimum alveolar anesthetic concentration in rats. *Anesth Analg* 2008; **107**(2): 479–485.

96 Brosnan RJ. Does anesthetic additivity imply a similar molecular mechanism of anesthetic action at N-methyl-D-aspartate receptors? *Anesth Analg* 2011; **112**: 568–573.

97 Brosnan RJ. GABA-A receptor antagonism increases NMDA receptor inhibition by isoflurane at a minimum alveolar concentration. *Vet Anaesth Analg* 2011; **38**(3): 231–239.

98 Brosnan RJ. Increased NMDA receptor inhibition at an increased sevofurane MAC. *BMC Anesthesiol* 2012; **12**: 9.

99 Rampil IJ, Mason P, Singh H. Anesthetic potency (MAC) is independent of forebrain structures in the rat. *Anesthesiology* 1993; **78**: 707–712.

100 Antognini JF, Schwartz K. Exaggerated anesthetic requirements in the preferentially anesthetized brain. *Anesthesiology* 1993; **79**: 1244–1249.

101 Rampil IJ. Anesthetic potency is not altered after hypothermic spinal cord transection in rats. *Anesthesiology* 1994; **80**: 606–610.

102 Eger EI II, Xing Y, Pearce R, *et al.* Isoflurane antagonizes the capacity of flurothyl or 1,2-dichlorohexafluorocyclobutane to impair fear conditioning to context and tone. *Anesth Analg* 2003; **96**: 1010–1018.

103 Alkire MT, Nathan SV. Does the amygdala mediate anesthetic-induced amnesia? Basolateral amygdala lesions block sevoflurane-induced amnesia. *Anesthesiology* 2005; **102**: 754–760.

104 Perauansky M, Rau V, Ford T, *et al.* Slowing of the hippocampal theta rhythm correlates with anesthetic-induced amnesia. *Anesthesiology* 2010; **113**: 1299–1309.

105 Rau V, Iyer SV, Oh I, *et al.* Gamma-aminobutyric acid type A receptor alpha 4 subunit knowckout mice are resistant to the amnesic effect of isoflurane. *Anesth Analg* 2009; **109**: 1816–1822.

106 Rau V, Oh I, Liao M, *et al.* Gamma-aminobutyric acid type A receptor beta3 subunit forebrain-specific knowckout mice are resistant to the amnesic effect of isoflurane. *Anesth Analg* 2011; **113**: 500–504.

107 Zurek AA, Bridgwater EM, Orser BA. Inhibition of alpha5 gamma-aminobutyric acid type A receptors restores recognitoin memory after general anesthesia. *Anesth Analg* 2012; **114**: 845–855.

108 Melzack R, Casey KL. Sensory, motivational and control determinants of pain; a new conceptual model. In: Kenshalo D, ed. *The Skin Senses.* Tallahassee, FL: Thomas, 1967; 423–443.

109 O'Connor TC, Abram SE. Inhibition of nociception-induced spinal sensitization by anesthetic agents. *Anesthesiology* 1995; **82**: 259–266.

110 Mitsuyo T, Dutton RC, Antognini JF, Carstens E. The differential effects of halothane and isoflurane on windup of dorsal horn neurons selected in unanesthetized decerebrated rats. *Anesth Analg* 2006; **103**(3): 753–760.

111 Zhang Y, Eger EI, Dutton RC, Sonner JM. Inhaled anesthetics have hyperalgesic effects at 0.1 minimum alveolar anesthetic concentration. *Anesth Analg* 2000; **91**: 462–466.

112 Sonner J, Li J, Eger EI. Desflurane and nitrous oxide, but not nonimmobilizers, affect nociceptive responses. *Anesth Analg* 1998; **86**(3): 629–634.

113 Flood P, Sonner JM, Gong D, Coates MM. Isoflurane hyperalgesia is modulated by nicotinic inhibition. *Anesthesiology* 2002; **97**: 192–198.

114 Yamakura T, Harris RA. Effects of gaseous anesthetics nitrous oxide and xenon on ligand-gated ion channels. Comparison with isoflurane and ethanol. *Anesthesiology* 2000; **93**: 1095–1101.

115 Zhang C, Davies MF, Guo TZ, Maze M. The analgesic action of nitrous oxide is dependent on the release of norepinephrine in the dorsal horn of the spinal cord. *Anesthesiology* 1999; **91**: 1401–1407.

116 Dwyer RC, Rampil IJ, Eger EI II, Bennett HL. The electroencephalogram does not predict depth of isoflurane anesthesia. *Anesthesiology* 1994; **81**: 403–409.

117 Scheller MS, Tateishi A, Drummond JC, Zornow MH. The effects of sevoflurane on cerebral blood flow, cerebral metabolic rate for oxygen, intracranial pressure, and the electroencephalogram are similar to those of isoflurane in the rabbit. *Anesthesiology* 1988; **68**: 548–552.

118 Rampil IJ, Weiskopf RB, Brown JG, *et al.* I-653 and isoflurane produce similar dose-related changes in the electroencephalogram of pigs. *Anesthesiology* 1988; **69**: 298–302.

119 Rampil IJ, Lockhart SH, Eger EI II, *et al.* The electroencephalographic effects of desflurane in humans. *Anesthesiology* 1991; **74**: 434–439.

120 Neigh JL, Garman JK, Harp JR. The electroencephalographic pattern during anesthesia with Ethrane: effects of depth of anesthesia, PaCO2 and nitrous oxide. *Anesthesiology* 1971; **35**: 482–487.

121 Joas TA, Stevens WC, Eger EI II. Electroencephalographic seizure activity in dogs during anaesthesia: studies with Ethrane, fluroxene, halothane, chloroform, divinyl ether, diethyl ether, methoxyflurane, cyclopropane and forane. *Br J Anaesth* 1971; **43**: 739–745.

122 Todd MM, Drummond JC. A comparison of the cerebrovascular and metabolic effects of halothane and isoflurane in the cat. *Anesthesiology* 1984; **60**: 276–282.

123 Karasawa F. The effects of sevoflurane on lidocaine-induced convulsions. *J Anesth* 1991; **5**(1): 60–67.

124 Fukuda H, Hirabayashi Y, Shimizu R, *et al.* Sevoflurane is equivalent to isoflurane for attenuating bupivacaine-induced arrhythmias and seizures in rats. *Anesth Analg* 1996; **83**: 570–573.

125 Murao K, Shingu K, Tsushima K, *et al.* The anticonvulsant effects of volatile anesthetics on penicillin-induced status epilepticus in cats. *Anesth Analg* 2000; **90**(1): 142–147.
126 Murao K, Shingu I, Tsushima K, *et al.* The anticonvulsant effects of volatile anesthetics on lidocaine-induced seizures in cats. *Anesth Analg* 2000; **90**(1): 148–155.
127 Scheller MS, Nakakimura K, Fleischer JE, Zornow MH. Cerebral effects of sevoflurane in the dog: comparison with isoflurane and enflurane. *Br J Anaesth* 1990; **65**: 388–392.
128 Osawa M, Shingu K, Murakawa M, *et al.* Effect of sevoflurane on central nervous system electrical activity in cats. *Anesth Analg* 1994; **79**: 52–57.
129 Woodforth IJ, Hicks RG, Crawford MR, *et al.* Electroencephalographic evidence of seizure activity under deep sevoflurane anesthesia in a nonepileptic patient. *Anesthesiology* 1997; **87**: 1579–1582.
130 Komatsu H, Tale S, Endo S, *et al.* Electrical seizures during sevoflurane anesthesia in two pediatric patients with epilepsy. *Anesthesiology* 1994; **81**: 1535–1537.
131 Cucchiara RF, Theye RA, Michenfelder JD. The effects of isoflurane on canine cerebral metabolism and blood flow. *Anesthesiology* 1974; **40**: 571–574.
132 Lutz LJ, Milde JH, Milde LN. The cerebral functional, metabolic, and hemodynamic effects of desflurane in dogs. *Anesthesiology* 1990; **73**: 125–131.
133 Munro A. *Observations on the Structure and Functions of the Nervous System.* Edinburgh: William Creech, 1783.
134 Kellie G. Account of the appearances observed in the dissection of two of three individuals presumed to have perished in the storm of the 3rd, and whose bodies were discovered in the vicinity of Leith on the morning of the 4th, November 1821: with some reflections on the pathology of the brain. *Trans Medico-Chirurgical Soc Edinb* 1824; **1**: 84–169.
135 Manohar M, Parks CM. Porcine systemic and regional organ blood flow during 1.0 and 1.5 minimum alveolar concentrations of sevoflurane anesthesia without and with 50% nitrous oxide. *J Pharmacol Exp Ther* 1984; **231**(3): 640–648.
136 Drummond JC, Todd MM, Scheller MS, Shapiro HM. A comparison of the direct cerebral vasodilating potencies of halothane and isoflurane in the New Zealand white rabbit. *Anesthesiology* 1986; **65**(5): 462–468.
137 Artru AA. Relationship between cerebral blood volume and CSF pressure during anesthesia with halothane or enflurane in dogs. *Anesthesiology* 1983; **58**(6): 533–539.
138 Holmstrom A, Akeson J. Desflurane increses intracranial pressure more and sevoflurane less than isoflurane in pigs subjected to intracranial hypertension. *J Neurosurg Anesthesiol* 2004; **16**: 136–143.
139 Lam AM, Mayberg TS, Eng CC, *et al.* Nitrous oxide-isoflurane anesthesia causes more cerebral vasodilation than an equipotent dose of isoflurane in humans. *Anesth Analg* 1994; **78**: 462–468.
140 Fraga M, Rama-Macerias P, Rodino S, *et al.* The effects of isoflurane and desflurane on intracranial pressure, cerebral perfusion pressure, and cerebral arteriovenous oxygen content difference in normocapnic patients with supratentorial brain tumors. *Anesthesiology* 2003; **98**: 1085–1090.
141 Matta BF, Heath KJ, Tipping K, Summors AC. Direct cerebral vasodilatory effects of sevoflurane and isoflurane. *Anesthesiology* 1999; **91**: 677–680.
142 Moore LE, Kirsch J, Helfaer MA, *et al.* Nitric oxide and prostanoids contribute to isoflurane-induced cerebral hyperemia in pigs. *Anesthesiology* 1994; **80**: 1328–1337.
143 Iadecola C. Does nitric oxide mediate the increases in cerebral blood flow elicited by hypercapnia? *Proc Natl Acad Sci USA* 1992; **89**: 3913–3916.
144 Sjakste N, Baumane L, Meirena D, *et al.* Drastic increase in nitric oxide content in rat brain under halothane anesthesia revealed by EPR method. *Biochem Pharmacol* 1999; **58**: 1955–1959.
145 Todd MM, Wu B, Warner DS, Maktabi M. The dose-related effects of nitric oxide synthase inhibition on cerebral blood flow during isoflurane and pentobarbital anesthesia. *Anesthesiology* 1994; **80**: 1128–1136.
146 Kant GJ, Muller TW, Lenox RH, Meyerhoff JL. In vivo effects of pentobarbital and halothane anesthesia on levels of adenosine 3′,5′-monophosphate and guanosine 3′,5′-monophosphate in rat brain regions and pituitary. *Biochem Pharmacol* 1980; **29**: 1891–1896.
147 Strebel S, Lam AM, Matta B, *et al.* Dynamic and static cerebral autoregulation during isoflurane, desflurane, and propofol anesthesia. *Anesthesiology* 1995; **83**: 66–76.
148 Hoffman WE, Edelman G, Kochs E, *et al.* Cerebral autoregulation in awake versus isoflurane-anesthetized rats. *Anesth Analg* 1991; **73**: 753–757.
149 Albrecht RF, Miletich DJ, Madala LR. Normalization of cerebral blood flow during prolonged halothane anesthesia. *Anesthesiology* 1983; **58**(1): 26–31.
150 Boarini DJ, Kassell NF, Coester HC, *et al.* Comparison of systemic and cerebrovascular effects of isoflurane and halothane. *Neurosurgery* 1984; **15**(3): 400–409.
151 Warner DS, Boarini DJ, Kassell NF. Cerebrovascular adaptation to prolonged halothane anesthesia is not related to cerebrospinal fluid pH. *Anesthesiology* 1985; **63**(3): 243–248.
152 McPherson RW, Kirsch J, Tobin J, *et al.* Cerebral blood flow in primates is increased by isoflurane over time and is decreased by nitric oxide synthase inhibition. *Anesthesiology* 1994; **80**: 1320–1327.
153 Kuroda Y, Murakami M, Tsuruta J, *et al.* Blood flow velocity of middle cerebral artery during prolonged anesthesia with halothane, isoflurane, and sevoflurane in humans. *Anesthesiology* 1997; **87**: 527–532.
154 McPherson RW, Brian JE, Traysman RJ. Cerebrovascular responsiveness to carbon dioxide in dogs with 1.4% and 2.8% isoflurane. *Anesthesiology* 1989; **70**(5):843–851.
155 Nishiyama T, Matsukawa T, Yokoyama T, Hanaoka K. Cerebrovascular carbon dioxide reactivity during general anesthesia: a comparison between sevoflurane and isoflurane. *Anesth Analg* 1999; **89**: 1437–1441.
156 Adams RW, Cucchiara R, Gronert GA, *et al.* Isoflurane and cerebrospinal fluid pressure in neurosurgical patients. *Anesthesiology* 1981; **54**: 97–99.
157 Scheller MS, Todd MM, Drummond JC. Isoflurane, halothane, and regional cerebral blood flow at various levels of PaCO2 in rabbits. *Anesthesiology* 1986; **64**(5): 598–605.
158 Brosnan RJ, LeCouteur RA, Steffey EP, *et al.* Direct measurement of intracranial pressure in adult horses. *Am J Vet Res* 2002; **63**(9): 1252–1256.
159 Brosnan RJ, Steffey EP, LeCouteur RA, *et al.* Effects of body position on intracranial and cerebral perfusion pressures in isoflurane-anesthetized horses. *J Appl Physiol* 2002; **92**: 2542–2546.
160 Brosnan RJ, Steffey EP, LeCouteur RA, *et al.* Effects of ventilation and isoflurane end-tidal concentration on intracranial and cerebral perfusion pressures in horses. *Am J Vet Res* 2003; **64**(1): 21–25.
161 Brosnan RJ, Steffey EP, LeCouteur RA, *et al.* Effects of duration of isoflurane anesthesia and mode of ventilation on intracranial and cerebral perfusion pressures in horses. *Am J Vet Res* 2003; **64**(11): 1444–1448.
162 Brosnan RJ, Esteller-Vico A, Steffey EP, *et al.* Effects of head-down positioning on regional central nervous system perfusion in isoflurane-anesthetized horses. *Am J Vet Res* 2008; **69**(6): 737–743.
163 Brosnan RJ, Steffey EP, LeCouteur RA, *et al.* Effects of isoflurane anesthesia on cerebrovascular autoregulation in horses. *Am J Vet Res* 2011; **72**(1): 18–24.
164 Knill RL, Kieraszewicz HT, Dodgson BG, Clement JL. Chemical regulation of ventilation during isoflurane sedation and anaesthesia in humans. *Br J Anaesth* 1983; **49**: 957–963.
165 Fourcade HE, Stevens WC, Larson CP Jr, *et al.* The ventilatory effects of forane, a new inhaled anesthetic. *Anesthesiology* 1971; **35**: 26–31.
166 Hirshman CA, McCullough KE, Cohen PJ, Weil JV. Depression of hypoxic ventilatory response by halothane, enflurane and isoflurane in dogs. *Br J Anaesth* 1977; **49**: 947–962.
167 Knill RL, Manninen PH, Clement JL. Ventilation and chemoreflexes during enflurane sedation and anaesthesia in man. *Can Anaesth Soc J* 1979; **26**: 353–360.
168 Coon RL, Kampine JP. Hypocapnic bronchoconstriction and inhalation anesthetics. *Anesthesiology* 1975; **43**: 635–641.
169 Klide AM, Aviado DM. Mechanism for the reduction in pulmonary resistance induced by halothane. *J Pharmacol Exp Ther* 1967; **158**: 28–35.
170 Tobias JD, Hirshman CA. Attenuation of histamine-induced airway constriction by albuterol during halothane anesthesia. *Anesthesiology* 1990; **72**: 105–110.
171 Habre W, Petak F, Sly PD, *et al.* Protective effects of volatile agents against methacholine-induced bronchoconstriction in rats. *Anesthesiology* 2001; **94**: 348–353.
172 Hirshman CA, Bergman NA. Halothane and enflurane protect against bronchospasm in an asthma dog model. *Anesth Analg* 1978; **57**: 629–633.
173 Hirshman CA, Edelstein H, Peetz S, *et al.* Mechanism of action of inhalational anesthesia on airways. *Anesthesiology* 1982; **56**: 107–111.
174 Mazzeo AJ, Cheng EY, Bosnjak ZJ, *et al.* Differential effects of desflurane and halothane on peripheral airway smooth muscle. *Br J Anaesth* 1996; **76**: 841–846.
175 Wiklund CU, Lim S, Lindsten U, Lindahl SGE. Relaxation by sevoflurane, desflurane and halothane in the isolated guinea-pig trachea via inhibition of cholinergic neurotransmission. *Br J Anaesth* 1999; **83**(3): 422–429.
176 Doi M, Ikeda K. Airway irritation produced by volatile anaesthetics during brief inhalation: comparison of halothane, enflurane, isoflurane and sevoflurane. *Can J Anaesth* 1993; **40**: 122–126.
177 Eger EI II. *Desflurane (Suprane): a Compendium and Reference.* Rutherford, NJ: Healthpress Publishing Group, 1993.
178 Terriet MF, Desouza GJA, Jacobs JS, *et al.* Which is most pungent: isoflurane, sevoflurane or desflurane? *Br J Anaesth* 2000; **85**: 305–307.
179 Lockhart SH, Rampil IJ, Yasuda N, *et al.* Depression of ventilation by desflurane in humans. *Anesthesiology* 1991; **74**: 484–488.
180 Munson ES, Larson CP Jr, Babad AA, *et al.* The effects of halothane, fluroxene and cyclopropane on ventilation: a comparative study in man. *Anesthesiology* 1966; **27**(6): 716–728.
181 Larson CP Jr, Eger EI II, Muallem M, *et al.* The effects of diethyl ether and methoxyflurane on ventilation: II. A comparative study in man. *Anesthesiology* 1969; **30**(2): 174–184.

182 Doi M, Ikeda K. Respiratory effects of sevoflurane. *Anesth Analg* 1987; **66**: 241–244.
183 Calverley RK, Smith NT, Jones CW, *et al*. Ventilatory and cardiovascular effects of enflurane anesthesia during spontaneous ventilation in man. *Anesth Analg* 1978; **51**: 610–618.
184 Hodgson DS, Steffey EP, Grandy JL, Woliner MJ. Effects of spontaneous, assisted, and controlled ventilation in halothane-anesthetized geldings. *Am J Vet Res* 1986; **47**: 992–996.
185 Steffey EP, Wheat JD, Meagher DM, *et al*. Body position and mode of ventilation influences arterial pH, oxygen and carbon dioxide tensions in halothane-anesthetized horses. *Am J Vet Res* 1977; **38**: 379–382.
186 Brandstater B, Eger EI II, Edelist G. Constant-depth halothane anesthesia in respiratory studies. *J Appl Physiol* 1965; **20**(2): 171–174.
187 Steffey EP, Farver TB, Woliner MJ. Cardiopulmonary function during 7 h of constant-dose halothane and methoxyflurane. *J Appl Physiol* 1987; **63**: 1351–1359.
188 Fourcade HE, Larson CP Jr, Hickey RF, *et al*. Effects of time on ventilation during halothane and cyclopropane anesthesia. *Anesthesiology* 1972; **36**: 83–88.
189 Steffey EP, Hodgson DS, Dunlop CI, *et al*. Cardiopulmonary function during 5 hours of constant-dose isoflurane in laterally recumbent, spontaneously breathing horses. *J Vet Pharmacol Ther* 1987; **10**: 290–297.
190 Steffey EP, Kelly AB, Woliner MJ. Time-related responses of spontaneously breathing, laterally recumbent horses to prolonged anesthesia with halothane. *Am J Vet Res* 1987; **48**: 952–957.
191 Steffey EP, Kelly AB, Hodgson DS, *et al*. Effect of body posture on cardiopulmonary function in horses during five hours of constant-dose halothane anesthesia. *Am J Vet Res* 1990; **51**: 11–16.
192 France CJ, Plumer HM, Eger EI II, Wahrenbrock EA. Ventilatory effects of isoflurane (Forane) or halothane when combined with morphine, nitrous oxide and surgery. *Br J Anaesth* 1974; **46**: 117–120.
193 Eger EI II, Dolan WM, Stevens WC, *et al*. Surgical stimulation antagonizes the respiratory depression produced by Forane. *Anesthesiology* 1972; **36**: 544–549.
194 Steffey EP, Eisele JH, Baggot JD, *et al*. Influence of inhaled anesthetics on the pharmacokinetics and pharmacodynamics of morphine. *Anesth Analg* 1993; **77**: 346–351.
195 Steffey EP, Pascoe PJ. Xylazine blunts the cardiovascular but not the respiratory response induced by noxious stimulation in isoflurane anesthetized horses (abstact). Proceedings of the 7th International Congress of Veterinary Anaesthesia, 2000.
196 Steffey EP, Gillespie RJ, Berry JD, *et al*. Circulatory effects of halothane and halothane-nitrous oxide anesthesia in the dog: spontaneous ventilation. *Am J Vet Res* 1975; **36**(2): 197–200.
197 Steffey EP, Gillespie JR, Berry JD, Eger EI II. Cardiovascular effects with the addition of N2O to halothane in stump-tailed macaques during spontaneous and controlled ventilation. *J Am Vet Med Assoc* 1974; **165**: 834–837.
198 Steffey EP, Baggot JD, Eisele JH, *et al*. Morphine-isoflurane interaction in dogs, swine and rhesus monkeys. *J Vet Pharmacol Ther* 1994; **17**: 202–210.
199 Steffey EP, Eisele JH, Baggot JD. Interactions of morphine and isoflurane in horses. *Am J Vet Res* 2003; **64**(2): 166–175.
200 Bennett RC, Steffey EP, Kollias-Baker C, Sams R. Influence of morphine sulfate on the halothane sparing effect of xylazine hydrochloride in horses. *Am J Vet Res* 2004; **65**(4): 519–526.
201 Steffey EP, Howland D Jr. Potency of enflurane in dogs: comparison with halothane and isoflurane. *Am J Vet Res* 1978; **39**: 673–677.
202 Klide AM. Cardiovascular effects of enflurane and isoflurane in the dog. *Am J Vet Res* 1976; **37**: 127–131.
203 Steffey EP, Howland D Jr. Comparison of circulatory and respiratory effects of isoflurane and halothane anesthesia in horses. *Am J Vet Res* 1980; **41**: 821–825.
204 Eger EI II. New inhaled anesthetics. *Anesthesiology* 1994; **80**: 906–922.
205 Merin RG, Bernard JM, Doursout MF, *et al*. Comparison of the effects of isoflurane and desflurane on cardiovascular dynamics and regional blood flow in the chronically instrumented dog. *Anesthesiology* 1991; **74**(3): 568–574.
206 Weiskopf RB, Holmes MA, Eger EI II, *et al*. Cardiovascular effects of I-653 in swine. *Anesthesiology* 1988; **69**: 303–309.
207 Pagel PS, Kampine JP, Schmeling WT, Warltier DC. Comparison of the systemic and coronary hemodynamic actions of desflurane, isoflurane, halothane, and enflurane in the chronically instrumented dog. *Anesthesiology* 1991; **74**: 539–551.
208 Warltier DC, Pagel PS. Cardiovascular and respiratory actions of desflurane: is desflurane different from isoflurane? *Anesth Analg* 1992; **75**: S17–S31.
209 Steffey EP, Woliner MJ, Puschner B, Galey F. Effects of desflurane and mode of ventilation on cardiovascular and respiratory functions and clinicopathologic variables in horses. *Am J Vet Res* 2005; **66**(4): 669–677.
210 Picker O, Scheeren TWL, Arndt JO. Inhalation anaesthetics increase heart rate by decreasing cardiac vagal activity in dogs. *Br J Anaesth* 1988; **87**(5): 748–754.
211 Malan TP, DiNardo JA, Isner J, *et al*. Cardiovascular effects of sevoflurane compared with those of isoflurane in volunteers. *Anesthesiology* 1995; **83**: 918–928.
212 Mutoh T, Nishimura R, Kim HY, *et al*. Cardiopulmonary effects of sevoflurane, compared with halothane, enflurane, and isoflurane, in dogs. *Am J Vet Res* 1997; **58**(8): 885–890.
213 Pagel PS, Kampine JP, Schmeling WT, Warltier DC. Influence of volatile anesthetics on myocardial contractility in vivo – desflurane versus isoflurane. *Anesthesiology* 1991; **74**: 900–907.
214 Pagel PS, Kampine JP, Schmeling WT, Warltier DC. Evaluation of myocardial contractility in the chronically instrumented dog with intact autonomic nervous system function: effects of desflurane and isoflurane. *Acta Anaesthesiol Scand* 1993; **37**(2): 203–210.
215 Boban M, Stowe DF, Buljubasic N, *et al*. Direct comparative effects of isoflurane and desflurane in isolated guinea pig hearts. *Anesthesiology* 1992; **76**: 775–780.
216 Stevens WC, Cromwell TH, Halsey MJ, *et al*. The cardiovascular effects of a new inhalation anesthetic, Forane, in human volunteers at constant arterial carbon dioxide tension. *Anesthesiology* 1971; **35**: 8–16.
217 Weiskopf RB, Cahalan MK, Eger EI II, *et al*. Cardiovascular actions of desflurane in normocarbic volunteers. *Anesth Analg* 1991; **73**: 143–156.
218 Bernard JM, Wouters PF, Doursout MF, *et al*. Effects of sevoflurane and isoflurane on cardiac and coronary dynamics in chronically instrumented dogs. *Anesthesiology* 1990; **72**: 659–662.
219 Clarke KW, Alibhai HIK, Lee YHL, Hammond RA. Cardiopulmonary effects of desflurane in the dog during spontaneous and artificial ventilation. *Res Vet Sci* 1996; **61**: 82–86.
220 Price HL. The significance of catecholamine release during anesthesia. *Br J Anaesth* 1966; **38**: 705–711.
221 Katz RL, Epstein RA. The interaction of anesthetic agents and adrenergic drugs to produce cardiac arrhythmias. *Anesthesiology* 1968; **29**:763–784.
222 Raventos J. The action of fluothane: a new volatile anaesthetic. *Br J Pharmacol* 1956; **11**: 394–409.
223 Muir BJ, Hall LW, Littlewort MCG. Cardiac irregularities in cats under halothane anaesthesia. *Br J Anaesth* 1959; **31**: 488–489.
224 Ueda I, Hirakawa M, Arakawa K, Kamaya H. Do anesthetics fluidize membranes? *Anesthesiology* 1986; **64**: 67–72.
225 Joas TA, Stevens WC. Comparison of the arrhythmic doses of epinephrine during Forane, halothane, and fluroxene anesthesia in dogs. *Anesthesiology* 1971; **35**(1): 48–53.
226 Muir WW III, Hubbell JAE, Flaherty S. Increasing halothane concentration abolishes anesthesia-associated arrhythmias in cats and dogs. *J Am Vet Med Assoc* 1988; **192**: 1730–1735.
227 Moore MA, Weiskopf RB, Eger EI II, *et al*. Arrhythmogenic doses of epinephrine are similar during desflurane or isoflurane anesthesia in humans. *Anesthesiology* 1993; **79**(5): 943–947.
228 Munson ES, Tucker WK. Doses of epinephrine causing arrhythmia during enflurane, methoxyflurane and halothane anesthesia in dogs. *Can Anaesth Soc J* 1975; **22**: 495–501.
229 Navarro R, Weiskopf RB, Moore MA, *et al*. Humans anesthetized with sevoflurane or isoflurane have similar arrhythmic response to epinephrine. *Anesthesiology* 1994; **80**: 545–549.
230 Weiskopf RB, Eger EI II, Holmes MA, *et al*. Epinephrine-induced premature ventricular contractions and changes in arterial blood pressure and heart rate during I-653, isoflurane, and halothane anesthesia in swine. *Anesthesiology* 1989; **70**: 293–298.
231 Johnston RR, Eger EI II, Wilson C. A comparative interaction of epinephrine with enflurane, isoflurane and halothane in man. *Anesth Analg* 1976; **55**: 709–712.
232 Hikasa Y, Okabe C, Takase K, Ogasawara S. Ventricular arrhythmogenic dose of adrenaline during sevoflurane, isoflurane, and halothane anaesthesia either with or without ketamine or thiopentone in cats. *Res Vet Sci* 1996; **60**: 134–137.
233 Tucker WK, Rackstein AD, Munson ES. Comparison of arrhythmic doses of adrenaline, metaraminol, ephedrine, and phenylephrine, during isoflurane and halothane anesthesia in dogs. *Br J Anaesth* 1974; **46**: 392–396.
234 Maze M, Smith CM. Identification of receptor mechanisms mediating epinephrine-induced arrhythmuas during halothane anesthesia in the dog. *Anesthesiology* 1983; **59**: 322–326.
235 Light GS, Hellyer PW, Swanson CR. Parasympathetic influence on the arrhythmogenicity of graded dobutamine infusions in halothane-anesthetized horses. *Am J Vet Res* 1992; **53**(7): 1154–1160.
236 Lemke KA, Tranquilli WJ, Thurmon JC, *et al*. Alterations in the arrhythmogenic dose of epinephrine after xylazine or medetomidine administration in halothane-anesthetized dogs. *Am J Vet Res* 1993; **54**: 2132–2138.
237 Lemke KA, Tranquilli WJ, Thurmon JC, *et al*. Alterations in the arrhythmogenic dose of epinephrine after xylazine or medetomidine administration in isoflurane-anesthetized dogs. *Am J Vet Res* 1993; **54**: 2139–2144.
238 Robertson BJ, Clement JL, Knill RL. Enhancement of the arrhythmogenic effect of hypercarbia by surgical stimulation during halothane anaesthesia in man. *Can Anaesth Soc J* 1981; **28**: 342.

239 Gelman S, Fowler KC, Smith LR. Liver circulation and function during isoflurane and halothane anesthesia. *Anesthesiology* 1984; **61**(6): 726–731.
240 Bernard JM, Doursout MF, Wouters P, *et al.* Effects of enflurane and isoflurane on hepatic and renal circulations in chronically instrumented dogs. *Anesthesiology* 1991; **74**(2): 298–302.
241 Bernard JM, Doursout MF, Wouters P, *et al.* Effects of sevoflurane and isoflurane on hepatic circulation in the chronically instrumented dog. *Anesthesiology* 1992; **77**(3): 541–545.
242 Frink EJ Jr, Morgan SE, Coetzee A, *et al.* The effects of sevoflurane, halothane, enflurane, and isoflurane on hepatic blood flow and oxygenation in chronically instrumented greyhound dogs. *Anesthesiology* 1992; **76**: 85–90.
243 Steffey EP, Farver TB, Woliner MJ. Circulatory and respiratory effects of methoxyflurane in dogs: comparison of halothane. *Am J Vet Res* 1984; **45**: 2574–2579.
244 Steffey EP, Howland D Jr. Isoflurane potency in the dog and cat. *Am J Vet Res* 1977; **38**: 1833–1836.
245 Steffey EP, Gillespie JR, Berry JD, *et al.* Circulatory effects of halothane and halothane–nitrous oxide anesthesia in the dog: controlled ventilation. *Am J Vet Res* 1974; **35**: 1289–1293.
246 Steffey EP, Howland D Jr. Cardiovascular effects of halothane in the horse. *Am J Vet Res* 1978; **39**: 611–615.
247 Pypendop BH, Ilkiw JE. Hemodynamic effects of sevoflurane in cats. *Am J Vet Res* 2004; **65**(1): 20–25.
248 Steffey EP, Gillespie JR, Berry JD, *et al.* Cardiovascular effect of halothane in the stump-tailed macaque during spontaneous and controlled ventilation. *Am J Vet Res* 1974; **35**: 1315–1319.
249 Stoelting RK. *Inhaled Anesthetics. Pharmacology and Physiology in Anesthetic Practice*, 3rd edn. Philadelphia: Lippincott-Raven, 1999; 36–76.
250 Wolfson B, Hebrick WD, Lake CL, Silar ES. Anesthetic indices – further data. *Anesthesiology* 1978; **48**: 187–190.
251 Wolfson B, Kielar CM, Lake C, *et al.* Anesthetic Index – a new approach. *Anesthesiology* 1973; **38**: 583–586.
252 Cullen DJ, Eger EI II. Cardiovascular effects of carbon dioxide in man. *Anesthesiology* 1974; **41**: 345–349.
253 Grandy JL, Hodgson DS, Dunlop CI, *et al.* Cardiopulmonary effects of halothane anesthesia in cats. *Am J Vet Res* 1989; **50**: 1729–1732.
254 Bahlman SH, Eger EI II, Halsey MJ, *et al.* The cardiovascular effects of halothane in man during spontaneous ventilation. *Anesthesiology* 1972; **36**: 494–502.
255 Cromwell TH, Stevens WC, Eger EI II, *et al.* The cardiovascular effects of compound 469 (Forane) during spontaneous ventilation and CO2 challenge in man. *Anesthesiology* 1971; **35**(1): 17–25.
256 Cullen LK, Steffey EP, Bailey CS, *et al.* Effect of high PaCO2 and time on cerebrospinal fluid and intraocular pressure in halothane-anesthetized horses. *Am J Vet Res* 1990; **51**: 300–304.
257 Smith NT, Eger EI II, Stoelting RK, *et al.* The cardiovascular and sympathomimetic response to the addition of nitrous oxide to halothane in man. *Anesthesiology* 1970; **32**(5): 410–421.
258 Yamashita K, Tsubakishita S, Futaoka S, *et al.* Cardiovascular effects of medetomidine, detomidine and xylazine in horses. *J Vet Med Sci* 2000; **62**(10): 1025–1032.
259 Yasuda N, Weiskopf RB, Cahalan MK, *et al.* Does desflurane modify circulatory responses to stimulation in humans. *Anesth Analg* 1991; **73**: 175–179.
260 Zbinden AM, Petersenfelix S, Thomson DA. Anesthetic depth defined using multiple noxious stimuli during isoflurane/oxygen anesthesia. II. hemodynamic responses. *Anesthesiology* 1994; **80**(2): 261–267.
261 Antognini JF, Berg K. Cardiovascular responses to noxious stimuli during isoflurane anesthesia are minimally affected by anesthetic action in the brain. *Anesth Analg* 1995; **81**: 843–848.
262 March PA, Muir WW, III. Minimum alveolar concentration measures of central nervous system activation in cats anesthetized with isoflurane. *Am J Vet Res* 2003; **64**(12): 1528–1533.
263 Love L, Egger C, Rohrbach B, *et al.* The effect of ketamine on the MACBAR of sevoflurane in dogs. *Vet Anaesth Analg* 2011; **38**(4): 292–300.
264 Yamashita K, Frukawa E, Itami T, *et al.* Minimum alveolar concentratin for blunting adrenergic responses (MAC-BAR) of sevoflurane in dogs. *J Vet Med Sci* 2012; **74**(4): 507–511.
265 Hofmeister EH, Brainard BM, Sams LM, *et al.* Evaluation of induction characteristics and hypnotic potency of isoflurane and sevoflurane in healthy dogs. *Am J Vet Res* 2008; **69**(4): 451–456.
266 Schmeling WT, Ganjoo P, Staunton M, *et al.* Pretreatment with dexmedetomidine: altered indices of anesthetic depth for halothane in the neuraxis of cats. *Anesth Analg* 1999; **88**: 625–632.
267 Eger EI II, Smith NT, Stoelting RK, *et al.* Cardiovascular effects of halothane in man. *Anesthesiology* 1970; **32**(5): 396–409.
268 Eger EI II, Bowland T, Ionescu P, *et al.* Recovery and kinetic characteristics of desflurane and sevoflurane in volunteers after 8-h exposure, including kinetics of degradation products. *Anesthesiology* 1997; **87**(3): 517–526.
269 Tayefeh F, Larson MD, Sessler DI, *et al.* Time-dependent changes in heart rate and pupil size during desflurane or sevoflurane anesthesia. *Anesth Analg* 1997; **85**(12): 1362–1366.
270 Cullen BF, Eger EI II, Smith NT, *et al.* Cardiovascular effects of fluroxene in man. *Anesthesiology* 1970; **32**(3): 218–230.
271 Libonati M, Cooperman LH, Price HL. Time-dependent circulatory effects of methoxyflurane in man. *Anesthesiology* 1971; **34**: 439–444.
272 Gregory GA, Eger EI II, Smith NT. The cardiovascular effects of diethyl ether in man. *Anesthesiology* 1971; **34**(1): 19–24.
273 Dunlop CI, Steffey EP, Miller MF, Woliner MJ. Temporal effects of halothane and isoflurane in laterally recumbent ventilated male horses. *Am J Vet Res* 1987; **48**: 1250–1255.
274 Steffey EP, Dunlop CI, Cullen LK, *et al.* Circulatory and respiratory responses of spontaneously breathing, laterally recumbent horses to 12 hours of halothane anesthesia. *Am J Vet Res* 1993; **54**: 929–936.
275 Yamanaka T, Oku K, Koyama H, Mizuno Y. Time-related changes of the cardiovascular system during maintenance anesthesia with sevoflurane and isoflurane in horses. *J Vet Med Sci* 2001; **63**(5): 527–532.
276 Whitehair KJ, Steffey EP, Willits NH, Woliner MJ. Recovery of horses from inhalation anesthesia. *Am J Vet Res* 1993; **54**: 1693–1702.
277 Steffey EP, Woliner MJ, Dunlop C. Effects of five hours of constant 1.2 MAC halothane in sternally recumbent, spontaneously breathing horses. *Equine Vet J* 1990; **22**: 433–436.
278 Shimosato S, Yasuda I. Cardiac performance during prolonged halothane anaesthesia in the cat. *Br J Anaesth* 1978; **50**: 215–219.
279 Price HL, Skovsted P, Pauca AL, Cooperman LH. Evidence for b-receptor activation produced by halothane in normal man. *Anesthesiology* 1970; **32**(5): 389–395.
280 Steffey EP, Howland D Jr. Potency of halothane-N_2O in the horse. *Am J Vet Res* 1978; **39**: 1141–1146.
281 Bahlman SH, Eger EI II, Smith NT, *et al.* The cardiovascular effects of nitrous oxide–halothane anesthesia in man. *Anesthesiology* 1971; **35**(3): 274–255.
282 Eisele JH Jr. Cardiovascular effects of nitrous oxide. In: Eger EI II, ed. *Nitrous Oxide/N2O*. New York: Elsevier, 1985; 125–156.
283 Steffey EP, Eger EI II. Nitrous oxide in veterinary practice and animal research. In: Eger EI II, ed. *Nitrous Oxide/N2O*.New York: Elsiever, 1984; 305–312.
284 Grandy JL, Hodgson DS, Dunlop CI, *et al.* Cardiopulmonary effects of ephedrine in halothane-anesthetized horses. *J Vet Pharmacol Ther* 1989; **12**: 389–396.
285 Dyson DH, Pascoe PJ. Influence of preinduction methoxamine, lactated ringer solution, or hypertonic saline solution infusion or postinduction dobutamine infusion on anesthetic-induced hypotension in horses. *Am J Vet Res* 1990; **51**(1): 17–21.
286 Swanson CR, Muir WW, III, Bednarski RM, *et al.* Hemodynamic responses in halothane-anesthetized horses given infusions of dopamine or dobutamine. *Am J Vet Res* 1985; **46**: 365–371.
287 Priano LL, Marrone B. Effect of halothane on renal hemodynamics during normovolemia and acute hemorrhagic hypovolemia. *Anesthesiology* 1985; **63**(4): 357–364.
288 Gelman S, Fowler KC, Smith LR. Regional blood flow during isoflurane and halothane anesthesia. *Anesth Analg* 1984; **63**(6): 557–566.
289 Steffey EP, Zinkl J, Howland D Jr. Minimal changes in blood cell counts and biochemical values associated with prolonged isoflurane anesthesia of horses. *Am J Vet Res* 1979; **40**(11): 1646–1648.
290 Steffey EP, Farver T, Zinkl J, *et al.* Alterations in horse blood cell count and biochemical values after halothane anesthesia. *Am J Vet Res* 1980; **41**(6): 934–939.
291 Stover SM, Steffey EP, Dybdal NO, Franti CE. Hematologic and biochemical values associated with multiple halothane anesthesias and minor surgical trauma of horses. *Am J Vet Res* 1988; **49**: 236–241.
292 Steffey EP, Giri SN, Dunlop CI, *et al.* Biochemical and haematological changes following prolonged halothane anaesthesia in horses. *Res Vet Sci* 1993; **55**: 338–345.
293 Nunez E, Steffey EP, Ocampo L, *et al.* Effects of alpha-2 adrenergic receptor agonists on urine production in horses deprived of food and water. *Am J Vet Res* 2004; **65**(10): 1342–1346.
294 Pedersoli WM. Blood serum inorganic ionic fluoride tetracycline and methoxyflurane anesthesia in dogs. *J Am Anim Hosp Assoc* 1977; **13**: 242–246.
295 Mazze RI, Trudell JR, Cousins MJ. Methoxyflurane metabolism and renal dysfunction: clinical correlation in man. *Anesthesiology* 1971; **35**: 247–252.
296 Leiman BC, Katz J, Stanley TH, Butler BD. Removal of tracheal secretions in anesthetized dogs: balloon catheters versus suction. *Anesth Analg* 1987; **66**: 529–533.
297 Mazze RI, Calverley RK, Smith NT. Inorganic fluoride nephrotoxicity: prolonged enflurane and halothane anesthesia in volunteers. *Anesthesiology* 1977; **46**: 265–271.
298 Kharasch ED, Hankins DC, Thummel KE. Human kidney methoxyflurane and sevoflurane metabolism – intrarenal fluoride production as a possible mechanism of methoxyflurane nephrotoxicity. *Anesthesiology* 1995; **82**(3): 689–699.

299 Morio M, Fujii K, Satoh N, *et al.* Reaction of sevoflurane and its degradation products with soda lime. *Anesthesiology* 1992; **77**: 1155–1164.

300 Gonsowski CT, Laster MJ, Eger EI II, *et al.* Toxicity of compound A in rats: effect of a 3-hour administration. *Anesthesiology* 1994; **80**: 556–565.

301 Gonsowski CT, Laster MJ, Eger EI II, *et al.* Toxicity of compound A in rats: effect of increasing duration of administration. *Anesthesiology* 1994; **80**: 566–573.

302 Kandel L, Laster MJ, Eger EI II, *et al.* Nephrotoxicity in rats undergoing a one-hour exposure to compound A. *Anesth Analg* 1995; **81**: 559–563.

303 Frink EJ Jr, Malan TP Jr, Isner RJ, *et al.* Renal concentrating function with prolonged sevoflurane or enflurane anesthesia in volunteers. *Anesthesiology* 1994; **80**: 1019–1025.

304 Muir WW III, Gadawski JE. Cardiorespiratory effects of low-flow and closed circuit inhalation anesthesia, using sevoflurane delivered with an in-circuit vaporizer and concentrations of compound A. *Am J Vet Res* 1998; **59**(5): 603–608.

305 Reilly CS, Wood AJJ, Koshakji RP, Wood M. The effect of halothane on drug disposition: contribution of changes in intrinsic drug metabolizing capacity and hepatic blood flow. *Anesthesiology* 1985; **63**: 70–76.

306 Pearson GR, Bogan JA, Sanford J. An increase in the half-life of pentobarbitone with the administration of halothane in sheep. *Br J Anaesth* 1973; **45**: 586–591.

307 Steffey EP, Martucci R, Howland D, *et al.* Meperidine–halothane interaction in dogs. *Can Anaesth Soc J* 1977; **24**(4): 459–467.

308 Smith CM, Steffey EP, Baggot JD, *et al.* Effects of halothane anesthesia on the clearance of gentamicin sulfate in horses. *Am J Vet Res* 1988; **49**(1): 19–22.

309 White PF, Johnston RR, Pudwill CR. Interaction of ketamine and halothane in rats. *Anesthesiology* 1975; **42**: 179–186.

310 Subcommittee of the National Halothane Study of the Committee on Anesthesia NAoS-NRC. Summary of the National Halothane Study: possible association between halothane anesthesia and postoperative hepatic necrosis. *JAMA* 1966; **197**: 121–134.

311 Inman WHW, Mushin WW. Jaundice after repeated exposure to halothane: an analysis of reports to the Committee on Safety of Medicines. *BMJ J* 1974; **1**: 5–10.

312 Holmes MA, Weiskopf RB, Eger EI II, *et al.* Hepatocellular integrity in swine after prolonged desflurane (I-653) and isoflurane anesthesia: evaluation of plasma alanine aminotransferase activity. *Anesth Analg* 1990; **71**: 249–253.

313 Eger EI II, Johnson BH, Ferrell LD. Comparison of the toxicity of I-653 and isoflurane in rats: a test of the effect of repeated anesthesia and use of dry soda lime. *Anesth Analg* 1987; **66**: 1230–1233.

314 Strum DP, Eger EI II, Johnson BH, *et al.* Toxicity of sevoflurane in rats. *Anesth Analg* 1987; **66**: 769–773.

315 Eger EI II, Johnson BH, Strum DP, Ferrell LD. Studies of the toxicity of I-653, halothane, and isoflurane in enzyme-induced, hypoxic rats. *Anesth Analg* 1987; **66**: 1227–1230.

316 Ross JAS, Monk SJ, Duffy SW. Effect of nitrous oxide on halothane-induced hepatotoxicity in hypoxic, enzyme-induced rats. *Br J Anaesth* 1984; **56**(5): 527–533.

317 Shingu K, Eger EI II, Johnson BH. Hypoxia per se can produce hepatic damage without death in rats. *Anesth Analg* 1982; **61**: 820–823.

318 Shingu K, Eger EI II, Johnson BH. Hypoxia may be more important than reductive metabolism in halothane-induced hepatic injury. *Anesth Analg* 1982; **61**: 824–827.

319 Whitehair KJ, Steffey EP, Woliner MJ, Willits NH. Effects of inhalation anesthetic agents on response of horses to three hours of hypoxemia. *Am J Vet Res* 1996; **57**: 351–360.

320 Reynolds ES, Moslen MT. Liver injury following halothane anesthesia in phenobarbital-pretreated rats. *Biochem Pharmacol* 1974; **23**: 189–195.

321 Reynolds ES, Moslen MT. Halothane hepatotoxicity: enhancement by polychlorinated biphenyl pretreatment. *Anesthesiology* 1977; **47**(1): 19–27.

322 Cooperman LH, Warden JC, Price HL. Splanchnic circulation during nitrous oxide anesthesia and hypocarbia in normal man. *Anesthesiology* 1968; **29**: 254–258.

323 Johnson EE, Hedley-Whyte J. Continuous positive-pressure ventilation and choledochoduodenal flow resistance. *J Appl Physiol* 1975; **39**: 937–942.

324 Davis M, Eddleston ALWF, Neuberger JM, *et al.* Halothane hepatitis. *N Engl J Med* 1980; **303**(19): 1123–1124.

325 Kitteringham NR, Kenna JG, Park BK. Detection of autoantibodies directed against human hepatic endoplasmic reticulum in sera from patients with halothane-associated hepatitis. *Br J Clin Pharmacol* 1995; **40**(4): 379–386.

326 Farrell G, Prendergast D, Murray M. Halothane hepatitis: detection of a constitutional susceptibility factor. *N Engl J Med* 1985; **313**: 1310–1315.

327 Denborough MA, Forster JFP, Lovell RRH. Anaesthetic deaths in a family. *Br J Anaesth* 1962; **34**: 395–396.

328 Gronert GA, Antognini JF, Pessah IN. Malignant hyperthermia. In: Miller RD, ed. *Anesthesia*, 5th edn. Philadelphia: Churchill Livingstone, 2000; 1033–1052.

329 Hall LW, Woolf N, Bradley JWP, Jolly DW. Unusual reaction to suxamethonum chloride. *BMJ* 1966; **2**: 1305.

330 Kirmayer AH, Klide AM, Purvance JE. Malignant hyperthermia in a dog: case report and review of the syndrome. *J Am Vet Med Assoc* 1984; **185**: 978–983.

331 Deuster PA, Bockman EL, Muldoon SM. In vitro responses of cat skeletal muscle to halothane and caffeine. *J Appl Physiol* 1985; **58**: 521–528.

332 Bagshaw RJ, Cox RH, Knight DH, Detwiler DK. Malignant hyperthermia in a grayhound. *J Am Vet Med Assoc* 1978; **172**: 61.

333 Rosenberg H, Waldron-Mease E. Malignant hyperpyrexia in horses: anesthetic sensitivity proven by muscle biopsy (abstract). In: *Annual Meeting of the American Society of Anesthesiologists* 1977; 333–334.

334 Hildebrand SV, Howitt GA. Succinylcholine infusion associated with hyperthermia in ponies anesthetized with halothane. *Am J Vet Res* 1983; **44**: 2280–2284.

335 Short C, Paddleford RR. Malignant hyperthermia in the dog – letter. *Anesthesiology* 1973; **39**: 462–463.

336 deJong RH, Heavner JE, Amory DW. Malignant hyperpyrexia in the cat. *Anesthesiology* 1974; **41**: 608–609.

337 Aleman M, Brosnan RJ, Williams DC, *et al.* Malignant hyperthermia in a horse anesthetized with halothane. *J Vet Intern Med* 2005; **19**: 363–367.

338 Aleman M, Riehl J, Aldridge BM, *et al.* Association of a mutation in the ryanodine receptor 1 gene with equine malignant hyperthermia. *Muscle Nerve* 2004; **30**(3): 356–365.

339 Aleman M, Aldridge BM, Riehl J, *et al.* Equine malignant hyperthermia. *Proc Am Assoc Equine Pract* 2004; **50**: 51–54.

340 Epstein RM, Rackow H, Salanitre E, Wolf GL. Influence of the concentration effect on the uptake of anesthetic mixtures: the second gas effect. *Anesthesiology* 1964; **25**: 364–371.

341 Stoelting RK, Eger EI II. An additional explanation for the second gas effect: a concentrating effort. *Anesthesiology* 1969; **30**(3): 273–277.

342 Taheri S, Eger EI. A demonstration of the concentration and second gas effects in humans anesthetized with nitrous oxide and desflurane. *Anesth Analg* 1999; **89**: 774–780.

343 Fukunaga AF, Epstein RM. Sympathetic excitation during nitrous oxide–halothane anesthesia in the cat. *Anesthesiology* 1973; **39**: 23–36.

344 Pypendop BH, Ilkiw JE, Imai A, Bolich JA. Hemodynamic effects of nitrous oxide in isoflurane-anesthetized cats. *Am J Vet Res* 2003; **64**(3): 273–278.

345 Liu WS, Wong KC, Port JD, Aridriano KP. Epinephrine-induced arrhythmia during halothane anesthesia with the addition of nitrous oxide, nitrogen or helium in dogs. *Anesth Analg* 1982; **61**: 414–417.

346 Lampe GH, Donegan JH, Rupp SM, *et al.* Nitrous oxide and epinephrine-induced arrhythmias. *Anesth Analg* 1990; **71**: 602–605.

347 Philbin DM, Foex P, Drummond G, *et al.* Postsystolic shortening of canine left ventricle supplied by a stenotic coronary artery when nitrous oxide is added in the presence of narcotics. *Anesthesiology* 1985; **62**: 166–174.

348 Leone BJ, Philbin DM, Lehot JJ, *et al.* Gradual or abrupt nitrous oxide administration in a canine model of critical coronary stenosis induces regional myocardial dysfunction that is worsened by halothane. *Anesth Analg* 1988; **67**: 814–822.

349 Nathan HJ. Nitrous oxide worsens myocardial ischemia in isoflurane-anesthetized dogs. *Anesthesiology* 1988; **68**: 407–416.

350 Diedericks J, Leone BJ, Foex P, *et al.* Nitrous oxide causes myocardial ischemia when added to propofol in the compromised canine myocardium. *Anesth Analg* 1993; **76**: 1322–1326.

351 Saidman LJ, Hamilton WK. We should continue to use nitrous oxide. In: Eger EI II, ed. *Nitrous Oxide/N2O* New York: Elsevier, 1985; 345–353.

352 Eger EI II, Lampe GH, Wauk LZ, *et al.* Clinical pharmacology of nitrous oxide: an argument for its continued use. *Anesth Analg* 1990; **71**: 575–585.

353 Lampe GH, Wauk LZ, Whitendale P, *et al.* Nitrous oxide does not impair hepatic function in young or old surgical patients. *Anesth Analg* 1990; **71**: 606–609.

354 Brodsky JB. Toxicity of nitrous oxide. In: Eger EI II, ed. *Nitrous Oxide/N2O* New York: Elsevier, **1985**; 259–279.

355 Lampe GH, Wauk LZ, Donegan JH, *et al.* Effect on outcome of prolonged exposure of patients to nitrous oxide. *Anesth Analg* 1990; **71**: 586–590.

356 Waldman FM, Koblin DD, Lampe GH, *et al.* Hematologic effects of nitrous oxide in surgical patients. *Anesth Analg* 1990; **71**: 618–624.

357 Nunn JF, Chanarin I. Nitrous oxide inactivates methionine synthetase. In: Eger EI II, ed. *Nitrous Oxide/N2O* New York: Elsevier, 1985; 211–233.

358 Koblin DD, Tomerson BW, Waldman FM, *et al.* Effect of nitrous oxide on folate and vitamin B12 metabolism in patients. *Anesth Analg* 1990; **71**: 610–617.

359 Layzer RB, Fishman RA, Schafer JA. Neuropathy following abuse of nitrous oxide. *Neurology* 1978; **28**: 504–506.

360 Layzer RB. Myeloneuropathy after prolonged exposure to nitrous oxide. *Lancet* 1978; **2**: 1227–1230.

361 Hong K, Trudell JR, O'Neil JR, Cohen EN. Biotransformation of nitrous oxide. *Anesthesiology* 1980; **53**: 354–355.

362 Hong K, Trudell JR, O'Neil JR, Cohen EN. Metabolism of nitrous oxide by human and rat intestinal contents. *Anesthesiology* 1980; **52**: 16–19.

363 Weathersby PK, Homer LD. Solubility of inert gases in biological fluids and tissues: a review. *Undersea Biomed Res* 1980; **7**: 277–296.
364 Steffey EP, Johnson BH, Eger EI II, Howland D Jr. Nitrous oxide increases the accumulation rate and decreases the uptake of bowel gases. *Anesth Analg* 1979; **58**: 405–408.
365 Eger EI II, Saidman LJ. Hazards of nitrous oxide anesthesia in bowel obstruction and pneumothorax. *Anesthesiology* 1965; **26**(1): 61–66.
366 Steffey EP, Gauger GE, Eger EI II. Cardiovascular effects of venous air embolism during air and oxygen breathing. *Anesth Analg* 1974; **53**: 599–604.
367 Munson ES, Merrick HC. Effect of nitrous oxide on venous air embolism. *Anesthesiology* 1966; **27**: 783–787.
368 Davis I, Moore JRM, Lahiri SK. Nitrous oxide and the middle ear. *Anaesthesia* 1979; **34**: 147–151.
369 Perreault L, Normandin N, Plamondon L, *et al.* Middle ear pressure variations during nitrous oxide and oxygen anaesthesia. *Can Anaesth Soc J* 1982; **29**(5): 428–434.
370 Saidman LJ, Eger EI II. Change in cerebrospinal fluid pressure during pneumoencephalography under nitrous oxide anesthesia. *Anesthesiology* 1965; **26**(1): 67–72.
371 Stanley TH, Kawamura R, Graves C. Effects of N2O on volume and pressure of endotracheal tube cuffs. *Anesthesiology* 1974; **41**: 256–262.
372 Stanley TH. Effects of anesthetic gases on endotracheal tube cuff gas volumes. *Anesth Analg* 1974; **53**(3): 480–482.
373 Stanley TH. Nitrous oxide and pressures and volumes of high- and low-pressure endotracheal tube cuffs in intubated patients. *Anesthesiology* 1975; **42**: 637–640.
374 Bednarski RM. Advantages and guidelines for using nitrous oxide. *Vet Clin North Am Small Anim Pract* 1992; **22**: 313–314.
375 Klide AM, Haskins SC. Precautions when using nitrous oxide. *Vet Clin North Am Small Anim Pract* 1992; **22**: 314–316.
376 Linde HW, Bruce DL. Occupational exposure of anesthetists to halothane, nitrous oxide and radiation. *Anesthesiology* 1969; **30**: 363–368.
377 Whitcher CE, Cohen EN, Trudell JR. Chronic exposure to anesthetic gases in the operating room. *Anesthesiology* 1971; **35**: 348–353.
378 Ward GS, Byland RR. Concentrations of methoxyflurane and nitrous oxide in veterinary operating rooms. *Am J Vet Res* 1982; **43**: 360–362.
379 Ward GS, Byland RR. Concentrations of halothane in veterinary operating and treatment rooms. *J Am Vet Med Assoc* 1982; **180**: 174–177.
380 Milligan JE, Sablan JL, Short CE. A survey of waste anesthetic gas concentrations in U.S. Airforce veterinary surgeries. *J Am Vet Med Assoc* 1980; **177**: 1021–1022.
381 Dreesen DW, Jones GL, Brown J, Rawlings CA. Monitoring for trace anesthetic gases in a veterinary teaching hospital. *J Am Vet Med Assoc* 1981; **179**: 797–799.
382 Manley SV, McDonell WF. Recommendations for reduction of anesthetic gas pollution. *J Am Vet Med Assoc* 1980; **176**: 519–524.
383 Manley SV, Taloff P, Aberg N, Howitt GA. Occupational exposure to waste anesthetic gases in veterinary practice. *California Vet* 1982; **36**: 14–19.
384 Pfaffli P, Nikki P, Ahlman K. Halothane and nitrous oxide in end-tidal air and venous blood of surgical personnel. *Ann Clin Res* 1972; **4**: 273–277.
385 Corbett TH. Retention of anesthetic agents following occupational exposure. *Anesth Analg* 1973; **52**: 614–618.
386 Ad Hoc Committee on Effects of Trace Anesthetic Agents on Health of Operating Room Personnel. *Waste Anesthetic Gases in Operating Room Air: A Suggested Program to Reduce Personnel Exposure.* Park Ridge, IL: American Society of Anesthesiologists, 1983.
387 Cohen EN, Bellville JW, Brown BW. Anesthesia, pregnancy, and miscarriage: a study of operating room nurses and anesthetists. *Anesthesiology* 1971; **35**: 343–347.
388 Cohen EN, Brown BW Jr, Bruce DL, *et al.* A survey of anesthetic health hazards among dentists. *J Am Dental Assoc* 1975; **90**: 1291–1296.
389 Lecky JH. Anesthetic pollution in the operating room: a notice to operating room personnel. *Anesthesiology* 1980; **52**: 157–159.
390 Berry A, McGregor DG, Baden JM, *et al. Waste Anesthetic Gases: Information for Management in Anesthetizing Areas and The Postanesthetic Care Unit (PACU).* Park Ridge, IL: American Society of Anesthesiologists, 2005.
391 American College of Veterinary Anesthesiologists Ad Hoc Committee on Waste Anesthetic Gas Pollution and Its Control. Commentary and recommendations on control of waste anesthetic gases in the workplace. *J Am Vet Med Assoc* 1996; **209**: 75–77.
392 Sessler DI, Badgwell JM. Exposure of postoperative nurses to exhaled anesthetic gases. *Anesth Analg* 1998; **87**: 1083–1088.
393 Summer G, Lirk P, Hoerauf K, *et al.* Sevoflurane in exhaled air of operating room personnel. *Anesth Analg* 2003; **97**(4): 1070–1073.
394 Cicerone RJ, Stolarski RS, Walters S. Stratospheric ozone destruction by man-made chlorofluoromethanes. *Science* 1974; **185**(4157): 1165–1167.
395 Fox JWC, Fox EJ, Villanueva R. Stratospheric ozone destruction and halogenated anaesthetics. *Lancet* 1975; **1**: 864.
396 Sherman SJ, Cullen BF. Nitrous oxide and the greenhouse effect. *Anesthesiology* 1988; **68**(5): 816–817.
397 Rowland FS. Chlorofluorocarbons and the depletion of stratospheric ozone. *Am Sci* 1989; **77**: 36–45.
398 Rowland FS. Stratospheric ozone depletion. *Phil Trans R Soc London B Biol Sci* 2006; **361**(1469): 769–790.
399 Logan M, Farmer JG. Anaesthesia and the ozone layer. *Br J Anaesth* 1989; **63**(6): 645–647.
400 Ishizawa Y. General anesthetic gases and the global environment. *Anesth Analg* 2011; **112**(1): 213–217.
401 Langbein T, Sonntag H, Trapp D, *et al.* Volatile anaesthetics and the atmosphere: atmospheric lifetimes and atmospheric effects of halothane, enflurane, isoflurane, desflurane and sevoflurane. *Br J Anaesth* 1999; **82**(1): 66–73.
402 Sulbaek Andersen MP, Nielsen OJ, Wallington TJ, Karpichev B, Sander SP. Assessing the impact on global climate from general anesthetic gases. *Anesth Analg* 2012; **114**(5): 1081–1085.
403 Ravishankara AR, Daniel JS, Portmann RW. Nitrous oxide (N2O): the dominant ozone-depleting substance emitted in the 21st century. *Science* 2009; **326**: 123–125.
404 United Nations. *Montreal Protocol on Substances that Deplete the Ozone Layer.* http://ozone.unep.org/newsite/en/montrealprotocol.php (accessed 19 September 2014).
405 Ryan SM, Nielsen CJ. Global warming potential of inhaled anesthetics: application to clinical use. *Anesth Analg* 2010; **111**(1): 92–98.
406 Sulbaek Andersen MP, Sander SP, Nielsen O, *et al.* Inhalation anaesthetics and climate change. *Br J Anaesth* 2010; **105**(6): 760–766.
407 Ryan S. Sustainable anesthesia. *Anesth Analg* 2012; **114**(5): 921–923.
408 Mychaskiw G II, Eger EI II. A different perspective on anesthetics and climate change. *Anesth Analg* 2013; **116**(3): 734–735.
409 Sulbaek Andersen MP, Nielsen OJ, Karpichev B, *et al.* Atmospheric chemistry of isoflurane, desflurane, and sevoflurane: kinetics and mechanisms of reactions with chlorine atoms and OH radicals and global warming potentials. *J Phys Chem* 2012; **116**: 5806–5820.
410 Sherman J, Le C, Lamers V, Eckelman M. Life cycle greenhouse gas emissions of anesthetic drugs. *Anesth Analg* 2012; **114**(5): 1086–1089.
411 Karzai W, Haberstroh J, Muller W, Priebe HJ. Rapid increase in inspired desflurane concentration does not elicit a hyperdynamic circulatory response in the pig. *Lab Anim* 1997; **31**: 279–282.
412 Rodgers RC, Hill GE. Equations for vapour pressure versus temperature: derivation and use of the Antoine equation on a hand-held programmable calculator. *Br J Anaesth* 1978; **50**: 415–424.
413 Susay SR, Smith MA, Lockwood GG. The saturated vapor pressure of desflurane at various temperatures. *Anesth Analg* 1996; **83**: 864–866.
414 Eger EI II. Desflurane animal and human pharmacology: aspects of kinetics, safety, and MAC. *Anesth Analg* 1992; **75**: S3–S9.
415 Webb AI, Weaver BMQ. Solubility of halothane in equine tissues at 37°C. *Br J Anaesth* 1981; **53**: 479–486.
416 Kety SS, Harmel MH, Broomell HT, Rhode CB. The solubility of nitrous oxide in blood and brain. *J Biol Chem* 1948; **173**: 487–496.
417 Wahrenbrock EA, Eger EI II, Laravuso RB, Maruschak G. Anesthetic uptake – of mice and men (and whales). *Anesthesiology* 1974; **40**: 19–23.
418 Coburn CM, Eger EI II. The partial pressure of isoflurane or halothane does not affect their solubility in rabbit blood or brain or human brain: inhaled anesthetics obey Henry's law. *Anesth Analg* 1986; **65**(9): 960–963.
419 Soares JHN, Brosnan RJ, Fukushima FB, *et al.* Solubility of haloether anesthetics in human and animal blood. *Anesthesiology* 2012; **117**(1): 48–55.
420 Targ AG, Yasuda N, Eger EI II. Solubility of I-653, sevoflurane, isoflurane, and halothane in plastics and rubber composing a conventional anesthetic circuit. *Anesth Analg* 1989; **69**: 218–225.
421 Cascorbi HF, Blake DA, Helrich M. Differences in the biotransformation of halothane in man. *Anesthesiology* 1970; **32**: 119–123.
422 Shiraishi Y, Ikeda K. Uptake and biotransformation of sevoflurane in humans: a comparative study of sevoflurane with halothane, enflurane and isoflurane. *J Clin Anesth* 1990; **2**(6): 377–380.
423 Chase RE, Holaday DA, Fiserova-Bergerova V, *et al.* The biotransformation of ethrane in man. *Anesthesiology* 1971; **35**(3): 262–267.
424 Holaday DA, Fiserova-Bergerova V, Latto IP, Zumbiel MA. Resistance of isoflurane to biotransformation in man. *Anesthesiology* 1975; **43**: 325–332.
425 McMurphy RM, Hodgson DS. The minimum alveolar concentration of desflurane in cats. *Vet Surg* 1995; **24**: 453–455.
426 Barter LS, Ilkiw JE, Steffey EP, *et al.* Animal dependence of inhaled anaeshtetic requirements in cats. *Br J Anaesth* 2004; **92**(2): 275–277.
427 Webb AI, McMurphy RM. Effect of anticholinergic preanesthetic medicaments on the requirements of halothane for anesthesia in the cat. *Am J Vet Res* 1987; **48**: 1733–1736.

428 Ide T, Sakurai Y, Aono M, Nishino T. Minimum alveolar anesthetic concentrations for airway occlusion in cats: a new concept of minimum alveolar anesthetic concentration airway occlusion response. *Anesth Analg* 1998; **86**(1): 191–197.

429 Steffey EP, Gillespie JR, Berry JD, *et al.* Anesthetic potency (MAC) of nitrous oxide in the dog, cat and stumptail monkey. *J Appl Physiol* 1974; **36**: 530–532.

430 Drummond JC, Todd MM, Shapiro HM. Minimal alveolar concentrations for halothane, enflurane, and isoflurane in the cat. *J Am Vet Med Assoc* 1983; **182**: 1099–1101.

431 Ilkiw JE, Pascoe PJ, Fisher LD. Effect of alfentanil on the mimimum alveolar concentration of isoflurane in cats. *Am J Vet Res* 1997; **58**(11): 1274–1279.

432 Pypendop BH, Ilkiw JE. The effects of intravenous lidocaine administration on the minimum alveolar concentration of isoflurane in cats. *Anesth Analg* 2005; **100**(1): 97–101.

433 Doi M, Yunoki H, Ikeda K. The minimum alevolar concentration of sevoflurane in cats. *J Anesth* 1988; **2**: 113–114.

434 Steffey EP, Howland D Jr. Halothane anesthesia in calves. *Am J Vet Res* 1979; **40**: 372–376.

435 Cantalapierdra AG, Villanueva B, Pereira JL. Anaesthetic potency of isoflurane in cattle: determination of the minimum alveolar concentration. *Vet Anaesth Analg* 2000; **27**(1): 22–26.

436 Doorley MB, Waters SJ, Terrell RC, Robinson JL. MAC of I-653 in beagle dogs and New Zealand white rabbits. *Anesthesiology* 1988; **69**: 89–92.

437 Wang BG, Tang J, White PF, *et al.* The effect of GP683, an adenosine kinase inhibitor, on the desflurane anesthetic requirement in dogs. *Anesth Analg* 1997; **85**: 675–680.

438 Hammond RA, Alibhai HIK, Walsh KP, *et al.* Desflurane in the dog; minimum alveolar concentration (MAC) alone and in combination with nitrous oxide. *J Vet Anaesth* 1994; **21**: 21–23.

439 Eger EI II, Brandstater B, Saidman LJ, *et al.* Equipotent alveolar concentrations of methoxyflurane, halothane, diethyl ether, fluroxene, cyclopropane, xenon, and nitrous oxide in the dog. *Anesthesiology* 1965; **26**(6): 771–777.

440 Regan MJ, Eger EI II. Effect of hypothermia in dogs on anesthetizing and apneic doses of inhalation agents. Determination of the anesthetic index (apnea/MAC). *Anesthesiology* 1967; **28**(4): 689–700.

441 Kazama T, Ikeda K. Comparison of MAC and the rate of rise of alveolar concentration of sevoflurane with halothane and isoflurane in the dog. *Anesthesiology* 1988; **68**: 435–438.

442 Steffey EP, Eger EI II. Hyperthermia and halothane MAC in the dog. *Anesthesiology* 1974; **41**(4): 392–396.

443 Himez RS Jr, DiFazio CA, Burmey RC. Effects of lidocaine on the anesthetic requirements of nitrous oxide and halothane. *Anesthesiology* 1977; **47**: 437–440.

444 Schwieger IM, Szlam F, Hug CC. Absence of agonistic or antagonistic effect of flumazenil (Ro 15-1788) in dogs anesthetized with enflurane, isoflurane, or fentanyl-enflurane. *Anesthesiology* 1989; **70**(3): 477–481.

445 Schwartz AE, Maneksha FR, Kanchuger MS, *et al.* Flumazenil decreases the minimum alveolar concentration of isoflurane in dogs. *Anesthesiology* 1989; **70**(5): 764–767.

446 DeYoung DJ, Sawyer DC. Anesthetic potency of nitrous oxide during halothane anesthesia in the dog. *J Am Anim Hosp Assoc* 1980; **16**: 125–128.

447 Murat I, Housmans PR. Minimum alveolar concentrations of halothane, enflurane, and isoflurane in ferrets. *Anesthesiology* 1988; **68**(5): 783–787.

448 Imai A, Steffey EP, Farver TB, Ilkiw JE. Assessment of isoflurane-induced anesthesia in ferrets and rats. *Am J Vet Res* 1999; **60**(12): 1577–1583.

449 Hikasa Y, Okuyama K, Kakuta T, *et al.* Anesthetic potency and cardiopulmonary effects of sevoflurane in goats: comparison with isoflurane and halothane. *Can J Vet Res* 1998; **62**: 299–306.

450 Antognini JF, Eisele PH. Anesthetic potency and cardiopulmonary effects of enflurane, halothane, and isoflurane in goats. *Lab Anim Sci* 1993; **43**: 607–610.

451 Doherty TJ, Rohrbach BW, Geiser DR. Effect of acepromazine and butorphanol on isoflurane minimum alveolar concentration in goats. *J Vet Pharmacol Ther* 2002; **25**: 65–67.

452 Doherty TJ, Rohrbach BW, Ross L, Schultz H. The effect of tiletamine and zolazepam on isoflurane minimum alveolar concentration in goats. *J Vet Pharmacol Ther* 2002; **25**(3): 233–235.

453 Doherty TJ, Will WA, Rohrbach BW, Geiser DR. Effect of morphine and flunixin meglumine on isoflurane minimum alveolar concentration in goats. *Vet Anaesth Analg* 2004; **31**(2): 97–101.

454 Tendillo FJ, Mascias A, Santos M, *et al.* Anesthetic potency of desflurane in the horse: determination of the minimum alveolar concentration. *Vet Surg* 1997; **26**(4): 354–357.

455 Steffey EP, Willits N, Woliner M. Hemodynamic and respiratory responses to variable arterial partial pressure of oxygen in halothane-anesthetized horses during spontaneous and controlled ventilation. *Am J Vet Res* 1992; **53**: 1850–1858.

456 Pascoe PJ, Steffey EP, Black WD, *et al.* Evaluation of the effect of alfentanil on the minimum alveolar concentration on halothane in horses. *Am J Vet Res* 1993; **54**: 1327–1332.

457 Steffey EP, Pascoe PJ. Detomidine reduces isoflurane anesthetic requirement (MAC) in horses. *Vet Anaesth Analg* 2002; **29**(4): 223–227.

458 Steffey EP, Pascoe PJ, Woliner MJ, Berryman ER. Effects of xylazine hydrochloride during isoflurane-induced anesthesia in horses. *Am J Vet Res* 2000; **61**(10): 1225–1231.

459 Aida H, Mizuno Y, Hobo S, *et al.* Deterimination of the miniumum alveolar concentration (MAC) and physical response to sevoflurane inhalation in horses. *J Vet Med Sci* 1994; **56**: 1161–1165.

460 Tinker JH, Sharbough FW, Michenfelder TD. Anterior shift of the dominant EEG rhythm during anesthesia in the Java monkey. *Anesthesiology* 1977; **46**: 252–259.

461 Sonner JM, Gong D, Eger EI II. Naturally occurring variability in anesthetic potency among inbred mouse strains. *Anesth Analg* 2000; **91**: 720–726.

462 Mazze RI, Rice SA, Baden JM. Halothane, isoflurane, and enflurane MAC in pregnant and nonpregnant female and male mice and rats. *Anesthesiology* 1985; **62**: 339–342.

463 Deady JR, Koblin DD, Eger EI II, *et al.* Anesthetic potencies and the unitary theory of narcosis. *Anesth Analg* 1981; **60**: 380–384.

464 Quinlan JJ, Homanics GE, Firestone LL. Anesthesia sensitivity in mice that lack the b3 subunit of the g-aminobutyric acid type A receptor. *Anesthesiology* 1998; **88**: 775–780.

465 Dahan A, Sarton E, Teppema L, *et al.* Anesthetic potency and influence of morphine and sevoflurane on respiration in mu-opioid receptor knockout mice. *Anesthesiology* 2001; **94**: 824–832.

466 Miller KW, Paton WDM, Smith EB, Smith RA. Physiochemical approaches to the mode of action of general anesthetics. *Anesthesiology* 1972; **36**: 339–351.

467 Lerman J, Oyston JP, Gallagher TM, *et al.* The minimum alveolar concentration (MAC) and hemodynamic effects of halothane, isoflurane, and sevoflurane in newborn swine. *Anesthesiology* 1990; **73**: 717–721.

468 Tranquilli WJ, Thurmon JC, Benson GJ, Steffey EP. Halothane potency in pigs (Sus. scrofa). *Am J Vet Res* 1983; **44**: 1106–1107.

469 Weiskopf R, Bogetz MS. Minimum alveolar concentrations (MAC) of halothane and nitrous oxide in swine. *Anesth Analg* 1984; **63**: 529–532.

470 Lundeen G, Manohar M, Parks C. Systemic distribution of blood flow in swine while awake and during 1.0 and 1.5 MAC isoflurane anesthesia with or without 50% nitrous oxide. *Anesth Analg* 1983; **62**: 499–512.

471 Eisele PH, Talken L, Eisele JH Jr. Potency of isoflurane and nitrous oxide in conventional swine. *Lab Anim Sci* 1985; **35**: 76–78.

472 Tranquilli WJ, Thurmon JC, Benson GJ. Anesthetic potency of nitrous oxide in young swine (Sus scrofa). *Am J Vet Res* 1985; **46**: 58–61.

473 Gallagher TM, Burrows FA, Miyasaka K, *et al.* Sevoflurane in newborn swine: anesthetic requirements (MAC) and circulatory responses. *Anesthesiology* 1987; **67**: A503.

474 Hecker KE, Baumert JH, Horn N, *et al.* Minimum anesthetic concentration of sevoflurane with different xenon concentrations in swine. *Anesth Analg* 2003; **97**(5): 1364–1369.

475 Wear R, Robinson S, Gregory GA. Effect of halothane on baroresponse of adult and baby rabbits. *Anesthesiology* 1982; **56**: 188–191.

476 Davis NL, Nunnally RL, Malinin TI. Determination of the minimum alveolar concentration (MAC) of halothane in the white New Zealand rabbit. *Br J Anaesth* 1975; **47**: 341–345.

477 Sobair ATH, Cottrell DF, Camburn MA. Focal heat stimulation for the determination of the minimum alveolar concentration of halothane in the rabbit. *Vet Res Commun* 1997; **21**: 149–159.

478 Drummond JC. MAC for halothane, enflurane, and isoflurane in the New Zealand white rabbit: and a test for the validity of MAC determinations. *Anesthesiology* 1985; **62**(3): 336–339.

479 Imai A, Steffey EP, Ilkiw JE, Farver TB. Comparison of clinical signs and hemodynamic variables used to monitor rabbits during halothane- and isoflurane-induced anesthesia. *Am J Vet Res* 1999; **60**(10): 1189–1195.

480 McLain GE, Sipes IG, Brown B, Thompson MF. The noncompetitive N-methyl-D-aspartate receptor antagonist, MK-810 profoundly reduces volatile anesthetic requirements. *Neuropharmacology* 1989; **28**: 677–681.

481 Shi WZ, Fahey MR, Fisher DM, *et al.* Increase in minimum alveolar concentration (MAC) of halothane by laudanosine in rabbits. *Anesth Analg* 1985; **64**: 282.

482 Scheller MS, Saidman LJ, Partridge BL. MAC of sevoflurane in humans and the New Zealand white rabbit. *Can J Anaesth* 1988; **35**: 153–157.

483 Eger EI II, Johnson BH. MAC of I-653 in rats, including a test of the effect of body temperature and anesthetic duration. *Anesth Analg* 1987; **66**: 974–977.

484 Yost CS, Hampson AJ, Leonoudakis D, *et al.* Oleamide potentiates benzodiazepine-sensitive g-aminobutyric acid receptor activity but does not alter minimum alveolar anesthetic concentration. *Anesth Analg* 1998; **86**: 1294–1300.

485 Laster MJ, Liu J, Eger EI II, Taheri S. Electrical stimulation as a substitute for the tail clamp in the determination of minimum alveolar concentration. *Anesth Analg* 1993; **76**: 1310–1312.

486 Taheri S, Halsey MJ, Liu J, *et al.* What solvent best represents the site of action of inhaled anesthetics in humans, rats, and dogs? *Anesth Analg* 1991; **72**: 627–634.

487 Vitez TS, White PF, Eger EI II. Effects of hypothermia on halothane MAC and isoflurane MAC in the rat. *Anesthesiology* 1974; **41**: 80–81.

488 Cole DJ, Kalichman MW, Shapiro HM, Drummond JC. The nonlinear potency of sub-mac concentrations of nitrous oxide in decreasing the anesthetic requirement of enflurane, halothane, and isoflurane in rats. *Anesthesiology* 1990; **73**: 93–99.

489 Steffey MA, Brosnan RJ, Steffey EP. Assessment of halothane and sevoflurane anesthesia in spontaneously breathing rats. *Am J Vet Res* 2003; **64**(4): 470–474.

490 Crawford MW, Lerman J, Saldivia V, Carmichael FJ. Hemodynamic and organ blood flow responses to halothane and sevoflurane anesthesia during spontaneous ventilation. *Anesth Analg* 1992; **75**: 1000–1006.

491 White PF, Johnston RR, Eger EI II. Determination of anesthetic requirement in rats. *Anesthesiology* 1974; **40**: 52–57.

492 Strout CD, Nahrwold MC. Halothane requirement during pregnancy and lactation in rats. *Anesthesiology* 1981; **55**: 322–323.

493 Roizen MF, White PF, Eger EI II, Brownstein M. Effects of ablation of serotonin or norepinephrine brain-stem areas on halothane and cyclopropane MACs in rats. *Anesthesiology* 1978; **49**: 252–255.

494 Waizer PR, Baez S, Orkin LR. A method for determining minimum alveolar concentration of anesthetic in the rat. *Anesthesiology* 1973; **39**: 394–397.

495 Russell GB, Graybeal JM. Differences in anesthetic potency between Sprague–Dawley and Long–Evans rats for isoflurane but not nitrous oxide. *Pharmacology* 1995; **50**: 162–167.

496 Rampil IJ, Laster M. No correlation between quantitative electroencephalographic measures and movement response to noxious stimuli during isoflurane anesthesia in rats. *Anesthesiology* 1992; **77**(5): 920–925.

497 DiFazio CA, Brown RE, Ball CG, *et al.* Additive effects of anesthetics and theories of anesthesia. *Anesthesiology* 1972; **36**: 57–63.

498 Russell GB, Graybeal JM. Direct measurement of nitrous oxide mac and neurologic monitoring in rats during anesthesia under hyperbaric conditions. *Anesth Analg* 1992; **75**: 995–999.

499 Gonsowski CT, Eger EI II. Nitrous oxide minimum alveolar anesthetic concentration in rats is greater than previously reported. *Anesth Analg* 1994; **79**: 710–712.

500 Palahniuk RJ, Shnider SM, Eger EI II. Pregnancy decreases the requirement for inhaled anesthetic agents. *Anesthesiology* 1974; **41**: 82–83.

501 Rampil IJ, Lockhart SH, Zwass MS, *et al.* Clinical characteristics of desflurane in surgical patients – minimum alveolar concentration. *Anesthesiology* 1991; **74**: 429–433.

502 Miller RD, Wahrenbrock EA, Schroeder CF, *et al.* Ethylene–halothane anesthesia: addition or synergism? *Anesthesiology* 1969; **31**: 301–304.

503 Saidman LJ, Eger EI II. Effect of nitrous oxide and of narcotic premedication on the alveolar concentration of halothane required for anesthesia. *Anesthesiology* 1964; **25**: 302–306.

504 Gibbons RT, Steffey EP, Eger EI II. The effect of spontaneous versus controlled ventilation on the rate of rise of alveolar halothane concentration in dogs. *Anesth Analg* 1977; **56**: 32–34.

505 Saidman LJ, Eger EI II, Munson ES, *et al.* Minimum alveolar concentrations of methoxyflurane, halothane, ether and cyclopropane in man: correlation with theories of anesthesia. *Anesthesiology* 1967; **28**: 994–1002.

506 Stevens WC, Dolan WM, Gibbons RD, *et al.* Minimum alveolar concentrations (MAC) of isoflurane with and without nitrous oxide in patients of various ages. *Anesthesiology* 1975; **42**: 197–200.

507 Kimura T, Watanabe S, Asakura N, *et al.* Determination of end-tidal sevoflurane concentration for tracheal intubation and minimum alveolar anesthetic concentration in adults. *Anesth Analg* 1994; **79**: 378–381.

508 Katoh T, Ikeda K. The minimum alveolar concentration (MAC) of sevoflurane in humans. *Anesthesiology* 1987; **66**: 301–304.

509 Katoh T, Ikeda K. The effect of clonidine on sevoflurane requirements for anaesthesia and hypnosis. *Anaesthesia* 2005; **52**: 364–381.

510 Katoh T, Ikeda K. The effects of fentanyl on sevoflurane requirements for loss of consciousness and skin incision. *Anesthesiology* 1998; **88**: 18–24.

511 Katoh T, Kobayashi S, Suzuki A, *et al.* The effect of fentanyl on sevoflurane requirements for somatic and sympathetic responses to surgical incision. *Anesthesiology* 1999; **90**(2): 398–405.

512 Suzuki A, Katoh T, Ikeda K. The effect of adenosine triphosphate on sevoflurane requirements for minimum alveolar anesthetic concentration and minimum alveolar anesthetic concentration awake. *Anesth Analg* 1998; **86**(1): 179–183.

513 Hornbein TF, Eger EI II, Winter PM, *et al.* The minimum alveolar concentration on nitrous oxide in man. *Anesth Analg* 1982; **61**: 553–556.

514 Martin-Jurado O, Vogt R, Knutter APN, *et al.* Effect of inhalation of isoflurane at end-tidal concentrations greater than, equal to, and less than the minimum anesthetic concentration on bispectral index in chickens. *Am J Vet Res* 2008; **69**(10): 1254–1261.

515 Curro TG, Brunson DB, Paul-Murphy J. Determination of the ED50 of isoflurane and evaluation of the isoflurane-sparing effect of butorphanol in cockatoos (Cacatua spp.). *Vet Surg* 1994; **23**: 429–433.

516 Ludders JW, Rode J, Mitchell GS. Isoflurane anesthesia in sandhill cranes (Grus canadensis): minimal anesthetic concentration and cardiopulmonary dose-response during spontaneous and controlled breathing. *Anesth Analg* 1989; **68**: 511–516.

517 Ludders JW, Mitchell GS, Rode J. Minimal anesthetic concentration and cardiopulmonary dose response of isoflurane in ducks. *Vet Surg* 1990; **19**: 304–307.

518 Fitzgerald G, Blais D. Effect of nitrous oxide on the minimal anesthetic dose of isoflurane in pigeons and red-tailed hawks. In: *Proceedings of the 4th International Congress of Veterinary Anaesthesia*, Utrecht, Netherlands, 1991; 27.

519 Pavez JC, Hawkins MG, Pascoe PJ, *et al.* Effect of fentanyl target-controlled infusions on isoflurane minimum anaesthetic concentration and cardiovascular function in red-tailed hawks (Buteo jamaicensis). *Vet Anaesth Analg* 2011; **38**(4): 344–351.

520 Escobar A, Valadao CAA, Brosnan RJ, *et al.* Effects of butorphanol on the minimum anesthetic concentration for sevoflurane in guineafowl (Numida meleagris). *Am J Vet Res* 2012; **73**(2): 183–188.

521 Mercado JA, Larsen RS, Wack RF, Pypendop BH. Minimum anesthetic concentration of isoflurane in captive thick-billed parrots (Rhynchopsitta pachyrhyncha). *Am J Vet Res* 2008; **69**(2): 189–194.

522 Smith J, Mason DE, Muir WW III. The influence of midazolam on the minimum anesthetic concentration of isoflurane in racing pigeons. *Vet Surg* 1993; **22**(6): 546–547.

523 Cherkin A, Catchpool JF. Temperature dependence of anesthesia in goldfish. *Science* 1964; **144**: 1460–1462.

524 Shim CY, Andersen NB. The effects of oxygen on minimal anesthetic requirements in the toad. *Anesthesiology* 1971; **34**: 333–337.

525 Wouters P, Doursout MF, Merin RG, Chelly JE. Influence of hypertension on MAC of halothane in rats. *Anesthesiology* 1990; **72**: 843–845.

526 Zucker J. Central cholinergic depression reduces MAC for isoflurane in rats. *Anesth Analg* 1991; **72**: 790–795.

527 Stone DJ, Moscicki JC, DiFazio CA. Thiopental reduces halothane MAC in rats. *Anesth Analg* 1992; **74**: 542–546.

528 Doherty TJ, Geiser DR, Rohrbach BW. Effect of acepromazine and butorphanol on halothane minimum alveolar concentration in ponies. *Equine Vet J* 1997; **29**(5): 374–376.

529 Heard DJ, Webb AI, Daniels RT. Effect of acepromazine on the anesthetic requirement of halothane in the dog. *Am J Vet Res* 1986; **47**: 2113–2116.

530 Webb AI, Obrien JM. The effect of acepromazine maleate on the anesthetic potency of halothane and isoflurane. *J Am Anim Hosp Assoc* 1988; **24**(6): 609–615.

531 Matthews NS, Dollar NS, Shawley RV. Halothane-sparing effect of benzodiazepines in ponies. *Cornell Vet* 1990; **80**: 259–265.

532 Hellyer PW, Mama KR, Shafford HL, *et al.* Effects of diazepam and flumazenil on minimum alveolar concentrations for dogs anestetized with isoflurane or a combination of isoflurane and fentanyl. *Am J Vet Res* 2001; **62**(4): 555–560.

533 Perisho JA, Buechel DR, Miller RD. The effect of diazepam on minimum alveolar anesthetic requirement (MAC) in man. *Can Anaesth Soc J* 1971; **18**: 536.

534 Murphy MR, Hug CC Jr. The anesthetic potency of fentanyl in terms of its reduction of enflurane MAC. *Anesthesiology* 1982; **57**: 485–488.

535 Ewing KK, Mohammed HO, Scarlett JM, Short CE. Reduction of isoflurane anesthetic requirement by medetomidine and its restoration by atipamezole in dogs. *Am J Vet Res* 1993; **54**: 294–299.

536 Gross ME, Clifford CA, Hardy DA. Excitement in an elephant after intravenous administration of atropine. *J Am Vet Med Assoc* 1994; **205**(10): 1437–1438.

537 Melvin MA, Johnson BH, Quasha AL, Eger EI II. Induction of anesthesia with midazolam decreases halothane MAC in humans. *Anesthesiology* 1982; **57**(3): 238–241.

538 Lambert-Zechovsky N, Bingen E, Bourillon A, *et al.* Effects of antibiotics on the microbial intestinal ecosystem. *Dev Pharmacol Ther* 1984; **7**(1): 150–157.

539 Doherty TJ, McDonell WN, Dyson DH, *et al.* The effect of a 5-hydroxytryptamine antagonist (R51703) on halothane MAC in the dog. *J Vet Pharmacol Ther* 1995; **18**: 153–155.

540 Weiskopf RB, Holmes MA, Rampil IJ, *et al.* Cardiovascular safety and actions of high concentrations of I-653 and isoflurane in swine. *Anesthesiology* 1989; **70**: 793–799.

17 Local Anesthetics

Eva Rioja Garcia
School of Veterinary Science, University of Liverpool, Leahurst Campus, UK

Chapter contents

Introduction

Local anesthetics reversibly block the generation and propagation of electrical impulses in nerves, thereby causing sensory and motor blockade. Their use dates from the late 1880s when cocaine was first used for ophthalmologic procedures by Carl Köller and Sigmund Freud. However, cocaine was found to be highly toxic and addictive. Since then, new agents with better pharmacologic profiles and less potential for systemic toxicity have been developed. Today, local anesthetics are widely used for local and regional anesthetic techniques. These techniques cause desensitization of a localized area of the body, which allows surgical procedures to be performed in the conscious animal. Alternatively, these techniques may be performed in the anesthetized animal where they decrease the need for general anesthetics and promote greater cardiorespiratory stability. Sustained analgesia when a long-acting local anesthetic is used is also beneficial in the recovery period. Additionally, the local anesthetic lidocaine may also be administered systemically for a variety of indications including management of ventricular arrhythmias, augmentation of intestinal motility, reduction in general anesthetic requirements, and analgesia.

Pharmacology

Molecular mechanism of action

Local anesthetics are considered primarily ion channel blockers, acting mainly on voltage-gated Na^+ channels. However, they also block voltage-dependent K^+ and Ca^{2+} channels, though with lower affinity [1–5]. Some studies also suggest that local anesthetics act on intracellular sites involved in the signal transduction of G-protein coupled receptors [6]. This range of molecular targets may explain some of the adverse and toxic effects that this group of drugs produces on various organ systems.

The most important mechanism of action leading to local anesthesia involves the blockade of inward Na^+ currents through voltage-gated Na^+ channels, thereby impeding membrane depolarization and nerve excitation and conduction [7]. The Na^+ channel is a multimolecular complex with a large α-subunit composed of almost 2000 amino acids that traverses the cell membrane several times. This subunit forms the channel's pore and gating apparatus [7]. Some smaller auxiliary β-subunits influence the activation-inactivation states of the channel [8]. The α-subunit consists of four domains (DI to DIV), each containing six helical segments (S1 to S6). The binding site for local anesthetic, antiarrhythmic and anticonvulsant drugs is located on the DIV S6 segment of the α-subunit [8]. It appears that this binding site is localized within the pore of the Na^+ channel and therefore is only accessible from the intracellular side [9].

The channel is a gated conduit for Na^+ ions and exists in three different gating states: resting (closed), open, and inactivated (Fig. 17.1), depending on the membrane potential and time. At resting membrane potential, the channel is predominantly in its resting state. During depolarization, the channel opens to allow passage of Na^+ ions and, after a few milliseconds, it spontaneously closes into an inactivated state to allow repolarization of the membrane. After repolarization the channel reverts to a resting state [8,10].

There is evidence that local anesthetics may interact with the lipid membrane, altering its fluidity, causing membrane expansion, and thus reducing Na^+ conductance [11]; however, this does not

Veterinary Anesthesia and Analgesia: The Fifth Edition of Lumb and Jones.
Edited by Kurt A. Grimm, Leigh A. Lamont, William J. Tranquilli, Stephen A. Greene and Sheilah A. Robertson.

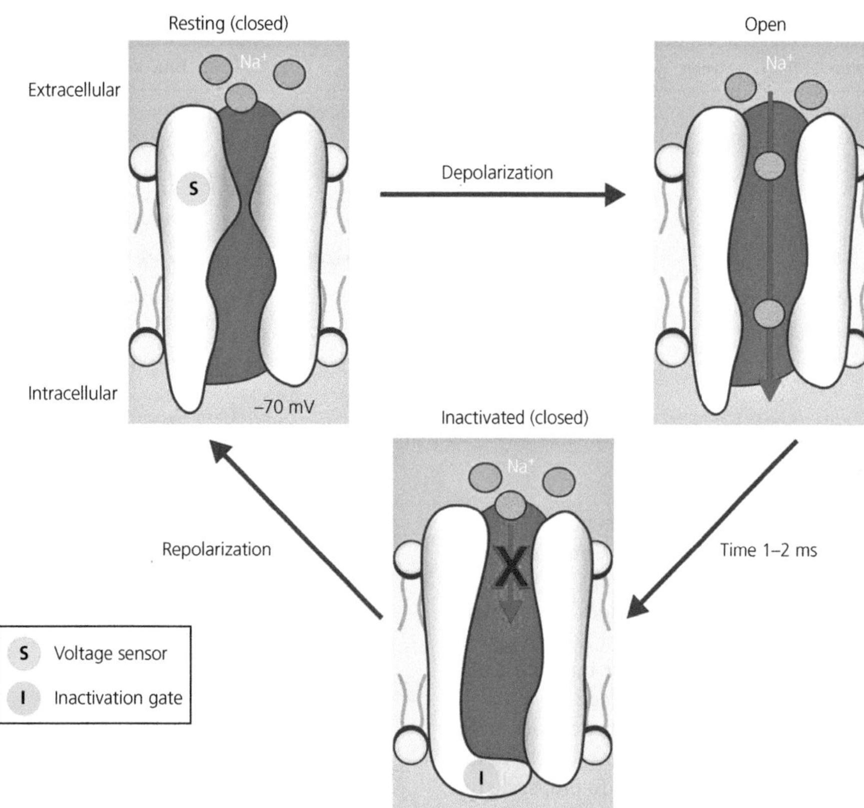

Figure 17.1 The Na+ channel has two gates: an activation ('voltage sensor') and an inactivation gate. At resting membrane potential the channel exists in its resting (closed) state. Depolarization of the membrane is 'sensed' by the voltage sensor and the channel opens, allowing Na+ ions to flow intracellularly. Within 1-2 ms the inactivation gate closes automatically (inactivated channel), allowing repolarization to occur. Repolarization leads to conformation changes with closure of the activation gate and opening of the inactivation gate within 2-5 ms (=refractory period). After repolarization, the channel is in a resting state again.

completely explain the mechanism of action of modern clinically used local anesthetics.

The 'modulated-receptor hypothesis' proposes that local anesthetics have high binding affinity for the Na+ channel in its open and inactivated states, but low affinity for the resting state [7,12]. Lipid-soluble drug forms are thought to enter and leave the receptor via a hydrophobic region of the membrane, while charged less lipid-soluble forms pass via a hydrophilic region (the inner channel pore) [12]. The hydrophilic pathway is open only when the gates of the channel are open, which causes cumulative binding of local anesthetics to the Na+ channel when the channels are active. The 'guarded-receptor hypothesis' proposes that the receptor for local anesthetics is located inside the channel and that the drug binds to this receptor with constant affinity [13]. Access to the receptor is regulated by the channel gates and therefore the channel needs to be open for the receptor to be accessible to the local anesthetic. Increasing the frequency of stimulation increases the number of Na+ channels in the open and inactive states, which increases the binding of local anesthetics.

Both hypotheses explain the property of tertiary amine local anesthetics whereby the depth of the block increases with repetitive membrane depolarization, which has been termed 'use-dependent block' or 'phasic block' [14,15]. On the other hand, blockade obtained on unstimulated nerves is constant, which is termed 'tonic block' [14,15].

Mechanism of blockade of neural tissue

Local anesthetics show a differential pattern of sensory and motor blockade that can be observed clinically when applied to peripheral nerves and the central neuraxis [16,17]. Vasodilation occurs first, followed by loss of sensation of temperature, sharp pain, light touch, and finally loss of motor activity (Table 17.1) [18]. This property is called 'differential block' and was first described by Gasser and Erlanger in 1929 when they observed that, within myelinated A fibers, cocaine reduced compound action potentials from slower and smaller fibers more rapidly than from faster and larger fibers [19]. However, this differential block *in vivo* cannot be simply explained by the size of the fiber, but rather is influenced by numerous factors including type of fiber (size and myelination), frequency of stimulation, length of nerve exposed to the local anesthetic, and choice and concentration of local anesthetic drug.

Initially it was hypothesized that the differential block produced by local anesthetics when applied to peripheral nerves was due to a greater susceptibility of small, unmyelinated C fibers compared to larger, myelinated A fibers. However, *in vitro* [20] and *in vivo* studies [14,21] have shown that A fiber susceptibility to phasic and tonic block is actually greater than that of C fibers, with the order of blockade from fastest to slowest being $A\gamma > A\delta = A\alpha > A\beta > C$. This would suggest that motor and proprioceptive deficits should occur prior to loss of nociception, but this is opposite to what is clinically observed.

Anatomic features such as myelination may also account for some differences in susceptibility, since myelin can effectively pool anesthetic molecules close to the axon membrane [22]. Experimental studies have found that unmyelinated fibers are less sensitive to lidocaine than myelinated fibers [23]. This is contrary to clinical observations of differential block which is manifested by the loss of small fiber-mediated sensation (e.g., temperature) two or more dermatomes beyond the sensory limit for large fiber-mediated sensations.

Table 17.1 Classification of nerve fibers and order of blockade.

Classification	Diameter (μM)	Myelin	Conduction (m/s)	Location	Function	Order of blockade
A-α	15–20	+++	30–120	Afferent/efferent for muscles and joints	Motor and proprioception	5
A-β	5–15	++	30–70	Efferent to muscle Afferent sensory nerve	Motor function and sensory (touch and pressure)	4
A-γ	3–6	++	15–35	Efferent to muscle spindle	Muscle tone	3
A-δ	2–5	+	5–25	Afferent sensory nerve	Pain (fast), touch, temperature	2
B	1–3	+	3–15	Preganglionic sympathetic	Autonomic function	1
C	0.4–1.5	–	0.7–1.3	Postganglionic sympathetic	Autonomic function, pain (slow), temperature	2

Adapted from references 15 and 36.

Exposure length of the nerve to the local anesthetic may in part explain differential block *in vivo*, as smaller fibers need a shorter length exposed than larger fibers for block to occur [24]. This has been called the 'critical length' to completely block conduction, which in myelinated fibers corresponds to three or more nodes of Ranvier [25]. Therefore, larger fibers with greater internodal distances are less susceptible to local anesthetic blockade.

Another important mechanism of local anesthetic blockade is the phenomenon of decremental conduction, which describes the diminished ability of successive nodes of Ranvier to propagate the impulse in the presence of a local anesthetic [26]. This principle explains why the propagation of an impulse can be stopped even if none of the nodes has been rendered completely inexcitable [25], as occurs for example with low concentrations of local anesthetics. Concentrations of local anesthetic that block 74–84% of the sodium conductance at successive nodes cause a progressive decrease in amplitude of the impulse, until it eventually decays below the threshold [25]. Higher concentrations that block greater than 84% of the sodium conductance at three consecutive nodes will prevent impulse propagation completely [25]. This explains why blocks of greater extent and duration result from injection of small-volume/high-concentration solutions versus large-volume/low-concentration solutions, despite the same total drug dose [27].

Some authors suggest that a large portion of the sensory information transmitted by peripheral nerves is carried via coding of electrical signals in after-potentials and after-oscillations [28]. Sub-blocking concentrations of local anesthetics can suppress these intrinsic oscillatory after-effects of impulse discharge without significantly affecting action potential conduction [29]. Thus, another possible mechanism of blockade of nerve function, especially at low concentrations of local anesthetics, is by disruption of coding of electrical information [15].

When local anesthetics are administered in the central neuraxis (epidurally or intrathecally) or systemically, they may possess other mechanisms of analgesic action at the level of the spinal cord in addition to the previously discussed ones. Local anesthetics inhibit other ion channels such as K^+ or Ca^{2+} channels at the level of the dorsal horn of the spinal cord. This may affect central neuroprocessing of sensory information, thereby contributing to their antinociceptive effects [30–32]. In addition to ion channels, nociceptive transmission is mediated by several neurotransmitters in the dorsal horn, such as the tachykinins (e.g., substance P). Local anesthetics have been shown to inhibit substance P binding and evoked increases in intracellular Ca^{2+} [33]. Additionally, local anesthetics also inhibit glutamatergic transmission in spinal dorsal horn neurons, reducing *N*-methyl-D-aspartate (NMDA)- and neurokinin-mediated postsynaptic depolarizations [34,35].

When nerve trunks or large nerves are targeted (e.g., brachial plexus), the somatosensory arrangement of the nerve fibers also affects the progression of the block (Fig. 17.2) [36].

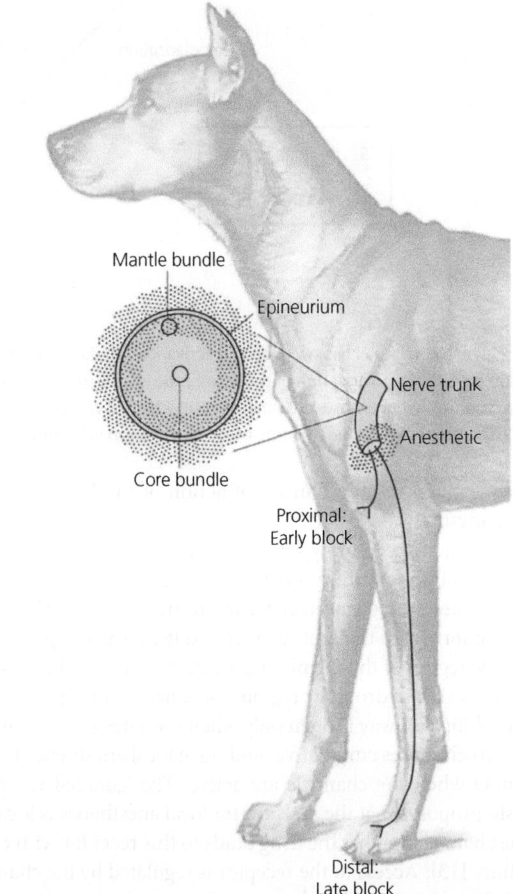

Figure 17.2 Nerve fibers in the mantle or peripheral bundles innervate primarily motor fibers of the proximal limb, whereas nerve fibers in the core or center bundles mainly innervate the sensory fibers of the distal foot. Therefore, the concentration gradient that develops during initial diffusion of local anesthetic into the nerve trunk causes onset of anesthesia to proceed from proximal to distal. Recovery from anesthesia also proceeds from proximal to distal because of absorption of local anesthetic into the circulation surrounding the nerve trunk. Source: Adapted from [36].

Chemical structure

Clinically useful local anesthetic drugs are composed of a lipophilic, benzene ring with different substitutions (aromatic ring) and a hydrophilic amine group (tertiary or quaternary amine), which are linked through an intermediate chain, either an ester or an amide. Depending on the type of link, local anesthetics are classified as amino-esters, hydrolyzed by plasma cholinesterases, or amino-amides, metabolized by the liver.

Physicochemical properties

The physicochemical properties influencing local anesthetic activity include molecular weight, pKa, lipid solubility, and degree of protein binding (Table 17.2) [37,38].

The molecular weight of clinically used local anesthetics is very similar, ranging between 220 and 288 Da. The diffusion coefficient is thus not significantly affected and molecular weight seems not to be an important factor determining differences in activity of local anesthetics [37]. However, changes in molecular weight due to alkyl substitutions may influence other properties such as lipid solubility and pKa.

All clinically useful local anesthetics are weak bases, and as such they exist in equilibrium between the neutral, non-ionized, lipid-soluble form (B) and the ionized (charged), water-soluble form (BH^+). They are formulated as acidic solutions of hydrochloride salts (pH 4–7), which are more highly ionized and thus water soluble.

The receptor for local anesthetics appears to be located within the pore of the Na^+ channel close to the cytoplasm [9] and only the ionized, charged form of the local anesthetic can interact with this receptor [39]. However, the main access of local anesthetics to the cell is by penetration of the lipophilic neutral form through the lipid membrane (Fig. 17.3).

Table 17.2 Physicochemical properties and relative potencies of clinically used local anesthetics.

Local anesthetic	pKa[a]	% Ionized (at pH 7.4)	Lipid solubility[b]	% Protein binding	Relative anesthetic potency[c]	Relative potency for CNS toxicity[d]	CV:CNS ratio[e]
Ester linked							
Low potency, short duration							
Procaine	8.89	97	100	6	1	0.3	3.7
Chloroprocaine	9.06	95	810	7	1	0.3	3.7
High potency, long duration							
Tetracaine	8.38	93	5822	94	8	2	ND
Amide linked							
Intermediate potency and duration							
Lidocaine	7.77	76	366	64	2	1	7.1
Mepivacaine	7.72	61	130	77	2	1.4	7.1
Prilocaine	8.02	76	129	55	2	1.2	3.1
Intermediate potency, long duration							
Ropivacaine	8.16	83	775	94	6	2.9	2
High potency, long duration							
Bupivacaine	8.1	83	3420	95	8	4	2
Levobupivacaine	8.1	83	3420	>97	8	2.9	2
Etidocaine	7.87	66	7317	94	6	2	4.4

[a] Measured with spectrophotometric method at 36°C, except prilocaine and ropivacaine measured at 25°C.
[b] Partition coefficients expressed as relative concentrations (mol/L) in octanol and buffer at 36°C, except prilocaine and ropivacaine measured at 25°C.
[c] Potency relative to procaine.
[d] Potency relative to lidocaine.
[e] Cardiovascular to central nervous system toxicity ratio. CV denotes the disappearance of pulse and CNS denotes the onset of seizures.
Data obtained from references 36, 38, and 40. ND = no data.

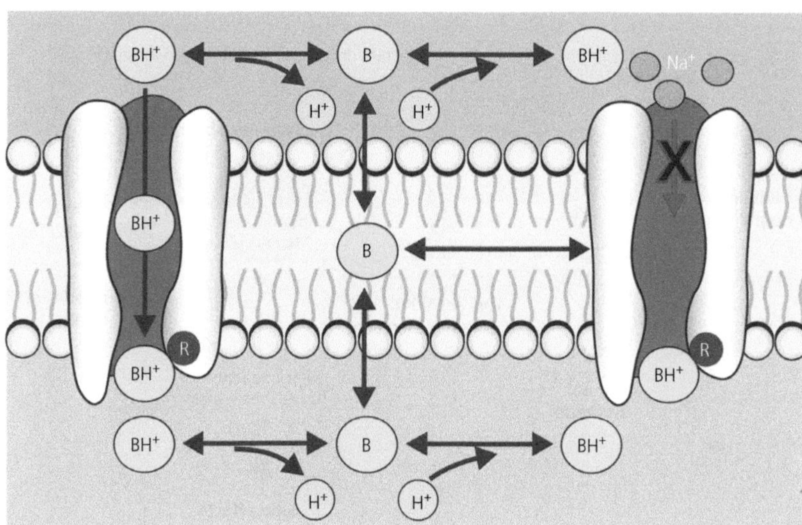

Figure 17.3 The cell membrane lipid bilayer with the Na^+ channel. Local anesthetics exist as a neutral base (B) and an ionized form (BH^+) in equilibrium. The neutral form is lipid soluble and easily crosses the cell membrane. The ionized form is more water soluble and can cross through the open channel. The neutral form can cause membrane expansion and closure of the Na^+ channel. The ionized form interacts with its receptor on the intracellular side of the Na^+ channel.

The pKa of a drug is the pH at which the two forms exist in equal amounts and is alkaline (pH >7.4) for all clinically used local anesthetics.

$$pKa = pH - \log([B]/[BH^+])$$

The higher the pKa, the greater the degree of ionization or proportion of local anesthetic in the ionized, charged hydrophilic form at physiologic pH (7.4), and the slower the onset of action. On the other hand, a local anesthetic with a low pKa will have a greater proportion of the non-ionized lipid-soluble form at physiologic pH and a more rapid onset of action.

Lipid solubility is the main determinant of intrinsic local anesthetic potency and it will determine the clinically relevant concentrations needed to produce effective conduction blockade [40–42]. Increasing lipid solubility facilitates the penetration through lipid membranes, potentially hastening onset of action; however, highly lipid-soluble agents will also become sequestered within the myelin and other lipid compartments. Thus, the net effect of increasing lipid solubility is delayed onset of action of local anesthetics [43]. On the other hand, sequestration of local anesthetic in myelin and other lipid compartments creates a depot for slow release of the drug, increasing the duration of the effect [43].

The degree of protein binding also influences activity of local anesthetics, as only the unbound, free fraction is pharmacologically active. Higher protein binding is associated with increased duration of action. This cannot be explained by slower dissociation kinetics from the Na^+ channel, as this dissociation occurs within seconds regardless of the degree of protein binding [44]. Increased duration of action of highly protein-bound local anesthetics is probably associated with other membrane or extracellular proteins [45].

Most clinically available local anesthetics are racemic mixtures of the *R*- and *S*-enantiomers in a 50:50 mixture. The exceptions are lidocaine, procaine, and tetracaine, which are achiral, and levobupivacaine and ropivacaine, which are the pure *S*-enantiomers or levoisomers [37,46]. Although both enantiomers have the same physicochemical properties, they have different affinities for the ion channels of Na^+, K^+ and Ca^{2+}, with the *R*-enantiomer having greater *in vitro* potency and thus greater therapeutic efficacy but also greater potential for systemic toxicity [47,48]. There is less potential for nervous and cardiac toxicity with the *S*-enantiomer compared with the *R*-enantiomer or the racemic mixture [49].

Studies *in vitro* have characterized the relative potencies of local anesthetic agents, which depend on their physicochemical properties (i.e., lipid solubility) but also the individual nerve fibers and frequency of stimulation [50]. However, *in vivo* potencies do not necessarily correlate with *in vitro* studies [51], because of the complex interaction of factors including site of administration, dose and volume of local anesthetics, and other environmental factors.

Local anesthetics with an amide group, high pKa, and lower lipid solubility show greater differential blockade, with more potent blockade of C fibers than of fast-conducting A fibers [43,52]. This is believed to be due to the slower diffusion across permeability barriers present in A fibers. The relative order of differential rate of blockade is chloroprocaine > ropivacaine > bupivacaine, levobupivacaine > lidocaine, mepivacaine > etidocaine [53,54]. This is especially true at low concentrations and the differential rate of blockade tends to disappear as local anesthetic concentrations increase.

Clinical pharmacology

Pharmacokinetics

Absorption

Disposition of local anesthetics within the body after local administration is governed by several competing factors including bulk flow, diffusion and binding to neural and non-neural structures, and vascular uptake (Fig. 17.4). The rate and extent of systemic absorption of the local anesthetic are important as toxic plasma concentrations may be achieved. Therefore, local anesthetics with lower systemic absorption will have a greater margin of safety. Systemic absorption depends on several factors including the site of

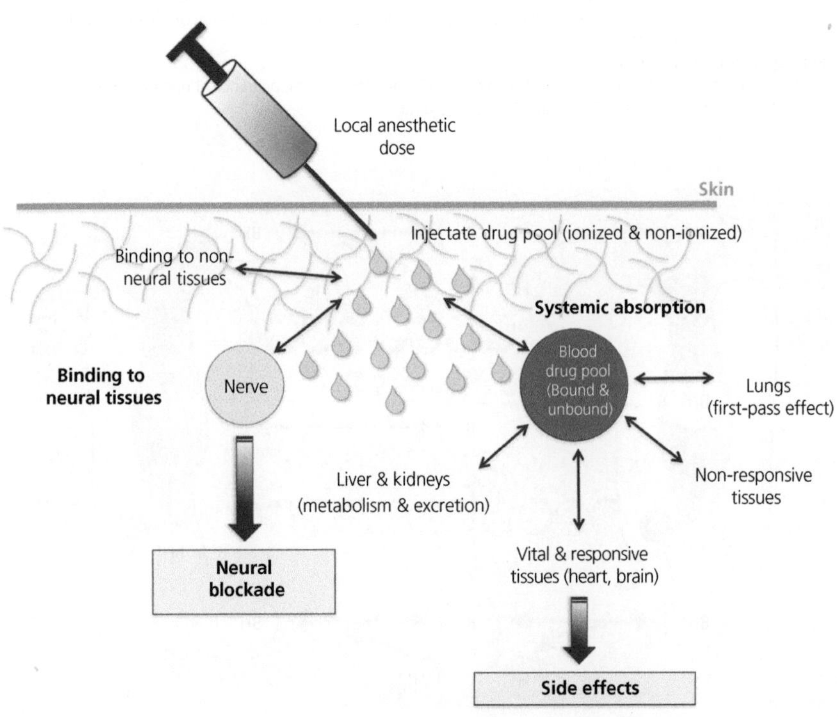

Figure 17.4 Disposition of local anesthetics within the body following peripheral administration.

injection (i.e., vascularity), the intrinsic lipid solubility and vasoactivity of the agent, the dose administered, the presence of additives such as vasoconstrictors, other formulation factors that modify local drug residence and release, the influence of the nerve block in the region (i.e., vasodilation), and the (patho)physiologic state of the patient [37].

In general, areas with greater vascularity will have a more extensive and rapid systemic absorption than areas with more fat, regardless of the agent used [15]. Areas with greater vascularity will have a greater peak plasma concentration (C_{max}) and a shorter time to peak plasma concentration (T_{max}). In an experimental study in pigs, lidocaine rate of absorption following subcutaneous administration was highest in the pectoral region, followed by the face and neck, with the slowest being the abdomen [55]. With regard to specific blocks, the degree of systemic absorption is as follows, in decreasing order: intercostal > epidural > brachial plexus > sciatic/femoral [56]. Following administration of lidocaine via inverted L nerve block in cows, the serum C_{max} was 572 ng/mL which occurred at T_{max} 0.52 h, while lidocaine via a caudal epidural block was undetectable in serum [57]. Systemic absorption of local anesthetic drugs is much lower after spinal (intrathecal) than after epidural administration [58,59]. Normally, the greatest risk of systemic toxicity coincides with T_{max} in arterial blood, which will vary from 5 to 45 min after injection, depending on the site of the block, speed of injection, and drug injected [37]. However, T_{max} is independent of the dose injected [60]. Faster speed of injection is associated with greater C_{max}, and therefore with increased risk of systemic toxicity [61].

Physicochemical properties of local anesthetics will also influence systemic absorption. In general, drugs with greater lipid solubility and protein binding will result in lower systemic absorption and C_{max} [37]. Therefore, shorter-acting amide drugs such as lidocaine and mepivacaine will be absorbed into the systemic circulation more readily than the long-acting bupivacaine, ropivacaine and levobupivacaine, probably because of binding of the latter to neural and non-neural lipid-rich tissues [15]. Another factor influencing the rate of absorption is the intrinsic vasoactivity of the local anesthetic. Most clinically used local anesthetics cause vasodilation when applied locally, with the exceptions of ropivacaine and levobupivacaine [62,63]. The vasoconstrictive activity of ropivacaine and levobupivacaine results in slower absorption and therefore longer T_{max} values [64,65].

Addition of a vasoconstrictor, such as epinephrine, will counteract the inherent vasodilating effects on the local vasculature of most agents, delaying their systemic absorption. Hyaluronidase is another additive sometimes added to local anesthetics to improve their anesthetic effect by causing depolymerization of interstitial hyaluronic acid and thus increasing the permeability of the tissues; however, it also enhances systemic absorption and the risk of systemic toxicity (see section on Additives later in this chapter).

Some new formulations, such as local anesthetic-loaded liposomes, polylactide microspheres or cyclodextrin inclusion complexes, among others, are designed to cause a slow release of the drug, providing a local depot of local anesthetic, which will significantly decrease systemic absorption and prolong the duration of effect [60,66,67]. When liposome-encapsulated lidocaine was administered epidurally to dogs the C_{max} was lower, while the T_{max} and the duration of effect (170 versus 61 min) were significantly longer compared to regular lidocaine [66]. In sheep, intercostal administration of bupivacaine-dexamethasone microspheres prolonged the duration of the block up to 13 days, with plasma concentrations remaining ten times below the convulsive concentration [68]. Liposome-encapsulated lidocaine has also been administered topically to cats at a dose of 15 mg/kg, which proved to be safe, with C_{max} well below the toxic plasma levels for that species [69]. Administration of different slow-release lidocaine formulations for sciatic nerve block in postoperative pain models in rats produced analgesia from 3 days up to 1 week and inhibited the development of hyperalgesia [70,71].

Distribution

After absorption into the bloodstream, amino-ester local anesthetics are rapidly hydrolyzed by plasma pseudocholinesterases and their distribution into body tissues is limited. Amino-amide local anesthetics are widely distributed into different body organs and tissues. The degree of tissue distribution and binding is normally represented by the pharmacokinetic parameter known as the apparent volume of distribution at steady state (Vd_{ss}), which is usually paralleled by the degree of protein binding [37]. Only the free, active fraction of the drug, and not the protein-bound fraction, governs tissue concentration and degree of entry into the central nervous system [72]. Amide-type local anesthetics bind primarily to α_1-acid glycoprotein (AAG) in the plasma and to a lesser extent to albumin [73,74]. In dogs, increasing concentrations of AAG caused an increase in total serum concentration but a decrease in the free fraction, Vd_{ss}, and elimination half-life of lidocaine [72,75]. Because AAG is an acute phase protein, its circulating levels will be increased during trauma, surgery, cancer or any inflammatory state. Therefore, although the total concentration of local anesthetic in plasma will be greater, reflecting the increase in AAG, the unbound (active) drug fraction will remain similar [37,76].

Amide-type local anesthetics in venous blood undergo first-pass pulmonary uptake, which effectively decreases the plasma concentration of the drug temporarily [77,78]. Consequently, the lungs are able to attenuate the toxic effects after accidental intravenous injections of local anesthetics. In animals with right-to-left cardiac shunts the pulmonary first-pass effect is absent and there is an increased risk of toxicity. The pulmonary uptake of a local anesthetic is mostly dependent on its physicochemical properties, mainly lipid solubility and pKa. More lipid-soluble agents undergo greater pulmonary uptake and those with lower pKa values will have a greater fraction of unionized base form, which is the form that accumulates in the lung [79]. Decreasing blood pH (i.e., acidemia) decreases the degree of pulmonary uptake of local anesthetics, which may contribute to increased plasma concentrations and promote toxicity [77,79]. The rank order of pulmonary uptake in rat lung slices was found to be bupivacaine > etidocaine > lidocaine [79]. Others have also found greater uptake of prilocaine compared to bupivacaine and mepivacaine in isolated perfused rat lungs, with little evidence of pulmonary metabolism [80]. The mean pulmonary uptake of lidocaine after IV administration in dogs has been calculated to be 63.6% [78]. There is evidence of a pulmonary contribution to lidocaine metabolism using rat pulmonary microsomes *in vitro* [81]. After an intravenous bolus injection in rabbits, the pulmonary uptake of levobupivacaine was greater than that of ropivacaine (31% versus 23%) [82].

Local anesthetic agents also distribute rapidly and extensively into milk and muscle at concentrations proportional to those in the bloodstream. Drugs that diffuse most readily into milk are those that are relatively lipophilic, unionized, not strongly protein bound, and with low molecular weights [83]. Following an inverted L nerve block with 100 mL of 2% lidocaine in adult Holstein cows, the lidocaine C_{max} in milk was 300 ng/mL compared with serum C_{max} of 572 ng/mL; T_{max} in milk was 1.75 h compared with serum T_{max} of 0.52 h [57]. The last measurable time of lidocaine detection in milk was 32.5 h with a mean concentration of 46 ng/mL [57]. The current Food Animal Residue Avoidance Database (FARAD) withdrawal recommendations for lidocaine are 24 h for meat and milk, which seem too short based on this study. On the other hand, following caudal epidural administration of 0.22 mg/kg of lidocaine there was no detectable lidocaine concentration present in any serum or milk sample [57]; therefore, a 24 h withdrawal time would be appropriate for this route and dose.

Local anesthetic drugs also cross the placenta and appear in the fetus following administration to the pregnant animal. Ester-linked local anesthetic agents are rapidly metabolized and placental transfer is limited [37]. Amide-linked local anesthetic agents can become 'trapped' in their ionized forms on the more acidotic fetal side of the placenta, and therefore their net transfer across the placenta is increased [84]. In pregnant ewes, as fetal blood pH decreased from 7.35 to 7.10, the fetal-maternal ratio (F:M) for lidocaine increased from 0.76 to 1.21 [84]. Apart from the pH, the degree of local anesthetic binding to both maternal and fetal plasma proteins is also an important determinant of placental transfer of local anesthetics, as only the unbound, free drug crosses the placenta [85]. Since fetal AAG content and binding are less than maternal [86], the F:M of highly protein-bound local anesthetics such as bupivacaine (F:M = 0.36) is lower than less protein-bound drugs such as lidocaine (F:M = 1) [85,87]. The placental transfer of levobupivacaine and ropivacaine is similar to bupivacaine in pregnant ewes [88].

An important consideration when choosing a local anesthetic agent in the pregnant animal is the ability of the neonate to metabolize and excrete the drug after birth. Studies in sheep show that back-transfer of bupivacaine, but not of lidocaine, from the fetus to the mother occurs [85,87]. Lidocaine and its metabolites monoethylglycinexylidide (MEGX) and glycinexylidide (GX) were detected in fetal urine within 1–2 h following intravenous infusion of lidocaine to pregnant ewes [85]. These studies suggest that lidocaine might be a better option in pregnant animals since the fetus/neonate will be able to readily eliminate the drug. They also suggest that if high plasma concentrations of local anesthetic in maternal blood are likely (i.e., large volumes used for local blockade or inadvertent intravenous administration), it would be beneficial to delay delivery in the case of bupivacaine, but there would be no benefit in doing so in the case of lidocaine [85].

Metabolism

Ester-linked local anesthetics are cleared mainly in the blood by non-specific plasma pseudocholinesterases, where they undergo ester hydrolysis. Esterases present in the liver, red blood cells, and synovial fluid also contribute to the clearance of these drugs [89–91]. Among the ester agents, chloroprocaine is cleared most rapidly due to its faster hydrolysis rate. *In vitro* half-lives tend to be very short for the ester-linked drugs, ranging from 11 s for chloroprocaine in human plasma [92] to 9 s and 12 s for procaine in equine whole blood and plasma, respectively [89], and up to several minutes for tetracaine [37]. *In vivo* terminal half-lives are typically longer, probably reflecting slow uptake from the site of administration and/or wide distribution within the body [37,93]. The terminal half-life of procaine in horses after intravenous administration is 50 min with an apparent volume of distribution of 6.7 L/kg [93]. The hydrolysis products of procaine, chloroprocaine, and tetracaine appear to be pharmacologically inactive. Procaine and benzocaine are hydrolyzed to para-aminobenzoic acid (PABA) which may, however, cause rare allergic reactions [37].

Cocaine undergoes ester hydrolysis in plasma and liver, but also *N*-demethylation in the liver to norcocaine, which subsequently undergoes further hydrolysis [91]. Cocaine is rarely used in veterinary medicine, but illegal use in horses or dogs before races to increase performance and delay the time to exhaustion is possible [94]. Procaine also possesses central nervous system stimulatory effects and its use is banned in racehorses [93].

Amide-linked local anesthetics are almost exclusively metabolized in the liver by microsomal enzymes (CYP450). Phase I reactions involve hydroxylation, *N*-dealkylation and *N*-demethylation, followed by Phase II reactions where the metabolites are conjugated with amino acids or glucuronide into less active and inactive metabolites. Clearance values differ among species, but typically the rank order of clearance is prilocaine > etidocaine > lidocaine > mepivacaine > ropivacaine > bupivacaine [37]. In humans, prilocaine is cleared most rapidly, with blood clearance values that exceed liver blood flow, indicating extrahepatic metabolism in this species [37]. Hydrolysis of prilocaine produces orthotoluidine (O-toluidine), a metabolite that oxidizes hemoglobin to methemoglobin [95].

Lidocaine undergoes hydroxylation and *N*-demethylation in the liver. Its two main metabolites are monoethylglycinexylidide (MEGX) and glycinexylidide (GX) in dogs [96], rabbits [97], rats [98], cats [99], horses [100,101], goats [102], and chickens [103], but these metabolites have not been detected in cows [104]. Of these metabolites, especially MEGX has significant activity (approximately 70% that of lidocaine) and could potentially contribute to its toxicity during prolonged intravenous infusions [37,101]. Other amides such as mepivacaine, bupivacaine, and ropivacaine undergo mainly *N*-dealkylation and hydroxylation. These agents produce the less toxic metabolite pipecoloxylidide (PPX) [105]. The *N*-dealkylated metabolite of bupivacaine, *N*-desbutylbupivacaine, is about half as cardiotoxic as bupivacaine, but less toxic to the central nervous system in rat studies [106]. Some amide metabolites are further conjugated to glucuronide before they are eliminated in the urine or bile [107].

Excretion

Local anesthetics are poorly water soluble, which limits renal excretion of the unchanged drug. The hydrolysis metabolites of ester-linked local anesthetics are mainly excreted in urine [108]. Similarly, the metabolites of amide-linked local anesthetics are eliminated in urine or bile. A small portion of amide-type local anesthetics is excreted unchanged in urine (4–7% for lidocaine, 6% for bupivacaine and 16% for mepivacaine in humans; 1.7–2.9% for lidocaine in horses) [109–111].

Factors affecting pharmacokinetics and activity

Patient factors, such as age, may influence the pharmacokinetics of local anesthetics. Absorption of lidocaine from laryngeal spray was higher in dogs less than 20 days of age compared to 2–3-month old puppies [112]. The volume of distribution and the elimination half-life of lidocaine were greater in neonatal lambs compared with adult sheep [113]. In a pharmacokinetic study of lidocaine in puppies, the elimination rate constant from the central compartment (K10) was lower and the elimination half-life longer in 3–16-day old compared with 6-month old puppies [114]. When comparing neonatal lambs with adult sheep, hepatic clearance of lidocaine was similar but renal clearance of unchanged drug was greater in the neonate, probably due to decreased protein binding, lower urine pH and decreased tubular reabsorption because of higher urine flow rates [113]. Plasma hydrolysis of ester-linked local anesthetics is also affected by age, as observed in human neonates and infants where plasma cholinesterase activity was half that of adults [115]. In geriatric animals, hepatic clearance of local anesthetics may be decreased and half-life increased [116,117].

Increased nerve sensitivity to local anesthetics seems to be present during pregnancy with faster onset of conduction blockade [118]. Acute progesterone treatment had no effect on bupivacaine-induced conduction blockade in the isolated rabbit vagus nerve; therefore, this effect is unlikely to be a direct effect of progesterone on the cell membrane but may involve hormonal effects on protein synthesis [119]. Pregnant ewes were found to clear lidocaine more rapidly, but bupivacaine and ropivacaine more slowly than non-pregnant ewes [120,121]. This difference may be explained by lidocaine's more dependent clearance on hepatic blood flow, which is increased during pregnancy, whereas clearance of bupivacaine and ropivacaine is more dependent on the hepatic enzymatic activity which may be inhibited during pregnancy [37].

Hepatic disease can decrease the rate of metabolism of amide-linked local anesthetics. Plasma pseudocholinesterase activity is also reduced in the presence of liver disease and during pregnancy, which will decrease the rate of hydrolysis of ester-linked local anesthetics [122,123]. In general, standard doses may be administered to animals with hepatic disease for single-dose neural blockade but repeated doses, dosing intervals, and continuous rate infusions need to be adjusted to avoid accumulation and toxicity [37]. A decrease in hepatic blood flow, as can occur during general anesthesia, cardiac disease, or any condition decreasing cardiac output, will decrease hepatic clearance of local anesthetics, especially those more dependent on hepatic blood flow such as lidocaine [37,124]. The Vd_{ss} and clearance (Cl) of intravenous lidocaine were significantly decreased in anesthetized compared to awake horses (0.4 vs 0.79 L/kg and 15 vs 29 mL/kg/min, respectively) [125], and in anesthetized compared to awake cats (1.4 vs 1.9 L/kg and 21 vs 26 mL/kg/min, respectively) [99]. Hepatic clearance of other amide-linked local anesthetics like mepivacaine or bupivacaine is more dependent on activity of hepatic enzymes and the effect of reduced hepatic blood flow is less pronounced.

Renal failure decreases plasma pseudocholinesterase activity by 40% in humans [126]. Amino-amides are excreted mainly as water-soluble metabolites, which may accumulate in animals with renal failure and contribute to central nervous system toxicity if they are active (e.g., MEGX and GX) [124].

Fasting has been shown to decrease hepatic clearance of lidocaine in horses [111]. Gastrointestinal disease (e.g., equine colic) may also affect clearance of amino-amide local anesthetics that depend mainly on hepatic blood flow, like lidocaine, especially if cardiac output is significantly reduced. However, pharmacokinetic parameters of intravenous lidocaine in horses undergoing abdominal surgery for colic are similar to those of healthy, awake horses, with Vd_{ss} and Cl values of 0.7 L/kg and 25 mL/kg/min [127]. It was hypothesized that the cardiac output of the horses included in that study might have been increased, rather than decreased [127].

Interestingly, diabetes mellitus increases hepatic clearance of lidocaine, although the excretion of the metabolite MEGX is impaired [128,129].

Concomitant administration of local anesthetics with other drugs may affect their distribution and elimination kinetics. Drugs that decrease plasma or red cell esterase activity, such as neostigmine or acetazolamide, will prolong half-life of ester-linked local anesthetics [130,131]. When CYP1A2 and CYP3A4 inhibitors, such as erythromycin, are co-administered with amino-amide local anesthetics, their hepatic clearance may decrease [132]. β-Adrenergic receptor blocking drugs reduce liver perfusion and inhibit the activity of hepatic microsomal metabolizing enzymes responsible for the metabolism of amino-amide local anesthetics; hence, greater plasma concentration and decreased elimination will occur when these drugs are co-administered [133].

Co-administration of different classes of local anesthetics may also affect their pharmacokinetic parameters. The rate of hydrolysis of chloroprocaine is reduced by concomitant administration of bupivacaine or etidocaine, but not when it is co-administered with lidocaine or mepivacaine [130,134].

Temperature may also affect the pharmacokinetics and pharmacodynamics of local anesthetics. Lidocaine's ability to block nerve impulses, both *in vitro* and *in vivo,* is potentiated by cooling [135,136]. Conversely, lidocaine uptake by mammalian sciatic nerve is reduced by cooling, with a 45% decrease when the temperature falls from 37°C to 20°C [137]. Some clinical studies in humans have observed an increase in the speed of onset of various types of blocks when the temperature of the local anesthetic solution was increased to 37°C [138–141], although this effect has not been consistent [142,143]. Cooling of the local anesthetic solution increases the pKa and the relative amount of ionized active form, while warming the solution decreases the pKa and increases the amount of non-ionized lipid-soluble form [137]. These pKa changes may explain the increased potency of local anesthetics with cooling and the hastening of onset of action with warming.

Baricity is one of the most important physical properties of local anesthetics during subarachnoid or intrathecal administration as it will affect the distribution and spread of the solution, and therefore impact the characteristics of the block [144]. Baricity of a local anesthetic solution is the calculated ratio of the density of the solution to the density of the cerebrospinal fluid (CSF), both measured at the same temperature, which is normally 37°C. Density is the weight in grams of 1 mL of the solution, and it is inversely related to its temperature [145]. An isobaric solution has a baricity ratio of 1. If the ratio is >1, the solution is hyperbaric, and if it is <1, it is hypobaric. At room temperature, most commercially available local anesthetic solutions are isobaric with respect to the CSF, but when they are warmed to body temperature they become hypobaric [145]. The densities of commercial 2% lidocaine and 0.5% and 0.75% bupivacaine are lower than that of human CSF at 37°C, which makes them relatively hypobaric [146]. Dilution of these solutions with water makes them increasingly hypobaric [146]. When local anesthetics are mixed with dextrose or hypertonic saline, the resulting solution is hyperbaric [145,147]. Neurotoxicity has been observed with hyperbaric bupivacaine when high concentrations and doses are administered intrathecally in dogs (≥10 mg of 1% or 2% bupivacaine in 10% glucose solution), but not with low concentrations and doses (5 mg of 0.5% bupivacaine in 10% glucose solution) [148]. High concentrations and doses of hypobaric bupivacaine (20 mg of 2% bupivacaine in water) were not associated with neurotoxicity when administered intrathecally to dogs [148].

Hypobaric solutions, when injected into the subarachnoid space, will migrate to non-dependent areas, because their density is lower than that of the CSF, while hyperbaric solutions will migrate to dependent areas. This migration allows preferential blockade to occur on the surgical side, with unilateral spinal anesthesia being possible when low doses of local anesthetics are used [149]. Isobaric solutions will migrate to both sides of the spinal cord, causing bilateral spinal block. In humans, it is reported that unilateral spinal block results in a four-fold reduction of the incidence of clinically relevant hypotension with more stable cardiovascular parameters as compared with conventional bilateral spinal block [150]. Because only small amounts of local anesthetic solution are injected, the extent of spinal block is reduced and the resolution of the sensory and motor blocks is faster [150].

Mixtures of local anesthetic agents with additives such as solvents or vasoconstrictors, or with other drugs such as opioids, may alter the density and baricity of the solution. When 0.125–0.5% bupivacaine solutions are mixed with fentanyl (0.005%), sufentanil (0.005%) or morphine (0.1%) the resultant solutions are hypobaric [151]. The mixture of 2% lidocaine and epinephrine (1:200 000) results in a hyperbaric solution [151].

There is some variation in the density of the CSF among individuals [152]. Density of the CSF may also be influenced by physiologic status of the animal (e.g., density is decreased during pregnancy in humans) [153]. Therefore, there may be some interindividual variation in clinical response to intrathecal solutions, especially with those that are marginally hypo- or hyperbaric [144].

Additives

Epinephrine has been used as an adjunct to local anesthetics for more than a century. The rationale behind its use is that it causes vasoconstriction and therefore decreases the systemic absorption of the local anesthetic agent, which decreases the dose of local anesthetic required and prolongs its duration of effect [154,155]. Decreased systemic absorption also reduces the local anesthetic C_{max}, which decreases the probability of systemic toxicity. Several studies have demonstrated decreased C_{max} of local anesthetics when administered with epinephrine both in peripheral and neuraxial blocks [155–158]. In general, the greatest effects are observed with shorter-acting rather than with longer-acting agents.

In addition to this pharmacokinetic interaction, epinephrine seems to have analgesic effects on its own when administered epidurally or intrathecally by stimulating α_2-adrenergic receptors, thereby inhibiting presynaptic neurotransmitter release from C and Aδ fibers in the substantia gelatinosa of the spinal cord dorsal horn [159–161]. It has also been shown that α_2-adrenergic receptors can modify certain K^+ channels in the axons of peripheral nerves, potentiating the impulse-blocking actions of local anesthetics [162,163]. A later study in rats also showed that local infiltration of epinephrine causes cutaneous anesthesia mediated by activation of local α_1-adrenergic receptors [164]. Therefore, it seems that pharmacokinetic and pharmacodynamic interactions between epinephrine and local anesthetics are responsible for the increased duration and intensity of the block when administered in combination.

A potential concern when epinephrine is co-administered with local anesthetics is a decrease in peripheral nerve or spinal cord blood flow, which could cause nerve or spinal cord ischemia. However, research studies with radiolabeled microspheres in dogs and cats show that epinephrine injected intrathecally causes regional dural vasoconstriction but does not reduce spinal cord or cerebral blood flow [165,166]. This is supported by many years of clinical experience using epinephrine-containing solutions for neuroaxial anesthesia and the absence of observed detrimental effects on spinal cord function [163,167]. *In vitro* studies in rats showed that sciatic nerve blood flow is reduced by injection of lidocaine without epinephrine, but that the reduction is more pronounced when epinephrine (5 μg/mL) is added [168]. However, a more recent *in vivo* rat study using radiolabeled microspheres showed that lidocaine with or without epinephrine (10 μg/mL) does not reduce sciatic nerve or surrounding skeletal muscle blood flow [169]. The authors of this study concluded that mechanisms other than local vasoconstriction might contribute to the prolongation of lidocaine peripheral nerve blockade by epinephrine.

Systemic absorption of epinephrine administered in combination with local anesthetics can also cause cardiovascular effects characterized by an increase in heart rate, stroke volume, and cardiac output, and a decrease in peripheral vascular resistance [170]. A study in humans also showed an improvement of left ventricular diastolic function with epinephrine added to local anesthetics, in contrast with norepinephrine, which impaired it [170]. Excessive plasma concentrations of epinephrine could precipitate tachycardia and arrhythmias.

The recommended concentrations of epinephrine for addition to local anesthetic solutions for clinical use range between 1:400 000 (1 mg/400 mL or 2.5 μg/mL) and 1:200 000 (1 mg/200 mL or 5 μg/mL] [163]. A 1:200 000 concentration can be obtained by adding 0.1 mL of a 1:1000 epinephrine solution (0.1 mg) into 20 mL of local anesthetic solution. Concentrations in excess of 5 μg/mL do not provide any additional decrease in C_{max} and should therefore be avoided in light of the potential for systemic side-effects [37]. Market preparations of local anesthetics that contain epinephrine have lower pH values than do plain or freshly prepared solutions. The lower pH of these epinephrine-containing preparations could potentially decrease the amount of unionized form, thereby slowing the onset of action.

Other vasoconstrictors such as phenylephrine or methoxamine may be added to prolong the duration of the effect of local anesthetics by decreasing their systemic absorption [171]. Some degree of pharmacodynamic interaction may also exist as the infiltration of these α_1-adrenergic receptor agonists caused cutaneous anesthesia in rats [164]. But in contrast with epinephrine, these other agents lack α_2-adrenergic receptor effects and, therefore, potential interactions with local anesthetics mediated by these receptors are not possible. Moreover, phenylephrine, but not epinephrine, caused a significant decrease in sciatic nerve and skeletal muscle blood flow when administered in combination with lidocaine [169], which could potentially cause complications due to nerve ischemia.

Vasoconstrictors should be avoided for blockade of areas with erratic blood supply or without good collateral perfusion (e.g., intravenous regional anesthesia, teat blocks, or large areas of skin) because of the possibility of vasoconstriction-induced tissue ischemia and necrosis.

Phentolamine, a non-selective α-adrenergic receptor antagonist, has been shown to reverse prolonged local anesthetic-induced block when administered in combination with vasoconstrictors [172]. A commercial preparation of phentolamine mesylate (OraVerse®) has been approved for the reversal of soft tissue anesthesia and the associated functional deficits resulting from local dental anesthesia in humans.

Hyaluronidase, an enzyme that depolymerizes hyaluronic acid, the main cement of the interstitium, may be added to local anesthetics to improve tissue penetration and thereby shorten onset and increase spread of the block [173]. Addition of hyaluronidase raises the pH of the anesthetic solution to a slightly more physiologic level, which may contribute to the shortening of onset by increasing the amount of unionized drug. However, local anesthetic C_{max} and the risk of systemic toxicity may also increase. Human and animal studies show diverse results with respect to improved efficacy. Some human studies show better quality of peribulbar or retrobulbar block and shorter onset of action when hyaluronidase is added at concentrations as low as 3.5 IU/mL to mixtures of 0.5% or 0.75% bupivacaine and 2% lidocaine [174–176], while others show no benefit when hyluronidase is added at concentrations as high as 150 IU/mL to a mixture of 0.75% bupivacaine and 2% lidocaine for peribulbar block [177,178]. Hyaluronidase added to bupivacaine with epinephrine (1:200 000) for brachial plexus block did not increase the speed of onset of anesthesia or reduce the incidence of inadequate nerve block [179]. In a recent study in dogs, the addition of 400 IU of hyaluronidase to 1.06 mg/kg of 0.5% levobupivacaine for lumbosacral epidural block decreased the onset from 15 to five min, but it also decreased the duration of block, while dermatomal spread was unchanged [180]. When used in infiltration anesthesia, hyaluronidase added at 15 IU/mL to 1% lidocaine increased the area of desensitized skin, but pain on injection also increased compared with plain 1% lidocaine [181]. The addition of hyaluronidase to lidocaine for infiltration block does not delay wound healing [182]. The addition of hyaluronidase seems particularly advantageous in ophthalmic blocks, as it has been shown to limit the acute intraocular pressure increase secondary to periocular injection and seems to have a protective effect against local anesthetic-induced myotoxicity resulting in postoperative strabismus [183].

The pH of commercially available local anesthetic solutions is normally acidic to enhance stability and solubility and extend shelf-life [184,185]. Alkalinization of the solution by addition of sodium bicarbonate causes an increase in the amount of local anesthetic in the unionized form, which is the lipid-soluble fraction able to cross the axonal membrane, thereby shortening the onset of the block. The intensity and duration of the block may also increase due to an increase in the transmembrane pH gradient, causing ion trapping of the ionized active form inside the nerve. The efficacy of alkalinization depends on the local anesthetic solution, the site of the block, and the concurrent addition of epinephrine.

Buffering of 1% lidocaine, 1% mepivacaine or 0.5% bupivacaine with sodium bicarbonate for intradermal administration does not affect the onset, extent, and duration of skin anesthesia in humans [186,187]. Addition of bicarbonate to lidocaine for median nerve block in humans increased the rate of motor block without changing the onset or extent of sensory block [188]. Similarly, alkalinization of 1% lidocaine or 0.25% bupivacaine to a pH of 7.4 did not prolong infraorbital nerve block duration in rats [189]. Studies using buffered local anesthetics during epidural anesthesia show controversial results. Some studies show shorter onset of epidural block when 1.5–2% lidocaine, 2% mepivacaine or 0.5% bupivacaine is alkalinized with bicarbonate [190–192], while others show no shortening of onset with buffered 2% lidocaine or 0.5% bupivacaine [193–195]. The alkalinization of 0.75% ropivacaine solution does not decrease sensory or motor block onset, but increases the duration of the epidural block [196]. In femoral and sciatic nerve blocks, the effects of alkalinization on the onset of sensory analgesia and motor block were more evident with 2% mepivacaine, but for brachial plexus axillary block, the greatest effect was observed with 2% lidocaine [192]. Nonetheless, in studies where hastening of block onset occurred with alkalinization, the decrease was less than 5 min when compared with commercial preparations. In addition, it seems that the effect of alkalinization is mainly observed when epinephrine is also added to the solution [197]. Thus, the value of alkalinization of local anesthetics appears debatable as a clinically useful tool to improve anesthesia [15].

Alkalinization has a greater effect when the local anesthetic is administered into an acidic environment, as with intravesicular instillation where the urine is normally acidic. Intravesicular instillation of 5% lidocaine buffered with an equal volume of 8.4% sodium bicarbonate to a pH of 8.0 provided local anesthesia of the bladder submucosa as indicated by the rapid decrease in pain scores in human patients with interstitial cystitis [198]. However, intravesicular administration of alkalinized lidocaine for up to three consecutive days had no apparent beneficial effect on decreasing recurrence rate and severity of clinical signs in cats with obstructive idiopathic lower urinary tract disease [199].

Buffered local anesthetics also have a greater effect when topically administered to the cornea. The corneal permeability of topically applied lidocaine increased when the pH of the solution was buffered from 5.2 to 7.2, with greater concentrations of lidocaine found in the aqueous humor [200,201].

Buffering of the local anesthetic solution with bicarbonate decreases pain on injection when administered subcutaneously and also decreases pain when an epidural catheter is inserted [184,185,202]. Reduction of pain on injection seems to be enhanced by additional warming of the solution to body temperature [202].

The most common dose of sodium bicarbonate used is 0.1 mEq per mL of local anesthetic solution. The addition of bicarbonate may cause precipitation of the solution, especially with bupivacaine and etidocaine when the pH rises above 7.0 [203]. Mepivacaine may also precipitate at a pH above neutral within 20 min [204]. Therefore, it is recommended to use the mixed solution immediately after the addition of sodium bicarbonate.

Carbonation of local anesthetics by adding carbon dioxide (CO_2) is sometimes used to decrease onset and improve quality of the block. Addition of CO_2 to a solution of lidocaine decreased the amount of lidocaine needed to achieve conduction block *in vitro* [205]. This potentiation of local anesthetic block is possibly due to a decreased intracellular pH, causing ion trapping. Carbonated lidocaine administered epidurally shortened the onset and improved the block in humans [206,207]; however, it did not offer any advantage over the hydrochloride salt for caudal epidural anesthesia in horses [208].

The addition of α_2-adrenergic receptor agonist drugs to local anesthetics during regional blocks is being increasingly used in veterinary medicine. Clonidine has been extensively used in humans to prolong the duration of intrathecal, epidural, and peripheral nerve blocks. Meta-analyses and systematic reviews clearly show an analgesic benefit from the addition of clonidine to local anesthetics [209]. In large animals, epidural or intrathecal xylazine has been used in combination with lidocaine since the early 1990s to prolong the analgesic effect [210]. Medetomidine administered either perineurally or systemically (0.01 mg/kg) in combination with mepivacaine for radial nerve block in dogs prolonged the duration of sensory and motor blockade, with residual sensory blockade persisting beyond the observable sedative effects [211]. Dexmedetomidine has been recently introduced as an adjuvant to regional anesthesia in humans and animals. Studies in rats have shown that administration of dexmedetomidine in combination with bupivacaine or ropivacaine enhances sensory and motor blockade in sciatic nerve block without inducing neurotoxicity [212,213]. Clinical studies in humans show a shorter onset, longer duration of sensory and motor block, enhanced block quality, lower pain scores, and decreased systemic opioid requirements when dexmedetomidine is added to bupivacaine or levobupivacaine for various blocks [214–217]. Addition of dexmedetomidine to lidocaine for intravenous regional anesthesia improved the quality of anesthesia and decreased analgesic requirements, but had no effect on the extent of sensory and motor blockade, or on onset and regression times [218,219].

The increased duration of analgesia caused by adding clonidine or dexmedetomidine to local anesthetics is due to hyperpolarization of C fibers through blockade of the so-called hyperpolarization-activated cation current [220,221]. α-Adrenergic receptors do not seem to be implicated as administration of α-adrenergic receptor antagonists does not reverse the conduction block nor decrease the duration of the block [220–222].

Mixtures of local anesthetics

Local anesthetic mixtures of amino-amide agents consisting of an intermediate acting agent, such as lidocaine or mepivacaine, combined with a long-acting agent, such as bupivacaine, are used in the belief that the combination will provide a shorter block onset and a similar duration than the long-acting agent administered alone. However, these mixtures produce unpredictable and variable clinical results. Clinical studies in humans using a 50:50 mixture of lidocaine or mepivacaine with bupivacaine or ropivacaine for peripheral nerve blocks show a shorter onset of effect, but also a shorter duration of action, compared with the administration of bupivacaine or ropivacaine alone [223–225]. The epidural or intrathecal combination of lidocaine and bupivacaine in cows [226], cats [227], and humans [228–231] produced similar sensory block onset than either agent alone, and the duration was intermediate between the two agents or similar to bupivacaine.

When chloroprocaine, a short onset, short duration of action amino-ester local anesthetic, is administered prior to bupivacaine, the duration of bupivacaine-induced blockade is decreased. This may be due to an inhibitory effect caused by chloroprocaine metabolites on the Na^+ channel receptor site for bupivacaine [232]. Mixing commercial preparations of chloroprocaine and bupivacaine resulted in a pH of 3.6 and nerve blockade with characteristics of a chloroprocaine block [233]. When the pH of the mixture was increased to 5.56, the nerve block resembled that of bupivacaine. Therefore, mixing commercially available solutions of local anesthetics results in unpredictable blockade that will depend on a number of factors including the pH of the final mixture [233]. Furthermore, local anesthetic toxicity of combinations of drugs is additive [234].

Tachyphylaxis

Tachyphylaxis to local anesthetics is defined as a decrease in duration, segmental spread, or intensity of a regional block despite repeated constant dosages [235]. In 1969, Bromage described that repeated injection of a constant dose of epidural lidocaine led to a reduction in both the number of dermatomes blocked and the duration of the block [236]. The incidence of this phenomenon in veterinary medicine is unknown, and probably is largely unrecognized. Tachyphylaxis appears neither to be linked to structural or pharmacologic properties of the local anesthetics, nor to the technique or mode of administration, as it can occur with both ester- and amide-linked local anesthetics and with either neuraxial or peripheral nerve blocks [236–239]. Bromage found that tachyphylaxis to local anesthetics is promoted by longer interanalgesic intervals between injections [236]. If local anesthetic injections were repeated at intervals short enough to prevent return of pain or at intervals with pain of less than 10 min duration, tachyphylaxis did not occur and augmentation of the analgesic effect was noted. Conversely, if the patient experienced pain between local anesthetic administrations for more than 10 min, tachyphylaxis occurred more rapidly.

The mechanisms underlying tachyphylaxis may involve both pharmacokinetic and pharmacodynamic aspects. Suggested pharmacokinetic mechanisms include local edema, increased epidural protein concentration, changes in local anesthetic distribution in the epidural space, a decrease in perineural pH (limiting the diffusion of local anesthetic from the epidural space to binding sites at the Na^+ channel), an increase in epidural blood flow, or an increase in local metabolism (favoring clearance of local anesthetics from the epidural space) [235]. Other factors of pharmacodynamic origin have also been suggested, such as antagonistic effects of nucleotides or increased Na^+ concentration, increased afferent input from nociceptors, or receptor downregulation of Na^+ channels [235]. A human study with repeated injections of epidural lidocaine showed lack of changes in the distribution or rate of elimination of lidocaine from the epidural space [239] and another study in rats failed to show an effect of tissue pH on the development of tachyphylaxis to bupivacaine [237].

Tachyphylaxis to local anesthetics does not result from reduced drug effectiveness at the nerve itself [240], but it seems to be mainly mediated by a spinal site of action [241]. Tachyphylaxis and central hyperalgesia seem to be related, as evidenced by studies in rats, where tachyphylaxis occurred only under conditions where they concurrently developed hyperalgesia in the tested paw [242]. If only non-noxious motor tests were used to test the duration of the block, tachyphylaxis did not occur. Moreover, it has been shown that drugs that prevent hyperalgesia at spinal sites, such as NMDA receptor antagonists [242] and NO-synthase inhibitors [243], prevent the development of tachyphylaxis. Therefore, it seems that a spinal nitric oxide pathway is involved in the development of tachyphylaxis to local anesthetics [241]. Additionally, descending pathways do not seem necessary for the development of tachyphylaxis since it occurs even after spinal cord transection at the tenth thoracic level in rats [241].

Local anesthetic switching has also been proposed when tachyphylaxis to a local anesthetic agent develops. This approach has been successful in humans with cancer-related pain in whom intrathecal morphine and bupivacaine were not effective and substitution of bupivacaine with lidocaine improved analgesia [244].

Specific drugs and clinical uses

Amino-esters

Procaine

This agent has a quick onset and short duration of effect (30–60 min) because of its rapid hydrolysis in blood [15]. Epinephrine may be added to prolong its duration of effect. Its potential for systemic toxicity is minimal, but it occasionally causes allergic reactions due to a hydrolysis metabolite (PABA).

Procaine is used in veterinary medicine for infiltration and nerve blocks at concentrations of 1–2% [245]. It is rarely used for topical anesthesia, as it is not very effective via this route [245]. In humans, it is sometimes administered intrathecally for short procedures [246].

Intravenous procaine is a central nervous system stimulant in horses [93]. Because of this property, and its analgesic effect when used for peripheral nerve blocks, it has been illegally used in racehorses [245]. Procaine is sometimes added to drug formulations (i.e., procaine penicillin) to prolong duration of effect.

Benzocaine

This agent is also a fast-acting and short-lasting local anesthetic, available exclusively for topical anesthesia. It causes methemoglobinemia in several animal species and therefore it is no longer used in clinical practice. Benzocaine is also an anesthetic for fish when added to water [247].

Chloroprocaine

This agent is similar to procaine, with a fast onset and short duration of action (30–60 min). It is available in concentrations of 1% to 3%. It is not widely used in veterinary medicine, but in humans its use has re-emerged for short-duration epidural and intrathecal anesthesia because it is associated with a lower incidence of transient neurologic symptoms compared with lidocaine [248]. It may also be used for local infiltration blocks when a short duration of effect is required.

Tetracaine

Tetracaine is also called amethocaine. It is rarely used in veterinary medicine. In humans it is most commonly used for intrathecal anesthesia because it has a fast onset (3–5 min) and its effect lasts 2–3 h [249]. It is rarely used for other forms of regional anesthesia due to its extremely slow onset and potential for systemic toxicity [249]. It is an excellent topical anesthetic and because of this property it is included in topical anesthetic solutions. However, the absorption of tetracaine from mucous membranes is very rapid and several fatalities have been reported after its use for endoscopic procedures in humans [250]. Human studies have shown that tetracaine topical preparations, including a lidocaine/tetracaine patch (Synera®, Rapydan®), provide faster and better dermal anesthesia than the eutectic mixture of lidocaine and prilocaine (EMLA® cream) [251,252].

Amino-amides

Lidocaine

Lidocaine remains the most versatile and most widely used local anesthetic in veterinary medicine because of its fast onset, moderate duration of effect, and moderate toxicity. It is available as 0.5%, 1%, 1.5%, and 2% solutions. Lidocaine is used for infiltration anesthesia, peripheral nerve blocks, epidural and intrathecal blocks, and intravenous regional anesthesia. The duration of plain lidocaine is approximately 1 h, which can be prolonged up to 3- h with the addition of epinephrine [15]. It is also commonly used topically for laryngeal desensitization before tracheal intubation (2%, 4% or 10% spray solution). For dermal anesthesia it is available in different formulations such as the eutectic mixture with prilocaine (2.5% EMLA® cream), as patches of lidocaine alone (5% Lidoderm®) or mixed with tetracaine (Synera®, Rapydan®).

Lidocaine has numerous non-anesthetic uses when administered intravenously. It is a Class Ib antiarrhythmic drug. It also reduces the requirements for inhalational anesthetics when administered intravenously in different species including dogs [253–255], cats [256], goats [102], horses [257,258], and calves [259]. It is also an analgesic drug for different types of pain when administered systemically, as shown in human patients [260,261] and experimental studies in laboratory animals [262,263]. Administration of intravenous lidocaine (2 mg/kg bolus followed by 0.05 mg/kg/min) produced thermal antinociception in horses [264]. However, it did not affect the thermal threshold in cats (plasma concentrations up to 4.3 μg/mL) [265], or the electrical threshold in dogs (2 mg/kg IV bolus followed by an infusion of up to 0.1 mg/kg/min) [266].

The mechanism by which systemically administered lidocaine produces analgesia is uncertain but is thought to include action at

Table 17.3 Pharmacokinetic parameters (mean ± SD) of intravenous lidocaine in domestic species.

	$T_{1/2}$ (min)	Vd_{ss} (L/kg)	Cl (mL/kg/min)
Dog [273]	68.1 ± 10.9	1.38 ± 0.08	27.5 ± 6
Cat [99]	100 ± 28	1.39 ± 0.37	26 ± 2.7
Horse [125]	79 ± 41	0.79 ± 0.16	29 ± 7.6
Cattle [104]	63.6 ± 42	3.3 ± 1.6	42.2 ± 20.5
Sheep [113]	30.9	NA	41.2

$T_{1/2}$ = terminal half-life; Vd_{ss} = apparent volume of distribution in steady state; Cl = total body clearance.

Na^+, Ca^{2+}, and K^+ channels and the NMDA receptor [30–32,34,35]. Lidocaine also possesses anti-inflammatory effects, which may be important in producing analgesia because inflammatory mediators augment neuronal excitability [267]. In addition, some studies show that lidocaine may improve intestinal motility and prevent development of postoperative ileus in horses [268–271], especially in those with reperfusion injury [272].

The disposition of lidocaine after intravenous administration has been described for sheep [113], dogs [96,114,273], cats [99], horses [125], cows [104], and chickens [103] (Table 17.3).

Mepivacaine

This agent has a pharmacologic profile very similar to lidocaine, with a slightly longer duration of effect (up to 2 h), probably because of slightly less intrinsic vasodilatory properties. It is available at concentrations from 0.5% to 2%. Its use in clinical practice is similar to lidocaine, except that it is not routinely used for intravenous regional anesthesia or for obstetric procedures because its metabolism is very slow in the fetus and newborn [249]. Unlike lidocaine, mepivacaine is not an effective topical anesthetic [249]. It is the preferred agent for diagnostic peripheral nerve blocks in horses because of its lower neurotoxicity compared with other local anesthetics [274].

Bupivacaine

This is a highly lipophilic agent, about four times as potent as lidocaine, and with slow onset of action (20–30 min) and a long duration of effect (3–10 h) [249]. It is used in concentrations ranging from 0.125% to 0.75%. Its clinical uses include infiltrative, peripheral nerve, epidural, and intrathecal blocks. Bupivacaine is not used for topical anesthesia and it is not recommended for intravenous regional anesthesia because of its high cardiotoxicity potential. It possesses intrinsic differential blocking properties, especially at low concentrations, and therefore is indicated when sensory blockade accompanied by minimal motor dysfunction is desired.

Levobupivacaine

This is the levoisomer or *S*-enantiomer of bupivacaine, with slightly less cardiotoxic potential than the racemic mixture. Its physicochemical properties and clinical uses are the same as bupivacaine.

Ropivacaine

This agent is structurally related to mepivacaine and bupivacaine, but it is marketed as the pure *S*-enantiomer to reduce the cardiotoxicity associated with the *R*-enantiomer. It is slightly less potent than bupivacaine and is available in concentrations of up to 1%. Its clinical uses are the same as bupivacaine, with similar onset of effect, a marginally shorter sensory blockade (up to 6 h) and a slightly lower degree of motor blockade at equipotent doses [249]. It has a

Table 17.4 Clinically relevant local anesthetic commercial names, indications, and doses.

Local anesthetic	Commercial name	Indications	Doses
Procaine	Novocaine, Procasel, Adrenacaine, Dalocain, Isocain (with epinephrine)	Infiltration Nerve blocks	Maximum 2–4 mg/kg
Lidocaine	Topical: EMLA cream (with prilocaine), Xylocaine, Intubeaze, Lidoderm patches Injectable: Lidocaine HCl, Lignocaine, Xylocaine (some with epinephrine)	Topical (dermal, mucous membranes) Infiltration Nerve blocks Interpleural Epidural Intrathecal[a] Intravenous (IV)	Maximum doses: 6–10 mg/kg (Ca), 3–5 mg/kg (Fe), 6 mg/kg (Eq, Bo, Ov, Cp, Sw) Epidural: 4 mg/kg of 2% sol. (0.2 mL/kg) (Ca, Fe, Ov, Cp, Sw), 6 mL total (Eq, Bo) IV intraoperative: 1–2 mg/kg bolus, 50–100 μg/kg/min (Ca), 25–50 μg/kg/min (Eq, Bo)
Mepivacaine	Carbocaine, Intra-Epicaine, Vetacaine	Infiltration Nerve blocks Interpleural Epidural Intrathecal[a] Intra-articular	Maximum dose: 5–6 mg/kg (Ca, Eq, Bo, Ov, Cp, Sw), 2–3 mg/kg (Fe) Intra-articular: 1–2 mg/kg
Bupivacaine	Marcaine	Infiltration Nerve blocks Interpleural Epidural Intrathecal[a]	Maximum dose: 2 mg/kg (Ca, Eq, Bo, Ov, Cp, Sw), 1–1.5 mg/kg (Fe) Epidural: 1 mg/kg of 0.5% sol. (0.2 mL/kg) (Ca, Fe, Ov, Ca, Sw), 6 mL total (Eq, Bo)
Levobupivacaine	Chirocaine	Infiltration Nerve blocks Interpleural Epidural Intrathecal[a]	Maximum dose: 3 mg/kg (Ca, Eq, Bo, Ov, Cp, Sw), 1.5 mg/kg (Fe) Epidural: 1 mg/kg of 0.5% sol. (0.2 mL/kg) (Ca, Fe, Ov, Cp, Sw), 6 mL total (Eq, Bo)
Ropivacaine	Naropin	Infiltration Nerve blocks Interpleural Epidural Intrathecal[a]	Maximum dose: 3 mg/kg (Ca, Eq, Bo, Ov, Cp, Sw), 1.5 mg/kg (Fe) Epidural: 1 mg/kg of 0.5% sol. (0.2 mL/kg) (Ca, Fe, Ov, Cp, Sw), 6 mL total (Eq, Bo)

[a] Intrathecal dose is 1/10th of epidural dose.
Ca Canine, Fe Feline, Eq Equine, Bo Bovine, Ov Ovine, Cp Caprine, Sw Swine.

biphasic effect on peripheral vasculature, causing vasoconstriction at concentrations below 0.5% and vasodilation at concentrations over 1% (Table 17.4) [275].

Adverse effects

Systemic toxicity

Local anesthetic drugs may cause central nervous system (CNS) and cardiac toxicity at high plasma concentrations. Plasma concentrations are determined by the rate of drug absorption into the systemic circulation, but the most common reason for excessive plasma concentrations is the inadvertent direct intravascular injection of the local anesthetic solution while performing peripheral or neuraxial blocks. Local anesthetics vary considerably in their potency at causing systemic toxic reactions, and generally this potency follows the same rank order as their potency at producing nerve blockade [276]. More lipid-soluble drugs (i.e., bupivacaine) are more potent at causing systemic toxicity than less lipid-soluble agents (i.e., lidocaine or mepivacaine), and the *S*-enantiomers or levoisomers (i.e., levobupivacaine or ropivacaine) are less toxic than the *R*-enantiomers or dextroisomers, or than the racemic mixture of both [277–280].

The dose of a local anesthetic causing systemic toxicity will depend on the route and speed of administration (rapid intravenous administration will be more likely to cause high plasma levels), the species involved, and patient factors (such as acid–base balance, serum potassium levels and whether the animal is under anesthesia).

The clinical incidence of systemic toxicity in domestic animals is unknown. The incidence of systemic toxicity associated with regional anesthetic blocks in humans is estimated to be around 1 in 10 000, with peripheral blocks having the highest incidence (7.5 in 10 000) [281,282].

Central nervous system toxicity

Central nervous system toxic signs follow a progression as the plasma concentration of local anesthetic increases (Fig. 17.5). At low doses, all local anesthetics are effective anticonvulsants, and they also have sedative effects [283]. In conscious, unsedated humans, the initial signs of local anesthetic CNS toxicity include tongue numbness, light-headedness, dizziness, drowsiness, paresthesia of sight and sound, and acute anxiety or even fear of death [284]. In horses, this has been described as alteration in visual function, rapid eye blinking, anxiety, mild sedation, and ataxia [268,269,285]. As the plasma level rises, local anesthetics inhibit inhibitory cortical neurons in the temporal lobe or the amygdala, allowing facilitatory neurons to function in an unopposed fashion, resulting in increased excitatory activity, which first leads to muscle twitching followed by grand mal seizures [276,283]. As the plasma concentration increases further, local anesthetics can inhibit both inhibitory and facilitatory pathways, resulting in CNS depression, unconsciousness, and coma [276,283].

Not all local anesthetics produce signs of aura, such as drowsiness or excitement, before the onset of seizures. With the highly lipophilic, highly protein-bound agents such as bupivacaine, the excitement phase can be brief and mild and the first signs may be bradycardia, cyanosis, and unconsciousness [286].

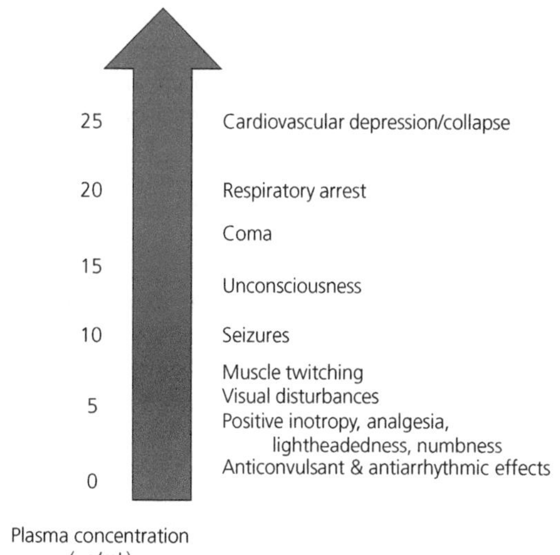

Figure 17.5 Progressive signs of lidocaine systemic toxicity with increasing plasma concentrations. Note: concentrations are approximate and depend on various factors (see text).

Central nervous system toxicity is generally assumed to precede cardiovascular toxicity. This derives from studies in conscious sheep where the doses and plasma drug concentrations associated with cardiovascular collapse (CV, defined as the disappearance of pulsatile blood pressure) and CNS toxicity (signified by the onset of seizures) were calculated as the CV:CNS ratio. Values for the CV:CNS ratio for various local anesthetics in conscious sheep are much greater than 1, supporting this notion [278,287].

In humans, the frequency of seizures and accompanying cardiovascular changes associated with various regional block techniques has been reviewed. There is a significant difference between the rate of seizure development with caudal > brachial plexus > epidural blocks, with no adverse cardiovascular or pulmonary effects occurring during seizures [288].

In conscious dogs, the mean cumulative dose required for convulsive activity was 4 mg/kg for tetracaine, 5 mg/kg for bupivacaine, 8 mg/kg for etidocaine, and 22 mg/kg for lidocaine in one study [9]. In another study, administration of intravenous infusions of lidocaine (8 mg/kg/min), bupivacaine (2 mg/kg/min), or ropivacaine (2 mg/kg/min) caused generalized seizures at an average dose of 21 mg/kg of lidocaine, 4 mg/kg of bupivacaine, and 5 mg/kg of ropivacaine in conscious dogs [289]. The first seizure activity observed with lidocaine toxicity in dogs was tonic extension at an infused dose of 12 mg/kg, followed by running activity after 23 mg/kg, and with tonic-clonic seizures occurring at an infused dose of 33 mg/kg [290]. The plasma concentration of lidocaine causing muscle tremors was 2.7 μg/mL after administration of a total dose of 11.1 mg/kg IV to conscious dogs [291]. The onset of seizures occurred when lidocaine plasma concentrations reached 8.2 μg/mL in another study involving awake dogs [292].

In conscious horses the mean toxic plasma concentration of lidocaine causing muscle fasciculations was determined to be 3.24 μg/mL (range 1.85–4.53 μg/mL), and it did not change regardless of speed of administration [285]. Such plasma concentrations may be achieved during prolonged lidocaine IV infusions of greater than 12 h in postcolic surgery horses [293,294].

In lightly anesthetized and ventilated cats, seizures occurred after administration of 12 mg/kg of lidocaine and 5 mg/kg of bupivacaine given at intravenous infusion rates of 16 mg/kg/min and 4 mg/kg/min, respectively [295]. The CV:CNS toxicity ratio for drug dosage was 4.0 with lidocaine and 4.8 with bupivacaine [295].

In conscious sheep, the doses of infused lidocaine, bupivacaine, and ropivacaine necessary to produce convulsions were 6.8 mg/kg, 1.6 mg/kg, and 3.5 mg/kg, respectively [296]. Therefore, the ratio of the mean convulsant doses (lidocaine/bupivacaine/ropivacaine) was approximately 5:1:2 [296].

There is an inverse relationship between the seizure threshold dose of local anesthetics and the arterial carbon dioxide tension [297]. This may be due to an increase in cerebral blood flow during hypercapnia causing increased delivery of drug to the brain and/or a decrease in plasma protein binding of local anesthetics causing an increase in free drug [298]. Hypoxemia also increases the CNS and cardiovascular toxicity of local anesthetics [299].

Cardiovascular toxicity

At low concentrations, most local anesthetics have an antiarrhythmic effect, but at higher concentrations, they produce cardiac toxicity. Local anesthetics block cardiac Na^+ channels and decrease the maximum rise of Phase 0 of the action potential, leading to a pronounced and evolving inhibition of cardiac conduction [300]. Electrocardiographic changes include prolonged PR and QRS intervals and a prolonged refractory period [300–302]. The cardiovascular effects of local anesthetics are complex and non-linear, involving direct effects on cardiac conduction and contractility and on vascular smooth muscle and also indirect effects mediated by the CNS [276].

All local anesthetics cause myocardial depression with small intravenous doses that cause no overt CNS toxicity [280,303]. At subconvulsant doses, heart rate may increase slightly and the QRS complex may widen, but there are no major effects on blood pressure and cardiac output [280,303]. These effects are mild and rapidly reversed, with no qualitative differences among local anesthetics [280]. At the onset of convulsions, there is a profound sympathetic response associated with all local anesthetics, which reverses the induced myocardial depression causing tachycardia and increased blood pressure and cardiac output [279,280,296]. Convulsant doses of all longer acting local anesthetics cause marked arrhythmias, typically ventricular tachycardia, that may progress to ventricular fibrillation or cardiovascular collapse [279,304]. Supraconvulsant doses of lidocaine cause profound hypotension, bradycardia, decreases in myocardial contractility, respiratory arrest, and ultimately asystole [279,296].

It has been postulated that the CNS toxic effects may be involved in the production of serious cardiotoxicity because of the onset of respiratory failure accompanied by hypoxia, bradycardia, hypercapnia, and acidosis [283].

While all local anesthetics cause direct negative inotropic effects, the shorter acting local anesthetics such as lidocaine and mepivacaine are less arrhythmogenic than the longer acting ones, such as bupivacaine or ropivacaine [279,304]. These differences are caused by differences in the kinetics of binding and unbinding from various ion channels [305,306]. While both shorter and longer acting agents have similar rates of binding to cardiac Na^+ channels, the longer acting agents have slower unbinding rates, hence predisposing to cardiac arrhythmias [276]. The *R*-enantiomers of the more lipophilic local anesthetics have slower unbinding rates than the *S*-enantiomers, thereby making them even more arrhythmogenic [305,306].

No ventricular arrhythmias were observed with cardiotoxic doses of lidocaine in conscious dogs [279]. Ventricular tachycardia with no hemodynamic impairment was observed in only one of eight conscious sheep with lidocaine and one of seven with mepivacaine [304]. In contrast, ventricular arrhythmias occurred in one of six conscious dogs with cardiotoxic doses of ropivacaine and five of six with bupivacaine [279]. Polymorphic ventricular tachycardia accompanied by decreased cardiac output occurred in seven of ten conscious sheep receiving bupivacaine, 4 of 11 with levobupivacaine and 5 of 12 with ropivacaine [304]. Even though the newer local anesthetics ropivacaine and levobupivacaine appear to be less cardiotoxic than bupivacaine (judging by the larger doses tolerated before the onset of serious arrhythmias), they must not be regarded as totally safe [307].

General anesthesia has a substantial impact on toxicity, mortality, and pharmacokinetics of various local anesthetics and distorts pharmacokinetic-pharmacodynamic relationships. In a study in halothane-anesthetized sheep, the pre-existing myocardial depression from halothane was markedly exacerbated by infusions of lidocaine, mepivacaine, prilocaine, bupivacaine, levobupivacaine or ropivacaine [304]. The cardiovascular toxic effects of each local anesthetic were also prolonged in anesthetized sheep compared with conscious sheep, and concurrently, the blood drug concentrations were markedly increased under general anesthesia. However, no serious arrhythmias occurred in any anesthetized sheep. Despite the exaggerated cardiovascular effects of the local anesthetics when the sheep were anesthetized, none of them died, whereas approximately 15% died from fatal cardiac arrhythmias when conscious [304].

As the K^+ gradient across cardiac myocyte membranes is the most important factor in establishing the membrane potential, hyperkalemia can markedly increase local anesthetic toxicity. Under conditions of hyperkalemia (5.4 mEq/L) in dogs, the cardiotoxic doses of both lidocaine and bupivacaine were halved compared to conditions of normokalemia, while the seizure-inducing doses did not change for either agent [308]. Conversely, hypokalemia decreases local anesthetic cardiotoxicity [308].

Treatment of systemic toxicity

When signs of systemic toxicity are noted, the administration of local anesthetic should be discontinued. Treatment of systemic toxicity is primarily supportive (Box 17.1). Oxygenation and ventilation are the main goals. It may be necessary to intubate the trachea and mechanically ventilate the animal to avoid or reverse hypoxemia, hypercapnia, and acidosis, all of which promote toxicity. If grand mal seizures are present, an anticonvulsant drug may be administered. If cardiovascular depression is also present, barbiturates or propofol are not recommended and treatment with a benzodiazepine is preferable.

Box 17.1 Guidelines for treatment of local anesthetic systemic toxicity.

CNS toxicity

1. Intubate trachea, administer O_2 and ventilate.
2. Treat seizures with a benzodiazepine.

Cardiac arrest

1. Start basic cardiopulmonary resuscitation.
2. Administer epinephrine at low doses (≤1 μg/kg IV).
3. AVOID lidocaine, vasopressin, calcium channel blockers, and β-blockers.
4. Administer a 20% lipid emulsion IV.
   - Initial bolus 1.5–4 mL/kg over 1 min.
   - Continue with CRI at 0.25 mL/kg/min for 30–60 min.
   - If non-responsive administer additional boluses of 1.5 mL/kg (up to maximum 7 mL/kg).
   - CRI may be continued at 0.5 mL/kg/h until clinical signs improve (24 h maximum).

Data obtained from references 309 and 319.

Cardiovascular toxicity induced by lidocaine or mepivacaine is usually mild and reversible with the use of positive inotropic drugs and fluid support [15]. Cardiac arrhythmias produced by longer acting local anesthetics such as bupivacaine (i.e., ventricular tachycardia or fibrillation) are usually malignant and refractory to routine treatment. In these cases, cardiopulmonary resuscitation should be immediately instituted and defibrillation initiated if necessary. In humans, the guidelines of the American Society of Regional Anesthesia and Pain Medicine recommend using low doses of epinephrine (<1 μg/kg) and avoiding vasopressin [309]. Calcium channel blockers should not be administered as their cardiodepressant effects are exaggerated [310]. Amiodarone rather than lidocaine is indicated to treat ventricular arrhythmias in this setting [310]. In cases of refractory cardiac arrest, it is recommended to use an intravenous lipid emulsion (i.e., Intralipid® 20%), which has been shown to reverse refractory arrhythmias caused by highly lipophilic local anesthetics in different experimental models [311,312] and in human clinical reports [313–315].

In a rodent model of bupivacaine-induced asystole in animals pretreated with an intravenous lipid solution, the median lethal dose (LD_{50}) of bupivacaine increased by 48% [311]. In a dog model of bupivacaine-induced cardiotoxicity (10 mg/kg IV), cardiopulmonary resuscitation was instituted for 10 min and then dogs received similar volumes of either intravenous saline fluid or a 20% lipid solution (4 mL/kg over 2 min, followed by 0.5 mL/kg/min over 10 min) [312]. Notably, all dogs in the saline control group failed to regain spontaneous circulation and died, while all dogs treated with the lipid solution survived, achieving near baseline blood pressure and heart rate values within 30 min of its administration [312]. Later studies in rats have demonstrated the potential adverse effects of epinephrine administered at high doses during lipid emulsion rescue with a higher incidence of ventricular arrhythmias, hyperlactatemia, hypoxia, acidosis, and pulmonary edema [316,317]. Another study in rats also demonstrated worse outcomes when vasopressin was administered alone or in combination with epinephrine compared with a lipid emulsion [318].

The exact mechanism of action of lipid emulsions is unknown and is likely multifactorial, but it is thought to be related to improved myocardial performance and a 'lipid sink' effect, which postulates that the lipophilic local anesthetic is sequestered into a lipid compartment within the bloodstream [319].

Propofol should not be administered as a substitute for intravenous lipid emulsions as its lipid content is too low (10%) and the large doses required would induce profound cardiovascular depression.

Local toxicity

Neurotoxicity

Exposure of the peripheral or central nervous systems to local anesthetics can cause direct damage, although this complication is rare. Mechanisms of local anesthetic neurotoxicity remain speculative, but some studies suggest injury to Schwann cells, which is time and concentration dependent [320], inhibition of fast axonal transport, disruption of the blood–nerve barrier, decreased neural blood flow with associated ischemia [321], and disruption of cell membrane integrity due to a detergent property of local anesthetics [322].

All local anesthetics are potentially neurotoxic and neurotoxicity parallels anesthetic potency. The *in vitro* rank order of potency for cytotoxicity is procaine ≤ mepivacaine < lidocaine < chloroprocaine < ropivacaine < bupivacaine, based on the LD_{50} for neuronal cells [274]. Neurotoxicity is also related to the concentration of local anesthetic. Clinically relevant concentrations of local anesthetics are considered safe for peripheral nerves [323]. The spinal cord and nerve roots, on the other hand, are more prone to injury [15]. Intrathecal administration of 8% lidocaine, 2% bupivacaine, and 1% tetracaine, but not of 2% chloroprocaine and 2% ropivacaine, caused histopathologic changes in the spinal cord and neurologic deficits in rabbits [324]. The cytotoxic effect of lidocaine and bupivacaine is concentration dependent, with higher concentrations causing death of all cells in culture. In contrast, mepivacaine, ropivacaine, procaine, and chloroprocaine did not kill all cells even at very high concentrations [274].

The effects of local anesthetics on spinal cord blood flow appear to be benign, and do not seem responsible for spinal cord neurotoxicity. Intrathecal administration of lidocaine, mepivacaine, bupivacaine, and tetracaine cause vasodilation and increase spinal cord blood flow, whereas ropivacaine causes vasoconstriction and decreases spinal cord blood flow, with both effects being concentration dependent [63].

The incidence of long-term neurologic injury in human patients undergoing spinal anesthesia is 0-0.02% [282]. Therefore, it seems to be a relatively safe technique in clinical practice if properly performed using clinically appropriate local anesthetic concentrations.

Myotoxicity

Local anesthetics can cause toxicity to skeletal muscle. Experimentally, all local anesthetics have the potential for myotoxicity at clinically relevant concentrations. Myotoxicity is concentration dependent, as observed in a study in rabbits where extraocular muscle injection with 0.75% bupivacaine caused acute myonecrosis and degeneration, compared with only scattered and significantly fewer areas of mild muscle fiber degeneration with 0.38% bupivacaine, and no muscle degeneration observed when the injection was with 0.19% bupivacaine [325]. Bupivacaine seems to be more myotoxic than other local anesthetics as judged by the larger extent of muscle lesions observed [326]. The mechanism of local anesthetic-induced muscle toxicity is likely to be related to dysregulation of intracellular calcium concentration and/or alterations in mitochondrial bioenergetics [327].

In most cases, local anesthetic-induced myonecrosis appears to be regenerative and clinically imperceptible. However, bupivacaine and ropivacaine produced irreversible skeletal muscle damage characterized by calcific myonecrosis observed 4 weeks after peripheral nerve blockade in a study in pigs [326].

Clinically relevant myopathy and myonecrosis have been described in humans after receiving continuous peripheral blocks, infiltration of wound margins, trigger point injections, and peri- and retrobulbar blocks [328].

Chondrotoxicity

Local anesthetics are sometimes injected intra-articularly in clinical practice. Local anesthetic chondrotoxicity has been demonstrated both *in vivo* and *in vitro* in both animal and human cartilage [329–332]. Clinically, chondrolysis has been associated with the use of intra-articular local anesthetic pain pumps in humans [333,334].

The chondrotoxicity exhibited by local anesthetics is time and concentration dependent. *In vitro* bovine chondrocyte viability decreased after just 15 min of exposure to 1% lidocaine, and longer exposures to 1% and 2% lidocaine further reduced chondrocyte viability [330]. Chondrocyte viability was reduced to a larger extent when exposed to 2% lidocaine than to 1% lidocaine [330]. This study also showed that the intact articular surface is not protective against local anesthetic chondrotoxicity [330].

In vitro exposure of equine chondrocytes to 0.5% bupivacaine, 2% lidocaine, or 2% mepivacaine for 30 or 60 min revealed that bupivacaine is the most chondrotoxic of the three local anesthetics and that mepivacaine is the least toxic [331]. Ropivacaine is also significantly less toxic than bupivacaine and lidocaine in both intact human articular cartilage and chondrocyte culture [335,336]. The marked chondrotoxicity exhibited by bupivacaine and lidocaine is mainly due to necrosis rather than apoptosis [331].

In conclusion, evidence suggests that there is a greater risk for chondrolysis with a longer exposure to a higher concentration of local anesthetic, such as with a pain pump, than with a single injection, and that mepivacaine seems to be the least toxic and consequently the preferred drug for intra-articular administration at the present time.

Methemoglobinemia

Methemoglobin (MHb) formation may be induced by certain local anesthetics in several animal species and in humans. Methemoglobin is produced by oxidative damage to the hemoglobin molecule. Specifically, the iron of the heme group is oxidized to the ferric (Fe^{3+}) form. In this state, it cannot bind oxygen (O_2) and therefore blood oxygen-carrying capacity is decreased. The physiologic range of MHb in the blood is 0–2% [337]. Concentrations of MHb of 10–20% are tolerated well, but higher levels are often associated with clinical signs, and levels above 70% may cause death [337]. Oxidative denaturation of hemoglobin can cause Heinz body formation (precipitated hemoglobin or globin subunits), which is irreversible and decreases the lifespan of red blood cells and causes hemolysis.

The local anesthetics more often associated with MHb formation are the ester-type benzocaine and the amide-type prilocaine. Administration of a 2 s spray of benzocaine (estimated dose 56 mg) to the mucous membranes of the nasopharynx of dogs, cats, ferrets, monkeys, rabbits, and miniature pigs induced MHb formation ranging from 3.5% to 38% 15–60 min after administration in more than 95% of the animals tested [338]. In sheep, intranasal administration of topical benzocaine for 2 s caused MHb in half of the animals tested, ranging from 16% to 26%, and a 10 s spray caused MHb levels of up to 50.5% [339,340]. Dermal administration of benzocaine has also been implicated in clinical cases of methemoglobinemia in dogs and cats [341,342]. An *N*-hydroxy metabolite of benzocaine (i.e., O-toluidine) is the likely active MHb-forming substance [339]. Prilocaine has been implicated in cases of methemoglobinemia in mothers and fetuses following epidural administration for labor [343] and following topical administration for dental procedures in humans [337]. Topical lidocaine did not induce MHb formation in sheep or monkeys, but it may be associated with MHb formation in cats and humans [339,344].

When MHb levels are 30% or higher, clinical signs of tissue hypoxia occur including cyanosis, dyspnea, nausea, vomiting, and tachycardia [337,341]. Lethargy, stupor, and shock occur when MHb levels approach 55% [337,342]. Animals with chronic methemoglobinemia may only present with Heinz body anemia and lethargy [342]. Chocolate brown-colored blood together with clinical signs that are not responsive to O_2 therapy are suggestive of methemoglobinemia. Definitive diagnosis is made by measuring the MHb concentration with co-oximetry or spectrophotometry. Blood smears will reveal the presence of Heinz bodies in the red blood cells.

Traditional first-line therapy of methemoglobinemia consists of slow intravenous administration of 1% methylene blue solution (4 mg/kg in dogs, 1–2 mg/kg in cats) [36]. The action of methylene blue depends on the availability of reduced nicotinamide adenine dinucleotide phosphate (NADPH) within red blood cells [337]. This dose can be repeated in dogs, but caution should be exercised in cats as repeated injections of methylene blue can markedly aggravate subsequent hemolysis without further lowering MHb content [345]. Dextrose should also be administered because it is the major source of reduced nicotinamide adenine dinucleotide (NADH) in red blood cells, which is necessary to form NADPH, which is in turn needed for methylene blue to be effective [337]. In severe cases a blood transfusion may be required.

Toxicosis (Oral ingestion)

Topical preparations containing lidocaine, benzocaine, and tetracaine are found in many prescription and non-prescription products, such as ointments, teething gels, suppositories, and aerosols. These topical local anesthetic preparations can be hazardous if ingested or inappropriately applied to animals. Between 1995 and 1999 the American Society for the Prevention of Cruelty to Animals (ASPCA) Animal Poison Control Center (APCC) consulted on more than 70 cases of local anesthetic toxicosis in a variety of animal species [346]. Benzocaine toxicosis cases reported to the ASPCA APCC involved either ingestion of topical preparations or application of a laryngeal spray before endotracheal intubation. Clinical signs in cats and ferrets with benzocaine toxicosis included varying degrees of vomiting, depression, cyanosis, dyspnea, and tachypnea [346]. Other signs observed with local anesthetic toxicosis in different species include prolonged sedation, vasodilation (leading to hypotension), cardiac arrhythmias, respiratory depression, tremors and seizures, and death [346].

Allergic reactions

Ester-type local anesthetics (e.g., procaine) are associated with a higher incidence of allergic reactions due to a p-aminobenzoic acid (PABA) metabolite. Amide-type agents do not undergo such metabolism and rarely cause allergic reactions. However, preservative compounds (i.e., methylparaben, sodium metabisulfite) used in preparations of amide-type local anesthetics are metabolized to PABA and may cause allergies [347,348]. Therefore, it is recommended that animals known to be allergic to ester-type local anesthetics be treated with a preservative-free amide-type agent [347].

Allergic reactions of dogs and cats treated with amide-type local anesthetics are very rare when compared with humans, which is probably because of their different metabolism and breakdown products [36].

Anaphylactic reactions are characterized by bronchospasm, upper airway edema, vasodilation, increased capillary permeability, and cutaneous wheal and flare [36]. Rapid intervention with airway maintenance, O_2 therapy, epinephrine administration, and volume expansion is essential to avoid a fatal outcome.

References

1 Komai H, McDowell TS. Local anesthetic inhibition of voltage-activated potassium currents in rat dorsal root ganglion neurons. *Anesthesiology* 2001; **94**: 1089–1095.

2 Olschewski A, Hempelmann G, Vogel W, *et al.* Blockade of Na+ and K+ currents by local anesthetics in the dorsal horn neurons of the spinal cord. *Anesthesiology* 1998; **88**: 172–179.

3 Xiong ZL, Strichartz GR. Inhibition by local anesthetics of Ca2+ channels in rat anterior pituitary cells. *Eur J Pharmacol* 1998; **363**: 81–90.

4 Sugiyama K, Muteki T. Local anesthetics depress the calcium current of rat sensory neurons in culture. *Anesthesiology* 1994; **80**: 1369–1378.

5 Scholz A. Mechanisms of (local) anaesthetics on voltage-gated sodium and other ion channels. *Br J Anaesth* 2002; **89**: 52–61.

6 Hollmann MW, Wieczorek KS, Berger A, *et al.* Local anesthetic inhibition of G protein-coupled receptor signaling by interference with Galpha(q) protein function. *Mol Pharmacol* 2001; **59**: 294–301.

7 Fozzard HA, Lee PJ, Lipkind GM. Mechanism of local anesthetic drug action on voltage-gated sodium channels. *Curr Pharm Des* 2005; **11**(21): 2671–2686.

8 Catterall WA. From ionic currents to molecular mechanisms: the structure and function of voltage-gated sodium channels. *Neuron* 2000; **26**(1): 13–25.

9 Narahashi T, Frazier DT. Site of action and active form of local anesthetics. *Neurosci Res* 1971; **4**: 65–99.

10 Wann KT. Neuronal sodium and potassium channels: structure and function. *Br J Anaesth* 1993; **71**(1): 2–14.

11 Yun I, Cho ES, Jang HO, *et al.* Amphiphilic effects of local anesthetics on rotational mobility in neuronal and model membranes. *Biochim Biophys Acta* 2002; **1564**(1): 123–132.

12 Hille B. Local anesthetics: hydrophilic and hydrophobic pathways for the drug-receptor reaction. *J Gen Physiol* 1977; **69**(4): 497–515.

13 Starmer CF, Grant AO, Strauss HC. Mechanisms of use-dependent block of sodium channels in excitable membranes by local anesthetics. *Biophys J* 1984; **46**(1): 15–27.

14 Huang JH, Thalhammer JG, Raymond SA, *et al.* Susceptibility to lidocaine of impulses in different somatosensory afferent fibers of rat sciatic nerve. *J Pharmacol Exp Ther* 1997; **292**: 802–811.

15 Liu SS, Joseph RS. Local anesthetics. In: Barash PG, Cullen BF, Stoelting RK, eds. *Clinical Anesthesia*, 5th edn. Philadelphia: Lippincott Williams & Wilkins, 2006; 453–471.

16 Stevens RA, Bray JG, Artuso JD, *et al.* Differential epidural block. *Reg Anesth* 1992; **17**: 22–25.

17 Sakura S, Sumi M, Yamada Y, *et al.* Quantitative and selective assessment of sensory block during lumbar epidural anaesthesia with 1% or 2% lidocaine. *Br J Anaesth* 1998; **81**: 718–722.

18 Nathan PW. Observations on sensory and sympathetic function during intrathecal analgesia. *J Neurol Neurosurg Psychiatry* 1976; **39**: 114–121.

19 Gasser HS, Erlanger J. Role of fibre size in the establishment of nerve block by pressure or cocaine. *Am J Physiol* 1929; **88**: 581–591.

20 Gissen AJ, Covino BG, Gregus J. Differential sensitivities of mammalian nerve fibers to local anesthetic agents. *Anesthesiology* 1980; **53**: 467–474.

21 Gokin AP, Philip B, Strichartz GR. Preferential block of small myelinated sensory and motor fibers by lidocaine: in vivo electrophysiology in the rat sciatic nerve. *Anesthesiology* 2001; **95**: 1441–1454.

22 Strichartz G, Pastijn E, Sugimoto K. Neural physiology and local anesthetic action. In: Cousins MJ, Carr DB, Horlocker TT, Bridenbaugh, eds. *Cousins & Bridenbaugh's Neural Blockade in Clinical Anesthesia and Pain Medicine*, 4th edn. Philadelphia: Lippincott Williams & Wilkins, 2009; 26–47.

23 Jaffe RA, Rowe MA. Differential nerve block. Direct measurements on individual myelinated and unmyelinated dorsal root axons. *Anesthesiology* 1996; **84**: 1455–1464.

24 Raymond SA, Steffensen SC, Gugino LD, *et al.* The role of length of nerve exposed to local anesthetics in impulse blocking action. *Anesth Analg* 1989; **68**: 563–570.

25 Fink BR. Mechanisms of differential axial blockade in epidural and subarachnoid anesthesia. *Anesthesiology* 1989; **70**: 851–858.

26 Condouris GA, Goebel RH, Brady T. Computer simulation of local anesthetic effects using a mathematical model of myelinated nerve. *J Pharmacol Exp Ther* 1976; **196**: 737–745.

27 Nakamura T, Popitz-Bergez F, Birknes J, *et al.* The critical role of concentration for lidocaine block of peripheral nerve in vivo. Studies of function and drug uptake in the rat. *Anesthesiology* 2003; **99**: 1187–1197.

28 Waikar SS, Thalhammer JG, Raymond SA, *et al.* Mechanoreceptive afferents exhibit functionally-specific activity dependent changes in conduction velocity. *Brain Res* 1996; **721**: 91–100.

29 Raymond SA. Subblocking concentrations of local anesthetics: effects on impulse generation and conduction in single myelinated sciatic nerve axons in frog. *Anesth Analg* 1992; **75**: 906–921.

30 Olschewski A, Wolff M, Bräu ME, *et al.* Enhancement of delayed-rectifier potassium conductance by low concentrations of local anaesthetics in spinal sensory neurones. *Br J Pharmacol* 2002; **136**: 540–549.

31 Olschewski A, Schnoebel-Ehehalt R, Li Y, *et al.* Mexiletine and lidocaine suppress the excitability of dorsal horn neurons. *Anesth Analg* 2009; **109**: 258–264.

32 Ku WH, Schneider SP. Multiple T-type Ca^{2+} current subtypes in electrophysiologically characterized hamster dorsal horn neurons: possible role in spinal sensory integration. *J Neurophysiol* 2011; **106**: 2486–2498.

33 Li YM, Wingrove DE, Too HP, *et al.* Local anesthetics inhibit substance P binding and evoked increases in intracellular Ca^{2+}. *Anesthesiology* 1995; **82**: 166–173.

34 Nagy I, Woolf CJ. Lignocaine selectively reduces C fibre-evoked neuronal activity in rat spinal cord in vitro by decreasing N-methyl-D-aspartate and neurokinin receptor-mediated post-synaptic depolarizations: implications for the development of novel centrally acting analgesics. *Pain* 1996; **64**: 59–70.

35 Furutani K, Ikoma M, Ishii H, *et al.* Bupivacaine inhibits glutamatergic transmission in spinal dorsal horn neurons. *Anesthesiology* 2010; **112**: 138–143.

36 Skarda RT, Tranquilli WJ. Local anesthetics. In: Tranquilli WJ, Thurmon JC, Grimm KA, eds. *Lumb and Jones' Veterinary Anesthesia and Analgesia*, 4th edn. Ames, IA: Blackwell Publishing, 2007; 395–418.

37 Mather LE, Tucker GT. Properties, absorption and disposition of local anesthetic agents. In: Cousins MJ, Carr DB, Horlocker TT, Bridenbaugh, eds. *Cousins & Bridenbaugh's Neural Blockade in Clinical Anesthesia and Pain Medicine*, 4th edn. Philadelphia: Lippincott Williams & Wilkins, 2009; 48–95.

38 Liu SS. Local anesthetics and analgesia. In: Ashburn MA, Rice LJ, eds. *The Management of Pain*. New York: Churchill Livingstone, 1997; 141–170.

39 Butterworth JF, Strichartz GR. Molecular mechanisms of local anesthetics: a review. *Anesthesiology* 1990; **72**: 711–734.

40 Strichartz GR, Sanchez V, Arthur R, *et al.* Fundamental properties of local anesthetics II. Measured Octanol:Buffer partition coefficients and pKa, values of clinically used drugs. *Anesth Analg* 1990; **71**: 158–170.

41 Brau ME, Vogel W, Hempelmann G. Fundamental properties of local anesthetics: half-maximal blocking concentrations for tonic block of Na^+ and K^+ channels in peripheral nerve. *Anesth Analg* 1998; **87**: 885–889.

42 Covino BG, Wildsmith JAW. Clinical pharmacology of local anesthetic agents. In: Cousins MJ, Bridenbaugh PO, eds. *Neural Blockade in Clinical Anesthesia and Management of Pain*, 3rd edn. Philadelphia: Lippincott-Raven, 1998; 97–128.

43 Gissen AJ, Covino BG, Gregus J. Differential sensitivity of fast and slow fibers in mammalian nerve II. Margin of safety for nerve transmission. *Anesth Analg* 1982; **61**: 561–569.

44 Ulbricht W. Kinetics of drug action and equilibrium results at the node of Ranvier. *Physiol Rev* 1981; **61**: 785–828.

45 Salinas FV, Liu SL, Scholz AM. Ion channel ligands, sodium channel blockers, local anesthetics. In: Evers AS, Maze M, eds. *Anesthetic Pharmacology, Physiologic Principles and Clinical Practice*. Philadelphia: Churchill Livingstone, 2004; 507–537.

46 Leone S, di Cianni S, Casati A, *et al.* Pharmacology, toxicology and clinical use of new long acting local anesthetics, ropivacaine and levobupivacaine. *Acta Biomed* 2008; **79**: 92–105.

47 Aberg G. Toxicological and local anesthetic effects of optically active isomers of two local anesthetic compounds. *Acta Pharmacol Toxicol Scand* 1972; **31**: 273–286.

48 Lee-Son MB, Wang GK, Concus A, *et al.* Stereoselective inhibition of neuronal sodium channels by local anesthetics. *Anesthesiology* 1992; **77**: 324–335.

49 Huang YF, Pryor ME, Veering BT, *et al.* Cardiovascular and central nervous system effects of intravenous levobupivacaine and bupivacaine in sheep. *Anesth Analg* 1998; **86**: 797–804.

50 Wildsmith JA, Brown DT, Paul D, *et al.* Structure–activity relationships in differential nerve block at high and low frequency stimulation. *Br J Anaesth* 1989; **63**: 444–452.

51 Pateromichelakis S, Prokopiou AA. Local anaesthesia efficacy: discrepancy between in vitro and in vivo studies. *Acta Anaesthesiol Scand* 1988; **32**: 672–675.

52 Wildsmith JA, Gissen AJ, Takman B, *et al.* Differential nerve blockade: esters v. amides and the influence of pKa. *Br J Anaesth* 1987; **59**: 379–384.

53 Ford DJ, Raj PP, Singh P, *et al.* Differential peripheral nerve block by local anesthetics in the cat. *Anesthesiology* 1984; **60**: 28–33.

54 Markham A, Faulds D. Ropivacaine. A review of its pharmacology and therapeutic use in regional anaesthesia. *Drugs* 1996; **52**: 429–449.

55 Mottura AA, Procickieviez O. The fate of lidocaine infiltrate during abdominoplasty and a comparative study of absorption of local anesthetic in 3 different regions: experimental studies in a porcine model. *Aesthet Surg J* 2001; **21**: 418–422.

56 Tucker GT, Moore DC, Bridenbaugh PO, *et al.* Systemic absorption of mepivacaine in commonly used regional block procedures. *Anesthesiology* 1972; **37**: 277–387.

57 Sellers G, Lin HC, Riddell MG, *et al.* Pharmacokinetics of lidocaine in serum and milk of mature Holstein cows. *J Vet Pharmacol Ther* 2009; **32**: 446–450.

58 Sum DC, Chung PC. Plasma lidocaine level during spinal or epidural anesthesia in geriatric patients. *Ma Zui Xue Za Zhi* 1993; **31**: 59–63.

59 Clement R, Malinovsky JM, Le Corre P, *et al.* Cerebrospinal fluid bioavailability and pharmacokinetics of bupivacaine and lidocaine after intrathecal and epidural administrations in rabbits using microdialysis. *J Pharmacol Exp Ther* 1999; **289**: 1015–1021.

60 Estebe JP, Le Corre P, du Plessis L, *et al.* The pharmacokinetics and pharmacodynamics of bupivacaine-loaded microspheres on a brachial plexus block model in sheep. *Anesth Analg* 2001; **93**: 447–455.

61 Jiang X, Wen X, Gao B, *et al.* The plasma concentrations of lidocaine after slow versus rapid administration of an initial dose of epidural anesthesia. *Anesth Analg* 1997; **84**: 570–573.

62 Johns RA, DiFazio CA, Longnecker DE. Lidocaine constricts or dilates rat arterioles in a dose-dependent manner. *Anesthesiology* 1985; **62**: 141–144.

63 Iida H, Ohata H, Iida M, *et al.* The differential effects of stereoisomers of ropivacaine and bupivacaine on cerebral pial arterioles in dogs. *Anesth Analg* 2001; **93**: 1552–1556.

64 Ala-Kokko TI, Partanen A, Karinen J, *et al.* Pharmacokinetics of 0.2% ropivacaine and 0.2% bupivacaine following caudal blocks in children. *Acta Anaesthesiol Scand* 2000; **44**: 1099–1102.

65 Karmakar MK, Aun CS, Wong EL, *et al.* Ropivacaine undergoes slower systemic absorption from the caudal epidural space in children than bupivacaine. *Anesth Analg* 2002; **94**: 259–265.

66 Mashimo T, Uchida I, Pak M, *et al.* Prolongation of canine epidural anesthesia by liposome encapsulation of lidocaine. *Anesth Analg* 1992; **74**: 827–834.

67 Tofoli GR, Cereda CM, de Araujo DR. Pharmacokinetic and local toxicity studies of liposome-encapsulated and plain mepivacaine solutions in rats. *Drug Deliv* 2010; **17**: 68–76.

68 Dräger C, Benziger D, Gao F, *et al.* Prolonged intercostal nerve blockade in sheep using controlled-release of bupivacaine and dexamethasone from polymer microspheres. *Anesthesiology* 1998; **89**: 969–979.

69 Fransson BA, Peck KE, Smith JK, *et al.* Transdermal absorption of a liposome-encapsulated formulation of lidocaine following topical administration in cats. *Am J Vet Res* 2002; **63**: 1309–1312.

70 Tobe M, Obata H, Suto T, *et al.* Long-term effect of sciatic nerve block with slow-release lidocaine in a rat model of postoperative pain. *Anesthesiology* 2010; **112**: 1473–1481.

71 Wang CF, Pancaro C, Gerner P, Strichartz G. Prolonged suppression of postincisional pain by a slow-release formulation of lidocaine. *Anesthesiology* 2011; **114**: 135–149.

72 Marathe PH, Shen DD, Artru AA, *et al.* Effect of serum protein binding on the entry of lidocaine into brain and cerebrospinal fluid in dogs. *Anesthesiology* 1991; **75**: 804–812.

73 Shand DG. Alpha 1-acid glycoprotein and plasma lidocaine binding. *Clin Pharmacokinet* 1984; **9**: 27–31.

74 Tucker G. Pharmacokinetics of local anaesthetics. *Br J Anaesth* 1986; **58**: 717–731.

75 De Rick AF, Belpaire FM, Dello C, Bogaert MG. Influence of enhanced alpha-1-acid glycoprotein concentration on protein binding, pharmacokinetics and antiarrhythmic effect of lidocaine in the dog. *J Pharmacol Exp Ther* 1987; **241**: 289–293.

76 Belpaire FM, de Rick A, Dello C, *et al.* Alpha 1-acid glycoprotein and serum binding of drugs in healthy and diseased dogs. *J Vet Pharmacol Ther* 1987; **10**: 43–48.

77 Palazzo MG, Kalso EA, Argiras E, *et al.* First pass lung uptake of bupivacaine: effect of acidosis in an intact rabbit lung model. *Br J Anaesth* 1991; **67**: 759–763.

78 Krejcie TC, Avram MJ, Gentry WB, *et al.* A recirculatory model of the pulmonary uptake and pharmacokinetics of lidocaine based on analysis of arterial and mixed venous data from dogs. *J Pharmacokinet Biopharm* 1997; **25**: 169–190.

79 Post C, Andersson RG, Ryrfeldt A, *et al.* Physico-chemical modification of lidocaine uptake in rat lung tissue. *Acta Pharmacol Toxicol (Copenh)* 1979; **44**: 103–109.

80 Geng WP, Ebke M, Foth H. Prilocaine elimination by isolated perfused rat lung and liver. *Naunyn Schmiedebergs Arch Pharmacol* 1995; **351**: 93–98.

81 Aoki M, Okudaira K, Haga M, *et al.* Contribution of rat pulmonary metabolism to the elimination of lidocaine, midazolam, and nifedipine. *Drug Metab Dispos* 2010; **38**: 1183–1188.

82 Ohmura S, Sugano A, Kawada M, *et al.* Pulmonary uptake of ropivacaine and levobupivacaine in rabbits. *Anesth Analg* 2003; **97**: 893–897.

83 Puente NW, Josephy PD. Analysis of the lidocaine metabolite 2,6-dimethylaniline in bovine and human milk. *J Anal Toxicol* 2001; **25**(8): 711–715.

84 Biehl D, Shnider SM, Levinson G, *et al.* Placental transfer of lidocaine: effects of fetal acidosis. *Anesthesiology* 1978; **48**: 409–412.

85 Kennedy RL, Bell JU, Miller RP, *et al.* Uptake and distribution of lidocaine in fetal lambs. *Anesthesiology* 1990; **72**: 483–489.

86 Hamshaw-Thomas A, Reynolds F. Placental transfer of bupivacaine, pethidine and lignocaine in the rabbit. Effect of umbilical flow rate and protein content. *Br J Obstet Gynaecol* 1985; **92**: 706–713.

87 Kennedy RL, Miller RP, Bell JU, *et al.* Uptake and distribution of bupivacaine in fetal lambs. *Anesthesiology* 1986; **65**: 247–253.

88 Santos AC, Karpel B, Noble G. The placental transfer and fetal effects of levobupivacaine, racemic bupivacaine, and ropivacaine. *Anesthesiology* 1999; **90**: 1698–1703.

89 Tobin T, Blake JW, Sturma L, *et al.* Pharmacology of procaine in the horse: procaine esterase properties of equine plasma and synovial fluid. *Am J Vet Res* 1976; **37**: 1165–1170.

90 Calvo R, Carlos R, Erill S. Effects of disease and acetazolamide on procaine hydrolysis by red blood cell enzymes. *Clin Pharmacol Ther* 1980; **27**: 179–183.

91 Matsubara K, Kagawa M, Fukui Y. In vivo and in vitro studies on cocaine metabolism: ecgonine methyl ester as a major metabolite of cocaine. *Forensic Sci Int* 1984; **26**: 169–180.

92 Kuhnert BR, Kuhnert PM, Philipson EH, *et al.* The half-life of 2-chloroprocaine. *Anesth Analg* 1986; **65**: 273–278.

93 Tobin T, Blake JW. A review of the pharmacology, pharmacokinetics and behavioral effects of procaine in thoroughbred horses. *Br J Sports Med* 1976; **10**: 109–116.

94 McKeever KH, Hinchcliff KW, Gerken DF, *et al.* Effects of cocaine on incremental treadmill exercise in horses. *J Appl Physiol* 1993; **75**: 2727–2733.

95 Hjelm M, Ragnarsson B, Wistrand P. Biochemical effects of aromatic compounds. 3. Ferrihaemoglobinaemia and the presence of p-hydroxy-o-toluidine in human blood after the administration of prilocaine. *Biochem Pharmacol* 1972; **21**: 2825–2834.

96 Wilcke JR, Davis LE, Neff-Davis CA, Koritz GD. Pharmacokinetics of lidocaine and its active metabolites in dogs. *J Vet Pharmacol Ther* 1983; **6**: 49–57.

97 Kammerer RC, Schmitz DA. Lidocaine metabolism by rabbit-liver homogenate and detection of a new metabolite. *Xenobiotica* 1986; **16**: 681–690.

98 Oda Y, Imaoka S, Nakahira Y, *et al.* Metabolism of lidocaine by purified rat liver microsomal cytochrome P-450 isozymes. *Biochem Pharmacol* 1989; **38**: 4439–4444.

99 Thomasy SM, Pypendop BH, Ilkiw JE, *et al.* Pharmacokinetics of lidocaine and its active metabolite, monoethylglycinexylidide, after intravenous administration of lidocaine to awake and isoflurane-anesthetized cats. *Am J Vet Res* 2005; **66**: 1162–1166.

100 Valverde A, Gunkelt C, Doherty TJ, *et al.* Effect of a constant rate infusion of lidocaine on the quality of recovery from sevoflurane or isoflurane general anaesthesia in horses. *Equine Vet J* 2005; **37**: 559–564.

101 Dickey EJ, McKenzie HC III, Brown KA, *et al.* Serum concentrations of lidocaine and its metabolites after prolonged infusion in healthy horses. *Equine Vet J* 2008; **40**: 348–352.

102 Doherty T, Redua MA, Queiroz-Castro P, *et al.* Effect of intravenous lidocaine and ketamine on the minimum alveolar concentration of isoflurane in goats. *Vet Anaesth Analg* 2007; **34**: 125–131.

103 Da Cunha AF, Messenger KM, Stout RW, *et al.* Pharmacokinetics of lidocaine and its active metabolite monoethylglycinexylidide after a single intravenous administration in chickens (Gallus domesticus) anesthetized with isoflurane. *J Vet Pharmacol Ther* 2012; **35**: 604–607.

104 Cox S, Wilson J, Doherty T. Pharmacokinetics of lidocaine after intravenous administration to cows. *J Vet Pharmacol Ther* 2012; **35**: 305–308.

105 Webb AI, Pablo LS. Local anesthetics. In: Riviere JE, Papich MG, eds. *Veterinary Pharmacology and Therapeutics*, 9th edn. Ames, IA: Wiley-Blackwell, 2009; 381–400.

106 Rosenberg PH, Heavner JE. Acute cardiovascular and central nervous system toxicity of bupivacaine and desbutylbupivacaine in the rat. *Acta Anaesthesiol Scand* 1992; **36**: 138–141.

107 Harkins JD, Karpiesiuk W, Tobin T, *et al.* Identification of hydroxyropivacaine glucuronide in equine urine by ESI+/MS/MS. *Can J Vet Res* 2000; **64**: 178–183.

108 O'Brien JE, Abbey V, Hinsvark O, *et al.* Metabolism and measurement of chloroprocaine, an ester-type local anesthetic. *J Pharm Sci* 1979; **68**: 75–78.

109 Reynolds F. Metabolism and excretion of bupivacaine in man: a comparison with mepivacaine. *Br J Anaesth* 1971; **43**: 33–37.

110 Rowland M, Thomson PD, Guichard A, Melmon KL. Disposition kinetics of lidocaine in normal subjects. *Ann N Y Acad Sci* 1971; **179**: 383–398.

111 Engelking LR, Blyden GT, Lofstedt J, *et al.* Pharmacokinetics of antipyrine, acetaminophen and lidocaine in fed and fasted horses. *J Vet Pharmacol Ther* 1987; **10**: 73–82.

112 Hastings CL, Brown TC, Eyres RL, *et al.* The influence of age on plasma lignocaine levels following tracheal spray in young dogs. *Anaesth Intensive Care* 1985; **13**: 392–394.

113 Morishima HO, Finster M, Pedersen H, *et al.* Pharmacokinetics of lidocaine in fetal and neonatal lambs and adult sheep. *Anesthesiology* 1979; **50**: 431–436.

114 Hastings CL, Brown TC, Eyres RL, *et al.* The influence of age on lignocaine pharmacokinetics in young puppies. *Anaesth Intensive Care* 1986; **14**: 135–139.

115 Zsigmond EK, Downs JR. Plasma cholinesterase activity in newborns and infants. *Can Anaesth Soc J* 1971; **18**: 278–285.

116 Abernethy DR, Greenblatt DJ. Impairment of lidocaine clearance in elderly male subjects. *J Cardiovasc Pharmacol* 1983; **5**: 1093–1096.

117 Veering BT, Burm AG, van Kleef JW, *et al.* Epidural anesthesia with bupivacaine: effects of age on neural blockade and pharmacokinetics. *Anesth Analg* 1987; **66**: 589–593.

118 Datta S, Lambert DH, Gregus J, *et al.* Differential sensitivities of mammalian nerve fibers during pregnancy. *Anesth Analg* 1983; **62**: 1070–1072.

119 Bader AM, Datta S, Moller RA, *et al.* Acute progesterone treatment has no effect on bupivacaine-induced conduction blockade in the isolated rabbit vagus nerve. *Anesth Analg* 1990; **71**: 545–548.

120 Santos AC, Pedersen H, Morishima HO, *et al.* Pharmacokinetics of lidocaine in nonpregnant and pregnant ewes. *Anesth Analg* 1988; **67**: 1154–1158.

121 Santos AC, Arthur GR, Lehning EJ, *et al.* Comparative pharmacokinetics of ropivacaine and bupivacaine in nonpregnant and pregnant ewes. *Anesth Analg* 1997; **85**: 87–93.

122 Gentz HD, Schlicht I, Wiederholt W. Pseudocholinesterase in patients with and without liver diseases. *Med Klin* 1978; **73**: 1422–1426.

123 Venkataraman BV, Iyer GY, Narayanan R, Joseph T. Erythrocyte and plasma cholinesterase activity in normal pregnancy. *Indian J Physiol Pharmacol* 1990; **34**: 26–28.

124 Waller ES. Pharmacokinetic principles of lidocaine dosing in relation to disease state. *J Clin Pharmacol* 1981; **21**: 181–194.

125 Feary DJ, Mama KR, Wagner AE, *et al.* Influence of general anesthesia on pharmacokinetics of intravenous lidocaine infusion in horses. *Am J Vet Res* 2005; **66**: 574–580.

126 Calvo R, Carlos R, Erill S. Procaine hydrolysis defect in uraemia does not appear to be due to carbamylation of plasma esterases. *Eur J Clin Pharmacol* 1983; **24**(4): 533–535.

127 Feary DJ, Mama KR, Thomasy SM, *et al.* Influence of gastrointestinal tract disease on pharmacokinetics of lidocaine after intravenous infusion in anesthetized horses. *Am J Vet Res* 2006; **67**: 317–322.

128 Peeyush M, Ravishankar M, Adithan C, *et al.* Altered pharmacokinetics of lignocaine after epidural injection in type II diabetics. *Eur J Clin Pharmacol* 1992; **43**: 269–271.

129 Gawrońska-Szklarz B, Musiał DH, Pawlik A, *et al.* Effect of experimental diabetes on pharmacokinetic parameters of lidocaine and MEGX in rats. *Pol J Pharmacol* 2003; **55**: 619–624.

130 Raj PP, Ohlweiler D, Hitt BA, *et al.* Kinetics of local anesthetic esters and the effects of adjuvant drugs on 2-chloroprocaine hydrolysis. *Anesthesiology* 1980; **53**: 307–314.

131 Calvo R, Carlos R, Erill S. Effects of disease and acetazolamide on procaine hydrolysis by red blood cell enzymes. *Clin Pharmacol Ther* 1980; **27**: 179–183.

132 Olkkola KT, Isohanni MH, Hamunen K, *et al.* The effect of erythromycin and fluvoxamine on the pharmacokinetics of intravenous lidocaine. *Anesth Analg* 2005; **100**: 1352–1356.

133 Tesseromatis C, Kotsiou A, Tsagataki M, *et al.* In vitro binding of lidocaine to liver tissue under the influence of propranolol: another mechanism of interaction? *Eur J Drug Metab Pharmacokinet* 2007; **32**: 213–217.

134 Lalka D, Vicuna N, Burrow SR, *et al.* Bupivacaine and other amide local anesthetics inhibit the hydrolysis of chloroprocaine by human serum. *Anesth Analg* 1978; **57**: 534–539.

135 Rosenberg PH, Heavner JE. Temperature-dependent nerve-blocking action of lidocaine and halothane. *Acta Anaesthesiol Scand* 1980; **24**: 314–320.

136 Butterworth JF, Walker FO, Neal JM. Cooling potentiates lidocaine inhibition of median nerve sensory fibers. *Anesth Analg* 1990; **70**: 507–511.

137 Sanchez V, Arthur GR, Strichartz GR. Fundamental properties of local anesthetics. I. The dependence of lidocaine's ionization and octanol:buffer partitioning on solvent and temperature. *Anesth Analg* 1987; **66**: 159–165.

138 Heath PJ, Brownlie GS, Herrick MJ. Latency of brachial plexus block. The effect on onset time of warming local anaesthetic solutions. *Anaesthesia* 1990; **45**: 297–301.

139 Han SS, Lee SC, Ro YJ, *et al.* Warming the epidural injectate improves first sacral segment block: a randomised double-blind study. *Anaesth Intensive Care* 2010; **38**: 690–694.

140 Liu FC, Liou JT, Day YJ, *et al.* Effect of warm lidocaine on the sensory onset of epidural anesthesia: a randomized trial. *Chang Gung Med J* 2009; **32**: 643–649.

141 Lee R, Kim YM, Choi EM, *et al.* Effect of warmed ropivacaine solution on onset and duration of axillary block. *Korean J Anesthesiol* 2012; **62**: 52–56.

142 Chilvers CR. Warm local anaesthetic – effect on latency of onset of axillary brachial plexus block. *Anaesth Intensive Care* 1993; **21**: 795–798.

143 Kristoffersen E, Sloth E, Husted JC, *et al.* Spinal anaesthesia with plain 0.5% bupivacaine at 19 degrees C and 37 degrees C. *Br J Anaesth* 1990; **65**: 504–507.

144 Greene NM. Distribution of local anesthetic solutions within the subarachnoid space. *Anesth Analg* 1985; **64**: 715–730.

145 Imbelloni LE, Moreira AD, Gaspar FC, *et al.* Assessment of the densities of local anesthetics and their combination with adjuvants: an experimental study. *Rev Bras Anestesiol* 2009; **59**: 154–165.

146 Horlocker TT, Wedel DJ. Density, specific gravity, and baricity of spinal anesthetic solutions at body temperature. *Anesth Analg* 1993; **76**: 1015–1018.

147 McLeod GA. Density of spinal anaesthetic solutions of bupivacaine, levobupivacaine, and ropivacaine with and without dextrose. *Br J Anaesth* 2004; **92**: 547–551.

148 Ganem EM, Vianna PT, Marques M, *et al.* Neurotoxicity of subarachnoid hyperbaric bupivacaine in dogs. *Reg Anesth* 1996; **21**: 234–238.

149 Kaya M, Oguz S, Aslan K, *et al.* A low-dose bupivacaine: a comparison of hyperbaric and hypobaric solutions for unilateral spinal anesthesia. *Reg Anesth Pain Med* 2004; **29**: 17–22.
150 Casati A, Fanelli G. Unilateral spinal anesthesia. State of the art. *Minerva Anestesiol* 2001; **67**: 855–862.
151 Richardson MG, Wissler RN. Densities of dextrose-free intrathecal local anesthetics, opioids, and combinations measured at 37 degrees C. *Anesth Analg* 1997; **84**: 95–99.
152 Lui AC, Polis TZ, Cicutti NJ. Densities of cerebrospinal fluid and spinal anaesthetic solutions in surgical patients at body temperature. *Can J Anaesth* 1998; **45**: 297–303.
153 Richardson MG, Wissler RN. Density of lumbar cerebrospinal fluid in pregnant and nonpregnant humans. *Anesthesiology* 1996; **85**: 326–330.
154 Bernards CM, Kopacz DJ. Effect of epinephrine on lidocaine clearance in vivo: a microdialysis study in humans. *Anesthesiology* 1999; **91**: 962–968.
155 Kuchembuck NL, Colahan PT, Zientek KD, *et al.* Plasma concentration and local anesthetic activity of procaine hydrochloride following subcutaneous administration to horses. *Am J Vet Res* 2007; **68**: 495–500.
156 Burm AG, van Kleef JW, Gladines MP, *et al.* Epidural anesthesia with lidocaine and bupivacaine: effects of epinephrine on the plasma concentration profiles. *Anesth Analg* 1986; **65**: 1281–1284.
157 Karmakar MK, Ho AM, Law BK, *et al.* Arterial and venous pharmacokinetics of ropivacaine with and without epinephrine after thoracic paravertebral block. *Anesthesiology* 2005; **103**: 704–711.
158 Ratajczak-Enselme M, Estebe JP, Rose FX, *et al.* Effect of epinephrine on epidural, intrathecal, and plasma pharmacokinetics of ropivacaine and bupivacaine in sheep. *Br J Anaesth* 2007; **99**: 881–890.
159 Reddy SV, Maderdrut JL, Yaksh TL. Spinal cord pharmacology of adrenergic agonist-mediated antinociception. *J Pharmacol Exp Ther* 1980; **213**: 525–533.
160 Collins JG, Kitahata LM, Matsumoto M, *et al.* Spinally administered epinephrine suppresses noxiously evoked activity of WDR neurons in the dorsal horn of the spinal cord. *Anesthesiology* 1984; **60**: 269–725.
161 Sonohata M, Furue H, Katafuchi T, *et al.* Actions of noradrenaline on substantia gelatinosa neurones in the rat spinal cord revealed by in vivo patch recording. *J Physiol* 2004; **555**: 515–526.
162 Sinnott CJ, Cogswell III LP, Johnson A, *et al.* On the mechanism by which epinephrine potentiates lidocaine's peripheral nerve block. *Anesthesiology* 2003; **98**: 181–188.
163 Niemi G. Advantages and disadvantages of adrenaline in regional anaesthesia. *Best Pract Res Clin Anaesth* 2005; **19**: 229–245.
164 Shieh JP, Chu CC, Wang JJ, *et al.* Epinephrine, phenylephrine, and methoxamine induce infiltrative anesthesia via alpha1-adrenoceptors in rats. *Acta Pharmacol Sin* 2009; **30**: 1227–1236.
165 Kozody R, Palahniuk RJ, Wade JG, *et al.* The effect of subarachnoid epinephrine and phenylephrine on spinal cord blood flow. *Can Anaesth Soc J* 1984; **31**: 503–508.
166 Porter SS, Albin MS, Watson WA, *et al.* Spinal cord and cerebral blood flow responses to subarachnoid injection of local anesthetics with and without epinephrine. *Acta Anaesthesiol Scand* 1985; **29**: 330–338.
167 Neal JM. Effects of epinephrine in local anesthetics on the central and peripheral nervous systems: neurotoxicity and neural blood flow. *Reg Anesth Pain Med* 2003; **28**: 124–134.
168 Myers RR, Heckman HM. Effects of local anesthesia on nerve blood flow: studies using lidocaine with and without epinephrine. *Anesthesiology* 1989; **71**: 757–762.
169 Palmer GM, Cairns BE, Berkes SL, *et al.* The effects of lidocaine and adrenergic agonists on rat sciatic nerve and skeletal muscle blood flow in vivo. *Anesth Analg* 2002; **95**: 1080–1086.
170 Niwa H, Hirota Y, Sibutani T, *et al.* The effects of epinephrine and norepinephrine administered during local anesthesia on left ventricular diastolic function. *Anesth Prog* 1991; **38**: 221–226.
171 Henslee TM, Hodson SB, Lamy CJ, *et al.* Vasoconstrictive agents commonly used in combination with local anesthetics: a literature review. *J Foot Surg* 1987; **26**: 504–510.
172 Yagiela JA. What's new with phentolamine mesylate: a reversal agent for local anaesthesia? *SAAD Dig* 2011; **27**: 3–7.
173 Kirby CK, Eckenhoff JE, Looby JP. The use of hyaluronidase with local anesthetic agents in nerve block and infiltration anesthesia. *Surgery* 1949; **25**: 101–104.
174 Dempsey GA, Barrett PJ, Kirby IJ. Hyaluronidase and peribulbar block. *Br J Anaesth* 1997; **78**: 671–674.
175 Nicoll JM, Treuren B, Acharya PA, *et al.* Retrobulbar anesthesia: the role of hyaluronidase. *Anesth Analg* 1986; **65**: 1324–1328.
176 Kallio H, Paloheimo M, Maunuksela EL. Hyaluronidase as an adjuvant in bupivacaine-lidocaine mixture for retrobulbar/peribulbar block. *Anesth Analg* 2000; **91**: 934–937.
177 Crawford M, Kerr WJ. The effect of hyaluronidase on peribulbar block. *Anaesthesia* 1994; **49**: 907–908.
178 Brydon CW, Basler M, Kerr WJ. An evaluation of two concentrations of hyaluronidase for supplementation of peribulbar anaesthesia. *Anaesthesia* 1995; **50**: 998–1000.
179 Keeler JF, Simpson KH, Ellis FR, *et al.* Effect of addition of hyaluronidase to bupivacaine during axillary brachial plexus block. *Br J Anaesth* 1992; **68**: 68–71.
180 DeRossi R, de Barros AL, Silva-Neto AB, *et al.* Hyaluronidase shortens levobupivacaine lumbosacral epidural anaesthesia in dogs. *J Small Anim Pract* 2011; **52**: 195–199.
181 Nevarre DR, Tzarnas CD. The effects of hyaluronidase on the efficacy and on the pain of administration of 1% lidocaine. *Plast Reconstr Surg* 1998; **101**: 365–369.
182 Wohlrab J, Finke R, Franke WG, *et al.* Clinical trial for safety evaluation of hyaluronidase as diffusion enhancing adjuvant for infiltration analgesia of skin with lidocaine. *Dermatol Surg* 2012; **38**: 91–96.
183 Etesse B, Beaudroit L, Deleuze M, *et al.* Hyaluronidase: here we go again. *Ann Fr Anesth Reanim* 2009; **28**: 658–665.
184 Morris R, McKay W, Mushlin P. Comparison of pain associated with intradermal and subcutaneous infiltration with various local anesthetic solutions. *Anesth Analg* 1987; **66**: 1180–1182.
185 McKay W, Morris R, Mushlin P. Sodium bicarbonate attenuates pain on skin infiltration with lidocaine, with or without epinephrine. *Anesth Analg* 1987; **66**: 572–574.
186 Christoph RA, Buchanan L, Begalla K, *et al.* Pain reduction in local anesthetic administration through pH buffering. *Ann Emerg Med* 1988; **17**: 117–120.
187 Jones JS, Plzak C, Wynn BN, *et al.* Effect of temperature and pH adjustment of bupivacaine for intradermal anesthesia. *Am J Emerg Med* 1998; **16**: 117–120.
188 Ririe DG, Walker FO, James RL, *et al.* Effect of alkalinization of lidocaine on median nerve block. *Br J Anaesth* 2000; **84**: 163–168.
189 Buckley FP, Duval Neto G, Fink BR. Acid and alkaline solutions of local anesthetics: duration of nerve block and tissue pH. *Anesth Analg* 1985; **64**: 477–482.
190 Capogna G, Celleno D, Varrassi G, *et al.* Epidural mepivacaine for cesarean section: effects of a pH-adjusted solution. *J Clin Anesth* 1991; **3**: 211–214.
191 Benzon HT, Toleikis JR, Dixit P, *et al.* Onset, intensity of blockade and somatosensory evoked potential changes of the lumbosacral dermatomes after epidural anesthesia with alkalinized lidocaine. *Anesth Analg* 1993; **76**: 328–332.
192 Capogna G, Celleno D, Laudano D, *et al.* Alkalinization of local anesthetics. Which block, which local anesthetic? *Reg Anesth* 1995; **20**: 369–377.
193 Stevens RA, Chester WL, Grueter JA, *et al.* The effect of pH adjustment of 0.5% bupivacaine on the latency of epidural anesthesia. *Reg Anesth* 1989; **14**: 236–239.
194 Verborgh C, Claeys MA, Camu F. Onset of epidural blockade after plain or alkalinized 0.5% bupivacaine. *Anesth Analg* 1991; **73**: 401–404.
195 Gaggero G, Meyer O, van Gessel E, *et al.* Alkalinization of lidocaine 2% does not influence the quality of epidural anaesthesia for elective caesarean section. *Can J Anaesth* 1995; **42**: 1080–1084.
196 Ramos G, Pereira E, Simonetti MP. Does alkalinization of 0.75% ropivacaine promote a lumbar peridural block of higher quality? *Reg Anesth Pain Med* 2001; **26**: 357–362.
197 Sinnott CJ, Garfield JM, Thalhammer JG, *et al.* Addition of sodium bicarbonate to lidocaine decreases the duration of peripheral nerve block in the rat. *Anesthesiology* 2000; **93**: 1045–1052.
198 Henry R, Patterson L, Avery N, *et al.* Absorption of alkalized intravesical lidocaine in normal and inflamed bladders: a simple method for improving bladder anesthesia. *J Urol* 2001; **165**: 1900–1903.
199 Zezza L, Reusch CE, Gerber B. Intravesical application of lidocaine and sodium bicarbonate in the treatment of obstructive idiopathic lower urinary tract disease in cats. *J Vet Intern Med* 2012; **26**: 526–531.
200 Zehetmayer M, Rainer G, Turnheim K, *et al.* Topical anesthesia with pH-adjusted versus standard lidocaine 4% for clear corneal cataract surgery. *J Cataract Refract Surg* 1997; **23**: 1390–1393.
201 Fuchsjäger-Mayrl G, Zehetmayer M, Plass H, *et al.* Alkalinization increases penetration of lidocaine across the human cornea. *J Cataract Refract Surg* 2002; **28**: 692–696.
202 Nakayama M, Munemura Y, Kanaya N, *et al.* Efficacy of alkalinized lidocaine for reducing pain on intravenous and epidural catheterization. *J Anesth* 2001; **15**: 201–203.
203 Mader TJ, Playe SJ, Garb JL. Reducing the pain of local anesthetic infiltration: warming and buffering have a synergistic effect. *Ann Emerg Med* 1994; **23**: 550–554.
204 Peterfreund RA, Datta S, Ostheimer GW. pH adjustment of local anesthetic solutions with sodium bicarbonate: laboratory evaluation of alkalinization and precipitation. *Reg Anesth* 1989; **14**: 265–270.
205 Bokesch PM, Raymond SA, Strichartz GR. Dependence of lidocaine potency on pH and PCO2. *Anesth Analg* 1987; **66**: 9–17.

206 Bromage PR, Burfoot MF, Crowell DE, *et al.* Quality of epidural blockade. 3. Carbonated local anaesthetic solutions. *Br J Anaesth* 1967; **39**: 197–209.
207 Gosteli P, van Gessel E, Gamulin Z. Effects of pH adjustment and carbonation of lidocaine during epidural anesthesia for foot or ankle surgery. *Anesth Analg* 1995; **81**: 104–109.
208 Schelling CG, Klein LV. Comparison of carbonated lidocaine and lidocaine hydrochloride for caudal epidural anesthesia in horses. *Am J Vet Res* 1985; **46**: 1375–1377.
209 Brummett CM, Williams BA. Additives to local anesthetics for peripheral nerve blockade. *Int Anesthesiol Clin* 2011; **49**: 104–116.
210 Grubb TL, Riebold TW, Huber MJ. Comparison of lidocaine, xylazine, and xylazine/lidocaine for caudal epidural analgesia in horses. *J Am Vet Med Assoc* 1992; **201**: 1187–1190.
211 Lamont LA, Lemke KA. The effects of medetomidine on radial nerve blockade with mepivacaine in dogs. *Vet Anaesth Analg* 2008; **35**: 62–68.
212 Brummett CM, Norat MA, Palmisano JM, *et al.* Perineural administration of dexmedetomidine in combination with bupivacaine enhances sensory and motor blockade in sciatic nerve block without inducing neurotoxicity in rat. *Anesthesiology* 2008; **109**: 502–511.
213 Brummett CM, Padda AK, Amodeo FS, *et al.* Perineural dexmedetomidine added to ropivacaine causes a dose-dependent increase in the duration of thermal antinociception in sciatic nerve block in rat. *Anesthesiology* 2009; **111**: 1111–1119.
214 Obayah GM, Refaie A, Aboushanab O, *et al.* Addition of dexmedetomidine to bupivacaine for greater palatine nerve block prolongs postoperative analgesia after cleft palate repair. *Eur J Anaesthesiol* 2010; **27**: 280–284.
215 Esmaoglu A, Yegenoglu F, Akin A, *et al.* Dexmedetomidine added to levobupivacaine prolongs axillary brachial plexus block. *Anesth Analg* 2010; **111**: 1548–1551.
216 Gupta R, Verma R, Bogra J, *et al.* A Comparative study of intrathecal dexmedetomidine and fentanyl as adjuvants to bupivacaine. *J Anaesthesiol Clin Pharmacol* 2011; **27**: 339–343.
217 Ammar AS, Mahmoud KM. Ultrasound-guided single injection infraclavicular brachial plexus block using bupivacaine alone or combined with dexmedetomidine for pain control in upper limb surgery: a prospective randomized controlled trial. *Saudi J Anaesth* 2012; **6**: 109–114.
218 Memiş D, Turan A, Karamanlioğlu B, *et al.* Adding dexmedetomidine to lidocaine for intravenous regional anesthesia. *Anesth Analg* 2004; **98**: 835–840.
219 Esmaoglu A, Mizrak A, Akin A, *et al.* Addition of dexmedetomidine to lidocaine for intravenous regional anaesthesia. *Eur J Anaesthesiol* 2005; **22**: 447–451.
220 Kroin JS, Buvanendran A, Beck DR, *et al.* Clonidine prolongation of lidocaine analgesia after sciatic nerve block in rats is mediated via the hyperpolarization-activated cation current, not by alpha-adrenoreceptors. *Anesthesiology* 2004; **101**: 488–494.
221 Brummett CM, Hong EK, Janda AM, *et al.* Perineural dexmedetomidine added to ropivacaine for sciatic nerve block in rats prolongs the duration of analgesia by blocking the hyperpolarization-activated cation current. *Anesthesiology* 2011; **115**: 836–843.
222 Leem JW, Choi Y, Han SM, *et al.* Conduction block by clonidine is not mediated by alpha-2-adrenergic receptors in rat sciatic nerve fibers. *Reg Anesth Pain Med* 2000; **25**: 620–625.
223 Ribotsky BM, Berkowitz KD, Montague JR. Local anesthetics. Is there an advantage to mixing solutions? *J Am Podiatr Med Assoc* 1996; **86**: 487–491.
224 Cuvillon P, Nouvellon E, Ripart J, *et al.* A comparison of the pharmacodynamics and pharmacokinetics of bupivacaine, ropivacaine (with epinephrine) and their equal volume mixtures with lidocaine used for femoral and sciatic nerve blocks: a double-blind randomized study. *Anesth Analg* 2009; **108**: 641–649.
225 Gadsden J, Hadzic A, Gandhi K, *et al.* The effect of mixing 1.5% mepivacaine and 0.5% bupivacaine on duration of analgesia and latency of block onset in ultrasound-guided interscalene block. *Anesth Analg* 2011; **112**: 471–476.
226 Vesal N, Ahmadi M, Foroud M, *et al.* Caudal epidural anti-nociception using lidocaine, bupivacaine or their combination in cows undergoing reproductive procedures. *Vet Anaesth Analg* 2013; **40**(3): 328–332.
227 Lawal FM, Adetunji A. A comparison of epidural anaesthesia with lignocaine, bupivacaine and a lignocaine-bupivacaine mixture in cats. *J S Afr Vet Assoc* 2009; **80**: 243–246.
228 Seow LT, Lips FJ, Cousins MJ, *et al.* Lidocaine and bupivacaine mixtures for epidural blockade. *Anesthesiology* 1982; **56**: 177–183.
229 Kaukinen S, Kaukinen L, Eerola R. Epidural anaesthesia with mixtures of bupivacaine-lidocaine and etidocaine-lidocaine. *Ann Chir Gynaecol* 1980; **69**: 281–286.
230 Magee DA, Sweet PT, Holland AJ. Epidural anaesthesia with mixtures of bupivicaine and lidocaine. *Can Anaesth Soc J* 1983; **30**: 174–178.
231 Jacobsen J, Husum B, von Staffeldt H, *et al.* The addition of lidocaine to bupivacaine does not shorten the duration of spinal anesthesia: a randomized, double-blinded study of patients undergoing knee arthroscopy. *Anesth Analg* 2011; **113**: 1272–1275.
232 Corke BC, Carlson CG, Dettbarn WD. The influence of 2-chloroprocaine on the subsequent analgesic potency of bupivacaine. *Anesthesiology* 1984; **60**: 25–27.
233 Galindo A, Witcher T. Mixtures of local anesthetics: bupivacaine-chloroprocaine. *Anesth Analg* 1980; **59**: 683–685.
234 Mets B, Janicki PK, James MF, *et al.* Lidocaine and bupivacaine cardiorespiratory toxicity is additive: a study in rats. *Anesth Analg* 1992; **75**: 611–614.
235 Kottenberg-Assenmacher E, Peters J. Mechanisms of tachyphylaxis in regional anesthesia of long duration. *Anasthesiol Intensivmed Notfallmed Schmerzther* 1999; **34**: 733–742.
236 Bromage PR, Pettigrew RT, Crowell DE. Tachyphylaxis in epidural analgesia: I. Augmentation and decay of local anesthesia. *J Clin Pharmacol J New Drugs* 1969; **9**: 30–38.
237 Baker CE, Berry RL, Elston RC. Effect of pH of bupivacaine on duration of repeated sciatic nerve blocks in the albino rat. Local Anesthetics for Neuralgia Study Group. *Anesth Analg* 1991; **72**: 773–778.
238 Wang C, Liu H, Wilder RT, *et al.* Effects of repeated injection of local anesthetic on sciatic nerve blocks response. *J Huazhong Univ Sci Technolog Med Sci* 2004; **24**: 497–499.
239 Mogensen T, Simonsen L, Scott NB, *et al.* Tachyphylaxis associated with repeated epidural injections of lidocaine is not related to changes in distribution or the rate of elimination from the epidural space. *Anesth Analg* 1989; **69**: 180–184.
240 Lipfert P, Holthusen H, Arndt JO. Tachyphylaxis to local anesthetics does not result from reduced drug effectiveness at the nerve itself. *Anesthesiology* 1989; **70**: 71–75.
241 Wang C, Sholas MG, Berde CB, *et al.* Evidence that spinal segmental nitric oxide mediates tachyphylaxis to peripheral local anesthetic nerve block. *Acta Anaesthesiol Scand* 2001; **45**: 945–953.
242 Lee KC, Wilder RT, Smith RL, *et al.* Thermal hyperalgesia accelerates and MK-801 prevents the development of tachyphylaxis to rat sciatic nerve blockade. *Anesthesiology* 1994; **81**: 1284–1293.
243 Wilder RT, Sholas MG, Berde CB. NG-nitro-L-arginine methyl ester (L-NAME) prevents tachyphylaxis to local anesthetics in a dose-dependent manner. *Anesth Analg* 1996; **83**: 1251–1255.
244 Mercadante S, Villari P, Ferrera P, *et al.* Local anesthetic switching for intrathecal tachyphylaxis in cancer patients with pain. *Anesth Analg* 2003; **97**: 187–189.
245 Mama KR, Steffey EP. Local anesthetics. In: Adams HR, ed. *Veterinary Pharmacology and Therapeutics*, 8th edn. Ames, IA: Blackwell, 2001; 343–359.
246 Axelrod EH, Alexander GD, Brown M, *et al.* Procaine spinal anesthesia: a pilot study of the incidence of transient neurologic symptoms. *J Clin Anesth* 1998; **10**: 404–409.
247 Heo GJ, Shin G. Efficacy of benzocaine as an anaesthetic for Crucian carp (Carassius carassius). *Vet Anaesth Analg* 2010; **37**: 132–135.
248 Forster JG, Rosenberg PH. Revival of old local anesthetics for spinal anesthesia in ambulatory surgery. *Curr Opin Anaesthesiol* 2011; **24**: 633–637.
249 Butterworth JF. Clinical pharmacology of local anesthetics. In: Cousins MJ, Carr DB, Horlocker TT, Bridenbaugh, eds. *Cousins & Bridenbaugh's Neural Blockade in Clinical Anesthesia and Pain Medicine*, 4th edn. Philadelphia: Lippincott Williams & Wilkins, 2009; 96–113.
250 Patel D, Chopra S, Berman MD. Serious systemic toxicity resulting from use of tetracaine for pharyngeal anesthesia in upper endoscopic procedures. *Dig Dis Sci* 1989; **34**: 882–884.
251 Lander JA, Weltman BJ, So SS. EMLA and amethocaine for reduction of children's pain associated with needle insertion. *Cochrane Database Syst Rev* 2006; **19**(3): CD004236.
252 Sawyer J, Febbraro S, Masud S, *et al.* Heated lidocaine/tetracaine patch (Synera, Rapydan) compared with lidocaine/prilocaine cream (EMLA) for topical anaesthesia before vascular access. *Br J Anaesth* 2009; **102**: 210–215.
253 Muir WW, Wiese AJ, March PA. Effects of morphine, lidocaine, ketamine, and morphine-lidocaine-ketamine drug combination on minimum alveolar concentration in dogs anesthetized with isoflurane. *Am J Vet Res* 2003; **64**: 1155–1160.
254 Valverde A, Doherty TJ, Hernandez J, *et al.* Effect of lidocaine on the minimum alveolar concentration of isoflurane in dogs. *Vet Anaesth Analg* 2004; **31**: 264–271.
255 Wilson J, Doherty TJ, Egger CM, *et al.* Effects of intravenous lidocaine, ketamine, and the combination on the minimum alveolar concentration of sevoflurane in dogs. *Vet Anaesth Analg* 2008; **35**: 289–296.
256 Pypendop BH, Ilkiw JE. The effects of intravenous lidocaine administration on the minimum alveolar concentration of isoflurane in cats. *Anesth Analg* 2005; **100**: 97–101.
257 Dzikiti TB, Hellebrekers LJ, van Dijk P. Effects of intravenous lidocaine on isoflurane concentration, physiological parameters, metabolic parameters and stress-related hormones in horses undergoing surgery. *J Vet Med A Physiol Pathol Clin Med* 2003; **50**: 190–195.

258 Rezende ML, Wagner AE, Mama KR, *et al.* Effects of intravenous administration of lidocaine on the minimum alveolar concentration of sevoflurane in horses. *Am J Vet Res* 2011; **72**: 446–451.
259 Vesal N, Spadavecchia C, Steiner A, *et al.* Evaluation of the isoflurane-sparing effects of lidocaine infusion during umbilical surgery in calves. *Vet Anaesth Analg* 2011; **38**: 451–460.
260 Yardeni IZ, Beilin B, Mayburd E, *et al.* The effect of perioperative intravenous lidocaine on postoperative pain and immune function. *Anesth Analg* 2009; **109**: 1464–1469.
261 Swenson BR, Gottschalk A, Wells LT, *et al.* Intravenous lidocaine is as effective as epidural bupivacaine in reducing ileus duration, hospital stay, and pain after open colon resection: a randomized clinical trial. *Reg Anesth Pain Med* 2010; **35**: 370–376.
262 Ness TJ. Intravenous lidocaine inhibits visceral nociceptive reflexes and spinal neurons in the rat. *Anesthesiology* 2000; **92**: 1685–1691.
263 Smith LJ, Shih A, Miletic G, *et al.* Continual systemic infusion of lidocaine provides analgesia in an animal model of neuropathic pain. *Pain* 2002; **97**: 267–273.
264 Robertson SA, Sanchez LC, Merritt AM, *et al.* Effect of systemic lidocaine on visceral and somatic nociception in conscious horses. *Equine Vet J* 2005; **37**: 122–127.
265 Pypendop BH, Ilkiw JE, Robertson SA. Effects of intravenous administration of lidocaine on the thermal threshold in cats. *Am J Vet Res* 2006; **67**: 16–20.
266 MacDougall LM, Hethey JA, Livingston A, *et al.* Antinociceptive, cardiopulmonary, and sedative effects of five intravenous infusion rates of lidocaine in conscious dogs. *Vet Anaesth Analg* 2009; **36**: 512–522.
267 Doherty TJ, Seddighi MR. Local anesthetics as pain therapy in horses. *Vet Clin North Am Equine Pract* 2010; **26**: 533–549.
268 Brianceau P, Chevalier H, Karas A, *et al.* Intravenous lidocaine and small-intestinal size, abdominal fluid, and outcome after colic surgery in horses. *J Vet Intern Med* 2002; **16**: 736–741.
269 Malone E, Ensink J, Turner T, *et al.* Intravenous continuous infusion of lidocaine for treatment of equine ileus. *Vet Surg* 2006; **35**: 60–66.
270 Rusiecki KE, Nieto JE, Puchalski SM, *et al.* Evaluation of continuous infusion of lidocaine on gastrointestinal tract function in normal horses. *Vet Surg* 2008; **37**: 564–570.
271 Torfs S, Delesalle C, Dewulf J, *et al.* Risk factors for equine postoperative ileus and effectiveness of prophylactic lidocaine. *J Vet Intern Med* 2009; **23**: 606–611.
272 Guschlbauer M, Feige K, Geburek F, *et al.* Effects of in vivo lidocaine administration at the time of ischemia and reperfusion on in vitro contractility of equine jejunal smooth muscle. *Am J Vet Res* 2011; **72**: 1449–1455.
273 Ngo LY, Tam YK, Tawfik S, *et al.* Effects of intravenous infusion of lidocaine on its pharmacokinetics in conscious instrumented dogs. *J Pharm Sci* 1997; **86**: 944–952.
274 Perez-Castro R, Patel S, Garavito-Aguilar ZV, *et al.* Cytotoxicity of local anesthetics in human neuronal cells. *Anesth Analg* 2009; **108**: 997–1007.
275 Cederholm I, Evers H, Lofstrom JB. Skin blood flow after intradermal injection of ropivacaine in various concentrations with and without epinephrine evaluated by laser Doppler flowmetry. *Reg Anesth* 1992; **17**: 322–328.
276 Mather LE. The acute toxicity of local anesthetics. *Expert Opin Drug Metab Toxicol* 2010; **6**: 1313–1332.
277 Aberg G. Toxicological and local anesthetic effects of optically active isomers of two local anesthetic compounds. *Acta Pharmacol Toxicol Scand* 1972; **31**: 273–286.
278 Santos AC, DeArmas PE. Systemic toxicity of levobupivacaine, bupivacaine, and ropivacaine during continuous intravenous infusion to nonpregnant and pregnant ewes. *Anesthesiology* 2001; **95**: 1256–1264.
279 Feldman HS, Arthur GR, Covino BG. Comparative systemic toxicity of convulsant and supraconvulsant doses of intravenous ropivacaine, bupivacaine, and lidocaine in the conscious dog. *Anesth Analg* 1989; **69**: 794–801.
280 Rutten AJ, Nancarrow C, Mather LE, *et al.* Hemodynamic and central nervous system effects of intravenous bolus doses of lidocaine, bupivacaine, and ropivacaine in sheep. *Anesth Analg* 1989; **69**: 291–299.
281 Faccenda KA, Finucane BT. Complications of regional anaesthesia: incidence and prevention. *Drug Saf* 2001; **24**: 413–442.
282 Auroy Y, Benhamou D, Bargues L, *et al.* Major complications of regional anesthesia in France: the SOS Regional Anesthesia Hotline Service. *Anesthesiology* 2002; **97**: 1274–1280.
283 Cox B, Durieux ME, Marcus MAE. Toxicity of local anaesthetics. *Best Pract Res Clin Anaesth* 2003; **17**: 111–136.
284 Marsch S, Schaefer H, Castelli I. Unusual psychological manifestation of systemic local anaesthetic toxicity. *Anesthesiology* 1998; **88**: 532–533.
285 Meyer GA, Lin HC, Hanson RR, *et al.* Effects of intravenous lidocaine overdose on cardiac electrical activity and blood pressure in the horse. *Equine Vet J* 2001; **33**: 434–437.
286 Rosenberg P, Kalso E, Tuominen M, *et al.* Acute bupivacaine toxicity as a result of venous leakage under the tourniquet cuff during a bier block. *Anesthesiology* 1983; **58**: 95–98.
287 Morishima HO, Pedersen H, Finster M, *et al.* Bupivacaine toxicity in pregnant and nonpregnant ewes. *Anesthesiology* 1985; **63**: 134–139.
288 Brown DL, Ransom DM, Hall JA, *et al.* Regional anesthesia and local anesthetic-induced systemic toxicity: seizure frequency and accompanying cardiovascular changes. *Anesth Analg* 1995; **81**: 321–328.
289 Liu PL, Feldman HS, Giasi R, *et al.* Comparative CNS toxicity of lidocaine, etidocaine, bupivacaine, and tetracaine in awake dogs following rapid intravenous administration. *Anesth Analg* 1983; **62**: 375–379.
290 Hofman WF, Jerram DC, Gangarosa LP. Cardiorespiratory and behavioral reactions to the lidocaine-induced convulsions in the dog. *Res Commun Chem Pathol Pharmacol* 1977; **16**: 581–591.
291 Lemo N, Vnuk D, Radisic B, *et al.* Determination of the toxic dose of lidocaine in dogs and its corresponding serum concentration. *Vet Rec* 2007; **160**: 374–375.
292 Wilcke JR, Davis LE, Neff-Davis CA. Determination of lidocaine concentrations producing therapeutic and toxic effects in dogs. *J Vet Pharmacol Ther* 1983; **6**: 105–111.
293 Milligan M, Kukanich B, Beard W, *et al.* The disposition of lidocaine during a 12-hour intravenous infusion to postoperative horses. *J Vet Pharmacol Ther* 2006; **29**: 495–499.
294 Navas de Solis C, McKenzie HC. Serum concentrations of lidocaine and its metabolites MEGX and GX during and after prolonged intravenous infusion of lidocaine in horses after colic surgery. *J Equine Vet Sci* 2007; **27**: 398–404.
295 Chadwick HS. Toxicity and resuscitation in lidocaine- or bupivacaine-infused cats. *Anesthesiology* 1985; **63**: 385–390.
296 Nancarrow C, Rutten AJ, Runciman WB, *et al.* Myocardial and cerebral drug concentrations and the mechanisms of death after fatal intravenous doses of lidocaine, bupivacaine, and ropivacaine in the sheep. *Anesth Analg* 1989; **69**: 276–283.
297 Heavner JE, Badgwell JM, Dryden CF Jr, *et al.* Bupivacaine toxicity in lightly anesthetized pigs with respiratory imbalances plus or minus halothane. *Reg Anesth* 1995; **20**: 20–26.
298 Burney RG, DiFazio CA, Foster JA. Effects of pH on protein binding of lidocaine. *Anesth Analg* 1978; **57**: 478–480.
299 Heavner JE, Dryden CF Jr, Sanghani V, *et al.* Severe hypoxia enhances central nervous system and cardiovascular toxicity of bupivacaine in lightly anesthetized pigs. *Anesthesiology* 1992; **77**: 142–147.
300 Beecroft C, Davies G. Systemic toxic effects of local anaesthetics. *Anaesth Intensive Care Med* 2010; **11**: 98–100.
301 Mazoit JX, Boico O, Samii K. Myocardial uptake of bupivacaine: II. Pharmacokinetics and pharmacodynamics of bupivacaine enantiomers in the isolated perfused rabbit heart. *Anesth Analg* 1993; **77**: 477–482.
302 Chang DH, Ladd LA, Wilson KA, *et al.* Tolerability of large-dose intravenous levobupivacaine in sheep. *Anesth Analg* 2000; **91**: 671–679.
303 Huang YF, Upton RN, Runciman WB. I.V. bolus administration of subconvulsive doses of lignocaine to conscious sheep: myocardial pharmacokinetics. *Br J Anaesth* 1993; **70**: 326–332.
304 Copeland SE, Ladd LA, Gu SQ, *et al.* The effects of general anesthesia on the central nervous and cardiovascular system toxicity of local anesthetics. *Anesth Analg* 2008; **106**: 1429–1439.
305 Valenzuela C, Snyders DJ, Bennett PB, *et al.* Stereoselective block of cardiac sodium channels by bupivacaine in guinea pig ventricular myocytes. *Circulation* 1995; **92**: 3014–3024.
306 Valenzuela C, Delpon E, Tamkun MM, *et al.* Stereoselective block of a human cardiac potassium channel (Kv1.5) by bupivacaine enantiomers. *Biophys J* 1995; **69**: 418–427.
307 Mather L, Chang D. Cardiotoxicity with modern local anaesthetics: is there a safe choice? *Drugs* 2001; **61**: 333–342.
308 Avery P, Redon D, Schaenzer G, *et al.* The influence of serum potassium on the cerebral and cardiac toxicity of bupivacaine and lidocaine. *Anesthesiology* 1984; **61**: 134–138.
309 Neal JM, Mulroy MF, Weinberg GL. American Society of Regional Anesthesia and Pain Medicine checklist for managing local anesthetic systemic toxicity: 2012 version. *Reg Anesth Pain Med* 2012; **37**: 16–18.
310 Weinberg GL. Current concepts in resuscitation of patients with local anesthetic cardiac toxicity. *Reg Anesth Pain Med* 2002; **27**: 568–575.
311 Weinberg GL, VadeBoncouer T, Ramaraju GA, *et al.* Pretreatment or resuscitation with a lipid infusion shifts the dose-response to bupivacaine-induced asystole in rats. *Anesthesiology* 1998; **88**: 1071–1075.
312 Weinberg G, Ripper R, Feinstein DL, *et al.* Lipid emulsion infusion rescues dogs from bupivacaine-induced cardiac toxicity. *Reg Anesth Pain Med* 2003; **28**: 198–202.

313 Rosenblatt MA, Abel M, Fischer GW, *et al.* Successful use of a 20% lipid emulsion to resuscitate a patient after a presumed bupivacaine-related cardiac arrest. *Anesthesiology* 2006; **105**: 217–218.

314 Warren JA, Thoma RB, Georgescu A, *et al.* Intravenous lipid infusion in the successful resuscitation of local anesthetic-induced cardiovascular collapse after supraclavicular brachial plexus block. *Anesth Analg* 2008; **106**: 1578–1580.

315 Sonsino DH, Fischler M. Immediate intravenous lipid infusion in the successful resuscitation of ropivacaine-induced cardiac arrest after infraclavicular brachial plexus block. *Reg Anesth Pain Med* 2009; **34**: 276–277.

316 Weinberg GL, di Gregorio G, Ripper R, *et al.* Resuscitation with lipid versus epinephrine in a rat model of bupivacaine overdose. *Anesthesiology* 2008; **108**: 907–913.

317 Hiller DB, Gregorio GD, Ripper R, *et al.* Epinephrine impairs lipid resuscitation from bupivacaine overdose: a threshold effect. *Anesthesiology* 2009; **111**: 498–505.

318 Gregorio G, Schwartz D, Ripper R, *et al.* Lipid emulsion is superior to vasopressin in a rodent model of resuscitation from toxin-induced cardiac arrest. *Crit Care Med* 2009; **37**: 993–999.

319 Fernandez AL, Lee JA, Rahilly L, *et al.* The use of intravenous lipid emulsion as an antidote in veterinary toxicology. *J Vet Emerg Crit Care* 2011; **21**: 309–320.

320 Yang S, Abrahams MS, Hurn PD, *et al.* Local anesthetic Schwann cell toxicity is time and concentration dependent. *Reg Anesth Pain Med* 2011; **36**: 444–451.

321 Kalichman MW. Physiologic mechanisms by which local anesthetics may cause injury to nerve and spinal cord. *Reg Anesth* 1993; **18**: 448–452.

322 Kitagawa N, Oda M, Totoki T. Possible mechanism of irreversible nerve injury caused by local anesthetics: detergent properties of local anesthetics and membrane disruption. *Anesthesiology* 2004; **100**: 962–967.

323 Selander D. Neurotoxicity of local anesthetics: animal data. *Reg Anesth* 1993; **18**: 461–468.

324 Yamashita A, Matsumoto M, Matsumoto S, *et al.* A comparison of the neurotoxic effects on the spinal cord of tetracaine, lidocaine, bupivacaine, and ropivacaine administered intrathecally in rabbits. *Anesth Analg* 2003; **97**: 512–519.

325 Zhang C, Phamonvaechavan P, Rajan A, *et al.* Concentration-dependent bupivacaine myotoxicity in rabbit extraocular muscle. *J AAPOS* 2010; **14**: 323–327.

326 Zink W, Bohl JR, Hacke N, *et al.* The long term myotoxic effects of bupivacaine and ropivacaine after continuous peripheral nerve blocks. *Anesth Analg* 2005; **101**: 548–554.

327 Nouette-Gaulain K, Sirvent P, Canal-Raffin M, *et al.* Effects of intermittent femoral nerve injections of bupivacaine, levobupivacaine, and ropivacaine on mitochondrial energy metabolism and intracellular calcium homeostasis in rat psoas muscle. *Anesthesiology* 2007; **106**: 1026–1034.

328 Zink W, Graf BM. Local anesthetic myotoxicity. *Reg Anesth Pain Med* 2004; **29**: 333–340.

329 Gomoll AH, Kang RW, Williams JM, *et al.* Chondrolysis after continuous intra-articular bupivacaine infusion: an experimental model investigating chondrotoxicity in the rabbit shoulder. *Arthroscopy* 2006; **22**: 813–819.

330 Karpie JC, Chu CR. Lidocaine exhibits dose- and time-dependent cytotoxic effects on bovine articular chondrocytes in vitro. *Am J Sports Med* 2007; **35**: 1621–1627.

331 Park J, Sutradhar BC, Hong G, *et al.* Comparison of the cytotoxic effects of bupivacaine, lidocaine, and mepivacaine in equine articular chondrocytes. *Vet Anaesth Analg* 2011; **38**: 127–133.

332 Dragoo JL, Braun HJ, Kim HJ, *et al.* The in vitro chondrotoxicity of single-dose local anesthetics. *Am J Sports Med* 2012; **40**: 794–799.

333 Hansen BP, Beck CL, Beck EP, *et al.* Postarthroscopic glenohumeral chondrolysis. *Am J Sports Med* 2007; **35**: 1628–1634.

334 Rapley JH, Beavis RC, Barber FA. Glenohumeral chondrolysis after shoulder arthroscopy associated with continuous bupivacaine infusion. *Arthroscopy* 2009; **25**: 1367–1373.

335 Piper SL, Kim HT. Comparison of ropivacaine and bupivacaine toxicity in human articular chondrocytes. *J Bone Joint Surg Am* 2008; **90**: 986–991.

336 Grishko V, Xu M, Wilson G, *et al.* Apoptosis and mitochondrial dysfunction in human chondrocytes following exposure to lidocaine, bupivacaine, and ropivacaine. *J Bone Joint Surg Am* 2010; **92**: 609–618.

337 Rehman HU. Methemoglobinemia. *West J Med* 2001; **175**: 193–196.

338 Davis JA, Greenfield RE, Brewer TG. Benzocaine-induced methemoglobinemia attributed to topical application of the anesthetic in several laboratory animal species. *Am J Vet Res* 1993; **54**: 1322–1326.

339 Guertler AT, Lagutchik MS, Martin DG. Topical anesthetic-induced methemoglobinemia in sheep: a comparison of benzocaine and lidocaine. *Fundam Appl Toxicol* 1992; **18**: 294–298.

340 Lagutchik MS, Mundie TG, Martin DG. Methemoglobinemia induced by a benzocaine-based topically administered anesthetic in eight sheep. *J Am Vet Med Assoc* 1992; **201**: 1407–1410.

341 Wilkie DA, Kirby R. Methemoglobinemia associated with dermal application of benzocaine cream in a cat. *J Am Vet Med Assoc* 1988; **192**: 85–86.

342 Harvey JW, Sameck JH, Burgard FJ. Benzocaine-induced methemoglobinemia in dogs. *J Am Vet Med Assoc* 1979; **175**: 1171–1175.

343 Poppers PJ, Mastri AR. Maternal and foetal methaemoglobinaemia caused by prilocaine. *Acta Anaesthesiol Scand Suppl* 1969; **37**: 258–263.

344 Martin DG, Watson CE, Gold MB, *et al.* Topical anesthetic-induced methemoglobinemia and sulfhemoglobinemia in macaques: a comparison of benzocaine and lidocaine. *J Appl Toxicol* 1995; **15**: 153–158.

345 Harvey JW, Keitt AS. Studies of the efficacy and potential hazards of methylene blue therapy in aniline-induced methaemoglobinaemia. *Br J Haematol* 1983; **54**: 29–41.

346 Welch SL. Local anesthetic toxicosis. *Vet Med* 2000; **95**: 670–673.

347 Eggleston ST, Lush LW. Understanding allergic reactions to local anesthetics. *Ann Pharmacother* 1996; **30**: 851–857.

348 Dooms-Goossens A, de Alam AG, Degreef H, *et al.* Local anesthetic intolerance due to metabisulfite. *Contact Derm* 1989; **20**: 124–126.

SECTION 3

Body Fluids and Thermoregulation

18 Acid–Base Physiology

William W. Muir
VCPCS, Columbus, Ohio, USA

Chapter contents

Introduction

A fundamental principle of physiology is homeostasis: the maintenance of constant conditions through dynamic equilibrium of the body's internal environment. One of the many processes that maintain homeostasis is the regulation of acid–base balance, a term introduced by L.J. Henderson [1]. Current understanding of acid–base physiology continues to evolve aided by new and improved technologies that permit the determination of heretofore unmeasurable ionic substances that contribute to acid–base equilibrium. Historical dogma and analytical innovations continue to influence clinical interpretation of acid–base disorders. What once was a purely descriptive science has become far more quantitative and mechanistically based, contributing significantly to a more comprehensive understanding of the multiple factors responsible for acid–base regulation in health and disease.

Central to all schemes of acid–base balance is the understanding that normal oxygen-dependent metabolism of food (carbohydrates, fats, and proteins) results in the predictable production of work, heat, and waste. Indeed, normal metabolic processes are responsible for the production of thousands of millimoles of carbon dioxide (CO_2; volatile acid) and potentially hundreds of milliequivalents of non-volatile hydrogen ions (fixed acid) daily. Individual differences in the amount of CO_2 and hydrogen ion (H^+) produced are influenced by diet, cellular basal metabolic rate, and body temperature. Animals consuming high-protein diets produce CO_2 and excess quantities of H^+ precursors, whereas animals consuming diets high in plant material produce CO_2 and excess quantities of bicarbonate ion (HCO_3^-) precursors. The CO_2 that is produced is combined with water and is catalyzed by carbonic anhydrase (CA) to form carbonic acid (H_2CO_3). The formation of carbonic acid from CO_2 and water (H_2O) (eqn 18.1) and the subsequent generation of H^+ and HCO_3^- (eqn 18.2) provide a focal point for almost all discussions of acid–base balance.

Historically, in the 1950s, plasma hydrogen ion concentration ($[H^+]$) and CO_2 content were the only relevant acid–base quantities that could be conveniently determined. Henderson's studies emphasized that large quantities of CO_2 are produced by metabolizing cells and that CO_2 is in equilibrium with H^+ and HCO_3^- ion.

$$CO_2 + H_2O = H_2CO_3 \tag{18.1}$$

$$H_2CO_3 \rightleftharpoons H^+ + HCO_3^- \tag{18.2}$$

Combining eqns. 7.1 and 7.2 yields:

$$CO_2 + H_2O \rightleftharpoons H_2CO_3 \rightleftharpoons H^+ + HCO_3^- \tag{18.3}$$

Once more, it is important to emphasize that current-day technologies have advanced the science of acid–base homeostasis far beyond that of the 1950s and Henderson's introduction of the term acid–base balance. Regardless, the central importance of H^+

Veterinary Anesthesia and Analgesia: The Fifth Edition of Lumb and Jones.
Edited by Kurt A. Grimm, Leigh A. Lamont, William J. Tranquilli, Stephen A. Greene and Sheilah A. Robertson.

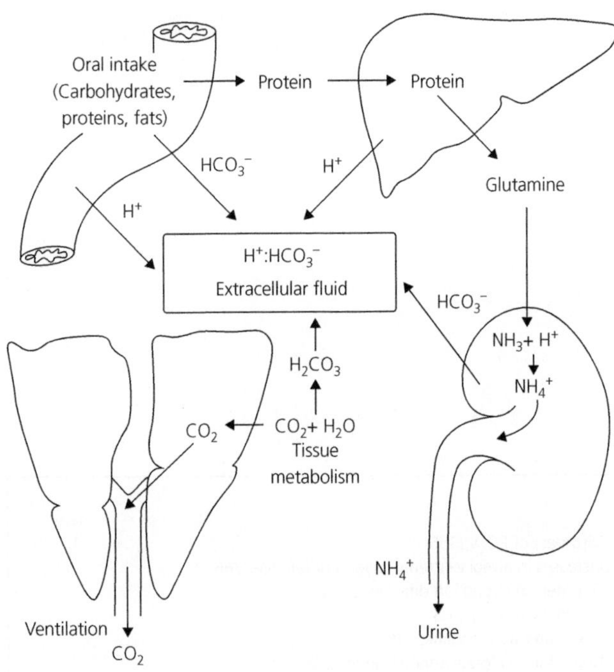

Figure 18.1 The gut, liver, lung, and kidney aid in acid–base homeostasis.

regulation to cell function and animal health cannot be overemphasized and led A.B. Hastings to state: 'Tiny though it is, I suppose no constituent of living matter has so much power to influence biological behavior' [2].

Acid–base homeostasis ([H$^+$] regulation) involves the integrated normal activity of the lungs, kidney, liver, and gastrointestinal tract (Fig. 18.1). The lung removes CO_2, the kidneys remove H$^+$ as fixed acid, the liver metabolizes protein, and the gut regulates the absorption of water and nutrients and eliminates wastes. This chapter reviews the basic principles that determine acid–base balance and their integration into both descriptive and quantitative approaches to acid–base abnormalities in animals. Other more specific texts should be consulted for a more comprehensive review of the subject [2–8].

Acids, bases, pH, pK, and the Henderson–Hasselbalch equation

Most formal definitions of acids or bases when applied to biologic solutions utilize the Bronsted–Lowery concept, which classifies acids as proton donors and bases as proton acceptors. A more appropriate working definition, however, may be that acids are substances that increase H$^+$ concentration ([H$^+$]), a term used synonymously with protons in aqueous solutions [9]. The strength of an acid and resultant acidity of a solution are determined by its activity coefficient, a factor influenced by temperature that determines the degree of dissociation. Since, by definition, a base is a H$^+$ (proton) acceptor, each acid dissociates into H$^+$ and a potential H$^+$ acceptor or conjugate base. For example, H_2CO_3 in aqueous solution dissociates into H$^+$ and its conjugate base HCO_3^-. Substances that are strong acids have weak conjugate bases and vice versa. Interestingly, water, the most abundant solvent in the body, can function as both an acid (H_3O^+; proton donor) or a base (H_2O; proton acceptor) depending on local conditions ($H^+ + H_2O \leftrightarrow H_3O^+$). At normal pH (7.40) and temperature (37–38 °C), water is the most abundant base in the body.

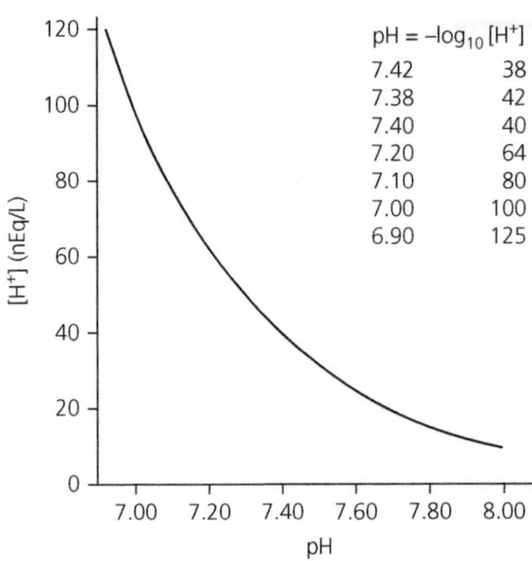

Figure 18.2 Relationship between [H$^+$] and pH. The relationship is not linear.

Physiologically and clinically, the formation of acids and therefore H$^+$ production are emphasized because the end-product of oral intake, tissue metabolism, and many pathophysiologic processes is the production and release of hydrogen ion. The concept of pH ($-\log_{10}$[H$^+$]) was developed in order to simplify the notation necessary to describe the large amounts of H$^+$ produced and the changes of [H$^+$] observed in nature and chemical experiments. This notation, although cumbersome mathematically, converts [H$^+$] to pH by the formula (Fig. 18.2):

$$pH = -\log_{10}[H^+] = \log_{10}(1/[H^+]) \tag{18.4}$$

Regardless of conversion issues and the relatively narrow range (20–150 nEq/L) over which changes in [H$^+$] occur in biologic fluids, the concept of pH has persisted and is routinely reported on most pH and blood gas analyzers. Conversion formulas for pH to [H$^+$] have been developed:

$$\text{if pH} > 7.40 \text{ then } [H^+] = (pH_m - 7.40)(40)(0.8) \tag{18.4a}$$

$$\text{If pH} < 7.40 \text{ then } [H^+] = (7.40 - pH_m)(40)(1.25) \tag{18.4b}$$

where pH_m is the measured pH. The development of the pH conversion in conjunction with the theory of acid–base balance and the introduction of methods to measure pH in blood by Hasselbalch (1912) led to the development of the Henderson–Hasselbalch equation and the characterization of acid–base disturbances as being either respiratory or metabolic (non-respiratory) in origin. The presence of many chemical equilibriums in blood (e.g., phosphates, sulfates) and the law of mass action produce many potential equilibrium equations that could be used to explain acid–base balance. The reasons why the carbonic acid equilibrium equation (eqns 18.1 and 18.2) was chosen to describe acid–base balance are (a) historical (methods were available to determine CO_2 content); (b) the finding that, other than water, HCO_3^- is the major base in the extracellular fluid and H_2CO_3 the major acid; and (c) the carbonic acid equation incorporates both volatile and non-volatile (fixed) substances. The law of mass action states that the rate (velocity) of a reaction is proportional to the concentration of the reactants and the dissociation constant (K) for the reaction. The rate of dissociation (r) for an acid can be characterized by:

$$[HA] \rightarrow [H^+] + [A^-] \quad (18.5)$$

using the dissociation constant K_1,

$$r_1 = K_1[HA] \quad (18.6)$$

Similarly:

$$[H^+] + [A^-] \rightarrow [HA] \quad (18.7)$$

and:

$$r_2 = K_2[H^+][A^-] \quad (18.8)$$

which at equilibrium results in $r_1 = r_2$, or:

$$K_2/K_1 = K_a = [H+][A-]/[HA] \quad (18.9)$$

where K_a is the dissociation constant for the acid HA. Applying this law to carbonic acid, Henderson derived:

$$[H+] = K_a[CO_2]/HCO_3^- \quad (18.10)$$

Henderson used the concentration of dissolved molecular CO_2 instead of H_2CO_3 because H_2CO_3 could not be measured. Hasselbalch then introduced PCO_2 into Henderson's equation and put the equation into logarithmic form, producing the now universally applied Henderson–Hasselbalch equation:

$$pH = pK_a + \log_{10}\left([HCO_3^-]/[s \times PCO_2]\right) \quad (18.11)$$

where pH is $-\log_{10}[H^+]$, pK_a is $= \log_{10}K_a$, and s is the solubility of CO_2. This equation is frequently rewritten for explanatory purposes as:

$$pH = pKa + \log\{[base]/[acid]\} = \text{kidney function/lung function} \quad (18.12)$$

Henderson deliberately applied the law of mass action to the equilibrium of carbonic acid. The Henderson–Hasselbalch equation indicates the amount of H^+ available to react with bases. Since acids and bases are charged particles, the application of this equation to biologic fluids assumes that:

1 mass is conserved: the concentration of all substances can be accounted for as the sum of the concentrations of dissociated and undissociated forms
2 all dissociation constants for all incompletely dissociated substances (weak acids or bases) are satisfied
3 electroneutrality is preserved: all positive charges must equal all negative charges.

These assumptions have particular relevance to the application of acid–base principles and to the interpretation of acid–base imbalances. The preservation of electroneutrality (anions = cations) serves as the basis for always integrating electrolyte (Na^+, K^+, Cl^-, etc.) concentrations into the diagnosis and interpretation of acid–base imbalances.

Body buffering systems

The body uses three principal mechanisms to minimize or buffer changes in $[H^+]$ [6,7]. Blood chemical buffers act within seconds to resist or reduce changes in $[H^+]$ and are the first line of defense against changes in pH. The respiratory system responds within minutes to resist changes in $[H^+]$ by regulating the partial pressure of CO_2 (physiologic buffering) and eliminating excess CO_2 molecules caused by an increase in H^+ production (chemical buffering).

$$\uparrow H + HCO_3^- \rightarrow H_2CO_3 \rightarrow H2O + CO_2 \text{(increased minute volume)} \quad (18.13)$$

Finally, H^+ that is produced by non-respiratory mechanisms (metabolic or non-respiratory acidosis) is excreted by the kidney in the urine over a period of hours or days (Fig. 18.3).

Chemical buffers

Chemical buffers are substances that minimize changes in the $[H^+]$ or the pH of a solution when an acid or base is added [10,11]. A buffer solution consists of a weak acid and its conjugate base and is most effective when the pH is within 1.0 pH units of its dissociation constant (pK_a) (Table 18.1). Alterations in blood, interstitial, and intracellular fluid $[H^+]$ are immediately modified by chemical buffer systems. The ratio of the anion $[A^-]$ form of the buffer to its conjugate acid [HA] is a function of its dissociation constant (pK_a) and the $[H^+]$. For weak acids, as $[H^+]$ increases, $[A^-]$ decreases and [HA] increases by equal amounts, keeping the total amount of A_{TOT} ($A_{TOT} = HA + A^-$) the same. The principal chemical H^+ buffers are the bicarbonate (HCO_3^-/H_2CO_3), phosphate (HPO_4^-/H_2PO_4), and protein ($Prot^-$/H Prot) buffer systems. Bone can contribute calcium carbonate and calcium phosphate to the extracellular fluid, thereby increasing the buffering capacity. Indeed, bone may account for up to 40% of the buffering of an acute acid load. Functionally, anytime there is an increase in $[H^+]$ in the body, the anion form of the buffer (HCO_3^-, HPO_4^-, and $Prot^-$) accepts the excess proton, converting the buffer to its conjugate acid (H_2CO_3, H_2PO_4, and H Prot). Because the body can have only one $[H^+]$, the ratio of the acid to salt forms of the various buffer pairs in solution can always be predicted by the Henderson–Hasselbalch equation (isohydric principle), providing their concentration and dissociation constant (pK_a) are known. With knowledge of the behavior of one buffer pair, one can

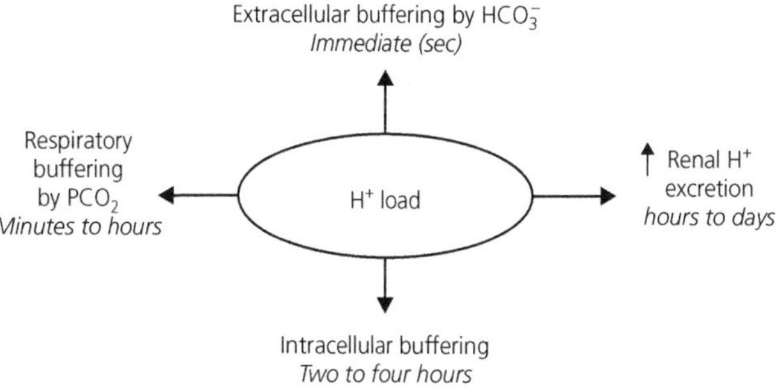

Figure 18.3 Body buffering mechanisms.

Table 18.1 pK_a values of important chemical buffers.[a]

Compound	pK_a
Lactic acid	3.9
3-Hydroxybutyric acid	4.7
Creatinine	5.0
Organic phosphates	6.0–7.5
Carbonic acid	6.1
Imidazole group of histidine	6.4–6.7
Oxygenated hemoglobin	6.7
Inorganic phosphates	6.8
α-Amino (amino terminal)	7.4–7.9
Deoxygenated hemoglobin	7.9
Ammonium	9.2
Bicarbonate	9.8

[a]Compounds with pK_a values in the range of 6.4 to 8.4 are most useful as buffers in biological systems. The pK_a values for the imidazole group of histidine and for α-amino (amino terminal) groups are for those side groups in proteins. The pK_a range for organic phosphates refers to such intracellular compounds as ATP. ADP. and 2.3-DPG.

Table 18.2 Major body buffers.

	pK_a	Compartment pH	Basis of Effectiveness	Weakness
ECF				
HCO_3^-	6.1	7.4	CO_2 removal by the lungs Quantity depends on lungs	Distance of pH from pK
ICF[a]				
Imidazole	Close to 7	7.0	Exceedingly large quantity	Changes charge on ICF proteins[b]
HCO_3^-	6.1	7.0	Relatively large quantity	Depends on lungs for CO_2 removal
Urine				
Inorganic phosphate	6.8	5–7	pK higher than urine pH	Little capacity to increase excretion rate

ECF. extracellular fluid: ICF. intracellular fluid; and HCO_3^-, sodium bicarbonate ion.
[a]Although ICF creatine phosphate is not a buffer, during acidemia it is hydrolyzed, rendering it capable of H^+ binding.
[b]This change in charge on ICF proteins can have important effects on enzyme activities, transporters, and ICF volume.

predict the behavior of all the other buffer pairs in solution. As pointed out above, the HCO_3^-/H_2CO_3 buffer pair is most frequently used to determine acid–base status in clinical practice because it is the most prominent chemical buffer in the extracellular fluid and in the presence of carbonic anhydrase, carbonic acid forms CO_2, which is eliminated by alveolar ventilation. Thus, during normal conditions, the body can be considered an 'open' system.

Approximately 60% of the body's chemical buffering capacity occurs by intracellular phosphates and proteins. Inorganic and organic (ATP, ADP, and 2,3-DPG) phosphates possess pK_a values that range from 6.0 to 7.5, making them ideal chemical buffers over a wide range of potential intracellular pH values. Inorganic phosphate (pK_a 6.8) is the major buffer in urine because renal tubular pH (6.0–7.0) includes the pK_a of the HPO_4^-/H_2PO_4 buffer pair.

Intracellular pH regulation depends on the activity of two cell membrane ion transport systems: the Na^+-H^+ and Cl^--HCO_3^- antiporters (chloride pump), and intracellular proteins. Proteins are by far the most important intracellular buffers. Hemoglobin contributes approximately 80% of the non-bicarbonate buffering capacity of whole blood and with other intracellular proteins is responsible for three-fourths of the chemical buffering power of the body. The most important intracellular protein-dissociable group is the imidazole ring of histidine (pK_a 6.4–6.7). The α-amino groups of proteins (pK_a 7.4–7.9) play a secondary but important role in intracellular buffering. Plasma proteins, particularly albumin, also contain histidine and α-amino groups, and collectively are responsible for 20% of the non-bicarbonate buffering capacity of whole blood (Table 18.2).

Respiratory system

The respiratory system provides a route by which [H^+] can be regulated by varying the partial pressure of carbon dioxide (PCO_2) (see Fig. 18.1). Chemoreceptors throughout the body, but particularly those located in the medulla and carotid body, monitor changes in [H^+] and PCO_2 and adjust breathing (tidal volume and frequency) to maintain a normal [H^+]. The association of H^+ with HCO_3^- and the subsequent formation of CO_2 and H_2O is an example of very rapid chemical buffering (closed system), whereas subsequent elimination of CO_2 by the lung via increased ventilation (open physiologic system) requires longer response time (usually in minutes). Changes in blood CO_2 also have important consequences for hemoglobin's affinity for oxygen and its buffering capacity. Increases in PCO_2 increase blood [H^+] and decrease hemoglobin affinity for oxygen (Bohr effect: shifting the oxygen-hemoglobin curve to the right). This decrease in the oxygen affinity of hemoglobin is advantageous in tissues, allowing hemoglobin to release more oxygen for metabolism. Non-oxygenated hemoglobin in turn can transport more CO_2 in the form of hemoglobin carbamino compounds (H^+-$Prot^-$) to the lungs (Haldane effect). It is important to realize that anytime there is a change in PCO_2, there is a relatively greater change in [H^+] than in [HCO_3^-], because [HCO_3^-] is measured in milliequivalents per liter and [H^+] in nanoequivalents per liter. Importantly, maintenance of [H^+] within a narrow range of values is vital to normal tissue enzyme activity and cell viability.

Renal system

The synthesis of new HCO_3^- and excretion of excess H^+ emphasizes the role of the kidneys in both chemical and physiologic buffering (see Fig. 18.1) [12]. Although relatively slow (hours or days), compared with the lungs (minutes) and chemical buffering (seconds), the kidney serves as the principal means by which acids, that are produced by metabolic processes (not owing to CO_2 production), are ultimately eliminated (see Fig. 18.3). All hydrogen ions produced by metabolic processes are excreted in the urine in combination with weak anions (titratable acidity), primarily phosphate and ammonium salts. The term *titratable acidity* may be considered synonymous with urinary phosphate concentration but actually represents all weak acids, including creatinine and urate. Net acid excretion by the kidney includes the titratable acidity and ammonium minus the HCO_3^- eliminated in the urine. Ammonium (NH_4^+) is produced in the proximal tubule primarily from glutamine metabolism to α-ketoglutarate and NH_3, a process that simultaneously generates HCO_3^-. Increases in H^+ production can increase the rate of ammonium salt excretion by five-fold during severe metabolic acidosis (Fig. 18.4).

It is important to note that potassium loss from cells can lead to intracellular H^+ or Na^+ accumulation in order to maintain electric neutrality. This effect in renal tubular cells can lead to increased H^+ excretion (aciduria) and HCO_3^- reabsorption ('paradoxical aciduria') [13]. Renal tubular cell acidosis may also augment glutamine metabolism and NH_3 production, leading to enhanced NH_4^+ excretion. Alkalemia and paradoxical aciduria are known to occur in people, rats, and ruminants. Their importance in dogs and cats is not well documented.

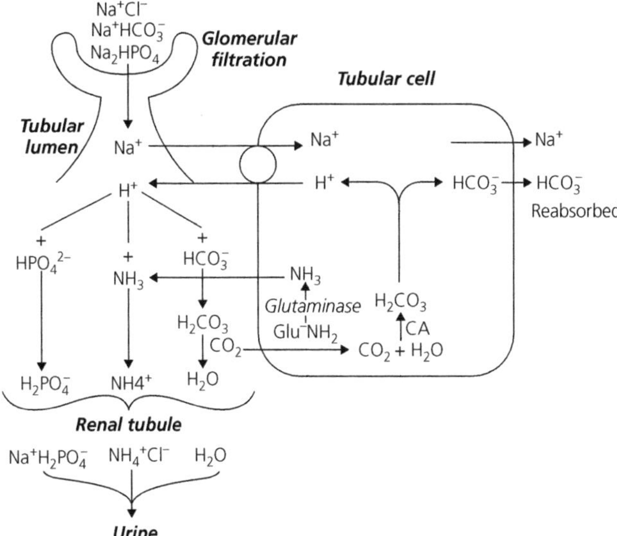

Figure 18.4 Reabsorption and regeneration of sodium bicarbonate ion (HCO_3^-) in the renal tubules. Bicarbonate reabsorption in the proximal tubule coincides with H^+ secretion. Bicarbonate regeneration in the renal tubules coincides with titration of phosphate by H^+ and ammonium formation.

Temperature effects on acid–base balance

Increases or decreases in body temperature are frequently encountered in animals during anesthesia and surgery. Increases in body temperature may be caused by stress, increases in skeletal muscle activity (inadequate relaxation), systemic disease, and/or infectious and genetic disorders (malignant hyperthermia). Hypothermia is a common consequence of anesthesia and surgery and is much more profound in small animals (<8 to 10 kg) because of their larger body surface area to body mass ratio. Decreases in body temperature are potentiated by cleaning solutions (water or alcohol), cold exposure (steel tables), illness (shock), drugs that cause vasodilation (phenothiazine drugs, inhalant anesthesia), and muscle relaxants (neuromuscular blocking drugs). Changes in body temperature affect the $[H^+]$ of all body fluids. Increases in body temperature decrease pH (increase $[H^+]$) and vice versa such that blood pH changes by 0.015–0.02 units/°C. Changes in $[H^+]$ and pH with body temperature are expected because of known temperature-induced changes on dissociation constants (pK_a) and the solubility of CO_2 in blood. For example, as body temperature decreases, the pK_a and blood solubility of CO_2 increase, producing an increase in pH and decrease in PCO_2 (Table 18.3). These temperature-dependent changes in both intracellular and extracellular pH are believed to be important in maintaining an OH^-/H^+ (relative alkalinity) ratio of 16:1 throughout the body [14]. A constant relative alkalinity of 16:1 for OH^- and H^+ is known to be optimal for cellular enzyme systems to function normally. The most important of the dissociable groups responsible for the maintenance of a constant OH^-/H^+ ratio is the imidazole ring of the histidine residues of hemoglobin. The fractional dissociation of imidazole-histidine remains constant as temperature changes and varies with pH during isothermal conditions. This regulation of imidazole-histidine dissociation to maintain acid–base balance is termed *alpha-stat* regulation in contrast to the *pH-stat* regulation concept wherein pH values are maintained constant (Table 18.4) [14].

Table 18.3 Effect of temperature on PO_2, PCO_2, and pH.

Temp °C	PO_2	PCO_2	pH
20	27	19	7.65
25	37	24	7.58
30	51	30	7.50
35	70	37	7.43
36	75	38	7.41
37	80	40	7.40
38	85	42	7.39
39	91	44	7.37
40	97	45	7.36

Both the alpha-stat and pH-stat concepts of acid–base balance have been used to interpret pH and blood gases in humans with body temperatures higher or lower than normal [15]. Proponents of the pH-stat hypothesis argue that it is important to maintain a constant pH of 7.40 and PCO_2 of 40 mmHg at any temperature, whereas proponents of the alpha-stat strategy attempt to keep a constant ratio of $[H^+]$ to $[OH^-]$ of 1:16. Proponents of the pH-stat strategy realize that if the pH and PCO_2 were kept constant at pH of 7.40 and PCO_2 of 40 mmHg during hypothermia, the animal would be acidotic, but they argue that pH-stat oriented therapy reduces morbidity [16]. Proponents of alpha-stat oriented therapy argue similarly and point out that blood flow to vital organs, particularly cerebral blood flow, becomes pressure dependent (loss of autoregulation) with pH-stat management. From a practical standpoint, pH and PCO_2 need not be corrected for temperature unless absolute values at the animal's current temperature are required. Determining the pH and blood gases (PO_2, PCO_2) from a blood sample taken from a hypothermic animal (the temperature at which most blood gas machines are calibrated is either 37 °C or 38 °C) enables interpretation of acid–base abnormalities for appropriate therapeutic decisions. This last statement is made with the knowledge that the pH and blood gas values obtained are correct only at 37 °C or 38 °C and do not represent the actual values at the animal's current body temperature (unless it is 37 °C or 38 °C). Therefore, both corrected and uncorrected blood gas values may be of questionable utility in animals with significant deviations from normal body temperature.

Acid–base terminology

Three approaches to acid–base physiology using different but inter-related variables have evolved to assess changes in acid–base balance (Fig. 18.5) [11]. As described above, traditional descriptions of acid–base balance and acid–base abnormalities are based on the Bronsted–Lowery definition (proton donor) of an acid and base and the Henderson–Hasselbalch equation to determine the pH and proton concentration. The terms *acidosis* and *alkalosis*, for example, are used to describe the abnormal or pathologic (-osis) accumulation of acid $[H^+]$ or alkali $[OH^-]$ in the body [6]. The terms *acidemia* and *alkalemia* are used to describe whether the blood pH is acid or alkaline, respectively. The Henderson–Hasselbalch equation characterizes all acid–base disturbances as being either respiratory or metabolic (non-respiratory) because of the body's production and elimination of volatile (dissolved CO_2, H_2CO_3) and non-volatile or fixed (e.g., lactic and phosphoric) acids, respectively. Therefore, only four primary acid–base abnormalities are possible: respiratory acidosis, metabolic acidosis, respiratory alkalosis, and metabolic alkalosis (Table 18.5).

Table 18.4 Comparison of pH-stat and alpha-stat acid–base regulation.

Concept	Purpose	Total CO_2	pH and $PaCO_2$ Maintenance	Intracellular state	α-Imidazole and buffering	Enzyme structure and function
pH-stat	Constant pH	Increases	Normal corrected values	Acidotic (excess H^+)	Excess (+) charge, buffering decreased	Altered and activity decreased
Alpha-stat	Constant OH^-/H^+	Constant	Normal uncorrected values	Neutral ($H^+ = OH^-$)	Constant net charge, buffering constant	Normal and activity maximal

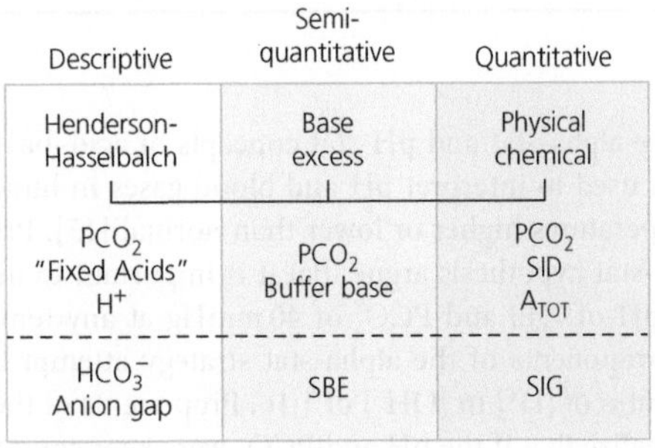

Figure 18.5 Three approaches used to describe acid–base imbalance. pCO_2 = partial pressure of carbon dioxide; SBE = standard base excess; SID = strong ion difference; A_{TOT} = total weak acid; SIG = strong ion gap.

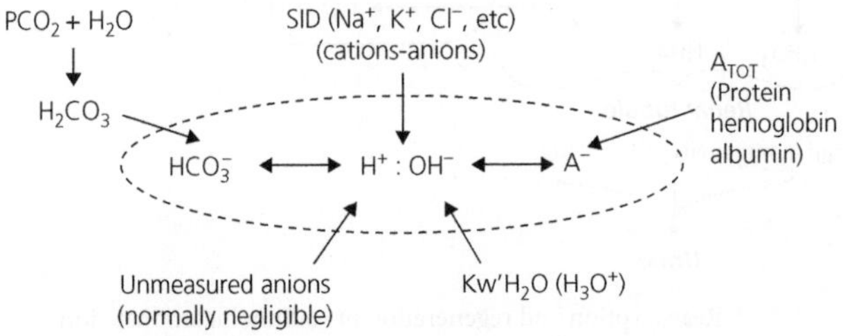

Figure 18.6 Independent variables responsible for acid–base balance. The dependent variables (H + and OH^-) are enclosed by the dashed line. SID = strong ion difference.

Table 18.5 Traditional characteristics of primary acid–base disturbances.

Disorder	pH	$[H^+]$	Primary disturbance	Compensatory response
Non-respiratory acidosis	↓	↑	↓ $[HCO_3^-]$	↓ PCO_2
Non-respiratory alkalosis	↑	↓	↑ $[HCO_3^-]$	↑ PCO_2
Respiratory acidosis	↓	↑	↑ $[PCO_2]$	↑ $[HCO_3^-]$
Respiratory alkalosis	↑	↓	↓ $[PCO_2]$	↓ $[HCO_3^-]$

Non-respiratory is used in preference to metabolic. HCO_3^-, sodium bicarbonate ion.

Clinically, the terms *respiratory* and *metabolic* have been used to imply the involvement of the lung and kidney in acid–base regulation:

$$pH = HCO_3^- / PaCO_2 = \text{kidney function(fixed acids)} / \text{lung function(volatile acids)} \tag{18.14}$$

The term *non-respiratory* frequently replaces metabolic in many discussions of acid–base imbalance because it incorporates all mechanisms responsible for acid–base imbalance other than the production of CO_2 and carbonic acid (H_2CO_3). These mechanisms include alterations in the concentrations of strong (fully dissociated) ions as assessed by the anion gap and strong ion difference (SID), non-volatile plasma buffers (primarily serum proteins; A_{TOT}), and the ionic strength (dissociation constants; pK_a) of the solution (Fig. 18.6). Note that metabolic or non-respiratory acid–base disturbances can be brought about by changes in strong ions or weak ions. These ions can be routinely measured (e.g., Cl^-) or not (e.g., lactate, ketones). Those that are not routinely measured are referred to as 'unmeasured ions.'

In summary, acid–base disorders are caused by four independent factors (PCO_2, SID, A_{TOT}, and pK_a) that can change $[H^+]$. Each term is regulated and can be changed independently of the others and result in changes in $[H^+]$ [7,8]. It should be noted, however, that changes in temperature can affect all the independent variables, a consideration that has special importance during surgery and anesthesia, especially in poikilotherms [14]. Primary abnormalities in acid–base balance can arise from disturbances in any one or several of the independent variables (see Fig. 18.6). Simple acid–base abnormalities are said to occur only when one independent variable is responsible for the acid–base disturbance. Mixed acid–base abnormalities are caused by disturbances in two or more of the independent variables. Mixed acid–base abnormalities may be additive (respiratory and non-respiratory acidosis) or offsetting (respiratory alkalosis and non-respiratory acidosis) with regard to their ability to influence $[H^+]$ measured as pH (Table 18.6) [17]. Offsetting mixed acid–base abnormalities occur when two primary acid–base abnormalities produce opposite effects on plasma $[H^+]$. Animals with offsetting mixed acid–base abnormalities have both acidosis and alkalosis but do not necessarily demonstrate acidemia or alkalemia, because the blood pH may be normal. Blood chemical observations that should lead to suspicions of a mixed acid–base disturbance when evaluating blood gas results include [17]:

- the presence of a normal pH with abnormal PCO_2 and/or $[HCO_3^-]$
- a pH change in a direction opposite to that predicted for the known primary disorder
- PCO_2 and $[HCO_3^-]$ changing in opposite directions.

Mixed acid–base disorders can be classified based on the origin of the primary disturbances as mixed respiratory disturbances, mixed non-respiratory and respiratory disturbances, mixed non-respiratory disturbances, and triple disorders. They also can be classified based on their effect on an animal's pH in additive combinations, offsetting combinations, and triple disorders (see Table 18.6). In additive combinations, both primary disorders tend to change pH in the same direction (e.g., respiratory acidosis and non-respiratory acidosis), whereas in offsetting combinations, the primary disorders tend to change the pH in opposite directions (e.g., respiratory alkalosis and non-respiratory acidosis). The final pH reflects the dominant of the two offsetting disorders in offsetting combinations [2]. Detailed reviews of mixed acid–base disorders in domestic animals have been presented elsewhere [4,5,17].

Secondary or compensatory (adaptive) acid–base changes frequently occur in response to most primary acid–base abnormalities and aid in buffering or minimizing changes in plasma [H^+]. Respiratory acid–base abnormalities, for example, are generally compensated for by controlled, oppositely directed changes in non-respiratory function (Table 18.7). In simple acid–base abnormalities such as primary respiratory acidosis caused by hypoventilation, the kidney compensates by producing non-respiratory alkalosis (see Table 18.5).

Respiratory compensation for non-respiratory acidosis is accomplished by increasing alveolar ventilation and CO_2 excretion by the lungs. Non-respiratory acidosis is characterized by an increase in [H^+], a decrease in blood [HCO_3^-] and pH, and a decrease in PCO_2 (respiratory alkalosis), caused by secondary hyperventilation whereas non-respiratory alkalosis is characterized by a decrease in [H^+], increase in blood [HCO_3^-] and pH, and an increase in PCO_2, owing to compensatory hypoventilation (respiratory acidosis) (see Table 18.5).

Table 18.6 Classification of mixed acid–base disorders.

Classification	Effect on the pH
Mixed respiratory disorders	
Acute and chronic respiratory acidosis	Additive
Acute and chronic respiratory alkalosis	Additive
Mixed respiratory and non-respiratory disorders	
Respiratory acidosis and non-respiratory acidosis	Additive
Respiratory acidosis and non-respiratory alkalosis	Offsetting
Respiratory alkalosis and non-respiratory acidosis	Offsetting
Respiratory alkalosis and non-respiratory alkalosis	Additive
Mixed non-respiratory disorders	
Non-respiratory acidosis and non-respiratory alkalosis	Offsetting
Normal plus high anion gap non-respiratory acidosis	Additive
Mixed high anion gap non-respiratory acidosis	Additive
Mixed normal anion gap non-respiratory acidosis	Additive
Triple disorders	
Non-respiratory acidosis, non-respiratory alkalosis, and respiratory acidosis	Final pH is function of relative dominance of acidifying and alkalinizing processes
Non-respiratory acidosis, non-respiratory alkalosis, and respiratory alkalosis	

In respiratory acid–base disorders, the compensation occurs in two phases. The first phase consists of titration by non-bicarbonate buffers, and the second phase reflects renal compensation of the acid–base disorder, by increasing or decreasing HCO_3^- and Cl^- excretion in the urine (Fig. 18.7). Respiratory acidosis is characterized by increased PCO_2, increased [H^+], decreased pH, and an associated increase in blood [HCO_3^-]. CO_2 accumulation is caused by alveolar hypoventilation. Renal compensation occurs by titration of non-bicarbonate buffers, increase in net acid and Cl^- excretion, and increase in HCO_3^- reabsorption by the kidneys [6,12]. Respiratory alkalosis is characterized by decreased PCO_2, decreased [H^+], increased pH, and a compensatory decrease in blood [HCO_3^-]. The initial compensation in respiratory alkalosis is caused by release of H^+ from non-bicarbonate buffers within cells. The second phase is mediated by a compensatory decrease in net acid excretion by the kidneys [12].

When analyzing secondary changes in a given acid–base disorder, it is important to remember the following.

1 With the exception of chronic respiratory alkalosis, compensation does not return the pH to normal. The pH almost always trends toward the primary condition.
2 Overcompensation does not occur.
3 Sufficient time must elapse for compensation to reach a steady state, at which time the expected compensation can be estimated (see Table 18.7).

The question that often arises when analyzing simple acid–base abnormalities that demonstrate both respiratory acidosis and non-respiratory alkalosis is, 'Which is the primary problem and is there a secondary and/or compensatory event?' The answer is not always obvious, although simple primary acid–base abnormalities generally change pH in the direction of the primary disorder. For example, an animal with respiratory acidosis and compensatory non-respiratory alkalosis would have a pH that tended to be acidotic (below normal,

Table 18.7 Compensatory responses in primary acid–base disorders.

Disorder	Primary change	Expected range of compensation
Non-respiratory acidosis	↓ [HCO_3^-]	PCO_2 = last 2 digits of pH × 100 $\Delta PCO_2 = 1–1.13\ (\Delta[HCO_3^-])$ $PCO_2 = [HCO_3^-] + 15$ $PCO_2 = 0.7\ [HCO_3^-] \pm 3$ (dogs)
Non-respiratory alkalosis	↑ [HCO_3^-]	PCO_2: variable increase PCO_2 = increases of 0.6 mmHg for each new 1 mEq/L increase in [HCO_3^-] $PCO_2 = 0.7\ [HCO_3^-] \pm 3$ (dogs)
Respiratory acidosis		
Acute	↑ PCO_2	Acute [HCO_3^-] increases 1 mEq/L and pH decreases 0.05 units for every 10 mmHg increase in PCO_2 $[HCO_3^-] = 0.15\ PCO_2 \pm 2$ (dogs)
Chronic	↑ PCO_2	[HCO_3^-] increases 3.5 mEq/L and pH decreases 0.07 units for every 10 mmHg increase in PCO_2 $[HCO_3^-] = 0.35\ PCO_2 \pm 2$ (dogs)
Respiratory alkalosis		
Acute	↓ PCO_2	[HCO_3^-] falls 2 mEq/L and pH increases 0.1 units for each 10 mmHg fall in PCO_2 $[HCO_3^-] = 0.25\ PCO_2 \pm 2$ (dogs)
Chronic	↓ PCO_2	[HCO_3^-] falls 5 mEq/L and pH increases 0.15 units for each 10 mmHg fall in PCO_2 $[HCO_3^-] = 0.55\ PCO_2 \pm 2$ (dogs)

HCO_3^-, sodium bicarbonate ion.

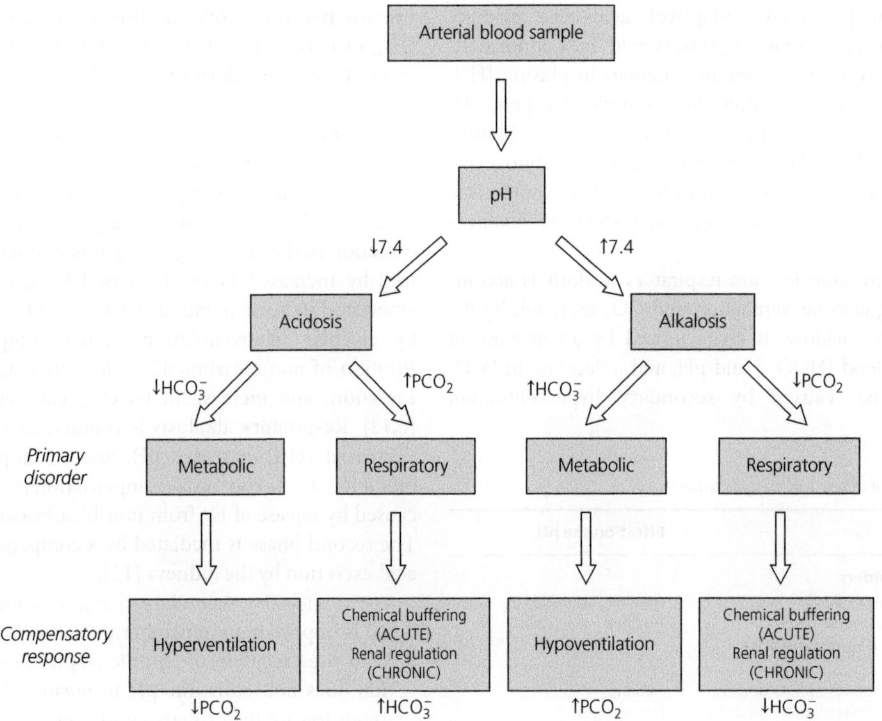

Figure 18.7 Analysis of simple acid–base disorders according to the traditional approach.

e.g., a pH of 7.31). Mixed respiratory and non-respiratory acid–base abnormalities are much more difficult to decipher, and like simple acid–base abnormalities must be carefully evaluated in the context of an animal's disease, and other available diagnostic information.

Because non-respiratory acidosis is so frequently associated with disease processes in animals, indices of acid–base balance have evolved that enable the non-respiratory component of acid–base abnormality to be evaluated quantitatively. The standard bicarbonate is the concentration of bicarbonate in plasma after the whole blood sample has been equilibrated to a PCO_2 of 40 mmHg at the species normal body temperature (many standard values from blood gas machines intended for use with human patients use normal human body temperature, 37 °C). Ruminants tend to have greater standard bicarbonate values. This index quantifies the non-respiratory component of any acid–base abnormality, because differences in the standard bicarbonate from normal (for the species in question, e.g., 23–28 mEq/L) cannot be caused by changes in PCO_2, which is held constant at 40 mmHg at the species normal body temperature. Similarly, the base excess (BE) quantitates the number of milliequivalents per liter of acid or base required to titrate 1 L of blood to pH 7.40 while the PCO_2 is held constant at 40 mmHg at the species normal body temperature. If BE is calculated from pH and PCO_2 as above, but at a hemoglobin concentration of 5 g/dL, total extracellular buffering can be determined. BE calculated in this fashion is termed the standard BE (SBE). The difference between BE and SBE is small, leading to few studies where SBE is reported. Both the standard bicarbonate and BE (or deficit) can be determined from nomograms. The BE has a normal value of zero (±2–3) and is changed only by non-volatile acids, thereby indicating non-respiratory acidosis. The numerical magnitude of the BE is a guide to therapy:

$$\text{Base } (Na^+HCO_3^-) \text{ needed} = (0.3) \times (BE) \times (\text{body weight [kg]}) \quad (18.15)$$

where 0.3 = % body weight that is extracellular water.

Most modern automated blood gas analyzers report an SBE value calculated from human data. While a canine SBE nomogram has been developed, it is rarely used because commercial blood gas analyzers are programmed specifically for human blood. In a broader sense, the base excess approach to acid–base analysis has met with criticism because the SBE parameter represents the net effect of all ongoing non-respiratory or metabolic acid–base abnormalities. In the case of coexisting metabolic acidosis and alkalosis, SBE alone may fail to identify any acid–base abnormality as these two disturbances could cancel each other out.

Anion gap

The anion gap (AG) is a useful tool to assess mixed acid–base disorders [18,19]. Chemically, there is no AG because electroneutrality must be maintained and the 'anion gap' actually is the difference between the unmeasured anions (UA^-) and unmeasured cations (UC^+). Following the law of electroneutrality:

$$([Na^+]+[K^+]+[UC^+])-([Cl^-]+[HCO_3^-]+[UA^-])=0 \quad (18.16)$$

or, when applied clinically:

$$AG=([Na^+]+[K^+])-([Cl^-]+[HCO_3^-])=[UA^-]-[UC^+] \quad (18.17)$$

Based on eqn 18.16, every time there is a decrease in $[HCO_3^-]$, either $[Cl^-]$ or $[UA^-]$ must increase to maintain electroneutrality. When titrated HCO_3^- is replaced by Cl^- in non-respiratory acidosis, the difference ($[UA^-]$ – $[UC^+]$; and consequently the AG) will remain the same (called hyperchloremic or normal AG acidosis). When titrated HCO_3^- is replaced by UA^-, the difference ($[UA^-]$ – $[UC^+]$; i.e., the AG) will increase while $[Cl^-]$ remains the same (called normochloremic or high AG acidosis) [20,21].

Table 18.8 Primary non-respiratory acid–base disorders and respiratory compensation.

Non-respiratory disorder	Na^+–Cl^-	AG	TCO_2	Respiratory compensation	Biochemical profile
Alkalosis					
Hypoalbuminemia	N	N,↓	↑	No	↓ Albumin
Hypochloremia	↑	N	↑	No	↓ $[Cl^-]$ corrected
Concentration	↑	N	↑	Yes	↑ $[Na^+]$
Acidosis					
Hyperalbuminemia	N	N,↑	↓	No	↑ Albumin
Hyperphosphatemia	N	N,↑	↓	No	↑ Inorganic phosphate
Hyperchloremia	↓	N	↓	Yes	↑ $[Cl^-]$ corrected
Dilution	↓	N	↓	Yes	↓ $[Na^+]$
Organic	N	↓	↓	Yes	Specific assays required

$Na^+ - Cl^-$ difference between sodium and chloride concentration: AG. anion gap: TCO_2. total CO_2; ↑. increase: N. normal: and ↓, decrease. See the text for limitations in using $Na^+ - Cl^-$ difference and AG.
Adapted from de Morais HAS, Muir WW. Strong ions and acid-base disorders. In: Bonagura JD, Kirk RW, eds. ***Kirk's Current Veterinary Therapy***, 12th edn. Philadelphia: WB Saunders, 1995; 121–127.

Negatively charged proteins, phosphates, sulfates, and organic acids (e.g., lactate, ß-hydroxybutyrate, acetoacetate, and citrate) constitute the UA^- [22]. Usually an increase in AG implies an accumulation of organic acids in the body [23]. An increase in AG also occurs in alkalemia caused by an increase in the net negative charge on serum proteins or in situations where concomitant non-respiratory or respiratory alkalosis over-rides a high AG non-respiratory acidosis [24,25]. Hypoalbuminemia probably is the only important cause of a decrease in AG, and each decrease in albumin concentration by 1 g/dL generally produces a decrease of approximately 3 mEq/L in the AG. A patient with concurrent lactic acidosis and hypoalbuminemia may have a normal calculated AG. Thus, AG alone can be clinically misleading in elucidating some complex mixed acid–base disorders.

The AG concept has some limitations and various corrections (AGc) have emerged to account for its inaccuracies [11,19]. The summation of $[Cl^-]$ and $[HCO_3^-]$ is not acceptable based upon their activity coefficients and the fact that HCO_3^- is not an independent variable [26]. Each of these anions has a different activity coefficient partially because they are present in extracellular fluid at concentrations that differ by a factor of more than 5 (i.e., $[Cl^-] = 110$ mEq/L vs $[HCO_3^-] = 21$ mEq/L) [26]. Regardless, the AG is helpful clinically. The AG does not account for the contribution of albumin and phosphate in acid–base balance and can change because of excessive exposure of serum to air, resulting in changes of 6.5 ± 2.3 mEq/L after 2h [19,27]. These changes are more pronounced in animals with respiratory acidosis [26].

Like AG, the $[Na^+]$ - $[Cl^-]$ difference (average normal value = 36 mEq/L) is potentially useful for initial assessment of those non-respiratory acid–base disturbances not associated with an increase in unmeasured anions (Table 18.8) [28]. If $[Na^+]$ is normal, an increase in this value is caused by hypochloremia and is an indication of metabolic alkalosis, whereas a decrease in the $[Na^+]$ - $[Cl^-]$ gradient is an indication of hyperchloremic acidosis [8]. In addition, chloride to sodium (Cl^-:Na^+) ratio (normal range 0.75–0.79) serves as a simple method to quantify the role of hyperchloremia in acid–base disturbances. A increased Cl^-:Na^+ ratio (>0.79) has an acidifying effect and a decreased ratio (<0.75) has an alkalinizing effect. Animals with metabolic acidosis and an increased Cl^-:Na^+ generally have hyperchloremia as the cause of acidosis. A normal Cl^-:Na^+ and metabolic acidosis indicate a mixed acidosis. The $[Na^+]$ - $[Cl^-]$ and Cl^-:Na^+ can be used in conjunction with the AG to identifying disorders in hydration and acid–base balance (Box 18.1).

Box 18.1 Relative changes in $[NA^+]_0$ and $[Cl^-]_0$ as an index of disorders in hydration or acid–base balance or both.

a Proportionate change in $[Na^+]_0$ and $[Cl^-]_0$ are always due to the disturbances of hydration alone.
Dehydration
$[Na^+]_0$ ↑ and $[Cl]_0$ ↑
Overhydration
$[Na^+]_0$ ↓ and $[Cl]_0$ ↓
b Changes in $[Cl^-]_0$ without any change in $[Na^+]_0$ is always due to disturbances of acid-base alone.
Respiratory acidosis or non-respiratory alkalosis
$[Na^+]_0$ and $[Cl^-]_0$ ↓
Respiratory alkalosis or hypercholemic acidosis
$[Na^+]_0$ and $[Cl]_0$ ↑
c Disproportionate changes in $[Na^+]_0$ and $[Cl^-]_0$ are due to disturbances in both hydration and acid-base balance.
Dehydration plus respiratory acidosis or non-respiratory alkalosis
$[Na^+]_0$ ↑ and $[Cl^-]_0$
Dehydration plus respiratory alkalosis or non-respiratory acidosis
$[Na^+]_0$ ↑ and $[Cl^-]_0$ ↑↑
Overhydration plus respiratory alkalosis or hyperchloremic acidosis
$[Na]_0$ ↓ and $[Cl^-]_0$
Overhydration plus respiratory acidosis or non-respiratory alkalosis
$[Na^+]_0$ ↓ and $[Cl^-]$ ↓↓

Modified from Emmett M, Seldin DW. Evaluation of acid-base disorders from plasma composition. In: Seldin DW, Giebisch G, eds. *The Regulation of Acid–Base Balance*. New York: Raven, 1989; 259–268.

Strong ion difference

An alternative theory of acid-base regulation was proposed in the early 1980s [3,29]. This theory questioned the limitations of using changes in bicarbonate to quantify acid–base abnormalities since, as suggested earlier, changes therein are not capable of quantifying the amount of acid or base that has been added to the plasma unless PCO_2 is held constant [10]. The theory is based upon the physicochemical properties of water-based solutions (see Fig. 18.5).

- The separation of the ionic components of a solute. Strong ions completely dissociate in solution and weak acids only partially dissociate in solution, existing in both the anionic dissociated form (A^-) and the undissociated form (HA) ($A_{TOT} = A^- + HA$).
- The sum of all positively charged ions in any compartment (solution) must equal the sum of all negatively charged ions. Pure water is a neutral solution because the H^+ and the OH^- concentrations are equal. As stated earlier, the concentration of

Table 18.9 Comparative normal values for pH, PCO_2, $[A_{TOT}]$ and [SID].

Animal	pH	PCO_2	$[A_{TOT}]$	[SID]	Comments
Human	7.37	45	17.2	37	SID ↑ Non-resp. alkalosis
Horse	7.43	44	14.0	40	
Cow	7.43	43	22.9	44	SID ↓ Non-resp. acidosis
Dog	7.40	37	17.4	27	
Cat	7.35	30	24.3	30	A_{TOT} ↑ Non-resp. acidosis
Pigeon	7.43	41	7.8	34	A_{TOT} ↓ Non-resp. alkalosis

Modified from Constable PD. Comparative animal physiology and adaptation. In: Kellum JA, Elbers PWG, eds. *Stewart's Textbook of Acid-Base Physiology*. www.Lulu.com, USA, 2009: 305–320.

these ions is determined by a temperature-sensitive dissociation constant.

- The amount of a substance remains constant unless it is added, removed, produced, or destroyed.

According to this theory, HCO_3^- is not a strong ion and $[HCO_3^-]$ and pH ($[H^+]$) are dependent variables determined by the independent variables PCO_2, $[A_{TOT}]$ (composed mostly of albumin and inorganic phosphates), and the difference between the strong cations and the strong anions (strong ion difference, SID; see Fig. 18.6) [30–33]. Normal values for these various independent variables have been derived for mammals (Table 18.9) [34]. Strong ions are substances that are completely dissociated in plasma at body pH.

$$SID = [Na^+ + K^+ + Ca^{+2} + Mg^{+2}] - [Cl^- + lactate]$$

The most important strong ions in plasma are Na^+, K^+, Ca^{2+}, Mg^{2+}, Cl^-, lactate, ß-hydroxybutyrate, acetoacetate, and sulfate. The influence of strong ions on pH and $[HCO_3^-]$ can always be expressed in terms of the SID. An increase in SID correlates with non-respiratory alkalosis, whereas a decrease in SID correlates with non-respiratory acidosis. In summary, SID and $[A_{TOT}]$ variables provide independent measures of the metabolic component of plasma pH. Therefore, when using a strong ion approach for acid–base analysis, there are four possible primary metabolic acid–base disorders. Metabolic acidosis is further defined by being either a (1) decreased SID or (2) increased $[A_{TOT}]$ acidosis, whereas metabolic alkalosis is characterized by an (3) increased SID or (4) decreased $[A_{TOT}]$ (Tables 18.9 and 18.10).

Clinical acid–base disturbances

Acid–base disturbances occur when an abnormality in one of the principal independent determinants of $[H^+]$ (e.g., PCO_2, SID, or $[A_{TOT}]$) occurs (see Table 18.9) [5,11,26,29,33,34]. So-called 'simple' acid–base disturbance includes both the primary process and the compensatory response. That is, if a sustained primary disturbance occurs in PCO_2, a compensatory change of regulated magnitude normally occurs in the SID and vice versa. If the primary disturbance results from a change in $[A_{TOT}]$, however, renal or ventilatory compensation does not occur [33–37]. Therapeutic success or failure depends on interventions that adjust the independent variables [33,35,37].

Disorders of PCO_2

The PCO_2 is an important variable in the determination of alveolar ventilation, pH and alveolar oxygen (P_AO_2) [$P_AO_2 = FiO_2(P_B-47) - 1.2(PaCO_2)$]. Primary respiratory disturbances result from increases (respiratory acidosis) or decreases (respiratory alkalosis) in PCO_2. Carbon dioxide tension can be changed by alveolar ventilation, which has a profound effect on $[H^+]$, and both together can be used to make descriptive decisions regarding acid–base and abnormalities (Table 18.11). Because $PaCO_2$ is inversely related to alveolar ventilation, measurement of $PaCO_2$ provides direct information about the adequacy of alveolar ventilation. Respiratory acidosis is therefore caused by and synonymous with hypoventilation, whereas respiratory alkalosis is caused by and synonymous with hyperventilation. The principal disorders associated with respiratory acidosis are airway obstruction, respiratory center depression (e.g., drugs or neurologic disorders), cardiopulmonary arrest ($PaCO_2$ may be below normal during cardiopulmonary resuscitation), neuromuscular diseases, diaphragmatic hernia, chest wall trauma, and inadequate mechanical ventilation. Therapy for respiratory acidosis should be directed toward elimination of the underlying cause of alveolar hypoventilation. Ventilatory assistance should be provided when necessary. Respiratory acidosis is not an indication for bicarbonate therapy. Administration of sodium bicarbonate will decrease $[H^+]$ and decrease ventilatory drive, thus worsening hypoxemia and hypercapnia. Treatment for hypercapnia in animals with chronic pulmonary disease should be directed toward the underlying disease.

The principal causes of respiratory alkalosis are hypoxia, low cardiac output, severe anemia, pulmonary disease (stimulation of peripheral reflexes, e.g., pneumonia), hyperventilation mediated by the central nervous system (e.g., drugs, central nervous system inflammation or tumor, liver disease, fear, or pain), and overzealous mechanical ventilation. Hypocapnia itself is not a major threat to the well-being of animals with respiratory alkalosis. The arterial pH in chronic primary respiratory alkalosis is usually normal or slightly alkalemic owing to efficient renal compensation in this setting. Therapy for the underlying disease responsible for hypocapnia should be the primary focus in animals with respiratory alkalosis. Notably, PCO_2 is a primary determinant of cerebral blood flow. Overventilation and low PCO_2 reduce cerebral blood flow and predispose to cerebral ischemia [38,39].

Increases in alveolar-arterial oxygen difference

The alveolar-arterial oxygen difference [$P(A\text{-}a)O_2$ gradient] may be useful in differentiating intrinsic pulmonary disease from extrapulmonary disease in animals with hypoxemia. Hypoxemia (decreased blood oxygen content) will, in turn, result in tissue hypoxia, and lactic (non-respiratory) acidosis. The $P(A\text{-}a)O_2$ gradient estimates the difference between the PO_2 in the alveoli and the arterial blood [38]. $P(A\text{-}a)O_2$ can be calculated clinically as (A-a) gradient = $(150 - 1.25 \times PaCO_2) - PaO_2$. In normal animals at sea level, the $P(A\text{-}a)O_2$ gradient should be less than 15 mmHg, although values up to 25 mmHg are considered normal when the FiO_2 is increased by administering supplemental oxygen (flow-by or oxygen cage) to awake patients. Even higher $P(A\text{-}a)O_2$ gradients may be normal when inhalant anesthetics are administered in very high (>0.9) FiO_2 mixtures.

Hypoxia can be caused by hypoventilation, decreased partial pressure of inspired O_2 (PiO_2), diffusion impairment, ventilation-perfusion mismatch (occasionally referred to as pseudoshunt), and right-to-left (vascular) shunts. The $P(A\text{-}a)O_2$ gradient will be

Table 18.10 Causes of metabolic acid–base abnormalities classified according to the strong ion approach.

SID acidosis (↓ SID)	SID alkalosis (↑ SID)

Dilution acidosis (↓ Na^+)
• With hypervolemia
  ○ Severe liver disease
  ○ Congestive heart failure
  ○ Nephrotic syndrome
• With normovolemia
  ○ Psychogenic polydipsia
  ○ Hypotonic fluid infusion
• With hypovolemia
  ○ Vomiting
  ○ Diarrhea
  ○ Hypoadrenocorticism
  ○ Third space loss
  ○ Diuretic administration
Hyperchloremic acidosis (↑ Cl^-_{corr})
• Loss of Na^+ relative to Cl^-
  ○ Diarrhea
• Gain of Cl^- relative to Na^+
  ○ Fluid therapy (0.9% NaCl, 7.2% NaCl, KCl-supplemented fluids
• Cl^- retention
  ○ Renal failure
  ○ Hypoadrenocorticism
Organic acidosis (↑ unmeasured strong ions)
• Uremic, keto- or lactic acidosis
• Toxicities
  ○ Ethylene glycol
  ○ Salicylate
A_{TOT} acidosis (↑ A_{TOT})
Hyperalbuminemia
• Water deprivation
Hyperphosphatemia
• Translocation
  ○ Tumor cell lysis
  ○ Tissue trauma/rhabdomyolysis
• Increased intake
  ○ Phosphate-containing enemas
  ○ Intravenous phosphate
• Decreased loss
  ○ Renal failure
  ○ Urethral obstruction
  ○ Uroabdomen
	Concentration alkalosis (↑ Na)
	• Pure water loss
	  ○ Water deprivation
	  ○ Diabetes insipidus
	• Hypotonic fluid loss
	  ○ Vomiting
	  ○ Non-oliguric renal failure
	  ○ Postobstructive diuresis
	Hypochloremic alkalosis (↓ Cl^-_{corr})
	• Gain of Na^+ relative to Cl^-
	  ○ Isotonic or hypertonic $NaHCO_3$ administration
	• Loss of Cl^- relative to Na^+
	  ○ Vomiting of stomach contents
	  ○ Thiazide or loop diuretics
	A_{TOT} alkalosis (↓ A_{TOT})
	Hypoalbuminemia
	• Decreased production
	  ○ Chronic liver disease
	  ○ Acute phase response to inflammation
	  ○ Malnutrition/starvation
	• Extracorporeal loss
	  ○ Protein-losing nephropathy
	  ○ Protein-losing enteropathy
	• Sequestration
	  ○ Inflammatory effusions
	  ○ Vasculitis

Modified from Constable PD. Comparative animal physiology and adaptation. In: Kellum JA, Elbers PWG, eds. ***Stewart's Textbook of Acid-Base Physiology***. www.Lulu.com, USA, 2009: 305–320.

Table 18.11 Primary processes associated with changes in $PaCO_2$ and pH.

$PaCO_2$	pH	Primary process
Normal	Normal	None
Normal	High	Metab. alkalosis, resp. alkalosis
Normal	Low	Metab. acidosis, resp. acidosis
High	Normal	Resp. acidosis, metab. alkalosis
High	High	Metab. alkalosis
High	Low	Resp. acidosis
Low	Normal	Chronic resp. alkalosis
Low	High	Resp. alkalosis
Low	Low	Metab. acidosis

normal in animals with either hypoventilation or decreased PiO_2 (e.g., residence at high altitude) because they still have normal lung function. Animals with hypoventilation have an increase in PCO_2, whereas animals breathing air with a low PiO_2 have a below-normal PCO_2 (hyperventilating). In contrast, the $P(A\text{-}a)O_2$ gradient is increased in animals with diffusion impairment (rarely recognized in veterinary medicine), ventilation-perfusion mismatch, and right-to-left shunt. Decreases in blood oxygenation can result in decreased oxygen delivery to tissues, anaerobic metabolism, and lactic acidosis (metabolic acidosis) [40]. The administration of 100% oxygen will usually improve hypoxemia in animals with ventilation-perfusion mismatch, but produces no or minimal effect in animals with significant right-to-left shunt.

Disorders in strong ion difference

Changes in SID are usually recognized by changes in $[HCO_3^-]$ or BE [26,30–33]. A decrease in SID is associated with non-respiratory acidosis, whereas an increase in SID is associated with non-respiratory alkalosis (see Table 18.9). There are three general mechanisms by which SID can change (Table 18.12): (a) changing the free-water content of plasma, (b) changing the Cl^- concentration, and (c) increasing the concentration of unidentified strong anions $[XA^-]$. The selection of intravenous fluids during anesthesia should always consider the SID although conventional rates of fluid administration (10 mL/kg/h) for up to 3 h do not affect

Table 18.12 Causes for changes in strong ion differences (SID).

Free-water abnormalities	
Increase in [Na^+]	→ Concentration alkalosis
Decrease in [Na^+]	→ Dilution acidosis
Chloride abnormalities	
Decrease in [Cl^-] corrected	→ Hypochloremic alkalosis
Increase in [Cl^-] corrected	→ Hyperchloremic acidosis
Unmeasured strong anion abnormalities	
Increase in [XA^-]	→ Organic acidosis

[XA^-]. unidentified strong anions.

acid–base balance [41,42]. Intravenous infusion of larger volumes at faster rates (>30 mL/kg/h) of either a crystalloid or synthetic colloid (hydroxyethyl starch) forces the SID and A_{TOT} of the extracellular fluid toward the SID and A_{TOT} of the fluid being administered. The ideal SID of a 'balanced' crystalloid solution should be approximately 24 mEq/L in order to counteract the A_{TOT} dilutional alkalosis produced by the fluid being administered: commercial crystalloids do not contain A_{TOT} [41,43]. The addition of weak organic ions like *l*-lactate do not contribute to the fluid SID and are metabolized on infusion. Notably the SID of 0.9% saline is 0 and infusions of large volumes of this fluid can produce hyperchloremic non-respiratory acidosis [41].

Disorders in [A_{TOT}]

Albumin and inorganic phosphate are non-volatile weak acids and collectively are the major contributors to [A_{TOT}] (see Fig. 18.6) [8,22,31,44]. Consequently, changes in their concentrations will change [H^+]. Hypoalbuminemia will tend to decrease [A_{TOT}] and cause a non-respiratory alkalosis (see Table 18.9). Although rare, an increase in albumin concentration can cause non-respiratory acidosis, owing to an increase in [A_{TOT}]. Phosphate is the second most important component of [A_{TOT}] and is normally present in plasma at a low concentration. Severe hyperphosphatemia can cause a large increase in [A_{TOT}], which can result in non-respiratory acidosis. The treatment for hyperphosphatemic acidosis, hyperalbuminemic acidosis, and hypoalbuminemic alkalosis should be directed at the underlying cause. The administration of sodium bicarbonate shifts phosphorus into cells and can be used as adjuvant therapy in patients with hyperphosphatemic acidosis [45].

Free-water abnormalities

Changing the water content of body fluid compartments will dilute or concentrate both strong anions and cations [8,26,33]. Consequently, SID will change by the same proportion. Changes in free water can be identified by evaluating the [Na^+]. An increase in SID caused by water loss increases in [Na^+] and results in concentration alkalosis, whereas a decrease in SID caused by decreases in [Na^+] results in dilutional acidosis. It has been suggested that changes in extracellular fluid (ECF) volume alone lead to acid–base disturbances; however, change in ECF volume by itself does not change SID, PCO_2, or [A_{TOT}] and therefore cannot change acid–base status [4]. The so-called contraction alkalosis believed to be caused by a decrease in ECF volume is in reality caused by a primary decrease in [Cl^-] [8,29,30]. The principal causes of free-water abnormalities are listed in Box 18.2. Therapy for dilution acidosis and concentration alkalosis should be directed at the underlying cause responsible for changing [Na^+]. If necessary, [Na^+] and osmolality should be corrected [46,47].

Box 18.2 Principal causes of free-water abnormalities.

- Concentration alkalosis (↑[Na^+])
  - Pure-water deficit
    - Primary hypodipsia
    - Diabetes Insipidus
    - Fever
    - Inadequate access to water
    - High environmental temperature
  - Hypotonic fluid loss
    - Vomiting
    - Peritonitis
    - Pancreatitis
    - Non-oliguric renal failure
    - Postobstructive diuresis
  - Sodium gain
    - Salt poisoning
    - Hypertonic fluid administration (e.g., hypertonic saline, sodium bicarbonate)
    - Hyperaldosteronism
    - Hyperadrenocorticism
- Dilution acidosis (↓[Na^+])
  - Severe liver disease
  - Nephrotic syndrome
  - Advanced renal failure
  - Congestive heart failure
  - Psychogenic polydipsia
  - Excessive sweating in horses
  - Hypotonic fluid administration (e.g., 0.45% sodium chloride solution)
  - Vomiting
  - Diarrhea
  - Uroabdomen
  - Hypoadrenocorticism
  - Diuretic administration

Adapted from de Morais HAS, Muir WW. Strong ions and acid-base disorders. In: Bonagura JD, Kirk RW, eds. *Kirk's Current Veterinary Therapy*, 12th edn. Philadelphia: WB Saunders, 1995; 121–127.

Isonatremic chloride abnormalities

If there is no change in the water content of plasma, plasma [Na^+] will be normal. Other strong cations (e.g., K^+) are regulated for purposes other than acid–base balance, and their concentration never changes sufficiently to affect SID substantially [20,21]. Consequently, SID changes only as a result of changes in strong anions when water content is normal. If [Na^+] remains constant, changes in [Cl^-] can substantially increase or decrease SID [46,47]. Evaluation of [Cl^-] must be considered in conjunction with the [Na^+] because [Cl^-] can change for reasons other than a change in water balance (see Box 18.1) [20]. The animal's [Cl^-] is therefore 'corrected' for changes in [Na^+], applying a formula developed for use in people and adapted for use in small and large animals:

$$[Cl^-]corrected = [Cl^-] \times [Na^+]normal/[Na^+] \tag{18.18}$$

where [Cl^-] and [Na^+] are the animal's Cl^- and Na^+ concentrations. The ideal [Na^+] is the normal Na^+ concentration for the species being evaluated. Suggested normal values for [Na^+] in dogs are 146 and 147 mEq/L, whereas for cats they range from 150 to 156 mEq/L [36]. In large animals, normal [Na^+] is approximately 136 mEq/L in horses and 144 mEq/L in cattle [44]. Normal [Cl^-] is approximately 107–113 mEq/L for dogs, 117–123 mEq/L for cats, 97–103 mEq/L for horses, and 101–107 mEq/L for cattle [36,48,49]. These values may vary for

Box 18.3 Principal causes of chloride abnormalities.

Hypochloremic alkalosis[a] (↓[Cl⁻] corrected)
- Excessive loss of chloride relative to sodium
  - Vomiting of stomach contents
  - Gastric reflux in horses with ileus
  - Abomasum torsion (ruminants)
  - Vagal indigestion with internal vomiting (ruminants)
  - Therapy with thiazides or loop diuretics
  - Hyperadrenocorticism
- Excessive gain of sodium relative to chloride
  - Sodium bicarbonate therapy

Hyperchloremic acidosis[b] (↑[Cl⁻] corrected)
- Excessive loss of sodium relative to chloride
  - Diarrhea
- Excessive gain of chloride relative to sodium
  - Fluid therapy (e.g., 0.9% NaCl, KCl supplemental fluids)
  - Salt poisoning
  - Total parenteral nutrition
  - Ammonium chloride or potassium chloride therapy
- Chloride retention
  - Renal failure
  - Renal tubular acidosis
- Hypoadrenocorticism
- Diabetes mellitus
- Drug induced (e.g., acetazolamide, spironolactone)

[a]Chronic respiratory acidosis will cause a compensatory decrease in corrected [Cl⁻].
[b]Chronic respiratory alkalosis will cause a compensatory increase in corrected [Cl⁻].
Adapted from de Morais HAS, Muir WW. Strong ions and acid-base disorders. In: Bonagura JD, Kirk RW, eds. *Kirk's Current Veterinary Therapy*, 12th edn. Philadelphia: WB Saunders, 1995; 121–127.

different laboratories and different analyzers. An increase or decrease in corrected [Cl⁻] indicates that Cl⁻ is responsible at least in part for the changes in SID. An increase in corrected [Cl⁻] (i.e., an increase in [Cl⁻] relative to [Na⁺]) results in a hyperchloremic non-respiratory acidosis, whereas a decrease in corrected [Cl⁻] (i.e., a decrease in [Cl⁻] relative to [Na⁺]) results in hypochloremic non-respiratory alkalosis. A [Cl⁻] corrected to normal in the presence of abnormal observed [Cl⁻] indicates that SID changes are caused by dilution acidosis or concentration alkalosis.

The principal causes of hyperchloremic acidosis and hypochloremic alkalosis are listed in Box 18.3. Treatment of hyperchloremic acidosis should be directed at correction of the underlying disease. Administration of $NaHCO_3$, when pH values are lower than the acceptable <7.20 will tend to correct hyperchloremic acidosis because this solution has an SID greater than plasma.

Chloride-responsive hypochloremic alkalosis can be caused by excessive loss of Cl⁻ relative to Na⁺ or by administration of substances containing more Na⁺ than Cl⁻ compared with ECF (e.g., $NaHCO_3$). The former can occur following the administration of diuretics that cause Cl⁻ loss (e.g., furosemide) or when the lost fluid has a low or negative SID, (e.g., acute vomiting). Chloride administration is essential for the treatment of chloride-responsive hypochloremic alkalosis. Renal Cl⁻ conservation is ordinarily enhanced in hypochloremic states and renal Cl⁻ reabsorption does not return to normal until plasma Cl⁻ concentration is restored to normal or near normal [26]. In situations where expansion of extracellular volume is desired, intravenous infusion of 0.9% NaCl is the treatment of choice. This solution has an SID of 0 and will decrease plasma SID [5]. If hypokalemia is present, KCl should be added to the fluid. If volume expansion is not necessary, Cl⁻ can be administered using salts without Na⁺ (e.g., ammonium chloride, potassium chloride, calcium chloride, and magnesium chloride). These salts should correct the alkalosis because Cl⁻ is given together with cations that are regulated within narrow limits for purposes unrelated to acid–base balance [5]. Chloride-resistant hypochloremic alkalosis can occur in animals by hyperadrenocorticism and primary hyperaldosteronism. Increased mineralocorticoid activity causes sodium retention and urinary chloride loss in these diseases and both will increase SID. Administration of chloride will not correct the metabolic alkalosis because of chloruresis. Fortunately, metabolic alkalosis in these animals is usually very mild.

Table 18.13 Principal disorders of the unidentified strong ions.

Disorder	Strong anions
Uremic acidosis	SO_4^{2-} and other anions of renal failure
Diabetic ketoacidosis, ketosis, pregnancy toxemia	Acetoacetate, ß-hydroxybutyrate
Lactic acidosis	Lactate
Salicylate intoxication	Salicylate
Ethylene glycol toxicity	Glycolate
Methanol toxicity	Formate

[XA⁻]. unidentified strong anions.
Adapted from de Morais HAS, Muir WW. Strong ions and acid-base disorders. In: Bonagura JD, Kirk RW, eds. *Kirk's Current Veterinary Therapy*, 12th edn. Philadelphia: WB Saunders, 1995; 121–127.

Isonatremic organic acid abnormalities

Accumulation of metabolically produced organic anions (e.g., lactate, acetoacetate, citrate, or ß-hydroxybutyrate) or addition of exogenous organic anions (e.g., salicylate, glycolate from ethylene glycol poisoning, and formate from methanol poisoning) can cause non-respiratory acidosis because these strong anions decrease SID [26]. Addition of some inorganic strong anions (e.g., SO_4^{2-} during renal failure) will resemble organic acidosis because SID decreases without changing electrolytes. The most frequently encountered causes of organic acidosis are listed in Table 18.13.

Treatment of organic acidosis should be directed toward the primary disorder and stabilization of the animal. Sodium bicarbonate should be used cautiously because metabolism of accumulated organic anions will normalize SID and increase [HCO_3^-]. The initial goal in animals with severe organic acidosis is to raise systemic pH to an acceptable value of >7.20 and treat the primary disease.

Estimation of strong anion concentration: strong Ion Gap

The AG, like SID, is calculated on the basis of the principle of electroneutrality and is used clinically to estimate the concentration of UA⁻. Organic acidosis increases the AG, whereas hyperchloremic acidosis does not. Unfortunately, UA⁻ includes strong anions [XA⁻] which AG accounts for and weak (variable charges of albumin and phosphates) unmeasured anions which it does not. The AG, like SID, actually changes secondary to changes in PCO_2, SID, or [A_{TOT}] and therefore does not always reflect the quantitative changes in UA⁻ even in the presence of organic acidosis [5]. The corrected AG (AGc) was formulated to correct this problem and changes in the baseline AGc (ΔAGc) are tightly correlated to the strong ion gap (SIG) (Fig. 18.8) [5,19,46].

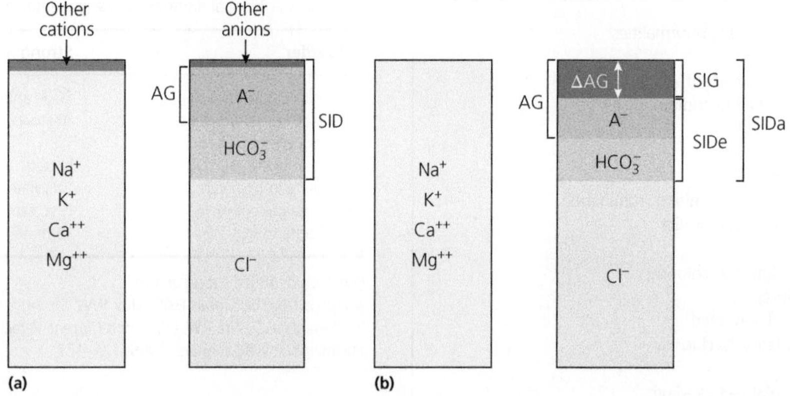

Figure 18.8 (A) Gamblegrams can be used to illustrate the relationship among the anion gap (AG) strong ion difference (SID) and strong ion gap (SIG). B. They can also be used to illustrate the difference between an abnormal and baseline AG (ΔAG). The ΔAG is quantitatively similar to the strong ion gap (SIG) or difference between the SID apparent (SIDa) and SID effective (SIDe): SIG = SIDa–SIDe.

The SIG represents the quantity of unmeasured anions other than lactate [19,31,50]. It can be quantified by the difference between the apparent SID (SIDa) and the effective SID (SIDe):

$$SIDa = (Na^+ + K^+ + Ca^{+2} + Mg^{+2}) - (Cl^- + lactate^-)$$
$$SIDe = CO_2 + A_{TOT}$$
$$SIG = SIDa - SIDe$$

The SIG is normally near zero; that is, the net negative charge of CO_2 and weak acids (A_{TOT}) counterbalances the net positive charge of the SIDa. The SIG indicates if either strong or weak ions or both are present but does not tell which. A metabolic acidosis with an increased SIG may occur in diabetic ketoacidosis where the SIG quantitatively reflects plasma ketone concentration. Studies conducted in humans suggest that SIG predicts mortality better than blood lactate, pH, or injury severity scores [31].

Evaluations of acid–base balance

A systematic stepwise approach should be followed in all animals with suspected acid-base disorders [37,46]. The first step is to determine the pH and the nature of the primary disorder from the blood gas analysis results. The possibility of a mixed respiratory and non-respiratory acid–base disorder should be assessed by calculating the expected compensation (see Table 18.7). If a non-respiratory acid–base disorder is present, it should be determined whether it is caused by a change in [A_{TOT}], SID, UA^- (the strong anions [XA^-] and weak unmeasured anions) or a combination of these factors [37,47]. Unfortunately, evaluation of changes in SID caused by increases in [XA^-] is not straightforward [11,32]. An increase in [XA^-] may be suspected in acidotic animals with diseases known to be associated with organic acidosis (e.g., renal failure and diabetic ketoacidosis) [45,46]. Measurement of lactate concentration enables one of the many XA^- to be quantified. When blood gas results are not available, the biochemical profile may help in determining the non-respiratory abnormalities present (see Table 18.8). The determination of XA^- obtained using a quantitative mathematical model is not constrained by the limitations mentioned earlier. However, calculation of SID_e in this model is not always simple and can be clinically impractical although various calculators have been developed to simplify the process [32,47,51]. General anesthesia produces dose-dependent respiratory and cardiovascular depression, thereby predisposing animals to the development of respiratory and non-respiratory acidosis which can exaggerate or complicate acid–base status. The application of quantitative methods for the analysis, diagnosis, and treatment of acid-base disorders compels clinicians to consider a more comprehensive set of potential causes for acid–base disturbances and by doing so, focuses diagnostic approaches and refines therapeutic decisions.

References

1 Henderson LJ. The theory of neutrality regulation in the animal organism. *Am J Physiol* 1908; **21**:427–448.
2 Hastings AB. Acid–base measurements in vitro. *Ann N Y Acad Sci* 1966; **133**: 15–24.
3 Stewart PA. *How to Understand Acid–Base: A Quantitative Acid–Base Primer for Biology and Medicine.* New York: Elsevier, 1981.
4 Fencl V, Rossing TH. Acid–base disorders in critical care medicine. *Annu Rev Med* 1989; **40**:17–29.
5 Jones NL. *Blood Gases and Acid–Base Physiology.* New York: Thieme, 1987.
6 Rose BD, Post TW. Acid–base physiology. *Clinical Physiology of Acid–Base and Electrolyte Disorders*, 5th edn. New York: McGraw-Hill, 2001; 299–324.
7 Dibartola SP. Metabolic acidosis. In: Dibartola SP, ed. *Introduction to Acid–Base Disorders*, 3rd edn. New York: Saunders Elsevier, 2006; 229–251.
8 Kellum JA, Elbers PWG. *Stewart's Textbook of Acid–Base. Lulu Enterprises*, 2009. www.Lulu.com
9 Corey HE. Fundamental principles of acid–base physiology. *Crit Care* 2005; **9**: 184–192.
10 Siggaard-Andersen O, Fogh-Andersen N. Base excess or buffer base (strong ion difference) as a measure of a non-respiratory acid–base disturbance. *Acta Anesthesiol Scand* 1995, **39**: 123–128.
11 Kellum JA. Clinical review: reunification of acid–base physiology. *Crit Care* 2005; **9**: 500–507.
12 Goraya N, Wesson DE. Acid–base status and progression of chronic kidney disease. *Curr Opin Nephrol Hypertens* 2012; **21**: 552–556.
13 Gingerich DA, Murdick PW. Experimentally induced intestinal obstruction in sheep: paradoxical aciduria in metabolic alkalosis. *Am J Vet Res* 1975; **36**: 663–668.
14 Nattie EE. The alpha-stat hypothesis in respiratory control and acid–base balance. *J Appl Physiol* 1990; **69**: 1201–1207.
15 Settergren G. pH-stat, alpha-stat versus temperature correction. *J Cardiothorac Anesth* 1989; **3**: 526–527.
16 Murkin JM, Martzke JS, Buchan AM, *et al.* A randomized study of the influence of perfusion technique and pH management strategy in 316 patients undergoing coronary artery bypass surgery. I. Mortality and cardiovascular morbidity. *J Thorac Cardiovasc Surg* 1995; **110**: 340–348.
17 Adams LG, Polzin DJ. Mixed acid–base disorders. *Vet Clin North Am Small Anim Pract* 1989; **19**: 307–326.
18 Reddy P, Mooradian A. Clinical utility of the anion gap in deciphering acid–base disorders. *Int J Clin Pract* 2009; **63**: 1516–1525.

19 Kellum JA. Acid-base disorders and strong ion gap. *Contrib Nephrol* 2007; **156**: 158–166.
20 Constable PD. Hyperchloremic acidosis: the classic example of strong ion acidosis. *Anesth Analg* 2003; **96**: 919–922.
21 Handy JM, Soni N. Physiological effects of hyperchloraemia and acidosis. *Br J Anaesth* 2008; **101**: 141–150.
22 Figge J, Mydosh T, Fencl V. Serum proteins and acid-base equilibria: a follow-up. *J Lab Clin Med* 1992; **120**: 713–719.
23 Gabow PA. Disorders associated with high altered gap. *Kidney Int* 1985; **27**: 472–483.
24 Goodkin DA, Krishna GG, Narins RG. The role of the anion gap in detecting and managing mixed metabolic acid-base disorders. *Clin Endocrinol Metab* 1984; **13**: 333–349.
25 Natelson S. On the significance of the expression 'anion-gap.' *Clin Chem* 1988; **29**: 283–284.
26 Constable PD. Clinical assessment of acid–base status: comparison of the Henderson–Hasselbalch and strong ion approaches. *Vet Clin Pathol* 2000; **29**: 115–128.
27 Nanji A, Blank D. Spurious increases in the anion gap due to exposure of serum to air. *N Engl J Med* 1982; **307**: 190–191.
28 Emmett M, Seldin DW. Evaluation of acid–base disorders from plasma composition. In: Seldin DW, Giebisch G, eds. *The Regulation of Acid–Base Balance.* New York: Raven, 1989; 259–268.
29 Stewart PA. Modern quantitative acid–base chemistry. *Can J Physiol Pharmacol* 1983; **61**: 1444–1461.
30 Fencl V, Leith DE. Stewart's quantitative acid–base chemistry: applications in biology and medicine. *Respir Physiol* 1993; **91**: 1–16.
31 Kellum JA, Kramer DJ, Pinsky MR. Strong ion gap: a methodology for exploring unexplained anions. *J Crit Care* 1995; **10**: 51–55.
32 Effros RM. Stewart approach is not always a practical clinical tool. *Anesth Analg* 2004; **98**: 271; author reply 271–272.
33 Wooten EW. Science review: Quantitative acid–base physiology using the Stewart model. *Crit Care* 2004; **8**: 448–452.
34 Constable PD. Comparative animal physiology and adaptation. In: Kellum JA, Elbers PWG, eds. *Stewart's Textbook of Acid-Base Physiology*. Lulu Enterprises, 2009; 305–320. www.Lulu.com
35 Morgan, JT. The Stewart approach – one clinician's perspective. *Clin Biochem Rev* 2009; **30**: 41–54.
36 Whitehair KJ, Haskins SC, Whitehair JG, Pascoe PJ. Clinical applications of quantitative acid–base chemistry. *J Vet Intern Med* 1995; **9**: 1–11.
37 Story DA, Morimatsu H, Bellomo R. Strong ions, weak acids and base excess: a simplified Fencl–Stewart approach to clinical acid–base disorders. *Br J Anaesth* 2004; **92**: 54–60.
38 Raichle ME, Plum F. Hyperventilation and cerebral blood flow. *Stroke* 1972; **3**: 566–575.
39 Yoon S, Zuccarello M, Rapoport RM. PCO_2 and pH regulation of cerebral blood flow. *Front Physiol* 2012; **3**: 365.
40 Habler OP, Messmer KF. The physiology of oxygen transport. *Transfus Sci* 1997; **18**: 425–435.
41 Morgan JT. The meaning of acid–base abnormalities in the intensive care unit: Part III: effects of fluid administration. *Crit Care* 2005; **9**: 204–211.
42 Valverde A, Hatcher ME, Stampfli HR. Effects of fluid therapy on total protein and its influence on calculated unmeasured anions in the anesthetized dog. *J Vet Emerg Crit Care* 2008; **18**: 480–487.
43 Kim JY, Lee D, Lee KC, *et al.* Stewart's physicochemical approach in neurosurgical patients with hyperchloremic metabolic acidosis during propofol anesthesia. *J Neurosurg Anesthesiol* 2008; **20**: 1–7.
44 Staempfli HR, Constable PD. Experimental determination of net protein charge and A(tot) and K(a) on nonvolatile buffers in human plasma. *J Appl Physiol* 2003; **95**: 620–630.
45 Barsotti G, Lazzeri M, Cristofano C, *et al.* The role of metabolic acidosis in causing uremic hyperphosphatemia. *Miner Electrolyte Metab* 1986; **12**: 103–106.
46 Rastegar A. Clinical utility of Stewart's method in diagnosis and management of acid–base disorders. *Clin J Am Soc Nephrol* 2009; **4**: 1267–1274.
47 Lloyd P. Strong ion calculator – a practical bedside application of modern quantitative acid–base physiology. *Crit Care Resus* 2004; **6**: 285–294.
48 McCullough SM, Constable PD. Calculation of the total plasma concentration of nonvolatile weak acids and the effective dissociation constant of nonvolatile buffers in the plasma for use in the strong ion approach to acid–base balance in cats. *Am J Vet Res* 2003; **64**: 1047–1051.
49 Constable PD. A simplified strong ion model for acid–base equilibria: application to horse plasma. *J Appl Physiol* 1997; **83**: 297–311.
50 Kaae J, de Morais HAS. Anion gap and strong ion gap: a quick reference. *Vet Clin Small Anim* 2008; **38**: 111–117.
51 Kurtz I, Kraut J, Ornekian V, Nguyen MK. Acid–base analysis: a critique of the Stewart and bicarbonate-centered approaches. *Am J Renal Physiol* 2008; **294**: F1009–F1031.

19 Perioperative Thermoregulation and Heat Balance

Kurt A. Grimm
Veterinary Specialist Services, PC, Conifer, Colorado, USA

Chapter contents

Introduction

Perianesthetic hypothermia, and less commonly hyperthermia, occur in almost all patients undergoing anesthesia. Despite the common occurrence of body temperature changes, few anesthetists understand the complex patterns of heat transfer and the multitude of factors which influence the rate and extent to which it occurs. This chapter will address these factors, the techniques used to limit heat loss, and the impact of hypo- and hyperthermia on patient morbidity.

Thermodynamics

Thermodynamics is the study of the transfer of heat and work between systems. In biology, the thermodynamic laws can be applied to explain many phenomena, but of interest to the anesthetist is the analysis of the transfer of body heat, clinically measured as core body temperature, to the external environment. The reverse (e.g., heat transfer from the external environment to the patient) is also of interest since an understanding of the process will allow a safe and effective means of maintaining or increasing patient temperature during the perianesthetic period. The heat transfer and storage properties of materials which contact the patient are also important since they often present hazards to the patient in the form of potential sources of burns. Fortunately, a detailed knowledge of the application of the laws of thermodynamics is not necessary to understand heat balance; however, a general understanding of conservation of energy (the first law of thermodynamics) and the heat flow to establish an equilibrium between systems (the second law of thermodynamics) will be useful.

Thermoregulation

An organism possesses heat energy which is conveniently measured as body temperature. The total amount of heat energy is a function of the temperature and the mass of the patient, just as kinetic energy is a function of the velocity (speed) of an object and its mass. In most domestic mammalian species the amount of heat energy (temperature) is relatively constant (homeothermic) despite continual metabolic heat production, and environmental heat gain and losses. The amount of body heat can be described using the terms normothermia (euthermia), hypothermia, and hyperthermia which refer to normal, decreased, and increased amounts of body heat respectively. Hyperthermia is an increase in temperature, but usually occurs in response to increased environmental temperature or altered thermoregulation. Pyrexia (i.e., fever) is similar in that it is an abnormal increase in temperature but it is due to an increase in the set-point, often related to immune response to pathogens. Hypothermia is the opposite condition and is most commonly associated with heat loss in excess to metabolic production or decreased thermoregulatory set-point which delays shivering or other homeostatic mechanisms.

Measured temperature values corresponding to these different states depend on the species since the normal ranges of

Veterinary Anesthesia and Analgesia: The Fifth Edition of Lumb and Jones.
Edited by Kurt A. Grimm, Leigh A. Lamont, William J. Tranquilli, Stephen A. Greene and Sheilah A. Robertson.

core body temperature can vary. Additionally, temperature can fluctuate with the time of day (or time of year for hibernating animals), hormonal influences, and activity levels, although these variations are usually minor compared to the changes induced by anesthesia. Additionally some species (especially amphibians, reptiles, and some fish) are normally subject to significant environmental temperature influences (poikilothermic) and definition of normal body temperature becomes problematic. Interestingly, the naked mole rat is the only known mammal to exhibit poikilothermic responses to environmental temperature changes as an adult [1].

Body temperature is sensed by temperature-responsive cells throughout the body. There are distinct populations of peripheral nerve endings (receptors) in the skin which discharge when their thermal thresholds are reached. Most receptors appear to utilize ion channels that belong to the transient receptor potential (TRP) family of cation channels [2]. There are also visceral receptors which are found generally in the brain (especially the anterior hypothalamus and preoptic area), spinal cord, and abdominal structures such as the gastrointestinal tract and urinary bladder [2]. The afferent input to the central nervous system (CNS) is carried by different nerve fiber types (e.g., A-δ and C-fibers) depending on whether the input is cold, hot, or noxious. These signals traverse ascending tracts of the spinal cord and eventually reach the hypothalamus where the signals are integrated and responses issued. Since local temperature can vary depending on the tissue type and metabolic activity, the thermal input to the CNS is a summary of multiple core and peripheral sensors. This 'averaging' of temperature allows the body to maintain a narrow thermal set-point which is associated with an interthreshold range (temperature variation where no compensatory responses [e.g., shivering, sweating, vasoconstriction or vasodilation] occur) of approximately ± 0.2 °C (Fig. 19.1). Anesthetic drugs can alter thermoregulatory thresholds for compensatory responses which is why perioperative patients often fail to shiver even though they are mildly hypothermic. The increase in the interthreshold range (approximate range of 3.5 °C) caused by drugs such as opioids, sedatives, and anesthetics is to some degree drug and dose dependent and reduces the patient's ability to tightly regulate core body temperature.

Core-to-periphery gradient

It is important to understand that body heat is not uniformly distributed throughout the organism. For example, the core body temperature is often several degrees (2–4 °C) higher than skin temperature (Fig. 19.2) [3]. There is also significant longitudinal variation in temperature in the limbs with the core-to-skin difference being greater the further the measurement is made from the trunk. This temperature gradient is maintained by the autonomic nervous system through mechanisms which regulate peripheral blood flow [4].

The majority of heat transfer between the core and periphery occurs via blood-borne convection (with some due to tissue-to-tissue conduction). Factors which influence the distribution of blood include arteriovenous anastomoses, cutaneous vasoconstriction or dilation, and countercurrent vascular heat exchange [3]. Sweating (in those species which possess this capability) and environmental temperature will also modify the redistribution of heat [3]. Additional

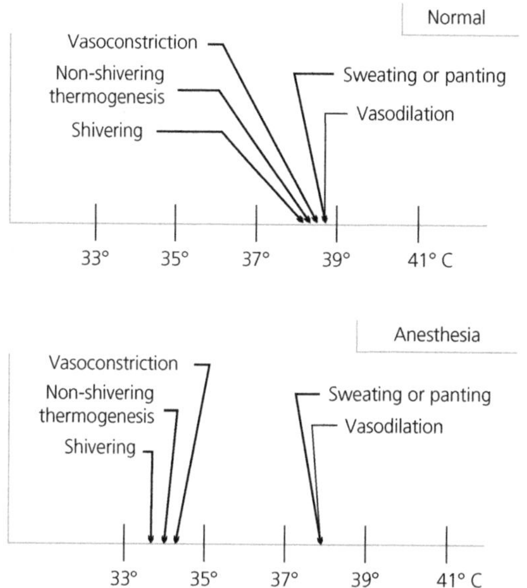

Figure 19.1 Thermoregulation is tightly controlled in healthy, unmedicated individuals. Many drugs used during the perianesthetic period (e.g., opioids and inhalant anesthetics) can alter the range over which compensatory responses to altered environmental and core body temperature occur.

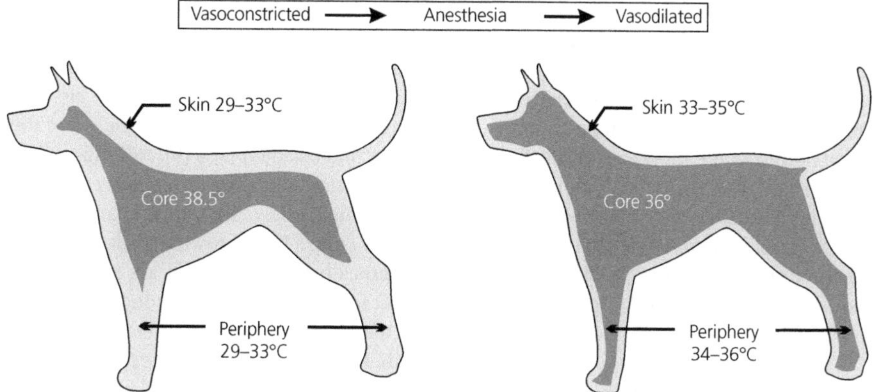

Figure 19.2 A temperature gradient normally exists between the skin surface and the body's core. The gradient is maintained by physiologic mechanisms such as peripheral vasoconstriction and altered blood flow distribution. Many anesthetics which cause indiscriminate vasodilation result in mixing of core and peripheral blood, leading to a lessening of the gradient and ultimately a decrease in core body temperature.

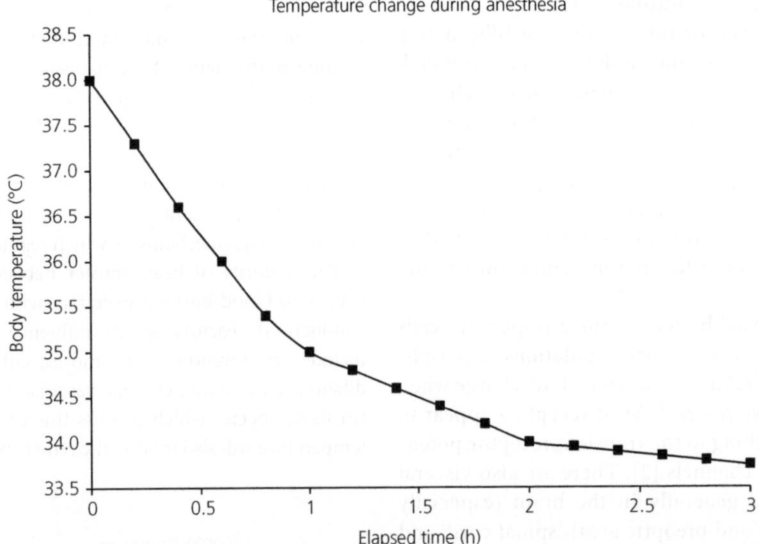

Figure 19.3 The hypothetical pattern of body temperature decrease during general anesthesia of a canine patient with minimal or no external heat support. During the first hour, core temperature usually decreases 1–1.5 °C. A second slower phase follows which represents less influence of core-skin blood redistribution and more dependence on environmental heat loss. Eventually patients reach a psuedoequilibrium with the environment and heat loss is minimal. Patients with a greater surface area-to-mass ratio (e.g., cats or small dogs) will experience faster changes while larger patients (e.g., horses) will experience slower changes. Use of supplemental heat sources in the perioperative period will tend to slow the rate of decrease of body temperature and elevate the minimum temperature reached. The surgical or diagnostic procedure being performed can also modify the rate of heat loss.

mechanisms exist such as panting or shivering which can modify heat loss and gain, although these mechanisms more directly affect the core temperature rather than the skin-to-core temperature gradient.

Interestingly, in humans about 95% of metabolically generated heat is lost to the environment via transfer across the skin with only about 5% lost through the respiratory tract. This implies that heat conservation devices such as airway heat exchangers will have minimal influence on the rate of change of core temperature during anesthesia [5–7]. Since human skin and hair density is significantly different from that of many domestic species, the importance of cutaneous heat loss may vary, but in general it remains a major mechanism contributing to perianesthetic hypothermia.

The reason why it is important to understand the skin-to-core temperature gradient is that it helps explain why anesthetized patients undergo a rapid decrease in body temperature following administration of anesthetic drugs, especially those which cause profound peripheral vasodilation (e.g., acepromazine and inhalant anesthetics). Drugs which cause less peripheral vasodilation often result in a less rapid decrease in temperature (e.g., total intravenous anesthesia with propofol or following premedication with dexmedetomidine) [8].

Most of the clinical research into anesthesia-associated body temperature change has been performed with human subjects. It should be remembered that body size and more specifically the surface area-to-mass ratio (alternatively the core-to-peripheral compartment ratio) can greatly influence the rate of change of core body temperature. The typical pattern of perianesthetic hypothermia has been described as having three phases: an initial rapid hypothermic phase, the linear decrease, and the plateau phase (Fig. 19.3).

Mechanisms of heat transfer

Heat energy that has reached the patient's body surface is transferred to the environment via four main mechanisms: radiation, conduction, convection, and evaporation. Radiation of heat is the electromagnetic (photon) transfer of energy between surfaces. It does not depend upon the temperature of the air around the patient, but does depend on the emissivity of the involved surfaces and their temperature difference (in °K) raised to the fourth power. Emissivity is an object's capacity to exchange heat, with a value of 1.0 being a perfect absorber of heat and 0 being a perfect reflector. Human skin has been described as having an emissivity of 0.95 (regardless of pigmentation) for infrared light [3]. Radiation has been identified as the most important mechanism resulting in heat loss and perianesthetic hypothermia [3] and of note, it is not significantly inhibited by common methods used to limit patient hypothermia (e.g., cloth blankets, circulating water blankets, forced warm air heaters).

Conduction and convection share a common theme in that heat energy flows from a warmer to a cooler surface. Conduction is usually direct transfer between two adjacent surfaces whereas convection is facilitated via an intermediary (e.g., moving air or flowing liquid). Transfer of heat via conduction is proportional to the difference between two surface temperatures and can be inhibited by placing insulation between them. With convection, the movement of air ('wind chill') increases heat loss proportional to the square root of the air velocity. Use of an air-trapping sheet or blanket around the patient will limit air flow and thus reduce the effects of convection by about 30% [9]. Adding additional layers does little to reduce heat loss from convection, emphasizing the importance of decreasing air flow rather than focusing on the insulating capability of the cover. Using towels, pads, or circulating water blankets underneath the patient will act as a layer of insulation and limit direct transfer of heat via conduction.

One important species difference to consider when interpreting studies of heat loss in domestic mammals compared to human subjects is the insulating effect of fur on conduction and convection. Convection is generally regarded as the second most important cause of intraoperative heat loss in humans, but can become the most important in environments with high air flow.

Evaporation of liquids from the skin or body cavity surface results in patient heat loss due to the 'donation' of heat energy required to vaporize the liquid. It is recognized that heat loss is greater with surgeries requiring large incisions with exposure of internal surfaces than with small incisions or non-invasive procedures. Evaporative losses can reach 50% of the total heat loss for smaller animal patients (rabbits) with large surgical fields [10], but has been estimated to be less relative to skin loss with larger animals (swine) [11]. Another source of evaporative heat loss is associated with use of water- or alcohol-based solutions to prepare the surgical site. Heat loss has been suggested to be less with water-based solutions than with alcohol [12]. Relative to other sources of heat loss, evaporative losses due to surgical site preparation tend to be small but significant.

Decreased core body temperature has long been associated with the intravenous administration of fluid therapy. The magnitude of this effect is a function of the temperature of the fluids being administered and their volume relative to the patient's body mass. When fluids are introduced at less than blood temperature, heat energy is transferred to the solution to increase the temperature until it reaches equilibrium with the patient's blood. Warming intravenous fluid can minimize this source of heat loss, but a medical fluid warming device should be used to avoid accidental overheating which could result in blood protein and enzyme damage. Many commercial devices limit fluid temperature to 104 °F (40 °C) which is approximate to the blood temperature of a febrile patient. Important limitations of fluid warmers include the rate of fluid flow and distance they can be positioned from the patient. Many fluid warmers have a specified range of fluid flow rates where the fluid they output will be at or near the indicated temperature. If flow rates are too high, there is inadequate time to absorb heat and reach equilibrium with the warmer surface resulting in cooler than indicated fluid. If flow rates are too low, the fluid loses significant heat to room air on its way to the patient. Long fluid lines positioned between the warmer and the patient will have a similar effect. Under clinical conditions, the amount of perianesthetic heat loss prevented by warming intravenous fluids is minor relative to other routes [13,14].

Active patient warming

Although patient heat loss cannot be completely prevented during anesthesia, several methods have succeeded in replacing heat losses or limiting their magnitude. The first phase of heat loss is the result primarily of the transfer of core heat to the periphery due to vasodilation (see Fig. 19.2). This phase is nearly impossible to prevent by application of an external heat source after induction. The most effective strategy is prewarming the skin and peripheral tissues to minimize the thermal gradient between the skin and the core so that once blood flow increases to the periphery, the heat energy required to re-establish equilibrium is minimal. This strategy is employed on some human patients, but has obvious limitations in veterinary patients. It is often impossible to restrain the patient to apply a warming device, but some species can be placed into warm ambient environments prior to induction. A major downside to this approach is that the patient will often respond by attempting to maintain a normal core temperature by panting, sweating, or other compensatory mechanisms.

Once anesthesia is induced, the focus is on limiting heat loss and maximizing safe heat supplementation. Use of blankets over the patient can reduce convective losses by approximately 30%, and placing insulation or circulating warm water blankets under all points where the patient contacts the surgery table or positioning devices will reduce conductive losses. However, the mainstay of limiting perianesthetic hypothermia is application of an external heat source (forced air unit, circulating warm water blanket, or resistive foam electrical unit).

Numerous methods to supply supplemental heat have been tried over the years by veterinarians during hospitalization or recovery from anesthesia. These have included using electric heating coils (e.g., farrowing heat pads), containers filled with warm water (e.g., latex gloves, bleach bottles, IV fluid bags), and bags filled with various cereal grains which can be microwaved [15,16]. None of these methods should be used during anesthesia due to the relatively high potential for causing skin burns to patients [17]. Conscious patients are able to sense impending thermal injury and will usually move away from a heat source. They also alter their body position frequently to limit the exposure of one area to pressure or heat. These innate protective mechanisms are abolished by general anesthesia, placing responsibility for protecting the patient from burns on the anesthetist. A complicating factor is peripheral blood flow to the skin, since lower blood flow allows accumulation of heat energy at the skin surface, increasing the risk of thermal injury. Since the previously mentioned methods of heat supplementation were not designed for use in anesthetized patients, they can be hazardous. Their main limitation is the heat content of solids and liquids is great enough that if left in contact with skin for a prolonged period, there can be enough heat transfer to cause a burn.

Forced air units circumvent this problem because the heat content of air is low (unless a hair dryer is used instead of a patient warmer). By using large volumes of warm air (containing relatively little heat energy), the risk of injury is less. However, if an object made of metal, water, or plastic is in contact with both the warmed air and skin, there is a potential to concentrate the heat energy and cause a burn, especially if an appropriate forced warm air blanket is not used to distribute the air flow.

Circulating warm water blankets reduce the risk of thermal injury by limiting the water temperature and distributing the water flow to areas of the pad which are not under significant pressure. Pressure points created by patient contact with the underlying table or positioning devices can create local areas of relative skin hypoperfusion. This local decrease in blood flow allows heat to accumulate in the hypoperfused tissue, increasing the risk of a burn.

Inexpensive electric heating pads do not redistribute heat delivery away from areas of pressure and hypoperfusion which is why they should never be used on anesthetized or recovering patients. Resistive foam electric heating pads are available and designed for use in anesthetized patients. The main difference is that the system reduces heat delivery when pad resistance is increased. Systems designed for anesthetized patients will be discussed in more detail below.

It should be apparent that the efficiency of heat transfer is directly related to the proportion of body surface which can be exposed to the external heat source. Also important is the surface-to-mass ratio of the area being warmed. Heat loss (and gain) is usually greatest in areas with a large blood flow and low mass such as the limbs. Use of insulation (e.g., bubblewrap) around legs has been suggested to slow heat loss while application of heat to the limbs versus the trunk has been shown to result in more effective warming [18]. While dentistry patients may have 80–90% of their body surface covered, abdominal and thoracic surgery patients are often only covered 50% or less due to the need for surgical access. This fact, coupled with increased evaporative losses due to large incisions and body cavity exposure, can result in significant hypothermia in small patients.

Forced warm air units

Many different models of forced warm air heating units are available. These are distinctly different from other sources of forced warm air which may have historically been used on veterinary patients such as hair dryers. The heat output of the unit is a function of the air temperature and the air flow volume at the hose end. However, the efficacy of the system to warm patients is mainly a function of the design of the blanket [19]. Important considerations are that the blanket should have minimal temperature differences between the warmest and coolest areas and that the effectiveness is a function of the temperature difference between the patient and the blanket. Patient coverage by the blanket is also a critical factor. With this knowledge, it would seem ill advised to save money by making home-made blankets out of items such as pillowcases. Additionally, the use of a blanket is important for even distribution of heat. 'Hosing' patients (aiming the blanket-end of the hose toward the patient) is inefficient and may result in overheating of plastic, metal, or other objects in direct contact with the patient's skin. Forced air warming units and their blankets are engineered as a system and when utilized as such can be effective [20,21].

Circulating warm water systems

One of the older systems designed for use with anesthetized patients consists of a water reservoir/heater/pump unit and a replaceable blanket/pad [22]. Key features of the pump are the incorporation of electrical safety features, since water and electricity are in close proximity, and the ability to limit the temperature of the water delivered to the patient (usually around 104 °F [40 °C]). Most units can be attached to several sizes and shapes of blankets and have internal features to warn of low water levels. Blankets are available in many sizes and shapes which is useful to maximize the body contact area.Water circulates through the blanket in channels formed between the plastic layers. Occlusion of some of the channels by patient pressure results in shunting of flow around that area, reducing the risk of heat accumulation at pressure points.

While circulating warm water systems are generally less expensive than other systems designed for anesthetized patients, there are some drawbacks. Usually the blanket is placed between the patient and the table. If more patient coverage is desired, additional blankets or units are needed. Also, failure or leakage of a blanket can result in drenching of the patient, causing significantly increased heat loss due to evaporation during transport and recovery. While circulating water blankets are more effective than no external heat support, they are usually less effective than forced warm air units [23]. Many anesthetists choose to use a circulating warm water blanket under the patient in combination with a forced warm air unit placed over or around the patient.

Resistive polymer electric heating

Resistive polymer heating systems (e.g., HotDog Patient Warming System, Augustine Biomedical + Design, Eden Prairie, MN; Inditherm, Inditherm plc, Rotherham, UK) differ from forced air and circulating warm water in that they are conductive rather than convective heat delivery devices. The major concern limiting the use of electric heating pads during anesthesia and recovery has been (and remains) the concern for thermal injury. Polymer heating differs from other electric heating pads in that the polymer heats evenly, limiting hot spots. The resistance to electrical flow (which is related to production of heat) is monitored by the controller, thereby regulating heat delivery. In addition, temperature sensors located in the pad independently monitor the temperature as a redundant system check.

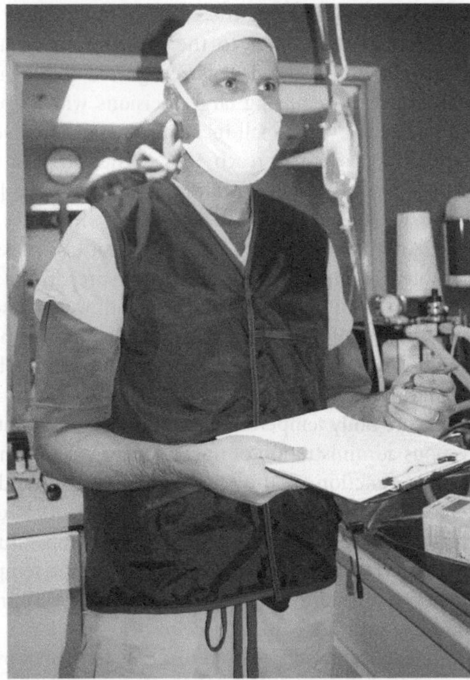

Figure 19.4 Optional vest which can be attached to a HotDog patient warmer control unit (Augustine Biomedical + Design, Eden Prairie, MN) or which can function with a stand-alone power supply. The vest makes very cold operating rooms comfortable for the anesthetist. Source: Dr JoAnna Anzelmo-Rump. Reproduced with permission.

Pad construction consists of several layers composed of the polymer, padding, waterproofing, and a protective layer. The integrity of the pad construction appears to be important since moisture inside the pad can alter function and heat delivery characteristics of the system and has been associated with thermal injury to patients. Additionally, the temperature sensing units inside the pad are located in discrete areas and ideally should be placed in contact with the patient's skin if an accurate measure of the contact point temperature is to be obtained.

Advantages of this system include less concern for surgical site contamination due to air flow (forced warm air systems)[24], lower disposable costs (forced warm air and circulating warm water systems), quiet solid-state functioning, and a simple direct current electrical cord connection between the pad and the controller unit. An additional benefit of this system to the anesthetist is the availability of a vest which can be plugged into the unit (or a stand-alone power supply) that can be worn by the anesthetist in cold operating rooms (Fig. 19.4). Potential downsides to the system include a relatively large initial purchase price and concern for thermal injury when the pad is damaged without obvious external signs. Many users (especially for dental procedures) wrap the pad around the patient, but a safer approach may be to place the pad over the patient to limit pressure points. Effectiveness of resistive polymer heating has been compared to forced warm air and other methods. Generally, the resistive polymer system is similar or somewhat more effective [25–29]. However, the major limitation with heat transfer and patient temperature maintenance remains the amount of body surface which can contact the pad.

Hyperthermia

Hyperthermia is rare during anesthesia. When it does occur, it is usually due to iatrogenic causes (e.g., too much heat gain from warming devices), large heavy-coated animals undergoing diagnostic procedures associated with little heat loss (e.g., a Newfoundland dog undergoing magnetic resonance imaging), or metabolic derangement or disease (e.g., malignant hyperthermia or suspected serotonin syndrome). When recognized, hyperthermia should be evaluated as to the clinical significance and a differential list of causes should be formulated. Transient mild hyperthermia (up to 104 °F [40 °C]) is seldom a risk to the patient and usually responds to remedying the suspected cause (turn off or turn down the heat support). If hyperthermia is associated with other signs of hypermetabolism (increased end-tidal CO_2, metabolic acidosis, hypoxia), malignant hyperthermia or some variant of hypermetabolic disease should be suspected and treated aggressively. Malignant hyperthermia has been reported in several species including humans, cats, dogs, horses, and swine [30–41]. Similar hypermetabolic syndromes have also been reported during capture of free-ranging wildlife.

A confounding factor of diagnosing the cause of hyperthermia, especially in cats, is the association of opioid administration with perianesthetic hyperthermia [42,43]. This effect appears to be related to opioid-altered thermoregulation in the central nervous system. Most other companion animal species experience hypothermia perianesthetically following opioid administration although there appear to be exceptions (e.g., Greyhounds) [31]. More detailed species-specific discussions of malignant hyperthermia appear elsewhere in this text.

Clinical significance of hypothermia

The first obstacle to a meaningful discussion of the significance of anesthetic-related hypothermia is defining at what patient temperature hypothermia occurs. Strictly speaking, it would be at any temperature below the patient's normal temperature. However, practical experience tells us that mild hypothermia is seldom associated with significant long-term complications; therefore many choose to define mild hypothermia as a body temperature between the patient's normal euthermic temperature and approximately 96.8 °F (36 °C), the temperature below which risk of complications is thought to increase in most species. It should be apparent that decreasing body temperature is a continuum and the risk of adverse outcomes is usually multifactorial. Therefore, defining at what temperature hypothermia is significant depends on the individual patient and comorbidities present. In general, it can be assumed that the risk of adverse outcomes increases as body temperature decreases, but accurately predicting the breakpoints at which an individual patient will have complications is impossible.

Anesthetic-related hypothermia in veterinary medicine is very common. Usually larger animals (equine and bovine species) will experience some degree of hypothermia, but the magnitude is usually small due to the large body mass-to-surface ratio, and potentially the high frequency of use of α_2-adrenergic receptor agonists as preanesthetics. Even though hypothermia may be classified as mild, there are several studies which have associated hypothermia in horses with longer times to standing [21,44]. Smaller species, including dogs and cats, often have mild-to-moderate hypothermia, even when supplemental heat sources are used. However, the reported incidence varies greatly depending on what temperature is used to define its onset [45–49].

The incidence and magnitude of hypothermia are highly correlated with several non-temperature-dependent risk factors for postanesthetic complications, including anesthetic duration, ASA status, patient size, patient age, surgical site, and reason for surgery [50,51]. Common complications usually attributed to hypothermia include increased risk of anesthetic overdose [52], prolonged recovery from anesthesia [53], postoperative wound infection, impairment of coagulation [54,55], increased shivering and discomfort during recovery, increased blood viscosity, and cardiac complications including arrhythmias and arrest [56]. While *in vitro* measures of coagulation and platelet function are temperature dependent and generally are impaired by hypothermia-associated temperatures, *in vivo* effects of hypothermia on coagulation can be variable depending on many patient and surgical factors.

Cardiac arrest is the most extreme example of increased mortality from hypothermia but does not usually occur until core temperature is below approximately 70 °F (20–23 °C) [56]. Other cardiovascular complications can occur at much higher body temperatures (e.g., hypotension, myocardial ischemia and arrhythmias due to increased oxygen demands secondary to shivering in recovery), but are of greater concern in patients with pre-existing cardiac disease than in normal healthy patients.

Postoperative wound infections have been demonstrated to be more common when mild hypothermia occurs during anesthesia [57], but others have found little difference when studying the rate of infection in clean wounds and instead suggest surgery time is more important [58]. Proposed mechanisms include decreased peripheral tissue blood flow during recovery and decreased function of T cells and neutrophils [57]. However, other factors, especially surgery time, surgery location, underlying health of the patient, and anesthesia-associated hypoxemia (relatively common in horses), should also be considered since these also correlate with wound infection rates [59–61]. Controlled hypothermia can be protective for some patients. The decreased rate of cellular metabolism associated with hypothermia may be protective in some conditions such as neurologic disease [62–64], myocardial ischemia[56], and tissue hypoxia [65].

Perianesthetic management of hypothermia

No formal guidelines exist for the management of body temperature during anesthesia of veterinary patients. However, body temperature monitoring in the perioperative period is recommended in the American College of Veterinary Anesthesia and Analgesia Monitoring Guidelines so that 'patients do not encounter serious deviations from normal body temperature' [66]. It should be appreciated that monitoring patient temperature does not alter heat balance changes associated with anesthesia. Application of appropriate external heat sources can alter but seldom prevents changes in temperature during the operative period unless patients can be in contact with the source over a large portion of their skin surface area and for a sufficient time to absorb adequate heat energy.

Management of patient temperature is a series of compromises made between the anesthetist, surgeon, and other personnel involved in the perioperative care of the patient. All anesthetists would like to have their patients wake up euthermic if possible since feeling cold can be uncomfortable. However, surgical, patient transport, and recovery logistics are often at odds with maintenance of euthermia. For example, dentistry patients can often be warmed by covering 80–90% of their skin surface area, and may be extubated at or near normal body temperature. However, a surgeon cannot gain access to the abdomen for an exploratory laparotomy with heating devices draped over the caudal half of the patient, so a significant decrease in heat transfer is mandated by surgical needs. Additionally, surgeons often expose abdominal contents during laparotomy, further decreasing patient heat balance through increased losses. Operating room temperature could be increased to minimize the temperature differential between the patient and environment but most surgeons prioritize their own comfort and keep operating room temperatures cool. Even with the limitations imposed by surgical needs, reasonable efforts should be made to apply effective means of heat supplementation to anesthetized patients, especially if the surgery is invasive or anesthesia time longer than a few minutes.

Since the majority (in some cases over 90%) of heat loss occurs through radiation, conduction, and convection of heat from the skin, focus should be placed on limiting these losses. Placing patients on insulating pads will slow conductive losses into the surgery table. Placing warming devices specifically designed for anesthetized patients over as much skin surface as reasonably possible will decrease the skin-to-environment temperature gradient and further slow or reverse loss. Placing one layer of material over or around the patient can limit air circulation and slow convective loss. Some have used radiant heat lamps over the patient to limit or reverse radiant heat loss (a significant proportion of overall loss) but this is not common practice and may be difficult to control.

Other methods of patient warming or heat loss prevention have been studied. In general, they are effective at addressing the intended mechanism, but often those mechanisms are relatively minor and do not have a major impact on overall heat loss. These include use of fluid warmers, airway humidifiers and heaters [67], use of water-based versus alcohol-based surgical preparation solutions, and additional insulation or blanket layers (e.g., bubblewrap on the feet). When considering the utility of these techniques, there should be thoughtful discussion about their effectiveness and potential to complicate or delay the anesthetic and surgical procedure.

Significant hypothermia in patients arriving in recovery is common, especially in small animal species after surgeries lasting 30 min or longer. The drugs used for premedication and anesthesia can significantly influence the observed body temperature decrease since vasoconstrictors (e.g., α_2-adrenergic receptor agonists) tend to limit cutaneous blood flow and heat transfer while vasodilators (e.g., acepromazine and inhalant anesthetics) tend to increase both [8]. While the amount of vasoconstriction or vasodilation can modify the rate at which heat is lost, they can also modify the rate at which externally applied supplemental heat sources can warm a patient in recovery. It can be more difficult to raise body temperature in an animal with profound peripheral vasoconstriction (due to normal response to hypothermia or pharmacologically induced). In some cases it may be reasonable to administer an antagonist to the drugs responsible for delaying patient warming (e.g., α_2-adrenergic receptor antagonists or opioid antagonists) to help restore cutaneous blood flow and central thermoregulatory responses. However, this is not frequently done following major surgery due to the loss of sedative and analgesic actions following reversal. Additionally, rapid increases in oxygen demands will follow onset of shivering. If the patient cannot increase oxygen delivery (diminished cardiovascular function or anemia) or has marginal blood oxygenation (respiratory disease), rapid tissue hypoxia may follow.

While hypothermia has been associated with several postoperative complications (e.g., increased wound infections, decreased coagulation and hemostasis, etc.), it seldom represents a true anesthetic emergency, even when severe. Therefore personnel should initially focus on critical parameters such as cardiovascular function (heart rate, blood pressure, cardiac output) and pulmonary function (end-tidal CO_2, oxyhemoglobin saturation, airway management) before addressing patient rewarming when patients present to recovery. Once the patient's vital functions are being monitored and supported, heat support can be applied. During the early recovery period when patients are unconscious or heavily sedated, the same concerns exist as during anesthesia with respect to placing heat sources not designed for anesthetized patients near or on the patient.

References

1 Daly TJ, Williams LA, Buffenstein R. Catecholaminergic innervation of interscapular brown adipose tissue in the naked mole-rat (Heterocephalus glaber). *J Anat* 1997; **190**: 321–326.

2 Morrison SF, Nakamura K. Central neural pathways for thermoregulation. *Front Biosci* 2011; **16**: 74–104.

3 Sessler DI. Perioperative heat balance. *Anesthesiology* 2000; **92**(2): 578–596.

4 Kurz A, Sessler DI, Christensen R, *et al.* Thermoregulatory vasoconstriction and perianesthetic heat transfer. *Acta Anaesthesiol Scand Suppl* 1996; **109**: 30–33.

5 Raffe MR, Martin FB. Effect of inspired air heat and humidification on anesthetic-induced hypothermia in dogs. *Am J Vet Res* 1983; **44**(3): 455–458.

6 Hofmeister EH, Brainard BM, Braun C, Figueiredo JP. Effect of a heat and moisture exchanger on heat loss in isoflurane-anesthetized dogs undergoing single-limb orthopedic procedures. *J Am Vet Med Assoc* 2011; **239**(12): 1561–1565.

7 Goldberg ME, Epstein R, Rosenblum F, *et al.* Do heated humidifiers and heat and moisture exchangers prevent temperature drop during lower abdominal surgery? *J Clin Anesth* 1992; **4**(1): 16–20.

8 Vainionpää M, Salla K, Restitutti F, *et al.* Thermographic imaging of superficial temperature in dogs sedated with medetomidine and butorphanol with and without MK-467 (L-659'066). *Vet Anaesth Analg* 2013; **40**(2):142–148.

9 Sessler DI, McGuire J, Sessler AM. Perioperative thermal insulation. *Anesthesiology* 1991; **74**(5):875–879.

10 Roe CF. Effect of bowel exposure on body temperature during surgical operations. *Am J Surg* 1971; **122**(1): 13–15.

11 English MJ, Papenberg R, Farias E, *et al.* Heat loss in an animal experimental model. *J Trauma* 1991; **31**(1): 36–38.

12 Sessler DI, Sessler AM, Hudson S, Moayeri A. Heat loss during surgical skin preparation. *Anesthesiology* 1993; **78**(6): 1055–1064.

13 Atayde IB, Franco LG, Silva MAM, *et al.* Fluid Heating System (SAF): effects on clinical and biochemistry parameters in dogs submitted to inhalatory anesthesia. *Acta Cirúrgica Bras Soc Bras Para Desenvolv Pesqui Em Cir* 2009; **24**(2): 144–149.

14 Chiang V, Hopper K, Mellema MS. In vitro evaluation of the efficacy of a veterinary dry heat fluid warmer. *J Vet Emerg Crit Care* 2011; **21**(6): 639–647.

15 Dyson D, Stoate C. Combating hypothermia, including recommendations for the use of oat bags. *Can Vet J* 1997; **38**(8): 517–518.

16 Jirapaet K, Jirapaet V. Assessment of cereal-grain warming pad as a heat source for newborn transport. *J Med Assoc Thail Chotmaihet Thangphaet* 2005; **88**(Suppl 8): S203–210.

17 Dunlop CI, Daunt DA, Haskins SC. Thermal burns in four dogs during anesthesia. *Vet Surg* 1989; **18**(3): 242–146.

18 Cabell LW, Perkowski SZ, Gregor T, Smith GK. The effects of active peripheral skin warming on perioperative hypothermia in dogs. *Vet Surg* 1997; **26**(2): 79–85.

19 Bräuer A, Quintel M. Forced-air warming: technology, physical background and practical aspects. *Curr Opin Anaesthesiol* 2009; **22**(6): 769–774.

20 Machon RG, Raffe MR, Robinson EP. Warming with a forced air warming blanket minimizes anesthetic-induced hypothermia in cats. *Vet Surg* 1999; **28**(4): 301–310.

21 Tomasic M. Temporal changes in core body temperature in anesthetized adult horses. *Am J Vet Res* 1999; **60**(5): 556–562.

22 Evans AT, Sawyer DC, Krahwinkel DJ. Effect of a warm-water blanket on development of hypothermia during small animal surgery. *J Am Vet Med Assoc* 1973; **163**(2): 147–148.

23 Clark-Price SC, Dossin O, Jones KR, *et al.* Comparison of three different methods to prevent heat loss in healthy dogs undergoing 90 minutes of general anesthesia. *Vet Anaesth Analg* 2013; **40**(3): 280–284.

24 Dasari KB, Albrecht M, Harper M. Effect of forced-air warming on the performance of operating theatre laminar flow ventilation. *Anaesthesia* 2012; **67**(3): 244–249.
25 Kibanda JO, Gurney M. Comparison of two methods for the management of intraoperative hypothermia in dogs. *Vet Rec* 2012; **170**(15): 392.
26 HotDog Patient Warming. www.vetwarming.com (accessed 22 September 2014).
27 Brandt S, Oguz R, Hüttner H, *et al.* Resistive-polymer versus forced-air warming: comparable efficacy in orthopedic patients. *Anesth Analg* 2010; **110**(3): 834–838.
28 Kimberger O, Held C, Stadelmann K, *et al.* Resistive polymer versus forced-air warming: comparable heat transfer and core rewarming rates in volunteers. *Anesth Analg* 2008; **107**(5): 1621–1626.
29 Hasegawa K, Negishi C, Nakagawa F, *et al.* [The efficacy of carbon-fiber resistive-heating in prevention of core hypothermia during major abdominal surgery]. *Masui* 2003; **52**(6): 636–641.
30 Chohan AS, Greene SA. Anesthesia case of the month. Malignant hyperthermia. *J Am Vet Med Assoc* 2011; **239**(7): 936–940.
31 Court MH. Anesthesia of the sighthound. *Clin Tech Small Anim Pract* 1999; **14**(1): 38–43.
32 Roberts MC, Mickelson JR, Patterson EE, *et al.* Autosomal dominant canine malignant hyperthermia is caused by a mutation in the gene encoding the skeletal muscle calcium release channel (RYR1). *Anesthesiology* 2001; **95**(3): 716–725.
33 Cosgrove SB, Eisele PH, Martucci RW, Gronert GA. Evaluation of greyhound susceptibility to malignant hyperthermia using halothane–succinylcholine anesthesia and caffeine-halothane muscle contractures. *Lab Anim Sci* 1992; **42**(5): 482–485.
34 Cornick JL, Seahorn TL, Hartsfield SM. Hyperthermia during isoflurane anaesthesia in a horse with suspected hyperkalaemic periodic paralysis. *Equine Vet J* 1994; **26**(6): 511–514.
35 De Jong RH, Heavner JE, Amory DW. Malignant hyperpyrexia in the cat. *Anesthesiology* 1974; **41**(6): 608–609.
36 Otto K. [Malignant hyperthermia as a complication of anesthesia in the dog]. *Tierärztl Prax* 1992; **20**(5): 519–522.
37 Kirmayer AH, Klide AM, Purvance JE. Malignant hyperthermia in a dog: case report and review of the syndrome. *J Am Vet Med Assoc* 1984; **185**(9): 978–982.
38 Bagshaw RJ, Cox RH, Knight DH, Detweiler DK. Malignant hyperthermia in a Greyhound. *J Am Vet Med Assoc* 1978; **172**(1): 61–62.
39 Klein L, Ailes N, Fackelman GE, *et al.* Postanesthetic equine myopathy suggestive of malignant hyperthermia. A case report. *Vet Surg* 1989; **18**(6): 479–482.
40 Bellah JR, Robertson SA, Buergelt CD, McGavin AD. Suspected malignant hyperthermia after halothane anesthesia in a cat. *Vet Surg* 1989; **18**(6): 483–488.
41 Adami C, Axiak S, Raith K, Spadavecchia C. Unusual perianesthetic malignant hyperthermia in a dog. *J Am Vet Med Assoc* 2012; **240**(4): 450–453.
42 Posner LP, Gleed RD, Erb HN, Ludders JW. Post-anesthetic hyperthermia in cats. *Vet Anaesth Analg* 2007; **34**(1): 40–47.
43 Niedfeldt RL, Robertson SA. Postanesthetic hyperthermia in cats: a retrospective comparison between hydromorphone and buprenorphine. *Vet Anaesth Analg* 2006; **33**(6): 381–389.
44 Voulgaris DA, Hofmeister EH. Multivariate analysis of factors associated with post-anesthetic times to standing in isoflurane-anesthetized horses: 381 cases. *Vet Anaesth Analg* 2009; **36**(5): 414–420.
45 Waterman A. Accidental hypothermia during anaesthesia in dogs and cats. *Vet Rec* 1975; **96**(14): 308–313.
46 Redondo JI, Suesta P, Gil L, *et al.* Retrospective study of the prevalence of postanaesthetic hypothermia in cats. *Vet Rec* 2012; **170**(8): 206.
47 Redondo JI, Suesta P, Serra I, *et al.* Retrospective study of the prevalence of postanaesthetic hypothermia in dogs. *Vet Rec* 2012; **171**(15): 374.
48 Redondo JI, Rubio M, Soler G, *et al.* Normal values and incidence of cardiorespiratory complications in dogs during general anaesthesia. A review of 1281 cases. *J Vet Med A Physiol Pathol Clin Med* 2007; **54**(9): 470–477.
49 Kennedy KC, Tamburello KR, Hardie RJ. Peri-operative morbidity associated with ovariohysterectomy performed as part of a third-year veterinary surgical-training program. *J Vet Med Educ* 2011; **38**(4): 408–413.
50 Brodbelt DC, Pfeiffer DU, Young LE, Wood JL. Results of the confidential enquiry into perioperative small animal fatalities regarding risk factors for anesthetic-related death in dogs. *J Am Vet Med Assoc* 2008; **233**(7): 1096–1104.
51 Brodbelt DC, Blissitt KJ, Hammond RA, *et al.* The risk of death: the confidential enquiry into perioperative small animal fatalities. *Vet Anaesth Analg* 2008; **35**(5): 365–373.
52 Regan MJ, Eger EI II. Effect of hypothermia in dogs on anesthetizing and apneic doses of inhalation agents. Determination of the anesthetic index (Apnea/MAC). *Anesthesiology* 1967; **28**(4): 689–700.
53 Pottie RG, Dart CM, Perkins NR, Hodgson DR. Effect of hypothermia on recovery from general anaesthesia in the dog. *Aust Vet J* 2007; **85**(4): 158–162.
54 Park KH, Lee KH, Kim H. Effect of hypothermia on coagulatory function and survival in Sprague–Dawley rats exposed to uncontrolled haemorrhagic shock. *Injury* 2013; **44**(1): 91–96.
55 Taggart R, Austin B, Hans E, Hogan D. In vitro evaluation of the effect of hypothermia on coagulation in dogs via thromboelastography. *J Vet Emerg Crit Care* 2012; **22**(2): 219–224.
56 Fujiki M, Misumi K, Sakamoto H, Kanemoto I. Circulatory arrest under hypothermic anesthesia using abdominal cavity cooling. *J Vet Med Sci* 1998; **60**(11): 1237–1242.
57 Putzu M, Casati A, Berti M, *et al.* Clinical complications, monitoring and management of perioperative mild hypothermia: anesthesiological features. *Acta BioMedica Atenei Parm* 2007; **78**(3): 163–169.
58 Beal MW, Brown DC, Shofer FS. The effects of perioperative hypothermia and the duration of anesthesia on postoperative wound infection rate in clean wounds: a retrospective study. *Vet Surg* 2000; **29**(2): 123–127.
59 Sturgeon C, Lamport AI, Lloyd DH, Muir P. Bacterial contamination of suction tips used during surgical procedures performed on dogs and cats. *Am J Vet Res* 2000; **61**(7): 779–783.
60 Brown DC, Conzemius MG, Shofer F, Swann H. Epidemiologic evaluation of postoperative wound infections in dogs and cats. *J Am Vet Med Assoc* 1997; **210**(9): 1302–1306.
61 Nicholson M, Beal M, Shofer F, Brown DC. Epidemiologic evaluation of postoperative wound infection in clean-contaminated wounds: a retrospective study of 239 dogs and cats. *Vet Surg* 2002; **31**(6): 577–581.
62 Steen PA, Newberg L, Milde JH, Michenfelder JD. Hypothermia and barbiturates: individual and combined effects on canine cerebral oxygen consumption. *Anesthesiology* 1983; **58**(6): 527–532.
63 Wass CT, Lanier WL, Hofer RE, *et al.* Temperature changes of > or = 1 degree C alter functional neurologic outcome and histopathology in a canine model of complete cerebral ischemia. *Anesthesiology* 1995; **83**(2): 325–335.
64 Michenfelder JD, Milde JH. The relationship among canine brain temperature, metabolism, and function during hypothermia. *Anesthesiology* 1991; **75**(1): 130–136.
65 Ohta S, Yukioka T, Wada T, *et al.* Effect of mild hypothermia on the coefficient of oxygen delivery in hypoxemic dogs. *J Appl Physiol* 1995; **78**(6): 2095–2099.
66 ACVAA Small Animal Monitoring Guidelines. www.acvaa.org (accessed 22 September 2014).
67 Kelly CK, Hodgson DS, McMurphy RM. Effect of anesthetic breathing circuit type on thermal loss in cats during inhalation anesthesia for ovariohysterectomy. *J Am Vet Med Assoc* 2012; **240**(11): 1296–1299.

20 Treatment of Coagulation and Platelet Disorders

Benjamin M. Brainard

Department of Small Animal Medicine and Surgery, College of Veterinary Medicine, University of Georgia, Athens, Georgia, USA

Chapter contents

Introduction

Interest in the process of both normal and disordered hemostasis in the veterinary patient has experienced resurgence in recent years. This is due in part to the availability of newer tests and techniques that can better illustrate the process and products of coagulation. At the same time, new understanding of the formation of clots *in vivo* has made it clear that traditional testing provides only a limited view into the actual mechanisms and pathophysiology of clot formation and platelet function.

The cell-based model of hemostasis

The cell-based model of hemostasis provides a framework for understanding the complex interactions between cellular components, soluble factors, and the vascular endothelium in the formation of a clot. In some cases this model explains why certain conditions (e.g. factor deficiencies) have a particular hemostatic phenotype. Coagulation as described by this model consists of three phases: initiation, amplification, and propagation [1].

The vast majority of coagulation *in vivo* occurs as a result of tissue factor (TF, factor III) initiation of the extrinsic coagulation cascade as opposed to contact activation via the intrinsic coagulation cascade [2]. Tissue factor is exposed following intimal injury of a blood vessel, and may also be present and available for coagulation on the surface of circulating cells and microparticles. These microparticles are small membrane blebs released from activated endothelial cells, platelets, or leukocytes. The other important player for initiation of coagulation is the platelet. Following activation, the platelet undergoes a shape change and rearrangement of the phospholipids on the surface of the outer platelet membrane. Anionic phospholipids such as phosphatidyl serine are exposed and provide a procoagulant surface for the assembly of constructs of coagulation factors to support propagation of coagulation [3]. The first complex formation occurs when exposed TF comes into contact with activated factor VII (fVIIa). This complex results in the generation of a small amount of thrombin (factor IIa) following activation of factor X and the formation of a TF-fVIIa-fXa complex [1].

The small amount of thrombin released in the initiation step promotes the amplification stage, where additional platelets as well as coagulation factors V and VIII and XI are activated [2]. Additional thrombin formation in the propagation phase will proceed using these factors and the platelet membrane. The tenase complex, composed of factors IXa, VIIIa, and calcium, plays a key step in thrombin formation during the propagation phase. The tenase complex activates coagulation factor X. The presence of factor Xa then allows formation of the prothrombinase complex, which is composed of factors Xa, Va, and calcium. The prothrombinase complex is an extremely efficient complex for the formation of thrombin (factor IIa) from prothrombin, which then catalyzes the formation of fibrin from fibrinogen [4].

Endogenous coagulation inhibitors are present at each stage of the coagulation process to prevent excessive thrombin formation. Tissue factor pathway inhibitor (TFPI) is a potent inhibitor of the TFfVIIa-Xa complex [1]. Antithrombin acts to inhibit factors Xa and IIa. The protein C/protein S system supports the inhibition of factors Va and VIIIa. Patients with urinary losses of antithrombin and humans with congenital low concentrations of protein C are thought to have an increased risk of the development of thromboembolism [5]. Dogs with sepsis have decreased activities of protein C and antithrombin [6]. Dogs with sepsis have also been reported to have increased thrombin-activatable fibrinolysis inhibitor (TAFI)

Veterinary Anesthesia and Analgesia: The Fifth Edition of Lumb and Jones.
Edited by Kurt A. Grimm, Leigh A. Lamont, William J. Tranquilli, Stephen A. Greene and Sheilah A. Robertson.

activity [7]. Other compounds outside the coagulation cascade help to support coagulation or stabilize the formed clot such as TAFI.

Coagulation and platelet function testing

The complex physiology of clot formation *in vivo* is very difficult to mimic *in vitro*. Most laboratory tests of coagulation function are focused on individual aspects of the coagulation cascade. Platelet function may be assessed using tools such as optical or impedance aggregometry which document the response of platelets (in platelet-rich plasma or whole blood, respectively) to discrete agonists such as adenosine diphosphate (ADP), collagen, or arachidonic acid [8].

Platelet function testing (primary hemostasis)

Most aggregometry testing is performed under a low shear condition, with gentle stirring which does not necessarily reflect the *in vivo* conditions of platelets associating with areas of endothelial injury under the high-shear conditions of flowing blood. The PFA-100 (Siemens-Dade Behring) is a whole blood test that aspirates blood through a small aperture using a vacuum [9]. The aperture is coated with a combination of either epinephrine and collagen or ADP and collagen. As platelets pass through the coated aperture, they are activated by the agonists and form a plug, stopping the flow of blood. The time it takes for this to occur is termed the 'closure time' and is measured in seconds. In dogs with von Willebrand disease (which impairs the ability of platelets to tether and adhere to sites of vascular injury) and in animals treated with drugs which decrease platelet activity, the closure time is prolonged [10]. This is a rapid, benchtop test that can be used to assess an animal's risk of bleeding due to platelet function abnormalities. It should be noted that low hematocrits and platelet counts less than 90,000/μL may cause prolonged closure times unrelated to platelet function.

Buccal mucosal bleeding time (BMBT) is another test that has been used to diagnose platelet function abnormalities. It is simple and can be done rapidly as part of a presurgical screen. To perform this test, the buccal mucosa is exposed and a standard incision (5 mm long and 1 mm deep) is made using a simplate device [11]. Once the incision is made, the area is observed for the formation of a gel-like platelet plug. The bleeding time is defined as the time until bleeding has ceased, and is between 3–5 min in normal animals. Because cats have a small buccal surface, the oral mucosal bleeding time (OMBT) is performed instead, by making the incision in the gums above the upper canine tooth [12]. Cats generally need to be sedated or anesthetized for this test. Like the PFA, the BMBT will be abnormally prolonged if patients have thrombocytopenia ($<75 \times 10^9$ platelets/L).

Coagulation testing

Assessment of coagulation factor activity is generally performed using citrated plasma but may also be assessed in whole blood systems. Most tests monitor the formation of a fibrin clot by exposing citrated plasma to calcium in combination with an activating substance and report the time until clot formation (which may be sensed optically or mechanically) as the clotting time [13]. The prothrombin time (PT) is initiated using a mixture of tissue factor and phospholipid and primarily assesses the extrinsic and common pathway of coagulation. Activated partial thromboplastin time (aPTT) is initiated with a strong contact activator such as kaolin, and reflects activity in the intrinsic and common pathways. The thrombin time is dependent on the blood fibrinogen concentration, and assesses only the formation of fibrin in the common pathway following the addition of thrombin. Modifications of both PT and aPTT have been developed to use citrated whole blood for coagulation testing as well [5]. The activated clotting time (ACT) adds whole blood to diatomaceous earth (a strong contact activator), and measures the time until it forms into a clot. The values for coagulation times of normal animals will vary depending on methodology and technique.

Viscoelastic coagulation testing using techniques such as thromboelastography (TEG), rotational thrombelastometry (ROTEM) or Sonoclot use citrated whole blood to evaluate both primary and secondary hemostasis, in addition to fibrinolysis [14]. Viscoelastic testing displays the change in viscosity as blood gels into a clot, and can identify both hypocoagulable and hypercoagulable states. Viscoelastic techniques have been described in dogs, cats, and horses [15–17].

Anticoagulant therapy

Classically, arterial thromboses are thought to result from activation or hyperactivity of platelets, as they are more likely to be activated by the shear stress of arterial blood flow. Venous thrombosis or thromboembolism is more associated with blood stasis and activation of coagulation factors [18]. While these two pathophysiologic consequences dictate different treatment approaches, the reality in veterinary medicine balances the need for patient safety and ease of administration by the owner. For this reason, most anticoagulants used in veterinary medicine are antiplatelet agents that can be administered orally. Injectable anticoagulants that target aspects of the coagulation cascade are also used, especially in hospitalized patients, and newer oral anticoagulants may provide a safer approach to providing adequate anticoagulation in veterinary patients.

Antiplatelet drugs

Platelet activation results in a series of events that make the platelet able to adhere to sites of vascular damage (tethered by molecules such as vWF and collagen), and also cause the release of agonist molecules that support coagulation and activate other platelets in the immediate area through specific receptors on the platelet surface. Molecules that are released from activated platelets include ADP, thromboxane, serotonin, and calcium. Because there are specific receptors for many of these agonists, antiplatelet agents have been designed to affect the binding or release of these agonists.

Aspirin (acetylsalicylic acid, ASA) is one of the agents most commonly used to decrease platelet responsiveness and has been evaluated in most domestic species. Aspirin exerts an antiplatelet effect by irreversible inhibition of platelet cyclo-oxygenase (COX), which produces thromboxane A_2 (TXA_2) from arachidonic acid in response to platelet activation [19,20]. TXA_2 is a potent vasoconstrictor and platelet activator, although platelet responses vary between species and individuals. In dogs, ASA at various doses has been recommended to decrease platelet activity in patients with immune-mediated hemolytic anemia (IMHA) and other diseases which are associated with hypercoagulable states (e.g., protein-losing nephropathy) [6]. In many of these cases, a low dose of ASA (0.5–1.0 mg/kg PO q 12 h) has been recommended, although the efficacy of these lower doses on platelet aggregation has recently been questioned. Interestingly, certain breeds or families of dogs may not be as responsive to ASA-mediated platelet inhibition [21]. The same may be true in humans, and a syndrome of 'aspirin resistance' has been described

[22]. In cats, ASA has been recommended for thromboprophylaxis in animals with hypertrophic cardiomyopathy, although efficacy for inhibition of platelet aggregation or for prevention of intracardiac thrombus formation has not been definitively demonstrated [20,23]. Apirin has been used to treat horses with jugular venous thrombosis.

Clopidogrel (Plavix®, Sanofi Synthelabo, New York) is another antiplatelet drug that has been investigated in veterinary species. Clopidogrel is an irreversible antagonist of the platelet $P2Y_{12}$ ADP receptor, one of two ADP receptors on the platelet surface. Pharmacodynamics of clopidogrel have been described in dogs, cats, and horses, where the drug effectively decreases platelet aggregation in response to ADP [12,24,25]. Because clopidogrel is a prodrug, it requires hepatic biotransformation to the active compound. Drugs that affect the hepatic P450 enzyme system may alter the pharmacokinetics of clopidogrel. However, recent studies do not indicate a clinically relevant interaction with proton pump inhibitors [26]. As with ASA, human patients have been identified who do not respond to clopidogrel therapy with a significant decrease in ADP-induced platelet aggregation. The mechanism may be altered hepatic processing or variations of platelet receptor affinity [27]. Veterinary patients with variable responses to clopidogrel therapy have not yet been identified, but are likely present.

Because both ASA and clopidogrel result in irreversible inhibition of platelet function, it is necessary for patients to form new platelets to regain platelet function. In animals with normal bone marrow, a new platelet population is generally present 5–7 days after cessation of antiplatelet medications. Aspirin and clopidogrel are frequently prescribed for veterinary patients with possible hypercoagulable conditions as they are generally well tolerated, easily administered at home, and associated with limited chance for significant hemorrhage as a result of therapy when used individually. When clopidogrel and ASA were used together in human patients, the antithrombotic effects were more pronounced, but there was also an increased incidence of gastrointestinal bleeding [28].

Coagulation inhibitors

The only currently available oral drug that affects the coagulation cascade is warfarin. It acts as a vitamin K epoxide reductase antagonist and prevents the recycling of vitamin K. It impairs the production of vitamin K-dependent coagulation factors (i.e., II, VII, IX, and X) [29]. Warfarin is very difficult to titrate. Clinical use requires weekly measurements of PT, a tightly regulated diet, and strict dosing schedule to minimize the chances for catastrophic hemorrhage. Warfarin therapy has been used as a component of medical management in dogs with venous thrombi [30] and was also utilized in a small number of cats with hypertrophic cardiomyopathy. However, in those cats its use was associated with a shorter survival time [23]. The effects of warfarin can be antagonized using either oral vitamin K (phytonadione) therapy or by transfusions of fresh frozen or stored plasma [31]. Despite the fact that warfarin is administered orally, it is not frequently used in veterinary medicine due to the severity of potential complications and difficulty in insuring owner compliance. Other oral anticoagulant medications such as rivaroxaban (Xarelto®, Bayer Healthcare) and apixaban (Eliquis®, Pfizer/Bristol-Myers Squibb) have recently been introduced for human patients [32,33]. These drugs are inhibitors of activated coagulation factor X (Xa) and have shown equivalent or superior effect to warfarin in a number of human studies. Studies of these drugs in animals are ongoing but if the drugs prove efficacious, they may finally provide a safe option for oral anticoagulation in veterinary patients.

Heparins are the other class of drugs commonly used for anticoagulation in veterinary species. The use of both unfractionated heparin (UFH) and low molecular weight heparins (LMWH) has been described in many animal species. They have been used to treat many conditions associated with potential or actual thrombosis [34, 35]. All heparins are injectable drugs and may be given by either the intravenous or subcutaneous route. Heparins enhance the inhibitory effect of antithrombin on activated coagulation factors X and II. Low molecular weight heparin is a smaller molecule, and is unable to inactivate factor IIa, only exerting an effect on factor Xa. Heparins are indicated for anticoagulation in patients with gross thrombosis, or for those in danger of thrombotic complications, especially in the perioperative period [36].

Unfractionated heparin has been used to treat dogs with IMHA, pulmonary thromboembolism, and occasionally for animals diagnosed to be in the hypercoagulable phase of disseminated intravascular coagulation (DIC) [36]. There is no evidence to support preincubation of fresh frozen plasma with UFH in the context of DIC, and this practice may actually decrease the amount of available antithrombin in the plasma. In addition, UFH is frequently used for anticoagulation during cardiopulmonary bypass procedures and other advanced techniques (e.g., hemodialysis). Postoperative UFH administration has been described in dogs following adrenal gland resection[37] and may be used for other vascular procedures. In horses, UFH may result in anemia caused by agglutination of red blood cells. This adverse event is rapidly reversed following the cessation of UFH therapy [38]. In humans, heparin-induced thrombocytopenia (HIT) is a significant concern, resulting from the generation of antibodies against heparin bound to platelet factor 4, leading to platelet activation and consumption, resulting in thrombocytopenia and thrombosis in some patients [39]. Heparin-induced thrombocytopenia is more likely to occur in patients receiving UFH, compared to those receiving LMWH [40]. HIT has not been reported in veterinary species.

In people, LMWH has a more favorable pharmacokinetic profile (once-daily dosing) and a decreased risk of hemorrhage compared to UFH. It may be safer in perioperative patients for this reason, although this has not been specifically studied in veterinary patients. Of the LMWHs available, dalteparin (Fragmin®, Pfizer) and enoxaparin (Lovenox®, Sanofi) have been most studied in veterinary medicine. Direct comparisons between these and UFH have been performed in cats[35] and dogs,[41] with more focused studies available in horses[42] and other species. Although the pharmacokinetics in humans are amenable to once-daily dosing, the pharmacodynamic studies available for veterinary species suggest that multiple doses may be required to maintain anti-factor Xa activity in the therapeutic range. The utility of LMWH versus UFH for thromboprophylaxis in veterinary medicine is also not clear. The use of a newer synthetic LMWH, fondaparinux, was recently described in cats (Table 20.1) [43].

Human guidelines for dosing of heparin are based on anti-Xa activity (aXa), and targets vary for prophylactic or therapeutic dosing. Target therapeutic aXa levels for UFH (measured at 4 h after administration of a dose) are 0.35–0.7 U/mL, while prophylactic levels are approximately 10% of these [44,45]. Low molecular weight heparin targets for therapeutic aXa levels are 0.5–1.0 U/mL and 0.1–0.3 U/mL for prophylaxis. In dogs, due to limited availability of rapid aXa testing, UFH is usually dose adjusted by measuring serial aPTT until the aPTT is extended to 1.5–2 times the normal

Table 20.1 Doses of anticoagulant and antiplatelet drugs used in veterinary medicine.

Drug	Species	Dose	Comments
Aspirin	Dog	5 mg/kg PO q24 h [19]	Analgesic dose higher
	Cat	81 mg/cat PO q48–72 h [23]	Questionable efficacy at either dose
	Horse	5 mg/kg PO q48 h [20]	No decrease in platelet function
		5 mg/kg PO q24 h [24]	Effective; single dose
		10 mg/kg [60]	
Clopidogrel	Dog	1 mg/kg PO q24 h [25]	
	Cat	18.75 mg/cat PO q24 h [12]	
	Horse	2 mg/kg PO q24 h [24]	
Warfarin	Dog	0.22 mg/kg PO q12–24 h [61]	Adjust using PT or INR
	Cat	0.06–0.09 mg/kg PO q24 h [62]	Monitor PT
Unfractionated heparin (UFH)	Dog	150–300 U/kg SC q8 h [15,34] 30–50 U/kg/h IV	Adjust to target aPTT or anti-Xa levels
	Cat	150–300 U/kg SC q6–8 h [35]	May result in anemia
	Horse	40–150 U/kg SC q12 h [63]	
Low molecular weight heparin	Dog	Dalteparin 150 U/kg q8 h [64,65]	Optimal dosing interval unknown
	Cat	Enoxaparin 0.8 mg/kg SC q6 h [66]	Single dose only
	Horse	Dalteparin 100–200 IU/kg SC q6–8 h [35,67]	
		Enoxaparin 1 mg/kg SC q6–12 h [35,68]	
		Dalteparin 50 U/kg SC q12 h [69]	
		Enoxaparin 40–80 U/kg [70]	

aPTT = activated partial thromboplastin time; INR = international normalized ratio; PO = per os; PT = prothrombin time; SC = subcutaneous.

value [46]. These guidelines will vary depending on the type of machine used to measure aPTT, and using some methodologies, a prolongation closer to 1.2–1.5 times normal aPTT may be indicated [15]. Dosing regimens for UFH and LMWH in dogs and cats have been recently reviewed [36].

Fibrinolytic drugs

In animals that have developed venous or arterial thrombi, blood flow and oxygen delivery may be restored through the use of fibrinolytic drugs that encourage the dissolution of clots *in vivo*. The primary drugs that have been used for clot dissolution are tissue plasminogen activator (tPA) and streptokinase. Streptokinase is no longer available commercially in the United States. Tissue plasminogen activator is a potent activator of plasmin, which acts to break down fibrin into fibrinopeptides A and B. If the fibrin has been cross-linked by activated factor XIII, dissolution by plasmin also results in the generation of d-dimers [47]. Systemic administration of tPA can be associated with hemorrhage, and rapid reperfusion of thrombosed areas following tPA administration may lead to reperfusion injury. Because of these side-effects when administered systemically, more recent investigations have reported on the local administration of tPA using catheter-guided delivery. When used for clot dissolution in cats with aortic thromboembolism, approximately 50% of cats experienced rapid reperfusion of thrombosed limbs [48]. This percentage is similar to that reported for cats receiving supportive care (treatment of congestive heart failure, analgesia) without specific fibrinolytic therapy, and most cats experienced side-effects including azotemia, neurologic signs, and sudden death [48]. Tissue plasminogen activator usage has been infrequently reported in clinical dogs, although it has been used experimentally in a number of different circumstances [49]. Prior reports of streptokinase in cats with aortic thromboembolism resulted in similar survival and reperfusion rates [50].

Protein C, in conjunction with cofactor protein S, is a potent endogenous anticoagulant protein. Due to the hypercoagulability recognized in human patients with severe sepsis, an activated protein C (aPC) product (Xigris®, Eli Lilly) was released for clinical usage. This compound was to be administered to patients with severe sepsis and septic shock. Initial results were promising and suggested a positive effect on the survival statistics [51]. However, these results were not upheld in more recent trials and the drug was discontinued in 2012 [52]. Although aPC was tested in dogs, the short duration of effect, possible immunogenicity of a human protein, and cost limited its use.

Procoagulant therapies

There are very few procoagulant therapies available to the veterinarian. The majority are topical products including hemostatic gels and solubilized liquid thrombin which are applied directly to the source of hemorrhage. In patients with hemorrhage due to clotting factor deficiency, products such as fresh frozen plasma or stored plasma may be appropriate to restore clotting function. In patients with anticoagulant rodenticide toxicosis or some forms of hepatic disease (especially in cats), the administration of vitamin K (phytonadione) at 1–5 mg/kg/day either PO or SC may allow the body to restart production of necessary factors.

Another drug that is available to human medicine and which has been used in dogs to a small degree is recombinant activated factor VII (fVIIa; Novoseven®, Novo Nordisk, Denmark). Its mechanism is explained as follows: although physiologic levels of fVIIa only result in small amounts of thrombin, the larger dose used with rfVIIa results in sufficient thrombin formation to allow coagulation to proceed. Activated factor VII is indicated for the cessation of bleeding in patients with hemophilia or other coagulation factor deficiencies and has been used to correct hemostatic testing abnormalities in fVII-deficient Beagles [53]. In addition to these labeled human uses, fVIIa has also been used to stop bleeding in patients with severe trauma and coagulopathy [54]. In this context, it has been shown to be effective to stop or slow bleeding without a concomitant increase in the incidence of thrombosis. While this represents a possible indication for use of fVIIa in veterinary patients, the effectiveness of therapy and immunogenicity of the compound itself have not been extensively studied.

If an iatrogenic coagulopathy has developed secondary to the use of heparin molecules, protamine may be used to reverse the effects of heparin. Protamine forms 1:1 complexes with heparins (UFH more so than LMWH). When administered in excess, it may cause anticoagulation. Dosing recommendations are 1–1.5 mg of protamine per 100 units of heparin administered. Because heparin is rapidly metabolized, if 30 min have elapsed following heparin administration, the protamine dose is halved and then subsequently halved 30 min later [55]. Protamine may cause histamine release and hypotension or bradycardia if administered rapidly IV, and has sometimes been reported to cause fatal anaphylactic reactions in humans, which may be related to prior exposure to protamine-containing insulin products (e.g., protamine-zinc insulins) [56]. Although these reactions have not been reported in veterinary medicine, protamine should be administered slowly, especially in patients who may have prior sensitization.

Drugs that support coagulation

Other drugs may be used to augment coagulation by strengthening the fibrin clot. The lysine analogues aminocaproic acid (Amicar, Immunex) and tranexamic acid (Cyklokapron, Pfizer) are classified as antifibrinolytic agents because of their ability to limit clot breakdown in normal and pathologic circumstances. Both of these drugs work by occupying the lysine binding site on plasmin. This prevents its association with fibrin and consequently stabilizes the clot (plasmin binds to lysine residues on fibrin to initiate fibrinolysis). In the context of an overdose of fibrinolytic agents, lysine analogues may help to stabilize or prevent hemorrhage.

Antifibrinolytics (especially aminocaproic acid) are frequently used in equine nasal surgery, where extensive hemorrhage can occur [57]. Other authors have considered their use in dogs with hemoperitoneum or other conditions where the maintenance of clot integrity is critical [58]. Recent studies in Greyhounds have described the use of aminocaproic acid following elective surgeries due to the tendency of this breed to develop postoperative hemorrhage 48–72 h following surgery [59]. The authors hypothesized, based on the onset of hemorrhage, that the bleeding occurs due to breakdown of formed clots, and that Greyhounds may be hyperfibrinolytic in some circumstances. Further research is needed to define an effective dose and dosage regimen in small animal medicine.

References

1 McMichael M. New models of hemostasis. *Top Companion Anim Med* 2012; **27**: 40–45.
2 Smith SA. The cell-based model of coagulation. *J Vet Emerg Crit Care* 2009; **19**: 3–10.
3 Mann KG, Krishnaswamy S, Lawson JH. Surface-dependent hemostasis. *Semin Hematol* 1992; **29**: 213–226.
4 Kalafatis M. Coagulation factor V: a plethora of anticoagulant molecules. *Curr Opin Hematol* 2005; **12**: 141–148.
5 Dixon-Jimenez AC, Brainard BM, Cathcart CJ, *et al.* Evaluation of a point-of-care coagulation analyzer (Abaxis VSPro) for identification of coagulopathies in dogs. *J Vet Emerg Crit Care* 2013; **23**: 402–407.
6 De Laforcade AM. Diseases associated with thrombosis. *Top Companion Anim Med* 2012; **27**: 59–64.
7 Jessen LR, Wiinberg B, Kjelgaard-Hansen M, *et al.* Thrombin-activatable fibrinolysis inhibitor activity in healthy and diseased dogs. *Vet Clin Pathol* 2010; **39**: 296–301.
8 Born G, Patrono C. Antiplatelet drugs. *Br J Pharmacol* 2006; **147(Suppl 1)**: S241–251.
9 Jandrey KE. Assessment of platelet function. *J Vet Emerg Crit Care* 2012; **22**: 81–98.
10 Callan MB, Giger U. Assessment of a point-of-care instrument for identification of primary hemostatic disorders in dogs. *Am J Vet Res* 2001; **62**: 652–658.
11 Brooks M, Catalfamo J. Buccal mucosa bleeding time is prolonged in canine models of primary hemostatic disorders. *Thromb Haemost* 1993; **70**: 777–780.
12 Hogan DF, Andrews DA, Green HW, *et al.* Antiplatelet effects and pharmacodynamics of clopidogrel in cats. *J Am Vet Med Assoc* 2004; **225**: 1406–1411.
13 Babski DM, Brainard BM, Krimer PM, *et al.* Sonoclot evaluation of whole blood coagulation in healthy adult dogs. *J Vet Emerg Crit Care* 2012; **22**: 646–652.
14 Ganter MT, Hofer CK. Coagulation monitoring: current techniques and clinical use of viscoelastic point-of-care coagulation devices. *Anesth Analg* 2008; **106**: 1366–1375.
15 Babski DM, Brainard BM, Ralph AG, *et al.* Sonoclot(R) evaluation of single- and multiple-dose subcutaneous unfractionated heparin therapy in healthy adult dogs. *J Vet Intern Med* 2012; **26**: 631–638.
16 Epstein KL, Brainard BM, Lopes MA, *et al.* Thrombelastography in 26 healthy horses with and without activation by recombinant human tissue factor. *J Vet Emerg Crit Care* 2009; **19**: 96–101.
17 Banerjee A, Blois SL, Wood RD. Comparing citrated native, kaolin-activated, and tissue factor-activated samples and determining intraindividual variability for feline thromboelastography. *J Vet Diagn Invest* 2011; **23**: 1109–1113.
18 Mackman N. Triggers, targets and treatments for thrombosis. *Nature* 2008; **451**: 914–918.
19 Brainard BM, Meredith CP, Callan MB, *et al.* Changes in platelet function, hemostasis, and prostaglandin expression after treatment with nonsteroidal anti-inflammatory drugs with various cyclooxygenase selectivities in dogs. *Am J Vet Res* 2007; **68**: 251–257.
20 Cathcart CJ, Brainard BM, Reynolds LR, *et al.* Lack of inhibitory effect of acetylsalicylic acid and meloxicam on whole blood platelet aggregation in cats. *J Vet Emerg Crit Care* 2012; **22**: 99–106.
21 Johnson GJ, Leis LA, King RA. Thromboxane responsiveness of dog platelets is inherited as an autosomal recessive trait. *Thromb Haemost* 1991; **65**: 578–580.
22 Berent R, Sinzinger H. "Aspirin – resistance"? A few critical considerations on definition, terminology, diagnosis, clinical value, natural course of atherosclerotic disease, and therapeutic consequences. *Vasa* 2011; **40**: 429–438.
23 Smith SA, Tobias AH, Jacob KA, *et al.* Arterial thromboembolism in cats: acute crisis in 127 cases (1992–2001) and long-term management with low-dose aspirin in 24 cases. *J Vet Intern Med* 2003; **17**: 73–83.
24 Brainard BM, Epstein KL, LoBato D, *et al.* Effects of clopidogrel and aspirin on platelet aggregation, thromboxane production, and serotonin secretion in horses. *J Vet Intern Med* 2011; **25**: 116–122.
25 Brainard BM, Kleine SA, Papich MG, *et al.* Pharmacodynamic and pharmacokinetic evaluation of clopidogrel and the carboxylic acid metabolite SR 26334 in healthy dogs. *Am J Vet Res* 2010; **71**: 822–830.
26 Douglas IJ, Evans SJ, Hingorani AD, *et al.* Clopidogrel and interaction with proton pump inhibitors: comparison between cohort and within person study designs. *BMJ* 2012; **345**: e4388.
27 Vadasz D, Sztriha LK, Sas K, *et al.* Aspirin and clopidogrel resistance: possible mechanisms and clinical relevance. Part I: Concept of resistance. *Ideggyogy Sz* 2012; **65**: 377–385.
28 Palacio S, Hart RG, Pearce LA, *et al.* Effect of addition of clopidogrel to aspirin on mortality: systematic review of randomized trials. *Stroke* 2012; **43**: 2157–2162.
29 Waddell LS, Poppenga RH, Drobatz KJ. Anticoagulant rodenticide screening in dogs: 123 cases (1996–2003). *J Am Vet Med Assoc* 2013; **242**: 516–521.
30 Winter RL, Sedacca CD, Adams A, *et al.* Aortic thrombosis in dogs: presentation, therapy, and outcome in 26 cases. *J Vet Cardiol* 2012; **14**: 333–342.
31 Logan JC, Callan MB, Drew K, *et al.* Clinical indications for use of fresh frozen plasma in dogs: 74 dogs (October through December 1999). *J Am Vet Med Assoc* 2001; **218**: 1449–1455.
32 Brainard BM, Cathcart CJ, Dixon AC, *et al.* In vitro effects of rivaroxaban on feline coagulation indices (abstract). *J Vet Intern Med* 2011; **25**: 697.
33 Conversy B, Blais MC, Gara-Boivin C, *et al.* In vitro evaluation of the effect of rivaroxaban on coagulation parameters in healthy dogs (abstract). *J Vet Intern Med* 2012; **26**: 776.
34 Pittman JR, Koenig A, Brainard BM. The effect of unfractionated heparin on thrombelastographic analysis in healthy dogs. *J Vet Emerg Crit Care* 2010; **20**: 216–223.
35 Alwood AJ, Downend AB, Brooks MB, *et al.* Anticoagulant effects of low-molecular-weight heparins in healthy cats. *J Vet Intern Med* 2007; **21**: 378–387.
36 Brainard BM, Brown AJ. Defects in coagulation encountered in small animal critical care. *Vet Clin North Am Small Anim Pract* 2011; **41**: 783–803.
37 Kyles AE, Feldman EC, de Cock HE, *et al.* Surgical management of adrenal gland tumors with and without associated tumor thrombi in dogs: 40 cases (1994–2001). *J Am Vet Med Assoc* 2003; **223**: 654–662.
38 Moore JN, Mahaffey EA, Zboran M. Heparin-induced agglutination of erythrocytes in horses. *Am J Vet Res* 1987; **48**: 68–71.
39 Cuker A, Gimotty PA, Crowther MA, *et al.* Predictive value of the 4Ts scoring system for heparin-induced thrombocytopenia: a systematic review and meta-analysis. *Blood* 2012; **120**: 4160–4167.

40 Junqueira DR, Perini E, Penholati RR, *et al.* Unfractionated heparin versus low molecular weight heparin for avoiding heparin-induced thrombocytopenia in postoperative patients. *Cochrane Database Syst Rev* 2012; **9**: CD007557.
41 Morris TA, Marsh JJ, Konopka R, *et al.* Anti-thrombotic efficacies of enoxaparin, dalteparin, and unfractionated heparin in venous thrombo-embolism. *Thromb Res* 2000; **100**: 185–194.
42 Schwarzwald CC, Feige K, Wunderli-Allenspach H, *et al.* Comparison of pharmacokinetic variables for two low-molecular-weight heparins after subcutaneous administration of a single dose to horses. *Am J Vet Res* 2002; **63**: 868–873.
43 Fiakpui NN, Hogan DF, Whittem T, *et al.* Dose determination of fondaparinux in healthy cats. *Am J Vet Res* 2012; **73**: 556–561.
44 Monagle P, Chalmers E, Chan A, *et al.* Antithrombotic therapy in neonates and children: American College of Chest Physicians Evidence-Based Clinical Practice Guidelines (8th Edition). *Chest* 2008; **133**: 887S–968S.
45 Hirsh J, Bauer KA, Donati MB, *et al.* Parenteral anticoagulants: American College of Chest Physicians Evidence-Based Clinical Practice Guidelines (8th Edition). *Chest* 2008; **133**: 141S–159S.
46 Breuhl EL, Moore G, Brooks MB, *et al.* A prospective study of unfractionated heparin therapy in dogs with primary immune-mediated hemolytic anemia. *J Am Anim Hosp Assoc* 2009; **45**: 125–133.
47 Griffin A, Callan MB, Shofer FS, *et al.* Evaluation of a canine D-dimer point-of-care test kit for use in samples obtained from dogs with disseminated intravascular coagulation, thromboembolic disease, and hemorrhage. *Am J Vet Res* 2003; **64**: 1562–1569.
48 Welch KM, Rozanski EA, Freeman LM, *et al.* Prospective evaluation of tissue plasminogen activator in 11 cats with arterial thromboembolism. *J Feline Med Surg* 2010; **12**: 122–128.
49 Hong TT, Huang J, Lucchesi BR. Effect of thrombolysis on myocardial injury: recombinant tissue plasminogen activator vs. alfimeprase. *Am J Physiol Heart Circ Physiol* 2006; **290**: H959–967.
50 Moore KE, Morris N, Dhupa N, *et al.* Retrospective study of streptokinase administration in 46 cats with arterial thromboembolism. *J Vet Emerg Crit Care* 2000; **10**: 245–257.
51 Vincent JL, Angus DC, Artigas A, *et al.* Effects of drotrecogin alfa (activated) on organ dysfunction in the PROWESS trial. *Crit Care Med* 2003; **31**: 834–840.
52 Marti-Carvajal AJ, Sola I, Gluud C, *et al.* Human recombinant protein C for severe sepsis and septic shock in adult and paediatric patients. *Cochrane Database Syst Rev* 2012; **12**: CD004388.
53 Callan MB, Aljamali MN, Margaritis P, *et al.* A novel missense mutation responsible for factor VII deficiency in research Beagle colonies. *J Thromb Haemost* 2006; **4**: 2616–2622.
54 Sorensen B, Fries D. Emerging treatment strategies for trauma-induced coagulopathy. *Br J Surg* 2012; **99**(Suppl 1): 40–50.
55 Plumb DC. *Veterinary Drug Handbook*, 5th edn. Ames, IA: Blackwell, 2005.
56 Weiler JM, Freiman P, Sharath MD, *et al.* Serious adverse reactions to protamine sulfate: are alternatives needed? *J Allergy Clin Immunol.* 1985; **75**: 297–303.
57 Ross J, Dallap BL, Dolente BA, *et al.* Pharmacokinetics and pharmacodynamics of epsilon-aminocaproic acid in horses. *Am J Vet Res* 2007; **68**: 1016–1021.
58 Kelmer E, Marer K, Bruchim Y, *et al.* Retrospective evaluation of the safety and efficacy of tranexamic acid (Hexacapron) for the treatment of bleeding disorders in dogs (abstract). *J Vet Emerg Crit Care* 2011; **21**: S7.
59 Marin LM, Iazbik MC, Zaldivar-Lopez S, *et al.* Retrospective evaluation of the effectiveness of epsilon aminocaproic acid for the prevention of postamputation bleeding in retired racing Greyhounds with appendicular bone tumors: 46 cases (2003–2008). *J Vet Emerg Crit Care* 2012; **22**: 332–340.
60 Segura D, Monreal L, Espada Y, *et al.* Assessment of a platelet function analyser in horses: reference range and influence of a platelet aggregation inhibitor. *Vet J* 2005; **170**: 108–12.
61 Neff-Davis CA, Davis LE, Gillette EL. Warfarin in the dog: pharmacokinetics as related to clinical response. *J Vet Pharmacol Ther* 1981; **4**: 135–140.
62 Smith SA, Kraft SL, Lewis DC, *et al.* Pharmacodynamics of warfarin in cats. *J Vet Pharmacol Ther* 2000; **23**: 339–344.
63 Feige K, Schwarzwald CC, Bombeli T. Comparison of unfractioned and low molecular weight heparin for prophylaxis of coagulopathies in 52 horses with colic: a randomised double-blind clinical trial. *Equine Vet J* 2003; **35**: 506–513.
64 Mischke R, Grebe S, Jacobs C, *et al.* Amidolytic heparin activity and values for several hemostatic variables after repeated subcutaneous administration of high doses of a low molecular weight heparin in healthy dogs. *Am J Vet Res* 2001; **62**: 595–598.
65 Mischke R, Grebe S. The correlation between plasma anti-factor Xa activity and haemostatic tests in healthy dogs, following the administration of a low molecular weight heparin. *Res Vet Sci* 2000; **69**: 241–247.
66 Lunsford KV, Mackin AJ, Langston VC, *et al.* Pharmacokinetics of subcutaneous low molecular weight heparin (enoxaparin) in dogs. *J Am Anim Hosp Assoc* 2009; **45**: 261–267.
67 Mischke R, Schmitt J, Wolken S, *et al.* Pharmacokinetics of the low molecular weight heparin dalteparin in cats. *Vet J* 2012; **192**: 299–303.
68 Van de Wiele CM, Hogan DF, Green HW , *et al.* Antithrombotic effect of enoxaparin in clinically healthy cats: a venous stasis model. *J Vet Intern Med* 2010; **24**: 185–191.
69 Whelchel DD, Tennent-Brown BS, Giguere S, Epstein KL. Pharmacodynamics of multi-dose low molecular weight heparin in healthy horses. *Vet Surg* 2013; **42**(4): 448–454.
70 Schwarzwald CC, Feige K, Wunderli-Allenspach H, *et al.* Comparison of pharmacokinetic variables for two low-molecular-weight heparins after subcutaneous administration of a single dose to horses. *Am J Vet Res* 2002; **63**: 868–873.

21 Clinical Pharmacology and Administration of Fluid, Electrolyte, and Blood Component Solutions

Amandeep S. Chohan[1] and Elizabeth B. Davidow[2]

[1]Veterinary Teaching Hospital, Washington State University, Pullman, Washington, USA
[2]ACCES BluePearl, Seattle, Washington, USA

Chapter contents

Physiology of body fluids

The body is principally composed of water, a triatomic molecule composed of two hydrogen molecules bound by covalent bonds to one oxygen molecule (H-O-H). Water behaves like a charged molecule; a dipole created by negatively charged oxygen and positively charged hydrogen. This polarity is responsible for imparting many of water's chemical and physical properties such as high surface tension, high specific heat, high heat of vaporization, low vapor pressure, and a high boiling point. Because of water's ionizing nature, substances dissolved in water segregate into individual components. Water also exists in an ionized form, composed of a negatively charged hydroxyl ion (OH^-) and a positively charged protonated ion (H_3O^+). The aqueous milieu created by water provides the framework where all the metabolic and enzymatic processes take place.

Total body water

Water is the single most abundant compound in the body, making up the majority of body weight. On average, water constitutes approximately 60% of adult mammalian body weight. Age, body composition, and sex can influence total body water (TBW). Neonatal animals have greater TBW compared to adults (80% vs 60%) and an age-related decrease has been described in companion animals during the first six months of age [1]. Adipose tissue has less water content compared to lean body tissues like muscle, so estimation of TBW needs to consider body condition since obesity can lead to overestimation.

To understand distribution of body water, the body fluids can be thought of as existing in two major compartments (i.e., intracellular [ICF] and extracellular [ECF] fluid compartments). Extracellular fluid can be further divided into two compartments: the interstitial fluid (ISF; that surround the cells) and intravascular fluid (IVF; fluid contained within the vessels) compartments. The largest volume of water in the body is contained within the cells, making ICF the largest contributor to body weight. Of TBW, about two-thirds (i.e., 40% of body weight) is ICF. The remaining one-third of TBW (i.e., 20% of body weight) is ECF where it is distributed between ISF and IVF in a ratio of 3:1. About three-quarters of ECF (i.e., 15% of body weight) is ISF that bathes the cells and one-quarter of ECF (i.e., 5% of body weight) is IVF (i.e., plasma volume).

Solute composition of various body fluid compartments

In addition to water, body fluid compartments also contain varying concentrations of different solutes (Table 21.1). This heterogeneity is because the membranes separating fluid compartments have different permeability characteristics for various solutes. The ICF and ECF are separated by cell membranes, while capillary endothelium separates

Veterinary Anesthesia and Analgesia: The Fifth Edition of Lumb and Jones.
Edited by Kurt A. Grimm, Leigh A. Lamont, William J. Tranquilli, Stephen A. Greene and Sheilah A. Robertson.

Table 21.1 Solute composition of various body compartments.

Ions (mEq/L)	Extracellular (ECF)		Intracellular (ICF)
	Interstitial (ISF)	Intravascular (plasma, IVF)	
Na^+	145	142	12
K^+	4	5	140
Ca^{2+}	2	2	4
Mg^{2+}	2	2	34
Cl^-	112	104	4
HCO_3^-	27	24	12
HPO_4^{2-}, $H_2PO_4^-$	2	2	40
Protein⁻	1	14	50

ISF and IVF. Endothelium is freely permeable to water and various ionic solutes and the concentration of these is similar in ISF and IVF. On the other hand, the cell membrane is freely permeable to water but by utilizing various carrier proteins, active transport and passive diffusion mechanisms maintain a specific intracellular milieu, resulting in very different solute concentrations in ICF compared to ECF (Table 21.1). Gibbs–Donnan equilibrium results in slightly different concentrations of cations and anions in the ISF and IVF (i.e., plasma) but clinically this difference is negligible and plasma concentration of various ions is considered a reflection of ECF solute concentrations. The major cation in ECF is Na^+ with Cl^- and HCO_3^- being the most abundant anions. In contrast, the major cations in ICF are K^+ and Mg^{2+} and most common anions are organic phosphates and proteins.

Movement of water between intracellular (ICF) and extracellular (ECF) fluid compartments

Movement of water between ICF and ECF is governed by the osmotic gradient created by the differing concentrations of solutes between these two fluid compartments. The different concentrations of solutes within a solution determine osmolality. It is dependent only on the number of particles in solution and not on their chemical formula, valence, molecular weight or size. Osmotic pressure due to solutes is expressed as milliosmoles per kilogram of water (mOsm/kg). In biologic fluids, difference between osmolarity and osmolality is not significant and the milliosmolar concentration of a solution can be expressed as milliosmolarity or milliosmolality of solution.

Osmolality (i.e., the number of osmotically active particles) in part determines the volume of water in ECF and ICF. Solutes that cannot cross cell membrane contribute to effective osmolality (or tonicity) and are called 'effective osmoles.' On the other hand, solutes that can freely diffuse across the cell membrane (like urea) are called 'ineffective osmoles' and do not contribute to fluid shifts across cell membranes since they are in equilibrium on both sides of the semi-permeable membrane. Osmosis is the movement of water across the semi-permeable membrane from an area of lower (low solute concentration) to higher (high solute concentration) osmotic pressure.

In both the plasma and interstitial fluid, osmolality is mainly the result of ions such as Na^+, K^+, Cl^-, HCO_3^-, glucose, and urea. Large molecules like albumin, though a hugely important component of colloid osmotic pressure (COP), contribute little to the osmolality. Being the most abundant cation in ECF, Na^+ and its associated anions are the major players responsible for ECF osmolality. Glucose constitutes another effective osmole by not being freely permeable through cell membranes, but urea is not an effective osmole because it is freely permeable across cell membranes. ECF osmolality (essentially the plasma osmolality) can be estimated by using the following formula:

$$\text{Plasma osmolaity (mOsm/kg)} = 2[(\text{Na+}) + (\text{K+})] + [(\text{Glucose})/18 + [\text{BUN}]/2.8$$

When the concentrations of various solutes on either side of the cell membrane are not disturbed (e.g., equilibrium), the fluid is in osmotic equilibrium (same osmolality) and there is no gradient for the movement of water between the two fluid compartments. If there is extracellular loss of free water, the concentration of solutes increases in the ECF, leading to generation of higher osmolality (i.e., osmotic pressure) compared to ICF, resulting in osmotic pull causing net movement (osmosis) of water through the cell membrane into the ECF until a new osmotic equilibrium is achieved. Hence water is lost from the ICF to replace ECF free water deficit.

Osmolality can be either measured or calculated (as described earlier). Osmolality is measured clinically by freezing point depression of a serum sample. Normal serum osmolality is around 300 mOsm/kg. Clinically, the measured osmolality may not be equal to the calculated value and the difference between the two (osmolal gap) can be used to predict the presence of unmeasured solutes.

Fluid shifts between intravascular (IVF; plasma) and interstitial (ISF) fluid compartments

Fluid shifts between IVF (plasma) and ISF compartments occur at the level of capillaries. The fundamental principles that govern movement were described by Starling in 1896 [2]. Fluid movement across the capillary wall is determined by the imbalance between the osmotic absorption pressure created by plasma proteins [colloid osmotic pressure (COP)] and the capillary hydrostatic pressure. The capillary endothelial barrier slowly leaks plasma proteins into ISF. Staverman's osmotic reflection coefficient, σ, can be used to quantify the degree of leakiness of capillary membrane to any particular solute. It ranges from 1 (i.e., 100% reflection or not permeable) to 0 (i.e., no reflection or completely permeable). For a membrane separating solutions of a single solute at two different concentrations, the principle of irreversible thermodynamics states that:

$$\frac{Jv}{A} = Lp[\Delta P - \sigma\Delta\Pi]$$

where Jv is the volume filtration rate per unit membrane area A, Lp represents the hydraulic permeability, ΔP the difference in hydrostatic pressures, and $\Delta\Pi$ the difference in osmotic pressures across the membrane.

Intravascular fluid and ISF each contain many solutes (species 'n'). Therefore, to describe the movement of fluid across the capillary wall, the above equation can be written as:

$$\frac{Jv}{A} = Lp[\Delta P - \sum_{i=1}^{n} \sigma n \Delta\Pi n]$$

where $\sum_{i=1}^{n} \sigma n \Delta\Pi n$ represents the sum of the difference in osmotic pressure exerted across the capillary wall by all the solutes in IVF and ISF. In the above equation ΔP describes the difference between local capillary blood pressure (Pc) and ISF hydrostatic pressure (Pi). In most microvascular beds the capillary wall is freely permeable to water and other ionic solutes like Na^+, K^+ and glucose because of their very small σ of ≤ 0.1. In other words, they are ineffective osmoles in this scenario and do not contribute to water distribution between ISF and IVF. Only the macromolecular solutes (like proteins) with high σ, and which are present in significantly different concentrations across the capillary wall, will contribute towards generation of osmotic gradients ($\sigma\Delta\Pi$). If Πp is the osmotic pressure generated by plasma proteins (COP) in IVF and Πi is the osmotic pressure generated by macromolecules in ISF then the above equation can be written as the conventional expression for Starling's equation as below:

$$\frac{Jv}{A} = Lp\,[(Pc - Pi) - \sigma\,(\Pi p - \Pi i)]$$

Under normal circumstances Pc is much greater than Pi, producing a hydrostatic pressure gradient at the arterial end that favors movement of fluid out of the capillary into the interstitium. Pc is decreased from arteriolar to venous end of the capillary while the Πp stays almost the same, resulting in an oncotic pressure gradient that favors the movement of fluid from the interstitium into the capillaries at the venous end [3]. Altogether there is a net filtration pressure that is responsible for the movement of water out of the capillaries into the interstitium. Some of the filtered fluid is normally returned back to the circulation via the lymphatic system.

Endothelial glycocalyx model of transvascular fluid exchange and modification of starling's equation

As the understanding of microcapillary structure has evolved, it has been proposed that the filtration properties of the capillary wall actually reside in an endothelial glycocalyx layer (EGL) that is a matrix of molecular fibers. The matrix covers the intercellular clefts and the endothelial cells on the luminal side of the capillaries [4, 5]. Traditional Starling's forces describe that the fluid filtered at the arteriolar end of the capillary is absorbed back into the circulation at the venous end under the influence of the dominant osmotic pressure gradient generated by the difference, $\Pi p - \Pi i$. Recently it was shown that the effect of Πi on fluid exchange at the capillary level is much less than predicted by Starling's original equation. It is now established that many capillaries filter fluid into the ISF throughout their length and absorption at the venous end of the capillaries does not take place. Plasma protein oncotic pressure (COP) opposes this filtration but does not change the direction of net filtration (i.e., filtration is always occurring towards the ISF). Most of the filtered fluid returns to the circulation via lymphatics. The endothelial glycocalyx layer separates plasma from a subglycocalyx space that contains a very small amount of protein. This subglycocalyx COP (Πg) should replace Πi in the Starling's equation to determine the transcapillary flow (Jv):

$$\frac{Jv}{A} = Lp\,[(Pc - Pi) - \sigma\,(\Pi p - \Pi g)]$$

Low protein concentration in the subglycocalyx space results in a low value of Πg causing a higher value for ($\Pi p - \Pi g$), in other words a bigger opposing force against the transcapillary flow (Jv) that occurs under the influence of difference in hydrostatic pressures around the capillary membrane (Pc – Pi). The fact that the low value of Πg results in low Jv, combined with the importance of lymph flow in various tissues as a major factor to return fluid back into circulation, are two critical features on which the glycocalyx model of transvascular fluid exchange is based.

An index of vascular permeability is transcapillary escape rate of albumin (TCERA). In humans it is about 5% of the plasma albumin per hour. This rate could double during surgery or increase 20% or more in septic patients. Evidence points to a compromised EGL in those patients. Loss of plasma albumin causes reduction in Πp leading to increase in Jv. Increasing the Πp (COP) in septic patients with colloids will decrease Jv and prolongs vascular expansion compared to crystalloids.

Different types of fluids used in clinical practice

Crystalloids

Crystalloid solutions are prepared by dissolving crystalline compounds in water. Most of the clinically used crystalloids are either polyionic sodium-based or dextrose solutions in water. Crystalloids are classified mostly based on their tonicity relative to plasma.

Isotonic crystalloids have similar tonicity/osmolality compared to the plasma. This means that administration of isotonic fluids will not cause any change in the solute concentration of the extracellular fluid. There will not be any alteration in the net osmotic forces that might trigger the water movement between ICF and ECF. Hence, the isotonic crystalloid fluid will stay within the ECF and no alteration in ICF volume will take place unless previous free water loss occurred from the ICF compartment. After intravenous administration, isotonic crystalloids stay within the ECF and redistribute into the IVF and ISF. This redistribution occurs according to the normal fluid distribution in the body so that within 30–60 min post infusion only about one-quarter of the administered amount remains intravascular and the rest moves out to the ISF [6,7]. The most commonly used isotonic fluids and their constituents can be found in Table 21.2.

Isotonic fluids contain mixtures of various electrolytes found in plasma in combination with or without components which affect the acid–base status of the patient. Some of these crystalloids contain dextrose. Except for physiological saline (0.9% NaCl) most of the

Table 21.2 Characteristics of various isotonic crystalloids compared to plasma.

Fluid (isotonic, replacement)	Electrolytes (mEq/L)					Buffers (mEq/L)			Osmolarity (mOsm/L)	pH
	Na^+	Cl^-	K^+	Ca^{2+}	Mg^{2+}	Lactate	Acetate	Gluconate		
0.9% NaCl	154	154	0	0	0	0	0	0	308	5.0
Lactated Ringer's solution	130	109	4	3	0	28	0	0	272	6.5
Plasmalyte148®	140	98	5	0	3	0	27	23	294	5.5
Normosol-R®	140	98	5	0	3	0	27	23	294	6.4
Plasma-Lyte A®	140	98	5	0	3	0	27	23	294	
Plasma	142	104	5	5	3		$HCO_3^- = 24$		300	7.4

commonly used crystalloids contain a precursor for bicarbonate production such as lactate or acetate and gluconate ions (lactated Ringer's solution [LRS] or Normosol® and Plasmalyte®, respectively). Lactate ions undergo either oxidation or gluconeogenesis primarily in the liver, although kidneys and muscle tissues also participate to some extent. During glycogenesis lactate is converted to glucose via pyruvate and this process utilizes H^+. So lactate also has a bicarbonate-sparing effect. Acetate is metabolized mostly in muscles and gluconate can be metabolized by most tissues. Because these crystalloids increase bicarbonate level in the plasma they have been called 'alkalinizing fluids.' 0.9% sodium chloride, on the other hand, is an 'acidifying solution' due to plasma bicarbonate dilution (dilutional acidosis) and high Cl^- content that can decrease strong ion difference and cause hyperchloremic metabolic acidosis [8–10]. Composition of some of these crystalloids more closely matches plasma (e.g., LRS, Plasmalyte 148®, Normosol-R®) compared to others (e.g., 0.9% NaCl) and they are considered balanced isotonic crystalloids in comparison to unbalanced crystalloids. Another way of looking at these crystalloids is from the standpoint of their clinical use. Most of the isotonic crystalloids, because of their similar osmolality and solute composition to plasma, do not cause osmotic water shift from blood cells to plasma and can be used for emergency volume resuscitation and are therefore called 'replacement fluids.'

To understand the clinical use of various crystalloids, it is imperative to understand which body compartment is deficient in the fluid (perfusion vs hydration) [11]. When isotonic crystalloids are used for replenishment of intravascular fluid and electrolyte deficits, about 75% of the fluid redistributes to ISF. Therefore relatively large volumes are usually administered to replenish intravascular deficits. In dogs Silverstein *et al.* demonstrated the potential of isotonic fluids to increase the blood volume [12]. Immediately following the infusion of fluid the blood volume increased by 76%, more than 3–4.5 times the increase following hypertonic fluid and colloids. However, at 30 min post infusion the increase was only 35%. The initial increase in blood volume was attributed to the greater volume of isotonic crystalloids administered. More importantly, the authors also calculated the efficacy ratio (ER; increase in blood volume compared to the volume of fluid infused) and isotonic fluid had an ER of only 0.4 at 30 min post infusion. Typically 3–4 times the volume of fluids is recommended to replenish the intravascular deficit.

Shock, hemorrhage, and severe volume deficit due to diarrhea, vomiting, excessive diuresis or third spacing constitute common scenarios when these fluids are administered. Crystalloids are also administered during most elective surgery procedures in healthy patients. It is often recommended that patients with shock should receive up to one blood volume (e.g., 80–90 mL/kg in dogs) in an hour, starting with one-quarter to one-third of the shock dose given incrementally with constant monitoring for desired endpoints to guide fluid therapy further (i.e., goal-directed fluid therapy). A typical fluid rate used for patients under general anesthesia is 5–10 mL/kg/h [13,14], although recent trends have been to reduce these rates further in patients without risk factors for perioperative fluid loss.

Slight variability in composition and concentration of various solutes (electrolytes and buffers) in different isotonic crystalloids (see Table 21.2) may make administration of one solution preferable in certain clinical situations. Patients with hypochloremic metabolic alkalosis and hypercalcemia may benefit from the use of 0.9% saline [15,16]. Alkalinizing fluids are not used very commonly in adult dehydrated cattle because metabolic acidosis is not a common occurrence except in cases of grain overload, hepatic lipidosis, chronic ketosis or kidney disease [17,18]. Patients that are acidotic may benefit from the use of alkalinizing fluids. Lactated Ringer's solution can contain either a racemic mixture of L- and D-lactate or just L-lactate. Fluids containing acetate might have a more profound alkalinizing effect, as dogs cannot metabolize D-lactate as readily [15].

Various isotonic crystalloids have different Na^+ ion concentrations, giving them a range of osmolalities (see Table 21.2). In severe electrolyte disturbances it is recommended to use a fluid with Na^+ concentration closest to the patient's for resuscitation to avoid rapid changes in Na^+ ion concentration (Na^+ concentration should not change more than 0.5–1 mEq/L/h). While resuscitating patients with head trauma or cerebral edema, replacement crystalloid solutions with the highest Na^+ concentration (i.e., 0.9% NaCl) will be least likely to reduce plasma osmolality that might favor the movement of water into brain cells. With a Na^+ content of 130 mEq/L, LRS is relatively hypotonic compared to plasma and has been associated with increased ICP in some models of traumatic brain injury [19,20].

Interstitial fluid accumulation/edema can occur after excessive fluid administration, especially in patients suffering from oliguric renal failure, cardiac insufficiency, head trauma, pulmonary contusions or decreased colloidal osmotic pressure. In clinical scenarios characterized by active intracavitary (abdominal or thoracic) or intracranial bleeding, aggressive fluid administration to achieve normotensive resuscitation endpoints before surgical control of bleeding is achieved could lead to increased hydrostatic pressure that might lead to disruption of blood clots and worsening of bleeding. 'Hypotensive' fluid resuscitation is often advocated in these patients, aiming to achieve the lower limit of clinically acceptable mean arterial pressure (60 mmHg, corresponding to perfusion pressure of various vital organ systems). Others suggest delayed fluid resuscitation until hemostasis is achieved; however, the risk of anesthetizing hemodynamically unstable patients should be weighed against the perceived risk of volume resuscitation. The veterinarian should also be cognizant of the possibility of excessive hemodilution of clotting factors, platelets, plasma protein, and red blood cells when large volumes of fluid are administered [6,7,21]. This may be even more relevant in patients undergoing surgical procedures associated with more blood loss or patients that already have pre-existing coagulopathies, hypoproteinemia or anemia.

Due to the presence of Ca^{2+} ions in LRS, it is recommended that blood products not be administered in the same fluid line since Ca^{2+} may antagonize common anticoagulants, leading to microemboli. Studies have concluded that rapid transfusion rates for whole blood (WB) or packed red blood cells (PRBCs) can be safely used with LRS [22] and that LRS can be safely used to dilute citrate phosphate dextrose (CPD) preserved PRBCs in emergency settings [23]. Because of the liver's major contribution to lactate metabolism, there has been some concern about use of LRS in patients with hepatic insufficiency. However, studies have failed to show any increase in blood lactate levels after LRS administration [24,25]. Hyperlactatemia is common in cancer patients due to use of anaerobic glycolysis by neoplastic cells, but a study in dogs suffering from lymphoma showed only a transient increase in lactate levels that became normal after 2 h of infusion [26]. Large quantities of rapidly administered acetate solutions can cause vasodilation due to release of adenosine from muscles that could cause hypotension, especially in hypovolemic patients [27–29].

Hypertonic crystalloids

Hypertonic solutions have an increased tonicity/osmolality compared to plasma. Administration of hypertonic fluids will increase osmotic pressure in the IVF and sets up a gradient for the movement of water from ISF as well as ICF (with lesser osmotic pressure; lower solute concentration). The most commonly used hypertonic fluids in clinical practice are hypertonic saline solutions (HSS; Table 21.3). The reflection coefficient of Na^+ for cell membrane is maintained close to 1, probably by the constant actions of the Na^+/K^+ ATPase pump whereas the reflection coefficient of the endothelial membrane is only 0.1. This means that most of the movement of water after HSS administration is from the ICF rather than ISF [30]. Hence, fluid is pulled out of the cells (cellular dehydration) and interstitium into the intravascular space. Analysis of transcapillary driving pressures (governed by Starling's forces) supports an immediate plasma volume expansion under the effect of HSS that rapidly reverses the transcapillary pressure gradient from a small filtration force under normal physiologic conditions to a large absorptive force (osmotic pressure gradient). Due to a very low reflection coefficient of capillary endothelium for Na^+, the generated osmotic pressure is transmitted across the capillary endothelium to the cell membrane and is responsible for pulling the water out of cells. As HSS itself does little to address TBW deficits, it is imperative that hypertonic therapy should be followed by administration of appropriate follow-up fluids (isotonic crystalloids, colloids or blood products). In cattle it was recommended that after using hypertonic fluids it is important to administer fluids oro-ruminally if the animal does not consume more than 5 gallons of fluid orally [17,31]. HSS are unbalanced crystalloids and are available in various concentrations having very high osmolality compared to plasma (see Table 21.3). Clinically 7.5% HSS is most commonly used. Although mannitol is also another hyperosmotic agent, its osmotic effects are typically delayed by 15–30 min [32] and effects are not as profound as 7.5% NaCl because its osmolarity is only half (1250 mOsm/L for 25% mannitol) as much. The discussion here will focus on HSS only.

In hypovolemic animals (hemorrhagic shock models) plasma volume expansion at the end of a HSS bolus/infusion given over 1–10 min at a dose of 4–8 mL/kg varied from 10 to 21 mL/kg with higher doses causing more volume expansion. However, HSS quickly equilibrated within ECF so that after 1–3 h there was minimal plasma volume expansion [33–36]. In normovolemic dogs Silverstein *et al.* showed that the efficacy ratio (defined as relative increase in blood volume in relation to the volume infused) was maximum with HSS immediately post infusion (2.7 ± 0.5; approximately three times that of other fluid types) and was still higher at 30 min post infusion compared to isotonic crystalloids and synthetic colloids [12]. In order to prolong the duration of effect, HSS was combined with a colloid (6% dextran 70 [HSD]) that not only increased the extent of immediate plasma volume expansion but

Table 21.3 Characteristics of various hypertonic saline solutions compared to plasma.

Composition	Hypertonic saline solutions					Normal saline	Plasma
	3%	5%	7.2%	7.5%	23%	0.9%	
Na^+ (mEq/L)	513	856	1232	1283	4004	154	142
Cl^- (mEq/L)	513	856	1232	1283	4004	154	104
Osmolarity (mOsm/L)	1026	1712	1464	2566	8008	308	300

the plasma volume expansion persisted 3 h later [34,35]. Other available colloids like hydroxyethyl starch (HES) can also be combined with HSS. This hypertonic-hyperoncotic combination constitutes 'small-volume fluid resuscitation' [17]. Usually it is constituted by diluting 23.4% HSS with the colloid in the ratio of 1:2.5 or the two can be used separately (2–6 mL/kg of 7% HSS + 4–10 mL of colloid) [17,31].

Cardiovascular effects of HSS administration are characterized by increase in preload, heart rate, and myocardial contractility and decrease in systemic vascular resistance, all of which work together to increase cardiac output [37–39]. Beneficial immunomodulatory effects have been described characterized by decreased interaction of neutrophils with endothelial cells, reduced neutrophilic activation and improved activity of lymphocytes and natural killer T cells [40–42]. HSS has also been shown to reduce cytotoxic edema and improve splanchnic and muscle capillary perfusion in animal injury models of soft tissue contusions, hemorrhagic shock, and superior mesenteric artery occlusion [43–47].

Most of the clinical and experimental literature on HSS/HSD suggests its application in the management of hemorrhagic hypovolemic shock [33–36,48,49]. Another area where HSS has been shown to be beneficial is in the management of intracranial hypertension. Although brain trauma management foundation guidelines [50] still recommend mannitol as the hyperosmolar therapy of choice (Level II evidence), new evidence has been emerging that shows hypertonic saline to be a better choice [51–56]. Benefits of hypertonic resuscitation have also been documented in the canine model of gastric dilation/volvulus-induced obstructive shock [57], canine model of bile-induced pancreatitis [58], and murine models of acute pancreatitis [59,60]

Large animal practice has found HSS/HSD to be particularly helpful where the patient's large blood volume makes volume expansion challenging. Oral rehydration therapy has been suggested as acceptable if the calf or cattle is <8% dehydrated, but a combination of HSS intravenous therapy plus oral rehydration was shown to be successful if dehydration was ≥8% [17,31]. Use of hypertonic-hyperoncotic resuscitation has been described in horses with endotoxemia [61,62], in calves with endotoxemia [63], diarrhea [64–66] and in adult endotoxemic cattle [67].

Use of HSS in patients with uncontrolled hemorrhage can lead to increased bleeding and worsened outcome compared to isotonic resuscitation. However, studies demonstrate that if the hemorrhage is controlled then HSS can improve hemodynamic variables and final outcomes [68–70]. It has been shown that if a bolus of hypertonic-hyperoncotic fluid (4 mL/kg) is administered slowly (over about 12 min) compared to 1 min, blood loss was significantly reduced and survival improved [69,71].

Pre-existing dehydration has been suggested as a contraindication to administration of HSS because a dehydrated intracellular environment could decrease the efficacy of intravascular hypertonic fluid resuscitation. Studies performed in dehydrated hemorrhagic swine [72] and sheep [73,74] models with preinfusion plasma osmolalities of 325–340 mOsm/L showed that administration of 4 mL/kg of 7.5% NaCl achieved hemodynamic stability and increase in plasma volume similar to euvolemic animals. When a rapid onset of action is desired, HSS in fact can be considered as an adjunct with isotonic resuscitation to correct hypovolemia in dehydrated patients. A recent study in endurance horses showed that horses resuscitated with 2 liters of HSS followed by 5 liters of isotonic saline achieved normal PCV and TP compared to horses that received 7 liters of 0.9% sodium chloride alone and had a residual hemoconcentration [75]. Keeping in mind the diuresis that occurs after HSS administration and mobilization of intracellular fluid to intravascular space with the potential to be filtered, the possibility of subsequent dehydration must be considered in veterinary patients, especially when appropriate follow-up fluid administration is delayed or impossible (e.g., some field conditions).

Hypertonic saline solution has been associated with cardiac arrhythmias, bradycardia, hypotension, and volume overload. Such effects are noted mostly when high doses of higher concentration HSS are administered at a very fast rate [76]. The recommended administration regimen of 7.5% NaCl at a dose of 4–6 mL/kg given at a rate no faster than 1 mL/kg/min is not usually associated with complications. Use of recommended doses rarely causes any consistent blood chemistry abnormalities but the potential for hypernatremia, hyperchloremic metabolic acidosis, hyperosmolar renal failure, and hypokalemia should be considered especially if pre-existing electrolytic abnormalities or repeated dosing with HSS are considered [8–10,21]. Ajito *et al.* [77] administered doses of 2.5, 5, and 15 mL/kg of 7.2% NaCl at a rate of 1.6 mL/kg/min to anesthetized beagle dogs. Administering 5 mL/kg caused only transient elevations in Na^+ (153 at 3 min; 165 at 5 min; baseline 142) that stayed below 160 mEq/L at the end of infusion whereas a dose of 15 mL/kg lead to consistent hypernatremia (161 to 174 mEq/L) from 10 min to 90 min after initiation of infusion. A study conducted in dogs showed that the maximum tolerated dose of 7.5% NaCl was 20 mL/kg, although that dose caused transient neurological signs like pacing and lethargy which resolved within 24 h [78].

Hypotonic crystalloids

Hypotonic crystalloid solutions have lower tonicity/osmolality than plasma (Table 21.4). Dextrose in water is a source of free water because the dextrose is metabolized leaving water which is free of osmotic particles. Dextrose administration decreases ECF solute concentration compared to ICF, creating an osmotic pressure gradient for movement of water from the ECF to ICF (cellular swelling). Less than 10% of infused hypotonic fluid remains in the IVF space after 30–60 min. Due to their large volume of distribution and potential for cellular swelling, hypotonic fluids are not indicated for intravenous volume replenishment. They are used mostly to replenish maintenance needs of patients in which water intake is absent because they are anorexic (no feed intake), unable to drink and/or fluid losses are not beyond normal physiologic losses (unlike vomiting, diarrhea, etc.) [79].

Maintenance fluid requirements can be calculated in several ways [80,81]. The simple empirical formula of 40 mL/kg/day (in large dogs) or 60 mL/kg/day (small dogs and cats) can be used. Since water requirements are tied to metabolism, daily maintenance energy expenditure (and water requirement) may be calculated as 140 kcal × body weight $(kg)^{0.75}$ [80]. Another formula used to calculate maintenance water requirement is [30 × body weight (kg)] + 70 but if the patient weight is less than 2 kg or more than 50 kg then it is proposed to use the caloric requirement to calculate the maintenance fluid requirements [80,81]. One milliliter of water is required for every kcal of energy consumed. The ongoing physiologic fluid losses may consist of insensible (feces, saliva, skin, and respiratory tract) and/or sensible (urinary) losses. These losses are typically hypotonic in nature with low Na^+ and high K^+ compared to that of ECF [81]. Hypotonic fluids are manufactured to match this composition (Table 21.4). In patients with normal renal function, isotonic replacement fluids with some added K^+ can also be used for maintenance purposes because kidneys can excrete excess electrolytes. Other major indications involve free water supplementation (e.g., hypernatremia, diabetes insipidus) and dextrose supplementation during hypoglycemia.

It is important to administer these fluids at a slower rate so that sudden and excessive dilution of plasma solutes is avoided as the reduced ECF osmolality could cause cellular swelling (cerebral edema). It is advisable to monitor electrolytic concentrations in patients receiving hypotonic fluids.

Synthetic colloids

Colloids are composed of macromolecular particles suspended in a crystalloid fluid solution. In the absence of increased microvascular permeability, their movement is limited across the endothelium and they are less able to accumulate in the interstitium. This results in a longer dwell time within the IVF compartment compared to crystalloids, and they can pull fluid into the IVF compartment based on their oncotic properties. Colloidal oncotic pressure is the osmotic pressure generated by the colloids in solution and is determined by the number of particles rather than their size. In clinical practice colloids are mostly used in patients requiring oncotic support (hypoproteinemia) to prevent interstitial fluid accumulation or in hypovolemic patients as a resuscitative fluid [82–87]. Colloidal preparations can be classified as consisting of blood component products or synthetic compounds composed of three major groups: the HES derivatives, dextrans, and gelatins. Most of the following discussion revolves around hydroxyethyl starch solutions due to their common use in clinical practice, but some basics about dextrans and gelatins have also been presented.

Table 21.4 Characteristics of commonly available hypotonic crystalloids compared to plasma.

Fluid	Electrolytes (mEq/L)					Buffers (mEq/L)			Osmolarity (mOsm/L)	pH	Glucose (g/L)
	Na^+	Cl^-	K^+	Ca^{2+}	Mg^{2+}	Lactate	Acetate	Gluconate			
0.45 % NaCl	77	77	0	0	0	0	0	0	154	5.0	0
0.45 % NaCl with 2.5% dextrose	77	77	0	0	0	0	0	0	280	4.5	25
Plasmalyte-M® with 5% dextrose	40	40	16	5	3	12	12	0	376	5.5	50
Normosol-M® with 5% dextrose	40	40	13	0	3	0	16	0	364	5.5	50
Dextrose 5%	0	0	0	0	0	0	0	0	252	4.0	50
Plasma	142	104	5	5	3		HCO_3^- = 24		300	7.4	

Hydroxyethyl starches

Hydroxyethyl starches (HES) are the synthetic colloid preparations most commonly used in both human and veterinary medicine. Chemically HES preparations are modified polymers of amylopectin, a polysaccharide very similar to glycogen. The polymers are suspended in saline or a balanced electrolyte crystalloid solution. Different preparations of HES with variable structural characteristics (Table 21.5) have different physicochemical properties governed by three main variables: mean molecular weight (MW), molar substitution (MS), and C2:C6 ratio. It is important to understand these differences in order to appreciate the clinical variability with respect to pharmacokinetics, pharmacodynamics and adverse effect profile of various HES preparations [88–90]. HES are typically identified by three numbers (e.g., 6% HES 130/0.4). The first number dictates the concentration of the solution, the second represents the manufactured mean MW in kilodaltons (kDa), and the third indicates the MS.

The concentration influences the initial volume expansion. 6% solutions are iso-oncotic and 10% solutions are hyperoncotic with considerably more volume expansion. Molecular weight is the weight-averaged (Mw) or number-averaged (Mn) size of the polymers. Since the polymers actually are of varying length (ranging from a few thousand to few million daltons) this parameter is only an average. HES are arbitrarily classified by the manufactured mean molecular weight into high MW (>400 kDa), medium MW (200–400 kDa), and low MW (<200 kDa) preparations. As Mw takes into account the individual weights of different particles, it is influenced by the presence of large molecules in the system and will give a larger value compared to the Mn that represents the total weight of all the molecules divided by the number of molecules. The ratio Mw:Mn provides an index of the polydispersity. It is important to understand that the given MW applies to the colloidal preparation *in vitro* because soon after these fluids are administered to a patient, the low molecular weight fraction is excreted by the renal route and larger molecules are progressively hydrolyzed by serum α-amylase, resulting in narrow distribution of molecular weights with an *in vivo* mean MW that is lower than the mean MW of the infused preparation. The decrease in COP after initial excretion of small molecular weight fraction is partly compensated by the availability of a greater number of small molecular weight molecules created by metabolism (cleavage) of larger molecules.

Molar substitution describes the degree of substitution of glucose molecules with hydroxyethyl groups. This substitution increases the polymer solubility and inhibits the metabolism of the polymer by amylase. The degree of MS can be calculated in two ways. One method, termed the degree of substitution (DS), is calculated by the number of substituted glucose residues divided by the total number of glucose residues. With the second method, MS is calculated as the average number of hydroxyethyl residues per glucose unit. More than one substitution can occur at each glucose residue so the MS could be higher than the DS. The value of 0.4 in the 6% HES 130/0.4 indicates that there are four hydroxyethyl residues on average per 10 glucose subunits. Based on degree of substitution, HES have been referred to as hetastarch (≥0.7), hexastarch (0.6), pentastarch (0.5), and tetrastarch (0.4). The greater the MS, the harder it is to metabolize the HES.

The C2:C6 ratio describes the pattern of hydroxyethylation and also impacts the pharmacokinetics of HES preparations. Hydroxyethyl groups at position C2 of the glucose molecule inhibit the access of α-amylase to the substrate more efficiently than the C6 position. HES products with high molecular weight, larger C2:C6 ratio and greater MS are metabolized slowly and have prolonged persistence in plasma. Based on these physicochemical properties, HES preparations can be classified in a more clinically relevant way as slowly degradable (e.g., hetastarch) or rapidly degradable (e.g., Voluven® or Vetstarch®) preparations (see Table 21.5).

Pharmacokinetics and pharmacodynamics of various HES preparations are complex in part due to their polydisperse nature [91]. After IV administration, particles having molecular weights below the renal threshold (45–60 kDa) are quickly filtered into the urine. Additionally, small amounts diffuse into the interstitium of tissues, eventually redistribute and are subsequently eliminated. A transient proportion is stored in tissues and degraded by the reticuloendothelial system. Larger molecules are retained in the plasma for a variable period of time subject to their metabolism by α-amylase. Metabolism is in turn influenced by the physicochemical properties of the particular HES preparations as described earlier [88–90]. The resulting smaller fractions after metabolism are further excreted in urine. Studies in animals and humans have demonstrated significantly more accumulation of slowly degradable HES preparations compared to rapidly degradable preparations, especially after repeated administrations [91]. Clearance of tetrastarches has been shown to be about 23 times faster than hetastarch and five times greater than pentastarch. Pharmacokinetics of HES has been described in dogs and horses [92–94]. Species-specific differences in plasma amylase activity have also been documented and contribute to the variable half-life of HES in different species. Relative to humans, amylase activity has been shown to be higher in dog plasma [92] and less in equine plasma [93].

The pharmacodynamics of fluids is related to the volume and duration of intravascular volume expansion and may be influenced by many factors including dose, speed of administration, specific colloid preparation, microvascular permeability, species of animal, and preinfusion intravascular volume status [88–91,95]. Iso-oncotic (6%) preparations of HES have been associated with similar increase

Table 21.5 Characteristics of hydroxyethyl starch preparations commonly used in veterinary anesthesia.

Type of HES	HES product	Physicochemical properties					Carrier	COP (mmHg)	Osmolarity (mOsm/L)	Plasma volume expansion (%)
		Conc.	Weight (kDa)		MS	C2:C6				
			Molecular	Number avg						
Rapidly degradable	Tetrastarch (Voluven®, Vetsrach®)	6%	130	70–80	0.4	9:1	Saline	High 30s	308	130
Slowly degradable	Hetastarch (Hextend®)	6%	670		0.75	4–5:1	Balanced	Low 30s	307	100
	Hetastarch (Hespan®)	6%	450	69	0.7	4:1	Saline	Low 30s	309	100

in intravascular volume compared to the volume administered while the hyperoncotic preparations (10%) can expand volume up to 145% by pulling fluid from the interstitial space [88,89]. The initial increase in plasma volume is the result of COP of the colloidal preparation administered and is mostly attributed to the large number of small molecular weight particles. As these smaller molecules are removed from the circulation during the first few hours, a significant decrease in COP occurs, translating clinically into reduced effect on plasma volume expansion over time. Due to the presence of the remaining large molecular weight particles in the plasma, the concentration of the colloidal preparation (mass per unit volume) may still be quite high but the COP will be low.

Slowly degradable preparations have a longer plasma half-life but it has been shown not to translate into increased duration of volume expansion. In spite of minimal plasma accumulation of tetrastarch the studies in orthopedic [96,97] and cardiac [98] surgeries have demonstrated its duration of effect (at similar concentration) to be comparable to pentastarch [99] and hetastarch [96,100]. It is important to understand that though the clearance and residual plasma concentration of HES are affected by their physicochemical properties (mainly MS and C2:C6 ratio [101]), the COP depends upon the number of osmotically active particles and not on the concentration of HES [88–90,95]. In a given volume of HES solution there will be more particles of lower molecular weight product compared to a HES preparation with higher molecular weight translating into a greater COP at similar plasma concentrations.

The effect of hetastarch on COP has been described in healthy ponies and horses, hypoproteinemic dogs and horses, hypovolemic and hypotensive dogs under anesthesia, and dogs undergoing orthopedic surgery [82,83,102–107]. Effects of various HES preparations on COP do not seem to last beyond 24 h. It is important to remember that variables like health status [104,105], pre-existing volume status [82,91,95], concurrent fluid therapy [106,108], dose [107], type of preparation [83,93,102], and anesthesia [109] all have the potential to influence plasma COP, meaning that results of different studies must be evaluated carefully. In a recently published study in horses, compared to 0.9% sodium chloride COP was higher in the group receiving tetrastarch (130/0.4) compared to hetastarch (600/0.75) but returned to baseline at 24 h [83]. Due to its ability to provide colloidal oncotic support and prolonged intravascular retention, HES has proven to be better at providing intravascular support and improvement in hemodynamic indices compared to crystalloids [82–87].

Adverse events have been associated with HES use in clinical patients. It is important to point out that results from *in vitro* studies cannot be directly extrapolated to clinical scenarios (*in vivo*) as side-effect profile is heavily impacted by the *in vivo* pharmacokinetic behavior of various HES products and slowly degradable preparations (hetastarch and pentastarch) carry more risk compared to rapidly degradable preparations (tetrastarches) [88–90].

All types of fluids have the potential to cause dilutional coagulopathy, but the HES solutions also impact hemostasis directly by altering both the primary and secondary hemostasis [88]. HES decreases the expression of platelet surface GP IIb-IIIa complex and also physically coats the surface of platelets, causing decreased interaction of agonists like soluble fibrinogen and von Willibrand factor (vWF) with this receptor, thus preventing platelet aggregation. HES also decreases FVIII/vWF complex concentration, possibly due to accelerated elimination of this complex after binding to HES. These adverse effects have clinically translated into increased blood loss perioperatively. Use of rapidly degradable HES preparations (HES 130/0.4) caused lower blood loss in various types of surgeries in humans compared to slowly degradable HES preparations (HES 200/0.5, HES 450/0.7, and HES 600/0.75) [96, 110,111]. Desmopressin has been suggested as a treatment option for mild coagulopathy associated with HES administration [112]. Veterinary studies in dogs [103,106,113–118] and horses [62, 83, 102,107,119] have also reported dose-related effects [107,116, 117,119,120] of hetastarch and tetrastarch on platelet function and FVIII/vWF complex[115–117,119–121] *in vitro* and *in vivo* but have failed to document increases in clinical bleeding at the dosages studied [103,106,113]. Several of these studies documented less impact on hemostasis when tetrastarches are used [83,107,116, 121]. Human studies [122,123] have shown that HES preparations formulated in balanced carrier solution containing Ca^{2+} ions cause less impairment of hemostasis compared to 0.9% sodium chloride-based formulations. Similar *in vitro* comparisons in dogs [115] and horses [119] did not show any better platelet function as assessed by estimation of platelet closure times. Concerns about hyperchloremic metabolic acidosis with 0.9% sodium chloride formulations have also been expressed [88].

A recent multicenter blinded trial in severely septic human patients revealed that HES 130/0.42 was associated with more mortality and need for renal replacement therapy compared to the Ringer's acetate group [124]. A recent meta-analysis in humans revealed increased risk of acute kidney injury in critically ill patients receiving HES preparations [125]. Studies documenting renal toxicity in veterinary patients are lacking.

Reports indicating a low incidence of anaphylactoid reactions, increases in α-amylase level and tissue accumulation of slowly degradable preparations causing pruritus in humans have been published [88,90]. In cats, hetastarch has been associated with vomiting if administered too rapidly.

Most of the dosage recommendations in veterinary patients are extrapolated from manufacturer's and human literature rather than veterinary-specific studies. The present recommendations dictate not to exceed a 20 mL/kg/day dose for hetastarch while tetrastarch doses could go as high as 50 mL/kg/day. Increased blood loss was reported in dogs where >30 mL/kg dose of hetastarch was used [126,127]. A few studies in horses have suggested a hetastarch dose of 10 mL/kg/day is well tolerated [62,93].

Dextrans

Dextrans are linear polysaccharide molecules and include a low (10% dextran 40) and high (6% dextran 70) molecular weight preparation in 0.9% saline. Smaller molecules are removed by glomerular filtration with bigger molecules staying in circulation longer and eventually being metabolized by dextranase enzyme systems in the kidney, liver, and spleen to produce carbon dioxide and water. Due to the importance of glomerular filtration in excretion of dextrans, half-life can be increased in patients with renal insufficiency. Dextrans are hyperoncotic compared to plasma and cause plasma volume expansion that can be more than the volume infused (dextran 40 > dextran 70).

Dextrans have been used to improve microcirculatory blood flow (especially dextran 40) and prevent deep vein thrombosis and thromboprophylaxis in humans. Complications associated with their use include anaphylactic reactions, renal function impairment (especially with dextran 40), and impaired hemostasis (inhibited platelet aggregation, dose-dependent hyperfibrinolysis, decreased levels of vWF and FVIII:C activity) [127–132]. They can also coat the surface of red blood cells, interfering with cross-matching procedures. A maximum dose of 10–20 mL/kg/day in dogs and 5–10 mL/kg/day in cats has been suggested to minimize adverse effects.

Gelatins

Gelatins are large molecular weight polydisperse proteins formed by hydrolysis of bovine collagen. Three modified newer generation gelatin preparations are succinylated or modified fluid gelatins, urea-cross-linked gelatins and oxy-cross-linked gelatins (oxypolygelatins). Gelatin preparations have similar average molecular weights (30– 35 kDa) and are supplied in concentrations of 3.5–5.5% [133]. The small size of gelatin molecules makes them liable to glomerular filtration which is their main route of elimination. Half-life of oxypolygelatin has been suggested at 2–4 h in dogs [129]. The distribution of total dose administered by 24 h is 71% in urine, 16% extravascular, and 13% remains in the plasma [133]. Rapid renal excretion means less plasma retention, and though similar side-effects on coagulation compared to other synthetic colloids are reported, their magnitude is less [129,134,135]. Urea-cross-linked gelatins have been associated with anaphylactoid reactions due to histamine release that were blocked by prophylactic use of histamine blockers [136]. Although there are no standard guidelines for gelatin dosages in veterinary species, a dose of 5 mL/kg for oxypolygelatin in dogs has been recommended [129].

Clinical implications of synthetic colloid use in veterinary medicine

Most of the studies in veterinary medicine have looked at the effect of HES, dextrans, and gelatins in healthy animals and have documented dose-related deterioration in both primary and secondary hemostasis but failed to show exacerbation of clinical bleeding. As effects of synthetic colloids on hemostasis are directly linked to their plasma concentration, it is reasonable to assume that if they are used in dosages higher than the maximum recommended, are used repeatedly, are used when there is decreased clearance (e.g., renal impairment) or are used in patients with pre-existing bleeding diathesis, the potential to increase clinical bleeding does exist. Similarly, though there is a lack of veterinary data documenting the effect of synthetic colloids on renal function, we know that renal filtration is the major route of excretion and urine osmolality and specific gravity is increased in dogs administered HES 600/0.75 [137]. Hyperviscosity of the urine after glomerular filtration of colloid molecules theoretically causing tubular obstruction due to stasis of urine flow seems the most likely mechanism of renal impairment [90,131,132]. So the possibility of renal dysfunction may exist, especially in critically ill patients with pre-existing renal compromise, warranting renal function monitoring (urine output, creatinine, blood urea nitrogen, etc.) and use of minimal amounts of synthetic colloids in such scenarios. Also hyperoncotic preparations seem to potentiate this issue so it might be advisable to use iso-oncotic preparations of synthetic colloids when possible [90,131,132].

Perioperative fluid therapy

The objective of perioperative fluid therapy is to maintain circulatory volume so that end-organ perfusion and oxygen delivery are not compromised. The traditional approach to achieving this goal entails administration of replacement crystalloids at a dose rate that could vary between 5 and 20 mL/kg/h [13,14]. This high rate of fluid administration was expected to offset the transient intraoperative hypovolemia due to fluid deprivation during preoperative fasting, vasodilation associated with anesthetic drugs, third spacing of intravascular fluids, insensible fluid losses, and intraoperative fluid or blood loss [138,139]. With emerging evidence, most of these theories are being proved wrong. Present perioperative patient management does not advocate prolonged fasting times [140], with patients usually having access to water up until the time of surgery. Additionally, blood volume has been shown to stay normal even after prolonged fasting [141]. The concept of third spacing of fluids during surgery [142] and fluid loading of normovolemic patients to prevent intraoperative hypotension [143] has also been questioned.

Stress associated with surgery and anesthesia leads to neuroendocrine responses mediated by stimulation of the hypothalamic pituitary adrenal axis, renin angiotensin and aldosterone system activation, atrial natriuretic peptide, and vasopressin release. All of these compensatory mechanisms can alter fluid dynamics independent of renal function [144]. In dogs, antidiuretic hormone concentration increased [145] and urine production decreased after morphine premedication [146] and did not change during anesthesia and surgery when patients received conventional fluid therapy [147] or increased crystalloid fluid administration [7].

Anesthesia- and surgery-related physiological effects cease or decrease at the end of surgery, resulting in a patient who has been given a relatively large quantity of fluids. Postoperatively such patients end up gaining body weight [147,148]. This positive fluid balance and weight gain mostly occurs in the ECF and has been shown to be associated with a host of abnormalities including increased lung water, decreased pulmonary function, increased infection rate, reduced gut motility, decreased PCV, decreased total protein, and a decrease in body temperature eventually translating into increased morbidity and mortality [148–151]. The Confidential Inquiry into Perioperative Small Animal Fatalities (CEPSAF) revealed that cats receiving fluids (likely not goal-directed dosing) were four times more likely to die and the authors speculated that excessive fluid administration causing fluid overload could be a cause [152]. Restrictive intraoperative fluid administration could improve postoperative pulmonary function and hypoxemia [153–155]. It was also observed that cats being monitored with pulse oximetry during anesthesia were 3–4 times less likely to die, although how that relates to fluid administration is unclear from this study [152].

Evidence from human anesthesia suggests that low-risk patients undergoing low to moderate risk surgery benefit from liberal intraoperative fluid therapy (20–40 mL/kg total dose) resulting in reduced postoperative complications like dizziness, pain, nausea, vomiting, drowsiness, and reduced hospital length of stay [155–157]. However, no compromise in renal function was noticed with restrictive fluid therapy in humans [154]. No impact on systolic blood pressure was noticed in dogs receiving fluid rates between 0 and 15 mL/kg/h [158] and increasing fluid rates from 0 to 30 mL/kg/h did not cause any change in urine production or oxygen delivery under anesthesia [7]. High-risk human patients undergoing major abdominal surgeries benefit from restrictive fluid therapy [159,160] though this has not been a universal finding.

What constitutes restrictive or liberal fluid therapy is still a question of debate because different randomized controlled trials in humans have used different fluid regimens [161]. Recently AAHA/AAFP fluid therapy guidelines in dogs and cats [162] have suggested initially starting fluid administration at 3 mL/kg/h in cats and 5 mL/kg/h in dogs, although these recommendations were not based on any specific clinical evidence and are not universally accepted.

Monitoring fluid balance

Measurement of ICF and ISF is not easily done and estimation of IVF volume is undertaken mostly in clinical practice. There is no single variable that could assess the intravascular volume status which creates some difficulties for application of goal-directed fluid therapy. Furthermore, it is important to do serial evaluations of a patient to optimize volume status. Clinical examination (mucous membrane color, capillary refill time, pulse rate and quality, temperature of extremities, mentation, skin turgor, moistness of mucous membranes, peripheral edema, thoracic auscultation for any crackles, papilledema, respiration rate, pulse oximetry, blood pressure, urine output), invasive hemodynamic monitoring to obtain objective data (direct blood pressure monitoring, cardiac output monitoring, cardiac filling pressures including central venous pressure and pulmonary artery occlusion pressure, pulse pressure and stroke volume variation, transesophageal echocardiography) and laboratory data (arterial and venous blood gases, electrolyte status, renal function evaluation) all should be used in conjunction to estimate the volume status. Information on various macrovascular (central venous pressure, arterial blood pressure, urine output) and microvascular (lactate concentration and clearance, base excess, mixed or central venous oxygen saturation) perfusion parameters help dictate the state of critical oxygen delivery to the tissues [163,164]. Early goal-directed therapy (EGDT) to normalize some of these endpoints has been shown to improve outcomes [165].

Therapy with synthetic colloids should ideally be monitored using colloid osmometry to measure COP rather than relying on the refractometric analysis because the relationship between COP and refractive index may be different for plasma proteins vs synthetic colloid [166]. There is a poor correlation between the changes in COP and total protein as measured by a refractometer after administration of hetastarch and dextran 70. Both of these synthetic colloids push the refractometric reading towards 4.5 g/dL [167]. Refractometric total solids readings typically decrease after colloid administration due to dilutional effects and these drops could be falsely interpreted as a need for additional colloidal support, leading to fluid overload [95].

Individualized goal-directed fluid therapy

It is important to realize that not all patients respond to fluid administration equally. It was shown that only 50% of critically ill patients have adequate cardiac preload reserve for response to volume expansion by increasing cardiac output [168]. So it is important to recognize patients that are fluid responsive to avoid ineffective or deleterious fluid overloading [169]. Although no standard fluid therapy guidelines have been devised as yet, an individualized fluid therapy approach called 'individualized goal-directed therapy' based on objective feedback from a patient's fluid responsiveness has been shown to improve outcome in perioperative settings [170–172].

Use of conventional static preload indices to guide intravascular volume therapy involves measurement of cardiac filling pressures (central venous pressure, pulmonary capillary wedge pressure, end-diastolic ventricular pressure) and has been shown to be an unreliable and generally late indicator of fluid overload, alterations in blood volume, and fluid responsiveness [169,173]. Originally, pulmonary artery catheterization (PAC) was used to guide optimal oxygen delivery in high-risk surgical patients but, due to morbidity and mortality increases associated with the use of the PAC itself, and failure to show any clear benefit, it fell out of favor in human medicine [174].

Monitoring fluid responsiveness has evolved into minimally invasive, dynamic flow-based hemodynamic monitoring techniques like transesophageal Doppler echocardiography and use of dynamic preload indices like systolic pressure variation (SPV), pulse pressure variation (PPV), stroke volume variation (SVV), and plethysmographic waveform variations [169,175–179]. These dynamic indices evaluate the cyclical changes in preload or venous return in response to fluid therapy and have been shown to be more reliable predictors of fluid responsiveness in an individual patient [169,175–179].

Both PPV and SVV occur due to cyclic changes in the intrathoracic pressure caused by mechanical ventilation [169,176,180]. Reduction in venous return during inspiration with positive pressure ventilation is the major determinant of this variation. According to the Frank–Starling principle, diastolic filling of the ventricles determines the myocardial stretch and hence stroke volume as related to myocardial contractility. In hypovolemic states, the SVV is high and the left ventricular contractility depends on the preload to a greater extent. In other words, the ventricle operates on the ascending limb of the Frank–Starling curve. As the volume expands, the left ventricular function shifts in the rightward direction on the Frank–Starling curve and causes an observed decrease in SVV [169,176,180]. Both PPV and SVV have been shown to be sensitive markers of ventricular responsiveness to the fluid loading.

Dynamic preload assessment can be performed in clinical patients that are monitored using direct blood pressure, are mechanically ventilated and have no arrhythmias [169,176]. Recently, plethysmograph variability index (PVI) and PPV have been assessed in a dog hemorrhagic shock model as predictors of volume changes [178,179]. The authors concluded that PVI derived from a pulse oximeter successfully detected hypovolemia and return to normovolemia but was not able to detect hypervolemia [178]. Similarly, they concluded that PPV was a reliable indicator of hypovolemia in a mechanically ventilated model of hemorrhagic shock in dogs [179]. In that study, the baseline PPV (%) was 10.1 ± 2.9, increased to 30 ± 8.3 after inducing hemorrhage, and normalized to 8.5 ± 3.7 after retransfusion. Transesophageal Doppler monitoring helps quantify preload either by measuring and calculating left ventricular end-diastolic area (LVEDA) or volume (LVEDV). In major abdominal surgeries, use of esophageal Doppler was associated with fewer postoperative complications, reduced admission to intensive care units, faster return of gastrointestinal function, and decreased length of hospital stay [181].

The question about the type of fluid (crystalloids or colloids) to be used for volume expansion has been debated for a long time. Colloids have been shown to be more efficacious in restoring intravascular volume [82,84–87] but in the absence of any clear-cut benefit on mortality, the human literature does not advocate the use of one over another [182].

Electrolytes

Sodium

Sodium is the most abundant cation in the ECF (see Table 21.1). In the cell membrane, Na^+/K^+ ATPase maintains a relatively low intracellular concentration of Na^+. The concentration of Na^+ in the serum is a reflection of the amount of Na^+ relative to total ECF and does not provide any indication about the content of total body sodium. Disorders of sodium are mostly the result of changes in the amount of body water so changes in Na^+ concentration should be viewed as changes in free water content of the body. The volume and tonicity of body fluids are maintained by regulation of Na^+ and water balance. In response to changes in intravascular volume, antidiuretic hormone (ADH), signals from baroreceptors and osmoreceptors, thirst mechanisms, renin-angiotensin-aldosterone system (RAAS), and atrial natriuretic peptide (ANP) all act accordingly to promote homeostasis [183].

Various disease processes can cause hypernatremia. It could result from hypotonic dehydration (resulting in hypovolemic hypernatremia), loss of free water (resulting in normovolemic hypernatremia) or ingestion or iatrogenic administration of high sodium-containing fluids (resulting in hypervolemia) [183]. Hypernatremia results in cellular dehydration (especially brain cells) as water moves from the ICF to the ECF. Shrinking of brain tissue can cause tearing of blood vessels, resulting in subarachnoid and intracerebral hemorrhage [184].

The pathophysiological consequences of hypernatremia are determined mainly by the rapidity of onset of hypernatremia rather than the absolute value. Under chronic circumstances (>2–3 days), the brain cells increase intracellular osmolality by accumulation of osmotically active solutes called 'idiogenic osmoles' [185,186]. Lien *et al.* [187] found that hypernatremia in rats increased concentrations of myoinositol, bataine, glycerophosphorylcholine, phosphocreatine, glutamine, glutamate, and taurine in the brain. Idiogenic osmoles help maintain intracellular volume and prevent efflux of fluid. Hence, in chronic hypernatremia, rapid correction of sodium level could decrease extracellular osmolality and cause movement of water into brain cells, causing cerebral edema. If hypernatremia is of relatively acute onset (<24 h), rapid correction is better tolerated because idiogenic osmoles are not yet present.

Intracranial hemorrhage and neuronal dehydration could result in muscle weakness, lethargy, ataxia, seizure, coma, and death [184]. Treatment should involve correction of the underlying problem and using fluids to replenish free water content. In hypovolemic patients, intravascular volume deficit should be corrected using a fluid that is isotonic to the patient followed by correction of free water deficit with fluids like 5% dextrose or 2.5% dextrose in 0.45% saline [188]. The formula given below could be used to calculate free water deficit:

$$[(\text{Serum Na}^+/140)-1]\times \text{Body weight (kg)}\times 0.6$$

It is recommended that in cases of chronic hypernatremia, the patient's water deficits should be corrected slowly over 48–72 h so that Na^+ concentration does not decrease at a rate that exceeds 0.5 mEq/L/h.

Hyponatremia can result from gain of free water or loss of sodium. It could occur in the presence of euvolemia (associated with normal osmolality and characterized by normal water and Na^+ content, pseudohyponatremia), dehydration (associated with hyperosmolality) or hypervolemia (associated with hypo-osmolality, seen most commonly clinically) [188]. Hyponatremia with hypo-osmolality could be further divided into hyponatremia with hypovolemia, hypervolemia or euvolemia depending on the underlying disease process. A syndrome of inappropriate secretion of ADH (SIADH) has been described in people and dogs that leads to hyponatremia with hypo-osmolality and euvolemia [189,190]. It is characterized by secretion of ADH in the absence of low osmolality or hypovolemia and could cause hyponatremia. In perioperative settings SIADH has been associated with the use of various anesthetic drugs including narcotics [189,191]. Sympathetic stimulation due to pain associated with surgical procedures can also cause ADH release in the absence of volume contraction. All these factors can lead to renal retention of water and development of hyponatremia in surgical patients [183]. Transurethral resection of prostate (TURP) syndrome is an established cause of hyponatremia in human anesthetic patients due to intravascular absorption of irrigation fluids causing hypotonic hyponatremia [192]. However, a case series describing a small number of dogs undergoing this procedure did not show hyponatremia [193].

Pathophysiological consequences of hyponatremia also depend on its rate of development. Decrease in serum sodium concentration can generate an osmotic gradient across the blood–brain barrier that would cause movement of water into brain cells causing cerebral edema. Signs typically do not develop unless the concentration drops below 125 mEq/L and include ataxia, vomiting, depression, seizures, and coma [194]. During chronic hyponatremia, the recommended Na^+ correction rate is not more than 0.5 mEq/L/h. If correction is faster, higher plasma osmolality can cause efflux of water from brain cells (cellular dehydration), producing the clinical syndrome of osmotic demyelination or central pontine myelenosis [195,196]. Treatment of hyponatremia will partly depend upon the volume status of the patient. An approach using 3% saline has been described for correction of hyponatremia [189].

Calcium

Calcium is a very important divalent cation that is involved in many biologic processes, out of which its effects on cardiac smooth muscle, vascular smooth muscle and blood coagulation are particularly important to the anesthesiologist [197]. In addition, calcium is involved in skeletal muscle contraction, neuronal conduction, synaptic transmission, and hormone secretion and acts as a major intracellular messenger required for many cellular functions. Approximately 99% of the total body calcium is stored as hydroxyapatite in the skeletal tissue and the rest is divided between the ICF and ECF compartments. Calcium exists in three biologic forms: in plasma as ionized or free calcium (iCa^{2+}); complexed or chelated to phosphate, sulphate, bicarbonate, citrate ,and lactate; and protein-bound calcium [198]. The biologically active form is the iCa^{2+} that is involved in various functions described earlier. The serum level of calcium is controlled by parathyroid hormone, calcitonin and calcitriol (1,25-dihydroxycholecalciferol). These hormones act at the level of bone, kidneys, and gastrointestinal tract to regulate calcium homeostasis [197].

Hypocalcemia is common in critically ill small animal patients, in horses suffering from colic, and sick cattle. It has been shown to carry a poor prognosis [18,31,61,199,200]. Also, inhalant anesthesia has been shown to decrease total and ionized calcium concentrations in horses [201,202]. Hypocalcemia could occur due to impaired parathyroid hormone (PTH) release (primary and secondary hypoparathyroidism, post thyroidectomy, post parathyroidectomy), impaired calcitriol synthesis (acute or chronic renal failure, malabsorptive syndromes, liver insufficiency, etc.) and chelation of serum calcium (sodium phosphate enemas, bicarbonate therapy, blood products containing citrate, ethylene glycol toxicity, saponification of fat in pancreatitis or steatitis, etc.) [197,200,203]. Hypoalbuminemia/hypoproteinemia could affect (decrease) total calcium concentration and formulas traditionally used to correct total calcium concentration for changes (decrease) in albumin concentration have been shown to be erroneous and it is advisable to always measure iCa^{2+} concentration [204].

The severity of clinical signs depends upon the magnitude and the rapidity of onset of hypocalcemia. Pathophysiological consequences are due to a decrease in threshold membrane potential resulting in increased membrane excitability as neural membranes become more permeable to sodium. Hyperkalemia and hypomagnesemia potentiate the cardiac and neuromuscular effects of hypocalcemia [188]. Clinical signs are attributable to neuromuscular irritability and could be characterized by tetany, seizures, restlessness or excitation, facial rubbing, muscle tremors, tachycardia, hyperthermia, hypotension, and cardiopulmonary arrest [188]. The electrocardiogram may reveal a prolonged QT interval. Symptomatic acute hypocalcemia should be treated with calcium gluconate (10% solution at a dose of 0.5–1.5 mL/kg), administered intravenously slowly over 15–20 min with continuous heart rate monitoring.

Hypercalcemia could result from increased resorption of calcium from bones (hyperparathyroidism, hypercalcemia of malignancy, etc.), increased absorption from the gastrointestinal tract (hypervitaminosis D, granulomatous diseases, antipsoriasis creams, vitamin D rodenticides, etc.) or decreased renal excretion (acute or chronic renal failure) [188]. Hydrogen ions can compete with iCa^{2+} for binding sites on albumin, hence acidemia can increase ionized calcium concentration [205]. Hypercalcemia can result in neuromuscular, cardiovascular, gastrointestinal, renal and skeletal muscle abnormalities [188,197]. Clinical signs may be characterized by nausea, anorexia, constipation, abdominal pain, polyuria, polydipsia, and soft tissue mineralization [188]. Electrocardiographic changes are characterized by QT interval shortening, prolonged PR interval and wide QRS complex.

Treatment of hypercalcemia should involve correction of dehydration, promoting calciuresis, inhibition of bone resorption, and treatment of underlying disease process [188,197]. Calcium-free fluids, especially 0.9% NaCl, are preferred as they competitively inhibit renal tubular calcium reabsorption [188]. Once the patient is properly hydrated, use of a loop diuretic (furosemide) can be considered to promote calciuresis with regular monitoring of serum electrolytes. Additionally glucocorticoids, bisphosphonates (pamidronate, etidronate disodium, etc.), and calcitonin could be used to treat some tumor-associated hypercalcemias and decrease bone resorption [188,197]. Effects of various drugs used during anesthesia, especially inhalant anesthetics, local anesthetics and non-depolarizing muscle relaxants, can be influenced by changes in calcium concentration [197].

Potassium

Potassium is the most abundant intracellular cation (see Table 21.1). About 95% of it is present intracellularly with only 5% present in the extracellular fluid. So, clearly the routine measurement of plasma potassium concentration gives little indication of total body potassium content. The normal high gradient between ICF and ECF potassium is maintained by the Na^+/K^+-ATPase pump. In the resting stage, permeability of the cell membrane is approximately 100 times higher for K^+ than Na^+ ions. Most of the effects seen due to alterations in ECF K^+ concentration are the result of alterations in resting membrane potential, which are particularly noticeable in excitable cell membranes like cardiac tissue. Potassium concentration is a reflection of intake (nutrition), gastrointestinal loss, renal function, and transcellular potassium shifts [206].

The major causes of hyperkalemia involve increased intake (mostly iatrogenic overadministration of potassium-containing fluids), decreased renal excretion (urethral obstruction, ruptured bladder, anuric or oliguric renal failure, hypoadrenocorticism, drugs, etc.), translocation from ICF to ECF (acute mineral acidosis, insulin deficiency, tumor lysis syndrome, drugs, etc.) and pseudohyperkalemia (hemolysis, thrombocytosis and sample collected in Na^+/K^+ EDTA) [206,207].

Hyperkalemia can decrease the resting membrane potential (makes it less negative) and could make the membranes hyperexcitable in the beginning but as the potassium concentration escalates further a point is reached when the resting membrane potential exceeds the threshold membrane potential, causing depolarization, but repolarization does not take place and the cell loses its excitability. Clinical signs include muscle weakness and cardiac toxicity that is especially apparent at concentrations >7.5 mEq/L. Concurrent hypocalcemia, hyponatremia, acidemia, and hypovolemia can exacerbate the cardiac deterioration at lower concentrations [188, 206,208]. Changes in the electrocardiogram due to hyperkalemia have been described [208]. As the concentration of potassium in ECF increases from mild to severe, changes in the electrocardiogram are characterized by increasing amplitude and narrowing of the T wave (tenting), shortening of the QT interval, prolongation of the PR interval, widening of the QRS complex, decreasing amplitude and widening of the P wave, disappearance of the P wave, atrial standstill, extreme bradycardia, sinoventricular rhythm and eventually sine wave appearance of the QRS complex followed by ventricular fibrillation or ventricular asystole. These ECG changes are inconsistent and influenced by other variables including acid–base balance, rate of K^+ increase, and concurrent electrolytic anomalies [208,209].

Treatment involves use of calcium salts for cardiac protection, initiating movement of potassium from ECF to ICF, bicarbonate therapy, diuresis with fluids and relieving urinary obstruction if present [206]. Peritoneal dialysis or hemodialysis are viable options for refractory hyperkalemia [188]. Although it is suggested to use fluids containing no potassium in patients with hyperkalemia, it has been shown that in cats with urethral obstruction, there was no difference in the rate of reduction of potassium with either Normosol-R® or 0.9% sodium chloride [210]. Intravenous administration of calcium raises the threshold membrane potential so that the gradient between resting and threshold membrane potential is re-established, resulting in restoration of membrane excitability. Calcium therapy starts to work within minutes and the response typically last anywhere between 30 and 60 min [206]. A slow bolus administration (10–20 min) of 10% calcium gluconate at a dose of 50–150 mg/kg (0.5–1.5 mL/kg) with continuous monitoring of ECG should be considered as fast administration could cause bradycardia. Approximately one-third of the dose should be administered if calcium chloride is used [188].

Calcium administration does not do anything to lower the potassium concentration. To actually move the potassium intracellularly and decrease the serum potassium concentration, intravenous dextrose can be administered with or without insulin. Insulin facilitates the movement of glucose into the cells and potassium moves in the same direction (intracellularly), though an independent mechanism resulting in Na^+/K^+-ATPase pump activation (especially in the muscles) has been suggested [211]. Regular crystalline insulin should be used at a dose of 0.25–0.5 U/kg of body weight. Dextrose (dilute 50%) at a dose of 2g (4 mL) per unit of insulin administered should be given simultaneously. Onset of treatment effect is about 30 min and it could last for about an hour [188]. Potential for iatrogenic hypoglycemia exists with insulin-dextrose therapy and once initial stabilization is achieved, dextrose supplementation may be required until euglycemia is reached. Intravenous administration of sodium bicarbonate results in alkalosis that in turn causes hydrogen ions to move from ICF to ECF and potassium moves into the ICF. The recommended dose is 1–2 mEq/kg but concerns about paradoxical cerebrospinal acidosis, hyperosmolality, and the patient's ability to ventilate should be weighed up beforehand. Also bicarbonate therapy will cause hypocalcemia that may be counterproductive if calcium salts have been used for their cardioprotective effects [188]. Therapy takes effect in about 15 min and could last for an hour. Use of β_2-agonist has been described to treat hyperkalemia by stimulating the Na^+/K^+-ATPase pump that occurs independent of insulin [212].

Hypokalemia is the result of dilution (from potassium-depleted fluids), decreased dietary intake, increased urinary excretion (chronic renal failure, postobstructive diuresis, diuretics, mineralocorticoid excess, etc.), increased gastrointestinal loss (vomiting, diarrhea), and intracellular shift (alkalosis, glucose/insulin-containing fluids, β-agonists, etc.) [188,206,213]. Refractory hypokalemia could occur in the presence of hypomagnesemia [186]. Clinical signs of hypokalemia are characterized by neuromuscular function disturbances due to hyperpolarization, especially when the concentration goes below 2.5 mEq/L, and could be characterized by cervical ventroflexion, respiratory paralysis, anorexia, vomiting, decreased gastrointestinal motility, and lethargy [188,214]. Electrocardiographic abnormalities could include ST segment depression, decreased amplitude or inversion of T wave, increased P wave amplitude and prolonged PR and QRS intervals but life-threatening arrhythmias are uncommon [188]. Treatment involves parenteral supplementation with potassium chloride or potassium phosphate as additives to the crystalloids. It is important to remember that potassium supplementation rate should not exceed more than 0.5 mEq/kg/h because of cardiotoxic effects of potassium on cardiac conduction [188]. If potassium-supplemented fluids are used during anesthesia it is important to have another catheter placed with a second fluid bag attached without additional potassium in case there is a need for fluid bolus administration.

Transfusion therapy

While crystalloids and synthetic colloids can provide cardiovascular support by improving hemodynamic variables, in situations of significant blood loss or coagulopathy, blood products become necessary. However, blood products are costly, have a more limited shelf-life, need specific storage conditions and are highly immunogenic due to presence of biologic products like proteins and cells. Thus, it is important to adequately determine when a transfusion is necessary, which components are needed and how to best deliver the blood safely. There are limited publications in the veterinary literature specifically about use of transfusions in the perioperative period and during anesthesia. However, an understanding of available blood components and their usage, indications for autologous transfusions, and new information about transfusions in situations of massive blood loss can help guide practice.

Blood component therapy

Red blood cell (RBC) products are indicated in anemic patients to improve their oxygen-carrying capacity. Oxygen delivery can be estimated by the following equation:

$$DO_2(\text{Delivery of oxygen}) = CO(\text{Cardiac output}) \times \text{Oxygen content of arterial blood}(CaO_2)$$

where $CaO_2 = (PaO_2 \times 0.003) + (SaO_2 \times Hb \times 1.34)$, PaO_2 is partial pressure of oxygen in arterial blood, and SaO_2 is saturation of hemoglobin with oxygen in arterial blood.

The transfusion trigger is the concentration of hemoglobin below which the DO_2 decreases to an extent that anaerobic metabolism starts. Although there is still a deficiency of literature defining a transfusion trigger in human surgical patients with substantial blood loss, in stable anemic patients RBC administration is recommended when the hemoglobin concentration falls below 6 g/dL (approx. 18% PCV) [215]. In small animals it has been suggested that a PCV of 15–18% may be a reasonable transfusion trigger [216]. In euvolemic cattle, a hemoglobin level of 5 g/dL (approx. PCV 15%) is recommended and in cattle undergoing surgery, having pulmonary disease or in late pregnancy, a transfusion trigger value of 7 g/dL (approx. PCV 21%) has been suggested [217]. A PCV of 20% has been suggested as the transfusion trigger in horses [218].

However, the use of only hemoglobin level as a transfusion trigger should be avoided and any decision to transfuse should be based on an individual patient's intravascular volume status, evidence of shock, duration (acute vs chronic), extent of anemia, and cardiopulmonary physiologic parameters. In acute settings, animals lack the compensatory changes that occur during chronic anemia such as right-shifted oxyhemoglobin dissociation curve due to increased synthesis of 2,3-DPG (facilitating oxygen release to tissues), diversion of blood flow away from skeletal, skin, and splanchnic circulation towards coronary and cerebral circulations secondary to alterations in sympathetic tone, and recruitment of capillaries to facilitate tissue oxygen extraction [219].

Intraoperatively it is important to monitor the amount of blood loss. This can be done by visual assessment of the surgical field, estimating the amount of blood on drapes and floor, and collecting and weighing the gauze and lap sponges. The amount of blood on gauze and lap sponges can be estimated by subtracting the weight of dry gauze and lap sponges from the weight of blood-soaked ones (assuming 1 g weight = 1 mL of blood). If no lavage fluid is used, the volume of blood collected in the suction bottle can be measured directly. If the bottle contains a mixture of blood and fluid, the following formula can be used to estimate blood loss [220]:

$$\text{Blood loss(mL)} = \frac{\text{PCV of suctioned fluid} \times \text{Volume in canister(mL)}}{\text{Preoperative patient PCV}}$$

It is also helpful to look at blood loss as a percentage of the total blood volume to estimate severity, as animals under anesthesia are often not able to compensate for significant blood loss as an awake patient can. Profound hemodynamic changes occur in anesthetized animals when approximately 15–20% of their blood volume is acutely lost and its impact on oxygen delivery may be more profound because of depressed cardiovascular reflexes under anesthesia [82,221].

Traditional transfusion triggers are based on PCV, intraoperative changes in PCV, and total solids (TS) and can be difficult to interpret in the face of intraoperative fluid therapy and the timing of measurement after blood loss. When whole blood is lost acutely, the ratio of red blood cells to plasma stays the same. The PCV only begins to decline after intraoperative fluid administration or after intravascular fluid shifts and other compensatory mechanisms result in plasma volume expansion and hemodilution [217]. Often a drop in TS will be the first sign of acute blood loss as splenic contraction may maintain the hematocrit initially. Alternatively, a decrease in PCV and TS due to fluid administration in a surgery without significant hemorrhage may represent hemodilution and a better estimate of actual blood loss may be obtained by rechecking the values after fluid redistribution has occurred (often several hours later).

Monitoring for indices of inadequate perfusion and oxygenation should not only involve standard intraoperative monitoring like blood pressure, heart rate, electrocardiography, and pulse oximetry but should also encompass indices of microvascular perfusion parameters like lactate, base excess, mixed venous saturation/central venous saturation, and echocardiography when applicable [163,164,215]. It has been shown that blood loss under anesthesia may decrease cardiac output more profoundly compared to changes in blood pressure and many times heart rate [221]. Thus, these standard cardiovascular parameters monitored in veterinary anesthesia may not identify the severity of blood loss but careful monitoring of physical blood loss as described above in conjunction with perfusion parameters like lactate and base excess could yield a better perspective on compromised oxygen delivery and need for improved oxygen-carrying capacity.

Various reasons for transfusion of whole blood or PRBC in veterinary patients include anemia due to blood loss, hemolysis, and erythropoietic failure [222–228]. Once the decision has been made to provide red blood cells, there are several products that can be chosen. **Fresh whole blood (FWB)** is commonly used in clinical veterinary medicine due to its ready availability from in-house donors. It has all the components of blood including RBC, plasma proteins, platelets and labile and stable coagulation factors. It should be used within 8 h of collection due to the potential for bacterial growth [229]. Its use should be restricted to patients with massive blood loss or those that are missing multiple components. Whole blood can be transfused at varying rates depending on the rate of blood loss and size of the volume deficit, but an initial dose of 10–22 mL/kg or a dose based on the required increase in PCV can be calculated as follows [229]:

$$\text{FWB(mL)} = [\text{PCV(required)} - \text{PCV(recipient)} \times \text{Wt(kg)} \times \text{Blood volume(mL/kg)}]/\text{PCV(Donor)}$$

If not used within 8 h, FWB can be stored in a refrigerator at 1–6°C for 28 days if CPDA-1 is used as a preservative or 30 days if acid citrate dextrose (ACD) is used.

Stored whole blood differs from FWB in that it lacks functional platelets and labile clotting factors (factors V and VIII). It can be used for supplementing oxygen-carrying capacity in a hypoproteinemic patient or a patient with lost circulatory blood volume. The dose can be calculated as for FWB.

Packed red blood cells are prepared by separating the red blood cells from plasma using a hard spin in a refrigerated centrifuge. PRBCs contain RBCs, a small amount of plasma, white blood cells (WBCs), platelets, and a small amount of anticoagulant. A unit of PRBC obtained from a unit of whole blood contains approximately the same oxygen-carrying capacity as a unit of whole blood but in a smaller volume. PRBC transfusion is indicated in patients that need improvement in their oxygen-carrying capacity but are otherwise normovolemic and have no clotting abnormalities. In severe thrombocytopenia risk of bleeding is also affected by degree of anemia. RBCs can reduce the risk of bleeding in such patients by scavenging nitric oxide, leading to an increase in platelet activity. The higher hematocrit following PRBC administration can push the platelets towards the endothelial wall to improve contact and increase production of thromboxane by platelets at the injury site, and help reduce shear stress [230,231]. If initial collection of PRBC is done in CPDA-1, the product can be stored at 4°C for approximately 20 days. If nutrient additive solutions are added, the storage time can be extended (35 days with Nutricel® or Optisol® and 37 days with Adsol®) [229]. The hematocrit of PRBC products can vary considerably, but if the PCV of PRBC is approximately 60% then the volume required to raise the recipient PCV can be calculated as below [232]:

$$\text{PRBC(mL)} = 1.5\text{mL} \times \text{desired \% increase in PCV} \times \text{Wt(kg)}$$

Plasma products are indicated perioperatively to treat significant coagulopathy. These may be used prophylactically in patients with known coagulopathies or perioperatively if active bleeding occurs. The type of product used depends on the coagulopathy being treated.

Fresh frozen plasma (FFP) is plasma separated by a hard spin from whole blood that is frozen within 8 h of collection. In addition to plasma proteins and clotting factors, FFP is rich in labile clotting factors V and VIII and vWF. FFP can be stored up to 1 year in a freezer maintained at -20°C to -30°C. FFP can be used prophylactically prior to surgery in patients with known significant inherited or acquired coagulopathies and can also be used perioperatively if active bleeding due to coagulopathy occurs and PT is greater than 1.5 times normal, APTT is greater than 2 times normal or INR is greater than 2 [215]. FFP can be thawed at room temperature or in a warm water bath maintained at 37°C. It should be placed in a sealed plastic bag before putting it in the water bath to prevent contamination of the ports. The recommended dosage for treatment of vitamin K antagonist rodenticide toxicity is 10–20 mL/kg [233] and 15-30 mL/kg is required to treat coagulopathy associated with hemophilia A or von Willebrand disease [234].

If FFP is stored for more than 1 year it is called **frozen plasma (FP)**. If at initial separation from whole blood it is not frozen within 8 h or if the FFP is thawed and refrozen, it is also called FP. It differs from FFP in the lack of labile clotting factors V and VIII and vWF. FP can be kept frozen at -20°C for 5 years from the date of collection. Though the labile clotting factors and anticoagulant proteins are not active, stored frozen plasma (SFP) can be used for treatment of vitamin K-dependent (factors II, VII, IX, and X) coagulopathies like rodenticide toxicity [229]. Also it can potentially be used as a source of albumin to provide COP support.

Cryoprecipitate (cryo) can be prepared from FFP within 12 months of collection. It is formed by slow thawing at 0°C to 6°C. A white precipitate forms and both the plasma and precipitated fractions are separated by centrifugation and refrozen. The precipitated fraction is called cryoprecipitate and serves as a concentrated source of labile factors V and VIII, vWF, and fibrinogen. It should be used within 10 months from the date of initial blood draw. Cryoprecipitate is the treatment of choice for prophylaxis or active bleeding in dogs with hemophilia A or vWD, although availability may sometimes be an issue [234,235]. Recommended dosing for cryoprecipitate is 1 unit per 10 kg of body weight.

The supernatant produced in the process of procuring cryo is called **cryo-poor plasma (CPP)**. CPP lacks labile clotting factors but still contains the non-labile factors II, VII, IX, and X so it can be used for the treatment of coagulopathies associated with rodenticide toxicity.

Albumin constitutes 50–60% of the total plasma protein and provides 75–80% of COP in healthy animals. It also has other important physiologic functions including transport of various substrates and drugs, buffer capacity, scavenging of free radicals, mediation of coagulation, and wound healing [236]. Many critically ill patients suffer from hypoalbuminemia that could result in complications like interstitial fluid accumulation including pulmonary edema, impaired wound healing, improper transport of various anesthetic drugs, hypercoagulability, and systemic organ dysfunction [237,238]. Hypoalbuminemia has been associated with poor prognosis in both human and veterinary patients. In critically ill patients, the relationship between albumin and COP is not predictable as expected and edema formation results from complex pathophysiological processes involving changes in capillary permeability, lymphatic function, plasma COP, albumin kinetics and extracellular matrix structure. The most common form of species-specific albumin supplementation for COP support has been in the form of plasma transfusions. However, a large volume of plasma will be required to supply a relatively small amount of albumin; it is estimated that 22.5 mL/kg of plasma will be required to raise the albumin level by 0.5 g/dL [239]. Consequently a large amount of fluid will accompany the plasma transfusion that potentially could lead to transfusion-associated circulatory overload (TACO). Two concentrated forms of albumin, **human serum albumin (HSA)** and **canine serum albumin (CSA)**, have been used as sources of albumin in veterinary species. Use of bovine serum albumin in dogs has also been described [240].

Use of human serum albumin has been reported mostly in small animal patients though its use in horses has also been described [241–244]. Use of 25% hyperoncotic (COP) and 5% iso-oncotic (COP) preparations has been described in retrospective studies in critically ill small animal patients [241–243] and prospectively in healthy animals [245–247].

A few prospective studies [245–247] have been undertaken in healthy dogs to study any potential adverse effects with the use of HSA. In these studies, a few dogs developed immediate hypersensitivity reactions (anaphylactoid reactions) characterized by vomiting, facial edema, tachypnea, collapse, and hypotension. In addition, some dogs developed delayed hypersensitivity reactions 5–13 days after the initial transfusion characterized by facial edema, limb edema, pruritus, shifting limb lameness, vomiting, lethargy, inappetance, ecchymoses, lymphadenopathy, diarrhea, and cutaneous lesions indicative of vasculitis. Two of the dogs in one study suffered fatal consequences [245]. The delayed hypersensitivity was shown to be characterized by antigen–antibody complex deposition in various tissues, a characteristic of type III hypersensitivity [245,248]. Also HSA transfusion lead to a prolonged IgE immune response in healthy dogs as shown by positive intradermal testing [247].

Interestingly, retrospective studies conducted in critically ill small animal patients receiving HSA showed fewer adverse reactions. In a study conducted by Mathews & Barry [241], out of 64 dogs and two cats, facial edema was reported in only two dogs while transfusing HSA, but no information was available about delayed reactions. Another study conducted in 73 critically ill dogs showed no fulminant anaphylaxis but minor complications in 27% animals characterized by tachypnea, tachycardia, increased body temperature, peripheral edema, and ventricular arrhythmias [242]. Delayed reactions were seen in three dogs 5–14 days after administration characterized by edema, urticaria, lameness, pyrexia, vomiting, cutaneous lesions, and generalized pain. A recent study in 418 dogs and 170 cats using 5% HSA showed diarrhea, hyperthermia or tremors in 43.5% dogs and 36.5% cats but there were no severe hypersensitivity reactions [243]. It has been suggested that the reason for this dichotomy in response is the inability of critically ill hypoalbuminemic patients to mount a good immune response [242,243]. It was shown that the healthy dogs had produced high levels of IgG antibodies at 10–14 days post infusion while it took 4–6 weeks for the critically ill animals to reach the peak IgG production [245–247]. Given the severe sequelae in relatively healthy patients, HSA should only be considered in severely compromised small animal patients where other options have been exhausted.

Fortunately, CSA has recently been introduced in the commercial market (lyophilized canine albumin, Animal Blood Resources International, Dixon, CA). The product is derived from canine source donor plasma using a heat shock process. It is available as a lyophilized preparation in 5 g vials that can be reconstituted with sodium chloride solution. It can be used either as a hyperosmotic 16% solution (166 mg/mL) or an iso-osmotic 5% (50 mg/mL) preparation. It can be administered as a 16% solution in hypotensive patients with low albumin concentrations with a goal of achieving acute volume expansion and maintenance of intravascular volume.

A recent clinical study documented the use of CSA in postoperative management of dogs after source control surgery for septic peritonitis [249]. Fourteen dogs were divided into two groups with one group receiving CSA and the other group receiving clinician-directed therapy (CDT). They used 800 mg/kg of 5% CSA for 6 h in the CSA group. Doppler blood pressure, albumin concentration, and COP were significantly higher at 2 h post infusion in the CSA group. Albumin concentration was significantly higher at 24 h post infusion in the CSA group compared to the CDT group, though no difference was noticed in COP at the 24 h time point. Both groups received similar amounts of crystalloids and synthetic colloids during their hospitalization. The authors speculated that HES (COP 32.7 mmHg) administration during subsequent hospitalization masked the effect of 5% CSA (COP 22 mmHg) on COP.

Another observational study in six hypoalbuminemic dogs with septic peritonitis used 800–884 mg/kg CSA [250]. This study also showed a significant increase in albumin and COP at 2 and 24 h compared to baseline but did not show any increase in systolic blood pressure at 2 h post infusion. None of the clinical studies showed any adverse reactions to administration of CSA, neither immediate nor late (6–8 weeks post transfusion). Only one dog showed an increase in respiration rate during the transfusion that resolved following the slowing of administration rate. A safety study was conducted by the manufacturer in healthy purpose-bred Beagle dogs which were given a dose of 1 g/kg over a period of 1 h repeated once weekly for 4 weeks [251]. All dogs tolerated the infusion well except one that, during the second weekly infusion, developed pallor and prolonged capillary refill time that resolved on slowing the infusion. The investigators concluded that healthy dogs tolerated the repeated infusion well without any evidence of physical or biochemical abnormality.

In spite of the favorable experimental data and physiologic benefits from the use of albumin, literature in human medicine has not been able to demonstrate significant benefits with its use over sodium chloride solution in terms of improvement in morbidity and mortality [252,253]. In trauma patients, the use of albumin may actually be a detriment over the use of crystalloids alone [252]. However, in subset analysis, there may be a small benefit to the use of albumin in those critically ill patients with sepsis or acute respiratory distress syndrome (ARDS) [252,254,255]. Similar studies are lacking in veterinary medicine. However, based on the available human literature, risk of HSA in animals and cost of CSA, the authors recommend that the use of species-specific albumin only be considered in animals with acute respiratory distress syndrome or severe sepsis with concurrent severe hypoalbuminemia (less than 1.3 g/dL).

Platelet transfusions in human patients are done for prophylactic as well as therapeutic purposes. A prospective study in humans revealed that out of 7401 platelet transfusions performed in 503 patients, about 74% were prophylactic in nature, 18% were therapeutic and 8% were administered prior to surgery or invasive procedures in patients with coagulopathy or at high risk of bleeding [256]. In the perioperative setting, prophylactic platelet transfusion should be considered if the platelet count is $<50\times10^9$/L [215]. The need for therapy, including any prophylactic treatment in patients with platelet counts in the range 50–100 $\times10^9$/L, should be based on potential for platelet dysfunction, anticipated or ongoing hemorrhage, and the risk of bleeding in a confined space (e.g., brain) [215]. Platelet transfusion may be indicated in patients with normal platelet count if there is suspected or known platelet dysfunction (e.g., antiplatelet drug exposure or congenital thrombopathies).

Outside the need for an invasive procedure with risk of bleeding, in humans, platelets are recommended for prophylaxis only if the count is $<10\times10^9$/L [257,258]. In actively bleeding patients therapeutic platelet transfusion is warranted if the count is $<20\times10^9$/L [257,258].

Fresh whole blood is the most readily available blood product that serves as a source of platelets and should be used within 8 h of collection. It should ideally be used in a patient that is anemic and also has thrombocytopenia or thrombocytopathia. A dose of 10 mL/kg is expected to raise the platelet count by 10,000/µL [259, 260]. In non-anemic patients, this amount of transfused RBCs may lead to polycythemia and volume overload. Advantages of using FWB are that no platelets are lost during the processing and there is less activation of platelets than if they were obtained by centrifugation [260].

Platelet-rich plasma (PRP) is produced from FWB using a 'soft spin' centrifugation. The supernatant plasma contains the platelets and is separated from the PRBCs [259]. The recommended dose of PRP is 1 unit per 10 kg of body weight. Use of whole blood to produce PRP has also been described in cattle and horses [261].

Platelet concentrate (PC) can be prepared from PRP by 'hard spin' centrifugation. The supernatant (platelet-poor plasma) is expressed into another satellite bag attached to the PRP bag, leaving about 35–70 mL of concentrated platelets. It is also stored in a fashion similar to PRP. A canine study revealed a mean platelet yield of 8×10^{10} per unit of PC and that about 25% of platelets are lost during the process of making PC from FWB [262]. Use of automated blood cell separators for canine plateletpheresis has been described that gave a mean platelet yield of 3.3×10^{11} platelets in a mean collected volume of 246 mL [263]. The recommended dose of PC is 1 unit per 10 kg of body weight and a maximum rise in platelet count by 40,000/µL is expected [259]. Fresh platelet products are stored at 20–24°C with gentle continuous or intermittent agitation for 5 days when prepared using a closed collection system [259].

Frozen platelet concentrate can be made by stabilizing apheresed platelets with 6% dimethyl sulfoxide (DMSO) or 2% DMSO and ThromoboSol® (a mixture of amiloride, adenosine, and sodium nitroprusside, second messenger effectors that inhibit platelet function) [264]. Valeri *et al.* showed that canine platelets preserved with 6% DMSO and kept at −80°C for 1 year had a 70% recovery rate with a half-life of 2 days versus 3.5 days for fresh platelets [265]. Further, the platelets were effective in stopping the bleeding in thrombocytopenic dogs [266]. A more recent canine study revealed 49% platelet recovery when preserved with 6% DMSO compared to 44% with 2% DMSO and ThromboSol® and the half-life was approximately 2 days compared to mean 3.8 days for fresh platelets [264]. Because the platelets retained the ability to be activated with a reasonable half-life, they still hold promise for the management of life-threatening bleeding in severely thrombocytopenic or thrombocytopathic dogs. Cryopreserved platelets with 6% DMSO are available in the veterinary market (leukoreduced frozen canine platelet concentrate, Animal Blood Resources International, Dixon, CA). The recommended dose is 1 unit/10 kg body weight given over 4 h. Studies evaluating this commercial product indicated a decreased recovery rate of platelets at 59% and increased activation of platelets as indicated by flow cytometry and aggregometry [267,268].

Lyophilized platelets (LYO) are stabilized using an aldehyde cross-linking of membrane proteins and lipids and then lyophilized. LYO can be stored in a refrigerator for up to 2 years and can be reconstituted with 0.9% sodium chloride immediately before administration [269]. Experimental data show that LYO act like normal platelets (as demonstrated by binding to collagen, damaged endothelium, vWF, and the cell membrane receptors), are activated normally, and bind fibrinogen [270,271]. In an experimental canine model of thrombocytopenia and platelet dysfunction induced by cardiac bypass, an infusion of LYO led to improvement in venous bleeding times that peaked at 20–30 min after infusion compared to the control group [272]. A prospective multicenter trial comparing LYO and fresh platelet concentrate (FRESH) in dogs with thrombocytopenia and evidence of active bleeding has been completed [273]. Out of the 37 dogs enrolled, 22 received LYO and 15 received FRESH; the incidence of transfusion reactions was low in both groups and there was no difference in hospitalization time and mortality between groups. There is also potential for LYO to be used as hemostatic agents even if the platelet count and function are normal. In a swine model of liver injury, administration of LYO lead to 80% survival compared to 20% in the placebo group [274]. One of the pigs in the LYO group had evidence of thrombi in other locations on necropsy indicating the risk of thromboembolic potential. Canine LYO are still experimental and are not yet commercially available.

Transfusion compatibility testing

Once the decision has been made to transfuse, compatibility testing should be undertaken if the transfusion is not an emergency or the patient is at high risk for an adverse reaction. If excessive bleeding is a risk, typing and cross-matching should be considered prior to the surgical procedure.

Blood typing

Blood groups have clinical significance because transfusion reactions are likely if an unmatched transfusion is administered in some situations. The number and type of significant blood groups vary between different domestic animal species. In dogs, recognized blood types include dog erythrocytic antigen (DEA) 1.1, 1.2, 3, 4, 5, and 7 [229,275,276]. The DEA 1 system, with its allelic subtypes (i.e., DEA 1.1, DEA 1.2, and possibly DEA 1.3), is the most antigenic. Due to the absence of naturally occurring isoantibodies, the first transfusion from a DEA 1.1-positive donor to a DEA 1.1-negative recipient should not cause an immune reaction to the erythrocytes. However, the second such transfusion will often lead to a severe hemolytic reaction if enough time has elapsed to allow an immune response to develop [277]. It has been shown that naturally occurring isoantibodies are present in some dogs for DEA 3, DEA

5, and DEA 7 [229,278,279]. These isoantibodies can result in transfusion reactions that are usually mild or delayed and a significantly shorter half-life of transfused RBCs may be noticed [280]. At present, a dog is considered a universal donor if it is DEA 4 positive and negative for all the other DEA antigens. "Dal", a newly discovered antigen, exists at a high frequency in dogs but is missing in some Dalmations [281]. *In vitro* antibodies against Dal induce a strong agglutination reaction and could cause a severe transfusion reaction. Based on population prevalence, it has been speculated that with DEA 1.1 compatibility testing the acute transfusion reaction risk could be decreased by 24% and by decreasing exposure to other DEA systems, the risk of acute and delayed transfusion reactions can be further reduced by an additional 8% [229]. In-house blood typing kits are available for DEA 1.1 and are recommended for dogs prior to transfusion in most circumstances.

Cats may be of blood group type A, B or AB. An additional feline blood group antigen "Mik" has also been identified [282]. Distribution of these blood types varies geographically with the highest prevalence of type B reported in Australia (36% of the population) [283]. Blood group B is more prevalent amongst some pure-bred cats, including Birman (18%), Devon Rex (41%), Cornish Rex (31%), British Shorthair (36%) and Scottish Fold (19%) [284]. Originally it was reported that 97% cats in the United States were type A and only 0.3% of cats in the north-east US were type B. However, a 1989 study revealed an incidence of 6% for type B in the US [285]. Type AB has been reported to occur in less than 1% of the general cat population, although this incidence may be higher as new typing methodologies appear better at identifying these cats [286]. Cats with blood group type A may have natural alloantibodies in low titers that can cause shortened RBC survival if type B blood is given. On the other hand, type B cats have naturally occurring isoantibodies against type A in high titers and that can cause a fatal reaction even if 1 mL of type A blood is transfused [287,288]. Type AB cats have neither alloantibody but should receive either AB or A type blood products because of the strong anti-A isoantibodies present in type B blood products. Most cats have the Mik antigen but in cats without Mik, naturally occurring isoantibodies can lead to a hemolytic transfusion reaction even without having received a previous transfusion [289]. In simple terms, the likelihood of incompatibility transfusion reaction is much higher in cats compared to dogs if an unmatched transfusion is performed. In-house typing kits are readily available for cats and it is strongly recommended that all cats are typed prior to transfusion.

In horses, there are no naturally occurring blood type alloantibodies. The Aa and Qa equine blood types are considered most antigenic [290]. Chances of adverse reactions increase if either the donor or recipient is a mare that has been bred previously. Thus, it is recommended to use blood from male horses or mares that have never been pregnant as preferred sources for unmatched transfusions. Also it is preferable to consider donors that are negative for factors Aa and Qa to prevent sensitization of brood mares against the two most common alloantigens involved in neonatal isoerythrolysis. It has been shown that quarter horses, standardbreds and Morgan horse breeds have Aa and Qa negative genotypes and should be evaluated as universal donor candidates [290]. Most horses without previous transfusions may receive one or multiple transfusions safely over a 3–4-day period from an unmatched donor as it takes 5–7 days for antibody production [291]. Blood typing for horses is available through only a few diagnostic laboratories because blood typing antiserum is not readily available [292].

In cattle, the likelihood of reaction during first transfusion is low due to a lack of naturally occurring isoantibodies or low titers in the serum. However, cows with J-negative antigen on the RBCs may have J antibodies that may cause a reaction on first transfusion if J-positive donor cells are used [293]. Although this reaction seems to be of minor clinical significance, the ideal donor cow should have J-negative RBCs.

Cross-matching

This procedure determines the serological compatibility between the recipient and donor blood and is based on an agglutination reaction. It allows detection of naturally occurring alloantibodies or alloantibodies produced as a result of previous exposure to incompatible blood products. The 'major cross-match' evaluates the compatibility between donor RBCs and recipient plasma/serum. The 'minor cross-match' is an assessment of compatibility between the recipient's RBCs and donor plasma/serum. In dogs, cross-matching is recommended if transfusion history is unknown, if hemolytic reaction is noticed during the first transfusion, if more than 7 days have lapsed between administration of transfusion or if the donor's DEA 7 type is unknown [277,294]. In cats, both typing and cross-matching should be strongly considered before an initial transfusion because of identification of the Mik antigen with naturally occurring alloantibodies and the potential for a fatal transfusion reaction [287–289]. In horses, cross-matching is recommended if a second transfusion is needed more than 4–7 days after a first transfusion or if any reaction is noted during the first transfusion. Cattle serum carries minimal agglutinating antibodies and cross-match is usually of little benefit in predicting a transfusion reaction unless a hemolytic test using complement is performed [217]. Standard cross-matching procedures [295] can be found in many texts. A gel cross-match kit is now available for dogs and cats that simplifies the procedure (RapidVet®-H, DMS Laboratories Inc., Flemington, NJ).

Transfusion considerations for massive blood loss

Massive transfusion (MT) involves administration of whole blood or blood components in an amount that is more than the patient's blood volume in 24 h or more than half of the blood volume in 3 h [296]. Conventional guidelines in human medicine regarding management of uncontrolled bleeding and excessive hemorrhage involved early administration of crystalloid and colloid fluid resuscitation to maintain arterial blood pressure and perfusion of tissues followed by 10 or more units of PRBC in the first 24 h to restore oxygenation of the tissues [297]. Both these processes are dilutive in nature and administration of PRBCs has also been considered proinflammatory. Recent human studies have shown that increasing the ratios of plasma and platelets relative to PRBCs early in the resuscitation phase leads to improvement in outcome [298–300]. Due to these new developments, some MT protocols (also known as substantial bleeding protocols [SBP] or trauma exsanguination protocol [TEP]) have been developed [301]. One study revealed that using a TEP, delivery of fixed component protocol (10 units of PRBCs, 4 units of FFP and 2 units of platelets) led to a drop in odds of mortality by 74%, decreased 30-day mortality (51% vs 66%) and overall consumption of blood products [302]. Also, there is evidence that the ratios of blood products at 6 h are more predictive of improved outcome than ratios at 24 h [303,304]. Earlier mathematical models to simulate exsanguinating patients revealed underutilization of clotting factor replacements [305,306]. One model [305] advocated an FFP:PRBC ratio of 2:3 and a platelet to PRBC ratio of 8:10 to prevent effects of hemodilution and coagulopathy, while the other model [306] advocated a ratio of 1:1:1 for platelets, plasma, and PRBCs, approximating the delivery of whole blood. Data from military and civilian studies and pooled analysis report a significant reduction in mortality when higher FFP:PRBC ratios are used [298–300].

There are no prospective randomized controlled trials that specify the optimal ratio of blood products for substantial bleeding trauma patients but based on the present evidence, it seems that delivery of platelets, FFP, and PRBCs in a ratio approaching 1:1:1 may provide better hemostatic resuscitation as part of damage control resuscitation (DCR) [307].

In line with human literature, one veterinary canine study with MT had a high mortality rate of 74% with 100% mortality in dogs with elevated clotting times [296]. Another study in three cats that received MT revealed 67% survival [225]. A dog with aortic laceration that received MT and 5 units of PRBCs, 3 units of FFP, and 1.2 L of autotransfused blood survived [308].

Blood administration

Due to the higher viscosity of PRBCs, administration can be facilitated by diluting the cells with warm 0.9% sodium chloride and using the largest possible catheter for venous access. RBC products can be warmed by wrapping in a sealed plastic bag and putting in a water bath maintained at 37°C. No other type of fluid or drugs except 0.9% sodium chloride should be routinely administered in the same line as blood products, especially calcium-containing fluids. The optimal route of administration is intravenous but the intraosseous route may be used in neonates and animals with difficult vascular access. In healthy dogs more than 90% RBCs can be seen in the peripheral circulation after intraosseous delivery [309]. The initial rate of administration is usually 0.25 mL/kg over the first 30 min to monitor for any adverse effects of transfusion. Rate can be increased to 10–20 mL/kg/h if no adverse effects are detected. In patients with heart disease, the rate should be less and in cats rates of 4 mL/kg/h, 10 mL/kg/h, and 60 mL/kg/h have been described in cardiovascular anomalies, normovolemia, and hypovolemic shock, respectively [222]. Ideally, blood transfusion is finished within 4 h due to the potential risk of bacterial overgrowth in blood maintained at room temperature. In settings of substantial bleeding or trauma, blood can be given as rapidly as possible. This is facilitated by using short length and larger gauge catheters.

Different types of pumps are available to allow administration of a specified volume over a specific time but this delivery technique can potentially influence the half-life of transfused RBCs. In dogs, use of a syringe pump was associated with significantly lower survival (24 h) of transfused RBCs compared to gravity flow techniques [310]. In cats, use of a syringe pump and a microaggregate filter (18 micron) did not result in any difference in short-term (12 h) or long-term (6 weeks) survivability of cells compared to the gravity flow technique [311]. The effect may not only be related to the use of a pump, but also the flow rate, tubing configuration, and other variables which can damage cells. All plasma products (FFP, FP, CPP, PRP, PC) should also be administered through a filter.

Adverse effects of transfusion

Transfusion reactions are categorized as immune mediated or non-immunologic as well as acute or chronic [312]. Immunologic reactions are often against RBCs, plasma proteins, WBCs or platelet antigens. Acute hemolytic transfusion reactions (AHTR), febrile non-hemolytic reactions (FNHTR) and allergic reactions make up most of the immediate reactions. Non-imunologic reactions can be related to administration, contamination, additives, and storage.

Acute hemolytic transfusion reactions are characterized by intravascular hemolysis and are antigen–antibody, type II hypersensitivity reactions primarily mediated by IgG. They occur due to sensitized alloantibody-mediated incompatibilities (such as a DEA 1.1-negative dog sensitized after receiving DEA 1.1-positive blood) or due to the presence of natural alloantibodies (like naturally occurring anti-A antibodies in a type B cat). The antigen–antibody interaction causes activation of complement and cytokines and can result in a systemic inflammatory response [313].

Febrile non-hemolytic transfusion reactions (FNHTR) are defined as a temperature increase of more than 1°C within 1–2 h of transfusion without other explanation [229,312]. These reactions are mostly associated with leukocyte-derived cytokines and/or circulating antileukocyte antibodies in the recipient against donor leukocytes. Use of leukoreduction filters while collecting blood components decreases the incidence of these reactions [229]. It is important to carefully monitor the patients because fever may also be due to bacterial contamination of the unit. If such a reaction is noticed, then the transfusion should be slowed or stopped. If fever is the only sign seen, it may be restarted slowly and non-steroidal anti-inflammatory drug administration could be considered.

Allergic reactions are the result of an IgE antibody-mediated type I hypersensitivity reaction and are caused by soluble substances in the donor plasma that bind to preformed IgE antibodies on mast cells in the recipient, causing release of histamine. These reactions can range from mild hives to severe anaphylaxis causing hypotension and shock. If only hives are seen, the transfusion can be temporarily interrupted and an antihistamine administered [312]. If the reaction is more severe, the transfusion should be discontinued and the patient treated as required with fluids and/or vasoactive drugs.

Transfusion-related acute lung injury (TRALI) is defined as respiratory distress with bilateral lung infiltrates, hypoxemia ($PaO_2/FiO_2 < 300$ mmHg) that occurs within 6 h of transfusion, with clinical exclusion of cardiac failure and other diseases [313]. In humans, the TRALI incidence has been reported to be between 0.08% and 15% [314]. A recent study in small animals reported the incidence of veterinary acute lung injury after transfusion (VetALI) to be 3.7% [315], similar to the incidence of acute lung injury in critically ill dogs. It has been reported with all types of blood products but FFP has been implicated most frequently.

Two theories have been proposed to explain the pathophysiology of TRALI [316,317]. The first one suggests it to be an antibody-mediated reaction in which antigranulocyte antibodies from the donor plasma agglutinate the donor leukocytes. This antigen–antibody interaction can cause complement activation, causing pulmonary sequestration and activation of neutrophils that leads to endothelial damage and capillary leakage. The second theory postulates TRALI as a result of two events ('two-hit' hypothesis). The first event is the clinical condition of the patient that causes endothelial activation and sequestration of neutrophils. The second event is the result of transfusion of biologically active mediators like lipids and cytokines that activate neutrophils already sequestered in the lungs, causing release of oxidases and proteases that leads to endothelial cell damage and capillary leakage, resulting in TRALI. The clinical picture of TRALI is very similar to ARDS with signs and symptoms including tachypnea, fever, tachycardia, and hypoxemia with no evidence of circulatory overload. Differentials include TACO, AHTRs, anaphylactoid reactions, and bacterial contamination.

Treatment is mainly supportive and may include only oxygen supplementation in minor cases or mechanical ventilation in severe cases. TRALI is usually self-limiting and human patients usually recover within 96 h.

In human medicine, development of TRALI has been particularly associated with plasma transfusion from parturient female donors, and use of plasma from male and non-parturient female donors decreases the incidence of TRALI significantly [318]. RBC alloantibodies are not increased in dogs with repeated pregnancies but WBC alloantibodies have not been studied [319].

Acute non-immunologic transfusion reactions can include sepsis, circulatory overload, problems with massive transfusion, and storage issues. In human medicine, bacterial contamination of blood components is considered one of the most common causes of morbidity and mortality, ranging from 100 to 150 transfused individuals each year [320]. Bacteria can originate from inadequately screened donors or from the venepuncture site. In a case series of 14 cats, contamination of blood products was linked to *Serratia marcescens* contamination of a jar containing alcohol-soaked cotton balls and a bag of saline solution used during venepuncture [321]. Signs of sepsis in six cats in this report included vomiting, diarrhea, collapse, and acute death. If sepsis is suspected, the transfusion should be stopped immediately and a Gram stain and blood culture should be obtained directly from the unit and the patient.

Blood products have significant colloidal potential and administration to normovolemic animals or animals with compromised cardiac or pulmonary function predisposes them to hypervolemia, known as **transfusion-associated circulatory overload (TACO)**. Clinical signs include dyspnea, cyanosis, pulmonary edema, increased central venous pressure, and pulmonary venous distension on thoracic radiographs. Treatment involves discontinuing the transfusion, oxygen supplementation, and diuretics.

Metabolic and hemostatic complications similar to humans have been described in dogs after massive transfusions that included hypocalcemia, hypomagnesemia, thrombocytopenia, elevations in clotting times (PT and APTT), and hypothermia [296]. Thrombocytopenia and dilutional coagulopathy occur from dilution of clotting factors and platelets with factor-depleted stored blood, resulting in prolongation of coagulation times. Elevation in clotting times was a poor prognostic indicator in the above study in dogs with MT. Hypocalcemia and hypomagnesemia likely arise from binding of anticoagulant citrate to ionized calcium and magnesium. Following transfusion, citrate is usually metabolized quite fast by the liver but under circumstances of rapid administration, could cause hypocalcemia. In addition, citrate metabolism may be slowed in patients with poor liver function, hypothermia or decreased perfusion to the liver. Symptomatic hypocalcemia (muscle tremors, arrhythmias, hypotension, etc.) should be treated using calcium gluconate (50–150 mg/kg of 10% solution) or calcium chloride (5–10 mg/kg of 10% solution). Stored blood usually is at a temperature of 4°C and if administered without warming could potentially cause arrhythmias and decreased cardiac output initially in addition to the hypothermia, although these adverse effects also depend on the rate of administration [322].

During storage, RBCs undergo a series of biologic and biochemical changes collectively referred to as 'the storage lesions.' There is progressive depletion of ATP and 2,3-DPG, decreased deformability of RBCs, decrease in the pH of stored units due to glycolysis and increased potassium content of the unit due to RBC lysis. In humans, transfusion-associated hyperkalemia can occur but RBCs from most dog breeds (except some like Akitas and Shiba Inus) are low in intracellular potassium so hyperkalemia from stored RBC products is less of a problem in most dogs [323]. Hyperkalemia has been reported in 20% (2/10) of dogs with MT and also in one dog that was given 28-day-old PRBCs [296,323]. During storage, formation of clots or introduction of air into the bag could potentially cause air embolism. Blood transfusion administration sets with a typical filter size of 170 micron are used to help remove the clots and debris.

Non-immune-mediated hemolysis can happen because of overheating, freezing of blood bag or mixing with hypotonic fluids. Signs of hemoglobinemia and/or hemoglobinuria can be noticed during transfusion without other associated signs of acute hemolytic transfusion reaction. In dogs, the incidence of transfusion-related adverse effects has been reported to range from 3.3% to 13% [227,228]. Clinical signs described in dogs may include fever, tachycardia, tachypnea, dyspnea, muscle tremors, vomiting, weakness, collapse, restlessness, and salivation. Hemoglobinemia and hemoglobinuria can also be observed in acute hemolytic transfusion reactions. In cats, the incidence of transfusion reaction has been reported to range from 1.2% to 8.7% [222–224]. Most adverse effects were FNHTRs. Other reported clinical signs included face rubbing, vomiting, salivation, and volume overload. Signs related to acute hemolytic transfusion reaction included pigmenturia, fever, and tachypnea. One study reported the incidence of adverse reactions to blood products to be 16% (7/44) in horses that included urticaria, anaphylaxis (characterized by acute colic, dyspnea, and excitation), and hemolysis [226]. One of the horses experiencing acute anaphylactic reaction had to be euthanized. Incidence of transfusion reactions to commercial equine plasma has been reported to be 8.7% in foals and 0% in adult horses and included fever, tachycardia, tachypnea, and colic [324]. Serum hepatitis has also been reported with commercial equine plasma. Non-commercial frozen equine plasma was associated with 10% adverse reactions that were mild in nature and included hives, tachycardia, pyrexia, tachypnea, severe pruritus, and swollen eyes [325].

The adverse effects reported in cattle include trembling, hives, edema, piloerection, stertorous breathing, tachycardia, tachypnea, dyspnea, and violent movements [217,326]. Regardless of the species, transfusion reaction signs typical for conscious animals may be masked or absent in anesthetized patients.

In cats, the half-life of transfused RBCs is approximately 35–38 days for compatible transfusions and decreases to only 1–2 h if a type B cat receives type A blood and approximately 2 days when type B blood is given to a type A cat [229]. The half-life of allogenic transfused RBCs in cattle has been shown to be 2–4 days with a rapid loss of 10–15% cells occurring in the first 24 h [217]. Previous studies using radioactive RBC labeling techniques have reported that transfused RBCs survive less than a week in the horse and sometimes less than 2 days, but a recent study using biotin-labeled RBCs reported an average lifespan of 20 days in allogenic RBC transfusions [327].

When patients are under anesthesia, adverse effects associated with transfusion reactions can be masked. American Society of Anesthesiologists practice guidelines recommend that patients should be monitored carefully for urticaria, hypotension, tachycardia, increased peak airway pressure, hyperthermia, hemoglobinuria, decreased urine output, and evidence of increased microvascular bleeding [215]. If any of these are seen, transfusion should be stopped and appropriate diagnostic testing should be ordered.

Alternatives to allogenic blood transfusions

Because of the potential complications associated with the use of allogenic blood products and to help conserve blood products, alternative strategies have been examined to reduce the need for blood products in the perioperative settings.

Autologous transfusion

Autologous transfusion involves administering blood to a patient that was previously collected from that patient. By using one's own blood, the risks associated with the transmission of infectious diseases or transfusion reactions are minimized. Three forms of autologous transfusion strategies have been explored. **Preoperative autologous blood donation (PABD)** provides a supply of safe blood for patients planned to undergo an elective surgical procedure that could potentially be associated with significant blood loss. Patients donate their own blood in advance which is stored for their own use. Data from human meta-analyses on PABD revealed a 63% reduction in allogenic blood transfusions but an increased overall transfusion of RBCs by 30% (both allogenic and autologous) in patients that undertook the donation. A decline in patient's hemoglobin by an average 1.23 g/dL from before PABD to immediately prior to surgery was reported [328–330]. Use of PABD has been described especially in total joint replacement surgeries in humans [331]. In veterinary medicine, PABD has been described in horses that were scheduled for sinus surgeries and in cats that underwent craniotomies [332,333]. In cats, the median time from donation until surgery was 12 days. The predonation median PCV was 30% (approximately 10 g/dL hemoglobin) and the PCV before surgery was 26% (approximately 8.7 g/dL hemoglobin), a drop (1.3 g/dL) similar to that reported in humans [328,333]. Preoperatively, mild anemia was noticed in 3/15 cats. Eleven of 15 cats that received an autologous transfusion perioperatively did not require an allogenic transfusion. Some inherent limitations to this technique would include need for advanced planning, cost, need for sedation in veterinary patients, risk of bacterial contamination and some patients may experience perioperative anemia and increased likelihood of transfusion need. In addition, waste of unneeded PABD units of blood products has been reported to vary from 18% to above 50% in humans [334,335]. Waste may be decreased by using the PABD unit for other animals but this would require infectious disease screening, blood typing and cross-matching, all of which add to the expense.

Acute normovolemic hemodilution (ANH) involves removal of a patient's whole blood before anticipated surgical blood loss. It is performed shortly before or after induction of anesthesia. The circulating blood volume is restored by using crystalloids or colloids in a ratio of 3:1 or 1:1 respectively. The blood is collected in standard blood collection bags and stored in the operating room at room temperature. Collected blood is administered within 6–8 h so that there is little deterioration of platelets and clotting factors. The main benefit of ANH is reduction in RBC losses when whole blood with lower PCV is lost after ANH is completed. A decrease in blood viscosity caused by hemodilution decreases peripheral resistance and cardiac output can be increased. Although arterial oxygen content (CaO_2) is decreased, DO_2 is maintained by the increase in cardiac output. When performing ANH, a target PCV of 25% is usual but should be dictated by the anticipated blood loss, pre-existing volume status, type of surgical procedure, PCV before ANH, presence of any other comorbidities and institutional policies. In order to calculate the amount of blood that could be collected to achieve a desired PCV, the following formula may be used:

$$\text{Collected blood(mL)} = \frac{[\text{EBV} \times (H_o - H_f)]}{H_{av}}$$

where EBV is effective circulating blood volume calculated as body weight (kg) times the volume of blood (mL/kg), H_o is the original PCV of the patient before ANH, H_f is the targeted PCV and H_{av} is the average of H_o and H_f. In humans, ANH has been successfully utilized during surgical procedures for radical prostatectomy, hip and knee arthroplasty and vascular surgeries. A relative drop of 31% in the frequency of allogenic transfusion has been reported [328,336–339].

Autologous transfusion using cell salvage methodology is a technique by which blood lost intra- or postoperatively is collected, washed, and administered to the patient. Relatively simple methods of blood salvage involve using sterile vacuum suction tips or a syringe and tubing system for blood aspiration connected to an attached reservoir for collection. If the blood has been in contact with serosal surfaces for more than an hour, defibrination occurs that precludes the need for an anticoagulant but when blood is collected from a site of fresh and rapid hemorrhage, anticoagulant will be required. The blood collected via these methods should be transfused within 4–6 h of collection compared to ANH which can be kept for up to 8 h.

Use of a semi-automated autotransfusion cell separator system (Electa Autotransfusion Cell Separator, Dideco, Mirandola, Italy) was described in a case series of dogs with hemoabdomen [340]. Blood is directly suctioned from the surgical field into a reservoir where automatic mixing with the anticoagulant takes place. It is then moved to a centrifugation bowl system, a process called 'priming' followed by 'washing' to remove plasma, activated clotting factors, anticoagulants, complement, and systemic medications. After completion of the washing phase, the 'emptying' phase moves the blood to a reinfusion bag. The authors speculated that by using the above technique, they were able to reduce the transfusion requirement. Meta-analysis in humans has shown that cell salvage techniques lead to 38% relative and 21% absolute reduction in the risk of exposure to allogenic RBC transfusion [341].

An in-line leukoreduction filter is used during transfusion of salvaged cells to reduce the nucleated cell count and bacterial load delivered to the patient. In humans, salvaged cell solutions used for administration are equal or superior to blood bank units with regard to cell morphology, pH, red cell osmotic resistance, and levels of 2,3-DPG [342,343]. The contraindication often given to using these techniques is in patients with neoplasia, to avoid iatrogenic hematogenous spread. However, this risk is reduced as the process of cell salvage and use of leukoreduction filters remove tumor cells. Studies in humans have failed to document increase in any adverse outcomes when cell salvage techniques were employed in perioperative oncologic settings [343–346]. Septicemia does not appear to be a major complication of cell salvaging [344,347]. If less sophisticated methods of autotransfusion are used and enteric contamination is suspected or hemoabdomen is from a suspected splenic hemangiosarcoma, autotransfusion should be avoided. To avoid hemolysis as a result of collection technique, it is recommended to keep the needle or suction tip below the surface of the blood to avoid air interface damage and to keep the maximum vacuum settings between 100 and 300 mmHg [348]. 'Cell salvage syndrome' could be a consequence of inadequate washing of RBCs and retention of plasma proteins, inflammatory cytokines, complement, free hemoglobin and fibrin degradation products that could cause disseminated intravascular coagulation, ARDS, acute kidney injury, and death [349].

Blood substitutes

Use of oxygen-carrying solutions as an alternative to blood transfusion has been researched for decades. Early versions of **hemoglobin-based oxygen carriers (HBOC)** were associated with nephrotoxic effects and a short intravascular half-life [350]. These were improved by ultrapurification to remove RBC stromal elements and polymerization of hemoglobin units with glutaraldehyde (Oxyglobin®, HBOC-200, Biopure Corporation, Cambridge, Mass) [351,352]. Oxyglobin® is the only clinically approved product for use in dogs and it is an ultrapurified glutaraldehyde-polymerized bovine-derived hemoglobin solution [352]. It is supplied as a sterile purple-colored colloid solution in a 60 mL or 125 mL package that contains 13 g/dL hemoglobin concentration in a modified Ringer's solution with a pH of 7.8 and osmolality of 300 mOsm/kg. Approximately 50% Hb polymers have molecular weight between 65 and 130 kDa with only 10% having molecular weight above 500 kDa and average molecular weight is 200 kDa.

Studies of the pharmacokinetics of Oxyglobin® in dogs revealed a dose-dependent plasma terminal half-life of 18–43 h for a dose varying between 10 and 30 mL/kg [353]. Administration to healthy dogs at a dose of 8.5 mL/kg, 21 mL/kg, and 42.5 mL/kg at a rate of 7 mL/kg/h revealed a mean elimination half-life of 22, 30, and 38 h respectively. Plasma clearance and volume of distribution were also dose related and clearance of individual plasma Hb components was inversely proportional to size (dimer > tetramer > octamer) [354, 355]. Most of the dose is cleared from plasma within 5–9 days after infusion. The pharmacokinetics of Oxyglobin® have been described in horses after a single dose of 250 mL (32.5 g) with median elimination half-life of 1.3 h for small aggregates and 12 h for large aggregates of hemoglobin [356]. The reticuloendothelial system is responsible for metabolizing Oxyglobin® and unstable tetramer and dimers that constitute less than 5% of Oxyglobin® are excreted by the kidneys.

Oxyglobin® has a higher P_{50} (34 mmHg) compared to canine blood, which is approximately 28 mmHg, and lower viscosity (1.3 versus 3.5 centipoise) compared to whole blood. The Oxyglobin® dissociation curve lies to the right of the canine hemoglobin dissociation curve, leading to improved oxygen offloading to the tissues with Oxyglobin®. After acute isovolemic hemodilution in dogs, administration of HBOC-201 (Hemopure®, a similar product studied for human patient use) led to a higher oxygen extraction ratio compared to autologous RBC transfusion [357]. Administration of HBOC-201 also restored the skeletal muscle oxygen tension to near baseline in a dog model of artificial arterial stenosis [358]. Bovine hemoglobin utilizes Cl^- instead of 2,3-DPG as an allosteric modulator to modify transport and affinity of oxygen, carbon dioxide and hydrogen ions, providing another advantage over stored blood that is typically low in 2,3-DPG.

Oxyglobin® has vasopressor properties due to scavenging of nitric oxide, upregulation of endothelins and improved arteriolar autoregulation due to increases in oxygen delivery [359]. The increase in systemic vascular resistance has been reported in dogs and ponies [360,361]. In a model of canine hemorrhagic shock, compared to hetastarch the administration of 30 mL/kg of HBOC led to faster reversal of tissue hypoxia characterized by reversal of splanchnic and systemic metabolic acidosis and resolution of lactatemia, but no increase in systemic and mesenteric oxygen delivery was noticed. This rapid reversal of anaerobic metabolism despite the lack of increase in oxygen delivery is potentially due to facilitation of oxygen delivery by HBOC at the level of the microcirculation rather than an increase in oxygen content and bulk delivery of oxygen to the microcirculation [362]. Clear-cut advantages of Oxyglobin® involve a wide range of storage temperature (2–30°C), a long shelf-life of 3 years from the date of manufacture and no need for a cross-match. Because of the absence of antigenic RBC membrane no antigenic response to its administration is expected. Oxyglobin® administered at a dose of 10 mL/kg produced IgG antibodies in dogs by 6 weeks that reached the highest titer by 10 weeks after the third transfusion, but no selective antibody deposition was noticed in the liver or kidneys and circulating antibodies did not diminish the ability of Oxyglobin® to transport oxygen [363]. In human surgical patients, HBOCs have been shown to decrease allogenic blood transfusions [364,365].

Oxyglobin® is approved for the treatment of anemia in dogs [366, 367] but has been used off-label for the treatment of same in cats [368–370] and its use in ponies [361] has been described. In cats, the off-label use was prompted by unavailability of feline blood products, unavailability of compatible blood donors and difficulties in blood typing due to RBC agglutination [368,369]. The side-effects observed in cats included tachypnea, mucous membrane discoloration, pigmenturia, vomiting, neurologic abnormalities, pulmonary edema, and pleural effusion [368,369]. Some cats [368] experiencing pulmonary edema or pleural effusions had prior presence of pleural effusions or pulmonary edema and in another study [369], all the cats that experienced pulmonary edema had evidence of cardiac pathology. In the initial study [368], cats that developed circulatory overload received a median Oxyglobin® dose of 20.6 mL/kg while cats with cardiac pathology [369] that received 12.3 mL/kg in 24 h experienced circulatory overload. Oxyglobin® should be used cautiously in cats as many cats with cardiomyopathy may not display overt clinical signs. In addition, monitoring central venous pressure, respiratory rate and jugular venous distension as general indicators of circulatory overload is recommended [368,369]. Out of seven ponies given Oxyglobin®, one experienced an anaphylactoid reaction characterized by intense pruritus, tachycardia, and tachypnea [361].

The recommended dose rate in dogs is 10–30 mL/kg with a rate not exceeding 10 mL/kg/h and in cats the recommendation is to keep the rate at 5 mL/kg/h or below to minimize the risk of circulatory overload.

Less than 5% of Oxyglobin® is present as unstable dimers and tetramers that are rapidly excreted in the urine. Their elimination may give the urine a reddish/orange tinge for 4–6 h after administration. During this time dipstick measurements of urine parameters (e.g., pH, protein, glucose, ketones) are unreliable. Also transient discoloration of sclera and skin can occur. Serum biochemistry tests that rely on colorimetric measurements are typically invalid. An opened bag should be used within 24 h because of the potential formation of methemoglobin and bacterial contamination.

Strategies to minimize perioperative blood loss

Selective and non-selective inhibitors of cyclo-oxygenase (COX) enzyme including carprofen, meloxicam, deracoxib, and aspirin can impair hemostasis by inhibiting platelet function to variable extents [371–373]. In addition, antiplatelet drugs such as clopidogrel also inhibit platelet function with effects in cats lasting for approximately 7 days after stopping drug administration [374]. If clinically acceptable, administration of these drugs should be discontinued preoperatively. For elective surgery, American Society of Anesthesiologists practice guidelines recommend discontinuing anticoagulation therapy if possible and/or delaying surgery long enough to decrease drug effects [215]. Desmopressin can improve hemostasis under invasive procedures such as biopsy and surgery. Use of desmopressin acetate (DDAVP) has been shown to improve primary hemostasis in dogs with aspirin-induced platelet dysfunction, von Willebrand's disease, and chronic liver disease [375,376].

Antifibrinolytic drugs prevent the breakdown of clots. In humans, their use has been associated with significant reduction in blood loss during and after surgery [377,378]. Aprotinin reduced the probability of RBC transfusion requirement by a relative 34% and appeared more effective than lysine analogs epsilon-aminocaproic acid and tranexamic acid. In the veterinary literature, two studies [379,380] demonstrated the use of epsilon-aminocaproic acid in retired running Greyhounds undergoing amputation and gonadectomy and its use was associated with significantly lower postoperative blood loss. American Society of Anesthesiologists practice guidelines do not recommend routine use of these agents but suggest that they can be used for reducing the need for allogenic blood transfusion for patients at high risk of excessive bleeding [215].

Maintenance of near-normothermia is important in the perioperative period because hypothermia can increase surgical blood loss [381]. In elective hip arthroplasty procedures, a drop in core body temperature of 1.6°C resulted in a 500 mL increase in blood loss and a significant increase in need for allogenic blood transfusion [382,383]. Hypothermia can influence both platelet function and clotting factor activity adversely [384,385]. It is important to remember that many factors other than body temperature can interact to increase operative blood loss.

Transfusions in the perioperative setting can be life saving when used correctly. It is crucial to pick the appropriate components, to use typing and cross-matching to minimize the risk of reactions, to monitor carefully for other reactions, and to use adjunctive techniques to reduce the need for allogenic transfusion. Use of autologous transfusion and cell salvage may improve our ability to improve oxygen delivery.

References

1 MacIntire DK. Pediatric fluid therapy. *Vet Clin Small Anim* 2008; **38**: 621–627.

2 Starling EH. On the absorption of fluids from the connective tissue spaces. *J Physiol* 1896; **19**: 312–326.

3 Landis EM, Pappenheimer JR. Exchange of substances through capillary walls. In: Hamilton WF, Dow P, eds. *Handbook of Physiology, Section 2: Circulation II*. Washington DC: American Physiological Society, 1963: 961–1034.

4 Woodcock TE, Woodcock TM. Revised Starling equation and the glycocalyx model of transvascular fluid exchange: an improved paradigm for prescribing intravenous fluid therapy. *Br J Anaesth* 2012; **108**: 384–394.

5 Levick JR, Michel CC. Microvascular fluid exchange and revised Starling principle. *Cardiovascular Res* 2010; **87**: 198–210.

6 Valverde A, Gianotti G, Rioja-Garcia E, *et al.* Effects of high volume, rapid fluid therapy on cardiovascular function and hematological values during isoflurane-induced hypotension in healthy dogs. *Can J Vet Res* 2012; **76**: 99–108.

7 Muir WW, Kitjawornrat A, Ueyama Y, *et al.* Effects of intravenous administration of lactated Ringer's solution on hematologic, serum biochemical, rheological, hemodynamic, and renal measurements in healthy isoflurane-anesthetized dogs. *J Am Vet Med Assoc* 2011; **239**: 630–637.

8 Kolsen-Peterson JA, Nielsen JO, Tonnesen E. Acid base and electrolyte changes after hypertonic saline (7.5%) infuaion: a randomized controlled clinical trial. *Scand J Clin Lab Invest* 2005; **65**: 13–22.

9 Hopper K, Epstein SE. Incidence, nature, and etiology of metabolic acidosis in dogs and cats. *J Vet Intern Med* 2012; **26**: 1107–1114.

10 Handy JM, Soni N. Physiological effects and hyperchloremia and acidosis. *Br J Anaesth* 2008; **101**: 141–150.

11 Tonozzi CC, Rudloff E, Kirby R. Perfusion versus hydration: impact on the fluid therapy plan. *Compend Contin Edu Vet* 2009; E1–E14.

12 Silverstein DC, Aldrich J, Haskins SC, *et al.* Assessment of changes in blood volume in response to resuscitative fluid administration in dogs. *J Vet Emerg Crit Care* 2005; **15**: 185–192.

13 Kudnig ST, Mama K. Guidelines for perioperative fluid therapy. *Compend Contin Edu Pract Vet* 2003; **25**: 102–111.

14 Bednarski R, Grimm K, Harvey R, *et al.* AAHA anesthesia guidelines for dogs and cats. *J Am Anim Hosp Assoc* 2011; **47**: 377–385.

15 Schenck PA, Chew DJ, Nagode LA, *et al.* Disorders of calcium: hypercalcemia and hypocalcemia. In: Dibartola SP, ed. *Fluid, Electrolyte, and Acid-Base Disorders in Small Animal Practice*. 4th edn. St Louis, Missouri: Elsevier, 2012; 120–194.

16 Schaer M. Therapeutic approach to electrolyte emergencies. *Vet Clin Small Anim* 2008; **38**: 513–533.

17 Smith GW. Supportive therapy of the toxic cow. *Vet Clin Food Anim* 2005; **21**: 595–614.

18 Roussel AJ, Cohen ND, Holland PS, *et al.* Alterations in acid–base and serum electrolyte concentrations in cattle: 632 cases (1984–1994). *J Am Vet Med Assoc* 1998; **212**: 1769–1775.

19 Pinto FC, Capone-Neto A, Prist R, *et al.* Volume replacement with lactated Ringer's or 3% hypertonic saline solution during combined experimental hemorrhagic shock and traumatic brain injury. *J Trauma* 2006; **60**: 758–764.

20 Ramming S, Shackford SR, Zhuang J, *et al.* The relationship of fluid balance and sodium administration to cerebral edema formation and intracranial pressure in a porcine model of brain injury. *J Trauma* 1994; **37**: 705–713.

21 Schmall LM, Muir WW, Robertson JT. Haematological, serum electrolyte and blood gas effects of small volume hypertonic saline in experimentally induced hemorrhagic shock. *Equine Vet J* 1990; **22**: 278–283.

22 Lorenzo M, Davis JW, Negin S, *et al.* Can Ringer's lactate be used safely with blood transfusions? *Am J Surg* 1998; **175**: 308–310.

23 Cull DL, Lally KP, Murphy KD. Compatibility of packed erythrocytes and Ringer's lactate solution. *Surg Gynecol Obstet* 1991; **173**: 9–12.

24 Goldstein SM, MacLean LD. Ringers lactate infusion with severe hepatic damage: effect on arterial lactate level. *Can J Surg* 1972; **15**: 318–321.

25 Didwania A, Miller J, Kassel D, *et al.* Effect of intravenous lactated Ringer' solution infusion on the circulating lactate concentration: Part 3. Results of a prospective, randomized, double-blind, placebo-controlled trial. *Crit Care Med* 1997; **25**: 1851–1854.

26 Vall DM, Ogilvie GK, Fettman MJ, *et al.* Exacerbation of hyperlactatemia by infusion of lactated Ringer's solution in dogs with lymphoma. *J Vet Intern Med* 1990; **4**: 228–232.

27 Steffen RP, McKenzie JE, Bockman EL, *et al.* Changes in dog gracilis muscle adenosine during exercise and acetate infusion. *Am J Physiol* 1983; **244**: H387–H395.

28 Saragoca MA, Bessa AM, Mulinari RA, *et al.* Sodium acetate, an arterial vasodilator: haemodynamic characterization in normal dogs. *Proc Eur Dial Transplant Assoc* 1985; **21**: 221–224.

29 Keshaviah PR. The role of acetate in the etiology of symptomatic hypotension. *Artif Organs* 1982; **6**: 378–387.

30 Strandvik GF. Hypertonic saline in critical care: a review of literature and guidelines for use in hypotensive states and raised intracranial pressure. *Anaesthesia* 2009; **64**: 990–1003.

31 Constable P. Fluid and electrolyte therapy in ruminants. *Vet Clin Food Anim* 2003; **19**: 557–597.

32 Barry KG, Berman AR. Mannitol infusion. Part III. The acute effect of the intravenous infusion of mannitol on blood and plasma volume. *N Engl J Med* 1961; **264**: 1085–1088.

33 Velasco IT, Pontieri V, Rocha e Silva M, *et al.* Hyperosmotic NaCl and severe hemorrhagic shock. *Am J Physiol* 1980; **239**: H664–H673.

34 Smith GJ, Kramer GC, Perron P, *et al.* A comparison of several hypertonic solutions for resuscitation of bled sheep. *J Surg Res* 1985; **39**: 517–528.

35 Velasco IT, Rocha e Silva M, Oliveira MA, *et al.* Hypertonic and hyperoncotic resuscitation from severe hemorrhagic shock in dogs: a comparative study. *Crit Care Med* 1989; **17**: 261–264.

36 Schertel ER, Valentine AK, Rademakers AM, *et al.* Influence of 7% NaCl on the mechanical properties of the systemic circulation in hypovolemic dogs. *Circ Shock* 1990; **31**: 203–214.

37 Wildenthal K, Mierzwiak DS, Mitchell JH. Acute effects of increased serum osmolality on left ventricular performance. *Am J Physiol* 1969; **216**: 898–904.

38 Kien ND, Kramer GC. Cardiac performance following hypertonic saline. *Braz J Med Biol Res* 1989; **22**: 245–248.

39 Gazitua MC, Scott JB, Swindall B. Resistance responses to local changes in plasma osmolality in three vascular beds. *Am J Physiol* 1971; **220**: 384–391.

40 Pascual JL, Khwaja KA, Chaudhury P, *et al.* Hypertonic saline and microcirculation. *J Trauma* 2003; **54**: S133–S140.

41 Ciesla DJ, Moore EE, Silliman CC, *et al.* Hypertonic saline attenuation of polymorphonuclear cytotoxicity: timing is everything. *J Trauma* 2000; **48**: 388–395.

42 Hirsh M, Dyugovaskaya L, Bashenko Y, *et al.* Reduced rate of bacterial translocation and improved variables of natural killer cell and T-cell activity in rats surviving controlled hemorrhagic shock and treated with hypertonic saline. *Crit Care Med* 2002; **30**: 861–867.

43 Rocha e Silva M, Poli de Figueiredo LF. Small volume hypertonic resuscitation of circulatory shock. *Clinics* 2005; **60**: 159–172.

44 Vajda K, Szabo A, Boros M. Heterogeneous microcirculation in the rat small intestine during hemorrhagic shock: quantification of the effects of hypertonic-hyperoncotic resuscitation. *Eur Surg Res* 2004; **36**: 338–344.

45 Zhao L, Wang B, You G, *et al.* Effects of different resuscitation fluids on the rheologic behavior of red blood cells, blood viscosity and plasma viscosity in experimental hemorrhagic shock. *Resuscitation* 2009; **80**: 253–258.

46 Jonas J, Heimann A, Strecker U, *et al.* Hypertonic/hyperoncotic resuscitation after intestinal superior mesenteric artery occlusion: early effects on circulation and intestinal reperfusion. *Shock* 2000; **14**: 24–29.

47 Mittlmeier T, Vollmar B, Menger MD, *et al.* Small volume hypertonic hydroxyethyl starch reduces acute microvascular dysfunction after closed soft tissue trauma. *J Bone Joint Surg* 2003; **85B**: 126–132.

48 Schmall LM, Muir WW, Robertson JT. Haematological, serum electrolyte and blood gas effects of small volume hypertonic saline in experimentally induced hemorrhagic shock. *Equine Vet J* 1990; **22**: 278–283.

49 Wade CE, Grady JJ, Kramer GC. Efficacy of hypertonic saline dextran fluid resuscitation for patients with hypotension from penetrating trauma. *J Trauma* 2003; **54**: S144–S148.

50 Bratton SL, Chestnut RM, Ghajar J, *et al.* Brain trauma foundation guidelines for the management of severe traumatic brain injury. II Hyperosmolar therapy. *J Neurotrauma* 2007; **24(S1)**: S14–S21.

51 Zornow MH, Todd MM, Moore SS. The acute cerebral effects of changes in plasma osmolality and oncotic pressure. *Anesthesiology* 1987; **67**: 936–941.

52 Qureshi AI, Silson DA, Traystman RJ. Treatment of elevated intracranial pressure in experimental intracerebral hemorrhage: comparison between mannitol and hypertonic saline. *Neurosurgery* 1999; **44**: 1055–1063.

53 Kamel H, Navi BB, Nakagawa K, *et al.* Hypertonic saline versus mannitol for the treatment of elevated intracranial pressure: a meta-analysis of randomized clinical trials. *Crit Care Med* 2011; **39**: 554–559.

54 Mortazavi MM, Romeo AK, Deep A, *et al.* Hypertonic saline for treating intracranial pressure: literature review with meta-analysis *J Neurosurg* 2012; **116**: 210–221.

55 Shackford SR, Schmoker JD, Zhuang J. The effect of hypertonic resuscitation on pial arteriolar tone after brain injury and shock. *J Trauma* 1994; **37**: 899–908.

56 Doyle JA, Davis DP, Hoyt DB. The use of hypertonic saline in the treatment of traumatic brain injury. *J Trauma* 2001; **50**: 367–383.

57 Schertel ER, Allen DA, Muir WW, *et al.* Evaluation of a hypertonic saline-dextran solution for treatment of dogs with shock induced by gastric-dilation-volvulus. *J Am Vet Med Assoc* 1997; **210**: 226–230.

58 Horton JW, Dunn CW, Burnweit CA, *et al.* Hypertonic saline-dextran resuscitation of acute canine bile-induced pancreatitis. *Am J Surg* 1989; **158**: 48–56.

59 Machado MC, Coelho AM, Pontieri V, *et al.* Local and systemic effects of hypertonic solution (NaCl 7.5%) in experimentally acute pancreatitis. *Pancreas* 2006; **32**: 80–86.

60 Shields CJ, Sookhai S, Ryan L, *et al.* Hypertonic saline attenuates end organ damage in experimental model of acute pancreatitis. *Br J Surg* 2000; **87**: 1336–1340.

61 Pantaleon LG, Furr MO, McKenzie HC, *et al.* Cardiovascular and pulmonary effects of hetastarch plus hypertonic saline solutions during experimental endotoxemia in anesthetized horses. *J Vet Intern Med* 2006; **20**: 1422–1428.

62 Pantaleon LG, Furr MO, McKenzie HC, *et al.* Effects of small- and large-volume resuscitation on coagulation and electrolytes during experimental endotoxemia in anesthetized horses. *J Vet Intern Med* 2007; **21**: 1374–1379.

63 Constable PD, Schmall LM, Muir WW, *et al.* Hemodynamic responses of endotoxemic calves to treatment with small-volume hypertonic saline solution. *Am J Vet Res* 1991; **52**: 990–998.

64 Constable PD, Gohar HM, Morin DE, *et al.* Use of hypertonic saline-dextran solution to resuscitate hypovolemic calves with diarrhea. *Am J Vet Res* 1996; **57**: 97–104.

65 Koch A, Kaske M. Clinical efficacy of intravenous hypertonic saline solution or hypertonic bicarbonate solution in the treatment of inappetent calves with neonatal diarrhea. *J Vet Intern Med* 2008; **22**: 202–211.

66 Senturk S. Effects of a hypertonic saline solution and dextran 70 combination in the treatment of diarrheic dehydrated calves. *J Vet Med A Physiol Pathol Clin Med* 3003; **50**: 57–61.

67 Tyler JW, Welles EG, Erskine RJ, *et al.* Clinical and clinicopathologic changes in cows with endotoxin-induced mastitis treated with small volumes of isotonic or hypertonic sodium chloride administered intravenously. *Am J Vet Res* 1994; **55**: 278–287.

68 Gross D, Landau EH, Klin B, *et al.* Treatment of uncontrolled hemorrhagic shock with hypertonic saline solution. *Surg Gynecol Obstet* 1990; **170**: 106–112.

69 Bruttig SP, O'Benar J, Wade CE, *et al.* Benefit of slow infusion of hypertonic saline/dextran in swine with uncontrolled aortotomy hemorrhage. *Shock* 2005; **24**: 92–96.

70 Landau EG, Gross D, Assalia A, *et al.* Treatment of uncontrolled hemorrhagic shock with hypertonic saline and external counter pressure. *Ann Emerg Med* 1989; **18**: 1039–1043.

71 Stern SA, Kowalenko T, Younger J, *et al.* Comparison of the effects of bolus vs. slow infusion of 7.5% NaCl/6% dextran-70 in a model of near-lethal uncontrolled hemorrhage. *Shock* 2000; **14**: 616–622.

72 McKirnan MD, Williams RL, Limjoco U, *et al.* Hypertonic saline/dextran vs. lactated Ringer's treatment for hemorrhage in dehydrated swine. *Circ Shock* 1994; **44**: 238–246.

73 Ho HS, Sondeen JL, Dubick MA, *et al.* The renal effects of 7.5% NaCl-6% dextran-70 versus lactated Ringer's resuscitation of hemorrhage in dehydrated sheep. *Shock* 1996; **5**: 289–297.

74 Sondeen JL, Gunther RA, Dubick MA. Comparison of 7.5% NaCl/6% dextran-70 resuscitation of hemorrhage between euhydrated and dehydrated sheep. *Shock* 1995; **3**: 63–68.

75 Fielding CL, Magdesian KG. A comparison of hypertonic (7.2%) and isotonic (0.9%) saline for fluid resuscitation in horses: a randomized, double-blinded, clinical trial. *J Vet Intern Med* 2011; **25**: 1138–1143.

76 Kramer GC. Hypertonic resuscitation: physiologic mechanisms and recommendations for trauma care. *J Trauma* 2003; **54**: S89–S99.

77 Ajito T, Suzuki K, Iwabuchi S. Effect of intravenous infusion of 7.2% hypertonic saline solution on serum electrolytes and osmotic pressure in healthy Beagles. *J Vet Med Sci* 1999; **61**: 637–641.

78 Dubick MA, Zaucha GM, Korte DW Jr, *et al.* Acute and subacute toxicity of 7.5% hypertonic saline-6% dextran-70 (HSD) in dogs. 2.Biochemical and behavioral responses. *J Appl Toxicol* 1993; **13**: 49–55.

79 Mensack S. Fluid therapy: options and rational administration. *Vet Clin Small Anim* 2008; **38**: 575–586.

80 Wellman ML, DiBartola SP, Kohn CW. Applied physiology of body fluids in dogs and cats. In: Dibartola SP, ed. *Fluid, Electrolyte, and Acid-Base Disorders in Small Animal Practice*, 4th edn. St Louis, Missouri: Elsevier, 2012; 2–25.

81 Silverstein DC. Daily intravenous fluid therapy. In: Silverstein D, Hopper K, eds. *Small Animal Critical Care Medicine*. St Louis, Missouri: Saunders, 2009; 271–275.

82 Muir WW, Wiese AJ. Comparison of lactated Ringer's solution and physiologically balanced 6% hetastarch plasma expander for the treatment of hypotension induced via blood withdrawal in isoflurane anesthetized dogs. *Am J Vet Res* 2004; **65**: 1189–1194.

83 Epstein KL, Bergren A, Giguere S, *et al.* Cardiovascular, colloid osmotic pressure, and hemostatic effects of 2 formulations of hydroxyethyl starch in healthy horses. *J Vet Intern Med* 2014; **28**: 223–233.

84 Aarnes TK, Bednarski RM, Lerche P, *et al.* Effect of intravenous administration of lactated Ringer's solution or hetastarch for the treatment of isoflurane induced hypotension in dogs. *Am J Vet Res* 2009; **70**: 1345–1353.

85 Hallowell GD, Corley KT. Preoperative administration of hydroxyethyl starch or hypertonic saline to horses with colic. *J Vet Intern Med* 2006; **20**: 980–986.

86 Hiltebrand LB, Kimberger O, Arnberger M, *et al.* Crystalloids versus colloids for goal-directed fluid therapy in major surgery. *Crit Care* 2009; **13**: R40–R53.

87 Mcllory DR, Kharasch ED. Acute intravascular volume expansion with rapidly administered crystalloid or colloid in the setting of moderate hypovolemia. *Anesth Analg* 2003; **96**: 1572–1577.

88 Westphal M, James MFM, Kozek-Langenecker S, *et al.* Hydroxyethyl starches, different products-different effects. *Anesthesiology* 2009; **111**: 187–202.

89 Kozek-Langenecker S. Effects of hydroxyethyl starch solutions on hemostasis. *Anesthesiology* 2005; **103**: 654–660.

90 Boldt J. Modern rapidly degradable hydroxyethyl starches: current concepts. *Anesth Analg* 2009; **108**: 1574–1582.

91 Jungheinrich C, Neff TA. Pharmacokinetics of hydroxyethyl starch. *Clin Pharmacokinet* 2005; **44**: 681–699.

92 Yacobi A, Gibson TP, McEntegrat CM, *et al.* Pharmacokinetics of high molecular weight hydroxyethyl starch in dogs. *Res Commun Chem Pathol Pharmacol* 1982; **36**: 199–204.

93 Meiseter D, Hermann M, Mathis GA. Kinetics of hydroxyethyl starch in horses. *Schweiz Arch Tierheilkd* 1992; **134**: 329–339.

94 Thompson WL, Fukushima T, Rutherford RB, *et al.* Intravascular persistence, tissue storage, and excretion of hydroxyethyl starch. *Surg Gynecol Obstet* 1970; **131**: 965–972.

95 Hughes D. Fluid therapy with artificial colloids: complications and controversies. *Vet Anaesth Analg* 2001; **28**: 111–118.

96 Gandhi SD, Weiskopf RB, Jungheinrich C, *et al.* Volume replacement therapy during major orthopaedic surgery using Voluven (hydroxyethyl starch 130/0.4) or hetastarch. *Anesthesiology* 2007; **106**: 1120–1127.
97 Langeron O, Doelberg M, Ang ET, *et al.* Voluven®, a lower substituted novel hydroxyethyl starch (HES 130/0.4) causes fewer effects on coagulation in major orthopaedic surgery than HES 200/0.5. *Anesth Analg* 2001; **92**: 855–862.
98 Gallandat Huet RC, Siemons AW, Baus D, *et al.* A novel hydroxyethyl starch (Voluven®) for effective perioperative plasma volume substitution in cardiac surgery. *Can J Anaesth* 2000; **47**: 1207–1215.
99 Ickx BE, Bepperling F, Melot C, *et al.* Plasma substitution effects of a new hydroxyethyl starch HES 130/0.4 compared with HES 200/0.5 during and after extended acute normovolaemic hemodilution. *Br J Anaesth* 2003; **91**: 196–202.
100 James MF, Latoo MY, Mythen MG, *et al.* Plasma volume changes associated with two hydroxyethyl starch colloids following acute hypovolaemia in volunteers. *Anaesthesia* 2004; **59**: 738–742.
101 Madjdpour C, Dettori N, Frascarol P, *et al.* Molecular weight of hydroxyethyl starch: is there an effect on blood coagulation and pharmacokinetics? *Br J Anaesth* 2005; **94**: 569–576.
102 Jones PA, Tomasic M, Gentry PA. Oncotic, hemodilutional, and hemostatic effects of isotonic saline and hydroxyethyl starch solutions in clinically normal ponies. *Am J Vet Res* 1997; **58**: 541–548.
103 Smiley LE, Garvey MS. The use of hetastarch as adjunct therapy in 26 dogs with hypoalbuminemia: a phase two clinical trial. *J Vet Intern Med* 1994; **8**: 195–202.
104 Moore LE, Garvey MS. The effect of hetastarch on serum colloid oncotic pressure in hypoalbuminemic dogs. *J Vet Intern Med* 1996; **10**: 300–303.
105 Jones PA, Bain FT, Byars TD, *et al.* Effect of hydroxyethyl starch infusion on colloid oncotic pressure in hypoproteinemic horses. *J Am Vet Med Assoc* 2001; **218**: 1130–1135.
106 Chohan AS, Greene SA, Grubb TL, *et al.* Effects of 6% hetastarch (600/0/75) or lactated Ringer's solution on hemostatic variables and clinical bleeding in healthy dogs anesthetized for orthopedic surgery. *Vet Anaesth Analg* 2011; **38**: 94–105.
107 Viljoen A, Page PC, Fosgate GT, *et al.* Coagulation, oncotic and haemodilutional effects of a third-generation hydroxyethyl starch (130/0.4) solution in horses. *Equine Vet J* 2013; 1–6 (epub ahead of print).
108 Wendt-Hornickle EL, Snyder LBC, Tang R, *et al.* The effects of lactated Ringer's solution (LRS) or LRS and 6% hetastarch on colloid osmotic pressure, total protein and osmolality in healthy horses under general anesthesia. *Vet Anaesth Analg* 2011; **38**: 336–343.
109 Wright BD, Hopkins A. Change in colloid osmotic pressure as a function of anesthesia and surgery in the presence and absence of isotonic fluid administration in dogs. *Vet Anaesth Analg* 2008; **35**: 282–288.
110 Kozek-Langenecker SA, Jungheinrich C, Sauermann W, *et al.* The effects of hydroxyethyl starch 130/0.4 (6%) on blood loss and use of blood products in major surgery: a pooled analysis of randomized clinical trials. *Anesth Analg* 2008; **107**: 382–390.
111 Gandhi S, Warltier D, Weiskopf R, *et al.* Volume substitution with HES 130/0.4 (Voluven) versus HES 450/0.7 (hetastarch) during major orthopedic surgery. *Crit Care* 2005; **9(Suppl 1)**: P206.
112 Conroy JM, Fishman RL, Reeves ST, *et al.* The effects of desmopressin and 6% hydroxyethyl starch on factor VIII:C. *Anesth Analg* 1996; **83**: 804–807.
113 Zoran DL, Jergens AE, Riedesel DH, *et al.* Evaluation of hemostatic analytes after use of hypertonic saline solution combined with colloids for resuscitation of dogs with hypovolemia. *Am J Vet Res* 1992; **53**: 1791–1796.
114 Smart L, Jandrey KE, Wierenga JR, *et al.* The effect of hetastarch (670/0.75) in vivo on platelet closure time in the dog. *J Vet Emerg Crit Care* 2009; **19**: 444–449.
115 Wierenga JR, Jandrey KE, Haskins SC, *et al.* In vitro comparison of the effects of two forms of hydroxyethyl starch solutions on platelet function in dogs. *Am J Vet Res* 2007; **68**: 605–609.
116 McBride D, Hosgood GL, Mansfield CS, *et al.* The effect of hydroxyethyl starch 130/0.4 and 200/0.5 on canine platelet function in vitro. *Am J Vet Res* 2013; **74**: 1133–1137.
117 McBride D, Hosgood G, Smart L, *et al.* Platelet closure time in dogs with hemorrhagic shock treated with hydroxyethyl starch 130/0.4 or 0.9% NaCl. In: *Proceedings of the 18th International Veterinary Emergency and Critical Care Society Meeting*, 2012; 701.
118 Gauthier V, Bersenas A, Holowaychuk M, *et al.* Effect of synthetic colloid administration of coagulation in dogs with systemic inflammation. In: *Proceedings of the 18th International Veterinary Emergency and Critical Care Society Meeting*, 2012; 697.
119 Blong AE, Epstein KL, Brainard BM. In vitro effects of hydroxyethyl starch solutions on coagulation and platelet function in horses. *Am J Vet Res* 2013; **74**: 713–720.
120 Classen J, Adamik KN, Weber K, *et al.* In vitro effect of hydroxyethyl starch 130/0/42 on canine platelet function. *Am J Vet Res* 2012; **73**: 1908–1912.
121 Bacek LM, Martin LG, Spangler EA, *et al.* Determination of the in vitro effects of two forms of hydroxyethyl starch solutions on thromboelastography and coagulation parameters in healthy dogs. In: *Proceedings of the 17th International Veterinary Emergency and Critical Care Society Meeting*, 2011; 732.
122 Boldt J, Haish G, Suttner S, *et al.* Effects of a new modified, balanced hydroxyethyl starch preparations (Hextend) on measures of coagulation. *Br J Anaesth* 2002; **89**: 722–728.
123 Deusch E, Thaler U, Kozek-Langenecker SA. The effects of high molecular weight hydroxyethyl starch solutions on platelet function. *Anesth Analg* 2004; **99**: 665–668.
124 Perner A, Hasse N, Guttormsen AB, *et al.* Hydroxyethyl starch 130/0.42 versus Ringer's acetate in severe sepsis. *N Engl J Med* 2012; **73**: 124–134.
125 Zarychanski R, Abou-Setta AM, Turgeon AF, *et al.* Association of hydroxyethyl starch administration with mortality and acute kidney injury in critically ill patients requiring volume resuscitation: a systematic review and meta-analysis. *JAMA* 2013; **309**: 678–688.
126 Garzon AA, Cheng C, Lerner B, *et al.* Hydroxyethyl starch (HES) and bleeding: an experimental investigation of its effect on hemostasis. *J Trauma* 1967; **7**: 757–766.
127 Thompson WL, Gadsen RH. Prolonged bleeding time and hypofibrinogenemia in dogs after infusion of hydroxyethyl starch and dextran. *Transfusion* 1965; **5**: 440–446.
128 Concannon KT, Haskins SC, Feldman BF. Hemostatic defects associated with two infusion rates of dextran 70 in dogs. *Am J Vet Res* 1992; **53**: 1369–1375.
129 Glowaski MM, Massat-Moon PF, Erb HN, *et al.* Effects of oxypolygelatin and dextran 70 on hemostatic variables in dogs. *Vet Anaesth Analg* 2003; **30**: 202–210.
130 Heath MF, Evans RJ, Hayes LJ. Dextran-70 inhibits equine platelet aggregation induced by PAF but not by other agonists. *Equine Vet J* 1998; **30**: 408–411.
131 Mailloux L, Swartz CD, Dappizzi R, *et al.* Acute renal failure after administration of low-molecular weight dextran. *N Engl J Med* 1967; **277**: 1113–1118.
132 Zwaveling JH, Meulenbelt J, van Xanten NH, *et al.* Renal failure associated with the use of dextran-40. *Neth J Med* 1989; **35**: 321–326.
133 Mitra S, Khandelwal P. Are all colloids same? How to select the right colloid? *Ind J Anaesth* 2009; **53**: 592–607.
134 de Jonge E, Levi M, Berends F, *et al.* Impaired haemostasis by intravenous administration of a gelatin-based plasma expander in human subjects. *Thromb Haemost* 1998; **79**: 286–290.
135 Mortelmans YJ, Vermaut G, Verbruggen AM, *et al.* Effects of 6% hydroxyethyl starch and 3% modified fluid gelatin on intravascular volume and coagulation during intraoperative hemodilution. *Anesth Analg* 1995; **81**: 1235–1242.
136 Lorenz W, Duda D, Dick W, *et al.* Incidence and clinical importance of perioperative histamine release: randomized study of volume loading and antihistamines after induction of anesthesia. *Lancet* 1994; **343**: 933–940.
137 Smart L, Hopper K, Aldrich J, *et al.* The effect of hetastarch (670/0.75) on urine specific gravity and osmolality in the dog. *J Vet Intern Med* 2009; **23**: 388–391.
138 Shires T, Williams J, Broen F. Acute changes in extracellular fluids associated with major surgical procedures. *Ann Surg* 1961; **154**: 803–810.
139 Virtue RW, LeVine DS, Aikawa JW. Fluid shifts during the surgical period: RISA and S35 determinations following glucose, saline or lactate infusions. *Ann Surg* 1965; **163**: 523–528.
140 Savvas I, Rallis T, Raptopoulos D. The effect of pre-anesthetic fasting time and type of food on gastric content volume and acidity in dogs. *Vet Anaesth Analg* 2009; **36**: 539–546.
141 Jacob M, Chappel D, Conzen P, *et al.* Blood volume is normal after pre-operative overnight fasting. *Acta Anesthesiol Scand* 2008; **52**: 522–529.
142 Brandstrup B, Svensen C, Engquist A. Hemorrhage and operation cause a contraction of the extracellular space needing replacement – evidence and implications? A systematic review. *Surgery* 2006; **139**: 419–432.
143 Jackson R, Reid JA, Thorburn J. Volume preloading is not essential to prevent spinal-induced hypotension at Caesarean section. *Br J Anaesth* 1995; **75**: 262–265.
144 Iijima T. Complexity of blood volume control system and its implications in perioperative fluid management. *J Anesth* 2009; **23**: 534–542.
145 Hauptman JG, Richter MA, Wood SL, *et al.* Effects of anesthesia, surgery, and intravenous administration of fluids on antidiuretic hormone concentration in healthy dogs. *Am J Vet Res* 2000; **61**: 1273–1276.
146 Robertson SA, Hauptman JG, Nachreiner RF, *et al.* Effects of acetylpromazine or morphine on urine production in halothane-anesthetized dogs. *Am J Vet Res* 2001; **62**: 1922–1927.
147 Boscan P, Pypendop BH, Siao KT, *et al.* Fluid balance, glomerular filtration rate, and urine output in dogs anesthetized for an orthopedic surgical procedure. *Am J Vet Res* 2010; **71**: 497–596.
148 Rahbari NN, Zimmermann JB, Schmidt T, *et al.* Meta-analysis of standard, restrictive and supplemental fluid administration in colorectal surgery. *Br J Surg* 2009; **96**: 331–341.
149 Chappell D, Jacob M, Hoffmann-Kiefer K, *et al.* A rational approach to perioperative fluid management. *Anesthesiology* 2008; **109**: 723–740.

150 Holte K, Sharrock NE, Kehlet H. Pathophysiology and clinical implications of perioperative fluid excess. *Br J Anaesth* 2002; **89**: 622–632.

151 Cotton BA, Guy JS, Morris JA, *et al.* The cellular, metabolic, and systemic consequences of aggressive fluid resuscitation strategies. *Shock* 2006; **26**: 115–121.

152 Brodbelt DC, Pfeiffer DU, Young LE, *et al.* Risk factors for anaesthetic-related death in cats: results from the Confidential Enquiry into Perioperative Small Animal Fatalities (CEPSAF). *Br J Anaesth* 2007; **99**: 617–623.

153 Holte K, Foss NB, Anderson J, *et al.* Liberal or restrictive fluid administration in fast-track colonic surgery: a randomized double-blinded study. *Br J Anaesth* 2007; **99**: 500–508.

154 Brandstrup B, Tonnesen H, Beier-Holgersen R, *et al.* Effect of intravenous fluid restrictions on postoperative complications: comparison of two perioperative fluid regimens: a randomized assessor-blinded multicenter trial. *Ann Surg* 2003; **238**: 641–648.

155 Yogendran S, Asokumar B, Cheng DC, *et al.* A prospective randomized double blinded study of the effect of intravenous fluid therapy on adverse outcome on outpatient surgery. *Anesth Analg* 1995; **80**: 682–686.

156 Lambert KG, Wakim JH, Lambert NE. Preoperative fluid bolus and reduction of postoperative nausea and vomiting in patients undergoing laproscopic gynecologic surgery. *AANA J* 2009; **77**: 110–114.

157 Holte K, Klarskov B, Christensen DS, *et al.* Liberal versus restrictive fluid administration to improved recovery after laproscopic cholecystectomy: a randomized, double blinded study. *Ann Surg* 2004; **240**: 892–899.

158 Gaynor JS, Wertz EM, Kesel LM, *et al.* Effect of intravenous administration of fluids on packed cell volume, blood pressure, total protein and blood glucose concentration in healthy halothane anesthetized dogs. *J Am Vet Med Assoc* 1996; **208**: 2013–2015.

159 Nisanevich V, Felsenstein I, Almogy G, *et al.* Effect of intraoperative fluid management on outcome after intraabdominal surgery. *Anesthesiology* 2005; **103**: 25–32.

160 Joshi GP. Intraoperative fluid restriction improves outcome after major elective gastrointestinal surgery. *Anesth Analg* 2005; **101**: 601–605.

161 Bundgaard-Nielson M, Secher NH, Kehlet H. 'Liberal' vs. 'Restrictive' perioperative fluid therapy – a critical assessment of the evidence. *Acta Anaesthesiol Scand* 2009; **53**: 843–851.

162 Davis H, Jensen T, Johnson A, *et al.* 2013 AAHA/AAFP fluid therapy guidelines for dogs and cats. *J Am Anim Hosp Assoc* 2013; **49**: 149–159.

163 Butler AL. Goal-directed therapy in small animal critical care. *Vet Clin Sm Anim* 2011; **41**: 817–838.

164 Hayes GM, Mathews K, Boston S, *et al.* Low central venous oxygen saturation is associated with increased mortality in critically ill dogs. *J Small Anim Pract* 2011; **52**: 433–440.

165 Rivers E, Nguyen B, Havstad S, *et al.* Early goal-directed therapy in the treatment of severe sepsis and septic shock. *N Engl J Med* 2001; **345**: 1368–1377.

166 Concannon KT. Colloid osmotic pressure and the clinical use of colloidal solutions. *J Vet Emerg Crit Care* 2002; **3**: 49–62.

167 Bumpus SE, Haskins SC, Kass PH. Effect of synthetic colloids on refractometric readings of total solids. *J Vet Emerg Crit Care* 1998; **8**: 21–26.

168 Michard F, Teboul JL. Predicting fluid responsiveness in ICU patients: a critical analysis of the evidence. *Chest* 2002; **121**: 2000–2008.

169 Renner J, Scholz J, Bein B. Monitoring fluid therapy. *Best Pract Res Clin Anesthesiol* 2009; **23**: 159–171.

170 Kehlet H, Bundgaard-Nielson M. Goal-directed perioperative fluid therapy. *Anesthesiology* 2009; **110**: 453–455.

171 Vallet B, Futier E, Robin E. Tissue oxygenation parameters to guide fluid therapy. *Transfusion Alter Transfusion Med* 2010; **11**: 113–117.

172 Brandstrup B, Svendsen PE, Fasmussen M, *et al.* Which goal for fluid therapy during colorectal surgery is followed by best outcome: near maximal stroke volume or zero fluid balance? *Br J Anaesth* 2012; **109**: 191–199.

173 Marik PE, Baram M, Vahid B. Does central venous pressure predict fluid responsiveness? A systematic review of literature and the tale of seven mares. *Chest* 2008; **134**: 172–178.

174 Harvey S, Harrison DA, Singer M, *et al.* Assessment of clinical effectiveness of pulmonary artery catheters in management of patients in intensive care (PAC-Man): a randomized controlled trial. *Lancet* 2005; **366**: 472–477.

175 Marik PE, Cavallazi R, Vasu T, *et al.* Dynamic changes in arterial waveform derived variables and fluid responsiveness in mechanically ventilated patients: a systematic review of literature. *Crit Care Med* 2009; **37**: 2642–2647.

176 Thiele R, Durieux ME. Arterial waveform analysis for the anesthesiologist: past, present, and future concepts. *Anesth Analg* 2011; **113**: 766–776.

177 Forget P, Lois R, de Kock M. Goal directed fluid management based on the pulse oximeter-derived Pleth variability index reduces lactate levels and improves fluid management. *Anesth Analg* 2010; **111**: 910–914.

178 Ricco C, Henao-Guerrero N, Shih A, *et al.* Pleth variability index derived from the radical-7 Masimo pulse oximeter as a non-invasive indicator of circulating volume changes in dogs. In: *Proceedings of the 18th International Veterinary Emergency and Critical Care Society Meeting*, 2012; 732.

179 Ricco C, Henao-Guerrero N, Shih A, *et al.* Pulse pressure variation in a model of hemorrhagic shock in mechanically ventilated dogs. In: *Proceedings of the 18th International Veterinary Emergency and Critical Care Society Meeting*, 2012; 732.

180 Michard F. Changes in arterial pressure during mechanical ventilation. *Anesthesiology* 2005; **103**: 419–428.

181 Abbas SM, Hill AG. Systematic review of the literature for the use of esophageal Doppler monitor for fluid replacement in major abdominal surgery. *Anaesthesia* 2008; **63**: 44–51.

182 Perel P, Roberts I, Ker K. Colloids versus crystalloids for fluid resuscitation in critically ill patients. *Cochrane Database Syst Rev* 2013; **2**: CD000567.

183 Dibartola SP. Disorders of sodium and water: hypernatremia and hyponatremia. In: Dibartola SP, ed. *Fluid, Electrolyte and Acid-Base Disorders in Small Animal Practice*, 4th edn. St Louis, Missouri: Elsevier, 2012; 45–79.

184 Androgue HJ, Madias NE. Hypernatremia. *N Engl J Med* 2000; **342**: 1493–1499.

185 Pollock AS, Arieff AI. Abnormalities of cell volume regulation and their functional consequences. *Am J Physiol* 1980; **239**: F195–F205.

186 Willard M. Therapeutic approach to chronic electrolyte disorders. *Vet Clin Small Anim* 2008; **38**: 535–541.

187 Lien YH, Shapiro JI, Chan L. Effects of hypernatremia on organic brain osmoles. *J Clin Invest* 1990; **85**: 1427–1435.

188 Schaer M. Therapeutic approach to electrolyte emergencies. *Vet Clin Small Anim* 2008; **38**: 513–533.

189 Ellison DH, Berl T. The syndrome of inappropriate antidiuresis. *N Engl J Med* 2007; **356**: 2064–2072.

190 Houston DM, Allen DG, Kruth SA, *et al.* Syndrome of inappropriate antidiuretic hormone secretion in a dog. *Can Vet J* 1989; **30**: 423.

191 Kokko H, Hall PD, Afrin LB. Fentanyl associated syndrome of inappropriate antidiuretic hormone secretion. *Pharmacotherapy* 2002; **22**: 1188–1192.

192 Demirel I, Ozer AB, Bayar MK, *et al.* TRUP syndrome and severe hyponatremia under general anesthesia. *BMJ Case Rep*, Nov 12, 2012 (epub ahead of print).

193 Liptak JM, Brutsher SP, Monnet E, *et al.* Transurethral resection in the management of urethral and prostatic neoplasia in 6 dogs. *Vet Surg* 2004; **33**: 505–516.

194 Toll J, Barr SC, Hickford FH. Acute water intoxication in a dog. *J Vet Emerg Crit Care* 1999; **9**: 19–22.

195 O'Brien DP, Kroll RA, Johnson GC, *et al.* Myelinolysis after correction of hyponatremia in two dogs. *J Vet Intern Med* 1994; **8**: 40–48.

196 Churcher RK, Wason ADJ, Eaton A. Suspected myelinolysis following rapid correction of hyponatremia in a dog. *J Am Anim Hosp Assoc* 1999; **35**: 492–497.

197 Aguilera IM, Vaughan RS. Calcium and the anesthetist. *Anaesthesia* 2000; **55**: 779–790.

198 Schenck PA, Chew DJ. Calcium: total or ionized? *Vet Clin Sm Anim* 2008; **38**: 497–502.

199 Holowaychuk MK, Martin LG. Review of hypocalcemia in septic patients. *J Vet Emerg Crit Care* 2007; **17**: 348–358.

200 Borer KE, Corley KTT. Electrolyte disorders in horses with colic. Part 2: calcium, sodium, chloride and phosphate. *Equine Vet Educ* 2006; **18**: 320–325.

201 Grubb TL, Benson GJ, Foreman JH, *et al.* Hemodynamic effects of ionized calcium in horses anesthetized with halothane or isoflurane. *Am J Vet Res* 1999; **60**: 1430–1435.

202 Gasthuys F, de Moor A, Parmentier D, *et al.* Cardiovascular effects of low dose calcium chloride infusions during halothane anesthesia in dorsally recumbent ventilated ponies. *J Am Vet Med Assoc* 1991; **38**: 728–736.

203 Dhupa N, Proulx J. Hypocalcemia and hypomagnesemia. *Vet Clin Sm Anim Pract* 1998; **28**: 587–608.

204 Sharp CR, Kerl ME, Mann FA. A comparison of total calcium, corrected calcium, and ionized calcium concentrations as indicators of calcium homeostasis among hypoalbuminemic dogs requiring intensive care. *J Vet Emerg Crit Care* 2009; **19**: 571–578.

205 Brennan SF, O'Donovan J, Mooney CT. Changes in canine ionized calcium under three storage conditions. *J Small Anim Pract* 2006; **47**: 383–386.

206 Dibartola SP, de Morais HA. Disorders of potassium: hypokalemia and hyperkalemia. In: Dibartola SP, ed. *Fluid, Electrolyte and Acid–Base Disorders in Small Animal Practice*, 4th edn. St Louis: Missouri: Elsevier, 2012; 92–119.

207 Kablack KA, Embertson RM, Bernard WV, *et al.* Uroperitoneum in the hospitalized equine neonates: retrospective study of 31 cases. *Equine Vet J* 2000; **32**: 505–508.

208 Tag TL, Day TK. Electrocardiographic assessment of hyperkalemia in dogs and cats. *J Vet Emerg Crit Care* 2008; **18**: 61–67.

209 Parks J. Electrocardiographic abnormalities from serum electrolyte imbalance due to feline urethral obstruction. *J Am Anim Hosp Assoc* 1975; **11**: 102–109.

210 Drobatz KJ, Cole SG. The influence of crystalloid type on acid–base and electrolyte status of cats with urethral obstruction. *J Vet Emerg Crit Care* 2008; **18**: 355–361.

211 Ho K. A critically swift response: insulin-stimulated potassium and glucose transport in skeletal muscle. *Clin J Am Soc Nephrol* 2011; **6**: 1513–1516.

212 Carvalhanna V, Burry L, Lapinsky SE. Management of severe hyperkalemia without hemodialysis: case report and literature review. *J Crit Care* 2006; **21**: 316-321.

213 Borer KE, Corley KTT. Electrolyte disorders in horses with colic. Part 1: potassium and magnesium. *Equine Vet J* 2006; **18**: 266–271.

214 Haldane S, Graves TK, Bateman S, *et al.* Profound hypokalemia causing respiratory failure in a cat with hyperaldosteronism. *J Vet Emerg Crit Care* 2007; **17**: 202-207.

215 American Society of Anesthesiologists. Practice guidelines for perioperative blood transfusion and adjuvant therapies: an updated report by the American Society of Anesthesiologists task force on perioperative blood transfusion and adjuvant therapies. *Anesthesiology* 2006; **105**: 198–208.

216 Davidow B. Transfusion medicine in small animals. *Vet Clin Small Anim* 2013; **43**: 735–756.

217 Divers TJ. Blood component transfusion. *Vet Clin Food Anim Pract* 2005; **21**: 615–622.

218 David JB. Blood-donor horses and wholeblood transfusion in private practice. In: Robinson NE, Sprayberry K, eds. *Current Therapy in Equine Medicine*, Vol**ume 6**. St Louis, Missouri: Saunders Elsevier, 2009; 224–226.

219 Herbert P, van der Linden P, Biro G, *et al.* Physiologic aspects of anemia. *Crit Care Med* 2004; **20**: 187–212.

220 Jutkowitz LA. Blood transfusion in the perioperative period. *Clin Tech Small Anim Pract* 2004; **2**: 75–82.

221 Teixeira Neto FJ, Luna S, Cruz MA, *et al.* A study of the effect of hemorrhage on the cardiorespiratory actions of halothane, isoflurane and sevoflurane in the dog. *Vet Anaesth Analg* 2007; **34**: 107–116.

222 Weingart C, Giger U, Kohn B. Whole blood transfusion in 91 cats: a clinical evaluation. *J Fel Med Surg* 2004; **6**: 139–148.

223 Klaser DA, Reine NJ, Hohenhaus AE. Red blood cell transfusion in cats: 126 cases (1999). *J Am Vet Med Assoc* 2005; **226**: 920–923.

224 Castellanos I, Couto CG, Gray TL. Clinical use of blood products in cats: a retrospective study (1997–2000). *J Vet Intern Med* 2004; **18**: 529–532.

225 Roux FA, Deschamps JY, Blais MC, *et al.* Multiple red cell transfusion in 27 cats (2003–2006). *J Fel Med Surg* 2008; **10**: 213–218.

226 Hurcombe SD, Mudge MC, Hinchcliff KW. Clinical and clinicopathologic variables in adult horses receiving blood transfusion. *J Am Vet Med Assoc* 2007; **231**: 267–274.

227 Kerl ME, Hohenhaus AE. Packed red blood cell transfusions in dogs: 131 case (1989). *J Am Vet Med Assoc* 1993; **202**: 1495–1499.

228 Callan MB, Oakley DA, Shofer ES, *et al.* Canine red blood cell transfusion practice. *J Am Anim Hosp Assoc* 1996; **32**: 303–311.

229 Day MJ, Barbara K, eds. *BSAVA Manual of Canine and Feline Haematology and Transfusion Medicine*, 2nd edn. Gloucester, UK: British Small Animal Veterinary Association, 2012.

230 Valeri CR, Khuri S, Ragno G. Nonsurgical bleeding diathesis in anemic thrombocytopenic patients: role of temperature, red blood cells, platelets, and plasma-clotting proteins. *Transfusion* 2007; **47**: 206S–248S.

231 Valeri CR, Cassidy G, Pivacek LE, *et al.* Anemia-induced increase in the bleeding time: implications for treatment of nonsurgical blood loss. *Transfusion* 2001; **41**: 977–983.

232 Sort JL, Diehl S, Seshadri R, *et al.* Accuracy of formulas used to predict post-transfusion packed cell volume rise in anemic dogs. *J Vet Emerg Crit Care* 2012; **22**: 428–434.

233 Brooks MB, Wardrop KJ. Stability of hemostatic proteins in canine fresh frozen plasma units. *Vet Clin Pathol* 2001; **30**: 91–95.

234 Stokol T, Parry B. Efficacy of fresh-frozen plasma and cryoprecipitate in dogs with von Willebrand's disease or hemophilia A. *J Vet Intern Med* 1998; **12**: 84–92.

235 Ching YNLH, Meyers KM, Brassard JA, *et al.* Effect of cryoprecipitate and plasma on plasma von Willebrand factor multimers and bleeding time in Doberman Pinschers with type-I von Willebrand's disease. *Am J Vet Res* 1994; **55**: 102–110.

236 Throop JL, Kerl ME, Cohn LA. Albumin in health and disease: protein metabolism and function. *Comp Cont Educ Vet* 2004; **26**: 932–939.

237 Mazzaferro EM, Rudloff E, Kirby R. The role of albumin replacement in the critically ill veterinary patient. *J Vet Emerg Crit Care* 2002; **12**: 113–124.

238 Vigano F, Perissinotto L, Bosco V. Administration of 5% human serum albumin in critically ill small animal patients with hypoalbuminemia: 418 dogs and 170 cats (1994–2008). *J Vet Emerg Crit Care* 2010; **20**: 237–243.

239 Wardrop KJ. Canine plasma therapy. *Vet Forum* 1997; **14**: 36–40.

240 Mosley CAE, Matthews KA. The use of concentrated serum albumin in canines. *Vet Anesth Analg* 2005; **32**: 14–15.

241 Mathews K, Barry M. The use of 25% human serum albumin: outcome and efficacy in raising serum albumin and systemic blood pressure in critically ill dogs and cats. *J Vet Emerg Crit Care* 2005; **15**: 110–118.

242 Trow A, Rozanski E, de Laforcade A, *et al.* Evaluation of the use of human albumin in critically ill dogs: 73 cases (2003–2006). *J Am Vet Med Assoc* 2008; **233**: 607–612.

243 Vigano F, Perissinotto L, Bosco V. Administration of 5% human serum albumin in critically ill small animal patients with hypoalbuminemia: 418 dogs and 170 cats (1994–2008). *J Vet Emerg Crit Care* 2010; **20**: 237–243.

244 DeWitt SF, Paradis MR. Use of human albumin as a colloidal therapy in the hypoproteinemic equine (abstract). *J Vet Intern Med* 2004; **14**: S8.

245 Francis AH, Martin L, Haldorson GJ, *et al.* Adverse reactions suggestive of type iii hypersensitivity in six healthy dogs given human albumin. *J Am Vet Med Assoc* 2007; **320**: 873–879.

246 Cohn LA, Kerl ME, Lenox CE, *et al.* Response of healthy dogs to infusion of human serum albumin. *Am J Vet Res* 2007; **68**: 657–663.

247 Martin LG, Luther TY, Alperin DC, *et al.* Serum antibodies against human albumin in critically ill and healthy dogs. *J Am Vet Med Assoc* 2008; **232**: 1004–1009.

248 Powell C, Thompson L, Murtaugh RJ. Type III hypersensitivity reaction with immune complex deposition in 2 critically ill dogs administered human serum albumin. *J Vet Emerg Crit Care* 2013; **23**: 598–604.

249 Craft EM, Powell LL. The use of canine-specific albumin in dogs with septic peritonitis. *J Vet Emerg Crit Care* 2012; **22**: 631–639.

250 Craft EM, de Laforcade A, Rozanski E, *et al.* The effect of transfusion with canine specific albumin in dogs with septic peritonitis. International Veterinary Emergency and Critical Care Symposium 2010; **631**.

251 Smith CL, Ramsey NB, Parr AM, *et al.* Evaluation of a novel canine albumin solution in normal Beagles (abstract). *J Vet Emerg Crit Care* 2009; **19(Suppl)**: A3

252 Finfer S, Bellomo R, Boyce N, *et al.* A comparison of albumin and saline for fluid resuscitation in the intensive care unit. *N Engl J Med* 2004; **350**: 2247–2256.

253 Roberts I, Blackhall K, Alderson P, *et al.* Human albumin solution for resuscitation and volume expansion in critically ill patients. *Cochrane Database Syst Rev* 2011; **11**: CD001208.

254 Delaney AP, Dan A, McCaffrey J, *et al.* The role of albumin as a resuscitation fluid for patients with sepsis: a systematic review and meta-analysis. *Crit Care Med* 2011; **39**: 386–391.

255 Martin GS, Mangialardi RJ, Wheeler AP, *et al.* Albumin and furosemide therapy in hypoproteinemic patients with acute lung injury. *Crit Care Med* 2002; **30**: 2175–2182.

256 Greeno E, McCullough J, Weisdorf D. Platelet utilization and the transfusion trigger: a prospective analysis. *Transfusion* 2007; **47**: 201–205.

257 Petrides M, Stack G, Cooling L, *et al.* *Practical Guide to Transfusion Medicine*. Bethesda, Maryland: AABB Press, 2007.

258 Callow CR, Swindell R, Randall W, *et al.* The frequency of bleeding complications in patients with haematological malignancy following the introduction of a stringent prophylactic platelet transfusion policy. *Br J Haematol* 2002; **118**: 677–682.

259 Abrams-Ogg AC. Triggers for prophylactic use of platelet transfusions and optimal platelet dosing in thrombocytopenic dogs and cats. *Vet Clin North Am Small Anim Pract* 2003; **33**: 1401–1418.

260 Callan MB, Appleman EH, Sachais BS. Canine platelet transfusions. *J Vet Emerg Crit Care* 2009; **19**: 401–415.

261 Clemmons RM, Bliss EL, Dorsey-Lee MR, *et al.* Platelet function, size and yield in whole blood and in platelet-rich plasma prepared using different centrifugation force and time in domestic and food-producing animals. *Thromb Haemost* 1983; **50**: 838–843.

262 Abrams-Ogg ACG, Kruth SA, Carter RF, *et al.* Preparation and transfusion of canine platelet concentrates. *Am J Vet Res* 1993; **54**: 635–642.

263 Callan MB, Appleman EH, Shofer FS, *et al.* Clinical and clinicopathologic effects of plateletpheresis on healthy donor dogs. *Transfusion* 2008; **48**: 2214–2221.

264 Appleman EH, Sachais BS, Patel R, *et al.* Cryopreservation of canine platelets. *J Vet Intern Med* 2009; **23**: 138–145.

265 Valeri CR, Feingold H, Marchionni LD. A simple method for freezing human platelets using 6 per cent dimethylsulfoxide and storage at -80 degrees C. *Blood* 1974; **43**: 131–136.

266 Valeri CR, Feingold H, Melaragno AJ, *et al.* Cryopreservation of dog platelets with dimethyl sulfoxide: therapeutic effectiveness of cryopreserved platelets in the treatment of thrombocytopenic dogs, and the effect of platelet storage at -80 degrees C. *Cryobiology* 1986; **23**: 387–394.

267 Guillaumin J, Jandrey KE, Norris JW, *et al.* Assessment of a dimethyl-sulfoxide-stabilized frozen canine platelet concentrate. *Am J Vet Res* 2008; **69**: 1580–1586.

268 Guillaumin J, Jandrey KE, Norris JW, *et al.* Analysis of a commercial dimethyl-sulfoxide-stabilized frozen canine platelet concentrate by turbidimetric aggregometry. *J Vet Emerg Crit Care* 2010; **20**: 571–577.

269 Bode AP, Fischer TH. Lyophilized platelets: fifty years in the making. *Artif Cells Blood Substit Immobil Biotechnol* 2007; **35**: 125–133.

270 Read MS, Reddick RL, Bode AP, *et al.* Preservation of hemostatic and structural properties of rehydrated lyophilized platelets: potential for long-term storage of dried platelets for transfusion. *Proc Natl Acad Sci USA* 1995; **92**: 397–401.

271 Fischer TH, Merricks EP, Bode AP, *et al.* Thrombus formation with rehydrated, lyophilized platelets. *Hematology* 2002; **7**: 359–369.

272 Bode AP, Lust RM, Read MS, *et al.* Correction of the bleeding time with lyophilized platelet infusions in dogs on cardiopulmonary bypass. *Clin Appl Thromb Hemost* 2008; **14**: 38–54.

273 Davidow EB, Brainard B, Martin LG, *et al.* Use of fresh platelet concentrate or lyophilized platelets in thrombocytopenic dogs with clinical signs of hemorrhage: a preliminary trial in 37 dogs. *J Vet Emerg Crit Care* 2012; **22**: 116–125.

274 Hawksworth JS, Elster EA, Fryer D, *et al.* Evaluation of lyophilized platelets as an infusible hemostatic agent in experimental non-compressible hemorrhage in swine. *J Thromb Haemost* 2009; **7**: 1663–1671.

275 Symons M, Bell K. Canine blood groups: description of 20 specificities. *Anim Genet* 1992; **23**: 509–515.

276 Symons M, Bell K. Expansion of the canine A blood group system. *Anim Genet* 1991; **22**: 227–235.

277 Giger U, Gelens CJ, Callan MB, *et al.* An acute hemolytic transfusion reaction caused by dog erythrocyte antigen 1.1 incompatibility in a previously sensitized dog. *J Am Vet Med Assoc* 1995; **206**: 1358–1362.

278 Kessler RJ, Reese J, Chang D, *et al.* Dog erythrocyte antigens 1.1, 1.2, 3, 4, 7, and Dal blood typing and cross-matching by gel column technique. *Vet Clin Pathol* 2010; **39**: 306–316.

279 Callan MB, Jones LT, Giger U. Hemolytic transfusion reactions in a dog with an alloantibody to a common antigen. *J Vet Intern Med* 1995; **9**: 277–279.

280 Swisher SN, Young LE, Trabold N. In vitro and in vivo studies of the behavior of canine erythrocyte-isoantibody systems. *Ann N Y Acad Sci* 1962; **97**: 15–25.

281 Blais MC, Berman L, Oakley DA, *et al.* Canine Dal blood type: a red cell antigen lacking in some Dalmatians. *J Vet Intern Med* 2007; **21**: 281–286.

282 Weinstein NM, Blais MC, Harris K, *et al.* A newly recognized blood group in domestic shorthair cats: the Mik red cell antigen. *J Vet Intern Med* 2007; **21**: 287–292.

283 Malik R, Griffin DL, White JD, *et al.* The prevalence of feline A/B blood types in the Sydney region. *Aust Vet J* 2005; **83**: 38–44.

284 Giger U, Bucheler J, Patterson DF. Frequency and inheritance of A and B blood types in feline breeds of the United States. *J Hered* 1991; **82**: 15–20.

285 Giger U, Kilrain CG, Filippich LJ, *et al.* Frequencies of feline blood groups in the United States. *J Am Vet Med Assoc* 1989; **195**: 1230–1232.

286 Proverbio D, Spada E, Baggiani L, *et al.* Comparison of gel column agglutination with monoclonal antibodies and card agglutination methods for assessing the feline AB group system and a frequency study of feline blood types in northern Italy. *Vet Clin Pathol* 2011; **40**: 32–39.

287 Giger U, Bucheler J. Transfusion of type-A and type-B blood to cats. *J Am Vet Med Assoc* 1991; **198**: 411–418.

288 Giger U, Akol KG. Acute hemolytic transfusion reaction in an Abyssinian cat with blood type B. *J Vet Intern Med* 1990; **4**: 315–316.

289 Weinstein NM, Blais MC, Harris K, *et al.* A newly recognized blood group in domestic shorthair cats: the Mik red cell antigen. *J Vet Intern Med* 2007; **21**: 287–292.

290 Slovis NM, Murray G. How to approach whole blood transfusions in horses. In: *Proceedings of the Annual Convention of the AAEP*, 2001; **47**: 266–269.

291 Wong PL Nickel L, Bowling AT, *et al.* Clinical survey of antibodies against red blood cells in horses after homologous blood transfusion. *Am J Vet Res* 1986; **47**: 2566–2571.

292 Tocci LJ, Ewing PJ. Increasing patient safety in veterinary transfusion medicine: an overview of pretransfusion testing. *J Vet Emerg Crit Care* 2009; **19**: 66–73.

293 Stormont CJ. Blood groups in animals. *Adv Vet Sci Comp Med* 1991; **36**: 9–55.

294 Young LE, O'Brien WA, Swisher SN, *et al.* Blood groups in dogs – their significance to the veterinarian. *Am J Vet Res* 1952; **13**: 207–213.

295 Lanevschi A, Wardrop KJ. Principles of transfusion medicine in small animals. *Can Vet J* 2001; **42**: 447–454.

296 Jutkowitz LA, Rozanski EA, Moreau JA, *et al.* Massive transfusion in dogs: 15 cases (1997–2001). *J Am Vet Med Assoc* 2002; **220**: 1664–1669.

297 Seghatchian J, Samama MM. Massive transfusion: an overview of the main characteristics and potential risks associated with substances used for correction of a coagulopathy. *Transfusion Apheresis Sci* 2012; **47**: 235–243.

298 Holcomb JB, Wade CE, Michalek JE, *et al.* Increased plasma and platelet to red blood cell ratios improves outcome in 466 massively transfused civilian trauma patients. *Ann Surg* 2008; **248**: 447–458.

299 Zink KA, Sambasivan CN, Holcomb JB, *et al.* A high ratio of plasma and platelets to packed red blood cells in the first 6 h of massive transfusion improves outcomes in a large multicenter study. *Am J Surg* 2009; **197**: 565–570.

300 Shaz BH, Dente CJ, Nicholas J, *et al.* Increased number of coagulation products in relationship to red blood cell products transfused improves mortality in trauma patients. *Transfusion* 2010; **50**: 493–500.

301 Nunez TC, Young PP, Holcomb JB, Cotton BA. Creation, implementation, and maturation of a massive transfusion protocol for the exsanguinating trauma patient. *J Trauma* 2010; **68**: 1498–1505.

302 Cotton BA, Gunter OL, Isbell J, *et al.* Damage control hematology: the impact of a trauma exsanguination protocol on survival and blood product utilization. *J Trauma* 2008; **64**: 1177–1182.

303 Gonzalez EA, Moore FA, Holcomb JB, *et al.* Fresh frozen plasma should be given earlier to patients requiring massive transfusion. *J Trauma* 2007; **62**: 112–119.

304 Sisak K, Soeyland K, McLeod M, *et al.* Massive transfusion in trauma: blood product ratios should be measured at 6 h. *ANZ J Surg* 2012; **82**: 161–167.

305 Hirshberg A, Dugas M, Banez EI, *et al.* Minimizing dilutional coagulopathy in exsanguinating hemorrhage: a computer simulation. *J Trauma* 2003; **54**: 454–463.

306 Ho AM, Karmakar MK, Dion PW. Are we giving enough coagulation factors during major trauma resuscitation? *Am J Surg* 2005; **190**: 479–484.

307 Spinella PC, Holcomb JB. Resuscitation and transfusion principles for traumatic hemorrhagic shock. *Blood Rev* 2009; **23**: 231–240.

308 Buckley GJ, Aktay SA, Rozanski EA. Massive transfusion and surgical management of iatrogenic aortic laceration associated with cystocentesis in a dog. *J Am Vet Med Assoc* 2009; **235**: 288–291.

309 Clark CH, Woodley CH. The absorption of red blood cells after parentral injection at various sites. *Am J Vet Res* 1959; **10**: 1062–1066.

310 McDevitt RI, Ruaux CG, Baltzer WI. Influence of transfusion technique on survival of autologous red blood cells in the dog. *J Vet Emerg Crit Care* 2011; **21**: 209–216.

311 Heikes B, Ruaux CG. Syringe and aggregate filter administration does not effect survival of transfused autologous feline red blood cells. *J Vet Emerg Crit Care* 2014; **24**: 162–167

312 Tocci LJ. Transfusion medicine in small animal practice. *Vet Clin Small Anim* 2010; **40**: 485–494.

313 Toy P, Popovsky MA, Abraham E, *et al.* Transfusion-related acute lung injury: definition and review. *Crit Care Med* 2005; **33**: 721–726.

314 Vlaar APJ, Juffermans NP. Transfusion related acute lung injury – clinical review. *Lancet* 2013; **382**: 984–994.

315 Thomovsky E, Bach J. Incidence of acute lung injury in dogs receiving transfusion. *J Am Vet Med Assoc* 2014; **244**: 170–174.

316 Marik PE, Corwin HL. Acute lung injury flowing blood transfusion: expanding the definition. *Crit Care Med* 2008; **36**: 3080–3084.

317 Gajic O, Rana R, Winters JL, *et al.* Transfusion-related acute lung injury in the critically ill. *Am J Respir Crit Care Med* 2007; **176**: 886–891.

318 Palfi M, Berg S, Ernerudh J, Berlin G. A randomized controlled trial of transfusion-related acute lung injury: is plasma from multiparous blood donors dangerous? *Transfusion* 2001; **41**: 317–322.

319 Blais MC, Rozanski EA, Hale AS, *et al.* Lack of evidence of pregnancy-induced alloantibodies in dogs. *J Vet Intern Med* 2009; **23**: 462–465.

320 Hillyer CD, Josephson CD, Blajchman MA, *et al.* Bacterial contamination of blood components: risks, strategies, and regulation: joint ASH and AABB educational session in transfusion medicine. *Hematology Am Soc Hematol Edu Program* 2003; **575–589**.

321 Hohenhaus AE, Drustin LM, Garvey MS. *Serratia marcescens* contamination of feline whole blood in a hospital blood bank. *J Am Vet Med Assoc* 1997; **210**: 794–798.

322 Maxwell MJ, Wilson MJA. Complications of blood transfusion. *Contin Educ Anaesth Crit Care Pain* 2006; **6**: 225–229.

323 Nickel JR, Shih A. Anesthesia case of the month. *J Am Vet Med Assoc* 2011; **239**: 1429–1431.

324 Hardefeldt LY, Keuler N, Peek SF. Incidence of transfusion reactions to commercial equine plasma. *J Vet Emerg Crit Care* 2010; **20**: 421–425.

325 Wilson EM, Holcombe SJ, Lamar A, *et al.* Incidence of transfusion reactions and retention of procoagulant and anticoagulant factor activities in equine plasma. *J Vet Intern Med* 2009; **23**: 323–328.

326 Soldan A. Blood transfusion in cattle. *In Pract* 1999; **21**: 590–595.

327 Mudge MC, Walker NJ, Borjesson DL, *et al.* Post-transfusion survival of biotin-labeled allogenic RBCs in adult horses. *Vet Clin Pathol* 2012; **41**: 56–62.

328 Forgie MA, Wells PS, Laupacis A, *et al.* Preoperative autologous donation decreased allogeneic transfusion by relative 63 percent, but increases exposure to all red blood cell transfusion by 30 percent: results of a meta-analysis. International Study of Perioperative Transfusion (ISPOT) Investigators. *Arch Int Med* 1998; **158**: 610–616.

329 Henry DA, Carless PA, Moxey AJ, *et al.* Pre-operative autologous donation for minimizing perioperative allogeneic blood transfusion. *Cochrane Database Syst Rev* 2002; 2: CD003602.

330 Carless P, Moxey A, O'Connell D, *et al.* Autologous transfusion techniques: a systematic review of their efficacy. *Transfusion Med* 2004; **14**: 123–144.

331 Sinclair KC, Clarke HD, Noble BN. Blood management in total knee arthroplasty: a comparison of techniques. *Orthopedics* 2009; **32**: 19.

332 Mudge MC, Macdonald MH, Owens SD, *et al.* Comparison of 4 blood storage methods in a protocol for equine pre-operative autologous donation. *Vet Surg* 2004; **33**: 475–486.

333 Fusco JV, Hohenhaus AE, Aiken SW, *et al.* Autologous blood collection and transfusion in cats undergoing partial craniectomy. *J Am Vet Med Assoc* 2000; **216**: 1584–1588.

334 Mijovic A, Britten C, Regan F, *et al.* Preoperative autologous blood donation for bone marrow harvests: are we wasting donors' time and blood? *Transfus Med* 2006; **16**: 57–62.

335 Bess RS, Lenke LG, Bridwell KH, *et al.* Wasting of preoperatively donated autologous blood in the surgical treatment of adolescent idiopathic scoliosis. *Spine* 2006; **31**: 2375–2380.

336 Monk TG, Goodnough LT, Brecher ME, *et al.* A prospective randomized comparison of three blood conservation strategies for radical prostatectomy. *Anesthesiology* 1999; **91**: 24–33.

337 Monk TG, Goodnough LT, Pulley DD, *et al.* Acute normovolemic hemodilution can replace preoperative autologous blood donation as a standard of care for autologous blood procurement in radical prostatectomy. *Anesth Analg* 1997; **85**: 953–958.

338 Oishi CS, d'Lima DD, Morris BA, *et al.* Hemodilution with other blood reinfusion techniques in total hip arthroplasty. *Clin Orthop* 1997; **339**: 132–139.

339 Schmied H, Schiferer A, Sessler DI, Meznik C. The effects of red-cell scavenging, hemodilution, and active warming on allogeneic blood requirements in patients undergoing hip or knee arthroplasty. *Anesth Analg* 1998; **86**: 387–391.

340 Hirst C, Admantos S. Autologous blood transfusion following red blood cell salvage for the management of blood loss in 3 dogs with hemoperitoneum. *J Vet Emerg Crit Care* 2012; **22**: 355–360.

341 Carless PA, Henry DA, O'Connell D, *et al.* Cell salvage for minimizing perioperative allogenic blood transfusion. *Cochrane Database Syst Rev* 2010; **4**: CD001888.

342 Serrick CJ, Scholz M, Melo A, *et al.* Quality of red blood cells using autotransfusion devices: a comparative analysis. *J Extra Corpor Technol* 2003; **35**: 28–34.

343 Kirkpatrick UJ, Adams RA, Lardi A, *et al.* Rheological properties and function of blood cells in stored bank blood and salvaged blood. *Br J Haematol* 1998; **101**: 364–368.

344 Esper SA, Waters JH. Intra-operative cell salvage: a fresh look at the indications and contraindications. *Blood Transfus* 2011; **9**: 139–147.

345 Catling S, Williams S, Freites O, *et al.* Use of a leucocyte filter to remove tumour cells from intra-operative cell salvage blood. *Anaesthesia* 2008; **63**: 1332–1338.

346 Waters JH, Donnenberg AD. Blood salvage and cancer surgery: should we do it? *Transfusion* 2009; **49**: 2016–2018.

347 Waters JH, Tuohy MJ, Hobson DF, *et al.* Bacterial reduction by cell salvage washing and leukocyte depletion filtration. *Anesthesiology* 2003; **99**: 652–655.

348 Gregoretti S. Suction-induced hemolysis at various vacuum pressures: implications for intraoperative blood salvage. *Transfusion* 1996; **36**: 57–60.

349 Bull BS, Bull MH. The salvaged blood syndrome: a sequel to mechanochemical activation of platelets and leukocytes? *Blood Cells* 1990; **16**: 5–20.

350 Reid TJ. Hb-based oxygen carriers: are we there yet? *Transfusion* 2003; **43**: 280–287.

351 Haney CR, Buehler PW, Gulati A. Purification and chemical modifications of hemoglobin in developing hemoglobin based oxygen carriers. *Adv Drug Deliv Rev* 2000; **40**: 153–169.

352 Muir WW, Wellman LM. Hemoglobin solutions and tissue oxygenation. *J Vet Intern Med* 2003; **17**: 127–135.

353 Oxyglobin® solution package insert. Cambridge: Biopure, 2000.

354 Rentko VT, Pearce LB, Moon-Massat PF, *et al.* Pharmacokinetics of a hemoglobin-based O2 carrier in dogs (abstract). *J Vet Intern Med* 2003; **17**: 407.

355 Rentko VT, Pearce LB, Moon-Massat PF, *et al.* Pharmacokinetics of low doses of a hemoglobin-based O2 carrier in dogs with normovolemic anemia (abstract). *J Vet Intern Med* 2003; **17**: 407.

356 Soma LR, Uboh CE, Guan F, *et al.* The pharmacokinetics of hemoglobin-based oxygen carrier hemoglobin glutamer-200 bovine in the horse. *Anesth Analg* 2005; **100**: 1570–1575.

357 Standl T, Horn P, Wilhelm S, *et al.* Bovine haemoglobin is more potent than autologous red blood cells in restoring muscular tissue oxygenation after profound isovolaemic haemodilution in dogs. *Can J Anaesth* 1996; **43**: 714–723.

358 Horn EP, Standl T, Wilhelm S, *et al.* Bovine hemoglobin increases skeletal muscle oxygenation during 95% artificial arterial stenosis. *Surgery* 1997; **121**: 411–418.

359 Spahn DR. Current status of artificial oxygen carriers. *Adv Drug Deliv Rev* 2000; **40**: 143–151.

360 Driessen B, Jahr JS, Lurie F, *et al.* Arterial oxygenation and oxygen delivery after hemoglobin-based oxygen carrier infusion in canine hypovolemic shock: a dose-response study. *Crit Care Med* 2003; **31**: 1771–1779.

361 Belgrave RL, Hines MT, Keegan RD, *et al.* Effects of polymerized ultrapurified bovine hemoglobin blood substitute administrated to ponies with normovolemic anemia. *J Vet Intern Med* 2002; **16**: 396–403.

362 Driessen B, Jahr JS, Lurie F, *et al.* Effects of isovolemic resuscitation with hemoglobin-based oxygen carrier Hemoglobin glutamer-200 (bovine) on systemic and mesenteric perfusion and oxygenation in a canine model of hemorrhagic shock: a comparison with 6% hetastarch solution and shed blood. *Vet Anesth Analg* 2006; **33**: 368–380.

363 Hamilton RG, Kelly N, Gawryl MS, *et al.* Absence of immunopathology associated with repeated IV administration of bovine Hb-based oxygen carrier in dogs. *Transfusion* 2001; **41**: 219–225.

364 Levy JH, Goodnough LT, Greilich PE, *et al.* Polymerized bovine hemoglobin solution as a replacement for allogeneic red blood cell transfusion after cardiac surgery: results of a randomized, double-blind trial. *J Thorac Cardiovasc Surg* 2002; **124**: 35–42.

365 Sprung J, Kindscher JD, Wahr JA, *et al.* The use of bovine hemoglobin glutamer-250 (Hemopure) in surgical patients: results of a multicenter, randomized, single blinded trial. *Anesth Analg* 2002; **94**: 799–808.

366 Rentko VT, Wohl J, Murtaugh R, *et al.* A clinical trial of hemoglobin-based oxygen-carrying (HBOC) fluid in the treatment of anemia in dogs. *J Vet Intern Med* 1996; **10**: 177.

367 Zambelli AB, Leisewitz AL. A prospective, randomized comparison of Oxyglobin (HB-200) and packed red blood cell transfusion for canine babesiosis. *J Vet Emerg Crit Care* 2009; **19**: 102–112.

368 Gibson GR, Callan MB, Hoffmann V, *et al.* Use of hemoglobin based oxygen carrying solutions in cats: 72 cases (1998–2000). *J Am Vet Med Assoc* 2002; **221**: 96–102.

369 Weingart C, Kohn B. Clinical use of a hemoglobin-based oxygen carrying solution (Oxyglobin) in 48 cats (2002–2006). *J Feline Med Surg* 2008; **10**: 431–438.

370 Wehausen CE, Kirby R, Rudloff E. Evaluation of the effects of bovine hemoglobin glutamer-200 on systolic arterial blood pressure in hypotensive cats: 44 cases (1997–2008). *J Am Vet Med Assoc* 2011; **238**: 909–914.

371 Brainard BM, Meredith CP, Callan MB, *et al.* Changes in platelet function, hemostasis, and prostaglandin expression after treatment with nonsteroidal anti-inflammatory drugs with various cyclooxygenase selectivities in dogs. *Am J Vet Res* 2007; **68**: 251–257.

372 Blois SI, Allen DG, Wood D, *et al.* Effects of aspirin, carprofen, deracoxib, and meloxicam on platelet function and systemic prostaglandin concentrations in healthy dogs. *Am J Vet Res* 2010; **71**: 349–358.

373 Mullins KB, Thomason JM, Lunsford KV, *et al.* Effects of carprofen, meloxicam and deracoxib on platelet function in dogs. *Vet Anaesth Analg* 2012; **39**: 206–217.

374 Hogan DF, Andrews DA, Green HW, *et al.* Antiplatelet effects and pharmacodynamics of clopidogrel in cats. *J Am Vet Med Assoc* 2004; **225**: 1406–1411.

375 Callan MB, Giger U. Effect of desmopressin acetate administration on primary hemostasis in Doberman Pinschers with type-1 von Willebrand disease as assessed by a point-of-care instrument. *Am J Vet Res* 2002; **63**: 1700–1706.

376 Sakai M, Watari T, Miura T, *et al.* Effects of DDAVP administration subcutaneously in dogs with aspirin induced platelet dysfunction and hemostatic impairment due to chronic liver disease. *J Vet Med Sci* 2003; **65**: 83–86.

377 Henry DA, Carless PA, Moxey AJ, *et al.* Anti-fibrinolytic use for minimizing perioperative allogenic blood transfusion. *Cochrane Database Syst Rev* 2011; **16**: CD001886.

378 Berenholtz SM, Pham JC, Garrett-Mayer E, *et al.* Effect of epsilon aminocaproic acid on red-cell transfusion requirements in major spinal surgery. *Spine* 2009; **34**: 2096–2103.

379 Marin LM, Iazbik MC, Zaldivar-Lopez S, *et al.* Retrospective evaluation of epsilon aminocaproic acid for the prevention of postamputation bleeding in retired racing Greyhounds with appendicular bone tumors: 46 cases (2003–2008). *J Vet Emerg Crit Care* 2012; **22**: 332–340.

380 Marin LM, Iazbik MC, Zaldivar-Lopez S, *et al.* Epsilon aminocaproic acid for the prevention of delayed postoperative bleeding in retired racing Greyhounds undergoing gonadectomy. *Vet Surg* 2012; **41**: 594–603.

381 Rajagopalan S, Mascha E, Na Jie, *et al.* The effects of mild perioperative hypothermia on blood loss and transfusion requirement. *Anesthesiology* 2008; **108**: 71–77.

382 Schmied H, Kurz A, Sessler DI, *et al.* Mild intraoperative hypothermia increases blood loss and allogeneic transfusion requirements during total hip arthroplasty. *Lancet* 1996; **347**: 289–292.

383 Schmied H, Schiferer A, Sessler DI, *et al.* The effects of red-cell scavenging, hemodilution, and active warming on allogeneic blood requirement in patients undergoing hip or knee arthroplasty. *Anesth Analg* 1998; **86**: 387–391.

384 Felfernig M, Blaicher A, Kettner SC, *et al.* Effects of temperature on partial thromboplastin time in heparinized plasma in vitro. *Eur J Anaesthesiology* 2001; **18**: 467–470.

385 Shimokawa M, Kitaguchi K, Kawaguchi M, *et al.* The influence of induced hypothermia for hemostatic function on temperature-adjusted measurements in rabbits. *Anesth Analg* 2003; **96**: 1209–1213.

SECTION 4

Cardiovascular System

22 Cardiovascular Physiology

William W. Muir

VCPCS, Columbus, Ohio, USA

Chapter contents

Introduction

The terms *circulatory system* and *cardiovascular system* are used to encompass an organ system that consists of the heart, blood and lymph vessels, and blood and lymph. The purpose of the cardiovascular system is to circulate blood and other essential materials, especially oxygen, to cells and remove waste products. Oxygen is the fuel that sustains life, and all tissues. The heart and brain, are particularly dependent upon continual oxygen availability in order to maintain normal metabolic function and cellular activities. Relatively brief periods (2–3 min) of cerebral or cardiac anoxia, for example, can produce devastating consequences that threaten life, even if blood flow is restored. More specifically, the principal function of (1) the heart is to pump blood; (2) the vasculature is to carry blood and to facilitate tissue perfusion and cellular exchange processes; (3) the blood is to transport (oxygen, carbon dioxide, nutrients, waste, hormones), regulate (pH, temperature, fluid balance) and protect (clotting mechanisms, immune response) the body from blood loss and foreign invaders; and (4) the lymph is to return filtered plasma to the circulation, defend against antigens, and transport fluid and fat from the intestine. Schematically, the cardiovascular system of mammals is a circuit comprised of two circulations (systemic and pulmonary) in series (Fig. 22.1). Oxygenated blood returning from the lungs enters the left atrium and then the left ventricle. Blood is then pumped into the aorta, which, in conjunction with an elaborate array of large conduits (arteries), distributes blood throughout the body. The terminal ends of these large arteries, the arterioles, differentially regulate blood flow and oxygen delivery based upon the tissues' oxygen requirements and give rise to smaller vessels, the capillaries, which are the principal sites for oxygen and nutrient transfer to tissues and the removal of the by-products of cellular metabolism. Capillaries, in turn, coalesce to form venules and small veins returning blood to larger veins that eventually empty into the right atrium and then the right ventricle. Blood is then pumped into the lungs, completing the circuit.

The circulation of blood depends on a functional heart, normal blood vessels, and an adequate blood volume, and functions to maintain a constant internal environment (interior milieu) for all living cells. Since blood flow is responsible for the uptake, delivery, and elimination of all anesthetic drugs, a fundamental understanding and appreciation of cardiovascular function and circulatory dynamics are required for safe anesthetic practice. This chapter reviews the anatomy and physiology of the cardiovascular system of mammals and describes or summarizes the general effects of anesthesia and anesthetic drugs when appropriate. A description of the structure, function, and physiology of the heart, blood and lymph vessels, and blood is followed by a review of hemorrheology, hemodynamics, local and neurohumoral control mechanisms, and the balance between oxygen delivery and oxygen consumption. A brief review of the circulatory system of exotic species is included for comparison and because of their increasing prevalence as pets.

Veterinary Anesthesia and Analgesia: The Fifth Edition of Lumb and Jones.
Edited by Kurt A. Grimm, Leigh A. Lamont, William J. Tranquilli, Stephen A. Greene and Sheilah A. Robertson.

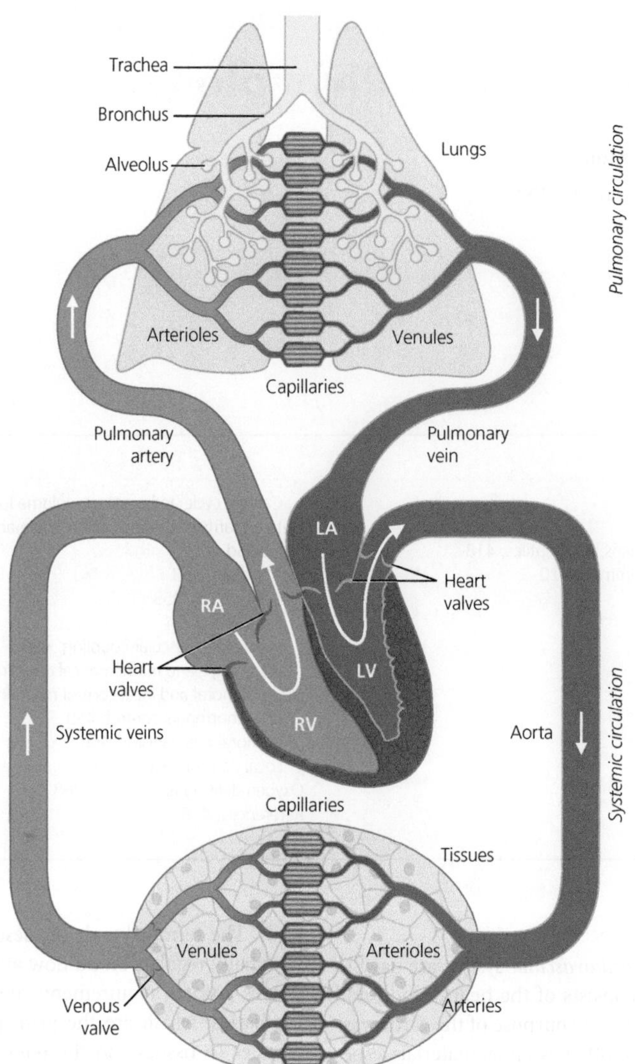

Figure 22.1 The cardiovascular system is comprised of the heart, blood, and two circulations (pulmonary and systemic). Pulmonary circulation: the pulmonary artery carries blood from the right ventricle (RV) to the lungs, where carbon dioxide is eliminated and oxygen is taken up. Oxygenated blood returns to the left atrium (LA) via the pulmonary veins. Systemic circulation: blood is pumped by the left ventricle (LV) into the aorta, which distributes blood to peripheral tissues. Oxygen and nutrients are exchanged for carbon dioxide and other by-products of tissue metabolism in capillary beds. Blood is returned to the right atrium (RA) by systemic veins. Source: modified from [55].

Circulatory system

All animals have a circulatory system, although this can vary substantially among genera. The American Veterinary Medical Association (AVMA) lists fish, ferrets, rabbits, hamsters, birds, gerbils, rodents, frogs, turtles, snakes, and lizards, among others, as exotic species. Several of these species have a unique circulatory system and not all have a four-chambered heart (Fig. 22.2). A discussion of current opinions regarding circulatory system architectures, 'open' or 'closed,' and each species' unique circulatory characteristics is beyond the scope of this chapter; however, the view that the hearts and circulations of amphibians and reptiles (three chambers; cardiac and vascular shunts) are functionally inefficient intermediate steps to the four-chambered hearts of birds and mammals is now considered antiquated [1,2]. It is more likely that cardiac and vascular shunts represent an adaptive phenotypic trait providing reptiles with the ability to regulate blood flow depending upon respiratory needs. A brief overview of the cardiovascular system of fish, amphibians, and reptiles follows.

Cardiovascular system: fish, amphibians, and reptiles

The fish heart pumps blood in a single loop throughout the body. They are considered to have a single-cycle (one 'circulation') or closed-loop circulatory system. The heart consists of four parts: two primary chambers, an entrance, and an exit (Fig. 22.2). Amphibians and most reptiles have a three-chambered heart and are considered to have a 'double' circulatory system (arterial and venous). The ventricle is incompletely separated into two pumps. Blood returning to the heart is pumped to the lungs, skin, and systemic circulation. Thus a mixture of oxygenated and deoxygenated blood is pumped into the systemic circulation.

The heart of many reptiles, including turtles, snakes, and lizards, consists of two atria and a single ventricle with a distinctive yet incomplete muscular ridge that acts to divide the ventricle into two major chambers and minimize the mixing of oxygenated and deoxygenated blood [2,3]. The pulmonary artery and right and

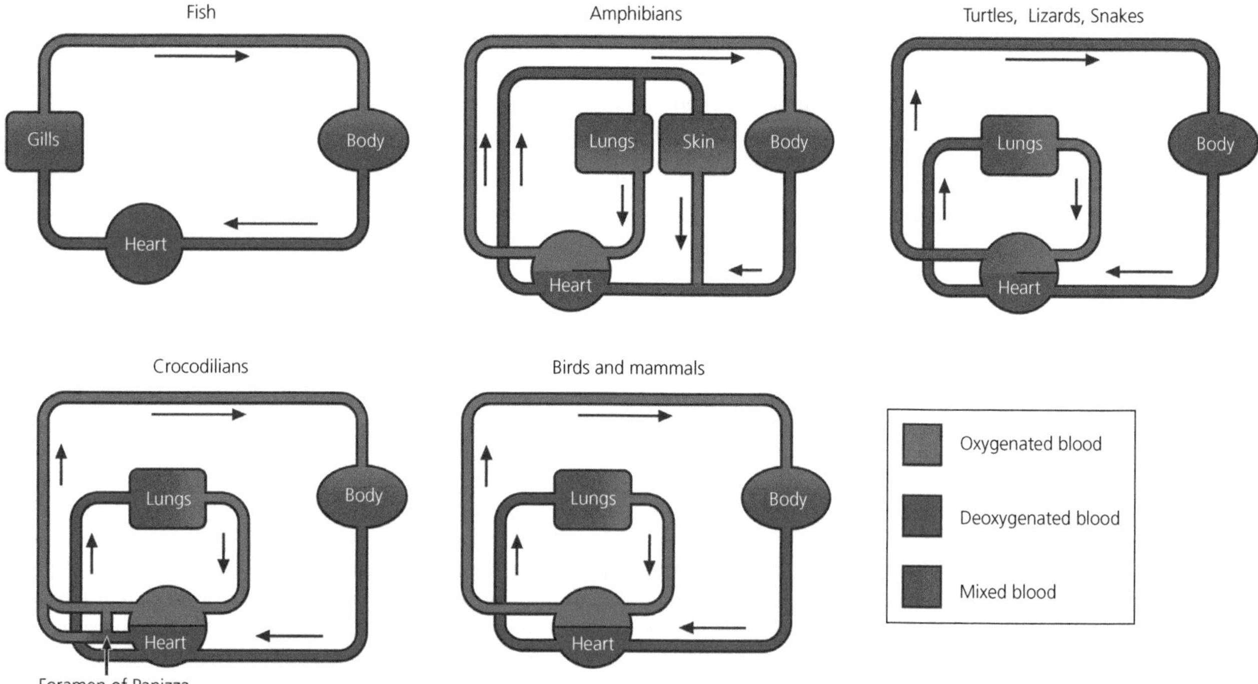

Figure 22.2 Comparative aspects of different circulatory systems. Note the foramen of Panizza in crocodilians. Source: modified from [2]. Reproduced with permission of the American Physiological Society.

left aortic arches originate from specific anatomic sites (cavum pulmonale; cavum venosum of the "single" ventricle; not shown) (Fig. 22.2). The sinus venosus is occasionally considered to be an additional chamber classifying the non-crocodilian heart as an atypical 'four-chambered' organ [4]. The pulmonary artery is equipped with a muscular sphincter that when contracted diverts blood flow through the incomplete ventricular septum into the left ventricle and out the aorta, producing a right-to-left (R–L) shunt estimated to equal 60–70% of the venous return. Both the pulmonary and systemic arterial vascular resistance and the degree of development of the muscular ridge control the magnitude and direction of cardiac shunting in reptiles [2]. For example, during diastole, deoxygenated blood mixes with oxygenated blood, but not during systole, when the contraction process causes the ventricle to function as a dual-chamber pressure pump. The above anatomic features determine the direction in which the blood flow is shunted and are believed to have important physiologic functions, including R–L shunting during diving and breath holding (Table 22.1). Both diving and breath holding increase peripheral vascular resistance, resulting in bradycardia, a normal response, in reptiles leading to the redirection of blood flow to the brain and heart. Reptiles switch from aerobic to anaerobic glycolysis during extended breath holding, resulting in acidemia, restricted pulmonary blood flow, and R–L shunting of blood in order to ensure that blood flow continues to the systemic circulation [3]. The resumption of normal breathing reverses these events, decreasing pulmonary resistance, increasing heart rate, and reducing R–L shunting. The described physiologic changes can be induced pharmacologically by dissociative anesthetics (ketamine, tiletamine), α_2-adrenergic receptor agonsists (medetomidine, dexmedetomidine), or propofol and should be anticipated [3]. Positive-pressure ventilation may help to minimize R–L shunting and maintain adequate tissue oxygenation.

Table 22.1 Hypothesized physiological functions of cardiac shunting

Physiological Function	Direction of Shunt
Saves cardiac energy	R-L
"Meters" lung oxygen stores	R-L
Reduces CO_2 flux into the lungs	R-L
Reduces plasma filtration into lungs	R-L
Facilitates warming	R-L
Triggers hypometabolism	R-L
Facilitates stomach acid secretion and digestion	R-L
Facilitates CO_2 elimination into lung*	L-R
Minimizes V/Q mismatching*	L-R
Improves systemic O_2 transport*	L-R
Myocardial oxygenation*	L-R

R-L, right-to-left (pulmonary bypass); L-R, left-to-right (systemic bypass).
*Hypothesized functions for L-R shunt apply only to turtles, snakes, and lizards. Crocodilian reptiles cannot develop L-R shunts due to anatomy; see text for details.

The systemic circulation of reptiles, as in other vertebrates, consists of arterial, venous, and lymphatic vessels. Snakes possess a vertebral venous plexus (VVP) comprised of a network of spinal veins located within and around the vertebral column. The plexus is supported by the surrounding bones, providing a route for venous return and maintenance of cerebral blood supply [3]. A renal–portal system is found in birds, amphibians, reptiles, and fish, but not in mammals. In species with a renal-portal system, venous blood returning from the tail and hindlimbs can be filtered through the kidneys and liver. Valves located between the abdominal and femoral veins regulate blood flow through the kidneys, especially during times of water conservation. Parenteral drug administration of potentially nephrotoxic drugs into the tail or caudal extremities is generally not recommended [4]. The administration of non-nephrotoxic drugs into the caudal extremities, however, does not pose a risk [5]. Reptiles have a lymphatic system but lack lymph nodes. The lymph vessels have muscular dilations referred to as 'lymph hearts' that propel the fluid into the venous system [4,5].

The circulatory anatomy of crocodilians is unique among reptiles and similar to that of birds and mammals (four separate chambers), thus preventing intracardiac R–L shunting. However, crocodilians retain the dual aortic arch system found in many reptiles [2]. The left aortic arch originates from the right ventricle next to the pulmonary artery and the right aortic arch originates from the left ventricle. Importantly, the left and right aortic arches of crocodilians communicate via the foramen of Panizza located close to the heart and via an arterial anastomosis in the abdomen (Fig. 22.2). This anatomic arrangement permits systemic venous blood to bypass the pulmonary circulation.

As suggested above, the consequences of R–L and left to right (L–R) shunts can have important anesthetic consequences (Table 22.1). An R–L shunt bypasses the lungs, diverting deoxygenated blood back into the systemic circulation, whereas an L–R shunt recirculates pulmonary venous (oxygenated) blood back into the pulmonary circulation. Physiologic L–R shunting in reptiles is not thought to contribute to overload of the pulmonary circulation due to the ability of blood to be shunted either L–R or R–L, although it can contribute to pulmonary over-circulation in mammals. Autonomic tone, neurohumoral substances, and the activity of pulmonary stretch and chemoreceptors control pulmonary and systemic vascular resistances in reptiles, which in turn control heart rate, ventricular blood volume, and ventricular contractility. Together, these factors determine the direction and magnitude of cardiac shunting. Ventilatory status (particularly in diving animals), thermoregulation, feeding, and digestion also influence cardiac shunting, although to what extent is not fully understood. For example, most reptiles breathe intermittently with long periods of apnea. Parasympathetic tone increases during apnea, resulting in bradycardia and increased pulmonary vascular resistance, promoting the development of R–L shunting [2]. Tachycardia, decreased pulmonary vascular resistance, and an increase in L–R shunting coincide with periods of ventilation [2].

Intrapulmonary or intracardiac (congenital malformation) shunts may affect the onset and termination of anesthetic drug effects, particularly if inhalant anesthetics are administered. The speed of inhalant anesthetic induction is determined by how fast the anesthetic partial pressure is reached in the brain, which is determined by the rate of anesthetic inflow into the lungs, the rate of anesthetic transfer to the blood, and the rate of anesthetic transfer from the arterial blood to the brain. An L–R shunt has minimal or no effect on the onset or elimination of inhalant anesthetics in mammals (Box 22.1). The speed of inhalant anesthetic induction is unchanged even though recirculation of blood through the lungs promotes a more rapid rate of rise in alveolar partial pressure. The speed of induction may be increased following the administration of an intravenous anesthetic due to the immediate transfer of the injectable drug to the systemic circulation and brain. An R–L shunt should slow the rate of inhalant anesthetic induction and elimination, and this effect should be more pronounced with less soluble anesthetics (isoflurane, sevoflurane, desflurane) than a more soluble anesthetic (halothane). This occurs because of the dilutional effect of shunted blood, which contains no volatile anesthetic, on the anesthetic partial pressure coming from ventilated alveoli. The alveolar uptake of highly soluble volatile anesthetics, however, is sufficient to offset partially the dilutional effect. Anesthetics with a low blood:gas partition coefficient (low solubility) are generally expected to produce a more rapid induction and recovery in normal mammals without R–L shunting. For example, anesthetic induction and washout in healthy pigs is more rapid with the less-soluble desflurane than with sevoflurane, which is more rapid than with isoflurane [6]. The rate of anesthetic uptake and speed of induction in animals with naturally occurring intracardiac shunts, however, should be delayed, as should the rate of elimination. A study comparing the effects of isoflurane, sevoflurane and desflurane in green iguanas (*Iguana iguana*) (60–70% R–L shunt), however, was unable to demonstrate significant differences in the pharmacokinetics for any induction or recovery event for isoflurane, sevoflurane, or desflurane and suggested that more favorable pharmacokinetics can be obtained by altering body temperature, cardiac preload, vagal tone, ventilation pattern, and the partial pressure of oxygen in the blood in order to decrease R–L shunt fraction [7].

Box 22.1 Effect of intracardiac shunts on anesthetic induction.

L–R shunt:
- IV anesthetic: little effect on induction
- Volatile anesthetic: little effect on induction

R–L shunt:
- IV anesthetic: rapid induction; blood bypasses lungs and goes to brain
- Right to left (volatile): slower induction

Cardiovascular system: birds and mammals

The heart of birds and mammals is composed of four chambers: two thin-walled atria separated by an interatrial septum, and two thick-walled ventricles separated by an interventricular septum. The unique respiratory system of birds, including the presence of air sacs, facilitates gas exchange throughout the respiratory cycle and has important inhalant anesthetic implications that are discussed elsewhere in this text. The following discussion focuses on the cardiovascular anatomy of mammals.

Heart: Anatomy

The boundaries of the cardiac chambers in mammals are easily defined by the great veins (cranial and caudal vena cava), which return blood to the right atrium; the smaller pulmonary veins, which return oxygenated blood from the lung to the left atrium; the coronary sulcus, which demarcates the atria from the ventricles; and the interventricular (longitudinal) sulci, which separate the right and left ventricles (Fig. 22.3).

All four chambers of the heart are easily visualized and interrogated by echocardiographic techniques, limited only by the animal's size and heart rate. The paraconal branch of the left main coronary artery, occasionally referred to as the left anterior descending coronary artery in humans, provides blood supply to the ventricular septum and left ventricular free wall. The subsinuosal coronary artery, generally an extension of the left circumflex coronary artery (the other major branch of the left main coronary artery), and occasionally a branch off the right coronary artery, provides blood supply to the majority of the left ventricle. The right coronary artery provides blood supply to the right ventricular free wall and portions of the left ventricle (Fig. 22.3b). The left coronary artery is generally dominant. The right coronary artery is more frequently dominant in cats and horses. Blood returning from the systemic circulation (venous return) and pulmonary circulation empties into the right and left atrium, respectively. The ventricles, the major pumping

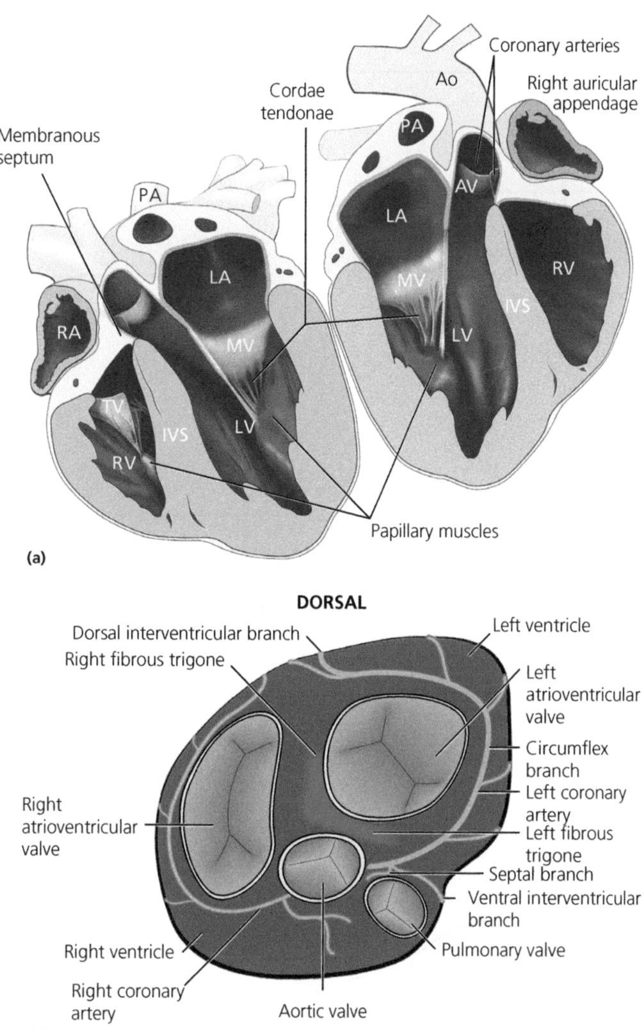

Figure 22.3 (a) The heart in mammals is a four-chambered pump comprised of two thin-walled and two thick-walled chambers and a highly reactive and diffuse vascular network (coronary circulation). The thin-walled right atrium (RA) and left atrium (LA) are separated from each other by a membranous septum (between the right and left atria). The interventricular septum (IVS) lies between the right and left ventricles. The tricuspid valve (TV) and mitral valve (MV) lie between the RA and RV and the LA and LV, respectively. The pulmonary and aortic (AV) valves separate the RV and LV from the pulmonary artery (PA) and aorta (Ao), respectively. (b) A fibrous trigone located at the center of the heart provides the scaffolding to which the heart valves, atria, and ventricles are attached. The right and left coronary arteries emerge from the root of the aorta to supply blood to all the chambers of the heart, including the heart valves.

chambers of the heart, are separated from the atria by atrioventricular valves. The tricuspid valve is located between the right atrium and right ventricle and the mitral valve between the left atrium and left ventricle. The ventricles receive blood from their respective atria and eject it across semilunar valves: the pulmonic valve is located between the right ventricle and pulmonary artery and the aortic valve between the left ventricle and aorta.

Once the process of cardiac contraction is initiated, almost simultaneous contraction of the atria is followed by nearly synchronous contraction of the ventricles, which results in a pressure differences between the atria, ventricles, and pulmonary and systemic circulations. Cardiac contraction produces differential pressure changes that are responsible for atrioventricular and semilunar valve opening and closing and the production of heart sounds (S1, S2, S3, and S4; see Hemodynamics). Chordae tendinea originating from papillary muscles located on the inner wall of the ventricular chambers are attached to the free edges of the atrioventricular valve leaflets and help to maintain valve competence by restraining their prolapse into the atria, thereby preventing regurgitation of blood into the atrium during ventricular contraction (Fig. 22.3a). Alteration in heart chamber geometry (e.g., stretch, dilation, or hypertrophy) produced by changes in blood volume, deformation (pericardial tamponade), or disease (tumors, scarring) can have profound effects on myocardial function, as do the effects produced by neurohumoral, metabolic, and pharmacological perturbations.

Heart: Metabolism

The maintenance of normal cardiac activity depends on the metabolic pathways by which ATP is generated. Even a superficial description of these pathways is far beyond the scope and purpose of this chapter and they are more appropriately described in reviews specifically designed to discuss this subject [8]. The heart generates

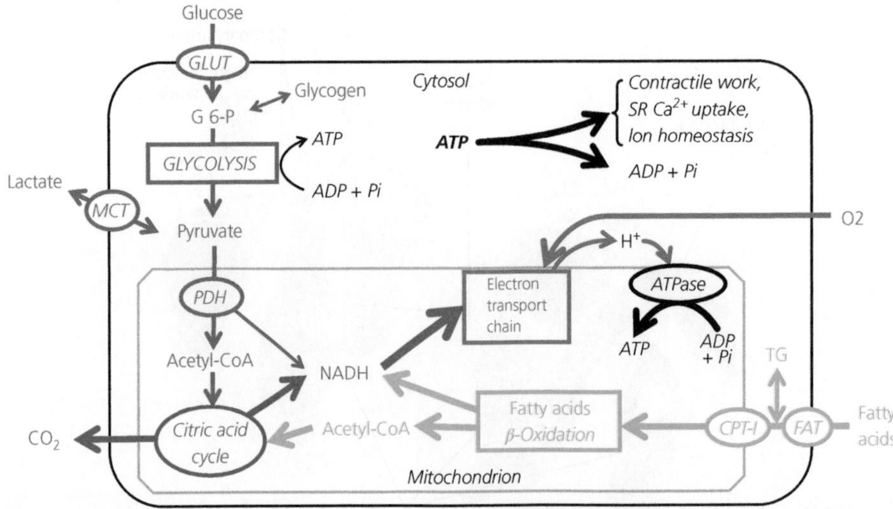

Figure 22.4 Linkages between cardiac power, ATP hydrolysis, oxidative phosphorylation, and NADH generation by dehydrogenases in metabolism. SR, sarcoplasmic reticulum. CPT-I, carnitine palmitoyltransferase-I; FAT, fatty acid transporter/CD36; G 6-P, glucose 6-phosphate; GLUT, glucose transporters; MCT, monocarboxylic acid transporters; PDH, pyruvate dehydrogenase. Source: modified from [8]. Reproduced with permission of the American Physiological Society.

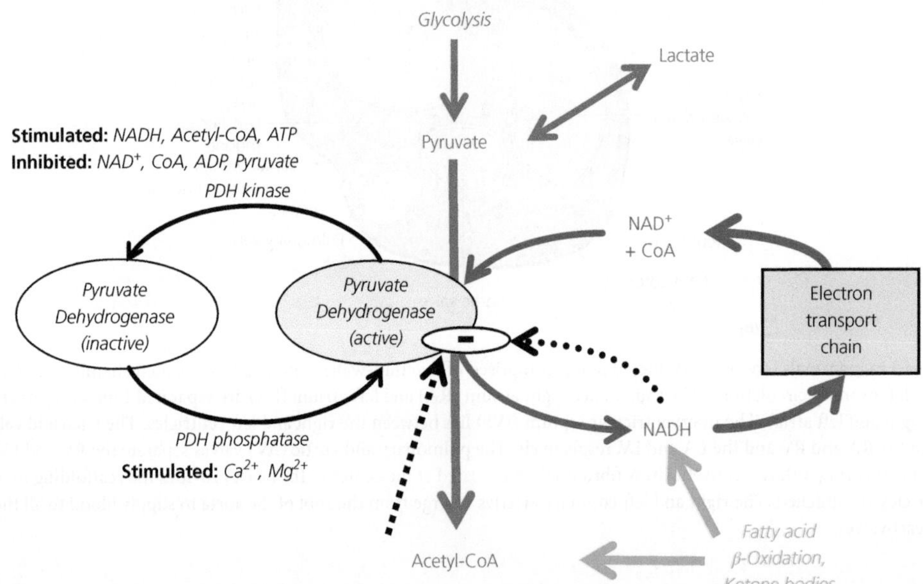

Figure 22.5 Regulation of the oxidation of glucose and lactate by pyruvate dehydrogenase (PDH). The activity of PDH is inhibited by product inhibition from acetyl-CoA and NADH (dashed arrows), and by phosphorylation by PDH kinase and dephosphorylation by PDH phosphatase. Modified from [8]. Reproduced with permission of the American Physiological Society.

ATP by two primary methods: oxidative phosphorylation and glycolysis (Fig. 22.4). Oxidative phosphorylation in the mitochondria is responsible for approximately 95% of ATP formation in the heart during normal non-ischemic conditions, with the remainder derived from glycolysis and GTP formation from the citric acid cycle. The heart utilizes all myocardial ATP in approximately 10 s during normal resting conditions, emphasizing the requirement for continuous production. Approximately 60–70% of ATP hydrolysis is utilized in cardiac contraction and the remaining 30–40% is used to maintain the function of ion pumps and sarcoplasmic reticulum Ca^{2+}-ATPase. The rate of oxidative phosphorylation is directly linked to the rate of ATP hydrolysis so that the ATP content remains constant during intense exercise or changes in blood catecholamine concentrations.

Mitochondrial oxidative phosphorylation is dependent upon the electron transport chain that generates nicotinamide adenine dinucleotide (NADH) and flavin adenine dinucleotide ($FADH_2$) produced primarily by the fatty acid oxidation pathway, the citric acid cycle, and the pyruvate dehydrogenase reaction and glycolysis (Fig. 22.5). The regulation of myocardial metabolism is linked to arterial carbon substrate concentration, hormone concentrations, coronary flow, inotropic state, and the nutritional status of the tissue [9,10]. The citric acid cycle is dependent upon acetyl-CoA formed from decarboxylation of pyruvate and the oxidation of fatty acids (Fig. 22.5). The reducing equivalents NADH and $FADH_2$ that are generated by dehydrogenases of glycolysis, the oxidation of lactate and pyruvate and fatty acid oxidation, or the citric acid cycle deliver electrons to the electron transport chain, resulting in ATP formation by oxidative phosphorylation. These processes are continually modified by the energy requirements of the cell and by neural and hormonal inputs. The ATP produced supplies energy for cardiac contraction, relaxation, and related activities.

Heart: Electrophysiology

The purpose of the heart is to pump blood in quantities sufficient to meet the body's oxygen demands. A highly integrated series of electrochemical followed by metabolic and mechanical events are required to achieve normal cardiac contractile function (excitation–contraction coupling). Notably, myocardial contraction is preceded by, and will not occur without, electric activation, although normal or near-normal electric activity is possible without myocardial contraction [electric–mechanical uncoupling; electric–mechanical dissociation (EMD); pulseless electrical activity (PEA)]. Pulseless electrical activity is the clinical term used to describe EMD and is defined as the lack of palpable pulse in the presence of organized cardiac electrical activity other than ventricular fibrillation or ventricular tachycardia.

The cardiac cell membrane (sarcolemma) is a highly specialized lipid bilayer that contains protein-associated channels, pumps, enzymes, and exchangers in an architecturally sophisticated yet fluid (reorganizable and movable) medium. The molecular composition and fluidity of cardiac membranes determine their ion transport and membrane-associated electric properties. The unequal distribution of various ions, especially sodium, potassium, and chloride, is responsible for the development of the resting membrane potential within cardiac cells as estimated by the Nernst equation or, more accurately, by the Goldman–Hodgkin–Katz constant-field equation [11,12].

Nernst equation for potassium ions:

$$E = \frac{RT}{zF}\ln\frac{[K^+]}{[K^+]}$$

$$-61 = 2.303RT/F$$

$$E_K = \frac{-61}{z}\log\frac{[K^+]_i}{[K^+]_o} = -96\text{ mV}$$

where E = electromotive force; $[K^+]_i$ and $[K^+]_o$ = intracellular and extracellular potassium concentration in mM, C_i and C_o = ion concentration inside (i) and outside (o) the cell membrane; z = valence of the ion, in this case 1; R = gas constant; T = absolute temperature; F = Faraday constant; and 2.303 = conversion of ln to log10; mV = millivolts at 37°C.

Goldman–Hodgkin–Katz equation:

$$E_m = -61\text{ mV}\log\frac{P_{K^+}[K^+]_o + P_{Na^+}[Na^+]_o + P_{Cl^-}[Cl^-]_i}{P_{K^+}[K^+]_i + P_{Na^+}[Na^+]_i + P_{Cl^-}[Cl^-]_o}$$

where E_m = resting membrane potential and "P" is the relative permeability of membrane Na, K and Cl in myocardial cells.

The transmembrane electric potential generated by cardiac cells is the result of transmembrane ion fluxes (active properties) which generate currents through 'gated' membrane pores or channels (Fig. 22.6; Table 22.2) [11]. The term *gated* refers to the opening (activation) or closing (by deactivation or inactivation) of ion channels. Ion channels are characterized by their ionic selectivity, conductance, gating characteristics, and density. The channel-gating mechanisms control ion passage and are composed of both activation and inactivation gates, which are voltage and frequently time dependent. The functional configuration of the gates determines the channel state: activated or open, inactivated or closed, and resting (capable of being activated). The directional movement (inward or outward) of the various ions ultimately depends on the channel state and the electrochemical driving force (equilibrium potential minus membrane potential) for each ion. The electrochemical driving force, as illustrated by the Nernst equation, is composed of an electric force and a concentration gradient. It should be noted that in the presence of many anesthetic drugs, particularly local anesthetics (lidocaine, bupivacaine), and inhaled anesthetics (halothane, isoflurane, sevoflurane), these same channels demonstrate use-dependent block [13–15]. Use-dependent block is the phenomenon exhibited by cardiac cells wherein, in the presence of a drug, increases in stimulation rate (e.g., heart rate) produce a more pronounced drug effect on the electrophysiologic properties of the heart than during slower rates of stimulation.

Excitability, or the ability of the cardiac cell membrane to generate and propagate an electric potential (action potential), is a fundamental intrinsic property of cardiac cells [11]. The cardiac action potential (AP) varies considerably from that of nerves and skeletal muscle and, as discussed earlier, is dependent upon the transmembrane flux of multiple ions (Table 22.3). The cardiac AP arises from a more negative membrane potential (90 vs 65 mV), is greater in magnitude (130 vs 80 mV), and is much longer in duration (150–300 vs 1–3 ms) than AP's recorded from nerve and skeletal muscle.

Five characteristic phases of the cardiac AP are discernible in most cardiac cells: phase 0, or the phase of rapid depolarization, is caused by the rapid and relatively large influx of sodium ions (fast inward current) into the cell; phase 1, the early phase of repolarization, is caused by the transient outward movement of potassium ions; phase 2, the plateau phase, is attributed to the continued, but decreased, entry of sodium ions and a large, but slow, influx of calcium ions (slow inward current) into cells; phase 3 is the phase of repolarization during which the membrane potential returns to its resting value because of potassium efflux (outward current) from the cell; and phase 4 is a resting phase in atrial and ventricular muscle cells prior to the initiation of the next AP (Fig. 22.7; Table 22.3). Notably, a great deal of interest has been focused upon repolarization currents (I_k) due to their importance in determining AP duration (long and short) and their involvement in what is termed long QT (LQT) syndrome. Long QT syndrome is an uncommon condition in humans in which delayed repolarization of the heart increases the risk of torsade de pointes predisposing to ventricular fibrillation. hERG (the human Ether-à-go-go-Related Gene or KCNH2) is a gene that codes for the potassium channel and forms the major portion of one of the ion channel proteins [the 'rapid' delayed

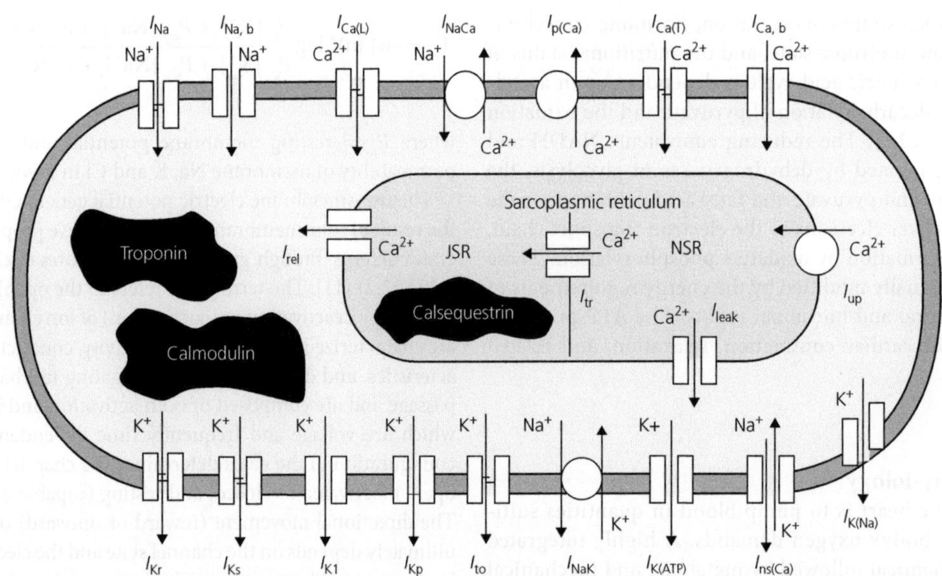

Figure 22.6 Schematic diagram of a myocardial cell channels and currents. I_{Na}, fast sodium current; $I_{Ca(L)}$, calcium current through L-type calcium channels; $I_{Ca(T)}$, calcium current through T-type calcium channels; I_{Kr}, rapid delayed rectifier potassium current; I_{Ks}, slow delayed rectifier potassium current; I_{to}, transient outward current; I_{Kl}, inward rectifier potassium current; $I_{K(ATP)}$, ATP-sensitive potassium current; I_{Kp}, plateau potassium current; $I_{K(Na)}$, sodium-activated potassium current (activated under conditions of sodium overload); $I_{ns(Ca)}$, non-specific calcium-activated current (activated under conditions of calcium overload); $I_{Na,b}$, sodium background current; $I_{Ca,b}$, calcium background current; I_{NaK}, sodium–potassium pump current; I_{NaCa}, sodium–calcium exchange current; $I_{P(Ca)}$, sarcolemnal calcium pump; I_{up}, calcium uptake from the myoplasm to the network sarcoplasmic reticulum (NSR); I_{rel}, calcium release from junctional sarcoplasmic reticulum (JSR); I_{leak}, calcium leakage from NSR to the myoplasm; I_{tr}, calcium translocation from NSR to JSR. Calmodulin and troponin are calcium buffers in the myoplasm. Calsequestrin is a calcium buffer in the JSR. Source: adapted from [12]. Reproduced with permission from Wiley.

Table 22.2 Currents associated with the cardiac action potential.

Current	Abbreviation	Qualities
Fast inward sodium current	I_{Na}	Responsible for upstroke of action potential; abolished by tetrodotoxin; inhibited by class I antiarrhythmic agents
Slow inward calcium current	I_{Ca}, I_{si}	Important for plateau phase of cardiac action potential; involved in excitation-contraction coupling; increased by β-stimulation; inhibited by calcium antagonists
Subtype T	$I_{Ca(t)}$	Transient calcium current, opening at low voltages (–60 to –50 mV); may be important in sinus node depolarization
Subtype L	$I_{Ca(l)}$	Long-duration calcium current, inhibited by calcium antagonists
Background potassium current (inward rectifier)	I_{K1} or I_{Kir}	Help to maintain resting membrane potential (RMP)
Voltage-gated delayed rectifier potassium currents	I_K (includes K_r and K_s)	Time-dependent outward potassium current; activated by depolarization (fully active at +10 mV) and deactivated by repolarization; voltage-gated; responsible for repolarization in nodal cells and contributes to spontaneous depolarization; divided into I_{Kr} (r = rapid) and I_{Ks} (s = slow). The hERG channel mediates the repolarizing I_{Kr} current in the cardiac AP
Early transient outward potassium current	I_{to}	Transient outward early potassium current, previously called *chloride current;* prominent in epicardial ventricular cells, Purkinje fibers and atrial cells; causes phase 1; may also shorten action potential duration
Other currents		
Diastolic pacemaker current in SA node and Purkinje fibers	I_f or I_h	Produces automaticity in SA node and Purkinje fibers
Sodium–calcium exchange current	$I_{Na/Ca}$	Contributes to late phase of the cardiac action potential
Chloride current	I_{Cl}	Activated by cAMP; shortens action potential duration during adrenergic stimulation
Ligand-operated G-dependent K currents		
Acetylcholine sensitive	I_{KACh}	Activated by acetylcholine muscarinic receptors in nodal, Purkinje, and atrial cells; not in ventricles; time independent; when current is switched on in nodal cells, spontaneous depolarization is delayed
Adenosine sensitive	I_{KADO}	Probably the same as I_{KACh}; adenosine stimulates time-independent background potassium current
ATP regulated	I_{KATP}	Lack of ATP activates (e.g., ischemia); inhibited by sulfonylureas, activated by K-channel activators (pinacidil)

Source: modified from Opie LH. *The Heart: Physiology and Metabolism*, 3rd edn. Philadelphia: Lippincott-Raven, 1998; 91–97.

rectifier current (I_{Kr})] that conducts potassium ions (K^+) out of cardiac muscle cells. This current is critical for returning the membrane potential to the resting state (repolarization). Although interesting physiologically and important for screening drug arrhythmogenic potential in humans, there is no convincing evidence that this gene, although present in most mammals (except rodents), contributes to the development of arrhythmias in animals [16].

The speed of conduction of the cardiac electrical impulse is determined by the magnitude and rate of sodium influx into cardiac cell, which in turn determines magnitude and rate of

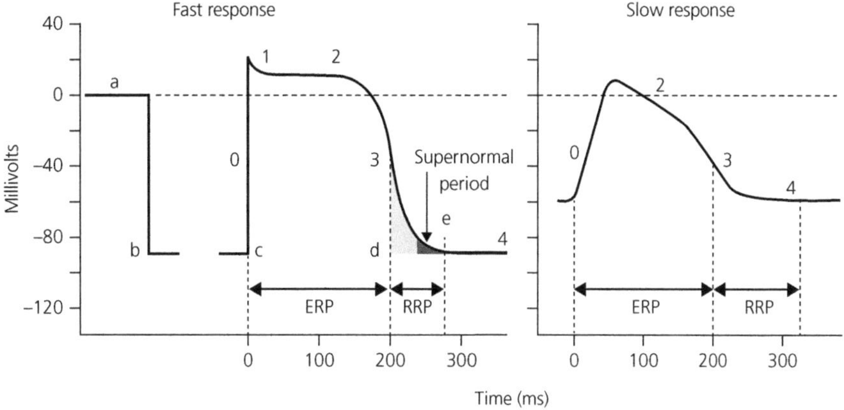

Figure 22.7 Cardiac action potential: transmembrane potential changes associated with fast-response and slow-response action potentials. Note that slow-response action potentials originate from a less negative resting membrane potential and have a much slower rate of rise (phase 0). During the supernormal period, a subthreshold stimulus can elicit a normal action potential. a-b: resting membrane potential; inside negative: c-d: ERP: cell stimulation does not produce a new action potential; d-e: RRP: a greater than normal stimulus can produce an action potential. See the text for an explanation of the action-potential phases 1–4. ERP, effective refractory period; RRP, relative refractory period.

Table 22.3 Major ion fluxes during the cardiac action potential.

Name	Ion	Movement	Current	Phase of Action Potential
I_{Na}	Na^+	In	Inward	0 (depolarization)
I_{to1}	K^+	Out	Outward	1 (early repolarization)
I_{to2}	Cl^-	In	Outward	1 (early repolarization)
I_{Ca}	Ca^{2+}	In	Inward	2 (plateau)
I_{K1}	K^+	In	Inward	inward-rectifying; resting membrane potential
(I_{kr}, I_k)	K^+	Out	Outward	3 (repolarization)
I_f	Na^+	In	Inward	4 (depolarization in automatic cells)

Open I_{K1} channels in resting cells are the major contributor to the equilibrium responsible for the Nernst potential during phase 4 (resting potential).
Source: modified from Katz AM. *Physiology of the Heart*, 3rd edn. Philadelphia: Lippincott Williams & Wilkins, 2001; **499**.

change in transmembrane potential (dV/dt) during phase 0 of the cardiac AP (Fig. 22.7). For a single cardiac cell, the change (d) in transmembrane potential (V) is related to the transmembrane ionic current (I_{ion}) and the membrane capacitance (C; 1 μF/cm^2) provided by the charge separation across the lipid bilayer:

$$dV/dt = 1/C \times I_{ion}$$

This equation states that changes in V occur due to displacement of charge on the membrane by the movement of ions across the cell membrane. This movement occurs due to the activity of voltage-gated ion channels, pumps, and exchangers, and I_{ion} represents its sum total.

A negative I_{ion} (movement of positive ions into the cell) produces a positive dV/dt, which elevates (i.e., depolarizes, makes more positive) the membrane potential. A positive I_{ion} indicates an outward flow of positive ions and acts to reduce (repolarize) the membrane potential by generating a negative dV/dt. The generation of the cardiac AP results from the time-, voltage-, and concentration-dependent evolution of I_{ion}, and represents the contribution of multiple ion-selective mechanisms for ion movement across the cardiac cell membrane (Fig. 22.7) [17]. Current flows from a depolarized cell to its neighboring less depolarized cells via intercellular resistive pathways known as gap junctions. The transmembrane current and the axial current that flows between cells in a linear cell chain can be described by

$$C_m\left(\frac{\partial V_m}{\partial t}\right) + I_{ion} = \left(\frac{a}{2r_i}\right)\left(\frac{\partial^2 V_m}{\partial r^2}\right)$$

where a is the fiber radius and r_i is the axial resistance per unit length. V_m is a function of both time (t) and space (x), hence the use of the partial derivative symbol ∂ indicating its first derivative in time ($\partial V_m/\partial t$) or its second derivative in space ($\partial^2 V_m/\partial x^2$). This equation states that the net change in axial current must be accounted for by the current that crosses the membrane. Notably, voltage-gated ionic channels are inhibited by anesthetic drugs. Intercellular channels (gap junctions) are also depressed (resistance increased) by anesthetic drugs through direct interaction with some of their protein subunits [18]. Thus, anesthetic drugs can produce several effects on specific membrane proteins, thereby interfering with cardiac excitability and transmission and propagation of electrical impulses.

The greater the dV_m/dt, the more rapid are the transmission and conduction of the cardiac impulse through cardiac tissue [12]. Cardiac cells that normally possess a more negative membrane potential (atrial and ventricular muscle cells and Purkinje cells) demonstrate greater excitability and a more rapid conduction velocity than those with less negative membrane potentials (sinoatrial and atrioventricular nodes and diseased myocardium) [11,12]. Calcium entry into cardiac cells during phase 2 triggers intracellular calcium release, which is important for normal cellular contraction and, with potassium, determines AP duration in atrial and ventricular myocytes. Since calcium enters the cell slowly and at a less negative membrane potential, cardiac cells with a reduced resting membrane potential (sinoatrial and atrioventricular nodes) demonstrate a considerably smaller phase 0 dV_m/dt and slow conduction velocity compared with atrial and ventricular muscle and Purkinje cells (Fig. 22.7) [12]. Potassium efflux from cardiac cells is controlled by a variety of mechanisms, including concentration differences across the membrane and the changing permeability (diffusional) characteristics of the cell membrane to potassium (Table 22.2). Collectively, the channels responsible for repolarization (phase 3) are also the major determinants of cardiac AP duration, cardiac cell refractoriness, and the duration of the supernormal period (Fig. 22.7). The duration of the cardiac AP has important clinical implications relative to the amount of calcium entry and the potential for arrhythmia development [11]. Longer cardiac APs permit more calcium entry into the cell and prolong cellular refractoriness. Arrhythmias develop if there are large disparities or inhomogeneities in AP duration and refractoriness of adjacent cardiac cells because of re-entry of electrical impulses into rapidly repolarized tissues and re-excitation [19]. Cardiac cells with particularly long-duration APs are thought to increase the likelihood of long QT intervals, afterdepolarizations and dispersion in AP refractoriness, thereby predisposing to cardiac arrhythmias from spontaneous activity or the development of reentrant electrical circuits (re-entry) in the heart.

Phase 4 diastolic depolarization (pacemaker potential) imparts the unique property of automaticity to the heart and occurs in the sinoatrial and atrioventricular nodes and specialized atrial and ventricular (Purkinje network) muscle fibers [11]. The resting membrane potential depolarizes towards a threshold potential which, when reached, triggers the development of an AP. The ionic processes responsible for phase 4 or diastolic depolarization vary between the various specialized tissues of the heart, primarily because of differences in their resting membrane potential and cell type (e.g., sinoatrial node versus atrioventricular node versus Purkinje cell). Cells in the sinoatrial and atrial ventricular nodes have comparatively less negative maximum diastolic potentials (–65 mV) than do Purkinje cells and depend on the entry of calcium ions (slow inward current) and a progressive decrease in membrane permeability to potassium efflux for their automaticity (Fig. 22.7) [11,12]. Automatic cells in atrial specialized pathways and the ventricular Purkinje network have a more negative maximum diastolic potential (–90 mV) and depend on a hyperpolarizing-induced 'funny' inward current, termed I_f, carried mainly by sodium ions and a decrease in potassium efflux for their automaticity (Table 22.2). Because potassium ions normally leave cardiac cells in order to restore or maintain the resting membrane potential, any decrease in potassium efflux facilitates depolarization. The principal mechanisms responsible for altering automaticity are changes in the threshold potential, the rate of phase 4 depolarization, and the maximum diastolic potential following repolarization. The cardiac tissue with the most rapid rate of phase 4 depolarization (normally the sinoatrial node) is termed the pacemaker and determines the heart rate. The cardiac pacemaker normally depresses the automaticity of slower or subsidiary pacemakers (overdrive suppression), preventing more than one pacemaker from controlling heart rate. Overdrive suppression in subsidiary pacemakers is due to activation of the sodium–potassium (Na^+–K^+) pump, leading to membrane hyperpolarization and a longer time to reach threshold (Fig. 22.8) [12]. Subsidiary pacemakers are most suppressed at fast heart rates because the Na^+–K^+ pump is more active at faster rates, resulting in a more negative maximum diastolic potential. Clinically, the administration of an antimuscarinic can produce increases in sinus rate that can eliminate (overdrive suppress) infrequent or slower ventricular arrhythmias. Automaticity is also influenced by local factors, including temperature, pH, and blood gases (PO_2 and PCO_2), extracellular potassium concentration, catecholamines, and various hormones (Fig. 22.9).

The sum of all the APs produced by each cardiac cell following activation by the sinoatrial node is responsible for the body surface electrocardiogram (ECG) (Fig. 22.10). Initiation of an electric impulse in the sinoatrial node is followed by rapid electric transmission of the impulse through the atria, giving rise to the P wave. Repolarization of the atria gives rise to the Ta wave, which although absent in most smaller animal ECGs is often obvious in large animals (horses and cattle), where the total atrial tissue mass is substantial enough to generate sufficient electromotive force to be electrocardiographically recognizable. Repolarization of the atria in smaller species (dogs and cats) and depolarization of the sinoatrial and atrioventricular nodes do not generate a large enough electric potential to be recorded at the body surface except in cases of sinus tachycardia. Once the wave of depolarization reaches the atrioventricular node, conduction is slowed because of the atrioventricular node's low resting membrane potential (approximately –60 mV) and the relatively depressed rate of phase 0 (decremental conduction). Increased parasympathetic tone can produce marked slowing of atrioventricular nodal conduction, leading to first-, second-, and, rarely, third-degree atrioventricular block. Many drugs used in anesthesia, including opioids, α_2-adrenergic receptor agonists, and occasionally acepromazine, increase parasympathetic tone, causing heart block and bradyarrhythmias. The use of antimuscarinic drugs is generally effective therapy in these situations but not for atrioventricular block caused by structural disease (e.g., inflammation, fibrosis, or calcification). Careful consideration is indicated when atropine or glycopyrrolate is coadministered with α_2-adrenergic receptor agonists due to the potential to produce or exacerbate cardiac arrhythmias and is most likely due to the development of marked changes in autonomic tone (dysautonomia) and increased strain (increased afterload) on the heart [20].

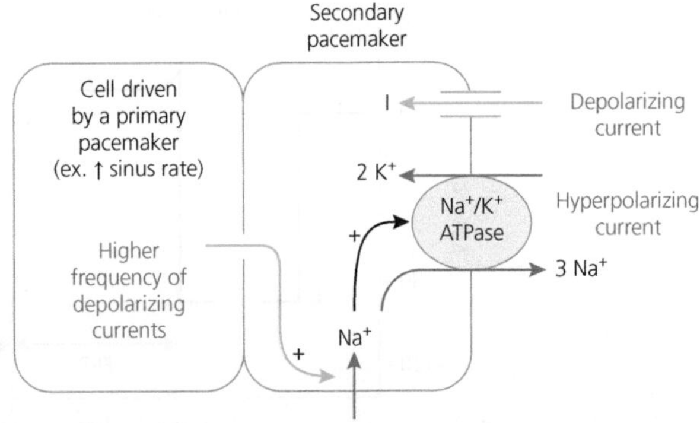

Figure 22.8 Overdrive suppression: activation of the Na^+–K^+ pump hyperpolarizes the cell membrane prolonging the time for the membrane potential to reach threshold, thereby potentially eliminating secondary (subsidiary) pacemaker activity. Primary pacemaker activity activates the secondary pacemaker resetting the depolarization process.

Under normal conditions, conduction of the electric impulse through the atrioventricular node produces the PR or PQ interval of the ECG and provides time for the atria to contract prior to activation and contraction of the ventricles (Fig. 22.10). This delay is functionally important, particularly at faster heart rates, because it enables atrial contraction to contribute to ventricular filling. It is worth remembering that cells of the atrioventricular node are extremely dependent on calcium ion for the generation of an AP and conduction of the electric impulse. Thus, cells of the atrioventricular node are extremely sensitive to drugs that block trans-sarcolemmal calcium flux, including excessive doses of anesthetics (inhalant and injectable anesthetics) and calcium channel antagonists (verapamil, diltiazem). These drugs and cardiac disease can produce atrioventricular block and postrepolarization refractoriness that are not responsive to the administration of antimuscarinics. Postrepolarization

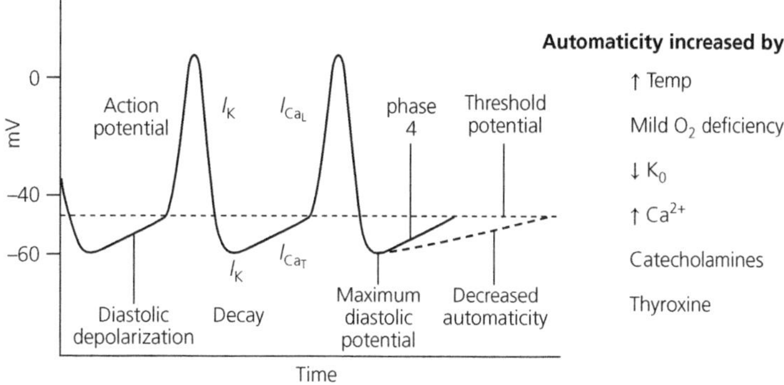

Figure 22.9 Automaticity: the sinoatrial node (pacemaker tissue) is characterized by a less negative maximum diastolic potential that moves toward threshold (phase 4 diastolic depolarization), a slow phase 0 caused primarily by activation of I_{Ca_L}, and a relatively rapid repolarization due to I_K. The rate of phase 4 diastolic depolarization (automaticity) can be increased by increases in heart rate, temperature, calcium, catecholamines, and thyroxine and decreases in oxygen tension and extracellular potassium concentration.

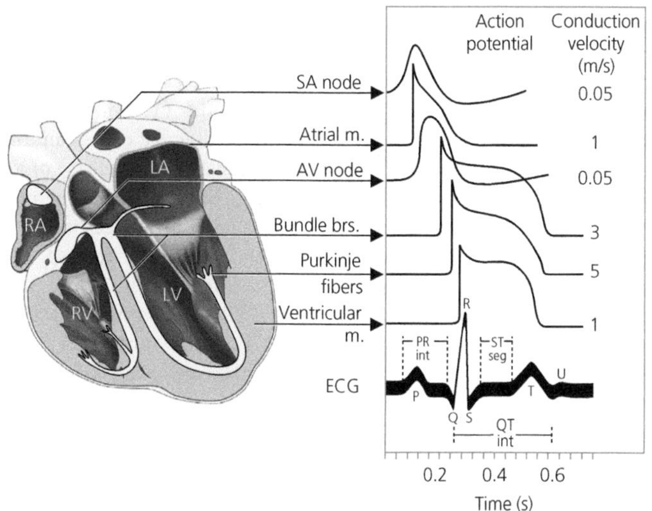

Figure 22.10 Cardiac APs recorded from the various tissues of the heart summate to produce the P–QRS–T complex of the electrocardiogram (ECG) recorded at the body surface. AV, atrioventricular node; brs, branches; int, interval; LA, left atrium; LV, left ventricle; m, muscle; RA, right atrium; RV, right ventricle; SA, sinoatrial node; seg, segment.

refractoriness is the phenomenon wherein cardiac cells remain refractory to electric activation after complete repolarization [21]. This phenomenon is most likely to produce atrioventricular block as the rate of atrial depolarization is increased. Increases in parasympathetic tone, particularly in the presence of drugs or disease (ischemia) that interfere with conduction of the electric impulse through the atrioventricular node, can lead to ECG evidence of first-degree (prolonged PR interval), second-degree (blocked P-wave conduction resulting in no QRS complex), or third-degree (dissociation of P and QRS complex) atrioventricular block.

Once the electrical impulse has traversed the atrioventricular node, it is rapidly transmitted to the ventricular muscle by specialized cardiomyocytes commonly referred to as Purkinje fibers. Bundles of Purkinje cells (the right and left bundle branches) transmit the electric impulses to the ventricular septum and to the right and left ventricular free walls, respectively, via the moderator band in the right ventricle and the left anterior and posterior divisions of the left bundle branch in the left ventricle. Purkinje cells and the so-called M or midmyocardial cells located at the terminal ends of the ventricular bundle branches and in the middle of the ventricular walls, respectively, have the longest AP and therefore serve as physiological 'gates' preventing the re-entry and recycling of electric impulses in the ventricular myocardium [22]. The relatively long duration of M-cell AP is believed to be responsible, in part, for the development of U waves in the ECG. Purkinje fibers conduct the electric impulse at relatively rapid speeds (3–5 m/s). Their distribution accounts for differences in the pattern of the ECG (ventricular depolarization) among species.

It is important to remember that, although the transmission of the electric impulse has, by analogy, been compared to dropping a pebble in water, thereby producing a concentric wavefront, the conduction of the electric impulse in the heart ultimately depends on spatial variation in myocardial cell refractoriness and uniform (isotropic) cell-to-cell resistive and capacitative (passive) membrane properties that are largely determined by low-resistance gap (nexus) junctions between cells [23,24].

The interval beginning immediately after the S wave of the QRS complex (J point) and preceding the T wave is referred to as the

ST segment. Elevation or depression of the ST segment (±0.2 mV or greater) from the isoelectric line is usually an indication of myocardial hypoxia or ischemia, low cardiac output, anemia, pericarditis, or cardiac contusion, and suggests the potential for arrhythmia development. The ST segment is followed by, or often slurs into, the T wave. The configuration and magnitude of the T wave vary considerably among species and are influenced by changes in heart rate, blood temperature, and the extracellular potassium concentration. Hyperkalemia, for example, produces an increase in membrane conductance to potassium. This shortens repolarization and produces T waves that are of large magnitude, generally spiked or pointed, and of short duration (short QT interval). Rarely, U waves can be distinguished immediately following the completion of the T wave and are believed to represent repolarization of M cells and possibly Purkinje cells (Fig. 22.10) [22]. Like Ta waves, U waves are more frequently observed in larger species of animals (horses and cattle) during electrolyte imbalances (hypokalemia or hypocalcemia) or following the administration of drugs that are occasionally used to treat heart disease (quinidine or digitalis).

Classically, several inhalant anesthetic drugs (chloroform, halothane) are known to sensitize the myocardium to catecholamines, resulting in the development of cardiac arrhythmias [25]. Similar observations have been reported for thiobarbiturates and to a minor (clinically irrelevant) extent for propofol or ketamine during isoflurane anesthesia [26–28]. This effect is likely produced by drug-related alterations on intracellular calcium cycling, resulting in alterations in electrical impulse propagation and cardiac cell excitability. Anesthetic drugs, particularly volatile anesthetics, are also known to interact with multiple cardiac ion channels. Experimental evidence suggests that volatile anesthetics, at concentrations of 1–2 MAC (minimum alveolar concentration), modify repolarizing cardiac potassium channels hERG and I_{Ks} [29]. Lower concentrations of volatile anesthetics prime the activation of sarcolemmal and mitochondrial K_{ATP} channels by stimulation of adenosine receptors and subsequent activation of protein kinase C (PKC) and by increased formation of nitric oxide and free oxygen radicals. Opioids activate δ- and κ-opioid receptors, leading to activation of PKC. The open state of the mitochondrial K_{ATP} channel and sarcolemmal K_{ATP} channel ultimately induces cytoprotection by decreasing Ca^{2+} overload in the cytosol and mitochondria, a phenomenon termed 'ischemic preconditioning' [30]. At slightly higher concentrations (i.e., at ≥2 MAC), calcium and sodium channels become involved. These effects alter the duration and shape (triangulation) of the AP, effective refractory period, and impulse conduction velocity, resulting in regional heterogeneous differences that promote re-entrant excitation. Triangulation, that is, slowing of repolarization, and slowing of conduction are the two most proarrhythmic changes in the cardiac AP [31,32]. Triangulation allows for reactivation of calcium current, more time for Na^+–Ca^{2+} exchange current, reactivation of sodium current, reduced synchronization of APs, and facilitation of re-excitation predisposing to the generation of early afterdepolarizations (EADs) [32]. Altered conduction, particularly slowed conduction, is an important parameter for determining the product of conduction velocity times refractory period (λ), which determines whether re-entry is impossible (λ > available length of excitable tissue) or possible (λ < available length of excitable tissue). When λ is shortened in combination with triangulation, the heart almost always goes into multifocal ventricular tachycardia or ventricular fibrillation. Generalized autonomic imbalance with both sympathetic and parasympathetic components may produce a neural stimulus that predisposes to subsequent cardiac repolarization and conduction abnormalities and coronary vasospasm. This may be responsible for the cardiac arrhythmias and warnings regarding the concurrent administration of an antimuscarinic and α_2-adrenergic receptor agonists [20].

In summary, the cardiac cell membrane possesses both active (ion movement) and passive (resistive and capacitive) properties that determine the heart's excitability, automaticity, rhythmicity, refractoriness, and ability to conduct an electric impulse. Anesthetic drugs, via their effects on both the active and passive properties of the heart, can produce significant alterations in cardiac excitability and conduction of the electric impulse, potentially predisposing animals to cardiac arrhythmias and mechanical contraction abnormalities [25–29,31–34].

Heart: excitation–contraction coupling

Excitation–contraction coupling refers to the process wherein electrical activation of the heart is transformed into muscle contraction [35,36]. The process begins with depolarization of the cardiac cell membrane and ends with the interaction of the contractile proteins in the individual sarcomeres. The normal extracellular $[Ca^{2+}]$ is 10^{-3} M compared with an intracellular $[Ca^{2+}]$ of 10^{-7} M. The electrical activation of the sarcolemma and transverse tubules (T tubule: deep invagination of the sarcolemma) by the cardiac AP causes an influx of a small quantity of calcium ions triggering the release of a much greater quantity of calcium (calcium-induced calcium release: CICR) from calsequestrin-bound calcium sources in the sarcoplasmic reticulum. Calcium-induced calcium release raises the intracellular calcium concentration from 10^{-7} to 10^{-5} M, causing cellular contraction (Fig. 22.11). The importance of calcium influx during phase 2 of the AP in the contractile process of cardiac muscle compared with other muscles (skeletal and smooth) cannot be overemphasized, because cardiac contraction is more dependent on, and responds instantaneously to, changes in the extracellular calcium concentration. Most calcium ions entering the cardiac cell do so through voltage-dependent calcium channels, although some calcium ions enter via the calcium–sodium exchange reaction [37].

Calcium channels are located throughout the T-tubule system, which penetrates deep into the cell interior. The T tubules abut large terminal cisternae, which are the terminal portion of a diffuse intracellular longitudinal tubular system: the sarcoplasmic reticulum. Voltage-dependent calcium channels are of two types (Table 22.2): a slow, long-lasting (L-type) channel that is opened by complete cellular depolarization, and a fast but transient (T-type) channel that is activated earlier than L-type channels and at more negative potentials (Fig. 22.11). The exact mechanism whereby the calcium channels (both L- and T-type) of the T tubules communicate with the calcium-release channels of the sarcoplasmic reticulum remains controversial [35]. The majority of calcium entering the cardiac cell during each AP does so through the L-type channel, also termed the dihydropyridine (DHP) receptor because of its sensitivity to specific types of calcium antagonists (verapamil, diltiazem, and nifedipine-like compounds) [37]. The rate of change of intracellular calcium concentration is the most effective activator of intracellular calcium release from the sarcoplasmic reticulum. This observation suggests that the rapid T-type channels may be important in the excitation–contraction process. T-type channels activate at more negative potentials than L-type channels and are insensitive to sodium channel blockers (e.g., lidocaine or tetrodotoxin) and calcium antagonist drugs [37]. The T-type channels,

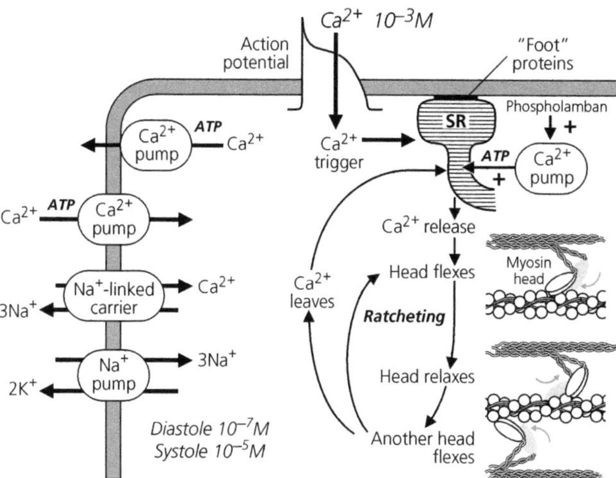

Figure 22.11 Calcium enters the cardiac cell during the cardiac action potential (phase 2). Increases in intracellular calcium trigger calcium release from the sarcoplasmic reticulum (SR) by a process termed calcium-induced calcium release (CICR). Increases in intracellular calcium (10^{-7}–10^{-5} M) in the vicinity of the contractile proteins cause the myosin heads to flex, resulting in sarcomere shortening. The utilization of adenosine triphosphate (ATP) and formation of adenosine diphosphate and inorganic phosphate, in combination with reuptake of calcium by the SR, cause the intracellular calcium concentration to decrease and the myosin head to relax. Phospholamban regulates the pump responsible for the reuptake of calcium into the SR.

therefore, account for the early phase of calcium channel opening and may be important in initiating intracellular calcium release and electric depolarization of less polarized tissues, such as the sinoatrial and atrioventricular nodes [17]. The L-type channels are more prevalent in atrial and ventricular muscle cells than are T-type channels, open at less negative potentials, and may account for the latter phases of calcium channel opening [36]. Both channels are physiologically linked via specialized bridging or spanning ('foot') proteins connecting them to the calcium-release mechanism in the sarcoplasmic reticulum. The foot proteins are a part of a high molecular weight protein complex in the sarcoplasmic reticulum, termed the ryanodine receptor (RyR) because of its affinity for the insecticide ryanodine [38]. Low concentrations of ryanodine enhance calcium release, whereas high concentrations inhibit calcium release from the sarcoplasmic reticulum. Ryanodine receptors are similar to the inositol triphosphate (IP_3) receptors, transport Ca^{2+} into the cytosol by recognizing Ca^{2+} on its cytosolic side, thus establishing a positive feedback mechanism; a small amount of Ca^{2+} in the cytosol near the receptor will cause it to release even more Ca^{2+} (e.g., CICR). Notably, there are multiple RyR isoforms and cardiac RyRs are of the RyR2 type [38]. Any drug that prolongs channel openings triggered by cytoplasmic Ca^{2+} will also promote RyR activation by luminal Ca^{2+}. For example, mutations in the skeletal muscle isoform (RyR1) of the ryanodine receptor Ca^{2+}-release channel is responsible for susceptibility to malignant hyperthermia, which may be triggered by inhalant anesthetics such as halothane [39]. The inositol 1,4,5-triphosphate receptors (IP_3R) provide a second pathway for internal Ca^{2+} release [40]. Their subcellular localization in cardiac myocytes is similar in atrial and ventricular myocytes and Purkinje fibers. They are believed to modulate transcription, amplify RyR2 Ca^{2+} signals, and provide independent cellular activation through diverse pathways that generate IP_3. The expression of this receptor is about 50-fold less than RyR2s in ventricular myocytes. The activation of IP_3Rs (mainly type 2 in atrial and ventricular myocytes and type 1 in Purkinje myocytes) by certain agonists (e.g., angiotensin II, endothelin, and norepinephrine) is believed important in development of hypertrophy and heart failure [40].

Summarizing, normal cardiac function is dependent upon the coupling of functionally related ion channels and transporters in the sarcolemma with calcium-release channels (RyR2) in the sarcoplasmic reticulum (SR), the intracellular Ca^{2+} storage organelle. Cardiac excitation–contraction (EC) coupling is initiated by an AP and membrane depolarization that activates voltage-gated L-type Ca^{2+} channels in the sarcolemma. The small increase in $[Ca^{2+}]_i$ due to the Ca^{2+} flux through the plasma membrane Ca^{2+} channels, is detected by nearby clusters of RyR2s in the junctional SR that produce Ca^{2+} sparks that amplify CICR. IP_3Rs serves as a second pathway for internal Ca^{2+} release. The synchronization of Ca^{2+} sparks by the AP produces the cell-wide $[Ca^{2+}]_i$ transient that activates contraction. Instability in cardiac Ca^{2+} management can be caused by altered RyR2 sensitivity, altered spatial organization of local Ca^{2+} release sites, or mutations and variants of the RyR2 and IP_3R proteins. Abnormal cardiac Ca^{2+} signaling results in defects in myocyte electrical activity and multiple cardiac disease phenotypes, resulting in arrhythmia, myopathy, heart failure, and a predisposition to anesthetic-associated drug toxicity.

Heart: contraction and relaxation

Cardiac myocytes are composed of contractile units termed sarcomeres, which contain thick (myosin) and thin (actin) contractile proteins, regulatory proteins (troponin and tropomyosin), and various structural proteins [37,41,42]. The thick myosin filaments are composed of approximately 300 molecules, each ending in a bilobed head (Fig. 22.12). Half (150) of the myosin bilobed heads are located at each end of the sarcomere and project from the thick filament towards the thin filaments (crossbridges). The thin filaments are attached at one end to structural proteins (Z line) that separate each sarcomere. Each thin filament contains two helical strands of actin intertwined with tropomyosin, which has periodic troponin complexes (Fig. 22.12).

Increases in intracellular calcium initiated during phase 2 of the cardiac AP are amplified by subsequent CICR and serve as the catalyst for actin–myosin interaction and sarcomere shortening. More specifically, calcium ions bind to the regulatory protein troponin C (C for calcium), which removes the inhibitory function of troponin I (I for inhibitor) on the chemical interaction between actin and myosin. Transformation of chemical energy into sarcomere shortening and mechanical work is dependent upon ATP hydrolysis and myosin ATPase. Hydrolysis of ATP to adenosine diphosphate (ADP) with the release of inorganic phosphate (P_i) produces a strong attachment between actin and myosin and a conformational change in the bilobed myosin head that causes the head to flex and the actin filaments to move centrally. The result of these changes is a movement ('ratcheting') between the myosin heads and the actin, such that the actin and myosin filaments slide past each other, resulting in sarcomere shortening and/or tension (Fig. 22.11) [41]. Ratcheting cycles occur as long as the cytosolic calcium remains elevated. Increases in intracellular calcium facilitate this chemical process by increasing myosin ATPase activity. Therefore, by combining with troponin C and increasing intracellular myosin ATPase activity, calcium serves as the principal factor in determining the rate at which crossbridges attach and detach.

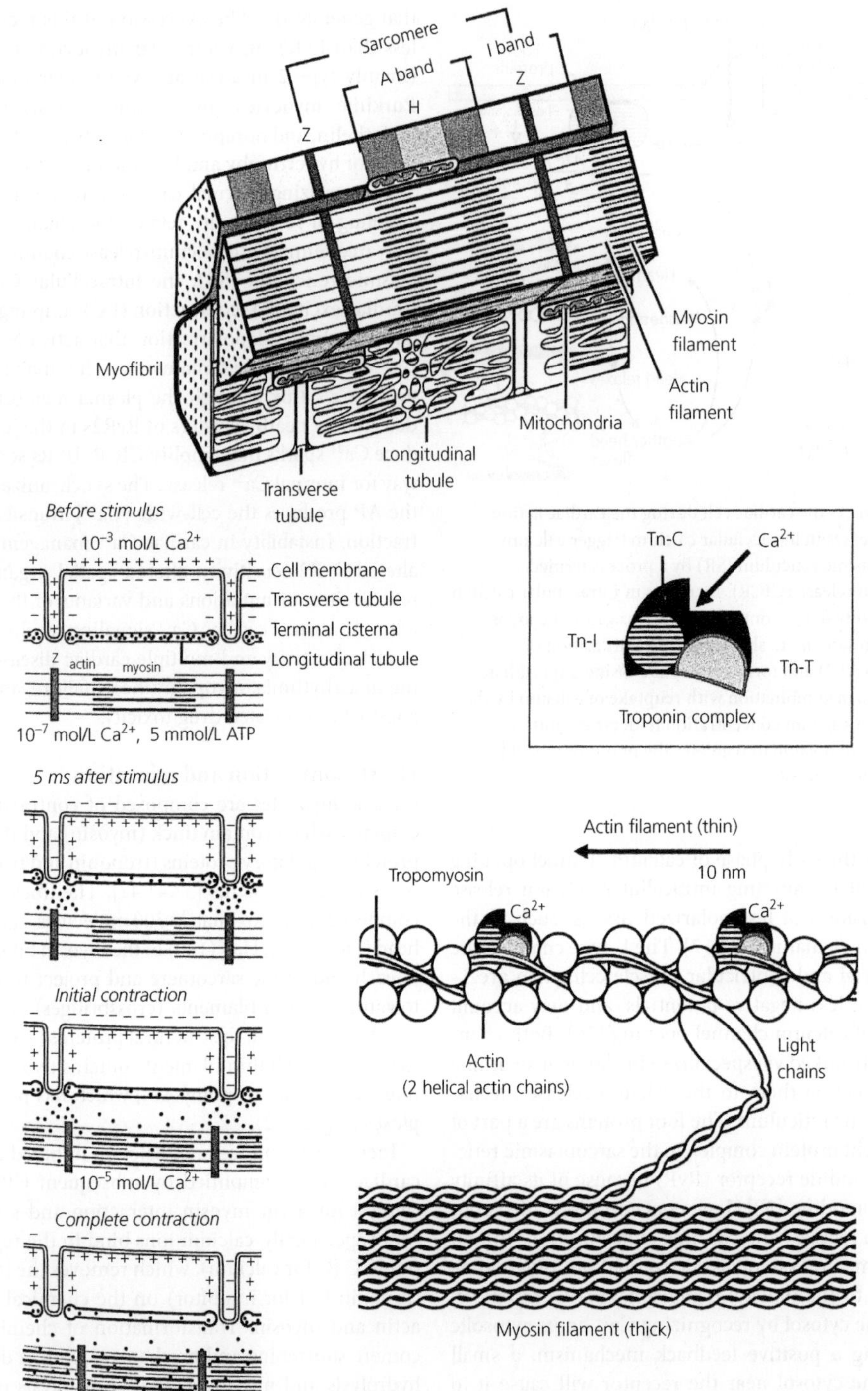

Figure 22.12 Cardiac muscle fibers contain an overlapping array of thin (actin) and thick (myosin) contractile proteins that produces various bands (A, H, I, and Z) within each sarcomere when viewed microscopically. Note that both the transverse tubule (T tubule) and longitudinal tubule systems facilitate the presence of relatively large amounts of extracellular calcium (10^{-3} M) in the vicinity of the contractile proteins (top). Membrane depolarization initiates calcium entry into the cardiac cell, contractile protein interaction, and sarcomere shortening (left). More specifically, the binding of calcium with troponin C (Tn-C) removes the inhibitory function of troponin I (Tn-I) on actin–myosin interaction. Troponin T (Tn-T) links the troponin complex to tropomyosin (right).

The rate of crossbridge interaction is the basis for the force–velocity relationship in isolated tissue experiments studying cardiac muscle contractile activity [42]. The rate of crossbridge attachment determines the velocity of sarcomere shortening and has been termed cardiac contractility [43]. Furthermore, by increasing the number of interacting crossbridges, intracellular calcium increases the maximum force attainable. Clinically, the rate of pressure change (dP/dt) and the rate of force development (dF/dt) in animals have been used as indirect, albeit rate and load-dependent, measures of cardiac contractility [43].

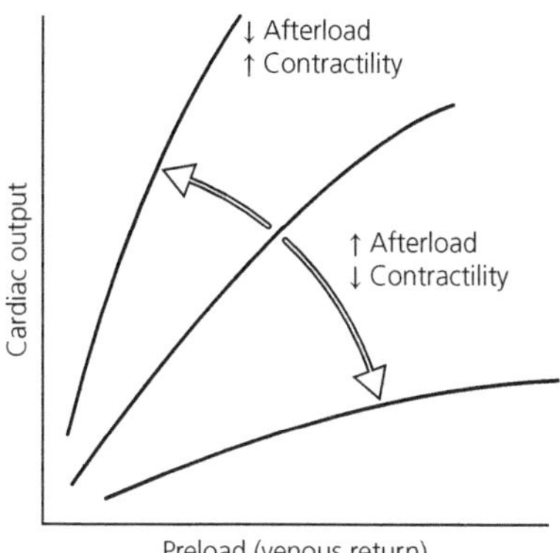

Figure 22.13 Starling's law of the heart: the concept of optimal sarcomere lengthening relative to the velocity of sarcomere shortening when translated to the intact heart predicts that increases in ventricular volume (increased preload) should increase cardiac output.

Optimal sarcomere length for actin–myosin interaction *in vitro* is approximately 2.2 μm. Lengths shorter or greater than this were once thought to decrease the force of cardiac contraction by theoretically decreasing the number of available myosin heads for interaction with actin [42]. The concept of optimal sarcomere length relative to the velocity of sarcomere shortening serves as the explanation for the Frank–Starling law of the heart (also known as Starling's law), which predicts an increase in contractile force when sarcomeres are stretched (increased end-diastolic ventricular volume) to their optimal length (Fig. 22.13). It is unlikely, however, that this explanation is totally correct, since sarcomeres rarely change in length (or only minimally so) when loaded, even during dilated forms of heart failure [37]. The more probable explanation for Starling's law of the heart is that sarcomere loading increases troponin C's affinity for calcium, leading to increased activation of the myofilament and sarcomere shortening without increases in sarcomere length or additional increases in intracellular calcium [37]. Most intravenous anesthetic drugs (e.g., barbiturates, ketamine, and propofol), and in particular the inhalation anesthetics, produce dose-dependent decreases in cardiac contractility by decreasing calcium influx through L-type channels, decreasing calcium release from the sarcoplasmic reticulum, and decreasing troponin C's sensitivity to calcium [44–54]. Mechanisms that enhance the concentration of cytosolic calcium increase the amount of ATP hydrolyzed and the force generated by the interaction of actin and myosin filaments and the velocity of shortening. Sympathetic activation of β-adrenergic receptors, for example, increases cAMP, which in turn activates protein kinase to increase calcium entry through L-type calcium channels [36]. Activation of the IP_3 signal transduction pathway also stimulates the release of calcium by the SR through IP_3 receptors located on the SR. Activation of the cAMP-dependent protein kinase phosphorylates phospholamban on the SR that normally inhibits calcium uptake. This disinhibition of phospholamban leads to increases in the rate of calcium uptake by the SR. Therefore, β-adrenergic receptor agonists increase the force and shortening velocity of contraction (i.e., positive inotropy), and increases the rate of relaxation (i.e., positive lusitropy).

The effects of both injectable and inhalant anesthetics on the sensitivity of troponin C for calcium remain to be clarified. Notably, halothane (and other inhalants), ischemia, catecholamines, and acidosis interfere with the reuptake of calcium by the sarcoplasmic reticulum, thereby interfering with the relaxation process and ultimately leading to intracellular calcium depletion [36]. Sympathetic activation of β-adrenergic receptors by endogenous (norepinephrine, epinephrine) or exogenous (dopamine, dobutamine) adrenergic agonists can be administered to increase cardiac contractile performance (inotropy) and accelerate relaxation (lusitropy) (Fig. 22.14). β-Adrenergic receptor stimulation activates a GTP-binding protein (G_S), which stimulates adenylyl cyclase (AC) to produce cAMP, which activates PKA, thereby phosphorylating proteins involved in excitation–contraction coupling (phospholamban, L-type Ca^{2+} channels, RyR, troponin I, and myosin-binding protein C).

Decreased interaction between actin and myosin filaments signals the beginning of the actin–myosin uncoupling process and myocardial relaxation, and is directly related to a decrease in intracellular calcium ion concentration [36,42]. Three principal mechanisms are important in reducing intracellular calcium ion concentration and the subsequent decrease in cardiac contractile force. The depolarization-triggered increases in intracellular calcium increase the activity of the calcium regulatory protein calmodulin. Calmodulin serves as an intracellular calcium sensor and, when activated (calmodulin–calcium complex), stimulates the active extrusion of calcium by pumps in the sarcolemma, increases the activity of a phospholamban-modulated calcium pump (increasing calcium uptake by the sarcoplasmic reticulum), and enhances the activity of the sodium-calcium exchanger (Fig. 22.11) [36]. Calcium sequestered by the SR by an ATP-dependent calcium pump (SERCA: sarco/endoplasmic reticulum calcium-ATPase) lowers the cytosolic calcium concentration and removes calcium from the troponin C. The reduced intracellular calcium induces a conformational change in the troponin complex, leading to troponin I inhibition of the actin binding site [42]. At the end of the cycle, a new ATP binds to the myosin head, displacing the ADP, and the initial sarcomere length is restored.

The Vascular System

The purpose of the vascular system (arteries, capillaries, and veins) is to transport blood, thereby facilitating the uptake and exchange of nutrients and the elimination of waste products. Larger blood vessels (>100–200 μm) are considered to comprise the macrocirculation and smaller vessels (≤100 μm) the microcirculation. Most large vessels are not embedded in organs and function to deliver blood to and from the heart and peripheral tissues. Most small vessels are embedded in organs and are actively involved in exchange processes and regulating blood flow. The circulatory system is comprised of two circulations connected in series: pulmonary and systemic (Fig. 22.1). The pulmonary artery and aorta deliver blood to the pulmonary and systemic circulations, respectively. The pulmonary circulation receives the majority of its blood supply from the right ventricle, perfuses the lung, and empties into the left atrium. The systemic circulation receives its blood supply, via the aorta, from the left ventricle. The aorta and other large arteries comprise the high-pressure portion of the systemic circulation. The systemic circulation perfuses most of the body's organs and tissues, and ultimately empties into the right atrium. More specifically, the vessels of the systemic circulation (like the pulmonary) undergo repeated division into smaller and smaller parallel vascular beds that terminate in arterioles (the smallest arteries), which further subdivide to form capillaries. The overall cross-sectional area of the circulation increases dramatically with each division, reaching a maximum in the capillaries (Fig. 22.15) [55].

From a purely functional standpoint, vessels can be categorized as primarily elastic Windkessel-type conduits (large arteries),

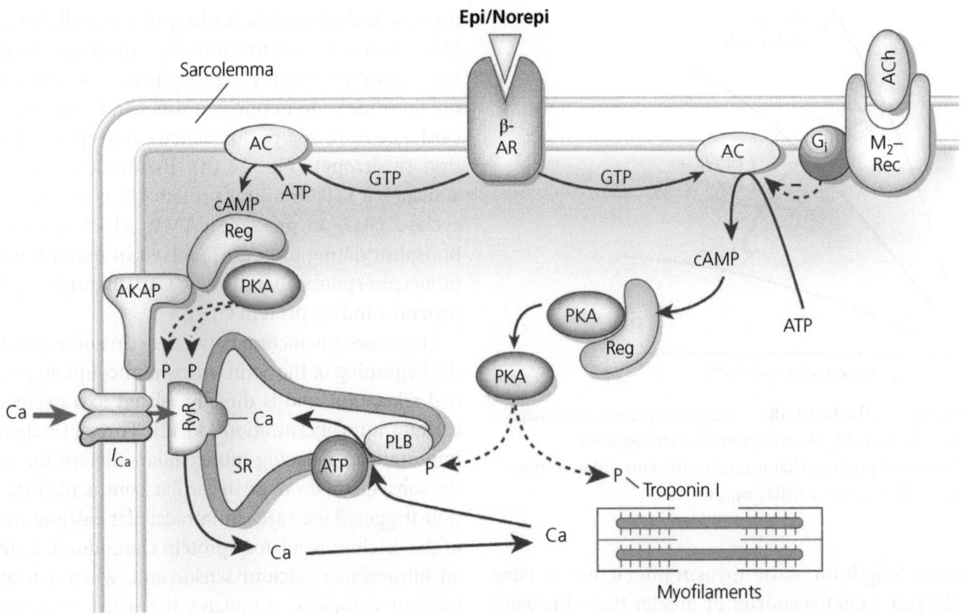

Figure 22.14 Adrenergic receptor activation and phosphorylation and excitation–contraction coupling. AC, adenylyl cyclase; ACh, acetylcholine; AKAP, a kinase anchoring protein; β-AR, β-adrenergic receptor and subunits; M2-Rec, M2-muscarinic receptor and subunits; PLB, phospholamban; Reg, PKA regulatory subunit; RyR, ryanodine receptor; SR, sarcoplasmic reticulum. Source: [36]. Reproduced with permission of *Nature*.

resistance vessels (small arteries), sphincter vessels (arterioles), exchange vessels (capillaries), capacitance vessels (venules and veins), large conduits (veins), and shunt vessels (arteriovenous anastomoses). Structurally, all blood vessels contain an endothelial layer (tunica intima) on their inner surface that provides a smooth surface and prevents clotting. All but capillaries also contain varying proportions of elastic fibers, smooth muscle, and collagen (Fig. 22.16). These three tissue types comprise the tunica media, which is composed mostly of smooth muscle and elastic connective tissue, and the tunica externa (adventitia), which contains fibrous collagen fibers. The proportion of elastic connective tissue to smooth muscle determines the vessel's principal function (i.e., conduit, resistive, or capacitive). Larger arteries possess a high proportion of elastic tissue in comparison with smooth muscle and fibrous tissues and are relatively stiff compared with veins. This structural difference enables the aorta to stretch following ventricular contraction and the ejection of blood. The potential (stored) energy imparted to the stretched aorta following cardiac contraction is returned as kinetic (motion) energy and blood flow as the ventricle starts to relax and the aortic valve closes. The highly elastic architecture of the aorta facilitates the continuous, albeit non-uniform, flow of blood (Windkessel effect) to peripheral tissues throughout the cardiac cycle (contraction–relaxation–rest). The Windkessel effect is believed to be responsible for as much as 50% of peripheral blood flow in most animals during normal heart rates. Cardiac arrhythmias, especially tachyarrhythmias, and vascular diseases (stiff non-elastic vessels) reduce the Windkessel effect and produce distinctive changes in the arterial pressure waveform.

A single layer of endothelial cells lines the entire vascular system and is a key factor in the maintenance of vessel wall structural and functional integrity. The endothelium acts as a semipermeable membrane that regulates the transfer of small and large molecules. Endothelial cells are dynamic and have both metabolic and synthetic functions exerting autocrine, paracrine, and endocrine actions that modulate smooth muscle contraction and relaxation, thrombosis, thrombolysis, and platelet and leucocyte adherence. Endothelial cells generate and maintain an endothelial surface layer (ESL), the glycocalyx [56]. The endothelial glycocalyx is a carbohydrate-rich layer composed of a negatively charged network of proteoglycans, glycoproteins, and glycolipids lining the vascular endothelium throughout capillaries (microvascular beds), arteries, and veins (macrovessels) [57]. It constitutes a voluminous intravascular compartment that plays an important role in maintaining vascular wall homeostasis by regulating blood flow, red and white blood cell movement, and vessel wall permeability in capillaries [57]. Pathologic loss of the glycocalyx initiates breakdown of the vascular barrier and has been linked to ischemia, systemic inflammatory response, sepsis, and volume overload [58,59].

Large arteries

Large arteries near the heart and throughout the extremities are highly elastic tubes that serve as conduits through which blood is transported to the periphery. The elasticity of large arteries opposes the stretching effect that the blood pressure produces following ventricular contraction. For example, the initial stretching of the aorta produced by ventricular ejection is opposed by the elastic tissue in the vessel walls, which returns the aorta and large arteries to their original dimension (Fig. 22.16). This squeezing phenomenon of large arteries is termed the Windkessel effect (see above) and helps to convert the discontinuous (cyclic or phasic) flow of arterial blood associated with ventricular pumping into a continuous, although somewhat non-uniform (pulsatile), flow to the peripheral arteries. The extent to which the larger arteries can be stretched depends on the ratio of elastic to collagen fibers. Large elastic arteries are not easily distended. Systemic arteries are in general 6–10 times less distensible than systemic veins. The pulmonary artery is about half as distensible as systemic or pulmonary veins (Fig. 22.17) [60].

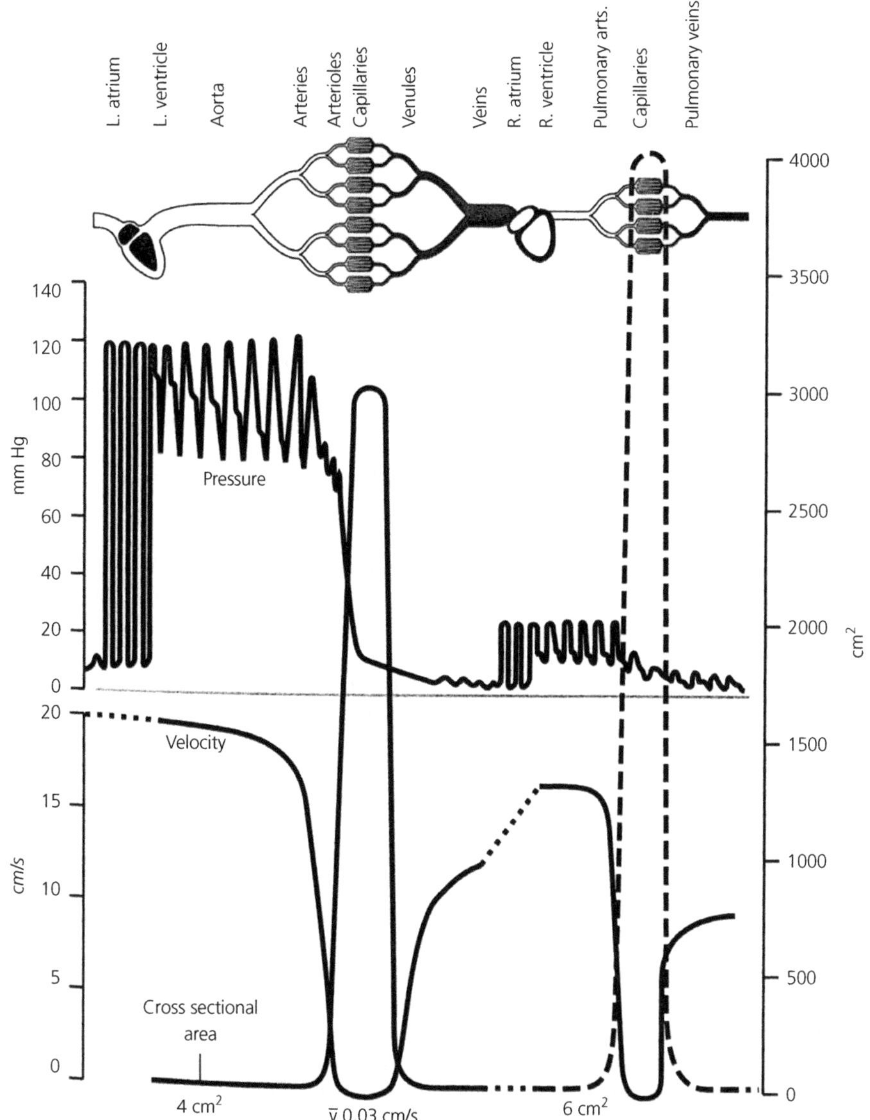

Figure 22.15 Relationship between blood pressure, blood flow velocity, and cross-sectional area of the cardiovascular system. Note that, as blood approaches the capillaries, blood pressure and blood flow velocity decrease and cross-sectional area increases. Source: modified from Witzleb Z. Functions of the vascular system. In: Schmidt RF, Thews G, eds. *Human Physiology*. New York: Springer, 1983; 408.

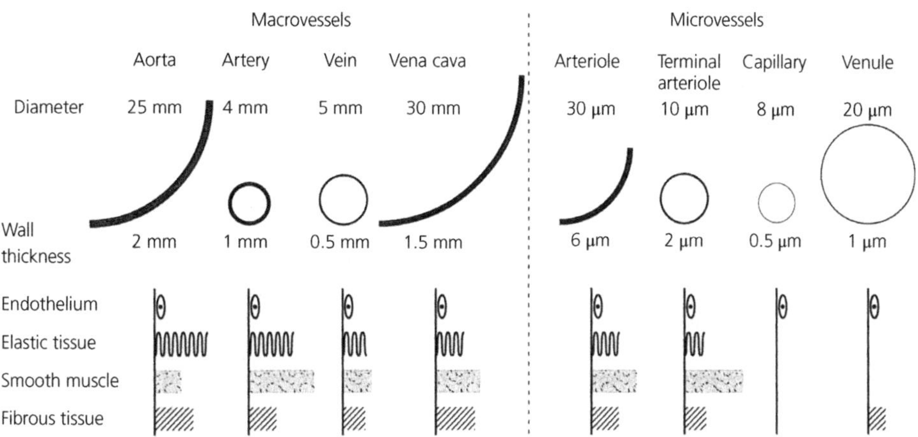

Figure 22.16 Components: elastic, smooth muscle, and fibrous tissue in blood vessels of the circulation. Note the relative absence of smooth muscle in capillaries and venules. Source: modified from Berne RM, Levy MN. *Principles of Physiology*, 1st edn. St Louis, MO: Mosby, 1990; **195**.

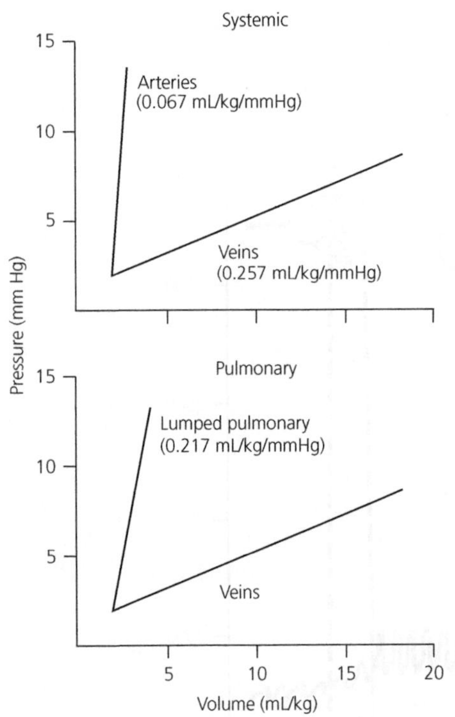

Figure 22.17 Compliance (volume–pressure) relationship for systemic arteries and veins and the lumped pulmonary vascular bed. Note that a small increase in volume causes a much larger increase in arterial pressure than venous pressure, suggesting a much lower compliance (greater elastance). Source: modified from [60]. Reproduced with permission of Lippincott Williams & Wilkins.

Small arteries

Peripheral larger arteries contain greater percentages of smooth muscle compared with elastic tissue, thereby providing greater control over vessel diameter, vascular resistance, and the regulation of blood flow. The amount of smooth muscle determines the vessel's resting tone, myogenic basal tone (spontaneous contractions), and the amount of stress relaxation (delayed capacitance) and reverse stress relaxation exhibited by the vessel. Stress relaxation is characterized by a rapid initial increase in resting tone caused by an increase in vascular volume that declines gradually during the next several minutes. Pressure decreases because of smooth muscle myofilament rearrangement. Reverse stress relaxation is the reverse of this process.

The most distal branches of peripheral (small) arteries terminate in arteries that are collectively considered as 'resistance vessels' since they control the distribution of tissue blood flow. These vessels contain a predominance of smooth muscle, are densely innervated, and include arterioles, metarterioles, and arteriovenous anastomoses. Notably, approximately 80% of the pressure drop between the aorta and large veins (vena cava) occurs across the arterioles (Fig. 22.15).

Resistance vessels

Resistance vessels include the terminal branches of small arteries, arterioles, metarterioles ('sphincter vessels': short vessel(s) that link arterioles and capillaries), and arteriovenous anastomoses (AVAs). Under normal conditions, the arterioles provide over 50% of the total systemic vascular resistance, whereas large and small arteries account for 20%, capillaries 25%, and veins 5%. Functionally, sphincter vessels help to regulate the number of open capillaries and therefore the size of the capillary bed that is available for exchange processes. The relatively thick-walled muscular arterioles and sphincter vessels are regulated by a variety of neural, humoral, and local metabolic factors, and are the principal determinants of both the volume and distribution of blood flow to all tissues of the body. Arteriovenous anastomoses bypass the capillary by connecting arterioles to venules, thereby permitting the shunting of blood from arterioles to venules. These vessels can reduce or totally interrupt blood flow to capillaries and are densely innervated by both α_1- and α_2-adrenergic receptors [61]. Arteriovenous anastomoses are found in the greatest numbers in the skin and extremities (ears, feet, and hooves) of most species and were originally thought to be primarily involved in thermoregulation [61,62]. They possess smooth muscle cells throughout their entire length and are located in most, if not all, tissue beds. More recently, their identification and verification in the intestinal wall, kidney, liver, and skeletal muscles have increased interest in their role as a separate blood flow regulatory mechanism for controlling nutrient blood flow to these tissues [60]. The influence of anesthetic drugs, particularly α_2-adrenergic receptor agonists on AVAs is unresolved but known to cause considerable redistribution of blood flow and cardiac output, predominantly reducing flow to less vital organs and shunt flow [63].

Capillaries

The microcirculation includes the smallest blood vessels in the body and consists of the terminal arterioles (~100 μm), the capillary network (4–8 μm) and venules (≤100 μm). The microcirculation is embedded within organs and responsible for regulating blood flow to the tissues and for exchange processes between blood and tissue. Capillaries separate the intravascular volume from the interstitial fluid volume. The capillary wall is a three-layered structure in most capillaries, consisting of the glycocalyx on the luminal surface, the basement membrane on the abluminal surface, and the endothelial cell in between. The intravascular volume therefore actually consists of the glycocalyx volume, plasma volume, and red cell volume. The glycocalyx is normally the dynamic and active interface between plasma and the capillary wall and can be visualized as a web of membrane-bound glycoproteins and proteoglycans on the luminal side of endothelial cells (Fig. 22.18) [56]. It acts as a semi-permeable molecular sieve with respect to anionic macromolecules such as albumin and other plasma proteins, whose size and structure appear to determine their ability to penetrate the layer. The normal ESL is impermeable to red blood cells and molecules larger than 70 kDa and semi-permeable to albumin (molecular weight ≈ 69 kDa; diameter ≈ 7 nm; reflection coefficient = 0.79–0.9) [64]. Functionally, amphipathic molecules such as albumin help to sustain and regulate the permeability of the glycocalyx [65,66].

There are three types of capillaries: continuous non-fenestrated, fenestrated, and discontinuous or sinusoidal (Fig. 22.19) [66]. All capillaries are variably porous and are found in varying numbers in different tissue beds, depending on tissue metabolism (O_2 requirements) and the importance of fluid exchange. Continuous non-fenestrated capillaries with tight junctions are located in all tissues of the body except epithelia and cartilage. They have a functional pore size of approximately 5 nm that permits the diffusion of water, small solutes, and lipid-soluble materials into the surrounding interstitial fluid, but the glycocalyx prevents the loss of larger molecules (>70 kDa) and blood cells [64].

Specialized continuous non-fenestrated capillaries are found throughout most of the central nervous system, enteric nervous system, retina, and thymus. The endothelial cells are bound together

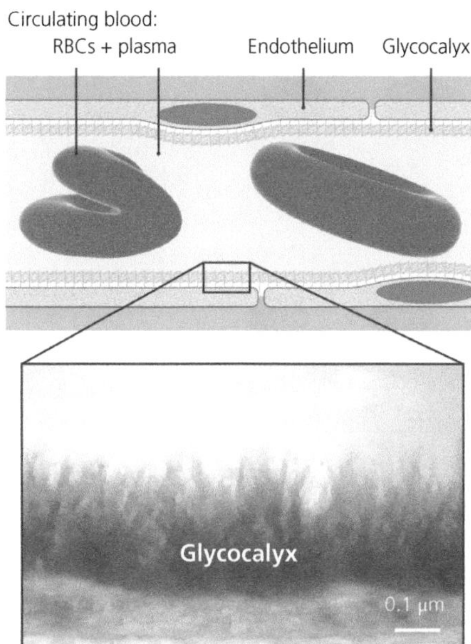

Figure 22.18 The glycocalyx is a web of membrane-bound glycoproteins and proteoglycans on the luminal side of endothelial cells. Source: adapted from [56].

by tight junctions with an effective pore size of <1 nm [66]. The endothelial cells of the brain and spinal cord are tightly opposed by zona occludens tight junctions with few breaks in the capillary wall and are responsible for the anatomic blood–brain barrier. The blood–brain barrier is only permeable to the smallest non-lipid-soluble molecules. Breaks within the inter-endothelial cell junctions produced by trauma or inflammation are the primary path for transvascular fluid filtration and increased porosity. Aquaporins, the water channel protein, are present within continuous, but not fenestrated, vascular endothelial cells [67]. Aquaporins selectively facilitate the rapid transport of fluid across epithelial and endothelial cells, but are also found in other tissue types, such as muscle and nerve cells. At the cellular level, aquaporins mediate osmotic water transport across cell plasma membranes and facilitate transepithelial fluid transport, cell migration, and neuroexcitation. There are at least 11 known members of the mammalian aquaporin gene family, which encode proteins that function as membrane channels, for water alone or for water plus small molecules [67].

Fenestrated capillaries with diaphragm fenestrae are present in skin, connective tissue, kidney, intestinal mucosa, endocrine and exocrine glands, and the choroid plexus, and can absorb interstitial fluid into plasma. The basement membrane of these capillaries is continuous, and their diaphragmed fenestrations are induced by vascular endothelial growth factors. Their upper pore size is in the range 6–12 nm [66]. Fenestrated capillaries with open fenestrae are capillaries that contain 'windows,' or pores, that span the endothelial lining. The pores permit the rapid exchange of water and solutes. Open fenestrated capillaries are present in the kidney cortex and medulla, the gastrointestinal mucosa, and the lymph nodes. The ESL serves as the major barrier to transcapillary flow of macromolecules larger than 15 nm [64].

Sinusoids (channels) resemble fenestrated capillaries, but in contrast they are discontinuous and are characterized by gaps between adjacent endothelial cells. The basement membrane and the ESL are lacking within the fenestrae and interstitial fluid is essentially part of the plasma volume in sinusoidal tissues (spleen, liver, bone marrow, endocrine organs). Plasma proteins (e.g., albumin) secreted by liver cells easily pass through sinusoids and into the bloodstream through pores as large as 200–280 nm [66]. Phagocytic cells monitor the passing blood in sinusoidal tissues, engulfing damaged red blood cells, pathogens, and cellular debris.

Regardless of the type of capillary examined, the exchange of fluid, nutrients, and cellular waste products between blood and interstitial fluid is their primary function. Capillary exchange is governed by two primary processes: diffusion and filtration. Fick's law of diffusion describes solute exchange (J_s) as

$$J_s = DAD_c / M_T$$

where D is the diffusion coefficient, A is the capillary surface area, M_T is the membrane thickness, and D_C is the concentration gradient or difference. The diffusion coefficient is determined by the diffusion medium and qualities characteristic of the diffusion particle such as molecular weight, ionic charge, and lipid solubility. Exchange by filtration is determined by four primary factors (P_c, P_i, π_c, and π_i) according to a dynamic equilibrium equation, first proposed by Starling and Landis (Starling's law of the capillary) and modified by Pappenheimer and Soto-Rivera:

$$Jv = K_f\left[\left(P_c - P_i\right) - \sigma\left(\pi_p - \pi_i\right)\right]$$

where Jv is fluid flux across the capillary (positive for filtration and negative for reabsorption), P_c and P_i are capillary and interstitial hydrostatic pressures, π_p and π_i are the plasma in the capillary and interstitial colloid osmotic pressures of proteins, K_f is the capillary filtration coefficient, and σ is the osmotic reflection coefficient for all plasma proteins [68,69]. The filtration coefficient (K_f) indicates the resistance of the capillary wall to fluid flow and is determined by the surface area, the number and radius of capillary pores, the capillary wall thickness, and the viscosity of the fluid being filtered. The osmotic reflection coefficient (σ) is an indicator of transvascular protein transport and is usually assumed to be very high (1 or close to 1) in normal animals, since most capillary beds are impermeable to colloids. Provided that all factors can be measured, calculated, or estimated in Starling's equation, the net fluid flux across the capillary wall can be quantitated accurately [69]. Conceptually, these factors were once believed to explain fluid filtration at the arterial end of the capillary and fluid reabsorption at the venous end of the capillary. Lymph vessels carried excess fluid away. It is now appreciated that non-fenestrated capillaries normally filter fluid to the interstitial fluid (ISF) throughout their entire length, that fluid flux to the interstitial space is under a dominant hydrostatic pressure gradient (capillary pressure P_c minus ISF pressure P_i), and that the effect of π_c on transvascular fluid exchange is much less than predicted (Fig. 22.20) [57].

The colloidal osmotic pressure (COP) difference that determines fluid exchange is that across the semi-permeable glycocalyx. The low protein concentration within the subglycocalyx intercellular spaces accounts for the low transcapillary flow (Jv) and lymph flow in most tissues. Absorption through venous capillaries and venules does not occur except in disease states. Under normal conditions, π_c opposes, but does not reverse, filtration and most of the filtered fluid returns to the circulation as lymph. The endothelial surface layer covers the endothelial intercellular clefts in fenestrated capillaries, separating plasma from an almost protein-free subglycocalyx space (Fig. 22.19). The COP (π_g) replaces π_i as a determinant of Jv. The fluid at the abluminal side of the glycocalyx is separated from

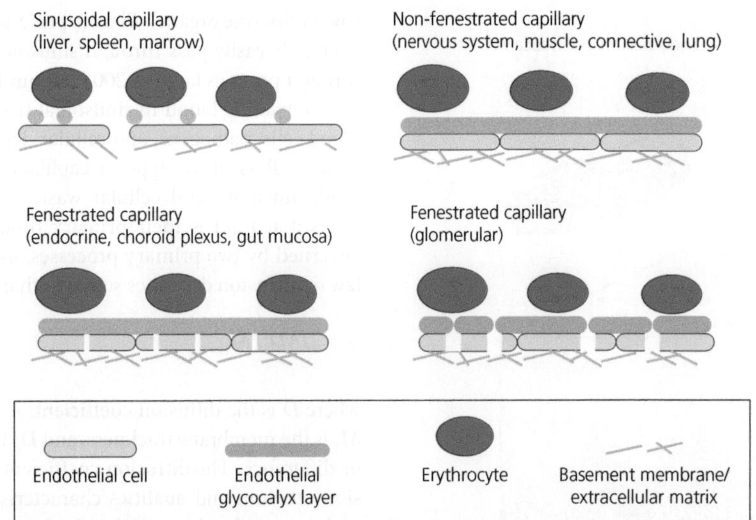

Figure 22.19 Illustration of the anatomic differences between various types of capillaries. Red blood cells are excluded from the glycocalyx layer. Source: [64]. Reproduced with permission of Oxford University Press.

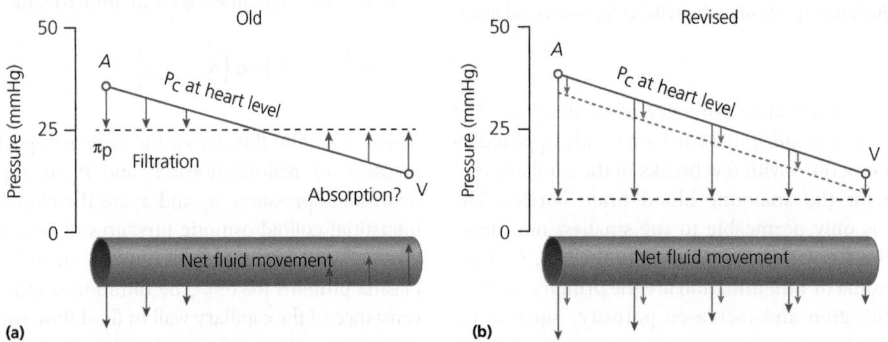

Figure 22.20 Imbalance of the classical Starling pressures when all four terms are measured in the same tissue. Part (a) shows the traditional filtration–reabsorption model proposed in most textbooks. Part (b) shows current evidence wherein fluid leaves the capillary throughout its entire length due to hydrostatic pressure and the influence on an intact glycocalyx; interstitial terms are considered negligible. The black arrows indicate net force imbalance and hence the direction and the magnitude of fluid exchange. The dot-dashed line (red) illustrates qualitatively the much smaller net filtration force predicted by the glycocalyx-cleft model. See Figure 22.21. Source: [57]. Reproduced with permission of Oxford University Press.

the pericapillary ISF by the tortuous path through the intercellular clefts. Plasma proteins, including albumin, escape to the interstitial space through the intercellular clefts (large pores), which are responsible for the increased *Jv* observed during inflammation. Importantly, *Jv* can be modified by many factors, including drugs and intravenous fluid replacement therapies. The revised Starling equation should be written as

$$Jv = K_f\left[\left(P_c - P_i\right) - \sigma\left(\pi_p - \pi_g\right)\right]$$

where π_g is the COP of the ultrafiltrate on the underside of the glycocalyx (Fig. 22.21). π_g can be very low, for two reasons: σ is high, or the outward flow of the ultrafiltrate prevents protein diffusion equilibrium between the subglycocalyx fluid and the pericapillary ISF.

Transcapillary fluid filtration provides the medium for diffusional flux of oxygen and nutrients required for cellular metabolism and removal of metabolic byproducts and influences vascular smooth muscle tone in arterioles, hydraulic conductivity in capillaries, and neutrophil transmigration across postcapillary venules. The redistribution of fluid across the microvascular endothelial barrier constitutes the primary mechanism for removal of excess fluid from the bloodstream and for the formation of lymph, particularly during vascular volume overload. Increases in P_c (volume overload, venous obstruction, and heart failure) and K_f (histamine, cytokines, and kinins) or decreases in π_p (hypoproteinemia) cause excess fluid to accumulate in the interstitial space, resulting in edema. Interstitial (or cellular) edema increases the diffusion distance for oxygen and other nutrients and collapses capillaries in swollen tissue (capillary no-reflow), especially in encapsulated organs (e.g., brain, kidney), compromising cellular metabolism and impairing nutritive tissue perfusion. Edema formation and capillary no-reflow also act to limit the diffusional removal of potentially toxic by-products of cellular metabolism. Edema is due not only to an increase in P_c but also to degradation of the ESL. Excessive fluid accumulation in the lung, intestine, and liver (so-called overflow organs) can result in fluid collection in the alveoli, intestinal lumen, and peritoneal cavity. Decreases in P_c (hypotension and hypovolemia) and increases in π_p (hyperproteinemia and dehydration) favor reabsorption of interstitial fluid into the vascular compartment (autotransfusion), reducing the potential for fluid to accumulate in the interstitial space. Anesthesia, anesthetic drugs, quantity and type of fluid administered, and the type of anesthetic techniques used can have important

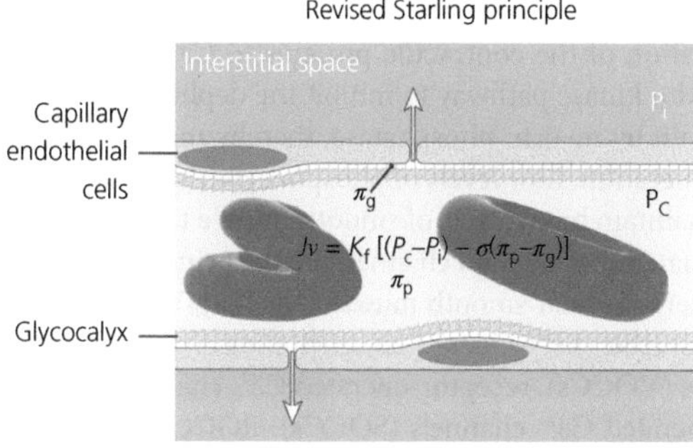

Figure 22.21 Revised Starlings law of the capillary. The 'double-barrier concept' recognizes the space beneath the endothelial glycocalyx to be almost protein-free (π_g). This changes the inwardly directed oncotic gradient suggested by Ernest Starling to the luminal side of the vessel wall. Transcapillary fluid loss is limited by an oncotic pressure gradient across the endothelial glycocalyx, and not across the whole anatomic vessel wall.

Box 22.2 Causes of increased interstitial fluid volume and edema.

- Increased filtration pressure
  - Arteriolar dilation
  - Venule constriction
  - Increased venous pressure (heart failure, incompetent valves, venous obstruction, increased total extracellular fluid volume, effect of gravity, etc.)
- Decreased osmotic pressure gradient across capillary
  - Decreased plasma protein level
  - Accumulation of osmotically active substances in interstitial space
- Increased capillary permeability
  - Substance P
  - Histamine and related substances
  - Kinins, etc.
- Inadequate lymph flow

effects on the Starling forces and the ESL [56,65,69]. For example, most anesthetic drugs and anesthetic techniques decrease P_c, causing net fluid reabsorption from the interstitial space and hemodilution. If the anesthetic drug or technique produces mild small artery vasodilation, P_c may increase, resulting in interstitial fluid accumulation (e.g., edema). Several anticancer (doxorubicin) and anesthetic drugs (e.g., morphine and meperidine) or drug diluents (Chremophor EL) cause histamine release, thereby increasing K_f. Fluid overload degrades the ESL, resulting in interstitial fluid accumulation (Box 22.2) [70–73].

Venules and Veins

Postcapillary venules are composed of an endothelial lining and fibrous tissue and function to collect blood from capillaries (Fig. 22.16). Like capillaries, the walls of the smallest venules are very porous and serve as major sites for fluid exchange. Fluid and macromolecular exchange occur most prominently at venular junctions where phagocytic white blood cells emigrate from the blood into inflamed or infected tissues. Some venules act as postcapillary sphincters, and all venules merge into small veins. Sympathetic innervation of larger venules can alter venular tone and plays an important function in regulating capillary hydrostatic pressure. Small and larger veins contain increasing amounts of fibrous tissue in addition to smooth muscle and elastic tissue, although their walls are much thinner than comparably sized arteries. Many veins contain valves that act in conjunction with external compression (contracting muscles and pressure differences in the abdominal and thoracic cavities) to facilitate the return flow of blood to the right atrium [74]. The venous system is a major blood reservoir containing 60–70% of the blood volume during resting conditions (Fig. 22.22). Veins are 30 times more compliant (distensible) than arteries (Fig. 22.17). Splanchnic and cutaneous veins have a high population of α_1- and α_2-adrenergic receptors, which when activated help to mobilize blood into the circulation when needed (see splanchnic circulation). Importantly, the heart cannot pump more blood into the circulation than it receives; therefore, venomotor tone (venous resistance) is a principal determinant of venous return and cardiac output.

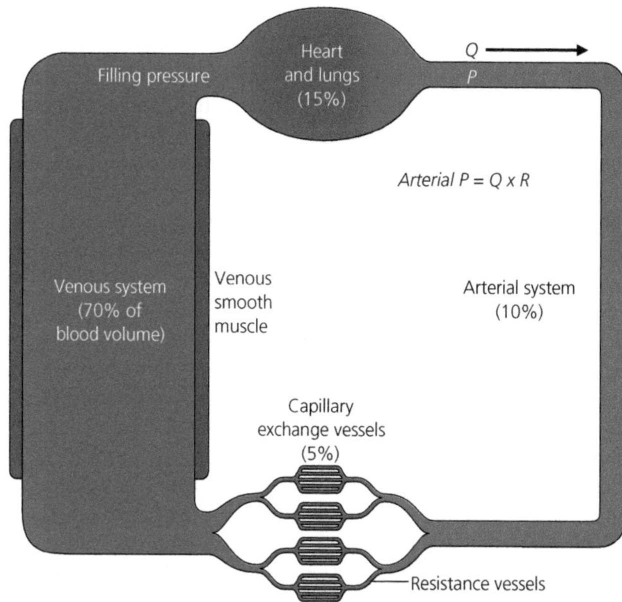

Figure 22.22 Blood is unevenly distributed throughout the circulatory system. The largest portion of the blood volume is contained within the systemic veins. Relatively small changes in venous capacity can alter the heart's filling pressure dramatically, causing predictable changes in cardiac output (*Q*), peripheral vascular resistance (*R*), and arterial blood pressure (*P*). Decreases in filling pressure, for example, decrease *Q* and *P* and increase *R*. Source: modified from [54].

Smooth muscle metabolism

Vascular smooth muscle metabolism of carbohydrates and fatty acids is compartmentalized and is characterized by a substantial production of lactic acid even under fully oxygenated conditions [75,76]. The role that the aerobic production of lactate plays in the energetics of smooth muscle has not been completely defined and likely serves as a mechanism affording optimal coordination and modulation of glucose supply and linking oxidative energy production with energy demand. The vascular smooth muscle membrane contains microdomains (caveolae) and ion channels that regulate cellular metabolism and cellular function. These include but are not limited to a host of receptors (nitric oxide, prostacyclin, endothelin, serotonin, vasopressin, adenosine, muscarinic receptors, adrenergic receptors), second messenger generators (adenylate cyclase, phospholipase C), G-proteins (RhoA, Gα), kinases (rho kinase, protein kinase C, protein kinase A), ion channels (L-type calcium channels, K_{ATP} channels, calcium-sensitive channels) in close proximity that regulate vascular smooth muscle function [75,76].

Smooth muscle contraction

Smooth muscle is an involuntary non-striated muscle that is fundamentally different from skeletal muscle and cardiac muscle in terms of structure, function, regulation of contraction, and excitation–contraction coupling. Vascular smooth muscle is divided into two subgroups: the single unit (unitary) and multiunit smooth muscle. Unitary vascular smooth muscle predominates at precapillary sphincter sites and is characterized by spontaneous activity initiated by pacemaker areas that is activated by stretch. Unitary vascular smooth muscle operates to maintain a constant local blood flow despite changing perfusion pressures [75]. Multiunit smooth muscle fibers do not usually respond to stretch, are present in larger arteries and veins, are under central nervous system control, and over-ride unitary smooth muscle in order to regulate the distribution of total body blood flow [75–77]. Smooth muscle cell contraction is regulated by receptor and mechanical (stretch) activation of the contractile proteins actin and myosin. A change in membrane potential initiated by action potentials can also trigger contraction. All three mechanisms lead to increases in cytosolic Ca^{2+} ($[Ca^{2+}]_i$) [76]. Increases in cytosolic Ca^{2+} increases Ca^{2+} release from intracellular stores (sarcoplasmic reticulum) and from the extracellular space through Ca^{2+} channels (receptor-operated Ca^{2+} channels). Contractile activity in smooth muscle is determined primarily by the phosphorylation of the light chain of myosin. Receptor or stretch activation increases intracellular Ca^{2+} that combines with the protein calmodulin. The Ca^{2+}–calmodulin complex activates myosin light-chain kinase (MLC kinase) to phosphorylate the light chain of myosin, resulting in the interaction of myosin with actin and contraction (Fig. 22.23). Energy released from ATP results in the cycling of the myosin crossbridges with actin for contraction. Sensitization of the contractile proteins to Ca^{2+} is signaled by the RhoA/Rho kinase pathway to inhibit the dephosphorylation of the light chain by myosin phosphatase, thereby maintaining sustained force generation. Low levels of phosphorylation of the myosin light chain maintain basal levels of smooth muscle tone [77,78].

Plasmalemmal calcium channels are the principal routes whereby Ca^{2+} enters vascular smooth muscle cells [78]. Various types of Ca^{2+} channels have been identified, including voltage-operated Ca^{2+} channels (VOCCs), receptor-operated Ca^{2+} channels (ROCCs), and store-operated Ca^{2+} channels (SOCCs). ROCCs are further subdivided into ligand-gated Ca^{2+} channels and second messenger-operated Ca^{2+} channels (SMOCCs) [79]. ROCCs can be blocked by calcium antagonists (e.g., verapamil, diltiazem, or nifedipine). All play a role in increasing intracellular Ca^{2+} concentration but VOCCs are believed to be crucial in the physiologic regulation of vascular smooth muscle tone. Cytosolic Ca^{2+} concentrations are reduced by plasma membrane Ca^{2+}-ATPase (PMCA), sarcoplasmic reticulum Ca^{2+}-ATPase (SERCA), the Na^+/Ca^{2+} exchanger, and cytosolic Ca^{2+}-binding proteins. Both PMCA-mediated Ca^{2+} extrusion and SERCA-mediated Ca^{2+} uptake play major roles in decreasing Ca^{2+} in vascular smooth muscle cells [78]. Various agonists (norepinephrine, epinephrine, angiotensin II, endothelin, etc.) can induce smooth muscle contraction by binding to G-protein coupled receptors that stimulate phospholipase C activity, which activates the membrane lipid phosphatidylinositol 4,5-bisphosphate (PIP_2) to catalyze the formation of two second messengers: IP_3 and diacylglycerol (DAG). Activation of IP_3 receptor channels is believed to play a primary physiologic role in intracellular Ca^{2+} mobilization. The binding of

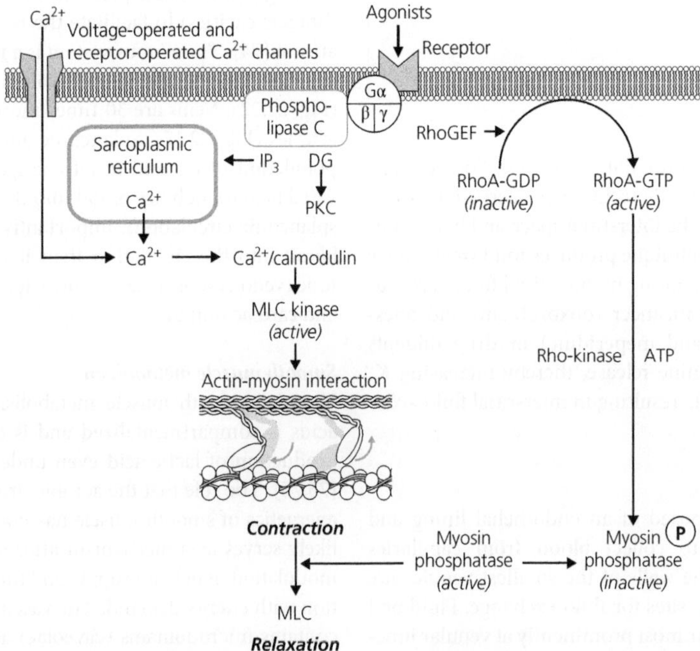

Figure 22.23 Excitation–contraction coupling in vascular smooth muscle: Calcium enters cardiac cells through two types of voltage-dependent calcium channels (L and T) and several types of receptor-operated channels. Not shown is that some agonists act on smooth muscle membrane receptors to stimulate phosphatidylinositol turnover and the production of inositol triphosphate (IP_3) and diacylglycerol (DG). IP_3 releases calcium from the SR and DAG activates protein kinase C, which stimulates the activity of the voltage-dependent slow calcium channels. Calcium entry into the cell triggers the release of intracellular calcium (calcium-induced calcium release) from the sarcoplasmic reticulum (SR). Increases in intracellular calcium also interact with calmodulin to form a calcium–calmodulin complex stimulating myosin light-chain kinase, which together with intracellular calcium facilitates actin–myosin interaction. Contraction terminates when myosin light-chain phosphatase dephosphorylates the myosin light chain and intracellular calcium is reduced by sarcolemmal (SL) and SR reuptake, intracellular calcium–extracellular sodium exchange, and the turning off of the slow calcium channels.

IP_3 to receptors on the sarcoplasmic reticulum results in the release of Ca^{2+} into the cytosol. Notably, these calcium induced calcium release (CICR) mechanisms are considered essential for normal cellular Ca^{2+} homeostasis in vascular smooth muscle cells [78,79].

In addition to the Ca^{2+}-dependent activation of MLC kinase, myosin light-chain phosphorylation is also regulated by MLC phosphatase (dephosphorylation), which removes high-energy phosphate from the light chain of myosin to promote smooth muscle relaxation (Fig. 22.23) [75–78]. Smooth muscle relaxation occurs as a result of removal of the contractile stimulus, decreases in intracellular Ca^{2+} concentration, an increased MLC phosphatase activity, or the direct action of a substance that inhibits contractile mechanism. A decrease in the intracellular Ca^{2+} concentration by Ca^{2+} uptake into the sarcoplasmic reticulum is dependent on ATP hydrolysis. Sarcoplasmic Ca^{2+} binding proteins also contribute to decreased intracellular Ca^{2+} concentrations. The plasma membrane also contains Na^+/Ca^{2+} exchangers and Ca^{2+}–Mg^{2+}-ATPases, providing an additional mechanism for reducing the concentration of activator Ca^{2+} inside the cell [77].

Most volatile and intravenous anesthetics inhibit vascular smooth muscle contractile activity. This response occurs at clinically relevant concentrations for volatile anesthetics and at the upper end or higher than clinically relevant anesthetic concentrations for injectable anesthetics [78,79]. Vasoconstriction to many common endogenous and exogenous receptor agonists including epinephrine, norepinephrine, dopamine, dobutamine, and phenylephrine is blunted by anesthetic drugs [79]. Receptor-operated activation, VOCCs, SERCA, and myofilament Ca^{2+} sensitivity is inhibited by volatile and injectable anesthetics. Isoflurane, sevoflurane, propofol, and benzodiazepines inhibit smooth muscle contraction by decreasing intracellular Ca^{2+} concentration; this effect is mediated by blocking calcium channels, especially the VOCCs, and by raising the intracellular cyclic AMP and cyclic GMP levels. Volatile anesthetic-induced suppression of smooth muscle contraction is also attributable to mechanisms independent of $[Ca^{2+}]_i$, which involve the depression of Ca^{2+} sensitization mediated by protein kinase C [79]. ATP-sensitive potassium channels (K_{ATP}) present in vascular smooth muscle cells play an important role in the vascular responses to a variety of pharmacologic and endogenous vasodilators [80]. The K_{ATP} channels are inhibited by intracellular ATP and by sulfonylurea agents. Pharmacological vasodilators used to lower arterial blood pressure (cromakalim, pinacidil) and many anesthetics, including isoflurane, sevoflurane, and propofol, directly activate K_{ATP} channels, resulting in exit of K^+ from the cell and membrane hyperpolarization [79–81]. The associated membrane hyperpolarization closes voltage-dependent Ca^{2+} channels, which leads to a reduction in intracellular Ca^{2+} and vasodilation [81]. Isoflurane activates K_{ATP} channels via protein kinase A (PKA) activation. By contrast, hypotension after systemic propofol administration is mainly caused by its direct relaxation effect on vascular smooth muscle [82]. Notably, K_{ATP} channels are activated during hypoxia, ischemia, acidosis, and septic shock [80].

Blood

Blood is a unique and complex fluid with many properties and functions that remain to be elucidated. Composed of approximately 60% plasma and 40% cells, blood is responsible for carrying oxygen, nutrients, and other substances (cells, platelets, clotting factors, electrolytes, proteins, hormones, etc.) to tissues and for transporting carbon dioxide, the by-products of cellular metabolism, and foreign substances (e.g., anesthetic drugs) to the organs of elimination. This suspension of red and white blood cells and platelets in plasma is responsible for maintaining a normal internal environment (homeostasis), defending against foreign substances (immunity), and preventing or limiting hemorrhage (hemostasis) [83]. The most essential function of blood is to deliver oxygen to tissues. Oxygen is relatively insoluble in plasma (93–95% water by volume): 0.003 mL O_2 per 100 mL of plasma per 1 mmHg partial pressure of oxygen (PO_2) or approximately 0.3 mL per 100 mL at a PO_2 equal to 100 mmHg. Hemoglobin (Hb) contained within erythrocytes (red blood cells: RBCs) transports much larger amounts of oxygen than can be carried by plasma. Encapsulation of Hb within RBCs has important biological consequences, including the rate of Hb saturation with oxygen, its intravascular half-life, prevention of renal toxicity, and maintenance of colloid osmotic pressure. The PO_2 at which Hb is 50% saturated with oxygen is termed the P_{50} (Fig. 22.24). In most species, the high concentration of 2,3-diphosphoglycerate within RBCs compared with plasma facilitates the release of oxygen from Hb and helps maintain a physiologically relevant P_{50} (26–28 mmHg). The amount of O_2 that can be carried by blood is dependent upon the amount of Hb per unit of blood. Hemoglobin exists as a tetramer (molecular weight 64 kDa) consisting of two α and two β polypeptide chains. Each polypeptide chain contains heme and a central iron molecule that can bind oxygen [83]. The affinity of Hb for oxygen depends on the PCO_2, pH, body temperature, the intraerythrocyte concentration of 2,3-diphosphoglycerate, and the chemical structure of Hb (Fig. 22.24) [3]. Heme must be in the reduced or ferrous state (Fe^{2+}) to bind oxygen. Each gram of Hb can carry approximately 1.34 mL of oxygen (oxygen capacity). Oxygen capacity does not include oxygen dissolved in plasma. This means that the amount O_2 carried by 15 g/dL Hb at sea level will be approximately 20 mL/100 mL (15 g/dL × 1.34 mL = 20.1 mL/100 mL). The total (dissolved in plasma; bound to Hb) amount of O_2 carried by blood is termed the oxygen content and is determined by the Hb oxygen capacity, percentage saturation (%Sat) of Hb, the Hb concentration, and the partial pressure of oxygen. The oxygen content of blood when the PO_2 is 100 mmHg and the Hb is 15 g/dL is 20.8 mL [$(1.34 \times Hb \times \%Sat) + (0.003 \times PO_2)(0.003 \times PO_2) = 20.8$ mL], emphasizing the importance of Hb's role as an oxygen carrier.

Methemoglobin is formed when the iron contained within the Hb molecule is oxidized to the ferric state (Fe^{3+}), and this form of Hb cannot bind oxygen. Hemoglobin is maintained in the Fe^{2+} state inside RBCs by reduced nicotine adenine dinucleotide (NADH)–methemoglobin reductase. Carboxyhemoglobin, sulfhemoglobin, and cyanmethemoglobin are other Hbs that are not capable carrying oxygen. The binding of oxygen to Hb has an important vasoregulatory role by promoting the binding of nitric oxide (NO), forming *S*-nitrosohemoglobin (SNO) [84,85]. Nitric oxide plays a central role in vascular physiology as an autocrine and paracrine vasodilator molecule that maintains basal vasomotor tone, mediates flow-mediated vasodilation, and inhibits platelet aggregation and endothelium adhesion molecule expression [86,87]. Current evidence suggests that deoxygenation of Hb is accompanied by an allosteric transition in *S*-nitrosohemoglobin [from the R (oxygenated) to the T (deoxygenated) structure] that releases the NO group [88]. *S*-Nitrosohemoglobin contracts blood vessels and decreases perfusion in the R structure, and relaxes vessels to improve blood flow in the T structure [88,89]. Thus, by sensing the physiologic oxygen gradient in tissues, Hb exploits conformation-associated changes in SNO to bring local blood flow into line with oxygen requirements (Fig. 22.25).

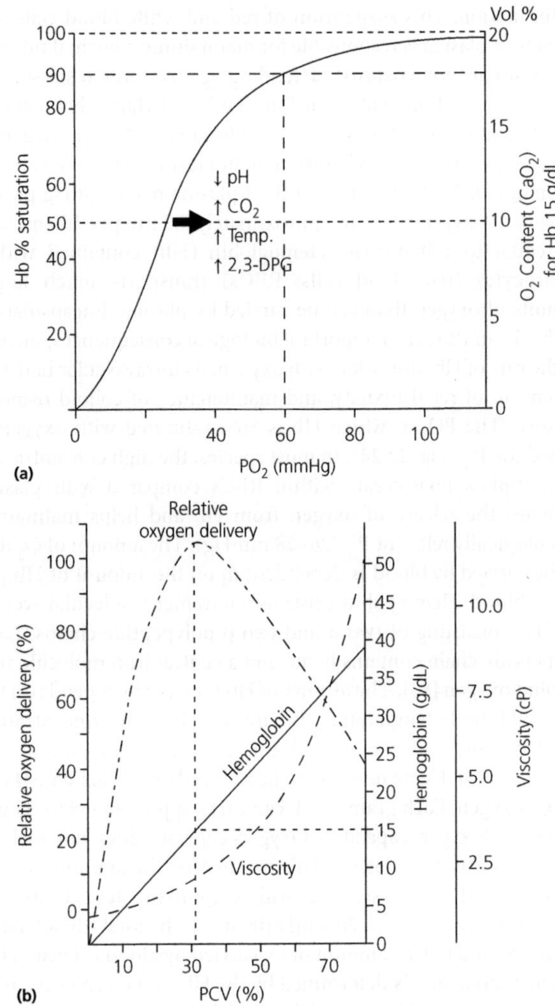

Figure 22.24 (a) The oxyhemoglobin dissociation curve: the blood partial pressure of oxygen (PO_2) is plotted against the saturation of hemoglobin (Hb) with oxygen (O_2). The curve is right shifted (Hb has less affinity for O_2) by acidosis (↓pH) and increases in carbon dioxide concentration [CO_2]), body temperature, and 2,3-diphosphoglycerate (2,3-DPG). This effect helps to unload O_2 from Hb in metabolizing tissues and increases Hb affinity for O_2 in the lungs. (b) The Hb concentration and the blood viscosity (μ) determine oxygen delivery to tissues. There is an 'ideal' Hb or packed cell volume (PCV) (3 × Hb = PCV) at which oxygen delivery to tissues is optimized. cP, centipoise.

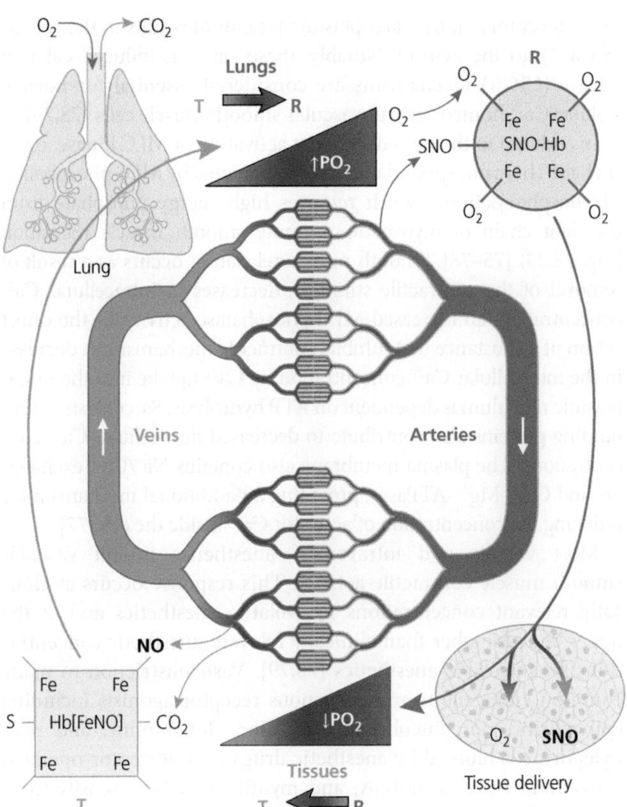

Figure 22.25 Simplified model of the respiratory cycle: a three-gas system involving NO, CO_2, and O_2. O_2 and CO_2 govern the equilibrium between the R and T structures of Hb, which in turn dictates whether NO bioactivity is dispensed to dilate blood vessels; dynamic and graded changes in arteriolar tone couple blood flow to metabolic demand ('hypoxic vasodilation and hyperoxic vasoconstriction'). NO bioactivity is linked to equilibrium between SNOs (*S*-nitrosylated hemoglobin) in the blood and tissues, the position of which is regulated by the allosteric state of hemoglobin. Source: [88]. Reproduced with permission of *Nature*.

Some of the carbon dioxide produced by metabolizing tissues binds to deoxygenated Hb and is eliminated by the lungs during the Hb oxygenation process prior to the blood returning to the systemic circulation and the cycle repeating itself. Free plasma Hb (hemolysis) is maintained in the ferrous (Fe^{2+}) redox state, which reacts with NO in a near-diffusion-limited reaction to inhibit NO signaling [89]. Extravasation of Hb into the subendothelial space and reductive recycling back to the ferrous state may enhance this effect. Oxidation of cell-free Hb from the ferric (Fe^{3+}) to the ferryl (Fe^{4+}) state acts as a potent proinflammatory agonist initiating oxidative cellular injury [90]. Free heme and iron promote inflammatory injury via activation of innate immune responses in macrophages and monocytes. Compensatory pathways that normally control these NO deoxygenation and oxidation reactions include haptoglobin- and hemopexin-mediated sequestration of Hb dimer and heme, respectively [90]. Hemoxygenase and biliverdin reductase signaling detoxify heme and iron and provide catalytic antioxidant, antiproliferative, and anti-inflammatory protective signaling. When protective Hb scavenging mechanisms are saturated, levels of cell-free Hb increase in the plasma, resulting in the consumption of nitric oxide. Since nitric oxide plays a major role in vascular homeostasis and is known to be a critical regulator of basal and stress-mediated smooth muscle relaxation and vasomotor tone, endothelial adhesion molecule expression, and platelet activation and aggregation, overconsumption can produce dire clinical consequences, including dystonias involving the gastrointestinal, cardiovascular, pulmonary, and urogenital systems, and clotting disorders. In addition, depletion of haptoglobin leads to clearance of free Hb dimers by the kidneys [86,87]. Furthermore, renal clearance of large quantities of Hb dimers can result in their precipitation in the proximal tubules, leading to renal tubular damage and renal failure [91]. Free Hb also increases the colloid osmotic pressure of whole blood. Collectively, this is an active area of current investigation and central to the development, clinical efficacy, and safety of Hb-based oxygen carriers. There is little if any information regarding the effects of anesthetic drugs on Hb oxygen-carrying capacity although several local anesthetics (e.g., prilocaine, benzocaine) and solution incipients (e.g., benzyl alcohol) are known to predispose to methemoglobinemia, especially in cats.

Lymphatic System

The peripheral lymphatic system is not anatomically part of the blood circulatory system and consists of a dense network of channels that function in conjunction with the circulatory system for the one-way transport of interstitial fluid, proteins, lipids, and waste products back to the blood circulation, via the thoracic duct (Fig. 22.26). It is integrally involved in maintaining normal circulatory dynamics, especially interstitial fluid volume (approximately 10% of the capillary filtrate). Lymphatic capillaries (lacteals) collect interstitial fluid (lymph) mainly in the form of chylomicrons (triglycerides, phospholipids, cholesterol, and proteins) that are eventually returned to the cranial vena cava and right atrium after passing through a series of lymph vessels and lymph nodes [93]. Lymph vessels have smooth muscle within their walls and contain valves similar to those in veins and are responsible for lymph flow [94].

The lymphatic system plays a critical role in tissue fluid homoeostasis, immune defense, and metabolic maintenance. Lymphatic vessels transport lymph, proteins, immune cells, and digested lipids, allowing fluid and proteins to be returned to the bloodstream, lipids to be stored, and antigens to be detected in lymph nodes. Lymphatic drainage is mainly driven by NO-dependent rhythmic constrictions of lymph vessel smooth muscle and skeletal muscle contraction (lymphatic pump) in conjunction with lymphatic valves (Fig. 22.26) [95]. Interstitial fluid balance (accumulation) is critically modulated by interstitial fluid pressure and inflammatory mediators. Lymph nodes filter the interstitial fluid and break down bacteria, viruses, and waste. Lymphatic capillaries exist in all vascularized organs and tissues except retina, bone, and brain. Lymphatic capillaries do not have a basement membrane but are lined with a single layer of partly overlapping lymphatic endothelial cells (LECs) [93,95]. The LECs are anchored to the extracellular matrices and function as primary valves that unidirectionally control lymph fluid drainage when the interstitial pressure increases. Lymphatic endothelial cells modulate the inflammatory response by secreting chemokines for recruitment of immune (dendritic) cells into the lymphatic system. Furthermore, proteins important in the innate immune response [e.g., Toll-like receptor (TLR-4)] are highly expressed in LECs and contribute to lipopolysaccharide (LPS)-induced lymphangiogenesis by chemotactic recruitment of macrophages [96,97]. Interestingly, morphine and other opioids are TLR-4 agonists. TLR-4 receptor activation has been linked to behavioral changes and long-term side-effects caused by opioids, including tolerance, hyperalgesia, and allodynia [98,99].

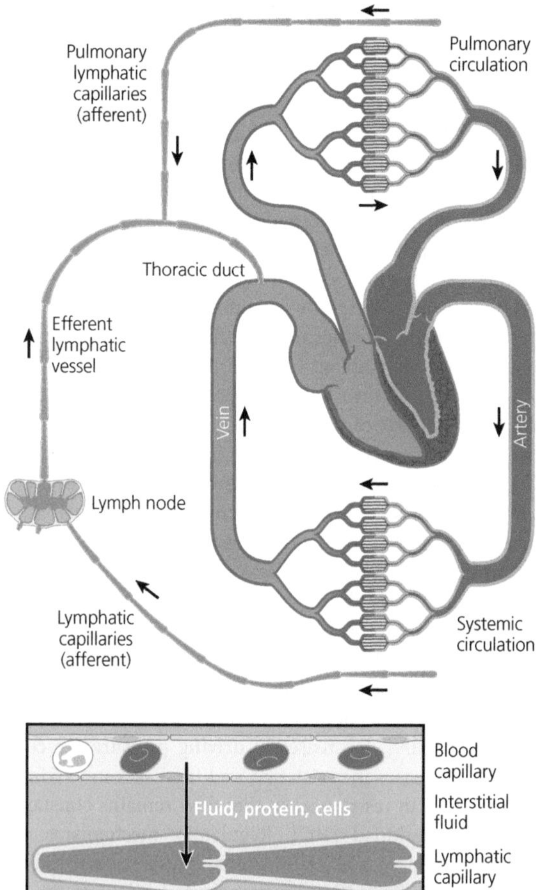

Figure 22.26 The lymphatic system (green) is a linear system in which the lymphatic capillaries in peripheral tissues drain lymph and transport it back to the blood vascular system through the thoracic duct.

Special circulations

The circulations of specific organ systems (brain, kidney, liver, etc.) are discussed in more detail in other chapters describing their physiology and anatomy. Three circulations, however, deserve special mention: coronary, pulmonary, and splanchnic. Myocardial blood flow and oxygen delivery are critical to the prevention of myocardial ischemia and maintenance of normal cardiac function. The pulmonary and splanchnic circulations receive all or a large proportion of the cardiac output, respectively, and are essential blood reservoirs. Anesthetic drugs and anesthesia blunt normal compensatory responses and autoregulatory mechanisms that mobilize and redistribute blood to tissues that are in highest demand. These effects are primarily due to their vasodilatory effects and depression of sympathoadrenal activation.

Coronary circulation

The heart has the highest oxygen consumption per unit of tissue mass of all the major organs in the body. Myocardial arterial oxygen extraction is 70–80%, compared with approximately 25% for most other organs. The heart receives approximately 5% of cardiac output (0.8 mL/min per gram of heart muscle) and possesses a rich capillary network, three to four times denser than that of skeletal muscle to achieve such high extraction [100–103]. Anatomic differences in the anatomy of the coronary circulation among species accounts for dissimilarities in the source and distribution of myocardial blood flow (Fig. 22.3b). The left anterior descending coronary artery and its diagonal branches supply a larger mass of myocardium than the circumflex in humans, swine, rats, and nonhuman primates. The circumflex artery supplies the largest mass of cardiac muscle in dogs, cats, horses, and cattle, although there is considerable individual animal variation [104]. Dogs have an extensive collateral circulation whereas pigs and primates do not [105]. Cardiac veins empty into the great cardiac vein, which empties into the right atrium via the coronary sinus and accounts for over 90% of the venous return from the heart [105]. Small capillary-like vessels (Thebesian veins) are present throughout the heart and drain directly into the cardiac chambers, accounting for approximately 4% of the venous return [106]. Flow across the resting myocardium is usually taken to be the pressure gradient between the aortic root (coronary driving pressure) and the right atrium, although coronary perfusion pressure in the left ventricle is more accurately determined as the difference between the aortic diastolic pressure and left ventricular end-diastolic pressure (LVEDP) [100]. Under normal conditions, the driving pressure is fully maintained along epicardial conduit vessels with little if any pressure loss in the distal epicardial arteries. Intra-coronary arterial pressure declines in the microvasculature (<100 μm), reaching a value of 20–30 mmHg across the capillaries [103]. Blood flow to the heart occurs mainly during diastole and decreases by more than 50% during isovolumic contraction in intramyocardial vessels compared with epicardial arteries, with mid-systolic flow becoming retrograde [103]. Blood flow resumes during isovolumic relaxation and diastole.

The principal determinant of blood flow resistance in the myocardium includes extravascular compression of intramural coronary vessels (30–40% of total resistances), the contractile state of the myocardium, and heart rate [101]. In addition, systolic ventricular torsion also increases coronary resistance, such that systolic flow within the myocardium may be zero or negative during systole. Coronary blood flow is mainly determined by local oxygen demand [107]. Autoregulatory mechanisms coordinate the interaction between intracoronary driving pressure and microvascular resistance in order to maintain adequate flow across the capillaries for substrate delivery and metabolite removal. The vascular endothelium is the final common pathway controlling vasomotor tone (coronary autoregulation) and, as with all other vessels, NO plays a major role [108,109]. Decreases in driving pressure are compensated for by decreases in resistance, and increases in driving pressure by increases in resistance, so that flow remains constant for a given cardiac workload [107]. Regulatory mechanisms operate within the physiologic range of arterial pressures but fail during hypotension when flows become strongly dependent on the driving pressure. Coronary arteries receive their innervation through bilateral vagal (parasympathetic) fibers from the cardiac plexus at the base of the aorta and sympathetic nerves arise from the stellate ganglion [110]. Parasympathetic fibers innervate primarily supraventricular cardiac structures, especially the SA and AV nodes. Factors that lower arterial blood pressure (hypovolemia), increase ventricular diastolic pressure (heart failure), or decrease diastolic time (tachycardia) lower the subendocardial to subepicardial flow ratio and can result in subendocardial ischemia and ST–T changes in the ECG. Increases in heart rate impinge on diastolic time more than systolic time, thereby decreasing perfusion time, and should be avoided [101]. Anesthesia and anesthetics drugs can also decrease myocardial perfusion by increasing right atrial or end diastolic pressure when myocardial function is impaired.

Pulmonary circulation

The pulmonary circulation receives the entire output of the right heart (total cardiac output), contains approximately 10–15% of the total blood volume, and serves as an important blood reservoir stabilizing left ventricular stroke volume and systemic blood volume [110]. The primary purpose of the pulmonary circulation is gas exchange. The right ventricle (RV) and the lungs are in series with the left ventricle and the systemic circulation, and the entire cardiac output passes through the lungs (Fig. 22.1). Pulmonary artery compliance buffers flow during RV ejection, reducing pulmonary artery pulse pressure. Similarly to the left ventricle, changes in right ventricular function can be described by load-dependent changes in developed pressure or load-independent changes in ventricular elastance, similarly to the left ventricle (see Hemodynamics). The right ventricle and pulmonary circulation buffer dynamic changes in blood volume and flow resulting from respiration, positional changes, and changes in left ventricular cardiac output. Pulmonary vascular pressures and pulmonary vascular resistance are much lower than those of the systemic circulation [111]. This low-pressure system has only limited ability to control the regional distribution of blood flow within the lungs, resulting in the most unique feature of the pulmonary circulation: the potential for the pulmonary capillaries to collapse. Mild increases in pulmonary arterial blood pressure normally distend and recruit pulmonary capillaries, decreasing pulmonary vascular resistance [110]. The low pressure of the pulmonary circulation, however, makes it susceptible to extravascular pressure and pulmonary blood flow is often described in terms of a 'Starling resistor' where the pressure surrounding a collapsible tube influences the passage of fluid through it. Pulmonary blood flow and blood flow distribution are determined by the difference between inflow pressure and outflow pressure, but in the lung outside pressure (alveolar pressure) and gravity often influence the regional distribution of pulmonary blood flow [110]. Low inflow pressure predisposes the lung to the so-called 'waterfall effect' wherein pulmonary venous pressure is below alveolar pressure and has no influence on blood flow or the determination of pulmonary vascular resistance. Whenever the surrounding pressure (mechanical ventilation) is greater than outflow pressure then blood flow is determined by the difference between inflow pressure and the surrounding pressure. Excessive and prolonged inspiratory pressure, for example, can markedly reduce or stop pulmonary blood flow, leading to marked reductions in blood flow to the left ventricle, cardiac output, and arterial blood pressure. Importantly, large increases in pulmonary artery blood pressure can overwhelm the pulmonary vascular bed's ability to be recruited and distend, resulting in pulmonary edema and/or ascites.

Another unique feature of the pulmonary circulation is vasoconstriction in response to hypoxic conditions. Hypoxic pulmonary vasoconstriction (HPV) functions as a negative feedback mechanism for matching ventilation and perfusion and is likely linked to local nitric oxide (vasodilator) production [112]. Alveolar hypoxia is the most important stimulus to hypoxic pulmonary vasoconstriction and the site of action seems to be in small extra-alveolar vessels. Under normal (non-hypoxic) conditions, circulating oxygen regulates its own uptake by adjusting local perfusion to match local ventilation. During hypoxic conditions, however, the pulmonary vessels constrict, increasing pulmonary arterial pressure. This response distends and recruits under perfused pulmonary vessels, effectively shunting blood to better ventilated alveoli, resulting in an improvement in the ventilation:perfusion ratio. Hypoxic pulmonary vasconstriction is minimally inhibited by most anesthetic drugs, including propofol [113,114].

Splanchnic circulation

The splanchnic circulation includes multiple organs, receives approximately 25% of cardiac output, and contains approximately 20% of total blood volume (Fig. 22.27a) [115]. Splanchnic veins are highly compliant and serve as one of the body's largest blood volume reservoirs. Splanchnic veins and the spleen contain a high population of α_1- and α2-adrenergic receptors and are highly sensitive to adrenergic stimulation or blockade (Fig. 22.27b) [115]. Depending upon the species, the spleen can be a significant reservoir of blood. The volume of blood mobilized from the spleen, liver, and intestine of dogs ranged from 6 to 30% and from 55 to 81% of their blood volumes following moderate (9 mL/kg) and severe (33 mL/kg) hemorrhage, respectively [116].

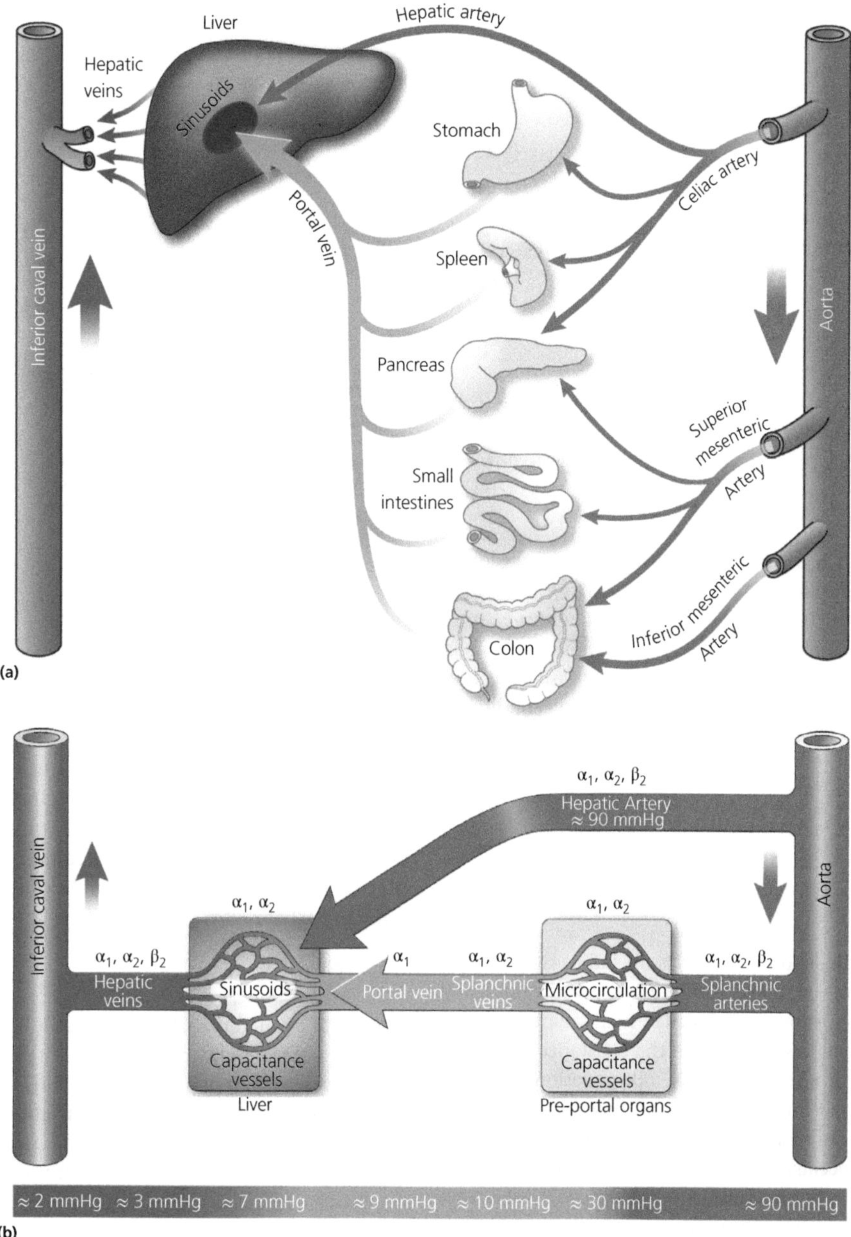

Figure 22.27 (a) The splanchnic circulation contains approximately 25% of the blood volume. Splanchnic arteries represent all arterial vessels of the preportal organs; splanchnic veins represent the pooled venous blood from all these organs. (b) The distribution of adrenoceptor subtypes (α_1, α_2, β_2) and approximate intravascular pressures (bottom bar) for corresponding segments of the splanchnic vasculature. Source: [115]. Reproduced with permission of Lippincott Williams & Wilkins.

During physiologic conditions, a change in splanchnic arterial flow produces a proportional change in the pressure within splanchnic capacitance vessels: the volume of blood in the splanchnic capacitance vessels is linearly related to the transmural pressure. If blood flow decreases, the blood volume and pressure within the veins decrease. The veins recoil, helping to maintain the intramural pressure and providing a driving force for expulsion of intravenous volume to the systemic circulation [117]. If arterial blood pressure decreases substantially, sympathoadrenal stimulation causes splanchnic arterial constriction that increases the pressure in capacitance vessels, expelling splanchnic blood into the systemic circulation [117]. Volume mobilization is the result of active venoconstriction and passive elastic recoil of the splanchnic veins secondary to decreased arterial inflow [115]. These processes deliver blood to the systemic circulation, effectively compensating for up to 50–60% of the volume lost following mild to moderate hemorrhage. Active mobilization of splanchnic blood volume is almost entirely the result of β_2- and α-adrenergic receptor activation [115]. Both β_2- and α-adrenergic receptors act in concert to shift blood maximally from the splanchnic vasculature into the systemic circulation by producing vasoconstriction, decreasing splanchnic vascular capacitance, and decreasing intrahepatic vascular resistance. Anesthesia and anesthetic drugs including benzodiazepines blunt, if not abolish, the ability of the splanchnic circulation to mobilize blood [117,118]. This effect may be as important as or more important than the arterial vasodilatory or negative myocardial contractile effects of anesthetic drugs when considering the potential causes of arterial hypotension and/or low cardiac output during anesthesia.

Hemorrheology

Hemorrheology is the study of blood flow in the vascular system and naturally includes an understanding of pressure and resistance [119]. Current flow (I) in electric circuits is determined by the electromotive force or voltage (E) and the resistance to current flow (R) according to Ohm's law:

$$I = E / R$$

Similarly, the flow of fluids (Q) through non-distensible tubes is determined by the driving pressure (P) and the resistance to flow (R):

$$Q = P / R$$

The resistance to blood flow is determined by blood vessel geometry (radius, length, morphology) and characteristics of the fluid medium, key among which is blood viscosity (η). The steady, non-pulsatile, laminar flow of Newtonian fluids (homogeneous fluids in which viscosity does not change with flow velocity or vascular geometry), such as water, saline, and, under physiological conditions, plasma, can be described by the Hagen–Poiseuille law, which states

$$Q = \frac{(P_1 - P_2) r^4 \pi}{8L\eta}$$

$$R = \frac{8L\eta}{r^4 \pi}$$

where $P_1 - P_2$ is the pressure difference, r^4 is the radius to the fourth power, L is the length of the tube, η is the viscosity of the fluid, and $8/\pi$ is a constant of proportionality [120]. The maintenance of laminar flow is a fundamental assumption of the resistance offered to steady-state fluid flow in the Hagen–Poiseuille equation. This law, although frequently used for assessing blood flow in the vascular system, is descriptive only and must be kept in perspective when considering real life, because blood is not a homogeneous fluid, blood flow is not steady, but pulsatile, and blood flow is not always laminar. These differences from the idealized steady laminar flow of Newtonian fluids through non-distensible tubes of constant radius have important consequences on the quantity of blood flow to peripheral tissue beds, oxygen delivery, and the distribution of blood flow among tissue beds. Distending pressure is a key factor in the determination of vessel or chamber wall tension and directly related to smooth muscle or myocardial oxygen consumption.

The relationship between vessel or chamber (when considering the heart) pressure, vessel diameter and wall thickness, versus tension in the vessel wall is described by Laplace's law:

$$P = \frac{2Th}{r} \text{ or } T = \frac{Pr}{2h}$$

where T is wall tension, P is developed pressure, r is the internal radius, and h is the wall thickness. This relationship is extremely important because it relates pressure, vessel dimension, and wall thickness to changes in tension development, which is known to be an important determinant of ventricular–vascular coupling (afterload), myocardial work, and myocardial oxygen consumption (Box 22.3) [121].

Box 22.3 Determinants of myocardial oxygen consumption.

1 Tension development
2 Heart rate
3 Contractile state
4 Basal cost (ion movements; membrane pumps)
5 Depolarization
6 Activation
7 Maintenance of active state
8 Shortening against a load (Fenn effect)
9 Direct metabolic effect of catecholamines

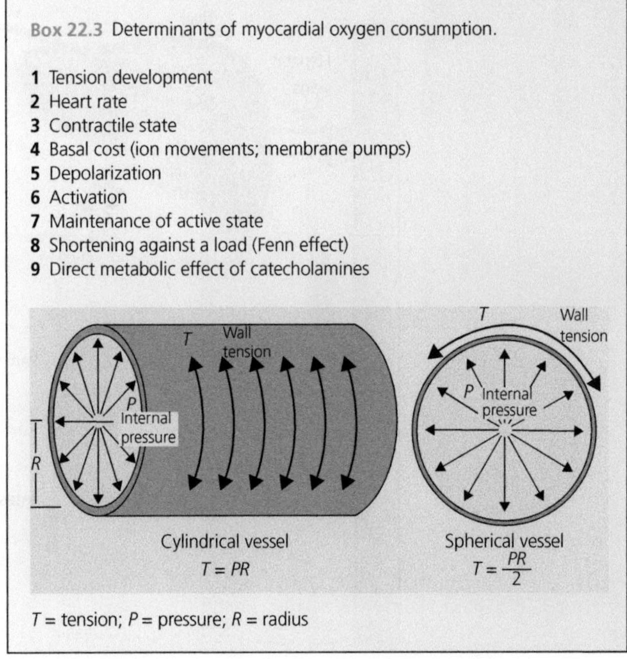

T = tension; P = pressure; R = radius

Blood is a non-Newtonian fluid that is delivered through progressively narrowing blood vessels in a pulsatile non-laminar or even turbulent manner. The major factors influencing blood flow resistance (R) are blood viscosity (η), which is largely determined by RBC concentration (HCT) and impedance [Z: dynamic (pulsatile) resistance: R_p], and collectively can be considered vascular hindrance [122]:

$$R_p = \eta \times Z$$

It should be noted that R_p (p = pulsatile) is principally dependent upon vessel geometry and is not the same as R in Ohm's law or the equivalent thereof in the Hagen–Poiseuille equation ($8L\eta/r^4\pi$), but represents the resistance to pulsatile, oscillatory, or, simply stated, physiological blood flow. The resistance (R) term in the Hagen–Poiseuille equation is more correctly thought of in terms of a non-pulsatile, a non-oscillatory, and more importantly a non-physiological system.

The viscosity term (η), although of lesser importance than Z in determining R_p, is primarily dependent upon the RBC concentration (hematocrit), RBC deformability and aggregability, plasma viscosity, temperature, and blood flow conditions (Fig. 22.24b) [123]. The rheological term that characterizes blood flow conditions is shear rate, which is a function of blood flow velocity and vascular geometry. The viscosity of blood is shear rate dependent. Viscosity decreases as shear rate increases according to

$$\eta = \text{shear stress}\left(\text{dyn/cm}^2\right) / \text{shear rate}\left(\text{s}^{-1}\right)$$

where shear stress is the force applied during pulsatile blood flow between theoretical layers of blood in the blood vessel [124,125]. Importantly, shear rate is the principal determinant of NO concentration, a potent local vasodilator [126]. Nitric oxide relaxes vascular smooth muscle by binding to the heme moiety of cytosolic guanylate cyclase, activating guanylate cyclase, and increasing intracellular levels of cyclic guanosine 3′,5′-monophosphate (cyclic GMP), resulting in vasodilation. It is interesting that shear rate gradually increases and blood viscosity decreases as large arteries become smaller, and is greatest in the capillaries regardless of low flow rates. This phenomenon (decreased viscosity in smaller vessels), known as the Fahraeus–Lindquist effect, is attributed to the centralization of RBCs, reduced RBC numbers (Fahraeus effect) at the vessel wall ('plasma skimming'), and RBC deformability, that is, viscosity in capillaries is low because RBCs may only be able to pass through capillaries in single file [123,127]. Summarizing, as the diameter of the vessel decreases, the concentration of RBCs (Fahraeus effect) and the viscosity decrease (Fahraeus–Lindquist effect).

The optimum hematocrit for transporting the most oxygen per unit time to tissues varies among species because of differences in anatomy and circulatory dynamics, but generally ranges between 30 and 45% [128]. Dogs and horses can contract their spleen, providing additional RBCs (raising the hematocrit) and oxygen-carrying capacity during times of stress or exercise. High hematocrits (polycythemia; >65%), low blood flow conditions (shock), increased RBC aggregability, rouleaux formation (sepsis), and hyperproteinemia (dehydration) all cause the viscosity to increase, resulting in a decrease in oxygen delivery to tissues (Fig. 22.28). High hematocrits result in sludging of blood in capillaries and venules and dramatically increase blood viscosity and the work of pumping blood. Hemodilution (fluid administration) can be beneficial in treating these conditions and has been used during anesthesia to reduce RBC loss and improve oxygen delivery [129,130]. Moderate levels of hemodilution reduce systemic hematocrit but compensate for a decrease in blood viscosity by increasing blood flow velocity (cardiac output), resulting in augmented or maintained oxygen delivery to tissue. If, however, the hematocrit is reduced to 40% of normal or less, the decrease in blood hemoglobin concentration jeopardizes blood oxygen content and tissue oxygenation. Under these conditions, oxygen delivery to tissue hinges on increasing oxygen extraction and maintaining the surface area for exchange, which is determined by the functional capillary density (FCD) [131]. Blood viscosity is mainly determined by hematocrit in larger vessels, whereas the shear rate at the wall in smaller vessels (<100–400 μm) is a function of the plasma viscosity. The viscous properties of plasma and plasma layer-vessel wall shear stress are both important in determining FCD in the microcirculation. Viscosity and flow velocity of plasma define shear stress in small vessels and are directly related to the production of vasodilatory substances such as prostacyclin and NO, key factors in determining FCD [126,131].

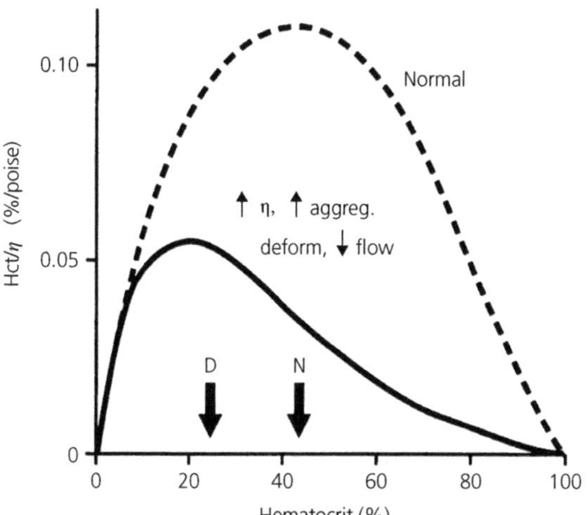

Figure 22.28 Effect of hematocrit (% Hct) on oxygen transport (Hct/η). The arrow marked N represents a relatively normal Hct. The arrow marked D represents an animal with anemia or hemodilution. The dashed line represents the normal situation when Hct is the only variable. The solid line represents the response to changes in Hct when plasma viscosity (η) is increased, red cell aggregation (aggreg) is increased, red cell deformability (deform) is decreased, or blood flow rate is decreased. Source: modified from [123].

Impedance

The second key factor in determining blood flow in pulsatile systems is impedance (Z) [132,133]. Quantitatively, impedance is the relationship between pulsatile pressure and pulsatile flow in arteries:

$$Z_L = \frac{P_1 - P_2}{Q} \qquad (Z_L = R_P + R)$$

where Z_L represents longitudinal impedance, which is the sum of the pulsatile (R_p) and steady non-pulsatile resistive (R) components of longitudinal arterial resistance. Under normal (non-stressed) conditions, the steady non-pulsatile resistive component represents 90% of the total impedance to blood flow and the pulsatile component comprises 10%. This fact (R = 90% of Z_L) is the principal reason why so many investigators and clinicians calculate vascular resistance from Ohm's law. The components of Z_L may change considerably, however, in diseased animals or during pharmacological manipulation, with R_p becoming much more important. Impedance is determined by the various frequency components that comprise the arterial pressure and flow velocity waveforms, is measured by applying a Fourier or harmonic analysis to these waveforms, and is expressed as a ratio or modulus and phase (Fig. 22.29), the key point being that impedance is a frequency-dependent, not time-dependent, index. Input impedance (Z_i), the ratio of pressure and flow at an arterial site that is considered to be the input to the vascular tree (e.g., the aortic root), depends on local arterial properties (e.g., elastance or compliance), the properties of all the vessels beyond the point of measurement down to the points where pulsations and pulse wave reflections from narrowing arteries (particularly arterioles) and vessel bifurcations disappear [132,133]. Impedance to blood flow, therefore, is viewed as having a resistive (steady-state) component due primarily to the arterioles and a reactive (pulsatile) component due to vessel wall properties (compliance, elastance, and pulse-wave reflection).

Low systolic arterial pressure permits more complete ventricular ejection, maintains low myocardial oxygen demands, and provides little stimulus for hypertrophy. High diastolic pressure ensures adequate coronary blood flow and myocardial perfusion because the majority of myocardial blood flow occurs during ventricular relaxation. Increases in arterial stiffness increase pulse-pressure amplitude and systolic pressure and decrease diastolic pressure. Poorly timed wave reflections generally increase diastolic pressure (increase Z_0: characteristic impedance). The totality of these effects increases myocardial work, oxygen consumption, and energy requirements, and decreases myocardial perfusion [121]. Ideally, the best match between the heart's pumping activity and the vascular response to the ejection of blood (ventricular–vascular coupling) is obtained when myocardial work is kept as low as possible (low systolic pressure) while adequate perfusion of the heart and peripheral tissues (high diastolic pressure) is maintained [134]. Anesthesia and fluid therapy produce variable effects on hematocrit, RBC

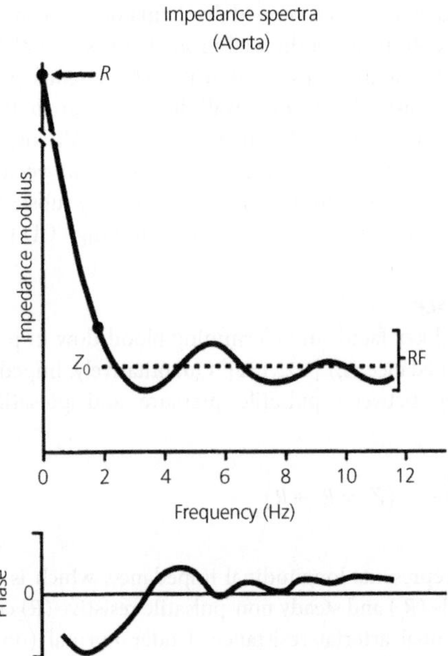

Figure 22.29 The hydraulic load (afterload) presented to the left ventricle by the systemic circulation can be characterized by expressing pressure–flow relationships in the ascending aorta as input impedance, the impedance modulus and phase of the aortic impedance spectra. The impedance modulus at 0 Hz (*R*, peripheral vascular resistance) decreases to a low value that oscillates around a characteristic value (Z_0) because of pulse-wave reflections (RF). Negative phase values indicate that flow harmonics precede pressure harmonics and vice versa.

deformability, and plasma protein concentrations, leading to alterations in η, which, when combined with changes in *Z*, may favorably affect ventricular–vascular coupling, provided that hypotension (mean arterial pressure less than 50–60 mmHg) does not occur [135,136].

Turbulence

Pulsatile blood flow may be laminar with a longitudinal velocity that takes the form of a parabola or may be irregular or turbulent (Fig. 22.30). More pressure, myocardial release of energy, and work are required to pump blood when the flow is turbulent. The potential for turbulence to develop in blood vessels can be predicted by a dimensionless number called the Reynolds number (*RN*) [137]:

$$RN = \frac{\rho D v}{\eta}$$

where ρ is fluid density, D is vessel diameter, and v is the mean blood flow velocity (Fig. 22.30). The blood viscosity (η) is inversely proportional to the Reynolds number and is an important determinant of turbulent blood flow. Turbulence usually produces periodic wave fluctuations and vibrations of the surrounding tissue structures, leading to murmurs and, with time, vascular dilation caused by weakening of the supporting elements of the vessel wall. Chronic or acute hemodilution (fluid therapy) reduces hematocrit, and therefore η, leading to an increase in Reynolds number and the production of 'physiologic' cardiac murmurs. Furthermore, flow restriction caused by congenital disease (aortic or pulmonic stenosis) or blood vessel narrowing leads to an increase in the velocity of blood flow, as predicted by the continuity equation, which states that blood flowing through different areas of a continuous intact vascular system must be equal; therefore, blood flow through a narrowing or narrowed orifice must increase. The flow downstream from the obstruction or narrowing is usually turbulent with multiple velocities and directions. Cardiac diseases (pulmonic and aortic stenosis) and vascular diseases (thrombophlebitis) that narrow valve openings or blood vessels increase velocity and are important causes of murmurs. Blood flow velocity measurements can be assessed clinically by Doppler echocardiography and the modified Bernoulli equation, $\Delta P = 4v^2$, with the assumption that velocity distal to the obstruction is significantly greater than the velocity proximal to the obstruction and therefore may be ignored [137].

Hemodynamics

Blood pressure in arteries, whether measured directly or indirectly, is frequently assessed during anesthesia. Arterial blood pressure measurement in particular is one of the fastest and most informative means of assessing cardiovascular function. When measured correctly and frequently, arterial blood pressure provides an accurate indication of drug effects, surgical events, and hemodynamic trends. The most important vascular determinant of arterial blood pressure is arteriolar tone, which can be modified by almost all anesthetic drugs [138,139]. The factors that ultimately determine arterial blood pressure are heart rate, stroke volume, vascular resistance, arterial compliance, and blood volume. The volume of blood in the vascular system is one of the major variables affecting arterial blood pressure and determines the mean circulatory filling pressure (MCFP), which is defined as the equilibrium pressure of the circulation when blood flow is zero [140]. The MCFP is approximately 7 mmHg when blood volume is normal (70–80 mL/kg). Increases in MCFP augment ventricular filling, cardiac output, and arterial blood pressure and decreases in MCFP have the opposite effect.

Arterial blood pressure is a key component in determining perfusion pressure and the adequacy of tissue blood flow. Perfusion pressures greater than 60 mmHg are generally thought to provide adequate tissue blood flow. The heart (coronary circulation), lung (pulmonary circulation), kidneys (renal circulation), abdominal structures (splanchnic circulation), and the fetus (fetal circulation) contain special circulations where changes in perfusion pressure can have immediate effects on organ function (see Special Circulations). For example, perfusion pressure in the coronary circulation is determined by the difference between arterial diastolic and ventricular end-diastolic pressure. If this pressure decreases, subendocardial ischemia develops.

Clinically, arterial blood pressure is generally measured and discussed in terms of mean arterial pressure realizing that both systolic and diastolic arterial pressures provide additional clinically useful information. When mean arterial blood pressure cannot be directly assessed, it is estimated by the equation

$$P_m = P_d + \frac{1}{3}(P_s - P_d) \quad \text{or} \quad P_m = \left(\frac{2}{3} \times P_d\right) + \left(\frac{1}{3} \times P_s\right)$$

where P_m, P_s, and P_d are mean (m), systolic (s), and diastolic (d) blood pressures, respectively (Fig. 22.31a) [141]. P_m, P_s, and P_d can be measured, calculated, or estimated using invasive (direct) arterial catheterization or non-invasive (indirect) Doppler or oscillometric techniques. Most drugs used to produce anesthesia decrease peripheral vascular resistance and arterial blood pressure. α_2-Adrenergic receptor agonists and dissociative anesthetics (ketamine, tiletamine) can increase peripheral vascular resistance, potentially increasing arterial blood pressure but decreasing cardiac output.

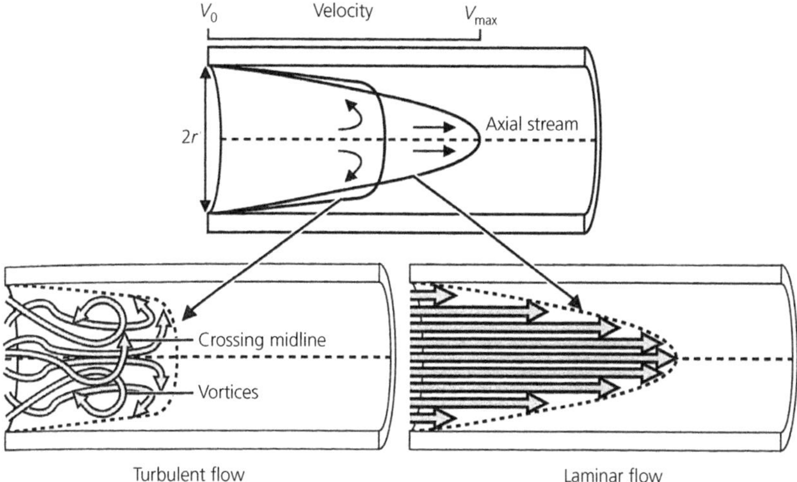

Figure 22.30 Velocity profiles for laminar and turbulent blood flow. Turbulence increases the energy required for blood flow because turbulence increases the loss of energy in the form of friction. Vortices develop during turbulent blood flow and both axial and mean velocities are lower than during laminar flow. V_{max} = maximum velocity.

The arterial pulse pressure ($P_s - P_d$) and pulse-pressure waveform provide valuable information regarding changes in vascular compliance (compliance = SV/aortic PP) and vessel tone [141]. Both the pressure and pressure waveform morphology change as the pressure wave travels peripherally: systolic pressure increases and mean pressure decreases; diastolic pressure decreases minimally (Fig. 22.32). Generally, drugs (phenothiazines) or diseases (septic shock) that produce marked arterial dilating effects increase vascular compliance, causing a rapid rise, short duration, and rapid fall in the arterial waveform while increasing the arterial pulse pressure [141]. Situations that produce vasoconstriction decrease vascular compliance, producing a longer duration pulse waveform and a slower fall in the systolic blood pressure to diastolic values. The pulse pressure may contain secondary and sometimes tertiary pressure waveforms, particularly if the measuring site is in a peripheral artery some distance from the heart [139]. Secondary and tertiary pulse waves are an indication of normal or elevated vascular tone in response to sympathetic nervous system stimulation or the vascular effects of drugs (e.g., ketamine, dexmedetomidine, or catecholamines).

Traditionally, both arterial and central venous pressures, waveform morphology, and waveform analysis have been used to assess cardiovascular status during anesthesia [142–146]. Emphasis is placed upon maximum and minimum acceptable values, pressure waveform morphology, and expected changes associated with anesthetic drugs and various therapies (vasopressors, fluid). Caution should be exercised when interpreting either of these variables, however, since increases in arterial blood pressure are not always associated with an increase in tissue perfusion and vice versa. Even greater caution is advised when assessing central venous pressure owing to its dependence on other variables (blood volume, heart rate, venous return, right ventricular function) [117,145]. Similarly, changes in waveform morphology are subject to many modifying variables (e.g., location within the arterial network, hemorrhage, sympathetic tone), several of which can produce acute changes in arterial or venous waveform morphology.

Cardiac cycle and pressure–volume loop

Cartoons of the cardiac cycle are used to illustrate the temporal relationships among its various components, including the electrical (ECG), mechanical (pressure, volume, and flow), and acoustic (heart sound) events associated with cardiac contraction and relaxation (Fig. 22.33a). Just as important (but not as descriptive) as the time-varying components of the cardiac cycle is the time-independent representation: the ventricular pressure–volume loop (Fig. 22.33b). The pressure–volume loop is a 'load-independent' index of ventricular systolic and diastolic performance and is also used to assess ventricular vascular interaction (coupling), and myocardial energetics. Changes in the pressure–volume loop illustrate and quantitate the determinants of changes in cardiac function: preload, afterload, and cardiac contractility [147,148]. The various qualitative components of the cardiac cycle and pressure–volume loop are essentially identical for both the right and left ventricles, although the sequence of electric activation, the pressure changes, and their morphology differ.

Because electrical activity precedes mechanical activity, the P wave of the surface ECG is a reasonable starting point to begin a description of the cardiac cycle (Fig. 22.33a). Electrical activation of the atria produces the P wave of the ECG and, due to rapid interatrial transmission of the electrical impulse (Bachmann's bundle), causes almost simultaneous contraction of the atria. Biphid P waves representing electrical activation of the right and left atria are frequently observed in ECGs obtained from large horses due to the increased muscle mass, relatively slow heart rate, and time needed for atrial electrical activation. Atrial contraction increases intra-atrial pressure, producing the 'a' wave of the atrial pressure curve. The atria (both right and left) function as blood reservoirs and conduits for blood transfer and, upon contraction, prime the ventricles contributing approximately 10–30% (more at faster heart rates) of the blood volume that fills the ventricles. The atrial 'kick' brings the atrioventricular valves into relatively close apposition prior to ventricular contraction and is responsible for the fourth heart sound (S_4). Ventricular contraction is signaled by the R wave of the ECG and begins after a variable delay (PR interval) during which the electric impulse traverses the atrioventricular node and Purkinje network. Once the ventricular pressure has increased to a value greater than that in the atrium, the atrioventricular valves close, actually bulging into their respective atria and giving rise to the 'c' wave of the atrial pressure curve. The atrioventricular valves are prevented from completely prolapsing into the

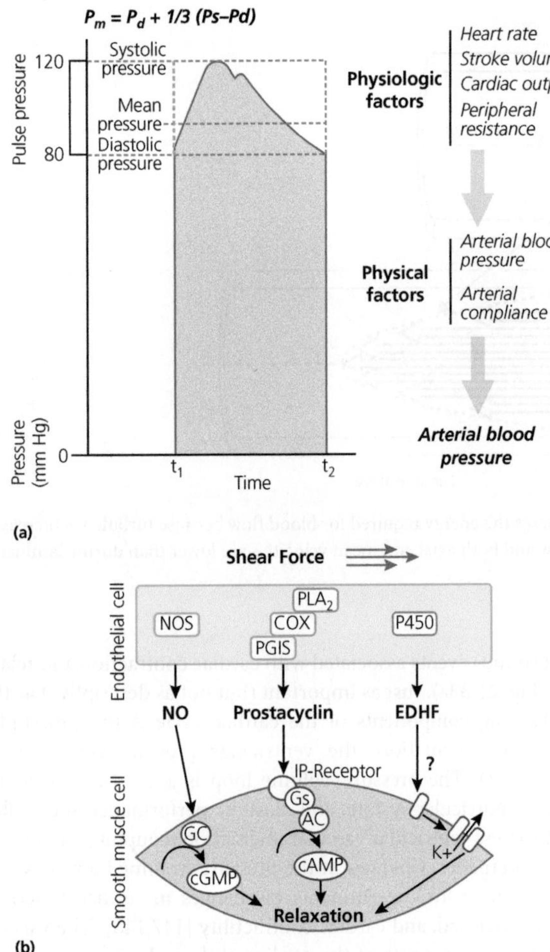

Figure 22.31 Arterial blood pressure and local control of blood flow. (a) Arterial blood pressure is determined by physiologic and physical factors. The mean arterial pressure (P_m) represents the area under the arterial pressure curve divided by the duration of the cardiac cycle and can be estimated by adding one-third the difference between the systolic arterial pressure (*Ps*) and diastolic arterial pressure (P_d) to P_d. $P_s - P_d$ is the pulse pressure. (b) Factors regulating peripheral resistance. Resistance to flow is determined by blood viscosity and vascular hindrance, which varies inversely with the number and radius of blood vessels, the latter being dependent upon blood flow and sheer force. Shear force acts on endothelial cells releasing nitric oxide (NO), prostacyclin, and EDHF (endothelium-derived hyperpolarizing factor), which cause the relaxation of vascular smooth muscle. NOS, NO synthase; PLA_2, phospholipase A_2; COX, cyclooxygenase; PGIS, prostacyclin synthase; P450, cytochrome P-450; AC, adenyl cyclase. Source: part (b) modified from [76].

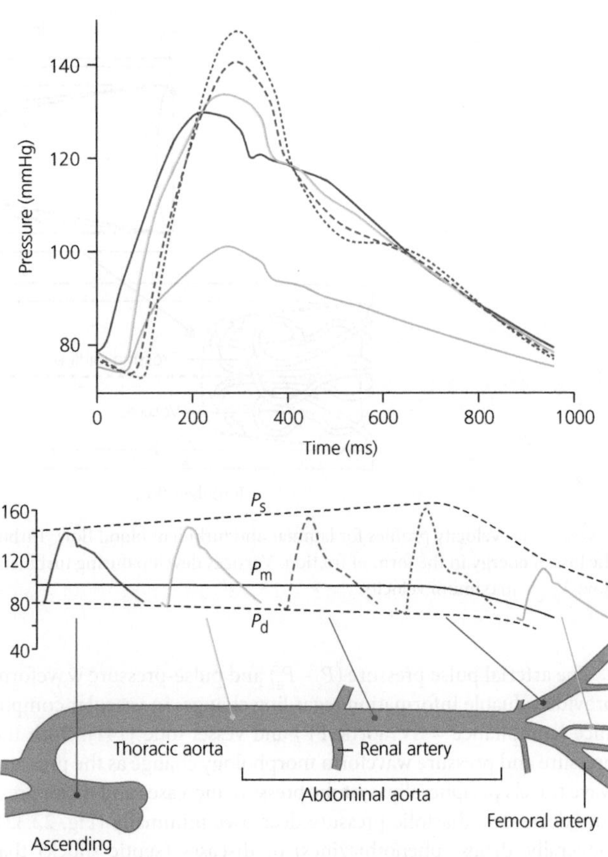

Figure 22.32 Arterial pressure waveform morphology moving distally in the arterial vasculature. The mean arterial pressure decreases progressively from the aorta toward the peripheral branches, reflecting the energy dissipation in flow. The large and medium-sized arteries have a slightly lower mean pressure but a slightly higher systolic pressure in comparison with the root of the aorta. The higher systolic pressure in the large and medium-sized arteries is explained by the reflection of pressure waves from the small arteries. The diastolic pressure shows a continuous decrease from the aorta towards the periphery. The pulse pressure ($P_s - P_d$) gradually increases from the aorta towards the medium-sized arteries. Source: modified from [132]. Reproduced with permission of Wiley.

atrial chambers by chordae tendineae, which are cord-like tendons that connect ventricular papillary muscles to the tricuspid valve and the mitral valve leaflets. The sudden development of tension in the contracting myocardium and tensing of the chordae tendineae coincident with atrioventricular valve closure are responsible for the first heart sound (S_1; Fig. 22.33a). The rapid increase in ventricular pressure while both the atrioventricular (mitral and tricuspid) and semilunar (aortic and pulmonic) valves are closed is termed isovolumic contraction because the volume of the ventricle remains constant (Fig. 22.33a,b). Once the ventricular pressure exceeds that in the aorta or pulmonary artery, the semilunar valves open and ejection begins (Fig. 22.33a,b). The ejection phase of the cardiac cycle is characterized by slowing of ventricular developed pressure, after the semilunar valves open, and an abrupt decrease in ventricular volume. These changes coincide with a large increase in aortic flow velocity and a decrease in the venous pressure curve as the atrioventricular valves are drawn towards the apex of the heart. Ventricular pressure exceeds aortic pressure during the first one-third of ventricular ejection (rapid ejection period), reaches equilibrium with aortic pressure, and thereafter, because of the onset of ventricular relaxation, declines more rapidly than aortic pressure (Fig. 22.33a). Blood continues to be ejected from the ventricle until the semilunar valves close. Closure of the semilunar valves marks the end of ventricular systole (by most definitions) and is associated with the development of the second heart sound (S_2). The second heart sound is composed of both aortic (A_2) and pulmonic (P_2) components and is frequently split (10–15 ms) during slow heart rates and in larger species (horses and cattle) [149]. The volume of blood ejected [stroke volume (SV)] by the normal ventricle is generally between 50 and 60% [ejection fraction (EF)] of its total volume.

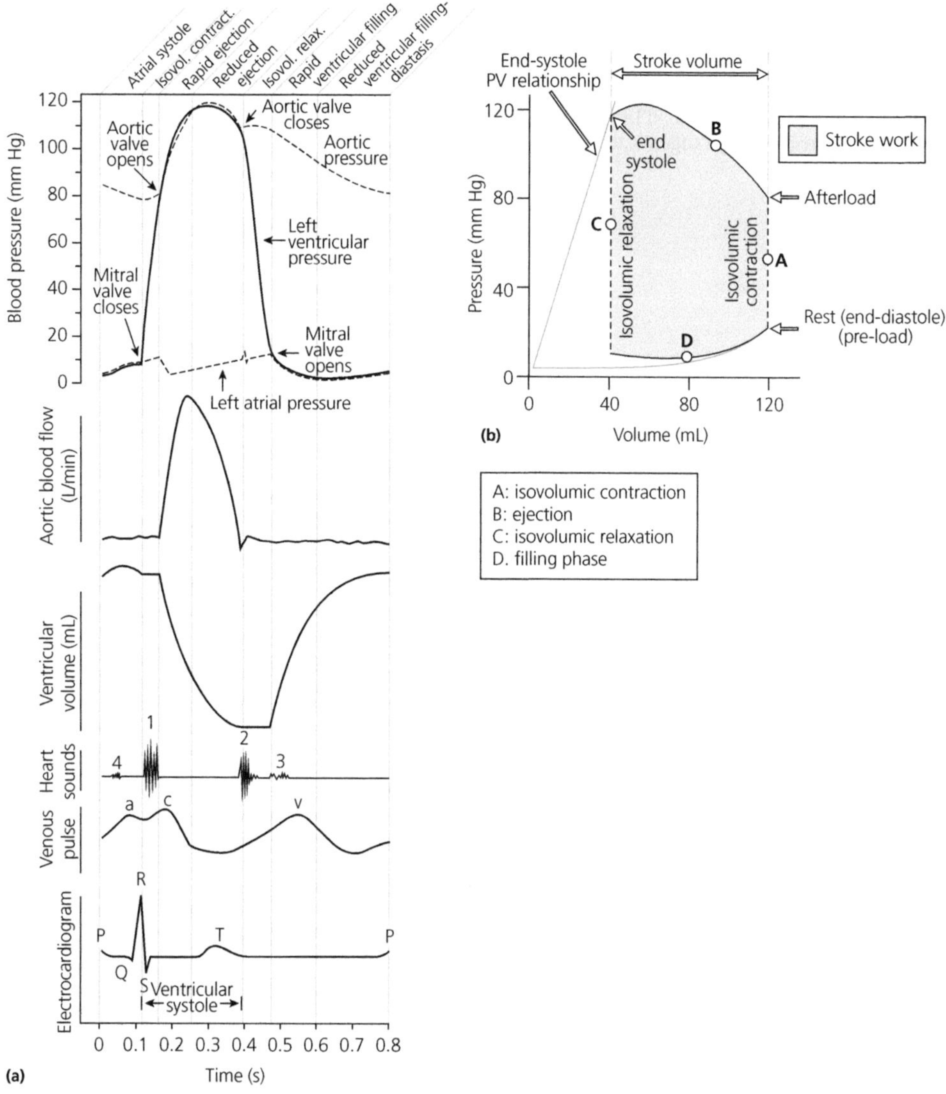

Figure 22.33 The cardiac cycle (a) illustrates the relationship among mechanical, acoustic, and electrical events in the heart as a function of time. The pressure–volume (PV) loop (b) is a time-independent illustration of the cardiac cycle that can be used to illustrate key events (e.g., end-systole; end-diastole), quantitate stroke volume, and derive load-independent indices of cardiac function. Isovol, isovolumic.

The period between closure of the semilunar valves and opening of the atrioventricular valves is termed isovolumic relaxation and marks the beginning of ventricular relaxation (Fig. 22.33a,b). Isovolumic relaxation is characterized by a rapid decrease in ventricular pressure and no change in ventricular volume, and coincides with the V wave of the atrial pressure curve (Fig. 22.33a). Once the ventricular pressure has fallen below the atrial pressure, the atrioventricular valves open, initiating the phase of rapid ventricular filling (possibly facilitated by ventricular suction) and producing the third heart sound (S_3). The third heart sound is believed to be caused by vibrations when the ventricular walls reach their elastic limit during ventricular filling, is relatively easily heard in larger species (horses and cattle), and gives rise to the characteristic ventricular gallop in dogs and cats with dilated forms of cardiac disease and increases in left atrial pressure [150]. Some cats can have gallops without having cardiac disease. Ventricular filling proceeds more gradually after the initial rapid filling phase, whereas ventricular pressure and volume increase non-linearly during late diastole (Fig. 22.33b). The slope of the pressure–volume curve (dP/dV; Fig. 22.33b) during ventricular filling is an index of ventricular stiffness, and its inverse (dV/dP) is used to assess ventricular compliance [148]. The slow mid-diastolic ventricular-filling phase continues as blood returns to the atria from the systemic and pulmonary circulations until the cardiac cycle is reinitiated by the next electric impulse.

A pressure–volume (PV; Fig. 22.34) loop is basically an irregular rectangle, inscribed in a counterclockwise fashion, in which intraventricular pressure is plotted on the y-axis against ventricular volume on the x-axis. Analysis of the PV loop begins at point B and occurs at end-diastole (onset of systole; heralded by closure of the AV valves and the first heart sound (Fig. 22.34). The coordinates of this point are end-diastolic volume (EDV) and end-diastolic pressure (EDP). The ratio of EDV to EDP is a measure of static ventricular compliance (C_{static}); the ratio of EDP to EDV is a measure of static ventricular stiffness. The relative flatness of the slope of the loop from A to B, as the ventricle fills, is an estimate of dynamic ventricular compliance ($C_{dynamic}$), and, like static ventricular stiffness, the steepness of the slope is a measure of dynamic stiffness. Thus lusitropy (ease of ventricular filling) may be expressed by the flatness of the slope of A to B of the PV loop and by the EDV:EDP ratio. Since A to B is not a straight line with a constant slope, a single slope may be either approximated, or slopes may be measured by constructing tangents to the line at any or all points.

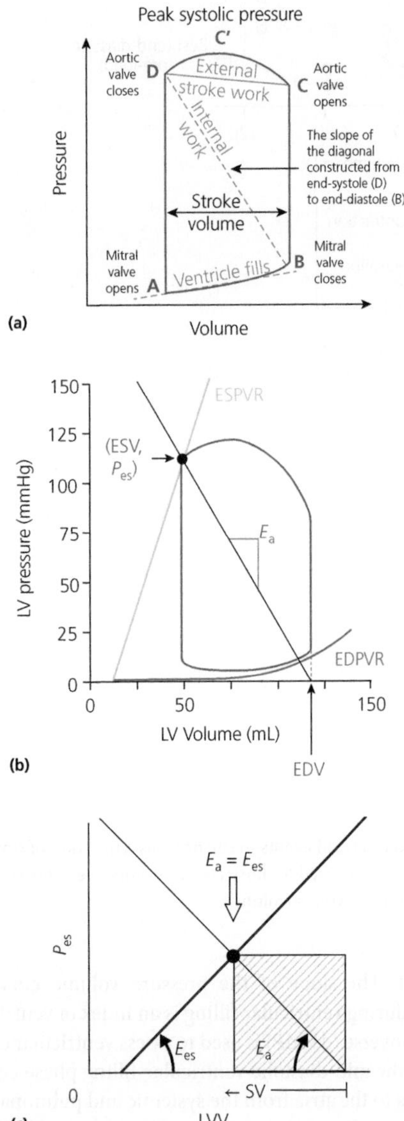

Figure 22.34 The pressure–volume relationship and E_{es}/E_a. (a) A single left ventricular pressure–volume loop provides load-independent information about ventricular systolic and diastolic function and ventricular–vascular coupling. The ventricular end-diastolic pressure at point B is an estimate of static ventricular compliance. The slope of the line from point A to point B expresses ventricular dynamic compliance. Maximum afterload occurs at point c (aortic valve opening). The aortic valve closes at point D [P_{es} in (b)] and is used to determine the end systolic pressure–volume relationship (ESPVR), used to determine the end-systolic elastance [E_{es} in (c)]. The slope of the diagonal from point D to point B expresses the arterial elastance [E_a in (b)]. (b) The ESPVR and end-diastolic pressure–volume relationship (EDPVR) are used to determine E_{es} and E_a. (c) The ratio of E_a to E_{es} expresses ventricular–vascular coupling ($E_a/E_{es} \approx 1$).

Ventricular pressure increases rapidly from B to C but there is no change in volume (isovolumetric contraction) until the semilunar valve opens (at C) and blood begins to be ejected into the aorta. Ventricular pressure changes minimally from C to D but ventricular volume decreases (isotonic contraction). The horizontal distance (BC to DA) represents the stroke volume (SV), and the ratio [(BC–DA):BC] times 100 is the ejection fraction (EF). The percentage of EDV represented by SV is considered a 'gold standard' for the general health of the cardiovascular system.

Point D of the PV loop occurs at the end of systole (ES) when ejection ceases and, soon thereafter, the semilunar valve closes. The coordinates for point D are end-systolic volume (ESV) and end-systolic pressure (ESP), and their ratio (EDP:EDV) is termed end-systolic elastance (E_{es}) or stiffness. Connecting many E_{es} values obtained from a family of PV loops produces a line termed the end-systolic pressure–volume relationship (ESPVR) or time-varying elastance, the slope of which represents myocardial contractility. The PV loop falls quickly from D to A. This constitutes the period of isovolumetric relaxation when pressure falls but ventricular volume does not change. At A, the AV valve opens, and isotonic relaxation begins as ventricular filling begins.

The total area within the PV loop represents the total work performed by the ventricle against the hindrance to ejection imposed by the arterial pressure. Total work is comprised of both internal work (caused by cycling of heavy meromyosin heads and stretching the series elastic elements) and external (i.e., moving a volume of blood against a resistance). Total work is a measure of myocardial oxygen demand (MVO_2) and, along with myocardial oxygen delivery (DO_2), can be used to estimate energetic balance (DO_2 - MVO_2).

Thus a single PV loop of the left ventricle allows the calculation of (1) lusitropy (dynamic and static diastolic function), (2) myocardial contractility, (3) stroke volume, and (4) myocardial oxygen demand. Furthermore, the ratio [(C′–DC):(BC–DA)] of pulsatile aortic pressure (C′–DC) to stroke volume (BC–DA) is the ratio of pulsatile pressure to pulsatile flow, used as an estimate of aortic input impedance, a useful monitor of ventricular–vascular coupling.

Determinants of cardiac performance and cardiac output

Cardiac performance is generally described in terms of the heart's five basic properties: chronotropy (rate), bathmotropy (excitability), dromotropy (conduction velocity), inotropy (contractility), and lusitropy (relaxation). The cardiac cycle and pressure–volume loop illustrate the temporal hemodynamic events that occur during cardiac contraction and relaxation. Clinically, M-mode echocardiography and spectral doppler are used to assess ventricular function. These techniques provide a dynamic temporal representation of cardiac function and, when coupled with hemodynamic computer software analysis systems, a pictorial and quantitative assessment of cardiac performance (Fig. 22.35).

The oxygen requirements of tissues are met by the continuous adjustment of cardiac output (CO), which is the product of heart rate (HR) and the volume of blood pumped by the heart during each cardiac cycle (stroke volume [SV]):

$$CO = HR \times SV$$

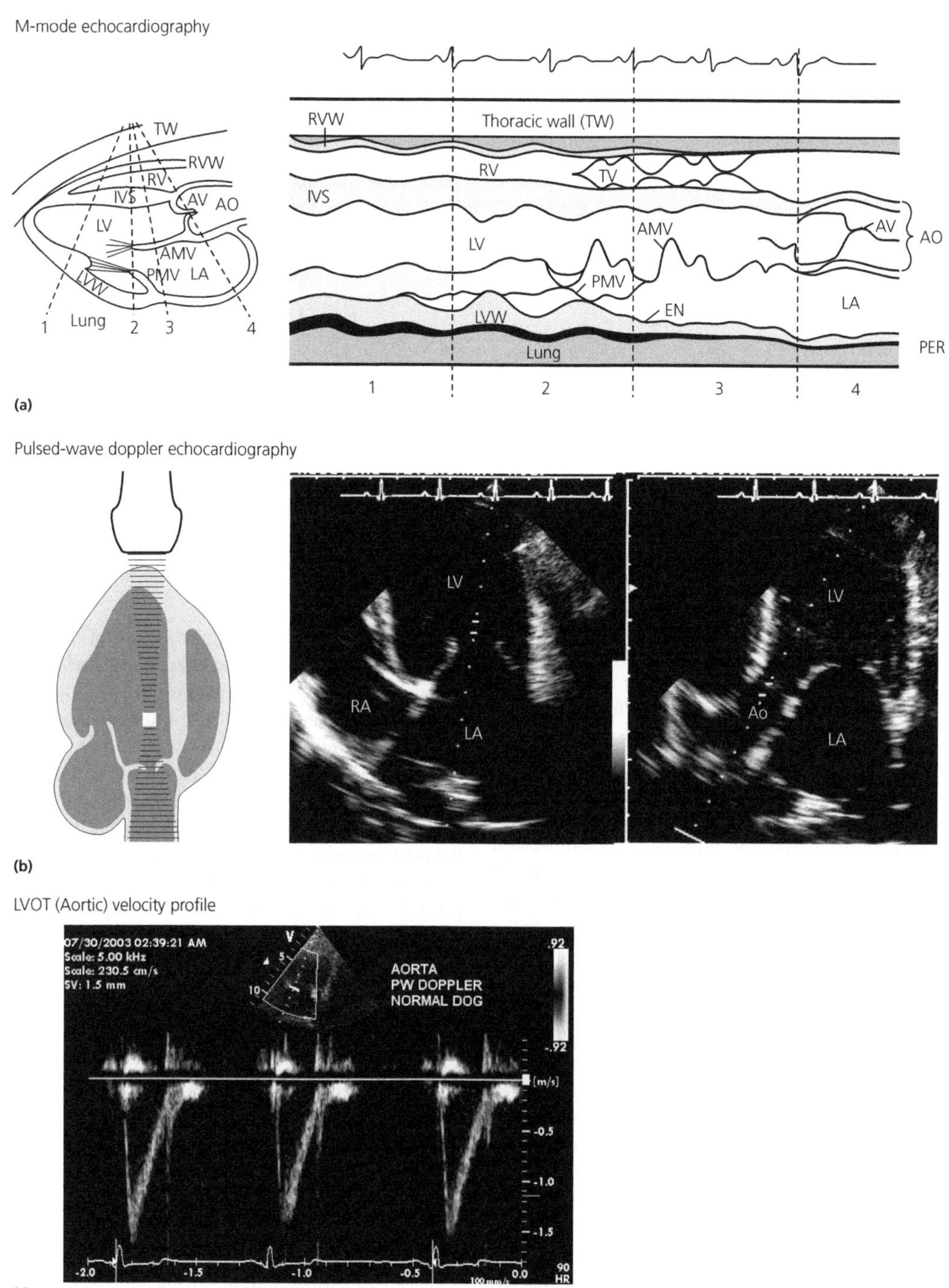

Figure 22.35 M-mode (a) and Doppler echocardiography (b and c) illustrate dynamic real-time relationships in cardiac function in animals. RVW, right ventricular wall; RV, right ventricle chamber; TV, tricuspid valve; IVS, interventricular septum; LV, left ventricular chamber; AMV, anterior mitral valve; PMV, posterior mitral valve; AV, aortic valve; AO, aorta; EN, endocardium; LVW, left ventricular wall.

Decreases in ventricular filling time and increases in total peripheral vascular resistance (TPR) limit cardiac output particularly at faster heart rates [151]:

$$CO = (MAP - CVP) / TPR$$

where MAP is mean arterial blood pressure, CVP is central venous pressure, and CO is cardiac output. Injectable anesthetics (barbiturates and propofol) and inhalant anesthetics (halothane, isoflurane, and sevoflurane) all have the potential to decrease heart rate, stroke volume, total peripheral vascular resistance, arterial blood pressure and cardiac output (Box 22.3). Stroke volume represents the difference between the end-diastolic and end-systolic ventricular volumes (SV = EDV − ESV; Fig. 22.33b). Traditionally, stroke volume has been considered to be primarily determined by cardiac contractility, and two vascular coupling factors, preload and afterload [152]. The refinement and development of more descriptive methods for the assessment of cardiac function, however, have led to

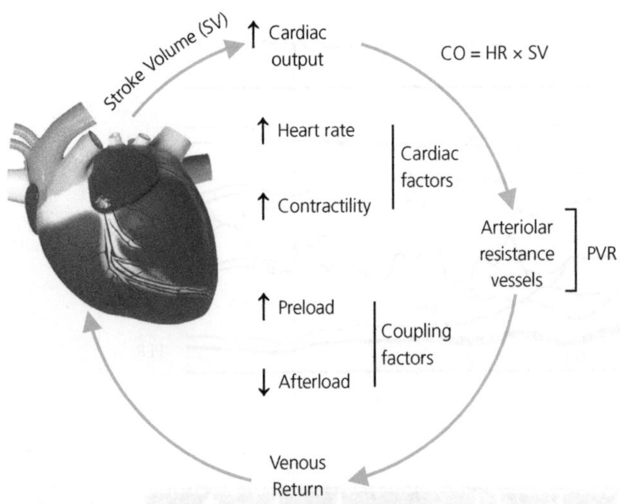

Figure 22.36 Cardiac output is equal to heart rate (HR) multiplied by stroke volume (SV), or arterial blood pressure (BP) divided by peripheral vascular resistance (PVR). Increases in heart rate, cardiac contractility, and preload and decreases in afterload can increase cardiac output. Preload and afterload are considered to be coupling factors and are modified by vascular resistance, capacitance, and compliance.

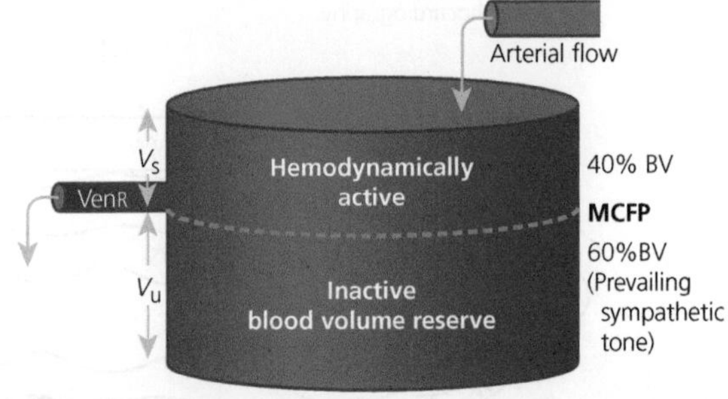

Figure 22.37 Stressed (V_s) and unstressed (V_u) volumes. Total blood volume can be divided into V_s and V_u. Blood below the venous return (VenR) hole does not affect venous return but serves as a reserve and can be mobilized by vasoconstriction. The height of the column of blood above VenR and the diameter of the hole (venous resistance) determine the rate of venous return (VR). The mean equilibration pressure when the heart is stopped is called the mean circulatory filling pressure (MCFP; 5–12 mmHg). VR = (MCFP – CVP)/venous resistance. The main determinant of the MCFP is V_s. Cardiac output (CO) is determined by VR, which is primarily determined by MCFP and CVP (MCFP – CVP). Constriction of the splanchnic veins, for example, increases MCFP, MCFP – CVP, VR, and CO.

focused consideration of relaxation (lusitropic) effects on stroke volume [153,154]. Lusitropic (compliance = 1/stiffness) properties are those that are responsible for ventricular chamber stiffness (dP/dV) or its inverse, compliance (dV/dP). It should be remembered that changes in preload, afterload, or cardiac contractile (inotropic) and relaxant (lusitropic) properties can influence one another and therefore influence stroke volume. These factors in turn are all modified by changes in heart rate, leading to a complex (mathematically coupled) interplay of variables that collectively determine cardiac output (Fig. 22.36) [151].

The terms preload and afterload, described earlier in this section as two vascular coupling determinants of cardiac output, originated from isolated muscle experiments in which preload represented the original load, length, or stretch placed on the muscle prior to its stimulation and contraction, and afterload represented the force or tension developed before the ventricle ejects. Isolated cardiac muscle studies (Langendorff system) continue to be essential for understanding and describing cardiac muscle physiology, metabolism, and muscle responses to various perturbations (hypoxia, ischemia, and drugs), and are usually presented as three-dimensional plots of force, velocity, and length [43]. Cardiac function in intact animals, however, is unlike isolated cardiac muscle, because, in addition to intrinsic factors, ventricular performance is determined by venous and arterial vascular coupling that are modulated by neurohumoral effects, pericardial and intrathoracic constraints, and atrial and ventricular contraction patterns [133,134]. Regardless, the terms preload and afterload remain popular jargon when describing ventricular performance in intact animals.

Preload

Preload is the hemodynamic load or stretch on the myocardial wall at the end of diastole just before contraction begins. There are several possible measures of preload: end-diastolic pressure (EDP), end-diastolic volume (EDV), wall stress at end-diastole, and end-diastolic sarcomere length. The EDV is directly related to the degree of stretch of myocardial sarcomeres [43]. Sarcomere length provides the most meaningful measure of muscle preload, but is impossible to measure in the intact heart. Preload in intact animals is usually explained in terms of the Frank–Starling relationship or as heterometric autoregulation: autoregulation of the strength of ventricular contraction that occurs in direct relation to the end diastolic fiber length [152]. Whether or not individual sarcomeres actually increase in length (stretch) with increases in ventricular volume is controversial (see the section Heart: Contraction and Relaxation); more likely, myofilaments simply develop an increased sensitivity to calcium, resulting in an increase in contractile force [36,42]. The Frank–Starling relationship serves as an important compensatory mechanism for maintaining stroke volume when ventricular contractility and afterload are acutely changed (Fig. 22.13). Preload is determined by venous return (VR) and venous return is dependent upon the mean circulatory filling pressure (MCFP: the pressure in all parts of the circulatory system when the heart is stopped and pressure equilibrates), the central venous pressure (CVP), and venous resistance [117,140]:

$$\text{VR} = (\text{MCFP} - \text{CVP}) / \text{venous resistance}$$

According to Gelman, Guyton, and co-workers, the main determinant of VR is MCFP (Fig. 22.37) [117,155,156]. Importantly, increases in cardiac output during fluid administration are more likely due to an increase in the MCFP and subsequent increase in VR than to increased cardiac contractility [117]. Because of the difficulty in accurately determining MCFP and ventricular volume in the clinical setting, ventricular diameter (echocardiography), ventricular EDP (cardiac catheterization), pulmonary capillary wedge pressure, and occasionally mean atrial pressure are used as estimates of preload [154]. End diastolic pressure can be assessed clinically by measuring the pulmonary capillary wedge pressure (PCWP) using a Swan–Ganz catheter that is placed through the right ventricle into the pulmonary artery. The substitution of pressure for volume, although common, must be done with the understanding that there are many instances (open-chest procedures and stiff or non-compliant hearts) when pressure does not accurately represent changes in ventricular volume and therefore is not an accurate index of preload.

Afterload

Afterload is the hydraulic load imposed on the ventricle during ejection and the term most commonly used to describe the force opposing ventricular ejection [151]. One major reason for the great interest in this physiological determinant of cardiac function is its inverse relationship with stroke volume and its direct correlation with myocardial oxygen consumption [121]. Although conceptually straightforward, clinical descriptions and use of the term afterload have suffered from multiple definitions and an incomplete understanding of what the term actually represents [157]. Afterload in isolated tissues is the force generated after the preload in order for the muscle to shorten [43]. The total load in isolated muscle experiments is therefore represented by the preload plus the afterload. In contrast to isolated muscle, afterload in intact animals changes continuously throughout ventricular ejection and is more accurately described by the tension (stress) developed by the left ventricular wall during ejection or as the arterial input impedance (Z_i) (Fig. 22.29) [158]. Ventricular wall stress or tension (T) is determined by the Laplace relationship ($T = Pr/2h$: T = tension; r = radius; h = wall thickness) [159]. In addition to ventricular wall stress, afterload in intact animals has been defined as the ventricular pressure at the end of systole (ESP), TPR, and arterial impendence. The ESP is estimated from the arterial pressure at the time of outlet valve closure and can be approximated by the mean pulmonary or arterial pressure for their respective ventricles.

A much more accurate, yet technically challenging, method for assessing afterload in intact animals is to measure ventricular–vascular coupling [134,160,161]. Arterial input impedance is an expression of the arterial system's response to pulsatile blood flow and is a function of arterial pressure, arterial wall elasticity, vessel dimensions down to the point where pulsations are attenuated, and blood viscosity (see Hemorrheology). Arterial input impedance incorporates time-varying resistance components (pressure and flow) and reactance components (elastance). The measurement of arterial input impedance requires the simultaneous and instantaneous measurement of aortic root pressure and flow [158]. Both waveforms are subjected to a Fourier transformation from which a series of sine waves and frequencies are derived. The characteristic impedance (Z_0) can be determined by averaging the impedance moduli at high frequencies (Fig. 22.29). The characteristic impedance is the pressure–flow relationship where pressure and flow waves are not influenced by wave reflection (it approximates input impedance during maximum vasodilation). Characteristic impedance is approximately 5% of the total arterial resistance and is generally a sensitive indicator of vessel wall elasticity or compliance. The impedance modulus at zero frequency (non-pulsatile flow) is equivalent to vascular resistance (R) and is usually described as TPR. Although much less accurate than the determination of impedance moduli, particularly when assessing the progression of cardiac disease or drugs that change both cardiac and vascular properties simultaneously, the measurement of TPR is used clinically as a measure of afterload and vascular tone because it is technically simple to obtain and intuitively easier to understand.

Contractility

Cardiac contractility (inotropy) is the intrinsic ability of the heart to generate force and, as such, relates directly to physicochemical processes and the availability of intracellular calcium (see Heart: Excitation–Contraction Coupling) [37]. Homeometric autoregulation is the term frequently applied to those factors, other than muscle fiber length, that influence the force of cardiac contraction. Contractility is generally described in isolated muscle preparations by shifts of the force–velocity–length relationship or in intact animals by shifts in the ventricular function curve (e.g., shifts in the Frank–Starling relationship) (Fig. 22.13) [43]. Notably, these methods are so-called 'load dependent,' implying that changes in other factors (heart rate, preload, afterload) influence the results obtained. A decrease in cardiac contractility is a key factor that can decrease cardiac output and potentially induce heart failure in animals with cardiac disease or following the administration excessive amounts of an anesthetic drug [162–164].

Ideally, indices of cardiac contractility should be load independent: changes in heart rate, preload, afterload, and cardiac size. Many indices of contractility have evolved in an attempt to develop a truly load-independent measure of cardiac contractile activity. These indices vary considerably in their load dependency, sensitivity, and specificity as measures of cardiac contractility, and generally fall into one of four broad categories: (1) isovolumic contraction phase indices, (2) ejection phase indices, (3) pressure–

Box 22.4 Hemodynamic indices of systolic and diastolic function.

Systolic function

1 Isovolumic indices
   - a Echocardiographic assessment (M-mode, two-dimensional, Doppler)
   - b dP/dt_{max} dP/dt_{40}, and $dP/dt/V_{ed}$
   - c V_{max}
   - d Power; rate of charge of power
2 Ejection-phase indices
   - a Echocardiographic assessment (M-mode, two-dimensional, Doppler)
   - b Cardiac output
   - c Ejection fraction, (EDV – ESV)/EDV
   - d Stroke work
   - e Maximum velocity of circumferential shortening
   - f Left ventricular ejection time
   - g Preejection period
3 Pressure-volume indices
   - a Echocardiographic assessment (M-mode, two-dimensional, Doppler)
   - b E_{es} and E_{max}
   - c End-systolic pressure-volume ratios
   - d T_{max} (time to E_{max})
4 Stress-strain indices
   - a Elastic stiffness (stress/strain)
   - b End-systolic stress-volume ratio

Diastolic function

1 Isovolumic relaxation indices (pressure derived)
   - a Echocardiographic assessment (M-mode, two-dimensional, Doppler)
   - b dP/dt_{min}
   - c Time constant of left ventricular pressure fall (T)
   - d Relaxation time
   - e $-dT/dt$ (tension fall)
2 Diastolic filling indices
   - a dP/dV
   - b Peak filling rate (dV/dt_{max})
   - c Chamber stiffness (dP/dV vs. P)
3 End-diastolic indices
   - a End-diastolic pressure
   - b End-diastolic P/V ratio
4 Interval-derived indices
   - a Echocardiographic assessment (M-mode, two-dimensional, Doppler)
   - b Time to $-dP/dt_{min}$; time to 50% $-dP/dt_{min}$
   - c Diastolic filling time
   - d Isovolumic relaxation period
   - e Time from minimal left ventricular dimension to mitral valve opening

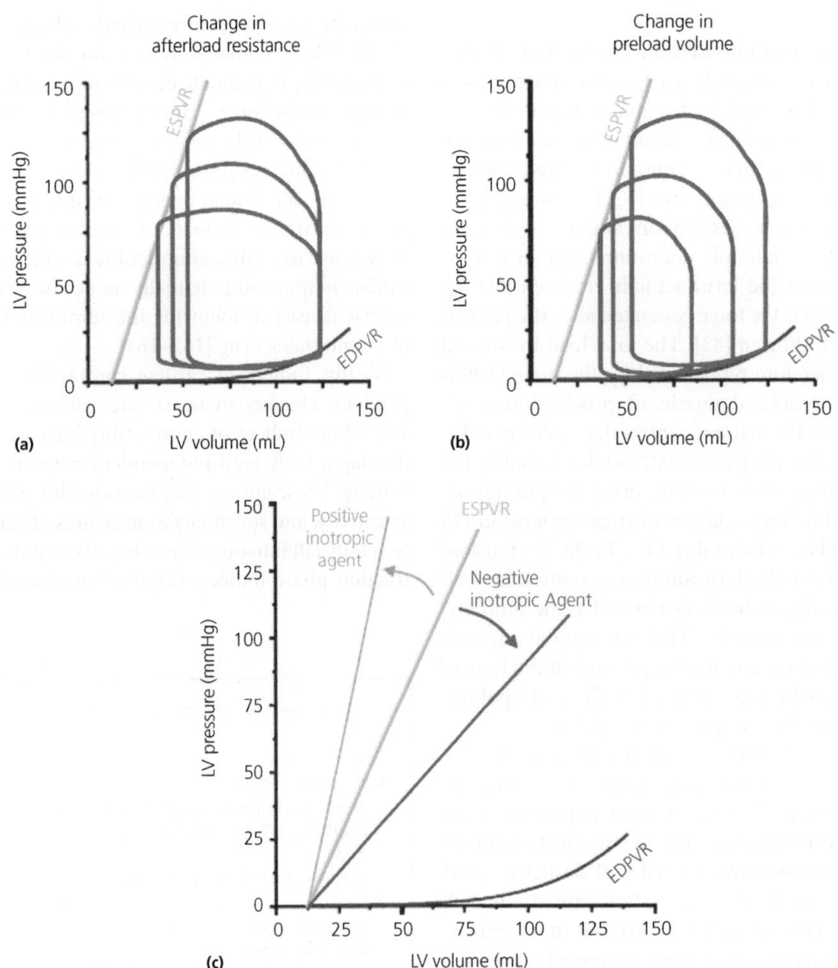

Figure 22.38 (a) Three PV loops with the same EDV but different aortic pressures: the total peripheral resistance was increased. The upper left-hand corner of each loop falls on the ESPVR; the bottom right part of the loop falls on the EDPVR (see Fig. 22.34). (b) Three different loops are shown that have different EDVs and different aortic pressures. The loops were obtained by decreasing venous return. (c) Changes in contractility change ventricular pressure generation and stroke volume. Drugs that increase the slope of the ESPVR increase E_{es}. E_{es} is the slope of the linear relation or end-systolic elastance. E_{es} is considered to be a reliable and accurate index of ventricular contractility because E_{es} varies with ventricular contractility but is not affected by changes in arterial system properties or changes in EDV. The pressure at end systole is the P_{es} [$P_{es} = E_{es}(V - V_0)$]. P_{es} is the end-systolic pressure, V_0 is the ventricular volume when $P = 0$, and V is the volume of interest.

volume relationship indices, and (4) stress–strain relationship indices (Box 22.4). Although many approaches for assessing cardiac contractility are useful experimentally and clinically, only the isovolumic phase indices (because of their ease of measurement), the pressure–volume relationship indices (because of their load independence), and the ejection phase index (preload recruitable stroke work: area enclosed within the LV pressure–volume loop plotted against the EDV) have gained acceptance. Additionally, the measurement of the pressure–volume relationship can be used to assess the systolic, diastolic, and myocardial energetic properties of the heart [165].

The slope of the end-systolic pressure–volume relationship (ESPVR) and end-systolic elastance (E_{es}) can be determined, under a constant level of contractility, by measuring the change in ESV (produced by partial venous occlusion) at several magnitudes of ESP (Figs 22.34a and 22.38a,b). The slope of the ESPVR is the most useful and accurate load-independent estimate of inherent cardiac contractility currently available (Fig. 22.38c).

Relaxation

Lusitropy refers to the ability of the myocardium to relax following excitation–contraction coupling and is fundamentally important to an understanding of cardiac performance [153]. The most popular and clinically relevant definition of diastole states that relaxation begins with the closure of the aortic valve, which is heralded by the second heart sound [S_2 (Fig. 22.33a)] [166]. Diastole is thereafter divided into four phases: (1) isovolumic relaxation, (2) early rapid ventricular filling, (3) slow ventricular filling (diastasis), and (4) atrial systole (during sinus rhythm). Mechanical factors, loading factors, inotropic activity, heart rate, and asynchronicity (patterns of relaxation) are the major determinants of lusitropy. Factors and interventions that specifically alter the relaxation properties of the heart are of special interest because of their importance in determining ventricular compliance or stiffness. A partial list of methods used to quantitatively describe relaxation includes pressure, volume-derived, and interval indices (Box 22.4). Indices of isovolumetric relaxation [rate of ventricular pressure decline (–d*P*/d*t*) and

Table 22.4 Pharmacologic effects of clinically relevant doses of commonly administered anesthetic drugs[a]

Drug	HR	Rhythm	ABP	CO	Cardiac Contractile Force	MCFP	Vessel Tone	Baroreceptor Reflex Activity	Sympathetic Nerve Activity	Splanchnic Venous Capacitance	Venous Return
Inhalant anesthetic	↑↓±	+	↓↓	↓↓	↓	↓↓	↓↓	↓↓	↓↓	↑↑	↓↓
Injectable hypnotic											
Propofol	±↓	+	↓↓	↓	↓	↓	↓	↓	↓	↑↑	↓↓
Etomidate	±	0	↓	↓	↓	±↓	±↓	±↓	±↓	↑	±↓
Barbiturate	±↑	+	±	↓	↓	±↓	↓	↓	↓	↑	↓
Neurosteroid	±↓	+	↓	↓	±↓	±↓	±↓	↓	↓	↑	↓
Chloralose	↓	0	±	±	±	±	±	±	±	±	±
Dissociative											
Ketamine	↑	+	↑	↑±	↑±	0	0	0	0↑	0	0
Tileatimine	↑	+	↑	↑±	↑±	0	0	0	0↑	0	0
Opioid											
Morphine	↓	0	–↓	–↓	0↓	0	0	0↓	0↓	0	0↓
Hydromorphone	↓	0	–↓	–↓	0↓	0	0	0↓	0↓	0	0↓
Fentanyl	↓	0	–↓	–↓	0↓	0	0	0↓	0↓	0	0↓
α_2-Agonist	↓↓	+	↑→↓	↓↓	0↓	↑→↓	↑→↓	0↓	0	↓→↑	↑→↓
Benzodiazepine											
Diazepam	0↑	0	0	0↓	0	0↓	0↓	0	0↓	0↓	0↓
Midazolam		0									
Phenothiazine											
Acepromazine	±↓	0	↓	0↓	0↓	↓	↓	↓	↓	↑	↓
Local anesthetic											
Lidocaine	±↑	–	↓	0↓	0↓	↓	↓	0	↓	↑	↓
Bupivacaine	±↑	–	↓	0↓	0↓	↓	↓	0	↓	↑	↓

[a]Clinicvally relevant dosages are generally equal to or less than those recommended by the manufacturer. Idealized effects expected from normal healthy dogs; ↑ = increase; ↓ = decrease; ± = increase or decrease; 0 = little or no change; ↑→↓ = increase followed by decease; ↓→↑ = decrease followed by increase; + = potentially arrhythmogenic; – = anti-arrhythmic

the time constant for relaxation (τ)] are useful for measuring the active phase of relaxation and reflect the dissociation of actin–myosin linkages because of reuptake of cytoplasmic calcium by the sarcoplasmic reticulum. Both indices are influenced by myocardial systolic function, ventricular loading conditions (preload and afterload), and heart rate and are therefore considered to be load dependent.

Regardless of the care in picking an index to evaluate cardiac systolic, diastolic, or contractile performance, it is clear that even greater thought must be given to the factors (determinants of performance) that influence the selected index. Drugs used as preanesthetic medication or for intravenous or inhalation anesthesia can produce profound effects on the cardiovascular system and indices of cardiac performance. Furthermore, greater consideration should be given to the effects of anesthetic drugs on venous function, MCFP, and VR. The venous vascular effects of anesthetics on the effective circulating blood volume are much more complex than originally surmised and can be responsible for precipitous and dramatic decreases in cardiac output (Table 22.4).

Ventricular–vascular coupling

Measures of both systolic and diastolic function have been expressed (both correctly and incorrectly) by many methods (e.g., maximal rates of rise and fall of intraventricular pressure, ratio of stroke volume to end-diastolic volume); however, the 'gold standard' (most correct) is to analyze plots of left ventricular pressure versus left ventricular volume (pressure–volume loops) from a family of pressure–volume loops obtained during a stepwise decrement in preload, usually achieved by occlusion of the caudal vena cava. It is important to determine both the systolic (force-generating ability) and diastolic (lusitropic or filling properties) function of the ventricle, and how the ventricle interacts with the arterial tree (ventricular–vascular coupling). This is relevant both to the pathogenesis of disease and to how therapy may remediate disease.

Venous return curve

The modern concept of ventricular–vascular coupling has been popularized by Guyton and co-workers, who used the vascular function curve, and more precisely the venous-return curve ('Guyton diagram') and cardiac (ventricular) function curve, to predict changes in cardiac output (Fig. 22.39) [155,156]. Guyton's ventricular–vascular coupling diagrams emphasized that the important independent variables for determination of cardiac output are the sums of vascular resistances and capacitances and cardiac contractility [155]. The 'Guyton diagram' illustrates the inverse relationship between venous pressure (CVP) and cardiac output (Fig. 22.39). The horizontal (abscissa) intercept of the venous-return curve or the venous pressure at zero cardiac output is MCFP, which is a function of venous capacitance and the total blood volume and has been directly correlated with survival from hemorrhagic and septic shock [167]. Variations in the venous-return curve can be produced by altering venous resistance, capacitance, or blood volume (Fig. 22.37). Equilibrium of the venous return–ventricular function curve is reached when venous return at a given pressure is matched by the ability of the ventricle to pump the blood returning to the heart (venous return). Thus, if venous pressure is increased (rapid fluid administration), cardiac output increases during the next cardiac cycle. Increases in cardiac output in turn transfer blood from the venous to the arterial circulation, thereby decreasing venous pressure. This process continues in progressively decreasing steps until a new equilibrium for cardiac output and venous return is reached, realizing that only one equilibrium point for cardiac output and venous return exists. Similar rationalizations can be used for other perturbations: changes in blood volume, arterial resistance, and cardiac contractility [157,165,167].

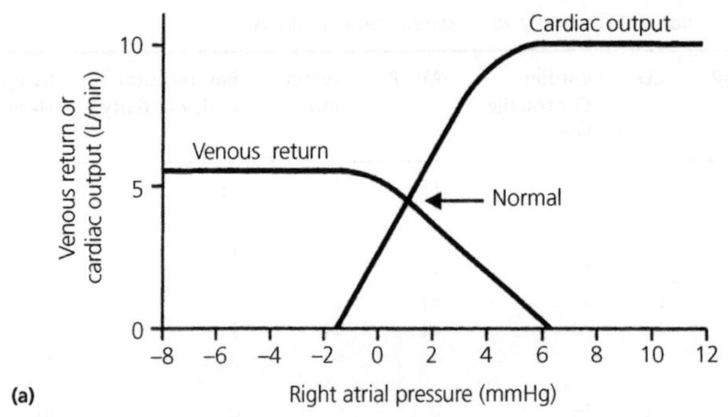

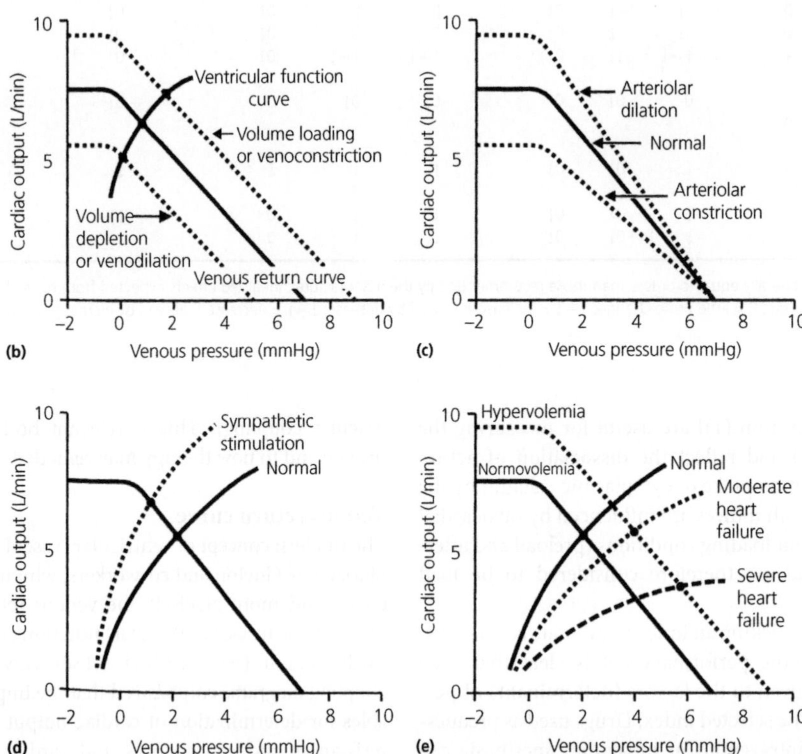

Figure 22.39 Venous return curves curves (Guyton diagrams). (a) Venous return and cardiac output (Guyton curves) are determined by the opposing effects of right atrial pressure. For example, increases in right atrial pressure increase cardiac output, but decrease venous return. Alterations in (b) blood volume, (c) sympathetic tone, (d) vascular tone, and (e) cardiac function produce predictable effects upon the coupling of venous return to cardiac output at a given venous pressure. Note that during moderate heart failure (e), cardiac output is preserved at the expense of increases in venous pressure.

It can be argued that this type of presentation of hemodynamics and cardiovascular function results in circular reasoning (mathematical coupling), since a change in cardiac output can be used to explain the change in venous return and vice versa. Indeed, since both venous return and cardiac output are dependent upon the flow around the circuit, the equilibrium point at which a given cardiac output is produced is a function of venous and arterial capacitance and resistance, blood volume, and cardiac contractility.

Ventricular–arterial coupling

Arterial constructs of ventricular–vascular coupling focus on the left ventricular pressure–volume relationship and the ejection of blood into the ascending aorta (ventricular–arterial coupling; Fig. 22.34b) [13,147,152,168,169]. The power of this approach stems from its capability to detect cardiovascular disease and identify probable causes for the pathogenesis of disease and the ability to derive a multitude of important indices for assessing cardiovascular function in intact animals [165].

The inscription of the instantaneous pressure–volume loop permits the calculation of load-dependent and -independent measures of cardiac contractility, myocardial oxygen requirements, and myocardial efficiency [152]. For example, the ratio of ventricular pressure to ventricular volume (dP/dV: time-varying elastance) varies throughout the cardiac cycle and inscription of the pressure–volume loop. Acute reductions in preload are used to produce progressively smaller pressure–volume loops and construct a straight line by connecting all of the end-systolic points. This line is known as the end-systolic pressure–volume relationship, as previously stated, the slope of which is the end-systolic ventricular elastance (E_{es}), a load-independent index directly proportional to ventricular contractility (Fig. 22.38a,b). The mechanical work [stroke work (SW)] performed by the heart is proportional to the pressure–volume area (PVA: area within the pressure-volume curve), which is linearly related to myocardial oxygen consumption (MVO_2), and which, when plotted against the end-diastolic volume, derives another sensitive and load-independent index of cardiac contractility termed preload recruitable stroke work (PRSW). Mechanical efficiency (ME) of the heart is the ratio of SW to MVO_2 and is derived by dividing SW by PVA (ME = SW/PVA).

The ejection of blood into the ascending aorta is governed by the same resistive and reactive (viscoelastic) properties that govern venous return. These arterial loading properties (afterload) influence stroke volume [55]. The difference between the end-diastolic and end-systolic volumes of the pressure–volume relationship is stroke volume, which, when plotted versus end-systolic pressure (P_{es}) during decreases in stroke volume, renders a line, the slope of which is the effective arterial elastance (E_a) (Fig. 22.34a,b). In practice, E_a is generally approximated by the ratio of P_{es} to stroke volume ($P_{es}/SV = E_a$). This parameter is particularly powerful because it incorporates the principal elements of vascular load (afterload), including peripheral resistance, total vascular compliance, characteristic impedance (see the section Determinants of Cardiac Performance and Cardiac Output), and alterations induced by heart rate changes. It is noteworthy that the purely resistive components of vascular load are adequately accounted for by determining the steady-state or non-pulsatile parameter, total peripheral resistance, which accounts for approximately 90% of vascular load under normal conditions. The pulsatile or dynamic component of vascular load generally accounts for approximately 10% of vascular load under normal conditions, adds to the resistive component, and becomes increasingly important during cardiovascular disease, changes in blood volume, or following the administration of drugs that affect the cardiovascular system [154,162–164]. Other methods for accurately analyzing arterial afterload have been described (see the section Determinants of Cardiac Performance and Cardiac Output).

Because both E_{es} and E_a have the measurement of P_{es} and ventricular volume in common, they can be plotted on a single graph to yield the 'ideal' ventricular-arterial coupling point for any set of cardiovascular circumstances (Fig. 22.34b). Stated another way, if end-diastolic volume (preload), E_a, and E_{es} are known, stroke volume and therefore cardiac output (CO = SV × HR) can be predicted. Furthermore, this analysis predicts that SW should be maximized when this relationship is equal to one ($E_{es} = E_a$) and that maximal mechanical efficiency (ME) is attained when $E_a = E_{es}/2$, since ME = SW/PVA = $1/(1 + E_a/E_{es}/2)$ [170].

The ideal ventricular-arterial coupling point in intact animals occurs when mean arterial pressure is adequate for organ flow (approximately 60–70 mmHg) and, as stated earlier, systolic pressure is low while diastolic pressure is high (small pressure pulse). Low systolic pressure facilitates maximal ventricular ejection and low oxygen demands by the myocardium, whereas high diastolic pressure ensures adequate coronary perfusion. Ideal ventricular arterial interaction is impaired by anything that decreases cardiac contractility (decreased E_{es}) or increases arterial stiffness (increased E_a). Increases in arterial stiffness increase pulse amplitude, increasing systolic pressure and thereby decreasing stroke volume for a given cardiac contraction while increasing MVO_2. Diastolic pressure usually falls, thereby reducing coronary blood flow and myocardial perfusion. Furthermore, alterations in the timing of pulse-wave reflection, principally initiated by increases in arteriolar tone, could augment systolic pressure and reduce diastolic pressure, exacerbating the situation [10,55,65].

Physiologic and Mathematical Coupling

Safe anesthetic practice is dependent upon accurate monitoring of anesthetic drug-related effects. This generally entails methods (corneal, palpebral reflexes, jaw tone) and techniques (physical, mechanical, electrical) for determining the level of consciousness (qualitative, categorical) and quantitatively assessing cardiorespiratory variables. Most experimental studies detailing anesthetic drug effects in humans and animals frequently include additional derived or calculated variables (cardiac output, vascular resistance, cardiac work, oxygen delivery and consumption) in order to provide more detailed information on drug-related effects. This information is then used to clarify and justify interpretations of drug actions. Since all data are subject to statistical analysis, it is beneficial to know if the variable under consideration is a dependent ('effect,' 'response,' 'output') or independent ('controlled,' 'manipulated') variable. A dependent variable may be a measured variable, such as directly measured rate, pressure, or flow, or a calculated variable whose value is determined by independent variables. For example, changes in heart rate (dependent variable) are often explained by drug-induced changes in arterial blood pressure (independent variable). The description of data describing anesthetic drug-induced effects, therefore, must be done carefully since any variable can be considered to be dependent upon something else. Arterial blood pressure, for example, can be considered a dependent variable, since its value depends on the instant of time at which it is measured and the position in the arterial or venous system that it is measured. Thus, it depends on the independent variables of time and position. Anesthetic drug-induced changes in arterial blood pressure are also often explained as a function of two other dependent variables, vascular resistance and cardiac output. These variables are all physiologically coupled. Furthermore, it is known that vascular resistance depends directly on blood viscosity – the higher the viscosity the higher is the resistance – and since viscosity depends on hematocrit, the higher the hematocrit the higher is the viscosity. Therefore, it is not surprising to find a relationship indicating that increases in peripheral vascular resistance are associated with increasing hematocrit and vice versa.

This is an example of physiologic coupling and is predictable because of the known dependence of vascular resistance on viscosity and the dependence of viscosity on hematocrit. Physiologic coupling between two dependent variables means that there is a common component variable upon which they both depend. Physiologic coupling must be considered when interpreting cardiorespiratory anesthetic drug-related effects and emphasizes the importance of identifying independent and dependent variables. Physiologic coupling is further complicated in many studies investigating the cardiovascular effects of anesthetic drugs by mathematical coupling, which leads to even greater errors in data analysis and interpretation. Mathematical coupling occurs when the relationship between two variables is due to a common component, where one of the variables is contained in the other variable or a third dependent variable is common to both variables [171,172]. For example, the product of cardiac output and arterial–venous oxygen difference can be used to calculate oxygen consumption using the Fick principle. This approach is frequently adopted to determine the critical point at which oxygen consumption becomes oxygen supply dependent. Mathematical coupling occurs because cardiac output and arterial oxygen content are used to calculate both variables (i.e., oxygen consumption and oxygen delivery). When variables with shared components are plotted, mathematical coupling of the random errors in both variables produces bias that confounds the true physiologic relationship.

Neurohumoral and local control mechanisms

Anesthesia is dependent upon the uptake or absorption, distribution, and elimination of anesthetic drugs. The diverse tissue volumes and their blood flows, drug tissue solubilities, and mechanisms of metabolism determine drug plasma concentration and final drug effects. Drugs are delivered to the various tissues of the body based upon the distribution of cardiac output (Table 22.5). On a per unit tissue volume basis, however, a greater portion of the cardiac output and therefore drug is distributed to 'vessel-rich' group (VRG: heart, brain, liver, kidney, splanchnic bed) tissues than to muscle group (MG: muscle, skin) or vessel-poor group (VPG: fat, bone, cartilage) tissues [173]. The distribution and regulation of blood flow, therefore, are a key factor in the onset, magnitude, and duration of drug effect. The regulatory control of the cardiovascular system and tissue blood flow is integrated through the combined effects of the central and peripheral nervous systems, the influence of circulating (humoral) vasoactive substances, and local tissue mediators [173–175]. These regulatory processes maintain blood flow at an appropriate level while distributing blood to meet the needs of tissue beds that have the greatest oxygen demand. Most organs compensate for changes in arterial blood pressure over the physiologic range by autoregulation. Autoregulation is defined as the physiologic maintenance of a constant flow over a moderate range of perfusion pressures. Notably, anesthesia depresses autoregulatory mechanisms [176].

Tissue blood flow is regulated by the integration of supraregional [central nervous system (CNS)], regional, and local factors. Together these factors coordinate immediate and long-term adjustments in cardiac output, total peripheral vascular resistance, vascular capacitance, and blood volume [117,174,175]. Higher brain centers, including the hypothalamus (pain and temperature) and cerebral cortex (emotions: vigilance and fear), facilitate or modify cardiovascular responses. Continuous adjustments in cardiovascular system function and reflex responses to both mechanical and chemical stimuli help to buffer significant changes in arterial blood pressure and intravascular volume and sustain oxygen and nutrient delivery to tissues (Box 22.5).

The autonomic nervous system exerts a major influence on the regulation of cardiovascular function [177,178]. Peripheral receptors, including baroreceptors, mechanoreceptors, and chemoreceptors, respond to changes in blood pressure, volume, or gas tensions, respectively, and send information to the CNS through afferent nerves [174]. These sensory signals are integrated, in 'control centers' located in the hypothalamus, pons, and medulla, into responses carried by efferent sympathetic or parasympathetic nerves to the periphery. The autonomic nervous system also modulates the release of various peptides providing a generalized humoral influence on cardiac contractile performance and vascular tone [177,178]. Minute-to-minute changes in blood flow are regulated by local control mechanisms, which are somewhat independent from nervous system input [179]. Vasodilator substances, primarily the by-products of tissue metabolism, act on small vessels, producing vasodilation proportional to the amount of metabolite produced. In addition, the vascular endothelium is known to modulate both local and neural control mechanisms through the release of prostaglandins and endothelium-derived factors, such as nitric oxide (Fig. 22.31b). Anesthetic drugs can and do interfere with the sensory (input), neural integration (processing), and effector

Table 22.5 Distribution of cardiac output.

Organ	% of Total
1. Heart	4
2. Brain	14
3. Kidneys	20
4. Gastrointestinal tract	22
5. Resting skeletal muscle	20
6. Skin	8
7. Other organs	12

Box 22.5 Cardiovascular and pulmonary reflexes and effects.

1. Anrep effect: increases in aortic pressure result in a positive inotropic effect, augmented resistance to outflow in the heart.
2. Branham's sign: slowing of the heart rate following compression or excision of an arteriovenous fistula (e.g., patent ductus arteriosus ligation).
3. Bainbridge reflex: an increase in heart rate caused by a rise in blood pressure in the great veins as they enter the right atrium.
4. Bezold–Jarisch reflex: afferent and efferent pathways in the vagus nerve – stimulation of cardiac, primarily ventricular, chemoreceptors or stretch receptors (mechanoreceptors) induces sinus bradycardia, hypotension, and peripheral vasodilation. Stretch of ventricular mechanoreceptors is responsible for syncope when standing.
5. Bayliss effect: stretch of vascular smooth muscle causes muscle contraction and increased resistance, which returns blood flow to towards normal.
6. High-pressure baroreceptor or pressoreceptor reflex: decreases in heart rate initiated by increases in arterial blood pressure. A decrease in arterial pressure produces hyperventilation.
7. Atrial stretch-receptor reflex: atrial distension causes the release of atrial natriuretic peptide (ANP) from the atria, resulting in diuretic activity, vasodilation, and aldosterone secretion. ANP is an endogenous antagonist of angiotensin II. Sinus and supraventricular tachycardias are common stimuli for this response.
8. Vasovagal reflex: initiated by a decrease in venous return to the heart (e.g., hypovolemia, orthostasis, compression of the inferior vena cava, and regional analgesia), causing sinus bradycardia and vasodilation. The term has come to include neurocardiogenic syncope, carotid sinus syndrome, and micturition syncope in human patients.
9. Craniocardiac reflex: stimulation of cranial nerves (olfactory, ophthalmic, and trigeminal), resulting in bradycardia and hypotension (depressor effects).
10. Abdominocardiac reflex: mechanical stimulation of the abdominal viscera causes changes in heart rate, usually slowing; rarely causes extrasystoles.
11. Oculocardiac reflex (Aschner's reflex): compression of the eyeball causes slowing of sinus heart rate.
12. Hering–Breuer reflex: effects of the vagus in the control of respiration – lung inflation arrests inspiration, and lung deflation initiates inspiration.
13. Pulmonary chemoreflex: stimulation of C-fiber endings [juxtapulmonary capillary receptors (J receptors)] by tissue damage, fluid accumulation and accumulation of cytokines produces sinus bradycardia, hypotension, shallow breathing and apnea, bronchoconstriction, and mucous secretion (e.g., isoflurane administration).
14. Venorespiratory reflex: increases in right atrial pressure stimulate increases in respiration.
15. Cough reflex: stimulation of the larynx, trachea, or main bronchi or chemical stimulation throughout the respiratory tree result in cough.
16. Vagovagal reflex: afferent and efferent pathways in the vagus nerve – stimulation or irritation of the larynx or trachea by a laryngoscope or endotracheal tube precipitates bradycardia.

Box 22.6 Factors that regulate arterial blood pressure and tissue perfusion.

Immediate (short term)
1 Autonomic nervous system (sympathetic and parasympathetic)
Regulates heart rate and vessel tone and capacity
2 Vascular baroreceptor or pressoreceptor reflexes (stretch receptors)
Regulate heart rate and vessel tone and capacity
3 Cardiac stretch receptors
Regulate heart rate and vessel tone and capacity
4 Chemoreceptor reflexes sense changes in oxygen and carbon dioxide (hydrogen ions)
Regulate heart rate and vessel tone
5 Bloodborne (humoral) responses (epinephrine and norepinephrine)
Regulate heart rate, vessel tone, and cardiac contractility
6 Local factors
Arteriolar oxygen partial pressure
Decreased oxygen produces vasodilatation and vice versa
Local metabolites
Increased production of carbon dioxide, hydrogen ions, and lactate
Myogenic autoregulation
Adjusts vessel tone to changes in blood pressure

Intermediate
1 Transcapillary fluid shifts (Starling's law of the capillary)
Regulate fluid filtration and reabsorption
2 Hormonal responses (renin and angiotensin)
Regulate vessel tone and salt and water retention

Long term
1 Oral fluid consumption
Regulates net fluid intake
2 Renal control system (vasopressin [ADH], aldosterone, and atrial natriuretic peptide)
Regulates total body water and renal fluid output

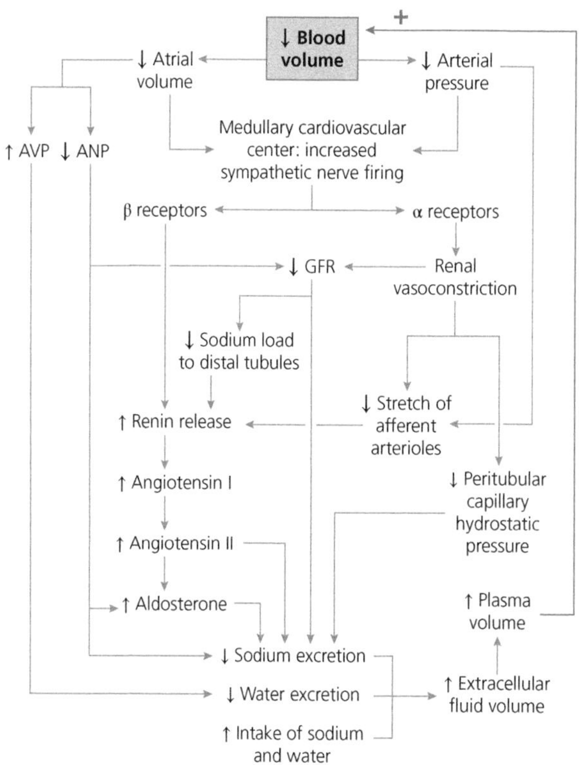

Figure 22.40 Neurohumoral response to a decrease in blood volume.

(output) mechanisms that control cardiovascular function [180–184]. Inhalation anesthetics in particular blunt compensatory responses to blood loss, trauma, fluid administration and resuscitative drugs (catecholamines, vasopressors) and if (when) administered in excessive amounts can totally abolish homeostatic control mechanisms [185]. Normally a decrease in arterial blood pressure in conscious animals is sensed by a variety of central and peripheral vascular baroreceptors, which are the most important short-term determinants of arterial blood pressure. Output from these receptors triggers readjustments in CNS autonomic output, which compensates for small changes in arterial blood pressure. Local myogenic autoregulation also helps to protect the brain, heart, liver, mesentery, and skeletal muscle from small changes in blood pressure. If arterial blood pressure is reduced to a point that tissue blood flow is negatively affected, CNS centers are activated, leading to substantial increases in heart rate, cardiac contractility, and vascular tone. Epinephrine and norepinephrine are released from the adrenal glands, which, combined with increases in sympathetic tone and activation of the renin–angiotensin system, intensify vasoconstriction (Box 22.6). Blood flow is redistributed to the lungs, heart, and brain and away from the skin, skeletal muscle, and kidney and splanchnic viscera. Additionally, peripheral chemoreceptors sense changes in the blood oxygen tension (PaO_2) and pH. The acute onset of hypoxemia or hypercarbia (acidemia) in conjunction with hypotension can induce peripheral vasoconstriction. If blood pressure is not restored, capillary hydrostatic pressure decreases, promoting the movement of fluid from the interstitial space into the capillaries, thus increasing intravascular volume. The intravascular shift of extravascular fluid can restore up to 50% of the intravascular volume in a relatively short period (hours) [117]. The constriction of the peripheral vasculature, centralization of blood volume, redistribution of the blood flow, and increase in cardiac output and arterial blood pressure are generally capable of restoring tissue perfusion, provided that the episode of hypotension or blood loss does not exceed the body's compensatory capabilities.

Neurohumoral control

Nervous system regulation of the cardiovascular system and blood volume depends on three components within the nervous system: afferent input, central integration and processing, and efferent output [177,178]. Neural and hormonal factors, including osmoreceptors in the hypothalamus, antidiuretic hormone released by neurons in the supraoptic and paraventricular nuclei, aldosterone and renin produced by the kidney, and the release of atrial natriuretic peptide (ANP) by atrial receptors sensitive to stretch, are all integrally involved in maintaining plasma and therefore blood volume. The one mechanism above all others, however, that dominates the control of plasma and blood volume is the effect of blood volume on arterial blood pressure and the consequences of arterial blood pressure on the urinary excretion of sodium and water (Fig. 22.40) [184]. Alterations in arterial blood pressure, therefore, can have profound effects on the differential distribution of blood flow among tissue beds, fluid exchange (gut, kidney), and blood volume (natriuresis and pressure diuresis). The interplay of these mechanisms ultimately controls hemodynamics, blood volume, extracellular fluid volume, and renal excretion of salt and water (Fig. 22.40).

Afferent input

Afferent input to the CNS is received from peripheral sensors that respond to acute changes in blood pressure, blood volume, and tissue metabolism (oxygenation). These peripheral sensors are the first step in a reflex arc in which the effector organs are the heart and vasculature. The reflex arc generally operates as a negative-feedback system designed to maintain a variable blood pressure at a fixed value, or set point [174].

Arterial baroreceptors are stretch receptors (mechanoreceptors) located in the carotid sinus and aortic arch that respond to increases in arterial blood pressure by incremental increases in the firing rate of sensory fibers, which are carried by the glossopharyngeal and vagus nerves. These impulses travel to the nucleus tractus solitarius within the CNS, are processed, and initiate an effector response that returns blood pressure to its normal range (Fig. 22.41). This response is accomplished by parasympathetic activation, which decreases heart rate and inhibition of sympathetic vasoconstrictor output to arterioles and veins. Baroreceptors become inoperative at an arterial blood pressure below 60 mmHg, but the frequency of nerve impulses increases progressively as the pressure rises above 60 mmHg, reaching a maximum at approximately 180 mmHg [174]. Most baroreceptors have a set point of approximately 100 mmHg. However, if arterial blood pressure changes to a new value and remains static, the baroreceptors can 'reset' to this new set point within 24–48 h. This is why baroreceptors are only effective for short-term control of blood pressure. Most, if not all, anesthetic drugs interfere with baroreceptor responsiveness. Inhalation anesthetics in particular depress normal baroreflex responsiveness and diminish sympathetic output from the CNS. The degree of baroreceptor depression depends on both the depth of anesthesia and the patient's physical status.

Cardiac mechanoreceptors are located in the right and left atria and ventricles and help to minimize changes in systemic blood pressure in response to changes in blood volume [184,185]. These cardiac stretch receptors differ from the baroreceptors in that the stretch receptors respond to comparatively small changes in stretch or pressure, as do pressure receptors within the pulmonary circulation. The atria contain two types of receptors located at the venoatrial junctions [174]. Atrial A receptors react primarily to changes in heart rate, whereas B receptors respond to short-term changes in atrial volume. An increase in atrial volume activates both the A and B atrial mechanoreceptors, sending impulses to the medulla via vagal afferents. Depending on the prevailing heart rate and arterial blood pressure, heart rate may increase (Bainbridge reflex) or decrease (baroreflex and activation of atrial depressor C fibers). Atrial distension also decreases sympathetic output to renal afferent arterioles, resulting in vasodilation, while the hypothalamus receives neural input, which decreases the release of vasopressin (antidiuretic hormone) that acts to increase urine flow [174].

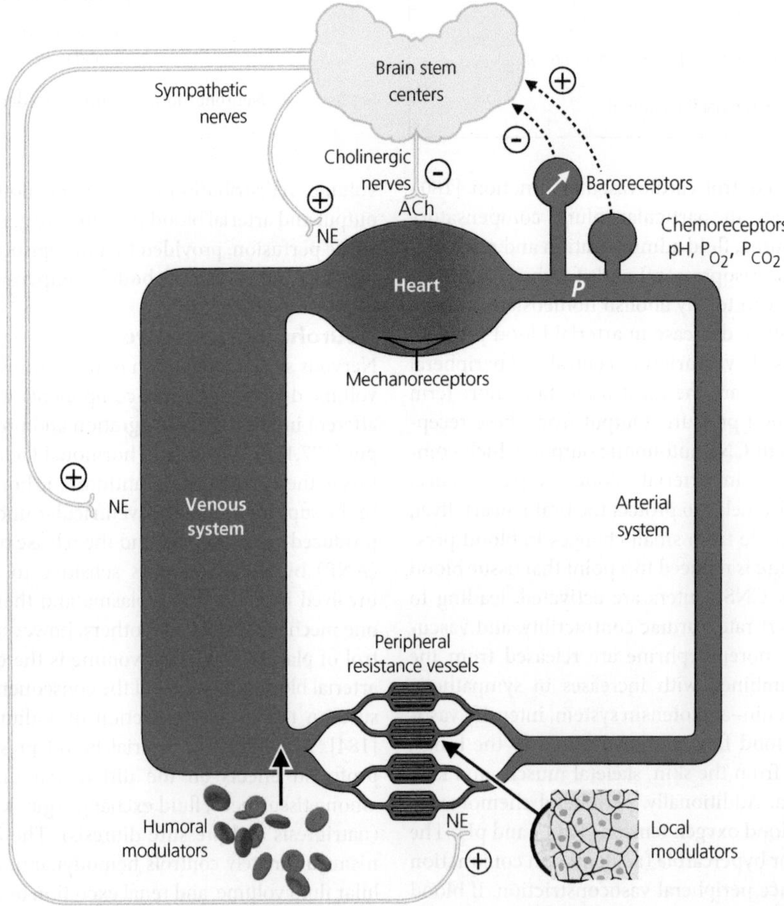

Figure 22.41 Nervous, humoral, and local (tissue) regulatory factors maintain blood flow and pressure within physiological limits. Mechanoreceptors and chemoreceptors sense changes in wall tension (stretch), pH, and blood gases [arterial oxygen partial pressure (PaO_2)] and partial pressure of carbon dioxide ($PaCO_2$), respectively. Metabolic products produced in peripheral tissues and released into the circulation modulate blood vessel tone and the distribution of blood flow. Nervous impulses generated by the heart, vasculature, and peripheral sensors are transmitted to and integrated in the brainstem, altering sympathetic and parasympathetic tone. The release of norepinephrine (NE) by sympathetic nerves stimulates the heart and constricts blood vessels. The release of acetylcholine (ACh) by parasympathetic nerves depresses the heart. +, stimulatory; –, inhibitory. Source: modified from [73].

A rapid loss of free water into the urine helps return circulating blood volume to normal values. In addition to these neural responses, ANP and brain natriuretic peptide (BNP) are released into the bloodstream [175]. Atrial natriuretic peptide and atrial natriuretic factor (ANF) are produced in atrial cardiomyocytes in response to atrial distension and increases sodium excretion by the kidney with an accompanying increase in water loss. Similarly, BNP, produced by ventricular muscle cells, depends on increases in ventricular filling pressures and myocardial stretch and becomes elevated during myocardial dysfunction [175].

Ventricular mechanoreceptors located in the ventricular endocardium discharge in parallel with changes in ventricular pressure and produce effects that help to regulate systemic blood pressure and myocardial work. Ventricular distension, however, also stimulates powerful depressor reflexes that decrease heart rate and peripheral vascular resistance, resulting in bradycardia and hypotension (Bezold–Jarisch reflex) [186,187]. The activation of ventricular non-myelinated C fibers serves as the basis for this reflex response. Impulses initiated by either ventricular distention or the injection of certain chemicals (e.g., capsaicin or serotonin) into the coronary arteries can produce the Bezold–Jarisch reflex, which is also called the coronary chemoreflex [187].

The carotid artery and aortic arch contain specialized sensory chemoreceptors termed the carotid and aortic bodies (Fig. 22.41) [174]. The carotid and aortic bodies receive the highest blood flow per gram of tissue weight of any organ within the body. These chemoreceptors are sensitive to changes in arterial oxygen and carbon dioxide tension, hydrogen ion concentration (pH), and temperature. The chemoreceptors of the carotid and aortic bodies help to regulate respiratory function in response to decreases in pH and the arterial partial pressure of oxygen and increases in the arterial partial pressure of carbon dioxide. Afferent activity from the carotid body is carried by the glossopharyngeal nerve and from the aortic body by the vagus nerve. These sensors are most sensitive to changes in hydrogen ion concentration and respond proportionally to the magnitude of the change from their set point. The set point for activation is a pH below 7.40. The approximate set point for carbon dioxide is 40 mmHg and for oxygen 80 mmHg. Increases in afferent activity from the chemoreceptors increase minute ventilation, restoring arterial blood pH, carbon dioxide, and/or oxygen to normal. Hypoxia, hypercarbia, and non-respiratory acidosis may cause bradycardia, coronary vasodilation, and an increase in systemic arteriolar resistance. This effect is pronounced if the normal increase in ventilation is prevented, for example, during anesthesia. Chemoreceptors located in the ventricular epicardium respond to hypoxia or ischemia by initiating the coronary chemoreflex (Bezold–Jarisch reflex), producing bradycardia and hypotension [187].

Efferent output

When afferent impulses from peripheral sensors arrive in the brain, they are integrated to produce a neural and/or humoral response. The nucleus tractus solitarius (NTS) in the medulla serves as a relay station for afferent impulses from peripheral sensors (Fig. 22.42a,b). Neurons originating in the NTS send information to the vagal nucleus and to various regions collectively referred to as the vasomotor center. Vagal nuclei send nerve fibers directly to the heart. Nerve cell bodies for the sympathetic nervous system are located in the thoracolumbar spinal cord and are linked to the NTS through axons traveling in the bulbospinal tract (Fig. 22.42a). The bulbospinal tract contains both excitatory and inhibitory axons that cause either increases or decreases in sympathetic output [175].

Centers in the hypothalamus link the somatic and autonomic responses necessary for animals to adapt to their environment. The centers initiate adrenergic constriction of resistance and capacitance vessels and cholinergic dilation of vessels supplying skeletal and cardiac muscle during the fight-flight response. Hypothalamic centers modulate the cardiovascular response (cutaneous vasoactivity) to body temperature changes during shivering, sweating, or panting. The hypothalamus also modulates the cardiovascular response to exercise and may be involved in blood pressure regulation. The autonomic nervous system, which is the efferent link between the CNS and the cardiovascular system, provides rapid control of both blood pressure and blood flow [174]. Efferent impulses are transmitted by both sympathetic and parasympathetic nerves. Adrenergic and cholinergic receptors in target organs initiate the intracellular changes that produce a cellular response to the signals arriving from the CNS.

Sympathetic nervous system

Sympathetic pathways originate in the intermediolateral columns of the thoracolumbar segments of the spinal cord [174,175]. Both inhibitory and excitatory input arrive at preganglionic sympathetic nerve cell bodies via axons traveling in the bulbospinal tract (Fig. 22.43). Descending inhibitory pathways are serotoninergic; descending excitatory pathways are adrenergic. The balance between these two types of input determines the prevailing level of sympathetic tone to the periphery.

Preganglionic sympathetic nerves send axons via the ventral roots of the spinal cord to paravertebral ganglia located just outside the vertebral column (Fig. 22.42a). Many of the preganglionic fibers ascend the paravertebral chains and synapse with postganglionic neurons in the cranial, middle, and caudal (stellate) cervical ganglia (Fig. 22.42a). Here they synapse with postganglionic sympathetic neurons, which send their fibers to the heart, blood vessels, and viscera. Postganglionic cardiac sympathetic nerve fibers innervate the sinoatrial node, the atrioventricular node, the atria, and the myocardium (Fig. 22.42a). Postganglionic sympathetic nerve fibers release the neurotransmitter norepinephrine, which binds to adrenoreceptors on cardiac cell membranes.

Postganglionic sympathetic nerve fibers also leave the paravertebral ganglia via spinal nerves to innervate vessels throughout the body. Normally, sympathetic tone maintains a partial state of contraction in vascular smooth muscle, providing the resistance necessary to maintain adequate systemic blood pressure and aid in the control of the fractional distribution of cardiac output to body tissues. The extent of innervation to the resistance vessels (arterioles) varies with tissue type. The kidney, spleen, gastrointestinal tract, and skin are extensively innervated by the sympathetic nervous system. Redistribution of blood flow away from these tissues during times of crisis preserves blood flow to the brain, heart, and skeletal muscle.

Sympathetic neurotransmission

Most sympathetic postganglionic fibers are adrenergic, releasing norepinephrine at their neuroeffector junctions [177]. The amino acid tyrosine is the substrate used by these nerves to produce norepinephrine. Tyrosine is actively transported across the nerve cell membrane into the neural axoplasm, where it is converted by tyrosine hydroxylase and decarboxylation to dopamine, which is stored in vesicles within the nerve. Inside the storage vesicles, a final hydroxylation step takes place to produce the neurotransmitter norepinephrine (Fig. 22.44).

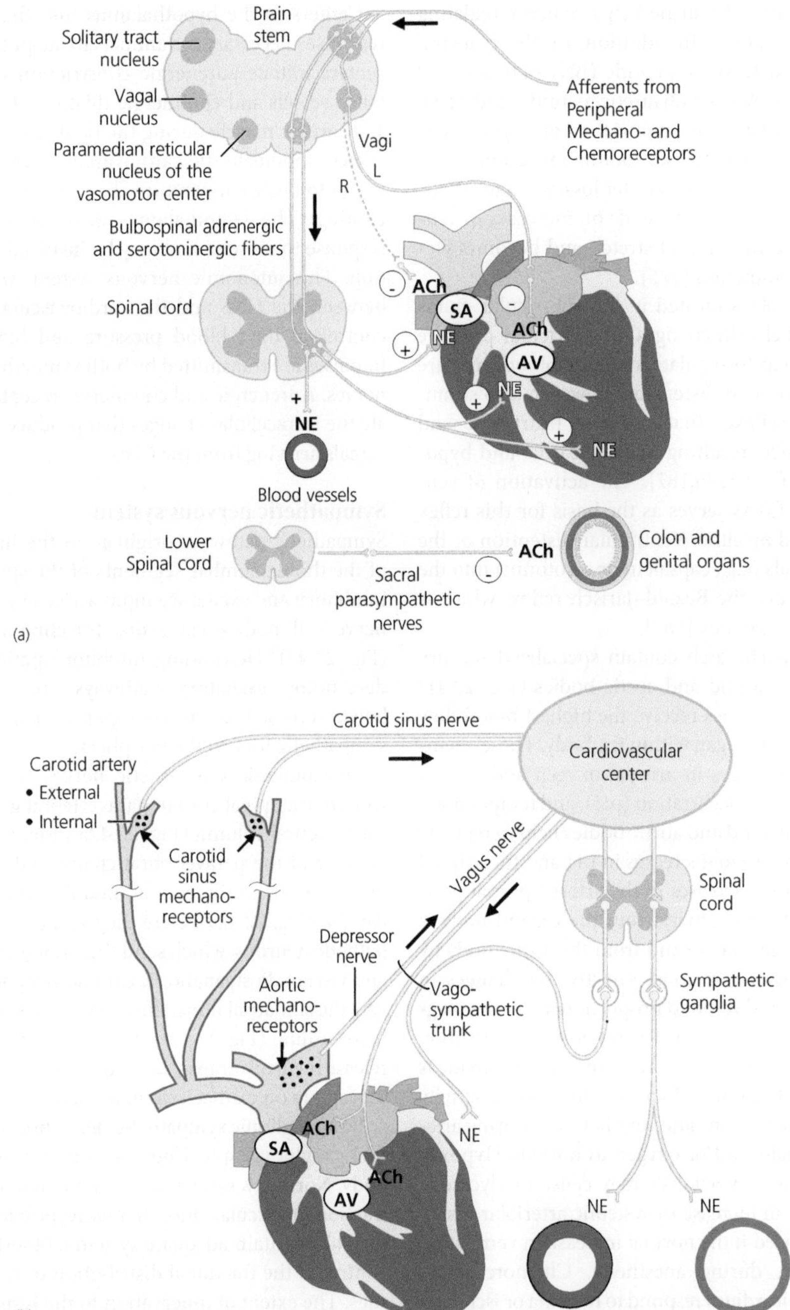

Figure 22.42 (a) Distribution of sympathetic and parasympathetic nerves to the cardiovascular system. The solitary-tract nucleus is the main receiving point in the brainstem for afferent input arriving from peripheral sensors and higher centers in the brain. Interneurons connect the solitary tract nucleus to the vasomotor center and bulbospinal tract fibers that descend to the spinal cord and synapse with preganglionic sympathetic nerves to the heart and blood vessels. Interneurons also connect the solitary-tract nucleus to the vagal nucleus in the brainstem, where neurons synapse with preganglionic parasympathetic nerve fibers carried by the vagus nerve to the heart. (b) Mechanoreceptors in the carotid sinus and aortic arch send impulses via the carotid sinus nerve, a branch of the glossopharyngeal nerve, and the vagosympathetic trunk, respectively, to the solitary tract nucleus in the brainstem (cardiovascular centers). Changes in the activity of these mechanoreceptors caused by changes in arterial blood pressure result in adjustments in sympathetic and parasympathetic outflow to the heart and resistance (arterial) and capacitance (veins) vessels. Ach, acetylcholine; AV, atrioventricular node; L, left vagus; NE, norepinephrine; R, right vagus; SA, sinoatrial node. Source: modified from [73]. Reproduced with permission of Springer.

Nerve action potentials increase intracellular calcium, causing the vesicles to fuse with the nerve cell membrane and release norepinephrine into the synaptic cleft, where it binds to a variety of adrenoreceptors (Table 22.6). There are presynaptic receptors on the nerve cell membrane and postsynaptic receptors on the effector organ. Postsynaptic receptor binding of norepinephrine triggers a cascade of intracellular events that ultimately produce a cellular action. The effective half-life of norepinephrine after release into the synaptic cleft is very short. Norepinephrine is degraded locally at the neuroeffector junction by the enzymes, monoamine

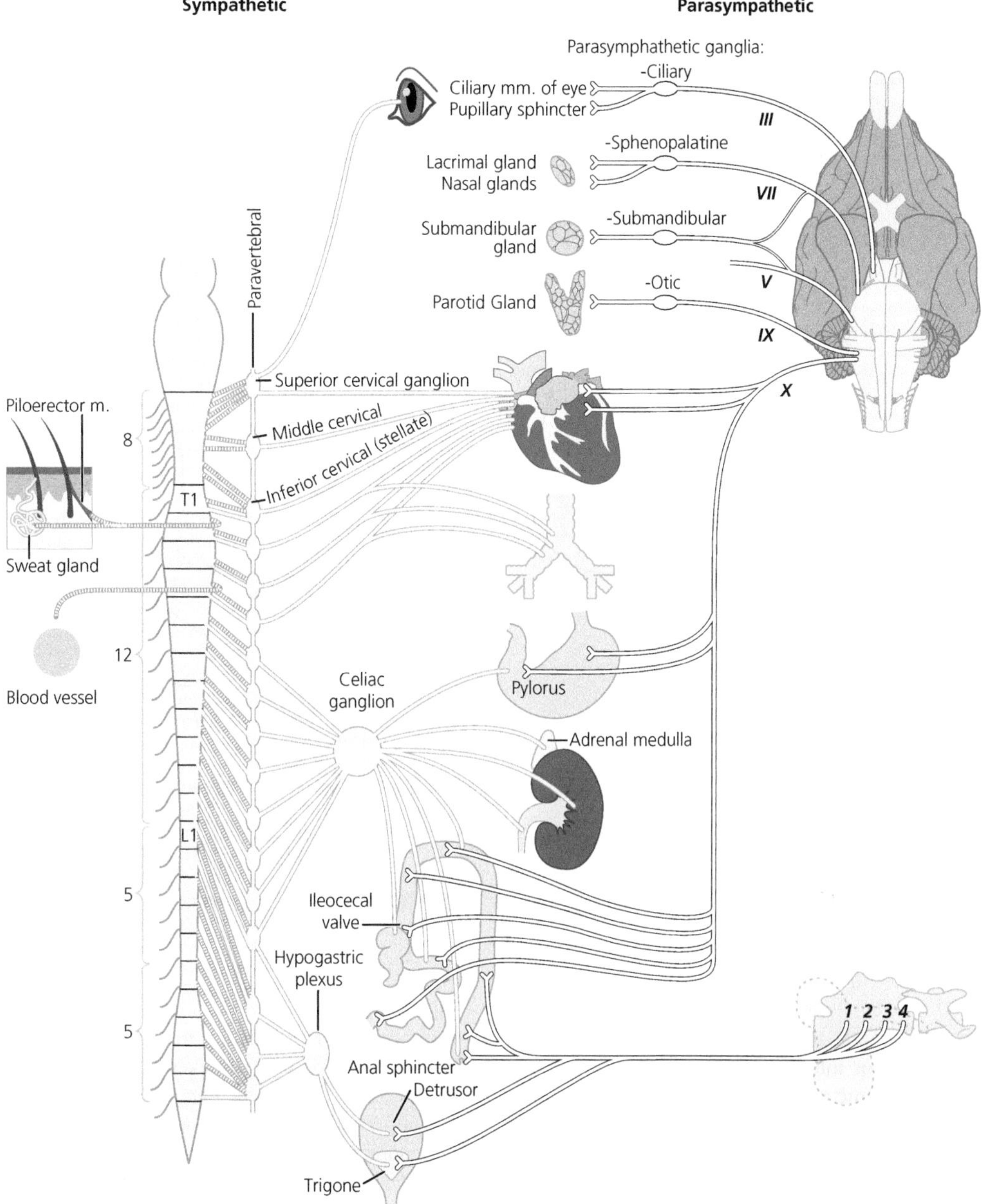

Figure 22.43 The autonomic nervous system.

oxidase (MAO) and catechol-*O*-methyltransferase (COMT) (Fig. 22.44). Most of the norepinephrine released into the synaptic cleft undergoes reuptake into adrenergic nerve terminals, where it re-enters storage vesicles. This neuronal amine-uptake system is designated uptake 1 and has a high affinity for norepinephrine, a lower affinity for epinephrine, and little affinity for the synthetic β-adrenergic agonist isoproterenol. Norepinephrine rapidly diffuses out of the synaptic cleft, where it undergoes reuptake at extraneuronal sites or is carried into the venous blood and metabolized in the lung. The extraneuronal reuptake pathway has been designated uptake 2 and has a low affinity for norepinephrine, a higher affinity for epinephrine, and a very high affinity for isoproterenol. Uptake 2 is of the greatest physiological significance in the elimination of circulating catecholamines, primarily epinephrine, released by the adrenal gland, and has little physiological significance for norepinephrine released at postganglionic sympathetic nerve terminals.

Adrenoreceptors

The sequence of intracellular events initiated by receptor binding of norepinephrine is determined by the type of adrenoreceptor stimulated. The classification of adrenoreceptors continues to evolve based on both pharmacological and molecular criteria (Table 22.6) [83–87]. All adrenoreceptors have a similar homology of structure and produce intracellular events by binding to membrane guanine nucleotide-regulatory proteins (G-proteins) [177]. The structure of the G-protein coupled receptor consists of a single-subunit protein with seven hydrophobic transmembrane segments, three hydrophilic extracellular sequences, and three hydrophilic intracytoplasmic loops. These membrane-associated regulatory proteins serve to

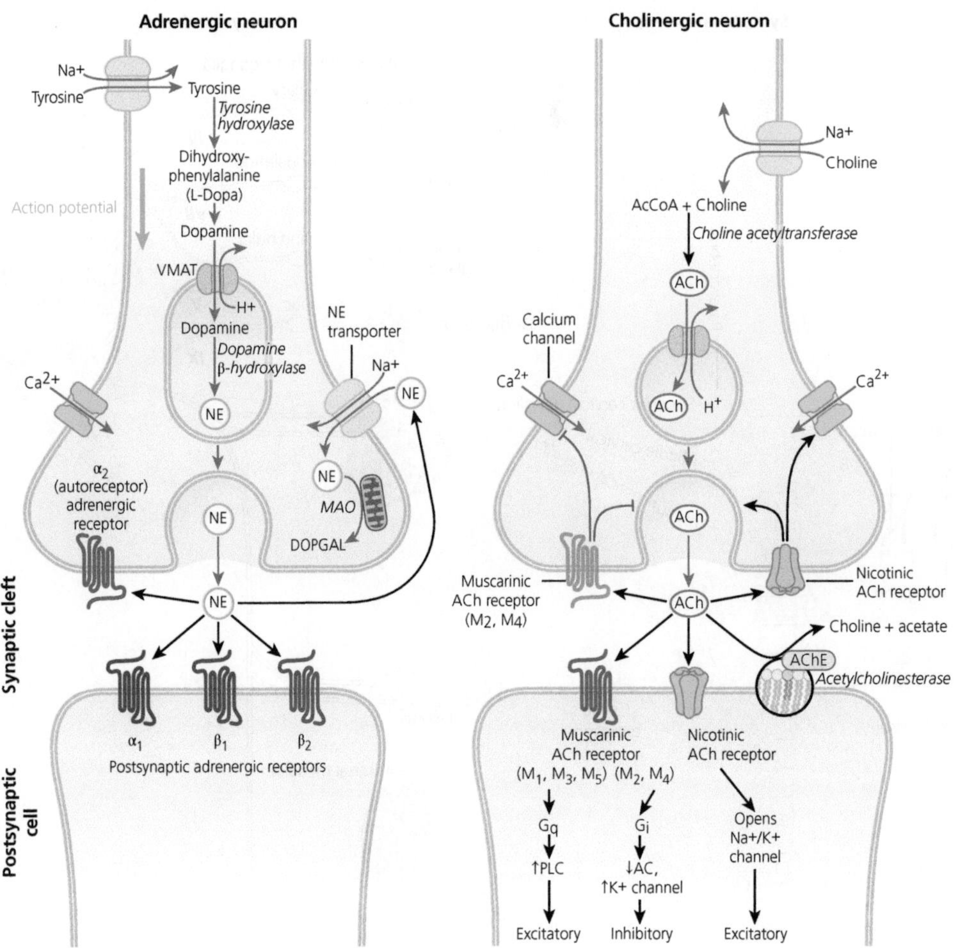

Figure 22.44 Neurochemical processes in adrenergic and cholinergic neurons.

convert the signal arriving at the cell membrane into a specific enzyme system response or ion-channel activity that produces a cellular response. Autonomic transmission in the cardiovascular system is initiated by stimulation of three different G-proteins: G_s stimulates adenylate cyclase, causing a rise in intracellular cAMP; G_i inhibits adenylate cyclase, decreasing the concentration of intracellular cAMP (Table 22.6); and G_p activates phospholipase C, which hydrolyzes phosphoinositol to inositol triphosphate (IP_3) and diacylglycerol (DAG). IP_3 causes the release of calcium ions (Ca^{2+}) from the sarcoplasmic reticulum. DAG activates protein kinase C, which phosphorylates contractile proteins in the myocardium and vascular smooth muscle.

β-Adrenergic receptors are classified pharmacologically into three types β_1, β_2, and β_3 based on their relative affinities for various agonists (Table 22.6) [177]. The physiological significance of the β_3 receptor is unclear, but it appears to be involved in regulation of metabolism and energy regulation. The β_1- and β_2-adrenoreceptor subtypes, when activated by norepinephrine, epinephrine, or other β-adrenergic agonists, stimulate the formation of the enzyme adenylate cyclase through the G_s-protein, causing an increase in intracellular cAMP. β-Adrenoreceptors also activate L-type Ca^{2+} channels in myocardial and vascular tissue, thereby increasing intracellular calcium concentration. Both β_1- and β_2-adrenoreceptors are found in the heart and are responsible for increases in heart rate and contractility during sympathetic stimulation (Table 22.7). β-Adrenoreceptor stimulation increases the slope of phase 4 diastolic depolarization in pacemaker tissues and subsidiary automatic cells. Increases in intracellular cAMP and Ca^{2+} increase cardiac contractility and facilitate cardiac relaxation. Although both β_1- and β_2-adrenoreceptors are present in the heart, β_1-adrenoreceptors predominate during health, especially in the ventricular myocardium.

β_2-Adrenoreceptors relax smooth muscle in vascular, bronchial, gastrointestinal, and genitourinary tissues. β_2-Adrenoreceptors in the vasculature are not innervated and therefore produce vasodilation in response to circulating catecholamines or drugs. Their location in specific vascular beds suggests a role in the distribution of blood flow, especially during exercise.

Three α_1-receptor subtypes have been classified according to their affinity to adrenergic agonists [177]. The receptor subtypes are designated α_{1A}, α_{1B}, and α_{1C}, but their distribution is not universal across species or within specific tissue beds. All α_1-adrenoreceptor subtypes currently identified produce their intracellular effect by activation of the enzyme phospholipase C via the G_p-protein. Phospholipase C hydrolyzes phosphoinositol and releases Ca^{2+} from intracytoplasmic stores, causing the contractile response seen in myocardial or vascular smooth muscle cells (Table 22.6).

Three subtypes of α_2-adrenoreceptors, α_{2A}, α_{2B}, and α_{2C}, have been identified by pharmacologic studies, although the tissue distribution of these subtypes is unclear [177]. α_2-Adrenoreceptors inhibit adenylate cyclase through the G_i-protein. Inhibition of adenylate cyclase

Table 22.6 G–coupled receptor superfamily of genes and gene products in cardiac tissue

Receptor Type and Subtype	Location	G Protein	Biological Response
Adrenergic			
β_1	Myocardium	G_s	AC stimulation, positive inotropic and chronotropic responses
	Coronary vascular	G_s	AC stimulation, vasodilation(?)
β_2	Myocardium	G_s	AC stimulation, positive inotropic and chronotropic responses
	Coronary vasculature(?)	G_s	AC stimulation, vasodilation(?)
α_1			
	Myocardium	G_p	PI hydrolysis stimulation, positive inotropic response(?)
	Coronary vasculature	G_p	PI stimulation, vasoconstriction
Muscarinic			
M_2	Myocardium	G_i	Shorten atrial action potential; slow sinus rate: slow AV conduction; AC inhibition, negative inotrope. and chronotrope
M_3	Coronary smooth muscle	G_p(?)	PI stimulation, vasoconstriction
M_3	Coronary endothelium	G_p(?)	EDRF production, GC stimulation, vasodilation

AC. adenylate cyclase: EDRF. endothelium-derived relaxing factor or nitric oxide: GC. guanylate cyclase: PI. phosphatidylinositol.
Modified from Opie.106 p. 164.
Source: modified from Opie LH. *The Heart: Physiology and Metabolism*, 3rd edn. Philadelphia: Lippincott-Raven, 1998; 91–97.

Table 22.7 Pharmacology of autonomic nervous system

	Sympathetic		Parasympathetic	
Organ	**Main receptor type**	**Response**	**Main receptor type**	**Response**
Heart				
1. SA Node	β_1	↑ *HR*	M_2	↓ *HR*
2. Atria	β_1	↑ *conductivity*	M_2	↑ *conductivity*
3. AV Node	β_1	↑ *conductivity*	M_2	↓ *conduction velocity (AV block)*
4. Ventricular muscle	β_1	↑ *contractility* ↑ *conductivity* ↑ *automaticity*	M_2	*No effect*
Blood vessels:				
Arterioles				
1. Sk. muscle	β_2	*Vasodilatation*	M_3	*No effect*
2. Skin & mucous membranes	α_1	*Vasoconstriction*	M_3	*No effect*
Veins	α_1 β_2	*Vasoconstriction* *Vasodilatation*	M_3	*No effect*
Bronchial Smooth muscle	β_2	*Relaxation*	M_3	*Contraction*
GI				
1. Smooth muscle.	α, β_2	↓ *Motility*	M_3	↑ *motility*
2. Sphincters	α_1	*Contraction*	$M2, M_3$	*Relaxation*
3. Glands	-	*No effect*	M_3	↑ *secretion*
Urinary Bladder				
Detrusor	β_2	*Relaxation*	M_3	*Contraction*
Trigone & sphincter	α_1	*Contraction*	M_2, M_3	*Relaxation*
Eye				
Radial muscle	α_1	*Contraction (active mydriasis)*	–	–
Circular muscle	–	–	M_3	*Contraction (Miosis)*
Ciliary muscle			M_3	*Contraction (accommodation for near vision)*
Male sex organs	α	*Ejaculation*	*M*	*Erection*
Salivary glands	α, β	*Thick viscous secretion*	M_3	*Profuse watery secretion*
Kidney	β_1	*Renin secretion*	–	*No effect*
Liver	β_2	*Glycogenolysis Gluconeogenesis*	–	*Effect*

attenuates cAMP production in target cells. This mechanism is important in platelets and renal tubules; however, in vascular smooth muscle, an alternative signal transduction mechanism is responsible for the vasoconstrictor response. α_2-Adrenoreceptors are located presynaptically and extrasynaptically in vascular smooth muscle. Stimulation of extrasynaptic α_2-adrenoreceptors by α-adrenergic agonists (norepinephrine, phenylephrine) activates a receptor-operated calcium channel that increases the concentration of calcium intracellularly, producing vascular smooth muscle contraction that complements the contractile effect of α_1-adrenoreceptors activated by stimulation of sympathetic nerves. Because of their extrasynaptic location, α_2-adrenoreceptors respond to circulating catecholamines, such as epinephrine and norepinephrine, and aid in maintaining generalized sympathetic vasoconstriction in response to catecholamine output from the adrenal gland. This later response is important in the fight-flight response that occurs in crisis situations such as trauma or hemorrhage.

The α_1- and α_2-adrenoreceptors coexist in the vasculature as described earlier [177]. There is a greater response to α_2 stimulation on the venous side of the circulation compared with the arterial side. Therefore, α_2-adrenoreceptor-mediated vasoconstriction may be most important in mobilizing blood volume from veins, leading to an increase in cardiac filling, which is an important first step in increasing cardiac output during stress situations such as exercise or hemorrhage [117]. The administration of an α_2-adrenergic receptor agonist (dexmedetomidine) produces generalized vasoconstriction of both arterial and venous vessels, resulting in increases in arterial blood pressure, systemic vascular resistance, venous return and right atrial pressure. Cardiac output, however, may not increase due to decreases in heart rate and increases in afterload (see Afterload) [188].

The α_1- and α_2-adrenoreceptors can cause complementary or antagonistic responses, depending on their location. For example, norepinephrine stimulates α_1-adrenoreceptors located on the postsynaptic cell membrane, causing contraction of vascular smooth muscle and vasoconstriction. Norepinephrine also binds to presynaptic α_2-adrenoreceptors, producing a negative-feedback effect that decreases the release of norepinephrine from the nerve terminal. Thus, α_2-adrenoreceptors help to modulate the vasoconstrictor response initiated by α_1-postsynaptic receptor stimulation. The α_2-adrenoreceptors help to ensure that only a short-term vasoconstrictor response occurs after sympathetic nerve stimulation.

Stimulation of postganglionic sympathetic fibers supplying vascular smooth muscle causes not only the release of the neurotransmitter norepinephrine, but also the release of the cotransmitter neuropeptide Y [177,189]. Neuropeptide Y is present in vesicles contained in postganglionic sympathetic nerve terminals, is synergistic with the effects of norepinephrine on the peripheral vasculature, and produces vasoconstriction. Neuropeptide Y is also found in the adrenal medulla. Circulating levels of neuropeptide Y inhibit renin release and stimulate the release of ANP. The role of neuropeptide Y in cardiovascular regulation has not been fully characterized; however, it may be an important mediator in the central control of blood pressure.

Sympathetic cholinergic nerve fibers originate in the cerebral cortex and send descending fibers to the spinal cord. These nerve fibers synapse in the sympathetic ganglia and send postganglionic fibers to precapillary vessels in skeletal muscle [83]. Postganglionic cholinergic sympathetic nerve fibers are activated only during times of high sympathetic tone (fear, pain, or exercise) and release acetylcholine, which produces vasodilation in skeletal muscle.

Parasympathetic neurotransmission

The parasympathetic nervous system (PNS) originates from two sites within the CNS: cervical spinal cord and sacral spinal cord (Fig. 22.43). Long preganglionic parasympathetic nerve fibers located in the CNS synapse with relatively short postganglionic parasympathetic neurons in ganglia located in the target organ. The cranial portion of the parasympathetic nervous system originates in the medulla oblongata. Axions travel via the vagus nerve to synapse with postganglionic parasympathetic nerves that terminate in the heart and blood vessels [174,177].

Acetylcholine is the neurotransmitter released at autonomic ganglia and from postganglionic parasympathetic nerves (Fig. 22.44). Cholinergic nerves actively transport choline from the extracellular fluid into the neural axoplasm, where it is acted upon by the enzyme choline acetyltransferase, combined with acetyl coenzyme A, and converted to acetylcholine, which like norepinephrine is stored in vesicles within the nerve (Fig. 22.44). Cholinergic nerve action potentials increase intracellular calcium, causing vesicular and nerve cell membrane fusion and the release of acetylcholine into the synaptic cleft. Acetylcholine binds to specific muscarinic receptors (M_1–M_5), mediating a cellular response that varies with the tissue innervated and the type of cholinergic receptor involved (Table 22.7). M_4 and M_5 receptors are preferentially expressed in the CNS [177]. The actions of acetylcholine are rapidly terminated by hydrolysis into choline and acetic acid by the enzyme acetylcholinesterase. The acetylcholine that diffuses out of the synaptic cleft and into the extracellular fluid or plasma is hydrolyzed by plasma butyrylcholinesterase (pseudocholinesterase). The choline produced from this metabolism is rapidly taken up by the nerve cell and used in the resynthesis of acetylcholine.

Cholinergic receptors are classified as either nicotinic or muscarinic (Table 22.6). Nicotinic receptors are located in autonomic ganglia, in the adrenal medulla, and at the neuromuscular junction of skeletal muscle. Muscarinic receptors are located at postganglionic parasympathetic nerve terminals [190].

Nicotinic receptors are pentameric membrane proteins that form a non-selective ion channel in the cell membrane. Postsynaptic nicotinic receptors, located in the autonomic ganglia or the neuromuscular junction, when stimulated by acetylcholine, open their ion channel, allowing the flow of cations into the nerve or muscle cell, resulting in depolarization and ultimately nerve cell transmission of an electric impulse or muscular contraction. Nicotinic receptors are subclassified into N_G receptors, located at autonomic ganglia, and N_S receptors, located in the neuromuscular junction and within the CNS [177].

Muscarinic receptors are located in the autonomic effector organs of the parasympathetic nervous system, for example, the heart, smooth muscle, and the exocrine glands (Table 22.7) [177]. They are G-protein coupled and show more homology to adrenergic and dopaminergic receptors than to the nicotinic cholinergic receptors.

The vagus nerve innervates the sinoatrial node, the atrial myocardium, the atrioventricular node, and to a much lesser extent the ventricular myocardium (Fig. 22.42b). Stimulation of M_2 receptors by acetylcholine activates several different membrane G-proteins, resulting in inhibition of adenylate cyclase, activation of potassium channels, and activation of phospholipase C, which hydrolyzes phosphoinositol. These effects cause a decrease in the slope of phase 4 diastolic depolarization in pacemaker and subsidiary automatic tissues, and hyperpolarization of cardiac cell membranes through activation of membrane potassium channels. Heart rate is decreased, as are the rate of conduction of impulses through the atrioventricular node and cardiac contractility. High levels of parasympathetic tone can produce atrioventricular block (first-degree, second-degree, and third-degree heart block) and temporary cardiac asystole. The right vagus nerve sends the majority of its fibers to the sinoatrial node and stimulation is more apt to produce sinus bradycardia and sinus arrest whereas stimulation of the left vagus nerve blocks conduction in the atrioventricular node. Stimulation of the parasympathetic nervous system produces minimal effects on most peripheral blood vessels (Table 22.7). Systemically admininistered acetylcholine, however, binds to M_2 receptors in vessels, which mediates an endothelium-dependent vasorelaxation [191].

The sacral division of the parasympathetic nervous system has preganglionic nerve cell bodies located in the intermediolateral column of the spinal cord [174,177]. Parasympathetic nerves in this region congregate to form the pelvic nerves that innervate the intestines, colon, rectum, bladder, and genitalia (Fig. 22.43). Stimulation of the parasympathetic nerves also causes increased blood flow to salivary glands and genital erectile tissue.

Humoral mechanisms

The autonomic nervous system functions to produce acute changes in cardiovascular function that can be large in magnitude, but are generally brief. More sustained changes in cardiopulmonary function are produced by humoral mechanisms (Box 22.6). The adrenal medulla is a modified sympathetic ganglion innervated by preganglionic sympathetic fibers and is part of the sympathetic nervous system. The neuronal cells of the adrenal medulla, rather than sending axons to target organs, release the neurotransmitters epinephrine and norepinephrine into the circulation. Precipitating factors for the release of catecholamines from the adrenal medulla include pain, trauma, hypovolemia, hypotension, hypoxia, hypothermia, hypoglycemia, exercise stress, and fear (fight-flight). Circulating catecholamines produce a variety of effects, including increases in metabolic rate, glycogenolysis in the liver and skeletal muscle, gluconeogenesis in the liver, and an increase in the availability of free fatty acids, an important nutrient source for the myocardium. Circulating catecholamines also increase heart rate and cardiac contractility, dilate vascular beds in skeletal and cardiac muscle, and constrict splanchnic and cutaneous arterioles, diminishing blood supply to organs that are less essential during a fight-flight response and rediverting blood to the heart, lung and brain. The actions of the adrenal medulla are complementary to the effects of sympathetic nerve stimulation. Together, the autonomic nervous system and humoral mechanisms provide both rapid (nervous system) and sustained (humoral) responses to stressful situations [174].

The kidney is the major site for activation of the renin–angiotensin system [192,193]. Renin is produced in the kidney during sodium depletion, hypotension, decreases in extracellular fluid volume, or increases in sympathetic output (Box 22.6). Secretion of renin into the systemic circulation converts circulating angiotensinogen, produced by the liver, to angiotensin I. Angiotensin I is converted to angiotensin II by an angiotensin-converting enzyme that is present in pulmonary vascular endothelium. Angiotensin II produces arteriolar constriction, producing increases in blood pressure, and stimulates the adrenal cortex to release aldosterone, a hormone that causes renal reabsorption of Na^+ and water, effectively increasing thirst and the extracellular fluid volume (Fig. 22.40).

The hypothalamus is directly involved in the central neural control of cardiovascular responses, but it also plays an important role in the humoral regulation of cardiovascular function. Arginine vasopressin [antidiuretic hormone (ADH)] is produced in the hypothalamus and is transported through nerve cell axons to the posterior pituitary [194]. Under normal circumstances, the pituitary releases vasopressin in response to increases in plasma solute, resulting in an increase in circulating vasopressin (Box 22.6). Vasopressin acts on the collecting ducts of the kidney, where it stimulates water conservation, thereby returning plasma osmolality (and volume) to normal. Vasopressin is a vasoconstrictor, especially in mesenteric vessels; therefore, the presence of circulating vasopressin is influential in the redistribution of systemic blood flow (Fig. 22.40). Vasopressin release by the pituitary can also occur in the absence of changes in plasma osmolality. Examples of non-osmotic stimuli that cause the release of vasopressin are pain, stress, hypoxia, heart failure, and vascular volume depletion. A number of anesthetic drugs are associated with increased circulating levels of arginine vasopressin, including opioids (morphine and meperidine) and barbiturates [75].

Local control systems

Autoregulation is the ability of blood vessels to adjust blood flow in accordance with metabolic need and to maintain blood flow despite extreme changes in tissue perfusion pressure (Fig. 22.45) [195,196]. Most tissues can regulate their own blood flow during physiological changes in perfusion pressure. Neurogenic basal tone exists in many vessels. Non-neurogenic (intrinsic) basal tone is additive to neurogenic basal tone and is present in vessels of the skin and skeletal muscle. A reduction in vasomotor tone in these vessels usually represents a reduction in the neurogenic component. Active dilation is a term applied when vascular tone decreases below the non-neurogenic basal level and is the result of two major components, a pressure-sensitive mechanism termed the myogenic component and a metabolic mechanism that is influenced by local oxygen tension [197]. Both mechanisms are linked to the release of local vasodilatory mediators. This phenomenon, also termed reactive hyperemia, occurs in arterioles less than 25 μm in diameter [198]. The myogenic mechanism is responsible for reactive hyperemia after short periods (<30 s) of ischemia. As flow returns to the previously occluded arteriole, blood flow velocity increases, which increases wall shear stress, causing the release of nitric oxide from the vascular endothelium [191]. The metabolic component of reactive hyperemia occurs after longer periods of occlusion (>30 s). Decreases in oxygen tension release a vasodilatory prostaglandin that maintains blood flow until normal oxygen tension is re-established. Endothelial damage in small arterioles eliminates the reactive hyperemic response altogether, since both nitric oxide and prostaglandins are products of vascular endothelial cells. Stretch of vascular smooth muscle opposes the myogenic vasodilator response seen in larger vessels (Bayliss effect: increased blood pressure stretches the blood vessel, causing it to constrict) [197]. The proposed mechanism for the Bayliss effect is a pressure-induced depolarization of the endothelial cell mediated through an inwardly

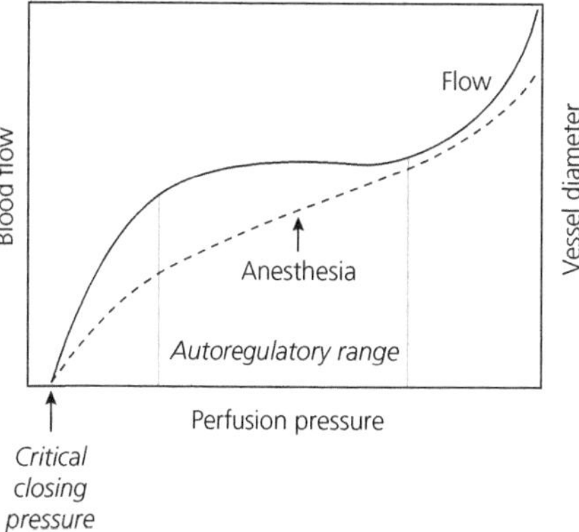

Figure 22.45 Autoregulation. The relationship between blood flow and perfusion pressure in peripheral vascular beds (excluding CNS) is characterized by the pressure range over which blood flow changes very little. The normal autoregulatory range for most vascular beds ranges between 60 and 180 mmHg. Some vascular beds (brain, gut, and skeletal muscle) close when the the perfusion pressure approximates 15–30 mmHg (critical closing pressure). Source: modified from [73].

rectifying potassium channel. The effects of anesthetic drugs on reactive hyperemia and the Bayliss effect remain to be resolved.

As previously discussed, capillary blood flow is linked to multiple factors including, but not limited to, the perfusion pressure, blood flow rate, tissue metabolic rate, oxygen tension, and plasma viscosity (see Hemorrheology) [92,199–201]. Collectively, these factors determine the number of perfused (RBC-containing) capillaries [131,200]. Under resting, baseline conditions, only a fraction (about one-third to half) of the capillaries in a given tissue are being perfused at any given moment. During times of increased oxygen demand (e.g., exercise), more capillary pathways can be opened to flowing red blood cells. Whether a given capillary is open or closed depends on the contractile state of a region of smooth muscle (probably a terminal arteriole) located near the entrance to a capillary. The number of open precapillary sphincters is approximately proportional to tissue metabolic activity and local hematocrit. As metabolic activity increases, the local oxygen tension decreases until a critical level of tissue hypoxia occurs, inducing vasodilation [92].

Current evidence also suggests that blood and plasma viscosity plays a pivotal role in determining the diameter, geometry, and perfusion of the microcirculation and functional capillary density (FCD) [202,203]. FCD, defined as the number of capillaries with passage of RBCs per unit surface area, is directly linked to survival. As previously indicated, increasing blood and plasma viscosity increases FCD, an effect that is attributed to microvascular vasodilation brought about by shear stress-induced release of nitric oxide. Furthermore, blood vessel geometry (i.e., shape and diameter) is not rigidly fixed and can be altered in response to changes in viscosity. This change can be reflected by changes in vascular hindrance (VH), or the contribution of vascular geometry to flow resistance. As blood viscosity increases, VH decreases and tissue perfusion improves. Hemorrhage and conventional fluid therapy result in hemodilution and a decrease in blood and plasma viscosity, negatively impacting the microcirculation and FCD. Maintaining or increasing the viscosity of resuscitation fluids in order to sustain plasma viscosity could lead to improved microvascular perfusion and improved long-term survival.

Peptides and other substances are important in regulating tissue blood flow (Table 22.8). The actions of local enzymes produce kinins such as bradykinin from the substrate kallikrein. Kinins

Table 22.8 Summary of factors affecting the caliber of the arterioles

Constriction	Dilation
Increased noradrenergic discharge	Decreased noradrenergic discharge
Circulating catecholamines (except epinephrine in skeletal muscle and liver)	Circulating epinephrine in skeletal muscle and liver
	Circulating atrial natriuretic peptide
Circulating angiotensin II	Activation of cholinergic dilators in skeletal muscle
Circulating arginine vasopressin	Bradykinin
Locally released serotonin	Histamine
Endothelin I	Substance P (axon reflex)
Neuropeptide Y	Nitric oxide and endothelium-derived relaxing factor
Circulating Na^+-K^- ATPase inhibitor	Prostacyclin and prostaglandin E_2
Decreased local temperature	Increased carbon dioxide tension
	Decreased pH
	Lactate, potassium ions, adenosine, etc.
	Increased local temperature

produce vasodilatory effects that are short lived because of rapid inactivation by peptidases in the plasma. Arachidonic acid metabolism produces a variety of prostaglandins that tend to be compartmentalized and produce very specific local effects. Renal hypoperfusion initiates the production of PGI_2, which acts to restore renal blood flow, urine volume, and sodium excretion. The preanesthetic administration of non-steroidal anti-inflammatory drugs (NSAIDs) may interfere with the production of these important prostaglandins by inhibiting cyclooxygenase enzyme activity. There are specific receptor sites on vascular endothelium for a variety of agonists (including acetylcholine, bradykinin, and histamine) that, when bound by the appropriate agonist, induce the formation and release of nitric oxide [191]. Vascular endothelial cells also produce a potent vasoconstrictor substance known as endothelin that acts upon endothelin receptors on vascular smooth muscle cells [204]. Endothelin is released by the endothelium in response to increased intraluminal pressure, contributing to the Bayliss effect (increase in smooth muscle myogenic tone), and is selective for certain vascular beds, including coronary vessels, renal afferent arteries, and venous capacitance vessels. It is both a positive inotrope and a chronotrope. Endothelin increases plasma levels of other humoral mediators, such as atrial natriuretic factor, renin, aldosterone, and circulating catecholamines (Table 22.8).

Oxygen delivery and uptake

Maintaining adequate tissue oxygenation depends on oxygen uptake by the lungs and oxygen delivery (DO_2) to metabolizing tissues. The importance of adequate DO_2 cannot be overemphasized, because reduced oxygen consumption (VO_2) and the development of increasing oxygen debt (O_2D) are known to be directly linked to increased morbidity and mortality [205–207]. Once DO_2 and tissue oxygenation fall below the minimum threshold for the oxidative metabolic requirements of the various cellular organs, an oxygen supply–demand imbalance occurs (Fig. 22.46). Inadequate DO_2 increases oxygen debt and promotes anaerobic metabolism. The severity of oxygen debt and anaerobic metabolism can be quantitated by their metabolic correlates: lactic acid and negative base excess (base deficit: BD). Lactate (La) accumulation and BD can be used clinically to quantitate accurately the onset and severity of oxygen debt, the probability of death, and the odds of therapeutic reversal [207,208]. Oxygen consumption is determined by the metabolic machinery within cells.

To summarize, the factors that determine the supply of oxygen to tissues are Hb concentration, the affinity of Hb for oxygen (P_{50}), the

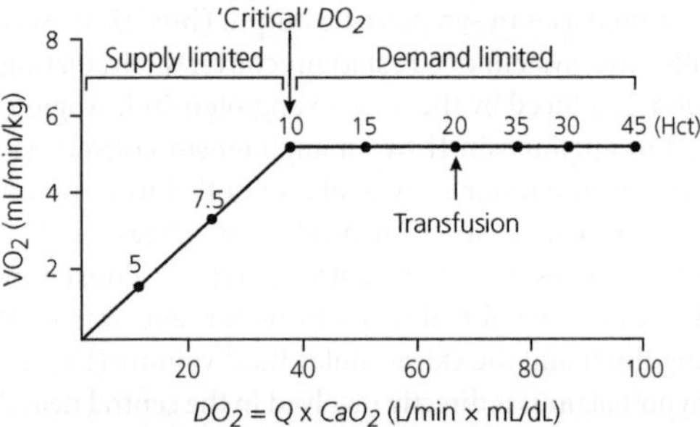

Figure 22.46 Oxygen consumption (VO_2) is normally potentially limited by oxygen delivery ($DO_2 = CO \times CaO_2$) and oxygen extraction ($OE = CaO_2 - CvO_2$). Decreases in cardiac output (blood flow) to critical values (DO_{2crit}) produce situations where VO_2 becomes dependent on DO_2 supply. Decreases in DO_2 below DO_{2crit} lead to the accumulation of oxygen (DO_2) (anaerobic metabolism) and the generation of lactic acid, resulting in metabolic acidosis. CaO_2, arterial oxygen content; CO, cardiac output; CvO_2, venous oxygen content.

saturation of Hb with oxygen (SaO_2), the arterial oxygen partial pressure (PaO_2), and cardiac output (CO). The VO_2 can be determined by the Fick, or oxygen consumption, equation [$VO_2 = CO(CaO_2 - CvO_2)$] [209]. The Fick equation can be rearranged to derive oxygen delivery ($DO_2 = CO \times CaO_2$), oxygen extraction ($OE = CaO_2 - CvO_2$), and the oxygen extraction ratio ($OER = CaO_2 \times CvO_2/CaO_2$), noting that all of the equations contain the term CaO_2 and are therefore mathematically coupled. Arterial blood oxygen content (CaO_2) is calculated as ($Hb \times 1.35 \times SaO_2$) + ($PaO_2 \times 0.003$). Arterial blood (Hb = 15 g/dL; PCV = 45%), for example, contains approximately 20–21 mL of oxygen/dL blood when SaO_2 = 100% and PaO_2 = 100 mmHg (room air). The venous blood oxygen content (CvO_2) is generally 14–15 mL/dL, yielding an OER of 0.2–0.3 (20–30%). Decreased hemoglobin concentrations (parasitism, hemorrhage, and hemodilution) cause oxygen extraction to increase in order to maintain the requisite oxygen delivery required by metabolizing tissues. The critical Hb concentration, DO_{2Crit}, and OER_{Crit} are approximately 4 g/dL, 5.0–7 mL/kg/min, and 0.6 (60%), respectively in normal healthy dogs (Fig. 22.46) [210–212].

Most anesthetics are known to decrease O_2 extraction and increase DO_{2Crit} in a dose-dependent manner while increasing blood lactate, an effect that has been explained by anesthetic-induced alterations in blood flow distribution (maldistribution) among organ systems [213,214]. These known effects emphasize the need for continuous monitoring methodologies and individualized goal-directed anesthetic techniques and protocols.

References

1 Reiber CL, McGaw IJ. A review of the "open" and "closed" circulatory systems: new terminology for complex invertebrate circulatory systems in light of current findings. *Int J Zool* 2009; **2009**: 301284.

2 Hicks JW. The physiological and evolutionary significance of cardiovascular shunting patterns in reptiles. *News Physiol Sci* 2002; **17**: 241–245.

3 Kik MJL, Mitchell MA. Reptile cardiology: a review of anatomy and physiology, diagnostic approaches, and clinical disease. *Semin Avian Exotic Pet Med* 2005; **14**: 52–60.

4 Girling SJ, Hynes B: Cardiovascular and haemopoietic systems. In Girling SJ, Raiti P, eds. *BSAVA Manual of Reptiles*, 2nd edn. Gloucester: BSAVA, 2004; 243–260.

5 Holz PH, Burger JP, Pasloske K, *et al.* Effect of injection site on carbenicillin pharmacokinetics in the carpet python, *Morelia spilota*. *J Herp Med Surg* 2002; **12**(4): 12–16.

6 Yasuda N, Targ AG, Eger EI II, *et al.* Pharmacokinetics of desflurane, sevoflurane, isoflurane, and halothane in pigs. *Anesth Analg* 1990; **71**: 340–348.
7 Brosnan RJ, Pypendop PH, Barter LS, *et al.* Pharmacokinetics of inhaled anesthetics in green iguanas (*Iguana iguana*) *Am J Vet Res* 2006; **67**: 1670–1674.
8 Stanley WC, Recchia FA, Lopaschuk GD. Myocardial substrate metabolism in the normal and failing heart. *Physiol Rev* 2005; **85**: 1093–1129.
9 Opie LH. Fuels: aerobic and anaerobic metabolism. In: Opie LH, ed. *Heart Physiology: from Cell to Circulation*, 4th edn. Baltimore: Lippincott Williams & Wilkins, 2004; 306–354.
10 Taegtmeyer H. Energy metabolism of the heart: from basic concepts to clinical applications. *Curr Prob Cardiol* 1994; **19**: 59–113.
11 Opie LH. Channels, pumps, and exchangers. In: Opie LH, ed. *Heart Physiology: from Cell to Circulation*, 4th edn. Baltimore: Lippincott Williams & Wilkins, 2004; 73–118.
12 Kleber AG, Rudy Y. Basic mechanisms of cardiac impulse propagation and associated arrhythmias. *Physiol Rev* 2004; **84**: 431–488.
13 Scholz A. Mechanisms of (local) anaesthetics on voltage-gated sodium and other ion channels. *Br J Anaesth* 2002; **89**: 52–61.
14 Turner LA, Polic S, Hoffmann RG, *et al.* Actions of volatile anesthetics on ischemic and nonischemic Purkinje fibers in the infracted canine heart: regional action potential characteristics. *Anesth Analg* 1993; **76**: 726–733.
15 Weigt HU, Kwok WM, Rehmert GC, *et al.* Voltage-dependent effects of volatile anesthetics on cardiac sodium current. *Anesth Analg* 1997; **84**: 285–293.
16 Möller C. Keeping the rhythm: hERG and beyond in cardiovascular safety pharmacology. *Expert Rev Clin Pharmacol* 2010; **3**: 321–329.
17 Rudy Y. The cardiac ventricular action potential. In: *The Handbook of Physiology. The Cardiovascular System. The Heart.* Bethesda, MD: American Physiological Society, 2002; Sect. 2, Vol. **I**, 531–547.
18 Burt JM, Spray DC. Volatile anesthetics block intercellular commnunication between neonatal rat myocardial cells. *Circ Res* 1989; **65**: 829–836.
19 Task Force of the Working Group on Arrhythmias of the European Society of Cardiology. The 'Sicilian Gambit': a new approach to the classification of antiarrhythmic drugs based on their actions on arrhythmogenic mechanisms. *Eur Heart J* 1991; **12**: 1112–1131.
20 Congdon JM, Marquez M, Niyom S, *et al.* Evaluation of the sedative and cardiovascular effects of intramuscular administration of dexmedetomidine with and without concurrent atropine administration in dogs. *J Am Vet Med Assoc* 2011; **239**: 81–89.
21 Koller BS, Karasik PE, Solomon AJ, *et al.* Relation between repolarization and refractoriness during programmed electrical stimulation in the human right ventricle implications for ventricular tachycardia induction. *Circulation* 1995; **91**: 2378–2384.
22 Antzelevitch C, Shimizu W, Yan GX, *et al.* The M cell: its contribution to the ECG and to normal and abnormal electrical function of the heart. *J Cardiovasc Electrophysiol* 1999; **10**: 1124–1152.
23 Spach MS, Dolber PC. Discontinuous anisotropic propagation. In: Rosen MR, Janse MJ, Wit AL, eds. *Cardiac Electrophysiology: a Textbook.* Mount Kisco, NY: Futura, 1990; 517–534.
24 Spach MS, Dolber PC, Heidlage JF. Influence of the passive anisotropic properties on directional differences in propagation following modification of the sodium conductance in human atrial muscle: a model of re-entry based on anisotropic discontinuous propagation. *Circ Res* 1988; **62**: 811–832.
25 Reynolds AK. On the mechanism of myocardial sensitization to catecholamines by hydrocarbon anesthetics. *Can J Physiol Pharmacol* 1984; **62**: 183–198.
26 Hayashi Y, Kamibayashi T, Sumikawa K, *et al.* Adrenoceptor mechanism involved in thiopental–epinephrine-induced arrhythmias in dogs. *Am J Physiol Heart Circ Physiol* 1993; **265**: H1380–H1385.
27 Kamibayashi T, Hayashi Y, Sumikawa K, *et al.* Enhancement by propofol of epinephrine-induced arrhythmias in dogs. *Anesthesiology* 1991; **75**: 1035–1040.
28 Bednarski RM, Majors LJ. Ketamine and the arrhythmogenic dose of epinephrine in cats anesthetized with halothane and isoflurane. *Am J Vet Res* 1986; **47**: 2122–2125.
29 Himmel HM. Mechanisms involved in cardiac sensitization by volatile anesthetics: general applicability to halogenated hydrocarbons? *Crit Rev Toxicol* 2008; **38**: 773–803.
30 Inagaki Y. Cardiac preconditioning by anesthetic agents: roles of volatile anesthetics and opioids in cardioprotection. *Ynago Acta Med* 2007; **50**: 45–55.
31 Hondeghem, LM. Relative contributions of TRIaD and QT to proarrhythmia. *J Cardiovasc Electrophysiol* 2007; **18**: 655–657.
32 Grant AO, Tranquillo J. Action potential and QT prolongation not sufficient to cause Torsades de Pointes: role of action potential triangulation. *J Cardiovasc Electrophysiol* 2007; **18**: 204–205.
33 Baum VC. Distinctive effects of three intravenous anesthetics on the inward rectifier (IK1) and the delayed rectifier (IK) potassium currents in myocardium: implications for the mechanism of action. *Anesth Analg* 1993; **76**: 18–23.
34 Hatakeyama N, Ito Y, Momose Y. Effects of sevoflurane, isoflurane, and halothane on mechanical and electrophysiologic properties of canine myocardium. *Anesth Analg* 1993; **76**: 1327–1332.
35 Greenstein JL, Winslow RL. Integrative systems models of cardiac excitation–contraction coupling. *Circ Res* 2011; **108**: 70–84.
36 Bers DM. Cardiac excitation–contraction coupling. *Nature* 2002; **415**: 198–205.
37 Opie LH. Excitation–contraction coupling and calcium. In: Opie LH, ed. *Heart Physiology: from Cell to Circulation*, 4th edn. Baltimore: Lippincott Williams & Wilkins, 2004; 159–185.
38 Laver DR. $Ca2^+$ stores regulate ryanodine receptor $Ca2^+$ release channels via luminal and cytosolic $Ca2^+$ sites. *Clin Exp Pharmacol Physiol* 2007; **34**: 889–896.
39 Diaz-Sylvester PL, Porta M, Copello JA. Halothane modulation of skeletal muscle ryanodine receptors: dependence on $Ca2^+$, $Mg2^+$ and ATP. *Am J Physiol Cell Physiol* 2008; **294**: C1103–C1112.
40 Hund TJ, Ziman AP, Lederer WJ, *et al.* The cardiac IP3 receptor: uncovering the role of "the other" calcium release channel. *J Mol Cell Cardiol* 2008; **45**: 159–161.
41 Katz AM. Structure, biochemistry, and biophysics; contractile proteins In: Katz AM, ed. *Physiology of the Heart*, 5th edn. Baltimore: Lippincott Williams & Wilkins, 2011; 88–106.
42 Opie LH. Myocaridal contraction and relaxation. In: Opie LH, ed. *Heart Physiology: from Cell to Circulation*, 4th edn. Baltimore: Lippincott Williams & Wilkins, 2004; 221–246.
43 Knowlen GG, Olivier NF, Kittleson ME. Cardiac contractility. *J Vet Int Med* 1987; **1**: 188–198.
44 Gelissen HP, Epema AH, Henning RH, *et al.* Inotropic effects of propofol, thiopental, midazolam, etomidate, and ketamine on isolated human atrial muscle. *Anesthesiology* 1996; **84**: 397–403.
45 Blanck TJJ, Chiancone E, Salviati G, *et al.* Halothane does not alter $Ca2^+$ affinity of troponin C. *Anesthesiology* 1992; **76**: 100–105.
46 Bosnjak ZJ, Supan FD, Rusch NJ. The effects of halothane, enflurane, and isoflurane on calcium current in isolated canine ventricular cells. *Anesthesiology* 1991; **74**: 340–345.
47 Bosnjak ZJ, Aggarwal A, Turner LA, *et al.* Differential effects of halothane, enflurane, and isoflurane on $Ca2^+$ transients and papillary muscle tension in guinea pigs. *Anesthesiology* 1992; **76**: 123–131.
48 Frazer MJ, Lynch C. Halothane and isoflurane effects on $Ca2^+$ fluxes of isolated myocardial sarcoplasmic reticulum. *Anesthesiology* 1992; **77**: 316–323.
49 Kongsayreepong S, Cook DJ, Housmans PR. Mechanism of the direct, negative inotropic effect of ketamine in isolated ferret and frog ventricular myocardium. *Anesthesiology* 1993; **79**: 313–322.
50 Pagel PS, Kampine JP, Schmeling WT, Warltier DC. Reversal of volatile anesthetic-induced depression of myocardial contractility by extracellular calcium also enhances left ventricular diastolic function. *Anesthesiology* 1993; **8**: 141–154.
51 Rusy BF, Komai H. Anesthetic depression of myocardial contractility: a review of possible mechanisms. *Anesthesiology* 1987; **67**: 745–766.
52 Schmidt U, Schwinger RHG, Uberfuhr P, *et al.* Evidence for an interaction of halothane with the L-type $Ca2^+$ channel in human myocardium. *Anesthesiology* 1993; **79**: 332–339.
53 Wilde DW, Davidson BA, Smith MD, Knight PR. Effects of isoflurane and enflurane on intracellular $Ca2^+$ mobilization in isolated cardiac myocytes. *Anesthesiology* 1993; **79**: 73–82.
54 Wheeler DM, Katz A, Rice RT, Hansford RG. Volatile anesthetic effects on sarcoplasmic reticulum Ca content and sarcolemmal Ca flux in isolated rat cardiac cell suspensions. *Anesthesiology* 1994; **80**: 372–382.
55 Shepard JT, Vanhoutte P. Components of the cardiovascular system: how structure is geared to function. *The Human Cardiovascular System: Facts and Concepts.* New York: Raven Press, 1979; 5–8.
56 Chappell D, Jacob M, Becker BF, *et al.* Expedition glycocalyx. A newly discovered "Great Barrier Reef". *Anaesthesist* 2008; **57**: 959–969 (in German).
57 Levick RJ, Michel CC. Microvascular fluid exchange and the revised Starling principle. *Cardiovasc Res* 2010; **87**: 198–210.
58 Chappell D, Westphal M, Jacob M. The impact of the glycocalyx on microcirculatory oxygen distribution in critical illness. *Curr Opin Anaesthesiol* 2010; **22**: 155–162.
59 Rodrigues SE, Granger DN. Role of blood cells in ischemia–reperfusion induced endothelial barrier failure *Cardiovasc Res* 2010; **87**: 291–299.
60 Green JR. Circulatory mechanics. *Fundamental Cardiovascular and Pulmonary Physiology*, 2nd edn. Philadelphia: Lea and Febiger, 1987; 59–80.
61 Roosterman D, George T, Schneider SW, *et al.* Neuronal control of skin function: the skin as a neuroimmunoendocrine organ. *Physiol Rev* 2006; **86**: 1300–1370.
62 Molyneux GS, Haller CJ, Mogg K, *et al.* The structure, innervation and location of arteriovenous anastomoses in the equine foot. *Equine Vet J* 1994; **26**: 305–312.
63 Lawrence CJ, Prinzen FW, de Lange S. The effect of dexmedetomidine on nutrient organ blood flow. *Anesth Analg* 1996; **83**: 1160–1165.

64 Woodcock TE, Woodcock TM. Revised Starling equation and the glycocalyx model of transvascular fluid exchange: an improved paradigm for prescribing intravenous fluid therapy. *Br J Anaesth* 2012; **108**: 384–394.
65 Becker B, Chappell D, Bruegger D, *et al.* Therapeutic strategies targeting the endothelial glycocalyx: acute deficits, but great potential. *Cardiovasc Res* 2010; **87**: 300–310.
66 Sarin H. Physiologic upper limits of pore size of different blood capillary types and another perspective on the dual pore theory of microvascular permeability. *J Angiogenes Res* 2010; **11**: 2–14.
67 Verkman AS. Aquaporins in clinical medicine. *Annu Rev Med* 2012; **63**: 303–316.
68 Pappenhiemer JR, Soto-Rivera A. Effective osmotic pressure of the plasma proteins and other quantities associated with the capillary circulation in the hindlimbs of cats and dogs. *Am J Physiol* 1948; **152**: 471–491.
69 Taylor AE. Capillary fluid filtration: Starling forces and lymph flow. *Circ Res* 1981; **49**: 557–575.
70 Eschalier A, Lavarenne J, Burtin C, *et al.* Study of histamine release induced by acute administration of antitumor agents in dogs. *Cancer Chemother Pharmacol.* 1988; **21**: 246–250.
71 Robinson EP, Faggella AM, Henry DP, *et al.* Comparison of histamine release induced by morphine and oxymorphone administration in dogs. *Am J Vet Res.* 1988; **49**: 1699–1701.
72 Guedes AG, Papich MG, Rude EP, *et al.* Comparison of plasma histamine levels after intravenous administration of hydromorphone and morphine in dogs. *J Vet Pharmacol Ther* 2007; **30**: 516–522.
73 Lorenz W, Schmal A, Schult H, *et al.* Histamine release and hypotensive reactions in dogs by solubilizing agents and fatty acids: analysis of various components in cremophor EL and development of a compound with reduced toxicity. *Agents Actions* 1982; **12**: 64–80.
74 Caggiati A, Phillips M, Lametschwandtner A, *et al.* Valves in small veins and venules. *Eur J Vasc Endovasc Surg* 2006; **32**: 447–452.
75 Webb RC. Smooth muscle contraction and relaxation. *Adv Physiol Educ* 2003; **27**: 201–206.
76 Clifford PS. Local control of blood flow. *Adv Physiol Educ* 2011; **35**: 5–15.
77 Akata T. Cellular and molecular mechanisms regulating vascular tone. Part 1: basic mechanisms controlling cytosolic $Ca2^+$ concentration and $Ca2^+$-dependent regulation of vascular tone. *J Anesth* 2007; **21**: 220–231.
78 Akata T. Cellular and molecular mechanisms regulating vascular tone. Part 2: regulatory mechanisms modulating $Ca2^+$ mobilization and/or myofilament sensitivity in vascular smooth muscle cells. *J Anesth* 2007; **21**: 232–242.
79 Akata T. General anesthetics and vascular smooth muscle: direct actions of general anesthetics on cellular mechanisms regulating vascular tone. *Anesthesiology* 2007; **106**: 365–391.
80 Bryden JE. Funtional roles of KATP channels in vascular smooth muscle. *Clin Exp Pharmacol Physiol* 2002; **29**: 312–316.
81 Tanaka A, Kawano T, Nakamura A, *et al.* Isoflurane activates sarcolemmal adenosine triphosphate-sensitive potassium channels in vascular smooth muscle cells: a role for protein kinase A. *Anesthesiology* 2007; **106**: 984–991.
82 Chang KSK, Davis RF. Propofol produces endothelium-independent vasodilation and may act as a $Ca2^+$ channel blocker. *Anesth Analg* 1993; **76**: 24–32.
83 Burton AC. Composition of blood. *Physiology and Biophysics of the Circulation*, 2nd edn. Chicago: Year Book Medical Publishers, 1972; 15–21.
84 Lima B, Forrester MT, Hess DT, Stammler JS. *S*-Nitrosylation in cardiovascular signaling. *Circ Res* 2010; **106**: 633–646.
85 Doctor A, Stamler JS. Nitric oxide transport in blood: a third gas in the respiratory cycle. *Compr Physiol* 2011, **1**: 541–568.
86 Schechter AN, Gladwin MT. Hemoglobin and the paracrine and endocrine functions of nitric oxide. *N Engl J Med* 2003; **348**: 1483–1485.
87 Chen K. Pittman RP, Popel AS. Nitric oxide in the vasculature: where does it come from and where does it go? A quantitative perspective. *Antioxid Redox Signal* 2008; **10**: 1185–1198.
88 McHahon, TH, Moone RE, Luschinger BP, *et al.* Nitric oxide in the human respiratory cycle. *Nat Med* 2002; **8**: 711–717.
89 Sonveaux P, Lobysheva II, Renon O, *et al.* Transport and peripheral bioactivities of nitrogen oxides carried by red blood cell hemoglobin: role in oxygen delivery. *Physiology* 2007; **22**: 97–112.
90 Rifkind JM, Nagababu E, Ramasamy S. The quaternary hemoglobin conformation regulates the formation of the nitrite-induced bioactive intermediate and the dissociation of nitric oxide from this intermediate. *Nitric Oxide* 2011; **24**: 102–109.
91 Silva G, Jeney V, Chora A, *et al.* Oxidized hemoglobin is an endogenous proinflammaotry agonist that targets vascular endothelial cell. *J Biol Chem* 2009; **284**: 29582–20595.
92 Vandergriff KD, Winslow RM. A theoretical analysis of oxygen transport: a new strategy for the design of hemoglobin-based red cell substitutes. In: Winslow RM, Vandergriff KD, Intaglieta M, eds. *Blood Substitutes: Physiological Basis of Efficacy.* Boston: Birkhauser, 1995; 143–154.
93 Choi I, Lee S, Hong YK. The new era of the lymphatic system: no longer secondary to the blood vascular system. *Cold Spring Harb Perspect Med* 2012; **2**: 1–23.
94 Margaris KN, Black RA. Modelling the lymphatic system: challenges and opportunities. *J R Soc Inerface* 2012; **9**: 601–612.
95 Kesler CT, Liao S, Munn LL *et al.* Lymphatic vessels in health and disease. *WIREs Syst Biol Med* 2013, **5**: 111–124.
96 Kang S, Lee SP, Kim KE, *et al.* Toll-like receptor 4 in lymphatic endothelial cells contributes to LPS-induced lymphangiogenesis by chemotactic recruitment of macrophages. *Blood* 2009; **113**: 2605–2613.
97 Hemmi H, Akira S. TLR signalling and the function of dendritic cells. *Chem Immunol Allergy* 2005; **86**: 120–135.
98 Hutchinson MR, Zhang Y, Shridhar M, *et al.* Evidence that opioids may have toll like receptor 4 and MD-2 effects. *Brain Behav Immun* 2010; **24**: 83–95.
99 Shavit Y, Wolf G, Goshen I, *et al.* Interleukin-1 antagonizes morphine analgesia and underlies morphine tolerance. *Pain* 2005; **115**: 50–59.
100 Ramanathan T, Skinner H. Coronary blood flow *Contin Educ Anaesth Crit Care Pain* 2005; **5**: 61–64.
101 Rowe GG. Responses of the coronary circulation to physiologic changes and pharmacologic agents. *Anesthesiology* 1974; **41**: 182–196.
102 Mirvis DM, Ramanathan KB. Alterations in transmural blood flow and body surface ST segment abnormalities produced by ischemia in the circumflex and left anterior descending coronary arterial beds of the dog. *Circulation* 1987; **76**: 697–704.
103 Schelbert HR. Anatomy and physiology of coronary blood flow. *J Nucl Cardiol* 2010; **17**: 545–554.
104 Christensen GC, Campeti FD. Anatomic and functional studies of the coronary circulation in the dog and pig. *Am J Vet Res* 1959; **20**: 18–23.
105 Sethna DH, Moffitt EA. An appreciation of the coronary circulation. *Anesth Analg* 1986; **65**: 294–305.
106 Esperança Pina JA, Correia M, O'Neill JG. Morphological study on the thebesian veins of the right cavities of the heart in the dog. *Acta Anat (Basel)* 1975; **92**: 310–320.
107 Moffitt EA, Sethna DH. The coronary circulation and myocardial oxygenation in coronary artery disease. *Anesth Analg* 1986; **65**: 395–401.
108 Tune JD, Richmond KN, Gorman MW, *et al.* Role of nitric oxide and adenosine in control of coronary blood flow in exercising dogs. *Circulation* 2000; **101**: 2942–2948.
109 Denn MJ, Stone HL. Autonomic innervation of dog coronary arteries. *J Appl Physiol* 1976; **41**: 30–35.
110 Greyson CR. The right ventricle and pulmonary circulation: basic concepts. *Rev Esp Cardiol* 2010; **63**: 81–95.
111 Naeije R. Pulmonary circulation at exercise. *Compr Physiol* 2012; **2**: 711–714.
112 Nagendran J, Stewart K, Hoskinson M, *et al.* An anesthesiologist's guide to hypoxic pulmonary vasoconstriction: implications for managing single-lung anesthesia and atelectasis. *Curr Opin Anaesthesiol* 2006; **19**: 34–43.
113 Van Keer L, Van Aken H, Vandermeersch E, *et al.* Propofol does not inhibit hypoxic pulmonary vasoconstriction in humans. *J Clin Anesth* 1989; **1**: 284–288.
114 Benumof JL. Isoflurane anesthesia and arterial oxygenation during one-lung ventilation. *Anesthesiology* 1986; **64**: 419–422.
115 Gelman S, Mushlin PS. Catecholamine-induced changes in the splanchnic circulation affecting systemic hemodynamics. *Anesthesiology* 2004; **100**: 434–439.
116 Carneiro JJ, Donald DE. Blood reservoir function of the dog spleen, liver and intestine. *Am J Physiol Circ Physiol* 1977; **232**: H67–H72.
117 Gelman S. Venous function and central venous pressure. *Anesthesiology* 2008; **108**: 735–748.
118 Gelman S, Reves JG, Harris D. Circulatory responses to midazolam anesthesia: emphasis on canine splanchnic circulation. *Anesth Analg* 1983; **62**: 135–139.
119 Baskurt OK, Meiselman HJ. Blood rheology and hemodynamics. *Semin Thromb Hemost* 2003; **5**: 435–450.
120 Sutera SP, Skalak R.. The history of Poiseuille's law. *Ann Rev Fluid Mech* 1993; **25**: 1–19.
121 Sonneblick EH, Braunwald JR. Oxygen consumption of the heart: newer concepts of its multifactorial determination. *J Am Coll Cardiol* 1999; **34**: 1365–1368.
122 O'Rourke MF, Pauca A, Jiang XJ. Pulse wave analysis. *Br J Clin Pharmacol* 2001; **51**: 507–522.
123 Lasala PA, Chien S, Michelsen CB. Hemorrheology: what is the ideal hematocrit? In: Askanasi J, Starker RM, Weissman C, eds. *Fluid and Electrolyte Management in Critical Care.* Boston: Butterworth, 1986; 203–213.
124 Hightower CM, Salazar Vázquez BY, Woo Park S, *et al.* Integration of cardiovascular regulation by the blood/endothelium cell-free layer. *Wiley Interdiscip Rev Syst Biol Med* 2011; **3**: 458–470.
125 Reinhart WH. Molecular biology and self-regulatory mechanisms of blood viscosity: a review. *Biorheology* 2001; **38**: 203–212.
126 Tsai AG, Acero C, Nance PR, *et al.* Elevated plasma viscosity in extreme hemodilution increases perivascular nitric oxide concentration and microvascular perfusion. *Am J Physiol Heart Circ Physiol* 2004; **288**: 1730–1739.

127 Pries AR, Secomb TW, Gaehtgens P, Gross JF. Blood flow in microvascular networks: experiments and simulation. *Circ Res* 1990; **67**: 826–834.
128 Crowell JW, Smith EE. Determinants of the optimal hematocrit. *J Appl Physiol* 1967; **22**: 501–504.
129 Chapler CK, Cain SM. The physiologic reserve in oxygen carrying capacity: studies in experimental hemodilution. *Can J Physiol Pharmacol* 1986; **64**: 7–12.
130 Leone BJ, Spahn DR. Anemia, hemodilution, and oxygen delivery. *Anesth Analg* 1992; **75**: 651–653.
131 Carbrales P, Tsai AG, Intaglietta M. Microvascular pressure and functional capillary density in extreme hemodilution with low- and high-viscosity dextran and a low-viscosity Hb-based O_2 carrier. *Am J Physiol Heart Circ Physiol* 2004; **287**: H363–H373.
132 O'Rourke MF, Pauca A, Jiang XJ. Pulse wave analysis. *Br J Clin Pharmacol* 2001; **51**: 507–522.
133 O'Rourke MF. Vascular impedance in studies of arterial and cardiac function. *Physiol Rev* 1982; **62**: 570–617.
134 Little WC, Cheng C. Left ventricular–arterial coupling in conscious dogs. *Am J Physiol* 1991; **261**: H70–H76.
135 Kouraklis G, Karayannacos P, Sechas M, *et al.* The influence of hemodilution on left ventricular function. *Int Angiol* 1990; **9**: 38–42.
136 Wood NB. Aspects of fluid dynamics applied to the larger arteries. *J Theor Biol* 1999; **199**: 137–161.
137 Yoganathan AP, Cape EG, Sung HW. Review of hydrodynamic principles for the cardiologist: applications to the study of blood flow and jets imaging techniques. *J Am Coll Cardiol* 1988; **12**: 1344–1253.
138 London GM, Pannier B. Arterial functions: how to interpret the complex physiology. *Nephrol Dial Transplant* 2010; **25**: 3815–3823.
139 Thiele RH, Durieux ME. Arterial waveform analysis for the anesthesiologist: past, present, and future concepts. *Anesth Analg* 2011; **113**: 766–776.
140 Rothe CF. Mean circulatory filling pressure: its meaning and measurement. *J Appl Physiol* 1993; **74**: 499–509.
141 Lamia B, Chemla D, Richard C, *et al.* Clinical review: interpretation of arterial pressure in shock states. *Crit Care* 2005; **9**: 601–606.
142 Barbeito A, Mark JB. Arterial and central venous pressure monitoring. *Anesthesiol Clin* 2006; **24**: 717–735.
143 London GM, Pannier B. Arterial functions: how to interpret the complex physiology. *Br J Clin Pharmacol* 2010; **51**: 507–522.
144 Montenij LJ, de Waal EE, Buhre WF. Arterial waveform analysis in anesthesia and critical care. *Curr Opin Anaesthesiol* 2011; **24**: 651–656.
145 Marik, PE, Baram M, Vahid B. Does central venous pressure predict fluid responsiveness? A systematic review of the literature and the Tale of the Seven Mares. *Chest* 2008; **134**: 172–178.
146 Marik PE. Nonivasive cardiac output monitors: a state-of-the-art review. *J Cardiothorac Vasc Anesth* 2013; **27**: 121–134.
147 Sagawa K. The end-systolic pressure–volume relation of the ventricle: definition, modifications and clinical use. *Circulation* 1981; **63**: 1223–1227.
148 Burkhoff D, Mirsky I, Hiroyuki S. Assessment of systolic and diastolic ventricular properties via pressure–volume analysis: a guide for clinical translational, and basic researchers. *Am J Physiol Heart Circ Physiol* 2005; **289**: H501–H512.
149 Welker FH, Muir WW. An investigation of the second heart sound in the normal horse. *Equine Vet J* 1990; **22**: 403–407.
150 Ettinger SJ, Suter PF. Heart sounds and phonocardiography. Canine Cardiology. *Philadelphia: WB Saunders*, 1970; **12–39**.
151 Pappano AJ, Wier WG. *Cardiovascular Physiology*. Philadelphia: Elsevier Mosby, 2013; 69–116.
152 Suga H, Igarashi Y, Yamada O, Goto Y. Mechanical efficiency of the left ventricle as a function of preload, afterload, and contractility. *Heart Vessels* 1985; **1**: 3–8.
153 Brutsaert DL, Rademakers FE, Sys SU, *et al.* Analysis of relaxation in the evaluation of ventricular function of the heart. *Prog Cardiovasc Dis* 1985; **28**: 143–163.
154 Pagel PS, Grossman W, Haering M, *et al.* Left ventricular diastolic function in the normal and diseased heart: perspecitives for the anesthesiologist. *Anesthesiology* 1993; **79**: 836–854.
155 Guyton AC, Richardson TQ, Langston JB. Regulation of cardiac output and venous return. *Clin Anesth* 1964; **3**: 1–34.
156 Beard DA, Feigl EO. Understanding Guyton's venous return curves. *Am J Physiol Heart Circ Physiol* 2011; **301**: H629–H633.
157 Rothe C. Toward consistent definitions for preload and afterload – revisited. *Adv Physiol Educ* 2003; **27**: 44–45.
158 Milnor WR. The normal hemodynamic state: vascular impedance and wave reflection. In: Milnor WR, ed. *Hemodynamics*, 2nd edn. Baltimore: Williams & Wilkins, 1989; 142–224.
159 Zhong L, Ghista DN, Tan RS. Left ventricular wall stress compendium. *Comput Methods Biomech Biomed Eng* 2012; **15**: 1015–1041.
160 Nichols WW, O'Rourke FO, Auolio AP, *et al.* Age-related changes in left ventricular/arterial coupling. In: Yin FCP, ed. *Ventricular/Vascular Coupling: Clinical, Physiological, and Engineering Aspects*. New York: Springer, 1987; 79–114.
161 Hayashida K, Sunagawa K, Noma M, *et al.* Mechanical matching of the left ventricle with the arterial system in exercising dogs. *Circ Res* 1992; **71**: 481–489.
162 Swanson CR, Muir WW. Simultaneous evaluation of left ventricular end-systolic pressure–volume ratio and time constant of isovolumic pressure decline in dogs exposed to equivalent MAC halothane and isoflurane. *Anesthesiology* 1988; **68**: 764–770.
163 Pagel PS, Kampine JP, Schmeling WT, Warltier DC. Comparison of the systemic and coronary hemodynamic actions of desflurane, isoflurane, halothane, and enflurane in the chronically instrumented dog. *Anesthesiology* 1991; **74**: 539–551.
164 Pagel PS, Schmeling WT, Kampine JP, Warltier DC. Alteration of canine left ventricular diastolic function by intravenous anesthetics in vivo: ketamine and propofol. *Anesthesiology* 1992; **76**: 419–425.
165 Sagawa K. The end-systolic pressure–volume relation of the ventricle: definition, modifications and clinical use. *Circulation* 1981; **63**: 1223–1227.
166 Little WC, Downes TR. Clinical evaluation of left ventricular diastolic performance. *Prog Cardiovasc Dis* 1990; **32**: 273–290.
167 Bressack, MA, Raffin TA. Importance of venous return, venous resistance, and mean circulatory pressure in physiology and management of shock. *Chest* 1987; **92**: 906–912.
168 Freeman GL, Colston JT. Role of ventriculovascular coupling in cardiac response to increased contractility in closed-chest dogs. *J Clin Invest* 1990; **86**: 1278–1284.
169 Hayashida K, Sunagawa K, Noma M, *et al.* Mechanical matching of the left ventricle with the arterial system in exercising dogs. *Circ Res* 1992; **71**: 481–489.
170 Westerhof N. Cardiac work and efficiency. *Cardiovasc Res* 2000; **48**: 4–7.
171 Archie JP. Mathematical coupling of data: a common source of error. *Ann Surg* 1980; **193**: 296–303.
172 Walsh TS, Lee A. Mathematical coupling in medical research: lessons from studies of oxygen kinetics. *Br J Anaesth* 1998; **81**: 118–120.
173 Eger EI. Tissue groups arranged by solubility and perfusion characteristics. *Anesthetic Uptake and Action*. Baltimore: Williams & Wilkins, 1974; 88–94.
174 Shepherd JT, Vanhoutte PM. Neurohumoral regulation. *The Human Cardiovascular System: Facts and Concepts*. New York: Raven Press, 1979; 107–155.
175 Mohrman DE, Heller LJ. Regulation of arterial pressure. *Cardiovascular Physiology* 6th edn. New York: McGraw-Hill, 2006; 161–184.
176 Armagan D, Lam AM. Cerebral autoregulation and anesthesia. *Curr Opin Anaesthesiol* 2009; **22**: 547–552.
177 Westfall TC, Westfall DP. Neurotransmission: the autonomic and somatic motor nervous systems. In: Brunton LL, Lazo JS, Parker KL, eds. *Goodman & Gilman's The Pharmacologic Basis of Therapeutics*, 11th edn. New York: McGraw-Hill, 2006; 137–181.
178 McCorry LK. Physiology of the autonomic nervous system. *Am J Pharm Educ* 2007; **71**: 1–11.
179 Segal SS. Regulation of blood flow in the microcirculation. *Microcirculation* 2005; **12**: 33–45.
180 Arimura H, Bosnjak ZJ, Hoka S, Kampine JP. Modifications by halothane of responses to acute hypoxia in systemic vascular capacitance, resistance, and sympathetic nerve activity in dogs. *Anesth Analg* 1991; **73**: 319–326.
181 Hart JL, Jing M, Bina S, *et al.* Effects of halothane on EDRF/cGMP-mediated vascular smooth muscle relaxations. *Anesthesiology* 1993; **79**: 323–331.
182 McCallum JB, Stekiel TA, Bosnjak ZJ Kampine JP. Does isoflurane alter mesenteric venous capacitance in the intact rabbit? *Anesth Analg* 1993; **76**: 1095–1105.
183 Toda H, Nakamura K, Hatano Y, *et al.* Halothane and isoflurane inhibit endothelium-dependent relaxation elicited by acetylcholine. *Anesth Analg* 1992; **75**: 198–203.
184 Isbister JP. Physiology and pathophysiology of blood volume regulation. *Transfus Sci* 1997; **18**: 409–432.
185 Ickx BE, Rigolet M, Van der Linder PJ. Cardiovascular and metabolic response to acute normovolemic anemia: effects of anesthesia. *Anesthesiology* 2000; **93**: 1011–1016.
186 Kinsella SM, Tuckey JP. Perioperative bradycardia and asystole: relationship to vasovagal syncope and the Bezold–Jarisch reflex. *Br J Anaesth* 2001; **86**: 859–868.
187 Campagna JA, Carter C. Clinical relevance of the Bezold–Jarisch reflex. *Anesthesiology* 2003; **98**: 1250–1260.
188 Maze M, Tranquilli W. Alpha-2 adrenoceptor agonists: defining the role in clinical anesthesia. *Anesthesiology* 1991; **74**: 581–605.
189 Gehler DR. Introduction to the reviews on neuropeptide Y. *Neuropeptides* 2004; **38**: 135–140.
190 Hosey MM. Diversity of structure, signaling and regulation within the family of muscarinic cholinergic receptors. *FASEB J* 1992; **6**: 845–852.
191 Calver A, Collier J, Vallance P. Nitric oxide and cardiovascular control. *Exp Physiol* 1993; **78**: 303–326.
192 Mirenda JV, Grissom TE. Anesthetic implications of the renin–angiotensin system and angiotensin-converting enzyme inhibitors. *Anesth Analg* 1991; **72**: 667–683.
193 Colson, P, Ryckwaert F, Coriat P. Renin angiotensin system antagoninsts and anesthesia. *Anesth Analg* 1999; **89**: 1143–1155.

194 Maybauer MO, Maybauer DM, Enkhbaatar P, *et al.* Physiology of the vasopressin receptors. *Best Pract Res Clin Anaesthesiol* 2008; **22**: 253–263.
195 Olsson RA. Local factors regulating cardiac and skeletal muscle blood flow. *Annu Rev Physiol* 1981; **43**: 385–395.
196 Lipowsky HH. Microvascular rheology and hemodynamics. *Microcirculation* 2005; **12**: 5–15.
197 Davis MJ, Hill MA. Signaling mechanisms underlying the vascular myogenic response. *Phyisol Rev* 1999; **79**: 387–423.
198 Pyke KE, Tschakovsky ME. Peak vs. total reactive hyperemia: which determines the magnitude of flow-mediated dilation? *J Appl Physiol* 2007; **102**: 1510–1519.
199 Popel AS, Johnson PC. Microcirculation and hemorheology. *Annu Rev Fluid Mech* 2005; **37**: 43–69.
200 Sriram K, Salazar Vázquez BY, Tsai AG, *et al.* Autoregulation and mechanotransduction control the arteriolar response to small changes in hematocrit. *Am J Physiol Heart Circ Physiol* 2012; **303**: H1096–H1106.
201 Cabrlaes P, Tsai AG. Plasma viscosity regulates systemic and microvascular perfusion during acute extreme anemic conditions. *Am J Physiol Heart Circ Physiol* 2006; **291**: H2445–H2452.
202 Késmárky G, Kenyeres P, Rábai M, *et al.* Plasma viscosity: a forgotten variable. *Clin Hemorheol Microcirc* 2008; **39**: 243–246.
203 Tsai AG, Friesenecker B, McCarthy M, *et al.* Plasma viscosity regulates capillary perfusion during extreme hemodilution in hamster skinfold model. *Am J Physiol Heart Circ Physiol* 1998; **275**: H2170–H2180.
204 Watts SW. Endothelin receptors: what's new and what do we need to know? *Am J Physiol Regul Integr Comp Physiol* 2010; **298**: R254–R260.
205 Dunham CM, Siegel JH, Weireter L, *et al.* Oxygen debt and metabolic acidemia as quantitative predictors of mortality and the severity of the ischemic insult in hemorrhagic shock. *Crit Care Med* 1991; **19**: 231–243.
206 Shoemaker WC, Appel PL, Kram HB. Role of oxygen debt in the development of organ failure sepsis, and death in high-risk surgical patients. *Chest* 1992; **102**: 208–215.
207 Rixen D, Siegel JH. Bench-to-bedside review: oxygen debt and its metabolic correlates as quantifiers of the severity of hemorrhagic and post-traumatic shock. *Crit Care* 2005; **9**: 441–453.
208 Siegel JH, Fabian M, Smith JA, *et al.* Oxygen debt criteria quantify the effectiveness of early partial resuscitation after hypovolemic hemorrhagic shock. *J Trauma* 2003; **54**: 862–880.
209 Geerts BF, Aarts LP, Jansen JR. Methods in pharmacology: measurement of cardiac output. *Br J Clin Pharmacol* 2011; **71**: 316–330.
210 Schumacker PT, Cain SM. The concept of a critical oxygen delivery. *Intens Care Med* 1987; **13**: 223–229.
211 Van der Linden P, Schmartz D, De Groote F, *et al.* Critical haemoglobin concentration in anaesthetized dogs: comparison of two plasma substitutes. *Br J Anaesth* 1998; **81**: 556–562.
212 Cain SM. Oxygen delivery and uptake in dogs during anemic and hypoxic hypoxia. *J Appl Physiol* 1977; **42**: 228–234.
213 Van der Linden P, Gilbart E, Engelman E, *et al.* Effects of anesthetic agents on systemic critical O_2 delivery. *J Appl Physiol* 1994; **71**: 83–93.
214 Van der Linden P, De Hert S, Mathieu N *et al.* Tolerance to acute isovolemic hemodilution. *Anesthesiology* 2003; **99**: 97–104.

23 Cardiac Output Measurement

Alessio Vigani
Department of Clinical Sciences, College of Veterinary Medicine, North Carolina State University, Raleigh, North Carolina, USA

Chapter contents

Introduction

Cardiac output is the volume of blood ejected from each of the ventricles per minute, usually reported in L/min, and is the product of the heart rate and stroke volume. Cardiac index is the cardiac output referenced to the body surface area, or body weight, of the patient, and is expressed in L/min/m^2 and L/min/kg, respectively. (Table 23.1) Cardiac output is determined by five primary variables: heart rate, rhythm, preload, contractility, and afterload [1].

Cardiac output summarizes in a single value the contribution of the cardiovascular system to the global oxygen delivery from the heart to the body. It therefore appears reasonable to monitor cardiac output in the assessment of cardiovascular insufficiency in any critical patient undergoing anesthesia. Unfortunately, no definitive studies have shown that the determination of cardiac output or its changes in response to therapy is superior to standard hemodynamic monitoring in terms of outcome [2]. In fact, there is lack of evidence of improved outcomes in acutely ill patients with the use of any specific monitoring device, not only cardiac output monitors [3]. Moreover, cardiac output should not be evaluated as a sole variable in a clinical setting. For instance, if metabolic rate is increased or blood flow distribution is abnormal in septic patients, they often have a normal or even increased cardiac output and may still be in circulatory failure [4].

This raises the question, why do we measure cardiac output? There is clear evidence that persistence of a low cardiac output state has significant detrimental effects on organ perfusion and oxygenation [5]. In critically ill human patients, a low cardiac output with sustained lack of response to therapy has been associated with a high mortality rate [6]. Therefore, at least in some specific patients, the measurement of cardiac output may represent a supplemental aid to assess the adequacy of therapy and to guide targeted therapeutic interventions (e.g., goal-directed fluid therapy) [2]. More specifically, in a hypotensive patient, whenever the clinical signs are difficult to interpret, or the cause of hypotension is not obvious and likely multifactorial (including anesthetic drug effects), the use of cardiac output monitoring should be considered. In this regard, estimation of cardiac output is a useful tool for patient management during anesthesia.

Measuring cardiac output is advantageous in monitoring anesthetic-related hemodynamic changes and also in assessing effectiveness of resuscitation of trauma and critically ill patients [7]. Monitoring the extent of the relative changes in cardiac output, for example, following fluid resuscitation in hypovolemic patients, allows the anesthetist to assess the effectiveness of the intervention and to separate fluid responders from non-responders [8–10]. In different scenarios, following patient trends in cardiac output rather than blood pressure, such as during dobutamine or a nitroprusside infusion, gives more meaningful information about the hemodynamic response to therapy [11].

Importantly, the determination of absolute values of cardiac output is often less important than following trends. The assessment of relative changes in cardiac output following the challenge of the cardiovascular system, with fluid loading or medications, is referred to as 'functional cardiac output monitoring' [12]. Once it has been determined that assessing cardiac output may be indicated for a given circumstance, then it is also important that its measurement is accurate enough to identify clinically relevant changes in response to therapy. An acute increase in cardiac output of 20–25% is usually accepted as clinically relevant to identify a positive response, because such a change corresponds to the limit of accuracy of current measuring techniques [13].

Veterinary Anesthesia and Analgesia: The Fifth Edition of Lumb and Jones.
Edited by Kurt A. Grimm, Leigh A. Lamont, William J. Tranquilli, Stephen A. Greene and Sheilah A. Robertson.

Table 23.1 Examples of typical cardiac output indices reported in veterinary species.

Species	SVI (mL/kg/beat)	HR (beats/min)	CI (mL/min/kg)
Cat	0.90–1.0	180	160–180
Cattle	0.7–0.8	60	35–50
Dog	1.6–1.9	120	190–230
Goat	1.1–1.3	80	85–100
Horse	2.6–3.0	45	115–135
Mouse	1.5–1.8	400	600–720
Rabbit	0.4–0.6	250	100–150
Rat	1–1.2	300	300–360
Sheep	0.7–0.9	80	55–70
Swine	1.2–1.4	100	120–140

SVI, stroke volume index; HR, heart rate; CI, cardiac index.

The ideal cardiac output monitoring technique would provide accurate, interpretable, and reproducible measurements, be user friendly, and be readily available. The ideal device should also be safe for the patient, be operator independent, provide a rapid response time, and be cost-effective. Ultimately, the results obtained should be clinically relevant to guide therapy. To be useful in the management of the hemodynamically unstable patient, the technique should rapidly allow cardiac output to be taken repetitively [14]. At present, there is no available device that meets all these criteria.

Basic principles of cardiac output monitoring

Veterinary anesthesiologists now have available an increasing number of techniques and measuring devices to assess cardiac output, and each technique has its own strengths and limitations [15]. As for the selection of monitoring systems for any other physiologic parameter, the following general principles can serve as guidelines to decide the more suitable cardiac output monitoring technique for use.

No hemodynamic monitoring technique can improve outcome by itself: estimating cardiac output is not an exception. Three fundamental conditions must be met for hemodynamic monitoring to affect outcome positively: (1) the results obtained must be of clinical relevance to the patient, (2) the data obtained must be sufficiently accurate and precise to trigger a therapeutic intervention, and (3) the therapeutic intervention must improve outcome. If the information obtained is inaccurate, or interpreted or applied incorrectly, the resultant intervention will be unlikely to improve the patient's condition and may potentially be detrimental [3,13].

The choice of monitoring system depends on the patient (species, size) and often on the availability of devices and expertise at a specific hospital or institution. The expertise and familiarity of the operator represent a critical factor in obtaining reliable results with many cardiac output monitoring devices. A typical example of high operator dependency is represented by echocardiography compared with other automatic devices that consistently produce results with low inter-operator variability [13].

As with any other monitored parameter, it is critical to integrate cardiac output data with other physiologic variables from multiple sources. The patient's blood pressure is important complementary information. A low cardiac output in a hypotensive patient will likely indicate hypovolemia or decreased cardiac function, whereas a high cardiac output in a hypotensive patient would suggest decreased vascular resistance [12].

In the clinical setting, cardiac output is estimated, not measured [16]. The only technique that allows its user to measure cardiac output directly is electromagnetic flowmetry, which requires the surgical implantation of a flow probe circumferentially to the main pulmonary artery. This technique is considered the gold standard in the research setting, but it is, for obvious reasons, impractical for clinical applications [17]. All values from bedside techniques are estimates of cardiac output based on assumptions and algorithms. Because of this estimation, comparison of results from different techniques often produces relatively poor agreement and significant bias [16]. In humans, the invasive pulmonary artery catheter (PAC) thermodilution technique is generally considered as the 'reference' standard for clinical purposes, but has its own limitations [8]. A measurement obtained by a less invasive technique may be preferable if it can be obtained more rapidly and easily, even if it is slightly less accurate. In veterinary medicine, an example of this is the utilization of the lithium dilution cardiac output technique as a suitable reference method in horses for comparison of other cardiac output monitoring devices [15,18–20].

Non-invasiveness of the technique should not be the priority. Although obviously preferable, being non-invasive is not always possible and may even be counterproductive. For instance, the real advantage of echocardiography over other cardiac output techniques is not its non-invasiveness but the peculiarity of providing a direct evaluation of cardiac function [21,22]. A completely non-invasive technique such as bioimpedance, despite being found reliable in healthy human individuals, has proved inconsistent when applied to critically ill patients or when used in other species [13,23].

History of cardiac output measurement

The first technique for the calculation of cardiac output was described by Adolph Fick in 1870. Fick described the calculation of cardiac output from the measurement of the oxygen content of arterial and mixed venous blood as well as oxygen consumption [24]. The Fick technique requires catheterization of the pulmonary artery for mixed venous blood sampling. This was first performed experimentally in live dogs in 1886 by Grehant and Quinquaud [25], and then by Zuntz and Hagemann in a horse in 1898 [26]. Its clinical use in humans did not occur for almost another 50 years. Measurement of oxygen consumption has always represented a significant challenge, and this remains a major limitation of the Fick technique [27]. For this reason, the use of estimates of oxygen consumption was introduced and the method was referred to as the modified Fick technique. The Fick technique became the standard for the measurement of cardiac output until the development of dye dilution techniques.

The dye dilution technique of cardiac output determination is based on the independent work of Stewart and Hamilton in the late nineteenth and early twentieth centuries [28]. The equation they derived allowed for the estimation of cardiac output by knowing the amount of an injected indicator and calculating the area under its dilution curve measured downstream. Dye dilution techniques were repeatedly shown to be as reliable as the Fick technique and of better suitability in the clinical setting [29–31]. Thus, dye dilution rapidly became the 'accepted method of reference' for cardiac output measurement [32].

Thermodilution, first described by Fegler in 1954, uses heat as an indicator, and relies on the same principles of dye dilution [33]. The landmark article on right heart catheterization with a balloon-tipped catheter by Swan *et al.* in 1970 [34] finally set the stage for the widespread clinical use of cardiac output monitoring [35]. Since then, the accuracy of thermodilution-based cardiac output measurements has been assessed in hundreds of studies. Interestingly, all of these studies have in common a major limitation represented by the lack of a gold standard for comparison. Over time, PAC-based thermodilution showed good agreement with direct Fick calculations and dye dilution techniques in a wide range of clinical conditions, and this, combined with the relative ease of insertion of a PAC in humans, has made this technique the clinical 'gold standard' for comparison with all new cardiac output monitors [32,36,37].

Despite the widespread use of PAC thermodilution, many studies have questioned the effectiveness and safety of this technology [38–43]. This has driven the recent interest in the development of alternative technologies that can measure cardiac output less invasively [44–46].

Techniques of determination of cardiac output

The development and validation of new technologies to measure cardiac output represent great opportunities for veterinary clinical and research application. Many of the techniques described in this chapter are currently used or will eventually be suitable for use in veterinary medicine.

The Fick principle

Cardiac output can be elegantly estimated by using the Fick principle. The technique is based on the law of conservation of mass [27]. The principle states that over a given time period, the quantity of O_2 or CO_2 entering or leaving the lungs is equal to the quantity of the gas taken up or expelled by the blood flowing in the pulmonary circulation. In mathematical terms, Fick principle-derived cardiac output equals the patient's oxygen uptake (VO_2) divided by the difference between arterial and mixed venous oxygen content (CaO_2 - CvO_2) [47]:

$$\text{cardiac output} = \frac{VO_2}{CaO_2 - CvO_2}$$

This is true only assuming the absence of any cardiopulmonary shunting [47]. Determining cardiac output using this method requires catheterization of both a peripheral artery and the main pulmonary artery for arterial and mixed venous blood sampling, respectively [27]. The measurement of VO_2 also requires accurate collection and analysis of exhaled gases or determination via closed-circuit techniques. The measurement of VO_2 is the most problematic step of the Fick method that has ultimately limited its use for clinical purposes [47].

An indirect Fick method known as the partial rebreathing technique has been developed to eliminate the need for pulmonary artery catheterization and invasive blood gas sampling. The NICO® monitor (Novametrix Medical Systems, Wallingford, CT, USA) applies the indirect Fick principle to elimination of carbon dioxide (CO_2) rather than uptake of oxygen [48]. This technology uses intermittent periods of partial rebreathing to allow the minimally invasive estimation of arterial and mixed venous CO_2 content. The monitor consists of a carbon dioxide sensor, a disposable airflow sensor connected to a closed loop system, and a pulse oxymeter. The NICO monitor estimates arterial and mixed venous CO_2 contents from measurements of end-tidal CO_2 partial pressure ($P_{ET}CO_2$) during normal breathing and rebreathing maneuvers. VCO_2 is calculated from minute ventilation and its carbon dioxide content. The arterial dioxide content ($CaCO_2$) is estimated from end-tidal carbon dioxide during periods of ventilation. Intermittent phases of partial rebreathing allow estimation of mixed venous CO_2 partial pressure ($PvCO_2$), from which CO_2 content ($CvCO_2$) is calculated. As the patient rebreathes, the level of $P_{ET}CO_2$ rises to a plateau level corresponding to the partial pressure of CO_2 in the blood entering the lungs (or mixed venous blood). At this equilibrium point, the CO_2 elimination from the lungs approaches zero and the partial pressure of CO_2 in the end pulmonary capillary blood (mixed venous blood) can be assumed to be equal to $P_{ET}CO_2$ [49].

Each cardiac output determination requires about 4 min. Every 3 min, a rebreathing valve that prevents normal volumes of CO_2 from being eliminated is activated and the patient's inhaled and exhaled gases are diverted through the NICO loop for 50 s [48]. As a result, the elimination of CO_2 drops and the concentration of CO_2 in the pulmonary artery increases. It is assumed that cardiac output remains unchanged under normal (N) and rebreathing conditions (R). To compensate for the presence of shunted blood, cardiopulmonary shunting is estimated by the use of pulse oximetry and F_IO_2 [49]. The general equation at the base of the technique is

$$\text{cardiac output} = \frac{VCO_2N - VCO_2R}{(CvCO_2N - CaCO_2N) - (CvCO_2R - CaCO_2R)}$$

where VCO_2, $CvCO_2$, and $CaCO_2$ are CO_2 consumption, venous CO_2 concentration, and arterial CO_2 concentration, respectively.

Because the diffusion rate of carbon dioxide is 20 times higher than that of oxygen, it is assumed that no difference in venous CO_2 ($CvCO_2$) will occur, whether under normal or rebreathing conditions. Hence the above equation is simplified to

$$\text{cardiac output} = \frac{VCO_2N - VCO_2R}{CaCO_2N - CaCO_2R}$$

Partial CO_2 rebreathing cardiac output showed sufficient reliability for clinical application in adult and pediatric human patients [50–52]. However, the accuracy of the NICO device in critical patients has been questioned [53]. The NICO monitor has been tested in veterinary species, including dogs and horses [53–55]. The need for endotracheal intubation and mechanical ventilation limits the use of this device to the intraoperative period. In validation studies in humans and in dogs, a tidal volume of 12 mL/kg produced cardiac output determinations that correlated well with measurements obtained by both thermodilution and lithium dilution techniques [55–57]. The need for constant CO_2 elimination precludes the use of the NICO monitor during spontaneous breathing in small animals, owing to the variability of the tidal volume [55].

Pulmonary artery catheter thermodilution

The traditional intermittent thermodilution technique uses as an indicator a bolus of ice-cold sterile saline injected into the right atrium via a pulmonary artery catheter (Swan–Ganz catheter). The change over time in the temperature of the blood in the main pulmonary artery is then used to calculate cardiac output [36].

A saline bolus of known volume and temperature is injected into the right atrium via the proximal port of a Swan–Ganz catheter [58]. The saline solution can be cooled in ice or injected at room temperature, and can be administered in a volume of either 5 or 10

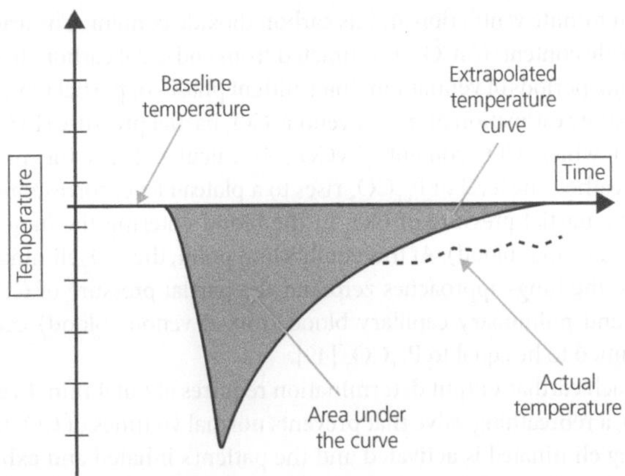

Figure 23.1 Graphical representation of the dilution curve for cardiac PAC thermodilution cardiac output.

mL. As a general rule, higher volumes and lower temperatures produce the most accurate results. The saline mixes with the blood as it passes through the right ventricle and the pulmonary artery, thus decreasing the temperature of the blood. The changes in blood temperature are detected by a thermistor at the distal end of the catheter, which lies within the main pulmonary artery, and a computer acquires the thermodilution curve over time (Fig. 23.1) [33]. The cardiac output computer then calculates flow (cardiac output from the right ventricle) using the acquired blood temperature information, and the starting temperature and volume of the injected saline bolus. The injection is normally repeated at least twice and the measurements are averaged. Because cardiac output changes during the respiratory cycle, it is important to inject the saline during a consistent phase of respiration. Conventionally this is done at the end of expiration [37].

As with all of the indicator-dilution methods, the measurement of thermodilution cardiac output is based on the Stewart–Hamilton equation:

$$\text{cardiac output} = \frac{\text{volume of indicator} \times \left(\text{Temp}_{\text{patient}} - \text{Temp}_{\text{indicator}}\right)}{\int \Delta\text{Temp}\, dt}$$

The denominator is a mathematical integration defined by the integral sign ∫ and ΔTemp is the gradient in temperature and represents the integral in the function. The d*t* indicates that time (*t*) is the variable of integration. The domain of the integration is from $t = 0$ to $t = \infty$. The function is then defined as the area under the curve bounded by the graph of ΔTemp, the time axis, and the vertical lines $t = 0$ and $x = \infty$. The temperature curve does not actually return to the baseline because of recirculation; the computer accounts for this in the calculation of the area under the curve, by extrapolating the projected return to baseline of the temperature.

Cardiac output is inversely proportional to ∫ΔTemp d*t*; therefore, when cardiac output is high, the indicator crosses the temperature sensor quickly, producing a small area under the ΔTemp curve. Conversely, when cardiac output is low, the bolus of cold saline diffuses in the right ventricle and pulmonary artery over a relatively long time, causing the area under the temperature versus time curve to be larger (Fig. 23.2).

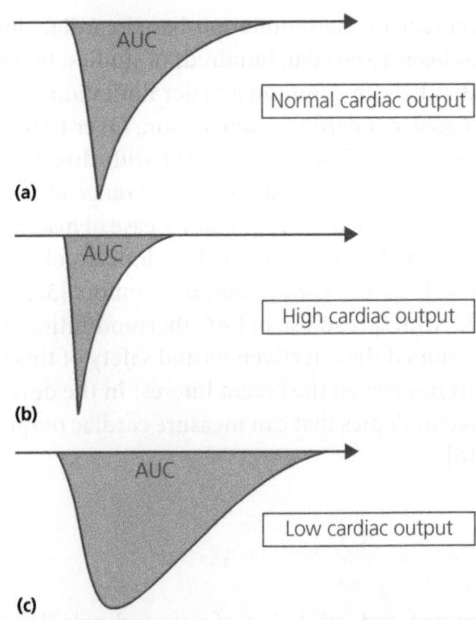

Figure 23.2 (a) Graphical representation of a normal cardiac output thermodilution curve; (b) high cardiac output thermodilution curve; (c) low cardiac output thermodilution curve. To be noted is the inverse relationship between the area under the curve (AUC) and cardiac output.

A modification of the original Swan–Ganz catheter includes a proximal thermal coil to warm blood in the cranial vena cava. The changes in blood temperature are then detected at the PAC's distal end using a thermistor. This method allows the continuous estimation of cardiac output, with the displayed values representing the average value of repeated determinations over the previous 10 min [58,59]. The use of averaged values of cardiac output corrects the inaccuracy of thermodilution associated with possible arrhythmias. The main disadvantage of this method is not being able to produce real-time values, thus limiting its usefulness in rapidly recognizing cardiac output changes in hemodynamically unstable patients.

Pulmonary artery catheterization allows simultaneous measurements of other hemodynamic parameters in addition to cardiac output, including pulmonary artery pressures, right- and left-sided filling pressures, and mixed venous oxygen saturation (SvO_2) [37].

There are some important sources of error with thermodilution measurements that need to be considered. If the volume injected is lower than that entered into the computer, the detected area under the curve will be artificially small and the calculated cardiac output will be falsely high. Also, if the temperature of the injected saline is lower than expected (e.g., using iced rather than room-temperature saline), the temperature change will be artificially large and the estimated cardiac output will be erroneously low [38].

Significant complications have been associated with the use of PACs and several reports have described the intrinsic risk of morbidity and mortality [39–43]. The PAC Man study in human patients recorded the occurrence of complications in 10% of insertions. The most common were arrhythmias, heart block, rupture of the right heart or pulmonary artery, thromboembolism, pulmonary infarction, valvular damage, and endocarditis. Similar endocardial and valvular lesions were also described in horses after the use of PACs [60]. Therefore, the use of the PAC should be restricted to selected patients where the benefit of its use may substantially outweigh the risks. Current recommendations for humans justify the use of a PAC only in patients with severe right ventricular failure and in patients requiring intensive monitoring of pulmonary vascular resistance during vasodilator therapy. Moreover, the use of a PAC and PAC thermodilution necessitate appropriate training as placement errors and misinterpretation of data are common.

In veterinary patients, there is limited clinical experience with the clinical use of PACs and PAC thermodilution [61–64]. This is mainly due to the invasiveness and the difficulty of placing and maintaining the catheter in the appropriate location. In addition, the PACs available on the market are specifically sized and designed for use in humans and are often inadequate for direct use in other species owing to morphological differences. In small dogs (less than 5 kg) and cats, for example, a standard PAC designed for adult human use, once advanced into the main pulmonary artery, would likely have the proximal port located in the jugular vein. The injection of the indicator in this location, rather than in the right atrium, will create loss and delayed mixing, with significant error in the estimation of cardiac output. The opposite scenario occurs in horses, where adult human PACs are too short. The proximal opening would be located in the right ventricle, instead of its proper place in the right atrium, significantly altering the estimation of cardiac output. However, pediatric human PACS and custom-designed PACs of appropriate size for veterinary species have been made, and are often used for research purposes.

Transpulmonary thermodilution and ultrasound indicator dilution

The basic principles of PAC thermodilution also apply to newer cardiac output monitoring systems that do not require the use of an actual pulmonary arterial catheter. Examples of these systems are the PiCCO® (Pulsion Medical Systems, Munich, Germany) and COstatus® (Transonic Systems, Ithaca, NY, USA), which allow cardiac output to be estimated by using a central venous and an arterial catheter only [65,66]. The basis of estimation of cardiac output by these systems is still the Stewart–Hamilton equation.

The PiCCO system is based on transpulmonary thermodilution for cardiac output determination and requires dedicated femoral artery access for measurements. PiCCO estimates cardiac output using central venous injections of ice-cold intravenous fluid as an indicator and measuring the changes in temperature over time by an arterial thermistor-tipped catheter placed in the femoral artery [65].

COstatus estimates cardiac output by using ultrasound technology to measure changes in blood ultrasound velocity following an injection of a small saline bolus (0.5–1 mL/kg) warmed to body temperature (37°C). To obtain measurements, a roller pump circulates blood through a disposable extracorporeal arteriovenous (AV) loop interposed between the peripheral arterial catheter and the distal lumen of the central venous catheter. Two reusable sensors that measure changes in blood ultrasound velocity and blood flow in the AV loop are clamped on to the arterial and venous limbs of the loop. The venous sensor detects the injection of saline and records the time and volume of injection. The arterial sensor then measures the changes in concentration of saline in the blood as a dilution, and also records the indicator travel time through the cardiopulmonary system. Stroke volume is then derived from the dilution curves obtained [67].

The agreement of cardiac output values measured using transpulmonary and ultrasound indicator dilution techniques with those measured using PAC thermodilution was shown to be adequate for clinical use in humans [68–71]. Moreover, both technologies provide volumetric variables in addition to cardiac output, such as global end-diastolic volume and measurements of extravascular lung water. These variables have been investigated as possible indicators of fluid responsiveness, with promising results [72,73].

PiCCO and COstatus appear significantly more practical and user friendly than PAC thermodilution. In addition, they do not require any specific customization for use in veterinary species. COstatus has been shown to be accurate and safe in very small patients (1 kg or less) [70]. All of these factors may allow the wider use of the these systems in veterinary medicine, especially in small animals, compared with PAC thermodilution [74,75].

Lithium dilution

The LiDCO™ system (LiDCO, London, UK) is an example of dye dilution cardiac output monitoring, based on intravascular injection of a minute amount of an isotonic lithium chloride solution (0.002–0.004 mmol/kg) used as an indicator [76]. These lithium doses are too small to exert any pharmacological or toxic effects. The lithium concentration in the blood is determined by a lithium-selective electrode connected to a peripheral arterial catheter. An advantage of the lithium indicator dilution cardiac output technique is that no central venous line is necessary for the injection of the indicator, which can be given via a regular peripheral line [77]. The lithium concentration versus time curve is recorded by withdrawing blood (4.5 mL/min) through a special disposable sensor, attached to the patient's arterial line. The voltage signal across the lithium-selective membrane is converted to lithium concentration by a computer. Cardiac output is calculated according to the equation [76]

$$\text{cardiac output} = \frac{\text{LiCl} \times 60}{\text{AUC} \times (1 - \text{PCV})}$$

where LiCl is the lithium chloride dose expressed in mmol, AUC is the area under the primary dilution curve and PCV is the packed cell volume. A correction for PCV is necessary to transform plasma flow into total blood flow because lithium is distributed only in the plasma. The lithium dilution technique has been shown to be at least as accurate as PAC thermodilution, but with the advantages of being simple to set up and operate. This system also conveniently uses catheters likely already to be in place in a critically ill patient. The system requires some familiarity to set up, but is relatively quick and user friendly. Similarly to thermodilution, the LiDCO performs poorly in the presence of tachyarrhythmias [76].

The LiDCO system has now become widely used in veterinary medicine in both the clinical and research setting. Good agreement with PAC thermodilution was found in dogs, cats, and horses, with the advantage of being less invasive, less expensive, and more user friendly [78–81]. In pigs, lithium dilution performed even better than PAC thermodilution when compared with electromagnetic flowmetry. In one study, cardiac output by lithium dilution, using a central venous catheter for injection, showed better agreement with electromagnetic flowmetry than PAC thermodilution [82]. Notably, although correlation studies of the LiDCO system with electromagnetic flowmetry (direct measurement of cardiac output) are lacking for many veterinary species, LiDCO is often arbitrarily used in the research setting as a reference system for comparison of other cardiac output monitoring systems [15,18–20,83,84]. This approach may potentially produce inaccurate conclusions.

The main disadvantage of lithium dilution is the blood loss associated with withdrawal of arterial blood for the determination of lithium concentration. Although the loss associated with a single measurement is minimal, it should be considered when applied to small animals, if a large number of determinations are to be performed.

Arterial waveform analysis

Arterial pressure waveform analysis allows the continuous determination of cardiac output [85]. In addition to the intermittent dilution cardiac output measurement discussed above, the PiCCO and LiDCO systems are also integrated with arterial pressure waveform analysis functions [59,86]. PiCCO uses arterial pulse contour analysis whereas LiDCO uses pulse power analysis for the beat-to-beat estimation of cardiac output [87]. Both methods require calibration before measurement of cardiac output based on the assumption that stroke volume is equal to the sum of systolic and diastolic flows, which are proportional to systolic and diastolic areas in the arterial pressure waveform (Fig. 23.3). The PiCCO system uses transpulmonary thermodilution for the calibration procedure, whereas LiDCO is calibrated using lithium dilution [88]. Repeated calibrations of the arterial pulse contour analysis systems are required in order to obtain adequate estimation of cardiac output. Recalibration is also needed whenever there is a change in vasomotor tone or any other significant change in the patient's clinical condition [89,90].

Other cardiac output devices based on arterial waveform analysis, such as the FloTrac/Vigileo (Edwards Lifesciences, Irvine, CA, USA), are available. These devices reportedly do not require baseline calibration and calculate stroke volume empirically [91]. However, the accuracy and precision of these methods are still questioned by many investigators [92]. Moreover, arterial pulse contour analysis is highly prone to technical difficulties related to damping and resonance within the measurement system [93]. For these reasons, further investigation of arterial waveform analysis techniques in different species and clinical scenarios is needed to define indications and recommendations for clinical use.

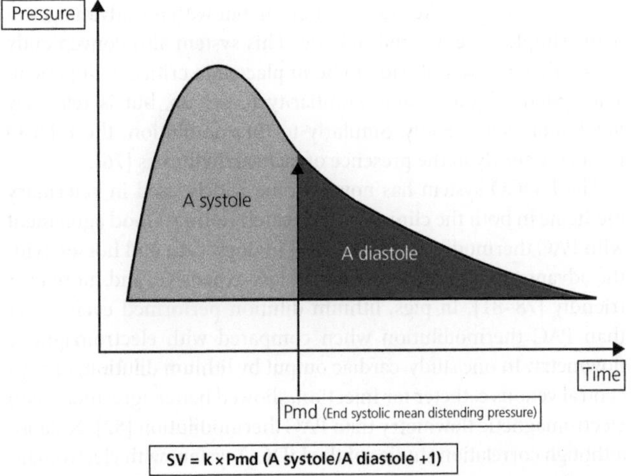

Figure 23.3 Arterial waveform analysis. Components in the arterial waveform used by the 'area under the curve' method. SV is the sum of systolic and diastolic flows, which are proportional to their respective areas under the arterial pressure curve; Pmd is the increment in mean arterial pressure at the end of systole, and is used for calculating diastolic flow; k is the calibration factor and is measured by calibrating against a known stroke volume, for example using transpulmonary thermodilution. Once k is known, beat-to-beat stroke volume can be calculated.

Echocardiography and echo-Doppler

Cardiac output can be determined with echocardiography using non-Doppler or Doppler-based methods [94,95]. A great advantage of echocardiography over other monitoring techniques is the large amount of hemodynamic information obtained beyond just cardiac output. Cardiac contractility and chamber filling can be rapidly assessed, and valves and pericardium can be directly visualized [21,22].

Non-Doppler techniques are based on approximate volumetric reconstructions of the left ventricular chamber. The most common method is based on Simpson's rule, wherein the left ventricle is divided into a series of disks stacked from base to apex. Two orthogonal planes are needed to construct the disks, and left ventricular volume is calculated by summing the approximated volumes of the individual disks. Stroke volume is calculated by determining the difference in volume between diastole and systole [94]. The time-consuming nature of the non-Doppler technique can make cardiac output estimation inadequate for a rapid assessment in emergency situations. Difficulty with endocardial border definition can also produce largely inaccurate results. For these reasons, non-Doppler techniques are rarely used for clinical purposes.

When an ultrasound beam is directed along the aorta, part of the ultrasound signal is reflected back by the moving red blood cells at a different frequency. The resultant shift in the signal's frequency, referred to as the Doppler effect, is used to determine the flow velocity. This represents the basic principle behind echo-Doppler cardiac output determination. Echo-Doppler cardiac output monitoring may be performed either transthoracically or transesophageally [96,97].

The determination of cardiac output begins with the measurement of the cross-sectional area (CSA) of the left ventricular outflow tract (LVOT). The reason for choosing this location is that the cross-section of the LVOT is essentially a circle and its area can be easily determined as πr^2. CSA can also be more accurately measured by tracing the boundary of the LVOT (Fig. 23.4a).

Following the CSA determination, a sample volume for pulse wave Doppler is placed at the location where area was determined. In small animals, the subcostal echocardiographic view is recommended for this assessment. Subcostal views of the heart can be obtained with the patient in right- or left-sided recumbency, and are relatively easy to obtain. These views usually are three- or four-chambered (left ventricle, portions of the right ventricle or atrium, portions of the left atrium, and LVOT with aorta), and allow the operator to obtain nearly perfect parallel alignment of the Doppler cursor with the LVOT. The pulse wave Doppler window can be placed just below the aortic valve plane, and this view allows for good flow tracings and measurements to be obtained. A profile of velocity over time is generated by this Doppler interrogation using the equation

$$V = \frac{f_d c}{2 f_i \cos\theta}$$

where V is erythrocyte velocity, f_d is Doppler shift, c is the velocity of the ultrasound wave, f_i is ultrasound frequency, and θ is the angle at which the ultrasound waves penetrate the vessel.

The tracing of the boundary of the velocity profile allows the determination of its integral over time. The velocity time integral (VTI) essentially represents the distance that blood travels during one beat and is referred to as 'stroke distance.' Multiplying VTI by

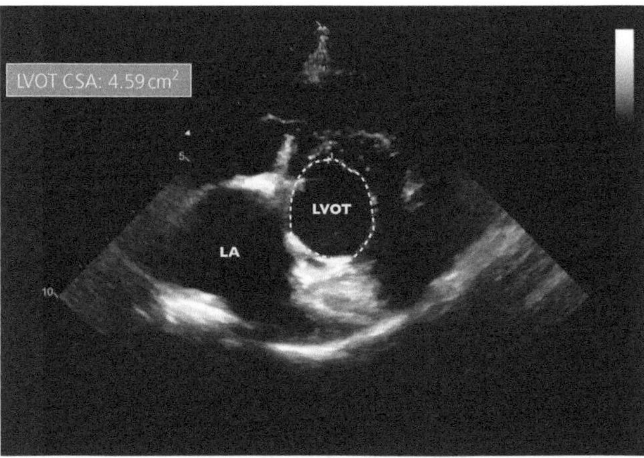

(a)

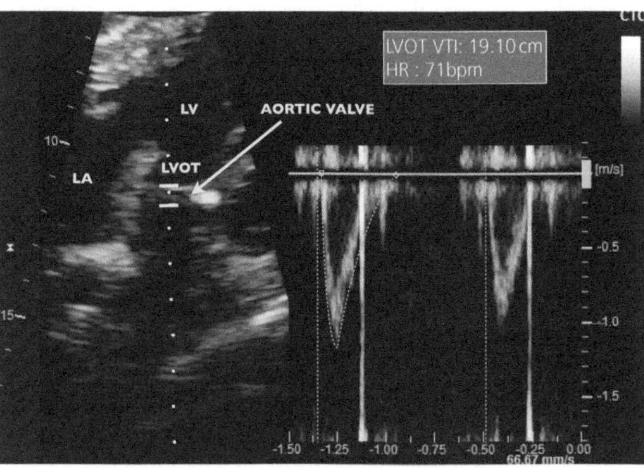

(b)

Figure 23.4 Transthoracic echo-Doppler estimation of cardiac output in a 27 kg dog. (A) Short-axis view for determination of cross-sectional area (CSA) of left ventricular outflow tract (LVOT). The dashed yellow line represents the tracing of the boundary of LVOT. LA, left atrium. (B) Subcostal view of left ventricle (LV) and LVOT. A pulse wave Doppler window is placed just below the aortic valve plane to obtain flow tracings and calculation of the velocity time integral (VTI) of LVOT. HR, heart rate. Cardiac output equals VTI × CSA × HR. The estimated patient's cardiac output is 6.224 L/min.

the cross-sectional area (CSA) of LVOT yields the stroke volume, which, this multiplied by heart rate (HR), determines cardiac output (Fig. 23.4b):

$$\text{cardiac output} = \text{HR} \times \text{CSA} \times \text{VTI}$$

This technique requires knowledge and skills to avoid pitfalls and to recognize inaccurate results [98]. Overall, Doppler-based cardiac output determination appears to be an acceptable alternative to thermodilution for clinical purposes, if performed correctly [99–101]. Important factors that can significantly affect accuracy are image quality, sample site, angle of insonation, the velocity signal-to-noise ratio, the possibility of measuring the diameter of the LVOT, and the shape of the aortic valve.

A described complication associated with the use of esophageal probes is heat-induced injury. Transesophageal echocardiography probes generate a certain amount of heat and for this reason are not suited for continuous cardiac output assessment [102].

Echocardiography instrumentation and expertise are rarely available to veterinary anesthesiologists. Currently, this remains the domain of veterinary cardiologists, who must be available to perform the procedure. There is significant evidence for the accuracy and practical applicability of echocardiography for cardiac output determination in many veterinary species, which will likely result in a wider range of uses for clinical purposes [103–106].

Thoracic bioimpendance and bioreactance

Bioimpedance uses the changes in conductivity of a high-frequency, low-magnitude alternating current passing across the thorax to derive stroke volume [107]. The changes in electrical conductivity are produced by the variations of intrathoracic blood flow during each cardiac cycle. A series of ECG-type electrodes are placed on the thorax and neck. A small, non-painful current is passed between the electrodes and the changes in voltage, also termed bioimpedance, are measured. The value of bioimpedance is converted to stroke volume using mathematical algorithms. Several patented algorithms based on different mathematical models of the thorax have been described [108,109].

The SV is generally calculated using the equation

$$\text{stroke volume} = \rho \times \frac{L^2}{Z_0^{\ 2}} \times \left(\frac{\mathrm{d}Z}{\mathrm{d}t}\right)_{\max} \times VET$$

where ρ is the resistivity of blood, L is the mean distance between the inner electrodes (the thoracic length), VET is the ventricular ejection time, $(\mathrm{d}Z/\mathrm{d}t)_{\max}$ is the maximum value of the first derivative during systole, and Z_0 is the basal thoracic impedance. Bioimpedance provides real-time estimation of stroke volume and cardiac output, along with measures of thoracic fluid content, left ventricular ejection time, systemic vascular resistance, and left cardiac work index [108].

Bioreactance has been developed from the bioimpedance technique but measures changes in frequency of electrical currents, rather than voltage, potentially making it less prone to noise-derived errors [110]. Both techniques are non-invasive and can be applied quickly. However, the greatest concern with these techniques is the accuracy and precision of the measurements. Physiologic studies in healthy humans showed good reliability of the results, but this was not consistent in critically ill patients, particularly in the presence of pulmonary edema and/or pleural effusion. In addition, electrical interference may also occur from other anesthesia monitoring devices connected to the patient [111–113].

Little or no evidence exists on the accuracy and reliability of these techniques in veterinary species [114,115]. Therefore, bioimpedance and bioreactance cardiac output determination should not be considered as a valid and reproducible method at present. A shortcoming of both bioimpedance and bioreactance mathematical models is the approximation of the shape of the chest as a cylinder or a cone for stroke volume determination. These represent oversimplifications of the electrical events occurring inside the thorax during the cardiac cycle and are sources of technique inaccuracy. It seems unlikely that the algorithms designed for human patients would be sufficiently accurate for use in various veterinary species.

Standard capnography as indicator of cardiac output

A simple and practical indicator of cardiac output in any anesthetized patient is end-tidal carbon dioxide (CO_2) measured by capnography. Assuming stable conditions of patient minute ventilation and body temperature, and in the absence of airway obstruction or extra-metabolic sources of CO_2 (laparoscopic surgery or sodium bicarbonate administration), a sudden change in end-tidal CO_2 has been shown to reflect a linearly proportional alteration in cardiac output. [116,117]. Therefore, the concurrent decrease in blood pressure and end-tidal CO_2 in an anesthetized patient may reflect a primary reduction in cardiac output. In such conditions, if sinus rhythm and normal heart rate are confirmed, therapeutic interventions should be focused on the optimization of preload and myocardial contractility to support stroke volume. In contrast, a decrease in blood pressure with no reduction in end-tidal CO_2 will likely indicate a decrease in systemic vascular resistance that may be readily controlled with a vasopressor agent.

References

1 Hall JE. Cardiac output, venous return, and their regulation. *Guyton and Hall Textbook of Medical Physiology*, 12th edn. Philadelphia: Saunders Elsevier, 2011; 229–240.

2 Della Rocca G, Pompei L. Goal-directed therapy in anesthesia: any clinical impact or just a fashion? *Minerva Anestesiol* 2011; **77**: 545–553.

3 Ospina-Tascon GA, Cordioli RL, Vincent JL. What type of monitoring has been shown to improve outcomes in acutely ill patients? *Intensive Care Med* 2008; **34**: 800–820.

4 Kehlet H, Bundgaard-Nielsen M. Goal-directed perioperative fluid management: why, when, and how? *Anesthesiology* 2009; **110**: 453–455.

5 Pinsky MR. Why measure cardiac output? *Crit Care* 2003; **7**: 114–116.

6 Pinsky MR. Hemodynamic evaluation and monitoring in the ICU. *Chest* 2007; **132**: 2020–2029.

7 Bilovski RN, Rivers EP, Horst HM. Targeted resuscitation strategies after injury. *Curr Opin Crit Care* 2004; **10**: 529–538.

8 Alhashemi JA, Cecconi M, Hofer CK. Cardiac output monitoring: an integrative perspective. *Crit Care* 2011; **15**: 214.

9 Rex S, Brose S, Metzelder S *et al.* Prediction of fluid responsiveness in patients during cardiac surgery. *Br J Anaesth* 2004; **93**: 782–788.

10 Reuter DA, Geopfert MS, Goresch T, *et al.* Assessing fluid responsiveness during open chest conditions. *Br J Anaesth* 2005; **94**: 318–323.

11 García X, Mateu L, Maynar J, *et al.* Estimating cardiac output. Utility in the clinical practice. Available invasive and non-invasive monitoring. *Med Intensiva* 2011; **35**: 552–561 (in Spanish).

12 Pinsky MR, Payen D. Functional hemodynamic monitoring. *Crit Care* 2005; **9**: 566–572.

13 Vincent JL, Rhodes A, Perel A, *et al.* Clinical review: update on hemodynamic monitoring – a consensus of 16. *Crit Care* 2011; **15**: 229.

14 Geerts BF, Aarts LP, Jansen JR. Methods in pharmacology: measurement of cardiac output. *Br J Clin Pharmacol* 2011; **71**: 316–330.

15 Corley KTT, Donaldson LL, Durando MM, *et al.* Cardiac output technologies with special reference to the horse. *J Vet Intern Med* 2003; **17**: 262–272.

16 Pugsley J, Lerner AB. Cardiac output monitoring: is there a gold standard and how do the newer technologies compare? *Semin Cardiothorac Vasc Anesth* 2010; **14**: 274–282.

17 Tabrizchi R, Iida N. Electromagnetic blood flow measurements. In: Moore J, Zouridakis G, eds. *Biomedical Technology and Devices Handbook*. Boca Raton, FL: CRC Press LLC, 2003, 3-1–3-20.

18 Shih A, Giguère S, Sanchez LC, *et al.* Determination of cardiac output in neonatal foals by ultrasound velocity dilution and its comparison to the lithium dilution method. *J Vet Emerg Crit Care* 2009; **19**: 438–443.

19 Valverde A, Giannotti G, Roja E, *et al.* Comparison of cardiac output determined by arterial pulse pressure waveform analysis method (FloTrac/Vigileo) versus lithium dilution method in anesthetized dogs. *J Vet Emerg Crit Care* 2011; **21**: 328–334.

20 Valverde A, Giguère S, Morey TE, *et al.* Comparison of noninvasive cardiac output measured by use of partial carbon dioxide rebreathing or the lithium dilution method in anesthetized foals. *Am J Vet Res* 2007; **68**: 141–147.

21 Cheung AT, Savino JS, Weiss SJ, *et al.* Echocardiographic and hemodynamic indexes of left ventricular preload in patients with normal and abnormal ventricular function. *Anesthesiology* 1994; **81**: 376–387.

22 Thys DM, Hillei Z. Left ventricular performance indices by transesophageal Doppler. *Anesthesiology* 1988; **69**: 728–733.

23 Silver MA, Cianci P, Brennan S, *et al.* Evaluation of impedance cardiography as an alternative to pulmonary artery catheterization in critically ill patients. *Congest Heart Fail* 2004; **10**: 17–21.

24 Fick A. Über die Messung des Blutquantums in den Herzventrikeln. *Sitzber Phys Med Ges Wurzburg* 1870; **36**: 290–291.

25 Grehant H, Quinquaud CE. Recherches expérimentales sur la mesure du volume de sang qui traverse les poumons en un temps donné. *C R Sci Soc Biol* 1886; **30**: 159.

26 Zuntz N, Hagemann O. Untersuchungen über den Stoffwechsel des Pferdes bei Ruhe und Arbeit. *Landwirtschaftl Jahrb Z Wiss Land-wirtschaft* 1898; **27**(3): 1–450.

27 Laszlo G. Respiratory measurements of cardiac output: from elegant idea to useful test. *J Appl Physiol* 2004; **96**: 428–437.

28 Stewart GN. Researches on the circulation time and on the influences which affect it. IV. The output of the heart. *J Physiol* 1897; **22**: 159–183.

29 Hamilton WF, Riley RL, Attyah AM, *et al.* Comparison of the Fick and dye injection methods of measuring the cardiac output in man. *Am J Physiol* 1948; **153**: 309–321.

30 Werko L, Lagexlof H, Bucht H, *et al.* Comparison of Fick and Hamilton methods for determination of cardiac output in man. *Scand J Clin Lab Invest* 1949, **1**: 109.

31 Miller DE, Gleason WL, MCintosh HD. A comparison of the cardiac output determination by the Fick method and dye dilution method using indocyanine green dye and a cuvette densitometer. *J Lab Clin Med* 1962; **59**: 345.

32 Venkataraman K, De Guzman MF, Khan AH, Haywood LJ. Cardiac output measurement: a comparison of direct Fick, dye dilution and thermodilution methods in stable and acutely ill patients. *J Natl Med Assoc* 1976; **68**: 281–284.

33 Fegler G. Measurement of cardiac output in anesthetized animals by a thermodilution method. *Q J Exp Physiol* 1954; **39**: 153–164.

34 Swan HJ, Ganz W, Forrester J, *et al.* Catheterization of the heart in man with use of a flow- directed balloon-tipped catheter. *N Engl J Med* 1970; **283**: 447–453.

35 Ganz W, Donoso R, Marcus HS, *et al.* A new technique for measurement of cardiac output by thermodilution in man. *Am J Cardiol* 1971; **27**: 392–396.

36 Weisel RD, Berger RL, Hectman HB. Measurement of Cardiac Output by Thermodilution. *N Engl J Med* 1975; **292**: 682.

37 Reuter DA, Huang C, Edrich T, *et al.* Cardiac Output Monitoring Using Indicator-Dilution Techniques: Basics, Limits, and Perspectives. *Anesth Analg* 2010; **110**(3): 799–811.

38 Tournadre JP, Chassard D, Muchada R. Overestimation of low cardiac output measured by thermodilution. *Brit J Anaesth* 1997; **79**: 514–516.

39 Harvey S, Harrison DA, Singer M, *et al.* Assessment of the clinical effectiveness of pulmonary artery catheters in management of patients in intensive care (PAC Man): a randomised controlled trial. *Lancet* 2005; **366**: 472–477.

40 Shah MR, Hasselblad V, Stevenson LW, *et al.* Impact of the Pulmonary Artery Catheter in Critically Ill Patients - Meta-analysis of Randomized Clinical Trials. *JAMA* 2005; **294**(13): 1664–1670.

41 Coonors AF Jr, Speroff T, Dawson NV, *et al.* The effectiveness of right heart catheterization in the initial care of critically ill patients. SUPPORT Investigators. *JAMA* 1996; **276**: 889–897.

42 Polanczyk CA, Rohde LE, Goldman L, *et al.* Right heart catheterization and cardiac complications in patients undergoing noncardiac surgery. *JAMA* 2001; **286**: 309–314.

43 Elliott CG, Zimmerman GA, Clemmer TP. Complications of pulmonary artery catheterization in the care of critically ill patients. A prospective study. *Chest* 1979; **76**: 647–652.

44 Cholley BP, Payen D. Noninvasive technique for measurements of cardiac output. *Curr Opin Crit Care* 2005; **11**: 424–429.

45 Parmley CL, Pousman RM. Noninvasive cardiac output monitoring. *Curr Opin Anaesthesiol* 2002; **15**: 675–680.

46 Botero M, Labato EB. Advances in noninvasive cardiac output monitoring: an update. *J Cardiothorac Vasc Anaesth* 2001; **15**: 631–640.

47 Haryadi DG, Orr JA, Kuck K, *et al.* Partial CO_2 rebreathing indirect Fick technique for non-invasive measurement of cardiac output. *J Clin Monit Comput* 2000; **16**: 361–374.

48 Jaffe MB. Partial CO_2 rebreathing cardiac output – operating principles of the NICO system. *J Clin Monit Comput* 1999; **15**: 387–401.

49 Haryadi DG, Orr JA, Kuck K, *et al.* Partial CO_2 rebreathing indirect Fick technique for non-invasive measurement of cardiac output. *J Clin Monit Comput* 2000; **16**: 361–374.

50 van Heerden PV, Baker S, Lim SI, *et al.* Clinical evaluation of the non-invasive cardiac output (NICO) monitor in the intensive care unit. *Anaesth Intensive Care* 2000; **28**: 427–430.

51 Levy RJ, Chivacci RM, Nicolson SC, *et al.* An evaluation of a noninvasive cardiac output measurement using partial carbon dioxide rebreathing in children. *Anesth Analg* 2004; **99**: 1642–1647.

52 Nilsson LB, Eldrup N, Berthelsen PG. Lack of agreement between thermodilution and carbon dioxide-rebreathing cardiac output. *Acta Anaesthesiol Scand* 2001; **45**: 680–685.

53 Giguère S, Bucki E, Adin DB, *et al.* Cardiac output measurement by partial carbon dioxide rebreathing, 2-dimensional echocardiography, and lithium-dilution method in anesthetized neonatal foals. *J Vet Intern Med* 2005; **19**: 737–743.

54 Gedeon A, Krill P, Kristensen J, *et al.* Noninvasive cardiac output determined with a new method based on gas exchange measurements and carbon dioxide rebreathing: a study in animals/pigs. *J Clin Monit* 1992; **8**: 267–278.

55 Gunkel CI, Valverde A, Morey TE, *et al.* Comparison of non-invasive cardiac output measurement by partial carbon dioxide rebreathing with the lithium dilution method in anesthetized dogs. *J Vet Emerg Crit Care* 2004; **14**: 187–195.

56 Berton C, Cholley B. Equipment review: new techniques for cardiac output measurement – oesophageal Doppler, Fick principle using carbon dioxide and pulse contour analysis. *Crit Care* 2002; **6**: 216–221.

57 Forrester JS, Ganz W, Diamond G, *et al.* Thermodilution cardiac output determination with a single flow directed catheter. *Am Heart J* 1972; **83**: 306–311.

58 Mathews L, Singh RK. Swan Ganz catheter in haemodynamic monitoring. *J Anaesth Clin Pharmacol* 2006; **22**: 335–345.

59 Della Rocca G, Costa MG, Pompei L, *et al.* Continuous and intermittent cardiac output measurement: pulmonary artery catheter versus aortic transpulmonary technique. *Br J Anaesth* 2002; **88**: 350–356.

60 Schlipf JW, Dunlop CI, Getzy DM, *et al.* Lesions associated with cardiac catheterization and thermodilution cardiac output determination in horses. In: *Proceedings of the 5th International Congress of Veterinary Anesthesia*, 1994; 71–72.

61 Muir WW, Skarda RT, Milne DW. Estimation of cardiac output in the horse by thermodilution techniques. *Am J Vet Res* 1976; **37**: 697–700.

62 Mizuno Y, Aida H, Hara H, *et al.* Comparison of methods of cardiac output measurements determined by dye dilution, pulsed Doppler echocardiography and thermodilution in horses. *J Vet Med Sci* 1994; **56**: 1–5.

63 Hendriks FFA, Schipperheyn JJ, Quanjer PH. Thermal dilution measurement of cardiac output in dogs using an analog computer. *Basic Res Cardiol* 1978; **73**: 459–468.

64 Dyson DH, McDonell WN, Horne JA. Accuracy of thermodilution measurement of cardiac output in low flows applicable to feline and small canine patients *Can J Comp Med* 1984; **48**: 425–427.

65 von Spiegel T, Wietasch G, Bursch J, *et al.* Cardiac output determination with transpulmonary thermodilution: an alternative to pulmonary artery catheterization? *Anaesthetist* 1996; **45**: 1045–1050.

66 Crittendon I III, Dreyer WJ, Decker JA, *et al.* Ultrasound dilution: an accurate means of determining cardiac output in children. *Pediatr Crit Care Med* 2012; **13**: 42–46.

67 de Boode WP, van Heijst AF, Hopman JC, *et al.* Application of the ultrasound dilution technology for cardiac output measurement: cerebral and systemic hemodynamic consequences in a juvenile animal model. *Pediatr Crit Care Med* 2010; **11**: 616–623.

68 Della Rocca G, Costa MG, Coccia C, *et al.* Cardiac output monitoring: aortic transpulmonary thermodilution and pulse contour analysis agree with standard thermodilution methods in patients undergoing lung transplantation. *Can J Anaesth* 2003; **50**: 707–711.

69 Sakka SG, Reinhart K, Meier-Hellmann A. Comparison of pulmonary artery and arterial thermodilution cardiac output in critically ill patients. *Intensive Care Med* 1999; **25**: 843–846.

70 de Boode WP, van Heijst AF, Hopman JC, *et al.* Cardiac output measurement using an ultrasound dilution method: a validation study in ventilated piglets. *Pediatr Crit Care Med* 2009; **11**:103–108.

71 Ballestero Y, Urbano J, López-Herce J, *et al.* Pulmonary arterial thermodilution, femoral arterial thermodilution and bioreactance cardiac output monitoring in a pediatric hemorrhagic hypovolemic shock model. *Resuscitation* 2012; **83**: 125–129.

72 Vigani A, Shih A, Queiroz P, *et al.* Quantitative response of volumetric variables measured by a new ultrasound dilution method in a juvenile model of hemorrhagic shock and resuscitation. *Resuscitation* 2012; **83**: 1031–1037.

73 Galstyan G, Bychynin M, Alexanyan M, *et al.* Comparison of cardiac output and blood volumes in intrathoracic compartments measured by ultrasound dilution and transpulmonary thermodilution methods. *Intensive Care Med* 2010; **36**: 2140–2144.

74 Shih A, Maisenbacher HW, Bandt C, *et al.* Assessment of cardiac output measurement in dogs by transpulmonary pulse contour analysis. *J Vet Emerg Crit Care* 2011; **21**: 321–327.

75 Shih A, Giguère S, Vigani A, *et al.* Determination of cardiac output by ultrasound velocity dilution in normovolemia and hypovolemia in dogs. *Vet Anaesth Analg* 2011; **38**: 279–285.

76 Linton RA, Band DM, Haire KM. A new method in measuring cardiac output in man using lithium dilution. *Br J Anaesth* 1993; **71**: 262–266.

77 Mason DJ, O'Grady M, Woods JP, *et al.* Comparison of a central and a peripheral (cephalic vein) injection site for the measurement of cardiac output using the lithium-dilution cardiac output technique in anesthetized dogs. *Can J Vet Res* 2002; **66**: 207–210.

78 Mason DJ, O'Grady M, Woods JP, *et al.* Assessment of lithium dilution cardiac output as a technique for measurement of cardiac output in dogs. *Am J Vet Res* 2001; **62**: 1255–1261.

79 Beaulieu KE, Kerr CL, McDonell WN. Evaluation of a lithium dilution cardiac output technique as a method for measurement of cardiac output in anesthetized cats. *Am J Vet Res* 2005; **66**: 1639–1645.

80 Linton RA, Young LE, Marlin DJ, *et al.* Cardiac output measured by lithium dilution, thermodilution, and transesophageal Doppler echocardiography in anesthetized horses. *Am J Vet Res* 2000; **61**: 731–737.

81 Corley KT, Donaldson LL, Furr MO. Comparison of lithium dilution and thermodilution cardiac output measurements in anaesthetised neonatal foals. *Equine Vet J* 2002; **34**: 598–601.

82 Kurita T, Morita K, Kato S, *et al.* Comparison of the accuracy of the lithium dilution technique with the thermodilution technique for measurement of cardiac output. *Br J Anaesth* 1997; **79**: 770–775.

83 Corley KT, Donaldson LL, Furr MO. Comparison of lithium dilution and thermodilution cardiac output measurements in anaesthetised neonatal foals. *Equine Vet J* 2002; **34**: 598–601.

84 Schauvliege S, Van den Eede A, Duchateau L, *et al.* Comparison between lithium dilution and pulse contour analysis techniques for cardiac output measurement in isoflurane anaesthetized ponies: influence of different inotropic drugs. *Vet Anaesth Analg* 2009; **36**:197–208.

85 Jansen JR, Schreuder JJ, Mulier JP, *et al.* A comparison of cardiac output derived from the arterial pressure wave against thermodilution in cardiac surgery patients. *Br J Anaesth* 2001; **87**: 212–222.

86 Jonas MM, Tanser SJ. Lithium dilution measurement of cardiac output and arterial pulse waveform analysis: an indicator dilution calibrated beat-by-beat system for continuous estimation of cardiac output. *Curr Opin Crit Care* 2002; **8**: 257–261.

87 Thiele RH, Durieux ME. Arterial waveform analysis for the anesthesiologist: past, present, and future concepts. *Anesth Analg* 2011; **113**: 766–776.

88 Ambrisko TD, Coppens P, Kabes R, *et al.* Lithium dilution, pulse power analysis, and continuous thermodilution cardiac output measurements compared with bolus thermodilution in anaesthetized ponies. *Br J Anaesth* 2012; **109**: 864–869.

89 Rhodes A, Sunderland R. Arterial pulse power analysis, the LiDCO™ plus system. In: Pinsky MR, Pyen D, eds. *Functional Hemodynamics.* Berlin: Springer, 2005; 183–192.

90 Buhre W, Weyland A, Kazmaier S, *et al.* Comparison of cardiac output assessed by pulse contour analysis and thermodilution in patients undergoing minimally invasive direct coronary artery bypass grafting. *J Cardiothorac Vasc Anaesth* 1999; **13**: 437–440.

91 Manecke GR Jr, Auger WR. Cardiac output determination from the arterial pressure wave: clinical testing of a novel algorithm that does not require calibration. *J Cardiothorac Vasc Anaesth* 2007; **21**: 3–7.

92 Compton FD, Zukunft B, Hoffmann C, *et al.* Performance of a minimally invasive uncalibrated cardiac output monitoring system (Flotrac/Vigileo) in haemodynamically unstable patients. *Br J Anaesth* 2008; **100**: 451–456.

93 Singer M, Allen MJ, Webb AR, *et al.* Effects of alterations in left ventricular filling, contractility and systemic vascular resistance on the ascending aortic blood velocity waveform of normal subjects. *Crit Care Med* 1991; **19**: 1138–1145.

94 Uehara Y, Koga M, Takahashi M. Determination of cardiac output by echocardiography. *J Vet Med Sci* 1995; **57**: 401–407.

95 Madan AK, UyBarreta VV, Aliabadi-Wahle S, *et al.* Esophageal Doppler ultrasound monitor versus pulmonary artery catheter in the hemodynamic management of critically ill surgical patients. *J Trauma* 1999; **46**: 607–612.

96 Josephs SA. The use of current hemodynamic monitors and echocardiography in resuscitation of the critically ill or injured patient. *Int Anesthesiol Clin* 2007; **45**: 31–59.

97 Gouveia V, Marcelino P, Reuter DA. The role of transesophageal echocardiography in the intraoperative period. *Curr Cardiol Rev* 2011; **7**: 184–196.

98 Lefrant JY, Bruelle P, Aya AG, *et al.* Training is required to improve the reliability of esophageal Doppler to measure cardiac output in critically ill patients. *Intensive Care Med* 1998; **24**: 347–352.

99 Su NY, Huang CJ, Tsai P, *et al.* Cardiac output measurement during cardiac surgery: oesophageal Doppler versus pulmonary artery catheter. *Acta Anaesthesiol Scan* 2002; **40**: 127–133.

100 Chew MS, Poelaert J. Accuracy and repeatability of pediatric cardiac output measurement using Doppler: 20 year review of literature. *Intensive Care Med* 2003; **29**: 1889–1894.

101 Perrino AC Jr, Harris SN, Luther MA. Intraoperative determination of cardiac output using multiplane transesophageal echocardiography: a comparison to thermodilution. *Anesthesiology* 1998; **89**: 350–357.

102 Urbanowicz JH, Kernoff RS, Oppenheim G, *et al.* Transesophageal echocardiography and its potential for esophageal damage. *Anesthesiology* 1990; **72**: 40–43.

103 Blissit KJ, Young LE, Jones RS, *et al.* Measurement of cardiac output in standing horses by Doppler echocardiography and thermodilution. *Equine Vet J* 1997; **29**: 18–25.

104 Young LE, Blissit KJ, Bartram DH, *et al.* Measurement of cardiac output by transoesophageal Doppler echocardiography in anaesthetized horses: comparison with thermodilution. *Br J Anaesth* 1996; **77**: 773–780.

105 Lopes PC, Sousa MG, Camacho AA, *et al.* Comparison between two methods for cardiac output measurement in propofol-anesthetized dogs: thermodilution and Doppler. *Vet Anaesth Analg* 2010; **37**: 401–408.

106 White SW, McRitchie RJ, Porges WL. A comparison between thermodilution, electromagnetic and Doppler methods for cardiac output measurement in the rabbit. *Clin Exp Pharmacol Physiol* 1974; **1**: 175–182.

107 Kubicek WG, Karnegis JN, Patterson RP, *et al.* Development and evaluation of an impedance cardiac output system. *Aerosp Med* 1966; **37**: 1208–1212.

108 Bernstein DP. Continuous non-invasive real time monitoring of stroke volume and cardiac output by thoracic electrical bioimpedance. *Crit Care Med* 1986; **14**: 898–903.

109 Van De Water JM, Miller TW. Impedance cardiography: the next vital sign technology. *Chest* 2003; **123**: 2028–2033.

110 Heerdt PM, Wagner CL, DeMais M, Savarese JJ. Noninvasive cardiac output monitoring with bioreactance as an alternative to invasive instrumentation for preclinical drug evaluation in beagles. *J Pharmacol Toxicol Methods* 2011; **64**: 111–118.

111 Albert N, Hail M, Li J, *et al.* Equivalence of bioimpedance and thermodilution methods in measuring cardiac output in patients with advanced, decompensated chronic heart failure hospitalized in critical care. *J Am J Crit Care* 2004; **13**: 469–479.

112 Sagemam WS, Riffenburgh RH, Spiess BD. Equivalence of bioimpedance and thermodilution in measuring cardiac index after cardiac surgery. *J Cardiothorac Vasc Anaesth* 2002; **16**: 8–14.

113 Yung GL, Fedullo PF, Kinninger K, *et al.* Comparison of impedance cardiography to direct Fick and thermodilution cardiac output determination in pulmonary arterial hypertension. *Congest Heart Fail* 2004; **10**: 7–10.

114 Tibballs J, Hochmann M, Osborne A, *et al.* Accuracy of the BoMED NCCOM3 bioimpedance cardiac output monitor during induced hypotension: an experimental study in dogs. *Anaesth Intensive Care* 1992; **20**: 326–331.

115 Yamashita K, Ueyama Y, Miyoshi K, *et al.* Minimally invasive determination of cardiac output by transthoracic bioimpedance, partial carbon dioxide rebreathing, and transesophageal Doppler echocardiography in beagle dogs. *J Vet Med Sci* 2007; **69**: 43–47.

116 Shibutani K, Muraoka M, Shirasaki S, *et al.* Do changes in end-tidal pCO_2 quantitatively reflect changes in cardiac output? *Anesth Analg* 1994; **79**: 829–833.

117 Wahba RW, Tessler MJ, Kleiman SJ. Changes in pCO_2 with acute changes in cardiac index. *Can J Anaesth* 1996; **43**: 243–245.

24 Anesthesia for Cardiopulmonary Bypass

Khursheed R. Mama
Department of Clinical Sciences, Colorado State University, Fort Collins, Colorado, USA

Chapter contents

Introduction

The term cardiopulmonary bypass is broadly applied to the procedure by which blood is diverted away from the heart and lungs while also providing oxygenated blood to other organs to sustain viability. There is a long history of the use of animals, predominantly pigs and sheep, for cardiovascular surgical training and research. Additionally, over the past two decades, animals, most notably dogs (albeit there are occasional reports of cats [1]) have been anesthetized with varying frequency in the clinical arena to facilitate surgical procedures involving the heart (and lungs) [2–15]. Although perioperative morbidity is common (e.g., dysrhythmias, bleeding, phrenic nerve damage, hypoventilation, hypoxemia), acute survival (off pump to recovery) percentages from the aforementioned reports are generally high, even 100%. Longer term survival, however, is variable, with wide-ranging complications including hemorrhage, thromboembolism, pleural effusion, heart failure, and sudden death being reported.

The focus of this chapter is to introduce the reader to cardiopulmonary bypass as used to facilitate cardiac surgery in canine patients. Challenges associated with this as a clinical tool have recently been reviewed [16]. Although anesthesia management is reviewed here, much of the chapter is devoted to introducing the basics of circuitry and instrumentation used to facilitate cardiopulmonary bypass and the considerations (e.g., cardiac protection, management of coagulation) that arise as a result. As the reader is no doubt aware, many cardiac procedures may be performed on the beating heart, sometimes with the added utilization of inflow occlusion and hypothermia. This chapter is limited to a discussion of the management of clinical canine patients where cardiopulmonary bypass is necessary to facilitate cardiac surgery.

The circuitry and patient cannulation

The external circuit

The circuit external to the patient consists of a reservoir for blood and fluids used to prime the pump, a membrane (versus bubble) [17] oxygenator of appropriate size (pediatric size is commonly used for small- to medium-sized dogs), ventilating system, pumps (roller or centrifugal) [18,19] of varying number (three to five) to facilitate circulation of blood, a heat exchanger and circulating heating/cooling water-bath to permit initial cooling and subsequent warming of the patient (Fig. 24.1). Tubing appropriate to the patient's size (so that excessive hemodilution resulting from excessive prime volume, exposure to circuit components, and subsequent red blood cell trauma can be minimized) connects these parts and is attached to lines from/to the patient. As the lung is no longer functional during this process, an oxygen flowmeter (or oxygen and air flowmeters along with an oxygen blender to vary the oxygen fraction) and vaporizer are connected to the circuit to facilitate the delivery of inhaled anesthetic as needed. Maintenance of anesthesia with parenterally administered injectable drugs has also been described [14]. Newer bypass circuits have an independent pump and tubing mechanism for delivery of cardioplegic solutions, and also in-line monitors (to record temperature, hematocrit,

Veterinary Anesthesia and Analgesia: The Fifth Edition of Lumb and Jones.
Edited by Kurt A. Grimm, Leigh A. Lamont, William J. Tranquilli, Stephen A. Greene and Sheilah A. Robertson.

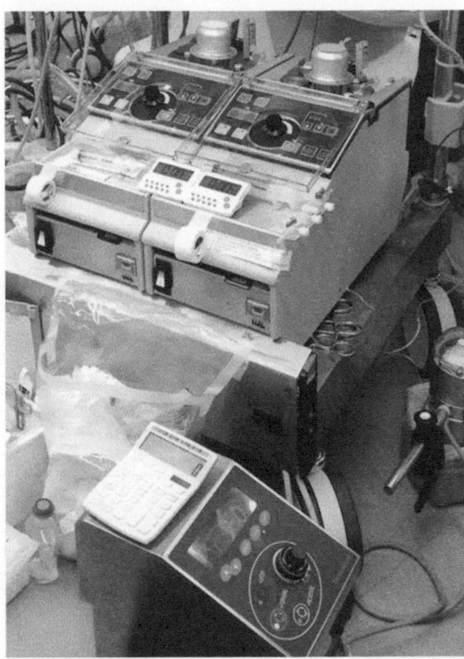

Figure 24.1 Standard and pediatric cardiopulmonary bypass pumps.

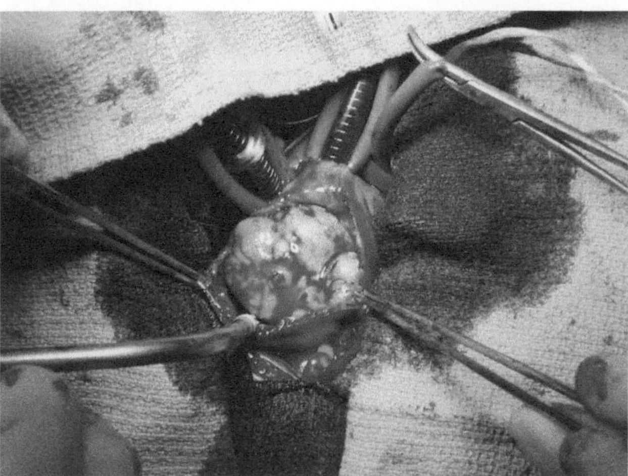

Figure 24.2 Bicaval cannulation for removal of a right atrial mass (in the center of the picture). The caudal vena cava is in the 11 o'clock position and cranial vena cava in the 1 o'clock position. Tape ties are pulled up around each cava, to prevent blood leakage into the right atrium. The cardiotomy sucker in the 7 o'clock position is in place to drain any coronary sinus flow.

saturation, etc.) on the arterial and/or venous side and safety devices (e.g., bubble detector and flow sensors). A more complete description and diagram of bypass circuitry available for human cardiopulmonary bypass are available in other medical texts [20].

Although the personnel responsible for the anesthetic management of the patient should have a general understanding of the external circuitry used, the author's experience has been that an individual with specialized training in perfusion should be responsible for ensuring functionality of the external circuitry and bypass equipment. The anesthesia personnel will, however, need to be in constant communication and provide the perfusionist with patient-specific information, such as the hematocrit and calculated blood volume. This information will be used to determine the pump prime volume with a target hematocrit of 25–30% to optimize capillary flow and oxygen-carrying capacity during bypass when hypothermia causes an increase in blood viscosity [21]. The perfusionist may request crystalloid fluids, synthetic colloids, blood or packed red cells (usually in smaller patients), and additives such as mannitol, sodium bicarbonate, and heparin to add to the pump prime. Steroids are added to the pump prime in some circumstances. The perfusion team may also request a vaporizer and inhalant anesthetic consistent with what the anesthesia team is using for the patient. Additional details regarding types and sizes of oxygenators, calculation of pump prime volume, components of prime solution, types and sizes of tubing, etc. may be found elsewhere [21–23].

Patient cannulation

Patient cannulation is performed by the surgical team. A lateral thoracotomy is the preferred approach in the dog if the cardiac procedure to be performed allows for this; a median sternotomy approach is a feasible alternative. Commonly, arterial (oxygenated) blood is actively returned (using a pump) to the patient via a cannula placed in the femoral artery; the carotid artery is more commonly used in smaller dogs. It is important that the anesthesia team is aware of which site will be used, and specifically for the femoral vessels, which limb will be utilized so they do not place the arterial catheter to monitor systemic arterial blood pressure in the same limb. The arterial cannula is either placed first or at the same time as the thoracotomy is performed if there are two surgeons. Early placement facilitates a quicker connection to the bypass circuitry if the patient's status deteriorates during placement of the venous cannula(e).

Bicaval or atrial venous cannulation is performed by the surgical team depending on the procedure to be performed. For procedures involving the right heart, bicaval cannulation is preferred to minimize blood in the surgical field and minimize compromise to venous drainage if the heart is retracted during the procedure (Fig. 24.2). The venous line connected to the cannula passively drains the majority of blood returned to the heart into the reservoir of the bypass circuit. Blood returning from the thebesian veins, coronary sinus, and systemic collaterals can usually be drained by appropriate (depending on the nature of the surgery) placement of these cannulas to reduce the risk of right ventricular distention. As this is a gravity-dependent process, the height of the patient above the reservoir is an important consideration. Suction may be cautiously applied to venous drainage if needed. An additional left ventricular vent line may be placed to minimize left ventricular distention and warming resulting from drainage of systemic, pericardial, and bronchopulmonary collaterals and thebesian veins [20]. A surgical suction cannula is also available and may be connected with a line to the reservoir.

Placement of the aforementioned cannulas facilitates extracorporeal circulation and a bloodless surgical field but does not offer a mechanism for myocardial protection. An additional cannula is therefore placed for administration of cardioplegia. This cannula may be placed such that flow of cardioplegic solution is anterograde via an aortic root cannula located on the cardiac side of the aortic cross clamp or retrograde via a balloon catheter in the coronary sinus. Cardioplegic solutions are administered to stop cardiac activity once the aortic cross clamp is placed to reduce energy requirements, protect myocardial cells, and scavenge free radicals. Cardioplegic solutions may be blood based (sanguineous) or crystalloid based, with additives for cardiac protection (e.g., mannitol or lidocaine) and high levels of potassium to stop electrical activity. Sanguineous solutions are thought to provide better oxygen delivery and scavenging of free radicals, especially for longer procedures [20,23]. Additional myocardial protection is achieved using systemic and/or local hypothermia (using iced saline slush around the heart if appropriate and with adequate protection of the phrenic nerve).

Systemic responses – pathobiology

Although cardiopulmonary bypass offers ideal conditions for surgical intervention, the processes involved also generate real or potential negative effects on a multitude of organ systems. These have been reviewed extensively and many continue to form the basis of ongoing study [24–27]. Briefly, contact of blood components with the cardiopulmonary bypass circuitry (tubing, pump, oxygenator) rapidly results in significant activation of the inflammatory cascade not dissimilar to that occurring in sepsis. Surgical processes also contribute and together these result in platelet, white blood cell, complement, and cytokine activation. The consequences of this inflammatory response can be far reaching, influencing coagulation, which in turn can increase microemboli and bleeding and result in organ dysfunction. This is therefore an area of significant investigation both into how anesthetic drugs or/and modifications in circuit components (e.g., heparin-bonded circuits) might favorably modulate these responses to benefit the patient. A few of the common medications and strategies that aim to maximize patient outcome in light of these changes are presented in the next section.

Drugs and interventions used during cardiopulmonary bypass

Antibiotics

Owing to the invasive nature of the surgical procedure and inflammatory changes resulting from bypass, a broad-spectrum antibiotic is administered prior to and at fixed intervals during surgery.

Steroids

Because of the many cellular and humoral changes that occur during cardiopulmonary bypass, steroid use has been advocated. Although steroid administration is associated with an increase in blood glucose, which in turn is associated with a poor neurologic outcome, considerations such as improved hemodynamic stability and reduced myocardial injury and inflammation generally outweigh concerns [28–30]. It has been our practice to administer a single dose of dexamethasone (1 mg/kg, IV) prior to initiating bypass.

Antifibrinolytics

Both lysine analogs (e.g., ε-aminocaproic acid and tranexamic acid) that inhibit proteases through antagonism of free plasmin and non-specific protease (or plasmin) and kalikrein inhibitors (e.g., aprotinin) have been used preoperatively with to the aim of reducing the need for post-bypass transfusion in human patients [31–33]. The lysine analogs act as antifibrinolytics and help prevent dissolution of the clot, while aprotinin has both antifibrinolytic and anti-inflammatory actions. The questionable efficacy in reducing transfusion requirements, cost, and potential for adverse effects has raised concerns with regard to their routine use for cardiac surgery. Limited numbers of dogs have received both ε-aminocaproic acid and aprotinin during clinical management, and data on benefits or side-effects for cardiovascular surgery are limited.

Anticoagulation and reversal

Heparin is approved and routinely utilized in human patients for anticoagulation during cardiopulmonary bypass despite the large individual variability in its actions. An initial dose of 300–400 IU/kg of unfractionated heparin has been recommended for human patients and has also been used in clinical canine patients. In the author's experience, the activated clotting time (ACT) following administration of this dose to dogs is typically greater than 1000 s when blood is sampled approximately 10 min after administration; an ACT greater than 400–480 s (in hypothermic patients) is considered by most to be adequate to initiate bypass. Repeated (often partial) dosing is considered necessary if ACT values approach this while the patient is still connected to the bypass circuit. With the availability of heparin-coated circuits, both initial and repeat dosing may need to be adjusted.

Low molecular weight heparin (e.g., dalteparin, enoxaparin) and also other anticoagulants (argatroban, dabigratran) with different mechanisms (e.g., direct thrombin inhibition) of action, in addition to antiplatelet medications (e.g., clopidogrel), are increasingly available for use in the management of (anti)coagulation in humans. Some of these have been studied and used in dogs and cats, but specific studies of their use during cardiopulmonary bypass are lacking [34,35].

The effects of heparin are reversed with protamine sulfate at the conclusion of cardiopulmonary bypass. As discussed later, slow administration is advised as protamine is reported to cause significant hypotension in dogs when administered rapidly [36].

Hypothermia

This is a strategy commonly used during cardiopulmonary bypass to reduce metabolic rate and oxygen consumption. Hypothermia preserves high-energy phosphate stores and reduces excitatory neurotransmitter release, calcium-mediated enzyme induction, and cell destruction [37,38]. The reduction in oxygen demand allows for lower pump flow rates, which in turn reduce cell trauma and embolic events and provide better surgical visualization. However, it is not without negative aspects. These include, but are not limited to, changes in drug disposition, coagulation, acid–base and electrolyte values, and increases in blood glucose, viscosity, and cardiac arrhythmogenicity.

Of significant importance to the anesthesia team is how pH and blood gas values are managed with body temperature changes. Recall that the solubility of carbon dioxide (and oxygen) in blood increases with hypothermia while its content remains constant. Hence the pCO_2 value decreases and pH increases. The influence of temperature on pH results from a change in carbon dioxide solubility (as stated above) and another mechanism that is independent of solubility. The latter mechanism by which pH is influenced is related to the fact that water, a weak solution of acid and base, is a primary solvent in body systems and its dissociation is directly influenced by temperature. As body temperature decreases, the tendency of water to dissociate to its ionized components (H^+ and OH^-) decreases. Changes in blood pH parallel temperature-related changes for water, but are tempered by the buffering capability of the amino acid histidine (and its five-membered imidazole ring). Hence blood pH remains higher than the pH of neutrality for water at a given temperature [21,38,39].

Alpha-stat management of acid–base balance allows pH and carbon dioxide tensions to follow thermodynamic dissociation changes but keeps the total carbon dioxide constant. The term alpha refers to the ratio of unprotonated to protonated histidine. Relevant to the clinician, pH and blood gas values are not corrected for body temperature, but interpreted and managed as they would be at 37°C. Conversely, pH-stat management consists of holding temperature-corrected values at normal (at 37°C) as the patient is cooled. In adult human patients, for various reasons including better maintenance of cerebral auto-regulation and prevention of stroke, alpha-stat management is most common, and this has also been the management strategy with which the author is familiar for dogs [21,22]. In young children, where the risk for microemboli to cause stroke is negligible, it has been suggested that pH-stat management may improve outcomes by increasing cerebral perfusion. A prospective study in children less than 9 months of age at the time of surgery, however, did not show any difference in neurologic development at either a 2- or 4-year follow-up. Interestingly, a trend to lower postoperative morbidity was observed [40].

Preanesthetic preparation

Patient evaluation

In addition to an accurate body weight and routine physical assessment and laboratory evaluation (of a complete blood count, serum chemistry profile, and urinalysis), the patient should have a coagulation profile and activated clotting time assessed and a blood type (and/or) cross-match performed. A complete cardiac evaluation and medication history should also be available. This information forms the basis of discussion among team members of any special considerations for the patient. For example, it may be in the patient's best interest to have certain medications discontinued in advance of anesthesia and surgery. Similarly, if a patient presents with abdominal or pleural effusion, drainage of the same may be considered.

Anesthesia setup

A small-animal anesthesia machine and ventilator should be checked for functionality and absence of leaks. Standard catheterization (arterial, venous and central venous – multi-lumen or Swan–Ganz catheter if desired) and intubation equipment in appropriate sizes should be available. As the patient will be anticoagulated, atraumatic catheter placement is followed by wrapping the catheter sites. A physiologic monitor with the capability to monitor heart rate and rhythm, direct arterial blood pressures, central venous/pulmonary artery pressures, end-tidal carbon dioxide, oxygen saturation and both rectal and esophageal temperature should be available. A tool to monitor the neuromuscular junction (e.g., peripheral nerve stimulator), coagulation status [ACT block or PT/INR (prothrombin time/international normalized ratio)], and urinary catheter and collection system should also be readied. It is the author's preference also to have a Doppler blood pressure monitor, respirometer, and PEEP (positive end-expiratory pressure) valves available. Multiple syringe pumps, intravenous fluids, colloids, blood product and medication/administration supplies, blood gas syringes, pressure bags, etc., are also best kept in an easily accessed location.

Additional supplies that should be available include a pacing unit and leads, defibrillator with both external and internal paddles, and tracheostomy supplies (in the event of need for postanesthesia ventilation). An epidural catheter may be considered (generally after coagulation status is normalized) to assist in postoperative pain management.

Medications

In addition to drugs used for anesthesia (Table 24.1), numerous other medications (Tables 24.2 and 24.3) should be available and in some cases drawn up. These include anticholinergics, inotropes, vasopressors, antiarrhythmics, dexamethasone, furosemide, electrolytes, sodium bicarbonate, heparin, an antifibrinolytic, a neuromuscular blocking agent, and protamine. Insulin may be necessary for treatment of hyperglycemia. Although it is our practice to use an opioid, benzodiazepine, inhaled anesthetic and neuromuscular blocking agent or balanced anesthesia plan, other anesthesia techniques have also been described [13,14].

Table 24.1 Suggested anesthesia drugs for dogs undergoing cardiopulmonary bypass.

Drug	Dose (mg/kg or as noted)
Premedication (SC/IM)	
Hydromorphone	0.1
Midazolam	0.1
Atropine	0.02
Anesthesia induction (IV)	
Fentanyl	0.01
Midazolam	0.2
Etomidate	0.5
Anesthesia maintenance (IV/CRI or inhaled)	
Fentanyl	0.35–0.7 μg/kg/min
Midazolam	0.35–0.7 μg/kg/min
Isoflurane	Dosed to effect
Atracurium	0.1–0.25

Table 24.2 Anticholinergics, inotropes, vasopressors, and antiarrhythmic medications for dogs anesthetized for cardiopulmonary bypass.

Drug	Bolus Dose (mg/kg)	Infusion Dose (μg/kg/min)
Atropine	0.02–0.04	
Lidocaine	1–3	80–100
Esmolol	0.1	70–100
Diltiazem	0.5–1.0 slowly	1–5
Dobutamine	NA	5–10
Dopamine	NA	2–10
Milrinone	0.05	0.5
Epinephrine	0.005–0.05	0.05–0.2
Phenylephrine	0.002–0.005	1–3
Norepinephrine	NA	0.1–0.2

Table 24.3 Adjunct drug doses for dogs undergoing anesthesia for cardiopulmonary bypass.

Drug	Dose (IV)
Heparin	300–400 IU/kg
Dexamethasone sodium phosphate	1 mg/kg
Cefoxitin	22 mg/kg every 90 min
ε-Aminocaproic acid	100 mg/kg loading dose slowly 10–15 mg/kg/h, CRI
Furosemide	0.5–2.0 mg/kg
Protamine (administer slowly)	3 mg/kg or 1.3 mg/mg heparin

The sequence of events and terminology

Much of what is described here is experientially based from work in two institutions. The author recognizes that other approaches are viable and better suited to other environments.

Following a quick assessment on the morning of surgery and confirmation of the medication and fasting status, the dog is premedicated. Premedication is administered subcutaneously or intramuscularly and generally consists of a non-histamine-releasing opioid such as hydromorphone or methadone. Midazolam and an anticholinergic may be concurrently administered. After approximately 30 min, during which time the anesthesia equipment has been checked for function and drug infusions verified, the dog is brought to the anesthesia induction area and instrumented with an ECG, Doppler, and cephalic intravenous catheter. Oxygen, intravenous fluids, and anesthesia drug infusions (which in our practice consist of fentanyl and midazolam) are started. As many dogs are being treated for heart failure, intravenous fluid administration is conservatively maintained in the range 1–2 mL/kg/h. Anesthesia is induced with intravenous fentanyl and midazolam along with a low dose of a hypnotic agent (e.g., etomidate or propofol) if needed. Following endotracheal intubation and connection to the anesthesia machine, additional equipment, including a pulse oximeter, capnograph, and esophageal temperature probe, are placed. Additional catheters to facilitate arterial and central venous blood pressure measurements and blood sampling for pH, blood gas, glucose, acid–base status, electrolyte, PCV/TP (packed cell volume/total protein), and ACT/PT (activated clotting time/prothrombin time) are placed. Support at this stage may consist of an inotrope to maintain blood pressure and an antiarrhythmic if arrhythmias are observed and of consequence to the patient. The patient is ventilated to maintain a normal arterial carbon dioxide tension, which is verified with a blood gas sample taken after the arterial catheter is in place. If other abnormalities are noted in pH, blood gas, acid–base, electrolyte, or glucose values, attempts are made to correct these. External heat is typically not provided in these patients at this stage since patient cooling will occur with initiation of bypass.

While the surgical site is being clipped, dexamethasone and antibiotics are administered (prophylactic antibiotics are repeated at 90 min intervals during anesthesia). If an antifibrinolytic agent is to be administered, it is also started at this time.

Following movement of the dog into the operating room and appropriate positioning, a rectal temperature probe and peripheral nerve stimulator (PNS) are placed and the central venous line is connected for monitoring. A baseline ACT or PT is taken prior to administration of heparin and commonly another blood sample is taken for measurement of pH, blood gases, electrolytes, glucose, lactate, PCV and TP. The patency of the urine collection system bag is verified and the bag emptied if necessary.

The surgeons begin working on placement of the femoral cannula and may simultaneously or subsequently begin the thoracotomy. This is usually a good time to have internal defibrillator paddles set up on the surgical table. Heparin is given and the ACT or PT is rechecked within 10 min following administration. A loading dose of the neuromuscular blocking agent is given slowly intravenously after assessing the patient's response to the thoracotomy incision and depending on the drug and anesthesiologist preference a constant-rate infusion (CRI) or repeat bolus administration is continued during the procedure and monitored using the PNS. Fentanyl and midazolam infusions are continued, and isoflurane and inotropes are adjusted as necessary to normalize blood pressure while maintaining an appropriate anesthetic plane. As surgeons manipulate the heart to place the cannulas, hypotension resulting from changes in cardiac filling and arrhythmias may be seen and are treated as necessary to minimize influence on blood pressure and/or chance of premature fibrillation. Positive end-expiratory pressure (PEEP) at 2.5–5.0 cmH_2O is applied after the chest is open in an effort to maintain oxygenation if it does not impair visualization by the surgeon [41,42]. Alternatively, it may be applied once the pericardial sling is in place.

Occasionally, a dog may lose blood or fibrillate during cannula placement. Treatment is appropriate to the cause and in some cases might include a rapid transfer to extracorporeal circulation. If the process goes uneventfully, then the planned transition to partial bypass is initiated by unclamping the venous lines (connected to the venous cannulas) and starting the arterial pump. It should be kept in mind that flow is no longer pulsatile so monitors will tend to record only a mean value once the heart stops ejecting. It is common for blood pressure to decrease significantly during this transition to extracorporeal circulation. This is thought to be due in part to abrupt changes in volume, hematocrit, colloid oncotic pressure, and viscosity. The perfusionist will adjust the pump flow to vary the mean arterial pressure with the traditional goal in adult humans being to maintain pressure between 40 and 70 mmHg [20]; recently, higher pressures have been suggested in human patients due to the beneficial impact on neurological outcome. The perfusionist may request a vasoconstrictor such as phenylephrine to assist in maintenance of blood pressure if the pump flow rate is deemed to be adequate for the size of the patient.

This is also the time when the perfusionist starts to take over the administration of the inhaled anesthetic, and mechanical ventilation may be reduced or stopped as the heart stops ejecting blood. PEEP is maintained as it has been shown in dogs to benefit oxygenation at least transiently without negative impact on cardiac output [41–43]. Injectable anesthetic infusions are frequently decreased as the patient is cooled. This is done despite demonstrated decreases in concentrations resulting from hemodilution and pump sequestration for drugs such as fentanyl due to the decrease in metabolic rate with hypothermia (which in turn decreases anesthetic requirements) and changes in protein binding (which increase the free drug fraction) [44,45]. If atracurium or cisatracurium is used for neuromuscular blockade, significant increases in dosing interval will be noted with hypothermia. Antifibrinolytic medications, when used, are usually continued until conclusion of bypass. Blood for pH, blood gases, acid–base, blood glucose and electrolyte values, ACT/PT, and PCV/TP may be obtained from the perfusionist, who is also able to administer medications (e.g., antibiotics, neuromuscular blocking agents) as necessary; IV lines may continue to be used but it should be noted that vascular flow patterns are altered and this may have an additional influence on drug kinetics. Peripheral vasoconstriction resulting from hypothermia is also common.

As the patient cools, the cardiac rhythm, if not already altered from primary disease and manipulation, will often change and ventricular fibrillation may be noted. Although one can attempt to defibrillate electrically at this time, success is limited in profoundly hypothermic patients. Hence it is best to place the patient on total bypass as soon as feasible. To do this, the surgeon places the aortic cross clamp and administers cardioplegic solution as previously described to stop electrical activity. Once the aortic cross clamp has been placed, the ventilator is turned off if this was not done previously. The perfusionist now assumes full responsibility for patient management while the surgical team works on the heart. The anesthesia team serves a supportive role during this period.

As the cardiac procedure is reaching its end, the anesthesia, surgical, and perfusion teams must be in communication to transition the patient off bypass successfully. It is worthwhile to check blood values just prior to coming off the pump. It should be kept in mind that potassium values may be abnormally high due to the administration of cardioplegic solution, but no intervention is necessary as this effect will resolve once cardiac circulation resumes. Infusions of antiarrhythmic, inotropic, and vasoactive drugs are usually started at this time in an effort to load them prior to coming off bypass; bolus doses may be used as needed. Although epinephrine or a combination of dobutamine and dopamine has been successfully used, the author's preference has been to transition the dog off bypass with dobutamine and phenylephrine. It has further been our experience that dogs do not typically require antihypertensive medications such as nitroprusside. However, these should be available as their necessity has been described by others. The perfusionist will also start to warm the patient at this time in anticipation of transitioning off bypass.

Ventricular fibrillation may be noted during this period or after removal of the aortic cross clamp. If defibrillation is unsuccessful after a few attempts, it may be wise to let the heart rest and warm, while the dog is still on partial bypass. Although there is no absolute guideline, clinical experience suggests that if defibrillation attempts are unsuccessful during weaning from the pump, warming the patient to between 33 and 35°C usually results in success. On rare occasions, the dog may need to be paced temporarily. The patient may also spontaneously resume a normal electrical rhythm and gradually begin to eject blood with cardiovascular support as warming continues. The surgeon will ask the anesthesia team to help de-air the heart by using the ventilator to give a large breath or series of breaths and move blood into the heart. Transesophageal echocardiography may also be used to verify the absence of air in the left heart prior to cardiac closure. Ventilation is resumed once the heart begins to eject blood as noted by return of pulsatile flow on the arterial line. The perfusionist will gradually decrease the pump's contribution to circulation as the heart resumes function.

Once the heart is pumping adequately, cannulas can be removed and protamine administration started. Doses between 2 and 6 mg/kg or 1.3 mg/mg heparin have been described. Selection of dose should be made after consideration of duration of heparin administration, ACT/PT values, and body temperature. Significant hypotension may be seen with protamine administration in dogs, which is thought to be primarily associated with histamine release, but increased central nitric oxide release has also been implicated [36, 46]. With slow administration, anaphylactoid reactions are still possible and in part are thought to be due to excessive complement activation resulting from the formation of heparin–protamine complexes. In some patients, anaphylactoid reactions may be mediated via IgE antibodies. The responses can be immediate or delayed. Protamine has also been reported to affect platelet number and function, enhance fibrinolysis, and decrease clot strength, which in turn can contribute to bleeding [47–49]. Given that there may be other causes of hypotension (e.g., surgical bleeding) during this period, communication between the surgical and anesthesia teams is critical to determine the cause and extent. pH, blood gases, blood glucose, acid–base status and electrolytes, PCV/TP, and ACT are checked as needed during this period and abnormal values are addressed. Urine output is also assessed at this time, keeping in mind that it is not unusual to see discoloration related to hemolysis following bypass. It is fairly common, despite the use of high potassium-containing cardioplegic solutions, to see potassium values decrease during this phase. Calcium values also tend to be low and supplementation may help correct protamine-induced hypotension. Although magnesium may be used in a patient where difficulty is encountered during defibrillation attempts, treatment is usually deferred until the patient is in the critical care unit owing to the potential for hypotension with administration. Fresh whole blood can be administered concurrently with or after protamine to provide platelets and coagulation factors.

The closure of the chest wall is managed as for any thoracotomy; a chest drain is placed. If blood gases are suggestive of hypoxemia relative to the F_IO_2, furosemide may be administered. The team may also elect to maintain these patients on a ventilator for the immediate postoperative phase either via the oro-tracheal tube or, if less sedation is desirable, a tracheotomy. Typically, anesthesia infusions are reduced during body wall closure. The supportive infusions and intravenous fluids (crystalloid, colloid, blood products) are titrated as necessary. If available, a cell saver can be a useful tool to conserve blood. At the conclusion of surgery, the critical care team verifies and rewraps all catheters, the chest tube, etc., and the patient is then transitioned to them for postoperative care.

Conclusion

Given the complexity of the process and relatively infrequent nature with which cardiopulmonary bypass is currently performed in veterinary medicine, it is imperative that lines of communication between the anesthesia, perfusion, surgery, and critical care teams are maintained to maximize the possibility of a successful outcome.

References

1 Brourman JD, Schertel ER, Holt DW, Olshove VA. Cardiopulmonary bypass in the cat. *Vet Surg* 2002; **31**: 412–417.

2 Klement P, Feindel CM, Scully HE, *et al.* Mitral valve replacement in dogs. Surgical technique and post operative management. *Vet Surg* 1987; **16**: 231–237.

3 Kombtebedde J, Ilkiw JE, Follette DM, *et al.* Resection of subvalvular aortic stenosis. Surgical and perioperative management in seven dogs. *Vet Surg* 1993; **22**: 419–430.

4 Monnet E, Orton EC, Gaynor JS, *et al.* Open resection of subvalvular aortic stenosis in dogs. *J Am Vet Med Assoc* 1996; **209**: 1255–1261.

5 Monnet E, Orton E, Gaynor J, *et al.* Diagnosis and surgical repair of partial atrioventricular septal defects in two dogs. *J Am Vet Med Assoc* 1997; **211**: 567–572.

6 Orton EC, Herndon GD, Boon JA, *et al.* Influence of open surgical correction on intermediate-term outcome in dogs with subvalvular aortic stenosis: 44 cases (1991–1998). *J Am Vet Med Assoc* 2000; **216**: 364–367.

7 Lew LJ, Fowler JD, Egger CM, *et al.* Deep hypothermic low flow cardiopulmonary bypass in small dogs. *Vet Surg* 1997; **26**: 281–289.

8 Orton EC, Mama K, Hellyer P, *et al.* Open surgical repair of tetralogy of Fallot in two dogs. *J Am Vet Med Assoc* 2001; **219**: 1089–1093.

9 Martin JM, Orton EC, Boon JA, *et al.* Surgical correction of double-chambered right ventricle in dogs. *J Am Vet Med Assoc* 2002; **6**: 770–774.

10 Griffiths LG, Orton EC, Boon JA. Evaluation of techniques and outcomes of mitral valve repair in dogs. *J Am Vet Med Assoc* 2004; **224**: 1941–1945.

11 Orton EC, Hackett TB, Mama K, Boon JA. Technique and outcome of mitral valve replacement in dogs. *J Am Vet Med Assoc* 2005; **226**: 1508–1511.

12 Tanaka R, Shimizu M, Hoshi K, *et al.* Efficacy of open patch-grafting under cardiopulmonary bypass for pulmonic stenosis in small dogs. *Aust Vet J* 2009; **87**: 88–92.

13 Kanemoto I, Taguchi, D, Yokoyama S, *et al.* Open heart surgery with deep hypothermia and cardiopulmonary bypass in small and toy dogs. *Vet Surg* 2010; **39**: 674–679.

14 Uechi M, Mizukoshi T, Mizuno T, *et al.* Mitral valve repair under cardiopulmonary bypass in small-breed dogs: 48 cases (2006–2009). *J Am Vet Med Assoc* 2012; **240**: 1194–2012.

15 Rodriguez AL, Mama KR, Wagner AE, *et al.* Retrospective evaluation of plasma biochemical values in dogs anesthetized for cardiopulmonary bypass and influence on anesthetic mortality. In: *Proceedings of the 9th World Congress of Veterinary Anesthesia 2006, Santos, Brazil*, **2006**; 131.

16 Pelosi A, Anderson LK, Paugh J, *et al.* Challenges of cardiopulmonary bypass – a review of the veterinary literature. *Vet Surg* 2013; **42**: 119–136.

17 Iwahashi H, Yuri K, Nose Y. Development of the oxygenator: past, present and future. *J Artif Organs* 2004; **7**: 111–120.

18 Nishinaka T, Nishida H, Endo M, *et al.* Less blood damage in the impeller centrifugal pump. A comparative study with the roller pump in open heart surgery. *Artif Organs* 1996; **20**: 707–710.

19 Linneweber J, Chow TW, Kawamura M, *et al.* In vitro comparison of blood pump induced platelet microaggregates between a centrifugal and roller pump during cardiopulmonary bypass. *Int J. Artif Organs* 2002; **25**: 549–555.
20 Nyhan D and Johns RA. Anesthesia for cardiac surgery procedures. In: Miller RD, ed. *Miller's Anesthesia*, 6th edn. Philadelphia: Elsevier Churchill Livingstone, 2005; 1941–2004.
21 Nussmeier NA, Hauser MC, Sarwar MF, *et al.* Anesthesia for cardiac surgical procedures. In: Miller RD, Eriksson LI, Fleisher LA, *et al.*, eds. *Miller's Anesthesia*, 7th edn. Philadelphia: Elsevier Churchill Livingstone, 2010; 1889–1975.
22 Greeley WJ, Berkowitz DH, Nathan AT. Anesthesia for pediatric cardiac surgery. In: Miller RD, Eriksson LI, Fleisher LA, *et al.*, eds. *Miller's Anesthesia*, 7th edn. Philadelphia: Churchill Livingstone Elsevier, 2010; 2599–2652.
23 Orton EC. Inflow occlusion and cardiopulmonary bypass. *Small Animal Thoracic Surgery*. Baltimore: Williams & Wilkins, 1995: 185–201.
24 Gravlee GP, Davis RE, Utley JR, eds. *Cardiopulmonary Bypass: Principles and Practice*. Baltimore: Williams & Wilkins, 1993.
25 Knudsen F, Andersen LW. Immunological aspects of cardiopulmonary bypass. *J Cardiothorac Anesth* 1990; **4**: 245–258.
26 Hirai S. Systemic inflammatory response syndrome after cardiac surgery under cardiopulmonary bypass. *Ann Thorac Cardiovasc Surg* 2003; **9**: 365–370.
27 Hammon JW Jr, Edmunds HL Jr. Extracorporeal circulation: organ damage. In: Cohn LH, Edmunds LH Jr, eds. *Cardiac Surgery in the Adult*. New York: McGraw Hill, 2003; 361–368.
28 Aarts LP, Boonstra PW, Rakhorst G, *et al.* Prophylactic use of dexamethasone in cardiopulmonary bypass. *Chest* 2004; **126**: 854S.
29 Engleman RM, Rousou JA, Flack JE, *et al.* Influence of steroids on complement and cytokine generation after cardiopulmonary bypass. *Ann Thorac Surg* 1994; **60**: 801–804.
30 Tilman VS, Savvas G, Gotz JKW, *et al.* Effects of dexamethasone on intravascular and extravascular fluid balance in patients undergoing coronary bypass surgery with cardiopulmonary bypass. *Anesthesiology* 2002; **96**: 827–834.
31 Troianos CA, Sypula RW, Lucas DM, *et al.* The effect of prophylactic epsilon-aminocaproic acid on bleeding, transfusions, platelet function and fibrinolysis during coronary artery bypass grafting. *Anesthesiology* 1999; **91**: 430–435.
32 American Society of Anesthesiologists Task Force on Perioperative Blood Transfusion and Adjuvant Therapies. Practice guidelines for perioperative blood transfusion and adjuvant therapies: an updated report by the American Society of Anesthesiologists Task Force on Perioperative Blood Transfusion and Adjuvant Therapies. *Anesthesiology* 2006; **105**: 198–208.
33 Kovesi T, Royston D. Pharmacological approaches to reducing allogenic blood exposure. *Vox Sang* 2003; **84**: 2–10.
34 Brainard BM, Kleine SA, Papich MG, *et al.* Pharmacodynamic and pharmacokinetic evaluation of clopidogrel and the carboxylic acid metabolite SR 26334 in healthy dogs. *Am J Vet Res* 2010; **71**: 822–830.
35 Mischke R, Schmitt J, Wolken S, *et al.* Pharmacokinetics of low molecular weight heparin dalteparin in cats. *Vet J* 2012; **192**: 299–303.
36 Stoelting RK, Henry DP, Verburg KM, *et al.* Haemodynamic changes and circulating histamine concentrations following protamine administration to patients and dogs. *Can Anaesth Soc J* 1984; **5**: 534–540.
37 Little DM. Hypothermia. *Anesthesiology* 1959; **20**: 842–877.
38 Davies LK. Hypothermia: physiology and clinical use. In: Gravlee GP, Davis RE, Utley JR, eds. *Cardiopulmonary Bypass: Principles and Practice*. Baltimore: Williams & Wilkins, 1993: 140–154.
39 Alston, TA. Blood gases and pH during hypothermia: the "-stats." *Int Anesthesiol Clin* 2004; **42**: 73–80.
40 Bellinger DC, Wypij D, du Plessis AJ, *et al.* Developmental and neurologic effects of alpha-stat versus pH-stat strategies for deep hypothermic cardiopulmonary bypass in infants. *J Thorac Cardiovasc Surg* 2001; **121**: 374–383.
41 Rustomjee T, Wagner A, Orton EC. Effect of 5 cm of water positive end-expiratory pressure on arterial oxygen tension in dogs during and after thoracotomy. *Vet Surg* 1994; **4**: 307–310.
42 Kudnig ST, Monnet E, Riquelme M, *et al.* Effect of positive end-expiratory pressure on oxygen delivery during 1-lung ventilation for thoracoscopy in normal dogs. *Vet Surg* 2006; **35**: 534–542.
43 Riquelme M, Monnet E, Kudnig ST, *et al.* Cardiopulmonary effects of positive end-expiratory pressure during one-lung ventilation in anesthetized dogs with a closed thoracic cavity. *Am J Vet Res* 2005; **66**: 978–983.
44 Mets B. The pharmacokinetics of anesthetic drugs and adjuvants during cardiopulmonary bypass. *Acta Anaesthesiol Scand* 2000; **44**: 261–273.
45 Hall RI. Cardiopulmonary bypass and the systemic inflammatory response: effects on drug action. *J Cardiothorac Vasc Anesth* 2002; **18**: 83–98.
46 Hamada Y, Kameyama Y, Narita H, *et al.* Protamine after heparin produces hypotension resulting from decreased sympathetic outflow secondary to increased nitric oxide in the central nervous system. *Anesth Analg*, 2005; **100**: 33–37.
47 Lindblad B, Wajefuield TW, Whitehouse WM, Stanley JC. The effect of protamine sulfate on platelet function. *Scand J Thorac Cardiovasc Surg* 1988; **22**: 55–59.
48 Nielsen VG. Protamine enhances fibrinolysis by decreasing clot strength: role of tissue factor-initiated thrombin generation. *Ann Thorac Surg* 2006; **81**: 1720–1727.
49 Bailey CJ, Koenigshof, AM. The effects of protamine sulfate on clot formation time and clot strength thromboelastography variables for canine blood samples. *Am J Vet Res* 2014; **75**: 338–343.

25 Cardiac Pacemakers and Anesthesia

Barret J. Bulmer
Tufts Veterinary Emergency Treatment and Specialties, Walpole, Massachusetts, USA

Chapter contents

Introduction

Cardiac anesthesia and surgery can generally be described as high risk, high reward. Pacemaker implantation exemplifies this since no other group of patients has such a high risk of sudden asystole and death, but yet can have a dramatic improvement in quality of life with successful implantation. The anesthetist can have a significant impact on the management of perioperative risk through understanding the surgical procedure and the needs of the cardiologist, selecting drugs and techniques that minimize the effects on heart rhythm and function, and having an emergency plan should severe bradycardia or asystole occur. Since pacemaker implantation can extend the lifespan of many animals, it is becoming more common to perform non-cardiac elective and emergency procedures on animals with pacemakers.

Since the first report of pacemaker implantation in a dog with complete heart block [1], artificial pacemakers have become a mainstay for dogs, and less commonly cats, for bradyarrhythmia management. Because of the increasing number of pacemaker implantations, there are two common scenarios that will be encountered by the anesthetist: (1) anesthesia for pacemaker implantation in a patient with a bradyarrhythmia, or (2) anesthesia of a patient with a previously implanted and functional artificial pacing system undergoing an unrelated medical or surgical procedure.

Artificial pacemakers

Permanent transvenous artificial pacemakers are comprised of one or more pacing leads and a pulse generator (Fig. 25.1). The pacing lead wire delivers the electrical impulses to the heart and serves as the sensing electrode to detect native electrical activity. The lead consists of three parts: (1) the conductor (a coil of wire that conducts the electrical current), (2) lead insulation, and (3) a lead connector. Attachment of a transvenous pacemaker lead to the endocardial surface is most often accomplished using either passive (e.g., tined) or active fixation (e.g., fixed or retractable helical screw) leads (Fig. 25.2). Many leads incorporate a steroid eluting reservoir in an attempt to reduce scar tissue formation, which, if it were to occur, could contribute to unacceptably high pacing thresholds.

The pacemaker lead is the weakest link of the implantable artificial pacemaker system. It serves a passive function to deliver current developed from the pulse generator to the heart and to relay signals from the heart to the pulse generator. At a stimulus rate of 70 beats/min the heart contracts 36.8 million times per year. Respiration, along with motion induced by ventricular and atrial contraction and closure of the tricuspid valve, exposes transvenous leads to profound mechanical stresses of flexion, torsion, and elongation that must be combated. Despite ever-improving lead technology, failure related to conductor fracture, insulation breakage, or lead dislodgement and failure at the header remain recognized complications (Fig. 25.3) [2].

The pulse generator contains the battery and computer circuitry controlling the timing of electrical impulses sent to the heart, the sensing threshold of the pacing lead, and the response to sensed electrical activity. Pulse generator technology has progressed with the incorporation of advanced circuitry and microprocessors providing telemetrically programmable pacing parameters and a wealth of diagnostic data to help monitor and manage arrhythmias [3]. These advancements have allowed the development of more sophisticated and physiologic pacing modalities.

Veterinary Anesthesia and Analgesia: The Fifth Edition of Lumb and Jones.
Edited by Kurt A. Grimm, Leigh A. Lamont, William J. Tranquilli, Stephen A. Greene and Sheilah A. Robertson.

Pacemaker modalities

Pacemakers implanted in dogs most often employ a single lead that paces the apex of the ventricle (e.g., right ventricle for a single transvenous lead) irrespective of atrial activity. More advanced pacing systems may employ a single-lead physiologic pacemaker (e.g., coordinates native atrial depolarization with ventricular stimulation) [4], a dual-lead system to pace the atria and ventricles, or a three-lead system to pace the atria along with simultaneous activation of the right and left ventricles [5]. Programmed pacemaker modalities are most often described using a five-letter code (Table 25.1). The NBG coding system is a joint project between the **N**orth American Society of Pacing and Electrophysiology (NASPE) and the **B**ritish Pacing and Electrophysiology **G**roup (BPEG). Although some newer pulse generators defy description by the NBG code, most pacemakers implanted in veterinary patients employ only the first three or four letters. However, with a potential increase in implantation of cardiac defibrillators in dogs [6,7], veterinary medicine may have need of the complete five-letter NBG code.

The first position in the code indicates the chamber paced, the second indicates the chamber sensed, the third indicates the response to spontaneous depolarizations, and the fourth commonly describes rate modulation. Hence a VVIR pacemaker paces and senses only the ventricle. In response to a sensed impulse, a VVIR pacemaker is inhibited until there is another period of quiescence in the sensed chamber. If no impulse is detected in a VVIR pacemaker at the end of a programmable lower rate interval, a ventricular stimulus will be delivered. The fourth position, most commonly an R, represents

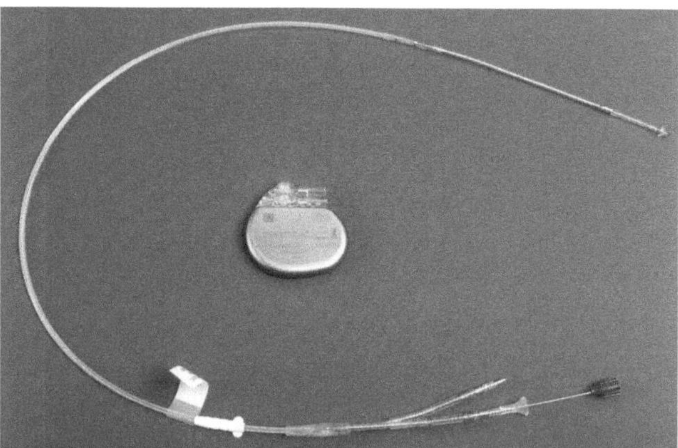

Figure 25.1 A dual-chamber pulse generator (both atrial and ventricular ports are present) along with a transvenous pacemaker lead. This particular lead has two floating atrial electrodes which enables atrioventricular (AV) sequential pacing in dogs with AV block using only a single pacemaker lead.

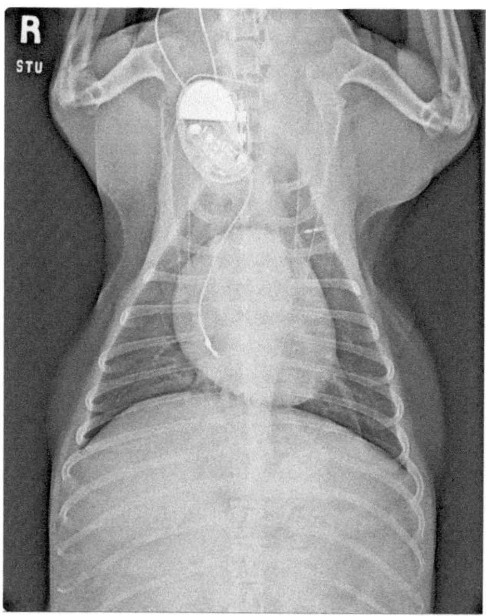

Figure 25.3 Radiograph from a dog that had loss of pacemaker capture on a recheck examination. Failure to pace was related to fracture of the pacing lead at its junction with the header.

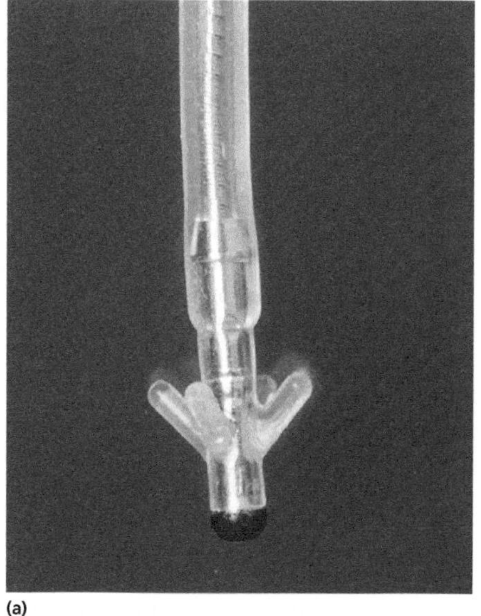

(a)

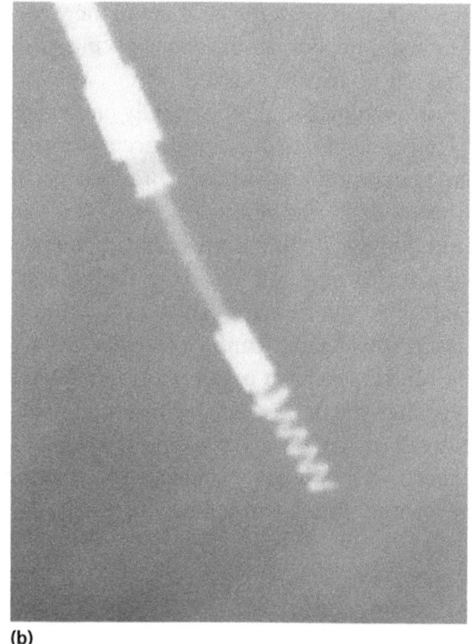

(b)

Figure 25.2 (a) Tined (passive) pacemaker leads employ small plastic 'fins' to entangle within the trabeculae carneae to enhance short-term lead security. (b) Active fixation leads have either a fixed or a retractable helical screw to penetrate and adhere to the myocardium.

Table 25.1 The five-letter NBG coding system description of pacemaker modalities.

I Chamber paced	II Chamber sensed	III Response to a sensed impulse	IV Programmable functions/Rate modulation	V Anti-tachycardia function
V = ventricle A = atrium D = dual (V and A) O = none	V = ventricle A = atrium D = dual (V and A) O = none	I = inhibited T = triggered D = dual (I and T) O = none	P = programmable M = multiprogrammable C = communicating R = rate modulation O = none	P = pacing S = shock D = dual (P and S) O = none

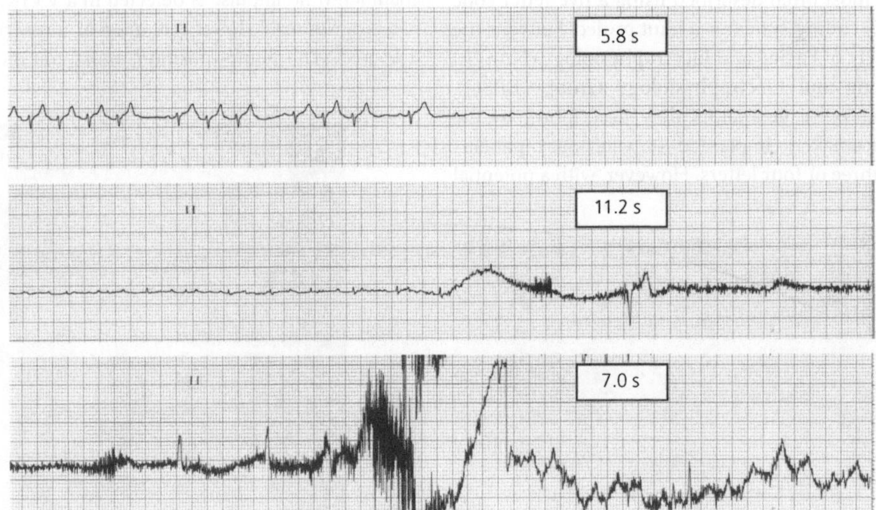

Figure 25.4 Continuous lead II ECG (25 mm/s) from a cat that presented for acute onset 'seizure-like' activity. The episodes were triggered by intermittent, sustained atrioventricular (AV) block with lack of a stable ventricular escape focus. In this particular ECG, an absence of AV conduction or stable ventricular escape focus persisted for approximately 24 s. The artifact in the ECG was produced by movement accompanying the syncopal episode. Emergency pacemaker implantation was performed and the cat survived without recurrence of episodes for more than 2 years.

rate modulation wherein an activity sensor (e.g., accelerometer, respiratory rate, QT interval) is able to increase the programmed heart rate during activity. A VDD pacemaker paces only the ventricle, but it senses both the atrium and ventricle. Delivery of a stimulating electrical impulse to the ventricle is triggered by a sensed atrial impulse and it is inhibited by a sensed ventricular impulse. A DDD pacemaker is able to sense and pace both the atrium and the ventricle. Biventricular (BiV) pacing implies simultaneous pacing of the right ventricular apex and left ventricular free wall.

Most pacemakers are programmed to discharge only on demand (synchronous pacing). However, on rare occasions pacemakers may be programmed (often temporarily) to an asynchronous pacing mode (e.g., VOO). In this modality, the ventricle is paced at a fixed rate independent of the underlying rhythm. Depending on the pulse generator, placement of a strong magnetic field over the generator may change the programming from synchronous to asynchronous. If the installed unit is an implantable cardioverter defibrillator, placement of a magnet over the generator usually turns off defibrillation. Asynchronous pacing can increase the likelihood that a pacemaker impulse may fall on the T-wave of a spontaneous beat, causing an R on T event, which may lead to ventricular fibrillation. The avoidance of asynchronous pacing will reduce this risk.

Anesthetic management

The most common indications for pacemaker implantation in dogs and cats are high-grade second- and third-degree atrioventricular (AV) block, sick sinus syndrome (SSS), and persistent atrial standstill. In humans, pacemaker implantation for these indications is usually performed on an outpatient basis with local anesthetic techniques, limiting the need for an anesthesiologist's involvement. However, to facilitate cooperation by veterinary patients, most artificial pacing systems are placed during general anesthesia [8,9]. Currently, there is no evidence that anesthetics alter the stimulation threshold of pacemakers [10]; therefore, the primary considerations when formulating an anesthetic plan are focused on (1) the utility of placing a temporary pacing system and (2) selection of anesthetic drug and techniques that do not adversely affect the animal's underlying cardiac status during the implantation procedures.

Patient evaluation

Patients may have considerable variability in their ventricular rate and underlying rhythm. Atropine response tests are often performed during initial patient workup and provide guidance as to whether anticholinergics will be beneficial. Cats with third-degree AV block have ventricular escape rates that far exceed those seen in most dogs [11]. The median heart rate reported in 21 cats with third-degree AV block was 120 beats/min (range 80–140) [11]. In the author's experience, cats with intermittent high-grade AV block (as opposed to sustained third-degree AV block) are the most unstable, often exhibiting ventricular asystole presumably related to overdrive suppression of ventricular escape foci (Fig. 25.4). The intermittent nature of AV block can also make diagnosis more challenging as the presence of sinus rhythm on examination does not exclude an intermittent arrhythmogenic cause for 'seizure-like' activity [12].

Additional testing such as blood chemistries and complete blood counts are also useful in helping identify primary or secondary changes such as renal insufficiency or electrolyte abnormalities. It should be emphasized that blood collection via jugular venipuncture should not be performed in these patients. Hematoma formation can delay or prevent successful transvenous lead placement, especially when transvenous temporary pacing is employed wherein both jugular veins are commonly used. Patients with a previously implanted transvenous pacing lead should never be injected or bled from that jugular vein since accidental damage to the pacing lead could result.

Temporary pacemaker implantation

Despite the increasing frequency of pacemaker implantation, anesthetic and procedural times remain long enough that animals with symptomatic bradyarrhythmias may become unstable with irreversible asystole. A recent report from an experienced veterinary cardiology center reported mean procedural times of 94.9 and 133.5 min and mean anesthesia times of 137.9 and 179.1 min for implantation of single- and dual-chamber pacing systems, respectively [13]. Therefore, placement of a temporary pacing system in the event that a ventricular escape focus becomes unstable, or a prolonged period of sinus arrest occurs, would seem prudent.

Either a transvenous or transthoracic [14] method is most often used to achieve temporary cardiac pacing. Pacing or electrophysiologic catheters placed transesophageal may capture the atria but would be less suitable for temporary pacing in dogs with AV block [15,16]. Prior to beginning the procedure, intravenous antibiotics are administered to reduce the risk of lead contamination, vegetative endocarditis, and phlebitis. Transvenous pacing requires placement of a catheter introducer into the jugular (or lateral saphenous) vein under mild sedation or local anesthesia. If local anesthetics (e.g., lidocaine or bupivacaine) are used in animals with an escape rhythm, the smallest dose possible is recommended owing to the potential inhibition of myocardial sodium channels and inadvertent suppression of the escape rhythm. Fluoroscopic guidance can be used to maneuver a temporary pacing lead, via the catheter introducer, through the right atrium, across the tricuspid valve, and into the right ventricle. After appropriate positioning, the temporary pacing lead is connected to an external temporary pulse generator and artificial pacing can commence. This permits control of heart rate during induction and prevents anesthetic drug-induced alterations. Transvenous pacing, in comparison with transthoracic pacing, has the advantage of myocardial stimulation without pain or thoracic skeletal muscle stimulation [14]. The disadvantages include the technical skill needed for placement of the catheter introducer and lead (especially if the patient is only lightly sedated), risk for vascular/cardiac perforation or infection, risk for lead dislodgement/loss of ventricular capture with lack of resumption of the ventricular escape focus leading to asystole, and the need for an external cardiac pulse generator and sterile temporary pacing lead.

Transthoracic temporary cardiac pacing generally employs an external cardiovertor defibrillator with pacing capabilities and a pair of disposable transthoracic patch electrodes. The left and right precordia are shaved, conductive paste is placed on the surface of the electrodes, and the adhesive patches are placed on the left and right side of the chest directly over the precordial impulse [14]. Often the electrodes are secured with elastic non-adhesive bandaging material to maintain skin contact during muscle contraction and patient movement. In most cases, anesthesia with rapid-acting injectable anesthetics is subsequently induced and testing for ventricular capture is performed. The disadvantages of transthoracic temporary pacing are the requirement for higher current output in comparison with transvenous pacing, the need for general anesthesia because of the pain induced by a required higher current output, thoracic skeletal muscle stimulation during cardiac pacing that may make permanent pacemaker placement more challenging, the potential risk in very large dogs of incomplete ventricular capture, and the need for a defibrillator with pacing capabilities. To avoid skeletal muscle stimulation when using transthoracic pacing, the cardiologist may test for ventricular capture and then turn off temporary pacing unless hemodynamically significant bradyasystole develops. Alternatively, neuromuscular junction-blocking drugs may be administered, requiring the availability of controlled ventilation methods. Neuromuscular junction-blocking drugs may not abolish all muscle activity since the pacing current may be high enough to cause direct muscle depolarization.

Temporary pacing systems should not be used without concurrent careful patient monitoring. If the temporary pacing lead were to dislodge from the endocardial surface or if the transthoracic electrodes failed to capture the ventricle, the ECG monitor will often still record the pacing spike in the absence of myocardial stimulation. Detection of a QRS complex following the pacing spike and monitoring of the arterial pulse allow confirmation of cardiac contraction. Temporary pacemakers should be viewed as a backup should asystole occur and not be relied upon to replace careful patient monitoring.

Permanent pacemaker implantation

Permanent pacemaker system implantation is usually performed under general anesthesia. Protocols may vary, but the over-riding goal is to maintain the intrinsic heart rate until the pacemaker can be activated. After the pacemaker has become active, protocol choice is of minimal importance. The most common transvenous technique involves identification, isolation, and incision of the jugular vein. The pacemaker lead, often with the help of a stylet and fluoroscopic guidance, is advanced through the cranial vena cava and right atrium, across the tricuspid valve, and into the apex of the right ventricle. A pulse generator pocket is often formed in the neck or dorsally between the scapula and, if necessary, the lead is tunneled under the skin to connect to the pulse generator. Following connection/activation of permanent pacing, threshold testing to ensure good ventricular capture is often performed, the lead and generator are secured in place, and the incision(s) are closed. Alternative techniques are available for placement of epicardial pacemaker leads [17,18] in cases of pacemaker revision or for the initial implantation in very small dogs, cats, and puppies.

Considerations for anesthesia

The use of anticholinergic drugs should be carefully considered based on the type of underlying rhythm, the expected response (as many animals with high-grade AV block have no meaningful increase in heart rate), and the cardiologist's preferences. The use of atropine or glycopyrrolate may increase the sinus rate in animals with responsive AV block or SSS. If responsive, these animals may develop tachyarrhythmias where the heart rate exceeds the upper limit of the pulse generator. Although this is not a problem for the patient, it may make it difficult to determine if the lead placement is suitable, and if the pulse generator settings are adequate to take over pacing when the effects of the anticholinergic eventually wane. Anticholinergics can also cause an initial transient increase in vagal tone, which may cause a temporary worsening of the underlying rhythm before any beneficial response is seen.

Anesthetic drug selection often incorporates classes that are thought to have minimal, or manageable, effects on conduction and heart rate. Dissociative anesthetics such as ketamine typically cause an increased heart rate through increased sympathetic nervous system activity. However, in animals with maximally stimulated sympathetic nervous systems, significant myocardial depression may occur [19]. Benzodiazepine premedication may provide some reduction in anesthetic dose requirements but excitation may be induced in some animals.

Hypnotic drugs such as propofol, alphaxalone, and barbiturates have been used with varying success. Propofol infusion is a technique that allows titration of depth of anesthesia without excessive depression of conduction. With all intravenous drug administration it should be remembered that animals with extremely low heart rates usually have low cardiac output and prolonged drug distribution (onset of effect), and doses result in higher initial plasma concentrations. Slower, careful administration is required when dosing to effect.

Opioid drugs have been used for sedation and analgesia prior to pacemaker implantation. They are reversible with specific antagonists and generally have minimal effects on myocardial contractility. However, most opioids, especially at higher doses, can enhance vagal tone and promote AV blockade. Anticholinergics will often minimize these effects.

Inhalant anesthetics allow the rapid titration of anesthetic depth. Many pacemakers have been placed during inhalant anesthesia, but effects on Ca^{2+} currents and other ion fluxes, with effects on conduction, have cautioned some to avoid inhalant administration until temporary or permanent pacing is established.

Following anesthesia, sedation is often desirable to facilitate a smooth recovery and minimize risk of lead dislodgement. α_2-Adrenergic receptor agonists are not recommended for pacemaker placement, but acepromazine, benzodiazepines, and sedating opioids have all been used successfully.

Complications

Severe bradyarrhythmia or hypotension during pacemaker implantation requires rapid treatment. The use of β_1-adrenergic receptor agonists such as isoproterenol, dobutamine, dopamine, or epinephrine may improve dromotropy and stimulate escape rates. However, the routine use of positive dromotropes may also potentiate mechanically triggered ventricular early depolarizations, which may lead to ventricular tachycardia or fibrillation. Drugs and equipment should be readied for administration, but withheld until clearly needed.

Ventricular arrhythmias during lead placement typically indicate that the lead has traversed the tricuspid valve. Treatment of ventricular early depolarizations with antiarrhythmic drugs such as lidocaine is often reserved for those patients with severe arrhythmias, and who are not relying on a ventricular escape rhythm for sustaining life.

Pacemaker patients undergoing non-cardiac procedures

Often the anesthetist is called upon to anesthetize patients with pacemakers for other emergent and elective procedures. Consultation with a cardiologist is advisable to assess the adequacy of the programmed parameters and battery life, the expected response to atrial, ventricular, or ectopic complexes, the severity of myocardial or valvular dysfunction, and recommendations for perioperative antibiotic prophylaxis. If possible, anesthesia should be performed in the same facility where the pacemaker programmer is located so that changes in pacing rate, threshold, or sensing algorithm can be made, if necessary. A contemporary ECG recording with the planned surgical procedure is recommended prior to induction of anesthesia.

Patients with rate-responsive, ventricular demand pacemakers (e.g., VVIR) often have a programmed lower rate limit at or below 80 beats/min. This may not be adequate to maintain arterial blood pressure in the face of inhalant anesthetic vasodilation (e.g., isoflurane). It is often advantageous to increase the minimum rate to a level appropriate for anesthesia (e.g., 120 beats/min). If the surgery also has a high likelihood of producing significant chest wall movement, it may be necessary to turn off rate responsiveness to avoid inappropriate pacemaker-derived tachycardia.

In most instances, artificial pacemakers are incompatible with magnetic resonance imaging. Similarly, high-frequency signals accompanying electrocautery may produce numerous complications with implanted pacemakers, including induction of arrhythmias, increased pacing rate in rate-responsive pacemakers, asynchronous pacing, inhibition of pacing, or electrical resetting. Therefore, monopolar electrocautery should ideally be avoided in pacemaker patients unless the pulse generator documentation specifically allows it. Some precautions that may be useful if electrocautery cannot be avoided include pacemaker reprogramming, using short, intermittent bursts at the lowest energy level, avoiding contact between the electrocautery probe and the pacemaker, placement of the return electrode as far from the pulse generator as possible, ensuring that the current pathway does not intersect the pulse generator, and the use of bipolar electrocautery.

Antimicrobial prophylaxis is important in pacemaker patients undergoing procedures associated with bacteremia (e.g., dental cleaning). Various protocols exist, but the goal is to reduce the risk associated with bacterial seeding of the transvenous lead and subsequent phlebitis and endocarditis, which may require surgical removal of the pacing lead.

Conclusion

Anesthesia delivery to patients requiring, or having had, pacemaker implantation can be challenging. By better understanding implantation procedures, the function of pacemakers, and interactions of anesthetic and hemodynamic supportive drugs, overall anesthetic risk can be reduced.

References

1 Buchanan JW, Dear MG, Pyle RL, Berg P. Medical and pacemaker therapy of complete heart block and congestive heart failure in a dog. *J Am Vet Med Assoc* 1968; **152**(8): 1099–1109.

2 Borek PP, Wilkoff BL. Pacemaker and ICD leads: strategies for long-term management. *J Interv Card Electrophysiol* 2008; **23**(1): 59–72.

3 Ohm OJ, Danilovic D. Improvements in pacemaker energy consumption and functional capability: four decades of progress. *Pacing Clin Electrophysiol* 1997; **20**(1 Pt 1): 2–9.

4 Bulmer BJ, Sisson DD, Oyama MA, *et al.* Physiologic VDD versus nonphysiologic VVI pacing in canine 3rd-degree atrioventricular block. *J Vet Intern Med* 2006; **20**(2): 257–271.

5 Estrada AH, Maisenbacher HW III, Prosek R, *et al.* Evaluation of pacing site in dogs with naturally occurring complete heart block. *J Vet Cardiol* 2009; **11**(2): 79–88.

6 Nelson OL, Lahmers S, Schneider T, Thompson P. The use of an implantable cardioverter defibrillator in a Boxer dog to control clinical signs of arrhythmogenic right ventricular cardiomyopathy. *J Vet Intern Med* 2006; **20**(5): 1232–1237.

7 Pariaut R, Saelinger C, Vila J, *et al.* Evaluation of shock waveform configuration on the defibrillation capacity of implantable cardioverter defibrillators in dogs. *J Vet Cardiol* 2012; **14**(3): 389–398.

8 Musselman EE, Rouse GP, Parker AJ. Permanent pacemaker implantation with transvenous electrode placement in a dog with complete atrioventricular heart block, congestive heart failure and Stokes–Adams syndrome. *J Small Anim Pract* 1976; **17**(3): 149–162.

9 Sisson D, Thomas WP, Woodfield J, *et al.* Permanent transvenous pacemaker implantation in forty dogs. *J Vet Intern Med* 1991; **5**(6): 322–331.

10 Veve I, Melo L.F. Anesthesia for pacemaker insertion. *Semin Cardiothorac Vasc Anesth* 2000; **4**(3): 138–143.

11 Kellum HB, Stepien RL. Third-degree atrioventricular block in 21 cats (1997–2004). *J Vet Intern Med* 2006; **20**(1): 97–103.

12 Penning VA, Connolly DJ, Gajanayake I, *et al.* Seizure-like episodes in 3 cats with intermittent high-grade atrioventricular dysfunction. *J Vet Intern Med* 2009; **23**(1): 200–205.

13 Genovese DW, Estrada AH, Maisenbacher HW, *et al.* Procedure times, complication rates, and survival times associated with single-chamber versus dual-chamber pacemaker implantation in dogs with clinical signs of bradyarrhythmia: 54 cases (2004–2009). *J Am Vet Med Assoc* 2013; **242**(2): 230–236.

14 DeFrancesco TC, Hansen BD, Atkins CE, *et al.* Noninvasive transthoracic temporary cardiac pacing in dogs. *J Vet Intern Med* 2003; **17**(5): 663–667.

15 Sanders RA, Green HW III, Hogan DF, *et al.* Efficacy of transesophageal and transgastric cardiac pacing in the dog. *J Vet Cardiol* 2010; **12**(1): 49–52.

16 Chapel EH, Sanders RA. Efficacy of two commercially available cardiac pacing catheters for transesophageal atrial pacing in dogs. *J Vet Cardiol* 2012; **14**(3): 409–414.

17 Fox PR, Matthiesen DT, Purse D, Brown NO. Ventral abdominal, transdiaphragmatic approach for implantation of cardiac pacemakers in the dog. *J Am Vet Med Assoc* 1986; **189**(10): 1303–1308.

18 Nelson DA, Miller MW, Gordon SG, *et al.* Minimally invasive transxiphoid approach to the cardiac apex and caudoventral intrathoracic space. *Vet Surg* 2012; **41**(8): 915–917.

19 Chamberlain JH, Seed RG, Undre N. Myocardial depression by ketamine. Haemodynamic and metabolic observations in animals. *Anaesthesia* 1981; **36**(4): 366–370.

26 Pathophysiology and Anesthetic Management of Patients with Cardiovascular Disease

Sandra Z. Perkowski[1] **and Mark A. Oyama**[2]

[1]Department of Clinical Studies-Philadelphia, School of Veterinary Medicine, University of Pennsylvania, Philadelphia, Pennsylvania, USA
[2]Department of Clinical Studies-Philadelphia, University of Pennsylvania, Philadelphia, Pennsylvania, USA

Chapter contents

Introduction

In animals with suspected cardiac disease, care must be taken both prior to and during anesthesia to assess the heart's ability to (1) provide adequate cardiac output and tissue perfusion, (2) maintain low venous pressures and prevent congestion, and (3) avoid arrhythmias. The preanesthetic database should include the medical history and physical examination, with particular attention to cardiac and pulmonary auscultation, inspection of the jugular veins, and palpation of peripheral arterial pulses. Commonly considered diagnostics include electrocardiography (ECG), thoracic radiography, echocardiography, and non-invasive blood pressure measurement. Recently, the use of cardiac-specific blood-based markers such as N-terminal pro-B-type natriuretic peptide (NT-proBNP) and cardiac troponin I (cTnI) as part of the preanesthetic work-up in animals with suspected cardiac disease has been contemplated. The decision regarding if and how to anesthetize patients with cardiac disease relies on the appropriate selection and interpretation of these and other diagnostic tests.

Preanesthetic evaluation

Electrocardiography

Electrocardiography is the gold standard for the evaluation of cardiac arrhythmias. However, in the absence of arrhythmias, the sensitivity of ECG to detect underlying cardiac dysfunction and disease is relatively poor. The ECG should be evaluated for heart rate, mean electrical axis (when applicable), rhythm, and criteria for cardiac chamber enlargement. The reader is referred to several excellent reviews of ECG interpretation for further information [1–3]. ECG findings that most commonly impact anesthesia include abnormalities of rate (either bradycardia or tachycardia) or criteria for chamber enlargement. In cats, abnormalities of mean electrical axis are occasionally detected with underlying structural disease, such as cardiomyopathy.

Clinically important bradycardias include second- or third-degree atrioventricular nodal (AV) block, sinus arrest or block, sinus bradycardia, and, less commonly, atrial standstill. The presence of AV block, sinus arrest/block, and sinus bradycardia is often challenged by administration of vagolytic agents such as atropine or glycopyrrolate. Complete resolution of the bradycardia following challenge usually indicates that the bradycardia is due to physiologic high-resting vagal tone, and bradycardia occurring while under anesthesia can be effectively treated with repeated administration of atropine or glycopyrrolate. Incomplete resolution or absence of response to vagolytic challenge often indicates injury or disease of the cardiac conduction system and additional diagnostics, such as thoracic radiography, echocardiography, serial ECG or 24 h ambulatory ECG (Holter) monitoring, should be pursued prior to anesthesia. Depending on the response to vagolytic challenge, some dogs with partial responses can be safely anesthetized with proper selection of anesthetic agents, monitoring, and/or availability of temporary artificial cardiac pacing. Most instances of sinus block/arrest or sinus bradycardia that is part of a pronounced respiratory sinus arrhythmia are vagally mediated and present little risk for anesthesia. In contrast, most cases of high-grade second-degree AV block, third-degree

Veterinary Anesthesia and Analgesia: The Fifth Edition of Lumb and Jones.
Edited by Kurt A. Grimm, Leigh A. Lamont, William J. Tranquilli, Stephen A. Greene and Sheilah A. Robertson.

AV block, and atrial standstill indicate the presence of either primary cardiac disease or severe electrolyte or acid–base disturbances and are associated with a significant increase in anesthetic risk. Various forms of bradycardia can also be present in patients with sick sinus syndrome wherein intermittent periods of bradycardia and tachycardia both occur.

Clinically important tachycardias include supraventricular or ventricular tachycardia and atrial fibrillation (AF) or flutter. Sinus tachycardia due to pain, hyperthyroidism, congestive heart failure, drugs/toxins (e.g., theophylline, terbutaline, theobromine) can also be present. The impact of tachyarrhythmias on anesthesia depends on the rate, frequency, and duration of such arrhythmias. Very rapid, frequent, and sustained tachyarrhythmias decrease diastolic filling time and cardiac output while increasing myocardial oxygen demand. Tachyarrhythmias such as sustained supraventricular or ventricular tachycardia and AF are often associated with clinically significant primary cardiac disease, such as degenerative mitral valve disease in the dog or various forms of cardiomyopathy in both the dog and cat. Ventricular arrhythmias are also common in dogs with extra-cardiac disease, especially disease of the abdomen such as splenic or hepatic neoplasia or gastric dilation/volvulus. Thus, further diagnostics such as thoracic radiography, echocardiography, abdominal ultrasound, and serum chemistry are usually pursued in animals with tachyarrhythmias. In cases wherein arrhythmias appear to be due solely to extra-cardiac causes such that echocardiography reveals normal cardiac structure and function, anesthesia often can be achieved with minimal additional risk.

Thoracic radiography

Thoracic radiography is an extremely useful tool in assessing patients with cardiac disease. Cardiac disease results in activation of neurohormonal responses that serve to increase cardiac preload via renal retention of fluid and sodium. The resultant volume overload produces eccentric cardiac hypertrophy, the severity of which reflects the degree of injury and neurohormonal activity. Thus, radiographic heart size is an excellent surrogate marker of disease severity and risk for congestive heart failure. Evaluation of radiographic heart size is confounded by variables such as radiographic technique, patient body weight, chest conformation, and breed. Standardized measurement techniques such as the vertebral heart size (VHS) are useful to minimize variability and increase diagnostic value. The VHS system has been extensively reviewed elsewhere [4–6]. Briefly, the long and short axis of the heart are measured from the right or left lateral projection and these measurements are indexed to the number of vertebral bodies starting from the cranial aspect of the fourth thoracic vertebra (Fig. 26.1). The sum of the vertebral length and width of the heart represents the VHS. The range of VHS in healthy dogs and cats is 8.5–10.5 and 6.9–8.1 vertebra, respectively. Although these ranges are generally regarded as applicable across a wide range of breeds and ages, some reports indicate slightly different ranges, although only two of the studies had at least 100 subjects (Table 26.1). As a preanesthetic test, VHS is useful in determining the severity of canine degenerative mitral valve disease in geriatric patients with the typical left-sided systolic murmur. In the authors' experience, regardless of the intensity of the murmur, dogs with VHS <11.0–11.5 are at low risk for spontaneous development of congestive heart failure (CHF), whereas those with VHS >11.5–12.0 are at higher risk. Coupled with inspection of the pulmonary veins and pulmonary parenchymal pattern, VHS helps assess the risk of induced CHF secondary to IV fluid administration (at 5–10 mL/kg/h) while under anesthesia.

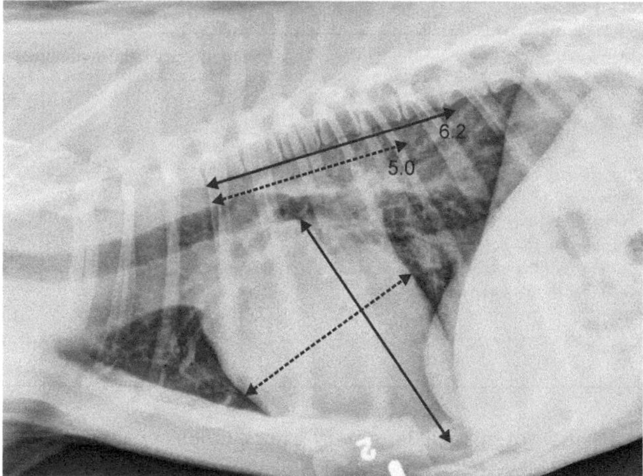

Figure 26.1 Right lateral thoracic radiograph from a 13-year-old female spayed Toy Poodle demonstrating the vertebral heart size (VHS) measurement technique. The length of the cardiac silhouette is measured from a point ventral to the carina of the trachea to the apex of the heart and the width of the silhouette is measured along the widest portion of the heart perpendicular to the long axis. The ventral border of the caudal vena cava is often used as the starting point for the width measurement. The length and width measurements are compared with the number of vertebral bodies starting from the cranial aspect of the fourth vertebral body. In this instance, the length of the silhouette is 6.2 vertebra and the width is 5.0 vertebra, yielding an overall VHS of 11.2.

Table 26.1 Reported mean (SD) radiographic vertebral heart size from various studies in dogs and cats.

Species/Breed	*n*	Mean (SD)	Comments
Canine/Beagle [7]	19	10.3 (0.4)	
Canine/Greyhound [8]	42	10.5 (0.1)	
Canine/Whippet [9]	44	11.0 (0.5)	Right lateral recumbency
		11.3 (0.5)	Left lateral recumbency
Canine/Rottweiler [9]	38	9.8 (0.1)	
Canine/Cavalier King Charles Spaniel [6]	10	10.8 (0.49)	
Canine/mixed [10]	63	9.8 (0.6)	Right lateral recumbency
		9.5 (0.8)	Left lateral recumbency
Canine/puppies [11]	11	10.0 (0.5)	3 months
		9.8 (0.4)	6 months
		9.9 (0.6)	12 months
	6	10.3 (0.6)	36 months
Canine/Boxer [12]	20	11.6 (0.8)	
Canine/Labrador Retriever [12]	25	10.8 (0.6)	
Canine/German Shepherd [12]	20	9.7 (0.7)	
Canine/Doberman [12]	20	10.0 (0.6)	
Canine/Cavalier King Charles Spaniel [12]	20	10.6 (0.5)	
Canine/Yorkshire Terrier [12]	22	9.7 (0.5)	
Canine/mixed [4]	100	9.7 (0.5)	
Feline/mixed [13]	50	7.3 (0.49)	Right lateral recumbency
		7.3 (0.55)	Left lateral recumbency
Feline/mixed [5]	100	7.5 (0.3)	

In species and diseases other than canine degenerative mitral valve disease, the authors regard VHS as a useful means to assess the risk of induced or spontaneous CHF in dogs with dilated cardiomyopathy and cats with hypertrophic or restrictive cardiomyopathy.

Table 26.2 Common echocardiographic measurements and calculations.

Measurement	Commonly used abbreviation(s)
Left ventricle at end-diastole	
Left ventricular end-diastolic dimension	LVEDD, LVIDd, LVd
Thickness of the left ventricular posterior wall	LVPWd
Thickness of the interventricular septum	IVSd
Left ventricle at end-systole	
Left ventricular end-systolic dimension	LVESD, LVIDs, LVs
Thickness of the left ventricular posterior wall	LVPWs
Thickness of the interventricular septum	IVSs
Diameter of the aortic root	AoD
Diameter of the left atrium	LAD
Fractional shortening [(LVEDD – LVEDSD)/LVEDD] × 100%	FS%

In instances of suspected canine or feline cardiomyopathy, detailed evaluation of systolic and diastolic function can be achieved using echocardiography in addition to VHS.

Echocardiography

Echocardiography represents the gold standard for the clinical evaluation of cardiac structure and function. It is less useful than thoracic radiography in trying to determine the presence or likelihood of CHF manifested as pulmonary edema. Echo provides data regarding ventricular and atrial chamber dimensions, thickness of the ventricular walls and interventricular septum, pattern of blood flow through the heart and proximal portions of the great vessels, myocardial contractility, and morphology of valve structure (Table 26.2). Echo should be performed by individuals not only proficient in image acquisition but also with an adequate familiarity of the pathophysiology of the most common cardiac diseases, since interpretation of the echocardiography-derived data is necessary to assess the impact of changes on anesthetic risk. Measurements from individual animals are interpreted using reference ranges from healthy animals indexed to body weight. The most accurate reference ranges utilize indices indexed to the body weight raised to the power of 1/3, providing a single range of values applicable across all body weights (Table 26.3) [14].

Diseases that result in volume overload (e.g., eccentric hypertrophy) such as canine mitral valve disease, dilated cardiomyopathy (DCM), and patent ductus arteriosus (PDA), result in increased diastolic chamber dimensions, whereas diseases that result in concentric hypertrophy such as feline hypertrophic cardiomyopathy (HCM), systemic hypertension, and congenital subaortic stenosis, result in increased diastolic and systolic ventricular wall thickness. Diseases that produce decreased contractility, such as DCM, result in increased systolic chamber dimensions. Interpretation of the echocardiogram relies on both subjective and objective evaluation. Because of many breed peculiarities with respect to chest conformation and imaging planes, objective data should always be compared against the subjective evaluation of the sonographer. In fact, subjective estimation of cardiac function by experienced echocardiographers possesses better correlation with angiographic evaluation than do many of the routine objective calculations [15]. Thus, objective measurements should align closely with the trained echocardiographer's subjective assessment of cardiac morphology and function, and discrepancies between the two often indicate measurement errors due to suboptimal imaging planes.

Echocardiographic studies are typically obtained by imaging through the thorax, but images can also be obtained with the use of an intraesophageal probe or transesophageal echocardiography (TEE). TEE, by virtue of its closer proximity to the heart, renders highly detailed views of the heart and great vessels and is often used in patients whose chest conformation or body weight precludes high-quality transthoracic imaging. The high resolution and visual acuity of TEE images facilitates cardiac catheterization procedures, such as device occlusion of PDA or balloon valvuloplasty of valvular pulmonic stenosis. The TEE probe consists of a flexible and steerable shaft (similar to an endoscope) with a phased array ultrasound transducer at its tip. Biplane TEE utilizes two transducers positioned at right-angles from each other whereas multiplane TEE utilizes a single transducer that can be rotated within the scope's housing to permit imaging along any plane from 0° to 180°. In veterinary patients, TEE examination is performed under general anesthesia or heavy sedation and the TEE probe is inserted through a mouth gag into the patient's oropharynx and esophagus. The probe is positioned over the heart base and multiple imaging planes of the heart can be obtained by switching between the two transducers (biplane) or by rotating the transducer within the probe housing (multiplane) (Fig. 26.2). Excellent reviews of biplane TEE imaging technique and planes in the dog and cat are available [16,17].

Table 26.3 Upper and lower bounds of the 95th percentile interval for indexed echocardiographic formula constants in healthy dogs. The constants multiplied by the body weight (BW in kg) raised to an exponential power provide a single reference range across all body weights for the indicated measurements.

Measurement	95% CI boundary	Formula (BW in kg)
iLVIDd	1.35–1.73	iLVIDd = LVIDd × $BW^{0.294}$
iLVIDs	0.79–1.14	iLVIDs = LVIDs × $BW^{0.315}$
iIVSd	0.33–0.52	iIVSd = IVSd × $BW^{0.241}$
iIVSs	0.48–0.71	iIVSs = IVSs × $BW^{0.240}$
iLVPWd	0.33–0.53	iLVPWd = LVPWd × $BW^{0.232}$
iLVPWs	0.53–0.78	iLVPWs = LVPWs × $BW^{0.222}$
iLAD	0.64–0.90	iLAD = LAD × $BW^{0.345}$
iAoD	0.68–0.89	iAoD = AoD × $BW^{0.341}$

Source: adapted from [14]. Reproduced with permission of Wiley.

Blood-based cardiac markers

The heart is an active endocrine organ. In the case of the sympathomimetic and renin–angiotensin–aldosterone systems, the heart is an end-organ target of neurohormonal activity, whereas in the case of atrial and B-type natriuretic peptide (ANP, BNP), the heart is a source of neurohormonal production. Measurement of ANP, BNP, and NT-proBNP (a precursor of BNP) can help differentiate cardiac versus respiratory etiology of respiratory signs, detect occult cardiomyopathy, and provide prognostic information [18–21]. In the setting of anesthesia, the natriuretic peptides, in addition to markers of cardiac tissue injury, such as cTnI, are probably most useful in helping to ascertain the risk of occult cardiomyopathy in cats during the preanesthetic work-up. In selected populations of cats that are at high risk for cardiomyopathy, such as adult cats with a heart murmur, gallop, or arrhythmia, NT-proBNP assay detects clinically significant occult cardiomyopathy with moderate sensitivity and specificity [19,20]. Elevated values warrant additional diagnostics such as echocardiography to achieve a definitive diagnosis and help formulate anesthetic recommendations. Natriuretic or troponin assay as part of the preanesthetic work-up prior to routine elective surgery (e.g., spay or neuter) is not currently recommended as the low prevalence of cardiomyopathy in these populations will result in many false-positive results.

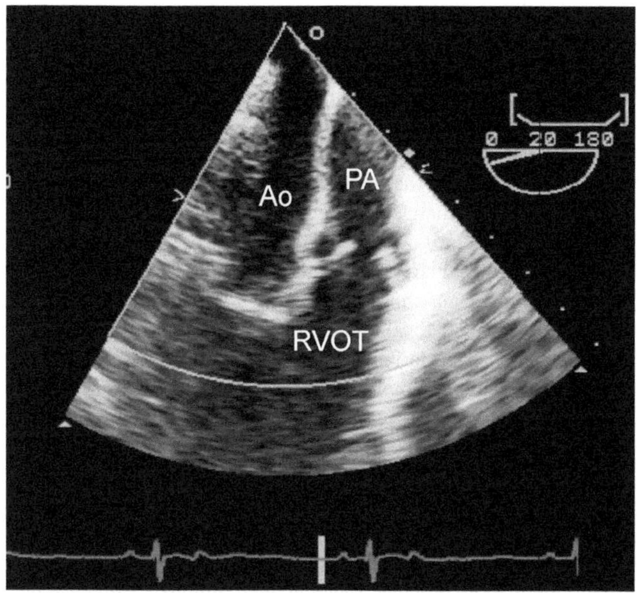

(a)

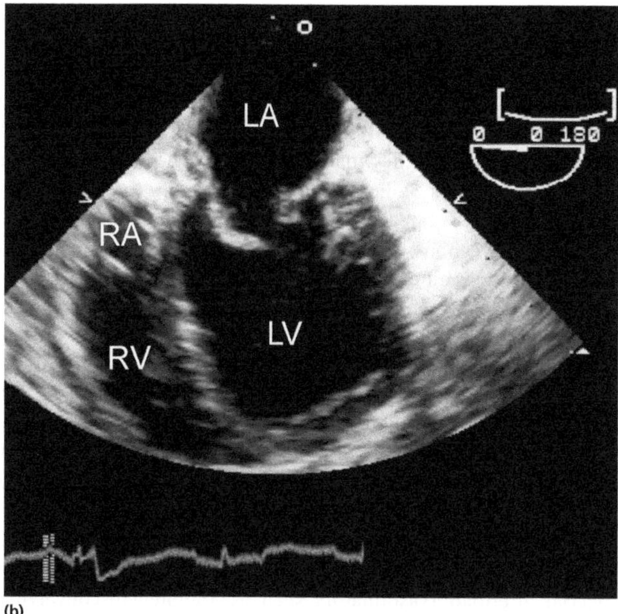

(b)

Figure 26.2 Transesophageal echocardiography (TEE) in (a) a dog with congenital pulmonic stenosis showing the incomplete opening and abnormal thickness of the pulmonic valve leaflets from the cranial transverse probe position (RVOT, right ventricular outflow tract; Ao, aorta; PA, pulmonary artery) and (b) a dog with congenital mitral stenosis showing incomplete opening of the mitral valve leaflets and from the middle transverse position (LA, left atrium; LV, left ventricle; RV, right ventricle; RA, right atrium).

Anesthesia for specific conditions

When anesthetizing any animal with cardiovascular disease, maintaining cardiac output and tissue perfusion is a primary goal. How that goal is best achieved, however, will differ depending on the underlying cardiac condition.

Cardiac output is the product of stroke volume and heart rate, and decreases in either of these can lead to a low output state. Conversely, fast heart rates, either atrial (e.g., AF) or ventricular in origin, can also lead to a low output state, since diastolic filling times are decreased and/or the atrial contribution (atrial 'kick') to ventricular filling is decreased. To determine accurately the reasons for a decrease in stroke volume, it is important to ascertain whether it is due to a change in preload, afterload [increased systemic vascular resistance (SVR)], and/or contractility of the left ventricle. All of these variables are interdependent. For example, chronic excess preload can cause ventricular over-distension and systolic dysfunction. Myocardial contractility and stroke volume also may be affected by indirect causes such as pericardial effusion, inflammatory cytokines, and anesthetic agents.

Valvular heart lesions and/or septal defects lead to changes in the loading conditions of the heart and the approach to the patient changes accordingly. For example, the left ventricle is volume overloaded in mitral regurgitation and pressure overloaded in subaortic stenosis. Compensatory mechanisms differ between conditions and can include chamber enlargement, myocardial hypertrophy, changes in vascular tone, and alterations in sympathetic activity. Changes in myocardial compliance and chronic myocardial dysfunction may follow. Anesthetic management requires an understanding of the alterations in loading conditions so that compensatory mechanisms may be preserved and problems may be anticipated and avoided before they occur.

Volume overload conditions

Mitral valve insufficiency/regurgitation

Pathophysiology

Mitral valve regurgitation (MR) can be caused by primary incompetence of the valve leaflets [e.g., myxomatous mitral valve degeneration (MMVD), bacterial endocarditis, congenital malformation] or secondarily to dilation of the annular ring in diseases that cause eccentric hypertrophy secondary to systolic dysfunction (e.g., DCM). MMVD is the most common cause of MR, having a prevalence of approximately 30% in small breed dogs over the age of 10 years. Regardless of the initial cause, the presence of MR induces further eccentric hypertrophy and annular dilation in a vicious cycle wherein 'MR begets further MR.'

Mitral regurgitation results in volume overload of the left ventricle and left atrium. With incompetence of the mitral valve, the outflow of the left ventricle is divided between the high-pressure/low-compliance outflow tract through the aorta and arterial tree, and the low-pressure/high compliance outflow route across the incompetent mitral valve into the left atrium. This mismatch in afterload conditions can result in MR volumes representing a high percentage of total stroke volume. This so-called regurgitant fraction can be as high as 50–70% of total stroke volume, and highlights the often severe degree of volume overload within the left ventricle and atrium. Thoracic radiography is particularly useful in dogs with MMVD such that the radiographic heart size is proportional to the severity of MR. In many cases of uncomplicated MMVD, radiographic inspection of the cardiac silhouette, pulmonary vessels, and pulmonary parenchyma provides sufficient information regarding severity of disease and risk for CHF and helps guide the need for chronic medical therapy.

Although the volume work of the left ventricle is increased, left ventricular systolic wall tension is minimally increased, as the high-compliance route allows a large percentage of the work to be done at low pressure. Thus, in most small breed dogs (body weight <15 kg) with MR, systolic contractility often appears normal or even hypercontractile when assessed by echocardiography. In larger breed dogs, systolic dysfunction secondary to MR is much more common, for reasons that are poorly understood. Thus, preanesthetic echocardiography to detect systolic dysfunction is often of greater value in large than small breed dogs.

The time course for the development of MR influences the severity of symptoms. If the MR develops slowly over time, the left atrium compensates with gradual dilation, and some dogs with severe amounts of MR can be asymptomatic. However, if the MR occurs acutely, as in the case of bacterial endocarditis or acute ruptured chordae tendineae, the sudden volume overload can lead to a rapid increase in left atrial pressures and severe pulmonary congestion.

Chronic medical therapy for MR involves reduction in preload (diuretics such as furosemide and spironolactone), reduction in arterial afterload [vasodilators such as angiotensin-converting enzyme inhibitors (ACEIs) and pimobendan], and maintenance of adequate systolic contractility (positive inotropes such as pimobendan). Initiation of medical therapy prior to elective anesthesia should be considered for newly diagnosed cases of MR.

Anesthetic considerations

The primary goal of anesthesia in the patient with mitral regurgitation is to maintain forward aortic flow while minimizing regurgitant flow. The volume of regurgitant flow across the mitral valve is related to the size of the regurgitant orifice (which is related to ventricular size), the time available for retrograde flow, and the pressure gradient across the dysfunctional valve [22]. Patients with chronic, compensated MR will be sensitive to changes in ventricular loading conditions and preload should generally be maintained during anesthesia [23]. Overzealous fluid administration should be avoided, however, to avoid ventricular distension and resultant changes in regurgitant flow. Preload reduction may be helpful in some cases. Heart rates should be maintained at a normal or slightly above normal rate to help maintain smaller left ventricular volumes and minimize MR secondary to annular dilation. Bradycardia also increases the duration of systolic contraction and time available for regurgitant flow.

Most patients with MR benefit greatly from afterload reduction. By reducing afterload, the left ventricular systolic pressures required for ejection from the ventricle to the aorta and arterial vasculature decrease, optimizing forward flow. This, in turn, decreases the pressure gradient from the left ventricle to the left atrium during systole and decreases regurgitant flow. Adequate depth of anesthesia and anesthetic agents that promote arteriolar dilation and maintenance of heart rate are generally recommended. In contrast, administration of drugs that cause marked increases in systemic blood pressure and afterload (e.g., α_2-adrenergic receptor agonists) can impair forward flow, increase regurgitant flow, and cause rapid deterioration of patients with MR. In early compensated MR, LV contractility may be preserved, but patients with significant MR may benefit from inotropic support with a drug such as dobutamine (Table 26.4).

Premedication may be required in some cases to decrease the anxiety of the animal and stress during patient handling, minimizing catecholamine release, tachycardia, and increased myocardial work. Ideally, patients should receive supplemental oxygen after receiving sedative medication, but the stress of restraint for oxygen administration should be considered. If preoperative sedation is necessary, opioid receptor agonists are generally the drug class of choice since they usually cause minimal cardiovascular depression; with left ventricular contractility, cardiac output, and systemic blood pressure being well maintained. In healthy animals, opioids cause behavioral changes ranging from sedation to excitement; however, in depressed or critically ill patients, opioids usually cause sedation. Opioids may cause bradycardia. Heart rate should be monitored and an anticholinergic such as glycopyrrolate or atropine administered if beneficial. Some animals with MR may also have pulmonary hypertension and right heart failure. Increased carbon dioxide secondary to opioid-induced hypoventilation can increase pulmonary pressures and may be of concern in those animals with pulmonary hypertension.

A combination of an opioid receptor agonist (e.g., fentanyl, oxymorphone, or hydromorphone) or agonist/antagonist (e.g., butorphanol) and a benzodiazepine tranquilizer (diazepam or midazolam) may be used to sedate patients for chest radiographs or echocardiography. This combination provides sedation with minimal cardiovascular depression [24–26]. Reversal may be accomplished by using an opioid receptor antagonist such as naloxone and/or a benzodiazepine antagonist such as flumazenil. Phenothiazine tranquilizers such as acepromazine in low doses may be beneficial in some patients with MR because they calm the patient [27], decrease afterload, and decrease the incidence of arrhythmias. Acepromazine should only be used after careful consideration, however, since α_1-adrenergic receptor antagonism may not only decrease afterload, resulting in increased forward blood flow, but also lead to venodilation and decreased preload.

In general, a carefully titrated induction is preferred in the cardiac patient with continuous monitoring of cardiovascular parameters. Although no one best technique exists, a high-dose opioid technique with or without etomidate, alphaxalone, or low-dose propofol is often advocated for induction to maintain systolic function in patients with severe myocardial dysfunction [28–37]. MR patients with minimal systolic dysfunction may be anesthetized with other protocols using propofol, alphaxalone, or etomidate (remembering to avoid excessive increases in systemic vascular resistance).

Most opioid receptor agonists, with the exception of meperidine, lack negative inotropic effects in clinically used doses. Rapid IV administration of morphine can cause histamine release, venodilation, and hypotension, hence this route is not routinely used [38]. Oxymorphone, hydromorphone, methadone, fentanyl, or some of the newer synthetic fentanyl derivatives such as remifentanil [39–41] are usually preferred. μ-Opioid receptor agonists such as fentanyl and its analogs, although relatively free of direct cardiovascular effects, can cause a significant vagally mediated bradycardia that would result in decreased cardiac output [42]. The extent of the bradycardia is dependent on the dose and rate of drug administration, and the use of any opioid in high doses can produce excessive bradycardia. Some anesthesiologists prefer to administer anticholinergics such as glycopyrrolate prior to high-dose opioids used during induction to avoid extreme swings in heart rate. Other adjunctive drugs often used include benzodiazepine tranquilizers such as midazolam or diazepam.

Etomidate is a useful anesthetic induction agent in any animal with cardiac disease associated with poor systolic function [43]. Left ventricular pressures, mean aortic pressure, and coronary blood flow do not change significantly in healthy dogs receiving up

Table 26.4 Inotropic and vasopressor drugs, receptor binding and standard dose range for dogs and cats.

Drug	α_1	α_2	β_1	β_2	Dose	Comments
Epinephrine	5+	3+	4+	2+	0.01–1 μg/kg/min	Primarily β effects at lower doses, increasing α effects at higher doses
					0.02–0.2 mg/kg bolus	For cardiac arrest
Norepinephrine	5+	5+	3+	0(+)	0.01–0.1 μg/kg/min	β_2 effect not seen clinically
Dobutamine	0(+)	0	4+	2+	1–20 μg/kg/min	
Phenylephrine	5+	2+	0	0	0.2–2 μg/kg/min	
Dopamine	1–5+	2+	3+	2+		Actions are dependent on dose
					1–3 μg/kg/min	Acts primarily on dopamine-1 receptors in renal and splanchnic vasculature to produce vasodilation
					5–10 μg/kg/min	Primarily β effects
					>10 μg/kg/min	Primarily α effects
Ephedrine	2+	+	3+	+	0.05–0.5 mg/kg	Primary action by an indirect effect. Direct and indirect effects (NE release)

to 2.5 mg/kg for induction. Etomidate is not arrhythmogenic and may also be useful in animals with cardiac conduction abnormalities. Rapid administration of large doses of propofol are generally to be avoided, owing to potentially profound cardiovascular effects, including vasodilation, decreased cardiac contractility, and hypotension. However, a low dose given as a slow infusion may be useful as an adjunct to aid intubation and maintain anesthesia. Alphaxalone has a rather large therapeutic index and can also be used to induce animals with heart disease, although adverse effects can be seen after larger doses given rapidly.

Maintenance of anesthesia can be achieved with an opioid and/or propofol infusion, with or without inhalational agent. Etomidate infusions are not recommended owing to the potential for hemolysis associated with the high osmolality of the commercially available formulations [44] and also concerns related to prolonged adrenocortical suppression. A single bolus injection of 2 mg/kg etomidate reduces the adrenocortical response to anesthesia and surgery for 2–6 h [45]. However, longer term infusions have been associated with prolonged adrenocortical suppression and higher mortality rates in critically ill multiple-trauma patients [46,47]. Most commonly used inhalational agents (e.g., isoflurane, sevoflurane, and desflurane) tend to preserve myocardial contractility at light anesthetic planes. Mild decreases in SVR coupled with adequate systolic function may reduce regurgitant fraction and are goals of anesthetizing patients with MR. Decreased preload and decreased systolic function associated with deep planes of inhalant anesthesia are not recommended; therefore, multimodal 'balanced' anesthetic techniques are often advocated.

Patients on medication for heart disease are generally continued on their medications (especially diuretics, calcium channel blockers, antiarrhythmics, and inotropic drugs) until the time of surgery. However, hypotension may be more pronounced under anesthesia in patients receiving angiotensin-converting enzyme inhibitors such as enalapril. It is always prudent to have inotropic and venoconstrictor agents immediately available for management of intraoperative hypotension since fluid administration is often contraindicated.

Dilated cardiomyopathy

Dilated cardiomyopathy (DCM) is defined as idiopathic systolic dysfunction and is accompanied by eccentric dilation and volume overload as the heart's generation of normal forward stroke volume decreases. The resulting left ventricular dilation involves the mitral valve annulus dilation and the resulting secondary MR further contributes to volume overload. DCM is common in large breed dogs, and in particular the Doberman Pinscher, Irish Wolfhound, and Great Dane. DCM is relatively uncommon in cats following the recognition of taurine deficiency and subsequent reformulation of commercial diets. Taurine deficiency is occasionally seen in dogs, and in particular the Cocker Spaniel.

DCM predisposes to congestive heart failure in addition to ventricular arrhythmias. In most cases, the heart failure is left-sided (pulmonary edema) but can occasionally be right-sided (ascites, pleural effusion). Frequent ventricular arrhythmias can cause activity intolerance, syncope, and sudden cardiac death. A combination of echocardiography, thoracic radiography, and ECG is typically used to diagnose and stage severity of DCM. Holter monitoring is commonly performed to screen at-risk dogs for ventricular premature beats, which is an early sign of disease. Chronic therapy is targeted towards reduction of preload (diuretics such as furosemide and spironolactone), reduction of afterload (ACEIs, pimobendan), and increased contractility (positive inotropes such as pimobendan and digoxin). Suppression of ventricular arrhythmias is performed acutely using lidocaine or procainamide continuous-rate infusion (CRI), and chronically using sotalol or amiodarone. Beta-blockers are occasionally used as an adjunctive ventricular antiarrhythmic but, owing to their negative inotropic effects, caution should be exercised in animals with severe systolic dysfunction or active congestive heart failure.

Many cases of DCM are further complicated by the development of AF. AF is particularly common in Great Danes, Mastiffs, Irish Wolfhounds, and other giant breed dogs with DCM. The rapid ventricular rate associated with AF increases myocardial oxygen demand and reduces cardiac output as diastolic filling time decreases. Hence therapy of AF involves reduction of atrioventricular nodal conduction and slowing of ventricular heart rate. The most common agents used include digoxin, calcium channel blockers (e.g., diltiazem), and beta-blockers.

Many dogs with early DCM are asymptomatic. Older, large breed dogs that have occasional ventricular early depolarizations (VPCs) before or during anesthesia, which do not resolve following anesthesia, may benefit from examination by a cardiologist. Some cases of occult DCM are only diagnosed after unexplained VPCs are noticed during and after anesthesia, prompting consultation with a cardiologist.

Anesthetic Considerations

Anesthetic considerations are similar to those of animals with MR, with the added concerns of decreased systolic function, congestive heart failure, and increased incidence of cardiac arrhythmias. Additionally, dogs with cardiomyopathy often have a significant downregulation of β-adrenergic receptors in the heart, although receptor affinity does not change [48], making these animals more resistant to treatment with a positive inotrope. Dogs with significant systolic dysfunction probably benefit from inotropic drug (e.g., dobutamine or dopamine) support during anesthesia.

Ventricular arrhythmias can be seen during anesthesia in animals with DCM. Antiarrhythmic drugs such as lidocaine and procainamide should be available, but are often reserved for cases where the frequency of abnormal beats creates significant blood pressure or cardiac output decreases. Although often unnecessary, esmolol, a short-acting beta-blocker, may be given as an infusion as indicated (0.5 mg/kg loading bolus followed by an infusion of 0.01–0.2 mg/kg/min to reduce the frequency of ventricular premature contractions associated with sympathetic stimulation). The dose rate may be adjusted as needed to minimize any negative inotropic effects from use of a beta-blocker.

In dogs with concurrent DCM and AF, electrocardioversion may be considered (if the patient is a candidate) at the beginning of anesthesia. The increased ventricular filling following resynchronization of the atria and ventricles can improve cardiac output. Alternatively, drugs that slow the sinus rate and conduction through the AV node, such as fentanyl, can be used during anesthesia. Anticholinergic agents are to be avoided in dogs with AF, but may be useful for dogs with DCM without AF that are bradycardic under anesthesia. Fentanyl at a dose of 5–40 μg/kg/h can be an effective anesthetic in sick dogs when used as a primary agent in combination with oxygen and ventilation in those animals that do not tolerate inhalant anesthetics. Remifentanil has an elimination half-life shorter than that of fentanyl, with rapid recovery times regardless of the duration of infusion, although either opioid is suitable for an infusion technique. Infusion of 0.25–0.5 μg/kg/min remifentanil with 0.2 mg/kg/min propofol produces little change in mean arterial blood pressures in healthy dogs, although the heart rate decreases with increasing doses of remifentanil [41].

Left-to-right shunting congenital defects

Ventricular septal defect and patent ductus arteriosus

Both ventricular septal defect (VSD) and patent ductus arteriosus (PDA) permit left-to-right shunting, which produces volume overload of the pulmonary circulation and left heart. As the physiologic response to the increased pulmonary circulation progresses, pulmonary and right ventricular pressures may increase, resulting in minimal or reverse flow (right-to-left shunt). Anesthesia without consideration of drug selection and patient management on systemic vascular resistance (and blood pressure) and pulmonary and right ventricular pressure may result in reverse shunt flow and rapid deterioration of the patient's condition. Careful echocardiographic evaluation prior to anesthesia and careful perianesthetic monitoring of patients can facilitate anesthetic management of patients with cardiovascular shunts.

Many VSDs in dogs and cats are relatively small and the volume of the shunt is not sufficient to cause congestive heart failure. In contrast, the majority of animals with PDA will suffer from left-sided heart failure within the first year of life if the defect is not corrected. PDA is common in dogs and less so in cats, whereas VSD is more common in cats than in dogs. Both PDA and VSD generate characteristic murmurs that often permit a tentative diagnosis based on the physical examination findings alone. In both diseases, a combination of echocardiography and thoracic radiography facilitate a definitive diagnosis and also assessment of shunting volume and risk for heart failure. In general, the extent of left ventricular eccentric hypertrophy and degree of left atrial dilation reflect the magnitude of the shunt. The extent of shunting depends not only the cross-sectional area of the lesion, but also on the relative pressures and compliance of the right and left portions of the circulation. Low pressure and compliance of the pulmonary circulation and right ventricle relative to the systemic circulation and left ventricle promote left-to-right shunting. Interventions that either increase right-sided pressure or decrease left-sided pressure decrease the shunt severity. Hence systemic arterial vasodilators can be used to reduce the shunt volume, as can surgical interventions such as pulmonary artery banding, which increase pressure within the right ventricle.

Anesthetic considerations

In animals with VSD or PDA, the degree and magnitude of shunt flow are dependent upon relative outflow resistances. With simple left-to-right shunting, pulmonary blood flow is increased and the right ventricle and pulmonary vasculature can be pressure or volume overloaded and some degree of pulmonary hypertension may be present. Further increases in pulmonary blood flow are avoided by preventing increases in SVR. In addition, manipulations that decrease pulmonary vascular resistance (PVR) (hypocapnia, alkalemia, spontaneous ventilation, deep anesthesia) can also increase the magnitude of left-to-right shunt flow.

In many cases, heart failure is not yet present and the animal is relatively young and active and may become excited with restraint. Almost any anesthetic agent that does not significantly alter SVR may be used safely for premedication, induction, or maintenance. Drugs that significantly increase SVR, including the α_2-adrenergic receptor agonists (e.g., dexmedetomidine) should be avoided.

In those cases in which some degree of congestive heart failure is present, considerations are similar to those in other patients with volume overload (see earlier). An opioid-based induction technique with benzodiazepine tranquilizer and etomidate, alphaxalone, or propofol followed by inhalation anesthesia or propofol infusion or combination of fentanyl/remifentanil and propofol infusion can all be used [41]. Propofol can result in clinically significant changes in cardiac shunt direction and arterial desaturation, however, due to a decrease in SVR [49]. This decrease is usually dependent on the dose and rapidity with which the propofol is given.

Diastolic pressures are often low in these patients owing to shunting of blood to the lower resistance pulmonary circulation. A characteristic change in the arterial waveform may be seen with ligation of the PDA, including a decrease in the pulse pressure, increase in mean and diastolic pressure, and reappearance of a dicrotic (reflected) wave (Fig. 26.3). Hypotension may be pronounced in some patients due to the low diastolic pressures and is generally treated with the use of an inotrope such as dobutamine (see Table 26.4), which helps maintain myocardial function and heart rate while avoiding increases in SVR. However, significant decreases in SVR must also be avoided, especially in those patients with significant pulmonary hypertension in which shunt flows may reverse in the face of inhalant anesthetic-associated arteriolar dilation. These patients will benefit from the administration of a vasoconstrictor (e.g., dopamine or phenylephrine; see Table 26.4) to maintain baseline SVR. A sudden decrease in arterial oxygen saturation due to venous admixture as monitored with a pulse oximeter or arterial blood gas may be an early indicator of shunt reversal.

If surgery is to be performed on a relatively young animal for repair of a congenital heart defect, the progressive maturation of the autonomic nervous system and cardiovascular responses must be taken into account. In puppies, the adrenergic vasoconstrictor

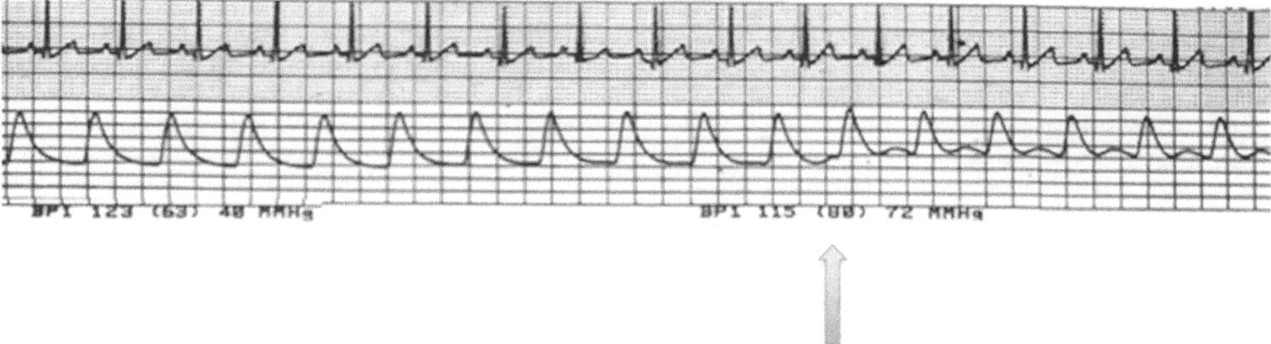

Figure 26.3 Output from a patient monitor during occlusion of a patent ductus arteriosus (PDA) showing the electrocardiogram and arterial pressure waveform. Notice the rapid increase in diastolic arterial blood pressure and the appearance of a dicrotic (reflected) wave during diastole immediately following occlusion (blue arrow). These changes are characteristic of decreased flow through the PDA and can be used to help identify the vessel during surgery.

response is not fully developed until after 8 weeks of age [50]. Similarly, although chronotropic responsiveness is apparent at 1 week, the inotropic response to sympathetic stimulation does not fully develop until after 8 weeks of age [51]. Neonatal patients typically have a higher heart rate and lower arterial blood pressure and systemic vascular resistance than adults. In addition, the cardiovascular response to sympathomimetic agents may be less pronounced in the neonate or pediatric patient than the adult animal of similar species [52–54].

Right-to-left shunting congenital defects

Tetralogy of Fallot and reverse patent ductus arteriosus

Tetralogy of Fallot (TF) and reverse patent ductus arteriosus (rPDA) are uncommon congenital heart defects in the dog and very rare in cats. The pathophysiology of both TF and rPDA involves right-to-left shunting and systemic hypoxemia. In the case of rPDA, concurrent pulmonary hypertension (PHT) is present. TF is caused by defects in the fetal conotruncal formation resulting in a dextro- or rightward-positioned aortic root, VSD, PS/pulmonic hypoplasia, and secondary right ventricular concentric hypertrophy. The presence of the pulmonic lesion creates pressure overload of the right ventricle sufficient to cause right ventricular to left ventricular shunting through the VSD. The dextropositioned aorta further contributes to admixture of unoxygenated blood into the systemic circulation. rPDA is characterized by a large cylindrical ductus arteriosus and development of progressive PHT over the animal's first 6–8 months of life. The PHT increases pulmonary artery pressures sufficiently to 'reverse' the flow through the ductus arteriosus and shunt blood from the pulmonary circulation to the systemic circulation. Animals with TF or rPDA often display poor growth, activity intolerance, weakness, fainting, and cyanosis. Echocardiography and radiography help provide a definitive diagnosis and assessment of disease severity. ECG abnormalities commonly include right axis shift, interventricular conduction abnormalities, ST segment changes, and occasionally ventricular arrhythmias. The degree of hypoxemia can be assessed through pulse oximetry or arterial blood gas analysis. Chronic hypoxemia stimulates red blood cell production and polycythemia is an important component of the pathophysiology of right-to-left defects. Clinical signs in animals with TF or rPDA are usually due to the hypoxemia and polycythemia, and congestive heart failure is very rare in both conditions. A packed cell volume (PCV) as high as 70–75% is not uncommon, and activity intolerance, organ dysfunction, and clotting abnormalities commonly occur at these extreme values. Periodic phlebotomy is used to maintain PCV at or below 65%.

The balance between the right- and left-sided pressures affects the extent of shunting, and interventions that lower systemic vascular resistance such as arterial vasodilators can potentiate signs. Signs of weakness or cyanosis are common during attempted exercise as systemic arterial vasodilation to the animal's skeletal muscle occurs. Affected animals are sometime prescribed non-selective beta-blockers such as propranolol to try and limit the amount of β_2-adrenergic receptor-mediated vasodilation during activity.

Anesthetic considerations

Goals of anesthesia for the patient with TF or other reverse shunt disorders are to maintain systemic vascular resistance and arterial pressures while minimizing changes in PVR and pulmonary pressures. As right-to-left shunting increases, so does arterial oxygen desaturation. Patients with significant pulmonary hypertension can be sensitive to changes in preload. Hypotension secondary to hypovolemia or vasodilation should be avoided and treated immediately if it occurs.

Premedication with an intramuscular opioid may be useful as struggling and sympathetic stimulation with restraint can increase right-to-left flow. These drugs should be used judiciously, however, as hypoventilation can lead to hypercarbia and respiratory acidosis, which can increase PVR and reverse shunting. Hypoxemia and hypotension can occur quickly in these patients, Preoxygenation prior to induction of anesthesia is extremely important, not only to address the underlying chronic hypoxemia that occurs in these animals, but also as a means of decreasing PVR. Other manipulations that can help decrease PVR include lowering of the hematocrit to <60% prior to anesthesia and hyperventilation with the maintenance of relative hypocarbia and respiratory alkalosis during anesthesia. Care must be taken with controlled ventilation, as increases in intrathoracic pressure with mechanical ventilation or the use of positive end expiratory pressure can increase PVR and the magnitude of right-to-left shunt flow.

Ketamine and midazolam may be used for induction, although patients with TF often have a dynamic component to the stenotic lesion and increases in heart rate may exacerbate the pulmonary outflow obstruction and reverse shunting [23]. An opioid-based induction technique is often used with or without etomidate, although significant decreases in heart rates should be avoided, especially if fentanyl or remifentanil is being used. All catheters and injection ports should be cleared of bubbles to avoid systemic air embolization.

Systemic vascular resistance must be maintained in these patients, as excessive hypotension will increase the right-to-left flow. Phenylephrine, an α-adrenergic receptor agonist causing arterial and venous vasoconstriction, can be useful in reversing right-to-left shunting during anesthesia, although other pressor agents such as dopamine may be used.

Conditions associated with pressure overload

Subaortic stenosis and pulmonic stenosis

Subaortic stenosis (SAS) and pulmonic stenosis (PS) are common congenital valvular defects in the dog. SAS and PS lead to a chronic systolic pressure increase in the left or right ventricle, respectively, with a resultant increase in wall tension and a compensatory increase in ventricular wall thickness or concentric hypertrophy. The increase in ventricular muscle mass and the increase in myocardial work required to generate increased systolic pressures result in an increased demand for coronary blood flow and myocardial oxygen delivery. In theory, the resulting risk for ischemia is greatest during periods of tachycardia and leads to myocardial necrosis, replacement fibrosis, and development of ventricular arrhythmias. In young dogs with severe SAS, the risk for syncope or sudden arrhythmic death in dogs is high, whereas risk of left-sided congestive heart failure is typically only seen in much older dogs. Right ventricular concentric hypertrophy, even in cases of severe PS, appears to be better tolerated than cases of left ventricular hypertrophy. Sudden death in dogs with severe PS is relatively uncommon, although clinical signs such as activity intolerance or syncope occur. In the authors' experience, congestive heart failure, in the form of ascites, is more common in dogs with PS.

Chronic medical management of severe SAS or PS often involves beta-blockers to reduce heart rate and myocardial oxygen demand. Echocardiography is an extremely useful modality to assess the severity of the SAS or PS lesion and extent of concentric hypertrophy. ECG and 24 h ambulatory ECG (Holter) monitoring is useful to evaluate cardiac rhythm and to detect ST segment elevation or depression, which is suggestive of myocardial ischemia. In both SAS and PS, arterial vasodilators should be used with caution as a decrease in arterial blood pressure increases the pressure gradient across the stenotic valve and can lead to increased myocardial work, severe hypotension, and decreased coronary perfusion pressure.

Anesthetic considerations

Patients with SAS or PS often have poor ventricular compliance and it is critically important to maintain adequate preload in these animals. Maintaining an adequate venous return by insuring a full intravascular volume to fill the non-compliant ventricular chamber will help optimize diastolic filling and cardiac output, although volume overload should be avoided. In addition, these patients are dependent on maintenance of a normal sinus rhythm and atrial 'kick' to optimize ventricular filling. Tachycardia must be avoided to limit myocardial oxygen deficit.

Afterload is elevated, but relatively fixed due to the stenosis at the level of the valve. Vasodilation and reductions in vascular tone generally do little to relieve the fixed afterload from a stenotic valve, but rather decrease preload and reduce coronary perfusion pressure.

When managing the patient with SAS or PS, it is important to minimize hypotension and treat aggressively if it develops. Volume is the first treatment for hypotension in these patients, followed by the use of a vasoconstrictor such as phenylephrine (see Table 26.4). Contractility is generally maintained, although inotropes may be helpful in patients with severe SAS or PS with ventricular dysfunction. Dopamine may be preferred to dobutamine since the former will maintain or increase SVR and may be more effective at treating inhalant anesthetic-associated hypotension [55,56], whereas dobutamine maintains or decreases SVR such that the mean arterial pressure changes little despite an increase in cardiac contractility [57–59]. In some patients with SAS or PS, the obstruction also has a dynamic component, which may be accentuated by reductions in ventricular size, as occurs with increases in heart rate or contractility or decreases in preload or afterload. In patients with PS, increases in PVR may be minimized by maintaining a high F_IO_2 and low $PaCO_2$.

Premedication of patients with SAS or PS may decrease the anxiety of the animal and stress during patient handling and help prevent unnecessary increases in heart rate. Care must be taken, however, to ensure adequate venous return (preload) and optimal diastolic filling. Ideally, patients should receive supplemental oxygen after receiving any medication. If preoperative sedation is necessary, opioids are generally the drug of choice since they cause minimal cardiovascular depression, although hypoventilation may be of concern in patients with PS. Antiarrhythmic therapy should be instituted to maintain a normal sinus rhythm as needed [60].

Diastolic dysfunction-associated diseases

Hypertrophic cardiomyopathy and restrictive cardiomyopathy pathophysiology

Hypertrophic cardiomyopathy (HCM) and restrictive cardiomyopathy (RCM) are common cardiomyopathies of the cat but are extremely rare in the dog. Both HCM and RCM are characterized by diastolic dysfunction as opposed to DCM, which is primarily a disease of systolic function. The pathophysiology of HCM involves idiopathic concentric hypertrophy of the left ventricle, increased myocardial oxygen demand, myocardial ischemia, and development of left ventricular outflow tract (LVOT) obstruction due to systolic anterior motion (SAM) of the mitral valve leaflets. The pathophysiology of RCM involves idiopathic fibrosis of the left ventricle muscle with resultant diastolic dysfunction in the absence of appreciable concentric hypertrophy. Thus, while the gross appearance of the left ventricle is different between HCM and RCM, the underlying pathophysiology involving diastolic performance is similar.

Diastolic dysfunction results in the inability of the ventricle to properly relax during diastole. The 'stiff' left ventricle requires increased pressure to fill properly and the resultant increase in left atrial pressure and volume overload predisposes to congestive heart failure. In cats, left-sided congestive heart failure can manifest as either pulmonary edema, pleural effusion, or both. Both ventricular arrhythmias due to suspected ischemia and also systemic thromboembolism are common in cats with HCM or RCM. It is prudent to evaluate any cat for cardiomyopathy that has unexplained ventricular premature contractions during the perianesthetic period.

The presence of SAM in cases of HCM is multifactorial and incompletely understood. Likely mechanisms for development of SAM include abnormal mitral leaflet morphology, interventricular septal hypertrophy, misalignment of the papillary muscle and chordae tendineae apparatus due to concentric hypertrophy, and increased flow rates through the narrowed LVOT which 'pulls' the mitral leaflets into the outflow tract. HCM with LVOT obstruction due to SAM is often termed hypertrophic obstructive cardiomyopathy (HOCM), and HOCM makes up as much as 50% of all HCM cases. The presence of the LVOT obstruction is akin to animals with subaortic stenosis. The resulting left ventricular pressure overload further stimulates concentric hypertrophy and increased myocardial oxygen demand. Therapy for HOCM involves reductions in ventricular contractility, heart rate, and outflow tract pressure gradient, which reduce the degree of SAM. Commonly used agents include beta-blockers such as atenolol or calcium channel blockers such as diltiazem. Systemic hypertension secondary to chronic kidney disease and hyperthyroidism are common comorbidities in geriatric cats with HCM or HOCM. Overly aggressive arterial vasodilators should be avoided as a reduction in systemic vascular resistance will increase the pressure gradient across the LVOT, potentiate SAM, and increase myocardial oxygen demand. Chronic therapy of HCM, HOCM, and RCM includes reduction in preload using diuretics, heart rate control using beta-blockers or calcium channel blockers, and antithrombosis using aspirin or clopidogrel. ACEIs are also often prescribed but used with caution due to their arterial vasodilatory potential.

Anesthetic considerations

Anesthesia in cats with HCM is directed at optimizing diastolic filling, both by maintaining relatively low heart rates and by avoiding drugs that may increase cardiac contractility. Optimizing preload and ventricular filling can be useful. Afterload reduction may worsen the obstruction and marked decreases in arterial pressures are poorly tolerated. Decreases in aortic pressure will contribute to inadequate coronary perfusion and potential myocardial ischemia. In contrast, increasing afterload may decrease SAM and outflow tract obstruction. One study found complete resolution of dynamic outflow obstruction in cats with HCM or SAM receiving medetomidine [61]. Medetomidine, an α_2-adrenergic receptor agonist, causes vasoconstriction and increased SVR, both potentially desirable with HCM with LVOT obstruction. However, systolic function should be carefully evaluated prior to administration of α_2-adrenergic receptor agonists, and ultimately drugs that can be titrated carefully (e.g., phenylephrine) may be better choices during the anesthetic period [62].

Positive inotropic activity can potentially increase dynamic outflow tract obstruction in addition to myocardial oxygen consumption. Ketamine or tiletamine can cause uncontrolled catecholamine release, tachycardia, and increased myocardial contractility and oxygen consumption [35,63–65]. These agents may also predispose to arrhythmias. Therefore, other anesthetic agents are usually preferred. Low doses of an opioid such as fentanyl, methadone, or oxymorphone may be given as part of the induction technique. Induction with etomidate, which has a minimal effect on cardiovascular contractility, and a benzodiazepine tranquilizer such as midazolam or diazepam is often used when venous access is available. Decreased systemic vascular resistance due to decreased sympathetic nervous system activity which accompanies loss of consciousness should be anticipated with any anesthetic protocol and appropriate contingency measures considered before induction.

Hypotension occurs with relative frequency in healthy cats anesthetized with inhalation anesthetics. Pressure support for cats with HCM under anesthesia usually involves the use of vasopressors such as phenylephrine, an α_1-adrenergic receptor agonist with little or no β-activity. Phenylephrine increases SVR with little direct effect on the myocardium. Wiese *et al.* [62] compared the cardiorespiratory effects of phenylephrine and dopamine in cats with HCM without LVOT anesthetized with isoflurane. Both agents increased systemic and arterial blood pressure, although only dopamine increased cardiac index. Plasma levels of cTnI were measured as a marker of cardiac injury and increased in response to hypotension but were not different between the two groups. Phenylephrine may still be preferred in those cases with LVOT.

Pericardial effusion

The pericardium encloses the heart within the sheet of fibroelastic tissue and the space between the epicardial surface of the heart and the parietal pericardium normally contains a small volume of fluid, the purpose of which is to lubricate the heart and provide a friction-free environment. Pericardial effusion is the abnormal accumulation of large volumes of fluid within the pericardial space, which exerts external compressive forces on the heart. The term *cardiac tamponade* is used to describe situations in which the volume of pericardial effusion is sufficient to decrease cardiac filling markedly, leading to poor cardiac output. In the case of pericardial effusion, the diastolic dysfunction that occurs is not due to an intrinsic abnormality of the myocardium but rather external compression and restriction of diastolic filling of the heart. Common causes of pericardial effusion include cardiac neoplasia and idiopathic pericarditis in the dog, and congestive heart failure and feline infectious peritonitis in the cat. Less common is infectious pericarditis or uremic pericarditis.

Common clinical findings in animals with cardiac tamponade include muffled heart sounds, dyspnea, weakness, collapse, pallor, hypotension, tachycardia, and right heart failure (typically ascites or chylothorax). ECG and thoracic radiography can reveal low-amplitude QRS complexes and electrical alternans and a globoid cardiac silhouette, respectively. Echocardiography is particularly useful in confirming the presence of pericardial effusion and detecting heart base masses. Hemangiosarcoma of the right atrium/auricle or chemodectoma associated with the aortic root are two common tumors associated with pericardial effusion.

Therapy involves pericardiocentesis, which provides immediate relief and improvement in cardiac output. Animals with pericardial effusion are very sensitive to changes in preload and diuresis should not be routinely performed unless the animal is volume overloaded, as this can worsen tamponade, further reduce cardiac output, and aggravate clinical signs. In cases with severe ascites, abdominocentesis can be performed to improve respiration and comfort. Chronic pericardial effusion often necessitates surgical pericardiectomy; however, the decision whether to pursue this course is influenced by the etiology of the effusion.

Anesthetic considerations

In the presence of tamponade, intrapericardial pressures determine venous return and the ventricle can become small and underloaded despite a compensatory increase in right and left ventricular filling pressures to maintain cardiac filling. Stroke volume becomes limited and cardiac output becomes dependent on compensatory mechanisms including peripheral vasoconstriction to maintain venous return, tachycardia, and increased contractility.

The goal of anesthesia is to select agents that will preserve these compensatory mechanisms and maintain forward flow. Intravenous fluids should be administered prior to induction of anesthesia to optimize preload and maintain cardiac filling pressures. Small (2–5 mL/kg) boluses of crystalloid or colloids at induction given to optimize preload can offset anesthetic-associated venodilation while avoiding the worsening of pericardial effusion that can occur with longer term fluid therapy. Drugs that cause myocardial depression, bradycardia, or vasodilation should be avoided. Ketamine, because of its sympathomimetic effects, may be helpful in preserving heart rate and blood pressure [63–65]. However, larger doses can induce hypotension in those animals that are already under maximum sympathetic stress or in critically ill patients [66, 67]. An opioid technique can be used, although anticholinergics may be required to preserve heart rate. Regardless of anesthetic technique, it is often beneficial to use a multimodal approach with careful monitoring and titration of drug effect.

Any manipulation that may decrease venous return should be avoided. Controlled positive-pressure ventilation with large tidal volumes may significantly decrease preload and cardiac output. Since thoracotomy for pericardectomy is usually the surgical treatment for pericardial effusion, positive-pressure ventilation using smaller volumes (lower peak inspiratory pressure) with a higher respiratory rate should be used. Pericardiocentensis may be indicated prior to induction of anesthesia in some animals with severe hemodynamic compromise.

Diseases associated with arrhythmias

Arrhythmogenic diseases resulting in tachycardia

Common tachycardias and associated cardiac diseases include ventricular tachycardia (VT) [seen in Boxer arrhythmogenic right ventricular cardiomyopathy (ARVC), feline cardiomyopathy, DCM, and SAS], AF (see in MMVD and DCM), supraventricular tachycardia (SVT) (seen in DCM and MMVD), and accessory pathway-mediated SVT in Labrador Retrievers. Common to all pathological tachycardias is the increase in myocardial oxygen demand and progressive decrease in diastolic filling time. The exact heart rate at which a tachycardia goes from beneficial to detrimental is dependent on many factors, including the origin of the tachycardia (i.e., sinus versus ectopic), species, breed (primarily related to body size), underlying systolic and diastolic function of the heart, and presence of eccentric or concentric hypertrophy. In general, ectopic heart rates >250 bpm in cats and small breed dogs and >200 bpm in large breed dogs are regarded as sufficiently tachycardic to warrant intervention. Clinical findings associated with tachycardia include signs of diminished cardiac output, such as weakness, syncope, pallor, disorientation, hypothermia, or cold extremities. Arterial blood pressure may be normal during tachycardia and reduced cardiac output, but it is due to compensatory arteriolar constriction. Anesthesia with subsequent arteriolar dilation may result in profound hypotension even though the heart rate does not decrease significantly. Tachycardias, especially VT, can predispose to ventricular fibrillation and sudden death.

Treatment is centered on addressing any underlying cardiac disease or heart failure, and administration of specific antiarrhythmic agents. Commonly used agents for acute treatment of ventricular arrhythmias during anesthesia include lidocaine, procainamide, and short-acting parenteral beta-blockers such as esmolol. Acute therapy for AF or SVT includes parenteral esmolol or calcium channel blockers such as diltiazem. Chronic therapy of ventricular arrhythmias often uses sotalol or mexiletine or less commonly amiodarone, and chronic therapy of AF or supraventricular arrhythmias uses oral digoxin, diltiazem and/or beta-blockers, and occasionally sotalol. Owing to the potential for side-effects, lidocaine and procainamide are uncommonly used in cats. Electrocardioversion of tachyarrhythmias may be appropriate for some patients and is often performed just after induction of anesthesia.

Arrhythmogenic diseases resulting in bradycardia

Common bradycardias include second and third (complete) AV nodal block, sick sinus syndrome (SSS), and atrial standstill. Bradycardia is relatively uncommon in cats but does occur. All cases of bradycardia detected with auscultation during the preanesthetic physical examination should be further evaluated with an ECG and other diagnostics as indicated. SSS is commonly seen in Miniature Schnauzers, whereas AV nodal block is often detected in larger breed dogs, such as the Labrador Retriever. Bradycardia can be detected in association with underlying structural heart disease, but often occurs in isolation, and is thought to represent primary disease of the cardiac conduction system. Idiopathic degeneration of the sinus node, AV node, and other conduction tissue is often assumed. In some cases, acute inflammatory injury to the heart (i.e., myocarditis) is suspected. Bradycardia secondary to electrolyte abnormalities such as severe hyperkalemia can occur in cases of renal disease, uncontrolled hyperadrenocorticism, soft tissue injury, and other conditions.

The exact heart rate at which a bradycardia becomes clinically significant depends on the underlying cardiac function, species, and breed. Periods of asystole lasting >5–8 s are usually sufficient to cause weakness or syncope. Chronic bradycardia with heart rates <50 bpm are often associated with activity intolerance, lethargy, weakness, or syncope in dogs. It should be remembered that resting heart rates during sleep can be relatively low to normal values during normal activity. However, the rate during sleep may be a better indicator of the patient's acceptable heart rate during anesthesia. Any time arterial blood pressure becomes heart rate dependent during anesthesia, intervention to increase the heart rate should be considered because it represents a point where stroke volume cannot increase further to maintain cardiac output. In rare instances, congestive heart failure due to excessively slow rates occurs. In the authors' experience, chronic symptomatic bradycardia in the cat is rare as most cats maintain escape rates at or near 100 bpm, which are sufficient to maintain an acceptable quality of life.

Therapy of bradycardia includes correction of underlying electrolyte abnormalities and support of heart rate through parenteral or oral parasympatholytic (e.g., atropine, glycopyrrolate, propantheline bromide) or sympathomimetic (e.g., isoproterenol, terbutaline, theophylline) agents. Standard diagnostics performed in animals with bradycardia include bloodwork, ECG, echocardiography, and radiography. Commonly, the influence of native vagal tone on the bradycardia is determined by ECG examination before and after administration of atropine, with the presumption that early or mild conduction system disease (such as asymptomatic intermittent second-degree AV block) can be differentiated from high resting vagal tone by an abnormal response to atropine. Rarely do cases of symptomatic AV block or SSS demonstrate a normal response to atropine, indicating the presence of structural disease of the conduction system.

In cases that are poorly responsive to medical therapy, artificial pacing can be performed. Permanent transvenous or epicardial pacemaker implantation is considered in animals with bradycardia sufficient to cause clinical signs. Temporary transvenous or transthoracic artificial pacing can also be performed in instances where temporary worsening of relatively benign bradycardia could occur, for instance, during anesthesia.

Anesthetic considerations

The goal of anesthesia in the patient with a known cardiac rhythm disturbance is to avoid further deterioration of the rhythm. Arrhythmias should be evaluated prior to anesthesia in terms of both their electrical stability (or lack thereof) and their hemodynamic consequences. Any electrolyte abnormalities should be corrected prior to induction. Stress during restraint of the animal should be minimized if at all possible. Very low doses of acepromazine in combination with an opioid may be helpful as a premedication in some animals with ventricular arrhythmias. In the case of tachycardias that are ventricular in origin, drugs such as propofol, alphaxalone or etomidate, which have little to no effect of cardiac conduction, may be preferred for induction. An opioid and/or benzodiazepine may also be used as part of the induction technique. A single dose of lidocaine can be given prior to induction to determine the efficacy of this agent in suppressing the ventricular arrhythmia and is occasionally continued as a CRI throughout the procedure, depending on the severity of the arrhythmia. As an alternative, procainamide may also be given intravenously and has a longer duration of action than lidocaine. Drugs such as ketamine that can cause catecholamine release and increased heart rate are usually avoided.

SVT can be difficult to differentiate from VT. In those patients with known SVT, vagomimetic drugs such as fentanyl or a fentanyl analog such as remifentanil may be useful, as these drugs can cause a pronounced decrease in sinus rate mediated through the vagus nerve [68–70]. In these patients, drugs that increase AV nodal conduction (e.g., anticholinergics) are generally avoided. In the case of severe SVT, esmolol may be loaded intravenously and given as a CRI, although the β-receptor blockade can also lead to negative inotropic effects.

For the patient with SSS or heart block, the goal of anesthesia is to prevent worsening of the bradycardia (e.g., asystole) with drug administration. A relatively high dose of atropine is often given prior to anesthesia to avoid the consequences of a sudden increase in vagal tone. Ketamine/benzodiazepine, propofol, and etomidate may all be used for induction. Drugs known to cause bradyarrhythmias, such as α_2-adrenergic receptor agonists, should be avoided. A temporary transvenous pacemaker may be placed prior to induction of anesthesia or transthoracic artificial pacing pads may be used as needed. Heart rates can decrease dramatically upon induction with the relative decrease in sympathetic tone. Dobutamine, dopamine, or isoproterenol infusions [71] should be readied prior to anesthetic induction if a temporary pacemaker has not been placed.

Hypotension

Systemic blood pressure is dependent on cardiac output and SVR and must be maintained above the minimum level required to maintain cerebral, coronary, and renal perfusion. Mean arterial blood pressures less than 65–70 mmHg are generally considered inadequate for maintaining optimal blood flow to tissues. In patients that are hypovolemic and hemodynamically unstable, neural and neurohormonal mechanisms can increase SVR and minimize apparent changes in blood pressure, while decreasing blood flow and oxygen delivery to the tissues. Patients that are compensating by increasing SVR can have a precipitous decrease in blood pressure following induction of anesthesia.

Cardiac output is determined by stroke volume and heart rate, although stroke volume can also be affected by changes in vascular resistance. Decreases in stroke volume may be seen secondary to decreased venous return (decreased preload), often caused by underlying fluid deficits or peripheral vasodilation (decreased SVR), leading to a relative fluid deficit. In addition, stroke volume may be decreased due to decreased myocardial contractility, increased SVR (increased afterload), and/or cardiac arrhythmias. Induction of anesthesia and the subsequent decreases in sympathetic stimulation can lead to decreases in heart rate, preload, and cardiac contractility, all of which will affect cardiac output. Similarly, administration of vagomimetic opioids (e.g., fentanyl) can reduce heart rate and affect blood pressure, although they are frequently recommended for use as adjunct anesthetics in cardiovascularly compromised patients to reduce inhalant anesthetic requirements.

Duration of hypotension is important in determining ultimate clinical outcome in both cardiac and non-cardiac patients [72], so early recognition is important. Methods for recognition of hypotension can include monitoring changes in heart rate and rhythm, measuring decreases in mean arterial pressure below 60–65 mmHg, and/or assessing changes in tissue perfusion. Tachycardia is generally considered a major compensatory response to fluid/blood loss and hypovolemia, although increases in heart rate may also be seen due to inadequate anesthesia, hypercarbia, hypoxemia, or drug administration (e.g., anticholinergics). In addition, the use of vagomimetic drugs such as fentanyl may mask the early compensatory increase heart rate in response to changes in preload.

Arterial blood pressure may be measured using non-invasive measuring techniques, including Doppler ultrasonographic flow probes and oscillometric measuring devices, or by direct arterial blood pressure measurements. Central venous pressure (CVP) is often used as an indicator of volume status in a given patient. However, a review of the literature found a very poor relationship between CVP and blood volume and also the inability of CVP change to predict the hemodynamic response to a fluid challenge [73]. Changes in parameters related to tissue oxygenation such as lactate, blood pH and base deficit, and central venous oxygen saturation are being used with increasing frequency to assess the adequacy of fluid resuscitation and inotropic and/or pressor support.

In any animal, the underlying cause of hypotension should be identified and corrected as rapidly as possible. Hypotension is common during anesthesia due to inadequate preoperative fluid replacement, failure to keep up with intraoperative fluid and/or blood loss, and dose-dependent effects of anesthetics on cardiac output and SVR. Rapid administration of high volumes of crystalloid fluid (e.g., Plasma-Lyte and lactated Ringer's solution) has a minimal effect in improving arterial blood pressure during isoflurane-induced hypotension in normovolemic dogs unless the anesthetic plane is also lightened [74,75]. Although cardiac output and stroke volume improve, arterial blood pressure does not change significantly due to decreases in SVR. Colloid administration using relatively large volumes of hetastarch (HES; hydroxyethyl starch) or dextran 70 [74,76] may increase both cardiac index and blood pressure in anesthetized animals. The underlying disease process, evaluation of ongoing losses and changes in volume status, and close monitoring of changes in PCV, total solids, and determinants of tissue oxygenation should all be used in determining the rate and type of fluids administered to the patient.

Higher fluid rates are usually needed in emergent patients with pre-existing deficits or ongoing blood losses. Low diastolic pressures (<40 mmHg), large position-associated changes in blood pressure, or difficulty in tolerating positive-pressure ventilation may all alert the clinician to the presence of inadequate volume. In some cases, maintenance of anesthesia may need to be changed from an inhalant to an injectable technique, which causes less myocardial depression and vasodilation than most inhalant techniques.

Pharmacological support

Pharmacological support may be required if hypotension is severe and does not respond to fluid therapy or changes in anesthetic depth. In addition, patients with cardiovascular disease may not tolerate fluid administration. Drugs are selected for cardiovascular support based on the patient's condition and underlying hemodynamic disturbance, the physiologic response desired, the pharmacology of the available drugs, and clinician experience and opinion. The principal effects include changes in heart rate (chronotropism), contractility (inotropism), myocardial conduction velocity (dromotropism), rhythm, and peripheral vasodilation or vasoconstriction, which influences preload and afterload. For many years, the choice of agent was made depending primarily on its effects on myocardial function and vascular resistance as determinants of blood pressure. More recently, attention has also been focused on changes in venous capacitance and preload and also the distribution of blood flow to the various organs. Changes in blood lactate, pH, and base deficit are often used clinically to help determine what changes in flow are occurring at the tissue level. Drugs used to treat hypotension are discussed in other chapters.

Shock

The therapeutic priority in patients with circulatory shock is oxygen delivery to the tissues. Sequelae to decreased cardiac output, decreased systemic vascular resistance, and/or decreased blood oxygen content include tissue hypoxia, systemic inflammation, and organ dysfunction. In order to achieve this goal, fluid resuscitation, including blood transfusion, and the use of vasopressors (see Table 26.4) may be required, although the optimal strategy including choice of fluid for resuscitation and hemodynamic goals are still controversial in both the human and the veterinary literature.

Selection of target indices for monitoring the hemodynamic response to therapy has changed over the last several years. Blood pressure is relatively easy to measure and is often used as a primary measurement for evaluating the severity of circulatory shock and the adequacy of resuscitation. Blood pressure is also a major criterion used in separating septic syndrome from septic shock [77]. Blood pressure monitoring has serious limitations, however, as it assumes that changes in blood pressure values are directly related to altered blood flow (i.e., SVR is unchanged). In the early stages of hemorrhage, neurohormonal mechanisms may maintain blood pressure near normal (at the expense of perfusion to selected tissues) by increasing SVR.

Shoemaker and colleagues first introduced the concept of goal-directed resuscitation in the 1980s, after noting that survivors of high-risk surgical procedures had a higher cardiac index and oxygen delivery in concert with an increased oxygen demand compared with non-survivors [78,79]. Changes in mean arterial pressure lagged behind changes in cardiac index, and by the time hypovolemia and low flow to the tissues were of sufficient magnitude to produce severe hypotension, the deteriorating circulatory condition was well advanced [80].

Early goal-directed therapy, involving manipulation of cardiac preload, afterload, and contractility to balance oxygen delivery with oxygen demand, has been used in human patients with systemic inflammatory response syndrome as a means to slow the progression to severe sepsis and septic shock. The systemic inflammatory response syndrome is a continuum, with circulatory abnormalities including intravascular volume depletion, peripheral vasodilation, myocardial depression, and increased tissue metabolic needs causing an imbalance between systemic oxygen delivery and oxygen demand. Changes in vital signs, central venous pressure, and urinary output have proven to be poor indicators of effective hemodynamic resuscitation and fail to detect tissue hypoxia. More recently, researchers have chosen alternative targets to monitor successful therapy [81], including normalized values for mixed venous oxygen saturation (as a substitute for cardiac index as a target of hemodynamic therapy), arterial lactate concentration, base deficit, and pH. Rivers *et al.* [81] found that, during the first 6 h of therapy, there was no significant difference in mean heart rate or central venous pressure between the early goal-directed therapy group and standard therapy group. Mean arterial pressure was maintained at ≥65 mmHg in both groups with the use of vasopressors and CVP was maintained at ≥8 mmHg with the use of crystalloid fluid boluses. However, patients in the early goal-directed groups first received red blood cells to maintain a hematocrit of ≥30% if the central venous oxygen saturation (venous blood gas from jugular central line) fell below 70%, and then received dobutamine to improve cardiac contractility if central venous oxygen saturation remained below 70%. Choice of the alternative target indices in the early stages of treatment improved survival rates by 16% in human patients with severe sepsis and served as the basis for recommendations made following the Surviving Sepsis Campaign in 2004 and 2008 [82,83]. Recommendations also included either dopamine or norepinephrine as a first-line vasopressor, although vasopressin or phenylephrine may also be used.

In terms of the type and amount of fluid used for resuscitation, no definitive proof can be found in the recent literature that supports the superiority of one type of fluid over another for fluid resuscitation in the acute trauma or septic patient [84–86]. An important advantage that colloids have over crystalloids is that they can induce a more rapid and persistent plasma expansion due to the larger increase in colloid oncotic pressure. In addition, resuscitation with large volumes of crystalloids has been associated with tissue edema and hyperchloremic metabolic acidosis. However, crystalloids are cheaper and research findings have shown no survival benefit when colloids are administered.

A review of critically ill human patients [87] with trauma or burns or after surgery found no evidence that resuscitation with colloids reduced the risk of death compared with resuscitation with crystalloids. Rather, impaired coagulation, an increase in clinical bleeding, and acute kidney injury are frequently reported with some types of HES used in humans [88,89]. In addition, recent reports in the human literature, including the VISEP (Efficacy of Volume Substitution and Insulin Therapy in Severe Sepsis) study [90], found that patients receiving HES for resuscitation had lower survival rates and more pronounced kidney dysfunction than patients resuscitated with crystalloids. Perner *et al.* [91] showed an increased risk of death (at day 90) in patients with severe sepsis who received fluid resuscitation with 6% HES in Ringer's acetate compared with patient resuscitated with Ringer's acetate alone (6S trial). Renal dysfunction was also more pronounced in the HES group. How these findings relate to fluid resuscitation in the septic or bleeding patient in the acute perioperative period is unknown, but HES has recently been removed from the human market in Europe and is currently under review in the United States.

Other colloids may be used for resuscitation. Whole blood, red blood cells, and fresh frozen plasma may all be used to expand intravascular volume and provide colloidal support. In addition, administration of whole blood or red blood cells can restore oxygen-carrying capacity in patients that are bleeding or anemic for other reasons. Risk of red blood cell administration includes transfusion reaction and many patients are blood typed or cross-matched prior to transfusion. Human serum albumin (HSA, 25%) has also been used in canine patients with markedly varied success. In human patients, the SAFE study found no difference in the overall mortality rates of ICU patients treated with albumin and saline [92]. However, in a subgroup of patients with brain injury, relative risk was higher in patients assigned to the albumin-treated group than the saline-treated group. One of the first retrospective reports of HSA administration in critically ill canine and feline patients [93] found that administration of an average of 5 mL/kg increased albumin levels and systemic blood pressure. However, two of the 64 dogs developed facial edema and five animals died during or immediately after transfusion. In healthy dogs receiving HSA, three of nine dogs developed facial edema and urticaria within days of receiving the transfusion and two dogs developed severe hypertension [94]. One of the nine dogs developed a severe anaphylactoid reaction within 10 min of receiving the infusion. Two out of two dogs receiving a second infusion had a similar severe anaphylactoid reaction. Martin *et al.* [95] found that administration of HSA resulted in antibody formation in both healthy and critically ill patients, with the onset time being shorter in the healthy dogs. Interestingly, two of the 57 control dogs also had anti-HSA antibodies, despite never having received an infusion. Canine albumin is also commercially available in the United States, although availability is limited. Allergic reactions occur with some regularity, but tend to be less severe than those seen with HSA.

References

1 Tilley LP, Burtnick NL. *ECG for the Small Animal Practitioner*. Jackson, WY: Teton NewMedia, 1999.

2 Fuentes VL, Johnson LR, Dennis D, eds. *Canine and Feline Cardiorespiratory Medicine*, 2nd edn. Quedgeley, Gloucester: British Small Animal Veterinary Association, 2013.

3 Tilley LP, Smith FW, Oyama MA, Sleeper MM, eds. *Manual of Canine and Feline Cardiology*, 4th edn. St. Louis, MO: Saunders Elsevier, 2013.

4 Buchanan JW, Bucheler J. Vertebral scale system to measure canine heart size in radiographs. *J Am Vet Med Assoc* 1995; **206**: 194–199.

5 Litster AL, Buchanan JW. Vertebral scale system to measure heart size in radiographs of cats. *J Am Vet Med Assoc* 2000; **216**: 210–214.

6 Hansson K, Haggstrom J, Kvart C, Lord P. Interobserver variability of vertebral heart size measurements in dogs with normal and enlarged hearts. *Vet Radiol Ultrasound* 2005; **46**: 122–130.

7 Kraetschmer S, Ludwig K, Meneses F, *et al.* Vertebral heart scale in the Beagle dog. *J Small Anim Pract* 2008; **49**: 240–243.

8 Marin LM, Brown J, McBrien C, *et al.* Vertebral heart size in retired racing Greyhounds. *Vet Radiol Ultrasound* 2007; **48**: 332–334.

9 Bavegems V, Van Caelenberg A, Duchateau L, *et al.* Vertebral heart size ranges specific for whippets. *Vet Radiol Ultrasound* 2005; **46**: 400–403.

10 Greco A, Meomartino L, Raiano V, *et al.* Effect of left vs. right recumbency on the vertebral heart score in normal dogs. *Vet Radiol Ultrasound* 2008; **49**: 454–455.

11 Sleeper MM, Buchanan JW. Vertebral scale system to measure heart size in growing puppies. *J Am Vet Med Assoc* 2001; **219**: 57–59.

12 Lamb CR, Wikeley H, Boswood A, Pfeiffer DU. Use of breed-specific ranges for the vertebral heart scale as an aid to the radiographic diagnosis of cardiac disease in dogs. *Vet Rec* 2001; **148**: 707–711.

13 Ghadiri A, Avizeh R, Rasekh A, Yadegari A. Radiographic measurement of vertebral heart size in healthy stray cats. *J Feline Med Surg* 2008; **10**: 61–65.

14 Cornell CC, Kittleson MD, Della TP, *et al.* Allometric scaling of M-mode cardiac measurements in normal adult dogs. *J Vet Intern Med* 2004; **18**: 311–321.

15 Mueller X, Stauffer JC, Jaussi A, *et al.* Subjective visual echocardiographic estimate of left ventricular ejection fraction as an alternative to conventional echocardiographic methods: comparison with contrast angiography. *Clin Cardiol* 1991; **14**: 898–902.

16 Loyer C, Thomas WP. Biplane transesophageal echocardiography in the dog: technique, anatomy, and imaging planes. *Vet Radiol Ultrasound* 1995; **36**: 212–226.

17 Kienle RD, Thomas WP, Rishniw M. Biplane transesophageal echocardiography in the normal cat. *Vet Radiol Ultrasound* 1997; **38**: 288–298.

18 Fox PR, Oyama MA, Reynolds C, *et al.* Utility of plasma N-terminal pro-brain natriuretic peptide (NT-proBNP) to distinguish between congestive heart failure and non-cardiac causes of acute dyspnea in cats. *J Vet Cardiol* 2009; **11**(Suppl 1): S51–S61.

19 Fox PR, Rush JE, Reynolds CA, *et al.* Multicenter evaluation of plasma N-terminal probrain natriuretic peptide (NT-pro BNP) as a biochemical screening test for asymptomatic (occult) cardiomyopathy in cats. *J Vet Intern Med* 2011; **25**: 1010–1016.

20 Wess G, Daisenberger P, Mahling M, *et al.* Utility of measuring plasma N-terminal pro-brain natriuretic peptide in detecting hypertrophic cardiomyopathy and differentiating grades of severity in cats. *Vet Clin Pathol* 2011; **40**: 237–244.

21 Hezzell MJ, Boswood A, Chang YM, *et al.* The combined prognostic potential of serum high-sensitivity cardiac troponin I and N-terminal pro-B-type natriuretic peptide concentrations in dogs with degenerative mitral valve disease. *J Vet Intern Med* 2012; **26**: 302–311.

22 Yoran C, Yellin EL, Becker RM, *et al.* Dynamic aspects of acute mitral regurgitation: effects of ventricular volume, pressure and contractility on the effective regurgitant orifice area. *Circulation* 1979; **60**: 170–176.

23 Nussmeier NA, Hauser MC, Sarwar MF, *et al.* Anesthesia for cardiac surgical procedures. In: Miller RD, Eriksson LI, Fleisher LA, *et al.*, eds. *Miller's Anesthesia*, 7th edn. Philadelphia: Churchill Livingstone Elsevier, 2010; 2599–2652.

24 Flacke JW, Davis LJ, Flacke WE, *et al.* Effects of fentanyl and diazepam in dogs deprived of autonomic tone. *Anesth Analg* 1985; **64**: 1053–1059.

25 Grimm KA, Tranquilli WJ, Gross DR, *et al.* Cardiopulmonary effects of fentanyl in conscious dogs and dogs sedated with a continuous rate infusion of medetomidine. *Am J Vet Res* 2005; **66**: 1222–1226.

26 Machado CG, Dyson DH, Mathews KA. Evaluation of induction by use of a combination of oxymorphone and diazepam or hydromorphone and diazepam and maintenance of anesthesia by use of isoflurane in dogs with experimentally induced hypovolemia. *Am J Vet Res* 2005; **66**: 1227–1237.

27 Smith LJ, Yi JK, Bjorling DE, Waller K. Effects of hydromorphone or oxymorphone, with or without acepromazine, on preanesthetic sedation, physiologic values, and histamine release in dogs. *J Am Vet Med Assoc* 2001; **218**: 1101–1105.

28 Nagel ML, Muir WW, Nguyen K. Comparison of the cardiopulmonary effects of etomidate and thiamylal in dogs. *Am J Vet Res* 1979; **40**: 193–196.

29 De Hert SG, Vermeyen KM, Adriaensen HF. Influence of thiopental, etomidate, and propofol on regional myocardial function in the normal and acute ischemic heart segment in dogs. *Anesth Analg* 1990; **70**: 600–607.

30 Pascoe P, Ilkiw J, Haskins S, Patz JD. Cardiopulmonary effects of etomidate in hypovolemic dogs. *Am J Vet Res* 1992; **53**: 2178–2182.

31 Coetzee A, Fourie P, Coetzee J, *et al.* Effect of various propofol plasma concentrations on regional myocardial contractility and left ventricular afterload. *Anesth Analg* 1989; **69**: 473–483.

32 Ismail EF, Kim S, Ramez Salem M, Crystal GJ. Direct effects of propofol on myocardial contractility in *in situ* canine hearts. *Anesthesiology* 1992; **77**: 964–972.

33 Nakaigawa Y, Akazawa S, Shimizu R, *et al.* Effects of graded infusion rates of propofol on cardiovascular haemodynamics, coronary circulation and myocardial metabolism in dogs. *Br J Anaesth* 1995; **75**: 616–621.

34 Ilkiw JE, Pascoe PJ, Haskins SC, Patz JD. Cardiovascular and respiratory effects of propofol administration in hypovolemic dogs. *Am J Vet Res* 1992; **53**: 2323–2327.

35 Pagel PS, Schmeling WT, Kampine JP, Warltier DC. Alteration of canine left ventricular diastolic function by intravenous anesthetics *in vivo*: ketamine and propofol. *Anesthesiology* 1992; **76**: 419–425.

36 Psatha E, Alibhai HI, Jimenez-Lozano A, *et al.* Clinical efficacy and cardiorespiratory effects of alfaxalone, or diazepam/fentanyl for induction of anaesthesia in dogs that are a poor anaesthetic risk. *Vet Anesth Analg* 2011; **38**: 24–36.

37 Rodríguez JM, Muñoz-Rascón P, Navarrete-Calvo R, *et al.* Comparison of the cardiopulmonary parameters after induction of anaesthesia with alphaxalone or etomidate in dogs. *Vet Anaesth Analg* 2012; **39**: 357–365.

38 Robinson EP, Faggella AM, Henry DP, *et al.* Comparison of histamine release induced by morphine and oxymorphone administration in dogs. *Am J Vet Res* 1988; **49**: 1699–1701.

39 Michelsen LG, Salmenpera M, Hug CC, *et al.* Anesthetic potency of remifentanil in dogs. *Anesthesiology* 1996; **84**: 865–872.

40 Gimenes AM, de Araujo Aguiar AJ, Perri SHV, de Paula Nogueira G. Effect of intravenous propofol and remifentanil on heart rate, blood pressure and nociceptive

response in acepromazine premedicated dogs. *Vet Anaesth Analg* 2011; **38**: 54–62.

41 Musk GC, Flaherty DA. Target-controlled infusion of propofol combined with variable rate infusion of remifentanil for anaesthesia of a dog with patent ductus arteriosus. *Vet Anaesth Analg* 2007; **34**: 359–364.

42 Reitan JA, Stengert KB, Wymore MI, Martucci RW. Central vagal control of fentanyl-induced bradycardia during halothane anesthesia. *Anesth Analg* 1978; **57**: 31–36.

43 Gooding JM, Weng JT, Smith RA, *et al.* Cardiovascular and pulmonary responses following etomidate induction of anesthesia in patients with demonstrated cardiac disease. *Anesth Analg* 1979; **58**: 40–41.

44 Moon PF. Acute toxicosis in two dogs associated with etomidate-propylene glycol infusion. *Lab Anim Sci* 1994; **44**: 590–594.

45 Dodam JR, Kruse-Elliott KT, Aucoin DP, Swanson CR. Duration of etomidate-induced adrenocortical suppression during surgery in dogs. *Am J Vet Res* 1990; **51**: 786–788.

46 Wagner RL, White PF, Kan PB, *et al.* Inhibition of adrenal steroidogenesis by the anesthetic etomidate. *N Engl J Med* 1984; **310**: 1415–1421.

47 Ledingham IM, Watt I. Influence of sedation on mortality in critically ill multiple trauma patients. *Lancet* 1983; **1**(8336): 1270.

48 Badino P, Odore R, Re G. Are so many adrenergic receptor subtypes really present in domestic animal tissues? A pharmacological perspective. *Vet J* 2005; **170**: 163–174.

49 Williams GD, Jones TK, Hanson KA, Morray JP. The hemodynamic effects of propofol in children with congenital heart disease. *Anesth Analg* 1999; **89**: 1411–1416.

50 Boatman DL, Shaffer RA, Dixon RL, Brody MJ. Function of vascular smooth muscle and its sympathetic innervation in the newborn dog. *J Clin Invest* 1965; **44**: 241–246.

51 Boatman DL, Brody MJ. Cardiac responses to adrenergic stimulation in the newborn dog. *Arch Int Pharmacodyn Ther* 1967; **170**: 1–11.

52 Driscoll DJ, Gillette PC, Lewis RM, *et al.* Comparative hemodynamic effects of isoproterenol, dopamine, and dobutamine in the newborn dog. *Pediatr Res* 1979; **13**: 1006–1009.

53 Park IS, Michael LH, Driscoll DJ. Comparative response of the developing canine myocardium to inotropic agents. *Am J Physiol* 1982; **242**: H13–H18.

54 Manders WT, Pagani M, Vatner SF. Depressed responsiveness to vasoconstrictor and dilator agents and baroreflex sensitivity in conscious, newborn lambs. *Circulation* 1979; **60**: 945–955.

55 Rosati M, Dyson DH, Sinclair MD, Sears WC. Response of hypotensive dogs to dopamine hydrochloride and dobutamine hydrochloride during deep isoflurane anesthesia. *Am J Vet Res* 2007; **68**: 483–494.

56 Pascoe PJ, Ilkiw JE, Pypendop BH. Effects of increasing infusion rates of dopamine, dobutamine, epinephrine and phenylephrine in healthy anesthetized cats. *Am J Vet Res* 2006; **67**: 1491–1499.

57 Abdul-Rasool IH, Chamberlain JH, Swan PC, *et al.* Cardiorespiratory and metabolic effects of dopamine and dobutamine infusions in dogs. *Crit Care Med* 1987; **15**: 1044–1050.

58 Vatner SF, McRitchie RJ, Braunwald E. Effects of dobutaine on left ventricular performance, coronary dynamics and distribution of cardiac output in conscious dogs. *J Clin Invest* 1974; **53**: 1265–1273.

59 Orchard CH, Chakrabarti MK, Sykes MK. Cardiorespiratory responses to an i.v. infusion of dobutamine in the intact anaesthetized dog. *Br J Anaesth* 1982; **54**: 673–679.

60 De Moraes AN, Dyson DH, O'Grady MR, *et al.* Plasma concentrations and cardiovascular influence of lidocaine infusions during isoflurane anesthesia in healthy dogs and dogs with subaortic stenosis. *Vet Surg* 1998; **27**: 486–497.

61 Lamont LA, Bulmer BJ, Sisson DD, *et al.* Doppler echocardiographic effects of medetomidine on dynamic left ventricular outflow tract obstruction in cats. *J Am Vet Med Assoc* 2002; **221**: 1276–1281.

62 Wiese AJ, Barter LS, Ilkiw JE, *et al.* Cardiovascular and respiratory effects of incremental doses of dopamine and phenylephrine in the management of isoflurane-induced hypotension in cats with hypertrophic cardiomyopathy. *Am J Vet Res* 2012; **73**: 908–916.

63 White PF, Way WL, Trevor AJ. Ketamine – its pharmacology and therapeutic uses. *Anesthesiology* 1982; **56**: 119–136.

64 Haskins SC, Farver TB, Patz JD. Ketamine in dogs. *Am J Vet Res* 1985; **46**: 1855–1860.

65 Pascoe PJ, Ilkiw JE, Craig C, Kollias-Baker C. The effects of ketamine on the minimum alveolar concentration of isoflurane in cats. *Vet Anaesth Analg* 2007; **34**: 31–39.

66 Lippman M, Appel PL, Mok MS, *et al.* Sequential cardiorespiratory patterns of anesthetic induction with ketamine in critically ill patients. *Crit Care Med* 1983; **11**: 730–734.

67 Jacobson JD, Hartsfield SM. Cardiovascular effects of intravenous bolus administration and infusion of ketamine–midazolam in isoflurane-anesthetized dogs. *Am J Vet Res* 1993; **54**: 1715–1720.

68 Joshi GP, Warner DS, Twersky RS, *et al.* A comparison of remifentanil and fentanyl adverse effect profile in a multicenter phase IV study. *J Clin Anesth* 2002; **14**: 494–499.

69 Nosier RK, Ficke DJ, Kundu A, *et al.* Sympathetic and vascular consequences from remifentanil in humans. *Anesth Analg* 2003; **96**: 1645–1650.

70 Allweiler S, Broadbelt DC, Borer K, *et al.* The isoflurane-sparing and clinical effects of a constant rate infusion of remifentanil in dogs. *Vet Anaesth Analg* 2007; **34**: 388–393.

71 Overgaard CB, Dzavik V. Inotropes and vasopressors. Review of physiology and clinical use in cardiovascular disease. *Circulation* 2008; **118**: 1047–1056.

72 Walsh M, Devereaux PJ, Garg AX, *et al.* Relationship between intraoperative mean arterial pressure and clinical outcomes after noncardiac surgery: towards an empirical definition of hypotension. *Anesthesiology* 2013; **119**: 507–515.

73 Marik PE, Baram M, Vahid B. Does central venous pressure predict fluid responsiveness? A systematic review of the literature and the tale of seven mares. *Chest* 2008; **134**: 172–178.

74 Aarnes TK, Bednarski RM, Lerche P, *et al.* Effect of intravenous administration of lactated Ringer's solution or hetastarch for the treatment of isoflurane-induced hypotension in dogs. *Am J Vet Res* 2009; **70**: 1345–1353.

75 Valverde, A, Gianotti G, Rioja-Garcia E, Hathaway A. Effects of high-volume, rapid-fluid therapy on cardiovascular function and hematological values during isoflurane-induced hypotension in healthy dogs. *Can J Vet Res* 2012; **76**: 99–108.

76 Sinclair MD, Dyson DH. The impact of acepromazine on the efficacy of crystalloid, dextran or ephedrine treatment in hypotensive dogs under isoflurane anesthesia. *Vet Anaesth Analg* 2012; **39**: 563–573.

77 Bone RC, Balk RA, Cerra FB, *et al.* Definitions for sepsis and organ failure and guidelines for the use of innovative therapies in sepsis. The ACCP/SCCM Consensus Conference Committee, American College of Chest Physicians/Society of Critical Care Medicine. *Crit Care Med* 1992; **20**: 864–874.

78 Shoemaker WC, Appel PL, Kram HB. Hemodynamic and oxygen transport responses in survivors and nonsurvivors of high-risk surgery. *Crit Care Med* 1983; **21**: 977–990.

79 Shoemaker WC, Appel P, Blamd R. Use of physiologic monitoring to predict outcome and to assist in clinical decision in critically ill postoperative patients. *Am J Surg* 1983; **146**: 43–50.

80 Wo CC, Shoemaker WE, Appel PL, *et al.* Unreliability of blood pressure and heart rate to evaluate cardiac output in emergency resuscitation and critical illness. *Crit Care Med* 1993; **21**: 218–223.

81 Rivers E, Nguyen B, Havstad S, *et al.* Early goal-directed therapy in the treatment of severe sepsis and septic shock. *N Engl J Med* 2001; **345**: 1368–1377.

82 Dellinger RP, Carlet JM, Masur H, *et al.* Surviving Sepsis Campaign: guidelines for management of severe sepsis and septic shock. *Crit Care Med* 2004; **32**: 858–873.

83 Dellinger RP, Levy MM, Carlet JM, *et al.* Surviving Sepsis Campaign: international guidelines for management of severe sepsis and septic shock. *Crit Care Med* 2008; **36**: 296–327.

84 Bouglé A, Harrois A, Duranteau J. Resuscitative strategies in traumatic hemorrhagic shock. *Ann Intensive Care* 2013; **3**: 1.

85 The National Heart, Lung, and Blood Institute Acute Respiratory Distress Syndrome (ARDS) Clinical Trials Network. Comparison of two fluid-management strategies in acute lung injury. *N Engl J Med* 2006; **354**: 2564–2575.

86 Mapstone J, Roberts I, Evans P. Fluid resuscitation strategies: a systematic review of animal trials. *J Trauma* 2003; **55**: 571–589.

87 Perel P, Roberts I. Colloids versus crystalloids for fluid resuscitation in critically ill patients. *Cochrane Database Syst Rev* 2011; (3): CD000567; update: Perel P, Roberts I, Ker K. *Cochrane Database Syst Rev* 2013; (2): CD000567.

88 Groeneveld AB, Navickis RJ, Wilkes MM. Update on the comparative safety of colloids: a systematic review of clinical studies. *Ann Surg* 2011; **253**: 470–483.

89 Choi SJ, Ahn HJ, Chung SS, *et al.* Hemostatic and electrolyte effects of hydroxyethyl starches in patients undergoing posterior lumbar interbody fusion using pedicle screws and cages. *Spine* 2010; **35**: 829–834.

90 Brunkhorst FM, Engel C, Bloos F, *et al.* Intensive insulin therapy and pentastarch resuscitation in severe sepsis. *N Engl J Med* 2008; **358**: 125–139.

91 Perner A, Haase N, Guttormsen AB, *et al.* Hydroxyethyl starch 130/0/42 versus Ringer's acetate in severe sepsis. *N Engl J Med* 2012; **367**: 124–134.

92 Finfer S, Bellomo R, Boyce N, *et al.* A comparison of albumin and saline for fluid resuscitation in the intensive care unit. *N Engl J Med* 2004; **350**: 2247–2256.

93 Mathews KA, Barry M. The use of 25% human serum albumin: outcome and efficacy in raising serum albumin and systemic blood pressure in critically ill dogs and cats. *J Vet Emerg Crit Care* 2005; **15**: 110–118.

94 Cohn LA, Kerl ME, Lenox CE, *et al.* Response of healthy dogs to infusions of human serum albumin. *Am J Vet Res* 2007; **68**: 657–663.

95 Martin LG, Luther TY, Alperin DC, *et al.* Serum antibodies against human albumin in critically ill and healthy dogs. *J Am Vet Med Assoc* 2008; **232**: 1004–1009.

SECTION 5

Respiratory System

27 Physiology, Pathophysiology, and Anesthetic Management of Patients with Respiratory Disease

Wayne N. McDonell and Carolyn L. Kerr

Department of Clinical Studies, Ontario Veterinary College, University of Guelph, Guelph, Ontario, Canada

Chapter contents

Introduction

Maintenance of adequate respiratory function is a prime requirement for safe anesthesia. Inadequate tissue oxygenation may lead to an acute cessation of vital organ function, especially of the brain or myocardium, and an anesthetic fatality. Excessive elevations in arterial carbon dioxide (CO_2) tensions [arterial CO_2 partial pressure ($PaCO_2$)] or sustained moderate hypoxemia may produce some level of organ dysfunction, which contributes to a less than optimum postanesthetic recovery. Delayed recovery of consciousness, postanesthetic myopathy in large animals, and postanesthetic renal, hepatic, or cardiac insufficiency can all originate from inadequate respiratory function during anesthesia.

During general anesthesia, there is always a tendency for arterial oxygen tensions [arterial oxygen partial pressure (PaO_2)] to be less than observed with the same species while conscious and breathing the same fraction of inspired-oxygen (F_IO_2) [1–5]. There is also a tendency for $PaCO_2$ to be elevated above the conscious resting values if the anesthetized animal is breathing spontaneously, and for increases in airway resistance to occur unless an endotracheal tube is used. Some differences are seen depending on the actual anesthetic regimen used, but the depth of anesthesia is often more of a factor. Species and breed differences exist, and some of these are illustrated in this chapter. Positioning during anesthesia, concurrent drug use, and the magnitude of preanesthetic cardiorespiratory dysfunction all affect respiratory function.

Respiratory dysfunction during general anesthesia and the postoperative period is caused by the disruption of many physiologic mechanisms and, in the larger species especially, an exaggeration of anatomic and mechanical factors [1,4]. An understanding of respiratory function as it relates to anesthesia requires consideration of (1) the neural control of respiration and its effect on alveolar ventilation (V_A); (2) the influence of anesthesia on the airway, chest wall, and lung volumes; and (3) the alterations in ventilation–perfusion (V/Q) relationships during anesthesia [2–5].

It is assumed that readers are already reasonably knowledgeable regarding basic pulmonary physiology, which is considered in detail elsewhere [5,6]. The review by Robinson is particularly useful for undergraduate readers [6]. Much of the information that is

Veterinary Anesthesia and Analgesia: The Fifth Edition of Lumb and Jones.
Edited by Kurt A. Grimm, Leigh A. Lamont, William J. Tranquilli, Stephen A. Greene and Sheilah A. Robertson.

available about the effects of anesthesia on respiration comes from studies in humans, and this information is summarized in a recent review at a level of complexity suitable for individuals in a specialist training program [5]. There are important differences, however, in the manner by which veterinarians generally administer anesthetics to animals compared with anesthesia of people. In veterinary practice, intravenous anesthetics are often used without oxygen supplementation, at least under field conditions. There is much less use of peripheral-acting muscle relaxants in veterinary anesthesia and, generally, intermittent positive-pressure ventilation (IPPV) is used on an 'as needed' rather than routine basis. During general anesthesia with inhalants, 100% oxygen is usually used as the carrier gas, whereas a 2:1 mixture of air, nitrogen, or nitrous oxide with oxygen is commonly used as the carrier gas in human anesthesia. Dogs and cats have frequently been used for investigations of neural control and mechanical alterations associated with anesthesia, but often under experimental situations that differ markedly from how anesthetics are administered to clinical patients. In addition, the range of body weight and size and, in many instances, unique physiologic adaptations of domestic and non-domestic animals undergoing anesthesia mean that the respiratory response to anesthesia may well be different from that classically described for people.

Definitions

Respiration is the total process whereby oxygen is supplied to and used by body cells and CO_2 is eliminated by means of gradients. *Ventilation* is the movement of gas in and out of alveoli. The ventilatory requirement for homeostasis varies with the metabolic requirement of animals, and it therefore varies with body size, level of activity, body temperature, and depth of anesthesia. Pulmonary ventilation is accomplished by expansion and contraction of the lungs. Several terms are used to describe the various types of breathing that may be observed:

1 *Eupnea* is ordinary, quiet breathing.
2 *Dyspnea* is labored breathing.
3 *Tachypnea* is increased respiratory rate.
4 *Hyperpnea* is fast and/or deep respiration, indicating 'over-respiration.'
5 *Polypnea* is a rapid, shallow, panting type of respiration.
6 *Bradypnea* is slow, regular respiration.
7 *Hypopnea* is slow and/or shallow breathing, possibly indicating 'under-respiration.'
8 *Apnea* is transient (or longer) cessation of breathing.
9 *Cheyne–Stokes respirations* increase in rate and depth, and then become slower, followed by a brief period of apnea.
10 *Biot's respirations* are sequences of gasps, apnea, and several deep gasps.
11 *Kussmaul's respirations* are regular, deep respirations without pause.
12 *Apneustic respiration* occurs when an animal holds an inspired breath at the end of inhalation for a short period before exhaling.

To describe the events of pulmonary ventilation, air in the lung has been subdivided into four different volumes and four different capacities (Fig. 27.1). Only tidal volume and functional residual capacity can be measured in conscious uncooperative animals:

1 *Tidal volume* (V_T) is the volume of air inspired or expired in one breath.
2 *Inspiratory reserve volume* (IRV) is the volume of air that can be inspired over and above the normal tidal volume.
3 *Expiratory reserve volume* (ERV) is the amount of air that can be expired by forceful expiration after a normal expiration.
4 *Residual volume* (RV) is the air remaining in the lungs after the most forceful expiration.

Another term frequently used is the minute respiratory volume or *minute ventilation* (V_{Emin}), which is equal to V_T times the *respiratory frequency* (*f*). Occasionally, it is desirable to consider two or more of the aforementioned volumes together. Such combinations are termed pulmonary capacities:

1 *Inspiratory capacity* (IC) is the tidal volume plus the inspiratory reserve volume. This is the amount of air that can be inhaled starting after a normal expiration and distending the lungs to the maximum amount.
2 *Functional residual capacity* (FRC) is the expiratory reserve volume plus the residual volume. This is the amount of air remaining in the lungs after a normal expiration. From a mechanical viewpoint, at FRC the inward 'pull' of the lungs due to their elasticity equals the outward 'pull' of the chest wall.

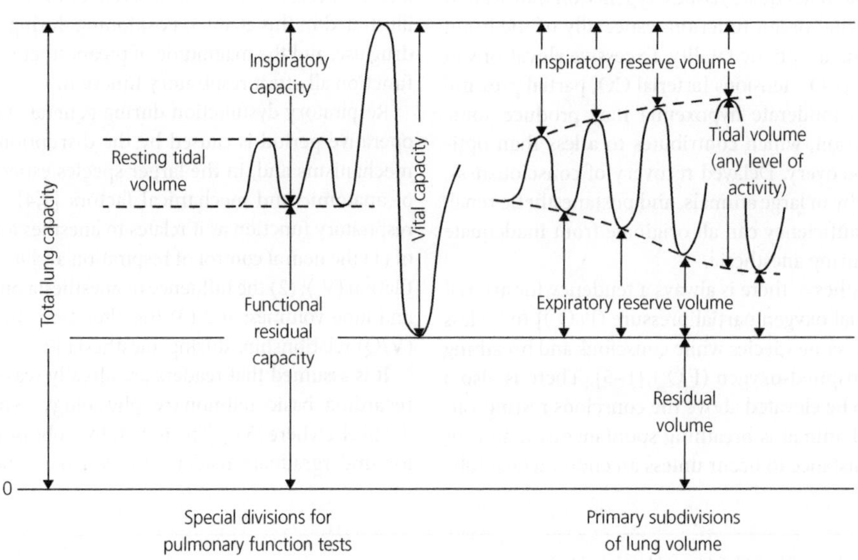

Figure 27.1 Lung volumes and capacities. Only tidal volume and functional residual capacity can be measured in conscious animals since the other measurements require cooperation of the subject being studied or general anesthesia.

3 *Vital capacity* (VC) is the inspiratory reserve volume plus the tidal volume plus the expiratory reserve volume. This is the maximum amount of air that can be expelled from the lungs after first filling them to their maximum capacity.
4 *Total lung capacity* (TLC) is the inspiratory reserve volume plus the tidal volume plus the expiratory reserve volume plus the residual volume, or the maximum volume to which the lungs can be expanded with the greatest possible inspiratory effort (or by full inflation to 30 cmH_2O airway pressure when a patient is anesthetized).

Respiratory function in conscious normal animals

From an anesthetist's viewpoint, it is useful to consider the respiratory system in terms of its major components: neural control, the bellows mechanism (chest wall and diaphragm), upper airway, and lung parenchyma (Fig. 27.2). Alterations of (1) the neural control of ventilation by sedative, opioid, or anesthetic depression; (2) upper airway or lower airway patency by muscle relaxation or spasm; or (3) the bellows mechanism of the thorax through neuromuscular paralysis, space-occupying lesions of the thorax, or a change in the diaphragm shape, location, or function may all appreciably affect ventilation adequacy and the efficiency of gas exchange. Within the parenchyma, less than optimum matching of fresh alveolar gas with pulmonary capillary blood will produce blood-gas alterations, particularly with regard to PaO_2.

Control of respiration

With the aid of the circulation, respiration regulates the oxygen, CO_2, and hydrogen ion environment of the cell. Respiratory function is controlled by central respiratory centers, central and peripheral chemoreceptors, pulmonary reflexes, and non-respiratory neural input. Control of respiration has been described as an integrated feedback control system [6]. The central neural 'controller' includes specialized groups of neurons located in the cerebrum, brainstem, and spinal cord that govern both voluntary and automatic ventilation through regulation of the activity of the respiratory muscles. The respiratory muscles by contracting produce alveolar ventilation, and changes in alveolar ventilation affect blood-gas tensions and hydrogen ion concentration. Blood-gas tensions and hydrogen ion concentrations are monitored by peripheral and central chemoreceptors that return signals to the central controller to provide necessary adjustments in ventilation. Mechanoreceptors in the lungs and stretch receptors in the respiratory muscles monitor, respectively, the degree of expansion or stretch of the lungs and the 'effort' of breathing, feeding back information to the central controller to alter the pattern of breathing. Adjustments also occur

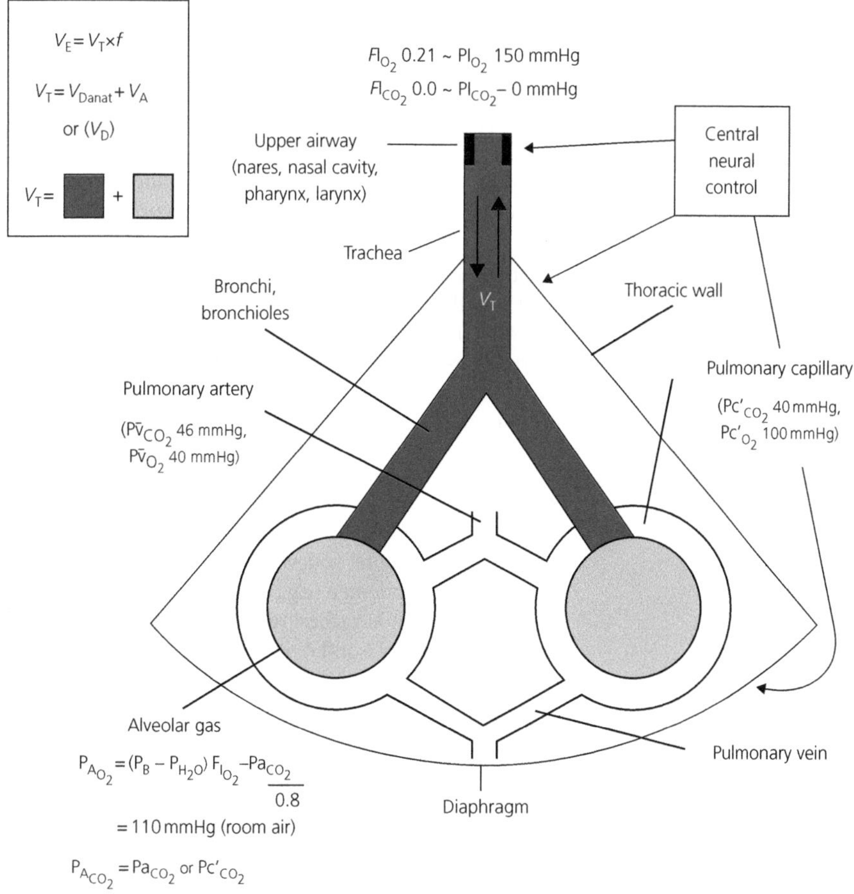

Figure 27.2 Diagrammatic representation of the neural control, bellows mechanism (diaphragm and thoracic wall), and matching of pulmonary artery blood and alveolar gas in the lung. Tidal volume (V_T), anatomic deadspace (V_{Danat}) (colored dark blue), alveolar ventilation (V_A) (colored light blue), and representative inspired (P_I), alveolar (P_A), and end-capillary (Pc') partial pressures of oxygen and carbon dioxide are also illustrated. See the text for a detailed explanation.

to accommodate non-respiratory activities such as thermoregulation and vocalization.

Overall, this complex control system produces a combination of respiratory frequency and depth that is best suited for optimum ventilation with minimal effort for the particular species, and that adjusts oxygen supply and CO_2 elimination so as to maintain homeostasis (reflected by stable arterial blood-gas levels) over a wide range of environmental and metabolic conditions. Sedatives, analgesics, anesthetics, and the equipment used for inhalational anesthesia may profoundly alter respiration and the ability of an animal to maintain cellular homeostasis. The alteration of respiratory control with anesthetics and perianesthetic agents is considered in more detail later in this chapter.

Mechanical factors

Transfer of gases to and from the lungs depends on developing a pressure gradient between the atmosphere and the alveoli, and is modified by the resistance to flow between these two regions and the elasticity of the lungs and chest wall. With spontaneous respiration, during inspiration active muscular effort serves to enlarge the pleural cavity through expansion of the thoracic wall and contraction of the diaphragm (Fig. 27.2). Intrapleural pressure is thereby reduced to a more subatmospheric pressure, and a mouth/nostril–alveolar pressure gradient is established. In contrast to inspiration, expiration is normally passive and depends on the return of the chest wall and lungs to a resting position, that is, to FRC. The horse is a notable exception in that abdominal muscle contraction plays a part in normal expiratory activity, producing a biphasic mode of exhalation [4,6]. As the size of the pleural space decreases, intrapleural and consequently alveolar pressures are elevated, and the pressure gradient is reversed so that air flows from the alveoli to the atmosphere. Thus, fluctuating pressure gradients between the atmosphere and the alveoli cause air to flow in and out of the lungs. The factors that contribute to these pressure gradients and the measurement of their magnitude are referred to as *pulmonary mechanics.*

During assisted or controlled artificial or mechanical ventilation, atmospheric to alveolar pressure gradients also occur, but mouth pressure is more positive than alveolar pressure on inspiration: hence the term *positive-pressure ventilation*. This has important circulatory consequences which will be considered in more detail later. Both the lungs and chest wall provide an elastic resistance to expansion on inspiration. The relationship between the pressure gradient (P) and the resultant volume (V) increase in liters (L) of the lungs and thorax is known as *total compliance* (C_T) [5,7]:

$$C_T\left(\mathrm{L/cmH_2O}\right)=\frac{\Delta V(\mathrm{L})}{\Delta P\left(\mathrm{cmH_2O}\right)}$$

The relationship of C_T to the individual compliance of the lungs (C_L) and chest wall (C_{CW}) is additive, because the lungs and chest wall are arranged concentrically and can be expressed as

$$\frac{1}{C_T}=\frac{1}{C_L}+\frac{1}{C_{CW}}$$

To measure C_T, V and the transthoracic pressure (that is, the pressure at the alveolus minus ambient pressure) must be known. In anesthetized animals, this is often estimated by measuring the inspiratory volume delivered from a ventilator bellows or rebreathing bag while recording the change in airway (taken to be alveolar) pressure between end-exhalation and end-inspiration. In recent years, automated spirometry systems using in-line gas flow measurement devices and side-stream gas analysis have made breath-by-breath monitoring of respiratory mechanics feasible during clinical anesthesia, at least when mechanical ventilation is being used [7]. These monitoring systems require flow sensors that remain accurate despite humidity and water vapor changes and that produce a linear response over the V_T being measured: hence different sensors are needed for small, middle-sized and large animals. The monitoring devices are generally capable of providing either flow/volume or pressure/volume loops over the course of each tidal volume, or sequential values for compliance and airway resistance. They therefore provide useful comparative data over the course of an anesthetic. The compliance values they provide are usually a measure of the lung and chest wall elasticity combined.

Dynamic C_T is the volume change divided by the transthoracic pressure change at the point of zero airflow (end inspiration) at a time when the previous inflow of air has been sufficiently rapid for dynamic factors to influence the distribution of air throughout the lung. For practical purposes, dynamic C_T is equal to the tidal volume divided by the peak airway pressure. *Static* C_T is determined when the preceding inflow of air has been sufficiently slow for distribution throughout the lung to be solely in accord with regional elasticity. Under these conditions, gas distribution to alveoli with faster and slower filling rates is equivalent, and as a result the static C_T (or C_L) value is usually greater than dynamic C_T (or C_L).

To determine the elasticity of the lung *per se* (C_L), V and the transpulmonary pressure gradient (that is, pressure at the alveolus minus pressure at the pleural space) must be known. This measurement is harder to determine accurately. In practice, the transpulmonary pressure gradient is generally determined by using a differential pressure transducer to determine mouth (considered equal to alveolar) and pleural pressure changes simultaneously. Pleural pressure changes are estimated from intrathoracic esophageal pressure swings recorded with a balloon-tipped catheter. Lungs develop a low compliance (become stiffer) with a reduction in lung volume or regional atelectasis; as a result of pulmonary edema or fibrosis, and, in the case of dynamic C_L, with regional differences in airway resistance.

If the lungs and/or chest wall are less compliant (i.e., stiffer), then higher transthoracic pressures are required to deliver a given tidal volume. Experienced anesthetists can often sense this change as an increased force required to squeeze mechanically a set volume from a rebreathing bag by hand. This may provide the first clue that an animal is developing a space-occupying problem in the thorax or abdomen (e.g., accumulation of air or blood), or that the end of the endotracheal tube has become repositioned in one main bronchus and is inflating only one lung.

For air to flow into the lungs, a pressure gradient must also be developed to overcome the non-elastic (airway) resistance to airflow. The relationship between the pressure gradient across the pulmonary system (P_L) and the rate of airflow (usually expressed in liters per second, L/s) is known as *airway resistance* (R_L) (expressed in $\mathrm{cmH_2O/L/s}$) [5–7]:

$$R_L\left(\mathrm{cmH_2O/L/s}\right)=\Delta P_L\left(\mathrm{cmH_2O/L/s}\right)$$

The caliber of the airway and the rate and pattern of airflow all contribute to the pressure gradient along the airway. According to the Hagen–Poiseuille law, for laminar gas flow through a tube the resistance to flow can be expressed as

$$\text{resistance to flow}\left(\text{cmH}_2\text{O/L/s}\right)=\frac{8\times\text{fluid or air viscosity}\times\text{tube length}}{\left(\text{tube radius}\right)^4}$$

The significance of this equation relative to anesthesia is to realize that changes in airway (or apparatus) diameter may markedly affect the resistance to airflow. For instance, if the diameter of the airway is reduced by 50% by using too small an endotracheal tube, the resistance increases 16-fold.

At higher flow rates that exceed the critical velocity of the system, or in the face of sudden changes in airway diameter, airflow will no longer be laminar and becomes turbulent. The significance of a transition from laminar to turbulent flow is illustrated by the fact that, at rates approximating critical flow, the resistance to flow increases by about 50% if the flow becomes turbulent. Airway resistance is measured by a variety of methods, most of which involve the simultaneous determination of instantaneous airflow with a pneumotachograph and of transpulmonary pressure (P_L) using a differential transducer.

Airway resistance increases with the rate of respiration and with narrowing of the airway by reflex contraction of the bronchiolar muscles, with small airway disease where there is edema of the airway wall and mucous accumulation, with a reduction in lung volume, or through aspiration of foreign material. Airway resistance during anesthesia can be minimized by using an airway that is as wide as possible and in which sudden alterations in direction or diameter are minimized. Increases in inspiratory airway resistance are of far more consequence than increases in expiratory airway resistance, since expiration is normally achieved by the elastic recoil of the lung and chest wall without a requirement for work by the respiratory muscles. This is why there is good tolerance of low levels (2–5 mmHg) of positive end-expiratory pressure (PEEP) whether employed as a means to prevent alveolar collapse or as a consequence of partially closing a pop-off valve to prevent collapse of a rebreathing bag.

Pulmonary ventilation

The important factor in pulmonary ventilation is the rate at which *alveolar air* is exchanged with atmospheric air. This is not equal to the minute ventilation volume because a large portion of inspired air is used to fill the respiratory passages, rather than alveoli, and no significant gaseous exchange occurs in this air (Fig. 27.2). The *respiratory frequency* (f) and volume of each breath, *tidal volume* (V_T), determine the *minute ventilation* (V_{Emin}). The portion of each V_T that reaches only the upper airway and tracheobronchial tree fills the *anatomic deadspace* and is referred to as *deadspace volume* (V_{Danat}). V_{Danat} is fairly constant; therefore, slow, deep breathing is more effective than rapid, shallow breathing. This is especially so during general anesthesia and with IPPV. The 'effective' volume, or the portion of V_T that contributes to gas exchange, is the *alveolar volume* (V_A), usually referred to as *minute alveolar ventilation* (V_{Amin}). There is some mixing between the gas in the anatomic deadspace and the alveolar gas due to the movement created by the beating heart [5]. This 'mixing' action probably explains why $PaCO_2$ levels are usually not all that elevated in smaller dogs or cats showing a very shallow tachypneic breathing pattern wherein V_T must be near V_{Danat}. It probably also explains why in an emergency situation insufflation of 15 L/min oxygen deep into the trachea in an apneic horse will maintain PaO_2 values in the 50–60 mmHg range (personal observation).

Non-perfused alveoli do not contribute to gas exchange and constitute the *alveolar deadspace* (V_{Dalv}). In conscious healthy animals, V_{Dalv} is minimal, whereas during general anesthesia it may increase owing to a fall in cardiac output (Q) and/or pulmonary artery blood pressure. *Physiological deadspace* (V_D) includes V_{Danat} and V_{Dalv} (Fig. 27.2), and is usually expressed as a minute value (V_{Dmin}) along with V_{Amin}, or as the ratio V_D/V_T. In unsedated tracheostomized dogs breathing quietly through a standard endotracheal tube, V_D was 5.9 mL/kg and V_D/V_T was 35% [8]. This V_D/V_T ratio is similar to that found in humans, but the V_D value is larger, reflecting the increased V_{Danat} in dogs on a body-weight basis. During methoxyflurane anesthesia with spontaneous respiration, V_D increased very little (about 0.5 mL/kg), but V_D/V_T increased to over 50% because V_T decreased. Others have reported similar results with other anesthetics. In larger species such as horses and cows, the V_D/V_T ratio in conscious animals is about 50% [9]. Higher proportions of deadspace have been reported, but such values probably reflect a tachypneic state or failure to subtract the added deadspace associated with the use of the mask in gas collection. In unsedated cows V_D is about 3.7 mL/kg and in horses about 5.2 mL/kg [9]. Representative normal ventilation, blood-gas, and acid–base values for a range of species are given in Tables 27.1 and 27.2.

Lung volumes

The subdivisions of lung volume are shown in Fig. 27.1. Most of these volumes cannot be measured in conscious animals, because to do so requires cooperation of the test subject. Measurements of V_T and FRC can be obtained in conscious animals; TLC is generally estimated by inflation of the lung to above 30 cmH_2O inflation pressure in anesthetized animals. Values for TLC are reasonably similar among the domestic species when compared on a body-weight basis, but the total volume varies from less than 2.0 mL in mice to over 45 L in horses and cows (Table 27.3). This factor and the variation in V_T observed across species (Table 27.1) have significant implications relative to the design of suitable inhalant anesthetic apparatus and the relative importance of added mechanical deadspace. One liter of apparatus deadspace in a healthy conscious horse or cow constitutes only a small proportion of the V_T and has little effect on V_A or blood gases [38], whereas a deadspace of even 15 mL in a cat amounts to 50% of V_T and will likely alter alveolar ventilation and $PaCO_2$ levels. In the smallest mammals, virtually all mask systems will lead to some rebreathing of CO_2 during anesthesia, unless a loose-fitting mask is used with a flow-through system.

The volume of gas remaining in the lungs at the end of a normal expiration (that is, the FRC) varies considerably as the position of the diaphragm, in particular, changes. Abdominal tympany from any source (e.g., near-term gravid uterus, bowel distension, obesity, or tumor) will tend to move the diaphragm forward and lessen the FRC. Few actual measurements have been made of this phenomenon in relation to animals, but the consequences for ventilation and respiratory function during anesthesia are consistent with a decrease in FRC [36,37].

Intrapulmonary matching of blood and gas

Matching of alveolar gas and pulmonary capillary blood flow is influenced by gravitational factors and by the pulmonary artery circulation being a low-pressure system. Intrapleural pressure is more subatmospheric in the uppermost part of the thorax than in the lowermost portion [39], partly because of the weight of the lung in

Table 27.1 Breathing frequency (*f*), tidal volume (V_T), and minute ventilation ($\dot{V}_E$) for various species.

Species	Mean Body Wt (kg)	*n*	Conditions[a]	*f* (breaths/min)	V_T		$\dot{V}_E$		Ref.
					mL	mL/kg	mL/min	mL/kg/min	
Mice	0.02	NS	Awake, prone	163.4	0.15	7.78	24.5	1239	10
	0.032	NS	Anesthetized	109	0.18	5.63	21.0	720	10
Rats	0.113	NS	Awake, prone	85.5	0.87	7.67	72.9	646	10
	0.305	NS	Awake, pleth	103	2.08	6.83	213	701	10
Cats	3.8	4	Unanesthetized, pleth	22	30	7.9	664	174	11
	3.7	NS	Anesthetized	30	34	9.2	960	310	10
Dogs	18.6	6	Awake, prone, chronic trach, intubated	13	309	16.6	3818	205	12
	18.8	8	Awake, standing, chronic trach, intubated	16.5	314	16.9	4963	264	8
Sheep	32–37	4	Awake, standing, mask	38	289	8.3	10400	297	13
Goats	36.3	3	Awake, standing, mask	13.6	470	12.9	6313	174	14
Pigs	46.4	6	Awake, standing, mask	26	483	10.4	11900	256	15
	47.6	6	Awake, standing, mask	17.6	602	12.6	10540	221	16
	12.9	4	Awake, standing	13.1	209	15.9	2731	208	17
Cows	517 Holstein	7	Awake, standing, mask	23.7	3676	7.1	85977	166	9
	405 Jersey	11	Awake, standing, mask	28.6	3360	8.3	94870	234	18
Calves	43–73 Hereford	8	4–6 weeks old, standing, sling	26.7	403	15.1	10290	385	19
Horses	402	6	Awake, standing, mask	11.8	4253	10.6	49466	123	9
	483	6	Awake, standing, mask	15.5	4860	10.1	74600	154	20
	486	15	Awake, standing, mask (some sedated) (mask V_D not removed)	10	7300	15.0	79000	163	21
Ponies	147	19	Awake, standing, mask	19.0	1370	9.3	26380	180	22

NS, not specified.
[a]pleth, whole-body plethysmograph; trach, tracheostomy.

Table 27.2 Arterial blood-gas and acid–base values for various species.

Species	Body Wt (kg)	*n*	Conditions	pHa	$PaCO_2$ (mmHg)	PaO_2 (mmHg)	HCO_3^- (mEq/L)	Ref.
Rats	0.207	10	Awake, chronic catheter	7.44	32.7		21.5	23
	0.305	8	Awake, prone, chronic catheter	7.467	39.8		28.7	24
Rabbits	3.1	NS	Awake, catheter	7.388	32.8	86	21	25
	3.5	20	Awake, catheter	7.47	28.5	89.2	20.2	26
Cats	2.5–5.1	8	Unsedated, chronic catheter, prone	7.41	28.0	108	18	27
	3–8	10	Unsedated, not restrained, chronic catheter	7.426	32.5	108	22.1	28
Dogs	18.8	8	Chronic tracheostomy, catheter, unsedated, standing	7.383	39.0	103.8	22.1	8
	12.2	22	Chronic catheters, lateral recumbency	7.40	35	102	21	29
Sheep	33	NS	Awake, catheter	7.44	40.9	96	27.6	25
	24.5	11	Unsedated, prone, carotid loop	7.48	33	92		30
Goats	18	6	Unsedated, standing	7.46	36.5	101		14
	47.6	6	Unsedated, standing, catheter	7.45	35.3	94.5	24.1	16
	46.6	6	Unsedated, standing	7.45	41.1	87.1	27.6	15
Calves	31–57	4	Standing, unsedated, aortic catheter	7.39	40	81	24	31
	48–66	20	Unanesthetized, catheter	7.37	42.8	93.6	23.6	32
Cows	517	7	Awake, unsedated, standing	7.40	39.6	83.1	24.4	9
	641	7	Awake, unsedated, standing	7.435	38.7	95.1	25.5	[a]
Horses	402	6	Awake, unsedated, standing	7.39	41.1	80.7	24.5	9
Ponies	147	19	Standing, aortic catheter	7.40	40	88.7	24.4	22

NS, not specified.
[a]R. Warren and W.N. McDonell, unpublished observations.

the thorax. Alveolar size is largest in the uppermost areas of the lung and smallest in the ventral regions. Since the larger alveoli have a lower compliance (they are less distensible), they expand less on inspiration, and air preferentially enters the more compliant lower alveoli, producing a vertical gradient of ventilation in standing animals breathing quietly [40–42]. This tendency for preferential ventral ventilation in the lung may also be associated with regional chest wall and diaphragmatic movement. During anesthesia, the distribution of ventilation becomes more uneven and may even reverse so that the uppermost lung of a laterally recumbent horse is receiving most of the ventilation.

For many years, it was believed that gravity was a primary determinant of pulmonary blood flow, producing a vertical perfusion gradient of blood flow with the lower lung regions being perfused more, and that this situation was present in both conscious and anesthetized animals and also both biped and quadruped species [42,43]. However,

Table 27.3 Lung volumes for various mammalian species.

Species	Body Wt (kg)	*n*	Conditions	TLC		FRC (mL/kg)	RV (mL/kg)	Ref.
				mL	mL/kg			
Mice	0.020	NS	Anesthetized	1.57	78.5	25.0	19.5	10
Rats	0.31	NS	Anesthetized, prone	12.2	39.4	6.8	4.2	10
Rabbits	3.14	NS	Anesthetized, supine	111	35.4	11.6	6.4	10
Cats	3.7	4	Anesthetized			17.8		33
Dogs	18.6	6	Awake, prone	2090	112.4	53.6	16.7	12
	9.2	140	Unsedated, 1 year old			44.8		34
Sheep	24.5	4	Unsedated, prone, nasal endotracheal tube			45.3		30
Goats	46.4	6	Unsedated, standing, face mask			49.6		15
Cows	517	7	Awake, standing			39.4		35
	537	5	Anesthetized, prone	45377	84.5	31.9	16.1	35
Horses	485		Anesthetized, prone	44800	92.4	36.3	19.0	36
	402	6	Awake, standing			51.3		35
	394	4	Anesthetized, prone, lung inflated to 35–40 cmH_2O, starved 18 h	45468	115.4	37.9		35
	450–822	6	Conscious, standing			35.6		37
Ponies	164–288	8	Conscious, standing			39.9		37

NS, not specified.

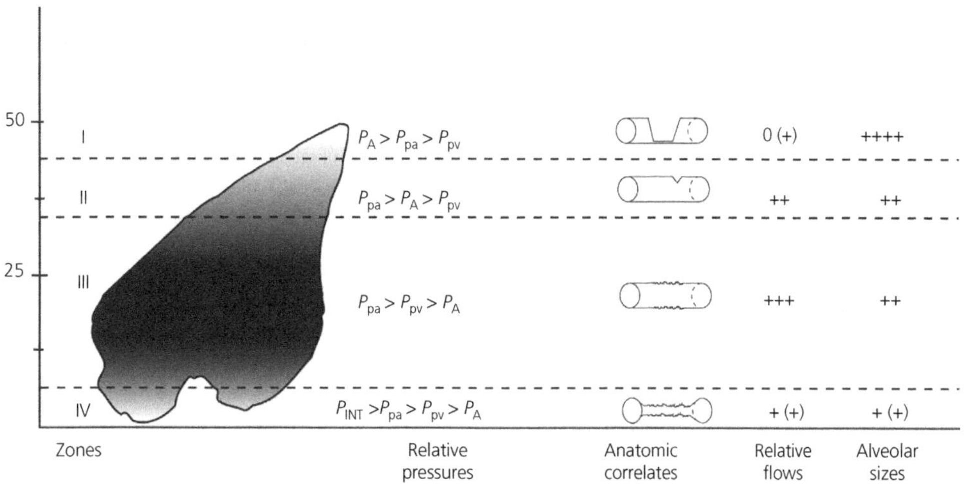

Figure 27.3 Diagrammatic illustration of pulmonary artery (P_{pa}), pulmonary vein (P_{pv}), pulmonary interstitial (P_{INT}), and alveolar (P_A) pressure–flow relationships in the lung. See the text for a detailed explanation. Source: modified from [43]. Reproduced with permission of Taylor & Francis.

more recent investigations suggest that there are other factors such as the branching pattern of the pulmonary artery and regional differences in resistance involved, and that the end result (in quadrupeds at least) is that there is considerable vertical uniformity of blood flow within the lung, or even greater dorsal perfusion [4,44–46].

The distribution of pulmonary blood flow in anesthetized animals is not as well understood and there are conflicting findings depending on the methods employed and the species studied [44,47–50]. General anesthesia, in addition to a change in body position, also produces alterations of cardiac output, drug-induced changes in pulmonary resistance and pulmonary vessel reactivity to hypoxia, and changes in lung volume and regional pleural pressure. These factors may result in gravity becoming a significant factor in the distribution of pulmonary blood flow, especially in lateral and dorsal recumbency in larger animals. Hence it is worth considering the historical gravitation based model of blood flow.

The gravitational effects on distribution of lung perfusion have been commonly divided, and functionally described as a three- or four-zone system [42,43]. At rest, the uppermost alveoli may be minimally perfused (Fig. 27.3, zone I), with alveolar pressure (P_A) greater than pulmonary artery (P_{pa}) and vein (P_{pv}) pressures. In zone II, P_{pa} is greater than P_A, and the difference between the two is the driving pressure for blood flow at the front end of the capillaries. The relationship between P_A and P_{pv} governs flow through the terminal aspect of the capillaries. In zone III, P_{pa} and P_{pv} both exceed P_A, and the vessels are fully distended, with the perfusion being determined by the pressure difference between P_{pa} and P_{pv}. In zone IV, the lung weight increases the interstitial pressure to a point that blood flow is reduced toward that of zone II, or less. These factors are important during anesthesia in that cardiac output is often reduced and P_{pa} may decrease. Until the recent research mentioned above, it was thought that when the body position was altered and an animal became recumbent, pulmonary blood flow would realign along gravitational lines consistent with the new body position [1,42,43]. However, as explained above, these relationships are not necessarily straightforward, especially in the larger species, perhaps because of the large decrease in FRC that accompanies recumbency and the generation of a larger zone IV area in the thorax.

Figure 27.4 provides an illustration of the non-gravitational distribution of blood flow in a halothane-anesthetized dog as measured by the injection of radioactive microspheres while positioned in dorsal (supine) or sternal (prone) body positions [44]. It is evident that there is a low-flow zone (zone IV) near the most dorsal and the most ventral parts of the lung in both sternal and dorsal body positions, and that the dorsal part of the lung receives proportionally more blood flow than the ventral aspect, irrespective of the body position. Similar findings have been presented for sheep and ponies [49,50].

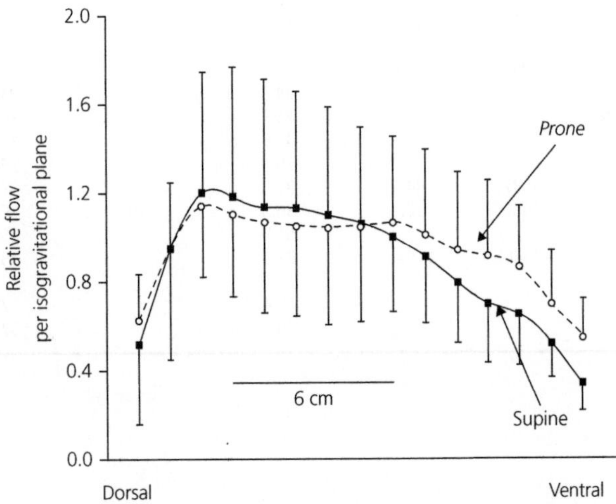

Figure 27.4 Relative pulmonary blood flow per isogravitational plane in a halothane-anesthetized dog while positioned in sternal (prone) or dorsal (supine) recumbency. Note the similarity of the gradient of blood flow in either body position, and the reduction of relative blood flow in the uppermost or lowermost sections of the lung in either body position. The error bars represent the heterogeneity of flow within isogravitational planes. Source: modified from [44]. Reproduced with permission of the American Physiological Society.

A simplified diagrammatic representation of altered *alveolar ventilation in relation to alveolar perfusion* (V/Q) is shown in Fig. 27.5. One extreme is to have a perfused alveolus or area of the lung with no ventilation so that the blood is not oxygenated while passing the region [3]. Other extremes are for the alveolus to be ventilated but not perfused, or alternatively for an alveolus or region to be neither ventilated nor perfused. Often the alteration of V/Q within the lung is somewhere in between these extremes and is characterized by alveoli throughout the lung that are only relatively under-ventilated or under-perfused, producing an increase in the alveolar–arterial oxygen gradient. Since CO_2 is more diffusible across the alveolar capillary membrane, diffusion and V/Q problems commonly lead to decreased PaO_2 levels before there is a change in $PaCO_2$ levels.

It is possible to compensate for non-ventilation of portions of the lung through increased ventilation of the rest of the lung in terms of CO_2 clearance, as occurs with tachypneic, pneumonic animals. However, the same increase in ventilation of 'good' lung areas will never compensate completely for areas where there is inadequate oxygen uptake. The hemoglobin oxygen-saturation curve is sigmoid shaped (Fig. 27.6), and hemoglobin is nearly fully saturated with oxygen at a PaO_2 of 90–100 mmHg. Consequently, an increase in ventilation to the 'good' areas of the lung cannot increase the

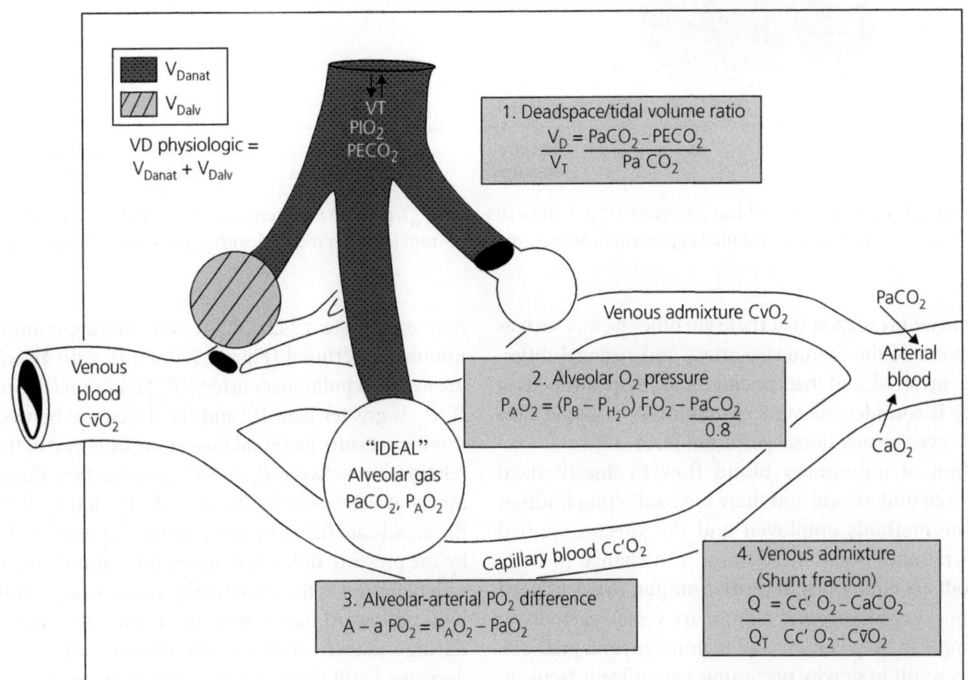

Figure 27.5 Schematic of uneven ventilation and blood flow. The alveolus on the left is ventilated, but not perfused, and hence is considered to be alveolar deadspace, whereas the alveolus on the right is perfused but not ventilated, and thus contributes to venous admixture or so-called shunt flow. The center alveolus is perfused and ventilated equally and thus would have a V/Q ratio of 1.0. Relevant equations are shown as eqns 1–4 for calculation of the deadspace/tidal volume ratio, the alveolar partial pressure of oxygen (P_AO_2), the alveolar-to-arterial partial pressure of oxygen (A – aPO_2) difference, and the venous admixture (Q/Q_T) fraction, respectively. Source: [4]. Reproduced with permission of Elsevier.

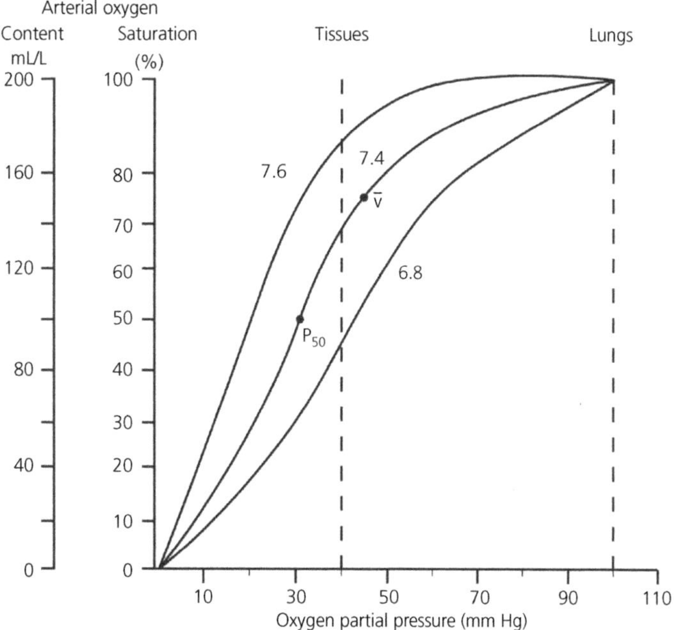

Figure 27.6 Oxygen–hemoglobin dissociation curves. The center curve represents the relationship between the partial pressure of oxygen and the percentage hemoglobin saturation at normal body temperature and blood pH, and shows the arterial partial pressure of oxygen (PaO_2) and percentage saturation as the blood goes through the lungs and tissues. The normal mixed venous PO_2 and the oxygen saturation values are shown ($\bar{v}$) along with the P_{50} value, which is the PO_2 at which the hemoglobin of a particular species is 50% saturated with oxygen. There is a shift of the hemoglobin dissociation curve to the right with acidemia (e.g., pH 6.8) or an increase in temperature, whereas there is a shift to the left with alkalemia (e.g., pH 7.6) or a lower body temperature. The oxygen content values on the left represent the blood oxygen content that would be expected if the hemoglobin concentration was the theoretical normal level of 150 g/L and body temperature and pH levels were also normal.

oxygen content of blood very much, even though the alveolar partial pressure of oxygen (P_AO_2) increases. The clinical significance of this is that many pulmonary problems present as hypoxemia rather than hypercapnia.

Effect of altered alveolar ventilation

For any given metabolic output, $PaCO_2$ and V_A are directly and inversely related: if V_A falls by 50%, $PaCO_2$ doubles; whereas, if V_A is increased by 100% (say, by IPPV), $PaCO_2$ levels will fall by 50% once equilibrium is established (Fig. 27.7). This is an important concept to grasp in that it explains how an experienced anesthetist can make fairly good approximations about the resultant $PaCO_2$ level he or she will produce when an animal is put on a volume-limited ventilator at a particular *f* and V_T setting. For instance, in most anesthetized dogs with a body weight that is average for the breed, $PaCO_2$ will be near eucapnic levels when *f* is set at 8–10/min and V_T at 15–20 mL/kg. In anesthetized adult horses and cows, a comparative eucapnic setting would be *f* at 5/min and V_T at 15 mL/kg.

Hyperventilation occurs when V_A is excessive relative to metabolic rate; as a result, $PaCO_2$ is reduced. Hyperventilation may or may not be accompanied by an increased respiratory rate, referred to as tachypnea. *Hypoventilation* is present when V_A is low relative to metabolic rate, and $PaCO_2$ rises: hypoventilation may be accompanied by a slow (bradypnea), normal, or rapid *f*. A lowered $PaCO_2$ level is referred to as *hypocapnia* and an elevated level as *hypercapnia*, whereas normal $PaCO_2$ is termed *eucapnia*. Most, but not all, of the common mammalian species have a normal resting $PaCO_2$ level close to 40 mmHg (Table 27.2). Hypercapnia and hypocapnia produce *respiratory acidosis* and *alkalosis*, respectively, because CO_2 in the body is in dynamic equilibrium with carbonic acid (H_2CO_3) and, ultimately, hydrogen ion concentration [H^+]:

$$CO_2 + H_20 \rightleftharpoons H_2CO_3 \rightleftharpoons H^+ + HCO_3^-$$

Acidemia and *alkalemia* are defined as a plasma pH significantly below or above, respectively, the normal arterial or venous value for the species in question. Concurrent metabolic acid–base disturbances and the presence or absence of compensation through renal excretion will determine the actual degree of pH change accompanying hypocapnia or hypercapnia. During general anesthesia, hypoventilation and hypercapnia are far more likely to occur in spontaneously breathing animals, whereas hyperventilation and hypocapnia most often occur when tidal volumes are too large in smaller animals during IPPV.

The relationship between V_A and oxygen saturation (and, in turn, the oxygen content of arterial blood) is not linear because of the sigmoid shape of the hemoglobin-saturation curve (Fig. 27.6). This factor has important clinical applications for anesthetists. With a 50% decrease in V_A, hemoglobin is still 80% saturated, and the actual oxygen content of blood (if the hemoglobin concentration is 15 g/dL) will have fallen only from 21.2 to 16.8 mL/dL (Fig. 27.7). Such an animal would not likely demonstrate cyanotic mucous membranes or even cardiovascular signs (tachycardia, bradycardia, or increased/decreased blood pressure) associated with respiratory insufficiency. However, as the level of V_A decreases further, there is a sharp and potentially catastrophic decrease in the oxygen content of arterial blood so that, at a V_A that is 40% of normal, hemoglobin saturation is 50% and the oxygen content has decreased to 7.04 mL/dL. This degree of hypoxemia may well lead to sudden cardiorespiratory

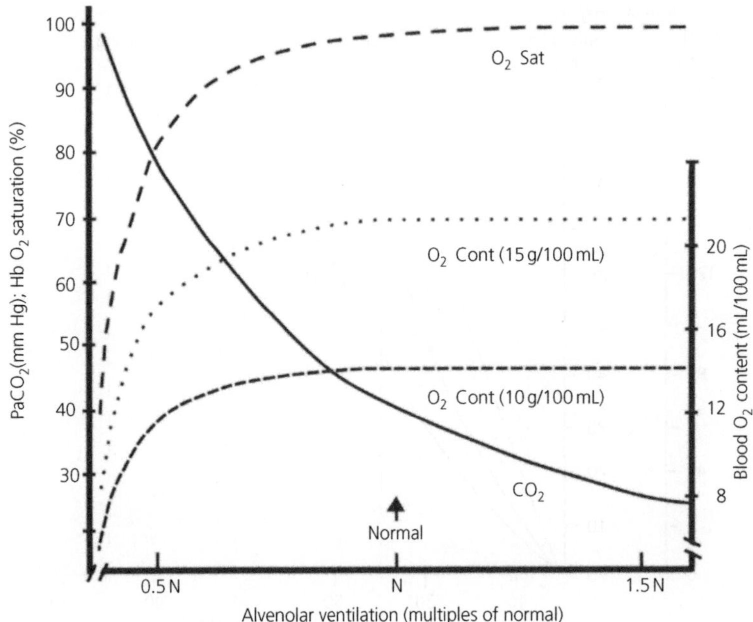

Figure 27.7 Effect of altered alveolar ventilation on hemoglobin saturation, blood oxygen content, and arterial carbon dioxide ($PaCO_2$) levels. As alveolar ventilation is halved, the $PaCO_2$ level doubles, illustrating the inverse and direct relationship between alveolar ventilation and carbon dioxide clearance. Note the difference in oxygen content with anemia (hemoglobin 10 g/100 mL instead of 15 g/100 mL), and the eventual sharp decrease in hemoglobin oxygen saturation and oxygen content as alveolar ventilation decreases to less than 50% of the normal value. See the text for further explanation.

collapse. An understanding of this non-linear effect of V_A deficiency on oxygen content helps to explain why an apparently 'O.K.' animal on an intravenous general anesthetic and breathing room air can suddenly stop breathing or go into cardiovascular collapse without any apparent change in the depth of anesthesia.

Figure 27.7 illustrates the important interrelationship between a lower hemoglobin level (e.g., 10 g/dL) and blood oxygen content with altered ventilation homeostasis. The blood oxygen content is reduced by nearly 7 mL/dL with a decrease in hemoglobin from 15 to 10 g/dL, even when hemoglobin saturation is 100%, and dangerously low blood oxygen contents occur with further ventilation depression.

Hypoxia refers to any state in which the oxygen in the lung, blood, and/or tissues is abnormally low, resulting in abnormal organ function and/or cellular damage. *Hypoxemia* refers to insufficient oxygenation of blood to meet metabolic requirements. In spontaneously breathing animals, hypoxemia is characterized by PaO_2 levels lower than the normal for the species. Resting PaO_2 levels in domestic species generally range from 80 to 100 mmHg in healthy, awake animals (Table 27.2). Some clinicians consider a PaO_2 below 70 mmHg (~94% hemoglobin saturation) as hypoxemia in animals at or near sea level, although the clinical significance of this degree of blood oxygen tension would vary depending on factors such as the health and age of the animal, hemoglobin concentration, and the duration of low oxygen tension in relation to the rate of tissue metabolism (e.g., hypothermic patients would be at less risk).

Oxygen transport

Under normal conditions, oxygen is taken into the pulmonary alveoli and CO_2 is removed from them at a rate that is sufficient to maintain the composition of alveolar air at a relatively constant concentration of gases. In the lung, gas is exchanged across both the alveolar and the capillary membranes [4,6]. The total distance across which exchange takes place is less than 1 μm; therefore, it occurs rapidly. Other than at high exercise levels, equilibrium almost develops between blood in the lungs and air in the alveolus, and the partial pressure of oxygen (PO_2) in the blood almost equals the PO_2 in the alveolus. While diffusion of oxygen across the alveolar-capillary space is a theoretical barrier to oxygenation, it is seldom a practical problem during veterinary anesthesia unless considerable pulmonary edema is present.

Table 27.4 Composition of respiratory gases during air breathing and while breathing 100% oxygen.

Air or Oxygen Breathing	Gas	Inspired Gas (%)	Expired Gas (%)	Alveolar Gas (%)
Air	Oxygen	20.95	16.1	14.0
Air	Carbon dioxide	0.04	4.1	5.6
Air	Nitrogen	79.0	79.2	80.0
Oxygen	Oxygen	~100[a]	~94[a]	~95[a]
Oxygen	Carbon dioxide	~0[a]	4.1	5.6
Oxygen	Nitrogen	~0[a]	~0[a]	~0[a]

[a]These values are approximate as it is uncommon for the inspired oxygen percentage to be completely 100%, or for the nitrogen gas to be completely 'washed out' from the lungs and body stores.

There is a relatively steep concentration or *partial pressure gradient* of oxygen from room air to the various body tissues: nasal air = 160, alveolar air = 100, arterial blood = 90–95, interstitial fluid = 30, intracellular fluid = 10, and venous blood = 40 mmHg. Little oxygen is lost in large blood vessels, and normally a continuous pressure gradient is present from the alveolus to the tissue cell.

The normal average alveolar compositions of respiratory gases in humans and most other species are given in Table 27.4 for air and oxygen breathing.

At body temperature, alveolar air is saturated with water vapor, which has a pressure at 37°C of 48 mmHg. If the barometric pressure in the alveolus is 760 mmHg (sea level), then the pressure due to dry air is 760 – 48 = 712 mmHg. Knowing the composition of alveolar air, one can calculate the partial pressure of each gas in the alveolus:

$$O_2 = (760 - 48) \times 0.14 = 100\text{mmHg}$$

$$CO_2 = (760 - 48) \times 0.056 = 40\text{mmHg}$$

$$N_2 = (760 - 48) \times 0.80 = 570\text{mmHg}$$

The oxygen partial pressure in the lungs at sea level is thus approximately 100 mmHg at 37–38°C. Under these conditions, 100 mL of plasma will hold 0.3 mL of oxygen dissolved in solution. Whole blood, under the same conditions, will hold nearly 21 mL of oxygen per 100 mL of blood, or about 60 times as much as plasma; CO_2 is similarly held by blood. It is apparent that oxygen and CO_2 in blood are transported largely in chemical combination with hemoglobin. Mammalian hemoglobin consists of four-unit molecules. The unit molecules each contain a heme, which is a protoporphyrin consisting of four pyrroles with a central ferrous ion (Fe^{2+}). Oxygen combines reversibly with the ferrous ion in proportion to the oxygen tension. At complete saturation, each gram of hemoglobin combines with 1.36–1.39 mL of oxygen. This is the total carrying capacity of hemoglobin, or four oxygen molecules combined with each hemoglobin molecule. The ability of hemoglobin to combine with oxygen depends on the PO_2 in the surrounding environment. The degree to which it will become saturated at various oxygen partial pressures varies considerably (Fig. 27.6). It is adjusted so that, even when ventilation is inefficient or the supply of oxygen is sparse as at higher altitudes, the degree of saturation still approaches 100%. For instance, although it is probably not fully saturated until it is exposed to a PO_2 of 250 mmHg, hemoglobin is approximately 94% saturated when the PO_2 is only 70 mmHg.

Although there is relatively little change in hemoglobin saturation between 70 and 250 mmHg PO_2, a marked change occurs between 10 and 40 mmHg, a PO_2 characteristic of actively metabolizing tissues. Thus, as hemoglobin is exposed to tissues having partial pressures of oxygen within this range, it will yield its oxygen to the tissues. The lower the PO_2 of these tissues, the greater is the amount of oxygen that hemoglobin will yield. The degree to which hemoglobin yields its oxygen is influenced by environmental pH, PCO_2, and temperature – all mechanisms that protect the metabolizing cell. As the pH decreases and the PCO_2 and local temperature increase, at any given PO_2 value, especially in the range 10–40 mmHg, hemoglobin releases oxygen to the surrounding environment more readily (Fig. 27.6). It is also interesting to note that Nature has adapted for the relatively lower oxygen environment of the fetus, because fetal hemoglobin carries a greater percentage of oxygen at a lower partial pressure.

Certain enzyme systems aid the dissociation of oxygen from hemoglobin, the most completely studied being the enzyme system producing 2,3-diphosphoglycerate (2,3-DPG). This system enhances the dissociation of oxygen from hemoglobin by competing with oxygen for the binding site. A lowered level of this enzyme, as occurs with stored blood used for transfusion, increases the affinity of hemoglobin for oxygen and thus acts as though the dissociation curve is shifted to the left. The oxygen tension at which 50% saturation of hemoglobin is achieved (P_{50}) provides a comparative measure of the affinity of hemoglobin for oxygen, and this value varies between species. Also, P_{50} is reduced in septic patients and in carbon monoxide poisoning, whereas the reverse has been encountered in chronic anemia. Since tissues require a given volume of oxygen per unit time, the hemoglobin concentration of blood has a significant influence on oxygen content and delivery to the tissues.

Although an increase in the P_AO_2 above normal causes only a small increase in the oxygen-carrying capacity of hemoglobin, plasma carries oxygen in an amount directly proportional to the PO_2 in the alveoli. At normal atmospheric pressure, when the animal is breathing air at 38°C, 0.3 mL of oxygen is carried in solution in 100 mL of blood. If pure oxygen is administered, the PO_2 in the alveoli is raised from 100 to almost 650 mmHg. Plasma oxygen is thus elevated almost sixfold, that is, from 0.3 to 1.8 mL per 100 mL of blood. The result is an increase of about 10% in the oxygen content of the blood, which may be of clinical significance in severely anemic animals. The PaO_2 level is also of some importance because oxygen transfers from blood to tissues by diffusion, and the process occurs at a rate proportional to the difference in oxygen tension between plasma and body tissues.

A common misconception is that oxygenation of patients can be improved by increasing the physical (airway) pressure at which oxygen is administered. Except in hyperbaric chambers, oxygenation of patients is improved not by increasing the barometric pressure of the gas mixture, but by increasing the *proportion* of PO_2 in the mixture. One apparent exception to this is the temporary use of increased inflation pressure to re-expand collapsed alveoli (recruitment maneuver) during prolonged anesthesia, although in this instance the improvement in PaO_2 is due to improved V/Q matching rather than increase oxygen pressure *per se*. At a positive alveolar pressure exceeding 40 mmHg, the capillary circulation in the lungs is inhibited; therefore, it is not practical to administer oxygen at an inflation pressure exceeding this pressure. During anesthesia, hypoxemic episodes are best handled by reducing the level of inhalant anesthetic in the mask or rebreathing bag along with ensuring there is a high inspired-oxygen concentration, while instituting IPPV at a normal *f*, V_T, and inflation pressure (12–15 mmHg in small animals and 20–25 mmHg in horses and cows).

In conscious, healthy animals, there is considerable capacity to increase the rate of oxygen supply to, and CO_2 removal from, the body tissues, with up to 30-fold increases seen in exercising horses. The gas transport is increased in conscious horses by a fivefold increase in cardiac output, a 50% increase in hemoglobin concentration, and a fourfold increase in the extraction of oxygen from the blood traversing skeletal muscle capillaries [6]. The capacity for increasing oxygen supply is considerably less in more sedentary species.

During general anesthesia, these adaptive mechanisms to increase systemic oxygen supply are markedly compromised. Anesthetized animals are not likely to be able to appreciably increase their V_{min} or cardiac output, the spleen is often dilated and incapable of contracting to increase hemoglobin levels, and a key muscle (myocardium) cannot extract a greater proportion of oxygen from the blood going through the capillaries in response to an increase in demand or decrease in oxygen supply.

Carbon dioxide transport

Arterial CO_2 levels are a function of both CO_2 elimination and production, and under normal circumstances $PaCO_2$ levels are maintained within narrow limits. During severe exercise, the production of CO_2 is increased enormously, whereas during anesthesia, production likely decreases. Elimination of CO_2 depends on pulmonary blood flow (cardiac output) and V_A. Normally, the production of CO_2 parallels the oxygen consumption according to the respiratory quotient: $R = V_{CO_2} / V_{O_2}$. Although the value varies depending on the diet, usually $R = 0.8$ at steady state. Due to the blood buffer systems, CO_2 transport to the lungs for excretion occurs with little change in blood pH. The importance of the lungs in excreting this volatile acid is illustrated by the fact that, in humans, the kidneys eliminate 40–80 mEq of hydrogen ions per day, whereas the lungs eliminate 13,000 mEq per day as CO_2.

A CO_2 pressure gradient, opposite to that of oxygen and much smaller, exists from the tissues to the atmospheric air: tissues = 50 mmHg (during exercise, this may be higher); venous blood = 46 mmHg; alveolar air = 40 mmHg; expired air = 32 mmHg; atmospheric air = 0.3 mmHg; and arterial blood = 40 mmHg (equilibrium with alveolar air). Carbon dioxide is carried from the mitochondria to the alveoli in a number of forms (Fig. 27.8). In the plasma, some CO_2 is transported in solution (5%), and some combines with water and forms carbonic acid, which in turn dissociates into bicarbonate and hydrogen ions (5%) [3]. Most (about 90%) of the CO_2 diffuses into the red blood cells, where it is either bound to hemoglobin or transformed (reversibly) to bicarbonate and hydrogen ions through the action of the enzyme carbonic anhydrase. The formation of bicarbonate in the red blood cells is accompanied by the chloride shift (this accounts for approximately 63% of the total CO_2 transport). The excellent buffering capacity of hemoglobin enables changes in hydrogen ion content to occur during this process with minimal change in pH. Under ordinary circumstances, the pH of venous blood is only 0.01–0.03 units lower than that of arterial blood. Carbon dioxide is also carried in the red blood cells in the form of carbamino compounds. Amino acids and aliphatic amines combine with CO_2 to form unstable carbamino compounds. Hemoglobin is the main protein acting in this manner, although many can do so. The efficiency of this reaction is greater with hemoglobin than with hemoglobin-bound oxygen. Thus, as hemoglobin and oxygen dissociate, hemoglobin's capacity to carry CO_2 increases.

The mechanisms of CO_2 and oxygen transport are integrated in the blood in at least three ways: (1) the acidity of carbonic acid produced in the tissues favors release of oxygen without a change in oxygen tension, whereas the release of CO_2 in the lungs favors oxygen uptake (Bohr effect); (2) release of oxygen favors CO_2 uptake and vice versa in the carbamino mechanism; upon the release of oxygen, hemoglobin becomes a weaker acid and is more capable of accepting hydrogen ions, thereby facilitating its buffering effect (Haldane effect); (3) the two acid forms of the hemoglobin molecule favor dissociation by shifting from one form to the other; oxygen uptake favors CO_2 loss and vice versa.

Just as the amount of oxygen transported by the blood depends on the PO_2 to which the blood is exposed, so is CO_2 transport likewise affected; however, the CO_2 dissociation curve is more or less linear. Thus, in contrast to the minimal effects on oxygen content (Fig. 27.6), hyperventilation and hypoventilation may have marked effects on CO_2 content of blood and tissues.

Respiratory function in the anesthetized animal

Upper airway obstruction

Under normal conscious conditions, the nasal cavity, pharynx, and larynx are responsible for more than 50% of the total airway resistance to breathing. With the onset of general anesthesia, the nasal alar and pharyngeal musculature relaxes and, in deeper planes, the cough reflex is abolished. The net effect is to predispose patients towards upper airway obstruction. This is particularly evident in brachycephalic dogs suffering from stenotic nares, an elongated soft palate, everted lateral laryngeal ventricles, and/or a hypoplastic trachea. In these animals, the onset of general anesthesia may produce serious and potentially fatal upper airway obstruction unless the trachea is intubated. Experience has shown that it is preferable to perform endotracheal intubation in all anesthetized dogs, partly to protect against upper airway obstruction, but also to protect against possible aspiration of secretions or refluxed gastric contents from the stomach. It is important, however, that the endotracheal intubation be done without producing any trauma. For most species, routine use of a laryngoscope reduces trauma during intubation. Use of a laryngoscope also facilitates a complete examination of the

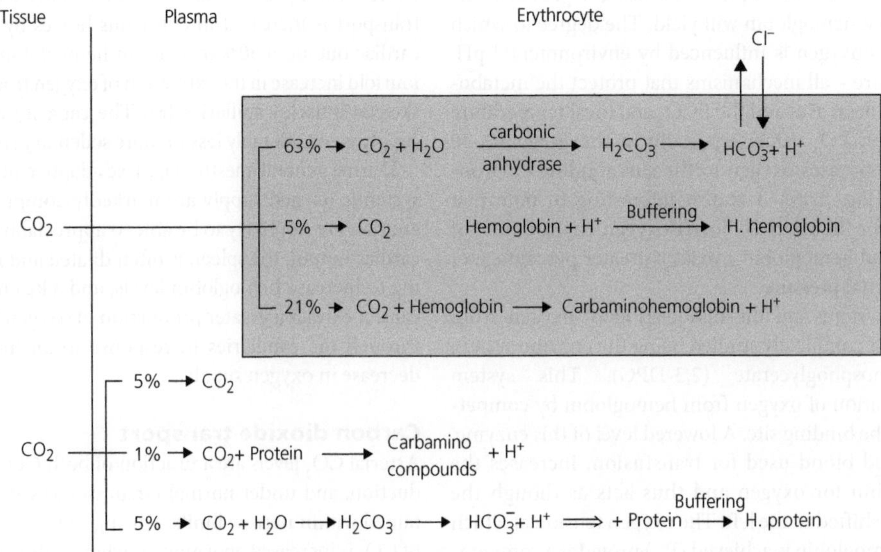

Figure 27.8 Transport of carbon dioxide in the blood. Carbon dioxide defuses out of the tissues into the plasma and erythrocyte, undergoing a variety of reactions that result in the production of bicarbonate and hydrogen ions. The hydrogen ions are then buffered either by proteins in the plasma or by hemoglobin, minimizing the pH change. In the lung, all of the reactions that are shown in this figure are reversed. Source: [4]. Reproduced with permission of Elsevier.

oropharyngeal cavity, which is a component of airway assessment and management. In many domestic and laboratory species, the decision on whether to use an endotracheal tube is a risk–benefit decision that must be determined based on the species involved, the anesthetic regimen employed, the experience of the anesthetist, the intended operation, the health of the animal, and the duration of anesthesia.

In ruminants, endotracheal intubation is required for all but the shortest-acting anesthetics, such as diazepam premedication with low-dose ketamine in sheep, calves, and goats, which only lasts about 5 min. The prime reason for endotracheal intubation is to protect against aspiration of rumen contents after active or passive regurgitation. In swine, endotracheal intubation is comparatively difficult and requires experience and care if trauma is to be avoided. Swine have inherently small airways and are more likely to develop apnea than other domestic species. Nevertheless, for most brief surgeries (e.g., hernia repair or cryptorchidectomy), the risk–benefit balance is often better served by not intubating swine, but instead by paying careful attention to the depth of anesthesia and to the character of respiration and head position so as to minimize the chance of serious upper airway obstruction. In most species, the best airway is provided when the head is kept in a somewhat extended position; pigs are unusual in that the best airway is provided with the head at a normal angle to the neck.

If significant upper airway obstruction occurs in any species, and the depth of anesthesia is not excessive, the animal usually develops an exaggerated respiratory effort that is primarily abdominal in character. The chest wall may even move inward on inspiration (paradoxical respiration) if the degree of upper airway obstruction is moderate or severe. The only other clinical situation that produces this subtle, but distinctive, change in the character of respiration is extremely deep anesthesia. This usually occurs at an anesthetic plane just before complete cessation of respiratory drive (apnea) ensues.

In rodents, such as mice, gerbils, hamsters, and guinea pigs, and in rabbits, endotracheal intubation may be difficult unless the anesthetist is experienced with the technique and has special equipment. In these species, longer, well-controlled periods of anesthesia for experimental purposes may well require endotracheal intubation. Shorter procedures in a veterinary practice may often be performed without using an endotracheal tube. A suitable face mask and non-rebreathing administration system may be used for oxygen administration (in the case of injectable anesthesia) or for administration of an oxygen-inhalant regimen using a precision vaporizer. When the anesthetist is capable of performing non-traumatic endotracheal intubation and has suitably small tubes (3–4 mm), it is preferable to intubate ferrets and rabbits, because surgical anesthetic planes produce considerable respiratory depression in both species, and it is much easier to deal with apnea if an endotracheal tube is already in place.

There is some controversy as to whether an endotracheal tube should always be placed in cats for shorter procedures (e.g., neutering). Cats tend to maintain a patent airway somewhat more effectively than do other species, unless drugs are used (e.g., ether) that increase the incidence of secretions and/or laryngospasm. Laryngospasm is comparatively rare when halothane, isoflurane, or sevoflurane is administered by mask, or when ketamine or propofol is used along with diazepam, acepromazine, or low-dose α_2-adrenergic receptor agonist sedation for injectable anesthesia. Moreover, endotracheal intubation requires a deeper level of anesthesia than is needed for some minor surgical or diagnostic procedures. Laryngospasm is more likely to occur after anesthesia when the larynx has been traumatized during intubation or when the endotracheal tubes have been cleaned with detergent or disinfectant between animals without adequate rinsing. In a recent review of a number of morbidity and mortality studies of feline anesthesia, the highest incidence of mortality was reported to be in the early recovery period [51]. The complication was commonly associated with postanesthetic airway obstruction and with trauma during insertion or maintenance of an endotracheal tube. On the other hand, there can be no denying the many advantages associated with endotracheal intubation in cats, as with other species. A patent airway is immediately available if the animal needs IPPV because of apnea or respiratory insufficiency, the risk of aspiration of gastric contents is markedly reduced, and it is easier to scavenge anesthetic waste gases if an inhalant anesthetic is being used. In cats, laryngeal desensitization with lidocaine may help to reduce spasm and trauma associated with the placement of a tube. Endotracheal tube placement should be based on a preanesthetic assessment of risk in an individual patient for airway compromise, and for the potential benefits of having a patent airway. If the patient is not intubated, the anesthetist should assure that an emergency airway and oxygen are readily available and the patency of the airway is being continuously monitored.

Veterinary anesthesia textbooks have hitherto placed little emphasis on the need to provide for a secure airway in horses, primarily because regurgitation is very rare. Although it is true that short-duration, injectable, field anesthetic techniques have been performed for many years without the use of an endotracheal tube, a considerable degree of upper airway obstruction does occur in horses (Fig. 27.9), primarily because their nostrils no longer flare during inspiration. Therefore, placement of an endotracheal tube may be considered desirable in most circumstances [52].

This tendency towards upper airway obstruction increases when a horse has been anesthetized for longer than 1–2 h, especially when placed in dorsal recumbency [53]. It is thought that passive congestion and tissue swelling occur because the nasopharynx structures are lower than the heart in anesthetized animals, and that this predisposes animals to airway obstruction in the recovery period when the endotracheal tube is removed. As a result, many equine anesthetists now secure an orotracheal, nasotracheal, or nasopharyngeal airway during the recovery process whenever horses have been anesthetized for any extended length of time (e.g., over 30–45 min) [54,55]. Clinically, it appears that ensuring an adequate diameter patent airway while a horse is trying to stand up (and is breathing vigorously) prevents the panic associated with partial or complete airway obstruction and leads to more controlled recoveries. There is still a need for large-scale morbidity and mortality studies that address the issue of when and where endotracheal tubes should be used during routine veterinary anesthesia, especially in a practice setting.

Anesthetic alteration of the control of ventilation

Respiratory drive and the adjustment in f, V_T, and V_A are achieved in conscious animals through a complex neural regulatory mechanism. Respiratory rhythm originates in the medulla and is modified by inputs from higher brain centers and the activity of chemoreceptor, pulmonary, and airway receptors. The central neural control mechanisms regulate the activity of the primary and accessory respiratory muscles, producing gas movement into and out of the lung and tracheobronchial tree. These control mechanisms are described in detail elsewhere [4,5,56]. Although there is certainly a similarity

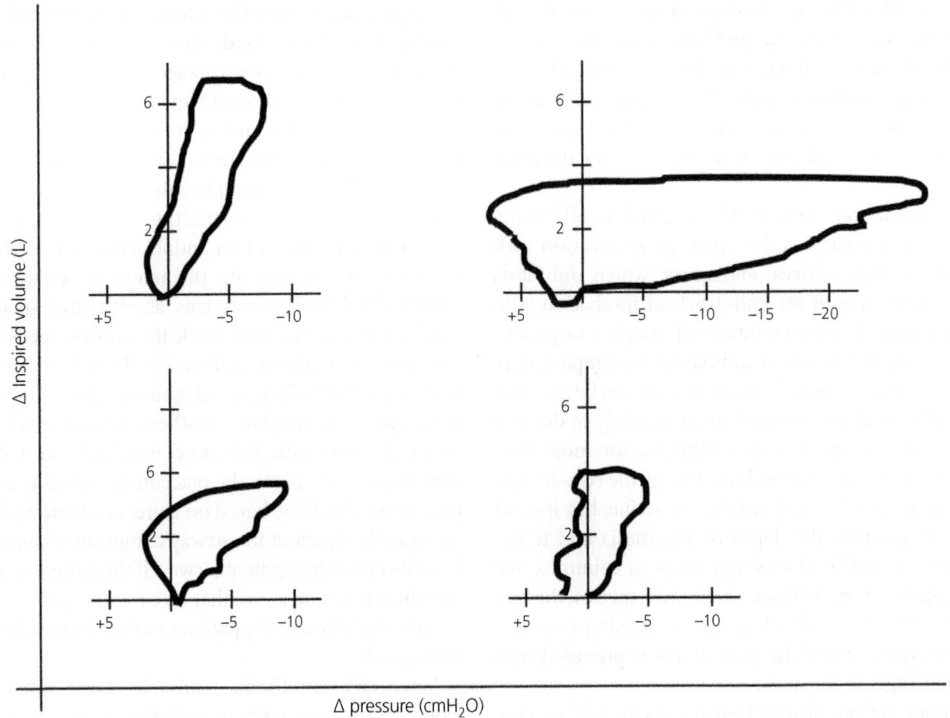

Figure 27.9 Changes in non-elastic work of breathing with the onset of general anesthesia (thiobarbiturate) in a spontaneously breathing horse. The change in transpulmonary pressure (airway opening to esophageal balloon) is shown as the abscissa and the change in volume (tidal volume) is shown on the ordinate scale. The area within the loops is a measure of the non-elastic work of breathing, and is a reflection of the airway resistance as well as a small component of tissue resistance. The *top-left loop* was obtained from the conscious horse breathing quietly; the *top-right loop* was obtained after 15 min of anesthesia with the horse in lateral recumbency and breathing without an endotracheal tube in place; the *bottom-left loop* is after the horse was intubated with a 25 mm tube; and the *bottom-right loop* was obtained once the horse stood in recovery with the tube removed. Note the large increase in non-elastic work of breathing during anesthesia until an endotracheal tube is inserted, and that fairly high negative pressures (10–15 cmH_2O) must be generated before there is an appreciable volume of inspired gas. This is indicative of upper airway obstruction. Source: W.N. McDonell, unpublished observations.

in the respiratory control mechanism between species, it is important to realize that various components may assume greater importance in different species.

While the detailed information referred to above is important in helping us understand the respiratory adaptations to high altitude, disease, and exercise, for the successful management of clinical anesthesia a much simplified understanding of the control of respiration will suffice (Fig. 27.10). In conscious animals, V_{Emin} and V_{Amin} are primarily determined by central chemoreceptor responsiveness to $PaCO_2$ levels. The *central chemoreceptors*, located on the ventral surface of the medulla and bathed by cerebrospinal fluid, are exquisitely sensitive to changes in $PaCO_2$ levels because CO_2 is readily diffusible into cerebrospinal fluid and the central chemoreceptor cell. The changes in $PaCO_2$ are probably ultimately detected as a change in the pH within the chemoreceptor cell. This ventilatory response to CO_2 is often presented as a response curve wherein V_{Amin} or V_{Emin} is plotted against the $PaCO_2$, the alveolar partial pressure of carbon dioxide (P_ACO_2), the end-tidal CO_2 partial pressure ($P_{ET}CO_2$), or the inspired-CO_2 level (Fig. 27.11a). An increase in $PaCO_2$ of 3–5 mmHg will produce a rapid doubling or tripling of V_{Amin} in an effort to return $PaCO_2$ to eucapnic levels. This response is slightly less sensitive in horses [57,58] and much less sensitive in burrowing and diving mammals [59]. In ruminants, the gas produced in the rumen may consist of more than 60% CO_2, and when it is eructated a significant proportion of this gas is inhaled, contributing to a cyclic breathing pattern [60]. A decrease in arterial pH will also stimulate respiration through the central and peripheral chemoreceptors, as seen with metabolic acidosis: this response is slower. The central chemoreceptors are not responsive to alterations in PaO_2 levels.

The *peripheral chemoreceptors*, which are located in the carotid and aortic bodies, generally play a significant part in respiratory drive only when PaO_2 levels fall below 60 mmHg [4,56]. This is illustrated in Fig. 27.11b, drawn from a study on conscious horses [61]. As the F_IO_2 was decreased from 1.0 (100% inspired oxygen) down to 0.16, there was no change in V_{Emin}. At an F_IO_2 of 0.16, the alveolar oxygen tension (P_AO_2) would be 60–65 mmHg at sea level. In sheep, goats, calves, and ponies, however, carotid body denervation causes some hypoventilation, hypoxemia, and hypercapnia, and it is estimated that carotid body receptor activity is responsible for up to 30% of the resting V_A drive in calves at sea level and up to 40% in miniature pigs [17,62]. During inhalant [63,64] or intravenous [65] anesthesia in horses, $PaCO_2$ levels will increase by 5–10 mmHg if the inspired gas is changed from room air (21% oxygen) or 50% oxygen to a 90–100% oxygen mixture. This may occur because peripheral chemoreceptors are partially responsible for the stimulus to ventilation under such situations, with high oxygen levels essentially blocking the stimulus. Nevertheless, the slight hypercapnia during oxygen administration is of much less consequence to the anesthetic safety than is the degree of hypoxemia that can occur with air breathing.

The activity of the central neural systems and the level of ventilatory drive are also influenced by the general level of central nervous

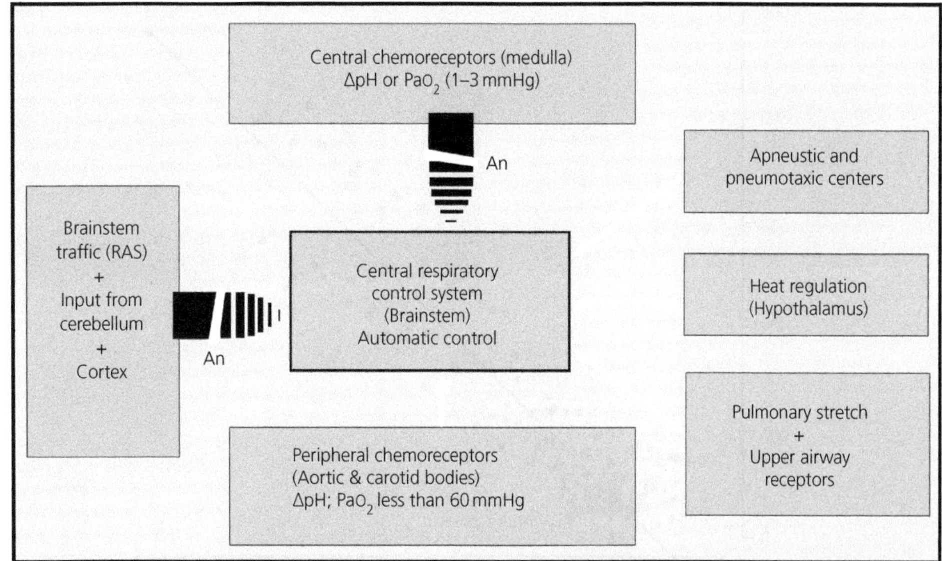

Figure 27.10 Schematic diagram of the control of ventilation in conscious and anesthetized animals. In the conscious animal, the level of alveolar ventilation is primarily determined by the arterial carbon dioxide ($PaCO_2$) level (as sensed by the central chemoreceptors) and the level of brainstem traffic. The apneustic and pneumotaxic centers and the stretch receptors adjust the relationship between tidal volume and frequency to achieve the required alveolar ventilation, usually while minimizing the work of breathing. General anesthesia (An) reduces brainstem traffic and the chemoreceptor response to carbon dioxide leading to an increase in $PaCO_2$. In most species, the peripheral chemoreceptors begin to influence the level of alveolar ventilation if PaO_2 falls below 60 mmHg. ΔpH, change of pH; RAS, reticular activating system.

system activity, especially by traffic through the reticular activating system (RAS). This is evidenced by the decrease in V_{Amin} and the small increase in $PaCO_2$ that accompany sleep, and by the fact that exercising animals commonly become hypocapnic even if tissue oxygen delivery is adequate. Anesthetists make good use of this link between RAS activity and respiratory drive by using an increase in sensory stimulation (limb flexion, twisting a horse's ear, rolling a dog or cat over, or vigorously rubbing the body surface) to increase ventilatory drive during emergence from inhalation anesthesia, thereby speeding inhalant drug elimination and recovery.

The apneustic and pneumotaxic centers, and pulmonary and airway receptors, are primarily responsible for adjusting the balance between *f* and V_T to achieve a given level of V_{Amin}, usually in a way that minimizes the energy cost of breathing. Although the function of these receptors is generally not considered to be greatly influenced by the action of anesthetic and perianesthetic agents, they may play a part in some of the species differences that we see in response to a particular drug or group of drugs [56]. For instance, as the inhaled dose of isoflurane is increased, *f* remains stable or increases in ferrets, whereas it decreases in rats and rabbits [66,67]. In dogs and cats, as the dose of an inhalant agent increases, *f* often remains constant or increases [68,69], although there is some variation in response between drugs [70]. In horses, *f* remains more or less constant with increasing inhalant anesthetic doses [71–73]. The respiratory rate is usually less with isoflurane, sevoflurane, or desflurane than with halothane at an equipotent dose, whereas V_T is larger [71,73]. The barbiturates usually decrease *f* and V_T as the dose is increased, whereas the primary response to increasing inhalant doses is to reduce V_T (ether is an exception). In ruminants, general anesthesia is often associated with tachypnea and very shallow breathing [74,75]. All of these differences might well originate from species and/or drug differences in the central inspiratory–expiratory switching mechanisms or lung receptor activity (stretch receptors, irritant receptors, and C-fibers), but so far the evidence is primarily speculative.

Irritant airway receptor activity, especially in the larynx and tracheal regions, appears to differ markedly between species. Horses, for instance, have a weak laryngeal reflex, so it is rather easy to insert a nasoendotracheal tube in a conscious horse, even without the aid of local anesthesia. In contrast, swine and cats have a strong laryngeal reflex, and fairly deep anesthesia is required for easy endotracheal intubation unless local desensitization is produced using a topical anesthetic. The response of dogs is intermediate.

Apneic threshold

The *apneic threshold* is the $PaCO_2$ level at which ventilation becomes zero; that is, where spontaneous ventilatory effort ceases (Fig. 27.11a) due to loss of central respiratory drive [e.g., low PCO_2 or high pH (relative to the set-point) at the medullary respiratory centers]. A $PaCO_2$ reduction of 5–9 mmHg from normal values through voluntary hyperventilation (a conscious human), or by artificial ventilation of sedated or anesthetized animals, produces apnea. The distance between the resting $PaCO_2$ level and the apnea threshold is relatively constant (i.e., 4–6 mmHg) irrespective of the anesthetic depth [56,76]. Veterinary anesthetists use the apneic threshold to control respiration (i.e., abolish spontaneous efforts) when putting an animal on a ventilator, or to provide temporarily for a quiet surgical field without having to resort to the use of muscle relaxant drugs. The fact that apnea develops with any depth of anesthesia and any anesthetic when $PaCO_2$ levels are lowered appreciably means that so-called 'assisted ventilation' soon becomes 'controlled ventilation' once the hypercapnia is corrected. A common clinical manifestation of this idea is the lack of efficacy when the anesthetist attempts to lower end-tidal CO_2 levels by intermittently 'bagging' the patient. Temporary improvement can be achieved, but the animal will become apneic once the apenic threshold has been reached (which is usually elevated from the desired end point such as 50 versus 40 mmHg). Spontaneous respiration will not resume until the apneic threshold is again crossed,

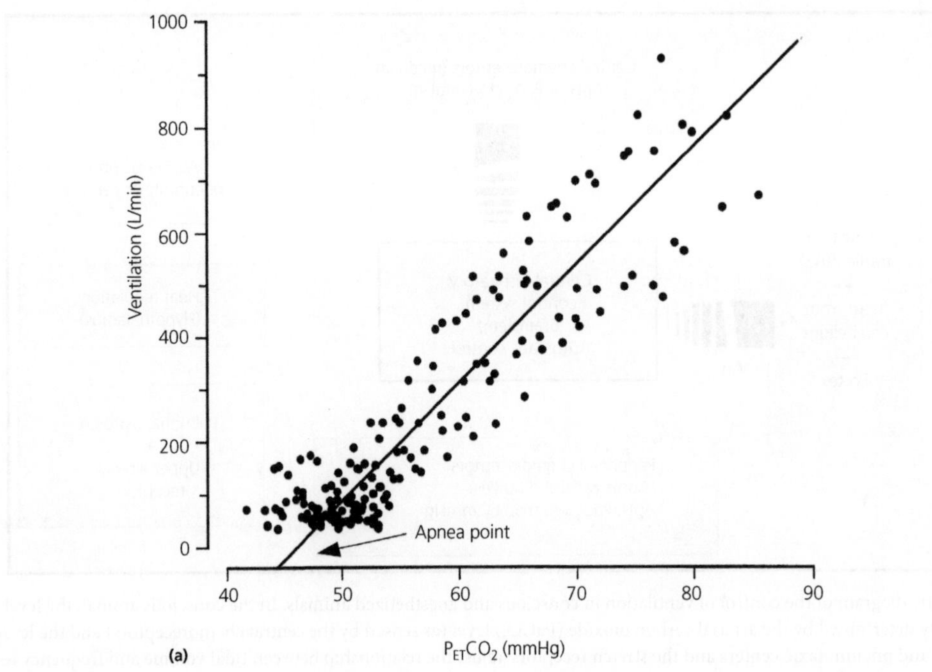

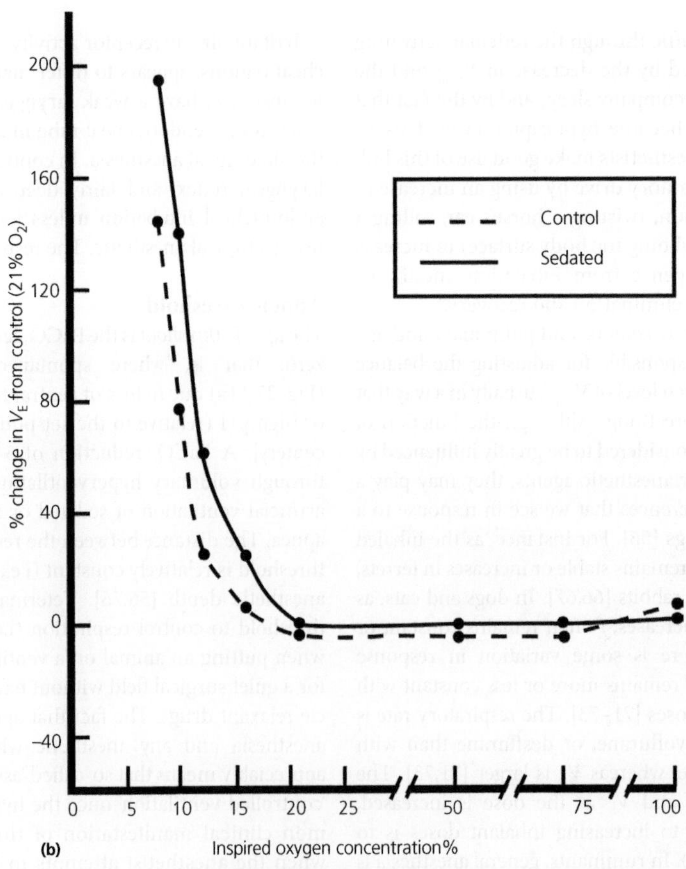

Figure 27.11 (a) This carbon dioxide response curve for six horses shows individual data points, the regression line, and the theoretical apnea point. Minute ventilation is plotted against end-tidal carbon dioxide. The horses were permitted to rebreathe CO_2 from a large spirometer filled with 30% oxygen. Source: data modified from [57]. (b) An oxygen response curve for non-sedated horses and for horses sedated with acepromazine. The percentage change in ventilation is plotted against the inspired oxygen concentration. Source: data modified from [61].

but at a level that usually represents hypercapnea. It should be apparent that controlled ventilation is usually a more effective strategy to maintain eucapnea during prolonged anesthesia or when respiratory depressant drugs are used.

Another clinically relevant feature of the apneic threshold relates to the return of spontaneous ventilation in the mechanically ventilated animal. Body CO_2 stores must accumulate to return $PaCO_2$ levels towards the apneic threshold level (which may be elevated from conscious levels due to anesthetic drugs) before spontaneous ventilation will resume. Hence the duration of apnea required before the animal commences spontaneous ventilation is proportional to the anesthetic depth, and also to the degree of hypocapnia produced during the period of IPPV. Recognizing this fact, most veterinary anesthetists will reduce both the inhaled anesthetic concentration and the frequency of breathing before trying to switch an animal from IPPV to spontaneous ventilation.

Drug effect on control of ventilation

Anesthetics and some perianesthetic drugs alter the central and peripheral chemoreceptor response to CO_2 and oxygen in a dose-dependent manner, as illustrated in Figs 27.12 and 27.13 [56,76–81]. This drug effect has important clinical implications in terms of

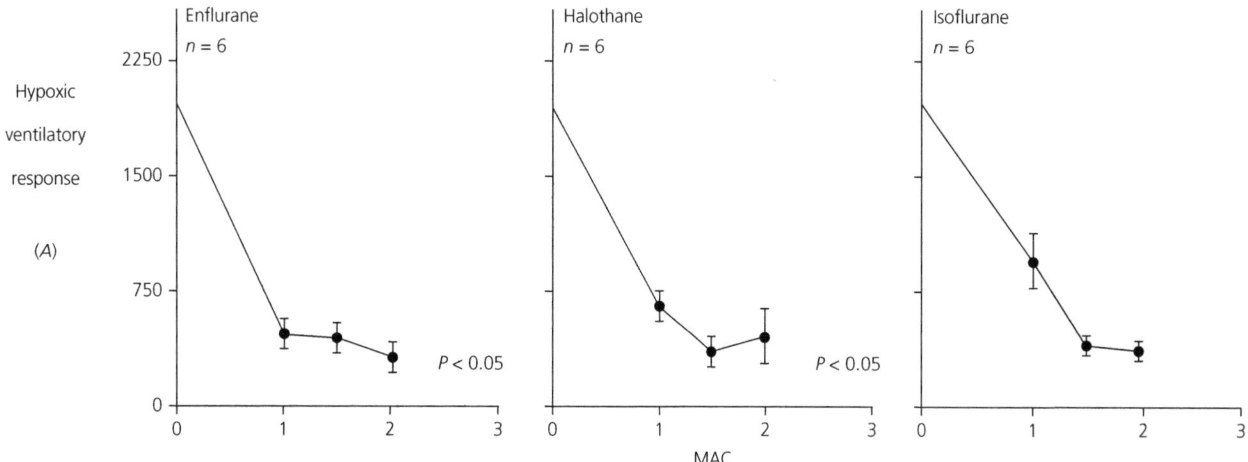

Figure 27.12 Change in the ventilation response to breathing hypoxic gas mixtures in conscious dogs and during 1.0, 1.5 and 2.0 minimal alveolar concentration (MAC) levels of enflurane, halothane, and isoflurane anesthesia. The value (*A*) describes the shape of the hyperbolic hypoxic ventilatory response, such that the greater the value for *A* the greater the response to hypoxia. The determination of *A* was made using curve-fitting and a least-squares regression plot of V_E against $1/(P_AO_2\text{-}3.5)$. Note the greatly reduced response in the hypoxic drive at even 1.0 MAC anesthesia with all three agents, and the virtually flat response at 1.5 and 2.0 MAC. Source: [78]. Reproduced with permission of Oxford University Press.

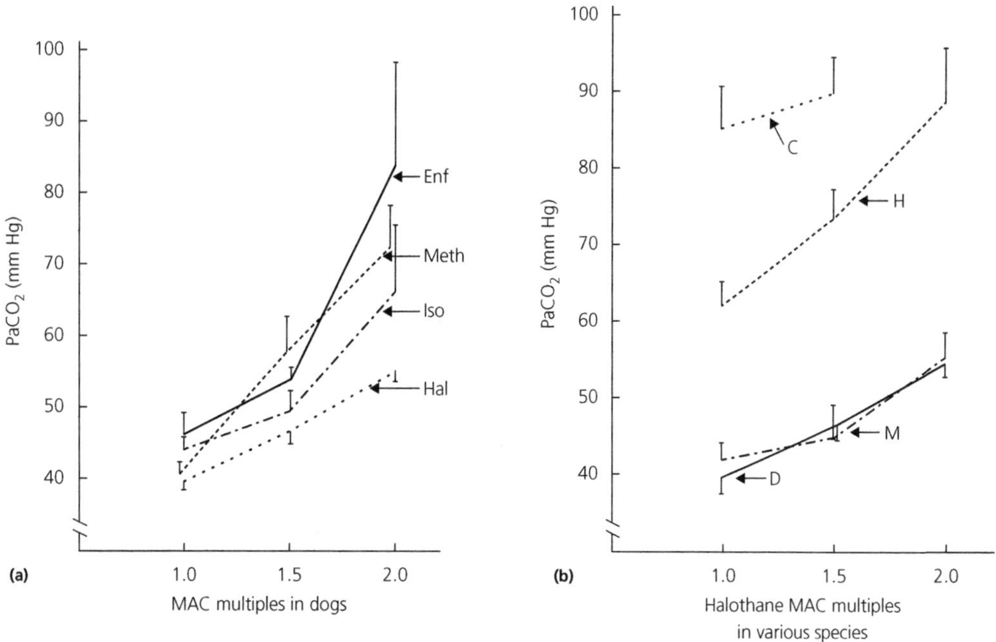

Figure 27.13 (a) Influence of increasing anesthetic dose (multiples of minimal alveolar concentration, MAC) on arterial carbon dioxide ($PaCO_2$) levels in spontaneously breathing dogs anesthetized with enflurane (Enf), methoxyflurane (Meth), isoflurane (Iso), or halothane (Hal).
Source: data compiled from a series of studies by Steffey and co-workers [68, 83, 84]. (b) Differences in the $PaCO_2$ with spontaneous breathing and increasing halothane levels (multiples of MAC) in calves (C), horses (H), monkeys (M), and dogs (D).
Source: data compiled from a series of studies by Steffey and co-workers [85–87].

maintaining homeostasis during the perioperative period. There will also be a diminution of external signs in hypoxemic or hypercarbic anesthetized animals, and perhaps during the recovery period [82]. Whereas non-sedated animals usually demonstrate obvious tachypnea and an increase in V_T or respiratory effort in response to serious hypoxemia or hypercapnia, these external signs of an impending crisis may well be absent or greatly diminished in anesthetized animals. Fortunately, it does seem that anesthetic-related depression of the peripheral chemoreceptor response to hypoxia is not as marked in dogs and cats as in humans [79–81]. The response in other species has not been studied.

Inhalant and injectable drugs

All of the general anesthetic agents in current use produce a dose-dependent decrease in response to CO_2 [4,56,76]. With commonly used inhalant agents, the CO_2 response is almost flat at a minimum alveolar concentration of 2.0 [78,79]. The reduced sensory input and central sensitivity to CO_2 produce a marked fall in V_{Amin}, usually through a dose-related fall in V_T, with *f* being reasonably well maintained. A proportional increase in V_D/V_T occurs, because V_{Danat} is more or less constant. As a result of these changes, $PaCO_2$ levels increase as the anesthetic dose is increased when animals breathe spontaneously (Fig. 27.13a) [68,83,84]. In light anesthetic planes (e.g., a minimum alveolar concentration of 1.2), $PaCO_2$ will generally remain moderately elevated, but stable, over many hours of anesthesia, whereas at higher concentrations or in ruminants, $PaCO_2$ increases progressively over time. The degree of hypercarbia at equipotent doses of inhalant (and intravenous) anesthetic agents varies with the species and the degree of surgical stimulation (Fig. 27.13b) [84–87]. Of the commonly used inhalant anesthetics, halothane produces the least increase in $PaCO_2$ during spontaneous respiration, whereas, at equipotent doses, isoflurane, sevoflurane, and desflurane produce somewhat higher and similar $PaCO_2$ levels in most species [70–73,88].

In ruminants, the degree of hypercarbia is greater with equipotent inhalant anesthetic doses than for horses, and horses show more respiratory depression than monkeys or dogs (Fig. 27.13b). Clinically, swine, ferrets, and rabbits also seem to be more prone to hypercarbia, whereas deep-diving seals may become totally apneic during light levels of anesthesia or with opioid-only sedation [89].

During surgery, the level of respiratory depression is usually less and the differences between drugs may disappear. For example, in dorsally recumbent, spontaneously breathing pregnant mares induced with xylazine and thiamylal sodium and maintained on halothane or isoflurane for laparotomy surgery, $PaCO_2$ levels increased from 53.8 to 58.3 mmHg during halothane anesthesia and were 60.7–63.5 mmHg during isoflurane anesthesia. There was no significant difference in $PaCO_2$ (or PaO_2) levels with the two agents from 30 to 90 min, although *f* was lower (4–5/min) with isoflurane than with halothane (8–10/min) [90].

Barbiturates, propofol, and the cyclohexamines (ketamine, phencyclidine, and tiletamine) also produce a similar dose-related alteration in the CO_2 response, which may, in the case of barbiturates, considerably outlast the period of actual anesthesia [91]. Although it is generally considered that ketamine is not as much of a respiratory depressant as the barbiturates [77], clinical experience and survey studies have shown that clinically effective doses of ketamine may induce apnea in some individuals. The typical response to increasing doses of barbiturates is for both V_T and *f* to decrease. When injectable anesthetics are used before inhalation agents, as is commonly done in clinical veterinary anesthesia, the respiratory-depressant effects of both drugs are at least additive [56,91].

Although the control of ventilation during anesthesia is primarily determined by a central (albeit reduced) CO_2 responsiveness, during very deep barbiturate anesthesia CO_2 ventilatory drive may disappear and the drive may become hypoxic. Hypoxic drive sensitivity is also lessened appreciably by general anesthetics (at least inhalants) in a dose-related manner (Fig. 27.12) [77–81]. It is interesting to note that, although the peripheral chemoreceptor response to PaO_2 at physiological levels (80–110 mmHg) is virtually non-existent in conscious animals, in anesthetized horses and ducks the $PaCO_2$ levels are greater at F_IO_2 1.0 than at F_IO_2 0.3 [63,92]. Therefore, the high oxygen levels used in most inhalant regimens might contribute somewhat to depression of ventilation while helping to ensure that the level of oxygenation is adequate.

Opioids

When given alone, opioids shift the CO_2 response curve to the right with little change in slope, except at very high doses. This means that the resting $PaCO_2$ level might be slightly higher in an animal receiving a therapeutic dose of an opioid for premedication or postoperative recovery, but that the response to further CO_2 challenge (from metabolism, airway obstruction, etc.) will not be abolished. Clinically, when opioids are used at high doses as part of a balanced anesthetic regimen, there is an additive effect of the opioid depression of the respiratory center and the general anesthetic, and considerable hypercarbia or even apnea may be produced [93,94]. In addition, the μ-opioids in particular tend to produce rapid, shallow breathing in dogs (especially before a surgical plane of anesthesia is obtained) [95], which may interfere with the subsequent uptake of an inhalant anesthetic.

At the doses commonly employed for routine opioid premedication or postoperative analgesia in veterinary practice, significant respiratory depression is rarely seen, at least in terms of producing hypercapnia [95–97]. Changes in ventilation pattern can occur and may range from a rapid shallow breathing to decreased frequency of ventilation owing to a decrease in apprehension. Interestingly, effective alveolar ventilation may well improve when opioid analgesics are employed for postoperative pain relief, especially with thoracic surgery [98]. The postoperative use of opioids has been implicated in the development of an increased incidence of postoperative atelectasis and hypoxemia in human patients, especially during sleep [99]. Clinical evidence suggests that the incidence of similar problems in veterinary patients is rare, but it is an area that warrants further study.

The historical tendency to minimize the use of opioids for postoperative analgesia because of the fear of serious respiratory problems is simply not based on facts, as is now well recognized [100]. However, some individual patients (e.g., intracranial hypertensive subjects) may experience significant respiratory depression therefore careful observation and monitoring of ventilation is advised, especially during recovery. There is a ceiling effect and less respiratory depression associated with opioid agonists/antagonists (e.g., pentazocine, butorphanol, nalbuphine, and buprenorphine) when used at high doses than with the pure μ-agonists (meperidine, morphine, and oxymorphone) [100,101]. Using the epidural route of administration helps to ensure that there is minimal postoperative respiratory depression with high-risk cases [102,103].

Tranquilizers

The phenothiazine and benzodiazepine sedatives often reduce the respiratory rate, especially if an animal is somewhat excited prior to administration, but they do not appreciably alter arterial blood-gas tensions [96,104,105]. There have been few studies of the effect of these drugs on CO_2 responsiveness, especially in animals. Horses sedated with acepromazine (0.65 mg/kg, IV) responded similarly, in terms of V_{Emin} change, to unsedated horses until the level of hypoxia or hypercapnia was quite severe (F_IO_2 of 0.1 or F_ICO_2 of 0.06), at which time the response was lessened [61]. When used alone, diazepam (0.05–0.4 mg/kg, IV) did not produce significant changes in PaO_2 or $PaCO_2$ in horses [106]. The respiratory-protective nature of these drugs is such that when they are combined with a general anesthetic, and the required dose of the general anesthetic is thereby lessened, ventilation is better than when an equipotent higher concentration of the general anesthetic (barbiturate or inhalant) is used alone. This may be one of the reasons why phenothiazine and benzodiazepine tranquilizers are widely employed as preanesthetic drugs in clinical practice.

Sedatives and Hypnotics

The α_2-adrenergic receptor agonists produce a more complicated effect on respiration. The usual clinical doses of xylazine and detomidine produce laryngeal relaxation in horses and alter pulmonary mechanics (dynamic compliance and pulmonary resistance) [107,108]. Some, but not all, of this effect is produced by the change in position of the horse's head with sedation [109]. Certainly, the degree of laryngeal dysfunction produced by α_2-adrenergic receptor agonist sedation in horses precludes the use of this type of sedation when carrying out diagnostic examination of the larynx. Although most studies have failed to demonstrate a significant increase in $PaCO_2$ levels after sedation of horses with xylazine, detomidine, or romifidine,[110,111]. a decrease in PaO_2 of 10–20 mmHg is often observed [107,109,110].

In sheep, it is apparent that clinically useful sedative doses of xylazine and other α_2-adrenergic receptor agonists produce significant hypoxemia, as illustrated in Fig. 27.14, without producing hypoventilation [112,113]. Sheep remain eucapnic or even become hypocapnic from the hypoxic stimulus. This response is associated with tachypnea, a fall in dynamic compliance of the lung (i.e., an increased stiffness), and an increase in the maximum change in transpulmonary pressure and pulmonary resistance during tidal breathing [112–114]. This response can occur with even subsedative doses [114], and the hypoxemia can last longer than the period of sedation [112,113]. On conventional and electron microscopic histological examination, the initial response appears to be associated with internalization of the surface coat and activation of the pulmonary intravascular macrophages found in sheep (and possibly other ruminants) [115]. It is hypothesized that these reactive cells release inflammatory mediators that lead to the rapid onset of bronchoconstriction and to leakage of the pulmonary vascular bed. By 10 min, there is obvious evidence of intra-alveolar edema and hemorrhage after clinical sedative doses of xylazine (Fig. 27.15) or medetomidine, and even after administration of the peripherally acting non-sedative α_2-adrenergic receptor agonist ST-91 [115].

It is unclear whether this adverse response also occurs in other ruminants, partly because the effect of a change in body position or the concurrent use of other drugs is difficult to differentiate. In calves, PaO_2 levels decreased from 88 to 55 mmHg after xylazine sedation and in goats a decrease from 90 to 65 mmHg was observed

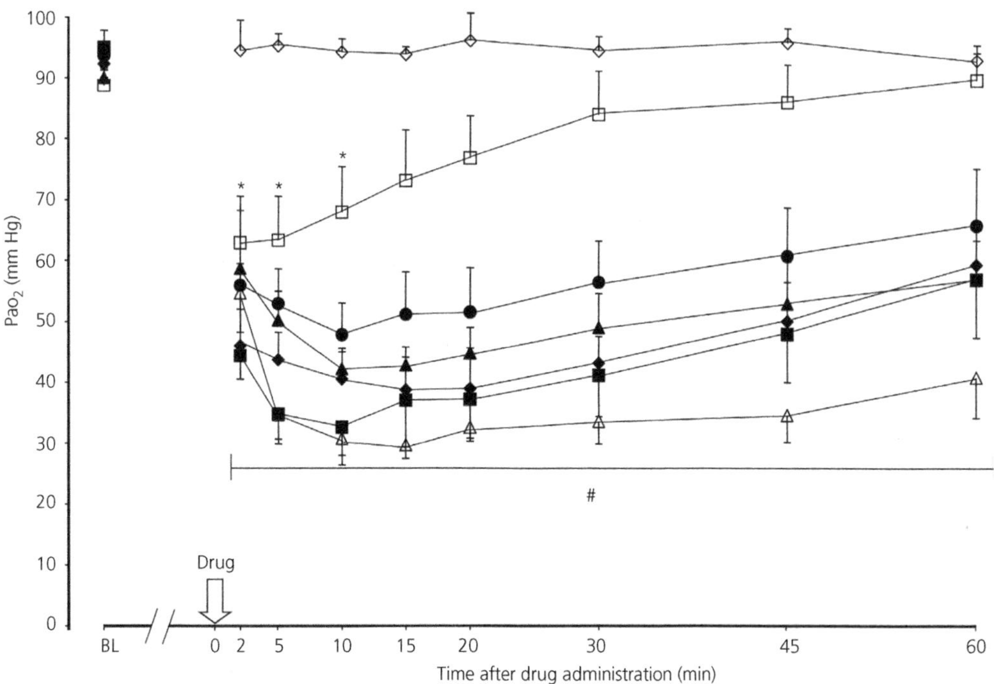

Figure 27.14 Arterial oxygen partial pressure (PaO_2) in sheep after intravenous saline, diazepam, or α_2-adrenergic receptor agonist administration in healthy adult sheep maintained in sternal recumbency. Baseline (BL) values and the values over 60 min are shown for saline (◊), diazepam (□) (0.4 mg/kg), xylazine (■) (150 μg/kg), romifidine (Δ) (50 μg/kg), detomidine (▲) (30 μg/kg), medetomidine (♦) (10 μg/kg), and the peripheral-acting experimental non-sedative α_2-adrenergic receptor agonist ST-91 (●) (30 μg/kg). Significant differences ($p \leq 0.05$) from placebo treatment for diazepam (*) and all other α_2-adrenergic receptor agonists (#) are shown. Note the marked degree of hypoxemia with PaO_2 values well below normal venous levels, and also the persistence of the hypoxemia over the full 60 min. This was well past the actual duration of sedation for a number of the agents. Source: data modified from [112, 113].

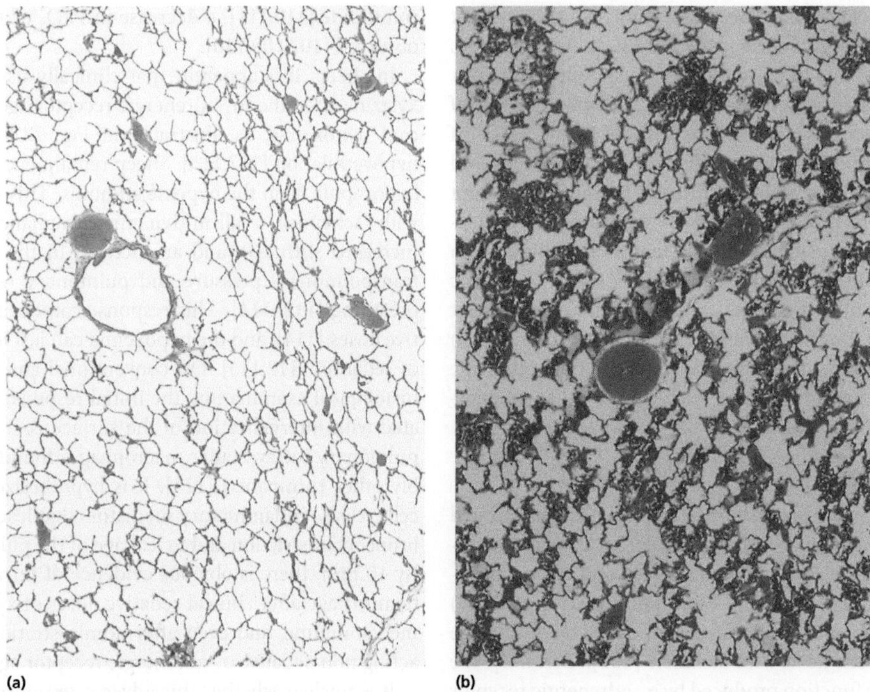

Figure 27.15 Histology of sheep lungs 10 min after administration of (a) intravenous saline or (b) 150 μg/kg of xylazine. Note the degree of alveolar hemorrhage and edema present after xylazine administration. Euthanasia and fixation as reported elsewhere [115]. Source: C. Celly, Ontario Veterinary College, University of Guelph, Guelph, Ontario, Canada. Reproduced with permission of C. Celly.

[116,117]. When seven healthy adult Holstein cows positioned in left lateral recumbency (on a tilt table) were given 0.2 mg/kg xylazine IV, mean PaO_2 levels decreased from 79.0 ± 4.5 (SEM) mmHg to 54.5 ± 2.7 mmHg at 5 min and to 58.4 ± 2.6 mmHg at 15 min after xylazine administration. $PaCO_2$ levels also increased significantly from 34.9 ± 2.0 mmHg to more normal levels of 45.0 ± 2.1 and 45.6 ± 1.4 mmHg at 5 and 15 min, respectively (R. Warren and W.N. McDonell, unpublished data).

Hypoxemia is a significant problem when wild deer, bison, and wapiti are immobilized using drug combinations containing α_2-adrenergic receptor agonists (or opioids) [118–120]. Treatment with supplemental oxygen is recommended and will increase PaO_2 to safer levels [120].

When used alone at sedative doses, the α_2-adrenergic receptor agonists exhibit little evidence of true respiratory depression in healthy dogs or cats [121–125]. There may be a decrease in respiratory rate and perhaps a small increase in $PaCO_2$ levels, but PaO_2 levels are well maintained. The peripheral cyanosis that has been reported in up to one-third of dogs sedated with medetomidine is believed to be caused by the low blood flow (with subsequent increased oxygen extraction) through peripheral capillary beds and venous desaturation, rather than a fall in arterial saturation [126].

It is important to appreciate, however, that the degree of respiratory depression produced by any α_2-adrenergic receptor agonist will be increased (often substantially) when the agonist is given along with other sedatives or anesthetic agents. A number of studies have clearly demonstrated that medetomidine or dexmedetomidine produce elevated $PaCO_2$ levels and lowered PaO_2 levels to mildly hypoxic values (i.e., 60–70 mmHg) when combined with either μ-or κ-opioid agonists, or with propofol or ketamine, at clinical doses in healthy animals. The decrease in PaO_2 levels is due in part to some degree of hypoventilation and to an increase in V/Q scatter, as described in the next section. Therefore, it is recommended that oxygen should be administered by face mask or endotracheal intubation whenever α_2-adrenergic receptor agonists are used in combination with other sedatives or injectable anesthetics [126]. This is especially true when dealing with geriatric or ill animals.

Other pulmonary consequences associated with anesthesia

General anesthetics, especially inhalant anesthetics, interfere with airway cilia activity and mucous clearance, both during the actual anesthetic period and also in the postanesthetic period [56]. It is not entirely clear how much of this effect is due to the anesthetic drug *per se*, to changes in airway humidity, or to the effect of concurrent oxygen administration. The anesthetic abolishment of the periodic normal physiologic 'sigh' associated with conscious ventilation, and the effect of changes in tidal volume with mechanical ventilation, may also be contributing factors. There is also a reduction in the normal pulmonary system resistance to infection, which may be of consequence in the immune-deficient animal or if there is an underlying clinical or subclinical pulmonary infection [56].

Changes in ventilation–perfusion relationships during anesthesia

The onset of general anesthesia [1–5] or, in the case of larger animals, even a change in body position [127–130] often produces lower PaO_2 levels than expected for the delivered concentration of inspired oxygen. This change can occur even without hypoventilation and during both spontaneous and controlled breathing. Lower PaO_2 is produced by altered ventilation/perfusion ratios within the lung. Much of what we know about this phenomenon of altered gas exchange is derived from studies of the human response to anesthesia, some experiments in dogs, and many studies on anesthetized horses. It is obvious when one looks at the collective results that there are important species differences, although the reason(s) for these differences are not always obvious.

Ventilation–perfusion scatter under normal conditions

To understand how anesthesia alters ventilation–perfusion (or V/Q) relationships, it is first necessary to appreciate the scatter of V/Q ratios in the normal lung of conscious animals and to appreciate the mechanisms by which regional matching of pulmonary blood flow and alveolar ventilation is optimized [6,42,43]. Figure 27.16 is a schematic representation of V/Q relationships in conscious and anesthetized animals.

Intrapleural pressure is more subatmospheric over the uppermost areas of the lung than adjacent dependent regions because of the 'weight' of the lung within the thoracic cavity [39,131]. Partly because of differences in lung density among species and partly because of differences in chest wall configuration, the total vertical gradient of intrapleural pressure over the whole lung apparently does not differ much among species, despite large differences in lung size and height. This is fortuitous, because otherwise there would be a tendency for too great a discrepancy between the size of the uppermost and lowermost alveoli. The gradient of intrapleural pressure means that in non-anesthetized animals the uppermost alveoli (A in Fig. 27.16) are larger than alveoli in the middle and lower regions of the lung (C and D). Since the pressure–volume curve of the lung is sigmoid, the larger alveoli tend to be on the flat part of the curve and thus distend less for any given change of intrapleural pressure during inspiration [3–5,132]. Thus, the more dependent alveoli (D) receive proportionally more of an inspired tidal volume, unless a disease process (e.g., chronic airway obstruction or pneumonia) or a decrease in lung volume leads to intermittent or complete airway closure (E and F) or actual atelectasis (G).

At the same time, there is a vertical gradient of pulmonary blood flow, because the pulmonary artery is a low-pressure system affected by hydrostatic pressure [42,133]. Some alveoli may receive no perfusion (A in Fig 27.16) and constitute an alveolar deadspace, whereas alveolus D receives more perfusion than alveolus B. In most species, the increased ventilation of alveolus D is not sufficient to match the higher perfusion, and the V/Q ratio of alveolus D is 0.7, compared with 1.7 for alveolus B. Overall, the collective scatter of V/Q ratios for the normal lung in resting individuals is 0.8–0.9.

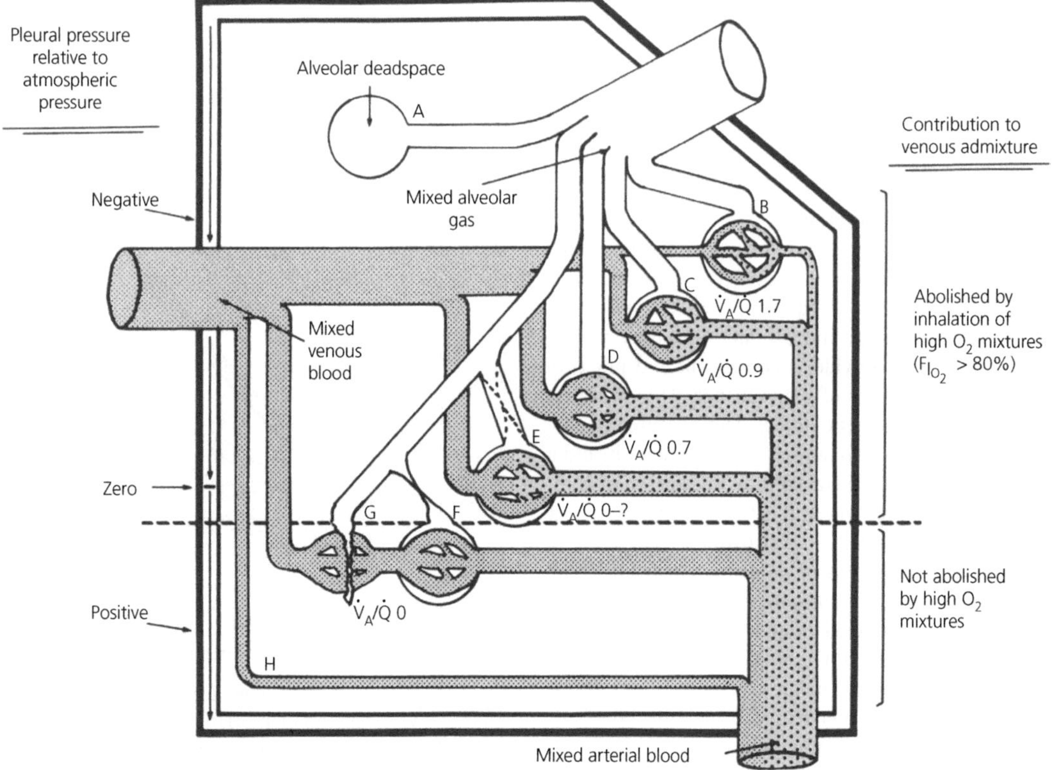

Figure 27.16 Schematic diagram of ventilation–perfusion (V/Q) relationships in the lung and the primary mechanisms whereby venous admixture and the alveolar-to-arterial [$P_{(A-a)}O_2$] gradient increases during anesthesia. The gradient of pleural pressure is shown with the dorsal aspect of the pleural space more subatmospheric than the dependent region, which may even become positive relative to the atmosphere if the lung volume decreases enough. The inflow of gas is represented by the *non-shaded area* in the tracheobronchial tree. This inspired gas may reach alveoli that are not perfused (A), alveoli that are variably perfused (B–D), or intermittently reach alveoli (E) through airways that only open later during the inspiration. Non-ventilated alveoli (F) will usually become atelectatic (G), especially when high inspired oxygen levels are used. The *finely shaded area* (blue) represents the flow of mixed venous blood from the pulmonary artery, and the *coarsely shaded area* (pink) represents postcapillary oxygenated blood. Blood flow from alveoli with low V/Q ratios (E), from non- ventilated alveoli (F, G), or from anatomic shunt areas (H) will all contribute to the venous admixture effect and increase the $P_{(A-a)}O_2$ gradient. The venous admixture effect of low V/Q areas is abolished when high-oxygen mixtures are inhaled, as even poorly ventilated alveoli will have sufficient oxygen to oxygenate the blood going past.

Based on radioisotope-distribution evidence, the vertical gradient of perfusion and ventilation is minimal in standing dogs with a horizontal lung [44,134], and matching of vertical perfusion and ventilation gradients in conscious horses is such that there is little difference in V/Q in different lung regions [45,135]. More recent studies using a multiple inert-gas washout method in horses suggest that the scatter of V/Q ratios in conscious horses is very similar to that seen in people [136]. No regions of low V/Q were identified, but a minor shunt component (less than 3% of cardiac output) was observed. A high V/Q area was observed (constituting 3–17% of the total), and the extent of this area was correlated with lower pulmonary artery pressures [136].

When pulmonary artery blood flows through vascular channels not adjacent to alveoli (H in Fig. 27.16) or passes non-ventilated alveoli (G and F), unoxygenated blood will pass from the right side of the circulation into the left side, leading to a lower PaO_2.

In conscious animals, if regional ventilation is decreased, a local vasoconstriction [hypoxic pulmonary vasoconstriction (HPV)] tends to divert blood flow away from underventilated areas of the lung [56,133]. An HPV response develops when the alveolar tension falls to less than 100 mmHg in the normal lung, and the response is maximal when the oxygen tension is approximately 30 mmHg [56]. There is an apparent difference in the strength of the HPV response to whole lung hypoxia in various species [137], based on high-altitude and excised lung studies [138–140]. Cattle and swine have a strong reflex, whereas ponies, cats, and rabbits have an intermediate response. Sheep, cats, and dogs show less response. It appears, however, that under normal conditions even species with a weak hypoxic pulmonary reflex are capable of considerable blood flow diversion in response to regional areas of low alveolar oxygen content [137,140].

Measurement of V/Q mismatch

When the barometric pressure, inspired-oxygen concentration, $PaCO_2$, and respiratory quotient are known, the P_AO_2 can be calculated by using one form of the alveolar air equation (Figs 27.2 and 27.5). The difference between this value and the PaO_2 [i.e., the *alveolar-to-arterial gradient*, $P_{(A-a)}O_2$] provides a convenient and practical measure of the relative efficiency of gas exchange. This measurement is commonly used in anesthetic studies. The measured $P_{(A-a)}O_2$ value increases as F_IO_2 increases for any given V/Q situation, and it is imperative that the F_IO_2 level be taken into account when comparisons are made. In practice, most $P_{(A-a)}O_2$ determinations are made at oxygen concentrations of 21% or near 100%.

The amount of *venous admixture* or *pulmonary-shunt flow* can be determined if mixed venous (pulmonary artery) and arterial blood oxygen contents are obtained along with a measurement of cardiac output and calculated P_AO_2 [141]. The terms venous admixture and shunt flow do not mean exactly the same thing, although they are often used interchangeably in the literature, which causes some confusion. Venous admixture refers to the degree of admixture of mixed venous blood with pulmonary end-capillary blood that would be required to produce the observed difference between the arterial and the end-capillary PO_2 [4,5]. The end-capillary PO_2 is assumed to equal the alveolar PO_2. Venous admixture is a calculated amount (i.e., a proportion of cardiac output) and includes the PaO_2-lowering effect of low V/Q areas, blood flow past non-ventilated areas, and true anatomic shunt flow (bronchial and thebesian venous blood flow). When the inspired-oxygen level is high, blood passing low-V/Q areas will be oxygenated (Fig. 27.16), and the $P_{(A-a)}O_2$ gradient and determination of venous admixture are a measure of all the total blood flow not contributing to gas exchange, hence the term pulmonary-shunt flow. Note that this flow includes both anatomic shunt flow and flow past non-ventilated or collapsed alveoli.

If one knows the inspired-oxygen concentration and the PaO_2, and assumes that the arterial–venous oxygen extraction is normal, an isoshunt diagram can be used to provide a convenient and reasonably accurate estimate of the magnitude of pulmonary-shunt flow (Fig. 27.17) [142]. Figure 27.17 also illustrates the poor response, in terms of improving PaO_2, that will occur with increased inspired-oxygen concentrations when shunt flows are over 30%.

Effect of positional changes

Very few thorough studies of the respiratory consequences of positional changes in conscious domestic animals have been completed because of the technical difficulties in carrying out such studies with uncooperative animals. In conscious human patients positioned in lateral recumbency, there is proportionately more ventilation to the lowermost lung [143]. There is a slight fall in FRC, but in individuals with normal lungs and body confirmation there is little change in PaO_2. Conscious dogs positioned in sternal (prone), lateral, and dorsal (supine) recumbency showed no positional change in FRC (Fig. 27.18) [144]. Unsedated sheep [127], cattle [129,130], and

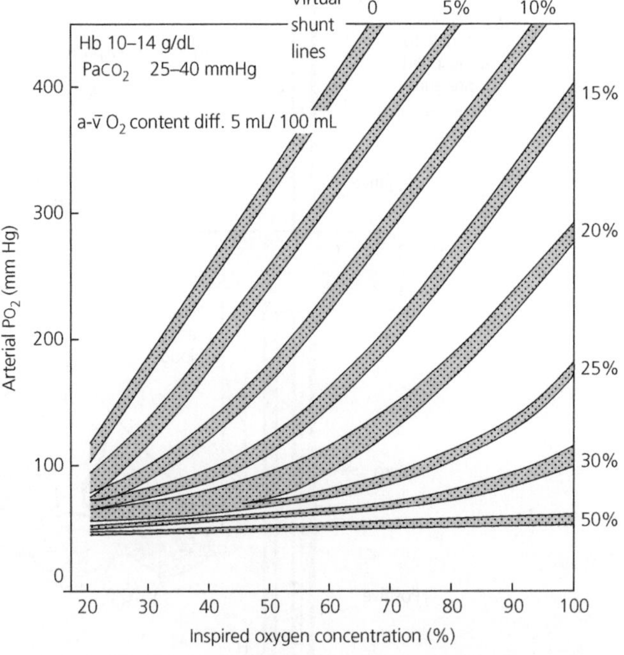

Figure 27.17 An isoshunt diagram depicting the relationship between inspired-oxygen concentration, arterial oxygen partial pressure (PO_2) and various degrees of venous admixture or pulmonary shunt. Shunt flow is expressed as a percentage of cardiac output, ranging from 0 to 50%. The arteriovenous (a-v) oxygen content difference is assumed to be 5.0 mL per 100 mL of blood, reflecting a normal cardiac output. The shunt bands have been drawn to include the range of hemoglobin (Hb) and arterial carbon dioxide partial pressure ($PaCO_2$) levels shown. Note that at the higher levels of shunt flow (30–50%) there is little improvement in arterial oxygen levels even when the inspired oxygen concentration is 100%. Also note that if the inspired oxygen concentration and PaO_2 are known, it is possible to obtain a quick estimate of the degree of venous admixture or shunt flow. Source: redrawn from [142]. Reproduced with permission of Oxford University Press.

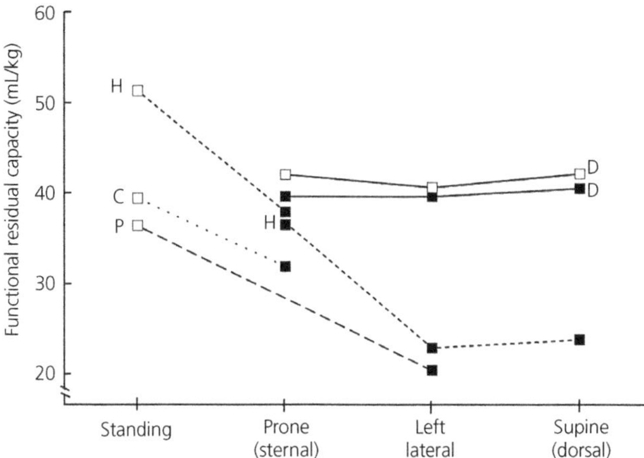

Figure 27.18 Effect of positional changes and general anesthesia on functional residual capacity (FRC) in dogs (D), cattle (C), ponies (P), and horses (H). FRC in the conscious state is shown by the open symbol and in the anesthetized state by a closed symbol. All measurements were obtained during barbiturate anesthesia. Note that FRC does not change appreciably in anesthetized dogs with positional changes and decreases markedly with the onset of anesthesia and recumbency in the larger species. In horses, FRC is markedly less in dorsal or lateral recumbency, compared with sternal recumbency. Source: data taken from various studies [35–37, 144].

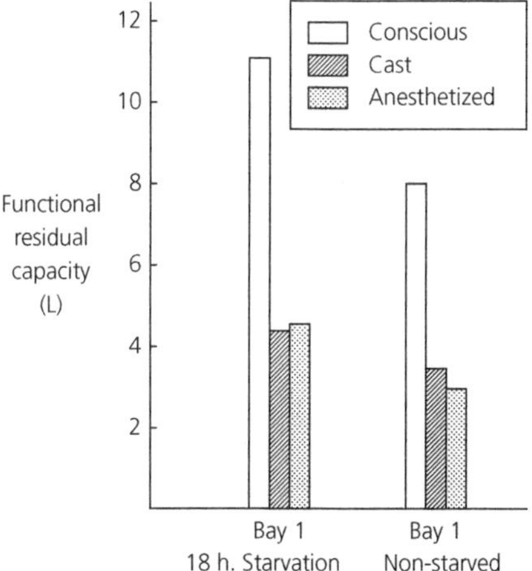

Figure 27.19 Functional residual capacity in a xylazine-sedated pony (273 kg) while standing (conscious), after positioning in left lateral recumbency with hobbles (cast), and following induction of anesthesia with thiopental (anesthetized). The study was performed twice, once after an 18 h period of starvation and once without starvation. FRC was measured by helium dilution [173].

ponies [128] developed some degree of hypoxia when put into lateral recumbency, although this finding was not present in another group of ponies [145]. Mean PaO_2 levels in non-sedated adult cattle positioned in dorsal recumbency are in the range 60–70 mmHg, with some animals experiencing marked hypoxemia [129,130].

Although the evidence in conscious animals is mainly circumstantial and meager, it does appear that the main determinant of the lower oxygen tensions is a decrease in lung volume (FRC) in recumbent animals (Fig. 27.19), as has been reported in anesthetized animals [36,37]. Interestingly, when conscious, sedated, 1400–4000 kg elephants voluntarily moved from a standing position to left lateral recumbency, PaO_2 levels only decreased from 96.2 to 83.8 mmHg (at 10 min) [146]. This relative protection against positional hypoxemia may be related to anatomic differences in the lung parenchyma, chest wall, and lung adhesion to the chest wall [147].

In standing cows and sheep, rumen distension and the associated increase in abdominal pressure produce a decrease in PaO_2, and at very high rumen pressures a reduction in V_{Emin} and cardiac output [148,149]. In four standing ponies (two fasted for 18 h and two non-fasted), FRC as measured by helium dilution decreased by 13.4% (range 11.6–14.7%) after sedation with 0.04 mg/kg of acepromazine given intramuscularly. In another study, overnight fasting increased the FRC of five standing, unsedated ponies by about 16% [37].

Effect of anesthesia and species differences

As mentioned earlier, deep sedation and general anesthesia commonly produce a fall in PaO_2 levels even in healthy animals. Some of this decrease can be associated with hypoventilation (Fig. 27.13), but even when $PaCO_2$ levels are eucapnic, PaO_2 is generally decreased. The anesthetic-induced change in PaO_2 is associated with increases in the scatter of V/Q ratios, $P_{(A\text{-}a)}O_2$ gradient, and the level of venous admixture [2,4,5]. In the case of larger mammals, there may even be gross V/Q mismatch [1,4,150]. It is generally appreciated that $P_{(A\text{-}a)}O_2$ gradients are always increased during general anesthesia in horses [1,151,152]. In a study of 160 clinical cases, the increase in $P_{(A\text{-}a)}O_2$ gradient was considerably greater in dorsally recumbent than laterally recumbent horses, and in spontaneously breathing versus mechanically ventilated horses [153]. During intravenous anesthesia, healthy horses positioned in lateral recumbency and breathing air consistently have PaO_2 levels in the 60–70 mmHg range, and depending on the drug mixture (or individual horse) may even have PaO_2 values as low as 50 mmHg [65,154,155]. In horses with diseased lungs or depressed cardiopulmonary function (e.g., anesthesia), it may be impossible to maintain PaO_2 levels above 70 mmHg even with 100% inspired oxygen and IPPV [156]. The same response to 100% oxygen administration may be observed in adult cattle [75].

Recumbency *per se* does not produce significant hypoxemia in healthy dogs, cats, or people, and in the case of larger mammals produces less of an increase in the $P_{(A\text{-}a)}O_2$ gradient than is seen after the onset of anesthesia. What are the factors that produce hypoxemic changes in anesthetized animals? Research on the respiratory effects of anesthetics has been focused on their influence on (1) the hypoxic pulmonary reflex (HPV); (2) lung volume, chest wall, and pulmonary mechanical factors; and (3) the resultant distribution of regional pulmonary blood and gas flow.

Hypoxic pulmonary vasoconstriction (HPV)

It appears that this important protective mechanism to optimize V/Q in the lung is obtunded by many anesthetics. In studies using excised lungs from dogs, cats, and rats most, if not all, inhalational agents reduced HPV, and none of the injectable agents examined (narcotics, barbiturates, propofol, and benzodiazepines) had any detectable effect [133]. The situation in intact anesthetized animals is less clear [56]. In pentobarbital-anesthetized dogs subjected to one-lung hypoxia, 0.5–1.5% halothane did not alter the response to hypoxia [157], whereas isoflurane at 1.0% increased the pulmonary shunt flow to the hypoxic lung by 22% [158]. In another *in vivo* canine study, neither sevoflurane nor desflurane anesthesia altered the pulmonary vasoconstriction associated with bilateral lung hypoxia [159]. A similar negative effect on HPV has been demonstrated with sevoflurane anesthesia in intact piglets [160]. The extent to which HPV is altered by inhalation and intravenous anesthetics in other species is not known.

The end result of any anesthetic-induced interference with HPV would be to increase the degree to which the PaO_2 is reduced with any given level of altered intrapulmonary gas distribution, whether caused by reduced lung volume, intermittent airway closure, or regional atelectasis. With an animal breathing 100% oxygen and HPV abolished, it can be estimated that PaO_2 will only be 100 mmHg with 30% of the lung atelectatic, compared with a PaO_2 level of over 400 mmHg with the same degree of atelectasis and an intact HPV response [140]. Few clinically relevant, controlled comparisons of $P_{(A\text{-}a)}O_2$ gradients have been performed using intravenous anesthesia compared with inhalational anesthesia in veterinary patients. In one study, PaO_2 was better maintained in horses when a xylazine–ketamine–guaifenesin infusion was used instead of halothane to maintain anesthesia [161], whereas in another study, no difference in PaO_2 levels or the pulmonary shunt fraction was observed when romifidine–ketamine–guaifenesin anesthesia and halothane were compared [162].

In anesthetized horses, there is evidence that pulmonary perfusion does not increase linearly from the uppermost to the lowermost lung areas solely on a gravitational basis, even if HPV is abolished [163,164]. It has been demonstrated that the gravity-dependent pulmonary blood flow of conscious horses is altered when they are positioned in sternal, lateral, or dorsal recumbency during halothane anesthesia [47]. There was a reduction in blood flow to the cranio-ventral areas of the lung and a proportional increase in flow to dorso-caudal regions, irrespective of body position. A non-gravitational pulmonary blood flow pattern in pentobarbital-anesthetized ponies has been demonstrated [49]. At least some of this diversion of pulmonary blood flow from the most dependent areas of the horse lung might be related to creation of a zone IV area of blood flow from reduced lung volume and an increase in interstitial fluid pressure (Fig. 27.3). This sort of diversion has been observed in persons at low lung volumes [165] and in dogs when interstitial fluid pressures were elevated [166]. Whatever the cause, in laterally recumbent horses, the redistribution of pulmonary blood flow away from relatively non-ventilated lower lung to better-ventilated upper lung has a beneficial effect in reducing the degree of venous admixture [164]. It is important to appreciate that redistribution is far from complete, and venous admixture or shunt flows in healthy horses often exceed 20%, and in diseased horses in dorsal recumbency may exceed 40% of cardiac output.

Functional residual volume

In recumbent humans, FRC is reduced by about 0.5 L with the induction of general anesthesia [132], which is 15–20% of the normal FRC. The mechanisms underlying this reduction in FRC remain unclear. Atelectasis, increased thoracic or abdominal blood volume, and loss of some inherent tone in the diaphragm at end-exhalation all seem to be involved [99,132,143]. Irrespective of the cause, there is evidence of a correlation between changes in FRC and the $P_{(A\text{-}a)}O_2$ gradient after induction of anesthesia [167]. Airway closure, atelectasis, and dependent regions of poorly aerated lung tissue have been demonstrated by using inert-gas elimination and computed tomographic techniques [2,5,168,169].

There is little information regarding FRC changes in dogs and cats, but in one well-controlled study the onset of general anesthesia did not alter FRC significantly in sternal, lateral, or dorsally recumbent dogs (Fig. 27.18) [144]. These were medium-sized mongrel dogs (13–28 kg), and larger dogs might show a different response. Differences in V/Q ratios during anesthesia have been noted between Beagles and Greyhound-type dogs [170].

In horses and cows, the decrease in FRC with the onset of recumbency and general anesthesia may be marked, as much as 50–70% (Fig. 27.18). This has been demonstrated radiographically [171,172] and directly measured by helium dilution [37,173] and nitrogen washout [36]. The change in FRC seems to be primarily related to the positional change from an upright posture to recumbency (Fig. 27.19) and, in horses at least, is greater in lateral or dorsal recumbency than when prone (Fig. 27.18) [36]. In laterally recumbent animals, the dependent lung is poorly aerated radiographically [171,172] and has a smaller FRC (as measured by helium dilution) (Fig. 27.20). Studies using nuclear scintigraphy and computed tomography have clearly demonstrated that there is markedly less ventilation of the dependent lung of horses in lateral recumbency during anesthesia [150,174]. This reduction in lower lung volume is accompanied by actual atelectasis (Fig. 27.21) and may be influenced by the degree of obesity or body conformation [175]. High oxygen concentrations in the inspired gas will lead to more alveolar atelectasis in horses, as observed in humans [2,5,65].

The FRC of anesthetized horses can be increased and the $P_{(A\text{-}a)}O_2$ gradient reduced through the use of high (20–30 cmH_2O) PEEP [156,175,176]. If PEEP of this magnitude is introduced, there is a marked decrease in venous return to the heart and in cardiac output. The mechanism by which PEEP reduces the $P_{(A\text{-}a)}O_2$ gradient and venous admixture is likely through increasing total and/or regional FRC, with subsequent prevention of the intermittent airway closure and reversal of the atelectasis that is represented diagrammatically by alveoli F and G in Fig. 27.16. Moens and colleagues used a double-lumened endotracheal tube and differential IPPV (higher V_T and PEEP of 10–20 cmH_2O) to the lowermost lung of fairly large laterally recumbent horses (420–660 kg) [177]. This technique increased PaO_2 levels by over 100% and decreased pulmonary-shunt perfusion by 33%. Similar beneficial effects have been reported using PEEP and selective mechanical ventilation of dependent areas of the lungs in dorsally recumbent horses (Fig. 27.22) [178,179]. With the onset of general anesthesia and positioning in lateral recumbency, PaO_2 levels were elevated to only about 250 mmHg, rather than the expected >500 mmHg that should have occurred if there was no problem with gas exchange. When the horses were moved into dorsal recumbency, their mean PaO_2 level decreased to below 100 mmHg. Conventional IPPV of the whole lung did little to improve PaO_2, whereas selective mechanical ventilation of the dependent areas of the lung with 20 cmH_2O restored PaO_2 to the level measured in lateral recumbency.

Chest wall and pulmonary mechanics changes

The evidence implicating alteration of chest wall (including diaphragm) and lung mechanical factors as causative agents in the increase in $P_{(A\text{-}a)}O_2$ during anesthesia is often conflicting. Certainly, there is a difference in the chest wall mechanics between people and dogs during general anesthesia [132]. It appears that most dog breeds (and probably cats) have a more compliant lateral chest wall that tends to contribute relatively little to the inspiratory effort, compared with the diaphragm, with clinical doses of most anesthetics. In all species, dangerously deep planes of anesthesia are commonly associated with flaccidity of the thoracic wall and paradoxical inward movement during inspiration (paradoxical inspiration). If one watches closely, this same type of respiration may be seen in cats, ferrets, and other small mammals, even with light levels of anesthesia.

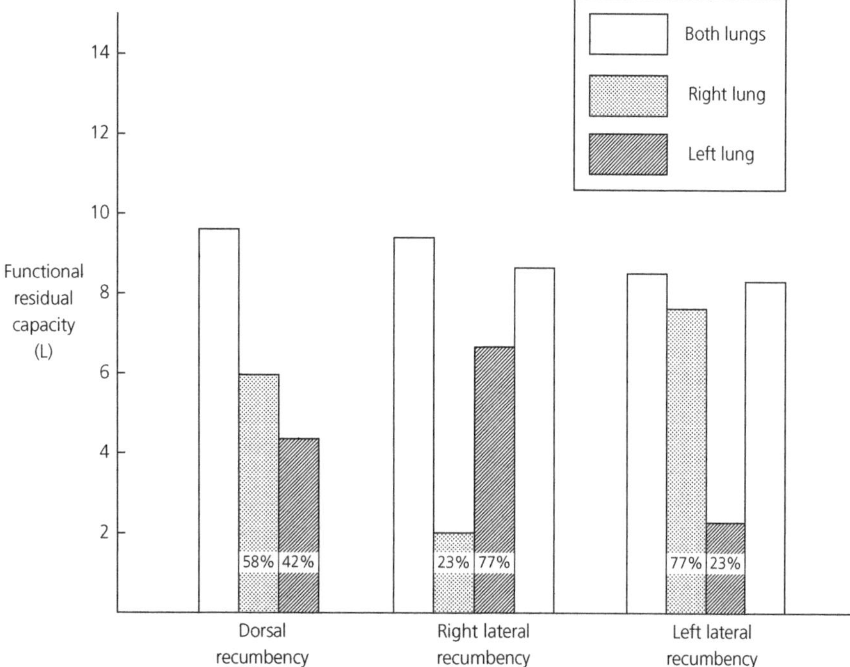

Figure 27.20 Functional residual capacity (FRC) of the left and right lungs, and both lungs, in a horse positioned in dorsal, and right and left lateral recumbency. The horse was maintained under stable intravenous anesthesia, and FRC was determined by helium dilution using a double-lumen endotracheal tube to separate the two lungs [173]. Note that the FRC of the dependent lung decreases from the proportion measured during dorsal recumbency and becomes a small percentage of the total FRC, irrespective of which lung is dependent.

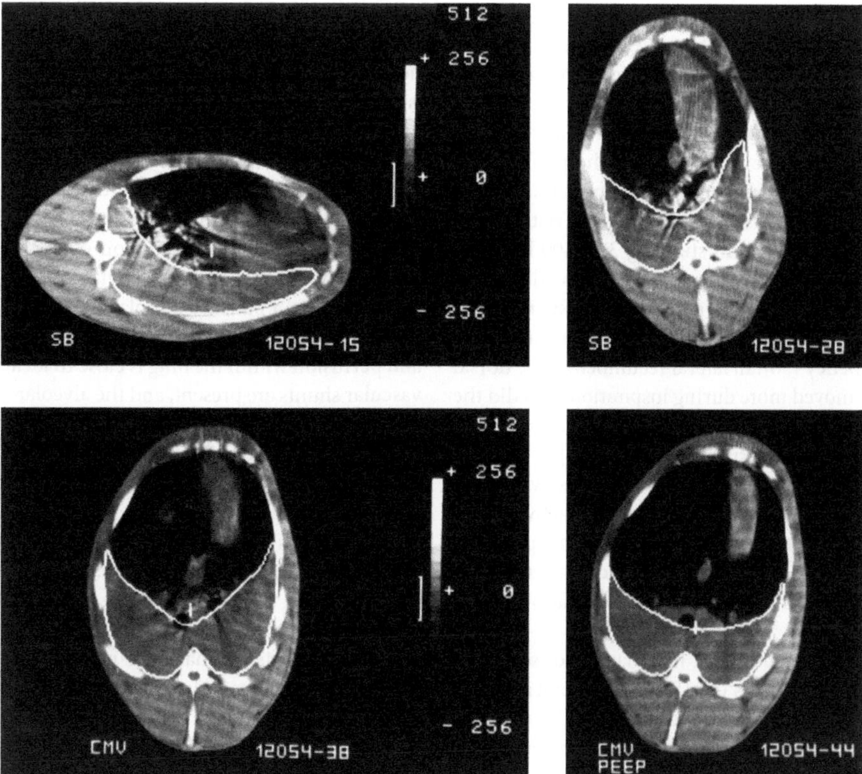

Figure 27.21 Transverse computed tomography scans of the thorax of a pony during anesthesia with thiopental/halothane in left lateral recumbency (top left), and in dorsal recumbency during spontaneous respiration (top right), mechanical ventilation (bottom left), and mechanical ventilation with PEEP of 10 cmH_2O (bottom right). Note the appearance of large dense areas encircled by a white line in dependent lung regions. The heart is visible as a white area in the middle of the thorax. Source: [174]. Reproduced with permission of Wiley.

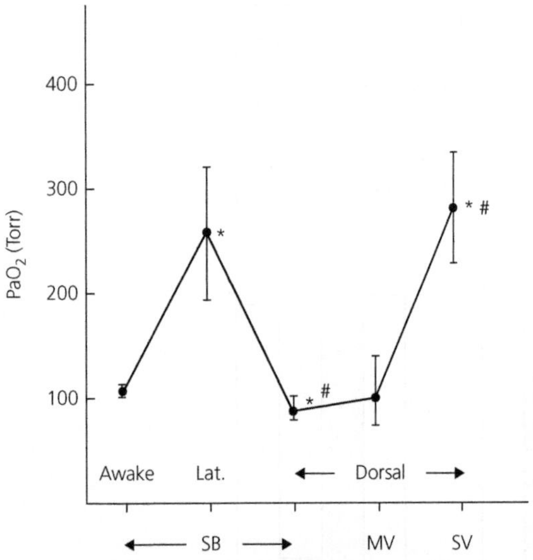

Figure 27.22 Arterial oxygen partial pressure (PaO_2) levels (mean ± SEM) in an awake standing horse breathing air ($F_IO_2 = 0.21$), and during anesthesia in lateral (Lat) and dorsal recumbent positions with high inspired oxygen levels ($F_IO_2 > 0.92$). SB = spontaneous breathing; MV = general mechanical ventilation; SV = selective mechanical ventilation of dependent lung regions with a positive end-expiratory pressure (PEEP) of 20 cmH_2O; * = significantly different from awake value; # = significantly different from the previous value. Source: [179]. Reproduced with permission of Oxford University Press.

In horses and cows, with the onset of anesthesia and movement into lateral recumbency, there is radiographic evidence of a marked change in the two-dimensional lung silhouette and the position of the diaphragm [171,172]. In ponies anesthetized with halothane, the diaphragmatic outline moved forward rather uniformly in sternal (prone) or lateral recumbency, but the forward shift was considerably greater in lateral recumbency [171]. When the ponies were positioned in dorsal (supine) recumbency, the diaphragmatic outline sagged towards the now dependent spine region. With minor variations, observations by Watney in studying 315–400 kg cattle were very similar [172]. The positional alteration of the diaphragmatic silhouette agrees nicely with the reduction in FRC noted by Sorenson and Robinson when ponies were moved from sternal to lateral or dorsal recumbency [36]. In lateral recumbency, the dorsal areas of the diaphragm moved more during inspiration than did the more ventral sternal area, while the uppermost crural movement exceeded that of the lowermost crural segment [180]. This is in contrast to awake and anesthetized recumbent persons, where the most dependent portions of the diaphragm are most active [181]. The tonic activity of the lateral chest wall, especially that provided by the serratus ventralis muscle, is greatly decreased in anesthetized horses, and it is postulated this reduces the stabilization of the lateral chest wall [182].

Although it is generally accepted that halothane and isoflurane produce bronchodilation in humans [56,183,184], general anesthesia produces an apparent increase in the elastic recoil of the lung [132]. In anesthetized ponies, halothane, isoflurane, and enflurane had a mild bronchodilating effect [185], whereas in cows [186,187] and in standing horses at subanesthetic concentrations [188], halothane did not produce bronchodilation. Interpretation of measurements of pulmonary resistance and compliance during anesthesia are made difficult because changes in lung volume *per se* will alter these values [6,183], as was demonstrated when non-fasted cows were studied over a 3 h anesthetic period [189]. It would appear, however, that the chest wall and lung volume changes play a much larger part in the generation of increased $P_{(A-a)}O_2$ gradients during anesthesia than any true alteration of lung mechanics.

Oxygen therapy and mechanical ventilation

As outlined earlier, sedation and general anesthesia can produce profound changes in a patient's respiratory function, with the degree of change depending on the drugs employed, the species involved, the depth of anesthesia, the surgical procedure, and the health of the animal. Of greatest concern are significant reductions in gas exchange causing inadequate oxygen delivery to vital tissues and/or CO_2 removal from the body. Oxygen therapy and/or mechanical ventilation support are therefore commonly used during the perioperative period in most veterinary species to alter a patient's oxygenation, ventilation, and/or work of breathing. Various physiologic and pathophysiologic factors can influence the degree to which a patient responds to such therapy. In addition, these interventions have physiologic consequences that extend beyond their desired outcomes. As such, prior to their use it is important for the clinician to understand the physiologic effects of oxygen therapy and mechanical ventilation in addition to their indications and contraindications.

Physiologic effects of oxygen therapy

The inspired oxygen fraction can be increased above 0.3 by administering oxygen at the level of the nares (face mask, nasal prongs), nasopharynx, or trachea [190–192]. When a patient is connected to an anesthetic machine with a sealed (cuffed) tracheal tube in place and oxygen is the sole fresh gas supply, it is possible to have the fraction of inspired oxygen exceed 0.95 within 5–20 min if the oxygen is delivered at flow rates recommended based on the particular breathing circuit [193].

The major physiologic effect of oxygen supplementation, and its primary reason for use, is to increase a patient's PaO_2; however, it may also impact a patient's ventilation and the morphology of their lung. In general, supplementation of inspired gases with oxygen, either alone or when associated with ventilation support, results in an increase in a patient's alveolar oxygen content, as described by the alveolar gas equation (Fig. 27.5). When matching of ventilation and perfusion within the lung is close to ideal, minimal right-to-left vascular shunts are present, and the alveolar–capillary membrane is normal, a patient's alveolar and arterial oxygen partial pressures will rise proportionately to the concentration of oxygen in the inspired gas (Fig. 27.23) [194].

Healthy dogs and cats typically have relatively low levels of venous admixture (less than 10%) from V/Q mismatching during general anesthesia and, as a consequence, oxygen supplementation results in measured PaO_2 values approaching theoretical P_AO_2 levels. Although inspired oxygen fractions are rarely measured, studies evaluating the respiratory effects of inhalant or injectable anesthetics in spontaneously breathing dogs and cats receiving only oxygen as the carrier or inspired gas, have reported PaO_2 levels greater than 450 mmHg [68,70,83,195–199]. Additionally, PaO_2 levels tend to remain stable over clinically relevant time frames in dogs and cats under general anesthesia. Although the low $P_{(A-a)}O_2$ gradient in these species brings into question the need for oxygen supplementation during heavy sedation or general anesthesia, a minimum inspired oxygen fraction of 0.3 is still recommended to minimize the risk of

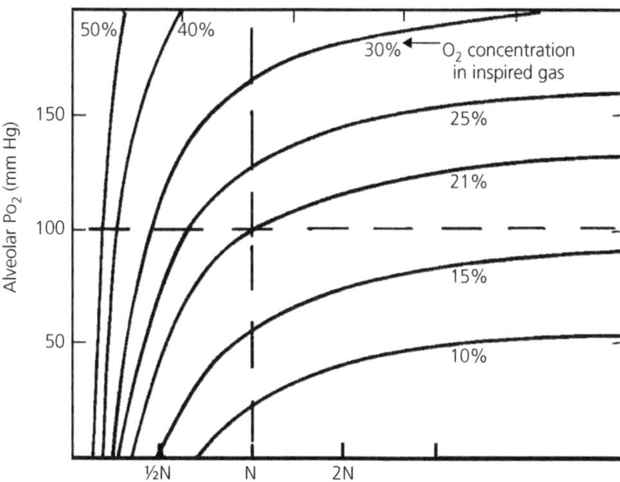

Figure 27.23 Protective effect of increased inspired oxygen concentrations with various degrees of alveolar hypoventilation and hyperventilation. A normal ventilation level such as to produce eucapnia is shown on the abscissa line as N, along with half normal ventilation (1/2N) and twice normal ventilation (2N). With 30% inspired oxygen alveolar PO_2 levels are above 100 mmHg even when alveolar ventilation is half normal. Source: modified from [194]. reproduced with permission of Elsevier.

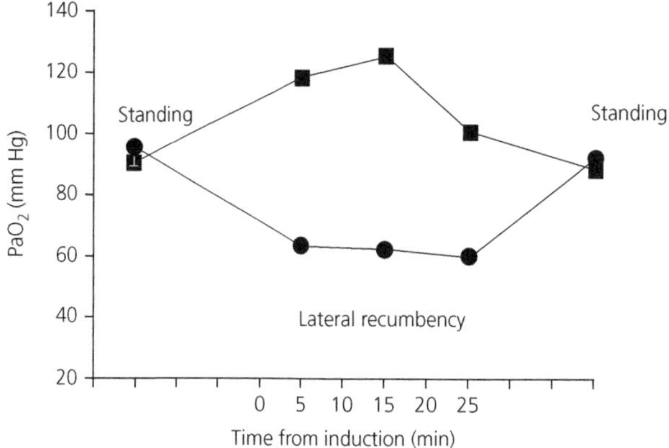

Figure 27.24 Mean arterial oxygen partial pressure (PaO_2) in 12 horses before anesthesia (standing), while anesthetized with xylazine–ketamine in lateral recumbency breathing room air, and after standing in recovery (●). Comparative PaO_2 levels in six horses also anesthetized with xylazine–ketamine, while receiving 15 L/min oxygen insufflation into the mid-tracheal location (■). Note the increase in PaO_2 levels to over 90 mmHg with the oxygen administration. Source: data taken from [155, 207].

hypoxemia due to hypoventilation and increases in V/Q mismatching relative to values in the conscious animal. Evidence to support this recommendation includes reports of impaired oxygenation as reflected by PaO_2 values below 65 mmHg in dogs sedated with an α2-adrenergic receptor agonists either alone or in combination with an opioid, and also reports of cyanosis and similarly low PaO_2 values during induction of anesthesia with injectable anesthetics when supplemental oxygen is not provided [104,200–202].

In some animals receiving oxygen supplementation, PaO_2 may not increase proportionally with P_AO_2. Patients with pulmonary parenchymal disease typically have clinically significant alveolar capillary diffusion barriers, V/Q mismatching, and increased shunt fractions. These patients typically have lower than expected increases in PaO_2 associated with oxygen therapy [203–206].

As discussed previously, recumbency and general anesthesia of mature large animal patients commonly produce significant V/Q mismatch and intrapulmonary shunting of blood. Thus, despite normal lung parenchyma prior to anesthesia, these patients have a reduced and variable response to oxygen supplementation when recumbent. Horses breathing room air while recumbent with an intravenous anesthetic regime commonly have PaO_2 values in the range 50–70 mmHg during the duration of recumbency. Tracheal (not nasal or nasopharyngeal) oxygen insufflation with 15 L/min will usually produce PaO_2 values greater than 90 mmHg (Fig. 27.24).

During inhalational anesthesia with 100% oxygen as the carrier gas, laterally recumbent spontaneously breathing healthy horses have PaO_2 values that typically range from 300 to 350 mmHg; horses in dorsal recumbency typically have lower levels, ranging from 200 to 300 mmHg [153]. Unlike the dog and cat, where PaO_2 levels remain stable over time during general anesthesia with an $F_IO_2 > 0.95$, PaO_2 values typically decrease over time in the equine, particularly when they are positioned in dorsal recumbency, or if they have not been held off-feed for at least 12 h prior to anesthesia [63,153,208–210].

While oxygen supplementation is generally administered to reduce the risk of hypoxemia, high inspired oxygen fractions delivered during general anesthesia (to either spontaneously breathing or mechanically ventilated patients) contribute to the development of atelectasis in numerous species, including dogs, cats, sheep, horses, and humans [65,211–217]. Absorption of alveolar gas, which is more soluble with higher oxygen contents, is responsible for the loss of functional alveolar volume. If the degree of atelectasis resulting from absorption is significant, it can contribute to an increase in the $P_{(A-a)}O_2$ gradient. As mentioned previously, under clinical conditions with typical anesthetic durations, PaO_2 levels tend to stay constant in dogs and cats, implying a relatively minor impact of absorption atelectasis on gas exchange in these species. In larger species such as the horse, the contribution of absorption of alveolar gases relative to the development of atelectasis as a consequence of compression of alveoli by abdominal contents may be relatively minor, but its significance may vary with body position and the specific inspired oxygen level [64,218]. In humans, atelectasis attributed to high F_IO_2 values has been associated with an increased incidence of postoperative hypoxemia and respiratory complications [219]. The presence of atelectasis has been associated with progression of lung injury in human patients and in numerous experimental animal models of lung injury receiving ventilatory support (see below).

In veterinary species, the clinical significance of anesthesia-associated atelectasis without hypoxemia on lung health in the patient with no pre-existing pulmonary disease is as yet undetermined. Irrespective of the impact on the creation or progression of lung injury, the presence of atelectasis may affect the quality of thoracic imaging and may warrant consideration of obtaining images while the animal is exposed to a lower F_IO_2, or following application of specific ventilator strategies aimed at maintaining lung volume [220]. In humans, until recently, administration of 100% oxygen via face mask prior to and during the induction of general anesthesia (e.g., preoxygenation) has been a relatively standard procedure to increase the time to hemoglobin desaturation once oxygen is withdrawn, as occurs during orotracheal intubation. However, this technique is now being called into question as it has been shown to result in a greater degree of atelectasis compared with inspiring lower oxygen fractions such as 60 or 80% [216]. Although preoxygenation is not a standard procedure in veterinary medicine, it is recommended in some cases in which a prolonged time from induction of anesthesia to achievement of a secure airway is anticipated, or with respiratory disease. Relative to the situation in human anesthesia, when oxygen is administered via face mask to veterinary species in the clinical setting it is unlikely that F_IO_2 values will be greater than 0.8 unless an unusually tight-fitting face mask is being utilized [191].

Although patient oxygenation is generally the focus when administering oxygen supplementation, the latter may also alter a patient's ventilatory drive. As discussed, anesthetics and several perianesthetic drugs alter the central and peripheral response to carbon dioxide and oxygen. The net effect of any given agent on respiratory drive may vary depending on the inspired oxygen fraction. Specifically, spontaneously breathing anesthetized patients receiving oxygen supplementation may experience a higher $PaCO_2$ level than animals breathing either room air or an $F_IO_2 < 0.5$. In particular, horses anesthetized with halothane receiving an F_IO_2 of 0.3 versus >0.85 had significantly lower $PaCO_2$ levels [63]. Similar findings have been reported in horses under injectable anesthesia [65]. Dogs that were preoxygenated prior to induction of anesthesia also had a tendency towards an increased $PaCO_2$ compared with dogs breathing room air [191]. Depression of the respiratory control mechanisms by high F_IO_2 levels or alteration in the affinity of hemoglobin for carbon dioxide with changing oxygen saturation have been suggested as potential mechanisms responsible for a greater degree of hypoventilation with oxygen supplementation in anesthetized patients [191,221].

Oxygen toxicity

It has long been recognized that high inspired oxygen levels (over 70%) when administered for prolonged periods will produce pulmonary dysfunction and even death in previously healthy laboratory and domestic animals. There is a recent excellent review of this condition, now termed *hyperoxic acute lung injury* [222]. The onset of the pulmonary damage seems to require F_IO_2 values >0.7, producing PaO_2 values in excess of 450 mmHg and a 'prolonged' exposure, certainly longer than the period usually associated with clinical veterinary anesthesia. As such, it seems that oxygen toxicity is more of a theoretical problem than a real consideration for veterinary anesthesia, despite the nearly universal use of 100% oxygen as the carrier gas during inhalational anesthesia. In the critical care situation, if prolonged mechanical ventilation is employed, the general approach is only to increase the F_IO_2 to the point where PaO_2 levels are in the range 90–100 mmHg with hemoglobin oxygen saturation levels close to or over 90%. With severe pulmonary parenchymal injury in humans, there is current discussion of targeting some degree of 'permissive hypoxia' [223,224]. However, to date there have not been any substantive clinical trials to validate such an approach, and the approach in a veterinary intensive care setting is still likely to be one of targeting normoxia.

Physiologic effects of mechanical ventilation

Current mechanical ventilation strategies all use positive pressure to expand the lung and promote gas exchange. Periodic delivery of a positive-pressure breath to a spontaneously breathing patient is termed intermittent positive-pressure ventilation (IPPV), whereas with continuous or conventional mechanical ventilation (CMV) the ventilator is set to deliver a tidal volume breath at a preset frequency, independent of the patient's ventilatory efforts. The latter is the most commonly employed mode of mechanical ventilation associated with anesthesia [225–227].

The use of mechanical ventilation in an anesthetized patient directly alters the patient's inspired gas content, gas exchange, and work of breathing. In addition, other systems, most importantly the cardiovascular system, are significantly impacted by ventilatory support and will be discussed.

Anesthesia ventilators are designed to be compatible with inhalant anesthetic delivery systems. Unlike critical care ventilators, where the F_IO_2 is controlled at the level of the ventilator, when using a ventilator designed for use in conjunction with an anesthetic machine, the content of the inspired gases are controlled at the level of the anesthetic machine (flow meter). At the present time in the clinical setting, oxygen is generally the sole carrier gas used and patients receiving ventilatory support are receiving an $F_IO_2 > 0.95$. When a patient receives this level of inspired oxygen during ventilatory support, P_AO_2 are at levels similar, if not above (due to lower $PaCO_2$ levels), those observed in the spontaneously breathing patient with an equivalent F_IO_2 level. In healthy dogs and cats receiving ventilatory support with an $F_IO_2 > 0.95$, PaO_2 values reach levels predicted by the alveolar gas equation, with values typically exceeding 450 mmHg. With healthy small ruminants, calves, and foals, PaO_2 values are usually 350–450 mmHg [228].

As with spontaneous breathing, the PaO_2 in some patients receiving mechanical ventilation can be less than the P_AO_2 since altered V/Q matching, intrapulmonary shunting, and the status of the alveolar capillary membrane can impact the efficacy of gas exchange. In the adult equine, if ventilatory support is initiated soon after induction of anesthesia, PaO_2 is generally maintained at higher levels than if the horses are permitted to ventilate spontaneously for a period of time following induction of anesthesia [153]. Even when mechanical ventilatory support is initiated immediately following induction of anesthesia, PaO_2 values vary with body position, being lowest in dorsal recumbency. Although several authors have reported improvements in PaO_2 in horses transferred from spontaneous ventilation to mechanical ventilation, others have reported inconsistent responses, with some horses showing no improvement and some showing a decrease in PaO_2 [179,210,229,230]. Most importantly, once hypoxemia is present in the spontaneously breathing equine, oxygenation is not consistently improved with conventional mechanical ventilation [153].

In humans with V/Q mismatch due to atelectasis secondary to underlying pulmonary disease, ventilator strategies that minimize lung over-distention and recruit atelectatic areas of the lung improve patient outcome compared with traditional ventilatory strategies [5]. Specifically, strategies that employ a low tidal volume and a variable degree of PEEP that minimizes loss of alveolar volume and/or recruits previously atelectatic lung are superior to approaches that use larger tidal volumes and low PEEP. The ability to measure lung mechanical properties is helpful in guiding lung recruitment during ventilator support and is key to the success of the low tidal volume strategy in the lung-injured patient [231]. A reduction in cyclic opening and closing of the lung units along with reduced shear forces between aerated and atelectatic lung are currently believed to be the main mechanisms responsible for the minimization of progression of lung injury [232]. Based on these findings, the focus of ventilator support for the lung-injured human patient has been on the long-term recruitment of lung versus the short-term maximization of oxygenation [231]. Although there have been no large randomized clinical trials in veterinary medicine to support the low tidal volume lung recruitment strategy for lung-injured patients, the evidence in animals from experimental work supports this approach and is currently recommended.

In the equine with no pre-existing lung pathology but compression atelectasis associated with general anesthesia and recumbency, the use of PEEP during CMV has variable effects on oxygenation, even when initiated early in the anesthetic period [176,234,235]. However, when PEEP is used with inotropic support, oxygenation can be improved [234,235]. The use of PEEP in combination with recruitment maneuvers has also been shown potential to increase PaO_2 values in the equine [236]. Unfortunately, once an equine patient has a significant degree of atelectasis, as evidenced by hypoxemia, it is unknown if oxygenation can be improved significantly, irrespective of the ventilatory strategy used. At present, the use of PEEP with lung recruitment maneuvers is feasible in small patients with critical care ventilators. In contrast, the ability to recruit collapsed lung areas without instituting other changes such as body position or altering the degree of abdominal tympany is limited in mature large animals in the clinical setting due to current commercially available ventilator limitations.

Although specific levels of PaO_2 may not be achievable by manipulating ventilatory support techniques in large animals, $PaCO_2$ levels can be manipulated by adjusting the ventilatory rate or tidal volume delivered by the ventilator in all species. The target or optimum $PaCO_2$ under general anesthesia varies depending on the species and the presence of underlying disease, in particular conditions with associated changes in arterial blood pH. As will be discussed, the cardiovascular side effects of positive-pressure ventilation also factor into the target $PaCO_2$ recommendations. In dogs and cats, recommended $PaCO_2$ levels are close to physiologic levels, with recommended target $PaCO_2$ values ranging from 35 to 45 mmHg. In large animals, striving for normocapnia is generally not recommended, unless required because of neurologic disease or to maintain blood pH >7.2. The rationale for permitting an above-normal $PaCO_2$ (permissive hypercapnea) is to minimize the direct cardiovascular depressant effects of positive-pressure ventilation (discussed below) and to maintain the indirect stimulatory effects of moderate increases in $PaCO_2$ on the cardiovascular system. In a study evaluating the cardiovascular effects of ventilatory support in halothane-anesthetized horses, a ventilatory strategy that resulted in normocapnia resulted in a greater negative impact on cardiac output than horses ventilated with a strategy resulting in a $PaCO_2$ in the 50–60 mmHg range [237]. This may be due to a reduced impact on intrathoracic pressure changes resulting from the lower end-expiratory pressures, or secondary to the effects of CO_2 on the cardiovascular system. Under experimental conditions in which horses were ventilated with a constant minute ventilation and $PaCO_2$ was adjusted by altering the inspired CO_2 concentration, moderate levels of hypercapnia ($PaCO_2 \approx 80$ mmHg) were shown to increase systemic arterial blood pressure and cardiac output, while heart rate remained at baseline levels [238]. It is also easier and faster to re-establish spontaneous respiration at the end of the anesthetic period when $PaCO_2$ is elevated versus eucapnia or below-normal $PaCO_2$ levels.

As discussed in the section Pulmonary Ventilation, it is alveolar ventilation that determines $PaCO_2$ and not minute ventilation. As anatomic deadspace is constant, ventilatory strategies that use lower tidal volumes will require a higher respiratory rate or minute ventilation setting to maintain target $PaCO_2$ levels. For example, healthy Beagle dogs ventilated with a constant minute ventilation and tidal volumes ranging from 6 to 15 mL/kg had higher $PaCO_2$ values when receiving the lower tidal volumes [239]. Adjustments in minute ventilation may also be necessary in patients with increased physiologic deadspace, as occurs in patients with increased V/Q mismatching, to achieve target $PaCO_2$ levels.

As with oxygen supplementation, mechanical ventilation can alter lung morphology. Specifically, the use of high F_IO_2 values during mechanical ventilation can also lead to the development of atelectasis. In a recent study, dogs anesthetized with a propofol infusion and ventilated with a relatively low V_T (12 mL/kg) for 40 min had mean PaO_2 values close to 450 mmHg, and the mean PaO_2 increased to 560–580 mmHg after an alveolar recruitment maneuver regime (lung inflation to 40 cmH_2O) [220]. When 5 cmH_2O PEEP was instituted after the alveolar recruitment maneuver, PaO_2 values remained at 570 mmHg, indicating the usefulness of low levels of PEEP in companion animals.

Although there is no doubt that mechanical ventilation support can induce lung injury when strategies that use excessive tidal volumes are used, there is a little evidence that normal tidal volume ventilation for short duration in animals with no pre-existing lung injury contributes to lung injury. In the lung injured animal, low tidal volume ventilation with end-expiratory pressures that minimize lung collapse are recommended [203,204].

One of the major factors to consider when implementing ventilatory support is the impact of positive-pressure ventilation on cardiovascular function. Both spontaneous and mechanical ventilation alter cardiovascular function by changing the intrathoracic pressure and lung volume, which in turn impact the cardiovascular system directly by altering preload, afterload, and/or heart rate [240–242]. Ventilation can also alter cardiovascular performance indirectly, by altering $PaCO_2$ or PaO_2 levels [237,238]. The relative significance of the direct versus indirect effects of ventilation on the cardiovascular system varies by species and health status of the patient. In particular, hypovolemic patients are particularly susceptible to the negative hemodynamic side-effects associated with ventilatory support [242,243]. Although there have been no detailed clinical investigations in small animals, numerous experimental studies in small animals and clinical studies in the equine have shown the potential negative impact of mechanical ventilatory support relative to spontaneous breathing on cardiovascular performance during anesthesia [73,230,244–246].

In-depth physiologic experiments using animals and also data collected from human patients have elucidated many of the mechanisms responsible for the cardiovascular depression associated with positive-pressure ventilatory support and the reader is directed to several excellent reviews [240,241,247]. Of the effects associated with physiologic tidal volume positive-pressure ventilation, the effect on right ventricular preload is likely the predominant factor influencing cardiovascular performance in patients with normal myocardial function. With spontaneous ventilation, air moves into the lungs due to a decrease in the intrapleural pressure and the creation of a negative pressure gradient between the mouth/nostril and alveoli. Due to the pressure gradient between the peripheral and intrathoracic venous system, blood flow into the thorax and right atrium increases. With the increase in flow, right atrial blood volume or preload is increased. As the latter is the major determinant of cardiac output in patients with normal myocardial contractility, stroke volume and cardiac output increase. In contrast, with positive-pressure ventilation, intrapleural pressure increases during inspiration, leading to a decrease in venous return and right ventricular output. The magnitude of the decrease in right ventricular preload is dependent on the degree and duration of intrapleural pressure change. Specifically, strategies that result in a greater increase in intrapleural pressure over a respiratory cycle, such as ventilatory strategies that use large tidal volumes, PEEP, or short expiratory times, have a greater negative impact on venous return and right ventricular preload. While left ventricular preload increases initially with lung inflation due to compression of pulmonary capillaries, the reduced right-sided preload and subsequent reduced right ventricular output in turn reduce left atrial volume or preload within several heartbeats [248].

In addition to the effect on right and left ventricular preload, delivery of a positive-pressure breath also alters ventricular afterload [240]. As lung volume increases, total pulmonary vascular resistance increases secondary to compression of intra-alveolar capillaries. Since pulmonary vascular resistance is the major determinant of right ventricular afterload, the latter also increases with increases in lung volume above FRC. With normal tidal volume breathing, this effect is minimal; however, the impact can be clinically significant when lung volumes are well above FRC for a large proportion of the respiratory cycle, such as occurs with alveolar recruitment maneuvers or strategies that use high PEEP. With respect to left ventricular afterload, during spontaneous ventilation and decreases in intrapleural pressure, left ventricular afterload increases due to an increase in transmural pressure of the aorta. The effect of ventilation on the left ventricular afterload is thought to be minimal in patients with normal myocardial function. In patients with left ventricular failure, however, positive-pressure ventilation may in fact improve hemodynamic stability by reducing left ventricular afterload.

The heart rate changes with respiration due to cyclic fluctuations in autonomic nervous system activity on the heart associated with lung inflation. The changes, however, are different if the patient is breathing spontaneously or if they are receiving ventilatory support. Specifically, during a spontaneous inspiratory breath vagal tone is reduced and heart rate increases; however, during positive-pressure ventilation, if the lungs are hyperinflated, as can occur during positive-pressure ventilation with excessive tidal volumes, heart rate decreases owing to increased vagal tone and reduced sympathetic input. The contribution of changes in heart rate to the reduced cardiac output observed with positive-pressure ventilation is likely minor during normal tidal volume ventilation. In contrast, if an excessively large tidal volume is delivered, such as during a recruitment maneuver or sigh, the heart rate may be temporarily but significantly reduced.

Although there have been no clinical trials comparing the impact of different ventilation strategies on cardiopulmonary performance in healthy small animal patients under routine anesthesia, the specific ventilatory strategy employed during anesthesia has been shown to impact cardiovascular performance in anesthetized horses. In particular, in horses maintained under halothane anesthesia positioned in lateral recumbency, a pressure-targeted ventilatory mode with a peak inspiratory pressure of 20 cmH_2O resulted in superior cardiovascular performance compared with a strategy that used a peak inspiratory pressure of 25 cmH_2O [243]. As minute ventilation was not controlled in this study, horses in the high peak inspiratory pressure group had a lower $PaCO_2$, which may have also contributed to the lower measured cardiac output. Consistent with the finding of a greater negative effect of higher peak inspiratory pressures are numerous studies showing reduced hemodynamic performance in experimental investigations of alveolar recruitment maneuvers, particularly in the presence of hypovolemia [249–252].

Clinical implications of altered respiration during anesthesia

The complexity of the respiratory response to anesthesia in veterinary patients may seem more than a little daunting to novice anesthetists and to veterinary practitioners of necessity functioning without the benefit of appreciable advanced training in the discipline. This is made so, in part, because of the variety of species that we attend to, and the wide range of drugs and environments in which veterinarians find that they must sedate, chemically restrain, or anesthetize animals. In this section, we summarize the most important clinical considerations regarding respiratory management on a species basis for typical relatively healthy patients. This overview is based to a large extent on personal experience and on discussions over the years with academic colleagues and practicing veterinarians. Unfortunately, there are exceedingly few morbidity and mortality surveys of relevant case material upon which one might base more objective conclusions. It is important to appreciate that exceptions to these generalizations may exist, based on the inherent health of the animal being treated, and because the anesthetic response in an individual animal is not always 'typical.' There is simply no safe alternative other than ongoing careful monitoring of the respiratory system during anesthesia.

Humans

Since so much of our knowledge of the altered physiology of anesthesia is derived from the literature on human patients, it helps to understand how human anesthesia differs from veterinary anesthesia. In anesthetized humans, alveolar deadspace increases by about 70 mL, and venous admixture constitutes approximately 10% of the cardiac output, compared with 2–3% in unanesthetized individuals [5]. With this degree of venous admixture, an inspired-oxygen concentration of about 35% will usually restore a normal PaO_2 (Fig. 27.17). Thus, the upper limit for nitrous oxide or nitrogen in an oxygen–nitrous oxide or oxygen–nitrogen mixture is commonly 66%; hence a 1:2 ratio of O_2 to N_2O or of O_2 to N_2 is used. Muscle relaxants and comparatively high doses of opioids (on an 'effect,' not milligrams per kilogram, basis) are commonly incorporated into the anesthetic regimen, so CMV is very commonly employed [3,5,7]. The target when ventilating anesthetized patients is usually to produce eucapnia or slight hypocapnia. This was originally done because of an apparent potentiation effect of the anesthetic dose, but now is done primarily to prevent sympathetic stimulation with resultant tachycardia and hypertension, both of which are dangerous in a patient population prone to atherosclerotic disease. Eucapnia also minimizes the risk of increased intracranial or intraocular pressure, which is especially important in trauma patients, the elderly, or those with ocular and/or central nervous system disease.

Some form of airway protection (oropharyngeal or endotracheal tube) is almost always used, and continuous monitoring of airway pressure is employed to ensure that there is no inadvertent disconnection from the anesthetic circuit of a paralyzed patient that cannot breathe spontaneously. Continuous end-tidal CO_2 and hemoglobin saturation monitoring is now widely employed, using capnography and non-invasive pulse oximetry, respectively [253]. The reasons for the increased use of these monitoring devices are that the equipment is now cost-effective and user friendly, provides medicolegal protection, and provides an early warning system of cardiorespiratory failure that decreases the mortality rate associated with general anesthesia [254,255].

Over the past decade in the field of human anesthesia, there has been considerable interest in the relationship between variable oxygen mixtures used for preoxygenation and during anesthesia and the development of atelectasis in the lung [216,217]. The usefulness of PEEP and/or forced vital capacity maneuvers (sighs or purposeful expansion of the lung) are being evaluated and debated in terms of the effect on the circulation of compromised patients, efficacy, and duration of effect [256–259]. The applicability of these findings is likely to vary among species, especially those that differ markedly in body mass from humans, or with increased communication (e.g., dogs) or decreased communication (e.g., ruminants) between alveoli through alveolar ducts or pores of Kohn [137]. In particular, it would be of great interest to know the highest F_IO_2 that it is possible to administer during general anesthesia in cattle and horses without contributing to additional atelectasis beyond that produced by position-related changes in FRC.

Dogs and cats

In reasonably healthy dogs and cats, the $P_{(A\text{-}a)}O_2$ gradient and the degree of venous admixture are less than in humans. Perhaps this is due to the smaller lungs in these species or to the difference in the chest wall changes during anesthesia [132], or perhaps because there is excellent collateral pulmonary ventilation in these species [137]. A high degree of collateral ventilation means that if an alveolus is not ventilated via the airway, it may well receive gas exchange through passages (pores of Kohn) leading to other alveoli that are ventilated.

Despite the relatively favorable situation in regard to V/Q mismatch in these species, a minimum inspired-oxygen level of 30–35% is still recommended. For the first few minutes after a barbiturate induction, PaO_2 may be as low as 50 mmHg in non-ventilated healthy dogs [260], with less change in cats [261]. The degree of hypoxemia is somewhat lower after a ketamine induction, but venous admixture still may be 20–25% for a few minutes after induction [104,105]. Obese, deeply anesthetized animals, animals with a distended abdomen (e.g., pregnancy or bowel obstruction), or those with pulmonary disease or space-occupying lesions of the thorax (tumor, pneumothorax, hemothorax, or diaphragmatic hernia) are particularly at risk. Oxygen supplementation is needed nearly as much in deeply sedated animals as in those receiving a general anesthetic (intravenous or inhalant). As can be seen in Fig. 27.23, increasing the inspired oxygen level also provides protection against hypoxemia caused by hypoventilation and, again, adequate protection is generally achieved with a venous admixture of 30–35%. This is why simple maneuvers such as placing a face mask with oxygen on a high-risk patient before and during induction or the use of a nasal oxygen catheter in the postoperative period are beneficial.

When 100% oxygen mixtures are used with the common inhalant anesthetics in dogs and cats free from serious cardiopulmonary disease, the arterial PaO_2 level is generally 450–525 mmHg whether the animal is breathing spontaneously or being ventilated, irrespective of body position [68,83,262]. With such high inspired-oxygen levels, hypoxemia usually occurs only through disconnection of the animal from the anesthetic machine, or with faulty placement of the endotracheal tube, cardiac arrest, or total apnea for over 5 min. Nevertheless, even with such high PaO_2 levels, tissue hypoxia can occur if hemoglobin levels are low or circulation is inadequate (low cardiac output).

The decision to institute assisted or controlled mechanical ventilation (CMV) is generally made to prevent or treat hypercapnia, rather than to achieve oxygenation. Nearly all spontaneously breathing dogs and cats show some degree of hypoventilation and hypercapnia ($PaCO_2$ 45–55 mmHg). The clinical importance of this in non-neurological cases is open to debate. Dogs and cats do not have atherosclerosis, and over the years hundreds of thousands of dogs and cats have been successfully anesthetized in practice while breathing spontaneously. From a practical viewpoint, with short-duration anesthetics (anesthesia of less than 1 h) in relatively healthy animals, the important aspects are to ensure that the airway is patent, that the animal is oxygenated, and that the animal does not become apneic; the development of moderate levels of hypercapnia is likely to be well tolerated. The need for IPPV increases as the depth of anesthesia has to be increased for certain types of surgery, such as hip replacement, unless local supplementation is used (e.g., epidural opioid or local anesthetic). It also increases when opioids are used as a major component of the anesthetic regimen, for obese, neonate, geriatric, or neurological patients, with certain body positions (e.g., perineal hernia repair or dorsal laminectomy), with prolonged operations, or when dealing with poor-risk patients.

A few guidelines relative to the respiratory component of anesthesia for dogs and cats are listed below:

1 Nearly all canine anesthetics are better administered with an endotracheal tube in place, and in many situations cats should be intubated.
2 Use at least 30–35% inspired oxygen in all anesthetized dogs and cats, even those on an injectable anesthetic mixture, or when deeply sedated.
3 Hypoxemia is rare in spontaneously breathing dogs and cats if breathing an oxygen mixture approaching 100%. However, oxygenation problems that are not apparent during anesthesia may become life threatening during recovery unless oxygen supplementation is continued.
4 After a prolonged period of anesthesia in cats and smaller dogs, and with shorter anesthetics in larger dogs with deep chests, it is advisable to inflate the lungs to 30 cmH_2O of airway pressure (i.e., to 'sigh' the lungs) periodically and at the end of anesthesia. The use of 5 cmH_2O PEEP will prevent most absorption atelectasis.
5 Prolonged immobility and excessive fluid administration can lead to increased venous admixture and a fall in PaO_2 in addition to that produced by anesthesia *per se* [263].

Small ruminants and swine

Ruminants are especially prone to develop regurgitation and aspiration, along with tachypnea and hypoventilation, during general anesthesia [74,75]. For shorter procedures (45–60 min), mild hypoventilation and hypercapnia often may be safely ignored if an adequate oxygen supply is maintained. Sedation and local analgesia techniques are often used for anesthesia as a means of maintaining a secure airway and adequate respiration [264]. During clinical anesthesia in pigs, especially if a barbiturate is used in a field situation, particular care must be taken to ensure that the airway is patent and that apnea does not occur.

The degree of V/Q mismatch and venous admixture is intermediate in these animals, and of such a magnitude that virtually all anesthetized animals breathing room air will have PaO_2 levels below normal. In dorsally recumbent, ventilated sheep anesthetized with pentobarbital–halothane, atelectasis of the dependent lung regions developed fairly quickly [265]. The magnitude of this atelectasis was much less than the same group observed in ponies [174]. Pulmonary disease is common in small ruminants and swine, and will lead to V/Q mismatch in addition to that induced by anesthesia, lowering PaO_2 levels further. Abdominal distension caused by the development of rumenal tympany or, in the case of swine, a full stomach will add to the degree of pulmonary dysfunction.

During inhalation anesthesia with 100% oxygen, PaO_2 is usually in the range 200–350 mmHg, well within acceptable limits [85,228]. In spontaneously breathing sheep, changes in body position (dorsal and left and right lateral) do not seem to alter the PaO_2 appreciably, and the $P_{(A\text{-}a)}O_2$ gradient is fairly constant when the sheep are sighed every 3–5 min [228]. Clinical experience suggests that the situation is similar in goats and pigs. The following are guidelines for respiratory management during anesthesia:

1 General anesthesia in sheep, goats, and calves with a developed rumen (i.e., by 2–4 weeks) requires placement of an endotracheal tube if protection against regurgitation and aspiration is to be ensured. This is best done for all but the shortest and lightest anesthetics.
2 Endotracheal intubation is not advised for swine unless the operation is complex or prolonged, or the operator is skilled with the technique.
3 During intravenous anesthesia of more compromised animals, application of a face mask or insertion of a nasal or tracheal oxygen catheter and insufflation of 2–5 L/min of oxygen will help to ensure that hypoxemia does not occur.
4 Ketamine-based anesthesia is less likely to lead to apnea or severe respiratory depression than is propofol or barbiturate anesthesia, but it can occur, so emergency support should be prepared.
5 Prolonged inhalation anesthesia (longer than 45–60 min) may require CMV to prevent hypercapnia and may be required to maintain a stable plane of anesthesia because of the tachypneic breathing pattern.
6 Mild to moderate hypercapnia is well tolerated, and serious hypoxemia is rare if inhalation anesthesia with 100% oxygen is used.
The combination of progressive abdominal tympany (even in animals fasted for up to 24 h) and the rapid, shallow respiration tend to produce a progressive increase in $P_{(A-a)}O_2$ gradients. Periodic sighing of the lungs (every 10–15 min) by inflating them to 30 cmH_2O seems to minimize the progressive increase in venous admixture and is particularly advisable at the end of an operation before extubation and return to a room-air environment. Placement in sternal recumbency during recovery benefits pulmonary function and, in the case of ruminants, helps to protect against regurgitation and aspiration.

Adult cattle and horses

Adult cattle [189,266] and horses [1,152,208] develop very significant increases in $P_{(A-a)}O_2$ gradients and venous admixture when they are anesthetized and become recumbent. On the basis of inspired-oxygen concentration and PaO_2 levels, it can be calculated that spontaneously breathing halothane-anesthetized horses have pulmonary shunt flows of 20–25%, with a reduction to about 15% in ventilated horses [208]. These were healthy horses, positioned in lateral recumbency and subjected to no surgery. Over the intervening 25 years, others have reported PaO_2 levels and $P_{(A-a)}O_2$ gradients from many studies in other healthy horses that are reflective of pulmonary shunt flows of at least the same magnitude [65,174,267]. The degree of V/Q mismatch is greater in dorsal than in lateral recumbency, in larger horses, and perhaps in older horses [153,210,229,244,268,269]. Researchers have consistently noted that the actual variability between PaO_2 levels in similar horses receiving similar anesthetics is fairly large (Fig. 27.25) [64,209]. The reasons for this variability are not clear, but probably relate to body conformation and perhaps the level of abdominal distension caused by obesity, gas distension, or ingesta in the large bowel. The $P_{(A-a)}O_2$ gradient in healthy, fasted animals does not generally increase greatly over time [209,244], but the PaO_2 will progressively decrease if the degree of abdominal distension increases. This was clearly illustrated in an interesting study of fed and non-fed cows, where the failure to fast the cows before the general anesthetic led to a progressive increase in $P_{(A-a)}O_2$ and pulmonary resistance, and a decrease in PaO_2 and dynamic compliance (Fig. 27.26a and b) [189].

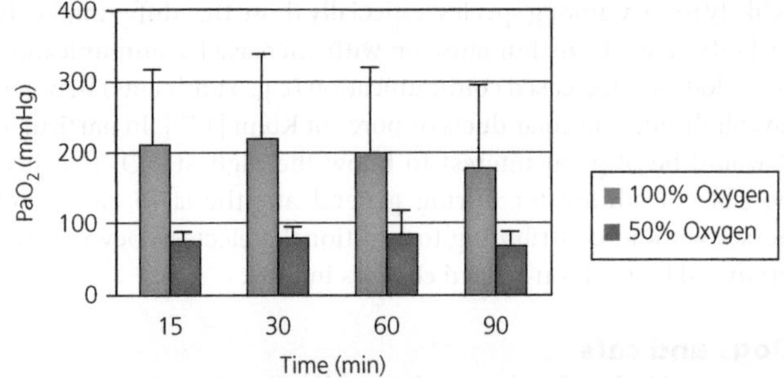

Figure 27.25 Arterial PO_2 values in eight spontaneously breathing, normal horses positioned in dorsal recumbency while anesthetized with isoflurane in either 50 or 100% oxygen. Note the low mean arterial partial pressure (PaO_2) levels in both groups considering the inspired oxygen levels and the wide standard deviation reflecting considerable variation in response between individual horses. In the 50% inspired oxygen group, PaO_2 levels ranged from a low of 46 to a high of 104 mmHg at the 90 min period of anesthesia and 3/8 horses were hypoxic ($PaO_2 \leq 60$ mmHg) at that time period. In the 100% inspired group, PaO_2 levels ranged from 72 to 401 mmHg after 90 min of anesthesia. Source: data from [64]. Image and details relative to individual horse differences provided by Crumley and co-authors and used with permission.

When an anesthetized horse (usually during colic surgery or cesarean section) inhales 100% oxygen and has a resultant PaO_2 value of less than 70 mmHg, it is clear from Fig. 27.17 that over 50% of the cardiac output is being shunted through the lungs without contributing to gas exchange. Although adult cattle also demonstrate fairly large $P_{(A-a)}O_2$ gradients during inhalational anesthesia, serious hypoxemia seems to be confined to very large animals, especially if they must be positioned in dorsal recumbency. Chronic pulmonary disease and lung consolidation are relatively common in cattle as an aftermath of juvenile respiratory disease. It is surprising that such animals do not demonstrate large increases in $P_{(A-a)}O_2$ levels during inhalant anesthesia, perhaps because pulmonary blood flow is also decreased in the non-ventilated lung areas.

When adult cattle are positioned in dorsal recumbency by using rope restraint, with or without sedation (e.g., casting), some of them become hypoxemic [129,130]. Horses anesthetized with the common injectable mixtures for brief field anesthesia also commonly have PaO_2 levels in the range 55–65 mmHg [154,155]. Admittedly, most animals so anesthetized survive with no obvious adverse after-effects. This is more a credit to the inherent safety reserve that the animals have relative to oxygen supply and to the underlying good health status of most patients than to the anesthetic regimens *per se*. Nasotracheal oxygen insufflation (15 L/min) markedly improves the safety factor in restraining and anesthetizing such animals (see Fig. 27.24), and is always desirable if circumstances permit such treatment. Some guidelines relative to respiratory support of anesthetized adult cattle and horses include the following:

1 General anesthesia requires endotracheal intubation in adult cattle because the risk of regurgitation and aspiration is high, even with prior fasting. There is some risk of regurgitation and aspiration when cattle are restrained in a recumbent position with sedatives, including xylazine. The incidence of regurgitation, however, is fairly low, and routine intubation of non-anesthetized cattle is not practical.
2 Longer anesthesia in horses is better performed with an endotracheal tube in place, and this also facilitates oxygen insufflation.

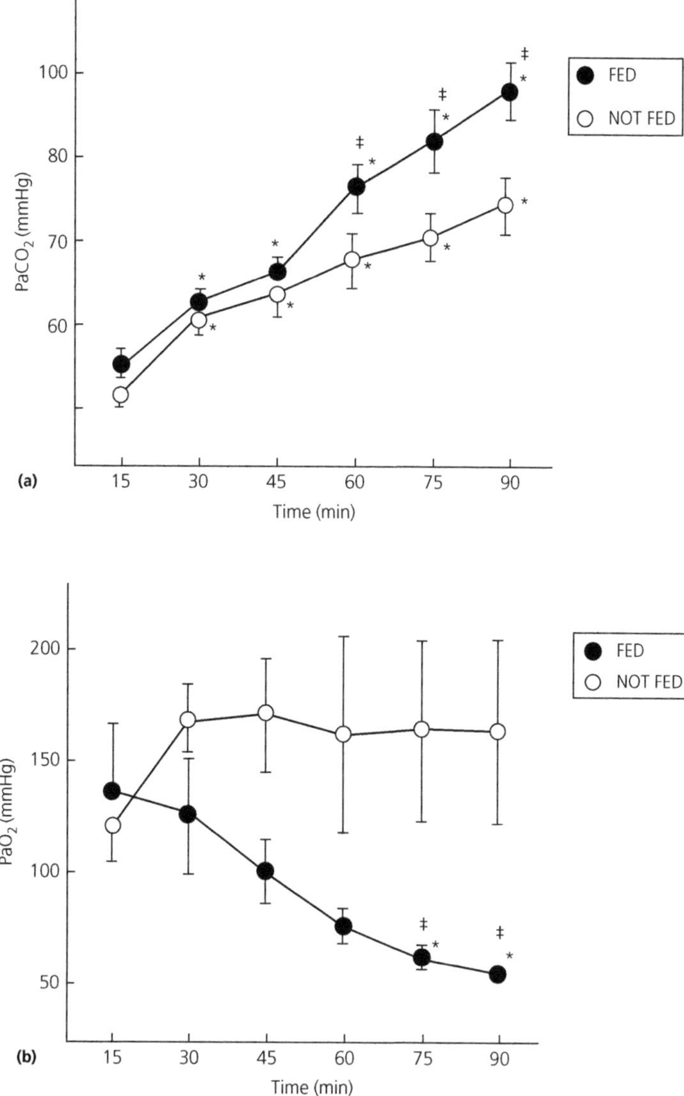

Figure 27.26 Change in (a) arterial carbon dioxide partial pressure ($PaCO_2$) and (b) arterial oxygen partial pressure (PaO_2) levels in spontaneously breathing cows with and without prior starvation. Note the greater degree of hypercapnia in the fed animals and the progressively lower PaO_2. This change was accompanied by an increase in the alveolar-to-arterial oxygen gradient [$P_{(A-a)}O_2$], an increase in airway resistance, and a decrease in compliance. These changes were probably associated with a decrease in lung volume from the development of abdominal tympany. Source: [189]. Reproduced with permission of AVMA.

3 Oxygen insufflation with 15 L/min, especially if the tip of the oxygen catheter tube is placed in the trachea, will usually prevent any serious hypoxia in relatively healthy horses and cattle during general anesthesia or recovery. This flow rate down the trachea will even maintain sufficient oxygenation to keep apneic animals alive for at least 10 min [270].
4 If oxygen supplementation is not possible, adult cattle and horses are better positioned in lateral than in dorsal recumbency (if the surgery permits the choice).
5 When preoperative starvation can be used, it is desirable, because it improves ventilation and oxygenation after the induction of anesthesia.
6 Nitrous oxide use is generally not advisable for cattle or in dorsally recumbent horses and, if used to supplement analgesia for orthopedic surgery in laterally recumbent horses, should not exceed an inspired concentration of 50% (e.g., 4 L of oxygen per 4 L of nitrous oxide) [271].
7 Inhalant general anesthetics lasting longer than 45 min in cattle almost always require CMV to prevent excessive $PaCO_2$ elevations. In horses, operations lasting over 1–2 h will generally need CMV if the need has not developed earlier. It should be appreciated that in dorsally recumbent horses breathing spontaneously, arterial hypoxemia is not always improved with initiation of CMV, which may actually decrease PaO_2 and seriously decrease oxygen delivery to tissues [153]. Moderate increases in $PaCO_2$ levels may actually produce useful hemodynamic stimulation without apparent adverse effects and seem to be well tolerated [237].
8 Although theoretically a reduction in F_IO_2 from the usual ~1.0 should lead to less ongoing alveolar collapse and absorption atelectasis in horses, experiments carried out recently using 50% inspired oxygen have not really improved the degree of V/Q mismatch, and a number of horses receiving 50% oxygen were hypoxic ($PaO_2 < 60$ mmHg) [64,218]. Hence the current

recommendation is still to use 100% oxygen as the carrier gas during equine (and bovine) inhalational anesthesia.

9 Treatment of low PaO_2 levels with high levels of PEEP (20–30 cmH_2O) is feasible if the blood volume is adequate and inotropic support is used [234,235]. Although differential lung ventilation with PEEP reduces hypoxemia experimentally [178,179], it is hard to see how this can be used clinically on those animals that actually need treating.

10 Periodic sighing of the lungs in adult cattle and horses probably does no harm, nor does it probably do much good. Full inflation of the lungs after the abdomen has been decompressed surgically, or when animals are positioned in sternal recumbency in recovery, can be useful in restoring adequate PaO_2 levels.

Exotic species

It is very difficult to generalize how best to optimize respiratory function during anesthesia for the diverse range of exotic animals. Even if not used routinely, supplemental oxygenation and the means to establish an airway should be available, if at all possible. Chemical stimulation of respiration (e.g., with doxapram) or the availability of receptor-specific antagonist drugs can be lifesaving in the case of an inadvertent anesthetic overdose, but should not be routinely relied upon to manage anesthesia in these species. Respiration is generally better supported with dissociatives than with propofol or barbiturate anesthetics. The larger the species, the more likely recumbency and positional changes may seriously interfere with cardiopulmonary homeostasis, although exceptions may exist (e.g., elephants). In general, it is desirable to keep larger terrestrial mammals in sternal rather than lateral or dorsal recumbency during restraint and/or anesthesia, unless such positioning will lead to excessive pressure on the limbs for a prolonged period.

Anesthesia for animals with respiratory disease or dysfunction

Upper airway disease or dysfunction

Patients with upper airway disease or dysfunction may present to the practitioner for procedures requiring anesthesia related or unrelated to their airway disease/dysfunction. Brachycephalic airway obstructive syndrome, laryngeal paralysis, collapsing trachea, foreign bodies and intraluminal masses are a few of the more common upper airway conditions that can result in a decrease in upper airway function. Although less common, abnormalities extrinsic to the airway (e.g., extrapharyngeal mass or abcess) can also create challenges related to upper airway management during the perioperative period.

Although the pathophysiology of the underlying conditions resulting in alterations in respiratory function must be considered, the approach to the anesthetic management of patients with upper airway disease is often similar irrespective of species, as outlined below. Although anesthetic drug choices are often of primary concern, it is likely the supportive measures and plans for airway management during the entire perianesthetic period that have the greatest impact on patient outcome [272].

In addition to patient-related concerns, the anesthetist must also consider the impact of the procedure being performed on their ability to provide optimal care during the anesthetic period. For example, access to the patient's head during the evaluation of the upper airway and subsequent procedures of the upper airway may be limited. This impacts the ability to monitor the patient's airway directly. In general, proactive consideration of possible complications and challenges will increase preparedness for untoward circumstances and improve patient outcome.

Brachycephalic canine breeds, including English and French Bulldogs, Pugs, Boston Terriers, Shih Tzu, Pekingese and Boxers, may or may not have marked symptomatic respiratory disease at rest. Abnormalities associated with the brachycephalic airway obstructive syndrome in dogs include stenotic nares, elongated soft palate, everted lateral laryngeal ventricules, everted tonsils, laryngeal collapse, and hypoplastic trachea [272–274]. In brachycephalic cats (Persian, Himalayan and Bermese breeds), similar pathology can exist. Irrespective of the species, upper airway abnormalities result in a reduction in airway diameter and an associated increase in upper airway resistance. To compensate for the latter, a greater negative intrathoracic pressure is created to generate adequate inspiratory airflow. In addition to the increase in the work of breathing, the dynamic pressure changes can further exacerbate the collapse of upper airway structures into the air passages and further increase the airway resistance. In severe cases, airway dysfunction is associated with inflammation and edema of the pharyngeal tissues. In addition to the respiratory system, cardiovascular and gastrointestinal abnormalities may be present in brachycephalic animals. Specifically, brachycephalic dogs have been shown to have a higher resting vasovagal tone than dogs of other breeds, which may predispose them to bradycardia [275]. In addition, dogs with the brachycephalic airway obstructive syndrome may also have functional and anatomic abnormalities of the gastrointestinal tract, which may predispose them to regurgitation or vomiting in the perioperative period [274]. The postoperative surgical complication rate of brachycephalic dogs in the perioperative period has been reported to be as high as 12%, with 5% developing severe dyspnea or death [273]. Overall, the major concerns related to anesthesia of the patient with brachycephalic airway syndrome are the development of airway obstruction (partial or complete) at any time in the anesthetic period (from preoperative sedation to full recovery) and the predisposition to bradycardia and regurgitation [272].

Both congenital and acquired laryngeal paralysis have been described in the canine [276]. Irrespective of the etiology, the condition is characterized by impaired abduction and adduction of the arytenoid cartilages and vocal folds, either unilaterally or bilaterally. As with the brachycephalic syndrome, the severity of symptoms associated with laryngeal paralysis can vary tremendously, with symptoms in some dogs limited to an increase in inspiratory noise with exercise whereas others may present with nearly complete airway obstruction. Hypoxemia may be present in moderately to severely affected dogs. Aspiration pneumonia may also be present as swallowing is impaired and, in severe cases, pulmonary edema can develop. The presence of underlying respiratory disease, potential for airway obstruction, and aspiration during recovery are the major anesthetic concerns for patients with laryngeal paralysis.

Equine laryngeal dysfunction is a relatively common upper airway disorder of unknown etiology. Generally, larger horses are affected unilaterally on the left side. Laryngeal paralysis secondary to guttural pouch mycosis, cervical trauma, neoplasia or inflammatory processes have been described, although these conditions are relatively rare relative to the idiopathic condition. Poor exercise tolerance and an increase in exercise-related upper airway noise are typical clinical signs [277]. Unfortunately both α_2-adrenergic receptor agonists and acepromazine influence the scoring of laryngeal dysfunction via endoscopy [278]. Intubation is rarely difficult in horses with unilateral laryngeal paralysis; however, the anesthetist should be prepared to use a smaller endotracheal tube to minimize trauma of the laryngeal structures during intubation in patients with severe clinical signs. The anesthetist should also be prepared to extubate temporarily the patient intraoperatively to permit visualization of arytenoid position.

Patients may present for general anesthesia to remove foreign bodies or luminal masses within the upper airways. The presence and impact of concurrent disease should be considered prior to anesthesia in addition to the surgical/procedural approach. The latter will impact airway management, oxygen delivery, and anesthesia maintenance.

Abnormalities extrinsic to the airway can also create upper airway management that is challenging during the perioperative period. For example, disease of the temporomandibular joint or oral masses can impair the anesthetist's ability to visualize the larynx adequately and perform orotracheal intubation. Extra-oral diseases such as salivary gland mucocoeles or neoplasia may also impair the ability to achieve orotracheal intubation using standard techniques.

A general approach to the patient with upper airway disease/dysfunction is as follows:

1 Preanesthetic diagnostics. A careful history and thorough physical examination should be employed with all patients, with particular attention to the patient's respiratory function during rest and exercise. The subsequent diagnostic plan should be tailored to the individual patient with consideration of the potential for concurrent disease and the need for evaluation prior to anesthesia. For example, in the case of laryngeal paralysis in the canine, a thoracic radiograph is recommended to screen for aspiration pneumonia and/or the presence of intrathoracic masses, particularly in older patients. In addition, a thyroid panel and measurement of acetylcholine receptor antibodies are recommended to rule out myasthenia gravis.
2 Preoperative preparation. If systemic abnormalities are present that may influence the response to anesthesia, they should be corrected if possible prior to induction of anesthesia. In particular, the patient's hydration status should be normalized. Hypoxemia should be addressed with oxygen therapy preoperatively.
3 Standard food withdrawal is generally appropriate for patients presenting with upper airway conditions.
4 Sedation. In small animal patients, standard sedation protocols should be adjusted in patients with significant upper airway disease. The administration of anticholinergic agents as part of the premedication regime in small animal patients with upper airway disease is somewhat controversial [272]. As vagal tone tends to be elevated in brachycephalic patients, personal preference is to include an anticholinergic agent when opioid drugs are used for premedication in this group of patients. Choice of premedication agents is again subject to personal preference and individual patient characteristics; however, the use of drugs that carry little risk of vomiting is recommended (e.g., buprenorphine rather than morphine). Additionally, antiemetic drugs can be used prophylactically to reduce further the risk of vomiting and aspiration. Options include use of an opioid alone or an opioid in combination with acepromazine. Although α_2-adrenergic receptor agonists are reversible, they are associated with considerable upper airway muscle relaxation and respiratory depression, in addition to their potential to induce vomiting when used in combination with μ-agonist opioids. Their use is therefore is not recommended in patients with significant upper airway obstruction. Similarly, acepromazine at high doses is not recommended owing to its prolonged duration of action.

   In large animal patients, α_2-adrenergic receptor agonists increase the work of breathing due to an increase in upper airway resistance, which is attributed to relaxation of the upper airways [109]. Although these agents are still routinely used in the horse with upper airway disease, the anesthetist should pay attention to the patient's head position following sedation prior to induction of anesthesia and the establishment of an airway, as dropping of the head or hyperflexion of the neck can impair airflow. Following sedation, all animals with upper airway disease should be kept under close observation.
5 Intravenous access should be secured in patients as soon as possible to facilitate an intervention should the animal experience an acute deterioration in airway patency.
6 Oxygenation and airway management. If the patient is not unduly stressed, preoxygenation is recommended in small animals with upper airway disease to increase the time to desaturation in the event that the time to secure an airway is prolonged [191]. In small animals, if orotracheal intubation is planned, a stylet and laryngoscope with varying sized blades should be available to facilitate direct visualization. The anesthetist should also plan to have endotracheal tubes of varying size available. When orotracheal intubation is not feasible or desired, alternatives should be considered in advance. Insufflation of oxygen via a catheter placed in the trachea may be a suitable approach in some cases. Use of a laryngeal mask or supraglottic airway device has been described in the dog, cat, and rabbit but may be of limited value depending on the pathology present [279–281]. Orotracheal intubation may also be performed in any species with the aid of an endoscope. In large animal species, nasotracheal intubation may be a suitable alternative. Tracheostomy is an alternative means of securing an airway in all species.
7 Analgesic plan. In small animal patients where there is risk of airway obstruction on recovery, avoid non-steroidal anti-inflammatory drugs (NSAIDs) prior to full recovery if possible, as corticosteroids may be required postoperatively to reduce airway edema and inflammation, particularly if surgery of the airway has occurred. As with all patients, a multimodal approach to analgesia should be taken with consideration of local anesthetic techniques in addition to the use of systemic analgesics.
8 Anesthetic induction. While the specific choice of injectable agent to use for induction of anesthesia in small animal patients with upper airway disease may vary depending on the need for assessment of laryngeal function, induction of anesthesia using inhalant anesthetics is not recommended owing to the prolonged duration of induction. One exception to this may be when the ability to intubate is seriously in doubt due to pathology (e.g., mass or web at the glottis) and apnea associated with injectable drugs could be fatal. Use of appropriate premedicants can greatly facilitate inhalant induction in these patients. A decision about the use of inhalant versus injectable techniques should be based on the patient, an understanding of the presumed pathology, and the risk–benefit analysis of the different options. In dogs, studies evaluating the suitability of different induction techniques with regard to the subsequent ability to assess oropharyngeal and laryngeal function have shown that the combination of ketamine and diazepam was less ideal than propofol or thiopental owing to lack of muscle relaxation [282]. Of note, in the latter study, dogs did not receive a sedative, which may have contributed to the lack of muscle relaxation. A second study reported thiopental as superior to propofol and ketamine–diazepam for the evaluation of laryngeal motion during laryngoscopy [283].

In large animals, standard injectable anesthetic-based induction techniques are generally appropriate.

9 Maintenance of anesthesia. In general, inhalant anesthetics are suitable for the maintenance protocol for most patients. If the airway cannot be sealed with a cuffed endotracheal tube, maintenance with injectable anesthetic agent(s) via a variable-rate infusion is recommended. In small animals, propofol is suitable whereas in large animals a mixture of ketamine, α_2-adrenergic receptor agonist, and guaifenesin is a commonly used alternative to inhalant-based anesthesia.
10 Ventilation. The resistance to breathing is dependent on the diameter of the airway; therefore, if a smaller than standard endotracheal tube or an alternative means of securing the airway results in a reduced airway diameter, the patient's work of breathing will be increased. As a result, the patient will have a greater probability of requiring ventilatory support. Means to support ventilation should be prepared prior to induction of anesthesia. This may involve having adequate personnel to provide manual ventilation or having a mechanical ventilator available and prepared for use.
11 Monitoring. Capnography is particularly useful in patients with airway disease. Inclusion of capnography will indicate the patency of the airway, detect early disconnections, and trend the adequacy of ventilation. Capnography is particularly useful if the anesthetist's access to the airway is reduced. Pulse oximetry is also a valuable monitoring tool in the small animal patient with upper airway dysfunction, particularly during the recovery phase after extubation when the animal must maintain its own airway patency and the risk for obstruction is increased.
12 Anesthetic recovery. Prior to recovery, a thorough airway examination should be performed. Debris and fluid in the oropharynx should be removed using suction or gentle swabbing. During recovery, oxygen should be provided for as long as possible. This is generally performed by insufflation of oxygen from an overhead source in large animals or via the breathing circuit in small animals. Extubation should only be performed once a strong swallow reflex is present and the animal will no longer tolerate the orotracheal tube. As airway obstruction is a risk, the anesthetist should be prepared to quickly reanesthetize and reintubate the patient if necessary. Oxygen supplementation well into the recovery period is often of benefit and the temporary use of an oxygen cage maybe of value in animals that resent restraint.
13 Postoperative considerations. Intensive postanesthetic monitoring should be adopted in patients with upper airway disease until normal mentation has returned and the animal is showing adequate oxygenation with minimal upper airway obstruction. Aspiration pneumonia is of particular concern postlaryngeal tie back and in brachycephalic breeds [276,284]. The use of analgesics associated with a low risk of vomiting, administration of antiemetic drugs, and early detection and aggressive treatment will likely improve outcome.

Lower airway and pulmonary parenchymal disease

Animals with lower airway disease may require anesthesia to permit diagnostic sample collection or to permit the performance of procedures unrelated to their lung disease. The diseases most commonly encountered in small animals include feline asthma, pneumonia, pulmonary masses, contusions, and atelectasis [272]. In large animal species, chronic obstructive pulmonary disease in adult horses and pneumonia in foals and calves are common. As with upper airway dysfunction, the pathophysiology of the individual conditions should be considered; however, the major concerns during the perianesthetic period are similar.

A General approach to the patient with lower airway and pulmonary parenchymal disease is as follows:

1 Preanesthetic diagnostics. At the minimum, a thorough physical examination should be performed immediately prior to anesthesia of patients with lung disease. Hypoxemia, hypercarbia, and hydration deficits will predispose patients to acid–base and electrolyte disturbances and measurement of blood-gas partial pressures and electrolytes is warranted if possible, particularly in the symptomatic patient presenting for anesthesia. In small animals, a preoperative thoracic radiograph should be considered to provide baseline status of lung parenchymal disease prior to anesthesia.
2 Preoperative preparation. As in the patient with upper airway disease, if systemic abnormalities are present, they should be corrected prior to anesthesia if possible. Oxygen and, in some cases, ventilatory support under heavy sedation may be required prior to anesthesia. In patients with airway disease, medical management should be instituted and the patient's condition optimized before elective procedures are undertaken.
3 Standard food withdrawal periods are generally appropriate.
4 Sedation. In adult equine patients with airway disease, standard sedation protocols are appropriate, as the sedative agents typically used do not impair oxygenation and ventilation and may in fact improve respiratory mechanics. In foals with pneumonia, doses of sedatives can generally be reduced and titrated to effect. In ruminants with pneumonia, alternatives to the α_2-adrenergic receptor agonists, such as benzodiazepines, are generally recommended to avoid profound sedation, hypoxemia, and hypercarbia.

   In small animal patients with reactive airway disease, the inclusion of an anticholinergic at the time of premedication may be advantageous owing to their bronchodilating effect, although their use is controversial. Acepromazine may be beneficial in these patients owing to its effects on inhibiting histamine release. Opioids with the potential to increase histamine release, such as intravenous meperidine, should be avoided.

   If a patient is hypoventilating prior to sedation, the anesthetist should be extremely cautious in using sedatives and opioid analgesics prior to induction of anesthesia and establishment of an airway owing to the potential for worsening of hypoventilation or even apnea with these agents. In these cases, it is prudent to induce anesthesia first and add opioid analgesics to the protocol once ventilation is supported.
5 Intravenous access. As with upper airway disease, establishment of intravenous access as early as possible is recommended to permit interventions if necessary.
6 Oxygenation and airway management. Irrespective of species, preoxygenation is warranted in any patient exhibiting hypoxemia prior to induction of anesthesia provided that the restraint needed does not create unacceptable distress. In those cases, alternatives to mask or flow by oxygen should be investigated. Plans to supplement oxygen and, if required, equipment available to secure the airway and maximize the delivery of oxygen should be available in the event that it is required at any point in the perioperative period. Ventilatory support may be required to maintain oxygenation during anesthesia. In cats with reactive airway disease, topical lidocaine can be used prior to intubation and may minimize the risk of bronchospasm.
7 Analgesic plan. As mentioned, if opioid analgesics are to be included in the analgesic plan, their effect on ventilation should

be considered. In the patient with inadequate ventilation prior to sedation, opioid administration can be delayed until ventilatory support measures are instituted prior to surgery. If a patient is receiving corticosteroids, NSAIDs should be avoided.

8 Induction of anesthesia and maintenance of anesthesia. In small animals with reactive airway disease, induction of anesthesia with ketamine or propofol is recommended over thiopental or etomidine owing to their relative bronchodilating effects. Dissociative anesthetics may offer the additional benefit of acting as sympathomimetics in most animals, which would also tend to increase lower airway diameter through indirect activation of β_2-adrenergic receptors. Caution should be exercised when using neuromuscular blockers and anticholinesterases as the latter may induce bronchoconstriction.

9 Ventilation. Hypoventilation is common in all patients under general anesthesia; however, inadequate ventilation may be more profound in patients with lower respiratory disease and/or it may result in impairment of oxygenation, particularly when receiving a low F_IO_2. When instituting ventilatory support in a patient with parenchymal lung disease, the goal should be to minimize the progression of lung injury. As discussed in the section Oxygen Therapy and Mechanical Ventilation, minimization of lung over-distention can be achieved by using low tidal volume strategies. In cases with severe lung injury, PEEP may be required to recruit the lung and minimize atelectasis. This may require the use of a critical care ventilator and therefore maintenance of anesthesia with injectable agents.

In patients with airway disease, a ventilatory strategy that uses slow inspiratory time and long expiratory time will permit full exhalation and prevent air trapping.

10 Monitoring. Capnography, pulse oximetry, and arterial blood-gas analysis are all recommended in the patient with severe respiratory disease.

11 Recovery. Prior to complete withdrawal of ventilatory support, aggressive monitoring of adequacy of ventilation should be verified with capnography or blood-gas analysis. Similarly, supplemental oxygen should only be withdrawn while monitoring oxygenation.

Anesthetic management of the patient with intrathoracic or chest wall disease

Numerous extra-pulmonary factors may influence a patient's respiratory function, including the presence of air or fluid in the thoracic cavity, a disruption in the normal chest wall or diaphragm anatomy (penetrating chest wound or a diaphragmatic hernia), or excessive chest wall rigidity due to abdominal distension. Animals with pleural space disease or traumatic disruption of the chest wall or diaphragm frequently have concurrent pulmonary parenchymal disease. In addition to the strategies listed above, preoperative preparation should include removal of pleural fluid or air prior to induction of anesthesia. Additionally, owing to the increased work of breathing associated with extra-pulmonary diseases, the anesthetist should be prepared to provide ventilatory support immediately after induction of anesthesia. Low tidal volume ventilatory strategies will minimize the increase in intrathoracic pressures and the subsequent cardiopulmonary effects of ventilatory support.

Some patients with chronic pleural space disease (e.g., chronic diaphragmatic hernia or chylothorax) may have lung lobe damage, which will be worsened by rapid re-expansion during surgery. The pathophysiology of pulmonary re-expansion injury (i.e., re-expansion pulmonary edema) appears complex but seems to involve changes in vascular integrity, infiltration of immune cells, and mechanical stresses. Edema has been observed in some individuals in the early postoperative period, which has led to various recommendations such as limited crystalloid volume administration, use of colloids, administration of diuretics, and administration of corticosteroids. Others have advocated using minimal airway pressure during CMV and waking the patient without trying to re-expand the lung lobes affected, rather relying on slow gradual re-expansion during the recovery period. This condition is seen in both human and veterinary patients and large clinical trials are necessary to provide definitive evidence on the best management practices.

One-Lung Ventilation

In human anesthetic practice, one-lung ventilation (OLV) has become fairly common as a means to facilitate the ease of surgery by providing a better visualization of the operating field and to isolate bronchial communications of diseased from healthy lung lobes during surgery. This applies to a number of thoracic procedures, including lung, esophageal, aortic, or mediastinal surgery. The potential for the development of hypoxemia during OLV in humans, along with methods of preventing and treating such hypoxemia, has been reviewed fairly recently [285]. One major source of hypoxemia is related either to faulty placement of the endobronchial blocker or double-lumen tube used to separate the lungs, or to accidental displacement of the tube during patient positioning for surgery. For this reason, both initial and re-examination of the tube positioning using endoscopy are highly recommended.

While one lung is ventilated during OLV, both lungs remain perfused, with the degree of perfusion of the non-ventilated lung depending on many factors [285]. These factors include the degree of collapse of the non-ventilated lung (which affects pulmonary resistance), the previous health of the non-ventilated lung, the degree to which cardiovascular function is impaired by the anesthetic, the ventilation regime used, and the degree to which the anesthetic regime used reduces the hypoxic pulmonary vasoconstrictor (HPV) response to local or regional (that is, lung lobe) hypoxemia. Perfusion of the non-ventilated or collapsed and non-ventilated lung inevitably leads to some degree of transpulmonary shunting and impairment of oxygenation. When an F_IO_2 level of 0.5 is used, as is common with human anesthesia, the development of hypoxemia is always a possibility and the oxygenation level must be diligently and continuously monitored [285]. The incidence of hypoxemia is higher when human patients are in dorsal recumbency or in left lateral recumbency, versus right lateral recumbency [285]. The difference in lateral recumbency occurs as the right lung is larger (about 55% of the total volume) than the left lung (45%); therefore, having the larger lung dependent and ventilated usually leads to better oxygenation. Surprisingly, there is no real evidence that intravenous anesthetic techniques lead to better oxygenation than inhalational methods, or that there is any real difference between the various inhalational anesthetics when used in clinical situations.

Until recently, there has not been wide usage of OLV anesthesia in veterinary anesthesia. With the advancements in endoscopic and thoracoscopic instrumentation and methods suitable for companion animals, reports of OLV are now appearing in the literature [286–291]. In some of these reports, a guide wire was used to insert an endobronchial blocker in the non-ventilated lung, and in some reports double-lumen endotracheal tubes designed for humans were used. There has been a recent evaluation of three different double-lumen devices for use in dogs, inserted using blind thoracoscopic assistance, and checked via endoscopy [292]. The study confirmed the importance of endoscopic confirmation of tube location in dogs, as is the situation in humans. Inadvertent stapling of an endobronchial blocker tip has also been reported [293].

Since the surgical approach in the dog and cat often occurs with the animal in lateral recumbency and the F_IO_2 level used generally will be close to 1.0, the risk of serious hypoxemia developing during OLV is likely to be minimal. That assumes that the tube placement is correct, the depth of anesthesia is appropriate, and the ventilation of the dependent lung is done properly so as to maintain eucapnia and dependent lung expansion. Use of a low level of PEEP (3–5 cmH_2O) during ventilation of the dependent lung will minimize the development of atelectasis in that lung. The need for surgical exposure will likely dictate whether or not some inflation of the nonventilated uppermost lung is maintained.

Investigations of the cardiopulmonary effects of closed-thorax OLV have been carried out in healthy experimental dogs anesthetized with isoflurane, with and without PEEP of the dependent ventilated lung [294,295]. These studies found that tissue oxygen supply was not significantly different during OLV versus the control bilateral lung ventilation, despite the large increase in $P_{(A-a)}O_2$ gradients, and presumably the level of venous admixture. The maintenance of tissue oxygen supply occurred because cardiac output was maintained and because the use of 100% oxygen as the inhalational carrier gas resulted in PaO_2 levels during OLV that were high enough to produce nearly full hemoglobin oxygen saturation, despite the increase in $P_{(A-a)}O_2$ gradient. This fortuitous situation may not be the case when OLV is used in diseased animals or if the circulatory status is compromised. Therefore, continuous monitoring of the oxygen saturation level and circulatory status is highly recommended.

References

1 Wagner AE. The importance of hypoxemia and hypercapnia in anaesthetized horses. *Equine Vet Educ* 1993; **5**: 207–211.

2 Hedenstierna G. Gas exchange during anaesthesia. *Br J Anaesth* 1990; **64**: 507–514.

3 Bigatello LM. Respiratory physiology: gas exchange and respiratory mechanics. *ASA Refresher Courses Anesthesiol* 2010; **38**: 1–7.

4 Robinson NE. The respiratory system. In: Muir WW, Hubbell JAE, eds. *Equine Anesthesia: Monitoring and Emergency Therapy*, 2nd edn. St Louis, MO: Saunders Elsevier, 2009; 11–36.

5 Hedenstierna G. Respiratory physiology. In: Miller RD, Eriksson LI, Fleisher LA, *et al.*, eds. *Miller's Anesthesia*, 7th edn. Philadelphia: Churchill Livingstone Elsevier, 2010; 361–391.

6 Robinson NE. Respiratory function. In: Klein BG, ed. *Cunningham's Textbook of Veterinary Physiology*, 5th edn. St Louis, MO: Saunders Elsevier, 2013; 495–548.

7 Lucangelo U, Bernabe MD, Blanch L. Respiratory mechanics derived from signals in the ventilator circuit. *Respir Care* 2005; **50**: 55–67.

8 McDonell WN. Ventilation and acid–base equilibrium with methoxyflurane anesthesia in dogs. MSc thesis, University of Guelph, 1969.

9 Gallivan GJ, McDonell WN, Forrest JB. Comparative ventilation and gas exchange in the horse and cow. *Res Vet Sci* 1989; **46**: 331–336.

10 Lai Y-L. Comparative ventilation of the normal lung. In: Parent RA, ed. *Treatise of Pulmonary Toxicology. Vol. 1: Comparative Biology of the Normal Lung*. Boca Raton, FL: CRC Press, 1992; 219–224.

11 Fordyce WE, Tenney SM. Role of carotid bodies in ventilatory acclimation to chronic hypoxia by the awake cat. *Respir Physiol* 1984; **58**: 207–221.

12 Gillespie DJ, Hyatt RE. Respiratory mechanics in the unanesthetized dog. *J Appl Physiol* 1974; **35**: 98–102.

13 Hales JRS, Webster MED. Respiratory function during thermal tachypnoea in sheep. *J Physiol (Lond)* 1967; **190**: 241–260.

14 Bakima M, Gustin P, Lekeux P, *et al.* Mechanics of breathing in goats. *Res Vet Sci* 1988; **45**: 332–336.

15 Mesina JE, Bisgard GE, Robinson GM. Pulmonary function changes in goats given 3-methylindole orally. *Am J Vet Res* 1984; **45**: 1526–1531.

16 Forster HV, Bisgard GE, Klein JP. Effect of peripheral chemoreceptor denervation on acclimatization of goats during hypoxia. *J Appl Physiol* 1981; **50**: 392–398.

17 Verbrugghe C, Laurent P, Bouvert P. Chemoreflex drive of ventilation in the awake miniature pig. *Respir Physiol* 1982; **47**: 379–391.

18 Keith IM, Bisgard GE, Manohar M, *et al.* Respiratory effects of pregnancy and progesterone in Jersey cows. *Respir Physiol* 1982; **50**: 351–358.

19 Bisgard GE, Ruis AV, Grover RF, *et al.* Ventilatory control in the Hereford calf. *J Appl Physiol* 1973; **35**: 220–226.

20 Willoughby RA, McDonell WN. Pulmonary function testing in horses. *Vet Clin North Am Large Anim Pract* 1979; **1**: 171–196.

21 Gillespie JR, Tyler WS, Eberly VE. Pulmonary ventilation and resistance in emphysematous and control horses. *J Appl Physiol* 1966; **21**: 416–422.

22 Orr JA, Bisgard GE, Forster HV, *et al.* Cardiopulmonary measurements in nonanesthetized, resting normal ponies. *Am J Vet Res* 1975; **36**: 1667–1670.

23 Libermann IM, Capano A, Gonzalez F, *et al.* Blood acid–base status in normal albino rats. *Lab Anim Sci* 1973; **23**: 862–865.

24 Lai Y-L, Tsuya Y, Hildebrandt J. Ventilatory response to acute CO_2 exposure in the rat. *J Appl Physiol* 1978; **45**: 611–618.

25 Lahiri S. Blood oxygen affinity and alveolar ventilation in relation to body weight in mammals. *Am J Physiol* 1975; **229**: 529–536.

26 Neutze JM, Wyler F, Rudolph AM. Use of radioactive microspheres to assess cardiac output in rabbits. *Am J Physiol* 1968; **215**: 486–495.

27 Dyson DH, Allen DG, Ingwersen W, *et al.* Effects of saffan on cardiopulmonary function in healthy cats. *Can J Vet Res* 1987; **51**: 236–239.

28 Herbert DA, Mitchell RA. Blood gas tensions and acid–base balance in awake cats. *J Appl Physiol* 1971; **30**: 434–436.

29 Horwitz LD, Bishop VS, Stone HL, *et al.* Cardiovascular effects of low-oxygen atmospheres in conscious and anesthetized dogs. *J Appl Physiol* 1969; **27**: 370–373.

30 Wanner A, Reinhart ME. Respiratory mechanics in conscious sheep: response to methacholine. *J Appl Physiol* 1978; **44**: 479–482.

31 Bisgard GE, Vogel JHK. Hypoventilation and pulmonary hypertension in calves after carotid body excision. *J Appl Physiol* 1971; **31**: 431–437.

32 Donawick WJ, Baue AE. Blood gases, acid–base balance, and alveolar–arterial oxygen gradient in calves. *Am J Vet Res* 1968; **29**: 561–567.

33 Crosfill ML, Widdicombe JG. Physical characteristics of the chest and lungs and the work of breathing in different mammalian species. *J Physiol (Lond)* 1961; **158**: 1–14.

34 Mauderly JL. Effect of age on pulmonary structure and function of immature and adult animals and man. *Fed Proc* 1979; **38**: 173–177.

35 Gallivan GJ, McDonell WN, Forrest JB. Comparative pulmonary mechanics in the horse and the cow. *Res Vet Sci* 1989; **46**: 322–330.

36 Sorenson PR, Robinson NE. Postural effects on lung volumes and asynchronous ventilation in anesthetized horses. *J Appl Physiol* 1980; **48**: 97–103.

37 McDonell WN, Hall LW. Functional residual capacity in conscious and anaesthetized horses. *Br J Anaesth* 1974; **46**: 802–803.

38 Gallivan GJ, Bignell W, McDonell WN, *et al.* Simple nonrebreathing valves for use with large mammals. *Can J Vet Res* 1989; **53**: 143–146.

39 Derksen FJ, Robinson NE. Esophageal and intrapleural pressures in the healthy conscious pony. *Am J Vet Res* 1980; **41**: 1756–1761.

40 Amis TC, Pascoe JR, Hornof W. Topographic distribution of pulmonary ventilation and perfusion in the horse. *Am J Vet Res* 1984; **45**: 1597–1601.

41 Schramel J, Nagel C, Palm F, *et al.* Distribution of ventilation in pregnant Shetland ponies measured by electrical impedance tomography. *Respir Physiol Neurobiol* 2012; **180**: 258–262.

42 West JB. Ventilation–perfusion relationships. *Am Rev Respir Dis* 1977; **116**: 919–943.

43 Porcelli RJ. Pulmonary hemodynamics. In: Parent RA, ed. *Treatise on Pulmonary Toxicology. Vol. 1: Comparative Biology of the Normal Lung*. Boca Raton, FL: CRC Press, 1992; 241–270.

44 Glenny RW, Lamm WJE, Albert RK, *et al.* Gravity is a minor determinant of pulmonary blood flow distribution. *J Appl Physiol* 1991; **71**: 620–629.

45 Hlastra MP, Bernard SL, Erikson HH, *et al.* Pulmonary blood flow distribution in standing horses is not dominated by gravity. *J Appl Physiol* 1996; **81**: 1051–1061.

46 Pelletier N, Robinson NE, Kaiser L, *et al.* Regional differences in endothelial function in horse lungs: possible role in blood flow distribution? *J Appl Physiol* 1998; **85**: 537–542.

47 Dobson A, Gleed RD, Meyer RE, *et al.* Changes in blood flow distribution in equine lungs induced by anaesthesia. *Q J Exp Physiol* 1985; **70**: 283–297.

48 Glenny RW, Polissar L, Robertson HT. Relative contribution of gravity to pulmonary perfusion heterogeneity. *J Appl Physiol* 1991; **71**: 2449–2452.

49 Jarvis KA, Steffey EP, Tyler WS, *et al.* Pulmonary blood flow distribution in anesthetized ponies. *J Appl Physiol* 1992; **72**: 1173–1178.

50 Walther SM, Domino KB, Glenny RW, *et al.* Pulmonary blood flow distribution in sheep: effects of anesthesia, mechanical ventilation, and changes in posture. *Anesthesiology* 1997; **87**: 335–342.

51 Brodbelt D. Feline anesthetic deaths in veterinary practice. *Top Companion Anim Med* 2010; **25**: 189–194.

52 Daunt DA. Supportive therapy in the anesthetized horse. *Vet Clin North Am Equine Pract* 1990; **6**: 557–573.

53 Wagner AE. Complications in equine anesthesia. *Vet Clin North Am Equine Pract* 2008; **24**: 735–752.

54 Kelly AB, Steffey EP. Inhalation anesthesia: drugs and techniques. *Vet Clin North Am Equine Pract* 1981; **3**: 59–71.

55 McDonell WN, Dyson DH. Management of anesthetic emergencies. In: White NA, Moore JN, eds. *Current Practice of Equine Surgery*. Philadelphia: JB Lippincott, 1990: 103–114.

56 Farber NE, Pagel PS, Warltier DC. Pulmonary pharmacology. In: Miller RD, Eriksson LI, Fleisher LA, *et al.*, eds. *Miller's Anesthesia*, 7th edn. Philadelphia: Churchill Livingstone Elsevier, 2010; 155–189.

57 Gauvreau GM, Wilson BA, Schnurr DL, *et al.* Oxygen cost of ventilation in the horse. *Res Vet Sci* 1995; **59**: 168–171.

58 Muir WW, Moore CA, Hamlin RL. Ventilatory alterations in normal horses in response to changes in inspired oxygen and carbon dioxide. *Am J Vet Res* 1975; **36**: 155–159.

59 Boggs DF. Comparative control of respiration. In: Parent RA, ed. *Treatise on Pulmonary Toxicology. Vol. 1: Comparative Biology of the Normal Lung*. Boca Raton, FL: CRC Press, 1992; 314–315.

60 Lekeux P, Rollin F, Art T. Control of breathing in resting and exercising animals. In: Lekeux P, ed. *Pulmonary Function in Healthy, Exercising and Diseased Animals*. Gent: Flemish Veterinary Journal (Special Issue) 1993; 123–145.

61 Muir WW, Hamlin RL. Effects of acetylpromazine on ventilatory variables in the horse. *Am J Vet Res* 1975; **36**: 1439–1442.

62 Bisgard GE, Vagel JH. Hypoventilation and pulmonary hypertension in calves after carotid body excision. *J Appl Physiol* 1971; **31**: 431–437.

63 Cuvelliez SG, Eicker SW, McLauchlan C, *et al.* Cardiovascular and respiratory effects of inspired oxygen fraction in halothane-anesthetized horses. *Am J Vet Res* 1990; **51**: 1226–1231.

64 Crumley MN, McMurphy RM, Hodgson DS, *et al.* Effects of inspired oxygen concentration on ventilation, ventilator rhythym, and gas exchange in isoflurane-anesthetized horses. *Am J Vet Res* 2013; **74**: 183–190.

65 Marntell S, Nyman G, Hedenstierna G. High inspired oxygen concentrations increase intrapulmonary shunt in anesthetized horses. *Vet Anaesth Analg* 2005; **32**: 338–347.

66 Imai A, Steffey EP, Farver TB, *et al.* Assessment of isoflurane-induced anesthesia in ferrets and rats. *Am J Vet Res* 1999; **60**: 1577–1583.

67 Imai A, Steffey EP, Ilkiw JE, *et al.* Comparison of clinical signs and hemodynamic variables used to monitor rabbits during halothane- and isoflurane-induced anesthesia. *Am J Vet Res* 1999; **60**: 1189–1195.

68 Steffey EP, Farver TB, Woliner MJ. Circulatory and respiratory effects of methoxyflurane on dogs: comparison of halothane. *Am J Vet Res* 1984; **45**: 2574–2579.

69 Gautier H, Bonora M, Zaoui D. Influence of halothane on control of breathing in intact and decerebrated cats. *J Appl Physiol* 1987; **63**: 546–553.

70 Mutoh T, Nishimura R, Kim HY, *et al.* Cardioplumonary effects of sevoflurane, compared with halothane, enflurane, and isoflurane, in dogs. *Am J Vet Res* 1997; **58**: 885–890.

71 Steffey EP, Howland D. Comparison of circulatory and respiratory effects of isoflurane and halothane anesthesia in horses. *Am J Vet Res* 1980; **41**: 821–825.

72 Grosenbaugh DA, Muir WW. Cardiorespiratory effects of sevoflurane, isoflurane, and halothane in horses. *Am J Vet Res* 1998; **59**: 101–106.

73 Steffey EP, Woliner MJ, Puschner B, *et al.* Effects of desflurane and mode of ventilation on cardiovascular and respiratory function and clinicopathologic variables in horses. *Am J Vet Res* 2005; **66**: 669–677.

74 Trim CM. Sedation and general anesthesia in ruminants. *Calif Vet* 1981; **35**: 29–36.

75 Steffey EP. Some characteristics of ruminants and swine that complicate management of general anesthesia. *Vet Clin North Am Food Anim Pract* 1986; **2**: 507–516.

76 Hornbein TF. Anesthetics and ventilatory control. In: Covino BG, Fozzard HA, Rehder K, Strichartz G, eds. *Effects of Anesthesia*. Bethesda, MD: American Physiological Society, 1985; 75–90.

77 Hirshman CA, McCullough RE, Cohen PJ, *et al.* Hypoxic ventilatory drive in dogs during thiopental, ketamine, or pentobarbital anesthesia. *Anesthesiology* 1975; **43**: 628–634.

78 Hirshman CA, McCullough RE, Cohen PJ, *et al.* Depression of hypoxic ventilatory response by halothane, enflurane and isoflurane in dogs. *Br J Aneath* 1977; **49**: 957–963.

79 Knill RL, Gelb AW. Ventilatory response to hypoxia and hypercapnia during halothane sedation and anesthesia in man. *Anesthesiology* 1978; **49**: 244–251.

80 Sluth EA, Dogas Z, Krolo M, *et al.* Dose-dependent effects of halothane on the phrenic nerve responses to acute hypoxia in vagotomized dogs. *Anesthesiology* 1997; **87**: 1428–1439.

81 Sluth EA, Dogas Z, Krolo M, *et al.* Effects of halothane on the phrenic nerve responses to carbon dioxide mediated by carotid body chempreceptors in vagotomized dogs. *Anesthesiology* 1997; **87**: 1440–1449.

82 Sarton E, Dahan A, Tepperma L, *et al.* Acute pain and central nervous system arousal do not resolve impaired ventilator response during sevoflurane sedation. *Anesthesiology* 1996; **85**: 295–303.

83 Steffey EP, Howland D. Isoflurane potency in the dog and cat. *Am J Vet Res* 1977; **38**: 1833–1836.

84 Steffey EP, Howland D. Potency of enflurane in dogs: comparison with halothane and isoflurane. *Am J Vet Res* 1978; **39**: 573–577.

85 Steffey EP, Howland D. Halothane anesthesia in calves. *Am J Vet Res* 1979; **40**: 372–376.

86 Steffey EP, Gillespie JR, Berry JD, *et al.* Cardiovascular effects of halothane in the stump-tailed macaque during spontaneous and controlled ventilation. *Am J Vet Res* 1974; **35**: 1315–1319.

87 Steffey EP, Howland D, Giri S, *et al.* Enflurane, halothane, and isoflurane potency in horses. *Am J Vet Res* 1977; **38**: 1037–1039.

88 Steffey MA, Bresnan RJ, Steffey EP. Assessment of halothane and sevoflurane anesthesia in spontaneously breathing rats. *Am J Vet Res* 2003; **64**: 470–474.

89 McDonell W. Anesthesia of the harp seal. *J Wildl Dis* 1972; **8**: 287–295.

90 Daunt DA, Steffey EP, Pascoe JR, *et al.* Actions of isoflurane and halothane in pregnant mares. *J Am Vet Med Assoc* 1992; **201**: 1367–1374.

91 Brandstater B, Eger EI, Edelist G. Constant depth halothane anesthesia in respiratory studies. *J Appl Physiol* 1965; **20**: 171–174.

92 Seaman GC, Ludders JW, Erb HN, *et al.* Effects of low and high fractions of inspired oxygen on ventilation in ducks anesthetized with isoflurane. *Am J Vet Res* 1994; **55**: 395–398.

93 Nolan AM, Reid J. The use of intraoperative fentanyl in spontaneously breathing dogs undergoing orthopaedic surgery. *J Vet Anaesth* 1991; **18**: 30–39.

94 Steffey EP, Eisele JH, Baggot JD. Interactions of morphine and isoflurane in horses. *Am J Vet Res* 2003; **64**: 166–175.

95 Copeland VS, Haskins SC, Patz DJ. Oxymorphone: cardiovascular, pulmonary, and behavioral effects in the dog. *Am J Vet Res* 1987; **48**: 1626–1630.

96 Turner DM, Ilkiw JE, Rose RJ, *et al.* Respiratory and cardiovascular effects of five drugs used as sedatives in the dog. *Aust Vet J* 1974; **50**: 260–265.

97 Berg RJ, Orton EC. Pulmonary function in dogs after intercostal thoracotomy: comparison of morphine, oxymorphone, and selective intercostal nerve block. *Am J Vet Res* 1986; **47**: 471–474.

98 Katz J, Kavanagh BP, Sandler AN. Preemptive analgesia: clinical evidence of neuroplasty contributing to post-operative pain. *Anesthesiology* 1992; **77**: 439–446.

99 Jones JG, Sapsford DJ, Wheatley RG. Post-operative hypoxaemia: mechanisms and time course. *Anaesthesia* 1990; **45**: 566–573.

100 Taylor PM, Houlton JEF. Post-operative analgesia in the dog: a comparison of morphine, buprenorphine, and pentazocine. *J Small Anim Pract* 1984; **25**: 437–451.

101 Jacobson JD, McGrath CJ, Smith EP. Cardiorespiratory effects of induction and maintenance of anesthesia with ketamine–midazolam combination, with and without prior administration of butorphanol or oxymorphone. *Am J Vet Res* 1994; **55**: 543–550.

102 Popilskis S, Kohn D, Sanchez JA, *et al.* Epidural versus intramuscular oxymorphone analgesia after thoracotomy in dogs. *Vet Surg* 1991; **20**: 462–467.

103 Pascoe PJ, Dyson DH. Analgesia after lateral thoracotomy in dogs: epidural morphine versus intercostal bupivacaine. *Vet Surg* 1993; **22**: 141–147.

104 Haskins SC, Farver TB, Patz JD. Cardiovascular changes in dogs given diazepam and diazepam–ketamine. *Am J Vet Res* 1986; **17**: 795–798.

105 Farver TB, Haskins SC, Patz JD. Cardiopulmonary effects of acepromazine and of the subsequent administration of ketamine in the dog. *Am J Vet Res* 1986; **47**: 631–635.

106 Muir WW, Sams RA, Huffman RH, *et al.* Pharmacodynamic and pharmacokinetic properties of diazepam in horses. *Am J Vet Res* 1982; **43**: 1756–1762.

107 Reitemeyer H, Klein HJ, Deegen E. The effect of sedatives on lung function in horses. *Acta Vet Scand* 1986; **82**: 111–120.

108 Lavoie JP, Pascoe JR, Kurpershoek CJ. Effects of xylazine on ventilation in horses. *Am J Vet Res* 1992; **53**: 916–920.

109 Lavoie JP, Pascoe JR, Kurpershoek CJ. Effect of head and neck position on respiratory mechanics in horses sedated with xylazine. *Am J Vet Res* 1992; **53**: 1653–1657.

110 Wagner AE, Muir WW, Hinchcliff KW. Cardiovascular effects of xylazine and detomidine in horses. *Am J Vet Res* 1991; **52**: 651–657.

111 Clarke KW, England GCW, Goossens L. Sedative and cardiovascular effects of romifidine, alone and in combination with butorphanol, in the horse. *J Vet Anaesth* 1991; **18**: 25–29.

112 Celly CS, McDonell WN, Young SS, *et al.* The comparative hypoxaemic effect of four alpha 2 adrenoceptor agonists (xylazine, romifidine, detomidine and medetomidine) in sheep. *J Vet Pharmacol Ther* 1997; **20**: 461–464.

113 Celly CS, McDonell WN, Black WD, *et al.* Cardiopulmonary effects of clonidine, diazepam, and the peripheral alpha-2 adrenoceptor agonist ST-91 in conscious sheep. *J Vet Pharmacol Ther* 1997; **20**: 472–478.

114 Celly CS, McDonell WN, Black WD. Cardiopulmonary effects of the α_2-adrenoceptor agonists medetomidine and ST-91 in anesthetized sheep. *J Pharmacol Exp Ther* 1999; **289**: 712–720.

115 Celly CS, Atwal OS, McDonell WN, *et al.* Histopathological alterations induced by α_2 adrenoceptor agonists in the lungs of sheep. *Am J Vet Res* 1999; **60**: 154–161.

116 Doherty TJ, Ballinger JA, McDonell WN, *et al.* Antagonism of xylazine induced sedation by idazoxan in calves. *Can J Vet Res* 1987; **51**: 244–248.

117 Kumar A, Thurmon JC. Cardiopulmonary, hemocytologic and biochemical effects of xylazine in goats. *Lab Anim Sci* 1979; **29**: 486–491.

118 Caulkett NA, Cattet MR, Cantwell S, *et al.* Anesthesia of wood bison with medetomidine–zolazepam/tiletamine and xylazine–zolazepam/tiletamine combinations. *Can Vet J* 2000; **41**: 49–53.

119 Caulkett NA, Cribb PH, Haigh JC. Comparative cardiopulmonary effects of carfentanil–xylazine and medetomidine–ketamine used for immobilization of mule deer and mule deer/white-tailed deer hybrids. *Can J Vet Res* 2000; **64**: 64–68.

120 Read MR, Caulkett NA, Symington A, *et al.* Treatment of hypoxemia during xylazine–tiletamine–zolazepam immobilization of wapiti. *Can Vet J* 2001; **42**: 861–864.

121 Allen DG, Dyson DH, Pascoe PJ, *et al.* Evaluation of a xylazine–ketamine hydrochloride combination in the cat. *Can Vet Res* 1986; **50**: 23–26.

122 Nguyen D, Abdul-Rasool I, Ward D, *et al.* Ventilatory effects of dexmedetomidine, atipamezole, and isoflurane in dogs. *Anesthesiology* 1992; **76**: 573–579.

123 Ko JCH, Bailey JE, Pablo LS, *et al.* Comparison of sedative and cardiorespiratory effects of medetomidine and medetomidine–butorphanol combination in dogs. *Am J Vet Res* 1996; **57**: 535–540.

124 Ko JCH, Fox SM, Mandsager RE. Sedative and cardiorespiratory effects of medetomidine, medetomidine–butorphanol, and medetomidine–ketamine in dogs. *J Am Vet Med Assoc* 2000; **216**: 1578–1583.

125 Lamont LA, Bulmer BJ, Grimm KA, *et al.* Cardiopulmonary evaluation of the use of medetomidine hydrochloride in cats. *Am J Vet Res* 2001; **62**: 1745–1749.

126 Sinclair M. A review of the physiological effects of α_2-agonists related to the clinical use of medetomidine in small animal practice. *Can Vet J* 2002; **44**: 885–897.

127 Mitchell B, Williams JT. Respiratory function changes in sheep associated with lying in lateral recumbency and with sedation by xylazine. *Proc Assoc Vet Anaesth Gr Br Ir* 1977; **6**: 32–36.

128 Hall LW. Cardiovascular and pulmonary effects of recumbency in two conscious ponies. *Equine Vet J* 1984; **16**: 89–92.

129 Klein L, Fisher H. Cardiopulmonary effects of restraint in dorsal recumbency on awake cattle. *Am J Vet Res* 1988; **49**: 1605–1608.

130 Wagner AE, Muir WW, Grospitch BJ. Cardiopulmonary effects of position in conscious cattle. *Am J Vet Res* 1990; **51**: 7–10.

131 Agostoni E. Mechanics of the pleural space. *Physiol Rev* 1972; **52**: 57–128.

132 Rehder K. Anesthesia and the mechanics of respiration. In: Covino BG, Fozzard HA, Rehder K, Strichartz G, eds. *Effects of Anesthesia.* Bethesda, MD: American Physiological Society, 1985; 91–106.

133 Marshall BE, Marshall C. Anesthesia and pulmonary circulation. In: Covino BG, Fozzard HA, Rehder K, Strichartz G, eds. *Effects of Anesthesia.* Bethesda, MD: American Physiological Society, 1985; 121–136.

134 Amis TC, Jones HA, Hughes JMB. A conscious dog model for study of regional lung function. *J Appl Physiol* 1982; **53**: 1050–1054.

135 Amis TC, Pascoe JR, Hornof W. Topographic distribution of pulmonary ventilation and perfusion in the horse. *Am J Vet Res* 1984; **45**: 1597–1601.

136 Hedenstierna G, Nyman G, Kvart C, *et al.* Ventilation–perfusion relationships in the standing horse: an inert gas elimination study. *Equine Vet J* 1987; **19**: 514–519.

137 Robinson NE. Some functional consequences of species differences in lung anatomy. *Adv Vet Sci Comp Med* 1982; **26**: 1–33.

138 Tucker A, McMurtry IF, Reeves JT, *et al.* Lung vascular smooth muscle as a determinant of pulmonary hypertension at high altitude. *Am J Physiol* 1975; **228**: 762–767.

139 Elliott AR, Steffey EP, Jarvis KA, *et al.* Unilateral hypoxic pulmonary vasoconstriction in the dog, pony and miniature swine. *Respir Physiol* 1991; **85**: 355–369.

140 Marshall BE, Marshall C, Benumof J, *et al.* Hypoxic pulmonary vasoconstriction in dogs: effects of lung segment size and oxygen tension. *J Appl Physiol* 1981; **51**: 1543–1551.

141 Araos JD, Larenza P, Boston RC, *et al.* Use of the oxygen content-based index, Fshunt, as an indicator of pulmonary venous admixture at various inspired oxygen fractions in anesthetized sheep. *Am J Vet Res* 2012; **73**: 2013–2020.

142 Benatar SR, Hewlett AM, Nunn JF. The use of iso-shunt lines for control of oxygen therapy. *Br J Anaesth* 1973; **45**: 711–718.

143 Froese AB. Effects of anesthesia and paralysis on the chest wall. In: Covino BG, Fozzard HA, Rehder K, Strichartz G, eds. *Effects of Anesthesia.* Bethesda, MD: American Physiological Society, 1985; 107–120.

144 Lai YL, Rodarte JR, Hyatt RE. Respiratory mechanics in recumbent dogs anesthetized with thiopental sodium. *J Appl Physiol* 1979; **46**: 716–720.

145 Rugh KS, Garner HE, Hatfield DG, *et al.* Arterial oxygen and carbon dioxide tensions in conscious laterally recumbent ponies. *Equine Vet J* 1984; **16**: 185–188.

146 Honeyman VL, Pettifer GR, Dyson DH. Arterial blood pressure and blood gas valves in normal standing and laterally recumbent African (*Loxodonta africana*) and Asian (*Elephas maximus*) elephants. *J Zoo Wildl Med* 1992; **23**: 205–210.

147 Engel S. The respiratory tissue of the elephant (*Elephas indicus*). *Acta Anat (Basel)* 1963; **5**: 105–111.

148 Ungerer T, Orr JA, Bisgard GE, *et al.* Cardiopulmonary effects of mechanical distension of the rumen in nonanesthetized sheep. *Am J Vet Res* 1976; **37**: 807–810.

149 Musewe VO, Gillespie JR, Berry JD. Influence of ruminal insufflation on pulmonary function and diaphragmatic electromyography in cattle. *Am J Vet Res* 1979; **40**: 26–31.

150 Hornof WJ, Dunlop CI, Prestage R, *et al.* Effects of lateral recumbency on regional lung function in anesthetized horses. *Am J Vet Res* 1986; **47**: 277–282.

151 Thurmon JC. General clinical considerations for anesthesia in the horse. *Vet Clin North Am Equine Pract* 1990; **6**: 485–494.

152 Stegman GF. Pulmonary function in the horse during anesthesia: a review. *J S Afr Vet Assoc* 1986; **57**: 49–53.

153 Day TK, Gaynor JS, Muir WW, *et al.* Blood gas values during intermittent positive pressure ventilation and spontaneous ventilation in 160 anesthetized horses positioned in lateral and dorsal recumbency. *Vet Surg* 1995; **24**: 266–276.

154 Wan PY, Trim CM, Mueller PO. Xylazine–ketamine and detomidine–tiletamine–zolazepam anesthesia in horses. *Vet Surg* 1992; **21**: 312–318.

155 Kerr CL, McDonell WN, Young SS. A comparison of romifidine and xylazine when used with diazepam/ketamine for short duration anesthesia in the horse. *Can Vet J* 1996; **37**: 601–609.

156 Wilson DV, McFeely AM. Positive end-expiratory pressure during colic surgery in horses: 74 cases (1986–1988). *J Am Vet Med Assoc* 1991; **199**: 917–921.

157 Sykes MK, Gibbs JM, Loh L, *et al.* Preservation of the pulmonary vasoconstrictor response to alveolar hypoxia during the administration of halothane to dogs. *Br J Anaesth* 1978; **50**: 1185–1196.

158 Domino KB, Borowec l, Alexander CM, *et al.* Influence of hypoxic pulmonary vasoconstriction in dogs. *Anesthesiology* 1986; **64**: 423–429.

159 Levsitsky MA, Davis S, Murray PA. Preservation of hypoxic pulmonary vasoconstriction during sevoflurane and desflurane anesthesia compared to the conscious state in chronically instrumented dogs. *Anesthesiology* 1998; **89**: 1501–1508.

160 Kerbaul F, Bellezza M, Guidon C, *et al.* Effects of sevoflurane on hypoxic pulmonary vasoconstriction in anaesthetized piglets. *Br J Anaesth* 2000; **85**: 440–445.

161 Young LE, Bartram DH, Diamond MJ, *et al.* Clinical evaluation of an infusion of xylazine, guaifenesin and ketamine for maintenance of anaesthesia in horses. *Equine Vet J* 1993; **25**: 115–119.

162 McMurphy RM, Young LE, Marlin DJ, *et al.* Comparison of the cardiopulmonary effects of anesthesia maintained by continuous infusion of romifidine, guaifenesin, and ketamine with anesthesia maintained by inhalation of halothane in horses. *Am J Vet Res* 2002; **63**: 1655–1661.

163 Staddon GE, Weaver BMQ. Regional pulmonary perfusion in horses: a comparison between anesthetized and conscious standing animals. *Res Vet Sci* 1981; **30**: 44–48.

164 Stolk PWT. The effect of anesthesia on pulmonary blood flow in the horse. *Proc Assoc Vet Anaesth Gr Br Ir* 1982; **10**: 119–129.

165 Hughes JMB, Glazier JB, Maloney JE, *et al.* Effect of lung volume on the distribution of pulmonary blood flow in man. *Respir Physiol* 1968; **4**: 58–72.

166 Hughes JMB, Glazier JB, Maloney JE, *et al.* Effect of extra-alveolar vessels on distribution of blood flow in the dog lung. *J Appl Physiol* 1968; **25**: 701–712.

167 Hewlett AM, Hulands GH, Nunn JF, *et al.* Functional residual capacity during anesthesia. III. Artificial ventilation. *Br J Anaesth* 1974; **46**: 495–503.

168 Reber A, Engberg G, Sporre B, *et al.* Volumetric analysis of aeration in the lungs during general anesthesia. *Br J Anaesth* 1996; **76**: 760–766.

169 Rothen U, Sporre B, Engberg G, *et al.* Airway closure, atelectasis and gas exchange during general anaesthesia. *Br J Anaesth* 1998; **81**: 681–686.

170 Clerex C, Van den Brom WE, de Vries HW. Comparison of inhalation-to-perfusion ratio in anesthetized dogs with barrel-shaped thorax vs dogs with deep thorax. *Am J Vet Res* 1991; **52**: 1097–1103.

171 McDonell WN, Hall LW, Jeffcott LB. Radiographic evidence of impaired pulmonary function in laterally recumbent anaesthetized horses. *Equine Vet J* 1979; **11**: 24–32.

172 Watney GCG. Radiographic evidence of pulmonary dysfunction in anesthetized cattle. *Res Vet Sci* 1986; **41**: 162–171.

173 McDonell WN. The effect of anesthesia on pulmonary gas exchange and arterial oxygenation in the horse. PhD dissertation, University of Cambridge, 1974.

174 Nyman G, Funkquist B, Kvart C, *et al.* Atelectasis causes gas exchange impairment in the anaesthetised horse. *Equine Vet J* 1990; **22**: 317–324.

175 Moens Y, Lagerweij E, Gootjes P, *et al.* Distribution of inspired gas to each lung in anaesthetized horses and influence of body shape. *Equine Vet J* 1995; **27**: 110–116.

176 Wilson DV, Soma LR. Cardiopulmonary effects of positive end-expiratory pressure in anesthetized, mechanically ventilated ponies. *Am J Vet Res* 1990; **51**: 734–739.

177 Moens Y, Lagerweij E, Gootjes P, *et al.* Influence of tidal volume and positive pressure on inspiratory gas distribution and gas exchange during mechanical ventilation in horses positioned in lateral recumbency. *Am J Vet Res* 1998; **59**: 307–312.

178 Moens Y, Largerweij E, Gootjes P, *et al.* Differential artificial ventilation in anesthetized horses positioned in lateral recumbency. *Am J Vet Res* 1994; **55**: 1319–1326.

179 Nyman G, Frostell C, Hedenstierna G, *et al.* Selective mechanical ventilation of dependent lung regions in the anesthetized horse in dorsal recumbency. *Br J Anaesth* 1987; **59**: 1027–1034.

180 Benson J, Manohar M, Kneller SK, *et al.* Radiographic characterization of diaphragmatic excursion in halothane-anesthetized ponies: spontaneous and controlled ventilation systems. *Am J Vet Res* 1982; **43**: 617–621.

181 Froese AB, Bryan AC. Effects of anesthesia and paralysis on diaphragmatic mechanics in man. *Anesthesiology* 1974; **41**: 242–255.

182 Hall LW, Aziz HA, Groenendyk J, *et al.* Electromyography of some respiratory muscles in the horse. *Res Vet Sci* 1991; **50**: 328–333.

183 Aviado DM. Regulation of bronchomotor tone during anesthesia. *Anesthesiology* 1975; **42**: 68–80.

184 Heneghan CPH, Bergman NA, Jordan C, *et al.* Effect of isoflurane on bronchomotor in man. *Br J Anaesth* 1986; **58**: 24–28.

185 Watney GCG, Jordan C, Hall LW. Effect of halothane, enflurane and isoflurane on bronchomotor tone in anaesthetized ponies. *Br J Anaesth* 1987; **59**: 1022–1026.

186 Watney GCG. Effects of xylazine/halothane anaesthesia on the pulmonary mechanics of adult cattle. *J Assoc Vet Anaesth* 1986; **14**: 16–28.

187 Watney GCG. Effect of halothane on bronchial caliber of anaesthetized cattle. *Vet Rec* 1987; **20**: 9–12.

188 Hall LW, Young SS. Effect of inhalation anesthetics on total respiratory resistance in conscious ponies. *J Vet Pharmacol Ther* 1992; **15**: 174–179.

189 Blaze CA, LeBlanc PH, Robinson NE. Effect of withholding feed on ventilation and the incidence of regurgitation during halothane anesthesia of adult cattle. *Am J Vet Res* 1988; **49**: 2126–2129.

190 Edwards LM. Transtracheal catheterization for oxygen therapy. *Vet Tech* 1998; **9**: 26–32.

191 McNally EM, Robertson SA, Pablo LS. Comparison of time to desaturation between preoxygenated and nonpreoxygenated dogs following sedation with acepromazine maleate and morphine and induction of anesthesia with propofol. *Am J Vet Res* 2009; **70**: 1333–1338.

192 Wong DM, Alcott CJ, Wang C, *et al.* Physiologic effects of nasopharyngeal administration of supplemental oxygen at various flow rates in healthy neonatal foals. *Am J Vet Res* 2010; **71**: 1081–1088.

193 Solano AM, Brosnan RJ, Steffey EP. Rate of change of oxygen concentration for a large animal circle anesthetic system. *Am J Vet Res* 2005; **66**: 1675–1678.

194 Nunn JF. *Applied Respiratory Physiology*, 3rd edn. London: Butterworth, 1987.

195 Ko JC, Thurmon JC, Benson GJ, *et al.* Hemodynamic and anesthetic effects of etomidate infusion in medetomidine-premedicated dogs. *Am J Vet Res* 1994; **55**: 842–846.

196 Ambros B, Duke-Novakovski T, Pasloske KS. Comparison of the anesthetic efficacy and cardiopulmonary effects of continuous rate infusions of alfaxalone-2-hydroxypropyl-β-cylodextrin and propofol in dogs. *Am J Vet Res* 2008; **69**: 1391–1398.

197 Hihasa Y, Kawanabe H, Takase K, *et al.* Comparisons of sevoflurane, isoflurane, and halothane anesthesia in spontaneously breathing cats. *Vet Surg* 1996; **25**: 234–243.

198 Pypendop BH, Ilkiw JE. Hemodynamic effects of sevoflurane in cats. *Am J Vet Res* 2004; **65**: 20–25.

199 Ingwerson W, Allen DG, Dyson DH, *et al.* Cardiopulmonary effects of a halothane/oxygen combination in healthy cats. *Can J Vet Res* 1988; **52**: 386–391.

200 Enouri SSE, Kerr CL, McDonell WN, *et al.* Cardiopulmonary effects of anesthetic induction with thiopental, propofol, or a combination of ketamine hydrochloride and diazepam in dogs sedated with a combination of medetomidine and hydromorphone. *Am J Vet Res* 2008; **69**: 586–595.

201 Rolfe NG, Kerr CL, McDonell WN. Cardiopulmonary and sedative effects of the peripheral α_2-adrenoceptor antagonist MK 0467 administered intravenously or intramuscularly concurrently with medetomidine in dogs. *Am J Vet Res* 2012; **73**: 587–594.

202 Smith JA, Gaynor JS, Bednarski RM, Muir WW. Adverse effects of administration of propofol with various preanesthetic regimes in dogs. *J Am Vet Med Assoc* 1993; **202**: 1111–1115.

203 Hopper K, Haskins SC, Kass PH, *et al.* Indications, management, and outcome of long-term positive-pressure ventilation in dogs and cats: 148 cases (1990–2001). *J Am Vet Med Assoc* 2007; **230**: 64–75.

204 Campbell VL, King LG. Pulmonary function, ventilator management, and outcome of dogs with thoracic trauma and pulmonary contusions: 10 cases (1994–1998). *J Am Vet Med Assoc* 2000; **217**: 1505–1509.

205 Lee JA, Drobatz KJ, Koch MW, *et al.* Indications for and outcome of positive-pressure ventilation in cats: 53 cases (1993–2002). *J Am Vet Med Assoc* 2005; **226**: 924–931.

206 Palmer JE. Ventilatory support of the critically ill foal. *Vet Clin North Am Equine Pract* 2005; **21**: 457–486.

207 Kerr CL, McDonell WN, Young SS. Cardiopulmonary effects of romifidine/ketamine or xylazine/ketamine when used for short duration anesthesia in the horse. *Can J Vet Res* 2004; **68**: 274–282.

208 Hall LW, Gillespie JR, Tyler WS. Alveolar–arterial oxygen tension differences in anaesthetized horses. *Br J Anaesth* 1968; **40**: 560–568.

209 Steffey EP, Kelly AB, Woliner MJ. Time-related responses of spontaneously breathing, laterally recumbent horses to prolonged anesthesia with halothane. *Am J Vet Res* 1987; **48**: 952–957.

210 Gleed RD. Improvement in arterial oxygen tension with change in posture in anaesthetized horses. *Res Vet Sci* 1988; **44**: 255–259.

211 Staffieri F, Franchini D, Carella GL, *et al.* Computed tomographic analysis of the effects of two inspired oxygen concentrations on pulmonary aeration in anesthetized and mechanically ventilated dogs. *Am J Vet Res* 2007; **68**: 925–931.

212 Staffieri F, Bauquier SH, Moate PF, *et al.* Pulmonary gas exchange in anaesthetized horses mechanically ventilated with oxygen or a helium/oxygen mixture. *Equine Vet J* 2009; **41**: 747–752.

213 Staffieri F, De Monte V, De Marzo C, *et al.* Effects of two fractions of inspired oxygen on lung aeration and gas exchange in cats under inhalant anaesthesia. *Vet Anaesth Analg* 2010; **37**: 483–490.

214 Staffieri F, Driessen B, De Monte V, *et al.* Effects of positive end-expiratory pressure on anesthesia-induced atelectasis and gas exchange in anesthetized and mechanically ventilated sheep. *Am J Vet Res* 2010; **71**; 867–874.

215 Martell S, Nyman G, Hedenstierna G. High inspired oxygen concentrations increase intrapulmonary shunt in anaesthetized horses. *Vet Anaesth Analg* 2005; **32**: 338–347.

216 Edmark L, Kostova-Aherdan K, Enlund M, *et al.* Optimal oxygen concentration during induction of general anesthesia. *Anesthesiology* 2003; **98**: 28–33.

217 Hedenstierna G, Edmark L. Mechanisms of atelectasis in the perioperative period. *Best Pract Res Clin Anaesthesiol* 2010; **24**: 157–169.

218 Hubbell JAE, Aarnes TK, Bednarski RM, *et al.* Effect of 50% and maximal inspired oxygen concentrations on respiratory variables in isoflurane-anesthetized horses. *BMC Vet Res* 2011; **7**: 23–33.

219 Duggan M, Kavanagh BP. Pulmonary atelectasis. A pathogenic perioperative entity. *Anesthesiology* 2005; **102**: 838–854.

220 De Monte V, Grasso S, De Marzo C, *et al.* Effects of reduction of inspired oxygen fraction or application of positive end-expiratory pressure after an alveolar recruitment maneuver on respiratory mechanics, gas exchange, and lung aeration in dogs during anesthesia and neuromuscular blockade. *Am J Vet Res* 2013; **74**: 25–33.

221 Marshall EK, Rosenfeld M. Depression of respiration by oxygen. *J Pharmacol Exp Ther* 1936: **57**: 437–457.

222 Kaller RH, Matthay MA. Hyperoxic acute lung injury. *Respir Care* 2013; **58**: 123–141.

223 MacIntyre NR. Supporting oxygenation in acute respiratory failure. *Respir Care* 2013; **58**: 142–150.

224 Martin DS, Grocott NP. Oxygen therapy in critical illness: precise control of arterial oxygenation and permissive hypoxemia. *Crit Care Med* 2013; **41**: 423–432.

225 Kerr CK, McDonell WN. Oxygen supplementation and ventilatory support. In Muir WW, Hubbell JAE, eds. *Equine Anesthesia: Monitoring and Emergency Therapy*, 2nd edn. St Louis, MO: Saunders Elsevier, 2009: 332–352.

226 Dyson DH. Positive pressure ventilation during anesthesia in dogs: assessment of surface area derived tidal volume. *Can Vet J* 2012; **53**: 63–66.

227 Hopper K, Powell LL. Basics of mechanical ventilation for dogs and cats. *Vet Clin North Am Small Anim Pract* 2013; **43**: 955–969.

228 Fujimoto JL, Lenchan TM. The influence of body position on the blood gas and acid–base status of halothane anesthetized sheep. *Vet Surg* 1985; **14**: 169–172.

229 Steffey EP, Wheat JD, Meagher DM, *et al.* Body position and mode of ventilation influence arterial pH, oxygen and carbon dioxide tensions in halothane-anesthetized horses. *Am J Vet Res* 1977; **38**: 379–382.

230 Edner A, Nyman G, Essen-Gustavsson B. The effects of spontaneous and mechanical ventilation on central cardiovascular function and peripheral perfusion during isoflurane anaesthesia in horses. *Vet Anaesth Analg* 2005; **32**: 136–146.

231 Henderson WR, Sheel AW. Pulmonary mechanics during mechanical ventilation. *Respir Physiol Neurobiol* 2012; **180**: 162–172.

232 DeProst N, Dreyfuss D. How to prevent ventilator-induced lung injury? *Minerva Anesthesiol* 2012; **78**: 1054–1066.

233 Fan E, Villar J, Slutsky AS. Novel approaches to minimize ventilator-induced lung injury. *BMC Med* 2013; **11**: 85.

234 Wilson DV, McFeely AM. Positive end-expiratory pressure during colic surgery in horses: 74 cases (1986–1988) *J Am Vet Med Assoc* 1991; **199**: 917–921.

235 Swanson CR, Muir WW. Hemodynamic and respiratory responses in halothane-anesthetized horses exposed to positive pressure end-expiratory pressure alone and with dobutamine. *Am J Vet Res* 1988; **49**: 539–542.

236 Hopster K, Kastner SBR, Rohn K, *et al.* Intermittent positive pressure ventilation with constant positive end-expiratory pressure and alveolar recruitment manoeuvre during inhalation anaesthesia in horses undergoing surgery for colic, and its influence on the early recovery period. *Vet Anaesth Analg* 2011; **38**: 169–177.

237 Wagner AE, Bednarski RM, Muir WW. Hemodynamic effects of carbon dioxide during intermittent positive-pressure ventilation in horses. *Am J Vet Res* 1990; **51**: 1922–1929.

238 Khanna AK, McDonell WN, Dyson DH, *et al.* Cardiopulmonary effects of hypercapnia during controlled intermittend positive pressure ventilation in the horse. *Can J Vet Res* 1995; **59**: 213–221.

239 Oura T, Rozanski RA, Buckley G, *et al.* Low tidal volume ventilation in healthy dogs. *J Vet Emerg Crit Care* 2012; **22**: 368–371.

240 Shekerdemian L, Bohn D. Cardiovascular effects of mechanical ventilation. *Arch Dis Child* 1999; **80**: 475–480.

241 Pinsky MR. Cardiovascular issues in respiratory care. *Chest* 2005; **128**: 592S–597S.

242 Pinsky MR. Heart lung interactions during mechanical ventilation. *Curr Opin Crit Care* 2012; **18**: 256–260.

243 Oliveira RH, Azevedo LCP, Park M, *et al.* Influence of ventilatory settings on static and functional haemodynamic parameters during experimental hypovolaemia. *Eur J Anaesthesiol* 2009; **26**: 66–72.

244 Hodgson DS, Steffey EP, Grandy JL, Woliner MJ. Effects of spontaneous, assisted, and controlled modes in halothane-anesthetized geldings. *Am J Vet Res* 1986; **47**: 992–996.

245 Mizuno Y, Aida H, Hara H, Fujinaga T. Cardiovascular effects of intermittent positive pressure ventilation in the anesthetized horse. *J Vet Med Sci* 1994; **56**: 39–44.

246 Steffey EP, Kelly AB, Hodgson DS, *et al.* Effect of body posture on cardiopulmonary function in horses during five hours of constant-dose halothane anesthesia. *Am J Vet Res* 1990; **51**: 11–16.

247 Pinsky MR. The hemodynamic consequences of mechanical ventilation: an evolving story. *Intensive Care Med* 1997; **21**: 493–503.

248 Wallis TW, Robotham JL, Compean R, *et al.* Mechanical heart–lung interaction with positive end-expiratory pressure. *J Appl Physiol* 1983; **54**: 1039–1047.

249 Neilsen J, Nilsson M, Fredin F, *et al.* Central hemodynamics during lung recruitment maneuvers at hypovolemia, normovolemia and hypervolemia. A study by echocardiography and continuous pulmonary artery flow measurements in lung-injured pigs. *Intensive Care Med* 2006; **32**: 585–594.

250 Odenstedt H, Aneman A, Karason S, *et al.* Acute hemodynamic changes during lung recruitment in lavage and endotoxin-induced ALI. *Intensive Care Med* 2005; **31**: 112–120.

251 Lim SC, Adams AB, Simonson DA, *et al.* Transient hemodynamic effects of recruitment maneuvers in three experimental models of acute lung injury. *Crit Care Med* 2004; **32**: 2378–2384.

252 Fujino Y, Goddon S, Dolhnikoff M, *et al.* Repetitive high-pressure recruitment maneuvers required to maximally recruit lung in a sheep model of acute respiratory distress syndrome. *Crit Care Med* 2001; **29**: 1579–1586.

253 Barker SJ, Tremper KK. Respiratory monitoring, blood-gas measurement, oximetry, and pulse oximetry. *Curr Opin Anaesthesiol* 1992; **5**: 816–825.

254 Cullen DJ, Nemeskal AR, Cooper JB, *et al.* Effect of oximetry, age, and ASA physical status on the frequency of patients admitted unexpectedly to a postoperative intensive care unit and severity of their anesthetic-related complications. *Anesth Analg* 1992; **74**: 181–188.

255 Cote CJ, Rolf N, Lui LM, *et al.* A single blind study of combined pulse oximetry and capnography in children. *Anesthesiology* 1991; **74**: 980–987.

256 Rothen HU, Neumann P, Berglund JE, *et al.* Dynamics of re-expansion of atelectasis during general anaesthesia. *Br J Anaesth* 1999; **82**: 551–556.

257 Magnusson L, Tenling A, Lemoine R, *et al.* The safety of one, or repeated, vital capacity maneuvers during general anesthesia. *Anesth Analg* 2000; **91**: 702–707.

258 Oczenski W, Schwarz S, Fitzgerald RD. Vital capacity manoeuver in general anaesthesia: useful or useless? *Eur J Anaesthesiol* 2004; **21**: 253–254.

259 Neumann P, Rothen HU, Berglund JE, *et al.* Positive end-expiratory pressure prevents atelectasis during general anaesthesia even in the presence of high inspired oxygen concentrations. *Acta Anaesthesiol Scand* 1999; **43**: 295–301.

260 Turner DM, Ilkiw JE. Cardiovascular and respiratory effects of three rapidly acting barbiturates in dogs. *Am J Vet Res* 1990; **51**: 598–604.

261 Dyson DH, Allen DG, Ingwersen W, *et al.* Evaluation of acepromazine/meperidine/atropine premedication followed by thiopental anesthesia in the cat. *Can J Vet Res* 1988; **52**: 419–422.

262 Steffey EP, Farver TB, Woliner MJ. Cardiopulmonary function during 7 h of constant-dose halothane and methoxyflurane. *J Appl Physiol* 1987; **63**: 1351–1359.

263 Ray JF, Yost L, Moallem S, *et al.* Immobility, hypoxemia, and pulmonary arteriovenous shunting. *Arch Surg* 1974; **109**: 537–541.

264 Ewing KK. Anesthesia techniques in sheep and goats. *Vet Clin North Am Food Anim Pract* 1990; **6**: 759–778.

265 Hedenstierna G, Lundquist H, Lundh B, *et al.* Pulmonary densities during anaesthesia: an experimental study on lung morphology and gas exchange. *Eur Respir J* 1989; **2**: 528–535.

266 Semrad SD, Trim CM, Hardee GE. Hypertension in bulls and steers anesthetized with guaifenesin–thiobarbiturate–halothane combination. *Am J Vet Res* 1986; **47**: 1577–1582.

267 Nyman G, Hedenstierna G. Comparison of conventional and selective mechanical ventilation in the anaesthetized horse. *J Vet Med* 1988; **35**: 299–315.

268 Nyman G, Funkquist B, Kvart C. Postural effects on blood gas tension, blood pressure, heart rate, ECG and respiratory rate during prolonged anaesthesia in the horse. *J Vet Med* 1988; **35**: 54–62.

269 Stegmann GF, Littlejohn A. The effect of lateral and dorsal recumbency on cardiopulmonary function in the anaesthetized horse. *J S Afr Vet Assoc* 1987; **58**: 21–27.

270 Blaze CA, Robinson NE. Apneic oxygenation in anesthetized ponies and horses. *Vet Res Commun* 1987; **11**: 281–291.

271 Young LE, Richards DLS, Brearly JC, *et al.* The effect of a 50% inspired mixture of nitrous oxide on arterial oxygen tension in spontaneously breathing horses anaesthetized with halothane. *J Vet Anaesth* 1992; **19**: 37–40.

272 Grubb T. Anesthesia for patients with respiratory disease and/or airway compromise. *Topics Companion Anim Med* 2010; **25**: 120–132.

273 Fasanella FJ, Shivley JM, Wardlaw JL, *et al.* Brachycephalic airway obstructive syndrome in dogs: 90 cases (1991–2008). *J Am Vet Med Assoc* 2010; **237**: 1048–1051.

274 Mercurio A. Complications of upper airway surgery in companion animals. *Vet Clin Small Anim* 2011; **41**: 969–980.

275 Doxey S, Boswood A. Differences between breeds of dog in a measure of heart rate variability. *Vet Rec* 2004; **154**: 713–717.

276 Millard RP, Tobias KM. Laryngeal paralysis in dogs. *Compend Contin Educ Vet* 2009; **31**: 212–219.

277 Janicek JC, Ketzner KM. Performance-limiting laryngeal disorders. *Compend Contin Educ Equine* 2008; 416–428.

278 Lindegaard C, Husted L, Ullum H, *et al.* Sedation with detomidine and acepromazine influences the endoscopic evaluation of laryngeal function in horses. *Equine Vet J* 2007; **39**: 553–556.

279 Reed F, Iff I. Use of a laryngeal mask airway in a brachycephalic dog with masticatory myositis and trismus. *Can Vet J* 2012; **53**: 287–290.

280 Cassu RN, Luna SPL, Neto FJT, *et al.* Evaluation of laryngeal mask as an alternative to endotracheal intubation in cats anesthetized under spontaneous or controlled ventilation. *Vet Anaesth Analg* 2004; **31**: 213–221.

281 Crotaz IR. An observational clinical study in cats and rabbits of an anatomically designed supraglottic airway device for use in companion animal veterinary anaesthesia. *Vet Rec* 2013; **172**: 606.

282 Gross ME, Dodam JR, Pope ER, *et al.* A comparison of thiopental, propofol, and diazepam–ketamine anesthesia for evaluation of laryngeal function in dogs premedicated with butorphanol–glycopyrrolate. *J Am Anim Hosp Assoc* 2002; **38**: 503–506.

283 Jackson AM, Tobias K, Long C, *et al.* Effect of various anesthetic agents on laryngeal motion during laryngoscopy in normal dogs. *Vet Surg* 2004; **33**: 102–106.

284 Hammel SP, Hottinger HA, Novo RE. Postoperative results of unilateral arytenoid lateralization for treatment of idiopathic laryngeal paralysis in dogs: 39 cases (1996–2002). *J Am Vet Med Assoc* 2006; **228**: 1215–1220.

285 Karzai w, Schwarzkopf K. Hypoxemia during one-lung ventilation. *Anesthesiology* 2009; **110**: 1402–1411.

286 Mayhew PD, Friedberg JS. Video-assisted thoracoscpic resection of noninvasive thymomas using one-lung ventilation in two dogs. *Vet Surg* 2008; **37**: 756–762.

287 Mosing M, Iff I, Moens Y. Endoscopic removal of a bronchial carcinoma in a dog using one-lung ventilation. *Vet Surg* 2008; **37**: 222–225.

288 Mayhew KN, Mayhew PD, Sorrell-Raschi L. *et al.* Thoracoscopic subphrenic pericardectomy using double-lumen endobronchial intubation for alternating one-lung ventilation. *Vet Surg* 2009; **38**: 961–966.

289 Bauquier SH, Culp WT, Lin RC. *et al.* One-lung ventilation using a wire-guided endobronchial blocker for thoracoscopic pericardial fenestration in a dog. *Can Vet J* 2010; **51**: 1135–1138.

290 Adami C, Axiak S, Rytz U. *et al.* Alternating one lung ventilation using a double lumen endobronchial tube and providing CPAP to the non-ventilated lung in a dog. *Vet Anaesth Analg* 2011; **38**: 70–76.
291 Pelaez MJ, Jolliffe C. Thoracoscopic foreign body removal and right middle lung lobectomy to treat pyothorax in a dog. *J Small Anim Pract* 2012; **53**: 240–244.
292 Mayhew PD, Culp WT, Pascoe PJ. *et al.* Evaluation of blind thoracoscopic-assisted placement of three double-lumen endobronchial tube designs for one-lung ventilation in dogs. *Vet Surg* 2012; **41**: 664–670.
293 Levionnois OL, Bergadano A, Schatzmann U. Accidental entrapment of an endobronchial blocker tip by a surgical stapler during selective ventilation for lung lobectomy in a dog. *Vet Surg* 2008; **35**: 82–85.
294 Riquelme M, Monnet E, Kudnig ST. *et al.* Cardiopulmonary changes induced during one-lung ventilation in anesthetized dogs with a closed thoracic cavity. *Am J Vet Res* 2005; **66**: 973–977.
295 Riquelme M, Monnet E, Kudnig ST. *et al.* Cardiopulmonary effects of positive end-expiratory pressure during one-lung ventilation in anesthetized dogs with a closed thoracic cavity. *Am J Vet Res* 2005; **66**: 978–983.

SECTION 6

Nervous System

28 Physiology, Pathophysiology, and Anesthetic Management of Patients with Neurologic Disease

Klaus A. Otto

Institut für Versuchstierkunde und Zentrales Tierlaboratorium, Medizinische Hochschule Hannover, Hannover, Germany

Chapter contents

Introduction

The living organism is constantly exposed to external and internal stimuli [1]. Transduction, transmission, transformation (modulation), translation (perception), and the response to stimulation are ongoing processes that are essential for the adaptation of the organism to changing conditions and daily survival [1,2]. All of these processes require the specialized nervous system, which, along with the endocrine system, mediates the adjustments and reactions of the organism to its internal and external environments [3].

General anesthesia has been defined as a drug-induced, reversible state characterized by amnesia, unconsciousness, analgesia, immobility, and muscle relaxation [4–8]. In order to achieve these goals, anesthetic agents must alter function in numerous parts of the nervous system. Most general anesthetic agents exert their depressive effects by acting at different sites in the brain and spinal cord while the primary targets of local-regional anesthetic agents are the peripheral sensory receptors, afferent and efferent peripheral nerve fibers, and the spinal cord. Anesthetic adjunctive drugs such as neuromuscular blocking agents (NMBAs) produce skeletal muscle paralysis by interfering with impulse transmission at the neuromuscular junction whereas analgesic drugs may impede transduction, transmission, and perception of noxious stimuli at specialized peripheral receptors (nociceptors) and at synapses located at spinal, and at different brain levels.

Anatomy of the nervous system

The nervous system may be divided into two major divisions, the peripheral nervous system (PNS) (sensory and the motor portions) and the central nervous system (CNS), which includes the autonomic nervous system (ANS) [1,3,9]. The PNS and CNS can be functionally defined as the neurologic systems that together allow the individual to respond voluntarily to sensory signals consciously perceived from the external environment [10]. Signal transmission at the various sites within the nervous system (i.e., from the sense organ to the neuron, from neuron to neuron, or from neuron to effector) will be mediated by neurotransmitters such as norepinephrine, epinephrine, and acetylcholine [1].

Peripheral nervous system

The PNS consist of sensory receptors and specialized sensory organs that detect the state of the body or its surroundings [10]. It also is comprised of afferent and efferent nerve fibers that conduct

Veterinary Anesthesia and Analgesia: The Fifth Edition of Lumb and Jones.
Edited by Kurt A. Grimm, Leigh A. Lamont, William J. Tranquilli, Stephen A. Greene and Sheilah A. Robertson.

impulses between receptors and sensory organs, various parts of the CNS, and peripheral effectors (e.g., skeletal muscle).

Central nervous system

Traditionally, the brain and the spinal cord together form the CNS. The brain is capable of storing information, generating thoughts, creating ambition, and determining reactions in response to sensations. In the last case, signals will originate in motor nuclei and be transmitted through the motor tracts within the CNS to the motor portion of the PNS [9,10].

The brain is comprised of the (1) telencephalon (cerebrum) with its two hemispheres (including rhinencephalon, corpus callosum, limbic system, hippocampus, ventriculus lateralis, ventriculus III, and corpus amygdalloideum), (2) diencephalon (including hypothalamus and thalamus), (3) mesencephalon (including tegmentum mesencephali), (4) metencephalon (including ventriculus IV, pons, and cerebellum), and (5) myelencephalon (including medulla oblongata) [1]. The brain and spinal cord are covered by three meninges: pia mater (pia mater encephali, pia mater spinalis), arachnoidea (arachnoidea encephali, arachnoidea spinales), and dura mater (dura mater encephali, dura mater spinalis), of which the pia mater is in direct contact with the brain and spinal cord while the dura mater is the most superficial membrane, partly fused with the endocranium and the periosteum in the spinal canal [1,3].

The three meninges form different spaces: the subarachnoid space (between pia mater and arachnoidea), the subdural space (between arachnoidea and dura mater), and the epidural space (between dura mater and the ligamentum flavum in the spinal canal) (Fig. 28.1) [1,3,11]. The subarachnoid space is one space in the CNS containing cerebrospinal fluid (CSF). Whereas CSF collection may be performed at more cranial (spatium atlantooccipitale) or caudal sites (spatium lumbosacrale), subarachnoid (intrathecal) administration of analgesic and anesthetic drugs (e.g., local anesthetics and opioids) will be administered in veterinary patients more frequently at the level of the lumbosacral, caudosacral, or intercaudal spaces. The vessel-rich epidural space contains fat and connective tissue and is located between the dural sac (dura mater) and the ligamentum flavum [1,11].

The blood–brain barrier (BBB) is an anatomic and enzymatic separation that isolates cerebral blood from most brain parenchyma and CSF. It is located at the choroid plexus, brain parenchymal vessels, subarachnoid vessels, and arachnoid membrane [12]. It is composed of cells connected by tight junctions that restrict intercellular diffusion and thereby force solute exchange to occur through the cells. Normally, the tight intercellular junctions prevent the passage of small to moderate amounts of epinephrine, norepinephrine, dopamine, or serotonin from blood to brain [13]. Under these circumstances, circulating catecholamines do not significantly affect the cerebral metabolic rate for oxygen ($CMRO_2$). However, if the BBB permeability is increased (e.g., intracranial hypertension, inflammation, or osmotic disruption), epinephrine and norepinephrine can enter the brain, where they reversibly increase $CMRO_2$ [13].

The CSF provides hydromechanical protection of the CNS, plays a prominent role in brain development, and influences neuronal functioning via regulation of interstitial fluid homeostasis [14].

CSF is produced under enzymatic control of carbonic anhydrase predominantly by the choroid plexuses in the lateral, third, and fourth ventricles of the brain and is distributed in the brain ventricles, the spinal cord central canal, and the subarachnoid spaces (Fig. 28.2) [14–16]. A minor volume of CSF will be derived as a metabolic by-product of the metabolism in the brain and spinal cord [15]. The rate of CSF production ranges from 0.02 and 0.05 mL/min in cats [15] and dogs [17], respectively, to about 0.40 mL/min in humans [16]. Compared with plasma ultrafiltrate, CSF is characterized by higher concentrations of Na^+, Cl^-, and Mg^{2+} and lower concentrations of glucose, proteins, amino acids, K^+, bicarbonate, and phosphate, but has the same tonicity [16].

The predominant sites of CSF drainage include absorption via cranial and spinal arachnoid villi into the venous outflow system and via cranial and spinal nerve sheaths or via the adventitia of cerebral arteries into the lymphatic outflow system [14]. CSF flow dynamics and pressure depend largely on factors such as arterial pulse wave, respiratory waves, the posture of the animal, jugular venous pressure, and physical effort [14]. Arterial hypotension, a decrease in cerebral perfusion pressure (CPP), or an increase in intracranial pressure (ICP), for example, will reduce CSF

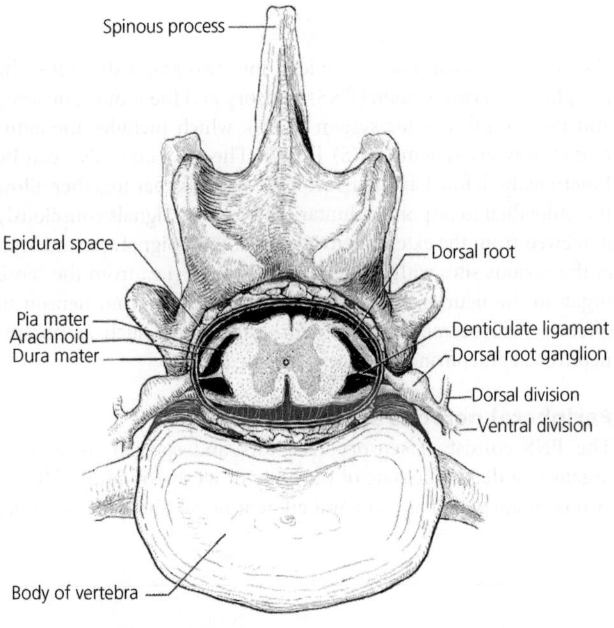

Figure 28.1 Transverse section of the spinal cord within the vertebral canal. Note the adipose tissue and blood vessels in the epidural space. Source: [360]. Reproduced with permission of John Wiley & Sons.

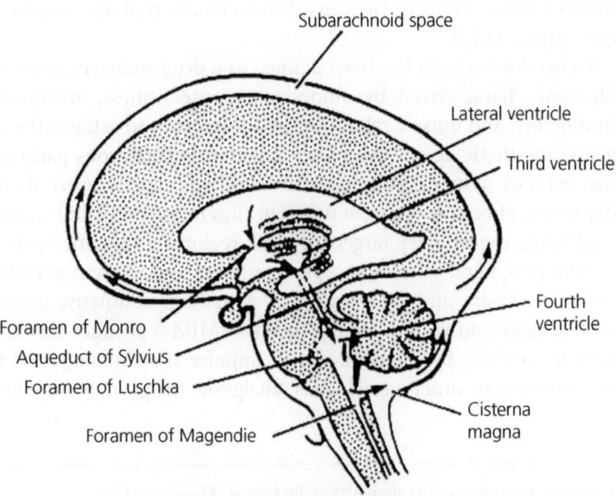

Figure 28.2 Circulation of cerebrospinal fluid in the human and subhuman primates. Non-primate mammals do not have the foramen of Magendie. Source: [361]. Reproduced with permission of John Wiley & Sons.

formation [16]. Pharmacologically, a reduction in CSF formation may be achieved by administration of diuretics (e.g., carbonic anhydrase inhibitor, furosemide), mannitol, and corticosteroids [16]. Anesthetics such as enflurane, ketamine, and halothane may increase or augment increased CSF formation whereas isoflurane and fentanyl might be preferable in patients with increased CSF volume [18–20].

Autonomic nervous system

The ANS regulates the body's internal environment and thus can be defined functionally as the neurologic system that acts to maintain homeostasis. Sensory neurons carry signals to integrative neurons within the spinal cord and the brain, which construct an appropriate response resulting in activation of effector organs. For the most part, the animal is unaware of ANS actions.

The ANS is a large segment of the nervous system, operates on a subconscious level, and controls the visceral functions of the internal organs. Visceral controls include maintenance of arterial blood pressure, gastrointestinal motility and secretion, urinary bladder emptying, and thermoregulation. One of the most striking characteristics of the ANS is the rapidity and intensity with which it can change visceral function. For instance, the arterial blood pressure can be doubled within 10–15 s [9,10].

The ANS is controlled mainly by centers located in the spinal cord, brainstem, and hypothalamus. In addition, portions of the limbic cortex can transmit impulses to lower centers and thereby influence autonomic control. Afferent signals entering the autonomic ganglia, spinal cord, brainstem, or hypothalamus can elicit appropriate reflex responses back to the visceral organs to control their activities. The efferent autonomic signals are transmitted to the body through the two major subdivisions of the ANS, called the sympathetic nervous system and the parasympathetic nervous system [9,10].

Sympathetic nervous system

The sympathetic nervous system is comprised of two paravertebral sympathetic chains of ganglia located on each side of the spinal column, two prevertebral ganglia (celiac and hypogastric ganglion), and nerve fibers extending from the ganglia to nerve endings in the internal organs. The sympathetic nerves originate in the spinal cord between segments T1 and L2 and pass first into the sympathetic chain and then to the tissues and organs (Fig. 28.3) [9,10].

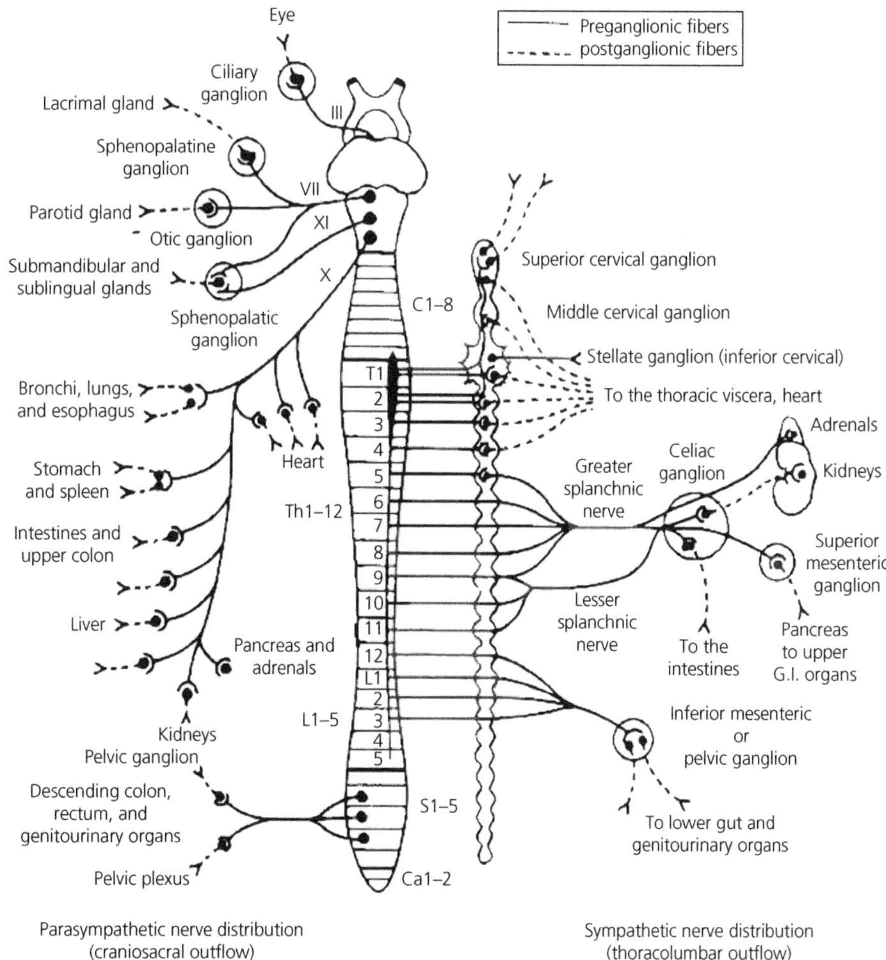

Figure 28.3 Schematic distribution of the craniosacral (parasympathetic) and thoracolumbar (sympathetic) nervous system. Parasympathetic preganglionic fibers pass directly to the organ that is innervated. Their postganaglionic cell bodies are situated near or within the innervated viscera. This limited distribution of the parasympathetic postganglionic fibers is consistent with the discrete and limited effect of parasympathetic function. The postganglionic sympathetic neurons originate in either the paired sympathetic ganglia or one of the unpaired collateral plexi. One preganglionic fiber influences many postganglionic neurons. Activation of the sympathetic nervous system produces a more diffuse physiologic response rather than discrete effects. G.I, gastrointestinal. Source: [362]. Reproduced with permission of John Wiley & Sons.

Unlike the skeletal motor nerve fibers, which are comprised of long, continuous neurons, each sympathetic nerve is composed of two neurons in series, one preganglionic and the other postganglionic. The cell body of each preganglionic neuron lies in the intermediolateral horn of the spinal cord and its fiber passes through a ventral spinal root into the corresponding spinal nerve. Immediately after the spinal nerve leaves the spinal column, the preganglionic sympathetic fibers leave the nerve and pass through the white ramus into one of the ganglia of the sympathetic chain. Thereafter, the fibers can (1) synapse with postganglionic neurons in the ganglion that it enters, (2) pass upwards or downwards in the chain and synapse in one of the other ganglia, or (3) pass for variable distances through the chain and then through one of the sympathetic nerves radiating outwards from the chain to terminate in one of the prevertebral ganglia. The postganglionic neuron originates either in one of the sympathetic chain ganglia or in one of the prevertebral ganglia. From either of these two sources, the postganglionic fibers travel to the various organs [9,10]. An exception to the two-neuron organization of the sympathetic nervous system is innervation of the adrenal medulla. Preganglionic nerve fibers pass without synapsing all the way from the intermediolateral horn cells of the spinal cord, through the sympathetic chains, through the splanchnic nerves, and finally into the adrenal medulla. There they end directly on modified neuronal cells that secrete epinephrine and norepinephrine into the bloodstream. These secretory cells are analogous to postganglionic neurons [9,10].

Parasympathetic nervous system

Fibers of the parasympathetic nervous system leave the CNS through the cranial nerves (CN) III, VII, IX, and X, the second and third sacral spinal nerves, and sometimes through the first and fourth sacral nerves (Fig. 28.4) [9,10]. About 75% of all parasympathetic nerve fibers are in the vagus nerves (CN X) and comprise a cranial, a cervical, and a thoracic part [1]. The vagus nerves supply parasympathetic fibers to the heart, lungs, esophagus, stomach, and other abdominal viscera. Parasympathetic fibers in CN III (oculomotor nerves) go to the pupillary sphincters and ciliary muscles of the eye, fibers in cranial nerve VII (facial nerves) pass to the lacrimal, nasal, and submandibular glands, and fibers from cranial nerve IX (glossopharyngeal nerves) pass to the parotid gland [9,10].

Both the parasympathetic and sympathetic systems have preganglionic and postganglionic neurons. The preganglionic parasympathetic fibers, however, pass uninterrupted all the way to the organ where the postganglionic neurons are located in the organ wall [9,10].

Autonomic nervous system neurotransmission

Synaptic transmission within the ANS utilizes acetylcholine (ACh) and norepinephrine (NE) (Table 28.1) [9,10,21,22]. All preganglionic sympathetic and parasympathetic neurotransmission is cholinergic. Postganglionic parasympathetic neurons are also cholinergic whereas postganglionic sympathetic neurons are noradrenergic (sometimes called adrenergic) (i.e., releasing NE) [9,10].

Acetylcholine activates two different types of cholinergic receptors, muscarinic (M) [23] and nicotinic (nAChR) receptors. In the group of G-protein coupled receptors, muscarinic receptors have attracted much attention as a possible target of some anesthetic and analgesic drugs [24]. Muscarinic ACh receptors have been found to be involved in various neuronal functions in the CNS and ANS [25]. Molecular cloning studies revealed the existence of five muscarinic receptor subtypes (M_{1-5}) [26]. Nicotinic receptors are found in the synapses between pre- and postganglionic neurons of both the sympathetic and the parasympathetic systems [9]. Nicotinic ACh receptors belong to a superfamily of ligand-gated ion channels that play key roles in synaptic transmission throughout the CNS [27]. Neuronal nicotinic receptors include many different subtypes constructed from a variety of nicotinic subunit combinations. The structural diversity and the presynaptic, axonal, and postsynaptic locations of nicotinic receptors contribute to the various roles that these receptors play in the CNS [27].

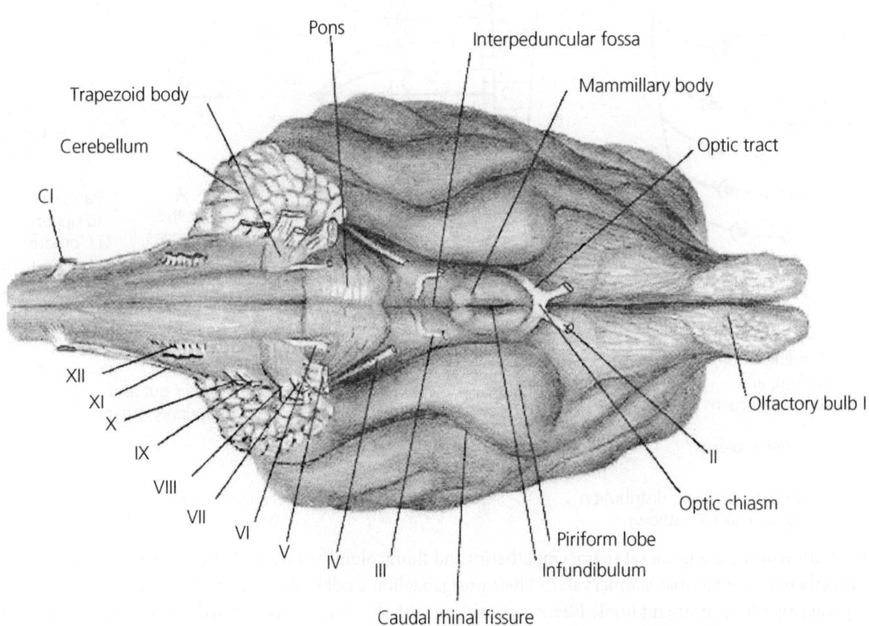

Figure 28.4 Ventral view of a canine brain and cranial nerves. Source: [360]. Reproduced with permission of Wiley.

Table 28.1 Selected effects of sympathetic (norepinephrine, NE) and parasympathetic (acetylcholine, ACh) nervous system activation.

Organ	Sympathetic Stimulation		Parasympathetic Stimulation	
	Transmitter	Effect, Receptor Type	Transmitter	Effect
Heart	NE	↑ Heart rate ($\beta_1>\beta_2$)	ACh	↓ Heart rate
		↑ Contractility ($\beta_1>\beta_2>\alpha_1$)		↓ Contractility
		↑ Conduction ($\beta_1>\beta_2$)		↓ Conduction
Arterioles	NE		ACh	
Coronary		Contraction/ dilation (α/β_2)		Vasodilation
Skin, mucosa		Contraction (α)		Vasodilation
Skeletal muscle		Contraction/ dilation (α/β_2)		Vasodilation
Cerebral		Contraction (α; slight)		Vasodilation
Pulmonary		Contraction/ dilation (α/β_2)		Vasodilation
Abdominal viscera		Contraction/ dilation (α/β_2)		–
Renal		Contraction/ dilation (α/β)		–
Veins (systemic)		Contraction/ dilation (α_1/β_2)		–
Lungs	NE		ACh	
Bronchiolar muscle		Contraction (α_1) Relaxation (β_2)		Contraction
Glands		↑ (β_2), ↓ (α) secretion	ACh	↑ Mucous secretion
Head	NE		ACh	
Lacrimal glands		(↑) Secretion		↑↑ Secretion
Salivary glands		↑ Blood flow		
Nasopharyngeal glands				
Eye muscles	NE		ACh	
Radial muscle (iris)		Contraction (mydriasis) (α_1)		
Pupillary sphincter muscle				Contraction (miosis)
Ciliary muscle		Relaxation (far vision) (β)		Contraction (near vision)
Gastrointestinal tract	NE		ACh	
Motility		↓ Motility (α_{1-2}, β_{1-2})		↑ Motility
Sphincter muscles		Contraction (α)		Dilation
Secretion		Inhibition (?)		↑ Secretion
Adrenal medulla	–		ACh	Secretion of Epi, NE

↑, Increase; ↓, decrease; (↑), minor effect; ↑↑, major effect; NE, norepinephrine; ACh, acetylcholine; Epi, epinephrine.
Source: adapted from [4,14,15].

Neuromuscular neurotransmission

Nicotinic receptors are also found in the membranes of skeletal muscle fibers at the neuromuscular junction [9]. The skeletal muscle fibers are innervated by large, myelinated nerve fibers that originate in the large motor neurons of the ventral horns of the spinal cord. Each nerve fiber normally branches many times and stimulates from three to several hundred skeletal muscle fibers. The nerve ending makes a synapse called the neuromuscular junction with only one such junction per muscle fiber.

The branching nerve terminals invaginate into the muscle fiber but lie entirely outside the plasma membrane. The entire structure is called the motor end plate. When a nerve impulse reaches the neuromuscular junction, ACh is released from the nerve terminals into the synaptic cleft [9]. ACh receptors in the muscle membrane are composed of five subunit proteins that form a tubular channel through the muscle membrane. Once ACh molecules have attached to one of the subunits, a conformational change opens the channel, allowing a predominant movement of Na^+ ions into the muscle cell, which is associated with a smaller K^+ outward current as the membrane is becoming progressively depolarized [9,28]. An action potential generated at the motor end plate spreads across the sarcolemma and down the invaginations (T-tubules) of this membrane, finally activating the contractile mechanism by Ca^{2+} release from the sarcoplasmic reticulum into the myoplasm, the so-called excitation–contraction coupling [28,29].

Physiology/pathophysiology of the central nervous system

Cerebral metabolism

Brain function is intimately related to both cerebral perfusion and metabolism [30]. The characteristic features of cerebral metabolism include (1) high cellular energy demands utilizing adenosine triphosphate (ATP) energy obtained from aerobic glucose oxidation, (2) no oxygen and minimal glucose and glycogen substrate reserves relative to consumption rates, and (3) low concentrations of high-energy phosphate compounds. All these characteristics render the brain highly dependent upon adequate blood flow for minute-to-minute delivery of oxygen and glucose [12,31,32].

The mean global $CMRO_2$ of the normal awake human brain is about 3.0–5.5 mL/100 g/min [33–38]. Approximately 60% of the available oxygen is expended in subserving the external work of the brain as represented in the electroencephalogram (EEG). In the absence of external work (i.e., an isoelectric EEG), the healthy normothermic brain will continue to consume about 40% of the normal energy and oxygen [38]. This basal metabolism is necessary for maintaining neuronal and glial cell integrity, including the energy requirements for maintaining ionic gradients, biosynthesis, and axonal transport [38]. The basal metabolic state can be reversibly produced by higher doses of anesthetic agents [39,40] and hypothermia [41].

At a surgical level of anesthesia in human patients, $CMRO_2$ decreased by 36–45% and EEG slowing and burst suppression pattern appeared at approximately 60% of the normal $CMRO_2$ [12]. Anesthetics (e.g., thiopental) may offer neuroprotection in pathologic states associated with cerebral hypoxia because they reduce O_2 requirements [42]. The decrease in $CMRO_2$ recorded with increasing anesthetic concentration in anesthetized dogs is non-linear for halothane, enflurane, and isoflurane [43]. The point at which the decline in the rate of $CMRO_2$ slows coincides with the change in EEG voltage dominance from posterior to anterior cerebral hemisphere [approximately 0.4 minimum alveolar concentration (MAC)] and indicates loss of consciousness (LOC) [43].

The functional and basal portion of $CMRO_2$, however, will be affected differently by general anesthetics and hypothermia. Whereas increasing doses of thiopental or isoflurane will reduce the functional portion of total $CMRO_2$ only, hypothermia will reduce both functional and basal $CMRO_2$ [38].

Among the volatile agents, isoflurane possesses some unique properties as it may produce an isoelectric EEG pattern at clinically relevant concentrations [40]. Isoflurane produces dose-related decreases in $CMRO_2$ but, once EEG isoelectricity and hence basal $CMRO_2$ have been reached, further increases in isoflurane concentration are not associated with further decreases in $CMRO_2$ [40]. Similarly to thiopental, the cerebral metabolic energy profile remains normal at EEG isoelectricity, suggesting that high concentrations of isoflurane are without toxic effects on oxidative phosphorylation [40], which makes isoflurane a relatively safe anesthetic even in the hypotensive patient [44].

Benzodiazepines such as diazepam and midazolam may also be used to decrease cerebral blood flow (CBF) and $CMRO_2$ [12,45–47].

Although global $CMRO_2$ is relatively stable, regional changes in $CMRO_2$ are continually occurring in the brain of awake organisms [38]. Because of the coupling of $CMRO_2$ and CBF, activation of one brain region will result in both increased metabolism and blood flow while simultaneous decreases may occur in unstimulated regions [48,49]. The net result will be a stable global $CMRO_2$ and any meaningful increase or decrease in global $CMRO_2$ in the awake brain should be viewed as pathologic in origin (e.g., seizure or stroke) [38].

Volatile anesthetic agents such as halothane, enflurane, and isoflurane, but not barbiturates, etomidate, or midazolam, may uncouple the tight relationship between CBF and $CMRO_2$, thus resulting in an increased blood flow despite a dose-related decrease the $CMRO_2$ [38,50]. Moreover, volatile anesthetic agents tend to attenuate autoregulation and at higher doses autoregulation may be lost, resulting in a CBF passively dependent upon CPP [38,51,52].

The normal cerebral metabolic rate for glucose consumption ($CMR_{glucose}$) approximates 4.5 mg/100 g/min [50]. The metabolic rate will be decreased during anesthesia, hypothermia, and/or hypercapnia [50–54].

Cerebral blood flow

The normal mean global CBF in humans is in the range 45–65 mL/100 g/min [33–37]. The cerebral circulation in most mammalian species includes two general types of arteries that supply the cerebral hemispheres: conducting vessels and penetrating vessels [12,55]. The conducting arteries essentially are non-resistance vessels and include the carotid, vertebral, occipital, and spinal artery together with their major and minor branches [1,12,55]. The penetrating or nutrient arterioles that enter the brain parenchyma at right-angles to the surface vessels are the resistance vessels and hence the site of primary CBF autoregulation [12,55]. Although the vessels receive autonomic innervation, neurogenic tone is not essential to normal CBF regulation [42,56]. There are, however, anatomic differences in the cerebral blood supply between species that may affect CBF and thus animal outcome [57–60]. Studies in cats revealed that wide opening of the jaw using a spring-held mouth gag may increase the risk of postanesthetic neurologic deficits, cortical blindness, and hearing deficits [59,60]. It could be shown that a maximally opened mouth in cats may be associated with a disrupted CBF and reduced direct blood flow to the retina or inner ear, most likely caused by stretching of the vasculature of the maxillary artery and adjacent muscles such as temporalis, masseter, and pterygoid muscles [59,60].

Cerebral blood flow autoregulation

CBF autoregulation refers to a multifactorial process that maintains constant CBF despite changes in systemic blood pressure and CPP over a wide range. CPP is the pressure difference between brain arteries and veins [42,61]. CBF autoregulation enables the brain to match the blood supply with its metabolic demand both regionally and globally [61]. CBF autoregulation usually is intact during light levels of general anesthesia but may be impaired or abolished during deep anesthesia [12]. Especially volatile anesthetic agents tend to attenuate autoregulation up to a point when CBF becomes passively dependent upon CPP [38,42,52].

The lower and upper limits of autoregulation in the typical normotensive patient are a mean arterial pressure (MAP) of about 60 and 130–150 mmHg, respectively [38,42,62,63]. Beyond these limits CBF becomes primarily flow dependent [12,61]. A decrease in MAP below the lower limit results in a CBF decrease and an increase in the arteriovenous oxygen difference [42]. At a MAP of 40 mmHg, symptoms of cerebral ischemia, including mental impairment, hyperventilation, and dizziness, occur [42]. Based upon the idealized autoregulation curve and on patients with normal cerebral vessels, CPP theoretically can decrease by approximately 30% before the lower limit of autoregulation is reached. This rule-of-thumb is useful clinically when planning the anesthetic management of a hypertensive or normotensive patient [12].

When MAP increases above the upper limit of autoregulation, blood flow exceeds the ability of the cerebral vasculature to constrict. Pronounced increases in CBF cause forced dilation of arterioles, which may be associated with disruption of the BBB and subsequent cerebral edema and/or hemorrhage [12,42].

The constancy of CBF is achieved by an active vascular response [42], thus rendering CBF directly proportional to CPP and inversely proportional to cerebrovascular resistance (CVR) [12]. For calculation of CPP, mean ICP (best approximation of true intracranial cerebral venous pressure) is subtracted from MAP ($CPP = MAP - ICP_{mean}$) [12]. An increase in perfusion pressure will elicit arteriolar constriction and a decrease in CPP is followed by arteriolar dilation. It is most likely that CBF autoregulation results from myogenic responses of smooth muscle cells of the arteriolar wall to the stretch caused by the distending transmural pressure [42] rather than by activation of the autonomic nerve fibers of perivascular nerves [64,65].

Although a network of sympathetic and parasympathetic nerve fibers supplies arteries on the brain surface and inside the brain tissue, no evidence of tonic autonomic control over pial arterial tone has been reported [42,66,67]. Moreover, changes in CBF subsequent to administration of angiotensin or trimetaphan are related to the drug effects on systemic arterial pressure rather than on cerebral vasculature [42].

Thin-walled, valveless cerebral veins drain blood into relatively thick-walled dural sinuses [12]. The site of entry of a cerebral vein into a dural sinus anatomically presents a relatively fixed orifice and physiologically presents a significant resistance to flow.

In chronic arterial hypertension, the cerebral vessels adapt to higher perfusion pressure by hypertrophy of the vessel wall, which in turn displaces the autoregulatory curve to the right [42,68]. Hence chronically hypertensive patients tolerate a high arterial pressure much better than do normotensive patients. However, displacement of the autoregulatory curve to the right also means that the lower limit is shifted to the right, which increases the risk of ischemia during systemic hypotension [42]. Therefore, chronically hypertensive patients do not tolerate the same acceptable lower limits (e.g., MAP of 60–70 mmHg) for arterial blood pressure as normotensive patients.

During hypovolemic hypotension, CVR will increase. The resultant increase in vessel tone results in a displacement of the autoregulatory curve to the right; subsequently, both the lower limit of CBF autoregulation and the lowest tolerated pressure are increased [42]. Therefore, during hemorrhagic hypotension, brain ischemia develops at a higher perfusion pressure than during pharmacologically induced hypotension where CVR is decreased.

Critical CBF is defined as the blood flow below which cerebral ischemia occurs. As CBF decreases further, a flow is reached below which cortical electrical function is abolished [12]. In normothermic, normocapnic, lightly anesthetized humans, the critical ischemic threshold of CBF is in the range 16–20 mL/100 g/min [42,69,70]. EEG evidence of cerebral ischemia invariably occurred at regional CBF (rCBF) below 10 mL/100 g/min, usually occurred at rCBF below 15 mL/100 g/min, and never occurred at rCBF above 24 mL/100 g/min. It was concluded that during normocapnia and general anesthesia with halothane or enflurane, critical rCBF is approximately 15 mL/100 g/min [70,71]. At a CBF of about 15 mL/100 g/min, the evoked electrocortical responses disappear completely, and at an even lower CBF of about 6–10 mL/100 g/min, a massive efflux of K^+ from and a Ca^{2+} influx into damaged cells occurs [30,69]. However, the critical ischemic threshold value of CBF may vary with different anesthetics and conditions [12].

Variations in partial pressure of arterial carbon dioxide ($PaCO_2$) exert the most profound influence on CBF regulation [42]. While hypercapnia can cause pronounced cerebral vasodilation, extreme hypocapnia can cause cerebral vasoconstriction up to the limit of ischemic brain hypoxia. Around the normal $PaCO_2$, CBF changes by about 4% [42] or 2 mL/100 g/min [51] for each 1 mmHg change in $PaCO_2$.

Carbon dioxide reactivity is mediated by pH variations in the CSF surrounding the arterioles [72]. The pH of CSF depends on the tension of freely diffusible CO_2 and the CSF bicarbonate concentration. This dual nature of the chemical control of CBF by $PaCO_2$ and CSF bicarbonate is also the basis for cerebral vasoparalysis in conjunction with brain tissue lactic acidosis [42]. $PaCO_2$-induced changes in CBF appear to subserve homeostasis of the pH in the brain, in that an increase in $PaCO_2$ is followed by an increase in CBF [42]. This will allow more efficient washout of metabolically produced CO_2, thereby damping the change in tissue PCO_2 and pH [42]. In addition to the maintenance of homeostasis of tissue PCO_2 and pH, CO_2-induced pH changes in CSF at the level of the brainstem will also affect pulmonary ventilation [42]. Cerebral blood flow and ventilation (both of which alter brain extracellular pH) in addition to metabolically induced bicarbonate changes protect brain tissue pH against both acute respiratory acidosis and alkalosis [42].

The value of inducing mild cerebral vasoconstriction by hyperventilation during neurosurgical procedures is well known [42]. Long-term hyperventilation over days produces a state of moderate hypocapnia but, as a result of the adaptation (normalization) of CSF pH and consequently of CBF to the lower PCO_2 value, hyperventilation-induced vasoconstriction will be of limited effect. Severe hypocapnia with $PaCO_2$ values below 20 mmHg will decrease CBF to such a so low value that the ischemic threshold for sustaining normal neuronal function can be reached; therefore, patient ventilation to $PaCO_2$ values of less than 25 mmHg is not recommended [42,73,74].

Moderate changes in PaO_2 during moderate arterial hypoxemia or arterial hyperoxemia do not exert a measurable influence on CBF [42]. An increase in CBF is not seen until PaO_2 decreases to below 50 mmHg [75], which is the same PO_2 value below which progressive brain tissue lactic acidosis appears [76]. These findings suggest that in hypoxia the CBF is regulated by the periarteriolar pH [42]. Anoxia or the combination of anoxia and hypercapnia may constitute pronounced cerebral vasodilation. Therefore, these conditions may produce a fatal increase in ICP and mass displacement (brain herniation) in patients with space-occupying intracranial lesions [42].

CBF autoregulation can be abolished by trauma, brain tumor, apoplexy, and noxious stimuli such as hypoxia and lactic acidosis [42,77,78]. Vasodilation or even complete vasomotor paralysis induced by lactic acid can readily over-ride the autoregulatory constrictor response to perfusion pressure increase. In such circumstances, any increase in MAP secondary to the intravenous injection of vasopressor drugs (e.g., norepinephrine, angiotensin) will increase CBF and result in cerebral hyperperfusion [77,78].

Cerebral vessels can synthesize prostaglandins and prostacyclin PGI_2 [79]. Prostacyclin is a vasodilator whereas thromboxane-A_2 is the most potent cerebral vasoconstrictor known [79,80].

Luxury perfusion or paradoxical response to $PaCO_2$

Pathologic conditions such as transient cardiac arrest, traumatic brain injury, brain tumor, or meningitis can cause inadequate cerebral perfusion and hypoxia, which in turn leads to severe tissue lactic acidosis, vasomotor paralysis, and increased ICP [42,81]. Vasomotor paralysis can occur within ischemic areas, around a tumor, in areas of infarction, or distal to vascular occlusions [50]. This means that loss of CBF autoregulation will not be restricted to the center of pathologic conditions but will also include surrounding areas with marginal perfusion [42,50]. Because of the loss of vessels' ability to respond to changes in either perfusion pressure or $PaCO_2$, rCBF is passively dependent on perfusion pressure. In this circumstance, normal or elevated perfusion pressure can produce blood flow that is 'supernormal' relative to the metabolic needs, a phenomenon termed *luxury perfusion syndrome* [12,82,83].

If CVR decreases in non-ischemic, normal regions of the brain (e.g., isoflurane anesthesia), blood may be shunted away from the area of vasomotor paralysis. This shunting is termed *intracerebral-steal syndrome* [12]. In contrast, an increase in CVR in normal cerebral regions will shunt blood into areas of vasomotor paralysis, a phenomenon referred to as the *inverse steal* or *Robin Hood syndrome* [12].

Spinal cord blood flow

As with cerebral circulation, spinal cord blood flow is maintained by autoregulation within certain MAP limits (e.g., 60–150 mmHg) [84,85]. Hypoxia produces vasodilation that overrides both the autoregulation and $PaCO_2$ effects on spinal cord blood flow [86]. Canine spinal cord blood flow increases sharply when PaO_2 declines to 60 mmHg and reaches a maximum at a PaO_2 of 30–40 mmHg [86]. Hypercapnia, on the other hand, produces a significant increase in spinal cord blood flow [84–86] and essentially abolishes autoregulation [85]. While hypoxia and hypercapnia markedly increase total spinal blood flow, the distribution of flow to gray and white matter will not be affected by changes in PaO_2 and $PaCO_2$, respectively [84].

The spinal cord gray matter seems to be especially vulnerable to damage by ischemia, owing to the high metabolic rate of neurons and associated high blood flow requirements [84]. This may be one major reason for the high incidence of paraplegia (0.9–6%) and mortality rate (9–22%) resulting from aneurysm repair of the thoracic aortic segment in humans [87].

Intraoperative loss of somatosensory-evoked potentials (SSEPs) has been used to predict loss of spinal cord function in humans [88]. For example, pronounced and progressive deterioration in SSEPs in a patient undergoing scoliosis repair returned to normal (control) values when deliberate hypotension was discontinued [89].

General anesthesia

The terms sedation and hypnosis describe states of mental depression in conjunction with diminished motor activity, anxiolysis, decreased arousal with slow incoherent responses to verbal commands, analgesia, and amnesia induced by a depressant drug [90–92]. Sedation (sometimes used as a synonym for hypnosis [90]) refers to a decreased level of arousal (i.e., long response times) resulting from sedative (subhypnotic) concentrations of a general anesthetic while hypnosis has been defined as unresponsiveness to verbal commands (in humans) [93].

Volatile and injectable anesthetic agents induce sedation or hypnosis by acting at different γ-aminobutyric acid type A ($GABA_A$) receptor subunits: acting at β_2-$GABA_A$ receptors produces sedation whereas binding to β_3-$GABA_A$ results in hypnosis [93]. However, no single anesthetic incorporates all the attributes of general anesthesia (e.g., sedation, hypnosis, amnesia, analgesia) to the same extent and, therefore, general anesthesia may be defined as amnesia and a reversible loss of and consciousness at low anesthetic concentrations and a loss of response to a painful stimulus at higher anesthetic concentrations [8,90].

Anesthetic-induced amnesia (loss of memory, absence of recall) will be primarily anterograde and can be assessed for both explicit (conscious) and implicit (unconscious) memory formation, respectively [90,93–96]. Data suggest that explicit memory seems to be the most sensitive target of inhaled general anesthetics [97] and that many anesthetic drugs already produce amnesia at concentrations well below those necessary for loss of consciousness [94,97]. At slightly higher doses, patients fail to move in response to a command and are considered unconscious, although clinical unresponsiveness is not necessarily synonymous with unconsciousness [91].

Loss of consciousness (LOC) can be defined as the reversible alteration of wakefulness and cognitive function of the brain (e.g., perception of the environment, thinking, attention, and memory) [98]. The primary end-points used in humans to determine LOC threshold during induction of anesthesia include the patient's inability to respond to non-noxious stimuli such as (1) cessation of counting [90], (2) loss of response to verbal command [99], (3) suppression of the eyelash reflex [100,101], (4) no response to calling out their name [102], (5) uninhibited release of a handheld object [103], or (6) no response to light tapping on the shoulder or light shaking [104]. In animals, loss of the righting reflex (LORR) has been used effectively as a surrogate measure for LOC [105]. Experimental data revealed a close correlation between LOC in humans and LORR in laboratory rodents (mouse and rat) over a range of anesthetic concentrations [105].

Immobility, another essential anesthetic goal, was established by Eger *et al.* in 1965 as a standard of anesthetic potency [106] because gross purposeful movement in response to a supramaximal noxious stimulus has been agreed upon to indicate inadequate anesthetic depth [107,108]. Immobility means the ablation of spontaneous or stimulus-induced movement by general anesthetic agents and is primarily mediated by decreasing the excitability of spinal neurons [93]. The fact that the anesthetic dose requirements for immobility are higher than those for producing unconsciousness suggests that the spinal cord and peripheral nervous system are less susceptible to depressive effects of general anesthesia [109,110].

The dose of propofol required to produce immobility during incision is more than four times higher than the dose leading to unconsciousness; therefore, propofol seems to be much more potent at producing unconsciousness than immobilization [97]. Similarly, the ratio of alveolar concentrations of volatile anesthetics producing immobility in contrast to unconsciousness has been reported to be in the approximate range 2–3 [97,111]. Consequently, anesthetic concentrations several-fold greater than those that produce immobility have been used to define the upper boundary of the clinically relevant concentration range [112].

Anatomic sites of anesthetic action

It has been postulated that general anesthetics act at multiple sites within the CNS by decreasing the transmission of information ascending from the spinal cord to the brain [113]. The major endpoints of general anesthesia such as amnesia and unconsciousness are most likely the result of anesthetic-impeded neurotransmission at supraspinal sites, including the brainstem [114], thalamus [6,105], and cerebral cortex [91,115–120]. Early studies revealed that direct electrical stimulation of the brainstem reticular formation (BSRF) in unanesthetized or lightly anesthetized animals led to cessation of synchronized discharge in the EEG and its replacement by a low-voltage, fast-wave EEG pattern (i.e., desynchronization). This response was blocked during deeper levels of general anesthesia [121–123]. These observations led to the concept of an ascending reticular activating system (ARAS) extending from the brainstem cholinergic nuclei [located in the caudal part of the midbrain reticular formation (MRF)], thence relayed through intralaminar thalamic nuclei to the cerebral cortex [124,125].

More detailed information on supraspinal features of general anesthesia have been provided by different functional monitoring techniques. Studies on the cerebral effects of thiopental [39], halothane [126], and isoflurane [40] revealed a dose-dependent decrease in global $CMRO_2$ and in EEG activity for thiopental and isoflurane. Increasing concentrations of thiopental or isoflurane resulted in a decrease in $CMRO_2$ until an isoelectric EEG or an isoelectric EEG pattern superimposed with spikes occurred, indicating extreme anesthetic depth. Neither continued administration of thiopental nor an increase in isoflurane concentration further affected the EEG pattern or the metabolic rate. Unlike the coupling between EEG and metabolic changes described for increasing concentrations of thiopental and isoflurane, doubling the halothane concentration produced a dose-related decrease in $CMRO_2$ that was unrelated to cortical electrical activity [126]. Halothane effects were examined in dogs in which systemic circulation was supported by extracorporeal circulation [126].

Recording electrical activity at different supraspinal sites in anesthetized goats revealed that a noxious stimulus (e.g., dew claw clamping) applied at 0.6 MAC of isoflurane resulted in an increase in electrical activity recorded at the caudal and rostral MRF, rostral thalamus, and cerebral cortex [127]. Increasing the isoflurane concentration to and above 1.1 MAC blunted the EEG response in terms of maintenance of a slow-wave, high-amplitude EEG pattern. These data suggest that isoflurane exerts its supraspinal effects by interfering with the transmission of sensory information through the MRF and thalamus [127]. EEG studies in anesthetized rodents further suggest depression of synaptic coupling between cortical structures [128] and of the hippocampus [129] by thiopental and isoflurane, respectively.

More recently, functional monitoring techniques such as positron emission tomography (PET) revealed that most general anesthetics produced a substantial decrease in neuronal activity in the cerebral cortex [115] that was associated with a dose-dependent decrease in the cerebral metabolism rate for glucose ($CMR_{glucose}$) [116,117]. Volatile [130,131], and injectable [116], anesthetic concentrations sufficient to produce loss of consciousness decreased cerebral metabolism by about 40–58% from the awake state. Changes in $CMR_{glucose}$ in subcortical areas such as the hippocampus, thalamus, midbrain, and cerebellum were less pronounced (48%) than in the cerebral cortex (58%) [116]. Unlike isoflurane and propofol, which caused fairly uniform metabolic changes throughout the various subcortical areas [130,131], halothane-induced depression in $CMR_{glucose}$ was most pronounced in areas such as the thalamus, limbic system, and locus ceruleus (LC) whereas the dorsal somatosensory cortex and parietal cortex were least affected [132].

Several studies suggest that the spinal cord is the major anatomic site where anesthetics predominantly cause immobility [133–135] and suppress hemodynamic responses [4] to noxious stimuli. Data indicate that halothane, enflurane, isoflurane, sevoflurane, and desflurane may produce immobility by direct spinal mechanisms such as diminishing α-motor neuron excitability as indicated by an F-wave depression [136–138] and/or a reduction in dorsal horn spontaneous activity [139]. Further evidence for spinally mediated suppression of movement responses is provided by the facts that neither acute precollicular decerebration [135] nor high thoracic spinal cord transection [134] altered the nature of the motor responses of isoflurane-anesthetized rats after tail clamping. Moreover, isoflurane's action on reflex-modulating neurons in the rostral ventromedial medulla (RVM) may be responsible, at least in part, for isoflurane-induced immobility [139–141].

Anesthetics can also modulate the level of consciousness indirectly by impeding the centripetal transfer of somatosensory information at the level of the spinal cord [113,125,142]. This theory is supported by the observations that anesthetic-induced cerebrocortical depression can be enhanced by additional suppression of centripetal impulse transmission by means of intrathecal administration of bupivacaine [143] or neuromuscular blockade using pancuronium [144].

Mechanisms of anesthetic actions

The exact mechanisms by which anesthetic agents produce the state of general anesthesia still remain unknown [96]. However, the fact that structurally and pharmacologically different drugs produce the same series of clinical end-points (e.g., sedation, amnesia, unconsciousness, and immobility) in a dose-dependent fashion led to the assumption that all these drugs produce the state of anesthesia by the same mechanisms. Claude Bernard formulated this 'unitary hypothesis' in 1875 [145]. In 1899, Hans Meyer reported on the correlation between the anesthetic potency and lipid solubility of chloroform [146]. The observation that the potency of anesthetics was correlated with lipid solubility led to the Meyer–Overton hypothesis [105]. This hypothesis was based on the assumption that anesthetics act by dissolving in the lipid bilayer of nerve membranes, thereby modifying membrane properties [105]. A non-specific physicochemical mechanism would result in the perturbation of membrane lipid bilayers of neuronal tissues [105,147,148]. Moreover, it was assumed that anesthesia commenced when a chemical substance had attained a certain molar concentration in the lipid constituents of the cell, independent of the drug structure [149].

Later, the critical volume hypothesis (i.e., lipid bilayer expansion hypothesis [150,151] or lateral pressure hypothesis[152]) was introduced as the physical mechanism of general anesthesia. It was assumed that anesthetic molecules, dissolved in the lipid bilayer, caused a modification of the dimensions of the cell membranes and, thereby, impeded the conduction of neuronal impulses. This hypothesis has been supported by study results where increases in ambient pressure could be successfully used to antagonize the anesthetic effects of liquid and gaseous anesthetics (i.e., pressure reversal) [151]. A pronounced increase in ambient pressure (6060–10 100 kPa) in animals anesthetized with urethane resulted in a decrease in anesthetic depth whereas reducing the ambient pressure deepened the level of anesthesia [153].

More recently, non-specific lipid-based theories of anesthetic mechanisms have gradually given way to the hypothesis that general anesthetics act via reversible effects on integral membrane proteins, particularly on ligand- and voltage-gated ion channels in the brain and spinal cord [112,154,155]. This hypothesis is supported by the discovery that a soluble, lipid-free protein such as firefly luciferase could be competitively inhibited by a chemically diverse range of simple anesthetics at inhibitory concentrations (IC_{50}) that closely mirrored *in vivo* potencies [156]. Moreover, the finding that isomers with the same lipid solubility may have different anesthetic potencies [157] cannot be explained by a correlation between lipid solubility and anesthetic potency. Finally, the discovery of stereoselectivity of general anesthetics (e.g., propofol [158] and isoflurane [159]) became the most definitive evidence that anesthetics act predominantly by binding directly to proteins [160].

Halogenated volatile anesthetic agents exert their anesthetic effects by enhancing inhibitory GABA and glycine receptors [97], by activation of 2P (two-pore domain) K^+ channels (e.g., TREK, TASK, TRESK) [161–163], by inhibition of excitatory glutamate receptors [164], and/or by acting on ion channels associated with nAChR [165] or serotonin subtype 3 receptors ($5\text{-}HT_3$) [166].

Unlike this multisite concept of anesthetic actions proposed for inhalant anesthetics, injectable anesthetics (e.g., propofol and etomidate) are assumed to exert sedation, hypnosis, and immobility predominantly by acting at inhibitory GABA receptors [93]. GABA is the most important inhibitory neurotransmitter in the mammalian brain and GABA receptors are found throughout the CNS [97,157,160]. The inhibitory GABA type A ($GABA_A$) receptor channel has long been considered a primary target for hypnotic drugs [96,160,167–172].

In addition to $GABA_A$ receptors, other ligand-gated chloride ion channel receptors have emerged as molecular targets of general anesthetics, including glycine receptors, $5\text{-}HT_3$ receptors, nACh receptors, and ionotropic glutamate receptors [97,112,160,173,174].

The three major types of ionotropic glutamate receptor channels are *N*-methyl-D-aspartate (NMDA), 2-carboxy-3-carboxymethyl-4-isopropenylpyrrolidine (kainate), and α-amino-3-hydroxy-5-methyl-4-isoxazolepropionic acid (AMPA) receptors [160,175], with NMDA receptors being known as an important target for ketamine and, to some extent, isoflurane [176–179].

Neurologic monitoring and testing

Neurologic monitoring during anesthesia primarily refers to monitoring of anesthetic depth, but may also include the detection and evaluation of neurologic disease states (e.g., seizure or brain ischemia) relevant for anesthetic management of the patient. Monitoring of anesthetic depth is primarily based on clinical signs and reflex response patterns first described by Arthur E. Guedel for ether anesthesia almost 100 years ago [180]. The shift from a mono-anesthetic approach to a balanced type of anesthesia, together with the marked progress in surgical techniques within the last century, supported the move to more sophisticated neurologic monitoring. This move was also accelerated by the recognition of the shortcomings of clinical signs used for monitoring anesthetic depth (e.g., blood pressure, heart rate) for detecting intraoperative awareness [181]. Therefore, EEG-based monitoring devices have become an integral part of monitoring anesthetic depth under specific circumstances in the medical and veterinary medical fields.

Electroencephalography

Electroencephalography (EEG) is the recording of spontaneous electrical brain activity from scalp electrodes [101,113,182]. Traditionally, the EEG has been recorded in the time domain from electrodes placed at standard positions according to the international 10–20 system [101,182,183]. The surface electrical signals represent the summation of the activity of millions of neurons in the cerebral cortex [101,184] and result from excitatory and inhibitory postsynaptic potentials (PSPs) in large pyramidal neurons located in the lower layers (e.g., layer V) of the cerebral cortex [122,184,185]. The EEG amplitude and frequency are modulated by afferent inputs from sensory-specific thalamic nuclei serving as gates between peripheral receptors and the cortex, and by epicenters within the cerebral cortex [186]. The EEG frequency bands utilized for assessment of anesthetic depth are the δ (0–4 Hz), θ (4–8 Hz), α (8–13 Hz), and β (13–30 Hz) bands [187,188].

In the 1930s, Hans Berger hypothesized that the appearance of α waves in the EEG may represent cerebrocortical events associated with consciousness in the awake man [189]. It has been generally accepted that the scalp-recorded rhythmic EEG activity associated with consciousness is generated from pacemaker neurons within the ARAS and mediated and modulated through thalamic connections [121,122,186,190,191]. These pacemaker neurons oscillate in the frequency range 8–12 Hz and synchronize the excitability of cells in the thalamocortical pathways. Small cerebrocortical areas seem also to act as epicenters from which alpha activity spreads through cortical neuronal networks and generates the α rhythm that dominates the resting EEG. In the awake state, consciousness is maintained by a circulating activity among ARAS, intralaminar nuclei, and the cerebral cortex [186]. Additional sensory stimulation will cause cortical arousal that is characterized by desynchronization of α oscillators with the appearance of a faster rhythm in the β frequency range (12–25 Hz) [186,191–194]. In general, desynchronization describes a shift in the EEG pattern from high-voltage, slow-wave activity to low-voltage, fast-wave activity [121,122,195].

During induction and maintenance of anesthesia, the progressive decrease in EEG frequency content (slowing) will be indicated by a shift from a low-voltage, fast-wave pattern to a high-voltage, slow-wave pattern [114,196–198]. Dose-dependent changes in EEG activity along with an increase in anesthetic depth were clearly demonstrated for many anesthetic agents [114,196]. As anesthetic depth increases, the predominant EEG pattern is characterized by a decrease in beta activity and a concomitant increase in both α and δ activity [199]. At LOC, EEG anteriorization occurs, which refers to an increase in alpha and delta activity in the anterior EEG leads relative to the posterior leads [6,199–201]. As anesthesia deepens further, EEG activity in the theta and delta frequency bands appears initially in centroposterior regions with subsequent anterior spread [201]. Finally, very deep levels of general anesthesia are first indicated by flat periods interspersed with periods of alpha and beta activity (burst suppression pattern) (Fig. 28.5), followed by a complete loss of electrical discharge (i.e., isoelectricity or electrical silence) [40,196,197]. As soon as the dose of the anesthetic agent has been reduced, these patterns reverse and lighter levels of anesthesia are indicated again by a decrease in amplitude and an increase in frequency content (Fig. 28.6). Controversy still exists as to whether anesthetic-induced

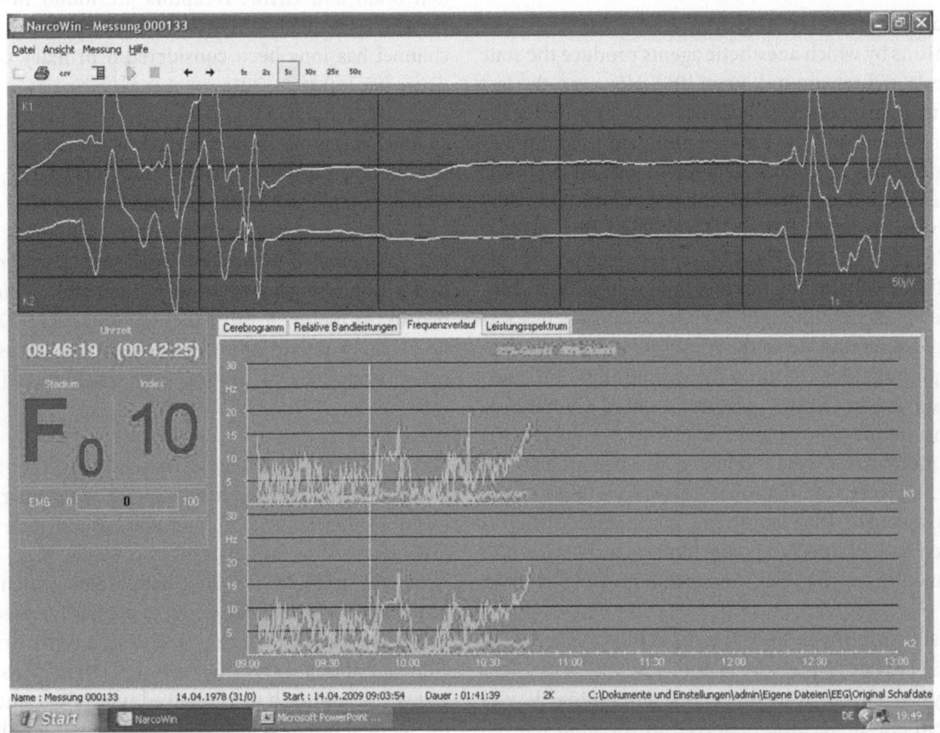

Figure 28.5 Narcotrend® two-channel EEG recording during hypothermic cardiopulmonary bypass surgery in sheep. Deep-level balanced anesthesia using isoflurane is indicated by (1) EEG burst suppression pattern in the analogous EEG (upper two curves), (2) Kugler stadium 'F_0,' and (3) low Narcotrend index '10.'

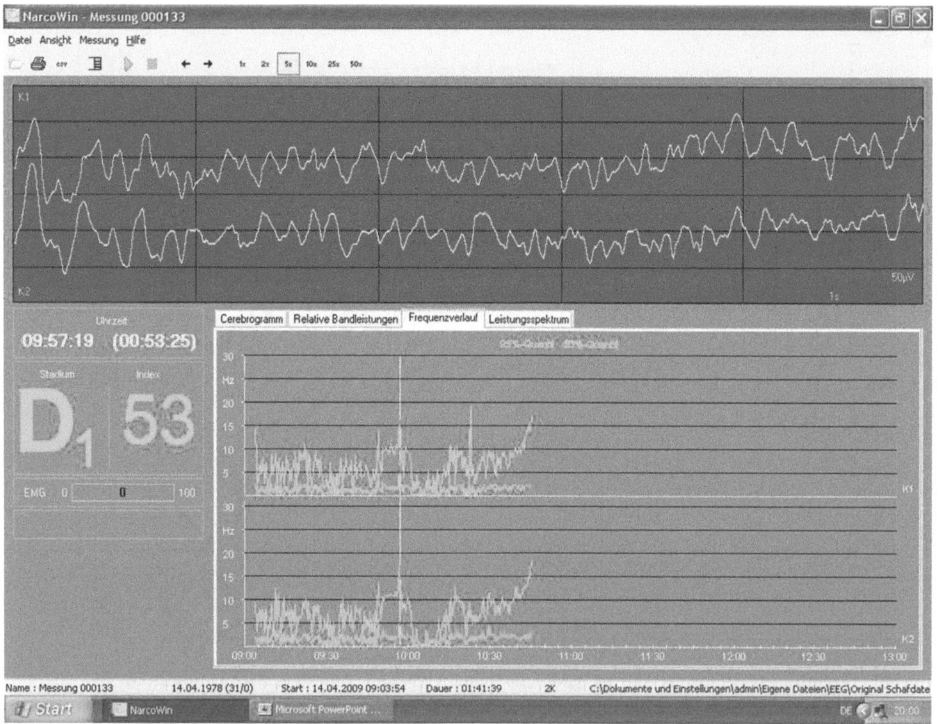

Figure 28.6 Narcotrend® two-channel EEG recording during hypothermic cardiopulmonary bypass surgery in sheep. Moderate level of anesthetic depth is indicated by (1) a shift from EEG burst suppression pattern to a low-voltage, fast-wave EEG pattern in the analogous EEG (upper two curves), (2) Kugler stadium 'D_1,' and (3) moderate Narcotrend index '53.'

unconsciousness results primarily from cortical or subcortical (thalamic) anesthetic actions [119,202–204].

In order to decrease the amount of EEG data traditionally recorded in the time domain, computer-processed EEG analysis (e.g., power spectrum analysis) was employed for intraoperative EEG monitoring more than 30 years ago [185,205–207]. The speed of data processing allows a minute-by-minute assessment of anesthetic depth [207,208]. By convention, the term power has been used as a measure of amplitude reflecting the origins of the Fourier analysis in radio engineering [186,207]. In order to summarize the most relevant information from an EEG sample, quantitative measures derived from power spectrum analysis have been devised [209]. These quantitative EEG (QEEG) variables include EEG median frequency (50%-quantile; MF) [210,211], spectral edge frequency (SEF) as the 80% [212,213], 90% [214], or 95% quantile [215,216], total power (μV^2) [188,217], percentage distribution of total power (relative power) into the δ, θ, α, and β frequency bands [5,211], and the power band ratios θ/δ, α/δ, and β/δ [210,217] derived from relative power. Reliable correlations between quantitative EEG variables and clinical signs demonstrate that certain aspects of brain electrical activity are sensitive to the level of consciousness. They provide practical clinical evidence that consciousness is a neurobiologic phenomenon that can be objectively quantified so that depth of anesthesia can be analyzed reliably using electrophysiologic variables. However, these variables provide relatively little insight into the mechanisms underlying both anesthesia and consciousness [186].

Another parameter frequently used for quantitative EEG analysis is the burst suppression ratio (BSR). EEG burst suppression pattern has been defined as an intermittent electrical activity interspersed with silence or as a near-complete depression of cortical electrical activity. Burst suppression indicates a non-specific (e.g., trauma, drugs, hypothermia) reduction in cerebral metabolic activity [185,218]. The burst suppression ratio has been calculated as the percentage of isoelectric periods occurring over a certain period of time [219].

The power spectrum calculated during anesthesia may be displayed in the compressed spectral array (CSA), where the component power is plotted as a function of frequency ($\mu V^2/Hz$) for each analyzed epoch (Fig. 28.7) [184,206,207]. The squared amplitudes are plotted as histogram and then smoothed to assist in its readability. The analysis of EEG epochs is repeated continuously with no loss of primary data while the resulting power spectra are plotted sequentially along the y-axis and the frequency range along the x-axis [206]. Hills and valleys in the CSA represent frequency bands with higher and lower power, respectively. EEG power spectrum analysis and display of data in the CSA format provide a simplified identification of small changes in the complex raw EEG [207].

EEG slowing during increasing depth of anesthesia is indicated by an increase in total power, an increase in relative power in the δ and θ frequency bands, and a decrease in α and β power and also in MF and SEF. These changes have been demonstrated in human patients and animals for a variety of anesthetic agents [188,210,213–215,220–222]. A decrease in anesthetic concentration will reverse EEG slowing and subsequent changes from deeper to lighter levels of anesthetic depth will be indicated by a shift in EEG power from the lower (δ and θ) to the higher (α and β) frequency ranges and by an increase in MF and SEF.

Studies in dogs revealed that EEG isoelectricity might be achieved with lower end-tidal isoflurane concentration compared with halothane [40,126]. These differential effects on EEG data also have been reported for studies in horses [213,223] and rats [224]. At

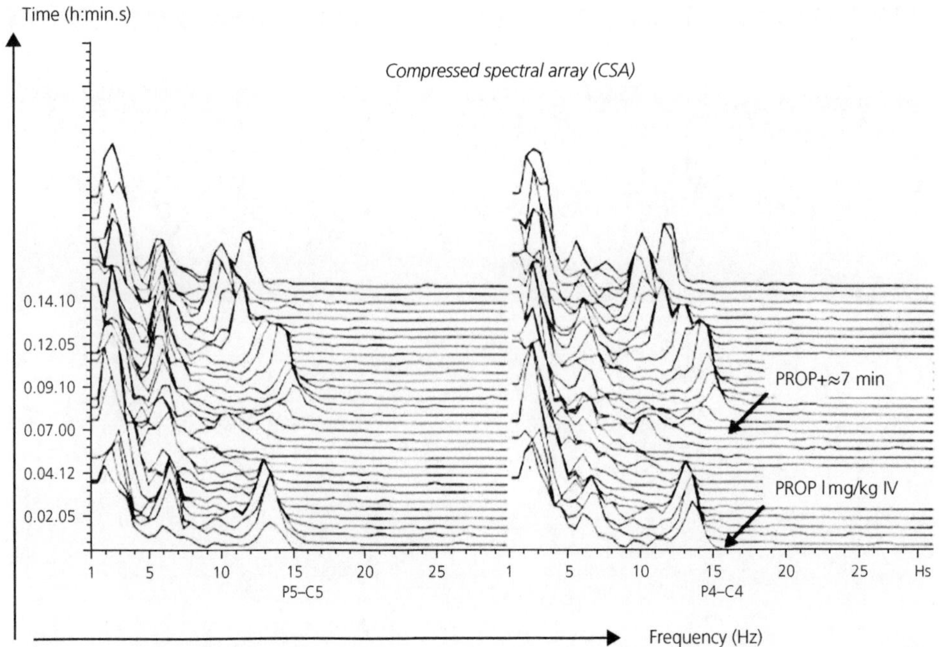

Figure 28.7 Two-channel EEG recording (CSA format) during halothane–fentanyl–N_2O–O_2 anesthesia for laminectomy in a dog. CSA format represents EEG slowing and activation following intravenous injection of propofol (1 mg/kg).

similar levels of anesthetic depth as determined by clinical signs or MAC multiples, animals anesthetized with isoflurane presented lower SEF, MF and/or β/δ ratio values but higher amplitude measures than those during halothane anesthesia. These results suggest that some anesthetic agents such as thiopental [196], isoflurane [114], and propofol [225] cause profound EEG suppression even at clinically relevant concentrations whereas others (e.g., halothane) [126] may not.

One major application of intraoperative EEG monitoring is the identification of EEG responses evoked by surgical stimuli [226]. Regardless of the site and type of stimulation, noxious stimuli may cause EEG desynchronization, indicated by replacement of predominant high-voltage, slow-wave activity by low-voltage, fast-wave activity, and increases in MF, SEF, and the power band ratios (θ/δ, α/δ, and β/δ) [5,121,210,227–230]. These changes in EEG pattern will occur during inadequate levels of anesthesia but will be depressed by increasing anesthetic depth.

EEG synchronization or paradoxical arousal is another form of EEG activation, which represents the opposite alteration in the cortical discharge in response to noxious stimulation (EEG slowing instead of increase in frequency content). The mechanism of this activation pattern is poorly understood [181,209,231]. Paradoxical arousal could falsely be interpreted as a deep level of anesthesia or brain hypoxia and has been reported in isoflurane-anesthetized human patients who underwent visceral urological, abdominal or, gynecological surgery [231,232], but also for different noxious stimuli applied during orthopedic surgery in isoflurane-anesthetized sheep [233]. In summary, the occurrence of intraoperative EEG arousal or paradoxical arousal may be affected by depth of anesthesia, intensity and type of noxious stimulation, individual differences, and age of the patient. The primary goal of intraoperative EEG monitoring is the maintenance of a high-voltage, slow-wave EEG pattern and to avoid changes in the EEG pattern in response to noxious stimulation.

In a number of studies, a close relationship between changes in the EEG pattern and simultaneously recorded autonomic variables in response to noxious stimulation could be clearly demonstrated. EEG desynchronization or synchronization during anesthesia were associated with changes in clinical signs such as mydriasis, hypertension, and/or tachycardia [122,228,231,233–236]. However, a poor correlation between EEG and hemodynamic responses to noxious stimulation has also been reported [212,217]. It was concluded that autonomic hemodynamic responses might be more closely related to neurophysiologic events in either the brainstem or spinal cord rather than to cortical events [213]. Similarly, a poor correlation between EEG and movement response to noxious stimulation has been noted in humans [218,237] and animals [135,238] anesthetized with isoflurane. Movement responses but no changes in the EEG pattern may be elicited by noxious stimuli, leading to the conclusion that the brain reacts more sensitively than the spinal cord to isoflurane [127,181].

Evoked potentials

Mid-latency auditory evoked potentials (MLAEPs) [239] and somatosensory-evoked potentials (SSEPs) [240] have been advocated for monitoring depth of anesthesia. SSEPs represent electrical signals generated by the nervous system following mechanical or electrical stimulation in the periphery and subsequent sequential activation of neuronal structures along the somatosensory pathways [105]. The averaged responses recorded from primary cortical receiving areas in response to electrical stimulation of peripheral nerves appear as negative waves or inflections [initial negative (Ni), second negative (Ns)] superimposed on a wave of surface positivity [initial positive (Pi), second positive (Ps)] [113].

For most anesthetics (except etomidate and propofol), an increase in anesthetic depth is indicated by an increase in latency and a decrease in the amplitude of Pi and Ni waves whereas arousal is associated with a decrease in latency and increase in amplitude

[96,113,153]. The effects of anesthetics on SSEPs in humans supports the idea that information transfer through the thalamus is disrupted, with the non-specific nuclei being most affected [105]. Neither MLAEPs nor EEG-derived variables can be used to predict movement response to noxious stimulation, thus limiting their use for intraoperative monitoring [237].

Bispectral index®

Bispectral index® (BIS®), like MF and SEF, is an index derived from raw EEG signal processing. Whereas MF and SEF extract frequency information from the EEG signal [241], BIS is composed of a combination of the time-domain, frequency-domain, and higher-order spectral subparameters and incorporates the degree of phase coupling between the component waves [185,242–244]. BIS is a dimensionless number intended to indicate the patient's level of consciousness [244]. BIS ranges from 100 (awake) to 0 (isoelectric EEG) [245]. A BIS of 55 in humans has been recommended as the upper limit that might assure adequate depth of surgical anesthesia [244,246].

Studies demonstrate dose-dependent decreases in BIS values with increasing end-tidal concentrations/doses of sevoflurane [247], isoflurane [248], and propofol [249]. When comparing the reliability of end-tidal anesthetic agent concentration (ETAC) and BIS for monitoring anesthetic depth in humans, data revealed that BIS monitoring conferred no benefit compared with ETAC monitoring with respect to avoidance of awareness [244,250,251]. With some awareness events apparently occurring with BIS values below the upper limit (e.g., 55–60), changing the volatile anesthetic concentration solely on the basis of a BIS value is not recommended [244]. Unlike ETAC, BIS was reported to be significantly more accurate than targeted or measured propofol concentrations during propofol sedation and hypnosis [103].

Like the poor correlation reported between changes in hemodynamic variables and spectral EEG parameters, several studies revealed that hemodynamic responses to noxious stimulation were not associated with concurrent changes in BIS [252–255]. In summary, EEG-derived depth of anesthesia monitors such as BIS are meant to supplement, but not to supplant, clinical decision-making [245].

Narcotrend® index

The Narcotrend® algorithm is based on pattern recognition of the raw EEG and classifies the EEG traces into different stages from A (awake) to F (burst suppression/isoelectricity) and into a dimensionless Narcotrend index (NI) ranging from 100 (awake) to 0 (isoelectricity) [256]. Both methods, BIS and NI, were considered equally effective in monitoring anesthetic depth during surgery in human patients [256–258].

A comparison of NI with clinical stages of anesthesia during experimental cardiac surgery in isoflurane-anesthetized sheep revealed a significant correlation between NI and increasing anesthetic depth as defined by clinical signs [259]. The most valuable information may be obtained from NI during cardiopulmonary bypass and the anesthetic period immediately following weaning the animal from the heart–lung machine when clinical signs are rarely available (Figs 28.8–28.11).

Entropy

EEG parameters based on the frequency spectrum analysis (e.g., MF, SEF) reflect only linear signal properties and therefore may be of limited value [210,260,261]. Non-linear EEG parameters (e.g., approximate entropy) may emphasize some additional characteristics of the EEG based on the non-linear chaotic behavior exhibited

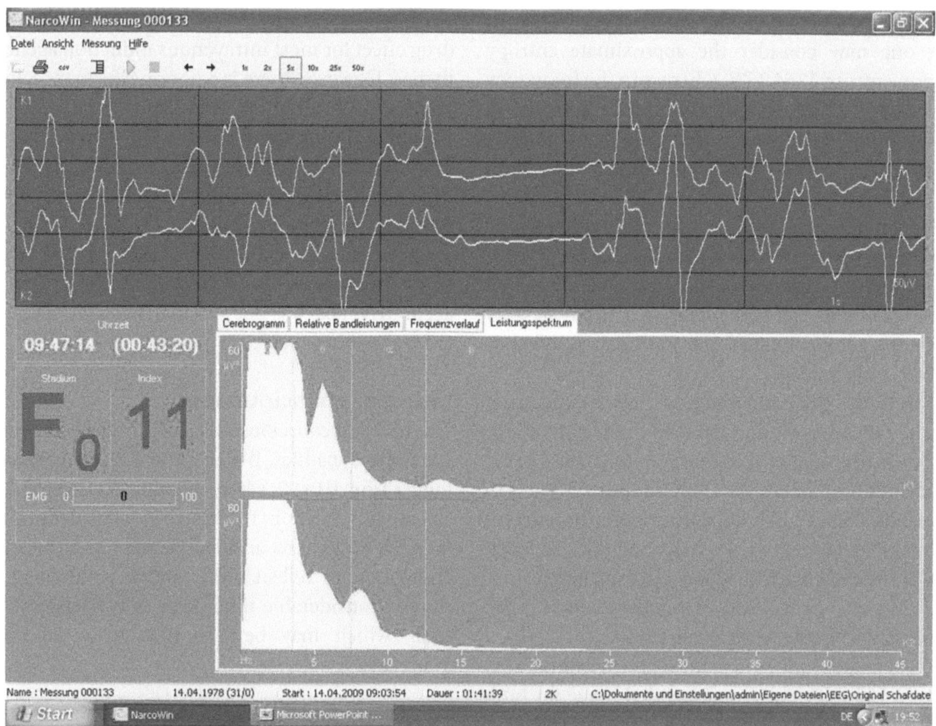

Figure 28.8 Narcotrend® two-channel EEG recording during hypothermic cardiopulmonary bypass surgery in sheep. Deep-level balanced anesthesia using isoflurane is indicated by (1) EEG burst suppression pattern in the analogous EEG (upper two curves), (2) Kugler stadium 'F_0,' and (3) low Narcotrend index '11.' Filled yellow curves (lower right part) indicate predominant EEG activity in the δ frequency band.

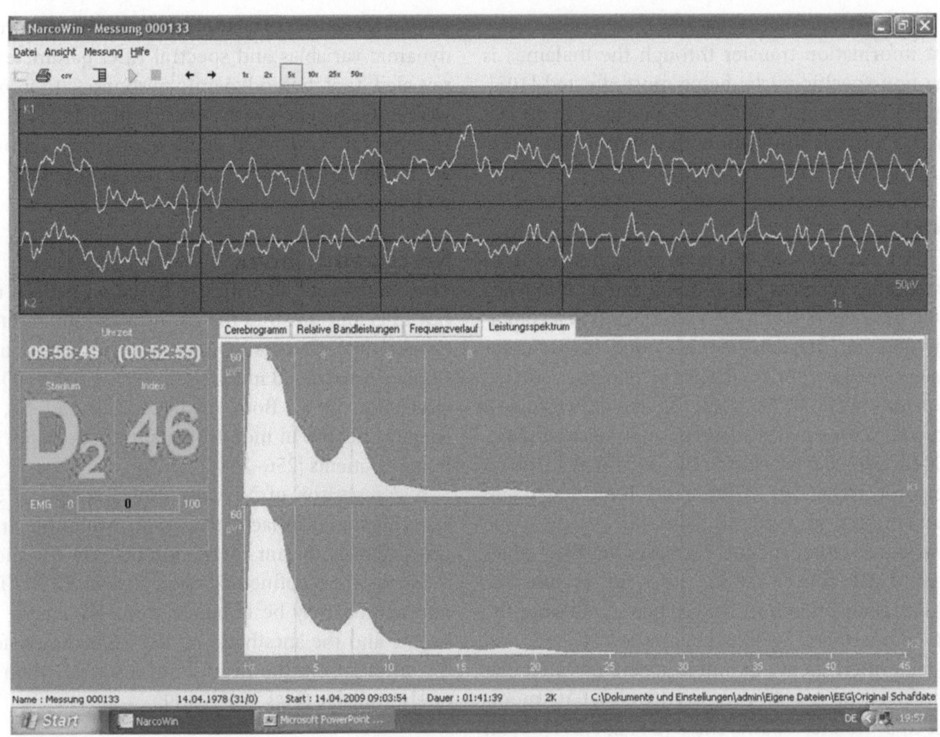

Figure 28.9 Narcotrend® two-channel EEG recording during hypothermic cardiopulmonary bypass surgery in sheep. Moderate-level balanced anesthesia using isoflurane is indicated by (1) low-voltage, fast-wave EEG pattern in the analogous EEG (upper two curves), (2) Kugler stadium 'D_2,' and (3) Narcotrend index '46.' Filled yellow curves (lower right part) indicate a shift in predominant EEG activity from the δ frequency band to higher frequency bands (α).

by neuronal systems [261–265]. Entropy analyzes the irregularity, complexity, and unpredictability of EEG signals [266].

There are different ways to compute the entropy of a signal. In the time domain, one may consider the approximate entropy [263,264] or Shannon entropy [264,267], whereas in the frequency domain, spectral entropy [268] may be computed. In order to optimize the speed at which information is derived from the EEG signal, it is desirable to construct a combination of time- and frequency-domain approaches [266].

State entropy (SE) and response entropy (RE) are another group of dimensionless numbers, which may be computed using the M-Entropy module of the S/5™ Anesthesia monitor. One important value is to separate EEG and electromyographic (EMG) activity [265], as the frequency composition of the EEG and EMG may overlap in the 30–50 Hz range [269].

SE is computed over the EEG-dominant part of the spectrum (0.8–32 Hz) primarily reflecting the cortical state of the patient. RE refers to the activity in the higher frequency range (0.8–47 Hz), which includes both EEG-dominant and EMG-dominant parts of the spectrum [265,270]. SE is intended to measure the current cortical state of the patient whereas RE, by reflecting EMG activity, is thought to be an indirect measure of adequacy of analgesia since EMG activity may increase as a result of intensive nociceptive stimulation and during decreasing levels of anesthesia.

Similarly to BIS, SE ranges from 91 (awake) to 0 (isoelectric EEG activity) and RE from 100 to 0. The recommended range for both parameters indicating adequate anesthesia is 40–60 [265,270]. Whenever SE increases above 60, anesthetic depth should be increased, but when RE exceeds the upper limit by 5–10 units, additional analgesics should be considered instead of deepening anesthesia [271]. At deeper levels of anesthesia, when EMG power is equal to zero, RE becomes equal to SE.

Generally, entropy values are suitable to quantify the anesthetic drug effect for most intravenous induction agents and volatile anesthetics. However, there is a poor performance during ketamine and nitrous oxide administration [265].

Numerous studies [261,272,273] consistently showed that permutation entropy could be used to discriminate efficiently between different levels of consciousness during anesthetic administration [274]. A multiple permutation measure, called composite multiscaler permutation entropy (CMSPE), could be used to detect subtle transitions between light and deep sevoflurane anesthesia accurately. This was not possible when the single-scale permutation entropy was used [275].

Index of consciousness

The index of consciousness (IoC) is derived from a combination of symbolic dynamics, β-ratio, and EEG suppression rate [270]. IoC ranges from 0 to 99, where 99 indicates an awake patient, 80 is associated with sedation, the range 40–60 is defined as the state recommended for general anesthesia, and 0 indicates isoelectric EEG. SE and IoC both reflect the hypnotic component of anesthesia and show a considerable time delay in reflecting the actual anesthetic level, which may be a limitation in detecting intraoperative awareness.

Cerebral state index

The Cerebral State Monitor™ (CSM) is another EEG-based monitor used to measure the depth of hypnosis during general anesthesia [276].

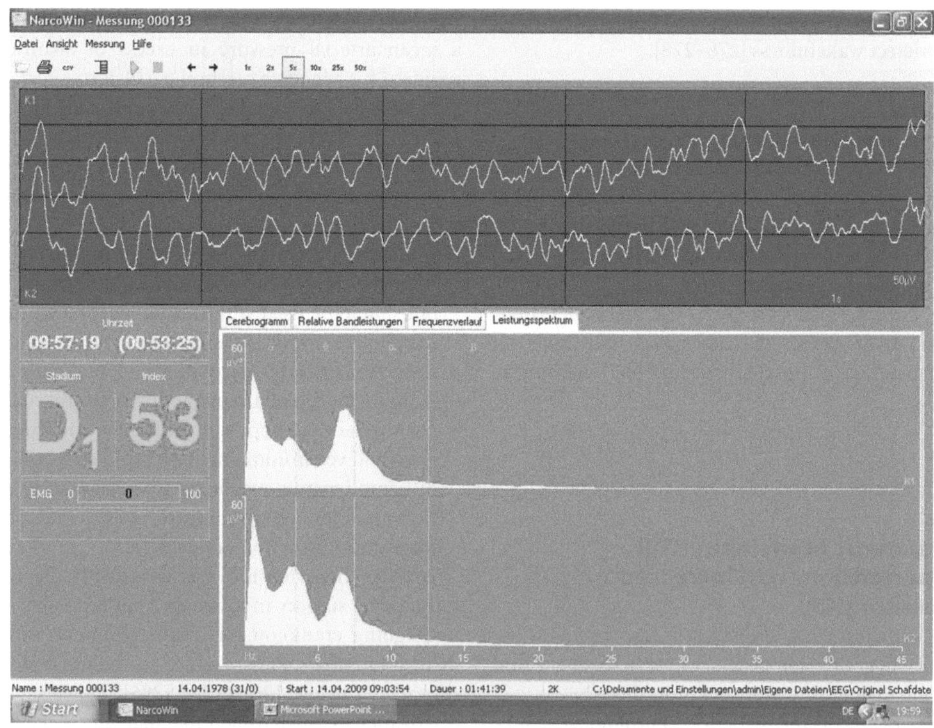

Figure 28.10 Narcotrend® two-channel EEG recording during hypothermic cardiopulmonary bypass surgery in sheep. Moderate-level balanced anesthesia using isoflurane is indicated by (1) low-voltage, fast-wave EEG pattern in the analogous EEG (upper two curves), (2) Kugler stadium 'D_1,' and (3) Narcotrend index '53.' Filled yellow curves (lower right part) indicate a shift in predominant EEG activity from the δ frequency band to higher frequency bands (α).

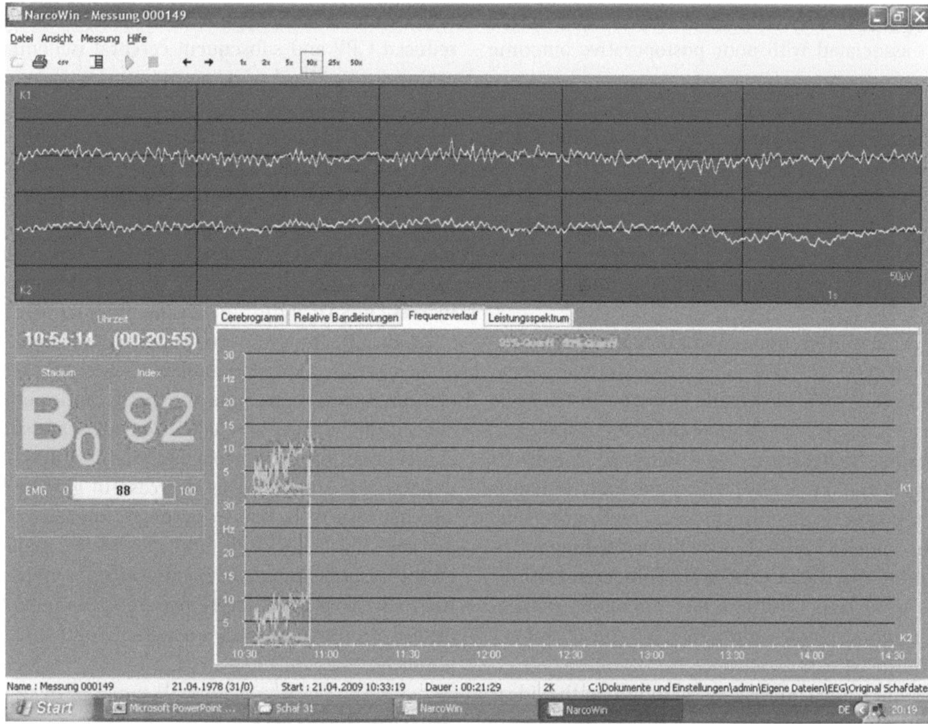

Figure 28.11 Narcotrend® two-channel EEG recording during emergence from anesthesia for hypothermic cardiopulmonary bypass surgery in sheep. Near-awakening is indicated by (1) low-voltage, fast-wave EEG pattern in the analogous EEG (upper two curves), (2) Kugler stadium 'B_0,' and (3) Narcotrend index '92' in conjunction with (4) a high EMG index '88.'

In summary, there are currently no EEG-based monitors available that can unfailingly detect wakefulness [276–278].

Electromyography

Electromyography is the measurement of electrical activity within the muscle [279,280]. Recordings are made with a needle inserted into a muscle. Analysis of the waveforms and firing rates of single or multiple motor units can give diagnostic information [279,280]. Clinical applications for EMG include the diagnostic of disorders of the spinal cord (e.g., acute disc herniation), disorders of peripheral nerves (e.g., traumatic neuropathies, polyneuritis), disorders of the neuromuscular junction (e.g., myasthenia gravis), and muscle disorders (e.g., myotonia, polymyositis) [281].

Management of selected nervous system disease states

Brain tumor, traumatic brain injury (TBI), Intracranial hypertension (ICH)/increased intracranial pressure (ICP)

In human patients with intracranial disease states, the following strategies have been suggested for perioperative assessment and protection of the brain during neurosurgical procedures:

1 Preoperative assessment of the patient's neurological status, including signs of mental depression (drowsiness, unconsciousness) and pupil size and reaction [282].
2 Documentation of signs and symptoms of raised intracranial pressure (e.g., vomiting, papilloedema, pupillary dilation) [282].
3 Perioperative blood pressure measurement in order to maintain adequate CPP [282,283].
4 Maintenance of euglycemia or slightly increased blood glucose levels (5.5–10 mmol/L) [282,283].
5 Avoid perioperative anemia (Hb ≥9–12 g/dL) as low Hb values have been associated with poor postoperative outcome [283,284].
6 Allow or produce mild hypothermia (32–35 °C) [283,285].

The intracranial space contains three components, brain tissue (80–85%), CSF (7–10%), and cerebral blood volume (CBV) (5–8%), and ICP represents the pressure caused by these three components within the non-distensible intracranial space [16]. The Monroe-Kelly hypothesis states that for ICP to remain normal, a volume increase in any one of the three components must be matched by a decrease in another [16].

Space-occupying brain tumors, traumatic brain injury (TBI), and subarachnoid hemorrhage (SAH) may all cause vasomotor paralysis and an increase in ICP with subsequent decrease in CBF and impaired O_2 delivery [12,286]. Rapidly increasing ICP is indicated by arterial hypertension, bradycardia, and respiratory irregularity ('vasopressor response') and frequently leads to cerebral herniation with brainstem compression, unconsciousness, and subsequent death [287]. This phenomenon is also known as the Cushing reflex, Cushing effect, Cushing reaction, Cushing phenomenon, Cushing response, Cushing's triad, and Cushing's law. Therefore, maintenance of adequate cerebral blood supply may be considered the major challenge in these patients.

Although there is still some controversy surrounding the 'ideal' CPP [288,289] and lower pressure limit for CBF autoregulation in patients with cerebral disorders [290], maintaining CPP above at least 60 [289,291] to 70 mmHg [292] has been recommended. Taking further into account that ICP may range from 10–15 mmHg (normal) [288] to approximately 20–30 mmHg (abnormal) [288,292], a mean arterial pressure in excess of 80 mmHg [283] may be required for adequate cerebral perfusion.

Additional therapeutic measures during elevated ICP may include the following [12,288,289,293–301]:

1 Adequate sedation and analgesia.
2 Improved cerebral venous drainage by elevating the head at a 15–30° angle.
3 Infusion of mannitol or hypertonic saline. Hypertonic saline may improve cerebral hemodynamics and brain tissue oxygenation but should be used with caution as it may cause hyperchloremic metabolic acidosis and subsequent renal impairment.
4 Induction of anesthesia with thiopental, propofol, or etomidate.
5 Administration of a rapid acting neuromuscular blocker (NMB) prior to laryngoscopy and endotracheal intubation. Both atracurium and vecuronium provide rapid onset of action. Suppression of hemodynamic responses to endotracheal intubation/extubation and subsequent increase in ICP may also be achieved by intravenous injection of lidocaine.

Arterial hypertension has frequently been reported during intracranial surgery in humans. Approximately 60–90% of patients undergoing craniotomy require treatment with antihypertensive medications [302,303] in order to maintain systolic arterial pressure (SAP) below 126 mmHg [286]. However, because of several disadvantages, including long half-life (e.g., labetol), minimum effect on elevated systemic vascular resistance (e.g., esmolol), and adverse effects on intracranial blood volume (e.g., sodium nitroprusside, hydralazine), cautious use of antihypertensive medications in humans has been recommended [303]. On the other hand, induction of transient arterial hypertension is required for vessel occlusion (e.g., temporary clipping, clamping, vasospasm) or alteration in cerebral autoregulation resulting from intracranial mass, hypertensive disease, or TBI [283].

Systemic arterial hypotension during anesthesia may result in reduced CPP and subsequent cerebral ischemia [286]. Therefore, perioperative blood pressure monitoring is essential for the detection and treatment of hypotension/hypertension. Arterial blood pressure should be measured before drug administration (if possible) and used as a guideline for intraoperative management. Additionally, measurement of changes in regional cerebral oxygen saturation (rSO_2) using near-infrared spectroscopy may help to identify cerebral O_2 desaturation (e.g., decrease in rSO_2 by >20% of baseline value). Measures to prevent desaturation may include increase in SAP and/or increasing the fraction of inspired O_2 [304].

After TBI, the brain may increase metabolic activity, which is often a ramification of glutamate release and excitotoxicity. In these circumstances, euglycemic or hypoglycemic patients' blood glucose concentrations may not allow for adequate substrate delivery to compensate for a hypermetabolic brain [305]. A metabolic crisis, defined as a simultaneous decrease in glucose below 0.7 mmol/L and increase in lactate-to-pyruvate ratio above 40 in the microdialyzate fluid may result [306]. Therefore, frequent measurements of the serum glucose concentration are important during neuroanesthesia as both severe hyperglycemia and hypoglycemia can have a profound impact on patient outcome after brain injury [286,305,307].

Seizure disorders

Seizure activity has been associated with marked increases in $CMRO_2$, CBF, and the potential risk for asphyxia in spontaneously breathing patients [42]. These changes may cause pronounced brain tissue lactic acidosis [308], as indicated by a sixfold increase in tissue lactate after only 5 s of seizure activity[309] and subsequent loss of CBF autoregulation [310]. Increases in cerebral energy requirements, arterial blood pressure, brain extracellular fluid (ECF) K^+ concentration, and/or ECF osmolality have been discussed as CBF-increasing factors during seizures [42]. Interestingly, an increase in cerebral venous PO_2 indicates that the accelerated utilization and production of ATP changes the balance between the initial (glycolytic) and the final (oxidative) breakdown of glucose, suggesting that hypoxia may not be the predominant cause of lactic acidosis [42].

Although seizure activity under general anesthesia is an uncommon phenomenon [311], patients with a history of seizures may require anesthesia for an elective and emergency surgery [312]. In these patients, preoperative considerations should include the history of incidence of seizures (e.g., increasing frequency), findings of previous diagnostics (e.g., magnetic resonance imaging studies ruling out space-occupying masses as a cause of seizures), and information on antiepileptic drug (AED) therapy [312]. Traditional AEDs exert antiseizure activity by (1) reducing the inward voltage-gated positive currents (Na^+, Ca^{2+}), (2) increasing inhibitory neurotransmitter activity (GABA), or (3) decreasing excitatory neurotransmitter activity (glutamate, aspartate) [312]. The older AEDs (e.g., carbamazepine, phenytoin, phenobarbital, primidone) may induce hepatic cytochrome P450 isoenzymes, leading to a reduction in the plasma concentration of some drugs (e.g., amiodarone, propranolol, verapamil, and pentobarbital) [313]. In patients with a history of well-controlled epilepsy, continuation of antiepileptic medication throughout the perioperative period has been recommended [312].

Seizure-like activity has been observed during the use of nitrous oxide (N_2O) in cats [312], administration of sevoflurane in children [314], or when high concentrations were used in conjunction with hypocapnia [315] and enflurane (humans, rats) [316,317]. Sustained EEG and motor evidence of seizure activity could also be induced by auditory stimuli in dogs anesthetized at concentrations of enflurane above 1 MAC. The seizure activity became particularly evident during hypocapnia [318].

Although seizure activity has been reported in one patient during isoflurane anesthesia [311], both isoflurane and desflurane have been recommended for anesthesia in refractory status epilepticus [319]. Similarly, the barbiturates (thiopental, methohexital, pentobarbital) and propofol are well established as agents for the treatment of refractory status epilepticus [312,320–322]. Although all agents have been reported to produce excitatory activity (e.g., myoclonus, opisthotonus), this does not usually represent seizure initiation and during subsequent induction of anesthesia with these agents at higher doses they act as anticonvulsants [323,324]. As with other intravenous anesthetic agents, low doses of ketamine may facilitate seizures, but at doses adequate to produce anesthesia, ketamine shows anticonvulsant properties in some species [325]. All benzodiazepines possess potent anticonvulsant properties [326]. Opioids such as fentanyl, alfentanil, sufentanil, and morphine have been reported to initiate generalized seizures and/or myoclonus after a low to moderate dose, particularly when administered intrathecally in humans [327–330].

Status epilepticus is a common medical emergency associated with increases in cerebral metabolism, CBF, catecholamine release, cardiac output, arterial and central venous pressure, and heart rate [331]. These changes need to be controlled rapidly in order to avoid loss of CBF autoregulation, cerebral hypoxia, cerebral edema, and intracranial hypertension [331].

Anesthesia with midazolam, propofol, or thiopental has been recommended for treatment of status epilepticus whereas opioids are usually avoided [312]. A study of humans subjected to cortical resection for the treatment of intractable epilepsy revealed that propofol (2 mg/kg IV) significantly decreased the median frequency of interictal spikes [332]. The authors concluded that the use of propofol in patients with epilepsy seems to be safe.

Acute spinal cord injury

The mechanisms and emergency care procedures for treatment of acute spinal cord injury in dogs and cats has been reviewed recently [333]. Spinal cord injuries are common in small animal species, are frequently associated with poor outcomes, and may result in euthanasia. The initial spinal cord trauma may be caused by acute intervertebral disk herniation, vertebral injuries, penetrating injuries, or by non-traumatic injuries such as fibrocartilage embolism. The initial trauma is often followed by a secondary injury to the spinal cord resulting from molecular and biochemical changes associated with the initial trauma (e.g., loss of spinal blood flow autoregulation, excessive release of aspartate and glutamate, intracellular Ca^{2+} accumulation, inflammation). The diagnosis of acute spinal cord injury is based on patient history and physical and neurologic examination [333]. Further diagnostic measures may include survey radiography and advanced imaging modalities such as myelography, computed tomography (CT), and magnetic resonance imaging (MRI) [333–335].

The initial emergency treatment of spinal cord injuries should focus on stabilization of the patient's cardiovascular and respiratory function in an effort to reduce spinal ischemia and hypoxia with subsequent progression of spinal cord injury [333]. While rapid expansion of the intravascular volume may be achieved by infusion of hypertonic crystalloid or synthetic colloid solutions, more specific treatment modalities, including the use of methylprednisolone, polyethylene glycol, antioxidant therapy, calcium-channel antagonists, 21-aminosteroids, opiate receptor antagonists, hyperbaric oxygen therapy, and/or therapeutic hypothermia, remain controversial in veterinary medicine. These various therapeutic measures have failed to achieve significant outcome improvement reliably or need additional research [333].

Spinal surgery techniques have inherent risks such as bleeding, infection, and the development of new neurological deficits, for example, respiratory muscle paralysis, blindness, and positioning-related injuries [286]. Surgery on the cervical spine by a ventral approach can be associated with recurrent laryngeal nerve injury caused by either direct pressure on the nerve during surgical retraction and/or compression of submucosal branches of the nerve by the endotracheal tube.

Myelomalacia

Myelomalacia is an ischemic or hemorrhagic necrosis of the spinal cord that can occur as a sequel to acute spinal cord injury [336,337]. Myelomalacia has been reported in dogs, cattle, goats, and horses [336,338,339]. In one case, a Quarter Horse underwent halothane anesthesia for castration and removal of a retained testicle [339]. After recovery from anesthesia, the horse was unable to rise. The next day, both hind legs knuckled when walking assisted. Patellar and flexor reflexes were reduced bilaterally and neither anal reflex nor tail tone was present. The horse died 8 days after surgery and necropsy revealed widespread bilaterally symmetrical necrosis of the gray matter most prominent in the ventral horns [338].

Neuronal anoxia/hypoxia seems to be the major cause of myelomalacia [340]. Therefore, manifold conditions, including embolization, thrombi, space-occupying lesions (e.g., protruded disk material, tumor, abscess), pronounced vasoconstriction following excessive hyperventilation, decreased spinal perfusion pressure and/or spinal venous congestion, may all result in histopathologic changes described for myelomalacia [336,338,339].

Myasthenia gravis

Myasthenia gravis (MG) is a neuromuscular disease caused by a deficiency of functional postsynaptic nAChRs at the neuromuscular junction [341–343]. MG may occur as both congenital and acquired disease in dogs and cats [341]. While the acquired form of MG is an autoimmune disease characterized by autoantibodies directed against nAChRs [9,341,342] and frequently associated with thymus disease (e.g., thymoma) [343,344], nAChR deficiency in congenital MG is not associated with an autoimmune response [341]. The decreased number of nAChRs causes a decreased capacity of the neuromuscular end plate to transmit the nerve signal adequately, leading to neuromuscular muscle weakness and fatigue [342,344,345]. Other clinical signs in dogs and cats may include bilateral facial weakness with decreased palpebral reflexes, marked skeletal muscle weakness at the pelvic limbs, inability to retract the claws, cervical ventroflexion, and megaesophagus [342,344]. Acute fulminating MG in dogs is often characterized by frequent regurgitation and aspiration of gastrointestinal tract contents and subsequent aspiration pneumonia. Rapid loss of muscle strength resulting in recumbency also commonly occurs [346]. Results of EMG and nerve conduction velocity tests in these dogs may not reveal abnormalities.

Patients with megaesophagus secondary to MG often require general anesthesia for other reasons (e.g., dental or orthopedic disease). These patients should be considered to be at higher anesthetic risk and require special attention to reduce aspiration. Rapid tracheal intubation, frequent esophageal suctioning, and use of antiemetics and prokinetic agents (e.g., maropitant, ondansetron, metoclopramide) have been recommended in addition to avoiding unnecessary perioperative medications associated with nausea and vomiting.

Because of the smaller number of normal nAChRs, MG patients often have an abnormal response to NMBAs. They are relatively resistant to succinylcholine (i.e., insufficient depolarization) and very susceptible to non-depolarizing neuromuscular blocking agents [343]. A reduction in the initial dose of atracurium and vecuronium in dogs to approximately one-sixth to one-fifth of the standard dose has been recommended [347,348].

When planning anesthesia in myasthenic patients, sedatives and/or opioid analgesics should be used with caution as the drugs may further deteriorate respiratory function, and some may increase the risk of perioperative nausea and vomiting [343]. On the other hand, emotional stress, pain, or surgery may induce a myasthenic crisis manifested as an exacerbation of clinical signs [349]. Therefore, cautious sedation combined with adequate analgesia (e.g., nonsteroidal anti-inflammatory drugs, regional anesthesia, or peripheral nerve blocks) and proactive monitoring and supportive care are indicated [343,344].

The maintenance of the daily dose of anticholinesterase medication (e.g., pyridostigmine) perioperatively in MG patients has been questioned, particularly since the drug may interfere with the metabolism of substrates of cholinesterase enzymes (e.g., mivacurium) [350]. Moreover, the more severe the disease and the higher the dose of pyridostigmine in humans, the more sensitive are patients towards non-depolarizing NMBAs such as vecuronium [351]. However, if neuromuscular blockade is not anticipated, the use of cholinesterase inhibitors should be considered.

Skeletal muscle weakness should encourage (or mandate) positive-pressure ventilation with or without administration of NMBAs [345]. Easy endotracheal intubation in myasthenic patients is usually possible without NMBA administration [352], and any use of NMBAs should include thorough neuromuscular monitoring [i.e., train-of-four (TOF) monitoring] in order to ensure full recovery (TOF >90%) at the end of anesthesia [343]. Sugammadex, a selective NMBA-binding agent specifically designed for inactivation of rocuronium by encapsulation of the agonist, was found to result in a faster reversal of the muscle paralysis with no postoperative complications [353].

Advanced imaging modalities (myelography, magnetic resonance imaging)

The potential complications and diagnostic value need to be considered when discussing neurologic imaging modalities. Postmyelographic complications such as bradycardia, asystole, seizures, hyperthermia, exacerbation of pre-existing signs of CNS dysfunction, hyperesthesia, vomiting, and aseptic meningitis (rare) have been reported. In addition, transient apnea during injection of the contrast medium into the cervical subarachnoid space and also prolonged anesthetic recovery and strenuous limb movements may occur [334,335]. These complications, in addition to the relatively poor ability to image soft-tissue changes, has resulted in decreased use of myelography in veterinary medicine.

Hyperosmolality and direct chemotoxicity of the contrast media have been identified as sources of neurotoxicity with the older media (e.g., iodinated oils, water-soluble iodinated ionic drugs) and has led to their limited use in myelography [335]. Second-generation non-ionic media including iohexol and iopamidol were developed to be less neurotoxic and became the drugs of choice in veterinary myelography. In addition to the use of less neurotoxic contrast media, postmyelographic complications can be minimized by careful subarachnoid puncture, good aseptic technique, slow injection of the contrast medium, adequate hydration of the patient, and postmyelographic contrast medium removal [335].

Because of the risk of postmyelographic seizures, drugs that by themselves may potentially increase seizure activity, including ketamine [354,355], N_2O [312], enflurane [316,317], and sevoflurane in conjunction with significant hypocapnia [315], should by avoided or used with caution and replaced by benzodiazepines [326], barbiturates [320,321], propofol [322], and isoflurane [319].

When comparing magnetic resonance imaging (MRI) with myelography in dogs with suspected cervical spondylomyelopathy (wobbler syndrome), three reviewers (100%) who independently evaluated the images agreed with the location of the most extensive lesion on MR images, while agreement using myelography was only 83% [356]. In addition, MRI provided information on lesion location because it allowed the direct examination of the spinal cord diameter and parenchyma. Myelography markedly underestimated the severity of the spinal cord compression in two dogs and failed to identify the cause of signs in another dog. The authors concluded that myelography can identify the location of the lesion in most patients, but MRI appears to be more accurate in predicting the site, severity, and nature of the spinal cord compression.

Diagnostic advantages of MRI over myelography have also been reported for the diagnosis of ischemia and spinal cord infarction [357]. Although MRI could not be used for a definite diagnosis of spinal cord infarction, the technique was effective in excluding extramedullary spinal lesions and supporting intramedullary infarction as a cause of acute neurologic signs. The indicated asymmetric lesions within the gray matter of the spinal cord correlated with the clinical neurolocalization and lateralization in each dog. Moreover, compressive myelopathy caused by acute hydrated nucleus pulposus extrusion (HNPE) will show characteristic MRI features with nuclear material of hydrated signal intensity immediately above the affected disc space [358].

When MRI was compared with radiography for the detection of vertebral fracture or subluxation in dogs with suspected vertebral instability, the data revealed identification of the disruption of supportive soft tissue structures, spinal cord compression, swelling, and intramedullary hemorrhage with MRI. These results led to the conclusion to establish MRI as the preferred preoperative diagnostic test for assessing spinal stability in dogs with spinal trauma and neurologic deficits [359]. For MRI studies in dogs, premedication with diazepam (0.23–0.32 mg/kg) or immediate induction with propofol to effect (up to 8 mg/kg IV) followed by maintenance of anesthesia with isoflurane has been suggested [357].

References

1 Seiferle E. Nervensystem, Sinnesorgane, endokrine Drüsen. In: Nickel R, Schummer R, Seiferle E, eds. *Lehrbuch der Anatomie der Haustiere*, Vol. **IV**. Berlin: Verlag Paul Parey, 1975; 3–188.

2 Waldvogel HH. *Analgetika, Antinozizeptiva, Adjuvanzien*. Berlin: Springer, 1996.

3 Dorland NW. *Dorland's Pocket Medical Dictionary*, 23rd edn. Philadelphia: WB Saunders, 1982; **663**.

4 Antognini JF, Berg K. Cardiovascular responses to noxious stimuli during isoflurane anesthesia are minimally affected by anesthetic action in the brain. *Anesth Analg* 1995; **81**: 843–848.

5 De Beer NAM, van Hooff JC, Cluitmans PJM *et al*. Haemodynamic response to incision and sternotomy in relation to auditory evoked potential and spontaneous EEG. *Br J Anaesth* 1996; **76**: 685–693.

6 Brown EN, Lydic R, Schiff ND. General anesthesia, sleep, and coma. *N Engl J Med* 2010; **363**: 2638–2650.

7 Zecharia AY, Franks NP. General anesthesia and ascending arousal pathways. Editorial views. *Anesthesiology* 2009; **111**: 695–696.

8 Franks NP, Zecharia AY. Sleep and general anesthesia. *Can J Anesth* 2011; **58**: 139–148.

9 Guyton AC. *Textbook of Medical Physiology*, 8th edn. Philadelphia: WB Saunders, 1991.

10 Wilson-Pauwels L, Stewart PA, Akesson EJ. *Autonomic Nerves*. Hamilton, ON: BC Decker, 1997.

11 Klide AM, Soma LR. Epidural analgesia in the dog and cat. *J Am Vet Med Assoc* 1968; **153**: 165–173.

12 Messick JM Jr, Newberg LA, Nugent M, *et al*. Principles of neuroanesthesia for the nonneurosurgical patient with CNS pathophysiology. *Anesth Analg* 1985; **64**: 143–174.

13 Artru AA, Nugent M, Michenfelder JD. Anesthetics affect the cerebral metabolic response to circulatory catecholamines. *J Neurochem* 1981; **36**: 1941–1946.

14 Sakka L, Coll G, Chazal J. Anatomy and physiology of cerebrospinal fluid. *Eur Ann Otorhinolaryngol Head Neck Dis* 2011; **128**: 309–316.

15 Thomas WB. Hydrocephalus in dogs and cats. *Vet Clin North Am Small Anim Pract* 2010; **40**: 143–159.

16 Fogarty-Mack P, Young WL. Neurophysiology. In: Hemmings H Jr, Hopkins P, eds. *Foundations of Anesthesia. Basic and Clinical Sciences*. London: Mosby, 2000; 201–212.

17 Oppelt WW, Patlak CS, Rall DP. Effect of certain drugs on cerebrospinal fluid production in the dog. *Am J Physiol* 1964; **206**: 247–250.

18 Artru AA, Nugent M, Michenfelder JD. Enflurane causes a prolonged and reversible increase in the rate of CSF production in the dog. *Anesthesiology* 1982; **57**: 255–260.

19 Artru AA. Relationship between cerebral blood volume and CSF pressure during anesthesia with halothane or enflurane in dogs. *Anesthesiology* 1983; **58**: 533–539.

20 Artru AA. Isoflurane does not increase the rate of CSF production in the dog. *Anesthesiology* 1984; **60**: 193–197.

21 Weiner N, Taylor P. Neurohumoral transmission: the autonomic and somatic motor nervous system. In: Goodman Gilman A, Goodman LS, Rall TW, Murad F, eds. *Goodman and Gilman's The Pharmacological Basis of Therapeutics*, 7th edn, New York: Macmillan, 1985; 66–99.

22 Palm D, Hellenbrecht D, Quiring K. Pharmakologie des noradrenergen Systems. Katecholamine, Adrenozeptor-Agonisten, Antisympathotonika und andere Antihypertensiva. Pharmakotherapie von Hypertonie, Hypotonie, obstruktiven Atemwegserkrankungen und vaskulären Kopfschmerzen. In: Forth W, Henschler D, Rummel W, eds. *Allgemeine und spezielle Pharmokologie und Toxikologie*, 5th edn. Mannheim: Wissenschaftsverlag, 1987; 124–168.

23 International Union of Basic and Clinical Pharmacology. IUPHAR/BPS Guide to Pharmacology. www.guidetopharmacology.org , accessed 23 September 2014.

24 Minami K, Uezono Y. The recent progress in research on effects of anesthetics and analgesics on G protein-coupled receptors. *J Anesth* 2013; **27**: 284–292.

25 Caulfield MP. Muscarinic receptors – characterization, coupling and function. *Pharmacol Ther* 1993; **58**: 319–379.

26 Wess J. Molecular biology of muscarinic acetylcholine receptors. *Crit Rev Neurobiol* 1996; **10**: 69–99.

27 Dani JA. Overview of nicotinic receptors and their roles in the central nervous system. *Biol Psychiatry* 2001; **49**: 166–174.

28 Prior CB, Marshall IG. Neuromuscular junction physiology. In: Hemmings H Jr, Hopkins P, eds. *Foundations of Anesthesia. Basic and Clinical Sciences*, 2nd edn. London: Mosby Elsevier, 2006; 435–443.

29 Hopkins PM. Voluntary motor systems – skeletal muscle, reflexes, and control of movement. In: Hemmings H Jr & Hopkins P (eds.) *Foundations of Anesthesia. Basic and Clinical Sciences*, 2nd edn. Elsevier Mosby: London, 2006: 421–433.

30 Astrup J, Symon L, Branston NM, et al. Cortical evoked potential and extracellular K^+ and H^+ at critical levels of brain ischema. *Stroke* 1977; **8**: 51–57.

31 Lassen NA. Cerebral blood flow and oxygen consumption in man. *Physiol Rev* 1959; **39**: 183–238.

32 Siesjö BK. Brain metabolism and anaesthesia. *Acta Anaesthesiol Scand* 1978; **70**(Suppl): 56–59.

33 Kety SS, Schmidt CF. The determination of cerebral blood flow in man by the use of nitrous oxide in low concentrations. *Am J Physiol* 1945; **143**: 53–66.

34 Scheinberg P, Stead EA Jr. The cerebral blood flow in male subjects as measured by the nitrous oxide technique. Normal values for blood flow, oxygen utilization, glucose utilization, and peripheral resistance, with observations on the effect of tilting and anxiety. *J Clin Invest* 1949; **28**: 1163–1171.

35 Sokoloff L, Perlin S, Kornetsky C, et al. The effects of D-lysergic acid diethylamide on cerebral circulation and over-all metabolism. *Ann NY Acad Sci* 1957; **66**: 468–477.

36 Lassen NA, Feinberg I, Lane MH. Bilateral studies of the cerebral oxygen uptake in young and aged normal subjects and in patients with organic dementia. *J Clin Invest* 1969; **39**: 491–500.

37 Cohen PJ, Alexander SC, Smith TC, et al. Effects of hypoxia and normocarbia on cerebral blood flow and metabolism in conscious man. *J Appl Physiol* 1967; **23**: 183–189.

38 Michenfelder JD. *Anesthesia and the Brain*. New York: Churchill Livingstone, 1988.

39 Michenfelder JD. The interdependency of cerebral functional and metabolic effects following massive doses of thiopental in the dog. *Anesthesiology* 1974; **41**: 231–236.

40 Newberg LA, Milde JH, Michenfelder JD. The cerebral metabolic effects of isoflurane at and above concentrations that suppress cortical electrical activity. *Anesthesiology* 1983; **59**: 23–28.

41 Steen PA, Newberg L, Milde JH, et al. Hypothermia and barbiturates: individual and combined effects on canine cerebral oxygen consumption. *Anesthesiology* 1983; **58**: 527–532.

42 Lassen NA, Christensen MS. Physiology of cerebral blood flow. *Br J Anaesth* 1976; **48**: 719–734.

43 Stullken EH Jr, Milde JH, Michenfelder JD, et al. The nonlinear responses of cerebral metabolism to low concentrations of halothane, enflurane, isoflurane, and thiopental. *Anesthesiology* 1977; **46**: 28–34.

44 Newman B, Gelb AW, Lam AM. The effect of isoflurane induced hypotension on cerebral blood flow and cerebral metabolic rate for oxygen in humans. *Anesthesiology* 1986; **64**(3): 307–310.

45 Cotev S, Shalit MN. Effects of diazepam on cerebral blood flow and oxygen uptake after head injury. *Anesthesiology* 1975; **43**: 117–122.

46 Nugent M, Artru AA, Michenfelder JD. Cerebral metabolic, vascular and protective effects of midazolam maleate. *Anesthesiology* 1982; **56**: 172–176.

47 Maekawa T, Sakabe T, Takeshita H. Diazepam blocks cerebral metabolic and circulatory responses to local anesthetic-induced seizures. *Anesthesiology* 1974; **41**: 389–391.

48 Kennedy C, Des Rossiers MH, Sakurada O, et al. Metabolic mapping of the primary visual system of the monkey by means of the autoradiographic [^{14}C]deoxyglucose technique. *Proc Natl Acad Sci U S A* 1976; **73**: 4230–4234.

49 Sokoloff L. Relation between physiological function and energy metabolism in the central nervous system. *J Neurochem* 1977; **29**: 13–26.

50 Smith AL, Wollman H. Cerebral blood flow and metabolism: effects of anesthetic drugs and techniques. *Anesthesiology* 1972; **36**: 378–400.

51 Shapiro HM. Anesthesia effects upon cerebral blood flow, cerebral metabolism, electroencephalogram, and evoked potentials. In: Miller RD, ed. *Anesthesia*, Vol. **2**. New York: Churchill Livingstone, 1986; 1249–1288.

52 Miletich DJ, Ivankovich AD, Albrecht RF, et al. Absence of autoregulation of cerebral blood flow during halothane and enflurane anesthesia. *Anesth Analg* 1976; **55**: 100–109.

53 Cohen PJ, Wollman H, Alexander SC, et al. Cerebral carbohydrate metabolism in man during halothane anesthesia: effects of $PaCO_2$ on some aspects of carbohydrate utilization. *Anesthesiology* 1964; **25**: 185–191.

54 Siesjö BK. Cerebral metabolic rate in hypercarbia – a controversy. *Anesthesiology* 1980; **52**: 461–465.

55 Sundt TN Jr, Siekert RG, Piepgras DG, et al. Bypass surgery for vascular disease of the carotid system. *Mayo Clin Proc* 1976; **51**: 677–692.

56 Rosendorff C, Mitchell G, Scriven DRL, et al. Evidence for dual innervation affecting local blood flow in the hypothalamus of the conscious rabbit. *Circ Res* 1976; **38**: 140–145.

57 Reiman C, Lluch S, Glick G. Develpoment and evaluation of an experimental model for the study of the cerebral circulation in the unanesthetized goat. *Stroke* 1972; **3**: 322–328.

58 Miletich DJ, Ivankovic AD, Albrecht RF, et al. Cerebral hemodynamics following internal maxillary artery ligation in the goat. *J Appl Physiol* 1975; **38**: 942–945.

59 Stiles J, Weil AB, Packer RA, et al. Post-anesthetic cortical blindness in cats: twenty cases. *Vet J* 2012; **193**: 367–373.

60 Barton-Lamb AL, Martin-Flores M, Scrivani PV, et al. Evaluation of maxillary arterial blood flow in anesthetized cats with the mouth closed and open. *Vet J* 2013; **196**: 325–331.

61 Jordan JD, Powers WJ. Cerebral autoregulation and acute ischemic stroke. *Am J Hypertens* 2012; **25**: 946–950.

62 Strandgaard S, Olesen J, Skinhøj E, Lassen NA. Autoregulation and brain circulation in severe arterial hypertension. *Br Med J* 1973; **i**: 507–510.

63 Paulson OB, Strandgaard S, Edvinsson L. Cerebral autoregulation. *Cerebrovasc Brain Metab Rev* 1990; **2**: 161–192.

64 Rapela CE, Green HD, Denison AB. Baroreceptor reflexes and autoregulation of cerebral blood flow in the dog. *Circ Res* 1967; **21**: 559–566.

65 Eklöf B, Ingvar DH, Kågström E, et al. Persistence of cerebral blood flow autoregulation following chronic bilateral cervical sympathectomy in the monkey. *Acta Physiol Scand* 1971; **82**: 172–176.

66 Edvinsson L, Nielsen KC, Owman C. Cholinergic innervation of choroid plexus in rabbits and cats. *Brain Res* 1973; **63**: 500–503.

67 Wahl M, Kuschinsky W, Bosse O, et al. Effect of *l*-norepinephrine on the diameter of pial arterioles and arteries in the cat. *Circ Res* 1972; **31**: 248–256.

68 Strandgaard S. Autoregulation of cerebral blood flow in hypertensive patients: the modifying influence of prolonged antihypertensive treatment on the tolerance to acute drug-induced hypotension. *Circulation* 1976; **53**: 720–727.

69 Astrup J, Siesjö BK, Symon L. Threshold in cerebral ischemia – the ischemic penumbra. *Stroke* 1981; **12**: 723–725.

70 Sharbrough FW, Messick JM Jr, Sundt TM Jr. Correlation of continuous electroencephalograms with cerebral blood flow measurements during carotid endarterectomy. *Stroke* 1973; **4**: 674–683.

71 Sundt TM Jr, Sharbrough FW, Piepgras DG, et al. Correlation of cerebral blood flow and electroencephalographic changes during carotid endarterectomy: with results of surgery and hemodynamics of cerebral ischemia. *Mayo Clin Proc* 1981; **56**: 533–543.

72 Lassen NA. Brain extracellular pH: The main factor controlling cerebral blood flow. *Scand J Clin Lab Invest* 1968; **22**: 247–251.

73 Harp JR, Wolman H. Cerebral metabolic effects of hyperventilation and deliberate hypotension. *Br J Anaesth* 1973; **45**: 256–262.

74 Alexander SC, Cohen PJ, Wollman H, et al. Cerebral carbohydrate metabolism during hypocarbia in man: studies during nitrous oxide anesthesia. *Anesthesiology* 1965; **26**: 624–632.

75 Kogure K, Scheinberg P, Reinmuth OM, et al. Mechanisms of cerebral vasodilatation in hypoxia. *J Appl Physiol* 1970; **29**: 223–229.

76 Siesjö BK, Nilsson L. The influence of arterial hypoxemia upon labile phosphates and upon extracellular and intracellular lactate and pyruvate concentrations in the rat brain. *Scan J Clin Lab Invest* 1971; **27**: 83–96.

77 Olesen J. Cerebral blood flow. Methods for measurement, regulation, effects of drugs and changes in disease. *Acta Neurol Scand Suppl* 1974; **57**: 1–134.

78 Lundgren O, Jodal M. Regional blood flow. *Annu Rev Physiol* 1975; **37**: 395–414.

79 Hallenbeck JM, Furlow TW Jr. Prostaglandin I_2 and indomethacin prevent impairment of postischemic brain reperfusion in the dog. *Stroke* 1979; **10**: 629–637.

80 Wolfe LS, Coceani F. The role of prostaglandin in the central nervous system. *Annu Rev Physiol* 1979; **41**: 669–684.

81 Olesen J. Total CO_2, lactate, and pyruvate in brain biopsies taken after freezing the tissue in situ. *Acta Neurol Scand* 1970; **46**: 141–148.

82 Lassen NA. The luxury-perfusion syndrome and its possible relation to acute metabolic acidosis localized within the brain. *Lancet* 1966; **ii**: 1113–1115.

83 Pálvölgyi R. Regional cerebral blood flow in patients with intracranial tumors. *J Neurosurg* 1969; **31**: 149–163.

84 Marcus ML, Heistad DD, Erhardt JC, et al. Regulation of total and regional spinal cord blood flow. *Circ Res* 1977; **41**: 128–134.

85 Griffiths IR. Spinal cord blood flow in dogs: the effect of blood pressure. *J Neurol Neurosurg Psychiatry* 1973; **36**: 914–920.

86 Griffiths IR. Spinal cord blood flow in dogs. 2. The effect of the blood gases. *J Neurol Neurosurg Psychiatry* 1973; **36**: 42–49.

87 Crawford ES, Walker HS III, Saleh SA, et al. Graft replacement of aneurysm in descending thoracic aorta: results without bypass or shunting. *Surgery* 1981; **89**: 73–85.

88 Grundy BL, Nelson PB, Doyle E, et al. Intraopertative loss of somatosensory-evoked potentials predicts loss of spinal cord function. *Anesthesiology* 1982; **57**: 321–322.

89 Grundy BL, Nash CL Jr, Brown RH. Arterial pressure manipulation alters spinal cord function during correction of scoliosis. *Anesthesiology* 1981; **54**: 249–253.

90 Campagna JA, Miller KW, Forman SA. Mechanism of actions of inhaled anesthetics. *N Engl J Med* 2003; **348**: 2110–2140.

91 Alkire MT, Hudetz AG, Tononi G. Consciousness and anesthesia. *Science* 2008; **322**: 876–880.

92 Brown EN, Purdon PL, Van Dort CJ. General anesthesia and altered states of arousal: a systems neuroscience analysis. *Annu Rev Neurosci* 2011; **34**: 601–628.

93 Grasshoff C, Rudolph U, Antkowiak B. Molecular and systemic mechanisms of general anaesthesia: the 'multi-site and multiple mechanisms' concept. *Curr Opin Anaesthesiol* 2005; **18**: 386–391.

94 ASA – American Society of Anesthesiologists Task Force on Intraoperative Awareness. Practice advisory for intraoperative awareness and brain function monitoring. *Anesthesiology* 2006; **104**: 847–864.

95 Dutton RC, Maurer AJ, Sonner JM, et al. Isoflurane causes anterograde but not retrograde amnesia for Pavlovian fear conditioning. *Anesthesiology* 2002; **96**: 1223–1229.

96 Mashour GA, Forman SA, Campagna JA. Mechanisms of general anesthesia: from molecules to mind. *Best Pract Res Clin Anaesthesiol* 2005; **19**: 349–364.

97 Forman SA, Chin VA. General anesthetics and molecular mechanisms of unconsciousness. *Int Anesthesiol Clin* 2008; **46**: 43–53.

98 Bonhomme V, Hans P. Monitoring depth of anaesthesia: is it worth the effort? *Eur J Anaesth* 2004; **21**: 423–428.

99 Dunnet JM, Prys-Roberts, Holland DE, et al. Propofol infusion and the suppression of consciousness: dose requirements to induce loss of consciousness and to suppress response to noxious and non-noxious stimuli. *Br J Anaesth* 1994; **72**: 29–34.

100 Forrest FC, Tooley MA, Saunders PR, et al. Propofol infusions and the suppression of consciousness: the EEG and dose requirements. *Br J Anaesth* 1994; **72**: 35–41.

101 Gugino LD, Aglio LS, Yli-Hankala A. Monitoring the electroencephalogram during bypass procedures. *Semin Cardiothorac Vasc Anesth* 2004; **8**: 61–83.

102 Glass PS, Bloom M, Kearse L, et al. Bispectral analysis measures sedation and memory effects of propofol, midazolam, isoflurane, and alfentanil in healthy volunteers. *Anesthesiology* 1997; **86**: 836–847.

103 Kearse LA Jr, Rosow C, Zaslavsky A, et al. Bispectral analysis of the electroencephalogram predicts conscious processing of information during propofol sedation and hypnosis. *Anesthesiology* 1998; **88**: 25–34.

104 Kodaka M, Johansen JW, Sebel PS. The influence of gender on loss of consciousness with sevoflurane or propofol. *Anesth Analg* 2005; **101**: 377–381.

105 Franks NP. General anaesthesia: from molecular targets to neuronal pathways of sleep and arousal. *Nat Rev Neurosci* 2008; **9**: 370–386.

106 Eger EI II, Saidman LJ, Brandstater B. Minimum alveolar anesthetic concentration: a standard of anesthetic potency. *Anesthesiology* 1965; **26**: 756–763.

107 Eger EI II, Koblin DD, Harris RA, et al. Hypothesis: inhaled anesthetics produce immobility and amnesia by different mechanisms at different sites. *Anesth Analg* 1997; **84**: 915–918.

108 Antognini JF, Carstens E. Measuring minimum alveolar concentration. More than meets the tail. *Anesthesiology* 2005; **103**: 679–680.

109 De Jong RH, Nace RA. Nerve impulse conduction during intravenous lidocaine injection. *Anesthesiology* 1968; **29**: 22–28.
110 Mashour GA, Orser BA, Avidan MS. Intraoperative awareness. From neurobiology to clinical practice. *Anesthesiology* 2011; **114**: 1218–1233.
111 Eger EI II. Age, minimum alveolar anesthetic concentration, and minimum alveolar anesthetic concentration-awake. *Anesth Analg* 2001; **93**: 947–953.
112 Krasowski MD, Harrison NL. General anaesthetic action on ligand-gated ion channels. *Cell Mol Life Sci* 1999; **55**: 1278–1303.
113 Angel A. Central neuronal pathways and the process of anaesthesia. *Br J Anaesth* 1993; **71**: 148–163.
114 Eger EI II, Stevens WC, Cromwell TH. The electroencephalogram in man anesthetized with forane. *Anesthesiology* 1971; **35**: 504–508.
115 Angel A. The G. L. Brown lecture. Adventures in anaesthesia. *Exp Physiol* 1991; **76**: 1–38.
116 Alkire MT, Haier RJ, Barker SJ, et al. Cerebral metabolism during propofol anesthesia in humans studied with positron emission tomography. *Anesthesiology* 1995; **82**: 393–403.
117 Fiset P, Paus T, Daloze T, et al. Brain mechanisms of propofol-induced loss of consciousness in humans: a positron emission tomography study. *J Neurosci* 1999; **19**: 5506–5513.
118 Purdon PL, Pierce ET, Bonmassar G, et al. Simultaneous electroencephalography and functional magnetic resonance imaging of general anesthesia. *Ann N Y Acad Sci* 2009; **1157**: 61–70.
119 Velly LJ, Rey MF, Bruder NJ, et al. Differential dynamic of action on cortical and subcortical structures of anesthetic agents during induction of anesthesia. *Anesthesiology* 2007; **107**: 202–212.
120 Ferrarelli F, Massimini M, Sarasso S, et al. Breakdown in cortical effective connectivity during midazolam-induced loss of consciousness. *Proc Natl Acad Sci U S A* 2010; **107**: 2681–2686.
121 Moruzzi G, Magoun HW. Brain stem reticular formation and activation of the EEG. *Electroencephalogr Clin Neurophysiol* 1949; **1**: 455–473.
122 Prince DA, Shanzer S. Effects of anesthetic upon the EEG response to reticular stimulation. Patterns of slow synchrony. *Electroencephalogr Clin Neurophysiol* 1966; **21**: 578–588.
123 Golovchinsky VB, Plehotkina SI. Difference in the sensitivity of the cerebral cortex and midbrain reticular formation to the action of diethyl ether and thialbarbital. *Brain Res* 1971; **30**: 37–47.
124 Kinomura S, Larsson J, Gulyás B, et al. Activation by attention of the human reticular formation and thalamic intralaminar nuclei. *Science* 1996; **271**: 512–515.
125 Steriade M. Arousal: revisiting the recticular activating system. *Science* 1996; **272**: 225–226.
126 Michenfelder JD, Theye RA. In vivo toxic effects of halothane on canine cerebral metabolic pathways. *Am J Physiol* 1975; **229**: 1050–1055.
127 Antognini JF, Carstens E. Isoflurane blunts electroencephalographic and thalamic-recticular formation responses to noxious stimulation in goats. *Anesthesiology* 1999; **91**: 1770–1779.
128 MacIver MB, Mandema JW, Stanski DR, et al. Thiopental uncouples hippocampeal and cortical synchronized electroencephalographic activity. *Anesthesiology* 1996; **84**: 1411–1424.
129 Simon W, Hapfelmeier G, Kochs E, et al. Isoflurane blocks synaptic plasticity in the mouse hippocampus. *Anesthesiology* 2001; **94**: 1058–1065.
130 Alkire MT, Haier RJ, Fallon JH. Toward a unified theory of narcosis: brain imaging evidence for a thalamocortical switch as the neurophysiologic basis of anesthetic-induced unconsciousness. *Conscious Cogn* 2000; **9**: 370–386.
131 Alkire MT, Haier RJ, Shah NK, et al. Positron emission tomography study of regional cerebral metabolism in humans during isoflurane anesthesia. *Anesthesiology* 1997; **86**: 549–557.
132 Alkire MT, Pomfrett CJD, Haier RJ, et al. Functional brain imaging during anesthesia in humans. Effects of halothane on global and regional cerebral glucose metabolism. *Anesthesiology* 1999; **90**: 701–709.
133 Antognini JF, Schwartz K. Exaggerated anesthetic requirements in the preferentially anesthetized brain. *Anesthesiology* 1993; **79**: 1244–1249.
134 Rampil IJ. Anesthetic potency is not altered after hypothermic spinal cord transection in rats. *Anesthesiology* 1994; **80**: 606–610.
135 Rampil IJ, Mason P, Singh H. Anesthetic potency (MAC) is independent of forebrain structures in the rat. *Anesthesiology* 1993; **78**: 707–712.
136 King BS, Rampil IJ. Anesthetic depression of spinal motor neurons may contribute to lack of movement in response to noxious stimuli. *Anesthesiology* 1994; **81**: 1484–1492.
137 Rampil IJ, King BS. Volatile anesthetics depress spinal motor neurons. *Anesthesiology* 1996; **85**: 129–134.
138 Antognini JF, Wang XW, Carstens E. Quantitative and qualitative effects of isoflurane on movement occurring after noxious stimulation. *Anesthesiology* 1999; **91**: 1064–1071.
139 Jinks SL, Carstens E, Antognini JF. Isoflurane differentially modulates on and off neurons while suppressing hind-limb motor withdrawals. *Anesthesiology* 2004; **100**: 1224–1234.
140 Vanegas H, Barbaro NM, Fields HL. Tail-flick related activity in medullospinal neurons. *Brain Res* 1984; **321**: 135–141.
141 Fields HL, Malick A, Burstein R. Dorsal horn projection targets of ON and OFF cells in the rostral ventromedial medulla. *J Neurophysiol* 1995; **74**: 1742–1759.
142 Kendig JJ. Spinal cord as a site of anesthetic action. *Anesthesiology* 1993; **79**: 1161–1162.
143 Eappen S, Kissin I. Effect of subarachnoid bupivacaine block on anesthetic requirements for thiopental in rats. *Anesthesiology* 1998; **88**: 1036–1042.
144 Schwartz AE, Navedo AT, Berman MF. Pancuronium increases the duration of electroencephalogram burst suppression in dogs anesthetized with isoflurane. *Anesthesiology* 1992; **77**: 686–690.
145 Mashour GA. Integrating the science of consciousness and anesthesia. *Anesth Analg* 2006; **103**: 975–982.
146 Meyer H. Zur Theorie der Alkoholnarkose. Erste Mitteilung. Welche Eigenschaft der Anästhesie bedingt ihre narkotische Wirkung? *Naunyn-Schmiedeberg's Arch Pharmacol* 1899; **42**(2-4): 109–118.
147 Miller KW. How do anesthetics work? *Anesthesiology* 1969; **30**: 127–128.
148 Franks NP, Lieb WR. Selectivity of general anesthetics: a new dimension. *Nat Med* 1997; **3**: 377–378.
149 Meyer KH. Contributions to the theory of narcosis. *Trans Faraday Soc* 1937; **33**: 1062–1064.
150 Mullins LJ. Some physical mechanisms of narcosis. *Chem Rev* 1954; **54**: 289–323.
151 Miller KW, Paton WDM, Smith RA, et al. The pressure reversal of general anesthesia and the critical volume hypothesis. *Mol Pharmacol* 1973; **9**: 131–143.
152 Cantor RS. The lateral pressure profile in membranes: a physical mechanism of general anesthesia. *Biochemistry* 1997; **36**: 2339–2344.
153 Angel A, Gratton DA, Halsey MJ, et al. Pressure reversal of the effect of urethane on the evoked somatosensory cortical response in the rat. *Br J Pharmacol* 1980; **70**: 241–247.
154 Franks NP, Lieb WR. Which molecular targets are most relevant to general anaesthesia? *Toxicol Lett* 1998; **100–101**: 1–8.
155 Garcia PS, Kolesky SE, Jenkins A. General anesthetic actions on $GABA_A$ receptors. *Curr Neuropharmacol* 2010; **8**: 2–9.
156 Franks NP, Lieb WR. Do general anaesthetics act by competitive binding to specific receptors? *Nature* 1984; **310**: 599–601.
157 Lambert DG. Mechanisms of action of general anaesthetic drugs. *Anaesth Intensive Care Med* 2010; **12**: 141–143.
158 Hales TG, Lambert JJ. The actions of propofol on inhibitory amino acid receptors of bovine adrenomedullary chromaffin cells and rodent central neurones. *Br J Pharmacol* 1991; **104**: 619–628.
159 Jones MV, Harrison NL. Effects of volatile anesthetics on the kinetics of inhibitory postsynaptic currents in cultured rat hippocampal neurons. *J Neurophysiol* 1993; **70**: 1339–1349.
160 Franks NP, Lieb WR. Molecular and cellular mechanisms of general anaesthesia. *Nature* 1994; **367**: 607–614.
161 Franks NP, Honoré E. The TREK K2P channels and their role in general anaesthesia and neuroprotection. *Trends Pharmacol Sci* 2004; **25**: 601–608.
162 Cull-Candy S, Brickley S, Farrant M. NMDA receptor subunits: diversity, development and disease. *Curr Opin Neurobiol* 2001; **11**: 327–335.
163 Krasowski MD, Hopfinger AJ. The discovery of new anesthetics by targeting $GABA_A$ receptors. *Expert Opin Drug Discov* 2011; **6**: 1187–1201.
164 Dildy-Mayfield JE, Eger EI II, Harris RA. Anesthetics produce subunit-selective actions on glutamate receptors. *J Pharmacol Exp Ther* 1996; **276**: 1058–1065.
165 Flood P, Role LW. Neuronal nicotinic acetylcholine receptor modulation by general anesthetics. *Toxicol Lett* 1998; **100–101**: 149–153.
166 Stevens RJN, Rüsch D, Davies PA, et al. Molecular properties important for inhaled anesthetic action on human 5-HT3A receptors. *Anesth Analg* 2005; **100**: 1696–1703.
167 MacDonald RL, Barker JL. Different actions of anticonvulsant and anesthetic barbiturates revealed by use of cultured mammalian neurons. *Science* 1978; **200**: 775–777.
168 Nicoll RA. Pentobarbital: differential postsynaptic actions on sympathetic ganglion cells. *Science* 1978; **199**: 451–452.
169 Leeb-Lundberg F, Snowman A, Olsen RW. Barbiturate receptor sites are coupled to benzodiazepine receptors. *Proc Natl Acad Sci U S A* 1980; **77**: 7468–7472.
170 Ferron J-F, Kroeger D, Chever O, et al. Cortical inhibition during burst suppression induced with isoflurane anesthesia. *J Neurosci* 2009; **29**: 9850–9860.
171 Rudolph U, Antkowiak B. Molecular and neuronal substrates of general anaesthetics. *Nat Rev Neurosci* 2004; **5**: 709–720.

172 Hemmings HC Jr, Akabas MH, Goldstein PA, et al. Emerging molecular mechanisms of general anesthetic action. *Trends Pharmacol Sci* 2005; **26**: 503–510.
173 Franks NP, Lieb WR. An anesthetic-sensitive superfamily of neurotransmitter-gated ion channels. *J Clin Anesth* 1996; **8**: 3S–7S.
174 Harris RA, Mihic SJ, Dildy-Mayfield JE, et al. Actions of anesthetics on ligand-gated ion channels: role of receptor subunit composition. *FASEB J* 1995; **9**: 1454–1462.
175 Kew JNC, Kemp JA. Ionotropic and metabotropic glutamate receptor structure and pharmacology. *Psychopharmacology* 2005; **179**: 4–29.
176 De Sousa SLM, Dickinson R, Lieb WR, et al. Contrasting synaptic actions of the inhalational general anesthetics isoflurane and xenon. *Anesthesiology* 2000; **92**: 1055–1066.
177 Flohr H, Glade U, Motzko D. The role of the NMDA synapse in general anesthesia. *Toxicol Lett* 1998; **100–101**: 23–29.
178 Yamakura T, Harris RA. Effects of gaseous anesthetics nitrous oxide and xenon on ligand-gated ion channels. Comparison with isoflurane and ethanol. *Anesthesiology* 2000; **93**: 1095–1101.
179 Hollmann MW, Liu HT, Hoenemann CW, et al. Modulation of NMDA receptor function by ketamine and magnesium. Part II. Interactions with volatile anesthetics. *Anesth Analg* 2001; **92**: 1182–1191.
180 Guedel AE. Third stage ether anesthesia: a sub-classification regarding the significance of the position and movements of the eyeball. *Pa Med Jl* 1921; **24**: 375–380.
181 Rampil IJ. Monitoring depth of anesthesia. *Curr Opin Anaesthesiol* 2001; **14**: 649–653.
182 Noachtar S, Binnie C, Ebersole J, et al. A glossary of terms most commonly used by clinical electroencephalographers and proposal for the report form for the EEG findings. *Klin Neurophysiol* 2004; **35**: 5–21 (in German).
183 Jasper HH. Report of the Committee on Methods of Clinical Examination in Electroencephalography. *Electroencephalogr Clin Neurophysiol* 1957; **10**: 370–375.
184 Tooley MA, Grant LJ, Davies AR. A micoprocessor based instrument for the spectral analysis of the EEG in anaesthesia. *Clin Phys Physiol Meas* 1984; **5**: 303–311.
185 Rampil IJ. A primer for EEG signal processing in anesthesia. *Anesthesiology* 1998; **89**: 980–1002.
186 John ER, Prichep LS. The anesthetic cascade. A theory of how anesthesia suppresses consciousness. *Anesthesiology* 2005; **102**: 447–471.
187 Kaieda R, Todd MM, Warner DS. The effects of anesthetics and $PaCO_2$ on the cerebrovascular, metabolic, and electroencephalographic responses to nitrous oxide in the rabbit. *Anesth Analg* 1989; **68**: 135–143.
188 Schwender D, Daunderer M, Mulzer S, et al. Spectral edge frequency of the electroencephalogram to monitor 'depth' of anaesthesia with isoflurane or propofol. *Br J Anaesth* 1996; **77**: 179–184.
189 Berger, H. Über das Elektroenzephalogramm des Menschen. Achte Mitteilung. *Arch Psychiat* 1934; **101**: 452–469.
190 Arduini A, Arduini MG. Effect of drugs and metabolic alterations on brainstem arousal mechanism. *J Pharmacol Exp Ther* 1954; **110**: 76–85.
191 Skinner JE, Lindsley DB. Electrophysiological and behavioral effects of blockade of the nonspecific thalamo-cortical system. *Brain Res* 1967; **6**: 95–118.
192 Hughes JR, John ER. Conventional and quantitative electroencephalography in psychiatry. *J Neuropsychiatry Clin Neurosci* 1999; **11**: 190–208.
193 John ER. A field theory of consciousness. *Conscious Cogn* 2001; **10**: 184–213.
194 John ER, Prichep LS, Knox W, et al. Invariant reversible QEEG effects of anesthetics. *Conscious Cogn* 2001; **10**: 165–183.
195 Kaada BR, Thomas F, Alnaes E, et al. EEG synchronization induced by high frequency midbrain reticular stimulation in anesthetized cats. *Electroencephalogr Clin Neurophysiol* 1967; **22**: 220–230.
196 Kiersey DK, Bickford RG, Faulconer A Jr. Electro-encephalographic patterns produced by thiopental sodium during surgical operations: description and classification. *Br J Anaesth* 1951; **23**: 141–152.
197 Clark DL, Rosner BS. Neurophysiologic effects of general anesthetics: I. The electroencephalogram and sensory evoked responses in man. *Anesthesiology* 1973; **38**: 564–582.
198 Keifer JC, Baghdoyan HA, Lydic R. Pontine cholinergic mechanisms modulate the cortical electroencephalographic spindles of halothane anesthesia. *Anesthesiology* 1996; **84**: 945–954.
199 Feshchenko VA, Veselis RA, Reinsel RA. Propofol-induced alpha rhythm. *Neuropsychobiology* 2004; **50**: 257–266.
200 Tinker JH, Sharborough FW, Michenfelder JD. Anterior shift of the dominant EEG rhythm during anesthesia in the Java monkey: correlation with anesthetic potency. *Anesthesiology* 1977; **46**: 252–259.
201 Gugino LD, Chabot RJ, Prichep LS, et al. Quantitative EEG changes associated with loss and return of consciousness in healthy adult volunteers anaesthetized with propofol or sevoflurane. *Br J Anaesth* 2001; **87**: 421–428.
202 Alkire MT, McReynolds JR, Hahn EL, et al. Thalamic microinjection of nicotine reverses sevoflurane-induced loss of righting reflex in the rat. *Anesthesiology* 2007; **107**: 264–272.
203 Antognini JF, Buonocore MH, Disbrow EA, et al. Isoflurane anesthesia blunts cerebral responses to noxious and innocuous stimuli: a fMRI study. *Life Sci* 1997; **61**: 349–354.
204 Hentschke H, Schwarz C, Antkowiak B. Neocortex is the major target of sedative concentrations of volatile anaesthetics: strong depression of firing rates and increase of $GABA_A$ receptor-mediated inhibition. *Eur J Neurosci* 2005; **21**: 93–102.
205 Fleming RA, Smith NT. An inexpensive device for analyzing and monitoring the electroencephalogram. *Anesthesiology* 1979; **50**: 456–560.
206 Myers RR, Stockard JJ, Fleming NI, et al. The use of on-line telephonic computer analysis of the E.E.G. in anaesthesia. *Br J Anaesth* 1973; **45**: 664–670.
207 Levy WL, Shapiro HM, Maruchak G, et al. Automated EEG processing for intraoperative monitoring: a comparison of techniques. *Anesthesiology* 1980; **53**: 223–236.
208 Walter DO. Introduction to computer analysis in electroencephalography. In: Niedermeyer E, Lopes da Silva F, eds. *Electroencephalography: Basic Principles, Clinical Applications, and Related Fields*, 2nd edn. Baltimore: Urban & Schwarzenberg, 1987; 863–870.
209 Kiyama S, Takeda J. Effect of extradural analgesia on the paradoxical arousal response of the electroencephalogram. *Br J Anaesth* 1997; **79**: 750–753.
210 Schwilden H, Stoeckel H. Untersuchungen über verschiedene EEG-Paramater als Indikatoren des Narkosezustands. Der Median als quantitatives Maß der Narkosetiefe. *Anästh Intensivther Notfallmed* 1980; **15**: 279–286.
211 Otto KA, Voigt S, Piepenbrock S, et al. Differences in quantitated electroencephalographic variables during surgical stimulation of horses anesthetized with isoflurane. *Vet Surg* 1996; **25**: 249–255.
212 White PF, Boyle WA. Relationship between hemodynamic and electroencephalographic changes during general anesthesia. *Anesth Analg* 1989; **68**: 177–181.
213 Otto K, Short CE. Electroencephalographic power spectrum analysis as a monitor of anaesthetic depth in horses. *Vet Surg* 1991; **20**: 362–371.
214 Schwender D, Daunderer M, Klasing S, et al. Power spectral analysis of the electroencephalogram during increasing end-expiratory concentration of isoflurane, desflurane and sevoflurane. *Anaesthesia* 1998; **53**: 335–342.
215 Hudson RJ, Stanski DR, Saidman LJ, et al. A model for studying depth of anesthesia and acute tolerance to thiopental. *Anesthesiology* 1983; **59**: 301–308.
216 Johnson CB, Young SS, Taylor PM. Analysis of the frequency spectrum of the equine electroencephalogram during halothane anaesthesia. *Res Vet Sci* 1994; **56**: 373–378.
217 Haga HA, Moerch H, Soli NE. Effects of intravenous infusion of guaifenesin on electroencephalographic variables in pigs. *Am J Vet Res* 2000; **61**: 1599–1601.
218 Dwyer RC, Rampil IJ, Eger EI II, et al. The electroencephalogram does not predict depth of isoflurane anesthesia. *Anesthesiology* 1994; **81**: 403–409.
219 Detsch O, Schneider G, Kochs E, et al. Increasing isoflurane concentration may cause paradoxical increases in EEG bispectral index in surgical patients. *Br J Anaesth* 2000; **84**: 33–37.
220 Schwilden H, Stoeckel H, Schüttler J. Closed-loop feedback control of propofol anaesthesia by quantitative EEG analysis in humans. *Br J Anaesth* 1989; **62**: 290–296.
221 Bergamasco L, Accatino A, Priano L. Quantitative electroencephalographic findings in beagles anaesthetized with propofol. *Vet J* 2003; **166**: 58–66.
222 Pichlmayr I, Lips U. Halothane-Effekte im Elektroenzephalogramm. *Anaesthesist* 1980; **29**: 530–538.
223 Johnson CB, Taylor PM. Comparison of the effects of halothane, isoflurane and methoxyflurane on the electroencephalogram of the horse. *Br J Anaesth* 1998; **81**: 748–753.
224 Antunes LM, Golledge HD, Roughan JV, et al. Comparison of electroencephalogram activity and auditory evoked responses during isoflurane and halothane anaesthesia in the rat. *Vet Anaesth Analg* 2003; **30**: 15–23.
225 Antunes LM, Roughan JV, Flecknell PA. Effects of different propofol infusion rates on EEG activity and AEP responses in rats. *J Vet Pharmacol Ther* 2003; **26**: 369–376.
226 Levy WJ. Power spectrum correlates of changes in consciousness during anesthetic induction with enflurane. *Anesthesiology* 1986; **64**: 688–693.
227 Kuramoto T, Oshita S, Takeshita H, et al. Modification of the relationship between cerebral metabolism, blood flow and electroencephalogram by stimulation during anesthesia in the dog. *Anesthesiology* 1979; **51**: 211–217.
228 Stanski DR, Vuyk J, Ausems M, et al. Can the EEG be used to monitor anesthetic depth for alfentanil with N_2O? *Anesthesiology* 1987; **67**: A401.
229 Freye E, Dehnen-Seipel H, Latasch L, et al. Slow EEG-power spectra correlate with haemodynamic changes during laryngoscopy and intubation following induction with fentanyl or sufentanil. *Acta Anaesthesiol Belg* 1999; **50**: 71–76.

230 Röpcke H, Rehberg B, Koenen-Bergmann M, et al. Surgical stimulation shifts EEG concentration–response relationship of desflurane. *Anesthesiology* 2001; **94**: 390–399.
231 Bischoff P, Kochs E, Droese D, et al. Topographisch-quantitative EEG-Analyse der paradoxen Arousalreaktion. EEG-Veränderungen bei urologischen Eingriffen unter Isofluran-/N_2O Narkose. *Anaesthesist* 1993; **42**: 142–148.
232 Bimar J, Bellville JW. Arousal reactions during anesthesia in man. *Anesthesiology* 1977; **47**: 449–454.
233 Otto KA, Mally P. Noxious stimulation during orthopaedic surgery results in EEG 'arousal' or 'paradoxical arousal' reaction in isoflurane-anaesthetised sheep. *Res Vet Sci* 2003; **75**: 103–112.
234 Oshima E, Shingu K, Mori K. EEG activity during halothane anaesthesia in man. *Br J Anaesth* 1981; **53**: 65–72.
235 Otto KA, Gerich T. Comparison of simultaneous changes in electroencephalographic and haemodynamic variables in sheep anaesthetised with halothane. *Vet Rec* 2001; **149**: 80–84.
236 Inada T, Shingu K, Nakao S, et al. Electroencephalographic arousal response during tracheal intubation and laryngeal mask airway insertion after induction of anaesthesia with propofol. *Anaesthesia* 1999; **54**: 1150–1154.
237 Kochs E, Kalkman CJ, Thornton C, et al. Middle latency auditory evoked responses and electroencephalographic derived variables do not predict movement to noxious stimulation during 1 minimum alveolar concentration isoflurane/nitrous oxide anesthesia. *Anesth Analg* 1999; **88**: 1412–1417.
238 Rampil IJ, Laster MJ. No correlation between quantitative electroencephalographic measurements and movement response to noxious stimuli during isoflurane anesthesia in rats. *Anesthesiology* 1992; **77**: 920–925.
239 Antognini JF, Wang XW. Isoflurane indirectly depresses middle latency auditory evoked potentials by action in the spinal cord in the goat. *Can J Anesth* 1999; **46**: 692–695.
240 Schwilden H, Kochs E, Daunderer M, et al. Concurrent recording of AEP, SSEP and EEG parameters during anaesthesia: a factor analysis. *Br J Anaesth* 2005; **95**: 197–206.
241 Sleigh JW, Donovan J. Comparison of bispectral index, 95% spectral edge frequency and approximate entropy of the EEG, with changes in heart rate variability during induction of general anaesthesia. *Br J Anaesth* 1999; **82**: 666–671.
242 Bruhn J, Bouillon TW, Radulescu L, et al. Correlation of approximate entropy, bispectral index, and spectral edge frequency 95 (SEF95) with clinical signs of 'anesthetic depth' during coadministration of propofol and remifentanyl. *Anesthesiology* 2003; **98**: 621–627.
243 Sigl JC, Chamoun NG. An introduction to bispectral analysis for the electroencephalogram. *J Clin Monit* 1994; **10**: 392–404.
244 Avidan MS, Zhang L, Burnside BA, et al. Anesthesia awareness and the bispectral index. *N Engl J Med* 2008; **358**: 1097–1108.
245 Crosby G. General anesthesia – minding the mind during surgery. *N Engl J Med* 2011; **365**: 660–661.
246 Serfontein L. Awareness in cardiac anesthesia. *Curr Opin Anesthesiol* 2010; **23**: 103–108.
247 Greene SA, Benson GJ, Tranquilly WJ, et al. Relationship of canine bispectral index to multiples of sevoflurane minimal alveolar concentration, using patch or subdermal electrodes. *Comp Med* 2002; **52**: 424–428.
248 Greene SA, Tranquilli WJ, Benson GJ, et al. Effects of medetomidine administration on bispectral index measurements in dogs during anesthesia with isoflurane. *Am J Vet Res* 2003; **64**: 316–320.
249 Martín-Cancho MF, Lima JR, Luis L, et al. Relationship of bispectral index values, haemodynamic changes and recovery times during sevoflurane or propofol anaesthesia in rabbits. *Lab Anim* 2006; **40**: 28–42.
250 Myles PS, Leslie K, McNeil J, et al. Bispectral index monitoring to prevent awareness during anaesthesia: the B-Aware randomised controlled trial. *Lancet* 2004; **363**: 1757–1763.
251 Avidan MS, Jacobsohn E, Glick D, et al. Prevention of intraoperative awareness in a high-risk surgical population. *N Engl J Med* 2011; **365**: 591–600.
252 Mi W-D, Sakai T, Takahashi S, et al. Haemodynamic and electroencephalographic responses to intubation during induction with propofol or propofol/fentanyl. *Can J Anaesth* 1998; **45**: 19–22.
253 Driessen JJ, Harbers JB, van Egmond J, et al. Evaluation of the electroencephalographic bispectral index during fentanyl–midazolam anaesthesia for cardiac surgery. Does it predict haemodynamic responses during endotracheal intubation and sternotomy? *Eur J Anaesthesiol* 1999; **16**: 622–627.
254 Kussman BD, Gruber EM, Zurakowski D, et al. Bispectral index monitoring during infant cardiac surgery: relationship of BIS to the stress response and plasma fentanyl levels. *Paediatr Anaesth* 2001; **11**: 663–669.
255 Nakayama M, Kanaya N, Edanaga M, et al. Hemodynamic and bispectral index responses to tracheal intubation during isoflurane or sevoflurane anesthesia. *J Anesth* 2003; **17**: 223–226.
256 Kreuer S, Wilhelm W. The Narcotrend monitor. *Best Pract Res Clin Anaesthesiol* 2006; **20**: 111–119.
257 Kreuer S, Bruhn J, Larsen R, et al. Application of Bispectral Index® and Narcotrend® index to the measurement of the electroencephalographic effects of isoflurane with and without burst suppression. *Anesthesiology* 2004; **101**: 847–854.
258 Kreuer S, Bruhn J, Stracke C, et al. Narcotrend or bispectral index monitoring during desflurane–remifentanil anesthesia: a comparison with a standard practice protocol. *Anesth Analg* 2005; **101**: 427–434.
259 Otto KA, Cebotari S, Höffler H-K, et al. Electroencephalographic Narcotrend index, spectral edge frequency and median power frequency as guide to anaesthetic depth for cardiac surgery in laboratory sheep. *Vet J* 2012; **191**: 354–359.
260 Rampil IJ, Sasse FJ, Smith NT, et al. Spectral edge frequency – a new correlate of anesthetic depth. *Anesthesiology* 1980; **53**: S12.
261 Jordan D, Stockmanns G, Kochs E, et al. Electroencephalographic order pattern analysis for the separation of consciousness and unconsciousness. *Anesthesiology* 2008; **109**: 1014–1022.
262 Fell J, Roschke J, Mann K, et al. Discrimination of sleep stages: a comparison between spectral and nonlinear EEG measures. *Electroencephalogr Clin Neurophysiol* 1996; **98**: 401–410.
263 Pincus SM, Gladstone IM, Ehrenkrank RA. A regularity statistic for medical data analysis. *J Clin Monit* 1991; **7**: 335–345.
264 Bruhn J, Röpcke H, Hoeft A. Approximate entropy as an electroencephalographic measure of anesthetic drug effect during desflurane anesthesia. *Anesthesiology* 2000; **92**: 715–726.
265 Bein B. Entropy. *Best Pract Res Clin Anaesthesiol* 2006; **20**: 101–109.
266 Viertiö-Oja H, Maja V, Särkelä M, et al. Description of the Entropy™ algorithm as applied in the Datex-Ohmeda S/5™ entropy module. *Acta Anaesthesiol Scand* 2004; **48**: 154–161.
267 Bruhn J, Lehmann LE, Röpcke H, et al. Shannon entropy applied to the measurement of the electroencephalographic effects of desflurane. *Anesthesiology* 2001; **95**: 30–35.
268 Inouye T, Shinosaki K, Sakamoto H, et al. Quantification of EEG irregularity by use of the entropy of the power spectrum. *Electroencephalogr Clin Neurophysiol* 1991; **79**: 204–210.
269 Greif R, Greenwald S, Schneitzer E, et al. Muscle relaxation does not alter hypnotic level during propofol anesthesia. *Anesth Analg* 2002; **94**: 604–608.
270 Kreuzer M, Zanner R, Pilge S, et al. Time delay of monitors of the hypnotic component of anesthesia: analysis of state entropy and index of consciousness. *Anesth Analg* 2012; **115**: 315–319.
271 Vakkuri A, Yli-Hankala A, Sandin R, et al. Spectral entropy monitoring is associated with reduced propofol use and faster emergence in propofol–nitrous oxide–alfentanil anesthesia. *Anesthesiology* 2005; **103**: 274–279.
272 Olofsen E, Sleigh JW, Dahan A. Permutation entropy of the electroencephalogram: a measure of anaesthetic drug effect. *Br J Anaesth* 2008; **101**: 810–821.
273 Silva A, Campos S, Monteiro J, et al. Performance of anesthetic depth indices in rabbits under propofol anesthesia. *Anesthesiology* 2011; **115**: 303–314.
274 Zanin M, Zunino L, Rosso OA, et al. Permutation entropy and its main biomedical econophysics applications: a review. *Entropy* 2012; **14**: 1553–1577.
275 Li D, Li X, Liang Z, et al. Multiscale permutation entropy analysis of EEG recordings during sevoflurane anesthesia. *J Neural Eng* 2010; **7**: 1–14.
276 Pilge S, Blum J, Kochs EF, et al. Does the cerebral state index separate consciousness from unconsciousness? *Anesth Analg* 2011; **113**: 1403–1410.
277 Zanner R, Pilge S, Kochs EF, et al. Time delay of the electroencephalogram index calculation: analysis of cerebral state, bispectral, and Narcotrend indices using perioperatively recorded electroencephalographic signals. *Br J Anaesth* 2009; **103**: 394–399.
278 Pilge S, Zanner R, Schneider G, et al. Time delay of index calculation: analysis of cerebral state, bispectral and Narcotrend indices. *Anesthesiology* 2006; **104**: 488–494.
279 Mills KR. The basics of electromyography. *J Neurol Neurosurg Psychiatry* 2005; **76**(Suppl 2): ii32–ii35.
280 Fors S. Neuromuscular manifestations of hypothyroidism in dogs. *Eur J Compan Anim Pract* 2007; **17**: 173–178.
281 Van Nes JJ. Clinical application of neuromuscular electrophysiology in the dog: a review. *Vet Q* 1986; **8**: 240–250.
282 Reddy U, Amin Y. Preoperative assessment of neurosurgical patients. *Anaesth Intensive Care Med* 2010; **11**:357–362.
283 Beheiry HE. Protecting the brain during neurosurgical procedures: strategies that can work. *Curr Opin Anesthesiol* 2012; **25**: 548–555.
284 Diedler J, Sykora M, Hahn P, et al. Low hemoglobin is associated with poor functional outcome after non-traumatic, supratentorial intracerebral hemorrhage. *Crit Care* 2010; **14**(2): R63.
285 Mackensen B, McDonagh DL, Warner DS. Perioperative hypothermia: use and therapeutic implications. *J Neurotrauma* 2009; **26**: 342–358.

286 Pasternak JJ, Lanier WL. Neuroanesthesiology update 2010. *J Neurosurg Anesthesiol* 2011; **23**: 67–99.

287 Fodstadt H, Kelly PJ, Buchfelder M. History of the Cushing reflex. *Neurosurgery* 2006; **59**: 1132–1137.

288 Girard F. Intracranial hypertension in the perioperative period. *Anesthesiol Rounds* 2003; **2**(4). http://www.anesthesiologyrounds.ca/crus/anestheng_0403.pdf (accessed 23 September 2014).

289 Robertson CS. Management of cerebral perfusion pressure after traumatic brain injury. *Anesthesiology* 2001; **95**: 1513–1517.

290 Drummond JC. The lower limit of autoregulation: time to revise our thinking? *Anesthesiology* 1997; **86**: 1431–1433.

291 Jellish WS. Anesthetic issues and perioperative blood pressure management in patients who have cerebrovascular diseases undergoing surgical procedures. *Neurol Clin* 2006; **24**: 647–659.

292 Rosner MJ, Rosner SD, Johnson AH. Cerebral perfusion pressure: management protocol and clinical results. *J Neurosurg* 1995; **83**: 949–962.

293 Hilgenberg JC. Comparison of the pharmacology of vecuronium and atracurium with that of other currently available muscle relaxants. *Anesth Analg* 1983; **62**: 524–531.

294 Sokoll MD, Gergis SD, Mehta M, et al. Safety and efficacy of atracurium (BW33A) in surgical patients receiving balanced or isoflurane anesthesia. *Anesthesiology* 1983; **58**: 450–455.

295 Morris RB, Cahalan MK, Miller RD, et al. The cardiovascular effects of vecuronium (ORG#NC45) and pancuronium in patients undergoing coronary artery bypass grafting. *Anesthesiology* 1983; **58**: 438–440.

296 Raisis AL, Leece EA, Platt SR, et al. Evaluation of an anaesthetic technique used in dogs undergoing craniectomy for tumor resection. *Vet Anaesth Analg* 2007; **34**: 171–180.

297 Kerwin AJ, Schinco MA, Tepas JJ III, et al. The use of 23.4% hypertonic saline for the management of elevated intracranial pressure in patients with severe traumatic brain injury: a pilot study. *J Trauma* 2009; **67**: 277–282.

298 Oddo M, Levine JM, Frangos S, et al. Effect of mannitol and hypertonic saline on cerebral oxygenation in patients with severe traumatic brain injury and refractory intracranial hypertension. *J Neurol Neurosurg Psychiatry* 2009; **80**: 916–920.

299 Qureshi AI, Suarez JI, Bhardwaj A, et al. Use of hypertonic (3%) saline/acetate infusion in the treatment of cerebral edema: effect on intracranial pressure and lateral displacement of the brain. *Crit Care Med* 1998; **26**: 440–446.

300 Schwarz S, Georgiadis D, Aschoff A, et al. Effects of hypertonic (10%) saline in patients with raised intracranial pressure after stroke. *Stroke* 2002; **33**: 136–140.

301 Wilcox CS. Regulation of renal blood flow by plasma chloride. *J Clin Invest* 1983; **71**: 726–735.

302 Bilotta F, Lam AM, Doronzio A, et al. Esmolol blunts postoperative hemodynamic changes after propofol–remifentanil total intravenous fast-track neuroanesthesia for intracranial surgery. *J Clin Anesth* 2008; **20**: 426–430.

303 Muzzi DA, Black S, Losasso TJ, et al. Labetol and esmolol in the control of hypertension after intracranial surgery. *Anesth Analg* 1990; **70**: 68–71.

304 Murphy GS, Szokol JW, Marymont JH, et al. Cerebral oxygen desaturation events assessed by near-infrared spectroscopy during shoulder arthroscopy in the beach chair and lateral decubitus positions. *Anesth Analg* 2010; **111**: 496–505.

305 Oddo M, Schmidt JM, Carrera E, et al. Impact of tight glycemic control on cerebral metabolism after severe brain injury: a microdialysis study. *Crit Care Med* 2008; **36**: 3233–3238.

306 Helbok R, Schmidt JM, Kurtz P, et al. Systemic glucose and brain energy metabolism after subarachnoid hemorrhage. *Neurocrit Care* 2010; **12**: 317–323.

307 Lanier WL, Stangland KJ, Scheithauer BW, et al. The effects of dextrose infusion and head position on neurologic outcome after complete cerebral ischemia in primates: examination of a model. *Anesthesiology* 1987; **66**: 39–48.

308 King LJ, Lowry OH, Passoneau JV, et al. Effects of convulsants on energy reserves in the cerebral cortex. *J Neurochem* 1967; **14**: 599–611.

309 Bolwig TG, Quistorff B. *In vivo* concentration of lactate in the brain of conscious rats before and during seizures: new ultra-rapid technique for the freeze-sampling of brain tissue. *J Neurochem* 1973; **21**: 1345–1348.

310 Plum F, Posner JB, Troy B. Cerebral metabolic and circulatory responses to induced convulsions in animals. *Arch Neurol* 1968; **18**: 1–13.

311 Hymes JA. Seizure activity during isoflurane anesthesia. *Anesth Analg* 1985; **64**: 367–368.

312 Perks A, Cheema S, Mohanraj R. Anaesthesia and epilepsy. *Br J Anaesth* 2012; **108**: 562–571.

313 Patsalos PN, Perucca E. Clinically important drug interactions in epilepsy: interactions between antiepileptic drugs and other drugs. *Lancet Neurol* 2003; **2**: 473–481.

314 Constant I, Seeman R, Murat I. Sevoflurane and epileptiform EEG changes. *Paediatr Anaesth* 2005; **15**: 266–274.

315 Mohanram A, Kumar V, Iqbal Z, et al. Repetitive generalized seizure activity during emergence from sevoflurane anesthesia. *Can J Anaesth* 2007; **54**: 657–661.

316 Modica PA, Tempelhoff R, White PF. Pro- and anticonvulsant effects of anesthetics (Part I). *Anesth Analg* 1990; **70**: 303–315.

317 Sleigh JW, Vizuete JA, Voss L, et al. The electrocortical effects of enflurane: experiment and theory. *Anesth Analg* 2009; **109**: 1253–1262.

318 Scheller M, Nakakimura K, Fleischer J. Cerebral effects of sevoflurane in the dog: comparison with isoflurane and enflurane. *Br J Anaesth* 1990; **65**: 388–392.

319 Mirsattari SM, Sharpe MD, Young R. Treatment of refractory status epilepticus with inhalational anesthetic agents isoflurane and desflurane. *Arch Neurol* 2004; **61**: 1254–1259.

320 Lowenstein D, Aminopff M, Simon R. Barbiturate anesthesia in the treatment of status epilepticus: clinical experience with 14 patients. *Neurology* 1988; **38**: 395–400.

321 Brown A, Horton J. Status epilepticus treated by intravenous infusion of thiopentone sodium. *Br Med J* 1967; **i**: 27–28.

322 Power KN, Flaatten H, Gilhus NE, et al. Propofol treatment in adult refractory status epilepticus. Mortality risk and outcome. *Epilepsy Res* 2011; **94**: 53–60.

323 Trzepacz PT, Weniger FC, Greenhouse J. Etomidate anesthesia increases seizure duration during ECT. A retrospective study. *Gen Hosp Psychiatry* 1993; **15**: 115–120.

324 Reddy R, Moorthy S, Dierdorf S, et al. Excitatory effects and electroencephalographic correlation of etomidate, thiopental, methohexital, and propofol. *Anesth Analg* 1993; **77**: 1008–1011.

325 Myslobodsky MS, Golovchinsky V, Mintz M. Ketamine: convulsant or anticonvulsant? *Pharmacol Biochem Behav* 1981; **15**: 27–33.

326 Modica PA, Tempelhoff R, White PF. Pro- and anticonvulsant effects of anesthetics (Part II). *Anesth Analg* 1990; **70**: 433–444.

327 Tortella F. Endogenous opioid peptides and epilepsy: quieting the seizing brain? *Trends Pharmacol Sci* 1988; **9**: 366–372.

328 Saboory E, Derchansky M, Ismaili M, et al. Mechanisms of morphine enhancement of spontaneous seizure activity. *Anesth Analg* 2007; **105**: 1729–1735.

329 Parkinson SK, Bailey SL, Little WL, et al. Myoclonic seizure activity in chronic high-dose spinal opioid administration. *Anesthesiology* 1990; **72**: 743–745.

330 Shih CJ, Doufas AG, Chang HC, et al. Recurrent seizure activity after epidural morphine in a post-partum woman. *Can J Anaesth* 2005; **52**: 727–729.

331 Kelso ARC, Cock HR. Status epilepticus. *Pract Neurol* 2005; **5**: 322–333.

332 Ebrahim ZY, Schubert A, Van Ness P, et al. The effect of propofol on the electroencephalogram of patients with epilepsy. *Anesth Analg* 1994; **78**: 275–279.

333 Park EH, White GA, Tieber LM. Mechanisms of injury and emergency care of acute spinal cord injury in dogs and cats. *J Vet Emerg Crit Care* 2012; **22**: 160–178.

334 Widmer WR. Iohexal and iopamidol: new contrast media for veterinary myelography. *J Am Vet Med Assoc* 1989; **194**: 1714–1716.

335 Widmer WR, Blevin WE. Veterinary myelography: a review of contrast media, adverse effects, and technique. *J Am Anim Hosp Assoc* 1991; **27**: 163–147.

336 Lu D, Lamb CR, Targett MP. Results of myelography in seven dogs with myelomalacia. *Vet Radiol Ultrasound* 2002; **43**: 326–330.

337 Platt SR, McConnell JF, Bestner M. Magnetic resonance imaging characteristics of ascending hemorrhagic myelomalacia in a dog. *Vet Radiol Ultrasound* 2006; **47**: 78–82.

338 Schatzmann U, Meister V, Frankhauser R. Akute Hämatomyelie nach längerer Rückenlage beim Pferd. *Schweiz Arch Tierheilkd* 1979; **121**: 149–155.

339 Zink C. Postanesthetic poliomyelomalacia in a horse. *Can Vet J* 1985; **26**: 275–277.

340 Gelfan S, Tarlov IM. Differential vulnerability of spinal cord structures to anoxia. *J Neurophysiol* 1955; **18**: 170–188.

341 Kirk RW, Bistner SI, Ford RB. *Handbook of Veterinary Procedures and Emergency Treatment*, 5th edn. Philadelphia: WB Saunders, 1990.

342 Richardson D. Acquired myasthenia gravis in a poodle. *Can Vet J* 2011; **152**: 169–172.

343 Blichfeldt-Lauridsen L. Hansen BD. Anesthesia and myasthenia gravis. *Acta Anaesthesiol Scand* 2012; **56**: 17–22.

344 Shilo Y, Pypendop BH, Barter LS, et al. Thymoma removal in a cat with acquired myasthenia gravis: a case report and literature review of anesthetic techniques. *Vet Anaesth Analg* 2011; **38**: 603–613.

345 Jones RS. The use of neuromuscular blocking agents for thymectomy in myasthenia gravis. *Vet Anaesth Analg* 2012; **39**: 220.

346 King LG, Vite CH. Acute fulminating myasthenia gravis in five dogs. *J Am Vet Med Assoc* 1998; **212**: 830–834.

347 Jones RS, Sharp NJH. Use of the muscle relaxant atracurium in a myasthenic dog. *Vet Rec* 1985; **117**: 500–501.

348 Jones RS, Brown A, Watkins PE. Use of the muscle relaxant vecuronium in a myasthenic dog. *Vet Rec* 1988; **122**: 611.

349 O'Riordan JI, Miller DH, Mottershead JP, et al. The management and outcome of patients with myasthenia gravis treated acutely in a neurological intensive care unit. *Eur J Neurol* 1998; **5**: 137–142.

350 Paterson IG, Hood JR, Russel SH, et al. Mivacurium in the myasthenic patient. *Br J Anaesth* 1994; **73**: 494–498.
351 Nilsson E, Meretoja OA. Vecuronium dose-response and maintenance requirements in patients with myasthenia gravis. *Anesthesiology* 1990; **73**: 28–32.
352 Kiran U, Choudhury M, Saxena N, et al. Sevoflurane as a sole anesthetic for thymectomy in myasthenia gravis. *Acta Anaesthesiol Scand* 2000; **44**: 351–353.
353 Petrun AM, Mekis D, Kamenik M. Successful use of rocuronium and sugammadex in a patient with myasthenia. *Eur J Anaesthesiol* 2010; **27**: 917–922.
354 Seamans J. Losing inhibition with ketamine. *Nat Chem Biol* 2008; **4**: 91–93.
355 Olney JW, Newcomer JW, Farber NB. NMDA receptor hypofunction model of schizophrenia. *J Psychiatr Res* 1999; **33**: 523–533.
356 Da Costa RC, Parent J, Dobson H, et al. Comparison of magnetic resonance imaging and myelography in 18 Doberman Pinscher dogs with cervical spondylomyelopathy. *Vet Radiol Ultrasound* 2006; **47**: 523–531.
357 Abramson CJ, Garosi L, Platt SR, et al. Magnetic resonance imaging appearance of suspected ischemic myelopathy in dogs. *Vet Radiol Ultrasound* 2005; **46**: 225–229.
358 Beltran E, Dennis R, Doyle V, et al. Clinical and magnetic resonance imaging feature of canine compressive cervical myelopathy with suspected hydrated nucleus pulposus extrusion. *J Small Anim Pract* 2012; **53**: 101–107.
359 Johnson P, Beltran E, Dennis R, et al. Magnetic resonance imaging characteristics of suspected vertebral instability associated with fracture or subluxation in eleven dogs. *Vet Radiol Ultrasound* 2012; **53**: 552–559.
360 Jenkins TJ. *Functional Mammilian Neuroanatomy*, 2nd edn. Philadelphia: Lea & Febiger, 1978.
361 Stoelting RK. *Pharmacology and Physiology in Anesthetic Practice*, 2nd edn. Philadelphia: JB Lippincott, 1991.
362 Barash PG, Cullen BF, Stoelting RK. *Clinical Anesthesia*. Philadelphia: JB Lippincott, 1989.

29 Nociception and Pain

Carolyn M. McKune[1], Joanna C. Murrell[2], Andrea M. Nolan[3], Kate L. White[4] and Bonnie D. Wright[5]

[1]Mythos Veterinary, LLC, Gainesville, Florida, USA
[2]School of Veterinary Sciences, University of Bristol, Langford, North Somerset, UK
[3]Edinburgh Napier University, Edinburgh, Scotland, UK
[4]School of Veterinary Medicine and Science, University of Nottingham, Nottingham, UK
[5]Fort Collins Veterinary Emergency and Rehabilitation Hospital, Fort Collins, Colorado, USA

Chapter contents

Introduction

Pain is a complex, multi-dimensional experience involving sensory and affective components. In layperson terms, 'pain is not just about how it feels, but how it makes you feel,' and it is the unpleasant feelings that cause the suffering we associate with pain. Pain is a uniquely individual experience in humans, the pain that one individual feels associated with an injury may differ in a major way from that experienced by another, both in its intensity and in how it is perceived and felt. This is evidenced from almost every clinical trial report of a new analgesic regimen, even when confounding factors are well controlled. Furthermore, the nature of pain is variable across many situations. The stories of pain experienced in

Veterinary Anesthesia and Analgesia: The Fifth Edition of Lumb and Jones.
Edited by Kurt A. Grimm, Leigh A. Lamont, William J. Tranquilli, Stephen A. Greene and Sheilah A. Robertson.

traumatic situations clearly illustrate that the time course of pain and its impact on our feelings and how we behave are not directly linked in time. This is well explored by Patrick Wall in *Pain: the Science of Suffering* [1]. Among many illustrations of the complexities of pain, he describes the experience of Harry Beecher, a young medical officer treating wounded troops admitted to a hospital on the beachhead at Anzio in 1944 during the Second World War. Seriously wounded soldiers admitted to the hospital over a period of 4 months were asked 'are you in pain; do you want something for it.' The answer was 'no' to both questions in 70% of cases. Later, after the War, he asked the same two questions of a group of age-matched men who had undergone surgery at the Massachusetts General Hospital in Boston and 70% answered 'yes' to both questions. He concluded that something about the context in which tissue damage occurred influenced the degree of pain suffered. The lack of pain in the early time course of some traumatic injuries is often followed by pain reports within 24 h; pain is rarely absent over time. The well-known phenomenon of phantom limb pain reveals the contrary position – in a large percentage of people who have amputations, pain is present chronically in the area of the amputated limb although healing is complete. Clearly, the onset of disease and pain as a consequence of this is less dramatic and immediate than in the traumatic situations described above and reflects the more common triggers and causes of pain in humans.

The nature of pain is equally complex in animals, although all aspects of its experience and expression are not likely to be identical. The physiology and pathophysiology of pain are remarkably similar and well conserved across mammalian species, and the capacity of animals to suffer as sentient creatures is well established and enshrined in law in many countries.

Pain and nociception

Embracing the many attributes of pain as an abstract construct into a definition is challenging. The official definition of pain by the International Association for the Study of Pain (IASP) is *an unpleasant sensory and emotional experience, associated with actual or potential tissue damage, or described in terms of such damage.* Thus the definition describes pain around experience. The conscious experience of pain defies precise anatomic, physiologic, and/or pharmacologic definition; furthermore, it can be experienced even in the absence of obvious external noxious stimulation, and it can be modified by behavioral experiences including fear, memory, and stress. Nociception is the *neural process of encoding noxious stimuli* [2], the consequences of which may be behavioral – either a simple motor withdrawal reflex or more complex avoidance behaviors – or autonomic (e.g., a rise in arterial blood pressure). Although pain is often the consequence of nociceptive activity, this is not necessarily always the case (e.g., rise in blood pressure in anesthetized animals during intense stimulation).

Pain classification

At its simplest, pain may be classified as either acute or chronic; however, the distinction between these states is not always clear. Acute pain largely occurs in response to tissue damage (generally acute) that resolves in a period of days, or possibly weeks. A good example is the time profile that normally occurs following an acute surgical stimulus [3]. Pain that is likely to be at its most intense in the first 24 h after surgery gradually declines over time, spontaneous pain disappearing initially and evoked pain thereafter. Within weeks, tissue healing is completed and pain has disappeared. Defining chronic pain is more arbitrary; it is clear that an animal suffering from osteoarthritis (OA) could be described as having a chronically painful condition. However, the point at which an acute condition that has become chronic (e.g., mastitis) becomes less clear. In practice, an arbitrary interval of time from onset of pain has been used; for example, pain of more than 3 months' duration can be considered to be chronic [4].

Acute pain is generally associated with tissue damage, or the threat of it, and serves the function of altering the animal's behavior in order to avoid or minimize damage and optimizing the conditions in which healing can take place. Acute pain varies in its severity from mild to excruciating. It is frequently associated with surgery, trauma, and/or some medical conditions. It is evoked by a specific disease or injury and it is self-limiting. Chronic pain lasts for longer periods and is classically associated with chronic inflammatory disease or a degenerative condition, or following nerve injury or damage. It can also represent pain that persists beyond the expected course of an acute disease process. It has no biological purpose and no clear end-point, and evidence from humans indicates that it can have a significant impact upon the quality of life of the sufferer. Chronic pain has been described in human medicine as *pain which persists beyond the normal time of healing, or as persistent pain caused by conditions where healing has not occurred or which remit and then recur* [2]. Thus acute and chronic pain are different clinical entities, and chronic pain may be considered as a disease state. Many animals suffer from long-term chronic disease and illness that is accompanied by chronic pain. During the lifetime of the animal, acute exacerbations of the chronic pain state may occur (breakthrough pain), or new sources of acute pain may occur independently (acute on chronic pain), jeopardizing effective pain management strategies.

Conscious perception of pain represents the final product of a complex neurologic information-processing system, resulting from the interplay of facilitatory and inhibitory pathways throughout the peripheral and central nervous systems. Several distinct types of pain exist, which may be classified as nociceptive (or physiologic pain), inflammatory, and neuropathic. Cancer pain often displays characteristics of both inflammatory and neuropathic pain. Inflammatory pain normally contributes to acute postoperative pain, until the wound has healed. It has a rapid onset and, in general, its intensity and duration are related to the severity and duration of tissue damage, The changes in the nociceptive system are generally reversible and normal sensitivity of the system should be restored as tissue heals. However, if the noxious insult was severe, or if a focus of ongoing irritation persists, then pain will persist, as is the case in animals with chronic inflammatory diseases such as OA.

Neuropathic pain is the pain that develops following injury to peripheral nerves or the central nervous system (CNS). There follows a plethora of changes in the peripheral nervous system, spinal cord, brainstem and brain as damaged nerves fire spontaneously and develop hyper-responsiveness to both inflammatory and normally innocuous stimuli (see later). In humans, neuropathic pain is commonly manifested in, for example, postamputation phantom limb pain and postherpetic neuropathy. It is surprising, therefore, that neuropathic pain is not described in animals more commonly, although clinicians are increasingly alert to its potential and to recognizing the presence of chronic pain. Persistent pain after surgery (postsurgical pain) remains a problem in humans, particularly following major surgery, with a minority of these patients experiencing severe chronic pain, often neuropathic in nature. The risk of persistent postsurgical pain in animals following surgery has not been quantified; however, it is likely to occur in some with the potential for this to impact adversely on quality of life.

There is good evidence from laboratory models indicating that the pathophysiology of different pain types, such as inflammatory, neuropathic, or cancer-related pain, is distinct from one another. For example, increases in substance P, calcitonin gene-related peptide (CGRP), protein kinase Cγ, and the substance P receptor were reported in the spinal cord in inflammatory pain [5], with significant decreases in substance P and CGRP and increases in galanin and neuropeptide Y in primary afferent neurons and the spinal cord in rodents with neuropathic pain. In cancer-related pain, there were no detectable changes in any of these markers in either primary afferent neurons or the spinal cord, although other changes were observed.

Pain physiology

The conscious experience of acute pain resulting from a noxious stimulus is mediated by a high-threshold nociceptive sensory system. In healthy animals, 'physiologic' pain is a term used to describe the pain normally associated with the presence of a potentially harmful stimulus. The physiology of pain has been well reviewed. In summary, there are distinct stages in the transmission of nociceptive information and distinct anatomic nociceptive pathways [6].

Nociceptors represent the free endings of primary sensory neurons. The primary afferent nerve fibers that carry information from these free nerve endings to their central location consist of two main types: unmyelinated C fibers and myelinated A-δ fibers. Unmyelinated C fibers, activated by intense stimuli, conduct impulses slowly (~0.5 m/s), and under normal conditions have no background discharge. They are broadly polymodal, i.e., they respond to different stimulus modalities. Stimulation thresholds of C fibers are higher than those of other types of afferent sensory fiber, requiring, for example, noxious thermal stimulation at temperatures above 45 °C to elicit a response [7]. It is worth noting that not all C fibers are nociceptors. Some respond to cooling and to innocuous stroking of haired skin [8]. A-δ fibers (type I and type II) transmit both non-noxious and noxious information under normal conditions, while non-noxious sensory information is transmitted by myelinated A-β fibers. Unmyelinated C fibers contribute to the 'slow burn' sensation of pain whereas A-δ fibers conduct impulses more quickly and contribute to the rapid 'stab' of the acute pain response. There is also a population of so-called 'silent nociceptors,' which are heat responsive but mechanically insensitive, that develop mechanical sensitivity probably when chemical mediators are released during inflammation or tissue damage [9]. C fibers may be further classified as peptidergic (those releasing neuropeptides, including substance P and CGRP) and non-peptidergic, which express the c-Ret neurotrophin receptor that is targeted by glial-derived neurotrophic factor. Nociceptors can also be distinguished according to their differential expression of channels that confer sensitivity to heat (TRPV1), cold (TRPM8), acidic environment (ASICs), and a range of chemical irritants (TRPA1) [10]. These different classes of nociceptors are associated with specific function in the detection of distinct pain modalities. Following tissue trauma, changes in the properties of nociceptors occur such that large-diameter A-β fibers may also transmit 'nociceptive information.'

Activation of specific receptors and ion channels (present in most tissues and organs) in peripheral unmyelinated nerve endings by chemical, mechanical, or thermal stimuli causes the initiation of action potentials that propagate the stimulus along the axons of primary afferent nerve fibers to synaptic sites in the dorsal horn of the spinal cord. This triggers the release of neurotransmitters, including glutamate and substance P, which activate neurons located in the spinal cord. The primary afferent fibers carrying impulses from these peripheral nociceptors can be divided into two types: unmyelinated C fibers and myelinated A-δ fibers; the A-δ fibers synapse in lamina I and V of the spinal cord and the C fibers largely in lamina II, also known as the substantia gelatinosa. The fibers of these second-order neurons project to various areas in the brain, both ipsilaterally and contralaterally to their site of origin, including to the periaqueductal gray (PAG) region in the spinomesencephalic tract, to the medial and ventrobasal thalamus in the spinothalamic tracts, and to the reticular formation (spinoreticular fibers). This activation pattern provides widespread positive and negative feedback loops by which information relating to noxious stimulation can be amplified or diminished. Sensory noxious input from the head region enters the cell bodies lying in the trigeminal ganglion and thereafter noxious information is conveyed to the nucleus caudalis (part of the trigeminal sensory complex). Descending axons of serotonergic and noradrenergic neurons from the brain synapse with inhibitory inter-neurons in the spinal cord to modify their function, and in healthy animals they are considered to be responsible for 'stress-induced analgesia.' In altered pain states, this effect may be blunted and there may be local disinhibition with the potential to increase pain perception.

As mentioned above, pain information is transmitted to higher brain centers through large tracts. The spinothalamic tract, originating from laminae I and V in the spinal cord, projects to the thalamus, the spinoreticular tract projects to the reticular formation, and the thalamus and the spinomesencephalic tract projects to the midbrain – the PAG region, the hypothalamus, and the limbic system. The perception of sensory information (processing, integration and recognition) occurs in multiple areas of the brain. The reticular activating system (in the brainstem) plays a key role in integrating information and both the subjective responses to pain through its projections to the thalamus and the limbic system, and the autonomic, motor, and endocrine responses. The PAG is significant in the descending inhibitory and facilitatory modulation of nociceptive information through its connections with the rostral ventromedial medulla and the medullary reticular formation. The thalamus relays information to the somatosensory cortex, which then projects information to other areas, including the limbic system. The cerebral cortex is the seat of conscious experience of pain; it exerts top-down control and can modulate the sensation of pain. Central pain associated with a cortical or subcortical lesion, which is not associated with any detectable pathology in the body, can be very severe.

Pain is considered to consist of three components: a *sensory-discriminatory* component (temporal, spatial, thermal/mechanical), an *affective* component (subjective and emotional, describing associated fear, tension, and autonomic responses), and an *evaluative* component, describing the magnitude of the quality (e.g., stabbing/pounding; mild/severe). Any mammal's pain experience is likely similarly composed, although our tendency is to focus on pain intensity alone.

Pain pathophysiology – clinical pain

It has been demonstrated that major surgical procedures are followed by an unpleasant sequence of events, including pain, reduced organ function, and prolonged hospital stay, despite the routine use of analgesics [11]. Moreover, a potential adverse and relatively common outcome from surgery in humans is the development of persistent or chronic pain [12], which can cause substantial distress in patients and have serious adverse effects on psychological, social and functional status, and quality of life [13].

It is widely recognized that peripheral tissue damage results in increased activation of peripheral nociceptors and an activity-dependent increase in central neuronal excitability, inducing peripheral and central sensitization [14]. The nociceptive sensory system is an inherently plastic system and, when tissue injury or inflammation occurs, the sensitivity of an injured region is enhanced. These changes contribute to postinjury hypersensitivity, which manifests as an increase in responsiveness to painful stimuli (hyperalgesia) and a decrease in pain threshold such that non-painful stimuli become painful (allodynia). The clinical hallmarks of sensitization of the nociceptive system are *hyperalgesia* and *allodynia*. Hyperalgesia is an exaggerated and prolonged response to a noxious stimulus, whereas allodynia is a pain response to a low-intensity, normally innocuous stimulus such as light touch to the skin or gentle pressure. Hyperalgesia and allodynia are a consequence of peripheral and central sensitization.

Sensitization

Peripheral sensitization is the result of changes in the environment bathing nociceptor terminals as a result of tissue injury or inflammation. Neurotransmitters and chemical mediators released by damaged cells may either directly activate the nociceptor or sensitize the nerve terminals, resulting in long-lasting changes in the functional properties of peripheral nociceptors. Trauma and inflammation can also sensitize nociceptor transmission in the spinal cord to produce *central sensitization*. This requires a brief, but intense, period of nociceptor stimulation (e.g., a surgical incision, intense input following tissue trauma, or intense input following nerve injury). As a result, the response threshold of the central neurons falls, their responses to subsequent stimulation are amplified, and their receptive fields enlarge to recruit additional previously 'dormant' afferent fibers into nociceptive transmission. Whereas primary hyperalgesia occurs in the periphery, secondary hyperalgesia occurs within the CNS (and precedes long-term central sensitization).

Peripheral changes

Maladaptive changes in ion channel expression can cause hyperexcitability of afferent pain-signaling neurons and their axons, thus resulting in pain [15]. Electrical activity of primary afferent neurons is primarily governed by the expression and function of ion channels that define the resting membrane potential, action potential initiation, and transmitter release from their terminals in the dorsal horn [16]. They include voltage-gated sodium channels, potassium and calcium channels, leak channels, and ligand-gated ion channels (e.g., acid-sensing ion channel, transient receptor potential channel). Those which have been implicated in pain signaling and which are providing useful targets for novel analgesic development include, for example, the NaV1.7 [17] and NaV1.8 [18] isoforms of voltage-gated sodium channels and the T-type calcium channels [15].

Voltage-gated sodium channels underlie action potential firing in excitable cells. Nine different channels are recognized (NaV1.1 to NaV1.9), which share a common overall structure but with different functional and pharmacologic profiles. Current non-specific sodium channel blockers used as analgesics are restricted in their applicability to pain management because they inhibit multiple channel isoforms, including those expressed in the brain and heart, and thus induce adverse effects. To date, research suggests that thee sodium channels, NaV1.7, NaV1.8, and NaV1.9, appear to be essential for inducing signals in peripheral nociceptors but are not essential for function of CNS neurons or myocytes [19,20]. Development of NaV1.7 blockers as potential analgesics agents is under way, with some promising results [21]. NaV1.8 channels have been linked to painful neuropathies in humans, and studies in rodents have provided supporting evidence of their role in neuropathic pain [22,23]. NaV1.9 (initially called NaN) is specifically expressed in dorsal root ganglion (DRG) and trigeminal ganglion neurons. NaV1.9 knockout mice display attenuated inflammatory pain behavior, suggesting a contribution to inflammatory pain [24]. Further work is required to elucidate the implications for analgesic drug development through targeting these and other peripheral ion channels.

Central changes

Many analgesic drugs in current use have a spinal site of action, highlighting the spinal cord's pivotal role in pain processing. Nociceptive inputs can trigger a prolonged increase in the excitability and synaptic efficacy of neurons in central nociceptive pathways, the phenomenon of central sensitization. Central sensitization manifests as pain hypersensitivity (tactile allodynia, secondary hyperalgesia, and enhanced temporal summation). Clinical studies in a range of disease/injury states have evidenced changes in pain sensitivity in patients with fibromyalgia, OA, musculoskeletal disorders, headache, temporomandibular joint disorders, dental pain, neuropathic pain, visceral pain hypersensitivity disorders, and post-surgical pain. The presence of hypersensitivity in syndromes that present in the absence of inflammation or a neural lesion, along with their similar pattern of clinical presentation and response to centrally acting analgesics, may reflect a common pathophysiology of central sensitization [25]. Many studies in animals have evidenced the development and presence of pain hypersensitivity, including in dogs and cats postoperatively [26–28] and in many animal species with acute and chronic inflammatory conditions [29–33].

The mechanisms of central sensitization have been studied and involve a range of excitatory and inhibitory interneurons, *N*-methyl-D-aspartate receptor activation, and descending influences from the brainstem, which can be both inhibitory and excitatory in nature. Prolonged firing of C fiber nociceptors causes release of glutamate from within the dorsal horn of the spinal cord, which acts on postsynaptic ionotropic glutamate receptors [*N*-methyl-D-aspartic acid (NMDA) and α-amino-3-hydroxy-5-methyl-4-isoxazolepropionic acid (AMPA) receptors], and the G-protein coupled metabotropic (mGLuR) family of receptors [34]. Glutamate release by sensory afferents acts on AMPA receptors if the impulse is short and acute. However, repetitive and high-frequency stimulus from C fibers induces amplification and prolongation of the response through activation of the NMDA receptor. This enhanced NMDA receptor activation (e.g., wind-up), facilitated by co-release of substance P and CGRP from C fibers [35], plays a role in inflammatory and neuropathic pain states and results in the activation and exacerbation of secondary hyperalgesia. Translational changes of the neurons in the dorsal horn of the spinal cord occur [36], which may contribute to the transition from persistent acute pain to chronic pain. NMDA receptors are also required for the descending inhibitory pathway of the CNS within the substantia gelatinosa. Hence this receptor plays a pivotal role in the induction and maintenance of pain. However, owing to adverse effects of the currently available drugs (ketamine, dextromethorphan, and memantine) and lack of specificity for the dorsal horn NMDA receptor (NR2B subtype), their clinical utility is constrained, although they may be effective as part of a multimodal approach to treating chronic pain.

Inflammation and nerve injury induce transcriptional changes in dorsal horn neurons, which includes the induction of cylooxygenase-2 (COX-2), mediated largely by interleukin-1β [37]. The CNS is a major target for pain control as upregulation of COX-2 expression leads to increased central sensitization and pain hypersensitivity. The downstream products of COX-2 activity in pain perception are largely linked to the CNS effects of PGE_2, which binds to prostaglandin E receptor subtypes EP1 or EP3 on sensory neurons and induces a range of effects that both reduce the threshold for sensory neuron activation and increase neuronal excitability.

There is a role for endocannabinoids in mediating central changes in neuronal activity and function [38]. Endocannabinoids, like prostaglandins, are derivatives of arachidonic acid; they act on cannabinoid receptors (CB1 and CB2), which are expressed in all nociceptive neuroanatomic pathways of the central (e.g., PAG) and peripheral nervous systems (e.g., peripheral nociceptors, dorsal root ganglion cells). Activation of the receptors reduces the release of neurotransmitters such as glutamate and they are involved in descending supraspinal inhibitory modulation via the PAG and rostral ventromedial medulla [39].

Cannabinoids possess antinociceptive properties in acute pain animal models and they display antihyperalgesic and antiallodynic properties in models of neuropathic pain, There are endogenous ligands, anandamide (activates CB1 and CB2 receptors), 2-arachidonoylglycerol (2-AG) (activates CB1 and CB2 receptors), and palmitoylethanolamide (activates CB2 receptors), which are produced in microglial cells during neuroinflammatory conditions. COX-2 can biotransform both anandamide and 2-AG to prostanoid compounds, hence during inflammation when COX-2 is unregulated the antinociceptive effects of the endocannabinoids can be lost and their metabolites can produce a pronociceptive effect.

Activation of CNS microglial cells (functionally equivalent to peripheral macrophages) plays a central role in pain [40]. Glial cells are activated by substances released from primary afferent terminals and from second-order transmission neurons (e.g., nitric oxide and prostaglandins). Activated glial cells upregulate cyclooxygenase-2 (COX-2) in dorsal root ganglion cells to produce prostaglandin E_2 and release additional neuroactive substances (cytokines), which increase the excitability of dorsal horn neurons and play a role in axonal sprouting, altered connectivity, and cell death (of, for example, inhibitory interneurons). This neuroplasticity leads to central sensitization with alterations in the phenotype of dorsal horn neurons and other neurons within the CNS. Hence persistent glial cell activity likely plays a role in the development of some chronic pain states [41].

Chronic pain

Arguably, understanding the factors associated with, and the causes of transitioning mechanisms from, acute to chronic pain is critical in advancing our knowledge and understanding of pain. Chronic pain accounts for a huge burden of suffering in humans and animal species. The role of acute and persistent pain in causing chronic pain is not fully evidenced but there are clearly many associated risk factors that contribute to this progression. In humans, there is work ongoing to identify whether some individuals have a higher inherited propensity for developing central sensitization than others and, if so, whether this conveys an increased risk in developing conditions with pain hypersensitivity, and the development of chronic pain. The links between acute and chronic pain were considered in a review by Voscopoulos and Lema [39], who concluded that the transition from acute to chronic pain occurs in discrete steps, initiated by the presence of persistent and intense stimuli.

There is strong evidence that certain groups of people are more vulnerable to developing chronic pain conditions (for a review, see Denk *et al.* [42]). In most conditions, only a proportion of patients will develop chronic pain (e.g., diabetic neuropathy and chronic pain postsurgery [43,44]). There appear to be a range of risk factors, including genetics, gender, age, and prior priming events, that may be associated with changes to the neuronal architecture and molecular processes. It is clear that previous pain history can predict future pain development, as will adverse life events such as stress and depressive illnesses. A study on neonatal pigs indicated that *in utero* stress can alter the immediate behavioral responses of piglets to tail-docking [45]. Understanding genetic vulnerability in different animal species will help to focus pain research and intervention strategies.

Models of nociception and analgesic testing

Although significant advances have been made in the basic understanding of pain processing and modulation in recent years, large gaps in our knowledge remain, particularly in the fields of anatomic, biochemical and physiologic mechanisms of pain. At the same time, unrelieved pain in humans remains a major healthcare issue, with approximately one-fifth of the adult population in Western countries suffering from chronic pain [46]. In the United States, the annual cost of medical treatment and lost productivity due to pain is $635 billion [47]. The current situation in animals with respect to adequacy of pain management is less well documented. Drugs with proven efficacy for the treatment of acute surgical pain are available for companion animals [e.g., licensed opioids and non-steroidal anti-inflammatory drugs (NSAIDs)]. However, with the exception of NSAIDs, the repertoire of licensed drugs for the management of chronic pain (e.g., pain caused by degenerative joint disease) in companion animals is very limited. Acute and chronic pain remain poorly treated in farm animals and exotic species.

It is widely accepted that research in animals is pivotal to an increased understanding of nociceptive and pain mechanisms and to the development of new analgesic drugs, for both humans and animals. Pain studies in humans generally focus on characterizing pain states, with few studies investigating underlying pain mechanisms, and studies in humans are inevitably hampered by ethical constraints. Although in humans the advent of advanced neuroimaging techniques allows the *in vivo* study of patterns of CNS activity concurrent with self-report of pain perception, ethical considerations surrounding induced pain models in humans, combined with current technological limitations, means that neuroimaging cannot replace the need for animal pain models [48,49]. In addition, neuroimaging lacks cellular resolution and poor temporal resolution; functional magnetic resonance imaging (fMRI) may not distinguish between very high levels of neuronal activity in the brain (and therefore may not be sensitive to different pain intensities) because the blood oxygen level-dependent (BOLD) signal can reach a ceiling. Neuroimaging does not allow the interrogation of small areas of the CNS such as the dorsal horn of the spinal cord or the peripheral nervous system with any precision, as the technique relies on integrating electrical signals across large sampling regions such as the brain.

Two main approaches have been adopted when studying pain in animals. The first approach is to study responses to brief noxious stimuli (defined as stimuli that are damaging to, or threaten to damage, normal tissues) in naive animals. In other words, brief phasic noxious thermal, electrical, or mechanical stimuli are delivered to healthy animals and the magnitude of the stimulus threshold required to elicit a response is measured (e.g., nociceptive threshold testing), or changes in neuronal activity, animal behavior, or body systems are studied during delivery of the stimulus. Response to brief phasic stimuli is commonly utilized as the outcome measure in analgesic drug testing (i.e., as an integral component of pain models), although it should be viewed as having limited applicability owing to the previously naive (normal) state of the nervous system and singular nociceptive modality (e.g., thermal nociceptors), which differs from most clinical pain syndromes.

The second approach is to induce pain in the animal by delivery of a tonic, sustained noxious stimulus that induces peripheral or central sensitization and subsequently to study pain mechanisms (e.g., by recording changes in behavioral or neuronal activity) or test analgesic drugs. In this chapter, the broad term 'pain model' is used to refer to the second approach. There is interest in using companion animals with naturally occurring disease conditions that cause pain (e.g., spontaneous OA in dogs) [50] to study pain mechanisms and evaluate analgesic drug efficacy for both humans and animals. However, there are disadvantages when using non-human subjects in analgesic studies, such as the lack of verbal feedback about the 'feelings' of the patient's pain and the vulnerability to observer bias.

Within any pain model, there are three distinct components that must be differentiated [51]. First, there is the study subject (variables include species, strain, sex, and age); second, there is the stimulus or type of tissue damage that is used to initiate pain (e.g., an injection of an irritant substance into a joint versus measuring cutaneous thermal threshold); and third, there is the outcome measure (e.g., behavior or physiological parameter) used as the surrogate biomarker for pain. Significant interest has arisen recently in trying to improve pain biomarkers in animal models with the recognition that end-points such as a tail flick in response to a noxious stimulus may be largely reflexive and not an indicator of higher brain perception. This is of particular relevance in the development of pain models for analgesic drug development.

Limitations of current animal models

Despite significant efforts in analgesic drug discovery, there has been limited success in developing and marketing new analgesic drugs with efficacy and acceptable adverse effect profiles for clinical patients with pain. Putative new analgesic drugs undergo screening and preclinical testing in animal models; therefore, it is important that the performance of a new analgesic in animal models is successfully translated to the human pain model and clinical patients. Although the reasons for failure of new drugs at the preclinical–clinical interface are multifactorial, there is a general agreement that limitations of current animal models play a major role in the current bottleneck in analgesic drug development [52]. Recognized general limitations of animal pain models occur at the level of the experimental animal (subject) and the pain assay or biomarker used to assess pain.

Experimental animal (subject)

The majority of preclinical pain research is carried out in young adult, healthy, intact male laboratory mice and rats of a specific strain. Although useful as a cost-effective and rapid screening method for *in vivo* testing of candidate molecules, this does not always translate well to the clinical population of pain patients. Therefore, it has been recommended [51] that pain studies include more diverse and heterogeneous groups of animals of both genders and of a variety of strains.

Nociceptive assay

A large number of nociceptive (pain) assays are currently available that aim to model nociceptive, inflammatory, and neuropathic pain. However, it is immediately apparent that there is a mismatch between the underlying pathophysiologic changes induced in experimental assays and the etiology of clinical pain conditions. For example, nerve ligation is commonly used as a model of neuropathic pain, yet diseases associated with neuropathic pain in humans rarely result from complete nerve ligation or nerve compression. There are often coexisting abnormalities that contribute to the perceived pain, such as coexisting neuropathy and inflammation. Most pain assays do not mimic the complexity of clinical pain states. Induced models of OA in rats and mice usually focus on the stifle joint and are induced by sterile inflammation or surgical disruption of the joint, leading to a rapid progression of OA that does not take into account the effect(s) of aging itself on perceived pain [53].

Biomarkers

Until recently, the majority of behavioral biomarkers used to measure analgesic drug effect in animal pain models relied on either evoked spinal reflexes (e.g., limb withdrawal from a von Frey filament) or innate behaviors such as vocalization or guarding that can also be performed by decerebrate animals [54]. Evoked withdrawal responses detect hyperalgesia and allodynia (although the two are difficult to distinguish from each other in animals) and therefore only provide information on the sensory and discriminative component of pain. They do not provide information about the emotional (affective) component, which is critical to the experience of pain in humans and animals, although more difficult to define in the latter. Although many patients with chronic neuropathic pain experience hyperalgesia and allodynia, they commonly report spontaneous pain (i.e., non-evoked pain) as the most debilitating and distressing aspect of their condition [55]. Therefore, unless biomarkers that evaluate spontaneous pain are employed in an assay, the effect on spontaneous pain may go undetected. New biomarkers sensitive to spontaneous pain that are able to detect changes in behavior associated with emotion are being developed.

Translational pain models

In recent years, the importance of translational approaches to animal research, which aim to bridge gaps between basic animal research and medical practice, has been recognized. As such, efforts are under way to develop assays and biomarkers that directly translate to experimental human pain models. This increases the likelihood that analgesics found effective in preclinical studies will remain efficacious in human clinical trials. Currently, there are very few assays that are translatable, although intradermal or cutaneous application of capsaicin and the UVb pain model are notable exceptions. The use of spontaneous disease models in companion animals is another approach to improving translatability of pain assays between humans and animals. Experimental pain studies in humans rely largely on psychophysics to quantify pain and therefore analgesic drug efficacy, but self-reporting of pain is inherently subjective. Commonly used behavioral biomarkers such as reflex withdrawal are also vulnerable to observer subjectivity. Considerable variability of reported results among researchers and laboratories is therefore common. Clearly, objective biomarkers directly translatable to humans that reflect the underlying neurobiology of perceived pain are needed to improve pain models.

Nociceptive and pain assays

In the following sections, the term pain is used to describe all assays carried out in awake animals; if the animal is anesthetized during the assay, the term nociception is used.

Phasic pain tests

Brief noxious (phasic) stimuli are widely used to elicit responses in order to study nociceptive pathways and increase the understanding of the neurobiology of pain in experimental animals and also for the purposes of analgesiometry (i.e., measuring changes in biomarkers to study the action of analgesic drugs). Broadly, nociceptive threshold testing (in animals) and quantitative sensory testing (QST) in humans are the terms used to describe the application of tests utilizing brief phasic stimuli. The stimuli might be applied to naive animals or to animals with induced pain, thus allowing the study of nociceptive pathways and drug efficacy in normal animals and animals with altered pain sensitivity caused by central and/or peripheral sensitization. For a complete review of phasic pain tests, see Le Bars *et al.* [56].

Beecher [57] was one of the first authors to set out ideal criteria for producing acute pain experimentally, and some of the optimal characteristics are as follows:

- The stimulus is applied to a body part where neurohistologic variations are at a minimum between different individuals and the stimulus can be measured and closely associated with the changes that produce pain.
- Quantitative data can be collected in response to a given stimulus under given conditions.
- There is little tissue damage at the pain threshold level and the hazard to the subject is small at high intensities.
- There is a relationship between the magnitude of the stimulus and the intensity of the pain experienced.
- It is possible to carry out repeat measurements without interfering with subsequent measurements.
- The stimulus is easy to apply and there is a clearly identifiable end-point.
- The test should be applicable to both humans and animals.

Stimulus modalities

Four modalities of noxious stimulation are commonly used in phasic acute nociceptive tests: electrical, thermal, mechanical, and chemical. The advantages and disadvantages of these different modalities when used to generate acute pain are shown in Table 29.1. Chemical stimulation is considered separately because it causes a slower, progressive, and non-escapable noxious stimulus. Commonly used phasic tests in awake animals are described in Table 29.2 (thermal stimuli), Table 29.3 (mechanical stimuli), and Table 29.4 (electrical stimuli).

Site of stimulus application

For practical reasons, phasic nociceptive stimuli are usually applied to the skin to activate cutaneous nociceptors, although stimuli are also applied to viscera in some models. The predominance of tests involving cutaneous nociceptors reflects the ease of access to the skin and the ability to stimulate the skin with minimal restraint of the animal. In awake laboratory animals, the plantar surface of the hind paw is often used as the site of stimulation because it is readily accessible for application of heat and mechanical stimuli. Awareness of the differences in cutaneous sensitivity between haired (found on most of the body) and glabrous skin (the plantar paw) in laboratory animals is important as it alters the translatability of pain tests between rats and humans [58]. The tail is commonly used as the site of stimulus application in acute pain tests in rats (e.g., thermal nociceptive stimuli). However, the tail is also essential for thermoregulation and balance, which can influence threshold responses measured following stimulation [56]. Concurrent noxious stimulation of more than one body part at the same time recruits endogenous inhibitory mechanisms and confounds measured threshold responses, so is best avoided [59]. Another consideration is the potential for repeated stimulation of the same body site to cause peripheral and central sensitization, thereby causing a reduction in threshold over time.

Outcome measures

Behavior

Laboratory animals generate a range of behavioral responses to delivery of phasic noxious stimuli classified by the underlying nociceptive pathways that are activated. The end-points classically used for each assay are detailed below; however, a few general comments are outlined here. Many phasic tests rely on the detection of motor withdrawal responses; therefore, impaired motor function (e.g., during administration of analgesic drugs that have concurrent effects on locomotion) will confound threshold responses. It is important to differentiate between withdrawal responses that are reflex (governed predominantly by spinal mechanisms) and more complex behaviors such as escape, avoidance, or licking of the body part where the stimulus was applied. The complexity of the end-point behavior will to some extent reflect recruitment of underlying nociceptive or pain mechanisms and therefore are commonly differentially sensitive to analgesic drugs [60]. End-point behaviors used in nociceptive tests should ideally be nociceptive specific, reliable, reproducible, and sensitive to administration of analgesic drugs.

Neurophysiologic end-points

Neurophysiologic techniques are increasingly important in studies to elucidate ascending pain pathways and cortical representation of pain [61–63]. Techniques that afford a direct window on the function of the CNS, such as electroencephalography, provide a unique insight into pain processing and how activation of nociceptive pathways results in pain perception in a conscious animal. The electroencephalogram (EEG) is the electrical activity recorded from electrodes placed at various locations on the scalp (human) or head (other species) [64]. It consists of the summated electrical activity of populations of neurons together with a contribution from the glial cells. Neurons are excitable cells with intrinsic electrical properties that result in the production of electrical and magnetic fields. These fields may be recorded at a distance from their sources and are termed 'far-field potentials.' Fields recorded a short distance from their source they are termed 'near-field' or local field potentials. Activity recorded from the surface of the cortex is described as the

Table 29.1 Advantages and disadvantages of different stimulus modalities used to study acute pain.

Stimulus Modality	Characteristics of the Stimulus	Advantages	Disadvantages
Electrical	Direct activation of all nerve fibers, thereby bypassing transduction mechanisms at the peripheral nociceptor	1. Quantifiable 2. Brief; controlled onset and offset 3. Reproducible 4. Non-invasive 5. Bypasses peripheral nociceptor transduction mechanisms that may be advantageous in the study of central pain mechanisms 6. Elicits a synchronized pattern of neuronal activity that is sufficient to generate reflex responses 7. Graded behavioral responses to increasing stimulus intensities 8. Translatable between humans and animals	1. Not a natural stimulus 2. Indiscriminate activation of all fiber types (therefore not selective for A-δ or C fibers) 3. Bypasses peripheral nociceptor transduction mechanisms, therefore of limited use for the study of peripheral pain mechanisms 4. Elicits a synchronized pattern of neuronal activity that does not replicate patterns of activity that occur in clinical pain states 5. Impedance of the tissue will determine the magnitude of the delivered stimulus – care must be taken to standardize the stimulus magnitude as much as possible
Thermal: general comments	Selective activation of cutaneous thermosensitive and nociceptive fibers. Rate of heating can be altered to selectively activate A-δ or C fibers	1. Natural stimulus 2. Most thermal stimuli deliver slow rates of heating of nociceptors and therefore selectively activate C fibers; efficient for revealing the activity of opioid analgesics	1. Surface skin temperature can be measured easily, but more difficult to measure the temperature at the level of the nociceptor. Thermocouples placed in the deeper tissues to measure temperature often disturb heat transfer 2. Thermal hyperalgesia is clinically less problematic than mechanical hyperalgesia in clinical pain patients
Thermal: radiant heat source	Conventional radiant heat sources emit light in the visible or adjacent infrared spectra	1. Easy to build 2. Selective; no concurrent stimulation of non-nociceptive neurons (e.g., low threshold mechanosensitive neurons)	1. Conventional radiant heat sources often lack power to cause synchronized neuronal activity and therefore generate reflex responses 2. Infrared light sources in the wavelengths generated by radiant heat sources are poorly absorbed by skin 3. Variability in stimulus magnitude determined by: (a) reflectance, transmittance and absorption properties of the skin and the electromagnetic spectrum emitted by the source of radiation. (b) conduction properties of the skin (c) initial temperature of the skin (d) the amount of caloric energy delivered to the surface of the skin
Thermal: contact thermode	Heat thermosensitive receptors by means of the conduction properties of the skin	1. Can deliver a slope of heating that grows linearly with time and can be precisely controlled 2. Difficult to secure to laboratory animals, widely used in companion and farm animals	1. Concurrent activation of low-threshold non-nociceptive nerves that exert and inhibitory influence on pain mechanisms 2. Thermode surface is usually flat and rigid and therefore does not conform very well to the skin surface 3. Rate of thermal transfer is dependent on the quality of the thermode-skin contact
Thermal: immersion in a thermostated water-bath		1. Rapid, although not instantaneous increase in skin temperature	
Thermal: CO_2 laser	Long-wavelength infrared source of radiation	1. Near total absorption of the light by the skin, irrespective of skin pigmentation or radiation from the skin surface 2. Thermal energy is maintained in the superficial surface of the skin where thermosensitive nerve terminals are located, limiting damage and therefore pain in deeper tissues 3. A highly focused beam can be generated, good spatial discrimination 4. Very rapid rates of heating can be achieved, allowing rapid onset and offset of the stimulus while meeting target temperature 5. No contact between the laser and the skin is necessary, therefore there is no concurrent activation of mechanosensitive non-nociceptive nerves	1. Expensive to buy 2. Safety precautions must be adopted during use (e.g., humans should wear protective eye goggles to prevent retinal damage from stray laser light)
Mechanical	Activation of A-δ and C fiber mechanoreceptors (e.g., von Frey filaments) Visceral pain can also be triggered by mechanical distension (e.g., colonic distension with a balloon)	1. Mechanical hyperalgesia is a cardinal feature chronic pain, therefore testing mechanical sensitivity is clinically relevant	1. Low-threshold mechanoreceptors are always co-stimulated, therefore the stimulus is not specific 2. Conventional mechanical stimuli, e.g., von Frey filaments, do not allow delivery of brief mechanical stimuli with a rapid onset and offset 3. Difficult to apply in a controlled manner to laboratory animals

Table 29.2 Phasic tests utilizing thermal stimuli.

Test	Brief Description of Methods Including Activation of Nociceptive/Pain Pathways	Species in Which Tests Are Commonly Applied	Behavioral End-Point	'Cut-Off'	Advantages	Disadvantages
Tail flick test (radiant heat)	Radiant heat applied to a small area on the tail; reaction time before a tail flick occurs is measured, 'tail-flick-latency.' Radiant heat emission can be controlled to adjust 'tail-flick latency' to alter sensitivity of the assay. A photoelectric cell timer switches off the lamp (heat source) when the tail is withdrawn. Selective activation of cutaneous thermosensitive and nociceptive fibers	Rodents	Tail-flick. Generally considered to be a spinal reflex when high-intensity power is used to generate the radiant heat and the tail flick latency is short. Will be subject to control by supraspinal structures. When the rate of heating is slower, then tail flick probably involves higher neural structures	Maximum latency (usually estimated to be 4–5 times the latency in naive animals)	Simple to carry out. Clearly identifiable end-point response, limits variability between animals under controlled experimental conditions	Tail is the predominant organ of thermoregulation in the rat. Factors that can affect tail flick latency and must be controlled for within an experiment include: 1. The rate of heating (determined by the power of the radiant heat source) 2. The area of tail stimulated (both site, proximal or distal, and total area). Prone to habituation (i.e., increase in latency) with shortened inter-stimulus interval and increased stimulus intensity
Tail flick test (immersion method)	Immersion of the tail in a hot liquid to produce a very rapid and linear increase in tail temperature. Greater area of the tail stimulated than for the radiant heat method. Latency to tail movement is measured A noxious cold stimulus can be used instead of a heat stimulus. Selective activation of cutaneous thermosensitive and nociceptive fibers	Rodents Monkey	Sudden movement of the tail that may be associated with whole-body movements	Maximum latency (see above)	Simple to carry out. Reflexes and higher neural structures generate the end point behavior Capability to change the temperature of the water-bath and therefore alter the sensitivity of the test (e.g., to study analgesics of different efficacies)	Tail is the predominant organ of thermoregulation in the rat. Latency will be modulated by the surface area of the tail stimulated
Paw withdrawal test	Radiant heat is applied to the plantar surface of the hind paw. Latency to paw-withdrawal is measured, a photoelectric cell timer switches off the lamp (heat source) when the paw is withdrawn. Termed the Hargreaves test when combined with inflammation to study hyperalgesia. Selective activation of cutaneous thermosensitive and nociceptive fibers	Rodents Dog	Paw withdrawal. Complex behavioral response	Maximum latency (see above)	Simple. Animal is freely moving, readily able to perform withdrawal responses	Baseline temperature of the skin will affect the latency to withdrawal. Freely moving animal, background level of activity in the flexor muscles of the leg varies with the position of the animal and this can alter speed of withdrawal response
Radiant heat	Heat source applied to a distinct body part on the animal, e.g., coronary band in horses, flank in pigs. Radiant heat may be generated by a light source or CO_2 laser. Selective activation of cutaneous thermosensitive and nociceptive fibers	Equidae Pig Cat	Withdrawal response to move the body part away from the stimulus, e.g., foot lift	Maximum latency (see above)	Simple	Some restraint is necessary to allow the heat to be focused on to the selected body part. Baseline temperature of the skin will affect the latency to withdrawal
Hot-plate test	Animal is introduced to an open-ended cylindrical space with a floor consisting of a metallic plate that is heated to a constant temperature (most commonly by a thermode). Reaction time (latency) to a behavioral response is measured. Activation of cutaneous thermosensitive and nociceptive fibers, co-activation of low-threshold mechanoreceptors	Rodents Birds (adapted, e.g., heated perch)	Paw licking. Jumping. Other complex behaviors such as sniffing or washing may be observed. Complex behavioral responses that are supraspinally integrated	Maximum latency (see above)	Various behavioral end-points may be differentially sensitive to analgesic drugs (increases sensitivity of the assay)	Stimulates all four limbs and tail simultaneously; may therefore recruit descending endogenous analgesia mechanisms. Complexity of behavioral responses that vary between animals can make it difficult to define the end-point. Reaction times decrease with increased testing of the same animal, therefore difficult to obtain a stable baselines
Contact thermode secured to the skin of the animal over a body part that is relatively flat to ensure sustained contact at the same pressure	Conventional thermodes have slow (<1 °C/s) rates of heating and selectively activate C fibers rather than A-δ fibers. Temperature at which a behavioral response occurs is the 'threshold' temperature. Activation of cutaneous thermosensitive and nociceptive fibers, co-activation of low-threshold mechanoreceptors	Equidae Cat Dog Birds Reptiles	*Nature* of the response varies between species, time of the response (early or late), and the site of application of the stimulus. Repertoire of behavioral end-points may be documented, e.g., skin twitch, head turn, movement to try to avoid the stimulus, leg lift (if stimulus is applied to the distal limb). Reflex and organized complex responses occur	Maximum temperature varies dependent on species and type of thermode	Equipment is relatively simple to build. Can apply to freely moving animal and well tolerated	*Nature* of the end-point may vary between animals, can be difficult to compare data between animals and between different experimenters. Limited sites of application of the thermode dependent on species. Threshold temperature affected by factors such as starting skin temperature and environmental temperature
Cold (rarely used in phasic tests of acute pain in naive animals, commonly used to assess neuropathic pain)	Application of a droplet of acetone or ethyl chloride spray to the hind paw to provide localized cooling of the skin. Use of ice–water baths (tail or foot immersion) or cold plates (e.g., Peltier cooled plate) on which the animal stands	Rodents Dog	Behavioral response (e.g., withdrawal) from the cold stimulus is typically observed, such as foot lifting, latency to lift the paw from a cold plate)	Maximum latency (usually estimated to be 4–5 times the latency in naive animals)	Abnormal sensory responses to cold are a common feature of clinical neuropathic pain states in humans	Magnitude of the cold stimulus is difficult to control and is affected by the ambient temperature and the temperature of the animal's skin

Table 29.3 Phasic tests utilizing mechanical stimuli.

Test	Brief Description of Methods Including Activation of Nociceptive/Pain Pathways	Species in Which Tests are Commonly Applied	Behavioral End-Point	'Cut-Off'	Advantages	Disadvantages
von Frey	von Frey filaments are blunt-ended plastic hairs of various diameters on fixed applicators. They are applied locally (most commonly to the plantar surface of the hind paw in rats) until they bend, at which point they exert a calibrated pressure. Filaments may also be used to assess responses to dynamic mechanical stimuli (e.g., brush allodynia). Automated and electronic von Frey devices are also available that provide a continuous scale of application (e.g., electronic asthesiometer). Site of application is variable in animals other than rodents. A-δ and C fibers (depending on filament diameter), co-activation of low-threshold mechanoreceptor	Rodents Dog Equidae Cattle Sheep	Withdrawal response to move away from the stimulus. May be accompanied by behaviors such as licking (e.g., of the paw) in animals with inflammatory or neuropathic pain arises from the stimulated area. The von Frey filament weight or the pressure applied by an electronic device required to elicit withdrawal is recorded	Manual von Frey filament systems do not employ a 'cut-off,' although this may be imposed by the experimenter. Automated devices allow a maximum preset pressure to be attained and the stimulus application is stopped. Maximum force (usually estimated to be 4–5 times the force in naive animals)	Easy to apply. May evaluate mechanical hyperalgesia and allodynia (although difficult to distinguish between them). Widely used, large body of published reference data	No 'gold standard' protocol for application, data generated between different experimenters and labs are very variable. Not nociceptive specific as co-activation of low-threshold mechanoreceptors. Debate about whether stimulus application elicits pain or nociception/mechanical sensations (e.g., touch) only. Rate of application of force not standardized in manual von Frey testing
Randall–Selitto test	Hind paw is placed between a fixed element (e.g., surface or blunt point) and a mobile blunt point exerting controlled pressure. The pressure is usually provided by a sliding counterweight system. Predominantly A-δ fibers, co-activation of low-threshold mechanoreceptor	Rat	Threshold (in grams) for appearance of a given behavior. The behavior may be a reflex withdrawal, struggling, or vocalization depending on the protocol	Imposed by the experimenter, should be below the level at which stimulus application causes tissue damage (usually estimated to be 4–5 times the force in naive animals)	When carried out correctly can give reproducible and reliable readings	Requires the animal to be restrained in an unnatural position, which requires training and prehabituation
Strain gauges	Strain gauges are fixed on blunt forceps. The animal is loosely restrained, the forceps are placed around the hind paw and an incremental force is applied until the paw is withdrawn. Predominantly A-δ fibers (dependent on probe type), co-activation of low-threshold mechanoreceptor	Rat	Withdrawal response	Imposed by the experimenter, should be below the level at which stimulus application causes tissue damage (usually estimated to be 4–5 times the force in naive animals)	When carried out correctly can give reproducible and reliable readings	Rate of application of force is variable depending on the experimenter; careful standardization is required
Mechanical devices used in species other than rodents	A variety of devices have been described. In general, force is applied to a body part via a blunt-ended pin/probe that is advanced against the skin and tissues using pneumatic devices that may be manually or electronically controlled. Nociceptive fiber activation will be determined by the type of pin/probe; sharp tips are more likely to activate A-δ fibers, larger diameter blunt-ended pins will more likely activate C fibers. Co-activation of low-threshold mechanoreceptors	Dog Cat Equidae Chicken	Withdrawal response; commonly the stimuli are applied to the limb, hence limb withdrawal is a common end-point	Imposed by the experimenter, should be below the level at which stimulus application causes tissue damage. Maximum latency (usually estimated to be 4–5 times the force in naive animals)	Devices are secured to the animal allowing it to be free moving. Well tolerated by animals. Rate of application of force can be controlled	Prehabituation may be required to give repeatable responses within the same individual. Repertoire of behavioral responses may be shown that signal the 'end-point' of the test, can lead to variability between different experimenters

Table 29.4 Phasic tests utilizing electrical stimuli.

Test	Brief Description of Methods Including Activation of Nociceptive/Pain Pathways	Species in Which Tests are Commonly Applied	Behavioral End-Point	'Cut-Off'	Advantages	Disadvantages
Application of long-lasting trains of electrical stimuli applied to the tail and/or paw	Electrical stimuli of gradually increasing intensities are delivered in trains lasting hundreds of milliseconds using subcutaneous electrodes or via the floor of a cage in which the animal is placed	Rodents	Sequence of responses depending on intensity from reflex movement/withdrawal, vocalization during stimulation, and vocalization that persists after the end of the stimulus. Responses are organized on a hierarchical basis dependent on the level of integration of the nociceptive and pain pathways	Maximum current intensity (estimated to be 4–5 times the intensity in naive animals)	Complex behavioral responses can be elicited	Concurrent stimulation of the paws and tail (electrical stimulation delivered through the floor) will likely recruit endogenous analgesia mechanisms
Use of single shocks or short chains of electrical stimulation of the tail	Threshold current intensity at which a defined behavioral response is displayed (±latency to the response). Stimuli delivered via subcutaneous electrodes	Rodents Monkeys	Sequence of behaviors; twitching, escape behaviors, vocalizations, and biting of the electrodes that are hierarchically organized (see above). Vocalizations may be recorded electronically and analyzed (e.g., spectrum, reaction time, threshold to vocalization)	Maximum current intensity (estimated to be 4–5 times the intensity in naive animals)	Complex behavioral responses can be elicited	
Electrical stimulation of the dental pulp	Some evidence to indicate that most of the afferent nerve fibers in dental pulp are nociceptive, thus allowing selective activation of nociceptive fibers using electrical stimuli. The experimental paradigm varies depending on the physiology of the tooth being stimulated (i.e., whether the tooth is continuously erupting, e.g., rat incisors, or has limited growth (e.g., cat and dog)	Rodents Dog Cat Monkeys	Disynaptic jaw-opening reflex that can be recorded electromyographically from the digastric muscle in awake animals. Coordinate behavioral responses such as licking, chewing, or changes in facial expression	Maximum current intensity (estimated to be 4–5 times the intensity in naive animals)	Reflex response is easily quantifiable. Can reveal the activity of non-opioid analgesics that cannot be detected by the hot-plate test	Debate over the selectivity of the electrical stimulus to activate nociceptive fibers. Not sensitive to the effects of NSAIDs

Table 29.5 Advantages and limitations of neurophysiologic techniques used to measure pain in awake animals.

Technique	Advantages	Limitations
Raw electroencephalogram	Flexible – the user can manipulate the recording equipment in order to optimize signal quality. All EEG data are retained, allowing comprehensive and detailed analysis. Data are recorded in real time rather than provision of discontinuous data points	Large quantities of data are generated that can hinder interpretation. Data require complex mathematical processing after collection; therefore, they cannot be immediately interpreted. Definition of an 'end-point' to a ramped stimulus is therefore problematic. A basic understanding of EEG recording is required. Subcutaneous needle electrodes or surface electrodes usually give a poor signal-to-noise ratio in awake animals; implantation of dural electrodes for awake recordings is invasive
Evoked potentials, e.g., somatosensory-evoked potentials (SEPs)	Evoked potentials generated from high-intensity noxious stimuli provide specific information on the neural processing of noxious stimuli. Targeted placement of electrodes at specific intracerebral loci allows the brain structures involved in the neural processing of pain to be identified. The SEP waveform is relatively easy to interpret	Signal averaging is required to generate a SEP; therefore, noxious stimuli must be repeatedly applied. The amplitude of the SEP signal is small compared with the EEG or electrical noise. Some skill is required to generate a SEP with an acceptable signal-to-noise ratio. The stimuli used to generate a SEP should only stimulate nociceptive fibers or the SEP will include non-nociceptive components. This is challenging and has only been achieved using radiant heat generated by lasers. Laser-evoked potentials reflect predominately A-δ fiber mediated activity rather than C fiber activity. Owing to the difficulties in generating a noxious stimulus that is time locked to allow EEG recording, SEPs are most commonly generated to heat (laser-evoked potentials) or electrical stimuli only.

electrocorticogram (ECoG), whereas electrical activity recorded from the scalp is the EEG. The EEG and ECoG are both far-field potentials. An evoked potential (EP) is generated by recording the EEG time locked to a sensory stimulus, such as presentation of an auditory tone. Averaging of the EEG over a sequence of responses allows the electrical activity specific to the stimulus to be extracted and presented by a plot of voltage (amplitude) against time. Somatosensory-evoked potentials (SEPs) recorded from the dura at various loci in animals in response to repetitive noxious stimuli are used extensively to study pain and analgesia [65–68]. Table 29.5 outlines the advantages and limitations of EEG and EPs in phasic pain tests.

Nociceptive withdrawal reflexes (NWRs) are an established neurophysiologic measure used in rodent models as a direct measure of spinal cord hyperexcitability and thus a biomarker of central sensitization [69,70]. They have also been translated to humans to quantify spinal cord excitability in patients with chronic pain, including pain caused by OA [71]. The NWR threshold is defined as the magnitude of the stimulus (e.g., electrical current) that is required to elicit an electromyographic (EMG) response remembering that central sensitization causes a decrease in this threshold. Temporal summation (amplification of the magnitude of the EMG signal in response to repetitive noxious stimulation) of the NWR is also measured to probe changes in the spinal nociceptive processing. Use of these techniques in rodents requires anesthesia. NWR thresholds and temporal summation have been measured in awake dogs and horses using electrical stimuli and used to characterize the antinociceptive effects of analgesic drugs [72–78].

The third major neurophysiologic end-point used in phasic pain tests in laboratory animals is direct recording of neuronal activity during stimulus application, for example, recording from peripheral afferent sensory fibers or from dorsal horn neurons using *in vivo* electrophysiology. These studies are usually carried out under terminal anesthesia.

Ethical considerations

It is widely acknowledged that studies in animals have played, and will continue to play, a pivotal role in advancing knowledge and developing new analgesic molecules in pain research. However, the majority of pain studies require the delivery of painful stimuli to the animal, and therefore are associated with ethical concerns and constraints that must be respected by the research community. The IASP published guidelines on the ethical use of animals in pain research [79], which are updated regularly and are a good reference source for people working in this field. The key points of the guidelines with respect to ethics in pain research are summarized as follows:

- Understand moral and ethical issues and arguments associated with the use of animals in experimentation.
- Understand how to design experiments that minimize the numbers of animals used, that maximize statistical inferences, and that maximize the recording of variables relevant to the assessment of pain experienced by animals.
- Know how to employ a nociceptive stimulus or condition that is minimal in intensity and duration (tested on the investigator when possible) so as to shorten the duration of an experiment consistent with the attainment of justifiable, ethical research objectives.
- Know reasons why unanesthetized animals should be minimally exposed to nociceptive stimuli from which they cannot escape or which they cannot avoid or terminate.
- Know reasons why pharmacologically paralyzed animals are anaesthetized or rendered neurosurgically insensate.

Maximum stimulus intensity

All phasic pain tests should incorporate a maximum stimulus intensity that is not exceeded in any test and is below the threshold intensity for that stimulus modality that is sufficient to cause lasting tissue damage. This is fundamental to carrying out pain experiments ethically in animals. It is important to maintain the physiologic well-being of the animal to ensure that collected data are valid, since tissue damage at the site of stimulation will induce peripheral and central sensitization that will result in a change in responsiveness in the pain test over time. The time interval between the application of each repeat test should be selected in order to prevent upregulation of nociceptive pathways. These factors are particularly important in tests involving the administration of analgesic drugs, where behavioral responses to the assay may be obtunded until high stimulus intensities would be otherwise attained.

Measurement of nociceptive withdrawal thresholds in companion animals

In recent years, numerous studies have been published in which nociceptive withdrawal thresholds were utilized to investigate the analgesic efficacy of drugs in companion animals [80–84] and to probe upregulation of nociceptive processes in clinical conditions causing pain (e.g., after surgery or as a result of chronic inflammatory diseases such as foot rot in sheep) [29,85–87]. Undoubtedly, measurement of nociceptive withdrawal thresholds to assess analgesic drug efficacy has a number of advantages. However, the effect of confounding factors must be understood in order to maximize the quality of the collected data. For example, environmental temperature, skin temperature, and level of distraction of the animal can all affect measured thresholds. Some advantages of the measurement of nociceptive withdrawal thresholds to quantify analgesic drug efficacy include the following:

- It is applied to naive animals to study the test drug in the target species.
- It is an objective measure of drug effect against a standardized noxious stimulus, thereby eliminating the variability associated with measuring drug effect in a clinical pain model.
- The methodology is ethically acceptable; imposing a maximum stimulus intensity below the level required to cause tissue damage prevents lasting harm.

However, there are a number of important limitations associated with the measurement of nociceptive withdrawal thresholds that must be considered during data interpretation:

- The technique relies on the detection of an end-point behavior that may be reflexive (e.g., skin twitch) or more complex (whole-body movement away from the stimulus). When measuring responses to analgesic drug administration, it is important that the end-point response is standardized to reduce variability in the collected data.
- It is problematic to relate a change in threshold to the clinical efficacy of the drug with any certainty.
- Owing to the requirement to impose a maximum stimulus intensity, data are very commonly censored following administration of an analgesic drug, so that the relative efficacies of different drugs (where censorship occurs for more than one drug) cannot be determined.
- There is a minimal time interval required between subsequent tests in order to prevent sensitization, which is problematic for pharmacokinetic–pharmacodynamic studies where frequent measurement of nociceptive thresholds is advantageous.
- Measurement of nociceptive withdrawal thresholds in naive animals allows the measurement of the analgesic effect of the drug (e.g., analgesic efficacy of opioids) but does not allow the assessment of the antihyperalgesic effects of drugs such as NSAIDs unless an inflammatory focus is introduced.

Pain models – tonic tests

Some pain models induce pain created by tissue or nerve injury and are therefore associated with medium- to long-lasting pain. Naturally occurring disease models of pain in animals are attractive because of their greater translatability to clinical pain conditions in humans; however, the number of conditions for which a well-characterized spontaneous pain model exists is currently limited.

Animal models of pain should fulfill a multidimensional set of criteria of validity to be considered relevant for human pathophysiology, of which face, mechanistic, and predictive validity are considered pivotal [88]. Face validity is the similarity of what is observed in the animal model to the human, and is considered in terms of both ethologic validity (i.e., similarity in behaviors) and biomarker validity (i.e., the function of the biomarker in representing underlying neurobiological mechanisms). Mechanistic validity assesses the similarity of the mechanism working in the animal model to the mechanism that is presumed to be working in the human disease, referring at the same time to the mechanism that is considered to produce changes in a biological biomarker and the mechanism that is sensitive to the action of effective therapeutic agents. Predictive validity is the performance of a therapeutic agent in the animal model compared with the therapeutic efficacy in clinical patients. It is widely acknowledged that current animal pain models fail to meet these criteria fully.

Induced pain models

A large number of different pain models have been developed with the primary aim of increasing understanding and treatment of clinical pain states. The majority of these have been developed in rodents, but some have been translated to companion and farm animals. Models are broadly divided into inflammatory or neuropathic pain models, although some newer models trigger both inflammatory and neuropathic pain mechanisms because it is recognized that many clinical pain conditions in humans have both a neuropathic and an inflammatory component [89]. Induced disease models have also been developed to replicate some disease conditions in humans, such as painful diabetic neuropathy and postherpetic neuralgia [90–92]. A large repertoire of biomarkers are used to assay pain in animal models. Broadly, these biomarkers can be classified based on whether the biomarker involves (1) measurement of phasic responses to acute noxious stimuli in awake animals (see above); (2) measurement of changes in spontaneous behavior; (3) assessment of affective state in more complex behavioral tests; or (4) measurements conducted in anesthetized animals (e.g., nociceptive withdrawal reflexes).

Models of inflammatory pain

Most models of inflammatory pain involve the injection of inflammatory mediators themselves or of chemical substances that provoke an immune response. The substances may be injected intradermally or subcutaneously, intraperitoneally, or into the joint capsule. Common cutaneous models of inflammatory pain and their advantages and disadvantages are shown in Table 29.6. Recognition that pain elicited from muscle has different characteristics from cutaneous pain has led to the development of models of muscle pain and hyperalgesia to understand better the mechanisms underlying the development of chronic muscle pain. Stimuli used to elicit muscle pain include injection of low-pH saline (pH 5.2–6.9), carrageenan, cytokines (e.g., tumor necrosis factor alpha and interleukin 6), mustard oil, zymogen, and hypertonic saline.

Arthritis is one of the most prevalent chronic health conditions and is a leading cause of disability in humans. Therefore, arthritis pain has long been a major area of research in biomedical science and different animal models of arthritis are available for the assessment of joint pain and analgesic drug effects. Commonly the knee (stifle) joint is studied in OA models. Animal models of OA include spontaneous OA in specific strains of mice and guinea pig, intra-articular injections of compounds to induce joint inflammation, or surgical disruption of the joint. Common models of arthritis (OA and rheumatoid arthritis) and their advantages and disadvantages are summarized in Table 29.7. Common methods of assessing arthritic knee joint pain are given in Table 29.8, including their advantages and disadvantages.

Models of neuropathic pain

Neuropathic pain is characterized by sensory abnormalities such as unpleasant abnormal sensation (dysesthesia), hyperalgesia, and allodynia. A battery of neuropathic pain models have been developed in animals in an attempt to simulate the diverse etiology of clinical neuropathic pain conditions in humans. These models cause substantial suffering to the animal, in terms of both pain severity and duration. As such, predefined end-points are usually imposed that can be used to indicate when euthanasia of the animal is required. These end-points are often relatively crude and relate to the general health status of the animal, for example, weight loss. There are no translational neuropathic pain models because the nerve damage required to produce neuropathic pain is irreversible. Table 29.9 gives an overview of the characteristics of commonly used models of neuropathic pain, with their advantages and disadvantages. Until recently, neuropathic pain in these models was most commonly assessed by application of phasic pain tests and assessment of behavior. For additional discussion, see the section Clinical Pain Assessment in Veterinary Medicine.

Models of visceral pain

Visceral pain, particularly arising from the bowel, is one of the most common reasons for medical presentation in humans and an area of unmet clinical need. Models of visceral pain in animals have been developed both to understand better the underlying neurophysiology of visceral pain pathways and to understand dysregulations of visceral hypersensitivity that occur with functional bowel disorders, such as irritable bowel syndrome (IBS). However, modeling IBS is particularly challenging because it is a functional disorder and therefore lacks significant pathology around which an animal model is based. An overview of methods used to induce visceral pain or visceral sensitivity in animals is given in Table 29.10. These methods are broadly divided into phasic stimuli that cause transient visceral stimulation (e.g., colorectal distension) and methods that produce tonic pain by inducing sensitization of the viscera (e.g., injection of irritant substances into the peritoneum or sensitization of the gut via instillation of irritant substances into the gut lumen). A range of different outcome measures are used to evaluate visceral pain in animals, ranging from behavior in awake animals to evoked reflexes and physiologic responses.

Behavior

Behavioral end-points that are species specific have been developed to quantify visceral nociception. The behavior of the rat has been scored during colorectal distension [93],where a graded score is given dependent on whether behavioral responses are confined to a brief head movement followed by immobility (score 1) through to body arching and lifting of pelvic structures (score 4). Referred somatic hyperalgesia associated with a noxious visceral stimulus is also used as a criterion for visceral pain, evaluated by, for example, application of von Frey hairs to the abdomen and scoring of subsequent behavioral responses. Owing to the prevalence of colic as a clinical manifestation of visceral pain in the horse, a number of methods are used to

Table 29.6 Common models of cutaneous inflammatory pain.

Name	Model Description	Species	Biomarker	Advantages	Disadvantages
Formalin test	0.5–0.15% formalin (37% formaldehyde) is injected intradermally (in rodents it is injected into the dorsal surface of the rat forepaw). Injection initially activates nociceptors (phase 1, 3 min after injection), the late phase (phase 2, 20–30 min after injection) involves a period of sensitization during which inflammatory phenomena (including paw edema) occur. Both phase 1 and 2 are considered to be triggered by peripheral mechanisms; phase 2 involves central sensitization	Rodents	Change in complex behaviors (licking, paw lifting). Behavioral reaction is biphasic accompanying the biphasic nature of the underlying neurophysiologic mechanisms that evoke pain. Application of phasic pain tests. Paw volume	Neurophysiology is well understood. Widely used as a pain assay, a large database to describe effects of different analgesics in the formalin model is available. Pain is of short duration (1–2 h) although inflammation may persist for a longer period	Difficult to quantify the pain-related behaviors, therefore outcome assessment can be variable between experimenters. Short-duration inflammatory pain model only
Carrageenan	Carrageenan is made from sulfated polysaccharides extracted from red seaweeds. It is injected to elicit localized inflammation through induction of an immune response and activation of nociceptors	Rodents (commonly injected intradermally in the paw). Cats, horses (tissue cage models)	Behavioral changes associated with inflammatory pain, generally less well defined than following injection of formalin. Application of phasic pain tests. Paw volume	Well established pain model Does not elicit a systemic immune response	Site of injection may remain thickened for a long duration, precluding repeat testing at the same site. Difficult to solubilize; thick, viscous substance that can make injection difficult
Complete Freund's adjuvant (CFA)	Suspension of heat-killed *Mycobacterium butyricum* or *Mycobacterium tuberculosum* in an adjuvant. Doses used in rodent pain models produce cutaneous inflammation that appears in minutes to hours and peaks within 5–8 h; duration of inflammation is ~24 h, hyperalgesia can persist for 1–2 weeks	Rodents (commonly injected intradermally in the paw)	See carrageenan	See carrageenan	See carrageenan
Mustard oil	Elicits inflammatory pain by activating transient receptor potential cation channel, subfamily A (TRPA1), an excitatory ion channel of primary afferent nociceptors. Usually applied topically to the skin; effects are of short duration	Rodents	See carrageenan		
Zymogen	A glucan from the cell walls of yeast; activates primary afferent nociceptors	Rodents	See carrageenan		
Kaolin	A suspension of kaolin is injected subcutaneously; may be mixed with carrageenan. Duration of inflammatory pain is ~1–2 days	Cats Rodents	Application of phasic pain tests	Well-established pain model	See carrageenan
Capsaicin	Pungent component of chilies that activates the transient receptor potential vanilloid type 1 (TRPV1), a heat-sensitive cation on nociceptor terminals. Used to study neurogenic inflammation and hyperalgesia. Intradermal injection of capsaicin results in a flare reaction (neurogenic inflammation), allodynia, and hyperalgesia, the areas of which extend beyond the injection site. Duration of thermal and mechanical hyperalgesia is dose dependent but can be up to 24 h	Rodents Humans	Application of phasic pain tests. Area of flare	Translational. Well-established pain model; the underlying neurophysiologic mechanisms are well described	Poor relationship between underlying pain mechanisms following capsaicin and clinical pain states. Repeated application of capsaicin results in desensitization of nociceptors to capsaicin and other noxious stimuli (which is reversible). At high concentrations capsaicin will cause sensory neuron toxicity and cell death
Skin incision	A surgical skin incision is used to generate inflammation	Rodents	Application of phasic pain tests. Behavioral changes associated with inflammatory pain	Triggers inflammatory pain mechanisms that are identical with those triggered by surgical trauma	Invasive. Cannot repeat in individual animals. Care must be taken to ensure asepsis
Surgery (e.g., castration and ovariohysterectomy)	Animals undergoing routine neutering are recruited for analgesia studies	Cats Dogs Equidae Deer (e.g., velvet antler removal)	Behavior. Application of phasic pain tests. EEG and EPs	Animals would be undergoing surgery anyway, therefore adheres to the experimental principle of reduction. Clinically relevant pain model to allow study of pain mechanisms and efficacy of analgesic drugs	Magnitude of the surgical stimulus may vary depending on patient factors and the skill of the surgeon. Requires case recruitment (i.e., owner consent)
UVb irradiation	Exposure to a UVb light source to produce a localized burn injury characterized by sterile inflammation	Rats Pigs	Application of phasic pain tests	Translational. Induces central and peripheral sensitization	Characteristics of the skin will affect the magnitude of the injury induced by a standardized exposure to UVb radiation

Table 29.7 Models of osteoarthritis and rheumatoid arthritis.

Name	Model Description	Species	Advantages	Disadvantages
Spontaneous OA in specific guinea pig strains, e.g., Hartley albino guinea pig	Bilateral disease of the knee joint that involves cartilage degeneration, subchondral sclerosis, and bone cysts. The pathogenesis is not fully understood	Guinea pig	Predictable onset and progression of the disease. Many similarities in disease progression to human OA	The strains of guinea pig are expensive to buy and must be housed for a long period before severe OA changes develop (up to 2 years)
Spontaneous OA in other laboratory animals	See above	Hamster Mouse	See above	See above, although progression of the disease will be more rapid in animals with a shorter life span, such as mice
Surgically induced OA	Surgically induced trauma to the joint caused by creation of a meniscal tear or menisectomy. Progressive changes in the knee joint occur relatively rapidly postsurgery	Rat Mouse Guinea pig Dog Rabbit	Reproducible. Mimics pathologic changes and pain of OA in humans	Depending on the size of the animal (species), the surgery can be technically challenging. Rapid progression of lesions after surgery, therefore insensitive in the detection of new compounds with protective effects against the development of OA
Intra-articular monosodium iodoacetate (MIA) injection into the knee	Induces degeneration of cartilage by inhibition of aerobic glycolysis, which kills chondrocytes. Joint pathology is characterized by chondrocyte necrosis resulting in decreased thickness of articular cartilage and fibrillation of the cartilage surface, separation of necrotic cartilage from the underlying bone, and exposure of subchondral bone	Can be induced in many species, commonly used in rats	Induced pathology is similar to human OA	Arthritic changes take several weeks to develop
Inflammatory monoarthritis (knee joint)	Injection of kaolin and carrageenan into the joint to produce an aseptic use-dependent monoarthritis with damage to the cartilage, inflammation of the synovia, and synovial fluid exudate. Other irritants that may be injected include zymosan and complete Freund's adjuvant (CFA)	Predominantly rat and mouse, cat, primate	Joint inflammation develops rapidly and persists for weeks. Large database relating to use of the model in laboratory animals	Only mimics the acute inflammatory phase of human OA
Rheumatoid arthritis	Polyarthritis induced by injection of immunogenic adjuvants (e.g., CFA). The adjuvant is usually injected intradermally or subcutaneously into the footpad or base of the tail to generate a polyarthritis	Predominantly rat and mouse	Well established and reproducible	Systemic nature of the arthritis can affect the overall condition and well-being of the animals and confound pain assessment
Rheumatoid arthritis	Immunogenic adjuvant arthritis induced by intradermal injection of cartilage-derived proteins	Rat Mouse	See above	See above
Rheumatoid arthritis	Non-immunogenic adjuvant arthritis induced by injection of compounds that do not contain major histocompatibility complex-binding peptides but involve T cell activation, e.g., mineral oil injected intradermally or subcutaneously	Rat Mouse	See above	See above
Gouty arthritis	Injection of monosodium urate crystals dissolved in saline or uric acid or suspended in mineral oil into the knee joint to produce acute inflammation	Rat Mouse Dog Chicken Cat	Acute synovitis generated within a few hours that resolves rapidly (within 3–7 days). No signs of systemic disease	

evaluate visceral pain in this species following visceral distension. End-point behaviors include expulsion of the balloon from the rectum (colorectal distension) associated with flank watching [94,95] and signs of abdominal pain such as pawing at the ground, kicking of the abdomen, and weight shifting of the hind limbs following duodenal distension [96]. Writhing (i.e., stereotyped abdominal contractions, movements of the whole body, twisting of the dorsoabdominal muscles, reduction in motor activity, and motor incoordination) are evoked in response to intraperitoneal administration of irritants and are collectively used as the outcome measure in the abdominal writhing test (rodents). The movements are considered reflex responses and are quantified in terms of their frequency. However, the frequency of cramps decreases spontaneously over time and therefore the writhing test is not used to assess the duration of action of putative analgesics. The number of cramps is also extremely variable between individual animals.

Abdominal muscle contraction

A common end-point in rodent studies of visceral nociception is contraction of the abdominal muscles in response to colorectal distension, usually recorded using electromyography in both awake (by prior implantation of EMG wires) and anesthetized animals [97,98]. There is a correlation between the distending pressure and the integrated electromyographic signal or the number of spike bursts during the period of distension. Electromyographic responses in neck muscles can also be recorded as a measure of nociceptive response to gastric distension. To avoid implanting EMG wires in muscles, abdominal contraction following balloon distension can be detected by amplifying rapid changes in pressure that are induced in the balloon.

Table 29.8 Common methods of assessing knee joint pain in arthritis.

Name	Brief Description of the Biomarker	Common Species in Which the Outcome Measure is Utilized	Advantages	Disadvantages
Weight bearing on the hind paws	Weight distribution between the two hind paws is measured as the force exerted by each hind limb on a transducer plate in the floor over a given period. Weight borne by each hind limb is expressed as a percentage of bodyweight. A weight-bearing deficit on the affected limb is taken as an indicator of pain	Rodents	Simple. Translational	Requires restraint of the animal and does not assess weight distribution to the forelimbs as occurs with hind limb arthritis. Indirect measure of knee pain
Weight bearing across all four paws	Weight load is detected while the animal is walking across four pairs of force sensor plates on the floor of an enclosed walkway	Rodents Dog Assessment of arthritis in other joints in chicken, cat, horse	Simple. Does not require restraint of the animal although a constant walking speed is usually necessary to facilitate data interpretation. Translational	Animals are required to move, which can be affected by motivation (and is integrally linked to pain)
Posture and gait analysis	Static and dynamic behaviors have been quantified using subjective rating scales. Gait analysis using kinematic techniques	Rodents Large animal species including dog, cat, horse, chicken	Subjective scales are simple to use and cheap. Gait analysis techniques are objective. Translational	Subjective scales are inherently variable and unvalidated. Gait analysis data can be difficult to interpret and require the animal to walk at a constant speed. Willingness to walk is affected by motivation (and is integrally linked to pain)
Spontaneous mobility	Automated systems are available (e.g., biotelemetry, activity boxes for rodents or continuous video of behavior and pattern recognition). Collar-mounted accelerometers to track movement over time along three axes. Assessment of willingness to perform spontaneous behavioral tasks, e.g., willingness of dogs to walk upstairs or cats to jump up or down from a raised surface	Rodents Large animal species including dog, cat, horse, chicken	Objective. Use of automated systems speeds and simplifies data analysis	Willingness to move is affected by motivation (and is integrally linked to pain)
Mechanical or heat sensitivity of the paw	See phasic pain tests (Tables 29.2 and 29.3)			
Mechanical sensitivity of the knee	Knee joint is compressed using calibrated forceps equipped with force transducers. Force required to evoke a reflex withdrawal is measured	Rat Mouse	Measures sensitivity of the knee joint that is not confounded by the hind paw Translational	Requires restraint of the animal
Struggling threshold angle of knee extension	Tibia is extended until the animal displays struggling behavior while the femur is held in position; the extension angle is then calculated	Rat	Measures sensitivity of the knee joint that is not confounded by the hind paw	Requires restraint of the animal
Vocalizations evoked by compression of the knee	Audible and ultrasonic vocalizations are measured, representing nociceptive and emotional–affective response, respectively	Rat Mouse	Ultrasonic vocalizations may give a better indication of joint pain than other reflexive measures such as withdrawal thresholds	Use of vocalizations has not been fully validated in rodent OA models
Neurophysiologic measures	Measurement of nociceptive withdrawal reflexes to electrical and mechanical stimuli in anesthetized animals to measure upregulation of central pain pathways. Direct recording from dorsal horn neurons to map peripheral receptive field size and neuronal activity (threshold and firing frequency) in response to non-noxious and noxious stimuli applied in the receptive field of the cell. Recording of spontaneous firing in peripheral sensory nerve fibers	Rat Mouse	Allows detailed investigation of the neurophysiologic changes accompanying pain caused by OA	Requires anesthesia; experiments are non-recovery. Technically challenging

Physiologic responses

In awake rats visceral distension causes an increase in blood pressure and tachycardia, whereas during deep, anesthesia a depressor response and bradycardia are generally noted (although the magnitude of the depressor/bradycardia response is modulated by the anesthetic agent used) [99].

Neuronal activity

The most direct approach to evaluate the effects of visceral distension is the recording of the neuronal activity of afferent or second-order neurons in anesthetized animals in acute electrophysiologic studies. Longer term neuronal responses are also evaluated by measuring c-fos expression in different areas of the spinal cord in response to mechanical distension. Visceral evoked potentials following colorectal distension are used to evaluate visceral nociception in awake rats [100,101].

Naturally occurring disease models

The study of naturally occurring or spontaneous diseases in animals has great potential because the underlying etiopathogenesis of the pain more likely replicates the mechanisms that result in clinical pain states in humans. With the exception of spontaneous

Table 29.9 Examples of common models of neuropathic pain, all of which are commonly induced in rat and mouse.

Name	Model Description	Induced Behavioral Changes	Advantages	Disadvantages
Peripheral nerve injury models				
Axotomy model	Complete transection of the sciatic nerve at the mid-thigh level combined with lesioning of the saphenous nerve to induce complete denervation of the hind limb. A neuroma develops at the proximal nerve stump	Pain is produced in the absence of any sensory input to the area. Autotomy is often observed, although whether this is an indication of spontaneous pain or a result of excessive grooming in the absence of sensory feedback is debated		Complete nerve transection is uncommon in humans. Severe ethical issues associated with autotomy
Chronic constriction injury	3–4 loose silk ligatures are placed around the sciatic nerve. Constriction of the sciatic nerve is associated with intraneural edema, focal ischemia, and Wallerian degeneration	Mild to moderate autotomy, guarding, excessive licking, and altered weight bearing. These features persist for at least 7 weeks after surgery	Clinical features correspond to complex regional pain syndrome in humans and the model has been used extensively for research on spontaneous pain and abnormal sensations	Variable outcome between different animals likely associated with the tightness of the ligatures placed around the nerve and type of suture material
Partial sciatic nerve ligation	Tight ligation of half to one-third of the sciatic nerve using a single ligature	Paw guarding and licking, not associated with autotomy	Immediate onset and long-lasting duration of allodynia and hyperalgesia parallel pain in humans with causalgia	
Spared nerve injury	The tibial and common peroneal nerves are tightly ligated followed by axotomy of the distal nerve, the sural nerve remains undamaged (hence spared nerve injury model). Allows the comparison of difference in mechanical and thermal sensitivities of non-injured skin territories adjoining denervated areas	See above	Surgical model is relatively easy to create compared with other models and lesser variability in the degree of damage. Allows simultaneous investigational changes in both injured primary sensory neurons and in unharmed sensory neurons so that their relative contribution to the pathophysiology of pain can be determined	
Sciatic inflammatory neuritis	A catheter is implanted around the sciatic nerve (under anesthesia), which is used to inject zymosan in awake, freely moving rats	See above	Human neuropathies are commonly caused by inflammation or infection rather than trauma, and inflammatory events occur after trauma. This model may better mimic many human conditions causing neuropathic pain	
Cuffing of the sciatic nerve	Placement of a polyethylene cuff around the sciatic nerve	See above	High reproducibility associated with a more consistent magnitude of nerve injury compared with nerve ligation or axotomy	
Central pain models				
Weight drop or contusion model	Spinal cord is exposed at the thoracolumbar level and a constant weight is dropped on the spinal cord to induce injury	Severe paraplegia and complete segmental necrosis. Dysthesia, spontaneous and evoked pain		Ethical considerations associated with paraplegia
Excitotoxic spinal cord injury	Intraspinal injections of excitatory amino acids to simulate injury induced elevations of excitatory amino acids	See above	Progressive pathologic changes associated with the injection closely resemble those induced by ischemic and traumatic spinal cord injury	
Spinal hemisection	Spinal cord is hemisected just cranial to L1 with a blade	See above	Numbers and types of injured fibers are controlled in each animal. The injured and intact sides of the animal are completely separated	
Drug-induced neuropathy models				
Drug-induced neuropathy	Systemic injection of drugs that induce neuropathy such as vincristine and cisplatin	Induce neuropathy; the clinical features are determined by the nerve type targeted by the drug	Non-surgical	Drugs often produce concurrent effects on the general health of the animal that can confound pain assessment
Disease-induced neuropathy models				
Diabetes-induced neuropathy	Diabetes is induced in the animal, for example, by administration of pancreatic β-cell toxins such as streptozotocin (STZ) or use of transgenic animals (mice) with type I and II diabetes	Induce a peripheral neuropathy with associated signs of neuropathic pain	Depending on the model can replicate clinical signs associated with painful diabetic neuropathy in humans	Animals develop other metabolic derangements associated with diabetes that can confound pain assessment
Cancer pain models, e.g., bone cancer pain	Bone cancer is induced by, e.g., inoculation of osteolytic fibrosarcoma cells into the femur of specific strains of mice	Produce behavioral changes attributed to neuropathic and inflammatory pain	Demonstrate the distinct pharmacologic and neurochemical aspects of cancer pain, suggesting the involvement of inflammatory, neuropathic and tumorigenic components in the pathogenesis of pain	May induce systemic changes in the animal associated with tumor growth that can compromise well-being and confound pain assessment

Table 29.10 Common models of visceral pain.

Name	Model description	Advantages	Disadvantages
Visceral distension	Overfilling the bladder with fluid, pressure distension of the colon, duodenum, esophagus, or ureter. Distension pressure is usually controlled by a barostat (computer-controlled pump)	'Natural' type of stimulus. Mechanical distension is relatively easy to control	Challenging to develop devices that provide a rapid distension (square-wave stimulus); increasing ramp distension profile is more common. Type and predictability of the distension predict outcome, independent of the distension pressure. Repeated distension does not result in visceral hypersensitivity, therefore cannot replicate pain and the heightened visceral sensitivity that occurs in people with inflammatory bowel disease (IBD)
Chemical irritation to induce hypersensitivity of the colon prior to mechanical distension	Application of chemical irritants to the colon (e.g., instillation of acetic acid, mustard oil, turpentine, zymosan)	Induce peripheral and central sensitization and increase responses to mechanical distension	Debate over whether chemical irritation prior to distension induces changes similar to the function changes that occur in people with IBD
Chronic irrigation of the bladder to induce cystitis using compounds such as mustard oil and cyclophosphamide	Acute or chronic instillation of compounds that are known irritants	Chronic administration of compounds causes histologic and neurophysiologic bladder changes that are similar to pathologic changes induced by clinical conditions resulting in chronic cystitis	
Intraperitoneal injections of irritant agents, e.g., acetic or hydrochloric acid, bradykinin, mustard oil		Well-established pain model	Parietal peritoneum receives somatic innervation, therefore model causes visceral and somatic pain. Latency to writhing and duration are dependent on the chemical properties of the injected irritant
Models of acute pancreatitis pain	Induction of pancreatic damage using systemic injection (IV) of dibutyltin dichloride; pancreatic injection of capsaicin or bradykinin	Histologic changes resembling acute pancreatitis in humans develop	There are almost no models of chronic pancreatitis

OA in some species of guinea pig and rodents, spontaneous disease models are most relevant to large animals. Spontaneous OA in the dog is a commonly used and appropriate (although perhaps not the best) model for translational and comparative studies based on animal size, anatomy, disease mechanisms, clinical similarities, and response to therapy. OA in dogs occurs as a result of trauma, degenerative changes, and overuse, as it does in humans [102]. There is also interest in exploiting naturally occurring OA in cats as a translational model for human OA. However, with the exception of OA in dogs, there are few other naturally occurring animal disease models that are validated as translatable pain models for human clinical pain conditions. Bone cancer pain (dogs) [103] and pain caused by idiopathic cystitis in cats [104] are notable exceptions. Using naturally occurring diseases in companion animals requires that validated outcome measures to assess pain are available (e.g., Canine Brief Pain Inventory) [103,105,106]. This approach overcomes the ethical considerations associated with creating experimental pain in animals. However, limitations include (1) ethical constraints imposed by studying pet dogs and (2) lack of homogeneity of the disease processes. Companion animal disease models are likely to be most useful as an intermediate step to study pain mechanisms or analgesic drug efficacy that sit between preclinical rodent models and experimental pain studies in humans.

Recent trends in pain evaluation in rodents

There is a growing trend in preclinical research to develop better methods for assessing pain, rather than nociception, in rodents, thus attempting to record and 'take into account' the affective or emotional component of pain in pain measurement. Although this area of research is still in its infancy, significant efforts have been made to develop novel measures of animal affect, many of them developed from the fields of ethology and animal welfare science. Some examples of new approaches to measuring pain in rodents are described below.

Place preference paradigm

The (conditioned) place preference paradigm is commonly used to evaluate the affective/motivational properties of drugs. The paradigm involves the pairing of a drug state with environments that have distinctive stimuli (i.e., a place). During a period of learning, the animal learns to associate one environment with treatment and the test drug and a second environment with a control treatment (e.g., saline). Subsequently, the animal's place preference is determined by allowing the animal to choose between these two environments, with the choice being made when the animal has not received the drug treatment. This paradigm is used to evaluate the effect of analgesic drugs in animals in chronic pain, with the underpinning rationale that animals in chronic pain should show a place preference for the environment that is paired with an analgesic drug. Place preference tests require animal training and must be carried out carefully to avoid confounding factors, for example, ensuring there are no factors inherent in the test environment that might induce a place preference other than the drug treatment. This type of test has been used to show the analgesic effects of different classes of drugs in the complete Freund's adjuvant (CFA) inflammatory pain model in rats [107] and analgesic effects of butorphanol in chickens with naturally occurring keel bone fractures [108].

Operant response paradigms

Operant response paradigms are commonly used in behavioral pharmacology and have been adapted to study the analgesic efficacy of different drugs in rodents. Operant conditioning relies on training animals to associate making a particular response with receiving either a reward (e.g., a sugar pellet) or a punishment (e.g., a foot shock). Operant paradigms allow the animal to exert control over the outcome, which is one of the key differences between operant and Pavlovian conditioning, where an outcome is associated with a stimulus over which the animal has no control. An example of an operant paradigm is one that gives a rat a choice between receiving a reward (e.g., sweet condensed milk) or preventing receiving an aversive painful stimulus [109–111]. To receive the reward, the animal must poke its nose through an opening equipped with a thermode, so that the aversive stimulus (e.g., heat or cold) is obtained at the same time as the reward. Reward-seeking behavior is reduced following peripheral inflammation, an observation that is reversed with analgesic drugs. The operant behavior paradigms allow the observation of more spontaneous types of behaviors when compared with stimulus evoked studies, but require considerable training and also have a motivational component that can complicate the interpretation of pain-related behavior.

Assessment of spontaneous behaviors

Quantification of spontaneous behavior has long been recognized as a useful tool for studying pain severity and analgesic drug efficacy in rodents [112]. However, traditional behavioral analysis is limited because it is extremely time consuming, so only a limited range of behaviors tend to be studied for a short period. The recent development of automated systems to quantify behaviors in rodents has significantly enhanced the capability of behavioral analysis in the study of pain. These systems have the capacity to collect data continuously and in a standardized way so that variation and error are minimized, to provide information about the movement of individual animals, and to track complex changes in behavior. Therefore, they offer the opportunity to detect very subtle changes in the behavior of individual animals, in terms of both mobility but also interactive behaviors such as play, nesting, and lying with cage mates. This significantly increases the sensitivity of behavioral assessment to detect pain and effects of analgesic drug administration.

Willingness to burrow (rats and mice) and to build nests in the home cage (mice) are used as pain bioassays in experimental models of pain in these species. These tests use the principle that rodents are highly motivated to perform these behaviors in their home cage if given the means to do so (i.e., burrowing and nesting substrate); therefore, quantifying an altered willingness to carry out these behaviors offers a means to probe changes in affective state following pain induction and subsequent administration of analgesic drugs. Spontaneous burrowing behavior in rats is reduced by peripheral nerve injury or inflammatory pain [113], an effect that is reversed by the administration of analgesic drugs, showing the utility of this assay in analgesic drug development. Similar studies have been carried out in mice using burrowing behavior [114–116] and nest building [117].

Facial expression

Emotions are associated with specific facial expression signatures in humans and this premise has been translated to animals to quantify changes in facial expression as a biomarker for pain. Langford and colleagues [118] were the first group to develop formally a facial coding scale for pain in mice [Mouse Grimace Scale (MGS)]. The scale was developed by capturing still images of mouse faces before and after induction of abdominal pain caused by peritoneal injection of acetic acid. Facial action units that were altered by pain included orbital tightening, nose bulge, cheek bulge, ear position, and whisker change. Importantly, following a formal training session, blinded observers were able to discriminate between 'in pain' and 'no pain' mice using the MGS. Langford and colleagues [118] applied the MGS to mice that had undergone different nociceptive tests and found that the MGS was sensitive for some nociceptive assays but not others. Noxious stimuli of moderate duration (10 min–4 h) were most likely to be associated with a 'pain face,' whereas very brief noxious stimuli (e.g., phasic pain tests) and neuropathic pain states were not detected by the MGS. This may reflect the nociceptive nature of phasic pain tests, and the fact that pain of a longer duration is not accompanied by a persistent change in facial expression. Importantly, chemical lesioning of the rostral anterior insula, a structure that is activated in humans by pain with an important emotional component, produced attenuation of the pain face. Pain scales using facial expression have been extended to other laboratory animals including the rat (Rat Grimace Scale) [119], rabbit (Rabbit Grimace Scale) [120], and horses [121].

Clinical pain assessment in veterinary medicine

The clinical assessment of pain remains a complex and challenging topic. Pain perception is not simply a function of detecting tissue-damaging stimuli (the sensory component) but also a function of the individual, both physiologically and emotionally. It is a unique personal experience that is difficult to assess in non-verbal patients. Whether animals 'suffer' differently to humans is still debated. Lack of the cognitive ability to understand or reason why the pain is occurring may, in some people's minds, make suffering worse in less intelligent and non-lingual patients. On the other hand, animals with highly developed brains are likely to have the capacity to 'think' and may possess a degree of self-awareness, making the pain they experience worse because of the emotional component [122]. Pain in more evolved animal species is likely a complex, multidimensional experience, dependent on the severity of the insult activating nociceptive pathways and its commensurate tissue damage, previous pain experiences, and social position within a flock, herd, or colony. Individual animals have different analgesic requirements following identical procedures and may show different endocrine and behavioral responses that can be related to age and gender [123–128]. Furthermore, other stressors [129,130] or experiences may modulate pain behaviors. Evidence also suggests that previous noxious insults modulate the stress axis and antinociceptive pathways. The effect on animals and humans of observing pain behaviors in others is also worth noting and in humans has been termed 'empathy.' This may not be expected in other species but parallels have been shown [131–133].

These individual variations are well documented and have challenged workers when developing valid and reliable methods of pain assessment. Assessment tools must accommodate these individual differences and enable analgesic regimes to be tailored to the individual [134,135].

Many investigators have used ethogram-based objective measurements of pain behaviors after a noxious stimulus to scale pain [136]. Furthermore, studies attempting to quantify 'event behaviors' rather than just record the time spent doing or not doing an activity found this to be a more sensitive indicator of assessing pain, for example, after castration in lambs [137]. Other studies have evaluated differences in activity budgets and event behaviors separately and in combination. One study evaluating pain following arthroscopy in horses found a significant difference in activity budgets between surgical and non-surgical horses, indicated by the time these horses spent eating, abnormally posturing, and residing at the front of the stable [138]. In this study, the activity budgets and postures appeared to be a more sensitive indicator of pain and likely are both species and noxious insult specific.

Advances in pain assessment represent a painstaking and time-consuming dedication to improving animal welfare. Attitudes towards pain assessment and treatment have changed dramatically over the past few decades, representing a shift in prioritizing analgesia in companion, farmed, and laboratory animals, which is important from an ethical and humanitarian standpoint.

Pain assessment is an important consideration in veterinary medicine for several reasons. The observation and assessment of pain lead to increased use of analgesic drugs. Ultimately, this trend should result in more appropriate prescribing of analgesic drugs rather than a 'one size fits all' approach, which leaves some patients under-treated for their pain. More judicious use of analgesics is only achieved if the assessment tools used for pain evaluation are well designed, validated, and appropriate for the type of pain or procedure. Pain behaviors are often subtle and observer practice is required to identify these signs in different species [139]. Finally, it is important to train all veterinary care providers to use pain assessment tools. Time for training and discussion must be created to ensure consistency, a process for audit, and gather ideas for improvement. Pain assessment of hospitalized patients and recording the data as one of the 'vital signs' is a positive step. The outcomes for prioritizing pain assessment are considerable for the many stakeholders involved in the process. Communicating to owners or caregivers about the pain assessment tools that the practice utilizes will optimize animal welfare, strengthen the human–animal bond, and ultimately improve the client–practice relationship and reputation. Professional, governmental, and various business entities along with research groups have provided training aids to assist in disseminating information and in making electronic versions easily accessible [140–145].

Quantification of pain

Quantifying pain is difficult because it is the perception of a multidimensional physiologic and emotional process. The quantification of pain includes its intensity, duration, frequency (constant or intermittent or associated with an activity or stressor), and quality [146]. It is also likely that some of the behaviors identified are similar to or identical with those displayed when the animal is stressed or distressed by factors other than pain.

As discussed previously, pain is often described as either acute or chronic. Acute pain will usually involve tissue damage and behavior to avoid further injury. Assessing chronic pain in humans demonstrates that there is a very obvious emotional component; depression, anger, and fear are common, and it is appropriate to discuss the patient's quality of life (QoL) rather than focus on the intensity of pain alone. As companion animals live longer, they are likely to suffer from chronic conditions such as OA, complex metabolic disease, and cancer. Quantifying pain and QoL in these individuals requires means of evaluation distinct from those commonly used to assess acute, protective, or physiologic pain [147].

Objective measures of acute pain

Physiologic variables

Most studies assessing pain in animals have focused on acute pain. There have been numerous studies evaluating the correlation between physiologic parameters such as heart rate, respiratory rate, pupil diameter, blood pressure, and acute pain scores [148]. Unsurprisingly, no physiologic parameter is reliable in isolation to indicate pain accurately [149,150]. These parameters are affected by many other factors, such as fear and stress, and at best may contribute to pain assessment in multifactorial scales [151]. There is a general consensus that the physiologic responses have a weak correlation with pain. However, one study investigating laminitis pain in horses examined the use of heart rate, heart rate variability (HRV), and behavioral and endocrine markers in evaluating the response to treatment. Although there was a poor correlation between pain behaviors and plasma concentrations of cortisol and catecholamines, the low- and high-frequency components of HRV did change significantly with treatment and behavioral indicators as measured by the Obel Laminitis Scale [152]. HRV is a useful tool for assessing pain in horses in conjunction with other methods; however, like other physiologic parameters, HRV is influenced by many other factors. Another study evaluating composite pain scales for the assessment of acute orthopedic pain in horses found that heart rate and respiratory rate were only moderately specific and sensitive indicators of orthopedic pain [153]. Evaluation of bowel sounds showed good to moderate specificity but only weak sensitivity. Interestingly, non-invasive blood pressure (NIBP), measured using an oscillometric device placed around the tail base, was a very specific and sensitive indicator of orthopedic pain [105].

Plasma cortisol, endorphins, and acute phase proteins

Changes in the plasma concentrations of hormones such as cortisol, β-endorphins and other acute phase proteins (APPs) have been measured as indicators of pain. Little correlation between behavioral indicators and elevations in these markers has been demonstrated. In fact, plasma cortisol has been demonstrated not to be a useful pain biomarker in the cat and dog [154]. These biomarkers may have other roles, such as categorizing the severity of disease, rather than retrospective indicators of pain [155]. The severity of inflammatory diseases such as bovine mastitis can be graded using the APP haptoglobin. Serum amyloid A and milk amyloid A measured in serum or milk are also diagnostic proteins for clinical and subclinical mastitis [156]. The relationship between inflammatory mastitis and pain remains undefined. Horses undergoing orthopedic procedures have demonstrated a correlation between blood cortisol concentrations and a composite pain score (CPS) [153]. For every incremental unit rise in blood cortisol, the CPS increased by 0.095 units, with the authors concluding that cortisol was a specific and sensitive indicator of orthopedic pain.

Behavior-based pain scoring

Veterinary patients are unable to self-report, hence clinicians are reliant on scoring systems that depend on the subjective assessment of pain by a proxy. Assessments are made by the owner or the attending veterinarian or nurse/technician, and all will have a degree of variability, subjectiveness, and bias when assessing the patient. The pain evaluation is affected by many observer-specific factors such as age, gender, clinical experience, year of graduation from veterinary school, and, perhaps most importantly, personal experience of painful procedures or conditions [157]. In 1985, Morton and Griffiths published a proposal to develop validated and robust pain scales [158]. Currently, there are still only a small number of validated scales available based on pain-specific behaviors.

One-dimensional scoring systems

Traditionally, acute pain assessment is performed using simple one-dimensional scales that assesses the intensity of pain (Fig. 29.1).

Simple descriptive scale

Simple descriptive scales are basic and highly subjective pain scales that typically have four or five descriptors. This scale type does not demonstrate sensitivity in detecting small changes in pain intensity. This type of scale has been used by Colorado State University (CSU)

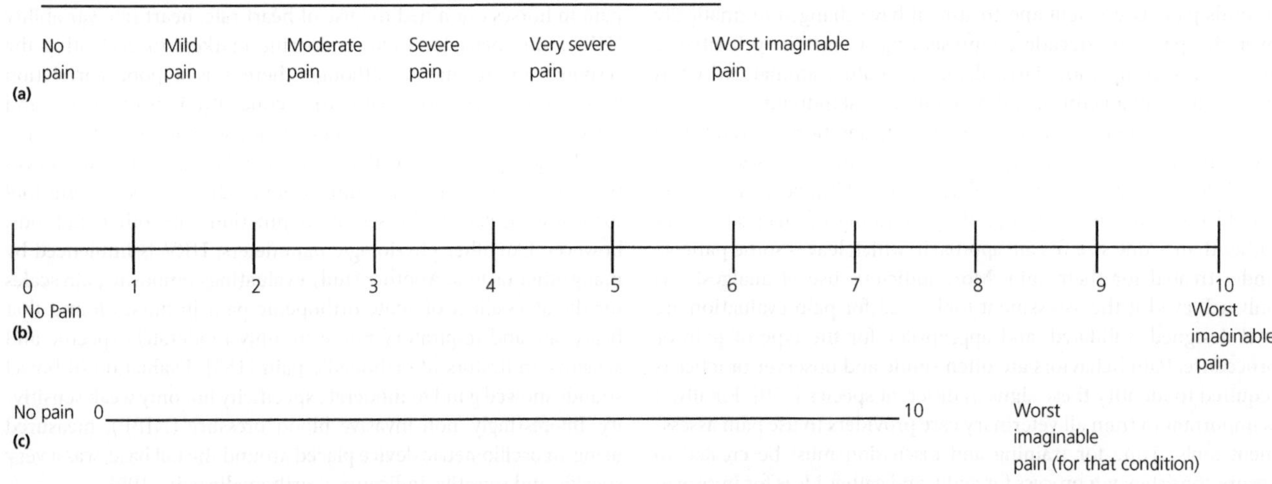

Figure 29.1 (a) A simple descriptive scale (SDS) consists of a scale with descriptors of the intensity of the pain. The descriptors can be single descriptive words or can be more detailed sentences. (b) A numeric rating scale (NRS) uses numbers rather than descriptors to score the pain. It is a discontinuous scale and the numbers are unequally weighted. In this example, 0 represents no pain and 10 represents the worst imaginable pain. (c) The visual analog scale (VAS) is a continuous scale that consists of a 10 cm line anchored at both ends by two verbal descriptors for the extremes of the particular condition. Intermediate numeric values or verbal descriptors are not recommended as this can encourage clustering of scores around the numbers or words.

and a version is reproduced in Fig. 29.2. Although still unvalidated, it undoubtedly represents a useful and freely available tool for pain assessment in cats.

Numerical rating scale

This scale uses numbers rather than descriptors to score pain. This scale type is discontinuous with unequal weighting between the categories (sometimes leading to incorrect statistical analysis of research data). It is often used when scoring individual behavioral characteristics in multidimensional scales. Multiple NRS scores have been used in horses following exploratory celiotomy to generate an overall behavior score [159].

Visual analog scale

This simple continuous scale is widely used and consists of a 100 mm line anchored at either end with (0) no pain and (100) worst imaginable pain (for this procedure). The observer marks on the line a point that correlates with the assessment of the pain. Training is necessary to reduce variation between assessors. One of the much-debated questions about the VAS is the linearity of the scale (e.g., does a score of 60 mm represent twice as much pain as 30 mm?). This is obviously important when determining an appropriate statistical test for evaluating the data generated. One survey demonstrated that approximately 50% of studies involving VAS measurements applied parametric statistics [160]. However, other researchers advocate the use of the non-parametric statistic for non-linear data. Use of confidence intervals may assist in the interpretation of the data from VAS but do not solve the problem of violation of the underlying assumptions of the statistical test [160,161].

Studies have shown significant observer variability with all three of the aforementioned scales [162]. Hewetson *et al.* investigated the use of an NRS and verbal rating scale to describe lameness and found 55–60% inter-observer variability with the two scales [163]. Intra-observer variability was of a similar magnitude of 58–60%. This highlights the subjective nature of the lameness examination and the variability that occurs when using these subjective scales. When one trained observer performs all observations, the NRS becomes a more reliable scale.

Lascelles *et al.* reported the refinement of the VAS, which involves a dynamic and interactive assessment of the patient (DIVAS). Numerous studies adopted this approach [164,165]. This additional component of the VAS involves observing the animal from a distance, then approaching and interacting with the patient and finally palpating the wound and surrounding area. VAS scales for questionnaires have also been investigated for assessing pain and lameness in dogs [166].

Multidimensional scoring systems

It is counterintuitive to assess something as multidimensional and complex as pain with a simple one-dimensional scale. In humans, however, multidimensional pain scales have been developed and validated. These scales incorporate questions to assess the affective component of pain and also intensity (sensory component) [167]. An argument can be made that the VAS combines behavioral and affective components of pain as a continuum and the assessor does not have to bother compartmentalizing pain components, and thus is somewhat of a holistic measure. Others would argue the continuum of VAS represents an undefined large number of categories covering multiple dimensions that the assessor is unaware of but nonetheless uses when assessing pain.

In all attempts to devise a valid and rigorous tool to assess pain involving behaviors, normal behaviors must be known and categorized. Fox *et al.* identified a comprehensive list of 166 behaviors associated with ovariohysterectomy in the dog. Incorporating all of these possible signs into a concise and easy to use pain assessment tool is a challenging task [168]. The Glasgow Composite Pain Scale identified 279 expressions or words associated with pain in the dog. This list was refined to 47 carefully considered well-defined descriptors in seven behavioral categories [169].

Bussières *et al.* [153] reported a pain scale based on a multifactorial NRS incorporating behavioral and physiologic data specific for equine orthopedic pain (Figure 29.3). Physiologic parameters included heart rate, respiratory rate, bowel sounds, and rectal temperature. Behavioral parameters included appearance (i.e., reluctance to move, restlessness, agitation, anxiety, and sweating), kicking at the abdomen, pawing or pointing limbs, and posture (i.e.,

Colorado State University

VETERINARY TEACHING HOSPITAL

Feline Acute Pain Scale

Date ______________________

Time ______________________

Rescore when awake	☐ **Animal is sleeping, but can be aroused - Not evaluated for pain** ☐ **Animal can't be aroused, check vital signs, assess therapy**

Pain Score	Example	Psychological & Behavioral	Response to Palpation	Body Tension
0	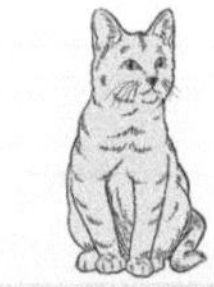	☐ **Content and quiet** when unattended ☐ **Comfortable** when resting ☐ Interested in or **curious** about surroundings	☐ **Not bothered** by palpation of wound or surgery site, or to palpation elsewhere	Minimal
1	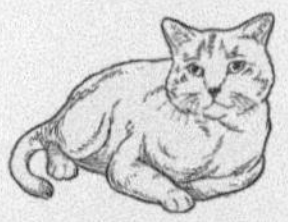	☐ **Signs are often subtle and not easily detected in the hospital setting**; more likely to be detected by the owner(s) at home ☐ Earliest signs at home may be **withdrawal from surroundings or change in normal routine** ☐ In the hospital, may be content or slightly unsettled ☐ **Less interested** in surroundings but will look around to see what is going on	☐ May or may not react to palpation of wound or surgery site	Mild
2	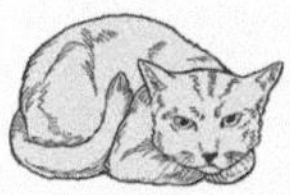	☐ Decreased responsiveness, **seeks solitude** ☐ **Quiet**, loss of brightness in eyes ☐ **Lays curled up or sits tucked up** (all four feet under body, shoulders hunched, head held slightly lower than shoulders, tail curled tightly around body) with eyes partially or mostly closed ☐ **Hair coat appears rough** or fluffed up ☐ May intensively groom an area that is painful or irritating ☐ Decreased appetite, **not interested in food**	☐ **Responds aggressively or tries to escape** if painful area is palpated or approached ☐ Tolerates attention, may even perk up when petted as long as painful area is avoided	Mild to Moderate **Reassess analgesic plan**
3	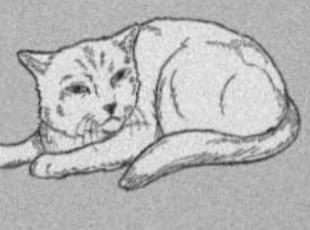	☐ Constantly **yowling, growling, or hissing** when unattended ☐ May bite or chew at wound, but **unlikely to move** if left alone	☐ **Growls or hisses at non-painful palpation** (may be experiencing allodynia, wind-up, or fearful that pain could be made worse) ☐ **Reacts aggressively** to palpation, **adamantly pulls away** to avoid any contact	Moderate **Reassess analgesic plan**
4	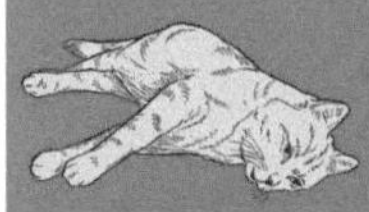	☐ Prostrate ☐ Potentially **unresponsive** to or unaware of surroundings, difficult to distract from pain ☐ Receptive to care (even aggressive or feral cats will be more tolerant of contact)	☐ **May not respond** to palpation ☐ **May be rigid to avoid painful movement**	Moderate to Severe **May be rigid to avoid painful movement** **Reassess analgesic plan**

RIGHT

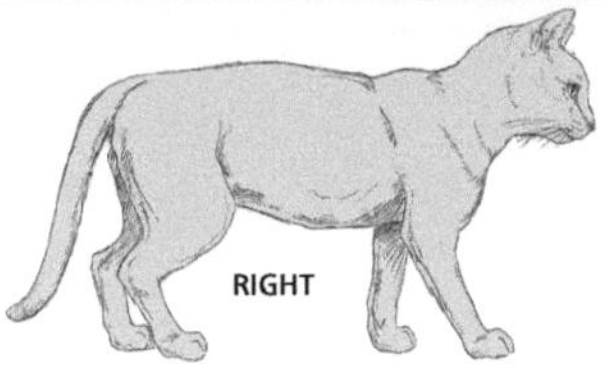

○ Tender to palpation
✕ Warm
■ Tense

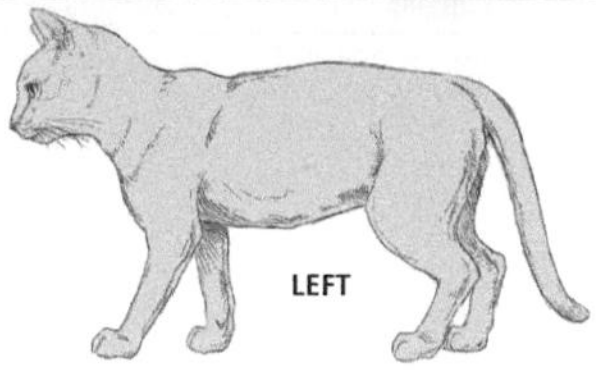

LEFT

Comments ____

Figure 29.2 Instructions for using the CSU Acute Pain Scale. The CSU Acute Pain Scale is intended primarily as a teaching tool and to guide observations of clinical patients. The scale has not been validated and should not be used as a definitive pain score. Use of the scale employs both an observational period and a hands-on evaluation of the patient. In general, the assessment begins with quiet observation of the patient in its cage at a relatively unobtrusive distance. Subsequently, the patient as a whole (wound as well as the entire body) is approached to assess reaction to gentle palpation, indicators of muscle tension and heat, response to interaction, etc. (1) The scale utilizes a generic 0–4 scale with quartermarks as its base along with a color scale as a visual cue for progression along the 5-point scale. (2) Realistic artist's renderings of animals at various levels of pain add further visual cues. Additional drawings provide space for recording pain, warmth, and muscle tension; this allows documentation of specific areas of concern in the medical record. A further advantage of these drawings is that the observer is encouraged to assess the overall pain of the patient in addition to focusing on the primary lesion. (3) The scale includes psychologic and behavioral signs of pain and also palpation responses. Further, the scale uses body tension as an evaluation tool, a parameter not addressed in other scales. (4) There is a provision for non-assessment in the resting patient. To the source authors' knowledge, this is the only scale that emphasizes the importance of delaying assessment in a sleeping patient while prompting the observer to recognize patients that may be inappropriately obtunded by medication or a more serious health concern. (5) Advantages of this scale include ease of use with minimal interpretation required. Specific descriptors for individual behaviors are provided which decreases inter-observer variability. Additionally, a scale is provided for both the dog and the cat. (6) A disadvantage of this scale is a lack of validation by clinical studies comparing it with other scales. Further, its use is largely limited to and is intended for use in acute pain. Source: Colorado State University: Veterinary Teaching College. © 2006 P.W. Hellyer, S.R. Uhrig, N.G. Robinson. Reproduced with permission.

Multifactorial numerical rating equine composite pain scale (ECPS)

General instructions

- Start performing the evaluation via distance observation, with the horse in the box.
- Spend 15 min at looking at the horse's behaviour.
- DO NOT physically push or pull the horse, nor guide it by a rope or halter, nor startle it, as these will interfere with natural movements.
- Score criteria in order, or according to convenience based on the horse's unsolicited movements.
- Next step is to complete a Physical examination of the horse
- Finally, characterize its Response to treatment, while scoring for its Interactive behaviour, as well as Response to palpation of the apparent painful area.
- NOTE: Although each of the following criteria has the potential to be expressed in painful horse, it is not expected that all will be present in a single animal

Evaluation procedure

1- Leave the horse in its box and observe its undisturbed behaviour (Appearance, Sweating), Posture, and Appetite. Assess posture both with the horse standing still and during locomotion.Stimulate appetite while proposing hay to the horse.

2- Spend 5 min to count for the number of Kicking at abdomen, Pawing on the floor, and Head movement. For the latter, look precisely to head movement, and lip curling.

3- Proceed to the physical examination of the horse while counting for its Heart rate, Respiratory rate, and recording Digestive sounds, and Rectal temperature.
In case, the situation does not allow to record initial physiological values, normal values for resting heart rate is 32–44 bpm in an adult, 50–70 bpm for a foal, for respiratory rate 8-14 bpm, and rectal temperature 37.5 (adult) - 38.5 °C (foal).

4 - Encourage the horse to interact with you and score for its Interactive behaviour, as well as its Response to palpation of the apparent painful area.

Multifactorial numerical rating equine composite pain scale (ECPS)

BEHAVIOUR	CRITERIA	SCORE/21
Appearance (reluctance to move, restlessness, agitation and anxiety)	Bright, lowered head and ears, no reluctance to move	0
	Bright and alert, occasional head movements, no reluctance to move	1
	Restlessness, pricked up ears, abnormal facial expressions, dilated pupils	2
	Excited, continuous body movements, abnormal facial expression	3
Sweating	No obvious signs of sweat	0
	Damp to the touch	1
	Wet to the touch, beads of sweat are apparent over the horse's body	2
	Excessive sweating, beads of water running off the animal	3
Posture (weight distribution, comfort)	Stands quietly, normal walk	0
	Occasional weight shift, slight muscles tremors	1
	Non-weight bearing, abnormal weight distribution	2
	Analgesic posture (attempts to urinate), prostration, muscles tremors)	3
Kicking at abdomen	Quietly standing, no kicking	0
	Occasional kicking at abdomen (1–2 times/5 min)	1
	Frequent kicking at abdomen (3–4 times/5 min)	2
	Excessive kicking at abdomen (>5 times/5 min), intermittent attempts to lie down and roll	3
Pawing on the floor (pointing, hanging limbs)	Quietly standing, no pawing	0
	Occasional pawing (1–2 times/5 min)	1
	Frequent pawing (3–4 times/5 min)	2
	Excessive pawing (>5 times/5 min)	3
Head movement	No evidence of discomfort, head straight ahead for most part	0
	Intermittent head movements laterally or vertically, occasional looking at flanks (1–2 times/5 min), lip curling (1–2 times/5 min)	1
	Intermittent and rapid head movements laterally or vertically, frequent looking at flank (3–4 times/5 min.), lip curling (3–4 times/5 min)	2
	Continuous head movements, excessive looking at flank (>5 times/5 min), lip curling (>5 times/5 min)	3
Appetite	Eats hay readily	0
	Hesitates to eat hay	1
	Shows little interest in hay, eats very little or takes hay in mouth but does not chew or swallow	2
	Neither shows interest in nor eat hay	3
PHYSIOLOGIC DATA	**CRITERIA**	**SCORE/12**
Heart rate	Normal compared to initial value (increase <10%)	0
	11–30% increase	1
	31–50% increase	2
	>50% increase	3
Respiratory rate	Normal compared to initial value (increase <10%)	0
	11–30% increase	1
	31–50% increase	2
	>50% increase	3
Digestive sounds (bowel movements)	Normal motility	0
	Decreased motility	1
	No motility	2
	Hypermotility	3
Rectal temperature	Normal compared to initial value (variation <0.5 °C)	0
	Variation les 1 °C	1
	Variation les 1.5 °C	2
	Variation ges 2 °C	3
RESPONSE TO TREATMENT	**CRITERIA**	**SCORE/06**
Interactive behaviour	Pay attention to people	0
	Exaggerated response to auditory stimulus	1
	Excessive-to-aggressive response to auditory stimulus	2
	Stupor, prostration, no response to auditory stimulus	3
Response to palpation of the painful area	No reaction to palpation	0
	Mild reaction to palpation	1
	Resistance to palpation	2
	Violent reaction to palpation	3
TOTAL ECPS		/39

Figure 29.3 Multifactorial numerical rating equine composite pain scale (ECPS). Source: Courtesy of Eric Troncy.

weight distribution, comfort, head movement, and appetite). This evaluation scheme also included response-to-treatment parameters: interactive behavior and response to palpation of the painful area. For all the parameters, a list of descriptors was devised to assist in assigning a score from 0 to 3, with 0 being normal and 3 being furthest from normal; the maximum total possible score is 39. There was good inter-observer repeatability with this multifactorial pain scale, with good specificity and sensitivity. In summary, the most specific and sensitive behavioral indicators of orthopedic pain in horses were response to palpation, posture, and pawing (to a lesser extent) [170].

Another study assessing pain in horses following arthroscopy used continuous videotaping, starting 24 h before and continuing for 48 h after surgery [138]. 'Activity budgets' were recorded based upon overall horse behavior and posture. Comparison of activity budgets identified a significant difference between surgical cases and control horses in the proportion of time spent eating, demonstrating abnormal postures, and positioning in the front of the box. Hunger/foraging and postanesthetic 'hangover' can potentially affect behaviors, especially overall level of activity, confounding the assessment. Horses were more restless postsurgery (i.e., spent less time in sternal recumbency), but it was difficult to detect by direct observation. Horses had less locomotion postsurgery, which could be considered a reluctance to move due to pain.

Surgical colic cases have been compared with horses undergoing MRI and with horses that underwent no treatment [159]. Physiologic data, gross pain behaviors using NRS, and activity budgets were compared. The 'time budget' was calculated by dividing the time spent exhibiting each behavior by the total time recorded. The behaviors recorded included activity, pain behaviors, locomotion, and rest. Within each of these categories existed further descriptors. After surgery, horses spent significantly less time moving. As expected, postsurgical patients demonstrated painful behaviors more than controls or non-surgical cases, but it was a small proportion of the total time under evaluation. The investigators concluded that following abdominal surgery in horses, reduced locomotion was a potential indicator of pain along with elevated cortisol concentration and heart rate.

Frequency and duration of pain assessment

The time spent assessing the animal is important as short, sporadic, and cursory examinations of patients will lead to missed pain behaviors. There are no guidelines for how long an animal should be observed, but intuitively the longer the better. In a pilot study, Raekallio *et al.* identified the challenges of assessing pain in horses [171]. In this study, horses were assessed following arthroscopy using a total postoperative pain severity index (TPPSI). This composite scale consisted of an NRS for a scoring pain, behavioral observations, physiologic measurements, and measurement of stress hormones. It was concluded that there was a poor correlation between the subjective and objective behavioral measures and that none of the behavioral signs were sensitive or reliable indicators of postoperative pain. A lack of power in this study could be due to the small numbers of horses evaluated, or the amount of time spent observing horses (two 1 min observations 5 min apart, which were averaged before surgery and at 2, 4, 6, 12, 24, 48, and 72 h after surgery). These time periods may be too short to detect behaviors associated with pain [172].

The presence of a person observing the animal may alter pain-associated behaviors. An undisturbed dog or cat may choose to curl up at the back of the cage, but when the assessor is present the patient may approach the front of the cage to seek attention or defend itself. This may also occur with larger animals; horses may interact with an observer or may show aversive behavior. Recent work has demonstrated the placebo effect that caregiver interaction can cause. It is wise to consider this potential impact when globally assessing pain [173].

Selection of assessment tool

In a busy practice environment, the method chosen for pain assessment should be user friendly. The Glasgow Composite Pain Scale has been refined to create a short form for this very reason and has been validated in assessing acute surgical pain in dogs [174].

Validated composite scales for acute pain in cats are still in their infancy but several recent studies show promise [175,176]. Items to be assessed must be collected and refined for inclusion in the questionnaire. Assessment forms must be scrutinized (face and content validity) and the scale must undergo test–retest reliability and validity testing [3,177].

The efficacy of subjective animal pain scoring systems can vary with type of pain assessed (e.g., acute or chronic pain), the scale used, the behaviors chosen for evaluation (dynamic or interactive), and the personnel involved [178]. Grooms, for example, can distinguish postsurgery horses from controls more successfully than veterinarians [138]. The grooms awarded higher pain scores to these horses, affirming the well-held belief that the owner/caregiver is the best individual to perform pain assessment as they are much more likely to detect subtle signs and deviations from normal behavior. Clinical experience also undoubtedly contributes to the reliability of the assessment [179].

Chronic pain

In 1986, the Association of Veterinary Teachers and Research Workers produced guidelines for overall pain assessment [180]. These guidelines suggested that observations be made by someone who can distinguish subtle changes in demeanor, behavior, and locomotion (in companion animals this is usually the owner), with subsequent interpretation of data by a person with knowledge and experience of pain assessment (i.e., a veterinarian). Three decades later, this approach is still in vogue; tools devised for assessment of chronic pain are heavily dependent on owner assessment with interpretation and decision-making done in conjunction with the veterinarian. In fact, recent studies demonstrate little correlation between the owner assessment and force plate gait analysis when evaluating response to treatment in osteoarthritic dogs [106]. This is not to suggest that sophisticated evaluation methods are not useful, but emphasizes that treatment efficacy in the eyes of the owners likely includes overall QoL [181].

A number of tools have been developed for the measurement of chronic pain and QoL in dogs [147,182]. These have been designed to some extent from existing QoL instruments for humans. QoL assessments aid in decision-making with respect to painful treatment interventions and the need for euthanasia [183,184]. QoL is an abstract construct used in human medicine that seems wholly appropriate when applied to the welfare of animals [185,186].

Since there is no 'gold standard' of chronic pain assessment with which to compare QoL scales, psychometric testing of various scales has been undertaken. The Liverpool Osteoarthritis in Dogs (LOAD) scale, the Helsinki Chronic Pain Index (HCPI), and the Canine Brief Pain Inventory (CBPI) were comparatively evaluated in 222 dogs with OA [177]. There were moderate correlations between all instruments, implying construct validity for all of them.

Significant but weak correlations were found between LOAD scores and 'symmetry index' (calculated from force-platform analysis for peak vertical force) and between CBPI scores and symmetry index. The CBPI is a multifactorial tool composed of a Pain Severity Score, Interference Score, and an Overall Quality of Life Score. Studies by Walton *et al.* [177] and others addressed criterion validity for the CPBI, as did a study by Brown *et al.* comparing the CPBI with force plate analysis [106].

The HCPI is an 11-item single-construct index of chronic pain [187]. Changes in the HCPI correlated well with change in QoL and with changes in the mobility VAS. It appears to provide a valid, reliable, and responsive method of assessing treatment response in osteoarthritic dogs. The HCPI has criterion validity on the basis of a correlation between HCPI and a QoL score on a VAS [188]. Interestingly, when the VAS and HCPI were compared using owner evaluation of pain in arthritic dogs, the conclusion was that a VAS was a poor tool for untrained owners because of poor face validity (i.e., owners could not identify their dogs' behavior as signs of pain). Only after the owners had seen pain diminish and then return (after completing a course of NSAIDs) did the VAS have face validity. The HCPI did not correlate with symmetry index from force plate analysis in the study undertaken by Walton *et al.* [177]. The reasons for this are unclear, but likely a function of wording and the weighting of descriptors.

A feline musculoskeletal pain index (FMPI) is a client questionnaire with good readability, internal consistency–reliability, and repeatability [189,190]. The FMPI did not demonstrate responsiveness or criterion validity in subsequent testing, however [191]. Responsiveness describes whether changes in a parameter can be detected following treatment, ideally in a blinded placebo-controlled design. The lack of responsiveness may have been as a result of many factors, such as a large placebo effect. In a novel study, Gruen *et al.* [192] used the FMPI and client-specific outcome measures (CSOM) and were able to circumvent the placebo effect by demonstrating recurrence of clinical signs after withdrawal of treatment compared with placebo. Criterion validity describes whether the results generated correlate with another validated measure. The FMPI did not show criterion validity either; however, this was correlating with activity measured by accelerometry [190]. This lack of correlation challenges the assumption that degenerative joint disease decreases activity, and that cats receiving NSAIDs are motivated to increase activity. Some owners are unconcerned about the activity levels *per se* in their elderly cats and are concerned about other potential indicators of pain. These findings highlight a need to include both active and non-active terms to assess cat pain and QoL better.

Web-based versions of these tools are available, facilitating easy and accessible recording for owners [193]. Multidimensional scales do not exist for all species and may not be appropriate in some cases. Even unidirectional scales have been used for chronic pain with some success. For example, Welsh *et al.* used the VAS and SDS to assess pain from 'footrot' lameness in sheep [194].

Pain faces

The function of pain is to demand attention and prioritize escape, recovery, and healing; where others can help achieve these goals, effective communication of pain is required [195]. Charles Darwin recognized that pain could be expressed in an animal's face [196]. Facial expression is used as a means of recognizing pain in infants and other non-verbal or cognitively impaired humans [197]. Benefits can occur in humans and some animals by displaying specific facial expressions for assistance or as a warning signal, whereas in some species, overt facial signaling more likely correlates with vulnerability. Consequently, some species may have adapted to their environments and circumstances over the eons by the diminishment of facial expressions [118,119,198,199].

Facial expressions associated with equine pain have been evaluated by the kinematic analysis of facial movements during a brief painful stimulus [200]. Facial expressions in horses that have undergone castration have also been described [121]. Being able to differentiate expressions from specific pain stimuli and intensities could potentially improve owners' and caregivers' ability to recognize specific painful experiences [201].

Eye contact in humans is particularly useful in conveying emotions [202]. Leach *et al.* used eye-tracking equipment to confirm the suspicion that observers, irrespective of gender or experience, spend the most time focused on the animal's face when assessing pain [203]. The technology involved in automated eye-tracking has been used to assess where people focus their attention in many activities, including observing attractiveness of other humans [204], driving [205], and using a computer or evaluating websites [206]. Automated eye-tracking technology can be applied to the caregiver's observation of an animal's behavior. Leach *et al.* [203]. identified a bias towards focusing on the face which then neglects other body clues associated with pain. Rabbits, for example, exhibit painful behaviors and postures primarily of the back and abdomen [207] (e.g., belly pressing, back arching, skin twitching along the back), and a bias towards facial expression may result in unrecognized pain. Similarly, castrated calves exhibited abnormal posture, abnormal walking, and licking associated with the surgical site [208]. Furthermore, signs typically waxed and waned, indicating that adequate observation time is required. Castrated or tail-docked lambs demonstrate behaviors predominately associated with the area of surgery and posture [209]. These reports simply re-emphasize the need to devise species-specific composite pain-assessment tools. It is generally agreed that the development of species-specific pain face measurements should improve pain assessment in many of our companion animal species.

In conjunction with the development and validation of pain tools, emphasis on appropriate training and audit of the use of pain assessment tools is also important. There is an assumption that all people working with animals automatically have the ability to assess pain and its severity. A survey of current methods used to recognize pain, suffering, and distress noted that the majority of research establishments use subjective assessment methods or scoring systems that are not validated (despite being confident that their pain assessment was adequate) [210]. Training should accompany the use of pain assessment measurements. Training personnel prior to employing behavioral evaluations such as is done with VAS scoring increased the percentage of animal caretakers identifying the need for analgesic therapy [211].

Functional measurements including force platform and pressure-sensitive platform assessment are used to study lameness in horses, dogs, cats, and sheep. These methods may also assist in clinical decision-making, for example, during the healing of bone fractures. Experimental data support the use of gait analysis in sheep that were recovering from tibial fractures as a non-invasive alternative to assessing bone healing [212]. Cats are more difficult to assess using these types of tools [213,214], as it is more challenging to get the cat to walk on the plate. However, limb function following onychectomy has been assessed with this technology [215,216]. The use of devices such as activity monitors or accelerometers may be more appropriate in cats [217]. Activity assessment as a means of evaluating the individual's overall QoL is potentially useful in dogs and cats. These electronic devices are attached to a collar or harness and indicate levels of activity that are often unobserved in the presence of humans. Careful placement is necessary to avoid erroneous activity recordings from eating and grooming movements. Comparison of accelerometer data with behavior indices associated with altered mobility would be further elucidating [218,219].

Summary of pain assessment methodology

Accurate and localized detection of pain remains a challenge in veterinary medicine because of the wide array of subtle behavioral changes observed among the various species of animals being evaluated. In addition to specific behaviors and postural alterations, subtle changes in time budget activities may be representative of pain type and severity. The recognition of chronic pain in animals has further challenged us to find better methods of assessing the overall QoL experienced by our patients [220].

Pharmacologic treatment of pain

Pharmaceuticals have been the cornerstone and often 'first-line' therapeutic intervention in successfully treating painful patients [221].

α_2-Adrenergic receptor agonists

α_2-Adrenergic receptor agonists have a wide range of effects on body systems, including the cardiovascular (CV), respiratory, endocrine, gastrointestinal (GI), and urogenital systems. The CNS is the primary site of analgesic action. Xylazine, detomidine, romifidine, medetomidine, and dexmedetomidine are commercially available veterinary α_2-adrenergic receptor agonists that provide analgesia to a variety of species [222–226]. However, these agents are not equal in their α_2-adrenergic receptor affinity. Of these drugs, dexmedetomidine is the most selective for the α_2-adrenergic receptor, with a relative binding affinity for α_2:α_1-receptors widely reported to be 1620:1, although the original source for this selectivity ratio actually gives 1620:1 as the affinity ratio of medetomidine [227], a drug that is a racemate of the stereoisomers levomedetomidine and dexmedetomidine. Because levomedetomidine is considered an inactive isomer, one can reasonably extrapolate that the selectivity ratios are similar.

Benefit versus risk is assessed before including these (or any) drugs in the pain management plan for a patient. Xylazine in the horse provides significant relief of visceral and somatic pain, perhaps even more so than opioids or NSAIDs [228–230]. Calves undergoing castration had a reduction in serum cortisol (one physiologic marker of pain) and improved behavior when a combination of low-dose xylazine and ketamine was administered prior to the procedure [231]. Antinociception occurred in llamas receiving tiletamine–zolazepam when xylazine was concurrently administered [232].

Sites of action

α_2-Adrenergic receptors are located within the CNS [233], peripherally [234], spinally [235], and supraspinally [236]. α_2-Adrenergic receptor agonists induce antinociception both by acting on the presynaptic terminals of primary afferent neurons and by direct inhibition of spinal cord neurons (likely via α_{2c}-receptors). Local infiltration induces analgesia, suggesting that peripheral α_2-adrenergic receptors also mediate analgesic action [237].

α_2-Adrenergic receptors

α-Adrenergic receptors have been described using a variety of classification schemes: location (i.e., pre- versus postsynaptic), response to activation or inhibition, and response to drug administration [238].

Receptor Subtypes

The α_2-adrenergic receptors can be subtype classified as α_{2a}, α_{2b}, or α_{2c}. It appears that the analgesic mechanism of action is mediated by G_i-protein activation of K^+ channels of the α_{2a}- and α_{2c}-receptor subtypes; analgesic α_{2a} activity is voltage dependent [235,239,240]. A high concentration of α_{2a}-receptors is present in the dorsal horn of the spinal cord, where most but not all of the analgesic effect is mediated (see below). Dexmedetomidine works preferentially at α_{2a}-receptors [241], although this preference is minor (10-fold) compared with its action at other receptor subtypes [242]. In addition to synergism (defined as greater than additive efficacy of an agent when administered together with another agent) between classes of drugs, there is also synergism between α_{2a}- and α_{2c}-receptor subtype agonists [243]. Synergism may also be present among drugs targeting a single receptor subtype [244].

Alternative receptors and synergism

Cannabinoid system

α_2-Adrenergic receptor agonists may target cannabinergic receptors to produce antinociception [245]. Additionally, there is some evidence in mice that synergism occurs between µ-opioid receptors, α_2-adrenergic receptor agonists, and cannabinoid receptors [246.

Muscarinic receptors

Work examining the role of muscarinic receptors in neuropathic pain suggests that a change in the noradrenergic–cholinergic axis of the spinal cord can occur. In a rat model of neuropathic pain, exposure to dexmedetomidine produced increases in acetylcholine concentration and decreased hyperalgesia, suggesting that dexmedetomidine may provide an analgesic benefit in this model [247].

Opioid receptors

Evidence of α_2-adrenergic receptor agonists enhancing opioid analgesia is evident in the literature for companion animal species [80,248,249]. However, very little information is available as to how this synergism occurs, perhaps due the complexity of the relationship. For example, synergism can be defined using isobolographic analysis [250]; however, this defines dose–response relationships, not underlying receptor interaction. It is clear that some µ-opioid agonists interact with α_2-adrenergic receptors, with possible preferential affinity for certain receptor subtypes (i.e., α_{2b} and α_{2c}) [251]. Certain disease states, such as inflammation, may favor the interaction of µ-opioid receptor agonists and the actions of α_2-adrenergic receptor agonists [252], but this remains controversial [253].

Local anesthetics

The only analgesic drugs that prevent nociceptive transmission are local anesthetics, which are used to facilitate a variety of veterinary procedures. This prevention of nociception is so effective that it is possible to substitute sedation and a local block for general anesthesia in some situations [254]. When compared with highly effective analgesic techniques, such as administration of an opioid and local anesthetic into the epidural space for hind limb orthopedic procedures, appropriate nerve blockade provides advantages such as less urine retention and reduced postoperative opioid consumption while providing a similar level of analgesia [255]. Local anesthetics are antinociceptive because they produce reversible neuronal conduction blockade, thus preventing transmission of noxious stimuli to the spinal cord and brain. Additionally, local anesthetics may produce dose-dependent anti-inflammatory effects as a result of physical changes (such as preservation of the endothelial barrier), in addition to direct effects on mediators of inflammation [256]. Local anesthetics appear both to inhibit proinflammatory mediator release and to alter proinflammatory mediator activity. Additionally, local anesthetics also appear to alter all stages of leukocyte migration to inflamed tissues, and may reduce free radical formation [257]. These effects would result in decreased nociception secondary to reduced inflammation.

In addition to local administration (e.g., regional nerve block or infiltration of tissue), systemic administration of local anesthetics for analgesia has been examined. Systemically administered lidocaine decreases minimum alveolar concentration values for inhaled anesthetics in many species, suggesting a possible role in modulation of noxious stimuli. However, conscious dogs tested with electrical cutaneous stimulation showed no change in nociceptive threshold with a variety of dosages of systemically administered lidocaine [258]. Certain clinical procedures, such as intraocular surgery, however, have yielded different results [259]. A study by Smith *et al.* [259] suggests that there is a benefit to the addition of intraoperative lidocaine. Similarly, work by Tsai *et al.* suggests that systemic administration of lidocaine provided comparable analgesia to meloxicam in clinical patients undergoing ovariohysterectomy [260].

Na^+ channels

The neuronal membrane has a resting potential between −60 and −90 mV that is maintained by active Na^+ transport out of the cell and K^+ transport into the cell. The membrane accomplishes this with an Na^+/K^+ ATPase pump. Because K^+ continually leaks from the membrane (via K^+-leak channels), and the membrane is relatively impermeable to Na^+, the membrane eventually becomes polarized. A noxious stimulus opens voltage-gated channels, allowing a massive Na^+ influx that results in depolarization and propagation of the action potential. Local anesthetics penetrate the nerve sheath, equilibrate, and bind to voltage-gated Na^+ channels to inhibit the conformational change that would otherwise occur in response to noxious stimuli. This prevents the channel from functioning. Local anesthetics do not affect resting membrane or threshold potential.

Nerve fibers

The type of nerve fiber that is affected makes a difference to the blockade achieved with a local anesthetic. Peripheral nerves vary in myelination, size, distance from stimuli, and depolarization threshold. Axons responsible for transmission of noxious stimuli are often small, with A-δ and C fibers providing the bulk of noxious transmission. A-δ fibers are myelinated whereas C fibers are not. In myelinated nerve fibers, Na^+ channels are concentrated in the nodes of Ranvier. To prevent transmission of stimuli, it is thought that it is necessary to block three consecutive nodes. Although, logically, it makes sense that blockade of smaller nerve fibers would occur first (secondary to a greater delivery of drug to nerve size), it is not necessarily true. This is due to the proportional relationship between conduction velocity and distance between action sites. Larger fibers having the greatest internodal distance and thus require less drug to provide blockade then smaller myelinated nerve fibers, which will have a smaller distance between internodal sites and thus require more drug to block all sites. Unmyelinated small nerves require the highest drug concentration as it is necessary to bathe essentially the entire nerve for blockade to occur [261].

Alternative receptors for local anesthetics

Local anesthetics may also block K^+ channels, although they have a much lower affinity for voltage-gated K^+ channels than for Na^+ channels [262]. Local anesthetics may also block Ca^{2+} channels [263,264], which is likely because of the structural similarity between Ca^{2+} channels and Na^+ channels. Modulation of *N*-methyl-D-aspartate receptors may also contribute to the antinociceptive action of certain local anesthetics [265].

N-Methyl-D-aspartate receptor antagonists

N-Methyl-D-aspartate (NMDA) receptor activation is critical in the processing of nociceptive signaling and, as a result, NMDA antagonists are unique in their ability to alter pain transmission. Ketamine has run the gamut of pain modulation applications, with reported use in acute, chronic, burn, cancer, and neuropathic pain settings [266–270]. Ketamine is often regarded as a more effective analgesic for somatic rather than visceral pain [271]. In people, the dose of ketamine required for analgesia is much lower than that required for anesthesia, especially if it is combined with an opioid [272]. These low doses did not appear effective in the cat or dog when assessed by laboratory methods of pain assessment [78,84]. Although the effectiveness of ketamine for acute pain is questionable based on laboratory studies, there is clinical evidence for the use of ketamine when hyperalgesia is likely to occur following tissue damage [273].

In the horse, subanesthetic doses of ketamine, when combined with tramadol, provided analgesia in cases of chronic laminitis [274], although caution is recommended when GI transit time is a concern [275]. There is some preclinical evidence that the (*S*)-ketamine enantiomer has more analgesic effects than the racemic mixture [276], but this is difficult to prove in clinical veterinary patients. Ketamine is often utilized as an adjunctive analgesic and its success as an analgesic drug is dependent on the type of pain that the patient is experiencing [277]. Ketamine can be a useful adjunct since there is usually a reduction in the amount of opioids that a patient requires for pain management when ketamine is incorporated in an analgesic regime. Additionally, ketamine's action as an NMDA antagonist may counter opioid-induced hyperalgesia [278,279]. Ketamine is not without adverse effects, however, and like other analgesic drugs its use should be based on a risk–benefit analysis.

Amantadine, an orally administered NMDA antagonist, may have some usefulness in the treatment of chronic pain associated with arthritis in dogs when used in conjunction with NSAIDs [280].

Effect of route of delivery

Although systemic administration of ketamine for antinociception remains the most common, other routes of administration have been explored. Similarly to local anesthetics, ketamine can produce an area of localized hypoalgesia. In fact, there is some suggestion that intravenous regional anesthesia can be improved with ketamine administration [281]. Human patients reported reduced radiation therapy-induced pain with the inclusion of topical ketamine on oral or skin mucosa [282].

Ketamine has also been administered via the epidural or subarachnoid route [283–285]. It is well absorbed from the epidural space, with a rapid onset and short but intense effect (the decrease in hyperalgesia may last longer). Ketamine does not come in a commercially available preservative-free formulation and comprehensive toxicity studies have not been completed.

Sites of action

Ketamine appears to have effects peripherally, within the dorsal horn of the spinal cord [286], and supraspinally in the limbic and thalamoneocortical systems [287]. NMDA receptors are located on the secondary afferent neurons (postsynaptically).

NMDA receptor structure and function

The NMDA receptor has a central ligand-gated ion channel surrounded by five subunits. It conducts multiple ions, including calcium, potassium, and sodium. Normally, the channel formed by these subunits is blocked by magnesium and does not allow ions to cross because the duration of depolarization is too short. However, glutamate with glycine (as an obligatory co-agonist) [288], activates the channel, usually associated with persistent nociceptive input. This activation results in stimulation of secondary messengers, enzymatic processes, and generation of nitric oxide, among other substances, resulting in central sensitization secondary to increased neuronal sensitivity. NMDA antagonists work by non-competitively binding the phencyclidine site of the NMDA receptor and antagonizing the effects of excitatory neurotransmitters. Antagonism can occur as the result of inhibition of receptor activation, potentiation of γ-aminobutyric acid (GABA) as an inhibitory neurotransmitter, and decreasing presynaptic release of glutamate.

NMDA antagonist antinociceptive effects

Opioid receptors

Undoubtedly, the analgesic effect of ketamine is mediated heavily by inhibition of the NMDA receptor, but a κ-opioid receptor effect cannot be excluded [289].

Monoaminergic receptors

There is potential involvement of the glutamate system in the mechanism of antidepressant drug action, suggesting that NMDA antagonists may be useful in the management of severe depression. The literature suggests improvement of pain symptoms in human patients when they were placed on NMDA antagonists for their depression [290]. The use of monoaminergic drugs in human pain management is common when treating depression as a common comorbidity to chronic pain (modulation of the emotional component of pain and dysinhibition).

Voltage-gated Na^+ channels and L-type Ca^{2+} channels

Na^+ and Ca^{2+} ion channels in the dorsal horn of the spinal cord are blocked with clinically relevant concentrations of ketamine when applied intrathecally [291]. This decrease in neuronal excitability likely also explains ketamine's efficacy following its epidural administration [292].

ATP-sensitive K^+ channels

ATP-sensitive K^+ channels (KATP) are activated through an increase in cyclic guanosine monophosphate (cGMP), via nitric oxide (NO). The stimulation of the NO/cGMP/KATP pathway is implicated as one of the molecular mechanisms responsible for the peripherally observed antinociception effects imparted by ketamine [293].

Neutrophil and cytokine suppression

Ketamine may reduce inflammation through its suppression of neutrophil production by inflammatory mediators, a reduction in cytokine production, and alteration of inflammatory cell recruitment [294].

Ketamine metabolites

Studies in rats suggest that norketamine, an active metabolite of ketamine, has analgesic effects [295]. However, this does not appear to be true in cattle, once again highlighting the importance of species-specific antinociceptive research [296].

Non-steroidal anti-inflammatory drugs (NSAIDs)

NSAIDs are typically used as long-acting, non-controlled, oral or injectable drugs for the management of pain. The AAHA/AAFP task force on pain management recommends NSAIDs as standard medications in the recovery period after elective procedures [297].

Damage to a cell's phospholipid membrane initiates the release or synthesis of inflammatory mediators that induce nociception. NSAIDs inhibit cyclooxygenase (COX) production of proinflammatory molecules from arachidonic acid, decreasing both prostaglandin (PG) formation and thromboxane (TX) production. COX isoenzymes are classified as either COX-1 or COX-2. As a generalization, COX-1 is considered a 'constitutive' enzyme. COX-2 is referred to as an 'inducible' (although there is some evidence for it being constitutive in the brain and kidney in some species) enzyme, and plays a role in the induction of pain, inflammation, and fever. The delineation between constitutive or inducible is an oversimplification; for example, when GI tissue is surgically damaged, COX-2 is likely necessary for healing [298]. Deleterious side-effects can result from inhibition of COX enzymes that play a role in basic homeostatic or compensatory functions.

In the horse, flunixin may provide a longer duration of postoperative analgesia than carprofen or phenylbutazone [299]. Flunixin is interesting among commonly used veterinary NSAIDs in that it appears to reduce visceral pain effectively [300]. NSAIDs as a class are usually most useful in somatic or integumentary pain where inflammation is a major component. NSAIDs are effective peripherally and topical application of 1% diclofenac has been shown to reduce inflammation (with the speculation that this would decrease pain) in horses undergoing regional limb perfusion [301]. In cattle undergoing dehorning and castration, postoperative average daily weight gain improved and cortisol concentrations (used as a physiologic pain marker) decreased when salicylates were included in the drinking water compared with cattle that underwent the same procedure but did not receive salicylates [302]. Pigeons, when appropriately dosed, had quantifiable analgesia from the inclusion of NSAID in their postoperative management plan [303].

Sites of action

NSAIDs produce analgesia by decreasing peripheral inflammatory COX enzyme conversion of arachidonic acid and, to some extent, reduce central pain transmission.

COX-1

There is evidence that the mechanism of action for the acute antinociceptive effects of NSAIDs at the level of the brain is in part mediated by COX-1 isoenzymes. It also appears that prostaglandins expressed in the neuronal tissue structures alter C fiber- rather than

A-δ fiber-mediated spinal nociception [304]. Expression of COX-1 mRNA is upregulated in the spinal cord in postoperative pain models, providing further evidence that COX-2 is not the only isoform contributing to spinal nociception [305].

COX-2

Inhibition of COX-2 isoenzymes is beneficial for animals with pain of inflammatory origin. It is believed that pain is suppressed by NSAID suppression of prostaglandin E_2 production (mediated by induced COX-2). Peripheral nociceptors are also upregulated in the presence of prostaglandin E_2 [306].

Because COX-1 inhibition is associated with many of the adverse effects of NSAIDs, it is sometimes recommended that NSAIDs that either preferentially or selectively target the COX-2 isoenzyme be used. However, it should be mentioned that no NSAID available in the veterinary market is without COX-1 effects (COX-1's neuronal involvement may be beneficial). Adverse effects in some organ systems can be minimized when COX-2 isoenzymes are targeted. It should also be noted that it is unlikely that COX-2 selective or preferential NSAIDs provide superior analgesia to their non-selective or non-preferential drugs [307]; their primary benefit is a reduction in the occurrence of some specific adverse GI effects and reduced bleeding associated with surgery.

Leukotrienes and 5-Lipoxygenase (5-LOX)

Eicosanoids, which are lipid mediators derived from arachidonic acid and released from the cell membrane by phospholipases, are the family to which leukotrienes belong. Leukotrienes are liberated by lipoxygenases (a proinflammatory mediator), and have a relatively poorly defined contribution to the nociceptive process (although in humans their inflammatory role in asthma is well characterized). There is some suggestion that 5-LOX inhibition suppresses mechanical allodynia and that leukotrienes themselves may play a role at the level of the spinal cord in neuropathic pain [308]. In the dog, expression of 5-LOX in osteosarcoma suggests that a dual inhibitor of 5-LOX/cyclooxygenase (e.g., tepoxalin) may have therapeutic benefit in addition to providing analgesia [309]. Osteoarthritic canine joints also express 5-LOX, suggesting that targeting this eicosanoid may improve analgesia in this condition [310]. Tepoxalin has been pharmacologically evaluated in the horse [311,312], but analgesic studies have not been performed. Tepoxalin has been use in the cat [313], and it appears to have an analgesic effect [314]. At the time of this writing, tepoxalin is no longer commercially available in the United States.

Opioids

Opioids remain the primary class of pharmacologic agents in treating acute severe pain. By mimicking the action of endogenous opioids (i.e., enkephalins, endorphins, and dynorphins) and binding their receptors, pain modulation occurs. Opioid receptors utilize G-protein inhibition of cyclic AMP to achieve their analgesic effect. This inhibition leads to increased K^+ conductance (which results in hyperpolarization of the second-order neuron) and to the inhibition of voltage-gated Ca^{2+} channels (neurotransmitter release from the first-order neuron is thus decreased), resulting in decreased neurotransmission of painful stimuli within the sensory afferent nervous system [315,316]. Inhibition of the release of other excitatory neurotransmitters such as substance P may occur through activation of peripheral opioid receptors [317]. It is important to note that opioids do not alter the conduction of impulses or the response of the nerve endings to noxious stimuli. Opioids are extremely effective at modulation of pain by raising the pain threshold, but they do not prevent the generation of noxious stimuli as local anesthetics and NSAIDs might. Important adverse effects of opioids, such as postoperative hyperthermia in cats [318] and dysphoria, warrant a review prior to their use. It should be mentioned that many adverse effects of opioids are diminished when an animal is in pain (as opposed to premedication in an animal that has not undergone an invasive procedure). Additionally, opioids generally have a high safety margin, and are reversible if deemed necessary.

Hypoalgesia imparted by opioids is not equally efficacious for all types of pain, and results may vary according to the research model used in assessing efficacy and also the species involved. For example, in the cat, visceral analgesia was obtained with butorphanol and nalbuphine, but when the same drugs were tested against an electrical stimulus in the cat, they were not as effective [319]. In the horse, response to thermal and electrical noxious stimuli is present after administration of morphine [320], yet when administered epidurally it appears effective in horses clinically [321,322]. Indeed, opioids such as remifentanil, which did not alter the minimal alveolar concentration (MAC) in anesthetized cats, induce an hypoalgesic effect in the same animals when conscious [323].

Sites of action

Opioids work peripherally, spinally, and supraspinally at stereospecific opioid receptors. These receptors occur both pre- and postsynaptically. Certain peripheral tissues, such as articular (synovium) tissue in the canine and equine species, can generate opioid receptors [324–326]. The peripheral action of opioids is more profound after an inflammatory event in articular or periarticular tissue, suggesting activation or upregulation of opioid receptors on primary afferent neurons locally [325]. Thus, intra-articular morphine is in part a suitable analgesic for conditions such as synovitis [327]. The corneal tissue generates opioid receptors in several species [328], and both topically applied tramadol and morphine have been used to provide analgesia of the cornea. Further evaluation of the effectiveness and toxicology of opioid-containing ophthalmic preparations is needed before prolonged routine use can be recommended [329,330].

Opioids produce postsynaptic inhibition of second-order neurons transmitting nociceptive information in the dorsal horn of the spinal cord. The presence of these receptors in the substantia gelatinosa accounts for the analgesic effects of epidurally administered opioids. Epidural administration allows the opioid to diffuse across the dura mater into the cerebrospinal fluid, which bathes the spinal cord. Drugs with low lipophilicity, such as morphine, have a longer duration of action as a result of a longer residence time. Although there have been many reports of various species benefiting from epidural opioid analgesia [331–333], the horse in particular should be mentioned. Although some questions remain concerning the adverse events associated with the singular systemic use of full μ-opioid agonists such as morphine in horses, epidural use is appears beneficial [321,334].

Supraspinally, there is a wide distribution of opioid receptors in the frontal cortex, amygdala, somatosensory cortex, colliculus, and cerebellum. However, this distribution likely varies greatly among species [335]. For example, species that tend to exhibit excitatory behavior in response to opioids (e.g., the cat and horse) have a lower concentration of opioid receptors in the amygdala and frontal cortex than species that typically become sedated (e.g., humans, dogs, and primates) [336]. This may explain the observed wide spectrum in altered mentation in differing species following specific opioid administration. Dogma suggests that birds show more κ-receptor expression, and therefore are more likely to respond to opioid drugs with κ-agonist activity. However, a few antinociceptive studies have suggested that μ-opioid agonists (e.g., hydromorphone) may also be effective (increased thermal threshold) in some species of birds [337,338].

The emotional component of pain is mediated via the limbic system, where opioids act to alter the motivation-affective component of perception (i.e., helping to make pain more tolerable). This effect in non-verbal species remains undefined but may be present in socially advanced species such as more highly evolved primates and aquatic mammals (porpoises and whales).

Opioid receptor classification

Opioid receptors have undergone various classification schemes. Currently, the International Union of Basic and Clinical Pharmacology (IUPHAR) classifies opioid receptors as δ, κ, μ, and nociception/orphanin FQ (NOP) [339]. Of these receptors, μ and κ are the main receptors involved in nociceptive modulation. The δ-receptor does not appear to play a role in acute analgesia. However, there appears a potential benefit to inducing δ-receptor agonist activity during some chronic pain states [340].

The μ-receptor gene has been identified and cloned and μ_1- and μ_2-opioid receptor subtypes have been identified [341,342]. Similarly, subtypes of δ (δ_1 and δ_2) and κ (κ_1, κ_2, and κ_3) receptors have been described. Until more information is available on the specific activity of each subtype, and clinically useful subtype selective agonists are developed, subtypes remain mostly of academic interest. The presence of specific opioid receptor subtypes suggest the possibility of developing more selective drugs with desirable analgesic qualities accompanied by fewer adverse effects.

Alternative mechanisms of actions

Monoaminergic receptors

Tramadol and its metabolites are relatively weak μ-receptor agonists, but tramadol also possesses both norepinephrine and serotonin reuptake inhibition [343,344]. Tapentadol's μ activity is greater than that of tramadol, with prominent norepinephrine reuptake inhibition and minimal serotonin effect. Tapentadol has greater opioid effect in humans than does tramadol because of better CNS penetration. Tramadol may be useful for mild pain, especially when combined with an NSAID [345]. Tapentadol has only recently been examined for veterinary use [346], but may prove more efficacious in some species.

Muscarinic receptors

Opioids can cause inhibition of acetylcholine release from nerve endings, which in addition to analgesia may explain some of the common side-effects of opioids (e.g., GI stasis, pupillary changes).

NMDA receptors

Opioid receptors may be uncoupled from downstream signaling pathways following protein kinase C activity as a result of excitatory amino acids binding to NMDA receptors. Prolonged opioid administration can ultimately result in reduced efficacy (i.e., tolerance) [347]. Hence it has been suggested that the inclusion of ketamine or methadone therapy, both of which have NMDA antagonist activity, may lessen the onset of opioid tolerance during longer term opioid therapy.

Adjunctive analgesics

Corticosteroids

Corticosteroids are anti-inflammatory drugs that reduce pain of inflammatory origin. They are available in a variety of forms, including topical, oral, and injectable. Most veterinarians choose an NSAID for reducing inflammation due to systemic adverse effects that can occur with longer term high-dose exogenous steroid administration (e.g., polyuria and polydipsia, gastrointestinal ulceration, iatrogenic Cushing's disease).

Site of action

The peripheral anti-inflammatory effects of glucocorticoids have been recognized for years. However, the role of the hypothalamic–pituitary–adrenocortical axis in pain modulation is less well understood, especially in companion animal species. There is some evidence in the rat that a central component is involved in the antinociceptive action of glucocorticoids [348].

Gabapentin and pregabalin

Gabapentin and pregabalin are commonly used in treating pain of neuropathic origin. These neuro-pharmaceutical compounds are structural analogs of GABA, although their mechanisms of action do not appear to result from any actual GABAergic receptor interaction. Gabapentin is widely used to treat a number of human neuropathic pain syndromes; however, evidence in non-verbal animals is less compelling [349]. Although pregabalin has undergone pharmacokinetic evaluations in companion animals, few data substantiating analgesic efficacy exist for companion animal species [350,351].

Sites of Action

The analgesic benefit of gabapentin and pregabalin occurs at spinal and supraspinal sites of actions. α_2-δ-Receptors associated with specific voltage-dependent calcium-channel blockade appear responsible for both the supraspinal action within the higher CNS and inhibition of the sensory afferent neurons within the peripheral nervous system [352].

Neurokinin (NK)-1 receptor antagonists

NK-1 receptors are activated by substance P. They are diffusely distributed in the body. Although the involvement of NK-1 receptors in nociception is still undergoing investigation, it appears that some may have a role in facilitating pain and hyperalgesia [353]. NK-1 receptors have been identified in the CNS and peripheral nervous system. Although maropitant is primarily used as an antiemetic, in a canine model of visceral nociception it decreased anesthetic requirement and noxious response to ovarian manipulation, suggesting a possible analgesic effect [354]. Much more work is necessary to determine if an analgesic effect of clinical significance can be achieved via CNS and peripheral nervous system NK-1 receptor antagonism [355,356].

Transient receptor potential vanilloid type 1 (TRPV 1) antagonists

TRPV1 receptors are upregulated in inflammation and also in certain neuropathic conditions [357]. Noxious stimuli, including capsaicin and heat, are integrated at the molecular level by this receptor. While agonists at TRPV1 sites may result in analgesia, the initial effect is considerable excitation which may result in neuronal damage and pain. Investigations of TRPV1 antagonists showed benefits for some pain states [358]. In a study of healthy pain-free dogs, nociceptive testing suggested superior analgesia with buprenorphine compared with ABT-116 (a TRPV1 antagonist) [359]. However, in dogs with chemically induced synovitis, analgesia occurred after the use of ABT-116 [360]. These drugs have some adverse effects, including hyperthermia and diarrhea [359]. More information on differences between species, dosage, and pain alleviated with this class of drugs is required before clinical recommendations can be made.

Site of action

TRPV1 receptors are ligand-gated nonselective cation channels that contribute to the regulation of intracellular calcium concentrations, and occur diffusely throughout the body.

Non-pharmacologic modifiers of pain

Physiology has provided a complex, multifaceted tapestry for both nociceptive sensing and modification of the transmitted signal. The term 'physical medicine' describes techniques and modalities that interact with physiologic processes of the body to exert effects on intrinsic healing mechanisms and homeostasis. Physical medicine techniques can interface with endogenous physiology in various ways via:

- temperature-related modalities
- tissue deformation
- peripheral neuromodulation
- spinal neuromodulation
- central neuromodulation
- kinematic modulation
- modulation of metabolism and blood flow
- muscle spasm and myofascial trigger points
- immune modulation.

Temperature-related modalities

Both hot and cold temperatures are detected by transient receptor potential (TRP) channels on nociceptive afferent neurons [361]. Different channel subtypes are specifically activated by some stimuli (hot or cold pain) and suppressed by others (analgesia) [362].

Cold can be analgesic, causing a decrease of pain signaling peripherally and spinally. It also decreases the migration of inflammatory cells to injured tissues, decreasing inflammation. Vasoconstriction reduces pain cascades (as both systems require a robust blood supply to amplify), reduces edema formation, and decrease inflammation. Cold decreases tissue metabolism and oxygen demand, and also reduces tissue distensibility [363]. Cold is frequently utilized in acute and inflammatory types of pain and to reduce secondary tissue injury attributed to inflammatory damage.

Warmth may be pain relieving or noxious depending on the condition of the tissue. Peripherally, warmth may inactivate and suppress TRP channels [361]. Centrally, heat provides competitive inhibition to nociceptive signals and releases antinociceptive neurotransmitters at the level of the thalamus, cerebral cortex, and spinal cord [363]. Heat increases tissue distensibility, tissue blood flow, and metabolism. By increasing blood flow, heat promotes edema formation in acutely injured tissue. However, by increasing venous dilation relative to arterial dilation, heat is useful in reducing previously established edema. Along with cold, heat reduces muscle spasm and, unlike cold, it also restores blood flow to hypoxic regions (myofascial trigger points). Increased tissue temperature also facilitate oxygen delivery by shifting the oxyhemoglobin dissociation curve in favor of unloading. In acute and inflammatory pain, heat amplifies pain signaling and is contraindicated. It is not applied during the acute inflammatory phase of injury, but plays an important long-term role in chronic pain and during the recovery phase of injury. Owing to the effects of tissue distensibility and trigger point deactivation, heat is an important precursor to stretching, range of motion manipulations, or exercises and massage.

Tissue deformation

Tissue deformation is a modulator of intrinsic healing in soft tissues such as skin, muscle, ligaments, tendons, fascia, cartilage, and periosteum. An integrated web is formed between muscle and fascia throughout the body, and this complex provides both active and passive tensile forces across the body [364]. Changes in the baseline tensile forces are associated with pain, and stretching of these soft-tissue components improves gait, mechanical pain, and local inflammation in rodents [365,366].

When this connective tissue complex is deformed, growth factors and a variety of proteins and neurotransmitters are released [367,368]. Fibroblasts in loose connective tissue respond to stretch within minutes, increasing ATP and cytoskeletal relationships with neighboring cells [369]. This cascade of events may lead to changes in nociceptive processing, metabolic processes, inflammation, blood flow, and healing capacity [370].

Modalities

A host of interventions predating modern pharmacology are utilized for the management of pain. Simple examples include various forms of massage (from extremely superficial lymphedema-type massage to deep-tissue massage), and various forms of activity such as exercise, stretching, and motion. More complex methods include joint mobilizations, acupuncture, and trigger-point release methods.

Acupuncture research demonstrates a significant impact of needling on mechanotransduction in the areolar connective tissue compartment [371]. Needle rotation triggers fibroblast spreading with an increase in cell body area within 30 min of a 720° rotation. This effect is blocked by pharmacologic inhibition of myosin contraction. The cytoskeletal response spreads centimeters from the original stimulus and leads to changes in phosphorylation, gene expression, protein synthesis, and extracellular milieu. Cumulative changes in fibroblast contraction, gene expression, and metabolism validate the observation that acupuncture effects amplify over time, and are persistent [372,373].

Shock-wave therapy applies the principles of tissue deformation to promote healing by use of sound waves to distort deep tissues. Deformation of deep tissues, especially at the junction of discrete tissue types (such as bone–tendon, periosteum–bone, and cartilage–bone) promotes healing in joints, deep tendon injuries, deep wounds, nerve injuries, and non-healing fractures [374]. Shock-wave therapy has demonstrated protective effects on cartilage in a cruciate injury model in rodents when used early in the degenerative process [375].

Neuromodulatory activities

Neuromodulatory modalities interact with the nervous system structures with the aim of restoring homeostasis. Neuromodulation modifies neurotransmitters in the skin, along axons, in the spinal cord, with interneurons, in the brain, and even in the supportive structures of the glia. These changes may be both short-term and long-standing.

Peripheral neuromodulation (mechano-transduction)

This technique utilizes a triad of peripheral pain-sensing components: the nerve ending, blood vessels (and circulating cells), and mast cells. When an acupuncture needle (or other form of stimulation) is applied, fibroblasts are wound around the tip of the needle, and mechano-transduction ensues. Mast cells release granules of mixed peptides and neurotransmitters, including opioid peptides, bradykinin, serotonin, and adenosine. Dilation of capillaries allows recruitment of inflammatory cells which release opioid peptides and other neurotransmitters. Receptor populations are altered to increase cannabinoid and opioid receptor populations on peripheral nerve endings, and transient receptor potential (TRP) channels undergo subtype changes. Interleukins and prostaglandins are altered at the location of needle entry, further promoting anti-inflammatory and analgesic activities (provided that severe tissue damage itself is not caused by employment of the technique) [376].

Spinal neuromodulation

Spinal neuromodulation can occur from altering a milieu of neurotransmitters including endogenous opioids, serotonin, norepinephrine, glutamate, and cytokines, and suppression of glial inflammation. It has long been recognized that inhibitors of opioid transmission reduce the efficacy of acupuncture-induced analgesia [377]. Addition of electrical impulses alters the type of opioids released from spinal cord segments, with low frequency (2–4 Hz) releasing endorphins and enkephalins and high frequency (100–200 Hz) releasing dynorphins [378].

Serotonin- and norepinephrine-releasing neurons projecting to the spinal cord are also implicated in neuromodulation associated with acupuncture and electro-acupuncture. A number of pharmacologic compounds target these receptor systems, and clinical data support that drug doses [opioids, selective serotonin reuptake inhibitors (SSRIs), serotonin–norepinephrine reuptake inhibitors (SNRIs)] are often reduced when combined with the use of various acupuncture modalities [376].

Glutamate and its receptors are major excitatory inputs at the level of the spinal cord. Phosphorylation of glutamate receptors is decreased with acupuncture, and inhibition of NMDA receptor activation has been suggested from the results of various studies [379].

Glial cells and cytokines

Acupuncture interferes with reactive oxygen species-induced activation of the microglial inflammatory cascades, potentially reducing pain after spinal cord injury [377,380]. Opioids are activators of microglia, and acupuncture changes that activation pattern [377,380]. Glia are also responsible for neurotrophic factors. Electrical stimulation and acupuncture may amplify nerve growth factors in glial cells that are known to influence CNS plasticity and sensitization [381].

Neurotrophic factors are released by a number of tissues associated with the peripheral and central nervous systems. As mentioned previously for peripheral mechano-transduction, growth factors released from these tissues may increase healing, modify the chemical milieu, and alter nerve growth, healing, and plasticity. Acupuncture may alter a number of these growth factors in each tissue location [382,383].

Central neuromodulation

Central neuromodulation serves to inhibit the sensory dimension of pain. Supraspinal structures associated with central neuromodulation from non-pharmacologic treatments include nuclei in the periaqueductal gray (PAG)–arcuate–nucleus raphe magnus–spinal pathway [384]. In addition to the hard-wired central modulatory pathways for pain, various environmental and behavioral factors influence pain processing [385]. Translational data show that laboratory rodents also experience behavioral alterations in pain sensation [386].

Physical medicine modalities obviously affect central neuromodulation [387]. This may augment the clinical effects of various physical medicine techniques, while also complicating the interpretation of physical medicine modalities in randomized clinical trials. Many physical medicine modalities show evidence for improvement compared with no treatment or standard pharmacologic treatment, but often do not show improvement over placebo [388]. Translating experimental findings from physical medicine modalities remains challenging when attempting to determine the exact physiologic and/or psychologic mechanisms associated with specific modality outcomes that are likely confounded by a significant placebo effect elicited through human–animal interaction itself (resulting in central neuromodulation) [389].

Kinematic training

Kinematic training includes both strength and function training, in addition to a form of neuromodulation, with the aim of improving neurologic function and outcomes. The nervous system is a use-dependent system, and by training with exercise, treadmills, and assistive devices, significant recovery from neurologic injury can be accomplished [390]. An animal may present anywhere on a continuum from minimally painful to extremely painful, and minimally functional to highly functional. Pain perceived and function do not necessarily match, increasing the need to evaluate each individual separately rather than focusing on a protocol-based approach to nerve injuries [391,392].

Stimulation of metabolism and blood flow

Stimulation of metabolic processes can play a role in augmenting many of the previous mentioned modalities and therapies. In recent years, laser therapy has become an increasingly utilized technique from within the physical medicine armamentarium that is available to veterinarians. Laser therapy contributes to neuromodulation and neuroprotection, in addition to having an effect of stimulating metabolism and cellular respiration via light energy [393]. There remain a number of unanswered questions about laser therapy (such as whether or not pulsing the light is important, the dose needed, and how quickly or slowly the dose is administered for best effect), but for painful conditions and wounds an increasing body of anecdotal clinical evidence has been established [394].

Muscle spasm, myofascial trigger points, and pain

Muscle spasm is a contributor to both acute and chronic pain. A significant percentage of acupuncture point locations are associated with regions that generate muscular dysfunction and pain, such as myofascial trigger points, musculotendinous junctions, and muscle motor points. Acupuncture needling techniques are standard practice in physical therapy (dry needling), osteopathic treatment of referred pain, and sports medicine practice [395,396]. The use of heat to disrupt trigger points was discussed under Temperature-Related Modalities. Massage also helps reduce myofascial trigger points and a variety of techniques have been established to address this particular component of a pain experience. Myofascial tension can result from stimuli arising in other locations (such as joints, spine, tendons), amplifies pain sensitization, and can damage local and regional tissues by creating excessive and persistent traction across joints and disk spaces. These actions, in turn, may contribute to intervertebral disk degeneration and rupture, OA, tendinopathies, and ligament rupture [397].

Immune modulation

Of the physical medicine modalities, acupuncture and exercise are the most extensively studied for their immune modulating effects [397]. Acupuncture has been demonstrated to have peripheral immune modulating actions such as modulating natural killer cell cytotoxicity and balancing T-cell subtypes that may favor healing versus lysing varieties. Furthermore, acupuncture has long been recognized to modulate centrally mediated neuroimmune communication [398]. Specific regions of neuroimmune modulatory activity include peripheral neurotransmitters (opioids, cannabinoids, serotonin, norepinephrine, etc.) that activate the autonomic nervous system in a spatiotemporal specific pattern and elicit measurable psychophysical responses such as analgesia, regulation of visceral function, and modified immune function. These circulating neurotransmitters modify the activity of a variety of immune cells. The steady state of the individual's immune system may alter the neural–immune signaling pathway. Centrally, acupuncture and exercise modalities affect the hypothalamus (and dorsal motor nucleus of the vagus), which is the primary center of neuroendocrine–immune modulation and also regulation of the autonomic nervous system [399].

Pain and immune states are intrinsically entwined, and the layers of these relationships are only gradually being realized. The utilization of various physical medicine modalities may alter both of these complex and interdependent systems simultaneously.

References

1 Wall PD. *Pain: the Science of Suffering*. New York: Columbia University Press, 2000.
2 IASP Taxonomy Working Group. *IASP Pain Terminology. Part III. Pain Terms. A Current List with Definitions and Notes on Usage*. Seattle, WA: IASP Press, 2011. http://www.iasp-pain.org/files/Content/ContentFolders/Publications2/ClassificationofChronicPain/Part_III-PainTerms.pdf (accessed 14 August 2014).
3 Morton C, Reid J, Scott E, *et al*. Application of a scaling model to establish and validate an interval level pain scale for assessment of acute pain in dogs. *Am J Vet Res* 2005; **66**(12): 2154–2166.
4 Mathews K, Kronen PW, Lascelles D, *et al*. Guidelines for recognition, assessment and treatment of pain. *J Small Anim Pract* 2014; **55**(6): E10–E68.
5 Honore P, Rogers SD, Schwei MJ, *et al*. Murine models of inflammatory, neuropathic and cancer pain each generates a unique set of neurochemical changes in the spinal cord and sensory neurons. *Neuroscience* 2000; **98**(3): 585–598.
6 Basbaum A, Jessell T. *The Perception of Pain*, 4th edn. New York: McGraw-Hill, 2000; 472–491.
7 Perl ER. Ideas about pain, a historical view. *Nat Rev Neurosci* 2007; **8**(1): 71–80.
8 Olausson H, Cole J, Rylander K, *et al*. Functional role of unmyelinated tactile afferents in human hairy skin: sympathetic response and perceptual localization. *Exp Brain Res* 2008; **184**(1): 135–140.
9 Schmidt R, Schmelz M, Forster C, *et al*. Novel classes of responsive and unresponsive C nociceptors in human skin. *J Neurosci* 1995; **15**(1 Pt 1): 333–341.
10 Julius D, Basbaum AI. Molecular mechanisms of nociception. *Nature* 2001; **413**(6852): 203–210.
11 Kehlet H, Holte K. Effect of postoperative analgesia on surgical outcome. *Br J Anaesth* 2001; **87**(1): 62–72.
12 Macrae WA. Chronic pain after surgery. *Br J Anaesth* 2001; **87**(1): 88–98.
13 Lerner RK, Esterhai JL Jr, Polomono RC, *et al*. Psychosocial, functional, and quality of life assessment of patients with posttraumatic fracture nonunion, chronic refractory osteomyelitis, and lower extremity amputation. *Arch Phys Med Rehabil* 1991; **72**(2): 122–126.
14 Woolf C, Chong M. Preemptive analgesia – treating postoperative pain by preventing the establishment of central sensitization. *Anesth Analg* 1993; **77**(2): 362–379.
15 Bourinet E, Altier C, Hildebrand ME, *et al*. Calcium-permeable ion channels in pain signaling. *Physiol Rev* 2014; **94**(1): 81–140.
16 Waxman SG, Zamponi GW. Regulating excitability of peripheral afferents: emerging ion channel targets. *Nat Neurosci* 2014; **17**(2): 153–163.
17 Dib-Hajj SD, Rush AM, Cummins TR, *et al*. Gain-of-function mutation in Nav1.7 in familial erythromelalgia induces bursting of sensory neurons. *Brain* 2005; **128**(Pt 8): 1847–1854.
18 Faber CG, Lauria G, Merkies IS, *et al*. Gain-of-function Nav1.8 mutations in painful neuropathy. *Proc Natl Acad Sci U S A* 2012; **109**(47): 19444–19449.
19 Nassar MA, Stirling LC, Forlani G, *et al*. Nociceptor-specific gene deletion reveals a major role for Nav1.7 (PN1) in acute and inflammatory pain. *Proc Natl Acad Sci U S A* 2004; **101**(34): 12706–12711.
20 Cox JJ, Reimann F, Nicholas AK, *et al*. An SCN9A channelopathy causes congenital inability to experience pain. *Nature* 2006; **444**(7121): 894–898.
21 Goldberg YP, Price N, Namdari R, *et al*. Treatment of Na(v)1.7-mediated pain in inherited erythromelalgia using a novel sodium channel blocker. *Pain* 2012; **153**(1): 80–85.
22 Jarvis MF, Honore P, Shieh CC, *et al*. A-803467, a potent and selective Nav1.8 sodium channel blocker, attenuates neuropathic and inflammatory pain in the rat. *Proc Natl Acad Sci U S A* 2007; **104**(20): 8520–8525.
23 Akopian AN, Souslova V, England S, *et al*. The tetrodotoxin-resistant sodium channel SNS has a specialized function in pain pathways. *Nat Neurosci* 1999; **2**(6): 541–548.
24 Priest BT, Murphy BA, Lindia JA, *et al*. Contribution of the tetrodotoxin-resistant voltage-gated sodium channel NaV1.9 to sensory transmission and nociceptive behavior. *Proc Natl Acad Sci U S A* 2005; **102**(26): 9382–9387.
25 Woolf CJ. Central sensitization: implications for the diagnosis and treatment of pain. *Pain* 2011; **152**(3 Suppl):S2–S15.
26 Lascelles BD, Cripps PJ, Jones A, Waterman AE. Post-operative central hypersensitivity and pain: the pre-emptive value of pethidine for ovariohysterectomy. *Pain* 1997; **73**(3): 461–471.
27 Lascelles B, Court M, Hardie E, Robertson S. Nonsteroidal anti-inflammatory drugs in cats: a review. *Vet Anaesth Analg* 2007; **34**(4): 228–250.
28 Lascelles BD, Cripps PJ, Jones A, Waterman AE. Post-operative central hypersensitivity and pain: the pre-emptive value of pethidine for ovariohysterectomy. *Pain* 1997; **73**(3): 461–471.
29 Ley SJ, Livingston A, Waterman AE. The effect of chronic clinical pain on thermal and mechanical thresholds in sheep. *Pain* 1989; **39**(3): 353–357.
30 Chambers JP, Livingston A, Waterman AE, Goodship AE. Analgesic effects of detomidine in thoroughbred horses with chronic tendon injury. *Res Vet Sci* 1993; **54**(1): 52–56.
31 Dolan S, Kelly JG, Huan M, Nolan AM. Transient up-regulation of spinal cyclooxygenase-2 and neuronal nitric oxide synthase following surgical inflammation. *Anesthesiology* 2003; **98**(1): 170–180.
32 Dolan S, Kelly JG, Monteiro AM, Nolan AM. Up-regulation of metabotropic glutamate receptor subtypes 3 and 5 in spinal cord in a clinical model of persistent inflammation and hyperalgesia. *Pain* 2003; **106**(3): 501–512.
33 Whay HR, Waterman AE, Webster AJF, O'Brien JK. The influence of lesion type on the duration of hyperalgesia associated with hindlimb lameness in dairy cattle. *Vet J* 1998; **156**(1): 23–29.
34 D'Mello R, Dickenson AH. Spinal cord mechanisms of pain. *Br J Anaesth* 2008; **101**(1): 8–16.
35 Suzuki R, Hunt SP, Dickenson AH. The coding of noxious mechanical and thermal stimuli of deep dorsal horn neurones is attenuated in NK1 knockout mice. *Neuropharmacology* 2003; **45**(8): 1093–1100.
36 Sandkuhler J, Chen JG, Cheng G, Randic M. Low-frequency stimulation of afferent Adelta-fibers induces long-term depression at primary afferent synapses with substantia gelatinosa neurons in the rat. *J Neurosci* 1997; **17**(16): 6483–6491.
37 Samad TA, Moore KA, Sapirstein A, *et al*. Interleukin-1β-mediated induction of Cox-2 in the CNS contributes to inflammatory pain hypersensitivity. *Nature* 2001; **410**(6827): 471–475.
38 Hosking RD, Zajicek JP. Therapeutic potential of cannabis in pain medicine. *Br J Anaesth* 2008; **101**(1): 59–68.
39 Voscopoulos C, Lema M. When does acute pain become chronic? *Br J Anaesth* 2010; **105**(Suppl 1): i69–i85.

40 Zhuang ZY, Wen YR, Zhang DR, *et al.* A peptide c-Jun N-terminal kinase (JNK) inhibitor blocks mechanical allodynia after spinal nerve ligation: respective roles of JNK activation in primary sensory neurons and spinal astrocytes for neuropathic pain development and maintenance. *J Neurosci* 2006; **26**(13): 3551–3560.

41 Bruce-Keller AJ. Microglial–neuronal interactions in synaptic damage and recovery. *J Neurosci Res* 1999; **58**(1): 191–201.

42 Denk F, McMahon SB, Tracey I. Pain vulnerability: a neurobiological perspective. *Nat Neurosci* 2014; **17**(2): 192–200.

43 Abbott CA, Malik RA, van Ross ER, *et al.* Prevalence and characteristics of painful diabetic neuropathy in a large community-based diabetic population in the U.K. *Diabetes Care* 2011; **34**(10): 2220–2224.

44 Kehlet H, Jensen T, Woolf C. Persistent postsurgical pain: risk factors and prevention. *Lancet* 2006; **367**(9522): 1618–1625.

45 Rutherford KM, Robson SK, Donald RD, *et al.* Pre-natal stress amplifies the immediate behavioral responses to acute pain in piglets. *Biol Lett* 2009; **5**(4): 452–454.

46 IASP. *Why Pain Control Matters in a World Full of Killer Diseases.* Seattle, WA: IASP Press, 2004. http://www.iasp-pain.org/files/Content/ContentFolders/GlobalYearAgainstPain2/20042005RighttoPainRelief/whypaincontrolmatters.pdf (accessed 14 August 2014).

47 Gaskin DJ, Richard P. The economic costs of pain in the United States. *J Pain* 2012; **13**(8): 715–724.

48 Wald LL. The future of acquisition speed, coverage, sensitivity, and resolution. *Neuroimage* 2012; **62**(2): 1221–1229.

49 Keedwell PA, Linden DE. Integrative neuroimaging in mood disorders. *Curr Opin Psychiatry* 2013; **26**(1): 27–32.

50 Garner BC, Stoker AM, Kuroki K, *et al.* Using animal models in osteoarthritis biomarker research. *J Knee Surg* 2011; **24**(4): 251–264.

51 Mogil JS. Animal models of pain: progress and challenges. *Nat Rev Neurosci* 2009; **10**(4): 283–294.

52 Rice AS, Cimino-Brown D, Eisenach JC, *et al.* Animal models and the prediction of efficacy in clinical trials of analgesic drugs: a critical appraisal and call for uniform reporting standards. *Pain* 2008; **139**(2): 243–247.

53 Vincent TL, Williams RO, Maciewicz R, *et al.* Arthritis Research UK Animal Models Working Group. Mapping pathogenesis of arthritis through small animal models. *Rheumatology (Oxford)* 2012; **51**(11): 1931–1941.

54 Matthies BK, Franklin KB. Effects of partial decortication on opioid analgesia in the formalin test. *Behav Brain Res* 1995; **67**(1): 59–66.

55 Backonja MM, Stacey B. Neuropathic pain symptoms relative to overall pain rating. *J Pain* 2004; **5**(9): 491–497.

56 Le Bars D, Gozariu M, Cadden SW. Animal models of nociception. *Pharmacol Rev* 2001; **53**(4): 597–652.

57 Beecher HK. The measurement of pain; prototype for the quantitative study of subjective responses. *Pharmacol Rev* 1957; **9**(1): 59–209.

58 Treede RD. Neurophysiological studies of pain pathways in peripheral and central nervous system disorders. *J Neurol* 2003; **250**(10): 1152–1161.

59 Villanueva L, Peschanski M, Calvino B, Le Bars D. Ascending pathways in the spinal cord involved in triggering of diffuse noxious inhibitory controls in the rat. *J Neurophysiol* 1986; **55**(1): 34–55.

60 Barrot M. Tests and models of nociception and pain in rodents. *Neuroscience* 2012; **211**: 39–50.

61 Valeriani M, Pazzaglia C, Cruccu G, Truini A. Clinical usefulness of laser evoked potentials. *Neurophysiol Clin* 2012; **42**(5): 345–353.

62 Baumgärtner U, Greffrath W, Treede RD. Contact heat and cold, mechanical, electrical and chemical stimuli to elicit small fiber-evoked potentials: merits and limitations for basic science and clinical use. *Neurophysiol Clin* 2012; **42**(5): 267–280.

63 Garcia-Larrea L. Objective pain diagnostics: clinical neurophysiology. *Neurophysiol Clin* 2012; **42**(4): 187–197.

64 Murrell JC, Johnson CB. Neurophysiological techniques to assess pain in animals. *J Vet Pharmacol Ther* 2006; **29**(5): 325–335.

65 Bromm B, Lorenz J. Neurophysiological evaluation of pain. *Electroencephalogr Clin Neurophysiol* 1998; **107**(4): 227–253.

66 van Oostrom H, Stienen PJ, van den Bos R, *et al.* Development of a rat model to assess the efficacy of the somatosensory-evoked potential as indicator of analgesia. *Brain Res Brain Res Protoc* 2005; **15**(1): 14–20.

67 van Oostrom H, Stienen PJ, van den Bos R, *et al.* Somatosensory-evoked potentials indicate increased unpleasantness of noxious stimuli in response to increasing stimulus intensities in the rat. *Brain Res Bull* 2007; **71**(4): 404–409.

68 Cruccu G, Aminoff MJ, Curio G, *et al.* Recommendations for the clinical use of somatosensory-evoked potentials. *Clin Neurophysiol* 2008; **119**(8): 1705–1719.

69 Kimura S, Tanabe M, Honda M, Ono H. Enhanced wind-up of the C fiber-mediated nociceptive flexor reflex movement following painful diabetic neuropathy in mice. *J Pharmacol Sci* 2005; **97**(2): 195–202.

70 Kelly S, Dobson KL, Harris J. Spinal nociceptive reflexes are sensitized in the monosodium iodoacetate model of osteoarthritis pain in the rat. *Osteoarthritis Cartilage* 2013; **21**(9): 1327–1335.

71 Courtney CA, Witte PO, Chmell SJ, Hornby TG. Heightened flexor withdrawal response in individuals with knee osteoarthritis is modulated by joint compression and joint mobilization. *J Pain* 2010; **11**(2): 179–185.

72 Peterbauer C, Larenza PM, Knobloch M, *et al.* Effects of a low dose infusion of racemic and S-ketamine on the nociceptive withdrawal reflex in standing ponies. *Vet Anaesth Analg* 2008; **35**(5): 414–423.

73 Spadavecchia C, Arendt-Nielsen L, Spadavecchia L, *et al.* Effects of butorphanol on the withdrawal reflex using threshold, suprathreshold and repeated subthreshold electrical stimuli in conscious horses. *Vet Anaesth Analg* 2007; **34**(1): 48–58.

74 Rohrbach H, Korpivaara T, Schatzmann U, Spadavecchia C. Comparison of the effects of the alpha-2 agonists detomidine, romifidine and xylazine on nociceptive withdrawal reflex and temporal summation in horses. *Vet Anaesth Analg* 2009; **36**(4): 384–395.

75 Levionnois OL, Menge M, Thormann W, *et al.* Effect of ketamine on the limb withdrawal reflex evoked by transcutaneous electrical stimulation in ponies anaesthetised with isoflurane. *Vet J* 2010; **186**(3): 304–311.

76 Bergadano A, Andersen OK, Arendt-Nielsen L, Spadavecchia C. Noninvasive assessment of the facilitation of the nociceptive withdrawal reflex by repeated electrical stimulations in conscious dogs. *Am J Vet Res* 2007; **68**(8): 899–907.

77 Bergadano A, Andersen OK, Arendt-Nielsen L, Spadavecchia C. Modulation of nociceptive withdrawal reflexes evoked by single and repeated nociceptive stimuli in conscious dogs by low-dose acepromazine. *Vet Anaesth Analg* 2009; **36**(3): 261–272.

78 Bergadano A, Andersen OK, Arendt-Nielsen L, *et al.* Plasma levels of a low-dose constant-rate-infusion of ketamine and its effect on single and repeated nociceptive stimuli in conscious dogs. *Vet J* 2009; **182**(2): 252–260.

79 IASP. *IASP Guidelines for the Use of Animals in Research.* Seattle, WA: IASP Press. http://www.iasp-pain.org/Education/Content.aspx?ItemNumber=1217 (accessed 14 August 2014).

80 Slingsby LS, Murrell JC, Taylor PM. Combination of dexmedetomidine with buprenorphine enhances the antinociceptive effect to a thermal stimulus in the cat compared with either agent alone. *Vet Anaesth Analg* 2010; **37**(2): 162–170.

81 Pypendop BH, Siao KT, Ilkiw JE. Thermal antinociceptive effect of orally administered gabapentin in healthy cats. *Am J Vet Res* 2010; **71**(9): 1027–1032.

82 Love EJ, Murrell J, Whay HR. Thermal and mechanical nociceptive threshold testing in horses: a review. *Vet Anaesth Analg* 2011; **38**(1): 3–14.

83 Hoffmann MV, Kästner SB, Kietzmann M, Kramer S. Contact heat thermal threshold testing in beagle dogs: baseline reproducibility and the effect of acepromazine, levomethadone and fenpipramide. *BMC Vet Res* 2012; **8**: 206.

84 Ambros B, Duke T. Effect of low dose rate ketamine infusions on thermal and mechanical thresholds in conscious cats. *Vet Anaesth Analg* 2013; **40**(6):e76–e82.

85 Ley SJ, Waterman AE, Livingston A. A field study of the effect of lameness on mechanical nociceptive thresholds in sheep. *Vet Rec* 1995; **137**(4): 85–87.

86 Slingsby LS, Jones A, Waterman-Pearson AE. Use of a new finger-mounted device to compare mechanical nociceptive thresholds in cats given pethidine or no medication after castration. *Res Vet Sci* 2001; **70**(3): 243–246.

87 Lascelles BD, Cripps PJ, Jones A, Waterman-Pearson AE. Efficacy and kinetics of carprofen, administered preoperatively or postoperatively, for the prevention of pain in dogs undergoing ovariohysterectomy. *Vet Surg* 1998; **27**(6): 568–582.

88 Willner P. The validity of animal models of depression. *Psychopharmacology (Berl)* 1984; **83**(1): 1–16.

89 Sacerdote P, Franchi S, Moretti S, *et al.* Cytokine modulation is necessary for efficacious treatment of experimental neuropathic pain. *J Neuroimmune Pharmacol* 2013; **8**(1): 202–211.

90 Fleetwood-Walker SM, Quinn JP, Wallace C, *et al.* Behavioral changes in the rat following infection with varicella-zoster virus. *J Gen Virol* 1999; **80**(Pt 9): 2433–2436.

91 Lee BH, Seong J, Kim UJ, *et al.* Behavioral characteristics of a mouse model of cancer pain. *Yonsei Med J* 2005; **46**(2): 252–259.

92 Lynch JL, Gallus NJ, Ericson ME, Beitz AJ. Analysis of nociception, sex and peripheral nerve innervation in the TMEV animal model of multiple sclerosis. *Pain* 2008; **136**(3): 293–304.

93 Al-Chaer ED, Kawasaki M, Pasricha PJ. A new model of chronic visceral hypersensitivity in adult rats induced by colon irritation during postnatal development. *Gastroenterology* 2000; **119**(5): 1276–1285.

94 Robertson SA, Sanchez LC, Merritt AM, Doherty TJ. Effect of systemic lidocaine on visceral and somatic nociception in conscious horses. *Equine Vet J* 2005; **37**(2): 122–127.

95 Sanchez LC, Merritt AM. Colorectal distention in the horse: visceral sensitivity, rectal compliance and effect of i.v. xylazine or intrarectal lidocaine. *Equine Vet J* 2005; **37**(1): 70–74.

96 Sanchez LC, Elfenbein JR, Robertson SA. Effect of acepromazine, butorphanol, or *N*-butylscopolammonium bromide on visceral and somatic nociception and duodenal motility in conscious horses. *Am J Vet Res* 2008; **69**(5): 579–585.
97 Willis WD, Al-Chaer ED, Quast MJ, Westlund KN. A visceral pain pathway in the dorsal column of the spinal cord. *Proc Natl Acad Sci U S A* 1999; **96**(14): 7675–7679.
98 Laird JM, Martinez-Caro L, Garcia-Nicas E, Cervero F. A new model of visceral pain and referred hyperalgesia in the mouse. *Pain* 2001; **92**(3): 335–342.
99 Ness TJ, Gebhart GF. Colorectal distension as a noxious visceral stimulus: physiologic and pharmacologic characterization of pseudaffective reflexes in the rat. *Brain Res* 1988; **450**(1–2): 153–169.
100 Hultin L, Nissen TD, Kakol-Palm D, Lindström E. Colorectal distension-evoked potentials in awake rats: a novel method for studies of visceral sensitivity. *Neurogastroenterol Motil* 2012; **24**(10): 964-e466.
101 Nissen TD, Brock C, Graversen C, *et al*. Translational aspects of rectal evoked potentials: a comparative study in rats and humans. *Am J Physiol Gastrointest Liver Physiol* 2013; **305**(2): G119–G128.
102 Cook JL, Kuroki K, Visco D, *et al*. The OARSI histopathology initiative – recommendations for histological assessments of osteoarthritis in the dog. *Osteoarthritis Cartilage* 2010; **18**(Suppl 3): S66–S79.
103 Brown DC, Boston R, Coyne JC, Farrar JT. A novel approach to the use of animals in studies of pain: validation of the canine brief pain inventory in canine bone cancer. *Pain Med* 2009; **10**(1): 133–142.
104 Hague DW, Stella JL, Buffington CA. Effects of interstitial cystitis on the acoustic startle reflex in cats. *Am J Vet Res* 2013; **74**(1): 144–147.
105 Brown DC, Boston RC, Coyne JC, Farrar JT. Ability of the Canine Brief Pain Inventory to detect response to treatment in dogs with osteoarthritis. *J Am Vet Med Assoc* 2008; **233**(8): 1278–1283.
106 Brown DC, Boston RC, Farrar JT. Comparison of force plate gait analysis and owner assessment of pain using the Canine Brief Pain Inventory in dogs with osteoarthritis. *J Vet Intern Med* 2013; **27**(1): 22–30.
107 Sufka KJ. Conditioned place preference paradigm: a novel approach for analgesic drug assessment against chronic pain. *Pain* 1994; **58**(3): 355–366.
108 Nasr MA, Murrell J, Nicol CJ. The effect of keel fractures on egg production, feed and water consumption in individual laying hens. *Br Poult Sci* 2013; **54**(2): 165–170.
109 Neubert JK, Widmer CG, Malphurs W, *et al*. Use of a novel thermal operant behavioral assay for characterization of orofacial pain sensitivity. *Pain* 2005; **116**(3): 386–395.
110 Nolan TA, Hester J, Bokrand-Donatelli Y, *et al*. Adaptation of a novel operant orofacial testing system to characterize both mechanical and thermal pain. *Behav Brain Res* 2011; **217**(2): 477–480.
111 Rossi HL, Vierck CJ, Caudle RM, Neubert JK. Characterization of cold sensitivity and thermal preference using an operant orofacial assay. *Mol Pain* 2006; **2**: 37.
112 Flecknell PA. Refinement of animal use – assessment and alleviation of pain and distress. *Lab Anim* 1994; **28**(3): 222–231.
113 Andrews N, Legg E, Lisak D, *et al*. Spontaneous burrowing behavior in the rat is reduced by peripheral nerve injury or inflammation associated pain. *Eur J Pain* 2012; **16**(4): 485–495.
114 Deacon RM. Burrowing in rodents: a sensitive method for detecting behavioral dysfunction. *Nat Protoc* 2006; **1**(1): 118–121.
115 Deacon RM. Digging and marble burying in mice: simple methods for in vivo identification of biological impacts. *Nat Protoc* 2006; **1**(1): 122–124.
116 Jirkof P, Cesarovic N, Rettich A, *et al*. Burrowing behavior as an indicator of post-laparotomy pain in mice. *Front Behav Neurosci* 2010; **4**: 165.
117 Deacon R. Assessing burrowing, nest construction, and hoarding in mice. *J Vis Exp* 2012; (**59**): e2607.
118 Langford DJ, Bailey AL, Chanda ML, *et al*. Coding of facial expressions of pain in the laboratory mouse. *Nat Methods* 2010; **7**(6): 447–449.
119 Sotocinal SG, Sorge RE, Zaloum A, *et al*. The Rat Grimace Scale: a partially automated method for quantifying pain in the laboratory rat via facial expressions. *Mol Pain* 2011; **7**: 55.
120 Keating SC, Thomas AA, Flecknell PA, Leach MC. Evaluation of EMLA cream for preventing pain during tattooing of rabbits: changes in physiological, behavioral and facial expression responses. *PLoS One* 2012; **7**(9): e44437.
121 Dalla Costa E, Minero M, Lebelt D, Stucke D, *et al*. Development of the Horse Grimace Scale (HGS) as a pain assessment tool in horses undergoing routine castration. *PLoS One* 2014; **9**(3): e92281.
122 Morton DB. Self-consciousness and animal suffering. *Biologist (London)* 2000; **47**: 77–80.
123 Aloisi AM, Albonetti ME, Carli G. Sex differences in the behavioral response to persistent pain in rats. *Neurosci Lett* 1994; **179**(1–2): 79–82.
124 Mogil JS, Chesler EJ, Wilson SG, *et al*. Sex differences in thermal nociception and morphine antinociception in rodents depend on genotype. *Neurosci Biobehav Rev* 2000; **24**: 375–389.
125 Gear RW, Miaskowski C, Gordon NC, *et al*. Kappa-opioids produce significantly greater analgesia in women than in men. *Nat Med* 1996; **2**: 1248–1250.
126 Wright-Williams SL, Courade J-P, Richardson CA, *et al*. Effects of vasectomy surgery and meloxicam treatment on faecal corticosterone levels and behavior in two strains of laboratory mouse. *Pain* 2007; **130**(1): 108–118.
127 Clark C, Mendl M, Jamieson J, *et al*. Do psychological and physiological stressors alter the acute pain response to castration and tail docking in lambs? *Vet Anaesth Analg* 2011; **38**(2): 134–145.
128 McCracken L, Waran N, Mitchinson S, Johnson CB. Effect of age at castration on behavioral response to subsequent tail docking in lambs. *Vet Anaesth Analg* 2010; **37**(4): 375–381.
129 Guesgen MJ, Beausoleil NJ, Stewart M. Effects of early human handling on the pain sensitivity of young lambs. *Vet Anaesth Analg* 2013; **40**(1): 55–62.
130 Sternberg WF, Ridgway CG. Effects of gestational stress and neonatal handling on pain, analgesia, and stress behavior of adult mice. *Physiol Behav* 2003; **78**: 375–383.
131 Loggia ML, Mogil JS, Bushnell MC. Empathy hurts: compassion for another increases both sensory and affective components of pain perception. *Pain* 2008; **136**(1–2): 168–176.
132 Mogil JS. The surprising empathic abilities of rodents. *Trends Cogn Sci* 2011; **16**(3): 143–144.
133 Langford DJ, Crager SE, Shehzad Z, *et al*. Social modulation of pain as evidence for empathy in mice. *Science* 2006; **312**(5782): 1967–1970.
134 Price J, Clarke N, Welsh EM, Waran N. Preliminary evaluation of subjective scoring systems for assessment of postoperative pain in horses. *Vet Anaesth Analg* 2003; **30**(2): 97.
135 Noonan GJ, Rand JS, Priest J, *et al*. Behavioral observations of piglets undergoing tail docking, teeth clipping and ear notching. *Appl Anim Behav Sci* 1994; **39**: 203–213.
136 Molony V, Kent JE. Assessment of acute pain in farm animals using behavioral and physiological measurements. *J Anim Sci* 1997; **75**(1): 266–272.
137 Molony V, Kent JE, McKendrick IJ. Validation of a method for assessment of an acute pain in lambs. *Appl Anim Behav Sci* 2002; **76**(3): 215–238.
138 Price J, Catriona S, Welsh EM, Waran NK. Preliminary evaluation of a behavior-based system for assessment of post-operative pain in horses following arthroscopic surgery. *Vet Anaesth Analg* 2003; **30**: 124–137.
139 Roughan JV, Flecknell PA. Behavioral effects of laparotomy and analgesic effects of ketoprofen and carprofen in rats. *Pain* 2001; **90**(1): 65–74.
140 Coulter CA, Flecknell PA, Richardson CA. Reported analgesic administration to rabbits, pigs, sheep, dogs and non-human primates undergoing experimental surgical procedures. *Lab Anim* 2009; **43**(3): 232–238.
141 Festing MFW. Principles: the need for better experimental design. *Trends Pharmacol Sci* 2003; **24**: 341–345.
142 Festing S. Opinion. Don't waste the animals. *New Sci* 2010; **206**: 22–23.
143 Richardson CA, Flecknell PA. Anaesthesia and post-operative analgesia following experimental surgery in laboratory rodents: are we making progress? *Altern Lab Anim* 2005; **33**(2): 119–127.
144 Cobos EJ, Portillo-Salido E. "Bedside-to-bench" behavioral outcomes in animal models of pain: beyond the evaluation of reflexes. *Curr Neuropharmacol* 2013; **11**(6): 560–591.
145 Eddie Clutton R, Clarke KW, Pascoe PJ. Animal welfare in biomedical publishing. *Vet Anaesth Analg* 2011; **38**(1): 1–2.
146 Ashley FH, Waterman-Pearson AE, Whay HR. Behavioral assessment of pain in horses and donkeys: application to clinical practice and future studies. *Equine Vet J* 2005; **37**(6): 565–575.
147 Wiseman-Orr ML, Nolan AM, Reid J, Scott EM. Development of a questionnaire to measure the effects of chronic pain on health-related quality of life in dogs. *Am J Vet Res* 2004; **65**: 1077–1084.
148 Cambridge AJ, Tobias KM, Newberry RC, Sarkar DK. Subjective and objective measurements of postoperative pain in cats. *J Am Vet Med Assoc* 2000; **217**(5): 685–690.
149 Holton L, Scott E, Nolan A, *et al*. Relationship between physiological factors and clinical pain in dogs scored using a numerical rating scale. *J Small Anim Pract* 1998; **39**(10): 469–474.
150 Smith J, Allen S, Quandt J, Tackett R. Indicators of postoperative pain in cats and correlation with clinical criteria. *Am J Vet Res* 1996; **57**(11): 1674–1678.
151 Firth A, Haldane S. Development of a scale to evaluate postoperative pain in dogs. *J Am Vet Med Assoc* 1999; **214**(5): 651–659.
152 Rietmann TR, Stauffacher M, Bernasconi P, *et al*. The association between heart rate, heart rate variability, endocrine and behavioural pain measures in horses suffering from laminitis. *J Vet Med A Physiol Pathol Clin Med* 2004; **51**(5): 218–225.
153 Bussières G, Jacques C, Lainay O, *et al*. Development of a composite orthopaedic pain scale in horses. *Res Vet Sci* 2008; **85**(2): 294–306.
154 Fox SM, Mellor DJ, Lawoko CR, *et al*. Changes in plasma cortisol concentrations in bitches in response to different combinations of halothane and butorphanol, with or without ovariohysterectomy. *Res Vet Sci* 1998; **65**(2): 125–133.

155 Eckersall PD, Bell R. Acute phase proteins: biomarkers of infection and inflammation in veterinary medicine. *Vet J* 2010; **185**(1): 23–27.

156 Eckersall PD, Young FJ, McComb C, *et al.* Acute phase proteins in serum and milk from dairy cows with clinical mastitis. *Vet Rec* 2001; **148**(2): 35–41.

157 Price J, Marques JM, Welsh EM, Waran NK. Pilot epidemiological study of attitudes towards pain in horses. *Vet Rec* 2002; **151**(19): 570–575.

158 Morton DB, Griffiths PH. Guidelines on the recognition of pain, distress and discomfort in experimental animals and an hypothesis for assessment. *Vet Rec* 1985; **116**(16): 431–436.

159 Pritchett LC, Ulibarri C, Roberts MC, *et al.* Identification of potential physiological and behavioral indicators of postoperative pain in horses after exploratory celiotomy for colic. *Appl Anim Behav Sci* 2003; **80**(1): 31–43.

160 Mantha S, Thisted R, Foss J, *et al.* A proposal to use confidence intervals for visual analog scale data for pain measurement to determine clinical significance. *Anesth Analg* 1993; **77**(5): 1041–1047.

161 Coulter CA, Flecknell PA, Leach MC, Richardson CA. Reported analgesic administration to rabbits undergoing experimental surgical procedures. *BMC Vet Res* 2011; **7**: 12.

162 Holton LL, Scott EM, Nolan AM, *et al.* Comparison of three methods used for assessment of pain in dogs. *J Am Vet Med Assoc* 1998; **212**(1): 61–66.

163 Hewetson M, Christley RM, Hunt ID, Voute LC. Investigations of the reliability of observational gait analysis for the assessment of lameness in horses. *Vet Rec* 2006; **158**(25): 852–858.

164 Lascelles B, Cripps P, Mirchandani S, Waterman A. Carprofen as an analgesic for postoperative pain in cats: dose titration and assessment of efficacy in comparison to pethidine hydrochloride. *J Small Anim Pract* 1995; **36**(12): 535–541.

165 Slingsby L, Waterman-Pearson A. Comparison of pethidine, buprenorphine and ketoprofen for postoperative analgesia after ovariohysterectomy in the cat. *Vet Rec* 1998; **143**(7): 185–189.

166 Hudson JT, Slater MR, Taylor L, *et al.* Assessing repeatability and validity of a visual analogue scale questionnaire for use in assessing pain and lameness in dogs. *Am J Vet Res* 2004; **65**: 1634–1643.

167 Melzack R. The McGill Pain Questionnaire: major properties and scoring methods. *Pain* 1975; **1**(3): 277–299.

168 Fox SM, Mellor DJ, Stafford KJ, *et al.* The effects of ovariohysterectomy plus different combinations of halothane anaesthesia and butorphanol analgesia on behavior in the bitch. *Res Vet Sci* 2000; **68**(3): 265–274.

169 Holton L, Reid J, Scott E, *et al.* Development of a behavior-based scale to measure acute pain in dogs. *Vet Rec* 2001; **148**(17): 525–531.

170 Van Loon JPAM, Back W, Hellebrekers LJ, Van Weeren PR. Application of a composite pain scale to objectively monitor horses with somatic and visceral pain under hospital conditions. *J Equine Vet Sci* 2010; **30**(11): 641–649.

171 Raekallio M, Taylor PM, Bennett RC. Preliminary investigations of pain and analgesia assessment in horses administered phenylbutazone or placebo after arthroscopic surgery. *Vet Surg* 1997; **26**(2): 150–155.

172 Wagner AE. Effects of stress on pain in horses and incorporating pain scales for equine practice. *Vet Clin North Am Equine Pract* 2010; **26**(3): 481–492.

173 Conzemius MG, Evans RB. Caregiver placebo effect for dogs with lameness from osteoarthritis. *J Am Vet Med Assoc* 2012; **241**(10): 1314–1319.

174 Reid J, Nolan A, Hughes J, *et al.* Development of the short-form Glasgow Composite Measure Pain Scale (GCMP-SF) and derivation of an analgesic intervention score. *Anim Welf* 2007; (16 s): 97–104.

175 Brondani JT, Luna SP, Padovani CR. Refinement and initial validation of a multidimensional composite scale for use in assessing acute postoperative pain in cats. *Am J Vet Res* 2011; **72**(2): 174–183.

176 McDowell NC. *Measuring Health: a Guide to Rating Scales and Questionnaires*, 3rd edn. New York: Oxford University Press, 2006.

177 Walton MB, Cowderoy E, Lascelles D, Innes JF. Evaluation of construct and criterion validity for the 'Liverpool Osteoarthritis in Dogs' (LOAD) clinical metrology instrument and comparison to two other instruments. *PLoS One* 2013; **8**: e58125.

178 Hielm-Björkman AK, Kuusela E, Liman A, *et al.* Evaluation of methods for assessment of pain associated with chronic osteoarthritis in dogs. *J Am Vet Med Assoc* 2003; **222**(11): 1552–1558.

179 Viñuela-Fernandez I, Jones E, McKendrick IJ, Molony V. Quantitative assessment of increased sensitivity of chronic laminitic horses to hoof tester evoked pain. *Equine Vet J* 2011; **43**(1): 62–68.

180 Association of Veterinary Teachers and Research Workers. Guidelines for the recognition and assessment of pain in animals. Prepared by a working party of the Association of Veterinary Teachers and Research Workers. *Vet Rec* 1986; **118**(12): 334–338.

181 Hercock CA, Pinchbeck G, Giejda A, *et al.* Validation of a client-based clinical metrology instrument for the evaluation of canine elbow osteoarthritis. *J Small Anim Pract* 2009; **50**(6): 266–271.

182 Brown DC, Boston RC, Coyne JC, Farrar JT. Development and psychometric testing of an instrument designed to measure chronic pain in dogs with osteoarthritis. *Am J Vet Res* 2007; **68**(6): 631–637.

183 Lynch S, Savary-Bataille K, Leeuw B, Argyle DJ. Development of a questionnaire assessing health-related quality-of-life in dogs and cats with cancer. *Vet Comp Oncol* 2011; **9**(3): 172–182.

184 Noli C, Colombo S, Cornegliani L, *et al.* Quality of life of dogs with skin disease and of their owners. Part 2: administration of a questionnaire in various skin diseases and correlation to efficacy of therapy. *Vet Dermatol* 2011; **22**(4): 344–351.

185 Birnbacher D. Quality of life – evaluation or description. *Ethical Theory Moral Pract* 1999; **2**(1): 25–36.

186 Wiseman-Orr ML, Scott EM, Reid J, Nolan AM. Validation of a structured questionnaire as an instrument to measure chronic pain in dogs on the basis of effects on health-related quality of life. *Am J Vet Res* 2006; **67**(11): 1826–1836.

187 Hielm-Björkman AK, Rita H, Tulamo RM. Psychometric testing of the Helsinki chronic pain index by completion of a questionnaire in Finnish by owners of dogs with chronic signs of pain caused by osteoarthritis. *Am J Vet Res* 2009; **70**(6): 727–734.

188 Hielm-Björkman AK, Kapatkin AS, Rita HJ. Reliability and validity of a visual analogue scale used by owners to measure chronic pain attributable to osteoarthritis in their dogs. *Am J Vet Res* 2011; **72**(5): 601–607.

189 Zamprogno H, Hansen BD, Bondell HD, *et al.* Item generation and design testing of a questionnaire to assess degenerative joint disease-associated pain in cats. *Am J Vet Res* 2010; **71**(12): 1417–1424.

190 Benito J, Depuy V, Hardie E, *et al.* Reliability and discriminatory testing of a client-based metrology instrument, feline musculoskeletal pain index (FMPI) for the evaluation of degenerative joint disease-associated pain in cats. *Vet J* 2013; **196**(3): 368–373.

191 Benito J, Hansen B, Depuy V, *et al.* Feline musculoskeletal pain index: responsiveness and testing of criterion validity. *J Vet Intern Med* 2013; **27**(3): 474–482.

192 Gruen ME, Griffith E, Thomson A, *et al.* Detection of clinically relevant pain relief in cats with degenerative joint disease associated pain. *J Vet Intern Med* 2014; **28**(2): 346–350.

193 Reid J, Wiseman-Orr ML, Scott EM, Nolan AM. Development, validation and reliability of a web-based questionnaire to measure health-related quality of life in dogs. *J Small Anim Pract* 2013; **54**(5): 227–233.

194 Welsh EM, Gettinby G, Nolan AM. Comparison of a visual analogue scale and a numerical rating scale for assessment of lameness, using sheep as a model. *Am J Vet Res* 1993; **54**(6): 976–983.

195 Williams AC. Facial expression of pain: an evolutionary account. *Behav Brain Sci* 2004; **25**(4): 439–455.

196 Darwin C. *The Expression of the Emotions in Man and Animals*. London: John Murray, 1872.

197 Lautenbacher S, Niewelt BG, Kunz M. Decoding pain from the facial display of patients with dementia: a comparison of professional and nonprofessional observers. *Pain Med* 2013; **14**(4): 469–477.

198 Matsumiya LC, Sorge RE, Sotocinal SG, *et al.* Using the Mouse Grimace Scale to reevaluate the efficacy of postoperative analgesics in laboratory mice. *J Am Assoc Lab Anim Sci* 2012; **51**(1): 42–49.

199 Leach MC, Klaus K, Miller AL, *et al.* The assessment of post-vasectomy pain in mice using behavior and the Mouse Grimace Scale. *PLoS One* 2012; **7**(4): e35656.

200 Love EJ, Gillespie L, Colborne GR. Facial expression of pain in horses. Presented at the Association of Veterinary Anaesthetists Spring Meeting, 13–16 April 2011, Bari, Italy.

201 Mogil JS, Crager SE. What should we be measuring in behavioral studies of chronic pain in animals? *Pain* 2004; **112**(1–2): 12–15.

202 Baron-Cohen S, Wheelwright S, Jolliffe T. Is there a "language of the eyes"? Evidence from normal adults, and adults with autism or Asperger syndrome. *Vis Cogn* 1997; **4**: 311–331.

203 Leach MC, Coulter CA, Richardson CA, Flecknell PA. Are we looking in the wrong place? Implications for behavioural-based pain assessment in rabbits (*Oryctolagus cuniculi*) and beyond? *PLoS One* 2011; **6**(3): e13347.

204 Dixson B, Grimshaw G, Linklater W, Dixson A. Eye-tracking of men's preferences for waist-to-hip ratio and breast size of women. *Arch Sex Behav* 2011; **40**(1): 43–50.

205 Sodhi M, Reimer B, Llamazares I. Glance analysis of driver eye movements to evaluate distraction. *Behav Res Methods Instrum Comput* 2002; **34**(4): 529–538.

206 Roth SP, Tuch AN, Mekler ED, *et al.* Location matters, especially for non-salient features – an eye-tracking study on the effects of web object placement on different types of websites. *Int J Hum Comput Stud* 2013; **71**(3): 228–235.

207 Leach MC, Allweiler S, Richardson C, *et al.* Behavioural effects of ovariohysterectomy and oral administration of meloxicam in laboratory housed rabbits. *Res Vet Sci* 2009; **87**(2): 336–347.

208 Molony V, Kent JE, Robertson IS. Assessment of acute and chronic pain after different methods of castration of calves. *Appl Anim Behav Sci* 1995; **46**(1–2): 33–48.

209 Kent JE, Molony V, Robertson IS. Changes in plasma cortisol concentration in lambs of three ages after three methods of castration and tail docking. *Res Vet Sci* 1993; **55**(2): 246–251.

210 Hawkins P. Recognizing and assessing pain, suffering and distress in laboratory animals: a survey of current practice in the UK with recommendations. *Lab Anim* 2002; **36**(4): 378–395.

211 Roughan JV, Flecknell PA. Training in behavior-based post-operative pain scoring in rats – an evaluation based on improved recognition of analgesic requirements. *Appl Anim Behav Sci* 2006; **96**(3–4): 327–342.

212 Seebeck P, Thompson MS, Parwani A, *et al.* Gait evaluation: a tool to monitor bone healing? *Clin Biomech* 2005; **20**: 883–891.

213 Lascelles BD, Findley K, Correa M, *et al.* Kinetic evaluation of normal walking and jumping in cats, using a pressure-sensitive walkway. *Vet Rec* 2007; **160**(15): 512–516.

214 Moreau M, Guillot M, Pelletier JP, *et al.* Kinetic peak vertical force measurement in cats afflicted by coxarthritis: data management and acquisition protocols. *Res Vet Sci* 2013; **95**(1): 219–224.

215 Romans CW, Conzemius MG, Horstman CL, *et al.* Use of pressure platform gait analysis in cats with and without bilateral onychectomy. *Am J Vet Res* 2004; **65**(9): 1276–1278.

216 Robinson DA, Romans CW, Gordon-Evans WJ, *et al.* Evaluation of short-term limb function following unilateral carbon dioxide laser or scalpel onychectomy in cats. *J Am Vet Med Assoc* 2007; **230**(3): 353–358.

217 Lascelles BDX, Hansen BD, Thomson A, *et al.* Evaluation of a digitally integrated accelerometer-based activity monitor for the measurement of activity in cats. *Vet Anaesth Analg* 2008; **35**: 173–183.

218 Hansen BD, Lascelles BDX, Keene BW, *et al.* Evaluation of an accelerometer for at-home monitoring of spontaneous activity in dogs. *Am J Vet Res* 2007; **68**(5): 468–475.

219 Dow C, Michel KE, Love M, Brown DC. Evaluation of optimal sampling interval for activity monitoring in companion dogs. *Am J Vet Res* 2009; **70**(4): 444–448.

220 Cockcroft P, Holmes MA. *The Handbook of Evidence-Based Veterinary Medicine.* Oxford: Blackwell, 2003.

221 Victoria NC, Inoue K, Young LJ, Murphy AZ. A single neonatal injury induces life-long deficits in response to stress. *Dev Neurosci* 2013; **35**(4): 326–337.

222 Valverde A. Alpha-2 agonists as pain therapy in horses. *Vet Clin North Am Equine Pract* 2010; **26**(3): 515–532.

223 Kästner SB. A2-agonists in sheep: a review. *Vet Anaesth Analg* 2006; **33**(2): 79–96.

224 Murrell JC, Hellebrekers LJ. Medetomidine and dexmedetomidine: a review of cardiovascular effects and antinociceptive properties in the dog. *Vet Anaesth Analg* 2005; **32**(3): 117–127.

225 Meyer H, Starke A, Kehler W, Rehage J. High caudal epidural anaesthesia with local anaesthetics or α_2-agonists in calves. *J Vet Med A Physiol Pathol Clin Med* 2007; **54**(7): 384–389.

226 Slingsby L, Taylor P, Monroe T. Thermal antinociception after dexmedetomidine administration in cats: a comparison between intramuscular and oral transmucosal administration. *J Feline Med Surg* 2009; **11**(10): 829–834.

227 Virtanen R. Pharmacological profiles of medetomidine and its antagonist, atipamezole. *Acta Vet Scand Suppl* 1989; **85**: 29–37.

228 Pippi NL, Lumb WV. Objective tests of analgesic drugs in ponies. *Am J Vet Res* 1979; **40**(8): 1082–1086.

229 Muir WW, Robertson JT. Visceral analgesia: effects of xylazine, butorphanol, meperidine, and pentazocine in horses. *Am J Vet Res* 1985; **46**(10): 2081–2084.

230 Hellyer PW, Bai L, Supon J, *et al.* Comparison of opioid and alpha-2 adrenergic receptor binding in horse and dog brain using radioligand autoradiography. *Vet Anaesth Analg* 2003; **30**(3): 172–182.

231 Coetzee JF, Gehring R, Tarus-Sang J, Anderson DE. Effect of sub-anesthetic xylazine and ketamine ('ketamine stun') administered to calves immediately prior to castration. *Vet Anaesth Analg* 2010; **37**(6): 566–578.

232 Seddighi R, Elliot SB, Whitlock BK, *et al.* Physiologic and antinociceptive effects following intramuscular administration of xylazine hydrochloride in combination with tiletamine–zolazepam in llamas. *Am J Vet Res* 2013; **74**(4): 530–534.

233 Paalzow L. Analgesia produced by clonidine in mice and rats. *J Pharm Pharmacol* 1974; **26**(5): 361–363.

234 Fehrenbacher JC, Loverme J, Clarke W, *et al.* Rapid pain modulation with nuclear receptor ligands. *Brain Res Rev* 2009; **60**(1): 114–124.

235 Ishii H, Kohno T, Yamakura T, *et al.* Action of dexmedetomidine on the substantia gelatinosa neurons of the rat spinal cord. *Eur J Neurosci* 2008; **27**(12): 3182–3190.

236 Guo TZ, Jiang JY, Buttermann AE, Maze M. Dexmedetomidine injection into the locus ceruleus produces antinociception. *Anesthesiology* 1996; **84**(4): 873–881.

237 Dogrul A, Coskun I, Uzbay T. The contribution of alpha-1 and alpha-2 adrenoceptors in peripheral imidazoline and adrenoceptor agonist-induced nociception. *Anesth Analg* 2006; **103**(2): 471–477.

238 Langer SZ. History and nomenclature of alpha-1 adrenoceptors. *Eur Urol* 1999; **36**(Suppl 1): 2–6.

239 Kohli U, Muszkat M, Sofowora GG, *et al.* Effects of variation in the human alpha2A- and alpha2C-adrenoceptor genes on cognitive tasks and pain perception. *Eur J Pain* 2010; **14**(2): 154–159.

240 Rinne A, Birk A, Bünemann M. Voltage regulates adrenergic receptor function. *Proc Natl Acad Sci U S A* 2013; **110**(4): 1536–1541.

241 Nazarian A, Christianson CA, Hua XY, Yaksh TL. Dexmedetomidine and ST-91 analgesia in the formalin model is mediated by α_2A-adrenoceptors: a mechanism of action distinct from morphine. *Br J Pharmacol* 2008; **155**(7): 1117–1126.

242 MacDonald E, Kobilka BK, Scheinin M. Gene targeting – homing in on alpha 2-adrenoceptor-subtype function. *Trends Pharmacol Sci* 1997; **18**(6): 211–219.

243 Graham BA, Hammond DL, Proudfit HK. Synergistic interactions between two alpha(2)-adrenoceptor agonists, dexmedetomidine and ST-91, in two substrains of Sprague–Dawley rats. *Pain* 2000; **85**(1–2): 135–143.

244 Fairbanks CA, Kitto KF, Nguyen HO, *et al.* Clonidine and dexmedetomidine produce antinociceptive synergy in mouse spinal cord. *Anesthesiology* 2009; **110**(3): 638–647.

245 Khodayar MJ, Shafaghi B, Naderi N, Zarrindast MR. Antinociceptive effect of spinally administered cannabinergic and 2-adrenoceptor drugs on the formalin test in rat: possible interactions. *J Psychopharmacol* 2006; **20**(1): 67–74.

246 Tham SM, Angus JA, Tudor EM, Wright CE. Synergistic and additive interactions of the cannabinoid agonist CP55,940 with mu opioid receptor and alpha2-adrenoceptor agonists in acute pain models in mice. *Br J Pharmacol* 2005; **144**(6): 875–884.

247 Kimura M, Saito S, Obata H. Dexmedetomidine decreases hyperalgesia in neuropathic pain by increasing acetylcholine in the spinal cord. *Neurosci Lett* 2012; **529**(1): 70–74.

248 Valtolina C, Robben J, Uilenreef J, *et al.* Clinical evaluation of the efficacy and safety of a constant rate infusion of dexmedetomidine for postoperative pain management in dogs. *Vet Anaesth Analg* 2009; **36**(4): 369–383.

249 Tranquilli W, Thurman JC, Turner TA, *et al.* Butorphanol tartrate as an adjunct to xylazine–ketamine in the horse. *Equine Pract* 1983; **5**: 26–29.

250 Fairbanks CA, Stone LS, Wilcox GL. Pharmacological profiles of alpha 2 adrenergic receptor agonists identified using genetically altered mice and isobolographic analysis. *Pharmacol Ther* 2009; **123**(2): 224–238.

251 Höcker J, Böhm R, Meybohm P, *et al.* Interaction of morphine but not fentanyl with cerebral α_2-adrenoceptors in α_2-adrenoceptor knockout mice. *J Pharm Pharmacol* 2009; **61**(7): 901–910.

252 Mansikka H, Zhou L, Donovan DM, *et al.* The role of mu-opioid receptors in inflammatory hyperalgesia and alpha 2-adrenoceptor-mediated antihyperalgesia. *Neuroscience* 2002; **113**(2): 339–349.

253 Lähdesmäki J, Scheinin M, Pertovaara A, Mansikka H. The α_2A-adrenoceptor subtype is not involved in inflammatory hyperalgesia or morphine-induced antinociception. *Eur J Pharmacol* 2003; **468**(3): 183–189.

254 Campoy L, Martin-Flores M, Ludders JW, Gleed RD. Procedural sedation combined with locoregional anesthesia for orthopedic surgery of the pelvic limb in 10 dogs: case series. *Vet Anaesth Analg* 2012; **39**(4): 436–440.

255 Campoy L, Martin-Flores M, Ludders JW, *et al.* Comparison of bupivacaine femoral and sciatic nerve block versus bupivacaine and morphine epidural for stifle surgery in dogs. *Vet Anaesth Analg* 2012; **39**(1): 91–98.

256 Joo JD, Choi JW, In JH, *et al.* Lidocaine suppresses the increased extracellular signal-regulated kinase/cyclic AMP response element-binding protein pathway and pro-inflammatory cytokines in a neuropathic pain model of rats. *Eur J Anaesthesiol* 2011; **28**(2): 106–111.

257 Swanton BJ, Shorten GD. Anti-inflammatory effects of local anesthetic agents. *Int Anesthesiol Clin* 2003; **41**(1): 1–19.

258 MacDougall LM, Hethey JA, Livingston A, *et al.* Antinociceptive, cardiopulmonary, and sedative effects of five intravenous infusion rates of lidocaine in conscious dogs. *Vet Anaesth Analg* 2009; **36**(5): 512–522.

259 Smith LJ, Bentley E, Shih A, Miller PE. Systemic lidocaine infusion as an analgesic for intraocular surgery in dogs: a pilot study. *Vet Anaesth Analg* 2004; **31**(1): 53–63.

260 Tsai TY, Chang SK, Chou PY, Yeh LS. Comparison of postoperative effects between lidocaine infusion, meloxicam, and their combination in dogs undergoing ovariohysterectomy. *Vet Anaesth Analg* 2013; **40**(6): 615–622.

261 Gissen AJ, Covino BG, Gregus J. Differential sensitivities of mammalian nerve fibers to local anesthetic agents. *Anesthesiology* 1980; **53**(6): 467–474.

262 Kindler CH, Paul M, Zou H, *et al.* Amide local anesthetics potently inhibit the human tandem pore domain background K^+ channel TASK-2 (KCNK5). *J Pharmacol Exp Ther* 2003; **306**(1): 84–92.

263 Sugiyama K, Muteki T. Local anesthetics depress the calcium current of rat sensory neurons in culture. *Anesthesiology* 1994; **80**(6): 1369–1378.

264 Xu L, Jones R, Meissner G. Effects of local anesthetics on single channel behavior of skeletal muscle calcium release channel. *J Gen Physiol* 1993; **101**(2): 207–233.

265 Furutani K, Ikoma M, Ishii H, *et al.* Bupivacaine inhibits glutamatergic transmission in spinal dorsal horn neurons. *Anesthesiology* 2010; **112**(1): 138–143.

266 Kosharskyy B, Almonte W, Shaparin N, *et al.* Intravenous infusions in chronic pain management. *Pain Physician* 2013; **16**(3): 231–249.

267 Elia N, Tramèr MR. Ketamine and postoperative pain – a quantitative systematic review of randomised trials. *Pain* 2005; **113**(1–2): 61–70.

268 White PF, Way WL, Trevor AJ. Ketamine – its pharmacology and therapeutic uses. *Anesthesiology* 1982; **56**(2): 119–136.

269 Bell RF. Ketamine for chronic non-cancer pain. *Pain* 2009; **141**(3): 210–214.

270 Leppert W. Ketamine in the management of cancer pain. *J Clin Oncol* 2013; **31**(10): 1374.

271 Alam S, Saito Y, Kosaka Y. Antinociceptive effects of epidural and intravenous ketamine to somatic and visceral stimuli in rats. *Can J Anaesth* 1996; **43**(4): 408–413.

272 Ahern TL, Herring AA, Stone MB, Frazee BW. Effective analgesia with low-dose ketamine and reduced dose hydromorphone in ED patients with severe pain. *Am J Emerg Med* 2013; **31**(5): 847–851.

273 Wagner A, Walton J, Hellyer P, *et al.* Use of low doses of ketamine administered by constant rate infusion as an adjunct for postoperative analgesia in dogs. *J Am Vet Med Assoc* 2002; **221**(1): 72–75.

274 Guedes AG, Matthews NS, Hood DM. Effect of ketamine hydrochloride on the analgesic effects of tramadol hydrochloride in horses with signs of chronic laminitis-associated pain. *Am J Vet Res* 2012; **73**(5): 610–619.

275 Elfenbein JR, Robertson SA, Corser AA, *et al.* Systemic effects of a prolonged continuous infusion of ketamine in healthy horses. *J Vet Intern Med* 2011; **25**(5): 1134–1137.

276 Pees C, Haas NA, Ewert P, *et al.* Comparison of analgesic/sedative effect of racemic ketamine and S(+)-ketamine during cardiac catheterization in newborns and children. *Pediatr Cardiol* 2003; **24**(5): 424–429.

277 Hocking G, Cousins MJ. Ketamine in chronic pain management: an evidence-based review. *Anesth Analg* 2003; **97**(6): 1730–1739.

278 Minville V, Fourcade O, Girolami JP, Tack I. Opioid-induced hyperalgesia in a mice model of orthopaedic pain: preventive effect of ketamine. *Br J Anaesth* 2010; **104**(2): 231–238.

279 Van Elstraete AC, Sitbon P, Trabold F, *et al.* A single dose of intrathecal morphine in rats induces long-lasting hyperalgesia: the protective effect of prior administration of ketamine. *Anesth Analg* 2005; **101**(6): 1750–1756.

280 Lascelles B, Gaynor J, Smith E, *et al.* Amantadine in a multimodal analgesic regimen for alleviation of refractory osteoarthritis pain in dogs. *J Vet Intern Med* 2008; **22**(1): 53–59.

281 Kumar A, Sharma D, Datta B. Addition of ketamine or dexmedetomidine to lignocaine in intravenous regional anesthesia: a randomized controlled study. *J Anaesthesiol Clin Pharmacol* 2012; **28**(4): 501–504.

282 Uzaraga I, Gerbis B, Holwerda E, *et al.* Topical amitriptyline, ketamine, and lidocaine in neuropathic pain caused by radiation skin reaction: a pilot study. *Support Care Cancer* 2012; **20**(7): 1515–1524.

283 Gómez de Segura IA, De Rossi R, Santos M, *et al.* Epidural injection of ketamine for perineal analgesia in the horse. *Vet Surg* 1998; **27**(4): 384–391.

284 DeRossi R, Benites A, Ferreira J, *et al.* Effects of lumbosacral epidural ketamine and lidocaine in xylazine-sedated cats. *J S Afr Vet Assoc* 2009; **80**(2): 79–83.

285 Rojas AC, Alves JG, Moreira E Lima R, *et al.* The effects of subarachnoid administration of preservative-free S(+)-ketamine on spinal cord and meninges in dogs. *Anesth Analg* 2012; **114**(2): 450–455.

286 Song XJ, Zhao ZQ. NMDA and non-NMDA receptors mediating nociceptive and non-nociceptive transmission in spinal cord of cat. *Zhongguo Yao Li Xue Bao* 1993; **14**(6): 481–485.

287 Duncan GE, Moy SS, Knapp DJ, *et al.* Metabolic mapping of the rat brain after subanesthetic doses of ketamine: potential relevance to schizophrenia. *Brain Res* 1998; **787**(2): 181–190.

288 Kohrs R, Durieux ME. Ketamine: teaching an old drug new tricks. *Anesth Analg* 1998; **87**(5): 1186–1193.

289 Hustveit O, Maurset A, Oye I. Interaction of the chiral forms of ketamine with opioid, phencyclidine, sigma and muscarinic receptors. *Pharmacol Toxicol* 1995; **77**(6): 355–359.

290 Mathew SJ, Shah A, Lapidus K, *et al.* Ketamine for treatment-resistant unipolar depression: current evidence. *CNS Drugs* 2012; **26**(3): 189–204.

291 Schnoebel R, Wolff M, Peters SC, *et al.* Ketamine impairs excitability in superficial dorsal horn neurones by blocking sodium and voltage-gated potassium currents. *Br J Pharmacol* 2005; **146**(6): 826–833.

292 DeRossi R, Frazílio FO, Jardim PH, *et al.* Evaluation of thoracic epidural analgesia induced by lidocaine, ketamine, or both administered via a lumbosacral approach in dogs. *Am J Vet Res* 2011; **72**(12): 1580–1585.

293 Romero TR, Duarte ID. Involvement of ATP-sensitive K^+ channels in the peripheral antinociceptive effect induced by ketamine. *Vet Anaesth Analg* 2013; **40**(4): 419–424.

294 Loix S, De Kock M, Henin P. The anti-inflammatory effects of ketamine: state of the art. *Acta Anaesthesiol Belg* 2011; **62**(1): 47–58.

295 Holtman JR, Crooks PA, Johnson-Hardy JK, *et al.* Effects of norketamine enantiomers in rodent models of persistent pain. *Pharmacol Biochem Behav* 2008; **90**(4): 676–685.

296 Gehring R, Coetzee JF, Tarus-Sang J, Apley MD. Pharmacokinetics of ketamine and its metabolite norketamine administered at a sub-anesthetic dose together with xylazine to calves prior to castration. *J Vet Pharmacol Ther* 2009; **32**(2): 124–128.

297 Hellyer P, Rodan I, Brunt J, *et al.* AAHA/AAFP pain management guidelines for dogs and cats. *J Feline Med Surg* 2007; **9**(6): 466–480.

298 Rushfeldt CF, Sveinbjørnsson B, Søreide K, Vonen B. Risk of anastomotic leakage with use of NSAIDs after gastrointestinal surgery. *Int J Colorectal Dis* 2011; **26**(12): 1501–1509.

299 Johnson CB, Taylor PM, Young SS, Brearley JC. Postoperative analgesia using phenylbutazone, flunixin or carprofen in horses. *Vet Rec* 1993; **133**(14): 336–338.

300 Jenkins WL. Pharmacologic aspects of analgesic drugs in animals: an overview. *J Am Vet Med Assoc* 1987; **191**(10): 1231–1240.

301 Levine DG, Epstein KL, Neelis DA, Ross MW. Effect of topical application of 1% diclofenac sodium liposomal cream on inflammation in healthy horses undergoing intravenous regional limb perfusion with amikacin sulfate. *Am J Vet Res* 2009; **70**(11): 1323–1325.

302 Baldridge SL, Coetzee JF, Dritz SS, *et al.* Pharmacokinetics and physiologic effects of intramuscularly administered xylazine hydrochloride–ketamine hydrochloride–butorphanol tartrate alone or in combination with orally administered sodium salicylate on biomarkers of pain in Holstein calves following castration and dehorning. *Am J Vet Res* 2011; **72**(10): 1305–1317.

303 Desmarchelier M, Troncy E, Fitzgerald G, Lair S. Analgesic effects of meloxicam administration on postoperative orthopedic pain in domestic pigeons (*Columba livia*). *Am J Vet Res* 2012; **73**(3): 361–367.

304 Leith JL, Wilson AW, Donaldson LF, Lumb BM. Cyclooxygenase-1-derived prostaglandins in the periaqueductal gray differentially control C- versus A-fiber-evoked spinal nociception. *J Neurosci* 2007; **27**(42): 11296–11305.

305 Prochazkova M, Dolezal T, Sliva J, Krsiak M. Different patterns of spinal cyclooxygenase-1 and cyclooxygenase-2 mRNA expression in inflammatory and postoperative pain. *Basic Clin Pharmacol Toxicol* 2006; **99**(2): 173–177.

306 Pateromichelakis S, Rood JP. Prostaglandin E2 increases mechanically evoked potentials in the peripheral nerve. *Experientia* 1981; **37**(3): 282–284.

307 Gilron I, Milne B, Hong M. Cyclooxygenase-2 inhibitors in postoperative pain management: current evidence and future directions. *Anesthesiology* 2003; **99**(5): 1198–1208.

308 Noguchi K, Okubo M. Leukotrienes in nociceptive pathway and neuropathic/inflammatory pain. *Biol Pharm Bull* 2011; **34**(8): 1163–1169.

309 Goupil RC, Bushey JJ, Peters-Kennedy J, Wakshlag JJ. Prevalence of 5-lipoxygenase expression in canine osteosarcoma and the effects of a dual 5-lipoxygenase/cyclooxygenase inhibitor on osteosarcoma cells in vitro and in vivo. *Vet Pathol* 2012; **49**(5): 802–810.

310 Lascelles BD, King S, Roe S, *et al.* Expression and activity of COX-1 and -2 and 5-LOX in joint tissues from dogs with naturally occurring coxofemoral joint osteoarthritis. *J Orthop Res* 2009; **27**(9): 1204–1208.

311 Giorgi M, Cuniberti B, Ye G, *et al.* Oral administration of tepoxalin in the horse: a PK/PD study. *Vet J* 2011; **190**(1): 143–149.

312 Giorgi M, Mengozzi G, Raffaelli A, Saba A. Characterization of in vivo plasma metabolites of tepoxalin in horses using LC-MS-MS. *J Pharm Biomed Anal* 2011; **56**(1): 45–53.

313 Goodman LA, Torres BT, Reynolds LR, Budsberg SC. Effects of firocoxib, meloxicam, and tepoxalin administration on eicosanoid production in target tissues of healthy cats. *Am J Vet Res* 2010; **71**(9): 1067–1073.

314 Charlton AN, Benito J, Simpson W, *et al.* Evaluation of the clinical use of tepoxalin and meloxicam in cats. *J Feline Med Surg* 2013; **15**(8): 678–690.

315 de Leon-Casasola OA, Lema MJ. Postoperative epidural opioid analgesia: what are the choices? *Anesth Analg* 1996; **83**(4): 867–875.

316 Atcheson R, Lambert DG. Update on opioid receptors. *Br J Anaesth* 1994; **73**(2): 132–134.

317 Beaudry H, Dubois D, Gendron L. Activation of spinal mu- and delta-opioid receptors potently inhibits substance P release induced by peripheral noxious stimuli. *J Neurosci* 2011; **31**(37): 13068–13077.

318 Posner L, Pavuk A, Rokshar J, *et al.* Effects of opioids and anesthetic drugs on body temperature in cats. *Vet Anaesth Analg* 2010; **37**(1): 35–43.

319 Sawyer D, Rech R. Analgesia and behavioral effects of butorphanol, nalbuphine, and pentazocine in the cat. *J Am Anim Hosp Assoc* 1987; **23**: 438–446.

320 Figueiredo JP, Muir WW, Sams R. Cardiorespiratory, gastrointestinal, and analgesic effects of morphine sulfate in conscious healthy horses. *Am J Vet Res* 2012; **73**(6): 799–808.

321 van Loon JP, Menke ES, L'Ami JJ, *et al.* Analgesic and anti-hyperalgesic effects of epidural morphine in an equine LPS-induced acute synovitis model. *Vet J* 2012; **193**(2): 464–470.
322 Van Hoogmoed LM, Galuppo LD. Laparoscopic ovariectomy using the endo-GIA stapling device and endo-catch pouches and evaluation of analgesic efficacy of epidural morphine sulfate in 10 mares. *Vet Surg* 2005; **34**(6): 646–650.
323 Brosnan R, Pypendop B, Siao K, Stanley S. Effects of remifentanil on measures of anesthetic immobility and analgesia in cats. *Am J Vet Res* 2009; **70**(9): 1065–1071.
324 Sheehy JG, Hellyer PW, Sammonds GE, *et al.* Evaluation of opioid receptors in synovial membranes of horses. *Am J Vet Res* 2001; **62**(9): 1408–1412.
325 Keates HL, Cramond T, Smith MT. Intraarticular and periarticular opioid binding in inflamed tissue in experimental canine arthritis. *Anesth Analg* 1999; **89**(2): 409–415.
326 Lindegaard C, Gleerup K, Thomsen M, *et al.* Anti-inflammatory effects of intra-articular administration of morphine in horses with experimentally induced synovitis. *Am J Vet Res* 2010; **71**(1): 69–75.
327 Santos LC, de Moraes AN, Saito ME. Effects of intraarticular ropivacaine and morphine on lipopolysaccharide-induced synovitis in horses. *Vet Anaesth Analg* 2009; **36**(3): 280–286.
328 Robertson SA, Andrew SE. Presence of opioid growth factor and its receptor in the normal dog, cat and horse cornea. *Vet Ophthalmol* 2003; **6**(2): 131–134.
329 Stiles J, Honda CN, Krohne SG, Kazacos EA. Effect of topical administration of 1% morphine sulfate solution on signs of pain and corneal wound healing in dogs. *Am J Vet Res* 2003; **64**(7): 813–818.
330 Clark JS, Bentley E, Smith LJ. Evaluation of topical nalbuphine or oral tramadol as analgesics for corneal pain in dogs: a pilot study. *Vet Ophthalmol* 2011; **14**(6): 358–364.
331 Aprea F, Cherubini GB, Palus V, *et al.* Effect of extradurally administered morphine on postoperative analgesia in dogs undergoing surgery for thoracolumbar intervertebral disk extrusion. *J Am Vet Med Assoc* 2012; **241**(6): 754–759.
332 Ambros B, Steagall PV, Mantovani F, *et al.* Antinociceptive effects of epidural administration of hydromorphone in conscious cats. *Am J Vet Res* 2009; **70**(10): 1187–1192.
333 Pablo LS. Epidural morphine in goats after hindlimb orthopedic surgery. *Vet Surg* 1993; **22**(4): 307–310.
334 Bennett R, Steffey E. Use of opioids for pain and anesthetic management in horses. *Vet Clin North Am Equine Pract* 2002; **18**(1): 47–60.
335 Thomasy SM, Moeller BC, Stanley SD. Comparison of opioid receptor binding in horse, guinea pig, and rat cerebral cortex and cerebellum. *Vet Anaesth Analg* 2007; **34**(5): 351–358.
336 Simon EJ. Opiate receptors in the central nervous system. *Curr Dev Psychopharmacol* 1977; **4**: 33–69.
337 Guzman DS, Drazenovich TL, Olsen GH, *et al.* Evaluation of thermal antinociceptive effects after intramuscular administration of hydromorphone hydrochloride to American kestrels (*Falco sparverius*). *Am J Vet Res* 2013; **74**(6): 817–822.
338 Geelen S, Sanchez-Migallon Guzman D, Souza MJ, *et al.* Antinociceptive effects of tramadol hydrochloride after intravenous administration to Hispaniolan Amazon parrots (*Amazona ventralis*). *Am J Vet Res* 2013; **74**(2): 201–206.
339 IUPHAR. *IUPHAR/BPS Guide to Pharmacology. Opioid Receptors*, 2013. http://www.guidetopharmacology.org/GRAC/FamilyDisplayForward?familyId=50&familyType=GPCRIASP (accessed 22 August 2014).
340 Gaveriaux-Ruff C, Nozaki C, Nadal X, *et al.* Genetic ablation of delta opioid receptors in nociceptive sensory neurons increases chronic pain and abolishes opioid analgesia. *Pain* 2011; **152**(6): 1238–1248.
341 Pasternak GW. Opioids and their receptors: are we there yet? *Neuropharmacology* 2014; **76**(Pt B): 198–203.
342 Hawley AT, Wetmore LA. Identification of single nucleotide polymorphisms within exon 1 of the canine mu-opioid receptor gene. *Vet Anaesth Analg* 2010; **37**(1): 79–82.
343 Raffa RB, Buschmann H, Christoph T, *et al.* Mechanistic and functional differentiation of tapentadol and tramadol. *Expert Opin Pharmacother* 2012; **13**(10): 1437–1449.
344 Pypendop B, Ilkiw J. Pharmacokinetics of tramadol, and its metabolite O-desmethyl-tramadol, in cats. *J Vet Pharmacol Ther* 2008; **31**(1): 52–59.
345 Flôr PB, Yazbek KV, Ida KK, Fantoni DT. Tramadol plus metamizole combined or not with anti-inflammatory drugs is clinically effective for moderate to severe chronic pain treatment in cancer patients. *Vet Anaesth Analg* 2013; **40**(3): 316–327.
346 Giorgi M, Meizler A, Mills PC. Pharmacokinetics of the novel atypical opioid tapentadol following oral and intravenous administration in dogs. *Vet J* 2012; **194**(3): 309–313.
347 Pockett S. Spinal cord synaptic plasticity and chronic pain. *Anesth Analg* 1995; **80**(1): 173–179.
348 Yarushkina NI, Bagaeva TR, Filaretova LP. Central corticotropin-releasing factor (CRF) may attenuate somatic pain sensitivity through involvement of glucocorticoids. *J Physiol Pharmacol* 2011; **62**(5): 541–548.
349 Aghighi SA, Tipold A, Piechotta M, *et al.* Assessment of the effects of adjunctive gabapentin on postoperative pain after intervertebral disc surgery in dogs. *Vet Anaesth Analg* 2012; **39**(6): 636–646.
350 Mullen KR, Schwark W, Divers TJ. Pharmacokinetics of single-dose intragastric and intravenous pregabalin administration in clinically normal horses. *Am J Vet Res* 2013; **74**(7): 1043–1048.
351 Salazar V, Dewey CW, Schwark W, *et al.* Pharmacokinetics of single-dose oral pregabalin administration in normal dogs. *Vet Anaesth Analg* 2009; **36**(6): 574–580.
352 Tanabe M, Takasu K, Kasuya N, *et al.* Role of descending noradrenergic system and spinal α_2-adrenergic receptors in the effects of gabapentin on thermal and mechanical nociception after partial nerve injury in the mouse. *Br J Pharmacol* 2005; **144**(5): 703–714.
353 Khasabov SG, Simone DA. Loss of neurons in rostral ventromedial medulla that express neurokinin-1 receptors decreases the development of hyperalgesia. *Neuroscience* 2013; **250**: 151–165.
354 Boscan P, Monnet E, Mama K, *et al.* Effect of maropitant, a neurokinin 1 receptor antagonist, on anesthetic requirements during noxious visceral stimulation of the ovary in dogs. *Am J Vet Res* 2011; **72**(12): 1576–1579.
355 Brain SD. Sensory neuropeptides: their role in inflammation and wound healing. *Immunopharmacology* 1997; **37**(2–3): 133–152.
356 Inoue M, Kobayashi M, Kozaki S, *et al.* Nociceptin/orphanin FQ-induced nociceptive responses through substance P release from peripheral nerve endings in mice. *Proc Natl Acad Sci U S A* 1998; **95**(18): 10949–10953.
357 Cortright DN, Szallasi A. Biochemical pharmacology of the vanilloid receptor TRPV1. An update *Eur J Biochem* 2004; **271**(10): 1814–1819.
358 Szallasi A. Small molecule vanilloid TRPV1 receptor antagonists approaching drug status: can they live up to the expectations? *Naunyn Schmiedebergs Arch Pharmacol* 2006; **373**(4): 273–286.
359 Niyom S, Mama KR, De Rezende ML. Comparison of the analgesic efficacy of oral ABT-116 administration with that of transmucosal buprenorphine administration in dogs. *Am J Vet Res* 2012; **73**(4): 476–481.
360 Cathcart CJ, Johnston SA, Reynolds LR, *et al.* Efficacy of ABT-116, an antagonist of transient receptor potential vanilloid type 1, in providing analgesia for dogs with chemically induced synovitis. *Am J Vet Res* 2012; **73**(1): 19–26.
361 Wang S, Lee J, Ro JY, Chung MK. Warmth suppresses and desensitizes damage-sensing ion channel TRPA1. *Mol Pain* 2012; **8**: 22.
362 White GE, Wells GD. Cold-water immersion and other forms of cryotherapy: physiological changes potentially affecting recovery from high-intensity exercise. *Extreme Physiol Med* 2013; **2**(1): 26.
363 Nadler SF, Weingand K, Kruse RJ. The physiologic basis and clinical applications of cryotherapy and thermotherapy for the pain practitioner. *Pain Physician* 2004; **7**(3): 395–399.
364 Masi AT, Nair K, Evans T, Ghandour Y. Clinical, biomechanical, and physiological translational interpretations of human resting myofascial tone or tension. *Int J Ther Massage Bodywork* 2010; **3**(4): 16–28.
365 Langevin HM, Fox JR, Koptiuch C, *et al.* Reduced thoracolumbar fascia shear strain in human chronic low back pain. *BMC Musculoskelet Disord* 2011; **12**: 203.
366 Corey SM, Vizzard MA, Bouffard NA, *et al.* Stretching of the back improves gait, mechanical sensitivity and connective tissue inflammation in a rodent model. *PLoS One* 2012; **7**(1): e29831.
367 Langevin HM, Bouffard NA, Badger GJ, *et al.* Dynamic fibroblast cytoskeletal response to subcutaneous tissue stretch ex vivo and in vivo. *Am J Physiol Cell Physiol* 2005; **288**(3): C747–C756.
368 Abbott RD, Koptiuch C, Iatridis JC, *et al.* Stress and matrix-responsive cytoskeletal remodeling in fibroblasts. *J Cell Physiol* 2013; **228**(1): 50–57.
369 Langevin HM, Fujita T, Bouffard NA, *et al.* Fibroblast cytoskeletal remodeling induced by tissue stretch involves ATP signaling. *J Cell Physiol* 2013; **228**(9): 1922–1926.
370 Langevin HM, Bouffard NA, Badger GJ, *et al.* Subcutaneous tissue fibroblast cytoskeletal remodeling induced by acupuncture: evidence for a mechanotransduction-based mechanism. *J Cell Physiol* 2006; **207**(3): 767–774.
371 Langevin HM, Churchill DL, Cipolla MJ. Mechanical signaling through connective tissue: a mechanism for the therapeutic effect of acupuncture. *FASEB J* 2001; **15**(12): 2275–2282.
372 Langevin HM, Bouffard NA, Churchill DL, Badger GJ. Connective tissue fibroblast response to acupuncture: dose-dependent effect of bidirectional needle rotation. *J Altern Complement Med* 2007; **13**(3): 355–360.
373 Groppetti D, Pecile AM, Sacerdote P, *et al.* Effectiveness of electroacupuncture analgesia compared with opioid administration in a dog model: a pilot study. *Br J Anaesth* 2011; **107**(4): 612–618.
374 Wang CJ. Extracorporeal shockwave therapy in musculoskeletal disorders. *J Orthop Res* 2012; **7**: 11.
375 Wang CJ, Sun YC, Wong T, *et al.* Extracorporeal shockwave therapy shows time-dependent chondroprotective effects in osteoarthritis of the knee in rats. *J Surg Res* 2012; **178**(1): 196–205.

376 Zhang R, Lao L, Ren K, Berman BM. Mechanisms of acupuncture–electroacupuncture on persistent pain. *Anesthesiology* 2014; **120**(2): 482–503.
377 He LF, Lu RL, Zhuang SY, *et al.* Possible involvement of opioid peptides of caudate nucleus in acupuncture analgesia. *Pain* 1985; **23**(1): 83–93.
378 Han JS. Acupuncture: neuropeptide release produced by electrical stimulation of different frequencies. *Trends Neurosci* 2003; **26**(1): 17–22.
379 Jang JY, Kim HN, Koo ST, *et al.* Synergistic antinociceptive effects of *N*-methyl-D-aspartate receptor antagonist and electroacupuncture in the complete Freund's adjuvant-induced pain model. *Int J Mol Med* 2011; **28**(4): 669–675.
380 Ando A, Suda H, Hagiwara Y, *et al.* Reversibility of immobilization-induced articular cartilage degeneration after remobilization in rat knee joints. *Tohoku J Exp Med* 2011; **224**(2): 77–85.
381 Wang TT, Yuan Y, Kang Y, *et al.* Effects of acupuncture on the expression of glial cell line-derived neurotrophic factor (GDNF) and basic fibroblast growth factor (FGF-2/bFGF) in the left sixth lumbar dorsal root ganglion following removal of adjacent dorsal root ganglia. *Neurosci Lett* 2005; **382**(3): 236–241.
382 Dong Z, Sun Y, Lu P, *et al.* Electroacupuncture and lumbar transplant of GDNF-secreting fibroblasts synergistically attenuate hyperalgesia after sciatic nerve constriction. *Am J Chin Med* 2013; **41**(3): 459–472.
383 Wang TH, Wang XY, Li XL, *et al.* Effect of electroacupuncture on neurotrophin expression in cat spinal cord after partial dorsal rhizotomy. *Neurochem Res* 2007; **32**(8): 1415–1422.
384 Zhang ZJ, Wang XM, McAlonan GM. Neural acupuncture unit: a new concept for interpreting effects and mechanisms of acupuncture. *Evid Based Complement Alternat Med* 2012; **2012**: 429412.
385 Miguez G, Laborda MA, Miller RR. Classical conditioning and pain: conditioned analgesia and hyperalgesia. *Acta Psychol (Amst)* 2014; **145**: 10–20.
386 Sikandar S, Ronga I, Iannetti GD, Dickenson AH. Neural coding of nociceptive stimuli-from rat spinal neurones to human perception. *Pain* 2013; **154**(8): 1263–1273.
387 Lee B, Sur BJ, Shim I, *et al.* Acupuncture stimulation attenuates impaired emotional-like behaviors and activation of the noradrenergic system during protracted abstinence following chronic morphine exposure in rats. *Evid Based Complement Alternat Med* 2014; **2014**: 216503.
388 Jensen KB, Kaptchuk TJ, Kirsch I, *et al.* Nonconscious activation of placebo and nocebo pain responses. *Proc Natl Acad Sci U S A* 2012; **109**(39): 15959–15964.
389 Raicek JE, Stone BH, Kaptchuk TJ. Placebos in 19th century medicine: a quantitative analysis of the BMJ. *BMJ* 2012; **345**: e8326.
390 Mannerkorpi K, Henriksson C. Non-pharmacological treatment of chronic widespread musculoskeletal pain. *Best Pract Res Clin Rheumatol* 2007; **21**(3): 513–534.
391 Feine JS, Lund JP. An assessment of the efficacy of physical therapy and physical modalities for the control of chronic musculoskeletal pain. *Pain* 1997; **71**(1): 5–23.
392 Labruyêre R, van Hedel HJA. Strength training versus robot-assisted gait training after incomplete spinal cord injury: a randomized pilot study in patients depending on walking assistance. *J Neuroeng Rehabil* 2014; **11**(1): 4.
393 Gonzalez-Lima F, Barksdale BR, Rojas JC. Mitochondrial respiration as a target for neuroprotection and cognitive enhancement. *Biochem Pharmacol* 2014; **88**(4): 584–593.
394 Chung H, Dai T, Sharma SK, Huang YY, *et al.* The nuts and bolts of low-level laser (light) therapy. *Ann Biomed Eng* 2012; **40**(2): 516–533.
395 Kalichman L, Vulfsons S. Dry needling in the management of musculoskeletal pain. *J Am Board Fam Med* 2010; **23**(5): 640–646.
396 Nieman DC. Exercise immunology: practical applications. *Int J Sports Med* 1997; **18**(Suppl 1): S91–S100.
397 Ge HY, Fernandez-de-Las-Peñas C, Yue SW. Myofascial trigger points: spontaneous electrical activity and its consequences for pain induction and propagation. *Chin Med* 2011; **6**: 13.
398 Kim SK, Bae H. Acupuncture and immune modulation. *Auton Neurosci* 2010; **157**(1–2): 38–41.
399 Takahashi T. Mechanism of acupuncture on neuromodulation in the gut – a review. *Neuromodulation* 2011; **14**(1): 8–12; discussion, 12.

SECTION 7

Hepatic System

30 Physiology, Pathophysiology, and Anesthetic Management of Patients with Hepatic Disease

Fernando Garcia-Pereira
Large Animal Clinical Sciences, College of Veterinary Medicine, University of Florida, Gainesville, Florida, USA

Chapter contents

Introduction

The liver is centrally located in the body, between the diaphragm and abdominal viscera, where it receives blood draining from the portal circulation. Blood arriving from the gastrointestinal tract is rich in proteins, fat, and carbohydrates, in addition to containing bacteria, drugs, and potential toxins. Besides the most obvious function, namely the hepatic participation in digestion (bile production, breakdown of nutrients, and elimination of bacteria from portal circulation), other more important functions to the anesthetist are the homeostasis of blood glucose, production of proteins needed for coagulation, production of albumin, biotransformation and excretion of drugs and their metabolites, and excretion of metabolic waste products.

Normal anatomy and physiology

The liver is the largest gland in the body. It comprises 1.5–4% of total body weight and is anatomically and physiologically similar among species. The liver can be divided into four main lobes (left, right, quadrate, and caudate lobes). The right and left lobes may be further subdivided into separate lateral and medial lobes. A gall bladder is present in most domestic species with the exception of the horse and the rat, in which large bile ducts compensate for the absence of the gall bladder. In some species the bile duct terminates directly on the duodenum (e.g., canine and bovine), but in others it shares a common duct with the pancreas (e.g., cat, horse, and small ruminants). This can be of importance, as some hepatobiliary diseases can also affect the pancreas of the those species [1]. Other less important anatomic differences are beyond the scope of this chapter.

Blood supply and structural organization

The arrangement of hepatic structures is centered on the caudal vena cava and portal vein. Blood returning from most of the gastrointestinal tract and spleen travels through the portal vein. The portal circulation supplies the majority of blood flow to the liver. A second blood supply is from the hepatic artery, which delivers highly oxygenated blood to help sustain hepatocellular function. Although the portal vein carries blood with a lower oxygen content than the hepatic artery, it plays an important role in the organ's oxygenation owing to the large volume of blood that it delivers.

The sinusoid is the functional unit of the liver and is organized around the hepatic vein similarly to the spokes on a wheel (Fig. 30.1). Hepatic artery blood enters the sinusoid either directly or through the peribiliary capillary plexus. It mixes with portal venous blood in the low-pressure sinusoid microvasculature. Sinusoidal hepatocytes can be divided in three different zones depending on their localization (Fig. 30.1). The periportal area, where blood flows into the organ, is called the zone 1 and the hepatocytes in this region have a large amount of mitochondria. This is where most oxidative processes occur. Zone 2 is a transitional some between zones 1 and 3. Zone 3 is located near the central veins (centrolobular), where blood will leave the organ and join the central

Veterinary Anesthesia and Analgesia: The Fifth Edition of Lumb and Jones.
Edited by Kurt A. Grimm, Leigh A. Lamont, William J. Tranquilli, Stephen A. Greene and Sheilah A. Robertson.

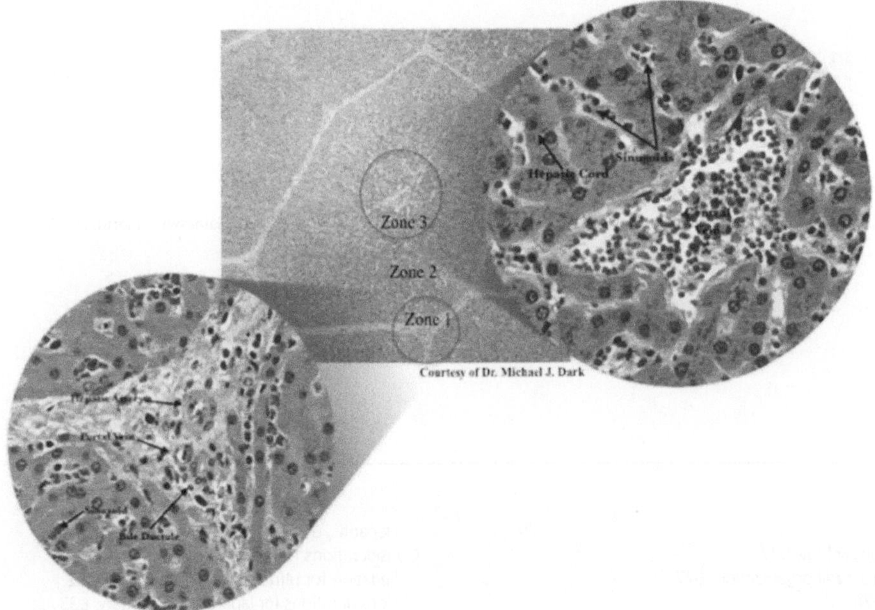

Figure 30.1 Microanatomy of the hepatic parenchyma. Zone 1, periportal; zone 3, centrolobular; zone 2, between zones 1 and 3. Source: Michael J. Dark, Department of Infectious Diseases and Pathology, College of Veterinary Medicine, University of Florida, Gainesville, FL, USA. Reproduced with permission of Michael J. Dark.

Box 30.1 Major functions of the liver.

Nutrient storage and supply
Plasma oncotic pressure
Lipid metabolism
Carbohydrate metabolism
Protein metabolism
Albumin
Coagulation protein
Cytokines
Fetal and extramedullary hematopoiesis
Biotransformation and biliary excretion
Ammonia removal and urea production
Clearance of plasma proteins

Source: adapted from [4]. Reproduced with permission of Wiley.

circulation. The hepatocytes of this region contain a large amount of smooth endoplasmatic reticulum and microsomal enzyme activity, and therefore play a major role in drug deactivation and metabolism. Knowledge of this arrangement becomes important in predicting hepatic areas that will be most affected by specific toxic metabolites.

An increase in portal pressure can promote neovascularization of splanchnic vasculature and development of acquired portosystemic shunts. Compensatory mechanisms must act so that an increase in portal flow minimally affects portal venous pressure. Several mechanisms are responsible for the maintenance of adequate sinusoidal perfusion pressure while maintaining low portal venous pressure, including low basal resistance, distensible pre- and postsinusoid resistance sites, highly compliant hepatic vasculature, and the hepatic artery buffer response (HABR) [2]. The HABR is mechanistically associated with adenosine because as portal blood flow decreases, adenosine accumulates, causing vasodilation of nearby hepatic arterioles. This dilation increases arterial blood flow and maintains hepatic perfusion [2,3].

Hepatic functions

The liver performs numerous functions affecting all systems of the body (Box 30.1) [4]. It plays a major role in protein synthesis and degradation, including albumin, coagulation proteins, and numerous peptides. Glycogen storage, nutrient metabolism, detoxification, and excretion of endogenous waste products and xenobiotics are other important functions.

Protein homeostasis

Normally, plasma protein availability is abundant relative to daily consumption. The protein concentration is decreased more often in chronic disease or severe loss. Albumin is the most abundant protein produced by the liver and is involved in several homeostatic processes. Notably, albumin is a major contributor to plasma oncotic pressure. Interestingly, albumin production is regulated (via feedback) in part through plasma oncotic pressure in addition to its plasma concentration [5]. Albumin is also a major plasma transport protein, binding to several substances, including some anesthetic drugs.

Several coagulation factors, such as fibrinogen, prothrombin, factors V, VII, IX, X, XI, XII, and XIII, prekallikrein, and high molecular weight kininogen are synthesized or activated by the liver [6]. The liver is also responsible for the synthesis of proteins that modulate coagulation, such as, plasminogen, plasminogen activator inhibitor-1, α_2-antiplasmin, antithrombin, and proteins C and S. Furthermore, it performs vitamin K-dependent carboxylation of prothrombin, factor VII, IX, and X, and proteins C and S [7].

Biotransformation and elimination of xenobiotics

The enzymatic systems involved in the biotransformation of substances are generally localized to the liver. However, other tissues, such as the lungs, kidneys, and gastrointestinal tract, have significant metabolic capabilities for some drugs. The route of administration and subsequent drug distribution to these sites must be considered when administering sedatives, analgesics, and anesthetics [8]. First-pass hepatic metabolism significantly reduces the bioavailability of several drugs, especially after enteral, and in some species rectal, administration.

Xenobiotic biotransformation can be divided into Phase I (oxidation, reduction, or hydrolysis) and Phase II (conjugation) reactions. Phase I transformation introduces a polar group (e.g., OH^- and NH_2^-) to the parent drug. These reactions often inactivate a drug. However, the addition of these functional radicals can result in active metabolites of some drugs, or cause the activation of a prodrug. One example of a prodrug is codeine, which is catalyzed by CYP2D6 and *O*-demethylated to form morphine. Codeine's analgesic activity seems to be related to *O*-demethylation of the drug locally in the central nervous system, explaining the low plasmatic concentration of morphine after an analgesic dose of codeine [7–9].

The cytochrome P450 system (CYPs) is the most important group of microsomal metabolizing enzymes of the body. They are found in several tissues, such as the liver, kidney, and intestines, and are responsible for the oxidation and reduction of xenobiotics and endogenous substances. These reactions convert relatively lipophilic compounds into hydrophilic metabolites to facilitate their elimination through the urine or bile. They are mostly carried out intracellularly in the microsomes of the smooth endoplasmatic reticulum (i.e., microsomal enzymes). Zone 3 hepatocytes have the highest content of cytochrome P450 enzymes. Their localization to where biotransformation is occurring is important in predicting the region where hepatic damage will be most evident when a drug is metabolized to toxic substances. An example is severe centrolobular necrosis and colangiohepatitis observed in some cats following administration of oral diazepam [10]. Although the same families and subfamilies of P450 enzymes are present in most domestic species, different individual enzymes might be encountered in each species. Additionally, the same enzyme may be present but act on a different substrate range compared with humans [11]. Therefore, it becomes problematic to extrapolate drug doses, intervals, effects and metabolic fate from human-derived data to veterinary species without supporting clinical data. Differences in CYP activity exist not only among species, but also among different breeds and genders. For example, Beagles have greater propofol hydroxylase activity (CYP2B) than Greyhounds [12]. Gender variability in dogs and cats for different CYP families has also been described [13].

Phase II reactions are responsible for conferring further hydrophilicity to a drug, facilitating its excretion. These reactions occur mostly in the cytosol. The domestic cat has been recognized to have a reduced ability to form glucuronide conjugates of many xenobiotics (e.g., propofol) [14]. Therefore, when low molecular weight phenolic derivatives are given to cats, they are biotransformed slowly, or are biotransformed and eliminated by other mechanisms [15,16]. Defects of the UGT1 A6 gene seems to be responsible for the poor glucuronidation of some drugs, such as acetaminophen [17]. However, cats have other UGT enzymes that can biotransform some other xenobiotics [18].

Some xenobiotics can induce CYP and glucuronosyltransferase activity. Ketamine can induce both enzyme types, contributing to the development of its own tolerance in rats [19]. Mutations can also affect drug elimination. An ATP-binding cassette (ABC) mutation in the gene ABCB1 causes MDR-1 (multidrug-resistant protein, formerly P-glycoproteins) efflux transporter deficiency. Reduced protein activity results in decreased removal of certain drugs from brain to blood, and from blood to bile on the hepatocellular surface in humans [20,21]. This may be related to some adverse effects of ivermectins and morphine-like derivatives from brain to systemic circulation in MDR-1 mutant dogs [22,23].

In the last two decades, a large amount of information on the metabolism and interaction of specific drugs in veterinary species has been published [24]. However, further research is warranted to characterize individual CYPs for each species and their substrates.

Immune and inflammatory response

The liver has a large role in host defense. Bacteria and toxins that gain access to the portal circulation are routinely phagocytized and processed by Kupffer cells in the sinusoids [25]. Kupffer cells are also scavengers of inflammatory mediators, appearing to play a major role in limiting the extent of the inflammatory response [26,27]. However, when an overwhelming amount of endotoxin is present, activated Kupffer cells can produce reductive oxygen radicals and cytokines. These processes allow Kupffer cells to signal hepatocytes and endothelial cells, changing their transcription products, in addition to recruiting circulating neutrophils. This hepatic immunologic response can be responsible for hepatocellular injury seen under some disease conditions. The close interaction between the inflammatory response and coagulation also plays a role in the pathogenesis of hepatic and multiorgan failure. For example, during endotoxemia and hypoperfusion, the activated hepatic cells (Kupffer, hepatocytes, and endothelial cells) promote inflammation and also a hypercoagulable state [28].

Testing and monitoring hepatic function

Liver function testing and liver enzyme interpretation

Biochemistry tests are often performed prior to sedation and anesthesia. Enzyme concentration abnormalities are common, but their relation to patient risk is often difficult to interpret. The serum concentration of alanine aminotransferase (ALT), aspartate aminotransferase (AST), alkaline phosphatase (ALP) and γ-glutamyl transpeptidase (GGT) are the most commonly measured hepatocellular enzymes in biochemical profiles. Hepatobiliary tissue damage can cause cellular leakage, resulting in increased plasma concentration of hepatocellular enzymes. However, this rise does not necessarily indicate the degree of hepatic dysfunction. This is especially true for chronic liver diseases, where reduced hepatocellular numbers secondary to fibrosis may result in near-normal liver enzyme values in the face of severely compromised function. Additionally, elevation of enzymes may represent cellular insult, but not correlate to interference with the ability to biotransform drugs used for anesthesia and pain management.

Substrate metabolism tests, such as pre- and postprandial bile acids or indocyanine green elimination, are better indicators of hepatic function [29]. A study evaluating the sensitivity and specificity of fasting ammonia and serum bile acids for diagnosis of portal systemic shunts in dogs and cats found the tests to have high sensitivity and specificity in both species [30]. Low serum concentrations of albumin, glucose, and urea nitrogen are usually present in liver dysfunction, but are not pathognomonic for liver diseases.

The position of the liver between the splanchnic and systemic circulation creates the potential for diseases of other organ systems to involve the liver, and consequently cause an increases in circulating liver enzymes. Additionally, several enzymes are found in tissue outside the liver (e.g., AST in skeletal muscle) and injury to these tissues may be falsely interpreted as hepatic injury. Elevation of enzymes, although highly sensitive to hepatic damage, is not specific to liver injury.

Common biochemical changes associated with liver pathology

The presence of liver dysfunction, independent of primary hepatic disease, can decrease the amount of several factors produced by the organ. Therefore, a biochemical profile, coagulation panel, and pre- and postprandial bile acids should be requested if the patient's hepatic function is questioned. A coagulation profile [e.g., prothrombin time (PT) and activated partial thromboplastin time (aPTT)] should be performed on all patients with liver disease undergoing a surgical procedure. Chronic hepatitis patients may show no clinical signs of a coagulopathy but can have a reduced amount of coagulation factors and be at a greater risk of coagulopathy after an insult such as surgery [31]. Blood typing and cross-matching may be warranted if the coagulation profile is abnormal or if a blood transfusion is anticipated. Plasma (fresh or fresh frozen) can be used to supplement coagulation factors in patients with many coagulation abnormalities.

The liver synthesizes several plasma proteins, including all serum albumin. Because the liver normally produces albumin at one-third of its capacity, hypoalbuminemia is seen only in severe cases of hepatic dysfunction or severe protein loss. Glomerular disease, protein-losing enteropathies and hemorrhage are non-hepatic causes and should be ruled out when hypoalbuminemia is present. Alpha- and beta-globulins are synthesized by the liver and their plasma concentration may be diminished with hepatic dysfunction. Reduction in plasma protein concentrations will decrease the bound fraction of some drugs, which can result in changes in volume of distribution, plasma concentration, and drug effect.

The liver plays a major role in glucose homeostasis. Patients with portosystemic shunts or acute hepatic failure are often hypoglycemic, or at risk for clinical hypoglycemia during the perianesthetic period. Mechanisms of hypoglycemia in hepatic dysfunction include one or a combination of the following: decreased gluconeogenesis, decreased glycogen storage, and diminished response to glucagon. Monitoring and maintenance of normoglycemia should be a priority during anesthesia. Dextrose solutions (1–5%) can be given in combination with other isotonic crystalloids during surgery as needed to maintain normoglycemia.

Drug biotransformation and elimination concerns with hepatic disease

Sedatives and anesthetics

Animals with liver disease that require anesthesia are often obtunded to some extent. Frequently, the administration of an opioid is sufficient to provide adequate sedation and analgesia for diagnostic and minor surgical procedures. Hydromorphone, oxymorphone, fentanyl, and methadone are full agonist opioids that provide good sedation and analgesia. Compared with morphine and meperidine, they present some potential advantages, as they are not associated with elevations in plasma histamine concentrations and decreased blood pressure after intravenous administration [32–34]. A decrease in systemic vascular resistance could possibly translate into a decrease in hepatic blood flow and subsequently decreased drug elimination capacity or further hepatic insult [35]. Opioids with short elimination half-lives such as fentanyl can be used as constant-rate infusions. Careful dose titration is important because the context-sensitive half-life of most opioids used in constant rate infusions will be longer than in normal patients [36]. Remifentanil is another opioid with a short elimination half-life that can be administered as an intravenous infusion. It is metabolized by plasma esterases and shows no accumulation after constant-rate infusion in humans presenting with severe liver disease [37].

Most sedatives used in veterinary medicine can be categorized into one of three groups: phenothiazines, benzodiazepines, and α_2-adrenergic receptor agonists. Acepromazine can be used in patients with liver disease but careful assessment of the patient is necessary. Acepromazine causes vasodilation due to its antagonistic effect at α_1-adrenergic receptors [38,39]. Acepromazine vasodilation may be beneficial to increase renal blood flow in anesthetized dogs [40], but experimental verification that it has the same effect on the hepatic circulation is lacking. When a patient has diminished intravascular oncotic pressure (e.g., hypoalbuminemia), hypovolemia and hypotension can be present even before sedation. In these cases, a combination of colloid (e.g., hydroxyethyl starch) and crystalloid fluid therapy may be necessary. Acepromazine is also known to affect platelet aggregation in dogs and should be avoided if significant coagulation abnormalities are present [41].

Benzodiazepine sedative drugs are often advocated in cases where there is significant disease because they tend to have fewer cardiovascular adverse effects. However, their use in patients with liver disease may be less advantageous. Advanced liver disease may result in hepatic encephalopathy (HE) due to accumulation of ammonium, NMDA hyperactivity, and decreased adenosine triphosphate, among other causes [42,43]. In humans, the benzodiazepine antagonist flumazenil is often used to minimize clinical signs associated with HE [44]. The use of benzodiazepines in veterinary patients presenting with HE is controversial as they may exhibit increased response to these drugs, resulting in aggravation of the HE [45].In the absence of HE, benzodiazepines can be used safely in patients with liver disease, although hepatic elimination is likely reduced and prolonged effects may occur [46,47]. Unwanted effects such as prolonged sedation can be antagonized by flumazenil if needed.

Dexmedetomidine provides excellent sedative and analgesic effects yet may be associated with significant cardiovascular depression characterized by decreases in cardiac output of as much as 50% [48,49]. Despite this, hepatic blood flow is unchanged in normal dogs after intravenous administration of up to 10 μg/kg, based on the radioactive microsphere method [50]. Medetomidine and dexmedetomidine have been shown to decrease hepatic enzymatic activity *in vitro*. It could be speculated that they would have clinically relevant pharmacokinetic drug interactions that would be more apparent in animals with liver disease. However, it is likely that their sparing effects on doses of other anesthetic agents (pharmacodynamic drug interaction) may be more clinically relevant than any direct effects on liver metabolic capacity [51]. Antagonism of α_2-adrenergic receptor agonists can speed recovery in animals with liver disease and would minimize the impact of impaired metabolism on the duration of α_2-adrenergic receptor agonist duration.

There have been numerous studies evaluating the effects of inhalant anesthetics on hepatic function and blood flow. However, relatively few studies have examined the impact of injectable anesthetics. Ketamine appears to cause a modest decrease in comparison with thiopental and etomidate [52,53]. Propofol has been shown to maintain hepatic blood flow via arterial vasodilation in dogs and thiopental appears to have similar effects [54,55]. In an ischemia/reperfusion rabbit model, propofol showed reduced hepatic reperfusion injury, in addition to oxidative radical formation [56,57].As a general rule, most agents have minimal direct effects on hepatic blood flow if systemic arterial blood pressure is maintained within normal limits. Propofol clearance exceeds hepatic blood flow, suggesting an extra-hepatic site of metabolism and making it a reasonable choice for patients with liver disease [58,59]. A retrospective study found no increase in morbidity or mortality in cats with hepatic lipidosis that were anesthetized with propofol for feeding tube placement [60]. However, like most anesthetic drugs, it has dose-dependent cardiac depressant and systemic vasodilatory effects that may alter hepatic blood flow in some cases [61].

Thiopental undergoes metabolism by the liver, has several active metabolites, and its administration may result in the induction of microsomal enzyme activity [62,63]. Termination of its anesthetic effects results mostly from redistribution to non-target tissues, suggesting that it may be acceptable to use it as a single bolus for induction.

Etomidate has been shown to cause minimal cardiovascular effects compared with propofol during anesthetic induction [61]. However, etomidate is in a propylene glycol-based vehicle. Propylene glycol is a hyperosmolar molecule and may cause erythrocyte rupture [64]. Because some patients presenting with hepatobiliary disease may have bilirubinemia and icterus due to biliary obstruction or decreased hepatic conjugation, the potential hemolysis caused by etomidate could further overload the liver. Although hemolysis does not appear to be significant in normal dogs after a single bolus, the clinical consequences in animals with liver disease have not been studied [65]. Etomidate clearance did not seem to change in human patients with hepatic cirrhosis compared with healthy patients, but the volume of distribution and elimination half-life doubled [66,67]. This increase in volume of distribution can mostly be explained by the inverse correlation between the plasmatic albumin concentration and protein binding, but may also be due to a slight decrease in albumin binding proprieties in the presence of hepatic cirrhosis or renal failure [68]. Etomidate has been demonstrated to inhibit cortisol synthesis by inhibiting 11β-hydroxylase and is generally not recommended in adrenal dysfunction seen in septic patients [69]. Although a subgroup of hepatic patients obviously fit such a group as septic bile peritonitis, a portion of human patients with non-septic acute and chronic liver diseases have shown a lower baseline and stimulated cortisol levels (hepatoadrenal syndrome) [69–71]. Furthermore, when ACTH stimulation tests were performed in these patients, the presence of etomidate in the anesthetic protocol increased the presence of adrenal insufficiency from 38 to 57% [69]. Hepatoadrenal syndrome has not yet been reported in the veterinary literature; however, care should be taken regarding the presence of concomitant adrenal insufficiency when using etomidate in liver patients. Etomidate is primarily metabolized by esterase hydrolysis in the rat. However, this route does not seem to play a significant role in the drug breakdown of several other species studied, pointing to a hepatic metabolism [72,73]. Its hepatic extraction ratio is 0.5, or 50% of the hepatic blood flow, which indicates that small changes in hepatic blood flow or function will have only moderate effects on etomidate clearance [74]. Overall, etomidate seems to be a good induction agent for the liver patient owing to its minimal cardiovascular effects, which preserve systemic and hepatic blood flow.

Dissociative anesthetics such as ketamine and tiletamine are reasonable choices for the induction of anesthesia in patients with hepatic disease. However, the co-administration of a benzodiazepine (e.g., zolazepam in tiletamine) may result in prolonged effects in animals with impaired hepatic function. In dogs, dissociative anesthetics are metabolized mostly by the liver; however, termination of effect would be expected to be minimally affected after administration of a single dose used for induction due to drug redistribution to muscular and adipose tissues [75]. A study in rats and a report in humans have shown ketamine infusions to cause hepatic injury after prolonged use, especially when repeated within a short interval between treatments [76,77]. The authors of the human report recommended that liver enzymes be routinely measured during chronic treatment using ketamine [76].

Inhalants

Inhalant anesthetics alter hepatic blood flow in a dose-dependent fashion. In general, inhalants impair autoregulatory mechanisms (i.e., HABR) that would otherwise maintain total hepatic blood flow. Studies in dogs have shown that isoflurane, sevoflurane, and desflurane better maintain total hepatic blood flow, oxygen supply, and delivery–consumption ratios than halothane or enflurane (Fig. 30.2) [78,79]. Although sevoflurane and desflurane appear to have the least effect on hepatic blood flow, it is important to note that, among the commonly used agents (isoflurane, sevoflurane, and desflurane), these effects are dose dependent. Consequently, efforts to reduce the dose administered will have a significantly greater impact than choice of inhalant anesthetic.

Isoflurane in a lipid emulsion was demonstrated to have a protective effect on hepatic ischemic/reperfusion (IR) injury when injected intravenously into rats. The mechanism for such protection seemed to be related to Kupffer cell inhibition [80]. Conversely, another study found protective effects of inhaling sevoflurane when given before, during, and after injury, but failed to find any beneficial effect of isoflurane administered by the same route on a rat model of IR injury [81]. Perhaps inhalant preconditioning may have beneficial effects during hepatic surgery if IR injury is predicted.

Neuromuscular blockers

The disposition of neuromuscular blocking drugs (NMBs) may be affected by liver disease. Vecuronium, rocuronium, and mivacurium all have increased volumes of distribution, prolonged elimination half-lives, and prolonged durations of effect in human patients with hepatic cirrhosis [82–84]. Atracurium and cis-atracurium undergo liver-independent elimination (by non-specific ester hydrolysis or Hofmann elimination) and have similar pharmacokinetics and pharmacodynamics in both healthy and liver-diseased patients [85–87]. A study evaluating cis-atracurium found no difference in onset and duration of action between healthy and portosystemic shunt-affected dogs [88].

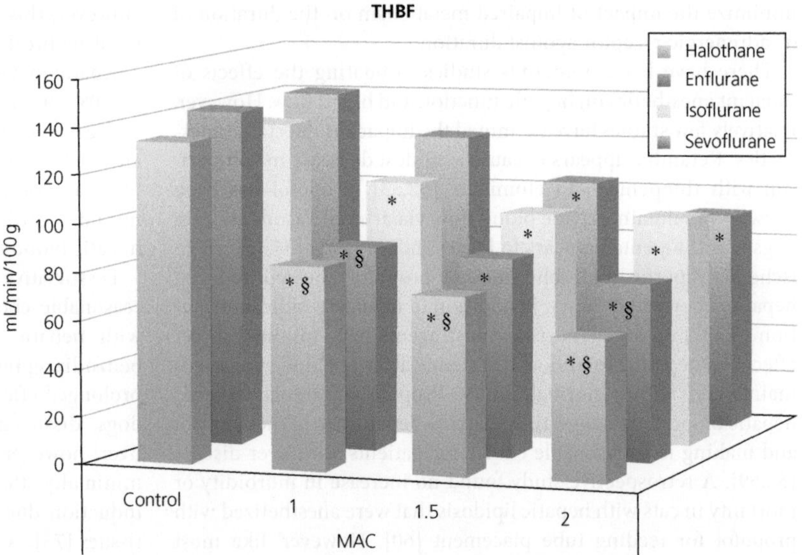

Figure 30.2 Effect of inhalant anesthetics on total hepatic blood flow (THBF) in Greyhound dogs. Bars marked with * are significantly different ($p < 0.05$) from their respective control group (awake dogs). Bars marked with § are significantly different ($p < 0.05$) from THBF values for isoflurane and sevoflurane at comparable minimum alveolar concentration (MAC) levels. Source: adapted from [78,79]. Reproduced with permission of Lippincott Williams & Wilkins and Springer.

Hepatic pathophysiology and approach to anesthetic management

Liver disease can have a significant impact on drug pharmacokinetics and pharmacodynamics depending on which hepatic functions are altered and the degree of insufficiency. Preanesthetic evaluation and diagnostic testing can help define the degree of impairment and provide information about how the anesthetic plan should be altered and how much anesthetic risk is increased.

Hepatitis

Patients with acute or chronic hepatitis can present clinical signs and laboratory abnormalities that may be correlated with prognosis. Generally, the clinical signs and laboratory results for patients with liver dysfunction are non-specific (e.g., anorexia, diarrhea, polyuria/polydipsia, and fatigue). Jaundice, hepatic encephalopathy, and ascites can also be present, representing significant hepatic insufficiency or greater disease severity. Ascites is a negative prognostic factor in dogs and humans with hepatitis [89,90]. Interestingly, one study found no relationship between the biochemical parameter results and severity of liver disease [91]. In another study investigating chronic hepatitis in Labrador Retrievers, it was demonstrated that 45% of these dogs presented with hyperbilirubinemia and 21% with hypoalbuminemia. Also, it was shown that prolongation of PT and aPTT, thrombocytopenia, anorexia, and hypoglobulinemia were associated with shorter survival times [31]. Another single-center study found that 57% of patients with hepatic diseases had least one abnormal coagulation parameter at presentation. Furthermore, the presence of cirrhosis in addition to chronic hepatitis was associated with the worst coagulation abnormalities among all liver diseases. Most of the coagulation abnormalities found in this study were related to a decrease in coagulation factor synthesis, not an increase in factors consumption [92]. Therefore, the simple presence of hepatic disease demonstrated by biochemical abnormalities with or without clinical signs should be taken into consideration by the anesthetist, independent of the degree of abnormality, as the latter does not correlate with disease severity. Also, in chronic hepatitis, coagulopathies are often absent, probably due to the balanced decrease in pro- and anticoagulant factors. However, in the presence of an insult, such as surgery, decompensation can occur and postoperative coagulopathy can result. This is particularly problematic in hypotensive patients where large volumes of fluid therapy are used to maintain perfusion. Volume expansion dilutes circulating coagulation factors and can cause decompensation and clinical abnormalities [93,94].

Considerations for diagnostic procedures

Liver biopsy may be necessary to determine the etiology and prognosis of hepatic disease. Samples can be obtained by ultrasound-guided biopsy instruments, laparoscopy, and laparotomy. Laparoscopy and laparotomy can also be used for the staging and resection of neoplasia or hepatobiliary repair. Knowledge of the specific implications of each technique can help the anesthetist prevent, anticipate, and resolve possible problems that may emerge during the procedure.

Sedation for ultrasound-guided biopsy

Biopsies can often be accomplished with sedation alone. For this technique, the patient needs to lie still and not react to sound or sensation of device activation. There is a chance that bleeding will occur after the biopsy, so the technique is not advisable in animals with significant coagulation abnormalities. The patient's clinical signs and laboratory results, in addition to its demeanor and mentation, will determine drug combination and dose selection. Benzodiazepines are often used in critically ill patients owing to their minimal cardiovascular effects, rapid elimination, and potential reversibility. Administration of an opioid alone or in combination with midazolam (0.2–0.5 mg/kg, IV or IM) or dexmedetomidine (2–10 μg/kg IV or IM) is often sufficient to facilitate ultrasound-guided biopsies from a range of mildly to severely obtunded patients. The opioids most commonly used in these combinations are butorphanol (0.2–0.4 mg/kg, IM or IV), methadone (0.3–0.5 mg/kg, IV), hydromorphone (0.05–0.2 mg/kg, IV or IM), oxymorphone (0.05–0.2 mg/kg, IV or IM), and fentanyl (5–15 μg/kg, IV). Although usually not necessary, flumazenil can be administered to reverse the sedative effects of benzodiazepines. When dexmedetomidine is used, atipamezole administration usually results in rapid and complete reversal of sedation and cardiovascular effects. In the absence of pain, naloxone may be administered to improve mentation and ventilation when opioid sedation is no longer required or desirable.

Monitoring during sedation is important because of the unpredictable changes in pharmacokinetics and drug effects with hepatic dysfunction, and oxygen supplementation may be advisable. Vasovagal hypotension during a few minutes after percutaneous liver biopsy has been reported [95]. Postprocedure monitoring for signs of hemorrhage (e.g., mucous membrane color, blood pressure, hematocrit, or repeat ultrasound) are warranted when the risk of bleeding is significant.

Considerations for laparoscopic surgery

Laparoscopy is commonly used for liver biopsy. In addition to the obvious possibility of bleeding and the difficulty in achieving hemostasis, this technique introduces a new set of problems related to insufflation of gases into the abdomen. The infusion of carbon dioxide to distend the abdomen and improve visualization can decrease cardiac venous return and impair ventilation. Cranial displacement of the diaphragm can make it more difficult for the spontaneously breathing animal to maintain adequate minute ventilation and will decrease pulmonary functional residual capacity. Intermittent positive-pressure ventilation (IPPV) may be required to maintain adequate oxygenation and ventilation. Positive-pressure ventilation can be effected manually or using a mechanical ventilator. The anesthetist should also monitor the intra-abdominal pressure, which should range from 10 to 16 mmHg with allowance for species differences [96]. In people, pneumoperitoneum was associated with an increase in hepatic blood flow provided that intra-abdominal pressures did not exceed 12 mmHg [97]. In dogs, pneumoperitoneum can cause transient increases in hepatic transaminases that lasted up to 48 h after desufflation. The increases in ALT and AST were directly proportional to the intra-abdominal pressure and duration of insufflation [98]. Positive-pressure ventilation has been shown to decrease hepatic blood flow, probably by decreasing venous return and cardiac output, so its use during abdominal insufflation should be closely monitored [78]. Monitoring of arterial blood pressure is important as an indirect predictor of tissue perfusion and assessment of the effect of intra-abdominal pressure on venous return. However, it should be noted that abdominal insufflation frequently results in an increase in arterial blood pressure that may not represent an increase in tissue perfusion. A reversed Trendelenburg position can help to minimize the effect of CO_2 infusion on ventilation; however, body position is usually dictated by the need of the surgeon to ensure adequate visualization. Capnography, although helpful, can be misleading because the difference between $ETCO_2$ and $PaCO_2$ can be significantly increased by ventilation/perfusion mismatching in some patients. Arterial blood-gas analysis may be more indicative of ventilation status.

Laparotomy

Laparotomy is the most traditional approach for hepatobiliary surgery. In addition to the concerns already mentioned for hepatic patients (e.g., hypoglycemia, hypoproteinemia, coagulopathies, and decreased drug metabolism), universal complications associated with any general anesthetic episode and open abdominal surgery must be taken into consideration. Hypothermia (which can exacerbate coagulopathies) is common in these cases and body temperature should be monitored and supportive measures taken.

Cholecystectomy and extrahepatic biliary tract obstruction

Extrahepatic biliary obstruction (EHBO) and cholecystectomy are associated with relatively high perioperative morbidity and mortality [99]. In one study, preoperative elevation of plasma creatinine and postoperative low mean arterial pressure were associated with increased mortality, especially in the presence of pancreatitis and septic bile peritonitis [100,101]. Hypercoagulability in dogs with naturally occurring EHBO has recently been demonstrated using thromboelastography [102]. It has been demonstrated that the earlier assumption of hypocoagulability in canine patients with EHBO should be re-evaluated. Likely, as in humans with EHBO, either hyper- or hypocoagulation can be present and should be investigated to provide the appropriate support or treatment [103]. In a study investigating the association of gall bladder mucoceles and endocrinopathies, dogs with hyperadrenocorticism were 29 times more likely to have a biliary mucocele [104]. These findings are important to the anesthesiologist as hyperadrenocorticism is also associated with hypercoagulable states [105].

Hepatic neoplasia

In addition to the concerns described for laparoscopic and laparotomic liver biopsies, severe and uncontrollable hemorrhage is a potential catastrophic complication during and following hepatic lobe resection. Immediate availability of blood products, including plasma, packed red blood cells, and whole blood, should be considered. Blood typing and cross-matching may be helpful in determining which donors are usable for emergency transfusion. Some neoplasia types are often associated with preoperative hemoabdomen and in those cases a preanesthetic transfusion maybe necessary and will improve the oxygen delivery to tissues during anesthesia. Quantification of the volume of blood lost before hemostasis is achieved may be helpful in determining the need for blood replacement, but the chronicity of blood loss will usually result in varying hemodynamic consequences. Therefore, decisions to transfuse are often based on several factors, including hematocrit, speed of blood loss, amount of blood loss, and hemodynamic stability.

Venous return should be evaluated by the anesthetist [using central venous pressure (CVP) or by evaluating the character of the arterial blood pressure (ABP) waveform] during hepatic retraction because compression of the major abdominal vessels by the surgeon is possible. Effective communication between the anesthetist and surgeon is extremely important to facilitate diagnosis of major hemodynamic complications verses temporary insults necessary for surgical access.

In a retrospective study evaluating clinical signs, diagnostic findings, and outcome of canine hepatocellular carcinoma, an increase in ALT and AST were associated with poorer prognosis. In general, the surgical outcome of hepatic lobectomies for hepatocellular carcinoma excision was reported to be excellent, with minimal postoperative mortality when preoperative values were not greatly deranged [106]. Coagulopathies and poor liver function are often confounding factors in these surgical cases and prognosis worsens as the percentage of hepatic mass excised increases.

Studies of the effects of general anesthesia and types of anesthetics on surgical outcomes are lacking. General anesthesia is known to cause dose-dependent cardiovascular and immune depression. In an attempt to minimize such complications, Yamamoto *et al.* reported a case series in which all patients had partial hepatectomies only under sedation and epidural anesthesia. After following 10 human patients, it was concluded that epidural techniques can be used for partial hepatectomies and also for other abdominal surgeries [107].

Portosystemic shunt

Portosystemic shunts are defined as anomalous vessels flowing from the portal circulation (e.g., stomach, intestines, pancreas, and spleen) to the central circulation (e.g., vena cava or azygous vein) without first passing through the liver [108]. The blood bypassing the liver allows substances normally metabolized there (e.g., ammonia, bile acids, short-chain fatty acids) to accumulate in the systemic circulation [109]. When shunts are present at birth, blood flow to the liver is decreased and hepatotropic substances are not effectively delivered. This results in a liver that fails to develop normally and that is often undersized with abnormal intrahepatic vascular structure.

Portosystemic shunt patients may present with non-specific signs such as hypoglycemia, hypoalbuminemia, coagulopathies, and altered response to substances metabolized and excreted by the liver [108–110]. Hypoglycemia and prolonged recoveries from anesthesia were reported in dogs with a congenital portosystemic shunt (cPSS) [111]. Many patients are undiagnosed until they are anesthetized for surgical sterilization at 6–12 months of age and fail to recover normally from anesthesia. It has been hypothesized that refractory hypoglycemia could be due to relative adrenal insufficiency, similar to that commonly seen with sepsis. In one study, no difference was found on preoperative baseline or post-ACTH stimulation testing among healthy ovariohysterectomy (OHE) and cPSS dogs. However, 30% of the cPSS dogs presented with preoperative hypoglycemia and over 40% developed hypoglycemia within 4 h after surgery. Although inadequate adrenal response was not found in this population of cPSS dogs, animals that presented with postoperative refractory hypoglycemia or prolonged anesthetic recoveries usually responded to the administration of dexamethasone (0.1 mg/kg, IV) [111]. Postoperative administration of acepromazine (0.05 mg/kg, IV) in that study could also have contributed to the prolonged recoveries seen in those patients.

HE and seizures may also be seen in portosystemic shunt cases [112]. Flumazenil has been used to improve mental status in humans with HE and it is hypothesized that intrinsic benzodiazepine-like compounds are important to this syndrome [113]. Whether similar improvements occur in veterinary HE patients following flumazenil administration has not been verified. Recently, C-reactive protein (CRP) plasma levels were shown to be elevated in cPSS dogs presenting with HE [112]. These findings reinforce the similarities in the pathogenesis of HE in humans and in cPSS dogs and the involvement of an inflammatory process in its pathogenesis [112].

Coagulation factors produced by the liver can be present at abnormal levels in PSS dogs. In a prospective study, platelet count, packed cell volume, and factor II, V, VII, and X concentrations were lower prior to surgery and aPTT was prolonged in PSS dogs compared with healthy dogs. The postoperative hemostatic profile revealed further alterations such as an increase in PT and decrease in factor I, IX, and XI concentrations. However, when postoperative hemostatic values were compared with those for a set of healthy patients undergoing ovariectomy, only PT and platelet count were significantly decreased. Additionally, even though the absolute activities of factors II, V, VII, and X were lower in the PSS group, the relative percentage changes from preoperative values were different only for platelet count and factor II activity [114]. Although the *in vitro* coagulation tests of PSS patients are commonly abnormal, clinical signs of bleeding disorders are uncommon in these dogs during and after shunt attenuation [114].

Preoperative mortality in cats and dogs undergoing surgical correction of PSS is reported to be low. However, postoperative outcomes have variable results in both species, including deterioration of patients' neurologic signs and death [115–118]. It is difficult to determine what role the anesthetic technique plays in postoperative outcomes. Many patients recover normally from anesthesia and begin to show signs of problems in the same time frame as the expected shunt closure, implying a greater role of altered blood flow in producing neurologic signs and death.

Interventional radiology

This technique uses fluoroscopy to guide an intravenous catheter to the site where the anomalous vessel (shunt) joins the systemic circulation. An expandable stent is placed in the caudal vena cava next to the anomaly insertion. This stent will prevent the thrombotic coils deployed into the shunt vessel from becoming lost in the systemic circulation if they dislodge [119]. The challenge for the anesthetist is to ensure complete immobilization of the patient at the critical stage of stent placement. During general anesthesia, an NMB can be administered to facilitate immobilization if mechanical ventilation is available. Atracurium and cis-atracurium can be used in boluses or constant-rate infusions to maintain paralysis. In some situations, the surgeon may require an inspiratory hold to decrease patient abdominal movement during critical periods (e.g., measuring the anomalous vessel and placement of the stent). Hypothermia is a common problem and the use of a radiolucent heating pad is essential. Monitoring of cardiovascular (ABP and CVP) and respiratory parameters ($ETCO_2$ and SpO_2) is necessary for the anesthetist and surgeon. Invasive ABP monitoring is ideal, but not mandatory, and CVP can be measured by connecting a sterile electronic transducer to the jugular catheter used by the surgeon to place the stent. The central venous catheter and pressure will help assess patient blood volume and guide fluid therapy, and also inform the surgeon of the abdominal caval pressure as catheter is advanced. As in other hepatic patients, colloidal and inotropic support may be needed. The anesthetist should be sure to restore vascular volume with crystalloids and colloids before inotropic administration. Dopamine (3–12 μg/kg/min) and dobutamine (2–10 μg/kg/min) are the most commonly used inotropes in veterinary medicine and can be used in these patients.

Hepatic lobe torsion

Hepatic lobe torsion has been described in dogs, horses, and cats [120–122]. The outcome is reported to be mostly favorable if recognition and surgical correction are made early. Canine patients may show relatively mild non-specific clinical signs such as increased liver enzymes [120]. Similarly to the dog, horses present with non-specific clinical signs and laboratory results, including peritoneal fluid accumulation, colic, inappetence, lethargy, and increased liver enzymes, which makes diagnosis difficult, potentially resulting in poor prognosis [123,124]. Surgical removal of the liver lobe is the usual treatment and is managed similarly to hepatic lobe resection for neoplasia.

Pain management in hepatobiliary diseases

Opioids are the mainstay of analgesia in the perioperative period. In humans, morphine can cause spasm of the common bile duct by constriction of the sphincter of Oddi, which increases the size and pressure in the gall bladder. This effect has not been demonstrated or observed in veterinary patients [125]. Since patients with liver dysfunction may take longer to metabolize opioids, their effects could last significantly longer than in a healthy patient [126,127]. Frequent assessments of analgesia are required to determine appropriate administration intervals. Sufentanil, alfentanil, fentanyl, and remifentanil are shorter acting opioids with pharmacokinetics that are minimally affected by liver disease [126,128]. Remifentanil, in particular, is rapidly hydrolyzed by plasma esterases, resulting in a high clearance and rapid elimination. The context-sensitive half-life seems to be independent of the dose or duration of infusions in human subjects with various degrees of liver dysfunction [37,126,129]. If a continuous infusion is not practical or desired, intermittent administration of hydromorphone, morphine, buprenorphine, methadone, and oxymorphone has been used, but a reduced dose or prolonged dosing interval may be needed.

Non-steroidal anti-inflammatory drugs (NSAIDs) are commonly used for acute and chronic pain management in dogs and cats. All NSAIDs have the potential to cause hepatic injury, either intrinsically (as is usually the case with aspirin and acetaminophen) or idiosyncratically (as tends to be the case with other NSAIDs, including the COX-2 selective agents). Idiosyncratic toxic reactions are rare, unpredictable, and not related to dose. Clinical signs include inappetence, vomiting, and icterus associated with elevations in serum hepatic enzymes and bilirubin. Any unexplained increase in these biochemical parameters after initiation of NSAID therapy should be investigated. Since there have been no large-scale prospective studies to evaluate the effects of NSAIDs on hepatic structure and function in animals with pre-existing liver disease, it is unknown whether or not this practice is safe. Additionally, NSAIDs may impair coagulation and hemostasis by affecting clot formation and platelet aggregation. Owing to the potential for adverse effects, the administration of NSAIDs to patients with hepatic dysfunction, especially those with coagulopathies, should be avoided or very closely monitored.

References

1 Weiss DJ, Gagne JM, Armstrong PJ. Relationship between inflammatory hepatic disease and inflammatory bowel disease, pancreatitis, and nephritis in cats. *J Am Vet Med Assoc* 1996; **209**(6): 1114–1116.

2 Lautt WW, Legare DJ, d'Almeida MS. Adenosine as putative regulator of hepatic arterial flow (the buffer response). *Am J Physiol* 1985; **248**(3 Pt 2): H331–H338.

3 Rocheleau B, Ethier C, Houle R, *et al.* Hepatic artery buffer response following left portal vein ligation: its role in liver tissue homeostasis. *Am J Physiol* 1999; **277**(5 Pt 1): G1000–G1007.

4 Hayes MF. Pathophysiology of the liver. In: Dunlop RH, Malbert, C.H., eds. *Veterinary Pathophysiology*, 1st edn. Ames, IA: Blackwell, 2004, 371–400.

5 Schreiber G, Urban J. The synthesis and secretion of albumin. *Rev Physiol Biochem Pharmacol* 1978; **82**: 27–95.

6 Brooks MB, DeLaforcade A. Acquired coagulopathies. In: Weiss DJ, Wardrop KJ, eds. *Schalm's Veterinary Hematology*, 6th edn. Ames, IA: Blackwell, 2010; 654–660.

7 Smith SA. Overview of hemostasis. In: Weiss DJ, Wardrop KJ, eds. *Schalm's Veterinary Hematology*, 6th edn. Ames, IA: Blackwell, 2010; 635–653.

8 Hunter RP, Mahmood I, Martinez MN. Prediction of xenobiotic clearance in avian species using mammalian or avian data: how accurate is the prediction? *J Vet Pharmacol Ther* 2008; **31**(3): 281–284.

9 Sindrup SH, Brosen K. The pharmacogenetics of codeine hypoalgesia. *Pharmacogenetics* 1995; **5**(6): 335–346.

10 Center SA, Elston TH, Rowland PH, *et al.* Fulminant hepatic failure associated with oral administration of diazepam in 11 cats. *J Am Vet Med Assoc* 1996; **209**(3): 618–625.

11 Shimada T, Mimura M, Inoue K, *et al.* Cytochrome P450-dependent drug oxidation activities in liver microsomes of various animal species including rats, guinea pigs, dogs, monkeys, and humans. *Arch Toxicol* 1997; **71**(6): 401–408.

12 Court MH, Hay-Kraus BL, Hill DW, *et al.* Propofol hydroxylation by dog liver microsomes: assay development and dog breed differences. *Drug Metab Dispos* 1999; **27**(11): 1293–1299.

13 van Beusekom CD, Schipper L, Fink-Gremmels J. Cytochrome P450-mediated hepatic metabolism of new fluorescent substrates in cats and dogs. *J Vet Pharmacol Ther* 2010; **33**(6): 519–527.

14 Capel ID, Millburn P, Williams RT. The conjugation of 1- and 2-naphthols and other phenols in the cat and pig. *Xenobiotica* 1974; **4**(10): 601–615.

15 Capel ID, French MR, Millburn P, *et al.* Species variations in the metabolism of phenol. *Biochem J* 1972; **127**(2): 25P–26P.

16 Capel ID, French MR, Millburn P, *et al.* The fate of [^{14}C]phenol in various species. *Xenobiotica* 1972; **2**(1): 25–34.

17 Court MH, Greenblatt DJ. Molecular basis for deficient acetaminophen glucuronidation in cats. An interspecies comparison of enzyme kinetics in liver microsomes. *Biochem Pharmacol* 1997; **53**(7): 1041–1047.

18 Ebner T, Schanzle G, Weber W, *et al. In vitro* glucuronidation of the angiotensin II receptor antagonist telmisartan in the cat: a comparison with other species. *J Vet Pharmacol Ther* 2013; **36**(2): 154–160.

19 Livingston A, Waterman AE. The development of tolerance to ketamine in rats and the significance of hepatic metabolism. *Br J Pharmacol* 1978; **64**(1): 63–69.

20 Huang L, Smit JW, Meijer DK, Vore M. Mrp2 is essential for estradiol-17β(β-D-glucuronide)-induced cholestasis in rats. *Hepatology* 2000; **32**(1): 66–72.

21 Lee J, Boyer JL. Molecular alterations in hepatocyte transport mechanisms in acquired cholestatic liver disorders. *Semin Liver Dis* 2000; **20**(3): 373–384.

22 Mealey KL, Bentjen SA, Gay JM, Cantor GH. Ivermectin sensitivity in collies is associated with a deletion mutation of the mdr1 gene. *Pharmacogenetics* 2001; **11**(8): 727–733.

23 Mealey KL, Northrup NC, Bentjen SA. Increased toxicity of P-glycoprotein-substrate chemotherapeutic agents in a dog with the MDR1 deletion mutation associated with ivermectin sensitivity. *J Am Vet Med Assoc* 2003; **223**(10): 1453–1455.

24 Fink-Gremmels J. Implications of hepatic cytochrome P450-related biotransformation processes in veterinary sciences. *Eur J Pharmacol* 2008; **585**: 502–509.

25 Laskin DL. Nonparenchymal cells and hepatotoxicity. *Semin Liver Dis* 1990; **10**(4): 293–304.

26 Katz S, Jimenez MA, Lehmkuhler WE, Grosfeld JL. Liver bacterial clearance following hepatic artery ligation and portacaval shunt. *J Surg Res* 1991; **51**(3): 267–270.

27 Mathison JC, Ulevitch RJ. The clearance, tissue distribution, and cellular localization of intravenously injected lipopolysaccharide in rabbits. *J Immunol* 1979; **123**(5): 2133–2143.

28 Dhainaut JF, Marin N, Mignon A, Vinsonneau C. Hepatic response to sepsis: interaction between coagulation and inflammatory processes. *Crit Care Med* 2001; **29**: S42–S47.

29 Center SA, Baldwin BH, Erb H, Tennant BC. Bile acid concentrations in the diagnosis of hepatobiliary disease in the cat. *J Am Vet Med Assoc* 1986; **189**(8): 891–896.

30 Ruland K, Fischer A, Hartmann K. Sensitivity and specificity of fasting ammonia and serum bile acids in the diagnosis of portosystemic shunts in dogs and cats. *Vet Clin Pathol* 2010; **39**(1): 57–64.

31 Shih JL, Keating JH, Freeman LM, Webster CR. Chronic hepatitis in Labrador Retrievers: clinical presentation and prognostic factors. *J Vet Intern Med* 2007; **21**(1): 33–39.

32 Guedes AG, Papich MG, Rude EP, Rider MA. Comparison of plasma histamine levels after intravenous administration of hydromorphone and morphine in dogs. *J Vet Pharmacol Ther* 2007; **30**(6): 516–522.

33 Robinson EP, Faggella AM, Henry DP, Russell WL. Comparison of histamine release induced by morphine and oxymorphone administration in dogs. *Am J Vet Res* 1988; **49**(10): 1699–1701.

34 Thompson WL, Walton RP. Elevation of plasma histamine levels in the dog following administration of muscle relaxants, opiates and macromolecular polymers. *J Pharmacol Exp Ther* 1964; **143**: 131–136.

35 Lagerkranser M, Andreen M, Irestedt L. Central and splanchnic haemodynamics in the dog during controlled hypotension with sodium nitroprusside. *Acta Anaesthesiol Scand* 1984; **28**(1): 81–86.

36 Hohne C, Donaubauer B, Kaisers U. Opioids during anesthesia in liver and renal failure. *Anaesthesist* 2004; **53**(3): 291–303 (in German).

37 Dershwitz M, Hoke JF, Rosow CE, *et al.* Pharmacokinetics and pharmacodynamics of remifentanil in volunteer subjects with severe liver disease. *Anesthesiology* 1996; **84**(4): 812–820.

38 Ludders JW, Reitan JA, Martucci R, *et al.* Blood pressure response to phenylephrine infusion in halothane-anesthetized dogs given acetylpromazine maleate. *Am J Vet Res* 1983; **44**(6): 996–999.
39 Hitt ME, Hanna P, Singh A. Percutaneous transabdominal hepatic needle biopsies in dogs. *Am J Vet Res* 1992; **53**(5): 785–787.
40 Bostrom I, Nyman G, Kampa N, *et al.* Effects of acepromazine on renal function in anesthetized dogs. *Am J Vet Res* 2003; **64**(5): 590–598.
41 Barr SC, Ludders JW, Looney AL, *et al.* Platelet aggregation in dogs after sedation with acepromazine and atropine and during subsequent general anesthesia and surgery. *Am J Vet Res* 1992; **53**(11): 2067–2070.
42 Aronson LR, Gacad RC, Kaminsky-Russ K, *et al.* Endogenous benzodiazepine activity in the peripheral and portal blood of dogs with congenital portosystemic shunts. *Vet Surg* 1997; **26**(3): 189–194.
43 Palomero-Gallagher N, Zilles K. Neurotransmitter receptor alterations in hepatic encephalopathy: a review. *Arch Biochem Biophys* 2013; **536**(2): 109–121.
44 Als-Nielsen B, Gluud LL, Gluud C. Benzodiazepine receptor antagonists for hepatic encephalopathy. *Cochrane Database Syst Rev* 2004; (**2**): CD002798.
45 Jones EA, Yurdaydin C, Basile AS. The role of endogenous benzodiazepines in hepatic encephalopathy: animal studies. *Alcohol Alcohol Suppl* 1993; **2**: 175–180.
46 Nishiyama T, Hirasaki A, Toda N, *et al.* Pharmacokinetics of midazolam in patients with liver damage for hepatectomy. *Masui* 1993; **42**(6): 871–875 (in Japanese).
47 Bozkurt P, Kaya G, Suzer O, Senturk H. Diazepam serum concentration–sedative effect relationship in patients with liver disease. *Middle East J Anesthesiology* 1996; **13**(4): 405–413.
48 Kuo WC, Keegan RD. Comparative cardiovascular, analgesic, and sedative effects of medetomidine, medetomidine–hydromorphone, and medetomidine–butorphanol in dogs. *Am J Vet Res* 2004; **65**(7): 931–937.
49 Flacke WE, Flacke JW, Bloor BC, *et al.* Effects of dexmedetomidine on systemic and coronary hemodynamics in the anesthetized dog. *J Cardiothorac Vasc Anesth* 1993; **7**(1): 41–49.
50 Lawrence CJ, Prinzen FW, de Lange S. The effect of dexmedetomidine on nutrient organ blood flow. *Anesth Analg* 1996; **83**(6): 1160–1165.
51 Baratta MT, Zaya MJ, White JA, Locuson CW. Canine CYP2B11 metabolizes and is inhibited by anesthetic agents often co-administered in dogs. *J Vet Pharmacol Ther* 2010; **33**(1): 50–55.
52 Thomson IA, Fitch W, Hughes RL, *et al.* Effects of certain i.v. anaesthetics on liver blood flow and hepatic oxygen consumption in the greyhound. *Br J Anaesth* 1986; **58**(1): 69–80.
53 Thomson IA, Fitch W, Campbell D, Watson R. Effects of ketamine on liver blood flow and hepatic oxygen consumption. Studies in the anaesthetised greyhound. *Acta Anaesthesiol Scand* 1988; **32**(1): 10–14.
54 Wouters PF, Van de Velde MA, Marcus MA, *et al.* Hemodynamic changes during induction of anesthesia with eltanolone and propofol in dogs. *Anesthes Analg* 1995; **81**(1): 125–131.
55 Haberer JP, Audibert G, Saunier CG, *et al.* Effect of propofol and thiopentone on regional blood flow in brain and peripheral tissues during normoxia and hypoxia in the dog. *Clin Physiol* 1993; **13**(2): 197–207.
56 Ye L, Luo CZ, McCluskey SA, *et al.* Propofol attenuates hepatic ischemia/reperfusion injury in an *in vivo* rabbit model. *J Surg Res* 2012; **178**(2): e65–e70.
57 Chan KC, Lin CJ, Lee PH, *et al.* Propofol attenuates the decrease of dynamic compliance and water content in the lung by decreasing oxidative radicals released from the reperfused liver. *Anesth Analg* 2008;**107**(4): 1284–1289.
58 Servin F, Farinotti R, Haberer JP, Desmonts JM. Propofol infusion for maintenance of anesthesia in morbidly obese patients receiving nitrous oxide. A clinical and pharmacokinetic study. *Anesthesiology* 1993; **78**(4): 657–665.
59 Zoran DL, Riedesel DH, Dyer DC. Pharmacokinetics of propofol in mixed-breed dogs and greyhounds. *Am J Vet Res* 1993; **54**(5): 755–760.
60 Posner LP, Asakawa M, Erb HN. Use of propofol for anesthesia in cats with primary hepatic lipidosis: 44 cases (1995–2004). *J Am Vet Med Assoc* 2008; **232**(12): 1841–1843.
61 Sams L, Braun C, Allman D, Hofmeister E. A comparison of the effects of propofol and etomidate on the induction of anesthesia and on cardiopulmonary parameters in dogs. *Vet Anaesth Analgesia* 2008; **35**(6): 488–494.
62 Taylor JD, Richards RK, Tabern DL. Metabolism of S35 thiopental (Pentothal); chemical and paper chromatographic studies of S35 excretion by the rat and monkey. *J Pharmacol Exp Ther* 1952; **104**(1): 93–102.
63 Sams RA, Muir WW. Effects of phenobarbital on thiopental pharmacokinetics in greyhounds. *Am J Vet Res* 1988; **49**(2): 245–249.
64 Nebauer AE, Doenicke A, Hoernecke R, *et al.* Does etomidate cause haemolysis? *Br J Anaesth* 1992; **69**(1): 58–60.
65 Moon PF. Acute toxicosis in two dogs associated with etomidate–propylene glycol infusion. *Lab Anim Sci* 1994; **44**(6): 590–594.
66 van Beem H, Manger FW, van Boxtel C, van Bentem N. Etomidate anaesthesia in patients with cirrhosis of the liver: pharmacokinetic data. *Anaesthesia* 1983; **38**(Suppl): 61–62.
67 Bonnardot JP, Levron JC, Deslauriers M, *et al.* Pharmacocinétique de l'étomidate en perfusion continue chez le patient cirrhotique [Pharmacokinetics of continuous infusion of etomidate in cirrhotic patients]. *Ann Fr Anesth Reanim* 1991; **10**(5): 443–449.
68 Carlos R, Calvo R, Erill S. Plasma-protein binding of etomidate in patients with renal-failure or hepatic cirrhosis. *Clin Pharmacokinet* 1979; **4**(2): 144–148.
69 Molenaar N, Bijkerk RM, Beishuizen A, *et al.* Steroidogenesis in the adrenal dysfunction of critical illness: impact of etomidate. *Crit Care* 2012; **16**(4): R121.
70 Kharb S, Garg MK, Puri P, *et al.* Assessment of adrenal function in liver diseases. *Indian J Endocrinol Metab* 2013; **17**(3): 465–471.
71 Hauser GJ, Brotzman HM, Kaufman SS. Hepatoadrenal syndrome in pediatric patients with end-stage liver disease. *Pediatr Crit Care Med* 2012; **13**(3): e145–e149.
72 Ghoneim MM, Van Hamme MJ. Hydrolysis of etomidate. *Anesthesiology* 1979; **50**(3): 227–229.
73 Calvo R, Carlos R, Erill S. Etomidate and plasma esterase activity in man and experimental animals. *Pharmacology* 1979; **18**(6): 294–298.
74 Van Hamme MJ, Ghoneim MM, Ambre JJ. Pharmacokinetics of etomidate, a new intravenous anesthetic. *Anesthesiology* 1978; **49**(4): 274–277.
75 Kaka JS, Hayton WL. Pharmacokinetics of ketamine and two metabolites in the dog. *J Pharmacokinet Biopharm* 1980; **8**(2): 193–202.
76 Noppers IM, Niesters M, Aarts LP, *et al.* Drug-induced liver injury following a repeated course of ketamine treatment for chronic pain in CRPS type 1 patients: a report of 3 cases. *Pain* 2011; **152**(9): 2173–2178.
77 Wai MS, Chan WM, Zhang AQ, *et al.* Long-term ketamine and ketamine plus alcohol treatments produced damages in liver and kidney. *Hum Exp Toxicol* 2012; **31**(9): 877–886.
78 Frink EJ Jr, Morgan SE, Coetzee A, *et al.* The effects of sevoflurane, halothane, enflurane, and isoflurane on hepatic blood flow and oxygenation in chronically instrumented greyhound dogs. *Anesthesiology* 1992; **76**(1): 85–90.
79 Hartman JC, Pagel PS, Proctor LT, *et al.* Influence of desflurane, isoflurane and halothane on regional tissue perfusion in dogs. *Can J Anaesth* 1992; **39**(8): 877–887.
80 Lu H, Yang LQ, Yu WF, *et al.* Protection of liver against ischemia/reperfusion injury by Kupffer cell mediated emulsified isoflurane preconditioning: experiment with rats. *Zhonghua Yi Xue Za Zhi* 2007; **87**(35): 2468–2471 (in Chinese).
81 Bedirli N, Ofluoglu E, Kerem M, *et al.* Hepatic energy metabolism and the differential protective effects of sevoflurane and isoflurane anesthesia in a rat hepatic ischemia-reperfusion injury model. *Anesth Analg* 2008; **106**(3): 830–837.
82 van Miert MM, Eastwood NB, Boyd AH, *et al.* The pharmacokinetics and pharmacodynamics of rocuronium in patients with hepatic cirrhosis. *Br J Clin Pharmacol* 1997; **44**(2): 139–144.
83 Lebrault C, Berger JL, D'Hollander AA, *et al.* Pharmacokinetics and pharmacodynamics of vecuronium (ORG NC 45) in patients with cirrhosis. *Anesthesiology* 1985; **62**(5): 601–605.
84 Devlin JC, Head-Rapson AG, Parker CJ, Hunter JM. Pharmacodynamics of mivacurium chloride in patients with hepatic cirrhosis. *Br J Anaesth* 1993; **71**(2): 227–231.
85 De Wolf AM, Freeman JA, Scott VL, *et al.* Pharmacokinetics and pharmacodynamics of cisatracurium in patients with end-stage liver disease undergoing liver transplantation. *Br J Anaesth* 1996; **76**(5): 624–628.
86 Ward S, Neill EA. Pharmacokinetics of atracurium in acute hepatic failure (with acute renal failure). *Br J Anaesth* 1983; **55**(12): 1169–1172.
87 Kisor DF, Schmith VD. Clinical pharmacokinetics of cisatracurium besilate. *Clinical Pharmacokinet* 1999; **36**(1): 27–40.
88 Adams WA, Senior JM, Jones RS, *et al.* cis-Atracurium in dogs with and without porto-systemic shunts. *Vet Anaesth Analg* 2006; **33**(1): 17–23.
89 Raffan E, McCallum A, Scase TJ, Watson PJ. Ascites is a negative prognostic indicator in chronic hepatitis in dogs. *J Vet Intern Med* 2009; **23**(1): 63–66.
90 Rahimi RS, Rockey DC. Complications and outcomes in chronic liver disease. *Curr Opin Gastroenterol* 2011; **27**(3): 204–209.
91 Fuentealba C, Guest S, Haywood S, Horney B. Chronic hepatitis: a retrospective study in 34 dogs. *Can Vet J* 1997; **38**(6): 365–373.
92 Prins M, Schellens CJ, van Leeuwen MW, *et al.* Coagulation disorders in dogs with hepatic disease. *Vet J* 2010; **185**(2): 163–168.
93 Stellingwerff M, Brandsma A, Lisman T, Porte RJ. Prohemostatic interventions in liver surgery. *Semin Thromb Hemost* 2012; **38**(3): 244–249.
94 Rogers CL, O'Toole TE, Keating JH, *et al.* Portal vein thrombosis in cats: 6 cases (2001–2006). *J Vet Intern Med* 2008; **22**(2): 282–287.
95 Proot SJ, Rothuizen J. High complication rate of an automatic Tru-Cut biopsy gun device for liver biopsy in cats. *J Vet Intern Med* 2006; **20**(6): 1327–1333.
96 Mayhew PD. Advanced laparoscopic procedures (hepatobiliary, endocrine) in dogs and cats. *Vet Clin North Am Small Anim Pract* 2009; **39**(5): 925–939.
97 Meierhenrich R, Gauss A, Vandenesch P, *et al.* The effects of intraabdominally insufflated carbon dioxide on hepatic blood flow during laparoscopic surgery assessed by transesophageal echocardiography. *Anesth Analg* 2005; **100**(2): 340–347.

98 Nesek-Adam V, Rasic Z, Kos J, Vnuk D. Aminotransferases after experimental pneumoperitoneum in dogs. *Acta Anaesthesiol Scand* 2004; **48**(7): 862–866.

99 Fahie MA, Martin RA. Extrahepatic biliary tract obstruction: a retrospective study of 45 cases (1983–1993). *J Am Anim Hosp Assoc* 1995; **31**(6): 478–482.

100 Mehler SJ, Mayhew PD, Drobatz KJ, Holt DE. Variables associated with outcome in dogs undergoing extrahepatic biliary surgery: 60 cases (1988–2002). *Vet Surg* 2004; **33**(6): 644–649.

101 Amsellem PM, Seim HB III, MacPhail CM, *et al.* Long-term survival and risk factors associated with biliary surgery in dogs: 34 cases (1994–2004). *J Am Vet Med Assoc* 2006; **229**(9): 1451–1457.

102 Mayhew PD, Savigny MR, Otto CM, *et al.* Evaluation of coagulation in dogs with partial or complete extrahepatic biliary tract obstruction by means of thromboelastography. *J Am Vet Med Assoc* 2013; **242**(6): 778–785.

103 Cakir T, Cingi A, Yegen C. Coagulation dynamics and platelet functions in obstructive jaundiced patients. *J Gastroenterol Hepatol* 2009; **24**(5): 748–751.

104 Mesich ML, Mayhew PD, Paek M, *et al.* Gall bladder mucoceles and their association with endocrinopathies in dogs: a retrospective case-control study. *J Small Anim Pract* 2009; **50**(12): 630–635.

105 Rose L, Dunn ME, Bedard C. Effect of canine hyperadrenocorticism on coagulation parameters. *J Vet Intern Med* 2013; **27**(1): 207–211.

106 Liptak JM, Dernell WS, Monnet E, *et al.* Massive hepatocellular carcinoma in dogs: 48 cases (1992–2002). *J Am Vet Med Assoc* 2004; **225**(8): 1225–1230.

107 Yamamoto K, Fukumori D, Yamamoto F, *et al.* First report of hepatectomy without endotracheal general anesthesia. *J Am Coll Surg* 2013; **216**(5): 908–914.

108 Center SA, Magne ML. Historical, physical examination, and clinicopathologic features of portosystemic vascular anomalies in the dog and cat. *Semin Vet Med Surg* 1990; **5**(2): 83–93.

109 Griffiths GL, Lumsden JH, Valli VEO. Hematologic and biochemical changes in dogs with portosystemic shunts. *J Am Anim Hosp Assoc* 1981; **17**(5): 705–710.

110 Gugler R, Lain P, Azarnoff DL. Effect of portacaval-shunt on disposition of drugs with and without first-pass effect. *J Pharmacol Exp Ther* 1975; **195**(3): 416–423.

111 Holford AL, Tobias KM, Bartges JW, Johnson BM. Adrenal response to adrenocorticotropic hormone in dogs before and after surgical attenuation of a single congenital portosystemic shunt. *J Vet Intern Med* 2008; **22**(4): 832–838.

112 Gow AG, Marques AI, Yool DA, *et al.* Dogs with congenital porto-systemic shunting (cPSS) and hepatic encephalopathy have higher serum concentrations of C-reactive protein than asymptomatic dogs with cPSS. *Metab Brain Dis* 2012; **27**(2): 227–229.

113 Aronson LR, Gacad RC, Kaminsky-Russ K, *et al.* Endogenous benzodiazepine activity in the peripheral and portal blood of dogs with congenital portosystemic shunts. *Vet Surg* 1997; **26**(3): 189–194.

114 Kummeling A, Teske E, Rothuizen J, Van Sluijs FJ. Coagulation profiles in dogs with congenital portosystemic shunts before and after surgical attenuation. *J Vet Intern Med* 2006; **20**(6): 1319–1326.

115 Havig M, Tobias KM. Outcome of ameroid constrictor occlusion of single congenital extrahepatic portosystemic shunts in cats: 12 cases (1993–2000). *J Am Vet Med Assoc* 2002; **220**(3): 337–341.

116 Lipscomb VJ, Jones HJ, Brockman DJ. Complications and long-term outcomes of the ligation of congenital portosystemic shunts in 49 cats. *Vet Rec* 2007; **160**(14): 465–470.

117 Tisdall PL, Hunt GB, Youmans KR, Malik R. Neurological dysfunction in dogs following attenuation of congenital extrahepatic portosystemic shunts. *J Small Anim Pract* 2000; **41**(12): 539–546.

118 Yool DA, Kirby BM. Neurological dysfunction in three dogs and one cat following attenuation of intrahepatic portosystemic shunts. *J Small Anim Pract* 2002; **43**(4): 171–176.

119 Bussadori R, Bussadori C, Millan L, *et al.* Transvenous coil embolisation for the treatment of single congenital portosystemic shunts in six dogs. *Vet J* 2008; **176**(2): 221–226.

120 Schwartz SG, Mitchell SL, Keating JH, Chan DL. Liver lobe torsion in dogs: 13 cases (1995–2004). *J Am Vet Med Assoc* 2006; **228**(2): 242–247.

121 Bentz KJ, Burgess BA, Lohmann KL, Shahriar F. Hepatic lobe torsion in a horse. *Can Vet J* 2009; **50**(3): 283–286.

122 Swann HM, Brown DC. Hepatic lobe torsion in 3 dogs and a cat. *Vet Surg* 2001; **30**(5): 482–486.

123 Tennent-Brown BS, Mudge MC, Hardy J, *et al.* Liver lobe torsion in six horses. *J Am Vet Med Assoc* 2012; **241**(5): 615–620.

124 Turner TA, Brown CA, Wilson JH, *et al.* Hepatic lobe torsion as a cause of colic in a horse. *Vet Surg* 1993; **22**(4): 301–304.

125 Flancbaum L, Alden SM, Trooskin SZ. Use of cholescintigraphy with morphine in critically ill patients with suspected cholecystitis. *Surgery* 1989; **106**(4): 668–673.

126 Tegeder I, Lotsch J, Geisslinger G. Pharmacokinetics of opioids in liver disease. *Clinical Pharmacokinet* 1999; **37**(1): 17–40.

127 Bower S, Sear JW, Roy RC, Carter RF. Effects of different hepatic pathologies on disposition of alfentanil in anaesthetized patients. *Br J Anaesth* 1992; **68**(5): 462–465.

128 Chauvin M, Ferrier C, Haberer JP, *et al.* Sufentanil pharmacokinetics in patients with cirrhosis. *Anesth Analg* 1989; **68**(1): 1–4.

129 Navapurkar VU, Archer S, Gupta SK, *et al.* Metabolism of remifentanil during liver transplantation. *Br J Anaesth* 1998; **81**(6): 881–886.

SECTION 8

Gastrointestinal and Endocrine Systems

31 Physiology, Pathophysiology, and Anesthetic Management of Patients with Gastrointestinal and Endocrine Disease

Jennifer G. Adams[1], Juliana Peboni Figueiredo[2] and Thomas K. Graves[3]

[1]Hull, Georgia, USA

[2]Small Animal Medicine and Surgery Academic Program, St. George's University – School of Veterinary Medicine, Grenada, West Indies

[3]College of Veterinary Medicine, Midwestern University, Glendale, Arizona, USA

Chapter contents

Introduction to the endocrine system

Hormones are substances secreted into the circulation in very small amounts to produce a biologic effect at distant target organs or cells. The endocrine system regulates the secretion of these hormones from several peripheral organs under the direction of the hypothalamus (HPT) in concert with the hypophysis or pituitary gland. The hypothalamus is a small area located in the ventral aspect of the diencephalon flanking each side of the third ventricle, almost directly above the caudal pharynx. In addition to endocrine control of metabolism, growth, and reproduction, the hypothalamus helps to coordinate other vital aspects of mammalian physiology, including the autonomic nervous system, behavior and emotion, and digestion [1,2].

The pituitary gland is located just below the hypothalamus, and is connected anatomically via the infundibular stalk. It has two main lobes, distinct in both anatomic composition and function. The adenohypophysis or anterior pituitary (AP) has three areas – the pars tuberalis, pars intermedia, and pars distalis. This lobe functions like a true endocrine gland, producing and secreting hormones that target the pancreas, thyroid glands, adrenal glands, reproductive organs, and the intestine. Secretion by the AP is controlled by releasing hormones from the HPT and feedback (usually negative) from serum levels of hormones produced by the target tissues, such as thyroxine, cortisol, and many others. The posterior pituitary (PP), also called the neurohypophysis, is composed of the pars nervosa and the infundibular stalk. Not a typical endocrine gland, the PP is actually an extension of the HPT, composed of the axons of neurons located in the supraoptic and paraventricular nuclei of the HPT that extend into the pars nervosa. These are neurosecretory neurons; they do not innervate cells in the PP – rather, they release hormones produced in the HPT (oxytocin and vasopressin or antidiuretic hormone) into the venous circulation of the PP. The PP is primarily a conduit between the HPT and the peripheral circulation [1,2]. One exception to the usual control of endocrine function by the hypothalamic–pituitary axis (HPA) is parathyroid hormone (PTH). There are no PTH 'releasing or stimulating' hormones; rather, PTH is secreted in response to serum calcium concentration, as described in the section Parathyroid Gland.

In patients with endocrine disorders, management of the endocrine disease is as important as the more usual aspects of anesthetic management (e.g., blood pressure, cardiac function, ventilation). This requires an understanding of the physiology and pathophysiology of endocrine function, which is challenging because of the complex relationships that exist between the HPT, the pituitary gland, and their peripheral target organs. This system coordinates and maintains homeostasis in addition to the overall functions of metabolism, growth, reproduction, and digestion.

In summary, the hypothalamus monitors homeostatic parameters and serum concentrations of numerous substances and secretes 'releasing' or 'inhibiting' hormones into a special portal circulation that is connected directly to the AP, and/or it activates neurons that stimulate secretion of hormones into the peripheral circulation via

Veterinary Anesthesia and Analgesia: The Fifth Edition of Lumb and Jones.
Edited by Kurt A. Grimm, Leigh A. Lamont, William J. Tranquilli, Stephen A. Greene and Sheilah A. Robertson.

the pars nervosa of the PP. The AP secretes trophic hormones into the peripheral circulation that stimulate target endocrine glands to produce and secrete other hormones that directly affect target tissues/cells. The function of the PP differs from that of the AP because it secretes hormones that directly affect target tissues, whereas the AP produces hormones that stimulate the production of other hormones [1].

Hormones are proteins (corticotropin, growth hormone, insulin), peptides (oxytocin, vasopressin), steroids (glucocorticoids, mineralocorticoids, sex hormones), or amines (dopamine, melatonin, epinephrine). Proteins and peptides are initially produced as large precursor molecules that are eventually cleaved to an active form and stored in secretory granules within cells. Steroid hormones are synthesized from cholesterol, which is produced by the liver. These are not stored, but are synthesized and released as needed. Proteins and peptides move through the circulation dissolved in the plasma, whereas steroid and thyroid hormones are transported bound to specific carrier molecules. Hormones must be in a free or unbound state to interact with a target cell, which usually occurs via two main mechanisms. Because steroids are lipophilic, they cross cell membranes without assistance and interact with structures inside the nuclei to alter cellular function. Peptides and proteins cannot cross cell membranes; these hormones attach to a membrane receptor, triggering a second messenger system that activates or inhibits cellular activities to produce a biologic effect [1].

The physiology and pathophysiology of the pancreas, thyroid, adrenal, and parathyroid glands are described below, followed by a discussion of the anesthetic management of the most common disorders of these organs seen in small animals. Although by no means a complete list, hormones of the endocrine system and their effects are summarized in Fig. 31.1 [1,2].

Pancreas

The pancreas is a nodular, bilobed gland located within the mesentery at the angle where the duodenum meets the stomach (Fig. 31.2). Two pancreatic ducts are usually found in the dog; the cat has only one. The pancreatic or dorsal duct drains the left lobe and joins the main bile duct before entering the duodenum at the major duodenal papilla; the ventral or accessory duct drains the right lobe into the duodenum at the minor duodenal papilla. The cat has only the dorsal duct to drain both areas [3].

Diabetes mellitus

The insulin-secreting beta cells of the pancreas are the most abundant cell type in the islets of Langerhans, but still make up only a very small proportion of the total pancreatic mass in dogs and cats. Diabetes mellitus (DM) occurs when there is inadequate insulin

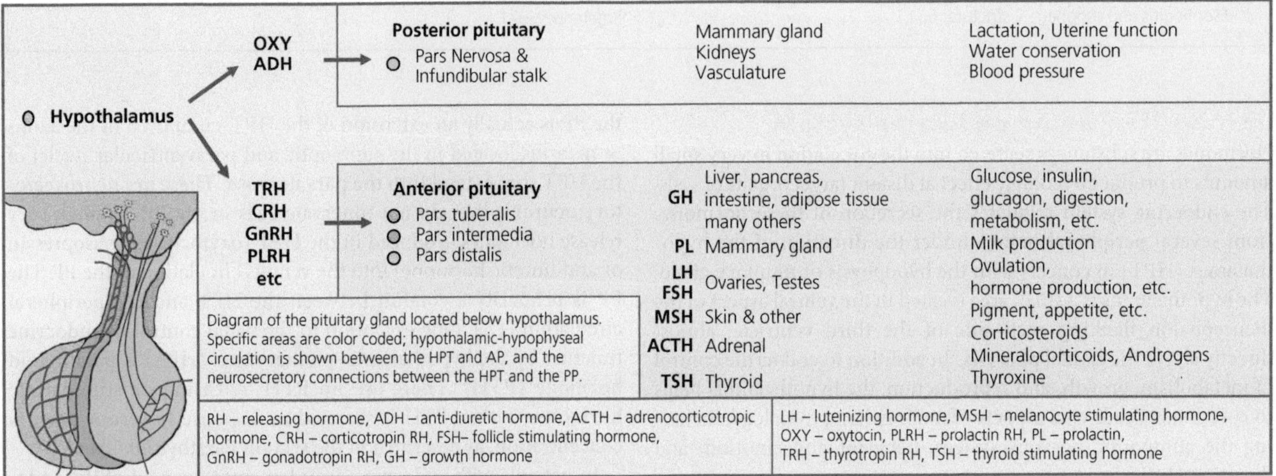

Figure 31.1 Summary of important hormones in the hypothalamic–pituitary axis (HPA) and their target tissues (pancreas, thyroid, reproductive, and adrenal glands). Note that the parathyroid gland and parathyroid hormone (PTH) are not affected by the HPA [1,2].

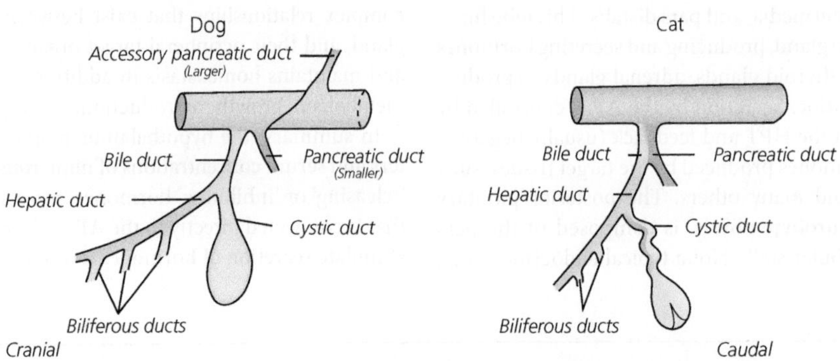

Figure 31.2 Anatomy of the pancreatic ducts of the dog and cat. Source: adapted from a drawing by Mr Joe Smith, Department of Veterinary Anatomy, University College Dublin, Dublin, Ireland. Reproduced with permission of Joe Smith.

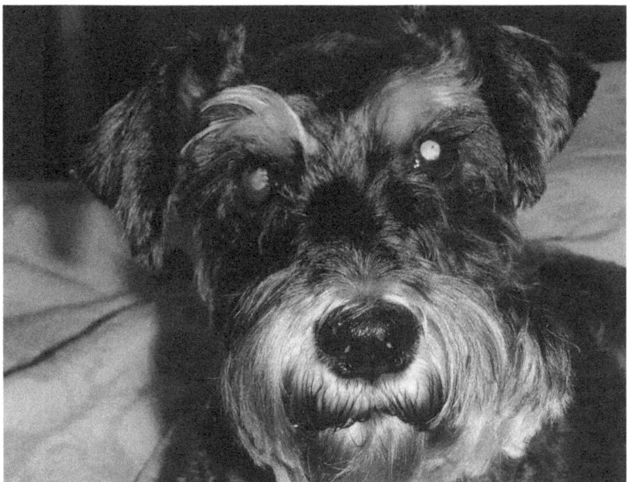

Figure 31.3 This 13-year-old Miniature Schnauzer had mature cataracts on both eyes (OU) due to DM. The dog underwent general anesthesia for removal of cataract on the right eye (OD). Mature cataract is still present on the left eye (OS), which may lead to a second anesthetic event.

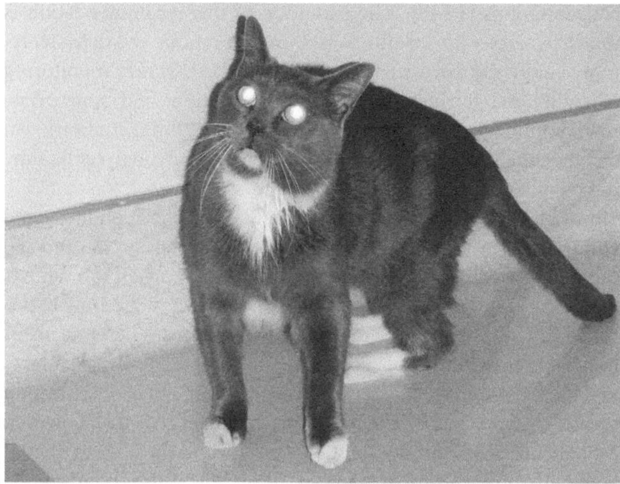

Figure 31.4 Plantigrade posture in a cat with DM is caused by peripheral neuropathy. The posture itself may not represent a complicating factor for anesthesia; however, it does suggest chronic and/or uncontrolled diabetes. Serial measurements of BG during anesthesia, ± insulin/dextrose administration, are warranted perioperatively. Source: Dr Todd Green, Department of Small Animal Medicine and Surgery, St George's University, St George's, Grenada. Reproduced with permission of Todd Green.

secretion to control hyperglycemia, but the pathophysiologic mechanisms are different between dogs and cats. The predominant form of DM in the dog is homologous to type 1 DM in people, with hyperglycemia due to deficiency in insulin secondary to beta cell destruction [4]. In cats, a homolog of human type 2 DM predominates. Type 2 diabetes results from insulin resistance and eventual exhaustion of beta cells [5,6]. There are several canine breeds at increased risk for DM, including the Australian Terrier, Miniature and Standard Schnauzers, Samoyed, Miniature and Toy Poodles, Cairn Terrier, Keeshond, Bichon Frise, and Finnish Spitz [7]. There are no feline breed predilections, but because cats primarily have the type 2 form, obesity increases the risk of diabetes dramatically in this species [8]. DM is diagnosed most frequently in middle-aged or older animals, and in dogs there is a female gender predilection.

In either species, clinical signs of DM occur due to the inability of cells to utilize carbohydrates as metabolic fuel, and the resultant hyperglycemia. When the concentration of glucose in the plasma exceeds the renal threshold for proximal tubular reabsorption of glucose from the filtrate, glucosuria ensues, causing osmotic diuresis and the common clinical signs of polyuria and polydipsia. Other clinical signs depend on the severity and chronicity of hyperglycemia, and include polyphagia and weight loss. Cataracts are common in dogs with DM (Fig. 31.3), and some cats with chronic DM develop a peripheral neuropathy that results in a plantigrade posture (Fig. 31.4). In severe forms of DM such as diabetic ketoacidosis (DKA) or hyperosmolar syndrome, patients can be in critical condition with clinical signs of vomiting, anorexia, severe dehydration, depression, coma, or death. For these reasons, animals with DKA are not good anesthetic candidates, although they rarely require anesthesia for diagnostic or surgical procedures.

The hallmarks of diagnosis of DM are the findings of hyperglycemia and glucosuria. Results of complete blood counts (CBCs) are often normal, but leukocytosis sometimes occurs in patients with concurrent infection, which is common in DM and DKA. In addition to hyperglycemia, serum chemistry analysis can show high liver enzyme activities, hypercholesterolemia, and, in dehydrated patients, azotemia and electrolyte disorders including hypokalemia, hypernatremia, hyponatremia, hypophosphatemia, and hypochloremia. In dogs and cats with DKA, blood-gas analysis reveals a low concentration of HCO_3^- and a high anion gap.

Treatment of DKA often requires hospitalization and critical care, including intravenous fluid therapy, constant-rate infusion (CRI) of insulin, and intensive monitoring of acid–base status, fluid balance, glucose, and electrolytes [9]. Most patients with DM, however, are not in a critical condition at diagnosis, and are treated on an outpatient basis [10]. In both dogs and cats, insulin is the mainstay of treatment. The range of available insulin preparations for use in dogs and cats is constantly changing, but at present most dogs are treated with either NPH (neutral protamine Hagedorn) or porcine lente insulin, and cats are treated with either porcine lente insulin, protamine zinc insulin, or one of the long-acting human recombinant insulin analogs such as insulin glargine or insulin detemir. Diet plays a role as in the management of DM. In cats, diets low in carbohydrates and higher in protein have been advocated [11]. Oral hypoglycemic drugs have been advocated to control hyperglycemia in diabetic cats, but the use of these drugs is not commonplace.

Monitoring of treatment is somewhat controversial, but measurement of serum fructosamine concentrations may be used to indicate long-term control of hyperglycemia. Although serial blood glucose (BG) curves have traditionally been recommended to assess the effects of insulin therapy, their use is called into question by studies in both dogs and cats showing the poor reliability of glucose curves for predicting glycemic control [12,13].

Anesthetic management

When dogs and cats with DM require anesthesia for medical and surgical procedures, these are usually not directly related to DM. For example, many diabetic dogs have cataracts that require removal via phacoemulsification under anesthesia [14]. Ideally, only well-regulated diabetic patients should be anesthetized, because patients with unregulated diabetes can have marked fluctuation of BG concentration. In poorly regulated patients, insulin administration prior to anesthesia may result in unpredictable perioperative BG concentrations [12,15]. The exception to this recommendation is intact females with insulin resistance that require ovariohysterectomy before the disease can be controlled [16]. Timely monitoring of serum BG during the perioperative period, and appropriate intervention (e.g., regular insulin or dextrose administration), can facilitate the prevention of extreme hyper- and hypoglycemia during the perioperative period.

In well-regulated diabetic dogs, the BG concentration measured within 1 h of insulin administration should be between 150 and 250 mg/dL. According to Feldman and Nelson [16], when the value is close to 150 mg/dL, a diabetic dog is more likely to become hypoglycemic later in the day when the patient is fasted. Therefore, insulin should be withheld or cautiously administered to these patients and the BG monitored closely. An early morning BG concentration greater than 300 mg/dL suggests poor control of glycemia; however, a single measurement does not confirm this. In these cases, inadequate glycemic control is more likely present if the fructosamine concentration is greater than 500 mg/dL [16]. Anesthesia for elective procedures should be delayed in these patients. Although rarely necessary, patients with DKA should not be anesthetized until the BG concentration decreases below 400 mg/dL. In hyperglycemic and DKA patients, meticulous attention to hydration status, acid–base status, and electrolyte imbalances is essential, because preoperative hyperglycemia may contribute to a hyperosmolar diuresis with subsequent dehydration and intraoperative hypotension [14,17,18]. In these patients, fluid therapy to correct water losses and electrolyte imbalances should be instituted before anesthesia.

For all patients with DM, elective anesthetic procedures should be performed as soon as possible in the morning after the first BG measurement. This reduces the need for a long period of fasting and allows the patient to resume normal activity more rapidly. Although continued insulin administration during preoperative fasting potentially increases the risk of hypoglycemia, insulin activity is important even during fasting to allow tissue uptake of nutrients. In addition, stress associated with anesthesia and surgery causes the release of hormones such as corticosteroids and catecholamines. These hormones promote glycogenolyis, gluconeogenesis, and ketogenesis, all of which increase the insulin requirement. Therefore, perioperative insulin administration is indicated to prevent severe hyperglycemia and minimize ketone formation perioperatively [16].

Although recommendations for preoperative fasting can vary, in general the day before surgery animals should be fed normally and insulin administered according to the usual regimen. Food should be withheld after 10 p.m. On the morning of surgery, BG should be measured before insulin administration and insulin should be given according to the patient's BG. Guidelines are presented in Table 31.1. No matter which protocol for feeding and insulin administration is recommended, communication between the owner, veterinarian, and anesthetist is important so that a clear history of insulin administration, feeding schedule, and patient health is shared.

Table 31.1 Guidelines for treatment of diabetic patients.

	Day Before Surgery	Morning of Surgery – a.m. Glucose Check		
		BG <100 mg/dL	BG 100–200 mg/dL	BG >200 mg/dL
Insulin	Normal regimen	None	¼ usual a.m. dose	½ usual a.m. dose
Comments	Fast after 10 p.m.	1–5% dextrose infusion[a]	1–5% dextrose infusion[a]	Withhold dextrose until BG <150 mg/dL

BG, blood glucose.
[a] This is part of the anesthetic maintenance fluid volume.
Source: modified from [16].

No absolute drug contraindications are imposed in diabetic patients. However, drugs with rapid elimination or that can be reversed may allow the diabetic patient to resume a normal feeding and insulin schedule sooner following anesthesia [14,19]. Vecuronium, an neuromuscular blocker commonly administered to produce centralization of the globe and immobilization during phacoemulsification, is reported to have a shorter duration of action in patients with DM [20]. The reason has yet to be elucidated, although this finding may have minimal clinical relevance.

During anesthetic maintenance of patients with DM, fluctuations of BG concentration are affected not only by the efficacy of current medical management, but also by the type and complexity of surgery, preoperative glucocorticoid administration, and the presence of infection [21]. Therefore, regardless of the initial BG, frequent perioperative monitoring of BG is recommended every 30–60 min [14,15]. Although the optimal target for BG in the perioperative period has not been defined, the administration of dextrose has been recommended when necessary to maintain the BG between 150 and 250 mg/dL during the intraoperative period and is continued throughout anesthetic recovery until the patient starts to eat. Dextrose should be stopped when/if the BG reaches 250 mg/dL in dogs or 300 mg/dL in cats, as this level is likely to promote glycosuria and diuresis [16,19]. Dextrose infusions are formulated by adding the appropriate amount of 50% dextrose to an isotonic fluid such as lactated Ringer's solution (LRS) to obtain a final concentration of 1–5% dextrose, and varied as needed for each patient. An intraoperative fluid rate of 5–10 mL/kg/h is usually adequate. If a BG concentration greater than 300 mg/dL persists, regular insulin may be administered IV or IM at 20% of the patient's usual dosage of long-acting insulin. Subsequent doses of regular insulin should be timed to avoid hypoglycemia and the dosage should be adjusted based on the effect of the first injection [16].

Diabetes is a risk factor for hypertension in dogs, although not in cats, and some may be on blood pressure medication. Many of these drugs produce vasodilation and may predispose patients to hypotension during anesthesia [21,22]. It has been suggested that diabetic dogs undergoing phacoemulsification are more likely to become hypotensive than non-diabetic dogs. The increased incidence and severity of intraoperative hypotension was likely attributable to hypovolemia secondary to hyperglycemia and the resultant osmotic diuresis and not to systemic medication [17]. In humans, the cardiovascular effects of autonomic diabetic neuropathy are well characterized and can predispose these patients to perioperative dysrhythmias and intraoperative hypotension [21]. In veterinary medicine, one study concluded that there were differences in vagal tone between diabetic and non-diabetic dogs [23]. However, whether this condition is associated with intraoperative hypotension or other cardiovascular complications in veterinary patients remains to be documented. For these reasons, blood pressure measurement is indicated [22].

Hypoglycemia or severe hyperglycemia can result in prolonged anesthetic recovery, central nervous system dysfunction, and DKA. Several of the clinical signs associated with these complications may go unnoticed until the end of anesthesia [14]. Although both hypo- and hyperglycemia are detrimental for the diabetic patient, a perioperative target BG associated with a positive postoperative outcome has not been established in veterinary medicine. In non-diabetic critically ill human patients, hyperglycemia (>180 mg/dL) has been associated with adverse outcomes. For this reason, tight glycemic control (80–110 mg/dL) has been advocated. However, this clinical approach has also been associated with increased hypoglycemic events and potentially worse outcomes [24]. In diabetic patients undergoing surgery, glycemic variability was associated with outcome; however, incremental decreases in intraoperative BG or euglycemia did not consistently reduce risk and may have worsened the postoperative mortality rate [25,26]. Conversely, severe intraoperative hyperglycemia is potentially associated with worse outcomes postoperatively [25], although hyperglycemic patients with diabetes had lower postoperative mortality than acutely hyperglycemic non-diabetic patients [26]. Therefore, in humans, recommendations of a moderate BG of 140–180 mg/dL appear most reasonable, in addition to avoidance of BG variability [27]. In veterinary medicine, such a recommendation has not been defined, but it seems reasonable to maintain a perioperative BG between 150 and 250 mg/dL with minimal fluctuations, as suggested by Feldman and Nelson [16].

The day after surgery, the diabetic dog or cat can usually return to their usual schedule of insulin administration and feeding. Patients that are not eating can be maintained with IV dextrose infusion and regular insulin injections given subcutaneously every 6–8 h [16].

Insulinoma

Insulinoma is the term for a functional tumor of pancreatic beta cells that constitutively secretes insulin and is unresponsive to changes in BG [28]. The resulting hypersecretion of insulin leads to chronic hypoglycemia and the accompanying clinical signs. Insulin-secreting tumors are uncommon and occur most commonly in middle-aged and older dogs [28]. They are extremely rare in cats [29]. These tumors, which are almost always malignant, tend to occur in either limb of the pancreas rather than in the body, and most have metastasized at the time of diagnosis [28,30]. The clinical signs observed in animals with insulinoma are the result of severe and prolonged hypoglycemia, and include seizures (most common sign), collapse, weakness, tremors, and ataxia, among others. Physical examination findings in dogs with insulinoma are usually unremarkable, although obesity is common.

With the exception of hypoglycemia, there are no markers for insulinoma on screening blood and urine tests. Diagnosis depends on the demonstration of fasting hypoglycemia with an inappropriately high serum concentration of insulin. Although formerly recommended, the insulin:glucose ratio is no longer used for the diagnosis of insulinoma because of poor diagnostic accuracy. Once insulinoma is suspected, abdominal ultrasound and/or computed tomography (CT) are indicated for the identification of a pancreatic tumor [31]. Thoracic radiographs should be taken to screen for pulmonary metastases, but the results are almost always normal.

Surgical removal of the primary tumor is usually recommended to help control hypoglycemia, but is rarely curative, as metastasis to lymph nodes and the liver is common. Even so, partial pancreatectomy improves survival, and average survival rates in dogs range from 7 to 42 months depending on the stage of disease and response to surgical treatment [30]. Survival rates for cats are thought to be considerably lower. In addition to surgery, medical therapy is necessary to prevent hypoglycemic crises in patients with insulinoma. It is important to consider that treatment of hypoglycemia with intravenous glucose may cause further insulin secretion and worsening of hypoglycemia. In a hypoglycemic crisis, there may be no choice but to give intravenous glucose; frequent monitoring is necessary to identify unpredictable changes in BG concentration. Intravenous infusion of glucagon has been reported to help stabilize BG concentrations in a dog with an insulinoma-associated hypoglycemic crisis [32]. Hypoglycemia may be prevented somewhat by feeding frequent small meals. If this strategy is ineffective, glucocorticoids are administered to antagonize the effects of insulin and increase gluconeogenesis. Prednisone is the most commonly used treatment for insulinoma, but other drugs have been used. Diazoxide is a benzothiadiazide that reduces insulin secretion by preventing closure of K^+-ATP channels on the beta cell plasma membrane, preventing depolarization of the cell. Gastrointestinal side-effects are common in dogs receiving diazoxide. Streptozotocin, a nitrosourea that is toxic to beta cells, has been used occasionally for the medical treatment of insulinoma in dogs [33]. Other treatment options include the use of somatostatin analogs, but these have not been evaluated for use in dogs with insulinoma.

Patients with insulinoma require medical management prior to surgery to control clinical signs and aid patient stability during anesthesia [28]. Preoperative fasting should be kept to a maximum of 8 h, and during this period the patient's BG should be monitored [34]. Glucose supplementation can be provided orally with corn syrup or intravenously with a 2.5–5% dextrose solution should clinical signs be observed [14]. The target BG concentration should be 50–60 mg/dL [14,35,36], although animals with insulinomas frequently tolerate resting BG concentrations of 30–40 mg/dL without clinical signs [18]. Preoperative hypoglycemia can also be managed with an intravenous infusion of glucagon at 5–40 ng/kg/min following a bolus of 50 ng/kg IV [32,37], or in conjunction with infusion of a low concentration of dextrose [34].

Anesthetic management

Clinical signs of hypoglycemia can be masked by general anesthesia and may only be detected following recovery [21]. Unless the BG concentration is monitored, it is unlikely that hypoglycemia will be identified during anesthesia [18,28], so the most important aspect of anesthetic management of insulinoma is serial monitoring of BG. Intraoperatively, the goal is not to correct hypoglycemia completely, but to maintain the BG concentration within the range that prevented clinical signs associated with neuroglycopenia prior to anesthesia [33,37,38]. BG should be measured especially during tumor manipulation because this can lead to insulin spikes and hypoglycemia intraoperatively [21]. Hyperglycemia should also be avoided so that the tumor is not stimulated to release excessive amounts of insulin, which can result in refractory hypoglycemia [14,18,28,32,37,38]. Fluid therapy during anesthesia should be gradually supplemented until the target BG is achieved, rather than administering large boluses of dextrose or a highly concentrated dextrose solution [36,37]. Dextrose supplementation greater than 5% is usually not needed and is not recommended [14]. To titrate the dextrose infusion rate, a bag of isotonic crystalloid fluid can be attached to a burette-type infusion set, where the crystalloid is mixed with dextrose to a desired concentration. Serial (i.e., every 30–60 min) measurement of BG allows the anesthetist to dilute or increase the dextrose concentration of the fluid as required. Alternatively, a separate infusion of dextrose can be given using an infusion pump or gravity flow. The volume of other fluids administered should be decreased to maintain the overall rate desired and avoid fluid overload.

The anesthetic protocol used for insulinoma patients should take into consideration the pain associated with major abdominal surgery, because the resultant sympathetic stimulation can cause hyperglycemia, with the potential for tumor stimulation and rebound hypoglycemia [28]. Pain management can be achieved with the administration of μ-opioid receptor agonists perioperatively as needed, both systemically and epidurally. Although α_2-adrenergic receptor agonists produce muscle relaxation and analgesia, and have an anesthetic-sparing effect [38], they have not been advocated for the anesthetic management of these patients owing to their inhibitory effect on the pancreatic beta cells and suppression of plasma insulin concentration [28,34]. However, in a recent study, when 5 μg/kg of medetomidine was administered with the preanesthetic medication to patients with insulinoma undergoing surgery, the usual response of pancreatic beta cells to α_2-adrenergic receptor agonists (i.e., decreased insulin plasma concentration) was seen. Medetomidine assisted in the maintenance of the BG concentration and decreased the amount of dextrose utilized during anesthesia. In addition, patients that received medetomidine had a more stable blood pressure throughout surgery, likely as a result of better analgesia [38]. It appears that a low dose of medetomidine (or other α_2-adrenergic receptor agonists) can be advantageous in patients with insulinoma provided that BG is monitored and dextrose infusion adjusted accordingly.

Pancreatitis is the second most common complication of partial pancreatectomy in patients with insulinoma. Although this is mostly a surgical complication, ensuring adequate perfusion to the pancreas throughout the perioperative period may reduce the risk. Maintenance of mean arterial pressure (MAP) above 60 mmHg and prevention of hypoxemia are ideal [36]. Serial BG measurement should be continued postoperatively. Transient hyperglycemia may occur due to atrophy of the normal pancreatic beta cells that remain; insulin administration may be necessary temporarily until the BG concentration stabilizes [28,36]. Dogs with gross metastasis at the time of surgery or with partially resected primary tumors are likely to have persistent signs of hypoglycemia postoperatively. Other potential postoperative complications include duodenal necrosis due to vascular compromise, ventricular arrhythmias, and central nervous system dysfunction secondary to prolonged hypoglycemia [34,36,39].

Pancreatitis

Pancreatitis occurs in both dogs and cats when digestive enzymes are activated within the pancreatic acinar cells [40–42]. The cause is generally unknown in veterinary patients, although ingestion of high-fat meals, various drugs, pancreatic trauma, pancreatic ischemia, pancreatic duct obstruction, and infection have been implicated in the dog. The cause of pancreatitis in the cat may be even less well understood, but the disease is seen in cats associated with hepatobiliary inflammation and/or inflammatory bowel disease [40–42].

Pancreatic enzymes are normally maintained as inactive forms called zymogens and sequestered in granules within acinar cells. When defense mechanisms are overwhelmed, these zymogens are activated and autodigestion of the pancreas ensues. Autodigestion leads to inflammatory infiltration of the pancreas and surrounding tissues. Pancreatitis occurs in acute or chronic forms. Acute pancreatitis is sometimes clinically very severe, but typically does not result in chronic changes to the pancreas, whereas chronic pancreatitis is often clinically vague, especially in cats, but results in irreversible changes to the pancreas, including atrophy and fibrosis.

Pancreatitis occurs most commonly in middle-aged and older dogs and cats [41,42]. Miniature Schnauzers have the highest rate of pancreatitis among dog breeds, and Shetland Sheepdogs, Yorkshire Terriers, and Poodles are also over-represented [43]. There is no established breed predilection for pancreatitis in cats. The clinical presentation of pancreatitis varies with the severity and chronicity of the condition. Dogs with pancreatitis typically show signs of depression, abdominal pain, fever, anorexia, vomiting, and diarrhea. The clinical presentation is more obscure in cats. Similarly to many feline diseases, anorexia and lethargy are common, making diagnosis difficult in some individuals. Classic signs of fever, abdominal pain, and vomiting are much less common in cats than in dogs. Mid-abdominal mass lesions, representing inflamed pancreas and surrounding tissues, may be palpable in either species. In severe forms of pancreatitis, life-threatening systemic complications such as respiratory distress syndromes, disseminated intravascular coagulation, and cardiac arrhythmia can occur.

There are no historical or physical examination findings that are pathognomonic for pancreatitis in either the dog or the cat. The CBC commonly reveals an inflammatory leukogram, sometimes with a left shift and toxic neutrophils. An increased hematocrit is found in dehydrated dogs, or a mild anemia associated with chronic inflammation may be present. Serum chemistry profiles may reveal evidence of dehydration with pre-renal azotemia, and increased liver enzyme activities may be seen. Pancreatitis is associated with hyperbilirubinemia, due to intrahepatic or posthepatic cholestasis, in cats more commonly than in dogs. Unfortunately, serum amylase and lipase tests are of no value in the diagnosis of pancreatitis in either species. Confirming a diagnosis of pancreatitis is often difficult. Over the past decade, tests for pancreatic lipase immunoreactivity have become available for both the dog and the cat [44–46]. Although these tests have some limitations in terms of diagnostic accuracy, they are superior to previously available tests, and are especially useful diagnostically when combined with pancreatic ultrasound and cytology of fine-needle aspirates of the pancreas.

Treatment of pancreatitis involves supportive care and pain management. Aggressive fluid therapy is necessary to correct dehydration and to maintain adequate perfusion of the pancreas. A balanced electrolyte solution is usually recommended for this purpose. Vomiting patients with pancreatitis should receive injectable antiemetic drugs. Metoclopramide has been used widely to treat vomiting in dogs with pancreatitis, but some clinicians question whether this drug may decrease gut perfusion, and it has fallen out of favor. Metoclopramide is less effective as an antiemetic drug in cats than in dogs. 5-HT_3 antagonists (e.g., ondansetron, dolasetron) are effective in treating emesis in both dogs and cats. Because maropitant may have some desired effects on visceral pain and, because it is an effective antiemetic in dogs and cats, it may be the antiemetic of choice in pancreatitis [47–49]. Alimentation is an important aspect of the treatment of pancreatitis. The traditional recommendation of withholding food from patients with pancreatitis has fallen out of favor in recent years, and the prevalent current opinion is that food should be withheld only if the patient is vomiting and there is risk of aspiration pneumonia. This is especially important in cats with pancreatitis because of the risk of hepatic lipidosis if food is withheld for long periods. Because high plasma lipids, obesity, and high-fat meals have been associated with pancreatitis, a low-fat diet is usually recommended. Fresh frozen plasma has been advocated for use in patients with pancreatitis, but studies of dogs and human patients have shown no benefit [50]. The use of antibiotics in treating pancreatitis is controversial. Pancreatitis is not typically a bacterial disease, although gut translocation of bacteria and sepsis could occur in severe cases. If sepsis is suspected, or if pancreatic fine-needle aspirates suggest infection, broad-spectrum antibiotics should be used.

Pancreatitis can occur following abdominal surgery in humans [51] and has been seen concurrently in dogs with other diseases such as diabetes mellitus, hyperadrenocorticism, renal failure, neoplasia, congestive heart failure, and autoimmune disorders [43].

Iatrogenic pancreatitis has been induced by drugs, including corticosteroids, nonsteroidal anti-inflammatory drugs (NSAIDs), organophosphates, thiazide diuretics, sulfonamides, tetracycline, azothioprine, furosemide, and estrogen [52]. Hence it is likely that animals with acute pancreatitis may be anesthetized for reasons unrelated to diagnosis or treatment of pancreatitis.

Surgical intervention is performed in patients with acute necrotizing pancreatitis, pancreatic abscess, pancreatic/bile duct obstruction, or evidence of infection or neoplasia or other mass lesions, and in those who fail to response to medical therapy. Endoscopic, surgical, or laparoscopic techniques may also be performed in patients with pancreatitis to place enterostomy tubes for enteral nutrition.

The choice of anesthetics for use in patients with pancreatitis is often based on other complicating factors, similar to those requiring exploratory laparotomy for gastrointestinal (GI) disease. Some patients may be severely compromised at presentation, but surgery is usually performed only after stabilization and generally only when medical therapy has failed.

Many opioids are known to stimulate contraction of the sphincter of Oddi, which increases pressure in the bile duct. Despite these concerns, since the pain caused by pancreatitis is frequently severe and sphincter contraction has likely already occurred, opioids are the mainstay of analgesic therapy in both humans and animals as they provide the best analgesia [53–55]. If vomiting is frequent, avoidance of premedication with α_2-adrenergic receptor agonists and opioids such as morphine or hydromorphone is prudent; however, the opioids may be used during maintenance. The profound cardiovascular effects, hyperglycemia, and hypoinsulinemia seen with α_2-adrenergic receptor agonists may also preclude their use in patients with pancreatitis. There is no clear best choice for the induction of anesthesia in patients with pancreatitis. Propofol has been associated with the development of pancreatitis in humans [56]. but this is not reported in dogs or cats. A retrospective evaluation of the use of propofol in 44 cats with primary hepatic lipidosis revealed no evidence of pancreatic dysfunction [57]. Halothane is not recommended in compromised patients, those with concurrent liver disease, or those with cardiac dysrhythmias. Maintenance of anesthesia with isoflurane or sevoflurane is preferred in such cases. In patients without coagulopathy, dermatitis, or sepsis, epidural administration of morphine provides good pain relief and can be used in addition to intravenous administration of other μ-agonist opioids. As always, the anesthetist should provide vigilant monitoring of anesthetic depth, maintain adequate vascular volume and perfusion, and prevent hypotension and hypoxemia.

Adrenal gland

The two adrenal glands are located retroperitoneally, with one gland craniomedial to each kidney. They are composed of a central medulla and outer cortex. Although located anatomically in a single gland, these areas are functionally distinct. The medulla originates from neural crest tissue of the embryonic ectoderm, whereas the cortex develops from the mesoderm. The medulla is densely innervated with preganglionic sympathetic fibers and is considered part of the autonomic nervous system. Its main cell type, the chromaffin cell, produces epinephrine and norepinephrine, and is important in emergent and stressful circumstances [58]. The adrenal cortex is an important endocrine organ, with three distinct zones that secrete different hormones in response to various stimuli. The most superficial zone, the zona glomerulosa, secretes mineralocorticoids, mainly aldosterone. Deep to this area is the zona fasciculata, which secretes glucocorticoid hormones, primarily cortisol in the dog and cat. The deepest zone of the adrenal cortex is the zona reticularis, which secretes sex hormones [59].

Hypoadrenocorticism

Diminished function of the adrenal cortex produces a condition called hypoadrenocorticism (HA) or Addison's disease. It occurs in most often in dogs, usually the result of immune-mediated destruction of the adrenal cortex [60,61]. HA can also result from pituitary adrenocorticotropic hormone (ACTH) deficiency (uncommon) or can be iatrogenic following treatment for Cushing's syndrome, or when high-dose steroid therapy is abruptly withdrawn. In its classic form, dogs present for complications of deficiency in both aldosterone and cortisol. A form of the disease in which signs of only cortisol deficiency are seen (termed 'atypical' hypoadrenocorticism) has been recognized [62]. Isolated aldosterone deficiency is rare in the dog, as is any form of HA in the cat [63]. Glucocorticoids exert multiple effects on the vasculature, affecting endothelial integrity, vascular permeability, and sensitivity to catecholamines. Consequently, they help maintain blood pressure. Aldosterone stimulates sodium and chloride reabsorption and potassium excretion in the cortical collecting duct of the renal tubules. Because water follows sodium, it is also reabsorbed, which promotes plasma volume expansion [37].

Among dog breeds, Standard Poodles, West Highland White Terriers, Bearded Collies, Nova Scotia Duck Tolling Retrievers, Great Danes, Rottweilers, Portuguese Water Dogs, and Leonbergers are predisposed to HA, and the disorder is more common in females. The disease can affect dogs of any age, but the median age is 4 years. There are no known breed predilections in cats, but most are middle-aged at the time of diagnosis [63].

Glucocorticoid deficiency is responsible for many of the vague, chronic, waxing and waning clinical signs of HA, including anorexia, lethargy, vomiting, diarrhea, and weight loss. Mineralocorticoid deficiency leads to potassium retention and urinary sodium and water loss. When severe, these changes result in dehydration, azotemia, hypotension, cardiac bradyarrhythmia, and collapse. Whenever a patient is presented with vague GI clinical signs and/or lethargy, HA should be suspected. Signs of the disease range from mild to severe, and those patients presenting in acute Addisonian crisis are at risk of death. Findings on a CBC can include anemia, lymphocytosis, or eosinophilia. The lack of a stress leukogram in an ill patient should also lead the clinician to suspect glucocorticoid deficiency [64]. Serum biochemistry findings include hyperkalemia, hyponatremia, hypoalbuminemia, mild hypercalcemia, and, in dehydrated patients, prerenal azotemia [64]. Even though the azotemia is prerenal in origin, the urine is not always concentrated, owing to the inability to retain sodium, and it is important not to assume a primary renal cause of azotemia because of a low urine specific gravity. Definitive diagnosis of HA requires measurement of serum concentrations of cortisol before and after stimulation with ACTH [65]. It has been reported that the finding of a normal or high basal cortisol concentration has a high negative predictive value for the diagnosis of HA, so ACTH stimulation testing is not always necessary [66]. Once the diagnosis of HA is made, treatment carries a good prognosis [67]. Dogs and cats in a non-critical condition are treated as outpatients with mineralocorticoid and glucocorticoid supplementation. Mineralocorticoid treatment can be in the form of either injectable desoxycorticosterone pivalate (DCP) or oral fludrocortisone. Fludrocortisone has mild glucocorticoid activity and glucocorticoid supplementation is not always needed with this drug. Patients treated with DCP should also receive very low maintenance doses of prednisone. Treatment of very sick Addisonian patients in adrenal crisis requires intravenous fluid therapy with normal saline and monitoring of electrolytes Treatment with steroids should be withheld initially pending adrenal function testing. Dogs in Addisonian crisis typically recover within a day of treatment, whereas cats are slower to recover.

Dogs and cats with acute HA rarely require anesthesia. Most patients with HA will undergo anesthesia for surgical procedures unrelated to the disease and should have been previously managed with medical therapy at the time of surgery [14,68]. In healthy patients, cortisol production increases by 5–10-fold after major surgery. Patients with HA have inappropriate responses to stress; consequently, glucocorticoid doses should be adjusted before surgery and anesthesia. Several preoperative glucocorticoid supplementation regimens in addition to baseline steroid therapy have been recommended for human patients with HA to prevent adrenal crisis and refractory hypotension in the perioperative period [21]. There have been no studies of steroid supplementation in dogs undergoing surgery; however, well-controlled dogs with HA should receive an extra dose of steroid before anesthesia in addition to their normal daily dose. Recommended doses of glucocorticoids include 0.1–2 mg/kg of dexamethasone sodium phosphate IV or 1–2 mg/kg of prednisolone sodium succinate IV and repeated as necessary [37,69]. Postoperatively, additional glucocorticoids are administered as needed [19]. Alternatively, an ACTH stimulation test prior to elective procedures may be useful to guide the need for supplementation [14].

If unstable HA patients require anesthesia for emergency procedures, they must be evaluated for hyperkalemia and hyponatremia, prerenal azotemia and hypovolemia, metabolic acidosis, and hypoglycemia. All these abnormalities should be managed prior to anesthesia. CBC and serum biochemistry are very useful when a diagnosis of HA is suspected; electrocardiography may show evidence of hyperkalemia when serum concentrations are >5.5 mEq/L, although this is fairly variable [70]. Volume replacement should be with intravenous isotonic crystalloid fluid, and may be all that is necessary to correct electrolyte abnormalities and stabilize vascular volume and blood pressure. If hyperkalemia persists, especially if an arrhythmia or bradycardia is present, specific therapy may be warranted to decrease serum potassium. Table 31.2 presents recommendations for the treatment of hyperkalemia [19,37,68].

Anesthetic management

The choice of anesthetic protocol in the patient with HA is not as critical as the perioperative medical management, and no specific drug is recommended. However, etomidate should be avoided in this patient population because it inhibits 11β-hydroxylase, an enzyme necessary for the synthesis of cortisol in dogs and cats, for 2–6 h after administration [71,72].

Since HA patients are more likely to become hypotensive during anesthesia and may not respond normally to the usual therapies, balanced electrolyte solution (e.g., LRS) should be administered intraoperatively at a rate of 5–10 mL/kg/h. This rate is adjusted or supplemental boluses may be administered depending on the patient's status [18,19]. Frequent blood pressure monitoring is warranted in these patients and hemodynamic support with positive inotropes may be necessary [18,21]. If invasive blood pressure is measured, variation in the amplitude of the systolic pressure waveform, especially following positive-pressure ventilation, may be seen when hypovolemia is present.

Hypercortisolism

Hypercortisolism (i.e., hyperadrenocorticism or canine Cushing's syndrome) results from excess circulating concentrations of cortisol [73]. In 80–85% of naturally occurring cases, the disease is the result of increased secretion of ACTH from an adenoma of the corticotrophs of the pars distalis of the pituitary, resulting in bilateral adrenocortical hyperplasia and excessive cortisol secretion [pituitary-dependent hypercortisolism (PDHC)]. Less commonly, hypercortisolism (HC) is caused by a cortisol-secreting tumor of the adrenal gland (ADHC). Iatrogenic Cushing's syndrome is caused by chronic administration of glucocorticoids. An 'atypical' form of Cushing's syndrome has also been described in which clinical signs are not associated with high cortisol concentrations, but rather from adrenal secretion of sex hormones. Whether this syndrome actually exists is the subject of controversy [74].

Excess cortisol leads to the clinical signs of Cushing's syndrome, including bilaterally symmetrical alopecia, comedones, dermal hyperpigmentation, dermal and muscle atrophy, polyuria/polydipsia (PU/PD), polyphagia, pendulous abdomen, hepatomegaly, panting, hypertension, and lethargy [73] (Fig. 31.5). Not all dogs with HC display all of these, but PU, PD, and dermatologic signs are

Table 31.2 Treatments for hyperkalemia.

Treatment	Dose	Mechanism	Comments
Replacement crystalloid fluids	Volume needed to treat hypovolemia	Dilution of K^+ and diuresis	Administer shock dose (90 mL/kg) in aliquots, e.g., ¼–⅓ of total dose; reassess patient status between doses; K^+ concentration in balanced replacement crystalloids is too low to worsen hyperkalemia
Calcium gluconate 10% solution	0.5–1.5 mL/kg over 10–20 min	Cardioprotective – increases the threshold potential, restoring potential difference	Does not lower K^+, protects heart temporarily and works quickly. Other therapies do reduce K^+; monitor ECG, slow or stop infusion if arrhythmias occur
Regular insulin	0.25–0.5 U/kg IV or IM, with dextrose bolus – 4 mL 50% dextrose IV per unit insulin	Stimulates transport of glucose and K^+ into cells	Rapid onset. Monitor BG levels. Supplement dextrose until insulin effect dissipates
Dextrose	0.5–1 mL/kg bolus followed by constant-rate infusion of 2.5%–5% dextrose solution	Stimulates endogenous insulin secretion, maintains BG following insulin administration	Also addresses hypoglycemia that is common with HA
Sodium bicarbonate	1–3 mEq/kg over 30 min	Increase pH – K^+ moves into the cell in exchange for hydrogen to maintain electrochemical balance	Slower onset of action, 1 h for distribution of bicarbonate

Source: modified from [37].

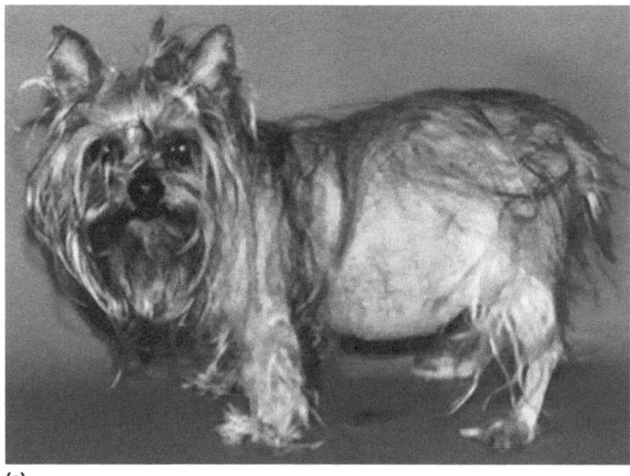

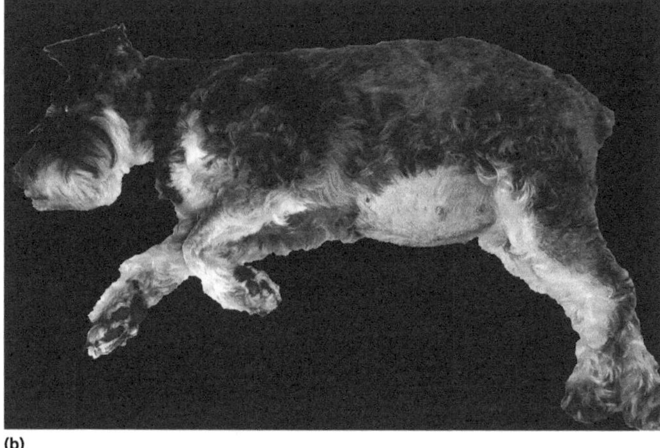

(a) (b)

Figure 31.5 (a) Dog with HC. Note alopecia, muscle atrophy in the rear limbs, and pendulous abdomen. Source: Dr Stephen DiBartola, Department of Veterinary Clinical Sciences, The Ohio State University, Columbus, OH, USA. Reproduced with permission of Stephen DiBartola. (b) Pendulous abdomen due to increased abdominal fat, hepatomegaly, and large bladder can impair ventilation and oxygenation in dogs with HC during anesthesia.

most common. When pituitary tumors become large enough, neurologic signs can be present, but this is not common.

Spontaneous Cushing's syndrome generally occurs in middle-aged and older dogs, but it is seen rarely in young dogs. There is no gender predilection for pituitary-dependent disease, but adrenal tumors may be more common in female dogs. Any pure-bred or mixed-breed dog can be affected, but Poodles, Boston Terriers, German Shepherds, Dachshunds, and Beagles are predisposed.

Dogs with HC show non-specific changes on CBC, most consistent with a stress response – neutrophilia, lymphopenia, and eosinopenia [73]. Routine serum biochemistry abnormalities include increased alkaline phosphatase activity (due to the presence of a steroid-induced isoform in the dog) in 90% or more of cases, increased alanine aminotransferase activity, hypercholesterolemia, and hyperglycemia [73]. Urinalysis typically reveals low specific gravity with or without mild proteinuria. Concurrent urinary tract infection is common in dogs with hypercortisolism [75].

When HC is suspected, the diagnosis is confirmed by one of several available screening tests [76,77]. The ACTH stimulation test, low-dose dexamethasone suppression test, urine cortisol:creatinine ratio, and dexamethasone-suppressed urine cortisol:creatinine ratio have all been studied. None of these tests are diagnostically perfect, and the most important screening test may well be the clinical index of suspicion, based on history and clinical signs, on the part of an astute clinician. It should be kept in mind that false-positive tests are common. In addition to screening tests for HC, tests to differentiate the cause of the condition are also recommended. High-dose dexamethasone suppression testing can confirm pituitary-dependent disease, and adrenal tumors can be investigated by abdominal ultrasound. The finding of a low plasma concentration of ACTH is consistent with an adrenal tumor, but ACTH assays are expensive and the hormone is unstable, so it is rarely measured. CT or MRI imaging can confirm the presence of a pituitary tumor. This may be especially useful in cases in which a pituitary macroadenoma is suspected based on the presence of neurologic signs.

Several treatment protocols are available for HC [78]. Most patients with pituitary-dependent disease are treated with either mitotane or trilostane [78,79]. The classic mechanism of mitotane is necrosis of the deeper zones of the adrenal cortex, sparing the superficial mineralocorticoid-producing zone. Other mechanisms inhibit steroid production without causing cellular damage. Trilostane causes a reversible, competitive inhibition of 3β-hydroxysteroid dehydrogenase, an enzyme necessary for the production of cortisol, aldosterone, and androgens in the adrenal cortex. Both of these drugs have benefits and drawbacks, but they are both effective in the majority of cases. Median survival times for dogs treated with mitotane or trilostane were reportedly 708 and 662 days, respectively [80]. Either drug can cause an acute Addisonian crisis. In addition to medical management, surgical resection of tumors by transsphenoidal hypophysectomy [81] or adrenalectomy [82]. has been successful.

Dogs with PDHC often require anesthesia for other concurrent diseases [14], and those with cortisol-secreting adrenocortical tumors may undergo adrenalectomy [68]. Dogs with PDHC treated with mitotane or trilostane may lack adequate functional adrenocortical reserve and may not handle stressful anesthetic or surgical events appropriately. Adequate adrenocortical reserve is indicated by a post-ACTH stimulation cortisol concentration of 2–5 μg/dL [34]. Patients with lower values should be managed as an iatrogenic Addisonian, requiring preoperative glucocorticoid supplementation as discussed above. In addition, sodium and potassium concentrations should be monitored in these patients [14,19]. Patients with both forms of HC are predisposed to hypertension and thrombus formation [83]. Hypertension should be managed with antihypertensive drugs (e.g., angiotensin-converting enzyme inhibitors) in conjunction with mitotane or trilostane prior to surgery [14,19]. Treatment with trilostane for 3–4 weeks before surgery can reverse the metabolic derangements of HC and minimize the risk of complications associated with adrenalectomy [84]. Goals of therapy are a post-ACTH serum cortisol concentration between 2 and 5 μg/dL and improvement of clinical signs [34].

Patients with ADHC are at increased risk of thromboembolic events [e.g., pulmonary thromboembolism (PTE)] perioperatively and may be on antithrombotic therapy (including heparin) before surgery. Regular measurement of activated partial thromboplastin time (APTT) may be indicated to ensure that the patient is receiving an appropriate dose and not at risk for excessive bleeding during surgery. The goal is an APTT that is increased by 1.5–2-fold, but no greater [14,19,85–88].

When ADHC is suspected, the extent of local vascular invasion should be determined with abdominal ultrasound and/or CT before surgery. If the tumor is in close proximity to or invades the aorta or vena cava, patients should be blood typed and/or cross-matched and blood or packed red blood cells (RBCs) should be available as excessive intraoperative hemorrhage is not uncommon [34,87].

Other clinical signs of HC, such as PU/PD, should also be evaluated in all patients with HC, including those receiving medical therapy. Patients that remain with PU/PD may dehydrate quickly with water restriction, and this should be considered in the preoperative preparation [14].

Anesthetic management

No specific anesthetic protocol is indicated or contraindicated for patients with HC; however, these patients may not require intense sedation, especially in those whose disease has not been well managed. Some patients are geriatric, and poor condition and lethargy are common [14]. The anesthetist should also consider that many HC patients require frequent short walks to promote blood flow when thrombosis is a concern. It may be beneficial to select drugs and dosages that allow the dog to be ambulatory within 4 h of surgery [83]. If HC is not well controlled, perioperative analgesia should be provided with opioids and local anesthetics. NSAIDs are often avoided in these cases owing to the potential risk of GI ulceration in dogs with a high endogenous cortisol concentration [14,89]. Dogs with HC commonly hypoventilate during anesthesia due to respiratory muscle weakness, increased abdominal fat, hepatomegaly, and bladder distension [14]. Hypoventilation may lead to respiratory acidemia and hypoxemia if oxygen is not supplemented, especially in recovery.

Monitoring of ventilation and oxygenation via end-tidal carbon dioxide, pulse oximetry, and/or arterial blood-gas analysis is warranted in patients with HC. Preoxygenation may be indicated in those patients with a large pendulous abdomen and care must be taken when positioning patients in dorsal recumbency to avoid compromise of ventilation. Controlled intermittent positive-pressure ventilation is frequently required in these patients. Direct blood pressure monitoring is helpful in patients anesthetized for adrenalectomy because the risk of rapid and excessive hemorrhage is high [14,19].

Following adrenalectomy, especially when invasion of the vena cava is/was present, patients are at even greater risk of thromboembolic complications, especially during anesthetic recovery. Clinical signs are non-specific and highly variable [90]; however, acute onset of dyspnea, tachypnea, cyanosis, and collapse should prompt suspicion of PTE. Blood-gas analysis usually reveals hypoxemia, hypocapnia, and increased alveolar to arterial oxygen gradient. Treatment is symptomatic and should be instituted immediately, with increased inspired oxygen fraction and cardiovascular support as needed [14].

Dexamethasone (0.05–0.1 mg/kg IV) should be administered postoperatively to adrenalectomy patients to prevent the development of hypoadrenocorticism. Sodium and potassium should also be monitored and mineralocorticoid therapy instituted if the sodium:potassium ratio decreases dramatically [34].

Pheochromocytoma

Pheochromocytoma (PHEO) is a catecholamine-secreting tumor that arises from chromaffin cells of the adrenal medulla. Reported in dogs, cats, humans, and other species, it can be malignant or locally invasive. Clinical signs can be dramatic but are often intermittent and paroxysmal due to the episodic release of catecholamines [68]. The most common signs are weakness, collapse, tachypnea, tachyarrhythmia, hypertension, and seizures [37]. Some overlap with clinical signs of HC also occurs. Concurrent hyperadrenocorticism and PHEO has been reported, so HC should be ruled out prior to surgery [91,92]. A minimum database consisting of CBC, serum chemistry profile, a baseline electrocardiogram (ECG), arterial blood pressure and thoracic radiographs should be evaluated. The basic evaluation will often be normal or may have changes related to catecholamine release. If HC is also present, liver enzymes may be elevated, and a stress leukogram may be present. Because excess production of catecholamines is diagnostic for PHEO, measurement of plasma and urine metanephrines is used for this diagnosis in humans [21]. Elevation of urinary catecholamine concentration (UCC) in animals may be supportive but can also be caused by excitement and other factors. Although some promise is seen for use in veterinary medicine, measurement of UCC is still not readily available [37] and diagnosis of an adrenal mass is most often detected via abdominal ultrasonography [93]. Identification as a PHEO can be determined via biopsy but this is rarely performed owing to the difficulty in obtaining good samples and the risk of hemorrhage or hypertensive crisis. However, the clinical signs of episodic weakness/collapse, arrhythmias, etc., are highly suggestive. The origin, architecture, vascularity, and invasiveness of the mass are best determined with CT or MRI. These examinations also help determine the feasibility of surgical removal in addition to the probable need for cross-matching and blood transfusion, although any time an adrenalectomy is scheduled, blood products should be immediately available [34,87,94,95]. Invasive PHEOs have been reported to affect not only the vena cava, but also the aorta, renal veins, and hepatic veins [37,95].

Anesthetic management

Preoperative management is very important in patients with suspected PHEO. Because of unpredictable tachyarrhythmia and hypertension, patients with PHEO are usually considered to be at high anesthetic risk. The best approach utilizes prolonged medical management to stabilize patients prior to surgical excision of the tumor. Medical therapy most often utilizes α-blockade with the goal of reducing catecholamine-induced hypertension. Phenoxybenzamine, a long-acting non-competitive α_1-adrenergic receptor antagonist with some α_2-receptor activity, is most frequently administered for 1–2 weeks before surgery. An oral dose of 0.25 mg/kg twice daily is often started, but in most cases is ineffective. As such, this dose should be increased during the course of the 2 weeks up to 2.5 mg/kg twice daily or until signs of hypotension are observed [34,37,87,95–98]. In dogs with PHEO, preoperative administration of phenoxybenzamine did not decrease the frequency or severity of perioperative hypertension, but improved the mortality rate from 43 to 13% [96]. Although phenoxybenzamine may not normalize perioperative blood pressure, the decrease in perioperative mortality is likely associated with decreased vasoconstriction and improvement of intravascular volume [96].

Atrial and ventricular tachycardias, and less often atrioventricular blocks, can occur with these tumors [14,19,95,99]. Preoperatively, severe tachycardia can be treated with oral β-adrenergic receptor antagonists, such as propranolol (0.2–1 mg/kg every 8 h) or atenolol (0.2–1 mg/kg every 12 h). However, better results are seen when α-blockade therapy is instituted first because β-receptor blockade alone may lead to unopposed α-receptor-mediated vasoconstriction, exacerbating hypertension [14,21,39,68,95].

Reflex bradycardia of vagal origin, although rare, may occur in dogs with PHEO due to hypertension. Preoperative management of hypertension should prevent bradyarrhythmias. Third-degree atrioventricular block in dogs with PHEO has also been related to myocardial damage and atrioventricular nodal fibrosis from chronic catecholamine exposure [99]. In this situation, evaluation of the heart condition is an important determinant of whether surgical treatment for PHEO should be pursued.

Chronic sympathetic stimulation and vasoconstriction seen with PHEO may cause intravascular volume depletion; hydration status should be assessed and corrected preoperatively [68,95]. Control of factors that stimulate catecholamine release is important in the anesthetic management of patients with PHEO, including fear, stress, pain, hypothermia, shivering, hypoxia, and hypercarbia. Although most anesthetic drugs have been used with some degree of success, those with sympathomimetic or vagolytic effects should be avoided in order to prevent possible adverse hemodynamic responses. Anticholinergic and ketamine administration is not usually recommended. Morphine and atracurium are also not good choices as histamine release may provoke the release of catecholamines from the tumor. Thiobarbiturates and halothane should be avoided owing to their tendency to cause ventricular arrhythmias, especially in the presence of excess catecholamines. Acepromazine may complicate treatment for hypotension, particularly if the patient has been pretreated with phenoxybenzamine [14,21,34,95]. An appropriate anesthetic protocol includes preanesthetic medication with an opioid that does not promote histamine release, such as oxymorphone, hydromorphone, methadone, or fentanyl, combined with a benzodiazepine and intravenous induction with propofol, alfaxalone or etomidate to facilitate endotracheal intubation [87,96,97]. Isoflurane or sevoflurane is preferred for anesthetic maintenance as opposed to desflurane, which can cause sympathetic stimulation. Inhalant agents should be supplemented with balanced anesthetic techniques using potent opioids such as fentanyl or remifentanil [14,95,96].

Multiple intravenous access sites and continuous electrocardiography and invasive arterial blood pressure monitoring during anesthesia are useful with PHEOs to identify and manage cardiac arrhythmias and abrupt changes in blood pressure promptly, and to manage blood loss [19,68,95]. Drugs to treat complications must be available for immediate administration when an emergency arises, especially during induction of anesthesia or manipulation of the tumor [91]. Sodium nitroprusside, a direct vasodilator, is the agent of choice to treat severe hypertension because of its potency, rapid onset, and short duration of action. Phentolamine, a short-acting competitive α-adrenergic antagonist and a direct vasodilator, when administered intravenously, is also an alternative for the treatment of hypertension during surgery [21,68,87,95,96]. During administration of these drugs, continuous blood pressure measurement helps find the most adequate infusion rate to avoid hypotension. In human medicine, magnesium sulfate ($MgSO_4$) has also been used for the treatment of hypertension and arrhythmias during anesthesia. $MgSO_4$ inhibits the release of catecholamines from the adrenal medulla and peripheral nerve terminals, reduces the sensitivity of α-adrenergic receptors to catecholamines, is a direct vasodilator, and has antiarrhythmic effects [21,37]. Although these antihypertensive medications have been used with success in patients with PHEO, hypertension may still occur during tumor manipulation, so careful surgical technique is warranted [21]. Tachyarrhythmias are managed with lidocaine or β-antagonists. Esmolol has a rapid onset and is short acting, which readily controls heart rate [14,21,37,68,95]. Table 31.3 provides drug dosages for antiarrhythmic therapy and pressure support.

Table 31.3 Treatments for complications seen during anesthesia in patients with pheochromocytoma [14, 37, 87, 95].

Problem	Drug	Dose	Comments
Hypertension	Nitroprusside	0.1–10 μg/kg/min IV	Dilates arterioles and veins. Monitor BP continuously, adjust rate as needed; light sensitive, cover infusion
	Phentolamine	Loading dose 0.1 mg/kg IV, with CRI at 1–2 μg/kg/min	Short-acting α-adrenergic blockade
	Magnesium sulfate	30 mg/kg over 10 min	May also help ventricular arrhythmia
Tachyarrhythmia	Lidocaine	Loading dose 2 mg/kg IV, with CRI at 50–75 μg/kg/min	Ventricular arrhythmia
	Esmolol	Loading dose 0.1–0.5 mg/kg IV, given over 1–2 min, with CRI at 50–70 μg/kg/min	Short-acting β-blockade; for sinus or supraventricular tachycardia
Refractory hypotension	Phenylephrine Norepinephrine Vasopressin	0.5–10 μg/kg/min IV 0.1–3 μg/kg/min IV 0.5–2 mU/kg/min IV	*Very* potent vasoconstrictors – use lowest effective dose; HR may slow

BP, arterial blood pressure; CRI, constant-rate infusion; HR, heart rate.

For any surgery involving the adrenal gland(s), there is significant potential for intraoperative blood loss, particularly for tumors involving the right adrenal gland because of its proximity to the caudal vena cava. Blood typing and/or cross-matching should be performed before surgery, and packed RBCs, fresh frozen plasma, or whole blood, should be available for immediate volume resuscitation if needed [14]. Surface-induced hypothermia to a temperature of 32°C (89.6°F) has been advocated for patients with a PHEO that invades the great vessels [87,96], to protect vital organs from reduced oxygen delivery during temporary vascular occlusion [100].

Intraoperative and postoperative hypotension following tumor excision is common. It is multifactorial, arising from a combination of an immediate decrease in catecholamine concentrations, vasodilation from residual α-blockade caused by phenoxybenzamine, impaired sympathetic reflexes, and hypovolemia. Treatment involves reduction of inhalant anesthetic concentration, reduction or discontinuation of phentolamine/nitroprusside, and volume expansion with isotonic crystalloid or colloid fluids; high volumes may be required. Vasopressor (e.g., phenylephrine, norepinephrine) and inotropic drugs are used to treat refractory hypotension, although patients treated with phenoxybenzamine may be less responsive to vasopressor therapy [14,19,21,68,95,101]. Treatment with a non-catecholamine pressor such as vasopressin may be necessary to maintain adequate blood pressure [101]. If bilateral adrenalectomy has been performed, glucocorticoid and mineralocorticoid replacement therapy will be necessary. In addition, BG should be monitored postoperatively, because hypoglycemia may occur when plasma catecholamine concentrations decrease suddenly. Continuous ECG and blood pressure measurement should be maintained for at least 24 h postoperatively [21,95].

Thyroid gland

The thyroid gland has two lobes, one on each side of the trachea, which may be connected via an isthmus. Each lobe is located distal to the larynx, ventrolateral to the trachea, and extending from the fifth to eighth tracheal rings. The thyroid gland is composed of numerous follicles lined by epithelial cells that produce and secrete hormone. These follicles serve as a storage area for precursors of thyroid hormones. Interspersed between the follicles, clusters of parafollicular or C cells are found that produce calcitonin. The parathyroid glands are also found in very close proximity to the thyroid glands [102,103].

Hypothyroidism

Hypothyroidism (HOT) occurs primarily in the dog, where it is most commonly an immune-mediated disease caused by lymphocytic infiltration of the thyroid gland with eventual destruction of functional thyroid tissue [104]. Idiopathic atrophy of the thyroid gland, in which no inflammatory component is found, is also described in the dog as a cause of clinical HOT [104]. Because thyroid hormone is responsible for maintenance of basal metabolism, the clinical signs of HOT are caused by a decrease in the metabolic rate. Multisystemic and vague, the most common clinical signs of HOT include weight gain, hair loss, dry skin and hair coat, and decreased activity [105,106]. Many other clinical signs, such as pyoderma, otitis, seizures, facial paralysis, laryngeal paralysis, and megaesophagus, have been attributed to HOT, but cause and effect have not been established and there are no data to support HOT as a cause of most of these signs. In severe forms of HOT, myxedema can develop. Myxedema occurs when abnormally high amounts of mucin accumulate in the skin and other tissues. The result is edematous skin (non-pitting, noticed especially on the head). Myxedema coma is a rare syndrome characterized by myxedema, severe lethargy, bradycardia, hypotension, hypoventilation, and hypothermia. Large breed dogs may be more likely to develop HOT. Doberman Pinschers, Great Danes, Irish Setters, English Setters, and Golden Retrievers are often cited as predisposed. There is no gender predilection, and the disease is typically diagnosed in middle-aged dogs.

The most common hematological and serum biochemical abnormalities in dogs with hypothyroid are hypercholesterolemia, hypertriglyceridemia, and mild normocytic normochromic anemia [105–107]. Confirming the diagnosis of HOT is not always straightforward. Because any concurrent illness and many drugs are associated with decreased total thyroxine (T4) concentrations, dogs may be mistakenly diagnosed with HOT if routine screening testing with total T4 is relied upon. Evaluation of serum concentrations of free T4 and canine thyrotropin (cTSH) have been advocated as the most accurate diagnostic strategy for HOT in the dog, but there is also considerable overlap of the results of these tests in dogs with HOT compared with dogs with non-thyroidal disease [108–110]. Circulating antibodies against thyroglobulin may be a marker for lymphocytic thyroiditis [107]. Previously, TSH stimulation testing was used to diagnose HOT in dogs, but the expense and unavailability of TSH have limited the use of this test.

Treatment of HOT is straightforward and involves daily supplementation with L-thyroxine. Follow-up measurement of total T4 approximately 6 h post-pill has been described to monitor treatment [105], but it may make more sense to monitor treatment based on clinical response and normalization of hematological and biochemical abnormalities.

Anesthetic Management

Untreated and inadequately treated HOT patients have a reduced metabolic rate and may recover more slowly from sedation or anesthesia [19]. Stabilization of the HOT state with hormone replacement therapy is therefore warranted prior to elective procedures [14]. CBC should be performed because mild to moderate anemia may be present, although in most cases anemia is not clinically significant [111]. Severe HOT (i.e., myxedema coma) is a rare condition and these patients should not be anesthetized unless an emergency situation exists that requires anesthesia. Bradycardia, hypotension, hypoventilation, hypothermia, and decreased level of consciousness are often present with myxedema coma and may complicate anesthesia [37,111]. In general, HOT patients present with muscle weakness and a frequently poor or obese body condition that compromises ventilation and oxygenation. Positioning of the patient in sternal recumbency is recommended [112]. Continuous monitoring of heart rate and rhythm, arterial blood pressure, ventilation, oxygenation, and temperature is important for the anesthetic management of these patients. Bradycardia and hypotension should be treated with anticholinergics, fluid therapy (crystalloids or synthetic colloids), and positive inotropes [14,37]. Slow rewarming of hypothermic patients is also indicated; this may also improve or correct bradycardia and hypotension. Patients with myxedema coma may require intravenous hormone replacement therapy with L-thyroxine postoperatively [19,21].

No specific anesthetic or anesthetic adjunct drug is contraindicated in dogs with HOT and studies have shown that the minimum alveolar concentrations (MACs) of halothane and isoflurane in euthyroid and hypothyroid dogs are clinically similar [113,114]. However, anecdotally, hypothyroid dogs appear to have reduced requirements for anesthetic drugs. This clinical impression can be partly explained as not being due to the thyroid state of the patient, but because hypothyroid dogs are more prone to hypothermia. Short-acting drugs that require minimal or no metabolism or that are readily antagonized are often preferred by many anesthetists. Opioids and benzodiazepines usually produce adequate preanesthetic sedation, especially in the lethargic elderly patient. Propofol and inhalant agents are often recommended for anesthetic induction and maintenance, although it is likely that most anesthetic agents have been used in HOT patients without any perceived increase in anesthetic risk [14,19]. Since the main mechanism for decreased cardiac output in HOT patients is a decrease in myocardium contractility, drugs that directly decrease contractility, such as halothane, should be avoided [14,115]. Isoflurane produces a similar cardiovascular response (dose-dependent decrease in cardiac output and blood pressure) in euthryroid and hypothyroid dogs. Thus, isoflurane is a suitable anesthetic for hypothyroid dogs and, as in any patient, cardiovascular depression can be minimized by using balanced anesthetic techniques [114].

Hyperthyroidism

Hyperthyroidism (HT) is one of the most common disorders of middle-aged and older cats and is usually caused by poorly controlled hypersecretion of thyroid hormone from autonomously hyperfunctional nodules of the thyroid gland [116]. The cause of this condition is unknown, but it is thought to be similar to toxic nodular goiter in human patients [117]. In people with this condition, activating mutations of the TSH receptor have been found. In rare cases, HT can be caused by thyroid carcinoma (1–2% of cats with thyrotoxicosis). HT is uncommon in dogs, and is seen in less than 20% of dogs with thyroid carcinoma [118]. In contrast to the cat, thyroid carcinomas are usually large and invasive in dogs.

The clinical signs of HT are caused by pathologically high overall metabolism due to sustained excessive circulating thyroid hormone concentrations [119]. Because of the nature of the disease, clinical signs are multisystemic. Excessive thyroid hormone causes hypertension, myocardial hypertrophy, chronic cellular malnutrition, hepatocellular stress, and decreased GI transit times. Thyrotoxicosis is also associated with an increased glomerular filtration rate that may mask underlying coexisting renal disease [120]. Historical findings include weight loss, polyphagia, vomiting, diarrhea, polyuria, polydipsia, hyperactivity, and behavioral changes that can range from depression to aggression. Physical examination findings include poor body condition, tachycardia, heart murmur, gallop rhythm, palpable thyroid nodules (unilateral or bilateral), and an unkempt hair coat (Fig. 31.6) [119].

The most common hematological abnormality in cats with HT is mild erythrocytosis (or a higher than expected normal RBC count) [119]. Increased alanine aminotransferase activity is the most common serum biochemical abnormality. Because of increased protein catabolism, there may be a mild or relative increase in blood urea nitrogen (BUN) concentration without a concurrent increase in the creatinine concentration. Increases in both BUN and creatinine typically signal the presence of concurrent renal disease, which complicates the treatment of HT [120].

Thoracic imaging (including echocardiography) may be useful in the assessment of cardiomegaly or associated congestive heart failure, or, in the case of dogs with HT, to investigate pulmonary metastases. Abdominal ultrasound may be performed in hyperthyroid cats to assess renal architecture and size, although further renal testing may better define renal function.

The finding of a high serum concentration of total thyroxine (T4) confirms the diagnosis in most cases [121], but some cats with HT have normal total T4 concentrations because of the presence of concurrent non-thyroidal disease or because of fluctuations in thyroid hormone concentrations. This condition is termed 'occult HT' [122] and can be diagnosed by several methods, including measurement of free T4 (which may be slightly more sensitive than total T4), repeat measurement of total T4, thyroid scintigraphy, or T3 suppression testing.

There are three main treatment options for feline HT. Radioiodine therapy is considered the treatment of choice because it is non-invasive, has few side-effects, and is effective in most cases [123]. Medical management of feline HT with methimazole or carbimazole is common, and is also effective [124]. Antithyroid drugs, however, often cause side-effects such as vomiting, self-induced facial excoriation, and anorexia. Life-threatening side-effects of antithyroid drugs are uncommon, and include thrombocytopenia, agranulocytosis, and hepatopathy. Surgical thyroidectomy is performed less commonly in cats than it was prior to the improved availability of radioiodine therapy, but it is still used in some cases [125]. Surgical complications include iatrogenic hypoparathyroidism, laryngeal paralysis, and HOT. Regardless of the mode of treatment, many cats with HT develop renal failure following treatment, and it is important that cats be monitored carefully in the post-treatment period [120].

Treatment of thyroid carcinoma in the dog depends on the size and stage of the tumor [118]. Small, non-invasive tumors may be treated with surgery alone, but most tumors are large and may not be surgically resectable. Radiation therapy (high doses of radioiodine or external beam radiation) and chemotherapy may be tried, but treatment is rarely curative. Many thyroid tumors are highly vascular and hemorrhage should be a consideration in the anesthetic planning.

Thyrotoxic storm, described as a syndrome of severe HT with exaggerated and life-threatening manifestations of the disease, occurs rarely in dogs and cats [126,127]. The condition has not been well described in veterinary patients, but it includes severe tachycardia, fever, GI signs, and central nervous system signs. The factors that precipitate a thyrotoxic storm are not well understood, and it is most commonly diagnosed in long-standing, previously

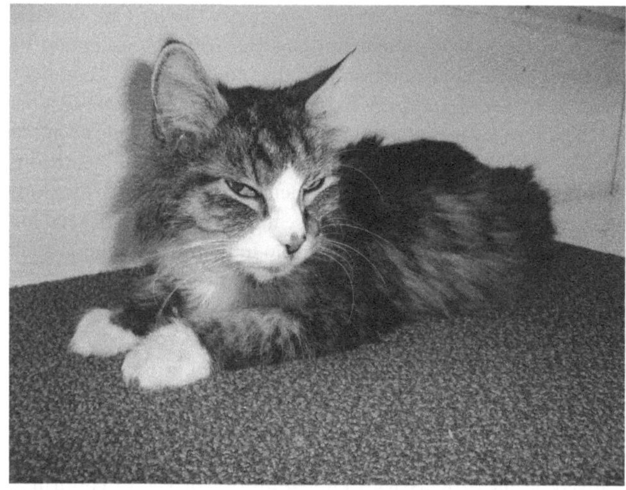

(a)

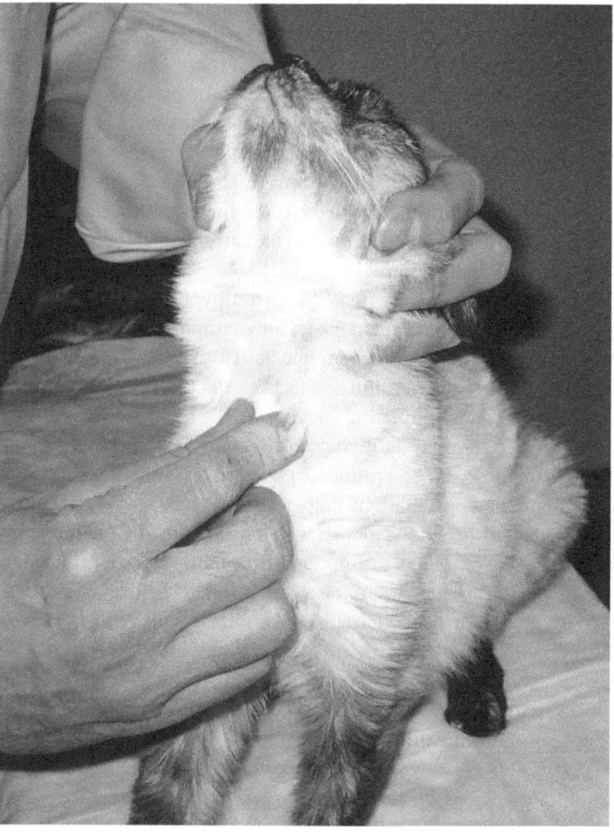

(b)

Figure 31.6 (a) A cat with HT, presented with weight loss and depression. These signs suggest poorly controlled HT and elective anesthesia should be delayed. Source: Dr Todd Green, Department of Small Animal Medicine and Surgery, St George's University, St George's, Grenada. Reproduced with permission of Todd Green. (b) Thyroid nodule palpation in a cat with HT. Source: Dr Thomas Graves, College of Veterinary Medicine, Midwestern University, Glendale, AZ, USA. Reproduced with permission of Thomas Graves.

undiagnosed, severe cases of HT. Laboratory findings are not dissimilar from typical presentations of HT with the exception of extremely high concentrations of thyroid hormone. Treatment involves the use of antithyroid drugs to decrease hormone synthesis, the use of iodine (oral potassium iodide, oral ipodate, or intravenous sodium iodide) to inhibit thyroid hormone secretion, treatment of hyperthermia, fluid therapy to correct dehydration, management of heart failure if present, β-adrenergic blockade for tachyarrhythmia, and corticosteroids to inhibit the peripheral conversion of T4 to the active hormone T3.

Anesthetic management

Attempts to make patients with HT euthyroid at the time of the anesthetic event are warranted in order to decrease the likelihood of tachycardia, hypertension, and increased myocardial work under anesthesia. Therefore, a thyroid panel should be performed preoperatively in all patients with known history of HT to confirm a euthyroid state. If total T4 or free T4 is above the reference range, treatment with carbimazole or methimazole for 6–12 weeks is indicated to minimize anesthetic (e.g., arrhythmias) and surgical complications [128]. In emergency cases, these patients should be stabilized before anesthesia as described in the previous section.

A thorough examination of the cardiovascular system is warranted in cats with HT as concurrent hypertrophic cardiomyopathy is common. A gallop rhythm, arrhythmia (e.g., ventricular tachycardia), or a systolic murmur may be detected on the physical examination. Preoperative arterial blood pressure measurement and renal testing should be performed in these cats [22].

Many cats with HT are treated with antihypertensive drugs [22]. β-Adrenergic receptor antagonists, for example, atenolol, are used to oppose the increased adrenergic activity seen with HT that is associated with hypertension and tachycardia [21,129]. Amlodipine or an angiotensin-converting enzyme (ACE) inhibitor may also be administered for their antihypertensive effects in hyperthyroid cats [129]. All these drugs produce significant vasodilation and may contribute to hypotension intraoperatively.

The goals of anesthesia for cats with lone HT are to avoid increases in myocardial oxygen consumption, hypertension, tachycardia, and arrhythmias. Stress should also be avoided before anesthesia. Acepromazine or benzodiazepines combined with opioids can be included in the preanesthetic medication [130]. Acepromazine reduces the sensitivity of the myocardium to catecholamines and blocks α-adrenergic receptors, hence it may help decrease the occurrence of catecholamine-induced arrhythmias and counteract hypertension. However, its use should be avoided when the patient is on antihypertensive medication or has cardiomyopathy. Opioids are desirable because generally they slow the heart rate and decrease myocardial oxygen consumption. Anticholinergics should not be routinely administered pre-emptively, as parasympathetic blockade can lead to an increase in myocardial oxygen consumption and increased arrhythmogenicity. Anticholinergics (preferably glycopyrrolate) may be cautiously administered when bradycardia and hypotension are present. Induction can be accomplished with propofol, alfaxalone, or etomidate. In the absence of an intravenous catheter, induction can be performed with inhalant anesthetics (isoflurane or sevoflurane) via a chamber, depending on the cat's temperament. It is important to keep in mind that stress associated with this technique, especially in a non-premedicated or aggressive cat, can be detrimental. Ketamine should be avoided because it stimulates sympathetic output and may cause an increase in heart rate and a decrease in ventricular filling [14,19,130].

For anesthetic maintenance, any of the potent inhalant anesthetic agents may be used. It is most important to establish and maintain adequate anesthetic depth to avoid exaggerated sympathetic nervous system responses [21]. The increased metabolic rate seen in hyperthyroid patients increases the demand for oxygen and glucose, and production of carbon dioxide. They are therefore more prone to hypoxemia and hypercarbia when ventilation is compromised. Cardiovascular (including arterial blood pressure and heart rhythm) and respiratory parameters should be monitored closely and ventilation controlled when necessary [19].

Cardiomyopathy caused by HT in cats is usually concentric, which decreases ventricular compliance and chamber size, leading to diastolic dysfunction. The goals of the anesthetic protocol used in cats with cardiomyopathy is to optimize ventricular filling by preventing stress, and maintaining a normal to low heart rate [131,132]. By maintaining good preload and a normal diastolic interval, ventricular filling, myocardial blood flow, and ventricular function are improved [19]. As for cats with lone HT, sedation in cats with cardiomyopathy is indicated in most cases and drugs that result in sympathetic stimulation (e.g., ketamine, nitrous oxide, desflurane) should be avoided. Although acepromazine decreases myocardial sensitivity to catecholamines, vasodilation and a decrease in systemic vascular resistance in cats with diastolic dysfunction could result in hypotension. In HT cats with hypertrophic obstructive cardiomyopathy, acepromazine may increase the gradient across the left ventricular outflow tract, worsening the obstruction. Therefore, acepromazine should be avoided. α_2-Adrenergic receptor agonists (medetomidine or dexmedetomidine) can be used as an alternative for preanesthetic medication of stressed cats with dynamic left ventricular outflow tract obstruction provided that systolic function is not reduced [132].

Although rare, untreated or poorly managed HT patients may develop thyrotoxic storm in the postoperative period. This is manifested by an increased heart rate, increased blood pressure, cardiac dysrhythmias, fever, and shock [19]. Monitoring of heart rate and rhythm, arterial blood pressure, and body temperature should be continued throughout recovery.

Thyroid neoplasia

In dogs, most thyroid tumors are non-functional and do not secrete excessive thyroid hormone. These tumors are usually carcinomas that may locally invade adjacent tissues – the larynx, trachea, cervical muscles, nerves, and esophagus. Pulmonary metastasis also often occurs [111].

Dogs with thyroid tumors usually present with a large space-occupying lesion on the ventral neck region (Fig. 31.7). Clinical signs are associated with the size of the tumor and secondary damage to the cervical tissues. Common clinical signs include airway compromise/obstruction, dyspnea, cough, vomiting, dysphagia, anorexia, and weight loss [19,111].

Diagnostics include biopsy of the mass and serum thyroid hormone concentrations. Thoracic radiographs may also be taken to identify pulmonary metastasis [111]. A CT or MRI scan of the neck is also useful to demonstrate anatomic abnormalities of the neoplastic and surrounding tissue [19]. The main treatment for thyroid carcinoma in dogs is excision of the tumor if pulmonary metastasis is not present. Radiation therapy can be effective in controlling tumors that cannot be completely excised [111].

Anesthetic management

Maintenance of a patent airway can represent the greatest challenge in the anesthetic management of dogs with large thyroid

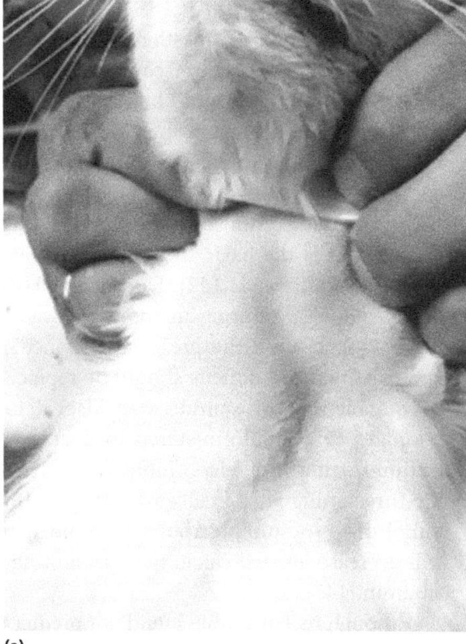

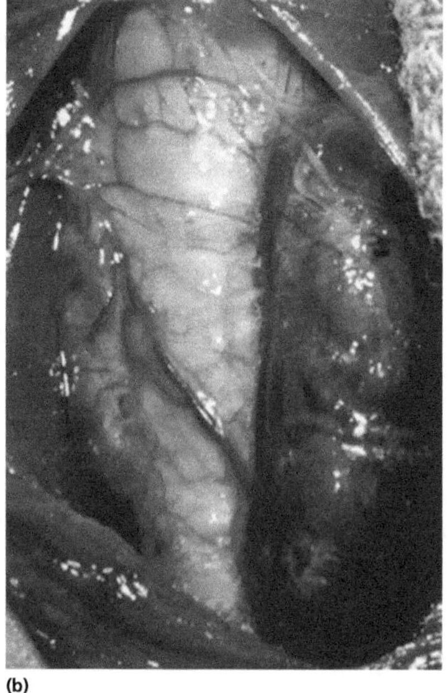

(a) (b)

Figure 31.7 (a) Although large thyroid masses are most common in dogs, cats may sometimes be diagnosed with this disease. Large space-occupying masses can be associated with respiratory distress prior to anesthesia and may represent a challenge for endotracheal intubation. Source: Dr Robert Sherding, Department of Veterinary Clinical Sciences, The Ohio State University, Columbus, OH, USA. Reproduced with permission of Robert Sherding. (b) Large mass in the ventral neck compressing the trachea. Airway obstruction may occur in recovery due to edema and hemorrhage. Source: Dr Stephen Birchard, Circle City Veterinary Specialty and Emergency Hospital, Carmel, IN, USA. Reproduced with permission of Stephen Birchard.

tumors. Any airway obstruction present in the awake patient will be exacerbated with sedation and anesthesia until an endotracheal tube is successfully placed across the obstruction. Obstruction can be caused by mechanical compression or nerve damage due to tumor invasion of surrounding tissues. Swelling and hemorrhage may also compromise respiration in recovery [19]. Any history of exercise intolerance or respiratory distress should be investigated. A thorough physical examination of the neck and close observation of respiratory effort should be performed. Potent sedatives such as α_2-adrenergic receptor agonists, although extremely useful to calm excitable dogs, can also produce intense neck muscle relaxation and may exacerbate any airway obstruction. If the patient would benefit from the calming effects of α_2-adrenergic receptor agonists, the anesthetist should not leave it unattended after drug administration, and induction drugs and intubation equipment should be readily available in case airway obstruction occurs. Preoxygenation is also recommended if the patient will tolerate it. Induction of anesthesia should be rapidly achieved without excitement. For this reason, an intravenous anesthetic technique (e.g., propofol) is the preferred method rather than mask induction with inhalant anesthetics. A preoperative history of dyspnea and/or exercise intolerance is predictive of possible airway obstruction during induction of anesthesia, and endotracheal intubation may be difficult. A tracheostomy pack should be available in case orotracheal intubation is not possible. Alternatively, orotracheal intubation can be performed with the aid of a fiber-optic bronchoscope, which can also be used to assess the degree of tracheal obstruction. If the thyroid mass is large, a reinforced endotracheal tube can help prevent obstruction of the tube. Intraoperatively, analgesics such as opioids (e.g., fentanyl, hydromorphone, methadone) and NSAIDs should be provided as indicated. In case of airway obstruction, both opioids and α_2-adrenergic receptor agonists can be readily reversed. However, caution should be exercised when NSAIDs are administered pre-emptively. Because thyroidectomy can potentially cause severe hemorrhage, some NSAIDs may reduce platelet function, resulting in impaired hemostasis. Additionally, impairment of renal autoregulation by NSAIDs can result in postoperative renal injury if hypovolemia is severe.

Postoperative complications from thyroidectomy include local hemorrhage and edema with tracheal compression, unilateral or bilateral damage to the recurrent laryngeal nerve, and inadvertent damage to or removal of the parathyroid glands [21,111]. Tracheal extubation should be performed with anticipation of complications and provisions for immediate reintubation [21]. If possible, extubation should be delayed until the patient is conscious and alert. Intravenous anesthetic, laryngoscope, and endotracheal tubes or a tracheostomy pack should be readily available in case of airway obstruction due to hematoma formation in the ventral neck or laryngeal paralysis. If airway obstruction occurs, the patient should be reanesthetized, a patent airway established, and oxygen and ventilation initiated. The cause of obstruction should be investigated. For example, the surgical wound should be evaluated and the patient may return to the operating room if a hematoma is palpated, and bleeding vessels should be secured to relieve airway obstruction.

Measurement of ionized calcium is also recommended postoperatively following bilateral thyroidectomy to identify damage to or loss of parathyroid function. Observation for clinical signs of hypocalcemia such as stiffness or tetany should be continued for at least 48 h postoperatively. Lastly, whenever a neck bandage is placed following surgery, it should be evaluated and monitored closely for effects on ventilation.

Parathyroid gland

Dogs and cats have four parathyroid glands, two embedded at the cranial pole of each lobe of the thyroid gland and two external to the gland. The structure of the parathyroid glands differs greatly from that of the thyroid gland, with densely packed cells surrounding capillary vessels [102]. Parathyroid hormone or parathormone (PTH) is produced and secreted by the parathyroid glands in response to calcium concentrations. PTH is very effective at increasing serum calcium via three main mechanisms: PTH (1) stimulates activity of osteoclasts to reabsorb bone, (2) encourages absorption of calcium from the gastrointestinal tract (GIT) via the activated form of vitamin D (produced in the kidney), and (3) discourages excretion of calcium in the urine [133]. When excessive amounts of PTH are produced, calcification of soft tissues occurs, with resultant dysfunction of the affected structures or organs.

Hyperparathyroidism

Primary hyperparathyroidism (PHPT) is an uncommon disorder of middle-aged and older dogs and is very rare in cats [134–136]. In most cases, PHPT is caused by a singular benign adenoma of an extracapsular parathyroid gland. These adenomas are small and usually non-palpable in the dog but may be palpable in the cat. Parathyroid adenocarcinomas are very rare. The present discussion is focused on PHPT in the dog.

Parathyroid adenomas autonomously secrete parathyroid hormone (PTH), causing hypercalcemia. In many cases of PHPT, the diagnosis is made after the investigation of a serendipitous finding of hypercalcemia because most dogs with PHPT show no clinical signs. Among those dogs showing clinical signs of hypercalcemia, PU/PD and signs of lower urinary tract inflammation are most common [136]. These signs are typically mild and are the direct result of hypercalcemia. Diagnosis of PHPT requires the demonstration of ionized hypercalcemia, a low or low-normal serum phosphorus concentration, and an inappropriately high concentration of PTH. It should be noted that a normal concentration of PTH in the face of hypercalcemia is inappropriate, and is indicative of PHPT [137]. Diagnostic investigation of PHPT may also include ultrasonography of the ventral cervical area to identify a parathyroid adenoma. Calcium-containing uroliths and associated urinary tract infections are fairly common in dogs with PHPT, so ultrasound of the urinary system, urinalysis, and bacterial culture of the urine are also important components of the diagnostic work-up [136].

Once diagnosed, PHPT is most often treated by surgical parathyroidectomy, which is curative. Other less invasive forms of treatment have been described, including percutaneous ultrasound-guided ablation using either heat or ethanol [138]. Intraoperative measurement of PTH, which has a serum half-life of approximately 2 min, has been used to indicate surgical cure [139]. The most common complication of treatment is postoperative hypocalcemia, which develops upon withdrawal of PTH-secreting tissue because the remaining non-adenomatous glands have atrophied due to chronic hypercalcemia. There are no known predictors of postoperative hypocalcemia, so ionized calcium concentrations must be monitored carefully in the postoperative period [140]. Clinical signs of hypocalcemia include anorexia, facial pruritis, GI signs, and neurological signs. Postoperative treatment of hypocalcemia requires administration of calcitriol and calcium supplementation. In such cases, normal parathyroid function will return, but the duration of treatment required is unpredictable.

Anesthetic management

The mainstay of the preanesthetic preparation of dogs with PHPT is to evaluate serum calcium concentration and treat symptomatic patients. Anesthesia should be delayed in patients when the total calcium (tCa) is greater than 15–16 mg/dL (3.75–4 mmol/L), because most dogs will have clinical signs when the tCa exceeds this concentration [19].

Intravenous administration of 0.9% sodium chloride (100–125 mL/kg/day) is the basic therapy to decrease tCa in symptomatic dogs with PHPT [141,142]. Dogs with PHPT may also be volume depleted due to vomiting and polyuria; water should be available to these patients until the preanesthetic medication is administered and existing fluid deficits should be replaced. Once the patient is normovolemic, furosemide, steroids, calcitonin, and/or bisphosphonates can be administered to decrease the calcium concentration further if needed (Table 31.4) [21,141,143]. In cases with life-threatening hypercalcemia [tCa >18–20 mg/dL (4.5–5.0 mmol/dL)], sodium bicarbonate, administered IV as a slow bolus, will decrease ionized calcium by promoting binding of calcium to albumin [141].

Although recent studies could not predict that a high serum ionized calcium present preoperatively is associated with postoperative hypocalcemia, some authors recommend treating dogs orally with active vitamin D metabolites such as calcitriol preoperatively, based on the presumption that a higher magnitude of preoperative hypercalcemia [total calcium >14–15 mg/dL (3.5–3.75 mmol/dL)] leads to more severe atrophy of the remaining parathyroid glands [141]. Calcitriol primes the gut for increased calcium absorption [141] and can be started 3–5 days prior to parathyroidectomy [34]. Careful monitoring of serum calcium and clinical signs should be continued during this period prior to surgery and calcitriol therapy discontinued if hypercalcemia worsens.

Chronic hypercalcemia can cause chronic kidney disease (CKD) in some dogs [21,144]; however, a definitive diagnosis of CKD may be challenging based on low urine specific gravity (USG) and azotemia owing to the diuretic effects of hypercalcemia. The presence or suspicion of CKD is another reason to maintain adequate hydration status before anesthesia [34].

There are no anesthetic drugs or techniques specifically indicated for dogs with primary hyperparathyroidism undergoing elective surgical treatment. Maintenance of hydration and urine output should continue during anesthesia, preferably with a calcium-free isotonic

Table 31.4 Treatments for hypercalcemia in hyperparathyroid dogs [141, 143].

Treatment	Dose	Comments
0.9% saline	90–120 mL/kg q 24 h IV	Volume expansion dilutes serum Ca^{2+}; extra Na^{+} in renal tubules ↓ Ca^{2+} reabsorption
Furosemide[a]	2–4 mg/kg q 8–12 h IV	↑ Ca^{2+} loss in urine ↓ reabsorption in bone
Prednisone	1–2 mg/kg q 12 h PO	↓ intestinal absorption
Dexamethasone	0.1–0.2 mg/kg q 12 h IV	↑excretion in urine
Calcitonin	4–6 IU/kg q 8–12 h SC	↓ activity of osteoclasts
Pamidronate	1.3–2 mg/kg in 150 mL 0.9% NaCl IV over 2–4 h	Inhibits osteoclast-mediated bone resorption ↑ Ca^{2+} uptake by bone
Sodium bicarbonate	1 mEq/kg IV slowly up to 4 mEq/kg	↑ binding of Ca^{2+} to albumin Emergency situations only

↑, increase; ↓, decrease; q, every.

[a]Not all diuretics are useful, e.g., avoid thiazides: they cause acidosis, which increases ionized Ca^{2+}.

crystalloid solution (e.g., 0.9% NaCl, Plasmalyte 148, or Normosol R) in patients with high ionized calcium. The existence of lethargy preoperatively may indicate that the patient's intraoperative anesthetic requirements could be decreased. Hypercalcemia might be expected to antagonize the effects of non-depolarizing muscle relaxants [21]; however, these agents are rarely administered to patients undergoing parathyroidectomy. The ECG should be monitored closely for bradycardia, prolonged PR interval, widened QRS complex, and shortened QT interval, although these are likely only in severely affected animals [141,143]. Periodic blood-gas analysis is warranted to monitor electrolytes and acid–base status, particularly if sodium bicarbonate has been administered to control hypercalcemia.

Following parathyroidectomy, there is risk of acute hypoparathyroidism due to atrophy of the remaining parathyroid glands. These dogs require frequent monitoring for hypocalcemia during the first 48 h postoperatively [19,141]. A central intravenous catheter is useful for frequent blood sampling and may be placed in recovery. Hypocalcemia without clinical signs usually does not require treatment unless the total serum calcium is <6 mg/d (<1.5 mmol/L) [141]. Intervention is also necessary when the total or ionized calcium concentration trend decreases suddenly [34]. These dogs should be monitored for excitement or anxiety, muscle tremors, and tetany. If clinical signs appear, intravenous calcium should be administered slowly to effect via a separate intravenous line. A loading dose of 10% calcium gluconate solution (9.3 mg calcium/mL) at 0.5–1.5 mL/kg (50–150 mg/kg) is administered IV over 10 min, followed by an infusion at 5–15 mg/kg/h (0.05–0.15 mL/kg/h). The heart rate should be monitored closely during the infusion of calcium. If it decreases markedly or if absolute bradycardia develops, the infusion should be stopped and then restarted at a slower rate after a few minutes. Progressive shortening of the QT interval on the ECG should also prompt a slower rate of calcium infusion. Oral calcitriol therapy and calcium supplements are also continued or started postoperatively [34]. Hemorrhage and airway compromise are always a concern when surgery is performed around the larynx/trachea, but may be less common with this procedure as parathyroid tumors are usually not very large. If a bandage is placed, it should be evaluated and monitored closely for effects on ventilation.

Anatomy of the gastrointestinal tract

The GIT of small animals is a continuous multilayered tube with variations in size, shape, and function for each organ. It includes the oropharynx, esophagus, stomach, small intestine, colon, and rectum. The liver, biliary tract, and exocrine pancreas are also part of the GIT; however, owing to the significant role that the liver plays in homeostasis (e.g., metabolism, excretion, coagulation factor synthesis, and albumin production), hepatic function and disease are addressed in a separate chapter (see Chapter 30). The intestinal wall has four main layers: (from inside to outside) a mucosa, submucosa, a muscularis with two layers of smooth muscle (an inner circular layer and outer longitudinal layer), and the serosa. The muscular layers of the esophagus are an exception to this basic structure. The entire esophagus of the dog has striated muscle, whereas the cat, horse, pig, and primates have striated muscle in the proximal two-thirds and smooth muscle in the distal portion, including the esophago-gastric junction. The composition of the specialized epithelium of the mucosal layer varies with each organ, but all organs perform digestive, secretory, and absorptive functions in addition to providing immune protection and surveillance. Contraction of the muscular layers mixes and transports ingesta throughout the GIT. The external serosal layer is a thin membrane made up of secretory cells that produce and secrete serous fluid. This fluid lubricates the surface, facilitating motility by decreasing friction due to contact with itself and other abdominal organs [145,146].

The enteric nervous system (ENS) has extrinsic and intrinsic components, both supplied with parasympathetic (PS) and sympathetic input via the autonomic nervous system. The intrinsic component (SMP) includes the myenteric and submucosal plexuses. The myenteric plexus, located between the circular and longitudinal muscle layers, controls intestinal motility. The submucosal plexus, found between the submucosa and the inner circular muscle layer, coordinates motion of the luminal epithelium. Other minor plexuses are also found within muscle and submucosal layers.

The extrinsic ENS consists of parasympathetic innervation to the upper and lower GIT via the vagus and pelvic nerves, respectively, and sympathetic innervation via spinal segments T1–L3. Both afferent and efferent nerve fibers are contained within the same nerves. Preganglionic PS neurons have long fibers that synapse with ganglia of the myenteric or submucosal plexuses within the GIT. Whereas preganglionic SMP fibers synapse with ganglia just outside the GIT, the postganglionic SMP neurons travel into the GIT itself, synapsing with the intrinsic plexuses and directly on to receptors in the intestine. Acetylcholine (ACh) is the neurotransmitter released by all preganglionic fibers. Postganglionic PS neurons may utilize ACh or various peptides such as substance P (SP), vasoactive intestinal peptide (VIP), neuropeptide Y (NPY), or gastrin-releasing peptide (GRP). Postganglionic SMP neurons release norepinephrine. In addition to the cholinergic, adrenergic, and peptidergic receptors, many other receptor types are found in the GIT that modify secretory, endocrine, and muscular activity. Receptors for μ- and δ-opioids, several serotonin types, and histamine are just a few [145–147].

Intestinal motility relies on two major patterns of muscular activity, the migrating motor complexes (MMC) seen during fasting, and a digestive pattern that begins when foodstuffs enter the stomach. MMCs are seen in dogs and humans, but motility in cats is controlled by a migrating spike complex pattern that is somewhat weaker than the MMC. The interstitial cells of Cajal, located within the myenteric plexuses, are specialized pacemaker cells that create and maintain MMCs. These are so-called 'slow waves' of depolarization that spread via gap junctions between smooth muscle cells over large sections of intestine but remain below the depolarization threshold for propulsive contractions. This activity provides a very effective housekeeping function for the intestine, moving residual fluid, mucus, bacteria, and cellular debris aborally during the interdigestive period. As a food bolus arrives, electrical activity increases and the digestive pattern begins. Sphincters and sections of intestine in the path of the bolus relax to allow entry as other sections contract in a segmental or propulsive fashion. Ingesta is mixed and moved along the GIT using the circular and longitudinal muscles, respectively. Feedback inhibition also occurs along the tract to 'brake' the intestine, providing longer and more thorough contact for digestion. Both the digestive and interdigestive patterns are controlled by the parasympathetic nervous system, with ACh and SP responsible for contraction and VIP and nitric oxide producing relaxation. Sympathetic input is primarily inhibitory, seen during times of stress, excitement, anxiety, fear, or pain. Numerous neurotransmitters and hormones are involved in the initiation and processing of the digestive phase, affecting motility, secretion, digestion, absorption, and blood flow [145,147–149].

Effects of anesthetic agents on gastrointestinal function

In healthy patients, the effects of most anesthetic agents on the GIT are usually short-lived as normal function returns with the decline of drug levels. Some adjunctive agents may have somewhat longer actions and decisions about their use should be made with an understanding of the primary GI problem, pre-existing or concurrent illness or organ dysfunction, and effects of surgery since these may obscure and/or compound the effects of the anesthetic drugs. Prolonged effects well into the postoperative period have the potential to affect outcome, especially in ruminant and equine patients where bloat and colic are significant risks following anesthesia and surgery.

Physiologic abnormalities encountered during anesthesia may produce signs of GI dysfunction and could be confused with direct effects of anesthetic drugs. These include dehydration, hypovolemia, hypotension, anemia, protein and electrolyte abnormalities, acid–base derangements, hypoxia, myocardial dysfunction, hypothermia, and changes in autonomic nervous system tone. Vomiting patients may be alkalotic due to loss of H^+ and Cl^- but eventually become acidotic with significant volume loss and/or tissue ischemia. As with all patients, preanesthetic evaluation of and treatment for any abnormalities of patient status are necessary to minimize the effects of anesthesia and maximize the potential for a positive outcome.

Effects of surgery that may significantly affect perioperative GI function (and sometimes anesthetic management) include manipulation/handling of intestine and/or abdominal masses, hemorrhage, and correction of the underlying GI problem (e.g., reperfusion of the stomach following derotation of a gastric dilation and volvulus). The surgeon should work together with anesthetist to minimize the effects of both surgery and anesthesia on perioperative GI function.

The effects of anesthetic agents on the GIT include changes in saliva production, nausea, vomiting, ileus, regurgitation, gastroesophageal reflux (GER), constipation, reduced secretion of digestive fluids, and aerophagia (associated with panting). Although there is considerable overlap of the effects of most drugs (e.g., opioids, α_2-adrenergic receptor agonists, anticholinergics, and inhalants all reduce motility), some effects tend to be more specific (e.g., anticholinergics reduce the volume of saliva but increase the viscosity). Ileus can result in tympany, especially if microbial gas production continues at a high rate as seen in ruminants and equine patients. In small animals, some suggest that this could be a contributing factor to the rare occurrence of gastric dilation or gastric dilation–volvulus (GDV) seen in dogs postoperatively.

Concurrent or chronic illness may complicate the clinical picture. For example, diabetic patients may suffer from gastroparesis and delayed gastric emptying secondary to autonomic neuropathy [150], and may be more likely to develop reflux, esophagitis, and/or vomiting postoperatively. Stress of disease and hospitalization also predispose patients to GI dysfunction, especially gastric ulceration and diarrhea. If anesthetic drugs are the primary cause of GI dysfunction in patients, many of these signs (e.g., ileus, nausea, vomiting) should resolve relatively quickly following cessation of drug administration. If they persist or are severe, further evaluation of the patient is warranted to ensure that another cause is not present (e.g., GI foreign body, GDV, or GI ulceration).

The most significant perianesthetic complications associated with GI dysfunction include pulmonary aspiration and/or esophagitis following vomiting, regurgitation, or GER, and postoperative ileus (POI). Aspiration may cause pneumonitis, pneumonia, and severe hypoxemia, which can result in cardiac arrest. Esophagitis, although common following anesthesia, when severe or untreated may result in stricture of the esophageal lumen, which can result in persistent vomiting, regurgitation, dysphagia, weight loss, and debilitation. POI greatly affects patient comfort following surgery and can affect outcome. It results in a greater incidence of nausea and vomiting, poor wound healing, delayed oral intake and mobility, increases the risk of respiratory and other system complications, and longer hospital stays with greater costs [151,152].

Nausea and vomiting

Nausea and vomiting are common adverse effects of anesthetic agents, especially in human patients. The underlying mechanisms of emesis are complex, as several emetic mechanisms result in vomiting. A humoral pathway is stimulated by blood-borne substances that affect the chemoreceptor trigger zone (CTZ) whereas a neural pathway activates the vomiting center (VC). Vomiting results when the VC is directly stimulated by one or more of several neurotransmitters. Histamine, acetylcholine, dopamine, serotonin (5HT and $5HT_3$), and neurokinin-1 (NK-1 or substance P) are important neurotransmitters in the VC. Dopamine, serotonin, and α_2-adrenergic receptors are found in the CTZ. Located outside the blood–brain barrier (BBB), the CTZ is sensitive to low levels of emetic agents in the circulation. Input from the cerebral cortex (anxiety, anticipation), the vestibular apparatus (motion sickness), and local damage to the GIT also directly stimulate the VC. Mucosal irritation and damage or distention of GI tissues results in emesis via the release of serotonin and/or stimulation of vagal afferent receptors [148,153–156].

While many opioids are associated with a high incidence of vomiting (e.g., morphine and hydromorphone), antiemesis has also been reported. This effect is thought to occur when increased numbers of opioid receptors in the VC are stimulated, as with very lipophilic opioids (fentanyl and congeners) or when given intravenously, especially at higher doses (butorphanol). This may also be the reason why vomiting is seen primarily after the first dose of opioids and is uncommon following subsequent doses [157,158].

The incidence of vomiting seen with anesthetic drugs is variable and depends on species, drugs used, dosage, route and timing of administration, presence/absence of pain, and concurrent medical problems. Aerophagia and repeated swallowing of blood and saliva (especially following dentistry procedures) can also significantly increase the risk of vomiting during recovery. Although dogs and cats occasionally vomit during recovery, most vomiting occurs with premedication in these species. Since vomiting is an active process, it usually does not occur during maintenance of surgical anesthesia, but can be seen during light planes or during intubation as the vomiting reflex in dogs and cats is not abolished until Stage III/Plane 2 [159]. Inhalant anesthetics are a significant cause of postoperative nausea and vomiting (PONV) in humans [160], but the incidence appears to be much lower in veterinary species. Vomiting occurs occasionally at induction with propofol [161] and etomidate [162], when used alone in dogs, and in recovery following continuous infusion of propofol [163]. A clinical study that compared the incidence of adverse effects in dogs maintained with propofol versus isoflurane after propofol induction reported a very low incidence of vomiting or retching, with 4/91 in the isoflurane group and 1/58 in the propofol group. However, a surprisingly high incidence of hypersalivation was seen in these dogs in recovery, in just over 20% of both groups. No other signs suggestive of nausea were seen, and the dogs did not appear to be suffering pain. The authors did not identify a cause for the salivation [164]. Another study reported salivation in 7/40 (17.5%) and vomiting during recovery in 6/40 (15%) when propofol was used for induction following four different premedication protocols. Most (12/13) of these were dogs not given acepromazine. The one dog given acepromazine presented for vomiting and had been anesthetized for gastroscopy [165]. Anti-cholinergics were not used in either study.

α_2-Adrenergic receptor agonists and μ-opioid receptor agonists cause vomiting in dogs and cats [157,166–171]. The incidence of vomiting clinically appears to be more common at higher doses and is generally greater in cats than dogs. Vomiting was not reported with continuous infusions of very low doses of dexmedetomidine or medetomidine in healthy dogs and cats [172–174]. There is minimal difference in the incidence of vomiting between the different α_2-adrenergic receptor agonists in dogs and cats; however, a significant difference is seen with different opioids. Morphine, meperidine, and hydromorphone (especially in cats), and to a lesser extent oxymorphone, are associated with the highest risk of vomiting. Vomiting is much less frequent with fentanyl and its derivatives, and is rare with methadone, butorphanol, and buprenorphine [157]. Vomiting is also less frequent with lower dosages and when patients are fasted prior to administration.

Acepromazine (ACP) has a mild antiemetic effect via dopamine antagonism in the chemoreceptor trigger zone. Its antihistamine effects may also contribute when morphine or meperidine is given concurrently [175,176].

Other drugs given during anesthesia may cause vomiting. Up to 75% of dogs administered a very high dose of lidocaine (200 μg/kg/min) as a continuous infusion during sevoflurane anesthesia vomited in recovery. When the dose was reduced (50 μg/kg/min) vomiting did not occur postoperatively [177]. In contrast, decreased nausea and vomiting were seen in humans treated with a lidocaine CRI for abdominal surgery [178,179].

Antiemetic therapy

Metoclopramide is a central dopamine (D_2) receptor antagonist that has been used for many years as an antiemetic in dogs. It also has prokinetic effects on the stomach, duodenum, and jejunum, and has some muscarinic and serotonin receptor ($5\text{-}HT_3$ antagonist/$5\text{-}HT_4$ agonist) actions at higher doses. The serotonin antagonist group (e.g., ondansetron, dolasetron, palonosetron) and the NK-1 antagonist maropitant have proven useful to prevent or decrease emesis caused by chemotherapeutic agents [180,181], α_2-adrenergic receptor agonists [182], and opioids [183,184].

Dexamethasone is an effective antiemetic in humans for the prophylactic treatment of PONV [185,186]. Its use decreases the frequency of vomiting in cats induced by xylazine, but high doses are necessary [187]. The anti-inflammatory, anti-immune, and adverse endocrine and GI effects probably preclude its routine use as a prophylactic antiemetic in veterinary patients.

Benzodiazepines, phenothiazines, and butyrophenones have been shown to have antiemetic effects in humans. Droperidol was formerly used frequently in small animals as a sedative, especially in combination with fentanyl (Innovar-Vet®). Droperidol is considered a highly effective antiemetic in humans; however, the risk of cardiac arrhythmias precluded its use for a time [185]. Adverse effects such as sedation, excitement, extrapyramidal effects, and the availability of better alternatives preclude the routine use of butyrophenones as antiemetics in veterinary medicine.

Gastroesophageal reflux

GER occurs commonly in dogs and cats under general anesthesia; incidence varies from 0 to 66% of cases. Numerous studies have investigated the occurrence of GER under many conditions and with numerous anesthetic agents (Table 31.5) [188–203].

Gastroesophageal reflux disease (GERD) is a common syndrome in humans, where it is reported to occur in 5–20% of adults, but may be as high as 40% in some areas [204,205]. The mechanisms of reflux in GERD include abnormally low lower esophageal sphincter (LES) pressure (LESP) and increased frequency and duration of transient lower esophageal sphincter relaxations (TLSRs). TLSRs are normal events that occur to vent gas formed in the stomach; they are most often seen following ingestion of food. TLSRs do not occur during general anesthesia in dogs and humans or deep sleep in humans [204,206–208].

Although the specific mechanism of anesthetic induced GER is unclear, reflux occurs when intragastric pressure exceeds or equals the LESP, and the barrier pressure (BP) normally present between the two areas is lost [204,206,207,209]. Intra-abdominal and intrathoracic pressure also contribute to LESP and the incidence of GER. The LES is actually a functional sphincter, an area of higher intraluminal pressure just above the cardia created by the circular arrangement of muscle layers in the distal esophagus in combination with the crura of the diaphragm. It remains in a tonically contracted state until stimulated to relax via relaxation of the upper esophageal sphincter and/or waves of peristaltic contractions higher in the esophagus. The anatomic position of the distal esophagus in relation to the right diaphragmatic crus results in an angled orientation to the stomach that also contributes to effective closure of the LES and prevention of retrograde flow of contents under normal conditions. Relaxation of the diaphragmatic crus and the LES must occur for TLSRs to take place in awake patients [204,206,207,210].

Although primarily controlled by the parasympathetic nervous system, numerous neurotransmitters and hormones are involved in regulation of LES tone (Table 31.6) [145,208].

Clinical GERD is much less common in dogs and cats than humans but has been identified in both species. Brachycephalic breeds may be predisposed [211]. It is likely underdiagnosed since mild cases may not result in clinical signs [212,213]. Numerous anesthetic drugs and

Table 31.5 Anesthetic protocols, procedures, and other factors associated with the incidence of regurgitation or GER in dogs except where specifically noted [188–203].

Increased Incidence of GER	Decreased Incidence of GER
Gastric acidity	Short fast, 3 h vs 10 h
Abdominal procedures	High-dose metoclopramide infusion
Orthopedic procedures	Meperidine vs morphine but poor sedation
Imaging studies	Diazepam vs atropine/propionylpromazine
Greater with propofol vs thiopental	No difference
Morphine, ↑ with higher doses also	Recumbency or head tilt
Medetomidine vs acepromazine/opioid	Halothane vs isoflurane vs ievoflurane
Older dogs, sicker dogs (ASA ≥3)	Vomiting following premedication
Longer anesthetic duration	Standard (17.3 h) vs short fast (4.7 h)
Prolonged fasting	
LMA vs endotracheal tube (kittens)	
Humans:	*Other factors*
Full stomach	Dogs that reflux early regurgitate more often
Late pregnancy	Prolonged fasting increases gastric acidity
Altered consciousness	Short fast (3 h) and half volume canned food
LMA (some types)	↑ gastric pH, no difference in volume

LMA, laryngeal mask airway.

Table 31.6 Neurotransmitters and hormones that affect lower esophageal sphincter (LES) pressure [145, 208].

Decrease LES Tone	Increase LES Tone
Nitric oxide and nitrates	Prostaglandin E
Vasoactive intestinal peptide	Muscarinic M_2, M_3 receptor agonists
Nicotine	Gastrin
β-Adrenergic agonists	Substance P
Dopamine	α-Adrenergic agonists
Cholecystokinin	Prostaglandin Fα
Secretin	Motilin
Calcitonin gene-related peptide	
Adenosine	

Table 31.7 Effects of anesthetic agents, analgesics, sedatives, adjunct medications, and miscellaneous factors on lower esophageal pressure in dogs, cats, and/or humans [209, 214–222].

Decrease LESP	Increase LESP	No Change
Inhalants Nitrous oxide* Atropine, glycopyrrolate Acepromazine	Acetylcholine Anticholinesterases Metoclopramide Domperidone	Nitrous oxide*
Dexmedetomidine (high doses) Xylazine		Dexmedetomidine
Benzodiazepines Morphine Meperidine Oxymorphone Fentanyl–droperidol Tricyclic antidepressants		Remifentanil
Propofol (high doses) Thiopental Alfaxalone Ketamine# Xylazine/ketamine#		Propofol
β-Adrenergic agonists Nitroprusside Calcium channel blockers Aminophyllines	α-Adrenergic stimulants	Propranolol Metropolol
Residual neuromuscular blockade (NMB)	Succinylcholine Pancuronium Vecuronium (small increase) Edrophonium Neostigmine	Atracurium NMB reversal with neostigmine and glycopyrrolate
Cisapride	Histamine Antacids	Histamine 2 blockers (H2B) cimetidine, ranitidine Proton pump inhibitors (PPIs)
Cricoid pressure Pregnancy Obesity Hiatal hernia Laryngeal mask airway Dorsal vs lateral recumbency Change from lateral to dorsal	Gastric acidification ↑ gastric or abdominal pressure	

*Conflicting results concerning nitrous oxide.
#Ketamine decreased LESP compared with awake values, but it remained much higher than that with other drugs.

adjunct medications, including sedatives, analgesics, induction agents, inhalants, and anticholinergics, have been shown to decrease LESP in humans, dogs, and cats, predisposing patients under general anesthesia to GER (Table 31.7) [209,214–222].

Although one group did not find a difference [188], others have identified a higher incidence of reflux with long durations of preoperative fasting in dogs. GER is more frequent with intra-abdominal and orthopedic procedures in dogs [191–194], and is seen more often in dogs than cats. Vomiting associated with premedication prior to anesthesia was not associated with increased GER in dogs [196,197]; however, the occurrence of GER under anesthesia is variable and unpredictable.

In spite of numerous investigations, the mechanism of GER seen with general anesthesia has not been proven. Loss of the barrier pressure between the distal esophagus and the cardia must occur [204,206,207,209], but it is not clear what specifically triggers this phenomenon. Increasing LESP tone with a high dose of metoclopramide given continuously decreased the incidence but did not completely prevent reflux in dogs [202].

Most cases of anesthesia-related GER in dogs develop fairly soon following induction, usually before 30 min. Choice of premedication plays a role, as has been demonstrated by higher doses of morphine causing more GER than lower doses [197]. Pharyngeal stimulation may also be a factor as it decreases both upper and lower esophageal pressures. Minor pharyngeal stimulation elicited relaxation of the LES more than 50% of the time in opossums anesthetized with pentobarbital [223]. Subthreshold stimulus of the pharynx produces longitudinal esophageal muscle contraction and LES relaxation in humans [224]. Interestingly, GER was seen in 50% of kittens managed with an LMA versus 14% with an endotracheal tube [200]. Perhaps the combination of pharyngeal stimulation at and following induction combined with the effects of multiple anesthetic drugs during the time of transition into deeper levels of anesthesia is significant; however, this does not explain episodes of reflux that occur later during anesthesia or in those without endotracheal intubation [195]. Many factors are likely involved; the specific triggers may be multiple and variable with patients, drugs used, and other circumstances.

In spite of the high frequency of GER detected using pH or impedance monitoring in dogs and cats, the incidence of visible regurgitation (i.e., oral drainage of fluid) is much lower. In a large study of 4257 dogs at a referral practice over a 2 year period, regurgitation was visually confirmed in only 27 or 0.63% of cases, with large dogs and orthopedic procedures at highest risk [192]. Regurgitation was observed in 75 or 1.3% of 5736 dogs in another large study [193], where greater risk was seen with an ASA status ≥3, abdominal and/or imaging procedures, long anesthetic duration, and larger size. Dogs anesthetized for all types of procedures regurgitated less than 1% of the time, even though GER was identified in 16.3 and 17.4% of cases in two other investigations [189,191]. Dogs anesthetized for orthopedic procedures (following administration of different premedications and injectable and inhalant anesthetics) regurgitated 0–16.7% of the time when GER was identified in 25–63% of the cases [194,197,198,201]. In cats, regurgitation was reported in 2% and 0 cases with an incidence of GER of 14 and 22.5% [195,200].

Prevention of GER in anesthetized dogs has been attempted with H_2 receptor antagonists, proton pump inhibitors (PPIs), and prokinetic drugs. Although famotidine does increase gastric pH more reliably than ranitidine, pH is not maintained as well with H_2 receptor antagonists as with PPIs [225,226]. Omeprazole (OME) given preoperatively to 47 dogs decreased the number of times that acidic reflux was identified (4 with OME vs 13 in the control group), but since lower esophageal pH was the only means utilized to identify reflux, some reflux events may have been missed [227]. Metoclopramide alone has been shown to decrease the incidence of GER, but did not completely prevent it in dogs. This effect was seen only when given via continuous infusion at a high dose [202]. Intravenous metoclopramide, and/or ranitidine prior to anesthesia followed by a metoclopramide infusion, did not decrease the incidence of GER in dogs anesthetized for ovariohysterectomy [228]. A recent study in 61 dogs using both impedance and pH monitors found that although esomeprazole alone increased pH, the addition of cisapride decreased the incidence of reflux significantly from 8/21 with placebo to 2/18 in the combination group [229].

The effect of several palliative treatments for GER was examined in ten dogs with regurgitation under anesthesia [230]. Removal of reflux fluid from the esophagus via suctioning did not significantly change the esophageal pH, lavage with tap water increased the pH to >4.0, and the infusion of a small volume of sodium bicarbonate increased the pH to >6.0, an effect that lasted from 1.5 to 3 h. Topical therapy does not prevent further reflux and many not help if non-acidic reflux occurs, but it may be useful for acidic reflux to reduce the risk or severity of esophagitis. Suctioning and lavage may also be useful in cases with a large volume of regurgitation.

Prolonged fasting times have been associated with an increased risk of reflux and a lower gastric pH in anesthetized dogs [188,189]. Gastric volume was not significantly different and the pH was higher in dogs fed canned food at half their daily energy requirement and fasted 3 h compared with those fasted for 10 h [199]. In light of the evidence presented above, it may be time to consider the recommendation of shorter fasting times for veterinary patients scheduled for elective anesthetic procedures. Guidelines used by the American Society of Anesthesiologists (ASA) for fasting in humans were recently decreased for both adults and children. Clear liquids are allowed up to 2 h prior to anesthesia, milk-type liquids are allowed up to 4–6 h, and a light meal is allowed up to 6 h in all patients [231].

Although prevention of GER is difficult, vigilant monitoring to identify when it has occurred and appropriate intervention will minimize complications. Management recommendations include the following:

1 Observe patients following premedication, especially with heavy sedation, drugs that cause emesis (e.g., morphine, α_2-adrenergic receptor agonists).
2 Attain a secure airway (AW) quickly following induction.
3 The endotracheal tube (ET):
   - Correctly sized.
   - Properly lubricated.
   - Appropriate cuff inflation.
4 Recheck tube placement and cuff inflation, especially with transport, positioning.
5 Keep head tipped down to encourage drainage of GER away from airway.
6 Have supplies close by for suctioning, cleaning of pharynx, esophagus.
7 If vomiting occurs – get head down.
8 Recovery
   - Examine pharynx before extubation.
   - Lavage esophagus when large-volume GER has occurred.
   - Extubate with cuff partially inflated.
   - Position with head/nose down, lower than shoulder at all times.

Esophagitis and esophageal stricture

Esophagitis can occur when the esophageal mucosa is exposed to caustic substances for prolonged periods and/or when esophageal defense mechanisms (EDMs) are impaired or overwhelmed. The EDMs include a superficial mucus/bicarbonate barrier, tight junctions between epithelial cells, and an intracellular and interstitial buffering capacity that is dependent on blood flow. Lack of clearance of esophageal contents via intermittent swallowing is also a factor in anesthetized patients. Saliva provides dilution, bicarbonate to neutralize acid, and volume to flush the lumen of the esophagus. Resistance to 30 min of exposure to acid has been demonstrated; however, pepsin, trypsin, bile salts, and possibly other irritating/caustic substances may be as important as acids in causing esophageal damage [204,212,232].

Reviews of esophageal disease in small animals list the causes of esophagitis and/or esophageal stricture as GER, vomiting and/or regurgitation, ingestion of foreign bodies or caustic substances (including some medications such as doxycycline), motility disorders, congenital or anatomic abnormalities (e.g., hiatal hernia), trauma, neoplasia, and infection [213,233–235]. Retrospective studies have examined the incidence, risk factors, and outcome of esophagitis or stricture in dogs and cats [194,236–241]. An episode of general anesthesia was a significant risk factor for many cases, presumably caused by anesthesia-related GER. Leib *et al* [213] identified 18 of 28 (64%), Adamama-Moraitou *et al.* [239] found 13 of 20 (65%), and Kushner and Shofer [240] reported 25 of 30 (83%) patients with esophageal stricture diagnosed soon following general anesthesia. Overall mortality in these reports was 21, 30, and 30%, respectively. Greater risk of esophagitis was seen in patients anesthetized for intra-abdominal procedures, especially ovariohysterectomy [239]. Manipulation of abdominal structures is presumed to increase gastric pressure versus LESP, which is further decreased by anesthetic agents. Progesterone levels in intact females has been suggested to contribute to the decrease in LESP; however, a study of barrier pressure and GER in female dogs anesthetized four times during different phases of their reproductive cycle showed no effect of hormone levels on the barrier pressure or the incidence of GER or esophagitis [242]. In contrast to dogs, a study of esophageal disease in cats over a 7.5 year period found anesthesia to be involved in only one of 33 cases [236].

A very low incidence of postanesthetic esophageal dysfunction has been reported when all cases presented for anesthesia were examined retrospectively. Twenty-five patients with esophageal stricture following anesthesia were identified over a 10 year period at one institution (0.1% of cases) [240], and three cases of esophagitis and ten cases of esophageal stricture (total 13 cases representing 0.07% of caseload) occurred over 8 years at another [241]. Mortality associated with the esophageal complications was 30 and 23%, respectively. Vomiting and regurgitation occurred postoperatively in most or all of these patients. Weight loss and chronic cough were also seen in some dogs (Fig. 31.8) [241].

Although esophageal dysfunction following anesthesia is uncommon, it is a devastating complication since mortality is frequently high. Any postoperative patient that exhibits vomiting, regurgitation, nausea, salivation, dysphagia, and/or anorexia should be monitored closely. Patients with persistent signs of dysphagia, vomiting, and/or regurgitation should be thoroughly evaluated for esophageal disease.

Aspiration

Aspiration of GI contents can occur perioperatively following GER, vomiting, and/or regurgitation. It can also occur during heavy sedation that impairs normally protective airway reflexes. Respiratory complications following aspiration include hypoventilation and/or hypoxemia, pneumonitis, bacterial pneumonia, and

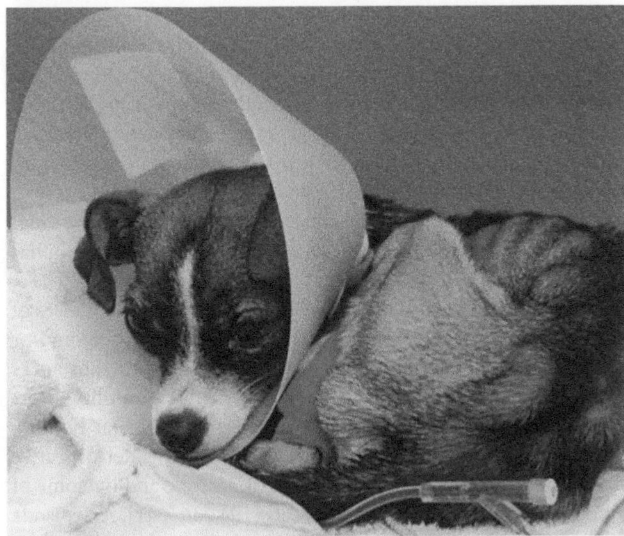

Figure 31.8 Patients with esophageal stricture may be debilitated due to dysphagia and aspiration pneumonia.

sometimes cardiac arrest. The extent of airway pathology depends on the volume and type of fluid aspirated. Three phases of damage have been identified: stage 1 is immediate – due to direct toxic damage to the epithelium. Depending on the volume of aspirated material, the end result is atelectasis, decreased compliance, ventilation/perfusion mismatch, and decreased oxygenation. Stage 2 follows within 4–6 h – an inflammatory reaction that causes pneumonitis. If not severe, this lesion may resolve. Stage 3 is seen when bacteria invade damaged tissue, producing aspiration pneumonia [243–245].

Early recognition and intervention are paramount to limiting the severity of aspiration pneumonia and its associated mortality. Signs of aspiration range from 'silent' with no apparent abnormalities to obvious airway obstruction following visible regurgitation of gastric contents. Unexplained oxygen desaturation, tachypnea, dyspnea or irregular respiratory patterns, auscultable abnormalities, and blanching of mucous membranes may be seen. Oxygen (100%) should be administered and the patient immediately positioned with the head down for drainage. Suction of the airways is necessary for liquid aspiration. Bronchoscopy may be required when particulate matter has been aspirated. Bronchodilator therapy and mechanical ventilation with positive end expiratory pressure may be needed to improve oxygenation. Prophylactic antibiotics are not usually recommended for pneumonitis cases owing to the potential for emergence of resistant bacteria [243,244,246]. Since bacterial colonization occurs later in the process, antibiotics are recommended only in those with confirmed infection, especially in otherwise healthy patients. However, patients with GI obstruction or on chronic antacid therapy may be an exception owing to the potential for enteric organisms to be found in reflux fluid [243,244,246].

A recent very large multicenter study evaluated the anesthesia caseload at six veterinary institutions over an 11 year period to determine the incidence and risk factors for aspiration pneumonia following anesthesia or sedation in dogs [247]. The criteria included radiographic or necropsy evidence of aspiration pneumonia within 72 h of sedation or general anesthesia. Multivariate analysis of numerous patient, procedure, and anesthetic factors was performed for 240 dogs identified along with 488 controls. The incidence of aspiration pneumonia varied significantly between institutions, from 0.04 to 0.26%, with an overall incidence of 0.17%. Of 12 dogs who were given sedation only, three developed aspiration pneumonia. Multivariate analysis revealed the following to be associated with anesthetic-related aspiration pneumonia: patient factors – megaesophagus and pre-existing respiratory or neurologic disease; procedures – upper airway surgery, endoscopy, thoracotomy, laparotomy, and neurosurgery; and anesthetic events – regurgitation during or after anesthesia and hydromorphone given intravenously at induction. Some factors were significantly associated with aspiration pneumonia but did not remain following the multivariate analysis [odds ratio (OR) <2]. These included the male gender and increasing ASA patient score, age, and body weight. Use of continuous infusion of analgesics or anesthetic agents was associated with a greater incidence of aspiration pneumonia (OR 1.8) when utilized during anesthesia but not when given postoperatively. Megaesophagus, in spite of a low occurrence, had the highest OR of 22.3, and upper airway surgery was next with OR 9.2. No specific breed was identified. Time of day, extubation during anesthesia, and the use of anticholinergics, positive-pressure ventilation, or epidural analgesia were not associated with aspiration pneumonia. Regurgitation was witnessed in only two cases with aspiration pneumonia. Forty-six of the 240 dogs (19.2%) were euthanized or died prior to discharge. However, an association of death with aspiration pneumonia could not be identified from the available data, so mortality was not determined [247].

Another retrospective case–control study examined aspiration pneumonia within 48 h of anesthesia in dogs anesthetized for repair of intervertebral disk disease. Significant risk factors for postoperative aspiration pneumonia included preanesthetic tetraparesis, a cervical lesion, MRI study, having more than one anesthetic procedure, longer duration of anesthesia, and postanesthetic vomiting or regurgitation [248].

Pre-existing neurologic and respiratory disorders, megaesophagus, perioperative vomiting/regurgitation, and anesthesia have been consistently identified in veterinary patients with aspiration pneumonia [248–251]. Even though the incidence of aspiration is low, predisposing factors are common and aspiration pneumonia carries a high risk of mortality. Vigilant monitoring for signs of aspiration is necessary, especially since most cases are subclinical, similarly to GER and esophagitis. Perioperative management to prevent these complications with appropriate intervention as soon as possible is always indicated.

Gastrointestinal motility/postoperative ileus

Some species appear to be especially sensitive to the effects of anesthetic agents on GI motility (e.g., rabbits, horses, ruminants, and humans). Postoperative nausea, vomiting, and ileus are very common in humans. Postoperative ileus (POI) is one of the most common reasons for prolonged hospitalization of humans [151,152,252]. Although most common following GI surgery, it is seen following other intra-abdominal procedures in humans and with many types of surgery in horses. POI is associated with increased mortality following colic surgery in horses [253], while colic in general and cecal impaction in particular are potentially serious complications seen following routine anesthesia and surgery in horses and may be associated with the development of ileus [254]. Rabbits are prone to GI stasis following stressful situations [255,256]. Other small animal species (e.g., dog and cat) certainly suffer from disruption of normal motility during anesthesia; however, related clinical problems are less common or perhaps less frequently recognized. Numerous researchers have used the dog as a model for the investigation of POI, but there are few specific reports of the incidence seen in clinical patients. In fact, it is rarely discussed in surgical textbooks or reviews of abdominal surgery in small animals. With the advent of intensive multimodal pain management protocols, the potential to affect motility has increased.

Intestinal function is temporarily eliminated or disrupted by most anesthetic/analgesic agents, including anticholinergics, μ-agonist opioids, α_2-adrenergic receptor agonists, inhalants, nitrous oxide, and induction agents other than ketamine [153,155,157,257–263]. Xylazine and medetomidine can inhibit motility of the stomach, small intestine [259,260], and colon [261] for hours in the dog. Anticholinergic drugs profoundly reduce GI motility in most species [264–270]. The effects of opioids on motility are many. μ-Agonists given systemically delay gastric emptying, increase sphincter tone, and variably affect intestinal smooth muscle contraction. Propulsive motility is inhibited and segmental contractions are enhanced, especially in the colon; absorption is increased while secretion is decreased. Constipation is a frequent complication with systemic opioids, from the combined effects on fluid transport and prolonged transit time [157,263,271]. In contrast, when morphine is administered epidurally, GI motility returns much faster in both dogs and humans [272,273]. Following general anesthesia in humans, motility generally returns to the small intestine first, then the stomach, and eventually the colon, which may require 5 days or more [274]. In experimental dogs with ileus, motility of the distal intestine and colon recovered first, followed by the proximal intestine and the stomach [275].

A recent investigation examined the effect of laparoscopy and prolonged sevoflurane anesthesia on propulsive motility and transit time in dogs anesthetized for ovariohysterectomy [276]. Following oral administration, a wireless sensor continuously measured intraluminal pressure, pH, and temperature as it traversed the GIT. Maximum and mean pressures created by gastric and small intestinal contractions and their frequency were recorded, and a motility index and a transit or emptying time were calculated. The frequency of contraction was not different from controls (awake dogs); however, changes in motility were seen quickly, within 20 min of induction. The motility index and the mean and maximum amplitudes of contraction of both the stomach and small bowel decreased significantly. Gastric emptying and small bowel transit times were prolonged, with means of 49 and 11.5 h and maxima of 59 and 14 h, respectively. No further effect of laparoscopy on motility was identified, but since it was performed in all the dogs, it is unclear what specific effects laparoscopy may have had on GI function. All the dogs were given hydromorphone and cephalexin for recovery, which may also have affected the postoperative results, especially the opioid. The results of this study showing a decrease in the force of intestinal contraction, inhibition of propulsive motility, and prolonged gastric emptying and small intestinal transit time provide excellent information for use in the design of further studies and evaluation of clinical patients in the future.

The mechanism of POI is multifactorial, with neural, hormonal, inflammatory, and pharmacologic components, but the inflammatory response seen in the muscularis externa is considered the most important and likely the primary cause of prolonged POI [149,263,274,277]. Activation of the sympathetic nervous system inhibits motility very soon following the surgical incision, but this effect is short-lived without other insult to the GIT. Handling of the intestine incites a local inflammatory response within the muscularis via activation of resident macrophages that is proportional to the intensity of intestinal damage. Influx of other leukocytes follows and release of inflammatory mediators is stimulated. Surgically induced peritoneal inflammation also occurs that contributes to the local and systemic effects seen. POI is further exacerbated by the effects of anesthetic agents on motility, and also the presence or development of peritonitis and sepsis [149,152,263,274,277–279].

Table 31.8 Recommendations for prevention of postoperative ileus in humans [149,152,252,258,272–274,279,280,320,321].

Maintain intestinal blood flow and oxygenation	Fluid therapy – goal oriented, restricted (avoid excessive volume)
	Avoid saline, use balanced solution, ± colloids
	Prevention, prompt treatment of hypotension
	Prevention, treatment of low protein, albumin
Perioperative analgesia	Systemic opioid-sparing protocols
	Thoracic epidural with local – block sympathetic input
	Epidural morphine – less inhibition of motility
	NSAIDs – COX-2 inhibitors – reduce inflammation, ketorolac
	Lidocaine infusion – anti-inflammatory, less/shorter POI
Surgical techniques	Minimize handling of intestine
	Laparoscopy whenever possible – less inflammation, shorter POI
	Helium is better – CO_2 promotes infection via tissue acidosis
	Air actually stimulates inflammation
Postoperative care	Enteral nutrition and ambulation as soon as possible; avoid nasogastric tubes
	Laxative therapy to treat, prevent constipation
	Peripheral opioid antagonists – alvimopam, methylnaltrexone
	Serotonin HT_4 agonists – cisapride, mosapride

Numerous interventions have been attempted in humans to reduce or ameliorate the incidence of POI. None have completely eliminated ileus, but improvements in patient comfort, shorter hospitalization, and better outcomes have been seen with the some interventions (Table 31.8).

Gastrointestinal conditions requiring anesthesia

Many patients that require anesthesia for GI disease are emergent and/or may be critically ill. Thorough preanesthetic evaluation and preparation prior to anesthesia help to minimize complications; however, this is not always possible in extremely emergent patients. Recommendations for a basic workup include measurement of hematocrit, total protein, BUN, creatinine, serum alkaline phosphatase (SAP), alanine aminotransferase (ALT), aspartate aminotransferase (AST), bilirubin, albumin, electrolytes, and total carbon dioxide. Blood-gas analysis and lactate are important in sick patients. Additional diagnostics appropriate to the problem at hand should be evaluated, such as radiographs or abdominal ultrasound.

General guidelines for the management of anesthesia for abdominal procedures are similar to recommendations for other disease conditions. Preservation of tissue oxygen delivery through the maintenance of blood flow and avoidance of hypoxemia are important. Additional consideration should be given to predictable complications (e.g., endotoxemia following reperfusion of damaged gut or cardiac dysrhythmias during splenectomy) and appropriate treatments planned. Finally, administration of adjunctive drugs to provide pain management, speed return of GI function, and limit adverse effects such as nausea and vomiting can improve patient care.

Laparotomy

The plan for an exploratory laparotomy often varies more with the patient's condition than with the primary GI problem. Some patients are healthy (e.g., gastropexy) and their management is similar to that for other elective abdominal procedures (e.g., ovariohysterectomy). Other patients may be severely ill and require laparotomy as a life-saving intervention. Fluid deficits and electrolyte abnormalities should be corrected as much as is reasonable prior to induction. Some patients may have pre-existing organ dysfunction that may or may not be related to the reason for the exploratory laparotomy. Ketamine, especially as a continuous infusion, should be used with caution in patients with renal dysfunction, especially cats since they excrete it and its metabolites to a significant extent in the urine. Thiopental should also be used with caution or avoided in debilitated patients and those with severe liver dysfunction. It should also be avoided in sighthounds. Both thiopental and propofol can sensitize the myocardium to catecholamine-associated arrhythmias and should be used carefully in patients with pre-existing dysrhythmias or cardiac disease, or when arrhythmias are highly likely such as GDV or splenic masses. Etomidate is useful for patients with pre-existing myocardial dysfunction (e.g., poor contractility) who are otherwise healthy as it has minimal effects on cardiovascular function. A dose of midazolam or diazepam, 0.2 mg/kg, just prior to injection of etomidate will improve muscle relaxation and facilitate intubation. However, etomidate is not recommended for very sick human patients, especially those with sepsis [281,282], as adrenal insufficiency and greater mortality has been reported in septic patients following induction of anesthesia with etomidate [283]. Some authors consider that the use of a single dose may not be harmful; however, further research is recommended. Inhalant induction is not recommended for patients with GI disease, especially those with emesis. Premedication with a benzodiazepine and an opioid is useful prior to exploratory laparotomy. Midazolam or diazepam with hydromorphone, oxymorphone, or fentanyl (or its congeners) is titrated intravenously to effect. To avoid traditional induction drugs entirely in compromised patients, additional doses of the benzodiazepine–opioid combination are administered until intubation is possible. Bradycardia and respiratory depression are sometimes significant following high doses of opioids used for induction, so preparations for intubation and ventilation should be made ready for use. Alternatively, a low dose of ketamine will often allow intubation following premedication. Fentanyl is easily continued as an infusion following induction.

Isoflurane, sevoflurane, or desflurane is preferred for maintenance of anesthesia for exploratory laparotomy over halothane as the latter sensitizes the myocardium to arrhythmias and decreases tissue blood flow to a greater extent. Nitrous oxide is not recommended as it will diffuse into the GIT, causing distention. The cardiovascular and respiratory effects of all the inhalants are more pronounced in debilitated patients; hypotension and hypoventilation are common. Because of pre-existing cardiovascular depression, sick patients frequently require lower levels of inhalant anesthetic. Vaporizer settings should be kept as low as possible to minimize hypotension, and occasionally discontinuation of inhalant anesthetic followed with injectable maintenance is necessary to maintain blood pressure with severe sepsis.

When anesthetic depth is inadequate, additional sedatives or analgesics are given intermittently or as a CRI. Continuous infusion provides a more constant level of drug delivery, and can reduce the level of inhalant anesthetic required. The infusion(s) is(are) are titrated to effect along with the inhalant setting to adjust anesthetic depth. Morphine or fentanyl, lidocaine, and/or ketamine are given as intravenous infusions in dogs [284–286]; lidocaine is not currently recommended for use in cats [287]. In patients without uncorrected hypovolemia, sepsis, coagulopathy, or dermatitis in the lumbosacral area, epidural administration of a local anesthetic with or without morphine can also provide intra- and postoperative analgesia.

Fluid therapy should be continued during anesthesia; the type of fluids and the rate necessary will vary depending on the patient's status. If hypotension persists despite correcting volume deficits, inotropes such as dobutamine and/or dopamine may increase cardiac output and improve blood pressure. Vasopressors may be necessary when decreased systemic vascular resistance is a significant component of the hypotension. Ephedrine is a sympathomimetic which can be given as a bolus; it is effective primarily for mild transient decreases in blood pressure. Phenylephrine, norepinephrine, vasopressin, and epinephrine are most often given as infusions and titrated to effect. These drugs are potent vasoconstrictors and should be used at the lowest effective dose to minimize tissue ischemia despite improved blood pressure.

Monitoring should continue throughout anesthesia and into recovery. Signs of anesthetic depth, heart and respiratory rate, mucous membrane color and capillary refill time, temperature, blood pressure, and electrocardiography are commonly evaluated parameters. Direct blood pressure is preferred for most laparotomies since changes in pressure can be rapid and severe. Pulse oximetry and capnography allow continuous real-time evaluation of ventilation and gas exchange and are commonly used. Arterial blood gas analysis is used to document respiratory and metabolic status and to evaluate periodically the success of therapy. Lactate measurement is an indirect estimate of tissue perfusion and oxygenation status [288]. Changes in lactate lag behind alterations of tissue metabolism, but are of some value in the evaluation of therapy and prognosis of patients with severe metabolic derangements (e.g., GDV). Although cardiac output (CO) monitors are less available, knowledge of the CO is very helpful in the assessment of the cardiovascular status in critical patients. When CO measurement is not available, variation in the arterial pressure waveform during mechanical ventilation may infer the presence of hypovolemia (Fig. 31.9). Close attention to volume loss and to the actions of the surgeon during laparotomy helps to avoid hemodynamic compromise by enabling the anesthetist to anticipate and treat problems in a timely fashion. For example, cardiovascular function is greatly affected by blood loss or removal of large volumes of effusion, and with handling of large masses; manipulation and derotation of ischemic bowel lead to the release of numerous inflammatory mediators that cause vasodilation and possibly cardiac dysfunction (Fig. 31.10).

Postoperative pain management is important for the comfort and outcome of patients with GI disease. Opioids are continued as intermittent boluses intravenously or intramuscularly, or via continuous infusion. Infusions of lidocaine and/or ketamine are also fairly effective. Lidocaine caused nausea and vomiting in dogs at high infusion rates [177], but is associated with improved outcome in humans following abdominal surgery [178,179], and in dogs with GDV [289]. Higher dosing of analgesics is usually required in the first 24 h postoperatively. These should be decreased as soon as possible so that enteral feeding can be instituted and to minimize the incidence of ileus. Infusions of low doses of α_2-adrenergic receptor agonists in patients with high analgesic requirements or opioid dysphoria are useful, but their adverse cardiovascular effects should be carefully considered in the individual patient.

NSAIDs are used frequently in human, ruminant, and equine patients following GI surgery with minimal complications [290–293]. However, dogs and cats are relatively sensitive to the GI side-effects of NSAIDs such as ulceration and hemorrhage [294–296]. Although they may be useful in healthy patients anesthetized for elective

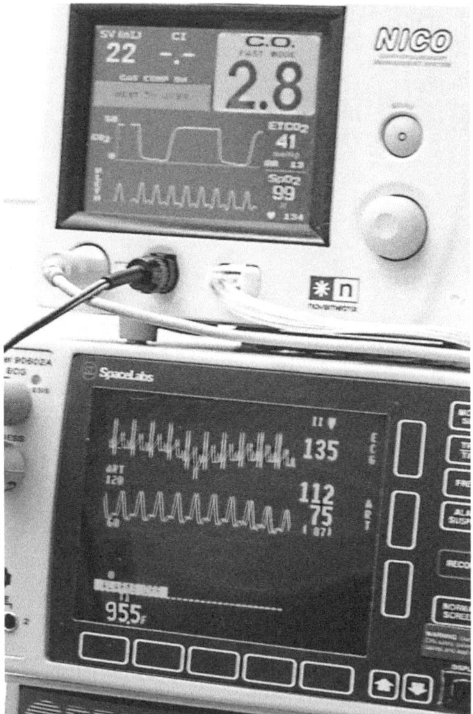

Figure 31.9 Monitoring of patients anesthetized for laparotomy includes ECG, blood pressure, pulse oximetry, and capnography. Non-invasive monitoring of cardiac output (NICO) is very useful in critical cases. This patient appears to be doing quite well with normal values for blood pressure, heart rate, end tidal CO_2, oxygen saturation, and cardiac output. However, a gradual variation in the systolic pressure wave infers that hypovolemia may be present.

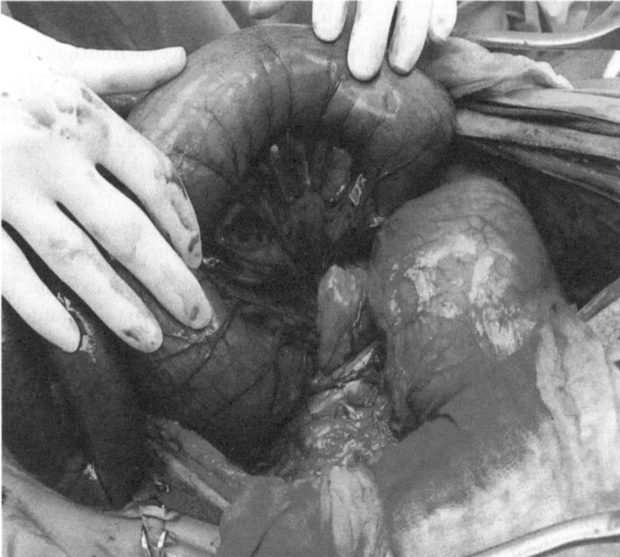

Figure 31.10 A mesenteric torsion in a German Shepherd dog presented for acute onset of abdominal discomfort and extreme depression.

procedures such as gastropexy, it may be best to avoid NSAIDs in patients with GI disease, renal compromise, hypotension, liver disease, coagulopathy, and other conditions that could be exacerbated by NSAID administration.

Megaesophagus

Megaesophagus is rare in cats but not uncommon in dogs. The most common cause in cats is dysautonomia, an acquired malfunction of the autonomic ganglia that leads to GI dysfunction. Congenital idiopathic megaesophagus has been reported in dogs and a few cats. It is presumed to be a defect of vagal sensory innervation where peristalsis of the esophagus does not occur because the dilation caused by a food bolus is not detected [212,297]. Acquired megaesophagus is frequently caused by mechanical obstruction. Vascular ring anomaly, esophageal stricture, hiatal hernia, tumor, granuloma, and foreign bodies are the more common causes. With time, the dilation of the esophagus proximal to the lesion becomes irreversible. Idiopathic megaesophagus is the most common cause of the acquired form in adult dogs, where loss of normal esophageal motility eventually results in dilation. Some cases of acquired megaesophagus are secondary to or associated with other disease conditions. Peripheral neuropathy, laryngeal paralysis, myasthenia gravis, severe esophagitis, lead poisoning, lupus myositis, and chronic or recurrent gastric dilation with or without volvulus were associated with an increased risk of megaesophagus in a retrospective study of 44 dogs. Hypothyroidism was not associated with megaesophagus in these dogs [297–300].

Patients with megaesophagus may be anesthetized for diagnostic tests or treatments such as endoscopy, electromyography, nerve conduction velocity, muscle and nerve biopsy, CT for mass lesions, bougienage, foreign body removal, and vascular ring anomaly correction. Megaesophagus may also be a concurrent disease in patients anesthetized for unrelated procedures such as dentistry. GER, regurgitation, and aspiration are the primary concerns when anesthetizing patients with megaesophagus. Prolonged fasting is not necessary or advised as the dysmotility and dilation prevent complete emptying of esophageal contents and an increased incidence of GER has been seen with long fasting times in normal dogs [189,190]. Some patients with chronic disease may be thin or debilitated due to malnutrition and some may be dehydrated if unable to retain adequate fluid intake. Many have repeated episodes of aspiration pneumonia and are at greater risk of hypoxemia perioperatively. These patients should be stabilized prior to anesthesia with IV fluid therapy and appropriate treatment for pneumonia. A dedicated anesthetist is very important in patients with megaesophagus, as airway management and constant monitoring for leakage of esophageal contents are necessary. Suction of esophageal contents should be performed immediately after intubation and just before discontinuation of anesthesia to reduce the risk of aspiration. Sternal recumbency and elevation of the neck with the nose tipped down may also help decrease the incidence. If regurgitation occurs, the nose and head should be lowered immediately to allow drainage. Pre-oxygenation is recommended for those with active pneumonia; these patients should be restrained cautiously to avoid struggling and excessive stress. Anesthetic drugs should be chosen based on the patient's status, with rapid IV induction and intubation necessary to secure a protected airway as quickly as possible. Avoidance of drugs that cause vomiting such as some opioids (e.g., morphine or hydromorphone) and α_2-adrenergic receptor agonists is also recommended.

Gastric dilation–volvulus

The GDV syndrome is an acute life-threatening disease seen most often in adult large or giant breed dogs, especially those with deep-chested conformation. However, it can occur in small breed dogs and puppies, and has even been reported in cats with coexisting diaphragmatic hernias [299,300]. Mortality rates of 33.3–60% [299,301] seen in the 1980s and earlier have improved but are still high. Recent studies have reported mortality rates of 10–26.8% [289,302–304]. Decreased mortality is likely associated with improvements in medical therapy, especially fluid resuscitation, decompression of the stomach whenever possible, and early surgical intervention. Mortality is correlated with the extent of damage to the stomach and surrounding organs, the presence of cardiac dysrhythmias pre- or postoperatively, both hypo- and hyperthermia at presentation, the development of postoperative acute renal failure, hypotension at any time during hospitalization, and the duration from onset to presentation or surgery and the time from presentation to surgery [302–305]. Reperfusion injury has also been implicated as a significant factor associated with mortality with GDV [306].

GDV is always an emergency. Blood flow to the stomach and surrounding organs is compromised and the caudal vena cava and portal vein become obstructed, greatly decreasing venous return to the heart and producing severe hypovolemic shock. Distention of the stomach also restricts ventilation via interference with diaphragmatic excursion. Early clinical signs of GDV include restlessness and anxiety, followed by hypersalivation, vomiting and/or retching, and distention of the abdomen. Eventually depression, weakness, and dyspnea develop if the distention is not relieved. Vomiting, salivation, and sequestration of hydrogen and chloride ions that occur with gastric outflow obstruction initially cause metabolic alkalosis. Metabolic acidosis develops later, secondary to the effects of ischemia, with increased lactate production and the release of inflammatory mediators. Endotoxemia can also develop with damage to the portal system. Reperfusion injury occurs when ischemia is reversed with gastric decompression/derotation and restoration of fluid volume.

Intravenous fluid therapy and gastric decompression should be initiated as quickly as possible. Baseline laboratory evaluation should include packed cell volume (PCV), total solids (TS), electrolytes, creatinine, and acid–base status. A clotting profile and venous lactate are useful to evaluate prognosis and guide therapy but generally should not delay surgical intervention if the owners would proceed regardless of the results. Gastric necrosis is likely present when more than one hemostatic test is abnormal and when lactate is greatly elevated at presentation and/or fails to decrease significantly with fluid resuscitation [307–310] predicting a poor outcome [309,310]. Radiography to distinguish between dilation and dilation–volvulus should be delayed until cardiovascular resuscitation is completed or well under way. Anesthetic personnel, equipment, and supplies should be made ready prior to arrival of the GDV so that surgical intervention may commence as soon as possible. Standard emergent therapy has been to give shock doses (80–90 mL/kg) of crystalloid solution via large-bore catheters, using the cephalic, saphenous, and/or jugular veins (Fig. 31.11). However, following goal-directed resuscitation guidelines to achieve appropriate clinical endpoints rather than a specific volume avoids hypervolemia and tissue edema and may improve outcome [281,282,311,312]. Clinical parameters to monitor include heart rate, arterial blood pressure, mucous membrane color and perfusion, tissue oxygenation, and mentation. PCV, TS or total protein, blood gases, and venous oxygen saturation should be measured as needed. Use of balanced crystalloid solutions is certainly effective; however, faster and longer lasting resuscitation is achieved with the addition of small volumes of hypertonic saline 7.5% (HS) at 2–4 mL/kg over 15 min, or colloids at 5–10 mL/kg over 30 min.

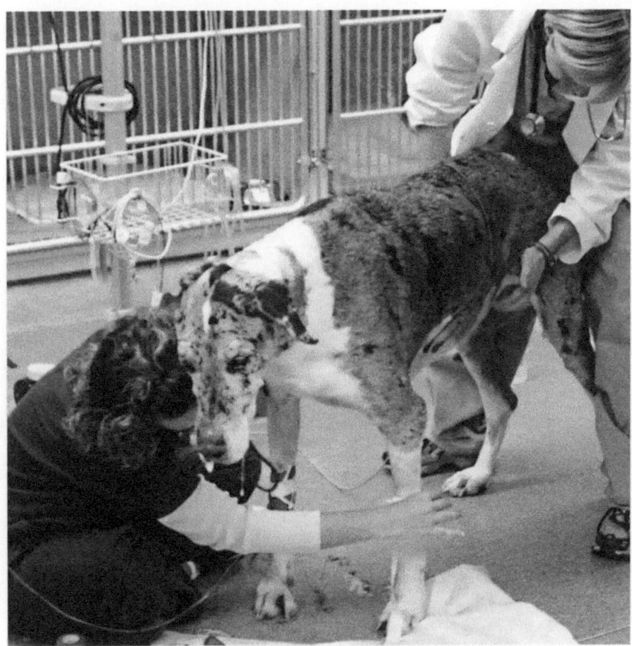

Figure 31.11 A Great Dane with GDV being prepared for anesthesia and surgery. Two intravenous catheters have been placed, one in each cephalic vein; ECG leads are attached to monitor cardiac rhythm. Note the salivation and depressed demeanor in this dog.

Alternatively, a combination of colloid and HS is given at 4–6 mL/kg. This simultaneous use of HS and colloid has been shown to improve cardiovascular status in both experimental and clinical cases of GDV [313,314].

Thoracic auscultation followed by electrocardiography should be performed soon following presentation, as cardiac arrhythmias are common with GDV and should be identified and treated prior to induction of anesthesia. They are usually ventricular in origin, but atrial fibrillation and sinus tachycardia also occur (Fig. 31.12) [315]. In some cases, antiarrhythmic agents may not be necessary, because the dysrhythmia is of minimal cardiovascular consequence or correction of hypovolemia, hypoxemia, hypercarbia, acid–base status, and/or electrolyte abnormalities provide resolution. Treatment of ventricular tachycardia may be necessary when extrasystoles are numerous or multifocal, when the sustained rate is very high (>160 beats/min), when extrasystoles are very early such that an 'R on T' phenomenon may occur, and always when hemodynamic status is affected by the arrhythmia. Lidocaine is given slowly IV as a 1–2 mg/kg bolus followed by an infusion at 25–100 μg/kg/min [316]. Postoperative treatment of cardiac arrhythmias may be necessary. A lidocaine CRI for dysrhythmias is also a useful adjunct to anesthesia as it decreases anesthetic requirements in dogs by as much as 37–43% [177,317]. Results of a recent study that used lidocaine preemptively in dogs with GDV showed significantly fewer cases with cardiac dysrhythmias, less renal impairment, and shorter hospitalization time compared with a historical control group [289]. Lidocaine has also been shown to have numerous anti-inflammatory effects [318–320] and may have prokinetic effects [178,321–323].

Gastric lavage may be necessary during correction of a GDV. Considerations for this procedure are similar to those for upper GI endoscopy and megaesophagus. Leakage of gastric contents is common and the endotracheal tube can be displaced. The head should be tipped downwards to help direct gastric contents away from the

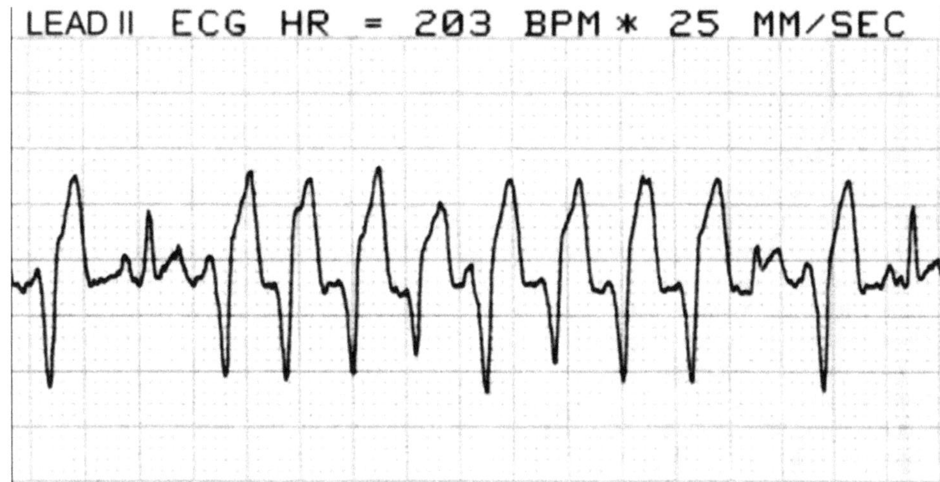

Figure 31.12 Ventricular tachycardia seen postoperatively in a dog anesthetized for correction of GDV.

pharynx. The pharynx should be examined and cleaned of any fluid or debris that may have leaked around the nasogastric tube prior to recovery.

In spite of much research devoted to the effects of ischemia reperfusion injury and its prevention or treatment, few therapies have been included in clinical practice. Avoidance of hyperoxia may be useful since greater damage has been seen following reperfusion in patients maintained at higher than normal PaO_2 levels [324]. Inhibition of oxygen radical formation with antioxidants and iron-chelating drugs such as deferoxamine has been shown to reduce reperfusion injury in dogs with GDV [306,325].

Hemoabdomen

Causes of hemorrhage into the peritoneal cavity are traumatic or atraumatic. Trauma is most often due to injury from impact with motor vehicles or penetrating objects. Abdominal organs, vasculature, and/or the abdominal wall may be affected. The larger parenchymal organs such as the liver and spleen are very often involved. Atraumatic lesions include hematoma or neoplasia of abdominal organs, organ displacement or torsion, and coagulation abnormalities (e.g., rodenticide toxicity). Neoplasia is very common, especially in dogs. Mass lesions of the liver, spleen, mesentery and adrenal glands are reported; the spleen is most commonly affected. Hemangiosarcoma is the most often identified neoplasm in both dogs and cats and usually affects the spleen or liver. Long-term prognosis is poor [326–328], but a high percentage of dogs with hemoperitoneum survive anesthesia and surgery to discharge. A retrospective investigation of spontaneous atraumatic hemoperitoneum in 65 cats found that 46% had abdominal neoplasia and 54% had non-neoplastic disease; hepatic necrosis and coagulopathy accounted for almost half of the latter. Only eight of the cats (12.3%) survived to discharge [329].

Hemorrhage into the abdomen can be gradual or sudden, and may quickly become life-threatening. Clinical signs are similar to blood loss from any cause with progressive signs of hypovolemic shock – increasing tachycardia, pale mucous membranes, weak pulses, decreased mentation, etc. Hypothermia is seen in dogs and is common in cats at presentation. Abdominal distention, a palpable fluid wave, abdominal pain, and subcutaneous discoloration at the umbilicus and scrotum are also sometimes seen. Radiography may show loss of abdominal detail with a 'ground-glass' appearance. Ultrasound will reveal the presence of free fluid and may reveal a mass or metastatic disease. Diagnostic peritoneal lavage may be necessary with smaller volumes of blood loss or when ultrasound is not available [326,328].

Anesthetic considerations for patients with hemoabdomen are potential respiratory compromise associated with large masses or fluid volumes pressing on the diaphragm, hypovolemia, anemia, and any organ dysfunction that may be present. Ideally, the patient is stabilized prior to surgery with intravenous fluids or blood transfusion. However, some prefer to replace erythrocyte losses after the source of the hemorrhage is stopped if the rate of loss is large. It is not necessary to correct the entire RBC deficit preoperatively; however, the patient should be treated to attempt to achieve normovolemia and a PCV ≥30% in dogs or 20% in cats, as oxygen delivery is usually adequate above these levels. Lower PCVs are often tolerated during anesthesia but are usually associated with slow or chronic blood loss rather than acute hemorrhage.

The volume of prior and ongoing blood loss must be estimated and replaced before hypovolemia severely affects cardiac output. Estimating loss is often difficult; techniques include weighing bloody sponges and towels, tracking the volume of lavage fluid used, and estimating the volume of blood and fluid collected in suction bottles.

Crystalloids are used for volume replacement assuming that an adequate number of erythrocytes remain to maintain oxygen delivery. The specific volume required is unknown and depends on the speed of loss, but several multiples of the volume lost are commonly recommended (e.g., three times the loss for acute hemorrhage up to eight times for gradual loss affecting the intracellular volume). When the intracellular volume is affected, replacement can proceed more slowly than when acute hemorrhage is present. Colloids are a rational replacement for plasma loss and are given at closer to a 1:1 ratio if PCV and protein levels are adequate. Losses greater than 20–30% of the patient's total blood volume should be replaced with whole blood, plasma or colloid, and packed RBCs, or an RBC substitute such as Oxyglobin®, to ensure adequate oxygen delivery. Autotransfusion may be useful in some cases but is not recommended with septic peritonitis, urinary rupture, and neoplastic lesions.

TS or total protein levels should be maintained at greater than 4–4.5 g/dL if possible. Serial PCV and TS measurements are helpful in determining the efficacy of therapy and the speed of blood loss, realizing that hemodilution will be present and that colloids will interfere with refractometer readings. Often response to volume restoration and increased oxygen-carrying capacity (e.g., normalization of heart rate and blood pressure) are more useful guides to fluid therapy during anesthesia. Lactate is a useful indicator of tissue oxygen delivery as it increases with severe hypovolemia and decreases as volume, cardiovascular function, and perfusion improve [288]. Although rapid volume replacement is sometimes necessary in extremely hypovolemic patients, large volumes can cause hypocoagulability (e.g., dilutional coagulopathy). Goal-directed fluid therapy utilizes smaller volume boluses with intermittent re-evaluation of cardiovascular status. Attainment of an acceptable arterial blood pressure and heart rate and improvement in clinical signs are recommended resuscitation endpoints [327].

Rapid evacuation of blood and manipulation of organs or large abdominal masses can cause significant hemodynamic instability (Fig. 31.13). Sequestration of a portion of the blood volume in the exteriorized tissues and/or redistribution of blood volume affects cardiac output and peripheral perfusion. In humans anesthetized for abdominal surgery, a syndrome of tachycardia, hypotension, and cutaneous hyperemia has been reported, called 'mesenteric traction syndrome' [203,330]. This has not been described or perhaps has not been investigated in animals, but release of prostacyclin, histamine, and other vasoactive substances is thought to cause the fluctuations in hemodynamic status when tension is placed on mesenteric vasculature.

Cardiac arrhythmias are common with splenic masses and other types of functional neoplasms (e.g., pheochromocytoma). Ventricular premature contractions and tachycardias are seen most often in dogs. The cause is uncertain and these arrhythmias are often difficult to eliminate until the mass has been removed. Predisposing factors such as hypovolemia, hypotension, hypoxemia, hypercarbia, and electrolyte abnormalities are other common causes of dysrhythmias under anesthesia.

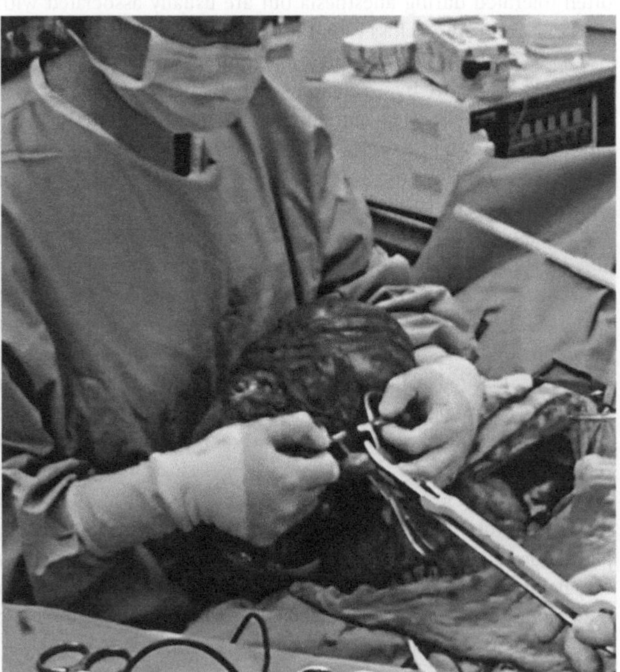

Figure 31.13 Manipulation of large abdominal masses can greatly affect cardiovascular stability under anesthesia.

Intestinal neoplasia

Lymphoma, carcinoma, leiomyoma, and gastrointestinal stromal tumors (GISTs) are common types of neoplasia found in the GIT of dogs and cats. Lymphoma is the most common intestinal neoplasia in the cat. Cats with GI lymphoma are usually negative for feline leukemia virus and feline immunodeficiency virus, unlike other types of lymphoma. GI lymphoma is also common in the dog; most are T cell in origin. A predisposition to intestinal carcinoma is reported in German Shepherd dogs and Siamese cats.

Esophageal neoplasia is rare in small animals. Squamous cell carcinoma (SCC), fibrosarcoma, osteosarcoma, and leiomyoma are seen. When it occurs in cats, SCC is most likely. Infection with *Spirocera lupi* is reported to cause fibrosarcoma, osteosarcoma, and other undifferentiated sarcomas. Melanoma is seen in the esophagus; it is more common in canine breeds with black mucous membranes.

Rare neuroendocrine tumors (or carcinoids) arise from enterochromaffin cells found in the mucosa of the GIT. Previously called APUDomas (amine precursor uptake and decarboxylation), carcinoids are rare in animals. Carcinoid syndrome occurs occasionally in humans; one report of ventricular tachycardia and melena in a boxer was associated with an intestinal carcinoid [331]. Serotonin, histamine, substance P, various kinins, catecholamines, and prostaglandins are just some of the chemicals secreted by carcinoid tumors. Usually, these substances are transported to the liver and metabolized; however, if they gain access to the circulation or the lumen of the bowel, clinical signs of hemodynamic instability and pulmonary and GI dysfunction follow. Arrhythmias, hypo- or hypertension, vasodilation, bronchospasm, diarrhea, and hypersecretion of intestinal fluid may occur. Anesthesia for such tumors should avoid the use of drugs that encourage histamine release such as morphine, atracurium, and succinylcholine. Dopamine, ephedrine, epinephrine, norepinephrine, histamine, and isoproterenol have been associated with carcinoid episodes in humans. Pretreatment with antihistamines and serotonin antagonists may be beneficial. Somatostatin receptors are found in some carcinoid tumors; the somatostatin analog octreotide is used to decrease secretion of serotonin and other substances. This has minimized clinical signs in humans and allowed the use of sympathomimetics under anesthesia [203,332].

Clinical signs of GI neoplasia usually reflect the area affected, but paraneoplastic syndromes are also seen with some tumors. Malaise, weight loss, and anorexia may be the only signs. Vomiting, diarrhea, and melena are also common with gastric and small intestinal lesions. Regurgitation is frequent with esophageal disease. Tenesmus, hematochezia, and constipation occur with lesions of the rectum. Abdominal pain, hemorrhage, obstruction, perforation, and intussusception also occur with GI neoplasia [333–337].

Anemia, hypoproteinemia, increased alkaline phosphatase and increased BUN are the most common laboratory abnormalities seen with neoplasia of the GIT. Anemia is often moderate, microcytic, and hypochromic due to chronic blood loss, but can also be normocytic and normochromic. Protein-losing enteropathy is common, causing hypoproteinemia due to hypoalbuminemia. BUN increases with chronic intraluminal blood loss due to recycling of protein [338].

Abdominal palpation may suggest the presence of neoplasia. Lesions are identified most often with radiography and ultrasonography. Aspirates and/or biopsies needed for definitive diagnosis are often obtained in conscious patients with ultrasound guidance; however, endoscopy and/or laparotomy under general anesthesia are sometimes necessary.

Paraneoplastic syndromes (PNSs) are caused by secretion of substances that affect tissues distant to the primary tumor. The syndromes possible with GI neoplasia are numerous, but not all patients exhibit signs of PNS. Hypercalcemia of malignancy occurs with lymphoma, is common with apocrine gland adenocarcinoma, but is less frequent with GI adenocarcinoma. Secretion of PTH or a PTH-related-peptide causes mobilization of calcium from bone, resulting in increased serum calcium and eventually mineralization of tissues, especially the kidney. Hypoglycemia with leiomyoma/leiomyosarcoma and lymphoma can be due to secretion of insulin, but it is often from excessive use of glucose by the tumor, and interference with gluconeogenesis and glycogenolysis. Thrombocytopenia and/or coagulopathy are seen with hemangiosarcoma, lymphoma, and mast cell tumors. Histamine release from mast cell tumors and gastrinomas can lead to gastric ulceration and hemorrhage. Histamine release can also occur under anesthesia, causing vasodilation and hypotension. Hypertrophic osteopathy is seen with esophageal tumors, thought to be caused by increased periosteal blood flow [331].

Anesthetic management for patients with GI neoplasia is similar to that described for laparotomy with attention to hypoproteinemia and therapy for paraneoplastic syndromes. Plasma and/or colloids are useful when total protein is <4.5 mg/dL or albumin is <2.0 mg/dL. Infusion of human albumin has been used but severe side-effects, including death, have been seen in some dogs [339–343]. Hypercalcemia may cause muscle tremors or weakness and arrhythmias. Correction of hypercalcemia in animals displaying clinical signs is likely beneficial prior to anesthesia; however, correction is usually not necessary in asymptomatic animals with minimal hypercalcemia. Therapy to decrease calcium levels relatively quickly prior to surgery includes dilution via fluid therapy using 0.9% sodium chloride, which also encourages renal excretion, diuresis with furosemide, and calcitonin to inhibit osteoclastic activity in bone. Glucocorticoids can also be given; biophosphonates are used for long-term management (see the earlier section Hyperparathyroidism) [124]. Glucose should be monitored in patients with GISTs and dextrose administered as needed to maintain serum glucose above 80 mg/dL.

Patients with mast cell tumors should be premedicated with antihistamines; avoidance of drugs that stimulate histamine release, such as morphine and meperidine, is recommended. Hemorrhage is common in patients with neoplasia, especially if tumors are large and management is described above in the section Hemoabdomen.

Septic peritonitis

Several authors have reviewed septic peritonitis in dogs [344,345], cats [346–349], or both [350–355]. It is categorized as localized or diffuse, and primary or secondary, depending on the extent of disease and source of infection, respectively. *Secondary* peritonitis is most common in dogs, due to perforation of or leakage from the GIT. Foreign bodies, perforating ulcers, rupture due to intestinal obstruction, ischemic lesions, abscess or infection of abdominal organs, neoplastic lesions, trauma caused by motor vehicle impact, and bite wounds or other penetrating injuries are causes of secondary septic peritonitis. Iatrogenic causes include dehiscence of surgical incisions, inadvertent puncture of intestine, leakage around feeding tubes, and contamination of the peritoneal space at surgery. In *primary* septic peritonitis, an intra-abdominal source of infection cannot be identified. This type is more common in cats [347,349,351,355,356]. Although somewhat variable, mortality reported in small animals with septic peritonitis is still high (31–64%), in spite of improvements in recognition and therapy [304,345,348,349]. Patients with secondary peritonitis treated surgically have higher survival rates than those treated medically or those with primary peritonitis [348,353]. Pre-existing peritonitis, low albumin and protein levels, and intraoperative hypotension are also risk factors for postoperative septic peritonitis and death [345].

Anorexia, lethargy, and vomiting are the most common clinical signs in dogs and cats. Diarrhea and abdominal pain are also seen in dogs; pain is vague or inapparent in cats. Signs of sepsis relate to the severity of abdominal contamination in most cases. Unlike dogs, bradycardia and hypothermia are frequently seen in cats with sepsis [346,347,349]. Diagnosis is suggested by history and physical examination. Abdominal radiographs and ultrasonography may reveal a specific lesion with or without effusion in cases with secondary peritonitis [357]. Pneumoperitoneum is diagnostic for intestinal leakage or infection with gas-forming bacteria [350,352,356,357]. A septic infiltrate seen on cytology of peritoneal effusion or lavage fluid confirms the diagnosis. Lactate is often increased in serum and/or in the abdominal fluid. Peritoneal lactate and the comparison of serum with peritoneal lactate were diagnostic in ≥90% of dogs, but were not accurate in cats [358]. Although factors identified with prognosis vary, hypotension, hypoalbuminemia, and hyperlactatemia are more consistently associated with mortality [344,347–349,353–355,358,359].

Patients with peritonitis are some of the most challenging cases presented for anesthesia. Although some patients may have a confirmed diagnosis of peritonitis prior to laparotomy, some procedures are diagnostic in addition to therapeutic. A thorough patient assessment should be performed to estimate the severity of cardiovascular compromise, as these patients are frequently very sensitive to the depressant effects of anesthetic agents and are likely to have the systemic inflammatory response syndrome (SIRS). SIRS can occur with any severe insult, including trauma, hemorrhage, and infection. Sepsis is the presence of SIRS in response to infection, most often bacterial, but fungal and protozoal infections also occur. Sepsis may progress to severe sepsis with organ dysfunction, poor perfusion, and hypotension; multiple organ dysfunction syndrome (MODS) is also seen in severely affected patients. Septic shock is present when hypotension persists following appropriate fluid resuscitation.

The pathophysiology of sepsis and septic shock is complex, involving numerous pathways in the body's attempts to restore oxygen delivery to vital tissues. In brief, sepsis begins when organisms and/or their toxins gain access to the circulation. The classic explanation involves the release of endotoxin from Gram-negative organisms and exotoxins or petidoglycans from Gram-positive organisms. Activation of white blood cells results in release of tumor necrosis factor-α, interleukins 1, 6, and 8, and a host of other proinflammatory mediators that include leukotrienes and prostaglandins, the potent vasodilator nitric oxide, oxygen radicals, platelet activating factor, and others. Damage to the microvascular endothelium causes loss of control of permeability, and coagulopathy also develops. To maintain homeostatic balance, the body generates an anti-inflammatory response. Initially, a 'hyperdynamic' stage is seen (in dogs) with increased cardiac output, tachycardia, vasodilation (bright red mucous membranes), and shortened capillary refill. As proinflammatory effects overwhelm the anti-inflammatory response, cardiovascular collapse ensues with continued vasodilation and myocardial dysfunction, poor perfusion, decreased capillary refill, bluish or pale mucous membranes, obtundation, and hypothermia. The end result is septic shock and multiple organ dysfunction [360–363].

The GIT plays an important role in the generation of SIRS and sepsis even when the intestinal serosa is intact and a primary source is located elsewhere. Inflammation damages the barrier function of the GI mucosal lining, allowing absorption of non-microbial factors into the lymphatic system, which eventually drain into the venous system via the thoracic duct. Ongoing SIRS is magnified, and respiratory dysfunction/distress and multiple organ failure can develop via this pathway. Translocation of bacteria and bacterial products is also thought to occur via the lymphatics rather than the portal system, but this is not necessary for the development of SIRS and MODS [364,365].

Early identification of SIRS/sepsis is vital to a positive outcome. SIRS is a clinical diagnosis, but signs are not always obvious in animals, especially cats. Abnormalities associated with SIRS in humans include tachycardia, tachypnea, leukocytosis or leucopenia, and hyper- or hypothermia. Suggested guidelines for the identification of SIRS in dogs and cats include at least two of the parameters in Table 31.9.

Prior to anesthesia, patients with SIRS/sepsis should be stabilized via vigorous fluid resuscitation and with vasopressors and/or inotropes when necessary to correct hypotension, improve perfusion, maintain tissue oxygen delivery, and prevent organ dysfunction. Goal-oriented therapy with clinical endpoints of fluid resuscitation has proven to be more successful than specific shock doses or volumes of fluid [366–370]. Use of the Surviving Sepsis Campaign (SSC) guidelines in humans has significantly improved mortality. A recent update of the human guidelines was released in 2012 [281,282]; veterinary guidelines are similar [356,368,371,372].

According to SSC guidelines, in addition to improvement in clinical signs, the goals of resuscitation therapy should be achieved within 6 h of admission (Table 31.10). Collection of samples for blood cultures is recommended prior to administration of broad-spectrum antibiotics, which ideally are given within the first hour. Efforts to identify the infective source should begin as soon as possible. Lactate should be measured at admission and followed intermittently to evaluate response to therapy. Measurement of $S_{cv}O_2$ is also recommended; however, this requires catheterization of the pulmonary artery, but the cranial vena cava is an acceptable alternative [373]. Lactate can substitute for $S_{cv}O_2$ as an estimate of oxygen delivery when central catheterization is not available.

Recent meta-analysis of the use of hetastarch (hydroxyethyl starch) in septic human patients has shown evidence of acute kidney injury (AKI) and greater mortality [374,375]. The use of 0.9% sodium chloride can cause hyperchloremic metabolic acidosis [376], so a balanced crystalloid electrolyte solution is the first choice for fluid therapy in humans. Infusion of albumin is recommended when hypoalbuminemia/hypoproteinemia is present, although human albumin use in dogs is not without significant risk, including death [339–343].

Table 31.9 Parameters for SIRS/sepsis in the dog and cat [366, 367, 371].

Parameter	Dog	Cat
Heart rate (beats/min)	>120	<140 or >225
Respiratory rate (breaths/min)	>40 or $PaCO_2$ <30 mmHg	>40
Temperature (°F)	<100.4 or >104.0	<100 or >104
Leukogram WBCs/µL	>18000 or <5000	>19000 or <5000

WBCs, white blood cells.

Table 31.10 Goals of therapy for sepsis [280–282, 370, 373].

Mean arterial pressure (MAP)	>65 mmHg
Central venous oxygen saturation ($S_{cv}O_2$)	>70%
Central venous pressure (CVP)	8–12 mmHg
Urine output	>0.5 mL/kg/h

Vasopressors are given when patients remain hypotensive following fluid resuscitation. Norepinephrine is the first choice in humans, followed by epinephrine, then vasopressin. Dopamine and phenylephrine are not recommended in humans, but no difference has been found with the use of various vasopressors in animals [368,371]. Vasopressors are very potent vasoconstrictors; they should be given at the lowest effective dose to avoid ischemia and masking of persistent hypovolemia. Inotropes are useful when myocardial dysfunction is identified or suspected; they are often necessary during anesthesia to offset the depressant effects of inhalants. Relative adrenal insufficiency occurs in sepsis [377]. As corticosteroids are necessary for the proper response to vasopressor therapy, physiologic doses are recommended for animals and humans who are still hypotensive following volume replacement and vasopressor therapy [281,282,377–379]. Hyper- or hypoglycemia is also seen in some septic patients. Maintenance of normal glucose levels in humans is recommended.

Anesthetic choices and management for patients with septic peritonitis are similar to those described above for exploratory laparotomy and GDV. Dosage requirements are greatly decreased in septic patients, and combinations of low levels of inhalant with intravenous agents and adjunctive medications (e.g., lidocaine) are utilized, titrating to effect at the lowest effective doses [380]. Close attention to clinical signs and measures of oxygenation and perfusion is always necessary in anesthetized patients, but anesthetic management can directly affect outcome in septic patients. Suggestions for monitoring are also described above; measurement of cardiac output when available is highly recommended in septic patients. Non-invasive methods utilizing the NICO or the LIDCO monitors have been shown to be reliable in larger dogs and could greatly aid the evaluation of therapy in these very sick patients.

Postoperatively, continuation of cardiovascular support is likely necessary, so monitors should be kept in place. Oxygenation should be evaluated closely in recovery (especially when switching to room air) to identify those patients that need oxygen support. Blood gases, electrolytes, glucose, and lactate should also be evaluated to reassess patient status and help determine supportive therapy needed postoperatively.

Foreign body removal and other abdominal procedures

Anesthetic considerations for intestinal obstruction, removal of abdominal masses or foreign bodies, biopsy of mass lesions and/or the intestine, and colectomy are similar to those for the general exploratory laparotomy discussed above. Hemorrhage is most often associated with removal of large abdominal masses as discussed above also; however, it may occur with dissection of adhesions or fibrous tissue contained in intestinal lesions. Foreign body removal and other lesions of the small or large intestine may be straightforward, but GI perforation and leakage are concerns. Duration may be long, as meticulous dissection of lesions and resection and anastamoses of the intestine may be required. Patients with prior leakage of intestinal contents or bile will have peritonitis and may also be septic.

References

1 Greco DS, Stabenfeldt GH. The endocrine system. In: Klein BG, ed. *Cunningham's Textbook of Veterinary Physiology*, 5th edn. St Louis, MO: Saunders Elsevier, 2013; 359–373.

2 Bowen R. The hypothalamus and pituitary gland. In: *Pathophysiology of the Endocrine System*. Colorado State University. http://www.vivo.colostate.edu/hbooks/pathphys/endocrine/index.html (accessed 18 February 2014).

3 Washabau RJ. Pancreas. In: Washabau RJ, Day MJ, eds. *Canine and Feline Gastroenterology*. St Louis, MO: Saunders Elsevier, 2013; 799–802.

4 Nelson RW. Canine diabetes mellitus. In: Ettinger SJ, Feldman EC, eds. *Textbook of Veterinary Internal Medicine*, 7th edn. St Louis, MO: Saunders Elsevier, 2010; 1782–1796.

5 Reusch C. Feline diabetes mellitus. In: Ettinger SJ, Feldman EC, eds. *Textbook of Veterinary Internal Medicine*, 7th edn. St Louis, MO: Saunders Elsevier, 2010; 1796–1816.

6 O'Brien TD. Pathogenesis of feline diabetes mellitus. *Mol Cell Endocrinol* 2002; **197**: 213–219.

7 Guptill L, Glickman L, Glickman N. Time trends and risk factors for diabetes mellitus in dogs: analysis of veterinary medical data base records (1970–1999). *Vet J* 2003; **165**: 240–247.

8 Rand JS, Fleeman LM, Farrow HA, *et al*. Canine and feline diabetes mellitus: nature or nurture? *J Nutr* 2004; **134**: 2072S–2080S.

9 O'Brien MA. Diabetic emergencies in small animals. *Vet Clin Small Anim Pract* 2010; **40**: 317–333.

10 Rucinsky R, Cook A, Haley S, *et al*. AAHA diabetes management guidelines. *J Am Anim Hosp Assoc* 2010; **46**: 215–224.

11 Frank G, Anderson W, Pazak H, *et al*. Use of a high-protein diet in the management of feline diabetes mellitus. *Vet Ther* 2001; **2**: 238–246.

12 Fleeman LM, Rand JS. Evaluation of day-to-day variability of serial blood glucose concentration curves in diabetic dogs. *J Am Vet Med Assoc* 2003; **222**: 317–321.

13 Alt N, Kley S, Haessig M, *et al*. Day-to-day variability of blood glucose concentration curves generated at home in cats with diabetes mellitus. *J Am Vet Med Assoc* 2007; **230**: 1011–1017.

14 Johnson C, Norman EJ. Endocrine disease. In: Seymour C, Duke-Novakovski T, eds. *BSAVA Manual of Canine and Feline Anaesthesia and Analgesia*, 2nd edn. Quedgeley: British Small Animal Veterinary Association, 2007; 274–284.

15 Kronen PWM, Moon-Massat PF, Ludders JW, *et al*. Comparison of two insulin protocols for diabetic dogs undergoing cataract surgery. *Vet Anaesth Analg* 2001; **28**: 146–155.

16 Feldman EC, Nelson RW. Canine diabetes dellitus. In: Feldman EC, Nelson RW, eds. *Canine and Feline Endocrinology and Reproduction*, 3rd edn. St Louis, MO: Saunders Elsevier, 2004; 486–538.

17 Oliver JA, Clark L, Corletto F, *et al*. A comparison of anesthetic complications between diabetic and nondiabetic dogs undergoing phacoemulsification cataract surgery: a retrospective study. *Vet Ophthalmol* 2010; **13**: 244–250.

18 Pascoe PJ. Perioperative management of fluid therapy. In: DiBartola SP, ed. *Fluid, Electrolyte, and Acid-Base Disorders in Small Animal Practice*, 4th edn. St Louis, MO: Saunders Elsevier, 2012; 405–435.

19 Harvey RC, Schaer M. Endocrine disease. In: Tranquilli WJ, Thurmon JC, Grimm KA, eds. *Lumb and Jones' Veterinary Anesthesia and Analgesia*, 4th edn. Ames, IA: Blackwell Publishing, 2007; 933–936.

20 Clark L, Leece EA, Brearley JC. Diabetes mellitus affects the duration of action of vecuronium in dogs. *Vet Anaesth Analg* 2012; **39**: 472–479.

21 Wall III RT. Endocrine Disease. In: Hines RL, Marschall KE, eds. *Stoelting's Anesthesia and Co-Existing Disease*, 6th edn. Philadelphia: Saunders Elsevier, 2012; 376–406.

22 Brown S. Hypertensive crisis. In: Silverstein D, Hopper K, eds. *Small Animal Critical Care Medicine*. St Louis, MO: Saunders Elsevier, 2009; 176–179.

23 Kenefick S, Parker N, Slater L, *et al*. Evidence of cardiac autonomic neuropathy in dogs with diabetes mellitus. *Vet Rec* 2007; **161**: 83–88.

24 Hwang JJ, Hwang DY. Treatment of endocrine disorders in the neuroscience intensive care unit. *Curr Treat Options Neurol* 2014; **16**: 271.

25 Duncan AE, Abd-Elsayed A, Maheshwari A, *et al*. Role of intraoperative and postoperative blood glucose concentrations in predicting outcomes after cardiac surgery. *Anesthesiology* 2010; **112**: 860–871.

26 Abdelmalak BB, Knittel J, Abdelmalak JB, *et al*. Preoperative blood glucose concentrations and postoperative outcomes after elective non-cardiac surgery: an observational study. *Br J Anaesth* 2014; **112**: 79–88.

27 Bilotta F, Rosa G. Glycemia management in critical care patients. *World J Diabetes* 2012; **3**: 130–134.

28 Goutal CM, Brugmann BL, Ryan KA. Insulinoma in dogs: a review. *J Am Anim Hosp Assoc* 2012; **48**: 151–163.

29 Greene SN, Bright RM. Insulinoma in a cat. *J Small Anim Pract* 2008; **49**: 38–40.

30 Hess RS. Insulin-secreting islet cell neoplasia. In: Ettinger SJ, Feldman EC, eds. *Textbook of Veterinary Internal Medicine*, 7th edn. St Louis, MO: Saunders Elsevier, 2010; 1779–1782.

31 Robben JH, Pollak YW, Kirpensteijn J, *et al*. Comparison of ultrasonography, computed tomography, and single-photon emission computed tomography for the detection and localization of canine insulinoma. *J Vet Intern Med* 2005; **19**: 15–22.

32 Fischer JR, Smith SA, Harkin KR. Glucagon constant-rate infusion: a novel strategy for the management of hyperinsulinemic-hypoglycemic crisis in the dog. *J Am Anim Hosp Assoc* 2000; **36**: 27–32.

33 Moore AS, Nelson RW, Henry CJ, *et al*. Streptozocin for treatment of pancreatic islet cell tumors in dogs: 17 cases (1989–1999). *J Am Vet Med Assoc* 2002; **221**: 811–818.

34 de Brito Galvão JF, Chew DJ. Metabolic complications of endocrine surgery in companion animals. *Vet Clin Small Anim Pract* 2011; **41**: 847–868.

35 Koenig A. Chapter 69: Hypoglycemia. In: Silverstein D, Hopper K, eds. *Small Animal Critical Care Medicine*. St Louis, MO: Saunders Elsevier, 2009; 295–298.

36 Reine NJ, Bonczynski J. Pancreatic beta cell neoplasia. In: Birchard SJ, Sherding RG, eds. *Saunders Manual of Small Animal Practice*, 3rd edn. St Louis, MO: Saunders Elsevier, 2006; 390–397.

37 Koenig A. Endocrine emergencies in dogs and cats. *Vet Clin Small Anim Pract* 2013; **43**: 869–897.

38 Guedes AG, Rude EP. Effects of pre-operative administration of medetomidine on plasma insulin and glucose concentrations in healthy dogs and dogs with insulinoma. *Vet Anaesth Analg* 2013; **40**: 472–481.

39 Shimada A, Morita T, Ikeda N, *et al*. Hypoglycaemic brain lesions in a dog with insulinoma. *J Comp Pathol* 2000; **122**: 67–71.

40 Xenoulis PG, Steiner JM. Current concepts in feline pancreatitis. *Top Companion Anim Med* 2008; **23**: 185–92.

41 Zoran DL. Pancreatitis in cats: diagnosis and management of a challenging disease. *J Am Anim Hosp Assoc* 2006; **42**: 1–9.

42 Armstrong PJ, Williams DA. Pancreatitis in cats. *Top Companion Anim Med* 2012; **27**: 140–147.

43 Cook AK, Breitschwerdt EB, Levine JF, *et al*. Risk factors associated with acute pancreatitis in dogs: 101 cases (1985–1990). *J Am Vet Med Assoc* 1993; **203**: 673–679.

44 McCord K, Morley PS, Armstrong J, *et al*. A multi-institutional study evaluating the diagnostic utility of the spec cPL™ and SNAP® cPL™ in clinical acute pancreatitis in 84 dogs. *J Vet Intern Med* 2012; **26**: 888–896.

45 Trivedi S, Marks SL, Kass PH, *et al*. Sensitivity and specificity of canine pancreas-specific lipase (cPL) and other markers for pancreatitis in 70 dogs with and without histopathologic evidence of pancreatitis. *J Vet Intern Med* 2011; **25**: 1241–1247.

46 Xenoulis PG, Steiner JM. Canine and feline pancreatic lipase immunoreactivity. *Vet Clin Pathol* 2012; **4**: 312–324.

47 Boscan P, Monnet E, Mama K, *et al*. Effect of maropitant, a neurokinin 1 receptor antagonist, on anesthetic requirements during noxious visceral stimulation of the ovary in dogs. *Am J Vet Res* 2011; **72**: 1576–1579.

48 Niyom S, Boscan P, Twedt DC, *et al*. Effect of maropitant, a neurokinin-1 receptor antagonist, on the minimum alveolar concentration of sevoflurane during stimulation of the ovarian ligament in cats. *Vet Anaesth Analg* 2013; **40**: 425–431.

49 Hickman MA, Cox SR, Mahabir S, *et al*. Safety, pharmacokinetics and use of the novel NK-1 receptor antagonist maropitant (Cerenia) for the prevention of emesis and motion sickness in cats. *J Vet Pharmacol Ther* 2008; **31**: 220–229.

50 Weatherton LK, Streeter EM. Evaluation of fresh frozen plasma administration in dogs with pancreatitis: 77 cases (1995–2005). *J Vet Emerg Crit Care* 2009; **19**: 617–622.

51 Estabrook SG, Levine EG, Bernstein LH. Gastrointestinal crises in intensive care. *Anesthesiol Clin* 1991; **9**: 367.

52 Bunch SE. The exocrine pancreas. In: Nelson RW, Couto CG , eds. *Small Animal Internal Medicine*, 3rd edn. St Louis, MO: Mosby, 2003; 552.

53 Gaynor AR. Acute pancreatitis. In: Silverstein DC, Hopper K, eds. *Small Animal Critical Care Medicine*. St Louis, MO: Saunders Elsevier, 2009; 537–541.

54 Thompson DR. Narcotic analgesic effects on the sphincter of Oddi: a review of the data and therapeutic implications in treating pancreatitis. *Am J Gastroenterol* 2001; **96**: 1266–1272.

55 Toouli J. Sphincter of Oddi: function, dysfunction, and its management. *J Gastroenterol Hepatol* 2009; **24**(S3): S57–S62.

56 Devlin JW, Lau AK, Tanios MA. Propofol-associated hypertriglyceridemia and pancreatitis in the intensive care unit: an analysis of frequency and risk factors. *Pharmacotherapy* 2005; **25**: 1348–1352.

57 Posner LP, Asakawa M, Erb HN. Use of propofol for anesthesia in cats with primary hepatic lipidosis: 44 cases (1995–2004). *J Am Vet Med Assoc* 2008; **232**: 1841–1843.

58 Bowen R. Functional anatomy of the adrenal gland. In: *Pathophysiology of the Endocrine System*. Colorado State University. http://arbl.cvmbs.colostate.edu/hbooks/pathphys/endocrine/adrenal/anatomy.html (accessed 2 February 2014).

59 Bowen R. Functional anatomy of the adrenal gland. Histology of the adrenal gland. In: *Pathophysiology of the Endocrine System*. Colorado State University. http://arbl.cvmbs.colostate.edu/hbooks/pathphys/endocrine/adrenal/histo.html (accessed 2 February 2014).

60 Klein SC, Peterson ME. Canine hypoadrenocorticism. Part I. *Can Vet J* 2010; **51**: 63–69.

61 Klein SC, Peterson ME. Canine hypoadrenocorticism. Part II. *Can Vet J* 2010; **51**: 179–184.

62 Thompson AL, Scott-Moncrieff JC, Anderson JD. Comparison of classic hypoadrenocorticism with glucocorticoid-deficient hypoadrenocorticism in dogs: 46 cases (1985–2005). *J Am Vet Med Assoc* 2007; **230**: 1190–1194.

63 Peterson ME, Greco DS, Orth DN. Primary hypoadrenocorticism in ten cats. *J Vet Intern Med* 1989; **3**: 55–58.

64 Peterson ME, Kintzer PP, Kass PH. Pretreatment clinical and laboratory findings in dogs with hypoadrenocorticism: 225 cases (1979–1993). *J Am Vet Med Assoc* 1996; **208**: 85–91.

65 Lathan P, Moore GE, Zambon S, *et al.* Use of a low-dose ACTH stimulation test for diagnosis of hypoadrenocorticism in dogs. *J Vet Intern Med* 2008; **22**: 1070–1073.

66 Lennon EM, Boyle TE, Hutchins RG, *et al.* Use of basal serum or plasma cortisol concentrations to rule out a diagnosis of hypoadrenocorticism in dogs: 123 cases (2000–2005). *J Am Vet Med Assoc* 2007; **231**: 413–416.

67 Kintzer PP, Peterson ME. Treatment and long-term follow-up of 205 dogs with hypoadrenocorticism. *J Vet Intern Med* 1997; **11**: 43–49.

68 Kintzer PP, Peterson ME. Diseases of the adrenal gland. In: Birchard SJ, Sherding RG, eds. *Saunders Manual of Small Animal Practice*, 3rd edn. St Louis, MO: Saunders Elsevier, 2006; 357–375.

69 Feldman EC, Nelson RW. Hypoadrenocorticism (Addison's disease). In: Feldman EC, Nelson RW, eds. *Canine and Feline Endocrinology and Reproduction*, 3rd edn. St Louis, MO: Saunders Elsevier, 2004; 394–439.

70 Miller MS, Tilley LP, Smith FWK, *et al.* Electrocardiography. In: Fox PR, Sisson D, Moise NS, eds. *Textbook of Canine and Feline Cardiology: Principles and Clinical Practice*, 2nd edn. Philadelphia: WB Saunders, 1999; 67–105.

71 Dodam JR, Kruse-Elliott KT, Aucoin DP, *et al.* Duration of etomidate-induced adrenocortical suppression during surgery in dogs. *Am J Vet Res* 1990; **51**: 786–788.

72 Moon PF. Cortisol suppression in cats after induction of anesthesia with etomidate, compared with ketamine–diazepam combination. *Am J Vet Res* 1997; **58**: 868–871.

73 Melian C, Perez-Alenza MD, Peterson ME. Hyperadrenocorticism in dogs In: Ettinger SJ, Feldman EC, eds. *Textbook of Veterinary Internal Medicine*, 7th edn. St Louis, MO: Saunders Elsevier, 2010; 1816–1840.

74 Behrend EN, Kennis R. Atypical Cushing's syndrome in dogs: arguments for and against. *Vet Clin Small Anim Pract* 2010; **40**: 285–296.

75 Forrester SD, Troy GC, Dalton MN, *et al.* Retrospective evaluation of urinary tract infection in 42 dogs with hyperadrenocorticism or diabetes mellitus or both. *J Vet Intern Med* 1999; **13**: 557–560.

76 Kooistra HS, Galac S. Recent advances in the diagnosis of Cushing's syndrome in dogs. *Vet Clin Small Anim Pract* 2010; **40**: 259–267.

77 Gilor C, Graves TK. Interpretation of laboratory tests for canine Cushing's syndrome. *Top Companion Anim Med* 2011; **26**: 98–108.

78 Brown CG, Graves TK. Hyperadrenocorticism: treating dogs. *Compend Contin Educ Vet* 2007; **29**: 132–134.

79 Barker EN, Campbell S, Tebb AJ, *et al.* A comparison of the survival times of dogs treated with mitotane or trilostane for pituitary-dependent hyperadrenocorticism. *J Vet Intern Med* 2005; **19**: 810–815.

80 Peterson ME. Medical treatment of canine pituitary-dependent hyperadrenocorticism (Cushing's disease). *Vet Clin Small Anim Pract* 2001; **31**: 1005–1014.

81 Meij B, Voorhout G, Rijnberk A. Progress in transsphenoidal hypophysectomy for treatment of pituitary-dependent hyperadrenocorticism in dogs and cats. *Mol Cell Endocrinol* 2002; **197**: 89–96.

82 Jiménez Peláez M, Bouvy BM, Dupré GP. Laparoscopic adrenalectomy for treatment of unilateral adrenocortical carcinomas: technique, complications, and results in seven dogs. *Vet Surg* 2008; **37**: 444–453.

83 Adin CA, Nelson RW. Adrenal Glands. In: Tobias KM, Johnston SA, eds. *Veterinary Surgery: Small Animal*. St Louis, MO: Saunders Elsevier, 2012; 2633–2042.

84 Vaughan MA, Feldman EC, Hoar BR, *et al.* Evaluation of twice-daily, low-dose trilostane treatment administered orally in dogs with naturally occurring hyperadrenocorticism. *J Am Vet Med Assoc* 2008; **232**: 1321–1328.

85 Scavelli TD, Peterson ME, Matthiesen DT. Results of surgical treatment for hyperadrenocorticism caused by adrenocortical neoplasia in the dog: 25 cases (1980–1984). *J Am Vet Med Assoc* 1986; **189**: 1360–1364.

86 Anderson CR, Birchard SJ, Powers BE, *et al.* Surgical treatment of adrenocortical tumors: 21 cases (1990–1996). *J Am Anim Hosp Assoc* 2001; **37**: 93–97.

87 Kyles AE, Feldman EC, De Cock HE, *et al.* Surgical management of adrenal gland tumors with and without associated tumor thrombi in dogs: 40 cases (1994–2001). *J Am Vet Med Assoc* 2003; **223**: 654–662.

88 Schwartz P, Kovak JR, Koprowski A, *et al.* Evaluation of prognostic factors in the surgical treatment of adrenal gland tumors in dogs: 41 cases (1999–2005). *J Am Vet Med Assoc* 2008; **232**: 77–84.

89 Trepanier LA. Drug interactions and differential toxicity of NSAIDs. In: *Proceedings of the 22nd Annual Veterinary Medical Forum – American College of Veterinary Internal Medicine*, 2004; 535–537.

90 Goggs R, Benigni L, Fuentes VL, *et al.* Pulmonary thromboembolism. *J Vet Emerg Crit Care (San Antonio)* 2009; **19**: 30–52.

91 von Dehn J, Nelson RW, Feldman EC, *et al.* Pheochromocytoma and hyperadrenocorticism in dogs: six cases (1982–1992). *J Am Vet Med Assoc* 1995; **207**: 322–324.

92 Barthez PY, Marks SL, Woo J, *et al.* Pheochromocytoma in dogs: 61 cases (1984–1995). *J Vet Intern Med* 1997; **11**: 272–278.

93 Besso JG, Penninck DG, Gliatto JM. Retrospective ultrasonographic evaluation of adrenal lesions in 26 dogs. *Vet Radiol Ultrasound* 1997; **38**: 448–455.

94 Maher ER Jr, McNeil EA. Pheochromocytoma in dogs and cats. *Vet Clin Small Anim Pract* 1997; **27**: 359–380.

95 Brainard BM. Pheochromocytoma. In: Silverstein D, Hopper K, eds. *Small Animal Critical Care Medicine*. St Louis, MO: Saunders Elsevier, 2009; 314–317.

96 Herrera MA, Mehl ML, Kass PH, *et al.* Predictive factors and the effect of phenoxybenzamine on outcome in dogs undergoing adrenalectomy for pheochromocytoma. *J Vet Intern Med* 2008; **22**: 1333–1339.

97 Massari F, Nicoli S, Romanelli G, *et al.* Adrenalectomy in dogs with adrenal tumors: 52 cases (2002–2008). *J Am Vet Med Assoc* 2011; **239**: 216–221.

98 Barrera J, Bernard F, Ehrhart EJ, *et al.* Evaluation of risk factors for outcome associated with adrenal gland tumors with or without invasion of the caudal vena cava and treated via adrenalectomy in dogs: 86 cases (1193–2009). *J Am Vet Med Assoc* 2013; **242**: 1715–1721.

99 Mak G, Allen J. Simultaneous pheochromocytoma and third-degree atrioventricular block in 2 dogs. *J Vet Emerg Crit Care* 2013; **23**: 610–614.

100 Moon PF, Ilkiw JE. Surface-induced hypothermia in dogs: 19 cases (1987–1989). *J Am Vet Med Assoc* 1993; **202**: 437–444.

101 Augoustides JG, Abrams M, Berkowitz D, *et al*: Vasopressin for hemodynamic rescue in catecholamine-resistant vasoplegic shock after resection of massive pheochromocytoma. *Anesthesiology* 2004; **101**: 1022–1024.

102 Bowen, R. Functional anatomy of the thyroid and parathyroid glands. In: *Pathophysiology of the Endocrine System*. Colorado State University. http://arbl.cvmbs.colostate.edu/hbooks/pathphys/endocrine/thyroid/anatomy.html (accessed 2 Feburary 2014).

103 VSSO Veterinary Society of Surgical Oncology. *Cancer Information: Thyroid Tumors*. http://www.vsso.org/Thyroid_Tumors_-_Canine.html (accessed 2 Feburary 2014).

104 Mooney CT. Canine hypothyroidism: a review of aetiology and diagnosis. *N Z Vet J* 2011; **59**: 105–114.

105 Scott-Moncrieff JCR. Hypothyroidism. In: Ettinger SJ, Feldman EC, eds. *Textbook of Veterinary Internal Medicine*, 7th edn. St Louis, MO: Saunders Elsevier, 2010; 1751–1761.

106 Panciera DL. Hypothyroidism in dogs: 66 cases (1987–1992). *J Am Vet Med Assoc* 1994; **204**: 761–767.

107 Ferguson DC. Testing for hypothyroidism in dogs. *Vet Clin Small Anim Pract* 2007; **37**: 647–669.

108 Peterson ME, Melián C, Nichols R. Measurement of serum total thyroxine, triiodothyronine, free thyroxine, and thyrotropin concentrations for diagnosis of hypothyroidism in dogs. *J Am Vet Med Assoc* 1997; **211**: 1396–1402.

109 Kantrowitz LB, Peterson ME, Melián C, *et al.* Serum total thyroxine, total triiodothyronine, free thyroxine, and thyrotropin concentrations in dogs with nonthyroidal disease. *J Am Vet Med Assoc* 2001; **219**: 765–769.

110 Scott-Moncrieff JC, Nelson RW, Bruner JM, *et al.* Comparison of serum concentrations of thyroid-stimulating hormone in healthy dogs, hypothyroid dogs, and euthyroid dogs with concurrent disease. *J Am Vet Med Assoc* 1998; **212**: 387–391.

111 Panciera DL, Peterson ME, Birchard SJ. Diseases of the thyroid gland. In: Birchard SJ, Sherding RG, eds. *Saunders Manual of Small Animal Practice*, 3rd edn. St Louis, MO: Saunders Elsevier, 2006; 327–342.

112 Sarlis NJ, Gourgiotis L. Thyroid emergencies. *Rev Endocr Metab Disord* 2003; **4**: 129–136.

113 Babad AA, Eger EI II. The effects of hyperthyroidism and hypothyroidism on halothane and oxygen requirement in dogs. *Anesthesiology* 1968; **29**: 1087–1093.

114 Berry SH, Panciera DL. The effect of experimentally induced hypothyroidism on the isoflurane minimum alveolar concentration in dogs. *Vet Anaesth Analg* 2014; doi: 10.1111/vaa.12156, Epub ahead of print 14 March 2014.

115 McMurphy RM, Hodgson DS, Bruyette DS, *et al.* Cardiovascular effects of 1.0, 1.5, and 2.0 minimum alveolar concentrations of isoflurane in experimentally induced hypothyroidism in dogs. *Vet Surg* 1996; **25**: 171–178.

116 Mooney CT. Hyperthyroidism. In: Ettinger SJ, Feldman EC, eds. *Textbook of Veterinary Internal Medicine*, 7th edn. St Louis, MO: Saunders Elsevier, 2010; 1761–1778.

117 Peterson ME, Ward CR. Etiopathologic findings of hyperthyroidism in cats. *Vet Clin Small Anim Pract* 2007; **37**: 633–645.

118 Barber LG. Thyroid tumors in dogs and cats. *Vet Clin Small Anim Pract* 2007; **37**: 755–773.
119 Broussard JD, Peterson ME, Fox PR. Changes in clinical and laboratory findings in cats with hyperthyroidism from 1983 to 1993. *J Am Vet Med Assoc* 1995; **206**: 302–305.
120 Graves TK. Hyperthyroidism and the kidneys. In: August JR, ed. *Consultations in Feline Internal Medicine*, 6th edn. St Louis, MO: Saunders Elsevier, 2010; 268–273.
121 Peterson ME. Diagnostic tests for hyperthyroidism in cats. *Clin Tech Small Anim Pract* 2006; **21**: 2–9.
122 Graves TK, Peterson ME. Diagnosis of occult hyperthyroidism in cats. *Probl Vet Med* 1990; **2**: 683–692.
123 Peterson ME. Radioiodine treatment of hyperthyroidism. *Clin Tech Small Anim Pract* 2006; **21**: 34–39.
124 Trepanier LA. Pharmacologic management of feline hyperthyroidism. *Vet Clin Small Anim Pract* 2007; **37**: 775–788.
125 Naan EC, Kirpensteijn J, Kooistra HS, *et al.* Results of thyroidectomy in 101 cats with hyperthyroidism. *Vet Surg* 2006; **35**: 287–293.
126 Tolbert MK, Ward CR. Feline focus – feline thyroid storm: rapid recognition to improve patient survival. *Compend Contin Educ Vet* 2010; **32**: E1–E6.
127 Klubo-Gwiezdzinska J, Wartofsky L. Thyroid emergencies. *Med Clin North Am* 2012; **96**: 385–403.
128 Birchard SJ. Thyroidectomy in the cat. *Clin Tech Small Anim Pract* 2006; **21**: 29–33.
129 Henik RA, Stepien RL, Wenholz LJ, *et al.* Efficacy of atenolol as a single antihypertensive agent in hyperthyroid cats. *J Feline Med Surg* 2008; **10**: 577–582.
130 Clutton RE. Cardiovascular disease. In: Seymour C, Duke-Novakovski T, eds. *BSAVA Manual of Canine and Feline Anaesthesia and Analgesia*, 2nd edn. Quedgeley: British Small Animal Veterinary Association, 2007; 200–219.
131 Bednarski RM. Anesthetic concerns for patients with cardiomyopathy. *Vet Clin Small Anim Pract* 1992; **22**: 460–465.
132 Lamont L, Bulmer B, Sisson D, *et al.* Doppler echocardiographic effects of medetomidine on dynamic left ventricular outflow tract obstruction in cats. *J Am Vet Med Assoc* 2002; **221**: 1276–1281.
133 Bowen R. Parathyroid hormone. In: *Pathophysiology of the Endocrine System*. Colorado State University. http://arbl.cvmbs.colostate.edu/hbooks/pathphys/endocrine/thyroid/pth.html (accessed 2 February 2014).
134 Schaefer C, Goldstein RE. Canine primary hyperparathyroidism. *Compend Contin Educ Vet* 2009; **31**: 382–390.
135 Bonczynski J. Primary hyperparathyroidism in dogs and cats. *Clin Tech Small Anim Pract* 2007; **22**: 70–74.
136 Feldman EC, Hoar B, Pollard R, *et al.* Pretreatment clinical and laboratory findings in dogs with primary hyperparathyroidism: 210 cases (1987–2004). *J Am Vet Med Assoc* 2005; **227**: 756–761.
137 Graves TK. When normal is abnormal: keys to laboratory diagnosis of hidden endocrine disease. *Top Companion Anim Med* 2011; **26**: 45–51.
138 Rasor L, Pollard R, Feldman EC. Retrospective evaluation of three treatment methods for primary hyperparathyroidism in dogs. *J Am Anim Hosp Assoc* 2007; **43**: 70–77.
139 Graham KJ, Wilkinson M, Culvenor J, *et al.* Intraoperative parathyroid hormone concentration to confirm removal of hypersecretory parathyroid tissue and time to postoperative normocalcaemia in nine dogs with primary hyperparathyroidism. *Aust Vet J* 2012; **90**: 203–209.
140 Arbaugh M, Smeak D, Monnet E. Evaluation of preoperative serum concentrations of ionized calcium and parathyroid hormone as predictors of hypocalcemia following parathyroidectomy in dogs with primary hyperparathyroidism: 17 cases (2001–2009). *J Am Vet Med Assoc* 2012; **24**: 233–236.
141 Schenk PA, Chew DJ. Diseases of the parathyroid gland and calcium disorders. In: Birchard SJ, Sherding RG, eds. *Saunders Manual of Small Animal Practice*, 3rd edn. St Louis, MO: Saunders Elsevier, 2006; : 343–356.
142 Schenk PA, Chew DJ, Nagode LA, *et al.* Disorders of calcium: hypercalcemia and hypocalcemia. In: DiBartola SP, ed. *Fluid, Electrolyte, and Acid-Base Disorders in Small Animal Practice*, 4th edn. St Louis, MO: Saunders Elsevier, 2012; 137–163.
143 Green T, Chew DJ. Calcium disorders. In: Silverstein D, Hopper K, eds. *Small Animal Critical Care Medicine*. St Louis, MO: Saunders Elsevier, 2009, 233–239.
144 Gear RN, Neiger R, Skelly BJ, *et al.* Primary hyperparathyroidism in 29 dogs: diagnosis, treatment, outcome and associated renal failure. *J Small Anim Pract* 2005; **46**: 10–16.
145 Washabau RJ. Integration of Gastrointestinal Function. In: Washabau RJ, Day MJ, eds. *Canine and Feline Gastroenterology*. St Louis, MO: Saunders Elsevier, 2013; 1–29.
146 Herdt TH, Sayegh AI. Regulation of the gastrointestinal functions, In: Klein BG, ed. *Cunningham's Textbook of Veterinary Physiology*, 5th edn. St Louis, MO: Saunders Elsevier, 2013; 263–273.
147 Bowen R. Control of digestive system function. In: *Pathophysiology of the Endocrine System*. Colorado State University. http://www.vivo.colostate.edu/hbooks/pathphys/digestion/basics/control.html (accessed September 2013).
148 Herdt TH, Sayegh AI. Motility patterns of the gastrointestinal tract. In: Klein BG, ed. *Cunningham's Textbook of Veterinary Physiology*, 5th ed. St Louis, MO: Saunders Elsevier, 2013; 274–285.
149 Luckey A, Livingston E, Tache Y. Mechanisms and treatment of postoperative ileus. *Arch Surg* 2003; **138**: 206–214.
150 Washabau RJ, Hall JA. Stomach: dysmotility. In: Washabau RJ, Day MJ, eds. *Canine and Feline Gastroenterology*. St Louis, MO: Saunders Elsevier, 2013; 630–634.
151 Grocott MP, Browne JP, Van der Meulen J, *et al.* The Postoperative Morbidity Survey was validated and used to describe morbidity after major surgery. *J Clin Epidemiol* 2007; **60**: 919–298.
152 Behm B, Stollman N. Postoperative ileus: etiologies and interventions. *Clin Gastroenterol Hepatol* 2003; **1**: 71–80.
153 Washabau RJ. Vomiting: pathophysiology and mechanisms. In: Washabau RJ, Day MJ, eds. *Canine and Feline Gastroenterology*. St Louis, MO: Saunders Elsevier, 2013; 167–169.
154 Bowen R. Physiology of vomiting. In *Pathophysiology of the Digestive System*. Colorado State University. http://www.vivo.colostate.edu/hbooks/pathphys/digestion/stomach/vomiting.html (accessed 10 August 2013).
155 Papich MG. Drugs affecting GI function. In: Riviere JE, Papich MG, eds. *Veterinary Pharmacology and Therapeutics*, 9th edn. Ames, IA: Wiley-Blackwell, 2009; 1247–1251.
156 Elwood C, Devauchelle P, Elliott J, *et al.* Emesis in dogs: a review. *J Small Anim Pract* 2010; **51**: 4–22.
157 KuKanich B, Papich MG. Opioid analgesic drugs. In: Riviere JE, Papich MG, eds. *Veterinary Pharmacology and Therapeutics*, 9th edn. Ames, IA: Wiley-Blackwell, 2009; 308–319.
158 Johnston KD. The potential for mu-opioid receptor agonists to be anti-emetic in humans: a review of clinical data. *Acta Anaesthesiol Scand* 2010; **54**: 132–140.
159 Muir WW III. General considerations for anesthesia. In: Tranquilli WJ, Thurmon JC, Grimm KA, eds. *Lumb and Jones' Veterinary Anesthesia and Analgesia*, 4th edn. Ames, IA: Blackwell Publishing, 2007; 13–14.
160 Apfel CC, Kranke P, Katz MH, *et al.* Volatile anaesthetics may be the main cause of early but not delayed postoperative vomiting: a randomized controlled trial of factorial design. *Br J Anaesth* 2002; **88**: 659–668.
161 Redondo JI. Clinical evaluation in dogs of a new formulation of propofol in a medium-chain and long-chain triglyceride emulsion. A multicentre study. Presented at the World Congress of Veterinary Anaesthesiology, Santos, Brazil, 12–16 September 2006.
162 Muir WW III, Mason DE. Side effects of etomidate in dogs. *J Am Vet Med Assoc* 1989; **194**: 1430–1434.
163 Hall LW, Chambers JP. A clinical trial of propofol infusion anaesthesia in dogs. *J Small Anim Pract* 1987; **28**: 623–637.
164 Tsai YC, Wang LY, Yeh LS. Clinical comparison of recovery from total intravenous anesthesia with propofol and inhalation anesthesia with isoflurane in dogs. *J Vet Med Sci* 2007; **69**: 1179–1182.
165 Smith JA, Gaynor JS, Bednarski RM, *et al.* Adverse effects of administration of propofol with various preanesthetic regimens in dogs. *J Am Vet Assoc* 1993; **202**: 1111–1118.
166 Vähä-Vahe T. Clinical evaluation of medetomidine, a novel sedative and analgesic drug for dogs and cats. *Acta Vet Scand* 1989; **30**: 267–273.
167 Cullen LK. Medetomidine sedation in dogs and cats: a review of its pharmacology, antagonism and dose. *Br Vet J* 1996; **152**: 519–535.
168 Sinclair MD. A review of the physiological effects of α_2-agonists related to the clinical use of medetomidine in small animal practice. *Can Vet J* 2003; **44**: 885–897.
169 Posner LP, Burns P. Sedative agents: tranquilizers, alpha-2 agonists and related agents. In: Riviere JE, Papich MG, eds. *Veterinary Pharmacology and Therapeutics*, 9th edn. Ames, IA: Wiley-Blackwell, 2009; 344.
170 Granholm M, McKusick BC, Westerholm FC, *et al.* Evaluation of the clinical efficacy and safety of dexmedetomidine or medetomidine in cats and their reversal with atipamezole. *Vet Anaesth Analg* 2006; **33**: 214–223.
171 Zoetis. Dexdomitor® (dexmedetomidine) package insert. https://online.zoetis.com/US/EN/Products/Pages/Dexdomitor/Default.aspx (accessed 18 September 2013).
172 Lamont L, Burton S, Caines D, *et al.* Effects of 2 different medetomidine infusion rates on selected neurohormonal and metabolic parameters in dogs. *Can J Vet Res* 2012; **76**: 143–148.
173 van Oostrom H, Doornenbal A, Schot A, *et al.* Neurophysiological assessment of the sedative and analgesic effects of a constant rate infusion of dexmedetomidine in the dog. *Vet J* 2010; **190**: 338–344.

174 Ansah OB, Raekallio M, Vainio O. Corrrelation between serum concentrations following continuous intravenous infusion of dexmedetomidine or medetomidine in cats and their sedative and analgesic effects. *J Vet Pharmacol Ther* 2000; **23**: 1–8.

175 Valverde A, Cantwell S, Hernandez J, *et al.* Effects of acepromazine on the incidence of vomiting associated with opioid administration in dogs. *Vet Anaesth Analg* 2004; **31**: 40–45.

176 Karaccas Y, Teixeira Neto FJ, Giordano T, *et al.* Incidence of emesis after different doses of morphine and the effects of three phenothiazine premedications on morphine induced vomiting in dogs. Presented at the World Congress of Veterinary Anaesthesiology, Santos, Brazil, 12–16 September 2006.

177 Matsubara LM, Oliva VN, Gabas DT, *et al.* Effect of lidocaine on the minimum alveolar concentration of sevoflurane in dogs. *Vet Anaesth Analg* 2009; **36**: 407–413.

178 McCarthy GC, Megalla SA, Habib AS. Impact of intravenous lidocaine infusion on postoperative analgesia and recovery from surgery: a systematic review of randomized controlled trials. *Drugs* 2010; **70**: 1149–1163.

179 Marret E, Rolin M, Beaussier M, *et al.* Meta-analysis of intravenous lidocaine and postoperative recovery after abdominal surgery. *Br J Surg* 2008; **95**: 1331–1338.

180 Rau SE, Barber LG, Burgess KE. Efficacy of maropitant in the prevention of delayed vomiting associated with administration of doxorubicin to dogs. *J Vet Intern Med* 2010; **24**: 1452–1457.

181 de la Puente-Redondo VA, Tilt N, Rowan TG, *et al.* Efficacy of maropitant for treatment and prevention of emesis caused by intravenous infusion of cisplatin in dogs. *Am J Vet Res* 2007; **68**: 48–56.

182 Santos LCP, Ludders JW, Erb HN, *et al.* A randomized, blinded, controlled trial of the antiemetic effect of ondansetron on dexmedetomidine-induced emesis in cats. *Vet Anaesth Analg* 2011; **38**: 320–327.

183 Hay Kraus BL. Efficacy of maropitant in preventing vomiting in dogs premedicated with hydromorphone. *Vet Anaesth Analg* 2013; **40**: 28–34.

184 Mathis A, Lee K, Alibhai HI. The use of maropitant to prevent vomiting induced by epidural administration of preservative free morphine through an epidural catheter in a dog. *Vet Anaesth Analg* 2011; **38**: 516–517.

185 Gan TJ, Diemunsch P, Habib AS, *et al.* Consensus guidelines for the management of postoperative nausea and vomiting. *Anesth Analg* 2014; **118**: 85–113.

186 Karanicolas PJ, Smith SE, Kanbur B, *et al.* The impact of prophylactic dexamethasone on nausea and vomiting after laparoscopic cholecystectomy: a systematic review and meta-analysis. *Ann Surg* 2008; **248**: 751–762.

187 Topal A, Gül NY. Effects of dexamethasone, metoclopramide or acepromazine on emesis in cats sedated with xylazine hydrochloride. *Acta Vet Brno* 2006; **75**: 299–303.

188 Wilson DV, Evans AT. Effect of a short preanesthetic fast on risk of gastroesophageal reflux during anesthesia in dogs. Presented at the Annual Meeting of the American College of Veterinary Anesthesiologists, Chicago, IL, 12–13 September 2006.

189 Galatos A, Raptopoulos D. Gastro-oesophageal reflux during anaesthesia in the dog: the effect of preoperative fasting and premedication. *Vet Rec* 1995; **137**: 479–483.

190 Savvas I, Raptopoulos D. Incidence of gastro-oesophageal reflux during anaesthesia, following two different fasting times in dogs. *Vet Anaesth Analg* 2000; **27**: 54–62.

191 Galatos A, Raptopoulos D. Gastro-oesophageal reflux during anaesthesia in the dog: the effect of age, positioning and type of surgical procedure. *Vet Rec* 1995; **137**: 513–516.

192 Lamata C, Loughton V, Jones M, *et al.* The risk of passive regurgitation during general anaesthesia in a population of referred dogs in the UK. *Vet Anaesth Analg* 2012; **39**: 266–274.

193 De Miguel García C, Pinchbeck GL, Dugdale A, *et al.* Retrospective study of the risk factors and prevalence of regurgitation in dogs undergoing general anaesthesia. *Open Vet Sci J* 2013; **7**: 6–11.

194 Wilson DV, Boruta DT, Dhanjal JK, *et al.* The prevalence of anesthetic-related gastroesophageal reflux during fracture repair in dogs. Presented at the American College of Veterinary Anesthesia Autumn Conference, International Veterinary Emergency and Critical Care Symposium, Phoenix, AZ, 18–21 September 2008.

195 Galatos AD, Savas I, Prassinos NN, *et al.* Gastro-oesophageal reflux during thiopentone or propofol anaesthesia in the cat. *J Vet Med A Physiol Pathol Clin Med.* 2001; **48**: 287–294.

196 Wilson DV. Peri-anesthetic gastroesophageal reflux. Presented at the International Veterinary Emergency and Critical Care Symposium, Nashville, TN, 14–18 September 2011.

197 Wilson DV, Evans AT, Miller R. Effects of preanesthetic administration of morphine on gastroesophageal reflux and regurgitation during anesthesia in dogs. *Am J Vet Res* 2005; **66**: 386–390.

198 Wilson DV, Evans AT, Mauer WA. Pre-anesthetic meperidine: associated vomiting and gastroesophageal reflux during the subsequent anesthetic in dogs. *Vet Anaesth Analg* 2007; **34**:15–22.

199 Savvas I, Rallia T, Raptopoulos D. The effect of pre-anaesthetic fasting time and type of food on gastric content volume and acidity in dogs. *Vet Anaesth Analg* 2009; **36**: 539–546.

200 Sideri AI, Apostolos D, Galatos AD, *et al.* Gastro-oesophageal reflux during anaesthesia in the kitten: comparison between use of a laryngeal mask airway or an endotracheal tube. *Vet Anaesth Analg* 2009; **36**: 547–554.

201 Wilson DV, Boruta DT, Evans AT. Influence of halothane, isoflurane, and sevoflurane on gastroesophageal reflux during anesthesia in dogs. *Am J Vet Res* 2006; **67**: 1821–1825.

202 Wilson DV, Evans AT, Mauer WA. Influence of metoclopramide on gastroesophageal reflux in anesthetized dogs. *Am J Vet Res* 2006; **67**: 26–31.

203 Ogunnaike BO, Whitten CW. Gastrointestinal disorders. In: Barash PG, Cullen BF, Stoelting RK, *et al.*, eds. *Clinical Anesthesia*, 6th edn. Philadelphia: Lippincott, Williams & Wilkins, 2009; 1221–1228.

204 Diamant NE. Pathophysiology of gastroesophageal reflux disease. *GI Motility Online*, 16 May 2006. http://www.nature.com/gimo/contents/pt1/full/gimo21.html (accessed 1 June 2013).

205 Richter JE. Gastrooesophageal reflux disease. *Best Pract Res Clin Gastroenterol* 2007; **21**: 609–631.

206 Holloway RH. The anti-reflux barrier and mechanisms of gastro-oesophageal reflux. *Clin Gastroenterol* 2000; **14**: 681–699.

207 Cox MR, Martin CJ, Dent J, *et al.* Effect of general anaesthesia on transient lower oesophageal sphincter relaxations in the dog. *Aust N Z J Surg* 1988; **58**: 825–830.

208 Hershcovici T, Mashimo H, R. Fass R. The lower esophageal sphincter. *Neurogastroenterol Motil* 2011; **23**: 819–830.

209 Cotton BR, Smith G. The lower oesophageal sphincter and anaesthesia. *Br J Anaesth* 1984; **56**: 37–46.

210 Martin CJ, Dodds WJ, Liem HH, *et al.* Diaphragmatic contribution to gastroesophageal competence and reflux in dogs. *Am J Physiol* 1992; **263**: G551–G557.

211 Poncet CM, Dupre GP, Freiche VG, *et al.* Prevalence of gastrointestinal tract lesions in 73 brachycephalic dogs with upper respiratory syndrome. *J Small Anim Pract* 2005; **46**: 273–279.

212 Washabau RJ. Esophagus. In: Washabau RJ, Day MJ, eds. *Canine and Feline Gastroenterology.* St Louis, MO: Saunders Elsevier, 2013; 580–594.

213 Leib MS, Dinnel H, Ward DL, *et al.* Endoscopic balloon dilation of benign esophageal strictures in dogs and cats. *J Vet Intern Med* 2001; **15**: 547–552.

214 Ogunnaike BO, Whitten CW. Gastrointestinal disorders. In: Barash PG, Cullen BF, Stoelting RK, *et al.*, eds. *Clinical Anesthesia*, 6th edn. Philadelphia: Lippincott, Williams & Wilkins, 2009; 1221–1228.

215 Open Anesthesia. ABA:Esoph Sphincter Tone – Anes Drugs. http://www.openanesthesia.org/index.php?title=Esoph_sphincter_tone:_Anes_drugs (accessed 7 January 2014).

216 Strombeck DR, Harrold D. Effects of atropine, acepromazine, meperidine and xylazine on gastroesophageal sphincter pressure in the dog. *Am J Vet Res* 1985; **46**: 963–965.

217 Hall JA, Magne ML, Twedt DC. Effect of acepromazine, diazepam, fentanyl-droperidol, and oxymorphone on gastroesophageal sphincter pressure in healthy dogs. *Am J Vet Res* 1987; **48**: 556–557.

218 Waterman AE, Hashim MA. Effects of thiopentone and propofol on lower oesophageal sphincter and barrier pressure in the dog. *J Small Anim Pract* 1992; **33**: 530–533.

219 van der Hoeven CW, Attia A, Deen L, *et al.* The influence of anaesthetic drugs on the LOS in propofol/nitrous oxide anaesthetized dogs. Pressure profilometry in an animal model. *Acta Anaesthesiol Scand* 1995; **39**: 822–826.

220 Hashim MA, Waterman AE. Effect of acepromazine, pethidine and atropine premedication on lower oesophageal sphincter pressure and barrier pressure in anaesthetized cats. *Vet Rec* 1993; **133**: 158–160.

221 Hashim MA, Waterman AE. Effects of thiopentone, propofol, alphaxalone-alphadolone, ketamine and xylazine–ketamine on lower oesophageal sphincter pressure and barrier pressure in cats. *Vet Rec*; **129**: 137–139.

222 Hashim MA, Waterman AE, Pearson H. Effect of body position on oesophageal and gastric pressures in the anaesthetized dog. *J Small Anim Pract* 1995; **36**: 196–200.

223 Paterson WG, Rattan S, Goyal RK. Experimental induction of isolated lower esophageal sphincter relaxation in anesthetized opossums. *J Clin Invest* 1986; **77**: 1187–1193.

224 Leslie E, Bhargava V, Mittal RK. A novel pattern of longitudinal muscle contraction with subthreshold pharyngeal stimulus: a possible mechanism of lower esophageal sphincter relaxation. *Am J Physiol Gastrointest Liver Physiol* 2012; **302**: G542–G547.

225 Mansfield CS, Hyndman T. Gastric cytoprotective agents. In: Washabau RJ, Day MJ, eds. *Canine and Feline Gastroenterology.* St Louis, MO: Saunders Elsevier, 2013; 500–504.

226 Tolbert K, Bissett S, King A, *et al.* Efficacy of oral famotidine and 2 omeprazole formulations for the control of intragastric pH in dogs. *J Vet Intern Med* 2011; **25**: 47–54.

227 Panti A, Bennett RC, Corletto F, *et al.* The effect of omeprazole on oesophageal pH in dogs during anaesthesia. *J Small Anim Pract* 2009; **50**: 540–544.

228 Favarato ES, Souza MV, Costa PR, *et al.* Evaluation of metoclopramide and ranitidine on the prevention of gastroesophageal reflux episodes in anesthetized dogs. *Res Vet Sci* 2012; **93**: 466–467.

229 Zacuto AC, Marks SL, Osborn J, *et al.* The influence of esomeprazole and cisapride on gastroesophageal reflux during anesthesia in dogs. *J Vet Intern Med* 2012; **26**: 518–525.

230 Wilson DV, Evans AT. The effect of topical treatment on esophageal pH during acid reflux in dogs. *Vet Anaesth Analg* 2007; **34**: 339–343.

231 American Society of Anesthesiologists Committee. Practice Guidelines for Preoperative Fasting and the Use of Pharmacologic Agents to Reduce the Risk of Pulmonary Aspiration: Application to Healthy Patients Undergoing Elective Procedures: an updated report by the American Society of Anesthesiologists Committee on Standards and Practice Parameters. *Anesthesiology* 2011; **114**: 495–511.

232 Evander A, Little AG, Riddell RH, *et al.* Composition of the refluxed material determines the degree of reflux esophagitis in the dog. *Gastroenterology* 1987; **93**: 280–286.

233 Glazer A, Walters P. Esophagitis and esophageal strictures. *Compend Contin Educ Vet* 2008; **30**: 281–292.

234 Han E. Diagnosis and management of reflux esophagitis. *Clin Tech Small Anim Pract* 2003; **18**: 231–238.

235 Sellon RK, Willard MD. Esophagitis and esophageal strictures. *Vet Clin Small Anim Pract* 2003; **33**: 945–967.

236 Frowde PE, Battersby IA, Whitley NT, *et al.* Oesophageal disease in 33 cats. *J Feline Med Surg* 2011; **13**: 564–569.

237 Bissett SA, Davis J, Subler K, *et al.* Risk factors and outcome of bougienage for treatment of benign esophageal strictures in dogs and cats: 28 cases (1995–2004). *J Am Vet Med Assoc* 2009; **235**: 844–850.

238 Han E, Broussard J, Baer KE. Feline esophagitis secondary to gastroesophageal reflux disease: clinical signs and radiographic, endoscopic, and histopathological findings. *J Am Anim Hosp Assoc* 2003; **39**: 161–167.

239 Adamama-Moraitou KK, Rallis TS, Prassinos NN, *et al.* Benign esophageal stricture in the dog and cat: a retrospective study of 20 cases. *Can J Vet Res* 2002; **66**: 55–59.

240 Kushner LI, Shofer FS. Incidence of esophageal strictures and esophagitis after general anesthesia. Presented at the World Congress of Veterinary Anaesthesiology, Knoxville, TN, 17–20 September 2003.

241 Wilson DV, Walshaw R. Postanesthetic esophageal dysfunction in 13 dogs. *J Am Anim Hosp Assoc* 2004; **40**(6): 455–460.

242 Anagnostou TL, Savvas I, Kazakos GM, *et al.* Effect of endogenous progesterone and oestradiol-17β on the incidence of gastro-oesophageal reflux and on the barrier pressure during general anaesthesia in the female dog. *Vet Anaesth Analg* 2009; **36**: 308–318.

243 Janda M, Scheeren TWL, Nöldge-Schomburg GF. Management of pulmonary aspiration. *Best Pract Res Clin Anaesthesiol* 2006; **20**: 409–427.

244 Marik PE. Pulmonary aspiration syndromes. *Curr Opin Pulm Med* 2011; **17**: 148–154.

245 Schulze HM, Rahilly LJ. Aspiration pneumonia in dogs: pathophysiology, prevention, and diagnosis. *Compend Contin Educ Vet* 2012; **34**(12): E5.

246 Schulze HM, Rahilly LJ. Aspiration pneumonia in dogs: treatment, monitoring, and prognosis. *Compend Contin Educ Vet* 2012; **34**(12): E1.

247 Ovbey DH, Wilson DV, Bednarski RM, *et al.* Prevalence and risk factors for canine post-anesthetic aspiration pneumonia (1999–2009): a multicenter study. *Vet Anaesth Analg* 2014; **41**: 127–136.

248 Java MA, Drobatz KJ, Gilley RS, *et al.* Incidence of and risk factors for postoperative pneumonia in dogs anesthetized for diagnosis or treatment of intervertebral disk disease. *J Am Vet Med Assoc* 2009; **235**: 281–287.

249 Alwood AJ, Brainard BM, LaFond E, *et al.* *Postoperative pulmonary complications in dogs undergoing laparotomy: frequency, characterization and disease-related risk factors.* 2006; **16**: 176–183.

250 Kogan DA, Johnson LR, Sturges BK, *et al.* Etiology and clinical outcome in dogs with aspiration pneumonia: 88 cases (2004–2006). *J Am Vet Med Assoc* 2008; **233**: 1748–1755.

251 Tart KM, Babski DM, Lee JA. Potential risks, prognostic indicators, and diagnostic and treatment modalities affecting survival in dogs with presumptive aspiration pneumonia: 125 cases (2005–2008). *J Vet Emerg Crit Care* 2010; **20**: 319–329.

252 Mythen MG. Postoperative gastrointestinal tract dysfunction: an overview of causes and management strategies. *Cleve Clin J Med* 2009; **76**(Suppl 4): S66–S71.

253 Morton AJ, AT Blikslager AT. Surgical and postoperative factors influencing short-term survival of horses following small intestinal resection: 92 cases (1994–2001). *Equine Vet J* 2002; **34**: 450–454.

254 Senior JM, Pinchbeck GL, Allister R, *et al.* Post anaesthetic colic in horses: a preventable complication? *Equine Vet J* 2006; **38**: 479–484.

255 Flecknell P. Analgesia and post-operative care. *Laboratory Animal Anesthesia*, 3rd edn. San Diego, CA: Elsevier Academic Press, 2009; 171–172.

256 Hawkins MG, Pascoe PJ. Anesthesia, analgesia and sedation of small mammals. In: Quesenberry KE, Carpenter JW, eds. *Ferrets, Rabbits, and Rodents Clinical Medicine and Surgery*, 3rd edn. St Louis, MO: Saunders Elsevier, 2012; 430, 445.

257 Healy TE, Foster GE, Evans EF, *et al.* Effect of some i.v. anaesthetic agents on canine gastrointestinal motility. *Br J Anaesth* 1981; **53**: 229–233.

258 Steinbrook RA. Epidural anesthesia and gastrointestinal motility. *Anesth Analg* 1998; **86**: 837–844.

259 Nakamura K, Hara S, Tomizawa N. The effects of medetomidine and xylazine on gastrointestinal motility and gastrin release in the dog. *J Vet Pharmacol Ther* 1997; **20**: 290–295.

260 Hsu WH, McNeel SV. Effect of yohimbine on xylazine-induced prolongation of gastrointestinal transit in dogs. *J Am Vet Med Assoc* 1983; **183**: 297–300.

261 Maugeri S, Ferrè JP, Intorre L, *et al.* Effects of medetomidine on intestinal and colonic motility in the dog. *J Vet Pharmacol Ther* 1994; **17**: 148–154.

262 Boscan P, Van Hoogmoed LM, Farver TB, *et al.* Evaluation of the effects of the opioid agonist morphine on gastrointestinal tract function in horses. *Am J Vet Res* 2006; **67**: 992–997.

263 Washabau RJ. Small intestine: dysmotility. In: Washabau RJ, Day MJ, eds. *Canine and Feline Gastroenterology.* St Louis, MO: Saunders Elsevier, 2013; 707–709.

264 Washabau RJ. Gastrointestinal motility disorders and gastrointestinal prokinetic therapy. *Vet Clin Small Anim Pract* 2003; **33**: 1007–1028.

265 Ali-Melkkilä T, Kanto J, Iisalo E. Pharmacokinetics and related pharmacodynamics of anticholinergic drugs. *Acta Anaesthesiol Scand* 1993; **37**: 633–642.

266 Eger EI II. Atropine, scopolamine, and related compounds. *Anesthesiology* 1962; **23**: 365–383.

267 Burger DM, Wiestner T, Hubler M, *et al.* Effect of anticholinergics (atropine, glycopyrrolate) and prokinetics (metoclopramide, cisapride) on gastric motility in Beagles and Labrador Retrievers. *J Vet Med A Physiol Pathol Clin Med* 2006; **53**: 97–107.

268 Braun U, Gansohr B, Haessig M. Ultrasonographic evaluation of reticular motility in cows after administration of atropine, scopolamine and xylazine. *J Vet Med A Physiol Pathol Clin Med* 2002; **49**: 299–302.

269 Teixeira Neto FJ, McDonell WN, Black WD, *et al.* Effects of glycopyrrolate on cardiorespiratory function in horses anesthetized with halothane and xylazine. *Am J Vet Res* 2004; **65**: 456–463.

270 Short, CE, Paddleford, RR, Cloyd GD. Glycopyrrolate or prevention of pulmonary complications during anesthesia. *Mod Vet Pract* 1974; **55**: 194–196.

271 DeHaven-Hudkins DL, DeHaven RN, Little PJ, *et al.* The involvement of the mu-opioid receptor in gastrointestinal pathophysiology: therapeutic opportunities for antagonism at this receptor. *Pharmacol Ther* 2008; **117**: 162–187.

272 Nakayoshi T, Kawasaki N, Suzuki Y, *et al.* Epidural administration of morphine facilitates time of appearance of first gastric interdigestive migrating complex in dogs with paralytic ileus after open abdominal surgery. *J Gastrointest Surg* 2007; **11**: 648–654.

273 Pöpping DM, Elia N, Van Aken HK, *et al.* Impact of epidural analgesia on mortality and morbidity after surgery: systematic review and meta-analysis of randomized controlled trials. *Ann Surg* 2014; **259**: 1056–1067.

274 Lubawski J, Saclarides T. Postoperative ileus: strategies for reduction. *Ther Clin Risk Manag* 2008; **4**: 913–917.

275 Yokoyama T, Kitazawa T, Takasaki K, *et al.* Recovery of gastrointestinal motility from post-operative ileus in dogs: effects of Leu13-motilin (KW-5139) and PGF2 alpha. *Neurogastroenterol Motil* 1995; **7**: 199–210.

276 Boscan P, Cochran S, Monnet E, *et al.* Effect of prolonged general anesthesia with sevoflurane and laparoscopic surgery on gastric and small bowel propulsive motility and pH in dogs. *Vet Anaesth Analg* 2014; **41**: 73–81.

277 Sido B, Teklote JR, Hartel M, *et al.* Inflammatory response after abdominal surgery. *Best Pract Res Clin Anaesthesiol* 2004; **18**: 439–454.

278 Bauer AJ, Boeckxstaens GE. Mechanisms of postoperative ileus. *Neurogastroenterol Motil* 2004; **16**(Suppl 2): 54–60.

279 van Bree SH, Nemethova A, Cailotto C, *et al.* New therapeutic strategies for post-operative ileus. *Nat Rev Gastroenterol Hepatol* 2012; **9**: 675–683.

280 Vather R, Bissett I. Management of prolonged post-operative ileus: evidence-based recommendations. *Aust N Z J Surg* 2013; **83**: 319–324.

281 Dellinger RP, Levy MM, Rhodes A, *et al.* Surviving Sepsis Campaign: international guidelines for management of severe sepsis and septic shock: 2012. *Crit Care Med* 2013; **41**: 580–637.

282 Chen G. Summary of the 2012 Surviving Sepsis Recommendations. Annotation of: Dellinger *et al.* Surviving Sepsis Campaign: international guidelines for management of severe sepsis and septic shock: 2012. *Crit Care Med.* 2013;**41**(2): 580–637. http://www.venturafamilymed.org/res/images/Documents/Inpatient_Medicine/2012%20Surviving%20Sepsis%20Recommendations.pdf (accessed 28 September 2014).

283 Chan CM, Mitchell AL, Shorr AF. Etomidate is associated with mortality and adrenal insufficiency in sepsis: a meta-analysis. *Crit Care Med* 2012; **40**: 2945–2953.

284 Aguado D, Benito J, Gómez de Segura IA. Reduction of the minimum alveolar concentration of isoflurane in dogs using a constant rate of infusion of lidocaine–ketamine in combination with either morphine or fentanyl. *Vet J* 2011; **189**: 63–66.

285 Muir WW III, Wiese AJ, March PA. Effects of morphine, lidocaine, ketamine, and morphine–lidocaine–ketamine drug combination on minimum alveolar concentration in dogs anesthetized with isoflurane. *Am J Vet Res* 2003; **64**: 1155–1160.

286 Wilson J, Doherty TJ, Egger CM, *et al.* Effects of intravenous lidocaine, ketamine, and the combination on the minimum alveolar concentration of sevoflurane in dogs. *Vet Anaesth Analg* 2008; **35**: 289–296.

287 Pypendop BH, Ilkiw JE. Assessment of the hemodynamic effects of lidocaine administered IV in isoflurane-anesthetized cats. *Am J Vet Res* 2005; **66**: 661–668.

288 Pang DS, Boysen S. Lactate in veterinary critical care: pathophysiology and management. *J Am Anim Hosp Assoc* 2007; **43**: 270–279.

289 Bruchim Y, Itay S, Shira BH, *et al.* Evaluation of lidocaine treatment on frequency of cardiac arrhythmias, acute kidney injury, and hospitalization time in dogs with gastric dilatation volvulus. *J Vet Emerg Crit Care* 2012; **22**: 419–427.

290 Anderson DE, Muir WW. Pain management in ruminants. *Vet Clin Food Anim Pract* 2005; **21**: 19–31.

291 PROSPECT. *Procedure Specific Postoperative Pain Management.* http://www.postoppain.org/frameset.htm (accessed 28 September 2014).

292 Robertson, SA, Sanchez LC. Treatment of visceral pain in horses. *Vet Clin Equine Pract* 2010; **26**: 603–617.

293 Leslie JB, Viscusi ER, Pergolizzi JV Jr, *et al.* Anesthetic routines: the anesthesiologist's role in GI recovery and postoperative ileus. *Adv Prev Med* 2011; **2011**: 976904.

294 KuKanich B, Bidgood T, Knesl O. Clinical pharmacology of nonsteroidal anti-inflammatory drugs in dogs. *Vet Anaesth Analg* 2012; **39**: 69–90.

295 Lascelles BD, Court MH, Hardie EM, *et al.* Nonsteroidal anti-inflammatory drugs in cats: a review. *Vet Anaesth Analg* 2007; **34**: 228–250.

296 Papich MG. An update on nonsteroidal anti-inflammatory drugs (NSAIDs) in small animals. *Vet Clin Small Anim Pract* 2008; **38**: 1243–1266.

297 Mace S, Shelton GD, Eddlestone S. Megaesophagus. *Compend Contin Educ Vet* 2012; **34**(2): E1–E8.

298 Gaynor AR, Shofer FS, Washabau RJ. Risk factors for acquired megaesophagus in dogs. *J Am Vet Med Assoc* 1997; **211**: 1406–1412.

299 Glickman L, Glickman NW, Perez CM. Analysis of risk factors for gastric dilatation and dilatation–volvulus in dogs. *J Am Vet Med Assoc* 1994; **204**: 1463–1471.

300 Formaggini L, Schmidt K, Lorenzi D. Gastric dilatation–volvulus associated with diaphragmatic hernia in three cats: clinical presentation, surgical treatment and presumptive aetiology. *J Feline Med Surg* 2008; **10**: 198–201.

301 Canine bloat panel offers research and treatment recommendations. *Friskies Res Dig* 1985; **24**: 1.

302 Beck J, Staatz A, Pelsue D, *et al.* Risk factors associated with short-term outcome and development of perioperative complications in dogs undergoing surgery because of gastric dilatation–volvulus: 166 cases (1992–2003). *J Am Vet Med Assoc* 2006; **229**: 1934–1939.

303 Buber T, Saragusty J, Ranen E, *et al.* Evaluation of lidocaine treatment and risk factors for death associated with gastric dilatation and volvulus in dogs: 112 cases (1997–2005). *J Am Vet Med Assoc* 2007; **230**: 1334–1339.

304 Mackenzie G, Barnhart M, Kennedy S, *et al.* A retrospective study of factors influencing survival following surgery for gastric dilatation–volvulus syndrome in 306 dogs. *J Am Anim Hosp Assoc* 2010; **46**: 97–102.

305 Brourman JD, Schertel ER, Allen DA, *et al.* Factors associated with perioperative mortality in dogs with surgically managed gastric dilatation–volvulus: 137 cases (1988–1993). *J Am Vet Med Assoc* 1996; **208**: 1855–1858.

306 Lantz GC, Badylak SF, Hiles MC, *et al.* Treatment of reperfusion injury in dogs with experimentally induced GDV. *Am J Vet Res* 1992; **53**:1594–1598.

307 Millis DL, Hauptman JG, Fulton RB Jr. Abnormal hemostatic profiles and gastric necrosis in canine GDV. *Vet Surg* 1993; **22**: 93–97.

308 de Papp E, Drobatz KJ, Hughes D. Plasma lactate concentration as a predictor of gastric necrosis and survival among dogs with GDV: 102 cases (1995–1998). *J Am Vet Med Assoc* 1999; **215**: 49–52.

309 Santoro Beer KA, Syring RS, Drobatz KJ. Evaluation of plasma lactate concentration and base excess at the time of hospital admission as predictors of gastric necrosis and outcome and correlation between those variables in dogs with gastric dilatation–volvulus: 78 cases (2004–2009). *J Am Vet Med Assoc* 2013; **242**: 54–58.

310 Zacher LA, Berg J, Shaw SP, *et al.* Association between outcome and changes in plasma lactate concentration during presurgical treatment in dogs with GDV: 64 cases (2002–2008). *J Am Vet Med Assoc* 2010; **236**: 892–897.

311 Muir WW. Fluid choice for resuscitation and perioperative administration. *Compend Contin Educ Vet* 2009; **31**(9):E1–E10.

312 Levinson AT, Casserly BP, Levy MM. Reducing mortality in severe sepsis and septic shock. *Semin Resp Crit Care Med* 2011; **32**: 195–205.

313 Allen DA, Schertel ER, Muir WW III, *et al.* Hypertonic saline/dextran resuscitation of dogs with experimentally induced gastric dilatation–volvulus shock. *Am J Vet Res* 1991; **52**: 92–96.

314 Schertel ER, Allen DA, Muir WW, *et al.* Evaluation of a hypertonic saline–dextran solution for treatment of dogs with shock induced by GDV. *J Am Vet Med Assoc* 1997; **210**: 226–230.

315 Muir WW, Lipowitz AJ. Cardiac dysrhythmias associated with gastric dilatation–volvulus in the dog. *J Am Anim Hosp Assoc* 1978; **172**: 683–689.

316 Cole S, Drobatz K. Emergency management and critical care. In: Tilley LP, Smith FWK Jr, Oyama MA, Sleeper MM, eds. *Manual of Canine and Feline Cardiology*, 4th edn. St Louis, MO: Saunders Elsevier, 2008; 352.

317 Valverde A, Doherty TJ, Hernández J, *et al.* Effect of lidocaine on the minimum alveolar concentration of isoflurane in dogs. *Vet Anaesth Analg* 2004; **31**: 264–271.

318 Cook VL, Jones Shults J, McDowell MR, *et al.* Anti-inflammatory effects of intravenously administered lidocaine hydrochloride on ischemia-injured jejunum in horses. *Am J Vet Res* 2009; **70**: 1259–1268.

319 Lahav M, Levite M, Bassani L, *et al.* Lidocaine inhibits secretion of IL-8 and IL-1β and stimulates secretion of IL-1 receptor antagonist by epithelial cells. *Clin Exp Immunol* 2002; **127**: 226–233.

320 Yardeni IZ, Beilin B, Mayburd E, *et al.* The effect of perioperative intravenous lidocaine on postoperative pain and immune function. *Anesth Analg* 2009; **109**: 1464–1469.

321 Rimbäck G, Cassuto J, Tollesson PO. Treatment of postoperative paralytic ileus by intravenous lidocaine infusion. *Anesth Analg* 1990; **70**: 414–419.

322 Malone E, Ensink J, Turner T, *et al.* Intravenous continuous infusion of lidocaine for treatment of equine ileus. *Vet Surg* 2006; **35**: 60–66.

323 Torfs S, Delesalle C, Dewulf J, *et al.* Risk factors for equine postoperative ileus and effectiveness of prophylactic lidocaine. *J Vet Intern Med* 2009; **23**: 606–611.

324 Kilgannon JH, Jones AE, Shapiro NI, *et al.* Association between arterial hyperoxia following resuscitation from cardiac arrest and in-hospital mortality. *J Am Med Assoc* 2010; **303**: 2165–2171.

325 Badylak SF, Lantz GC, Jeffries M. Prevention of reperfusion injury in surgically induced GDV in dogs. *Am J Vet Res* 1990; **51**: 294–299.

326 Vinayak A, Krahwinkel DJ. Managing blunt trauma–induced hemoperitoneum in dogs and cats. *Compend Contin Educ Vet* 2004; **26**: 276–291.

327 Lux CN, Culp WTN, Mayhew PD, *et al.* Perioperative outcome in dogs with hemoperitoneum: 83 cases (2005–2010). *J Am Vet Med Assoc* 2013; **242**: 1385–1391.

328 Herold LV, Devey JJ, Kirby R, *et al.* Clinical evaluation and management of hemoperitoneum dogs. *J Vet Emerg Crit Care* 2008; **18**: 40–53.

329 Culp WT, Weisse C, Kellogg ME, *et al.* Spontaneous hemoperitoneum in cats: 65 cases (1994–2006). *J Am Vet Med Assoc* 2010; **236**: 978–982.

330 Avgerinos DV, Theoharides TC. Mesenteric traction syndrome or gut in distress. *Int J Immunopathol Pharmacol* 2005; **18**: 195–199.

331 Tappin S, Brown P, Ferasin L. An intestinal neuroendocrine tumour associated with paroxysmal ventricular tachycardia and melena in a 10-year-old boxer. *J Small Anim Pract* 2008; **49**: 33–37.

332 Bergman PJ. Paraneoplastic syndromes. In: Withrow SJ, Wail DM, Page RL, eds. *Withrow and McEwen's Small Animal Clinical Oncology*, 5th edn. St Louis, MO: Saunders Elsevier, 2013; 83–97, 521.

333 Willard MD. Esophagus: neoplasia. In: Washabau RJ, Day MJ, eds. *Canine and Feline Gastroenterology.* St Louis, MO: Saunders Elsevier, 2013; 595–598.

334 Minami T. Stomach neoplasia. In: Washabau RJ, Day MJ, eds. *Canine and Feline Gastroenterology.* St Louis, MO: Saunders Elsevier, 2013; 634–637.

335 Bergman PJ. Small intestine neoplasia. In: Washabau RJ, Day MJ, eds. *Canine and Feline Gastroenterology.* St Louis, MO: Saunders Elsevier, 2013; 710–714.

336 Washabau RJ, Hall JA. Large intestine. In: Washabau RJ, Day MJ, eds. *Canine and Feline Gastroenterology.* St Louis, MO: Saunders Elsevier, 2013; 764–767.

337 Willard MD. Alimentary neoplasia in geriatric dogs and cats. *Vet Clin Small Anim Pract* 2012; **42**: 693–706.

338 Tripathi NK, Gregory CR, Latimer KS. Urinary system. In: Latimer KS, ed. *Duncan and Prasse's Veterinary Laboratory Medicine: Clinical Pathology*, 5th edn. Ames, IA: Wiley-Blackwell, 2011; 275.

339 Trow AV, Rozanski EA, Delaforcade AM, *et al.* Evaluation of use of human albumin in critically ill dogs: 73 cases (2003–2006). *J Am Vet Assoc* 2008; **233**: 607–612.

340 Mathews KA, Barry M. The use of 25% human serum albumin: outcome and efficacy in raising serum albumin and systemic blood pressure in critically ill dogs and cats. *J Vet Emerg Crit Care* 2005; **15**: 110–118.

341 Mathews KA. The therapeutic use of 25% human serum albumin in critically ill dogs and cats. *Vet Clin Small Anim Pract* 2008; **38**: 595–605.

342 Francis AH, Martin LG, Haldorson GJ, *et al.* Adverse reactions suggestive of type III hypersensitivity in six healthy dogs given human albumin. *J Am Vet Med Assoc* 2007; **230**: 873–879.
343 Powell C, Thompson L, Murtaugh RJ. Type III hypersensitivity reaction with immune complex deposition in 2 critically ill dogs administered human serum albumin. *J Vet Emerg Crit Care* 2013; **23**: 598–604.
344 Bentley AM, Otto CM, Shofer FS. Comparison of dogs with septic peritonitis: 1988–1993 versus 1999–2003. *J Vet Emerg Crit Care* 2007; **17**: 391–398.
345 Grimes JA, Schmiedt CW, Cornell KK, *et al.* Identification of risk factors for septic peritonitis and failure to survive following gastrointestinal surgery in dogs. *J Am Vet Med Assoc* 2011; **238**: 486–494.
346 Brady CA, Otto CM, Van Winkle TJ, *et al.* Severe sepsis in cats: 29 cases (1986–1998). *J Am Vet Med Assoc* 2000; **217**: 531–535.
347 Costello MF, Drobatz KJ, Aronson LR, *et al.* Underlying cause, pathophysiologic abnormalities, and response to treatment in cats with septic peritonitis: 51 cases (1990–2001). *J Am Vet Med Assoc* 2004; **225**: 897–902.
348 Parsons KJ, Owen LJ, Lee K, *et al.* A retrospective study of surgically treated cases of septic peritonitis in the cat (2000–2007). *J Small Anim Pract* 2009; **50**: 518–524.
349 Ruthrauff CM, Smith J, Glerum L. Primary bacterial septic peritonitis in cats: 13 cases. *J Am Anim Hosp Assoc* 2009; **45**: 268–276.
350 Kelmer E, Tobias KM. Septic peritonitis. *Stand Care* 2009; **11**(2): 6–11.
351 Ragetly GR, Bennett RA, Ragetly CA. Septic peritonitis: etiology, pathophysiology, and diagnosis. *Compend Contin Educ Vet* 2011; **33**(10): E1–E6.
352 Culp WT, Holt DE. Septic peritonitis. *Compend Contin Educ Vet* 2010; **32**(10): E1–E14.
353 Culp WT, Zeldis TE, Reese MS, *et al.* Primary bacterial peritonitis in dogs and cats: 24 cases (1990–2006). *J Am Vet Med Assoc* 2009; **234**: 906–913.
354 King LG. Postoperative complications and prognostic indicators in dogs and cats with septic peritonitis: 23 cases (1989–1992). *J Am Vet Med Assoc* 1994; **204**: 407–414.
355 Volk SW. Septic peritonitis. In: Silverstein DC, Hopper K, eds. *Small Animal Critical Care Medicine*. St Louis, MO: Saunders Elsevier, 2009; 579–583.
356 Boller EM, Otto CM. Sepsis. In: Silverstein DC, Hopper K, eds. *Small Animal Critical Care Medicine*. St Louis, MO: Saunders Elsevier, 2009; 454–458.
357 Anderson, KL, Feeney DA. Diagnostic imaging of the gastrointestinal tract. In: Washabau RJ, Day MJ, eds. *Canine and Feline Gastroenterology*. St Louis, MO: Saunders Elsevier, 2013; 205–244.
358 Levin GM, Bonczynski JJ, Ludwig LL, *et al.* Lactate as a diagnostic test for septic peritoneal effusions in dogs and cats. *J Am Anim Hosp Assoc* 2004; **40**: 364–371.
359 Kenney EM, Rozanski EA, Rush JE, *et al.* Association between outcome and organ system dysfunction in dogs with sepsis: 114 cases (2003–2007). *J Am Vet Med Assoc* 2010; **236**: 83–87.
360 Thomovsky E, Johnston PA. Shock pathophysiology. *Compend Contin Educ Vet* 2013; **35**(8): E1–E9.
361 Bonanno FG. Physiopathology of shock. *J Emerg Trauma Shock* 2011; **4**: 222–232.
362 Bulmer BJ. Cardiovascular dysfunction in sepsis and critical illness. *Vet Clin Small Anim Pract* 2011; **41**: 717–726.
363 Hotchkiss RS, Monneret G, Payen D. Sepsis-induced immunosuppression: from cellular dysfunctions to immunotherapy. *Nat Rev Immunol* 2013; **13**: 862–874.
364 Deitch EA. Gut lymph and lymphatics: a source of factors leading to organ injury and dysfunction. *Ann N Y Acad Sci* 2010; **1207**(S1): E103–E111.
365 Deitch EA. Gut-origin sepsis: evolution of a concept. *Surgeon* 2012; **10**: 350–356.
366 Purvis D, Kirby R. Systemic inflammatory response syndrome: septic shock. *Vet Clin Small Anim Pract* 1994; **24**: 1225–1247.
367 de Laforcade AM. Systemic inflammatory response syndrome. In: Silverstein DC, Hopper K, eds. *Small Animal Critical Care Medicine*. St Louis, MO: Saunders Elsevier, 2009; 46–49.
368 Butler AL. Goal-directed therapy in small animal critical illness. *Vet Clin Small Anim Pract* 2011; **41**: 817–838.
369 Rivers EP, Katranji M, Jaehne KA, *et al.* Early interventions in severe sepsis and septic shock: a review of the evidence one decade later. *Minerva Anestesiol* 2012; **78**: 712–724.
370 Conti-Patara A, de Araújo Caldeira J, de Mattos-Junior E, *et al.* Changes in tissue perfusion parameters in dogs with severe sepsis/septic shock in response to goal-directed hemodynamic optimization at admission to ICU and the relation to outcome. *J Vet Emerg Crit Care* 2012; **22**: 409–418.
371 Koenig A. Surviving sepsis: does anything make a difference? Presented at the ACVS 2011 Symposium, Chicago, IL, 1-5 November 2011.
372 Aldrich J. Shock fluids and fluid challenge. In: Silverstein DC, Hopper K, eds. *Small Animal Critical Care Medicine*. St Louis, MO: Saunders Elsevier, 2009; 276–280.
373 de Laforcade AM, Silverstein DC. Shock. In: Silverstein DC, Hopper K, eds. *Small Animal Critical Care Medicine*. St Louis, MO: Saunders Elsevier, 2009; 41–45.
374 Mutter TC, Ruth CA, Dart AB. Hydroxyethyl starch (HES) versus other fluid therapies: effects on kidney function. *Cochrane Database Syst Rev* 2013; (**7**): CD007594.
375 Haase N, Perner A, Hennings LI, *et al.* Hydroxyethyl starch 130/0.38–0.45 versus crystalloid or albumin in patients with sepsis: systematic review with meta-analysis and trial sequential analysis. *BMJ* 2013; **346**: f839.
376 Stephens R, Mythen M. Resuscitation fluids and hyperchloraemic metabolic acidosis. *Trauma* 2003; **5**: 141–147.
377 Martin LG. Critical illness-related corticosteroid insufficiency in small animals. *Vet Clin Small Anim Pract* 2011; **41**: 767–782.
378 Peyton JL, Burkitt JM. Critical illness-related corticosteroid insufficiency in a dog with septic shock. *J Vet Emerg Crit Care* 2009; **19**: 262–268.
379 Annane D, Bellissant E, Bollaert PE, *et al.* Corticosteroids in the treatment of severe sepsis and septic shock in adults: a systematic review. *JAMA* 2009; **301**: 2362–2375.
380 Eissa D, Carton EG, Buggy DJ. Anaesthetic management of patients with severe sepsis. *Br J Anaesth* 2010; **105**: 734–743.

SECTION 9

Urogenital System

32 Physiology, Pathophysiology, and Anesthetic Management of Patients with Renal Disease

Stuart C. Clark-Price[1] and Gregory F. Grauer[2]

[1]Department of Veterinary Clinical Medicine, College of Veterinary Medicine, University of Illinois, Urbana, Illinois, USA

[2]Department of Clinical Sciences, College of Veterinary Medicine, Kansas State University, Manhattan, Kansas, USA

Chapter contents

Introduction

The art and science of veterinary medicine continue to advance at a brisk pace and, as a result of improvement in life-prolonging therapies, clinicians will be exposed to increasing numbers of older patients and those with various managed illnesses that will require continued care. The kidney is an organ commonly associated with disease [i.e., chronic kidney disease (CKD)] in geriatric patients. Additionally, patients with acute diseases are managed more intensively than in previous years and clinicians are expected to be well versed in up-to-date techniques to provide quality medicine. Renal diseases in veterinary patients have various species prevalences, with feline patients being over-represented. In fact, up to 20% of cats will be affected with CKD during their lifetime and in cats older than 15 years of age, 31% have evidence of renal disease [1].

Equine and ruminant patients have a much lower overall prevalence of renal disease than cats and will be discussed less in this chapter. Although the total prevalence of renal disease in dogs is lower than in cats, advanced age also plays a role. Of dogs with azotemic CKD, 45% are older than 10 years of age [2]. Similarly to cats and dogs, the prevalence of CKD in horses increases with age. Horses older than 15 years of age have a prevalence of 0.23%, increasing to 0.51% in stallions older than 15 years of age [3].

Veterinary practitioners will anesthetize animals with renal diseases in the regular course of daily practice. Therefore, it is imperative that the veterinarian providing anesthesia has an understanding of renal physiology, renal pathophysiology, and the effects of sedative, analgesic, and anesthetic drugs on the kidney.

Normal anatomy and physiology

A complete in-depth overview of the anatomy and physiology of the renal system is beyond the scope of this chapter, and the reader is referred to medical anatomy and physiology text books for further detailed descriptions [4–6].

Anatomy of the urinary tract

Grossly, the urinary system can be divided into the kidneys, the ureters, the urinary bladder, and the urethra. The kidney can be further divided into the cortex, medulla, and renal pelvis. The renal pelvis is essentially the expanded proximal portion of the ureters, which carry urine from the kidney to the urinary bladder. Between species, there are several anatomic differences that exist within the kidney. Dogs, cats, horses, and small ruminants have unilobar kidneys that contain a renal crest or basin within the renal pelvis that collects urine and empties into the proximal urethra. Additionally, gland-like structures in the wall of the horse's renal pelvis secrete a mucous-like substance that is responsible for the cloudy and foamy nature of normal horse urine. Swine and bovine kidneys are multilobar kidneys that contain renal papillae (medullary extensions or pyramids) that

Veterinary Anesthesia and Analgesia: The Fifth Edition of Lumb and Jones.
Edited by Kurt A. Grimm, Leigh A. Lamont, William J. Tranquilli, Stephen A. Greene and Sheilah A. Robertson.

empty into cup-like calyces that then empty into the renal pelvis. The gross shape of the kidney is fairly similar in that most species have the classic kidney shape with a smooth surface and having two poles. The exceptions are the right kidney of the horse, which tends to have a heart-like shape, and the lobulated kidneys of the bovine species, due to incomplete fusion of the kidney lobes. The ureters are smooth muscle-lined tubes that carry urine from the kidney to the bladder. The urinary bladder can be anatomically divided into the body and the neck or trigone region. The body consists of a compliant three-layered muscular wall that can accommodate incoming urine for storage and later voiding. This allows the bladder to vary greatly in shape, size, and position within the pelvis and abdomen. The urethra is a muscular tube that connects the bladder to the genitals, allowing transit of urine from the bladder to the external environment. Anatomic variations of the urethra exist based on gender and species.

At the histological level, the kidney can be anatomically described by its functional unit, the nephron (Fig. 32.1). There are two types of nephrons, cortical and juxtamedullary, based on their location within the cortex and medulla. The nephron is composed of a renal corpuscle, made up of a glomerulus and Bowman's capsule, and the renal tubule, made up of the proximal convoluted tubule, loop of Henle, distal convoluted tubule, and the collecting duct.

Physiologic function

Physiologically, the kidneys play an important role in fluid, electrolyte, and acid–base regulation and also waste removal and hormone secretion. The main functions of the kidneys are filtration, reabsorption, and secretion. To accomplish these functions, the kidneys receive about 25% of the cardiac output via the renal arteries, which branch off directly from the caudal aorta. This high percentage of cardiac output is necessary to facilitate filtration and because the kidney is highly metabolically active (i.e., it has a very high oxygen and substrate consumption rate). Even short-term renal ischemia can lead to acute renal injury and failure. Renal blood flow (RBF) is regulated by extrinsic nervous and hormonal control and by intrinsic autoregulation. The renal vasculature is highly innervated by sympathetic constrictor fibers originating in the spinal cord segments between T4 and L1. The kidneys lack sympathetic vasodilating fibers and parasympathetic innervation. Dopamine receptors in the renal vasculature and tubules help regulate vasodilation and blood flow. There are two known subtypes of dopamine receptors, DA-1 and DA-2. Both of these receptors have been identified in dogs, rats, rabbits, and other animals. It was thought that cats did not possess renal dopamine receptors; however, in 2003, a D-1-like receptor was identified that is considered to be different from receptors found in rats, dogs, or humans [7]. Intrinsic autoregulation of RBF is demonstrated by a constant flow when the mean

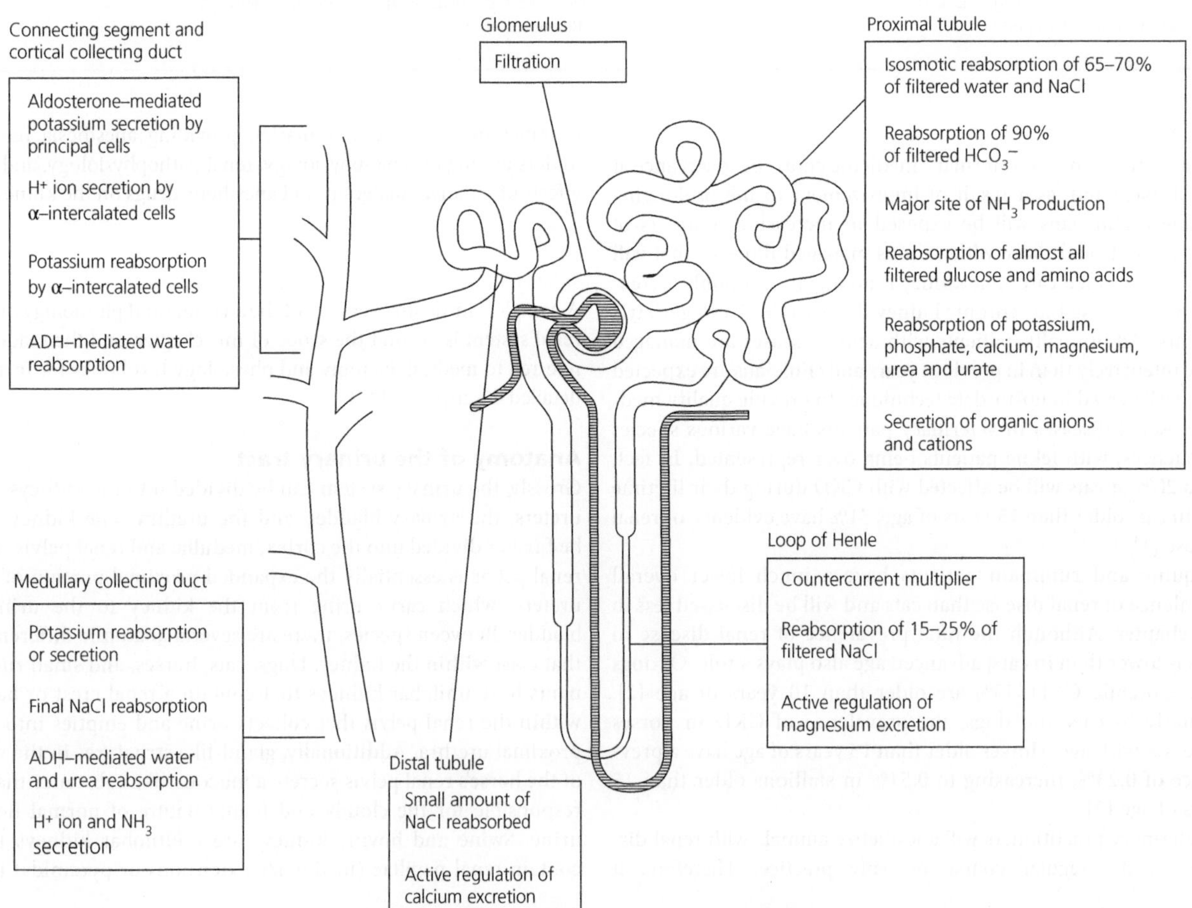

Figure 32.1 Anatomy and physiologic function of each portion of the nephron. Source: DiBartola SP. Applied renal physiology. In: DiBartola SP, ed. *Fluid, Electrolyte, and Acid–Base Disorders in Small Animal Practice*, 3rd edn. St. Louis, MO: Saunders Elsevier, 2006; 26–44. Reproduced with permission of Elsevier.

arterial blood pressure ranges from 80 to 180 mmHg. When the mean arterial blood pressure is in this range, the kidney can control blood flow via alteration of resistance in the glomerular afferent arterioles. Although the exact mechanism of renal autoregulation is not known, the phenomenon protects glomerular capillaries during hypertension and preserves renal function during hypotension. In addition to renal autoregulation, extrinsic forces (e.g., neural, hormonal, and pharmacologic) and intrinsic forces (e.g., kidney disease) may cause alterations in RBF. Catecholamines are major hormonal regulators of RBF. Epinephrine and norepinephrine cause dose-dependent changes in RBF. Low doses increase arterial blood pressure and increase RBF through increased cardiac output, whereas higher doses cause a decreased RBF through increased vascular resistance. The renin–angiotensin–aldosterone system is also an important regulator of RBF (see later). In addition, prostaglandins play an important role in the regulation of RBF. Prostaglandin (PG) E_2 and I_2 (prostacyclin) cause vasodilation within the kidney. Generation of PGE_2 and PGI_2 occurs through the upregulation of cyclooxygenase enzymes; in particular, the cyclooxygenase-2 (COX-2) enzyme plays a largely constitutive and protective role. The COX-2 enzyme is found mainly in the macula densa but can also be found in other areas of the cortex and the medulla. During low blood flow or hypotensive states, COX-2-derived PG promotes natriuresis, renin release, and vasodilation of afferent arterioles to preserve RBF.

Although the kidney receives a high percentage of the cardiac output, blood flow is not evenly distributed throughout the kidney. The renal cortex receives the majority of the blood (90–95%), thus leaving the medulla relatively hypoperfused and hypoxic. This dichotomous blood flow strategy maximizes flow-dependent activities in areas of the kidney that specialize in high-efficiency filtration.

Filtration occurs at the glomerulus, a network of specialized capillaries encapsulated in an epithelial structure called Bowman's capsule. Hydrostatic pressure drives plasma filtration across the glomerulus into the proximal convoluted tubules. The capillaries allow only fluid, very small proteins, and electrolytes to be filtered so that, with the exception of albumin and larger proteins, the glomerular filtrate is very similar in composition to plasma (Table 32.1). The glomerular capillaries are composed of a single layer of endothelial cells with small fenestrations that provide the filtration surface. Under these cells is an acellular basement membrane composed of various proteins such as collagen that provide a scaffold for the epithelial cells and also act as a charged membrane that enables or limits the passage of charged particles such as albumin. The rate of formation of the filtrate, or glomerular filtration rate (GFR), is a measurable parameter that can be evaluated clinically to determine renal excretory function. GFR is expressed as milliliters of glomerular filtrate per kilogram of body weight formed per minute (mL/kg/min). Blood flow into the glomeruli for filtration is under pressure and is regulated by afferent (preglomerular) and efferent (postglomerular) arterioles. The amount of filtrate formed is directly related to the pressure across the capillaries and this pressure can be described mathematically using the Starling's equation:

$$Q = K_f[(P_c - P_i) - \sigma(\Pi_c - \Pi_i)]$$

where Q is the net fluid movement across the capillaries, K_f is the filtration coefficient (which depends on the permeability and length of the filtration surface), P_c is the capillary hydrostatic pressure, P_i is the interstitial hydrostatic pressure, σ is the reflection or filtration coefficient, Π_c is the capillary oncotic pressure, and Π_i is the interstitial oncotic pressure. When measured at the afferent arteriole end of the glomerulus, the net filtration pressure is about 10 mmHg, resulting in a net outflow. When measured at the efferent arteriole end of the glomerulus, the net filtration pressure is about 0 mmHg, resulting in zero net outflow.

Similarly to RBF, GFR is maintained by an autoregulation system. The renin–angiotensin–aldosterone hormone system is particularly important for GFR and also plays a role in RBF. When blood pressure and subsequent renal perfusion decrease, renin is released from specialized juxtaglomerular cells. Renin is then responsible for the transformation of angiotensinogen (produced by the liver) to angiotensin I, which is subsequently converted to angiotensin II (AT-II, a potent vasoconstrictor) by angiotensin-converting enzyme (ACE) produced by the vascular endothelium (primarily from the lungs but also from other organ endothelium). AT-II directly increases blood pressure through constriction of smooth muscle in arterioles but also has multiple endocrine and paracrine effects. Locally within the kidney, AT-II activates sodium uptake in the tubules of the nephron, promoting fluid retention and increased blood volume. At the adrenal gland, AT-II increases release of the steroid hormone aldosterone, which also promotes sodium conservation, potassium elimination, and increased fluid retention and blood pressure. At the pituitary gland, AT-II enhances vasopressin (previously known as antidiuretic hormone) release, which increases water reabsorption in the kidneys through the insertion of water channels (aquaporin-2) in the membrane of the distal tubules of the nephron. Vasopressin also has direct vasoconstriction properties through G-protein coupled V receptors in vascular endothelium. Additionally, AT-II induces intrarenal release of the vasodilating prostaglandins PGE_2 and prostacyclin that counteract the vasoconstricting effects of AT-II, thereby preventing excessive intrarenal vascular resistance and local ischemia. A second intrinsic system, called tubuloglomerular feedback, also contributes to the autoregulatory system that helps maintain GFR. A distinct group of epithelial cells within the distal convoluted tubule (DCT), the macula densa, contact the glomerulus between the afferent and efferent

Table 32.1 Major activity and filtrate composition in the nephron.

Nephron Structure	Major Activity	Filtrate Composition	Comments
Glomerulus	Filtration of plasma	Isotonic	Cell-free filtrate containing only fluid, electrolytes, and small proteins
Proximal convoluted tubule	45–55% of filtrate is reabsorbed	Isotonic	90% of HCO_3^- is reabsorbed and filtrate becomes acidic
Descending loop of Henle	25–40% of filtrate H_2O is reabsorbed	Hypertonic	H_2O reabsorption via osmosis
Ascending loop of Henle	Major area of solute reabsorption	Hypotonic	Active transport via Na^-–K^+-ATPase, cells are impermeable to H_2O
Distal convoluted tubule	5% of filtrate is reabsorbed	Hypotonic	Less than 10% of originally filtered H_2O is present
Collecting duct	0.5 to 10% of H_2O reabsorption	Hyper-, iso-, or hypotonic (urine)	Under the influence of arginine vasopressin

arterioles as part of the juxtaglomerular apparatus (JGA). Osmoreceptors within the macula densa cells sense decreased sodium concentrations within the tubular lumen and initiate a cascade of events resulting in renin release from the juxtaglomerular cells. Alternatively, increased sodium chloride concentrations result in an undefined cascade of events that suppresses renin release and leads to production of vasoactive factors (nitric oxide, adenosine triphosphate, prostaglandins) that reduce GFR and promote free water conservation.

Filtered fluid that leaves the glomerulus next enters the proximal convoluted tubules (PCT). The major function of the PCT is to reabsorb the majority of the filtrate. In fact, more than 60% of the filtered substances are reabsorbed in the PCT. Transport across the PCT membrane into the interstitial tissues and then into the vascular space occurs via both active and passive transport with Starling's forces dictating the passive phases. The majority of ions filtered at the glomerulus (Na^+, K^+, Ca^{2+}, Cl^-, HCO_3^-) are reabsorbed in the PCT so that filtrate leaving the PCT and entering the loop of Henle has lower levels of electrolytes than plasma. Water passively follows the active reabsorption of electrolytes so that the osmolality of the tubular fluid is similar to that of plasma at both ends of the PCT. Organic low molecular weight proteins (insulin, glucagon, parathyroid hormone, etc.) that were filtered are also actively reabsorbed in the PCT. Secretion of substances also occurs in the PCT. Organic ionic wastes are eliminated via secretion into the filtrate and these include protein-bound exogenous substances that are not filtered at the glomerulus, for example, endotoxins, antibiotics, and anesthetic and analgesic drugs such as morphine and ketamine, and endogenous wastes such as bile salts, urates, and prostaglandins. PCT secretion is exceptionally important for endogenous waste removal in birds and reptiles. In mammals, one of the main waste products from muscle metabolism is urea, which is freely filtered at the glomerulus; however, uric acid is the waste product from muscle metabolism in birds and reptiles. Uric acid in not filtered at the glomeruli and its removal is dependent upon active mechanisms in the PCT in these species.

Next, the remaining filtrate enters the descending loop of Henle (DloH). Metabolic activity within the DloH is minimal and little to no active transport process occurs. Pure water reabsorption and minimal solute drag occur as the filtrate travels through the DloH to the highly active ascending (AloH) or thick portion of the loop of Henle.

The AloH is one of the most metabolically active parts of the tubule and the entire kidney. The endothelium is simple cuboidal with many mitochondria which provide the energy for high-capacity active transport. The filtrate is further modified as the majority of electrolyte reabsorption within the loop of Henle takes place in the AloH. An abundant concentration of Na^+–K^+-ATPase pumps can be found on the luminal surface of the tubules which are responsible for the active transport of Na^+, K^+, and Cl^- into the cell and out of the filtrate. Other ions such as Mg^{2+} and Ca^{2+} move down a cation-selective paracellular pathway into the interstitium. Particularly in the case of K^+, hyperkalemia can result in electrical conduction pathology and therefore both apical and basolateral K^+ channels exist to increase secretion into the filtrate for eventual removal in the urine. As the AloH is highly metabolically active, it has a high demand for substrates such as oxygen and therefore has increased sensitivity to damage during hypoxemia or hypotension. Additionally, several medications can exert their effects both therapeutically and pathologically at the AloH. For example, furosemide works as a diuretic by inhibiting Na^+–K^+-ATPase pumps and preventing electrolyte and fluid reabsorption and aminoglycoside antibiotics such as gentamicin can inhibit protein synthesis and result in acute tubular necrosis in the PCT and the AloH. The AloH is impermeable to water so that filtrate entering the DCT is hypotonic; this is in fact how the kidney forms dilute urine in the absence of ADH.

After the AloH, the highly modified hypotonic filtrate enters the distal convoluted tubules (DCT). Electrolyte and water reabsorption occurs to modify the filtrate further; however, K^+ and H^+ secretion is of major importance in the DCT. Because the majority of HCO_3^- was reabsorbed in the PCT, only a very small amount of HCO_3^- remains and therefore both K^+ and H^+ must be actively pumped into the lumen to counter an imbalance between negatively and positively charged ions. This can result in K^+ and H^+ competing with each other for secretion and is often the reason why hyperkalemia is associated with acidemia.

Finally, the filtrate enters the collecting duct, where it can be modified one more time before being classified as urine. Collecting duct tubular cells must be impermeable to water when patients are overhydrated and permeable to H_2O during dehydration. This is accomplished via the actions of the hormone vasopressin [antidiuretic hormone (ADH)]. When states of dehydration exist, vasopressin is released from the neurohypophysis, stimulated by increased plasma osmolality, and its presence at the level of the kidneys and induces the translocation and insertion of water channels called aquaporin-2 into the cells of the DCT and collecting duct. Water is then allowed to be reabsorbed, resulting in a more concentrated urine. Interestingly, α_2-adrenergic agonist drugs such as xylazine block the vasopressin receptors located within the collecting ducts, preventing water reabsorption. This can be observed clinically as animals voiding large amounts of dilute urine after sedation with an α_2-adrenergic agonist and can result in worsening dehydration in animals with a negative fluid balance.

On leaving the collecting duct, the filtrate is considered to be urine, where it is gathered in the renal pelvis and transported to the urinary bladder via the ureters for storage and voiding.

Testing and monitoring renal function

Canine and feline

Biochemical testing

Blood urea nitrogen (BUN) and serum creatinine (SC) concentrations provide a crude index of the GFR. As the SC concentration is influenced by fewer extrarenal variables and it is not resorbed by the renal tubules, it is a better index of GFR than is the BUN concentration. The sensitivity of elevated BUN and SC concentrations is an issue, however; azotemia resulting from impaired renal function is not detectable until approximately three-quarters of the nephrons in both kidneys are non-functional. This proportion may be even higher in dogs and cats with chronic progressive renal disease due to compensatory hypertrophy of remaining nephrons. Assessment of renal function by use of SC concentration can be improved by following three guidelines/recommendations. (1) Interpret SC concentrations in the light of potential prerenal (e.g., hydration status, cardiac output, and muscle mass) and postrenal (e.g., obstructive uropathies and rupture of urinary system) influences. (2) Consider employing tighter reference ranges. The International Renal Interest Society (IRIS) has recommended that SC values of 1.4 and 1.6 mg/dL be considered the upper limit of normal for most dogs and cats, respectively. Exceptions likely include heavily muscled dogs such as Greyhounds that may have higher normal SC concentrations. (3) Longitudinal monitoring of SC concentrations in the same patient facilitates detection of declining renal function, even if SC values remain within normal limits. For example, an SC concentration that increases from 0.6 to 1.2 mg/dL over time may indicate a ≥50% reduction in renal function (assuming that the muscle mass has not changed and the hydration status is normal).

Measurement of the specific gravity of urine is often used to assess renal tubular function; however, like BUN and SC, this measure of renal function is neither sensitive nor specific. In dogs, decreases in urine-concentrating ability are not detectable until approximately two-thirds of the nephrons are non-functional. In cats, this proportion is thought to be higher; it is not uncommon for cats with renal azotemia (more than three-quarters nephron loss) to retain the ability to produce hypersthenuric urine. In addition to this lack of sensitivity, non-renal influences can compromise urine-concentrating ability (e.g., decreased ADH concentrations and systemic diseases/disorders that can decrease kidney responsiveness to ADH such as hypercalcemia and hyperadrenocorticism).

As an alternative to standard clinicopathologic tests, the detection and quantification of urine enzymes (enzymuria) have been used to recognize early nephrotoxicity in the dog. As most serum enzymes are not filtered by the glomerulus because of their high molecular weight, enzymuria can be an indication of renal tubular leakage or necrosis. Several enzymes originate from specific cellular organelles and thus can serve as markers for damage to a specific site. For example, γ-glutamyl transpeptidase (GGT) originates from the proximal tubular brush border and *N*-acetylglucosaminidase (NAG) is a lysosomal enzyme. Enzymuria usually precedes azotemia and decreased urine-concentrating ability associated with nephrotoxic proximal tubular injury by several days. Urine GGT:creatinine and NAG:creatinine ratios have been shown to reflect accurately 24 h urine GGT and NAG excretion in dogs, if determined before the onset of azotemia [8]. Determination of baseline urine GGT:creatinine and NAG: creatinine ratios therefore should be considered in all dogs that are to receive potentially nephrotoxic drugs. Two- to threefold increases in the GGT:creatinine or NAG:creatinine ratio over the baseline are suggestive of clinically relevant tubular damage. Drug therapy should be discontinued if this occurs.

Proteinuria is another clinicopathologic finding that can help lead to a diagnosis of kidney disease. Renal proteinuria can be associated with increased filtration through damaged glomerular capillary walls (i.e., glomerular proteinuria) and/or decreased reabsorption by tubular epithelial cells (i.e., tubular proteinuria). Tubular lesions in patients with acute kidney injury/acute renal failure (AKI/ARF) may result in proteinuria; however, renal proteinuria is more commonly associated with CKD. The sensitivity of renal proteinuria as a marker of CKD is high, especially if species-specific albuminuria assays and/or the urine protein:creatinine ratio are monitored. The specificity of proteinuria for renal disease is relatively low. Pre- and postrenal causes of proteinuria need to be ruled out. Proteinuria of renal origin is persistent (multiple assessments separated by 7–14 days should be positive) and associated with a normal/inactive urine sediment.

Renal clearance and glomerular filtration rate

Given the lack of sensitivity of the BUN, SC, and urine specific gravity, assessment of GFR may be accomplished to provide more accurate information about renal excretory function, especially prior to the onset of persistent renal azotemia when early renal disease is suspected. Renal clearance is the rate at which a substance is completely cleared from a certain volume of plasma. Substances used to measure renal clearance must be freely filtered by the glomerulus (not protein bound) and not be affected by tubular reabsorption or secretion or by metabolism elsewhere in the body. In addition, the substance used must not alter renal function. Renal clearance of inulin is the gold standard method for the determination of GFR; however, it is difficult to measure inulin in plasma and urine. On the other hand, it is relatively easy to determine the renal clearance of creatinine, and therefore more practical. The renal clearance of endogenous creatinine can be calculated by multiplying the concentration of creatinine in urine by the rate of urine production and then dividing the product by the SC concentration:

$$\text{volume of plasma cleared (mL/min)} = \text{GFR (mL/min)} = \frac{\text{urine creatinine (mg/dL)} \times \text{urine volume (mL/min)}}{\text{SC (mg/dL)}}$$

For example, if the urine creatinine concentration is 60 mg/dL, urine production is 3 mL/min, and the SC concentration is 1.8 mg/dL, then 100 mL of plasma is cleared of creatinine per minute. This value is divided by the animal's body weight in kilograms and expressed in milliliters per minute per kilogram. Note that prerenal and postrenal factors, and also renal parenchymal lesions, will influence GFR. The major disadvantage of renal clearance studies is the requirement for timed urine collections.

From a clinical standpoint, plasma clearance studies are less invasive and less time consuming. For example, plasma clearance of iohexol, an iodinated radiographic contrast agent, has been shown to estimate GFR reliably in dogs and cats. Iohexol plasma clearance is ideally performed in patients that are well hydrated and fasted for 12 h prior to the study. Iohexol (Omnipaque 240 mg I/mL, GE Healthcare, Princeton, NJ, USA) is administered IV at dosage of 300 mg iodine/kg body weight and then blood samples are collected at 2,3, and 4 h after the IV injection from a separate vein. Serum from each blood sample is harvested (~1.5 mL of serum is needed per sample) and then transported either chilled or frozen to the specialized reference laboratory (e.g., Diagnostic Center for Population and Animal Health, Toxicology Section, Michigan State University) for measurement and calculation of GFR.

Renal scintigraphy using ^{99m}Tc-labeled diethylenetriamine-pentaacetic acid also allows the GFR to be measured and is available at several US universities and major referral centers. This is a quick, non-invasive method that does not require urine collection and has the advantage of being able to evaluate quantitatively individual kidney function. Disadvantages of this procedure include its limited availability, exposure of the animal to radioisotopes, the need for radioisotope disposal, and poorer correlation with inulin clearance compared with plasma iohexol clearance.

Urine output measurement

Measuring the volume of urine produced is most frequently used as an aid in determining the maintenance fluid requirements of dogs and cats with AKI/ARF. These patients may have large variations in their urine production, ranging from oliguria and anuria to polyuria. One of the major goals of fluid therapy in patients with AKI/ARF is to induce and maintain a diuresis. Fluid therapy should be tailored to match urine volume plus other losses, including insensible losses (e.g., water loss due to respiration) and continuing losses (e.g., fluid loss due to vomiting or diarrhea). Insensible losses are estimated at 20 mL/kg/day. Urine output is quantitated for 6–8 h intervals (often best accomplished with an indwelling or intermittent urinary catheter) and that volume plus insensible loss is replaced over an equivalent subsequent time period. The volume of fluid loss due to vomiting and/or diarrhea is estimated and that amount is added to the 24 h fluid needs of the patient. Fluid losses or gains can also be indirectly estimated by weighing the patient 2–3 times per day on the same scale.

Renal biopsy

Biopsy and histopathologic evaluation of renal tissue are a valuable diagnostic and prognostic tool. Renal biopsy should be considered if the diagnosis is in question (e.g., immune complex glomerulonephritis versus amyloidosis in dogs with proteinuria), if treatment may be altered on the basis of results (e.g., confirmation and culture of bacterial pyelonephritis), or if the prognosis may be altered on the basis of results (e.g., evidence of reversible tubular lesions in a dog or cat with acute tubular necrosis). A specific diagnosis is required in order to implement targeted treatment in most animals with renal disease and, for a specific diagnosis to be obtained, frequently a biopsy must be performed. In addition, the prognosis for animals with renal disease is most accurate if based on three variables: (1) the severity of dysfunction, (2) the response to treatment, and (3) the renal histopathologic findings. Renal biopsy should be considered only after less invasive tests have been carried out and coagulation/hemostasis have been assessed. Contraindications to renal biopsy include a solitary kidney, a coagulopathy, severe systemic hypertension, and renal lesions associated with fluid accumulation (e.g., hydronephrosis, renal cysts and abscesses). In addition, renal biopsy should not be attempted by inexperienced clinicians or in animals that are not adequately restrained. Renal biopsy specimens can be obtained percutaneously using the keyhole technique or under laparoscopic or ultrasonographic guidance. Frequently, the best way to obtain a specimen is at laparotomy when both kidneys can be visualized, because post-biopsy hemorrhage can then be accurately assessed and treated and an adequate biopsy specimen assured. The cortical region of the kidney should be biopsied to obtain an adequate number of glomeruli in the specimen and to avoid renal nerves and major vessels in the medullary region. Most animals will have microscopic hematuria for 1–3 days after the biopsy procedure, and overt hematuria is not uncommon. Severe hemorrhage occurs less than 3% of the time and is almost always the result of faulty technique. When possible, immunofluorescent or immunohistochemical techniques and electron microscopy should be used to maximize the information gained from the biopsy specimen. Communication with the laboratory pathologist prior to biopsy will help determine which fixatives should be used and will maximize the utility of the biopsy sample.

Equine

In a similar fashion to small animal patients, SC is a commonly used index to assess renal function (GFR). Similarly to small animals, it is expected that SC elevations associated with renal lesions will not be observed until approximately 75% of the nephrons become non-functional; and measurement of SC in early renal disease is of little value. BUN measurement as a single test of renal function in horses has minimal diagnostic value. In horses, BUN is reabsorbed after filtration at the collecting ducts in a rate-dependent manner based on the rate of fluid movement. As fluid rates and volumes increase in the collecting duct, less urea is reabsorbed, and as fluid rates decrease, more urea is reabsorbed independent of the filtration rate of urea. Therefore, fluid therapy in horses with renal disease may reduce BUN but not in a manner that reflects improvement in GFR. Because SC is not reabsorbed, it is the most commonly used single test of renal function in horses. Azotemia, elevated SC, and BUN can be further divided into prerenal, renal and postrenal in origin. The use of a BUN:SC ratio has been described for use in characterizing azotemia in horses and to separate acute and chronic forms of renal failure. The ratio is theoretically higher for prerenal azotemia because of increased urea reabsorption due to dehydration and low tubular flow rates compared with azotemia secondary to intrinsic renal disease. In horses with acute renal failure, BUN:SC ratios are less than 10:1, whereas in chronic disease, ratios can be expected to be greater than 10:1 [9].

GFR can also be measured in equine patients, providing a quantitative assessment of renal function; however, measurement of urine output is challenging in horses as an indwelling urinary catheter for urine collection is impractical.

Serum electrolyte concentration measurements should also be considered in the diagnostic plan for horses with renal disease. Na^+ and Cl^- levels are often decreased in horses with renal disease whereas K^+ can be elevated, decreased, or normal. Hyperkalemia is most often observed with disease states associated with urine outflow obstructions or urinary bladder ruptures and subsequent uroperitoneum. Serum Ca^{2+} should also be monitored as horses with AKI are often hypocalcemic whereas those with CKD are often hypercalcemic.

Urine samples should be obtained from horses with suspected renal disease for a complete urinalysis, including sediment examination. In a similar fashion to small animal patients, specific gravity should be measured along with microscopic examination for cells, casts, and crystals. The brush borders of the proximal tubular cells are rich in enzymes that play a role in the metabolic activity of the endothelium. Measured urinary GGT has been used, as a ratio with urine creatinine (UC), to determine and monitor the extent of acute tubular damage. GGT:UC ratios greater than 100 IU/g are considered to be clinically important but lower ratios should be interpreted with caution as GGT release from the proximal tubules can occur with minor insults that may be clinically irrelevant.

Fractional clearance of electrolytes may hold better diagnostic utility than urinary GGT for acute tubular damage [9]. The nephrons, as a collective group, work to conserve more than 99% of filtered Na^+ and Cl^- ions in the normal horse (supplemented salts or intravenous fluid administration will artificially increase the amount of excreted electrolytes in urine and thus complicate the utility of fractional clearance calculations). Increases in fractional clearance may be an indicator of early tubular damage. Serum and urine samples are collected simultaneously and Na^+, Cl^-, and creatinine levels are determined. Using the following equation, a clearance value can be determined for sodium and chloride:

$$Cl_A/Cl_{Cr} = \frac{\text{serum}[Cr]}{\text{urine}[Cr]} \times \frac{\text{urine}[A]}{\text{serum}[A]} \times 100$$

where Cl_A/Cl_{Cr} is the fractional clearance ratio, [A] is the measured electrolyte A (either Na^+ or Cl^-) and [Cr] is creatinine concentration.

Renal biopsy via ultrasound guidance is easily performed in horses and use of a needle biopsy instrument minimizes the risks (hemorrhage, bowel penetration, and peritonitis). Biopsy and histopathology can identify the type of lesion, location, and severity and provide guidance for prognosis.

Ruminant

Many of the same diagnostic procedures performed in small animals and horses can be performed in ruminant species. However, for economic concerns, renal function testing is often limited to findings on routine chemistry analysis and urinalysis strips.

Acute kidney injury/acute renal failure

Etiology and pathogenesis

The kidneys are highly susceptible to the effects of ischemia and toxicants because of their unique anatomic and physiologic features. For example, the large renal blood flow (approximately 20% of the cardiac output) results in the increased delivery of bloodborne toxicants to the kidney compared with that to other organs. The renal cortex is especially susceptible to toxicants because it receives 90% of the renal blood flow and contains the large endothelial surface area of the glomerular capillaries. Within the renal cortex, the epithelial cells of the proximal tubule and thick ascending loop of Henle are most frequently affected by ischemia and toxicant-induced injury because of their transport functions and high metabolic rates. Toxicants disrupt the metabolic pathways that generate ATP, and ischemia can rapidly deplete cellular ATP stores. With the resulting loss of energy, the sodium/potassium (Na^+/K^+) pump fails, leading to cell swelling and death. By resorbing water and electrolytes from the glomerular filtrate, tubular epithelial cells may be exposed to increasingly higher concentrations of toxicants within the tubular lumen. Toxicants that are either secreted or resorbed by tubular epithelial cells (e.g., gentamicin) may accumulate in high concentrations within these cells. Similarly, the countercurrent multiplier system may concentrate toxicants in the medulla. Finally, the kidneys also play a role in the biotransformation of many drugs and toxicants. This usually results in the formation of metabolites that are less toxic than the parent compound; however, in some cases (e.g., the oxidation of ethylene glycol to glycolate and oxalate), the metabolites are more toxic than the parent compound.

The two major causes of AKI/ARF are toxic and ischemic injury. Toxic insults to the kidney can often be caused by therapeutic agents, in addition to the better known nephrotoxicants such as ethylene glycol and aminoglycoside antibiotics. Similarly, ischemic insults to the kidney can occur in the hospital setting in conjunction with anesthesia and surgery or with the use of vasodilators or non-steroidal anti-inflammatory drugs (NSAIDs) [10]. Prolonged anesthesia with inadequate fluid therapy in older animals with pre-existing, subclinical CKD is a frequent cause of renal ischemia and AKI/ARF in the hospital setting. Normal kidneys can maintain adequate renal perfusion pressure by autoregulation provided that the mean arterial blood pressure exceeds approximately 60–70 mmHg. This autoregulation may be compromised in patients with pre-existing CKD, especially during anesthesia. The resulting decline in renal blood flow and perfusion pressure can adversely affect GFR and delivery of oxygen and nutrients to the metabolically active tubular epithelial cells. Tubular cell swelling secondary to decreased Na^+/K^+ pump activity occurs due to osmotic extraction of water from the extracellular space, which in turn can cause the amount of water in the plasma to decrease. The consequences of decreased plasma water in the renal vasculature are red blood cell aggregation and vascular congestion and stasis, which tend to potentiate and perpetuate decreased glomerular blood flow and decreased oxygen and nutrient delivery.

In ARF, dysfunction and reduced glomerular filtration occur at the individual nephron level as a result of a combination of tubular obstruction, tubular backleak, renal arteriolar vasoconstriction, and decreased glomerular capillary permeability. Specifically, cellular debris within the tubule may inspissate and obstruct the flow of filtrate through the nephron. Alternatively, interstitial edema may compress and obstruct renal tubules. Backleak (i.e., abnormal reabsorption of filtrate) occurs because of a loss of tubular cell integrity, allowing the glomerular filtrate to cross from the tubular lumen into the renal interstitium and subsequently the renal vasculature. Tubular backleak is enhanced by tubular obstruction and increased intratubular pressures proximal to the obstruction. The decreased reabsorption of solute and water by damaged proximal tubule segments results in the increased delivery of solutes and fluid to the distal nephron and macula densa in many nephrons, which causes afferent glomerular arteriole constriction. The exact mediators of this vasoconstriction are not known, but natriuretic factor, the renin–angiotensin system, and thromboxane may be involved. A decrease in the permeability of the glomerular capillary wall also leads to a reduction in glomerular filtration. The impaired glomerular capillary permeability that occurs in ARF often persists after vasoconstriction and renal blood flow have been corrected.

Acute tubular damage leading to ARF has three distinct phases: (1) initiation, (2) maintenance, and (3) recovery. During the initiation phase, therapeutic measures that reduce the renal insult can prevent the development of established ARF. In this initiation phase, individual tubules are damaged but overall renal function remains adequate. Acute tubular damage prior to the development of ARF is suggested by renal tubular epithelial cells and cellular or granular casts in the urine sediment. The maintenance phase is characterized by the development of tubular lesions and nephron dysfunction (i.e., renal azotemia and concurrent urine-concentrating deficits). Although therapeutic interventions during the maintenance phase may be lifesaving, they usually do little to diminish the severity of existing renal lesions, improve function, or hasten recovery. In the recovery phase, renal lesions are repaired and function improves. Tubular damage may be reversible if the tubular basement membrane is intact and viable epithelial cells are present. Although new nephrons cannot be produced and irreversibly damaged nephrons cannot be repaired, the functional hypertrophy of surviving nephrons may adequately compensate for the decrease in nephron numbers. Even if renal functional recovery is incomplete, adequate function may be re-established.

Clinical features and diagnosis

Clinical signs of AKI/ARF are often non-specific and include lethargy, depression, anorexia, vomiting, diarrhea, and dehydration; occasionally, uremic breath or oral ulcers may be present. A diagnosis of ARF is suspected if azotemia develops acutely and is associated with persistent isosthenuria or minimally concentrated urine. Prerenal dehydration and azotemia superimposed on an inability to concentrate urine (e.g., Addison's disease, hypercalcemia, or overzealous use of furosemide) initially mimics renal failure; however, in these prerenal cases, volume replacement results in resolution of the azotemia.

Acute renal failure occurs within hours or days of exposure to the insult. Unique clinical signs and clinicopathologic findings associated with ARF include enlarged or swollen kidneys, hemoconcentration, good body condition, active urine sediment (e.g., granular casts, renal epithelial cells), and relatively severe hyperkalemia and metabolic acidosis (especially in the face of oliguria/anuria). Clinical signs in an animal with ARF tend to be severe relative to those seen in an animal with CKD and similar magnitude of azotemia. Renal ultrasonographic findings in dogs and cats with ARF are usually non-specific, with diffusely normal to slightly hypoechoic renal cortices. In animals with calcium oxalate nephrosis associated with ethylene glycol ingestion, the renal cortices can be very hyperechoic. Doppler estimation of the resistive index (RI) in renal arcuate arteries is increased in many dogs with ARF; however, this method of evaluation must be more extensively correlated with the renal histopathologic changes before firm conclusions regarding the merits of the RI can be drawn.

Renal biopsy specimens from dogs and cats with ARF show proximal tubular cell degeneration, ranging from cloudy swelling to necrosis, with edema and mononuclear and polymorphonuclear leukocyte infiltration in the interstitium. Ethylene glycol and melamine-associated nephrotoxicity is frequently associated with intratubular crystals. Although toxicant-induced ARF cannot be differentiated histopathologically from ARF caused by ischemia in all cases, renal histologic findings are often helpful in establishing a prognosis. Evidence of tubular regeneration (e.g., flattened, basophilic epithelial cells with irregular nuclear size, mitotic figures, high nuclear to cytoplasmic ratios) and the finding of generally intact tubular basement membranes are good prognostic findings and may be observed as early as 3 days post-insult. Conversely, large numbers of granular casts, extensive tubular necrosis, and interstitial mineralization and fibrosis with disrupted tubular basement membranes are poor prognostic signs. In addition to the renal histopathologic changes, the degree of functional impairment and, even more important, the response to therapy should be considered when formulating a prognosis.

Chronic kidney disease

Etiology and pathogenesis

Unlike AKI/ARF, the cause of CKD is usually difficult to determine. Because of the interdependence of the vascular and tubular components of the nephron, the endpoint of irreversible glomerular or tubular damage is the same. A morphologic heterogeneity among nephrons exists in the chronically diseased kidney, with the changes ranging from severe atrophy and fibrous connective tissue replacement to marked hypertrophy. The histopathologic changes are not process specific and the underlying cause is therefore usually unknown. Nevertheless, recent studies have shown that primary glomerular disorders are a major cause of CKD in the dog. Because total glomerular filtration is uniformly reduced, CKD may be considered a single pathologic entity, although many diverse pathways can lead to this endpoint.

The pathophysiology of CKD can be considered at both the organ and systemic levels. At the level of the kidney, the fundamental pathologic change that occurs is a loss of nephrons and decreased GFR. Reduced GFR in turn results in increased plasma concentrations of substances that are normally eliminated from the body by renal excretion. Many substances have been shown to accumulate in the plasma in patients with CKD. The constellation of clinical signs known as the uremic syndrome is thought to occur, at least in part, as a result of increasing plasma concentrations of these substances. Components of the uremic syndrome include sodium and water imbalance, anemia, carbohydrate intolerance, neurologic disturbances, gastrointestinal tract disturbances, osteodystrophy, immunologic incompetence, and metabolic acidosis.

In addition to excreting metabolic wastes and maintaining fluid and electrolyte balance, the kidneys also function as endocrine organs and catabolize several peptide hormones. Therefore, hormonal disturbances also play a role in the pathogenesis of CKD. For example, the decreased production of erythropoietin and calcitriol in animals with CRF contributes to the development of non-regenerative anemia and hyperparathyroidism, respectively. Conversely, decreased metabolism and decreased excretion lead to increased concentrations of parathyroid hormone and gastrin, which contribute to the development of hyperparathyroidism and gastritis, respectively.

The pathophysiologic changes that occur in CKD are brought about in part by compensatory mechanisms. The osteodystrophy of CKD occurs secondary to hyperparathyroidism, which develops in an attempt to maintain normal plasma calcium and phosphorus concentrations. Similarly, the GFR of intact hypertrophied nephrons increases in animals with CKD in an attempt to maintain adequate renal function. However, proteinuria and glomerulosclerosis in these individual nephrons leading to additional nephron damage and loss may be consequences of this hyperfiltration.

Clinical features and diagnosis

In contrast to AKI/ARF, CKD develops over a period of months or years, and its clinical signs are often relatively mild for the magnitude of the azotemia. Unique signs of CRF include a long-standing history of weight loss, polydipsia/polyuria, poor body condition, non-regenerative anemia, and small and irregularly shaped kidneys. A diagnosis of CKD is usually based on a combination of compatible historical, physical examination, and clinicopathologic findings. Plain radiographs can confirm the presence of small kidneys in small animal patients but is usually not feasible in larger horses and ruminants. Renal ultrasonography will usually show diffusely hyperechoic renal cortices with loss of the normal corticomedullary boundary. The increased cortical echogenicity results from replacement of the irreversibly damaged nephrons with fibrous connective tissue. Radiographic studies and ultrasonography can also help identify or rule out potentially treatable causes of CKD, such as pyelonephritis and renal urolithiasis. Renal biopsy is not routinely performed in animals with CKD unless the diagnosis is in question. Renal histopathologic preparations will show some combination of a loss of tubules with replacement fibrosis and mineralization, glomerulosclerosis and glomerular atrophy, and foci of mononuclear cells (small lymphocytes, plasma cells, and macrophages) within the interstitium in association with fibrous connective tissue replacement.

Staging chronic kidney disease

Once a diagnosis of CKD has been established and fluid therapy has resolved any prerenal azotemia (i.e., the disease is stable), staging the kidney disease process can help clinicians focus their diagnostic and therapeutic efforts. Table 32.2 was developed by IRIS as a guide to staging canine and feline CKD. Serum creatinine concentrations must always be interpreted in light of the patient's urine specific gravity and physical examination findings in order to rule out pre- and postrenal causes of azotemia. The CKD stages are further classified by the presence or absence of proteinuria and systemic hypertension (Table 32.3). The classic diagnosis of renal failure based on renal azotemia (persistent azotemia superimposed on the inability to concentrate urine) pertains to CKD stages 2–4. Stage 1

Table 32.2 IRIS CKD staging system for cats and dogs.

Animal	Serum Creatinine Concentration (mg/dL)			
	Stage 1 Non-Azotemic CKD	Stage 2 Mild Renal Azotemia	Stage 3 Moderate Renal Azotemia	Stage 4 Severe Renal Azotemia
Cats	<1.6	1.6–2.8	2.9–5.0	>5.0
Dogs	<1.4	1.4–2.0	2.1–5.0	>5.0

Table 32.3 IRIS CKD substaging for proteinuria and hypertension for cats and dogs.

Parameter	Classification
Urine protein:creatinine ratio	
<0.2 (cats and dogs)	Non-proteinuric
0.2–0.4 (cats), 0.2–0.5 (dogs)	Borderline proteinuric
>.4 (cats), >0.5 (dogs)	Proteinuric
Systolic blood pressure (mmHg)	
<140	Normotensive
140–160	Borderline hypertensive
>160	Hypertensive

CKD (non-azotemic CKD) could be diagnosed in cats and dogs with persistent proteinuria of renal origin, urine-concentrating deficits due to renal parenchymal disease, increases in serum creatinine concentration over time (even if the values remain in the normal range), or abnormal renal palpation or renal imaging findings.

Further diagnostics and treatment

In general, the diagnostic approach to a patient once CKD has been identified and staged is focused on three areas: (1) characterization of the renal disease, (2) characterization of the stability of the renal disease and renal function, and (3) characterization of the patient's problems associated with the decreased renal function. Further definition of the renal disease (beyond a standard minimum database) could include quantification of proteinuria, measurement of blood pressure, urine culture, kidney imaging, and possibly kidney biopsy. The stability of the renal function may be assessed by serial monitoring of abnormalities identified during the initial evaluation of renal disease. This monitoring should always include serial serum biochemistry profiles, urinalyses, quantification of proteinuria [e.g., urine protein:creatinine (UPC) ratio], and measurement of blood pressure, but may also include follow-up urine cultures and ultrasonographic examinations. Characterization of the renal disease and its stability are most important in the earlier stages of CKD when appropriate treatment has the greatest potential to improve or stabilize renal function. Characterization of the patient's clinical sequela becomes more important in the later stages of CKD, when clinical signs tend to be more severe. In the later stages of CKD, diagnostic (and subsequent therapeutic) efforts should be directed at the anorexia, vomiting, acidosis, potassium depletion, hypertension, anemia, and so on that can adversely affect the patient's quality of life.

Similarly to the diagnostic approach to CKD, the therapeutic approach should also be tailored to fit the patient's stage of disease. For example, disease-specific treatments for nephroliths or bacterial pyelonephritis, and also treatments designed to slow the progression of renal disease (so-called renoprotective treatments) will be of most value in the earlier stages of CKD. Renoprotective treatments include dietary change designed to reduce serum

Table 32.4 Effects of anesthetics on renal blood flow (RBF) and glomerular filtration rate (GFR).

Drug	RBF	GFR
Isoflurane	Slight decrease	Decrease
Sevoflurane	Slight decrease	Decrease
Thiopental	No change	No change or slight decrease
Ketamine	Increase	Decrease or no change
Propofol	No change	No change
Etomidate	No change	No change

Source: adapted from Green SA, Grauer GF. 2007. Renal disease. In: Tranquilli WJ, Thurmon JC, Grimm KA, eds. *Lumb and Jones' Veterinary Anesthesia and Analgesia*, 4th edn. Ames, IA: Blackwell Publishing, 2007; 915–919. Reproduced with permission of Wiley.

phosphorus concentrations and ACE inhibitors designed to normalize systemic and intraglomerular blood pressures and reduce proteinuria. In the later stages of CKD, treatment tends to be focused on ameliorating the patient's clinical signs associated with the decreased renal function.

Anesthetic drugs and renal disease

Renal disease and injury can result in alterations in the pharmacokinetics and pharmacodynamics of drugs administered during the perianesthetic period. Many of the drugs (or their metabolites) commonly used have some degree of renal metabolism and/or excretion (e.g., ketamine, benzodiazepines, and some opioids) and potential alterations in pharmacokinetic parameters should be taken into account in the anesthetic plan for these patients. Additionally, comorbidities associated with renal diseases, including azotemia, acid–base disturbances, electrolyte imbalances, dehydration, anemia, coagulopathy, hypertension, and encephalopathy, should be considered and appropriate alterations made in drug and therapy choices.

Azotemia is often associated with a decrease in plasma pH and can decrease plasma protein binding of administered drugs, resulting in higher concentrations of active free drug and increased risk of relative overdose. However, the clinical significance of this effect may be of minor importance. Effects of anesthetics on RBF can be generally described as all anesthetics are likely to decrease the rate of glomerular filtration. Anesthetic drugs may directly affect RBF or they may indirectly alter renal function via changes in cardiovascular and/or neuroendocrine activity [11]. Sedative and analgesic drugs have varying effects on RBF and GFR and generally relate to individual drug effects on cardiac output and vasomotor tone. Most anesthetics that decrease GFR do so as a consequence of decreased RBF (Table 32.4). Anesthetics that alter catecholamine release and systemic concentrations may have variable effects on RBF and thus GFR and renal function. For example, intramuscular administration of a combination of medetomidine and butorphanol increased GFR in healthy dogs, whereas that of a combination of medetomidine, butorphanol, and atropine did not [12]. However, in another study, medetomidine significantly decreased GFR in healthy dogs, whereas a combination of xylazine, ketamine, and halothane or propofol did not affect GFR [13].

Knowledge of the adverse effects of drugs used in the perianesthetic period is essential; it is often the results of magnification of these side-effects in the face of renal disease that poses the greatest risk for these patients. Phenothiazine tranquilizers (e.g., acepromazine) produce dose-dependent hypotension by antagonism of vascular α-adrenergic receptors. Phenothiazines may also antagonize dopamine receptors and therefore may prevent dopamine-induced increases in RBF during surgery. However, RBF and GFR do not change significantly in the face of mild hypotension and may this may actually impart protection of renal function after low-dose acepromazine administration [14]. Additionally, the use of phenothiazines as a renal preconditioning agent reduced the histopathologic damage in kidneys subject to ischemia and reperfusion [15]. Conversely, one study reported significant variations in systemic blood pressure and renal ultrasound perfusion parameters after a relatively high dose of acepromazine (0.1 mg/kg) and concluded that acepromazine should be avoided in patients with nephropathy. A relatively low dose of acepromazine (0.01–0.02 mg/kg) in patients with stable kidney disease in which the use of dopamine is not planned has been recommended [16]. Acepromazine use should probably be restricted to patients with stable and compensated renal diseases and avoided in patients in acute crises or in which maintenance of adequate perfusion pressure during anesthesia is a concern.

α_2-Adrenergic agonist drugs such as dexmedetomidine and xylazine can have significant dose-dependent depressant effects on heart rate and cardiac output and increase systemic vascular resistance. These effects could be expected to reduce RBF and subsequently GFR; in fact, in a study using a short-term controlled-rate infusion, dexmedetomidine was shown to decrease RBF by up to 30% [17]. However, there is evidence that medetomidine in combination with anticholinergic and opioid drugs has minimal effects on GFR in dogs [12]. Additionally, dexmedetomidine may be renal protective in the face of ischemia and reperfusion injury. Dexmedetomidine reduced metabolic activity and demonstrated antioxidant effects in rabbits undergoing experimental renal ischemia and reperfusion injury [18]. For patients at risk for acute renal injury due to hypoperfusion, dexmedetomidine use may have some benefit, but α_2-adrenergic agonist administration is accompanied by profound diuresis. The mechanism is likely multifactorial, including inhibition of vasopressin (AVP) release, inhibition of cAMP formation in the kidney, redistribution of aquaporin-2 receptors, inhibition of renin release, increased atrial natriuretic peptide, inhibition of renal sympathetic activity, osmotic diuresis due to increased plasma glucose, and inhibition of tubular sodium reabsorption [19]. Interestingly, these mechanisms differ in importance between individual α_2-agonist drugs and species [19]. For instance, xylazine had a greater diuretic effect than medetomidine in dogs, and medetomidine decreased plasma AVP whereas xylazine did not [20]. The increased production of dilute urine may be detrimental in patients with postrenal urinary tract obstruction or dehydration and hypovolemia [21,22].

Benzodiazepines are a commonly used class of drugs within veterinary medicine, primarily for their muscle relaxant and mild sedative properties. Diazepam and midazolam have minimal effects on cardiac output, systemic vascular resistance, and blood pressure. Consequently, their use probably has little impact on RBF and GFR. However, benzodiazepines, similarly to most injectable anesthetic and analgesic drugs, are protein bound in the plasma and their use in azotemic patients may consequently have more active free drug. Reduction in initial dosage is probably warranted in patients with acute kidney disease or which are severely acidotic, azotemic, or hypoproteinemic. Patients with stable disease may not need any adjustment in dosage. Additionally, in patients with acute kidney injury, midazolam may have reduced hepatic metabolism. Through an unknown mechanism, as the severity and duration of acute kidney injury increases, the activity of CYP3A, an enzyme associated with the P450 system in the liver, is decreased, delaying metabolism and prolonging the effect of drugs such as midazolam [23]. Diazepam and lorazepam are not water soluble and therefore are delivered in propylene glycol for injection. Propylene glycol can induce proximal renal tubular cell injury and necrosis, particularly in drugs administered as infusions [24–26]. Midazolam is water soluble and delivered in an aqueous solution and may be a more appropriate benzodiazepine for use in patients with significant kidney disease.

Anesthetic and analgesic protocols for patients with kidney disease are often built around the use of opioids [16]. Opioids will provide sedation and analgesia to patients with minimal impact on cardiac output and thus RBF [27]. It should be noted, however, that the pharmacokinetics of opioids can be altered in patients with renal disease or failure [28]. Longer acting opioids with active metabolites, such as morphine and meperidine (pethidine), should be used with caution as the metabolites have a delayed clearance. In humans, it has been recommended to avoid the use of morphine, meperidine, and dextropropoxyphene altogether in patients with renal dysfunction to avoid prolonged narcosis [29]. However, species differences in the metabolism of morphine may reduce the risk of these drugs in veterinary patients. The pharmacokinetics of buprenorphine, alfentanil, sufentanil, and remifentanil, at least in human patients with renal dysfunction, are little changed. Fentanyl, administered as a single dose, shows little change in its pharmacokinetic profile; however, significant tissue accumulation and prolonged effect can occur with continuous infusion [29]. Remifentanil is a short-acting opioid that undergoes complete metabolism within the plasma and, although a metabolite, GR90291, can accumulate in patients with renal failure, it does not produce significant opioid effects. It is therefore one of the most recommended opioids for use in human patients with renal dysfunction [30]. Clinicians should also be cognizant of the fact that opioids can cause urine retention when administered systemically or as an epidural injection.

Injectable anesthetic agents can also have an effect on renal parameters. Thiobarbiturates increase systemic vascular resistance but decrease renal vascular resistance with no net change in RBF. A serious concern with barbiturates is the change in pharmacodynamics associated with this class of drugs in patients with renal disease. Barbiturates (like many other drugs) are highly protein bound, and this protein binding can be altered in states of severe azotemia. It is well documented that animals with azotemia have decreased protein binding of thiopental and are at a higher risk of relative overdose when using thiopental [31,32]. Additionally, the central nervous system of azotemic animals is more susceptible to the effects of thiopental when measured by electroencephalogram [33,34]. This is thought to occur from allosteric endogenous compounds that enhance thiopental effects that are normally inhibited in non-azotemic animals. It is probably best practice to avoid the use of thiopental in patients with azotemia or renal disease; however, if necessary, total dosages should be reduced.

Ketamine (and likely tiletamine) increases RBF and renal vascular resistance [35]. Even though there can be an increase in RBF, ketamine administration may result in an abnormal distribution of blood flow within the kidney. Additionally, as the dose of ketamine increases, renal sympathetic nerve activity increases, RBF decreases and renal vascular resistance increases [36]. Ketamine also directly inhibits dopamine transporter proteins in the kidney, but the clinical relevance of this is unclear [37]. Ketamine and its metabolites are highly dependent on renal excretion. In cats, it has been said that the majority of the drug is excreted unchanged and therefore should be avoided in cats with renal insufficiency [38]. However, in fact, ketamine is metabolized to norketamine, a first-step metabolite, in the liver of cats, but unlike in other species, norketamine is not further metabolized [39]. Ketamine is 53% protein bound and higher levels of free drug can be expected in azotemic animals, although the increase in free drug may be clinically unimportant [40]. Interestingly, in humans after long-term abuse, the development of two syndromes involving the urinary system, ketamine-induced ulcerative cystitis and ketamine-induced vesicopathy, have been reported [41,42].

Propofol is one of the most commonly used induction agents in human and veterinary anesthesia. Propofol demonstrates a dose- and rate-dependent reduction in arterial blood pressure. However, at moderate to low doses it has minimal effects on RBF and GFR and is frequently used for the induction of anesthesia in patients with kidney disease [43,44]. In sheep, propofol caused minor hemodynamic changes in RBF that were not considered to be clinically important [45], and GFR was not significantly affected in dogs administered propofol at clinically used dosages [13,46]. In human patients with chronic kidney disease and uremia, the pharmacokinetics of propofol were similar to those of healthy control patients [47] and recovery from propofol anesthesia was no different to that of controls [48]. Propofol is considered to be a suitable agent for induction and total intravenous anesthesia in human patients with uremia, although reduced doses may be required [49].

Etomidate is an anesthetic agent known for its minimal effects on heart rate, blood pressure, and cardiac output. Etomidate has also been shown to have no significant effect on renal function and urine output in anesthetized rats [50]. Like propofol, etomidate does not significantly affect GFR in dogs [47]. However, similarly to diazepam, propylene glycol is used as a solvent in most etomidate preparations.

Inhalant anesthetics can cause systemic hypotension, especially during excessive depth, which can result in renal ischemia secondary to reduced RBF and GFR. This is a result of one of the major side-effects of potent volatile anesthetics, peripheral vasodilation. Inhalant anesthetics also depress myocardial contractility and cardiac output in a dose-dependent manner. Concurrently, inhalation anesthetics also tend to decrease RBF and GFR in a dose-dependent manner. Light planes of inhalation anesthesia preserve renal autoregulation of blood flow, whereas deep planes are associated with depression of autoregulation and decreases in RBF. Although isoflurane has minor direct effects on RBF, it decreases GFR and urine output [51]. Sevoflurane, although not well studied, seems to have similar effects to isoflurane on RBF [52]. However, when in contact with carbon dioxide absorbents, sevoflurane degrades to a nephrotoxic substance called compound A. Compound A has been shown to cause permanent damage to the kidneys of rats but has not been shown to cause problems in humans with renal insufficiency or in dogs with normal renal function [53,54]. Desflurane has no effect on RBF at concentrations up to twice the minimal alveolar concentration (MAC), but it decreases renal vascular resistance at concentrations greater than 1.75 MAC [55]. For most human patients, and most likely for veterinary patients, the effects of inhaled anesthetics on renal function are reversed at the termination of anesthesia. However, some patients may not regain the ability to regulate urine production for several days [56]. Any patient that demonstrates postanesthetic oliguria should be evaluated immediately for AKI.

As stated previously, COX-1 and COX-2 are necessary for the normal functioning of the healthy kidney. In fact, of the two enzymes, COX-2 may be more important for renal development and preservation of RBF and GFR, particularly during hypovolemia [57]. NSAIDs exert their effects through suppression of these enzymes, reducing the production of proinflammatory prostaglandins. Unfortunately, NSAIDs also suppress the production of prostaglandins necessary for constitutive functions. NSAIDs that preferentially suppress COX-2 may be more detrimental to renal function than more mixed-profile NSAIDs in patients with kidney disease [57]. In healthy dogs, the use of perioperative carprofen or meloxicam did not result in adverse effects or alterations of renal function [58]. Additionally, in dogs undergoing repair for traumatic facture repair, the administration of perioperative carprofen did not cause any clinically relevant adverse effects. However, even in healthy patients, the use of NSAIDs may result in fatal renal injury in dogs and cats [59,60]. The use of NSAIDs in any patient with evidence of AKI or CKD should be avoided unless necessary for maintenance of quality of life. In those patients, informed owner consent and very thorough patient monitoring are essential.

Anesthesia and the stress associated with surgery can cause the release of aldosterone, vasopressin, renin, and catecholamines. Accordingly, RBF and GFR (and therefore urine production) are generally decreased with surgery in any patient. In fact, in the face of appropriate intravenous fluid administration (10 mL/kg/h) during anesthesia, dogs with normal kidney function will have a urine output less than the usual range of 1–2 mL/kg/h in awake animals [61]. Additionally, these dogs will have evidence of fluid retention that resolves over time after anesthesia. This decrease in urine output may be a normal compensatory mechanism that occurs during reduced metabolic activity of the kidney or during a period when the kidneys are working to conserve solutes and fluid during insults to the body. It is therefore recommended to use additional parameters rather than just urine output as an indicator of fluid balance and renal function in anesthetized animals [61].

Anesthetic management of patients with renal disease

Patients with suspected or known renal disease or dysfunction should have a complete physical examination, biochemical testing, baseline arterial blood pressure measurement, and renal function evaluation prior to any anesthetic event. Additionally, renal diseases are often accompanied by dysfunction of other organ systems and should be considered in any anesthetic plan. Concomitant drug therapy should also be accounted for and incorporated into the anesthetic plan. For example, cats with hyperthyroidism may have chronic kidney disease, hypertension, and hypertrophic cardiomyopathy. Antihypertensive and antiarrhythmic drugs can result in patients having an increased response to drugs that affect the central nervous system, leading to relative overdose.

Preanesthetic stabilization of patients with renal disease may be more critical to a successful outcome than the anesthetic drugs that are administered. Overall, the most important parameters for a patient with renal disease are hydration status and circulating blood volume. Maintaining RBF and GFR through adequate hydration will reduce the likelihood of further renal injury and preserve renal function [62]. Hydration has been shown to be effective in the treatment of renal injury and is a good strategy to prevent the progression of early-stage kidney disease to more advanced-stage kidney disease [63]. Azotemic patients can be administered intravenous fluids before surgery to achieve euhydration and diuresis. If azotemia is severe and is accompanied by electrolyte abnormalities

Table 32.5 Example of an anesthetic plan for a small animal patient with renal disease.

Drug	Dose	Route
Premedication:		
Opioid of choice:		
Butorphanol	0.2–0.4 mg/kg	Intramuscular
Hydromorphone	0.1–0.2 mg/kg	Intramuscular
Morphine	0.1 mg/kg (cats)	Intramuscular
	0.25–1.0 mg/kg (dogs)	Intramuscular
Midazolam[a]	0.2–0.4 mg/kg	Intramuscular
Induction:		
Propofol	4–6 mg/kg (to effect)	Intravenous
or		
Etomidate	1–2 mg/kg (to effect)	Intravenous
Maintenance:		
Isoflurane	1–2% (to effect)	Inhalation
or		
Sevoflurane	2–3% (to effect)	Inhalation
Adjunctive to maintenance:		
Remifentanil	0.005–0.02 mg/kg/h	Intravenous infusion
or		
Fentanyl	0.005–0.02 mg/kg/h	Intravenous infusion
Supportive treatments:		
Replacement crystalloid fluid (lactated Ringer's, Normosol-R, or Plasma-Lyte A)	10–20 mL/kg for first hour 5–10 mL/kg/h thereafter	
Mannitol (20–25% solution)[b]	Loading dose 500 mg/kg Infusion 1 mg/kg/min	

[a] In healthy cats and dogs, midazolam may elicit aggressive or excitable behavior and can be removed from the plan.
[b] Mannitol is prone to crystallization at room temperatures and should be warmed prior to administration and delivered through a filter.

or acid–base imbalances, hospitalization and diuresis can be performed over several hours prior to anesthesia. Anemic patients undergoing anesthesia and procedures with the potential for blood loss should have a red blood cell transfusion if the hematocrit is less than 18–20%.

Once a patient is deemed stable, anesthesia can be performed. A plan that uses anesthetic and analgesic drugs that have minimal effects on cardiac output, blood pressure, and perfusion when possible has been recommended [16]. Premedication in small animal patients can be achieved with an opioid–benzodiazepine combination and induction of anesthesia can be accomplished with propofol, thiopental, etomidate, benzodiazepine-dissociative, or benzodiazepine–opioid combinations (Table 32.5). It is important to remember that all of these anesthetic drugs can cause some degree of reduced RBF and/or GFR and that using these drugs 'to effect' is recommended. Anesthesia can be maintained with either isoflurane or sevoflurane. In addition, constant-rate infusions using opioid agonists such as remifentanil or fentanyl for inhalant anesthetic reduction will reduce the dose-dependent side-effects of inhalant anesthetics and may improve RBF and GFR. In adult horses, anesthetic premedication without an α_2-adrenergic agonist is impractical, hence using reduced doses and combining with butorphanol may allow for adequate sedation. Induction with a benzodiazepine–ketamine or benzodiazepine–thiopental combination can be performed. Using a reduced dose of ketamine or thiopental may limit the induction agent's adverse effects on RBF and GFR. In smaller horses or ponies, propofol can be used as an induction agent.

Continuing intravenous fluid therapy throughout the anesthetic period is recommended to maintain fluid volume and hydration. Initially a rate of 20 mL/kg for the first hour can be administered and thereafter a rate of 10 mL/kg/h should be maintained if the patient does not have heart disease, hypoproteinemia, or severe anemia. The choice of intravenous fluid is based on the animal's electrolyte and acid–base status. In general, animals with mild to moderate renal insufficiency/failure that are well prepared for surgery or anesthesia can be administered a replacement crystalloid intravenous fluid. If there is potential for urinary tract obstruction or the patient is anuric, intravenous fluids should be used cautiously to prevent fluid overload until the obstruction is relieved or the anuria resolves.

Vigilant monitoring of a patient will help the anesthetist to identify hypotension, arrhythmias, hypoxemia, or hypoventilation that could negatively impact renal function. Continuous electrocardiography (ECG) can detect changes in cardiac electrical activity that can be associated with electrolyte abnormalities such as hyperkalemia. Arterial blood pressure (ABP) should be measured to detect systemic hypotension and decreased renal perfusion pressure. Indirect ABP measurement can be easily performed with an oscillometric or Doppler technique; however, direct arterial catheterization is preferred as it is a more accurate and immediate measurement. Additionally, arterial blood gas samples can be obtained from the arterial catheter for analysis. Mean ABP should be maintained above 70–80 mmHg. In patients exhibiting hypertension when evaluated prior to anesthesia, maintenance of mean ABP closer to preanesthetic levels may be necessary to preserve renal perfusion. Pulse oximetry (S_pO_2) can be used to detect hemoglobin desaturation rapidly and alert the anesthetist to the potential for a decrease in tissue oxygen delivery. Continuous end-tidal carbon dioxide ($ETCO_2$) measurement can be used to detect hypoventilation and the need for assisted ventilation. Excessive arterial carbon dioxide can lead to acidemia, which may exacerbate acute renal disease [64]. Periodic arterial blood gas analysis can be useful for following trends in pH, oxygen content, and electrolytes. Advanced monitoring can be performed, particularly in critically ill animals. Central venous pressure (CVP) can be measured via a jugular catheter as an indirect measurement of blood volume to evaluate the rate of intravenous fluid administration. Normal CVP should be between 3 and 5 cmH_2O in dogs and cats. If the CVP rises more than 10 cmH_2O, fluid administration should be slowed or stopped.

If the CVP falls in response to the fluids being stopped, they may be resumed at a slower rate. An elevated CVP of more than 10 cmH_2O indicates inadequate myocardial function or volume overload. Cardiac output measurement can give indications of preload, stroke volume, system vascular resistance, and patient response to inotropic and pressor agents that can have an effect on RBF and GFR.

Adjunctive treatments for patients with renal disease

During the perianesthetic period, pharmacologic manipulation of cardiovascular and renal physiology may be beneficial in renal disease patients. Dopamine infusions (1–10 µg/kg/min) have long been considered useful in improving myocardial function and cardiac output. In human patients with renal disease, lower (e.g., renal) doses of dopamine (2 µg/kg/min) have been shown to increase urinary output but do not improve overall outcome compared with IV fluid therapy [63]. In dogs, low doses (1–3 µg/kg/min) are used to promote RBF and GFR, but studies showing benefit are lacking. Controversy exists regarding the use of dopamine to improve renal function in cats. Questions remain as to whether or not cats have appropriate dopamine receptors in their kidneys and low-dose dopamine has not been shown to have a diuretic effect in cats [65]. In fact, dopamine infusions of 10–100 µg/kg/min may increase urine output without changing GFR, suggesting that that diuresis is due to decreased tubular reabsorption and that dopamine receptors appear to have no role in RBF or GFR in cats [66]. Doses of dopamine above approximately 10 µg/kg/min may cause α-adrenergic renal vasoconstriction and decreased RBF and should be avoided. An alternative inotrope for use during anesthesia is dobutamine (2–20 µg/kg/min). Dobutamine can increase cardiac output and potentially blood pressure without significant vasoconstrictive and dopaminergic actions.

Furosemide has also been investigated during anesthesia in patients with renal dysfunction. As a loop diuretic, furosemide decreases the metabolic activity of the renal tubules; however, furosemide infusion has been shown to result in elevated creatinine levels in anesthetized human patients and its use is not recommended [63,67].

The osmotic diuretic mannitol has several potentially beneficial effects on the kidney. Mannitol is freely filtered and not reabsorbed by the kidney and therefore acts as an osmotic agent in the renal tubules and also in the systemic circulation. Administration of mannitol can induce renal arteriole dilation, decrease vascular resistance and blood viscosity, and scavenge oxygen free radicals [68]. Renal blood flow in cats may be improved by administering an intravenous loading dose of mannitol (500 mg/kg) and continuing a constant-rate infusion (1 mg/kg/min) during the anesthetic period [69]. In AKI, mannitol induced the redistribution of systemic blood flow to the kidneys and increased urine flow [70]. In an experimental model of hypoxia in rabbit kidneys, mannitol reduced tubular cell swelling and prevented proximal intratubular hypertension, resulting in improved blood flow [71]. Mannitol should be used cautiously in patients that are receiving other diuretics such as acetazolamide, as excessive use can result in hyponatremic acute renal failure [72].

Fenoldopam is a dopamine receptor agonist at the DA-1 receptor that has renal vasodilating properties. Fenoldopam has no effect on DA-2 or α-receptors that can cause vasoconstriction and result in decreased RBF and GFR. In fact, fenoldopam increases RBF and may assist in preserving renal function. Fenoldopam has been shown to decrease creatinine and improve renal function in humans at a dose of 0.1 µg/kg/min compared with dopamine infusion and may be effective in decreasing renal hypoperfusion [73]. In dogs, fenoldopam at a dose of 0.8 µg/kg/min resulted in a steady-state plasma concentration of 20 ± 17 ng/mL. Heart rate and systolic blood pressure were unaffected by the infusion in any of the dogs [74]. However, in a canine model of rhabdomyolysis, fenoldopam administration decreased creatinine clearance and increased the severity of renal injury [75]. In awake, healthy cats, fenodopam at 0.5 µg/kg/min increased urine output only after 6 h of infusion and increased sodium excretion. Additionally, fenoldopam administration had a biphasic effect on GFR, decreasing in the first 6 h and then increasing it subsequently [76].

Anesthetic management of patients with urethral obstruction

Species commonly presenting for obstruction and correction of urethral obstruction are cats, dogs, sheep, and goats; however, horses and cattle can also be affected. Patients with urethral obstruction often present with metabolic and acid–base abnormalities. These include hyperkalemia, azotemia, acidemia, hyperphosphatemia, hyperglycemia, hypocalcemia, hyponatremia, and hypochloremia. Hyponatremia and hypochloremia are often associated with urine leakage into the abdominal cavity, and any patient presenting with these abnormalities should be examined for urethral or urinary bladder rupture. Hyperkalemia is perhaps of greatest concern and should be addressed immediately. In general, patients having a serum potassium concentration greater than 5.5–6.0 mEq/L should not be anesthetized until the potassium levels can be normalized. ECG abnormalities are commonly observed with potassium concentrations exceeding 7 mEq/L. The presence of ECG abnormalities at a given plasma concentration can also be related to the chronicity of the change, suggesting that preanesthetic ECG may be of value any time potassium abnormalities are present. The resting membrane potential of cardiac muscle depends on the permeability and extracellular concentration of potassium (Fig. 32.2). During hyperkalemia, the membrane's resting potential is raised (partially depolarized), and fewer sodium channels are available to participate in the action potential. As the serum potassium concentration increases, repolarization occurs more rapidly and automaticity, conductivity, contractility, and excitability are decreased. These changes produce the classic ECG appearance of a peaked T wave

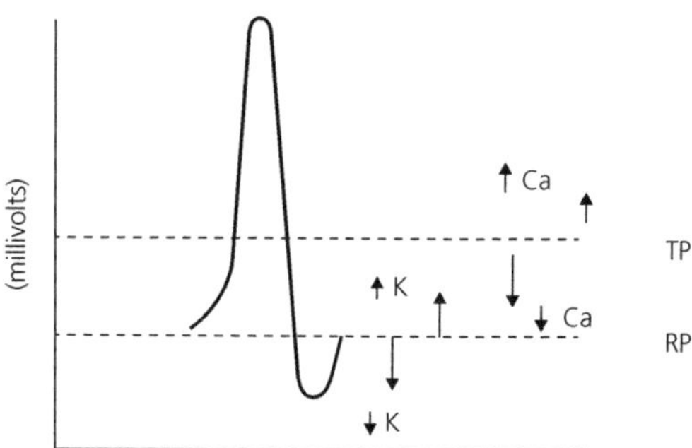

Figure 32.2 Relationships between extracellular concentrations of potassium) and calcium and the resting potential (RP) and threshold potential (TP). An action potential is generated when there is sufficient depolarization to reach the TP. Increased extracellular potassium will result in raised (less negative) RP, whereas increased extracellular calcium will result in raised TP.

Table 32.6 Treatment options for patients with hyperkalemia.

Treatment	Dosage	Use	Comments
Calcium chloride	0.1 mg/kg, IV	Raises threshold potential	Administer slowly. Works temporarily.
50% Dextrose	1–2 ml/kg, IV	Increases endogenous insulin release to drive K^+ into cells	Dilute to 5–10% solution to reduce osmotic damage
Regular insulin	0.25–1 U/kg, IV	Drives K^+ into cells	Administer with dextrose and monitor blood glucose to prevent hypoglycemia
Sodium bicarbonate	1–2 mEq/kg, IV	Increases pH to cause exchange of intracellular H^+ for K^+	Monitor ventilation; CO_2 retention can result in worsening of acidemia

with a prolonged PR interval progressing to wide QRS complexes and loss of P waves.

Mild chronic hyperkalemia may not require treatment prior to anesthesia. If treatment is instituted for chronic hyperkalemia, serum potassium should be lowered gradually to allow intracellular potassium time to re-establish physiological transmembrane concentration gradients. If hyperkalemia is acute or ECG abnormalities are noted, treatment should be initiated prior to induction of anesthesia. The most rapid treatment for the cardiac effects associated with hyperkalemia is 10% calcium chloride (0.1 mg/kg IV). Calcium will increase the membrane's threshold potential, resulting in increased myocardial conduction and contractility. Because increased serum potassium concentration causes the resting potential to be less negative (partially depolarized), the calcium ion-induced increase in threshold potential temporarily restores the normal gradient between resting and threshold potentials. It should be recognized that administration of calcium will not affect the serum potassium concentration, and its effects will therefore be short-lived. Regimens to decrease the serum potassium concentration by shifting potassium intracellularly include bicarbonate administration and combined infusion of glucose and insulin (Table 32.6). Because acidemia favors extracellular movement of potassium and worsens hyperkalemia, intermittent positive-pressure ventilation may be required to prevent anesthetic drug-induced hypercapnia and respiratory acidosis.

In some patients, percutaneous cystocentesis can be performed blindly or with ultrasound guidance to drain urine and reduce patient discomfort, although bladder injury and rupture and aortic laceration are a concern [77]. Intravenous fluid therapy should be instituted to correct dehydration and acid–base and electrolyte abnormalities. Once the patient is stabilized, anesthesia can be provided with a protocol similar to that in Table 32.5 in small animal patients and small ruminants and standard protocols for larger patients. Horses with urethral obstruction have been reported to rupture their bladder during induction of anesthesia, presumably due to increased abdominal compartment pressure from recumbency [78]. Perineal urethrosotomy can be performed in male horses using sedation and epidural anesthesia to relieve the obstruction. Intravenous fluid therapy using potassium-free fluids has been considered the treatment of choice for animals with urethral obstruction. However, particularly in cats, compared with physiologic saline (0.9% NaCl), lactated Ringer's solution is a better choice as animals have a decreased duration of metabolic and electrolyte imbalances after the obstruction is cleared [79].

In cats with mild or partial urethral obstruction, only sedation may be needed to facilitate passing a urethral catheter and clearing the obstruction. In these cases, after fluid therapy and stabilization, an opioid can be administered for analgesia followed by subanesthetic doses of propofol (0.25–1.0 mg/kg, IV) for sedation. Supplemental oxygen should be provided during propofol sedation. In male cats, intraurethral administration of 4 mL of diluted atracurium (0.5 mg/mL) significantly increased the chance and reduced the time necessary to remove an obstruction [80]. Another approach is the use of a coccygeal epidural with a local anesthetic such as lidocaine for reducing pain and discomfort during and after unblocking of the urethra [81]. However, intravesicular administration of lidocaine and sodium bicarbonate has no beneficial effects and does not reduce the recurrence rate or severity of clinical signs in cats with urethral obstruction [82].

Careful postanesthetic care of these patients is essential as prolonged diuresis after the obstruction has been relieved is common. Urine output of greater than 2 mL/kg/h can be expected in about 46% of cats within the first 6 h of treatment, which will require higher fluid therapy rates that should be tapered off over the following few days [83].

In sheep or goats with urethral obstruction, sedation or anesthesia may be needed to extrude the penis and examine the urethral process, one of the most common sites for urethral obstruction in these species. Preanesthetic stabilization to correct acid–base, fluid, and electrolyte imbalances should occur in a manner similar to that mentioned previously for small animal patients. α_2-Adrenergic receptor agonists, such as xylazine, should be avoided owing to their diuretic effects [84]. A benzodiazepine in combination with an opioid may provide adequate sedation for initial examination, particularly in painful animals. Anesthesia can be induced with propofol, benzodiazepine-dissociative, or mask with inhalant anesthetic. Additionally, adjunctive anesthesia can be provided with epidural administration of local anesthetic.

Anesthetic management of patients with urinary bladder rupture and uroabdomen

Uroabdomen is defined as urine in the peritoneal cavity and can occur in any species of animal. In small animals, uroabdomen is most commonly caused by vehicular trauma but can also result from rupture of ureters, bladder, or urethra secondary to obstruction or neoplasia, or from iatrogenic injury. In large animal species, uroabdomen is most commonly associated with urethral obstruction; however, in neonatal foals it most commonly found in males and is thought to occur when the foal passes through the birth canal with a full bladder or secondary to umbilical infection and necrosis of the urachus [85].

In any species, it is important to recognize that uroabdomen is not a surgical emergency. Correction of postrenal azotemia, acid–base, and electrolyte abnormalities is paramount and surgical correction can usually be delayed for several hours until the patient is stabilized [86]. Hyponatremia, hypochloremia, and hyperkalemia are common abnormalities. Hyponatremia and hypochloremia develop as a result of dilution from excess free water that is unable to be excreted and hyperkalemia develops because excess potassium is unable to be excreted in the face of liberation from intracellular stores, particularly during acidosis [87]. Fluid and electrolyte replacement therapy is recommended and hyperkalemia can be treated as previously indicated. Abdominocentesis can be performed to remove accumulating urine and reduce the azotemic and potassium loads. Peritoneal fluid creatinine can be compared with serum creatinine and ratios greater than 2:1 confirm uroperitoneum. Once a patient's serum abnormalities are normalized, and in particular potassium is reduced, animals can be anesthetized with previously mentioned protocols for surgical correction.

Postanesthesia oliguria and acute kidney injury

Decreased urine output and AKI are important complications that can develop after anesthesia and include the development of incidental kidney disease in addition to acute progression of CKD. Postanesthesia oliguria (<0.5 mL/kg/h) can occur in patients after prolonged anesthesia or after a major surgical procedure and should prompt consideration and evaluation of causes of oliguria or AKI [88]. Some degree of oliguria can be expected in patients that have fluid or blood loss and secondary to the stress response of the adrenal cortex. In human patients, increased aldosterone and vasopressin release has been documented in the first 24 h after surgery. These increases result in increased salt and water reabsorption, thereby reducing urine production. However, this oliguria should be temporary and generally does not last for more than 24 h.

Pathologic causes of postanesthesia oliguria and AKI can be divided into prerenal, renal, and postrenal categories [88]. Prerenal causes include hypotension and hypovolemia. Renal causes include acute tubular necrosis (ischemia and reperfusion) and acute interstitial nephritis (drug toxicity such as from NSAIDs, antibiotics, or diuretics). Postrenal abnormalities can result from physical obstruction of urine flow.

Techniques designed for the prevention of postanesthesia oliguria and AKI are recommended, particularly in high-risk patients. Physiologic monitoring of vital signs for identification of hypotension and decreased perfusion includes mucous membrane color, capillary refill time, measurement of blood pressure, pulse oximetry, $ETCO_2$, and electrocardiography. Advanced monitoring techniques such as CVP and cardiac output measurements may be warranted in critical patients. Administration of intravenous fluids to maintain or expand intravascular volume it the mainstay of therapy for the prevention of AKI [88]. Colloidal therapy such as the use of hydroxyethyl starch may be of benefit in maintaining vascular expansion; however, there is some evidence that it may be nephrotoxic [89]. As mentioned previously, the use of mannitol may be appropriate for maintenance of RBF and GFR during anesthesia in cases with high risk of postanesthetic oliguria or AKI. Techniques to maintain mean arterial pressure of greater than 60–65 mmHg in small animal patients and smaller horses and ruminants and greater than 70–75 mmHg in adult horses and ruminants are of paramount importance for adequate perfusion of the kidneys. The level of acceptable hypotension is dependent on baseline blood pressure and mean arterial pressures may need to be maintained at higher levels in animals with chronic hypertension [90]. In human patients, it is recommended that mean arterial pressure by maintained within 20% of awake baseline values, since this is within the range of blood pressure drop during sleep [88,91]. The use of inotropic agents or anesthetic sparing techniques (MAC reduction) to achieve these desired pressures should be standard practice for patients with conditions that predispose to AKI.

Management of the postanesthetic patient in which oliguria or AKI is diagnosed should start with determining the cause. Reversible causes such as obstruction, hypotension, and hypovolemia should be ruled out or corrected. Measurement of blood pressure and intravenous fluid challenges can be useful. If the oliguria is determined to be of renal origin (not pre- or postrenal), function and diagnostic testing as described previously should be performed.

Treatment of postanesthesia oliguria and AKI is centered on intravenous fluid and electrolyte therapy. The use of diuretic and vasoactive drugs is controversial. Dopamine has traditionally been used in patients with oliguria and AKI. Lower doses ranging from 1 to 3 μg/kg/min have been used to increase RBF, GFR, urine output, and sodium excretion and decrease renal vascular resistance in several species [92]. In humans, low-dose dopamine therapy in patients with renal dysfunction resulted in transient improvements in urine output and creatinine levels; however, mortality and long-term outcomes did not improve [93]. The use of diuretics such as furosemide have also failed to show any improvement in clinical outcomes and may even worsen renal injury [88]. In hypovolemic patients, furosemide may increase the nephrotoxicity of other drugs by increasing their contact time in the renal tubules [94]. Diuretics may be useful in patients that develop pulmonary edema and fluid overload secondary to AKI [95]. Mannitol, as stated previously, may have beneficial effects in patients with AKI and can also be used in patients with volume overload and pulmonary edema.

Once postanesthetic oliguria and AKI has been identified and reversible conditions have been treated, the goal of therapy is to minimize ongoing or long-term renal damage. Long-term monitoring of renal function may be necessary.

References

1 Boyd LM, Langston C, Thompson K, *et al.* Survival in cats with naturally occurring chronic kidney disease (2000–2002). *J Vet Intern Med* 2008; **22**(5): 1111–1117.

2 Polzin DJ, Osborne CA, Jacob F, *et al.* Chronic renal failure. In: Ettinger SJ, Feldman EC, eds. *Textbook of Veterinary Internal Medicine*, 5th edn. Philadelphia: WB Saunders, 2000; 1634–1662.

3 Schott HC. Examination of the urinary system. In: Reed SM, Bayly WM, Sellon DC, eds. *Equine Internal Medicine*, 3rd edn. St. Louis, MO: Saunders Elsevier, 2010; 1162–1176.

4 Rose DB, Post T, Stokes J. *Clinical Physiology of Acid–Base and Electrolyte Disorders*, 6th edn. New York: McGraw-Hill, 2013.

5 Hall JE. *Guyton and Hall Textbook of Medical Physiology*, 12th edn. Philadelphia: Saunders Elsevier, 2010.

6 DiBartola SP, ed. *Fluid, Electrolyte, and Acid–Base Disorders in Small Animal Practice*, 4th edn. St Louis, MO: Elsevier, 2011.

7 Flournoy WS, Wohl JS, Albrecht-Schmitt TJ, *et al.* Pharmacologic identification of putative D1 dopamine receptors in feline kidneys. *J Vet Pharmacol Ther* 2003; **26**(4): 283–290.

8 Grauer GF, Greco DS, Behrend EN, *et al.* Estimation of quantitative enzymuria in dogs with gentamicin-induced nephrotoxicosis using urine enzyme/creatinine ratios from spot urine samples. *J Vet Intern Med* 1995; **9**(5): 324–327.

9 Schott HC. Chronic renal failure. In: Reed SM, Bayly WM, Sellon DC, eds. *Equine Internal Medicine*, 3rd edn. St. Louis, MO: Saunders Elsevier, 2010; 1183–1198.

10 Surdyk KK, Sloan DL, Brown SA. Renal effects of carprofen and etodolac in euvolemic and volume-depleted dogs. *Am J Vet Res* 2012; **73**(9): 1485–1490.

11 Hall JA. Renal effects of the inhalation agents. In: Faust RJ, ed. *Anesthesiology Review*, 3rd edn. Philadelphia: Churchill Livingstone, 2002; 103–104.

12 Grimm JB, Grimm KA, Kneller SK. *et al.* The effect of a combination of medetomidine–butorphanol and medetomidine, butorphanol, atropine on glomerular filtration rate in dogs. *Vet Radiol Ultrasound* 2001; **42**(5): 458–462.

13 Fusellier M, Desfontis JC, Madec S, *et al.* Influence of three anesthetic protocols on glomerular filtration rate in dogs. *Am J Vet Res* 2007; **68**(8): 807–811.

14 Bostrom I, Nyman G, Kampa N, *et al.* Effects of acepromazine on renal function in anesthetized dogs. *Am J Vet Res* 2003; **64**(5): 590–598.

15 Pazoki-Toroudi HR, Ajami M, Habibey R. Premedication and renal preconditioning: a role for alprazolam, atropine, morphine and promethazine. *Fundam Clin Pharmacol* 2010; **24**(2): 189–198.

16 Weil AB. Anesthesia for patients with renal/hepatic disease. *Top Companion Anim Med* 2010; **25**(2): 87–91.

17 Lawrence CJ, Prinzen FW, de Lange S. The effect of dexmedetomidine on nutrient organ blood flow. *Anesth Analg* 1996; **83**(6): 1160–1165.

18 Kilic K, Hanci V, Selek S, *et al.* The effects of dexmedetomidine on mesenteric arterial occlusion-associated gut ischemia and reperfusion-induced gut and kidney injury in rabbits. *J Surg Res* 2012; **178**(1): 223–232.

19 Murahata Y, Hikasa Y. Comparison of the diuretic effects of medetomidine hydrochloride and xylazine hydrochloride in healthy cats. *Am J Vet Res* 2012; **73**(12): 1871–1880.

20 Talukder MH, Hikasa Y. Diuretic effects of medetomidine compared with xylazine in healthy dogs. *Can J Vet Res* 2009; **73**(3): 224–236.

21 Nunez E, Steffey EP, Ocampo L, *et al.* Effects of α_2-adrenergic receptor agonists on urine production in horses deprived of food and water. *Am J Vet Res* 2004; **65**(10): 1342–1346.

22 Saleh N, Aoki M, Shimada T, *et al.* Renal effects of medetomidine in isoflurane-anesthetized dogs with special reference to its diuretic action. *J Vet Med Sci* 2005; **67**(5): 461–465.

23 Kirwan CJ, MacPhee IA, Lee T, *et al.* Acute kidney injury reduces the hepatic metabolism of midazolam in critically ill patients. *Intensive Care Med* 2012; **38**(1): 76–84.

24 Yorgin PD, Theodorou AA, Al-Uzri A, *et al.* Propylene glycol-induced proximal renal tubular cell injury. *Am J Kidney Dis* 1997; **30**(1): 134–139.

25 Hayman M, Seidl EC, Ali M, *et al.* Acute tubular necrosis associated with propylene glycol from concomitant administration of intravenous lorazepam and trimethoprim–sulfaethoxazole. *Pharmacotherapy* 2003; **23**(9): 1190–1194.

26 Zar T, Yusufzai I, Sullivan A, *et al.* Acute kidney injury, hyperomolality and metabolic acidosis associated with lorazepam. *Nat Clin Pract Nephrol* 2007; 3(9): 515–520.

27 Lamont LA, Mathews KA. Opioids, nonsteroidal anti-inflammatories, and analgesic adjuvants. In: Tranquilli WJ, Thurmon JC, Grimm KA, eds. *Lumb and Jones' Veterinary Anesthesia and Analgesia*, 4th edn. Ames, IA: Blackwell Publishing, 2007; 241–271.

28 Hohne C, Donaubauer B, Kaisers U. Opioids during anesthesia in liver and renal failure. *Anaesthesist* 2004; **53**(3): 291–303.

29 Davies G, Kingswood C, Street M. Pharmacokinetics of opioids in renal dysfunction. *Clin Pharmacokinet* 1996; **31**(6): 410–422.

30 Hoke JF, Shulgman D, Dershwitz M, *et al.* Pharmacokinetics and pharmacodynamics of remifentanil in persons with renal failure compared with healthy volunteers. *Anesthesiology* 1997; **87**(3): 533–541.

31 Danhof M, Levy G. Kinetics of drug action in disease states. V. Acute effect of urea infusion on phenobarbital concentrations in rats at onset of loss of righting reflex. *J Pharmacol Exp Ther* 1985; **232**(2): 430–434.

32 Ghoneim MM, Pandya H. Plasma protein binding of thiopental in patients with impaired renal or hepatic function. *Anesthesiology* 1975; **42**(5): 545–549.

33 Srivastava K, Hatanaka T, Katayama K, *et al.* Influence of plasma dialysate from normal and renal dysfunction rats on the electroencephalogram and gamma-aminobutyric acid A receptor complex modulation of thiopental. *Biol Pharm Bull* 1999; **22**(3): 288–294.

34 Srirastava K, Hatanaka T, Katayama K, *et al.* Pharmacokinetic and pharmacodynamic consequences of thiopental in renal dysfunction rats: evaluation with electroencephalography. *Biol Pharm Bull* 1998; **21**(12): 1327–1333.

35 Priano LL. Alteration of renal hemodynamics by thiopental, diazepam, and ketamine in conscious dogs. *Anesth Analg* 1928; **61**(10): 853–862.

36 Chien CT, Cheng YJ, Chen CF, *et al.* Differentiation of ketamine effects on renal nerve activity and renal blood flow in rats. *Acta Anaesthesiol Taiwan* 2004; **42**(4): 185–189.

37 Nishimura M, Sato K. Ketamine stereoselectively inhibits rat dopamine transporter. *Neurosci Lett* 1999; **274**(2): 131–134.

38 Flecknell PA. Injectable anaesthetics. In: Hall LW, Taylor PM, eds. *Anaesthesia of the Cat*. London: Baillière Tindall, 1994; 129–156.

39 Waterman AE. Influence of premedication with xylazine on the distribution and metabolism of intramuscularly administered ketamine in cats. *Res Vet Sci* 1983; **35**(3): 285–290.

40 Baggott JD, Blake JW. Disposition kinetics of ketamine in the domestic cat. *Arch Int Pharmacodyn Ther* 1976; **220**(1): 115–124.

41 Morgan CJ, Curran HV. Ketamine use: a review. *Addiction* 2012; **107**(1): 27–38.

42 Middela S, Pearce I. Ketamine-induced vesicopathy: a literature review. *Int J Clin Pract* 2010; **65**(1): 27–30.

43 Wouters PF, Van de Velde MA, Marcus MA, *et al.* Hemodynamic changes during induction of anesthesia with eltanolone and propofol in dogs. *Anesth Analg* 1995; **81**(1): 125–131.

44 Shiga Y, Minami K, Uezono Y, *et al.* Effects of the intravenously administered anaesthetics ketamine, propofol, and thiamylal on the cortical renal blood flow in rats. *Pharmacology* 2003; **68**(1): 17–23.

45 Booke M, Armstrong C, Hinder F, *et al.* The effects of propofol on hemodynamics and renal blood flow in healthy and in septic sheep, and combined with fentanyl in septic sheep. *Anesth Analg* 1996; **82**(4): 738–743.

46 Chang J, Kim S, Jung J, *et al.* Evaluation of the effects of thiopental, propofol, and etomidate on glomerular filtration rate measured by the use of dynamic computed tomography in dogs. *Am J Vet Res* 2011; **72**(1): 146–151.

47 Kirvela M, Olkkola KT, Rosenberg PH, *et al.* Pharmacokinetics of propofol and haemodynamic changes during induction of anaesthesia in uraemic patients. *Br J Anaesth* 1992; **68**(2): 178–182.

48 Nathan N, Debord J, Narcisse F, *et al.* Pharmacokinetics of propofol and its conjugates after continuous infusion in normal and in renal failure patients: a preliminary study. *Acta Anaesthesiol Belg* 1993; **44**(3): 77–85.

49 de Gasperi A, Mazza E, Noe L, *et al.* Pharmacokinetic profile of the induction dose of propofol in chronic renal failure patients undergoing renal transpalantation. *Minerva Anestesiol* 1996; **62**(1): 25–31.

50 Petersen JS, Shalmi M, Christensen S, *et al.* Comparison of the renal effects of six sedating agents in rats. *Physiol Behav* 1996; **60**(3): 759–765.

51 Gelman S, Fowler KC, Smith LR. Regional blood flow during isoflurane and halothane anesthesia. *Anesth Analg* 1984; **63**(6): 557–565.

52 Bernard JM, Doursout MF, Wouters P, *et al.* Effects of sevoflurane and soflurane on hepatic circulation in the chronically instrumented dog. *Anesthesiology* 1992; **77**(3): 541–545.

53 Conzen PF, Kharasch ED, Czerner SFA, *et al.* Low-flow sevoflurane compared with low-flow isoflurane anesthesia in patients with stable renal insufficiency. *Anesthesiology* 2002; **97**(3): 578–584.

54 Sun L, Suzuki Y, Takata M, *et al.* Repeated low-flow sevoflurane anesthesia: effects on hepatic and renal function in beagles. *Masui* 1997; **46**(3): 351–357.

55 Merin RG, Bernard JM, Doursout MF, *et al.* Comparison of the effects of isoflurane and desflurane on cardiovascular dynamics and regional blood flow in the chronically instrumented dog. *Anesthesiology* 1991; **74**(3): 568–574.

56 Hayes MA, Goldenberg IS. Renal effects of anesthesia and operation mediated by endocrines. *Anesthesiology* 1963; **24**: 487–499.

57 Kramer BK, Kammerl MC, Komhoff M. Renal cyclooxygenase-2 (COX-2). Physiological, pathophysiological, and clinical implications. *Kidney Blood Press Res* 2004; **27**(1): 43–62.

58 Crandell DE, Mathews KA, Dyson DH. Effect of meloxicam and carprofen on renal function when administered to healthy dogs prior to anesthesia and painful stimulation. *Am J Vet Res* 2004; **65**(10): 1384–1390.

59 Pages JP. Néphropathies dues aux anti-inflammatoires non stéroïdiens (AINS) chez le chat: 21 observations (1993–2001). *Prat Méd Chir Anim Compagnie* 2005; **40**: 177–181.

60 Dyer F, Diesel G, Cooles S, *et al.* Suspected adverse reactions, 2009. *Vet Rec* 2010; **167**(4): 118–121.

61 Boscan P, Pypendop BH, Siao DT, *et al.* Fluid balance, glomerular filtration rate, and urine output in dogs anesthetized for an orthopedic surgical procedure. *Am J Vet Res* 2010; **71**(5): 501–507.

62 Wagener G, Brentjens TE. Anesthetic concerns in patients presenting with renal failure. *Anesthesiol Clin* 2010; **28**(1): 39–54.

63 Lassnigg A, Donner E, Grubhofer G, *et al.* Lack of renoprotective effects of dopamine and furosemide during cardiac surgery. *J Am Soc Nephrol* 2000; **11**(1): 97–104.

64 Kazory A, Ducloux D. Successful management of respiratory failure can improve renal function. *Am J Crit Care* 2009; **18**(1): 10–11.

65 Wohl JS, Schwartz DD, Flournoy S *et al.* Renal hemodynamic and diuretic effects of low-dosage dopamine in anesthetized cats. *J Vet Emerg Crit Care* 2007; **17**(1): 45–52.

66 Clark KL, Roberson MJ, Drew GM. Do renal tubular dopamine receptors mediate dopamine-induced diuresis in the anesthetized cat? *J Cardiovasc Pharmacol* 1991; **17**(2): 267–276.

67 Cowgill LD, Elliott DA. Acute renal failure. In: Ettinger SJ, Feldman EC, eds. *Textbook of Veterinary Internal Medicine*, 5th edn. Philadelphia: WB Saunders, 2000; 1615–1633.

68 Ho KM, Power BM. Benefits and risks of furosemide in acute kidney injury. *Anaesthesia* 2010; **65**(3): 283–293.

69 McClellan JM, Goldstein RE, Erb HN, *et al.* Effects of administration of fluids and diuretics on glomerular filtration rate, renal blood flow, and urine output in healthy awake cats. *Am J Vet Res* 2006; **67**(4): 715–722.

70 Braqadottir G, Redfors B, Ricksten SE. Mannitol increases renal blood flow and maintains filtration fraction and oxygenation in postoperative acute kidney injury: a prospective interventional study. *Crit Care* 2012; **16**(4): R159.

71 Bipat R, Steels P, Cuypers Y, *et al.* Mannitol reduces the hydrostatic pressure in the proximal tubule of the isolated blood-perfused rabbit kidney during hypoxic stress and improves its function. *Nephron Extra* 2011; **1**(1): 201–211.

72 Tsai SF, Shu KH. Mannitol-induced acute renal failure. *Clin Nephrol* 2010; **74**(1): 70–73.
73 Brienza N, Malcangi V, Dalfino L, *et al.* A comparison between fenoldopam and low-dose dopamine in early renal dysfunction of critically ill patients. *Crit Care Med* 2006; **34**(3): 707–714.
74 Bloom CA, Labato MA, Hazarika S, *et al.* Preliminary pharmacokinetics and cardiovascular effects of fenoldopam continuous rate infusion in six healthy dogs. *J Vet Pharmacol Ther* 2012; **35**(3): 224–230.
75 Murray C, Markos F, Snow HM, *et al.* Effects of fenoldopam on renal blood flow and its function in a canine model of rhabdomyolysis. *Eur J Anaesthesiol* 2003; **20**(9): 711–718.
76 Simmons JP, Wohl JS, Schwartz DD, *et al.* Diuretic effects of fenoldopam in healthy cats. *J Vet Emerg Crit Care* 2006; **16**(2): 96–103.
77 Buckely GJ, Aktay SA, Rozanski EA. Massive transfusion and surgical management of iatrogenic aortic laceration associated with cystocentesis in a dog. *J Am Vet Med Assoc* 2009; **235**(3): 288–291.
78 Pankowski RL, Fubini SL. Urinary bladder rupture in a two-year-old horse: sequel to a surgically repaired neonatal injury. *J Am Vet Med Assoc* 1987; **191**(5): 560–562.
79 Cunha MG, Freitas GC, Carregaro AB, *et al.* Renal and cardiorespiratory effects of treatment with lactated Ringer's solution or physiologic saline (0.9% NaCl) solution in cats with experimentally induced urethral obstruction. *Am J Vet Res* 2010; **71**(7): 840–846.
80 Galluzzi F, De Rensis F, Menozzi A, *et al.* Effect of intraurethral administration of atracurium besylate in male cats with urethral plugs. *J Small Anim Pract* 2012; **53**(7): 411–415.
81 O'Hearn AK, Wright BD. Coccygeal epidural with local anesthetic for catheterization and pain management in the treatment of feline urethral obstruction. *J Vet Emerg Crit Care* 2011; **21**(1): 50–52.
82 Zezza L, Reusch CE, Gerber B. Intravesical application of lidocaine and sodium bicarbonate in the treatment of obstructive idiopathic lower urinary tract disease in cats. *J Vet Intern Med* 2012; **26**(3): 526–531.
83 Francis BJ, Wells RJ, Rao S, *et al.* Retrospective study to characterize postobstructive diuresis in cats with urethral obstruction. *J Feline Med Surg* 2010; **12**(8): 606–608.
84 MacLeay JM. Urolithiasis. In: Smith BP, ed. *Large Animal Internal Medicine*, 4th edn. St. Louis, MO: Mosby Elsevier, 2009; 950–958.
85 Hardy J. Uroabdomen in foals. *Equine Vet Educ* 1998; **10**(1): 21–25.
86 Diver TJ. Urinary disorders in the foal. In: Smith BP, ed. *Large Animal Internal Medicine*, 4th edn. St. Louis, MO: Mosby Elsevier, 2009; 947–949.
87 Behr MJ, Hackett RP, Bentinck-Smith J, *et al.* Metabolic abnormalities associated with rupture of the urinary bladder in neonatal foals. *J Am Vet Med Assoc* 1981; **178**(3): 263–266.
88 Chenitz KB, Lane-Fall MG. Decreased urine output and acute kidney injury in the postanesthesia care unit. *Anesthesiol Clin* 2012; **30**(3): 513–526.
89 Groeneveld AB, Navickis RJ, Wilkes MM. Update on the comparative safety of colloids: a systemic review of clinical studies. *Ann Surg* 2011; **253**(3): 470–483.
90 Venkataraman R, Kellum JA. Prevention of acute renal failure. *Chest* 2007; **131**(1): 300–308.
91 Loredo JS, Nelesen R, Ancoli-Israel S, *et al.* Sleep quality and blood pressure dipping in normal adults. *Sleep* 2004; **27**(6): 1097–1103.
92 Schwartz LB, Bissell MG, Murphy M, *et al.* Renal effects of dopamine in vascular surgical patients. *J Vasc Surg* 1988; **8**(4): 367–374.
93 Friedrich JO, Adhikari N, Herridge MS, *et al.* Meta-analysis: low-dose dopamine increases urine output but does not prevent renal dysfunction or death. *Ann Intern Med* 2005; **142**(7): 510–524.
94 Stoelting RK, Hillier SC. Diuretics. In: Stoelting RK, Hillier SC, eds. *Pharmacology and Physiology in Anesthetic Practice*, 4th edn. Philadelphia: Lippincott Williams & Wilkins, 2006; 486–495.
95 Karajala V, Mansour W, Kellum JA. Diuretics in acute kidney injury. *Minerva Anestesiol* 2009; **75**(5): 251–257.

33 Anesthetic Considerations for Renal Replacement Therapy

Rebecca A. Johnson
School of Veterinary Medicine, University of Wisconsin, Madison, Wisconsin, USA

Chapter contents

Introduction

The kidneys are responsible for numerous essential biological functions, such as removing nitrogenous end-products from the blood, retaining solutes, proteins, and blood cells, maintaining acid–base balance, regulating electrolyte levels and erythropoiesis, and controlling systemic blood pressure. Acute kidney injury (AKI) and chronic kidney disease (CKD) are common clinical entities that are associated with impaired kidney function. Depending on etiology and chronicity, patients exhibit clinical signs such as vomiting, diarrhea, oral ulceration, anorexia, weight loss, polydipsia, and changes in urine output such as polyuria, oliguria, or anuria. Patients may also commonly present with electrolyte and acid–base disturbances (e.g., hyperkalemia, metabolic acidosis), and/or volume overload. To relieve these severe clinical signs, improve the quality of life, and extend lifespan in these patients, renal replacement therapies have recently become popular as treatment options to manage clinical signs of uremia in dogs and cats.

Renal replacement therapies include both extracorporeal techniques (hemodialysis and hemofiltration) and intracorporeal techniques (peritoneal dialysis and renal transplantation). Although these therapies are associated with significant financial, ethical, and emotional considerations, they have progressed from non-traditional, infrequent clinical entities to more common, progressive therapeutic options for companion animals with renal impairment. In this chapter, first the unique principles used in the critical anesthetic management of dogs and cats undergoing renal transplantation are discussed, followed by a discussion of specific dialysis techniques.

Renal transplantation

Introduction

In the mid-1950s, Guild and colleagues performed the first successful renal transplantation on identical twin humans [1]. However, only in the last few decades has renal transplantation gained popularity in clinical veterinary medicine as a therapy for companion animals with CKD. Morbidity and mortality rates associated with renal transplantation differ significantly between dogs and cats. For example, mean survival time for clinical canine patients is variable, reported to be from 18 days [2] up to 8 months [3]. In contrast, mean survival times in clinical feline patients are between 360 and 613 days, with 59–65% still alive after 6 months and 41–45% after 3 years [4–6]. The exact reasons for lower success rates in canine renal transplantation compared with the cat are not entirely clear. However, strong canine host immune responses require that potent immunosuppressive therapy is administered to prevent rejection, thereby increasing the possibility of adverse events [7–9]. Consistent with this hypothesis, a retrospective analysis of 26 canine renal transplants showed that 8 out of 12 necropsied dogs died from thromboembolic events [2]. Thromboembolism is associated with immunosuppression (among other factors) and is reported as a complication in human transplantation, but is infrequently seen in cats [9,10]. Although increasing age of both canine and feline patients is also identified as an important risk factor for increased mortality following transplantation in both dogs and cats [2,6], severe preoperative azotemia, hypertension, and cardiovascular disease are also associated with increased mortality solely in cats [6]. Thus, although renal transplantation appears to be a promising

Veterinary Anesthesia and Analgesia: The Fifth Edition of Lumb and Jones.
Edited by Kurt A. Grimm, Leigh A. Lamont, William J. Tranquilli, Stephen A. Greene and Sheilah A. Robertson.

treatment for CKD in dogs and cats, discriminant patient selection and preoperative risk assessment may enhance the survival of kidney transplant recipients.

Preoperative considerations

Many patients with CKD that present for renal transplantation will have acid–base and electrolyte abnormalities. Additional comorbidities such as hypertension and cardiovascular disease are also common and are associated with a higher postoperative mortality in feline patients [6]. Perioperative treatment of these disorders may reduce complication rates; therefore, patients should be medically managed before transplantation and coexisting problems corrected as much as possible. A complete blood count and serum biochemistry should be performed as the magnitude of the elevations in blood urea nitrogen (BUN) and creatinine levels is associated with increased mortality in cats [6], but not in dogs [2]. In addition, urinalysis and urine culture, blood typing, thoracic and abdominal radiographs, cardiac and abdominal ultrasound and systemic blood pressure measurements should be performed to screen for any pre-existing comorbidities and to ensure compatible blood types. Preoperative patient preparation includes placement of a double- or triple-lumen central venous catheter for chronic administration of balanced electrolyte solutions to correct electrolyte and acid–base abnormalities, to measure central venous pressure (CVP), and to facilitate blood sampling (Fig. 33.1). Immunosuppressive therapy may also be instituted and hemo- or peritoneal dialysis may be performed prior to transplantation (see below). A red blood cell transfusion or erythropoietin replacement therapy may also be administered to enhance oxygen-carrying capacity if the patient is severely anemic (PCV <20%). The transfusion trigger point for patients with chronic kidney disease is often lower than for healthier patients owing to compensatory mechanisms associated with chronic disease; therefore, patients should be assessed on an individual basis.

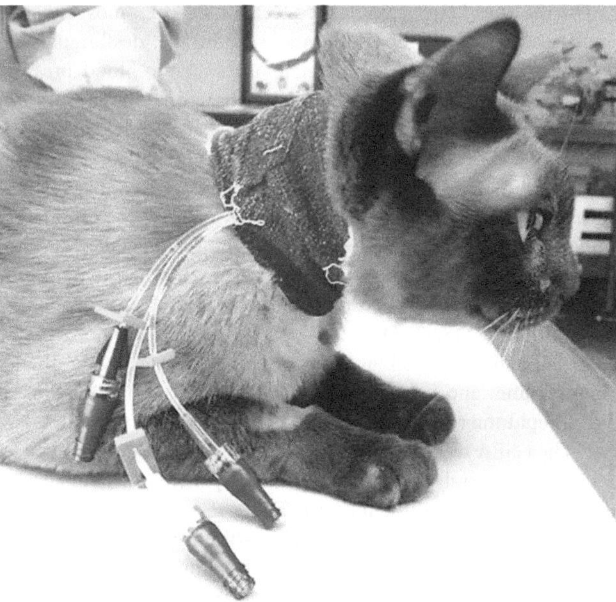

Figure 33.1 An example of one type of triple-lumen intravenous catheter inserted in the right jugular vein of a cat. These catheters should be placed preoperatively under sedation using the Seldinger technique and are subsequently used for CVP monitoring, fluid therapy, blood administration, and blood sampling perioperatively. They may also be used for hemodialysis techniques.

Anesthetic management

The ultimate goal of the anesthetic period is to provide acceptable anesthesia, analgesia, and muscle relaxation to patients without compromising remaining renal function or function of the new graft. Hence the anesthetic plan includes agents that have minimal cardiovascular depression, are not directly nephrotoxic, and minimally rely on the kidneys for their excretion.

Kidney donor management

Kidney donors are provided by the clients or are adopted by the recipient's owner prior to any surgical procedure. They are young, healthy animals with normal cardiovascular and renal function, hence the anesthetic procedures for kidney removal are routine and are chosen based on the individual donor's disposition and anesthetic needs. However, acepromazine is frequently used pre- or intraoperatively to promote renal vasculature dilation through α_1-adrenergic receptor blockade [11,12] and μ-opioid receptor agonists are commonly used as adjunctive analgesic agents.

Kidney recipient management

Kidney recipient patient anesthesia is handled similarly to that for other patients with CKD. However, recipients do present unique challenges as they accept a new kidney (graft) that has been removed from a donor and has been stored in hypoxic conditions for minutes to hours (Fig. 33.2A) (for microsurgical and storage techniques, see [2,13–16]). Although few currently used anesthetic agents are directly nephrotoxic, many alter renal function through decreases in cardiac output, systemic blood pressure, neuroendocrine status, and renal blood flow (RBF), which will subsequently affect the glomerular filtration rate (GFR). The stress response to surgery can release aldosterone, vasopressin, renin, and endogenous catecholamines, which can increase renal vascular resistance and subsequently reduce GFR [17–19]. Hence the objectives of the anesthetic period include reducing patient stress and maintaining systemic blood pressure (and therefore GFR) to the greatest extent possible via the use of anesthetic agents with minimal cardiovascular depression.

Anesthetic and analgesic agents must be chosen according to the individual patient's physiologic status and signalment as each transplant patient is unique; there is no universal protocol that can be used for every patient. However, preoperative medication using a combination of the μ-opioid receptor agonist fentanyl and a benzodiazepine is common since neither fentanyl nor the benzodiazepine class of drugs substantially affects cardiovascular function (Table 33.1) [20–23]. For example, fentanyl or a fentanyl analog (including sufentanil, alfentanil, and remifentanil) and midazolam are commonly used intravenously to facilitate anesthetic induction, provide analgesia, and reduce the stress response to surgery. Fentanyl is advantageous since it has a relatively short duration of action, which facilitates rapid adjustments, does not release histamine, and is minimally excreted (<10%) unchanged by the kidneys [24–26]. Although other opioids such as hydromorphone may be acceptable for use as analgesics, morphine is not recommended. Morphine administration increases plasma histamine levels, which can be associated with systemic hypotension [24]. In addition, morphine-6-glucuronide is an active metabolic product of morphine in dogs and humans and delayed elimination in patients with renal insufficiency may prolong drug effects [27–31]. Although cats have

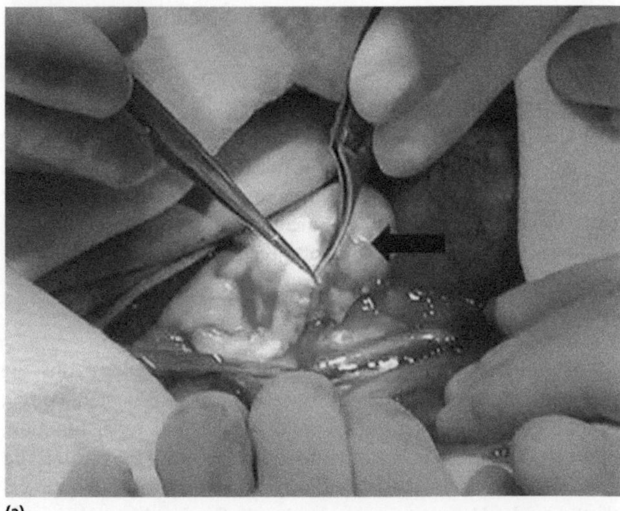
(a)

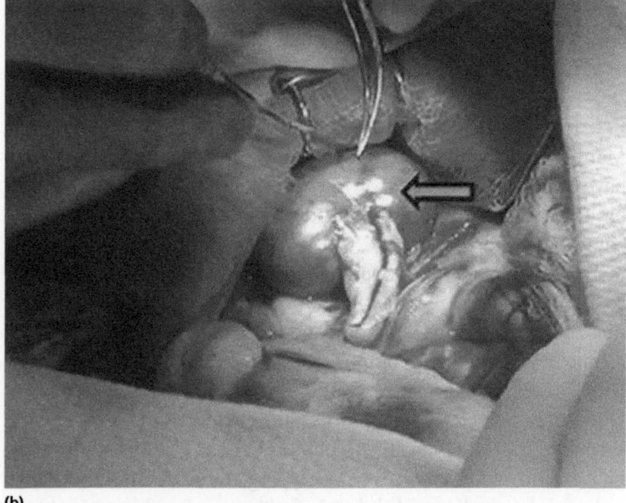
(b)

Figure 33.2 Intraoperative renal transplantation. (a) Donor kidney (dark arrow) placed in the abdomen of the recipient following extracorporeal storage. Note the pale color of the stored kidney as the anastomoses are not yet completed in this photograph. (b) Donor kidney (gray arrow) following renal artery and vein anastomoses and application of chlorpromazine to the renal artery. Note the pink (perfused) color of the kidney compared with the kidney in (a). Source: Dr Jon H. McAnulty, Department of Surgical Sciences, School of Veterinary Medicine, University of Wisconsin, Madison, Wisconsin, USA. Reproduced with permission of Jon McAnulty.

Table 33.1 Commonly used anesthetic/analgesic agents for renal replacement therapy recipients

Agent		Dose/Route
Premedicants/Sedatives/Analgesics		
Benzodiazepines	Midazolam	0.05-0.20 mg/kg IV, IM
	Diazepam	0.05-0.2 mg/kg IV
Opioids	Fentanyl	2-5 μg/kg IV
	Hydromorphone	0.05-0.1 mg/kg IV, IM
	Oxymorphone	0.05-0.1 mg/kg IV, IM
Induction Agents	Propofol	2-8 mg/kg to effect IV
Maintenance Agents		
Inhalants	Isoflurane	Minimal doses required
	Sevoflurane	
	Desflurane	
Opioids	Fentanyl	2-20 μg/kg/hr IV
Post-operative Analgesics		
Opioids	Buprenorphine	20-40 μg/kg IV, TM, IM
	Fentanyl	1-4 μg/kg/hr IV

low levels of glucuronyl transferase and morphine undergoes a different type of conjugation reaction in this species, the pharmacokinetics of morphine are somewhat similar to those of dogs and humans but clearance rates may be slightly slower [32–34]. Hence morphine administration in feline kidney recipients is not routinely recommended when other opioids are available. Similarly, α_2-adrenergic agonists such as dexmedetomidine should be avoided as they reduce cardiac output with increases in systemic vascular resistance [35–40]. Phenothiazines are also not recommended as a routine premedication since administration may result in lower systemic vascular resistance and potentially decreased arterial blood pressure in both conscious and anesthetized dogs and cats via peripheral α-adrenergic receptor blockade [12,41,42].

Anesthetic induction is accomplished with slow administration of small doses of propofol as it is rapidly metabolized by both hepatic and extra-hepatic means and RBF and GFR are minimally affected (Table 33.1) [43,44]. Although significantly metabolized in the liver, ketamine is usually avoided since its active metabolite, norketamine, is excreted unchanged by the kidney [45] and may contribute to prolonged drug effects in animals with decreased renal function. If ketamine is required as a premedication or induction agent (for example, due to animal behavior or lack of an alternative), doses should be reduced as much as possible by combination with appropriate coinduction agents. Etomidate is not routinely recommended since, although it has minimal cardiovascular effects, it induces adrenal suppression, which has been associated in some studies with increased postoperative mortality in critically ill humans [46,47].

During anesthetic maintenance (see Table 33.1), most inhalant anesthetics reduce GFR (isoflurane, sevoflurane, desflurane) and attempts to reduce levels and maintain systemic blood pressure should be made [44,48]. Therefore, it is common to use a constant-rate infusion of fentanyl or another fentanyl analog throughout the surgical procedure to reduce inhalant levels and enhance antinociception [49–51]. Although there have been concerns that sevoflurane may not be safe for use in AKI or CKD due to the production of potentially nephrotoxic compound A (at least in rodent species) and inorganic fluoride, no adverse effects have been shown in clinical patients and it can be used in these patients, as can isoflurane and desflurane [48,52–54].

In humans, regional anesthesia employing local anesthetics (bupivacaine) and opioids in spinal, epidural, or combinations of spinal–epidural (CSEA) anesthetic techniques have been used [55–58]. The CSEA technique is suggested to be a safe and useful alternative to general anesthesia in those patients where general anesthesia may be difficult, such as those with significant lung pathology or cardiovascular instability. Although the stress response on the renal vasculature would likely be diminished when using local anesthetics in these techniques and thus may promote increased renal blood flow to the graft, no significant differences were found in anesthesia time or duration, surgical conditions, hemodynamic stability, or early postoperative renal function when CSEA was compared with general inhalant anesthesia [55,56]. Currently, these techniques are not commonly used in veterinary patients owing to concern about neurological complications following neuraxial injections in heparinized and immunosuppressed patients.

Intraoperative anesthetic monitoring is essential for the risk management of renal transplant patients and includes pulse oximetry, capnometry, electrocardiography, and core body temperature. In addition, intraoperative hemodynamic monitoring and management are imperative to ensure reasonable organ perfusion pressure yet not subject the patient to fluid overload. Although CVP does not always correlate well with the general overall fluid status of the patient, acute changes in CVP may indicate impending fluid overload. However, this relationship is still debated [59]. Invasive blood pressure should be closely monitored since patients may experience normo-, hypo-, or hypertension throughout the procedure and into the postoperative period. An arterial catheter should be placed in the dorsal pedal or femoral artery contralateral to the side of transplantation if possible, since the aorta or its major branches may be occluded during renal artery anastomosis. Alternatively, the coccygeal artery may be used but may be difficult to keep clean and patent postoperatively. Care in handling these catheters is essential as patients may be purposely heparinized and excessive bleeding at the puncture site may occur. Alternatively, indirect blood pressures using an ultrasonic Doppler flow detector may be used if an artery cannot be catheterized, but can be less accurate depending on circumstances [60–64].

Intravenous fluid therapy should consist of a balanced electrolyte solution administered at a rate of 5–10 mL/kg/h based on the individual patient's needs and comorbidities (e.g., heart disease). In humans, 0.9% sodium chloride is not recommended owing to extracellular shifts in serum potassium, increases in serum chloride and a decrease in pH (hyperchloremic acidosis) [65–67]. Synthetic colloids such as hetastarch (hydroxyethyl starch) should be used with caution owing to potential adverse effects such as coagulopathies, reticuloendothelial system dysfunction, and impaired renal function [68]. Their use is reserved for situations that require colloid osmotic pressure increases, since complete data on the use of even medium molecular weight hetastarch on graft function are not fully available. If patients remain hypotensive under general anesthesia, β-adrenergic receptor agonists such as dobutamine can be used to increase cardiac output. The use of dopamine remains controversial because of species differences in receptor pharmacology and potential increase in systemic vascular resistance with higher doses [31]. If the patient cannot tolerate further fluid loading, vasopressors may be considered to treat hypotension, despite the risk of renal vasoconstriction. In humans, norepinephrine use does not have a negative effect on recipient graft function since the harmful effects of systemic hypotension likely outweigh the potential renal vasoconstriction caused by norepinephrine [69,70]. However, this has yet to be tested in clinical veterinary patients.

During surgery, mannitol (0.5–1.0 g/kg) may be administered intravenously as the vascular anastomosis is nearly completed to increase renal perfusion pressure, reduce ischemia-reperfusion injury, and diminish the delay in graft function [2,31,71]. Heparin may be administered once adequate hemostasis is maintained since patients are often prothrombotic due to hypercoagulability and hypofibrinolysis [10,72]. If the newly anastomosed renal artery exhibits profound vasoconstriction, chlorpromazine may be used topically as a peripheral α-adrenergic receptor antagonist and direct vascular smooth muscle relaxant to initiate vasodilation of the artery and likely enhance RBF (Fig. 33.2B) [73]. Prior to the end of the surgical procedure in cats, the fentanyl infusion may be discontinued and buprenorphine administered intravenously for postoperative analgesia (Table 33.1). Alternatively, fentanyl (or fentanyl analog) infusions may be titrated in cats and also in dogs at lower dosages for postoperative analgesia. Intensive postoperative cardiovascular monitoring is recommended if these agents are used. Non-steroidal anti-inflammatory agents (NSAIDs) are not recommended owing to their potential nephrotoxic, hepatotoxic, and gastrointestinal effects [74].

Recovery and complications

Hypertension can be present throughout the procedure or can occur as the vascular clamps are removed from the new kidney. It may persist or even worsen postoperatively [2,5,6,14,75,76]. The pathogenesis of hypertension is likely multifactorial, possibly due to a combination of primary renal disease, calcineurin inhibitors (such as the immunosuppressive agent cyclosporine), corticosteroid administration, and increased renin or angiotensin II levels originating within the graft [2,5,6,14,75,76]. Although intraoperative hypertension can be quickly managed with increasing inhalant concentrations and/or nitroprusside infusions, postoperative management is usually accomplished with the continued administration of antihypertensive agents such as nitroprusside, hydralazine, or amlodipine. Therefore, frequent arterial blood pressure monitoring is essential in the postoperative period, ideally with an arterial line. Indirect blood pressures using an ultrasonic Doppler flow detector may also be used if arterial catheterization is not possible or cannot be maintained [60–64]. Hypertension is a common risk factor for stroke in humans [77]. In addition, feline patients that have close monitoring and management of postoperative blood pressure have reduced rates of postoperative neurologic disease, including seizures, stupor, ataxia, and central blindness [78], although no link was found in one study between postoperative seizures and hypertension [6]. However, it is possible that postoperative ischemic events may be likely in postoperative hypertensive cats that lead to overt neurologic signs.

Postoperative complications are common and can include rejection, infection, thromboembolic disease, congestive heart failure, delayed graft function, acute postoperative neurologic disease, uroabdomen, gingival hyperplasia associated with cyclosporine, and intestinal intussusception [2,6]. In some cases, postoperative hemodialysis can be used to manage delayed graft function, acute rejection, pyelonephritis, and other complications until the problem is resolved [79]. Although significant complications are associated with renal transplantation in cats and dogs, surgical and anesthetic techniques are consistently improving as additional information regarding preoperative patient stabilization and treatment of complications becomes available. Dialysis techniques directed at reducing the circulating uremic products and correction of acid–base and electrolyte disturbance beforehand are discussed in the next section.

Peritoneal dialysis

Introduction

Peritoneal dialysis (PD) is an alternative renal replacement therapy used to remove temporarily solutes and excess fluid and to control electrolyte and acid–base balance until renal function recovers sufficiently. Comprehensive reviews of the techniques and equipment have been published recently [80,81]. In PD, the exchange of solutes and fluid occurs between two compartments: the peritoneal capillary blood and the dialyzate placed in the peritoneal cavity. Fluid and solutes are transported via diffusion and osmosis/

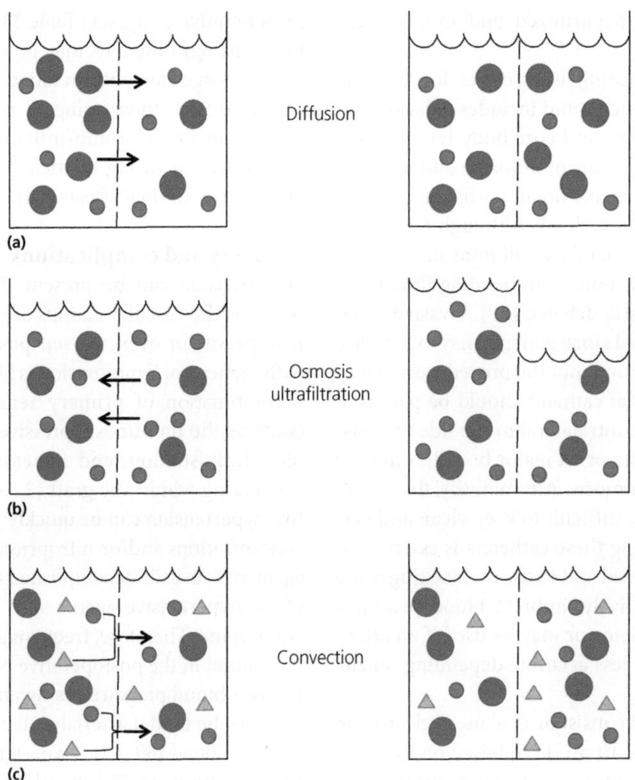

Figure 33.3 Schematic representation of processes involved in dialysis techniques. (a) *Diffusion.* Diffusion occurs when solutes travel across a semipermeable membrane based on their concentration gradient; solutes move from a higher concentration to areas with lower concentrations. (b) *Osmosis/ultrafiltration.* Osmosis is the net movement of water (solvent) across a semipermeable membrane into a region of higher solute concentration in an attempt to equalize the relative solute concentration. With ultrafiltration, hydrostatic pressure is used to force solvent across the membrane. (c) *Convection.* Convection occurs as the solute travels within the mass movement of the solvent.

ultrafiltration, with a minor role played by convection (Fig. 33.3) [82]. More specifically, solutes are removed as they diffuse across the semipermeable peritoneal membranes, the rate being determined by the membrane permeability of the molecules (size and charge), available surface area, and concentration gradient. Fluids are removed by osmosis/ultrafiltration as water moves from areas with low osmolar concentrations into the dialyzate, which has high osmolality (e.g., dextrose) or by using pressure gradients. Convection of solutes also occurs as they are trapped in the flow of water, although this process is more important in hemodialysis than in peritoneal dialysis [82]. Overall transport across the peritoneal membrane is commonly explained by the three-pore theory, where large pores (100–200 Å in diameter) allow the transport of macromolecules such as albumin, small pores (20–25 Å) allow low molecular weight substances such as urea, creatinine and glucose to pass and ultrasmall pores (4–6 Å) transport only water [83].

Case selection

Typically, PD is used for veterinary patients with AKI associated with oliguria or anuria refractory to fluid therapy and in patients with severe acute uremia with BUN >100 mg/dL or creatinine >10 mg/dL [84]. Peritoneal dialysis is also used for the treatment of exposure to diffusible toxins such as ethylene glycol and barbiturates, severe metabolic abnormalities (e.g., hypercalcemia, hyperkalemia), and extreme core body temperature derangements [83]. Although PD is less efficient than hemodialysis in reducing uremia [83], several case reports have shown the efficacy of PD in veterinary patients [85–88]. The advantages include minimal technical skill required, good cardiovascular tolerance, lack of expensive extracorporeal equipment, and decreased risk of bleeding [89]. However, it is not recommended for patients with severe coagulopathy, omental adhesions, peritonitis, diaphragmatic or abdominal hernias, or severe hypoalbuminemia [80].

Peritoneal dialysis procedures and equipment

Peritoneal dialysis is accomplished through a fill-and-drain system using an indwelling peritoneal catheter (Fig. 33.4). The catheter and its placement are absolutely critical for successful PD. The catheter should allow sufficient inflow and outflow volumes, be biocompatible, resist infection, and reduce leakage [83]. Catheters come in various brands and types and can be aseptically placed percutaneously using the Seldinger technique, through a mini-surgical approach, or by direct visualization through a laparotomy or laparoscopy [80–83]. When using the percutaneous or mini-surgical approach, patient sedation and a local anesthetic block of the skin ± peritoneum is required (Table 33.1). Commonly, a μ-opioid receptor agonist such as fentanyl with or without a benzodiazepine such as midazolam intravenously is adequate to complete the procedure. Buprenorphine may alternatively be used. Lidocaine infiltration around the tube insertion site is recommended. If surgical catheter implantation is required, animals can be managed similarly to other AKI cases, taking care to maintain blood pressure without further fluid overloading of the patient.

Following catheter placement, a variety of dialyzates can be used for the exchange procedures, each with their own advantages and disadvantages (for reviews, see: Bersenas [80], Cooper and Labato [81], and Ross and Labato [83]). The goal is not to normalize the azotemia immediately but gradually to correct the patient's hemodynamics and acid–base and electrolyte derangements while reducing BUN to 60–100 mg/dL and creatinine to 4.0–6.0 mg/dL over 24–48 h [84]. First, a small amount of fresh dialyzate is initially directed into the drainage bag and the peritoneal cavity is drained so that any contaminants introduced during the catheterization procedure are flushed into the drainage bag and not the peritoneal cavity. Warmed dialyzate solution is placed in the peritoneal cavity by gravity or infusion pump over 5–10 min, where it remains for approximately 30–45 min (the 'dwell time'). Following the exchange of fluid and solutes across the membrane, the dialysis fluid is removed over 15 min and discarded. This is repeated hourly until the patient stabilizes [80]. Initial infusion volumes are small (10–20 mL/kg) but may be increased after 24 h to 30–40 mL/kg. Once the goals have been met, patients are frequently changed to chronic dialysis protocols where the dialyzate remains in the peritoneal cavity for longer periods and 3–4 exchanges per day are performed [83]. Patients should be continuously monitored for acute blood volume and electrolyte changes. Catheter outflow obstructions are common and body weight, CVP, systemic arterial blood pressure, urine output, and pulmonary status are monitored extremely closely. Other complications also occur but are usually manageable, and include dialyzate retention, subcutaneous sequestration of dialyzate, hypoalbuminemia, peritonitis, and pleural effusion (for reviews, see: Bersenas [80] and Cooper and Labato [81]).

In summary, PD is an effective tool in managing AKI or dialyzable toxin exposure and may even be used in cases where hemodialysis and/or transplantation are not feasible. The PD procedures frequently require sedation and/or general anesthesia and patients should be treated similarly to others with renal impairment.

Hemodialysis

Introduction and case selection

The first attempt at hemodialysis was performed in 1914 by Abel and colleagues, who removed blood from animals, passed it through a device with semipermeable membranes, and then placed it back into the animal [90]. They termed this process *vividiffusion*, which has become the fundamental process upon which current hemodialysis techniques are based. Intermittent hemodialysis (IHD) is an extracorporeal renal replacement therapy that mainly uses the principle of diffusion to normalize acid–base and electrolyte abnormalities and to remove uremic toxins from the blood through a semipermeable membrane. Convection (also called solvent drag) and adsorption play a minor role. The solute concentration gradient, molecular weight, and membrane permeability all affect the rate of transfer across the dialysis membrane [91]. IHD is an excellent technique to remove low molecular weight substances (<500 Da) such as urea, creatinine, and electrolytes. In veterinary medicine, its primary application is in AKI, where conventional therapy fails to resolve the biochemical or clinical signs of uremia, and to prevent further patient deterioration prior to recovery of renal function [79,92]. It is also commonly used as an indefinite renal replacement therapy during CKD in the face of severe refractory uremia (BUN >90–100 mg/dL, creatinine >6–8 mg/dL), hyperkalemia, and fluid overload. Intermittent hemodialysis can be performed prior to renal transplantation to stabilize a high-risk patient further [91,93–95]. Modified current human dialysis techniques have been used in many diverse animal species, including tortoises, rabbits, sheep, and horses [96], but its clinical use in cats and dogs has only recently gained in popularity and feasibility.

Alternatively, a technique called continuous renal replacement therapy (CRRT) can be used in the treatment of AKI, in which renal function is expected to return quickly, or for patients who are to be transitioned to IHD [97]. The basic difference between the techniques is that CRRT is a continuous process that not only relies on diffusion through straw-like semipermeable membranes but also emphasizes convection and, to a lesser extent, adhesion, allowing for removal of higher molecular weight solutes compared with IHD. Continuous renal replacement therapy has multiple treatment modalities: continuous venovenous hemofiltration (CVVH; purely convective), continuous venovenous hemodialysis (CVVHD; diffusive modality), and continuous venovenous hemodiafiltration (CVVHDF; convection and diffusion) [98]. However, CRRT is relatively new and requires specialized training and continuous 24 h patient care. Although it has therapeutic advantages over IHD, its use is not widespread at present but it is appearing to show significant promise for the future treatment of patients with renal insufficiency.

Intermittent hemodialysis procedures and equipment

A reliable, double- or triple-lumen intravenous jugular catheter (preferably a dialysis catheter) is imperative for the success of IHD (Fig. 33.1). These catheters can be temporary or permanent and have been described in detail elsewhere [99]. Temporary (non-cuffed, non-tunneled) catheters are the most commonly used for IHD and are routinely placed employing the Seldinger technique using sedation and a local anesthetic block of the catheter site. Permanent catheters are often cuffed, with a portion located subcutaneously. Insertion often requires a short period of general anesthesia and patients are treated similarly to others with AKI or CKD (Table 33.1).

The dialyzer (i.e., artificial kidney) is a small, disposable, sealed compartment containing thousands of hollow straws (called the hollow fiber design) (Fig. 33.5A) [91]. The blood flows within the straws and the dialyzate flows in a concurrent or countercurrent direction around the straws. The membranes are semipermeable, allowing transfer of fluid and solutes by diffusion and convection [91]. There are many types of dialyzer units, differing in chamber, tubing, and pore size. The selection of the hemodialyzer is based on the amount of extracorporeal blood volume and also on its diffusive, connective, and biocompatibility features (Fig. 33.5B) [79].

Hemodialysis machines (Fig. 33.6) come in several brands, are fairly expensive, and have been reviewed elsewhere [100]. The machine allows manipulations of blood flow rate, dialyzate flow rate, direction of blood flow and dialyzate flow, dialyzate composition, treatment length, sodium profiling to regulate plasma osmolality, anticoagulant administration rate, temperature of returning blood, and fluid removal from the blood [91]. Although these machines can remove wastes extremely efficiently and fairly quickly, the goal is not to decrease BUN and creatinine rapidly but to return the patient's homeostasis gradually over multiple sessions. Sessions are usually planned at 2–3 times per week and are 1–6 h in length, but can be longer depending on patient need.

The ultimate goal for IHD is to prolong patient survival, since in most cases renal function does not recover without renal

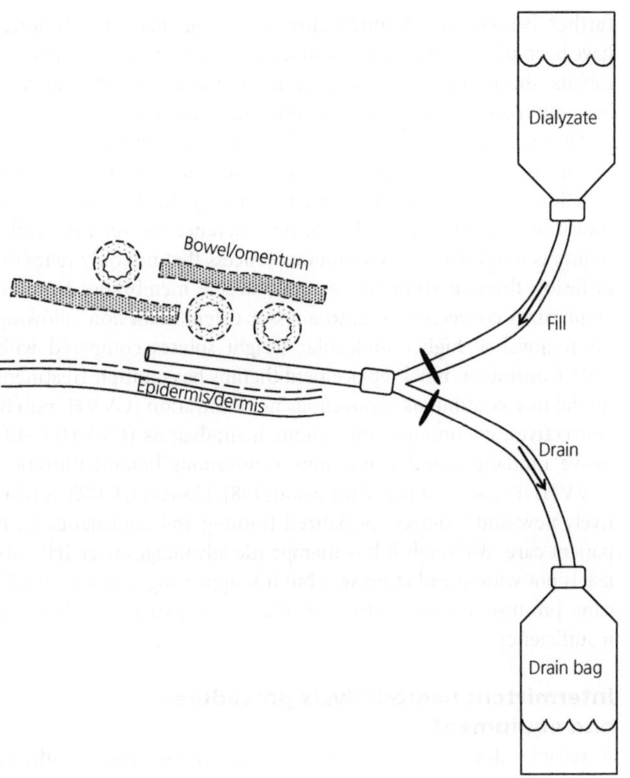

Figure 33.4 Drain-and-fill technique for peritoneal dialysis. The peritoneal cavity is initially infused by gravity or pump with fresh dialyzate through a preplaced peritoneal catheter. During the dwell time, neither the fresh dialyzate bag nor the drain bag is opened and fluids and solutes are exchanged from the blood within the peritoneal capillaries into the dialyzate across the semipermeable peritoneal membrane (dashed lines). The dialyzate is then drained from within the peritoneal cavity and discarded.

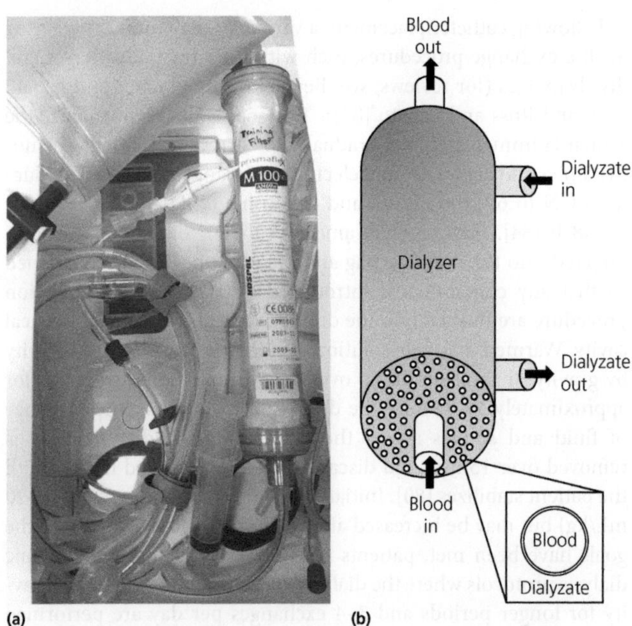

Figure 33.5 The hemodialyzer. (a) an example of a currently used hemodialyzer set (Prismaflex® System Hemofilter Set, Gambro, Lakewood, CO, USA). Sets are sterile and prepackaged with all the necessary filtration and tubing required by the hemodialysis machine. Multiple types are commercially available that can provide diffusion, convection and adsorption, depending on the dialysis prescription. (b) Schematic representation of the 'hollow-fiber' design within the hemodialyzer. It consists of numerous straws for blood transport separated from the dialyzate by a semipermeable membrane through which exchange of solutes and water occurs. Dialyzed blood is then returned back to the patient through a centrally placed intravenous catheter.

transplantation. Complications do occur with IHD, especially with methods of hemodialysis used early on in veterinary medicine. Dialysis disequilibrium (and corresponding neurologic dysfunction from cerebral edema) and hemorrhage associated with anticoagulation were common issues leading to mortality. With current techniques, complications are infrequently fatal, and although dialysis disequilibrium and hemorrhage may still occur, they mainly consist of hypotension, hypovolemia, venous thrombosis, pulmonary thromboembolism, pulmonary edema, pleural effusion, anemia, thrombocytopenia, leukopenia, nausea, vomiting, and inappetance [79,93,101–103]. Despite complications with the technique, IHD appears to be a viable treatment modality to improve outcomes in dogs and cats that do not respond adequately to medical management of their renal impairment.

Drug (anesthetic agent) clearance in dialysis

One goal of renal replacement therapy is to enhance the clearance of potential endogenous or exogenous toxins within the blood. However, plasma levels of drugs being administered to the patient can also be affected by these therapies and can make dosing protocols challenging. Although the type of dialysis technique chosen affects the extent of drug removal from the blood, other factors, such as membrane, solute, and patient characteristics, also affect drug clearance [98].

Membrane properties

The filter age, material, and surface area, and pore size influence drug filtration, with higher permeability filters and filters with larger surface areas allowing for more drug clearance in dialysis. The effects are more pronounced for intermediate molecular weight drugs [104]. In addition, the choice of dialysis technique will affect the amount of drug removal. The ultrafiltration rate, dialysis rate, blood flow rate, and, for convective processes, the selection of pre- versus post-dialyzer replacement fluids can also change drug clearance rates based on the protocol chosen for a specific patient [105].

Drug characteristics

The solubility, volume of distribution, molecular weight, protein binding, pK_a, and degree of renal and extrarenal elimination of the specific drug will affect its clearance rate [105]. For example, drugs with a large volume of distribution usually have a high affinity for tissues with a smaller proportion found in the intravascular space. The lower blood concentration results in a smaller concentration gradient to drive clearance by dialysis. In contrast, drugs with smaller volumes of distribution are more likely to remain intravascular and be quickly cleared by dialysis techniques [106,107]. Highly protein-bound drugs are less likely to be removed by dialysis than unbound drugs since bound drugs cannot cross dialysis membranes as easily as free drugs [107]. An important caveat is that disease states such as uremia, hypoalbuminemia, and nephrotic syndrome are associated with reduced protein binding of drugs, potentially allowing for more to be cleared by dialysis [108]. In

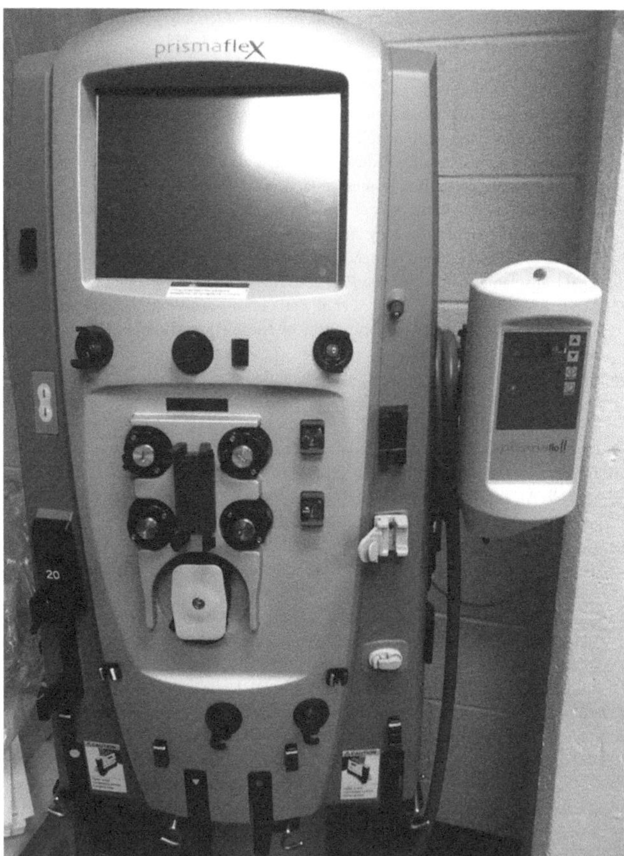

Figure 33.6 The hemodialysis machine. This is an example of one type of hemodialysis machine (Prismaflex® System, Gambro, Lakewood, CO, USA) that can accommodate the hemodialysis equipment described in Fig. 33.5. The machine should be able to deliver a wide range of extracorporeal blood purification therapies that can be individualized to each patient's needs and should be compatible with a range of hemofiltration sets supplied by the specific company.

addition, according to the Gibbs–Donnan effect, anionic proteins within the blood decrease the availability of cationic drugs available for clearance [106]. Therefore, if an anesthetic or analgesic drug has a relatively small volume of distribution (e.g., alfentanil versus fentanyl) and/or has relatively low protein binding (e.g., ketamine versus thiopental), its clearance may be hastened during dialysis.

Patient factors

Several patient factors affect drug clearance during dialysis. Patient age, gender, residual renal function, and cardiovascular and liver reserve function may directly or indirectly alter the amount of free drug available for filtration by dialysis [109]. In addition, changes in acid–base status of the animal that are associated with concurrent (renal) disease also affect the ionization of some pharmacologic agents, which can change the volume of drug distribution, protein binding, and renal or hepatic drug clearance [105].

Many data have been collected on drug protocols in patients undergoing renal replacement therapies, especially with regard to antibiotics (for a review, see Monaghan and Acierno [98]). However, studies on the disposition of anesthetic or analgesic agents, especially in veterinary patients, are lacking. Since most dialysis techniques in veterinary medicine are intermittent in nature (PD or IHD), it may be prudent to administer analgesic agents immediately after the dialysis treatment is completed to ensure that adequate levels are achieved before the next dialysis treatment and to try to extend the time between doses. Until detailed investigations on the pharmacokinetics of specific anesthetic and analgesic agents in veterinary patients undergoing dialysis have been performed, we must extrapolate our drug dosing schedules based on available human drug information, monitor the patient's status closely, and dose according to the individual patient's needs.

Conclusion

Feline renal transplantation appears to be an acceptable treatment option for patients with end-stage renal disease as it can extend lifespan and improve overall renal function and quality of life. Although morbidity and mortality rates in canine patients are significantly higher, newer immunosuppressive therapies and strategies to improve anticoagulation may greatly improve future results in this species. Renal transplantation in any species is not without complications, even though preoperative stabilization through techniques such as IHD can improve refractory azotemia, acid–base derangements, and electrolyte abnormalities. The anesthetic management of these patients can be complicated as metabolic, acid–base, and blood pressure derangements are complicated and frequent.

References

1 Merrill JP, Murray JE, Harrison JH, Guild WR. Successful homotransplantation of the human kidney between identical twins. *JAMA* 1956; **160**(4): 1364–1380.
2 Hopper K, Mehl ML, Kass PH, *et al.* Outcome after renal transplantation in 26 dogs. *Vet Surg* 2012; **41**(3): 316–327.
3 Mathews KA, Holmberg DL. Kidney transplantation in dogs with naturally occurring end-stage renal disease. *J Am Anim Hosp Assoc* 2000; **36**(6): 475.
4 Mathews KA, Gregory CR. Renal transplants in cats: 66 cases (1987–1996). *J Am Vet Med Assoc* 1997; **211**(11): 1432–1436.
5 Adin CA, Gregory CR, Kyles AE, Cowgill L. Diagnostic predictors of complications and survival after renal transplantation in cats. *Vet Surg* 2001; **30**(6): 515–521.
6 Schmeidt CW, Holzman G, Schwartz T, McAnulty JF. Survival, complications, and analysis of risk factors after renal transplantation in cats. *Vet Surg* 2008; **37**(7): 683–695.
7 Kyles AE, Gregory CR, Griffey SM, *et al.* Immunosuppression with a combination of the leflunomide analog, FK778, and microemulsified cyclosporine for renal transplantation in mongrel dogs. *Transplantation* 2003; **75**(8): 1128–1133.
8 Bernsteen L, Gregory CR, Kyles A, *et al.* Microemulsified cyclosporine-based immunosuppression for the prevention of acute renal allograft rejection in unrelated dogs: preliminary experimental study. *Vet Surg* 2003; **32**(3): 213–219.
9 Gregory CR, Kyles A, Bernsteen L, Mehl M. Results of clinical renal transplantation in 15 dogs using triple drug immunosuppressive therapy. *Vet Surg* 2006; **35**(2): 105–112.
10 Friedman GS, Meier-Kriesche HU, Kaplan B, *et al.* Hypercoagulable states in renal transplant candidates: impact of anticoagulation upon incidence of renal allograft thrombosis. *Transplantation* 2001; **72**(6): 1073–1078.
11 Popovic NA, Mullane JF, Yhap EO. Effects of acetylpromazine maleate on certain cardiorespiratory responses in dogs. *Am J Vet Res* 1972; **33**(9): 1819–1824.
12 Ludders JW, Reitan JA, Martucci R, *et al.* Blood pressure response to phenylephrine infusion in halothane-anesthetized dogs given acetylpromazine maleate. *Am J Vet Res* 1983; **44**(6): 996–999.
13 McAnulty JF. Hypothermic storage of feline kidneys for transplantation: successful ex vivo storage up to 7 hours. *Vet Surg* 1998; **27**(4): 312–320.
14 Bernsteen L, Gregory CR, Pollard RE, *et al.* Comparison of two surgical techniques for renal transplantation in cats. *Vet Surg* 1999; **28**(6): 417–420.
15 Bernsteen L., Gregory CR, Kyles A, *et al.* Renal transplantation in cats. *Clin Tech Small Anim Pract* 2000; **15**(1): 40–45.
16 Philips H, Aronson LR. Use of end-to-side arterial and venous anastomosis techniques for renal transplantation in two dogs. *J Am Vet Med Assoc* 2012; **240**(3): 298–303.
17 Hayes MA, Goldenberg IS. Renal effects of anesthesia and operation mediated by endocrines. *Anesthesiology* 1963; **24**: 487–499.

18 Walker LA, Buscemi-Bergin M, Gellai M. Renal hemodynamics in conscious rats: effects of anesthesia, surgery, and recovery. *Am J Physiol* 1983; **245**(1): F67–F74.

19 Koepke JP. Renal responses to stressful environmental stimuli. *Fed Proc* 1985; **44**(13): 2823–2827.

20 Chai CY, Wang CS. Cardiovascular actions of diazepam in the cat. *J Pharmacol Exp Ther* 1966; **154**(2): 271–280.

21 Freye E. Effect of high doses of fentanyl on myocardial infarction and cardiogenic shock in the dog. *Resuscitation* 1974; **3**(2): 105–113.

22 Liu W, Bidway AV, Stanley TH, Isem-Amaral J. Cardiovascular dynamics after large doses of fentanyl and fentanyl plus N_2O in the dog. *Anesth Analg* 1976; **55**(2): 168–172.

23 Jones DJ, Stehling LC, Zauder HL. Cardiovascular responses to diazepam and midazolam maleate in the dog. *Anesthesiology* 1979; **51**(5): 430–434.

24 Rosow CE, Moss J, Philbin DM, Savarese JJ. Histamine release during morphine and fentanyl anesthesia. *Anesthesiology* 1982; **56**(2): 93–96.

25 Peng P, Sandler AN. A review of the use of fentanyl analgesia in the management of acute pain in adults. *Anesthesiology* 1999; **90**(2): 576–599.

26 Stoelting RK, Hillier SC. Opioid agonists and antagonists. *Pharmacology and Physiology in Anesthetic Practice*, 4th edn. Philadelphia: Lippincott Williams & Wilkins, 2006; 104–109.

27 Chauvin M, Sandouk P, Scherrmann JM, *et al.* Morphine pharmacokinetics in renal failure. *Anesthesiology* 1987; **66**(3): 327–331.

28 Sear JW, Hand CW, Moore RA, McQuay HJ. Studies on morphine disposition: influence of general anesthesia on plasma concentrations of morphine and its metabolites. *Br J Anaesth* 1989; **62**(1): 22–27.

29 Sear JW, Hand CW, Moore RA, McQuay HJ. Studies on morphine disposition: influence of renal failure on the kinetics of morphine and its metabolites. *Br J Anaesth* 1989; **62**(1): 22–27.

30 Osborne R, Joel S, Grebenik K, *et al.* The pharmacokinetics of morphine and morphine glucuronides in kidney failure. *Clin Pharmacol Ther* 1993; **54**(2): 158–167.

31 Schmidt S, Jungwirth B. Anesthesia for renal transplant surgery: an update. *Eur J Anesthesiol* 2012; **29**(12): 552–558.

32 Davis LE, Donnelly EJ. Analgesic drugs in the cat. *J Am Vet Med Assoc* 1968; **153**(9): 1161–1167.

33 Faura CC, Collins SL, Moore RA, McQuay HJ. Systematic review of factors affecting the ratios of morphine and its major metabolites. *Pain* 1998; **74**(1): 43–53.

34 Taylor PM, Robertson SA, Dixon MJ, *et al.* Morphine, pethidine and buprenorphine disposition in the cat. *J Vet Pharmacol Ther* 2001; **24**(6): 391–398.

35 Lawrence CJ, Prinzen FW, de Lange S. The effects of dexmedetomidine on nutrient organ blood flow. *Anesth Analg* 1996; **83**(6): 1160–1165.

36 Ansah OB, Raekallio M, Vainio O. Comparison of three doses of dexmedetomidine with medetomidine in cats following intramuscular administration. *J Vet Pharmacol Ther* 1998; **21**(5): 380–387.

37 Pypendop BH, Verstegen JP. Hemodynamic effects of medetomidine in the dog: a dose titration study. *Vet Surg* 1998; **27**(6): 612–622.

38 Lamont LA, Bulmer BJ, Grimm KA, *et al.* Cardiopulmonary evaluation of the use of medetomidine hydrochloride in cats. *Am J Vet Res* 2001; **62**(11): 1745–1749.

39 Mendes GM, Selmi AL, Barbudo-Selmi GR, *et al.* Clinical use of dexmedetomidine as premedicant in cats undergoing propofol–sevoflurane. *J Feline Med Surg* 2003; **5**(5): 265–270.

40 Murrell JC, Hellebrekers LJ. Medetomidine and dexmedetomidine: a review of the cardiovascular effects and antinociceptive properties in the dog. *Vet Anaesth Analg* 2005; **32**(3): 117–127.

41 Colby ED, Sanford TD. Blood pressure and heart and respiratory rates of cats under ketamine/xylazine, ketamine/acepromazine anesthesia. *Feline Pract* 1981; **11**(5): 19–21.

42 Stepien RL, Bonagura JD, Bednarski RM, Muir WW III. Cardiorespiratory effects of acepromazine maleate and buprenorphine hydrochloride in clinically normal dogs. *Am J Vet Res* 1995; **56**(1): 78–84.

43 Shiga Y, Minami K, Uezono Y, *et al.* Effects of the intravenously administered anaesthetics ketamine, propofol and thiamylal on the cortical renal blood flow in rats. *Pharmacology* 2003; **68**(1): 17–23.

44 Greene SA, Grauer GF. Renal disease. In: Tranquilli WJ, Thurmon JC, Grimm KA, eds. *Lumb and Jones' Veterinary Anesthesia and Analgesia*, 4th edn. Ames, IA: Blackwell Publishing, 2007; 915–920.

45 Hanna RM, Borchard RE, Schmidt SL. Pharmacokinetics of ketamine HCl and metabolite I in the cat: a comparison of i.v., i.m., and rectal administration. *J Vet Pharmacol Ther* 1988; **11**(1): 84–93.

46 Kruse-Elliott KT, Swanson CR, Aucoin DP. Effects of etomidate on adrenocortical function in canine surgical patients. *Am J Vet Res* 1987; **48**(7): 1098–1100.

47 Albert SG, Ariyan S, Rather A. The effect of etomidate on adrenal function in critical illness: a systematic review. *Intensive Care Med* 2011; **37**(6): 901–910.

48 Stoelting RK, Hillier SC. Inhaled anesthetics. *Pharmacology and Physiology in Anesthetic Practice*, 4th edn. Philadelphia: Lippincott Williams & Wilkins, 2006; 69–72.

49 Murphy MR, Hug CC Jr. The anesthetic potency of fentanyl in terms of its reduction of enflurane MAC. *Anesthesiology* 1982; **57**(6): 485–488.

50 Ilkiw JE, Pascoe PJ, Fisher LD. Effect of alfentanil on the minimum alveolar concentration of isoflurane in cats. *Am J Vet Res* 1997; **58**(11): 1267–1273.

51 Murphy EJ. Acute pain management pharmacology for the patient with concurrent renal or hepatic disease. *Anaesth Intensive Care* 2005; **33**(3): 311–322.

52 Cronnelly R, Salvatierra O, Feduska NJ. Renal allograft function following halothane, enflurane, or isoflurane anesthesia. *Anesth Analg* 1984; **63**: 202.

53 Litz RJ, Hübler M, Lorenz W, *et al.* Renal responses to desflurane and isoflurane in patients with renal insufficiency. *Anesthesiology* 2002; **97**(5): 1133–1136.

54 Teixeira S, Costa G, Costa F, *et al.* Sevoflurane versus isoflurane: does it matter in renal transplantation? *Transplant Proc* 2007; **39**(8): 2486–2488.

55 Akpek EA, Kayhan Z, Dönmez A, *et al.* Early postoperative renal function following renal transplantation surgery: effect of anesthetic technique. *J Anesth* 2002; **16**(2): 114–118.

56 Hadimioglu N, Ertug Z, Bigat Z, *et al.* A randomized study comparing combined spinal epidural or general anesthesia for renal transplant surgery. *Transplant Proc* 2005; **37**(5): 2020–2022.

57 Bhosale G, Shah V. Combined spinal–epidural anesthesia for renal transplantation. *Transplant Proc* 2008; **40**(4): 1122–1124.

58 Nicholls AJ, Tucker V, Gibbs P. Awake renal transplantation; a realistic alternative to general anesthesia. *Transplant Proc* 2010; **42**(5): 1677–1678.

59 Marik PE, Baram M, Vahid B. Does central venous pressure predict fluid responsiveness? A systematic review of the literature and the tale of seven mares. *Chest* 2008; **134**(1): 172–178.

60 Grandy JL, Dunlop CI, Hodgeson DS, *et al.* Evaluation of the Doppler ultrasonic method of measuring systolic arterial blood pressure in cats. *Am J Vet Res* 1992; **53**(7): 1166–1169.

61 Binns SH, Sisson DD, Buoscio DA, Schaeffer DJ. Doppler ultrasonographic, oscillometric sphygmomanometric, and photoplethysmographic techniques for noninvasive blood pressure measurement in anesthetized cats. *J Vet Intern Med* 1995; **9**(6): 405–414.

62 Caulkett NA, Cantwell SL, Houston DM. A comparison of indirect blood pressure monitoring techniques in the anesthetized cat. *Vet Surg* 1998; **27**(4): 370–377.

63 Bosiack AP, Mann FA, Dodam JR, *et al.* Comparison of ultrasonic Doppler flow monitor, oscillometric, and direct arterial blood pressure measurements in ill dogs. *J Vet Emerg Crit Care (San Antonio)* 2010; **20**(2): 207–215.

64 Shih A, Robertson S, Vigani A, *et al.* Evaluation of an indirect oscillometric blood pressure monitor in normotensive and hypotensive anesthetized dogs. *J Vet Emerg Crit Care (San Antonio)* 2010; **20**(3): 313–318.

65 O'Malley CM, Frumento RJ, Hardy MA, *et al.* A randomized, double-blind comparison of lactated Ringer's solution and 0.9% NaCl during renal transplantation. *Anesth Analg* 2005; **100**(5): 1518–1524.

66 Hadimioglu N, Saadawy I, Saglam T, *et al.* The effect of different crystalloid solutions on acid–base balance and early kidney function after kidney transplantation. *Anesth Analg* 2008; **107**(1): 264–269.

67 Khajavi MR, Etezadi F, Moharari RS, *et al.* Effects of normal saline vs. lactated Ringer's during renal transplantation. *Ren Fail* 2008; **30**(5): 535–539.

68 Davidson IJ. Renal impact of fluid management with colloids: a comparative review. *Eur J Anaesthesiol* 2006; **23**(9): 721–738.

69 Bellomo R, Wan L, May C. Vasoactive drugs and acute kidney injury. *Crit Care Med* 2008; **36**(4 Suppl): S179–S186.

70 Kim JM, Kim SJ, Joh JW, *et al.* Is it safe to use a kidney from an expanded criteria donor? *Transplant Proc* 2011; **43**(6): 2359–2362.

71 Schnuelle J, Johannes van der Woude F. Perioperative fluid management in renal transplantation: a narrative review of the literature. *Transpl Int* 2006; **19**(12): 947–959.

72 Irish A. Hypercoagulability in renal transplant recipients. Identifying patients at risk of renal allograft thrombosis and evaluating strategies for prevention. *Am J Cardiovasc Drugs* 2004; **4**(3): 139–149.

73 Stoelting RK, Hillier SC. Drugs used for psychopharmacologic therapy. *Pharmacology and Physiology in Anesthetic Practice*, 4th edn. Philadelphia: Lippincott Williams & Wilkins, 2006; 412.

74 KuKanich B, Bidgood T, Knesl O. Clinical pharmacology of nonsteroidal anti-inflammatory drugs in dogs. *Vet Anaesth Analg* 2012; **39**(1): 69–90.

75 Kyles AE, Gregory CR, Wooldridge JD, *et al.* Management of hypertension controls postoperative neurologic disorders after renal transplantation in cats. *Vet Surg* 1999; **28**(6): 436–441.

76 Tutone VK, Mark PB, Stewart GA, *et al.* Hypertension, antihypertensive agents and outcomes following renal transplantation. *Clin Transplant* 2005; **19**(2): 181–192.

77 Ponticelli C, Campise MR. Neurological complications in kidney transplant recipients. *J Nephrol* 2005; **18**(5): 521–528.

78 Kyles AE, Gregory CR, Wooldridge JD, *et al.* Management of hypertension controls postoperative neurologic disorders after renal transplantation in cats. *Vet Surg* 1999; **28**(6): 436–441.

79 Cowgill LD, Francey T. Hemodialysis and extracorporeal blood purification. In: DiBartola SP, ed. *Fluid, Electrolyte, and Acid–Base Disorders in Small Animal Practice*, 4th edn. St Louis, MO: Saunders Elsevier, 2012; 680–709.
80 Bersenas AME. A clinical review of peritoneal dialysis. *J Vet Emerg Crit Care* 2011; **21**(6): 605–617.
81 Cooper RL, Labato MA. Peritoneal dialysis in veterinary medicine. *Vet Clin North Am Small Anim Pract* 2011; **41**(1): 91–113.
82 Blowey DL, Alon US. Dialysis principles for primary health-care providers. *Clin Pediatr* 2005; **44**(1): 19–29.
83 Ross LA, Labato MA. Peritoneal dialysis. In: DiBartola SP, ed. *Fluid, Electrolyte, and Acid–Base Disorders in Small Animal Practice*, 4th edn. St Louis, MO: Saunders Elsevier, 2012; 665–679.
84 Cowgill LD. Application of peritoneal dialysis and hemodialysis in the management of renal failure. In: Osborne CA, ed. *Canine and Feline Nephrology and Urology*. Baltimore, MD: Lee & Febiger, 1995; 573–584.
85 Fox LE, Grauer FG, Dubielzig RR, Bjorling DE. Reversal of ethylene glycol-induced nephrotoxicosis in a dog. *J Am Vet Med Assoc* 1987; **191**(11): 1433–1435.
86 Crisp MS, Chew DJ, DiBartola SP, Birchard SJ. Peritoneal dialysis in dogs and cats: 27 cases (1976–1987). *J Am Vet Med Assoc* 1989; **195**(9): 1262–1266.
87 Beckel NF, O'Toole TE, Rozanski EA, *et al*. Peritoneal dialysis in the management of acute renal failure in 5 dogs with leptospirosis. *J Vet Emerg Crit Care* 2005; **15**(3): 201–205.
88 Dorval P, Boysen SR. Management of acute renal failure in cats using peritoneal dialysis: a retrospective study of six cases (2003–2007). *Feline Med Surg* 2009; **11**(2): 107–115.
89 Gabriel DP, Nascimento GVR, Caramori JT, *et al*. Peritoneal dialysis in acute renal failure. *Renal Failure* 2006; **28**(6): 451–456.
90 Abel J, Rowntree L, Turner B. On the removal of diffusible substances from the circulating blood of living animals by dialysis. *J Pharmacol Exp Ther* 1914; **5**(3): 275–316.
91 Bloom CA, Labato MA. Intermittent hemodialysis for small animals. *Vet Clin North Am Small Anim Pract* 2011; **41**(1): 115–133.
92 Eatroff AE, Langston CE, Chalhoub S, *et al*. Long-term outcome of cats and dogs with acute kidney injury treated with intermittent hemodialysis: 135 cases (1997–2010). *J Am Vet Med Assoc* 2012; **241**(11): 1471–1478.
93 Elliott DA. Hemodialysis. *Clin Tech Small Anim Pract* 2000; **15**(3): 136–148.
94 Langston C. Hemodialysis in dogs and cats. *Compend Contin Educ Pract Vet* 2002; **24**(7): 540–549.
95 Groman R. Apheresis in veterinary medicine: therapy in search of a disease. In: *Proceedings of the Advanced Renal Therapies Symposium*. New York: Animal Medical Center, 2010; 26–32.
96 Cowgill LD, Langston CE. History of hemodialysis in dogs and companion animals. In: Ing TS, Rahman MA, Kjellstrand CM, eds. *Dialysis: History, Development and Promise*. Singapore: World Scientific, 2012; 901–914.
97 Acierno MJ. Continuous renal replacement therapy in dogs and cats. *Vet Clin North Am Small Anim Pract* 2011; **41**(1): 135–146.
98 Monaghan KN, Acierno MJ. Extracorporeal removal of drugs and toxins. *Vet Clin North Am Small Anim Pract* 2011; **41**(1): 227–238.
99 Chalhoub S, Langston CE. Vascular access for extracorporeal renal replacement therapy in veterinary patients. *Vet Clin North Am Small Anim Pract* 2011; **41**(1): 147–161.
100 Poeppel K, Langston CE, Chalhoub S. Equipment commonly used in veterinary renal replacement therapy. *Vet Clin North Am Small Anim Pract* 2011; **41**(1): 177–191.
101 Langston CE, Cowgill LD, Spano JA. Applications and outcomes of hemodialysis in cats: a review of 29 cases. *J Vet Intern Med* 1997; **11**(6): 348–355.
102 Fischer JR, Pantaleo V, Francey T, Cowgill LD. Veterinary hemodialysis: advances in management and technology. *Vet Clin North Am Small Anim Pract* 2004; **34**(4): 935–967.
103 Langston CE, Poeppel K, Mitelberg E. *AMC Dialysis Handbook. New York: Animal Medical Center*, 2010; **3**.
104 Joy MS, Matzke GR, Frye RF, Palevsky PM. Determinants of vancomycin clearance by continuous venovenous hemofiltration and continuous venovenous hemodialysis. *Am J Kidney Dis* 1998; **31**(6): 1019–1027.
105 Bouman CS. Antimicrobial dosing strategies in critically ill patients with acute kidney injury and high-dose continuous veno-venous hemofiltration. *Curr Opin Crit Care* 2008; **14**(6): 654–659.
106 Bugge JF. Pharmacokinetics and drug dosing adjustments during continuous venovenous hemofiltration or hemodiafiltration in critically ill patients. *Acta Anaesthesiol Scand* 2001; **45**(8): 929–934.
107 Churchwell MD, Mueller BA. Drug dosing during continuous renal replacement therapy. *Semin Dial* 2009; **22**(2): 185–188.
108 Choi G, Gomersall CD, Tian Q, *et al*. Principles of antibacterial dosing in continuous renal replacement therapy. *Crit Care Med* 2009; **37**(7): 2268–2282.
109 Bayliss G. Dialysis in the poisoned patient. *Hemodial Int* 2010; **14**(2): 158–167.

34 Anesthetic Considerations During Pregnancy and for the Newborn

Marc R. Raffe

Veterinary Anesthesia and Critical Care Associates LLC, St. Paul, Minnesota, USA

Chapter contents

Introduction

By their very nature, anesthetics, analgesics, tranquilizers, and sedatives cross the blood–brain barrier. The physicochemical properties that allow drugs to cross the blood–brain barrier also facilitate placental transfer. It is not possible to anesthetize the mother selectively because all agents that affect the maternal central nervous system will also affect the fetus, resulting in central nervous system depression and decreased viability at delivery.

The ideal anesthetic protocol for pregnancy or the peri-parturient period provides analgesia, muscle relaxation, and sedation/narcosis without unduly endangering either mother or fetus. Selection of an anesthetic protocol for cesarean section should be based on safety of the mother and fetus, patient comfort, and the veterinarian's familiarity with the anesthetic technique. Factors in decision-making regarding anesthesia protocol include altered physiology of the mother induced by pregnancy and labor, impact of selected drugs on the mother and fetus, carryover effects on the neonate following separation from the mother, and the risk of anesthetic-related complications. Irrespective of the technique used, a major goal of drug selection should be to minimize fetal depression. Fetal depression may be pre-existing due to prolonged labor prior to fetal delivery, and is due in part to decreases in placental perfusion, resulting in fetal hypoxemia, acidosis, and stress. Hence both mother and fetus may be in a physiologically compromised state. The veterinarian is faced with the dilemma of having to anesthetize a physiologically compromised mother without adversely affecting the fetus. A complete understanding of the physiologic changes present and the potential impact of anesthesia drugs in this patient population is essential to navigate both mother and fetus safely through the birthing period.

Pregnancy-associated changes in maternal physiology

Metabolic demands of gestation and parturition are met by altered physiologic function (Table 34.1). Most of the data describing physiologic alterations of pregnancy have been obtained from data collected in humans and ewes. Although little work has been done in other species, the changes should be comparable, if not greater, in magnitude. Birth weight expressed as a percentage of maternal weight for people, sheep, dogs, and cats is 5.7, 11.4, 16.1, and 13.2%, respectively [1]. This suggests that the physiologic burden and therefore physiologic alterations may actually be greater in animals than in women.

Cardiovascular

During pregnancy, maternal blood volume increases by approximately 40%; plasma volume increases more than red cell mass, resulting in decreased hemoglobin concentration and packed cell

Veterinary Anesthesia and Analgesia: The Fifth Edition of Lumb and Jones.
Edited by Kurt A. Grimm, Leigh A. Lamont, William J. Tranquilli, Stephen A. Greene and Sheilah A. Robertson.

Table 34.1 Physiological alterations induced by pregnancy

Variable	
Heart rate	↑
Cardiac output	↑
Blood volume	↑
Plasma volume	↑
Packed cell volume, hemoglobin, and plasma protein	↓
Arterial blood pressure	O
Central venous pressure	O, ↑ during labor
Minute volume of ventilation	↑
Oxygen consumption	↑
pHa and PaO_2	O
$PaCO_2$	↓
Total lung and vital capacity	O
Functional residual capacity	↓
Gastric emptying time and intragastric pressure	↑
Gastric motility and pH of gastric secretions	↓
Gastric chloride ion and enzyme concentration	↑
SGOT, LDH, and BSP retention time	↑
Plasma cholinesterase	↓
Renal plasma flow and glomerular filtration rate	↑
Blood urea nitrogen and creatinine	↓
Sodium ion and water balance	O

volume [2]. Increased heart rate and stroke volume cause cardiac output to increase 30–50% above normal [3,4]. Plasma estrogens decrease peripheral vascular resistance, resulting in an increase in cardiac output while systolic and diastolic blood pressures remain unchanged. During labor and the immediate postpartum period, cardiac output increases an additional 10–25% as a result of blood being extruded from the contracting uterus [5]. Cardiac output during labor is also influenced by body position, pain, and apprehension [2]. During labor, systolic pressure increases by 10–30 mmHg. Although central venous pressure does not change during pregnancy, because of increased venous capacity, it increases slightly (4–6 cmH_2O) during labor and has been reported to increase by up to 50 cmH_2O during painful fetal extraction [6]. The posterior vena cava and aorta can be compressed by the enlarged uterus and its contents during dorsal recumbency. This can cause decreased venous return and cardiac output with reductions in uterine and renal blood flow. Although this does not appear to be as serious a problem in dogs and cats, time spent restrained or positioned in dorsal recumbency should be kept to a minimum [7,8].

Because cardiac work is increased during pregnancy and parturition, cardiac reserve is decreased. Patients with previously well-compensated heart disease may suffer pulmonary congestion and heart failure caused by a gestation-induced increase in cardiac workload and increased hemodynamic demand secondary to parturition-associated pain [9]. In such patients, pain and anxiety control is a key component of successful patient management during the periparturient period. However, care must be taken to avoid additional cardiac depression and decompensation induced by excessive doses of sedatives or anesthetics. The use of ecbolic agents during or after parturition can adversely affect cardiovascular function. Oxytocin in large or repeated doses induces peripheral vasodilation and hypotension, which can adversely affect both mother and fetus through decreased tissue perfusion. Ergot derivatives used to control uterine bleeding can induce vasoconstriction and hypertension [10].

Pulmonary

During pregnancy, increased serum progesterone concentration increases respiratory center carbon dioxide ($PaCO_2$) sensitivity. As a result of increased ventilatory minute volume, $PaCO_2$ progressively decreases during gestation and approaches 30 mmHg at parturition. Because long-term renal compensation for respiratory alkalosis occurs, arterial pH remains within normal values. Hyperventilation may further be stimulated during labor by pain, apprehension, and anxiety. Oxygen consumption increases by 20% owing to the developing fetus, placenta, uterine muscle, and mammary tissue. Arterial oxygen tension remains unchanged [2].

Pregnancy also affects the mechanics of ventilation. Airway conductance is increased and total pulmonary resistance is decreased by progesterone-induced relaxation of bronchial smooth muscle. Lung compliance is unaffected. Functional residual capacity (FRC) is decreased by craniodorsal displacement of the diaphragm and abdominal organs by the gravid uterus. In addition, during labor FRC decreases further because of increased pulmonary blood volume subsequent to intermittent uterine contraction. Because of the decrease in FRC, small airway closure develops at end exhalation in approximately one-third of human parturients during tidal ventilation [2]. Total lung capacity and vital capacity are unaltered. Because FRC is decreased, hypoventilation induces hypoxemia and hypercapnia more readily in pregnant than non-pregnant patients. Hypoxemia is exacerbated by increased oxygen consumption during labor. Oxygen administration prior to anesthetic induction increases oxygen reserve by facilitating pulmonary denitrogenation. Preoxygenation is advisable if the patient is tolerant.

Induction of anesthesia with inhalation agents is more rapid in pregnant than non-pregnant patients. The equilibration rate between inspired and alveolar anesthetic partial pressure is accelerated by increased alveolar ventilation and decreased FRC. Additionally, increased progesterone and endorphin levels in the central nervous system decrease anesthetic requirements.

Gastrointestinal

A number of functional changes in gastrointestinal tract physiology occur with gestation and parturition. Physical displacement of the stomach by the gravid uterus, decreased gastric motility, and increased serum progesterone all contribute to delayed gastric emptying and are especially manifest during the last trimester. Acid, chloride, and enzyme concentrations in gastric secretions are increased due to altered hormone physiology during gestation. Lower esophageal sphincter tone is decreased, and intragastric pressure is increased. Pain and anxiety during labor have been shown to decrease gastric motility further [2].

As a result of altered gastric function, the risk of regurgitation (both active and passive) and aspiration is increased in parturients. Because increased gastric acidity and decreased gastric muscular tone may be present, metoclopramide and an H_2 receptor antagonist drug (cimetidine, ranitidine, or famotidine) may be administered as part of the preanesthetic protocol [11]. Frequently, patients presented for cesarean section have been fed or the time of the last feeding is unknown. Parturients should be regarded as having a full stomach, and anesthesia techniques should be selected that produce rapid airway management and control to prevent aspiration of foreign material. Risk of vomiting is increased by hypotension, hypoxia, and toxic reactions to local anesthetics. Because of these concerns, periparturient patients should be considered high risk and prophylactic measures are recommended. In companion animals, prophylactic administration of antiemetics such as maropitant and ondansetron are routinely considered. Smooth induction of general anesthesia and prevention of hypotension during epidural anesthesia will decrease the incidence of vomiting. Because silent regurgitation can occur when the intragastric pressure is high, a cuffed endotracheal tube is preferred for airway management during general anesthesia. Passive regurgitation can be induced by positive-pressure ventilation with a face mask or by manipulation of abdominal viscera. Atropine administration may increase gastroesophageal sphincter tone, thereby helping to prevent regurgitation, but may also inhibit the actions of metoclopramide that increase gastric motility and emptying by sensitizing gastric smooth muscle to acetylcholine [6,11].

Liver and kidney

Pregnancy induces minor alterations in hepatic function. The plasma protein concentration decreases slightly, but total plasma protein is increased because of the increase in blood volume. Bilirubin concentration is unaltered. Serum enzyme concentrations [serum alanine aminotransferase (SALT) and alkaline phosphatase] can be slightly increased, and sulfobromophthalein sodium retention is increased. The plasma cholinesterase concentration decreases, which may lead to prolonged action of succinylcholine in pregnant patients, particularly if they have been exposed recently to organophosphate parasiticides (e.g., anthelmintics, flea collars, or dips). Despite these alterations, overall liver function is generally well maintained [2].

Renal plasma flow and glomerular filtration rate are increased by approximately 60% in pregnant patients, so blood urea nitrogen and creatinine concentrations are lower than in non-pregnant patients [6]. Sodium and water balance are unaffected. Elevated blood urea nitrogen or creatinine levels may indicate renal pathology or compromise in parturient patients. In these patients, drugs with known nephrotoxic potential, such as methoxyflurane, aminoglycoside antibiotics, and non-steroidal anti-inflammatory drugs (NSAIDs), should be avoided.

Uterine blood flow

Stable uteroplacental circulation is important to fetal and maternal homeostasis and neonatal survival. Uterine blood flow is directly proportional to systemic perfusion pressure and inversely proportional to vascular resistance created in myometrial blood vessels. Placental perfusion is mainly dependent on uteroplacental perfusion pressure; however, placental vessels have rudimentary mechanisms for changing vascular resistance. Anesthesia may decrease uterine blood flow and thereby contribute to reduced fetal viability. In addition, uterine vascular resistance is indirectly increased by uterine contractions and hypertonia (oxytocic response). Placental hypotension is induced by hypovolemia, anesthetic-induced cardiovascular depression, or sympathetic blockade producing reduced uterine perfusion pressure. Uterine vasoconstriction is induced by endogenous sympathetic discharge or by exogenous sympathomimetic drugs having α_1-adrenergic effects (e.g., epinephrine, norepinephrine, methoxamine, phenylephrine, and metaraminol) [2,12,13]. Hypotension induced by adjunctive drugs combined with increased uterine tone induced by ecbolics should be avoided.

Summary

Parturients are at greater anesthetic risk than are healthy non-parturient patients because of pregnancy-associated physiologic alterations. Cardiac reserve diminishes during pregnancy, and high-risk patients can suffer acute cardiac decompensation or failure. Pregnant patients are prone to hypoventilation, hypoxia, and hypercapnia because of altered pulmonary function. Inhalation and local anesthetic requirement is decreased, thus increasing the likelihood of a relative overdose and excessive depression. Finally, emesis or regurgitation and aspiration can occur if induction is not immediately followed by rapid airway control.

Pharmacologic alterations induced by pregnancy

Pregnancy affects the uptake, distribution, and disposition of anesthetic agents and adjuncts. The concentration of free (non-ionized, unbound) drug in maternal plasma is affected by changes in protein binding, placental transfer, distribution in fetal tissues, and biotransformation by maternal and fetal liver. The effect of pregnancy on anesthetic agents has been studied. The rate of barbiturate biotransformation appears to be decreased in pregnancy [14]. Succinylcholine and procaine metabolism are decreased because of decreased plasma cholinesterase concentration [14]. Increased renal blood flow and glomerular filtration associated with pregnancy favor renal drug excretion. The inhalation anesthetic dose (MAC) is reduced for all agents. Minimum alveolar concentration values are reduced in pregnant compared with non-pregnant ewes. Thus, anesthetic induction may be extremely rapid, requiring as little as one-fourth to one-fifth of the time required for non-pregnant patients [15]. Care must be taken to prevent volatile-agent overdose in pregnant patients.

The placenta is highly permeable to anesthetic drugs, and anesthetic drugs administered to the mother usually induce fetal effects proportionate to those observed in the mother. Placental transfer of drugs can occur by several mechanisms, by far the most important being simple diffusion. Diffusion across the placenta is determined by molecular weight, the degree to which the drug is bound to maternal plasma proteins, lipid solubility, and degree of ionization. Drugs with low molecular weight (MW <500 Da), a low degree of protein binding, and high lipid solubility and that are mostly non-ionized at maternal blood pH diffuse rapidly across the placenta. Conversely, drugs that are larger (MW >1000 Da), are highly protein bound, have low lipid solubility, and are mostly non-ionized generally cross the placenta slowly. Most anesthetics and anesthetic adjuncts diffuse quickly across the placental barrier. The muscle-relaxant drugs are an exception because they are highly ionized and of low lipid solubility. Although they can be recovered from fetal blood, they are generally regarded as having minimal placental transfer and negligible fetal effect [14,16]. The placenta does not appear to metabolize anesthetics or anesthetic adjuncts.

Physiochemical properties and physiologic/pharmacokinetic events that occur within the fetus and mother also affect placental drug transfer [14]. The degree to which a drug is ionized is determined by its pK_a and the pH of the patient's body fluids. Drugs that are weak acids will be less ionized as pH decreases [16]. For example, thiopental is a weak acid with a pK_a of 7.6. In acidemic patients (pH <7.4), a greater proportion of the administered dose is in the non-ionized form. As the proportion of the non-ionized form of the drug increases, the drug fraction that is protein bound is reduced, thus effectively increasing the clinical response on a milligram basis. As a result, it is well recognized that acidemia decreases the required anesthetic dose of thiopental and other barbiturates. Weakly basic drugs such as opioids and local anesthetics are more highly ionized at pH values less than their pK_a [17]. Hence their effect on the mother and fetus is less on a milligram dose basis.

The distribution of a drug between mother and fetus is also influenced by the blood pH. Normally, the fetal pH is 0.1 unit less than that of the mother. hence weakly basic drugs with pK_a values near

7.4 (e.g., many opiates and local anesthetics) are found in higher concentration in fetal tissues and plasma than in those of the mother because of 'ion trapping.' Lower fetal pH increases ionized drug concentration, thereby reducing the maternal–fetal concentration gradient and non-ionized drug transfer across the placenta to the fetus [18].

Fetal drug concentration is also affected by redistribution, metabolism, and protein binding. The drug concentration in the umbilical vein is greater than in fetal organs (brain, heart, and other vital organs). As much as 85% of umbilical venous blood initially passes through the fetal liver, where drug may be sequestered or metabolized. In addition, umbilical venous blood containing drug enters the inferior vena cava via the ductus venosus and mixes with drug-free blood returning from the lower extremities and pelvic viscera (Fig. 34.1). Therefore, the fetal circulation buffers vital fetal tissues from sudden changes in drug concentration. Drug binding to fetal proteins may also reduce free-drug availability [14,16].

Drug concentration and effects in the fetus can be considerably higher and have longer presence than in the mother because fetal drug metabolism is not rapid as the mother's. The fetal microsomal enzyme system is not as active, which suggests a longer drug half-life. This is complicated by the fact that drugs will also redistribute out of the fetus into the mother as her plasma levels decrease, making clinical estimation of fetal plasma concentrations difficult. Fetal drug toxicity can be enhanced by fetal or maternal metabolism to more toxic metabolites and by drug–metabolite and drug–drug interactions [18].

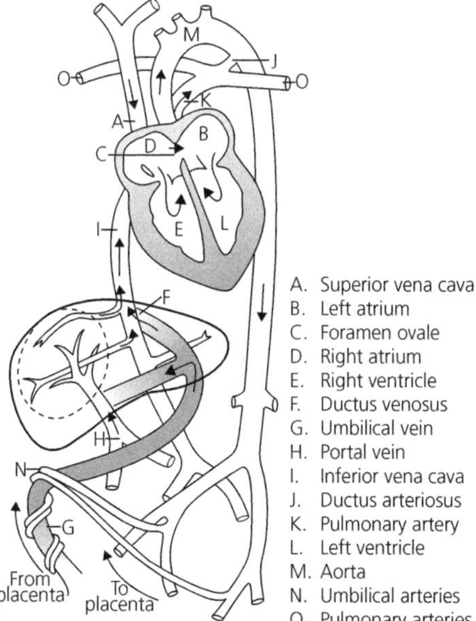

Figure 34.1 The direction of blood flow in the fetal vascular system is indicated by arrows. The darkened vascular segments represent the umbilical blood and its path of flow into the liver and inferior vena cava via the ductus venosus. Blood flow through the foramen ovale and ductus arteriosus provides a direct path to the arterial system, bypassing the lungs. In neonates, the ductus arteriosus and foramen ovale close shortly after birth. This functional closure results in blood flowing through the neonate's lungs, where it is arterialized as in the adult. The time required for anatomic closure of the foramen ovale in the foal may be as long as 12 months. Two months maybe required for permanent closure of the foramen ovale.

The administration of a fixed dose of drugs with rapidly decreasing plasma concentration (e.g., thiopental, propofol, or succinylcholine) briefly exposes the fetus and placenta to a high maternal blood drug concentration. This is in contrast to the sustained maternal blood levels of drugs administered by continuous infusion or inhalation, which result in continuous placental transfer of drug to the fetus [14,18].

Anesthesia during pregnancy

Maternal exposure to general anesthesia has potential consequences for the unborn fetus. The reported fetal risks that occur change during the gestation period and are categorized by gestational trimester. General anesthesia during the first trimester of pregnancy is associated with fetal teratogenesis, spontaneous abortion, and fetal death. Anesthesia exposure during the middle trimester is generally considered the safest period of gestation; however, spontaneous abortion and fetal death have been reported following general anesthesia during this period. Anesthesia exposure during the final trimester carries a risk of premature labor and fetal death. Most of the reported consequences are in the human literature since the veterinary medical literature is incomplete. There appears to be interspecies variability with respect to anesthesia-associated risk. This may be due to species specificity in uteroplacental perfusion, placentation anatomy, and maternal homeostasis. There does not appear to be a specific drug-linked risk associated with increased fetal morbidity/mortality. Care must be taken to assure that maternal physiology is maintained during the anesthesia episode. Maintaining maternal cardiorespiratory physiology, oxygen delivery, and acid–base balance assures uteroplacental perfusion and oxygen delivery, which are of paramount importance for postanesthetic fetal viability. In the human literature, it is recommended that NSAIDs be avoided after the first trimester in order to avoid premature closure of the ductus arteriosus [19].

Anesthetic drugs and cesarean section

Anesthetic drugs should be carefully chosen and properly administered in order to avoid excessive maternal depression and to maximize neonatal vigor and viability. As noted above, the specific characteristics that make a drug an excellent anesthetic agent are also those that facilitate rapid transplacental transfer and neonatal depression. Therefore, it is prudent to consider that no agent should be used unless distinctly indicated. A brief overview of anesthetic drug classes in periparturient anesthesia follows.

Anticholinergic agents

Anticholinergic drugs, such as atropine and glycopyrrolate, are historically used to decrease salivation and inhibit excessive vagal efferent activity that may occur when traction is applied to the uterus [20]. Their risk-reducing value varies with species; they are more effective in dogs and cats, with less impact in other species. Many parturients have eaten before delivery. The presence of gastric contents increases the likelihood of regurgitation, which is enhanced by hypoxia or hypotension. The influence of anticholinergics upon emesis is variable [6,20]. In women, atropine has not been shown to decrease the incidence of emesis at parturition [20]. Glycopyrrolate increases gastric pH, thus decreasing the severity of Mendelson's syndrome (i.e., chemical pneumonitis caused by aspiration of gastric contents during anesthesia, especially at parturition) should regurgitation and aspiration of vomitus occur [21]. Additionally, because glycopyrrolate does not readily cross the placenta, it does not affect the fetus to the same extent as atropine. Therefore, it may be a more appropriate anticholinergic for use in these patients.

Tranquilizers and sedatives

Because of their long duration of action, there are no indications for the routine use of these agents in parturient patients [6,17,18]. They should be restricted to markedly apprehensive or excited parturients and only in doses sufficient to induce a calming effect. Acepromazine can induce significant maternal and fetal depression even at relatively low doses. Diazepam and midazolam can induce neonatal depression characterized by the absence of vocalization and by lethargy, hypotonus, apnea, and hypothermia immediately following birth [22–24]. It has been suggested that these effects are dose related and can be minimized by administering low doses (<0.14 mg/kg IV), although no safe dose has been established in domestic animals [24]. Residual benzodiazepine-induced lethargy and muscle relaxation in either the mother or neonate can be antagonized with flumazenil, a specific benzodiazepine antagonist administered to effect [25].

α_2-Adrenergic agonists have significant effects on both maternal and fetal homeostasis. Xylazine rapidly crosses the placenta and induces both maternal and fetal respiratory and circulatory depression. Detomidine appears to be well tolerated when administered to pregnant mares at 20–60 μg/kg. Two studies demonstrated no increase in drug-related change in uterine activity or increased incidence of spontaneous abortion following repeated dosing [26,27]. Similar results have been reported in cattle [28]. Limited information is available regarding the effect of medetomidine on pregnancy. In dogs, there appears to be a dose-related effect on uterine muscle activity that was documented during the parturient and immediate postparturient period [29]. There are no reports characterizing the effect of dexmedetomidine on pregnancy or parturition in domestic species. There are case reports of its use in humans with good success [30]. Romifidine induces a transient increase in intrauterine pressure following administration [31].

When used with ketamine, xylazine produces significant and potentially life-threatening cardiopulmonary changes, resulting in decreased tissue perfusion in healthy dogs [32]. The use of xylazine or xylazine–ketamine combinations should be avoided in small animal patients presented for cesarean section. However, combined xylazine–ketamine has often been used in dystocia mares. Little information is available regarding the use of detomidine or medetomidine in companion animal cesarean section anesthesia. Their structural and pharmacologic similarities to xylazine suggest that similar precautions should be observed with their use.

Opioids

Opioids rapidly cross the placenta and can cause neonatal respiratory and neurobehavioral depression [18,33,34]. In addition, fetal elimination may require 2–6 days. It appears that equianalgesic doses of opioids induce an equal degree of CNS depression. Therefore, choice is based on the desired duration of opioid action. Commonly used μ-opioid receptor agonists include morphine, fentanyl, meperidine, oxymorphone, hydromorphone, and methadone [18]. Agents having opiate agonist–antagonist or partial agonist activity include butorphanol and buprenorphine. They reportedly induce less respiratory depression than do pure opiate agonists. Butorphanol provides mild to moderate levels of sedation in addition to its analgesic qualities. Buprenorphine produces mild sedation plus good to excellent analgesia.

One of the advantages of opioid agonists is that direct antagonists are available to reverse their action. Of the antagonist agents, naloxone (0.04 mg/kg IV) appears to be the most effective. It is a pure antagonist without agonist action. Nalorphine and levallorphan, two other antagonist agents, have opiate activity of their own and can increase respiratory depression induced by other non-opiate agents (e.g., barbiturates, phenothiazines, and inhalation agents). Because all opioid antagonists rapidly cross the placenta, maternal administration before delivery has been advocated to reverse opioid-induced neonatal depression. This technique deprives the mother of analgesia at the time when it is needed most. Therefore, these agents should be administered directly to neonates. Finally, because the action of naloxone is shorter than that of most opioid agonists, renarcotization may occur as naloxone is metabolized and excreted. Therefore, both mother and neonates should be carefully monitored for recurring signs of narcosis after opioid reversal with naloxone [18]. Should this occur, additional naloxone can be given.

Sedative-hypnotics

Thiopental has been used to produce rapid induction of basal narcosis for intubation and inhalation anesthesia. The pharmacologic effects of thiopental on cardiovascular and respiratory function include increased heart rate, decreased arterial pressure, and changes in peripheral vascular resistance. Apnea is common on induction. Recovery from thiopental is generally rapid because of redistribution and metabolism. Although thiopental rapidly crosses the placenta, it is also rapidly cleared from the neonatal circulation. Fetal metabolism may contribute to its rapid clearance *in utero*. Barbiturates can cause neonatal respiratory depression, sleepiness, and decreased activity. Suckling activity is decreased and has been reported to be depressed for 4 days in neonates [18]. These effects are reduced when thiopental is administered in lower doses (<4 mg/kg) [18].

The administration of propofol intravenously produces rapid induction of basal narcosis for intubation and inhalation anesthesia. The pharmacologic effects of propofol on cardiovascular and respiratory function are nearly identical with, but slightly greater than, those of thiopental. Recovery from propofol is prompt and smooth owing to rapid redistribution and metabolism. Metabolism occurs primarily in the liver, but extrahepatic metabolism also occurs. Although propofol rapidly crosses the placenta, it is rapidly cleared from the neonatal circulation.

Several studies have compared the use of propofol in companion animal cesarean section anesthesia with more traditional general anesthesia techniques. In dogs, propofol followed by isoflurane anesthesia resulted in newborn survival rates comparable to those with epidural anesthesia and superior to those with general anesthesia induced with thiopental [35]. Cohort retrospective studies by Moon and co-workers [23,24] indicated that administration of propofol intravenously followed by isoflurane increased puppy vigor, vocalization, and survival following surgery. Their findings were similar to those in a previously reported study [35]. Constant-rate infusion of propofol as a sole anesthetic agent in pregnant ewes demonstrated maternal hemodynamics superior to those of isoflurane anesthesia [35]. The uterine blood-flow profile was similar in both techniques. Propofol–sevoflurane anesthesia in pregnant ewes and goats demonstrated that fetal physiology was maintained following propofol administration, but hemodynamic indices decreased after exposure to sevoflurane [36,37]. These studies support the use of propofol in a balanced general anesthesia protocol for cesarean section. In dogs and cats, the induction dose of propofol is 4–8 mg/kg IV. Supplemental doses are 0.5–2.0 mg/kg IV.

Longer term constant-rate infusions of propofol to maintain anesthesia may result in some fetal depression, however. The induction dose in sheep and goats is 3–5 mg/kg IV.

Etomidate is a short-acting non-barbiturate hypnotic. In dosages suitable for anesthetic induction, etomidate induces rapid anesthesia with minimal cardiovascular effects in dogs [38,39]. Etomidate is rapidly redistributed and metabolized by hepatic microsomal enzymes and by plasma esterases. Fetal tissue perfusion is well maintained, as shown by more rapid initiation of neonatal spontaneous breathing and greater fetal vitality at delivery than with thiopental [35]. The induction dose of etomidate in non-premedicated dogs and cats is 1.0–3.0 mg/kg IV [39]. Based on its rapid elimination profile in cats, etomidate may be suitable for repeated intravenous administration in low doses in this species [38]. However, repeated administration of etomidate may also cause acute hemolysis, as has been reported in dogs [40]. Etomidate frequently causes pain on intravenous injection in non-premedicated patients. In addition, myoclonus or involuntary movements can occur upon injection, but can be prevented by premedication with benzodiazepines and/or opioids, both of which may exacerbate neonate depression.

Saffan® is a combination of two progesterone-like steroids (alfaxalone, 9 mg/mL, and alfadolone, 3 mg/mL). This agent can be administered intravenously or intramuscularly to cats. Anesthetic induction is smooth and rapid. Cardiovascular depression is proportionate to dose and similar to that of equivalent doses of thiopental or methohexital. Saffan induces less respiratory depression than barbiturates and is compatible with the commonly used preanesthetics, muscle relaxants, and inhalation anesthetics [41,42]. It has been shown to cross the placenta. Its use in dogs is not recommended because the solubilizing agent (cremaphore) causes severe histamine release. However, it has been used to induce anesthesia in dogs pretreated with antihistamines [39]. Alfaxan-CD has been applied in many countries as a short-acting anesthetic for use in dogs and cats. In this formulation, alfaxalone is solubilized in a cyclodextran carrier devoid of histamine-releasing properties. It has proved to be an effective short-acting anesthetic with minimal cardiopulmonary depression and few adverse effects. Because of these properties, its use for anesthesia in cesarean section surgery is acceptable.

Dissociatives

Ketamine has been used in general anesthesia for cesarean section. In women, doses of less than 1 mg/kg induced minimal neonatal depression [20,25]. Alternatively, thiopental (2–3 mg/kg) and ketamine (0.5 mg/kg) have been co-administered to induce anesthesia in parturient women. Low doses of ketamine (3–5 mg/kg IV in dogs, 2–4 mg/kg IV in cats, and 2 mg/kg IV in horses) may be used for anesthetic induction [43]. Because effective induction doses for these agents are higher in companion animals than humans, neonatal depression is more likely to be associated with their use. A retrospective cohort study in dogs indicated that ketamine use leads to increased puppy risk associated with respiratory depression, apnea, decreased vocalization, and increased mortality at birth [23,24]. For these reasons, ketamine should be used cautiously in this species. No data for comparative fetal viability are available in other species.

Little information is available regarding the use of tiletamine–zolazepam in cesarean section. Based on pharmacologic profile, the characteristics of this proprietary drug mixture are qualitatively similar to those of other dissociative–benzodiazepine tranquilizer mixtures. *In vivo* characteristics of these agents suggest that caution should be exercised in companion animal cesarean section anesthesia because of their rapid and extensive transplacental transfer and absence of specific antagonist agents.

Neuroleptanalgesia

The combination of opioid and tranquilizer class drugs can induce anesthesia effectively in depressed, exhausted parturients. As noted above, both opioids and tranquilizers extensively cross the utero-placental interface and may cause significant fetal depression. These agents are usually used as an anesthetic supplement following fetal removal, although they have been successfully used for induction and maintenance prior to fetal extraction. If fetal depression is noted after administration of these agents, sublingual or intranasal administration of naloxone (1–2 drops) rapidly reverses opioid effects in neonates. Continuous monitoring for neonatal renarcotization is warranted [43].

Inhalation agents

Inhalation anesthetics may be used to induce anesthesia in calm or depressed mothers. These agents readily cross the placenta with rapid fetal and maternal equilibration. The degree of neonatal depression is proportional to the depth of anesthesia induced in the mother. Deep levels of maternal anesthesia cause maternal hypotension, decreased uterine blood flow, and fetal acidosis. Isoflurane, sevoflurane, and desflurane are preferred because induction and recovery of mother and neonate are more rapid. Nitrous oxide can be used to potentiate their effect, thus decreasing the total amount of volatile agent administered. If nitrous oxide is administered at 60% or less, fetal depression is minimal and neonatal diffusion hypoxia does not occur upon delivery [18–20].

Skeletal muscle relaxants

Skeletal muscle relaxants cross the placenta to a very limited extent and have little effect on neonates when used in clinical doses. Because of this property, these drugs are very useful in balanced anesthesia techniques for cesarean section to facilitate rapid airway management and provide surgical site relaxation [16,19,20]. Because of its rapid onset of action and relatively brief duration, succinylcholine is a traditional choice when combined with an ultrashort-acting barbiturate or propofol for induction of anesthesia and airway control. Mivacurium has been used because of its rapid onset of effect and relatively brief duration of action (15–20 min). Atracurium and vecuronium provide an intermediate duration of action (20–35 min). Their characteristics make them attractive alternatives in longer procedures. The use of long-acting muscle relaxants, such as pancuronium (45 min) and doxacurium (1–3 h), is to be avoided because of their length of action compared with procedure time [18]. Any time skeletal muscle relaxants are administered, controlled positive-pressure ventilation must be utilized and reversal of non-depolarizing neuromuscular junction-blocking drugs with neostigmine or edrophonium can be performed when surgery times are short or respiratory depression is prolonged.

Guaifenesin has been used to relax skeletal muscle in horses, cattle, and small ruminants. Although reports are limited, clinical impressions indicate that transplacental transfer is minimal based on vigor of the newborn after delivery.

Local anesthetics

Local anesthetics are frequently used in combination with other agents or as the sole anesthetic agent for regional techniques. Esters of *p*-aminobenzoic acid (procaine or tetracaine) are metabolized by maternal and fetal pseudocholinesterase. Hence there is little accumulation of these agents in the fetus. Amide derivatives (e.g., lidocaine, mepivacaine, bupivacaine, etidocaine, and ropivacaine) are metabolized by hepatic microsomal enzymes. After absorption from the injection site, blood levels decrease slowly but can reach significant concentrations in the fetus. Neonatal blood concentrations in excess of 3 μg/mL of lidocaine or mepivacaine can cause neonatal depression at delivery. These concentrations rarely occur after epidural administration but can occur with excessive volumes of drug used for local infiltration [18].

Sympathetic blockade resulting in maternal hypotension and decreased uteroplacental perfusion may occur after epidural injection. This can be controlled by judicious administration of IV fluids to offset the increased capacity of the vascular system [18]. In addition to IV fluids, vasopressors can be used to treat maternal hypotension caused by sympathetic blockade. Because ephedrine acts centrally and has minimal arterial vasoconstrictor properties while increasing venous tone and thereby preload, it can be used to treat maternal hypotension, thus restoring uterine blood flow. Mephentermine acts in a similar manner. Other agents with α_1-adrenergic receptor activity increase maternal blood pressure by increasing systemic vascular resistance. This may cause the uterine blood flow to decrease, and fetal deterioration often occurs. In addition, these agents can stimulate hypertonic uterine contractions, further decreasing uteroplacental perfusion [18,20].

Supplemental agents

Concerns regarding emesis or passive regurgitation immediately following anesthesia induction have been reported in the human obstetric literature. This concern arises from recent food ingestion coupled with delayed gastrointestinal transit time noted with pregnancy. To reduce patient risk of regurgitation/aspiration, several drug classes have been recommended. The recommended drugs are targeted to modify one or more of the following: gastroesophageal sphincter tone, gastric pH, downstream movement of gastrointestinal contents, or vomiting reflex. Currently, human recommendations include administration of an H_2-receptor antagonist, non-particulate antacid, and a prokinetic prior to anesthesia induction of parturient patients. Recent reports suggest that maropitant, a central-acting antiemetic, is highly effective in reducing emesis in the perioperative period. Its application in veterinary obstetric anesthesia is still not defined [44].

Anesthetic techniques for cesarean section

General anesthesia

Cesarean section anesthesia can be accomplished by either regional or general anesthesia. General anesthesia is often selected for performing caesarian sections in dogs, cats, and horses. Advantages of general anesthesia include speed and ease of induction, reliability, reproducibility, and control. General anesthesia provides optimum operating conditions with relaxed immobile patients. Tracheal intubation ensures control of the maternal airway, thereby preventing aspiration of vomitus or regurgitated gastrointestinal tract contents. In addition, it provides a route for maternal oxygen administration, thereby improving fetal oxygenation. When general anesthesia is administered and monitored properly, maternal cardiopulmonary function is well maintained [20,43].

General anesthesia may be more appropriate than regional anesthesia in selected clinical situations. These include severe maternal hypovolemia, prolonged dystocia in which the mother is exhausted and the fetus is severely stressed, maternal cardiac disease or failure, morbid obesity, cases in which the mother is so aggressive or fractious as to preclude regional anesthesia, and brachycephalic dogs with upper airway obstruction. Additionally, if the safety or value of the mother is more important than that of the offspring to the client, general anesthesia will likely allow more intensive anesthetic management of maternal problems. Finally, most veterinarians are more confident of their ability to induce general anesthesia safely than to use regional anesthesia techniques.

General anesthesia does have certain disadvantages. It will likely produce greater neonatal depression than will regional anesthesia. Inadequate anesthetic plane causes maternal catecholamine release, which may result in hypertension and decreased uteroplacental perfusion, leading to both maternal and fetal stress and deterioration of cardiopulmonary function [13,14,27]. Loss of airway protective reflexes following anesthetic induction may produce aspiration and airway management challenges when the trachea is not properly intubated. Aspiration and inability to intubate the trachea successfully are the leading causes of maternal mortality associated with cesarean section in women [20,44]. Fortunately, dogs, cats, and horses are relatively easy to intubate because of their anatomic features. However, ruminants and swine are relatively difficult to intubate, and this presents problems for most veterinarians.

Horses

Dystocia in mares has a profound effect on the survival of foals [45,46]. Foals are normally delivered within 20–30 min after chorioallantoic membrane rupture. Few foals survive when the duration is increased to 40 min, and none are likely to survive when the duration is 90 min or longer [47,48]. The time from chorioallantoic rupture to delivery is significantly different in surviving (71.7 ± 34.3 min) versus non-surviving (85.3 ± 37.4 min) foals [45]. This makes dystocia in mares more of an emergency than it is for most species [45,49].

Physical examination, anesthetic induction, and delivery should be accomplished in the shortest period possible when there is the chance of delivering a live foal [45]. Time-consuming techniques for anesthetic induction should be abandoned in favor of methods that provide reliable sedation and smooth, controlled induction with favorable recoveries. Recommendations for anesthesia of term mares has been extrapolated from work done in other species and may not be relevant. Goals for delivering anesthesia are no different than for other species, but with a greater emphasis placed on rapid completion of the procedure. Laboring mares are typically agitated and distressed prior to anesthetic induction, and good sedation is therefore important to ensure a smooth and safe induction. Xylazine and detomidine will provide sufficient sedation and can be reversed in neonates after delivery. Detomidine may cause less increase in uterine tone than xylazine and has been suggested by some as the sedative of choice in mares [42]. When butorphanol is combined with xylazine or detomidine, reliable restraint and analgesia occur. The dose of xylazine or detomidine can be lowered when combined with butorphanol, minimizing potential side-effects of the α_2-adrenergic agonists.

Anesthesia induction can be rapidly achieved with xylazine (0.8 mg/kg IV) followed by induction with ketamine (2.2 mg/kg IV) and diazepam (0.08 mg/kg IV) (Table 34.2). Anesthesia is then maintained with isoflurane or sevoflurane in 100% oxygen [45]. While vaginal delivery is attempted, the ventral abdomen is clipped and prepped so that, if needed, cesarean section may be accomplished rapidly. In one report, this approach to dystocia resulted in 94% of vaginal delivery mares and 89% of cesarean section mares surviving

Table 34.2 Seelcted anesthesia techniques for elective and emergency cesarean section anesthesia in common domestic species.

Species	Drug or Technique		
	Elective Cesarean Section	**Emergency Cesarean Section**	**Comments**
Dog	1. Lumbosacral epidural 2. Anticholinergic Propofol, 4–8 mg/kg Isoflurane or sevoflurane Post-removal pain meds 3. Anticholinergic Fentanyl, 3 μg/kg Propofol, 4–8 mg/kg Isoflurane or sevoflurane	1. Lumbosacral epidural 2. Sevoflurane or isoflurane mask Induction 3. Anticholinergic Fentanyl, 3 μg/kg Propofol, 4–8 mg/kg Isoflurane or sevoflurane 4. Anticholinergic Fentanyl, 3 μg/kg Propofol, 4–8 mg/kg Line block Atracurium, 0.2 mg/kg	1. May require assistant to restrain epidural patients 2. Give oxygen to all patients as soon as possible 3. Monitor heart rate and redo anticholinergic if needed 4. Minimal Inhalant agent dose until all fetuses are removed 5. May need to reverse fentanyl with sublingual naloxone If fetus is depressed
Cat	1. Propofol, 4–8 mg/kg Laryngeal anesthesia Sevoflurane or isoflurane Additional analgesia following fetal removal 2. Fentanyl, 3–5 μg/kg Propofol, 4 mg/kg Laryngeal anesthesia Sevoflurane or isoflurane Additional analgesia following fetal removal	1. Ketamine, 3 mg/kg Fentanyl, 3–5 μg/kg Lumbosacral epidural 2. Ketamine, 3 mg/kg Fentanyl, 3–5 μg/kg Propofol, 2–4 mg/kg Sevoflurane or Isoflurane Additional analgesia following fetal removal	1. May require assistant to restrain epidural patients 2. Give oxygen to all patients as soon as possible 3. Minimal Inhalant agent dose until all fetuses are removed 4. May need to reverse fentanyl with sublingual naloxone if fetus is depressed
Horse	1. GGE to effect Ketamine, 2 mg/kg Isoflurane or sevoflurane Caudal epidural for pain management 2. GGE to effect Thiopental, 4–6 mg/kg Isoflurane or sevoflurane Caudal epidural for pain management 3. Xylazine, 0.8 mg/kg, IV premed followed by induction with Ketamine, 2.2 mg/kg Diazepam, 0.08 mg/kg	1. GGE to effect Ketamine, 2 mg/kg Isoflurane or sevoflurane Caudal epidural for pain management 2. Xylazine, 0.8 mg/kg, IV premed followed by induction with Ketamine, 2.2 mg/kg Diazepam, 0.08 mg/kg	1. Standing restraint not performed in horses for cesarean section anesthesia 2. Postoperative pain management similar to that for colic patients
Cattle	1. Xylazine, 10 mg Paravertebral block 2. Xylazine, 10 mg Inverted 'L' block 3. Incisional line block 4. Xylazine, 10 mg GGE to recumbency Isoflurane or sevoflurane following intubation	1. Xylazine, 10 mg Paravertebral block 2. Xylazine, 10 mg Inverted 'L' block 3. Incisional line block 4. Xylazine, 10 mg GGE to recumbency Isoflurane/sevoflurane following intubation	1. Avoid recumbency with regional techniques 2. Can reverse xylazine in newborns if depression Is noted 3. Supplemental analgesia in postoperative period as warranted 4. Caudal epidural to reduce post-parturient 'straining'
Sheep/Goat	1. Lumbosacral epidural Sedation 2. Incisional line block Sedation 3. Propofol, 4–6 mg/kg Isoflurane or sevoflurane	1. Lumbosacral epidural Sedation 2. Incisional line block Sedation 3. Propofol, 4–6 mg/kg Isoflurane or sevoflurane	1. Sheep have a high pain sensitivity 2. Variable and inconsistent response to opioids for pain management 3. α_2 Agents are frequently selected for supplemental analgesia
Pig	1. Lumbosacral epidural Sedation 2. Incisional line block Sedation 3. Propofol, 4–6 mg/kg Isoflurane or sevoflurane	1. Lumbosacral epidural Sedation 2. Incisional line block Sedation 3. Propofol, 4–6 mg/kg Isoflurane or sevoflurane	1. Will need sedation in addition to regional analgesia in elective section 2. Good response to opioid analgesic agents following fetal removal 3. NSAIDs are frequently used for pain management
Llama	1. GGE to effect 2. Propofol, 2–4 mg/kg 3. Isoflurane or sevoflurane	1. GGE to effect 2. Isoflurane or sevoflurane	1. Limited reports in literature 2. Pain management following fetal removal as per other procedures

to discharge with a 42% delivery of live foals. Nearly 30% of foals survived to discharge [45]. In this scenario, specific choice of anesthetic agent is probably less important than the time to induction and delivery of the foal. Studies have been carried out comparing the effects of isoflurane and halothane in pregnant mares, and no marked differences between the two were demonstrated [50]. Less soluble agents (such as isoflurane and sevoflurane) have the advantage of being more rapidly cleared from foals after delivery than halothane [51]. Studies in pony mares found that anesthesia maintenance with propofol or a combination of guaifenesin (GGE), ketamine, and detomidine (GKD) preserved cardiovascular function in both the mare and fetus [52,53]. This suggests that GKD could be suitable for anesthetic induction of term mares. In the field, where equipment is not readily available for delivering inhalation anesthesia, a guaifenesin–ketamine–xylazine mixture has been infused to effect for up to 1 h to maintain an adequate level of central nervous system depression [53].

Monitoring and support of an anesthetized pregnant mare are no different than for any anesthetized horse. Care should be taken to avoid maternal hypoxia in order to maintain fetal oxygenation until delivery. Mechanical ventilation should be considered to help offset the ventilation–perfusion mismatching that occurs. Arterial blood gases should be assessed shortly after initiating positive-pressure ventilation to ensure that the desired increase in PaO_2 is occurring.

Positive-pressure ventilation in a mare with severe abdominal distension has the potential to decrease cardiac output to all tissues drastically, including maternal circulation to the foal. Arterial blood pressure should be monitored directly and ideally kept above 70 mmHg by adjusting anesthetic depth and rate of fluid delivery and by administering inotropes and/or vasopressors.

Mares recovering from dystocia or cesarean section may have a difficult time regaining the strength needed to stand. Special attention should be given to the condition of the recovery area, and the floor should be cleaned of all obstetric lubricant and dried. Mares should be placed on a well-padded surface in a recovery area and may be rope assisted during recovery when necessary.

Dogs and cats

A range of general anesthesia techniques for cesarean section in dogs and cats have been reported to be satisfactory (Table 34.2) [54]. All reported techniques have common strategies for successful patient management, which include the following: (1) induction of anesthesia must be smooth and rapid, (2) intubation should be accomplished quickly and ventilation supported to ensure adequate oxygenation, and (3) drugs and technique selected should maintain fetal viability as much as possible.

As previously noted, studies have compared the outcome on maternal safety and fetal vitality of several commonly used anesthesia protocols used in caesarian section. The results of these studies indicated that, in dogs, propofol followed by isoflurane anesthesia resulted in newborn survival rates comparable to those using epidural anesthesia and superior to those with general anesthesia induced with thiopental [23,24,35]. Sevoflurane has also been reported to produce viable newborns when used in caesarian section anesthesia protocols. Comparable studies have not been performed in cats; however, their maternal–fetal anatomy and physiology support similar success with this strategy.

Supplemental oxygen administration can significantly increase fetal oxygen content and viability following surgical extraction. Administration of oxygen to the mother is not associated with a significant decrease in uterine blood flow or fetal acidosis [18]. Fetal red blood cells have a lower 2,3-diphosphoglycerate concentration than do adult red blood cells, hence fetal hemoglobin can carry more oxygen at low oxygen tensions than can adult hemoglobin. Physiologically, this is important because it ensures a higher level of hemoglobin saturation at the normally low oxygen partial pressures (PO_2 of umbilical vein 30 mmHg) to which the fetus is exposed [21,55]. Inspired oxygen concentrations of 50% or more during general anesthesia result in more vigorous neonates because of improved oxygenation [18]. Therefore, oxygen administration is indicated regardless of the anesthetic protocol.

Tidal and minute ventilation must be critically evaluated during the anesthetic period to avoid either hypoventilation or hyperventilation. The total effect of carbon dioxide on the fetus is not clear, but passive hyperventilation of the mother causes hypocapnia with decreased uterine artery blood flow. This decreased placental perfusion causes fetal hypoxia, hypercapnia, and acidosis. With adequate arterial oxygenation, a modest increase in $PaCO_2$ is well tolerated by the fetus [18]. Adequacy of ventilation and oxygenation may be assessed by observing rate of respiration, excursion of the chest wall and/or reservoir bag, and color of mucous membranes, by implementation of pulse oximetry and capnography, and by determination of $PaCO_2$ and PaO_2.

Maintaining hemodynamic perfusion indices is essential for the safety and vitality of both the mother and fetus. Arterial blood pressure should be monitored and kept above a mean arterial pressure of 70 mmHg by adjusting anesthetic depth and rate of fluid delivery, and by administering inotropes and vasopressors, as needed.

Regional anesthesia

Regional anesthesia techniques are well established for cesarean section [17]. There is increased response to, and distribution of, local anesthetic agents during gestation and parturition. As a result, the dose and volume of local anesthetic for epidural or spinal anesthesia can be reduced by approximately one-third in pregnant patients as compared with non-parturients. Regional anesthesia (epidural or subarachnoid) has the advantages of technique simplicity, minimal exposure of the fetus to drugs, less intraoperative bleeding, and, because the mother remains awake, minimal risk of aspiration [56]. In addition, muscle relaxation and analgesia are optimal. Caudal spinal anatomy in the lumbosacral region varies by species. The spinal cord terminates at the level of the sixth lumbar vertebra in dogs, reducing the risk of subarachnoid (true spinal) injection of the anesthetic agent. The spinal cord terminates variably between L_7 and mid-sacrum in cats, making subarachnoid injection a greater possibility [57]. In swine and ruminants, the spinal cord terminates at the mid-sacrum, making subarachnoid injection a possibility at the lumbosacral junction.

Dogs and cats

Epidural anesthesia has been successfully used in dogs and cats for cesarean section anesthesia. Traditionally, a short-acting local anesthetic (2% lidocaine) is administered at a dose of 1 mL per 3.25–4.5 kg of body weight in the epidural space to provide surgical site anesthesia. In recent years, epidurally administered drugs, including lidocaine and bupivacaine in a 1:1 volumetric mixture, have provided extended duration of surgical anesthesia and pain management in the early recovery period. This may be supplemented with epidural opioids and α_2-adrenergic agonists to extend the postoperative analgesic period.

Pigs, sheep, and goats

Spinal techniques work well in sows, sheep, and goats. The technique is well established and not difficult. When using this technique, it is sometimes necessary to restrain a sow's head and forelimbs. If sows are sedated and restrained in lateral recumbency with the head extended, the soft palate may occlude the airway and the patient may suffocate. Because cesarean section in swine is often viewed as a last-ditch effort by producers, it is often delayed until the sow's overall condition has severely deteriorated. Therefore, a high percentage of sows presented for cesarean section are hypovolemic and hypotensive. Fluids can be readily administered to sows via indwelling catheters placed into the ear veins prior to anesthetic administration. This will restore circulating volume and offset hypotension induced by spinal techniques.

Cattle

Epidural and spinal anesthesia often induces recumbency, which is undesirable in large ruminants. An alternative is to perform standing cesarean section in cattle using either a proximal or distal paralumbar block. In cows that are in poor condition, exhausted, or in shock, the distal technique is preferred because it does not induce a scoliosis-like position and the cow is more likely to remain standing throughout the procedure.

Disadvantages of epidural or subarachnoid anesthesia include hypotension secondary to sympathetic blockade. Hypotension induced by epidural anesthesia can be managed with IV fluid and catecholamine administration. Lactated Ringer's solution or 0.9 or 0.45% sodium chloride mixed with equal volumes of 5% dextrose solution can be administered at approximately 20 mL/kg over 15–20 min to maintain arterial blood pressure. When hypotension is severe, ephedrine may be administered (0.15 mg/kg IV). Hypotension and visceral manipulation during the procedure can cause nausea and vomiting. Because the mother remains conscious, the forelimbs and head often move. This precludes the use of a spinal technique in highly excited or fractious patients and in mares, because they become hysterical when they are unable to stand.

Local anesthesia

Local infiltration or field block may be used, but these techniques have several disadvantages compared with regional techniques. Infiltration requires larger amounts of anesthetic agent, which is systemically absorbed and can create fetal depression. In addition, muscle relaxation and analgesia are not as profound or as uniform compared with regional anesthesia. In many cases, field block is supplemented with heavy sedation or tranquilization to calm and stabilize a mother; these agents further contribute to maternal and fetal depression. For these reasons, field block is often abandoned for either general or epidural anesthesia.

Care of the newborn

Following delivery, the newborn's head is cleared of membranes and the oropharynx of fluid. The umbilical vessels should be milked toward the fetus to empty them of blood, clamped or ligated approximately 2–5 cm from the body wall, and severed from the placenta. Neonates can then be gently rubbed with a towel to dry them and stimulate breathing. Vigorous motion should be avoided because amniotic fluid is readily absorbed in the lungs and contributes to distribution of pulmonary surfactant in the alveoli. The head and neck should be supported to avoid whiplash and prevent injury [58]. Flow-by oxygen administration in the vicinity of the muzzle is helpful to increase heart rate and oxygen delivery to tissues in distressed, exhausted neonates. Reversal of opioids by sublingual or intranasal administration of 1–2 drops of naloxone is warranted in cases where opioids were administered as part of the general anesthesia technique. An oral dose of 2.5% dextrose (0.1–0.5 mL) is helpful to improve energy substrates required for initial breathing effort in stressed neonates. Finally, maintaining warmth is vital because hypothermia can occur rapidly after birth.

A small IV catheter may be used to intubate and support oxygen delivery in neonates that will not initiate breathing, and their breathing can be artificially supported by using a syringe and three-way valve attached to an oxygen source. As a final measure, doxapram can be used to stimulate breathing in neonates. In puppies, a dosage of 1–5 mg (approximately 1–5 drops from a 20–22-gauge needle) is topically administered to the oral mucosa or injected intramuscularly or subcutaneously. In kittens, the dosage is 1–2 mg (1–2 drops) [54]. Airways must be clear before doxapram administration. External thoracic compressions may be warranted if the heart rate is slow and does not respond to support measures. A rapid physical examination checking for genetic defects (cleft palate, chest deformity, or abdominal wall fusion) is also important to determine whether viability is present. Newborn puppy viability has been associated with umbilical vein blood lactate concentrations [59]. Umbilical vein lactate levels >5 mmol/L were correlated with increased neonate mortality within 48 h of delivery. Five minute Apgar scores have also been evaluated in puppies as a prognostic indicator of early survival [60]. Puppies that scored within the 7–10 range had greater 48 h survival than those scoring less.

When general anesthesia is used in ruminants or horses, the oropharynx can be cleared of fluid and the trachea intubated after the fetal head is delivered through the uterine incision. The fetus can then be delivered and the umbilicus severed. Because the uteroplacental and umbilical circulation is preserved until the airway is secured, hypoxia is prevented. Once the fetus is delivered, ventilation can be supported, if necessary, via a bag valve mask resuscitator.

After completion of surgery and recovery from anesthesia, the newborn can be introduced to their mother. If introduction is delayed, the neonates should be exposed briefly to the mother to provide colostrum and then kept in a warm environment until anesthesia recovery is complete to avoid accidental crushing. If regional anesthesia was used, they can be placed with their mother as soon as the surgery is complete.

Perioperative pain management

This represents a challenge in cesarean section patients because of concerns regarding transfer of anesthetic and analgesic drugs into milk and its impact on neonates. This area has been extensively studied in people and in food-producing species. Most of the current information is from humans and cattle; however, because of the similarity of the lactation process in all mammals, the information may be extrapolated to other species.

The phenothiazine tranquilizer chlorpromazine does not appear to transfer to milk at levels that cause fetal depression [53]. No corollary evidence is available for acepromazine, but similarity in molecular structure coupled with clinical experience supports a similar effect on newborns. The benzodiazepine class tranquilizer diazepam crosses significantly into milk and may cause lethargy, sedation, and weight loss in newborns [56]. Other class members, including clonazepam and alprazolam, induce drowsiness, hypotonia, and apnea in newborns after nursing episodes. The effects of lorazepam and midazolam are unknown; however, based on the effects attributed to other class members, they should be used with caution in lactating mothers. Xylazine transiently increases in milk and then decreases to non-detectable levels by 12 h after administration [61]. Detomidine (80 μg/kg) can be detected at a low level in milk after administration but is non-detectable by 23 h later [62].

Codeine, propoxyphene, and morphine are well tolerated by newborns when used in maternal pain management, even when repeat doses are administered over several days [63]. Meperidine (pethidine) has been reported to cause decreased suckling behavior and sedation when used in serial doses [63,64]. Fentanyl (100 μg) and sufentanil (10–50 μg) are not detectable in breast milk after epidural administration in humans [65].

Thiopental has been detected in colostrum and breast milk after a single bolus induction dose (5 mg/kg) in women [66]. Long-acting barbiturates such as phenobarbital are contraindicated because of their extensive presence in milk [67]. Propofol is detectable in colostrum and milk after a single-dose administration [68]. However, little clinical effect is noted based on excellent newborn vitality immediately after delivery [23,24]. The residual presence of inhalation anesthetic agents in milk is not known; however, clinical experience suggests that prolonged neonatal sedation following clinical recovery of mothers is not common.

Local anesthetic drugs (e.g., lidocaine and bupivacaine) and first-generation bupivacaine metabolites are excreted in milk after their epidural administration in humans. Although these agents are detectable in milk, their influence on neonates is negligible based on maximum Apgar (activity, pulse, grimace, appearance, and respiration) scores at delivery [69].

NSAIDs appear to reach only limited levels in milk after maternal administration. In humans, acetaminophen and aspirin are considered compatible with breast feeding [63]. Studies evaluating carprofen in cattle indicated that milk levels were below detectable limits (<0.022 μg/mL) after a single-dose administration. After experimental induction of mastitis, carprofen was detected at low levels (0.16 μg/mL) for 12 h following single-bolus administration and decreased to undetectable levels (<0.022 μg/mL) by 24 h [70]. Following a single dose of ketoprofen (3.3 mg/kg) in cattle, detectable but non-quantifiable concentrations were present in milk for only 2 h [71]. Similar results have been reported in lactating goats [72].

Based on current evidence, it appears that most commonly used analgesic drug classes may be safely administered during the lactation period without adverse effects on newborns.

References

1 Dawes GS. *Foetal and Neonatal Physiology*. Chicago: Year Book, 1968; **15**.

2 Shnider SM. The physiology of pregnancy. In: *Annual Refresher Course Lectures*. Park Ridge, IL: American Society of Anesthesiologists, 1978; 1251–1258.

3 Kerr MG. Cardiovascular dynamics in pregnancy and labour. *Br Med Bull* 1968; **24**: 19–24,.

4 Ueland K, Parer JT. Effects of estrogens on the cardiovascular system of the ewe. *Am J Obstet Gynecol* 1966; **96**: 400–406.

5 Ueland K, Hansen JM. Maternal cardiovascular dynamics. II. Posture and uterine contractions. *Am J Obstet Gynecol* 1969; **103**: 1–7.

6 James EM III. Physiologic changes during pregnancy. In: *Annual Refresher Course Lectures*. Park Ridge, IL: American Society of Anesthesiologists, 1980; 1251–1255.

7 Marx CE. Physiology of pregnancy: high risk implications. In: *Annual Refresher Course Lectures*. Park Ridge, IL, American Society of Anesthesiologists, 1979; 1251–1254.

8 Kerr MC, Scott DB. Inferior vena caval occlusion in late pregnancy. *Clin Anesth* 1973; **10**: 17–22.

9 Stoneham AE, Graham J, Rozanski EA, Rush JE. Pregnancy-associated congestive heart failure in a cat. *J Am Anim Hosp Assoc* 2006; **42**: 457–461.

10 Lipton B, Hershey SC, Baez S. Compatibility of oxytocics with anesthetic agents. *JAMA* 1962; **179**: 410–416.

11 Paddleford RR. Anesthesia for cesarean section in the dog. *Vet Clin North Am Small Anim Pract* 1992; **22**: 481–484.

12 Wright RC, Shnider SM, Levinsan G, *et al.* The effect of maternal stress on plasma catecholamines and uterine blood flow in the ewe [Abstract]. In: *Annual Meeting of the Society of Obstetric Anesthesia and Perinatology*, 1978; 17–20.

13 Morishema HO, Yeh M-N, James LS. The effects of maternal pain and hyperexcitability upon the fetus: possible benefits of maternal sedation [Abstract]. In: *Scientific Session of American Society of Anesthesiologists Annual Meeting, Atlanta, GA*, 1977.

14 Alper MH. Perinatal pharmacology. In: *Annual Refresher Course Lectures*. Park Ridge, IL: American Society of Anesthesiologists, 1979; 1261–1267.

15 Palahniuk RJ, Shnider SM, Eger EI III, Lopez-Manzanara P. Pregnancy decreases the requirements of inhaled anesthetic agents. *Anesthesiology* 1974; **41**: 82–83.

16 Einster M. Perinatal pharmacology. In: *Annual Refresher Course Lectures*. Park Ridge, IL: American Society of Anesthesiologists, 1980; 1261–1264.

17 Collins VI. *Principles of Anesthesiology*, 2nd edn. Philadelphia: Lea & Febiger, 1976; **199**.

18 Gutsche B. Perinatal pharmacology. In: *Annual Refresher Course Lectures*. Park Ridge, IL: American Society of Anesthesiologists, 1978; 1291–1299.

19 Theis JCW. Acetylsalicylic acid (ASA) and non-steriodal drugs (NSAIDS) during pregnancy: are they safe? *Can Fam Physician* 1996; **42**: 2347–2349.

20 Datta S, Alper MH. Anesthesia for cesarean section. *Anesthesiology* 1980; **53**: 142–160.

21 Goodger WJ, Levy W. Anesthetic management of the cesarean section. *Vet Clin North Am* 1973; **3**: 85–89.

22 Moon PF, Erb HN, Ludders JW, *et al.* Perioperative management and mortality rates of dogs undergoing cesarean section in the United States and Canada. *J Am Vet Med Assoc* 1998; **213**: 365–369.

23 Moon PF, Erb HN, Ludders JW, *et al.* Perioperative risk factors for puppies delivered by cesarean section in the United States and Canada. *J Am Anim Hosp Assoc* 2000; **36**: 359–368.

24 Moon-Massat PF, Erb HN. Perioperative factors associated with puppy vigor after delivery by cesarean section. *J Am Anim Hosp Assoc* 2002; **38**: 90–96.

25 Tranquilli WJ, Lemke K, Williams LL, *et al.* Flumazenil efficacy in reversing diazepam or midazolam overdose in dogs. *J Vet Anaesth* 1992; **19**: 65–68.

26 Terttu K, Oijala M. The effect of detomidine (Domosedan) on the maintenance of equine pregnancy and foetal development: ten cases. *Equine Vet J* 1988; **20**: 323–326.

27 Jedruch J, Gajewski Z, Kuussaari J. The effect of detomidine hydrochloride on the electrical activity of uterus in pregnant mares. *Acta Vet Scand* 1989; **30**: 307–311.

28 Pyörälä E, Koppinen J, Vainio O, Alanko M. Detomidine in pregnant cows. *Nord Vet Med* 1986; **38**: 237–240.

29 Jedruch J, Gajewski Z, Ratajska-Michalczak K. Uterine motor responses to an alpha 2-adrenergic agonist medetomidine hydrochloride in the bitches during the end of gestation and the post-partum period. *Acta Vet Scand Suppl* 1989; **85**: 129–134.

30 El-Tahan MR, Mowafi HA, Al Sheikh IH, *et al.* Efficacy of demedetomidine in suppressing cardiovascular and hormonal responses to general anaesthesia for caesarean section: a dose response study. *Int J Obstet Anesth* 2012; **21**: 222–229.

31 Schatzmann U, Josseck H, Stauffer J.-L, *et al.* Effects of α_2-agonists on intrauterine pressure and sedation in horses: comparison between detomidine, romifidine and xylazine. *J Vet Med Ser A* 1994; **41**: 523–529.

32 McDonnell W, Van Corder I. Cardiopulmonary effects of xylazine/ketamine in dogs [Abstract]. In: *Annual Scientific Meeting of the American College of Veterinary Anesthesiologists, Las Vegas, NV*, 1982.

33 Palahniuk RJ. Obstetric anesthesia in the healthy parturient. In: *Annual Refresher Course Lectures*. Park Ridge, IL: American Society of Anesthesiologists, 1979; 1271–1274.

34 Hodgkinson R, Bhatt M, Wang CN. Double-blind comparison of the neurobehaviour of neonates following the administration of different doses of meperidine to the mother. *Can Anaesth Soc J* 1978; **25**: 405–411.

35 Funkquist PM, Nyman GC, Lofgren AJ, Fahlbrink EM. Use of propofol–isoflurane as an anesthetic regimen for cesarean section in dogs. *J Am Vet Med Assoc* 1997; **211**: 313–317.

36 Gaynor JS, Wertz EM, Alvis M, Turner AS. A comparison of the haemodynamic effects of propofol and isoflurane in pregnant ewes. *J Vet Pharmacol Ther* 1998; **21**: 69–73.

37 Setoyama K, Shinzato T, Kazuhiro M, *et al.* Effects of propofol–sevoflurane anesthesia on the maternal and fetal hemodynamics, blood gases, and uterine activity in pregnant goats. *J Vet Med Sci* 2003; **65**: 1075–1081.

38 Nagel ML, Muir WW, Nguyen K. Comparison of the cardiopulmonary effects of etomidate and thiamylal in dogs. *Am J Vet Res* 1979; **40**: 193–196.

39 Muir WW, Swanson CR. Principles, techniques, and complications of feline anesthesia and chemical restraint. In: Sherding R, ed. *The Cat: Diseases and Clinical Management*. New York: Churchill Livingstone, 1989; 81–116.

40 Ko JCH, Thurmon JC, Benson GJ, Tranquilli WJ. Acute hemolysis with etomidate–propylene glycol infusion in the dog. *J Vet Anaesth* 1993; **20**: 92–94.

41 Hall LW. Althesin in the large animal. *Postgrad Med J* 1972; **48**(Suppl 2): 55–58.

42 Corbet HR. The use of Saffan in the dog. *Aust Vet Pract* 1977; **7**: 184–188.

43 Greene SA. *Veterinary Anesthesia and Pain Management Secrets*. Philadelphia: Hanley and Belfus, 2002; 229–231.

44 Hay Kraus, BL. Efficacy of maropitant in preventing vomiting in dogs premedicated with hydromorphone. *Vet Anes Analg* 2013; **40**: 28–34.

45 Byron CR, Embertson RM, Bernard WV, *et al.* Dystocia in a referral hospital setting: approach and results. *Equine Vet J* 2002; **35**: 82–85.

46 Abernathy-Young KK, LeBlanc MM, Embertson RM, *et al.* Survival rates of mares and foals and postoperative complications and fertility of mares after cesarean section: 95 cases (1986–2000). *J Am Vet Med Assoc* 2012; **241**: 927–934.

47 Youngquist RS. Equine obstetrics. In: Morrow DA, ed. *Current Therapy in Theriogenology*, 2nd edn. Philadelphia: WB Saunders, 1986; 693–699.

48 Freeman DE, Hungerford LL, Schaeffer D, *et al.* Caesarean section and other methods for assisted delivery: comparison of effects on mare mortality and complications. *Equine Vet J* 1999; **31**: 203–207.

49 Embertson RM. Dystocia and caesarian sections: the importance of duration and good judgement. *Equine Vet J* 1999; **31**: 179–180.

50 Daunt DA, Steffey EP, Pascoe JR, *et al.* Actions of isoflurane and halothane in pregnant mares. *J Am Vet Med Assoc* 1992; **201**: 1367–1374.

51 Wilson DV. Anesthesia and sedation for late-term mares. *Vet Clin North Am Equine Pract* 1994; **10**: 219–236.

52 Taylor PM, White KL, Fowden AL, *et al.* Propofol anaesthesia for surgery in late gestation pony mares. *Vet Anaesth Analg* 2001; **28**: 177–187.

53 Lin HC, Wallace RL, Harrison IW, Thurmon JC. A case report on the use of guaifenesin–ketamine–xylazine anesthesia for equine dystocia. *Cornell Vet J* 1994; **84**: 61–66.

54 Hellyer PW. Anesthesia for cesarian section: anesthetic considerations for surgery. In: Slatter D, ed. *Slatter's Textbook of Small Ani mal Surgery*, 2nd edn. Philadelphia: WB Saunders, 1991; 2300–2303.

55 Guyton AC. *Textbook of Medical Physiology*, 4th edn. Philadelphia: WB Saunders, 1971; **78**.

56 Iqbal MM, Sobhan T, Ryals T. Effects of commonly used benzodiazepines on the fetus, the neonate, and the nursing patient. *Psychiatr Serv* 2002; **53**: 39–49.

57 Hall LW, Taylor PM. *Anaesthesia of the Cat*. London: Baillière Tindall, 1994; **124**.

58 Goericke-Pesch S, Wehrend A. New method for removing mucus from the upper respiratory tract of newborn puppies following caesarean section. *Vet Rec* 2012; **170**: 289.

59 Groppetti D, Pecile A, Del Carro AP, *et al*. Evaluation of newborn canine viability by means of umbilical vein lactate measurement, Apgar score and uterine tocodynamometry. *Theriogenology* 2010; **74**: 1187–1196.

60 Veronesi MC, Panzani S, Faustini M, Rota A. An Apgar scoring system for routine assessment of newborn puppy viability and short-term survival prognosis. *Theriogenology* 2009; **72**: 401–407.

61 Delehant TM, Denhart JW, Lloyd WE, Powell JD. Pharmacokinetics of xylazine, 2,6-dimethylaniline, and tolazoline in tissues from yearling cattle and milk from mature dairy cows after sedation with xylazine hydrochloride and reversal with tolazoline hydrochloride. *Vet Ther* 2003; **4**: 128–134.

62 Salonen JS, Vaha-Vahe T, Vainio O, Vakkuri O. Single dose pharmacokinetics of detomidine in the horse and cow. *J Vet Pharmacol Ther* 1989; **12**: 65–72.

63 Bar-Oz B, Bukowstein M, Benyamini L, *et al*. Use of antibiotic and analgesic drugs during lactation. *Drug Saf* 2003; **26**: 925–935.

64 Wittels B, Glosten B, Faure EA, *et al*. Postcesarean analgesia with both epidural morphine and intravenous patient-controlled analgesia: neurobehavioral outcomes among nursing neonates. *Anesth Analg* 1997; **85**: 600–606.

65 Madej TH, Strunin L. Comparison of epidural fentanyl with sufentanil: analgesia and side effects after a single bolus dose during elective cesarean section. *Anaesthesia* 1987; **42**: 1156–1161.

66 Andersen LW, Qvist T, Hertz J, Mogensen F. Concentrations of thiopentone in mature breast milk and colostrum following an induction dose. *Acta Anaesthesiol Scand* 1987; **31**: 30–32.

67 Knowles JA. Effects on the infant of drug therapy in nursing mothers. *Drug Ther* 1973; **3**: 57–59.

68 Schmitt JP, Schwoerer D, Diemunsch P, Gauthier-Lafaye J. Passage of propofol in the colostrum: preliminary data. *Ann Fr Anesth Reanim* 1987; **6**: 267–268.

69 Ortega D, Viviand X, Loree AM, *et al*. Excretion of lidocaine and bupivacaine in breast milk following epidural anesthesia for cesarean delivery. *Acta Anaesthesiol Scand* 1999; **43**: 394–397.

70 Lohuis JA, van Werven T, Brand A, *et al*. Pharmacodynamics and pharmacokinetics of carprofen, a nonsteroidal anti-inflammatory drug, in healthy cows and cows with *Escherichia coli* endotoxin-induced mastitis. *J Vet Pharmacol Ther* 1991; **14**: 219–229.

71 De Graves FJ, Riddell MG, Schumacher J. Ketoprofen concentrations in plasma and milk after intravenous administration in dairy cattle. *Am J Vet Res* 1996; **57**: 1031–1033.

72 Musser JM, Anderson KL, Tyczkowska KL. Pharmacokinetic parameters and milk concentrations of ketoprofen after administration as a single intravenous bolus dose to lactating goats. *J Vet Pharmacol Ther* 1998; **21**: 358–363.

SECTION 10

Comparative Anesthesia and Analgesia

35 Comparative Anesthesia and Analgesia of Dogs and Cats

Peter J. Pascoe and Bruno H. Pypendop
Department of Surgical and Radiological Sciences, School of Veterinary Medicine, University of California, Davis, California, USA

Chapter contents

Dogs

Range of sizes

The domestic dog has been manipulated by selective breeding into a bewildering variety of shapes and sizes, originally with some functional purpose, but more recently with appearance as a major driving force of breed standards. This has led to an array of adult dog weights ranging from <1 kg (e.g., teacup Yorkshire Terrier) to >100 kg (e.g., St. Bernard). Clinical experience suggests that smaller dogs generally require larger doses, on an mg/kg basis. However, there is no validated scientific basis for calculating these relative dose rates.

While the validity of formulas used to adjust dose for body mass is debated, most scaling factors such as body surface area are actually irrelevant to allometric scaling. The relevant information is the slope of the relationship between mass (e.g., body weight [BW]) and the variable to be corrected (e.g., dose); this slope is determined by the exponent used, and therefore scaling to BW^x, where x is some exponent (e.g., $x = 0.67$). This relationship between body weight and dose would be as effective (provided that dose actually varies as a function of body size) as body surface area and avoids the criticism that body surface area may not be known. Table 35.1 shows how dose might be affected by scaling it to different tissues and activities.

Perhaps a more rational approach would be based on pharmacokinetics using pharmacokinetic parameters to describe the distribution of a drug in the body. Initial mixing of a drug with the plasma is in the central compartment and generally scales to (i.e., is a function of) body weight [1,2]. Based on this consideration, it would appear that dose calculations based on body weight raised to some factor (e.g., 0.67) are appropriate for rapid-acting anesthetic and analgesic drugs.

Obesity has been estimated to occur in over 30% of cats and dogs [3,4]. This presents a challenge for the anesthetist because there are no simple and accurate techniques to estimate lean weight to guide dosing. Although adipose tissue has a relatively low blood flow per gram of tissue, it will affect the distribution of some drugs (e.g., propofol). Experience in obese humans indicates that the dose of induction drug is greater than the dose expected for the predicted lean body weight but not as high as the dose required for actual body weight. For example, the total propofol dose in obese versus non-obese children was only 7% greater, even though average weight was 170% of non-obese children [5]. A recent study reported that the induction dose of propofol was larger, on a mg/kg basis, in dogs of normal weight than in overweight dogs [6]. However, a possible confounding factor in that study was the administration of medetomidine for premedication. All dogs receive the same dose, based on their total body mass. It is unknown if the anesthetic-sparing effect of medetomidine correlates better with total or lean body mass; if the latter is correct, medetomidine would be expected to produce a larger reduction in propofol requirement in the overweight dogs, because they would have received a larger relative effective dose. In any case, changes in dose of induction agent can be accounted for, in clinical practice, by titrating the drug to the desired effect. Obesity may have many other anesthetic management implications before and during anesthesia [7].

Veterinary Anesthesia and Analgesia: The Fifth Edition of Lumb and Jones.
Edited by Kurt A. Grimm, Leigh A. Lamont, William J. Tranquilli, Stephen A. Greene and Sheilah A. Robertson.

Table 35.1 Doses of a drug scaled to various metabolic activities or organ weights based on a 20 μg/kg dose for a 20 kg dog. BW = body weight in kg. The scaling factors are drawn from references 165–168. Note that the exponent (slope) contains the relevant information, as identical doses would be calculated by the relationships with similar exponents, regardless of the difference in the multiplier (e.g., kidney weight and liver weight doses).

kg	BSA dose (dose/kg)	BMR dose (dose/kg)	Renal clearance dose (dose/kg)	Kidney weight dose (dose/kg)	Hepatic blood flow dose (dose/kg)	Liver weight dose (dose/kg)	Hepatic function dose (dose/kg)	Heart weight dose (dose/kg)	Brain weight dose (dose/kg)
Formula	$0.0484 \times BW^{0.67}$	$3.8 \times BW^{0.734}$	$4.2 \times (BW \times 1000)^{0.69}$	$0.0212 \times (BW \times 1000)^{0.85}$	$0.0554 \times BW^{0.894}$	$0.037 \times BW^{0.849}$	$0.00816 \times BW^{0.885}$	$0.0066 \times (BW \times 1000)^{0.98}$	$39 \times BW^{0.27}$
1	54 (54)	44 (44)	51 (51)	31 (31)	27 (27)	31 (31)	28 (28)	21 (21)	178 (178)
5	158 (32)	145 (29)	154 (31)	123 (25)	116 (23)	123 (25)	117 (23)	103 (21)	275 (55)
10	251 (25)	240 (24)	248 (25)	222 (22)	215 (22)	222 (22)	217 (22)	203 (21)	332 (33)
20	400 (20)	400 (20)	400 (20)	400 (20)	400 (20)	400 (20)	400 (20)	400 (20)	400 (20)
30	525 (18)	539 (18)	529 (18)	565 (19)	575 (19)	564 (19)	573 (19)	595 (20)	446 (15)
50	739 (15)	784 (16)	753 (15)	872 (17)	907 (18)	871 (17)	900 (18)	982 (20)	512 (10)
80	1013 (13)	1107 (14)	1041 (13)	1300 (16)	1381 (17)	1298 (16)	1364 (17)	1556 (19)	582 (7)
100	1176 (12)	1303 (13)	1214 (12)	1571 (16)	1686 (17)	1569 (16)	1662 (17)	1937 (19)	618 (6)

To arrive at these values the scaled value was calculated for a 20 kg animal and the unit dose was then calculated based on 400 μg for that scaled animal. This unit dose was then multiplied by the scaled size for each body weight in the table.
BSA = body surface area; BMR = basal metabolic rate; BW = body weight in kg. The scaling factors are drawn from references 165–168.

Sighthounds

These are dogs that historically have hunted by sighting their prey rather than using scent. Phenotypically, sighthounds are deep chested, have long legs and relatively narrow bodies, and are very lean. Many people classify the Afghan, Borzoi, Saluki, Greyhound, Italian Greyhound, Whippet, Irish Wolfhound, Scottish Deerhound, Ibizan Hound, Basenji, and Rhodesian Ridgeback, as well as a number of other rarer breeds, as sighthounds [8]. However, based on genetic analysis, these breeds do not all share the same lineage [9]. The Afghan and Saluki are far closer to the wolf, on a genetic basis, than the Greyhound or Borzoi. Published studies related to anesthesia of sighthounds typically use the Greyhound breed and document that these breeds have a longer recovery time following thiobarbiturate anesthesia [10,11]. Studies also demonstrate slightly longer recoveries following both propofol and alfaxalone in Greyhounds [12,13]. These results were initially ascribed to the large muscle mass and minimal adipose tissue found in Greyhounds and hence generalized to all sighthounds. However, more recent data have demonstrated that the Greyhound breed may have relative deficiencies in hepatic metabolism [14,15]. Such a deficiency is unlikely in all sighthounds given the differences in genetic origins. There are also no published reports of delayed anesthetic recovery in sighthounds other than Greyhounds although there are many anecdotes regarding such events.

Other breed-associated anesthetic considerations

Some clients in veterinary practice have been advised by a breeder, or have looked up information on the internet which suggests that some breeds have 'sensitivities' to particular anesthetics [16]. The origin of this advice is often unclear and very few breed-related problems during anesthesia have been consistently reported by veterinarians. An abnormal response to an anesthetic could be related to an individual strain within a breed whereby a particular breeder or group of breeders have produced animals that have a characteristic that they want to promote at the expense of potentially propagating congenital, developmental, or genetic abnormalities (e.g., hydrocephalus or cardiomyopathy), resulting in alterations in response to anesthetics.

The MDR-1 or ABCB-1 gene polymorphism has been found in a number of herding breeds and some others. Proteins produced by this gene family (ATP binding cassette [ABC] family) are found in many areas of the body but their presence in the intestine and the blood–brain barrier is most important with respect to anesthetic and analgesic drugs. This gene is one of several that affect the brain concentrations reached by some drugs [17]. Experiments in MDR-1-deficient mice suggest that there is about a 25% increase in morphine and fentanyl neuronal cell concentrations and more than a two-fold increase in methadone. Meperidine does not appear to interact with p-glycoprotein. *In vitro* data would suggest that sufentanil, alfentanil, oxymorphone, and butorphanol [18,19] do not have significant interactions with p-glycoprotein. Buprenorphine appears to have minimal interaction with p-glycoprotein but its metabolite, norbuprenorphine, is removed in part from the brain by this transporter [20]. Anesthetic drugs commonly used for induction and maintenance do not appear to interact with p-glycoprotein.

Some breed-associated anesthetic concerns may be related to prevalent pathology within a breed. Anecdotally, Boxers have been reported to be at increased risk of adverse effects (e.g., collapse) following administration of acepromazine. Since this adverse effect is rare and difficult to study scientifically, it is not known if this is related to the prevalence of dilated cardiomyopathy in this breed or is an enhancement of a vagal response to the drug, as reported in a number of other brachycephalic breeds [21].

A number of breeds have emerged from morbidity/mortality studies as having higher anesthetic risk when analyzing data using univariate analysis. These effects do not appear when a more thorough multivariate analysis is performed, indicating that other factors influence the observed complication rate (e.g., a greater incidence of complications in small breed dogs) [22,23]. Despite the unreliability of internet reports of breed sensitivities, it is incumbent on the anesthetist to investigate specific concerns presented by an owner.

Histamine release

This appears to occur more in dogs than other species but the specific reason is unclear. One example is the release of histamine following the administration of Cremophor, the solvent used in some injectable anesthetics (e.g., Saffan®). This has resulted in the deaths of a number of dogs [24]. While not advised, some practitioners continued use in conjunction with antihistamines even though it was never approved for use in dogs [25]. Morphine and meperidine are associated with histamine release and although it is difficult to compare species, the plasma concentrations of histamine in dogs appear to be considerably higher than those found in humans [26–28].

Brachycephalic breeds

There are various degrees of the manifestation of the brachycephalic syndrome (e.g., stenotic nares, elongated soft palate, everted lateral ventricles, hypoplastic trachea, and bronchial collapse) [29]. Conchal shortening creating both rostral and caudal obstruction of the nasal passages has also been described [30]. This constellation of anatomic changes leads to an increased potential for airway obstruction, especially if the animal is not fully conscious [31]. The anesthetist should consider the following.

1 Use careful, conservative administration of sedatives.
2 Have a range of endotracheal tubes available since a hypoplastic trachea requires a much smaller tube size. For example, it is not unusual for a 25 kg English Bulldog to require a 6.5 mm endotracheal tube.
3 Preoxygenate the patient if possible without stressing the animal.
4 Use a rapid intravenous induction technique. Mask induction with an inhalant is not routinely recommended for these individuals.
5 Use induction and maintenance drugs that allow for a rapid return of consciousness. Reversible drugs may also be beneficial.
6 Maintain the airway for as long as practical. The dental occlusion of these animals is abnormal and it is rare for a brachycephalic dog to be able to significantly damage an endotracheal tube.
7 Observe the patient for breath sounds and paradoxical ventilation immediately after extubation to diagnose obstruction as quickly as possible. When the airway is obstructed, the thorax will collapse during inspiration while the abdomen expands. Monitoring hemoglobin saturation (e.g., pulse oximetry) continuously during recovery, especially following extubation, is strongly advocated for early detection of hypoxemia.
8 Attempt to open the upper airway by placing the animal in sternal recumbency and extending the head, opening the mouth and pulling the tongue forward. Sometimes just propping the head up so that the neck is extended will be enough to maintain an airway early after extubation.
9 If the animal obstructs, reanesthetize and reintubate, waiting again for consciousness to return before attempting endotracheal tube removal.

A brachycephalic dog that is to be anesthetized should have its upper airway examined immediately after induction and surgical correction performed if deemed necessary. Owners should be educated about surgical correction of palate elongation and everted laryngeal saccules (if needed), and how it may improve recovery from anesthesia.

Tracheal collapse

There is a breed predilection to the occurrence of tracheal collapse, with small breeds (e.g., Yorkshire Terriers, Chihuahuas, and Pomeranians) being over-represented. Tracheal collapse is commonly associated with collapse in the lower airways, making it more difficult to manage perioperatively [32,33]. Medical management of these patients prior to elective anesthesia is often possible, with antibiotics to treat respiratory infections, weight loss, bronchodilators, antisecretory agents, antitussives, anabolic steroids, and diuretics [34,35].

The anesthetic management of patients with tracheal collapse is in many ways similar to that used for brachycephalic breeds. In preparation, it is important to have endotracheal tubes available that are long enough to reach the carina if the potential for intrathoracic tracheal collapse exists. Recovery is the most dangerous period if the airway has not been stented as collapse may reoccur and cause airway obstruction. It is therefore important to try to provide a calm recovery so that there are no sudden increases in activity that require increased respiratory effort or stimulate coughing. Supplemental oxygen and sedatives can be very helpful following extubation. Recently, a technique for applying CPAP via face mask has been described which may prove useful during recovery for these patients [36].

Tracheal stents have been used in dogs with tracheal collapse [37]. With the placement of extraluminal stents, the anesthetic management is as above. For intraluminal stents, the dog is usually intubated initially for tracheal size measurement. In small patients it is not possible to deploy the stent through the endotracheal tube so the animal must be maintained on injectable anesthetics such as propofol or alfaxalone and supplemented with oxygen by insufflation or jet ventilation during placement.

Erythrocyte potassium

Dogs are unusual in that they have relatively low intraerythrocyte potassium concentrations. Concentrations around 5–6 mmol/L are usually found in most canine erythrocytes but there are a number of breeds (e.g., Akita, Shiba Inu and other breeds of Japanese origin) that have higher potassium concentrations. Potassium leakage from erythrocytes is of concern in other species when blood is stored for transfusion. In CPD-A1 stored canine blood, plasma potassium increased to over 8 mmol/L after 30 days of storage. In human stored red cells (where the erythrocytes contain higher concentrations of potassium) the plasma potassium increased to 30 mmol/L at 3 weeks and to 44 mmol/L by 6 weeks [38,39]. Even with these higher concentrations of potassium, it is unlikely to significantly raise plasma potassium during a single unit transfusion, but when multiple units are used it can result in hyperkalemia [40].

Cats

Handling and behavior

Recommendations for feline-friendly handling have been developed by the American Association of Feline Practitioners and the International Society of Feline Medicine, and endorsed by the American Animal Hospital Association [41]. In particular, handling the fearful or aggressive cat may be challenging. Recommendations for managing these cats include training prior to the visit, oral benzodiazepines (with the associated risk of disinhibition), use of towels, muzzles, nets, and/or cat bags. The authors specifically recommended against the use of acepromazine, based on its lack of anxiolytic effect and the potential to increase aggression [41].

Fractious cats may require sedation prior to handling. Several agents and combinations have been reported to be effective. In particular, α_2-adrenergic receptor agonists, alone or combined with opioids or dissociative anesthetics, and dissociative anesthetics, usually combined with acepromazine or a benzodiazepine, appear to produce consistent, dose-dependent sedation in cats [42–48]. α_2-Adrenergic receptor agonists alone or in combination with ketamine have been shown to be effective following oral or buccal administration [49–52].

Behaviors associated with pain may be difficult to detect in cats. Particular attention should be given to loss of normal behavior, such as decreased appetite, decreased grooming, or decreased activity; expression of abnormal behaviors, such as inappropriate elimination, vocalization, aggression, altered facial expression, or hiding; and reaction to touch or palpation of the painful area [53]. To date, there is no pain scoring system that has been validated for use in cats; this illustrates the difficulty of assessing pain in this species, and the need to carefully observe each individual and encourage owner observation and reporting for subtle changes in behavior.

Drug metabolism in cats

It has been well documented that important metabolic differences exist between cats, dogs, and humans; dose extrapolation from these latter species to cats should therefore be undertaken with caution. In particular, the activity of UDP-glucuronosyltransferase (UGT), an enzyme involved in the conjugation of many substrates, is much lower in cats than in dogs and humans [54–57]. This results, for example, in a low rate of elimination of acetaminophen and a high potential for toxicity. The genetic cause for this low enzymatic activity has been identified; cats have a non-functional pseudogene for UGT1A6 [55]. In addition, they may also have reduced Phase I metabolism (oxidation, reduction, hydrolysis) compared to other species, due to lower activity of some hepatic cytochrome P450 (CYP) enzymes. It has recently been reported that the activities of CYP1A, CYP2C, CYP2D, CYP2E, and CYP3A were lower in feline than in canine and human hepatic microsomes; the activity of CYP2B was comparable [58]. This may contribute to the differences in drug metabolism observed in cats, compared to dogs or humans. For example, in a study on the pharmacokinetics of tramadol, the rate at which *O*-desmethyltramadol (the metabolite likely responsible for the opioid effect of tramadol) was produced appeared to be similar to that of humans deficient in CYP2D6. These same humans appear to get less pain relief from this drug than the normal 'good metabolizers' [59].

Another important example of drug metabolism species variance is found with propofol. The total body clearance of propofol was reported to be at least twice as fast in dogs as in cats [60–62]. Propofol is metabolized through glucuronidation by UGT and hydrolysis by CYP2B6 and CYP2C in humans [63]; in dogs, the rate-limiting step is reported to be CYP2B11 activity [15]. It is therefore unclear, based on the study cited above reporting similar activities of CYP2B in dogs and cats, why cats clear propofol much more slowly than dogs; in any case, the differences in metabolism of propofol may have clinical consequences, as increasing the duration of propofol infusion has been reported to significantly prolong recovery in cats [64].

Inhalant anesthetics

The anesthetic potency of inhalant anesthetics, as characterized by their minimum alveolar concentration (higher MAC values), tends to be lower in cats than in many other species, including dogs and horses [65–77]. Nitrous oxide was found to decrease the MAC of halothane but when combined with isoflurane, the effect was inconsistent [66,77]. While, to the authors' knowledge, there is no study directly comparing the effects of inhalant anesthetics in dogs and cats, clinical experience suggests that at similar anesthetic depth, blood pressure tends to be lower in cats than in dogs. Some evidence for this can be found by comparing studies in which inhalant anesthetics were administered at similar multiples of their minimum alveolar concentration in both species. Such studies show that, at moderate inhalant anesthetic concentrations, blood pressure and cardiac index are more depressed in cats than in dogs [75,78–81].

Opioids

In cats, opioids cause pupillary dilation and sometimes excitation [82]. Opioid-induced manic (excitatory) behavior is usually only seen following administration of high doses [83]. At clinical doses, opioids cause analgesia and euphoria, sometimes dysphoria [84–87]. It has been suggested that the excitatory effects of high-dose morphine may be characterized by a non-opioid receptor-mediated effect [88]. There is evidence that the manic response in cats is not necessarily linked to their action at opioid receptors *per se*, but related to the release of monoamines [83].

Opioids may have biphasic effects on the cardiovascular system in cats. At low doses, they may lower heart rate and blood pressure, while large doses increase heart rate, cardiac output, and blood pressure [82,89]. These latter effects seem to be related to increased concentrations of circulating catecholamines, and do not occur in adrenalectomized cats [82,89]. Catecholamine-induced hemodynamic effects are probably centrally induced by an effect on opioid receptors, because they are prevented by naloxone [90].

Hyperthermia following opioid administration has been reported in cats [91–94]. The effect appears dose dependent and is consistent when high doses are administered. In a retrospective clinical study, the administration of hydromorphone at doses between 0.05 and 0.1 mg/kg was strongly associated with rectal temperatures >40°C; this association was confirmed in a prospective clinical study [91,92]. In the research setting, a prospective study showed that clinically relevant doses of several opioids result in increased body temperature; however, in that study, the increase was mild to moderate and body temperature remained <40°C in most cases [93].

Opioids decrease the dose of inhalant anesthetic required to produce immobility in cats [95]. However, the magnitude of the effect appears to be smaller in cats than in some other species, the largest reduction in MAC of an inhalant anesthetic induced by an opioid being approximately 35% following administration of alfentanil to produce very high plasma concentrations (500 ng/mL) [96]. For comparison, plasma alfentanil concentrations close to half the value targeted in the cat study (223 ng/mL) reduced MAC by 68.5% in dogs [97]. While different inhalant anesthetics were used in the dog and cat studies (enflurane and isoflurane, respectively), the difference in effect suggests a large difference in potency (measured as MAC reduction) of alfentanil in the two species. The variability in MAC reduction may also be larger in cats than in dogs, as illustrated by the fact that studies on the effect of the same opioid do not consistently detect a decrease in MAC [87,98]. A recent study comparing the effects of high plasma concentrations of fentanyl, alfentanil, and sufentanil on the MAC of isoflurane in cats found significant MAC reduction only with alfentanil; the effect was antagonized by administration of naltrexone, suggesting that it is mediated by opioid receptors [99].

Non-steroidal anti-inflammatory drugs (NSAIDs)

The use of NSAIDs in cats has been reviewed [84,100,101]. These drugs are commonly used in cats for their anti-inflammatory and analgesic properties but caution is recommended, since glucuronide conjugation is a major metabolic pathway for most of these drugs [101]. The incidence of adverse effects (renal injury, hepatotoxicity, gastrointestinal ulceration, abnormal hemostasis) in cats may therefore be higher than in some other species. Nevertheless, there is favorable evidence for the short-term, perioperative use of several NSAIDs in cats, including carprofen [102–109], ketoprofen [102,105,110–112], tolfenamic acid [102,113,114], meloxicam [102,113–118], and robenacoxib [110,111,119–121]. There is less evidence regarding the safety of chronic NSAID use in cats; recommendations have been issued by a panel of experts [100]. A recent retrospective study suggested that meloxicam could be administered long term to cats at 0.02 mg/kg once daily, even if they have stable chronic kidney disease [122]. In that study, there was less progression of the kidney disease in treated cats than in untreated cats. However, it should be remembered that the repeated dosing of meloxicam is proscribed in some jurisdictions (e.g., United States).

Endotracheal intubation

Tracheal intubation of cats remains essential to the maintenance of a patent airway during anesthesia. However, anesthetists should be aware that the Confidential Enquiry into Perioperative Small Animal Fatalities found that endotracheal intubation increased the odds of anesthetic-related death in cats by approximately two-fold [123]. Previous studies had also suggested that endotracheal intubation was associated with major complications in cats [124,125]. The reasons for these findings are not entirely clear; however, they may be related to the small size of the cat's upper airway and its laryngeal responsiveness to mechanical stimulation. Laryngeal spasm can be produced in anesthetized and decerebrate cats by mechanical stimulation of the soft palate, pharynx, larynx, and trachea [126,127]. It has been recommended to desensitize the larynx with a local anesthetic prior to intubation in cats in order to decrease the incidence of laryngeal spasm; nevertheless, it is possible that improper intubation technique would be more likely to cause complications in cats than in dogs.

Tracheal avulsion or rupture and bronchial rupture have been reported in cats [128–133]. In at least 36 cases, tracheal rupture was associated with intubation. It was hypothesized that cuff overinflation, possibly in combination with multiple position changes, was the mechanism responsible for the pathology observed. Associated clinical signs were subcutaneous emphysema, coughing, gagging, dyspnea, anorexia, and fever. Surgical and/or conservative management are usually successful unless the injury extended to the carina.

Postanesthetic cortical blindness

Postanesthetic cortical blindness has been reported in cats [134,135]. According to one case series, blindness is temporary in the majority of cases. The aggressive or excessive use of mouth gags (e.g., excess tension on the jaw muscles for prolonged periods) may be a risk factor for postanesthetic blindness. The cerebral perfusion of a cat is anatomically different from that of many other species and prolonged compression or tensioning of extracalvarial structures (e.g., muscles of mastication) can cause cerebral ischemia [134]. A recent study evaluating blood flow in the maxillary artery in anesthetized cats using imaging techniques showed that the use of spring-loaded mouth gags to open the mouth maximally resulted in alterations in both blood flow and the electroretinogram in some cats [136]. The authors concluded that mechanical occlusion of blood flow through the maxillary artery during maximal opening of the mouth may contribute to the pathogenesis of postanesthetic blindness due to reduced retinal blood flow. If a mouth gag is used, it therefore appears important to avoid large opening of the mouth and/or to limit the time during which it is applied.

Fluid therapy and blood volume

The Confidential Enquiry into Perioperative Small Animal Fatalities suggested that the administration of intravenous fluids to cats during anesthesia resulted in an approximately four-fold increase in the risk of death [123]. While the reasons for this finding are not entirely clear, excessive fluid administration resulting in fluid overload was suspected to be at least partly responsible. Cats may be at higher risk of fluid overload and/or excessive dilution of blood components than dogs, particularly when large amounts of fluids are rapidly administered, because their absolute blood volume is smaller. Blood volume in cats has been reported to be 56–67 mL/kg [137–139]. Rapid fluid administration during inhalant anesthesia may also be more frequent in cats than in dogs, since blood pressure tends to be lower at similar anesthetic concentrations (see Inhalant anesthetics above). Moreover, due to their small size and a relatively high incidence of undiagnosed (subclinical) cardiomyopathy, some cats are more prone to receiving excessive fluid volumes than are individuals of many larger species. Rate of fluid administration is typically based on body weight; based on the considerations above, it may be preferable to adjust these rates based on some fraction of blood volume.

Blood groups

Three blood groups have been identified in cats: A, B, and AB [140,141]. Cats with type B blood have naturally occurring, strong hemagglutinating antibodies against type A cells, whereas cats with type A blood have naturally occurring, weak hemolyzing and hemagglutinating antibodies against type B cells [142]. Severe transfusion reactions of the anaphylactic type, with almost immediate destruction of the transfused red blood cells, are therefore commonly observed if type A blood is transfused to a cat with type B blood; cats with type A blood receiving type B blood typically only develop mild transfusion reactions [142,143]. In addition, naturally occurring antibodies against a common antigen, *Mik*, may be involved in acute hemolytic transfusion reactions following an AB-matched transfusion [144].

Prevalence of the different blood types has been reported for various geographical locations [141,145–159]. Type A blood has the highest prevalence, ranging from 62% to 99.6%; in the US, close to 100% of domestic cats are type A. The prevalence of type B blood ranges from 0.4% to 36%, the latter being reported for the Sydney area of Australia. Cats with type AB blood are rare, representing 5% or less of the feline population (less than 0.2% in North America).

Prevalence of B blood is moderate to high (15–60%) in some cat breeds, including British Shorthair, Abyssinian, Birman, Devon Rex, Himalayan, Persian, Scottish Fold, Somali, Angora, and Turkish Van, whereas it is very low (close to 0%) in other breeds, including American Shorthair, Siamese, and Norwegian Forest [149,152,160].

Dopamine and dopamine receptors

Dopamine is commonly used in anesthetized cats to treat hypotension. Within the range of clinical doses, its effect is believed to be primarily due to an increase in cardiac contractility, mediated by activation of β_1-adrenergic receptors. A study has demonstrated increases in cardiac index without significant increase in vascular resistance at doses ranging from 2.5 to 20 μg/kg/min [161]. Another, more controversial indication for low doses of dopamine is to increase renal blood flow, particularly in acute renal failure. The effect is postulated to be due to activation of dopamine D_1 receptors, causing renal vasodilation and increased renal blood flow. It is unclear whether cats would respond to dopamine in that manner. D_1-like receptors have been identified in feline kidneys but they appear different from the human and canine D_1 receptor [162]. In any case, studies in humans have failed to demonstrate benefits of low-dose dopamine in acute renal failure, and suggest that some effects may actually be detrimental to renal function [163,164]. In cats with renal failure, the use of dopamine may be indicated at doses increasing cardiac output, particularly during hypotension, rather than at doses targeting D_1 receptors.

References

1 Mahmood I. Application of allometric principles for the prediction of pharmacokinetics in human and veterinary drug development. *Adv Drug Deliv Rev* 2007; **59**: 1177–1192.

2 Krejcie TC, Avram MJ. What determines anesthetic induction dose? It's the front-end kinetics, doctor! *Anesth Analg* 1999; **89**: 541–544.

3 McGreevy PD, Thomson PC, Pride C, *et al*. Prevalence of obesity in dogs examined by Australian veterinary practices and the risk factors involved. *Vet Rec* 2005; **156**: 695–702.

4 Scarlett JM, Donoghue S, Saidla J, Wills J. Overweight cats: prevalence and risk factors. *Int J Obes Relat Metab Disord* 1994; **18**(Suppl 1): S22–28.

5 Olutoye OA, Yu X, Govindan K, *et al*. The effect of obesity on the ED(95) of propofol for loss of consciousness in children and adolescents. *Anesth Analg* 2012; **115**: 147–153.

6 Boveri S, Brearley JC, Dugdale AH. The effect of body condition on propofol requirement in dogs. *Vet Anaesth Analg* 2013; **40**: 449–454.

7 Clutton RE. The medical implications of canine obesity and their relevance to anaesthesia. *Br Vet J* 1988; **144**: 21–28.

8 Court MH. Anesthesia of the sighthound. *Clin Tech Small Anim Pract* 1999; **14**: 38–43.

9 Parker HG, Kim LV, Sutter NB, *et al*. Genetic structure of the purebred domestic dog. *Science* 2004; **304**: 1160–1164.

10 Bogan J. Factors affecting duration of thiopentone anaesthesia in dogs, with particular reference to greyhounds. *Vet Anesth Analg* 1970; **1**: 18–24.

11 Sams RA, Muir WW, Detra RL, Robinson EP. Comparative pharmacokinetics and anesthetic effects of methohexital, pentobarbital, thiamylal, and thiopental in Greyhound dogs and non-Greyhound, mixed-breed dogs. *Am J Vet Res* 1985; **46**: 1677–1683.

12 Pasloske K, Sauer B, Perkins N, Whittem T. Plasma pharmacokinetics of alfaxalone in both premedicated and unpremedicated Greyhound dogs after single, intravenous administration of Alfaxan at a clinical dose. *J Vet Pharmacol Ther* 2009; **32**: 510–513.

13 Zoran DL, Riedesel DH, Dyer DC. Pharmacokinetics of propofol in mixed-breed dogs and greyhounds. *Am J Vet Res* 1993; **54**: 755–760.

14 Sams RA, Muir WW. Effects of phenobarbital on thiopental pharmacokinetics in greyhounds. *Am J Vet Res* 1988; **49**: 245–249.

15 Hay Kraus BL, Greenblatt DJ, Venkatakrishnan K, Court MH. Evidence for propofol hydroxylation by cytochrome P4502B11 in canine liver microsomes: breed and gender differences. *Xenobiotica* 2000; **30**: 575–588.

16 Hofmeister EH, Watson V, Snyder LB, Love EJ. Validity and client use of information from the World Wide Web regarding veterinary anesthesia in dogs. *J Am Vet Med Assoc* 2008; **233**: 1860–1864.

17 Tournier N, Decleves X, Saubamea B, *et al*. Opioid transport by ATP-binding cassette transporters at the blood–brain barrier: implications for neuropsychopharmacology. *Curr Pharmaceut Design* 2011; **17**: 2829–2842.

18 Dagenais C, Graff CL, Pollack GM. Variable modulation of opioid brain uptake by P-glycoprotein in mice. *Biochem Pharmacol* 2004; **67**: 269–276.

19 Groenendaal D, Freijer J, Rosier A, *et al*. Pharmacokinetic/pharmacodynamic modelling of the EEG effects of opioids: the role of complex biophase distribution kinetics. *Eur J Pharm Sci* 2008; **34**: 149–163.

20 Brown SM, Campbell SD, Crafford A, Regina KJ, Holtzman MJ, Kharasch ED. P-glycoprotein is a major determinant of norbuprenorphine brain exposure and antinociception. *J Pharmacol Exp Ther* 2012; **343**: 53–61.

21 Popovic NA, Mullane JF, Yhap EO. Effects of acetylpromazine maleate on certain cardiorespiratory responses in dogs. *Am J Vet Res* 1972; **33**: 1819–1824.

22 Brodbelt DC, Pfeiffer DU, Young LE, Wood JL. Results of the confidential enquiry into perioperative small animal fatalities regarding risk factors for anesthetic-related death in dogs. *J Am Vet Med Assoc* 2008; **233**: 1096–104.

23 Dyson DH, Maxie G, Schnurr D. Anesthetic related morbidity and mortality in small animals. *Vet Surg* 1997; **26**: 157–158.

24 Denton TG, du Toit DF, Reece-Smith H. Reactions to Althesin in dogs. *Anaesthesia* 1980; **35**: 615–616.

25 Corbett HR. The use of Saffan in the dog. *Aust Vet Pract* 1977; **7**: 184–188.

26 Robinson EP, Faggella AM, Henry DP, Russell WL. Comparison of histamine release induced by morphine and oxymorphone administration in dogs. *Am J Vet Res* 1988; **49**: 1699–1701.

27 Flacke JW, Flacke WE, Bloor BC, *et al*. Histamine release by four narcotics: a double-blind study in humans. *Anesth Analg* 1987; **66**: 723–730.

28 Philbin DM, Moss J, Rosow CE, *et al*. Histamine release with intravenous narcotics: protective effects of H1 and H2-receptor antagonists. *Klin Wochenschr* 1982; **60**: 1056–1059.

29 De Lorenzi D, Bertoncello D, Drigo M. Bronchial abnormalities found in a consecutive series of 40 brachycephalic dogs. *J Am Vet Med Assoc* 2009; **235**: 835–840.

30 Oechtering TH, Oechtering GU, Noller C. Structural characteristics of the nose in brachycephalic dog breeds analysed by computed tomography. *Tierarztliche Praxis Ausgabe K, Kleintiere/Heimtiere* 2007; **35**: 177–187.

31 Hoareau GL, Jourdan G, Mellema M, Verwaerde P. Evaluation of arterial blood gases and arterial blood pressures in brachycephalic dogs. *J Vet Intern Med* 2012; **26**: 897–904.

32 Johnson LR, Pollard RE. Tracheal collapse and bronchomalacia in dogs: 58 cases (7 /2001–1 /2008). *J Vet Intern Med* 2010; **24**: 298–305.

33 Pardali D, Adamama-Moraitou KK, Rallis TS, Raptopoulos D, Gioulekas D. Tidal breathing flow-volume loop analysis for the diagnosis and staging of tracheal collapse in dogs. *J Vet Intern Med* 2010; **24**: 832–842.

34 White RAS, Williams JM. Tracheal collapse in the dog – is there really a role for surgery? A survey of 100 cases. *J Small Anim Pract* 1994; **35**: 191–196.

35 Adamama-Moraitou KK, Pardali D, Athanasiou LV, *et al*. Conservative management of canine tracheal collapse with stanozolol: a double blinded, placebo control clinical trial. *Int J Immunopathol Pharmacol* 2011; **24**: 111–118.

36 Briganti A, Melanie P, Portela D, *et al*. Continuous positive airway pressure administered via face mask in tranquilized dogs. *J Vet Emerg Crit Care* 2010; **20**: 503–508.

37 Sun F, Uson J, Ezquerra J, *et al*. Endotracheal stenting therapy in dogs with tracheal collapse. *Vet J* 2008; **175**: 186–193.

38 Karon BS, van Buskirk CM, Jaben EA, *et al*. Temporal sequence of major biochemical events during blood bank storage of packed red blood cells. *Blood Transfus* 2012; **10**: 453–461.

39 Maede Y, Amano Y, Nishida A, *et al*. Hereditary high-potassium erythrocytes with high Na, K-ATPase activity in Japanese shiba dogs. *Res Vet Sci* 1991; **50**: 123–125.

40 Vraets A, Lin Y, Callum JL. Transfusion-associated hyperkalemia. *Transfus Med Rev* 2011; **25**: 184–196.

41 Rodan I, Sundahl E, Carney H, *et al*. AAFP and ISFM feline-friendly handling guidelines. *J Feline Med Surg* 2011; **13**: 364–375.

42 Biermann K, Hungerbuhler S, Mischke R, Kastner SB. Sedative, cardiovascular, haematologic and biochemical effects of four different drug combinations administered intramuscularly in cats. *Vet Anaesth Analg* 2012; **39**: 137–150.

43 Selmi AL, Mendes GM, Lins BT, *et al*. Evaluation of the sedative and cardiorespiratory effects of dexmedetomidine, dexmedetomidine-butorphanol, and dexmedetomidine-ketamine in cats. *J Am Vet Med Assoc* 2003; **222**: 37–41.

44 Nagore L, Soler C, Gil L, *et al*. Sedative effects of dexmedetomidine, dexmedetomidine-pethidine and dexmedetomidine-butorphanol in cats. *J Vet Pharmacol Ther* 2013; **36(3)**: 222–228.

45 Navarrete R, Dominguez JM, del Granados M, *et al*. Sedative effects of three doses of romifidine in comparison with medetomidine in cats. *Vet Anaesth Analg* 2011; **38**: 178–185.

46 Selmi AL, Barbudo-Selmi GR, Mendes GM, *et al*. Sedative, analgesic and cardiorespiratory effects of romifidine in cats. *Vet Anaesth Analg* 2004; **31**: 195–206.

47 Ansah OB, Raekallio M, Vainio O. Comparison of three doses of dexmedetomidine with medetomidine in cats following intramuscular administration. *J Vet Pharmacol Ther* 1998; **21**: 380–387.

48 Dyson DH, Pascoe PJ, Honeyman V, Rahn JE. Comparison of the efficacy of three premedicants administered to cats. *Can Vet J* 1992; **33**: 462–464.

49 Porters N, Bosmans T, Debille M, *et al*. Sedative and antinociceptive effects of dexmedetomidine and buprenorphine after oral transmucosal or intramuscular administration in cats. *Vet Anaesth Analg* 2014; **41**(1): 90–96.

50 Santos LC, Ludders JW, Erb HN, *et al*. Sedative and cardiorespiratory effects of dexmedetomidine and buprenorphine administered to cats via oral transmucosal or intramuscular routes. *Vet Anaesth Analg* 2010; **37**: 417–424.

51 Grove DM, Ramsay EC. Sedative and physiologic effects of orally administered alpha 2-adrenoceptor agonists and ketamine in cats. *J Am Vet Med Assoc* 2000; **216**: 1929–1932.

52 Wetzel RW, Ramsay EC. Comparison of four regimens for intraoral administration of medication to induce sedation in cats prior to euthanasia. *J Am Vet Med Assoc* 1998; **213**: 243–245.

53 Hellyer P, Rodan I, Brunt J, *et al*. AAHA/AAFP pain management guidelines for dogs and cats. *J Feline Med Surg* 2007; **9**: 466–480.

54 Van Beusekom CD, Fink-Gremmels J, Schrickx JA. Comparing the glucuronidation capacity of the feline liver with substrate-specific glucuronidation in dogs. *J Vet Pharmacol Ther* 2014; **37**(1): 18–24.

55 Court MH, Greenblatt DJ. Molecular genetic basis for deficient acetaminophen glucuronidation by cats: UGT1A6 is a pseudogene, and evidence for reduced diversity of expressed hepatic UGT1A isoforms. *Pharmacogenetics* 2000; **10**: 355–369.

56 Court MH, Greenblatt DJ. Molecular basis for deficient acetaminophen glucuronidation in cats. An interspecies comparison of enzyme kinetics in liver microsomes. *Biochem Pharmacol* 1997; **53**: 1041–1047.

57 Court MH, Greenblatt DJ. Biochemical basis for deficient paracetamol glucuronidation in cats: an interspecies comparison of enzyme constraint in liver microsomes. *J Pharm Pharmacol* 1997; **49**: 446–449.

58 Van Beusekom CD, Schipper L, Fink-Gremmels J. Cytochrome P450-mediated hepatic metabolism of new fluorescent substrates in cats and dogs. *J Vet Pharmacol Ther* 2010; **33**: 519–527.

59 Pypendop BH, Ilkiw JE. Pharmacokinetics of tramadol, and its metabolite O-desmethyl-tramadol, in cats. *J Vet Pharmacol Ther* 2008; **31**: 52–59.

60 Cleale RM, Muir WW, Waselau AC, *et al.* Pharmacokinetic and pharmacodynamic evaluation of propofol administered to cats in a novel, aqueous, nano-droplet formulation or as an oil-in-water macroemulsion. *J Vet Pharmacol Ther* 2009; **32**: 436–445.

61 Hughes JM, Nolan AM. Total intravenous anesthesia in greyhounds: pharmacokinetics of propofol and fentanyl – a preliminary study. *Vet Surg* 1999; **28**: 513–524.

62 Cockshott ID, Douglas EJ, Plummer GF, Simons PJ. The pharmacokinetics of propofol in laboratory animals. *Xenobiotica* 1992; **22**: 369–375.

63 Restrepo JG, Garcia-Martin E, Martinez C, Agundez JA. Polymorphic drug metabolism in anaesthesia. *Curr Drug Metab* 2009; **10**: 236–246.

64 Pascoe PJ, Ilkiw JE, Frischmeyer KJ. The effect of the duration of propofol administration on recovery from anesthesia in cats. *Vet Anaesth Analg* 2006; **33**: 2–7.

65 Brown BR Jr, Crout JR. A comparative study of the effects of five general anesthetics on myocardial contractility. *I. Isometric conditions. Anesthesiology* 1971; **34**: 236–245.

66 Steffey EP, Gillespie JR, Berry JD, *et al.* Anesthetic potency (MAC) of nitrous oxide in the dog, cat, and stump-tail monkey. *J Appl Physiol* 1974; **36**: 530–532.

67 Drummond JC, Todd MM, Shapiro HM. Minimal alveolar concentrations for halothane, enflurane, and isoflurane in the cat. *J Am Vet Med Assoc* 1983; **182**: 1099–1101.

68 Webb AI, McMurphy RM. Effect of anticholinergic preanesthetic medicaments on the requirements of halothane for anesthesia in the cat. *Am J Vet Res* 1987; **48**: 1733–1735.

69 Steffey EP, Howland D Jr. Isoflurane potency in the dog and cat. *Am J Vet Res* 1977; **38**: 1833–1836.

70 Doi M, Yunoki H, Ikeda K. The minimum alveolar concentration of sevoflurane in cats. *J Anesth* 1988; **2**: 113–114.

71 McMurphy RM, Hodgson DS. The minimum alveolar concentration of desflurane in cats. *Vet Surg* 1995; **24**: 453–455.

72 Barter LS, Ilkiw JE, Steffey EP, *et al.* Animal dependence of inhaled anaesthetic requirements in cats. *Br J Anaesth* 2004; **92**: 275–277.

73 Pypendop BH, Ilkiw JE. The effects of intravenous lidocaine administration on the minimum alveolar concentration of isoflurane in cats. *Anesth Analg* 2005; **100**: 97–101.

74 Reid P, Pypendop BH, Ilkiw JE. The effects of intravenous gabapentin administration on the minimum alveolar concentration of isoflurane in cats. *Anesth Analg* 2010; **111**: 633–637.

75 Pypendop BH, Ilkiw JE. Hemodynamic effects of sevoflurane in cats. *Am J Vet Res* 2004; **65**: 20–25.

76 Escobar A, Pypendop BH, Siao KT, *et al.* Pharmacokinetics of dexmedetomidine administered intravenously in isoflurane-anesthetized cats. *Am J Vet Res* 2012; **73**: 285–289.

77 Imai A, Ilkiw JE, Pypendop BH, *et al.* Nitrous oxide does not consistently reduce isoflurane requirements in cats. *Vet Anaesth Analg* 2002; **29**: 98.

78 Mutoh T, Nishimura R, Kim HY, *et al.* Cardiopulmonary effects of sevoflurane, compared with halothane, enflurane, and isoflurane, in dogs. *Am J Vet Res* 1997; **58**: 885–890.

79 Grandy JL, Hodgson DS, Dunlop CI, *et al.* Cardiopulmonary effects of halothane anesthesia in cats. *Am J Vet Res* 1989; **50**: 1729–1732.

80 Hodgson DS, Dunlop CI, Chapman PL, Grandy JL. Cardiopulmonary effects of anesthesia induced and maintained with isoflurane in cats. *Am J Vet Res* 1998; **59**: 182–185.

81 McMurphy RM, Hodgson DS. Cardiopulmonary effects of desflurane in cats. *Am J Vet Res* 1996; **57**: 367–370.

82 Wallenstein MC. Biphasic effects of morphine on cardiovascular system of the cat. *Eur J Pharmacol* 1979; **59**: 253–260.

83 Dhasmana KM, Dixit KS, Jaju BP, Gupta ML. Role of central dopaminergic receptors in manic response of cats to morphine. *Psychopharmacologia* 1972; **24**: 380–383.

84 Robertson SA. Managing pain in feline patients. *Vet Clin North Am Small Anim Pract* 2008; **38**: 1267–1290.

85 Lascelles BD, Robertson SA. Antinociceptive effects of hydromorphone, butorphanol, or the combination in cats. *J Vet Intern Med* 2004; **18**: 190–195.

86 Robertson SA, Wegner K, Lascelles BD. Antinociceptive and side-effects of hydromorphone after subcutaneous administration in cats. *J Feline Med Surg* 2009; **11**: 76–81.

87 Brosnan RJ, Pypendop BH, Siao KT, Stanley SD. Effects of remifentanil on measures of anesthetic immobility and analgesia in cats. *Am J Vet Res* 2009; **70**: 1065–1071.

88 Yaksh TL, Harty GJ, Onofrio BM. High dose of spinal morphine produce a nonopiate receptor-mediated hyperesthesia: clinical and theoretic implications. *Anesthesiology* 1986; **64**: 590–597.

89 Pascoe PJ, Ilkiw JE, Fisher LD. Cardiovascular effects of equipotent isoflurane and alfentanil/isoflurane minimum alveolar concentration multiple in cats. *Am J Vet Res* 1997; **58**: 1267–1273.

90 Gaumann DM, Yaksh TL, Tyce GM, Stoddard S. Sympathetic stimulating effects of sufentanil in the cat are mediated centrally. *Neurosci Lett* 1988; **91**: 30–35.

91 Niedfeldt RL, Robertson SA. Postanesthetic hyperthermia in cats: a retrospective comparison between hydromorphone and buprenorphine. *Vet Anaesth Analg* 2006; **33**: 381–389.

92 Posner LP, Gleed RD, Erb HN, Ludders JW. Post-anesthetic hyperthermia in cats. *Vet Anaesth Analg* 2007; **34**: 40–47.

93 Posner LP, Pavuk AA, Rokshar JL, *et al.* Effects of opioids and anesthetic drugs on body temperature in cats. *Vet Anaesth Analg* 2010; **37**: 35–43.

94 Clark WG, Cumby HR. Hyperthermic responses to central and peripheral injections of morphine sulphate in the cat. *Br J Pharmacol* 1978; **63**: 65–71.

95 Ilkiw JE, Pascoe PJ, Tripp LD. Effects of morphine, butorphanol, buprenorphine, and U50488H on the minimum alveolar concentration of isoflurane in cats. *Am J Vet Res* 2002; **63**: 1198–1202.

96 Ilkiw JE, Pascoe PJ, Fisher LD. Effect of alfentanil on the minimum alveolar concentration of isoflurane in cats. *Am J Vet Res* 1997; **58**: 1274–1279.

97 Hall RI, Szlam F, Hug CC Jr. The enflurane-sparing effect of alfentanil in dogs. *Anesth Analg* 1987; **66**: 1287–1291.

98 Ferreira TH, Aguiar AJ, Valverde A, *et al.* Effect of remifentanil hydrochloride administered via constant rate infusion on the minimum alveolar concentration of isoflurane in cats. *Am J Vet Res* 2009; **70**: 581–588.

99 Brosnan RJ, Pypendop BH. Personal communication.

100 Sparkes AH, Heiene R, Lascelles BD, *et al.* ISFM and AAFP consensus guidelines: long-term use of NSAIDs in cats. *J Feline Med Surg* 2010; **12**: 521–538.

101 Lascelles BD, Court MH, Hardie EM, Robertson SA. Nonsteroidal anti-inflammatory drugs in cats: a review. *Vet Anaesth Analg* 2007; **34**: 228–250.

102 Slingsby LS, Waterman-Pearson AE. Postoperative analgesia in the cat after ovariohysterectomy by use of carprofen, ketoprofen, meloxicam or tolfenamic acid. *J Small Anim Pract* 2000; **41**: 447–450.

103 Polson S, Taylor PM, Yates D. Analgesia after feline ovariohysterectomy under midazolam-medetomidine-ketamine anaesthesia with buprenorphine or butorphanol, and carprofen or meloxicam: a prospective, randomised clinical trial. *J Feline Med Surg* 2012; **14**: 553–559.

104 Taylor PM, Steagall PV, Dixon MJ, *et al.* Carprofen and buprenorphine prevent hyperalgesia in a model of inflammatory pain in cats. *Res Vet Sci* 2007; **83**: 369–375.

105 Tobias KM, Harvey RC, Byarlay JM. A comparison of four methods of analgesia in cats following ovariohysterectomy. *Vet Anaesth Analg* 2006; **33**: 390–398.

106 Mollenhoff A, Nolte I, Kramer S. Anti-nociceptive efficacy of carprofen, levomethadone and buprenorphine for pain relief in cats following major orthopaedic surgery. *J Vet Med A Physiol Pathol Clin Med* 2005; **52**: 186–198.

107 Al-Gizawiy MM, Rude E. Comparison of preoperative carprofen and postoperative butorphanol as postsurgical analgesics in cats undergoing ovariohysterectomy. *Vet Anaesth Analg* 2004; **31**: 164–174.

108 Balmer TV, Irvine D, Jones RS, *et al.* Comparison of carprofen and pethidine as postoperative analgesics in the cat. *J Small Anim Pract* 1998; **39**: 158–164.

109 Lascelles BD, Cripps P, Mirchandani S, Waterman AE. Carprofen as an analgesic for postoperative pain in cats: dose titration and assessment of efficacy in comparison to pethidine hydrochloride. *J Small Anim Pract* 1995; **36**: 535–541.

110 Sano T, King JN, Seewald W, *et al.* Comparison of oral robenacoxib and ketoprofen for the treatment of acute pain and inflammation associated with musculoskeletal disorders in cats: a randomised clinical trial. *Vet J* 2012; **193**: 397–403.

111 Giraudel JM, Gruet P, Alexander DG, *et al.* Evaluation of orally administered robenacoxib versus ketoprofen for treatment of acute pain and inflammation associated with musculoskeletal disorders in cats. *Am J Vet Res* 2010; **71**: 710–719.

112 Morton CM, Grant D, Johnston L, *et al.* Clinical evaluation of meloxicam versus ketoprofen in cats suffering from painful acute locomotor disorders. *J Feline Med Surg* 2011; **13**: 237–243.

113 Murison PJ, Tacke S, Wondratschek C, *et al.* Postoperative analgesic efficacy of meloxicam compared to tolfenamic acid in cats undergoing orthopaedic surgery. *J Small Anim Pract* 2010; **51**: 526–532.

114 Benito-de-la-Vibora J, Lascelles BD, Garcia-Fernandez P, *et al.* Efficacy of tolfenamic acid and meloxicam in the control of postoperative pain following ovariohysterectomy in the cat. *Vet Anaesth Analg* 2008; **35**: 501–510.

115 Ingwersen W, Fox R, Cunningham G, Winhall M. Efficacy and safety of 3 versus 5 days of meloxicam as an analgesic for feline onychectomy and sterilization. *Can Vet J* 2012; **53**: 257–264.

116 Gassel AD, Tobias KM, Egger CM, Rohrbach BW. Comparison of oral and subcutaneous administration of buprenorphine and meloxicam for preemptive analgesia in cats undergoing ovariohysterectomy. *J Am Vet Med Assoc* 2005; **227**: 1937–1944.

117 Carroll GL, Howe LB, Peterson KD. Analgesic efficacy of preoperative administration of meloxicam or butorphanol in onychectomized cats. *J Am Vet Med Assoc* 2005; **226**: 913–919.

118 Slingsby LS, Waterman-Pearson AE. Comparison between meloxicam and carprofen for postoperative analgesia after feline ovariohysterectomy. *J Small Anim Pract* 2002; **43**: 286–289.
119 Kamata M, King JN, Seewald W, *et al.* Comparison of injectable robenacoxib versus meloxicam for peri-operative use in cats: results of a randomised clinical trial. *Vet J* 2012; **193**: 114–118.
120 Pelligand L, King JN, Toutain PL, *et al.* Pharmacokinetic/pharmacodynamic modelling of robenacoxib in a feline tissue cage model of inflammation. *J Vet Pharmacol Ther* 2012; **35**: 19–32.
121 Giraudel JM, King JN, Jeunesse EC, *et al.* Use of a pharmacokinetic/pharmacodynamic approach in the cat to determine a dosage regimen for the COX-2 selective drug robenacoxib. *J Vet Pharmacol Ther* 2009; **32**: 18–30.
122 Gowan RA, Lingard AE, Johnston L, *et al.* Retrospective case-control study of the effects of long-term dosing with meloxicam on renal function in aged cats with degenerative joint disease. *J Feline Med Surg* 2011; **13**: 752–761.
123 Brodbelt DC, Pfeiffer DU, Young LE, Wood JL. Risk factors for anaesthetic-related death in cats: results from the confidential enquiry into perioperative small animal fatalities (CEPSAF). *Br J Anaesth* 2007; **99**: 617–623.
124 Dyson DH, Maxie MG, Schnurr D. Morbidity and mortality associated with anesthetic management in small animal veterinary practice in Ontario. *J Am Anim Hosp Assoc* 1998; **34**: 325–335.
125 Clarke KW, Hall LW. A survey of anaesthesia in small animal practice: AVA/BSAVA report. *J Assoc Vet Anaesth GB Ireland* 1990; **17**: 4–10.
126 Rex MA. Laryngospasm and respiratory changes in the cat produced by mechanical stimulation of the pharynx and respiratory tract: problems of intubation in the cat. *Br J Anaesth* 1971; **43**: 54–57.
127 Rex MA. A review of the structural and functional basis of laryngospasm and a discussion of the nerve pathways involved in the reflex and its clinical significance in man and animals. *Br J Anaesth* 1970; **42**: 891–899.
128 White RN, Oakley MR. Left principal bronchus rupture in a cat. *J Small Anim Pract* 2001; **42**: 495–498.
129 White RN, Burton CA. Surgical management of intrathoracic tracheal avulsion in cats: long-term results in 9 consecutive cases. *Vet Surg* 2000; **29**: 430–435.
130 Mitchell SL, McCarthy R, Rudloff E, Pernell RT. Tracheal rupture associated with intubation in cats: 20 cases (1996–1998). *J Am Vet Med Assoc* 2000; **216**: 1592–1595.
131 Hardie EM, Spodnick GJ, Gilson SD, *et al.* Tracheal rupture in cats: 16 cases (1983–1998). *J Am Vet Med Assoc* 1999; **214**: 508–512.
132 White RN, Milner HR. Intrathoracic tracheal avulsion in three cats. *J Small Anim Pract* 1995; **36**: 343–347.
133 Lawrence DT, Lang J, Culvenor J, *et al.* Intrathoracic tracheal rupture. *J Feline Med Surg* 1999; **1**: 43–51.
134 Stiles J, Weil AB, Packer RA, Lantz GC. Post-anesthetic cortical blindness in cats: twenty cases. *Vet J* 2012; **193**: 367–373.
135 Jurk IR, Thibodeau MS, Whitney K, *et al.* Acute vision loss after general anesthesia in a cat. *Vet Ophthalmol* 2001; **4**: 155–158.
136 Barton-Lamb A, Martin-Flores M, Ludders J, *et al.* Evaluation of maxillary arterial flow in cats with and without use of a spring loaded dental mouth gag. International Veterinary Emergency and Critical Care Symposiumm, 2012; San Antonio, TX.
137 Breznock EM, Strack D. Effects of the spleen, epinephrine, and splenectomy on determination of blood volume in cats. *Am J Vet Res* 1982; **43**: 2062–2066.
138 Breznock EM, Strack D. Blood volume of nonsplenectomized and splenectomized cats before and after acute hemorrhage. *Am J Vet Res* 1982; **43**: 1811–1814.
139 Spink RR, Malvin RL, Cohen BJ. Determination of erythrocyte half life and blood volume in cats. *Am J Vet Res* 1966; **27**: 1041–1043.
140 Eyquem A, Podliachouk L, Millot P. Blood groups in chimpanzees, horses, sheep, pigs, and other mammals. *Ann N Y Acad Sci* 1962; **97**: 320–328.
141 Griot-Wenk ME, Callan MB, Casal ML, *et al.* Blood type AB in the feline AB blood group system. *Am J Vet Res* 1996; **57**: 1438–1442.
142 Giger U, Bucheler J. Transfusion of type-A and type-B blood to cats. *J Am Vet Med Assoc* 1991; **198**: 411–418.
143 Lanevschi A, Wardrop KJ. Principles of transfusion medicine in small animals. *Can Vet J* 2001; **42**: 447–454.
144 Weinstein NM, Blais MC, Harris K, *et al.* A newly recognized blood group in domestic shorthair cats: the Mik red cell antigen. *J Vet Intern Med* 2007; **21**: 287–292.
145 Bagdi N, Magdus M, Leidinger E, *et al.* Frequencies of feline blood types in Hungary. *Acta Vet Hung* 2001; **49**: 369–375.
146 Medeiros MA, Soares AM, Alviano DS, *et al.* Frequencies of feline blood types in the Rio de Janeiro area of Brazil. *Vet Clin Pathol* 2008; **37**: 272–276.
147 Giger U, Kilrain CG, Filippich LJ, Bell K. Frequencies of feline blood groups in the United States. *J Am Vet Med Assoc* 1989; **195**: 1230–1232.
148 Zheng L, Zhong Y, Shi Z, Giger U. Frequencies of blood types A, B, and AB in non-pedigree domestic cats in Beijing. *Vet Clin Pathol* 2011; **40**: 513–517.
149 Giger U, Bucheler J, Patterson DF. Frequency and inheritance of A and B blood types in feline breeds of the United States. *J Hered* 1991; **82**: 15–20.
150 Hubler M, Arnold S, Casal M, *et al.* The blood group distribution in domestic cats in Switzerland. *Schweiz Arch Tierheilkd* 1993; **135**: 231–235.
151 Jensen AL, Olesen AB, Arnbjerg J. Distribution of feline blood types detected in the Copenhagen area of Denmark. *Acta Vet Scand* 1994; **35**: 121–124.
152 Knottenbelt CM, Addie DD, Day MJ, Mackin AJ. Determination of the prevalence of feline blood types in the UK. *J Small Anim Pract* 1999; **40**: 115–118.
153 Mylonakis ME, Koutinas AF, Saridomichelakis M, *et al.* Determination of the prevalence of blood types in the non-pedigree feline population in Greece. *Vet Rec* 2001; **149**: 213–214.
154 Ruiz de Gopegui R, Velasquez M, Espada Y. Survey of feline blood types in the Barcelona area of Spain. *Vet Rec* 2004; **154**: 794–795.
155 Silvestre-Ferreira AC, Pastor J, Sousa AP, *et al.* Blood types in the non-pedigree cat population of Gran Canaria. *Vet Rec* 2004; **155**: 778–779.
156 Malik R, Griffin DL, White JD, *et al.* The prevalence of feline A/B blood types in the Sydney region. *Aust Vet J* 2005; **83**: 38–44.
157 Arikan S, Gurkan M, Ozaytekin E, *et al.* Frequencies of blood type A, B and AB in non-pedigree domestic cats in Turkey. *J Small Anim Pract* 2006; **47**: 10–13.
158 Forcada Y, Guitian J, Gibson G. Frequencies of feline blood types at a referral hospital in the south east of England. *J Small Anim Pract* 2007; **48**: 570–573.
159 Marques C, Ferreira M, Gomes JF, *et al.* Frequency of blood type A, B, and AB in 515 domestic shorthair cats from the Lisbon area. *Vet Clin Pathol* 2011; **40**: 185–187.
160 Arikan S, Duru SY, Gurkan M, *et al.* Blood type A and B frequencies in Turkish Van and Angora cats in Turkey. *J Vet Med A Physiol Pathol Clin Med* 2003; **50**: 303–306.
161 Pascoe PJ, Ilkiw JE, Pypendop BH. Effects of increasing infusion rates of dopamine, dobutamine, epinephrine, and phenylephrine in healthy anesthetized cats. *Am J Vet Res* 2006; **67**: 1491–1499.
162 Flournoy WS, Wohl JS, Albrecht-Schmitt TJ, Schwartz DD. Pharmacologic identification of putative D1 dopamine receptors in feline kidneys. *J Vet Pharmacol Ther* 2003; **26**: 283–290.
163 Jones D, Bellomo R. Renal-dose dopamine: from hypothesis to paradigm to dogma to myth and, finally, superstition? *J Intensive Care Med* 2005; **20**: 199–211.
164 Schenarts PJ, Sagraves SG, Bard MR, *et al.* Low-dose dopamine: a physiologically based review. *Curr Surg* 2006; **63**: 219–225.
165 Davidson IW, Parker JC, Beliles RP. Biological basis for extrapolation across mammalian species. *Regul Toxicol Pharmacol* 1986; **6**: 211–237.
166 Adolph EF. Quantitative relations in the physiological constitutions of mammals. *Science* 1949; **109**: 579–585.
167 Boxenbaum H. Interspecies variation in liver weight, hepatic blood flow, and antipyrine intrinsic clearance: extrapolation of data to benzodiazepines and phenytoin. *J Pharmacokinet Biopharmaceut* 1980; **8**: 165–176.
168 Bronson RT. Brain weight-body weight scaling in breeds of dogs and cats. *Brain Behav Evol* 1979; **16**: 227–236.

36 Anesthesia and Pain Management of Shelter Populations

Andrea L. Looney
Massachusetts Veterinary Referral Hospital, IVG Hospitals,Woburn, Massachusetts, USA

Chapter contents

Introduction

Animals in shelters require sedation, anesthesia, and pain management for basic surgery, animal handling, and preservation of quality of life (QOL). Guidelines for shelter animal care have been written using the Five Freedoms for Animal Welfare as a basis [1]. Guidelines for high-volume surgery have also been developed [2]. A number of resources [3] provide recommendations for the care of patients within a shelter environment (Box 36.1). Various strategies to improve anesthetic care which are standard in private veterinary practice have been resisted in shelters out of concern that they will result in fewer surgical sterilizations and increased euthanasia of unwanted offspring. As such, most shelter anesthesia techniques are a compromise, accepting a higher morbidity/mortality rate.

Perioperative risk

A multicenter veterinary practice (not including shelters) study of anesthetic complications has reported the risk of anesthetic death is approximately 0.17% in dogs and 0.24% in cats [4]. Comparable rates of human anesthetic-related death range from 0.001% to 0.05% [5]. Shelter-related morbidity and mortality rates are slightly higher, with rates of 0.04–0.4% being reported by some groups. Animals that are feral, defensive, and stressed often mask illnesses and poor health, resulting in higher anesthetic risk than what a cursory physical exam and assignment of an American Society of Anesthesiologists (ASA) physical status might suggest. One cause of significant mortality that has been identified in shelters is failure to monitor and manage patient oxygenation (especially in cats) following sedation or intramuscular induction of anesthesia. Other causes include underlying occult cardiac disease and parasitism-related lung pathology [6]. These results suggest that placing heavily sedated/anesthetized animals in an area where close monitoring of breathing and oxygenation is available could significantly reduce shelter mortality.

Anesthetic and pain management considerations

Anesthetic protocols are often tailored to the specific shelter setting based on finances, staff numbers and training level, patient numbers, species, types of surgery, and available facilities. Perianesthetic practices in shelter medicine can often be improved through education, adherence to common basic perioperative care and safety principles, and outcomes analysis.

Protocols typically try to achieve rapid onset, consistency, and reversibility. Because there are so many different scenarios in shelter medicine, the basics of solid perioperative care, knowledge of drugs and consistency of their use, proper patient selection, troubleshooting and problem solving, objective monitoring, and outcomes assessment all help dictate the success of anesthesia/pain management more than does choice of a specific drug protocol.

Anesthetic plan

A licensed veterinarian should be responsible for performing a physical exam on the patient, determining the health status or problem list, and formulating a plan. Due to the large number of procedures in some shelters, anesthesia is often performed following a standard operating procedure based on physical status rather than

Veterinary Anesthesia and Analgesia: The Fifth Edition of Lumb and Jones.
Edited by Kurt A. Grimm, Leigh A. Lamont, William J. Tranquilli, Stephen A. Greene and Sheilah A. Robertson.

Box 36.1 Websites oriented to improvement of shelter animal medicine.

www.sheltervet.org
www.aspcapro.org
www.maddiesfund.org
www.sheltermedicine.com
www.sheltermedicine.vetmed.ufl.edu

being tailored to the individual patient. The standard anesthetic plan may be unalterable by staff; therefore, patient screening and selection for surgery and anesthesia are critical.

Most patients in a shelter will undergo sterilization; however, an increasing number undergo anesthesia for fracture repair, abdominal surgery, cystotomy, dental surgery, and mass removal in an attempt to increase adoptability. Factors to be considered when determining patient acceptance for anesthesia include the availability of referral to a more suitable facility, age, weight, health status, and overall anesthetic risk.

Client-owned pets (already adopted) are usually scheduled for surgery at 4 months of age (or older) to allow time for development of immunity following vaccination. In a shelter or trap-neuter-release (TNR) program, patients can be of any age, but sterilization prior to sexual maturity is ideal to prevent future births [7–10]. In adoption settings, immature animals generally undergo spay/neuter surgeries prior to adoption in order to ensure owner compliance for sterilization with the understanding that sexually intact animals have an increased risk of owner relinquishment [11–14]. Most high-volume spay neuter venues allow surgery on animals as early as 6 weeks of age that weigh more than 0.5–1 kg; however, body condition and physical exam should also be considered.

History about patient health which is readily available in a private practice (e.g., coughing sneezing, vomiting, diarrhea, prior vaccines, and illness) may not be available for shelter patients. When available, standardized intake forms can expedite history taking, and dictate whether individual patient risk assessment should be more thoroughly discussed. Client, guardian, caretaker or trapper consent to anesthesia and surgery should acknowledge the physical state of the animal (ASA class), risks inherent in anesthesia, and continued need for supervision and care postoperatively.

Patient factors

Patient selection for anesthesia has a default category that unless life-threatening illness is present (especially that related to cardiac, pulmonary or nervous systems), the animal will be anesthetized. Veterinarians must weigh the risks and benefits of anesthesia in patients with medical conditions such as upper respiratory infection, parasite infestation, endometritis, estrus, and heartworm disease. While some conditions may increase anesthetic risk, the benefits to society of surgical sterilization may outweigh any individual patient's risk of death or complications [15].

For higher risk patients, the owner/caretaker/trapper should be consulted. They should have the opportunity to consider adverse outcomes. In the case of non-elective surgery on higher ASA status patients, the doctor on duty (along with the custodian of the patient if known or present) must consent after considering the following.

1 Will surgery result in increased chance of adoptability?
2 What will be the public's perception of the disease, the surgery, and aftercare?
3 Can the anesthesia protocol be manipulated (dosage or agents changed) to improve safety?
4 If the protocol is modified, how will this affect 'work flow' (number of animals sterilized that day)?
5 What will be the required aftercare, especially for TNR patients, or need for hospitalization?

Physical status is clearly linked to anesthetic outcome Poor health when undergoing anesthesia and surgery is associated with increased probability of anesthetic death [16]. A recent study concluded that efforts must be directed towards patient evaluation and preanesthetic improvement of patient condition.

Patient examination

All patients should be screened thoroughly, yet as efficiently as possible. Further work-up of problems identified in the physical exam may not be possible given the time, finances, or staff available. However, a complete evaluation of preoperative patient condition (e.g., bloodwork, radiographs, ultrasound, echocardiogram) should be made if possible.

The physical examination should be performed by the veterinarian performing the surgery, or by trained staff with the veterinarian's oversight. A baseline pain and anxiety score should be recorded. This score can be a simple subjective visual analogue scale with 0 = no pain to 5 = very painful, and 0 = no anxiety to 5 = very anxious. The exam should be attempted prior to anesthesia, although anxiety, aggression or feral behavior may often prevent safe handling of unsedated patients. In these cases the decision about whether a physical examination is performed prior to or after drug administration should be at the discretion of the veterinarian.

Body weight should be determined as close to the time of surgery as possible to facilitate accurate dosing. An accurate weight is especially important for pediatric, neonatal, and exotic animals, all of whom can have significant increases or decreases in weight within hours. A scale with acceptable accuracy (e.g., gram, mail, or exotics scale) should be utilized for patients under 1 kg. A scale accurate to the 1/10th kg should be utilized for patients under 5 kg. When weighing is not feasible (e.g., intractable or feral animals) body weight should be estimated carefully.

Shelter animals are often grouped according to approximate weights or weight categories rather than dosed specifically on a per kilogram or pound dose. In many shelters this is considered acceptable for selecting anesthesia drug dosages, volumes, breathing circuits, and even need for perioperative fluids, supplemental heat, and dextrose administration. However, it should be remembered that small errors are of large significance when patient weights are low.

Body condition score assessment is important since obesity may impair ventilation during anesthesia and recovery [17]. Extreme body condition scores suggest that changes in drug dosages (including inhalants, fluids, temperature control) may be required and predict procedural difficulties.

Laboratory test selection should be based on findings of a thorough physical exam and history. A European study concluded that many abnormalities revealed by routine preoperative screening were usually of little clinical relevance and did not prompt major changes to the anesthetic technique [18]. In 84% of dogs, blood work was considered unnecessary or did not change anesthetic management. Of the remaining 16%, surgery in less than 1% of the cases would have been postponed, additional perioperative therapy would have been provided in 5% of the cases, and anesthesia protocol altered in 0.2%. The authors concluded that in dogs, routine preanesthetic lab work is unlikely to yield additional information relative to perioperative care or anesthesia drugs/techniques utilized.

These results certainly do not imply that preanesthesia testing in the shelter is not worthwhile. Blood work results frequently will not deter surgery but do allow modification of anesthetic protocol and prompt vigilant monitoring under anesthesia. Postoperatively, biochemical testing may identify those individuals at risk of organ failure and those in need of further care [19].

Available point-of-care testing (POCT) devices require minimal samples of blood to perform rapid biochemical analyses and make screening of shelter patients feasible. Alternatively, inexpensive minimum database tests such as packed cell volume (PCV), total solids, blood urea nitrogen, glucose (also known as the quick assessment tests or QATS), and urine specific gravity can be performed. Age, health status, and disease potential should dictate necessity of preoperative testing [18,20,21].

Patient preparation

Postponing surgery and stabilization of hydration status, nitrogen balance, oxygenation, electrolyte status, glucose control, blood cell counts, and central nervous system integrity will reduce morbidity and mortality and assist fluid and airway management, monitoring, and temperature control (Box 36.2). Subclinical dehydration is common in the shelter population, especially if animals are housed for more than 1–2 days prior to surgery. Preoperative fasting for dogs and cats is ideal, but withholding water prior to surgery is not usually necessary or recommended. Prolonged fasting for greater than 4–6h is not warranted, especially for pediatric or very small patients [22–25]. Prolonged fasting increases the chance of perioperative regurgitation, and postoperative renal, myocardial, and thromboembolic disease [24–26]. Pediatric animals should not be fasted for more than 2h prior to surgery. Exceptions for preoperative fasting may be made for feral cats in traps due to the safety risk of removing uneaten bait (27–31).

Some shelter animals are at risk of hypoglycemia (e.g., sick, parasitized, poor body condition, elderly, recently postweaning females, and those animals undergoing prolonged capture, restraint, stress, and fasting). If blood glucose testing is unavailable, oral transmucosal administration of 50% dextrose (0.5mL/10kg), dextrose-containing corn syrup, or molasses is advocated. If intravenous fluids are given, supplementation with 1–2.5% dextrose will similarly improve blood glucose [32].

Pediatric littermates or housemates may benefit from being housed together. Intractable or feral animals should be housed in traps or other enclosures to allow for the administration of anesthetic drugs without extensive handling and to minimize stress on the animal. These animals should be removed for surgery only after sedation and returned to the holding enclosure dependent on safety for human interaction or when considered adequately recovered. If possible, the most anxious/aggressive animals should be afforded a cool-down period prior to their anesthesia or, at a minimum, should be separated from other preanesthetic patients to avoid pheromone and other inhalant or visual stimuli, all of which are not conducive to sedation and anesthesia. Owned animals entering the shelter for surgery should be housed separately to minimize the risk of spreading infectious disease.

Box 36.2 Common conditions for which stabilization prior to anesthesia is critical.

1 Extreme stress and overhandling
2 Trauma
3 Extreme dermatologic conditions
4 Starvation
5 Severe dehydration
6 Known intestinal or urinary obstruction
7 Malnourishment or starvation
8 Severe parasitism
9 Toxicity
10 Life-threatening respiratory disease

Pediatric considerations

Elective surgery, particularly ovariohysterectomy and neutering, of pediatric dogs and cats (between 8 and 16 weeks of age) is supported by the American Veterinary Medical Association and is becoming increasingly common. With short surgery times the incidence of intra- and postoperative complications is low. Anesthetic recovery and healing time are also shorter [27,30,31,33].

Spay or neuter surgery can be performed on puppies and kittens at 5–6 weeks of age if weighing at least 1kg. Historically, pediatric surgery has focused on adverse physiologic effects such as obesity, stunted growth, musculoskeletal disorders, perivulvar dermatitis, puppy vaginitis, feline lower urinary tract disorder, and urinary incontinence. However, most of these fears appear to be unfounded [34–36]. Effects on development of other diseases (e.g., cancer) are still being debated.

Minimal preoperative waiting periods and stress reduction, including the allowance of litter play and nursing/feeding 1–2h before anesthesia, are routinely allowed in shelter situations. Accurate weighing immediately prior to induction, minimal fasting and premedication, judicious use of anticholinergics, and body heat support beginning at premedication are recommended. Surgical preparation includes adequate but not excessive surgical clipping, minimal use of alcohol to avoid hypothermia, and use of table covers to avoid chilling. Careful and cautious tissue handling, minimal surgical incision length, and fast surgical time lessen the impact of anesthesia and surgery [28,29,33].

Anesthesia equipment

Non-rebreathing systems rely on relatively high fresh gas flows to remove carbon dioxide. Most non-rebreathing circuits require 150–300mL/kg/min gas flows and as such, work best on patients under 3kg. Rebreathing circuits work for patients larger than 3kg, often existing in pediatric and adult diameters, and require oxygen flows of only 5–30mL/kg/min depending on their semi-closed/semi-open system configuration [37]. Pediatric rebreathing circuits can be used for patients as small as 1kg as long as tidal volume is sufficient to actuate the unidirectional valves. Non-rebreathing circuits are often bulkier, clumsier, and provide more points of error in attachment and integrity than do rebreathing circuits, particularly if caseload is heavy or staff are less experienced.

Carbon dioxide absorbents usually require changing in shelter populations once to twice a week depending on number of patients using the machine, size, and oxygen flow rates. Activated charcoal waste gas scavenging canisters are not recommended for use in shelter or elective high-volume/spay neuter operations due to the short useful life of the system. Lifespan typically ranges from 3 to 6h total (not per day) per canister. Exhaustion of the canister is indicated by increased weight as indicated on each canister [37,38]. Active scavenging systems rely on extractor fans or hospital vacuum systems to remove waste gases and are very efficient and cost-effective in the long run.

Standard procedures for controlling potential infectious disease spread via anesthesia equipment should be practiced [39,40]. In particular, shelter programs should include the following.

1 Staff should wash their hands or sanitize between patients and litters [41,42].
2 Examination surfaces and physical exam equipment should be cleaned and disinfected between patients using agents known to be effective against common pathogens [43,44].
3 All anesthesia equipment that has direct patient contact (e.g., endotracheal tubes, laryngoscope blades, pulse oximeter clips, esophageal stethoscope, thermometer, etc.) should be thoroughly cleaned in very mild soap and water, rinsed thoroughly, dried, and disinfected between patients [45].
4 A hot water and dilute soap cleaning and rinsing should be performed on all circuits and tracheal tubes prior to soaking in diluted chlorohexidene acetate (1:30 or greater dilution). Following the soaking, it is critical to rinse all circuits and tracheal tubes with water to avoid disinfectant residues known to elicit laryngospasm or tracheal necrosis. Breathing circuits (non- and rebreathing both) should be thoroughly cleaned, disinfected, rinsed and dried 1–2 times per week at minimum.
5 Drying (utilizing forced air or warm non-moist environments) of both circuits and tracheal tubes is highly recommended to avoid mold contamination. Blow dryers and forced hot air can assist with gross removal of moisture; these methods can, however, easily dry and make friable soft endotracheal tubes and cuffs, capable of injuring patients.
6 Endotracheal tube cuffs should be inflated during the processes of cleaning and drying. Examine all cuffs daily, rinse carefully, and not aggressively deflate (this forms rough cuff edges). Endotracheal tube cuffs should be deflated prior to insertion [46].
7 Laryngoscope blades, breathing circuits, endotracheal tubes, and bottle or tube cleaning brushes should be ideally divided into 2–4 'sets' and color or number coded accordingly. Sets should be rotated through weekly-biweekly uses. Ideally, the set that is utilized for each patient should be noted on the anesthesia record. If a hospital or shelter infection is suspected, color or number coding can assist in identifying possibly contaminated blades, tubes, breathing circuits, and brushes, and patient contact can be traced from the records [47].
8 Due to antimicrobial effects of CO_2 absorbers, patients rarely contaminate internal parts of the machine with bacteria. However, mold contamination is possible and as such, anesthesia machine unidirectional valves and domes as well as absorbent canisters should be disassembled, cleaned with mild detergent, wiped with alcohol, then left open to dry [45].
9 Regular culturing of breathing circuits, absorbent canisters, and rebreathing bags should be performed for both bacterial and fungal contaminants [48,49].
10 Surgery of infected animals should follow healthy animals within the day's schedule.

Recommendations for checkout of veterinary machines have been published and are available in this and a variety of other anesthesia manuals and texts [47,50]. Frequency and timing of checklist usage will depend on surgical caseload, technician availability, and experience. Daily or minimal weekly equipment checklists do not take the place of regular vaporizer and machine servicing, which normally is performed every 2–6 months by credentialed or certified technicians [49].

Anesthetic protocols

Selecting anesthetic protocols for each shelter, feral, TNR or high-volume spay/neuter program depends on many factors, including the daily number and type of patients, the skill and efficiency of available technical assistance, the timing and competence of surgical/anesthetic technique, and financial/medicolegal considerations within the program itself. The four criteria that form the basis of safe anesthesia are:

1 analgesia
2 anxiolysis
3 immobility and muscle relaxation
4 controlled reversible depression of the central nervous system (unconsciousness and amnesia).

The ideal shelter anesthesia protocol should have an acceptable risk (safety margin) for animals of all ages. The protocol must also be economical, easy to use with a small volume for injection, have rapid onset and recovery with a reasonable duration after a single administration, be predictable, and possess perioperative analgesic properties [51,52]. Though many shelter/feral/TNR venues will utilize inhalant isoflurane or sevoflurane, just as many utilize injectable anesthetic combinations. Some shelters routinely intubate and others do not.

Dozens of anesthetic protocols have been published for elective surgery [53–61]. Protocols with acceptable risk typically utilize:

- reversible agents (opioids, benzodiazepines, and α_2-adrenergic receptor agonists)
- doses based on accurate body weight rather than dosing based on volume per cat or dog or giving a 'hub' of drug
- use of the lowest possible doses of sedative/anesthetic
- minimal anticholinergics (except very young patients), and avoid inhalant-only protocols (except where necessary due to animal handling concerns).

Although shelter anesthesia differs from private practice, in either setting success depends more on the familiarity, competence, and speed of the individuals involved (technicians and veterinarians) than on choosing drug protocols.

Drug considerations

Anesthetic and analgesic drug usage in shelters is similar to use for dogs and cats in a private practice setting, with the emphasis on simplification to avoid accidents and adverse effects. Major differences are the heavy reliance on injectable anesthetic combinations over inhalant anesthetics for simplicity, and the use of simple local anesthetic techniques and partial agonist opioids for pain control due to concerns of some programs about handling schedule II narcotics.

For most dog spay or prescrotal incisions, a combination consisting of 0.3 mg/kg bupivicaine, 1–2 mg/kg lidocaine, and 1–2 mL saline can be used. A combination of local anesthetic employed for cat spay or neuter incisions is 0.5–1 mg bupivicaine, 2–4 mg lidocaine, and 0.1–0.2 mL saline for a 3–5 kg cat. The solution can be dripped onto the closed linea alba or into the scrotal incision [62,63]. Use of topical local anesthetics requires less technical skill than subcutaneous or compartmental administration and reduces the occurrence of inadvertent vascular or peritoneal injection.

μ-Opioid receptor agonists provide analgesia but the need for federal, state, and local narcotics licensing along with concern about diversion often intimidates shelter management into using mixed agonist (buprenorphine) or agonist-antagonist (butorphanol, nalbuphine) opioids. While these agents are sometimes considered less effective, combining them with an α_2-adrenergic receptor agonist produces more intense and longer lasting analgesia [64–67].

As with any sedative/anesthetic combination, the profound sedation and relaxation that α_2-adrenergic agonists produce can result in hypoxia associated with upper airway obstruction. In shelters, multiple animals are often injected with heavy sedatives/anesthetics and then left unobserved during the onset of drug action. The loss of airway patency may result from unusual body positioning and the animal's inability to correct it when obstruction occurs. Feral mature intact male cats are particularly prone to this phenomenon, as are larger dogs (mastiffs, pit bulls) and brachycephalic breeds. Staff should be positioned to observe the induction when intramuscular administration occurs and be sure that an airway is patent in every animal [51,52].

Glycopyrrolate (0.005–0.01 mg/kg) is often included in protocols for patients that are under 6 weeks of age because their ability to alter stroke volume is limited, making cardiac output more dependent on heart rate [68,69]. Careful consideration should be given to the significant increase in cardiac workload that may occur when using α_2-adrenergic receptor agonists and anticholinergic agents together [70–74].

Injectable drug administration should be limited to intravenous and intramuscular routes, avoiding intraperitoneal and subcutaneous routes. Choice of agent is based on cost, technical skill level for administration, animal's level of consciousness following premedication, diversion potential, and typical daily schedule. Often, a single injection can reduce patient pain and stress response. Injectable combinations usually include α_2-adrenergic receptor agonists, opioids, and dissociatives [53–59].

Sevoflurane and isoflurane are the two inhalant gases most widely used in shelter environments. Inhalant anesthesia is not as commonly used as injectable anesthesia in shelter environments for many reasons. First, most shelter surgical procedures are performed very quickly, often limiting the need for prolonged anesthesia. Second, the use of anesthesia equipment such as oxygen cylinders, machines, and breathing circuits often carries higher risk of technical problems, especially given the number of surgeries performed and the hectic nature of the environment. Finally, the mobile nature of many shelter or spay/neuter venues makes dealing with large pieces of equipment difficult. Most shelter operations are moving towards total injectable (non-inhalant) regimens for premed, induction, and maintenance of anesthesia. Processing of patients (surgery, tattooing, identification, microchipping, vaccination, infectious disease testing) becomes simpler, easier, and overall more efficient. Unfortunately, the ability to carefully titrate anesthetic depth is lessened with injectable protocols.

Anesthesia for higher risk patients

Certain precautions should be taken when anesthetizing a patient with severe upper airway, nasopharyngeal disease or overt obstruction (e.g., severe upper respiratory infection in cats). These points of care are listed in Box 36.3. Heart murmurs may be auscultated and can be caused by many conditions ranging from the benign to life-threatening (e.g., excitement, congenital disease, anemia, valvular disease, thyroid disease, hypertension, cardiomyopathy, etc.). Murmurs often indicate the need to further evaluate a patient, including obtaining a better history, blood work, blood pressure measurement, radiographs, electrocardiograms, or even echocardiograms. However, in the shelter environment patients are rarely afforded a work-up beyond auscultation.

Box 36.3 Points of care for shelter patients with severe upper respiratory disease.

- Avoid undue stress or excitement perioperatively since this increases respiratory effort.
- Premedication is indicated to relieve stress unless the patient is severely dyspneic; in the case of the latter, heavy sedation may cause obstruction. As such, control of the airway via quick IV induction and intubation followed by oxygen supplementation is the best anesthetic approach. Additional medications can then be administered after induction and intubation in these cases.
- Premedication with dexmedetomidine (cats: 5–10 µg/kg and dogs 3–5 µg/kg) and opioid is often utilized in patients with upper airway disease, as sedation will frequently allow airway cleaning and easier manipulation of the mouth, larynx, and pharynx at time of intubation. However, it is important to truly watch and critically inspect these patients once they are sedated to assure airway patency with such profound and sudden sedation, particularly in large male cats with excessive jowls and redundant pharyngeal tissue.
- Anticholinergic administration is not recommended unless severe vagal tone is induced by upper respiratory negative pressure generation, because of its effects on thickening of respiratory secretions.
- Oxygen supplementation should be provided prior to induction to allow for saturation of hemoglobin in the event of apnea following administration of induction agents [63].
- If intubation is performed (recommended), liberal use of lidocaine spray on the pharynx, larynx, and arytenoids may reduce laryngospasm. Attempts to intubate should be minimized as the larynx becomes extremely irritable and prone to spasm.
- Reversal of agents is not required but recoveries should be monitored for laryngospasm and airway obstruction.
- Patients with irritable, copious soft tissue, laryngeal and pharyngeal disease (classic upper respiratory disease cat) usually fare better with earlier tracheal tube removal and close observation for reobstruction or regurgitation during recovery.
- Frequent observation of the breathing pattern, oxygenation, and ventilation status as well as endotracheal tube patency for mucus plugging and obstruction is advised. Capnography is a useful tool in these patients.

Barring kittens and puppies likely to have an innocent murmur or a congenital defect, patients are likely to have some organic diastolic or systolic dysfunction. Mature cats with murmurs or gallops may have hypertension, anemia, hypertrophic cardiomyopathy, restrictive cardiomyopathy, congenital defects, thyroid disease, or pulmonary disease. Adult dogs may have undiagnosed congenital disease, pericardial or atrial disease, heartworm disease, dilative cardiomyopathy, or valvular disease. Points of care for patients with presumptive cardiac issues are listed in Box 36.4.

Anesthetic monitoring

The determination and assessment of trends in vital parameters are critical to accurate assessment of plane of anesthesia and early detection of potentially life-threatening complications [75,76]. Regardless of what monitoring is utilized, the caregiver should be informed about level of CNS depression, circulation, oxygenation, and ventilation. A record should be kept of significant events, recognition of worrisome trends, and drugs and supportive care given.

Electrocardiography should not be used as the sole monitor in any anesthetic setting because it can demonstrate normal electrical activity in a mechanically stopped heart. Pulse oximetry allows measurement of both pulse rate and patient oxygenation status [77,78]. Blood pressure measurement can be routinely performed in shelter situations. Recent studies have shown good agreement between high-definition oscillometry, Doppler, and invasive blood

Box 36.4 Points of care for patients with presumptive cardiac disease in the shelter environment.

- If the animal is dyspneic, coughing, open mouth breathing, aerophagic, or on physical exam, has pulmonary crackles, tachy- or bradyarrythmias, has poor hind leg pulse quality, jugular pulsations and distension, reduced lung auscultation, the possibility of serious underlying disease is high. These findings should dictate that the caretaker, guardian, adopter, or owner seek further diagnostic testing prior to undergoing anesthesia and elective surgery. If the surgery must be performed regardless of lack of work-up, the following suggestions can be utilized.
- Try to avoid stress (excessive handling, heavy restraint, squeeze cage, etc.), and allow plenty of air circulation/low humidity around these patients preanesthetically. In hot environments, use of a fan frequently keeps these patients from overt aerophagia as well as decreasing panting.
- Cats with murmurs and open mouth breathing should receive a chest tap and low-dose furosemide 2 mg/kg SC or IM once sedated from their premedication.
- Dogs with murmurs should be given low-dose furosemide (1–2 mg/kg SC or IM) and walked within ½ hour prior to premedication.
- Premedication with opioid and midazolam (0.3–0.5 mg/kg, IM).
- Once sedated, oxygenation by mask and during clipping and prep is advised.
- After premedication, cats can be induced with midazolam (0.2 mg/kg IV) followed by very slow intravenous propofol (2–3 mg/kg IV) to effect for intubation.
- Following preoxygenation in dogs, induction with heavy-dose midazolam (0.5 mg/kg IV) and ketamine (2 mg/kg IV) is given to effect.
- Once intubated and placed on oxygen and inhalant, heart rate and blood pressure should be monitored.
- Fluid therapy should be minimized (2–3 mL/kg/h) if given at all.

Note: Animals with severe respiratory and/or cardiovascular disease should be carefully evaluated for adoptability. Euthanasia may be the humane choice for patients that show signs of distress or severe disease. Use of the recommended points of care is not a substitute for further diagnostic testing (standard of veterinary medical care) or referral and they should only be used as a last resort in patients with the understanding that some forms of heart disease may be adversely affected by these recommendations.

pressure measurements [79,80]. Trends of blood pressure readings in anesthetized patients can identify the need for titration of anesthetic depth or for volume support (e.g., fluid bolus). Capnography allows evaluation of circulation, ventilation, and inhalant delivery systems [81,82].

Monitored parameters should be checked and recorded regularly in each surgery. Recording intervals of 5 or 10 min are desirable. The essential point of monitoring is that vigilance and timely interpretation are required. Ideally, monitoring should also provide reliable data for judging the quality of anesthesia delivered [83,84].

Anesthesia recovery

Shepherding a smooth transition from an anesthetized state to wakeful comfort requires practiced vigilance. Successful recoveries can be measured by minimal adverse patient events and staff satisfaction. Prompt attention and communication can minimize negative consequences [84,85]. Ensuring safe, comfortable recovery environments with appropriate heat, air circulation, and minimal noise is essential [86]. Caution is advised during recovery to avoid airway restriction (via simple head malpositioning) and sudden emergence delirium with subsequent caretaker injury. It is advisable to allow recovery on flat, steady surfaces such as flooring or cages. Recovery with siblings is recommended for pediatric patients to help provide warmth and familiarity with surroundings [87].

Body temperature should be preserved with individual surface and body coverage including paper, towels or blankets [88,89]. If needed, options for supplemental heat sources include convective warming (warm air), circulating hot water blankets, and heat lamps (vigilantly monitored) [90,91]. Anesthetized and heavily sedated animals are unable to move away from excessively hot sources. Use of heat support designed specifically for anesthetized patients is strongly recommended.

To protect against hypoglycemia, pediatric, geriatric, and frail patients should be offered small amounts of food as soon as possible when mentally appropriate as determined by adequate righting and swallowing reflexes. Neonatal patients should eat as soon as reasonable following surgery [69]. Small amounts of water should be offered as soon as patients are ambulatory. Caution should be exercised with postoperative feeding of brachycephalic patients as airway obstruction is more likely in this group of animals; regurgitation happens frequently and esophageal motility may not be optimum in these patients as well.

Oxygen supplementation is especially helpful to debilitated, dehydrated, nutritionally poor or traumatized patients. Oxygen supplementation helps to reduce the risk of cellular alveolar hypoxia which can lead to tissue hypoxia [78]. Ventilation is the process whereby the body exhales or otherwise gets rid of carbon dioxide and should be closely monitored in recovering animals.

Preparation for emergencies

Standard emergency and reversal drugs must be in ample supply and easily accessible. Periodic verification and documentation of expiry dates and volumes of emergency supplies are important [92,93]. A simple emergency chart should be clearly posted or readily available to allow for the rapid determination of drug dosages [94].

Regular drills or rounds are helpful, particularly in helping staff identify true arrests versus regular anesthetic respiratory and cardiovascular depression. Training may also include equipment checks, the institution of the ABCs of CPR, record keeping for emergencies, review of difficult cases, and morbidity/mortality rounds [93]. Recent guidelines have been developed to improve outcomes associated with anesthesia and non-anesthesia-related arrest situations [95].

References

1 Association of Shelter Veterinarians. Guidelines for standards of care in animal shelters. www.sheltervet.org/about/shelter-standards/ (accessed 26 September 2014).

2 Looney AL, Bohling MW, Bushby PA, *et al.* The association of shelter veterinarians veterinary medical care guidelines for spay–neuter programs. *J Am Vet Med Assoc* 2008; **233**(1): 74–86.

3 Miller L, Zawistowski S. *Shelter Medicine for Veterinarians and Staff*, 2nd edn. Ames, IA: John Wiley and Sons, 2012.

4 Brodbelt DC, Blissit KJ, Hammond RA *et al.* The risk of death: the Confidential Enquiry into Perioperative Small Animal Fatalities. *Vet Anaesth Analg* 2008; **35**(5): 365–373.

5 Li G, Warner M, Lang B, *et al.* Epidemiology of anesthesia-related mortality in the United States, 1999–2005. *Anesthesiology* 2009; **110**(4): 759–765.

6 Gerdin JA, Slater M, Makolinski K, *et al.* Post-mortem findings in 54 cases of anesthetic associated death in cats from two spay-neuter programs in New York State. *J Fel Med Surg* 2011; **13**(12): 959–966.

7 Manning AM, Rowan AN. Companion animal demographics and sterilization status: results from a survey in four Massachusetts towns. *Anthrozoos* 1992; **3**: 192–201.

8 Alexander SA, Shane SM. Characteristics of animals adopted from an animal control center whose owners complied with a spaying/neutering program. *J Am Vet Med Assoc* 1994; **205**: 472–476.

9 New JC, Kelch WJ, Hutchison JM, *et al.* Birth and death rate estimates of cats and dogs in US households and related factors. *J Appl Anim Welf Sci* 2004; **7**: 229–241.

10 Griffin B. Prolific cats: the impact of her fertility on the welfare of the species. *Compend Contin Educ Pract Vet* 2001; **23**: 1058–1067.

11 Moulton C. Early spay/neuter: risks and benefits for shelters. *Am Hum Shoptalk* 1990; **7**: 1–6.

12 Patronek GJ, Glickman LT, Beck AM, *et al.* Risk factors for relinquishment of cats to an animal shelter. *J Am Vet Med Assoc* 1996; **209**: 582–588.

13 Scarlett JM, Salman MD, New JG, *et al.* Reasons for relinquishment of companion animals in U.S. animal shelters: selected health and personal issues. *J Appl Anim Welf Sci* 1999; **2**: 41–57.

14 Mondelli F, Previde EP, Verga M, *et al.* The bond that never developed: adoption and relinquishment of dogs in a rescue shelter. *J Appl Anim Welf Sci* 2004; **7**: 253–266.

15 Ross AF, Tinker JH. Anesthesia risk. In: Miller RD, ed. *Anesthesia*, 4th edn. New York: Churchill Livingstone, 1994; 791.

16 Bille C, Auvigne V, Libermann S, *et al.* Risk of anaesthetic mortality in dogs and cats: an observational cohort study of 3546 cases. *Vet Anaesth Analg* 2012; **39(1)**: 59–68.

17 Laflamme DP. Development and validation of a body condition score system for dogs. *Canine Pract* 1997; **22**: 10.

18 Alef M, von Praun F, Oechtering G. Is routine pre-anaesthetic haematological and biochemical screening justified in dogs? *Vet Anaesth Analg* 2008; **35(2)**: 132–140.

19 Ross AF, Tinker JH. Anesthesia risk. In: Miller RD, ed. *Anesthesia*, 4th edn. New York: Churchill Livingstone, 1994; 791.

20 Gaynor JS, Dunlop CI, Wagner AE, *et al.* Complications and mortality associated with anesthesia in dogs and cats. *J Am Anim Hosp Assoc* 1999; **35**: 13–17.

21 Bille C, Auvigne V, Libermann S, *et al.* Risk of anaesthetic mortality in dogs and cats: an observational cohort study of 3546 cases. *Vet Anaesth Analg* 2012; **39(1)**: 59–68.

22 Miller M, Wishart HY, Nimmo WS. Gastric contents at induction of anaesthesia: is a 4-hour fast even necessary? *Br J Anaesth* 1983; **55**: 1185–1188.

23 Hardy JF, Lepage Y, Bonneville-Chouinard N. Occurance of gastroesophaeal reflux on induction of anaesthesia does not correlate with the volume of gastric contents. *Can J Anaesth* 1990; **37**: 502–508.

24 Strunin L. How long should patients fast before surgery? Time for new guidelines. *Br J Anaesth* 1993; **70**: 1–3.

25 Galatos AD, Raptopoulos D. Gastro-esophageal reflux during anaesthesia in the dog: the effect of pre-operative fasting and premedication. *Vet Rec*1994; **137**: 479–483.

26 Savas I, Raptopoulos D. The effect of fasting and type of food on the gastric content volume and ph at induction of anaesthesia in the dog. Proceedings of the 6th ICVA Meeting, Thessaloniki, Greece, 1997; 114.

27 Grandy JL, Dunlop CI. Anesthesia of pups and kittens. *J Am Vet Med Assoc* 1991; **198**: 1244–1249.

28 Faggella AM, Aronsohn MG. Anesthetic techniques for neutering 6- to 14-week-old kittens. *J Am Vet Med Assoc* 1993; **202**: 56–62.

29 Faggella AM, Aronsohn MG. Evaluation of anesthetic protocols for neutering 6- to 14-week-old pups. *J Am Vet Med Assoc* 1994; **205**: 308–314.

30 Howe LM. Prepubertal gonadectomy in dogs and cats – Part I. *Compend Contin Educ Pract Vet*1999; **21**: 103–111.

31 Howe LM. Prepubertal gonadectomy in dogs and cats – Part II. *Compend Contin Educ Pract Vet*1999; **21**: 197–201.

32 Moon PF. Fluid therapy and blood transfusion. In: Seymour C, Gleed RD, eds. *Manual of Small Animal Anaesthesia and Analgesia*. Cheltenham: British Small Animal Veterianary Association, 1999; 119–121.

33 Bushby PA. Pediatric spay and neuter. Proceedings of the Western Veterinary Conference, Las Vegas, 2012. www.wvc.org (accessed 25 September 2014).

34 Root MV, Johnston S, Johnston G, *et al.* The effect of prepuberal and postpuberal gonadectomy on penile extrusion and urethral diameter in the domestic cat. *Vet Radiol Ultrasound* 1996; **37(5)**: 363–366.

35 Salmeri KR, Bloomberg M, Scruggs S, Shille V. Gonadectomy in immature dogs: effects on skeletal, physical and behavioral development. *J Am Vet Med Assoc* 1991; **198(7)**: 1193–1203.

36 Stubbs WP, Bloomberg M, Scruggs S, *et al.* Prepubertal gonadectomy in the domestic feline: effects on skeletal, physical and behavioral development. *Vet Surg* 1993; **22**: 568–572.

37 Ludders JW, Stafford KL. Basic equipment for small animal anesthesia; use and maintenance, part II. *Compend Contin Educ Pract Vet* 1991; **12(1)**: 35–40.

38 Clutton RE. Anaesthetic equipment. In: Seymour C, Gleed RD, eds. *Manual of Small Animal Anaesthesia and Analgesia*. Cheltenham: British Small Animal Veterianary Association, 1999; 37–38.

39 McKelvey D, Hollingshead KW. *Small Animal Anesthesia and Analgesia*. St Louis, MO: Mosby, 2000.

40 Dorsch JA, Dorsch SE. Cleaning and sterilization. In: Dorsch JA, Dorsch SE, eds. *Understanding Anesthesia Equipment*, 4th edn. Baltimore, MD: Williams and Wilkins, 1999; 969–1013.

41 Bryce EA, Spencer D, Roberts FJ. An in-use evaluation of an alcohol-based pre-surgical hand disinfectant. *Infect Control Hosp Epidemiol* 2001; **22**: 635–639.

42 Knecht CD, Allen AR, Williams DJ, Johnson JH. Operating room conduct. In: Knecht CD, Allen AR, Williams DJ, Johnson JH, eds. *Fundamental Techniques in Veterinary Surgery*, 3rd edn. Philadelphia: WB Saunders, 1987; 74–103.

43 AORN. Recommended practices for sterilization in the perioperative practice setting association of operating room. *Nurses J* 2006; **83(3)**: 700–722.

44 Fossum TW. Sterilization and disinfection. In: Fossum TW, ed. *Small Animal Surgery*, 3rd edn. St Louis, MO: Mosby, 2007; 9–14.

45 George RH. A critical look at chemical disinfection of anaesthetic apparatus. *Br J Anaesth* 1975; **47**: 719–722.

46 Day TK. Endotracheal tubes and ancillary equipment for intubation. *Semin Vet Med Surg (Small Anim)* 1993; **8(2)**: 115–118.

47 Muir WW. Anesthesia machines and breathing systems. In: Muir WW, Hubbell JAE, Skarda RT, eds. *Handbook of Veterinary Anesthesia*, 3rd edn. St Louis, MO: Mosby, 2000; 210–229.

48 Postlethwait RW. Principles of operative surgery: antisepsis, technique, sutures, and drains. In: Sabiston DC, ed. *Textbook of Surgery*. Philadelphia: WB Saunders, 1972; 300–318.

49 Tamse JG. Preventive maintenance of medical and dental equipment. Association for the Advancement of Medical Instrumentation 13th Annual Meeting, Washington DC, 1978.

50 Mason DE. Anesthesia machine checkout and troubleshooting. *Semin Vet Med Surg (Small Anim)* 1993; **8**: 104.

51 Ko JCH, Berman AG. Anesthesia in shelter medicine. *Top Comp Anim Med* 2010; **25(2)**: 92–97.

52 Looney AL. Anesthesia and pain management in shelter populations. In: Miller L, Zawistowski S, eds. *Shelter Medicine*, 2nd edn. Ames, IA: Wiley-Blackwell, 2013.

53 Verstegen J, Fargetton X, Donnay I, *et al.* Comparison of the clinical utility of medetomidine/ketamine and xylazine/ketamine combinations for the ovariectomy of cats. *Vet Rec*1990; **127**: 424–426.

54 Williams LS, Levy JK, Robertson SA, *et al.* Use of the anesthetic combination of tiletamine, zolazepam, ketamine, and xylazine for neutering feral cats. *J Am Vet Med Assoc* 2002; **220(10)**: 1491–1495.

55 Robertson SA. Anesthesia protocols for early kitten sterilization and feral cat clinics. Proceedings of the Western Veterinary Conference, Las Vegas, 2005. www.wvc.org (accessed 25 September 2014).

56 Cistola AM, Golder FJ, Centonze LA *et al.* Anesthetic and physiologic effects of tiletamine, zolazepam, ketamine, and xylazine combination (TKX) in feral cats undergoing surgical sterilization. *J Feline Med Surg* 2004; **6(5)**: 297–303.

57 Harrison KA, Robertson S, Levy J, *et al.* Evaluation of medetomidine, ketamine and buprenorphine for neutering feral cats. *J Feline Med Surg* 2011; **13(12)**: 896–902.

58 Ko J, Austin B, Barletta M, *et al.* Evaluation of dexmedetomidine and ketamine in combination with various opioids as injectable anesthetic combinations for castration in cats. *J Am Vet Med Assoc* 2011; **239(11)**: 1453–1462.

59 Polson S, Taylor PM, Yates D. Analgesia after feline ovariohysterectomy under midazolam-medetomidine-ketamine anaesthesia with buprenorphine or butorphanol, and carprofen or meloxicam: a prospective, randomised clinical trial. *J Feline Med Surg* 2012; **14(8)**: 553–559.

60 Zaki S,Ticehurst K, Miyaki Y. Clinical evaluation of Alfaxan-CD(R) as an intravenous anaesthetic in young cats. *Aust Vet J* 2009; **87(3)**: 82–87.

61 O'Hagan BJ, Pasloske K, McKinnon C, *et al.* Clinical evaluation of alfaxalone as an anaesthetic induction agent in cats less than 12 weeks of age. *Aust Vet J* 2012; **90(10)**: 395–401.

62 Zilberstein LF, Moens YP, Leterrier E. The effect of local anaesthesia on anaesthetic requirements for feline ovariectomy. *Vet J* 2008; **178(2)**: 214–218.

63 Egger C, Love L. Local and regional anesthesia techniques, Part 1: Overview and five simple techniques. *Vet Med* 2009; **104(1)**: 24–40.

64 Kuo WC, Keegan RD. Comparative cardiovascular, analgesic, and sedative effects of medetomidine, medetomidine-hydromorphone, and medetomidine-butorphanol in dogs. *Am J Vet Res* 2004; **65(7)**: 931–937.

65 Girard NM, Leece EA, Cardwell JM. The sedative effects of low-dose medetomidine and butorphanol alone and in combination intravenously in dogs. *Vet Anaesth Analg* 2010; **37(1)**: 1–6.

66 Slingsby L, Murrell JC, Taylor PM. Combination of dexmedetomidine with buprenorphine enhances the antinociceptive effect to a thermal stimulus in the cat compared with either agent alone. *Vet Anaesth Analg*2010; **37**(**2**): 162–170.

67 Grimm KA, Tranquilli WJ, Thurmon JC, *et al.* Duration of nonresponse to noxious stimulation after intramuscular administration of butorphanol, medetomidine, or a butorphanol-medetomidine combination during isoflurane administration in dogs. *Am J Vet Res* 2000; **61**(**1**): 42–47.

68 Kampschmidt K. Drug use in the neonatal pediatric small animal patient. Proceedings of the Western Veterinary Conference, Las Vegas, 2006. www.wvc.org (accessed 25 September 2014).

69 Pascoe PJ, Moon PF. Periparturient and neonatal anesthesia. *Vet Clin North Am Small Anim Pract* 2001; **31**(**2**): 315–340.

70 Ko JC, Fox SM, Mandsager RE. Effects of preemptive atropine administration on incidence of medetomidine-induced bradycardia in dogs. *J Am Vet Med Assoc* 2001; **218**(**1**): 52–58.

71 Congdon JM, Marquez M, Niyom S, Boscan P. Evaluation of the sedative and cardiovascular effects of intramuscular administration of dexmedetomidine with and without concurrent atropine administration in dogs. *J Am Vet Med Assoc* 2011; **239**(**1**): 81–89.

72 Monteiro ER, Campagnol D, Parrilha LR, Furlan LZ. Evaluation of cardiorespiratory effects of combinations of dexmedetomidine and atropine in cats. *Feline Med Surg* 2009; **11**(**10**): 783–792.

73 Dobromylskyj P. Cardiovascular changes associated with anaesthesia induced by medetomidine combined with ketamine in cats. *J Small Anim Pract* 1996; **37**(**4**): 169–172.

74 Verstegen J, Fargetton X, Donnay I, *et al.* An evaluation of medetomidine/ketamine and other drug combinations for anaesthesia in cats. *Vet Rec* 1991; **128**: 32–35.

75 Haskins SC. Monitoring the anesthetized patient. In: Short CS, ed. *Principles and Practice of Veterinary Anesthesia*. Baltimore, MD: Williams and Wilkins, 1987; 455–477.

76 Haskins SC. Monitoring the anesthetized patient. In: Thurmon JC, Tranquilli WJ, Benson GJ, eds. *Lumb and Jones' Veterinary Anesthesia*, 3rd edn. Baltimore, MD: Williams and Wilkins, 1996; 409–424.

77 Burns PM, Driessen B, Boston R, *et al.* Accuracy of a third vs. first generation pulse oximeter in predicting arterial oxygen saturation and pulse rate in the anesthetized dog. *Vet Anaesth Analg* 2006; **33**(**5**): 281–295.

78 Robertson SA. Oxygenation and ventilation. In: Greene SA, ed. *Veterinary Anesthesia and Pain Management Secrets*. Philadelphia: Hanley and Belfus, 2002; 15–20.

79 Seliskar A. Comparison of high definition oscillometric and Doppler ultrasound devices with invasive blood pressure in anaesthetized dogs. *Vet Anaesth Analg* 2013; **40**(**1**): 21–27.

80 Chetboul V, Tissier R, Gouni V, *et al.* Comparison of Doppler ultrasonography and high-definition oscillometry for blood pressure measurements in healthy awake dogs. *Am J Vet Res* 2010; **71**(**7**): 766–772.

81 Moon RE, Camporesi EM. Respiratory monitoring. In: Miller RD, ed. *Anesthesia*, 3rd edn. New York: Churchill Livingstone, 1990; 1165–1184.

82 Grosenbaugh DA, Muir WM. Using end-tidal carbon dioxide to monitor patients. *Vet Med* 1998; **93**(**1**): 67–70.

83 Holden D. Postoperative care. In: Seymour C, Gleed RD, eds. *Manual of Small Animal Anaesthesia and Analgesia*. Cheltenham: British Small Animal Veterinary Association, 1999; 17–18.

84 Short CE. *Principles and Practice of Veterinary Anesthesia*. Baltimore, MD: Williams and Wilkins, 1987.

85 Hackett TB. The postoperative cat – monitoring, analgesia and nursing care. Proceedings of the Western Veterinary Conference, Las Vegas, 2002. www.wvc.org (accessed 25 September 2014).

86 Salmeri KR. Postoperative care of the small animal surgical patient. Proceedings of the Atlantic Coast Veterinary Conference, 2002. www.acvc.org (accessed 25 September 2014).

87 Macintire DK. Pediatric intensive care. *Vet Clin North Am Small Anim Pract* 1999; **29**: 971–988.

88 Insler SR, Sessler DI. Perioperative thermoregulation and temperature monitoring. *Anesthesiol Clin* 2006; **24**(**4**): 823–837.

89 Armstrong SR, Roberts BK, Aronsohn M. Perioperative hypothermia. *J Vet Emerg Crit Care* 2005; **15**(**1**): 32–37.

90 Harvey RC. Hypothermia. In: Greene SA, ed. *Veterinary Anesthesia and Pain Management Secrets*. Philadelphia: Hanley and Belfus, 2002; 149–152.

91 Machon RG, Raffe MR, Robinson EP. Warming with a forced air warming blanket minimizes anesthesia induced hypothermia in cats. *Vet Surg* 1999; **28**(**4**): 301–310.

92 Wingfield WE. Cardiopulmonary arrest. In: Wingfield WE, Raffe MR, eds. *The Veterinary ICU Book*. Jackson Hole, WY: Teton New Media, 2002; 421–452.

93 Cole SG, Otto CM, Hughes D. Cardiopulmonary cerebral resuscitation in small animals – a clinical practice review. part II. *J Vet Emerg Crit Care* 2003; **13**(**1**): 13–23.

94 Muir WW. Cardiovascular emergencies. In: Muir WW, Hubbell JAE, Bednarski, eds. *Handbook of Veterinary Anesthesia*, 4th edn. St Louis, MO: Mosby, 2007; 557–575.

95 www.acvecc-recover.org/ (accessed 25 September 2014).

37 Comparative Anesthesia and Analgesia of Equine Patients

Lori A. Bidwell
College of Veterinary Medicine, Michigan State University, East Lansing, Michigan, USA

Chapter contents

Introduction

Equine anesthesia has always been associated with greater patient risk compared to other common domestic species. Delivery of anesthesia is complicated by many factors including the large patient size range, the need to induce controlled recumbency during anesthetic induction, specialized equipment requirements, perfusion issues related to large body mass, and instinctive behaviors. In addition, drug dosages are often extrapolated from those of other species and many of the drugs are used in an extra-label manner. Understanding of the unique factors associated with equine anesthesia compared to other species is the first step in improving patient safety.

Anesthetic risk

The risk of anesthetic mortality is greater in equine species than other domestic animals. Studies have reported rates between 0.24% and 1.6% for horses [1–4] compared to dogs (0.05%) and cats (0.11%) [5]. A mortality rate of 1% is referenced in most surgical facilities when discussing risk of anesthesia with horse owners; however, the percentage can increase considerably with metabolically unstable patients such as those with colic. The primary complications associated with death are cardiac arrest, orthopedic injuries in recovery, and myopathy or neuropathy post anesthesia. Postanesthetic colic is an additional concern. The use of opioid analgesics, time of surgery, choice of anesthetics, and concurrent use of certain antibiotics have been implicated as risk factors for developing postoperative colic, although specific links have not been determined [6–11].

Variation in size

Horses come in a broad range of sizes. A miniature horse foal can weigh less than 10 kg while a draft horse used for competition pulling can weigh up to 1300 kg. Because of this size variation, specific equipment must be purchased to move these animals, deliver anesthetic, and assist or control ventilation. A small animal anesthetic machine can be used for most miniature horses, neonates, and foals up to 150 kg but large animal anesthetic systems must be purchased for older foals and horses. The limiting factor with small animal systems is the size of the sodasorb canister, the size of the rebreathing bag, and the size of the tubing and the connector that attaches to the endotracheal tube. Prices for equine anesthetic machines can range from $14 000 to $50 000 (2014 prices) depending on the model, inclusion of a ventilator, and construction of the breathing system. Endotracheal tubes, rebreathing bags, and anesthetic tubing are specifically made for equine patients and therefore more expensive than equipment used in small animal patients (much of which is repurposed from the human market). Much of the monitoring equipment designed for human patients can be adapted for use on larger species. One common problem is that human monitors often consider normal heart rates in adult horses to be bradycardic with default alarms set for rates below 40 beats per minute.

Surgical tables and hoisting mechanisms must be designed specifically for equine or large animal patients. If a practice regularly sees large draft breed horses, it is wise to purchase a 2 ton hoist rather than the typical 1 ton hoist as larger horses can overstress inappropriate equipment. In addition, the typical surgical table designed for an adult equine is not big enough to support the mass of a 1000 kg patient for a procedure requiring lateral recumbency.

Veterinary Anesthesia and Analgesia: The Fifth Edition of Lumb and Jones.
Edited by Kurt A. Grimm, Leigh A. Lamont, William J. Tranquilli, Stephen A. Greene and Sheilah A. Robertson.

Therefore, two surgical tables may need to be used together to provide adequate support. If two tables are not available, the use of stacked pads or mats can substitute under limbs, head, and neck. Many of the draft breeds do not have long enough tails to attach a rope for assisted recovery. Fortunately, most draft horses are relatively co-operative regarding recovery.

Size is also a factor in determining peripheral (skeletal muscle) perfusion. Mean arterial blood pressure requirements increase as muscle mass (and muscle compartment/compression pressure) increases. The risk of postanesthetic neuropathy and myopathy is higher in equine patients, particularly draft and large warmblood breeds. While recommendations on minimum mean arterial pressures during anesthesia vary, this author recommends a minimum mean arterial blood pressure in horses greater than 500 kg of at least 80 mmHg based on personal experience. Maintaining a mean arterial blood pressure of greater than 70 mmHg in normal adult horses has been shown to minimize postoperative complications associated with hypotension [12,13]. Neonates and foals have lower normal resting mean arterial blood pressure (47–50 mmHg in neonates and 55–70 mmHg in foals) but there has been a report of a neonate developing postanesthetic myositis after an anesthetic event with average mean arterial blood pressure between 45 and 65 mmHg [14]. Therefore, the goal with all ages and sizes of horses should be to maintain blood pressure above 60 mmHg in foals and 70–80 mmHg in adults depending on body size. Adjuncts to increase mean arterial blood pressure include inotropes, vasopressors, and catecholamines. Dobutamine is used most often in equine patients but dopamine, ephedrine, phenylephrine, vasopressin, norepinephrine, epinephrine, and calcium salts are alternative options if used appropriately. Of the inotropes, dobutamine has been found to be the most useful for increasing mean arterial blood pressure in neonates, foals, and adult horses under general anesthesia [15–17].

Cardiopulmonary resuscitation

Anatomic variation complicates cardiopulmonary resuscitation. An equine neonate or older foal can be managed similar to a canine but adult equine ribs are narrow and impossible to separate by hand if open chest cardiac compressions are required. A rib resection is required for open chest compressions and this is not practical in most situations. Therefore, chest compressions on an adult equine patient require use of the anesthetist's full body weight concentrated on either both knees or feet. External chest compressions must be performed at a minimum of 80 compressions/min in an adult to produce a cardiac output near 50% of that of a deeply anesthetized horse [18]. However, external compressions of 20/min in ponies have been shown to produce a cardiac output of approximately 50% normal baseline values [19]. As an alternative to external compressions, when a horse arrests under general anesthesia for abdominal exploration, the surgeon can make an incision through the diaphragm and perform direct cardiac compression.

Although cardiac arrhythmias are common in horses during exercise and after anesthesia, ventricular fibrillation is uncommon in horses prior to arrest [20–22]. Even if ventricular fibrillation is present, most electrical cardiac defibrillators are not designed to deliver a large enough electrical output required to defibrillate an adult equine heart.

Considerations for equine induction

Inducing recumbency in horses from the standing position can be dangerous. In order to minimize the risk, appropriate sedation and muscle relaxation should be administered prior to induction. Ketamine is one of the primary induction drug used in horses but it lacks any muscle relaxant properties. In fact, without premedication, induction with ketamine is physically dramatic. Muscle relaxation and induction can be improved by increasing the dose of premedication, adding an opioid or phenothiazine to an α_2-adrenergic receptor agonist, or adding a benzodiazepine to ketamine for induction [23,24].

There are differences in induction doses between horses, donkeys, and mules. Donkeys are typically less affected by premedication and induction drugs when compared to horses. Mules appear to be intermediate between donkeys and horses. Dosing drugs for donkeys should be based on 1.5 times the dose of a horse. The exception to this rule is guaifenesin, as donkeys are more sensitive to the central effects of the drug, resulting in hypotension and apnea with bolus administration. The difference in response to drugs in donkeys appears to be due to variation in body water distribution and drug metabolism [25,26].

Effect of recumbency in equine patients

Prolonged recumbency in equine patients is not benign. Ventilation/perfusion mismatch and shunting are inevitable when an equine patient is recumbent. Lateral recumbency results in atelectasis of the dependent lung and dorsal recumbency results in progressive atelectasis of the dorsal lung fields [27]. Controlled ventilation can improve arterial oxygenation but in a patient with abdominal distension associated with colic, ruptured bladder or pregnancy, cardiac output can be compromised during periods of high intrathoracic pressure. In contrast to small animal patients, a recent study performed with horses found that decreasing the inspired oxygen concentration to 50% from >95% resulted in significant reductions in arterial oxygen saturation; therefore, the use of lower inspired oxygen concentrations to reduce atelectasis is not recommended [28,29].

Heart rate considerations

Sedation with an α_2-adrenergic receptor agonist in horses results in bradycardia. This can be further compounded by the concurrent administration of many anesthetic drugs. However, the dissociative agent ketamine has sympathomimetic properties and its administration often produces transient increases in heart rate. Typically, once heart rate returns to baseline levels under anesthesia, there are no peaks or large changes in heart rate that are indicative of arousal as is seen in small animal patients. Increased heart rate in response to surgical stimulation is unusual in the healthy adult equine under general anesthesia.

Equine neonate versus foal

A neonate is less equipped to alter stroke volume in response to hypovolemia and bradycardia. In neonates, heart rate has a primary function in controlling cardiac output. The most commonly used premedication for horses are α_2-adrenergic receptor agonists and one effect associated with these drugs is bradycardia. Therefore, it seems prudent to minimize use of α_2-adrenergic receptor agonists in neonates or compromised older foals. Older foals can have variable responses to drugs and should be dosed individually based on behavior [30,31].

The pregnant mare

A pregnant mare presenting for an emergency procedure requiring general anesthesia has several physiologic differences that challenge the anesthetist. Vasodilation induced by inhalant anesthetic is enhanced by circulating hormones induced by pregnancy and parturition [32]. In human females, endothelial-derived hyperpolarization (EDH) and nitric oxide (NO) are responsible for decreased vascular tone [33]. Oxygenation in the mare is complicated by the gravid uterus and abdominal contents placing pressure on the diaphragm, resulting in reduced functional residual capacity. Controlled or assisted ventilation is often necessary to allow the mare to receive an appropriate tidal volume. Tipping the mare slightly off dorsal recumbency also facilitates venous return by reducing direct compression of the caudal vena cava. In order to appropriately ventilate the pregnant mare, airway pressures often exceed 30 cmH_2O, particularly when the mare is in the Trendelenburg position for manipulation of the fetus. In this situation, airway pressures reaching 60 cmH_2O are often required to deliver a tidal volume of 10 mL/kg. In addition to ventilation concerns, endotracheal intubation is recommended to prevent aspiration of gastrointestinal contents. Due to the emergency nature of dystocia or cesarean section, fasting prior to the procedure rarely occurs. In human medicine, elevated intragastric pressure, delayed gastric emptying, and circulating progesterone relaxing the gastroesophageal sphincter are blamed for the increased risk of aspiration pneumonia [34,35].

Fluid therapy considerations

A discussion involving fluid therapy in horses under general anesthesia can be controversial. The traditional thought process regarding fluid therapy involves administration of isotonic fluids at a rate of 5–15 mL/kg/h and bolusing fluids as needed during periods of hypotension. This rate of administration has been found to be ineffective in preventing hypotension induced by inhaled anesthetics [36]. The plasma volume expansion from crystalloids is less than 20–25% of the volume administered. In addition, the traditional practice of administering crystalloids for blood loss in a 3:1 ratio is not as effective as once thought. Rather than using a prescribed fluid rate for every patient, crystalloids and colloids should be administered on a patient-specific basis by using goal-directed fluid therapy endpoints (e.g., blood gases, capillary refill time, mucous membrane color, and pulse variation) for evaluation [37,38].

Recovery

The true challenge of equine anesthesia compared to other domestic species is safely returning the patient to the standing position without injury. The role of the anesthetist continues through the recovery period by appropriate selection of sedatives and often assisting the horse in attempts to stand. Horses have a flight instinct that prevents most of them from remaining recumbent in the recovery stall. In addition, some patients will prematurely attempt to stand because of the need to urinate following administration of large volumes of intravenous fluids and increased urine production following α_2-adrenergic receptor agonist administration.

The transition of a horse receiving anesthetic in 100% oxygen with vascular and ventilatory support to a recovery stall without monitoring or oxygen supplementation is not one in which heavy sedation is recommended. However, sedation may smooth the recovery from inhalant anesthesia. It is important to use a balance of technique and sedation for a safe recovery. Ideally, the adult horse should be maintained in recumbency until there is loss of nystagmus, response to sound, and return of menace and tongue tone in response to gentle traction. Menace response is a learned behavior, so foals typically will not respond to stimulation over the eye unless there is direct contact with the lids or cornea (the latter is not recommended unless in an emergency situation). Sedation can be administered just prior to moving the horse into recovery. Depending on the depth of anesthesia, 50–150 mg xylazine or 5–20 mg romifidine or detomidine with or without 2–5 mg acepromazine can be administered intramuscularly prior to moving the horse into recovery. An additional small dose of a sedative can be administered intravenously if needed [39–41]. A towel over the eyes and cotton in the ears aids in minimizing stimulation from outside the stall, particularly in horses that are sound sensitive.

There are several recovery techniques that can be utilized depending on the specific case: unassisted recovery or 'self recovery,' rope recovery utilizing ropes on the halter and tail as a pulley system through rings on the walls, pool recovery, sling recovery, and recovery on a tilt table [42]. Self recovery is practical for young healthy horses after elective procedures. Rope, pool, sling, and tilt table recovery are utilized for patients in whom instability or weakness is a concern. Rope recovery requires a stall with rings in the walls, strong cotton or web rope and two people to pull the ropes to assist the horse at the appropriate time. Some finesse is needed in that the head rope should be used for support and the tail rope is used for the majority of assistance (where the most effort is required by the handler). Horses need to have freedom in their front end to get momentum to stand; therefore, the head rope should not be pulled tightly until the horse is standing. Pool, sling, and tilt table recovery are typically reserved for fractures and horses with neurologic concerns. Recovering a foal from anesthesia is a very different process from that of adults. Foals should be assisted in recovery until approximately 5–6 months of age.

References

1 Johnston GM, Taylor PM, Holmes MA, *et al.* Confidential enquiry into perioperative equine fatalities (CEPEF-1): preliminary results. *Equine Vet J* 1995; **27**: 193–200.

2 Bidwell LA, Bramlage LR, Rood WA. Equine perioperative fatalities associated with general anesthesia at a private practice: a retrospective case series. *Vet Anaesth Analg* 2007; **34**: 23–30.

3 Johnston GM, Eastman JK, Wood JL, *et al.* The confidential enquiry into perioperative equine fatalities (CEPEF): mortality results of Phases 1 and 2. *Vet Anaesth Analg* 2002; **29**: 159–170.

4 Young SS, Taylor PM. Factors influencing the outcome of equine anaesthesia: a review of 1,314 cases. *Equine Vet J* 1993; **25**: 147–151.

5 Brodbelt DC, Bissitt KJ, Hammond RA, *et al.* The risk of death: the confidential enquiry into perioperative small animal fatalities. *Vet Anaesth Analg* 2008; **35**: 365–373.

6 Senior JM, Pinchbeck GL, Allister R, *et al.* Post anaesthetic colic in horses: a preventable complication? *Equine Vet J* 2006; **33**: 479–484.

7 Little D, Redding WR, Blikslager AT. Risk factors for reduced perioperative fecal output in horses: 37 cases (1997–1998). *J Am Vet Med Assoc* 2001; **218**: 414–420.

8 Mircica E, Clutton RE, Kyles KW, *et al.* Problems associated with perioperative morphine in horses: a retrospective cases analysis. *Vet Anaesth Analg* 2003; **30**: 147–155.

9 Senior JM, Pinchbeck G, Dugdale AHA, *et al.* A retrospective study of the risk factors and prevalence of colic in horses after orthopaedic surgery. *Vet Rec* 2004; **155**: 321–325.

10 Anderson MS, Clark L, Dyson S, *et al.* Risk factors for colic in horses after general anaesthesia for MRI or nonabdominal surgery: absence of evidence of effect from perianaesthetic morphine. *Equine Vet J* 2006; **38**: 368–374.

11 Mircica E, Clutton RE, Kyles KW, Blisset KJ. Problems associated with perioperative morphine in horses: a retrospective case analysis. *Vet Anaesth Analg* 2003; **30**: 147–155.

12 Duke T, Filzek U, Read MR, *et al.* Clinical observations surrounding an increased incidence of postanesthetic myopathy in halothane-anesthetized horses. *Vet Anaesth Analg* 2006; **33**: 122–127.

13 Grandy JL, Steffey EP, Hodgson DS, Wollner MJ. Arterial hypotension and the development of postanesthetic myopathy in halothane-anesthetized horses. *Am J Vet Res* 1987; **48**: 192–197.

14 Manning M, Dubielzig R, McGuirk S. Postoperative myositis in a neonatal foal: a case report. *Vet Surg* 1996; **24**: 69–72.

15 Craig CA, Haskens SC, Hildebrand SV. The cardiopulmonary effects of dobutamine and norepinephrine in isoflurane-anesthetized foals. *Vet Anaesth Analg* 2007; **34**: 377–387.

16 Valverde A, Giguere S, Sanchez LC, *et al.* Effects of dobutamine, norepinephrine and vasopressin on cardiovascular function in anesthetized neonatal foals with induced hypotension. *Am J Vet Res* 2006; **67**: 1730–1737.

17 deVries A, Brearly JC, Taylor PM. Effects of dobutamine on cardiac index and arterial blood pressure in isoflurane-anesthetized horses under clinical conditions. *J Vet Pharmacol Ther* 2009; **32**: 353–358.

18 Hubbell JA, Muir WW, Gaynor JS. Cardiovascular effects of thoracic compression in horses subjected to euthanasia. *Equine Vet J* 1993; **25**: 282–284.

19 Frauenfelder HC, Fessler JF, Latshaw HS, *et al.* External cardiovascular resuscitation of the anesthetized pony. *J Am Vet Med Assoc* 1981; **179**: 673–676.

20 Morgan RA, Raftery AG, Cripps P, *et al.* The prevalence and nature of cardiac arrhythmias in horses following general anaesthesia and surgery. *Acta Vet Scand* 2011; **23**: 53–62.

21 Buhl R, Meldgaard C, Barbesgaard L. Cardiac arrhythmias in clinically healthy showjumping horses. *Equine Vet J* 2010; **38(Suppl)**: 196–201.

22 Barbesgaard L, Buhl R, Meldgaard C. Prevalence of exercise-associated arrhythmias in normal performing dressage horses. *Equine Vet J* 2010; **38(Suppl)**: 202–207.

23 Mantrell S, Nyman G. Effects of additional premedication on romifidine and ketamine anesthesia in horses. *Acta Vet Scand* 1996; **37**: 315–325.

24 Hubbell JA, Hinchcliff KW, Schmall LM, *et al.* Anesthetic, cardiorespiratory and metabolic effects of four intravenous anesthetic regimens induced in horses immediately after maximal exercise. *Am J Vet Res* 2000; **61**: 1545–1552.

25 Maloiy GMO. Water economy of the Somali donkey. *Am J Physiol* 1970; **219**: 1522–1527.

26 Matthews NS, Taylor TS, Hartsfield SM, *et al.* Pharmacokinetics of ketamine in mules and mammoth asses premedicated with xylazine. *Equine Vet J* 1994; **26**: 241–243.

27 Nyman G, Funkquist B, Kyart C, *et al.* Atelectasis causes gas exchange impairment in the anaesthetized horse. *Equine Vet J* 1990; **22(5)**: 317–324.

28 Gonçalves Dias LG, Nunes N, Lopes PC, *et al.* The effects of 2 levels of inspired oxygen fraction in blood gas variables in propofol-anesthetized dogs with high intracranial pressure. *Can J Vet Res* 2009; **73**: 111–116.

29 Crumley MN, McMurphy RM, Hodgson DS, Kreider SE. Effects of inspired oxygen concentration in ventilation, ventilatory rhythm, and gas exchange in isoflurane-anesthetized horses. *Am J Vet Res* 2013; **74**: 183–190.

30 O'Connor SJ, Gardner DS, Ousey JC, *et al.* Development of baroreflex and endocrine responses to hypotensive stress in newborn foals and lambs. *Pflurgers Arch* 2005; **450**: 298–306.

31 Lombard CW, Evans M, Martin L, Tehrani J. Blood pressure, electrocardiogram and echocardiogram measurements in the growing pony foal. *Equine Vet J* 1984; **16**: 342–347.

32 Fowden AL, Forhead AJ, Ousey JC. The endocrinology of equine parturition. *Exp Clin Endocrinol Diabetes* 2008; **116**: 393–403.

33 Morton JS, Davidge ST. Arterial endothelium-derived hyperpolarization – potential role in pregnancy adaptations and complications. *J Cardiovasc Pharmacol* 2013; **61**: 197–203.

34 American College of Obstetricians and Gynecologists. ACOG Technical Bulletin: Pulmonary disease in pregnancy. *J Gynecol Obstet* 1996; **54**: 187–196.

35 Baggish MS, Hooper S. Aspiration as a cause of maternal death. *Obstet Gynecol* 1974; **43**: 327–336.

36 Valverde A, Gianotti G, Rioja-Garcia E, *et al.* Effects of high-volume, rapid fluid therapy on cardiovascular function and hematological values during isoflurane-induced hypotension in healthy dogs. *Can J Vet Res* 2012; **76**: 99–108.

37 Muir WW, Wiese AJ. Comparison of lactated ringers solution and a physiologically balanced 6% hetastarch plasma expander for the treatment of hypotension induced via blood withdrawal in isoflurane-anesthetized dogs. *Am J Vet Res* 2004; **65**: 1189–1194.

38 Jacob M, Chappell D, Homann-Kiefer K, *et al.* The intravascular volume effect of Ringer's lactate is below 20%: a prospective study in humans. *Crit Care* 2012; **16**: R86.

39 Oijala M, Katila T. Detomidine (Domosedan) in foals: sedative and analgesic effects. *Equine Vet J* 1988; **20**: 327–330.

40 Valverde A, Black B, Cribb NC, *et al.* Assessment of unassisted recovery from repeated general isoflurane anesthesia in horses following post-anesthetic administration of xylazine or acepromazine or a combination of xylazine and ketamine. *Vet Anaesth Analg* 2013; **40**: 3-12.

41 Woodhouse KJ, Brosnan RJ, Nguyen KQ, *et al.* Effects of postanesthetic sedation with romifidine or xylazine on quality of recovery from isoflurane anesthesia in horses. *J Am Vet Med Assoc* 2013; **15**: 242–244.

42 Banquler SH, Kona-Brown JJ. Comparison of the effects of xylazine and romifidine administered perioperatively on the recovery of anesthetized horses. *Can Vet J* 2011; **52(9)**: 987–993.

38 Comparative Anesthesia and Analgesia of Ruminants and Swine

HuiChu Lin
College of Veterinary Medicine, Auburn University, Auburn, Alabama, USA

Chapter contents

Introduction

General anesthesia in farm animals, like cattle, small ruminants (sheep and goats), camelids (llamas and alpacas), and pigs, requires special attention due to anatomic and physiologic differences from dogs, cats, and horses. Cattle, sheep, and goats have a stomach that is divided into four compartments, whereas llamas and alpacas have three compartments. Though anatomically different, the digestive system of these animals functions similarly. Significant size and body weight differences also exist, varying from 2–3 kg immediately after birth to 500–1000 kg when fully grown. Accurate dosing of injectable drugs and appropriate sized anesthetic equipment and accessories should be available. Ruminants (cattle, sheep, and goats) generally tolerate physical restraint and recumbency well. This behavior advantages local and/or regional anesthetic techniques, allowing many minor surgical procedures to be performed in the standing position. Because camelids and swine are less tolerant to physical restraint, general anesthesia is more frequently performed for even minor surgical procedures.

Farm animals share nociceptive pathway anatomy with other mammals, and therefore have the ability to process information similarly. Analgesia to prevent and reduce pain should be included as an essential part of surgery and anesthetic management. When surgical procedures require general anesthesia, balanced anesthetic techniques should be employed to provide narcosis, analgesia, and muscle relaxation. Minimizing the stress response induced by handling, surgery, and anesthesia is also important.

Anesthesia and surgery outside routine veterinary care can be costly relative to the value of the animal. Anesthetics/anesthetic adjuncts commonly used in farm animal practice may not have regulatory approval for use in ruminants, camelids, and swine [1,2]. In the United States the Animal Medicinal Drug Use Clarification Act (AMDUCA) of 1994 codifies the requirements for extra-label drug use (ELDU). In general, ELDU is permitted when animal health is threatened or death may result if a condition is untreated; however, the prescribing veterinarian is responsible for advising owners how to insure that no residual drug reaches processors or consumers [3]. Practitioners working outside the US should consult the appropriate regulations for their practice area to determine the specific requirements for drug use in animals intended for food production.

Anesthetics are usually only used for short durations and animals are unlikely to be marketed immediately after surgery. Furthermore, newer anesthetics tend to have very short plasma elimination half-lives ($t_{½}$) and are potent enough that only low tissue concentrations are required to produce general anesthesia. The possibility of anesthetic residues persisting in edible tissues after the surgical incision has healed, approximately 14 days, is low. Thus, problems with anesthetic drug residues appear to be rare [4]. Nevertheless, veterinarians should consult the Food Animal Residual Avoidance Databank (FARAD) for guidance on estimated meat and milk withdrawal intervals for ELDU of analgesics, tranquilizers, and injectable anesthetics as well as for updates on drugs prohibited from ELDU [1,2,5] (Table 38.1). Camelids are considered fiber animals, not food-producing animals, so concerns for violative drug residues and withdrawal times are minimal.

In addition to food, pigs are often used for a variety of medical research and other non-food-producing roles.

Veterinary Anesthesia and Analgesia: The Fifth Edition of Lumb and Jones.
Edited by Kurt A. Grimm, Leigh A. Lamont, William J. Tranquilli, Stephen A. Greene and Sheilah A. Robertson.

Table 38.1 The recommended withdrawal interval for ruminants for single and multiple treatments of anesthetic and analgesic drugs.

Drug	Species	Dose (mg/kg)	Milk withdrawal interval (hours)	Meat withdrawal interval (days)	Country
Acepromazine	Cattle Sheep Goats	≦0.13, IV ≦0.44, IM	48	7	US, FARAD
Acepromazine	Swine	≦0.055, IV ≦0.44, IM	–	7	US, FARAD
Acepromazine	Cattle	0.13, IV 0.27, IM	48	2	Australia
Acepromazine	Cattle	0.055, IV 0.13-0.44, IM 0.13-0.26, PO	48	7	Canada
Acepromazine	Swine	≦0.13, IM	–	7	Canada
Aspirin	Cattle Sheep Goats	≦100, BID	24	1	US, FARAD
Atropine	Cattle Sheep Goats	Anesthetic adjunct	24	7	US, FARAD
Atropine	Cattle Sheep	0.03–0.06, IV, IM, SC, SID 0.08–0.16, IV, IM, SC, SID Multiple dose, ≦0.2 mg/kg	72 144	14 28	United Kingdom Antidote
Atropine	Swine	0.02–0.04, IV, IM, SC, SID Multiple dose, ≦0.2 mg/kg	72 144	14 28	United Kingdom Antidote
Bupivacaine	Cattle Sheep Goats	0.05 1.5–1.8	Clear rapidly	Clear rapidly	Not yet established by FARAD
Butorphanol	Sheep	0.022–0.05, IV, IM	48	2	Not yet established by FARAD
Detomidine	Cattle Sheep Goats	≦0.08, IV or IM	72	3	US, FARAD
Detomidine	Cattle	0.02–0.08, IV or IM	72	1	Switzerland
DMSO	Cattle Sheep Goats	Not specified	96	4	US, FARAD
Fentanyl	Goats	50 μg/h, transdermal patch	48-96	2-4	Not yet established by FARAD
Guaifenesin	Cattle Sheep Goats	≦100, IV	48	3	US, FARAD
Guaifenesin	Cattle	60–100, IV	Not specified	Not specified	Switzerland
Ketamine	Cattle Sheep Goats	≦2, IV 10, IM	48	3	US, FARAD
Ketamine	Swine	≦10, IV or IM	–	2	US, FARAD
Ketamine	Cattle	5, IV 10–20, IM	0	0	France
Ketamine	Cattle	Adult: 2, IV Calves: ≦10, IV	72	1	Switzerland
Ketoprofen	Cattle Sheep Goats	≦3.3, SID, ≦3days	24	7	US, FARAD
Lidocaine (with epinephrine)	Cattle Sheep Goats	Infiltration Epidural	24	1	US, FARAD
Meloxicam	Cattle	0.5, IM, SC	120	15	European counties
Meperidine	Cattle Sheep Goats	2–4	48–96	2–4	Not yet established by FARAD
Morphine	Cattle Sheep Goats	0.1	Clear rapidly	Clear rapidly	Not yet established by FARAD
Phenylbutazone	Cattle Sheep Goats	Not recommended, prolonged excretion			US
Tolazoline	Cattle	2–4, IV	48	8	New Zealand US, FARAD
Ultra-short barbiturates	Cattle Sheep Goats	Thiamylal: ≦5.5 Thiopental: ≦9.4	24	1	US, FARAD
Xylazine	Cattle Sheep Goats	0.016–0.1, IV 0.05–03, IM 0–2, IM	72 24 120	5 4 10	US, FARAD
Xylazine	Cattle	0.11–0.33, IM	48	3	Canada
Xylazine	Cattle	0.025–0.15, IV 0.025–0.3, IM	0	2	France

Table 38.1 (*Continued*)

Drug	Species	Dose (mg/kg)	Milk withdrawal interval (hours)	Meat withdrawal interval (days)	Country
Xylazine	Cattle	0.016–0.1, IV 0.01–0.3, IM 1.2–2, IM	72 120	3 7	Germany
Xylazine	Cattle	0.05–0.4, IM	24	4	New Zealand
Xylazine	Cattle	0.016–0.1, IV 0.05–0.3, IM	72	3	Switzerland
Xylazine	Cattle	0.05–0.3, IM	48	14	United Kingdom
Yohimbine	Cattle Sheep Goats	≦0.3, IV	72	7	US, FARAD

IM = intramuscular; IV = intravenous; PO = per os; SC = subcutaneous.

References:

Coetzee JF. A review of pain assessment techniques and pharmacological approach to pain relief after bovine castration: practical implications for cattle production within the United States. *Appl Anim Behav Sci* 2011; **135**: 192–213.

Craigmill, AL, Rangel-Lugo M, Damien P, *et al.* Extralabel use of tranquilizers and general anesthetics. *J Am Vet Med Assoc* 1997; **211**: 302–304.

Fajt VR. Label and extralabel drug use in small ruminants. *Vet Clin North Am Food Anim Pract* 2001; **17**: 403–420.

Haskel SRR, Gehing R, Payne MA, *et al.* Update on FARAD food animal drug withholding recommendation. *J Am Vet Med Assoc* 2003; **223**: 1277–2003.

Valverde A, Doherty TJ. Pain management in cattle and small ruminants. In: Anderson DE, Rings DM, eds. *Current Veterinary Therapy: Food Animal Medicine*, 5th edn. St Louis, MO: Saunders/Elsevier, 2009; 534–574.

Pot-bellied pigs have become popular house pets in the last two decades. Although the commercial value of these pigs may not be extraordinary, their owners are usually willing to spend more for veterinary care.

There are many anatomic and physiologic characteristics of pigs that make anesthetic management challenging. Special considerations for laboratory swine are discussed extensively elsewhere [6,7].

Sites of drug administration

Oral administration of a tranquilizer or sedative is sometimes needed to facilitate capture and/or reduce stress associated with restraint. In ruminants and camelids, oral medication is absorbed primarily via the rumen into the circulation. Absorption and distribution of the drug are affected by motility and the pH of the ruminal fluid. Reticuloruminal motility is primarily controlled by the medullary gastric center in the brain. Physical conditions like CNS depression, pain, fear, excitement, pyrexia, endotoxemia, hypocalcemia, and extreme wall distension (e.g., rumen tympany) tend to reduce rumen motility. Analgesics and anesthetics like opioids, α_2-adrenergic receptor agonists, and general anesthetics decrease gastric motility, resulting in prolonged gastric emptying time and enhanced drug absorption [8]. The pH difference of saliva (8.2), plasma (7.4), and ruminal contents (5.5–6.5) also affects drug absorption and distribution by altering drug ionization. Ionization and the amount of drug in saliva, plasma, and rumen are constantly changing, making it difficult to predict bioavailability and distribution of orally administered drugs (e.g., tranquilizer, sedative, or injectable anesthetic) [8]. Intramuscular (IM) and intravenous (IV) administration are usually the preferred routes because they produce more predictable calming. In monogastric animals like pigs, the pH in the stomach is acidic (1.5–2.5) [9]. As a result, there is usually better and faster absorption from the gastrointestinal tract and greater bioavailability of orally administered sedative drugs.

The external jugular veins of ruminants are easily palpable and visualized when occluded. A 14 gauge, 2–3 inch needle can be placed in the jugular vein of adult cattle for administration of injectable anesthetics and fluids during surgery. A 14 gauge, 5¼ inch over-the-needle indwelling catheter may be placed and secured for longer duration IV medication or fluid therapy. A surgical cut-down can be performed to facilitate insertion of the catheter through the thick skin of adult cattle. A 16 or 18 gauge IV catheter is appropriate for calves and small ruminants. The technique for IV catheterization in smaller ruminant species is similar to that used in calves. However, skin incision is generally not needed in smaller ruminants and the jugular vein is easily visualized when occluded.

Venepuncture and catheterization can be difficult in camelids because these animals have thick fiber coats and neck skin. More importantly, they do not have a jugular furrow and the external jugular veins lie deep to the sternomandibularis and brachiocephalicus muscles, ventral to the cervical vertebral transverse processes, and superficial to the carotid artery and vagosympathetic trunk within the carotid sheath for most of their length [10–14]. External jugular veins of camelids are not always visible even with occlusion of the vessels, particularly in adult males. The right external jugular vein is preferred for venepuncture and catheterization to avoid damage to the esophagus which runs on the left side of the neck. The landmarks for easy venepuncture are the cranial portion of the neck at the level of the mandible, on the caudoventral aspect of the neck, medial to the fifth cervical vertebral transverse process [12] (Fig. 38.1).

Venous blood of camelids carries a high percentage of oxyhemoglobin and appears to be bright red, and thus may be mistaken for arterial blood [15]. In addition, the caudoventral site of the right external jugular vein is in close proximity to the carotid artery. Attention to an absence of characteristic pulsatile arterial flow will help prevent inadvertent carotid arterial injection [12]. A 14 gauge indwelling catheter is appropriate for adult camelids, and a 16 or 18 gauge catheter is suitable for crias. The catheter should be secured with suture or bandage. Skin cut-down is helpful in passing the catheter into the jugular vein [16,17]. Camelids, like other long-necked animals, have four or five jugular vein valves located at irregular intervals to prevent blood pooling in the head when the animal grazes. The presence of these valves can hinder the advancement of an IV catheter, even when correct catheter placement is confirmed by blood flowing into the stylet of the catheter. Distension of the jugular vein with

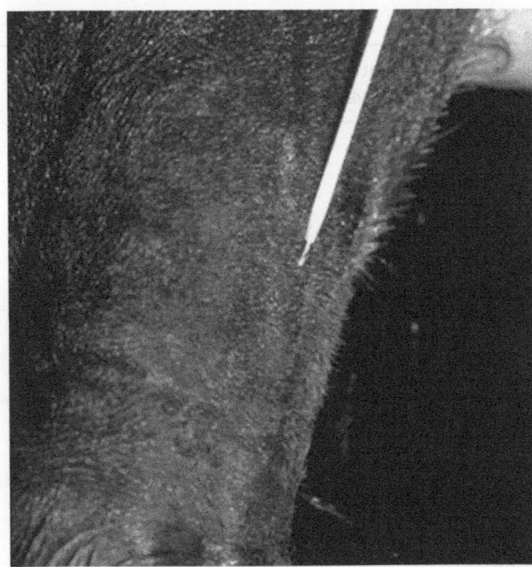

Figure 38.1 Intravenous catheterization in a llama. Source: HuiChu Lin, Department of Clinical Sciences, College of Veterinary Medicine, Auburn University, AL, USA.

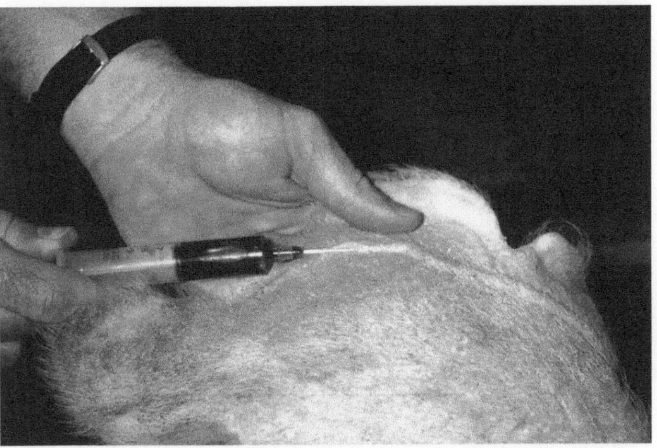

Figure 38.2 Intravenous catheterization in the auricular vein in a pig. Source: HuiChu Lin, Department of Clinical Sciences, College of Veterinary Medicine, Auburn University, AL, USA.

sterile saline facilitates advancement. If distension of the vessel is unsuccessful, relocate the placement site 1–2 cm cranially or caudally from the previous site [17]. An auricular (ear) vein is an alternative site for IV injection using a 25 gauge needle or butterfly catheter to deliver a small volume of sedative drug to cooperative camelids.

Pigs usually resist physical restraint. They are easily stressed when restrained and generally respond by constant struggling and vocalization [18–20]. Some pigs are susceptible to a genetic disorder, malignant hyperthermia (MH) or porcine stress syndrome, which is often fatal once triggered. Succinylcholine and halogenated inhalation anesthetics may trigger MH. Stressors like transportation or unfamiliar surroundings can also precipitate MH.

Preanesthetic physical examination and evaluation should be as stress free as possible. Rapid IM administration tends to be less stressful for pigs. Most pigs have a thick layer of subcutaneous fat, and more so for pot-bellied pigs. The adipose tissue layers in the neck and rump are particularly thick. Accurate deposition of preanesthetics or anesthetics into the muscle layer requires a needle with adequate length. Too short a needle will result in depositing the drug into the adipose tissue and slowed onset of action. It is recommended that IM injection be made at the semimembranosus and semitendinosus muscles located just above the hock or in the caudal portion of the biceps femoris muscle [18]. There is less fat in the area over these muscles, so muscle tissue can be reached with a 1½ inch needle. At the cervical or thoracic areas of the trapezius muscle, at least a 2 inch long needle will be required to ensure drug injection into muscle tissue. Inconsistent effects are observed more frequently if shorter needles are used in these areas [18]. Similar to other food-producing animals, IM injection into the gluteal 'ham' muscles is not recommended because of the potential for muscle inflammation and fibrosis [21].

Intravenous injection of preanesthetics or anesthetics in pigs can be very difficult, particularly in pot-bellied pigs, because of the lack of visible superficial veins. Generally, pigs do not tolerate physical restraint and often struggle throughout the procedure, increasing the risk of perivascular injection. On occasion, an auricular vein can be used for IV injection if the pig co-operates or is easily restrained (Fig. 38.2). Ideally, deep sedation and immobilization can be achieved with IM injection and anesthesia maintained with IV infusion, if needed. The jugular vein or anterior vena cava can be used for IV injection, but this technique is made difficult due to the thick neck and abundant jowls.

Auricular veins, especially lateral auricular veins, are common sites for IV injection because they are more superficial and easily accessible. However, in dark-colored ears IV injection remains challenging (e.g., pot-bellied pigs). In larger adults the central dorsal auricular vein is often utilized. An 18 or 20 gauge, 1–1½-inch hypodermic needle, indwelling, or butterfly catheter can be used, while a 21 or 23 gauge needle is suitable for smaller ears. A butterfly catheter has a shorter needle and tends to stay in the vessel better than hypodermic needles, especially when the animal struggles during the injection. An indwelling catheter should be placed if postoperative IV medication and/or fluid therapy are needed.

Intramedullary cannulation has been used for fluid and drug administration when other vascular access cannot be established. An 18 gauge cannula can be placed into either the greater tubercle of the humerus or the trochanteric fossa of the femur. Although this technique is performed easily in immature pigs, rate of fluid administration may be limited in older pigs due to the presence of fat and fibrosis of the medullary canal [22].

Positioning during anesthesia

Neuromyopathy has been associated with improper positioning and inadequate padding of the surgery table. Myopathy does not occur readily in large ruminants but nerve paralysis has been observed. Adult cattle should be placed on a 10 cm thick high-density foam pad, whereas a 5 cm thick foam pad is sufficient for calves, small ruminants, and camelids. When placing adult cattle in dorsal recumbency, the animal should be balanced squarely on its back with the gluteal areas bearing equal weight. All limbs should be flexed and relaxed. While in lateral recumbency, an automotive inner tube (valve stem pointed down) can be placed under the elbow of the dependent (lower) forelimb to prevent radial nerve paralysis. The dependent forelimb placed through the inner tube and the tube positioned directly under the shoulder, which prevents pressure on the radial nerve as it traverses the musculospiral groove of the humerus. The bony point of the shoulder should be positioned within the hollow center of the inner tube. Non-elastic or duct tape can be wrapped over the part of the inner tube not under the weight of the shoulder (opposite of valve stem) to prevent the tube from collapsing under the shoulder and ensure support.

Once the inner tube is in place, pull the dependent forelimb anteriorly so the weight of the thorax rests on the triceps but not the humerus. Both uppermost limbs (front and hindlimbs) should be elevated and parallel to the table surface to maintain venous drainage and prevent injury to the brachial plexus. These techniques minimize the pressure on the radial, femoral, or peroneal nerve of the dependent limb and prevent nerve paralysis. The head and neck should be at a slightly extended position (Figs 38.3 and 38.4). The dependent eye needs to be protected by administration of ophthalmic ointment and ensuring closure of the eye to minimize the risk of corneal ulcer [23,24]. For camelids, similar precautions should be instituted to prevent radial nerve paralysis. A padded, supporting 'H block' made of styrofoam with duct tape around the exterior can be used to support the upper, non-dependent limbs and keep pressure off the lower, dependent limbs. While in dorsal recumbency, overflexion or overstretching of the limbs to clear the limbs from the operative site with ropes should be avoided. Camelids have prominent eyes and administration of ophthalmic ointment and additional padding with gauze or soft towels under the dependent eye will minimize the potential for corneal laceration or ulceration [25].

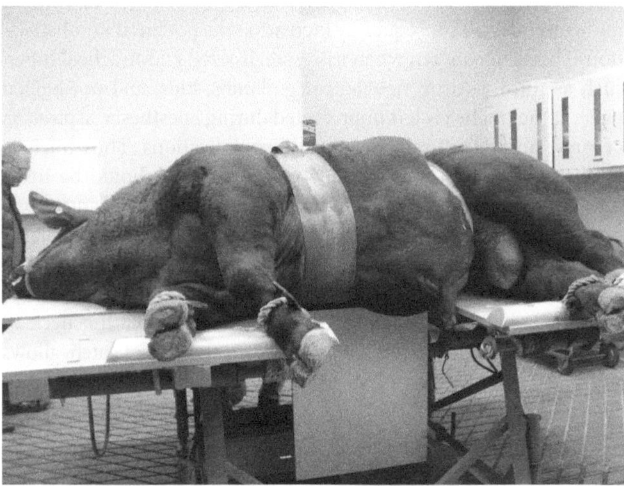

Figure 38.3 Positioning of the head and neck during lateral recumbency in a bull. Source: HuiChu Lin, Department of Clinical Sciences, College of Veterinary Medicine, Auburn University, AL, USA.

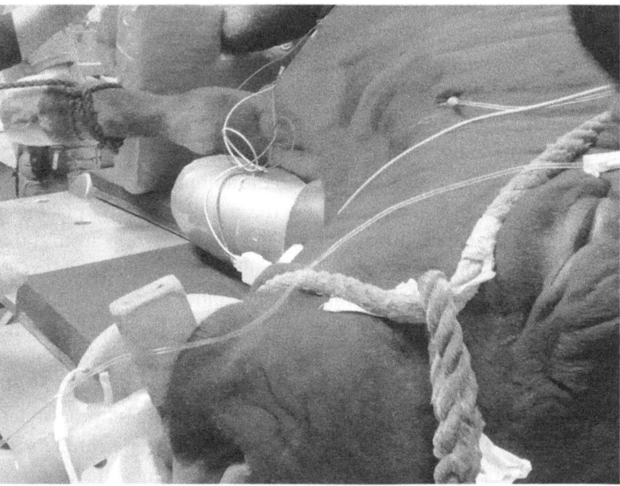

Figure 38.4 Supportive H-block and inner tube to prevent neuromyopathy during lateral recumbency in a bull. Source: HuiChu Lin, Department of Clinical Sciences, College of Veterinary Medicine, Auburn University, AL, USA.

Cardiopulmonary systems

Positional changes required for anesthesia and surgery can result in significant mismatching of ventilation and perfusion. This effect results from gravity and the weight of the chest wall on pulmonary blood flow and alveolar ventilation [26,27]. Normal, awake cattle breathe with smaller tidal volume and faster respiratory rate than do horses. Factors thought responsible for the observed smaller tidal volume and faster respiratory rate include smaller and completely separated bovine lung lobes[28]; lower work of breathing due to a greater maximum change in pleural pressure and the non-elastic work of breathing as well as lower dynamic lung compliance[29,30]; decreased breathing efficiency due to a diaphragm that is flatter and more vertical in conformation[31]; a large, easily expandable stomach which sits immediately caudal to the diaphragm and when filled to its maximum occupies three-quarters of the abdominal cavity[32–34]; and lastly, a tendency to greater alveolar ventilation and higher O_2 consumption[35]. As a result, cattle tend to have greater differences between alveolar and arterial O_2 partial pressure (PAO_2–PaO_2) than horses, particularly if placed in dorsal recumbency (even in the awake state) [26,27,36].

Lateral or dorsal recumbency causes the weight of the abdominal viscera to shift downward and forward, pushing the diaphragm further into the thoracic cavity, resulting in decreased functional residual capacity of the lung. The rumen of adult cattle is a big fermentation chamber with a capacity of 115–150 L or 250–300 g/kg of body weight. Preanesthetic fasting may reduce the degree of fermentation, but fermentation continues during anesthesia and gas accumulates in the rumen due to prohibition of eructation, resulting in increased intragastric pressure. As a result, lung compliance, tidal volume, and minute ventilation decrease significantly. This in turn increases the degree of ventilation/perfusion mismatch and the subsequent development of hypoventilation and hypoxemia [37,38].

Cardiopulmonary depression associated with commonly used anesthetics tends to exacerbate the severity of hypoventilation and hypoxemia [39]. Furthermore, compression of the great vessels such as the vena cava by the weight of abdominal viscera while in lateral or dorsal recumbency can result in decreased venous return, cardiac output, arterial blood pressures, and tissue perfusion [40]. Studies have shown that ventilation, cardiac output, and arterial blood pressure are better maintained when animals are positioned in sternal recumbency [37,38]. Unfortunately, many surgical procedures performed under general anesthesia require the animal to be placed in lateral or dorsal recumbency for easy surgical access. Nevertheless, arterial blood pressure in cattle in most instances is well maintained within acceptable limits during anesthesia [23].

Lateral recumbency has been reported to cause a significant decrease in PaO_2 in conscious sheep [41]. Severe hypoxemia and pulmonary edema have been implicated as the causes of death in sheep that die under anesthesia when xylazine has been administered [42–44]. Hypoxemia has also been observed in standing sheep during xylazine sedation [45,46]. All α_2-adrenergic receptor agonists cause significant decreases in PaO_2 without affecting $PaCO_2$ [47]. Increased airway pressure [48], severe pulmonary parenchymal damage [49], as well as bronchospasm and venospasm [50] occur as a result of peripheral α_2-adrenergic stimulation.

Gastrointestinal tract

Ruminal tympany

Ruminal tympany, regurgitation, and aspiration pneumonia are common problems associated with general anesthesia in ruminants. As mentioned previously, fermentation continues even in anesthetized animals. Postprandial gas production of an average of 30 L per hour has been reported in cattle [51]. Normal, awake animals are able to relieve the gas produced by fermentation through the esophagus. However, sedatives, anesthetics, and some body positions tend to inhibit gastrointestinal motility and inhibit eructation.

Regurgitation

Regurgitation and aspiration of stomach contents can occur in ruminants and camelids during anesthesia, particularly in non-fasted animals. The chance of regurgitation decreases significantly when water is restricted for 6–12 h and feed withheld for 12–24 h prior to anesthesia. Adult cattle have a large rumen that is usually full of liquid materials and does not empty completely even after 24–48 h of fasting. Regurgitation tends to occur more frequently when animals are in left lateral compared to right lateral recumbency. It can occur during either light (active regurgitation) or deep (passive regurgitation) anesthesia in spite of preanesthetic fasting and water withholding. Active regurgitation occurs during light anesthesia which is characterized by explosive discharge of large quantities of ruminal materials. Passive regurgitation occurs during deep planes of anesthesia when the esophageal muscles and transluminal pressure gradients relax as a result of anesthetic-induced muscle relaxation. If the airway is not protected, a large amount of ruminal material can be inhaled into the trachea and reach the small airways. Consequences of aspiration of acidic ruminal content may include aspiration pneumonia. Alveolar and capillary integrity are lost. Aspiration pneumonia is often characterized by reflex airway closure, bronchospasm, destruction of type II alveolar cells and pulmonary capillary lining cells, pulmonary edema and hemorrhage, dyspnea, hypoxemia, and cyanosis.

The prognosis following aspiration depends on the amount and the pH of the ruminal materials [51]. Pigs tend to have very acidic stomach contents with pH values as low as 1.5–2.5 [9] but pH values remain within 5.5–6.5 for the rumen [8] and 6.4–7.0 for the C-1 of camelids [25]. Thus, in ruminants and camelids the impact of aspiration depends more on the amount of bacterial microflora and solid food materials aspirated, whereas in pigs the acidity of the aspirate is more damaging to pulmonary tissues. Nevertheless, reflex airway constriction, mechanical airway obstruction, and aspiration of bacteria occur and can be life threatening in ruminants [51]. In extreme cases, the animal dies before an endotracheal tube can be placed to protect the airway. Preoperative withholding of feed and water and endotracheal intubation with immediate cuff inflation following induction are recommended in all anesthetized ruminants and camelids.

Pigs are monogastric and regurgitation does not occur as commonly as in ruminants. However, vomiting can result when pigs were not fasted before anesthesia and following administration of xylazine. In pigs, withholding food for 12 h and water for 6–8 h before anesthesia is sufficient for most elective surgeries [20,52]. It has been recommended to remove hay, alfalfa or straw from the diet and environment for a minimum of 2–3 days prior to anesthesia to avoid prolonged gastric emptying time.

Salivation

Ruminants normally salivate profusely during anesthesia. Total amounts of salivary secretion in conscious adult cattle and sheep have been reported to be 50 L and 6–16 L per 24 h, respectively [53,54]. In the past, antimuscarinics like atropine have been routinely administered as part of the anesthetic induction regimen in an attempt to prevent salivation. However, atropine is only able to reduce the water content of the saliva [55], causing it to become more viscous and subsequently increasing the potential for obstruction. This is of concern when using small-sized endotracheal tubes, such as those used in neonates (e.g., lambs, kids, and pot-bellied pigs). If the trachea is left unprotected during anesthesia, aspiration of large amounts of saliva can cause complications. Thus tracheal intubation with appropriate inflation of the cuff should be instituted immediately following induction. For large ruminants, positioning the animal on the surgery table in a way that the throat latch is elevated relative to the mouth and thoracic inlet helps to drain and prevent pooling of saliva and regurgitant in the oral cavity (see Fig. 38.4). Placing a sandbag or rolled towel under the neck of smaller ruminants or camelids to elevate the throat latch allows saliva and regurgitant to flow away from the airway opening [56] (Fig. 38.5).

Endotracheal intubation

Tracheal intubation is often difficult to accomplish in farm animals. Blind intubation as performed in horses is less likely to succeed. For large ruminants, this author's preference is to use the digital palpation technique to guide the endotracheal tube into the trachea with the animal in either sternal or lateral recumbency immediately following induction of anesthesia. Another technique is to use a stomach tube as stylet and, with the aid of digital palpation, to place the stomach tube in the trachea. The anesthetist then threads the endotracheal tube into the trachea and removes the stomach tube once the endotracheal tube is in place.

In calves, intubation is easier when the animal is placed in sternal recumbency and an assistant pulls the mouth open by placing a loop of gauze around the upper jaw and a second loop around the lower jaw and tongue. An assistant should lift the head up and keep the head and the neck in a straight line to allow visualization of the epiglottis and the larynx. If the larynx cannot be visualized, the neck should be extended further. A laryngoscope with a long blade (250–350 mm) can be used to depress the tongue base and the epiglottis to enable visualization of the larynx. A 'guide tube' or 'stylet' (preferably two 10 French, 22 inch long polyethylene canine urethral catheters taped together to make up three times the length of the endotracheal tube) can be used (Figs 38.6 and 38.7). A cuffed endotracheal tube will prevent regurgitation and aspiration of ruminal contents, and the calf should be maintained in sternal recumbency until the cuff is inflated.

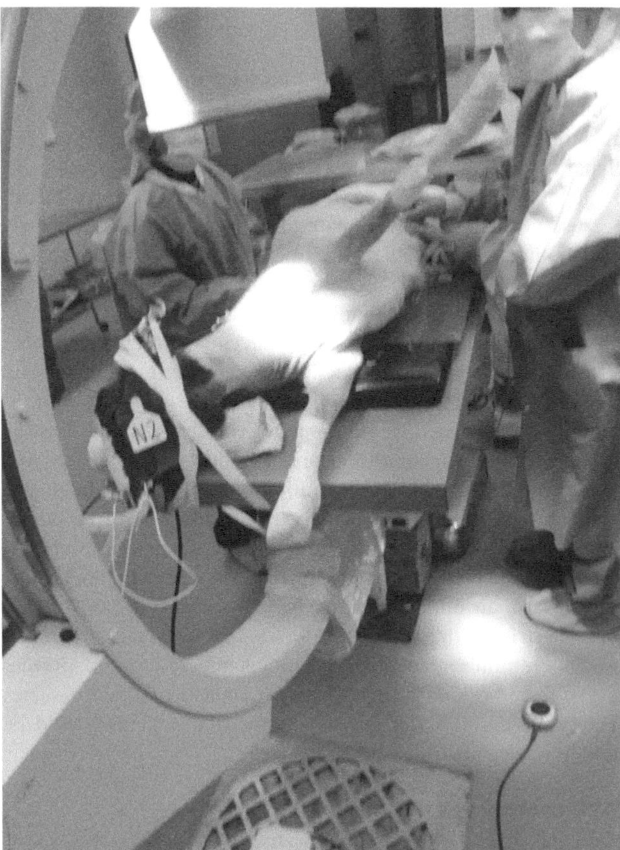

Figure 38.5 Elevation of the throat latch during lateral recumbency in a goat. Source: HuiChu Lin, Department of Clinical Sciences, College of Veterinary Medicine, Auburn University, AL, USA.

Intubation in small ruminants and camelids is more difficult when compared to carnivores, because their jaws cannot be opened as widely, their intermandibular space is narrow, and the laryngeal opening is invisible behind the thick base of the tongue. In addition, the elongated soft palate may be situated either ventral or dorsal to the epiglottis in llamas and alpacas. This adds to the difficulty of direct visualization of the larynx and correct endotracheal intubation [25]. In general, the technique used for tracheal intubation of small ruminants and camelids is similar to that used in calves. With the animal in sternal recumbency, intubation is accomplished with the help of a guide tube or stylet and a long-bladed laryngoscope (250–350 mm) as described for calves previously. Hyperextending the animal's neck is sometimes helpful in visualizing the larynx (see Figs 38.6, 38.7). If difficulty is encountered in advancing the endotracheal tube through the larynx into the trachea, repositioning of the head, fixing the larynx from the exterior, and gently rotating the tube 360° while advancing the tube are recommended. Most importantly, the animal must be adequately anesthetized (relaxed) to prevent spasms when threading the tube through the arytenoid cartilage into the trachea. Similar to calves, a cuffed endotracheal tube should be used and the animal should be maintained in sternal recumbency until the cuff is inflated appropriately. Blind intubation, similar to that used in horses, has been used for intubation in sheep and goats. However, this technique may require multiple attempts in order to successfully place the endotracheal tube in the trachea.

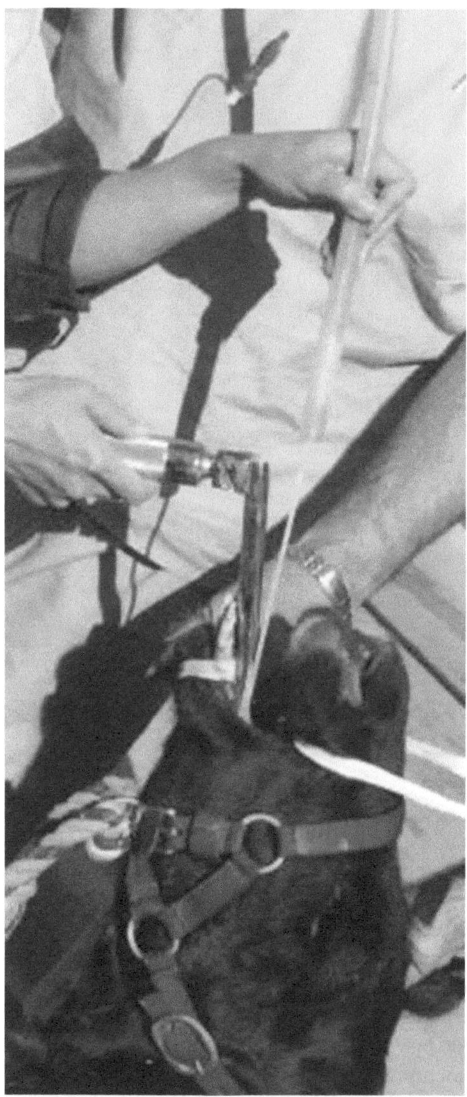

Figure 38.6 Endotracheal intubation of a llama. Source: HuiChu Lin, Department of Clinical Sciences, College of Veterinary Medicine, Auburn University, AL, USA.

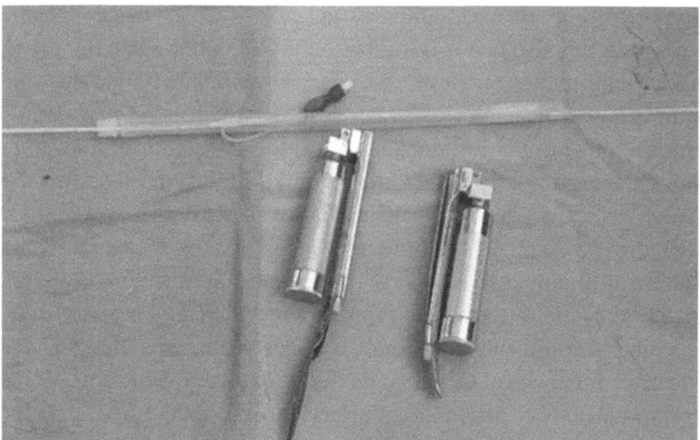

Figure 38.7 Endotracheal tracheal tube, 'guide tube' (stylet), and laryngoscope used for calves, small ruminants, camelids, and pigs. Source: HuiChu Lin, Department of Clinical Sciences, College of Veterinary Medicine, Auburn University, AL, USA.

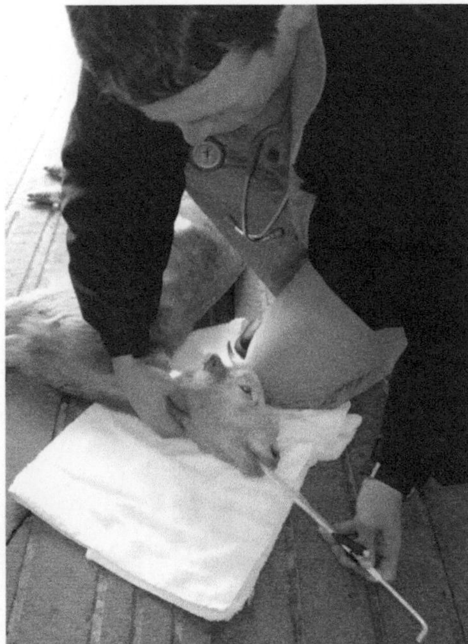

Figure 38.8 'Stick intubation' technique in a goat. Source: HuiChu Lin, Department of Clinical Sciences, College of Veterinary Medicine, Auburn University, AL, USA.

Another technique described as 'stick intubation' has been used effectively in small ruminants in the field. With the animal in lateral recumbency, a small diameter rod made of wood or stainless steel can be used as a stylet to stiffen the endotracheal tube, with one hand occluding the esophagus while the other hand manipulates the endotracheal tube into the trachea (Fig. 38.8). Care and gentle maneuvering should always be used to prevent laryngeal spasm and minimize trauma to the oral mucous membrane.

Of all domestic species, endotracheal intubation has proven to be most difficult in pigs because the mouth cannot be widely opened, the epiglottis is often entrapped behind the soft palate, the prominent dorsal protrusion of the base of the tongue obstructs the view for direct visualization of the larynx, the small larynx slopes downward, creating an acute angle to the tracheal opening (ventral floor fornix), and susceptibility to laryngeal spasm. Vomiting can also occur if intubation is attempted while the pig is under light planes of anesthesia, especially when the animal is not appropriately fasted prior to anesthesia. Application of a small amount of a local anesthetic (e.g., 2% lidocaine solution) to desensitize the larynx may reduce the potential for laryngeal spasm. In larger or adult pigs, tracheal intubation is easier to accomplish with the pig in sternal recumbency. Using the same technique as in small ruminants and camelids with the aid of laryngoscope and stylet, the epiglottis and laryngeal aperture can be visualized. Keeping in mind the acute angle between the larynx and tracheal opening, it is helpful to put some dorsal pressure at the end of the endotracheal tube as it enters the larynx. This technique keeps the tip of the tube slightly elevated as it advances into the trachea. Other helpful tips for successful endotracheal intubation in pigs are to spin the tube 180° or use a screw-like approach and advance it in a dorsal direction while the tube enters the arytenoid cartilages into the trachea [7,18,57,58].

Thermoregulation

Hypothermia

Decreased heat production as well as increased heat loss are the primary causes of significant decreases in body temperature and hypothermia observed during anesthesia and surgery [59]. Hypothermia is a common anesthetic complication in small companion animals, but is rarely an issue for adult cattle and camelids because of their large body mass to surface area ratio. The body temperature of adult cattle and camelids seldom drops more than 0.5°C during anesthesia if none of the major body cavities is opened. However, hypothermia can be a significant problem in small ruminants, particularly in pediatric patients. Hypothermia often results in significant reduction of anesthetic requirement and prolonged recovery [60]. Although often obese, pigs lack an insulating hair coat and thus are prone to hypothermia and must be protected from temperature extremes and insensible heat loss during anesthesia [20]. Long duration of anesthesia without supplemental heat in pediatric pigs has resulted in hypothermia with body temperature of 92°F and subsequent prolonged recovery has been observed by this author. Therefore, supplemental heat with a forced warm air unit, circulating warm water blanket, or resistive foam electric heating pad (e.g., Hot Dog Patient Warmer) can be used to minimize reduction of body temperature and prevent severe hypothermia during surgery. Supplemental heat sources specifically designed for use in anesthetized patients should be used to reduce the risk of thermal burns.

Malignant hyperthermia

Malignant hyperthermia, also referred to as 'porcine stress syndrome,' is a genetic disorder with mutation of the ryanodine receptor gene (RYR1), important for function of calcium channels in skeletal muscles [61–63]. The presence of mutated ryanodine receptors allows a massive amount of calcium to be released from the cells into the sarcoplasmic reticulum, resulting in excessive generalized skeletal muscle contraction [64]. Malignant hyperthermia has been reported in other animal species, but pigs and humans seem to be most susceptible [61,63,64]. Certain breeds of pigs like Pietrain, Poland China, and Landrace have a higher prevalence of this syndrome; Large White, Yorkshire, and Hampshire, on the other hand, much less so [52,65].

The clinical signs of malignant hyperthermia syndrome are manifested as a sudden and dramatic rise in body temperature and end-tidal CO_2 followed by excessive muscle fasciculation, muscle rigidity, tachypnea, tachycardia, arrhythmias, myoglobinuria, metabolic acidosis, renal failure, and often death. Prognosis is usually poor once the episode is initiated in spite of immediate aggressive treatments. The triggering agents of malignant hyperthermia include stress (induced by excitement, transportation, or preanesthetic handling and restraint), halogenated inhalation anesthetics (e.g., halothane, isoflurane, sevoflurane, and desflurane), and succinylcholine. Lidocaine and ketamine had been indicated as triggering agents, but there is no evidence to support this theory [66].

Halogenated inhalation anesthetics are a known trigger for malignant hyperthermia, and halothane is most frequently reported as an initiator in pigs [67]. Only one incidence of isoflurane-induced malignant hyperthermia has been reported in a pot-bellied pig [68]. There are no reports of isoflurane- or sevoflurane-induced malignant hyperthermia episodes in cattle. Analysis of muscular contracture in frogs showed that the augmentation of caffeine-induced contractures of sartorius muscle by isoflurane is three times, enflurane is four times, and halothane is 11 times baseline [69]. A human study showed that in a total of 75 malignant hyperthermia cases, 42 were isoflurane related, 12 were sevoflurane, 11 were halothane, and eight were enflurane related [70]. The lower incidence associated with halothane in humans likely represents its limited use in people.

Treatments for malignant hyperthermia are primarily symptomatic. Early recognition of symptoms (e.g., muscle rigidity, sudden rise in body temperature and end-tidal CO_2) and aggressive treatments (e.g., immediate discontinuation of inhalation anesthetics and institution of ice packs and alcohol baths) are the keys to better prognosis. Dantrolene sodium has been effective as a treatment (1–3 mg/kg IV) and prophylaxis (5 mg/kg PO) for malignant hyperthermia [22]. In 1981, McGrath *et al.* [71] reported that acepromazine at 1.1 mg/kg IM and 1.65 mg/kg IM reduced the incidence of malignant hyperthermia by 40% and 73%, respectively. A lower dose of 0.55 mg/kg IM was only able to delay but not prevent the onset of the episode.

Anesthetic requirements

Xylazine is a potent sedative, analgesic, and muscle relaxant that is frequently used as a preanesthetic or anesthetic adjunct in ruminants and camelids. Cattle require only one-tenth of the dose needed in horses to produce equipotent sedation [72]. It appears that Brahmans have the lowest dose requirement, Herefords are intermediate, and Holsteins are the least sensitive [73,74].

Administration of xylazine to pregnant ruminants in the final trimester may cause altered uterine motility and may be associated with premature parturition and retention of fetal membranes [75,76]. In pregnant dairy cows during late gestation, administration of xylazine (0.04 mg/kg IV) resulted in a significant increase in uterine vascular resistance (118–156%) and a decrease in uterine blood flow (25–59%) which resulted in a significant decrease in O_2 delivery (59%) [77]. Therefore, the use of xylazine during late gestation in pregnant ruminants is not routinely recommended to avoid detrimental effects to the fetus.

Pronounced and prolonged responses have been observed when xylazine was administered to cattle under high ambient temperature [78]. Interestingly, camelids require more xylazine than ruminants, so higher doses are required to produce similar sedation and the dose requirement is even higher for alpacas than llamas. Compared to other farm animal species, pigs have the highest dose requirement for α_2-adrenergic agonist-induced sedation. α_2 Adrenergic receptor agonists may not produce adequate sedation in some pigs. Pigs also appear less responsive to the pharmacologic effects of opioids [79,80]. Though benzodiazepines (e.g., diazepam and midazolam) often do not produce effective sedation in other species, they seem to produce reliable sedation in pigs [19].

Ruminants and camelids require less tolazoline (an α_2-adrenergic receptor antagonist) than other species [81,82]. Lower doses of tolazoline at 0.5–1.5 mg/kg IV are recommended for use in ruminants. Others have suggested that IV administration of tolazoline should be avoided, except in emergency situations, to prevent adverse effects such as hypotension and cardiac asystole [83].

Statements by owners and breeders regarding anesthetic management such as 'injectable anesthetics should not be used in young pigs' and 'ketamine in particular should not be used in pot-bellied pigs of any age' are common [84]. These statements are not supported by controlled, scientific studies. Furthermore, the clinical experiences of this author and most practicing veterinarians indicate otherwise.

Ruminants recover gradually but smoothly from Telazol® anesthesia as a result of the slower metabolism and longer lasting effect of zolazepam [85,86]. Pigs, on the other hand, often experience prolonged and rough recovery characterized by swimming motions with repeated attempts to right themselves when recovering from Telazol anesthesia, similar to that observed when ketamine is used alone [19,87]. Studies have shown that tiletamine and zolazepam are both eliminated more slowly in pigs than in other species [87] and tiletamine apparently has a longer effect than zolazepam in pigs [86].

Ruminants reportedly have extremely low levels of pseudocholinesterase, the enzyme responsible for metabolism and inactivation of depolarizing neuromuscular blocking drugs such as succinylcholine. Therefore, administration of succinylcholine to ruminants often results in prolonged duration of muscle paralysis and is contraindicated [88].

Airway management during recovery

Prior to removal of the endotracheal tube, manual removal of regurgitant and saliva from the buccal cavity or by lavaging with water may be performed. During recovery, displacement of the soft palate can occur in camelids, causing the soft palate to situate dorsally to the epiglottis and hinder air flow into the larynx. This is a serious condition and may result in upper airway obstruction and eventually cardiac arrest since camelids are obligate nasal breathers. If the animal has regained consciousness and swallowing reflex, the problem can be corrected by encouraging the animal to swallow. Otherwise, the animal needs to be reintubated until the swallowing reflex returns [89].

Prolonged duration of dorsal recumbency in camelids often results in severe nasal edema which can cause airway obstruction following extubation during recovery [90]. Keeping the animal's head high with the animal in sternal recumbency, administration of a nasal spray containing phenylephrine and providing O_2 insufflations with a demand valve should be instituted until the nasal edema diminishes and adequate air flow through the nasal cavity resumes.

Pigs are more difficult to intubate until one becomes accustomed to their anatomic differences. Laryngeal edema and laryngospasm caused by failed intubation attempts can potentially result in airway obstruction in lightly anesthetized pigs. Topical lidocaine applied to the larynx and adequate plane of anesthesia during the intubation process will allow smooth and successful intubation and minimize trauma to the larynx [91]. In sows receiving spinal anesthesia and placed in lateral recumbency for cesarean section, restraint of the head with rope may be necessary to prevent head movement. Care should be taken to avoid placing the head in extension. Unlike most other species, extension of the head can complicate rather than resolve upper airway obstruction in swine. Similar to camelids, dorsal displacement of soft palate resulting in airway obstruction and suffocation has been reported in swine due to their long soft palate engaging the larynx [91]. This complication occurs in non-intubated pigs during anesthesia or following extubation as a result of dorsal displacement of the long soft palate [89]. Noisy respiration after extubation indicates possible laryngeal spasm or upper airway obstruction and should be investigated immediately [18].

References

1 Craigmill AL, Rangel-Lugo M, Damian P, *et al.* Extralabel use of tranquilizers and general anesthetics. *J Am Vet Med Assoc* 1997; **211**: 302–304.

2 Davis JL, Smith GW, Baynes RE, *et al.* Update on drug prohibited for extralabel use in food animals. *J Am Vet Med Assoc* 2009; **235**: 528–534.

3 US FDA. Animal Medicinal Drug Use Clarification Act of 1994 (AMDUCA). www.fda.gov/AnimalVeterinary/GuidanceComplianceEnforcement/ActsRulesRegulations/ucm085377.htm (accessed 29 September 2014).

4 Papich MG. Drug residue considerations for anesthetics and adjunctive drugs in food-producing animals. *Vet Clin North Am Food Animal Pract* 1996; **12**: 693–706.

5 Fajt VR. Label and extralabel drug use in small ruminants. *Vet Clin North Am Food Anim Pract* 2001; **17**: 403–420.

6 Smith AC, Ehler W, Swindle MM. Anesthesia and analgesia in swine. In: Kohn DH, Wixson SK, White WJ, Benson GJ, eds. *Anesthesia and Analgesia in Laboratory Animals.* New York: Academic Press, 1997; 313–336.

7 Swindle MM. Anesthesia and analgesia. In: *Surgery, Anesthesia, and Experimental Techniques in Swine.* Ames, IA: Iowa State University Press, 1998; 33–63.

8 Hinchcliff KW, Jernigan AD, Upson DW, *et al.* Ruminant pharmacology. *Vet Clin North Am Food Animal Pract* 1991; **7**: 633–649.

9 DeRouchey J, Goodband B, Tokach M, *et al.* Digestive system of the pig – anatomy and function. *Proceedings of the North American Veterinary Conference*, 2009; **375–376.**

10 Fowler ME. The jugular vein (*Lama peruna*): a clinical note. *J Zoo Anim Med* 1983; **14**: 77–78.

11 Fowler ME. Anatomy information. *Camelid Medicine Workshop Syllabus* 1984: 5–16.

12 Amsel SI, Kainer RA, Johnson LW. Choosing the best site to perform venipuncture in a llama. *Vet Med* 1987; **82**: 535–536.

13 Riebold TW, Kaneps AJ, Schmotzer WB. Anesthesia in the llama. *Vet Surg* 1989; **18**: 400–404.

14 Pugh DG, Navarre CB, Ruffin DC, *et al.* A review of diagnostic procedures in llamas and alpacas. *Vet Med* 1999; **94**: 654–659.

15 Grint N, Dugdale A. Brightness of venous blood in South American camelids: implications for jugular catheterization. *J Anaesth Analg* 2009; **36**: 63–66.

16 Heath RB. Llama anesthetic programs. *Vet Clin North Am Food Anim Pract* 1989; **5**: 71–80.

17 Davis IA, McGaffin JR, Kuchinka GD. Intravenous catheterization of the external jugular vein in llamas. *Compend Contin Educ Pract Vet* 1996; **18**: 330–335.

18 Ko JCH, Thurmon JC, Tranquilli WJ, *et al.* Problems encountered when anesthetizing potbellied pigs. *Vet Med* 1993; **88**: 435–440.

19 Moon PF, Smith LJ. General anesthetic techniques in swine. *Vet Clin North Am Food Anim Pract* 1996; **12**: 663–691

20 Wolff P. Pet pig problems. *Proceedings of the North American Veterinary* Conference, 2009; 416–419.

21 Ivany JM, Muir WW. Farm animal anesthesia. In: Fubini SL, Ducharme NG, eds. *Farm Animal Surgery.* St Louis, MO: Saunders, 2004; 97–112.

22 Anderson DE, St Jean G. Anesthesia and surgical procedures in swine. In: Zimmerman JJ, Karriker LA, Ramirez A, Schwartz KJ, Stenson GW, eds. *Diseases of Swine,* 10th edn. Ames, IA: John Wiley, 2012; 119–140.

23 Thurmon JC, Benson GJ. Anesthesia in ruminants and swine. In: Howard JC, ed. *Current Veterinary Therapy: Food Animal Practice*, 3rd edn. Philadelphia: WB Saunders, 1993; 58–76.

24 Riebold TW. Ruminants. In: Tranquilli WJ, Thurmon JC, Grimm KA, eds. *Lumb and Jones' Veterinary Anesthesia and Analgesia*, 4th edn. Ames, IA: Blackwell Publishing, 2007; 731–746.

25 Fowler ME. Anesthesia. In: *Medicine and Surgery of Camelids*, 3rd edn. Ames, IA: John Wiley, 2010; 111–127.

26 McDonell W. Respiratory system. In: Thurmon JC, Tranquilli WJ, Benson GJ, eds. *Lumb and Jones' Veterinary Anesthesia*, 3rd edn. Baltimore, MD: Williams & Wilkins, 1996; 115–147.

27 Tagawa M, Okano S, Sako T, *et al.* Effect of change in body position on cardiopulmonary function and plasma cortisol in cattle. *J Vet Med Sci* 1994; **56**: 131–134.

28 McLaughlin RF, Tyler WS, Canada RO. A study of the subgross pulmonary anatomy in various mammals. *Am J Vet Res* 1961; **108**: 149–165.

29 Musewe VO. Respiration mechanics, breathing patterns, ventilation, and diaphragmatic electromyogram (EMG) in normal, unsedated adult, domestic cattle (*Bos Taurus*) breathing spontaneously in the standing and the sternal-recumbent body positions, and during inflation of the rumen with air. PhD thesis. Davis, CA: University of California Davis, 1978.

30 Gallivan GJ, McDonell WN, Forrest JB. Comparative pulmonary mechanics in the horse and the cow. *Res Vet Sci* 1989; **46**: 322–330.

31 Lumb AB. Pulmonary ventilation: mechanisms and the work of breathing. In: Lumb AB, ed. *Nunn's Applied Respiratory Physiology.* Oxford: Butterworth Heinemann, 2000; 112–137.

32 Dyce KM, Sack WO, Wensing CJG. The abdomen of the ruminants. In: *Textbook of Veterinary Anatomy.* Philadelphia: WB Saunders, 1987; 633–656.

33 Habel RE. Ruminant digestive system. In: Getty R, ed. *Sisson and Grossman's The Anatomy of the Domestic Animals*, 5th edn. Philadelphia: WB Saunders, 1975; 861–915.

34 Kesler EM, Ronning M, Knodt CB. Functional and structural development of the ruminant forestomach. *J Anim Sci* 1951; **10**: 969–975.

35 Gallivan GJ, McDonell WN, Forrest JB. Comparative ventilation and gas exchange in the horse and the cow. *Res Vet Sci* 1989; **46**: 331–336.

36 Wagner AE, Muir WW, Brospitch BJ. Cardiopulmonary effects of position in conscious cattle. *Am J Vet Res* 1990; **51**: 7–10.

37 Musewe VO, Gillepsie JR, Berry JD. Influence of ruminal insufflation on pulmonary function and diaphragmatic electromyography in cattle. *Am J Vet Res* 1979; **40**: 26–31.

38 Desmecht D, Linden A, Lekeux P. Pathophysiological response of bovine diaphragm function to gastric distension. *J Appl Physiol* 1995; **78**: 1537–1546.

39 Lin HC, Tyler JW, Welles EG, *et al.* Effects of anesthesia induced and maintained by continuous intravenous administration of guaifenesin, ketamine, and xylazine in spontaneously breathing sheep. *Am J Vet Res* 1993; **54**: 1913–1916.

40 Klein L, Fisher N. Cardiopulmonary effects of restraint in dorsal recumbency on awake cattle. *Am J Vet Res* 1988; **49**: 1605–1608.

41 Mitchell B, Williams JT. Respiratory function changes in sheep associated with lying in lateral recumbency and with sedation by xylazine. *Proceedings of the Association of Veterinary Anaesthetists of Great Britain and Ireland*, 1976–77; **6**: 30–36.

42 Hsu WH, Schaffer DD, Hanson CE. Effects of tolazoline and yohimbine on xylazine-induced central nervous system depression, bradycardia, and tachypnea in sheep. *J Am Vet Med Assoc* 1987; **190**: 423–426.

43 Hsu WH, Hanson CE, Hembrough FB, *et al.* Effects of idazoxan, tolazoline, and yohimbine on xylazine-induced respiratory changes and central nervous system depression in ewes. *Am J Vet Res* 1989; **50**: 1570–1573.

44 Lin HC, Tyler JW, Wallace SS, *et al.* Telazol and xylazine anesthesia in sheep. *Cornell Vet* 1993; **83**: 117–124.

45 Doherty TJ, Ballinger JA, McDonnell WN, *et al.* Antagonism of xylazine-induced sedation by a new alpha-2 adrenergic receptor antagonist idazoxan. *Can J Vet Res* 1987; **55**: 244–248.

46 Waterman AE, Nolan A, Livingston A. Influence of idazoxan on respiratory blood gas changes induced by alpha-2 adrenergic receptor adrenoceptor agonist drugs in conscious sheep. *Vet Rec* 1987; **121**: 105–107.

47 Celly CS, McDonell WN, Black WD. The comparative hypoxaemic effect of four alpha-2 adrenergic receptor adrenoceptor agonists (xylazine, romifidine, detomidine, and medetomidine) in sheep. *J Vet Pharmacol Ther* 1997; **20**: 464–471.

48 Nolan A, Livingston A, Waterman A. The effects of alpha-2 adrenoceptor agonists on airway pressure in anaesthetized sheep. *J Vet Pharmacol Ther* 1986; **9**: 157–163.

49 Celly CS, Atwal OS, McDonell WN, *et al.* The histopathologic alterations induced in the lungs of sheep by use of alpha-2 adrenergic receptor-adrenergic receptor agonists. *Am J Vet Res* 1999; **60**: 154–161.

50 Kästner SBR. Alpha-2 adrenergic receptor-agonists in sheep: a review. *Vet Anaesth Analg* 2006; **33**: 79–96.

51 Steffey EP. Some characteristics of ruminants and swine that complicate management of general anesthesia. *Vet Clin North Am Food Animal Pract* 1986; **2**: 507–516.

52 Thurmon JC, Benson GJ. Special anesthesia considerations of swine. In: Short CE, ed. *Principles & Practice: Veterinary Anesthesia.* Baltimore, MD: Williams & Wilkins, 1987; 308–322.

53 Somers M. Saliva secretion and its functions in ruminants. *Aust Vet J* 1957; **33**: 297–301.

54 Kay RNR. The rate of flow and composition of various salivary secretion in sheep and calves. *J Physiol* 1960; **150**: 515–537.

55 Weaver AD. Complications in halothane anesthesia of cattle. *Zentralb Veterinarmed A* 1971; **18**: 409–416.

56 Thurmon JC, Benson GJ. Anesthesia in ruminants. In: Howard JL, ed. *Current Veterinary Therapy: Food Animal Practice.* Philadelphia: WB Saunders, 1983; 58–81.

57 Swindle MM. *Anesthetic and Perioperative Techniques in Swine.* Andover, MA: Charles River Laboratories, 1991.

58 Wilbers AM. Routine veterinary care of pot-bellied pigs. *Proceedings of the North American Veterinary Conference*, 2009; 410–412.

59 Haskins SC. Monitoring the anesthetized patients. In: Short CE, ed. *Principles & Practice: Veterinary Anesthesia.* Baltimore, MD: Williams & Wilkins, 1987; 455–477.

60 Hall LW, Clarke KW. Accident and emergencies associated with anesthesia. In: *Veterinary Anaesthesia*, 8th edn. London: Baillière Tindall: London, 1983; 367–388.

61 Fuji J, Otsu K, Zorzato F, *et al.* Identification of a mutation in porcine ryanodine receptor associated with malignant hyperthermia. *Science* 1991; **253**: 448–451.

62 Geer R, Decanniere C, Ville H, *et al.* Identification of halothane gene carriers by use of an in vivo 3IP nuclear magnetic resonance spectroscopy in pigs. *Am J Vet Res* 1992; **53**: 1711–1714.

63 Houde A, Pomnier SA, Roy R. Detection of the ryanodine receptor mutation associated with malignant hyperthermia in purebred swine populations. *J Anim Sci* 1993; **71**: 1414–1418.

64 Stoelting RK, Dierdorf SF, McCammon RL. Pediatric patients. In: *Anesthesia and Coexisting Disease*, 2nd edn. New York: Churchill Livingstone, 1988; 807–883.

65 Jorgensen JS, Cannedy AL. Physiologic and pathologic considerations for ruminants and swine anesthesia. *Vet Clin North Am Food Anim Pract* 1996; **12**: 481–500.

66 Hildebrand SV. Hyperthermia, malignant hyperthermia, and myopathy. In: Short CE, ed. *Principles & Practice: Veterinary Anesthesia*. Baltimore, MD: Williams & Wilkins, 1987; 517–532.

67 Stoelting RK, Hillier SC. Inhaled anesthetics. In: *Pharmacology & Physiology in Anesthetic Practice*, 4th edn. Philadelphia: Lippincott Williams & Wilkins, 2005; 42–86.

68 Claxton-Gill MS, Cornick-Seahorn JL, Gamboa JC, *et al.* Suspected malignant hyperthermia syndrome in a miniature pot-bellied pig anesthetized with isoflurane. *J Am Vet Med Assoc* 1993; **203**: 1434–1436.

69 Reed SB, Strobel GE. An in vitro model of malignant hyperthermia: differential effects of inhalation anesthetics on caffeine-induced muscle contractures. *Anesthesiology* 1978; **48**: 254–259.

70 Hopkins PM. Malignant hyperthermia: pharmacology of triggering. *Br J Anaesth* 2011; **107**: 48–56.

71 McGrath CJ, Rempel WE, Addis PB, *et al.* Acepromazine and droperidol inhibition of halothane-induced malignant hyperthermia (porcine stress syndrome) in swine. *Am J Vet Res* 1981; **42**: 195–198.

72 Greene SA, Thurmon JC. Xylazine – a review of its pharmacology and use in veterinary medicine. *J Vet Pharmacol Ther* 1988; **11**: 295–313.

73 Raptopoulos D, Weaver BMQ. Observations following intravenous xylazine administration in steers. *Vet Rec* 1984; **114**: 567–569.

74 Trim CM. Special anesthesia considerations in the ruminant. In: Short CE, ed. *Principles & Practice: Veterinary Anesthesia*. Baltimore, MD: Williams & Wilkins, 1987; 285–300.

75 LeBlanc MM, Hubbell JAE, Smith HC. The effect of xylazine hydrochloride on intrauterine pressure in the cow and the mare. *Proceedings of the Annual Meeting of the Society of Theriogenology*, 1984; **211–220**.

76 Jansen CAM, Lowe KC, Nathanielsz PW. The effects of xylazine on uterine activity, fetal and maternal oxygenation, cardiovascular function, and fetal breathing. *Am J Obstet Gynecol* 1984; **148**: 386–390.

77 Hodgson DS, Dunlop CI, Chapman PL, *et al.* Cardiopulmonary effects of xylazine and acepromazine in pregnant cows in late gestation. *Am J Vet Res* 2002; **63**: 1695–1699.

78 Fayed AH, Abdalla EB, Anderson RR, *et al.* Effect of xylazine in heifers under thermoneutral or heat stress conditions. *Am J Vet Res* 1989; **50**: 151–153.

79 Steffey EP, Baggot JD, Eisele JH, *et al.* Morphine-isoflurane interaction in dogs, swine and Rhesus monkeys. *J Vet Pharmacol Ther* 1994; **17**: 202–210.

80 Moon PF, Scarlett JM, Ludders JW, *et al.* The effect of fentanyl on the minimum alveolar concentration of isoflurane in swine. *Anesthesiology* 1995; **83**: 535–542.

81 Read MR, Duke T, Towes AR. Suspected tolazoline toxicosis in a llama. *J Am Vet Med Assoc* 2000; **216**: 227–229.

82 Lin HC, Riddell MG. Tolazoline: dose responses and side effects in non-sedated Holstein calves. *Bov Practitioner* 2008; **42**: 86–92.

83 Anderson DE. New methods for chemical restraint and field anesthesia in cattle. *Proceedings of the North American Veterinary Conference*, 2011; **6–11**.

84 www.pigs4ever.com/pot_belly_pig_information (accessed 29 September 2014).

85 Lin HC, Thurmon JC, Benson GJ, *et al.* The hemodynamic response of calves to tiletamine-zolazepam anesthesia. *Vet Surg* 1989; **18**: 328–334.

86 Lin HC, Thurmon JC, Benson GJ, *et al.* Telazol – a review of its pharmacology and use in veterinary medicine. *J Vet Pharmacol Ther* 1992; **16**: 383–418.

87 Kumar AH, Mann J, Remmel RP. Pharmacokinetics of tiletamine and zolazepam (Telazol) in anesthetized pigs. *J Vet Pharmacol Ther* 2006; **129**: 587–589.

88 Adams HR. Cholinergic pharmacology: neuromuscular blocking agents. In: Booth NH, McDonald LE, eds. *Veterinary Pharmacology and Therapeutics*, 6th edn. Ames, IA: Iowa State University Press, 1998; 137–151.

89 Reibold TW. Management of intraoperative and postoperative anesthetic complications in ruminants and swine. *Vet Clin North Am Food Animal Pract* 1986; **2**: 665–676.

90 Abrahamsen EJ. Chemical restraint, anesthesia, and analgesia for camelids. *Vet Clin North Am Food Animal Pract* 2009; **25**: 455–494.

91 Benson GJ. Anesthetic management of ruminants and swine with selected pathophysiologic alteration. *Vet Clin North Am Food Anim Pract* 1986; **2**: 677–691.

39 Comparative Anesthesia and Analgesia of Laboratory Animals

Paul A. Flecknell[1] and Aurelie A. Thomas[2]

[1]Institute of Neuroscience, Newcastle University, Newcastle upon Tyne, UK
[2]Comparative Biology Centre, Newcastle University, Medical School, Newcastle upon Tyne, UK

Chapter contents

Introduction

With up to 100 million animals used in research annually worldwide, including 1 million animals anesthetized annually in the United Kingdom alone [1], laboratory animal medicine and anesthesia are an important area requiring veterinary involvement. With the implementation of the principles of the 3Rs – *Reduction, Replacement, Refinement* [2] – and increased awareness of the importance of the public's perception of the use of animal models for research, the involvement of veterinary anesthetists in this field has been steadily increasing. There is now a general acceptance of the need to refine experiments; that is, to reduce to a minimum the pain and distress that might be experienced when animals are used in research. However, a recent survey indicated that less than 25% of laboratory rodents received postoperative analgesics, while less than 40% were anesthetized with agents likely to have some analgesic properties [3]. Encouraging greater use of postoperative analgesics and implementing improvements in anesthesia and intraoperative care require veterinary anesthetists to become aware of the unique challenges posed by working in a research environment. In addition to working with less familiar species, under constraints that are specific to the research project and the local legislative framework, the anesthetist may also be asked to work with agents that are not usually encountered in clinical practice (e.g., chloralose, urethane); to advise researchers on the most appropriate anesthetic and analgesic protocols in light of study goals; to accommodate animals with appropriate anesthesia lasting as short as a few seconds or as long as a few days; and to provide expertise on the ethical aspects of research projects. Although dealing with these issues may seem daunting, the involvement of veterinary anesthetists is essential to help promote improvements in anesthesia and perioperative care as well as enhancing the standards of animal welfare.

Anesthetics and analgesics

Commonly used drug doses for laboratory animals are listed in Tables 39.1–39.3. Unless specified below, the reader should assume that the drugs' pharmacokinetics in laboratory animals are broadly similar to those described in companion animals. Some particularly relevant properties of commonly used sedative, anesthetic, and analgesic agents are described in this section.

Anesthetics

Inhalants (mainly isoflurane and sevoflurane) are becoming increasingly popular in laboratory animal anesthesia for a number of reasons. Their adverse effects are well documented, they can be used in all of the commonly used laboratory rodents, and one agent (isoflurane) undergoes virtually no biotransformation. As a consequence, they represent a good option for the most commonly used research protocols. Second, using inhalants allows rapid induction and easy adjustment of the anesthetic to a standard, predetermined level, therefore reducing the variation between subjects and subsequently minimizing the number of animals to be used in a particular study. Third, inhalants are commonly used for induction of small mammals in an anesthetic chamber (Fig. 39.1), a simple and easy method of anesthesia induction. Finally, recovery from isoflurane

Veterinary Anesthesia and Analgesia: The Fifth Edition of Lumb and Jones.
Edited by Kurt A. Grimm, Leigh A. Lamont, William J. Tranquilli, Stephen A. Greene and Sheilah A. Robertson.

Table 39.1 Commonly used drugs and dosages in commonly encountered small mammals.

	Mice	Rats	Guinea pigs	Rabbits	Comments
Acepromazine	2–5 mg/kg IP, SC	2.5 mg/kg IM, IP	0.5–1 mg/kg IM	1 mg/kg IM	
Alfaxalone			40 mg/kg IM, IP	9–12 mg/kg IM	
Atropine	0.04 mg/kg SC	0.05 mg/kg IP, SC	0.05 mg/kg IM, IP	50–250 μg/kg, IM, SC	
Dexmedetomidine	15–50 μg/kg SC	15–50 μg/kg SC	0.25 mg/kg IM, IP	50–250 μg/kg, IM, SC	
Diazepam	5 mg/kg IP	2.5–5 mg/kg IP	2.5 mg/kg IP, IM	1–2 mg/kg IM	
Fentanyl/fluanisone (Hypnorm)	0.5 mL/kg IP	0.2–0.5 mL/kg IM	0.8–1.0 mL/kg IM, IP	0.3 mL/kg IM	Analgesia and sedation
Fentanyl/fluanisone (Hypnorm) + diazepam	0.4 mL/kg + 5 mg/kg IM	0.6 mL/kg + 2.5 mg/kg IM	1.0 mL/kg + 2.5 mg/kg IM	0.3 mL/kg IM + + 2 mg/kg IM	Surgical plane of anesthesia
Glycopyrrolate	??	0.5 mg/kg IM		0.1 mg/kg IM mg/kg IV	
Ketamine	100–200 mg/kg IM	50–100 mg/kg IM, IP	40–100 mg/kg IM, IP	25–50 mg/kg IM	
Ketamine/acepromazine	100 mg/kg + 5 mg/kg IP	75 mg/kg + 2.5 mg/kg IP	100 mg/kg + 5 mg/kg IP	50 mg/kg + 1 mg/kg IM	Light anesthesia
Medetomidine	30–100 μg/kg SC	30–100 μg/kg SC	0.5 mg/kg IM, IP	0.1–0.5 mg/kg IM, SC	
Xylazine	5–10 mg/kg IP	1–5 mg/kg IP	5 mg/kg IP	2–5 mg/kg IM, SC	
Ketamine/ dexmedetomidine	100 mg/kg + 0.25 mg/kg IP	60–75 mg/kg + 0.125–0.25 mg/kg IP	40 mg/kg + 0.25 mg/kg IP	15 mg/kg SC + 0.12 5 mg/kg SC	Surgical plane of anesthesia, but more variable effects in mice
Urethane		1000 mg/kg IP	1500 mg/kg IV, IP	1000–2000 mg/kg IV	Non-recovery procedures only

IM = intramuscular; IP = intraperitoneal; IV = intravenous; SC = subcutaneous.

Table 39.2 Commonly used drugs and dosages for selected primate species.

	Macaque spp	Marmosets	Comments
Alfaxalone	1–3 mg/kg IV (after initial ketamine sedation)	10 mg/kg IM 2–5 mg/kg IV	Immobilization (IM), light–medium anesthesia
Atropine	0.04 mg/kg SC	0.05 mg/kg IP, SC	
Dexmedetomidine	15–50 μg/kg SC	15–50 μg/kg SC	
Diazepam	5 mg/kg IP	2.5–5 mg/kg IP	
Glycopyrrolate	??	0.5 mg/kg IM	
Ketamine	100–200 mg/kg IM	50–100 mg/kg IM, IP	Immobilization
Medetomidine	30–100 μg/kg SC	30–100 μg/kg SC	
Xylazine	5–10 mg/kg IP	1–5 mg/kg IP	
Ketamine/ dexmedetomidine	5–10 mg/kg and 0.01–0.03 mg/kg IM	5 mg/kg and 0.05 mg/kg IM	Light to moderate anesthesia
Ketamine/xylazine	10 mg/kg and 0.15–0.5 mg/kg IM	10 mg/kg and 0.15–0.5 mg/kg IM	Light to moderate anesthesia

IM = intramuscular; IP = intraperitoneal; IV = intravenous; SC = subcutaneous.

Table 39.3 Neuromuscular junction blocking agents and dosages for selected laboratory animal species.

	Mice	Rats	Guinea pigs	Rabbits	Non-human primates
Alcuronium	?	?	?	0.1–0.2 mg/ kg IV	0.1–0.2 mg/ kg IV
Atracurium	?	?	?	?	0.09–0.2 mg/ kg IV
Pancuronium	?	2 mg/kg IV	0.06 mg/kg IV	0.1 mg/kg, IV	0.04–0.1 mg/ kg IV
Succinylcholine	?	?	?	0.5 mg/kg, IV	?
Vecuronium	?	1 mg/kg IV	?	?	0.04–0.06 mg/ kg IV

IV = intravenous.

and sevoflurane anesthesia is usually rapid compared to injectable anesthetic combinations given by SC or IM injection.

Minimum alveolar concentration (MAC) values in smaller mammals are broadly similar to those in other species. Although modern inhalant agents are widely considered to be both effective and non-irritant [4,5], they vary in their pungency and this may affect an animal's willingness to breathe normally [6,7]. Apneic episodes

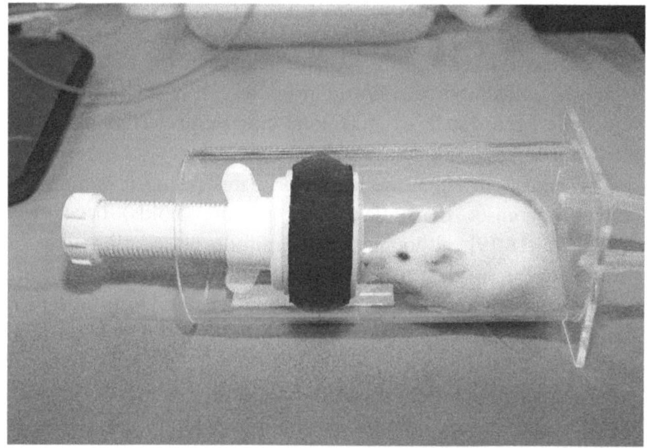

Figure 39.1 Induction chamber for use with small (<100 g) mammals. The chamber size is appropriate to the size of animal, allowing the concentration of anesthetic agent to be increased rapidly without the use of high fresh gas flows.

can occur in rabbits with all of the commonly used agents and this, coupled with possible catecholamine release, could increase the anesthetic risk and also introduce some intersubject variability. When inducing anesthesia in rabbits with a face mask, briefly removing the mask if an episode of apnea occurs and replacing the mask when respiration resumes will avoid the risks associated with prolonged breath holding. Some degree of aversion to volatile agents has been demonstrated in rats and mice, with isoflurane being more aversive than sevoflurane or halothane [8]. Isoflurane appears particularly irritant to guinea pigs, triggering pronounced ocular and nasal discharge. In the author's experience, sevoflurane appears less irritating but still causes lacrimation. Halothane is much less irritating in guinea pigs, but this needs to be balanced against the risk of other adverse effects [9,10]. In all species, stress associated with induction of anesthesia can be minimized by use of preanesthetic medication.

Ketamine remains the agent most widely used for anesthetizing laboratory rodents. It is most frequently used in combination with sedatives or sedative/analgesics, since when administered as the sole agent to rodents it does not produce even light anesthesia. In combination with xylazine and acepromazine, ketamine produces a safe, long-lasting (e.g., 54 min), and stable surgical plane of anesthesia in mice [11]. When ketamine is combined with either medetomidine or dexmedetomidine, the depth of anesthesia is less consistent than in other non-rodent species, but this is still a useful combination in many mouse strains [11,12]. The most reliable combination for producing a surgical plane of anesthesia in rats and most other rodents is ketamine in combination with an α_2-adrenergic receptor agonist [13].

Unlike in other species, ketamine used alone in non-human primates (NHP) produces heavy sedation (10 mg/kg) to light surgical anesthesia (25 mg/kg) [13] with good relaxation of skeletal and laryngeal muscles. Repeated use of ketamine in NHPs, however, raises a few concerns. First, ketamine has been shown to be associated with long-term cognitive impairment in NHPs, if administered during a sensitive period for brain development (*in utero* or during the first week of life) [14,15]. This is a significant concern given that most NHPs are used as animal models for neuroscience studies. Repeated ketamine administrations are associated with anesthetic tolerance. Anesthetic doses administered for three consecutive days are sufficient to increase the time to recumbency by approximately 35% [16], and this is comparable with human data. Ketamine has also been reported to cause local myotoxic effect in New World primates [17], such that other injectable agents such as alfaxalone may be preferred for intramuscular injection in these species.

Alternatives to ketamine use in primates (using α_2-adrenergic receptor agonists, benzodiazepines, and/or opioids) have been described [18,19], although the magnitude of sedation may be unsuitable for surgical procedures. It is of interest that NHP are notably resistant to sedation with benzodiazepines. Doses as high as 3 mg/kg, administered orally, merely produce mild sedation and anxiolysis, without inducing recumbency [19].

Most injectable anesthetic agents have similar properties in small rodents and companion animals and therefore are not discussed in depth here. One noteworthy difference relating to the use of injectable anesthetics in small rodents is the difficulty of obtaining intravenous access. This results in anesthetic combinations being administered as single injection by the intraperitoneal, subcutaneous, or intramuscular route, rather than intravenously, to effect. Although this is a simple and rapid means of producing anesthesia, it has inevitable consequences in relation to the safety of certain anesthetic agents, especially those with a narrow safety margin. Since there is considerable variation between different strains of rodents in their response to anesthetic agents, anesthetic combinations that have a broad safety margin or are wholly or partially reversible are preferred. If a neuroleptanalgesic-based combination is used (i.e., Hypnorm® [fentanyl and the butyrophenone fluanisone] combined with midazolam), fentanyl can be partially antagonized with small doses of buprenorphine, butorphanol or even nalbuphine instead of complete reversal with naloxone [20]. By doing so, respiratory depression and some sedative effect from the potent μ-opioid agonist are reversed, but some analgesia is preserved for the immediate recovery period.

Some injectable anesthetic agents remain in research settings due to scientific reasons or ease of use, but are no longer used in veterinary clinical practice. Urethane is an ethyl-carbamate producing long-lasting and stable (6–10 h) surgical anesthesia with little cardiovascular or respiratory adverse effects. Urethane is still used for non-recovery procedures involving the recording of some CNS responses and for neuropharmacology studies. Spinal reflexes are depressed but it has virtually no depressant action on the brain itself (EEG comparable to sleep patterns), and most autonomic reflexes are well preserved. It is a water-soluble compound metabolized by the liver into ethanol and carbamic acid, before renal excretion. Despite initial studies suggesting that urethane is mainly acting on $GABA_A$ receptors, it is now established that only 23% of urethane's action is $GABA_A$ mediated. Urethane interacts at a multitude of receptors including the α_1 glycine receptor (agonist, 33%), the NMDA and AMPA receptors (antagonist, 10% and 18% respectively), and possibly on acetylcholine receptors, but with only weak effects at each target [21]. When administered intraperitoneally, it has profound endocrine and metabolic effects, producing peritonitis, necrosis of the abdominal contents, and massive leakage of plasma into peritoneal cavity [22] so must only be used for non-recovery procedures. Urethane is a carcinogen and protective equipment should be worn when handled.

α-Chloralose is an anesthetic that has numerous dose-dependent CNS effects, both excitatory and inhibitory. It provides long-lasting light anesthesia, with minimal cardiovascular side-effects. However, induction and recovery are very prolonged, so the agent is usually restricted to terminal procedures, after induction of anesthesia with another agent (typically an inhalant). A further disadvantage of chloralose is that the anesthetic depth is not usually sufficient for surgical manipulations to be performed.

Chloral hydrate is used occasionally in rodent anesthesia for neuropharmacology studies. Surgical depth of anesthesia can be achieved [23] but in some strains of rats, chloral hydrate causes postanesthetic ileus that can be fatal [24]. Using a dilute solution of chloral hydrate may help reduce the incidence of ileus.

Tribromoethanol is used primarily in mice although its popularity has declined markedly because of undesirable side-effects. If incorrectly prepared or stored, administration is associated with high mortality. This can also occur when freshly prepared solutions are used [25]. It is clear that the incidence of adverse effects varies greatly in different research facilities, perhaps due to the agent itself not being supplied as a commercial pharmaceutical product. For this reason, decisions as to whether to use the agent should be made on a case-by-case basis. When used successfully, tribromoethanol produces 15–20 min of surgical anesthesia, with reasonably rapid recovery.

Analgesics

Opioids

Despite growing emphasis on animal welfare and refinement of animal models, less than 25% of laboratory rodents undergoing surgical procedure are given analgesic drugs (35% of those that are receive buprenorphine [3]). This might be partially explained by a number of largely unfounded concerns related to the potential interactions of opioids and other analgesics and specific types of research projects. For example, in spite of a lack of convincing clinical data in humans, opioids are commonly associated with immunodepression in critical care unit patients. This has led to concerns that use of these agents in a research setting could cause immunosuppression, and this could interact with some research models. In laboratory animals, not only is this phenomenon subject to major interstrain variability [26], but also immunodepression only occurs when animals receive dose rates of analgesics greatly in excess of those used for postoperative pain relief, for prolonged periods (e.g., 300 mg/kg morphine) [27–29]. Opioids have also been shown to have effects on tumor growth and metastasis, and this has been considered a contraindication to their use when implanting or transplanting tumors for cancer research studies. Published data are conflicting in this area, suggesting that morphine can either promote or slow down tumor growth and metastatic spread. The mechanisms involved remain poorly understood, and other than some possible immune-modulative effects, opioids may impact tumor cell aggressiveness and angiogenesis [30].

In each of these examples, a proper appraisal of the available literature, in consultation with the research workers involved, should lead to an evidence-based decision as to whether to use opioids or whether an alternative analgesic strategy should be adopted. When making these decisions, it is also important to include a consideration of the various effects of unalleviated pain. In the authors' experience, there are almost no circumstances in which an analgesic regimen of some type cannot be implemented.

Amongst the opioids, buprenorphine remains the analgesic agent most frequently administered to laboratory animals, both to rodents [3] and to larger species [31]. Buprenorphine is 35 times as potent as morphine when administered IM in rats [32], and has a long duration of action (3–5 h in mice, 6–8 h in rats). Its poor oral bioavailability (5–10%), coupled with a significant hepatic first-pass metabolism, renders oral administration of buprenorphine of limited value in rodents as its duration of action decreases to 1–2 h (0.5 mg/kg, rats) [33], although this may still provide sufficient analgesia following some surgical procedures [34]. Although use of buprenorphine in palatable oral formulations remains popular, we recommend it is only given by this route when effective methods of pain assessment are being used.

The ceiling effect, abundantly described in the literature, occurs only when doses exceeding approximately 3 mg/kg are administered in rats [35], and is therefore of little concern when using this agent for postoperative pain relief. Clinically relevant adverse effects of opioids are similar to those in other animal species. Interestingly, studies on rats showed that even at large IV doses, buprenorphine failed to produce clinically significant respiratory depression [36,37]. An unusual effect of opioids in rodents is the production of pica behavior. This is thought to be analogous to vomiting in other species, and has been reported following use of buprenorphine in rats [38]. The incidence of pica appears to be low, but if noted, analgesia should be provided using a non-opioid analgesic.

Other opioids can be used in laboratory animals as well. Methadone, for instance, has been shown to attenuate signs of neuropathic pain for 2 h in mice (3 mg/kg, SC) [39]. This effect may be due to μ-opioid receptor agonist action, but also, in part, to antagonism of NMDA receptors. Although species-specific studies documenting the efficacy of this agent in alleviating postsurgical pain are lacking, methadone has been used in NHPs (0.3–0.5 mg/kg, IM) when the surgical procedure renders the animal at risk of experiencing chronic or neuropathic pain. Compared to other full μ-opioid receptor agonists, methadone seems to produce less sedation and inappetence.

Managing pain in laboratory rodents can be difficult because of the large numbers of animals that may need to be treated (e.g., 20–30 animals all undergoing surgery in one day). In addition, the relatively short action of some analgesics requires repeated handling and injections, which in itself can be stressful. Possible approaches to these problems are the use of slow-release preparations and transdermal delivery (e.g., cutaneous patch) technology. Fentanyl patches or transdermal solutions can be used in larger laboratory animals, with the same concerns and indications for use as in other species. It is important to securely attach the patch to the animal to reduce the risk of ingestion. Ingestion of a patch can be fatal since fentanyl is readily absorbed by the oropharyngeal mucosa [40]. Alternatively, a rapid ingestion may not result in clinical signs since there appears to be a high first-pass metabolism following gastrointestinal absorption. The small size of laboratory rodents makes use of patches impractical in most circumstances. We would not recommend use of transdermal solutions of fentanyl in small rodents, since their small size would make accurate administration very difficult. Slow-release formulations of a number of analgesics have been compounded (e.g., Buprenorphine SR®, Veterinary Technologies, LLC, Windsor, Colorado). This formulation appears to provide sustained release up to 72 h in rats and mice. A preliminary study suggested up to 12 h of pain reduction can be provided in mice [41] and a longer duration in rats [42]. The latter study did not report any problems with pica but up to 40% of the rats developed some skin irritation following SC injection. A modified formulation appears to have resolved problems of irritancy following injection. Pharmacokinetic studies performed in NHPs suggest that Buprenorphine SR®™ plasma concentrations remain above a possible analgesic threshold for approximately 5 days, but no pharmacodynamics tests were performed [43].

Anti-inflammatory drugs

Non-steroidal anti-inflammatory drugs (NSAIDs) are the second most commonly administered agents for pain relief in rodents and other laboratory animal species [3,31]. All of the NSAIDs licensed for use in animals or people can be administered in laboratory rodent and NHP species. Of the agents available, the oral preparation of meloxicam is of particular value as it is highly palatable to many small rodents and to NHPs, particularly if added to their favorite foodstuff. The efficacy of NSAIDs in relieving postoperative pain in rodents has been widely reported [44–46] but their duration of action remains uncertain. Carprofen and meloxicam appear to have a duration of at least 8 and possibly 24 h. The general considerations related to their use in other veterinary species apply equally to laboratory animal species; however, since most laboratory animals undergoing surgery are young, healthy adults, concerns related to pre-existing diseases are usually reduced.

Specific concerns related to the use of NSAIDs in animal models are sparse and poorly understood. Given the link between inflammation and carcinogenesis, recent studies have attempted to categorize the relationship between NSAIDs and cancer models. The results suggest that in addition to the mechanism of action (degree of COX 1 vs COX 2 inhibition), the type of cancer as well as the dose and frequency of NSAID administration (U-shaped response curve) correlate to efficacy [47–49].

Recent meta-analysis of clinical studies suggested that steroids might be useful adjuncts to a multimodal analgesic approach to managing surgical pain. A single preoperative dose of dexamethasone, administered to people, contributed to a reduction in postoperative pain as well as opioid consumption, without any steroid-associated adverse effects [50]. The analgesic mechanism of dexamethasone remains obscure, and may be related to its general anti-inflammatory properties as well as interactions with opioid receptors [51]. Since steroids may be administered routinely to laboratory animals following neurosurgery procedures, it may be necessary to factor their potential analgesic effects into a postoperative care protocol. When not indicated for other purposes, steroids may not be a first-line choice of analgesia provision because of their negative effect on wound healing and immunomodulation [52].

Local and regional analgesia/anesthesia

Local anesthetic techniques are underutilized in laboratory species, and regional analgesia (spinal or epidural techniques) have been used primarily as research techniques [53]. The same general principles and approaches used in larger species can be applied in laboratory rodents, but their small size makes overdose more likely. Local anesthesia is most often used in conjunction with general anesthesia, since small rodents are likely to be stressed by the physical restraint needed if local anesthesia is used alone. Use of local anesthetics enables the dosage of general anesthetic agents to be reduced, usually minimizing adverse effects and potential interactions with research variables. Infiltration of the surgical site can be a means of prolonging the duration of surgical anesthesia, rather than administering additional doses of injectable anesthetic agents. Aside from local infiltration, topical local anesthesia (e.g., using EMLA cream) can be used to prevent pain or discomfort associated with venepuncture [54], or to provide anesthesia for minor procedures (e.g., ethyl chloride for tail biopsy in mice) [55]. Maximum safe doses of local anesthetics have not been well documented but as a guide, total dose should not exceed 10 mg/kg of lidocaine or 2 mg/kg of bupivacaine.

Gabapentin and pregabalin

Despite their abundant use in animal models of chronic pain, very few studies have looked at the benefit of gabapentin and pregabalin in laboratory animals as part of postsurgical pain management. A study anecdotally reports prolonged analgesia in a mouse model of fibromyalgia 4 days after gabapentin administration [56]. More recently, the MAC-sparing effect of gabapentin was demonstrated in rats with both sevoflurane and isoflurane [57,58]. There appear to be no reports of the use of these drugs for clinical pain relief in NHPs.

Laboratory rodents and lagomorphs

Anatomic and physiologic considerations

In order to anesthetize these species safely and effectively, and to manage their perioperative care, it is important to become familiar with their normal behavior, anatomy, and physiology. Rats, mice, and hamsters are active primarily during the dark phase of their photoperiod while rabbits are most active at dawn and dusk (i.e., crepuscular). This should be remembered when assessing normal behavior during what would usually be an inactive phase of their diurnal rhythm. Almost all feeding and drinking by rats and mice occurs during the dark phase and postsurgical pain or stress following procedures undertaken during the light phase can suppress these activities. Consequently, voluntary oral intake may not resume for 24 h or more. This can have significant detrimental effects in these small animals, since relatively short periods of fasting can result in hypoglycaemia and moderate dehydration. For similar reasons, preanesthetic fasting should be avoided and since these species do not vomit, fasting does not reduce the incidence of aspiration.

Witholding food from rabbits and guinea pigs should also be avoided, since it can result in gastrointestinal disturbances which can have serious consequences (e.g., alterations to gut flora, ileus, and production of enterotoxemia). Since these species do not vomit, there is no advantage to withholding food. All of these species exhibit a degree of neophobia, so postsurgically their normal diet should always be offered along with palatable high-energy and high-water content supplements. All of these species are coprophagic, a normal activity that is important for adequate nutrition. Inadvertent prevention of this activity by use of Elizabethan collars, to prevent interference with wounds, for example, should be avoided.

The small size of rodents makes clinical examination difficult, and since these species often regard people as a threat, they often show elevated heart and respiratory rates. These rates may exceed 200–250 breaths or heart beats per minute, so they are too fast to accurately record on clinical examination (Table 39.4). The small size also restricts venous access, except in the rabbit where access via the marginal auricular, saphenous or cephalic veins is relatively easy. The most important consequence of the small size of these animals is their high surface area to body weight ratio, which greatly increases heat loss during anesthesia. Even short periods of anesthesia are associated with significant cooling unless efforts are made to minimize hypothermia.

The metabolic rate of most species varies with body mass raised to the three-quarters power. Small mammals have a high metabolic rate resulting in a relatively high dose requirement of many of the agents commonly used in anesthesia and pain management. For example, the commonly recommended dose of buprenorphine in a dog is 0.005–0.03 mg/kg. In a mouse, the dose rate is 0.05–0.1 mg/kg [32]. Calculations of a dose for mice, based on the dose in dogs, using allometric scaling provides a similar dose (0.03 mg/kg). If a validated dose rate is not available, a calculation using allometric scaling is more likely to provide an appropriate dose than simple extrapolation.

Handling, restraint, and drug administration

General principles of good handling can be applied to rodents and lagomorphs. It is important that the anesthetist or an assistant is familiar with restraint for the safety and comfort of the animal. Illustrations of methods of restraint are widely available (e.g., www.procedureswithcare.org.uk). Drug administration is safer and easier if an assistant restrains the animal while a second person administers the drug. Intramuscular injections are best avoided if a large volume of agent is required since it can cause muscle damage [59].

Table 39.4 Normal physiologic parameter values for common laboratory animal species.

	Mice	Rats	Guinea pigs	Rabbits	Non-human primates (rhesus)
Heart rate	500–600 min^{-1}	350 min^{-1}	155 min^{-1}	220 min^{-1}	150 min^{-1}
Respiratory rate	180 min^{-1}	80 min^{-1}	120 min^{-1}	55 min^{-1}	35 min^{-1}
Body temperature	37 °C	38 °C	38 °C	38 °C	39 °C
Adult body weight	30–40 g	250–450 g	500–1500 g	0.5–8 kg	6–12 kg
Food consumption (complete pelleted diet)	10–20 g/100 g	10 g/100 g	6 g/100 g	5 g/100 g	–
Water consumption	10–20 mL/100 g	10–12 mL/100 g	100 mL/kg	120 mL/kg	50–100 mL/kg

Intraperitoneal administration of injectable anesthetics is widely practiced in research facilities. It is simple and convenient, but is associated with a relatively high failure rate because of inadvertent drug delivery into the fat, subcutaneous or gut tissue [60]. When possible, it is preferable to use the subcutaneous route, which is simple to undertake in all of these species. Common sites for subcutaneous injection are either in the scruff or the flank. As in other species, the volume administered should be the lowest possible, and suggested doses are listed in Table 39.1.

Airway management

In most research facilities, oxygen and volatile anesthetics are delivered to small rodents and rabbits using a face mask. This makes support of ventilation difficult to achieve, and where there is a need for this, endotracheal intubation should be considered. With practice, intubation is straightforward in rabbits [13], but more difficult in guinea pigs and small rodents. It is made easier if a purpose-designed apparatus is used (Figs 39.2 and 39.3) which allows direct visualization of the larynx during intubation.

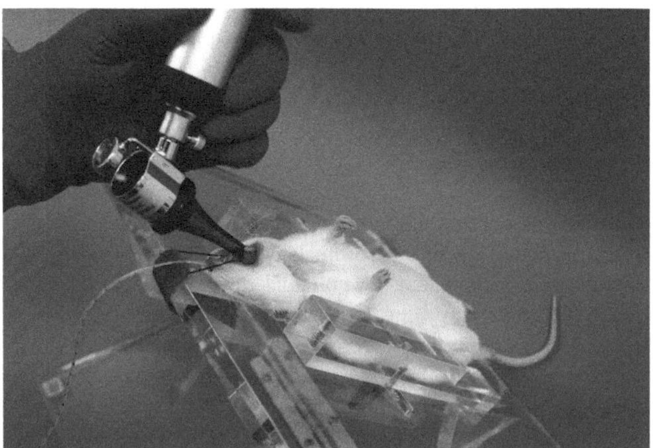

Figure 39.2 Visualization of the larynx in a rat using a modified otoscope speculum (Hallowell EMC) to enable intubation. A nasal catheter is used to deliver oxygen or volatile anesthetic during the procedure.

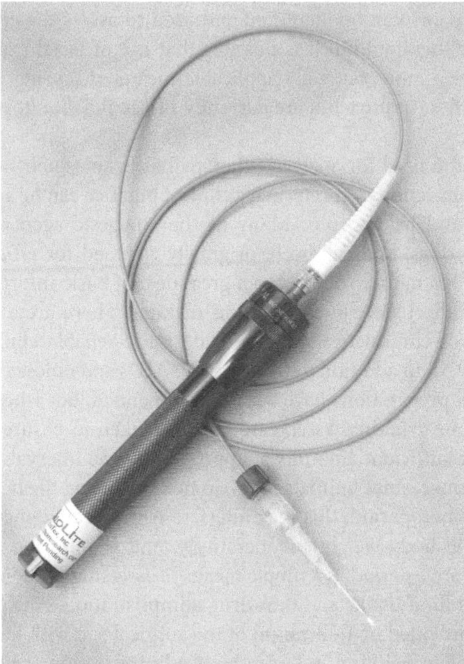

Figure 39.3 Fiberoptic guide for intubation of rats and mice (Kent Scientific). An intravenous catheter is used as the endotracheal tube.

Once intubated, the animal should be connected to a breathing system. Unmodified Bain's circuits and T-pieces can be used when animals are breathing spontaneously, but care must be taken to minimize equipment deadspace. It is reasonable to assume that tidal volume is approximately 5–10 mL/kg (e.g., a mouse will have a tidal volume of only 0.2–0.3 mL). Significant rebreathing of expired gases can only be avoided by constructing low-deadspace connectors for the breathing system.

Fresh gas flow rates needed to minimize rebreathing can be calculated for these breathing systems using standard formulas; however, in many research facilities, flow rates when using face masks are often greatly in excess of minima (e.g., 1–2 L/min for a mouse, rather than the 30–50 mL/min required). This may be because the vaporizer is not accurate at very low flows, but additional reasons include the use of active scavenging systems (Fig. 39.4) that overextract from the mask, drawing in room air. Delivered anesthetic gas (concentration) dilution results in animals becoming inadequately anesthetized at lower fresh gas flows. These problems can be avoided by using specifically designed low-flow, passive scavenged masks (Fig. 39.5) or purpose-designed equipment such as that shown in Fig. 39.6.

The low tidal volumes of rodents often require use of purpose-designed ventilators although "T-piece occluder" designs can function well. In larger species such as rabbits, ventilators and breathing systems used in cats can be used successfully. A wide range of rodent ventilators are available from specialist suppliers. As in other species, key factors to consider are the range of tidal volumes and respiratory frequencies that can be delivered, whether PEEP is required, whether the ventilator requires a compressed gas source to operate, whether it is mechanically driven, and what safety features and alarms are provided. As in other species, the ability to alter the inspiratory:expiratory (I:E) ratio is useful. When breathing normally, rodents have a 1:1 I:E ratio [61]; however, extending this to 1:2 or 1:3 to minimize the effects of positive pressure ventilation on the cardiovascular system can be an advantage.

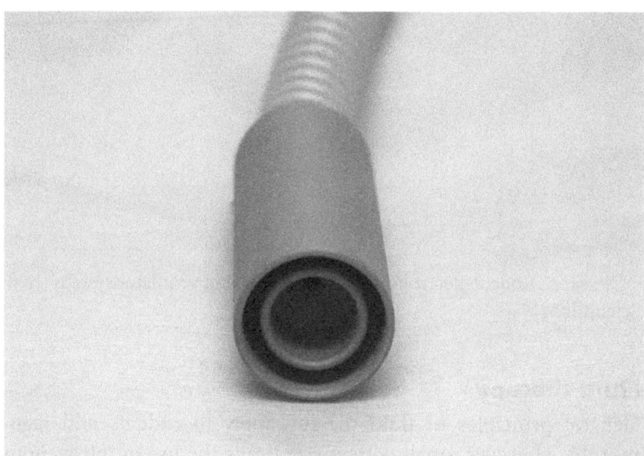

Figure 39.4 Rodent face mask with active scavenge system. The outer mask is attached to an extraction system.

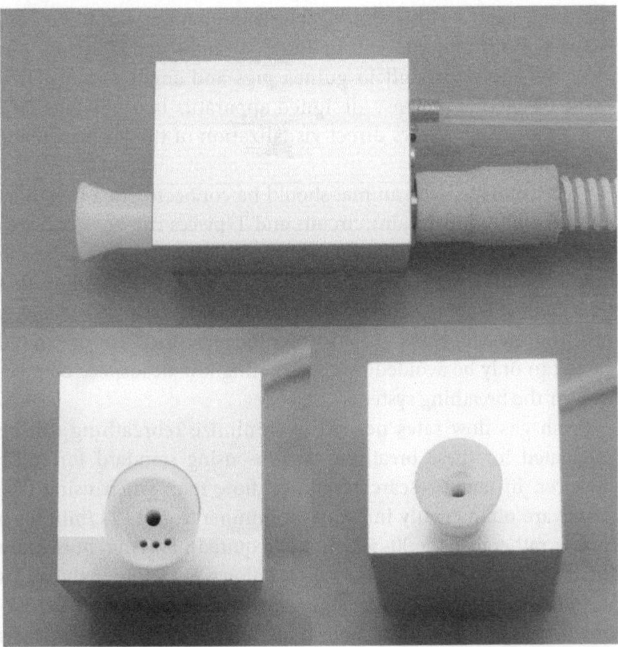

Figure 39.5 Low deadspace, passively scavenged rodent mask (AAS). (*Top*) Side-view showing metal block that stabilizes the mask, and provides warming of the anesthetic gases. (*Lower left*) View of mask to show gas delivery and scavenging ports. (*Lower right*) Mask with rubber membrane in place, to provide a seal around the mouse's nose.

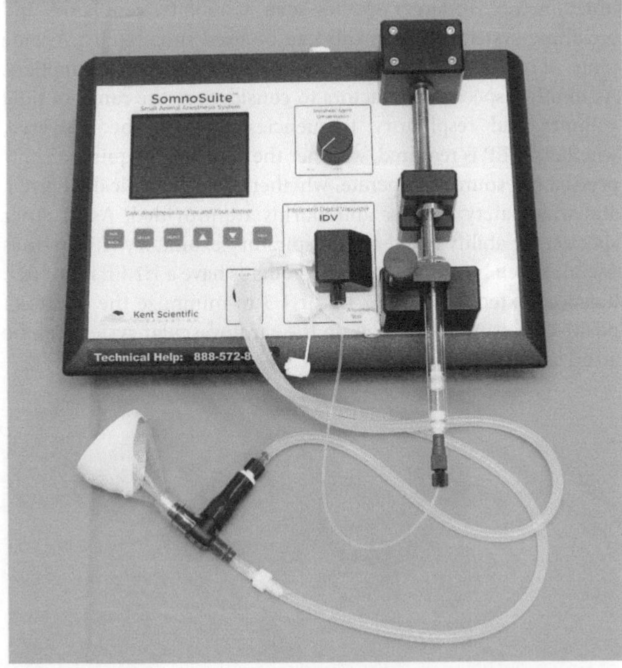

Figure 39.6 Rodent electronic vaporizer, mask, and ventilator system (Kent Scientific).

Fluid therapy

General principles of fluid therapy apply to rodents and lagomorphs. However, small patient size limits the use of intravenous fluid administration. If animals are not clinically dehydrated, then absorption of fluids following IP or SC administration occurs over 4–6 h. If more rapid fluid administration is needed, either a peripheral vein can be catheterized using an over-the-needle catheter or an intraosseous catheter can be placed [62]. Infusion pumps capable of delivering appropriate rates are readily available from a number of equipment manufacturers.

Maintenance of body temperature

Heating pads suitable for use in small rodents are available. Devices that adjust the temperature of the blanket depending upon the body temperature of the animal are preferred, but it is important to check that the temperature sensor probe tip is sufficiently small for use in rodents. It is also advisable to monitor the temperature of the blanket directly, using an additional thermometer. Both electric and circulating hot water systems are available. Forced air warming systems can be used in rabbits, but are usually impractical for use in mice and rats. Following anesthesia, animals should be placed in a suitable incubator to maintain body temperature during recovery.

Postoperative care

Postsurgical pain management, together with other supportive care, is essential if recovery from surgery and anesthesia is to be rapid and uneventful. When dealing with laboratory animals, anesthetists must be aware of the additional considerations that arise as a result of the particular use of these animals. When devising protocols for postoperative pain relief, the potential interactions of the agents chosen on research protocols can be minimized by use of appropriate dose rates, for an appropriate period of time. This requires accurate assessment of the degree of pain that is present and its duration, in order to determine the efficacy of analgesic therapy.

A number of pain assessment tools have been developed, including those which track simple clinical measures such as body weight and food and water consumption [63], complex behavioral measures such as nest building [64], specific pain-related behaviors [45,46] and changes in facial expression [65–67]. Pain assessment of laboratory animals is a rapidly developing area.

Following abdominal surgery in rats and mice, a series of abnormal behaviors can be identified and used to assess the efficacy of analgesic therapy [68]. It is possible that use of facial expressions may offer a more generally applicable means of scoring pain and both of these approaches are currently in use in laboratory animal facilities.

Once the need for analgesic therapy has been established, all of the options familiar in veterinary clinical practice can be applied in rodents and lagomorphs. Many of the analgesic agents used in humans, dogs, and cats were originally assessed for efficacy and safety in laboratory rodents, so a great deal of basic information is available to guide clinical decision making. There are a growing number of clinical trials that provide more reliable clinical data (Table 39.5). In addition to the use of NSAIDs and opioids by injection, oral preparations have been recommended, but when dosing via food or drinking water, care must be taken to ensure animals consume sufficient amounts at appropriate time intervals. As discussed above, since animals often do not eat during the light phase of their photoperiod, this may interfere with effective medication. Recording body weight preoperatively, and monitoring it in the postoperative period, is a simple means of assessing the adequacy of fluid and food intake and thus drug administration. Analgesia can also be provided by infiltration of the surgical site with local anesthetic, and by epidural and intrathecal administration of analgesics, although practical constraints may limit this approach in small rodents (see above).

Table 39.5 Analgesic drugs and dosages for common laboratory animal species.

	Mice	Rats	Guinea pigs	Rabbits	Non-human primates
Buprenorphine	0.1 mg/kg IP, SC, q6–8 h	0.05 mg/kg SC, IP q6–8 h	0.05 mg/kg SC, IP q6–8 h	0.01–0.05 mg/kg SC, IM q6–8 h	0.005–0.01 mg/kg SC, IM q6–8 h
Butorphanol	1–2 mg/kg IP, SC, q2 h	1–2 mg/kg IP, SC, q2 h	1–2 mg/kg IP, SC, q3 h	0.1–0.5 mg/kg SC, q3 h	0.1 mg/kg SC, IM q3 h
Carprofen	5 mg/kg SC or orally q12 h	5 mg/kg SC or orally q12 h	2.5 mg/kg SC q24 h	4 mg/kg SC q24 h	2–4 mg/kg SC q24 h
Meloxicam	5 mg/kg SC q24 h	0.5–1 mg/kg IP, SC or orally q24 h	0.5–1.0 mg/kg SC q24 h	0.6 mg/kg, IM, SC q24 h	0.2 mg/kg IP, SC or orally q24 h
Morphine	2–5 mg/kg IP, SC, q2–4 h	2–5 mg/kg IP, SC, q2–4 h	2–5 mg/kg IP, SC, q2–4	2–3 mg/kg, SC, IM q2–4 h	1–2 mg/kg SC, IM q2–4 h
Tramadol	5 -10 mg/kg IP, SC Q6–12 h	5–10 mg/kg IP, SC q6–12 h	?	?	1–2 mg/kg SC, IM q2–4 h, 2 mg/kg orally q12 h

IM = intramuscular; IP = intraperitoneal; SC = subcutaneous.

Non-human primates

A variety of NHPs are used worldwide for biomedical research. The species used range from New World primates (capuchins, marmosets, squirrel monkeys) to Old World primates (macaques, baboons, chimpanzees). Non-human primates are used in a wide range of biomedical studies, primarily for neuroscience, immunology, and infectious disease research. Given the highly sensitive nature of the use of NHPs for biomedical research, any proposed project should take particular care to apply the 3Rs principle to minimize the potential pain and distress caused by the experiments.

Anesthetic considerations

Handling any conscious NHP should be avoided not only because of the stress caused to the animal, but also because of the risk of physical injuries to the operator (mainly bites and scratches). In addition to the risk of traumatic injury, NHPs can carry a number of hazardous and in some cases potentially fatal zoonotic diseases (i.e., herpes B virus) [69]. Appropriate personal protective equipment, usually comprising gloves, eye protection, and laboratory coat or gown, should be worn when working with NHPs.

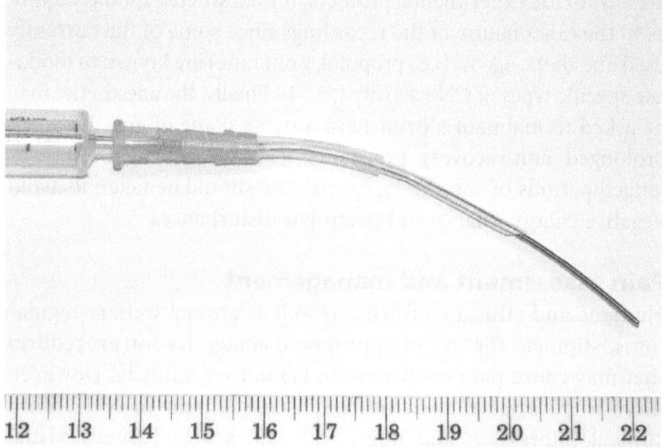

Figure 39.7 Modified catheter for intubation of marmosets or other small primates. The silastic tubing provides a seal at the larynx, and also reduces the risk of kinking of the catheter at the hub. A Seldinger catheter guidewire, anchored in a syringe, is used to aid intubation (Hallowell EMC).

Preanesthetic considerations

Primates are social animals and should be group housed whenever possible in a cage containing retreat areas. Assessing a freely moving primate in its home cage is difficult, reducing any preanesthetic examination to a simple visual check. As a consequence, the preanesthetic physical examination is commonly performed under sedation (usually ketamine based). Intravenous access is achieved via superficial veins (e.g., cephalic or saphenous veins) using 20–22 G catheters. The caudal (tail) vein is a more suitable option for New World monkeys using a 22–24 G catheter.

Endotracheal intubation

Primates should be fasted prior to anesthesia because of their ability to regurgitate or vomit. Following induction, intubation is recommended to prevent aspiration. Primates are capable of a wide range of vocalization. This is made possible by a caudal descent of the larynx, increasing its resonance capacity. Compared with other non-primate animals, the descent of the larynx causes a large part of the tongue to be in the hypopharynx, and this can restrict visualization of the entrance of the larynx. The larynx is richly vascularized and seems to be particularly prone to tissue trauma compared to non-primate species, so care should be taken while introducing the endotracheal tube. The diameter of the larynx and trachea is smaller in primates than in other species of equivalent weight. For instance, a 3–3.5 mm outer diameter (OD) endotracheal tube is appropriate for a 6 kg macaque, and a 5.5 mm OD tube would be suitable for an adult male macaque (15 kg). In New World monkeys, the animal is best placed in dorsal recumbency on a tilting table to maximize the alignment of the oral cavity with the larynx. Marmosets or capuchins are best intubated with a modified over-the-needle catheter mounted on a stylet (Fig. 39.7) [70]. Marmosets, like pigs, have a pronounced laryngotracheal angle and the tube should be gently rotated 180° once it has passed the vocal folds [70]. Lastly, special attention should be paid to the length of the tube, as NHPs have shorter tracheas than other species. The distal end of the tube should not be advanced past the points of the scapula on a macaque to avoid endobronchial intubation or trauma to the carina [71]. In marmosets, the length of the trachea can be predicted by multiplying the craniosacral length of the marmoset by a factor of 0.42 [70].

Equipment and monitoring

New World monkeys often appear heavier than they actually are (a few hundred grams). In these smaller species, a rodent ventilator and breathing system are appropriate. Larger primate species can easily be anesthetized with similar apparatus to that used in cats and small dogs.

Recovery

Recovery from anesthesia should be as rapid and smooth as possible. Larger animals will usually need to recover in a secure recovery box or cage because of the risk of them biting the anesthetist or nursing staff. Gentle extubation is usually performed as soon as protective reflexes begin to return and hemoglobin saturation remains within normal limits without supplemental oxygen. Primates are usually recovered in purpose-built cages at high ambient temperature.

NHPs in neuroscience

Most of the primates undergoing surgery are used for neuroscience research projects. Surgical procedures may involve craniotomies and implantation of permanent neuroelectrodes, with the inherent risk of CNS edema or seizure during the postoperative period. Any increase in intracranial pressure should be avoided by controlling the arterial partial pressure of CO_2 and the mean arterial pressure and the appropriate use of glucocorticoids (e.g., methylprednisolone) [72]. If electrical recordings from the CNS during anesthesia are part of the experimental protocol, the anesthetist should inquire as to the exact nature of the recordings since some of the currently used anesthetic agents (i.e., propofol, isoflurane) are known to modulate specific types of CNS activity [73,74]. Finally, the anesthetist may be asked to maintain a primate in a stable plane of anesthesia for prolonged non-recovery procedures (>24h). During these prolonged periods of anesthesia, special care should be taken to avoid negative energy balance and electrolyte disturbances.

Pain assessment and management

Humane and ethical concerns, as well as animal welfare regulations, stipulate the use of appropriate analgesics for procedures that may cause pain or distress to laboratory animals. However, there is no scale that definitively assesses pain in NHP. Both clinical impression and numerical pain scores (usually visual analogue or numerical rating scales) are used despite the paucity of validation studies. As in any other species, behavioral indicators of pain are expected (decreased food intake and activity) and are attenuated by administration of analgesics [75]. Primates tend to hide behavioral signs of mild or moderate pain from unfamiliar observers, so animals are best assessed by a familiar handler or remotely via cameras. Attempts are currently under way to develop cage-side pain scoring using facial expressions (Leech, personal communication).

All of the commonly available analgesics can be used in primates, but long-lasting drugs/formulations are preferred to avoid the stress induced by repeated physical restraint and drug injection (see Table 39.5). In the authors' experience, fentanyl patches can be applied to NHPs to provide relief from moderate to severe pain. If a patch is applied, the primate group should be closely monitored to avoid the risk of fentanyl overdose following oral ingestion of the patch [40]. As in other species, multimodal analgesic approaches, combining opioids and NSAIDs, appear to be particularly useful in controlling postsurgical pain.

References

1 Home Office. Statistics of Scientific Procedures on Living Animals. www.gov.uk/government/publications/user-guide-to-home-office-statistics-of-scientific-procedures-on-living-animals (accessed 29 September 2014).

2 Russel W, Burch L. *The Principles of Humane Experimental Technique*. London: Universities Federation for Animal Welfare, 1992.

3 Stokes EL, Flecknell PA, Richardson CA. Reported analgesic and anaesthetic administration to rodents undergoing experimental surgical procedures. *Lab Anim* 2009; **43**(2): 149–154.

4 Jones RM. Desflurane and sevoflurane: inhalation anaesthetics for this decade? *Br J Anaesth* 1990; **65**(4): 527–536.

5 Atkinson RS, Rushman GB, Davies N. *Lee's Synopsis of Anesthesia*. Oxford: Butterworth Heinemann, 1993.

6 Flecknell PA, Liles JH. Halothane anesthesia in the rabbit: a comparison of the effects of medetomidine, acepromazine and midazolam on breath-holding during induction. *Vet Anaesth Analg* 1996; **23**(1): 11–14.

7 Hedenqvist P, Roughan JV, Antunes L, Orr H, Flecknell PA. Induction of anesthesia with desflurane and isoflurane in the rabbit. *Lab Anim* 2001; **35**(2): 172–179.

8 Leach M, Bowell V, Allan T, Morton D. Measurement of aversion to determine humane methods of anesthesia and euthanasia. *Anim Welfare* 2004: S77–S86.

9 Furst S. Demonstration of a cellular immune response in halothane-exposed guinea pigs. *Toxicol Appl Pharmacol* 1997; **143**(2): 245–255.

10 Shenton JM, Chen J, Uetrecht JP. Animal models of idiosyncratic drug reactions. *Chemico-Biol Interact* 2004; **150**(1): 53–70.

11 Arras M, Autenried P, Rettich A, Spaeni D, Rülicke T. Optimization of intraperitoneal injection anesthesia in mice: drugs, dosages, adverse effects, and anesthesia depth. *Comp Med* 2001; **51**(5): 443–456.

12 Burnside WM, Flecknell PA, Cameron AI, Thomas ALA. A comparison of medetomidine and its active enantiomer dexmedetomidine when administered with ketamine in mice. *BMC Vet Res* 2013; **9**(1): 48.

13 Flecknell P. *Laboratory Animal Anesthesia*. Philadelphia: Academic Press, 2009.

14 Paule MG, Li M, Allen RR, *et al.* Ketamine anesthesia during the first week of life can cause long-lasting cognitive deficits in rhesus monkeys. *Neurotoxicol Teratol* 2011; **33**(2): 220–230.

15 Slikker W, Zou X, Hotchkiss CE, *et al.* Ketamine-induced neuronal cell death in the perinatal rhesus monkey. *Toxicol Sci* 2007; **98**(1): 145–158.

16 Settle TL, Rico PJ. The effect of daily repeated sedation using ketamine or ketamine combined with medetomidine on physiology and anesthetic characteristics in Rhesus Macaques. *J Med Primatol* 2010; **39**(1): 50–57.

17 Davy CW, Trennery PN, Edmunds JG, Altman JF, Eichler DA. Local myotoxicity of ketamine hydrochloride in the marmoset. *Lab Anim* 1987; **21**(1): 60–67.

18 Miyabe T, Nishimura R, Mochizuki M. Chemical restraint by medetomidine and medetomidine–midazolam and its reversal by atipamezole in Japanese macaques (Macaca fuscata). *Vet Anaesth Analg* 2001; **28**(3): 168–174.

19 Pulley ACS, Roberts JA, Lerche NW. Four preanesthetic oral sedation protocols for rhesus macaques (Macaca mulatta). *J Zoo Wildl Med* 2004; **35**(4): 497–502.

20 Hu C, Flecknell PA, Liles JH. Fentanyl and medetomidine anesthesia in the rat and its reversal using atipamazole and either nalbuphine or butorphanol. *Lab Anim* 1992; **26**(1): 15–22.

21 Hara K, Harris RA. The anesthetic mechanism of urethane: the effects on neurotransmitter-gated ion channels. *Anesth Analg* 2002; **94**(2): 313–318.

22 Maggi CA, Meli A. Suitability of urethane anesthesia for physiopharmacological investigations in various systems. Part 1: General considerations. *Experientia* 1986; **42**(2): 109–114.

23 Field KJ, White WJ, Lang CM. Anaesthetic effects of chloral hydrate, pentobarbitone and urethane in adult male rats. *Lab Anim* 1993; **27**(3): 258–269.

24 Fleischman RW, McCracken D, Forbes W. Adynamic ileus in the rat induced by chloral hydrate. *Lab Anim Sci* 1977; **27**(2): 238–243.

25 Lieggi CC, Artwohl JE, Leszczynski JK, Rodriguez NA, Fickbohm BL, Fortman JD. Efficacy and safety of stored and newly prepared tribromoethanol in ICR mice. *Contemp Top Lab Anim Sci* 2005; **44**(1): 17–22.

26 Eisenstein TK, Meissler JJ, Rogers TJ, Geller EB, Adler MW. Mouse strain differences in immunosuppression by opioids in vitro. *J Pharmacol Exp Ther* 1995; **275**(3): 1484–1489.

27 Chao CC, Hu S, Molitor TW, Zhou Y. Morphine potentiates transforming growth factor-beta release from human peripheral blood mononuclear cell cultures. *J Pharmacol Exp Ther* 1992; **262**(1): 19–24.

28 MacFarlane AS, Peng X, Meissler JJ, *et al.* Morphine increases susceptibility to oral Salmonella typhimurium infection. *J Infect Dis* 2000; **181**(4): 1350–1358.

29 Wang J, Barke RA, Charboneau R, Schwendener R, Roy S. Morphine induces defects in early response of alveolar macrophages to Streptococcus pneumoniae by modulating TLR9-NF-kappa B signaling. *J Immunol* 2008; **180**(5): 3594–3600.

30 Afsharimani B, Cabot P, Parat M-O. Morphine and tumor growth and metastasis. *Cancer Metastasis Rev* 2011; **30**(2): 225–238.

31 Coulter C, Flecknell P, Richardson C. Reported analgesic administration to rabbits, pigs, sheep, dogs and non-human primates undergoing experimental surgical procedures. *Lab Anim* 2009; **43**(3): 232.

32 Roughan JV, Flecknell PA. Buprenorphine: a reappraisal of its antinociceptive effects and therapeutic use in alleviating post-operative pain in animals. *Lab Anim* 2002; **36**(3): 322–343.

33 Leach MC, Forrester AR, Flecknell PA. Influence of preferred foodstuffs on the antinociceptive effects of orally administered buprenorphine in laboratory rats. *Lab Anim* 2010; **44**(1): 54–58.

34 Roughan JV, Flecknell PA. Evaluation of a short duration behaviour-based post-operative pain scoring system in rats. *Eur J Pain* 2003; **7**(5): 397–406.

35 Raffa RB, Ding Z. Examination of the preclinical antinociceptive efficacy of buprenorphine and its designation as full- or partial-agonist. *Acute Pain* 2007; **9**(3): 145–152.

36 Ohtani M, Kotaki H, Nishitateno K, Sawada Y, Iga T. Kinetics of respiratory depression in rats induced by buprenorphine and its metabolite, norbuprenorphine. *J Pharmacol Exp Ther* 1997; **281**(1): 428–433.

37 Gueye PN. Buprenorphine and midazolam act in combination to depress respiration in rats. *Toxicol Sci* 2002; **65**(1): 107–114.

38 Clark JA Jr, Myers PH, Goelz MF. Pica behavior associated with buprenorphine administration in the rat. *Lab Anim Sci* 1997; **47**(3): 300–303.

39 Erichsen HK, Hao J-X, Xu X-J, Blackburn-Munro G. Comparative actions of the opioid analgesics morphine, methadone and codeine in rat models of peripheral and central neuropathic pain. *Pain* 2005; **116**(3): 347–358.

40 Deschamps J-Y, Gaulier J-M, Podevin G, Cherel Y, Ferry N, Roux FA. Fatal overdose after ingestion of a transdermal fentanyl patch in two non-human primates. *Vet Anaesth Analg* 2012; **39**(6): 653–656.

41 Carbone ET, Lindstrom KE, Diep S, Carbone L. Duration of action of sustained-release buprenorphine in 2 strains of mice. *J Am Assoc Lab Anim Sci* 2012; **51**(6): 815–819.

42 Foley PL, Liang H, Crichlow AR. Evaluation of a sustained-release formulation of buprenorphine for analgesia in rats. *J Am Assoc Lab Anim Sci* 2011; **50**(2): 198–204.

43 Nunamaker EA, Halliday LC, Moody DE. Pharmacokinetics of 2 formulations of buprenorphine in macaques (Macaca mulatta and Macaca fascicularis). *J Am Assoc Lab Anim Sci* 2013; **52**(1): 48–56.

44 Roughan JV, Flecknell PA. Evaluation of a short duration behaviour-based post-operative pain scoring system in rats. *Eur J Pain* 2003; 7(5): 397–406.

45 Wright-Williams SL, Courade JP, Richardson CA. Effects of vasectomy surgery and meloxicam treatment on faecal corticosterone levels and behaviour in two strains of laboratory mouse. *Pain* 2007p; **130**(1-2): 108–118.

46 Roughan JV, Flecknell PA. Behavioural effects of laparotomy and analgesic effects of ketoprofen and carprofen in rats. *Pain* 2001; **90**(1-2): 65–74.

47 Nadda N, Setia S, Vaish V, Sanyal SN. Role of cytokines in experimentally induced lung cancer and chemoprevention by COX-2 selective inhibitor, etoricoxib. *Mol Cell Biochem* 2012; **372**(1-2): 101–112.

48 Williams JL, Ji P, Ouyang N, Liu X, Rigas B. NO-donating aspirin inhibits the activation of NF-kappaB in human cancer cell lines and Min mice. *Carcinogenesis* 2008; **29**(2): 390–397.

49 Shukoor MI, Tiwari S, Sankpal UT, *et al.* Tolfenamic acid suppresses cytochrome P450 2E1 expression in mouse liver. *Integr Biol* 2012; **4**(9): 1122.

50 De Oliveira GS, Almeida MD, Benzon HT, McCarthy RJ. Perioperative single dose systemic dexamethasone for postoperative pain: a meta-analysis of randomized controlled trials. *Anesthesiology* 2011; **115**(3): 575–588.

51 Pieretti S, di Giannuario A, Domenici MR, et al. Dexamethasone-induced selective inhibition of the central mu opioid receptor: functional in vivo and in vitro evidence in rodents. *Br J Pharmacol* 1994; **113**(4): 1416–1422.

52 Durmus M, Karaaslan E, Ozturk E, *et al.* The effects of single-dose dexamethasone on wound healing in rats. *Anesth Analg* 2003; **97**(5): 1377–1380.

53 Fairbanks CA. Spinal delivery of analgesics in experimental models of pain and analgesia. *Adv Drug Deliv Rev* 2003; **55**(8): 1007–1041.

54 Flecknell P, Liles J. The use of lignocaine-prilocaine local anaesthetic cream for pain-free venepuncture in laboratory animals. *Lab Anim* 1990; **24**(2): 142–146.

55 Jones CP, Carver S, Kendall LV. Evaluation of common anesthetic and analgesic techniques for tail biopsy in mice. *J Am Assoc Lab Anim Sci* 2012; **51**(6): 808–814.

56 Nishiyori M, Ueda H. Prolonged gabapentin analgesia in an experimental mouse model of fibromyalgia. *Mol Pain* 2008; **4**: 52.

57 Boruta DT, Sotgiu G, Golder FJ. Effects of intraperitoneal administration of gabapentin on the minimum alveolar concentration of isoflurane in adult male rats. *Lab Anim* 2012; **46**(2): 108–113.

58 Aguado D, Abreu M, Benito J, Garcia-Fernandez J. The effects of gabapentin on acute opioid tolerance to remifentanil under sevoflurane anesthesia in rats. *Anesth Analg* 2012; **115**(1): 40–45.

59 Smiler KL, Stein S, Hrapkiewicz KL, Hiben JR. Tissue response to intramuscular and intraperitoneal injections of ketamine and xylazine in rats. *Lab Anim Sci* 1990; **40**(1): 60–64.

60 Das RG, North D. Implications of experimental technique for analysis and interpretation of data from animal experiments: outliers and increased variability resulting from failure of intraperitoneal injection procedures. *Lab Anim* 2007; **41**(3): 312–320.

61 Schwarte LA, Zuurbier CJ, Ince C. Mechanical ventilation of mice. *Basic Res Cardiol* 2000; **95**(6): 510–520.

62 Briscoe JA, Syring R. Techniques for emergency airway and vascular access in special species. *Semin Avian Exotic Pet Med* 2004; **13**(3): 118–131.

63 Liles J, Flecknell P. The influence of buprenorphine or bupivacaine on the post-operative effects of laparotomy and bile-duct ligation in rats. *Lab Anim* 1993; **27**(4): 374–380.

64 Pham TM, Hagman B, Codita A, van Loo PLP, Strömmer L, Baumans V. Housing environment influences the need for pain relief during post-operative recovery in mice. *Physiol Behav* 2010; **99**(5): 663–668.

65 Langford DJ, Bailey AL, Chanda ML, *et al.* Coding of facial expressions of pain in the laboratory mouse. *Nat Methods* 2010; **7**(6): 1–6.

66 Keating SCJ, Thomas AA, Flecknell PA, Leach MC. Evaluation of EMLA cream for preventing pain during tattooing of rabbits: changes in physiological, behavioural and facial expression responses. *PLoS ONE* 2012; **7**(9): e44437.

67 Leach MC, Klaus K, Miller AL, di Perrotolo MS, Sotocinal SG, Flecknell PA. The assessment of post-vasectomy pain in mice using behaviour and the mouse grimace scale. *PLoS ONE* 2012; **7**(4): e35656.

68 Roughan JV, Flecknell PA. Behaviour-based assessment of the duration of laparotomy-induced abdominal pain and the analgesic effects of carprofen and buprenorphine in rats. *Behav Pharmacol* 2004; **15**(7): 461–472.

69 Locatelli S, Peeters M. Non-Human Primates, Retroviruses, and Zoonotic Infection Risks in the Human Population. *Nature Educ Knowledge* 2012; **3**(10): 62.

70 Thomas AA, Leach MC, Flecknell PA. An alternative method of endotracheal intubation of common marmosets (Callithrix jacchus). *Lab Anim* 2012; **46**(1): 71–76.

71 Murphy KL, Baxter MG, Flecknell PA. Anesthesia and analgesia in nonhuman primates. In: Abee CR, Mansfield K, Tardif SD, Morris T, eds. *Nonhuman Primates in Biomedical Research 1*. Philadelphia: Academic Press, 2012.

72 Bracken M. Steroids for acute spinal cord injury (review). *Cochrane Database Syst Rev* 2012; **1**: CD001046.

73 Antognini JF, Atherley R, Carstens E. Isoflurane action in spinal cord indirectly depresses cortical activity associated with electrical stimulation of the reticular formation. *Anesth Analg* 2003; **96**(4): 999–1003.

74 Mahon S, Deniau JM, Charpier S. Relationship between EEG potentials and intracellular activity of striatal and cortico-striatal neurons: an in vivo study under different anesthetics. *Cereb Cortex* 2001; **11**(4): 360–373.

75 Allison SO, Halliday LC, French JA, Novikov DD, Fortman JD. Assessment of buprenorphine, carprofen, and their combination for postoperative analgesia in olive baboons (Papio anubis). *J Am Assoc Lab Anim Sci* 2007; **46**(3): 24–31.

40 Comparative Anesthesia and Analgesia of Zoo Animals and Wildlife

Nigel Anthony Caulkett[1] and Jon M. Arnemo[2]

[1]Department of Veterinary Clinical and Diagnostic Science, University of Calgary, Calgary, Alberta, Canada

[2]Hedmark University College, Campus Evenstad, Norway, and Swedish University of Agricultural Sciences, Umeå, Sweden

Chapter contents

Introduction

Chemical immobilization of free-ranging wildlife can be challenging. The nature of the procedure dictates that veterinarians must alter or even ignore many of the principles that underlie good anesthetic practice in other settings. It is generally not possible to access the patients for a preanesthetic physical examination or laboratory work. Physical status of the patients cannot be accurately assessed, and animals are usually assumed to be healthy. Even if physical status and anesthetic risk could be determined, generally only a few effective protocols are available.

Induction of anesthesia in wildlife can be extremely stressful, and stress-related conditions or injuries can result. Free-ranging wildlife are subject to environmental hazards and are often at risk for hypothermia or hyperthermia. Appropriate supportive care, such as controlled ventilation, intravenous fluid therapy, or inotropic support, is often not possible in field situations. Veterinarians may be required to work on species for which there is very little information about their physiology or pharmacologic response to drugs. Extrapolation between similar species may be required, but can result in unexpected complications. Issues of human safety also must be considered. Given the challenges that are encountered during wildlife capture, it is not surprising that morbidity and mortality of animals can be high and injury to people engaged in the capturing procedure more common.

This chapter focuses on the major principles of wildlife capture and handling. It is beyond the scope of a single chapter to provide complete dose recommendations for terrestrial mammals. *The Handbook of Wildlife Chemical Immobilization* [1] and *Zoo Animal and Wildlife Anesthesia and Immobilization* [2] can be used to find detailed drug and dose information for individual species.

Field anesthesia

General considerations

Wildlife capture is often required for both research and management purposes. Capture events should be carefully planned because complications can often be anticipated and responses better prepared. Capture sites may be chosen based on their suitability and the timing chosen in an appropriate season of the year when environmental hazards are minimized. For example, ungulates may be captured in late winter or spring to decrease the risk of hyperthermia and enable tracking in snow or visualization of animals in deciduous forest. Often individual animals do not have to be targeted in management projects, and the capture team can

Veterinary Anesthesia and Analgesia: The Fifth Edition of Lumb and Jones.
Edited by Kurt A. Grimm, Leigh A. Lamont, William J. Tranquilli, Stephen A. Greene and Sheilah A. Robertson.

choose any animal in a relatively safe capture environment. It is generally possible to adhere to strict pursuit time limits. If it is not absolutely necessary to capture the target animal, pursuit can be terminated to decrease the risk of stress-related disease, such as exertional myopathy. Current literature and non-veterinary experts in the field can be consulted prior to the capture event to ensure the most suitable technique is used. It may also be possible to close areas to the public where wildlife are captured. Finally, appropriate equipment for monitoring and supportive care should be obtained and taken into the field when possible.

Weather

Weather conditions may dictate whether wildlife capture is possible. Safe helicopter flight is generally not possible in high winds or foggy conditions. Snow and rain can lead to hypothermia, particularly if wind is also present to enhance convective heat loss. Smaller mammals may be particularly prone to hypothermia. Hyperthermia is a serious complication that can be difficult to treat in field situations. Several of the drug regimens used for wildlife capture can impede thermoregulation and lead to hypothermia or hyperthermia [3,4]. When possible, captures should be planned for the cooler hours of the day during summer months. In remote locations, sudden changes in weather may also be a hazard to personnel. It is important to keep track of current and forecasted conditions during planned events. Capture for management purposes may occur at any time. Provisions should be made to prevent heat loss and actively cool animals, if required.

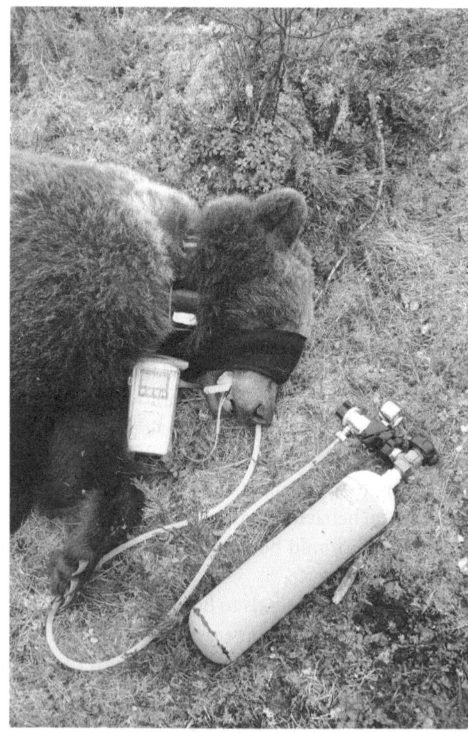

Figure 40.1 Oxygen delivery via intranasal cannulation in a brown bear.

Equipment

Logistics generally dictate what type of equipment can be carried in a field situation. It is often difficult to carry all but the most necessary pieces. Fortunately, there are compact ambulatory monitors suitable for field use.

Equipment should withstand field use and be as lightweight and compact as possible. Hypoxemia is a common complication of wildlife anesthesia, particularly with ruminants [5–11]. Oxygen is fundamental supportive care during field anesthesia. Aluminum E and D cylinders, combined with a sturdy regulator and flowmeter, are ideal for field use (Fig. 40.1). Recent reports have demonstrated the utility of portable oxygen concentrators in field situations [12]. Oxygen concentrators may provide an attractive alternative to compressed oxygen cylinders as they do not require refilling, and eliminate many of the risks of working with compressed gas (Fig. 40.2). Often, nasal insufflation of oxygen is adequate to treat hypoxemia. However, equipment for airway management and ventilatory support is recommended for many scenarios. It is difficult to carry a wide range of emergency drugs or an adequate volume of crystalloid fluids to treat shock, but a basic emergency kit containing epinephrine, atropine, lidocaine, and reversal agents should always be carried. Ruminants are predisposed to ruminal tympany so a suitably sized tube to desufflate the rumen should be available. Equipment should also be carried to treat lacerations and other incidental injuries during capture.

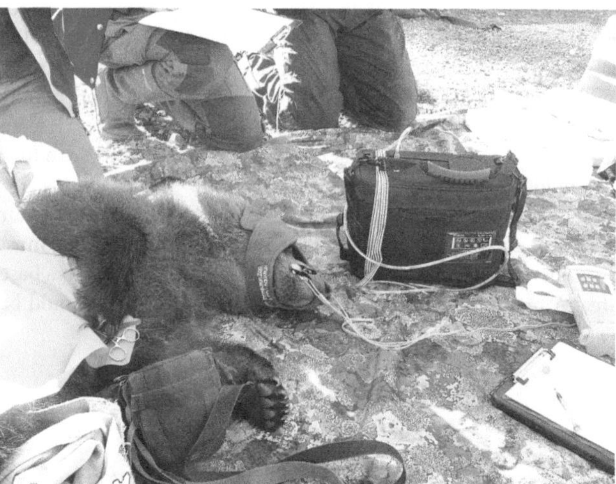

Figure 40.2 Portable oxygen concentrators can be used instead of compressed gas cylinders in field situations. They have some advantages for use in remote locations.

Capture technique

An animal may be captured initially by physical or chemical means. The choice of capture technique depends on the species, the terrain, the facilities, and the experience of the capture crew. Many species of ungulates can be effectively captured and handled by experienced teams with physical techniques such as net guns [13–15]. Physical restraint can be very stressful for wild animals, but sedatives or anesthetics can be used to decrease the stress of handling once animals have been netted [15].

Net gunning can cause high rates of mortality if it is performed by inexperienced personnel. The risk to capture personnel can also be high. During a 10-year period in New Zealand there were 127 helicopter crashes and 25 human fatalities during net gun capture of red deer [16]. These figures stress the need for experienced pilots and capture personnel.

The use of physical restraint will confine an animal's movements during the induction of anesthesia which may be a positive when terrain dictates a limited escape route. Physical restraint can induce greater stress than chemical restraint [17]. Generally, physical restraint should be of brief duration to avoid stress-related complications.

Hazards

A number of hazards can be encountered during anesthesia of free-ranging wildlife. It is important to perform a risk assessment prior to embarking on a project to identify and minimize the risks. The target species can pose a risk to personnel. There are the obvious risks of serious personnel injury from carnivores, but ungulates can also act aggressively. Many deer species undergo a period of rut during the breeding season, during which stags are often more aggressive. Injury may also occur from flailing limbs or heads in lightly anesthetized animals. It is important to know how a species will act in a stressful situation, and to leave an exit for the animal (and for the capture personnel) if things do not go according to plan. The best way to avoid injury is to work with people who are familiar with animal behavior. Many species carry zoonotic disease, so capture personnel should be aware of this potential and handle the animal appropriately.

During capture, the focus tends to be on the captured animal. It is always important to be aware of the surrounding environment because other animals may approach. This is particularly important with social carnivores, such as lions. It is also important with bears, particularly if members of a family group are captured. In these situations, an armed lookout should be posted to protect the capture team.

A firearm back-up is important with more dangerous species. The primary person performing the back-up should be trained and experienced in the use of firearms, and an appropriate firearm should be used. If firearms are commonly used, all members of the capture team should receive firearm safety training. Similar training is advisable for people using dart rifles or pistols. Pepper spray may be considered as a non-lethal alternative to firearms. Recent studies have demonstrated that pepper spray is as effective as a firearm in many situations [18] (Fig. 40.3).

The environment itself can be hazardous since capture may occur in remote and rugged locations. In these situations, personnel must be prepared to look after themselves if they cannot return to a base area. A method of communication with rescue services should be established. In some environments, weather can change rapidly and often dictates whether capture should take place. There are hazards specific to the terrain and region; for instance, capture personnel should receive avalanche training before working in mountainous regions during winter when there is an avalanche risk. It is important to anticipate risks in any environment.

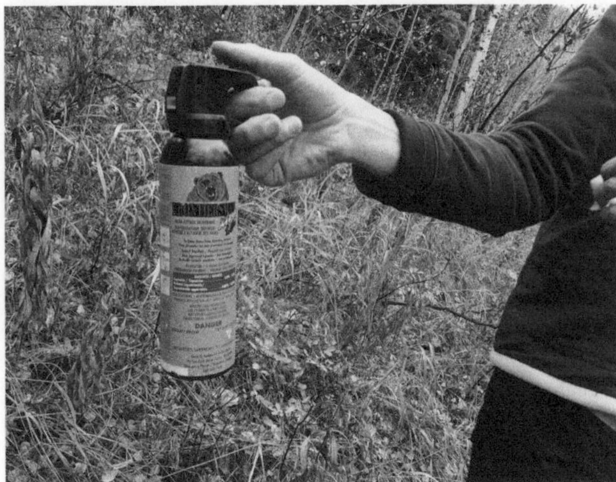

Figure 40.3 Pepper spray has been proven to effectively deter bear attacks; it is a potential less lethal option for personal defense against dangerous wildlife.

Pharmaceuticals used for wildlife immobilization and anesthesia can present a serious human health hazard because of their high potency and concentrated formulations. Handling of potent narcotics, such as carfentanil, etorphine, and thiafentanil, carries the risk of lethal toxicity in people [1,2,19]. These drugs must be handled with extreme caution. Protective clothing, such as disposable gloves or face shields, should be used to prevent skin or mucous membrane contact. A pharmacologic antagonist should be available to treat human exposure. Potent narcotics receive a great deal of attention, but any concentrated sedative or anesthetic must also be handled carefully. Medetomidine can be formulated at a concentration of 40 mg/mL for use in wildlife. Dexmedetomidine, which is used at a dose of 1–2 μg/kg in people [20], is approximately twice as potent as medetomidine [21]. This dose is equivalent to 2–4 μg of medetomidine per 1 kg of body weight or a total of 150–300 μg in a 75 kg person. The high end of this dose range is equivalent to a 0.0075 mL volume of concentrated medetomidine. Obviously, there is serious risk of toxicity from exposure to a very low volume of a 40 mg/kg medetomidine formulation. Tiletamine-zolazepam is another immobilizing mixture that can be delivered in a concentrated form and therefore must be handled with caution. Everyone working on a capture team should be trained in first aid, and equipment should be available to provide respiratory and airway support.

Wildlife anesthesia should never be performed by a single person. At least two trained people should be present whenever potent drugs are handled. Loading and charging of darts is a time of high risk for exposure to drugs, during which the use of face shields may be considered to prevent contamination of mucous membranes. Darts should be charged under a protective cover to decrease the risk of accidental drug exposure. Antagonists, such as naloxone, should always be immediately available in case of inadvertent human exposure.

Dart delivery equipment should be handled with care and only by trained individuals. Darts have the potential to induce significant tissue injury and death. Firearm safety rules apply to darting equipment, and individuals handling this equipment should be appropriately trained.

Helicopters present a significant hazard. Wildlife capture requires a very skilled pilot to decrease risk of injury to the target animal and the capture personnel [22]. Anyone working around a helicopter must receive training in helicopter safety.

Prior to any capture, it is advisable to meet with local medical personnel and discuss an evacuation and treatment plan in case of inadvertent human exposure. A meeting of this nature will familiarize physicians and emergency medical services personnel with the drugs that are being used and the potential treatments. In the event of an emergency, this can save valuable time and someone's life.

Remote drug delivery equipment

Wildlife capture often requires drug delivery over relatively long distances. Generally, it is difficult to deliver drugs accurately at distances greater than 40 m but there have been major advances in the equipment available for remote drug delivery. It is important to realize that these systems have the potential to produce serious injury or death if they are used inappropriately. The major sources of injury arise from dart impact trauma, high-velocity injection of dart contents, and inaccurate dart placement.

Dart impact trauma results from dispersion of energy on dart impact. Impact kinetic energy is represented by the following equation: $KE = 1/2M \times V^2$, where M = mass of the dart and V = velocity [1]. High velocity is the major factor that will cause trauma. A good general rule is to use the lowest velocity that will provide an accurate trajectory at a given distance. Practice with a darting system at a variety of distances is vital to minimize velocity. The other major factor is the mass of the dart. Darts with a lower mass will have less impact energy at a given velocity. This should be a consideration in the choice of a darting system, particularly when dealing with smaller animals that are more prone to trauma.

Inaccurate dart placement can cause injury. This most frequently occurs if the dart penetrates the abdomen, thorax, or other vital structures of the head and neck. The major factors that can lead to inaccurate dart placement include lack of practice with the darting system, an attempt to place a dart over an excessive range, and inherent inaccuracy of the darting system.

The final source of injury is related to high-velocity injection of dart contents. Systems that expel drug via an explosive charge can disrupt tissue and produce trauma. These systems should only be used on large, well-muscled animals (Fig. 40.4). Injection volume should be minimized to decrease the degree of tissue trauma. When possible, the use of darts that deliver their contents via compressed air should be considered. The choice of system depends on the range required, the dart size, and individual characteristics of the target animal. A more complete review and manufacturer information can be found elsewhere [1,2,22,23].

Darts

Darts must deliver their contents into a muscle group on impact for capture to be rapid and smooth. Choice of a system will depend on the situation and the size of the animal.

Explosive discharge mechanisms

Darts that use an explosive discharge mechanism can produce considerable muscle trauma and should be reserved for large, well-muscled animals. These darts have an aluminum or plastic body into which a small explosive cap is placed between the plunger and the tail. Upon impact, a firing pin inside the cap is forced forward, against the resistance of a spring, detonating the charge. The expanding gas pushes the plunger forward and the drug is expelled through the needle. The short duration of injection (e.g., 0.001 s) can result in high injectate velocity which may cause tissue damage [22]. The explosive caps are very sensitive to moisture and must be kept dry. When placed in the dart, the cap must have its open end against the tail. If it is turned around, detonation and expulsion of the drug will occur at the moment the projector is fired.

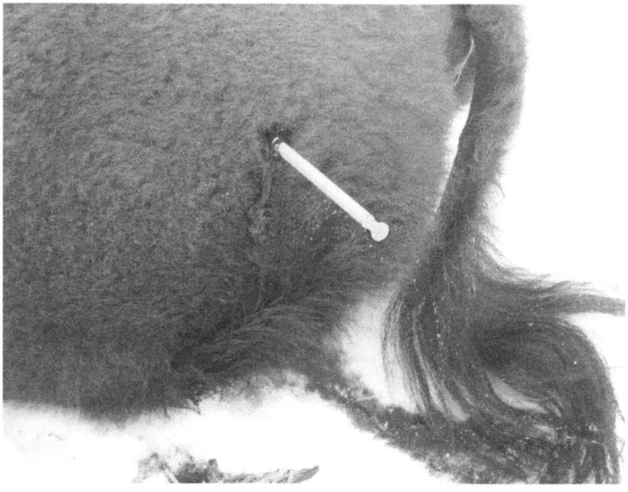

Figure 40.4 Dart-induced trauma in a bison. Explosive injection of dart contents has the potential to induce muscle trauma and hematoma.

If reusable darts are used, the fit of the dart should be tested by inserting the dart in the muzzle. If it slides in and out with ease, the dart is not significantly deformed and it can be reloaded. If the dart jams in the muzzle, the dart should not be reused. With repeated use, the dart barrel may expand to the point where the aluminum is weakened by the threads cut into it. This is caused by the high pressure created in the dart when gases from the explosive charge push the plunger forward.

All of the darts with explosive discharge mechanisms inject through the tip of the needle. The needle should be barbed so that it stays in the animal during injection. If there is no barb or if the barb is removed, the force of the frontal expulsion of the drug is often sufficiently powerful to drive the dart out of the animal, resulting in only partial injection.

Air-activated mechanisms

These darts consist of an aluminum or plastic body into which compressed air is introduced through a one-way valve in the tail piece. At impact, a silicone seal is displaced, exposing a port in the side of the needle. The plunger is pushed forward by air pressure and the drug is expelled through the open port. Depending on the type and usage, plastic darts can be used repeatedly, but will eventually begin to leak or lose air pressure. In extreme cold, the drug may freeze inside the dart; therefore, darts should be kept warm in a secure container placed in an inside pocket or in a heated vehicle or helicopter.

Pharmacology

Ideal drug combination for wildlife capture

Wildlife immobilization has progressed a great deal in recent years. A variety of drugs are available to facilitate capture and handling, and new techniques continue to develop. An ideal drug or combinations thereof would possess the following properties.

Rapid onset of activity

A rapid effect is one of the most important attributes required in a capture drug. The induction period is a hazardous time. Handlers and bystanders may be at risk of injury if induction is prolonged. Rapid onset will limit the risks of trauma, hyperthermia, and possibly capture myopathy. Ideally, the animal should be immobilized within 1–5 min after injection. Practically, most current combinations can take longer than 5 min to induce anesthesia.

High margin of safety

Drugs used for wildlife capture must have a high margin of safety. It is difficult to transport supportive equipment into the field so capture drugs should produce minimal cardiopulmonary depression. Wild animals are not weighed prior to capture, and it is common to overestimate weight. Capture drugs must have high safety margins or therapeutic index to decrease the risk of mortality from overdose.

Handler safety

Precautions must always be taken to avoid human exposure to drugs. Ideally, drugs should be relatively safe to handle, with minimum risks of intoxication if the handler contacts the drug. The ability to antagonize the effects of any drug is also desirable in field situations.

Small volume of delivery

Capture drugs should be potent and concentrated enough to facilitate delivery at low volumes, ideally less than 3 mL. This decreases the risk of injection trauma from high-velocity injection and facilitates accurate dart flight.

Level of CNS effect

The animal should rapidly lose motor function and ideally become unconsciousness and unaware of its surroundings.

Ability to antagonize immobilization

Free-ranging wildlife often live in an environment full of potential hazards, so they must be cared for until they are fully awake. A pharmacologic antagonist will speed recovery and is also of value in emergency situations. Because it can be difficult to provide supportive care, complications such as hyperthermia can quickly become life threatening and drug antagonism may be the only viable option in managing unexpected complications.

Species versatility

Wildlife managers often deal with a variety of species. Thus, an ideal drug or combinations thereof should have predictable effects in a wide range of species. This limits the number of drugs required to be kept on hand and familiarity of the drug or combination(s) used most commonly.

Drug stability

Wildlife capture may need to be performed in a wide range of ambient temperatures. Ideally, drugs should remain stable, in solution, over a wide range of temperatures.

Analgesia

In recent years, it has become more common to perform potentially painful procedures during wildlife handling. These procedures can include ear tagging, tooth removal, biopsies, and even surgery for abdominal or subcutaneous implant placement. These procedures dictate that appropriate intraoperative and postoperative analgesia be provided.

Opioids

A variety of opioids have been used for wildlife capture. Opioids can be used in a wide range of species, but are particularly effective in ungulates. The opioids produce analgesia and sedation, but lack muscle-relaxant properties. They have been used alone or, more often, with a neuroleptic agent, the inclusion of which potentiates the opioid's sedative effects, resulting in a smoother induction and decreased muscle rigidity. Opioids are predictable, act relatively fast, and can be reversed with the administration of a suitable antagonist. If not reversed, the duration of immobilization is lengthy, often several hours, during which the animal is at risk from opioid-induced respiratory depression and environmental hazards. Underdosing of opioids can result in a prolonged induction time characterized by CNS excitation which can cause hyperthermia, exhaustion, lost animals, and/or death of the animal. The adverse effects of opioid-induced immobilization include:

1 excitation after administration, resulting in aimless running, pacing, or walking, which may lead to hyperthermia or capture myopathy [24]
2 regurgitation of ruminal content or vomiting; the risk of regurgitation appears increased when carfentanil is combined with xylazine [25]
3 severe respiratory depression and hypoxemia [5,9]
4 muscle rigidity [24]
5 renarcotization [24–26].

Many of the opioids such as carfentanil, etorphine, and thiafentanil are several thousand times more potent than morphine in humans and must be handled carefully to avoid accidental exposure [1,2,19,22].

Carfentanil

Carfentanil has been used for wildlife capture since the early 1980s and is commercially available at a concentration of 3 mg/mL. It is particularly useful in ungulates, but has also been used in large carnivores [27–29]. Advantages of carfentanil include high potency, rapid onset of activity, reliability, and reversal with an appropriate antagonist. The use of carfentanil alone can cause muscle rigidity so it is often combined with a sedative agent with muscle-relaxant properties, such as xylazine [24]. Evidently, there are disadvantages of using this combination in moose, because the addition of xylazine to carfentanil reportedly produces an increased incidence of aspiration pneumonia [25].

Carfentanil has a relatively long effect. Carfentanil-induced immobilization should be antagonized with an appropriate antagonist once the procedure is completed. If the duration of the antagonist is shorter than that of carfentanil, renarcotization can result. Naltrexone is typically used for reversal of carfentanil. Renarcotization has been reported following antagonism with naloxone, diprenorphine, and nalmefene [26,27]. Other adverse effects of carfentanil-based combinations include respiratory depression, hypoxemia, hypertension, CNS excitation, and hyperthermia [5,9,30].

Etorphine

Etorphine hydrochloride has been used successfully in many species, but has been particularly effective in ungulates, rhinoceroses, and elephants. Etorphine can be used alone or in combination with a suitable neuroleptic agent. Induction course and immobilization duration are dose dependent. Underdosing can cause excitation with its associated problems. At optimum doses, the first effects may be observed 3–8 min after intramuscular injection. The full effect may be reached in 20–30 min. Recovery is slow (up to 7 or 8 h) if no antagonist is given. When an antagonist is administered, animals will recover in 1–3 min after intravenous injection and in 5–10 min following intramuscular injection. The most serious adverse effect is respiratory depression. For that reason, an animal should not be kept immobilized longer than necessary, and drug effect should be reversed as soon as possible. Other side-effects are often dose or species dependent and may include excitement, muscle tremors, convulsions, regurgitation, bloat, bradycardia, tachycardia, hypertension, hyperthermia, and renarcotization.

Thiafentanil

Thiafentanil has some potential advantages over both carfentanil and etorphine such as rapid induction, greater therapeutic index, shorter half-life, lower incidence of renarcotization and less respiratory and cardiac depression [31]. Thiafentanil is commercially available only in South Africa, but its use has been described in a variety of species [1,2,31]. It has been used alone or in combination with α_2-adrenergic receptor agonist. Reports have detailed the use of thiafentanil combined with medetomidine and ketamine [6,32]. This is a promising drug combination that appears to be efficacious and have fewer side-effects than does high-dose single narcotic immobilization [1,2,22,31].

Butorphanol

Several recently developed immobilizing combinations include butorphanol. It has been used to enhance sedation in combination with medetomidine and azaperone [33]. Butorphanol administered in combination with etorphine improved ventilatory function during immobilization of rhinos [34]. Butorphanol has agonist activity at the κ-opioid receptor and is generally antagonistic at μ-opioid receptors. It is commercially available in concentrations of 30 and 50 mg/mL. These high-concentration formulations greatly increase the utility of this drug for remote delivery.

Opioid antagonists

A major advantage of opioid-based immobilization is the ability to antagonize the opioid. To be effective, the antagonist's effect should outlast the agonist drug's sedation, and ideally be highly selective for the desired receptor type(s). The three drugs commonly used for this purpose are naltrexone, naloxone, and diprenorphine. Naltrexone is probably the most versatile drug, with the lowest risk of renarcotization. Naloxone and naltrexone are the preferred antagonists for opioid overdose in humans.

Naltrexone

Naltrexone is commercially available in a 50 mg/mL concentration. It is a pure opioid antagonist (i.e., it has no known agonistic properties) that will produce rapid antagonism of μ-opioid receptor agonists. The major advantage of naltrexone is that it will produce reliable antagonism of longer-acting opioids, such as carfentanil. A study comparing carfentanil reversal with nalmefene, diprenorphine, and naltrexone demonstrated renarcotization with diprenorphine and nalmefene [25]. Naltrexone has been recommended at a dose of 100 mg:1 mg for naltrexone-carfentanil and 10–30 mg:1 mg for naltrexone-thiafentanil. The drug is effective following intramuscular and intravenous administration. A more rapid antagonism will occur if it is administered intravenously.

Naloxone

Naloxone is also a pure narcotic antagonist. It may be used to reverse the effects of all the aforementioned opioids, and reversal occurs within 1–3 min of intravenous injection. Naloxone has a short half-life so animals may revert to a state of motor impairment within a few hours and require repeated treatment with naloxone. Renarcotization has been noted in field studies that used naloxone as an antagonist for carfentanil [26]. A low dose of naloxone (2 μg naloxone administered intravenously for every 1 μg carfentanil given) has been shown to improve oxygenation while maintaining immobilization in elk [5].

Diprenorphine

Diprenorphine is the antagonist used to reverse the effects of etorphine. While it does have agonistic properties of its own, when given following etorphine, diprenorphine acts as an antagonist. Reversal is rapid following intravenous injection, with animals becoming ambulatory in 1–3 min. If the antagonist is injected intramuscularly, reversal takes longer (up to 15–20 min). Adverse effects are rare, although overdosing may cause continued immobilization because of its partial agonist activity. Following accidental human exposure to etorphine, diprenorphine should not be used as an antagonist because of its agonist effects.

Cyclohexamines

This class of drugs produce a state of dissociative anesthesia. When used alone, the cyclohexamines produce muscle rigidity or twitching. Other adverse effects are hyperthermia, excessive salivation, catecholamine release, and convulsions. The cyclohexamines act fast, have a relatively wide margin of safety, and depress respiration and circulation only moderately at optimum doses. Laryngeal reflexes are somewhat preserved with these agents.

Cyclohexamines may be used alone in some species, but the addition of a benzodiazepine or α_2-adrenergic receptor agonist will be additive or synergistic, produce a smoother induction and recovery, and alleviate the muscle rigidity common with dissociative anesthesics [3]. The cyclohexamines have been used in a wide variety of species, but are particularly known for their effectiveness in carnivores, primates, and birds. There are no known antagonists for this class of drugs. The drugs in this category most utilized for immobilization include ketamine and the tiletamine-zolazepam combination.

Ketamine

Ketamine is commercially available in 10, 50, and 100 mg/mL aqueous solutions. Since these concentrations may be too low for efficient delivery to larger species, it may be lyophilized and reconstituted at 200 mg/mL. Ketamine should never be used as the sole immobilizing agent. A tranquilizer-sedative should be co-administered in almost all cases to reduce or prevent its hypertonic effects. Ketamine has been used successfully in many species, and doses vary widely from one species to another. Induction time and immobilization duration are dose and species dependent. At optimum doses, the first effects are observed in 2–5 min following intramuscular injection, with the full effects usually attained in 5–10 min. Immobilization usually lasts from 45 min to 2 h.

Adverse effects of ketamine may include convulsions, catatonia, apnea, excessive salivation, and hyperthermia. Many of these effects can be negated by adding a benzodiazepine or α_2-adrenergic receptor agonist. Medetomidine-ketamine combinations have some advantages over xylazine use because a lower dose of ketamine is usually required [1,2,35]. This will result in smaller injection volumes and the ability to antagonize medetomidine with fewer adverse side-effects from the remaining ketamine. It is noteworthy that ketamine-based combinations are unreliable in bears. Sudden recoveries have been encountered with xylazine-ketamine and medetomidine-ketamine in brown and polar bears [35,36].

Tiletamine-zolazepam

A commercial preparation of tiletamine (Telazol®), a dissociative anesthetic, and zolazepam, a benzodiazepine agonist, is available as a freeze-dried powder product. It is effective in a variety of species and at optimum doses its first effects may be noticeable within 1 or 2 min following intramuscular injection. Full effects can be reached within 15–30 min. The onset is usually smooth, with good muscle relaxation and somatic analgesia. The duration of effect, quality of emergence, and duration of recovery vary with species because tiletamine and zolazepam are metabolized at different rates in various species. Recovery occurs in 3–8 h in most cases, but may be prolonged in some species.

The tiletamine-zolazepam combination may cause hypertension and increase heart rate and cardiac output. Other effects are salivation, occasional muscle rigidity and ataxia, and hyperthermia (particularly if the mixture is combined with an α_2-adrenergic receptor agonist) [36–39]. Tiletamine-zolazepam has been used alone in a variety of species [40]. It is very effective in carnivores, and recovery tends to be smooth, but can be prolonged. The use of this combination alone in ungulates can result in rough recoveries. Reconstitution of tiletamine-zolazepam with an α_2-adrenergic receptor agonist will decrease the volume injected, enhance analgesia, and decrease recovery times following antagonism of the α_2-adrenergic receptor agonist [8,36–39,41,42].

α_2-Adrenergic receptor agonists

α_2-Adrenergic receptor agonists are CNS depressants with sedative, muscle relaxant, and analgesic properties. Used alone, α_2-adrenergic receptor agonists produce unreliable immobilization in most wild species. They are best used in combination with opioids or dissociative anesthetics. When used in high doses, α_2-adrenergic receptor agonists may critically depress respiration and circulation. Commonly encountered adverse effects include hypoxemia in ungulates and hypertension with or without bradycardia [7–10,35,37,38,43]. These agents can also contribute to ruminal tympany and regurgitation in ungulates [8,25]. In very excited animals (capture situations), they do not produce a predictable level of immobilization. They also disrupt thermoregulatory mechanisms, leading to hyperthermia or hypothermia [3,35,36]. Recovery without reversal from high doses is usually prolonged and difficult. In field situations, it is generally recommended that the effects of α_2-adrenergic receptor agonists be antagonized at the completion of the procedure to help minimize adverse physiologic actions and capture outcomes.

Xylazine

Xylazine is commonly available in 20 and 100 mg/mL aqueous solutions. It is also available in powder form and as a 300 mg/mL solution specifically for use in wildlife capture. The 20 mg/mL solution is too dilute to be useful for remote injection.

When administered alone, xylazine does not produce reliably immobilized free-ranging wildlife. It may appear to induce a recumbent, sleep-like state but stimulation may cause rapid arousal with defense responses intact. In calm animals, the initial sedative effect may be seen within 4–5 min of intramuscular injection, with full effect reached within 15–20 min. Adverse effects can include hypoxemia, bradycardia, hypotension, ruminal tympany, and decreased thermoregulatory ability.

Xylazine has been used effectively in combination with opioids and cyclohexamines. The response to high doses of xylazine may conceal a recovery from the primary immobilizing drug and place workers at risk if the animal is suddenly aroused by noises, touch, or other stimulation.

The effects of xylazine may be reversed with the administration of several α_2-adrenergic receptor antagonists. Approximately 1 mg of atipamezole administered intramuscularly is required to antagonize 10 mg of xylazine. If xylazine is used in combination with a cyclohexamine, its effects should not be reversed before the animal has metabolized a significant fraction of the latter in an attempt to minimize the adverse effects of the cyclohexamine.

Xylazine is typically used intramuscularly for wildlife immobilization. Intranasal administration can be beneficial to decrease stress and struggling following net gun capture [15]. This route has a relatively rapid onset of activity and is simple to administer in physically restrained animals [15].

Detomidine

Detomidine is commercially available in a 10 mg/mL solution. The effects of detomidine have been well studied in horses, but information on its use for immobilization of captive and free-ranging equids and wild animals is limited. It has been combined with etorphine in rhinoceros and has proven to be effective in zebras when combined with carfentanil and ketamine [44,45]. The action of detomidine is much like that of xylazine. Its effects may be reversed by an appropriate α_2-adrenergic receptor antagonist. In general, 5 mg (IM) of atipamezole should be used to antagonize 1 mg of detomidine.

Medetomidine

Medetomidine is a potent α_2-adrenergic receptor agonist that has proven useful for wildlife capture. The 1 mg/mL formulation suitable for use in small mammals is too dilute for use in larger species. Medetomidine is also commercially available in 10, 20, and 40 mg/mL concentrations, which are more adequate for capture of most large land mammals. Medetomidine will produce sedation, analgesia, and muscle relaxation. Medetomidine should not be used alone because, as with xylazine, immobilization is unreliable. Medetomidine can be combined with a low dose of ketamine or tiletamine-zolazepam. A relatively low dose of the dissociative drug is required in combination with medetomidine, and antagonism of medetomidine with atipamezole (at 3–5 times the medetomidine dose) will hasten recovery [1,33]. Similar to all α_2-adrenergic receptor agonists, adverse effects of medetomidine include hypertension, bradycardia, and hypoxemia [8,9,35,37,43,45]. Hypoxemia may be particularly pronounced in ruminants [8]. Medetomidine can also impair thermoregulatory ability, resulting in hyperthermia [36,37].

Dexmedetomidine

Dexmedetomidine is approximately twice as potent as medetomidine; currently it is available only in a relatively dilute form for small animal use. It can be used interchangeably with medetomidine at approximately half the dose (on a microgram basis). This drug has utility in small wildlife; it will have greater utility in larger species if a concentrated form becomes available to reduce volume requirements.

α_2-Adrenergic receptor antagonists

The utility of α_2-adrenergic receptor agonist-induced sedation is greatly increased by the availability of specific antagonists. Atipamezole is the most selective of the three currently available antagonists and can be used in all species. There are apparent species-dependent differences in response to yohimbine and tolazoline but less so with atipamezole [2]. Yohimbine, for example, is not particularly effective in wild bovids, and either tolazoline or atipamezole reversal is preferred in these species. Antagonists should generally be administered intramuscularly unless the situation is an emergency. Central nervous system excitement, tachycardia, and hypotension followed by hypertension may be seen with intravenous antagonist administration [35,46]. Animals may arouse rapidly and without warning from immobilization following intravenous administration of atipamezole [8,36,43]. With potentially dangerous species, this may not allow adequate time to retreat to a safe distance.

Neuroleptic drugs

Neuroleptic agents such as acepromazine and droperidol have been used as adjunctive agents in wildlife capture for many years. Typically, they have been used in combination with potent opioids such as etorphine. A more recent application of these agents is the use of long-acting tranquilizers to facilitate translocation of wild animals. Long-acting neuroleptics have been developed to treat human psychosis. Depending on the formulation, these drugs may have effects for days to weeks. They will produce an overall reduction in stress of handling, which should decrease the incidence of trauma and myopathy and facilitate adaptation to a novel environment. Typically, these agents are of the phenothiazine, butyrophenone, or benzodiazepine drug class [47,48]. A short-acting agent, such as haloperidol, may be combined with a long-acting agent, such as perphenazine enanthate, to produce rapid onset of action and prolonged activity [48].

Perphenazine enanthate

Perphenazine is a slow-onset, long-acting phenothiazine derivative formulated in a sesame oil vehicle. The onset of perphenazine is 12–16 h, and its effects can last up to 10 days. The use of this drug has been reported in a variety of species, including red deer and Przewalski's horses [49,50]. Flight distance is decreased in red deer, and animals maintain better body condition than controls during changes in environment [49]. In Przewalski's horses, the drug has been used to effectively decrease dominance aggression during the establishment of a bachelor herd [50].

Zuclopenthixol acetate

This drug is a thioxanthine derivative that has been used in a variety of species with effects lasting up to 3–4 days [49,51–53]. Treated animals have a decreased flight distance and are easier to manipulate. Animals spend more time eating and drinking compared with controls and spend less time pacing. A dose of 1 mg/kg IM has been used in most studies. Occasionally, extrapyramidal signs have been noted [53] but usually resolve without treatment [53].

Azaparone

This butyrophenone drug has classically been used for tranquilization of swine. It has been used in combination with α_2-adrenergic receptor agonists and opioids for anesthesia and immobilization of wild and farmed ungulates [47]. In pigs it has a duration of approximately 6 h. Its duration of action has not been reported in wildlife species. Azaperone has been used in wild ungulates to provide tranquilization for short translocations.

Drug combinations

As stated previously, it is uncommon to use single agents for wildlife capture. Typically, agents are combined either for their synergistic immobilizing effects or to counter adverse physiologic effects of singular agents. The combination of an opioid with an α_2-adrenergic receptor agonist has already been discussed. Xylazine-ketamine has been used for many years and has the advantage of versatility (i.e., it is effective in many ungulate and carnivore species). The major disadvantages of xylazine-ketamine combinations are the large volume required and the residual effects of ketamine if xylazine is antagonized soon after administration. Medetomidine-ketamine shares the versatility of xylazine-ketamine, with the advantages of decreased volume and lower ketamine requirement. Antagonism of medetomidine will likely cause fewer side-effects from residual ketamine, because its dose requirement is lower [1,2,35].

Medetomidine-ketamine is useful in a wide range of species [1,2]. Nevertheless, it should always be used cautiously. Its use is even avoided in bears, because sudden recoveries have been reported in brown and polar bears [35,36]. Xylazine-tiletamine-zolazepam and medetomidine-tiletamine-zolazepam can be delivered in small volumes and are useful in a wide range of wildlife species, as well. Antagonism of the α_2-adrenergic receptor agonist will hasten recovery. Time to sternal recumbency and standing is generally more rapid after antagonism of medetomidine compared with xylazine because of the lower dose requirement of tiletamine-zolazepam when combined with medetomidine [7,36–39].

A combination of butorphanol, azaperone, and medetomidine has been developed for wildlife capture. The mixture has been used to successfully capture a variety of wild and captive species [47]. Sedation is mostly reversible with atipamezole and naltrexone in combination. There will be residual tranquilization from azaperone, as no antagonist has been developed for this drug.

The capture event

Precapture planning

Before undertaking any wildlife capture, an appropriate plan of action must be devised. The target species should be researched to determine the most effective and current techniques. A decision needs to be made as to the use of physical or chemical restraint. Logistical considerations are important and include establishing communication and evacuation plans. Equipment must be carefully selected for use in the field. Drug needs must be anticipated, and it is generally wise to budget for at least 50% more drug than is actually needed. This will help to offset any drug wasted from lost darts or poor dart placement.

In the immediate precapture period, the target animal is located and weight is estimated. The terrain, weather, and other factors must be evaluated to determine whether capture should be attempted. Most commonly, the drug dart is loaded after the target animal has been located and observed; however, there may be times when it is more practical to load the darts beforehand. Drug doses may be calculated for specific sizes or age groups, and the darts are preloaded and marked accordingly. However, metal darts should not be kept loaded for longer than a 12 h period because of the possibility that corrosive action of the drugs may impair the injection mechanism. Preloaded darts with air-activated discharge mechanisms should not be pressurized because they have a tendency to lose pressure if armed for an extended period.

Generally, the animal will need to be approached to within a distance of 30–40 m for accurate dart delivery. There are many methods to facilitate approaching to within this distance. Animals may be stalked, baited, approached in a vehicle or helicopter, or trapped or snared prior to approach. Trapping has the advantage of limiting movement during the capture event, but it may prove to be more stressful than helicopter capture [17]. Pursuit of animals should generally be limited to no more than 2–5 min. The incidence of capture myopathy, hyperthermia, and trauma will increase with prolonged chase times. In management situations, pursuit may often be required until the animal is captured. It is beyond the scope of this chapter to thoroughly discuss species-specific considerations. It is advisable to include experienced personnel on the capture team and to consult with experienced wildlife managers, biologists, and veterinarians to determine anticipated complications, animal behavior when stressed, and the current approaches to dealing with the target species.

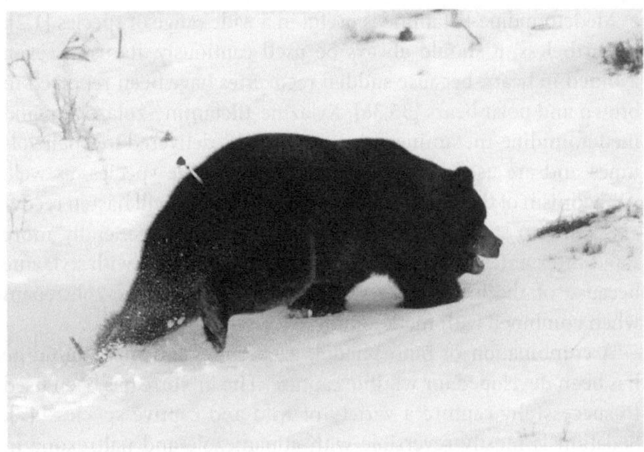

Figure 40.5 Correct dart placement in a brown bear. The dart has been placed into the well-muscled hindquarter of the bear.

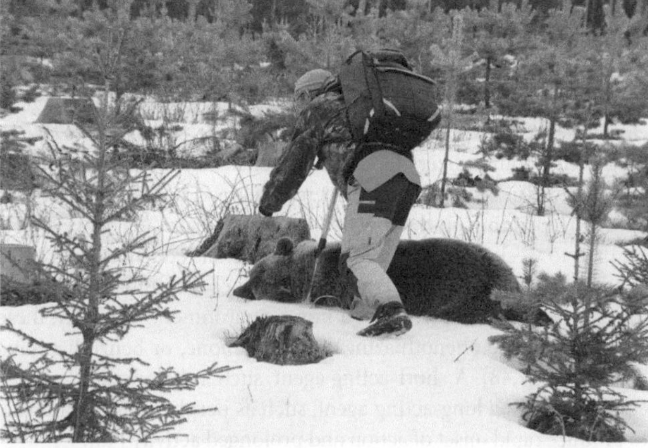

Figure 40.6 Cautious approach to a bear. It is important to extend your reach and have an escape route planned during initial approach to dangerous wildlife.

Induction

Many factors may influence induction time. These include the drug dose received, the animal's physical condition, its age and gender, and its sensitivity to the immobilizing drug. Dart placement is probably the most important determinant of induction time. To facilitate quick absorption of the drug, the muscle masses of the neck, shoulder, or hindquarter must be injected (Fig. 40.5). Animals that are excited or stressed can have induction times that are considerably longer than in calm animals.

Some animals will put on considerable fat deposits prior to denning and fasting and must be dealt with in a different manner during these periods of the year. Brown bears, for example, can generally be darted in the hindquarter when they emerge from spring dens. In the fall, these animals have considerable fat deposits overlying the rump and must be darted in the shoulder or neck. As soon as the dart is placed, the time should be recorded, and the animal must be carefully observed to ensure that it is not lost during the induction period.

The initial approach to a darted animal can be dangerous. The animal should be observed from a safe distance to determine that there is no purposeful movement. When α_2-adrenergic receptor agonist-based protocols are used (e.g., medetomidine-ketamine or xylazine-tiletamine-zolazepam), the animal's head or limbs should not move prior to approach. If tiletamine-zolazepam alone or narcotics are used, there may be some involuntary movement in adequately immobilized animals.

Once it has been determined that the animal is immobilized, it should be cautiously approached accompanied by a firearm backup if necessary. It is important to leave safe exits for the capture team and the animal. To gauge the animal's response, auditory stimulation such as clapping or shouting should be employed. If there is no response to auditory stimulation, the response to tactile stimulation should be gauged. It is advisable to use a stick or pole syringe to extend reach when stimulating the animal (Fig. 40.6). When it is safe, the palpebral reflex and airway can be checked. A set of vital signs, including rectal temperature, respiratory rate, and heart rate, should be monitored. The animal's eyes can be lubricated with an ophthalmic solution or gel, and a blindfold can be placed to decrease visual stimulation. At this point, hobbles may be considered to limit movement in the event of sudden recovery in ungulates.

Monitoring and supportive care

Following capture, the animal should be positioned to avoid pressure points and ensure optimum ventilation in a recumbent animal. Carnivores may be positioned in lateral or sternal recumbency, but ruminants should be positioned in sternal recumbency whenever possible. The head and neck should be extended to maintain a patent airway. A stretcher system may be employed to facilitate movement of the animal and to keep it elevated above the ground. Vital signs should be monitored every 5–10 min. Painful procedures such as tooth extraction or biopsies should be performed soon after induction when the animal is in the deepest plane of anesthesia. If animals are manipulated to determine body mass, it is best to do this during a deeper plane of immobilization-anesthesia because stimulus can hasten arousal [54].

Hypoxemia is common during wildlife immobilization and anesthesia [5–11,30,37,43]. Hypoxemia in the face of hyperthermia is particularly serious. Hyperthermia and increased metabolic rate increase tissue oxygen demand. This can increase the risk of inducing exertional myopathy or even cause acute mortality. Hypoxemia can often be prevented or treated in the field with the administration of supplemental oxygen. The animal should be monitored ideally with a pulse oximeter. Normal hemoglobin saturation should be 95–98%. A value below 85% is considered hypoxemic. If a pulse oximeter is not available, the mucous membranes should be monitored closely for cyanosis. Severely hypoxemic animals are often tachycardic. Tachycardia followed by severe bradycardia (heart rate <30 beats/min) is often a warning sign that hypoxemia is very severe. The occurrence of hypoxemia has been linked to prolongation of recovery times in ungulates [55,56].

Portable equipment is available to facilitate oxygen delivery. An ambulatory regulator and an aluminum D cylinder are lightweight, portable, and sturdy. They can provide a 10 L/min flow for up to 30 min. An E cylinder will provide this flow for 1 h or more. Portable oxygen concentrators have been used effectively as well. A nasal catheter can be used for insufflation in most animals. The catheter should be threaded as far as the medial canthus of the eye. The flow rate should be adjusted to maintain a saturation of greater than 95% (Fig. 40.7).

Heart rate and pulse quality should be monitored every 5–10 min. The auricular artery is easily palpated in many ungulate

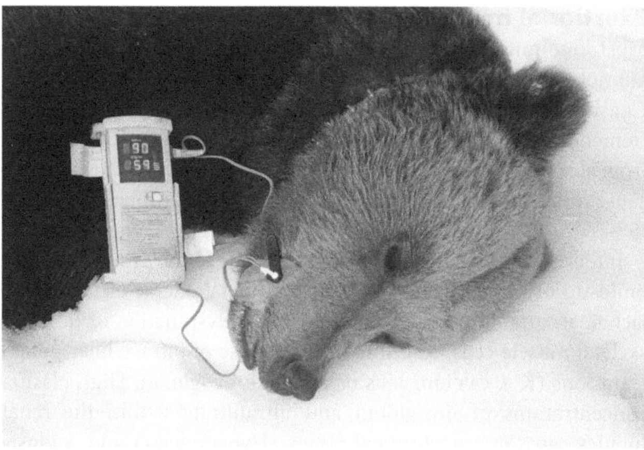

Figure 40.7 Pulse oximeter used to measure percent hemoglobin saturation in a brown bear.

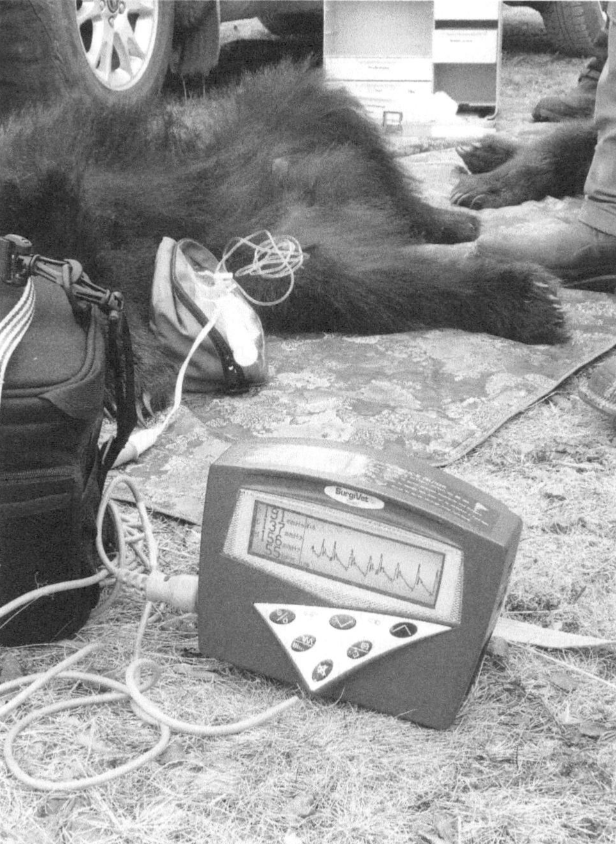

Figure 40.8 Direct blood pressure measurement in a brown bear. The arterial catheter has been placed in the femoral artery of the bear.

species but if it cannot be palpated, a femoral pulse can usually be used. Equipment is available to measure direct or indirect blood pressure and electrocardiographic status in the field (Fig. 40.8).

In ruminants, sternal recumbency will help to prevent ruminal tympany. If ruminal tympany is a problem, the animal may be rocked gently to stimulate eructation. A tube passed nasally or orally to the rumen can be used, but may predispose to regurgitation and aspiration. Generally, if ruminal tympany is severe, it is advisable to finish the procedure quickly and antagonize the anesthetic agents. If α_2-adrenergic receptor agonists have been used, the administration of tolazoline, yohimbine, or atipamezole will help to reinitiate ruminal activity and facilitate the correction of tympany.

Rectal temperature should be monitored every 5–10 min. Ungulates are particularly prone to hyperthermia, especially after a long chase. Planning immobilization during cooler periods of the day or at cooler times of the year should be considered. Rectal temperatures higher than 40°C are cause for concern, and attempts should be made to cool the animal. Cold water sprayed on the animal or snow packed into the inguinal and axillary regions may help lower body temperature. Rectal temperature higher than 41°C is an emergency and should be treated aggressively. It is difficult to cool large animals actively, and often the best option with severe hyperthermia is to antagonize the immobilizing agents and allow the animal to recover.

Loud noises increase the risk of sudden arousal, especially the vocalizations of distressed offspring. Other factors to consider are movement (i.e., changing the body position of a bear or location of the anesthetized animal) or degree of painful stimuli. Signs for assessing CNS depression will depend on the agent used. As drug effects lesson, spontaneous blinking will occur. Carnivores often develop chewing and paw movements. They will start to lift their head and may attempt to raise themselves with their forelimbs. Animals with significant head movement generally require a top-up dose of tiletamine-zolazepam or ketamine unless they are to be left to recover. Small additional doses of tiletamine-zolazepam can significantly prolong recovery and should be used only if longer than 30 min of additional immobilization is required. Ketamine is a better 'top-up' choice if only 5–20 min of additional time is needed.

With xylazine-ketamine or medetomidine-ketamine immobilization, head lifting or limb movement signals that the animal is minimally obtunded and should not be approached or manipulated. Increased intensity of the palpebral reflex or nystagmus are generally good indicators that CNS depression is lessening. When procedures are completed, the area should be cleared of equipment, and personnel should retreat to a safe area and observe the recovery.

Recovery

Considerations for recovery vary depending on the drugs used and the circumstances at hand. If a reversible drug combination was not used, the animal should be observed until it can ambulate. The animal should be placed in a comfortable position and its airway cleared. A final set of vital signs are obtained. Typically, two people remain with the animal to administer the reversal drug(s). Antagonists are typically administered intramuscularly unless there is an immediate physiologic need for rapid intravenous drug reversal.

Complications related to wildlife capture

Physical trauma

During immobilization and capture, physical injuries such as contusions, lacerations, abrasions, punctures, and fractures may occur. Minor injuries can be treated successfully in the field, but fractures and other serious conditions are difficult to treat effectively and often require that the animal be euthanized.

Minor lacerations may be cleaned, treated with a topical antibiotic ointment, and protected with an insect repellant. An appropriate antibiotic may be given intramuscularly to help prevent infection. Closure may be considered for large lacerations, which should be cleaned and debrided as much as possible. These lacerations are often contaminated and, if they are closed, appropriate drainage and administration of long-acting antibiotics must be considered.

The potential for physical trauma may be reduced by taking careful notice of any hazard in the environment that may increase the likelihood of injury during capture. Traps, snares, nets, or other forms of manual restraint should be appropriate for the species and set by trained individuals.

Hyperthermia

The most immediate sign is a critical rise in body temperature to above 40–41°C (depending on the species). Other symptoms include rapid shallow breathing, panting, and weak, rapid, or irregular heart rate. Treatment includes moving the animal into shade or spraying it with cold water. Packing ice or snow around the animal in the winter and/or cold water enemas may also be indicated.

The risk of hyperthermia may be reduced by avoiding warm days, limiting activities to the coolest part of the day, avoiding prolonged pursuits, and minimizing physical restraint (Fig. 40.9).

Hypothermia

Hypothermia is of most concern when ambient temperatures are low. It occurs most commonly in young animals, animals with small body mass, and those in poor body condition. Hypothermia is generally characterized by body temperature below 35°C. It may result in prolonged recovery, acidosis, coagulopathies, and arrhythmias. Supportive procedures consist of drying and covering the animal, and providing external heat sources such as hot water bottles.

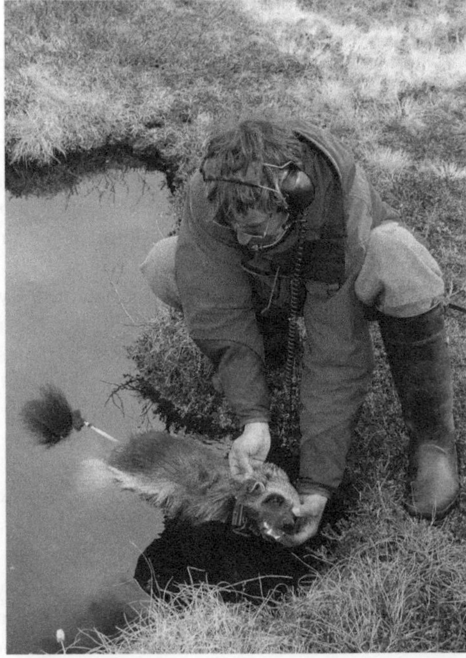

Figure 40.9 Active cooling of a hyperthermic wolverine. In a field situation, immersion in cold water can be a good option to treat severe hyperthermia in smaller wildlife species.

Exertional myopathy

Most free-ranging animals exert themselves infrequently. They are not conditioned for running at full effort over long distances. Chasing wild animals with a helicopter or motor vehicle imposes a tremendous amount of stress. The effects of sympathetic exhaustion from sustained stress combined with intense muscular exertion can cause a life-threatening syndrome known as exertional myopathy [57–59].

Intense sustained muscular exertion leads to the production and build-up of lactate in muscle cells and metabolic acidosis. Severe lactate accumulation may cause metabolic dysfunction or death of skeletal muscle cells, resulting in the release of intracellular potassium ions (K^+), calcium ions (Ca^{2+}), and myoglobin. High plasma concentrations of myoglobin and ultrafiltrate within the renal tubules can cause acute renal failure. Hyperkalemia and acidosis cause acute arrhythmias and circulatory failure.

Exertional myopathy is difficult to treat, so prevention is of the utmost importance. Chase time should be limited to 2 min and capture efforts not be resumed for at least 1 day, if failed. In situations where several individuals from the same herd require capture (often the situation with net gunning), it is advisable to have enough handlers to capture multiple individuals at the same time rather than repeatedly stressing the herd. Visual and auditory stimulation, handling, and restraint of the captured animal should be kept to a minimum. Four common clinical syndromes of exertional myopathy have been identified: acute death syndrome, delayed peracute death syndrome, ataxic-myoglobinuric syndrome, and muscle rupture syndrome.

Respiratory depression and hypoxemia

Major causative factors include immobilizing agents (particularly potent opioids), ventilation-perfusion mismatching, and airway obstruction.

The best technique for preventing hypoventilation is endotracheal intubation and controlled ventilation with supplemental inspired oxygen. This can be difficult in field situations, however, particularly with larger animals. The partial reversal of narcotics has been used to treat respiratory depression when intubation was impractical [5].

Hypoventilation and/or ventilation-perfusion mismatch generally respond to supplemental inspired oxygen delivery [7,10], although arterial CO_2 partial pressure and respiratory acidemia often remain [30]. The simplest way to reduce the incidence of hypoxemia is supplemental inspired oxygen via a nasal cannula [7]. The animal should be monitored with a pulse oximeter and oxygen flow adjusted to maintain hemoglobin saturation (SpO_2) greater than 95%. Other causes of acute respiratory compromise include aspiration and pneumothorax (secondary to dart penetration of the thoracic cavity). Pneumothorax requires thoracocentesis, so equipment to perform this procedure should be available if at all possible.

Capture-associated mortality

There is no doubt that the chemical immobilization of free-ranging mammals is a minimal form of veterinary anesthesia conducted under the most extreme circumstances. Anesthetic risk is influenced by the capture protocols chosen to meet the challenges unique to each species and its environment. Typically, most deaths are observed in the early phase of a large capture project before immobilization methods have been refined, drug doses have been adjusted, and team members are experienced.

Moreover, an increased risk of mortality accompanies health evaluation of animals under environmental or pathogenic stress. Overall, capture mortality of free-ranging mammals can be grouped into three categories:

- direct effects of the immobilizing drug itself (e.g., respiratory depression, shock, hyperthermia, and asphyxia caused by tympany or vomiting)
- indirect effects (e.g., drowning, pneumothorax due to misplacement of darts, and trauma from dart impact) or indirect consequences of the drug used (e.g., etorphine often induces hyperthermia, which may cause the animal to seek water for cooling, with drowning as a possible sequela)
- secondary effects caused by the capture process itself (e.g., trauma from traps, long-term effects from chasing or stress, separation of family groups, and various problems with radio collars or implantable transmitters). Secondary effects have nothing to do with the anesthetic risk *per se* and should be treated as a separate entity.

In his review of stress and capture myopathy in artiodactylids, Spraker [58] stated that a mortality rate greater than 2% during trapping is unacceptable. This should be the rule of thumb when a large number (n >100) of free-ranging animals are being anesthetized or captured (e.g., a mortality rate greater than 2% during chemical immobilization requires that the anesthetic protocol be re-evaluated). By using immobilizing drugs and doses with proven safety, proper remote drug delivery systems, and established capture methods and techniques, an experienced capture team decreases the risk of mortality.

Protocols and dosages

Readers are referred to the *Handbook of Wildlife Chemical Immobilization* and *Zoo Animal and Wildlife Anesthesia and Immobilization* for complete dosing information and a reference list by species [1,2]. It should be appreciated that, generally speaking, dosages required for immobilization of free-ranging animals are generally higher than those required in captive individuals [1,60]. This factor must be kept in mind when dosages are planned for wildlife capture, or a relative underdose may occur. Obviously, injection site and method of drug delivery also affect dose requirements. Comparison of hand injection versus dart delivery demonstrated that 50% more drug was required when animals were darted [61].

References

1 Kreeger TJ, Arnemo JM. *Handbook of Wildlife Chemical Immobilization*, 4th edn. Sybille, WY: published by author, 2012.
2 West G, Heard D, Caulkett NA, eds. *Zoo Animal and Wildlife Anesthesia and Immobilization*, 2nd edn. Ames, IA: Wiley-Blackwell, 2013.
3 Klein LV, Klide AM. Central α_2 adrenergic and benzodiazepine agonists and their antagonists. *J Zoo Wildl Med* 1989; **20**: 138–153.
4 Cattet MRL, Caulkett NA, Stenhouse GB. Anesthesia of grizzly bears using xylazine-zolazepam-tiletamine or zolazepam-tiletamine. *Ursus* 2003; **14:** 88–93.
5 Moresco AM, Larsen RS, Sleeman JM, *et al.* Use of naloxone to reverse carfentanil citrate-induced hypoxemia and cardiopulmonary depression in Rocky Mountain wapiti (Cervus elaphus nelsoni). *Zoo Wildl Med* 2001; **32**: 81–89.
6 Citino SB, Bush M, Grobler D, Lance W. Anaesthesia of roan antelope (Hippotragus equinus) with a combination of A3080, medetomidine and ketamine. *J S Afr Vet Assoc* 2001; **72**: 29–32.
7 Read MR, Caulkett NA, Symington A, Shury TK. Treatment of hypoxemia during xylazine-tiletamine-zolazepam immobilization of wapiti. *Can Vet J* 2001; **42**: 661–664.
8 Caulkett NA, Cattet MRL, Cantwell S, *et al.* Anesthesia of wood bison with medetomidine-Telazol and xylazine-Telazol combinations. *Can Vet J* 2000; **41**: 49–53.
9 Caulkett NA, Cribb PH, Haigh JC. Comparative cardiopulmonary effects of carfentanil-xylazine and medetomidine-ketamine in mule deer and mule deer/white-tailed deer hybrids. *Can J Vet Res* 2000; **64**: 64–68.
10 Read MR. A review of alpha-2 adrenoceptor agonists and the development of hypoxemia in domestic and wild ruminants. *J Zoo Wildl Med* 2003; **34**: 134–138.
11 Heard DJ, Olsen JH, Stover JS. Cardiopulmonary changes associated with chemical immobilization and recumbency in white rhinoceros (Ceratotherium simum). *J Zoo Wildl Med* 1992; **23**: 197–200.
12 Fahlman Å, Caulkett N, Arnemo JM, *et al.* Efficacy of a portable oxygen concentrator with pulsed delivery for treatment of hypoxemia during anesthesia of wildlife. *J Zoo Wildl Med* 2012; **43**: 67-76.
13 Kock MD, Jessup A, Clark RK, Franti CE. Effects of capture on biological parameters in free-ranging bighorn sheep (Ovis canadensis): evaluation of drop-net, drive-net, chemical immobilization and the net gun. *J Wildl Dis* 1987; **23**: 641–651.
14 Kock MD, Jessup A, Clark RK, *et al.* Capture methods in five subspecies of free-ranging bighorn sheep: an evaluation of drop-net, drive-net, chemical immobilization, and the net gun. *J Wildl Dis* 1987; **23**: 634–640.
15 Cattet MRL, Caulkett NA, Wilson C, *et al.* Intranasal administration of xylazine to reduce stress in elk captured by net gun. *J Wildl Dis* 2004; **40**: 562–565.
16 Jessup DA, Clark RK, Weaver RA, Kock MD. The safety and cost-effectiveness of net-gun capture of desert bighorn sheep (Ovis canadensis nelsoni). *J Zoo Anim Med* 1988; **19**: 208–213.
17 Cattet MRL, Christison K, Caulkett NA, Stenhouse GB. Physiologic responses of grizzly bears to different methods of capture. *J Wildl Dis* 2003; **39**: 649–654.
18 Smith T, Herrero S, Debruyn T, Wilder J. Efficacy of bear deterrent spray in Alaska. *J Wildl Man* 2008; **72**: 640–645.
19 Haymerle A, Fahlman Å, Walzer C. Human exposures to immobilizing agents: results of an online survey. *Vet Rec* 2010; **167**: 327-332.
20 Belleville JP, Ward DS, Bloor BC, Maze M. Effects of intravenous dexmedetomidine in humans. I. Sedation, ventilation, and metabolic rate. *Anesthesiology* 1992; **77**: 1125–1133.
21 Kallio A, Ponkilainen R, Scheinin H. Effects of dexmedetomidine, a selective alpha-2 adrenoceptor agonist on hemodynamic control mechanisms. *Clin Pharmacol Ther* 1989; **46**: 33–42.
22 Kock MD, Burroughs R, eds. *Chemical and Physical Restraint of Wild Animals. A Training and Field Manual for African Species.* 2nd edn. Greyton, South Africa: International Wildlife Veterinary Services, 2012.
23 Bush M. Remote drug delivery systems. *J Zoo Wildl Med* 1992; **23**: 159–180.
24 Haigh JC. Opioids in zoological medicine. *J Zoo Wildl Med* 1990; **21**: 391–413.
25 Kreeger TJ. Xylazine-induced aspiration pneumonia in Shira's moose. *Wildl Soc Bull* 2000; **28**: 751–753.
26 Allen JL. Renarcotization following carfentanil immobilization of nondomestic ungulates. *J Zoo Wildl Med* 1989; **20**: 423–426.
27 Kock MD, Berger J. Chemical immobilization of free-ranging North American bison in Badlands National Park, South Dakota. *J Wildl Dis* 1987; **23**: 625–633.
28 Haigh JC, Lee LJ, Schweinsburg RE. Immobilization of polar bears with carfentanil. *J Wildl Dis* 1983; **19**: 140–144.
29 Kreeger TJ, Bjornlie D, Thompson D, *et al.* Immobilization of Wyoming bears using carfentanil and xylazine. *J Wildl Dis* 2013; **49**: 674–678.
30 Schumacher J, Citino SB, Dawson R. Effects of a carfentanil-xylazine combination on cardiopulmonary function and plasma catecholamine concentrations in female bongo antelopes. *Am J Vet Res* 1997; **58**: 157–161.
31 Lance BR, Kenny DE. Thiafentanil oxalate (A3080) in domestic ungulate species. In: Miller RE, Fowler ME, eds. *Fowler's Zoo and Wild Animal Medicine*, vol. **7**. St Louis, MO: Elsevier, 2012; 589–595.
32 Grobler D, Bush M, Jessup D, Lance W. Anaesthesia of gemsbok (Oryx gazelle) with a combination of A3080, medetomidine and ketamine. *J S Afr Vet Assoc* 2001; **72**: 81–83.
33 Miller BF, Osborn DA, Lance WR, *et al.* Butorphanol-azaperone-medetomidine for immobilization of captive white-tailed deer. *J Wildl Dis* 2009; **45**: 457–467.
34 Miller M, Buss P, Joubert J, *et al.* Use of butorphanol during immobilization of free-ranging white rhinocerous (Ceratotherium simum) *J Zoo Wildl Med* 2013; **44**: 55–61.
35 Jalanka HH, Roeken BO. The use of medetomidine, medetomidine-ketamine combinations, and atipamezole in nondomestic mammals: a review. *J Zoo Wildl Med* 1990; **21**: 259–282.
36 Cattet MRL, Caulkett NA, Polischuk SC, Ramsay MA. Anesthesia of polar bears with zolazepam-tiletamine, medetomidine-ketamine, and medetomidine-zolazepam-tiletamine. *J Zoo Wildl Med* 1999; **30**: 354–360.
37 Caulkett NA, Cattet MRL, Caulkett JM, Polischuk SC. Comparative physiological effects of Telazol, medetomidine-ketamine, and medetomidine-Telazol in polar bears (Ursus maritimus). *J Zoo Wildl Med* 1999; **30**: 504–509.
38 Cattet MRL, Caulkett NA, Lunn NJ. Anesthesia of polar bears using xylazine-zolazepam-tiletamine or zolazepam-tiletamine. *J Wildl Dis* 2003; **39**: 655–664.
39 Cattet MRL, Caulkett NA, Stenhouse GB. Anesthesia of grizzly bears using xylazine-zolazepam-tiletamine or zolazepam-tiletamine. *Ursus* 2003; **14**: 88–93.
40 Schobert E. Telazol use in wild and exotic animals. *Vet Med* 1987; **82**: 1080–1088.

41 Murray SSL, Monfort SL, Ware L, *et al.* Anesthesia in female white-tailed deer using Telazol and xylazine. *J Wildl Dis* 2000; **36**: 670–675.

42 Millspaugh JJ, Brundige GC, Jenks JA, *et al.* Immobilization of rocky mountain elk with Telazol and xylazine hydrochloride, and antagonism by yohimbine hydrochloride. *J Wildl Dis* 1995; **31**: 259–262.

43 Caulkett NA, Cattet MRL. Physiological effects of medetomidine-zolazepam-tiletamine immobilization in black bears (Ursus americanus). *J Wildl Dis* 1997; **33**: 618–622.

44 Kock MD, Morkel P, Atkinson M, Foggin C. Chemical immobilization of free-ranging white rhinoceros (Ceratotherium simum simum) in Hwange and Matobo National Parks, Zimbabwe, using combinations of etorphine (M99), fentanyl, xylazine and detomidine. *J Zoo Wildl Med* 1995; **26**: 207–219.

45 Klein L, Citino SB. Comparison of detomidine/carfentanil/ketamine and medetomidine/ketamine anesthesia in Grevy's zebra. In: *Proceedings of the Joint Conference of the American Association of Zoo Veterinarians, Wildlife Disease Association, and American Association of Wildlife Veterinarians*, East Lansing, Michigan, 1995; 290–293.

46 Caulkett NA, Duke T, Cribb PH. Cardiopulmonary effects of medetomidine-ketamine in domestic sheep (Ovis ovis) maintained in sternal recumbency. *J Zoo Wildl Med* 1996; **27**: 217–226.

47 Bush M, Citino SB, Lance WR. The use of butorphanol in anesthesia protocols for zoo and wild mammals. In: Miller RE, Fowler ME, eds. *Fowler's Zoo and Wild Animal Medicine*, vol. 7. St Louis, MO: Elsevier, 2012; 596–603.

48 Ebedes H. The use of long-acting tranquilizers in captive wild animals. In: McKenzie A, ed. *The Capture and Care Manual: Capture, Care, Accommodation and Transportation of Wild African Animals.* Pretoria, South Africa: Wildlife Decision Services and the South African Veterinary Foundation, 1993; 71–99.

49 Diverio S, Goddard PJ, Gordon IJ, Elston DA. The effect of management practices on stress in farmed red deer (Cervus elaphus) and its modulation by long-acting neuroleptics: behavioural responses. *Appl Anim Behav Sci* 1993; **36**: 363–376.

50 Atkinson MW, Blumer ES. The use of a long-acting neuroleptic in the Mongolian wild horse (Equus przewalskii przewalskii) to facilitate the establishment of a bachelor herd. In: *Proceedings of the Annual Meeting of the American Association of Zoo Veterinarians*, Houston, Texas, 1997; 199–200.

51 Shury TK. Use of azaperone with zuclopenthixol acetate for tranquilization of free ranging wood bison and immobilization with carfentanil and xylazine. In: *Proceedings of the Annual Meeting of the American Association of Zoo Veterinarians*, Omaha, Nebraska, 1998; 408–409.

52 Clippinger TL, Citino SB, Wade S. Behavioral and physiologic response to an intermediate-acting tranquilizer, zuclopenthixol, in captive Nile lechwe (Kobus megaceros). In: *Proceedings of the Annual Meeting of the American Association of Zoo Veterinarians*, Omaha, Nebraska, 1998; **38–40**.

53 Read M, Caulkett N, McCallister M. Evaluation of zuclopenthixol acetate to decrease handling stress in wapiti. *J Wildl Dis* 2000; **36**: 450–459.

54 Cattet MRL, Caulkett NA, Streib KA, *et al.* Cardiopulmonary response of anesthetized polar bears to suspension by net and sling. *J Wildl Dis* 1999; **35**: 548–556.

55 Risling TE, Fahlman Å, Caulkett NA, Kutz S. Physiological and behavioral effects of hypoxemia in reindeer immobilized with xylazine-etorphine. *Anim Prod Science* 2011; **51**: 1-4.

56 Paterson JM, Caulkett NA, Woodbury MR. Physiologic effects of nasal oxygen or medical air administered prior to and during carfentanil-xylazine anesthesia in North American elk (Cervus canadensis manitobensis). *J Zoo Wildl Med* 2009; **40**: 39–50.

57 Harthoorn AM. Physical aspects of both mechanical and chemical capture. In: Nielsen L, Haigh JC, Fowler ME, eds. *Chemical Immobilization of North American Wildlife.* Milwaukee, WI: Wisconsin Humane Society, 1982; 63–71.

58 Spraker TR. Stress and capture myopathy in artiodactylids. In: Fowler ME, ed. *Zoo and Wild Animal Medicine: Current Therapy 3.* Philadelphia: WB Saunders, 1993; 481–488.

59 Williams ES, Thorne T, Exertional myopathy. In: Fairbrother A, Locke LL, Hoff GL, eds. *Noninfectious Diseases of Wildlife*, 2nd edn. London: Manson, 1996; 181–193.

60 Heard DJ. Chemical immobilization of felids, ursids, and small ungulates. *Vet Clin North Am Exot Anim Pract* 2001; **4**: 267–298.

61 Ryeng KA, Arnemo JM, Larsen S. Determination of optimal immobilizing doses of a medetomidine hydrochloride and ketamine hydrochloride combination in captive reindeer. *Am J Vet Res* 2001; **62**: 119–126.

41 Comparative Anesthesia and Analgesia of Aquatic Mammals

David B. Brunson
Zoetis, LLC, Florham Park, New Jersey, USA

Chapter contents

General considerations

Marine mammals, which are air-breathing animals that have evolved for a primarily aquatic environment, include seals, sea lions, walruses, whales, cetaceans, polar bears, sea otters, and manatees. These animals have highly adapted physiology that presents unique anesthetic challenges.

Drug delivery is difficult for several reasons. Animals that live in a cold aquatic environment have heavy fur coats, thick blubber, or fat layers for insulation. Remote drug delivery requires special considerations for the site, depth, and method of drug injection. Intravenous (IV) access is usually very limited even on immobilized or anesthetized animals.

The pulmonary systems are highly developed to facilitate rapid oxygen and carbon dioxide exchange, as well as breath holding. Marine mammals frequently have short upper airways with extensive cartilaginous support down to the small bronchioles. They also take large breaths (tidal volumes), which aids in rapid gas exchange.

Seals breathe episodically in sleep. Higher centers in the brain modulate the central rhythm generator both positively and negatively for breathing. During episodic breathing, these modulating influences alternate in a fashion that produces periods of apnea alternating with periods of relatively high-frequency ventilation [1]. If seals are awoken during high-frequency ventilation, their breathing immediately slows.

Marine mammals have a highly developed dive reflex. This is a complicated physiologic adaptation that is characterized by breath holding (apnea), decreased heart rate, and shunting of blood to critical aerobic organs. During a dive, peripheral tissues either reduce metabolic functions or function by hypoxic or anaerobic pathways. The implication for anesthesia is that absorption may be unpredictable or slower if central nervous system (CNS) depressants are administered intramuscularly during breath holding or during activation of the dive reflex. Once breathing is initiated, blood flows to the periphery. Darting or drug administration should be timed to occur during active ventilation and avoided during apnea.

Much is still unknown regarding specific marine mammal species and their physiologic adaptations. Most immobilization and anesthetic information is obtained through observations during field capture or during medical management of captive animals. Thus, much of what we know is anecdotal and observational rather than from blinded, well-controlled studies of the drugs and animal physiology. As a result, when an anesthetic technique works well, it is adopted and used repeatedly. On the other hand, when even a single immobilization or anesthetic management is associated with either ineffective or adverse effects, the drugs are frequently abandoned. This chapter attempts to provide guidance to readers on what has been used successfully and cautions where information is still limited. For each species and situation, chemical capture, restraint, and anesthetic procedures should be carefully researched, planned, and executed. Networking with individuals experienced with the species and working conditions will increase the chances of a successful outcome. Generally, marine mammals should not be darted with an anesthetic while remaining in their aquatic environment, because they can dive out of sight and drown.

Cetaceans

Porpoises and whales breathe through a modified nasal orifice, called the blowhole, located on the dorsum of the head just anterior to the cranial vault. It appears on the surface as a single, transversely crescentic opening with a forward-facing concavity. It is closed by a muscular nasal plug and opens through the action of forehead

Veterinary Anesthesia and Analgesia: The Fifth Edition of Lumb and Jones.
Edited by Kurt A. Grimm, Leigh A. Lamont, William J. Tranquilli, Stephen A. Greene and Sheilah A. Robertson.

muscles. Normally under water it remains closed. In porpoises, ventral to the blowhole are vestibular and tubular air sacs connected to the paired nares, which begin a few centimeters down the respiratory passage. A septum divides the nares for 10–12 cm, after which the respiratory passage becomes single again just above the glottis. The larynx forms an arytenoepiglottal tube giving a direct opening from the internal nares to the lungs, thus enabling the animal to breathe only through the blowhole (Fig. 41.1). Approximately 10 cm from the base of the larynx, the trachea branches into a separate right bronchus which, at about 15 cm, bifurcates into two main bronchi. It is important, when a porpoise is intubated, that the endotracheal tube not extend into the bronchus. To ensure proper placement, the tube should be measured and marked prior to placement.

Porpoises can take one full respiration in 0.3 s. With a tidal volume of 5–10 L, the flow rates through the air passages range from 30 to 70 L/s during expiration and inspiration. Porpoises breathe two or three times each minute. Each breath is deep (approximately 80% tidal air). After inspiration, the animal holds an apneustic plateau for 20–30 s, followed by rapid exhalation and inspiration.

Preanesthetic treatment with anticholinergics is recommended. Bradycardia, which is frequently observed during anesthesia, may be produced by strong parasympathetic stimulation or the effects of sedatives or analgesics. An IV or intramuscular (IM) dosage of atropine at 0.02 mg/kg is recommended.

Sedation and analgesia have been studied in porpoises to identify drugs that produce minimal respiratory depression. Sedation with diazepam has produced variable results. As in many mammalian species, benzodiazepines appear to have mild sedative effects, with minimal respiratory or cardiovascular depression. The primary use of these drugs should be for their antianxiety and synergistic effects with other CNS depressants, such as opioids. Diazepam or midazolam at 0.05–0.1 mg/kg IV has been used safely in cetaceans [2].

The relatively short-acting opioid meperidine provides moderate restraint in cetaceans, without obvious deleterious effects. Three dosages of meperidine have been studied in several species of cetaceans and pinnipeds. The IM dosages evaluated were 0.11, 0.23, or 0.45 mg/kg administered by hand syringe [3]. Restraint was achieved rapidly, with maximum effect occurring 20 min after IM injection and lasting for 2–3 h. Analgesia appeared to last as long as 4 h and was sometimes accompanied by restoration of appetite in animals suffering physical discomfort. The higher doses increased sedation and analgesia without noticeably depressing respiration. Based on the results of this study, the recommended initial dose of meperidine is 0.2 mg/kg IM when sedating cetaceans. If deemed necessary, higher dosages can be used safely, however.

Porpoises can be intubated while awake but intubation is more easily accomplished after sedation or induction of unconsciousness. Porpoises have relatively large airways. A 24–30 mm equine endotracheal tube with an inflatable cuff can be used. The mouth is held open with towels by assistants. The hand is inserted into the pharynx and grasps and pulls the larynx anteroventrally from the normal intranarial position. The endotracheal tube is then guided into the trachea by inserting two fingers into the glottis and passing the tube along the palm of the hand. A method of introducing the endotracheal tube through the blowhole has been described for use in smaller cetaceans, like *Delphinus delphis* and *Stenella styx* [4]. For induction without thiopental, 3.5% isoflurane or halothane is administered for 5–15 min via a mask or endotracheal tube, after which 1.0–1.25% is used to maintain surgical anesthesia. If thiopental is used to induce anesthesia before intubation, 1.5–2.0% isoflurane or halothane is sufficient for maintenance. Sevoflurane should be an excellent inhalant anesthetic for cetaceans. Because of its lower blood-gas solubility, it equilibrates faster than isoflurane, thus hastening induction and recovery. The lower potency of sevoflurane requires higher vaporizer settings for induction and maintenance. Expected settings would be 4.5–5.0% for mask induction and 2.25–2.75% for maintenance.

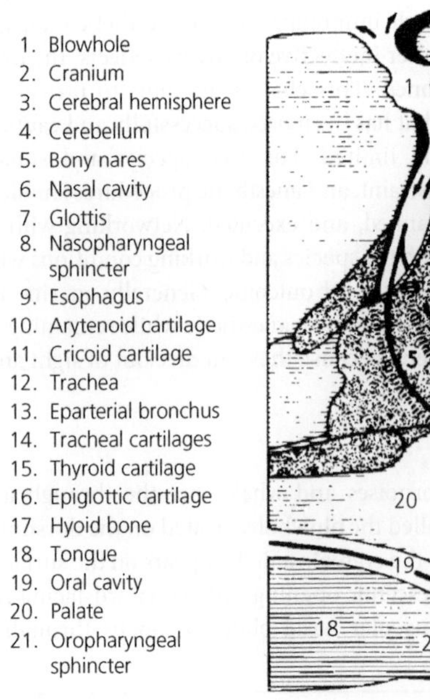

Figure 41.1 Sagittal view of the head and neck of the bottlenose dolphin. Source: Nagel *et al.* [41]. Reprinted with permission from AAAS.

Induction can be achieved by the IV administration of thiopental at 10 mg/kg or propofol at 4–6 mg/kg via one of the tail-fluke veins. These dosage recommendations are for unsedated animals. Lower dosages should be used if an animal is already sedated or debilitated. Injection of thiopental alone (10 mg/kg IV) produces 10–15 min of light anesthesia followed by 45 min of respiratory depression, during which the animal may require artificial ventilation. A dose of 15–25 mg/kg IV produces surgical anesthesia for 10–25 min, with respiratory depression lasting 1–2.5 h. Sensitivity to barbiturates has been further demonstrated following high doses of intraperitoneal pentobarbital (10–30 mg/kg), which has reportedly caused respiratory failure and death [5]. Consequently, this technique is no longer recommended. Likewise, because plasma cholinesterase levels may be extremely low or absent in bottlenose dolphins (*Tursiops truncatus*), the use of succinylcholine to induce muscular paralysis is not recommended.

The heart rate during general anesthesia is typically 100–120 beats per minute (bpm). During delivery of 100% oxygen, arterial pH averages 7.35, partial pressure of oxygen (PaO_2) is maintained at 100–200 mmHg, and partial pressure of carbon dioxide ($PaCO_2$) is 35–50 mmHg. In conscious cetaceans breathing ambient air, arterial PaO_2 reportedly ranges from 65 to 98 mmHg, and $PaCO_2$ ranges from 40 to 60 mmHg.

Cessation of tail-fluke movements indicates surgical anesthesia and occurs after loss of strong corneal and eyelid reflexes. The swimming reflex is considered the best criterion for assessing the depth of anesthesia. Reflexes typically observed when assessing depth of anesthesia in porpoises include (1) the palpebral reflex, (2) corneal reflex, (3) swallowing in response to tactile stimulation of the pharynx, (4) retraction of the tongue, (5) reflex movements of the body when the anus is distended, (6) tail movements, (7) movements of the pectoral flippers in response to surface stimulation, (8) movement of the blowhole after stimulation of the nares or vestibular sacs, and (9) vaginal or penile movements when the area is manipulated.

During the recovery period, the endotracheal tube is kept in position until the blowhole reflex returns. This usually requires 15–45 min after cessation of inhalant administration. Timing the removal of the endotracheal tube is critical. Extubation should occur only after the animal is capable of breathing on its own, as manifested by movements of the blowhole and thorax, and by struggling, coughing, and/or bucking. When the endotracheal tube is removed, the larynx must be placed in its normal intranarial position. If the animal does not exhale through the blowhole within 3 min or if the heart rate falls below 60 bpm, the endotracheal tube must be reinserted and the animal ventilated for a few more minutes. In water, porpoises are near neutral in buoyancy. Out of water, it is more difficult for them to breathe and maintain circulation. For this reason, animals should be returned to water as soon as possible following recovery from anesthesia.

Local anesthesia can be used to provide analgesia for minor painful procedures. Using structural landmarks, a method has been devised for anesthetizing the lower jaw of the bottlenose dolphin [6]. With this procedure, its teeth can be extracted and age determined by counting dentine layers in sections of etched teeth. The toxic doses of various local anesthetics have not been determined in cetaceans, so one should use the smallest dose necessary to desensitize tissues or structures prior to surgery or invasive diagnostic procedure.

Toothed and baleen whales

Chemical immobilization and anesthesia have been attempted in large cetaceans. Killer whales have been sedated with meperidine and midazolam for minor procedures coupled with local anesthesia. Sedation has been attempted in removing an embedded rope in a free-ranging North Atlantic right whale. The adult male was estimated to be 50 feet long and weigh 40 000 kg. Each attempt at sedation was separated by at least 2 weeks. The dosage was increased on each attempt, with the final attempt producing mild sedation. Based on killer whale experiences and initial ineffective attempts with lower dosages, the most effective dose of midazolam was determined to be 0.025 mg/kg IM. The meperidine dose was set at 0.17 mg/kg IM. Four doses were administered to the whale over 2 h 43 min for a total dose of 40 g of meperidine and 4 g of midazolam. Although the whale never stopped swimming, its respiratory frequency decreased and diving behavior ceased [7].

Pinnipedia

Pinniped species are made up of the otarids (eared seals), phocids (true seals), and odobenids (walruses). The physical characteristics vary widely among these groups. Size is especially variable, and body weight should be estimated carefully based on species, age, and gender. Perianesthetic mortality of California sea lions has been reported for free-ranging animals that underwent anesthesia following stranding [8]. Fatality rate during anesthesia was reported at 3.4% and it increased to 4.3% if deaths during the following 72 h were included. Euthanasia was not included in these numbers, suggesting that anesthetic mortality can be quite high, especially when the health status of the animal is poor.

As a group, these animals have highly efficient respiratory systems. The alveolar exchange in seals has been measured at approximately 46% as compared with terrestrial mammals, where the alveolar exchange is usually in the range of 12–16%. In species that can be physically restrained or sedated with benzodiazepine tranquilizers (diazepam or midazolam, 0.1 mg/kg IM), induction with gas anesthetics is recommended [9]. Mask inductions with isoflurane or sevoflurane can be very fast, occurring in as little as three to four breaths because of high alveolar exchange and the low solubility of these anesthetic gases. Respiratory monitoring used in domestic species such as end-tidal CO_2 have been demonstrated to be useful in pinnipeds [10].

Injectable anesthetic drug elimination during anesthesia may be more variable compared to other mammals. These changes may be due to physiologic changes related to adaptations to diving which can be invoked during daily life. There is evidence that the clearance of iohexol, a radiographic contrast agent used to measure glomerular filtration rate and renal blood flow in domestic species such as dogs and cats, is non-linear in healthy California sea lions. The non-linearity may be related to changes in renal blood flow which are more dynamic than in other species [11]. This may alter the pharmacokinetics of drugs which undergo significant renal excretion.

During anesthesia of pinnipeds, their temperature should be continuously monitored via esophageal or rectal probe. Hyperthermia or hypothermia can occur during physical restraint, sedation, anesthesia, and handling outside the normal aquatic environment. It is important to be prepared to support body temperature by either warming or cooling the animal, as necessary. Assessment of ventilation requires the use of both carbon dioxide monitoring and pulse oximetry. A Doppler flow detector can also be an important tool in assessing peripheral perfusion.

Odobenidae (walruses)

Walruses are very challenging to anesthetize. Adult males weigh up to 3000 pounds (1360 kg). High mortality rates have been reported with the use of opioids and dissociative anesthetics but are most likely the result of severe respiratory and circulatory compromise when the animals are out of the water and under anesthesia. Respiratory arrest has been commonly reported during immobilization with potent opioids. Even with ventilatory support, these large animals may develop circulatory failure during anesthesia.

Captive walruses have been immobilized with a combination of midazolam (0.1 mg/kg) and meperidine (2.2 mg/kg). To prevent vagal induced bradycardia, the use of atropine (0.04 mg/kg) is also recommended. The recommended injection sites for IM injections are the hip and epaxial muscles. A long needle (3–4 inches) must be used to ensure effective IM drug absorption.

Intravenous access is difficult, but vascular access can be obtained via the epidural venous sinus. Needle placement is identical to placement of epidural needles or catheters via the lumbosacral space. With the walrus in sternal recumbency, the wings of the ileums can be palpated. The needle should be perpendicular to the skin. For large walruses, a 6 inch-long spinal needle is required. Easy aspiration of blood with a syringe indicates proper depth and placement. Epidural IV access can be used for administration of fluid, emergency drugs, and anesthetics. Small boluses of propofol (40–60 mg) can be used to relax muscles and facilitate endotracheal intubation. During inhalant anesthesia, emergency drugs can be administered via the endotracheal tube when IV access is not available.

During the onset of immobilization and anesthesia, heart rate is usually between 80 and 100 bpm. As anesthesia deepens, heart rate slows to around 60 bpm. Apnea is common during anesthesia and immobilization. Ventilatory support is essential when working with walruses.

Intubation is easiest with the walrus in sternal recumbency with head extended. Despite their large size, walruses have small oral cavities. Digital palpation of the larynx and direct placement of the endotracheal tube is possible once the animal is relaxed and the mouth pulled open by an assistant.

Isoflurane can be used to maintain general anesthesia in walruses. Oxygen flow rates and vaporizer settings are similar to those recommended for equine anesthesia. The oxygen flow rate should be at least 4 L/min to ensure adequate delivery of anesthetic and oxygen.

When used alone, meperidine has been administered by IM injection at dosages ranging from 0.23 to 0.45 mg/kg. In this dose range, sedation/restraint is usually moderate, without apparent detrimental effects [3].

Otariidae (sea lions and fur seals)

Attempts to sedate seals and sea lions have met with variable success. As is the case for most wildlife, sedatives alone should not be relied on for immobilization. Additionally, species response may vary with the use of phenothiazine and benzodiazepine tranquilizers [12]. Nevertheless, the use of tranquilizers is beneficial in the overall management of Otariidae because tranquilizers decrease the overall anesthetic dose requirement and adverse side-effects when combined with dissociatives or opioids.

Ringed seals and sea lions have been immobilized with ketamine alone (4.5–11.0 mg/kg IM) [13]. However, because of the concern for excessive salivation, animals with respiratory problems should not be given high doses of ketamine alone. Atropine (total dose 0.3–0.6 mg) can be given concurrently to prevent excessive salivation. Phocid seals have been successfully anesthetized with a combination of ketamine (1.5 mg/kg) and diazepam (0.05 mg/kg) IM or IV [14]. This protocol is preferred over ketamine (2 mg/kg) alone because the ketamine dose can be decreased and induction and recovery are generally smoother. Apparently, Weddell seals (*Leptonychotes weddellii*) can be safely immobilized with relatively low doses of ketamine (2 mg/kg IM) prior to induction with a gas anesthetic [15].

Southern elephant seals (*Mirounga leonina*) are generally so lethargic that they can be injected at close range with a pole syringe [16]. A 16–18 gauge needle up to 4 inches long is needed to penetrate the skin and underlying blubber. Although succinylcholine (2.5 mg/kg) has been used to immobilize seals rapidly [16], it should not be used without concurrent analgesic or anesthetic drug administration and ventilatory support.

For IV injections, sea lions are best restrained in a squeeze cage to enable access to a protruding flipper. A vein on the ventral aspect of the flipper, approximately 3 cm anterior to its posterior edge, can be used for IV administration. Thiopental or thiamylal can be given at the rate of 2.2–4.4 mg/kg to produce anesthesia [17]. Barbiturates should be given rapidly to minimize struggling and to produce relaxation. Alternatively, isoflurane or halothane can be administered by means of a face mask to induce anesthesia. Sea lions can hold their breath for as long as 5 min. When they do breathe, their air intake is enormous and rapid. For this reason, the respiratory pattern during anesthetic induction is not an accurate gauge of CNS depression. Once the animal is induced, the trachea is easily intubated for further inhalant administration. Concentrations of 0.75–1.5% are usually sufficient to maintain anesthesia.

Northern sea lions have been successfully anesthetized with Telazol® (tiletamine-zolazepam). The recommended dose range is 1.8–2.5 mg/kg IM. The effective dose may vary from one animal to another. Tiletamine-zolazepam doses of more than 2.5 mg/kg IM can be fatal in sea lions. Hypothermia is commonly observed in animals that receive higher doses (2.5 mg/kg IM or larger) [18].

Several anesthetic regimens have been described for inducing anesthesia in California sea lions (*Zalophus californianus*) [19]. The first combination consists of atropine (0.02 mg/kg) given IM 10 min prior to medetomidine (0.14 mg/kg IM) and ketamine (2.5 mg/kg IM) administration. Sea lions of all ages and weights (13.5–145.0 kg) have been anesthetized with this mixture. Following IM injection, induction time ranges from 9 to 17 min, whereas anesthesia time ranges from 17 to 57 min [20]. It should be noted that the standard 1.0 mg/mL concentration of medetomidine is too dilute and expensive for this technique and may limit its use. Reversal with atipamezole at a dosage of 0.2 mg/kg IM can hasten and reduce recovery time [20].

In a similar study using 1.0 mg/kg IM of Telazol®, the medetomidine dosage was reduced by half to 0.07 mg/kg IM. Induction time was reduced to approximately 5 min, while anesthesia/immobilization with this mixture averaged nearly 30 min. The disadvantages of this anesthetic regimen include prolonged ataxia, weakness, and some disorientation during recovery. Typically, this combination will provide a rapid induction with a reliable plane of anesthesia. Recovery can be hastened with atipamezole at a dosage of 0.2 mg/kg IM [20].

Young California sea lion pups that are hand caught can be induced by mask technique alone using either isoflurane or sevoflurane. Induction and recovery times average under 10 min when using isoflurane alone to maintain anesthesia [21]. Relaxation is evident within a few minutes of administration of isoflurane by mask.

Premedication with IM meperidine (0.23–0.45 mg/kg) apparently provides little restraint of sea lions, while causing profound respiratory depression. Consequently, low dosages are advised when using meperidine for analgesia or as part of the immobilization technique in this species of seals [3].

Steller sea lions have been darted using Telazol® delivered via a carbon dioxide-powered blowpipe. The average dose administered was 2.3 mg/kg IM. Approximately one-third of the animals required additional CNS depression with isoflurane to achieve anesthesia. Following induction, all animals were intubated and maintained on isoflurane in oxygen. If apneustic breathing was observed after Telazol® injection, doxapram was used to stimulate breathing and aid in induction of inhalant anesthesia [22]. Young Steller sea lion pups and yearlings caught by trained scuba divers have become severely hypothermic (<90°F [<32°C]) when anesthetized immediately after snaring, emphasizing the importance of monitoring temperature closely when working with this species [22].

Both ketamine (2.1 mg/kg IM) and Telazol® (1.1 mg/kg IM) have been used to immobilize fur seals. Individual animal response to these drugs appears to be highly variable, however. The dose requirement for satisfactory levels of anesthesia and immobilization appears to be less than for most other species of seals. Few side-effects have been observed when using low doses of these drugs, aside from mild tremors caused by ketamine, and respiratory depression or prolonged apnea caused by tiletamine-zolazepam. When working with fur seals, relatively low doses of ketamine or Telazol® can be quite effective, especially for animals in good body condition [23].

Phocids (true seals)

Phocidae or true seals include northern hemisphere seals such as the harbor, gray, bearded, and hooded seals. The southern hemisphere seals include monk, crabeater, Weddell, leopard, Ross, and elephant seals. Many of these species have been studied in free-ranging environments and are commonly included in zoological parks and aquariums.

Southern elephant seals have been extensively studied, and multiple anesthetic techniques have been used successfully. Telazol® has been administered to over 1000 southern elephant seals without acute fatality. Older and better conditioned animals appear to have faster recoveries, and no gender differences have been noted. Apnea has been observed in some animals, but typically lasts less than 5 min [24]. A 1 mg/kg IM dose of Telazol® is considered both safe and effective in this species [25]. Telazol® administration at a dose under 0.5 mg/kg IV will produce anesthesia in 30 s or less. Anesthesia achieved with IV Telazol®, even at this low dose, will range from 15 to 20 min [26].

Ketamine alone can be administered to elephant seals at doses ranging from 2 to 8 mg/kg IM. At a dose of 8–9 mg/kg IM, immobilization should occur in 15 min. The dosage required depends greatly on which sedative is used in conjunction with ketamine. An IM dose of 0.4–0.5 mg/kg of xylazine has been combined with 5–6 mg/kg of ketamine for short periods of immobilization [27]. Alternatively, diazepam can be dosed at 0.3 mg/kg IM with 8 mg/kg IM of ketamine. Lower doses of xylazine (0.4 mg/kg) or diazepam (0.1 mg/kg) can also be given IV to supplement muscle relaxation during ketamine anesthesia. Medetomidine (0.013 mg/kg IM) has also been combined with ketamine (2 mg/kg IM) to enhance muscle relaxation during immobilization [28].

In a study on the use of antagonists and stimulants to reverse sedation in elephant seals, yohimbine (0.06 mg/kg IM) reversed xylazine sedation better than did doxapram, whereas 4-aminopyridine actually prolonged recovery [29]. Doxapram (0.5, 1, 2, and 4 mg/kg IV) caused a dose-dependent increase in the depth and rate of ventilation, which began within 1 min, peaked after 2 min, and lasted for up to 5 min. The 2 mg/kg dose appeared to be both safe and effective. Higher dosages (4 mg/kg) caused arousal and shaking in some seals. Administration of doxapram via the endotracheal tube was an unreliable route of drug delivery [30].

Butorphanol has been evaluated as an analgesic in young elephant seals at a dosage of 0.055 mg/kg IM [30]. The dosage was conservative and produced minimal observable effects. A complete evaluation of this opioid's analgesic efficacy in seals requires additional use and observation. Similarly, published reports of anesthetics in many phocids are sparse, making dosage recommendations based on efficacy and safety difficult. For example, when 30 Weddell seals were administered Telazol® at IM doses ranging from 100 to 300 mg, only 16 were fully immobilized, while seven were moderately sedated and seven were only lightly sedated. However, nearly 25% of the animals in the study died. The cause of mortality is unknown and likely not due solely to either the drugs or dosages used [31].

Several IM drugs or drug mixtures have been described for use in gray seals. These include ketamine (6 mg/kg) and diazepam (0.3 mg/kg), which produced adequate immobilization [32]; tiletamine-zolazepam (1 mg/kg); and carfentanil (0.01 mg/kg) with ketamine (5 mg/kg) and xylazine (1 mg/kg) [33]. Each of these drug combinations was reportedly effective in immobilizing gray seals. Weddell seals have been successfully immobilized under field conditions using approximately 2 mg/kg IM ketamine with 0.1 mg/kg IM midazolam. Additional doses of 0.5 mg/kg ketamine and 0.025 mg/kg midazolam given intramuscularly could prolong immobilization. This combination was reported to be adequate in 33/40 animals with onset of 12 min and duration of 38 ± 19 min [34].

Sirenia (manatees)

Many minor procedures can be performed with proper physical restraint. Local anesthetic infiltration should be used for procedures that are painful. Captive manatees are removed from the water by draining the pool or elevating the bottom of the holding tank. While out of the water, manatees should be sprayed with water to avoid skin drying and should be kept out of the sun to prevent skin burning. They should be held in sternal recumbency because the tail is potentially dangerous if placed in dorsal or lateral recumbency. The tail can be restrained by assistants and foam pads.

Sedation with midazolam generally works well. A dosage of 0.045 mg/kg IM is recommended. For light general anesthesia and restraint, the combination of midazolam (0.066 mg/kg IM) and meperidine (up to 1.0 mg/kg IM) is effective. Flumazenil and naloxone are effective antagonists for this combination [35].

Nasotracheal intubation is easily accomplished with the aid of a fiberoptic endoscope, which is placed in one nasal passage while the endotracheal tube is passed via the opposite nasal passage. Manual or mechanical ventilation is recommended to maintain the carbon dioxide level within normal limits during general anesthesia. Isoflurane or sevoflurane are appropriate anesthetics for maintenance with expected vaporizer settings of 1.5–2.5%.

Carnivora

Polar bears

Since polar bears can have substantial fat deposits throughout the year, the shoulder and neck are the best sites for IM drug delivery. Male polar bears can be large and heavy. Body weights of greater than 500 kg are not uncommon. Because of their large size and drug requirements, potent drug combinations are required to keep drug volume and dart size to a minimum. Immobilized polar bears should be positioned to avoid excessive pressure on limb muscles because such pressure has caused muscle swelling and lameness. During the summer, polar bears enter a hypometabolic state that is characterized by fasting and decreased body temperature (93–95°F [34–35°C]). Intramuscular mobilizing drug requirements may also be decreased during the summer. In areas where large numbers of polar bears congregate, reversible anesthetic protocols should be considered because they will decrease the risk of predation by other bears. Reversible protocols should also be considered for mother bears with cubs. Polar bears immobilized with Telazol® typically keep their heads out of the water better than bears immobilized with opioids. This is probably due to muscle extension with the use of dissociative anesthetic versus the relaxed curled body position associated with the use of carfentanil or etorphine.

Mature polar bears can be darted with 22 caliber blank powered projectors and explosive discharge darts. A needle up to 10 cm long is necessary to ensure the IM injection of drugs. Polar bears are notorious for pretending to be immobilized and have been known to awaken suddenly when approached. Always use caution when approaching this species.

Immobilization drug choices include dissociatives and opioids. Because Telazol® is available in a lyophilized form, it can be reconstituted with an α_2-adrenergic receptor agonist, keeping the total volume lower than with ketamine. Dosages of 8–10 mg/kg of Telazol® will produce reliable immobilization, but can also result in prolonged recoveries [36]. Used alone, the volume requirements are high, making the use of a large dart necessary. The greater mass of a large volume and the dart itself are more likely to produce excessive tissue trauma and animal injury when the projectile penetrates tissue. For this reason, an IM combination of xylazine (2 mg/kg) and Telazol® (3 mg/kg) is preferred as it has approximately half the volume requirement of Telazol® alone. Additionally, partial reversal can be accomplished by administration of either yohimbine or atipamezole. When rapid reversal of this mixture is not achieved, it is probably due to residual zolazepam sedation.

A similar anesthetic regimen consists of the IM injection of 75 μg/kg of medetomidine mixed with 2.2 mg/kg of Telazol® [37]. This combination has a rapid onset of action and can be delivered IM in a small volume to free-ranging polar bears. To reduce volume, medetomidine (1 mg/mL) can be lyophilized and reconstituted to a concentration of 6 mg/mL. The IM dosage range reported for this mixture was 1.2–7.7 mg/kg. In all bears, the total volume injected was always less than 10 mL. The average dose of medetomidine injected was 0.07 mg/kg, whereas the average dose of Telazol® injected was 2.3 mg/kg. This regimen resulted in an average anesthesia time of approximately 3 h. When medetomidine was reversed with atipamezole (0.24 mg/kg IM), recovery time was reduced to an average of 6 min [38]. Medetomidine co-administration substantially reduced the volume requirement of Telazol® while providing analgesia. If Telazol® is used alone, dosage requirement increases from under 2.5 to 5 mg/kg IM. With the medetomidine-tiletamine-zolazepam mixture, bears become ataxic in 1–3 min, typically sit in 4–5 min, and become recumbent shortly thereafter. Maximal effects are usually seen in 20 min. The duration is dose dependent, with recumbency lasting approximately 2 h [37]. Following immobilization, the suspension of polar bears in a cargo net can cause acute hypertension (up to a 50% increase in mean arterial pressure), hypoxemia, and evidence of stress. Cargo nets can restrict both ventilation and circulation. Bears should be transported on a rigid platform rather than lifted in a net [38].

Opioids can provide for some sedation and analgesia, as well as immobilization. Fentanyl, carfentanil, and etorphine have all been used to immobilize polar bears. The published mean IM dosage for fentanyl in polar bears is 0.44 mg/kg. Unless concentrated forms of fentanyl become available, the volume needed is usually too large for the practical use of this drug in adult bears. Fentanyl reportedly provides better muscle relaxation than etorphine. Naloxone can be dosed at 25 mg per 10 mg of fentanyl or 25 mg per 0.5 mg of etorphine for rapid reversal (within 10 min) [39].

Sea otters

Numerous combinations have been assessed in sea otters, including Telazol®, butorphanol-diazepam, oxymorphone-acepromazine-diazepam, azaperone-fentanyl-diazepam, medetomidine-ketamine, and fentanyl-diazepam. Of these, the most effective combinations appear to be fentanyl (0.1 mg/kg) with either acepromazine or diazepam (0.22 mg/kg IM) [40–42].

Manual restraint and nets are often effective for capture and examination. Hand injection can be used in these situations. If manual restraint is feasible, mask induction with either isoflurane or sevoflurane works well. Altered thermoregulation may cause body temperature to increase during capture. Otters should be transported in well-ventilated cages that are iced to help keep animals cool during transport.

Experience in sedating sea otters after the 1989 Valdez oil spill resulted in the recommendation of combined fentanyl (0.05–0.1 mg/kg IM) and diazepam (0.1 mg/kg IM) as the preferred technique in this species. It should be noted that many other immobilizing mixtures were used only a few times, and the mortality rate for all anesthetized sea otters was extremely high because of oil exposure [43].

Other drug combinations used successfully to sedate, immobilize, or anesthetize sea otters include Telazol® alone (2 mg/kg IM); ketamine (2.5 mg/kg IM) and medetomidine (0.25 mg/kg IM); ketamine (10 mg/kg IM) and midazolam (0.25 mg/kg IM); ketamine (1.5 mg/kg IM) and xylazine (1.5 mg/kg IM); and etorphine (0.03–0.05 mg/kg IM) with diazepam (0.06 mg/kg IM).

References

1 Milsom WK, Harris MB, Reid SG. Do descending influences alternate to produce episodic breathing? *Respir Physiol* 1997; **110**: 307–317.

2 Meshcherskii RM, Meniailov NV, Shepeleva IS, *et al.* Narcotization of dolphins without blocking their own respiration. *Zh Evol Biokhim Fiziol* 1978; **14**: 410–411 (in Russian).

3 Joseph BE, Cornell LH. The use of meperidine hydrochloride for chemical restraint in certain cetaceans and pinnipeds. *J Wildl Dis* 1988; **24**: 691–694.

4 Rieu M, Gautheron B. Preliminary observations concerning a method for introduction of a tube for anaesthesia in small delphinids. *Life Sci* 1968; **7**: 1141–1146.

5 Lily JC. *Man and Dolphin.* New York: Doubleday, 1961.

6 Ridgway SH, Green RF, Sweeney JC. Mandibular anesthesia and tooth extraction in the bottlenosed dolphin. *J Wildl Dis* 1975; **11**: 415–418.

7 Brunson DB, Rowles TK, Gulland FM, *et al.* Technique for drug delivery and sedation of a free-ranging North Atlantic Right Whale (Balenea glacialis). In: *Proceedings of the American Association of Zoo Veterinarians*, 2002; 320–322.

8 Stringer EM, van Bonn W, Chinnadurai SK, Gulland FM. Risk factors associated with perianesthetic mortality of stranded free-ranging California sea lions (Zalophus californianus) undergoing rehabilitation. *J Zoo Wildl Med* 2012; **43**(2): 233–239.

9 Yamaya Y, Ohba S, Koie H, *et al.* Isoflurane anaesthesia in four sea lions (Otaria byronia and Zalophus californianus). *Vet Anaesth Analg* 2006; **33**(5): 302–306.

10 Pang DS, Rondenay Y, Troncy E, *et al.* Use of end-tidal partial pressure of carbon dioxide to predict arterial partial pressure of carbon dioxide in harp seals during isoflurane-induced anesthesia. *Am J Vet Res* 2006; **67**(7): 1131–1135.

11 Dennison SE, Gulland FM, Braselton WE. Standardized protocols for plasma clearance of iohexol are not appropriate for determination of glomerular filtration rates

in anesthetized California sea lions (Zalophus californianus). *J Zoo Wildl Med* 2010; **41**(1): 144–147.

12 Hubbard RC, Poulter TC. Seals and sea lions as models for studies in comparative biology. *Lab Anim Care* 1968; **18**(Suppl): 288–297.

13 Beraci JR. An appraisal of ketamine as an immobilizing agent in wild and captive pinnipeds. *J Am Vet Med Assoc* 1973; **163**: 574–577.

14 Beraci JR, Skirnisson K, St Aubin DJ. A safe method for repeatedly immobilizing seals. *J Am Vet Med Assoc* 1981; **179**: 1192–1193.

15 Hochachka PW, Liggins GC, Quist J, *et al.* Pulmonary metabolism during diving: conditioning blood for the brain. *Science* 1977; **198**: 831–834.

16 Ling JK, Nicholls DG, Thomas CDB. Immobilization of southern elephant seals with succinylcholine chloride. *J Wildl Manage* 1967; **37**: 468–479.

17 Tidgway SH, Simpson JG. Anesthesia and restraint for the California seal lion, Zalophus californianus. *J Am Vet Med Assoc* 1969; **155**: 1059–1063.

18 Loughlin TR, Spraker T. Use of Telazol® to immobilize female northern sea lions (Eumetopias jubatus) in Alaska. *J Wildl Dis* 1989; **25**: 353–358.

19 Haulena M, Gulland FM, Calkins DG, Spraker TR. Immobilization of California sea lions using medetomidine plus ketamine with and without isoflurane and reversal with atipamezole. *J Wildl Dis* 2000; **36**: 124–130.

20 Haulena M, Gulland FM. Use of medetomidine-zolazepam-tiletamine with and without atipamezole reversal to immobilize captive California sea lions. *J Wildl Dis* 2001; **37**: 566–573.

21 Heath RB, DeLong R, Jameson V, Bradley D, Spraker T. Isoflurane anesthesia in free ranging sea lion pups. *J Wildl Dis* 1997; **33**: 206–210.

22 Dabin W, Beauplet G, Guinet C. Response of wild subantarctic fur seal (Arctocephalus tropicalis) females to ketamine and tiletamine-zolazepam anesthesia. *J Wildl Dis* 2002; **38**: 846–850.

23 Field IC, Bradshaw CJ, McMahon CR, Harrington J, Burton HR. Effects of age, size and condition of elephant seals (Mirounga leonine) on their intravenous anaesthesia with tiletamine and zolazepam. *Vet Rec* 2002; **151**: 235–240.

24 Baker JR, Fedak MA, Anderson SS, Arnbom T, Baker R. The use of a tiletamine-zolazepam mixture to immobilize wild grey seals and southern elephant seals. *Vet Rec* 1990; **126**: 75–77.

25 McMahon CR, Burton H, McLean S, Slip D, Bester M. Field immobilisation of southern elephant seals with intravenous tiletamine and zolazepam. *Vet Rec* 2000; **146**: 251–254.

26 Woods R, McLean S, Burton HR. Pharmacokinetics of intraven ously administered ketamine in southern elephant seals (Mirounga leonina). *Comp Biochem Physiol* 1999; **123**: 279–284.

27 Gales NJ, Burton HR. Prolonged and multiple immobilizations of the southern elephant seal using ketamine hydrochloride or ketamine hydrochloride-diazepam combinations. *J Wildl Dis* 1987; **23**: 614–618.

28 Woods R, McLean S, Nicol S, Burton H. Chemical restraint of southern elephant seals (Mirounga leonine): use of medetomidine, ketamine and atipamezole and comparison with other cyclohexamine-based combinations. *Br Vet J* 1996; **152**: 213–224.

29 Woods R, McLean S, Nicol S, Burton H. Antagonism of some cyclohexamine based drug combinations used for chemical restraint of southern elephant seals (Mirounga leonina). *Aust Vet J* 1995; **72**: 165–171.

30 Nutter F, Haulena M, Bai SA. Preliminary pharmacokinetics of single dose intramuscular butorphanol in elephant seals (Mirounga angustirostris). In: *Proceedings of the American Asso ciation of Zoo Veterinarians/American Association of Wildlife Veterinarians Joint Conference*, 1998; 372–373.

31 Phelan JR, Green K. Chemical restraint of Weddell seals (Leptonychotes weddellii) with a combination of tiletamine and zolazepam. *J Wildl Dis* 1992; **28**: 230–235.

32 Baker JR, Anderson SS, Fedak MA. The use of a ketamine-diazepam mixture to immobilize wild grey seals (Halichoerus grypus) and southern elephant seals (Mirounga leonina). *Vet Rec* 1988; **123**: 287–289.

33 Baker JR, Gatesman TJ. Use of carfentanil and a ketamine-xylazine mixture to immobilize wild grey seals (Halichoerus grypus). *Vet Rec* 1985; **116**: 208–210.

34 Mellish JA, Tuomi PA, Hindle AG, Horning M. Chemical immobilization of Weddell seals (Leptonychotes weddellii) by ketamine/midazolam combination. *Vet Anaesth Analg* 2010; **37**(2): 123–131.

35 Walsh M, Bossart G. Manatee medicine. In: Fowler ME, Miller E, eds. *Zoo and Wild Animal Medicine: Current Therapy*, 4th edn. Philadelphia: WB Saunders, 1999; 507–516.

36 Haigh JC, Stirling I, Broughton E. Immobilization of polar bears (Urus maritimus Phipps) with a mixture of tiletamine hydrochloride and zolazepam hydrochloride. *J Wildl Dis* 1985; **21**: 43–47.

37 Caulkett NA, Cattet MRL, Caulkett JM, Polischuk SC. Comparative physiologic effects of Telazol®, medetomidine-ketamine, and medetomidine-Telazol® in polar bears (Ursus maritimus). *J Zoo Wildl Med* 1999; **30**: 504–509.

38 Cattet MRL, Caulkett NA, Streib KA, Torske KE, Ramsay MA. Cardiopulmonary response of anesthetized polar bears to suspension by net and sling. *J Wildl Dis* 1999; **35**: 548–555.

39 Patenaude RP. Evaluation of fentanyl citrate, etorphine hydrochloride, and naloxone hydrochloride in captive polar bears. *J Am Vet Med Assoc* 1979; **175**: 1006–1007.

40 Sawyer DC, Williams TD. Chemical restraint and anesthesia of sea otters affected by the oil spill in Prince William Sound, Alaska. *J Am Vet Med Assoc* 1996; **208**: 1831–1834.

41 Nagel EL, Morgane PJ, McFarland WL. Anesthesia for the bottlenose dolphin Tursiops truncatus. *Science* 1964; **146**: 1591–1593.

42 Bauquier SH, Hinshaw KC, Ialeggio DM, *et al.* Reversible immobilization of giant otters (Pteronura brasiliensis) using medetomidine-ketamine and atipamezole. *J Zoo Wildl Med* 2010; **41**(2): 346–349.

43 Soto-Azat C, Boher F, Flores G, *et al.* Reversible anesthesia in wild marine otters (Lontra felina) using ketamine and medetomidine. *J Zoo Wildl Med* 2006; **37**(4): 535–538.

42 Comparative Anesthesia and Analgesia of Reptiles, Amphibians, and Fishes

Cornelia I. Mosley[1] and Craig A. Mosley[2]

[1] Ontario Veterinary College, University of Guelph, Canada

[2] Mosley Veterinary Anesthesia Services, Rockwood, Ontario, Canada

Chapter contents

Introduction

Reptiles, amphibians, and fishes are unique animal classes encountered in veterinary medicine and are very different in terms of anatomy, physiology, and behavioral adaptations from the more familiar mammals. Regardless of the differences among these animal classes, by using sound anesthetic principles reasonably safe and effective anesthesia can be performed, even in the absence of species-specific information. In the following sections, emphasis has been placed on providing comparative anatomic and physiologic information relevant to the anesthetic management of each class of animals. A comprehensive review of the anesthetic and analgesic literature is beyond the scope of this text, but is available elsewhere and should be consulted for additional detail [1–6].

Reptile anesthesia

Anesthetic management of reptiles is associated with many challenges. Reptilia represents a diverse class of animals in terms of size, environmental requirements, behavior, physiology, and anatomy. There are over 7800 species represented by four main orders (Crocodylia, Testudines, Squamata, and Rhynchocephalia). Compounding the difficulties created by these inherent species differences, there is relatively little peer-reviewed research investigating anesthesia and analgesia in reptiles and much of the earlier literature is anectodal in nature and persists as accepted fact despite contradictory evidence. Fortunately there has been considerable interest in this area recently and scientific studies investigating anesthesia and analgesia in reptiles are becoming more available.

Applying generalized anesthetic recommendations to such a large and varying group of animals is difficult. Clinical application of various techniques is often ascribed to one of the the three principal orders: the crocodilians (crocodiles and alligators), the chelonians (tortoises and turtles), and the squamates (snakes and lizards). An understanding of normal physiology, pathophysiology, the action and disposition of anesthetic and related drugs, and a familiarity with the design and use of related anesthetic equipment are important considerations. A thorough preanesthetic assessment and carefully designed anesthetic plan with attention to premedication, induction, maintenance, monitoring, supportive care, recovery, and ongoing postoperative support and analgesia all contribute to the reduction of risk associated with anesthesia.

Anatomy and physiology

Reptiles have long been considered to be the class of vertebrates that reflect the evolutionary transition between the aquatic and amphibious ectothermic vertebrates, and endothermic birds and mammals. However, most evolution of the vertebrates stems from several very ancient common ancestors and the major classes of extant vertebrates have subsequently evolved in parallel for millions of years, hence reptiles are not evolutionary predecessors of mammals. Reptiles arguably represent one of the most ancient, successful and well-adapted classes of animals, with some species surviving essentially unchanged for hundreds of millions of years. Recent investigations recognize reptilian physiologic evolutionary adaptations as 'optimal or advantageous,' enabling exothermic animals to inhabit almost all of the available non-polar ecologic niches.

Veterinary Anesthesia and Analgesia: The Fifth Edition of Lumb and Jones,
Edited by Kurt A. Grimm, Leigh A. Lamont, William J. Tranquilli, Stephen A. Greene and Sheilah A. Robertson.

Although many aspects of reptilian physiology are similar to those of endothermic vertebrates, significant differences are present. Such differences may alter both the action and disposition of anesthetics and analgesics.

Metabolism and thermoregulation

The ectothermic nature of reptiles and their generally lower metabolic rates are probably the two most striking differences between mammals and reptiles that impede extrapolation of anesthetic principles and practices between the two groups. Reptiles derive much of their body heat from the surrounding environment and use behaviors such as basking or burrowing to regulate their body temperatures. Reptiles can also alter their body temperature through changes in their cardiovascular physiology. During periods of warming some reptiles increase their heart rate and the degree of right-to-left cardiac shunting to increase the fraction of blood flow that is directed to the periphery for heating and ultimate return to the body core [7]. This adaptation facilitates more rapid and efficient warming of the animal.

Reptiles will tend to choose a preferred optimal temperature zone (POTZ) maintaining a body temperature that is presumably ideal for the animal. In most instances reptiles undergoing anesthesia should be maintained at the average or the high end of their POTZ to ensure optimal metabolic function. Species-specific ranges can often be found in general husbandry references or extrapolated from known species which are found in similar natural habitats. In general, 20–25 °C is recommended for most aquatic and temperate reptile species and 25–35 °C for most tropical species [8].

Although ambient temperature is one of the main determinants of metabolic rate in resting reptiles, and consequently the metabolism and excretion of drugs [9], there are significant interspecies and intraindividual variations. Minimum and maximum oxygen consumption rates of individual reptilian species range from almost zero to values similar to a resting mammal [10]. The oxygen consumption of any individual is a function of the species, the temperature, and the individual. In general, the varanid and lacertid lizards tend to have relatively high metabolic rates, and boid snakes and chelonians have lower rates. Surface-dwelling squamates have higher metabolic rates than burrowing species, and species of lizards that eat insects or other vertebrates have higher metabolic rates than do herbivorous species [11]. Those species with higher inherent metabolic rates may be expected to more rapidly metabolize and excrete drugs compared to those with lower metabolic rates, but this has not been conclusively demonstrated.

Cardiovascular system

The non-crocodilian reptile heart has three chambers: two completely separate atria and a single anatomically continuous ventricle. The crocodilian heart is more typical of that seen in mammals and birds with two completely divided atria and two ventricles. In the crocodilian heart, the foramen of Panizza allows for some intravascular shunting under circumstances of breath holding, such as diving. In non-crocodilian reptiles, the ventricle is divided into two main chambers by a septum-like structure called the Muskelleiste or muscular ridge (Fig. 42.1). This ridge originates from the ventral ventricular wall and runs from the ventricular apex to the base, dividing the ventricle into two anatomically defined but connected chambers: the cavum pulmonale and the cavum dorsale [12,13], comparable in function to the right and left ventricles of mammals, respectively. The cavum dorsale is sometimes further subdivided into the cavum venosum and cavum arteriosum. The

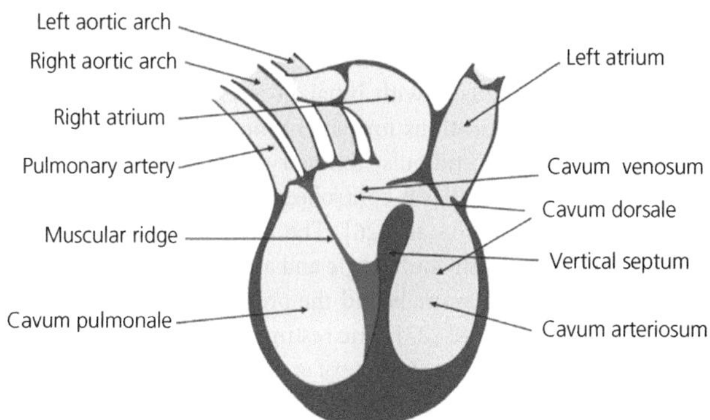

Figure 42.1 A generalized schematic demonstrating the anatomy and separation of blood flow in the non-crocodilian reptile heart. The cavum venosum is the region of the heart where mixing of oxygenated and deoxygenated blood may occur. Deoxygenated blood returning to the heart via the right atrium passes through the cavum venosum to the cavum pulmonale. The volume of blood remaining in the cavum venosum after the muscular ridge contacts the dorsal wall of the heart (during systole), relative to the volume of oxygenated blood in the cavum arteriosum, will determine the magnitude of the shunted fraction of blood. The shunt fraction is ultimately controlled by pressure differences between the systemic and pulmonary circulations resulting in larger or smaller volumes of deoxygenated blood remaining in the cavum venosum during systole.

dorsolateral border of the muscular ridge is free, permitting the flow of blood between the cavum pulmonale and cavum dorsale. However, during ventricular systole the muscular ridge presses against the dorsal wall of the ventricle and separates the cavum pulmonale from the cavum dorsale; thus in a functional sense, the heart is capable of acting as a two-circuit pump. The pulmonary artery arises from the cavum pulmonale and two aortic arches arise from the cavum venosum of the cavum dorsale. The left aortic arch becomes the dorsal aorta while the right aortic arch forms the subclavian and carotids and a third branch joins the dorsal aorta. However there is considerable anatomic variation among species.

Cardiac shunting occurs commonly in reptiles [14–16]. Cardiac shunts can occur in both directions, and under some circumstances may occur simultaneously in both directions [14,17,18]. The direction of the net shunt determines whether the systemic or pulmonary circulation receives the majority of the cardiac output. Intracardiac shunting has three important functions. First, shunting serves to stabilize the oxygen content of the blood during respiratory pauses. Second, the right-to-left shunt is partly responsible for facilitating heating by increasing systemic blood flow. Third, a right-to-left shunt directs blood away from the lungs during breath holding.

During anesthesia, cardiac shunting can affect systemic arterial oxygen content and the uptake and elimination of inhaled anesthetics. The size and direction of the shunts are ultimately controlled by pressure differences between the pulmonary and systemic circulations and the washout of blood remaining in the cavum venosum (an anatomic subchamber of the cavum dorsale described in many reptiles) [14,16,18,19]. The pressure differences are principally controlled by cholinergic and adrenergic factors that regulate the vascular resistance of the pulmonary and systemic circulation [14,20–25].

Large right-to-left shunts limit the amount of anesthetic uptake early in the anesthetic period and slow anesthetic elimination at the end of anesthesia. Such shunts can delay the induction to and recovery from inhaled anesthesia. Changes in the level and direction of shunts may account for the unexpected awakening seen in some reptiles anesthetized with inhalant anesthetics. Intracardiac shunts also have implications for patient monitoring, in particular airway gas monitoring and pulse oximetry.

Blood pressure in reptiles is controlled by mechanisms similar to those described in mammals [26]. The cardiovascular system of reptiles responds to both cholinergic and adrenergic stimulation in a manner similar to mammals and the presence of a baroreceptor reflex has been described [27]. The resting blood pressures of reptiles tend to be stable in the absence of external stimuli but may vary with temperature, activity or state of arousal [28,29]. In contrast to mammals, systemic arterial blood pressures vary greatly among various reptilian species, making it difficult to identify a 'normal' arterial blood pressure [26]. 'Normal' blood pressure in reptiles may be more profoundly affected by environmental stresses such as habitat and temperature, species activity level, and size compared to the role of these factors on influencing blood pressure in mammals. This greater variability may originate from a reptile's poor ability to regulate normal homeostasis independent of temperature and environment.

Chelonians tend to have the lowest mean arterial pressures (15–30 mmHg) while some varanids have resting arterial pressures similar to mammals (60–80 mmHg) [30]. In the green iguana, normal resting mean arterial blood pressures are reported to be in the range of 40–50 mmHg while mean pulmonary arterial pressures are in the range of 15–30 [30]. The systemic blood pressures in snakes correspond to the gravitational stress they are likely to experience [31–33]. Snakes from arboreal habitats tend to have higher arterial pressures than those that are primarily aquatic. An allometric relationship between arterial blood pressure and body mass has also been described in snakes. As body mass increases, so does blood pressure. Several anesthetics, such as sevoflurane, isoflurane, halothane, propofol, tiletamine-zolazepam, and ketamine, have been shown to induce cardiopulmonary changes in reptiles similar to those seen in mammals [34–42].

Pulmonary system

The most significant difference between the respiratory physiology of reptiles, mammals, and birds is the lower oxygen consumption rate of reptiles. This difference reflects the lower reptilian metabolic rate. Both reptile respiratory anatomy and physiology vary markedly across species. The lungs of non-crocodilian reptiles are suspended freely in the common pleuroperitoneal cavity and are not located in a closed pleural space. In reptiles, the lungs tend to be sac-like with varying degrees of partitioning (Fig. 42.2). Highly aerobic species such as the varanids tend to have highly partitioned lungs with numerous septae and invaginations that increase the surface area for gas exchange. Chelonians and lizards tend to have paired lungs while most snakes have a single functional right lung. The functional units of the lung are referred to as ediculi and faveoli which are structures analogous to mammalian alveoli. Most reptile lungs exhibit areas of both type of parenchyma. There is little detail regarding the trachea and extrapulmonary bronchial tree system in reptiles. The tracheal rings of chelonians tend to be complete, necessitating care when placing an endotracheal tube. In addition, the trachea may bifurcate quite proximally, so inadvertent endobronchial intubation may occur (Fig. 42.3). Many snakes also possess a tracheal lung, the significance of which is unclear. The lungs of reptiles tend to have a smaller respiratory surface area relative to lung volume.

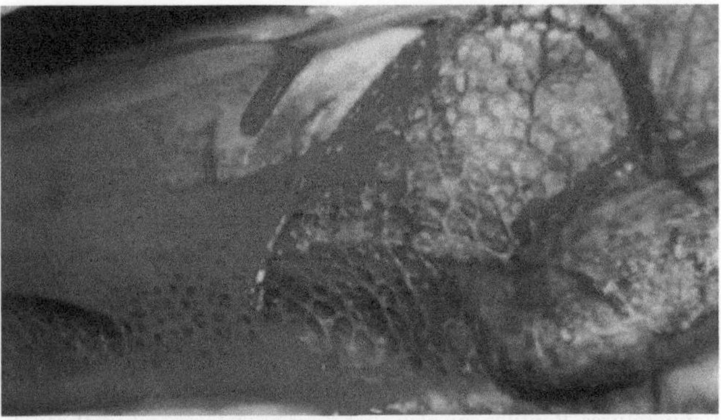

Figure 42.2 The lungs of many reptiles tend to be 'sac-like' with a comparatively low respiratory surface area relative to total lung volume. However, lung structure varies markedly among species with highly aerobic species having more partitions and invaginations to increase respiratory surface area. The image shows the dissection of the lung in a boid snake demonstrating the sac-like structure.

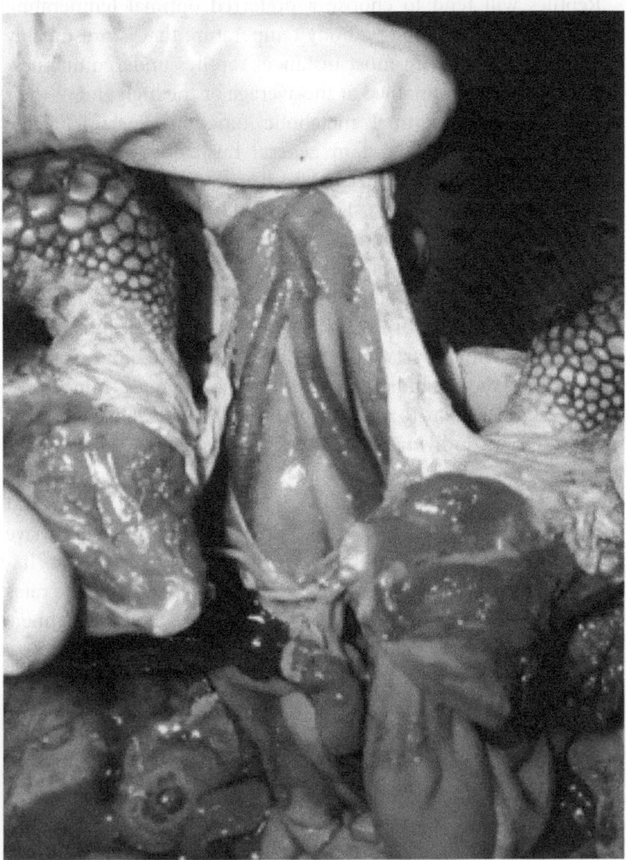

Figure 42.3 The trachea of many chelonians bifurcates quite proximally, increasing the risk of unilateral bronchial intubation.

Because reptiles lack a diaphragm, they rely on the thoracic musculature for ventilation. Both inspiration and expiration are active processes so the respiratory depression associated with anesthesia may be more profound than that observed in mammalian species where expiration is a passive process. Because the muscles of ventilation include many of the same muscles used for locomotion, these two functions are relatively incompatible. Chelonians are faced with additional respiratory challenges since expansion of the thoracic cavity by movement of the ribs is not possible. The dorsal surface of the lungs is attached to the carapace and the ventral surface is attached to the abdominal viscera. Inspiration is accomplished by enlarging the visceral cavity, and expiration occurs by forcing the viscera up against the lungs, driving air out. This is accomplished by contraction of various posterior abdominal muscles and several pectoral girdle muscles.

Control of respiration

The control of respiration in reptiles is poorly understood. Both peripheral receptor and centrally mediated control have been proposed. It seems most likely that there is an interaction between a central system which generates the pattern of respiration and afferent chemoreceptor input [43,44]. Both carbon dioxide partial pressure and pH appear important for stimulating normal ventilation but there is evidence that oxygen tension may play a role in normal ventilation, even under normoxic conditions [45]. Although there are some species variations, reptiles are generally viewed as episodic breathers [46–48]. Breathing occurs in respiratory "bursts" of activity followed by a pause of varying duration. Pulmonary vascular perfusion is also intermittent and changes in perfusion are in concert with respiratory rate and rhythm [22,49,50]. Ambient temperature has variable effects on the frequency, tidal volume, and minute ventilation [51] and due consideration should be given to maintaining the optimal temperature for a particular species.

Effects of inspired CO_2 and O_2

The response of reptiles to inspired CO_2 is quite variable. Inspiration of greater than 4% CO_2 in snakes and lizards produces an increase in tidal volume, a decrease in respiratory frequency, and an overall decrease in minute ventilation [52,53]. In turtles, specifically *Pseudemys scripta* and *Chrysemys picta*, the response to an increase in CO_2 is an increase in minute ventilation as a result of increases in both respiratory frequency and tidal volume [26,54–56]. In turtles, breathing less than 21% but more than 10% oxygen produces little change in the respiratory pattern. At fractional inspired oxygen concentrations below 10%, some species increase ventilation while others retain their resting minute ventilation. Others may decrease ventilation [48,52,57–59]. In those species in which minute ventilation decreases or remains unchanged, metabolic oxygen consumption decreases.

During anesthesia, most reptiles are maintained using an inhalant anesthetic delivered in nearly 100% oxygen. The delivery of a high oxygen concentration may further compound respiratory depression by blunting the contribution of oxygen for the stimulation of normal ventilation. In several reptiles species, exposure to 100% oxygen significantly decreases minute ventilation [52,54,60–62], suggesting that high inspired oxygen may be responsible for at least some of the respiratory depression seen during anesthesia. The magnitude of this effect is likely small compared to the effects of anesthetics on central control of respiration and the muscles of respiration. However, there is some evidence that in the green iguana, recoveries from isoflurane anesthesia may be faster when the animal is breathing room air rather than 100% oxygen, possibly by improving ventilation and the subsequent removal of the inhalant from the body [63]. Interestingly, in studies using Dumeril's monitors (*Varanus dumerili*) no significant differences in recovery times from either isoflurane or sevoflurane anesthesia were found between animals ventilated with room air or those ventilated with 100% oxygen [64]. This may reflect differences in study methods or species differences.

Renal system

Reptiles cannot produce urine more concentrated than plasma, making the excretion of nitrogenous wastes more challenging for terrestrial reptiles. Most reptiles excrete nitrogenous waste as uric acid (uricotelic). Some turtles and crocodilians can also excrete urea. Uric acid is produced in the liver and, unlike ammonia and urea, it is very insoluble in water and is excreted as a semi-solid in dilute urine. In the reptilian kidney tubule, urine is very dilute so uric acid remains in solution. The cloaca forms a common conduit for products of the urogenital and gastrointestinal systems. It is often described as three distinct compartments but the actual degree of anatomic separation of these compartments varies by species. The most craniad portion is the coprodeum which is a continuation of the terminal colon followed by the urodeum that receives connections from the urogenital system and urinary bladder (if present; not all reptiles have a urinary bladder, e.g., snakes) and the proctodeum which is the most caudal section also commonly described as the vent. Dilute urine empties into the urodeum and then into the bladder or large intestine (via the coprodeum) where water is reabsorbed causing the uric acid to precipitate. This results in the excretion of nitrogenous waste with relatively little water. The bladder of some reptiles can be used for the storage of water. Reptilian urine is not a good indicator of renal function.

Many reptiles also have specialized salt-excreting glands that allow for the excretion of very high concentrations of sodium, potassium, and chloride. Many reptiles living in extremely arid locations can tolerate the marked fluctuations in total body water and plasma osmolarity that can occur in these environments. When faced with limited water supplies, plasma osmolarity can rise to levels higher than those known in any other vertebrate species. Many reptiles also have a renal portal system where blood from the hind legs and tail will pass through the kidneys before returning to the heart [65]. The effect of this system on the pharmacokinetics of drugs seems to be of little clinical significance in healthy animals. However, it is probably still best to avoid injection of nephrotoxic drugs or those that are likely to be significantly metabolized by the kidney into the hindlimbs and tail of reptiles [66].

Hepatic system

The reptilian liver appears to be similar in structure and function to the liver of other vertebrates. Although there is little detail known about the reptilian liver, it is assumed that it probably plays important roles in tolerance to anaerobic metabolism, hypothermia, and adaptation to the physical environment. The liver of reptiles has a lower metabolic capacity compared to mammalian livers [67] and the metabolic rate is very sensitive to changes in temperature [68]. The lower metabolic rates for the reptilian liver probably account for at least some of the prolonged effects commonly seen with drugs such as antibiotics. The lower metabolic capacity of the liver may partly contribute to the prolonged anesthetic recoveries seen when using drugs that require extensive hepatic metabolism for termination of their clinical effect.

Clinical anesthesia

Detailed information regarding clinical anesthesia in reptiles has been reviewed elsewhere and the reader should consult these references for specific information on anesthetic and analgesic techniques, drugs, dosage, and patient monitoring recommendations [1–6]. A few general concepts regarding reptile anesthesia will be presented below.

Patient presentation/assessment

Regardless of species or procedure, a preanesthetic assessment should be performed on all patients. Patient assessment should include a complete history, species identification, and physical examination. Any additional diagnostic tests such as blood work and imaging should be performed as indicated. Because most anesthetics produce some degree of cardiopulmonary depression, animals should be physiologically stable prior to the induction of anesthesia if possible. In some reptiles the size, disposition or anatomy may prevent the performance of a physical examination. In these animals an assessment of body weight and general appearance may assist in determining the general health status of the animal. Species identification and information on their natural habitat may be useful. All animals should be kept at their preferred body temperature (PBT) throughout the anesthetic period and recovery. Performing anesthetic procedures early in the day allows animals predisposed to prolonged recoveries to recover during regular working hours rather than late into the night when support staff and patient supervision my be reduced.

Routes of drug administration

Intramuscular drug administration is most common in reptiles. Historically, hindlimb and tail sites have been avoided because of concerns related to the first-pass effect associated with passage of administered drug through the kidneys via the renal portal system during absorption. However, studies in some reptiles (turtles and green iguanas) suggest that this may be more of a theoretical than practical concern because only a small fraction of blood from the hindlimbs and tail passes through the kidney [65,66]. However, it is probably best to avoid hindlimb and tail administration of nephrotoxic drugs. The epaxial muscles provide a suitable injection site in most snakes. In lizards, the muscle mass of the forelimb (triceps and biceps), hindlimb (quadriceps, semimembranosus, and semitendinosus), and tail can be used. Caution should be used in species known to autotomize (drop) their tails (many geckos), because it is possible for an animal to 'shed' their tail during handling. In chelonians, injections are most often administered in the triceps muscle. The cranial surface of the foreleg should be avoided since the proximity of the radial nerve to injection sites in this area increases the risk of damage to this nerve. The pectoral muscles can also be used, though in many chelonian species there is a lack of significant muscle mass in this area.

While intravenous drug administration is not always feasible in reptiles, the combination of good technique, practice, appropriate patient selection, and skilled physical restraint can facilitate predictable access to the ventral coccygeal vein in even very small snakes and lizards and the dorsal coccygeal vein in tortoises and freshwater turtles. In sea turtles, the dorsal cervical sinus has also been used for intravenous administration of drugs [69]. Intravascular injection decreases the latency of onset of action of an administered drug. It also decreases the variability in uptake and tissue irritation that is associated with intramuscular injections in reptiles. Techniques for catheterization of the coccygeal vein in both lizards and crocodilians have been described [70].

Intravenous catheterization of the coccygeal or abdominal veins is most often performed without direct visualization. In some species of turtles and tortoises the jugular vein can be visualized but this technique often requires a skin incision and blunt dissection. Venous sinus sites are not ideal for intravenous catheter placement but over-the-needle catheters can be used. A small gauge wire stylet through a needle (Seldinger technique) can be used to facilitate difficult catheterization. When required, cut-down procedures should be performed in conjunction with a local or general anesthetic. Lidocaine diluted down to a 1% solution with sterile saline can be used for local infiltration. Although toxic doses have not been determined in reptiles it is probably best to use less than 8–10 mg/kg. The most common sites for vascular access and associated technical tips are presented in Box 42.1.

Intraosseous catheterization has been described in the green iguana (*Iguana iguana*), sea turtles, and desert tortoises [71–74]. Studies in green iguanas found similar renal uptake of the radioactive substance whether administered intraosseously or intravenously [71]. In desert tortoises the humerus provided delivery to the systemic circulation similar (84%) to jugular administration followed by the femur, plastocarpacial junction and the gular region of the plastron [74]. This suggests that intraosseous drug administration is a suitable alternative to intravenous administration. To the authors' knowledge, propofol is the only anesthetic drug that has been studied with intraosseous administration, but many other anesthetic and non-anesthetic drugs have been administered successfully via this route.

Endotracheal intubation

Intubation is easily accomplished in most reptiles because the glottis is in a relatively rostral position in the mouth at the base of the tongue. A small drop of lidocaine (diluted to 1%) can be used to desensitize the glottis and may facilitate tracheal intubation. In some aquatic reptiles anatomic modifications of glottal folds may obscure direct visualization. The animal should be intubated with the largest diameter tube that can be placed easily. The mucus of reptiles tends to be very viscous and mucoid plugs can form in endotracheal tubes during longer procedures. It is important that this be recognized quickly as an inability of the lungs to fully deflate during expiration will occur. The trachea of some chelonians bifurcates quite rostrally and endobronchial intubation is possible. The tracheal rings in chelonians and crocodiles are complete and in most reptiles cuffed endotracheal tubes are avoided to prevent accidental overinflation and damage to the tracheal structures.

Pain, nociception, and analgesia

Analgesic management of reptiles is challenging as a result of their unique physiologic, anatomic, and behavioral adaptations. Reptile pain and nociception have not been extensively studied, although there is compelling evidence that reptiles are capable of nociception. However, the sensory significance of nociception to the individual is poorly understood. Pain is normally defined as 'an unpleasant sensory and emotional experience associated with actual or potential tissue damage, or described in terms of such damage' [75]. Using this definition, pain is essentially an emotional experience. Arguably it is impossible to describe this experience in reptiles given our current level of understanding and available technology. However, undoubtedly reptiles experience noxious insults as some sort of negative event and modify their behavior to escape such insults. A more robust and inclusive definition of pain may be more appropriate when describing pain in non-human animals. For example, the following definition of pain would avoid the emotional aspects associated with the human definition and yet is suitably robust to encompass a range of experiences reasonably expected to result in what we might refer to as pain in a human: 'a sensory experience representing awareness of damage or the potential for tissue damage that results in a behavioral and physiologic response to minimize/prevent the

Box 42.1 Sites for intravascular access in reptiles.

Squamates (snakes)

- The coccygeal vein is located on the ventral midline of the tail. The needle should be inserted sufficiently caudal to the vent in order to avoid the hemipenes and anal sacs. The vessel is entered via a ventral midline approach and the needle is advanced with gentle suction until either the vein or the vertebral body is contacted.
- The jugular vein can be used but requires a skin incision to visualize. An incision is made 4–7 scutes cranial to the heart at the junction of the ventral scutes and lateral body scales. The vein is then identified using blunt dissection just medial to the tips of the ribs.
- The palatine vein is easily visualized in larger snakes and is located medial to the palatine teeth in the roof of the mouth. The technique is greatly facilitated by short-term anesthesia but it is possible to collect blood from these vessels in awake animals using a mouth speculum.
- Use of the heart for venepuncture is not recommended except for emergency situations.
- There are to our knowledge no intraosseous sites described for drug administration in snakes.

Squamates (lizards)

- The coccygeal vein is located on the ventral midline of the tail. The needle should be inserted sufficiently caudal to the vent in order to avoid the hemipenes. The vessel can be entered from either a ventral midline approach or laterally. The ventral approach is simple to perform: the needle is advanced with gentle suction until the vein or a vertebral body is contacted. The lateral technique involves inserting the needle just ventral to the transverse process of the vertebral body and walking the needle ventral until the vein is contacted.
- The ventral abdominal vein is located on the ventral midline of the abdomen and can be entered percutaneously or via a small skin incision for direct visualization of the vessel.
- The cephalic vein is located on the dorsal surface of the distal foreleg. A skin incision is generally required for visualization.
- The jugular vein is located on the lateral surface of the neck at about the level of the tympanum. It may be palpated in some species, but is generally difficult to visualize. A small skin incision is often required for direct visualization. The jugular veins tend to be located more dorsal than those in mammals. There is a large lymphatic sinus close to the vein and contamination with this lymph fluid occurs frequently.
- Intraosseous techniques have been described for the distal femur, proximal tibia, and proximal humerus. The techniques are similar to those described for other small animal patients.

Chelonians (turtles and tortoises)

- The dorsal coccygeal vein is located midline dorsal to the coccygeal vertebrae. It is a technique requiring minimal restraint. The needle is introduced in a craniad direction at a 45–90° angle from the skin.
- The dorsal cervical sinus (supravertebral) is located on the dorsolateral aspect of the neck in sea turtles. It is located one-third the distance from the carapace to the head, cranial to the cranial edge of the carapace. The head is directed forward and down and the needle is introduced lateral to the midline on either side.
- The occipital venous sinus has been described in freshwater turtles and is located midline below the occipitus. It requires that the head be restrained firmly and in an extended ventroflexed (45–90° angle from the carapace) position. The needle is then introduced midline just caudal to the occipitus and nearly perpendicular to the spine. Lymph contamination is a possibility.
- The subcarpacal sinus or supravertebral sinus is located under the carapace just caudal to the last cervical vertebra and craniad to the first thoracic vertebra. This sinus can be approached by pressing the head into the shell and palpating for the first thoracic vertebra (incorporated into the carapace). The needle should be directed through the skin just caudal to the juncture of the last cervical vertebra up towards the carapace and first thoracic vertebra.
- The jugular veins are located on the lateral sides of the neck at about the level of the tympanum. In some species venepuncture of the jugular vein is relatively straightforward and can be visualized or a small skin incision can be made to facilitate direct visualization. Unfortunately, this technique requires the neck to be fully extended and in unco-operative animals, a short-acting anesthetic or tranquilizer may be required.
- Intraosseous techniques have been described using the plastron/plastron bridge but needles/catheters may end up in an intracoelomic rather than intraosseous position. The technique is described as passing a needle at an angle through the bony bridge between the plastron and carapace.

recurrence and promote healing of damage' (modified from Molony [76]). The experience of pain in non-human animals may be similar to the experience in humans but it is important to consider that among classes and species of animals, pain may differ quantitatively and qualitatively.

There are many gaps present in our understanding of reptile nociception, pain, consciousness, and suffering and although tempting, extrapolation from other vertebrate lineages should be undertaken cautiously. Reptiles have undergone millions of years of independent biologic evolution, separate from other vertebrate classes. While it is appealing to assume that all lineages of vertebrates have evolved similar survival strategies, it may also be somewhat presumptuous. It is true that the ability to sense noxious stimulus or potentially damaging stimuli is arguably necessary for the survival of all animals (invertebrates and vertebrates) but it is the significance of this sensation to the individual that remains less clear. Does the ability to perceive and suffer from pain, as defined in human terms, offer an evolutionary or biologic advantage to all animals or only some animals (i.e., humans)? Unfortunately, this is a complex and elusive question but one that nonetheless merits investigation. Regardless of an animal's ability to experience pain and suffering as a negative emotional response, the aim should be to limit the biologic perturbations associated with the physiologic (nociceptive) processing accompanying a noxious stimulus.

Evidence for pain in reptiles

Various criteria have been used to evaluate the balance of evidence for the presence or absence of pain in animals. These criteria as they pertain to reptiles are briefly described below.

Presence of nociceptors

The origination of the sensation associated with a noxious stimulus, transduction, occurs in specialized sensory nerve endings called nociceptors. Primarily nociceptive neurons (slowly adapting polymodal C-fibers) have not been identified in reptiles. However, there is no evidence in the literature that they have been sought and not found but rather no one has looked specifically for these types of fibers. However, high-threshold A-δ mechanical nociceptors [77] and C-fiber mechanical nociceptors [78] have been identified in one species of snake. These fibers are nociceptors capable of transmitting nociceptive information.

Ascending transmission pathways

Spinothalamic projections analogous to the neospinothalamic (fast pain) and paleospinothalamic (slow pain) tracts have been identified [79] in reptiles and are presumed to be capable of transmitting nociceptive information from the body to the brain. Trigeminal tracts have also been identified [77,80] that may be capable of transmitting pain from the head to the brain. Unfortunately, there are no functional studies examining the role of these pathways in nociceptive processing.

Brain structures

Reptiles appear to possess brain structures necessary for experiencing pain (neocortex) and morphologically there are direct spinal connections to the brainstem and dorsal thalamus in the midbrain. However, once again functional studies are lacking and it is possible and even likely that brain processing of information may occur differently in different animals. For example, in some animals smell and vision are highly developed and vast regions of the brain are dedicated to these activities, possibly producing sensations far beyond those a human could experience or even imagine.

It has been suggested that differences in reptiles' brain systems compared to birds and mammals may be ones of degrees of elaboration rather than presence or absence [81]. It is possible that the response to a noxious stimulus in reptiles is associated with less fidelity and scope compared to mammals. Perhaps a reptile's 'emotions' and the experience of pain are an "all or none" phenomena (rage or no rage, pain or no pain) rather than the graded experiences of human emotions (rage, anger, irritation, discontent, neutral, happiness, etc.). Certainly humans describe a range of painful experiences from those that are simply a mild irritant to those that are intolerable.

Nociceptive receptors and substances

The opioid system has been well studied in reptiles and the presence of opioid receptors and endogenous opioids has been described [82–85]. Their exact role, receptor subtypes present, and their anatomic locations are somewhat less clear. Although opioids are important for modulating the neural processing of noxious stimuli, they also play roles in many other body systems, such as the reproductive, thermoregulatory, gastrointestinal, and circadian systems. In addition, several nociceptive-related neuropeptides (i.e., glutamate, substance-P, calcitonin gene-related peptide) have been identified in reptiles but their functions are not well elucidated.

Known analgesic actions on nociceptive or nocifensive behaviors

It is important to note that behavioral evidence does not always suggest awareness or conscious recognition of the nociceptive stimulus (i.e., pain perception). Many of the tests used to examine an animal's response to a known or presumptive analgesic are actually measuring the effect the substance has on the animal's nociceptive or nocifensive response. Nocifensive is a poorly defined term that is sometimes used to describe the unconscious withdrawal or movement away from a noxious stimulus. It is a response that can occur below the level of consciousness and hence differs from the response associated specifically with pain perception.

Several experimental studies have examined the response of reptiles to substances known to be analgesic in mammals, primarily the opioids. These studies have involved evaluating responses to various types of noxious stimuli including thermal, mechanical, and chemical irritation. In general, these studies suggest that opioids reduce the response to some of these stimuli although there is inconsistency among the different experimental nociceptive models used, the response of different reptile species to similar testing situations, and the drugs themselves.

It must be noted that the inability to demonstrate a reduction in the nociceptive responses of an animal when administered a substance known to be analgesic in humans, or other animals, does not necessarily mean the substance has no effect on nociception, only that it did not have an effect given the specific experimental design used. There are numerous factors (i.e., dose, specific nociceptive model used, species, personnel involved, experimental conditions, etc.) that can affect the results and broad generalizations based on a single experiment should be made cautiously. For example, when reptiles are in the presence of something or someone that might be perceived as a threat (e.g., human), the reptile may appear to 'ignore' or minimize the significance of the noxious stimulus (e.g., heat) and hence their measurable responses to this insult. Tonic immobility is often used to describe the antipredator behavior demonstrated by many prey species. This response is associated with modulation of ascending nociceptive pathways that appear to have an antinociceptive effect [86–88]. The lack of normal response to a noxious stimulus could certainly influence the results of an experiment and should be considered when designing and evaluating experiments. However, with accumulating work and evidence, some trends useful for clinical decision making are being discovered.

Avoidance learning

There are no known studies of avoidance learning in response to a noxious stimulus in reptiles.

Suspension of normal behavior

Although there are no specific studies that have examined the suspension of normal behaviors in reptiles experiencing what one might call pain, there is reasonable anecdotal information from clinicians and reptile owners. These experiences suggest that a reptile's normal behaviors (eating, basking, social interaction) are altered by animal pain and the provision of an appropriate analgesic will hasten the resumption of these normal behaviors compared to allowing the animal's discomfort to diminish naturally. Of course, this is anecdotal and the observations are undoubtedly influenced by preconceived biases and beliefs, including a belief that analgesics can hasten recovery from pain.

Amphibian anesthesia

Providing anesthesia and analgesia for amphibians is a challenge for most clinicians but due to the growing popularity of amphibians as pets, it is an increasingly needed service. Amphibians are also used extensively in laboratory research and display exhibitions and from an animal welfare aspect, it is necessary to provide this service with knowledge and skill. A solid understanding of anatomy and physiology of the wide variety of species in this group of animals is essential for providing good perioperative anesthesia care.

The class Amphibia has three orders with over 4500 species and newly discovered species are added every year [89,90]. The order Anura represents frogs and toads (over 3500 living species), the order Caudata (around 375 species) includes salamanders, newts, and sirens, and the order Gymnophiona includes the caecilians (88 species) [89]. Each species has its own anatomic and physiologically unique features and extrapolations from one species to the other are not always possible. In addition, there are a limited number of studies to help guide anesthesia and pain management in amphibians.

Anatomy and physiology

Metamorphosis

Amphibians change significantly throughout their life with a metamorphosis from strictly aquatic egg and larval stages to an adult stage that can be terrestrial, semi-aquatic or aquatic [91]. This metamorphosis includes the loss of the tail and gills, development of lungs, transformation from a two-chambered to a three-chambered heart, and development of four legs [91–93]. The unique features that stand out in amphibians are the multiple forms of breathing (gills, lungs, skin, and buccopharyngeal), the three-chambered heart, semi-permeable skin, a renal portal system, and ectothermic temperature regulation.

Metabolism and thermoregulation

Amphibians are ectotherms. Each species has a preferred optimum temperature and has limited tolerance to temperature changes. Changes will affect metabolism, fluid regulation, and activity levels [94]. In general, amphibians require cooler temperatures than reptiles and ambient temperatures of 23.8–26.7 °C (75–80 °F) are reported to be an acceptable range for most species during the perianesthetic period [92,94]. Species-specific needs (tropical vs subtropical species) should be identified and temperatures adjusted. To optimize ambient humidity, levels should be maintained above 70% [92].

Cardiovascular system

The cardiovascular system of adult amphibians is composed of a three-chambered heart, an arterial/venous vascular system and an extensive lymphatic system, in comparison to tadpoles that only have a two-chambered heart and a single loop circulation system, similar to fish [93]. The adult amphibian heart has two atria and one ventricle and is considered to have an incomplete double circulation [95,96]. The heart lies internally underneath the pectoral girdle and sternum and a heart beat can be visualized on the ventral surface (midline just caudal to the level of the animal's shoulder) [91,93]. The right atrium is larger than the left atrium in all amphibians and the ventricle is thick-walled with numerous tabercules found in many species [93]. In caudatas the interatrial septum can be incomplete (fenestrated) but in anurans it is complete [92,93].

All of the venous blood arrives at the sinus venosus and enters the right atrium [95,96]. The arterialized blood flows into the left atrium and both atria empty into the one ventricle. During ventricular systole, the blood is pumped into the bulbus cordis from where three main arteries leave (carotid artery, aorta, and pulmocutaneous artery) [95–97]. The carotid artery sends oxygenated blood to the head, the aorta sends oxygenated mixed blood to the body, and the pulmocutaneous artery sends mostly venous blood to skin and lungs to pick up oxygen [96–98]. The ventricle in frogs, toads, and salamanders is anatomically one ventricle but is functionally divided due to the slit-like trabercular meshwork, that keeps arterial (oxygenated) blood on the left side of the ventricle and venous (desaturated) blood on the right side by creating a laminar flow pattern and preventing mixing during contraction [96–100]. Additionally, a spiral valve in the bulbus cordis will create spiral streaming of blood flow and direction of more oxygenated blood to the carotid artery and aorta from the left side of the ventricle, while the pulmocutaneous arteries receive more venous blood [96]. The septa between the three different arteries also help guide the blood flow, depending on cardiac output [96,100].

The amphibian lymphatic system is characterized by a high rate of lymph production and circulation with the function of draining fluids from the tissue and returning it to circulation [101]. The lymphatic system includes lymph hearts that lie in junctions of veins and which beat irregularly or synchronically at 50–60 bpm depending on the fluid status of the animal [101]. Various numbers of lymph hearts are present depending on species. Frogs and salamanders have fewer (e.g., 4–20) than caecilians (e.g., 100–200) [93]. These lymph hearts function to preserve unidirectional flow of lymph back to the heart and to return proteins to the circulation [93,101]. Lymph is mainly formed from plasma filtration as well as transcutaneous water uptake. Lymph collects in large subcutaneous lymph sacs (especially in anurans) and flows through afferent pores into the lymph hearts [101]. The lymph sacs can give indications of disease and fluid load when enlarged [92,94,101].

Both salamanders and anurans have a renal portal system and a hepatic portal system [93,94,97,102]. For the renal portal system, the veins from the hindlegs of the animal unite into the Jacobson's veins, which are paired and flow through the kidneys before entering the postcaval vein. Blood that flows through the hepatic portal vein system will flow from the ventral abdominal vein through the liver before entering the postcaval vein and returning to the heart. The factors that regulate the renal portal system are not fully understood, but the renal portal and hepatic portal systems may impact the pharmacokinetics of drugs that are given in hindlegs or tail (first-pass effect) so anesthetics are in some instances are preferentially injected into the front end of the animal.

Specific vessels for venipuncture in amphibians are the ventral abdominal vein, the femoral and the lingual vein (lingual venous plexus on underside of tongue in anurans) and the tail vein in caudatas [90,103]. Depending on the size of the animal, these can be used for blood collection or administration of anesthetic agents.

Respiratory system

Adult amphibians have up to four different modes of respiration. Most prominent are pulmonic and cutaneous gas exchange and buccopharyngeal (gular or guttural) breathing [93]. Aquatic salamanders also breathe via external gills (branchial mode) [93]. The buccal cavity and pharynx is used for gas exchange and can either be viewed as an extension of cutaneous respiration or its own entity due to its specific muscular pumping activity and unique vascular supply [93]. Cutaneous respiration is possible due to a large surface area (often increased via skinfolds), a very thin and semi-permeable epidermis, and a dermis that is highly vascularized [93]. This form of breathing is important as it is an efficient form of respiration during anesthesia.

The anatomic lungs in amphibians come in various shapes and sizes from small simple sac-like structures (aquatic species) to sacculated forms with alveoli in the anterior lung area (terrestrial species) [93]. The lungs are located cranially in amphibians following a short trachea with cartilaginous rings. The lungs have pulmonic epithelium that can easily be damaged with overventilation or an endotracheal tube placed too far distally [91,104]. Endotracheal tubes should be placed just past the larynx [90,91,93,104]. The mode of respiration may change in various species depending on oxygen and carbon dioxide tension of the environment [103,105]. When administered 100% oxygen, the animal commonly stops breathing through their lungs or via the buccopharyngeal movements and is primarily relying on cutaneous respiration [103]. This complicates assessment of anesthetic depth, ventilation, and oxygenation. For cutaneous respiration to be efficient, the skin must be kept moist [94]. The permeability of the skin for gas exchange varies in different species (toads have thicker and less permeable skin).

Cutaneous system and fluid regulation

Amphibian skin is an important organ for immune functions and water regulation [92]. Evaporation through the skin is a major contributing factor of water loss (particularly on the dorsal surface) [92,94]. Uptake of water from the environment is managed from the ventral surface, including a functional structure in the pelvic area called the 'drinking patch' which contributes 80% of water uptake in anurans [94]. Only a very small percentage of water intake is from gastrointestinal uptake; therefore oral fluid supplementation will be less effective than keeping an animal moist by soaking in an appropriate fluid (e.g., isotonic or hypotonic water) [92,94]. Osmolality of the environmental fluid is particularly important in aquatic amphibians as the difference between external fluid and plasma osmolality will determine water regulation and movement. Amphibians can change the composition of their plasma to tolerate fluctuations in water osmolality, but an imbalance can lead to volume overload when the kidneys are compromised [94]. The high permeability of amphibian skin allows for absorption of exogenous compounds like drugs and toxic substances.

Clinical anesthesia

Preanesthetic considerations

Species-specific knowledge about the particular amphibian patient is helpful for anesthesia planning and delivery. Using hypothermia is outdated and providing adequate anesthesia and analgesia is the standard of care. There is still a need for species-specific studies for amphibians as well as clinical anesthesia publications.

Physical examination and restraint

The amphibian patient should be evaluated before anesthesia, similar to any other species, to detect abnormalities that may increase the risk of anesthetic complications. Observation in its enclosure will provide information on general activity level and demeanor, breathing pattern, and hydration. Due to the sensitivity of the amphibian skin, premoistened and talc-free latex gloves should be worn when handling to reduce the risk of skin damage and transfer of pathogens and toxins to or from both handler and animal [90,92,103]. Secretion of toxins from the skin is common in many amphibian species and can lead to irritation, various degrees of illness, and potentially death (some poisonous frogs can produce lethal toxins) [92,103]. Other skin secretions of some species can be gluey or foul-smelling, which are difficult to remove from the handler and cause discomfort [103]. Some species are able to expel their secretion over quite a distance and protective eyewear should be considered [103].

The water/fluids used to moisten the latex gloves and the water used to keep the animal wet should be distilled and dechlorinated to prevent chlorine uptake via the skin [90–92,103]. Some handlers also suggest coating the gloves with a non-toxic water-soluble gel to provide better skin protection in species with delicate skin [103].

Amphibians often show an instinctive flight response and should be gently restrained to prevent falling or escape. Restraint should be as brief, efficient, stress free, comfortable, and safe for the animal as possible. Some species struggle, others cease in resignation, although a potential sudden burst of activity to escape should always be anticipated [103]. In animals that seem very stressed and difficult to restrain, a clear plastic or glass jar or plastic bag can be used to facilitate the handling. Many anurans tend to fill themselves with air when they are stressed which can make a physical examination more difficult [92]. Often amphibians urinate when stressed or handled and the lack of this behavior may be an indication of dehydration [92]. Dehydrated amphibians show skin tenting and sunken eyes, feel tacky and show decreased activity and mentation, so rehydration is important before attempting anesthesia [92].

Restraint is successfully performed in caudatas by encircling the animal behind their forelimbs with the index finger and thumb with the remaining fingers enclosing the body [90,103]. Salamanders have a tail autotomy reflex so the tail should be handled with care [90,103]. Some anurans can bite and bigger species can be held by grasping them on a skinfold on their back behind the front legs or by holding them immediately anterior to the hindlegs with one hand and around the front legs with the second hand [90,103]. Sometimes chemical immobilization is necessary for a thorough physical examination.

Hypocalcemia is a common problem in amphibians and the hypocalcemic animal may present with tetany, muscle fasciculations, paresis, GI stasis, and bloating [94]. Hypocalcemia can be treated with calcium gluconate in a bath as calcium is readily taken up via the skin [92,94]. Blood chemistry analysis is not generally done before anesthesia to minimize stress of restraint but can be done after induction if a more thorough clinical evaluation is desired.

Fasting

In general, fasting is not necessary as amphibians can maintain a closed larynx and risk of aspiration is minimal. Fasting is reserved for species that eat large rodent prey and recommendations are to fast these species for 24–48 h prior to anesthesia to decrease risk of ileus and facilitate visualization during coelemic procedures [91].

Anesthetic agents

There are various anesthetic drugs that can be used with amphibians. Selection depends on the procedure to be performed, level of immobilization needed, and duration of anesthesia. Options include immersion in MS-222, clove oil or less commonly benzocaine. MS-222 is most commonly used and seems to have a wide margin of safety in most species, but does need buffering with sodium bicarbonate in amphibians [91,106,107]. Clove oil and its different compounds eugenol and isoeugenol have become popular throughout the last few years and show species-specific different responses in amphibians [108,109]. A common side-effect is a gastric prolapse, which might be due to the pungent taste of clove oil [110]. Clove oil is administered via immersion and might cause cutaneous necrosis in some species when administered directly on the skin of the animal [111].

Topical (cutaneous) administration of various agents like sevoflurane or isoflurane liquid mixed in KY jelly has been reported and seems to have species-specific variability in effect [112]. Isoflurane can also be bubbled through the water via an anesthetic delivery system (routine anesthesia machine) [112,113]. This method has the disadvantage of high exposure levels of waste gases for the humans in the surrounding environment. To decrease the risk, sealed containers should be used, which conversely makes handling of the patient difficult. Induction times are slow and recovery times rapid as soon as the patient is removed from the bath [91]. Parenteral injections of propofol, alfaxalone, ketamine or α_2-adrenergic receptor agonists have been reported, but show wide species-specific variability, unpredictable inductions and recoveries, and undesirable mortality rates [91,114]. Propofol can be used in the form of an immersion bath for chemical restraint and sedation (but not surgical anesthesia) [115]. Premedication can be done in some species but is not routinely performed. However, the administration of an analgesic with or without a sedative before induction may be beneficial, particularly in bigger species.

Monitoring

Heart rate (HR), respiration rate, and anesthetic depth are most commonly monitored during amphibian anesthesia. As normal heart rates differ from species to species, a baseline HR should ideally be obtained in the individual before anesthesia. If this is not practical due to stress on the animal, a baseline HR should be taken immediately after induction so a trend can be formed. Heart rate can be obtained by visualization or with the help of a small Doppler probe placed over the heart (at the xiphoid process of the sternum). An electrocardiogram can show good tracings of electrical events, but care should be taken to avoid skin damage with alligator clips or electrode patches. Hypodermic needles (27 gauge) can be inserted through the skin and alligator clips then fastened to the needles. The oesophageal ECG (single probe) is an excellent alternative to the external ECG set-up [107]. Knowledge about normal heart rate values in the different amphibian species is limited although the belief is that overall amphibians have relatively low HR values (approximately 50 bpm) [94].

Under anesthesia, HR trends will provide information about the animal's status. A sudden drop or slow decrease of HR over time will suggest an increase in depth and adjustments to anesthetic administration should be made. Adjustments are made by changing the anesthetic concentration of the bath (diluting or, in case of desired increase in depth, concentrating of the anesthetic agent in the solution). Alternatively, syringes filled with desired anesthetic concentrations can be premade and used as needed to lighten or deepen the anesthetic depth via flushing the solution over the skin of the amphibian [91].

The stages of anesthesia have been reported by various clinicians [91,103,104]. Cessation of movement and loss of the righting reflex is often the first indication that anesthetic induction is complete. A light stage is assumed when the righting reflex is lost and abdominal breathing movement stopped. Surgical anesthetic depth is reached when the withdrawal reflex is lost (e.g., no response to toe pinch in hindleg) and no gular respiration is present. Gular respiration can be visualized as the movement under the mandible and along the ventral neck. Although apnea is common (i.e., unable to visualize gular and/or abdominal breathing), cutaneous respiration is still present as long as the dermis is kept moist to enable gas exchange [91]. Intubation is commonly not necessary unless it is a larger species with poor permeability of the dermis or other concerns about oxygenation are present [91]. A narrow glottis can make intubation challenging [107]. Due to the short trachea, the endotracheal tube is placed not much further than just past the larynx. Pulse oximetry has not yet been validated in amphibians so it is primarily used to monitor trends. Intraoperative support is provided by assuring that adequate thermal support, adequate fluid uptake, and adequate analgesia for painful procedures are addressed.

Recovery

The recovery phase in amphibians can be prolonged and close monitoring may reduce complications. Any residual topical anesthetic should be rinsed off and the animal recovered on room air. The surface and skin should be kept moist with fluid. Withdrawal reflexes will return first with an increase of the gular respiration. The righting reflex should strengthen and the animals start moving around with improving co-ordination. Most recoveries are smooth and rather slow, but some amphibians may go through a phase of excitement and erratic movements that need to be monitored to prevent injuries. The animal should only be returned to its normal environment when fully recovered to prevent accidental drowning [90,107].

Analgesia is an important aspect of adequate anesthesia management in any species, including amphibians. Research has demonstrated that amphibians have a well-established endogenous opioid system and that opioids are effective in providing pain relief [116–119]. Behavior studies demonstrate an alteration of behavior and avoidance of painful stimuli, suggesting that amphibians have a sense of discomfort [120,121]. The presence of nociceptive structures and pathways in some amphibian species is comparable with mammalian pathways [122,123]. The afferent sensory fibers of frogs show the same characteristics as mammalian sensory afferent fibers: large and medium myelinated A-fibers, small myelinated B-fibers, and small unmyelinated C-fibers [121,122,124]. The sensory afferent fibers then connect in the dorsal area of the frog's spinal cord [122,125]. Neurotransmitters associated with nociceptive transmission (e.g., substance P, glutamate) and endorphinergic neurons to inhibit the release of substance P are also present in the amphibian spinal cord. It has also been recognized that peripheral sensitization to noxious stimuli can occur [121,126,127]. Opioid receptors and endogenous opioid peptides are highly evolved in amphibian brain and spinal cord [119,121,122,128].

Dermorphin is a potent amphibian-specific opioid compound that is present in the skin of certain South American frog species [121,129–131]. It is considered to be 40 time more potent than morphine with its main activity as a full μ-agonist [130]. Deltorphine is another endogenous opioid peptide produced in the skin of another frog genus, acting as a potent δ-receptor agonist [130]. The functional role of dermorphin in amphibians is not clear, but speculations have been made about its role as protection from predators, or playing a role in hibernation.

The ascending nociceptive pathways from the spinal cord to the brain are not fully understood in amphibians [122] and the projection to the telencephalon seems less organized, but is recognized [107]. The perception of pain and subsequent suffering in amphibians is an ongoing debate due to the lack of a cerebral and/or limbic cortex [121,122,124]. Independent of that debate, nociception appears to be well developed and analgesics should be used when painful procedures are performed to prevent any physiologic and pathophysiologic consequences of the upregulation of the nociceptive pathway, including a significant stress response.

Various studies have been performed to assess efficacy of different analgesic agents [92,120,123,132–136]. Most recommendations come from studies conducted with acetic acid applied to the skin as the noxious stimulus [123]. Very little research has focused on clinical analgesia, but some recommendations have been made by clinicians who perform amphibian anesthesia in clinical settings. It should be kept in mind that species-specific differences are likely present and that extrapolations from one species to the next may have varying effects in onset, duration, and efficacy.

All opioids (including butorphanol, morphine, buprenorphine, and fentanyl) seem to have a dose-dependent effect with relatively long durations and lower margins of safety at high doses compared to other domesticated species [92,120,123,132,133]. The α_2-adrenergic receptor agonists (e.g., xylazine and dexmedetomidine) also provide long-lasting analgesia and can be used without producing immobilization [123,134–136].

Fish anesthesia

Fish anesthesia has significantly improved over the past 10 years with the enhanced understanding of species-specific physiology in response to anesthesia [137,138]. To date, there are over 30 000 different species of fish with dissimilar anatomy and physiology and adapted to various diverse aquatic ecosystems. Their classification is constantly changing but currently 4500 genera, 515 families, and 62 orders are recognized.

The teleosts (jawed fish) are the biggest group among fish. Other less common groups are the ray-finned fishes (Acinopteryii), lobe-finned fishes (Sarcopterygii), and jawless fishes (Agnatha) [138,139]. A daunting number of differences in relation to water temperature, water quality and salinity, behavior and response to drugs make anesthesia in fish a challenge [138].

Anatomy and physiology

Respiratory system

Most fish use gills for respiration, but various adaptations have been made in many fish species depending on oxygen availability and demand. The gills are located behind the head in the buccal cavity and are covered by a sturdy flap (e.g., the operculum in bony fish) for protection. A gill consists of a gill arch, a filament, and a comprehensive vascular system. These highly folded, highly vascular, very thin membranes make for efficient gas exchange. The vascular anatomy consists of a branchial basket, that arises from the aorta, and afferent branchial arteries that branch off to supply the arch and bifurcate further into afferent filamental arteries which end at the tip of the filament [140]. Off the afferent filamental artery divert the afferent lamellar arterioles to supply the lamella. Blood flows through the lamella via various channels and blood gases (O_2 and CO_2) are exchanged in agreement with the concepts of maximal surface area contact, changes in blood flow velocity, and optimal O_2 gradient tensions. The short efferent lamellar arterioles arise and provide blood flow back into efferent filamental arteries and at the base of the filament the blood flows into the efferent branchial arteries that later form the lateral aorta [140]. These vessels are the arterio-arterial circulation. A countercurrent system to optimize oxygen uptake is present in many fish. The venous blood moves in the opposite direction to the water, to create a more favorable gradient between the oxygen in the blood and water to maximize uptake [140]. The fish will draw in water through its mouth (flap over the gills is closed) and the water is pushed out over the gills by closing the mouth and opening the gill cover. Some species force water over the gills to achieve more efficient ventilation for increased metabolic demand and varying degrees of this ram ventilation are used in specific species (rhythmic movements of lower jaw and opercula or consistent movement through water) [138,141]. The number of gills vary in different species (e.g., 3–7 arches). Additional functions of the gills include osmoregulation, nitrogen excretion, hormone metabolism, and acid–base regulation [140].

The skin also functions as a respiratory organ. Highly vascular skin, particularly in the young, can facilitate diffusion of gases. This ability is species dependent but can make up 30% of respiration in some [142]. Therefore skin should be handled carefully and with wet gloves to prevent damage. Various other modifications and adaptations have evolved in different fish species and a thorough knowledge of the species-specific respiratory functions is crucial for understanding the impact it may have on anesthesia [138].

Cardiovascular system

The cardiovascular system in fish is considered a single cycle closed-loop circulation system. This means that the four-chambered heart pumps blood in a single circuit through the body, picking up oxygen on the way through the gills. The heart itself consists of a sinus venosus, a single atrium, a ventricle, and a bulbus arteriosus. It is commonly referred to as a two-chambered heart or a four-chambered heart arranged in series [143]. Blood is pumped out of the single-chambered ventricle into the bulbus arteriosus through a pair of ventricular-bulbar valves at the ventricular–bulbar junction. The bulbus arteriosus is in most fish non-contractile but elastic and resembles a bulge at the base of the aorta [143]. In sharks this bulbus arteriosus is called the conus arteriosus with contractile cardiac muscle fibers and several rows of valves [143]. Blood flows from the aorta to the gills for oxygenation and then to the body. The hepatic and the common cardinal veins drain blood returning from the body into the sinus venosus (a sac-like contractile structure) [143] before blood flows into the atrium. At the sinoatrial junction the atrium and the sinus venosus are separated by a sinoatrial valve that regulates the flow into the atrium. From the thin-walled but muscular atrium, the blood is pumped back into the ventricle through a pair of atrioventricular valves at the atrioventricular junction. The valves ensure unidirectional blood flow [143].

On an ECG (pre- and postcordial leads), the P wave represents the onset of atrial (auricular) contraction. The QRS represents the invasion of the ventricle, with the P-R interval corresponding to the time for the impulse to cross the atrium and the atrioventricular junction. The T wave represents the repolarization of the ventricle [144]. Fish do seem to have a baroreceptor reflex that slows heart rate when arterial blood pressure increases [144]. A branchiocardiac reflex exists (increasing heart rate with increasing respiratory rate) to ensure optimal oxygen uptake. This reflex can be utilized with the described 'buccal flow/heart rate reflex' which increases heart rate by increasing water flow rate through the buccal cavity (either by moving fish through the water or flowing anesthetic-free water through the buccal cavity/gills to hasten elimination of anesthetics) [138,145,146].

Nervous system

Fish, like vertebrates, have a peripheral and a central nervous system. The peripheral nervous system can be functionally divided into a somatic division (responsible for motor and sensory activity) and an autonomic division, which includes a sympathetic, parasympathetic, and enteric nervous system [147]. The central nervous system includes a spinal cord, medulla oblongata and a brain, which has a telencephalon, diencephalon (epithalamus, thalamus, hypothalamus), mesencephalon, and a cerebellum. Fish possess an archipallium but, like amphibians, lack a neopallium in the cerebrum [147].

Fish are easily stressed, resulting in high morbidity and mortality [147–149]. Main stressors are water quality changes (e.g., temperature, pH, nitrogenous waste concentration), handling, transportation, disease, noise and light abnormalities, inadequate nutrition, stocking, and many more [147]. Fish react to stress via a neuroendocrine response that includes the adrenergic system and the hypothalamic-pituitary-inter-renal axis [147]. Various factors and neurotransmitters play a role including corticotropin-releasing factor, adrenocorticotropic hormone, catecholamines, etc. [147]. Fish show three stages of the stress response depending on duration and intensity of the stressing factor (e.g., primary, secondary and tertiary stress response) [147,150,151]. The primary response is similar to mammals via a neuroendocrine pathway resulting in fight or flight response through a catecholamine release [147,152]. With persistent stress, consistent circulation of cortisol and catecholamines will lead to the secondary response resulting in increase in cardiac output, metabolic rate, respiration, lactic acid, and fatty acids [147,153]. Continuing chronic stress leads to the tertiary stress response, which manifests as physiologic exhaustion, including decreased immune function, reproduction, growth rate, changes in behavior, and increased mortality [147,150,151,154].

Nociception in fish is considered a stress factor that elicits a strong response. After reception of nociceptive signals from nociceptors, signals travel via the peripheral nerves (C- or A-δ fibers, depending on species and pain stimulus) [147]. Similar to mammals, the signal is sent via the spinothalamic and trigeminal tracts to the brain. Fish have a functional endogenous opioid system and all four opioid receptor types have been identified [116,118,147,153,155–157]. An ongoing debate and current research are investigating if fish are able to experience pain or a pain-like state [147,158–163]. Even though this question remains unanswered, it is accepted that fish have a functional nociception system and are capable of nociception and respond with stress to a noxious stimulus [146,147,159]. Since this response to noxious stimulus is present, most scientists and clinicians should aim to provide analgesia to alleviate the stress response [147,164–166]. Recommendations have been published for analgesics used in fish that undergo surgical procedures. Focus has been on NSAIDs, local anesthetics, and opioids [104,138,147,148,167,168].

Thermoregulation

Almost all fish are ectothermic, meaning that anesthesia is impacted when water temperatures are outside their optimal temperature ranges. Induction time and recovery are usually prolonged in lower temperatures due to decreased respiratory rates and cardiac output, and slower metabolism [167,169]. Acidosis and hypercapnia occur at higher temperatures, leading to hyperventilation and subsequently decreased induction and recovery times [169]. Tuna and some shark species have developed the ability of endothermy by conserving heat and increasing body temperature above ambient water temperatures.

Overview of clinical anesthesia of fish

Neiffer has provided an excellent description of fish anesthesia in *Zoo Animal and Wildlife Immobilization and Anesthesia* [138], with detailed species-specific drug information. The following will provide a general overview of fish anesthesia and the reader is directed to Neiffer's chapter for specific details on bony fish anesthesia.

Considerations for fish anesthesia

All fish are anesthetized or sedated in water. Anesthesia is commonly performed via immersion in a water bath and subsequently maintained in flow-by systems. In larger species injectable anesthesia can be used to facilitate smooth induction. It is important that all water quality parameters are similar to the water of the fish's normal environment. This includes the water temperature, salinity, pH, and mineral composition (hardness) [166]. Water from the fish's tank (environment) is commonly used for induction and anesthesia.

The equipment, drug concentrations, and dosing depend on the species, size, and condition. Similar to mammals, bigger fish need less drug per unit weight.

Anesthetic drugs used for fish anesthesia include tricaine methanesulfonate (MS-222), benzocaine, metomidate, isoeugenol, 2-pheoxyethanol, and quinaldine. Simplistically, MS-222 is a local anesthetic which blocks the voltage-gated sodium channels leading to the inhibition of action potentials and nerve conduction [170]. Its anesthetic mechanism of action is not fully understood, but has been attributed to a peripheral and central effect by blocking Na^+ channels and to a lesser extent K^+ and Ca^{2+} channels as well as activation of secondary messenger via membrane-bound protein activation [170]. Muscle relaxation, sedation, and cardiovascular and respiratory depression occur in a dose-dependent manner. MS-222 is administered by immersion and uptake is via the gills and skin. MS-222 is rapidly biotransformed via acetylation into polar and non-polar metabolites [171] and excreted via gills and kidney. Continual administration of MS-222 via flow-through to the gills can be used to maintain anesthesia. The concentration can be changed to adjust depth of anesthesia. MS-222 is water soluble and the dissolution of the drug into water may decrease pH. Depending on the optimal water pH for a specific fish species, water may need to be buffered to assure ideal water quality. Buffer requirements depend on the anesthetic concentration used and the alkalinity of the water source [172]. Salt water usually is more alkaline and has a natural buffering capacity [168]. MS-222 is the only FDA-approved anesthetic for fish with a withdraw time of 21 days [173].

Benzocaine is also a local anesthetic but has the disadvantage that it needs to be dissolved in an organic solvent (ethanol or acetone) before addition to water and use as an immersion anesthetic. Metomidate is a non-barbiturate hypnotic that inhibits $GABA_A$ receptors. Metomidate decreases cortisol release by blocking the hypothalamus-pituitary-inter-renal axis activation [174]. Administration of metomidate is by immersion or oral administration. Isoeugenol is a compound of clove oil and has become a commonly used fish anesthetic (Aqui-S™). Its use is associated with cardiorespiratory depression and stress response and the agent has been controversial due to its potential carcinogenic properties.

Combinations of drugs have been explored to decrease the adverse effects associated with the use of a single anesthetic in higher doses. Adjunctive drugs that have been combined with the anesthetic agents include benzodiazepines, opioids, and NSAIDs. Morphine has been used as an analgesic in fish and shows promising effectiveness in some species. It appears to have a long duration of action [175–177]. Butorphanol and buprenorphine appear to have limited analgesic effects in the species studied [164,178].

Parenteral administration of anesthetic agents (intravenous, intramuscular, and intracoelomic) in addition to parenteral (oral) administration can be used as an alternative to immersion in some larger species. The most practical method with the least potential for damage is intramuscular administration. The ideal injection site in most species is the dorsal saddle area, which is located around the dorsal fin [137]. Problems associated with intramuscular anesthetic use include unreliable response, prolonged recovery, and the need for ventilatory support [146,168,179]. These problems may be influenced by health condition, age, stress, body condition and others, that can lead to varying degrees of response. This form of anesthetic administration can help in circumstances where tank induction is not practical (big species, big holding facilities, and personal safety requirements such as for sharks, rays, etc.) [179,180]. Injections can be performed with a pole syringe or an underwater dart gun, or by hand injection [181]. Injectable anesthetic agents used are species dependent and include azaperone, medetomidine or dexmedetomidine with ketamine, alfaxalone or propofol.

Preanesthetic considerations

Fasting fish for 12–24h is recommended when possible to reduce the amount of nitrogenous waste production (ammonia and nitrite). High levels of nitrogenous waste compounds may decrease oxygenation, lead to acidemia and methemoglobinemia, and may affect uptake and metabolism of anesthetic agents [146]. The risk of regurgitation can be reduced when the fish is fasted. Regurgitation can lead to obstruction of gills [146,182].

Anesthetic depth can be monitored by assessing muscle relaxation via jaw tone and body muscle tone in addition to monitoring heart rate and respiratory rate. Evaluating loss of righting reflex and responsiveness to stimuli is also important. Fish show similar signs and stages of anesthetic depth as mammals and various descriptions have been published throughout the literature [146,166,183].

In general, fish anesthesia is subdivided into three levels or stages (light, surgical, deep). Depending on the fish species, the characteristics of a specific level might have different attributes. Surgical anesthesia will be associated with a loss of equilibrium, loss of reaction to pressure on peduncle and loss of reaction to emersion with no activity and relaxed muscles. Respiratory rate and heart rate consistently decrease with increasing depth. Heart beats can be directly visualized in thin body-walled species but most species require a Doppler probe or an ECG to evaluate heart rate. The Doppler probe can be placed directly over the heart or into the opercular slit. ECG clips can be placed on the fins or attached to hypodermic needles placed through the skin. ECG electrode patches are not recommended due to concern for damaging the skin. Respiratory rate is monitored by observing gill movements. With increasing depth of anesthesia movements will become reduced. If cardiac output is adequate, flow-by of water through the gills will provide adequate gas exchange, but it is recommended to decrease the anesthetic concentration. Flowing water through the gills is easily achieved by moving the fish through the water, but in most situations where surgery is performed, a recirculating water system is required to allow procedures on the fish while it remains out of the water.

The technique for performing flow-by anesthesia of fish can vary with the available equipment, but in general fish are induced in a tank with anesthetic added to the water. After achieving adequate depth of anesthesia, the fish is taken out of the water tank and placed on an elevated foam holder or padded fenestrated shelf inside a container which can collect circulated water. The buccal cavity is intubated with a bifurcated plastic tube (size depending on species) and connected to a non-recirculating or recirculating system (dependent on fish size) to supply aerated water containing anesthetics. Recirculating systems will reuse the collected water via a submersible variable-flow aquarium pump or manually via a syringe.

An example for a non-recirculating system is an intravenous fluid bag filled with water which contains anesthetic and an air stone for aeration. The bag (reservoir) is connected with a drip-set to tubing inserted into the buccal cavity [104,138,139,146]. Recommended flow rates are influenced by drug concentration, but 1–3 L/kg/min is common to assure the gills stay wet for optimal gas exchange but prevents gastric dilation which can occur at higher flow [146]. The fish's skin and cornea remain moistened by gently spraying water over the fish with a syringe.

At the end of the procedure the depth of anesthesia is lightened. Providing the fish has strong pulses and is ventilating well by itself, it is placed into a dedicated aerated recovery tank void of any anesthetics. The fish is held in an upright position and moved through the water to provide flow of oxygenated water across the gills for washout. The fish will gradually be able to hold itself up and start swimming with decreasing degrees of incoordination. The fish should be monitored during recovery to prevent injury.

References

1 Sladky KK, Mans C. Clinical anesthesia in reptiles. *J Exot Pet Med* 2012; **21**: 17–31.

2 Fleming GJ. Crocodilians (crocodiles, alligators, caimans, gharial). In: West G, Heard DJ, Caulkett N, eds. *Zoo Animal and Wildlife Immobilization and Anesthesia*. Ames, IA: Blackwell Publishing, 2007; 223–231.

3 Bertelsen MF. Squamates (snakes and lizards). In: West G, Heard DJ, Caulkett N, eds. *Zoo Animal and Wildlife Immobilization and Anesthesia*. Ames, IA: Blackwell Publishing, 2007; 233–243.

4 Schumacher J. Chelonians (turtles, tortoises, and terrapins). In: West G, Heard DJ, Caulkett N, eds. *Zoo Animal and Wildlife Immobilization and Anesthesia*. Ames, IA: Blackwell Publishing, 2007; 259–266.

5 Schumacher J, Yelen T. Anesthesia and analgesia. In: Mader DR, ed. *Reptile Medicine and Surgery*, 2nd edn. St Louis, MO: Saunders Elsevier, 2006; 442–452.

6 Schumacher J, Mans C. Anesthesia. In: Mader DR, Divers SJ, eds. *Current Therapy in Reptile Medicine and Surgery*. St Louis, MO: Elsevier Saunders, 2014; 134–153.

7 Baker LA, White FN. Redistribution of cardiac output in response to heating in *Iguana iguana*. *Comp Biochem Physiol* 1970; **35**: 253–262.

8 Varga M. Captive maintenance and welfare. In: Girling SJ, Raiti P, eds. *BSAVA Manual of Reptiles*, 2nd edn. Gloucester, UK: BSAVA Press, 2004; 6–17.

9 Preston DL, Mosley CA, Mason RT. Sources of variability in recovery time from methohexital sodium anesthesia in snakes. *Copeia* 2010; **3**: 496–501.

10 Ultsch GR, Jackson DC. Long-term submergence at 3 degrees C of the turtle Chrysemys picta bellii in normoxic and severely hypoxic water. III. Effects of changes in ambient PO2 and subsequent air breathing. *J Exp Biol* 1982; **97**: 87–99.

11 Andrews RM, Pough FH. Metabolism of squamate reptiles: allometric and ecological relationships. *Physiol Zool* 1985; **58**: 214–231.

12 Van Mierop LHS, Kutsche M. Some aspects of comparative anatomy of the heart. In: Johansen K, Burggren WW, eds. *Cardiovascular Shunts: Phylogenetic, Ontogenic and Clinical Aspects*. Copenhagen, Denmark: Munksgaard, 1985; 38–56.

13 Van Mierop LHS, Kutsche M. Comparitive anatomy of the ventricular septum. In: Wenick ACG, ed. *The Ventricular Septum in the Heart*. Boston, MA: Martinus Nijhoff, 1981; 35–46.

14 Comeau SG, Hicks JW. Regulation of central vascular blood flow in the turtle. *Am J Physiol* 1994; **267**: R569–578.

15 Herman J, Wang T, Smits AW, *et al*. The effects of artificial lung inflation on pulmonary blood flow and heart rate in the turtle Trachemys scripta. *J Exp Biol* 1997; **200**: 2539–2545.

16 Hicks JW, Ishimatsu A, Molloi S, *et al*. The mechanism of cardiac shunting in reptiles: a new synthesis. *J Exp Biol* 1996; **199**: 1435–1446.

17 Ishimatsu A, Hicks JW, Heisler N. Analysis of intracardiac shunting in the lizard, Varanus niloticus: a new model based on blood oxygen levels and microsphere distribution. *Respir Physiol* 1988; **71**: 83–100.

18 Heisler N, Neumann P, Maloiy GM. The mechanism of intracardiac shunting in the lizard Varanus exanthematicus. *J Exp Biol* 1983; **105**: 15–31.

19 Hicks JW, Malvin GM. Mechanism of intracardiac shunting in the turtle Pseudemys scripta. *Am J Physiol* 1992; **262**: R986–992.

20 Luckhardt AB, Carlson AJ. Studies on the visceral sensory nervous system. *Am J Physiol* 1921; **56**: 72–112.

21 White FN. Circulation. In: Gans C, Dawson WR, eds. *Biology of the Reptilia, Physiology A*. New York: Academic Press, 1976; 275–334.

22 Burggren WW, Glass ML, Johansen K. Pulmonary ventilation: perfusion relationships in terrestrial and aquatic chelonian reptiles. *Can J Zool* 1977; **55**: 2024–2034.

23 Milsom WK, Langille BL, Jones DR. Vagal control of pulmonary vascular resistance in the turtle Chrysemys scripta. *Can J Zool* 1977; **55**: 359–367.

24 Berger PJ, Burnstock G. Autonomic nervous system. In: Gans C, ed. *Biology of the Reptilia*. New York: Academic Press, 1979; 1–57.

25 Lillywhite HB, Donald JA. Pulmonary blood flow regulation in an aquatic snake. *Science* 1989; **245**: 293–295.

26 Burggren W, Farrell A, Lillywhite HB. Vertebrate cardiovascular systems. In: Dantzler WH, ed. *Handbook of Physiology*. New York: Oxford University Press, 1997; 254–267.

27 Berger PJ. The reptilian baroreceptor and its role in cardiovascular control. *Am Zool* 1987; **27**: 111–120.

28 Stinner JN. Cardiovascular and metabolic responses to temperature in Coluber constrictor. *Am J Physiol* 1987; **253**: R222–227.

29 Stinner JN, Ely DL. Blood pressure during routine activity, stress, and feeding in black racer snakes (Coluber constrictor). *Am J Physiol* 1993; **264**: R79–84.

30 Farrell AP. Introduction to cardica scope in lower vertebrates. *Can J Zool* 1991; **69**: 1981–1984.

31 Seymour RS, Lillywhite HB. Blood pressure in snakes from different habitats. *Nature* 1976; **264**: 664–666.

32 Lillywhite HB, Pough FH. Control of arterial pressure in aquatic sea snakes. *Am J Physiol* 1983; **244**: R66–73.

33 Lillywhite HB, Gallagher KP. Hemodynamic adjustments to head-up posture in the partly arboreal snake, Elaphe obsoleta. *J Exp Zool* 1985; **235**: 325–334.

34 Bennett RA, Schumacher J, Hedjazi-Haring K, *et al*. Cardiopulmonary and anesthetic effects of propofol administered intraosseously to green iguanas. *J Am Vet Med Assoc* 1998; **212**: 93–98.

35 Schumacher J, Lillywhite HB, Norman WM, *et al*. Effects of ketamine HCl on cardiopulmonary function in snakes. *Copeia* 1997; 395–400.

36 Custer RS, Bush M. Physiologic and acid–base measures of gopher snakes during ketamine or halothane-nitrous oxide anesthesia. *J Am Vet Med Assoc* 1980; **177**: 870–874.

37 Bonath K. Halothane inhalation anaesthesia in reptiles and its clinical control. *International Zoo Yearbook* 1979; **19**: 112–125.

38 Rooney MB, Levine G, Gaynor J, *et al.* Sevoflurane anesthesia in desert tortoises (Gopherus agassizii). *J Zoo Wildl Med* 1999; **30**: 64–69.

39 Stirl R, Bonath KH. Cardiovascular, pulmonary and acid–base measurements in boa constrictors during tiletamine-zolazepam sedation. In: *Proceedings of the 5th International Congress of Veterinary Anesthesia*, 1994.

40 Arena PC, Richardson KC, Cullen LK. Anaesthesia in two species of large Australian skink. *Vet Rec* 1988; **123**: 155–158.

41 Anderson NL, Wack RF, Calloway L, *et al.* Cardiopulmonary effects and efficacy of propofol as an anesthetic in brown tree snakes (*Boiga irregularis*). *Bull Assoc Reptil Amphib Vet* 1999; **9**: 9–15.

42 Mosley CA, Dyson D, Smith DA. The cardiovascular dose–response effects of isoflurane alone and combined with butorphanol in the green iguana (Iguana iguana). *Vet Anaesth Analg* 2004; **31**: 64–72.

43 Milsom WK. Mechanoreceptor modulation of endogenous respiratory rhythms in vertebrates. *Am J Physiol* 1990; **259**: R898–910.

44 Smatresk NJ. Chemoreceptor modulation of endogenous respiratory rhythms in vertebrates. *Am J Physiol* 1990; **259**: R887–897.

45 Wang T, Smits AW, Burggren W. Pulmonary function in reptiles. In: Gans C, Gaunt AS, eds. *Biology of the Reptilia*. Ithaca, NY: Society for the Study of Amphibians and Reptiles, 1998; 319.

46 Wood SC, Lenfant CJM. Respiration: mechanics, control and gas exchange. In: Gans C, Dawson WR, eds. *Biology of the Reptilia, Physiology A*. New York: Academic Press, 1976; 225–274.

47 Shelton G, Jones DR, Milsom WK. Control of breathing in ectothermic vertebrates. In: Geiger SR, Widdicombe JG, eds. *Handbook of Physiology. Section 3: The Respiratory System*. Bethesda, MD: American Physiological Society, 1986.

48 Glass ML, Wood SC. Gas exchange and control of breathing in reptiles. *Physiol Rev* 1983; **63**: 232–260.

49 Johansen K, Hanson D, Lenfant C. Respiration in a primitive air breather, Amia calva. *Respir Physiol* 1970; **9**: 162–174.

50 Shelton G, Burggren W. Cardiovascular dynamics of the chelonia during apnoea and lung ventilation. *J Exp Biol* 1976; **64**: 323–343.

51 Perry SF. Structure and function of the reptilian respiratory system. In: Lenfant C, Wood CM, eds. *Comparative Pulmonary Physiology. Current Concepts*. New York: Marcel Dekker, 1989; 193–236.

52 Glass ML, Johansen K. Control of breathing in *Acrochordus javanicus*, an aquatic snake. *Physiol Zool* 1976; **49**: 328–340.

53 Templeton JR, Dawson WR. Respiration in the lizard *Crotaphytus collaris*. *Physiol Zool* 1963; **36**: 104–121.

54 Glass ML, Burggren W, Johansen K. Ventilation in an aquatic and a terrestrial chelonian reptile. *J Exp Biol* 1978; **72**: 165–179.

55 Jackson DC, Palmer SE, Meadow WL. The effects of temperature and carbon dioxide breathing on ventilation and acid–base status of turtles. *Respir Physiol* 1974; **20**: 131–146.

56 Jackson DC, Kraus DR, Prange HD. Ventilatory response to inspired CO2 in the sea turtle: effects of body size and temperature. *Respir Physiol* 1979; **38**: 71–81.

57 Boyer DR. Comparative effects of hypoxia on respiratory and cardiac function in reptiles. *Physiol Zool* 1966; **39**: 307–316.

58 Jackson DC. Ventilatory response to hypoxia in turtles at various temperatures. *Respir Physiol* 1973; **18**: 178–187.

59 Hitzig BM, Allen JC, Jackson DC. Central chemical control of ventilation and response of turtles to inspired CO2. *Am J Physiol* 1985; **249**: R323–328.

60 Benchetrit G, Armand J, Dejours P. Ventilatory chemoreflex drive in the tortoise, Testudo horsfieldi. *Respir Physiol* 1977; **31**: 183–191.

61 Benchetrit G, Dejours P. Ventilatory CO2 drive in the tortoise Testudo horsfieldi. *J Exp Biol* 1980; **87**: 229–236.

62 Frankel HM, Spitzer A, Blaine J, *et al.* Respiratory response of turtles (Pseudemys scripta) to changes in arterial blood gas composition. *Comp Biochem Physiol* 1969; **31**: 535–546.

63 Diethelm G. The effect of oxygen content of inspiratory air (FIO_2) on recovery times in the green iguana *(Iguana iguana)*. Doctor of Veterinary Medicine thesis, University of Zurich, 2001.

64 Bertelsen MF, Mosley CA, Crawshaw GJ, *et al.* Inhalation anesthesia in Dumeril's monitor (*Varanus dumerili*) with isoflurane, sevoflurane, and nitrous oxide: effects of inspired gases on inducion and recovery. *J Zoo Wildl Med* 2005; **36**: 62–68.

65 Holz P, Barker IK, Crawshaw GJ, *et al.* The anatomy and perfusion of the renal portal system in the red-eared slider (Trachemys scripta elegans). *J Zoo Wildl Med* 1997; **28**: 378–385.

66 Holz P, Barker IK, Burger JP, *et al.* The effect of the renal portal system on pharmacokinetic parameters in the red-eared slider (Trachemys scripta elegans). *J Zoo Wildl Med* 1997; **28**: 386–393.

67 Berner NJ. Oxygen consumption by mitochondria from an endotherm and an ectotherm. *Comp Biochem Physiol B Biochem Mol Biol* 1999; **124**: 25–31.

68 Penick DN, Paladino FV, Steyermark AC, *et al.* Thermal dependence of tissue metabolism in the green turtle (*Chelonia mydas*). *Comp Biochem Physiol* 1996; **113A**: 293–296.

69 Chittick EJ, Stamper MA, Beasley JF *et al.* Medetomidine, ketamine, and sevoflurane for anesthesia of injured loggerhead sea turtles: 13 cases (1996–2000). *J Am Vet Med Assoc* 2002; **221**: 1019–1025.

70 Wellehan JFX, Lafortune M, Gunkel C, *et al.* Coccygeal vascular catheterization in lizards and crocodilians. *J Herpetol Med Surg* 2004; **14**: 26–28.

71 Maxwell LK, Jacobson ER. Allometric scaling of kidney function in green iguanas. *Comp Biochem Physiol A Mol Integr Physiol* 2004; **138**: 383–390.

72 Bennett RA. Reptile anesthesia. *Semin Avian Exot Pet Med* 1998; **7**: 30–40.

73 Whitaker BR, Krum H. Medical management of sea turtles. In: Fowler ME, Miller RE, eds. *Zoo and Wild Animal Medicine*, 4th edn. Philadelphia: WB Saunders, 1999; 217.

74 Young BD, Stegeman N, Norby B, *et al.* Comparison of intraosseous and peripheral venous fluid dynamics in the desert tortoise (Gopherus agassizii). *J Zoo Wildl Med* 2012; **43**: 59–66.

75 IASP. IASP Taxonomy. www.iasp-pain.org/Education/Content.aspx?ItemNumber=1698 (accessed 1 October 2014).

76 Molony V. Comments on Anand and Craig, PAIN, 67 (1996) 3–6. *Pain* 1997; **70**: 293.

77 Liang YF, Terashima S, Zhu AQ. Distinct morphological characteristics of touch, temperature, and mechanical nociceptive neurons in the crotaline trigeminal ganglia. *J Comp Neurol* 1995; **360**: 621–633.

78 Terashima S, Liang YF. C mechanical nociceptive neurons in the crotaline trigeminal ganglia. *Neurosci Lett* 1994; **179**: 33–36.

79 Kevetter GA, Willis WD. Collateralization in the spinothalamic tract: new methodology to support or deny phylogenetic theories. *Brain Res* 1984; **319**: 1–14.

80 Desfilis E, Font E, Garcia-Verdugo JM. Trigeminal projections to the dorsal thalamus in a lacertid lizard, Podarcis hispanica. *Brain Behav Evol* 1998; **52**: 99–110.

81 Butler AB, Cotterill RM. Mammalian and avian neuroanatomy and the question of consciousness in birds. *Biol Bull* 2006; **211**: 106–127.

82 Reiner A. The distribution of proenkephalin-derived peptides in the central nervous system of turtles. *J Comp Neurol* 1987; **259**: 65–91.

83 De la Iglesia JA, Martinez-Guijarro FI, Lopez-Garcia C. Neurons of the medial cortex outer plexiform layer of the lizard Podarcis hispanica: Golgi and immunocytochemical studies. *J Comp Neurol* 1994; **341**: 184–203.

84 Lindberg I, White L. Reptilian enkephalins: implications for the evolution of proenkephalin. *Arch Biochem Biophys* 1986; **245**: 1–7.

85 Ng TB, Hon WK, Cheng CH, *et al.* Evidence for the presence of adrenocorticotropic and opiate-like hormones in the brains of two sea snakes, Hydrophis cyanocinctus and Lapemis hardwickii. *Gen Comp Endocrinol* 1986; **63**: 31–37.

86 Mauk MD, Olson RD, LaHoste GJ, *et al.* Tonic immobility produces hyperalgesia and antagonizes morphine analgesia. *Science* 1981; **213**: 353–354.

87 Porro CA, Carli G. Immobilization and restraint effects on pain reactions in animals. *Pain* 1988; **32**: 289–307.

88 Tambeli CH, Fischer L, Monaliza SL, *et al.* The functional role of ascending nociceptive control in defensive behavior. *Brain Res* 2012; **1464**: 24–29.

89 Wright KM. Taxonomy of amphibians kept in captivity. In: Wright KM, Whitaker BR, eds. *Amphibian Medicine and Captive Husbandry*. Malabar, FL: Krieger, 2001; 3–14.

90 Mitchell MA. Anesthetic considerations for amphibians. *J Exot Pet Med* 2009; **18**: 40–49.

91 Stetter MD. Amphibians. In: West G, Heard DJ, Caulkett N, eds. *Zoo Animal and Wildlife Immobilization and Anesthesia*. Ames, IA: Blackwell Publishing, 2007; 205–209.

92 Clayton LA, Gore SR. Amphibian emergency medicine. *Vet Clin North Am Exot Anim Pract* 2007; **10**: 587–620.

93 Wright KM. Anatomy for the clinician. In: Wright KM, Whitaker BR, eds. *Amphibian Medicine and Captive Husbandry*. Malabar, FL: Krieger, 2001; 15–30.

94 Wright KM. Applied physiology. In: Wright KM, Whitaker BR, eds. *Amphibian Medicine and Captive Husbandry*. Malabar, FL: Krieger, 2001; 31–34.

95 Haberich FJ. Demonstration of the functional separation of venous and arterial blood in the frog circulation by x-ray angiography. *Pflugers Arch Gesamte Physiol Menschen Tiere* 1967; **293**: 193–198.

96 Haberich FJ. The functional separation of venous and arterial blood in the univentricular frog heart. *Ann NY Acad Sci* 1965; **127**: 459–475.

97 Heinz-Taheny KM. Cardiovascular physiology and disease of amphibians. *Vet Clin Exot Anim* 2009; **12**: 39–50.

98 Langille BL, Jones DR. Dynamics of blood flow through the hearts and arterial systems of anuran amphibia. *J Exp Biol* 1977; **68**: 1–17.

99 Johansen K, Hanson D. Functional anatomy of the hearts of lungfishes and amphibians. *Am Zool* 1968; **8**: 191–210.
100 Johansen K. Cardiovascular dynamics in the amphibian *Amphiuma tridactylum Cuvier*. *Acta Physiol Scand* 1964; **217**: 1–82.
101 Jones JM, Wentzell LA, Toews DP. Posterior lymph heart pressure and rate and lymph flow in the toad Bufo marinus in response to hydrated and dehydrated conditions. *J Exp Biol* 1992; **169**: 207–220.
102 Duellman WE, Trueb L. *Biology of Amphibians*. Baltimore, MD: Johns Hopkins University Press, 1994.
103 Wright KM. Restraint techniques and euthanasia. In: Wright KM, Whitaker BR, eds. *Amphibian Medicine and Captive Husbandry*. Malabar, FL: Krieger, 2001; 111–122.
104 Stetter MD. Fish and amphibian anesthesia. *Vet Clin North Am Exot Anim Pract* 2001; **4**: 69–82.
105 West NH, van Vliet BH. Sensory mechanism regulaing the cardiovascular and respiratory systems. In: Feder ME, Burggren WW, eds. *Environmental Physiology of the Amphibians*. Chicago, IL: University of Chicago Press, 1992; 151–182.
106 Downes U. Tricaine (MS222) is a safe anesthetic compound compared to benzocaine and pentobarbital to induce anesthesia in leopard frogs (Rana pipiens). *Pharmacol Rep* 2005; **57**: 467–474.
107 Guenette SA, Giroux MC, Vachon P. Pain perception and anaesthesia in research frogs. *Exp Anim* 2013; **62**: 87–92.
108 Goulet F, Vachon P, Helie P. Evaluation of the toxicity of eugenol at anesthetic doses in African clawed frogs (Xenopus laevis). *Toxicol Pathol* 2011; **39**: 471–477.
109 Goulet F, Helie P, Vachon P. Eugenol anesthesia in African clawed frogs (Xenopus laevis) of different body weights. *J Am Assoc Lab Anim Sci* 2010; **49**: 460–463.
110 Mitchell MA, Riggs S, Singleton B. Evaluating the clinical and cardiopulmonary effects of clove oil and propofol in tiger salamanders (*Ambystoma tigrinum*). *J Exot Pet Med* 2009; **18**: 50–56.
111 Ross A, Guenette SA, Helie P, *et al.* Case of cutaneous necrosis in African clawed frogs Xenopus laevis after the topical application of eugenol. *Can Vet J* 2006; **47**: 1115–1117.
112 Stetter MD, Raphael B, Indiviglio F, *et al.* Isoflurane anesthesia in amphibians: comparison of five application methods. In: *Proceedings of the American Association of Zoo Veterinarians*, 1996; 255–257.
113 Smith JM, Stump KC. Isoflurane anesthesia in the African clawed frog (Xenopus laevis). *Contemp Top Lab Anim Sci* 2000; **39**: 39–42.
114 Posner LP, Bailey KM, Richardson EY, *et al.* Alfaxalone anesthesia in bullfrogs (Lithobates catesbeiana) by injection or immersion. *J Zoo Wildl Med* 2013; **44**: 965–971.
115 Guenette SA, Beaudry F, Vachon P. Anesthetic properties of propofol in African clawed frogs (Xenopus laevis). *J Am Assoc Lab Anim Sci* 2008; **47**: 35–38.
116 Rosenblum PM, Peter RE. Evidence for the involvement of endogenous opioids in the regulation of gonadotropin secretion in male goldfish, Carassius auratus. *Gen Comp Endocrinol* 1989; **73**: 21–27.
117 Stevens CW, Klopp AJ, Facello JA. Analgesic potency of mu and kappa opioids after systemic administration in amphibians. *J Pharmacol Exp Ther* 1994; **269**: 1086–1093.
118 Rosenblum PM, Callard IP. Endogenous opioid peptide system in male brown bullhead catfish, *Ictalurus nebulosus* lesueur: characterization of naloxone binding and the response to naloxone during the annual reproductive cycle. *J Exp Zool* 1988; **245**: 244–255.
119 Stevens CW. Opioid research in amphibians: an alternative pain model yielding insights on the evolution of opioid receptors. *Brain Res Brain Res Rev* 2004; **46**: 204–215.
120 Koeller CA. Comparison of buprenorphine and butorphanol analgesia in the eastern red-spotted newt (Notophthalmus viridescens). *J Am Assoc Lab Anim Sci* 2009; **48**: 171–175.
121 Machin KL. Amphibian pain and analgesia. *J Zoo Wildl Med* 1999; **30**: 2–10.
122 Stevens CW. Analgesia in amphibians: preclinical studies and clinical applications. *Vet Clin North Am Exot Anim Pract* 2011; **14**: 33–44.
123 Duncan A. Reptile and amphibian analgesia. In: Fowler ME, Miller RE, eds. *Zoo and Wild Animal Medicine*, 7th edn. Philadelphia: Elsevier, 2012; 247–253.
124 Machin KL. Fish, amphibian, and reptile analgesia. *Vet Clin North Am Exot Anim Pract* 2001; **4**: 19–33.
125 Nikundiwe AM, de Boer-van Huizen R, ten Donkelaar HJ. Dorsal root projections in the clawed toad (Xenopus laevis) as demonstrated by anterograde labeling with horseradish peroxidase. *Neuroscience* 1982; **7**: 2089–2103.
126 Echlin F, Propper N. 'Sensitization' by injury of the cutaneous nerve endings in the frog. *J Physiol* 1937; **88**: 388–400.
127 Habgood JS. Sensitization of sensory receptors in the frog's skin. *J Physiol* 1950; **111**: 195–213.
128 Stevens CW. Opioid antinociception in amphibians. *Brain Res Bull* 1988; **21**: 959–962.
129 Braga PC, Tiengo M, Biella G, *et al.* Dermorphin, a new peptide from amphibian skin, inhibits the nociceptive thalamic neurons firing rate evoked by noxious stimuli. *Neurosci Lett* 1984; **52**: 165–169.
130 Erspamer V. The opioid peptides of the amphibian skin. *Int J Devl Neuroscience* 1992; **10**: 3–30.
131 Stevens CW, Yaksh TL. Spinal action of dermorphin, an extremely potent opioid peptide from frog skin. *Brain Res* 1986; **385**: 300–304.
132 Mettam JJ, Oulton LJ, McCrohan CR, *et al.* The efficacy of three types of analgesic drugs in reducing pain in the rainbow trout, *Oncorhynchus mykiss*. *Appl Anim Behav Sci* 2011; **133**: 265–274.
133 Mohan S, Stevens CW. Systemic and spinal administration of the mu opioid, remifentanil, produces antinociception in amphibians. *Eur J Pharmacol* 2006; **534**: 89–94.
134 Brenner GM, Klopp AJ, Deason LL, *et al.* Analgesic potency of alpha adrenergic agents after systemic administration in amphibians. *J Pharmacol Exp Ther* 1994; **270**: 540–545.
135 Stevens CW, MacIver DN, Newman LC. Testing and comparison of non-opioid analgesics in amphibians. *Contemp Top Lab Anim Sci* 2001; **40**: 23–27.
136 Willenbring S, Stevens CW. Thermal, mechanical and chemical peripheral sensation in amphibians: opioid and adrenergic effects. *Life Sci* 1996; **58**: 125–133.
137 Neiffer DL, Stamper MA. Fish sedation, analgesia, anesthesia, and euthanasia: considerations, methods, and types of drugs. *ILAR J* 2009; **50**: 343–360.
138 Neiffer DL. Boney fish (lungfish, sturgeon, teleosts). In: West G, Heard DJ, Caulkett N, eds. *Zoo Animal and Wildlife Immobilization and Anesthesia.*. Ames, IA: Blackwell Publishing, 2007; 159–196.
139 Harms CA. Anesthesia in fish. In: Fowler ME, Miller RE, eds. *Zoo and Wild Animal Medicine*, 5th edn. St Louis, MO: WB Saunders, 2003; 2–20.
140 Olson KR. Vascular anatomy of the fish gill. *J Exper Zool* 2002; **293**: 214–231.
141 Bushnell PG, Jones DR. Cardiovascular and respiratory physiology of tuna: adaptations for support of exceptionaly high metabolic rates. *Environ Biol Fishes* 1994; **40**: 303–318.
142 Bruecker P, Graham M. The effects of the anesthetic ketamine hydrochloride on oxygen consumption rates and behaviour in the fish Heros (Cichlasoma) citrinellum. *Comp Biochem Physiol* 1993; **104C**: 57–59.
143 Sherrill J, Weber ES, Marty GD, *et al.* Fish cardiovascular physiology and disease. *Vet Clin North Am Exot Anim Pract* 2009; **12**: 11–38.
144 Satchell GH. The reflex co-ordination of the heart beat with respiration in the dogfish. *J Exp Biol* 1960; **37**: 719–731.
145 Ross L, Ross B. *Anaesthetic and Sedative Techniques for Aquatic Animals*, 3rd edn. Oxford: Wiley-Blackwell, 2008.
146 Neiffer DL, Stamper MA. Fish sedation, analgesia, anesthesia, and euthanasia: considerations, methods, and types of drugs. *ILAR J* 2009; **50**: 343–360.
147 Weber ES. Fish analgesia: pain, stress, fear aversion, or nociception? *Vet Clin North Am Exot Anim Pract* 2011; **14**: 21–32.
148 Weber EP III , Weisse C, Schwarz T, *et al.* Anesthesia, diagnostic imaging, and surgery of fish. *Compend Contin Educ Vet* 2009; **31**: E11.
149 Laitinen M, Valtonen T. Cardiovascular, ventilatory and total activity responses of brown trout to handling stress. *J Fish Biol* 1994; **45**: 933–942.
150 Barton BA, Iwama G. Physiological changes in fish from stress in aquaculture with emphasis on the response and effects of corticsterioids. *Annu Rev Fish Dis* 1991; **1**: 3–26.
151 Barton BA, Morgan JD, Vijayan MN. Physiological and condition-related indicators of environmental stress in fish. In: Adams SM, ed. *Biological Indicators of Aquatic Ecosystem Stress*. Bethesda, MD: American Fisheries Society, 2002; 111–148.
152 Donaldson EM. The pituitary–interrenal axis as an indicator of stress in fish. In: Pickering AD, ed. *Stress and Fish*. London: Academic Press, 1981; 11–47.
153 Ackerman PA, Forsyth RB, Mazur CF, *et al.* Stress hormones and the cellular stress response in salmonids. *Fish Physiol Biochem* 2000; **23**: 327–336.
154 Gregory TR, Wood CM. The effects of chronic plasma cortisol elevation on the feeding behavior, growth, competitive ability, and swimming performance of juvenile rainbow trout. *Physiol Biochem Zool* 1999; **72**: 286–295.
155 Dreborg S, Sundstrom G, Larsson TA, *et al.* Evolution of vertebrate opioid receptors. *Proc Natl Acad Sci USA* 2008; **105**: 15487–15492.
156 McDonald LK, Joss JM, Dores RM. The phylogeny of Met-enkephalin and Leu-enkephalin: studies on the holostean fish Lepisosteus platyrhincus and the Australian lungfish, Neoceratodus forsteri. *Gen Comp Endocrinol* 1991; **84**: 228–236.
157 Vallarino M. Occurrence of β-endorphin-like immunoreactivity in the brain of the teleost, *Boops boops*. *Gen Comp Endocrinol* 1995; **60**: 63–69.
158 Posner LP. Introduction: pain and distress in fish: a review of the evidence. *ILAR J* 2009; **50**: 327–328.
159 Sneddon LU. Pain perception in fish: indicators and endpoints. *ILAR J* 2009; **50**: 338–342.

160 Sneddon LU, Braithwaite VA, Gentle MJ. Do fishes have nociceptors? Evidence for the evolution of a vertebrate sensory system. *Proc Biol Sci* 2003; **270**: 1115–1121.
161 Sneddon LU. Evolution of nociception in vertebrates: comparative analysis of lower vertebrates. *Brain Res* 2004; **46**: 123–130.
162 Rose JD. The neurobehavioral nature of fishes and the question of awareness of pain. *Rev Fish Sci* 2002; **10**: 1–38.
163 Rose D, Woodbury CJ. Animal models of nociception and pain. In: Conn PM, ed. *Sourcebook of Models for Biomedical Research*. Totoway, NJ: Humana Press, 2008; 333–339.
164 Harms CA, Lewbart GA, Swanson CR, *et al.* Behavioral and clinical pathology changes in koi carp (Cyprinus carpio) subjected to anesthesia and surgery with and without intra-operative analgesics. *Comp Med* 2005; **55**: 221–226.
165 Smith SA. Pain and distress in fish. *ILAR J* 2009; **50**: 327–415.
166 Sneddon LU. Clinical anesthesia and analgesia in fish. *J Exot Pet Med* 2012; **21**: 32–43.
167 Neiffer DL, Stamper MA. Fish sedation, analgesia, anesthesia, and euthanasia: considerations, methods, and types of drugs. *ILAR J* 2009; **50**: 343–360.
168 Harms CA. Anesthesia in fish. In: Fowler ME, Miller RE, eds. *Zoo and Wild Animal Medicine, Current Therapy*, 4th edn. Philadelphia: WB Saunders, 1999; 158–163.
169 Aguiar LH, Kalinin AL, Rantin FT. The effects of temperature on the cardio-respiratory function of teh neotropical fish Piaractus mesopotamicus. *J Therm Biol* 2002; **27**: 299–308.
170 Butterworth JF IV , Strichartz GR. Molecular mechanisms of local anesthesia: a review. *Anesthesiology* 1990; **72**: 711–734.
171 Wayson KA, Downes H, Lynn RK, *et al.* Studies on the comparative pharmacology and selective toxicity of tricaine methanesulfonate: metabolism as a basis of the selective toxicity in poikilotherms. *J Pharmacol Exp Ther* 1976; **198**: 695–708.
172 Carter KM, Woodley CM, Brown RS. A review of tricaine methanesulfonate for anesthesia of fish. *Rev Fish Biol Fisheries* 2011; **21**: 51–59.
173 Rub AM, Jepsen N, Liedtke TL, *et al.* Surgical insertion of transmitters and telemetry methods in fisheries research. *Am J Vet Res* 2014; **75**: 402–416.
174 Davis KB, Griffin BR. Physiological responses of hybrid striped bass under sedation of several anesthetics. *Aquaculture* 2004; **233**: 531–548.
175 Baker TR, Baker BB, Johnson SM, *et al.* Comparative analgesic efficacy of morphine sulfate and butorphanol tartrate in koi (Cyprinus carpio) undergoing unilateral gonadectomy. *J Am Vet Med Assoc* 2013; **243**: 882–890.
176 Newby NC, Gamper AK, Stevens ED. Cardiorespiratory effects and efficacy of morphine sulfate in winter flounder (*Pseudopleuronectes americanus*). *Am J Vet Res* 2007; **68**: 592–597.
177 Newby NC, Wilkie MP, Stevens ED. Morphine uptake, disposition, and analgesic efficacy in the common goldfish (Carassius auratus). *Can J Zool* 2009; **87**: 388–399.
178 Davis MR, Mylniczenko N, Storm T, *et al.* Evaluation of intramuscular ketoprofen and butorphanol as analgesics in chain dogfish (*Scyliorhinus rotifer*). *Zoo Biol* 2006; **25**: 491–500.
179 Stamper MA. Elasmobranches (sharks, rays, and skates). In: West G, Heard DJ, Caulkett N, eds. *Zoo Animal and Wildlife Immobilization and Anesthesia*. Ames, IA: Blackwell Publishing, 2007; 197–203.
180 Flemming GJ, Heard DJ, Floyd RF, Riggs A. Evaluation of propfol and medetomidine-ketamine for short-term immobilization of Gulf of Mexico sturgeon (*Acipenser oxyrinchus de soti*). *J Zoo Wildl Med* 2003; **34**: 153–158.
181 Harvey B, Denny C, Kaiser S, *et al.* Remote intramuscular injection of immobilising drugs into fish using a laser-aimed underwater dart gun. *Vet Rec* 1988; **122**: 174–177.
182 Harms CA, Bakal RS. Techniques in fish anesthesia. *J Sm Exot Anim Med* 1995; **3**: 19–25.
183 Oikawa S, Takeda T, Itazawa Y. Scale effects of MS-222 on a marine teleost, porgy *Pagrus major*. *Aquaculture* 1994; **121**: 369–379.

43 Comparative Anesthesia and Analgesia of Birds

John W. Ludders
College of Veterinary Medicine, Cornell University, Ithaca, New York, USA

Chapter contents

Introduction

The class Aves consists of 27 orders, 168 families and approximately 10 000 species worldwide. Birds, regarded as the only clade of dinosaurs to have survived the Cretaceous–Paleogene extinction event 65.5 million years ago, inhabit every continent and live in a wide range of environmental niches. For example, emperor penguins (*Aptenodytes forsteri*) live in the Antarctic, and one study recorded an individual ocean dive record of 540 m (1772 ft) lasting 18 min [1]. A Ruppell's griffon (*Gyps rueppelli*), the highest flying bird, was sucked into a jet engine at 11,485 m (37,900 feet) over the west African country of Côte d'Ivoire. Bar-headed geese (*Anser indicus*) routinely fly over the Himalayas at more than 8481 meters (27 825 ft) when migrating between central and south Asia. The burrowing owl (*Athene cunicularia*) nests underground while wandering albatrosses spend most of their life in flight, landing only to breed. The weight and size of birds vary greatly. Bee hummingbirds (*Mellisuga helenae*) measure 5–6 cm (2–2.4 inches) in length and weigh 1.6–2 g while the ostrich (*Struthio camelus*) has a height of 2.75 m (9 feet) and weighs up to 145 kg.

Throughout time, humans have had a practical interest in birds as a source of food. In domesticating and selecting for desirable production characteristics, such as rapid weight gain or high egg production, a number of structural and functional changes have occurred in domesticated species that are not seen in their wild relatives. For example, domesticated turkeys and chickens have smaller lung volumes and less gas exchange surface area compared to their wild counterparts.

The tremendous diversity in form, function, and mode of life that exists across avian orders, and between wild and domesticated species, poses challenges to the anesthetic management of birds, but a challenge that can be lessened by considering and applying basic principles of avian anatomy, physiology, and pharmacology. Of crucial importance are the avian pulmonary and cardiovascular systems as they tend to be sources of frequent problems in the design and implementation of anesthetic protocols for birds. Much of this chapter focuses on these two systems.

Pulmonary system

The avian pulmonary system consists of two separate and distinct functional components: one for ventilation (trachea, bronchi, air sacs, thoracic skeleton, muscles of respiration) and one for gas exchange (parabronchial lung). These two components can be used to advantage when anesthetizing birds, especially when using inhalant anesthetics.

Ventilation components

Larynx, trachea, syrinx

The avian larynx is located at the base of the tongue and protrudes into the pharynx as a somewhat heart-shaped mound [2]. Birds do not have an epiglottis so when the tongue is pulled gently forward, the larynx is easily visualized in most birds (Fig. 43.1). A notable exception is the flamingo with its ventroflexed beak and large fleshy tongue that make it difficult to visualize the larynx.

Veterinary Anesthesia and Analgesia: The Fifth Edition of Lumb and Jones,
Edited by Kurt A. Grimm, Leigh A. Lamont, William J. Tranquilli, Stephen A. Greene and Sheilah A. Robertson.

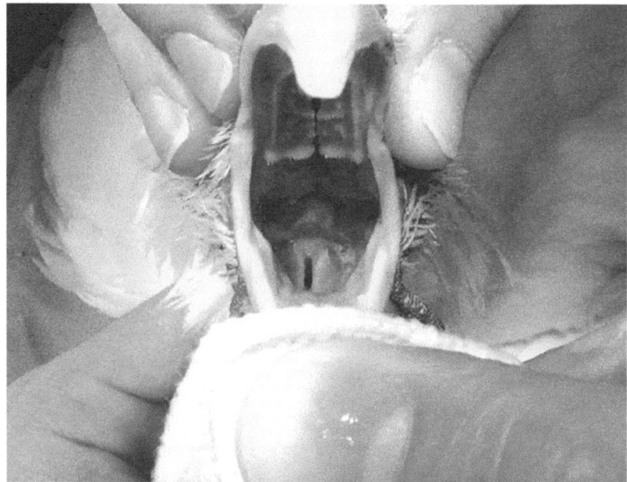

Figure 43.1 Larynx of a chicken.

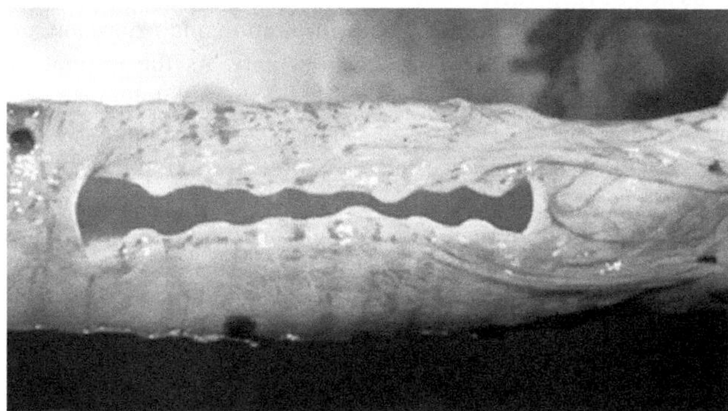

Figure 43.2 Tracheal slit of an emu (*Dromaius novaehollandiae*). Source: J. A. Smith, DVM, DACVAA, with permission.

The avian trachea, which consists of complete cartilaginous rings, conducts air from the nares and mouth to the bronchi while warming, moisturizing, and screening particulate matter from inspired gas [2]. From one avian class to another, there are tracheal anatomic differences that have significant implications for ventilation. For example, emu and ruddy ducks have an inflatable sac-like diverticulum that opens from the trachea. In the emu the sac arises from the ventral surface of the trachea approximately three-quarters of the way down the neck where the tracheal rings are incomplete and form a slit-like opening (Fig. 43.2) [2]. It is present in both sexes and is responsible for the characteristic booming call of the emu. In male ruddy ducks, the sac opens in a depression on the dorsal wall of the trachea immediately caudal to the larynx, thus lying between the trachea and esophagus [2]. The sac may act as a sounding board for the bill-drumming display of the males [2].

Some penguins and petrels possess a double trachea consisting of a median septum dividing part of the trachea into right and left channels [2]. In both groups of birds, the septum extends cranially from the bronchial bifurcation, but its length is quite variable. For example, in the jackass penguin (*Spheniscus demersus*) the septum extends to within a few centimeters of the larynx, whereas in the rockhopper penguin (*Eudyptes* spp.) it is only 5 mm in length [2].

Other classes of birds have complex tracheal loops or coils in the caudal neck, within the keel, or within the thorax and keel (Fig. 43.3). Studies in cranes (*Grus* spp.) have demonstrated that

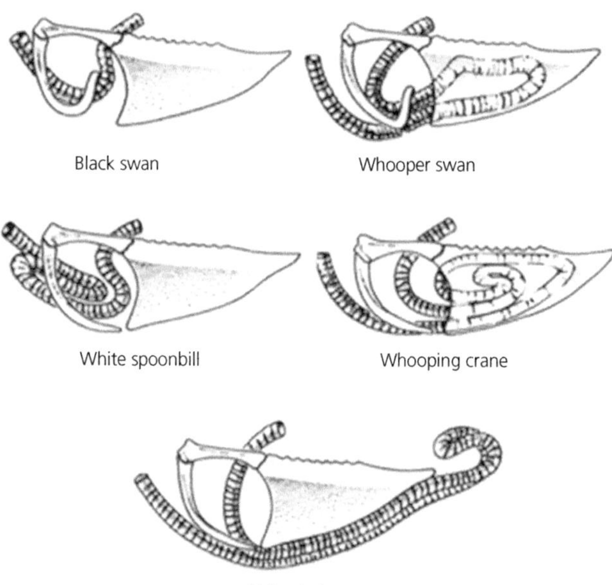

Figure 43.3 Different forms of tracheal loops: black swan (*Cygnus atratus*); whooper swan (*Cygnus cygnus*); white spoonbill (*Platalea leucorodia*); whooping crane (*Grus americana*); helmeted curassow (*Crax pauxi*). Source: Adapted from McLelland [2].

tracheal coiling enables these birds to produce extremely loud calls using very low driving pressures [3].

Birds generally have relatively long necks, not to mention tracheal loops and coils, which affects tracheal deadspace which is an important consideration during general anesthesia. The typical avian trachea is 2.7 times longer than that of comparably sized mammals, but it is 1.29 times wider, so tracheal resistance to gas flow is comparable in birds and mammals [2]. Tracheal deadspace volume in birds is about 4.5 times larger than that of comparably sized mammals, but the relatively low respiratory frequency, approximately one-third that of mammals, and larger tidal volume of birds ensure that the effect of the larger tracheal deadspace volume is decreased [2]. The net effect is that avian minute tracheal ventilation is only about 1.5–1.9 times that of mammals [2].

The syrinx, the sound-producing organ in birds, is located at the junction of the trachea and mainstem bronchi. Its location and structure explain why gas flowing through the trachea, especially during positive pressure ventilation, can produce sound in an anesthetized, intubated bird.

Bronchi and secondary bronchi

Mammals have 23 orders of bronchial branching leading to the gas exchange area of the lung (the alveoli), but birds have only three orders of branching before gas exchange tissue is reached [4]. The avian bronchial system consists of a primary bronchus (extra- and intrapulmonary), secondary bronchi, and tertiary bronchi (commonly referred to as parabronchi). The parabronchi and their surrounding mantle of tissue (the periparabronchial mantle) is where gas exchange occurs [4,5].

The primary bronchus enters the lung ventrally and obliquely at the junction of the cranial and middle thirds of the lung, then passes dorsolaterally to the lung surface, where it turns caudally in a dorsally curved direction until at the caudal lung margin it opens into the abdominal air sac [6]. The primary bronchi have low columnar,

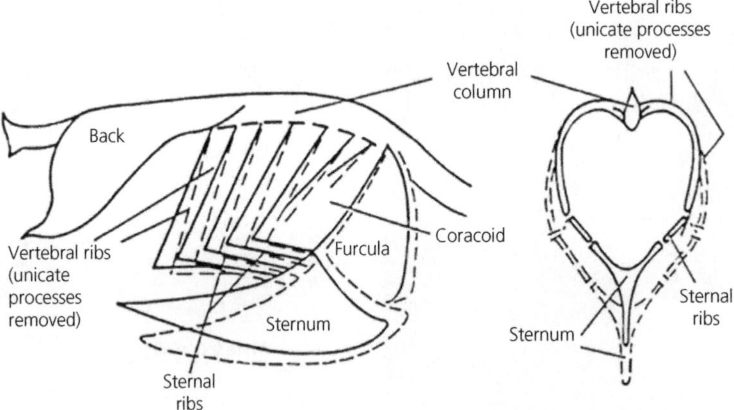

Figure 43.4 Changes in the position of the thoracic skeleton during breathing in a bird. The solid lines represent thoracic position at the end of expiration while the dotted lines show the thoracic position at the end of inspiration. Source: Fedde MR. Respiration. In: Sturkie PD, ed. *Avian Physiology*, 4th edn. New York: Springer, 1986; 191–220.

pseudostratified epithelium under which is a well-developed internal circular smooth muscle layer and longitudinally oriented smooth muscles [7] that can change the internal diameter of the primary bronchus. Acetylcholine, pilocarpine, and histamine contract bronchial smooth muscles; atropine blocks the effects of these drugs but has no effect when given alone [8].

A secondary bronchus is any bronchus arising from a primary bronchus. For a short distance, they have the same histologic structure as the primary bronchus, but subsequently develop simple squamous epithelium [9,10]. In most birds the secondary bronchi are arranged into four groups: medioventral, mediodorsal, lateroventral, and laterodorsal [5]. The medioventral secondary bronchi arise from the primary intrapulmonary bronchus close to where it enters the lung, and occupy the ventral surface of the lung [11]. The mediodorsal, lateroventral, and laterodorsal secondary bronchi arise from the caudal curved portion of the primary intrapulmonary bronchus. Many medioventral and lateroventral secondary bronchi open into the cervical, clavicular, cranial thoracic, or abdominal air sacs.

Air sacs

Birds have nine air sacs: two cervical, an unpaired clavicular, two cranial and two caudal thoracic, and two abdominal air sacs. The air sacs are thin-walled structures composed of simple squamous epithelium that is vessel poor; as such, air sacs do not significantly contribute to gas exchange [12,13]. Adrenergic and cholinergic nerve plexuses have been described in the walls of air sacs, and vasoactive intestinal polypeptide, and fibers containing substance P, somatostatin and enkephalin occur in the walls of the air sacs of chickens (*Gallus gallus*) [13]. To a varying extent, depending upon the species, diverticula from the air sacs aerate the cervical vertebrae, some of the thoracic vertebrae, vertebral ribs, sternum, humerus, pelvis, and head and body of the femur [5].

The air sacs functionally provide a tidal flow of air to the relatively rigid avian lung which changes in volume by only 1.6% [14,15]. Based on their bronchial connections, air sacs are grouped into a cranial group, consisting of the cervical, clavicular, and cranial thoracic air sacs, and a caudal group, consisting of the caudal thoracic and abdominal air sacs [16]. The volume is distributed approximately equally between the cranial and caudal groups [17]. During ventilation, all air sacs are effectively ventilated, with the possible exception of the cervical air sacs. The ratio of ventilation to volume is similar for each air sac [17].

Muscles of respiration and the thoracic skeleton

In birds, unlike in mammals, both inspiration and expiration are active processes requiring muscular activity. As the inspiratory muscles contract, the internal volume of the thoracoabdominal cavity increases (Fig. 43.4). Since air sacs are the only volume-compliant structures in the body cavity [17], pressure within the air sacs becomes negative relative to ambient atmospheric pressure, and air flows from the atmosphere into the pulmonary system, specifically into the air sacs and across the gas exchange surfaces of the lungs. During expiration, pressure within the air sacs becomes positive relative to ambient atmospheric pressure, and air flows from the air sacs and pulmonary system to the environment.

The ventilation components: Considerations for anesthesia

Endotracheal tubes and intubation

Birds larger than a cockatiel can be intubated, but intubation may be difficult in those species that have unique oropharyngeal anatomy, or in small birds [18]. For example, psittacine species, especially smaller birds such as budgerigar parakeets (*Melopsittacus undulatus*), can be difficult to intubate because of the difficult-to-visualize location of the glottis at the base of the humped, fleshy tongue [19]. Commercially manufactured endotracheal tubes for small birds do not exist and intravenous (IV) catheters have been used as endotracheal tubes [20]. Catheters can be an effective means for intubating and delivering inhalant anesthetics to small birds, but the nature of their design and construction may cause tracheal injury. While commercially available endotracheal tubes possess some degree of flexibility and thermoplasticity, IV catheters do not and thus may cause tracheal trauma (abrasion or puncture) if not inserted carefully. If an IV catheter is used for intubation it must be of appropriate circumference so as to allow some degree of gas leak between the tracheal wall and the catheter, thus avoiding air sac volotrauma or barotrauma to the lungs [20].

Another hazard of endotracheal tubes of small internal diameter is the resistance they impose on gas flow, a hazard that increases when they develop partial or complete obstructions as a result of mucus accumulation. Mucus production during anesthesia can be copious and the cold, dry fresh gases used in inhalant anesthesia have a drying effect that makes the mucus thick and tenacious. Endotracheal tube obstruction can be detected by observing the bird's pattern of ventilation. As the airway becomes progressively occluded, the expiratory phase becomes prolonged. Artificially sighing, the bird usually confirms the presence of an obstruction because the keel will move and the abdominal wall will expand in a seemingly normal manner, but they will return slowly or not at all to their end-expiratory positions. Airway noises, especially gurgling, may be heard as the tube becomes more obstructed with mucus. Airway obstructions must be corrected quickly either by extubating the bird, cleaning the tube and reinserting it, or by replacing it with a clean tube. An anticholinergic, such as atropine (0.04 mg/kg) or glycopyrrolate (0.01 mg/kg), administered intramuscularly, may reduce mucus production and lessen the risk of developing mucus plugs.

If an endotracheal tube has a cuff, either the cuff should not be inflated or it must be inflated with extreme caution; in small birds it is better not to inflate the cuff. Because of the complete cartilaginous tracheal rings, an overly inflated cuff will injure the tracheal mucosa or rupture the tracheal rings. When a cuff is overinflated the tracheal rings tend to rupture longitudinally rather than circumferentially. Intubation-induced tracheal trauma may not become evident for several days until the processes of healing and fibrotic narrowing of the trachea cause signs of dyspnea.

As mentioned previously, the flamingo with its ventroflexed beak and large fleshy tongue can be difficult to intubate. The key is to reduce the amount of equipment in the mouth. This can be accomplished by shining a transilluminator light from the outside of the mouth into the oral cavity and then using a cotton-tipped applicator to bring the tongue forward so that the larynx can be visualized and the endotracheal tube inserted (personal communication, Dr Noha Abou-Madi, Cornell University, November 2012).

Depending on their size, ostriches can be intubated with endotracheal tubes with internal diameters of 10–18 mm, while emus generally require endotracheal tubes measuring 9–14 mm [21]. Careful inflation of the cuff is usually necessary to allow good ventilation of adult ratites. The tracheal cleft in emus does not complicate intubation, but it does make effective positive pressure ventilation difficult; this problem can be overcome by placing a snug wrap around the distal third of the neck [21].

Body position and muscle relaxation

Depending on the species, a bird's body position during anesthesia may adversely affect ventilation, especially dorsal recumbency in chickens [22]. At least two factors may explain this phenomenon: the weight of the abdominal viscera may compress the abdominal air sacs, thereby effectively reducing a bird's tidal volume, and during anesthesia there is some degree of muscle relaxation such that a bird with large, heavy pectoral muscles may not be able to generate sufficient muscular effort to lift the keel against gravity, again reducing tidal volume. However, in red-tailed hawks (*Buteo jamaicensis*) anesthetized with isoflurane, dorsal recumbency did not compromise ventilation or oxygen transport more than when the birds were in lateral recumbency [23].

When considering sternal recumbency, it seems reasonable that anything which interferes with movement of the keel, including anesthesia-induced muscle relaxation, would compromise ventilation. In anesthetized, spontaneously breathing red-tailed hawks, volumetric analysis of computed tomographic images showed that sternal recumbency resulted in the greatest lung and air sac volumes and lowest lung density compared to right lateral or dorsal recumbency [24]. Although this study did not measure physiologic variables, such as $PaCO_2$ and PaO_2, to determine the effect of sternal recumbency on effective ventilation, the results suggest that in red-tailed hawks pulmonary function is not adversely affected by sternal recumbency. Nonetheless, as for any anesthetized patient, to overcome ventilation problems in birds associated with muscle relaxation it is reasonable to maintain as light a plane of anesthesia as possible.

Gas exchange component

Tertiary bronchi (parabronchi) and air capillaries

A tertiary bronchus or parabronchus and its mantle of surrounding tissue consisting of air capillaries and blood vessels is the basic unit of gas exchange. The parabronchi, which connect the two main sets of secondary bronchi, are long, narrow tubes that anastomose profusely (Fig. 43.5) [11,13]. There is a network of smooth

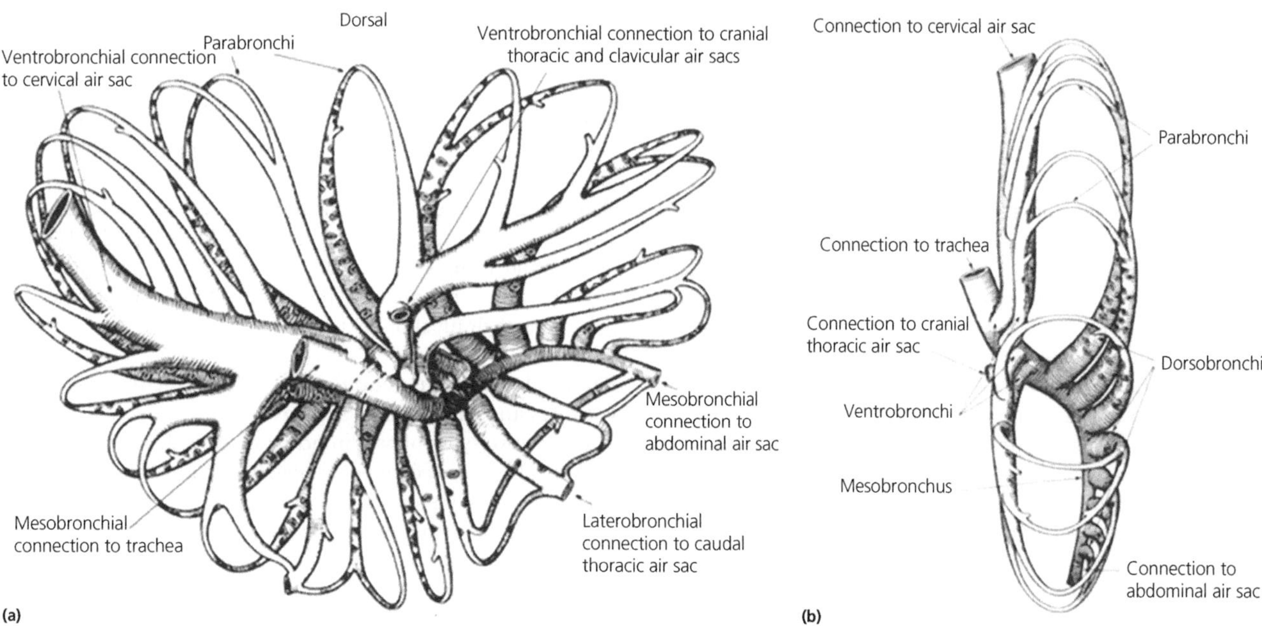

Figure 43.5 Two views of secondary bronchi and parabronchi in the right lung of a goose. (a) Medial view. (b) Dorsal view. Source: Brackenbury JH. Ventilation of the lung-air sac system. In: Seller TJ, ed. *Bird Respiration*, vol **I**. Boca Raton,FL: CRC Press, 1987, with permission.

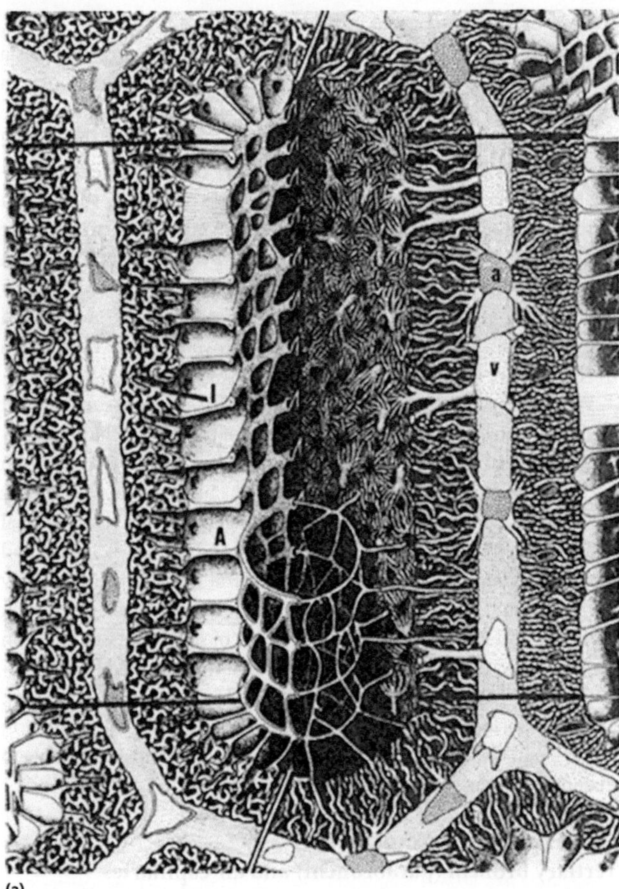

(a)

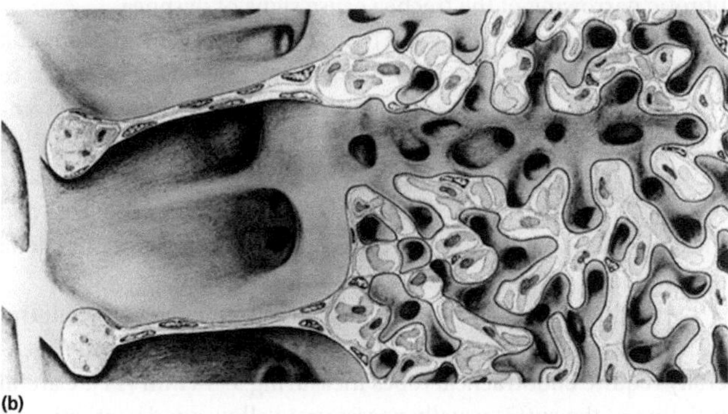

(b)

Figure 43.6 Three-dimensional diagrams of a parabronchus and an atrium. (a) Sagittal section of a parabronchus. On the left side are atria with infundibula departing from them and the three-dimensional air capillary meshwork arising from the infundibula. On the right side within the interparabronchial septa are the arterioles (*dense stippling*) from which the capillaries originate and run radially to the lumen. The infundibula lie between the capillaries which are surrounded by a well-developed three-dimensional air capillary network. (b) Atrium and infundibulum. At the left, two of the circular smooth muscle bundles surrounding the lumen of the parabronchus are shown in cross-section. The atria are separated by septa running horizontally and vertically. Originating from each atrium, a few infundibula pass perpendicularly into the parabronchial mantle. At the right an infundibulum is shown in longitudinal section with air capillaries arising from it at all levels. The air capillaries cross-link and interlace, making up a three dimensional meshwork around the blood capillaries. The very thin epithelium of the air capillaries and its surfactant film are shown as a single dark line. Source: [7]. Reproduced with permission from Elsevier Science and Professor Duncker; digital image kindly provided by Professor Duncker.

muscle surrounding the entrances to the parabronchi; with electric stimulation of the vagus nerve, the smooth muscle can contract and cause narrowing of parabronchial openings [25]. The inner surfaces of the tubular parabronchi are pierced by numerous openings into chambers called atria that are separated from each other by interatrial septa (Fig. 43.6) covered by a thin epithelial layer with a core of densely packed bundles of smooth muscle framing the atrial openings [5]. Since the avian lung is richly innervated with vagal and sympathetic nerves, it is possible that afferent and efferent neural pathways exist for controlling pulmonary smooth muscle, thus varying air flow through the parabronchial lung in response to a variety of stimuli [16]. Arising from the abluminal floor of each atria are funnel-shaped ducts (infundibula) that lead to air capillaries of 3–20 μm diameter that form an anastomosing three-dimensional network intimately interlaced with a similarly structured network of blood capillaries [6,26–28]; gas exchange occurs within this mantle of interlaced air and blood capillaries.

The law of Laplace ($P = \gamma/r$) where P is the opening pressure, γ surface tension, and r radius of tubule, when applied to tubules of small diameter, such as air capillaries, indicates that high surface tensions result and generate significant negative pressure across the blood–gas barrier that could lead to influx of fluid or collapse the tubules [29]. However, air and blood capillaries possess structural elements that preserve their anatomic and gas exchange integrity. These elements form an interdependent, tightly coupled network of tension and compression in the avian lung that gives the lungs rigidity while strengthening the air and blood capillaries, thus preserving their function [27].

Paleopulmonic and neopulmonic parabronchi: Lung volumes and direction of gas flow

There are two types of parabronchial tissue: paleopulmonic parabronchial tissue (paleopulmonic lung), found in all birds, consisting of parallel stacks of profusely anastomosing parabronchi (Fig. 43.7a), and neopulmonic parabronchial tissue (neopulmonic lung), a meshwork of anastomosing parabronchi located in the caudolateral portion of the lung; its degree of development is species dependent (Fig. 43.7b,c). Penguins and emus have only paleopulmonic parabronchi. Pigeons, ducks, and cranes have both paleopulmonic and neopulmonic parabronchi with the neopulmonic parabronchi

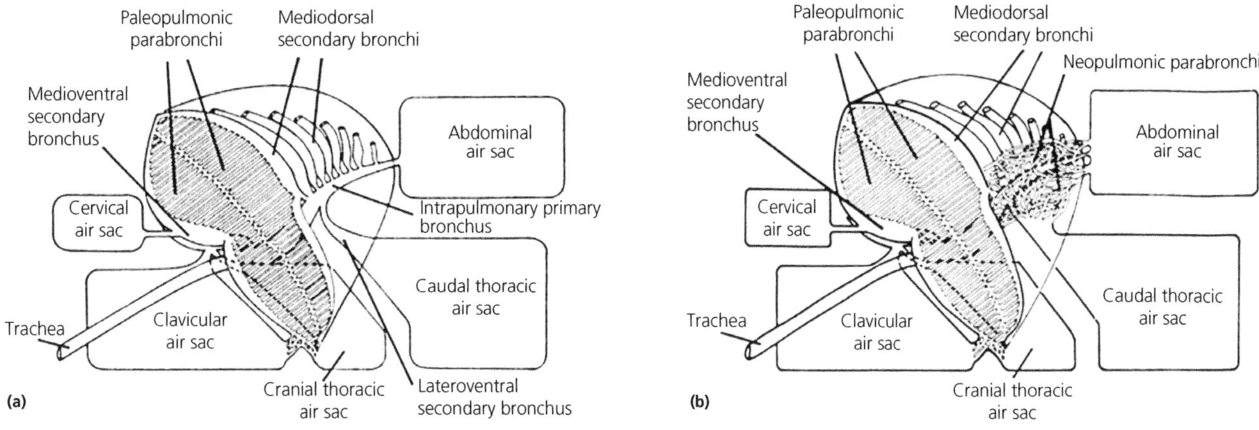

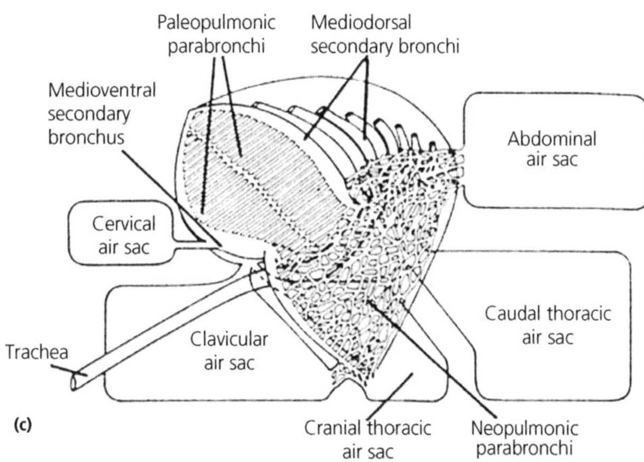

Figure 43.7 Diagram of paleopulmonic and neopulmonic lungs. (a) The paleopulmonic lung found in penguins and emus. (b) The paleopulmonic and neopulmonic lung found in storks, ducks, and geese. (c) The paleopulmonic and the more highly developed neopulmonic lung found in chickens, sparrows, and other song birds. Source: [16].

accounting for 10–12% of the total lung volume. In fowl-like birds and song birds, the neopulmonic parabronchi are more developed and may account for 20–25% of the total lung volume. Paleopulmonic and neopulmonic parabronchi are histologically indistinguishable from each other.

Compared to mammals, specific total lung volume in birds is about 27% smaller, but specific surface area of the blood–gas (tissue) barrier is ~15% greater; the ratio of the tissue surface area to the volume of the exchange tissue is 170–305% greater [30]. The harmonic mean thickness of the tissue barrier in birds is 56–67% less (less resistance to gas diffusion) and the pulmonary capillary blood volume is 22% greater. With the exception of specific total lung volume, these morphometric parameters favor the gas exchange capacity of birds [30].

The specific volume (respiratory gas volume per unit body mass) of the avian pulmonary system is between 100 and 200 mL/kg, but the volume of gas in the parabronchi and air capillaries accounts for only 10% of the total specific volume [17]. By comparison, a dog's specific volume is 45 mL/kg, and the pulmonary gas volume in the mammalian lung is 96% of the total specific volume. Because the ratio of residual gas volume (i.e., gas in the lungs) to tidal volume is so much smaller in birds than in mammals, it has been suggested that cyclic changes in parabronchial gas flow, such as reversal of gas flow, could produce significant and intolerable cyclic changes in gas exchange somewhat analogous to breath holding [15]. The unidirectional flow of gas within the paleopulmonic lung solves this problem.

Allometry, the scaling of selected physiologic variables to body mass, has been applied to avian species [31,32]. For a summary of respiratory variables covering a wide range of avian species and allometric equations relating body mass to respiratory variables, the reader is referred to an article by Frappell and co-workers [31].

Direction of gas flow

During a respiratory cycle, the direction of gas flow in the paleopulmonic parabronchi is unidirectional, whereas in the neopulmonic parabronchi it is bidirectional (Fig. 43.8) [16,17]. The unidirectional flow of gas through the paleopulmonic parabronchi is probably due to aerodynamic valves, not mechanical valves [13,33–40]. Although poorly understood, the mechanisms involved probably include the orientation of secondary bronchial and air sac orifices to the direction of gas flow, elastic pressure differences between the cranial and caudal group of air sacs, and gas convective inertial forces [13].

Cross-current model of gas exchange

The movement of gas within the parabronchi and outwards into the atria and infundibulae is by convective flow and then by diffusion into the air capillaries [28,41]. Blood flows from the periphery via the interparabronchial artery and arterioles, ultimately flowing into the blood capillaries where it meets the outward moving air. This

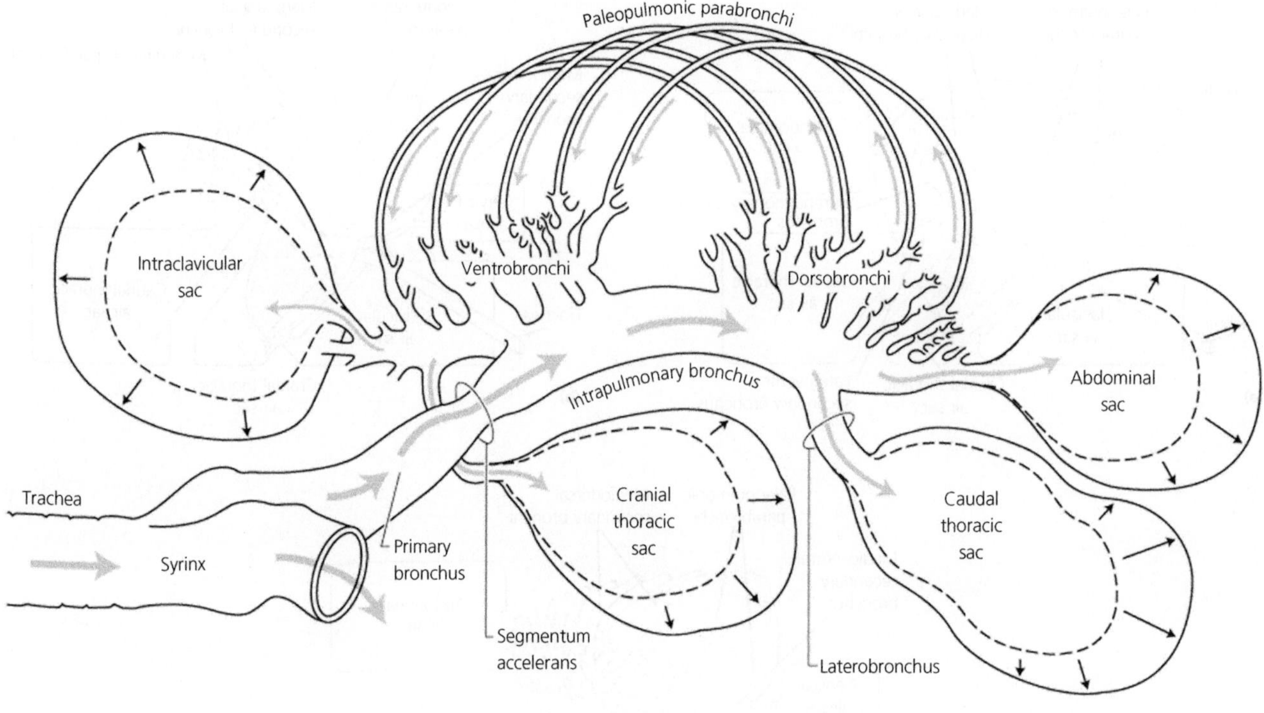

Figure 43.8 Schematic representation of the right paleopulmonic lung and air sacs of a bird and the pathway of gas flow through the pulmonary system during inspiration and expiration (the neopulmonic has been removed for purposes of clarity). (a) Inspiration. (b) Expiration. Source: Adapted from [4] and [16].

multicapillary serial arterialization system increases the duration over which the respiratory media (air and blood) are exposed to each other [13]. Within the cross-current design is a 'countercurrent' system created by the centripetal (inward) flow of the deoxygenated blood and the centrifugal (radial, outward) flow of air from the parabronchial lumen [13]. Thus there is no equivalent of alveolar gas because parabronchial gas continuously changes in composition as it flows along the length of the parabronchus [42].

The efficiency of the avian lung can be put into perspective by considering what happens to the partial pressures of carbon dioxide (CO_2) and oxygen (O_2) both in respired gas as it flows through the lung and in blood as it perfuses the lung. As gas flows along a parabronchus, it receives CO_2 and gives off O_2 so that at the inflow end of the parabronchus, gas has the lowest partial pressure of CO_2 while gas at the outflow end has the highest partial pressure of CO_2; the reverse is true for O_2. The overall result is that the partial pressure of CO_2 in end-parabronchial gas (P_ECO_2) can exceed the partial pressure of CO_2 in arterial blood ($PaCO_2$), and the partial pressure of O_2 in end-parabronchial gas (P_EO_2) can be lower than the partial pressure of O_2 in arterial blood (PaO_2) [43–45]. This potential overlap of blood and gas partial pressure ranges for both CO_2 and O_2 demonstrates the high gas exchange efficiency of the avian lung [43,44].

Control of ventilation

Birds have many of the same physiologic components for respiratory control as mammals, such as a central respiratory pattern generator, central chemoreceptors sensitive to PCO_2, and many similar peripheral chemoreceptors [46]. Birds have a unique group of peripheral receptors located in the lung called intrapulmonary chemoreceptors (IPCs) that are vagal respiratory afferents inhibited by high lung PCO_2 and excited by low lung PCO_2, thus providing phasic feedback for the control of breathing, specifically rate and depth of breathing [46–49]. They are not mechanoreceptors and are insensitive to hypoxia [50,51]. However, IPCs are not the sole receptors stimulated by inhaled gas containing low partial pressures of CO_2; arterial and central chemoreceptors are also stimulated [52].

There may be species differences in CO_2 responsiveness depending upon the ecologic niche a given species occupies. The CO_2 responsiveness of IPCs in chickens, ducks, emus, and pigeons is greater than that of IPCs of burrowing owls that live underground where the CO_2 concentration is higher than that of above ground-dwelling birds [53,54].

Gas exchange components and control of ventilation: considerations for anesthesia

Gas exchange in awake, healthy birds occurs through a process involving a wide range of integrated pulmonary and extrapulmonary factors that operate submaximally (a broad-based low-key strategy) [55]. Thus gas exchange efficiency is not usually apparent under resting conditions and certainly not during anesthesia. However, the gas exchange efficiency of the avian lung is real and is not limited just to O_2 and CO_2, but applies to the exchange of inhalant anesthetics as well.

The avian lung lacks a significant functional residual volume, a feature that limits how long a bird can remain apneic during anesthesia. This is a concern during induction of anesthesia of birds, especially waterfowl, because apnea and bradycardia can occur and may last for up to 5 min. Although referred to as a dive response, in diving ducks it is a stress response mediated by stimulation of trigeminal receptors in the beak and nares [56–59]. Anesthetic gases are not required to elicit this response as it can be triggered by placing a mask snugly over a bird's beak and face. During this stress response, blood flow is preferentially distributed to the kidneys, heart, and brain [60]. This response makes safe induction of anesthesia challenging, and raises the question whether premedicants, such as butorphanol, diazepam, or midazolam, ameliorate or eliminate the dive response and shorten the time to intubation in birds likely to experience a dive response, such as waterfowl. In non-divers, specifically parrots, butorphanol does not shorten the time between the start of induction and intubation. In a study involving adult Hispaniolan Amazon parrots (*Amazona ventralis*), there was not a significant difference in time between induction with sevoflurane to intubation of birds premedicated with butorphanol (2 mg/kg, IM) compared to birds not premedicated with butorphanol [61].

In mammalian species it is well recognized that anesthetics, through their effects on the central nervous system and peripheral chemoreceptors, significantly depress ventilatory responses to hypoxia and hypercapnia [62–64]. Since birds have many of the same mechanisms for controlling ventilation, one must assume that anesthetics will similarly depress avian ventilatory control mechanisms. A number of studies have shown that inhalants depress the responsiveness of a number of peripheral control mechanisms in birds, including IPCs, that directly or indirectly affect ventilation [65–67].

General anesthesia disrupts ventilatory control mechanisms in birds, so whenever possible a bird's ventilation should be assisted or controlled so as to minimize or prevent anesthesia-induced hypoventilation. During positive pressure ventilation, the direction of gas flow within the avian lung may be reversed, but the efficiency of the cross-current system is independent of the direction of air flow relative to blood flow [17,68]. Studies of mechanically, bidirectionally ventilated birds from which arterial blood samples were collected and analyzed did not show adverse effects of mechanical ventilation on gas exchange [69–71].

Because of the flow-through nature of the avian pulmonary system, it is possible to ventilate birds by flowing a continuous stream of gas through the trachea and lungs, and out through a ruptured or cannulated air sac [72,73]. It is also possible to cannulate an abdominal or caudal thoracic air sac and flow inhalant anesthetic through the air sac, across the lung and out via the trachea. This same technique can be used to induce and maintain anesthesia in birds,[72,74–77] and offers a unique, effective means by which to maintain anesthesia for procedures that require full, unimpeded access to the head. This technique has been used in birds as small as zebra finches [78]. In one study of ducks in which arterial blood gases were compared before and after cannulation of the clavicular air sac, both PaO_2 and $PaCO_2$ remained unchanged, but tidal volume increased and minute ventilation doubled [79]. However, a study involving sulfur-crested cockatoos (*Cacatua galerita*) reported that anesthesia could not be maintained in this species when isoflurane was insufflated through the clavicular air sac [75]. This suggests that there may be species differences as to which air sac is best cannulated for delivery of inhalant anesthetics.

Cardiovascular system

The avian heart is a four-chambered muscular pump that separates venous blood from arterial blood. Birds have larger hearts, larger stroke volumes, lower heart rates, and higher cardiac output than mammals of comparable body mass [80]. Birds also have higher blood pressures than do mammals [80,81]. The atria and ventricles are innervated by sympathetic and parasympathetic nerves [82] and norepinephrine and epinephrine are the principal sympathetic neurotransmitters while acetylcholine is the principal parasympathetic neurotransmitter.

The conduction system of the avian heart consists of the sinoatrial node, the atrioventricular node and its branches, and Purkinje fibers [82]. Two groups of animals can be identified by the depth

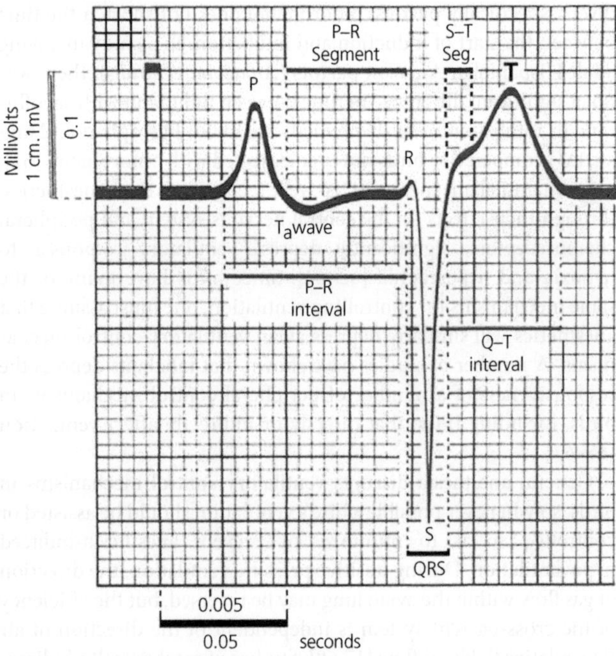

Figure 43.9 An ECG from a pigeon. The ECG trace from a normal bird may have the appearance of ventricular tachycardia primarily because of the large negative S wave. Source: [95].

and degree to which Purkinje fibers ramify within the ventricular myocardium, and the pattern of ramification is classified as type 1 or 2 [83]. The pattern of Purkinje fiber distribution within the ventricular myocardium is responsible for QRS morphology. In birds, Purkinje fibers completely penetrate the ventricular myocardium from endocardium to epicardium and the pattern of ventricular activation is described as type 2b, a pattern that may facilitate synchronous beating at high heart rates [84].

Cardiovascular system: Considerations for anesthesia

Excitement and handling can increase the concentration of norepinephrine and epinephrine, especially epinephrine, in the heart and blood of birds [81,85]. This has significant implications for the anesthetic management of birds because inhalant anesthetics, especially halothane, sensitize the myocardium to catecholamine-induced cardiac arrhythmias. Hypoxia, hypercapnia, and anesthetics, the last depending on the type and in a dose-dependent manner, depress cardiovascular function.

The morphometry of the normal avian ECG has been mistaken for ventricular tachycardia (Fig. 43.9) [84]. Electrocardiograms have been described for a number of avian species,[86–102] and the anesthetist must be familiar with them so as to be able to distinguish between normal and abnormal cardiac rhythms encountered during anesthesia.

General considerations for anesthesia

Physical examination

Every bird should be given a thorough physical examination prior to anesthesia. A number of excellent texts describe in detail the techniques for physical examination and what to look for in specific avian species [103–105]. In general, quiet observation of a bird in its cage will provide a great deal of information. A bird's awareness of and attention to its surrounding environment, body form and posture, feather condition, and respiratory rate provide clues to its physical condition. Birds should be removed from their cage and examined, with particular attention given to the nares and mouth. A stethoscope with a pediatric head for small species should be used to examine the heart and pulmonary system. The sharpness of the keel should be assessed as it is a good indicator of muscle mass and body fat.

Fasting

Withholding food from birds prior to anesthesia and surgery is controversial. Arguments against fasting stem from a concern that fasted birds will become hypoglycemic because of their high metabolic rate and poor hepatic glycogen storage [106,107]. However, because of the hazards associated with regurgitation in minimally fasted birds, some practitioners recommend that avian species, regardless of size, be fasted overnight [108]. A reasonable approach for healthy birds is to withhold food long enough for the upper GI tract to empty, usually overnight in large birds and 4–6 h in smaller birds [109]. In an emergency, a bird with a full crop should be held upright during induction with a finger positioned just below the mandible so as to block the esophagus [109]. Once the bird is anesthetized, the crop can be emptied by placing a finger covered with gauze over the choanal slits to prevent food from entering the nasal cavity and then milking the food contents out of the crop and esophagus [109]. At the end of anesthesia the oral cavity should be checked for and cleaned of food material to prevent aspiration.

Physical restraint

Physical restraint is a crucial aspect of the anesthetic management of any bird. Improper restraint can cause a variety of problems for a bird, including physical trauma (wing or leg fractures) or physiologic stress, the latter of which may predispose to cardiovascular instability. Because birds cannot dissipate heat through the skin, they can become stressed and easily overheated with prolonged restraint. For example, during 15 min of restraint the average cloacal temperature of Amazon parrots (*Amazona* spp.) increased significantly by 2.38 °C (4.28 °F) while mean respiratory rates increased significantly from 129 to 252 breaths/min [110]. These findings emphasize the importance of limiting restraint time and observing for tachypnea, even in healthy parrots, to avoid potentially life-threatening increases in body temperature [110]. In a study involving undisturbed geese, the humoral indices of stress (i.e., blood levels of catecholamines, corticosterone, and lactate) were as low or lower than the lowest values previously reported for birds [111]. In contrast, even though the birds looked calm during a 5 min routine handling procedure to which they had been conditioned for weeks, there was a significant increase in the level of stress-related humoral indices within 2 min after the start of restraint [111]. This clearly shows that the absence of stress cannot be deduced by only observing behavior [111]. A bird may appear calm when restrained, but in fact may be very stressed. Psittacine owners often judge the expertise of a veterinarian by his or her ability to restrain their bird without bruising it around the face. In general, a bird must be restrained so that the wings and legs are controlled and not allowed to flap or kick about. For long-necked birds such as herons and cranes, the neck must be gently controlled so that the bird does not suffer head, eye, or neck trauma; restraining the bird's head and neck also protects the handler.

Understanding the physical characteristics and mechanisms of defense that birds possess is crucial for effective restraint that protects both the bird and handler. Each avian species has its own unique and effective mechanisms for defense. Most birds of prey do not bite, but they can and will use their talons and beak to great effect. Their talons can inflict severe physical trauma on a handler or assistant and the risk of infection from such wounds is quite real. Psittacines have very strong beaks that can cause severe soft tissue injury. Cranes and herons use their long, pointed beaks in a spearing manner, and they tend to strike at eyes, a reason for wearing glasses or goggles when working with these birds. Cranes and ratites, such as emus and ostriches, will jump and strike forward with their legs and clawed feet; an adult ratite can produce a very powerful and dangerous strike-kick.

Injectable drugs for anesthesia and analgesia

Given that there are approximately 10 000 species of birds and that each species has species-specific pharmacokinetic and pharmacodynamic profiles for each injectable drug [85], the following discussion will highlight a few key issues that must be considered when planning to use injectable drugs in birds. For a thorough review of the pharmacology of analgesic drugs used in birds, the reader is encouraged to read the article by Hawkins and Paul-Murphy [85].

Injectable anesthetics are used frequently to produce anesthesia and analgesia in birds and there are many reasons for doing so, including low cost, ease of use, rapidity of anesthetic inductions, no need for expensive equipment to deliver or maintain anesthesia, and minimal if any anesthetic pollution of the work environment. There are, however, inherent disadvantages to using injectables, including significant variation among species and individual birds in terms of dose and response, difficulty in delivering a safe volume to small birds, ease of overdosing by any route, difficulty in maintaining surgical anesthesia without severe cardiopulmonary depression, and the potential for prolonged, violent recoveries [107].

Pharmacologic considerations

Pharmacologic principles applicable to mammals also apply to birds. The pharmacokinetic profile of a drug is described by protein binding, volume of distribution, biotransformation, and excretion, and it will differ from one avian species to another because the relationship between biotransformation and excretion is determined by metabolic factors and heredity [112]. A frequent assumption is that all birds are pharmacologically similar, but this misconception can lead to either limited efficacy or intoxication even among closely related species [112]. Allometric scaling has been used to determine safe, effective doses for drugs used in birds [112–115] and its general principles serve as a rational basis for understanding how body mass or metabolic rate may affect drug doses in some species and for some drugs. For example, a recommended dose for ketamine in a small psittacine weighing under 100 g is 0.07–0.10 mg/g IM, while a bird weighing over 500 g would receive 0.03–0.06 mg/g IM [116]. However, allometric scaling is not useful for extrapolating doses of non-steroidal anti-inflammatory drugs (NSAIDs) between avian species [117] and may not be useful for extrapolating doses of opioids.

There is very little information concerning the pharmacodynamics of drugs used in birds, but studies have shown there can be significant differences in response among avian species given the same drug [85,118,119]. For example, the commercially available form of ketamine consists of a racemic mixture of the *l*- and *d*+forms of ketamine. In great horned and snowy owls this racemic mixture produces chemical restraint and anesthesia of poor quality [119]. When great horned owls receive only the *d*+form of ketamine, anesthesia induction is smoother and there are fewer cardiac arrhythmias, whereas the *l*- form of ketamine is associated with inadequate muscle relaxation, cardiac arrhythmias, and excited behavior during recovery [119]. It is unknown whether these differences are due to differing metabolic pathways among birds, production of pharmacologically active metabolites, or differences in types of receptors or receptor sensitivity.

Pain, analgesics, and opioids

Assessing pain in birds is problematic because the signs of pain vary from one avian species to another [85]. Behavioral signs of pain may be cryptic and subtle, but may include crouching, immobility, failure to dust bathe, under- or overgrooming of feathers, or separation from the flock [85].

Opioids are a mainstay of analgesic therapy in mammals, but for a number of reasons, their use as analgesics in birds has not been straightforward. Many studies of opioids in birds have focused on their effects on learned behavior, motivation, or song production [120–127]. Neural systems involved in motivation and reward in song birds are neuroanatomically well positioned to influence the song control system [126] and motor control [123], findings that are consistent with a dynamic role for opioid receptors in adjusting social behavior and interactions [122,127]. In terms of motor function, a study in chickens indicated that motor deficits associated with the administration of morphine may mask its analgesic effects [128]. In male starlings (*Sturnus vulgaris*), a link was found between analgesia and song, an interaction indicating that distinct neural mechanisms regulate communication in different social contexts (breeding versus non-breeding seasons), a finding that strongly supports a hypothesis that certain types of song (general song versus female-directed song) are tightly linked to opioid release [129].

An early study mapping opioid receptors in the avian brain reported that κ-opioid receptors account for 76% of the radiolabeling of pigeon forebrain tissues [130]. This suggested that a κ-opioid receptor agonist, such as butorphanol, may be a more effective analgesic in birds than a μ-opioid, such as morphine. Indeed, the results of early studies evaluating the analgesic effects of morphine in birds were conflicting in that morphine produced hyperalgesia in one study [131] while producing analgesia in another [132]. These conflicting results probably reflect both species differences in response to morphine and dose-related effects.

A study of fentanyl in white cockatoos (*Cacatua alba*) demonstrated dose-related analgesic effects. Following injection with two different doses of fentanyl (0.02 mg/kg, IM or 0.2 mg/kg, SC), the low dose did not produce analgesia even though for 2 h plasma levels were at concentrations considered analgesic in humans [133]. The high dose provided significant analgesia in some birds, but required a large volume (approximately 2.3 mL per 572 g bird) and caused excitement in some birds [133]. In red-tailed hawks (*Buteo jamaicensis*) a constant rate infusion of fentanyl reduced isoflurane MAC by up to 55% while minimally affecting cardiovascular variables [134].

In African gray parrots, buprenorphine (0.1 mg/kg, IM) did not have analgesic effects when compared to saline [135]. In domestic fowl, the intra-articular application of buprenorphine (0.05–1 mg) to treat experimentally induced articular pain did not have any effect on pain behavior [136]. However, the time to foot withdrawal from a noxious stimulus was increased in pigeons (*Columba* spp.) given buprenorphine (0.25 and 0.5 mg/kg, IM) [85].

Butorphanol has been shown to produce analgesia in cockatoos and African gray parrots [135,137,138]. In guineafowl, butorphanol (2 mg/kg, IV) decreased the MAC of sevoflurane by 9 ± 3%, a clinically insignificant reduction, while a dose of 4 mg/kg reduced MAC, at 15 and 30 min following the injection, by 21 ± 4% and 11 ± 8%, respectively [139].

Injection sites

Subcutaneous injection sites include the area over the back between the wings, the wing web, and the skinfold in the inguinal region. The pectoral and thigh muscles can be used for intramuscular injections. The ulnaris vein, dorsal metatarsal vein, and jugular vein can be used for intravenous injections as well as for catheterization. The right jugular vein is larger and easier to visualize than the left jugular vein in many birds.

Local anesthetics

Local anesthetics have been used in birds with unfortunate consequences, including seizures and cardiac arrest due to the use of inappropriate doses in small birds [107,140]. For example, 0.1 mL of 2% lidocaine administered intramuscularly or subcutaneously to a 30 g parakeet is equivalent to 67 mg/kg, a toxic overdose for any animal. Lidocaine can be used in birds for local anesthesia, but the dose should not exceed 4 mg/kg, a dose difficult to achieve in very small birds unless the drug is diluted. Bupivacaine may be used, but its dose should not exceed 2 mg/kg. Lidocaine and bupivacaine have been assessed for their efficacy in producing brachial plexus blockade. In chickens, lidocaine or bupivacaine (1 mL/kg) was injected after plexus localization via nerve stimulator, but only 66% of 18 blocks produced sensory blockade [141]. In anesthetized female mallard ducks (*Anas platyrhynchos*), results were highly variable when either bupivacaine (2 or 8 mg/kg) or a combination of lidocaine (15 mg/kg) and epinephrine (3.8 μg/kg) was injected around the brachial plexus [142]. Although local anesthetics may yet be shown to provide sufficient local analgesia in birds, they do not relieve the stress associated with physical restraint of an awake bird.

Inhalant anesthetics

Isoflurane currently is considered the inhalant anesthetic of choice for use in birds, but sevoflurane may be supplanting it because of its faster induction and recovery characteristics [143]. Inhalant anesthetics possess several advantages for patient management, including rapid induction and recovery, easier control of anesthetic depth, concurrent use of oxygen that provides respiratory support, and recovery is not dependent on metabolic or excretory pathways. A disadvantage is the need for special equipment such as a source of oxygen, a vaporizer, a breathing circuit, and a mechanism for scavenging waste anesthetic gases.

Breathing circuits and fresh gas flows

Non-rebreathing circuits, such as the Bain circuit or Norman elbow, are ideal for use in birds <10 kg because they offer minimal resistance to patient ventilation. An additional advantage to the plastic Bain circuit is its light weight, a desirable feature when used in very small birds. Oxygen flow for a non-rebreathing circuit should be 150–200 mL/kg/min. For birds that weigh >10 kg, such as ratites, the breathing circuit should be commensurate with the size of the bird. Emus and ostriches under 130 kg can be maintained on a small animal breathing circuit while larger ostriches can be maintained on a large animal breathing circuit [21].

Induction methods

The number and variety of techniques for inducing gas anesthesia in birds are only limited by the anesthetist's imagination. Birds can be induced with commercially available small animal masks or with homemade masks fabricated from plastic bottles, syringe cases, syringes, or breathing hose connectors. Mask induction techniques can be used in a wide variety of sizes of birds, from the very small up to and including the emu. Mask inductions are unsatisfactory in adult ostriches because of the dangers in restraining large birds [21].

Other techniques include the use of plastic bags or chambers. Birds can be induced by inserting their heads into plastic bags (preferably clear plastic) into which oxygen and anesthetic vapor are introduced via a non-rebreathing circuit. Plastic bags have been used to completely enclose a bird cage in order to induce anesthesia in a bird that was difficult to handle [144].

An anesthetic chamber can be used to induce anesthesia. A disadvantage to this technique is that the anesthetist is not in physical contact with the bird and unable to get a feel for how the bird is responding to the anesthetic. In addition, birds can injure themselves as they pass through stage II (involuntary excitement) anesthesia.

Whatever technique is used, the anesthetist must take precautions to control and eliminate anesthetic gas pollution in the work environment. If a mask is used, it should fit snugly over the bird's beak and face, or over its entire head. If a plastic bag or chamber is used, it should be free of leaks. Once induction is completed, the bag or chamber must be removed from the area without the contents being released into the workplace environment.

Minimal anesthetic concentration

The concepts which guide our use of inhalant anesthetics are as applicable to birds as they are to mammals. One such concept is the minimum alveolar concentration (MAC) of an inhalant anesthetic that prevents gross purposeful movement in 50% of anesthetized mammals exposed to a maximal noxious stimulus. The MAC provides a description of concentration and effect (potency), allows us to quantify factors which influence anesthetic requirements, and is equally applicable to all inhalation anesthetics [145]. The term, as defined, is not appropriate for discussions concerning birds because they do not have an alveolar lung. For birds, MAC has been defined as the minimal anesthetic concentration required to prevent gross purposeful movement in response to a painful stimulus [69] and it is usually determined via a bracketing technique.

MAC values of halothane, isoflurane, and sevoflurane in birds are shown in Table 43.1; they are similar to MAC values reported for mammals [146,147]. This lends support to the observation that

Table 43.1 Minimum anesthetic concentration (MAC) for halothane, isoflurane, and sevoflurane in birds.

Bird	Halothane	Isoflurane	Sevoflurane
Chicken (*Gallus gallus*) [152,159,186]	0.85%	1.25%	2.21%
Cinereous vulture (*Aegypius monachus*) [187]	–	1.06%	–
Cockatoo (*Cacatua* spp.) [137]	–	1.44%	–
Duck (*Anas platyrhynchus*) [150,151]	1.05%	1.32%	–
Guineafowl (*Numida meleagris*) [139]	–	–	2.90%
Red-tailed hawk (*Buteo jamaicensis*) [134]	–	2.05%	–
Sandhill crane (*Grus canadensis*) [69]	–	1.35%	–
Thick-billed parrots (*Rhynchopsitta pachyrhyncha*) [188,189]	–	1.07%	2.39–3.94%*

*Not determined by bracketing technique.

different classes or species of animals do not show large variations in effective concentrations of inhalant anesthetics [145].

In general, halothane, isoflurane, and sevoflurane, in a dose-dependent manner, depress ventilation in birds [69,148–153]. Anesthetic index (AI), a measure of the tendency of an inhalant anesthetic to cause respiratory depression and apnea, is derived by dividing the end-tidal concentration of an anesthetic at apnea by the MAC for the anesthetic [154]. The lower the AI for an anesthetic, the greater its depressant effect on ventilation. In ducks anesthetized with halothane, the AI was 1.51 [150] and for isoflurane it was 1.65 [151]. The AI value for isoflurane is considerably lower than for dogs (2.5) [155], cats (2.4) [155], and horses (2.3) [151–156], suggesting that isoflurane depresses ventilation more in birds than in mammals.

The effect of halothane on blood pressure can be variable. In chickens and ducks, increasing concentrations of halothane can cause a decrease in mean arterial blood pressure [152,157] or no change [150]. In contrast, isoflurane appears to consistently cause a dose-dependent decrease in mean arterial blood pressure [69,151,157,158], possibly because of isoflurane-associated peripheral vasodilation. Sevoflurane has been reported to decrease blood pressure in chickens in a dose-dependent manner during controlled ventilation [153,159] but not during spontaneous ventilation, probably because of hypercapnia due to hypoventilation [153]. In crested caracara (*Caracara plancus*), sevoflurane moderately depressed blood pressure and did so without producing cardiac arrhythmias [148]. In red-tailed hawks anesthetized with sevoflurane, blood pressure was significantly lower compared to when they were awake and physically restrained [160].

In mammals, positive pressure ventilation depresses mean arterial blood pressure by creating positive intrathoracic pressures that compress the great vessels, thus impeding the venous return of blood to the heart. In sandhill cranes anesthetized with isoflurane, mean arterial blood pressure was higher during positive pressure ventilation than during spontaneous ventilation [69]. Such is not the case in chickens anesthetized with sevoflurane [153].

Hypoventilation not only makes it difficult to control the plane of anesthesia, but it can have a variety of adverse effects on cardiopulmonary function. For example, in ducks anesthetized and maintained at a constant end-tidal halothane concentration of 1.5%, and in which $PaCO_2$ was varied from 40 to 80 mmHg, unifocal and multifocal cardiac arrhythmias occurred in 50% of the ducks [156]. The mean $PaCO_2$ at which arrhythmias developed was 67 ± 12 mm Hg; in five of six ducks the arrhythmias disappeared after CO_2 inhalation was terminated [161]. To avoid the adverse effects of hypercarbia on cardiac function in anesthetized birds, ventilation should be supported by maintaining a light plane of anesthesia and, when possible, by assisting or controlling ventilation.

Adjuncts to general anesthesia

Fluids

Birds tend to have higher plasma sodium and osmolality compared to mammals [162–166]. For this reason, fluids with an osmolarity close to 300–320 mOsm/L, such as Normosol-R®, Plasmalyte-R®, Plasmalyte-A®, and NaCl 0.9%, have been recommended for fluid therapy in birds, specifically parrots [162], but this is a reasonable guideline for fluid support of any bird during anesthesia.

Nitrous oxide

Nitrous oxide can be used as an adjunct to general anesthesia, but it is not suitable as the sole anesthetic [167]. Nitrous oxide (50%) may decrease the concentration of isoflurane necessary to maintain a suitable plane of anesthesia by only 11% [168]. As with other anesthetic gases and vapors, nitrous oxide is not uniquely sequestered or concentrated in the air sacs. The considerations for using nitrous oxide are the same as for its use in mammals, such as adequate pulmonary function and delivery of sufficient oxygen to meet the patient's metabolic demands. Thirty percent oxygen is generally accepted as the minimum fraction of inspired oxygen that should be provided. Nitrous oxide may pose problems in some avian species. For example, diving birds such as pelicans have subcutaneous pockets of air that do not communicate with the respiratory system, and the use of N_2O in these birds can result in subcutaneous emphysema [169].

Muscle relaxants

Neuromuscular blocking drugs (NMBs) have two purposes in birds: whole-body skeletal muscle paralysis to facilitate surgical procedures, and to produce mydriasis. The neuromuscular and cardiovascular effects of atracurium, when used as a muscle paralytic, have been reported in chickens [170]. The effective dose associated with 95% twitch depression in 50% of the birds ($ED_{95/50}$) was 0.25 mg/kg IV, and $ED_{95/95}$ was calculated to be 0.46 mg/kg IV. The duration of action for the 0.25 mg/kg and 0.45 mg/kg doses was 34.5 ± 5.8 min and 47.8 ± 10.3 min, respectively; these durations of action are similar to those reported in dogs [171,172]. Edrophonium (0.5 mg/kg, IV) reversed muscle paralysis. There were small but statistically significant changes in cardiovascular variables in that heart rate decreased and blood pressure increased after atracurium was administered, but these changes were considered unimportant clinically [170].

Avian pupillary diameter is controlled by skeletal muscles and neuromuscular paralytics have been used to produce mydriasis. In adult cockatoos (*Cacatua sulphurea*), African gray parrots (*Psittacus erithacus*), and blue-fronted Amazon parrots (*Amazona aestivate*), vecuronium (injectable formulation; 0.8 mg/mL) diluted with sterile sodium chloride solution (NaCl, 0.9%) consistently produced the greatest pupillary dilation, and did so with few systemic side-effects, with one notable exception [173]: a cockatoo collapsed and died soon after a combination of vecuronium and saponin (a surface-acting penetrating agent) was dropped onto its eye. This suggests that for mydriasis, vecuronium should not be combined with an agent promoting corneal penetration, thus enhancing systemic uptake with potentially fatal effects. It also reinforces the reality that avian species differ significantly in their responses to any given drug. A contributing factor for variability in response to NMBs may be the tremendous interspecies variation in acetylcholinesterase levels: 0.87 μmol of substrate hydrolyzed/min/mL in cormorants to 7.89 μmol of substrate hydrolyzed/min/mL in mallard ducks [174].

In juvenile double-crested cormorants (*Phalacrocorax auritus*), vecuronium alone or in combination with atropine and phenylephrine was evaluated as a mydriatic [175]. The combination of vecuronium, atropine, and phenylephrine produced the most consistent and greatest dilation and longest average duration; no side-effects from vecuronium were observed [175]. In kestrels (*Falco tinnunculus*), rocuronium (0.12 mg in each eye) [176] or vecuronium (4 mg/mL; 2 drops in each eye, 3 times, at 15-min intervals)[177] are effective mydriatics. Rocuronium has also been shown to be effective in a number of raptorial species, including common buzzards (*Buteo buteo*; 0.40 mg of rocuronium in each eye), little owls (*Athene noctua*; 0.20 mg in each eye) [178] and tawny owls (*Strix aluco*; single topical administration of 0.35 mg in each eye) [179]. In some species, alcuronium and pancuronium have not been found to produce safe or consistently effective mydriasis [177]. None of the studies report corneal injuries following instillation of any neuromuscular paralytic injectable drugs.

Monitoring

Birds must be monitored during anesthesia. Physiologic variables to monitor include respiratory rate and tidal volume, oxygenation, heart rate and rhythm, body temperature, and muscle relaxation. Both respiratory rate and tidal volume should be monitored during anesthesia in an effort to assess the adequacy of ventilation and the depth of anesthesia. Respiratory frequency by itself can be misleading as to the adequacy of ventilation and anesthetic depth. High respiratory frequencies in an anesthetized bird do not necessarily indicate the bird is light and hyperventilating, but are more often associated with small tidal volumes and a greater proportion of deadspace ventilation than effective ventilation [69].

Ventilation can be monitored by watching the frequency and degree of motion of the sternum or movements of the breathing circuit reservoir bag. Capnography can be used to monitor ventilation in birds, but accurate sampling of airway gas may require adjustments in sampling flow rate or technique [180]. Respiratory pauses longer than 10–15 s should be treated by lightening the plane of anesthesia and, when possible, ventilating the bird by either periodically squeezing the reservoir bag or using a positive pressure mechanical ventilator. During positive pressure ventilation, airway pressure should not exceed 15–20 cmH_2O pressure to prevent volotrauma to the air sacs. Respiratory frequencies of 8–10 breaths/min and airway pressures of 10 cmH_2O generally achieve the desired goals of producing a stable plane of anesthesia and acceptable minute ventilation for oxygenation and elimination of CO_2. When it is not possible to measure airway pressure, as is often the case when using non-rebreathing circuits, one should strive for some degree of visible movement of the sternum (keel) and abdomen.

Pulse oximetry can be used to monitor oxygenation, but typical pulse oximeters are designed to measure oxygenated and deoxygenated mammalian hemoglobin, not avian hemoglobin. Critical incidents in birds, like dysrhythmias, severe blood loss, or movement artifacts, cause fluctuations and discontinuity of displayed values and failure to record actual values [181]. Oximeters also tend to underestimate oxygenation levels at high oxygen saturation levels and overestimate oxygenation levels at lower saturation levels [181]. The adequacy of cardiopulmonary function and oxygenation can also be assessed visually by noting the color and capillary refill time of mucous membranes, the color of the cere, beak, or bill, as well as coloration on the head where there is a lack of feathers.

The heart is an electromechanical pump. Its function can be assessed by monitoring mucous membrane color and refill time, palpating peripheral pulses, and monitoring the ECG and blood pressure either indirectly or directly. Standard bipolar and augmented limb leads can be used to monitor and record the avian ECG. To assure adequate skin contact for an interference-free signal, ECG clips can be attached to hypodermic needles inserted through the skin at the base of each wing and through the skin at the level of each stifle. An alternative technique is to attach the ECG clips to stainless steel wires that have been inserted through the prepatagium of each wing and the skin at the lateral side of each stifle. The wire size selected depends on the size of the bird. Twenty- or 22-gauge wire can be used in birds larger than 500 g. Appropriately sized hypodermic needles are used to insert the wires through the skin.

Blood pressure as an indicator of cardiac pump function can be assessed by directly monitoring arterial blood pressure in birds larger than 4 kg, but this technique is not feasible in smaller birds. The Doppler flow probe (Parks Electronics, Aloha, Oregon) is an effective device for monitoring blood flow in small birds, and blood flow or blood pressure in either moderate size or large birds. In awake birds representing 17 commonly kept psittacine species and weighing between 230 and 1263 g, the precision of the blood pressure measurements obtained indirectly with a Doppler device was poor [182]. In Hispaniolan Amazon parrots (*Amazona ventralis*) anesthetized with isoflurane, attempts to measure blood pressure with an oscillometric device proved unsuccessful [183]. In the same birds, there was substantial disagreement between indirect blood pressure measurements obtained with a Doppler device and directly measured systolic arterial blood pressure [183]. A study comparing Doppler and oscillometric methods of indirect arterial blood pressure with direct arterial measurements in anesthetized and awake red-tailed hawks found the oscillometric technique unreliable [160]. Using a Doppler device and a cuff of 40–50% of limb circumference, measurements obtained from either the pectoral or pelvic limb yielded values closer to mean arterial blood pressure than systolic arterial blood pressure [160].

Body temperature should be monitored. The stress associated with anesthesia and surgery is minimized when birds are maintained at or near their normal body temperature. During anesthesia, it is not unusual to see major fluctuations in body temperature, but hypothermia is the most common problem, decreasing the amount of anesthetic needed to maintain anesthesia, causing cardiac instability, and prolonging recovery. In well-insulated birds (feathers, drapes, heating pads) hyperthermia can also occur and cause cardiac instability and an increased oxygen demand. Body temperature can be monitored with an electronic thermometer and a long flexible thermistor probe inserted into the esophagus to the level of the heart. Temperature monitored via the cloaca can vary significantly over time owing to cloacal movements that affect the position of the thermometer or thermistor probe. The clinically acceptable range of core body temperatures is 38.3–40.6 °C [184]. A variety of warming devices and techniques have been evaluated in anesthetized birds, including foam padding or circulating warm water pad inserted between the bird and room-temperature table top, heating lamp, and airway gas warmer-humidifier [185]; only the heating lamp effectively maintained core body temperature. In Hispaniolan Amazon parrots (*Amazona ventralis*) the most effective method for maintaining body temperature was a forced-air warming device (Bair Hugger) at a medium setting (38 °C) [184]. Although this device did not prevent an initial drop in core body temperature, it maintained body temperature within a clinically acceptable range [184]. Additional strategies for controlling body temperature are to maintain a light plane of surgical anesthesia, raise or lower environmental temperature as needed, or wet the bird's legs with alcohol.

Recovery

Precautions should be taken to protect birds while they recover from anesthesia. Birds must be kept from flopping around, as this can lead to serious head, neck, wing, or leg injuries. Struggling and flopping behavior can be prevented by lightly wrapping a bird with a towel, but wrapping poses its own hazards. If a bird is wrapped too tightly, sternal movements will be impeded and breathing will be difficult if not impossible. Wrapping can lead to excessive retention of body heat and cause hyperthermia. If a bird has not been fasted prior to anesthesia, regurgitation can occur during recovery. Keeping a bird intubated during the recovery phase helps to maintain an open airway.

References

1 Handrich Y, Bevan RM, Charrassin JB, *et al.* Hypothermia in foraging king penguins. *Nature* 1997; **388**(6637): 64–67.

2 McLelland J. Larynx and trachea. In: King AS, McLelland J, eds. *Form and Function in Birds*. London: Academic Press, 1989; 69–103.

3 Gaunt AS, Gaunt SLL, Prange HD, Wasser JS. The effects of tracheal coiling on the vocalizations of cranes (*Aves; Gruidae*). *J Comp Physiol A* 1987; **161**: 43–58.

4 Brown RE, Brain JD, Wang N. The avian respiratory system: a unique model for studies of respiratory toxicosis and for monitoring air quality. *Environ Health Perspect* 1997; **105**(2): 188–200.

5 McLelland J. Anatomy of the lungs and air sacs. In: King AS, McLelland J, eds. *Form and Function in Birds*. London: Academic Press, 1989; 221–279.

6 Duncker H. Structure of avian lungs. *Respir Physiol* 1972; **14**: 44–63.

7 Duncker H. Structure of the avian respiratory tract. *Respir Physiol* 1974; **22**: 1–19.

8 King AS, Cowie AF. The functional anatomy of the bronchial muscle of the bird. *J Anat* 1969; **105**: 323–336.

9 Hodges RD. *The Histology of the Fowl*. London: Academic Press, 1974.

10 King AS, McLelland J, eds. *Birds – Their Structure and Function*, 2nd edn. London: Baillière Tindall, 1984.

11 Scheid P, Piiper J. Gas exchange and transport. In: Seller TJ, ed. *Bird Respiration*. Boca Raton, FL: CRC Press, 1987.

12 Magnussen H, Willmer H, Scheid P. Gas exchange in air sacs: contribution to respiratory gas exchange in ducks. *Respir Physiol* 1976; **26**: 129–146.

13 Maina JN. Development, structure, and function of a novel respiratory organ, the lung-air sac system of birds: to go where no other vertebrate has gone. *Biol Rev Camb Philos Soc* 2006; **81**(4): 545–579.

14 Jones JH, Effmann EL, Schmidt-Nielsen K. Lung volume changes during respiration in ducks. *Respir Physiol* 1985; **59**(1): 15–25.

15 Scheid P. Mechanisms of gas exchange in bird lungs. *Rev Physiol Biochem Pharmacol* 1979; **86**: 138–186.

16 Fedde MR. Structure and gas-flow pattern in the avian respiratory system. *Poultry Sci* 1980; **59**: 2642.

17 Scheid P, Piiper J. Respiratory mechanics and air flow in birds. Form and function. In: *Birds*. London: Academic Press, 1989; 369–391.

18 Klide AM. Avian anesthesia. *Vet Clin North Am* 1973; **3**(2): 175–186.

19 Sedgwick CJ. Anesthesia of caged birds. In: Kirk R, ed. *Current Veterinary Therapy VII*. Philadelphia: WB Saunders, 1980; 653–656.

20 Roberson DW, Alosi JA, Messana EP, *et al.* Endotracheal isoflurane anesthesia for chick auditory surgery. *Hearing Res* 2000; **141**: 165–168.

21 Ludders JW, Matthews N. Avian anesthesia. In: Thurmon J, Benson J, Tranquilli W, eds. *Lumb and Jones' Veterinary Anesthesia*, 3rd edn. Baltimore, MD: Williams and Wilkins, 1996; 645–669.

22 King AS, Payne DC. Normal breathing and the effects of posture in *Gallus domesticus*. *J Physiol* 1964; **174**: 340–347.

23 Hawkins MG, Malka S, Pascoe PJ, *et al.* Evaluation of the effects of dorsal versus lateral recumbency on the cardiopulmonary system during anesthesia with isoflurane in red-tailed hawks (*Buteo jamaicensis*). *Am J Vet Res* 2013; **74**(1): 136–143.

24 Malka S, Hawkins MG, Jones JH, *et al.* Effect of body position on respiratory system volumes in anesthetized red-tailed hawks (Buteo jamaicensis) as measured via computed tomography. *Am J Vet Res* 2009; **70**(9): 1155–1160.

25 Barnas GM, Mather FB, Fedde MR. Response of avian intrapulmonary smooth muscle to changes in carbon dioxide concentration. *Poultry Sci* 1978; **57**: 1400–1407.

26 Maina JN, Nathaniel C. A qualitative and quantitative study of the lung of an ostrich, *Struthio camelus*. *J Exp Biol* 2001; **204**: 2313–2330.

27 Maina JN, Jimoh SA, Hosie M. Implicit mechanistic role of the collagen, smooth muscle, and elastic tissue components in strengthening the air and blood capillaries of the avian lung. *J Anat* 2010; **217**(5): 597–608.

28 Woodward JD, Maina JN. Study of the structure of the air and blood capillaries of the gas exchange tissue of the avian lung by serial section three-dimensional reconstruction. *J Microsc* 2008; **230**: 84–93.

29 Bernhard W, Gebert A, Vieten G, *et al.* Pulmonary surfactant in birds: coping with surface tension in a tubular lung. *Am J Physiol Regul Integr Comp Physiol* 2001; **281**(1): R327–337.

30 Maina JN, King AS, Settle G. An allometric study of pulmonary morphometric parameters in birds, with mammalian comparisons. *Philos Trans R Soc Lond B Biol Sci* 1989; **326**(1231): 1–57.

31 Frappell PB, Hinds DS, Boggs DF. Scaling of respiratory variables and the breathing pattern in birds: an allometric and phylogenetic approach. *Physiol Biochem Zool* 2001; **74**(1): 75–89.

32 Pokras MA, Karas AM, Kirkwood JK, Sedgwick CJ. An introduction to allometric scaling and its use in raptor medicine. In: Redig PT, Hunter B, eds. *Raptor Biomedicine*. Minneapolis, MN: University of Minnesota Press, 1993; 211–228.

33 Banzett RB, Butler JP, Nations CS, *et al.* Inspiratory aerodynamic valving in goose lungs depends on gas density and velocity. *Respir Physiol* 1987; **70**(3): 287–300.

34 Banzett RB, Nations CS, Wang N, *et al.* Pressure profiles show features essential to aerodynamic valving in geese. *Respir Physiol* 1991; **84**(3): 295–309.

35 Brown R, Kovacs C, Butler J, *et al.* The avian lung: is there an aerodynamic expiratory valve? *J Exp Biol* 1995; **198**: 2349–2357.

36 Butler JP, Banzett RB, Fredberg JJ. Inspiratory valving in avian bronchi: aerodynamic considerations. *Respir Physiol* 1988; **72**(2): 241–255.

37 Jones JH, Effmann EL, Schmidt-Nielsen K. Control of air flow in bird lungs: radiographic studies. *Respir Physiol* 1981; **45**(2): 121–131.

38 Kuethe DO. Fluid mechanical valving of air flow in bird lungs. *J Exp Biol* 1988; **136**: 1–12.

39 Scheid P, Piiper J. Aerodynamic valving in the avian lung. *Acta Anaesthesiol Scand Suppl* 1989; **90**: 28–31.

40 Wang N, Banzett RB, Butler JP, Fredberg JJ. Bird lung models show that convective inertia effects inspiratory aerodynamic valving. *Respir Physiol* 1988; **73**(1): 111–124.

41 Crank WD, Gallagher RR. Theory of gas exchange in the avian parabronchus. *Respir Physiol* 1978; **35**(1): 9–25.

42 Scheid P, Piiper J. Analysis of gas exchange in the avian lung: theory and experiments in the domestic fowl. *Respir Physiol* 1970; **9**: 246–262.

43 Piiper J, Scheid P. Gas exchange in avian lungs: models and experimental evidence. In: Bolis L, Schmidt-Nielsen K, eds. *Comparative Physiology*. Amsterdam, Netherlands: North-Holland Publishing, 1973.

44 Powell FL, Scheid P. Physiology of gas exchange in the avian respiratory system. In: King AS, McLelland J, eds. *Form and Function in Birds*. London: Academic Press, 1989; 393–437.

45 Powell FL, Shams H, Hempleman SC, Mitchell GS. Breathing in thin air: acclimatization to altitude in ducks. *Respir Physiol Neurobiol* 2004; **144**(2–3): 225–235.

46 Gleeson M. Control of breathing. In: King AS, McLelland J, eds. *Form and Function in Birds*. London: Academic Press, 1989; 439–484.

47 Hempleman SC, Rodriguez TA, Bhagat YA, Begay RS. Benzolamide, acetazolamide, and signal transduction in avian intrapulmonary chemoreceptors. *Am J Physiol Regul Integr Comp Physiol* 2000; **279**(6): R1988–1995.

48 Hempleman SC, Adamson TP, Begay RS, Solomon IC. CO_2 transduction in avian intrapulmonary chemoreceptors is critically dependent on transmembrane Na^+/H^+ exchange. *Am J Physiol Regul Integr Comp Physiol* 2003; **284**(6): R1551–1559.

49 Shoemaker JM, Hempleman SC. Avian intrapulmonary chemoreceptor discharge rate is increased by anion exchange blocker 'DIDS'. *Respir Physiol* 2001; **128**(2): 195–204.

50 Barnas GM, Mather FB, Fedde MR. Are avian intrapulmonary CO_2 receptors chemically modulated mechanoreceptors or chemoreceptors? *Respir Physiol* 1978; **35**(2): 237–243.

51 Hempleman SC, Burger RE. Receptive fields of intrapulmonary chemoreceptors in the Pekin duck. *Respir Physiol* 1984; **57**(3): 317–330.

52 Fedde MR, Nelson PI, Kuhlmann WD. Ventilatory sensitivity to changes in inspired and arterial carbon dioxide partial pressures in the chicken. *Poultry Sci* 2002; **81**(6): 869–876.

53 Hempleman SC, Burger RE. Comparison of intrapulmonary chemoreceptor response to PCO2 in the duck and chicken. *Respir Physiol* 1985; **61**(2):179–184.

54 Kilgore DL, Faraci FM, Fedde MR. Static response characteristics of intrapulmonary chemoreceptors in the pigeon and burrowing owl, a species with a blunted ventilatory sensitivity to carbon dioxide. *Fed Proc* 1984; **43**: 638.

55 Figueroa D, Olivares R, Salaberry M, *et al.* Interplay between the morphometry of the lungs and the mode of locomotion in birds and mammals. *Biol Res* 2007; **40**(2): 193–201.

56 Butler PJ. The exercise response and the "classical" diving response during natural submersion in birds and mammals. *Can J Zool* 1988; **66**: 29–39.

57 Furilla RA, Jones DR. The contribution of nasal receptors to the cardiac response to diving in restrained and unrestrained redhead ducks (*Aythya americana*). *J Exp Biol* 1986; **121**: 227–238.

58 Jones DR, Furilla RA, Heieis MRA, *et al.* Forced and voluntary diving in ducks: cardiovascular adjustments and their control. *Can J Zool* 1988; **66**(1): 75–83.

59 Woakes AJ. Metabolism in diving birds: studies in the laboratory and the field. *Can J Zool* 1988; **66**: 138–141.

60 Jones DR. Regional distribution of blood flow during diving in the duck (*Anas platyrhynchos*). *Can J Zool* **57**(5): 995–1002.

61 Klaphake E, Schumacher J, Greenacre C, *et al.* Comparative anesthetic and cardiopulmonary effects of pre- versus postoperative butorphanol administration in Hispaniolan Amazon parrots (*Amazona ventralis*) anesthetized with sevoflurane. *J Avian Med Surg* 2006; **20**(1): 2–7.

62 Hirshman CA, McCullough RE, Cohen PJ, Weil JV. Hypoxic ventilatory drive in dogs during thiopental, ketamine, or pentobarbital anesthesia. *Anesthesiology* 1975; **43**(6): 628–634.

63 Hirshman CA, McCullough RE, Cohen PJ, Weil JV. Depression of hypoxic ventilatory response by halothane, enflurane and isoflurane in dogs. *Br J Anaesth* 1977; **49**(10): 957–963.

64 Pavlin EG, Hornbein TF. Anesthesia and the control of ventilation. In: Cherniak NS, Widdicombe JG, eds. *Handbook of Physiology: The Respiratory System.* Bethesda, MD: American Physiological Society, 1986; 972.

65 Bagshaw RJ, Cox RH. Baroreceptor control of heart rate in chickens (*Gallus domesticus*). *Am J Vet Res* 1986; **47**: 293–295.

66 Molony V. Classification of vagal afferents firing in phase with breathing in *Gallus domesticus*. *Respir Physiol* 1974; **22**: 57–76.

67 Pizarro J, Ludders JW, Douse MA, Mitchell GS. Halothane effects on ventilatory responses to changes in intrapulmonary CO_2 in geese. *Respir Physiol* 1990; **82**(3): 337–347.

68 Scheid P, Piiper J. Cross-current gas exchange in avian lungs: effects of reversed parabronchial air flow in ducks. *Respir Physiol* 1972; **16**(3): 304–312.

69 Ludders JW, Rode J, Mitchell GS. Isoflurane anesthesia in sandhill cranes (*Grus canadensis*): minimal anesthetic concentration and cardiopulmonary dose-response during spontaneous and controlled breathing. *Anesth Analg* 1989; **68**(4): 511–516.

70 Pettifer GR, Cornick-Seahorn J, Smith JA, *et al.* The comparative cardiopulmonary effects of spontaneous and controlled ventilation by using the Hallowell EMC Anesthesia WorkStation in Hispaniolan Amazon parrots (*Amazona ventralis*). *J Avian Med Surg* 2002; **16**(4): 268–276.

71 Piiper J, Drees F, Scheid P. Gas exchange in the domestic fowl during spontaneous breathing and artificial ventilation. *Respir Physiol* 1970; **9**: 234–245.

72 Burger RE, Lorenz FW. Artificial respiration in birds by unidirectional air flow. *Poultry Sci* 1960; **39**: 236–237.

73 Burger RE, Meyer M, Graf W, Scheid P. Gas exchange in the parabronchial lung of birds: experiments in unidirectionally ventilated ducks. *Respir Physiol* 1979; **36**(1): 19–37.

74 Jaensch SM, Cullen L, Raidal SR. Comparison of endotracheal, caudal thoracic air sac, and clavicular air sac administration of isoflurane in sulphur-crested cockatoos (*Cacatua galerita*). *J Avian Med Surg* 2001; **15**(3): 170–177.

75 Jaensch SM, Cullen L, Raidal SR. Air sac functional anatomy of the sulphur-crested cockatoo (Cacatua galerita) during isoflurane anesthesia. *J Avian Med Surg* 2002; **16**(1): 2–9.

76 Whittow GC, Ossorio N. A new technic for anesthetizing birds. *Lab Anim Care* 1970; **20**: 651–656.

77 Wijnberg I, Lagerweij E, Zwart P. Inhalation anesthesia in birds through the abdominal air sac, using a unidirectional, continuous flow. *Vet Anaesth Analg* 1991; **18**(Suppl 1): 249–253.

78 Nilson PC, Teramitsu I, White SA. Caudal thoracic air sac cannulation in zebra finches for isoflurane anesthesia. *J Neurosci Methods* 2005; **143**(2): 107–115.

79 Rode JA, Bartholow S, Ludders JW. Ventilation through an air sac cannula during tracheal obstruction in ducks. *J Assoc Avian Vet* 1990; **4**: 98–102.

80 Grubb BR. Allometric relations of cardiovascular function in birds. *Am J Physiol* 1983; **245**: H567–572.

81 Sturkie PD. Heart and circulation: anatomy, hemodynamics, blood pressure, blood flow. In: Sturkie PD, ed. *Avian Physiology*, 4th edn. New York: Springer, 1986.

82 Sturkie PD. Heart: contraction, conduction, and electrocardiography. In: Sturkie PD, ed. *Avian Physiology*, 4th edn. New York: Springer, 1986.

83 O'Callaghan MW. Regulation of heart beat. In: Phillipson AT, Hall LW, Pritchard WR, eds. *Scientific Foundations of Veterinary Medicine*. London: Heinemann, 1980.

84 Keene BW, Flammer K. ECG of the month. *J Am Vet Med Assoc* 1991; **198**(3): 408–409.

85 Hawkins MG, Paul-Murphy JR. Avian analgesia. *Vet Clin North Am Exot Anim Pract* 2011; **14**(1): 61–80.

86 Casares M, Enders F, Montoya JA. Comparative electrocardiography in four species of macaws (genera *Anodorhynchus* and *Ara*). *J Vet Med A Physiol Pathol Clin Med* 2000; **47**(5): 277–281.

87 Cinar A, Bagci C, Belge F, Uzun M. The electrocardiogram of the Pekin duck. *Avian Dis* 1996; **40**(4): 919–923.

88 Espino L, Suarez ML, Lopez-Beceiro A, Santamarina G. Electrocardiogram reference values for the buzzard in Spain. *J Wildl Dis* 2001; **37**(4): 680–685.

89 Hassanpour H, Hojjati P, Zarei H. Electrocardiogram analysis of the normal unanesthetized green peafowl (*Pavo muticus*). *Zoo Biol* 2011; **30**(5): 542–549.

90 Hassanpour H, Moghaddam AK, Bashi MC. The normal electrocardiogram of conscious golden eagles (*Aquila chrysaetos*). *J Zoo Wildl Med* 2010; **41**(3): 426–431.

91 Hassanpour H, Zarei H, Hojjati P. Analysis of electrocardiographic parameters in helmeted guinea fowl (*Numida meleagris*). *J Avian Med Surg* 2011; **25**(1): 8–13.

92 Kisch B. The electrocardiogram of birds (chicken, duck, pigeon). *Exp Med Surg* 1951; **9**: 103–124.

93 Lopez Murcia MM, Bernal LJ, Montes AM, *et al.* The normal electrocardiogram of the unanaesthetized competition "Spanish Pouler" pigeon (*Columba livia gutturosa*). *J Vet Med A Physiol Pathol Clin Med* 2005; **52**(7): 347–349.

94 Lumeij JT, Stokhof AA. Electrocardiogram of the racing pigeon (*Columba livia domestica*). *Res Vet Sci* 1985; **38**(3): 275–278.

95 Nap AMP, Lumeij JT, Stokhof AA. Electrocardiogram of the African grey (*Psittacus erithacus*) and Amazon (*Amazona* spp.) parrot. *Avian Pathol* 1992; **21**(1): 45–53.

96 Rezakhani A, Komali H, Mokhber-Dezfoul MR, *et al.* A preliminary study on normal electrocardiographic parameters of ostriches (Struthio camelus). *J S Afr Vet Assoc* 2007; **78**(1): 46–48.

97 Rodriguez R, Prieto-Montana F, Montes AM, *et al.* The normal electrocardiogram of the unanesthetized peregrine falcon (*Falco peregrinus brookei*). *Avian Dis* 2004; **48**(2): 405–409.

98 Talavera J, Guzman MJ, del Palacio MJ, *et al.* The normal electrocardiogram of four species of conscious raptors. *Res Vet Sci* 2008; **84**(1): 119–125.

99 Uzun M, Yildiz S, Onder F. Electrocardiography of rock partridges (*Alectoris graeca*) and chukar partridges (*Alectoris chukar*). *J Zoo Wildl Med* 2004; **35**(4): 510–514.

100 Zandvliet M. Electrocardiography in psittacine birds and ferrets. *Sem Avian Exotic Pet Med* 2005; **14**(1): 34–51.

101 Zenoble R, Graham D. Electrocardiography of the parakeet, parrot and owl. In: *Proceedings of the Annual Meeting of the American Association of Zoo Veterinarians*, 1979.

102 Zenoble RD. Electrocardiography in the parakeet and parrot. *Comp Cont Educ Pract Vet* 1981; **3**: 711–716.

103 Cooper JE. *Birds of Prey: Health and Disease*, 3rd edn. Oxford: Blackwell Science, 2002.

104 Miller RE, Fowler M, eds. *Fowler's Zoo and Wild Animal Medicine Current Therapy*, 7th edn. St Louis, MO: Elsevier/Saunders, 2012.

105 Ritchie BW, Harrison GJ, Harrison LR. *Avian Medicine: Principles and Application*. Lake Worth, FL: Wingers Publishing, 1994.

106 Altman RB. Avian anesthesia. *Comp Cont Educ Pract Vet* 1980; **2**: 38–43.

107 Franchetti DR, Klide AM. Restraint and anesthesia. In: Fowler ME, ed. *Zoo and Wild Animal Medicine*. Philadelphia: WB Saunders, 1978; 359–364.

108 Harrison GJ. Pre-anesthetic fasting recommended. *J Avian Med Surg* 1991; **5**: 126.

109 Sinn LC. Anesthesiology. In: Zantop DW, ed. *Avian Medicine: Principles and Application*. Lake Worth, FL: Wingers Publishing, 1997; 589–599.

110 Greenacre CB, Lusby AL. Physiologic responses of Amazon parrots (*Amazona* species) to manual restraint. *J Avian Med Surg* 2004; **18**(1): 19–22.

111 Le Maho Y, Karmann H, Briot D, *et al.* Stress in birds due to routine handling and a technique to avoid it. *Am J Physiol* 1992; **263**: R775–781.

112 Dorrestein GM. The pharmacokinetics of avian therapeutics. *Vet Clin North Am Small Anim Pract* 1991; **21**(6): 1241–1264.

113 Boxenbaum H. Interspecies scaling, allometry, physiological time, and the ground plan of pharmacokinetics. *J Pharmacokinet Biopharm* 1982; **10**(2): 201–227.

114 Schmidt-Nielsen K. *Scaling – Why Is Animal Size So Important?* Cambridge: Cambridge University Press, 1991.

115 Sedgwick C, Pokras M. Extrapolating rational drug doses and treatment periods by allometric scaling. In: *Proceedings of the 55th Annual Meeting of the American Animal Hospital Association*, 1988; 156–161.

116 McDonald S. Common anesthetic dosages for use in psittacine birds. *J Assoc Avian Vet* 1989; **3**: 186–187.

117 Baert K, de Backer P. Comparative pharmacokinetics of three nonsteroidal antiinflammatory drugs in five bird species. *Comp Biochem Physiol C Toxicol Pharmacol* 2003; **134**(1): 25–33.

118 Dorrestein GM, van Miert AS. Pharmacotherapeutic aspects of medication of birds. *J Vet Pharmacol Ther* 1988; **11**(1): 33–44.

119 Redig PT, Larson AA, Duke GE. Response of great horned owls given the optical isomers of ketamine. *Am J Vet Res* 1984; **45**(1): 125–127.

120 France CP, Woods JH. Morphine, saline and naltrexone discrimination in morphine-treated pigeons. *J Pharmacol Exp Ther* 1987; **242**(1): 195–202.

121 Herling S, Valentino RJ, Solomon RE, Woods JH. Narcotic discrimination in pigeons: antagonism by naltrexone. *Eur J Pharmacol* 1984; **105**: 137–142.

122 Kelm CA, Forbes-Lorman RM, Auger CJ, Riters LV. Mu-opioid receptor densities are depleted in regions implicated in agonistic and sexual behavior in male European starlings (*Sturnus vulgaris*) defending nest sites and courting females. *Behav Brain Res* 2011; **219**(1): 15–22.

123 Khurshid N, Agarwal V, Iyengar S. Expression of mu- and delta-opioid receptors in song control regions of adult male zebra finches (*Taenopygia guttata*). *J Chem Neuroanat* 2009; **37**(3): 158–169.

124 Leander JD, McMillan DE. Meperidine effects on schedule-controlled responding. *J Pharmacol Exp Ther* 1977; **201**(2): 434–443.

125 Leander JD. Opioid agonist and antagonist behavioural effects of buprenorphine. *Br J Pharmacol* 1983; **78**(4): 607–615.

126 Riters LV. Evidence for opioid involvement in the motivation to sing. *J Chem Neuroanat* 2010; **39**(2): 141–150.

127 Riters LV. Pleasure seeking and birdsong. *Neurosci Biobehav Rev* 2011; **35**(9): 1837–1845.

128 Rager DR, Gallup GG Jr. Apparent analgesic effects of morphine in chickens may be confounded by motor deficits. *Physiol Behav* 1986; **37**(2): 269–272.

129 Kelm-Nelson CA, Stevenson SA, Riters LV. Context-dependent links between song production and opioid-mediated analgesia in male European starlings (*Sturnus vulgaris*). *PLoS One* 2012; **7**(10): e46721.

130 Mansour A, Khachaturian H, Lewis ME, *et al.* Anatomy of CNS opioid receptors. *Trends Neurosci* 1988; **11**(7): 308–314.

131 Hughes RA. Codeine analgesic and morphine hyperalgesic effects on thermal nociception in domestic fowl. *Pharmacol Biochem Behav* 1990; **35**(3): 567–570.

132 Bardo MT, Hughes RA. Brief communication. Shock-elicited flight response in chickens as an index of morphine analgesia. *Pharmacol Biochem Behav* 1978; **9**(1): 147–149.

133 Hoppes S, Flammer K, Hoersch L, *et al.* Disposition and analgesic effects of fentanyl in white cockatoos (*Cacatua alba*). *J Avian Med Surg* 2003; **17**(3): 124–130.

134 Pavez JC, Hawkins MG, Pascoe PJ, *et al.* Effect of fentanyl target-controlled infusions on isoflurane minimum anaesthetic concentration and cardiovascular function in red-tailed hawks (*Buteo jamaicensis*). *Vet Anaesth Analg* 2011; **38**(4): 344–351.

135 Paul-Murphy JR, Brunson DB, V M. Analgesic effects of butorphanol and buprenorphine in conscious African grey parrots (*Psittacus erithacus erithacus* and *Psittacus erithacus timneh*). *Am J Vet Res* 1999; **60**(10): 1218–1221.

136 Gentle MJ, Hocking PM, Bernard R, Dunn LN. Evaluation of intraarticular opioid analgesia for the relief of articular pain in the domestic fowl. *Pharmacol Biochem Behav* 1999; **63**(2): 339–343.

137 Curro TG, Brunson DB, Paul-Murphy JR. Determination of the ED50 of isoflurane and evaluation of the isoflurane-sparing effect of butorphanol in cockatoos (*Cacatua* spp.). *Vet Surg* 1994; **23**(5): 429–433.

138 Paul-Murphy JR, Ludders JW. Avian analgesia. *Vet Clin North Am Exot Anim Pract* 2001; **4**(1): 35–45.

139 Escobar A, Valadao CA, Brosnan RJ, *et al.* Effects of butorphanol on the minimum anesthetic concentration for sevoflurane in guineafowl (*Numida meleagris*). *Am J Vet Res* 2012; **73**(2): 183–188.

140 Fedde MR. Drugs used for avian anesthesia: a review. *Poultry Sci* 1978; **57**(5): 1376–1399.

141 Figueiredo JP, Cruz ML, Mendes GM, *et al.* Assessment of brachial plexus blockade in chickens by an axillary approach. *Vet Anaesth Analg* 2008; **35**(6): 511–518.

142 Brenner DJ, Larsen RS, Dickinson PJ, *et al.* Development of an avian brachial plexus nerve block technique for perioperative analgesia in mallard ducks (*Anas platyrhynchos*). *J Avian Med Surg* 2010; **24**(1): 24–34.

143 Granone TD, de Francisco ON, Killos MB, *et al.* Comparison of three different inhalant anesthetic agents (isoflurane, sevoflurane, desflurane) in red-tailed hawks (*Buteo jamaicensis*). *Vet Anaesth Analg* 2012; **39**(1): 29–37.

144 Bednarski RM, Ludders JW, LeBlanc PH, *et al.* Isoflurane-nitrous oxide-oxygen anesthesia in an Andean condor. *J Am Vet Med Assoc* 1985; **187**(11): 1209–1210.

145 Quasha AL, Eger EI, Tinker JH. Determination and applications of MAC. *Anesthesiology* 1980; **53**(4): 315–334.

146 Eger EI. *Isoflurane: A Compendium and Reference*. Madison, WI: Anaquest, 1985.

147 Steffey EP. Inhalation anesthetics. In: Thurmon JC, Tranquilli WJ, Benson GJ, eds. *Lumb and Jones' Veterinary Anesthesia*, 3rd edn. Baltimore, MD: Williams and Wilkins, 1996, 297.

148 Escobar A, Thiesen R, Vitaliano SN, *et al.* Some cardiopulmonary effects of sevoflurane in crested caracara (*Caracara plancus*). *Vet Anaesth Analg* 2009; **36**(5): 436–441.

149 Jaensch SM, Cullen L, Raidal S. Comparative cardiopulmonary effects of halothane and isoflurane in galahs (*Eolophus roseicapillus*). *J Avian Med Surg* 1999; **13**(1): 15–22.

150 Ludders JW. Minimal anesthetic concentration and cardiopulmonary dose-response of halothane in ducks. *Vet Surg* 1992; **21**(4): 319–324.

151 Ludders JW, Mitchell GS, Rode J. Minimal anesthetic concentration and cardiopulmonary dose response of isoflurane in ducks. *Vet Surg* 1990; **19**(4): 304–307.

152 Ludders JW, Mitchell GS, Schaefer SL. Minimum anesthetic dose and cardiopulmonary dose response for halothane in chickens. *Am J Vet Res* 1988; **49**(6): 929–932.

153 Naganobu K, Ise K, Miyamoto T, Hagio M. Sevoflurane anaesthesia in chickens during spontaneous and controlled ventilation. *Vet Rec* 2003; **152**(2): 45–48.

154 Regan MJ, Eger EI. Effect of hypothermia in dogs on anesthetizing and apneic doses of inhalation agents. Determination of the anesthetic index (Apnea/MAC). *Anesthesiology* 1967; **28**(4): 689–700.

155 Steffey EP, Howland D. Isoflurane potency in the dog and cat. *Am J Vet Res* 1977; **38**(11): 1833–1836.

156 Steffey EP, Howland D, Giri S, Eger EI. Enflurane, halothane, and isoflurane potency in horses. *Am J Vet Res* 1977; **38**(7): 1037–1039.

157 Goelz MF, Hahn AW, Kelley ST. Effects of halothane and isoflurane on mean arterial blood pressure, heart rate, and respiratory rate in adult Pekin ducks. *Am J Vet Res* 1990; **51**(3): 458–460.

158 Greenlees KJ, Clutton RE, Larsen CT, Eyre P. Effect of halothane, isoflurane, and pentobarbital anesthesia on myocardial irritability in chickens. *Am J Vet Res* 1990; **51**(5): 757–758.

159 Naganobu K, Fujisawa Y, Ohde H, *et al.* Determination of the minimum anesthetic concentration and cardiovascular dose response for sevoflurane in chickens during controlled ventilation. *Vet Surg* 2000; **29**(1): 102–105.

160 Zehnder AM, Hawkins MG, Pascoe PJ, Kass PH. Evaluation of indirect blood pressure monitoring in awake and anesthetized red-tailed hawks (*Buteo jamaicensis*): effects of cuff size, cuff placement, and monitoring equipment. *Vet Anaesth Analg* 2009; **36**(5): 464–479.

161 Naganobu K, Hagio M, Sonoda T, *et al.* Arrhythmogenic effect of hypercapnia in ducks anesthetized with halothane. *Am J Vet Res* 2001; **62**(1): 127–129.

162 Beaufrere H, Acierno MJ, Mitchell M, *et al.* Plasma osmolality reference values in African grey parrots (*Psittacus erithacus erithacus*), Hispaniolan Amazon parrots (*Amazona ventralis*), and red-fronted macaws (*Ara rubrogenys*). *J Avian Med Surg* 2011; **25**(2): 91–96.

163 Chan FT, Lin PI, Chang GR, *et al.* Hematocrit and plasma chemistry values in adult collared scops owls (*Otus lettia*) and crested serpent eagles (*Spilornis cheela hoya*). *J Vet Med Sci* 2012; **74**(7): 893–898.

164 Lumeij JT, Overduin LM. Plasma chemistry references values in psittaciformes. *Avian Pathol* 1990; **19**(2): 235–244.

165 Lumeij JT, Remple JD, Remple CJ, Riddle KE. Plasma chemistry in peregrine falcons (*Falco peregrinus*): reference values and physiological variations of importance for interpretation. *Avian Pathol* 1998; **27**(2): 129–132.

166 Verstappen FA, Lumeij JT, Bronneberg RG. Plasma chemistry reference values in ostriches. *J Wildl Dis* 2002; **38**(1): 154–159.

167 Arnall L. Anaesthesia and surgery in cage and aviary birds (I). *Vet Rec* 1961; **73**: 139–142.

168 Korbel R, Burike S, Erhardt W, *et al.* Effects of nitrous oxide application in racing pigeons (*Columbia livia gmel.*, 1789, var. dom.). A study using the air sac perfusion technique. *Is J Vet Med* 1996; **51**: 133–139.

169 Reynold WT. Unusual anesthetic complication in a pelican. *Vet Rec* 1983; **113**: 204.

170 Nicholson A, Ilkiw JE. Neuromuscular and cardiovascular effects of atracurium in isoflurane-anesthetized chickens. *Am J Vet Res* 1992; **53**(12): 2337–2342.

171 Martin-Flores M, Lau EJ, Campoy L, *et al.* Twitch potentiation: a potential source of error during neuromuscular monitoring with acceleromyography in anesthetized dogs. *Vet Anaesth Analg* 2011; **38**(4): 328–335.

172 McMurphy RM, Davidson HJ, Hodgson DS. Effects of atracurium on intraocular pressure, eye position, and blood pressure in eucapnic and hypocapnic isoflurane-anesthetized dogs. *Am J Vet Res* 2004; **65**(2): 179–182.

173 Ramer JC, Paul-Murphy JR, Brunson D, Murphy CJ. Effects of mydriatic agents in cockatoos, African gray parrots, and blue-fronted Amazon parrots. *J Am Vet Med Assoc* 1996; **208**(2): 227–230.

174 Thompson HM. Avian serum esterases: species and temporal variations and their possible consequences. *Chem Biol Interact* 1993; **87**: 329–338.

175 Loerzel SM, Smith PJ, Howe A, Samuelson DA. Vecuronium bromide, phenylephrine and atropine combinations as mydriatics in juvenile double-crested cormorants (*Phalacrocorax auritus*). *Vet Ophthalmol* 2002; **5**(3): 149–154.

176 Barsotti G, Briganti A, Spratte JR, *et al.* Safety and efficacy of bilateral topical application of rocuronium bromide for mydriasis in European kestrels (*Falco tinnunculus*). *J Avian Med Surg* 2012; **26**(1): 1–5.

177 Mikaelian I, Paillet I, Williams D. Comparative use of various mydriatic drugs in kestrels (*Falco tinnunculus*). *Am J Vet Res* 1994; **55**(2): 270–272.

178 Barsotti G, Briganti A, Spratte JR, *et al.* Bilateral mydriasis in common buzzards (*Buteo buteo*) and little owls (*Athene noctua*) induced by concurrent topical administration of rocuronium bromide. *Vet Ophthalmol* 2010; **13**(Suppl): 35–40.

179 Barsotti G, Briganti A, Spratte JR, *et al.* Mydriatic effect of topically applied rocuronium bromide in tawny owls (*Strix aluco*): comparison between two protocols. *Vet Ophthalmol* 2010; **13**(Suppl): 9–13.

180 Edling TM, Degernes LA, Flammer K, Horne WA. Capnographic monitoring of anesthetized African grey parrots receiving intermittent positive pressure ventilation. *J Am Vet Med Assoc* 2001; **219**(12): 1714–1718.

181 Schmitt PPM, Gobel T, Trautvetter E. Evaluation of pulse oximetry as a monitoring method in avian anesthesia. *J Avian Med Surg* 1998; **12**(2): 91–99.

182 Johnston MS, Davidowski LA, Rao S, Hill AE. Precision of repeated, Doppler-derived indirect blood pressure measurements in conscious psittacine birds. *J Avian Med Surg* 2011; **25**(2): 83–90.

183 Acierno MJ, da Cunha A, Smith J, *et al.* Agreement between direct and indirect blood pressure measurements obtained from anesthetized Hispaniolan Amazon parrots. *J Am Vet Med Assoc* 2008; **233**(10): 1587–1590.

184 Rembert MS, Smith JA, Hosgood G, *et al.* Comparison of traditional thermal support devices with the forced-air warmer system in anesthetized Hispaniolan Amazon parrots (*Amazona ventralis*). *J Avian Med Surg* 2001; **15**(3): 187–193.

185 Phalen DN, Mitchell ME, Cavazos-Martinez ML. Evaluation of three heat sources for their ability to maintain core body temperature in the anesthetized avian patient. *J Avian Med Surg* 1996; **10**(3): 174–178.
186 Naganobu K, Hagio M. Dose-related cardiovascular effects of isoflurane in chickens during controlled ventilation. *J Vet Med Sci* 2000; **62**(4): 435–437.
187 Kim YK, Lee SS, Suh EH, *et al.* Minimum anesthetic concentration and cardiovascular dose-response relationship of isoflurane in cinereous vultures (*Aegypius monachus*). *J Zoo Wildl Med* 2011; **42**(3): 499–503.
188 Mercado JA, Larsen RS, Wack RF, Pypendop BH. Minimum anesthetic concentration of isoflurane in captive thick-billed parrots (*Rhynchopsitta pachyrhyncha*). *Am J Vet Res* 2008; **69**(2): 189–194.
189 Phair KA, Larsen RS, Wack RF, *et al.* Determination of the minimum anesthetic concentration of sevoflurane in thick-billed parrots (*Rhynchopsitta pachyrhyncha*). *Am J Vet Res* 2012; **73**(9): 1350–1355.

SECTION 11

Anesthesia and Analgesia for Domestic Species

44 Dogs and Cats

Richard M. Bednarski
College of Veterinary Medicine, The Ohio State University, Columbus, Ohio, USA

Chapter contents

Introduction

The selection of a particular anesthetic plan is predicated upon the patient's physical status and temperament, the type of procedure for which anesthesia is being considered, anticipation of perioperative pain, the familiarity of the anesthetist with the anesthetic drugs, the type of facility and equipment available, the personnel available for assistance, and the cost of anesthetic drugs [1]. There is no single best method for anesthetizing dogs or cats, and familiarity with just one anesthetic technique at best limits a veterinarian's ability to perform the myriad of surgical and diagnostic procedures commonly performed in a modern veterinary practice and at worst results in unnecessary risk to the patient. A debilitated dog or cat undergoing extensive repair of a fractured limb will require a different anesthetic regimen than one undergoing routine neutering, one requiring short-term restraint for radiography, or a geriatric patient requiring extensive dental manipulations.

General anesthesia is characterized by muscle relaxation, unconsciousness, amnesia, and analgesia. It is difficult for a single drug to provide all of these elements without causing significant disturbances to patient homeostasis. Inhalation anesthetics come closest to satisfying all of these conditions, but even they are more useful when co-administered with anesthetic adjunctive drugs such as sedatives, opioids, local anesthetics, or hypnotics. As a general rule, when formulating an anesthetic plan, it is best to consider using relatively low doses of several different drugs rather than a large dose of a single drug. For example, apnea resulting from a large bolus of propofol can be eliminated, or its duration shortened, by prior administration of acepromazine, opioids, or α_2-adrenergic receptor agonists, which allow administration of a lower propofol dose [2]. The opioid drugs, although important components of modern anesthetic regimens, by themselves do not produce general anesthesia [3]. Muscle rigidity, salivation, and long recoveries associated with large dosages of ketamine can be lessened when the latter is combined in reduced doses with opioids, α_2-adrenergic receptor agonists, and hypnotic drugs such as benzodiazepines [4].

Any chemical restraint or general anesthetic plan must include a provision to control pain if it is present or anticipated. A good analgesic regimen should include drugs sufficient to ensure analgesia during and after the procedure. The one aspect that should not vary among anesthetic procedures is the degree of vigilance associated with monitoring an anesthetized dog or cat. Early warning of impending anesthetic difficulty is the single most important factor responsible for decreasing anesthetic-related morbidity and mortality.

Preanesthetic considerations

Recording a thorough history and conducting the physical and laboratory evaluation are the most important components of a preanesthetic evaluation. Even young, seemingly healthy, animals presented for routine procedures such as neutering require both. These animals may have never been examined previously by a

Veterinary Anesthesia and Analgesia: The Fifth Edition of Lumb and Jones.
Edited by Kurt A. Grimm, Leigh A. Lamont, William J. Tranquilli, Stephen A. Greene and Sheilah A. Robertson.

veterinarian, and congenital disorders, severe parasitism, or heartworm disease may be discovered.

Signalment

Review of patient signalment is a key preanesthetic consideration (Box 44.1). Anesthesiologists are often questioned about 'sensitivity to anesthesia' in a variety of dog and cat breeds. Although several breed-associated anesthesia concerns (e.g., predisposition to hereditary diseases that increase anesthetic risk) have been documented, all breeds have been successfully anesthetized by using standard anesthetic regimens, and most reports of 'sensitivities' are anecdotal. One well-documented breed-associated anesthetic concern is the altered pharmacokinetics of barbiturates and propofol in sighthounds [5,6]. Another is brachycephalic breeds and their associated airway anatomic malformations. This presents a concern for ensuring a patent airway during the perianesthetic period. Also, there is evidence that these breeds possess a greater resting vagal tone, heightening a concern for anesthetic-induced bradycardia [7]. Since toy breeds have a greater surface area to body mass ratio and have a relatively greater metabolic rate, they require careful attention to maintenance of body heat and blood glucose concentrations. Additionally, they require a relatively greater dose of drugs on a per kilogram basis than larger dogs. Generally, there are no gender-related differences in the response to anesthesia. However, a history of the estrous cycle will often identify recent estrus and thus alert the clinician to the concerns associated with an enlarged and vascularized uterus. This would potentially cause concern regarding blood loss during an ovariohysterectomy. Additionally, the owner of an intact female animal should be queried about the possibility of their animal being pregnant because the stress of surgery and anesthesia may adversely affect the fetus(es).

Age is an important anesthetic consideration. Generally, the very young (less than 11 weeks) and the aged (more than 80% of the expected lifespan) do not biotransform anesthetic drugs as rapidly as do healthy adult animals [8]. Healthy geriatric patients may only require 25–50% of the dose of sedatives, hypnotics, tranquilizers, and opioids given to comparable young, healthy animals.

Box 44.1 Signalment and history, including questions of organ system function.

- **A** Signalment
  - **1** Age
  - **2** Breed
  - **3** Gender
- **B** Body weight
- **C** Duration of ongoing complaint
- **D** Concurrent medications
  - **1** Angiotensin-converting enzyme inhibitors
  - **2** H_2 blockers
  - **3** Antibiotics: aminoglycosides
  - **4** Cardiac glycosides
  - **5** Phenobarbital
  - **6** Non-steroidal anti-inflammatory drugs
  - **7** Calcium channel blockers
  - **8** Beta-blockers
  - **9** Tricyclic antidepressants
- **E** Signs of organ system disease
  - **1** Diarrhea
  - **2** Vomiting
  - **3** Polyuria-polydipsia
  - **4** Seizures and personality change
  - **5** Exercise intolerance
  - **6** Coughing and stridor
  - **7** Weight loss and loss of body condition
- **F** Previous anesthesia and allergies
- **G** Duration since last meal

History

In addition to questions concerning organ system function (Box 44.1), the owner should be questioned regarding any previous anesthetic episodes, past and present illnesses, and past and current medication history, including history of heartworm prophylaxis [9]. The time elapsed since the last feeding should be noted.

Physical examination

The preanesthetic physical examination should be thorough, with all body systems considered (Box 44.2). Any abnormality discovered by physical examination or suggested by the medical history should be followed with appropriate laboratory or other suitable diagnostic testing. The assessment of an animal's temperament is critical. Vicious or aggressive animals will require a different approach to anesthesia than quiet, relaxed individuals.

Laboratory evaluation

There is no objective evidence supporting age-based or American Society of Anesthesiologists (ASA) physical status-based (see below) minimum laboratory evaluation requirements [1]. Regardless, the minimum preanesthetic laboratory data suggested for young, healthy dogs are hematocrit and plasma protein. These tests are easy, quick, and inexpensive to perform. Hematocrit is an indicator of hemoglobin concentration, which directly relates to the ability of the blood to transport oxygen to tissues. As a general rule, a

Box 44.2 Preanesthetic physical examination.

- **A** Body weight and body condition
  - **1** Obesity
  - **2** Cachexia
  - **3** Dehydration
- **B** Cardiopulmonary
  - **1** Heart rate and rhythm
  - **2** Auscultation
    - **i** Heart sounds and murmurs
    - **ii** Breath sounds
  - **3** Capillary refill time
  - **4** Mucous membrane color
    - **i** Pallor
    - **ii** Cyanosis
  - **5** Pulse character
- **C** Central nervous system and special senses
  - **1** Temperament
  - **2** Seizure, coma, and stupor
  - **3** Vision and hearing
- **D** Gastrointestinal
  - **1** Parasites
  - **2** Abdominal palpation
- **E** Hepatic
  - **1** Icterus
  - **2** Abnormal bleeding
- **F** Renal
  - **1** Palpate kidneys and bladder
- **G** Integument
  - **1** Tumors
  - **2** Flea infestation
- **H** Musculoskeletal
  - **1** Lameness
  - **2** Fractures
- **I** Pain Assessment

Table 44.1 Physical status classification of veterinary patients.

ASA Physical Status[a]	Patient Description
I	Normal healthy patient
II	Non-incapacitating systemic disease (e.g., obesity, mild dehydration, and simple fractures)
III	Severe systemic disease not incapacitating (e.g., compensated renal insufficiency, stable congestive heart failure, controlled diabetes mellitus, or cesarean section)
IV	Severe systemic disease that is a constant threat to life (e.g., gastric dilation and volvulus)
V	Moribund, not expected to live 24h irrespective of intervention (e.g., severe uncompensated systemic disturbance)

ASA, American Society of Anesthesiologists.
[a]Procedures performed under emergency conditions are denoted by placing an *E* behind the physical status number.

hematocrit of less than 20% indicates the need for perioperative administration of blood. Hemoglobin concentration (g/dL) can be approximated by dividing the hematocrit by three.

For elective procedures in middle-aged to older animals, or animals treated chronically with medications that could alter liver or renal function [e.g., non-steroidal anti-inflammatory drugs (NSAIDs), phenobarbital, or antineoplastic chemotherapeutics], a complete blood count, urinalysis, and biochemistry profile is recommended. Other laboratory tests should be performed (e.g., thoracic radiographs and/or echocardiography) if the history or physical examination suggests specific organ system disease. A minimum laboratory database prior to emergency anesthesia for a debilitated dog or cat should include packed cell volume, total protein, and electrolytes (sodium, potassium, and chloride).

Physical status

Many factors (e.g., age, breed, concurrent disease, surgical procedure, surgeon skill, and available equipment) contribute to the overall anesthetic risk for a given patient. One risk factor is the physical status of the patient. A convenient system of status classification for veterinary patients has been adapted from the ASA [1]. In general, physical status I and II patients appear to be at less risk for anesthetic complications. Physical statuses III–V are usually at greater anesthetic risk. However, this is not to imply that category I and II patients are at no risk from unanticipated anesthetic mishaps (Table 44.1).

Patient preparation

Fasting

Healthy dogs and cats should be fasted for at least 6h prior to being anesthetized, if possible. Water can be allowed until just prior to anesthesia for most procedures. Dogs and cats less than 8 weeks old and those weighing less than 2kg should not be fasted longer than 1–2h, because they are at a greater risk for perianesthetic hypoglycemia. They should receive dextrose-containing intravenous fluids during any prolonged anesthesia (longer than 15min) and/or serial blood glucose measurements until fully recovered.

Patient stabilization

When possible, life-threatening physiological disturbances should be medically addressed prior to anesthesia (Box 44.3). However, this may not always be possible, and anesthesia should never be delayed if immediate surgical or medical intervention is needed to save the patient's life.

Box 44.3 List of conditions that should be corrected prior to anesthesia.

A Severe dehydration
B Anemia or hypoproteinemia
  1 Packed cell volume <20% with acute blood loss
  2 Serum albumin concentration <2.0 g/dL
C Acid-base and electrolyte disturbances
  1 pH <7.2
  2 Serum potassium concentration <2.5–3.0 or >6.0 mEq/L
D Pneumothorax
E Cyanosis
F Oliguria or anuria
G Congestive heart failure
H Severe, life-threatening cardiac arrhythmias

Box 44.4 Considerations for selecting an anesthetic plan.

A Procedure to be performed
  1 Duration
    i <15min
    ii 15min–1h
    iii >1h
  2 Type of procedure
    i Minor medical or surgical
    ii Major invasive surgery
  3 Anticipated perioperative pain
B Available assistance and equipment
  1 Assistance
    i Ventilatory assist or control
    ii Restraint
  2 Equipment
    i Anesthetic machine
  3 Type of inhalation anesthetic
  4 Appropriate monitoring devices
C Patient's temperament
  1 Quiet, relaxed, or calm
  2 Nervous and/or excitable
  3 Vicious
  4 Moribund or comatose
D Physical status
  1 ASA category I through V
E Breed
  1 Sight hound
  2 Brachycephalic
  3 Toy

Anesthetic and analgesic plan

Several aspects should be considered when formulating an anesthetic plan (Box 44.4). In general, the anesthetic or chemical restraint technique relies primarily on local anesthesia, injectable anesthesia, or inhalation anesthesia. Regardless, these primary techniques are typically supplemented with some degree of drug-induced sedation and systemically administered analgesics. Techniques frequently overlap. For example, inhalation anesthesia is usually initiated with injectable anesthetics. Local anesthetic nerve blocks are typically accompanied by general anesthesia or sedation.

The remainder of the discussion regarding the choice of anesthetic and analgesic drugs assumes that the reader has reviewed and has a familiarity with the pharmacology of the various anesthetic drugs [10,11]. Although the drug combinations described are suitable for a variety of patients, the reader should refer to the appropriate sections of this text or consult a veterinary anesthesiologist if questions remain about how to anesthetize and monitor specific patients. Drug availability can be an issue, so it is best to become familiar with a variety of techniques.

Short-term anesthesia (less than 15 minutes)

By themselves, sedative–opioid combinations are suitable for short-term restraint for minimally invasive procedures or those procedures not requiring general anesthesia such as radiography, or physical examination in an intractable animal (Tables 44.2 and 44.3). An advantage is that one or both of these components is reversible, allowing a rapid return to preanesthetic mentation and function (Table 44.4). Any of the short-term injectable drugs discussed below can be added to the sedative–opioid regimen when complete immobilization or general anesthesia is necessary. If potentially painful surgical procedures are attempted under heavy sedation (e.g., laceration repair following dexmedetomidine/butorphanol), a local anesthetic should be incorporated in the plan to reduce the risk of animal arousal due to surgical stimulation.

Several drugs are available for chemical restraint or short-term anesthesia (Tables 44.2, 44.3, 44.5, and 44.6). Immobilization for a short duration not requiring strong analgesia (radiography, suture removal, otoscopic examination, etc.) can be performed most simply with intravenous injectable drugs such as propofol, alphaxalone, ketamine–propofol, ketamine–midazolam, etomidate, or, less commonly, thiopental or methohexital. These drugs induce rapid and predictable short-term loss of consciousness. The duration of action following a single bolus dose of these drugs is generally less than 15 min with animals ambulatory within 30–60 min postadministration. Prior administration of sedative/tranquilizing drugs generally improves the quality of immobilization [12,13].

Table 44.2 Sedatives and tranquilizers for chemical restraint or premedication.

Drug	Dosage (mg/kg)[a]	Comments
Dexmedetomidine	Dogs, 0.002–0.02 IV, IM Cats, 0.02–0.04 IV, IM	Moderate to deep sedation Duration 60–180 min
Acepromazine	Dogs, 0.02–0.2 IV, IM, SC (3 mg max.) Cats, 0.02–0.2 IV, IM	Mild to moderate sedation Duration 30–90 min
Midazolam	Dogs, 0.1–0.3 IV, IM (7 mg max.) Cats, 0.1–0.2 IV, IM	Minimal sedation Most useful when combined with other sedatives, opioids, or ketamine

IM, intramuscular; IV, intravenous; SC, subcutaneous.
[a]Generally the low end of the dosage range is used IV and in sick or debilitated patients.

Table 44.3 Opioids and sedative–opioid combinations.

Drug(s)	Dosage (mg/kg)[a]	Comments
Morphine	0.2–0.5 IM, SC	Duration 3–5 h Vomiting Mild sedation Dysphoria can occur when used alone in young, healthy dogs or cats Can release histamine
Hydromorphone	0.1–0.2 IV, IM, SC	Duration 3–5 h Vomiting Mild sedation Dysphoria can occur when used alone in young healthy dogs or cats
Oxymorphone	0.05–0.1 IV, IM, SC	Same as for hydromorphone; less incidence of vomiting
Methadone	0.3–0.5 IV, IM, SC	Same as for oxymorphone; minimal incidence of vomiting
Butorphanol	0.2–0.4 IV, IM, SC	Duration 1 h in dogs and up to 2–3 h in cats Opioid agonist/antagonist Minimal sedation when used alone
Buprenorphine	0.005–0.02 IV, IM, SC, oral transmucosal (cats)	Duration 6–8 h Partial opioid agonist
Dexmedetomidine–opioid[b]	Dogs, 0.002–0.007 IV, IM Cats, 0.004–0.01 IV, IM	Duration of sedation 30 min–1 h Both drugs are reversible Observe for bradycardia Useful for immobilization of difficult to handle or vicious animals
Acepromazine–opioid[b]	Dogs, 0.02–0.1 IV, IM Cats, 0.02–0.2 IV, IM	Duration of sedation 15 min–1 h Can be combined in the same syringe Useful for immobilization of difficult to handle or vicious animals
Midazolam–opioid[b]	Dogs, 0.1–0.3 IV, IM Cats, 0.1–0.2 IV, IM	Duration of sedation 40 min Can be combined in the same syringe Generally produces poor results in young, healthy animals Not recommended for immobilization of vicious or difficult to handle animals Better quality restraint in older or debilitated animals

IM, intramuscular; IV, intravenous; SC, subcutaneous.
[a]Use low end of opioid dosage in cats.
[b]Use dosage ranges (lower end only for use in cats) for opioids listed above.

Table 44.4 Antagonists of various classes of anesthetic drugs.

Drug	Dosage (mg/kg)
α_2-Adrenergic	
Yohimbine	0.1 IV, IM
Atipamezole	Equal volume to administered dose of medetomidine or dexmedetomidine, IM[a]
Benzodiazepine	
Flumazenil	0.01–0.2 IV[b]
Opioid	
Naloxone	0.002–0.02 IV, IM[c]

IM, intramuscular; IV, intravenous.
[a]Dosage in milligrams is equal to five times the previously administered dosage of medetomidine or ten times the previously administered dosage of dexmedtomidine.
[b]Begin with lowest dosage and repeat, if necessary, to effect.
[c]Use lowest dosage for 'partial' reversal and highest dosage for complete reversal (see text for explanation).

Table 44.5 Injectable anesthetic drugs[a].

Drug	Dosage (mg/kg)	Comments
Propofol	4.0–6.0 IV CRI 0.2–0.8 mg/kg/min	Duration 5–10 min after single-bolus dose Apnea for several minutes with rapid injection
Alfaxalone	1.0–5.0 IV, IM CRI 0.1–0.2 mg/kg/min	Use lower end of dosage IV after premedication and for anesthetic induction Use larger dosages IM for longer term immobilization
Etomidate	0.5–2.0 IV	Duration 5–10 min Myoclonus, gagging/retching
Propofol–ketamine	2.0/2.0 IV	Duration 5–10 min after single bolus dose Less hypotension than with propofol alone
Thiopental	8.0–20.0 IV	Use lower dosage after premedication
Methohexital	3.0–8.0 IV	Duration 3–5 min Muscle rigidity Best if preceded by a tranquilizer or sedative

IM, intramuscular; IV, intravenous; CRI, constant-rate infusion.
[a]Injectable ketamine-based combinations for use in cats are listed in Table 44.8.

Table 44.6 Suggestions for premedication in healthy dogs and cats.[a]

Patient Type	Premedication
Young, normal, healthy	Acepromazine Dexmedetomidine Either of the above with an opioid agonist if moderate to severe perioperative pain is anticipated Either of the above with butorphanol or buprenorphine if less intense pain is anticipated or for moderate restraint
Aggressive/vicious[b]	Acepromazine–opioid agonist Dexmedetomidine–opioid agonist Xylazine–opioid agonist
Geriatric	Acepromazine (low end of dosage range) Midazolam–opioid
Painful procedures	Acepromazine–opioid agonist Dexmedetomidine–opioid agonist Midazolam–opioid agonist

[a]These drugs or drug combinations should be administered intramuscularly between 15 and 30 min prior to anesthetic induction.
[b]Can add ketamine 2–3 mg/kg IM for additional restraint.

Currently, propofol is widely used for short-term immobilization in cats and dogs. Because of its rapid plasma clearance, multiple boluses of propofol, or a propofol infusion, can be used to prolong the duration of restraint without significantly prolonging the duration of recovery [12]. Respiratory depression may be significant and ventilatory assistance should be available

A combination of ketamine and midazolam produces less muscle relaxation than propofol, alfaxalone, propofol–ketamine, or thiopental. In dosages typically used, ketamine–midazolam is also associated with increased salivation and dysphoria upon recovery [4]. However, dissociative–anesthetic combinations generally produce less respiratory and cardiovascular depression than other available short-acting injectable anesthetics. Muscle relaxation and recovery quality are improved and salivation is lessened when dissociatives are given with or preceded by a tranquilizer or sedative [4].

Thiopental (currently not available in the United States) is relatively inexpensive and is suitable for short-term restraint of most healthy dogs and cats. A disadvantage to its use as a sole anesthetic is that relatively large doses are required, full recovery can take up to 1 h, and recovery can be associated with ataxia and disorientation. These undesirable characteristics are reduced when its administration is preceded by a tranquilizer such as acepromazine or a sedative such as dexmedetomidine. Another disadvantage is that it must be administered intravenously, a problem with fractious or uncooperative animals. Perivascular thiopental administration is associated with local tissue inflammation, pain, and potential tissue necrosis. Perivascular administration should be attended to by infiltratng the area with a crystalloid fluid (e.g., 0.9% sodium chloride) at a volume equal to 3–5 times the volume of perivascularly administered thiopental. Additionally, a local anesthetic such as lidocaine and an anti-inflammatory (e.g., methylprednisolone) may be infiltrated near the site of perivascular injection. Another important side effect of thiopental is the significant respiratory depression that can accompany its use.

Alfaxalone is a neurosteroid anesthetic drug that produces hypnosis and muscle relaxation by enhancing conduction of the $GABA_A$ receptor ion. Immobilization is characterized by excellent muscle relaxation and hypnosis in dogs and cats. It can be administered intravenously or intramuscularly, and its duration of action is dose dependent. Like propofol, it is compatible for use following commonly used preanesthetic sedatives and tranquilizers to sustain general anesthesia [14–16]. However respiratory depression may be significant and ventilatory assistance should be available [15,16].

The relatively cumbersome nature of inhalation anesthetic delivery makes it inconvenient for use in very short procedures, and its use solely for routine induction of unconsciousness and anesthesia is not recommended. On occasion it can prove useful for chamber induction of feral or fractious cats. It can also be useful for short-term anesthesia in neonates or those animals with severe organ system compromise and a reduced ability to clear drugs through the kidney or liver. Mask induction with inhalant anesthetics should be preceded by preanesthetic administration whenever possible to reduce the stress and anxiety (and catecholamine release) associated with initial inspiration of high concentrations of inhalant anesthetics.

Intermediate-term anesthesia (15 minutes to 1 hour)

For procedures of intermediate duration that do not require significant analgesia, the previously discussed drugs suitable for short-term restraint can be used and redosed to effect. Typically, one-third to half of the induction dose is administered slowly to prolong the anesthetic effect. Thiopental and ketamine–midazolam should not be redosed multiple times. Their initial duration of action following bolus administration depends primarily on redistribution away from the brain to other tissues, such as muscle. However, when these tissues are saturated with drug, redistribution greatly slows, and metabolism becomes the rate-limiting factor for awakening. Propofol and alfaxalone, because of their relatively rapid clearances and large volumes of distribution, can be administered repeatedly to dogs by using small boluses or by constant-rate infusion (Table 44.5).

Invasive surgical procedures such as feline onychectomy or canine and feline gonadectomy typically require 15 min–1 h of anesthesia, accompanied by good perioperative analgesia. Several options are available. A combination of Telazol®, ketamine, and xylazine is suitable for cats, although its use has been associated with relatively prolonged recoveries [14]. An alternative is the combination of dexmedetomidine, ketamine, and an opioid agonist. Inclusion of dexmedetomidine in the combination suggests that antagonism of the anesthetic and analgesic effects with atipamezole is possible, if required. Inhalation anesthesia following sedation and induction of anesthesia with a rapidly acting injectable drug such as propofol is also appropriate for procedures of intermediate duration and may be the most convenient and most controllable. Inhalant anesthetic delivery of this duration usually requires intubation and careful monitoring, but has the benefit of enabling a rapid adjustment of the depth of anesthesia should anesthetic conditions change unexpectedly (e.g., loss of blood or respiratory arrest).

Long-term anesthesia (longer than 1 hour)

Long procedures are best managed by maintenance with inhalation anesthesia. Awakening from sevoflurane and isoflurane anesthesia is predictably rapid. Even sick and debilitated patients recover from prolonged periods of inhalation anesthesia relatively quickly, and liver or renal impairment does not preclude drug clearance. As an alternative, injectable anesthesia using intramuscularly or intravenously administered drugs has been described (see above) [15–21].

Those techniques which involve infusion of propofol or alfaxalone and opioid combinations along with reversible tranquilizers or sedatives are most suitable for prolonged anesthesia because of propofol's and alfaxalone's predictably rapid clearance. Those techniques involving non-reversible drugs, such as Telazol®, are less suited for prolonged immobilization because of the attendant prolonged recovery. Most anesthetic techniques are associated with some degree of respiratory depression and a loss of the protective swallowing reflex, so tracheal intubation and a means to assist ventilation are essential to reducing anesthetic risk.

Premedication

Inhalation anesthesia can be initiated without premedication; however, administration of a sedative, tranquilizer, opioid, or combination of these drugs is recommended prior to induction (Tables 44.2 and 44.3). Preanesthetic drugs aid in restraint, reduce apprehension, decrease the quantity of potentially more dangerous drugs used to produce general anesthesia, facilitate induction, enhance perioperative analgesia, and reduce arrhythmogenic autonomic reflex activity. Premedications are usually administered intramuscularly or subcutaneously 15–30 min before induction. The choice of premedication depends on signalment, temperament, physical status, concurrent disease, the procedure to be performed, and personal preference (Table 44.6). For procedures associated with postoperative pain, premedication should include an analgesic such as an opioid and possibly an NSAID. Fewer analgesics are typically needed postoperatively when analgesics are administered pre-emptively [22]. Repeated and frequent patient assessment following surgery is needed to assess the adequacy of analgesia. Additional analgesics should be administered when needed.

Induction

Induction is most easily accomplished in most animals with propofol, alfaxalone, ketamine–midazolam, propofol–ketamine, etomidate, or less commonly thiopental (Table 44.5). Advantages of an intravenous method of induction include rapid loss of consciousness and ability to intubate endotracheally quickly. Alternatives to these rapid intravenous induction protocols include administration of a higher dose intramuscular dissociative (cyclohexylamine) anesthetic–benzodiazepine combination (e.g., Telazol®), chamber or mask inhalant induction, or high-dose intravenous opioid induction. These techniques can be useful in special circumstances, but for routine use in healthy dogs and cats their disadvantages generally outweigh their advantages.

Chamber or mask inhalant induction

One disadvantage to chamber and mask induction is the associated waste-gas pollution. Another is the struggling and associated stress that some animals experience during the induction phase [23]. Mask induction is most easily accomplished in moribund animals and small tractable dogs. Prior tranquilization or sedation enhances the quality and speed of induction, as does the use of a non-rebreathing system to deliver the anesthetic agent initially [24]. Chamber induction is most useful in intractable cats and very small dogs. Isoflurane and sevoflurane are the most suitable inhalants for this because they produce a relatively rapid induction [25]. Relatively high oxygen flow rates (4 L/min for chamber and 3 L/min for mask) and vaporizer settings (3–5% isoflurane and 5–7% sevoflurane in healthy animals) are used. The use of nitrous oxide is not necessary during chamber or mask induction with currently used agents [26]. With chamber induction, once the animal has lost its righting reflex and is unresponsive to the chamber being tilted from side to side, it is removed from the chamber and induction is continued using an appropriately sized mask. Mask induction is begun by exposing the animal to the mask and oxygen. The inhalation concentration is slowly increased to 3–5% for isoflurane and 5–7% for sevoflurane. This is accomplished with a non-rebreathing or rebreathing circuit by gradually increasing the vaporizer setting over 2–4 min. Use of a non-rebreathing anesthetic system to deliver gas to the chamber or mask will facilitate rapid induction because exchange of the room air in the reservoir bag, breathing circuit, and carbon dioxide absorber with anesthetic-laden gas from the vaporizer is not necessary.

Intravenous high-dose opioid induction

A disadvantage to opioid induction is the attendant relatively slow loss of consciousness. Advantages include good cardiovascular stability (although severe bradycardia may be seen when anticholinergics are not co-administered) and the attenuation of the stress response associated with anesthesia and surgery. Opioid induction works best in debilitated dogs and is not recommended in cats or young, healthy dogs that are not well sedated. Incremental doses of an opioid agonist (Table 44.3) are alternated with small incremental doses of midazolam (Table 44.2) until the dog can be intubated.

Anesthetic maintenance

The maintenance phase of anesthesia begins when unconsciousness is induced and ends with discontinuation of anesthetic delivery. After the loss of consciousness, a properly sized cuffed endotracheal tube or alternative airway is usually inserted to allow assisted ventilation, if necessary, and protect against aspiration of oropharyngeal contents. Adequate cardiovascular function is rapidly verified and the anesthetic vaporizer turned on. The initial and subsequent anesthetic vaporizer settings (percentage concentration of inhalant) vary with the condition of the patient, the type of breathing circuit used, and the fresh-gas flow rate (Table 44.7). The relatively high fresh-gas flow rate and vaporizer setting that are initially used after induction are decreased to maintenance settings when the patient nears the desired anesthetic plane (usually when palpebral reflexes disappear and the heart rate begins to decrease). The vaporizer setting is adjusted according to signs of anesthetic depth. The most useful signs of anesthetic depth in dogs and cats include a combination of muscle tone (assessed by opening the mouth to its full extent), heart and respiratory rates, and systemic arterial blood pressure. Other monitors that may be used include a pulse oximeter and a capnometer. Pulse oximetry non-invasively provides an estimate of hemoglobin's oxygen saturation (normal is greater than 95%). This information along with packed cell volume or hemoglobin concentration indicates the oxygen content of arterial blood. A capnometer non-invasively assesses ventilation by monitoring respiratory rate and end-tidal expired (related to arterial) CO_2 partial pressure. End-tidal CO_2 monitors can also identify problems with the gas delivery system such as malfunctioning one-way valves

Table 44.7 Vaporizer settings[a].

Drug	Induction Phase (%)	Maintenance Phase (%)
Isoflurane	3	1–3
Sevoflurane	4–5	2–4

[a]Listed vaporizer settings assume a fresh-gas flow rate of 1–2 L/min during the induction phase (i.e., the first several minutes following induction with an injectable drug), and a fresh-gas flow rate of at least 10 mL/kg/min during the maintenance phase. Vaporizer settings for closed breathing systems are typically 1–2% higher. See the text for discussion of mask or chamber induction.

and exhausted CO_2 absorbent, especially when graphic display of the CO_2 time profile is provided (i.e., a capnogram).

The anesthetic record

This is part of the patient's permanent record and should include notation of patient status, the anesthetic drugs used including time of administration, dose and effect, duration of the surgery, and notation of significant perioperative events. Ideally, heart rate, respiratory rate, blood pressure, and any other variables monitored should be recorded at regular intervals (5–10 min). Recording these data at regular intervals creates a visual aid that assists in determining the change in patient status during the anesthetic period. For example, a steadily increasing heart rate accompanied by a steadily decreasing blood pressure during a 15 min interval could signal hypotension caused by fluid loss or excessive anesthetic depth. This is easily observed on the anesthetic record but may not be noticed without the visual prompt of the data recorded over time.

Perioperative analgesia

Concurrent administration of various analgesic drugs during inhalation anesthesia is useful to enhance intraoperative and postoperative analgesia. These drugs can be continued into the postanesthetic period to maintain analgesia. Infusions of low doses of ketamine, lidocaine, opioids, and their combinations have been described as adjuncts to inhalation anesthesia (Table 44.8) [27–29]. When using these drugs, the concentration of inhalant anesthetic can often be significantly reduced. Increased respiratory depression is a concern, and the adequacy of ventilation should be closely monitored and ventilation should be assisted as needed.

Recovery

Recovery begins when the procedure for which a patient has been anesthetized is finished and the anesthetic drugs have been discontinued. Patient status should be monitored regularly during recovery until the patient is conscious and extubated, and heart rate, respiratory rate, and body temperature have returned to normal. Young, healthy animals undergoing routine procedures usually do not need supplemental oxygen during recovery, although it should be immediately available. However, continuous use of pulse oximetry is helpful to identify unexpected postanesthetic hypoxemia.

Table 44.8 Drugs and drug combinations administered by constant-rate infusion to enhance intraoperative analgesia.

Drug(s)	Infusion Rate	Comments
Ketamine	0.6 mg/kg/h	Useful as an adjunct to other perioperative analgesics
Fentanyl	5–15 μg/kg/h	Useful alone or with other perioperative analgesics
Lidocaine[b]	3.0 mg/kg/h	Useful alone or with other perioperative analgesics; first administer loading dose of 2 mg/kg
Morphine–lidocaine[a]–ketamine	0.24/3.0/0.6 mg/kg/h[b]	Useful alone or with other perioperative analgesics; first administer loading dose of 2 mg/kg lidocaine and ketamine

[a]Avoid lidocaine in cats.
[b]To 1 L of crystalloid, add 48 mg of morphine, 600 mg of lidocaine, and 120 mg of ketamine. Administer at 5 mL/kg/h intraoperatively. Concentration can be adjusted to fit postoperative maintenance fluid rates.

Hypoxemia caused by respiratory depression, atelectasis-related ventilation/perfusion mismatch, and/or rapidly decreased fraction of inspired oxygen (e.g., near 100% oxygen to 21% room air) is easily addressed if detected early. If nitrous oxide was used during anesthetic maintenance, the breathing circuit should be repeatedly filled with oxygen and the patient allowed to breathe an oxygen-enriched gas mixture for 5–10 min after discontinuation of nitrous oxide. This helps prevent the diffusion hypoxia that can develop if the inspired oxygen concentration suddenly decreases while nitrous oxide is rapidly moving from the blood into the alveolar gas. Sick or debilitated dogs and cats benefit from supplemental oxygen during recovery, particularly if hypothermic, because shivering can significantly increase oxygen consumption. The endotracheal tube cuff should be partially deflated and endotracheal tube untied when a patient is disconnected from the anesthetic machine. This permits extubation in the event that the patient rapidly awakens and begins chewing, but care should be exercised when moving the animal to the recovery area so premature accidental extubation does not occur. At this time the animal's nose should be positioned slightly ventral to allow drainage of any accumulated oral or pharyngeal fluid that accumulated during the procedure. If an esophageal stethoscope or temperature probe was used, it should be removed at this time. Dogs and cats should be extubated as soon as swallowing occurs, unless there is a specific contraindication to removing the endotracheal tube at this time (e.g., brachycephalic airway syndrome). Dogs and cats should never be left to recover unobserved. Patients should recover in a well-ventilated area to minimize pollution of the workspace by exhaled anesthetic gas.

Occasionally, a dog or cat will suddenly awaken from anesthesia disoriented and will vocalize, paddle, and appear incoherent. This sudden arousal can be caused by emergence delirium, opioid dysphoria, or pain, and it is important to distinguish between them. Emergence delirium occurs most frequently in poorly or non-premedicated animals and in particular those awakening rapidly from inhalant anesthesia. With emergence delirium, the dog or cat will become quiet and more comfortable, usually within 10 min. A quiet, reassuring voice and gentle restraint can guide the animal through this period of excitement. Alternatively, a low dosage of IV propofol (0.25–1 mg/kg) can dramatically lessen the dysphoric behavior, allowing a smooth recovery. Occasionally, a low dose of dexmedetomidine (0.5–1 μg/kg IV) or acepromazine (0.01–0.05 mg/kg IV) is necessary to quiet an excited dysphoric animal. If pain is believed to be the cause of the rough recovery, rapid-acting opioid analgesics (e.g., fentanyl) should be administered intravenously. Postoperative pain control is managed best with preanesthetic analgesic administration of relatively long-lasting analgesics, perioperative analgesic infusion, local anesthetics, and attention to signs of pain. Dogs and cats can become dysphoric during recovery, related to perioperative opioid administration [30]. Opioid dysphoria can be diminished with partial opioid reversal using the opioid antagonist naloxone (1–2 μg/kg IV).

Dogs or cats receiving perioperative fluids can develop a fully distended or overdistended urinary bladder that can cause signs of discomfort. If a full bladder is palpated, it can be gently expressed before recovery.

Delayed anesthetic recovery

Occasionally, a dog or cat that received several drugs (especially opioids) during the anesthetic episode will remain mildly hypothermic and unresponsive. In these instances, consideration should be given to antagonism of reversible drugs (α_2-adrenergic receptor agonists or opioids) that were given as part of the anesthetic regimen. Relatively small IV boluses of naloxone (1–2 μg/kg) can be used to reverse the central nervous system (CNS) and thermoregulatory depression associated with the opioids while leaving opioid analgesia mostly intact. Atipamezole can be used to reverse α_2-adrenergic receptor agonist-related CNS depression.

Severe hypoglycemia is an easily corrected problem that can result in delayed anesthetic recovery. Blood glucose concentration should be measured if hypoglycemia is suspected, and intravenous dextrose-containing fluids given until blood glucose concentrations normalize. Arterial hypotension associated with blood loss or poor cardiac function can cause altered mentation and slow recovery. Periodic measurement of arterial blood pressure during recovery, especially in debilitated patients, is warranted. Hypercapnea ($PaCO_2$ approaching 100 mmHg) associated with respiratory-depressant anesthetic and adjunctive drugs may cause severe mental impairment and possibly respiratory arrest. Use of capnometry or arterial blood-gas analysis during the anesthetic and recovery period helps facilitate early detection and correction of respiratory depression. Occasionally, animals with undiagnosed, compensated CNS disease (e.g., hydrocephalus) may decompensate under anesthesia, resulting in impaired brain function. Prevention of hypercapnea, hypoxemia, and hypotension and rapid implementation of resuscitative measures (e.g., mannitol and controlled positive-pressure ventilation) may limit brain injury and speed recovery. Many problems that lead to delayed recovery from anesthesia can be prevented or otherwise managed with appropriate patient monitoring during and after anesthetic drug delivery.

References

1 Bednarski R, Grimm K, Harvey R, *et al.* AAHA anesthesia guidelines for dogs and cats. *J Am Anim Hosp Assoc* 2011; **47**: 377–385.

2 Kojima K, Nishimura R, Mutoh T, *et al.* Effects of medetomidine–midazolam, acepromazine–butorphanol, and midazolam–butorphanol on induction dose of thiopental and propofol and on cardiopulmonary changes in dogs. *Am J Vet Res* 2002; **63**: 1671–1679.

3 Hall R, Szlam F, Hug C. The enflurane sparing effect of alfentanyl in dogs. *Anesth Analg* 1987; **66**: 1287–1291.

4 Haskins S, Farver T, Patz J. Cardiovascular changes in dogs given diazepam and diazepam–ketamine. *Am J Vet Res* 1986; **47**: 795–798.

5 Robinson EP, Sams RA, Muir WW. Barbiturate anesthesia in greyhound and mixed breed dogs: comparative cardiopulmonary effects, anesthetic effects, and recovery rates. *Am J Vet Res* 1986; **47**: 2105–2112.

6 Hay Kraus BL,Greenblatt DJ, Venkatakrishnan K, Court MH. Evidence for propofol hydroxylation by cytochrome P4502B11 in canine liver microsomes: breed and gender differences. *Xenobiotica* 2000; **30**: 575–588.

7 Doxey S, Boswood A. Differences between breeds of dog in a measure of heart rate variability. *Vet Rec* 2004; **154**: 713–717.

8 Short C. Drug disposition in neonatal animals. *J Am Vet Med Assoc* 1984; **184**: 1161–1162.

9 Seahorn J, Robertson S. Concurrent medications and their impact on anesthetic management. *Vet Forum* 2002; **119**: 50–67.

10 Ilkiw J. Injectable anesthesia in dogs. Part I. Solutions, doses and administration. In: Gleed RD, Ludders JW, eds. *Recent Advances in Veterinary Anesthesia and Analgesia: Companion Animals*. Ithaca, NY: International Veterinary Information Service, 2002; www.ivis.org (accessed 1 October 2014).

11 Ilkiw J. Injectable anesthesia in dogs. Part 2. Comparative pharmacology. In: Gleed RD, Ludders JW, eds. *Recent Advances in Veterinary Anesthesia and Analgesia: Companion Animals*. Ithaca, NY: International Veterinary Information Service, 2002; www.ivis.org (accessed 1 October 2014).

12 Nolan AM, Reid J. Pharmacokinetics of propofol administered by infusion in dogs undergoing surgery. *Br J Anaesth* 1993; **70**: 546–551.

13 Smith JA, Gaynor JS, Bednarski RM, Muir WW. Adverse effects of administration of propofol with various preanesthetic regimens in dogs. *J Am Vet Med Assoc* 1993; **202**: 1111–1115.

14 Muir W, Lerche P, Wiese A, *et al.* The cardiorespiratory safety and anesthetic effects of alfaxan CD RTU when administered alone or in combination with preanesthetic medications in dogs [Abstract]. In: *Veterinary Midwest Anesthesia and Analgesia Conference, Indianapolis, IN*, 17–18 April 2004.

15 Suarez MA, Dzikit BT, Stegmann FG, Hartman M. Comparison of alfaxalone and propofol administered as total intravenous anesthesia for ovariohysterectomy in dogs. *Vet Anaesth Analg* 2012; **39**: 236–244.

16 Herbert GL, Bowlt KL, Ford-Fennah V, *et al.* Alfaxalone for total intravenous anesthesia in dogs undergoing ovariohysterectomy: a comparison of premedication with acepromazine and dexmedetomidine. *Vet Anaesth Analg* 2013; **40**: 124–133.

17 Williams LS, Levy JK, Robertson SA, *et al.* Use of the anesthetic combination of tiletamine, zolazepam, ketamine, and xylazine for neutering feral cats. *J Am Vet Med Assoc* 2002; **220**: 1491–1495.

18 Hughes JM, Nolan AM. Total intravenous anesthesia in greyhounds: pharmacokinetics of propofol and fentanyl – a preliminary study. *Vet Surg* 1999; **28**: 513–524.

19 Ilkiw JE, Pascoe PJ. Effect of variable-dose propofol alone and in combination with two fixed doses of ketamine for total intravenous anesthesia in cats. *Am J Vet Res* 2003; **64**: 907–912.

20 Ilkiw JE, Pascoe PJ. Cardiovascular effects of propofol alone and in combination with ketamine for total intravenous anesthesia in cats. *Am J Vet Res* 2003; **64**: 913–915.

21 Mendes G, Selmi A. Use of a combination of propofol and fentanyl, alfentanil, or sufentanil for total intravenous anesthesia in cats. *J Am Vet Med Assoc* 2003; **223**: 1608–1613.

22 Woolf CF, Chong M. Preemptive analgesia: treating postoperative pain by preventing the establishment of central sensitization. *Anesth Analg* 1993; **77**: 362–379.

23 Mutoh T, Nishimura R, Kim H. Rapid inhalation induction of anesthesia by halothane, enflurane, isoflurane, and sevoflurane and their cardiopulmonary effects in dogs. *J Vet Med Sci* 1995; **57**: 1007–1013.

24 Mutoh T, Nishimura R, Sasaki N. Effects of medetomidine–midazolam, midazolam–butorphanol, or acepromazine–butorphanol as premedicants for mask induction of anesthesia with sevoflurane in dogs. *Am J Vet Res* 2002; **63**: 1022–1028.

25 Lerche P, Muir WW, Grubb T. Mask induction of anaesthesia with isoflurane or sevoflurane in premedicated cats. *J Small Anim Pract* 2002; **43**: 12–15.

26 Mutoh T, Nishimura R, Sasaki N. Effects of nitrous oxide on mask induction of anesthesia with sevoflurane or isoflurane in dogs. *Am J Vet Res* 2001; **62**: 1727–1733.

27 Wagner A, Walaton J, Hellyer P, *et al.* Use of low doses of ketamine administered by constant rate infusion as an adjunct for postoperative analgesia in dogs. *J Am Vet Med Assoc* 2002; **221**: 72–75.

28 Muir W, Wiese A, March P. Effects of morphine, lidocaine, ketamine, and morphine–lidocaine–ketamine drug combination on minimum alveolar concentration in dogs anesthetized with isoflurane. *Am J Vet Res* 2003; **64**: 1155–1160.

29 Nunes de Moraes A, Dyson D, O'Grady M, *et al.* Plasma concentrations and cardiovascular influence of lidocaine infusions during isoflurane anesthesia in healthy dogs and dogs with subaortic stenosis. *Vet Surg* 1998; **27**: 486–497.

30 Becker WM, Mama KR, Rao S, *et al.* Prevalence of dysphoria after fentanyl in dogs undergoing stifle surgery. *Vet Surg* 2013; **42**: 302–307.

45 Canine and Feline Local Anesthetic and Analgesic Techniques

Luis Campoy[1], Matt Read[2] and Santiago Peralta[1]

[1] Department of Clinical Sciences, College of Veterinary Medicine, Cornell University, Ithaca, New York, USA
[2] Faculty of Veterinary Medicine, University of Calgary, Calgary, Alberta, Canada

Chapter contents

General considerations

Loco-regional anesthesia is used extensively in human medicine to provide intra- and postoperative pain control and involves injection of local anesthetic solutions around sensory neural tissue (centrally or peripherally) to prevent nerve conduction. There are numerous documented benefits to using regional anesthesia instead of, or in combination with, general anesthesia, and this has resulted in significant refinement of these techniques for use in people. Although local anesthetic techniques have been used for many years in veterinary medicine, advanced techniques are now being studied to facilitate the increasing number of invasive and painful surgical procedures performed. With a growing emphasis on improving pain management for animals, loco-regional anesthetic procedures originally described for use in people are now being adapted to different animal species [1–7].

Classification of loco-regional anesthesia

Topical or surface anesthesia

Topical or surface anesthesia has great appeal since transmission of sensory information can be blocked before it starts at the site of a superficial injury. Unfortunately, most local anesthetics are not readily absorbed across the skin surface, and special formulations are needed for them to be used in this way. Eutectic mixtures of local anesthetics comprised of 2.5% lidocaine and 2.5% prilocaine formulated as a cream have been used to decrease pain for a variety of dermal procedures in people, and has been studied in cats to minimize pain associated with jugular puncture [8]. These creams are indicated for dermal anesthesia and have been reported to be useful for preventing pain associated with percutaneous intravenous catheter placement, blood sampling, and superficial skin closure in people. When used according to directions, the cream is applied to the skin and covered with an occlusive dressing to facilitate

Veterinary Anesthesia and Analgesia: The Fifth Edition of Lumb and Jones.
Edited by Kurt A. Grimm, Leigh A. Lamont, William J. Tranquilli, Stephen A. Greene and Sheilah A. Robertson.

absorption of the local anesthetics. Local anesthetic efficacy is achieved after approximately 60 min and lasts for up to 2 h.

Originally developed for treating post-herpetic neuralgia pain in people, transdermal lidocaine patches (Lidoderm®, Endo Pharmaceuticals, Dublin, Ireland) contain 5% lidocaine and their use has been studied in horses, cats, and dogs [9–12]. The penetration of lidocaine into intact skin is sufficient to produce a local analgesic effect, but does not produce a complete sensory nerve block. Clinical trials in people have demonstrated that lidocaine patches placed near the site of incision can produce prolonged dynamic pain control and reduce the amount of systemic opioids required for postoperative analgesia [13,14]. Studies of lidocaine patches specific to veterinary species are lacking. Owing to differences in skin composition, extrapolation of human studies must be done with a great deal of caution until validation of results is completed in randomized blinded trials performed in the species of interest.

Infiltration anesthesia

Infiltration anesthesia involves the injection of local anesthetic solution into and around the planned surgical field, not specifically targeted near any particular nerve or nervous system structure. Many use the term *local anesthesia* as a synonym for infiltration anesthesia, although strictly speaking topical anesthesia would also be a form of local anesthesia. Several studies have reported incision infiltration in dogs and cats [15–17]. Development and use of wound infusion catheters have taken this technique a step further, allowing the continuous or intermittent delivery of local anesthetics into tissues surrounding surgical wounds without the need for repeated needle penetration for injection of analgesic drugs [18].

Regional or nerve (plexus) block anesthesia

Regional anesthesia refers to the injection of a local anesthetic solution adjacent to a peripheral nerve to temporarily block conduction and therefore sensory afferent and/or motor efferent activity in the anatomic region innervated by the nerve(s). These techniques are commonly used to provide intra- and postoperative analgesia in many parts of the body, including the head, limbs, and trunk.

Randomized controlled studies in humans suggest that regional anesthetic techniques contribute to superior pain relief, faster postoperative recoveries, and reduced hospital stays compared with systemic opioids [19]. Excellent texts [19] and other tools for teaching regional anesthesia are available for veterinary patients [1,2,20–34].

Neuraxial anesthesia

The administration of agents with anesthetic and/or analgesic properties via epidural or spinal routes can be effective at relieving pain [35–42]. Epidural anesthesia refers to the administration of drugs (usually a local anesthetic solution) into the epidural (extradural) space, whereas the administration of a drug into the subarachnoid space is known as spinal, subarachnoid, or intrathecal anesthesia. Opioids and other classes of analgesic agents can be administered by this route [43,44].

The site of action of drugs deposited in the epidural space is mainly the nerve roots as they leave the spinal cord and travel out from the intervertebral foramina. Dorsal and ventral spinal root transmission becomes inhibited when these structures are bathed by the local anesthetic solution [45,46]. Drug access to the site of action is largely dependent on the drug's physical and chemical properties, its effects with membranes that cover and protect the nervous tissue, volume of drug administered, and gravitational/concentration-dependent distribution of the solution.

Intra-articular analgesia

Local anesthetics, opioids, steroids, and other adjuvants are commonly administered into joints as a means of providing intra-articular analgesia. Intra-articular injection of local anesthetic provides analgesia for intra-articular structures only, and will not prevent pain arising from extra-articular structures such as subchondral bone, extra-articular soft tissue, or skin.

Recently, attention has been drawn to the possible toxic effects of local anesthetics on chondrocytes. Based on clinical experience, a single injection of low-concentration bupivacaine solution appears to be safe (gross observations), and the chondrotoxic effects of a single intra-articular injection of 0.5% bupivacaine appear minor (but statistically significant) and are unlikely to be detected clinically [47]. Repeated administration of bupivacaine via indwelling intra-articular catheters has been associated with chondromalacia and should be avoided. Ropivacaine is less chondrotoxic than bupivacaine [48]. and mepivacaine appears to have negligible effects *in vitro* and is therefore the drug of choice of many for intra-articular administration.

Since the discovery of opioid receptors on peripheral nerves and in joints, several studies have described the analgesic effect of opioids (mainly morphine) after arthroscopy or joint surgery in humans [49]. Low doses of intra-articular morphine will significantly reduce pain after knee surgery through an action on local opioid receptors that reaches its maximum effect 3–6 h after injection [49].

Intravenous regional anesthesia (IVRA)

Also referred to as a 'Bier block,' IVRA involves administration of a local anesthetic into a peripheral vein, where it is distributed to the tissues served by the local venous drainage, and provides surgical anesthesia for up to 90 min. Prior to drug administration, the limb is elevated and wrapped in a tight bandage to exsanguinate the distal extremity. A tourniquet is then applied proximal to the injection site, and the local anesthetic is injected into a vein. The tissues distal to the tourniquet will be desensitized. Care must be exercised so that limb ischemia time is kept at a minimum to avoid tissue damage. Additionally, early release of the tourniquet may result in transient increases in local anesthetic plasma concentrations, which can result in central nervous and myocardial system toxicities. IVRA has many applications for distal limb surgery of limited duration and remains a reliable, quick, and simple regional anesthetic technique for a variety of procedures on the distal extremities [50].

Patient preparation

To perform the majority of nerve blocks in dogs and cats they are either sedated or anesthetized. Patients should be relaxed, easy to manipulate and position, and be either minimally or completely unresponsive to needle advancement, electrolocation, and injection.

Patient positioning is an important aspect of any regional anesthetic procedure since nerves are flexible structures whose locations can vary depending on the patient's position. Recommended approaches for different nerve blocks may or may not be possible depending on the patient's position and, in some instances, patient positioning may also have an effect on the distribution of drugs following injection. Using described and standardized positioning may minimize complications.

Equipment

Most equipment is readily available from veterinary suppliers, but some specialized items (e.g., insulated needles and stimulating catheters, nerve stimulators) may be ordered from specialized medical equipment companies or suppliers to the human medical market. Recently, veterinary-specific products for regional anesthesia in dogs and cats have been developed. There are many different needles, catheters, pumps, and specialized pieces of equipment that can be used, each with inherent advantages and disadvantages depending on the specific species and procedure. Continued product development to improve patient safety and enhance utility for the anesthetist is likely.

Needles

Needles are generally selected based on their physical characteristics (e.g., tip design, length, gauge, absence or presence of insulation) and clinician preference and are typically designed for single use. Recently, several studies have investigated the effects of different needle types on nerve injury [51–53]. These studies showed that there is considerable post-traumatic inflammation and structural changes within nerves that have been impaled by needles. There were no overall differences between needle types (pencil-point, short-bevel or Tuohy) but, as could be expected, gross nerve injury scores were significantly lower with smaller-diameter needles. Smaller gauge needles are advisable for peripheral nerve blocks to minimize the risk of nerve injury in the rare event that a nerve is inadvertently perforated.

The design of the needle tip can affect the anesthetist's ability to appreciate the different tissue planes that are encountered as the needle is manipulated (Fig. 45.1). If several different tissue planes will be crossed during a particular regional block, either short-bevel or Tuohy needles may be useful (Fig. 45.1c–f). These 'blunt' needles convey more resistance to needle advancement and the anesthetist is more likely to detect changes in needle resistance as tissue planes are penetrated. Additionally, blunt (30–45° bevel, atraumatic) needle tips are less likely to penetrate the perineurium, especially if the needle approaches the nerve from a perpendicular orientation. Blunt needles can be used for both single injections and placement of indwelling catheters. For these reasons, blunt needles are typically chosen when performing regional anesthetic techniques.

The length of the needle depends on the anticipated depth of the target nerve. Longer needles are more difficult to manipulate once they are *in situ*, especially if they are of a small gauge. Larger gauge needles are less prone to deflection, and allow for easier aspiration and injection, better appreciation of resistance to injection, and the potential to pass an indwelling catheter. Smaller gauge needles tend to cause less pain in awake patients and have less risk of causing nerve trauma. Based on these considerations, small-gauge needles (25-, 27-gauge) are typically used for infiltration anesthesia (e.g., incision blocks) and superficial blocks (e.g., dental blocks), whereas larger gauge needles (19–22-gauge) are used for deeper tissue blocks (e.g., brachial plexus, lumbar plexus, epidural).

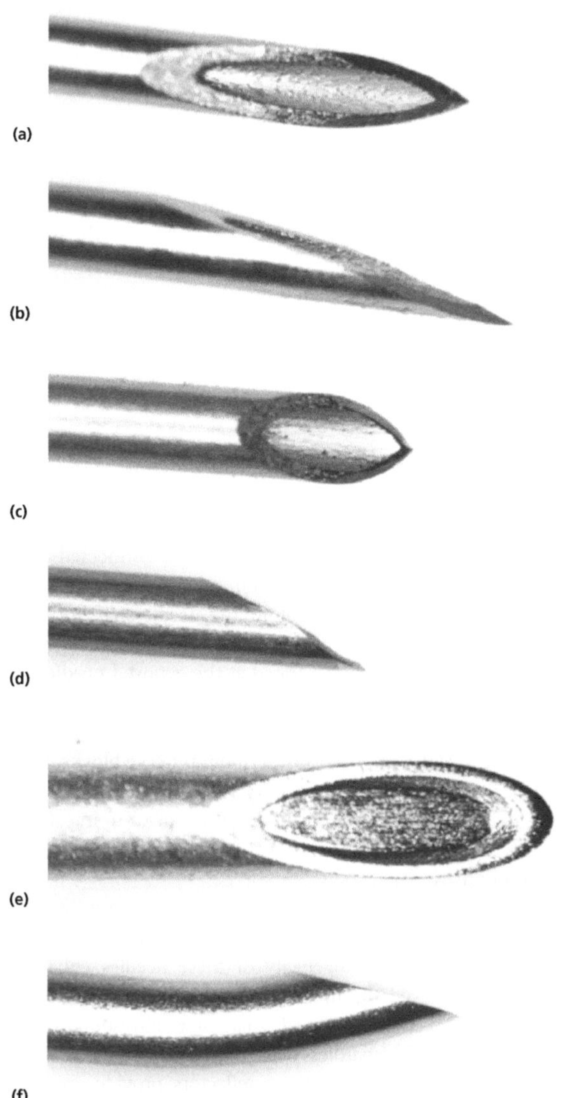

Figure 45.1 Needle tips at 25× magnification. (a), (b) 22-gauge hypodermic needle; (c), (d) 20-gauge insulated nerve block needle; (e), (f) 20-gauge Tuohy needle. Note the short bevel of the insulated needle and the round, blunt tip of the Tuohy needle when compared with the hypodermic needle.

Spinal needles

Spinal needles are manufactured with close-fitting, removable stylets that prevent tissue or fluid from entering the needle. Most spinal needles have short- or medium-blunt tips, blunter than that of a typical hypodermic needle while still allowing the needle to penetrate tissues easily. As a result, for certain blocks, Tuohy needles are preferred. Clear needle hubs allow the anesthetist to inspect visually for the presence of blood or cerebrospinal fluid (CSF) prior to drug administration.

Tuohy needles

Tuohy needles can be insulated or non-insulated and are curved at the distal tip (Fig. 45.1e,f). They can be used to perform single injections or to facilitate placement of indwelling epidural or perineural catheters. The curve at the distal tip helps to direct the catheter in a particular direction. The tips of Tuohy needles are not as sharp as hypodermic or spinal needles and, as a result, resistance is easily felt as multiple tissue planes are penetrated.

Uninsulated needles

Uninsulated needles (e.g., hypodermic and spinal needles) are bare metal along their entire length and, if used with a nerve stimulator, current is released along the entire needle shaft. As a result, uninsulated needles have a much larger conducting area and a higher threshold current is required to stimulate a peripheral nerve [54]. Since current is released along the entire shaft of an uninsulated needle, if the tip of the needle passes the target nerve it is still possible to stimulate the nerve if the shaft is in close proximity to it. Additionally, as the needle shaft passes through muscle tissue, nonspecific muscular twitch may occur, confusing the operator as to the location of the needle tip. In a study that compared the use of insulated and uninsulated needles for performance of nerve blocks in cats, researchers found that when uninsulated needles were used, the greatest degree of nerve stimulation occurred when the needle was already 0.5–1 cm past the target nerves. Depending on the volume of local anesthetic solution injected at that location, it would more than likely result in a failed nerve block.

Insulated needles

Insulated needles are coated with a thin layer of non-conducting material over the entire length of the needle except for a small area that is exposed at the tip (Fig. 45.1c,d). When connected to a peripheral nerve stimulator, the insulation on the needle prevents electric current from being leaked along the needle shaft into the surrounding tissues. As a result, the current conducts down the length of the needle and is concentrated at the exposed needle tip. Since the current is released only from the tip, high current density is achieved and the accuracy of needle placement improves [54]. When insulated needles are used for peripheral nerve blocks, low-intensity currents (0.2–0.5 mA) can be used to stimulate motor fibers, helping to identify target nerves successfully prior to injection.

Echogenic needles

Echogenic needles have been developed to facilitate ultrasound-guided needle placement in people. Although other needles will show up on ultrasound, the increased echogenicity of these needles enhances visibility. This is achieved through the addition of reflector surface angles along the distal end of the needle shaft. Since ultrasound waves are reflected off the needle regardless of its puncture angle and position relative to the ultrasound beam, these reflectors provide excellent visibility of the needle during ultrasound monitoring.

Catheters

Continuous delivery of local anesthetic drugs can be achieved by the use of perineural and epidural catheter placement. Using this technique, local anesthetics and adjunct medications (e.g., opioids and α_2-adrenergic receptor agonists) can be administered either as intermittent boluses or as continuous infusions for prolonged periods.

At its simplest, a catheter can be advanced through either a stimulating or non-stimulating needle into the target area (perineural or epidural) and secured in place for later use. Although this method is relatively easy to perform, it lacks a means of confirming correct catheter positioning close to a nerve and therefore has a lower success rate.

In people, the high failure rates associated with perineural catheters prompted the development of stimulating catheters. These special catheters allow for stimulation of the target nerve through the catheter, even after it has been *in situ* for an extended period (hours to days). This allows for repeated confirmation that the distal tip of the catheter is still adjacent to the desired nerves/plexus prior to subsequent drug administrations.

There are a variety of catheters for epidural or perineural use in dogs and cats. Most catheters are made from either Teflon or polyamide nylon, which makes them stiff enough to be used without a stylet, while also helping to prevent kinking or stretching. Catheters can be either closed-tip with multiple fenestrations along their distal end, or open-ended with a single opening at their distal tip. Fenestrated catheters are typically used for perineural placement since they disperse local anesthetic solutions over a wider area, whereas open-end uni-port catheters are most often used for continuous epidural drug administration.

Wound catheters

Wound catheters (also referred to as fenestrated catheters or diffusion catheters) have a closed tip and numerous fenestrations (small holes/microports) at regular intervals along their distal segment (Fig. 45.2). This design allows local anesthetic solutions to be infused directly into surgical sites or wounds either in areas of the body that cannot be blocked through specific regional anesthetic techniques, or for longer-term analgesia when the original block technique cannot easily be performed repeatedly [18].

When used for analgesia, a wound catheter should be placed in the deepest part of the surgical field, adjacent to exposed nerves if possible (Fig. 45.2c). Next, the catheter should be tunneled subcuta-

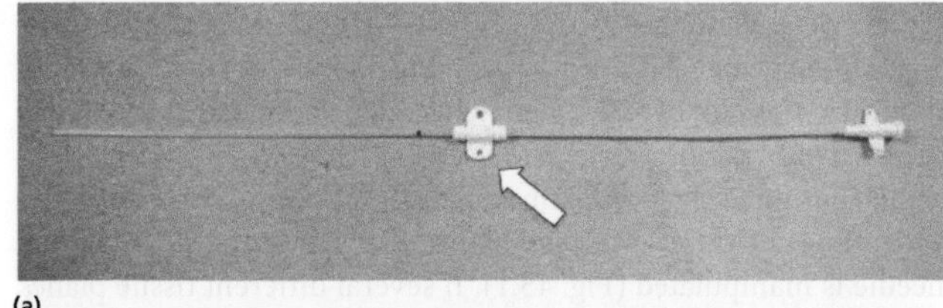
(a)

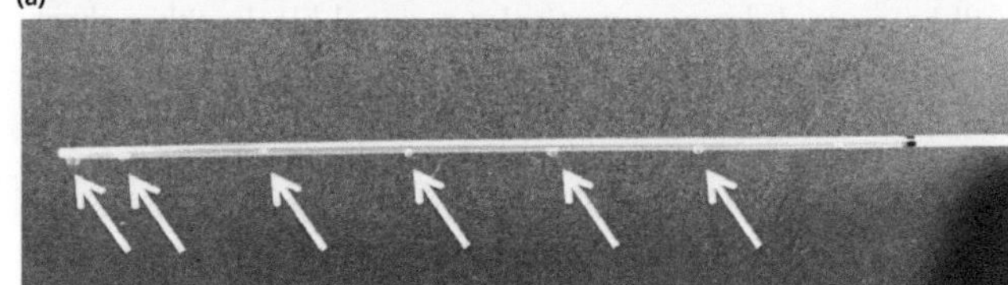
(b)

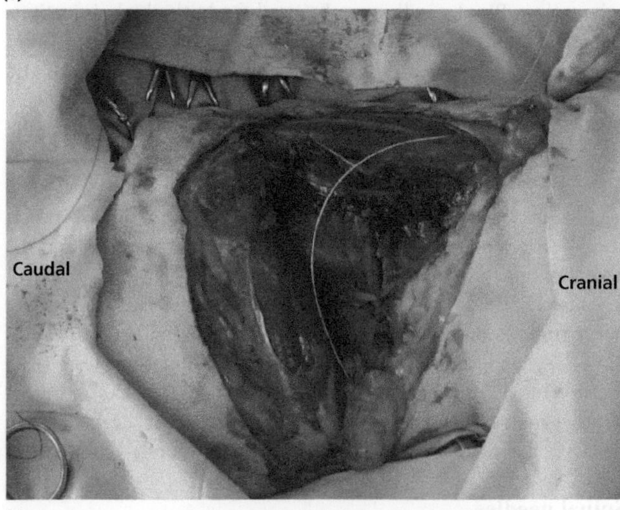

(c)

Figure 45.2 An example of a wound catheter. (a) Note the moveable 'suture wing' (arrow) that can be moved along the catheter to a convenient position for suturing to the skin. (b) Demonstration of a local anesthetic solution being injected through fenestrations in the catheter. (c) A wound catheter being placed into a large surgical defect in the right flank of a cat following resection of a neoplastic lesion.

neously away from the surgical site so that it exits the skin dorsal to the wound through a separate skin incision. Movable suture wings are used to anchor the catheter to the patient's skin, and can be positioned as needed along the catheter to prevent migration or dislodgment (Fig. 45.2a). If desired, an antibacterial filter can be attached to the proximal end of the catheter and a sterile dressing applied at the exit site. Wound catheters are usually maintained in patients for several days, allowing local anesthetics to be administered well into the postoperative period [18].

There is some degree of variability in the distribution of infused solutions when different infusion rates are used. There tends to be a more even distribution along all fenestrations when injection speeds mimic those that might be experienced during intermittent bolus administration, whereas there is an uneven distribution of drug flow when very slow rates (that would be associated with constant rate infusions with pumps) are used. Although wound soaker catheters can be effective for providing postoperative analgesia, variation based on catheter performance and individual animal responses is anticipated, hence catheters should not be relied upon solely [55].

Peripheral nerve stimulators

This device generates a square-wave electrical current (Fig. 45.3). Nerves are selectively stimulated depending on their size (large-diameter axons are more easily excited than smaller diameter fibers), which explains why motor nerves can be stimulated at lower currents than sensory nerves [56]. The closer the needle is to the target nerve, the lower is the electrical current required to elicit a muscle response. At sufficiently low currents (approximately 0.2–0.6 mA), if the stimulating needle is able to elicit contractions of the effector muscle or muscle group, it is assumed that the needle-to-nerve distance is small enough that when local anesthetic solution is injected, sensory block will occur.

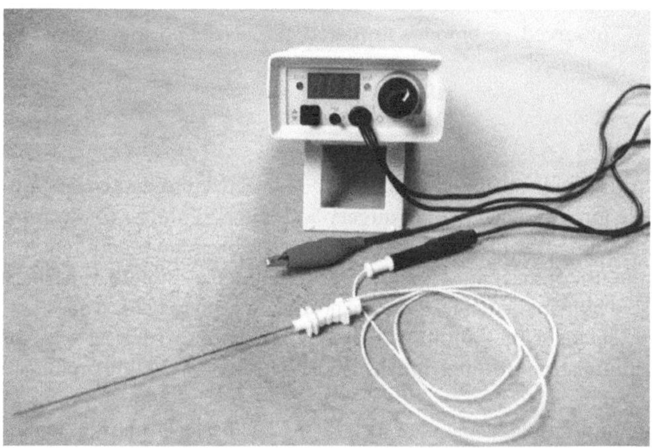

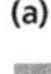

(a)

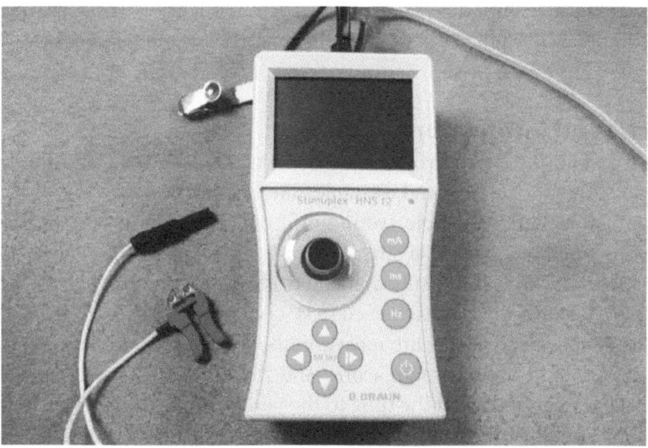

(b)

Figure 45.3 Examples of peripheral nerve stimulators. (a) Stimuplex® Dig RC; (b) Stimuplex® HNS12 (B. Braun Medical, Bethlehem, PA, USA).

For many years, anesthetists believed that using a peripheral nerve stimulator not only improved success rates, but that based on the minimum stimulating current (MSC) at which motor fibers could be depolarized, intraneural injections could be avoided. Fairly recent studies using ultrasound to visualize needles *in situ* during nerve blocks have determined that the level of current cannot be used to determine whether a needle tip is located extra- or intraneurally [57–60]. Chan *et al.* [58] evaluated stimulating currents associated with intraneural needle placement in the brachial plexus of pigs and found that the minimum current to elicit a motor response was 0.43 mA (0.12–1.8 mA) [median (minimum–maximum)], and concluded that a motor response above 0.5 mA does not necessarily exclude an intraneural injection. Kapur *et al.* [61] studied the neurological outcome after intraneural injections into sciatic nerves and found that the worst outcomes were associated with high injection pressures (20–38 psi, ~138–262 kPa) whereas intraneural injections at moderate pressures (<12 psi, 82.7 kPa) had a longer than expected duration, but no other adverse effects. All ultrasound-guided perineural injections were accompanied by low injection pressures (<5 psi, 34.5 kPa). The true incidence of intraneural injections is unknown, but long-term sequelae would appear to be relatively rare. Most blocks in veterinary medicine are still performed blindly (not ultrasound guided), yet few complications associated with intraneural injections have been reported.

Clinical use of peripheral nerve stimulation

Peripheral nerve stimulators should always be used in conjunction with insulated needles. The negative electrode serves as the searching electrode and is connected to the insulated needle. The positive (red) electrode is connected to the patient's skin. When used with this configuration, the current will induce depolarization of a target nerve, resulting in obvious muscle twitches. If the leads are reversed, twice the current is required to induce a motor response and the anesthetist may cause trauma as they search repeatedly for a nerve that will elicit the expected responses. Based on the arrangement of the electrodes, with newer nerve stimulators it is virtually impossible to connect the electrodes backwards (Fig. 45.3).

Features

Ideally, the anesthetist should be able to control the current (mA) and impulse frequency (Hz). Nerve stimulators should have an easily readable display that shows the current that is being delivered to the patient, and also some warning mechanism (audible alarm, visual indicator) if the dialed current is not being delivered to the patient (e.g., if the return electrode becomes disconnected from the patient). Ideally, the nerve stimulator should be designed to adjust the necessary settings without breaking sterile technique. Current can be adjusted by digital or analog dials and remote controllers (e.g., foot pedals, or hand-held remote controllers). Since effective current levels estimate the needle-to-nerve distance, the stimulator should allow for current intensity adjustments in small increments across the clinically useful range of 0.1–1.0 mA.

A pulse frequency of 2 Hz is optimal for peripheral nerve location during nerve blocks. Compared with a pulse frequency of 1 Hz, the anesthetist is less likely to pass the target nerve between consecutive impulses as they advance their needle. When using nerve stimulators only capable of 1 Hz, the needle must be advanced very slowly in order to avoid missing the nerve between consecutive pulses.

Clinical technique

1 The negative electrode should be connected to the insulated needle.
2 The positive electrode (red) is connected to the patient. The site placement of the positive electrode is irrelevant with modern stimulators provided that good contact is achieved [19].
3 The peripheral nerve stimulator should be turned on and the current set at 1.0–1.5 mA.
4 Using anatomic landmarks, the insulated needle is slowly advanced towards the desired nerve. When the nerve is exposed to enough current, depolarization of the nerve may occur, resulting in an observable or palpable muscle contraction.
5 If motor responses are not elicited, withdraw the needle to the level of the skin and redirect it.
6 Once a twitch is obtained, slowly decrease the current to zero, confirming that the twitches decrease in intensity.
7 Gradually increase the current from zero while making fine needle adjustments until a twitch is elicited at a final current of 0.5 mA or less. Document the 'minimum stimulating current' (MSC).
8 Aspirate using the syringe. If blood is aspirated, reposition the needle. If aspiration is negative, it does not completely rule out intravascular needle placement, but it does suggest that the needle is located in a safe location to inject.
9 Slowly inject the local anesthetic solution. As soon as the solution is injected, motor twitches will disappear when the local anesthetic (an electrolyte solution) expands the conductive area around the stimulating needle, making the low-level current less effective for stimulating the nerve [62].
10 Ensure that there is minimal resistance to injection of the local anesthetic solution.
11 Once the injection has been made, the patient should be monitored to ensure that no signs of local anesthetic systemic toxicity or other complications (hematoma, etc.) occur.

Ultrasound equipment

The combination of ultrasound technology and electrolocation is gaining popularity. Ultrasound allows for real-time visualization of the stimulating needle, and also identification of peripheral nerves and other important anatomic structures such as vessels, muscle bellies, and fasciae. Although ultrasound guidance and electrolocation can be used separately for performing nerve blocks, they are very useful when utilized together.

It is important to have the ability to obtain good-quality images of nerves of interest. The quality of the images that are obtained depends on the ultrasound machine, transducer selection, and the skill of the clinician. High-frequency linear array transducers (10–15 MHz) are most suitable for imaging superficial nerves that are less than 5 cm beneath the surface of the skin.

Clinical use of combined ultrasound-guided–peripheral nerve stimulation blocks

1 To begin the procedure, verify that the ultrasound machine settings are optimized for nerve imaging.
2 Set the nerve stimulator at a frequency of 1 Hz (for minimal disturbance of the ultrasound image) and a current of 0.4 mA (a typical threshold current).
3 Apply isopropyl alcohol (70%) to the area to be scanned. The alcohol will improve transducer-to-skin coupling, enhancing the quality of the ultrasound image.
4 Using your non-dominant hand, place the transducer over the relevant area. Glide, rotate, or tilt the transducer until the target nerve (or nearby structures) can be identified in its short axis.
5 Insert the stimulating needle. Note that the long axis of the needle should be placed directly beneath the long axis of the ultrasound beam. This is known as the 'in-plane' technique, and allows the needle shaft and tip to be visualized while being advanced under the ultrasound beam.
6 Advance the needle towards the nerve, keeping the needle tip in the field of ultrasound view at all times.
7 Watch for the characteristic contractions of the appropriate muscle as the stimulating needle approaches the nerve.
8 Before administering the local anesthetic, aspirate the syringe. Positive aspiration of blood suggests that the needle has inadvertently penetrated a vessel and must be repositioned prior to drug administration.
9 If no blood is observed on aspiration, slowly begin to inject the local anesthetic. As you inject, visualize fluid spreading around the nerve.
10 The anesthetic solution will appear as a hypoechoic (black) circumferential ring around the nerve. The visualization of solution around the nerve rules out intravascular, but not intraneural needle placement.
11 If at any point during the injection resistance is encountered, the presence of fluid accumulation around the nerve cannot be observed, or blood is aspirated, the needle position should be adjusted.

Local infiltration and wound infusions

Although local anesthetics have been injected into tissues as a simple form of analgesia for surgery and other painful procedures for decades, over the last few years there has been renewed interest in the use of local anesthetics at the surgical site. In both veterinary and human medicine, there are now many reports of local anesthetics being either infiltrated preoperatively into surgical sites or administered through indwelling catheters for providing prolonged pain relief.

Infiltrating the planned surgical field with a local anesthetic solution is an easy and inexpensive alternative to performing more advanced techniques. A promising new modality is the relatively simple technique of placing a multi-fenestrated (multi-holed) catheter (Fig. 45.2).

Wound infiltration

Wound infiltration involves the direct injection of a local anesthetic into the surgical field and is simple, safe, and inexpensive (Fig. 45.4). [15,16,63–66]. In people, wound infiltration has been used to provide operative analgesia since the early 1900s. Instillation of local anesthetic into skin, subcutaneous tissue, fascia, muscle, and/or parietal peritoneum is achieved [63]. Local anesthetics such as lidocaine and bupivacaine are most commonly utilized, and have been shown to (1) reduce pain scores and the need for supplementary analgesics, (2) extend the time to the patient's first request for analgesia, and (3) reduce the duration of hospital stays.

Several studies have reported the results of using incisional infiltration of local anesthesia for a variety of abdominal surgeries in animals [15–17,67]. Carpenter *et al.* [15] randomly administered

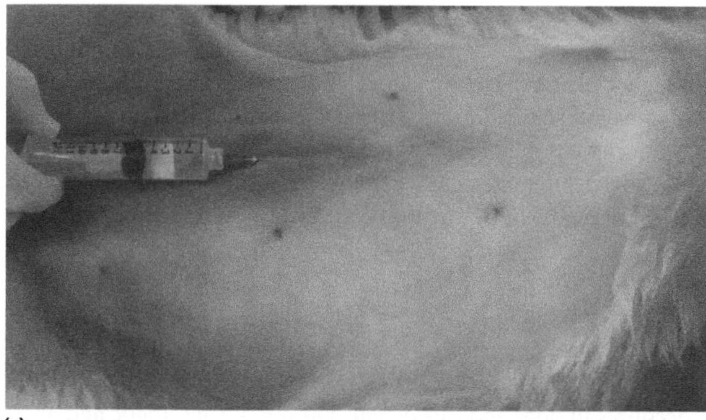

(a)

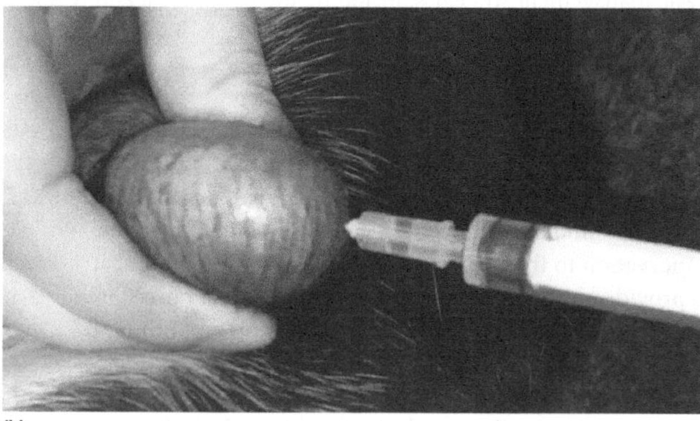

(b)

Figure 45.4 Examples of using local infiltration techniques to contribute to surgical analgesia. (a) Use of bupivacaine for incisional infiltration along the ventral abdomen of a dog scheduled for laparotomy surgery. (b) Use of a testicular block prior to castration surgery.

saline, lidocaine with epinephrine, or bupivacaine into the intraperitoneal space immediately prior to closure of the linea alba. A 'splash' block using either saline, lidocaine with epinephrine, or bupivacaine immediately prior to closure of the skin of each dog was also compared. Intraperitoneal and incisional bupivacaine provided effective analgesia following ovariohysterectomy. More dogs required supplemental analgesia in the saline control group than in the bupivacaine group, and bupivacaine-treated dogs had lower pain scores (using visual analog and composite pain scores) and were less sedate than control dogs [15].

Savvas *et al.* [16] compared saline and bupivacaine for pre- or postoperative incisional use. They administered the solutions both subcutaneously and intramuscularly at the proposed incision site either just before the start of, or at the end of surgery (following subcutaneous tissue closure). This study documented that preoperative administration of bupivacaine resulted in significantly lower pain scores and less frequent use of additional postoperative analgesia compared with the other groups (postoperative incisional infiltration with either bupivacaine or saline). None of the preoperative bupivacaine-treated dogs required additional postoperative analgesics, and it was concluded that this technique is a simple, attractive, and effective approach to reduce postoperative pain for at least 24 h after celiotomy in dogs.

Fitzpatrick *et al.* [17] compared either no incisional injection, preoperative infiltration with saline, preoperative infiltration using bupivacaine, or postoperative infiltration using bupivacaine along the superficial and deep tissues of the incision site. Dogs received various opioids for premedication, on recovery, and every 6 h for the first 24 h postoperatively along with carprofen. A blinded observer used a composite pain scale and a quantitative tool (von Frey filaments) to test peri-incisional analgesia for 24 h following surgery. No significant differences in pain scores, doses of rescue analgesics, and responses to von Frey filaments between the different treatment groups were found. Supplemental analgesia from the bupivacaine incisional block in dogs receiving multimodal analgesia was undetectable. None of the dogs required rescue analgesia, and incisional bupivacaine did not increase the incidence of complications.

Lykkegaard *et al.* [67] measured the effects of pre-emptive analgesic intervention on spinal nociception and activation of the hypothalamic–pituitary axis. Prior to surgery, the skin, muscle, and peritoneum of pigs was infiltrated with either saline or a mixture of lidocaine and bupivacaine. A third group was anesthetized but did not undergo surgery (sham group). Two hours after surgery, half of the pigs from each group were euthanized and gene expression was measured in the dorsal horn of the spinal cord. Gene expression is frequently used in laboratory studies as a marker of nociception and a measure of neuronal activity following various painful stimuli. The surviving pigs had blood collected at predetermined times postoperatively for determination of ACTH, cortisol, C-reactive protein and interleukin-6 concentrations. Compared with the saline infiltration group, the sham and local anesthetic groups had no increases in c-fos gene expression, whereas the saline infiltration group had dramatic increases in plasma ACTH and cortisol compared with the other two groups. It was concluded that preoperative incisional infiltration of a local anesthetic can have profound inhibitory effects on spinal nociception and HPA-axis activation caused by surgery, and the use of directly applied local anesthetics during surgery and other traumatic procedures was recommended.

Wound catheters

Wound catheters are highly effective when used in combination with systemically administered analgesic agents as part of a balanced analgesia plan. In many cases, wound catheters may be superior to other methods such as systemically administered opioids and non-steroidal analgesic drugs. In people, wound catheters are typically placed in incisions at the end of major surgery [68–70]. Catheters are placed in a variety of locations: subcutaneous, subfascial, intra-articular, periosteal, and peripleural [68]. In animals, wound catheters have been used for total ear canal ablation (minimal apparent benefits), amputation, oncologic surgery, and closure of large wounds [18,71–74]. Most veterinary reports describe using either bupivacaine in intermittent boluses or lidocaine as a continuous infusion in both dogs and cats, e.g., bupivacaine 0.5% administered at 1 mg/kg every 6–8 h [18,73] or lidocaine 2% administered as an infusion at 1.5–3 mg/kg/h [18,72].

In one study, bupivacaine was compared with saline for infusion through wound catheters in dogs [75]. Bupivacaine was administered at 2 mg/kg, followed by additional doses (1 mg/kg) every 6 h. Equivalent volumes of saline were administered to control dogs. Compared with saline, bupivacaine lowered the postoperative interventional and non-interventional pain scores in the dogs, decreased the need for other analgesics, and improved appetite. Wound sensitivity to palpation was not affected. Plasma bupivacaine levels were within acceptable and safe ranges.

Clinical use

The human literature documents benefits to the patient when continuous infusion or intermittent doses of local anesthetics are used for >24 h as opposed to administering only a single treatment

(Fig. 45.2c). If transected nerves can be visualized (e.g., following limb amputation), the catheter can be positioned in close proximity to the nerves, otherwise the catheter is simply positioned into the wound [18]. All of the catheter fenestrations should be located under the skin. Overall, the reported incidence of complications related to the use of wound catheters is relatively low in both the veterinary and the human literature. The complications described can be divided into two types:

1 Equipment-related complications include catheter dislodgement from the site of placement, catheter disconnection from the local anesthetic delivery system, catheter occlusion, and catheter breakage. These issues are generally considered to be minor and are more of an inconvenience to the veterinary staff than a danger to the patient.
2 Drug-related complications include local anesthetic toxicities that are the result of systemic absorption of the delivered anesthetic or inadvertent overdose. Calculating toxic doses of the local anesthetics to be used minimizes the potential for drug-related complications.

Most complications following the use of wound catheters are considered to be minor [18,68,72,73,76,77]. Radlinsky *et al.* [71] and Wolfe *et al.* [72] both reported on the use of wound catheters for local analgesia in dogs following total ear canal ablation. Catheter-related complications were uncommon and considered minor. Serious complications such as wound infection and dehiscence of the surgical site did not occur in either study. A retrospective study on the clinical use of wound soaker catheters in dogs [18] found that the most common complication was disconnection from the delivery system in cases where 'home-made' catheters were created from red rubber catheters versus the use of commercially available catheters. The incidence of wound infections was similar to the overall infection rate observed in comparable surgical cases without catheter placement. One dog developed signs of local anesthetic toxicity manifesting as tremors and ataxia, which resolved quickly when the lidocaine infusion was discontinued.

Dental blocks

Dental and oral diseases that require surgical intervention are highly prevalent in small animals [78]. Current standards for dental and oral procedures in dogs and cats dictate appropriate anesthetic and analgesic management strategies, including the use of local and regional blocks when indicated [79,80]. Common indications for dental and oral local and regional anesthesia in small animals include dental extractions, endodontic therapy, operative dentistry, periodontal surgery, maxillomandibular fracture repair, palatal defect repair, oral oncologic surgery, and biopsies of oral tissues [81–83].

The implementation of local and regional anesthesia requires a thorough understanding of the relevant anatomy. The sensory innervation to the oral cavity including all the intraoral structures is provided by the mandibular (V2) and maxillary divisions (V3) of the trigeminal nerve (V), and their corresponding branches (Fig. 45.5) [84].

Needles sizes ranging from 25- to 27-gauge have been recommended [83]; needles should be flexible and ideally have a short atraumatic bevel [85]. Because the tips of these needles easily

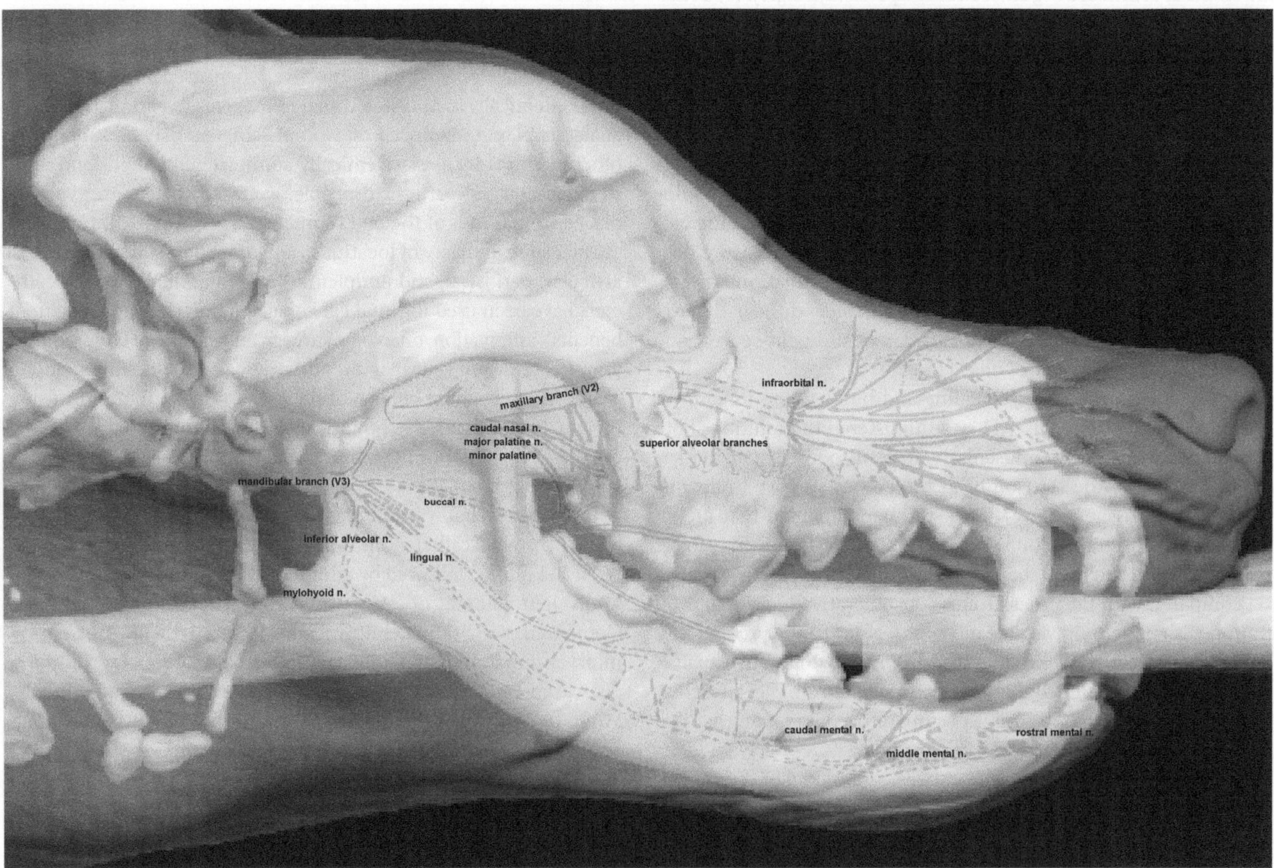

Figure 45.5 Distribution of the maxillary (V2) and mandibular (V3) branches of the trigeminal nerve (V).

become blunt or bent, the needle that is used to draw the anesthetic from the vial should not be used to administer the block [86]. Additionally, a new needle should be used for each site when performing more than one block.

Maxillary nerve block

Anatomy

The maxillary nerve provides sensory innervation to the maxillary teeth and associated hard and soft tissues, hard and soft palates, the nose and lower eyelids. It exits the cranium via the round foramen and courses rostrally along the dorsal surface of the medial pterygoid muscle towards the pterygopalatine fossa (Fig. 45.6). At that point, the zygomatic and pterygopalatine nerves arise, and the maxillary nerve continues its course as the infraorbital nerve, entering the infraorbital canal via the maxillary foramen. The pterygopalatine nerve gives rise to the minor and major palatine nerves. These emerge at the palatal area via the corresponding foramina, and provide innervation to the soft and hard palate, respectively [84,87].

The caudal, middle, and rostral superior alveolar nerves arise from the infraorbital nerve. The caudal superior alveolar nerves arise in the pterygopalatine fossa before the infraorbital nerve enters the canal, and supply the first and second molar teeth. Within the infraorbital canal, the middle and rostral superior alveolar nerves emerge; these nerves supply the rostral premolars via numerous foramina located on the floor of the canal, and the canine and incisor teeth via the incisivomaxillary canal. The infraorbital nerve exits the infraorbital canal via the infraorbital foramen, and gives rise to the external nasal, internal nasal and superior labial branches [84,87].

Indications

When the maxillary nerve is blocked, the whole ipsilateral maxillary quadrant is anesthetized, including all teeth, associated gingiva, alveolar bone, dental pulp, and the hard and soft tissues of the hard and soft palates. Other maxillofacial structures anesthetized include part of the nasal mucosa (excluding the septal mucosa served by the ethmoidal nerve) [84] and the upper lip [88,89]. The indications for a maxillary block include ipsilateral maxillary dental extractions, periodontal surgery, endodontic therapy, biopsies, maxillectomy, incisivectomy, rhinotomy, rhinoscopy, and palatal surgery [81,83,90].

Technique

Several techniques have been described to block the maxillary nerve; these are based on depositing a local anesthetic agent in or just caudal to the pterygopalatine fossa. Some of the techniques use an extraoral approach and some are based on an intraoral route [81–83,90]. The patient may be positioned in dorsal, sternal, or lateral recumbency. The puncture site is located on the ventral aspect of the rostral half of the zygomatic arch. The needle should be directed slightly rostrally towards the pterygopalatine fossa/maxillary foramen, where the anesthetic agent is deposited [81,83]. Salivary gland and maxillary artery damage may occur [89]. Another concern is that the tip of the needle approaches the nerve perpendicularly, increasing the risk of nerve damage [91].

The rostral branches of the maxillary nerve can be blocked using the infraobital approach. The infraorbital foramen may be palpated extra- or intraorally, using the non-dominant hand. In dogs, the foramen is consistently located dorsal to the maxillary third premolar tooth, and is easily palpated as an oval-shaped structure. In cats, the foramen is located immediately medial to the prominent rostral end of the zygomatic arch [83,90]. After the infraorbital foramen has been identified, the dominant hand is used to advance the needle caudally on a horizontal plane, maintaining it parallel to the hard palate (Fig. 45.7) [81,90]. In cats and brachycephalic dogs, a short needle is recommended. Larger dogs may have a canal longer than 2 cm, so a longer needle is necessary to reach the targeted area [83].

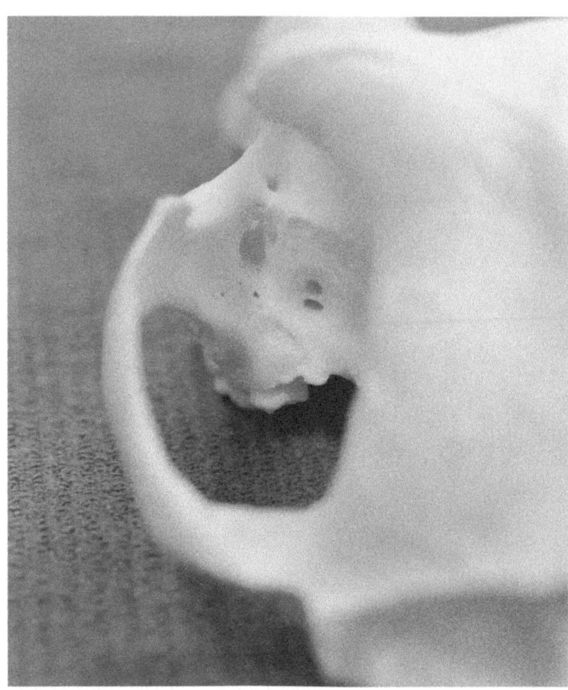

Figure 45.6 Caudal view of the pterygopalatine fossa. The maxillary foramen is the larger oval-shaped foramen in the center of the fossa and represents the caudal opening of the infraorbital canal.

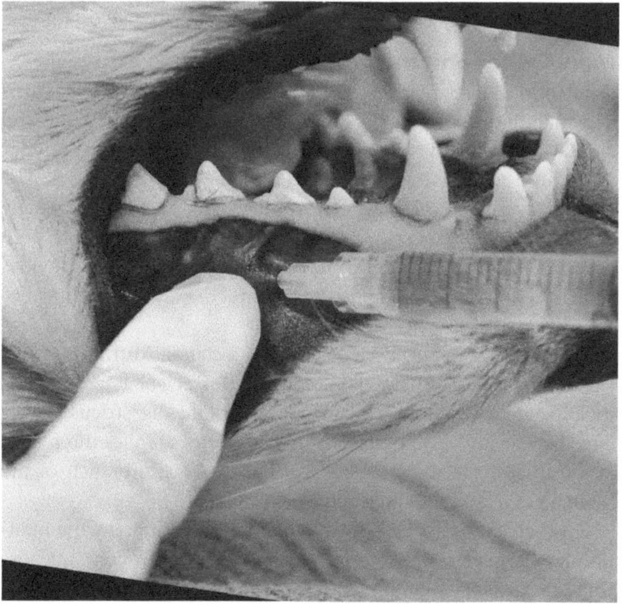

Figure 45.7 Maxillary nerve block being performed via the infraorbital canal. The needle is introduced into the canal via the infraorbital foramen and is advanced caudally towards the pterygopalatine fossa where the anesthetic agent will be deposited. Note that the patient is in dorsal recumbency.

The infraorbital approach offers several advantages over other techniques used to block the maxillary nerve. First, it ensures that the needle is advanced accurately to the desired location. Also, the tip of the needle advances parallel to nerves avoiding perpendicular contact, thus decreasing the risk of nerve damage. Moreover, because the canal guides the needle, damage to the zygomatic salivary gland is unlikely. Evidence suggests that this technique is safer and more effective than the lateral approach [89]. The infraorbital approach may not consistently anesthetize the maxillary molar area [83]. It is possible that this occurs if the anesthetic agent is deposited in the infraorbital canal and not in the pterygopalatine fossa. However, it is possible that this is due to collateral innervation to the associated alveolar mucosa and gingiva via the buccal nerve (branch of the mandibular nerve) [84]. A technique to block the buccal nerve in small animals has not been documented.

Hematoma formation at the infraorbital foramen area is a frequent but usually minor complication that results from accidental laceration of the infraorbital arteries or accompanying vein [83,90]. Immediate treatment is usually limited to applying manual pressure over the area to promote hemostasis.

The maxillary nerve can also be anesthetized via an intraoral caudal approach [81,83]. The technique consists of introducing a short needle just caudal to the maxillary tuberosity, directing it dorsally so that the tip lies close to the maxillary nerve. The patient should be in dorsal recumbency with the mouth completely open, avoiding delays and without using a mouth gag so the risk of altered blood flow via the maxillary artery is minimized, especially in cats. The use of mouth gags in cats has been associated with acute blindness and deafness due to possible compression of the maxillary artery by the angular process of the mandible [92,93]. One major concern when administering this block is accidental penetration of the orbit; other disadvantages include possible perpendicular contact with the maxillary nerve, and injury to the maxillary artery and zygomatic salivary gland. There are no clinical studies documenting the efficacy and safety of this particular technique.

Mandibular and inferior alveolar nerve block

Anatomy

The mandibular nerve exits the cranium via the oval foramen and courses rostrally on the medial aspect of the temporomandibular joint, and gives rise to the buccal and masticatory nerves. The masticatory nerve provides motor innervation to the rostral belly of the digastricus muscle; the buccal nerve crosses the pterygoid muscles towards the lateral aspect of the ramus, and provides sensory innervation to the vestibular mucosa and skin ventral to the zygomatic bone [84].

As the mandibular nerve continues its course rostrally, it gives rise to the lingual, mylohyoid, and inferior alveolar nerves. The mylohyoid nerve supplies the rostral belly of the digastricus muscle and the mylohyoid muscle. The lingual nerve supplies the rostral two-thirds of the tongue. The sublingual nerve, a branch of the lingual nerve, supplies the sublingual mucosa [84].

On the lateral aspect of the medial pterygoid muscle, the mandibular nerve becomes the inferior alveolar nerve, coursing rostrally towards the mandibular foramen. At that point, the inferior alveolar nerve penetrates into the mandibular canal via the mandibular foramen, where it provides sensory fibers to the teeth before further ramifying into the caudal, middle, and rostral mental nerves, which exit the mandibular canal via the corresponding mental foramina [84,87].

Indications

Blocking the inferior alveolar nerve provides regional anesthesia to the ipsilateral mandibular quadrant, including teeth, alveolar bone, and gingiva. The indications for an inferior alveolar nerve block include ipsilateral mandibular dental extractions, periodontal surgery, endodontic therapy, biopsies, and mandibulectomy [81,83,90]. The mental nerves supply the lower lip and rostral intermandibular area [84].

Technique

The mandibular foramen can be palpated intraorally using the index finger of the non-dominant hand (Fig. 45.8). The foramen is located on the medial and ventral portion of the ramus, between the third mandibular molar tooth and the angular process. Alternatively, gentle palpation can be used to identify the inferior alveolar nerve and artery before entering the canal [81,83].

While maintaining the index finger on the mandibular foramen, the other hand is used to advance the needle. The needle can be introduced intraorally under the mucosa, or extraorally through the skin of the ventral aspect of the mandible (Fig. 45.9). For both techniques, the needle must be slowly advanced along the medial aspect of the mandible until the tip is located over the mandibular foramen [83]. For the extraoral technique, the patient should be placed in dorsal or lateral recumbency. For the intraoral technique, the patient can be in dorsal or lateral recumbency with the mouth completely open.

Hematoma formation at the mandibular foramen may be a frequent but usually minor complication that results from accidental laceration of the local blood vessels [90]. Immediate treatment is usually limited to applying manual pressure over the area to promote hemostasis. Another reported, but apparently infrequent,

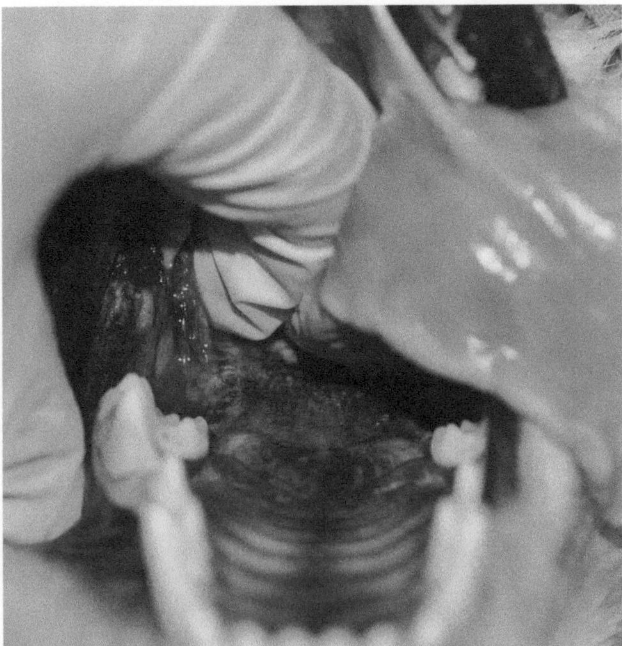

Figure 45.8 Palpation of the mandibular foramen of a dog cadaver. The index finger of the non-dominant hand is used to locate the foramen intraorally at a point between the mandibular third molar tooth and the angular process, on the medial aspect of the ramus.

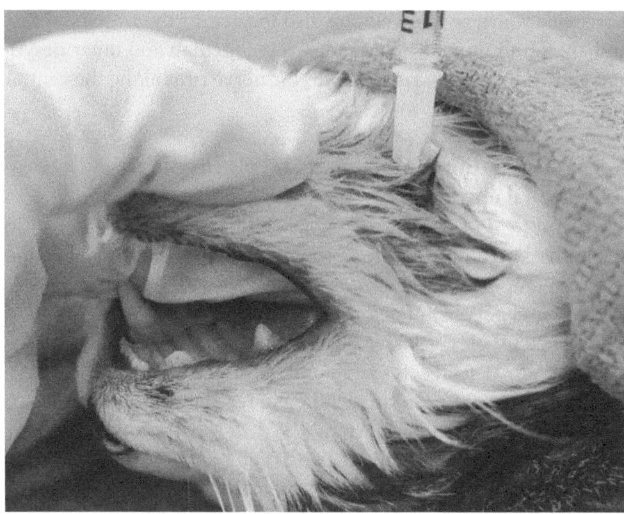

Figure 45.9 Extraoral caudal approach to the inferior alveolar nerve of a cat cadaver. The needle is introduced through the skin of the ventral mandibular area and is slowly advanced along the medial aspect of the ramus until towards the mandibular foramen, where the anesthetic agent will be deposited.

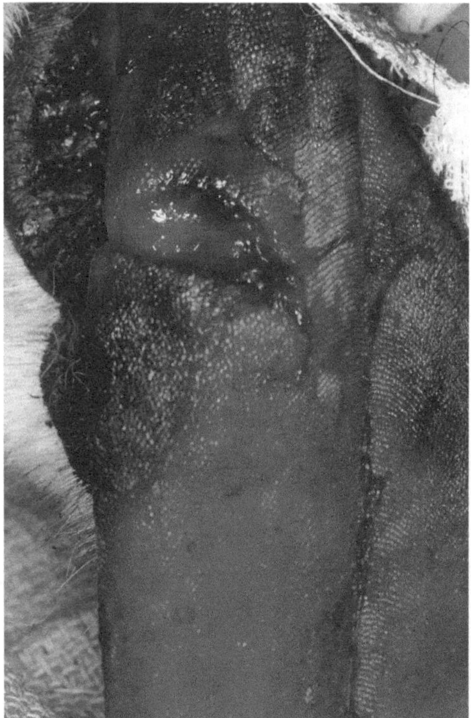

Figure 45.10 Self-inflicted wounds on the tongue of a dog that occurred during postanesthetic recovery. This patient had received bilateral inferior alveolar nerve blocks via a caudal approach.

complication is self-mutilation of the tongue during recovery from general anesthesia (Fig. 45.10) [90]. It has been suggested that this is due to diffusion of the local anesthetic solution onto the lingual nerve when attempting an inferior alveolar block using the caudal approach [83]. Deep and multiple tongue lacerations that may bleed profusely can occur very quickly, and the patient may require immediate surgical repair under general anesthesia.

The rostral approach consists of blocking the inferior alveolar nerve directly in the mandibular canal via the middle mental foramen [94–96]. First, the middle mental foramen is palpated using the non-dominant hand. The foramen is typically located between the roots of the canine and the first premolar teeth. Intraorally, the area is covered by the labial frenulum; it may be necessary to displace it rostrally or caudally. Extraoral palpation is an alternative. Owing to its small size, the middle mental foramen is generally not palpable in small dogs and cats. Once the foramen has been identified, a needle is introduced at a 45° angle and advanced until it is engaged in the mental foramen; this can be done intra- or extraorally. Significant needle manipulation may be necessary, and damage to the middle mental and inferior alveolar nerve and artery is possible [81]. The area anesthetized is variable and likely depends on how caudal within the canal the local anesthetic agent diffuses [94–96]. In general, the applicability of this technique may be limited to the rostral premolar, canine, and incisor teeth, and the rostral area of the lower lip.

Local tissue dental blocks

Local dental infiltrative blocks are routinely used in human dentistry either as the sole means to achieve anesthesia for dental and oral procedures or to supplement regional anesthesia techniques [97]. Common local block techniques include intraosseous, intraligamentary (periodontal ligament), supraperiosteal, and intrapulpal injection [81,83].

No published clinical data are available on the use of these techniques in dogs and cats. Some local block techniques (e.g., intraligamentary) have been tested in dogs under experimental conditions [98]; others (e.g., supraperiosteal) are hypothetically considered ineffective owing to the thickness of the associated cortical bone [81]. Some local blocks require specialized equipment, representing an additional cost [99]. Also, the duration of action of local blocks is shorter than that of regional blocks [81,97]. As a result, local blocks are infrequently used in dogs and cats. Local anesthesia for dental procedures in dogs and cats have been reviewed in several publications [100–102].

Thoracic limb blocks

The cervical paravertebral block [103,104] is a technique that can be used to provide anesthesia and analgesia to the proximal thoracic limb (including the humerus, shoulder, and distal scapula). Recently, ultrasound has been used to identify the roots of the brachial plexus [20]. Using this technique, proximal structures including the shoulder and humerus, and also those that are more distally located on the limb, can be identified. The traditional 'axillary' approach for performing brachial plexus blocks in small animal patients is performed at the level of the scapula–humeral joint, and will only provide anesthesia to the distal humerus and beyond [28,105]. The placement of perineural catheters adjacent to the brachial plexus is possible, but presents the challenge of keeping the catheter in the correct location and preventing early catheter displacement once patients become ambulatory [106,107]. Bupivacaine 0.5%, with or without the addition of dexmedetomidine (0.5–2 μg per mL of bupivacaine used), is most commonly used to provide surgical anesthesia [108–112].

Cervical paravertebral block

The cervical paravertebral block is an advanced-level technique [88]. In 2007, Hofmeister *et al.* performed an anatomic study using a blind approach to the nerves of dog cadavers, and reported a relatively low success rate (only three out of nine cadavers had successful staining of all four nerve roots) [103]. The following year, an updated and revised technique was described by Lemke and Creighton [104]. Rioja *et al.* [113] evaluated the use of methylene blue injections using a modification of Lemke and Creighton's technique. They used three different approaches to the nerves: blind, electrolocation using a nerve stimulator, and ultrasound-guided. The low overall success rate of the three techniques for staining the target nerves and the high incidence of potentially complications (dye staining of the cervical spinal cord) led them to suggest caution in using this block in clinical patients until further research has been completed.

Brachial plexus block

Anatomy

The brachial plexus of the dog is formed from the ventral branches of the C6, C7, C8, and T1 spinal nerves (Fig. 45.11). The most important nerves (moving from cranial to caudal) are the suprascapular, subscapular, axillary, musculocutaneous, radial, median, and ulnar nerves.

- The ventral root of C6, with some input from C7, is the main contributor to the suprascapular nerve.
- The ventral root of C7, with some input from C6, is the main contributor to the musculocutaneous nerve and subscapular nerve.
- The ventral root of C8, with some input from T1, is the main contributor to the radial nerve and axillary nerve.
- The ventral root of T1, with some input from C8, is the main contributor to the median nerve and ulnar nerve.

After the nerve roots emerge through the intertransversarius musculature, there is an exchange of nerve fibers between them. The four roots then cross the ventrolateral border of the scalenus muscle and divide to form the brachial plexus. After the roots cross the axillary space, the plexus divides to form the individual nerves.

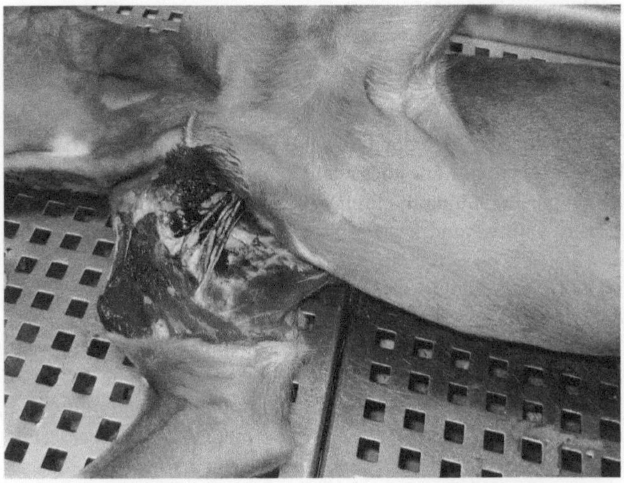

Figure 45.11 Dissection of the right axillary area of a dog in lateral recumbency showing the anatomy of the brachial plexus. Methylene blue dye has been used to stain the musculacutaneous and radial nerves. Note the intimate relationship of the radial, median and ulnar nerves immediately dorsal to the axillary artery and vein.

The axillary artery and vein are also located in the axillary space, and are found immediately caudal to the median and ulnar nerves and cranial to the first rib. The phrenic nerve runs along the ventral border of the scalenus muscle.

Nerve stimulation-guided brachial plexus block (traditional approach)

Technique

A standard regional anesthesia tray is prepared with the following specific equipment:

- Peripheral nerve stimulator.
- Insulated needle (22-gauge, 50 mm for cats and small and medium-sized dogs, 21-gauge, 100 mm for large dogs).

With the patient positioned in lateral recumbency and the leg to be blocked placed uppermost and held in a natural position perpendicular to the longitudinal axis of the body, palpate the major landmarks (scapulohumeral joint, acromion, greater tubercle, jugular vein). The puncture site is located cranial to the acromion and medial to the subscapularis muscle. Draw an imaginary line between the acromion and the cranial border of the greater tubercle. A second line is drawn perpendicular to the first, from the cranial border of the acromion. This line provides the direction of needle advancement (Fig. 45.12) [28].

Insert the needle and carefully advance it medial to the scapula in a caudal direction. Once the tip of the needle is near the musculocutaneous nerve, contractions of the biceps brachii muscle will result in flexion of the elbow. Extension of the elbow (radial nerve response) is also an acceptable endpoint. However, to stimulate the radial nerve, the tip of the needle will likely have already passed the more cranially located musculocutaneous nerve, so injection at this location will most likely miss the musculocutaneous nerve. Pronation of the extremity (median/ulnar nerve response) should not be considered an acceptable endpoint. This response suggests that the tip of the needle has passed the radial and musculocutaneous nerves, and is stimulating the median and ulnar nerves. Injection at this location will not block the entire brachial plexus and block failure will result. In addition, care must be taken if twitches involving the carpus are observed since the axillary vessels lie just ventral to the radial nerve and further caudal needle

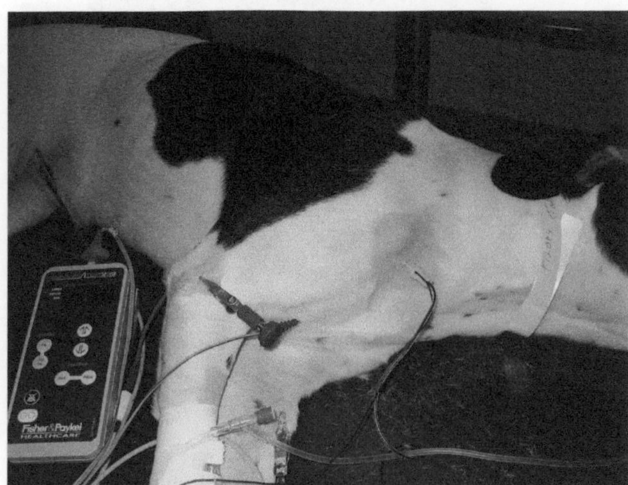

Figure 45.12 Needle position for performance of a brachial plexus block in a dog using nerve stimulation. The puncture site is located cranial to the acromion and medial to the subscapularis muscle.

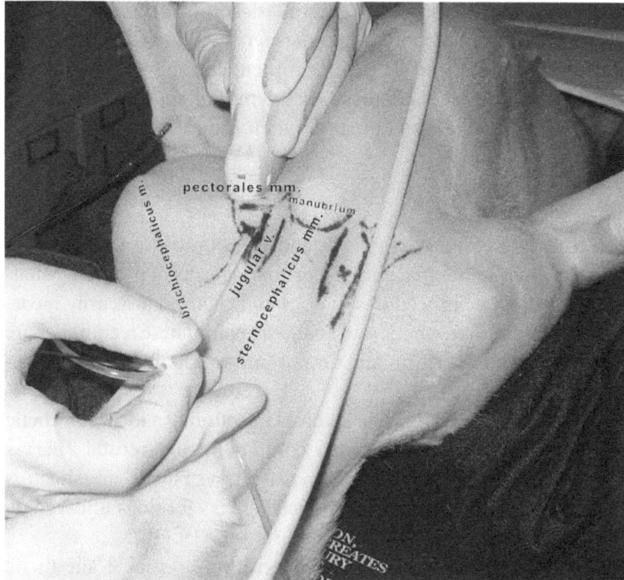

Figure 45.13 Dog in dorsal recumbency. The transducer is placed into the axillary region, in the space between the manubrium of the sternum and the supraglenoid tubercle of the scapula. The transducer is oriented in a parasagittal plane. The following landmarks were drawn on the skin: jugular vein, cranial border of pectorales muscles, medial border of brachiocephalicus muscle, and cranial border of sternum. The puncture site is shown as 'X'. Note that the stimulating needle is being advanced in a cranial to caudal direction in-plane with respect to the ultrasound transducer. Source: [20]. Reproduced with permission from Wiley.

advancement runs the risk of vascular puncture. The recommended volume of local anesthetic solution to be injected for a nerve-stimulator guided brachial plexus block is 0.25–0.3 mL/kg [2].

Combined ultrasonography–electrolocation-guided brachial plexus block

Technique[20].

A standard regional anesthesia tray is prepared with the following equipment:

- Ultrasound machine with a high-frequency (9–15 MHz) transducer.
- Peripheral nerve stimulator.
- Insulated needle (22-gauge, 50 mm for small dogs, 21-gauge, 100 mm for medium-sized and large dogs).

The patient should be positioned in dorsal recumbency with the thoracic limbs flexed in a natural position (Fig. 45.13). Place the transducer over the axillary region in the fossa that exists between the manubrium of the sternum and the supraglenoid tubercle of the scapula. The probe should be oriented in a parasagittal plane until an image of the axillary vessels ('double-bubble' sign) and the roots of the brachial plexus can be visualized in their short axis (Fig. 45.14). Once the root of C8 has been identified (found immediately dorsal to the axillary artery), insert the stimulating needle 'in-plane,' dorsal to the cranial edge of the pectoralis muscle and lateral to the jugular vein. Advance the needle in a cranial-to-caudal direction, keeping the needle tip in the field of ultrasound view at all times. Watch for the characteristic contractions of the triceps brachii muscle, resulting in elbow extension. The total volume of local anesthetic to be injected should be approximately 0.15–0.2 mL/kg. Stimulation of C6 will result in contraction of the supra- and infraspinatus muscles, resulting in shoulder rotation, flexion, or extension.

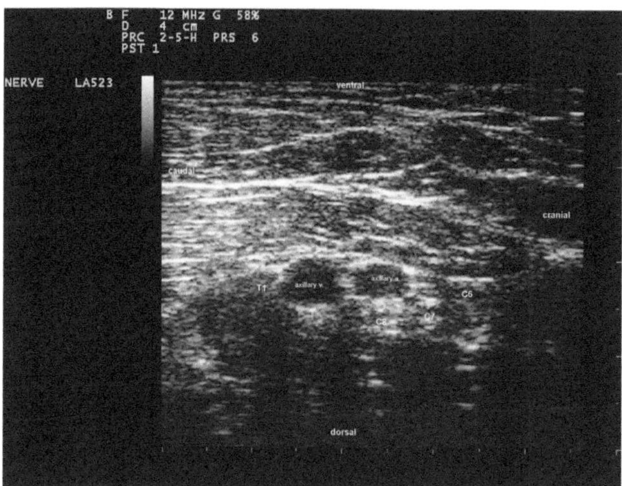

Figure 45.14 Ultrasound image of the axillary region. The roots of the brachial plexus are labeled C6, C7, C8 and T1. Note the location of C8 dorsal to the axillary artery.

Intra-articular analgesia

The intra-articular administration of local anesthetic agents has proven effective for knee arthroscopy in people [114], but pain control for shoulder surgery is more difficult to achieve [115]. Indications for intra-articular drug administration include the following:

- Surgical procedures involving the shoulder or elbow (mainly arthroscopic procedures).
- Osteoarthritis.
- Inflammatory arthritis.

The most obvious concerns about intra-articular injections are the risk of infection and the possibility for chondrotoxicity caused by local anesthetic solutions.

- Strict adherence to sterile technique is of utmost importance.
- The chondrotoxicity of local anesthetics appears to be dose and time dependent.

Prolonged intra-articular administration of high concentrations of local anesthetic solutions may result in adverse clinical effects (chondrolysis) [116]. A single injection of low-concentration mepivacaine or bupivacaine appears safer [117].

Elbow injection

With the patient in lateral recumbency and the limb to be blocked positioned uppermost, a finger is placed on the medial epicondyle and the limb is palpated distally until the approximate level of the joint is reached. The puncture site is slightly caudal to this location. To ensure placement within the joint, a syringe is attached to the needle and used to aspirate synovial fluid (Fig. 45.15a). The joint is filled with injectate until moderate pressure is felt against the plunger. Overfilling may lead to rupture of the joint capsule and loss of injectate into the peri-articular soft tissues. The elbow can also be approached medially in a similar manner, except with the affected leg down.

Shoulder injection

The patient should be positioned in lateral recumbency and the limb to be blocked positioned uppermost. The shoulder is palpated to locate the superior ridge of the greater tubercle. The acromion should also be located and the space craniodistal to its border

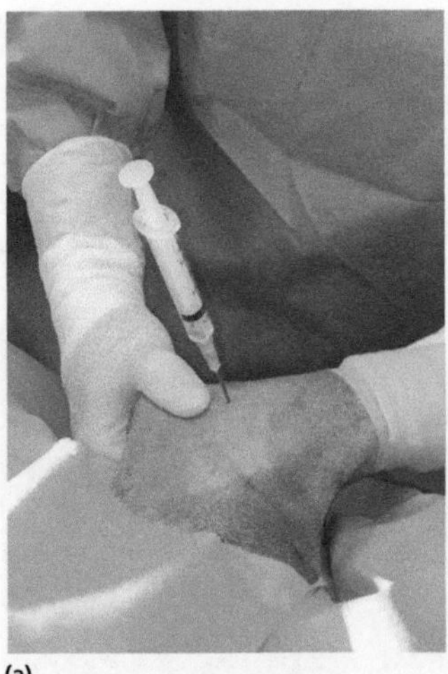
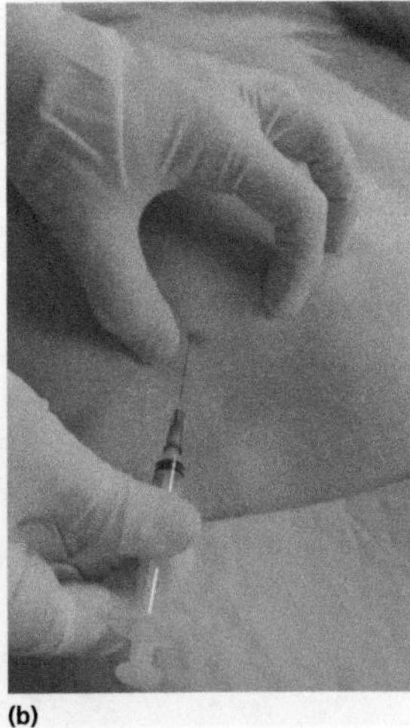

(a) (b)

Figure 45.15 (a) A needle has been placed into the elbow joint on the medial aspect of the left thoracic limb of a dog that is positioned in dorsal recumbency. (b) A needle is being placed into the right scapula–humeral joint of a dog that is positioned in left lateral recumbency.

palpated. The puncture site is located at the craniocaudal midpoint of the ridge (Fig. 45.15b). The needle should be directed caudally and medially at a 70° angle from perpendicular. Local anesthetics, opioids, steroids, and other adjuvants such as clonidine or dexmedetomidine have been administered for intra-articular pain relief.

Radial, median, musculocutaneous, and ulnar (RUMM) nerve block

Anatomy

The radial nerve emerges between the medial and lateral heads of the triceps and brachialis muscle in the caudolateral aspect of the mid-humerus. The musculocutaneous, median, and ulnar nerves run adjacent to the brachial artery on the medial aspect of the limb. There is some separation between the musculocutaneous nerve and median and ulnar nerves. At the level of the mid-humerus, these nerves are surrounded by connective tissue and fat.

Technique[118].

A standard regional anesthesia tray is prepared with the addition of the following specific equipment:

- Peripheral nerve stimulator.
- Insulated needle (22-gauge, 50 mm).

The patient should be positioned in lateral recumbency and the leg to be blocked uppermost (for the radial nerve block) or lowermost for the musculocutaneous, median, and ulnar nerve blocks. The puncture site for the radial nerve block is on the lateral side between the long head of the triceps and the brachialis muscle, caudal to the humerus, at the level between the middle and distal thirds of the humerus. The puncture site for the ulnar, median, and musculocutaneous nerves is on the medial side of the limb. The pulse of the brachial artery can be palpated just proximal to the elbow joint between the biceps brachialis and the medial head of the triceps. The puncture site will be mid-humerus, cranial and caudal to the brachial artery.

Insert the needle and advance it towards the target nerve(s). Once the tip of the needle is within appropriate range, stimulation of the radial nerve will result in extension of the carpus (extensor carpi twitch); stimulation of the median nerve will result in flexion and pronation of the antebrachium (flexor carpi, pronator teres twitch), and stimulation of the ulnar nerve will result in flexion of the forepaw (flexor carpi). The recommended volume to be injected for the radial nerve (lateral site) is 0.1 mL/kg and for the musculocutaneous, median, and ulnar nerves 0.15 mL/kg.

Thoracic blocks

Selective intercostal nerve block and infusion of local anesthetics into the interpleural space are the primary means of providing analgesia for thoracic procedures in dogs and cats and are easily incorporated into the anesthetic and analgesic plan. These techniques are relatively easy to perform and do not impose significant risk when performed correctly.

Intercostal nerve blockade involves injection of a local anesthetic solution adjacent to several contiguous intercostal nerves (Figs 45.16 and 45.17). Using intercostal nerve blocks, investigators have been able to document beneficial effects for dogs undergoing a variety of thoracic surgical procedures [43,119,120].

Interpleural analgesia involves deposition of a local anesthetic solution into the pleural space that exists between the parietal and visceral pleurae (Fig. 45.18). Multiple studies in dogs have shown that interpleurally administered local anesthetics works by gravity-dependent, multidermatomal blockade of intercostal nerves [121–123]. The local anesthetic diffuses across the parietal pleura to block the underlying intercostal nerves that course through the area. The distribution of interpleural nerve blockade corresponds with the lowermost part of pleural space where pooling of the local anesthetic solution occurs [124,125]. Interpleural administration of local anesthetics has proven useful for providing pain relief not only for thoracic surgeries, but also for painful disorders of the cranial abdomen (e.g., pancreatitis) [126].

With any of these techniques, it is important to calculate local anesthetic doses carefully and to dilute the drugs as needed to ensure adequate injectate volumes (e.g., in small patients).

Intercostal nerve blocks

Anatomy

The thoracic and cranial lumbar (L1, L2) spinal nerves are responsible for sensory innervation of the trunk [127]. The ventral branches of the thoracic spinal nerves (T2–T13) contribute to the peripheral nerves that are found within the intercostal spaces between adjacent ribs. Intercostal nerves lie immediately caudal to each rib and run in close proximity to the intercostal arteries and veins that lie beneath the parietal pleura along the caudal aspect of the associated ribs (Fig. 45.16). Together, the nerve, artery, and vein in each intercostal space course in a dorsal to ventral direction away from the vertebrae towards the sternum.

Intercostal nerves serve a dual purpose – some fibers provide motor function to the intercostal muscles, whereas others detach lateral branches to provide sensory innervation to the skin lying over the lateral and ventral aspects of the chest wall and abdominal floor. Although each intercostal space is associated with a specific nerve, there is significant overlap of sensory dermatomes and, for this reason, any regional anesthetic technique must take this sensory distribution into consideration [119,128].

Technique

The patient should be placed in lateral recumbency, with the operative side of the thorax positioned uppermost. The rib immediately cranial to the anticipated incision is palpated as far dorsally as

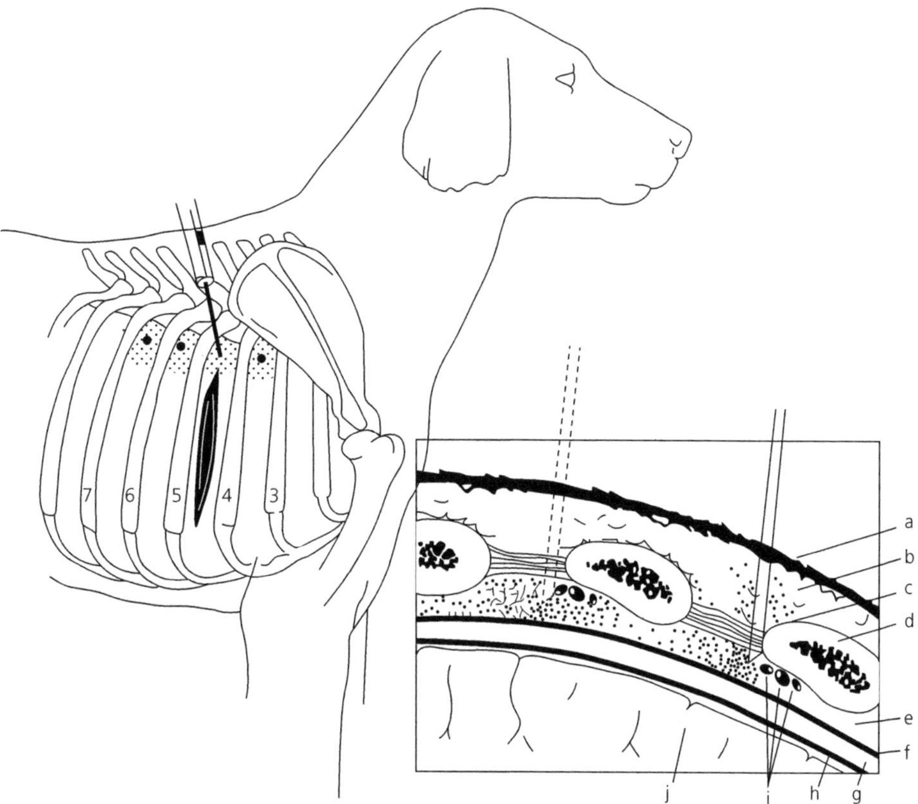

Figure 45.16 Needle placement for inducing intercostal nerve blocks in a dog, showing the lateral aspect and the sagittal section. Inset: (a) skin, (b) subcutaneous tissue, (c) intercostal muscles, (d) rib, (e) subcostal space, (f) parietal pleura and fascia, (g) interpleural space, (h) visceral pleura, (i) intercostal artery, vein, and nerve, and (j) lung.

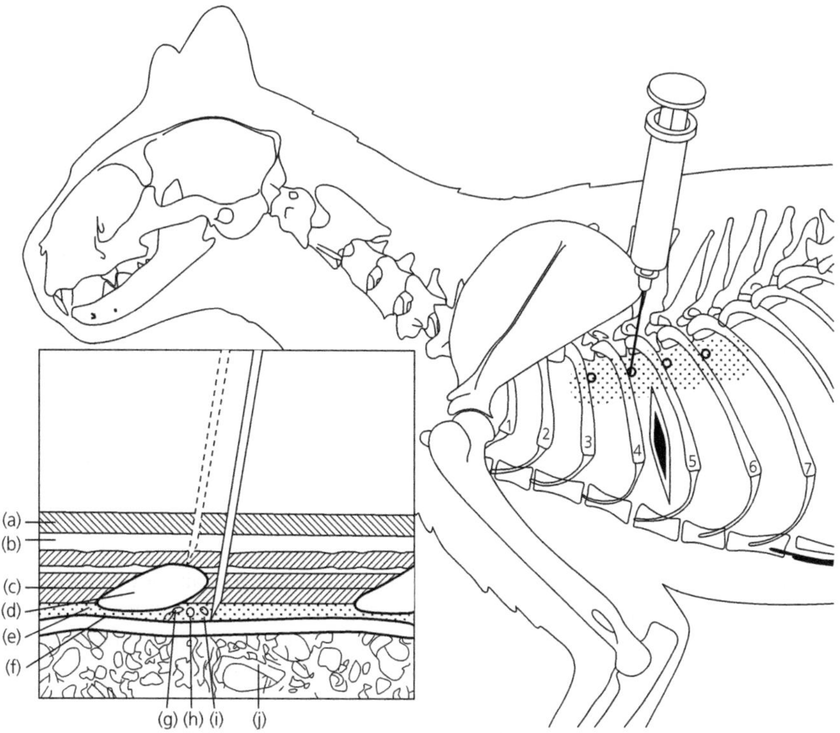

Figure 45.17 Needle placement for inducing intercostal nerve blocks in a cat, showing the lateral aspect and the sagittal section. Inset: (a) skin, (b) subcutaneous tissue, (c) intercostal muscles, (d) rib, (e) subcostal space, (f) parietal pleura and fascia, (g) intercostal vein, (h) intercostal artery, (i) intercostal nerve, and (j) lung.

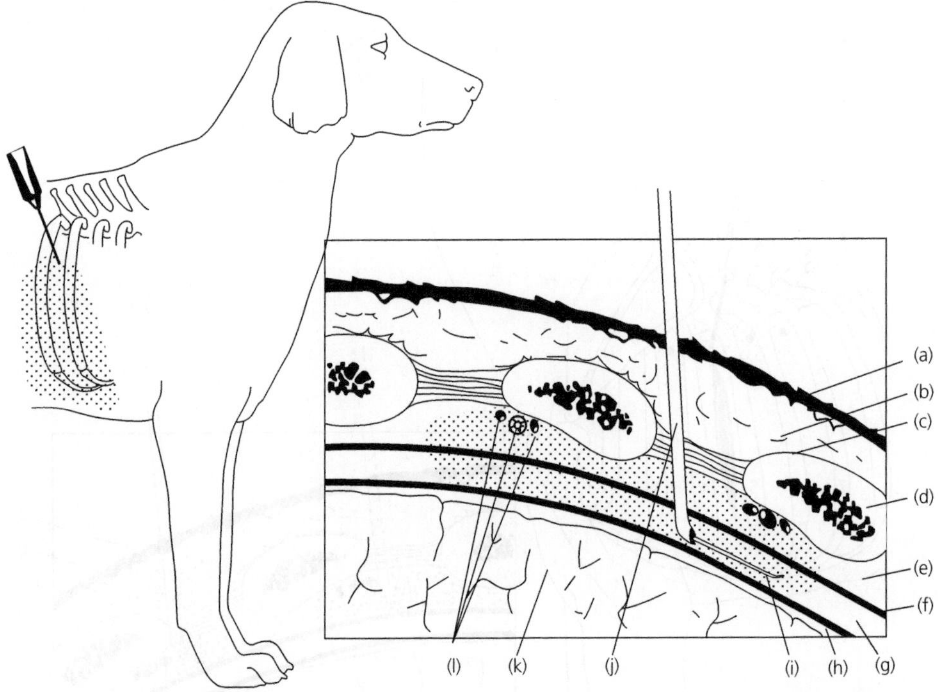

Figure 45.18 Interpleural catheter placement in a dog. Inset: (a) skin, (b) subcutaneous tissue, (c) intercostal muscles, (d) rib, (e) subcostal space, (f) parietal pleura and fascia, (g) interpleural space, (h) visceral pleura, (i) catheter, (j) Tuohy needle, (k) lung, and (l) intercostal artery, vein, and nerve.

possible so that its associated intercostal nerve can be targeted as proximally as possible. At the target site, a needle is advanced through the skin onto the lateral aspect of the rib. The needle tip is then 'walked off' the rib caudally into the intercostal space. Caution should be used to not advance the tip of the needle beyond the thickness of the intercostal muscle so that it penetrates the parietal pleura and enters the pleural space.

Once in the desired location, a syringe is used to aspirate for blood and air. Negative aspiration suggests that the needle tip is not placed intravascularly in an intercostal artery or vein (e.g., blood would be aspirated) or in the pleural space (e.g., air would be aspirated). After calculating the maximum dose to be used for the patient, an appropriate volume of local anesthetic (0.5–1.0 mL) is then slowly injected through the needle at the site on the caudal aspect of the rib to perform an individual intercostal nerve block. The technique is then repeated at two sites cranial and two sites caudal to the initial rib in order to block successfully adjacent dermatomes that will potentially be involved in the surgical field. Using a nerve stimulator, a low-level current (e.g., 0.5 mA) can be used to search for the nerve. When the needle is 'walked off' the caudal aspect of the rib, muscle twitches will be observed within the intercostal space with nerve stimulation. Nerve stimulation is particularly helpful for identifying the correct location in overweight animals when landmarks are not easily palpated and a blind approach might increase risk to the patient (e.g., inadvertent penetration of the pleural space, pneumothorax, or intravascular injection).

Inadvertent vascular puncture is not uncommon whereas puncture into the thoracic cavity is less common. If the pleural space is entered, an insignificant pneumothorax can potentially result but is usually detected upon aspiration of air into the needle.

Interpleural regional analgesia

Technique

The patient should be positioned in lateral recumbency. An over-the-needle catheter is connected to a syringe filled with 2–3 mL of saline via a three-way stopcock, and is advanced onto the lateral aspect of the seventh or eighth rib at its midpoint (as measured from the dorsal to ventral aspect of the thoracic cavity). The needle is then 'walked off' the cranial border of the rib until it can be advanced through the intercostal space. Entering the thorax at the cranial border of the rib helps minimize the risk of traumatizing the intercostal nerve and vascular bundle. Once the parietal pleura has been penetrated (often with a palpable 'pop' or 'click'), the column of saline in the syringe will slowly decrease in volume as the negative interpleural pressure aspirates the saline into the interpleural space. Once the needle tip has been confirmed to be in the interpleural space, the catheter is gently advanced off the needle stylet into the interpleural space. The preloaded syringe with local anesthetic solution is then switched with the saline and the calculated volume of local anesthetic is slowly injected over 1–2 min through the catheter and into the interpleural space. Following injection of the local anesthetic, the catheter is withdrawn and the patient is positioned with the operative side down for at least 10 min, allowing the local anesthetic to pool and block the underlying intercostal nerves. Alternatively, an indwelling catheter or chest tube can be placed into the interpleural space to facilitate repeated injections.

The large surface area of the pleura can potentially result in rapid absorption of the administered local anesthetic solution and high plasma levels of the local anesthetic can result, potentially leading to local anesthetic systemic toxicity [129]. No adverse cardiovascular effects were reported by Bernard *et al.* when local anesthetic was administered interpleurally to patients with or without an open pericardium [130]. A small volume of air can be aspirated into the pleural space due to the negative intrathoracic pressure. This can result in an insignificant pneumothorax and is not considered to be of clinical significance. Lung trauma is rarely an issue.

Catheter dislodgement can occur whenever an indwelling catheter is placed at any site in the body. After correctly positioning the catheter in the interpleural space, it should be secured to the patient by means of adhesive patches, tissue glue, suture, and/ or bandages. Subcutaneous tunneling of larger gauge interpleural catheters can be used as a further means to reduce the likelihood of dislodgment and to prevent air inadvertently entering the interpleural space around the catheter. A C-clamp or other similar device may be used to reduce the possibility of air being aspirated through the chest tube or catheter following inadvertent dislodgment or other issues.

Investigators observed a loss of diaphragmatic function on the injection side after administration of 1.5 mg/kg of interpleural bupivacaine [131]. Dogs that received bilateral blockade demonstrated paradoxical respirations and generated negative intra-abdominal pressures upon inspiration. Patients at increased risk of cardiovascular and respiratory complications may be better treated with alternative methods of pain relief (e.g., intercostal nerve blocks, thoracic epidural anesthesia).

Thoracic paravertebral block

Thoracic paravertebral blocks were first described in human patients in 1905 as a method to provide abdominal analgesia. They involve injection of local anesthetic within the thoracic paravertebral space to produce unilateral sensory, motor, and sympathetic block that is suitable for procedures of the lateral chest and abdomen [132,133]. Although there is a growing body of evidence to support the use of thoracic paravertebral blocks in people, few studies have been published to date that investigated or reported this technique in animals, although investigations are under way in dogs and cats [134].

Transversus abdominis plane (TAP) block

The TAP block was originally described in 2001 for use in people as an alternative method of providing complete sensory analgesia to the lateral and anterior abdominal wall [135].

The transversus abdominis plane (TAP) block involves deposition of a local anesthetic solution into a neuro-fascial plane, effectively blocking the nerves that supply the anterior abdominal wall that exists within the potential space between the transversus abdominis and internal abdominal oblique muscles. In people, TAP blocks have been used to provide sensory blockade of the lower thoracic and upper lumbar abdominal afferent nerves for a variety of abdominal procedures, including bowel resection via midline abdominal incision, cesarean delivery, abdominal hysterectomy via transverse abdominal incision, open appendectomy, and laparoscopic cholocystectomy with all four ports below the umbilicus. The block must be performed bilaterally if it is to be effective for providing analgesia across the patient's midline.

Anatomy

The abdominal wall consists of three muscle layers: the external abdominal oblique, the internal abdominal oblique, and the transversus abdominis, in addition to their associated fascial sheaths. The segmental ventral branches of the caudal thoracic and cranial lumbar nerves innervate the skin, muscles, and parietal peritoneum of the ventral abdominal wall. These branches leave their respective intervertebral foramina and pierce the musculature of the lateral abdominal wall to run ventrally through the fascial plane that exists between the internal abdominal oblique and transversus abdominis muscles. Cadaveric studies in people have shown extensive branching and communication of nerves within the fascial plane [136].

Technique

A standard regional anesthesia tray is prepared with the following equipment:

- Ultrasound machine with high-frequency (9–15 MHz) linear-array transducer.
- Tuohy or spinal needles.

Owing to the variability in body-wall thickness of dogs and cats, performing the TAP block blindly in small animals is unlikely to be successful and is therefore not recommended. An ultrasound-guided technique allows for direct visualization of the different layers of the body wall, increasing the chances of block success while decreasing chances of peritoneal puncture. Alternatively, the surgeon can place the block through the abdominal incision while visualizing the transverse abdominis muscle layer prior to body wall closure.

Using ultrasound, the patient is placed in lateral recumbency with the side to be blocked uppermost. The area of interest is found midway between the caudal aspect of the last rib and iliac crest, at the horizontal level corresponding to the patient's axilla. The lateral body wall between the caudal aspect of the last rib and the iliac crest is imaged and a clear image of the three muscle layers of the abdominal wall should be obtained prior to needle insertion. Using an 'in-plane' needling approach, the needle is advanced through the external and internal abdominal oblique muscles and into the fascial plane overlying the transversus abdominis muscle. A small (0.5–1.0 mL) test dose of local anesthetic solution is injected into the potential space between the transversus abdominis and the internal abdominal oblique muscles. The use of ultrasound allows for direct visualization of local anesthetic spread within the desired facial plane (Fig. 45.19). Once the needle is confirmed to be in the correct location within the fascial plane, the remainder of the diluted local anesthetic solution is injected up to a total volume of 1 mL/kg (ensuring that the patient does not receive more than 2 mg/kg of bupivacaine in total). Following performance of the TAP block on one side, the patient is turned over and the procedure is repeated using an additional 1 mL/kg of the diluted local anesthetic solution.

Schroeder *et al* [137] first reported the use of TAP blocks in animals, and reported perceived analgesia of 8–10 h duration in a Canadian lynx undergoing exploratory laparotomy. Two cadaveric studies of the block using medium-sized dogs suggested the potential

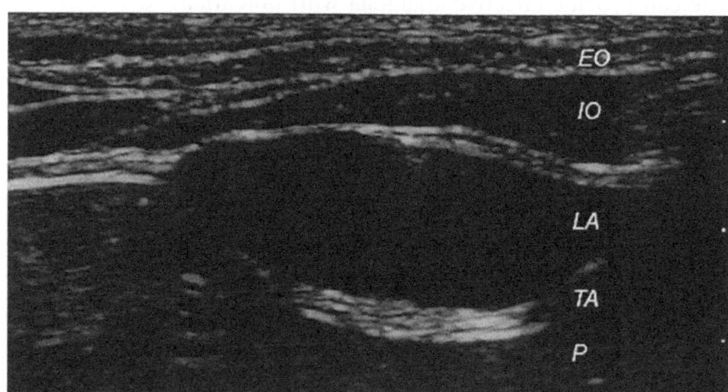

Figure 45.19 Ultrasonographic image postinjection of local anesthetic solution (5 mL of 0.125% bupivacaine) into the fascial plane overlying the transversus abdominis. Small dots on the right of the image indicate 1 cm depth markers. EO, external abdominal oblique; IO, internal abdominal oblique; LA, local anesthetic; TA, transversus abdominis; P, peritoneal cavity. Source: [139]. Reproduced with permission of Wiley.

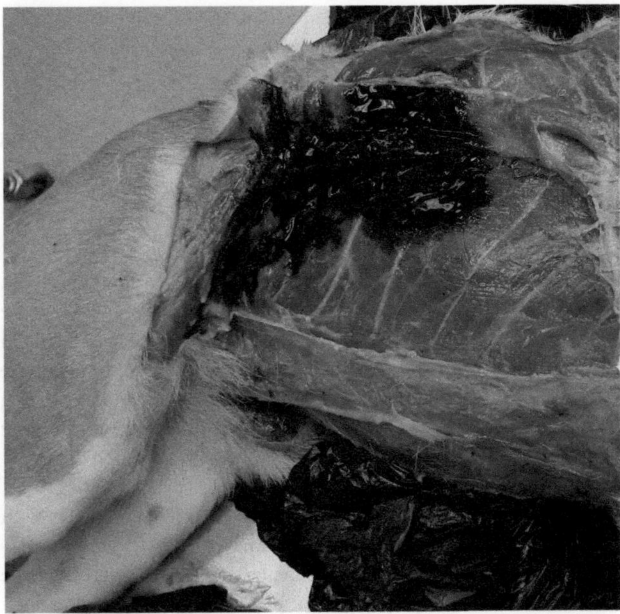

Figure 45.20 Dissection of the lateral abdominal wall showing T12–L3 spread of methylene blue solution following ultrasound-guided TAP block in a cadaver. Source: [139]. Reproduced with permission of Wiley.

utility of this block. Following ultrasound-guided injection, the spread of injectate in the canine cadavers was largely comparable to that in human cadavers (Fig. 45.20) [138–140]. Adequate coverage of the ventral nerve roots of T12–L2 was demonstrated following injection, so one would expect this block to provide adequate coverage for many canine abdominal wall procedures.

Placement of indwelling catheters into the TAP neuro-fascial space in people has recently been reported, and has been used to provide prolonged analgesia to patients over 3–4 days [141–143]. To date, there have been no reports of the use of TAP catheters in animals.

The pelvic limb

Until recently, local anesthetic techniques for the pelvic limb have been limited mainly to epidural approaches or intra-articular injections in small companion animals. However, peripheral nerve blockade can provide effective analgesia with potentially less morbidity than neuraxial anesthesia [21]. Interest in utilizing these blocks in dogs and cats is increasing [2,20–34].

Peripheral nerve blocks

The pelvic limb is supplied by two nerve plexuses (lumbar and sacral) that need to be partly or entirely blocked to provide surgical anesthesia and analgesia to the entire pelvic limb (including the hemipelvis). Blocking the femoral/saphenous nerve will provide anesthesia of the femur (mid-diaphysis to distal), femorotibial joint (medial aspect of the femorotibial joint capsule), femorotibial intra-articular structures, skin of the dorsomedial tarsus and first digit. The sciatic nerve block (if used alone) is sufficient to perform surgery of the foot and hock. Both nerves (femoral and sciatic) must be blocked for almost any stifle procedure.

A combination of bupivacaine 0.5% and dexmedetomidine (0.5–2 μg/mL of injectate solution) is commonly used by the authors to provide surgical anesthesia. For example, adding 50 μg of dexmedetomidine to a 50 mL vial of 0.5% bupivacaine will create a solution that contains bupivacaine 0.5% and dexmedetomidine at a concentration of 1 μg/mL.

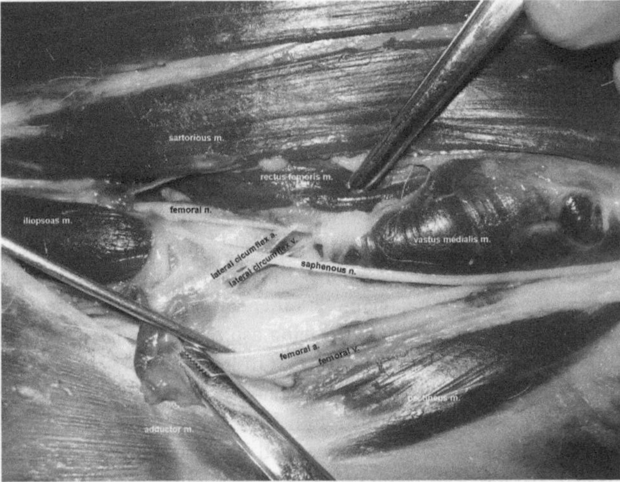

Figure 45.21 Dissection of the femoral triangle of the left pelvic limb of a dog cadaver. The caudal belly of the sartorius muscle has been displaced cranially to allow for visualization of the femoral nerve. Note the anatomic relationship of the femoral vessels to the femoral nerve.

There are many different approaches to blocking the nerves of the pelvic limb. A femoral triangle (inguinal) approach to the femoral nerve and a lateral approach (ischiatic tuberosity–greater trochanter line approach) for the sciatic nerve (described here) are considered to be of an intermediate level of difficulty, and are associated with low complication rates. Other approaches may be more challenging and success and complication rates may be largely linked to the clinician's experience.

Femoral/saphenous nerve block (femoral triangle/inguinal approach)

Anatomy

At the caudal aspect of the iliopsoas muscle, the femoral nerve exits the muscle and courses across the femoral triangle (Fig. 45.21). The femoral triangle is demarcated by the iliopsoas muscle proximally, the pectineus muscle caudally, and the sartorius muscle cranially. Within the triangle, the femoral nerve is located cranial to the femoral artery and vein, running deep to the caudal belly of the sartorius muscle. At this level, the femoral nerve gives rise to the saphenous nerve and the lateral circumflex vessels originate from the femoral artery and vein. These vessels cross the femoral triangle in a cranio-caudal direction, disappearing between the vastus medialis and rectus femoris muscles. The femoral nerve then continues distally, entering the quadriceps muscle between the vastus medialis and rectus femoris.

Technique

Nerve stimulation-guided femoral nerve block is performed using a standard regional anesthesia tray prepared with the following specific equipment:

- Peripheral nerve stimulator.
- Insulated needle (22-gauge, 50 mm).

With the patient positioned in lateral recumbency and the limb to be blocked positioned uppermost, abducted 90° and extended caudally, the pectineus and the iliopsoas muscles are located. The pulse of the femoral artery is palpated. In this position, the femoral

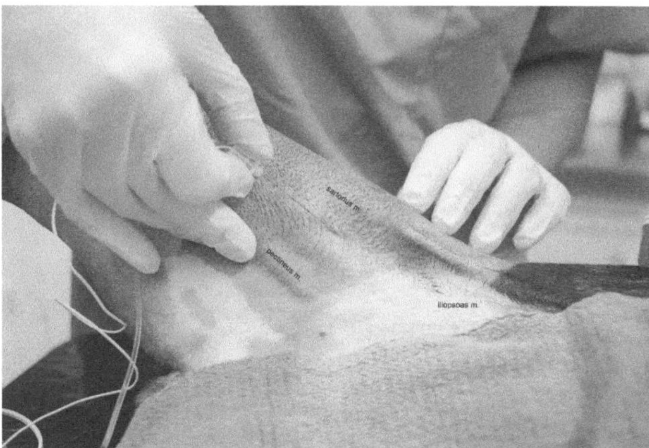

Figure 45.22 Performance of a right-sided femoral nerve block in a dog using a femoral triangle approach. The stimulating needle is inserted cranial to the femoral artery and advanced towards the iliopsoas muscle, maintaining a 20–30° angle to the skin.

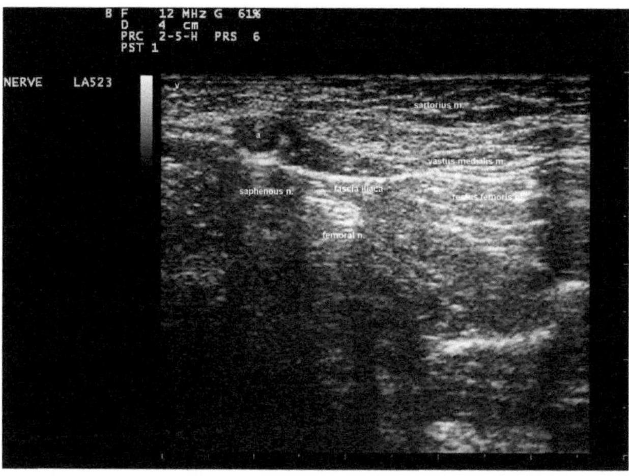

Figure 45.23 Ultrasonographic cross-section (short-axis) view of the femoral triangle of a dog.

nerve runs parallel to the femoral artery in a more cranial location. The puncture site is located within the femoral triangle, cranial to the femoral artery (Fig. 45.22).

A stimulating needle is inserted cranial to the femoral artery and advanced towards the iliopsoas muscle, maintaining a 20–30° angle with respect to the skin. As the needle is advanced, the fascia iliaca is penetrated (a 'pop' should be felt). Once the tip of the needle is near the femoral nerve, contractions of the quadriceps muscle will result in stifle extension. Bupivacaine 0.5% combined with dexmedetomidine (0.5 μg/mL) provides approximately 14 (6–24) h [(median (minimum–maximum)]of effect until rescue analgesia may be needed following stifle surgery [21]. The recommended volume to be injected is 0.1 mL/kg.

Combined ultrasonography–electrolocation-guided femoral nerve block

The combined block is performed using a standard regional anesthesia tray prepared with the following specific equipment:

- Ultrasound machine with a high-frequency (9–15 MHz) transducer.
- Peripheral nerve stimulator.
- Insulated needle (22-gauge, 50 mm for small dogs, 20-gauge, 100 mm for medium/large dogs).

The patient is positioned in lateral recumbency with the limb to be blocked positioned uppermost, abducted 90° and extended caudally. With the transducer placed over the femoral triangle, in a cranio-caudal direction, a short-axis view of the femoral vessels and the nerve should be obtained (since it is usually compressed by the pressure that is being exerted by the ultrasound transducer, the femoral vein is rarely seen adjacent to the artery) (Fig. 45.23). The femoral and saphenous nerves are located cranial and deep to the femoral artery; they are visible as nodular hyperechoic structures directly beneath the thin caudal belly of the sartorius muscle and the fascia iliaca (hyperechoic line, superficial to the femoral nerve). The rectus femoris muscle can be seen cranial to the femoral nerve. The puncture site is located in the proximal and cranial aspect of the thigh (cranial belly of the sartorius muscle) in-plane with the transducer (Fig. 45.24). The recommended volume to be injected is 0.1 mL/kg [20,23,33,144]. However, the final injection volume can be assessed by monitoring the ultrasound image.

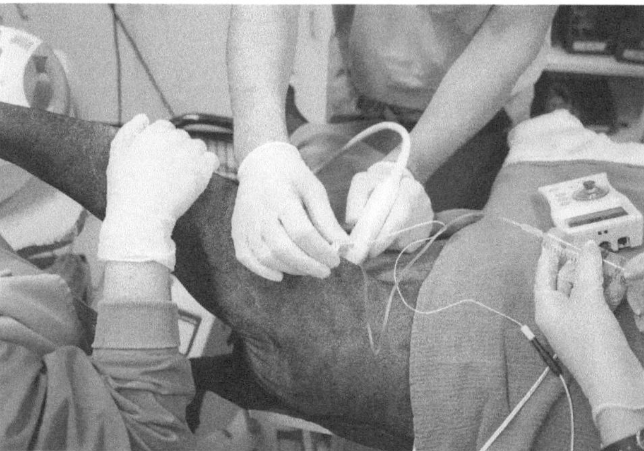

Figure 45.24 Performance of a left-sided femoral nerve block in a dog. The ultrasound transducer is positioned to visualize the femoral triangle in short-axis in the inguinal area, and the stimulating needle is advanced in-plane in a cranial-to-caudal direction through the sartorius and rectus femoris muscles towards the femoral nerve.

Sciatic nerve block

Anatomy

The sciatic nerve courses down the pelvic limb between the greater trochanter and the ischiatic tuberosity (Fig. 45.25). In this region, the sciatic nerve gives rise to the muscular branches that supply the hamstring muscles (semitendinosus and semimembranosus muscles). The caudal gluteal vessels lie just caudal to these muscular branches. Immediately distal to the greater trochanter and ischiatic tuberosity, the sciatic nerve lies between the biceps femoris muscle laterally and the semimembranosus muscle caudal and medially. The sciatic nerve then divides into its two branches, the tibial nerve medially and the common peroneal nerve laterally. The location of this division is variable and can occur anywhere from the level of the hip joint to just proximal to the stifle joint.

Nerve stimulation-guided sciatic nerve block

This block is performed using a standard regional anesthesia tray prepared with the following specific equipment [20,32,145]:

- Peripheral nerve stimulator.
- Insulated needle (22-gauge, 50 mm).

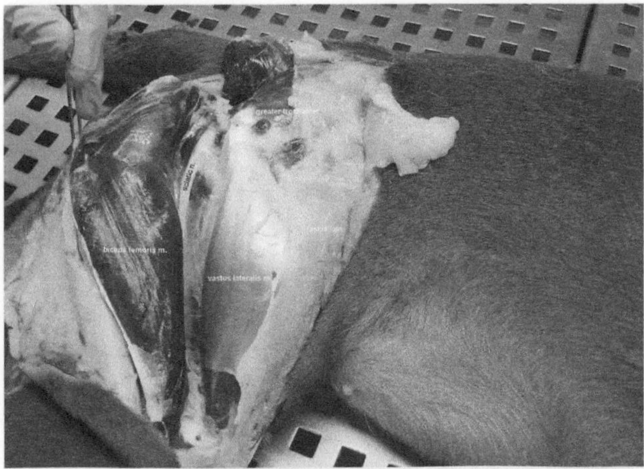

Figure 45.25 Dissection of lateral thigh of a canine cadaver showing the right sciatic nerve. The biceps femoris muscle has been reflected caudally and the gluteal muscle has been transected to allow for easier visualization of the sciatic nerve and its surrounding structures. Methylene blue dye has been used to stain the proximal aspect of the sciatic nerve.

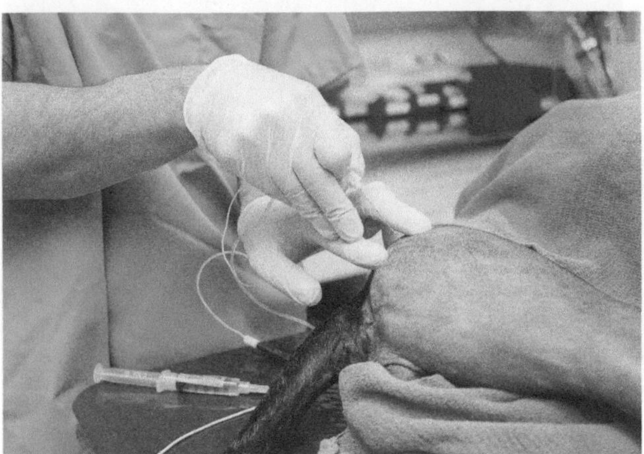

Figure 45.26 Performance of a right-sided sciatic nerve block in a dog using the lateral approach. The index and middle fingers of the non-dominant hand are used to palpate the greater trochanter and ischiatic tuberosity. The puncture site is located one-third of the distance from the greater trochanter to the ischiatic tuberosity.

The patient is positioned in lateral recumbency. The limb to be blocked is positioned uppermost and extended in a natural position (Fig. 45.26). Identify the greater trochanter and ischiatic tuberosity. The puncture site is located at the point between the cranial and the middle thirds of a line that is drawn between these two bony landmarks. The stimulating needle is inserted through the skin and is advanced in a 45° angle to the skin. Once the tip of the needle is near the sciatic nerve, dorsiflexion or plantar extension of the foot will be elicited. The recommended volume to be injected is 0.05–0.1 mL/kg [2].

Contractions of the semimembranosus or semitendinosus muscles should not be considered an acceptable endpoint. If stimulation of the hamstring muscles is observed without foot movement, the needle is likely to be stimulating the muscular branches of the sciatic nerve, and not the sciatic nerve itself. Injections in this location will miss the main sciatic nerve and may result in regional anesthetic block failure.

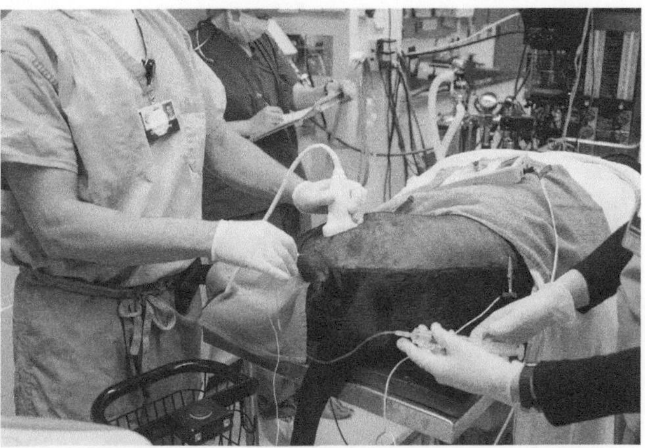

Figure 45.27 Performance of a left-sided sciatic nerve block in a dog. The ultrasound transducer is placed over the area immediately distal to the greater trochanter and ischiatic tuberosity. The stimulating needle follows a caudo-cranial direction towards the sciatic nerve through the semimembranosus muscle, medial to the fascia of the biceps femoris muscle.

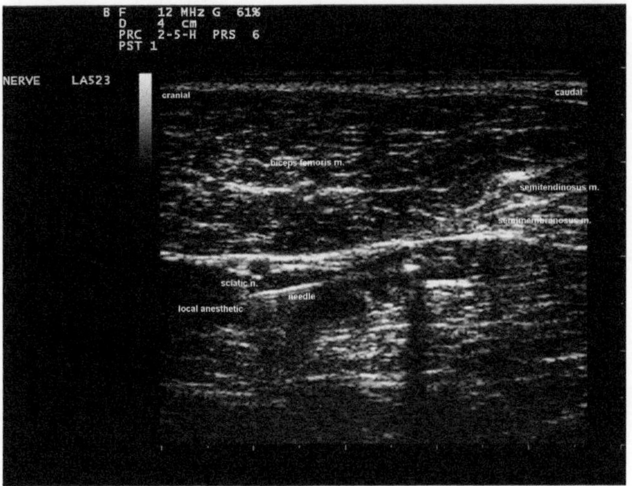

Figure 45.28 Ultrasonographic cross-section (short-axis) view of the sciatic nerve deep to the biceps femoris muscle.

Combined ultrasonography–electrolocation-guided sciatic nerve block

The combined block is performed using a standard regional anesthesia tray prepared with the following specific equipment [20,23,25,33,144]:

- Ultrasound machine with a high-frequency (9–15 MHz) transducer.
- Peripheral nerve stimulator.
- Insulated needle (22-gauge, 50 mm for small dogs, 20-gauge, 100 mm for medium/large dogs).

The patient is positioned in lateral recumbency with the limb to be blocked positioned uppermost and extended in a natural position (Fig. 45.27). With the transducer oriented in a craniocaudal position over the lateral aspect of the thigh and immediately distal to the ischiatic tuberosity, a short-axis view of the sciatic nerve is obtained (Fig. 45.28). The needle puncture site is located in the caudal aspect of the thigh immediately distal to the ischiatic tuberosity, in-plane with the ultrasound transducer. The stimulating needle is advanced in a caudo-cranial direction, guiding it through the semimembranosus muscle and medial to the fascia of the biceps femoris muscle towards the sciatic nerve, keeping the needle tip in the field of view at all times. Plantar extension or dorsiflexion of the foot will be elicited when the needle approaches the sciatic nerve. The recommended volume to be injected is 0.05–0.1 mL/kg [20,23,33]. The final injection volume should be assessed by monitoring the ultrasound image.

Intra-articular blocks

A commonly used strategy for pain management following joint surgery is the intra-articular administration of analgesics such as local anesthetics or opioids [146]. The intra-articular injection of local anesthetics desensitizes intra-articular structures only and may reduce the dose and interval for administrating supplemental analgesic therapy [146].

Stifle technique

The patient is positioned in dorsal or lateral recumbency. The stifle joint is held in a flexed position. The needle is inserted lateral to the patellar ligament, mid-way between the cranial pole of the patella and the tibial tuberosity and the hub of the needle is observed for the presence of synovial fluid (confirming correct needle position). However, absence of synovial fluid does not necessarily rule out correct needle location. Depending on the size of the patient, 1–6 mL of local anesthetic solution may be injected into the joint. Lack of resistance during injection confirms correct intra-articular position of the needle tip and excludes injection into periarticular soft tissue or a fat pad.

Coxofemoral joint technique

The patient should be positioned in lateral recumbency with the coxofemoral joint to be injected located uppermost. The limb is slightly flexed, with the stifle in a neutral position [147]. The puncture site is located cranial and proximal to the greater trochanter. Once the needle has entered the joint, the hub of the needle should be observed for evidence of synovial fluid (this would confirm correct needle positioning). However, absence of synovial fluid does not rule out correct needle positioning. Depending on the size of the patient, 1–6 mL of local anesthetic solution can be injected into the joint. Lack of resistance during injection confirms correct intra-articular position of the needle tip and excludes injection into periarticular soft tissue or a fat pad.

Epidural anesthesia

The administration of agents with analgesic properties via the epidural or spinal routes provides effective anesthesia and analgesia for procedures involving the pelvis and pelvic limbs, and also the tail, perineum and abdomen. Recently, the use of epidural anesthesia for blockade of thoracic segments in dogs has been reported [148]. Epidural analgesia can also be extended by using an indwelling catheter.

The lumbosacral approach (L7–S1) to performing epidural anesthesia in dogs and cats is technically easy to perform owing to the relatively wide intervertebral space at this location [41], although more cranial approaches in dogs have also been described [149,150]. A sacrococcygeal approach to the epidural space has been described in cats to minimize the risk of dural puncture and help facilitate urethral catheterization in blocked cats [151,152].

Anatomy

The vertebral canal contains the epidural space and the intrathecal structures. The roof of the canal is formed by the vertebral laminae and the interarcuate ligament or yellow ligament (ligamentum flavum). This ligament widens at the level of the intervertebral openings. The epidural space in the dog is largest at the lumbosacral level where the dural sac tapers (Fig. 45.29). At this level (L7–S1), the supraspinous and interspinous ligaments are relegated to the fibrous and connective tissue in between where the two epaxial muscles meet.

Caudally, the spinal cord tapers into a conical structure called the conus medullaris. In large dogs, the conus medullaris generally extends as far as the junction between the sixth and seventh lumbar vertebrae. In smaller dogs, the conus medullaris is located at the lumbosacral space. In dogs, the dural sac typically ends at the level

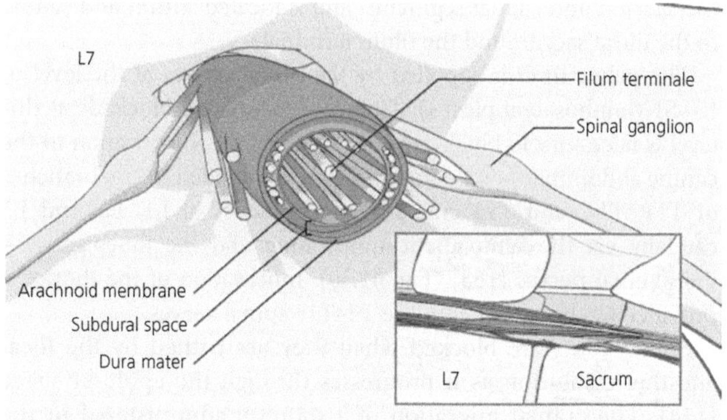

(a)

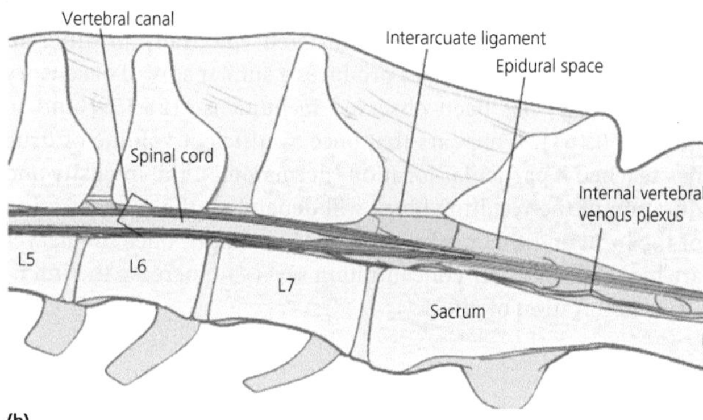

(b)

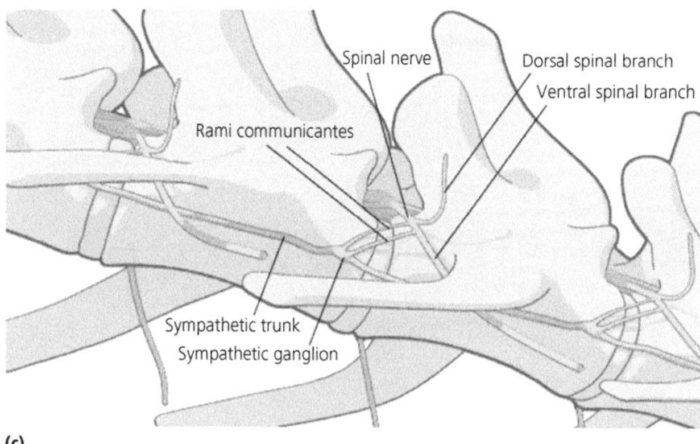

(c)

Figure 45.29 (a, b) Illustrations showing the spinal anatomy at the lumbosacral level. (c) Sympathetic trunk.

of L6–L7 whereas in cats the dural sac extends caudally as far as the first sacral segment.

The dorsal and ventral rootlets emerge bilaterally from each segment of the spinal cord. These rootlets bind together to form the dorsal and ventral roots. Each root progresses separately towards the intervertebral foramen, at which point the two (dorsal and ventral roots) merge to form the corresponding spinal nerve. The dura mater (dura mater spinalis) forms a cylindrical tube with lateral extensions accompanying the roots and spinal nerves as they exit the vertebral canal through the intervertebral foramina. Each spinal nerve divides into dorsal and ventral branches and, in the region of T1–L4, two rami communicantes that join the sympathetic trunk.

The epidural space is located between the dura mater and the boundaries of the vertebral canal. It contains adipose and connective tissue and the internal vertebral venous plexus. The cauda equina comprises a bundle of nerve fibers formed by the roots of the sacrum and caudal segments, and is located within and caudal to the dural sac, around the filum terminale.

The pelvic limb is supplied by the spinal nerves at the level of L3–S1 (lumbosacral plexus). Therefore, segmental blockade at this level is necessary to block the entire pelvic limb. Innervation to the canine abdominal wall and peritoneum is provided by the branches of T11, T12, and T13 cranially and branches of L1, L2, and L3 caudally via the sympathetic innervation and the ilioepigastric–ilioinguinal nerves [153] (Fig. 45.30). Innervation of the thorax is provided by the branches of the T2–T13 spinal nerves.

Spinal roots are blocked when they are bathed by the local anesthetic solution as it progresses through the epidural space [154]. The cranial migration of a solution administered in the epidural space is related to the injected volume of local anesthetic solution [155–157]. However, several studies have reported that the same total drug mass administered epidurally in different concentrations and volumes produces a similar spread of sensory blockade; this has been observed in humans [158,159] and in dogs [160,161]. It appears that once a sufficient volume of drug has reached a particular location (dermatome), the intensity and duration of the resulting block will depend on the concentration of the local anesthetic administered. Put simply, once the nerves are blocked, a greater concentration serves to increase the intensity and duration of effect.

The sympathetic chain arises from the T1–L4 segments of the spinal cord (outward and inward rami communicantes) (Fig. 45.29c). Preganglionic sympathetic blockade will result in vasodilation in the blocked dermatomes and, in some cases, may contribute to arterial hypotension. The degree of sympathetic nerve blockade caused by epidural anesthesia will be related to the extent of local anesthetic spread.

Technique

To perform an epidural injection, the animal may be placed in either sternal or lateral recumbency, depending on the patient's medical condition and the clinician's preference (Fig. 45.31). With respect to body position, Gorgi *et al.* found significantly greater migration of injectate on the right side in dogs that were maintained in right lateral recumbency for up to 40 min after injection, compared with dogs that were turned from left to right lateral recumbency after epidural injections [156]. Further studies are needed to evaluate the shortest amount of time required to achieve a significant laterality of the block, since a 40 min waiting period is unlikely to be acceptable in clinical situations.

The standard lumbosacral puncture site is located between the dorsal spinous processes of L7 and S1 (medial sacral crest) (Fig. 45.31). The needle is advanced through the skin and into the subcutaneous tissue (Fig. 45.32). Usually there should not be any resistance to needle advancement through these tissues. The needle is then advanced through the supraspinous and interspinous ligaments (Fig. 45.33). Resistance will be noted as the needle penetrates these ligaments. If during any of these manipulations the needle comes into contact with bony structures, it should be withdrawn slightly, and redirected cranial or caudal as appropriate in a gentle and controlled manner. Several methods have been developed for identifying the epidural space, including the use of a 'hanging drop,' 'loss of resistance,' and, more recently, electrostimulation.

Hanging drop

In dogs, pressure within the epidural space has been reported to be anywhere from –6 to +15 mmHg [162]. If a drop of saline or local anesthetic solution is placed in the hub of a Tuohy needle, as the needle penetrates into the epidural space it will usually be aspirated into the space. One study reported 100% false negatives

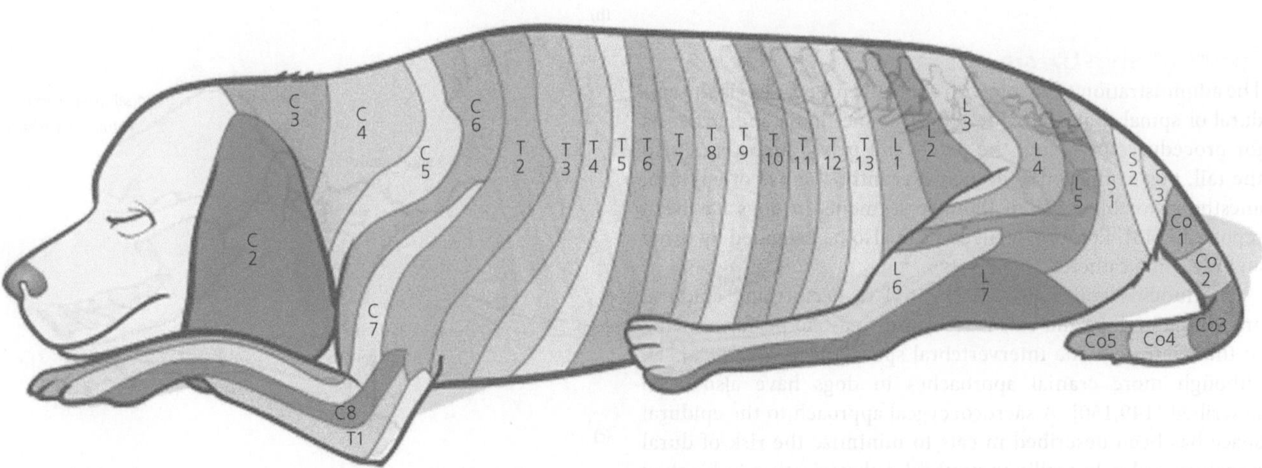

Figure 45.30 Dermatome map of sensory innervation to the skin in the dog.

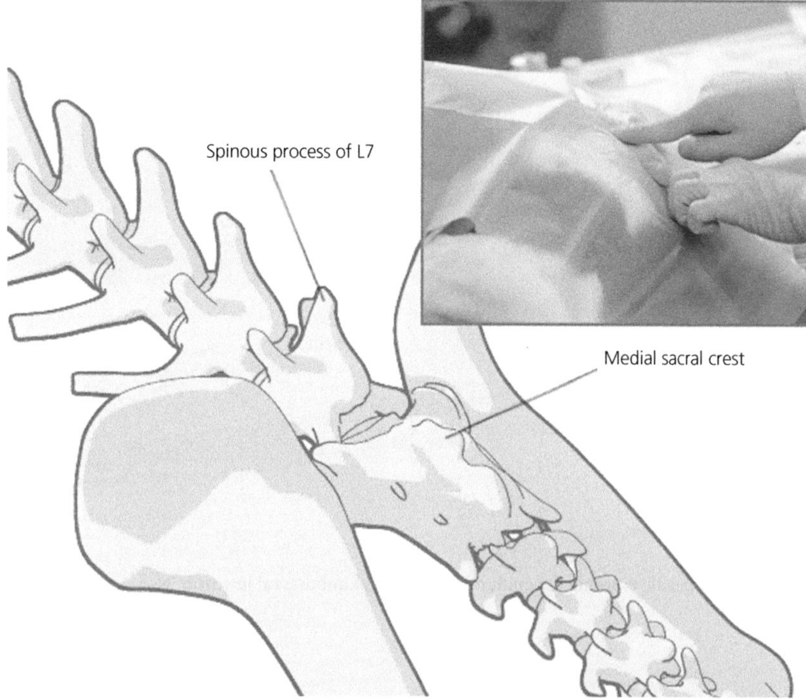

Figure 45.31 The typical puncture site for performing epidural anesthesia in the dog is located between the spinous process of L7 and the medial sacral crest of S1.

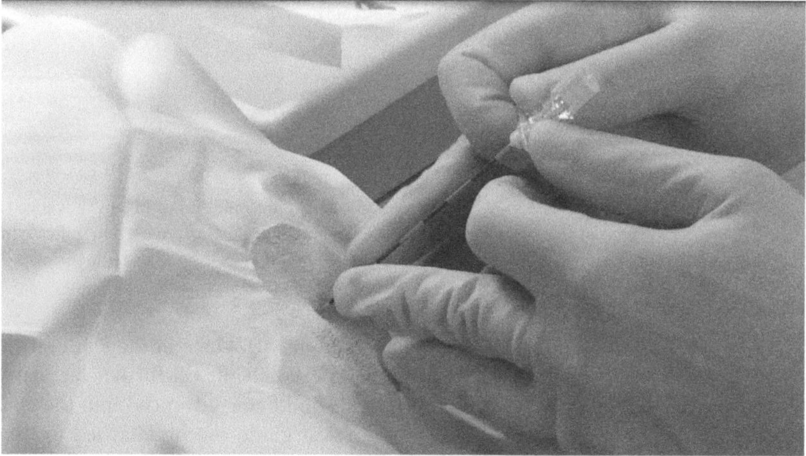

Figure 45.32 A Tuohy needle is advanced towards the epidural space at the lumbosacral space of a dog. Note that the index and thumbs of each hand are used to hold the wings while the middle fingers are used to stabilize the needle shaft.

(i.e., the needle tip is located within the epidural space but saline remains in the hub) with the hanging drop technique when the spinal needle was placed during lateral recumbency, compared with a positive aspiration in seven out of eight dogs positioned in sternal recumbency [163]. It seems that gravity and the possible subatmospheric pressure within the epidural space and mainly the recoil of the ligamentum flavum when pierced by a blunt needle such as a Tuohy needle may play a role in the efficacy of this technique.

Resistance to injection of air or fluid is felt while the needle is advanced through the intervertebral ligaments. If pressure is being applied to the plunger of a 'loss of resistance' (LOR) syringe, a sudden loss of resistance to injection will be appreciated when the needle punctures the ligamentum flavum and enters the epidural space (Fig. 45.34). A false-positive result may ensue if the needle is located within the intervertebral fat. It is also possible to obtain a false-negative result (correct placement but no LOR) if foreign material (blood clots, fat, periostium, skin) fills the needle bore and causes obstruction. If air is used for the LOR technique, a very small volume should be injected since the use of air (0.3 mL/kg) may be associated with significantly less spread of the injected solution, uneven cranial distribution of the solution, and occasional compression of the spinal cord [164].

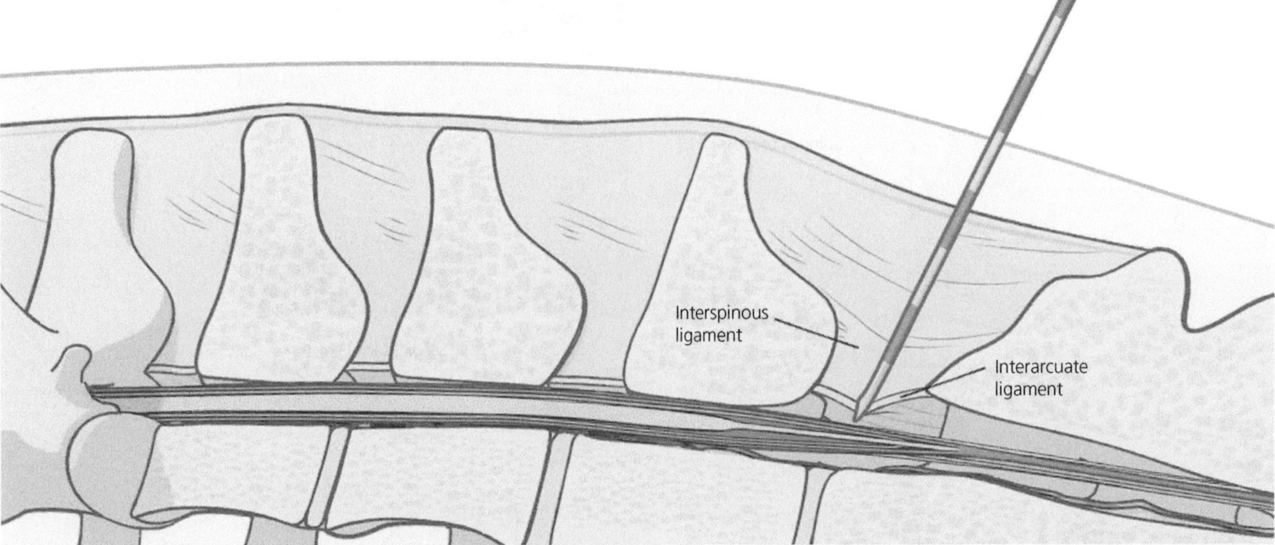

Figure 45.33 Illustration showing a Tuohy needle entering the epidural space at the lumbosacral junction. Note the recoil of the ligamentum flavum.

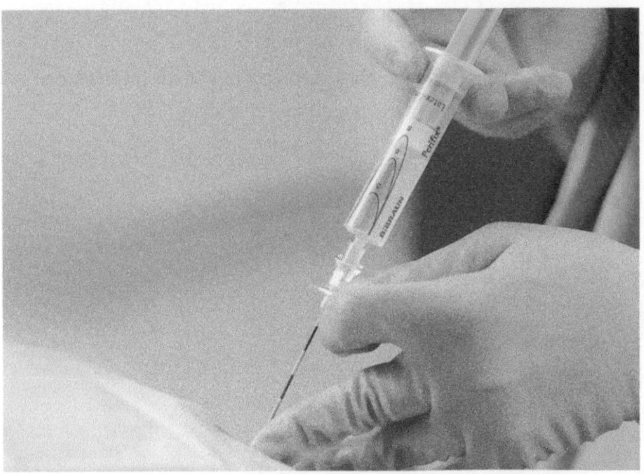

Figure 45.34 During performance of epidural anesthesia, a 'loss of resistance' (LOR) syringe can be used to identify when the epidural space is entered.

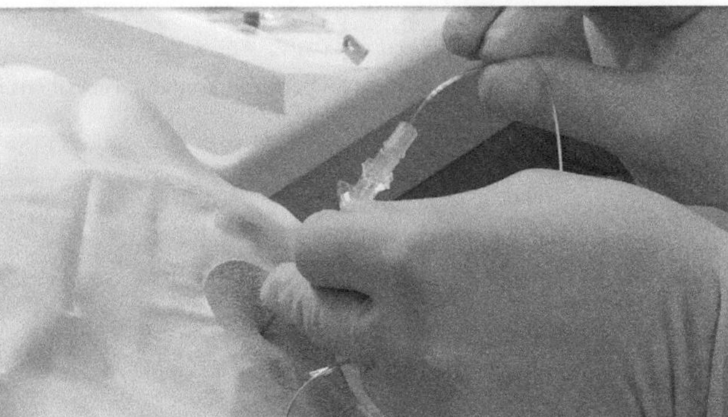

Figure 45.35 An epidural catheter is advanced into the hub of a Tuohy needle. Four solid marks are used to indicate the point at which the catheter should be exiting the needle tip.

Electrolocation

Several studies have demonstrated that each layer of the spinal cord requires a different threshold current to elicit a motor response [62,165]. Nerve stimulation is useful for identifying the epidural space in dogs, and when the needle tip is located in the epidural space, twitches in the pelvic limbs and tail will be observed [166,167].

After entering the epidural space, the needle hub should be inspected for the presence of CSF or blood. If either fluid is observed, the needle should be removed and the procedure should be repeated. If desired, an extension set can be attached to the needle to make drug administration easier. At this point, the calculated drug volume can be administered partially (if a catheter will subsequently be placed) or totally.

Catheter placement

The bevel of the Tuohy needle should be directed cranially to assist with placement of the catheter (see the earlier discussion on equipment). Once in the epidural space, if the needle hub is tipped caudally, it will further facilitate the catheter exiting the needle and being advanced into the epidural space. The threading assist guide can be attached to the needle hub to aid with catheter insertion. The epidural catheter should be threaded with the dominant hand through the needle, paying attention to the depth markings on the catheter (four solid marks indicate the point at which the catheter should be exiting the needle tip) (Fig. 45.35). Moderate pressure may be required to pass the catheter beyond the tip of the needle. Advance the catheter past the desired level (1 cm at a time) to account for needle withdrawal. In most cases, the catheter should not be advanced into the epidural space more than 5 cm owing to the risk of the catheter curling back on itself. The catheter should never be removed with the needle left in place owing to the risk of shearing the catheter with the bevel of the needle. If the catheter is accidentally sheared off or broken, it is usually left in place and surgical retrieval is not usually recommended.

To withdraw the needle, the catheter is held at its point of entry between the thumb and index fingers while the needle is removed. Subcutaneous tunneling of the catheter several centimeters away from its point of entry provides a good fixation and at the same time minimizes potential catheter site contamination. After having checked for the absence of spontaneous flow of CSF or blood from the catheter when the end of the catheter is held in a dependent position, a catheter connector can be attached, and also a bacterial filter. Following negative aspiration, the remainder of the initial bolus of solution can be administered.

Injection Volume

The typical doses that are recommended for epidural anesthesia in dogs and cats are presented in Tables 45.1 and 45.2.

Table 45.1 Volumes of local anesthetics used for epidural anesthesia in dogs.

Drug	Puncture Site	Dermatome	Volume (mL/kg)	Ref.
Bupivacaine 0.25%	Lumbosacral	L3	0.2	[146]
Bupivacaine 0.5%	Lumbosacral	Adequate for ovariohysterectomy[a]	0.36	[157]
Bupivacaine 0.25%	Lumbosacral	T9	0.4	[146]

[a]The ovaries are supplied by the sympatetic chain via the hypogastric nerves (T10–L1).

Table 45.2 Volumesof local anesthetics (based on dye-staining studies) used for epidural anesthesia in cats.

Drug	Puncture Site	Dermatome	Volume (mL/kg)	Ref.
Methylene blue solution	Lumbosacral	L1–L2	0.2	[144]
Methylene blue solution	Lumbosacral	Up to T7	0.3	[144]
Methylene blue solution	Lumbosacral	T6–T10	0.4	[144]

Drugs for continuous epidural anesthesia and analgesia

Analgesics most frequently used by the authors for continuous epidural anesthesia are bupivacaine (0.125–0.25%) with or without the addition of morphine (0.1 mg/kg per 12–24 h) or fentanyl (1–2 μg/mL of solution, 10–20 μg of fentanyl per 10 mL of bupivacaine mixed in the same syringe). The recommended infusion rate through the catheter is 0.02–0.05 mL/kg/h.

If analgesia is inadequate, a bolus of a more concentrated solution can be given (e.g., bupivacaine 0.5%) and the rate of the infusion can be increased while maintaining the original concentrations. If the extension of blockade is found to be excessive, the rate should be subsequently reduced. If signs of muscle weakness appear, the concentration is reduced while maintaining the same infusion rate. If signs of deep sedation appear, the opioid dose can be reduced.

Contraindications

There are several contraindications to the use of epidural anesthesia in small animal patients. Alternatives to epidural anesthesia should be considered in patients with bleeding disorders (thrombocytopenia, coagulation disorders). Since placing a needle in the vertebral canal can result in inadvertent puncture of an epidural venous sinus, hemorrhage may result in the formation of an epidural hematoma compressing the spinal cord. Epidural anesthesia using a local anesthetic should be avoided in patients with uncorrected hypovolemia and hypotension since they will be at further risk following sympathetic nerve blockade. Opioids may continue to be used in these patients. Finally, epidural anesthesia should be avoided in patients with skin infections or evidence of neoplasia at the site of injection. Alternative routes (e.g., sacrococcygeal route) or regional anesthetic techniques should be considered. Potential complications associated with neuraxial administration (single dose or continuous) and how to avoid them are summarized in Table 45.3.

Table 45.3 Potential complications associated with continuous epidural administration.

Complication	Possible explanation	Possible avoidance
Related to the technique		
Accidental drug administration		Correct syringe labeling and implementation of 'time-outs/check lists' are recommended to prevent this type of operator error from occurring
Neural damage/neurotoxicity		Appropriate technique and equipment should be used to minimize tissue trauma The use of preservative-free, 'for epidural use'-approved solutions is recommended
Infections		Strict adherence to best practice and standard of care in terms of skin preparation and technique is recommended
Inadvertent subarachnoid/spinal or subdural injection	Subarachnoid (intrathecal, spinal) needle location	Check for absence of CSF and deliver a test dose before delivering the full dose to rule out intrathecal or subdural needle insertion
Inadvertent intravascular injection	Intravascular needle location such as the ventral venous plexus	Check for absence of blood and deliver a test dose before delivering the full dose to rule out intravascular needle insertion
Related to local anesthetic solutions		
Hypotension/bradycardia	Sympathetic blockade	Intravenous fluids, vasopressors, and anticholinergic drugs should be used as needed
Horner's syndrome	Blockade of sympathetic trunk at cervical dermatomes	Can be observed if local anesthetic reaches cervical dermatomes
Respiratory depression	Extensive migration of the injectate, intercostal nerve blockade, and exceptionally, phrenic nerve paralysis, and circulatory insufficiency at the respiratory center	Avoid excessive cranial migration of local anesthetic Opioids can cause delayed respiratory depression
Total spinal anesthesia	Local anesthetic-induced depression of the cervical spinal cord and the brainstem Excessive spread of an intrathecal injection of local anesthetic Inadvertent spinal injection	Avoid excessive cranial migration of local anesthetic
Toxicity		See Section 2, Pharmacology, Chapter 11
Related to opioids		
Urinary retention	Detrusor muscle relaxation (interruption of sacral parasympathetic outflow?)	Patients should be monitored over the first 24–48 h following epidural morphine, and treated symptomatically as needed

Intravenous regional anesthesia (IVRA)

Intravenous regional anesthesia was first described for use in people by a German surgeon, August Bier. IVRA is relatively straightforward to perform: a tourniquet is applied to a limb proximal to the planned surgical site and a local anesthetic is injected intravenously distal to the tourniquet. Since blood vessels and nerves are typically found in close proximity in the extremities, following intravenous injection the local anesthetic spreads from the vessels into the nearby tissues to reach the nerve trunks [168]. IVRA can be used to provide analgesia and anesthesia for short surgical procedures involving the distal extremities (distal to the elbow and the hock) as an alternative to a ring block placed at a proximal level on the leg. Prolonged application of a tourniquet must be avoided owing to the potential for tissue ischemia underneath and distal to the tourniquet and possible ischemic pain associated with the compression of these tissues. For these reasons, IVRA is only recommended for use in procedures lasting less than 90 min [169]. In some instances, intravenous regional anesthesia can be used as the sole anesthetic technique for the procedure when combined with procedural sedation, however, in most cases, IVRA is used to provide the analgesic component of a balanced (multimodal) general anesthetic protocol.

The main advantage of IVRA is that since the technique involves exsanguination of the limb proximal to the surgical site, blood loss during the procedure is minimized. The major limitations of using IVRA are the longer time to perform versus a ring block, limited duration of the procedure due to tourniquet placement, and the lack of prolonged postoperative analgesia following tourniquet release. Studies conducted in people and dogs have demonstrated that IVRA and brachial plexus blocks provide comparable levels of intraoperative analgesia for the distal thoracic limb [170,171].

Lidocaine is the only local anesthetic that is recommended for use with IVRA in the veterinary literature, and has been used at doses of 2.5–5 mg/kg and at concentrations of 0.25–2% [171–174]. In dogs and cats, a 0.5% lidocaine solution up to a total injected volume of 0.6 mL/kg works well for most situations. Even though a tourniquet is used to keep the local anesthetic in the distal limb, there is always a possibility of leakage under the cuff [173]. For this reason, formulations that contain epinephrine or preservatives should be avoided. Bupivacaine has a very narrow therapeutic index and when used for IVRA in people is associated with severe complications, including death [175–177]. For this reason, bupivacaine should never be used for IVRA.

Prior to tourniquet application, the distal limb must be exsanguinated using a flexible bandage (Esmarch, flexible self-adhering bandaging tape). This prevents the injected local anesthetic solution from being diluted by blood, making it more effective for analgesia. The type of tourniquet used will contribute to both the success of the block and the overall safety of the procedure. If the tourniquet does not effectively prevent arterial blood flow from entering the distal limb or does not effectively prevent the injected local anesthetic from entering the systemic circulation, complications may occur [178]. There are two main types of tourniquets: non-pneumatic tourniquets that are made of rubber or elasticized cloth, and pneumatic cuff tourniquets inflated with air.

Esmarch bandages are more commonly used in small animals. The main disadvantage is the inability to measure the pressure created. As a result, patients may experience more pain from tourniquet-related ischemia and have an increased risk of tissue damage. A double tourniquet technique may be used to minimize this. Protecting the area where the tourniquet will be placed with soft padding can help in the prevention of compressive tissue damage. The upper limit for duration of tourniquet application must be strictly adhered to.

Pneumatic tourniquets are available with both single- or double-cuff configurations. All pneumatic tourniquets should have a pressure gauge (manometer) that indicates the pressure in the tourniquet cuff bladder. A less expensive alternative for use in small animal patients is to use a sphygmomanometer and a blood pressure cuff (after the cuff is first tested for leaks). The sphygmomanometer is used to inflate the blood pressure cuff and to monitor and adjust cuff pressure over time. Pressures 50–100 mmHg above the lower occlusion pressure (the pressure at which arterial pulses can no longer be detected distal to the cuff) are suggested to prevent arterial blood from entering the distal limb [7].

Technique

Using a standard technique, catheterize a vein in the distal limb using a small-gauge catheter (e.g., 24- or 22-gauge) (Fig. 45.36a). Depending on the patient's anatomy, the length of the catheter, and the location of skin puncture, the catheter can be directed either proximally or distally, although this may not be critical to success. Secure the catheter to prevent its dislodgement when the bandage exsanguinates the limb. Identify an arterial pulse in the distal limb and mark the area where the pulse is readily palpable with a pen. Following exsanguination of the limb and application of the tourniquet, pulse absence at this location verifies efficacy. It is useful first to determine the lower cuff occlusion pressure preventing arterial flow distal to the tourniquet. This measurement is not only different between patients, but also varies over the course of an anesthetic period due to changes in arterial blood pressure and limb movement. The tourniquet cuff pressure must be maintained above (usually 50–100 mmHg higher) the lower occlusion pressure throughout the procedure.

Prior to tourniquet application, an elastic bandage is applied concentrically around the limb from the distal to proximal end, while being careful not to dislodge the IV catheter (Fig. 45.36b). The tourniquet should then be applied to the limb. If a pneumatic tourniquet is used, the cuff should be inflated to a pressure 50–100 mmHg above the previously measured lower occlusion pressure (Fig. 45.36c). In the case of a non-pneumatic rubber tourniquet, the band should be placed above the elastic wrap that was used for exsanguination and secured tightly to prevent inadvertent release. Document the time of tourniquet application in the anesthetic chart. The remaining procedures (e.g., completion of IVRA, preparation for surgery, surgery) should be completed in less than 90 min to avoid ischemia of tissues under the tourniquet.

Once the tourniquet is in place, the elastic bandage should be carefully removed. Confirm that the previously identified peripheral pulse is now absent. Never proceed with the block if an arterial pulse is detected. If arterial blood is allowed to enter the distal limb while venous blood is being occluded, the limb will become edematous over the course of the procedure. The local anesthetic solution should be slowly injected over 2–3 min, avoiding high injection pressures that might increase venous pressure and cause leakage of the local anesthetic under the tourniquet (Fig. 45.36d). Document the time of local anesthetic injection and continually observe the patient for signs of systemic toxicity thereafter. Following injection, the catheter can be removed. At the end of the procedure, the tourniquet is removed slowly while the surgical site is closely evaluated for hemorrhage during initial re-perfusion (Fig. 45.37).

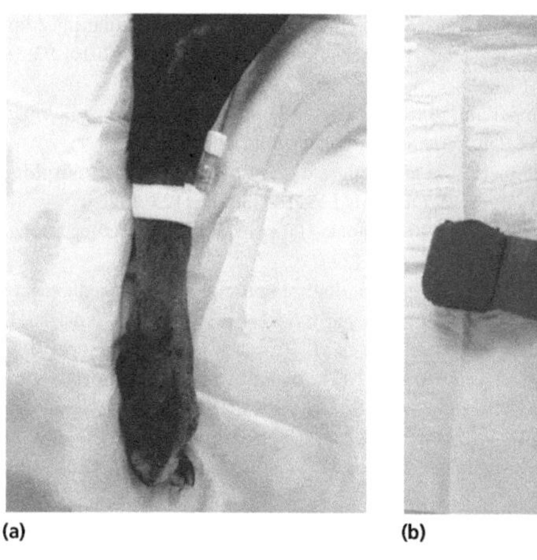
(a)

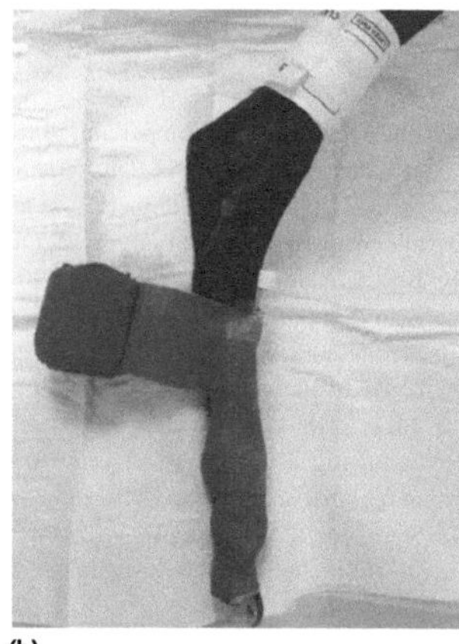
(b)

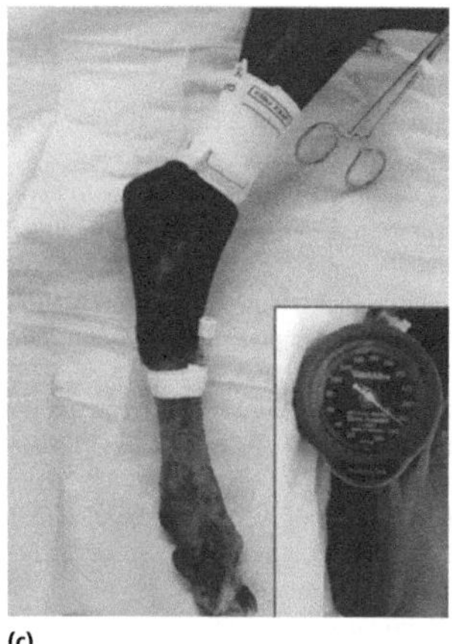
(c)

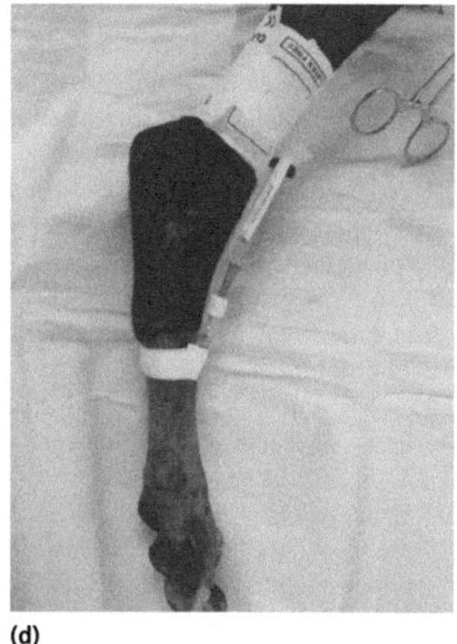
(d)

Figure 45.36 Photographs of the right pelvic limb of a dog scheduled for toe amputation. (a) An intravenous catheter has been placed in a distal vein and has been secured with tape. (b) A blood pressure cuff (serving as a pneumatic tourniquet) has been placed above the tarsus and the distal limb is being desanguinated by wrapping the leg with an elastic bandage (Vetrap®). (c) After the limb has been desanguinated, the blood pressure cuff is inflated using a sphygmomanometer and the elastic bandage is removed. (d) Lidocaine is being injected into the limb distal to the inflated tourniquet. Following injection, the catheter will be removed and the leg prepared for surgery.

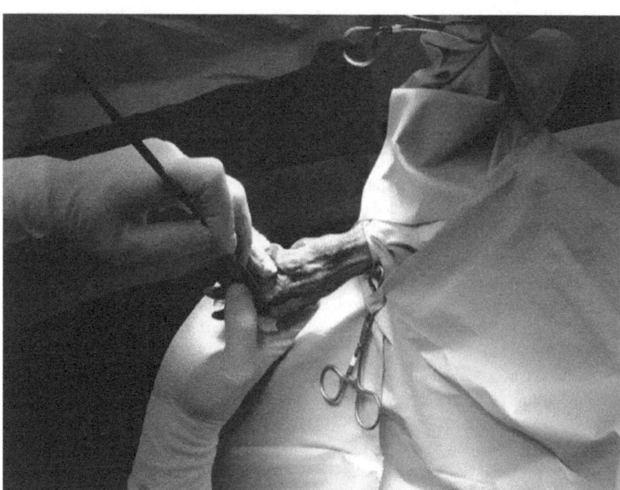

Figure 45.37 The distal pelvic limb of a dog undergoing amputation of a digit. IVRA has already been performed and a tourniquet has been applied proximally on the limb. Note the lack of bleeding as a result of the surgery.

If the block is not sufficient, it is useful to have a fast-acting analgesic (e.g., fentanyl) available, and equipment and drugs for induction of general anesthesia should be available. If lidocaine leakage occurs around the tourniquet, awake patients may have central nervous system side-effects such as tremors or seizures. If these occur, administration of a benzodiazepine or rapid-acting induction drug intravenous is helpful.

Because ischemic pain is one of the major limitations of IVRA, efforts have been made to limit its occurrence (co-administration of adjuncts with the local anesthetic solution, infiltration of the skin under the tourniquet with a local anesthetic, administration of systemic analgesic/hypnotic drugs, use of a double-cuff tourniquet). Use of a double-cuff tourniquet appears to be the most effective. In veterinary medicine, the upper time limit of 90 min should be strictly adhered to and systemic analgesics given if discomfort is evident.

In people, injury has been linked to tourniquet pressures greater than 400 mmHg (~7.5 psi, 52 kPa) [179]. If tourniquet pressure can be measured, the cuff pressure should not exceed 400 mmHg. Sensation will typically return within 15–30 min of tourniquet release.

References

1 Mosing M, Reich H, Moens Y. Clinical evaluation of the anaesthetic sparing effect of brachial plexus block in cats. *Vet Anaesth Analg* 2010; **37**(2): 154–161.

2 Campoy L, Martin-Flores M, Looney AL, *et al.* Distribution of a lidocaine–methylene blue solution staining in brachial plexus, lumbar plexus and sciatic nerve blocks in the dog. *Vet Anaesth Analg* 2008; **35**(4): 348–354.

3 Figueiredo JP, Cruz ML, Mendes GM, *et al.* Assessment of brachial plexus blockade in chickens by an axillary approach. *Vet Anaesth Analg* 2008; **35**(6): 511–518.

4 Zarucco L, Driessen B, Scandella M, *et al.* Sensory nerve conduction and nociception in the equine lower forelimb during perineural bupivacaine infusion along the palmar nerves. *Can J Vet Res* 2010; **74**(4): 305–313.

5 Watts AE, Nixon AJ, Reesink HL, *et al.* Continuous peripheral neural blockade to alleviate signs of experimentally induced severe forelimb pain in horses. *J Am Vet Med Assoc* 2011; **238**(8): 1032–1039.

6 Bardell D, Iff I, Mosing M. A cadaver study comparing two approaches to perform a maxillary nerve block in the horse. *Equine Vet J* 2010; **42**(8): 721–725.

7 Campoy L, Read RM. *Small Animal Regional Anesthesia and Analgesia.* Oxford: Wiley-Blackwell, 2013.

8 Wagner KA, Gibbon KJ, Strom TL, *et al.* Adverse effects of EMLA (lidocaine/prilocaine) cream and efficacy for the placement of jugular catheters in hospitalized cats. *J Feline Med Surg* 2006; **8**(2): 141–144.

9 Bidwell LA, Wilson DV, Caron JP. Lack of systemic absorption of lidocaine from 5% patches placed on horses. *Vet Anaesth Analg* 2007; **34**(6): 443–446.

10 Ko J, Weil A, Maxwell L, *et al.* Plasma concentrations of lidocaine in dogs following lidocaine patch application. *J Am Anim Hosp Assoc* 2007; **43**(5): 280–283.

11 Ko JC, Maxwell LK, Abbo LA, *et al.* Pharmacokinetics of lidocaine following the application of 5% lidocaine patches to cats. *J Vet Pharmacol Ther* 2008; **31**(4): 359–367.

12 Weil AB, Ko J, Inoue T. The use of lidocaine patches. *Compend Contin Educ Vet* 2007; **29**(4): 208–210.

13 Saber AA, Elgamal MH, Rao AJ, *et al.* Early experience with lidocaine patch for postoperative pain control after laparoscopic ventral hernia repair. *Int J Surg* 2009; **7**(1): 36–38.

14 Habib AS, Polascik TJ, Weizer AZ, *et al.* Lidocaine patch for postoperative analgesia after radical retropubic prostatectomy. *Anesth Analg* 2009; **108**(6): 1950–1953.

15 Carpenter RE, Wilson DV, Evans AT. Evaluation of intraperitoneal and incisional lidocaine or bupivacaine for analgesia following ovariohysterectomy in the dog. *Vet Anaesth Analg* 2004; **31**(1): 46–52.

16 Savvas I, Papazoglou LG, Kazakos G, *et al.* Incisional block with bupivacaine for analgesia after celiotomy in dogs. *J Am Anim Hosp Assoc* 2008; **44**(2): 60–66.

17 Fitzpatrick CL, Weir HL, Monnet E. Effects of infiltration of the incision site with bupivacaine on postoperative pain and incisional healing in dogs undergoing ovariohysterectomy. *J Am Vet Med Assoc* 2010; **237**(4): 395–401.

18 Abelson AL, McCobb EC, Shaw S, *et al.* Use of wound soaker catheters for the administration of local anesthetic for post-operative analgesia: 56 cases. *Vet Anaesth Analg* 2009; **36**(6): 597–602.

19 Hadzic A, Vloka JD. *Peripheral Nerve Blocks: Principles and Practice*. New York: McGraw-Hill, 2004.
20 Campoy L, Bezuidenhout AJ, Gleed RD, *et al.* Ultrasound-guided approach for axillary brachial plexus, femoral nerve, and sciatic nerve blocks in dogs. *Vet Anaesth Analg* 2010; **37**(2): 144–153.
21 Campoy L, Martin-Flores M, Ludders JW, *et al.* Comparison of bupivacaine femoral and sciatic nerve block versus bupivacaine and morphine epidural for stifle surgery in dogs. *Vet Anaesth Analg* 2012; **39**(1): 91–98.
22 Campoy L, Martin-Flores M, Ludders JW, *et al.* Procedural sedation combined with locoregional anesthesia for orthopedic surgery of the pelvic limb in 10 dogs: case series. *Vet Anaesth Analg* 2012; **9**(4): 436–440.
23 Costa-Farre C, Blanch XS, Cruz JI, *et al.* Ultrasound guidance for the performance of sciatic and saphenous nerve blocks in dogs. *Vet J* 2011; **187**(2): 221–224.
24 Dumas MP, Ravasio G, Carotenuto AM, *et al.* Post-operative analgesic effects, after orthopaedic surgery in the dog, of loco-regional ropivacaine and bupivacaine blockade using the nerve locator technique: 159 cases. *Vet Res Commun* 2008; **32**(Suppl 1): S283–S286.
25 Echeverry DF, Gil F, Laredo F, *et al.* Ultrasound-guided block of the sciatic and femoral nerves in dogs: a descriptive study. *Vet J* 2010; **186**(2): 210–215.
26 Echeverry DF, Laredo FG, Gil F, *et al.* Ventral ultrasound-guided suprainguinal approach to block the femoral nerve in the dog. *Vet J* 2012; **192**(3): 333–337.
27 Echeverry DF, Laredo FG, Gil F, *et al.* Ultrasound-guided 'two-in-one' femoral and obturator nerve block in the dog: an anatomical study. *Vet Anaesth Analg* 2012; **39**(6): 611–617.
28 Mahler SP, Adogwa AO. Anatomical and experimental studies of brachial plexus, sciatic, and femoral nerve-location using peripheral nerve stimulation in the dog. *Vet Anaesth Analg* 2008; **35**(1): 80–89.
29 Mahler SP. Ultrasound guidance to approach the femoral nerve in the iliopsoas muscle: a preliminary study in the dog. *Vet Anaesth Analg* 2012; **39**(5): 550–554.
30 Portela D, Melanie P, Briganti A, *et al.* Nerve stimulator-guided paravertebral lumbar plexus anaesthesia in dogs. *Vet Res Commun* 2008; **32**(Suppl 1): S307–S310.
31 Portela DA, Otero PE, Tarragona L, *et al.* Combined paravertebral plexus block and parasacral sciatic block in healthy dogs. *Vet Anaesth Analg* 2010; **37**(6): 531–541.
32 Portela DA, Otero PE, Briganti A, *et al.*Femoral nerve block: a novel psoas compartment lateral pre-iliac approach in dogs. *Vet Anaesth Analg* 2012; **40**(2): 194–204.
33 Shilo Y, Pascoe PJ, Cissell D, *et al.* Ultrasound-guided nerve blocks of the pelvic limb in dogs. *Vet Anaesth Analg* 2010; **37**(5): 460–470.
34 Vettorato E, Bradbrook C, Gurney M, *et al.* Peripheral nerve blocks of the pelvic limb in dogs: a retrospective clinical study. *Vet Comp Orthop Traumatol* 2012; **25**(4): 314–320.
35 Klide AM, Soma LR. Epidural analgesia in the dog and cat. *J Am Vet Med Assoc* 1968; **153**(2): 165–173.
36 Evers WH. Epidural anesthesia in the dog: a review of 224 cases with emphasis on cesarean section. *Vet Med Small Anim Clin* 1968; **63**(12): 1121–1124.
37 Acosta AD, Gomar C, Correa-Natalini C, *et al.* Analgesic effects of epidurally administered levogyral ketamine alone or in combination with morphine on intraoperative and postoperative pain in dogs undergoing ovariohysterectomy. *Am J Vet Res* 2005; **66**(1): 54–61.
38 Abelson AL, Armitage-Chan E, Lindsey JC, *et al.* A comparison of epidural morphine with low dose bupivacaine versus epidural morphine alone on motor and respiratory function in dogs following splenectomy. *Vet Anaesth Analg* 2011; **38**(3): 213–223.
39 Sarotti D, Rabozzi R, Corletto F. Efficacy and side effects of intraoperative analgesia with intrathecal bupivacaine and levobupivacaine: a retrospective study in 82 dogs. *Vet Anaesth Analg* 2011; **38**(3): 240–251.
40 Shaver SL, Hofmeister EH. What is the evidence? Combination of local analgesic and opioid epidural protocols. *J Am Vet Med Assoc* 2011; **238**(11): 1410–1411.
41 Valverde A. Epidural analgesia and anesthesia in dogs and cats. *Vet Clin North Am Small Anim Pract* 2008; **38**(6): 1205–1230.
42 Perez TE, Grubb TL, Greene SA, *et al.* Effects of intratesticular injection of bupivacaine and epidural administration of morphine in dogs undergoing castration. *J Am Vet Med Assoc* 2013; **242**(5): 631–642.
43 Pascoe PJ, Dyson DH. Analgesia after lateral thoracotomy in dogs. Epidural morphine vs. intercostal bupivacaine. *Vet Surg* 1993; **22**(2): 141–147.
44 Troncy E, Junot S, Keroack S, *et al.* Results of preemptive epidural administration of morphine with or without bupivacaine in dogs and cats undergoing surgery: 265 cases (1997–1999). *J Am Vet Med Assoc* 2002; **221**(5): 666–672.
45 Bernards CM, Shen DD, Sterling ES, *et al.* Epidural, cerebrospinal fluid, and plasma pharmacokinetics of epidural opioids (part 1): differences among opioids. *Anesthesiology* 2003; **99**(2): 455–465.
46 Bernards CM, Shen DD, Sterling ES, *et al.* Epidural, cerebrospinal fluid, and plasma pharmacokinetics of epidural opioids (part 2): effect of epinephrine. *Anesthesiology* 2003; **99**(2): 466–475.
47 Chu CR, Coyle CH, Chu CT, *et al.* In vivo effects of single intra-articular injection of 0.5% bupivacaine on articular cartilage. *J Bone Joint Surg Am* 2010; **92**(3): 599–608.
48 Piper SL, Kim HT. Comparison of ropivacaine and bupivacaine toxicity in human articular chondrocytes. *J Bone Joint Surg Am* 2008; **90**(5): 986–991.
49 Stein C, Comisel K, Haimerl E, *et al.* Analgesic effect of intraarticular morphine after arthroscopic knee surgery. *N Engl J Med* 1991; **325**(16): 1123–1126.
50 Brill S, Middleton W, Brill G, *et al.* Bier's block; 100 years old and still going strong! *Acta Anaesthesiol Scand* 2004; **48**(1): 117–122.
51 Steinfeldt T, Graf J, Schneider J, *et al.* Histological consequences of needle–nerve contact following nerve stimulation in a pig model. *Anesthesiol Res Pract* 2011; **2011**: 591851.
52 Steinfeldt T, Nimphius W, Werner T, *et al.* Nerve injury by needle nerve perforation in regional anaesthesia: does size matter? *Br J Anaesth* 2010; **104**(2): 245–253.
53 Steinfeldt T, Nimphius W, Wurps M, *et al.* Nerve perforation with pencil point or short bevelled needles: histological outcome. *Acta Anaesthesiol Scand* 2010; **54**(8): 993–999.
54 Ford DJ, Pither C, Raj PP. Comparison of insulated and uninsulated needles for locating peripheral nerves with a peripheral nerve stimulator. *Anesth Analg* 1984; **63**(10): 925–928.
55 Hansen B, Lascelles BD, Thomson A, *et al.* Variability of performance of wound infusion catheters. *Vet Anaesth Analg* 2013; **40**(3): 308–315.
56 Basser PJ, Roth BJ. New currents in electrical stimulation of excitable tissues. *Annu Rev Biomed Eng* 2000; **2**: 377–397.
57 Perlas A, Niazi A, McCartney C, *et al.* The sensitivity of motor response to nerve stimulation and paresthesia for nerve localization as evaluated by ultrasound. *Reg Anesth Pain Med* 2006; **31**(5): 445–450.
58 Chan VW, Brull R, McCartney CJ, *et al.* An ultrasonographic and histological study of intraneural injection and electrical stimulation in pigs. *Anesth Analg* 2007; **104**(5): 1281–1284.
59 Tsai TP, Vuckovic I, Dilberovic F, *et al.* Intensity of the stimulating current may not be a reliable indicator of intraneural needle placement. *Reg Anesth Pain Med* 2008; **33**(3): 207–210.
60 Sauter AR, Dodgson MS, Stubhaug A. Ultrasound controlled nerve stimulation in the elbow region: high currents and short distances needed to obtain motor responses. *Acta Anaesthesiol Scand* 2007; **51**(7): 942–948.
61 Kapur E, Vuckovic I, Dilberovic F, *et al.* Neurologic and histologic outcome after intraneural injections of lidocaine in canine sciatic nerves. *Acta Anaesthesiol Scand* 2007; **51**(1): 101–107.
62 Tsui BC, Wagner A, Cave D, *et al.* Threshold current for an insulated epidural needle in pediatric patients. *Anesth Analg* 2004; **99**(3): 694–696.
63 Moiniche S, Mikkelsen S, Wetterslev J, *et al.* Qualitative systematic review of incisional local anaesthesia for postoperative pain relief after abdominal operations. *Br J Anaesth* 1998; **81**(3): 377–383.
64 Campagnol D, Teixeira-Neto FJ, Monteiro ER, *et al.* Effect of intraperitoneal or incisional bupivacaine on pain and the analgesic requirement after ovariohysterectomy in dogs. *Vet Anaesth Analg* 2012; **39**(4): 426–430.
65 Moldal ER, Eriksen T, Kirpensteijn J, *et al.* Intratesticular and subcutaneous lidocaine alters the intraoperative haemodynamic responses and heart rate variability in male cats undergoing castration. *Vet Anaesth Analg* 2013; **40**(1): 63–73.
66 McMillan MW, Seymour CJ, Brearley JC. Effect of intratesticular lidocaine on isoflurane requirements in dogs undergoing routine castration. *J Small Anim Pract* 2012; **53**(7): 393–397.
67 Lykkegaard K, Lauritzen B, Tessem L, *et al.* Local anaesthetics attenuates spinal nociception and HPA-axis activation during experimental laparotomy in pigs. *Res Vet Sci* 2005; **79**(3): 245–251.
68 Liu SS, Richman JM, Thirlby RC, *et al.* Efficacy of continuous wound catheters delivering local anesthetic for postoperative analgesia: a quantitative and qualitative systematic review of randomized controlled trials. *J Am Coll Surg* 2006; **203**(6): 914–932.
69 Sidiropoulou T, Buonomo O, Fabbi E, *et al.* A prospective comparison of continuous wound infiltration with ropivacaine versus single-injection paravertebral block after modified radical mastectomy. *Anesth Analg* 2008; **106**(3): 997–1001.
70 Tirotta CF, Munro HM, Salvaggio J, *et al.* Continuous incisional infusion of local anesthetic in pediatric patients following open heart surgery. *Paediatr Anaesth* 2009; **19**(6): 571–576.
71 Radlinsky MG, Mason DE, Roush JK, *et al.* Use of a continuous, local infusion of bupivacaine for postoperative analgesia in dogs undergoing total ear canal ablation. *J Am Vet Med Assoc* 2005; **227**(3): 414–419.
72 Wolfe TM, Bateman SW, Cole LK, *et al.* Evaluation of a local anesthetic delivery system for the postoperative analgesic management of canine total ear canal ablation – a randomized, controlled, double-blinded study. *Vet Anaesth Analg* 2006; **33**(5): 328–339.
73 Davis KM, Hardie EM, Lascelles BD, *et al.* Feline fibrosarcoma: perioperative management. *Compend Contin Educ Vet* 2007; **29**(12): 712–714.

74 Davis KM, Hardie EM, Martin FR, *et al*. Correlation between perioperative factors and successful outcome in fibrosarcoma resection in cats. *Vet Rec* 2007; **161**(6): 199–200.

75 Hardie EM, Lascelles BD, Meuten T, *et al*. Evaluation of intermittent infusion of bupivacaine into surgical wounds of dogs postoperatively. *Vet J* 2011; **190**(2): 287–289.

76 Johnson DW, Hatton KW, Flynn JD. Continuous wound catheters: practical considerations for use. *Orthopedics* 2008; **31**(9): 865–867.

77 Kehlet H, Kristensen BB. Local anesthetics in the surgical wound – is the pendulum swinging toward increased use? *Reg Anesth Pain Med* 2009; **34**(5): 389–390.

78 Verstraete FJM, Lommer MJ, eds. *Oral and Maxillofacial Surgery in Dogs and Cats*. Edinburgh: Saunders Elsevier, 2012.

79 Holmstrom SE, Bellows J, Colmery B, *et al*. AAHA dental care guidelines for dogs and cats. *J Am Anim Hosp Assoc* 2005; **41**(5): 277–283.

80 Beckman BW. Pathophysiology and management of surgical and chronic oral pain in dogs and cats. *J Vet Dent* 2006; **23**(1): 50–60.

81 Rochette J. Regional anesthesia and analgesia for oral and dental procedures. *Vet Clin North Am Small Anim Pract* 2005; **35**(4): 1041–1058.

82 Lemke KA, Dawson SD. Local and regional anesthesia. *Vet Clin North Am Small Anim Pract* 2000; **30**(4): 839–857.

83 Pascoe PJ. Anesthesia and pain management. In: Verstraete FJM, Lommer MJ, eds. *Oral and Maxillofacial Surgery in Dogs and Cats*. Edinburgh: Saunders Elsevier, 2012; 23–42.

84 Evans HE, Kitchell RL. Cranial nerves and cutaneous innervation of the head. In: Evans HE, ed. *Miller's Anatomy of the Dog*, 3rd edn. Philadelphia: WB Saunders, 1993; 953–987.

85 Selander D, Dhunér KG, Lundborg G. Peripheral nerve injury due to injection needles used for regional anesthesia. An experimental study of the acute effects of needle point trauma. *Acta Anaesthesiol Scand* 1977; **21**(3): 182–188.

86 Rout PG, Saksena A, Fisher SE. An investigation of the effect on 27-gauge needle tips following a single local anaesthetic injection. *Dent Update* 2003; **30**(7): 370–374.

87 Evans HE. The skeleton. In: Evans HE, ed. *Miller's Anatomy of the Dog*, 3rd edn. Philadelphia: WB Saunders, 1993; 122–218.

88 Lemke KA, Dawson SD. Local and regional anesthesia. *Vet Clin North Am Small Anim Pract* 2000; **30**(4): 839–857.

89 Viscasillas J, Seymour CJ, Brodbelt DC. A cadaver study comparing two approaches for performing maxillary nerve block in dogs. *Vet Anaesth Analg* 2013; **40**(2): 212–219.

90 Woodward TM. Pain management and regional anesthesia for the dental patient. *Top Companion Anim Med* 2008; **23**(2): 106–114.

91 Macfarlane AJ, Bhatia A, Brull R. Needle to nerve proximity: what do the animal studies tell us? *Reg Anesth Pain Med* 2011; **36**(3): 290–302.

92 Barton-Lamb AL, Martin-Flores M, Scrivani PV, *et al*. Evaluation of maxillary arterial blood flow in anesthetized cats with the mouth closed and open. *Vet J* 2013; **196**(3): 325–331.

93 Stiles J, Weil AB, Packer RA, *et al*. Post-anesthetic cortical blindness in cats: twenty cases. *Vet J* 2012; **193**(2): 367–373.

94 Krug W, Losey J. Area of desensitization following mental nerve block in dogs. *J Vet Dent* 2011; **28**(3): 146–150.

95 Gross ME, Pope ER, O'Brien D, *et al*. Regional anesthesia of the infraorbital and inferior alveolar nerves during noninvasive tooth pulp stimulation in halothane-anesthetized dogs. *J Am Vet Med Assoc* 1997; **211**(11): 1403–1405.

96 Gross ME, Pope ER, Jarboe JM, *et al*. Regional anesthesia of the infraorbital and inferior alveolar nerves during noninvasive tooth pulp stimulation in halothane-anesthetized cats. *Am J Vet Res* 2000; **61**(10): 1245–1247.

97 Reader AW, Nusstein JM, Hargreave KM. Local anesthesia in endodontics. In: Hargreaves KM, Cohen S, eds. *Pathways of the Pulp*, 10th edn. Amsterdam: Elsevier, 2011; 691–719.

98 Roahen JO, Marshall FJ. The effects of periodontal ligament injection on pulpal and periodontal tissues. *J Endod* 1990; **16**(1): 28–33.

99 Moore PA, Cuddy MA, Cooke MR, *et al*. Periodontal ligament and intraosseous anesthetic injection techniques: alternatives to mandibular nerve blocks. *J Am Dent Assoc* 2011; **142**(Suppl 3): 13S–18S.

100 Tranquilli WJ, Grimm KA, Lamont LA. *Pain Management for the Small Animal Practitioner*, 2nd edn. Jackson, WY: Teton New Media, 2004.

101 Skarda RA, Tranquilli WJ. Local and regional anesthetic and analgesic techniques: dogs. In: Tranquilli WJ, Thurmon JC, Grimm KA, eds. *Lumb and Jones' Veterinary Anesthesia and Analgesia*, 4th edn. Ames, IA: Blackwell Publishing, 2007; 561–569.

102 Skarda RA, Tranquilli WJ. Local and regional anesthetic and analgesic techniques: cats. In: Tranquilli WJ, Thurmon JC, Grimm KA, eds. *Lumb and Jones' Veterinary Anesthesia and Analgesia*, 4th edn. Ames, IA: Blackwell Publishing, 2007; 595–604.

103 Hofmeister EH, Kent M, Read MR. Paravertebral block for forelimb anesthesia in the dog-an anatomic study. *Vet Anaesth Analg* 2007; **34**(2): 139–142.

104 Lemke KA, Creighton CM. Paravertebral blockade of the brachial plexus in dogs. *Vet Clin North Am Small Anim Pract* 2008; **38**(6): 1231–1241.

105 Futema F, Tabacchi D, Costa JO, *et al*. A new brachial plexus block technique in dogs. *Vet Anaesth Analg* 2002; **29**: 133–139.

106 Moens NM, Caulkett NA. The use of a catheter to provide brachial plexus block in dogs. *Can Vet J* 2000; **41**(9): 685–689.

107 Mahler SP, Reece JL. Electrical nerve stimulation to facilitate placement of an indwelling catheter for repeated brachial plexus block in a traumatized dog. *Vet Anaesth Analg* 2007; **34**(5): 365–370.

108 Brummett CM, Norat MA, Palmisano JM, *et al*. Perineural administration of dexmedetomidine in combination with bupivacaine enhances sensory and motor blockade in sciatic nerve block without inducing neurotoxicity in rat. *Anesthesiology* 2008; **109**(3): 502–511.

109 Brummett CM, Padda AK, Amodeo FS, *et al*. Perineural dexmedetomidine added to ropivacaine causes a dose-dependent increase in the duration of thermal antinociception in sciatic nerve block in rat. *Anesthesiology* 2009; **111**(5): 1111–1119.

110 Brummett CM, Amodeo FS, Janda AM, *et al*. Perineural dexmedetomidine provides an increased duration of analgesia to a thermal stimulus when compared with a systemic control in a rat sciatic nerve block. *Reg Anesth Pain Med* 2010; **35**(5): 427–431.

111 Brummett CM, Williams BA. Additives to local anesthetics for peripheral nerve blockade. *Int Anesthesiol Clin* 2011; **49**(4): 104–116.

112 Brummett CM, Hong EK, Janda AM, *et al*. Perineural dexmedetomidine added to ropivacaine for sciatic nerve block in rats prolongs the duration of analgesia by blocking the hyperpolarization-activated cation current. *Anesthesiology* 2011; **115**(4): 836–843.

113 Rioja E, Sinclair M, Chalmers H, *et al*. Comparison of three techniques for paravertebral brachial plexus blockade in dogs. *Vet Anaesth Analg* 2012; **39**(2): 190–200.

114 Reuben SS, Sklar J, El-Mansouri M. The preemptive analgesic effect of intraarticular bupivacaine and morphine after ambulatory arthroscopic knee surgery. *Anesth Analg* 2001; **92**(4): 923–926.

115 Singelyn FJ, Lhotel L, Fabre B. Pain relief after arthroscopic shoulder surgery: a comparison of intraarticular analgesia, suprascapular nerve block, and interscalene brachial plexus block. *Anesth Analg* 2004; **99**(2): 589–592.

116 Karpie JC, Chu CR. Lidocaine exhibits dose- and time-dependent cytotoxic effects on bovine articular chondrocytes in vitro. *Am J Sports Med* 2007; **35**(10): 1621–1627.

117 Webb ST, Ghosh S. Intra-articular bupivacaine: potentially chondrotoxic? *Br J Anaesth* 2009; **102**(4): 439–441.

118 Trumpatori BJ, Carter JE, Hash J, *et al*. Evaluation of a midhumeral block of the radial, ulnar, musculocutaneous and median (RUMM block) nerves for analgesia of the distal aspect of the thoracic limb in dogs. *Vet Surg* 2010; **39**(7): 785–796.

119 Berg RJ, Orton EC. Pulmonary function in dogs after intercostal thoracotomy: comparison of morphine, oxymorphone, and selective intercostal nerve block. *Am J Vet Res* 1986; **47**(2): 471–474.

120 Flecknell PA, Kirk AJ, Liles JH, *et al*. Post-operative analgesia following thoracotomy in the dog: an evaluation of the effects of bupivacaine intercostal nerve block and nalbuphine on respiratory function. *Lab Anim* 1991; **25**(4): 319–324.

121 Stobie D, Caywood DD, Rozanski EA, *et al*. Evaluation of pulmonary function and analgesia in dogs after intercostal thoracotomy and use of morphine administered intramuscularly or intrapleurally and bupivacaine administered intrapleurally. *Am J Vet Res* 1995; **56**(8): 1098–1109.

122 Dhokarikar P, Caywood DD, Stobie D, *et al*. Effects of intramuscular or interpleural administration of morphine and interpleural administration of bupivacaine on pulmonary function in dogs that have undergone median sternotomy. *Am J Vet Res* 1996; **57**(3): 375–380.

123 Conzemius MG, Brockman DJ, King LG, *et al*. Analgesia in dogs after intercostal thoracotomy: a clinical trial comparing intravenous buprenorphine and interpleural bupivacaine. *Vet Surg* 1994; **23**(4): 291–298.

124 Riegler FX, VadeBoncouer TR, Pelligrino DA. Interpleural anesthetics in the dog: differential somatic neural blockade. *Anesthesiology* 1989; **71**(5): 744–750.

125 VadeBoncouer TR, Riegler FX, Pelligrino DA. The effects of two different volumes of 0.5% bupivacaine in a canine model of interpleural analgesia. *Reg Anesth* 1990; **15**(2): 67–72.

126 Dravid RM, Paul RE. Interpleural block – Part 2. *Anaesthesia* 2007; **62**(11): 1143–1153.

127 Dyce KM, Sack WO, Wensing CJG. *Textbook of Veterinary Anatomy*, 4th edn. St Louis, MO: Saunders Elsevier, 2010.

128 Thompson SE, Johnson JM. Analgesia in dogs after intercostal thoracotomy. A comparison of morphine, selective intercostal nerve block, and interpleural regional analgesia with bupivacaine. *Vet Surg* 1991; **20**(1): 73–77.

129 Kushner LI, Trim CM, Madhusudhan S, *et al.* Evaluation of the hemodynamic effects of interpleural bupivacaine in dogs. *Vet Surg* 1995; **24**(2): 180–187.

130 Bernard F, Kudnig ST, Monnet E. Hemodynamic effects of interpleural lidocaine and bupivacaine combination in anesthetized dogs with and without an open pericardium. *Vet Surg* 2006; **35**(3): 252–258.

131 Kowalski SE, Bradley BD, Greengrass RA, *et al.* Effects of interpleural bupivacaine (0.5%) on canine diaphragmatic function. *Anesth Analg* 1992; **75**(3): 400–404.

132 Davies RG, Myles PS, Graham JM. A comparison of the analgesic efficacy and side-effects of paravertebral vs epidural blockade for thoracotomy – a systematic review and meta-analysis of randomized trials. *Br J Anaesth* 2006; **96**(4): 418–426.

133 Karmakar MK. Thoracic paravertebral block. *Anesthesiology* 2001; **95**(3): 771–780.

134 Portela DA, Otero PE, Sclocco M, *et al.* Anatomical and radiological study of the thoracic paravertebral space in dogs: iohexol distribution pattern and use of the nerve stimulator. *Vet Anaesth Analg* 2012; **39**(4): 398–408.

135 Rafi AN. Abdominal field block: a new approach via the lumbar triangle. *Anaesthesia* 2001; **56**(10): 1024–1106.

136 Rozen WM, Tran TM, Ashton MW, *et al.* Refining the course of the thoracolumbar nerves: a new understanding of the innervation of the anterior abdominal wall. *Clin Anat* 2008; **21**(4): 325–333.

137 Schroeder CA, Schroeder KM, Johnson RA. Transversus abdominis plane block for exploratory laparotomy in a Canadian lynx (*Lynx canadensis*). *J Zoo Wildl Med* 2010; **41**(2): 338–341.

138 Tran TM, Ivanusic JJ, Hebbard P, *et al.* Determination of spread of injectate after ultrasound-guided transversus abdominis plane block: a cadaveric study. *Br J Anaesth* 2009; **102**(1): 123–127.

139 Schroeder CA, Snyder LB, Tearney CC, *et al.* Ultrasound-guided transversus abdominis plane block in the dog: an anatomical evaluation. *Vet Anaesth Analg* 2011; **38**(3): 267–271.

140 Bruggink SM, Schroeder CA, Baker-Herman TL, Schroeder KM. Weight based volume of injection influences the cranial to caudal spread of local anesthetic solution in ultrasound guided transversus abdominis plane blocks in canine cadavers. In: *Abstracts of the American Society of Regional Anesthesia and Pain Medicine 36th Annual Regional Anesthesia Meeting and Workshops, Las Vegas, NV*, 5–8 May 2011.

141 Niraj G, Kelkar A, Fox AJ. Oblique sub-costal transversus abdominis plane (TAP) catheters: an alternative to epidural analgesia after upper abdominal surgery. *Anaesthesia* 2009; **64**(10): 1137–1140.

142 Gucev G, Yasui GM, Chang TY, *et al.* Bilateral ultrasound-guided continuous ilioinguinal–iliohypogastric block for pain relief after cesarean delivery. *Anesth Analg* 2008; **106**(4): 1220–1222.

143 Heil JW, Ilfeld BM, Loland VJ, *et al.* Ultrasound-guided transversus abdominis plane catheters and ambulatory perineural infusions for outpatient inguinal hernia repair. *Reg Anesth Pain Med* 2010; **35**(6): 556–558.

144 Costa-Farre C, Blanch XS, Cruz JI, *et al.* Ultrasound guidance for the performance of sciatic and saphenous nerve blocks in dogs. *Vet J* 2011; **187**(2): 221–224.

145 Mahler SP, Adogwa AO. Anatomical and experimental studies of brachial plexus, sciatic, and femoral nerve-location using peripheral nerve stimulation in the dog. *Vet Anaesth Analg* 2008; **35**(1): 80–89.

146 Day TK, Pepper WT, Tobias TA, *et al.* Comparison of intra-articular and epidural morphine for analgesia following stifle arthrotomy in dogs. *Vet Surg* 1995; **24**(6): 522–530.

147 Saunder WB, Hulse DA, Schulz KS. Evaluation of portal locations and periarticular structures in canine coxofemoral arthroscopy: a cadaver study. *Vet Comp Orthop Traumatol* 2004; **17**(4): 184–188.

148 Oliveira G, Vivan M, Diasj B. Evaluation of the extension and cardiorespiratory effects of thoracic epidural anesthesia in dogs (Abstract). *Vet Anaesth Analg* 2010; **37**(3): 44.

149 Zhang D, Nishimura R, Nagahama S, *et al.* Comparison of feasibility and safety of epidural catheterization between cranial and caudal lumbar vertebral segments in dogs. *J Vet Med Sci* 2012; **73**(12): 1573–1577.

150 Zhang D, Fujiwara R, Iseri T, *et al.* Distribution of contrast medium epidurally injected at thoracic and lumbar vertebral segments. *J Vet Med Sci* 2013; **75**(5): 663–666.

151 Maierl J, Reindl S, Knospe C. Observations on epidural anesthesia in cats from the anatomical viewpoint. *Tierarztl Prax* 1997; **25**(3): 267–270 (in German).

152 O'Hearn AK, Wright BD. Coccygeal epidural with local anesthetic for catheterization and pain management in the treatment of feline urethral obstruction. *J Vet Emerg Crit Care* 2011; **21**(1): 50–52.

153 Evans HE, ed. *Miller's Anatomy of the Dog*, 3rd edn. Philadelphia: WB Saunders, 1993.

154 Liu SS, Bernards CM. Exploring the epidural trail. *Reg Anesth Pain Med* 2002; **27**(2): 122–124.

155 Lee I, Yamagishi N, Oboshi K, *et al.* Distribution of new methylene blue injected into the lumbosacral epidural space in cats. *Vet Anaesth Analg* 2004; **31**(3): 190–194.

156 Gorgi AA, Hofmeister EH, Higginbotham MJ, *et al.* Effect of body position on cranial migration of epidurally injected methylene blue in recumbent dogs. *Am J Vet Res* 2006; **67**(2): 219–221.

157 Freire CD, Torres ML, Fantoni DT, *et al.* Bupivacaine 0.25% and methylene blue spread with epidural anesthesia in dog. *Vet Anaesth Analg* 2010; **37**(1): 63–69.

158 Nakayama M, Yamamoto J, Ichinose H, *et al.* Effects of volume and concentration of lidocaine on epidural anaesthesia in pregnant females. *Eur J Anaesthesiol* 2002; **19**(11): 808–811.

159 Duggan J, Bowler GM, McClure JH, *et al.* Extradural block with bupivacaine: influence of dose, volume, concentration and patient characteristics. *Br J Anaesth* 1988; **61**(3): 324–331.

160 Otero P, Tarragona L, Ceballos M, *et al.* Epidural cephalic spread of a local anesthetic in dogs: a mathematical model using the column length (Abstract). *Vet Anaesth Analg* 2010; **37**(3): 35.

161 Otero P, Tarragona L, Waxman Dova S. Effects of epidurally administered ropivacaine at three different concentrations in dogs (Abstract). *Vet Anaesth Analg* 2006; **34**(4): 69.

162 Iff I, Moens Y, Schatzmann U. Use of pressure waves to confirm the correct placement of epidural needles in dogs. *Vet Rec* 2007; **161**(1): 22–25.

163 Naganobu K, Hagio M. The effect of body position on the 'hanging drop' method for identifying the extradural space in anaesthetized dogs. *Vet Anaesth Analg* 2007; **34**(1): 59–62.

164 Iseri T, Nishimura R, Nagahama S, *et al.* Epidural spread of iohexol following the use of air or saline in the 'loss of resistance' test. *Vet Anaesth Analg* 2010; **37**(6): 526–530.

165 Tsui BC, Gupta S, Finucane B. Detection of subarachnoid and intravascular epidural catheter placement. *Can J Anaesth* 1999; **46**(7): 675–678.

166 Garcia-Pereira FL, Hauptman J, Shih AC, *et al.* Evaluation of electric neurostimulation to confirm correct placement of lumbosacral epidural injections in dogs. *Am J Vet Res* 2010; **71**(2): 157–160.

167 Read MR. Confirmation of epidural needle placement using nerve stimulation in dogs. *Vet Anaesth Analg* 2005; **32**(4): 13.

168 Lillie PE, Glynn CJ, Fenwick DG. Site of action of intravenous regional anesthesia. *Anesthesiology* 1984; **61**(5): 507–510.

169 Davis K, McConachie I. Intravenous regional anaesthesia. *Curr Anaesth Crit Care* 1998; **9**(5): 261–264.

170 Chan VW, Peng PW, Kaszas Z, *et al.* A comparative study of general anesthesia, intravenous regional anesthesia, and axillary block for outpatient hand surgery: clinical outcome and cost analysis. *Anesth Analg* 2001; **93**(5): 1181–1184.

171 De Marzo C, Crovace A, De Monte V, *et al.* Comparison of intra-operative analgesia provided by intravenous regional anesthesia or brachial plexus block for pancarpal arthrodesis in dogs. *Res Vet Sci* 2012; **93**(3): 1493–1497.

172 Webb AA, Cantwell SL, Duke T, *et al.* Intravenous regional anesthesia (Bier block) in a dog. *Can Vet J* 1999; **40**(6): 419–421.

173 Kushner L, Fan B, Shofer F. Intravenous regional anesthesia in isoflurane anesthetized cats: lidocaine plasma concentrations and cardiovascular effects. *Anesth Analg* 2002; **29**(3): 140–149.

174 Duke T. Local and regional anesthetic and analgesic techniques in the dog and cat. Part II. Infiltration and nerve blocks. *Can Vet J* 2000; **41**(12): 949–952.

175 Feldman HS, Arthur GR, Covino BG. Comparative systemic toxicity of convulsant and supraconvulsant doses of intravenous ropivacaine, bupivacaine, and lidocaine in the conscious dog. *Anesth Analg* 1989; **69**(6): 794–801.

176 Moore DC. Bupivacaine toxicity and Bier block: the drug, the technique, or the anesthetist. *Anesthesiology* 1984; **61**(6): 782.

177 William B, Archibald D, Rao G. Regional intravenous anesthesia with bupivacaine hydrochloride in dogs. *Cheiron* 1992; **21**: 153–154.

178 Hoffmann AC, van Gessel E, Gamulin Z, *et al.* Quantitative evaluation of tourniquet leak during i.v. regional anaesthesia of the upper and lower limbs in human volunteers. *Br J Anaesth* 1995; **75**(3): 269–273.

179 Fanelli G, Casati A, Garancini P, Torri G. Nerve stimulator and multiple injections technique for upper and lower limb blockade: failure rate patient acceptance and neurologic complications. *Anesth Analg* 1999; **88**(4): 847–852.

46 Horses

Regula Bettschart-Wolfensberger
Vetsuisse Faculty, Section Anaesthesiology, University of Zurich, Zurich, Switzerland

Chapter contents

Introduction

General anesthesia in horses is challenging and, despite using modern monitoring and anesthetics techniques, anesthesia of horses carries a high risk [1]. Since the first and only series of multicenter studies looking at perioperative fatalities was performed, more than 20 years have elapsed [2,3]. Despite the limited number of practical anesthetic techniques, few studies have directly compared the different available techniques in order to identify the least risky options for anesthetizing horses [4,5]. There are still many unstudied and unanswered questions about how to best perform equine anesthesia. This chapter aims to provide an overview of peculiarities associated with horses and a focus on management of anesthesia and solutions for common problems.

Preanesthetic considerations

Guidelines on how long an adult horse should be fasted before general anesthesia have varied and little scientific literature addressing this problem is available. When using a dissociative-based induction protocol (e.g., ketamine), regurgitation and aspiration of gastric contents are usually not a major concern. Fasting a horse longer than about 4 h increases the acidity and viscosity of the gastric contents, which may lead to an enhanced risk of acidic fluid aspiration and subsequent respiratory tract injury. Since horses typically browse for their food, prolonged fasting can cause stress in individual horses, which will negatively influence motility of the gastrointestinal tract [6] or potentiate ulceration in horses prone to it [7]. A negative energy balance might impair normal metabolism and derange oxygen–glucose physiology during the perioperative period, although this is usually not a major concern for healthy horses.

Preanesthetic fasting also has potential benefits. Less material in the gastrointestinal (GI) tract places less pressure on the major abdominal vessels and causes less cranial displacement of the diaphragm. This may reduce impairment of venous return to the heart and improve ventilation, likely providing better oxygenation and oxygen delivery to the tissues. Further, ongoing microbial gas production within the GI tract is probably decreased in fasted horses. Since postoperative colic can be a major complication following anesthesia and surgery in horses, reduced gas production can limit ileus. This effect on colic rates has been shown in fasted in comparison with unfasted horses [8]. However, the use of a muzzle to limit oral intake of solid feed has been associated with more postoperative colic than the simple avoidance of preoperative feeding while allowing the horse to consume some of its bedding [9]. Many anesthesiologists are convinced that preoperative overnight fasting for 8–12 h is beneficial for most horses. Easy access to water is important (no muzzle), but with some individuals this necessitates that the amount of edible bedding is limited.

Horses instinctively tend to flee when they are in threatened or frightened. Therefore, the periods immediately before losing and after regaining consciousness can be difficult to manage in horses unaccustomed to close human contact. Once a horse is excited or frightened it can be very difficult to calm it down again. Often, higher sedative dosages (with potentially more untoward side-effects) will

Veterinary Anesthesia and Analgesia: The Fifth Edition of Lumb and Jones.
Edited by Kurt A. Grimm, Leigh A. Lamont, William J. Tranquilli, Stephen A. Greene and Sheilah A. Robertson.

be needed. Therefore, it is beneficial to avoid excitement and reduce pain by the proper use of sedation and analgesic drugs before anesthesia induction and also during recovery.

In addition to the judicious use of sedatives, common principles of physical restraint should be applied to the handling of horses. Some degree of physical restraint, such as taking hold of the halter or lifting the patient's leg, is combined with appropriate sedatives to yield a tractable horse. The method of physical restraint will be based on a number of factors, including size and temperament of the horse, availability of personnel, and the duration or type of procedure.

Standing sedation

Sedation of horses for physical examination or standing procedures is commonly performed using readily available sedatives and analgesics (Table 46.1). Intravenous administration of α_2-adrenergic receptor agonists (e.g., xylazine, detomidine, romifidine, medetomidine, or dexmedetomidine) form the basis of most drug combinations used to achieve moderate or heavy sedation in horses. Sublingual administration of detomidine (Dormosedan Gel®; Zoetis, Florham Park, NJ, USA) may be useful for horses that cannot be given injections. For standing surgeries, use of sedation is combined with administration of both systemic and local analgesics. Epidural injection of local anesthetics in combination with xylazine at the first intercoccygeal space is recommended for perineal surgeries.

Table 46.1 Drugs used for standing chemical restraint, for analgesia, or as preanesthetics in horses.

Drug	Dose and Route	Onset of Optimal Effect	Comments
Acepromazine	0.02–0.05 mg/kg, IM, IV	30–40 min	Avoid use in neonates or stressed or hypotensive horses
Detomidine	0.01–0.02 mg/kg, IV	3–5 min	Ataxia, head-down posture
	0.02–0.04 mg/kg, IM	20 min	Start with low dose, repeat as needed (but not before 20 min)
			Allow adequate time to action; can be given orally
Dexmedetomidine	0.003–0.005 mg/kg, IV	5 min	Premedication dose, very short acting
	0.002 mg/kg/h, IV	5 min	Excellent analgesia during general anesthesia
			Markedly decreases anesthetic requirement
Romifidine	0.04–0.1 mg/kg, IV	5–10 min	Ataxia, head-down posture
	0.08–0.12 mg/kg, IM	15–25 min	Start with low dose, repeat as needed (but not before 30 min)
Xylazine	0.5–1.0 mg/kg, IV	3–5 min	Ataxia, head-down posture
Butorphanol	0.01–0.03 mg/kg, IV	3–5 min	Analgesic; usually given in combination with a sedative
Morphine	0.1–0.2 mg/kg, IM, IV	3–5 min	Analgesic; sedate with α_2-agonist prior to administration
			Has potential for excitation, especially in non-painful horses or at higher dose rates
Phenylbutazone	1.1–4.4 mg/kg, IV, PO	8–12 h	Analgesic; extreme perivascular irritant
Flunixin meglumine	1.1 mg/kg, IV, IM, PO	12–24 h	Analgesic; local tissue reactions IM
Meclofenic acid	2.2 mg/kg, PO	24 h	Analgesic; approved for horses

Preanesthetic sedation

For most cases, it is possible to catheterize a jugular vein using local anesthetic infiltration with or without prior administration of a sedative. Intramuscular acepromazine (e.g., 0.03–0.05 mg/kg) at least 30 min before placement of an intravenous catheter may help calm some horses [10]. Alternatively (or if additional sedation is needed), an α_2-adrenergic receptor agonist, with or without an opioid such as butorphanol, can be given intravenously or intramuscularly. As acepromazine is longer acting, cannot be antagonized, and the potential adverse effects are numerous, the anesthetist should avoid its use in cases of pre-existing hypotension, low hematocrit, or moderate to severe liver impairment. Following catheter placement, horses are ideally left undisturbed for at least 5–10 min. If not sedated prior to catheter placement, they can be sedated intravenously with about one-third of the total dose of the α_2-adrenergic receptor agonist of choice (Table 46.1). As soon as some sedation becomes apparent, horses can usually be walked into the anesthesia induction area with minimal resistance.

Once in the induction area, the remainder of the sedative is administered slowly to reach the desired depth of sedation (i.e., the horse becomes unresponsive to surrounding stimuli). In horses that do not become heavily sedated, the dose may be increased by about 25%, or co-administration of an opioid may enhance sedation and analgesia. Generally, reduction of the dose of α_2-adrenergic receptor agonists is reserved only for severely compromised horses that cannot be stabilized before anesthesia induction. In such patients, a higher dose of benzodiazepine during induction (0.06 instead of 0.02 mg/kg) may improve muscle relaxation.

Some veterinarians will prefer the induction of general anesthesia in horses using a co-induction with a shorter acting α_2-adrenergic receptor agonist such as xylazine (0.5–1.0 mg/kg), medetomidine (7 μg/kg) or dexmedetomidine (3–5 μg/kg). Their untoward cardiopulmonary effects are shorter lasting than those associated with detomidine or romifidine and peak intensity of adverse effects is less pronounced [11,12].

Some anesthetists prefer to combine sedatives with opioids. The combination of α_2-adrenergic receptor agonists with an opioid receptor agonist improves quality of sedation [13,14]. In horses, the minimal alveolar concentration (MAC) of inhaled anesthetics is not consistently decreased following opioids [15] and respiration during anesthesia might be more depressed [16]. Therefore, some anesthetists do not routinely administer opioids before induction and intraoperative analgesia is provided by other means.

In uncooperative animals where catheter placement is difficult, acepromazine alone at the above-mentioned dose rates does not usually result in adequate sedation. In those horses, it can be beneficial to sedate them with intramuscular injection of an α_2-adrenergic receptor agonist [e.g., romifidine (40 μg/kg) or detomidine (10 μg/kg)] in combination with an opioid such as butorphanol (0.02 mg/kg). Yearlings, thoroughbreds, and Arabians tend to need higher dosages and in very difficult horses, doubling the initial dose of the sedative will avoid the repetitive stress of injection and resulting stimulation. Most important is to leave horses given intramuscular detomidine at least 20 min and intramuscular romifidine 30 min in an undisturbed environment to allow peak effect to develop before attempting to handle the horse. If further doses of sedatives are needed to achieve satisfactory calming effects, long-lasting cardiopulmonary effects dominated by reduced cardiac output and severe peripheral vasoconstriction and reduced peripheral perfusion may result [17,18]. This might be detrimental in the case of general anesthesia. Myopathies and neuropathies, a consequence of inadequate tissue blood flow, contribute to a significant extent to the incidence of equine perioperative fatalities [3,19].

Induction of anesthesia

For many veterinarians, the preferred anesthetic induction agent in horses is ketamine. Other induction drugs are available and may be used in horses (Table 46.2). When used properly, they cause the horse slowly to assume sternal and then lateral recumbency. A significant disadvantage of ketamine in comparison with other alternatives (propofol, alphaxalone, barbiturates) is poor muscle relaxation and hypnosis when used alone. To minimize these undesirable attributes, horses should be deeply sedated before anesthesia induction with ketamine. Additionally, the use of centrally acting muscle relaxants significantly enhances the quality of equine induction. Guaifenesin (35–50 mg/kg) can be given intravenously to effect (until the horse becomes ataxic and buckles its knees) just prior to the bolus of ketamine (with or without additional muscle relaxants such as benzodiazepine, e.g., diazepam or midazolam). These muscle-relaxing agents reduce muscle hypertonus and reflex activity, which facilitates endotracheal intubation. Guaifenesin administration can be cumbersome in adult horses as effective dosages result in the need for relatively large volumes to be administered. Furthermore, it can cause phlebitis even if used at a relatively low concentration of 5% [20]. For this reason, many prefer to use a benzodiazepine for muscle relaxation. An additional advantage of benzodiazepine use is the availability of an antagonist, flumazenil. It has not been extensively studied or routinely used in equine anesthesia because of expense, but in cases of emergency a dose of 0.01 mg/kg IV can reverse the action of commonly used doses of benzodiazepines.

Most anesthetists prefer to keep the dose of the benzodiazepines for co-induction low (0.02 mg/kg), which minimizes the impact on respiration and reduces ataxia during recovery. An intravenous bolus of ketamine of 2–3 mg/kg in combination with diazepam or midazolam results in recumbency within 1.5–2 min and is associated with relatively deep anesthesia for about 8–15 min. If a surgical manipulation is not successfully performed within this time frame, or the trachea intubated and maintenance of anesthesia with an inhalation agent begun, additional ketamine (1–1.5 mg/kg, IV) may be administered. If a short-acting α_2-adrenergic receptor agonist was used for sedation (xylazine, medetomidine, or dexmedetomidine), it should also be readministered at 50% of the initial dose.

Following anesthesia induction with ketamine, some animals will have rapid nystagmus, limb movements, or muscle tremors. Under such circumstances, additional anesthetic drug(s) should be given without delay to prevent emergence from anesthesia during critical periods such as hoisting onto the surgical table. As barbiturates have the fastest onset of action, most anesthetists prefer thiopental for this purpose, when it is available. A dose of 0.5 mg/kg in most horses will relax muscles without causing apnea and intubation can be easily performed. Other alternatives to barbiturates that have been described for anesthesia in horses are alfaxalone and propofol. Propofol induction of an adult horse requires a large volume of drug that may prove cost prohibitive [21,22]. Alfaxalone (1 mg/kg, IV) has been compared with ketamine for induction of anesthesia in a study of six horses following xylazine and guaifenesin administration [23]. Induction and recovery times and qualities were similar, although the horses receiving alfaxalone had a higher incidence (5/6 horses) of muscle tremor during induction. Similarly to the use of propofol, alfaxalone induction requires a large volume and is prohibitively expensive.

Table 46.2 Drugs used for induction and maintenance of anesthesia in sedated horses.

Drug	Dose	Comments
Diazepam	0.02–0.06 mg/kg, IV	Used for muscle relaxation; combined with ketamine
Guaifenesin	50 mg/kg, IV to effect	Muscle relaxant, must be used in combination with anesthetics such as ketamine or propofol
Ketamine	2.0–3.0 mg/kg, IV	Requires maximum sedation prior to administration to induce anesthesia
Midazolam	0.02–0.06 mg/kg, IV	Used for muscle relaxation; combined with ketamine
Tiletamine–zolazepam	0.7–1.0 mg/kg, IV	Requires maximum sedation prior to administration to induce anesthesia; may be reconstituted with ketamine and either xylazine or detomidine in various combinations of 'TKX' or 'TKD'
'Triple drip'	1–2 mL/kg/h	Mixture of guaifenesin 5%, ketamine 0.1%, and xylazine 0.05% Do not use to induce anesthesia in adult horses Used for extending injectable anesthesia induced by xylazine/ketamine

Maintenance of general anesthesia

The use of several drugs in combination is called balanced anesthesia if their net effect is to produce unconsciousness, muscle relaxation, amnesia, and antinociception. In modern equine practice there appear to be numerous combinations that can achieve this balance. The use of inhalant-only anesthesia is being replaced by the use of inhalation anesthesia in combination with sedatives, analgesics, and muscle relaxants, given either by infusion or by repetitive bolus administration. This type of anesthesia is called partial intravenous anesthesia (PIVA). If no inhalation anesthesia is used but only intravenous drugs are administered, it is total intravenous anesthesia (TIVA).

The aim of PIVA is to provide analgesia and reduce inhalation anesthetic requirements. It is expected that with balanced anesthesia, cardiopulmonary function and intraoperative antinociception will be better, and postoperative pain reduced. Since most drugs used for PIVA also have effects on cardiopulmonary function, the net effect of PIVA remains to be tested for most combinations used and can vary depending on the health status of the animal. However, there is general agreement among practitioners that PIVA is, under most circumstances, better than the use of only inhalation anesthesia. One exception involves surgeries where the surgical field can be locally or regionally anesthetized. However, such techniques are more limited in horses than in other species because regional blocks of extremities persisting into the recovery phase can result in injuries during the horse's attempts to stand.

For PIVA, lidocaine, ketamine, different α_2-adrenergic receptor agonists, and various opioids (alone or in combination with each other) have been used in addition to inhalation anesthesia. Some anesthetists have also advocated additional midazolam or guaifenesin to enhance muscle relaxation, although the impact of muscle relaxants on recovery needs to be considered carefully. The problem with all these polypharmacy combinations is that the pharmacokinetic and pharmacodynamic interactions can be difficult to predict in individual animals [24]. During clinical anesthesia, plasma levels cannot be rapidly measured so some drugs with a narrow therapeutic window (e.g., lidocaine) might result in toxic levels when standard dose rates are used under certain circumstances [24,25].

Context-sensitive half-life (the half-life determining recovery following varying durations of infusion) can change with infusion time and pathophysiologic status of the horse. Differences in cardiac output and liver blood flow might further influence the plasma levels of drugs found in individual horses. Metabolites with pharmacological activity, such as norketamine, that are metabolized more slowly than the parent drug [26], can potentially accumulate and influence recovery after longer infusions. If PIVA is used, the anesthetist has to be aware of the effects of all the drugs used, and the patient closely monitored to avoid adverse drug interactions.

Several studies have favorably reported the use of PIVA [27–30]. A discussion of some of the drugs that are used for PIVA and important aspects of their use follows. Additional reviews, including dose rates for common drugs, are available [31].

α_2-Adrenergic receptor agonists

All available α_2-adrenergic receptor agonists have been used successfully for PIVA. They seem optimal in horses, as they cause reliable sedation, good analgesia, and inhalant anesthetic dose reduction. Accumulation will not lead to excitement in recovery, but to prolonged sedation, eventually leading to a smoother recovery phase. α_2-Adrenergic receptor agonists are used for sedation prior to anesthesia induction (achieving a loading dose) in almost all horses and therefore a steady state will be quickly achieved without intraoperative loading dose administration.

Medetomidine and dexmedetomidine are potent and shorter acting, making them better suited for titration of effect during PIVA [32,33]. Detailed reports of the safety and effectiveness of medetomidine and dexmedetomidine compared with other α_2-adrenergic receptor agonists registered for horses (xylazine, detomidine, romifidine) have been published [34–36]. Useful features of medetomidine infusions are that recovery is better compared with a lidocaine constant-rate infusion (CRI) alone [37,38] and that no accumulation of medetomidine or its metabolites has been noted. Medetomidine CRIs (3.5 μg/kg/h) have been used in horses for up to 9 h, resulting in recoveries (to standing) requiring no longer than 1.5 h. Clinical use of dexmedetomidine CRIs is similar (1–2 μg/kg/h), as a sedative/analgesic adjunct to inhalant anesthesia.

An intravenous bolus of an α_2-adrenergic receptor agonist causes vasoconstriction, bradycardia, and a decrease in cardiac output – adverse effects that can be undesirable during equine anesthesia. However, during CRI of lower doses, cardiopulmonary effects are minimized [39] and combination with inhalation anesthesia seems favorable [40]. Urine production is increased with administration of α_2-adrenergic receptor agonists; therefore, a urinary catheter during long surgeries is highly recommended to avoid over-distension of the bladder intraoperatively and to prevent urination during the critical recovery period. Replacement of fluids lost via increased urine production should be included in the fluid therapy plan.

Opioids have been used in combination with medetomidine and dexmedetomidine CRIs [41]. Whereas butorphanol (25 μg/kg IV loading dose followed by 25 μg/kg/h CRI) during isoflurane–medetomidine anesthesia failed to show any effect other than prolonged time to swallowing following anesthesia, morphine (0.15 mg/kg bolus followed by 0.1 mg/kg/h) in combination with dexmedetomidine CRI resulted in a decrease in requirement for an inhalant anesthetic of 67% [42].

Lidocaine

Lidocaine is frequently used as part of balanced anesthesia in horses due to its numerous useful effects [43]. Cardiovascular safety seems to be good, as the horse is not particularly prone to adverse cardiovascular effects of low-dose lidocaine [44]. The inhalant anesthetic requirement (MAC) decreases in a dose-dependent fashion [45], and at clinically used dose rates (1.2 mg/kg bolus given over 10 min, followed by 35–60 μg/kg/h) the MAC reduction is about 25–27% [46,47], with resultant plasma lidocaine levels of around 2000 ng/mL. Since plasma levels of 1850–4530 ng/mL have been associated with visual dysfunction, tremors, or ataxia [48], lidocaine administration should be stopped 30 min before the end of inhalation anesthesia to minimize problems in recovery [49]. Lidocaine clearance is reduced by general anesthesia and some disease processes [24,25], so careful or reduced dosing is advocated in compromised horses.

Ketamine

Ketamine is a dissociative anesthetic and analgesic that is a noncompetitive antagonist at NMDA receptors, and is therefore potentially useful as an analgesic in cases of chronic or neuropathic pain [50]. Ketamine can cause sympathetic nervous system stimulation rather than the depression that is seen with most other anesthetic drugs, and its use in cardiovascular compromised patients is reasonable in many cases. Ketamine in PIVA (0.6–1.0 mg/kg/h) can reduce inhalant requirements by up to 25%. A potential problem during prolonged infusions of ketamine (e.g., longer than 2 h) is the accumulation of active metabolites, including norketamine [26]. Even if the ketamine administration is stopped before the inhalation agent is turned off, some residual effects causing excitement during recovery might persist. The quality of recovery has been shown to be better if (*S*)-ketamine is used instead of racemic ketamine [51]; however, (*S*)-ketamine can still result in very rough recoveries following a long duration of administration and in animals that are not easily sedated by premedications. An inhalant anesthetic reduction of up to 49% has been achieved when ketamine is combined with lidocaine [27,30], although the influence on recovery following prolonged use (>2 h) remains to be tested.

Opioids

There is no doubt that μ-opioid agonists are analgesics in horses as in other species, but they do not provide a reliable intraoperative effect [15]. In one report, the use of fentanyl (at relatively high dose rates) resulted in a consistent MAC-reducing effect [52]; however this technique has never gained popularity in clinical practice, probably because another report showed no reliable MAC reduction but a very high incidence of poor recoveries [53]. Morphine has been shown to improve recovery [16] following orthopedic surgery, therefore some clinicians choose to administer morphine (0.1 mg/kg, IM) following arthroscopy before recovery. Intra-articular morphine may also be administered for postoperative pain relief following arthroscopic procedures.

Muscle relaxants: Benzodiazepines and guaifenesin

Various reports have included benzodiazepines or guaifenesin as adjuncts during equine anesthesia. Benzodiazepines provide MAC reduction [54], and intraoperative anesthesia is improved by muscle relaxation without the negative influences on cardiovascular function. Midazolam CRI (0.5 mg/kg/h) in combination with ketamine, medetomidine, and sevoflurane has been advocated because of its minimal effects on cardiopulmonary function compared with other protocols [29]. Guaifenesin, ketamine, and medetomidine in combination with sevoflurane have resulted in similar outcomes [55]. However, midazolam or guaifenesin CRIs during inhalation anesthesia may result in severe ataxia and difficult recoveries after prolonged surgeries (e.g., longer than 2 h).

Field anesthesia

Common protocols for providing anesthesia to horses and ponies under field conditions include combinations of ketamine and an α_2-adrenergic receptor agonist [56–60]. Topping off xylazine/ketamine anesthesia by administering one-quarter to half the induction doses of each is a common practice. Addition of butorphanol (0.02 mg/kg, IV) or an intravenous infusion of guaifenesin may aid in attaining appropriate levels of analgesia or skeletal muscle relaxation, respectively. Guaifenesin should not be given as the sole agent to horses because it provides no analgesic effect and has minimal hypnotic effect. Alternatively, diazepam (0.1 mg/kg, IV) and midazolam (0.1 mg/kg, IV) have been used to replace guaifenesin when enhanced skeletal muscle relaxation is desired.

The combination of guaifenesin, ketamine, and xylazine (often referred to as 'triple drip') has been described when intravenous maintenance of anesthesia is needed for a longer procedure [61]. Briefly, solutions of 0.1 or 0.2% ketamine, 0.05% xylazine, and 5% guaifenesin are prepared. The mixture is administered to horses already anesthetized with xylazine and ketamine (or a similar protocol using an α_2-adrenergic receptor agonist and ketamine) in order to extend the anesthesia following attainment of recumbency. Typical doses of triple drip for field anesthesia are 1–2 mL/kg/h, IV. Some anesthetists prefer to administer 50–100 mL of triple drip after every 7–10 min of anesthesia. If the respiration rate increases, it indicates that the anesthetic plane is lightening and a shorter interval between boluses is needed. Deeper or slower respirations indicate that the interval between boluses should be increased. For most horses weighing around 450 kg, approximately 1 h of general anesthesia is provided by 1 L of triple drip. For simple 'topping off' of xylazine/ketamine anesthesia, triple drip solution offers a satisfactory alternative. Intubation and availability of supplemental oxygen are prudent during triple drip anesthesia. Respiratory depression and bradycardia may occur during administration of triple drip, hence respiration and heart rate should be monitoring closely during anesthesia.

Monitoring

Monitoring of anesthesia in horses, distilled to its essence, consists of the collection of data that allow the anesthetist to judge whether the depth of anesthesia is sufficient and cardiopulmonary function (including oxygen delivery to tissues) is adequate. To know which level of anesthesia is ideal for an individual horse can be difficult since the two (anesthetic depth versus cardiopulmonary function) are often competing. Inhalation anesthetics dose-dependently depress cardiopulmonary function, which is why anesthetists attempt to maintain anesthesia at as light a level as possible. However, unstable anesthesia dominated by repetitive movement of the horse followed by hasty drug administration should be avoided. During inhalation-based anesthesia, a sluggish palpebral reflex should usually be present without nystagmus. However, some horses will not retain palpebral reflexes despite being at a light anesthetic level. In spontaneously breathing horses, respiration should be regular and not influenced by surgical stimulation. During TIVA with alfaxalone- or propofol-based protocols, judgment of depth of anesthesia is similar to that for inhalation anesthesia. To assess ketamine-based anesthesia is more difficult and depends on concurrently used drugs since reflexes often are stronger (spontaneous blinking) and the presence of nystagmus is not necessarily indicative of insufficient depth of anesthesia. Ketamine-anesthetized horses should show no reaction to surgical stimulation and should have a regular breathing pattern, although apneustic breathing may be seen immediately following bolus administration at induction.

Various parameters can be measured for assessment of cardiopulmonary function during anesthesia. The commonly monitored parameters include heart rate, arterial blood pressure, respiratory rate, hemoglobin saturation (measured by pulse oximetry), and end-tidal CO_2. Capillary refill time, mucous membrane color, heart rate, respiration rate, and pulse quality are also useful measures that can be easily checked, especially in field conditions where multiparameter monitors are unavailable. Arterial blood gases, pH, packed cell volume, plasma proteins, lactate, or relevant electrolytes can be measured repeatedly, especially during long or complicated anesthesia. Although these parameters have ranges that are considered clinically acceptable, none really indicate if oxygenation of vital tissues is adequate when taken alone. The measurement of cardiac output, intramuscular lactate [62], or peripheral tissue perfusion [63] is not currently routine, but improved technology may make them more useful in the future and may give more insight as to what is happening at the tissue level.

Adequate cardiovascular function and tissue oxygenation

It is well recognized that one of the most important aspects of equine anesthesia planning is maintenance of adequate cardiovascular function and tissue oxygenation. Optimal positioning of horses on soft padding will evenly distribute the horse's weight and prevent focal areas of hypoperfusion. Care should be taken to avoid positioning that might stretch or compress nerves (such as bending legs with tension or stretching the neck in dorsal recumbency). Most studies investigating factors affecting the development of postanesthetic myopathy were performed using halothane anesthesia [64–66]. From these studies, it was learned that minimal mean arterial blood pressures of ≥70 mmHg appear important to maintain perfusion of large muscles during recumbency. Since halothane is not a vasodilator like modern inhalation anesthetics (e.g., isoflurane and sevoflurane), tissue perfusion is likely maintained at slightly lower mean arterial blood pressures with the more modern agents provided that local compression of tissues does not prevent flow. This is logical since perfusion is also a function of cardiac output and vascular resistance, not blood pressure alone.

Under clinical circumstances, blood pressure is usually the major cardiovascular parameter measured, even though it does not allow direct assessment of tissue perfusion. This is due to the ease with which relatively accurate data can be gathered and the relationship they have to tissue blood flow (although many confounders exist). When mean arterial blood pressure is low (<50 mmHg), interventions are required in any case. However, if the mean blood pressure is 70 mmHg or greater, it does not assure that all tissues are well perfused and other parameters should be assessed to determine if the horse is doing well (color of mucous membranes, heart rate, serum lactate, fluid status).

Impaired cardiopulmonary function will result in decreased peripheral tissue oxygenation. Cardiopulmonary function is usually reduced more as the dose of inhalation agent used becomes greater [67]. Therefore, careful titration of inhalation anesthetics is warranted. Despite adequate fluid therapy and a light depth of anesthesia, perfusion may not be adequate, requiring sympathomimetics be used, especially in critically ill horses [68]. Dobutamine (up to 1.5 μg/kg/min) can increase blood pressure and cardiac output with minimal undesired effects such as tachyarrhythmias. Care must be taken if atropine is administered concurrently, as arrhythmogenicity and chronotropic effects of dobutamine are enhanced [69]. In the case of low systemic vascular resistance (e.g., endotoxemia), ephedrine (0.06 mg/kg), norepinephrine (1–3 μg/kg) or phenylephrine (1–6 μg/kg/min) is a reasonable option [65–68]. However, the use of vasoconstrictors without concurrent increases in cardiac output may raise blood pressure but decrease tissue perfusion, so careful titration and monitoring are important with their use.

Another important factor for the anesthetist to monitor and manage is ventilation. Adequate ventilation is crucial to maintain arterial oxygenation and elimination of carbon dioxide. However, indiscriminate use of mechanical ventilation may have detrimental cardiovascular ramifications. During spontaneous ventilation, mean intrapleural pressures are subatmospheric, which facilitates venous return, cardiac output, and oxygen delivery. In contrast, intermittent positive-pressure ventilation, especially using high airway pressure and short expiratory times, can induce the opposite.

Anesthesia of spontaneously ventilating horses often results in high arterial CO_2 partial pressures ($PaCO_2 > 70$ mmHg) [70]. The level of acceptable hypercapnia in horses is debatable and may depend on several factors, including cardiovascualar function and acid–base status. One study in mechanically ventilated horses reported beneficial cardiopulmonary stimulation with moderate ($PaCO_2 \sim 60$ mmHg) and severe ($PaCO_2 > 80$ mmHg) hypercapnia (i.e., permissive hypercapnia) [71]. However, other anesthetists have stated that a $PaCO_2$ above 70 mmHg is unacceptably high in most patients [72]. In a prospective study of elective clinical cases, no difference in cardiopulmonary function (including cardiac output measurements) between spontaneously and controlled ventilation groups could be demonstrated ($PaCO_2$ 50–60 mmHg in both groups) [73]. Yet others have reported cardiovascular function and muscle perfusion to be clearly worse with controlled ventilation in comparison with spontaneous breathing [74]. In clinical practice where cardiac output is usually not measured, it is sometimes difficult to decide whether controlled or spontaneous ventilation is best. In horses with poor cardiovascular function that cannot be stabilized before anesthesia, or in severely distended (and therefore suffering from reduced venous return anyhow) colic horses that are put in dorsal recumbency, it may be better to allow the horse to ventilate spontaneously and help maintain cardiac output. In athletic horses and thoroughbreds, mechanical ventilation is often necessary. Ventilation should be initiated soon after induction, with the goal of reducing the alveolar–arterial oxygen gradient change [75]. To optimize ventilation further, different positive end-expiratory pressure (PEEP) levels (10, 20 and 30 cmH_2O) have been used. Positive end-expiratory pressure reduced intrapulmonary shunt and increased functional residual capacity, but cardiac output was decreased and tissue oxygen delivery was lower when higher PEEP was used [76]. A more recent study combined PEEP (10 cmH_2O) with repetitive recruitment maneuvers (RM) in colic horses and compared it with IPPV ventilation without RM [77]. Arterial oxygenation was better with PEEP and RM but the influence of the technique on oxygen delivery was not evaluated as cardiac output was not measured. Continuous positive airway pressure (CPAP) in spontaneously breathing horses also increases arterial oxygenation, but its influence on oxygen delivery remains to be thoroughly evaluated [78].

Anesthesia recovery

Environmental considerations

For optimal recovery, it is important to provide the horse with a warm and quiet environment. For foals, the best recovery option may be in the stall with its mother (Fig. 46.1). It is usually not beneficial for horses to recover in a dimly lit recovery stall [79], but the eyes can be covered with a towel to reduce light stimuli if desired (Fig. 46.2). This allows the horse to see once it achieves sternal recumbency. Ear plugs (either commercially available or made of cotton) may reduce auditory stimuli or, more commonly, ambient noise is kept to a minimum. With the aid of a soft, deflatable pillow or mattress, horses can to some extent be discouraged from attempting to get up too early [80].

By allowing additional time for anesthetic drug elimination, better and more coordinated recoveries are usually achieved. Most horses do not tolerate well the endotracheal tube remaining in place once they regain consciousness, although different techniques have been used to attempt to maintain airway patency and allow oxygen administration during the recovery phase. Late extubation has some increased risk of laryngeal spasm and should be weighed against the benefit of maintaining an airway during recovery. In fasted horses, some clinicians prefer to extubate slightly before swallowing is expected (especially in young, difficult horses). The administration of 0.25% phenylephrine [81] into the nasal passages results in rapid local vasoconstriction, decongestion, and improved air flow. Upper airway obstruction may lead to pulmonary edema [82], possibly with fatal consequences. If there is any potential for upper airway obstruction (due to, for example, laryngeal surgery or

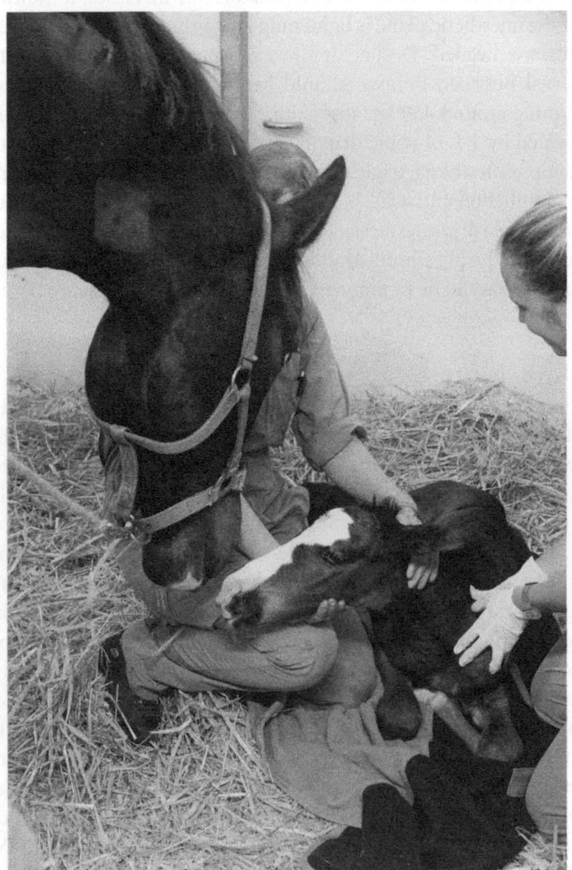

Figure 46.1 Foal recovering in the stall with its mother.

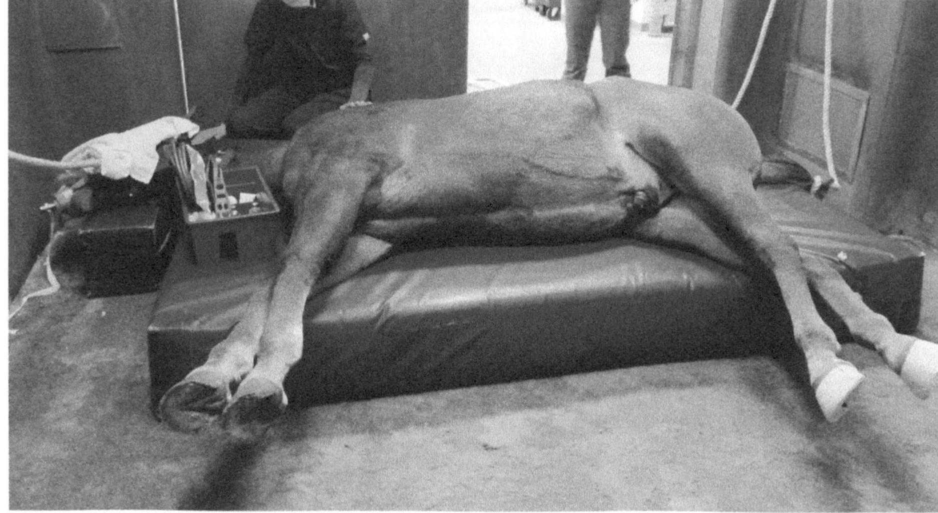

Figure 46.2 Horse positioned for recovery from general anesthesia. Source: Dr Tania Perez, Veterinary Teaching Hospital, Washington State University, Pullman, WA, USA. Reproduced with permission of Tania Perez.

long recumbency in combination with low plasma albumin concentration), the cuffed endotracheal tube can be fixed to the mandible and extubation takes place once the horse is standing. Care should be taken that nothing can be aspirated through the tube. If horses have a nasogastric tube in place (as is often the case with patients undergoing colic surgery), they should be removed before recovery to prevent complications [83].

Timing of recovery

The optimal timing of recovery is dependent on the anesthetic and the surgery performed. Recumbency is often irksome to the horse and is usually kept to a minimum. However, following anesthesia lasting 1 h or longer, a horse may take 30–45 min to eliminate the anesthetic adequately. Ideally, the horse assumes the sternal position and waits a further 10–15 min to stand up. If it chooses to remain in sternal recumbency longer, this is not harmful. However, if the horse is still in lateral recumbence after 60 min it should be carefully checked and necessary measures taken to minimize the risk of neuropathy or myopathy. If no reason is obvious why the horse is not getting up (or at least assuming a sternal position) by 60 min, hand clapping or other stimuli may persuade it to rise.

Additional sedation and analgesia

Optimal sedation and analgesia facilitate a good recovery. Even though all sedatives impair cardiopulmonary function to some extent, some horses will recover better with postanesthetic sedation. Most horses are not adversely affected by the cardiopulmonary effects of low doses of α_2-adrenergic receptor agonists, especially when administered as the effects of the anesthetics are rapidly disappearing. It has been clearly shown that α_2-adrenergic receptor agonists are beneficial [84] and the use of morphine (0.1 or 0.2 mg/kg, IM, given 20 min after anesthesia induction) also improves recovery quality [16]. Differences among recovery parameters between xylazine (0.1 mg/kg, IV), detomidine (2 μg/kg, IV), and romifidine (8 μg/kg, IV) were not demonstrated in one study utilizing research horses [84]. However, a clinical study in healthy horses comparing xylazine (0.1 or 0.2 mg/kg, IV) with romifidine (10 or 20 μg/kg, IV) following isoflurane anesthesia demonstrated that 20 μg/kg romifidine resulted in the best quality recoveries, and it was speculated that maybe even higher dose rates could be beneficial in difficult horses [85]. Some recent experimental studies have also investigated if a 15 30 min prolongation of anesthesia with ketamine or propofol in combination with xylazine after discontinuation of inhalant anesthetic administration would result in improved recovery [86–88]. In those studies, the use of injectable anesthesia at the end of anesthesia improved recovery quality; however, propofol combinations resulted in apnea and low arterial oxygenation, which was deemed a significant complication. A single bolus of xylazine in comparison with xylazine combined with ketamine following isoflurane anesthesia resulted in better recoveries in another group of experimental horses [5]. This study also tested acepromazine (0.02 mg/kg, IV), which resulted in a similar recovery quality to xylazine–ketamine. It remains to be studied scientifically in large numbers of clinical cases whether horses recover better with certain α_2-adrenergic receptor agonists or with injectable anesthetic combinations given towards the end of anesthesia. Such studies ideally would also include different dose ranges, ASA status groups, and surgery types.

The ideal time to administer the sedative is dependent on the drug used, as the time to achieve maximum effect of the different α_2-adrenergic receptor agonists differs (e.g., romifidine takes longer than xylazine) [89], the status and character of the horse, and the duration of anesthesia. If the sedative is given too early in recovery or at too high a dose (on top of significant levels of inhalant anesthetic that remain), spontaneous ventilation might be impaired. On the other hand, if a difficult horse has already started to move, it will be more difficult to prevent it from trying to get up with only a small bolus of an α_2-adrenergic receptor agonist. Of course, the optimum time point of administration of the sedative is also dependent on the inhalant anesthetic used, the use of other concurrent drugs, the duration and severity of the procedure, and the nature of the horse.

Following isoflurane or sevoflurane anesthesia, the horse can be allowed to breathe oxygen for about 3–5 min. When the first signs of a reduced depth of anesthesia become apparent (spontaneous blinking, slow nystagmus, increased respiratory rate), xylazine or medetomidine can be given. If romifidine is chosen, it is administered as soon as spontaneous breathing is present owing to the longer onset of effect. Horses that show nystagmus or limb movements can be given the sedative without delay.

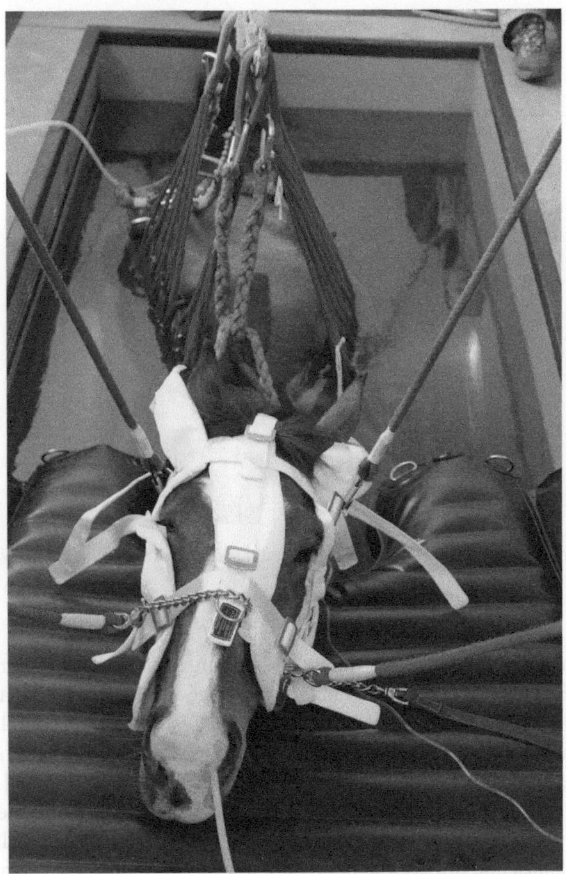

Figure 46.3 Horse recovering from general anesthesia in a hydropool.

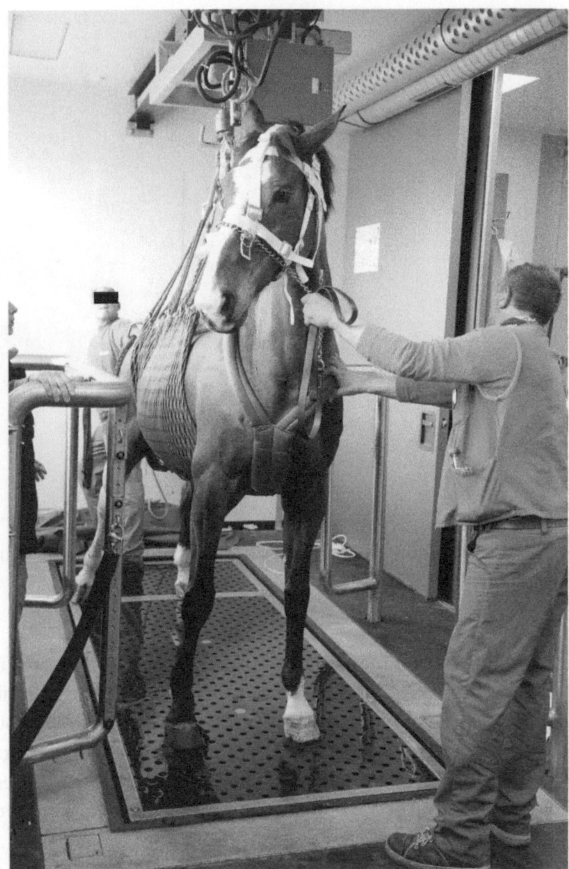

Figure 46.4 Standing horse after hydropool floor has been raised to ground level.

Morphine at a dose of 0.1 mg/kg also may improve recovery quality [16]. The administration of morphine intraoperatively does not consistently reduce inhalant MAC [15]. but can reduce arterial oxygenation in spontaneously breathing horses [16]. Therefore, some anesthetists prefer to administer morphine (0.1 mg/kg) intramuscularly 10 min before the end of surgery.

Recovery assist systems

Catastrophic injuries during recovery contribute about 30–50% of equine anesthetic fatalities. Horses with long bone fractures, very old horses, and exhausted horses (such as pregnant mares or horses with colic following extensive surgeries) often do not have the strength to get up on their feet safely and may require help. Several systems aimed at helping horses during this crucial phase have been tested. The decision whether to assist recovery or not should be made based on recovery box design, availability of trained personnel, availability of adequate assist systems, and on the horse itself.

Numerous systems have been described. Tail ropes with or without head ropes can be used to assist most horses [90]. Experienced personnel will aid in successful use since timing is important to avoid pulling the horse off balance. The ropes can be used to stabilize the horse, but should not be used to attempt to 'lift' it. For recovery of horses with specific concerns (e.g., long bone fractures), slings or nets have been used [91]. Ideally, the horses would be made accustomed to such devices before anesthesia to increase acceptance during recovery. The use of a tilt table has been described. This technique can be personnel and time intensive and not successful in every case [92]. Hydropools [93] (Figs 46.3 and 46.4) or pools with a raft system for the horse [94] are another option that is relatively safe for recovery of horses that are not capable of regaining a standing position without risk of severe injury.

References

1 Bidwell LA, Bramlage LR, Rood WA. Equine perioperative fatalities associated with general anaesthesia at a private practice – a retrospective case series. *Vet Anaesth Analg* 2007; **34**(1): 23–30.

2 Johnston GM. Confidential enquiry into perioperative equine fatalities. *Equine Vet Educ* 1991; **3**(1): 5–6.

3 Johnston GM. Findings from the CEPEF epidemiological studies into equine perioperative complications. *Equine Vet Educ* 2005; **15**(S7): 64–68.

4 Whitehair KJ, Steffey EP, Willits NH, Woliner MJ. Recovery of horses from inhalation anesthesia. *Am J Vet Res* 1993; **54**(10): 1693–1702.

5 Valverde A, Black B, Cribb NC, *et al.* Assessment of unassisted recovery from repeated general isoflurane anesthesia in horses following post-anesthetic administration of xylazine or acepromazine or a combination of xylazine and ketamine. *Vet Anaesth Analg* 2013; **40**(1): 3–12.

6 Hospes R, Bleul U. The effect of extended preoperative fasting in mares undergoing surgery of the perineal region. *J Equine Vet Sci* 2007; **27**(12): 542–545.

7 Murray MJ, Eichorn ES. Effects of intermittent feed deprivation, intermittent feed deprivation with ranitidine administration, and stall confinement with ad libitum access to hay on gastric ulceration in horses. *Am J Vet Res* 1996; **57**(11): 1599–1603.

8 Senior JM, Pinchbeck GL, Allister R, *et al.* Post anaesthetic colic in horses: a preventable complication? *Equine Vet J* 2006; **38**(5): 479–484.

9 Jones RS, Edwards GB, Brearley JC. Commentary on prolonged starvation as a factor associated with post operative colic. *Equine Vet Educ* 1991; **3**(1): 16–18.

10 Johnston GM, Eastment JK, Wood JLN, Taylor PM. The confidential enquiry into perioperative equine fatalities (CEPEF): mortality results of Phases 1 and 2. *Vet Anaesth Analg* 2002; **29**(4): 159–170.

11 Ringer SK, Schwarzwald CC, Portier KG, *et al.* Effects on cardiopulmonary function and oxygen delivery of doses of romifidine and xylazine followed by constant rate infusions in standing horses. *Vet J* 2013; **195**(2): 228–234.
12 Yamashita K, Tsubakishita S, Futaok S, *et al.* Cardiovascular effects of medetomidine, detomidine and xylazine in horses. *J Vet Med Sci* 2000; **62**(10): 1025–1032.
13 Ringer SK, Portier KG, Fourel I, Bettschart-Wolfensberger R. Development of a romifidine constant rate infusion with or without butorphanol for standing sedation of horses. *Vet Anaesth Analg* 2012; **39**(1): 12–20.
14 Ringer SK, Portier KG, Fourel I, Bettschart-Wolfensberger R. Development of a xylazine constant rate infusion with or without butorphanol for standing sedation of horses. *Vet Anaesth Analg* 2012; **39**(1): 1–11.
15 Bennett RC, Steffey EP. Use of opioids for pain and anesthetic management in horses. *Vet Clin North Am Equine Pract* 2002; **18**(1): 47–60.
16 Love EJ, Lane JG, Murison PJ. Morphine administration in horses anaesthetized for upper respiratory tract surgery. *Vet Anaesth Analg* 2006; **33**(3): 179–188.
17 Daunt DA, Dunlop CI, Chapman PL, *et al.* Cardiopulmonary and behavioral responses to computer-driven infusion of detomidine in standing horses. *Am J Vet Res* 1993; **54**(12): 2075–2082.
18 Edner A, Nyman G, Essén-Gustavsson B. The relationship of muscle perfusion and metabolism with cardiovascular variables before and after detomidine injection during propofol–ketamine anaesthesia in horses. *Vet Anaesth Analg* 2002; **29**(4): 182–199.
19 Raisis AL. Skeletal muscle blood flow in anaesthetized horses. Part II. Effects of anaesthetics and vasoactive agents. *Vet Anaesth Analg* 2005; **32**(6): 331–337.
20 Herschl MA, Trim CM, Mahaffey EA. Effects of 5% and 10% guaifenesin infusion on equine vascular endothelium. *Vet Surg* 1992; **21**(6): 494–497.
21 Muir WW, Lerche P, Erichson D. Anaesthetic and cardiorespiratory effects of propofol at 10% for induction and 1% for maintenance of anaesthesia in horses. *Equine Vet J* 2009; **41**(6): 578–585.
22 Brosnan RJ, Steffey EP, Escobar A, *et al.* Anesthetic induction with guaifenesin and propofol in adult horses. *Am J Vet Res* 2011; **72**(12): 1569–1575.
23 Keates HL, van Eps AW, Pearson MR. Alfaxalone compared with ketamine for induction of anaesthesia in horses following xylazine and guaifenesin. *Vet Anaesth Analg* 2012; **39**(6): 591–598.
24 Feary DJ, Mama KR, Wagner AE, Thomasy S. Influence of general anesthesia on pharmacokinetics of intravenous lidocaine infusion in horses. *Am J Vet Res* 2005; **66**(4): 574–580.
25 Feary DJ, Mama KR, Thomasy SM, *et al.* Influence of gastrointestinal tract disease on pharmacokinetics of lidocaine after intravenous infusion in anesthetized horses. *Am J Vet Res* 2006; **67**(2): 317–322.
26 Lankveld DP, Driessen B, Soma LR, *et al.* Pharmacodynamic effects and pharmacokinetic profile of a long-term continuous rate infusion of racemic ketamine in healthy conscious horses. *J Vet Pharmacol Ther* 2006; **29**(6): 477–488.
27 Enderle AK, Levionnois OL, Kuhn M, Schatzmann U. Clinical evaluation of ketamine and lidocaine intravenous infusions to reduce isoflurane requirements in horses under general anaesthesia. *Vet Anaesth Analg* 2008; **35**(4): 297–305.
28 Kempchen S, Kuhn M, Spadavecchia C, Levionnois OL. Medetomidine continuous rate intravenous infusion in horses in which surgical anaesthesia is maintained with isoflurane and intravenous infusions of lidocaine and ketamine. *Vet Anaesth Analg* 2012; **39**(3): 245–255.
29 Kushiro T, Yamashita K, Umar MA, *et al.* Anesthetic and cardiovascular effects of balanced anesthesia using constant rate infusion of midazolam–ketamine–medetomidine with inhalation of oxygen–sevoflurane (MKM-OS anesthesia) in horses. *J Vet Med Sci* 2005; **67**(4): 379–384.
30 Villalba M, Santiago I, Gomez de Segura IA. Effects of constant rate infusion of lidocaine and ketamine, with or without morphine, on isoflurane MAC in horses. *Equine Vet J* 2011; **43**(6): 721–726.
31 Valverde A. Balanced anesthesia and constant-rate infusions in horses. *Vet Clin North Am Equine Pract* 2013; **29**(1): 89–122.
32 Bettschart-Wolfensberger R, Jaggin-Schmucker N, Lendl C, *et al.* Minimal alveolar concentration of desflurane in combination with an infusion of medetomidine for the anaesthesia of ponies. *Vet Rec* 2001; **148**(9): 264–267.
33 Gozalo-Marcilla M, Hopster K, Gasthuys F, *et al.* Effects of a constant-rate infusion of dexmedetomidine on the minimal alveolar concentration of sevoflurane in ponies. *Equine Vet J* 2013; **45**(2): 204–208.
34 Devisscher L, Schauvliege S, Dewulf J, Gasthuys F. Romifidine as a constant rate infusion in isoflurane anaesthetized horses: a clinical study. *Vet Anaesth Analg* 2010; **37**(5): 425–433.
35 Wagner AE, Dunlop CI, Heath RB, *et al.* Hemodynamic function during neurectomy in halothane-anesthetized horses with or without constant dose detomidine infusion. *Vet Surg* 1992; **21**(3): 248–255.
36 Kuhn M, Köhler L, Fenner A, *et al.* Isofluran-Reduktion und Beeinflussung kardiovaskulärer und pulmonaler Parameter durch kontinuierliche Romifidin-Infusion während der Narkose bei Pferden – Eine klinische Studie. *Pferdeheilkunde* 2004; **20**(6): 511–516.
37 Ringer SK, Kalchofner K, Boller J, *et al.* A clinical comparison of two anaesthetic protocols using lidocaine or medetomidine in horses. *Vet Anaesth Analg* 2007; **34**(4): 257–268.
38 Valverde A, Rickey E, Sinclair M, *et al.* Comparison of cardiovascular function and quality of recovery in isoflurane-anaesthetised horses administered a constant rate infusion of lidocaine or lidocaine and medetomidine during elective surgery. *Equine Vet J* 2010; **42**(3): 192–199.
39 Bettschart-Wolfensberger R, Bettschart R, Vainio O, Marlin D. Cardiopulmonary effects of a two hour infusion of medetomidine and its reversal by atipamezole in horses and ponies. *Vet Anaesth Analg* 1999; **26**: 8–12.
40 Marcilla MG, Schauvliege S, Segaert S, *et al.* Influence of a constant rate infusion of dexmedetomidine on cardiopulmonary function and recovery quality in isoflurane anaesthetized horses. *Vet Anaesth Analg* 2012; **39**(1): 49–58.
41 Bettschart-Wolfensberger R, Dicht S, Vullo C, *et al.* A clinical study on the effect in horses during medetomidine–isoflurane anaesthesia, of butorphanol constant rate infusion on isoflurane requirements, on cardiopulmonary function and on recovery characteristics. *Vet Anaesth Analg* 2011; **38**(3): 186–194.
42 Gozalo-Marcilla M, Hopster K, Gasthuys F, *et al.* Minimum end-tidal sevoflurane concentration necessary to prevent movement during a constant rate infusion of morphine, or morphine plus dexmedetomidine in ponies. *Vet Anaesth Analg* 2014; **41**(2): 212–219.
43 Doherty TJ, Seddighi MR. Local anesthetics as pain therapy in horses. *Vet Clin North Am Equine Pract* 2010; **26**(3): 533–549.
44 Sinclair M, Valverde A. Short-term anaesthesia with xylazine, diazepam/ketamine for castration in horses under field conditions: use of intravenous lidocaine. *Equine Vet J* 2009; **41**(2): 149–152.
45 Doherty TJ, Frazier DL. Effect of intravenous lidocaine on halothane minimum alveolar concentration in ponies. *Equine Vet J* 1998; **30**: 300–303.
46 Dzikiti TB, Hellebrekers LJ, Dijk P. Effects of intravenous lidocaine on isoflurane concentration, physiological parameters, metabolic parameters and stress-related hormones in horses undergoing surgery. *J Vet Med A* 2003; **50**(4): 190–195.
47 Rezende ML, Wagner AE, Mama KR, *et al.* Effects of intravenous administration of lidocaine on the minimum alveolar concentration of sevoflurane in horses. *Am J Vet Res* 2011; **72**(4): 446–451.
48 Meyer GA, Lin HC, Hanson RR, Hayes TL. Effects of intravenous lidocaine overdose on cardiac electrical activity and blood pressure in the horse. *Equine Vet J* 2001; **33**(5): 434–437.
49 Valverde A, Gunkel C, Doherty TJ, *et al.* Effect of a constant rate infusion of lidocaine on the quality of recovery from sevoflurane or isoflurane general anaesthesia in horses. *Equine Vet J* 2005; **37**(6): 559–564.
50 Muir WW. NMDA receptor antagonists and pain: ketamine. *Vet Clin North Am Equine Pract* 2010; **26**(3): 565–578.
51 Larenza MP, Ringer SK, Kutter AP, *et al.* Evaluation of anesthesia recovery quality after low-dose racemic or S-ketamine infusions during anesthesia with isoflurane in horses. *Am J Vet Res* 2009; **70**(6): 710–718.
52 Thomasy SM, Steffey EP, Mama KR, *et al.* The effects of i.v. fentanyl administration on the minimum alveolar concentration of isoflurane in horses. *Br J Anaesth* 2006; **97**(2): 232–237.
53 Knych HKD, Steffey EP, Mama KR, Stanley SD. Effects of high plasma fentanyl concentrations on minimum alveolar concentration of isoflurane in horses. *Am J Vet Res* 2009; **70**(10): 1193–1200.
54 Matthews NS, Dollar NS, Shawley RV. Halothane-sparing effect of benzodiazepines in ponies. *Cornell Vet* 1990; **80**(3): 259–265.
55 Yamashita K, Satoh M, Umikawa A, *et al.* Combination of continuous intravenous infusion using a mixture of guaifenesin–ketamine–medetomidine and sevoflurane anesthesia in horses. *J Vet Med Sci* 2000; **62**(3): 229–235.
56 Valverde A. Balanced anesthesia and constant-rate infusions in horses. *Vet Clin North Am Equine Pract* 2013; **29**(1): 89–122.
57 McMurphy RM, Young LE, Marlin DJ, Walsh K. Comparison of the cardiopulmonary effects of anesthesia maintained by continuous infusion of romifidine, guaifenesin, and ketamine with anesthesia maintained by inhalation of halothane in horses. *Am J Vet Res* 2002; **63**(12): 1655–1661.
58 Taylor PM, Luna SP, Sear JW, Wheeler MJ. Total intravenous anaesthesia in ponies using detomidine, ketamine and guaiphenesin: pharmacokinetics, cardiopulmonary and endocrine effects. *Res Vet Sci* 1995; **59**(1): 17–23.
59 McCarty JE, Trim CM, Ferguson D. Prolongation of anesthesia with xylazine, ketamine, and guaifenesin in horses: 64 cases (1986–1989). *J Am Vet Med Assoc* 1990; **197**(12): 1646–1650.
60 Greene SA, Thurmon JC, Tranquilli WJ, Benson GJ. Cardiopulmonary effects of continuous intravenous infusion of guaifenesin, ketamine and xylazine in ponies. *Am J Vet Res* 1986; **47**(11): 2364–2367.
61 Davidson GS. Equine anesthesia: triple drip. *Int J Pharm Compd* 2008; **12**(5): 402–404.

62 Edner AH, Essén-Gustavsson B, Nyman GC. Metabolism during anaesthesia and recovery in colic and healthy horses: a microdialysis study. *Acta Vet Scand* 2009; **51**(1): 10.

63 Raisis AL. Skeletal muscle blood flow in anaesthetized horses. Part I: measurement techniques. *Vet Anaesth Analg* 2005; **32**(6): 324–330.

64 Duke T, Filzek U, Read MR, *et al.* Clinical observations surrounding an increased incidence of postanesthetic myopathy in halothane-anesthetized horses. *Vet Anaesth Analg* 2006; **33**(2): 122–127.

65 Dodman NH, Williams R, Court MH, Norman WM. Postanesthetic hind limb adductor myopathy in five horses. *J Am Vet Med Assoc* 1988; **193**(1): 83–86.

66 Grandy JL, Steffey EP, Hodgson DS, Woliner MJ. Arterial hypotension and the development of postanesthetic myopathy in halothane-anesthetized horses. *Am J Vet Res* 1987; **48**(2): 192–197.

67 Brosnan RJ. Inhaled anesthetics in horses. *Vet Clin North Am Equine Pract* 2013; **29**(1): 69–87.

68 Schauvliege S, Gasthuys F. Drugs for cardiovascular support in anesthetized horses. *Vet Clin North Am Equine Pract* 2013; **29**(1): 19–49.

69 Light GS, Hellyer PW. Effects of atropine on the arrhythmogenic dose of dobutamine in xylazine–thiamylal–halothane-anesthetized horses. *Am J Vet Res* 1993; **54**(12): 2099–2103.

70 Day TK, Gaynor J, Muir WW, *et al.* Blood gas values during intermittent positive pressure ventilation and spontaneous ventilation in 160 anesthetized horses positioned in lateral or dorsal recumbency. *Vet Surg* 1995; **24**: 266–276.

71 Khanna AK, McDonell WN, Dyson DH, Taylor PM. Cardiopulmonary effects of hypercapnia during controlled intermittent positive pressure ventilation in the horse. *Can J Vet Res* 1995; **59**(3): 213–221.

72 Moens Y. Mechanical ventilation and respiratory mechanics during equine anesthesia. *Vet Clin North Am Equine Pract* 2013; **29**(1): 51–67.

73 Kalchofner KS, Picek S, Ringer SK, *et al.* A study of cardiovascular function under controlled and spontaneous ventilation in isoflurane–medetomidine anaesthetized horses. *Vet Anaesth Analg* 2009; **36**(5): 426–435.

74 Edner A, Nyman G, Essén-Gustavsson B. The effects of spontaneous and mechanical ventilation on central cardiovascular function and peripheral perfusion during isoflurane anaesthesia in horses. *Vet Anaesth Analg* 2005; **32**(3): 136–146.

75 Nyman G, Funkquist B, Kvart C, *et al.* Atelectasis causes gas exchange impairment in the anaesthetised horse. *Equine Vet J* 1990; **22**(5): 317–324.

76 Wilson DV, Soma LR. Cardiopulmonary effects of positive end-expiratory pressure in anesthetized, mechanically ventilated ponies. *Am J Vet Res* 1990; **51**(5): 734–739.

77 Hopster K, Kastner SB, Rohn K, Ohnesorge B. Intermittent positive pressure ventilation with constant positive end-expiratory pressure and alveolar recruitment manoeuvre during inhalation anaesthesia in horses undergoing surgery for colic, and its influence on the early recovery period. *Vet Anaesth Analg* 2011; **38**(3): 169–177.

78 Mosing M, Rysnik M, Bardell D, *et al.* Use of continuous positive airway pressure (CPAP) to optimise oxygenation in anaesthetised horses – a clinical study. *Equine Vet J* 2013; **45**(4): 414–418.

79 Clark-Price SC, Posner LP, Gleed RD. Recovery of horses from general anesthesia in a darkened or illuminated recovery stall. *Vet Anaesth Analg* 2008; **35**(6): 473–479.

80 Ray-Miller WM, Hodgson DS, McMurphy RM, Chapman PL. Comparison of recoveries from anesthesia of horses placed on a rapidly inflating–deflating air pillow or the floor of a padded stall. *J Am Vet Med Assoc* 2006; **229**(5): 711–716.

81 Lukasik VM, Gleed RD, Scarlett JM, *et al.* Intranasal phenylephrine reduces post anesthetic upper airway obstruction in horses. *Equine Vet J* 1997; **29**(3): 236–238.

82 Senior M. Post-anaesthetic pulmonary oedema in horses: a review. *Vet Anaesth Analg* 2005; **32**(4): 193–200.

83 Veres-Nyéki KO, Graubner C, Aloisio F, Spadavecchia C. Pulmonary edema at recovery after colic operation with in-situ nasogastric tube in a horse. *Schweiz Arch Tierheilkd* 2011; **153**(9): 401–404.

84 Santos M, Fuente M, Garcia-Iturralde R, *et al.* Effects of alpha-2 adrenoceptor agonists during recovery from isoflurane anaesthesia in horses. *Equine Vet J* 2003; **35**(2): 170–175.

85 Woodhouse KJ, Brosnan RJ, Nguyen KQ, *et al.* Effects of postanesthetic sedation with romifidine or xylazine on quality of recovery from isoflurane anesthesia in horses. *J Am Vet Med Assoc* 2013; **242**(4): 533–539.

86 Wagner AE, Mama KR, Steffey EP, Hellyer PW. Evaluation of infusions of xylazine with ketamine or propofol to modulate recovery following sevoflurane anesthesia in horses. *Am J Vet Res* 2012; **73**(3): 346–352.

87 Wagner AE, Mama KR, Steffey EP, Hellyer PW. A comparison of equine recovery characteristics after isoflurane or isoflurane followed by a xylazine–ketamine infusion. *Vet Anaesth Analg* 2008; **35**(2): 154–160.

88 Steffey EP, Mama KR, Brosnan RJ, *et al.* Effect of administration of propofol and xylazine hydrochloride on recovery of horses after four hours of anesthesia with desflurane. *Am J Vet Res* 2009; **70**(8): 956–963.

89 Ringer SK, Portier K, Torgerson PR, *et al.* The effects of a loading dose followed by constant rate infusion of xylazine compared with romifidine on sedation, ataxia and response to stimuli in horses. *Vet Anaesth Analg* 2013; **40**(2): 157–165.

90 Wilderjans H. The 1 man rope assisted recovery from anaesthesia in horses. Presented at the 10th International Congress of the World Equine Veterinary Association, Moscow, 2008.

91 Steffey EP, Brosnan RJ, Galuppo LD, *et al.* Use of propofol–xylazine and the Anderson Sling Suspension System for recovery of horses from desflurane anesthesia. *Vet Surg* 2009; **38**(8): 927–933.

92 Elmas CR, Cruz AM, Kerr CL. Tilt table recovery of horses after orthopedic surgery: fifty-four cases (1994–2005). *Vet Surg* 2007; **36**(3): 252–258.

93 Picek S, Kalchofner KS, Ringer SK, *et al.* Anaesthetic management for hydropool recovery in 50 horses. *Pferdeheilkunde* 2010; **26**(4): 515–522.

94 Sullivan EK, Klein LV, Richardson DW, *et al.* Use of a pool–raft system for recovery of horses from general anesthesia: 393 horses (1984–2000). *J Am Vet Med Assoc* 2002; **221**(7): 1014–1018.

47 Horses with Colic

Cynthia M. Trim[1] **and Molly K. Shepard**[2]

[1]Department of Large Animal Medicine, College of Veterinary Medicine, University of Georgia, Athens, Georgia, USA
[2]University of Georgia, Athens, Georgia, USA

Chapter contents

Introduction

Colic has been defined as acute abdominal pain localized in a hollow organ and often caused by spasm, obstruction, or twisting. Although abdominal pain may have other etiologies, colic in horses most often refers to abdominal pain of gastrointestinal (GI) origin. An epidemiologic survey of colic in the United States from 1998 to 1999 documented an incidence of 4.2 colic events per 100 horses per year, amounting to an annual cost of approximately $115 300 000 [1].

This chapter discusses the anesthetic management of horses with colic using a combination of the authors' experiences and published information. Some information from publications before 2000 that were cited in the corresponding chapter (Chapter 51) in the previous edition of this book has been assigned a single reference [2].

Survival rates

Colic related to GI disease is one of the most significant causes of morbidity and mortality in horses, with a reported incidence from 3.5 to 10.6 cases per 100 horses per year [1,3,4]. Tinker *et al.* reported that colic was responsible for nearly one-third of all reported deaths in a population of 1427 horses [4]. Despite the grim statistics, published surveys have confirmed that survival rates of horses undergoing surgery for colic have improved over the past three decades [2,5].

Progress towards increased survival rates may be attributed to changes in medical, surgical, and anesthetic management. Horses with proximal duodenitis–jejunitis, for example, have been found to have a higher survival rate after medical management than after anesthesia and surgery [6]. Likewise, conservative treatment of horses with renosplenic entrapment resulted in a significantly higher survival rate than surgical treatment [7]. Removal of these horses from the surgical statistics contributes to improved short-term survival rates.

Higher mortality rates occur in horses with strangulating bowel disease compared with non-strangulating disease, and in horses with devitalized bowel compared with non-devitalized bowel [8–10]. The greater the length of non-viable small intestine that was resected, the higher was the mortality rate reported [11]. In one study, horses with non-strangulating lesions were 3.9 times more likely to survive anesthesia and recovery [12].

Persisting associations with decreased survival are the measurement of higher than normal packed cell volume (PCV) [8,10,11,13–16] or heart rate (HR) [14,17,18] before anesthesia, presumably reflections of the severity of the metabolic abnormalities. Elevated PCV and HR may be consequences of hypovolemia, endotoxemia, pain, anxiety, and/or splenic contraction. Endotoxin has been detected in plasma following small intestinal strangulation obstruction in anesthetized experimental ponies and in patients at hospital admission [2,19]. Endotoxin may also be released into the circulation during surgery [20].

Endotoxemia and the systemic inflammatory response

Endotoxin includes the lipid-A portion of lipopolysaccharide (LPS), a component of Gram-negative bacterial cell walls normally

Veterinary Anesthesia and Analgesia: The Fifth Edition of Lumb and Jones.
Edited by Kurt A. Grimm, Leigh A. Lamont, William J. Tranquilli, Stephen A. Greene and Sheilah A. Robertson.

found within the equine intestine. Disruption of GI mucosal barriers by ischemia leads to movement of LPS into the peritoneal cavity and eventually uptake into the systemic circulation. Endotoxin stimulates an acute phase response and the release of inflammatory mediators such as tumor necrosis factor (TNF-α), interleukin-1 (IL-1) and interleukin-6 (IL-6).

Significance of endotoxemia

Circulation of these toxins and inflammatory compounds represents an important risk factor for mortality in horses that develop colic [21]. Amplification of this process leads to a systemic inflammatory response syndrome (SIRS) manifested as tachycardia, tachypnea, alterations in body temperature, and leucopenia or leukocytosis. SIRS has been defined in foals as the presence of two or more of the following conditions: HR >120 beats/min, respiratory rate >30 breaths/min, rectal temperature >39.2°C (102.6°F) or <37.2°C (99.0°F), white blood cell (WBC) count >12 500 or <4000 cells/μL, or >10% immature 'band' neutrophils, and evidence of sepsis, cerebral ischemia or hypoxia, or trauma [22]. An adaptation has been used in adult horses: HR ≥60 beats/min, respiratory rate ≥30 breaths/min, body temperature ≥38.6°C (101.5°F), WBC count ≥12 500 or ≤4500 cells/μL, and ≥10% band neutrophils [23].

Additional clinical signs attributable to the inflammatory response depend on the magnitude of endotoxemia and the subsequent inflammatory cascade. Studies in many species have demonstrated that early septic shock is characterized by a hyperdynamic cardiovascular system, specifically tachycardia, vasodilation, and increased cardiac index (CI), whereas CI is decreased in more advanced (decompensated) septic shock [24–27]. Progression of SIRS in horses includes leak of protein from the vasculature into the abdominal cavity, which lowers the circulating colloid osmotic pressure (COP) and may contribute to decreased peripheral perfusion.

Coagulation abnormalities are common in horses with colic. Endotoxin activates circulating monocytes to release thromboplastin-like procoagulants that may initiate microvascular thrombi [2]. Coagulation abnormalities such as decreased antithrombin III (ATIII) activity, increased fibrinogen degradation product (FDP) titers, and thrombocytopenia occur in higher frequency in horses with small intestinal lesions compared with large intestinal lesions or those with colitis. Abnormalities of coagulation are more frequent in horses with devitalized bowel compared with horses without devitalized bowel [28].

Medical management of endotoxemia

While supportive therapy remains the mainstay for endotoxemia and SIRS, management of these horses may include treatments that specifically target endotoxin and the inflammatory cascade. Treatments include hyperimmune plasma, polymyxin B, flunixin meglumine, dimethyl sulfoxide, pentoxifylline, heparin, and lidocaine.

Hyperimmune plasma is an intravenous (IV) therapy containing a high concentration of antiendotoxin antibodies that directly bind endotoxin [29]. Polymyxin B is a bacterial antimicrobial with a predominantly Gram-negative spectrum of activity, which at lower doses also directly binds the lipid-A component of LPS. In an equine model of induced endotoxemia, polymyxin B decreased TNF-1α, fever, and tachycardia, whether administered before or after the administration of LPS [30]. Polymyxin B may be selected for horses with focal sources of LPS release, such as ischemic bowel, and ideally is administered before releasing strangulated bowel. Nephrotoxicity and neurotoxicity are potential side-effects [31], but the recommendation to withhold polymyxin B from azotemic horses remains controversial as many horses with endotoxemia have prerenal azotemia associated with hypovolemia. As no report exists substantiating these concerns, the recommendation is for cautious use of polymyxin B in azotemic horses with colic [30].

In addition to its efficacy as a visceral analgesic, flunixin meglumine inhibits cyclooxygenase, thereby decreasing the release of thromboxane and prostaglandin F-1α (PGF-1α). When administered prior to LPS in experimental endotoxemia in horses, flunixin decreased HR, rectal temperature, and attitude score compared with horses administered saline after LPS [2]. Unfortunately, flunixin appears to increase the permeability of ischemic-injured jejunum to LPS and impairs recovery of barrier function [32,33]. Deracoxib and firocoxib are non-steroidal anti-inflammatory drugs (NSAIDs) that may not inhibit the recovery of barrier function in the jejunum [33]. Experimental studies have also demonstrated that some NSAIDs, including flunixin, inhibit intestinal motility.

Pentoxifylline is a xanthine derivative with limited clinical effects in horses when administered alone prior to an *in vivo* LPS challenge. Pentoxifylline injected immediately after endotoxin in experimental horses resulted in significantly lower respiratory rates and rectal temperatures, and the whole blood recalcification time (a measure of endotoxin-related coagulopathy) was longer [2]. When paired with flunixin meglumine, however, pentoxifylline resulted in significantly lower leukocyte counts, in addition to rectal temperature, pulse rate, PGF-1α and thromboxane B_2 concentrations in models of induced endotoxemia [2].

Dimethyl sulfoxide (DMSO) is a colorless, organosulfur liquid used as a solvent in several medicinal preparations owing to its ability to dissolve both polar and non-polar compounds. Although it traditionally has been given to ameliorate reperfusion injury, no studies support its efficacy as a free radical scavenger. IV administration of DMSO reduced fever in horses with experimentally induced endotoxemia, but had no effect on plasma TNF-1α, glucose, or lactate concentrations, WBC count, or HR [34].

Administration of lidocaine by IV infusion is a useful adjunct therapy in horses with colic owing to its ability to scavenge free radical species and function as an anti-inflammatory agent to some extent. Lidocaine may be considered a specific treatment for postischemic reperfusion injury in horses with ischemic GI lesions. In one *in vitro* study in human patients, lidocaine inhibited the metabolic function of neutrophils in a dose-dependent manner, thereby inhibiting the inflammatory cascade [35]. More recent investigations of experimentally induced jejunal ischemia documented that lidocaine infusion during anesthesia reduced markers of inflammation, including PGE_2 concentration and mucosal COX-2 expression [32,36]. Lidocaine may also preserve GI motility by protecting smooth muscle against the deleterious effects of reperfusion injury [37,38].

When coagulation abnormalities are suspected, administration of heparin may be indicated for its ability to deactivate thrombin and factor Xa, an effect that may prevent fibrin formation and inhibit thrombin-induced activation of platelets and factors V and VIII. Unfractionated heparin therapy is not without adverse side-effects, as it decreases PCV, prolongs activated partial thromboplastin time (aPTT) and thrombin time (TT), and increases the prevalence of jugular vein thrombosis. Low molecular weight heparin, a compound with less antithrombin and more antifactor Xa activity, has been cited as a favorable, albeit costly, alternative with respect to potential side-effects [39].

Pattern recognition receptors (PRRs) include Toll-like receptors and others that are present on cell surfaces and in intracellular structures [40]. These receptors must be activated for bacterial infections to be eliminated but overstimulation leads to systemic inflammation. Toll-like receptor 4 (TLR4) plays a significant role in equine endotoxemia and it is possible that in the future antagonists of the TLR4–myeloid differentiation protein-2 (MD2) receptor complex may be developed for therapeutic use [40].

Influence of anesthesia and surgery

The duration of anesthesia has been inversely associated with survival rate in several investigations [8,13,41,42]. Horses that survived surgical treatment for colic had significantly shorter anesthesia times than horses that died or were subsequently euthanized. This association with outcome may reflect an adverse impact of anesthesia and/or increased complexity of the surgical procedure.

Pregnant mares

Management of pregnant mares with colic includes the added concern for fetal mortality. In a review of 228 pregnant Thoroughbred mares requiring surgery for colic, 152 (66.7%) had a live foal compared with 78.3% in mares without colic [43]. The prognosis for a live foal after colic surgery was significantly better in mares ≤15 years old or with ≥40 days of gestation. Live foals were less likely when the duration of colic before surgery was >5 h and anesthesia duration >3 h [5,42,44].

In another review of 153 pregnant mares, of light horse and draft breeds, 46 (30%) either aborted or delivered a dead foal after surgery, significantly more often than for mares medically treated for colic [44]. Intraoperative hypotension, mean arterial pressure (MAP) <70 mmHg, was associated with a higher foal mortality, particularly when the mare was in the last 60 days of gestation. Supplementation with progesterone after anesthesia had no association with foaling rate.

Effect of anesthetic agents on gastrointestinal function

The features and regulation of equine GI motility have been described in detail [45,46]. Investigations in horses have utilized a variety of techniques, including surgically implanted bipolar Ag/AgCl or stainless-steel electrodes sutured to the mucosa at various levels in the intestinal tract, insertion of catheters with pressure-tipped sensors through a gastric cannula and guided with an endoscope into the intestine, and measurement of pressure changes in intraluminal balloons. The duration of gastric emptying and intestinal transit time have been measured using timed movement of non-absorbable markers such as radiolabeled substances, barium-impregnated spheres, phenol red, and solubilized acetaminophen. The markers are instilled into the stomach via a nasogastric (NG) tube or chronically implanted gastric cannulas.

Some investigations have included collection of feces for several days after a specific treatment. Decreased fecal output may not be of great significance as it is not always associated with clinical signs of abdominal discomfort. Abdominal auscultation of intestinal motility or computer analysis of abdominal sounds and measurement of defecation frequency have been used in many investigations, although the techniques have considerable variability [46]. Drug effects on contractility of muscle strips of intestine *in vitro* have been studied but the results do not always predict the effects observed *in vivo*. Intestinal blood flow has been measured using ultrasonic blood flow probes implanted during a previous experimental surgery.

Interpretation of any experimental data is complicated by the fact that different parts of the GI tract respond differently to any given drug, and that treatment-induced effects in healthy experimental horses may not be the same as those in horses with GI disease.

Xylazine causes significant dose-dependent decreases in duodenal, jejunal, cecal, and colonic activity in horses [47–50], and this effect is magnified when xylazine is combined with either butorphanol or buprenorphine [49–51]. Detomidine decreases motility to a greater extent and for longer duration than xylazine [49]. Measurements of activity in the small intestine, cecum, and left ventral colon confirmed significantly decreased frequency of contractions for 30 min after romifidine at a dose of 0.08 mg/kg [52]. Butorphanol has a mild and transient effect on motility at low dosages; however, significantly decreased intestinal motility for 60 min and decreased GI transit time for several hours have been measured in healthy horses following a higher dosage (0.1 mg/kg) [53]. Butorphanol may be administered as a continuous infusion to maintain a steady state. Administration of a loading dose, 0.018 mg/kg, followed by continuous IV infusion at 0.024 mg/kg/h in healthy horses significantly slowed the GI transit time [poly(ethylene glycol) marker], and the horses passed significantly less feces in the 24 h of treatment and in the following 24 h than control horses [53].

In clinical practice, morphine administered as a single high dose, 0.6 mg/kg, with xylazine for sedation in standing horses results in ileus in some horses several hours later. Administration of naloxone IV results in return of intestinal sounds within 5 min. In healthy experimental horses, morphine administered at 0.5 mg/kg IV every 12 h for 6 days caused intestinal stasis and significantly decreased the number of bowel movements in the 6 h following administration, and decreased the volume of feces produced in 24 h [54]. Some horses showed signs of abdominal discomfort.

Lower doses of morphine, 0.1–0.2 mg/kg, are more commonly administered during anesthesia in horses. Morphine sulfate, 0.05 and 0.10 mg/kg, administered once IM or IV to healthy awake horses resulted in significantly decreased GI motility scores obtained by abdominal auscultation at 1 h after administration for all doses and for 2 h after 0.1 mg/kg IV, although no signs of discomfort were observed [55]. Retrospective studies of clinical patients anesthetized for procedures unrelated to GI disease both have [56] and have not [57] identified increased prevalence of colic after anesthesia in horses receiving morphine. One study reported that out of 496 anesthetic episodes, 14 horses developed colic within 7 days and all but one received morphine, 0.1 mg/kg, during anesthesia [56]. In another retrospective study of 533 anesthetics, 20 horses developed colic within 7 days [57]. Morphine, 0.1–0.15 mg/kg, was administered to 44% of all horses before or during anesthesia, including 14 of the horses that developed colic. Other potential risk factors for postanesthetic colic identified in this study, of which 62% involved anesthesia for magnetic resonance imaging (MRI) and 38% for non-abdominal surgery, included surgery and the use of isoflurane as a maintenance anesthetic agent (71% of total anesthetic episodes). The substantially lower prevalence of colic in horses anesthetized for MRI may have been due to the maintenance of a lighter plane of anesthesia and absence of pain in recovery. The results of these studies were likely influenced by other factors that predispose horses to colic, such as recent changes in diet or management, recent transport, pain or anxiety, other anesthetic agents, and NSAIDs.

Fentanyl may be administered by IV injection, by IV infusion, or from a transdermal patch. Fentanyl has a marked depressant effect on motility, an effect that may be due to its anticholinergic effects. Fentanyl, 0.01 and 0.05 mg/kg, IV induced a significant inhibition of propulsive activity at the cecocolic segment and closure of the cecocolic sphincter for 1–2 h [58].

Alvimopan is administered to human patients after intestinal resection and appears to shorten the time to return of normal GI function and decrease hospitalization time [59]. This peripherally acting μ-opioid antagonist does not cross the blood–brain barrier to alter centrally mediated analgesia but will antagonize peripheral opioid effects, such as depression of GI motility. A crossover study in healthy horses evaluated morphine, 0.5 mg/kg, administered IV every 12 h for six consecutive days with or without another peripherally acting opioid antagonist, *N*-methylnaltrexone, 0.75 mg/kg [60]. Barium spheres were used to facilitate the measurement of fecal production and confirmed that *N*-methylnaltrexone attenuated the GI depression from morphine. Similarly, a peripheral α_2-adrenergic receptor antagonist, MK-467, prevented decreased intestinal motility (determined by abdominal auscultation) without altering sedation induced by detomidine in healthy horses [61]. Further evaluation of the use of peripherally acting opioid and α_2-adrenergic antagonists in horses may provide useful information for the anesthetic management of horses with colic.

A difference between inhalation agents was detected in horses anesthetized for arthroscopic surgery where abdominal auscultation of intestinal sounds and evaluation of GI transit time using chromium markers revealed a more rapid return of GI motility after isoflurane than after halothane anesthesia [62]. In human patients undergoing laparoscopic surgery, when anesthetized with either sevoflurane or desflurane and a continuous infusion of remifentanil, hyperperistalsis that interfered with completion of intestinal anastomosis was observed during desflurane but not with sevoflurane anesthesia [63]. Studies evaluating the effects of inhalation agents on intestinal motility in horses are needed.

The published information concerning the effect of lidocaine on GI motility is conflicting. In healthy horses, administration of lidocaine, 1.3 mg/kg, followed by an IV infusion of 0.05 mg/kg/min, prolonged the intestinal transit time by several hours (barium-impregnated spheres) and fecal output was decreased in the first 24 h [64]. In a study of healthy horses with implanted Ag/AgCl electrodes on the jejunum, the same lidocaine dose rates did not change the duration of the migrating myoelectric complex or spiking activity [65]. However, increasing concentrations of lidocaine *in vitro* have improved the contractility of jejunum that had been subjected to 15 min of ischemia and increased intraluminal pressure *in vivo*. In addition, release of creatine kinase (CK) (a marker for cell membrane permeability) from handled normal jejunal smooth muscle was decreased and also from ischemic tissue [37,66]. These results indicate that damaged muscle may be more susceptible to the effects of lidocaine [37] and that lidocaine interacts with smooth muscle membranes and preserves cellular function [37,66]. One caveat is that the *in vitro* tissues were exposed to lidocaine concentrations exceeding concentrations measured in horses. Lidocaine may also attenuate the adverse effect of flunixin on mucosal barrier permeability [32]. It has been proposed that lidocaine therapy would, therefore, be beneficial for damaged intestine that remained in the abdomen after surgery, for example, after extensive handling, adjacent to an anastomosis, or a site that cannot be resected, minimizing the severity or occurrence of postoperative ileus.

Postoperative ileus

Ileus has been defined as a syndrome of functional inhibition of propulsive bowel motility [46]. Postoperative ileus (POI) is a causal reason for death or euthanasia in horses after surgery for colic [5,11]. The clinical signs are decreased or absent intestinal sounds, mild to no colic pain, large volumes of gastric reflux, increased PCV, and continued cardiovascular deterioration. A significant cause of increased morbidity in human patients after GI surgery, POI has been the subject of many publications. Mechanisms attributed to the occurrence of POI are (1) primary inflammation following hypoxic damage from increased intraluminal pressure and from surgical manipulation, with inflammation spreading throughout the GI tract even when only a small part has been manipulated, (2) a second immunologic phase that determines the extent and duration of POI, originating with infiltration of leukocytes in response to currently unknown triggers, and (3) further potentiation by intestinal edema from excessive IV fluid loading, decreased motility effects of opioids, α_2-adrenergic receptor agonists, and other drugs, and treatment-induced altered cellular metabolism [67,68]. Endotoxin and inflammation initiate inducible nitric oxide synthetase (iNOS) that releases NO. Nitric oxide has protective GI properties including antibacterial effect and vasodilation to counter decreased intestinal perfusion, but also is an inhibitory transmitter of GI motility. Many changes in anesthetic management are employed in the attempt to prevent or treat POI [69,70], and further information is provided in this chapter.

Preanesthetic considerations

Preanesthetic evaluation and preparation are important factors that influence successful outcome in horses with colic.

Patient characteristics

Horses of all ages, breeds, and reproductive stages may require surgery for colic, but patient characteristics (signalment) can be used to identify animals at risk for particular lesions or anesthetic complications. Breed and temperament may significantly influence the horse's behavior. Stallions, mares with foals, or animals that are not accustomed to handling may require additional sedation during induction and recovery, and these animals may be more likely to be excited when emerging from anesthesia. Fetal viability may be compromised by maternal hypotension or hypoxemia, or by the effects of α_2-adrenergic receptor agonists on intrauterine pressure [71].

The patient's clinical history may provide valuable information. Prolonged duration of colic prior to hospital presentation may result in significant fluid loss, electrolyte disturbances, especially hypocalcemia, self-inflicted injuries, and exhaustion of catecholamine stores. Colic occurring shortly after feeding may signify an increased risk for gastric bloat and rupture. A recent history of general anesthesia is important because it may provide insight into the horse's anticipated response to anesthesia and behavior in recovery [72].

Horses with strangulating lesions may develop significantly lower serum concentrations of ionized calcium and ionized magnesium than horses with non-strangulating GI obstructions [73]. Significant abdominal distention may accompany large intestinal displacement or volvulus, and may interfere with the horse's ventilation, oxygenation, and venous return, influencing systemic organ perfusion.

Patient evaluation and preparation

Preanesthetic evaluation of a horse with colic is a practice in multitasking, as data must be gathered and treatments initiated rapidly. Triage of these patients requires an accurate history, speedy but thorough physical examination, and ideally, a minimum clinicopathologic database, including measurements of PCV, total protein, serum electrolytes, lactate concentrations, markers of renal function, and ideally arterial or venous pH and blood-gas analysis.

Events that must occur immediately after the horse's arrival include jugular vein catheterization (one or two 10- or 14-gauge catheters or a 10-gauge catheter with arthroscopy tubing and no coil for rapid fluid infusion [74]), passage of an NG tube to decompress the stomach, a physical examination with emphasis on the cardiopulmonary and GI systems, and collection of blood for laboratory tests. An additional person should gather historical information supplied by the referring veterinarian and from the client, including deworming history, comorbidities, previous colic episodes (where, when), diet changes, recent water intake and appetite, duration of the colic, presence of gastric reflux, and the horse's normal activities or 'job' (Fig. 47.1).

Physical examination of the horse should include measurements of temperature, HR, respiratory rate, and arterial blood pressure (non-invasive, NIBP). Evaluation of the cardiovascular system should include assessment of skin turgor, mucous membrane color, capillary refill time (CRT), palpation of a pulse for rate, rhythm, and deficits, and auscultation of the heart and lungs. Shock or hypoperfusion may be recognized by tachycardia, tachypnea, prolonged CRT, bright red or dark or purple-tinged mucous membrane color, and depressed mentation. Hypertension or hypotension may be confirmed by NIBP measurement. When these findings are correlated with hyperlactatemia, or reduced central venous oxygen saturation (right atrium, $ScvO_2$), suggesting poor tissue perfusion, aggressive therapy should be initiated. The abdomen should be observed for distension. Details of the GI examination will be needed to complete the preanesthetic evaluation.

A recently constructed acute abdominal pain scale (EAAPS) for horses utilized behaviors associated with colic pain and identified rolling, pawing, kicking, and kicking the abdomen to be associated with need for surgical treatment [75]. Discomfort may also be displayed by restlessness and alteration in facial expression. Heart rate and respiratory rate have been found to have a poor correlation with pain behaviors. Donkeys do not display pain as horses do, exhibiting dullness and a depressed appetite as signs of abdominal pain [76].

A multimodal approach to pain management is recommended, including administration of an NSAID such as flunixin meglumine, an α_2-adrenergic receptor agonist such as xylazine or detomidine, and possibly an opioid such as butorphanol, with repeated re-evaluations at 20 min intervals (Fig. 47.1).

Significance of laboratory test results

Decreased survival has been associated with increased PCV, but PCV is also elevated by hypovolemia and stress-induced splenic contraction. Low total protein and albumin concentrations may be indicative of protein loss by vascular leakage. Hypoproteinemia increases the risk for hypotension during anesthesia, promotes tissue edema, and increases sensitivity to highly protein-bound drugs such as phenothiazines and benzodiazepines. Colloid fluid administration is indicated for horses with hypoproteinemia.

Commonly occurring electrolyte disturbances include hypocalcemia, hypomagnesemia, and less commonly hypokalemia. Normal reference ranges may vary between laboratories but in one equine study, the normal ionized serum calcium (*i*Ca) range was 1.61–1.68 mmol/L and ionized magnesium (*i*Mg) range 0.43–0.5 mmol/L [73]. Total Ca^{2+} and Mg^{2+} concentrations were not closely correlated with measurements of *i*Ca and *i*Mg. Calcium is essential for normal muscle function, including cardiac muscle and smooth muscle found in the GI tract and endothelium, thereby influencing cardiac contractility, widespread vascular tone (blood pressure), and GI motility. Magnesium is an important cofactor for many ion channels, including Na,K-ATPase, which regulates intracellular K^+ in addition to ATP production in many tissues. In one clinical trial of horses with colic, 88% were hypocalcemic on arrival [77]. In another, 86% and 54% of horses had abnormally low *i*Ca and *i*Mg, respectively, before undergoing exploratory laparotomy for colic [73]. Low *i*Ca or *i*Mg was significantly more prevalent among horses that had strangulating lesions compared with non-strangulating lesions, and horses that were euthanized intraoperatively had significantly lower *i*Mg than horses that recovered from anesthesia. Horses that developed POI also had significantly lower *i*Mg than those with normal motility. Neither *i*Mg nor *i*Ca predicted survival or hospitalization time in this patient population. Based on these findings, the authors recommended supplementing *i*Ca-deficient horses (*i*Ca <1.1 mmol/L) with 10 mg/kg calcium gluconate over 30–60 min and Mg supplementation in deficient horses with 25 mg/kg over 120 min. Additional measurements are used to guide further treatment.

Lactate is a by-product of glycolysis that accumulates in tissues when oxygen is unavailable. Hyperlactatemia occurs most commonly due to circulatory shock or arterial hypoxemia, and less commonly from increased systemic or localized production by the lungs, gut, or WBCs in inflammatory states, reduced metabolism by the liver, or cellular hypoxia during intoxications [73]. Hyperlactatemia is an indicator of non-survival in humans and horses with septic or endotoxemic shock [22,78–80]. Comparison of lactate concentrations in blood and abdominal fluid may predict whether the lesion is strangulating or non-strangulating. Lower venous lactate concentrations (1.01 ± 0.37 mmol/L) have been measured in healthy adult horses of non-miniature breeds than in neonatal foals <36 h of age (2.0 ± 0.7 mmol/L) and miniature horses [79,81]. Given the variability in reference ranges, interpretation of measured lactate concentrations is focused on trends over time rather than a single lactate concentration. Horses with colic that had a slow return of blood lactate concentration to normal over 72 h had a lower probability for survival than horses with a more rapid decrease in lactate [82]. Similarly, trends of serial lactate measurements in foals proved more predictive of survival than a single value [22,81]. The trends in lactate concentrations must be interpreted in conjunction with indicators of cardiovascular function and oxygen delivery (DO_2) to form therapeutic recommendations (Fig. 47.1).

Azotemia may represent a negative prognostic indicator for horses with colic, but should also be interpreted with caution, as many horses that survived colic surgery had prerenal azotemia. Tests of coagulation, platelet count, prothrombin time (PT), aPTT, or thromboelastography, may be advisable in horses with signs of SIRS or endotoxemia. In the presence of hypocoagulation or coagulation factor depletion, plasma may be administered intraoperatively. Hyperglycemia is a common finding in horses with colic before anesthesia but is likely the result of stress and administration of α_2-adrenergic receptor agonists. The importance of instituting therapy to maintain blood glucose within normal limits in horses is unknown. However, intensive insulin therapy in critically ill human patients was not supported by a meta-analysis based on mortality rates [83]. Ancillary diagnostic tests such as abdominocentesis and transabdominal ultrasound provide information on the progression of the disease that can be incorporated into the anesthetic management plan.

Fluid therapy

The goals of fluid resuscitation are restoration of organ perfusion, maintenance of microcirculation, delivery of oxygen and nutrients to tissues, and removal of waste products. Clinical trials and

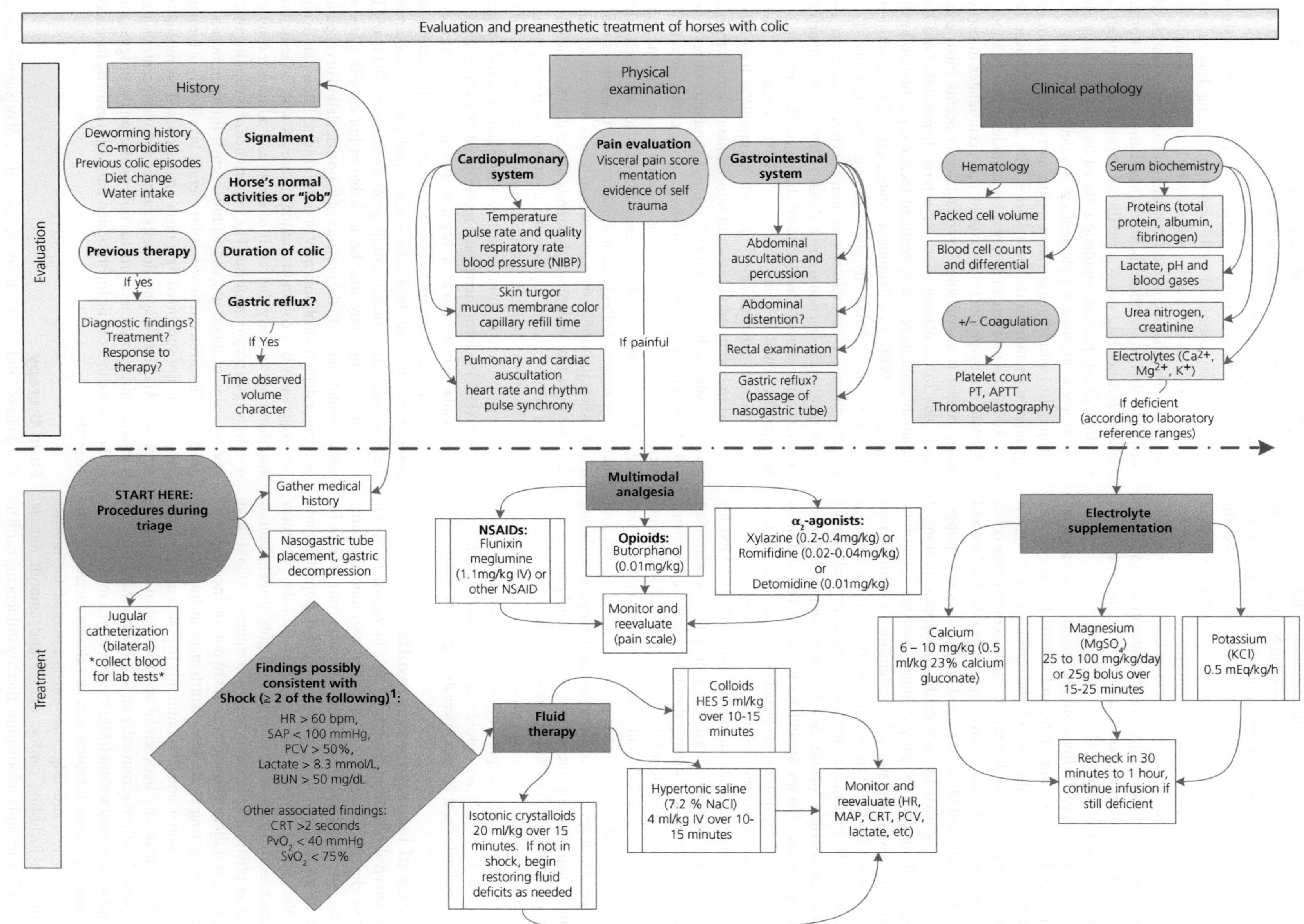

Figure 47.1 Recommended procedures for preanesthetic evaluation and treatment of horses requiring anesthesia for colic. Source: Grulke S, Olle E, Detilleux J, *et al.* Determination of gravity and shock score for prognosis in equine surgical colic. *J Vet Med A Physiol Pathol Clin Med* 2001; **48**: 465–473. Reproduced with permission of Wiley.

experimental studies have explored the effectiveness of various fluid strategies in horses, but have resulted in no consensus. Nevertheless, we aim to make our own recommendations based on this information.

Fluids commonly used for fluid resuscitation of horses include isotonic crystalloids, 7.5% hypertonic saline solution (HSS), and colloids. Crystalloids and colloids behave very differently following IV administration, particularly the newer generation colloids with lower molecular weight and molar substitution [84].

Evaluation of fluid strategies is complicated by the use of a multitude of therapeutic endpoints, for example, degree of plasma expansion, MAP >65 mmHg, cardiac output (CO), $ScvO_2$, central venous pressure (CVP) 8–12 cmH_2O, pulmonary arterial occlusion pressure (PAOP), urine output >0.5 mL/kg/h, and improved cardiovascular function 'shock reversal' (serum lactate <2.2 mmol/L and discontinuation of vasopressor therapy) [85], mixed venous oxygen tension (pulmonary artery, $P\bar{v}O_2$), oxygen extraction ratio (O_2ER), systolic or pulse pressure variation, microcirculation, and outcomes such as acute renal injury, hospital length of stay or mortality rate, and neurological outcome [86,87].

The Surviving Sepsis Campaign: 2012 [86], a compilation of evidence-based recommendations for management of human patients with septic shock, recommends that resuscitation should begin immediately on presentation at the hospital in patients with hypotension or elevated serum lactate concentration. Recommendations include infusion of crystalloid fluid to achieve target values for MAP, CVP, $ScvO_2$, and urine production, and administration of IV antibiotics as early as possible. Relatively healthy horses may not require urgent care but fluid therapy may be particularly important for horses with suspected ischemic bowel because these animals have a higher mortality rate. Urine production is not a helpful treatment indicator for horses given any α_2-adrenergic receptor agonist.

Although isotonic crystalloid fluid boluses are a traditionally accepted means of restoring vascular volume, this strategy alone may not be adequate in some horses with GI disease. According to Starling's law, of all the factors governing fluid movement across capillary membranes, the force most responsible for holding fluid within the capillary is intravascular COP. Several colloid products are available for IV fluid resuscitation, including hydroxyethyl starches (HESs), gelatins, and dextrans. Gelatin and dextran 40 have fallen out of favor for many veterinary professionals. The combination of HSS and dextran has been extensively investigated but is not currently recommended for treatment of trauma in humans [88].

HESs are synthetic colloids that are classified by five criteria: concentration, solvent, mean molecular weight (MW, in kDa), molar substitution (MS, hydroxyethyl residues per 10 glucose subunits) and C2/C6 ratio. More modern, 'third-generation' HES solutions (e.g., Voluven, Hospira, IL, USA) have lower MW (130 kDa) and lower MS (0.4). These products have higher concentrations of active oncotic particles, but show less accumulation in the circulation over time, and have minimal effect on coagulation, theoretically less effect on renal function, and improved tissue oxygenation and microcirculatory effects [89].

HES administered to horses maintains a colloid effect for up to 24 h. Horses administered two HES formulations, 10 mL/kg of low (6% hetastarch) or high (6% tetrastarch) MW and MS, had systolic arterial pressures (obtained by NIBP) higher than horses receiving an equal volume of 0.9% saline for up to 24 h [90]. In a related study, administration of 10 mL/kg boluses of 6% hetastarch (600/0.75) or 6% tetrastarch (130/0.4) significantly increased COP and MAP in healthy horses, with a more prolonged change in COP from tetrastarch (K. Epstein, personal communication). Although HES solutions may exert adverse coagulopathic effects, the low-MW tetrastarch exerted a significantly shorter duration of adverse effect on platelet function than hetastarch, based on automated platelet analysis, von Willebrand's factor (vWF) and factor VIII quantification [90]. Evaluation of renal function following administration of HES, pentastarch (HES 200/0.5) 10 mL/kg followed by lactated Ringer's solution (LRS) 10 mL/kg, in healthy horses, horses with surgical colic, and horses with acute colitis, revealed that all horses with colitis or large intestinal ileus experienced significant decreases in serum urea and creatinine concentrations within 24 h after colloid infusion [91]. Infusion of 10% pentastarch (HES with MS of 0.5) 4 mL/kg followed by LRS 20 mL/kg improved CI in horses undergoing colic surgery for up to 150 min after induction compared with horses given 7.5% saline 4 mL/kg followed by 20 mL/kg LRS [92].

In one single-center study, colloid–crystalloid combinations provided no benefit over crystalloid infusion alone for reversal of shock in human patients with severe sepsis [93]. Patients received 6% tetrastarch (130/0.4) plus crystalloid or only crystalloid fluid and there was no difference between treatments in the time to return of normal serum lactate concentration, MAP and $ScvO_2$, time to discontinuation of vasopressor therapy, or ICU and hospital mortality rates. Patients in the colloid group had significantly longer ICU hospitalization and longer mechanical ventilatory support than the crystalloid group, required more blood products, and had a significantly higher rate of acute kidney injury and renal replacement therapy [93]. Investigations comparing the efficacy of crystalloids and colloids in reversing septic shock and the impact on outcome in horses with colic are necessary.

HSS is a valuable, inexpensive option for rapid blood volume expansion and an important component of 'small-volume fluid resuscitation' that has been advocated for decades in the treatment of shock [94]. Administration of HSS may improve tissue perfusion by multiple mechanisms. HSS rapidly restores intravascular volume by influx of fluid from the interstitial space (the osmolality of HSS is approximately eight times that of plasma). HSS also reduces the expression of leukocyte surface adhesion molecules such as L-selectin and CD11b, thereby inhibiting endothelial–leukocyte interaction, subsequent release of toxic elastases and free radicals, decreasing vascular leakage, and improving preload [95]. HSS also improves myocardial contractility and microcirculation by reducing blood viscosity, dilating precapillary sphincters, and constricting postcapillary sphincters, facilitating perfusion to previously constricted capillary beds [95–97]. Experimental and clinical investigations in several species support the effectiveness of HSS [88]. It has been proposed that infusion of HSS and HES may support preload without creating volume overload. However, in one study of anesthetized horses given endotoxin to induce hyperdynamic shock, IV infusion of HSS (5 mL/kg) and HES (10 mL/kg) over 30 min failed to improve cardiovascular function as much as 60 mL/kg Normosol-R [98].

'Goal-directed fluid therapy' or the judicious administration of fluids according to certain monitoring endpoints used to assess perfusion or volume status has been advocated in human septic shock, with reasonable success [99]. A clinical study in anesthetized human patients showed that those receiving fluid volumes directed by changes in serial cardiac output (CO) measurements had significantly shorter hospital stays, less postoperative nausea and vomiting, and faster return to eating solid food than patients receiving non-goal-directed fluid therapy [99]. In another study, goal-directed therapy with 6% tetrastarch (HES 130/0.4) in anesthetized, mechanically ventilated pigs significantly increased microcirculation and oxygen tension in both healthy and perianastomotic colonic tissue compared with goal-directed crystalloid or restricted fluid therapy [100]. Interestingly, systemic indicators of hemodynamic stability (HR, MAP, CVP, CI, PAOP, arterial lactate) did not reflect the changes observed in microcirculation or tissue oxygenation. Given the derangements of splanchnic circulation in horses with colic, the consideration of GI microcirculation seems vital to fluid therapy decisions, although data have yet to be generated in support of its significance as a clinical endpoint in horses.

Fluid administration, general anesthesia, and surgical procedures significantly decrease plasma COP. COP decreases during inhalation anesthesia in healthy horses. In one study, COP decreased from 22.2 ± 2 to 15 ± 1.3 mmHg in healthy horses during inhalation anesthesia [101]. The COP returns to the preanesthetic value several hours after anesthesia in healthy horses given 10 mL/kg/h of crystalloid fluid (J.G. Adams, personal communication). Low COP, 18.7 ± 2.2 mmHg, has been measured in horses with colic before anesthesia with a further decrease to 11.6 ± 1.6 mmHg after administration of crystalloid fluid at 19.5 ± 3.9 mL/kg/h during anesthesia [102]. Fluid retention after anesthesia is of concern [103]. Surgical manipulation increases fluid accumulation in the interstitium of tissues, presumably via impairment of lymphatic drainage and subsequent inflammation. Reduced GI transit time and reductions in blood flow, disorders of motility, and leukocyte infiltration occur for at least 24 h after simple bowel manipulation [104,105]. Local inflammation and edema are greater following more invasive procedures such as resection and anastomosis of intestine. Aggressive therapy with crystalloid fluids may increase tissue edema and adversely affect outcome.

More clinical studies comparing the effects of fluid type and administration strategy on microcirculation, hemodynamic variables, shock reversal, and ultimate patient outcome in horses with colic are needed. Based on the recent literature concerning human and veterinary species, it is the authors' opinion that a combination of hypertonic saline (up to 4 mL/kg), isotonic crystalloid therapy (not excessive), and HES (particularly the more contemporary, low molar substitution fluids) should be utilized to stabilize these patients for anesthetic procedures (Fig. 47.1). A stronger emphasis on colloid therapy may be elected in cases with pre-existing hypoproteinemia. For horses with GI disease, the effects of aggressive perioperative crystalloid therapy on postoperative integrity of GI tissues may be a significant source of morbidity.

Equipment

The anesthesia machine and monitoring equipment should be assembled at all times, and especially at the end of the working day, to be ready for an emergency procedure. Check lists for equipment and procedures increase efficiency and safety.

The time from induction to attachment of all monitoring equipment and surgical incision can be shortened by preparation of the horse before induction of anesthesia, such as clipping hair overlying the facial arteries and abdominal surgical site, and placement of a second jugular catheter to facilitate multiple drug and fluid infusions. A functioning NG tube should be in place before induction of anesthesia because of the difficulty inserting a tube in an anesthetized horse. Attempts to remove fluid from the stomach should be made immediately before induction of anesthesia.

Preparation of the anesthetist should not be forgotten. Before starting to anesthetize each horse, the sequence of events from premedication to all the procedures to be performed when the horse is on the table should be imagined, including recall of all the potential problems associated with this specific horse, reviewing a plan of action to manage each one. 'Mental practice,' where one imagines an action without physically performing the action, is used extensively to improve performance in human athletes and for training of surgical techniques, but the value and optimal use in anesthetist training is still under investigation [106,107]. Nonetheless, we find the process to be a helpful, logical approach to streamlining technical procedures.

Anesthetic protocols

Many anesthetic agent combinations and dose rates are used to anesthetize healthy horses. The most frequently used combinations have changed over time. Personal choices are based on preferences of mentors modified by personal experience, which is in turn influenced by the nature and breed composition of the hospital caseload, since horses of different breeds and work use respond differently to anesthesia. Anesthetic agents may be chosen based on familiarity of use, available facilities, and preanesthetic evaluation of the individual patient. Sedative and analgesic agents may be administered before, during, and at the end of anesthesia to provide a balanced technique. The intended goals are unconsciousness and analgesia with the least physiologic deviations from the normal healthy conscious state followed by the best quality of recovery. Specific anesthetic agents have not been statistically associated with mortality outcome in horses with colic. These results may be influenced by confounding factors; for example, new agents with purportedly less adverse effects are commonly used initially only in the sickest patients. Logical reasoning suggests that agents that preserve CO and visceral and muscle blood flows are the best choices for sick patients.

Anesthetic agents and combinations

Currently, most horses with colic, except foals, are premedicated with an α_2-adrenergic receptor agonist with or without an opioid. Anesthesia is most frequently induced in all horses with ketamine (in combination with diazepam, midazolam, guaifenesin, or propofol) and maintained with an inhalation agent (Table 47.1).

The physical status of horses with colic varies from the relatively healthy ASA Class 3 patient to one that is moribund (Class 5E), making it necessary in some cases to modify the anesthetic protocols used for induction of anesthesia in healthy horses. Horses with colic may be tired and have many physiologic abnormalities that render them susceptible to greater cardiopulmonary depression

Table 47.1 Example of an anesthetic agent combination for general anesthesia in horses with colic.

Premedication[a]	Induction of Anesthesia	Maintenance of Anesthesia[b]
Xylazine (0.3–1.1 mg/kg) or romifidine (0.04–0.1 mg/kg) IV followed by butorphanol (0.02 mg/kg) IV	Ketamine[a] (1.0–2.3 mg/kg) IV, alone or preceded by diazepam (0.05 mg/kg), or guaifenesin (25–50 mg/kg), or propofol (0.4 mg/kg) IV	Isoflurane or sevoflurane with lidocaine (1.3–2.0 mg/kg over 15 min followed by 1.5–3.0 mg/kg/h) IV

[a] Dose rate should be adjusted for administration of sedatives or opioids in the hour(s) before anesthesia and for the horse's physical health.

[b] Additional drugs may be administered during anesthesia, such as boluses or continuous infusion of an opioid, an α_2-adrenergic receptor agonist, or a low dose of ketamine.

than usual. Preanesthetic evaluation should include an assessment of the horse's mental attitude towards physical restraint, the unaccustomed environment, and interaction with people. This information is based on observation of the horse's body stance, movements, and facial expression, and intuition, and should be incorporated into choice of anesthetic management during induction and recovery. In summary, preanesthetic evaluation must provide an assessment of each horse's likely response to anesthesia so that appropriate anesthetic agents and dose rates may be administered and complications anticipated.

Induction of anesthesia

Different methods are used to control horses during induction of anesthesia, influenced by the facilities available. Use of a moveable partition to hold the horse against a wall during loss of consciousness is common, but free fall, with or without human support and guidance, or use of a vertical tilting table are alternatives. One author's (C.M.T.) preference is to maintain the horse in sternal recumbency after induction of anesthesia until the trachea is intubated and the endotracheal tube cuff is inflated. The rationale is that extension of the head and neck for passage of the endotracheal tube is easier when the horse is in a sternal position, full extension is essential for rapid intubation with a straight endotracheal tube, and spontaneous reflux of gastric fluid appears to be less frequent than during lateral recumbency.

Artificial ventilation is begun immediately using a demand valve and oxygen, and continued while hobbles are applied and the horse is hoisted or ready for transportation. The endotracheal tube is connected to the anesthetic delivery system immediately after the horse is lifted onto the table.

Horses with excessive abdominal distension, hypoxemia, or poor cardiovascular function may benefit from intranasal administration of oxygen, 15 L/min, during induction of anesthesia. SpO_2 and MAP decrease when a horse is moved into dorsal recumbency and when lifted using a hoist [108,109]. Infusion of dobutamine IV during induction of anesthesia and transportation may provide cardiovascular support.

Management of foals

Foals should be prevented from nursing for 30 min before induction of anesthesia to minimize the risk of milk reflux when first anesthetized. The mare should accompany the foal to keep them calm until the foal is anesthetized. Sedation for the mare may be necessary after separation. Young foals are physically easier to restrain and are manually supported during the onset of anesthesia.

Gastric reflux into the oropharynx may occur even with an NG tube in place. Nasotracheal intubation is advisable before induction of anesthesia in a foal that is spontaneously refluxing. The nasotracheal tube in a foal with colic should not be changed for an orotracheal tube during anesthesia as gastric fluid reflux and aspiration may occur when the airway is unprotected. Ventilation should be controlled to prevent hypoventilation and to avoid excessive negative intrathoracic pressures on inspiration when the internal diameter of the nasotracheal tube is substantially smaller than would be used for orotracheal intubation.

The response of a neonatal foal <7 days of age is different from that of a foal aged 2–3 months. Anesthesia can be induced in very young foals with diazepam, 0.05 mg/kg, and ketamine, 1.0–2.0 mg/kg, with or without a low dose of opioid, and maintained with sevoflurane or isoflurane. The anesthetic requirement (MAC) of inhalation agents in foals is significantly decreased from that in adult horses. Older foals may tolerate the cardiovascular effects of an α_2-adrenergic receptor agonist, generally used at a low dose, before administration of diazepam (or midazolam) and ketamine for induction of anesthesia followed by inhalation anesthesia.

Maintenance of anesthesia

Total intravenous anesthesia (TIVA) with an α_2-adrenergic receptor agonist and ketamine is most commonly administered when a horse is to be rolled in an attempt to correct a left dorsal colon displacement. Phenylephrine or ephedrine at 0.06 mg/kg can be administered IV at the same time to decrease the size of the spleen and facilitate release of the entrapped bowel. Rarely, rolling the horse during anesthesia results in arterial rupture and massive intra-abdominal hemorrhage that is manifested by the horse showing initial signs of recovery from anesthesia, then weakening and death in the recovery stall.

Anesthesia for celiotomy is usually maintained with an inhalation agent, most commonly isoflurane or sevoflurane, and adjunct drugs. Administration of 100% inspired oxygen with controlled ventilation is usually necessary to maintain systemic arterial oxygenation and normocarbia by counteracting effects of dorsal recumbency, weight of ingesta in the intestines on the diaphragm, and increased intra-abdominal pressure. Of note, there is evidence that even in presence of adequate systemic PaO_2, the tissue oxygen tension in perianastomotic and intra-anastomotic colon tissue is increased when the inspired oxygen concentration is increased to near 100% [110].

Comparison of the cardiovascular effects of the inhalation agents in healthy experimental horses has revealed that, for equipotent concentrations, CO is higher during isoflurane anesthesia than during halothane. In another investigation, lower dobutamine infusion rates were required to maintain MAP >70 mmHg during sevoflurane anesthesia compared with isoflurane [111]. Adjunct agents may be administered to provide analgesia and sedation. Continuous IV infusions, with or without loading doses, of α_2-adrenergic receptor agonists, opioids (butorphanol, morphine, or remifentanil), ketamine, or lidocaine are administered singly or in combinations. Administration of an adjunct drug may allow a decrease in the inspired anesthetic concentration so that the plasma concentration decreases more rapidly at the end of anesthesia, potentially improving the quality of recovery through less ataxia. Depending on the pharmacodynamics of the adjunct agent, the decrease in inhalation agent concentration may or may not result in improved MAP, CO, or regional perfusion. The contribution of opioids to antinociception during anesthesia in horses is controversial.

Lidocaine is commonly administered for its anti-inflammatory effect starting soon after induction of anesthesia at a loading dose of 1.3–2.0 mg/kg infused over 15–20 min followed by a continuous infusion of 0.05 mg/kg/min (3 mg/kg/h). A loading dose of 2 mg/kg over 20 min achieved an average plasma lidocaine concentration of 920 ng/mL by 30 min that was sustained by the infusion of 0.05 mg/kg/min [112]. Lidocaine administered as an infusion of 0.05 mg/kg/min without a loading dose will achieve steady-state conditions and similar blood concentrations by 3 h [113]. Lidocaine infusion allows a significant reduction (27%) in the end-tidal inhalant concentration but without resulting in improved cardiovascular function [114]. Serum lidocaine concentrations are lower in awake horses than in anesthetized horses for the same infusion dose rate [115].

Anesthetic management

Anesthetic care goes beyond the simple administration of drugs and is an important component of preventing physiological abnormalities that may impact on outcome.

Monitoring

The horse should be positioned on a table that has adequate padding to avoid muscle damage from compression. The head must be elevated above heart level to minimize nasal mucosa congestion that will contribute to airway obstruction after tracheal extubation. Should gastric reflux occur around the NG tube, the head must be lowered to promote drainage and then the endotracheal tube retained during recovery from anesthesia. The pelvic limbs should not be frog-legged for the duration of anesthesia, unless essential for surgical exposure, to avoid induction of postanesthetic myopathy [116]. Limbs and muscles should be protected from excessive pressure by careful use of rope, leather, or webbing shackles, by insertion of padding, or by adjusting positioning.

Monitoring of inhalation anesthesia should include frequent evaluation of muscle relaxation (lack of response to surgery, eyeball position), reflexes (palpebral reflex), cardiovascular function and peripheral perfusion [heart rate and rhythm, mucous membrane color and CRT, peripheral pulse strength and rhythm, invasive blood pressure (IBP), and perfusion of the surgical site], adequacy of ventilation (rate and depth of breathing), and body temperature. Additional useful monitoring includes pulse oximetry, capnography, arterial pH and blood-gas analysis, $ScvO_2$, and inhalation agent analysis. Some hospitals are also equipped to perform cardiac output determinations. In certain situations during anesthesia, for example when a hyperkalemic periodic paralysis episode is suspected or after administration of calcium, there is a need to measure plasma electrolyte concentrations.

Depth of anesthesia

Muscle movement or a marked increase in HR or MAP in response to surgical manipulation, and the presence of a brisk palpebral reflex or wide-amplitude nystagmus, indicate a light plane of anesthesia. The palpebral reflex may be absent during moderate or excessive depth of anesthesia. Low MAP may reflect an increasing depth of anesthesia or an absolute or relative hypovolemia, hypoproteinemia, or endotoxemia.

Measurements of inspired and end-tidal inhalation agent concentrations provide useful information for maintaining a constant depth of anesthesia and some guidance against under- or overdosage. The anesthetic concentration in a large delivery circuit is less than the vaporizer setting, influenced by the rate of oxygen inflow and patient uptake, eliminating the usefulness of the vaporizer setting in assessing anesthetic delivery. Mean MAC values in healthy adult horses and ponies have been reported to be 0.97–1.31% for isoflurane, 2.31–2.84% for sevoflurane, 0.88–0.95% for halothane, and 7.6–8.06% for desflurane. Very young foals have decreased requirements for anesthetic agents and MAC values of 0.9% for isoflurane and 0.7% for halothane have been reported. An adequate depth of anesthesia for surgery is generally achieved at an end-tidal inhalant concentration of 1.0–1.5 × MAC when few other agents are administered. Anesthetic gas analysis for assessing depth is limited since MAC is not identical in every animal, mean MAC values determined in groups of experimental animals may vary with measurement techniques, and concurrent administration of other anesthetic agents and the patient's physiologic status decrease anesthetic requirement. Administration of sedatives and analgesic agents before and during anesthesia decreases anesthetic requirement (MAC) to varying extents, and the effects may be greater in sick than in healthy horses. Nonetheless, clinical experiences have confirmed the value of this measurement even when adjustments for the above factors are required [117].

Respiratory system

Measurement of end-tidal carbon dioxide partial pressure ($ETCO_2$) provides a reasonable estimate of adequacy of ventilation in healthy anesthetized horses during mechanical ventilation. Unfortunately, despite the use of intermittent positive-pressure ventilation (IPPV), the degree of lung collapse that is commonly present in horses anesthetized for colic surgery frequently results in discrepancies between $PaCO_2$ and $ETCO_2$. $PaCO_2$ has been reported to be on average 12 mmHg higher than $ETCO_2$ (range, 0–37.5 mmHg) for anesthetized horses with colic, compared with 5 mmHg in healthy horses [2,118]. Consequently, arterial blood-gas analysis should be performed early to determine the $ETCO_2$–$PaCO_2$ difference for that patient. Capnography can then be used to evaluate any trends during maintenance of anesthesia.

Identification of hypoxemia (PaO_2 < 60 mmHg, 8 kPa) is important. A peripheral measure of hemoglobin saturation using pulse oximetry (SpO_2) is a frequently used substitute for the measurement of PaO_2. Pulse oximeters have variable accuracy in different species, in foals and adult horses, and at different sites of the body. Attachment of the probe to the tongue has been reported to provide the highest correlation between SpO_2 and SaO_2 for several models in horses. Some pulse oximeters consistently underestimate the actual value for SaO_2 incorrectly identifying hypoxemia, whereas for others SpO_2 < 93% represents hypoxemia. Measurement of PaO_2 should be used to confirm suspected hypoxemia.

Cardiovascular system

Circulatory function is assessed using mucous membrane color, CRT, evaluation of peripheral pulse strength and rhythm, IBP and observation of the arterial waveform, analysis of the electrocardiogram (ECG) for dysrhythmias, and observation of the operative site for color and bleeding. Cardiopulmonary measurements in anesthetized horses are often decreased from values in the awake unsedated animal [119,120. and our recommended target values are given in Table 47.2.

NIBP can be used to provide an estimate of systolic arterial pressure (SAP) or MAP before anesthesia but is not sufficiently accurate for anesthetic management, especially of patients that are sick or undergoing laparotomy. Arterial pressures are measured by inserting a catheter in the facial or transverse facial artery with a transducer placed level with the thoracic inlet or point of the shoulder (assumed corresponding to the right atrium) for horses in dorsal recumbency.

Table 47.2 Target values for measured variables in anesthetized adult horses.

Measured Variable	Range	Units
Heart rate	>26 and <50	beats/min
Peripheral MAP	>70 and <120	mmHg
pHa	>7.30 and <7.50	–
$PaCO_2$	>33 and <50	mmHg
	>4.39 and <6.65	kPa
PaO_2	>80 (sea level)	mmHg
	>10.64	kPa
	Preferably higher	
Base excess	–6 to +10	mEq/L
Packed cell volume	>26 and <45	%

Hypotension frequently accompanies inhalation anesthesia in healthy and in sick horses. Hypotension is commonly defined as MAP <60–65 mmHg in other species; however, in anesthetized horses, MAP <70 mmHg warrants institution of treatment to support organ blood flow and autoregulation and to minimize the incidence of postanesthetic myopathy [121]. Whereas hypotension is a recognized indicator of decreased peripheral perfusion, MAP >65 mmHg is not, as other factors, including oxygen content of arterial blood, CO, and systemic vascular resistance (SVR), must be considered.

Observation of the arterial pressure waveform for cyclical variation in SAP and pulse pressures, 'cycling,' occurring in sequence with the cycles of the mechanical ventilator provides an indication of decreased CO and need for blood volume expansion. The increase in intrathoracic pressure during IPPV reduces venous return (decreased preload) and increases afterload. The reduction in ejection volume from the right ventricle leads to decreased left ventricular filling after a few beats, and subsequently decreased stroke volume. Variables evaluated are the systolic pressure variation (SPV) and pulse pressure variation (PPV). A simple analysis that is done in our practice is to observe the difference between the highest and lowest SAP or PPV within a respiratory cycle [122,123]. Small decreases in SAP are a normal consequence of IPPV but pronounced cycling is abnormal. Unfortunately, visual assessment provides only a rough estimate. Correlation was poor between SPV and PPV calculated manually over three respiratory cycles in horses anesthetized for elective and emergency procedures [124].

Currently in human medicine, differences in PPV (ΔPP) are calculated using monitors with advanced digital software that recognizes the respiratory cycles from capnography, measures ΔPP directly from the arterial waveform, and then averages multiple cycles [125,126]. Marked ΔPP has been identified as highly accurate in predicting that a fluid challenge will increase CO in critically ill human patients, HES being the most frequently reported fluid used for this purpose [125,126]. ΔPP is a better predictor of fluid responsiveness than static indicators (right atrial pressure or PAOP). The threshold for ΔPP that separates 'responders' from 'non-responders' varies between 6.5 and 12.5% and differences in reported threshold may be due to factors such as respiratory rate or left ventricular dysfunction. Guidelines for measuring ΔPP are that patients should be without cardiac arrhythmias and ventilation should be controlled with a tidal volume >7 mL/kg (human patients), although accuracy has also been confirmed in human septic patients ventilated at 6 mL/kg with positive end-expiratory pressure (PEEP) [126].

A variety of techniques are available for the measurement of CO. The lithium dilution technique is a relatively non-invasive method that utilizes arterial and venous catheters that are usually present in anesthetized horses with colic. Unfortunately, the sensor may not be accurate when the horse has received an α_2-adrenergic receptor agonist [127]. The non-invasive cardiac output technique involving CO_2 rebreathing (NICO) may be used in small foals as an approximation of CO and to monitor trends [128,129].

Placement of a pulmonary artery catheter allows the measurement of $P\bar{v}O_2$, which is representative of total body O_2 extraction. Mixed venous saturation ($S\bar{v}O_2$) is approximately 70–75% in healthy animals and a decrease to less than 65% is a significant value. A low $S\bar{v}O_2$ occurs in situations of low CO or MAP and increased O_2ER during sepsis. Elevated $S\bar{v}O_2$ may indicate high CO or decreased O_2ER, and may be present with hyperdynamic endotoxic shock, recognized in horses by bright red mucous membranes, rapid CRT, and bounding peripheral pulse. Insertion of a pulmonary artery catheter is costly and not recommended in patients with sepsis. Measurement of $ScvO_2$ in blood collected from a catheter with the tip in the right atrium may be used as a surrogate for $S\bar{v}O_2$ [130]. Blood must be sampled from the right atrium, or very close to it, for accuracy as overestimation of $ScvO_2$ will occur the further the tip is away from the right atrium. In the presence of adequate CO, $ScvO_2$ describes the adequacy of overall tissue oxygenation.

Temperature

Obtaining an accurate body temperature may be difficult in horses. Only a probe placed deep within the rectum may be accurate, as recording from just inside the anus may be altered by rectal palpation, and temperatures measured in the nasal cavity or ear are lower than the core temperature. Hypothermia may result in increased ataxia during recovery from anesthesia and increased catabolism in the days following anesthesia. Warming a horse during anesthesia is difficult, particularly in an air-conditioned room. Nonetheless, attempts should be made to slow the rate of heat loss by the use of warm IV fluids, application of a forced warm air blanket over the horse's head, neck, and thorax, and maintaining a warm recovery room.

Intraoperative complications

Since hypoventilation is so common in horses in dorsal recumbency with gas or fecal distension of the GI tract pressing on the diaphragm, it is our preference to begin IPPV at the start of anesthesia. Guidelines are 10 breaths/min and sufficient tidal volume to decrease $PaCO_2$ to <50 mmHg.

Hypotension

MAP should not be allowed to decrease below 70 mmHg, owing to the well-documented risk of myopathy. The urgency for treatment is greater when low arterial pressure is accompanied by a prolonged CRT, pale or gray gum color, pulse pressure cycling, PaO_2 < 60 mmHg (8 kPa), pale intestinal color, or ongoing moderate or rapid hemorrhage.

An acute decrease in MAP should first be verified by flushing the arterial catheter, observation of the arterial waveform, and palpation of a pulse to rule out cardiac arrest. An acute onset of hypotension may follow induction of anesthesia, a change of body position, administration of an anesthetic drug or antibiotic, and surgical manipulation or untwisting of the bowel. Surgical manipulation of an ischemic bowel may result in the release of endotoxin and inflammatory mediators into the circulation, sometimes resulting in an abrupt, dramatic decrease in MAP and pHa. Prompt treatment by discontinuing anesthetic administration and increasing administration of a vasoactive agent is essential. In some cases where there has been a severe decrease in pHa, administration of sodium bicarbonate, 1 mEq/L, is indicated in addition to addressing the underlying pathophysiology. Measurement of pH and blood gases, repeated 20 min later, is advisable to guide further management.

Treatment with a fluid challenge or vasoactive drugs will not effectively correct hypotension caused by aortocaval compression. Tachycardia is the main response to administration of increasing dose rates of inotropes or pressors in this scenario. MAP may be improved when abdominal pressure is decreased after abdominal incision. Diagnosis is confirmed by surgical elevation of the intestinal tract away from the aorta and caudal vena cava resulting in an immediate rebound in MAP.

Treatment based on abnormal measurements is outlined in the flow chart shown in Fig. 47.2a. Hypotension as the result of hypovolemia should be treated by IV administration of fluid challenges

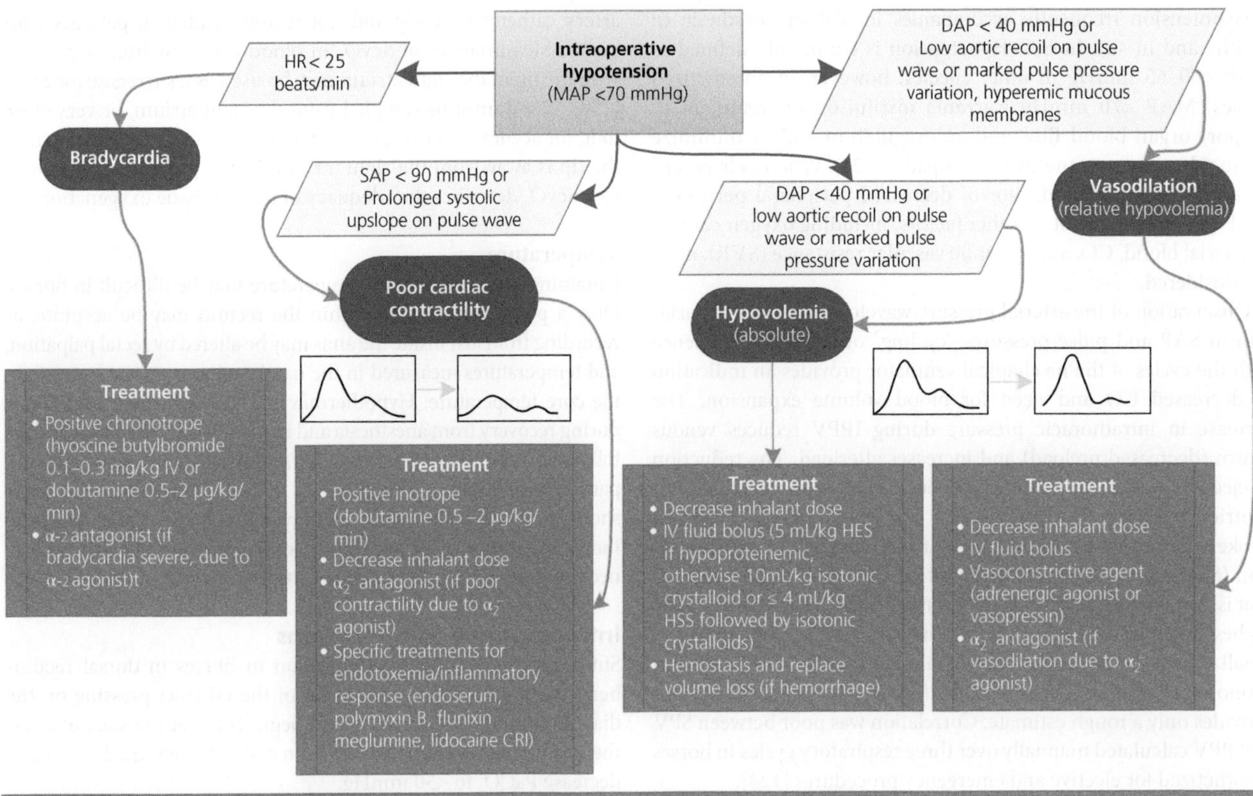

(a)

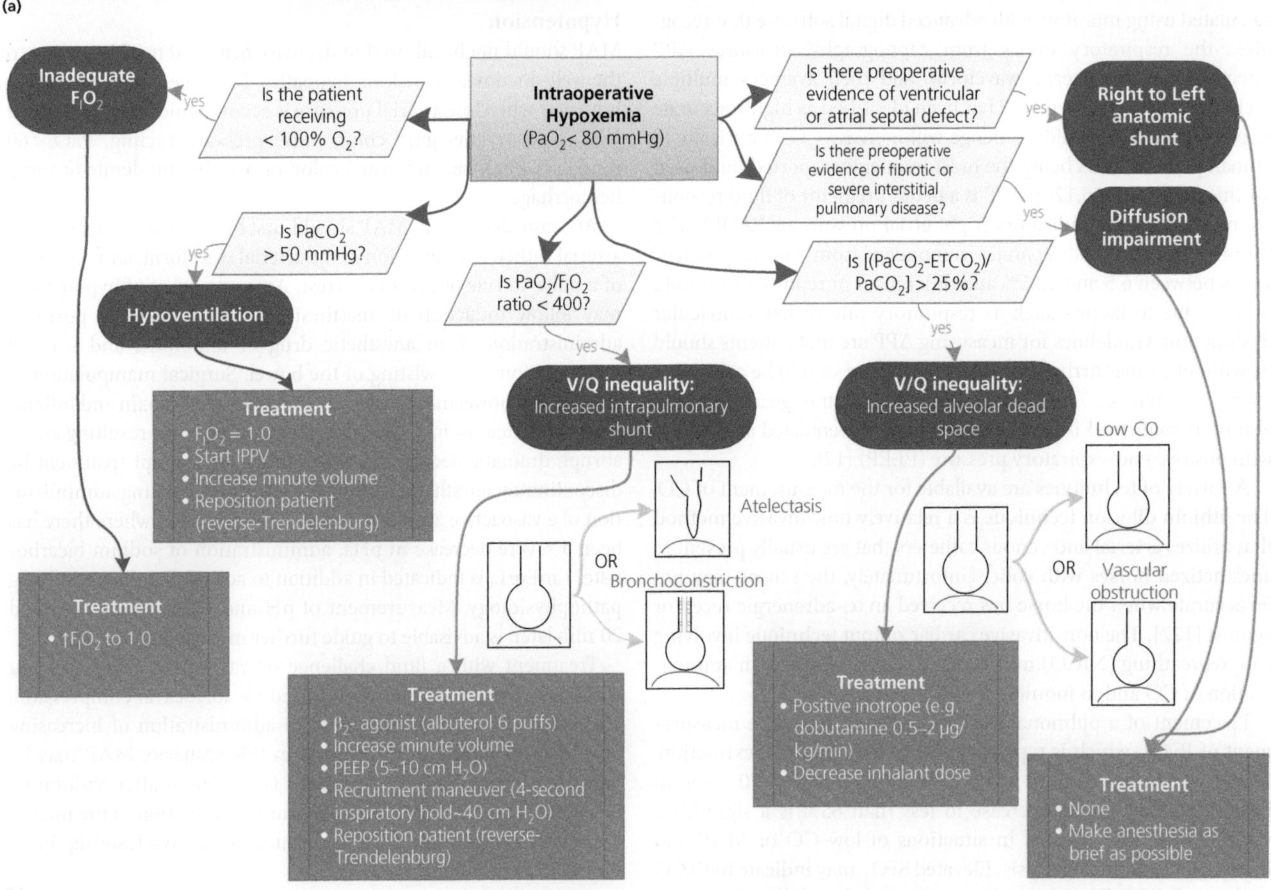

(b)

Figure 47.2 (a) Troubleshooting hypotension in anesthetized horses with colic, organized by probable etiology (oval boxes). Bulleted points are provided as treatment options. Pulse waveforms suggest general changes that correspond to etiology. (b) Troubleshooting hypoxemia in anesthetized horses with colic, organized by probable etiology (oval boxes) and information required to identify the etiology (diamond boxes). Alveolar diagrams provide examples of V/Q inequality.

to expand blood volume, initially crystalloid fluid in 5 mL/kg increments. In the absence of an improvement in MAP, or $ScvO_2$ if available, infusion of a colloid such as HES, dextran 70, or plasma may be effective (see earlier). HSS 7.5% administered IV at 2–4 mL/kg over 10 min often results in an increase in MAP. Calcium borogluconate (23% 0.5 mL/kg infused over 20 min) may increase MAP in horses with hypocalcemia or vasodilation. However, this should not be infused during a surgical anastomosis as the intestine may become hypermotile and the diameter of the intestine will decrease, resulting in loose sutures.

Administration of fluids to ensure normal blood volume does not always restore hemodynamic stability. The physiologic mechanisms that result in low MAP and decreased perfusion may be several, including vasodilation (inhalation agent, hypercarbia, or sepsis), decreased venous return (hypovolemia, excessive abdominal distension, change in body position, aortocaval compression, or hemorrhage), or decreased myocardial function (anesthetic agent depression, IV antibiotic, endotoxemia, acidemia, hypocalcemia, or cardiac disease and dysrhythmias). The causes of hypotension should be assessed and essential treatment directed to remove or counter the cause.

The choice of vasoactive drug for cardiovascular support should be based on the clinical situation, and more than one drug may be required to achieve optimum balance. Dobutamine is commonly used as a first-line vasoactive agent for the treatment of hypotension. Administered as a low dose, 0.1–0.5 μg/kg/min, dobutamine may increase MAP by a mild, non-statistically significant increase in SVR [131]. Higher dose rates of 3, 5, or 10 μg/kg/min significantly increase MAP and CI with a decrease in HR [132,133], although increased HR may be observed in some horses. Ephedrine increases MAP and CI, and may be administered alone or with dobutamine, by intermittent boluses or continuous infusion. Ephedrine, 0.06 mg/kg, injected IV as a bolus may increase HR and MAP with generally a slow onset (5 min) and duration of less than 30 min. Infusion of ephedrine, 0.02 mg/kg/min, for 10 min in healthy isoflurane-anesthetized horses increased CI, MAP, and SVR, with no change in HR, and these improvements persisted for 90 min [134]. Dopamine also increases cardiac contractility but causes vasodilation when infused at low dose rates, decreasing MAP. Dopamine is best reserved for treatment of severe second- or third-degree atrioventricular (AV) heart block and for treatment of cardiac arrest, when the infusion rate should be 7–10 μg/kg/min.

Vasodilation-induced hypotension attributed to the inhalation agent may be partly managed by reducing the inspired anesthetic concentration. The addition of lidocaine allows a decrease in the dose of inhalation agent required for anesthesia but may not result in improved MAP. Vasodilation may also be treated by administration of a vasopressor such as norepinephrine or phenylephrine. Infusions of norepinephrine, 0.05–0.4 μg/kg/min, in healthy conscious or anesthetized foals increased MAP dose dependently by inducing vasoconstriction, but decreased CI and HR [133,135,136]. In another study of healthy foals with isoflurane-induced hypotension, higher infusion rates of norepinephrine, 0.3 and 1.0 μg/kg/min, increased SVR, MAP, and CI with no change in HR [137].

Phenylephrine, 0.13–0.42 μg/kg/min, has been used to increase MAP during anesthesia of horses with colic [16]. In healthy experimental horses anesthetized with isoflurane, IV infusion of phenylephrine, 2 μg/kg/min for 10 min, significantly increased MAP by vasoconstriction but decreased CI and DO_2 [134]. A retrospective study of survival in horses after colic surgery found no association between the use of dobutamine and mortality; however, increased duration of phenylephrine administration was associated with increased intraoperative and overall deaths [138]. Phenylephrine may be directly implicated in influencing an adverse outcome or the results may be a reflection that phenylephrine was used to manage the sickest horses.

Endogenous vasopressin is released during stress and hypotension from anesthesia, hypovolemia, and hemorrhage, to cause vasoconstriction that may halt the decline of or improve MAP. Increased plasma concentrations of vasopressin were measured in eight healthy clinical horses after 1 h of anesthesia [16]. Plasma vasopressin concentrations were significantly greater in horses with colic than in healthy horses before anesthesia, with no further increase during anesthesia [16]. Human patients in advanced stages of septic shock develop resistance to catecholamines in the treatment of vasodilatory hypotension and coincidentally have low endogenous plasma concentrations of vasopressin [139,140]. Treatment with arginine vasopressin (AVP) is recommended when hypoperfusion persists despite adequate intravascular volume and infusion of norepinephrine and dobutamine [86]. The current consensus is that AVP is not the first line of vasoactive treatment. Both the role and dose rate of AVP are controversial.

Studies of AVP administration in horses are few. One retrospective study of septic neonatal foals that were hypotensive despite administration of fluids and dobutamine, with or without norepinephrine, were treated with either norepinephrine, 0.05–1.75 μg/kg/min, or AVP, 0.1–2.5 mU/kg/min, IV [141]. Both treatments significantly increased MAP but not all foals achieved a MAP of 65 mmHg.

The issues of induced vasoconstriction and the benefit of improved systemic pressure on GI function and mortality are not resolved. Increased MAP may be the result of increased SVR associated with decreased CO and decreased tissue blood flow. Intestinal perfusion might be decreased by peripheral vasoconstriction and improved systemic hemodynamic variables may provide a sense of false security and no indication of the status at the tissue level. In one study of anesthetized pigs receiving lactated Ringer's solution 3 mL/kg/h during laparotomy, treatment of hypotension with norepinephrine (mean values 0.035–0.12 μg/kg/min to achieve MAP 65 or 75 mmHg) did not adversely affect or increase hepatosplanchnic blood flow or oxygen tension in intestinal tissue [142]. Hypotension induced by deep isoflurane anesthesia in healthy neonatal foals was treated by IV infusion of norepinephrine, AVP, or dobutamine [137]. Only AVP decreased oxygen delivery and $CcvO_2$ (oxygen content of central venous blood), and gastric tonometry indicated a decrease in gastric mucosal blood flow. The authors suggested that lack of effect of AVP on MAP might be because healthy foals would not have had a decrease in endogenous vasopressin prior to administration of AVP. The mechanism of isoflurane-induced vasodilation is not the same as sepsis-induced vasodilation; consequently, responses to vasoactive drugs may vary according to the clinical condition.

Other studies of septicemia or endotoxemia have emphasized the lack of a relationship between systemic pressure and tissue blood flow. In human patients with septic shock, dobutamine (5 μg/kg/min) increased systemic hemodynamic variables but did not improve sublingual or hepatosplanchnic perfusion [143]. In conscious sheep with induced long-term endotoxemia (24 h), hyperdynamic shock was characterized by increased CO and hypotension, increased superior mesenteric artery blood flow, and decreased intestinal muscularis and mucosal blood flow [27]. Administration of norepinephrine increased CO and MAP but had no effect on mesenteric artery and intestinal blood flow. The ileal mitochondrial activity that had been decreased by endotoxemia was not significantly increased by infusion of norepinephrine. *Escherichia coli* endotoxemia in experimental pigs was associated with decreased jejunal mucosal tissue oxygenation [144]. Norepinephrine with or without AVP increased MAP, CO, and mesenteric arterial blood flow. However, although norepinephrine improved jejunal mucosal PO_2, simultaneous infusion of AVP resulted in a smaller improvement.

Dysrhythmias

Atrial fibrillation is commonly associated with arterial hypotension during anesthesia. Fortunately, the hypotension can often be treated satisfactorily by infusion of dobutamine. Atrial fibrillation spontaneously developing during anesthesia generally reverts to normal cardiac rhythm within a few hours after anesthesia.

Second-degree AV heart block (2° AV block) is an arrhythmia that frequently occurs in resting healthy conscious horses. This arrhythmia usually disappears during anesthesia, except when detomidine or an α_2-adrenergic receptor agonist infusion is administered. Treatment is unnecessary when HR and tissue perfusion are adequate and hypotension is not present. Bradycardia, with or without 2° AV block, is sometimes observed soon after starting a dobutamine infusion. If MAP decreases, the infusion rate of dobutamine should be decreased and a different vasoactive agent, such as ephedrine, administered to maintain MAP.

Third-degree AV heart block (3° AV block) rarely develops in anesthetized horses and must be treated as a cardiac arrest. Treatment includes immediate administration of dopamine, 7–15 μg/kg/min, IV, with or without atropine, and reduced or stopped anesthetic administration. If the 3° AV block is continuous (not interspersed with normal complexes), the horse should be repositioned in lateral recumbency for external cardiac massage. Lack of response to dopamine and cardiac massage should be followed by other components of cardiopulmonary cerebral resuscitation.

Bradycardia (<24 beats/min) associated with hypotension can be countered by administration of an anticholinergic agent, with varying responses depending on the agent administered. Both atropine, 0.02 mg/kg, and hyoscine, 0.2 mg/kg, IV induced tachycardia, hypertension, and increased CI in healthy horses sedated with detomidine, 0.02 mg/kg [145]. Glycopyrrolate, 0.005 mg/kg, administered IV in anesthetized horses increased HR, MAP, and CO for 75–105 min [146]. Hyoscine, 0.1 mg/kg, IV in anesthetized horses significantly increased HR and MAP for up to 10 min but did not reduce the amount of dobutamine required to maintain MAP >70 mmHg [147]. Decreased GI function is a potential adverse effect of the use of an anticholinergic agent. Hyoscine may cause the least effect and be best suited for horses with colic. Atropine can decrease GI motility after anesthesia for several hours and occasionally up to 2 days. Glycopyrrolate prolonged decreased intestinal motility (auscultation of abdominal sounds) in horses for 10 h after anesthesia [146]. Hyoscine did not prolong intestinal motility (auscultation of intestinal sounds) in experimental horses sedated with detomidine, and GI transit time (using the solid-phase marker chromium oxide) was the same for detomidine alone and detomidine with atropine or hyoscine [145].

Tachycardia, defined as HR >55 beats/min, may have many causes during anesthesia. High intra-abdominal pressure from intestinal distension or aortocaval compression can seriously reduce venous return, initiating a reflex tachycardia, although tachycardia does not always occur in response to hypotension during anesthesia. Excessive distension of the stomach or urinary bladder may be responsible for tachycardia. Cardiac effects of endotoxin, some vasoactive drugs such as dobutamine and ephedrine, and hypercarbia may cause tachycardia. Treatment should be directed at ruling out possible causes of tachycardia. Persisting tachycardia into the postanesthetic period has been associated with increased mortality.

Premature ventricular complexes (PVCs) may be associated with endotoxemia or sympathetic stimulation [148]. Isolated PVCs do not usually warrant treatment. Lidocaine, the accepted treatment for PVCs, may already have been chosen as an anesthetic adjunct drug for its anti-inflammatory and antiendotoxin effects.

Hypoxemia

Arterial oxygenation varies widely in anesthetized horses with colic. Hypoxemia, defined as $PaO_2 \leq 60$ mmHg (8 kPa), may develop at any point in the anesthetic period, with reported prevalence between 6 and 37.8% [13,149,150]. In one study, mean PaO_2 was numerically lower in 50 horses undergoing surgery for colic than in healthy anesthetized horses but the prevalence of hypoxemia was only 6% and was not correlated with outcome [149]. Thus far, a relationship between intraoperative arterial hypoxemia and negative outcome in horses with colic has not been established. Anecdotal experiences of horses with hypoxemia (PaO_2 38–45 mmHg; 5–6 kPa) for 3.5 h followed by uncomplicated recovery from anesthesia and discharge home alive are puzzling. One might expect that hypoxemia would influence the viability of intestine with already compromised blood flow. Survival after prolonged hypoxemia without obvious neurologic signs may be in part the result of cerebral blood flow maintained above the critical level by use of cardiovascular support, and in part by the protective effect of decreased cerebral metabolic rate by anesthetic agents and by hypothermia. An experimental study in healthy horses anesthetized with isoflurane or halothane identified that circulatory function was less depressed during induced hypoxemia (PaO_2 50 mmHg; 6.65 kPa) compared with normoxia for both agents [151]. CO was higher during isoflurane than halothane anesthesia, and although biochemical markers of muscle and hepatic injury increased after anesthesia, they were lower after isoflurane, suggesting that the potential for severe effects from hypoxemia may be less during isoflurane than halothane anesthesia.

Since pressure of the GI tract on the diaphragm is a cause of inadequate ventilation and lung collapse, as expected, PaO_2 may increase when the colon is exteriorized from the abdomen [149]. Several treatments have been tested for their abilities to reverse hypoxemia (Fig. 47.2b). The first step is to increase the inspired concentration of O_2 when a lower concentration has been used, and institution of IPPV, if not already started. Occasionally, IPPV may only further expand adequately expanded alveoli with no effect on collapsed alveoli, resulting in no change or a decrease in PaO_2.

A significant consequence of dorsal recumbency in anesthetized horses is the increased proportion of cardiac output perfusing non-ventilated regions of the dependent lung (shunt). Reduction in the shunt fraction may be achieved by recruitment of collapsed alveoli using PEEP, continuous positive airway pressure (CPAP), PEEP plus lung expansion to initially reopen collapsed areas of lung (recruitment), and by redistributing perfusion by administering a drug by inhalation that results in bronchodilation, such as albuterol (salbutamol), or vasodilation, such as nitric oxide (NO).

A mild CPAP maintained during inspiration and expiration helps to keep airways open. It is used by people with obstructive sleep apnea to breath more easily at night and for the treatment of premature infants with immature lungs. The Tafonius (Hallowell

EMC, Pittsfield, MA, USA and Vetronic Services, Abbotskerswell, UK) anesthesia machine incorporates a feature that will maintain CPAP for horses. CPAP was evaluated in a prospective clinical trial of healthy anesthetized horses breathing spontaneously [152]. A CPAP of 8 cmH_2O resulted in increased PaO_2. No significant differences in MAP or dobutamine requirements were recorded in horses with or without CPAP; CI was not measured.

Addition of PEEP to the delivery circuit increased PaO_2 in some anesthetized horses but may give inconsistent results [150,153]. Increasing PEEP in healthy isoflurane-anesthetized horses to 10 and 15 cmH_2O at 15 min intervals using respiratory rates of 9 breaths/min, an inspiratory:expiratory time ratio of 1:2, and peak inspiratory pressure (PIP) of 30–33 cmH_2O significantly increased PaO_2 without decreasing CO [154]. Horses with colic that were ventilated with 10 cmH_2O PEEP from the start of anesthesia had significantly higher PaO_2 than horses receiving IPPV with no PEEP [155].

The alveolar recruitment maneuver (ARM) is a ventilator strategy involving progressive increases in airway pressure that will open bronchioles and alveoli [153,156]. This maneuver is generally combined with PEEP to maintain the improvement in oxygenation. In a group of horses with colic anesthetized and ventilated at PIPs of 35–45 cmH_2O and 10 cmH_2O PEEP, ARM was applied by increasing PIP to 60, 80, and then 60 cmH_2O for three consecutive breaths, each held for 10 s [155]. The ARM was repeated if PaO_2 was not increased, on average three times (range 1–8), and resulted in increased PaO_2 compared with conventional IPPV.

Albuterol (salbutamol) causes bronchodilation by a direct β_2-adrenergic receptor agonist effect on bronchial smooth muscle and has been used to treat horses with recurrent airway obstruction (RAO) [157,158]. Albuterol (Ventolin®) is available in a metered-dose inhaler that delivers 90 μg of drug per actuation. The dose required to induce maximum bronchodilation in conscious horses was six actuations (540 μg albuterol), but there was a large variation between individuals [from two (180 μg) to ten (900 μg) actuations]. The bronchodilation induced by albuterol lasted 30–60 min [157]. Albuterol is easily administered to anesthetized horses by introduction into the breathing circuit through an adapter at the Y-piece. The drug is administered during inspiration to ensure delivery into the lungs using several actuations at a time. In the authors' experience, administration of albuterol resulted in improvement of PaO_2 in some horses. Albuterol, 2 μg/kg, administered by inhalation in horses anesthetized for colic surgery, resulted in a significant increase in PaO_2 by 20 min [159].

Nitric oxide (NO) delivered as a pulse during inspiration should result in preferential delivery of NO to well-ventilated alveoli, increasing local blood flow by vasodilation [160]. In experimental healthy horses spontaneously breathing isoflurane (end-tidal 1.5–1.7%, $F_IO_2 > 0.9$), NO delivered into the endotracheal tube during the first 30 or 43% of inspiration increased PaO_2 and $PaCO_2$ while decreasing venous admixture [160]. In a comparison of horses with and without NO during anesthesia, PaO_2 remained higher for 30 min into recovery in horses that had received NO [161]. Administration of NO is currently cumbersome and must be improved, and the treatment must be evaluated in anesthetized horses with colic.

Recovery from anesthesia

All the complications that occur during recovery from anesthesia in healthy horses occur in horses recovering from colic surgery; airway obstruction, pulmonary edema, excitement, excessively rapid or prolonged time to standing, myopathy, neuropathy, dislocation or long bone fracture, ataxia, and lacerations. A variety of recommendations for management at this time have been made in the previous chapter.

Recovery to standing

Continuing lidocaine infusion to the end of anesthesia may result in greater ataxia and adversely impact on the quality of recovery [162]. Consequently, it is common practice to discontinue lidocaine administration approximately 30 min before moving the horse into the recovery room.

There are some features of management that are specifically relevant to horses that have had colic surgery. The NG tube should be removed at the end of anesthesia to avoid complications during recovery. The NG tube increases the risk for nasal bleeding if jostled and the tube may pass over the larynx and cause airway obstruction after endotracheal extubation. The tube may closely adhere (stick) to the nasal mucosa after an hour or more of anesthesia due to drying of membranes and so should be removed slowly to minimize the risk of nasal mucosal tears and bleeding. The risk of bleeding is increased when the tube has been inserted into the dorsal nasal meatus instead of into the larger ventral meatus. Removing the tube in the operating room before the end of anesthesia is advisable so that the horse's head can be lowered in the event of severe hemorrhage, and treatment, such as nasal packing, is more easily implemented.

Anesthesiologists vary in their management preferences for the transitional period from controlled ventilation to spontaneous breathing. Since hypoxemia is prevalent in horses in the early recovery period as a result of changes in body position, decreased ventilation, and decreased inspired O_2 concentration, the authors prefer to defer weaning to spontaneous breathing until the horse is in the recovery stall. IPPV is discontinued immediately before transportation of the horse from the operating room and controlled ventilation is resumed with a demand valve after the horse has been placed in lateral recumbency on the recovery mat. Controlled ventilation with oxygen in early recovery not only maintains oxygenation [163] but also speeds elimination of the inhalation agent that would be causing respiratory depression and residual ataxia. The demand valve is activated to deliver 8–10 breaths/min for approximately 10 min before rate is slowed to 4 breaths/min and $PaCO_2$ allowed to increase, thereby stimulating spontaneous breathing.

Xylazine, 0.2 mg/kg, or romifidine, 0.02 mg/kg, is administered IV as the depth of anesthesia appears to lighten as judged by the strength of the palpebral reflex (5–10 min after the inhalation agent is discontinued). The timing of drug administration may be adjusted by assessment of depth of inhalation anesthesia, breed and individual temperament of the patient, and recovery facilities, for example, long transportation time between surgery room and recovery stall.

The decision to remove the endotracheal tube before the horse is standing will be influenced by hospital management for healthy horses and the status of each patient, such as the presence of nasal mucosal edema, gastric reflux, or nasal hemorrhage. The endotracheal tube can be (1) left in place and taped so that the tube exits from the mouth through the interdental space, or (2) removed and a slightly smaller tube inserted through the ventral nasal meatus and guided into the trachea for nasotracheal intubation, affixed by tape around the tube and around the horse's muzzle for security, or (3) removed completely after the horse is breathing spontaneously. In all horses, supplemental oxygen should be supplied through tubing inserted into the endotracheal tube, if present, or two-thirds of the way into the ventral nasal meatus. Oxygen flow is 5 L/min for foals and 15 L/min for adult horses.

As a general guideline, the authors recommend the use of a halter and rope assistance (head and tail, as the facility allows) for horses recovering from colic surgery that have experienced any of the following during anesthesia: hypoxemia, hypotension, hypothermia, moderate to severe hemorrhage, anesthesia duration >3 h, age >20 years, exhaustion from a prolonged colic episode, clinical indication suggestive of endotoxemia, or pre-existing lameness.

Postoperative care

Pain scoring scales have been developed specifically for horses after exploratory laparotomy [164,165]. The scales may be based on observation of behaviors when alone or in response to human approach [164], and may include physiologic variables and response to palpation [165]. The activities within the categories are assigned a numerical score from 1 to 4 or from 0 to 6, with a predetermined final score indicating severe pain. The residual effects of anesthesia must be taken into consideration when assessing behavior within 5 h of the end of anesthesia, such as a down ear position, droopy eyelids, and a decrease in hind limb weight bearing, although neck angle may be unchanged [166].

Postoperative pain management generally consists of administration of an NSAID, lidocaine, and an opioid. The contribution of lidocaine to analgesia may be related to the abdominal incision, as an experimental study in awake horses indicated that lidocaine may provide somatic analgesia but not visceral analgesia (determined by duodenal and colorectal distension pressure) [112]. Butorphanol administered by IV infusion for 24 h beginning after horses were returned to their stalls significantly delayed the time to first passage of feces [167]. However, an analgesic effect was suggested because during that time, compared with horses not receiving butorphanol, the behavior scores were better, plasma cortisol concentrations were decreased and weight loss was less.

Discussions in both veterinary and human medicine question the optimal perioperative management that will minimize long-term GI depression and facilitate GI recovery. Topics include evaluation of the impact of agents, such as α_2-adrenergic receptor agonists and opioids, when continued for analgesia for several days into the recovery.

In summary, anesthetic management of horses with colic is based on a thorough preanesthetic evaluation that is a guide for choice of appropriate preanesthetic treatment, anesthetic agents, and drug dosages, and plans for anticipated complications. Important aspects of management involve maintaining the patient's physiologic status as near normal as possible by adequate preoperative treatment and manipulation of anesthetic agents and adjunct drugs during anesthesia. A smooth recovery from anesthesia is always desirable and, although largely influenced by the patient's temperament, the final result is a combination of sedation and analgesia modified by the residual effects of the GI disease, anesthesia, and the surgical procedure. More studies are needed in horses to evaluate the impact of anesthetic agents, PaO_2, and fluid therapy on the GI microcirculation and tissue oxygenation.

References

1 Traub-Dargatz JL, Kopral CA, Seitzinger AH, *et al.* Estimate of the national incidence of and operation-level risk factors for colic among horses in the United States, spring 1998 to spring 1999. *J Am Vet Med Assoc* 2001; **219**: 67–71.

2 Trim CM, Moore JN. Horses with colic. In: Tranquilli WJ, Thurmon JC, Grimm KA, eds. *Lumb and Jones' Veterinary Anesthesia and Analgesia*, 4th edn. Ames, IA: Blackwell Publishing, 2007; 1019–1026.

3 Kaneene JB, Miller R, Ross WA, *et al.* Risk factors for colic in Michigan (USA) equine population. *Prev Vet Med* 1997; **30**: 23–36.

4 Tinker MK, White NA II, Lessard P, *et al.* Prospective study of equine colic incidence and mortality. *Equine Vet J* 1997; **29**: 448–453.

5 Mair TS, Smith LJ. Survival and complication rates in 300 horses undergoing surgical treatment of colic. Part 1. Short-term survival following a single laparotomy. *Equine Vet J* 2005; **37**: 296–302.

6 Underwood C, Southwood LL, McKeown KP, *et al.* Complications and survival associated with surgical compared with medical management of horses with duodenitis–proximal jejunitis. *Equine Vet J* 2008; **40**: 373–378.

7 Lindegaard C, Ekstrøm CT, Wulf SB, *et al.* Nephrosplenic entrapment of the large colon in 142 horses (2000–2009): analysis of factors associated with decision of treatment and short-term survival. *Equine Vet J* 2011; **43**(Suppl 39): 63–68.

8 Pascoe PJ, McDonell WN, Trim CM, *et al.* Mortality rates and associated factors in equine colic operations: a retrospective study. *Can Vet J* 1983; **24**: 76–85.

9 de Bont MP, Proudman CJ, Archer DC. Surgical lesions of the small colon and post operative survival in a UK hospital population. *Equine Vet J* 2013; **45**: 460–464.

10 Suthers JM, Pinchbeck GL, Proudman CJ, *et al.* Survival of horses following strangulating large colon volvulus. *Equine Vet J* 2013; **45**: 219–223.

11 Archer DC, Pinchbeck GL, Proudman CJ. Factors associated with survival of epiploic foramen entrapment colic: a multicentre, international study. *Equine Vet J* 2011; **43**(Suppl 39): 56–62.

12 Driscoll N, Baia P, Fischer AT Jr, *et al.* Large colon resection and anastomosis in horses: 52 cases (1996–2006). *Equine Vet J* 2008; **40**: 342–347.

13 Trim CM, Adams JG, Cowgill LM, *et al.* A retrospective survey of anaesthesia in horses with colic. *Equine Vet J* 1989; (Suppl 7): 84–90.

14 Proudman CJ, Dugdale AHA, Senior JM, *et al.* Pre-operative and anaesthesia-related risk factors for mortality in equine colic cases. *Vet J* 2006; **171**: 89–97.

15 McCarthy RN, Hutchins DR. Survival rates and post-operative complications after equine colic surgery. *Aust Vet J* 1988; **65**: 40–43.

16 Ludders JW, Palos H-M, Erb HN, *et al.* Plasma arginine vasopressin concentration in horses undergoing surgery for colic. *J Vet Emerg Crit Care* 2009; **19**: 528–535.

17 Furr MO, Lessard P, White NA II. Development of a colic severity score for predicting the outcome of equine colic. *Vet Surg* 1995; **24**: 97–101.

18 Fugaro MN, Coté NM. Survival rates for horses undergoing stapled small intestinal anastomosis: 84 cases (1988–1997). *J Am Vet Med Assoc* 2001; **218**: 1603–1607.

19 Senior JM, Proudman CJ, Leuwer ML, *et al.* Plasma endotoxin in horses presented to an equine referral hospital: correlation to selected clinical parameters and outcomes. *Equine Vet J* 2011; **43**: 585–591.

20 Trim CM, Barton MH, Quandt JE. Plasma endotoxin concentrations in anesthetized horses with colic (Abstract). *Vet Surg* 1997; **26**: 163.

21 Steverink PJGM, Sturk A, Wagenaar-Hilbers JPA, *et al.* Endotoxin, interleukin-6 and tumor necrosis factor concentrations in equine acute abdominal disease: relation to clinical outcome. *Innate Immun* 1995; **2**: 289–299.

22 Corley KT, Donaldson LL, Furr MO. Arterial lactate concentration, hospital survival, sepsis, and SIRS in critically ill neonatal foals. *Equine Vet J* 2005; **37**: 53–59.

23 Epstein KL, Brainard BM, Gomez-Ibanez SE, *et al.* Thromboelastography in horses with acute gastrointestinal disease. *J Vet Intern Med* 2011; **25**: 307–314.

24 Sennoun N, Montemont C, Gibot S, *et al.* Comparative effects of early versus delayed use of norepinephrine in resuscitated endotoxic shock. *Crit Care Med* 2007; **35**: 1736–1740.

25 Verdant CL, De Backer D, Bruhn A, *et al.* Evaluation of sublingual and gut mucosal microcirculation in sepsis: a quantitative analysis. *Crit Care Med* 2009; **37**: 2875–2881.

26 Ruiz C, Hernandez G, Godoy C, *et al.* Sublingual microcirculatory changes during high-volume hemofiltration in hyperdynamic septic shock patients. *Crit Care* 2010; **14**: R170.

27 Andersson A, Rundgren M, Kalman S, *et al.* Gut microcirculatory and mitochondrial effects of hyperdynamic endotoxaemic shock and norepinephrine treatment. *Br J Anaesth* 2012; **108**: 254–261.

28 Welch RD, Watkins JP, Taylor TS, *et al.* Disseminated intravascular coagulation associated with colic in 23 horses (1984–1989). *J Vet Intern Med* 1992; **6**: 29–35.

29 Sykes BW, Furr MO. Equine endotoxemia – a state-of-the-art review of therapy. *Aust Vet J* 2005; **83**: 45–50.

30 Barton MH, Parviainen A, Norton N. Polymyxin B protects horses against induced endotoxaemia *in vivo*. *Equine Vet J* 2004; **36**: 397–401.

31 MacKay RJ, Clark CK, Logdberg L, *et al.* Effect of a conjugate of polymyxin B–dextran 70 in horses with experimentally induced endotoxemia. *Am J Vet Res* 1999; **60**: 68–75.

32 Cook VL, Jones Shults J, McDowell M, *et al.* Attenuation of ischaemic injury in the equine jejunum by administration of systemic lidocaine. *Equine Vet J* 2008; **40**: 353–357.

33 Marshall JF, Blikslager AT. The effect of nonsteroidal anti-inflammatory drugs on the equine intestine. *Equine Vet J* 2011; **43**(Suppl 39): 140–144.

34 Kelmer G, Doherty TJ, Elliot S, *et al.* Evaluation of dimethyl sulphoxide effects on initial response to endotoxin in the horse. *Equine Vet J* 2008; **40**: 358–363.

35 Hyvonen PM, Kowolik MJ. Dose-dependent suppression of the neutrophil respiratory burst by lidocaine. *Acta Anaesth Scand* 1998; **42**: 565–569.

36 Cook VL, Jones Shults J, McDowell M, *et al.* Anti-inflammatory effects of intravenously administered lidocaine hydrochloride on ischemia-injured jejunum in horses. *Am J Vet Res* 2009; **70**: 1259–1268.

37 Guschlbauer M, Hoppe S, Geburek F, *et al.* In vitro effects of lidocaine on the contractility of equine jejunal smooth muscle challenged by ischaemia-perfusion injury. *Equine Vet J* 2010; **42**: 53–58.

38 Guschlbauer M, Feige K, Geburek F, *et al.* Effects of in vivo lidocaine administration at the time of ischaemia and reperfusion on in vitro contractility of equine jejunal smooth muscle. *Am J Vet Res* 2011; **72**: 1449–1455.

39 Feige K, Schwartzwald CC, Bombeli T. Comparison of unfractioned and low molecular weight heparin for prophylaxis of coagulopathies in 52 horses with colic: a randomised double-blind clinical trial. *Equine Vet J* 2003; **35**: 506–513.

40 Werners AH, Bryant CE. Pattern recognition receptors in equine endotoxemia and sepsis. *Equine Vet J* 2012; **44**: 490–498.

41 Morton AJ, Blikslager AT. Surgical and postoperative factors influencing short-term survival of horses following small intestinal resection: 92 cases (1994–2001). *Equine Vet J* 2002; **34**: 450–454.

42 Proudman CJ, Smith JE, Edwards GB, *et al.* Long-term survival of equine surgical colic cases. Part 2. Modelling post operative survival. *Equine Vet J* 2002; **34**: 438–443.

43 Drumm NJ, Embertson RM, Woodie JB, *et al.* Factors influencing foaling rate following colic surgery in pregnant Thoroughbred mares in central Kentucky. *Equine Vet J* 2012; **45**: 346–349.

44 Chenier TS, Whitehead AE. Foaling rates and risk factors for abortion in pregnant mares presented for medical or surgical treatment of colic: 153 cases (1993–2005). *Can Vet J* 2009; **50**: 481–485.

45 Koenig J, Cote N. Equine gastrointestinal motility – ileus and pharmacological modification. *Can Vet J* 2006; **47**: 551–559.

46 Hudson NPH, Merritt AM. Equine gastrointestinal motility research: where we are and where we need to go. *Equine Vet J* 2008; **40**: 422–428.

47 Adams SB, Lamar CH, Masty J. Motility of the distal portion of the jejunum and pelvic flexure in ponies: effects of six drugs. *Am J Vet Res* 1984; **45**: 795–799.

48 Clark ES, Thompson SA, Becht JL, *et al.* Effects of xylazine on cecal mechanical activity and cecal blood flow in healthy horses. *Am J Vet Res* 1988; **49**: 720–723.

49 Merritt AM, Burrow JA, Hartless CS. Effect of xylazine, detomidine, and a combination of xylazine and butorphanol on equine duodenal motility. *Am J Vet Res* 1998; **59**: 619–623.

50 Rutkowski JA, Ross MW, Cullen K. Effects of xylazine and/or butorphanol or neostigmine on myoelectric activity of the cecum and right ventral colon in female ponies. *Am J Vet Res* 1989; **50**: 1096–1101.

51 Cruz FSF, Carregaro AB, Machado M, *et al.* Sedative and cardiopulmonary effects of buprenorphine and xylazine in horses. *Can J Vet Res* 2011; **75**: 35–41.

52 Freeman SL, England GCW. Effect of romifidine on gastrointestinal motility, assessed by transrectal ultrasonography. *Equine Vet J* 2001; **33**: 570–576.

53 Sellon DC, Monroe VL, Roberts MC, *et al.* Pharmacokinetics and adverse effects of butorphanol administered by single intravenous injection or continuous intravenous infusion in horses. *Am J Vet Res* 2001; **62**: 183–189.

54 Boscan P, Van Hoogmoed LM, Farver TB, *et al.* Evaluation of the effects of the opioid agonist morphine on gastrointestinal tract function in horses. *Am J Vet Res* 2006; **67**: 992–997.

55 Figueiredo JP, Muir WW, Sams R. Cardiorespiratory, gastrointestinal, and analgesic effects of morphine sulfate in conscious healthy horses. *Am J Vet Res* 2012; **73**: 799–808.

56 Senior JM, Pinchbeck GL, Dugdale AHA, *et al.* Retropective study of the risk factors and prevalence of colic in horses after orthopaedic surgery. *Vet Rec* 2004; **155**: 321–325.

57 Andersen MS, Clark L, Dyson SJ, *et al.* Risk factors for colic in horses after general anaesthesia for MRI or nonabdominal surgery: absence of evidence of effect from perianaesthetic morphine. *Equine Vet J* 2006; **38**: 368–374.

58 Roger T, Bardon T, Ruckebusch Y. Comparative effects of mu and kappa opiate agonists on the cecocolic motility in the pony. *Can J Vet Res* 1994; **58**: 163–166.

59 Wang S, Shah N, Philip J, *et al.* Role of alvimopan (Entereg) in gastrointestinal recovery and hospital length of stay after bowel resection. *P T* 2012; **37**: 518–525.

60 Boscan P, Van Hoogmoed LM, Pypendop BH, *et al.* Pharmacokinetics of the opioid antagonist *N*-methylnaltrexone and evaluation of its effects on gastrointestinal tract function in horses treated or not treated with morphine. *Am J Vet Res* 2006; **67**: 998–1004.

61 Vainionpää MH, Raekallio MR, Pakkanen SAE, *et al.* Plasma drug concentrations and clinical effects of a peripheral alpha-2-adrenoceptor antagonist, MK-467, in horses sedated with detomidine. *Vet Anaesth Analg* 2013; **40**: 257–264.

62 Durongphongtorn S, McDonell WN, Kerr CL, *et al.* Comparison of hemodynamic, clinicopathalogic, and gastrointestinal motility effects and recovery characteristics of anesthesia with isoflurane and halothane in horses undergoing arthroscopic surgery. *Am J Vet Res* 2006; **67**: 32–42.

63 De Corte W, Delrue H, Vanfleteren LJ, *et al.* Randomized clinical trial on the influence of anaesthesia protocol on intestinal motility during laparoscopic surgery requiring small bowel anastomosis. *Br J Surg* 2012; **99**: 1524–1529.

64 Rusieki KI, Nieto JE, Puchalski SM, *et al.* Evaluation of continuous infusion of lidocaine on gastrointestinal tract function in normal horses. *Vet Surg* 2008; **37**: 564–570.

65 Milligan M, Beard W, KuKanich B, *et al.* The effect of lidocaine on postoperative jejunal motility in normal horses. *Vet Surg* 2007; **36**: 214–220.

66 Tappenbeck K, Hoppe S, Hopster K, *et al.* Lidocaine and structure-related mexiletine induce similar contractility-enhancing effects in ischaemia–reperfusion injured equine intestinal smooth muscle in vitro. *Vet J* 2013; **196**: 461–466.

67 van Bree SHW, Nemethova A, Cailotto C, *et al.* New therapeutic strategies for postoperative ileus. *Nat Rev Gastroenterol Hepatol* 2012; **9**: 675–683.

68 Wehner S, Vilz TO, Stoffels B, *et al.* Immune mediators of postoperative ileus. *Langenbecks Arch Surg* 2012; **397**: 591–601.

69 Doherty TJ. Postoperative ileus: pathogenesis and treatment. *Vet Clin North Am Equine Pract* 2009; **25**: 351–362.

70 Leslie JB, Viscusi ER, Pergolizzi JV Jr, *et al.* Anesthetic routines: the anesthesiologist's role in GI recovery and postoperative ileus. *Adv Prev Med* 2011; **2011**: 976904.

71 Schatzmann U, Josseck H, Stauffer JL, Goossens L. Effects of alpha 2-agonists on intrauterine pressure and sedation in horses: comparison between detomidine, romifidine and xylazine. *Zentralbl Veterinarmed A* 1994; **41**: 523–529.

72 Valverde A, Black B, Cribb NC, *et al.* Assessment of unassisted recovery from repeated general isoflurane anesthesia in horses following post-anesthetic administration of xylazine or acepromazine or a combination of xylazine and ketamine. *Vet Anaesth Analg* 2013; **40**: 3–12.

73 Garcia-Lopez JM, Provost PJ, Rush JE, *et al.* Prevalence and prognostic importance of hypomagnesemia and hypocalcemia in horses that have colic surgery. *Am J Vet Res* 2001; **62**: 7–12.

74 Nolen-Walston RD. Flow rates of large animal fluid delivery systems used for high-volume crystalloid resuscitation. *J Vet Emerg Crit Care* 2012; **22**: 661–665.

75 Sutton GA, Dahan R, Turner D, *et al.* A behaviour-based pain scale for horses with acute colic: scale construction. *Vet J* 2013; **196**: 394–401.

76 Ashley FH, Waterman-Pearson AE, Whay HR. Behavioural assessment of pain in horses and donkeys: application to clinical practice and future studies. *Equine Vet J* 2005; **37**: 565–575.

77 Delesalle C, Dewulf J, Lefebvre RA, *et al.* Use of plasma ionized calcium levels and Ca^{2+} substitution response patterns as prognostic parameters for ileus and survival in colic horses. *Vet Q* 2005; **27**: 157–172.

78 Moore JN, Owen RR, Lumsden JH. Clinical evaluation of blood lactate levels in equine colic. *Equine Vet J* 1976; **8**: 49–54.

79 Dunkel B, Kapff JE, Naylor RJ, Boston R. Blood lactate concentrations in ponies and miniature horses with gastrointestinal disease. *Equine Vet J* 2013; **45**, 666–670.

80 van den Boom R, Butler CM, van Oldruitenborgh-Oosterbaan MMS. The usability of peritoneal lactate concentration as a prognostic marker in horses with severe colic admitted to a veterinary teaching hospital. *Equine Vet Educ* 2010; **22**: 420–425.

81 Castagnetti C, Pirrone A, Mariella J, *et al.* Venous blood lactate evaluation in equine neonatal intensive care. *Theriogenology* 2010; **73**: 343–357.

82 Tennent-Brown BS, Wilkins PA, Lindborg S, *et al.* Sequential plasma lactate concentrations as prognostic indicators in adult equine emergencies. *J Vet Intern Med* 2010; **24**: 198–205.

83 Griesdale DEG, de Souza RJ, van Dam RM, *et al.* Intensive insulin therapy and mortality among critically ill patients: a meta-analysis including NICE-SUGAR study data. *Can Med Assoc J* 2009; **180**: 821–827.

84 Chappell D, Jacob M, Hoffmann-Kiefer K, *et al.* A rational approach to perioperative fluid management. *Anesthesiology* 2008; **109**: 723–740.

85 Bayer O, Reinhart K, Sakr Y, *et al.* Renal effects of synthetic colloids and crystalloids in patients with severe sepsis: a prospective sequential comparison. *Crit Care Med* 2011; **39**: 1335–1342.

86 Dellinger RP, Levy MM, Rhodes A, *et al.* Surviving Sepsis Campaign: International Guidelines for Management of Severe Sepsis and Septic Shock: 2012. *Crit Care Med* 2013; **41**: 580–637.

87 Vincent JL, Gerlach H. Fluid resuscitation in severe sepsis and septic shock: an evidence based review. *Crit Care Med* 2004; **32**(Suppl 11): S451–S454.

88 Santry HP, Alam HB. Fluid resuscitation: past, present, and the future. *Shock* 2010; **33**: 229–241.

89 Westphal M, James MF, Kozek-Langenecker S, *et al.* Hydroxyethyl starches: different products – different effects. *Anesthesiology* 2009; **111**: 187–202.

90 Epstein KL, Bergren A, Giguère S, Brainard BM. Cardiovascular, colloid osmotic pressure and hemostatic effects of 2 formulations of hydroxyethyl starch in healthy horses. *J Vet Intern Med* 2014; **28**: 223–233.

91 Schusser GF, Rieckhoff K, Ungemach FR, *et al.* Effect of hydroxyethyl starch solution in normal horses and horses with colic or acute colitis. *J Vet Med A Physiol Pathol Clin Med* 2007; **54**: 592–598.
92 Hallowell GD, Corley KT. Preoperative administration of hydroxyethyl starch or hypertonic saline to horses with colic. *J Vet Intern Med* 2006; **20**: 980–986.
93 Bayer O, Reinhart K, Kohl M, *et al.* Effects of fluid resuscitation with synthetic colloids or crystalloids alone on shock reversal, fluid balance, and patient outcomes in patients with severe sepsis: a prospective sequential analysis. *Crit Care Med* 2012; **40**: 2543–2551.
94 Oliveira RP, Velasco I, Soriano FG, *et al.* Clinical review: hypertonic saline resuscitation in sepsis. *Crit Care* 2002; **6**: 418–423.
95 Pascual JL, Khwaja KA, Chaudhury P, *et al.* Hypertonic saline and the microcirculation. *J Trauma* 2003; **54**(Suppl 5): S133–S140.
96 Oliveira RP, Weingartner R, Ribas EO, *et al.* Acute haemodynamic effects of a hypertonic saline/dextran solution in stable patients with severe sepsis. *Intensive Care Med* 2002; **28**: 1574–1581.
97 Kreimeier U, Thiel M, Peter K, *et al.* Small-volume hyperosmolar resuscitation. *Acta Anaesth Scand* 1997; **41**: 302–306.
98 Pantaleon LG, Furr MO, McKenzie HC II, *et al.* Cardiovascular and pulmonary effects of hetastarch plus hypertonic saline solutions during experimental endotoxemia in anesthetized horses. *J Vet Intern Med* 2006; **20**: 1422–1428.
99 Gan TJ, Soppitt A, Maroof M, *et al.* Goal-directed intraoperative fluid administration reduces length of hospital stay after major surgery. *Anesthesiology* 2002; **97**: 820–826.
100 Kimberger O, Arnberger M, Brandt S, *et al.* Goal-directed colloid administration improves the microcirculation of healthy and perianastomotic colon. *Anesthesiology* 2009; **110**: 496–504.
101 Boscan P, Watson Z, Steffey EP. Plasma colloid osmotic pressure and total protein trends in horses during anesthesia. *Vet Anaesth Analg* 2007; **34**: 275–283.
102 Boscan P, Steffey EP. Plasma colloid osmotic pressure and total protein in horses during colic surgery. *Vet Anaesth Analg* 2007; **34**: 408–415.
103 Brauer KI, Scensen C, Hahn RG, *et al.* Volume kinetic analysis of the distribution of 0.9% saline in conscious versus isoflurane-anesthetized sheep. *Anesthesiology* 2002; **96**: 442–429.
104 Kalff JC, Buchholz BM, Eskandari MK, *et al.* Biphasic response to gut manipulation and temporal correlation of cellular infiltrates and muscle dysfunction in rat. *Surgery* 1999; **126**: 498–509.
105 Behrendt FF, Tolba RH, Overhaus M, *et al.* Indocyanine green fluorescence measurement of intestinal transit and gut perfusion after intestinal manipulation. *Eur Surg Res* 2004; **36**: 210–218.
106 Moppett I, Sevdalis N. From pilots to Olympians: enhancing performance in anaesthesia through mental practice. *Br J Anaesth* 2013; **110**: 169–172.
107 Hayter MA, Bould MD, Afsari M, *et al.* Does warm-up using mental practice improve crisis resource management performance? A simulation study. *Br J Anaesth* 2013; **110**: 299–304.
108 Braun C, Trim CM, Maney JK, *et al.* Selected cardiopulmonary effects of hoisting anaesthetized horses (Abstract). Association of Veterinary Anaesthetists Spring Meeting, London, 10–12 April 2013.
109 Braun C, Trim CM, Eggleston RB. Effects of changing body position on oxygenation and arterial blood pressures in foals anesthetized with guaifenesin, ketamine, and xylazine. *Vet Anaesth Analg* 2009; **36**: 18–24.
110 Kimberger O, Fleischmann E, Brandt S, *et al.* Supplemental oxygen, but not supplemental crystalloid fluid, increases tissue oxygen tension in healthy and anastomotic colon in pigs. *Anesth Analg* 2007; **105**: 773–779.
111 Driessen B, Nann L, Benton R, *et al.* Differences in need for hemodynamic support in horses anesthetized with sevoflurane as compared to isoflurane. *Vet Anaesth Analg* 2006; **33**: 356–367.
112 Robertson SA, Sanchez LC, Merritt AM, *et al.* Effect of systemic lidocaine on visceral and somatic nociception in conscious horses. *Equine Vet J* 2005; **37**: 122–127.
113 Dickey EJ, McKenzie HC III, Brown JA, *et al.* Serum concentrations of lidocaine and its metabolites after prolonged infusion in healthy horses. *Equine Vet J* 2008; **40**: 348–352.
114 Wagner AE, Mama KR, Steffey EP, *et al.* Comparison of the cardiovascular effects of equipotent anesthetic doses of sevoflurane alone and sevoflurane plus an intravenous infusion of lidocaine in horses. *Am J Vet Res* 2011; **72**: 452–460.
115 Feary DJ, Mama KR, Wagner AE, *et al.* Influence of general anesthesia on pharmacokinetics of intravenous lidocaine infusion in horses. *Am J Vet Res* 2005; **66**: 574–580.
116 Dodman NH, Williams RN, Court MH, *et al.* Postanesthetic hind limb adductor myopathy in five horses. *J Am Vet Med Assoc* 1988; **193**: 83–86.
117 Parviainen AK, Trim CM. Complications associated with anaesthesia for ocular surgery: a retrospective study 1989–1996. *Equine Vet J* 2000; **32**: 555–559.
118 Koenig J, McDonell W, Valverde A. Accuracy of pulse oximetry and capnography in healthy and compromised horses during spontaneous and controlled ventilation. *Can J Vet Res* 2003; **67**: 169–174.
119 Grosenbaugh DA, Muir WW. Cardiorespiratory effects of sevoflurane, isoflurane, and halothane anesthesia in horses. *Am J Vet Res* 1998; **59**: 101–106.
120 Thomas WP, Madigan JE, Backus KQ, *et al.* Systemic and pulmonary haemodynamics in normal neonatal foals. *J Reprod Fertil* 1987; **35**(Suppl): 623–628.
121 Young SS, Taylor PM. Factors influencing the outcome of equine anaesthesia: a review of 1,314 cases. *Equine Vet J* 1993; **25**: 147–151.
122 Perel A, Pizov R, Cotev S. Systolic blood pressure variation is a sensitive indicator of hypovolemia in ventilated dogs subjected to graded hemorrhage. *Anesthesiology* 1987; **67**: 498–502.
123 Michard F, Chemla D, Richard C, *et al.* Clinical use of respiratory changes in arterial pulse pressure to monitor the hemodynamic effects of PEEP. *Am J Respir Crit Care Med* 1999; **159**: 935–939.
124 Fielding CL, Stolba DN. Pulse pressure variation and systolic pressure variation in horses undergoing general anesthesia. *J Vet Emerg Crit Care* 2012; **22**: 372–375.
125 Marik PE, Cavallazzi R, Vasu T, *et al.* Dynamic changes in arterial waveform derived variables and fluid responsiveness in mechanically ventilated patients: a systematic review of the literature. *Crit Care Med* 2009; **37**: 2642–2647.
126 Freitas FGR, Bafi AT, Nascente APM, *et al.* Predictive value of pulse pressure variation for fluid responsiveness in septic patients using lung-protective ventilation strategies. *Br J Anaesth* 2013; **110**: 402–408.
127 Ambrisko TD, Coppens P, Kabes R, *et al.* Lithium dilution, pulse power analysis, and continuous thermodilution cardiac output measurements compared with bolus thermodilution in anaesthetized ponies. *Br J Anaesth* 2012; **109**: 864–869.
128 Giguère S, Bucki E, Adin DB, *et al.* Cardiac output measurement by carbon dioxide rebreathing, 2-dimentional echocardiography, and lithium dilution method in anesthetized neonatal foals. *J Vet Intern Med* 2005; **19**: 737–743.
129 Valverde A, Giguère S, Morey TE, *et al.* Comparison of noninvasive cardiac output measured by use of partial carbon dioxide rebreathing or the lithium dilution method in anesthetized foals. *Am J Vet Res* 2007; **68**: 141–147.
130 Walley KR. Use of central venous oxygen saturation to guide therapy. *Am J Respir Crit Care Med* 2011; **184**: 514–520.
131 Raisis AL, Young LE, Blissitt KJ, *et al.* Effect of a 30-min infusion of dobutamine hydrochloride on hind limb blood flow and hemodynamics in halothane-anesthetized horses. *Am J Vet Res* 2000; **61**: 1282–1288.
132 Swanson CR, Muir WW III, Bednarski RM, *et al.* Hemodynamic responses in halothane-anesthetized horses given infusions of dopamine or dobutamine. *Am J Vet Res* 1985; **46**: 365–370.
133 Craig CA, Haskins SC, Hildebrand SV. The cardiopulmonary effects of dobutamine and norepinephrine in isoflurane-anesthetized foals. *Vet Anaesth Analg* 2007; **34**: 377–387.
134 Fantoni DT, Marchioni GG, Ida KK, *et al.* Effect of ephedrine and phenylephrine on cardiopulmonary parameters in horses undergoing elective surgery. *Vet Anaesth Analg* 2013; **40**: 367–374.
135 Hollis AR, Ousey JC, Palmer L, *et al.* Effects of norepinephrine and a combined norepinephrine and dobutamine infusion on systemic hemodynamics and indices of renal function in normotensive neonatal Thoroughbred foals. *J Vet Intern Med* 2006; **20**: 1437–1442.
136 Hollis AR, Ousey JC, Palmer L, *et al.* Effects of norepinephrine and combined norepinephrine and fenoldepam infusion on systemic hemodynamics and indices of renal function in normotensive neonatal foals. *J Vet Intern Med* 2008; **22**: 1210–1215.
137 Valverde A, Giguère S, Sanchez CL, *et al.* Effects of dobutamine, norepinephrine, and vasopressin on cardiovascular function in anesthetized neonatal foals with induced hypotension. *Am J Vet Res* 2006; **67**: 1730–1737.
138 Dugdale AHA, Langford J, Senior JM, *et al.* The effect of inotropic and/or vasopressor support on postoperative survival following equine colic surgery. *Vet Anaesth Analg* 2007; **34**: 82–88.
139 Bauer SR, Lam SW. Arginine vasopressin for the treatment of septic shock in adults. *Pharmacotherapy* 2010; **30**: 1057–1071.
140 Maybauer MO, Walley KR. Best vasopressor for advanced vasodilatory shock: should vasopressin be part of the mix? *Intensive Care Med* 2010; **36**: 1484–1487.
141 Dickey EJ, McKenzie HC III, Johnson A, *et al.* Use of pressor therapy in 34 hypotensive critically ill neonatal foals. *Aust Vet J* 2010; **88**: 472–477.
142 Hiltebrand LB, Koepfli E, Kimberger O, *et al.* Hypotension during fluid-restricted abdominal surgery. Effects of norepinephrine treatment on regional and microcirculatory blood flow in the intestinal tract. *Anesthesiology* 2011; **114**: 557–564.
143 Hernandez G, Bruhn A, Luengo C, *et al.* Effects of dobutamine on systemic, regional and microcirculatory perfusion parameters in septic shock: a randomized, placebo-controlled, double-blind, crossover study. *Intensive Care Med* 2013; **39**: 1435–1443.
144 Maier S, Hasibeder W, Pajk W, *et al.* Arginine-vasopressin attenuates beneficial norepinephrine effect on jejunal mucosal tissue oxygenation during endotoxinaemia. *Br J Anaesth* 2009; **103**: 691–700.

145 Pimenta ELM, Teixeira Neto FJ, Sá PA, *et al.* Comparative study between atropine and hyoscine-N-butylbromide for reversal of detomidine induced bradycardia in horses. *Equine Vet J* 2011; **43**: 332–340.
146 Teixeira Neto FJ, McDonell WN, Black WD, *et al.* Effects of glycopyrrolate on cardiorespiratory function in horses anesthetized with halothane and xylazine. *Am J Vet Res* 2004; **65**: 456–463.
147 Borer KE, Clarke KW. The effect of hyoscine on dobutamine requirement in spontaneously breathing horses anesthetized with halothane. *Vet Anaesth Analg* 2006; **33**: 149–157.
148 Nostell K, Bröjer J, Höglund K, *et al.* Cardiac troponin I and the occurrence of cardiac arrhythmias in horses with experimentally induced endotoxemia. *Vet J* 2012; **192**: 171–175.
149 McCoy AM, Hackett ES, Wagner AE, *et al.* Pulmonary gas exchange and plasma lactate in horses with gastrointestinal disease undergoing emergency exploratory laparotomy: a comparison with an elective surgery horse population. *Vet Surg* 2011; **40**: 601–609.
150 Wilson DV, McFeely AM. Positive end-expiratory pressure during colic surgery in horses: 74 cases (1986–1988). *J Am Vet Med Assoc* 1991; **199**: 917–921.
151 Whitehair KJ, Steffey EP, Woliner MJ, *et al.* Effects of inhalation anesthetic agents on response of horses to three hours of hypoxemia. *Am J Vet Res* 1996; **57**: 351–360.
152 Mosing M, Rysnik M, Bardell D, *et al.* Use of continuous positive airway pressure (CPAP) to optimise oxygenation in anaesthetised horses – a clinical study. *Equine Vet J* 2013; **45**: 414–418.
153 Moens Y. Mechanical ventilation and respiratory mechanics during equine anesthesia. *Vet Clin North Am Equine Pract* 2013; **29**: 51–67.
154 Ambrósio AM, Ida KK, Souto MTMR, *et al.* Effects of positive pressure titration on gas exchange, respiratory mechanics and hemodynamics in anesthetized horses. *Vet Anaesth Analg* 2013; **40**: 564–572.
155 Hopster K, Kästner SB, Rohn K, *et al.* Intermittent positive pressure ventilation with constant positive end-expiratory pressure and alveolar recruitment manoeuvre during inhalation anaesthesia in horses undergoing surgery for colic, and its influence on the early recovery period. *Vet Anaesth Analg* 2011; **38**: 169–177.
156 Tusman G, Böhm SH. Prevention and reversal of lung collapse during the intraoperative period. *Best Pract Res Clin Anaesthesiol* 2010; **24**: 183–197.
157 Derksen FJ, Olszewski MA, Robinson NE, *et al.* Aerosolized albuterol sulfate used as a bronchodilator in horses with recurrent airway obstruction. *Am J Vet Res* 1999; **60**: 689–693.
158 Bertin FR, Ivester KM, Couëtil LL. Comparative efficacy of inhaled albuterol between two hand-held delivery devices in horses with recurrent airway obstruction. *Equine Vet J* 2011; **43**: 393–398.
159 Robertson SA, Bailey JE. Aerosolized salbutamol (albuterol) improves PaO_2 in hypoxaemic anaesthetized horses – a prospective clinical trial in 81 horses. *Vet Anaesth Analg* 2002; **29**: 212–218.
160 Nyman G, Grubb TL, Heinonen E, *et al.* Pulsed delivery of inhaled nitric oxide counteracts hypoxemia during 2.5 hours of inhalation anaesthesia in dorsally recumbent horses. *Vet Anaesth Analg* 2012; **39**: 480–487.
161 Grubb T, Edner A, Frendin JHM, *et al.* Oxygenation and plasma endothelin-1 concentrations in healthy horses recovering from isoflurane anaesthesia administered with or without pulse-delivered inhaled nitric oxide. *Vet Anaesth Analg* 2013; **40**: e9–e18.
162 Valverde A, Gunkel C, Doherty TJ, *et al.* Effect of a constant rate infusion of lidocaine on the quality of recovery from sevoflurane or isoflurane general anaesthesia in horses. *Equine Vet J* 2005; **37**: 559–564.
163 Ida KK, Fantoni DT, Souto MTMR, *et al.* Effect of pressure support ventilation during weaning on ventilation and oxygenation indices in healthy horses recovering from general anesthesia. *Vet Anaesth Analg* 2013; **40**: 339–350.
164 Pritchett LC, Ulibarri C, Roberts MC, *et al.* Identification of potential physiological and behavioral indicators of postoperative pain in horses after exploratory celiotomy for colic. *Appl Anim Behav Sci* 2003; **80**: 31–43.
165 Graubner C, Gerber V, Doherr MG, *et al.* Clinical application and reliability of a post abdominal surgery pain assessment scale (PASPAS) in horses. *Vet J* 2011; **188**: 178–183.
166 Seibert LM, Parthasarathy V, Trim CM, *et al.* An ethogram of post-anesthetic recovery behaviors in horses: comparison of pre- and post-anesthetic behaviors. *Vet Anaesth Analg* 2003; **30**: 113.
167 Sellon DC, Roberts MC, Blikslager AT, *et al.* Effects of continuous rate intravenous infusion of butorphanol on physiologic and outcome variables in horses after celiotomy. *J Vet Intern Med* 2004; **18**: 555–563.

48 Equine Local Anesthetic and Analgesic Techniques

Rachael E. Carpenter[1] and Christopher R. Byron[2]

[1] Virginia-Maryland Regional College of Veterinary Medicine, Blacksburg, Virginia, USA

[2] Virginia-Maryland College of Veterinary Medicine, Virginia Tech, Blacksburg, Virginia, USA

Chapter contents

Introduction

In horses, many diagnostic and surgical procedures can be performed safely and humanely by combining local anesthetic techniques with sedation and/or physical restraint. In conjunction with a good physical examination, and thorough palpation of the limbs including tendons and joints, one of the most important techniques for the equine practitioner to master is local and regional anesthesia and analgesia of the limbs. Use of these techniques can aid in localizing lameness, provide analgesia and anesthesia for standing procedures or diagnostics, and provide intra- or postoperative analgesia. Mastery of other techniques (e.g., epidural and craniofacial nerve blocks) will facilitate procedures on standing patients, avoiding the relatively high morbidity and mortality associated with general anesthesia of the equine patient.

Choice of local anesthetic agent

The choice of which local anesthetic(s) to be used is usually made based on the onset and duration of action of the individual agent(s) and the desired result. Improper injection technique or misidentification of the landmarks can result in incomplete block and other complications. Aseptic preparation of the skin is recommended for local anesthetic injection sites, especially when injecting into a joint or the epidural or subarachnoid space. Desired anesthetic effects without complications are obtained by using proper techniques, including aspiration before injection to avoid intravenous or intra-arterial administration and avoidance of injections through or into inflamed tissues.

The blocks described in this chapter are most commonly accomplished with lidocaine (with the exception of the diagnostic blocks for lameness examination) unless specified otherwise. Lidocaine has a rapid onset of action and a relatively short duration of effect of about 1 h. Where a longer duration of action is desired (for analgesia), mepivacaine, bupivacaine, or ropivacaine may be substituted. Local anesthesia of the limbs for diagnostic nerve blocks is usually accomplished with mepivacaine because it has a slightly longer duration of effect than lidocaine (up to 2 h), but lidocaine may be substituted at the same volume if needed. For more in-depth information on the pharmacology (metabolism, elimination, toxicity, and individual medication profiles) of local anesthetics, see Chapter 17.

Anesthesia of the head

Local anesthesia of the head is most commonly used clinically for dental and sinus surgery, ocular examinations, and laceration repair.

Veterinary Anesthesia and Analgesia: The Fifth Edition of Lumb and Jones.
Edited by Kurt A. Grimm, Leigh A. Lamont, William J. Tranquilli, Stephen A. Greene and Sheilah A. Robertson.

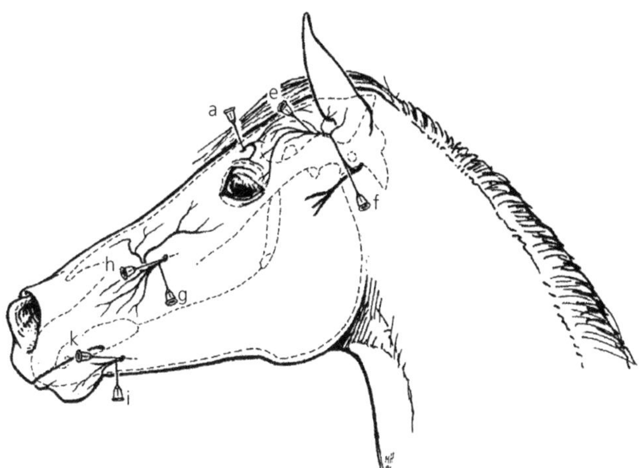

Figure 48.1 Sites for needle placement to desensitize the supraorbital (a), auriculopalpebral (e and f), infraorbital (g and h), mental (i), and alveolar mandibular (k) nerves.

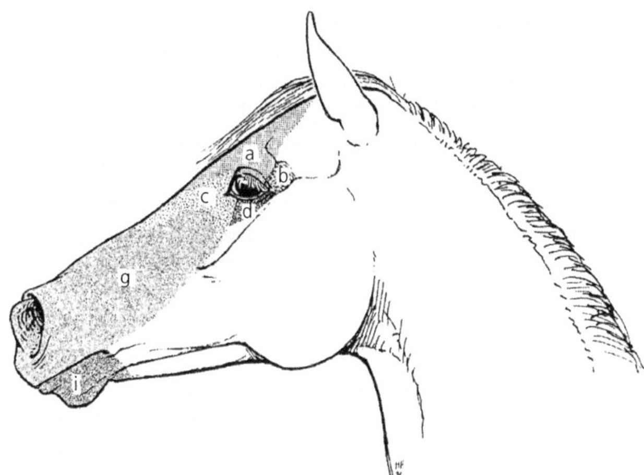

Figure 48.2 Area of skin desensitization after blocking the supraorbital (a), lacrimal (b), infratrochlear (c), zygomatic (d), infraorbital (g), and mental (i) nerves.

Infraorbital nerve block

The infraorbital nerve block facilitates surgery of the nasal area or incisors. Desensitization of the upper lip and nose is achieved by injecting 5 mL of local anesthetic with a 1 in (2.5 cm) 20 G needle over the infraorbital nerve as it emerges from the infraorbital canal (Fig. 48.1g). The infraorbital canal can be palpated after displacing the flat levator labi superioris muscle dorsally, and then palpating with the index finger approximately half the distance and 2.5 cm dorsal to a line connecting the nasomaxillary notch and the rostral end of the facial crest.

To desensitize the teeth as far as the first molar, the maxillary sinus, the roof of the nasal cavity, and the skin almost to the medial canthus of the eye, 5 mL of local anesthetic are deposited within the infraorbital foramen using a 2 in (5.0 cm) 20 G needle (Fig. 48.1h) [1]. The local anesthesia produced by this technique is generally not sufficient to allow standing extraction of the premolars or trephination of the maxillary sinus, but may be a useful adjunct to general anesthesia in those cases. A study using computed tomography (CT) and contrast injections examined two techniques for infiltration of the infraorbital nerve within the pterygopalatine fossa in the hopes of refining the technique for better analgesia of the cheek teeth [2].

Recent work has suggested that idiopathic head shaking may be a facial pain syndrome resulting from trigeminal neuropathy. Idiopathic head shaking is a diagnosis without a conclusive diagnostic test, but a recent study has suggested utilizing desensitization of the infraorbital nerve as a diagnostic tool for this disorder [3].

Maxillary nerve block

Desensitization of the maxilla, premaxilla, paranasal sinuses, and sinus cavity can be achieved by blocking the maxillary nerve at the pterygopalatine fossa (where the nerve enters the infraorbital canal). Two methods of infiltration have been described. In the first, a 3.5 in (8.9 cm) 20–22 G spinal needle is inserted on the ventral border of the zygomatic process of the temporal bone at the narrowest point of the zygomatic arch and directed rostromedially and ventrally in the direction of the sixth cheek tooth on the contralateral maxillary arcade [4]. The second approach is accomplished by inserting the needle at a 90° angle to the head so that it enters the pterygopalatine fossa just caudal to the maxillary tuberosity [5]. Recently, a cadaver study evaluated the accuracy of methods used to infiltrate the maxillary nerve, and determined that using an angulated needle placement or a perpendicular needle placement were equally accurate [6].

Mandibular nerve block

Blocking the mandibular nerve will desensitize the ipsilateral side of the mandible and the associated dental structures. The mandibular nerve can be blocked as it enters the mandibular canal at the mandibular foramen where it becomes the inferior alveolar nerve. The location of the mandibular foramen may be approximated using the intersection of a line passing vertically downwards from the lateral canthus of the eye and a line extending backwards from the table of the mandibular molar teeth. A 6 in (15.24 cm) 20–22 G needle is inserted at the ventral border of the ramus, just rostral to the angle of the mandible and then advanced to the location of the mandibular foramen. In that location, 15–20 mL of local anesthetic may be injected. The second approach involves inserting the needle at the caudal border of the ventral ramus of the mandible about 3 cm ventral to the temporomandibular joint and then advancing the needle to the approximate location of the mandibular foramen, taking care to stay as close to the medial aspect of the mandible as possible. To perform the block, 15–20 mL of local anesthetic are injected into the area. A recent study examined the accuracy of the two approaches to the inferior alveolar nerve block and found that both the traditional approaches were accurate, but that currently recommended doses of local anesthetics may be excessive [7].

Mental nerve block

To desensitize the lower lip, the mental nerve is blocked with 5 mL of local anesthetic rostral to the mental foramen (Figs 48.1i and 48.2i). After the tendon of the depressor labii inferioris is displaced, the lateral border of the mental foramen is palpated at the horizontal ramus of the mandible in the middle of the interdental space [8].

The lower incisors and premolars can be desensitized by inserting a 3 in (7.5 cm) 20 G spinal needle into the mental foramen as far as possible in a ventromedial direction and depositing 10 mL of local anesthetic to desensitize the mandibular alveolar nerve. This technique is difficult and is probably best used as an adjunct to general anesthesia for extraction of teeth.

Anesthesia for ocular procedures

Because of the strength with which the horse can close its eyelids and keep them closed, some form of sedation and local anesthesia is generally required for a complete ophthalmic examination. These same techniques will often allow satisfactory completion of minor diagnostic and surgical procedures. In addition to the specific blocks listed below, a line block (local anesthetic deposited along the superior and/or inferior orbital rims) and infiltration anesthesia may be used to facilitate surgical procedures and placement of subpalpebral lavage catheters.

Topical anesthesia

Topical anesthesia is usually required for examination of an eye that is a source of pain. In addition, topical anesthesia will facilitate minor diagnostic and surgical procedures of the cornea and conjunctiva such as collection of samples for cytologic examination, removal of superficial corneal foreign bodies, and subconjunctival injections.

Proparacaine and tetracaine are the most commonly used topical ophthalmic anesthetics. Preservative-free ophthalmic formulations are preferred for topical ocular use because preservatives can damage the corneal epithelium. Although proparacaine and tetracaine are generally interchangeable, tetracaine is more irritating to the cornea than proparacaine. Other local anesthetics that have been used topically include lidocaine, mepivacaine, and bupivacaine.

In humans, the onset of action of proparacaine is approximately 15 s, and the duration of action is approximately 15–30 min [9]. In horses, using two drops of 0.5% tetracaine increases the duration of maximal anesthetic effects from 5.5 to 16 min, and increasing the concentration to 1% tetracaine increases the duration of maximal anesthetic effects from 5.5 to 15.25 min [10]. A study in horses compared the efficacy and duration of topically applied proparacaine ophthalmic solution, lidocaine injectable solution, mepivacaine injectable solution, and bupivacaine injectable solution and concluded that bupivacaine may be most appropriate for procedures requiring longer periods of corneal anesthesia. In that study, corneal sensitivity was decreased for 35 min following topical application of 0.5% proparacaine and 2% mepivacaine, for 45 min following 2% lidocaine, and for 60 min following 0.5% bupivacaine [11].

Repeated use of topical anesthesia can reduce Schirmer tear test values, cause mild corneal epithelial damage, and suppress wound healing with prolonged use. Because of these potential adverse effects, topical anesthetics should not be prescribed as analgesic agents for painful ocular conditions.

Auriculopalpebral nerve block

The most important nerve block used in ocular examinations to prevent closure of the eyelid is the auriculopalpebral nerve block. This block primarily affects the motor innervation to the orbicularis oculi muscle, without affecting the sensory innervation to the eyelids.

The auriculopalpebral nerve is usually blocked where the nerve is easily palpable along the most dorsal aspect of the zygomatic arch (Fig. 48.3e) or the depression caudal to the mandible at the ventral edge of the temporal position of the zygomatic arch (Fig. 48.3f). In each location, the needle is placed subcutaneously in the area where the nerve is palpated and 1–2 mL of local anesthetic are injected over the nerve [8,12].

Auriculopalpebral blocks will diminish the blink reflex, so artificial tears should be applied to the cornea to prevent drying and care should be exercised to protect the eye from accidental trauma or debris until recovery is complete. Despite the suggestion that relaxation of the eyelid from auriculopalpebral nerve blocks would lower intraocular pressure (IOP) and interfere with the diagnosis of glaucoma, it has been shown that an auriculopalpebral nerve block has no effect on IOP [13].

Sensory nerve blocks

The supraorbital nerve block will desensitize the majority of the upper eyelid, and can be used to facilitate minor surgical procedures of the nasal portion of the upper lid. The nerve emerges through the supraorbital foramen, which can be easily palpated

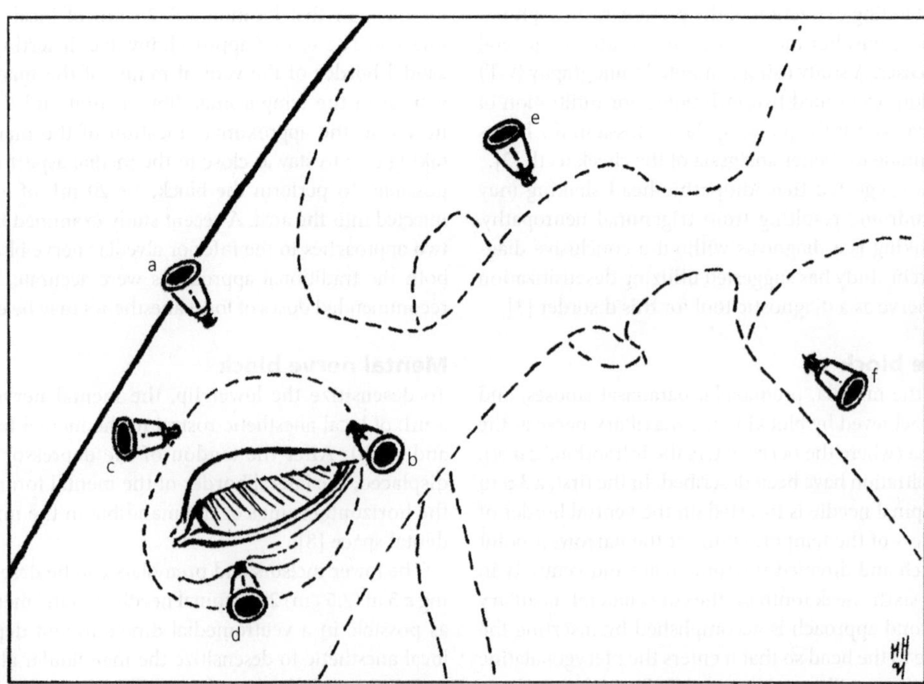

Figure 48.3 Needle placement to supraorbital (a), lacrimal (b), infratrochlear (c), zygomatic (d), and auriculopalpebral (e and f) nerves.

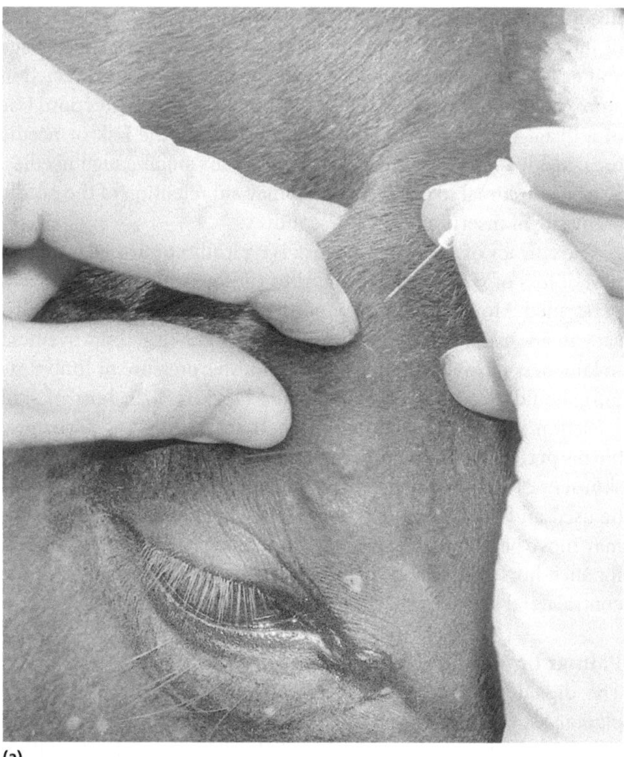

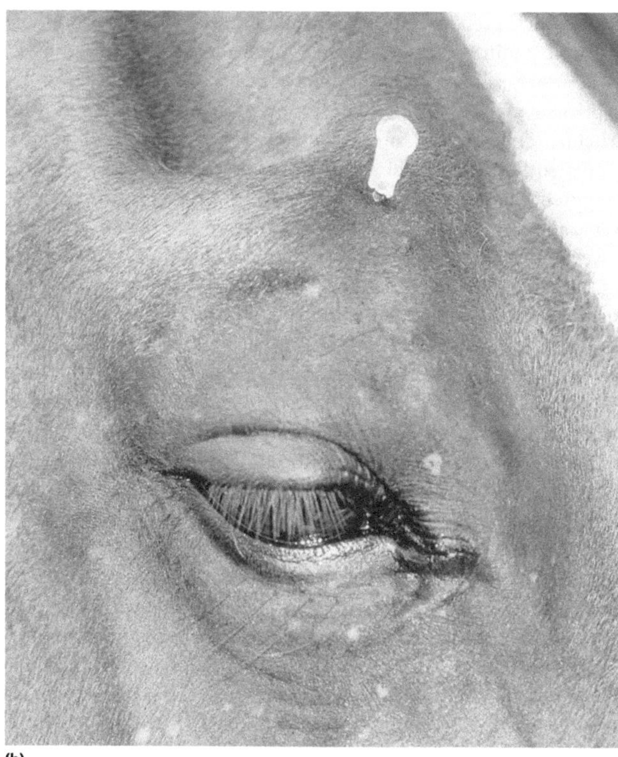

(a) (b)

Figure 48.4 (a) Palpation of the supraorbital nerve. (b) A 2.5 cm, 25 G needle is inserted into the supraorbital foramen.

with the index finger about 5–7 cm dorsal to the medial canthus and in the center of an imaginary triangle formed by grasping the supraorbital process of the frontal bone with the thumb and middle finger and sliding medially (Fig. 48.4a). Approximately 2 mL of local anesthetic are injected subcutaneously over the foramen, 1 mL as the needle is inserted into the foramen, and 2 mL as the needle is inserted to its full depth (2.5 cm) into the foramen (Fig. 48.4b). Successful completion of this block will desensitize the forehead, including the middle two-thirds of the upper eyelid, and since this block will also desensitize some of the terminal branches of the auriculopalpebral nerve, motor function of the orbicularis oculi muscle may be affected [14].

For more complete desensitization of the eyelids, the supraorbital block may be combined with techniques that block the lacrimal, infratrochlear, and zygomatic nerves. The lacrimal nerve is desensitized by inserting a needle percutaneously at the lateral canthus of the eye and directing it medially along the dorsal rim of the orbit (Fig. 48.3b). Deep injection of 2–3 mL of anesthetic at this site desensitizes the lateral canthus, lateral aspect of the upper eyelid, lacrimal gland, local connective tissue, and temporal angle of the orbit (Fig. 48.2b) [12,14].

Anesthesia of the medial canthus, lacrimal glands, nictitans, and connective tissues (Fig. 48.2c) is achieved by injecting 2–3 mL of local anesthetic around the infratrochlear nerve. The needle is inserted through the bony notch or the palpable irregularity on the dorsal rim of the orbit near the medial canthus (Fig. 48.3c) [12,14].

To infiltrate the zygomatic nerve and desensitize the lower two-thirds of the lower eyelid, skin, and connective tissue (Fig. 48.2d), the needle is placed subcutaneously on the lateral aspect of the bony orbit and supraorbital portion of the zygomatic arch and 3–5 mL of local anesthetic are injected (Fig. 48.3d) [12,14].

Standing enucleation may be accomplished with sedation in addition to blockade of the auriculopalpebral, infratrochelar, lacrimal, and zygomatic nerves [15], or with blockade of the supraorbital, infratrochlear, lacrimal, and zygomatic nerves [16]. If general anesthesia is contraindicated or financially undesirable, standing enucleation may be an option.

Local anesthesia of the limbs

Various techniques may be used to desensitize areas of limbs in horses for diagnostic or therapeutic purposes. These include perineural, intra-articular, and intrabursal injection techniques and local infiltration (e.g., ring blocks and line blocks) of local anesthetic. These techniques are frequently used therapeutically to provide temporary relief from pain or to facilitate procedures for treatment or diagnosis of diseases. In addition, local anesthesia techniques are an integral part of the procedures used to diagnose lameness in horses. The blocks used for therapeutic and diagnostic purposes are similar. However, clinicians should keep in mind that blocks performed for diagnosis of lameness should be carried out in a manner that desensitizes the most specific region possible (to allow identification of the affected structures with confidence), whereas blocks performed for therapeutic relief from pain or to allow performance of a procedure (e.g., surgery) may be applied so that a larger (i.e., less specific) area is desensitized. Therefore, the goal of the local anesthesia procedure should be considered when performing these techniques. In general, perineural injections performed as distally as possible and with the smallest effective amount of local anesthetic increase the specificity of such blocks.

Skin at injection sites should be cleaned and prepared prior to needle insertion to reduce the likelihood of infection of deeper tissues. Such preparation may include the use of alcohol only or povidone–iodine or chlorhexidine gluconate scrub followed by a sterile water, saline solution, or alcohol rinse. Skin should also be aseptically prepared prior to insertion of a needle in a synovial structure and the use of sterile gloves, syringes, needles, and unopened bottles of local anesthetic are recommended owing to the potential for septic arthritis. Clipping of hair prior to aseptic preparation for injection of synovial structures is often performed; however, clients may object to this. Removal of hair prior to preparing the skin may not be necessary; the number of bacterial colony-forming units on skin over midcarpal and distal interphalangeal joints after a povidone–iodine and 70% alcohol scrub is not significantly different between areas that are clipped and those that are not clipped to remove hair [17]. Removal of hair in horses with thick coats (hirsutitic horses or during cold weather), for horses with soiled coats, and to aid identification of landmarks for select injections may be warranted. Clipping of hair with an electric clipper and a size 40 clipper blade decreases contamination of joints with tissue debris and hair after needle insertion [18]. In addition, the use of stylets for spinal needles, 22 G needles rather than 20 G needles, and angled needle insertion reduces joint contamination when hair is not clipped [18]. Aseptic preparation is typically not necessary before performing perineural blocks; however, the skin should be clean and the area should be briefly scrubbed or wiped with alcohol. As a precaution, the skin should be thoroughly prepared whenever there is a risk of inadvertent puncture of a synovial structure. In addition, needles should only be handled on the outside surface of the hub when sterile gloves are not worn.

Depending on the block performed, injections may be performed with the limb in a weight-bearing or flexed position. Changes in position may aid the identification of anatomic landmarks before needle insertion. Restraint of the horse by a capable handler should be applied in all instances; the use of a twitch is typically warranted. The ipsilateral or a contralateral limb may be held by an assistant if the horse is reluctant to stand still during a block. However, the handler must exercise extreme care in such instances so that neither the clinician nor the assistant is injured; this is particularly important when the contralateral limb is held, and should not be attempted with fractious horses. Sedation may be necessary to perform a block; however, this should be avoided when the horse must be walked or trotted as part of a lameness examination. Sedation of horses with detomidine may not alter the severity of lameness but can alter the pattern of locomotion [19].

Intra-articular blocks may be best performed with mepivacaine, because the severity of toxic effects of that local anesthetic on equine articular chondrocytes is less than that with lidocaine and markedly less than that with bupivacaine [20].

Choice of needle gauge is based primarily on personal preference. However, 20 G needles are useful for a wide variety of injections. Use of smaller (22–25 G) needles can be advantageous for perineural injections and local anesthesia of superficial synovial structures in the distal aspects of limbs because they may reduce the horse's reaction and can be easier to place precisely. Use of larger (18 or 19 G) needles is typically warranted for injections performed with long [more than 1.5 in (3.8 cm)] needles, through thick fascia or muscle, or when movement of the horse may cause bending and breakage of the needle. Choice of needle length should be made with consideration of the location of the structure to be injected and the locations of other deeper structures that may sustain iatrogenic damage during needle insertion. For horses that are prone to move during an injection or in instances during which motion of the needle may cause deposition of local anesthetic outside the region of interest, extension set tubing may be used between the syringe and needle. For perineural injections, the needle may be directed in a proximal to distal direction or a distal to proximal direction. Use of a distal to proximal direction may decrease the risk of needle breakage if the horse moves, particularly for small-gauge needles. Use of a proximal to distal direction may aid retention of the needle at the site of insertion if the horse moves.

The efficacy of a perineural block is typically confirmed by detection of loss of skin sensation distal to the site where the block was performed. However, this may not be a reliable indication of efficacy in all instances, and the use of other signs (e.g., improvement in lameness or loss of response to hoof tester pressure or limb flexion) should also be used to assess the block further. Loss of skin sensation is not a reliable indicator of the efficacy of perineural blocks performed in the proximal aspect of a limb. When checking skin sensation, a blunt object that will not cause skin trauma should be used and light to moderate pressure should be applied. Horses may move because of the presence and movements of the clinician; for such horses, it may be helpful to check skin sensation from the contralateral side or to have an assistant cover the horse's eyes.

Palmar or plantar digital nerve block

The digital neurovascular bundles are located in the palmar or plantar aspect of the pastern region (between the coronary band and metacarpophalangeal joint) medial and lateral to the deep digital flexor tendon. The digital nerves are the most palmar or plantar structures in these neurovascular bundles (Figs 48.5a and 48.6a). Local anesthesia of these nerves may be performed with the limb in a weight-bearing or flexed position. Digital nerve blocks are typically performed with a 1 in (2.5 cm) 22 G needle or a ⅝ in (1.5 cm) 25 G needle. The needle is advanced through the skin and approximately 1.5 mL of local anesthetic are injected perineurally. The palmar or plantar aspect of the foot (including the heel bulbs, sole, and navicular bursa and associated structures) are desensitized starting within 5–10 min after performance of the block (Fig. 48.7a).

Digital nerve blocks do not significantly reduce the response of non-lame horses to flexion of the distal limbs [21]; therefore, clinicians should keep in mind that these blocks may not improve distal limb flexion responses in lame horses. Digital nerve blocks should be performed just proximal to the collateral cartilages of the foot to reduce the likelihood that proximal interphalangeal joint pain would be alleviated by the block [22]. Local anesthesia of palmar digital nerves may alleviate lameness attributable to pain of the sole of the foot [23] or the distal interphalangeal joint [24]. Palmar digital nerve blocks performed with mepivacaine are fully effective between 15 min and 1 h after the block, and effects may persist for more than 2 h [25]. Local anesthesia of palmar digital nerves affects kinematic gait analysis variables in horses with navicular disease [26].

Block of the dorsal branches of the digital nerves

Structures of the dorsal aspect of the foot and pastern region can be desensitized by blocking the medial and lateral dorsal branches of the palmar or plantar digital nerves (Figs 48.5b and 48.6b). This block is typically performed in addition to the digital nerve block; a 1–1.5 in (2.5–3.8 cm) 20 or 22 G needle is used to inject 1.5–3 mL of local anesthetic subcutaneously as the needle is passed in a dorsal direction from the site of injection of the palmar or plantar digital nerves; the needle should be inserted up to the hub. Performing the block in the proximal aspect of the pastern provides analgesia for a larger area than is provided when the block is performed in the

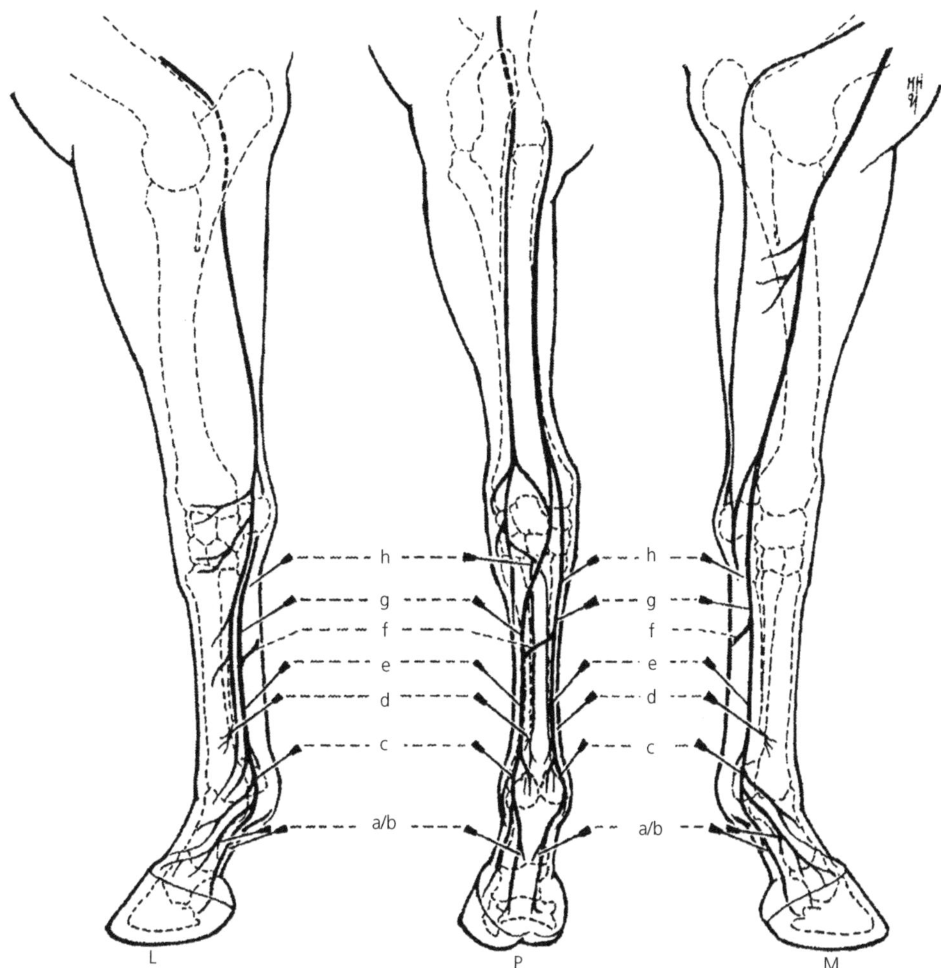

Figure 48.5 Needle placement for nerves of the distal part of the left thoracic limb of the horse, lateral (L), palmar (P), and medial (M) views: lateral and medial palmar digital nerves (a), dorsal branches (b), lateral and medial palmar digital nerves (base sesaboid) (c), lateral and medial palmar nerves (d and g), lateral and medial palmar metacarpal nerves (e), communicating branch (f), and location of high suspensory block (h).

distal aspect of the pastern; therefore, use of a distal location yields a block that is more specific for structures of the dorsal region of the foot and dorsodistal aspect of the pastern.

Abaxial sesamoid (basisesamoid) block

The medial and lateral palmar or plantar digital nerves (including dorsal branches) can be blocked at the level of the distal abaxial aspect of the proximal sesamoid bones (Figs 48.5c and 48.6c); 3–5 mL of local anesthetic are injected perineurally with a 1 in (2.5 cm) 22 G needle or a ⅝ in (1.5 cm) 25 G needle. Local anesthesia at this level provides analgesia of the foot and the palmar or plantar aspect of the pastern region. As with digital nerve blocks, abaxial sesamoid nerve blocks may not have an effect on lameness that is exacerbated by flexion of the distal aspect of a limb [21]. In a substantial number of horses, local anesthetic may diffuse proximally after this block [27].

Low palmar or plantar (low four-point) nerve block

The medial and lateral palmar or plantar nerves and palmar metacarpal or palmar metatarsal nerves are desensitized with this block (Figs 48.5d–e and 48.6d–e). For palmar or plantar nerves, local anesthetic is injected between the suspensory ligament and the deep digital flexor tendon; because of the proximity to the digital flexor tendon synovial sheath, the area should be thoroughly prepared, the hub of the needle should be checked to ensure that synovial fluid is not obtained, and the injection should be performed at a level approximately 1 cm proximal to the distal ends of the splint bones. For the palmar metacarpal or plantar metatarsal nerves, local anesthetic is injected between the third metacarpal or metatarsal bone and the suspensory ligament at a level just distal to the distal extent of the splint bones; because of the proximity to the palmar or plantar pouch of the fetlock joint, the area should be thoroughly prepared and the hub of the needle checked to ensure that synovial fluid is not obtained. If synovial fluid is obtained, the needle should be withdrawn and redirected. These blocks provide analgesia for most structures of the fetlock joint and structures distal to that joint (Fig. 48.7d). Subcutaneous injection of additional local anesthetic in a dorsal direction may be necessary to provide complete analgesia.

Local anesthetic diffusion in a proximal direction is minimal after performance of a low palmar nerve block [28], and diffusion is unlikely to cause a decrease in the severity of lameness attributable to pain in the proximal aspect of the metacarpal region [29].

Proximal metacarpal or metatarsal region blocks

The high palmar or plantar (high four-point) block desensitizes the medial and lateral palmar or plantar nerves and palmar metacarpal or plantar metatarsal nerves in the proximal aspect of the metacarpal

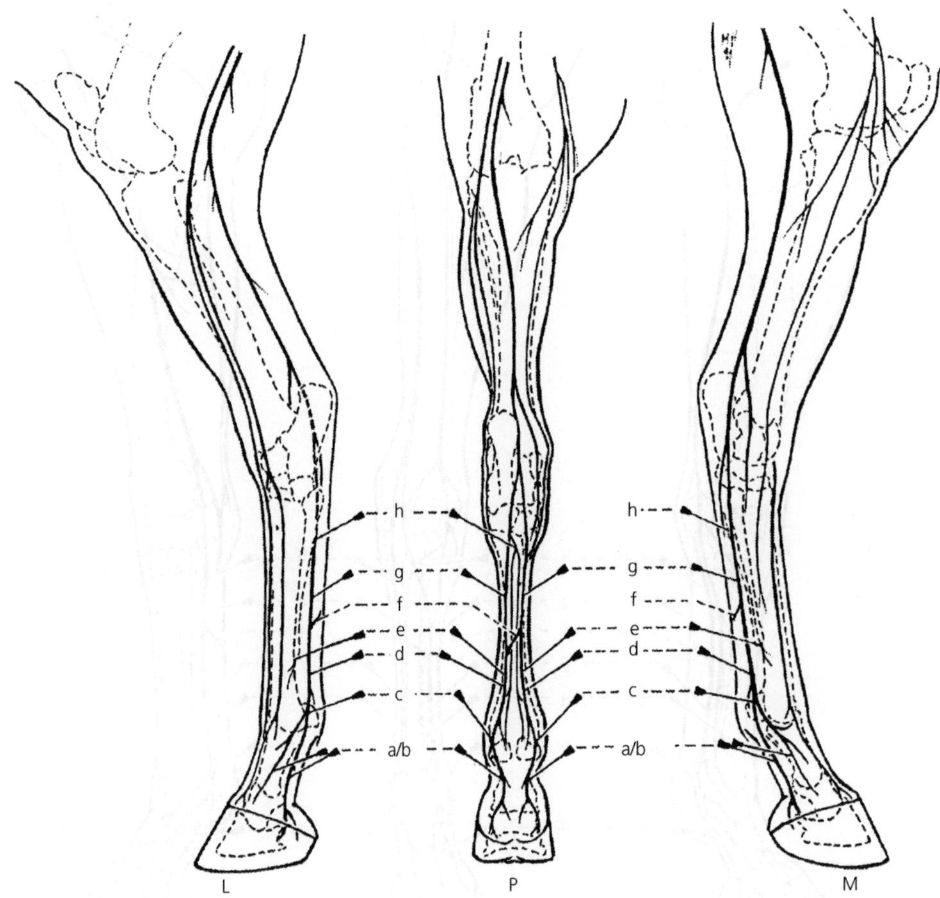

Figure 48.6 Needle placement for nerves of the distal part of the left pelvic limb of the horse, lateral (L), plantar (P), and medial (M) views: lateral and medial plantar digital nerves (a), dorsal branches (b), lateral and medial plantar digital nerves (base sesamoid) (c), lateral and medial plantar nerves (d and g), lateral and medial plantar metatarsal nerves (e), communicating branch (f), and location of high suspensory block (h).

region proximal to the communicating branch of the medial and lateral palmar or plantar nerves (Figs 48.5f–h and 48.6f–h). The palmar or plantar nerves are desensitized between the suspensory ligament and the deep digital flexor tendon; this area is typically easiest to palpate with the limb in a weight-bearing position. The palmar metacarpal or plantar metatarsal nerves are desensitized via injection of local anesthetic along the axial aspects of the splint bones; this is easiest to accomplish with the limb in a flexed position. For complete analgesia of the dorsal aspect of the limb in this region, local anesthetic should be injected subcutaneously in a ring block to the dorsal midline of the limb (Fig. 48.7). The palmar aspect of the carpometacarpal joint may be entered when performing this block [30]; therefore, the area should be thoroughly prepared and suction applied after connection of the syringe to the needle to ensure that synovial fluid is not obtained. Inadvertent injection of the carpometacarpal joint would provide anesthesia to the middle carpal joint, which could lead to erroneous conclusions during a lameness examination. The origin of the suspensory ligament may not be completely desensitized with this block. Gas may be introduced into tissues while performing this block and can temporarily interfere with ultrasonographic examination of structures of the proximal palmar metacarpal region [31].

The origin of the suspensory ligament may be desensitized via direct injection of the structure with local anesthetic. The block is performed with the limb in a flexed position. The needle is advanced into the proximal aspect of the suspensory ligament along the axial aspect of the splint bone, and local anesthetic is injected in several sites in a fan-shaped pattern. The injection may be performed from the medial and lateral aspects, or just the lateral aspect of the limb (particularly in hind limbs, where injection from the medial side may be difficult). Use of an 18 or 19 G needle may prevent inadvertent needle breakage if the horse moves while performing this block.

The lateral palmar nerve can be desensitized at the level of the accessory carpal bone to provide analgesia for the deep structures of the palmar aspect of the forelimb, including the proximal aspect of the suspensory ligament. The block can be performed from the lateral or medial aspect of the limb. For the lateral approach, local anesthetic is deposited perineurally between the distal aspect of the accessory carpal bone and the proximal aspect of the fourth metacarpal (lateral splint) bone; this can be performed with the limb in a weight-bearing position or with the carpus flexed. Use of a medial approach to the nerve may prevent inadvertent injection of the carpal synovial sheath [32]. This technique is performed with the limb in a weight-bearing position. A ⅝ in (1.5 cm) 25 G needle is inserted in a groove in the flexor retinaculum fascia at the palmaromedial aspect of the accessory carpal bone. The needle is directed in a mediolateral direction until it contacts bone, and then local anesthetic is injected.

Local anesthesia of the deep branch of the lateral plantar nerve provides analgesia of the proximal aspect of the suspensory ligament

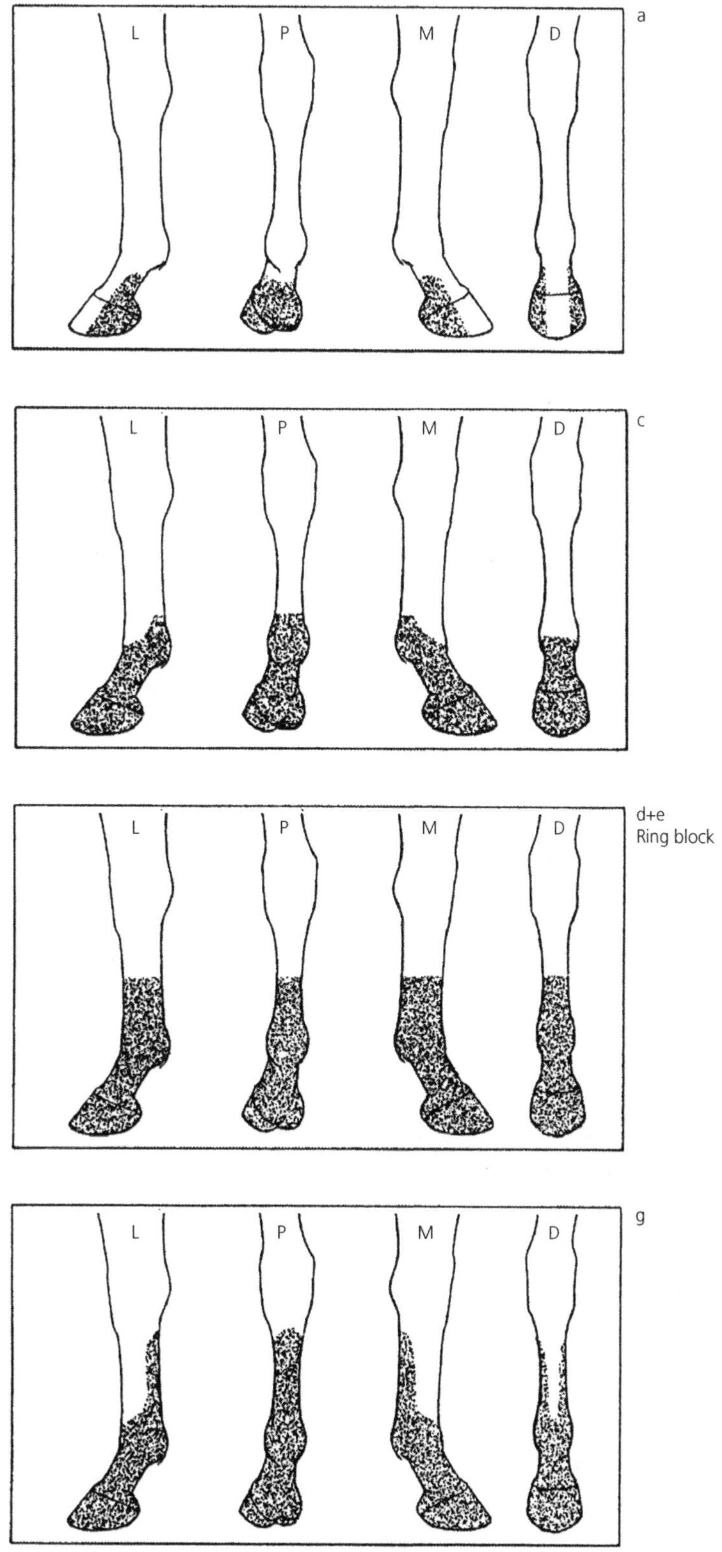

Figure 48.7 Desensitized subcutaneous area after a, d, d + e, and g blockade.

in the hind limb. A 1.5 in (3.8 cm) 18 or 19 G needle is inserted 1.5–2 cm distal to the head of the fourth metatarsal bone (lateral splint bone) and directed axial to that bone [33,34]. The needle may be directed either proximodorsally or dorsally; insertion of the needle in a proximodorsal direction may provide more specific local anesthesia of the deep branch of the lateral plantar nerve and lead to less diffusion of the local anesthetic versus insertion of the needle in a dorsal direction [34]. Because of a small risk of tarsometatarsal joint puncture, the skin should be thoroughly prepared before performance of the block.

Median, ulnar, and medial cutaneous antebrachial nerve blocks

Performance of these blocks in combination provides analgesia for structures of the antebrachium, carpus, and distal aspect of a forelimb. These blocks may be performed before a procedure or for diagnostic purposes. Local anesthesia of the median nerve is performed just distal to the superficial pectoral muscle at the caudomedial aspect of the radius, cranial to the flexor carpi radialis muscle (Fig. 48.8a); approximately 10 mL of local anesthetic are injected. The ulnar nerve is desensitized approximately 10 cm proximal to the accessory carpal bone at the caudal aspect of the limb in a palpable groove between the flexor carpi ulnaris and ulnaris lateralis muscles (Fig. 48.8b); a 1 in (2.5 cm) 20 G needle should be inserted to the hub and approximately 10 mL of local anesthetic injected as the needle is withdrawn. The medial cutaneous antebrachial nerve is desensitized just cranial to the cephalic vein at the dorsomedial aspect of the middle of the radius (Fig. 48.8c); approximately 5 mL of local anesthetic are injected. The medial cutaneous antebrachial nerve provides analgesia only for skin, so the block is not required for diagnostic purposes. The median and ulnar nerve blocks are not commonly performed for diagnostic purposes; however, these blocks can be very useful for determining a diagnosis in horses with forelimb lameness that is not affected by intra-articular blocks or perineural blocks of the distal aspect of a limb. As such, the median and ulnar nerve blocks can be useful for the diagnosis of problems causing pain in the carpal bones or the distal aspect of the radius and pain attributable to soft tissue problems between the distal aspect of the antebrachium and proximal aspect of the metacarpus.

Tibial, peroneal, and saphenous nerve blocks

Local anesthesia of the tibial and peroneal nerves desensitizes bone and soft tissues of the distal aspect of the tibia, the hock, and structures distal to the hock. For local anesthesia of the tibial nerve, a 1.5 in (3.8 cm) 20 G needle is inserted 10 cm proximal to the tuber calcis caudal to the deep digital flexor muscle (Fig. 48.9a); 15–20 mL of local anesthetic are injected. Although the nerve is located medially, the injection may be performed from the medial side or from the lateral side. When performing the block from the lateral side, the needle should be inserted to a depth sufficient to ensure deposition of local anesthetic perineurally without penetration of the skin on the medial side of the limb. Because it is difficult to maintain contact between the syringe and needle when the horse moves, it may be useful to connect extension set tubing between the needle and syringe. The superficial and deep peroneal nerves are desensitized by insertion of a to 3.5 in (8.9 cm) 18 G needle 10 cm proximal to the tuber calcis in a palpable groove between the long and lateral digital extensor muscles on the lateral aspect of the limb (Fig. 48.9c). The needle is inserted until the caudolateral edge of the tibia is contacted, and 20–30 mL of local anesthetic are injected as the needle is withdrawn to desensitize both the deep and superficial peroneal nerves. A subcutaneous ring block may be necessary to provide complete skin analgesia for surgery. After performing these blocks, horses may drag their toe; caution should be used during lameness examination of such horses. As for the median and ulnar nerve blocks in the forelimb, these blocks are not commonly performed but may help reach a diagnosis in horses with lameness that is not affected by intra-articular blocks or distal pernineural blocks.

The saphenous nerve is desensitized by injection of 5 mL of local anesthetic perineurally near the saphenous vein approximately 10 cm proximal to the tibiotarsal joint with a 1 in (2.5 cm) 20 or 22 G needle (Fig. 48.9b). This block is useful for providing analgesia to the skin of the medial aspect of the limb. It is not performed for diagnostic analgesia during a lameness examination.

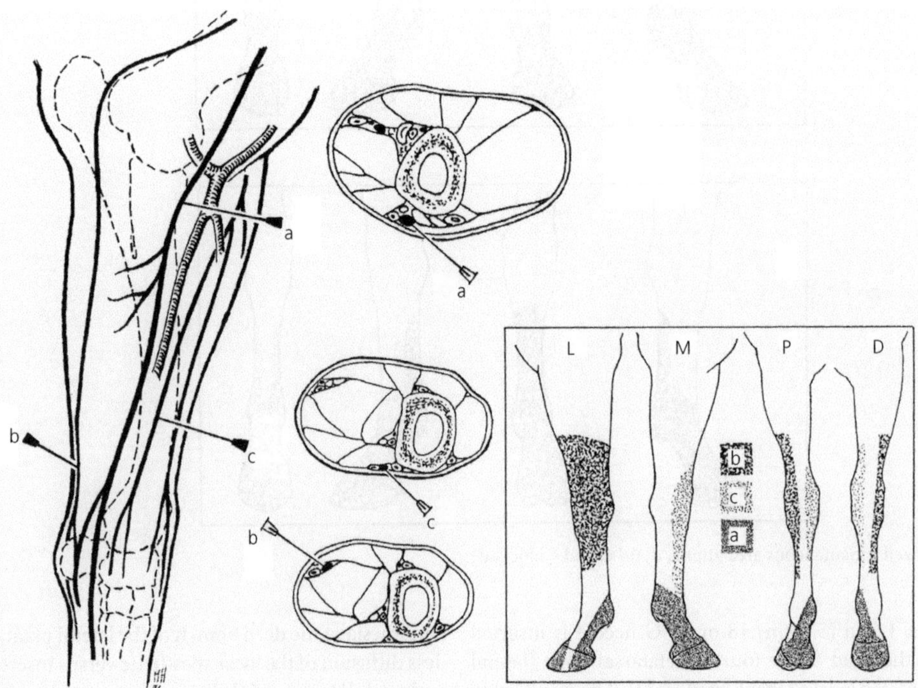

Figure 48.8 Needle placement for median nerve (a), ulnar nerve (b), and musculocutaneous nerve (c); cross-sections and desensitized subcutaneous areas of left forelimb. L, lateral; M, medial; P, palmar; and D, dorsal aspects.

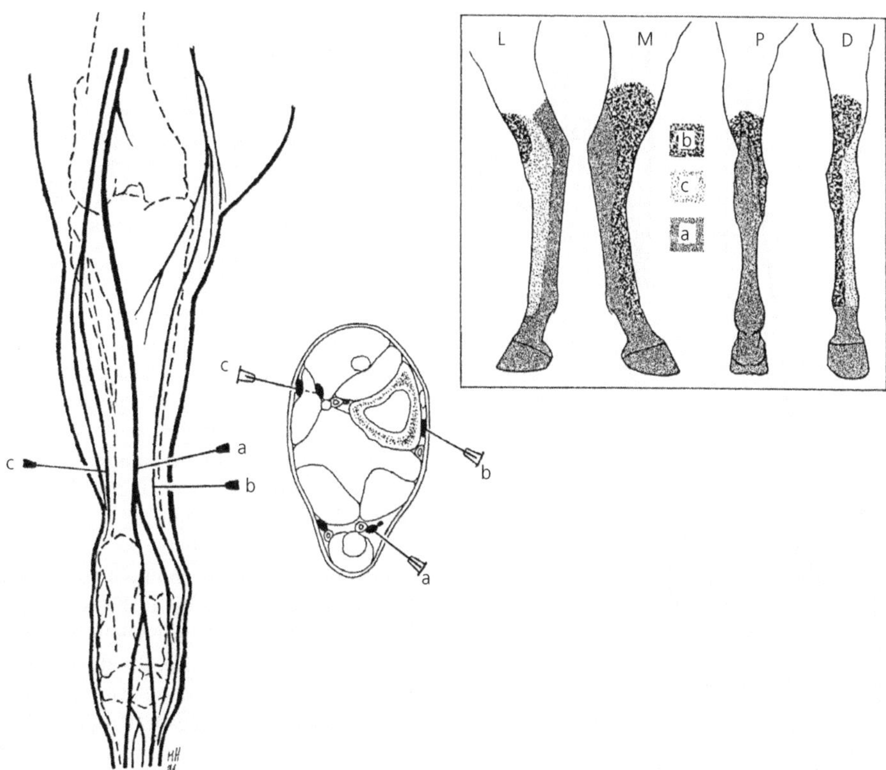

Figure 48.9 Needle placement for tibial nerve (a), saphenous nerve (b), and peroneal nerve (c); cross-sections and desensitized subcutaneous areas of left rear limb. L, lateral; M, medial; P, plantar; and D, dorsal aspects.

Intra-articular and intrabursal anesthesia of the limbs

Navicular bursa

Several techniques can be used for injection of the navicular bursa. However, an approach from the distal palmar aspect of the limb in which the position of the navicular bursa is determined on the basis of external anatomic landmarks may yield the highest success rate [35,36]. This technique is typically performed with the foot on an inclined wooden block to position the distal aspect of the limb in a flexed position. The position of the navicular bone can be predicted to be at a location 1 cm distal to the coronary band at the midpoint between the most dorsal and most palmar aspect of the coronary band. Injection of 1–2 mL of local anesthetic subcutaneously at the needle insertion site may decrease movement of the horse while performing this block. A 3.5 in (8.9 cm) 18–20 G needle is inserted at the midpoint between the heel bulbs just proximal to the coronary band and advanced toward the predicted position of the navicular bone (Fig. 48.10a). After the navicular bone is encountered, the needle is withdrawn slightly. Correct needle placement can be confirmed by aspiration of a small amount of synovial fluid (which is rarely obtained) or via radiography. Then, 3–5 mL of local anesthetic are injected. Improvement of lameness within 10 min after injection suggests that the lameness is caused by pain in the navicular bursa or associated structures [37,38]; however, distal interphalangeal joint pain may be improved by local anesthesia of the navicular bursa 20–30 min after injection [38]. Mepivacaine can diffuse between the navicular bursa and the distal interphalangeal joint [39]. Analgesia of the navicular bursa may improve lameness caused by pain in the dorsal aspect of the sole of the foot [40].

Coffin (distal interphalangeal) joint

For local anesthesia of the distal interphalangeal joint, a 1.5 in (3.8 cm) 20 G needle is inserted 1 cm proximal to the coronary band and 2 cm lateral to the dorsal midline aspect of the limb (Fig. 48.10b). The needle is directed distomedially toward the palmar or plantar lateral aspect of the extensor process of the third phalanx (coffin bone). Alternatively, the needle may be inserted into the dorsoproximal pouch of the joint on the dorsal midline aspect of the limb 1 cm proximal to the coronary band and directed in a palmar or plantar direction either parallel to the ground or distally toward the solar surface of the foot. The horse should be in a weight-bearing position while performing this block. Injection of 6 mL of local anesthetic into the distal interphalangeal joint may desensitize the dorsal aspect (toe) of the sole of the foot, whereas injection of 10 mL may also desensitize the angles (heel) of the sole [41]. Therefore, injection of a maximum of 6 mL is recommended to increase the specificity of the block when it is performed for diagnostic purposes. Because mepivacaine can diffuse between the distal interphalangeal joint and the navicular bursa [39], intra-articular distal interphalangeal joint blocks may not be specific for problems of that joint.

Proximal interphalangeal (pastern) joint

The proximal interphalangeal joint is desensitized via insertion of a 1.5 in (3.8 cm) 20 G needle into the palpable joint space under the extensor tendon on the dorsal aspect of the limb in a lateral to medial or medial to lateral direction (Fig. 48.10c). This approach is typically performed with the limb in a weight-bearing position. Alternatively, the joint may be entered at the palmar or plantar lateral aspect with the limb in a flexed position. The needle is inserted

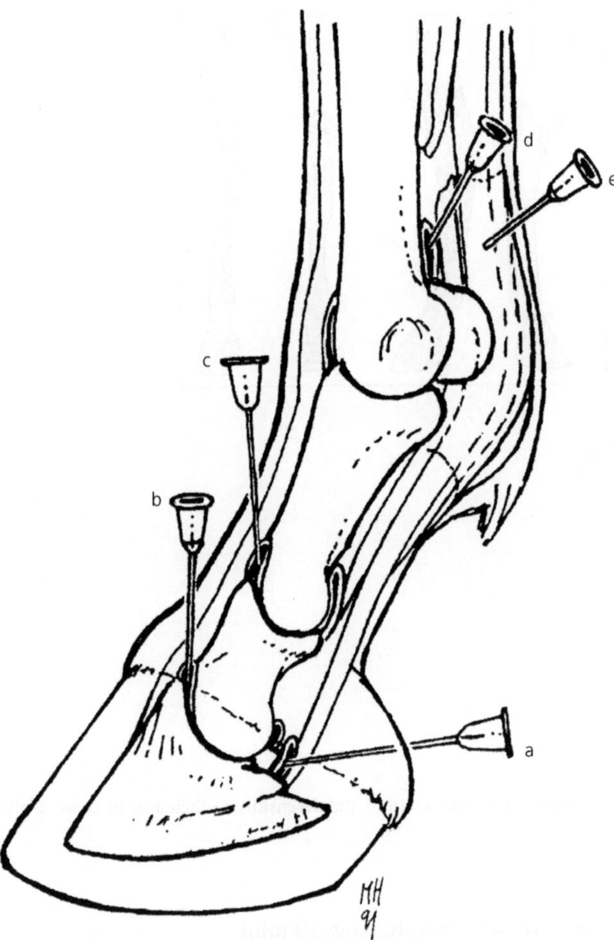

Figure 48.10 Needle placement into the podotrochlear bursa (a), coffin joint (b), pastern joint (c), volar pouch of the fetlock joint capsule (d), and digital flexor tendon sheath (e).

dorsal to the digital neurovascular bundle towards a palpable depression between the distal aspect of the first phalanx and the proximal aspect of the second phalanx; 5–10 mL of local anesthetic are injected.

Metacarpophalangeal or metatarsophalangeal (fetlock) joint

Fetlock joints may be injected via a dorsomedial or dorsolateral approach or various palmar or plantar approaches. For the dorsal approach, a 1.5 in (3.8 cm) 20 G needle is inserted into the palpable joint space proximal to the first phalanx under the extensor tendon; this approach is performed with the limb in a weight-bearing position. The palmar or plantar joint pouch may be entered from the lateral aspect of the limb in three locations. The proximal aspect of the palmar or plantar pouch may be entered in an area bound by the third metacarpophalangeal or metatarsophalangeal (cannon) bone dorsally, suspensory ligament (palmarly or plantarly), distal end of the splint bone (proximally), and apical aspect of the lateral proximal sesamoid bone distally (Fig. 48.10d). The palmar or plantar pouch may also be entered through the collateral ligament of the lateral proximal sesamoid bone between the cannon bone and the proximal sesamoid bone; this may be the easiest approach to obtain hemorrhage-free synovial fluid and inject the fetlock joint, particularly in a horse without synovial effusion. Alternately, the palmar or plantar aspect of the joint may be entered at the distolateral aspect in a space bounded by the digital neurovascular bundle (palmarly or plantarly), the distal aspect of the lateral proximal sesamoid bone (proximodorsally), and the proximal aspect of the proximal phalanx (distodorsally). The palmar or plantar approaches are best performed with the distal aspect of the limb in a flexed position. The fetlock joint is injected with 10 mL of local anesthetic.

Digital flexor tendon sheath

When distended with synovial fluid, the digital flexor tendon sheath can be desensitized via approaches to the proximal or distal aspects. For the proximal approach, a 1 in (2.5 cm) 20 G needle is inserted into the sheath 1 cm proximal to the palmar or plantar annular ligament and 1 cm palmar or plantar to the lateral branch of the suspensory ligament (Fig. 48.10e). For the distal approach, the needle is inserted into the sheath in the palmar or plantar aspect of the pastern between the proximal and distal digital annular ligaments; care should be taken to avoid puncture of the deep digital flexor tendon at this location. Those blocks may be performed with the limb in a weight-bearing or non-weight-bearing position. As an alternative, the distal aspect of the limb may be flexed and the needle can be inserted into the sheath on the palmaro- or plantarolateral aspect of the limb just distal to the lateral proximal sesamoid bone between the proximal annular ligament and proximal digital annular ligament. In addition, a palmar or plantar axial sesamoidean approach can be used [42]. The limb is held in flexion and a 1 in (2.5 cm) 20 G needle is inserted at the level of the middle aspect, 3 mm axial to the palmar or plantar border of the lateral proximal sesamoid bone and dorsal to the flexor tendons. The needle is directed at a 45° angle to the sagittal plane towards the inter-sesamoidean ligament. That technique is preferred for horses without substantial synovial effusion of the sheath. Local anesthesia of the digital flexor tendon sheath appears to be specific for that structure because it is unlikely to improve lameness attributable to pain in the sole of the foot, distal interphalangeal joint, or navicular bursa [43].

Carpal joint blocks

The radiocarpal (antebrachiocarpal) joint can be entered on the dorsal aspect with the limb lifted off the ground and the carpus flexed. A 1 in (2.5 cm) 20 G needle is inserted in the palpable depression of the joint either medial or lateral to the extensor carpi radialis tendon; 5–10 mL of local anesthetic are injected. Alternatively, the needle may directed into the palmar aspect of the joint between the lateral digital extensor and ulnaris lateralis tendons in a palpable V-shaped depression bordered by the caudolateral aspect of the radius and ulnar carpal bone and the proximal aspect of the accessory carpal bone with the limb in a weight-bearing position (Figs 48.11a and 48.12a, c).

The middle carpal joint can be entered on the dorsal aspect with the limb held off the ground with the carpus flexed. The needle is inserted on the medial or lateral side of the extensor carpi radialis tendon, in a manner similar to that for injection of the radiocarpal joint. Alternatively, the palmar aspect of this joint may be injected via insertion of the needle palmar to the articulation of the ulnar and fourth carpal bones and distal to the accessory carpal bone (Figs 48.11b and 48.12b, d). The middle carpal joint communicates with the carpometacarpal joint; therefore, both of these joints are desensitized.

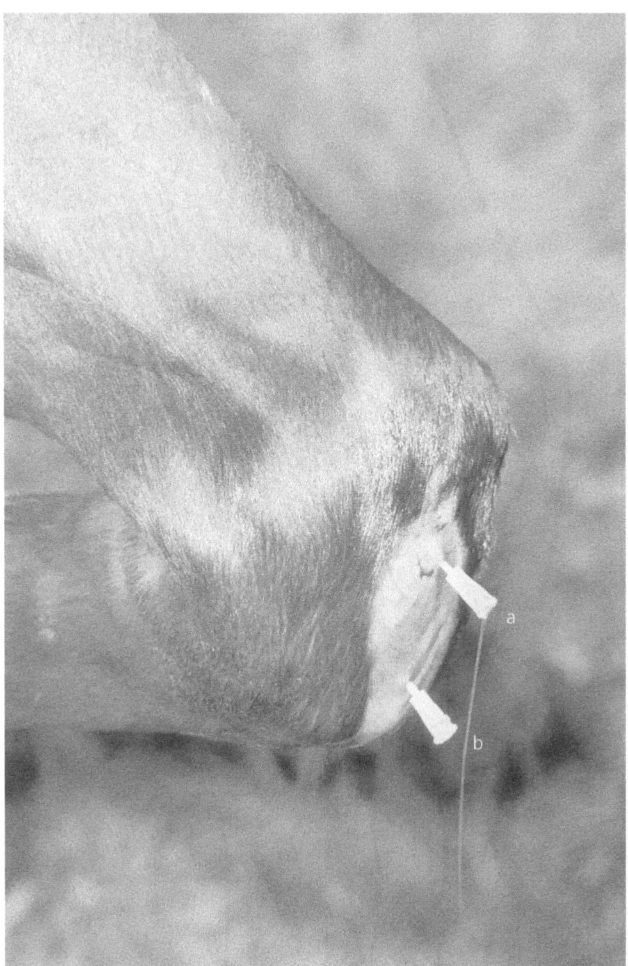

Figure 48.11 Needle placement into the radiocarpal joint (a) and intercarpal joint (b) of the right forelimb.

Carpal canal block

The carpal canal is most easily identified from the lateral aspect of the forelimb when synovial effusion is present. It is important to differentiate carpal sheath effusion from effusion of the carpal joints. The carpal sheath may be entered with a 1 in (2.5 cm) 20 G needle between the lateral digital extensor and ulnaris lateralis tendons 1–3 cm proximal to the accessory carpal bone; 15 mL of local anesthetic are injected. Another approach is to place the needle in the sheath 1.5 cm distal to the accessory carpal bone at the dorsolateral aspect of the deep digital flexor tendon.

Elbow joint block

The elbow joint may be blocked at the cranial or caudal edge of the lateral collateral ligament, two-thirds of the distance distally between the palpable lateral epicondyle of the humerus and the lateral tuberosity of the proximal aspect of the radius (Fig. 48.13a). A 1.5 in (3.8 cm) 18 or 20 G needle is inserted perpendicular to the skin and 20 mL of local anesthetic are injected. It is important to ensure that local anesthetic is injected into the joint; this is confirmed by aspirating synovial fluid prior to injection. Injection of local anesthetic periarticularly after insertion of the needle cranial to the lateral collateral ligament can lead to temporary radial nerve paralysis [44]. The caudal pouch of the elbow joint may also be entered with a 3.5 in (8.9 cm) 18–20 G needle inserted in a distal, cranial, and medial direction in the palpable depression bordered by the olecranon (caudally) and the distal aspect of the humerus (cranially).

Olecranon bursa block

The olecranon bursa is injected with a 1.5 in (3.8 cm), 20 G needle directed into the bursa over the caudal aspect of the olecranon (Fig. 48.13b). This block is rarely indicated.

Bicipital bursa block

For local anesthesia of the bicipital bursa, a 3.5 in (8.9 cm) 18 G needle is inserted at the cranial aspect of the humerus, 3.5 cm distal to the prominence on the craniolateral aspect of the greater tubercle

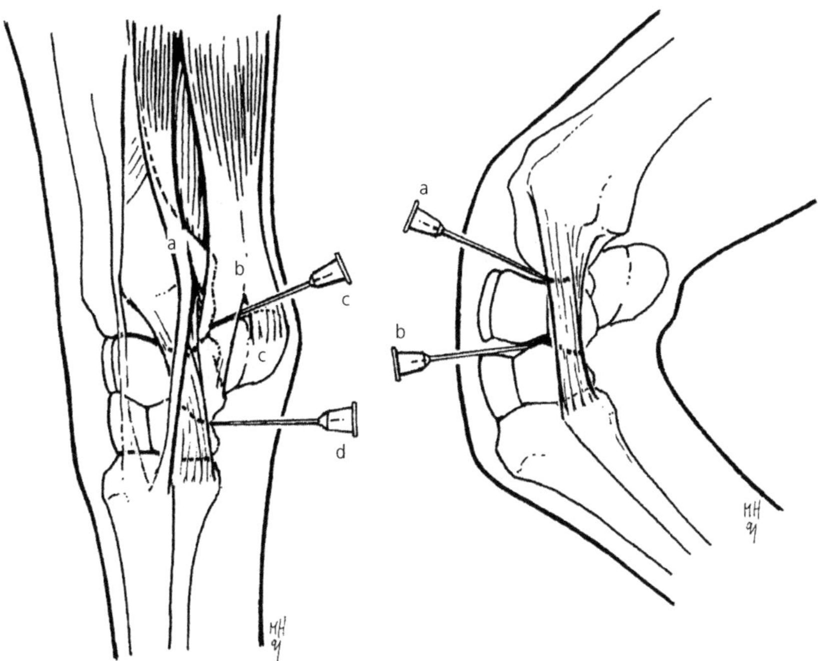

Figure 48.12 Needle placement into the radiocarpal (a and c) and intercarpal (b and d) joints of the left forelimb. a, Lateral digital extensor tendon; b, tendon of ulnaris lateralis muscle; c, accessory carpal bone.

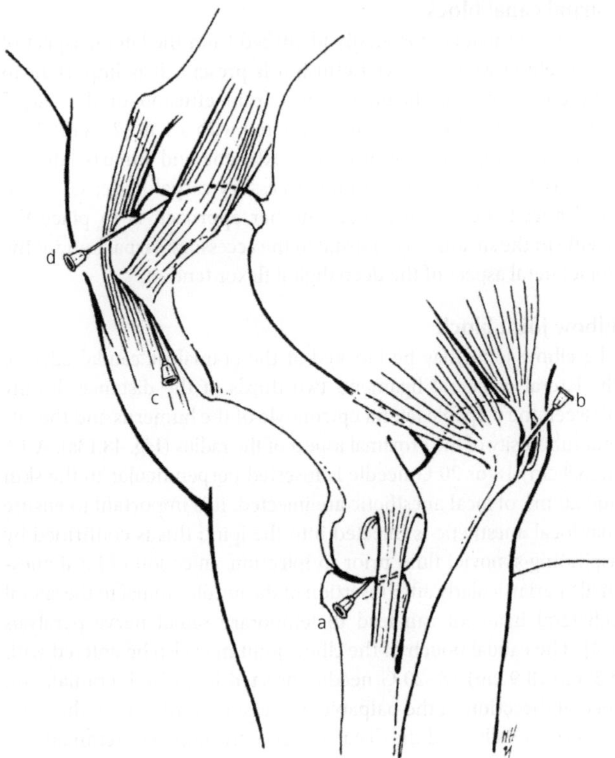

Figure 48.13 Needle placement into the elbow joint (a), olecranon bursa (b), bicipital bursa (c), and shoulder joint (d) of the left forelimb.

(Fig. 48.13c). The needle is directed along the cranial surface of the humerus in a proximomedial direction; 10–15 mL of local anesthetic are injected. Radiographic examination after injection of radiopaque contrast medium may be necessary to confirm successful entry into the bicipital bursa [45]. Ultrasonographic guidance may improve the accuracy of needle placement for local anesthesia of the bicipital bursa [46].

Shoulder joint block

For local anesthesia of the shoulder joint, the depression between the cranial and caudal prominences of the lateral tuberosity of the humerus is palpated cranial to the infraspinatus tendon. An 18 G needle at least 3.5 in (8.9 cm) long is inserted into the center of the depression and directed in a caudomedial direction at a 45° angle (Fig. 48.13d); 20 mL of local anesthetic are injected. Correct placement of the needle can typically be confirmed by aspiration of synovial fluid. Temporary suprascapular nerve anesthesia and subsequent supraspinatus and infraspinatus muscle dysfunction are a rare complication of this block [44]. Ultrasonographic guidance may improve the accuracy of needle placement in the shoulder joint [46].

Cunean bursa block

The cunean bursa may be desensitized by inserting a 1 in (2.5 cm) 22 G needle between the cunean tendon and the bones of the distal aspect of the tarsus (Figs 48.14a and 48.15). The needle is inserted from the distal aspect of the cunean tendon and 5–10 mL of local anesthetic are injected.

Tarsal joint blocks

Tarsal joints are typically injected with the limb in a weight-bearing position. The tarsometatarsal joint is most reliably entered from the plantarolateral aspect of the limb in a palpable depression 1 cm proximal to the head of the lateral fourth metatarsal (splint) bone

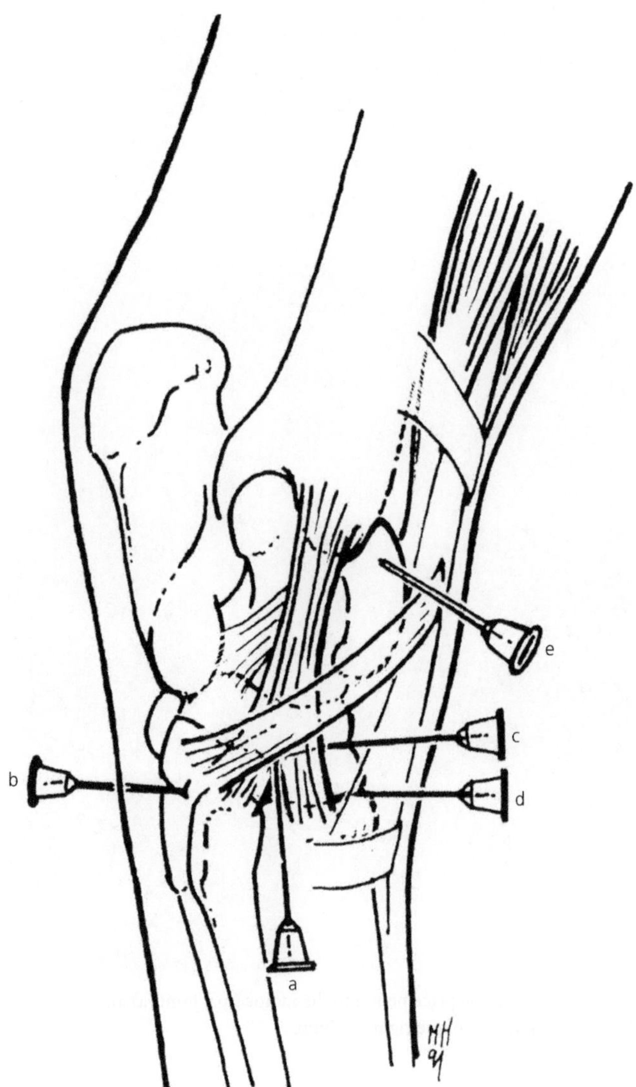

Figure 48.14 Needle placement into the cunean bursa (a), tarsometatarsal space (b and d), distal metatarsal space (c), and tibiotarsal space (e) of the left hock joint; medial aspect.

(Figs 48.14b and 48.16). A 1–1.5 in (2.5–3.8 cm) 20 G needle is directed in a distomedial direction. Synovial fluid is typically obtained and 3–4 mL of local anesthetic should be injected without substantial resistance. This joint may be entered from the dorsal aspect of the limb (Fig. 48.14d); however, this approach is typically only used if the plantarolateral approach is unavailable because of skin damage or if an additional portal is necessary for joint lavage. The distal intertarsal (centrodistal) joint is desensitized by inserting a 1 in (2.5 cm) 22 G needle in a small palpable joint depression on the medial aspect of the limb just ventral to the cunean tendon (Fig. 48.14c); 3–5 mL of local anesthetic are injected. The tibiotarsal (tarsocrural) joint is large and easily injected in the dorsomedial pouch 2–3 cm distal to the tibia and medial to the peroneus tertius and tibialis cranialis tendons (Fig. 48.14e); 15 mL of local anesthetic are injected. Care should be taken to avoid the saphenous vein, which typically courses over the center of the dorsomedial pouch of the joint. When synovial effusion is present, this joint can be approached from the plantarolateral aspect. For this approach, the needle is inserted in the center of the palpable distended joint pouch bordered by the tuber calcis (caudally), distal aspect of the

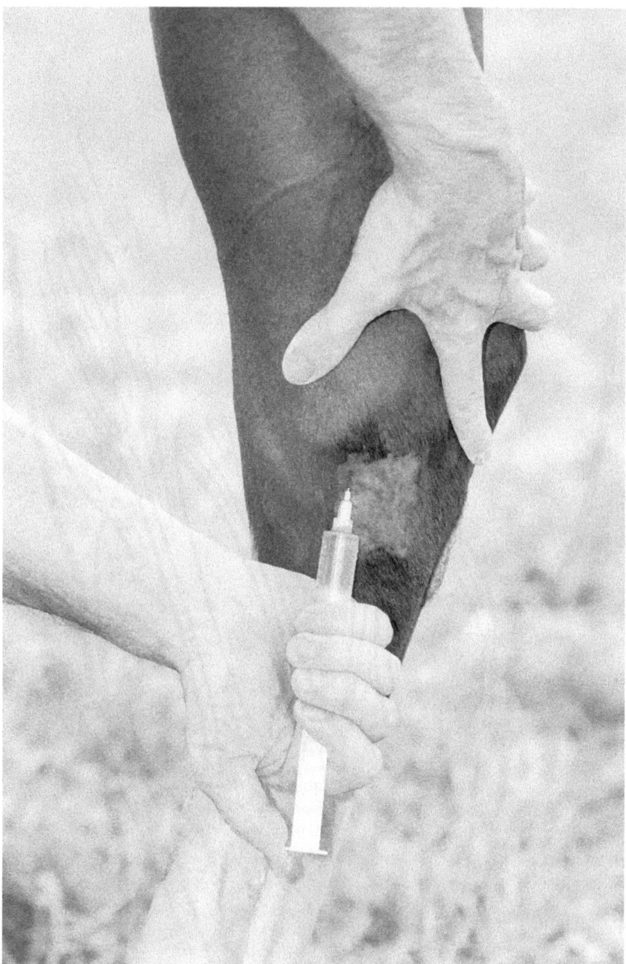

Figure 48.15 Injection of local anesthetic (10 mL) into the cunean bursa of the right rear limb; medial aspect.

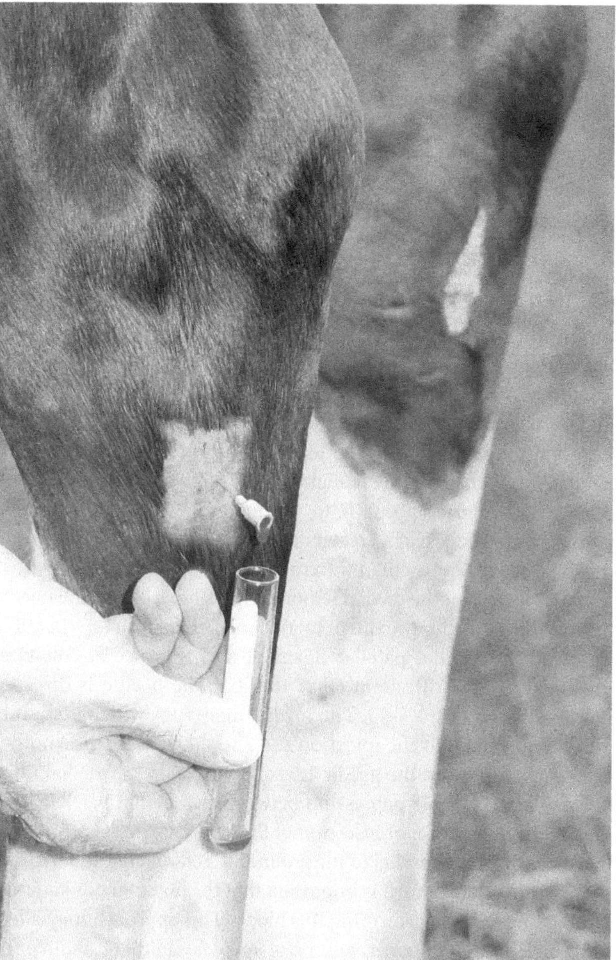

Figure 48.16 Collection of fluid from the tarsometatarsal joint (left rear leg).

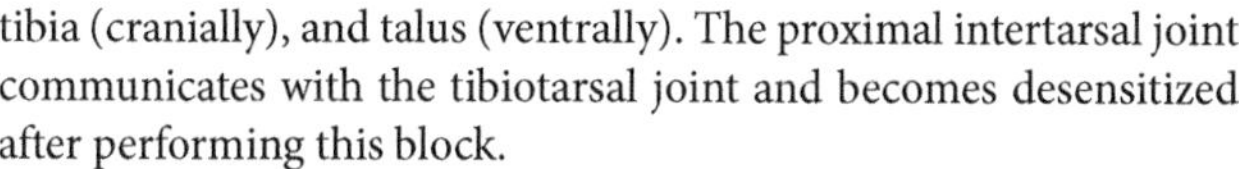

tibia (cranially), and talus (ventrally). The proximal intertarsal joint communicates with the tibiotarsal joint and becomes desensitized after performing this block.

Horses have variable communication among the tarsal joints. A substantial percentage (up to 38%) of horses have communication between the tarsometatarsal and distal intertarsal joints [47–50]. Infrequently, injection of the distal tarsal joints may cause entry of local anesthetic into the proximal intertarsal and tarsometatarsal joints [47] or the tarsal sheath [48]. High injection pressures may increase the frequency of tarsometatarsal and distal intertarsal joint communication [50].

Calcaneal bursae blocks

Calcaneal bursae in horses include the subcutaneous calcaneal bursa (subcutaneous superficial to the superficial digital flexor tendon plantar to the calcaneus), inter-tendinous calcaneal bursa (between the gastrocnemius and superficial digital flexor tendons), and gastrocnemius calcaneal bursa (just proximal to the calcaneus and dorsal to the gastrocnemius tendon) [51]. The intertendinous and gastrocnemius calcaneal bursae communicate; the subcutaneous bursa communicates with the other calcaneal bursae in 39% of studied limbs of horses. A 1.5 in (3.8 cm) 20 G needle may be inserted into the bursae, which are palpable when synovial effusion is present; 10 mL of local anesthetic are injected.

Tarsal sheath block

The tarsal sheath extends from the proximal aspect of the calcaneus to the proximal aspect of the metatarsal region. The sheath surrounds the deep digital flexor tendon as it courses over the sustentaculum tali of the calcaneus, medial to the body of the bone. The sheath is easiest to identify when it is distended with synovial fluid. The tarsal sheath may be desensitized at its proximal or distal aspects via insertion of a 1.5 in (3.8 cm) 20 G needle and injection of 15 mL of local anesthetic.

Stifle joint blocks

The stifle joint includes the femoropatellar and medial and lateral femorotibial articulations. In horses, communication among these joint compartments is variable. The most common communication is between the medial femorotibial and femoropatellar compartments, which is detected in 60–80% of limbs with normal stifle joints [52,53]. Communication among other stifle joint compartments is detected less frequently. The pattern of communication is typically bilaterally symmetrical; however, communication among compartments may be affected by joint disease and the location chosen for joint injection. Therefore, for diagnostic and therapeutic purposes, each compartment should be considered a separate entity and injected independently. However, clinicians should be aware that mepivacaine can diffuse among stifle joint compartments and detection of an improvement in lameness after local anesthesia of an individual articulation may not be specific [54]. Because lameness attributable to stifle joint problems may be caused by extra-synovial structures (such as collateral and cruciate ligaments), improvement may not be observed until 20 min or longer after injection of local anesthetic. Each compartment is typically desensitized with 20 mL of local anesthetic by use of a 1.5 in (3.8 cm) 18 G needle.

The femoropatellar compartment is injected distal to the patella, medial or lateral to the middle patellar ligament (Fig. 48.17a). The needle is advanced perpendicular to the skin or in a slightly proximal direction. Alternatively, the lateral cul-de-sac of the femoropatellar compartment may be injected [55]; the needle is inserted 5 cm proximal to the lateral tibial plateau caudal to the lateral patellar ligament and lateral trochlear ridge of the femur. The needle is directed perpendicular to the long axis of the femur until bone is contacted, then withdrawn slightly before injection of local anesthetic. The lateral approach to the femoropatellar compartment may allow collection of a greater amount of synovial fluid and result in less cartilage injury than the cranial approach [56].

For injection of the medial femorotibial compartment, the needle is inserted 1.5 cm proximal to the medial plateau of the tibia between the medial patellar ligament and the medial collateral ligament of the stifle joint (Fig. 48.17b). The needle is directed perpendicular to the skin. The medial meniscus, which is slightly distal and caudal to the injection site, should be avoided. Another approach is to insert the needle 1.5 cm proximal to the medial tibial plateau in a palpable depression between the medial patellar ligament and the tendon of insertion of the sartorius muscle [57]. The needle is directed parallel to the ground in a cranial to caudal direction in a sagittal plane. It is important that the horse stands squarely on the limb while performing this block. This approach may allow the collection of a greater volume of synovial fluid and reduce the risk of iatrogenic cartilage and medial meniscus injury compared with the approach between the medial patellar ligament and medial collateral ligament.

The lateral femorotibial compartment may be injected by various approaches. These include needle insertion sites caudal to the lateral patellar ligament and 1 cm proximal to the lateral tibial plateau (Fig. 48.17c); proximal to the tibia and caudal to the tendon of origin of the long digital extensor muscle; and between the long digital extensor tendon and the extensor groove at the proximal aspect of the tibia. However, insertion of the needle directly through the long digital extensor tendon 1–4 cm distal to the lateral tibial plateau is the most successful technique for injection of the lateral femorotibial compartment of the stifle joint [58].

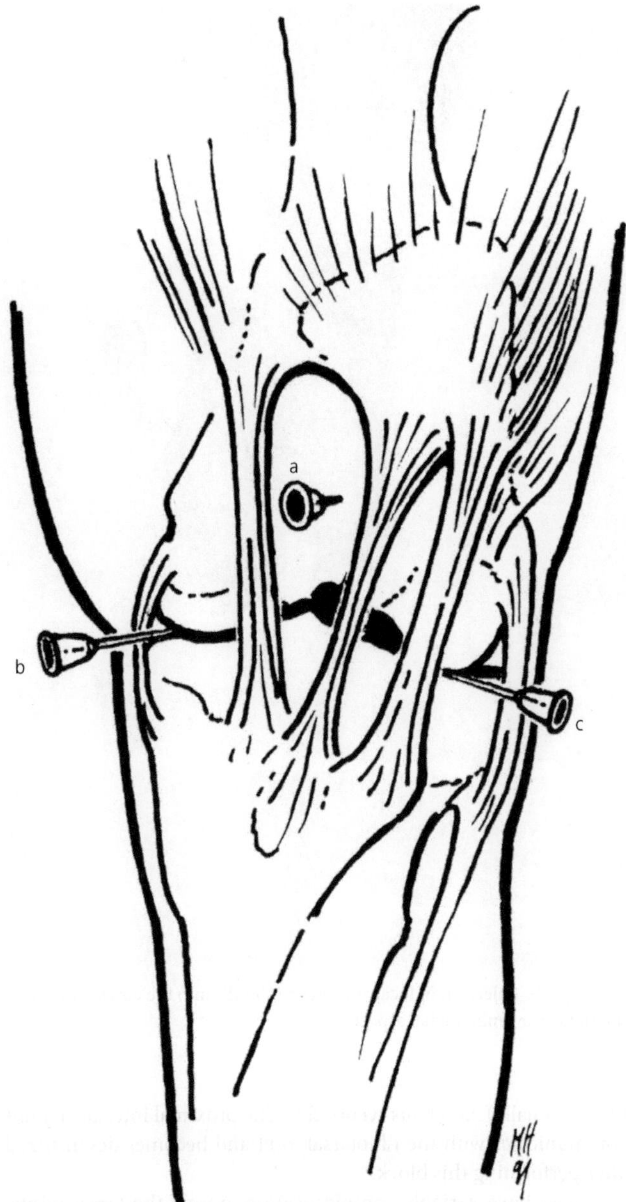

Figure 48.17 Needle placement into the femoropatellar pouch (a), medial femorotibial pouch (b), and lateral femorotibial pouch (c) of the stifle joint.

Coxofemoral (Hip) joint block

The coxofemoral joint is difficult to inject, particularly in large horses, because of the depth of the joint from the skin surface. Before insertion of the needle, it is important to ensure that the horse is standing squarely, with the limbs perpendicular to the ground. An 18 G needle at least 6 in (15 cm) long should be used. Because of the risk of needle breakage or bending attributable to the length of the needle and depth of the joint, adequate physical restraint is important and subcutaneous injection of local anesthetic at the needle insertion site and sedation of the horse may be necessary. The site of needle insertion is in a palpable depression between the large caudal and small cranial parts of the major trochanter of the proximal aspect of the femur (Fig. 48.18a). The needle is directed medially in a slightly cranioventral direction along the neck of the femur. Proper needle placement should be confirmed via aspiration of synovial fluid before injection; 20 mL of local anesthetic are injected. Ultrasonographic guidance may aid placement of the needle in the coxofemoral joint [59].

Trochanteric bursa block

The trochanteric bursa is located between the tendon of the medial gluteal muscle and the cranial part of the greater trochanter of the femur. The bursa is located via palpation of the greater trochanter and a 1.5–3.5 in (3.8–8.9 cm) 18 G needle is inserted perpendicular to the skin until bone is contacted (Fig. 48.18b); 5–10 mL of local anesthetic are injected. Positioning the limb caudally with the foot in a non-weight-bearing position on a block and use of ultrasonographic guidance may facilitate accurate insertion of the needle into the trochanteric bursa [60].

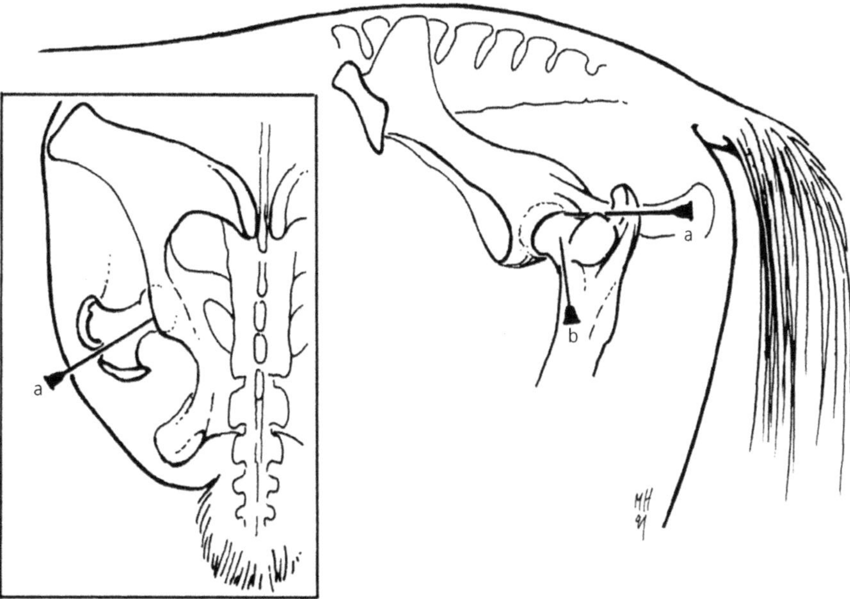

Figure 48.18 Needle placement into the coxofemoral joint (a) and the trochanteric bursa (b).

Regional anesthesia/analgesia

Regional anesthesia and analgesia can be used as adjuncts to general anesthesia to decrease anesthetic requirements, or can be used to facilitate standing procedures when combined with restraint and sedative/tranquilizers in the conscious horse.

Anesthesia for laparotomy/laparoscopy

Correction of uterine torsion is the most common procedure where standing laparotomy has historically been used, but it may also be useful for exploratory surgery when general anesthesia is not an option for financial or other reasons. Standing laparoscopy is now more commonly used for several standing abdominal procedures, including ovariectomy, nephrectomy, embryo transfer, castration of abdominal cryptorchids, and liver or kidney biopsy. Four techniques have been described for standing abdominal procedures: infiltration anesthesia, paravertebral thoracolumbar anesthesia, segmental dorsolumbar epidural anesthesia, and segmental thoracolumbar subarachnoid anesthesia. Segmental dorsolumbar epidural anesthesia and segmental thoracolumbar subarachnoid anesthesia are infrequently used and will not be discussed here; however, interested readers are directed to the previous edition of this book for complete and thorough descriptions [61].

Infiltration anesthesia

The most commonly used local anesthetic technique for standing abdominal procedures in horses is simple infiltration of the incision (line block). For most standing procedures, the incisions will be small, and infiltration anesthesia will be sufficient when combined with restraint and systemic sedation and analgesia. A 1 in (2.5 cm) 20 or 22 G needle is used to deposit 1 mL of local anesthetic for each centimeter of incision. For laparoscopy, the small incision sites required for insertion of the camera and instruments may be desensitized individually, whereas for laparotomy, a larger area of desensitization will be required.

Pain is minimized (and cooperation of the patient maximized) if the injections are slow and deliberate, and the needle is advanced through the edge of the desensitized skin. This technique assures that the horse senses only the initial needle insertion. A 10-15 mL injection of local anesthetic is usually sufficient for desensitization of the skin and subcutaneous tissues. Depending on the local anesthetic used, at least 15 min should be allowed for maximum anesthetic effect.

After the superficial structures are desensitized, the deeper layers of muscle and peritoneum can be desensitized with a 3–4 in (7.5–10 cm) 18 G needle; 50–150 mL of local anesthetic may be required depending on the area of desensitization needed. In an average 500 kg (1100 lb) adult horse, dosages of less than 250 mL of 2% lidocaine are not expected to cause toxicity [62].

Local infiltration is easy to perform and requires no knowledge about specific nerve location. Disadvantages include disruption of normal tissue architecture, incomplete anesthesia (especially of the peritoneum), incomplete muscle relaxation of the abdominal wall, toxicity after inadvertent injection into the peritoneal cavity, and increased cost and time involved with long incisions.

Paravertebral thoracolumbar anesthesia

When long incisions are required in patients where general anesthesia is not an option, paravertebral thoracolumbar anesthesia (paravertebral block) can be used as an alternative to infiltration anesthesia [63]. Even though this block is technically difficult, it can be performed in thin-muscled horses with easily palpable landmarks. To perform the block, the last thoracic (T18) and first and second lumbar (L1 and L2) spinal nerves are desensitized approximately 10 cm from the dorsal midline, after they have emerged from the intervertebral foramina and have split into their dorsal and ventral branches and medial and lateral ramifications, respectively (Fig. 48.19).

The sites for desensitization are palpated by locating the third lumbar transverse process, which is on a line between the most caudal extension of the last rib and perpendicular to the long axis of the spinal vertebrae. The distance between the injection sites is 3–6 cm (Fig. 48.20). After the skin is desensitized, the ventral branches of T18, L1, and L2 are blocked using a 3 in (7.5 cm) 18 G needle. The

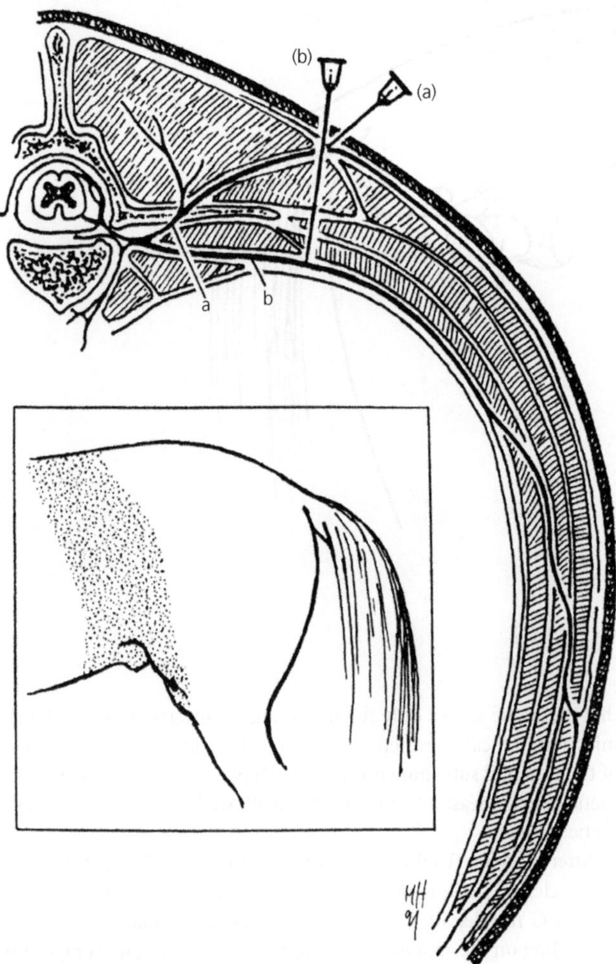

Figure 48.19 Needle placement for paravertebral nerve blockade. A cranial view of a transection of the first lumbar vertebra at the location of the intervertebral foramen: (a) subcutaneous infiltration and (b) retroperitoneal infusion. a, Dorsal branch and b, ventral branch of the L1 vertebral nerve). Inset: desensitized subcutaneous area after blockade of T18, L1, and L2 vertebral nerves.

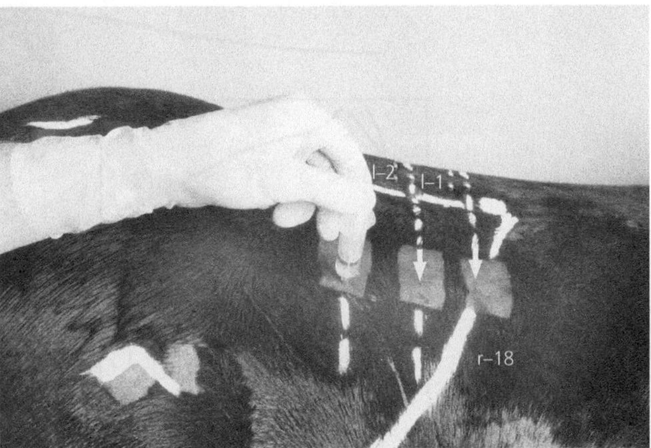

Figure 48.20 Right thoracolumbar area of a standing adult horse with injection sites (arrows) for distal paravertebral block. r-18, last rib; l-1 and l-2, spinous processes of first and second lumbar vertebrae. The dotted line transects the corresponding interspaces between spinous and transverse processes. Subcutaneous injection of l-2 is shown. Source: Skarda RT. Practical regional anesthesia. In: Mansmann RA, McAllister ES, Pratt PW, eds. *Equine Medicine and Surgery*, Vol. **1**, 3rd edn. Santa Barbara, CA: American Veterinary, 1982; 229–238.

needle is advanced to the peritoneum (where there will be a loss of resistance or a slight sucking sound as air enters the needle) and then withdrawn to a retroperitoneal position, where 15 mL of local anesthetic are injected (Fig. 48.19b) [63].

Advantages of paravertebral anesthesia over infiltration anesthesia include smaller doses of local anesthetic, a wide area of desensitization, muscle relaxation, and the absence of local anesthetic in the incision (minimizing hematomas, edema, and possible interference with healing). The main disadvantages are the difficulty in performing the block and the fact that in a horse with a good body condition score and muscle coverage the landmarks are extremely difficult to palpate. There is also a chance that the third lumbar spinal nerve may be inadvertently desensitized, which causes loss of motor control to the ipsilateral pelvic limb.

Anesthesia for reproductive procedures

Many reproductive procedures can be performed in the standing sedated horse. Castrations, episioplasty, repair of recto-vaginal fistulas, and perineal urethrostomy may all be completed with appropriate local anesthesia.

Anesthesia for castration

Castration is one of the most common surgical procedures performed in equine practice. For older horses or horses that are intractable, general anesthesia is generally recommended owing to potential complications such as hemorrhage. Even when general anesthesia is used, 15 mL of 2% lidocaine will decrease intraoperative blood pressure responses and cremaster muscle tension and can be a beneficial supplement to general anesthesia [64]. In another study, incisional, intratesticular and intrafunicular lidocaine was found to be an effective adjunct to intravenous anesthesia [65].

In standing horses, restraint of the horse's head and sedation are required in addition to local anesthesia. The use of stocks is generally not recommended for standing castration, owing to the potential for injury to the surgeon. A twitch may be used to aid restraint, and for safety reasons the person holding the twitch should stand on the same side as the surgeon. The skin of the scrotum and prepuce should be aseptically prepared and then the block can be done with one of three techniques.

In the most commonly used technique, a 3 in (7.5 cm) 20 G needle is inserted perpendicularly through the tensed skin of the scrotum and local anesthetic is injected until the testicle is turgid (approximately 20–30 mL) (Fig. 48.21). After approximately 10 min, the castration can usually be performed painlessly, with no further need for the twitch.

In the second technique, a 1 in (2.5 cm) 20 G needle may be inserted into the spermatic cord percutaneously as close to the external inguinal ring as possible. At that point, 20–30 mL of local anesthetic are injected in a fan-shaped manner without perforating the skin, spermatic artery, or vein. The incision site into the scrotum must still be infiltrated subcutaneously with 5–10 mL of local anesthetic since the skin of the scrotum is not desensitized by the deposition of the local anesthetic into the spermatic cord. The procedure must then be repeated on the other side. Infiltration of the spermatic cord is not as effective as infiltration directly into the testicle.

In the third technique, a 6 in (15 cm) 18 G needle is inserted into the testicle and directed into the spermatic cord while 30 mL of

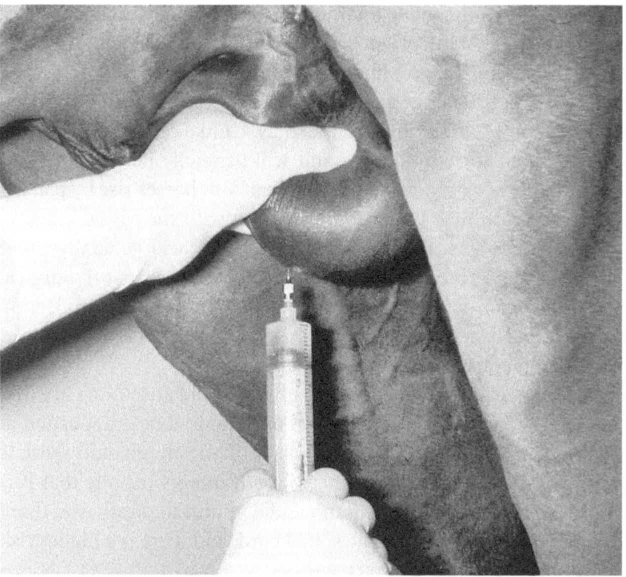

Figure 48.21 Needle placement for right intratesticular injection in a standing horse.

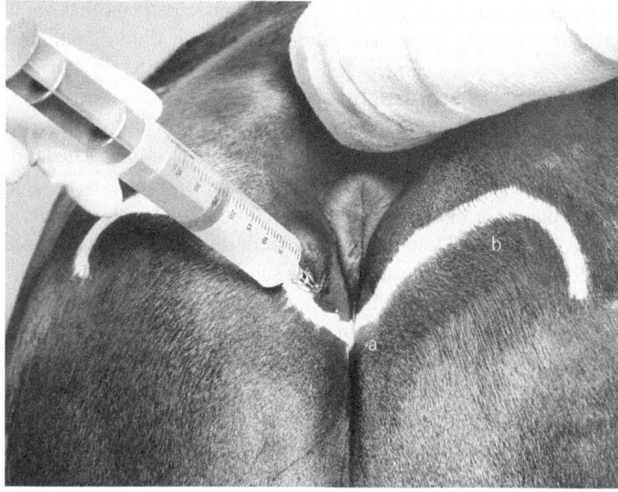

Figure 48.22 Topographic anatomy for perineal and pudendal nerve block. The palpable ischiatic arch (a) and ischiatic tuberosity (b) are marked. Infiltration of the left pudendal nerve with local anesthetic is shown. Source: Skarda RT. Practical regional anesthesia. In: Mansmann RA, McAllister ES, Pratt PW, eds. *Equine Medicine and Surgery*, Vol. **1**, 3rd edn. Santa Barbara, CA: American Veterinary, 1982; 229–238.

local anesthetic are being injected. Prior to beginning the surgery, the skin of the scrotum at the incision sites is also desensitized.

Cryptorchid castration is more commonly performed under general anesthesia by laparotomy or laparoscopy, but in a recent study intratesticular or mesorchial infiltration of lidocaine combined with administration of a non-steroidal anti-inflammatory drug (NSAID) and caudal epidural injection of detomidine provided adequate analgesia in standing stallions undergoing laparoscopic cryptorchidectomy [66].

Anesthesia of the perineum

While a caudal epidural is commonly used to allow perineal surgeries, including urethrostomy, to be performed in standing horses, regional anesthesia of the perineum may also be used. To perform regional anesthesia of the area, the superficial and deep (sub-fascial) branches of the perineal nerves must be desensitized. A 1 in (2.5 cm) 22 G needle is inserted approximately 2.5 cm dorsal to the ischial arch and 2.5 cm lateral to the anus so that 5 mL of local anesthetic may be injected subcutaneously. After directing the needle dorsally 0.5–1 cm, a deeper sub-fascial injection of 5–7 mL is made, and then the procedure is repeated on the opposite side [67].

Anesthesia of the penis or vulva

The penis may be desensitized by blocking the pudendal nerves at the ischium (Fig. 48.22). This will desensitize the penis and the internal lamina of the prepuce in addition to relaxing the penis and allowing it to be extruded. To perform the block, a 1.5 in (3.8 cm) 20 G needle is inserted on the right and left side of the anus about 2 cm dorsal to the ischial arch and lateral to the anus and is angled ventrally towards the midline. The needle is advanced until the point contacts the ischial arch where the pudendal nerves course around the ischium. Then 5 mL of local anesthetic are deposited adjacent to each nerve, which results in the penis being extruded within about 5 min of a successful block.

While a line block with local anesthetic is still commonly utilized for desensitization of the vulva, the technique described above may also be used. It is interesting to note that one study has suggested that use of lidocaine/prilocaine topical anesthetic cream is as effective as lidocaine infiltration in providing local anesthesia when performing episioplasty in mares and caused less anatomic disruption [68].

Epidural anesthesia/analgesia

In horses, epidural anesthesia combined with systemic sedation and standing restraint allows for regional anesthesia of the anus, perineum, rectum, vulva, vagina, urethra, and bladder. Additionally, epidural analgesia can provide good adjunctive analgesia for painful conditions of the stifles and hocks. In the horse, the spinal cord ends at the level of the caudal half of the second sacral vertebra, so caudal epidural injection may be performed without risk of spinal injection.

Indications/contraindications

The choice of drugs placed epidurally will dictate whether anesthesia or analgesia is produced, and the specific medication and volume chosen will determine the spread. Indwelling epidural catheters can also be placed when repeated administration of analgesic or anesthetic drugs are anticipated. Indications for epidural injection of drugs in horses include anesthesia of the perineum, rectum, anus, tail, urethra, bladder, vulva, or vagina for surgery in the standing horse. Other indications include relief of tenesmus and correction of uterine torsion, and also fetotomy. Additionally, epidural analgesia/anesthesia may be used as adjuncts to general anesthesia for surgery of these same structures and the hindlimbs to reduce the minimum alveolar concentration of inhalants [69,70]. Epidural analgesia can be used postoperatively for pain management of these same areas, as an adjunct to systemic medications, and for alleviation of pain related to septic joints.

Contraindications to epidurals in horses include infection at the puncture site, sepsis, uncorrected hypovolemia, bleeding disorders, anticoagulation therapy (potentially used in horses with laminitis), spinal cord disease, and anatomic abnormalities. This technique may also be contraindicated in weak or ataxic patients that are at risk for becoming recumbent after epidural drug administration.

Lumbosacral subarachnoid

The lumbosacral epidural space is technically difficult to access and requires a specialized catheter–stylet unit for injections. The landmarks for injection are difficult to determine and there is a risk of dural puncture and inadvertent injection into the subarachnoid space, which could lead to motor blockade and ataxia if the intended epidural dose is administered in the subarachnoid space. Catheters may be advanced from the lumbosacral epidural space for either caudal epidural, or rostrally for segmental thoracolumbar analgesia.

Much easier to master is either single injection or catheterization of the lumbosacral subarachnoid space [71]. The site for injection is the same as for collection of cerebrospinal fluid and may be palpated at the intersection of a line 1–2 cm caudal to each tuber coxae and the dorsal midline. The skin should be prepared using aseptic techniques. Systemic sedation will generally be needed to perform this procedure. The skin may be desensitized with 2–3 mL of 2% lidocaine to minimize discomfort from the passage of the spinal needle. A 6.8 in (17.5 cm) 17 G Huber-point Tuohy needle and stylet with the bevel directed cranially is advanced along the median plane perpendicular to the spinal cord and inserted into the subarachnoid space (Fig. 48.23). If bone is encountered before the subarachnoid space is entered, the needle should be redirected cranially or caudally, while staying on midline. Once the subarachnoid space is punctured, 2–3 mL of cerebrospinal fluid should be removed, and a small amount (approximately 2 mL) of local anesthetic can be injected. Injecting large amounts of local anesthetic will potentially cause motor blockade and recumbency. Unlike cattle, which rise by starting with their hindlimbs and will generally lie placidly until motor blockade of their hindlimbs wears off, horses rise by placing their forelimbs first and then pushing up with their hindlimbs, so motor blockade of the hind limbs in horses will generally cause them to panic and struggle until the blockade wears off. Surgical anesthesia can be maintained by placing a catheter and injecting approximately one-quarter of the original dose of local anesthetic at 30 min intervals, or as needed.

Advantages to thoracolumbar subarachnoid anesthesia are that it requires a small volume of local anesthetic that is deposited at the nerve roots, there is a rapid onset of anesthesia, and there is minimal physiologic disturbance. Disadvantages include that it is more technically difficult than caudal epidural anesthesia, there is potential for damage to the spinal cord, and there is a higher risk of motor blockade and ataxia.

Caudal epidural

Caudal epidural anesthesia and/or analgesia performed at the sacrococcygeal or the first coccygeal (Co1–Co2) space is the preferred and most commonly used technique in the horse as it is safer and

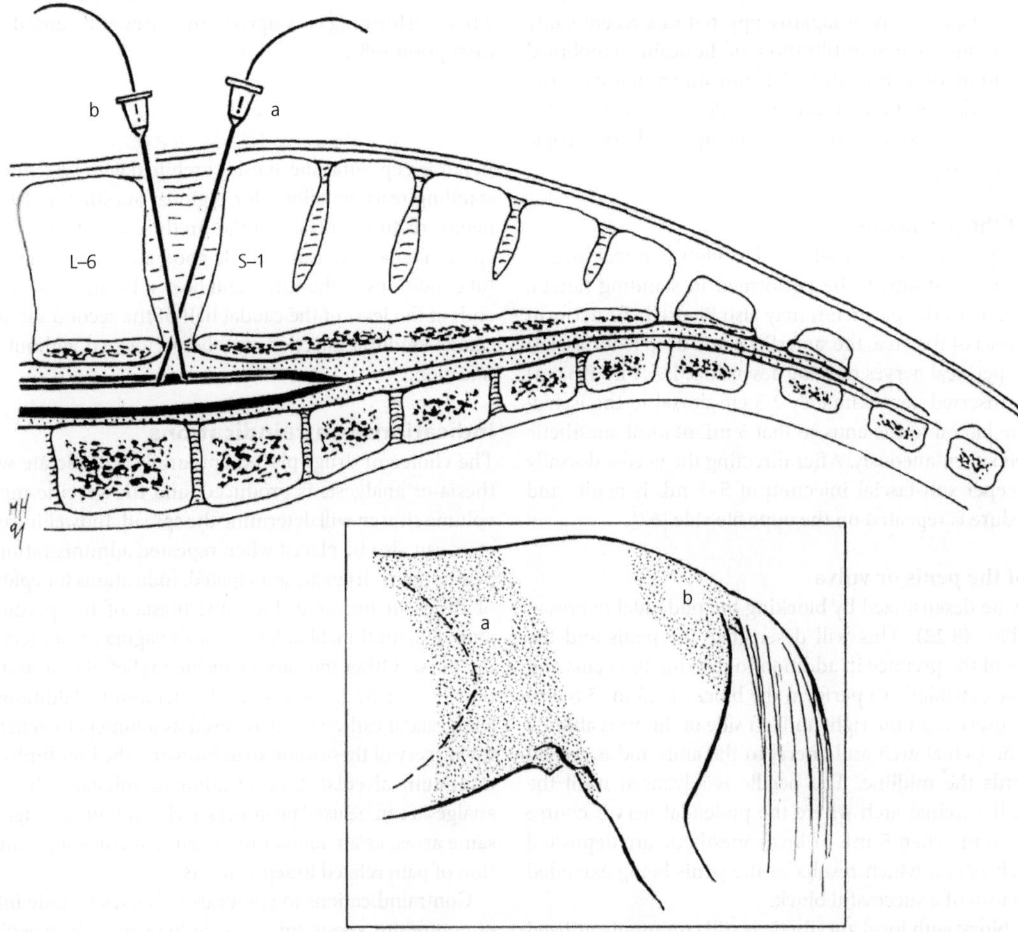

Figure 48.23 Needle and catheter placement for thoracolumbar subarachnoid anesthesia (a) and caudal subarachnoid anesthesia (b). Desensitized subcutaneous area after segmental (a) and caudal (b) blockade is applied.

easier to perform than lumbosacral subarachnoid anesthesia, and requires no specialized equipment.

The site for injection is either the sacrococcygeal or the first coccygeal space [72]. In some horses, the last sacral and first coccygeal vertebrae are fused and the first moveable space may be the first coccygeal interspace. The space is palpated while moving the tail up and down; it is the first moveable space caudal to the sacrum, which is generally 2.5–7.5 cm cranial to the origin of the tail hairs. The tail may be raised and lowered, or some people prefer a 'pump handle' motion to identify the space.

After aseptic preparation, 1 mL of 2% lidocaine may be injected to desensitize the skin if desired. There are two commonly used techniques for a one-time injection into the caudal epidural space. In the first, a 1.5 in (3.8 cm) 18 G needle is inserted at the center of the palpated space perpendicular to the skin (Fig. 48.24a). The 'hanging drop' technique can be utilized where the hub of the needle is filled with saline before advancing the needle and then when the needle enters the epidural space, the negative pressure will pull the drop into the epidural space. A slight popping may also be felt as the needle crosses the interarcuate ligament. The depth of the space from the skin is approximately 3.5–8 cm in adult horses. When the needle is thought to be in the epidural space, aspiration will confirm lack of blood or cerebrospinal fluid and a test dose of air or saline may be made to confirm loss of resistance to injection. In the second technique, a 5–7.5 in (12.7–19 cm) 18 G spinal needle is inserted at the caudal part of the interspace, at approximately 30° parallel to the horizontal plane (Fig. 48.24b). This technique can be useful for epidural injection if the horse has previously had epidural injections which can result in development of fibrous tissue.

Traditionally, epidural puncture has been confirmed by aspiration of a fluid drop (i.e., hanging drop), or lack of resistance on injection. These methods are not always useful and the human medical literature has described the use of acoustic devices to detect a pressure drop by means of an audible signal when the ligamentum flavum is perforated [73]. Recently, an acoustic device has been used to identify the extradural space in standing horses [74].

Continuous caudal epidural anesthesia

For repeated and long-term administration of epidural medications, epidural catheters are recommended. Epidural catheterization can be used successfully for repeated epidural delivery of analgesics and anesthetics in horses with various clinical conditions, including fractures, lacerations, septic arthritis, myositis, perineal injuries, and cellulitis [75]. One study showed that long-term epidural administration of a morphine–detomidine combination was not associated with adverse systemic effects in horses even though localized inflammation and fibrosis was seen [76].

After aseptic preparation and optional desensitization of the skin, the needle is introduced at an angle of approximately 45° to the skin (Fig. 48.24c). Once the needle is determined to be in the

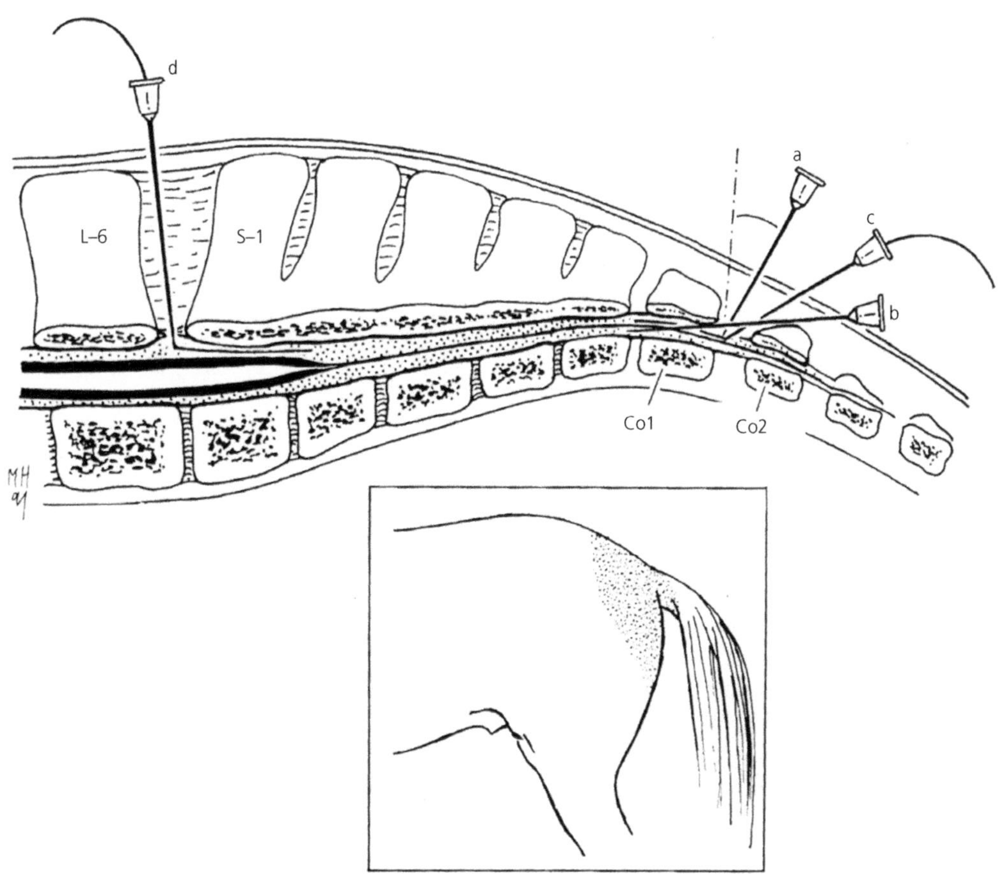

Figure 48.24 a and b, needle placement for caudal epidural anesthesia; c and d, catheter placement into sacral epidural space for continuous caudal epidural anesthesia. L-6, sixth lumbar; S-1, first sacral dorsal spinous process; Co1 and Co2, first and second coccygeal vertebrae. Desensitized subcutaneous area after caudal blockade is applied.

epidural space, the catheter may be introduced 10–30 cm into the epidural space by advancing it with the opening of the needle facing cranially. Once the catheter is placed, it is held in place while removing the needle, and then secured to the skin with adhesive and suture material; the entire catheter may then be covered with adhesive dressing. The injection port should be aseptically prepared prior to each injection and a bacterial filter may be used between the catheter and the injection port.

Epidural medications

Depending on the desired effect and duration of action, local anesthetics, α_2-adrenergic receptor agonists, opioids and other medications including ketamine, tramadol, and tiletamine–zolazepam (Telazol®) have been shown to be effective at providing anesthesia and analgesia when used epidurally.

Epidural local anesthetics

Epidural local anesthetics provide analgesia by preventing depolarization of the nerve membrane and conduction of nerve impulses. The most common local anesthetics used for epidural application in horses are 2% lidocaine and 2% mepivacaine.

Lidocaine is an effective epidural analgesic. The dose required to desensitize effectively the anus, perineum, rectum, vulva, vagina, urethra, and bladder is 6–8 mL of a 2% solution in a 450 kg mare (0.26–0.35 mg/kg). The cranial spread and intensity of analgesia are dose dependent, but generally, sensory and motor blockade ranging from the coccygeal to second lumbar vertebra is produced within 5–15 min and lasts 60–90 min. Redosing should be performed with caution since inadvertent overdose can cause profound ataxia, recumbency, and hypotension [77,78].

Mepivacaine (2%) acts very similarly to lidocaine when used as an epidural agent in horses. Similarly to lidocaine, the extent of the desensitized area is determined by the volume of local anesthetic injected (Fig. 48.25). Analgesia usually reaches peak effect in 20 min and lasts approximately 80 min [79].

Caudally injected hyperbaric bupivacaine (0.5%, 0.06 mg/kg) produces bilateral perineal analgesia in horses, with a rapid onset of action (<6 min) and a long duration of action (>5 h) [80]. Heart and respiratory rates, arterial blood pressure, and rectal temperature were not changed after epidural administration of bupivacaine.

Ropivacaine is the most recently investigated local anesthetic for local and regional anesthesia in horses. Various doses and concentrations have been investigated, ranging from 0.1 mg/kg of 0.5% ropivacaine (8 mL/500 kg) [81] to 0.02 mg/kg of 0.5% ropivacaine (5 mL/500 kg) [82]. Epidural ropivacaine has a rapid onset (approximately 10 min) and can last approximately 3 h. Recently, low-dose lumbosacral epidural ropivacaine was shown to provide effective analgesia in conscious and anesthetized ponies without affecting motor function to the pelvic limbs [83].

Epinephrine can be added to local anesthetic solutions at a concentration of 5 μg/mL (1:200 000) to hasten the onset, prolong the duration, and improve the quality of epidural anesthesia.

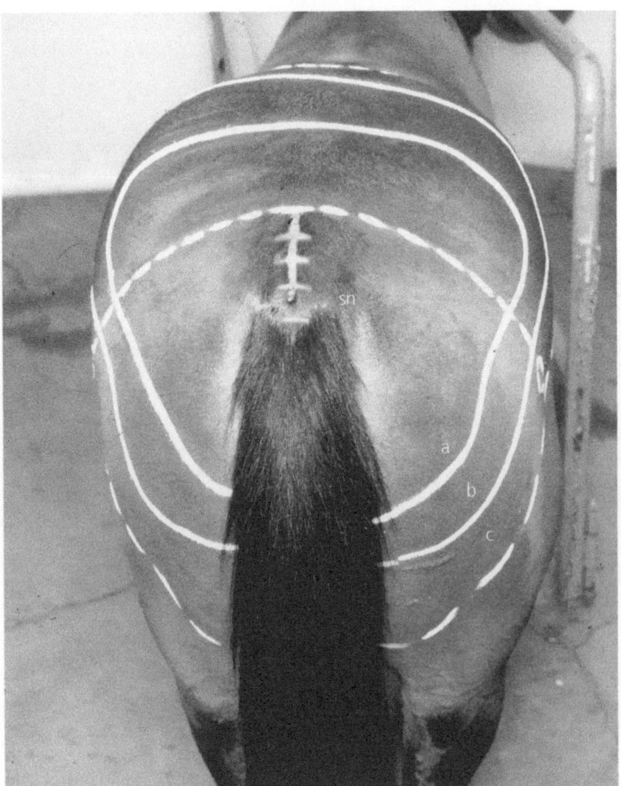

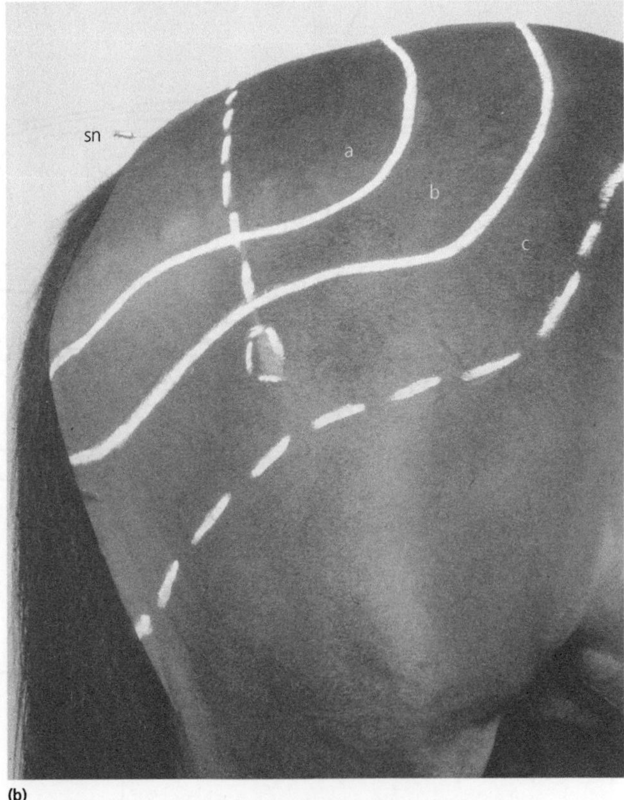

Figure 48.25 Desensitized skin area in a standing horse 20 min after epidural injection of (a) 6, (b) 8, and (c) 10 mL of 2% carbocaine via a 5.9 in (15 cm) 18 G spinal needle inserted at the third coccygeal interspace to its full length horizontally. sn, spinal needle with stylet. (a) Dorsocaudal and (b) lateral aspects. Source: Skarda RT. Practical regional anesthesia. In: Mansmann RA, McAllister ES, Pratt PW, eds. *Equine Medicine and Surgery*, Vol. 1, 3rd edn. Santa Barbara, CA: American Veterinary, 1982; 229–238.

Epidural α_2-adrenergic agonists

Following epidural administration, α_2-adrenergic receptor agonists bind to receptors in the substantia gelatinosa layer of the spinal cord and produce analgesia, which can be reversed by intravenous administration of α_2-adrenergic receptor antagonists such as atipamazole (0.1 mg/kg) [84] and yohimbine (0.05 mg/kg) [85]. α_2-adrenergic receptor agonists deposited as described for a caudal epidural must diffuse cranially to affect receptors in the spinal cord. If signs of ataxia or sedation develop after caudal epidural administration of α_2-adrenergic receptor agonists, the horse should be supported with a tail-tie or in stocks until normal motor function has been regained. Horses that become recumbent after epidural administration of α_2-adrenergic receptor agonists may require heavy sedation or general anesthesia to keep them from panicking until their motor function has returned.

As noted above, specific antagonists may be used to reverse undesirable effects of epidurally administered α_2-adrenergic receptor agonists. Intravenous yohimbine reduced epidural detomidine-induced perineal analgesia, reversed head ptosis, improved pelvic limb position, terminated sweating and diuresis, and antagonized detomidine-induced decreases in heart rate and cardiac output; but did not affect detomidine-induced decreases in respiratory rate [85].

Xylazine

Xylazine has been used at a dose of 0.17 mg/kg diluted to 10 mL with 0.9% saline [86]. The duration of analgesia is approximately 2.5 h and hindlimb ataxia is uncommon. Sedation is minimal and cardiovascular and respiratory variables and also core and rectal temperatures do not change appreciably [87].

In horses under general anesthesia, epidural xylazine (0.15 mg/kg) reduces the minimum alveolar concentration (MAC) of halothane by 35% to noxious stimulation of the thoracic limbs and by 40% in the pelvic limbs [70]. A second study did not reproduce this effect, but horses that had been given epidural xylazine (0.15 mg/kg diluted to 0.15 mL/kg with saline) required less halothane and inotropic support to maintain mean arterial blood pressure above 60 mmHg and had a higher cardiac index than horses anesthetized with halothane alone [88].

In general, xylazine is a more desirable α_2-adrenergic receptor agonist for epidural use than detomidine since it produces a more potent antinociceptive action in the perineal dermatomes, with minimal cardiovascular depression, head ptosis, changes in pelvic limb position, and diuresis [89].

Detomidine

Detomidine has been used in caudal epidurals at a dose of 60 μg/kg diluted to 10 mL with sterile water [90]. The analgesia from this technique can be variable, with bilateral spread from the coccyx to as far cranially as T14 in some horses. Analgesia is accompanied by mild ataxia, some buckling of the pelvic limbs and deep sedation. The onset of action is about 5 min and the duration is approximately 3 h. Because of the systemic side-effects, an initial dose of no more than 20 μg/kg should be used in debilitated horses.

Other α_2-adrenergic receptor agonists

Medetomidine (15 μg/kg diluted to 8 mL with 0.9% saline) and romifidine (80 μg/kg diluted to 8 mL with 0.9% saline) did not produce surgical analgesia in the perineal region of adult horses when injected into the caudal epidural space [91,92]. Based on these results, medetomidine and romifidine do not appear to be as effective as xylazine and detomidine.

Epidural opioids

Epidural opioids have been extensively studied and can produce long-lasting analgesia when used alone or in combination with local anesthetics, α_2-adrenergic receptor agonists, and/or ketamine. They have been used for acute and chronic pain and are effective when administered pre-emptively, intraoperatively, or postoperatively.

Morphine

Epidural morphine has long been considered a reasonable alternative for treating pain that does not respond to standard medication protocols such as systemic NSAIDs. In an early case report, epidural morphine was used to relieve the pain associated with a luxated fetlock and comminuted fracture of the first phalanx in a pregnant horse; the onset of action seemed to be approximately 30 min after injection and lasted for 8–16 h based on the behavior of the mare [93].

Morphine is commonly used at a dose of 0.1 mg/kg diluted to a volume of 20 mL with sterile water and administered as a caudal epidural for the relief of pain. It will induce segmental analgesia from the coccyx to the thoracic dermatomes [94]. The analgesic action is greatest at the dermatomes closest to the epidural injection site and lasts approximately 5 h [94].

In recent studies, morphine was shown to be an effective analgesic for experimentally induced forelimb pain [95]. It has also produced analgesic and antihyperalgesic effects in horses with acute synovitis [96]. In a study in mares undergoing laparoscopic ovariectomy, epidural morphine administration lowered the requirements for systemic sedation and local anesthesia [97]. Although there are concerns about systemic opioids and gastrointestinal side-effects in horses, epidural morphine did not cause clinical signs of colic, although it temporarily reduced gastrointestinal motility [98].

Hydromorphone

In one study, epidural administration of hydromorphone (0.04 mg/kg diluted to 20 mL with sterile saline) was shown to increase the avoidance threshold to noxious electrical stimulation in the perineal, lumbar, sacral, and thoracic regions in horses. The onset of action was approximately 20 min and the duration was 250 min after injection, and no significant sedation or ataxia was reported [99].

Methadone

When the effects of caudal epidural methadone (0.1 mg/kg) were compared with those of lidocaine (0.35 mg/kg) using a thermal stimulation model, perineal analgesia was apparent within 15 min after injection [100]. The perineal analgesia from methadone lasted 5 h after injection compared with 3 h with lidocaine. Unlike lidocaine, methadone did not cause ataxia. In a recent study, methadone (0.4 mg/kg) was used to validate lumbosacral spinal cord somatosensory evoked potentials as a tool to assess nociception in horses [101].

Meperidine

Meperidine (pethidine) is a synthetic opioid that has the strongest local anesthetic effect of the clinically used opioids. Caudal epidural injection of meperidine produces bilateral analgesia from the coccygeal to first sacral dermatomes with minimal sedation and ataxia. With a dose of 0.8 mg/kg (5% solution), the onset of action is 12 min with a duration from 4 to over 5 h [102]. A second study produced similar results: 0.6 mg/kg of a 5% solution produced bilateral perineal analgesia in less than 10 min with an average duration of 4 h [103].

Butorphanol

Despite the widespread use of butorphanol in horses as a systemic analgesic, it has not been shown to increase avoidance behavior to noxious stimuli [94] or to affect the MAC of halothane [69] after caudal epidural administration.

Other epidural medications

Ketamine

Ketamine produced analgesia of the tail, perineum, and upper hindlimb in horses in an experimental model [104]. Dosages of 0.5, 1 and 2 mg/kg ketamine (diluted to a total volume of 10 mL with 0.9% saline) provide analgesia of the tail and hindlimb for 30–80 min. There is also a dose-related sedative effect which peaks between 15 and 30 min after injection. Cardiovascular and respiratory variables are largely unchanged, but more investigation is needed to determine if the analgesia produced by epidural ketamine is sufficient for standing surgical procedures.

Tramadol

Tramadol is a centrally acting analgesic drug with opioid and non-opioid mechanisms of action. In horses, tramadol (1.0 mg/kg diluted to a total volume of 20 mL in sterile water) produced perineal and sacral analgesia within 30 min with a duration of action of up to 4 h [94]. Recently, the pharmacokinetics of epidural tramadol have been examined. After caudal epidural injection of 2 mg/kg, plasma metabolites were detectable from 5 min to 8 h in concentrations within the extrapolated therapeutic range for humans, suggesting that this compound warrants further investigation in horses [105].

Tiletamine–zolazepam

Epidural tiletamine–zolazepam (Telazol®) (0.5 and 1.0 mg/kg) produces a small increase in the tolerance to a noxious pressure stimulus (blunt tipped forceps) in horses, and could be indicated for short-term moderate epidural analgesia, but further studies examining the spinal toxicity should be completed before recommending the use of this technique clinically [106].

Epidural medication combinations

Xylazine and lidocaine

Xylazine (0.17 mg/kg of a 2% solution) and lidocaine (0.22 mg/kg of a 2% solution) can be safely used for long-lasting caudal epidural anesthesia in healthy adult horses [78]. The combination provides up to 5 h of perineal anesthesia whereas each drug alone has a duration of only about 3 h. There may be some ataxia with the combination, but heart and respiratory rates are minimally affected. Although there appears to be a large margin of safety with this combination, it is worth noting that there is one report of a Thoroughbred mare undergoing sudden collapse in the hindquarters 90 min after completion of the epidural injection for urogenital surgery [107].

Morphine and detomidine

Morphine and detomidine provided profound hindlimb analgesia in horses with experimentally induced lameness [108]. Epidural morphine (0.2 mg/kg) combined with detomidine (30 μg/kg) also significantly decreased lameness after bilateral stifle arthroscopy in horses [109]. A more recent study found that the analgesic effects of epidural buprenorphine (0.005 mg/kg) plus detomidine (0.15 mg/kg) were equivalent to those after epidural morphine plus detomidine in horses undergoing bilateral stifle arthroscopy [110].

Morphine and romifidine

Caudal epidural romifidine (30–60 μg/kg) combined with morphine (0.1 mg/kg) produces moderate analgesia for 60–90 min depending on the dose of romifidine used. Intense sedation, moderate ataxia of the hindlimb, and a decrease in heart and respiratory rates were noted during the 4 h observation period [111].

Fentanyl and romifidine

Caudal epidural fentanyl and romifidine were compared with romifidine alone in one study, and the onset of action of the combination was significantly faster and lasted significantly longer than with romifidine alone. Additionally, the quality of analgesia as assessed by the surgeon was significantly improved, and there was no difference in ataxia, sedation, or side-effects between groups [81].

Meperidine and lidocaine

In one study, caudal epidural anesthesia with a combination of meperidine (0.3 mg/kg) and lidocaine (0.2 mg/kg) was shown to prolong the duration of anesthesia compared with lidocaine or meperidine alone [103].

Tramadol and lidocaine

Tramadol (0.5 mg/kg) combined with lidocaine (0.2 mg/kg of a 2% solution) was shown to extend the duration of perineal analgesia, as measured using a pinprick and thermal stimulation, over lidocaine alone when used as a caudal epidural. The duration of action of lidocaine alone was 70 min and that of tramadol with lidocaine was 210 min [112].

Neostigmine and lidocaine

Addition of neostigmine to lidocaine for caudal epidural administration increased lidocaine's duration of action. Lidocaine (0.2 mg/kg of a 2% solution) was administered alone or combined with 1 or 2 μg/kg of neostigmine as a caudal epidural. Neostigmine combined with lidocaine induced perineal analgesia for 2.5 h with a low prevalence of adverse effects in standing horses [113].

Ketamine combinations

Ketamine (1.0 mg/kg) and xylazine (0.5 mg/kg) have been used in combination for caudal epidurals in horses and have been shown to produce good analgesia of the tail, perineal region, anus, and vulva [114]. The onset of action is 5–9 min and the duration is an average of 120 min. There is some systemic sedation with this combination.

Recently, epidural bupivacaine alone (0.02 mg/kg of a 0.25% solution), bupivacaine with morphine (0.02 mg/kg with 0.1 mg/kg) and bupivacaine with ketamine (0.02 mg/kg with 0.5 mg/kg) were compared for their ability to provide analgesia in conscious horses [115]. The onset of action was 5 min for bupivacaine, 10 min for bupivacaine with morphine and 15 min for bupivacaine with ketamine. The duration of action was 315 min for bupivacaine with morphine, 210 min for bupivacaine and 240 min for bupivacaine with ketamine. While morphine and ketamine may be effective adjuncts to bupivacaine for caudal epidurals, bupivacaine with morphine may be preferable to a high dose of bupivacaine alone or to bupivacaine with ketamine.

Complications

There are several reported complications to epidural injections. Poor technique, anatomic abnormalities, and previous epidurals causing development of fibrous tissue at the site can cause failure of analgesia/anesthesia. Overdose of local anesthetics and/or α_2-adrenergic receptor agonists can cause excessive ataxia and possibly recumbency.

If recumbency results from inadvertent overdose of epidural anesthetics, it may be necessary to keep the horse sedated or anesthetized until the motor function to the hindlimbs returns. Sedation and cardiovascular depression may be associated with systemic uptake of medications (especially α_2-adrenergic receptor agonists) used epidurally. Finally, there have been rare reports of systemic pruritis in horses after epidural morphine [116–118].

Novel regional analgesic techniques

Intra-articular morphine

Opioid receptors are present in synovial membranes of horses [119] and acute inflammation has been shown to upregulate these receptors [120]. Whereas the intra-articular use of morphine is widespread in human medicine, there have been few clinical studies evaluating the use of this technique in horses. In one study, 120 mg of morphine administered intra-articularly after lipopolysaccharide (LPS)-induced synovitis improved markers of inflammation and clinical lameness scores [121]. Another study found that 20 mg of intra-articular morphine in combination with 20 mg of ropivacaine produced an effective and prolonged analgesic effect, which may offer at least 24 h of pain relief for acute synovitis [122].

Abaxial nerve block with ketamine

Ketamine provided local analgesia when used to perform an abaxial sesamoid block (5 mL of 2 or 3% ketamine solution) with an onset of action of approximately 2 min and a duration of action of up to 15 min [123]. Alkalinization of a 1% ketamine solution provides more consistent and persistent local analgesia [124].

Topical application of lidocaine patches

In humans, lidocaine patches are widely used for the treatment of neuropathic pain and postherpetic neuralgia. Despite good results reported anecdotally by practitioners, clinical studies evaluating their efficacy are limited. One clinical study failed to show a local antinociceptive effect from application of lidocaine patches in horses [125]. There is a lack of systemic absorption of lidocaine from 5% patches placed above the carpus in horses, suggesting that any local analgesic response is not from systemic absorption [126].

Topical NSAIDs

Topical diclofenac had clinical sign-modifying and disease-modifying effects in an experimental osteoarthritis model [127]. In one study in horses undergoing intravenous regional limb perfusion, topical diclofenac reduced inflammation as judged by visual assessment and ultrasonography [128]. Despite encouraging research studies and anecdotal reports, results of the limited available clinical studies are mixed. One study showed safety and efficacy of topically applied 1% diclofenac liposomal cream for the relief of lameness in horses [129], whereas other studies showed a lack of effect in horses with osteoarthritis [130]. One reason for this may be that diclofenac has low percutaneous absorption in horses. Recent studies have examined penetration enhancers to improve absorption [131], which may improve clinical efficacy.

Continuous delivery of local anesthetics for lower limb analgesia

A technique has been described for the continuous delivery of local anesthetics for lower limb analgesia [132]. The technique for placement of the catheters was first developed in cadaver limbs with the catheter being inserted 2–4 cm distal to the accessory carpal bone medially and laterally, and then passing it so that the tip was adjacent to the communicating branch of the medial and lateral palmar nerves. The catheters were well tolerated by the test horses, but after 1–2 days there was significant limb swelling in horses receiving local anesthetic infusions, but not in the horses receiving saline infusion. A second study compared continuous peripheral neural blockade (CPNB) with bupivacaine with intermittent peripheral neural blockade (IPNB) with bupivacaine in experimentally induced tendonitis pain [133]. CPNB provided better analgesia than IPNB when lameness was scored and behavioral and physiologic signs of pain were monitored. This study used the CPNB catheters for 3 days, and further investigation is needed to determine if this technique is useful for longer term treatment.

References

1 Edwards JF. Regional anaesthesia of the head of the horse: an up-to-date survey. *Vet Rec* 1930; **10**: 873–975.

2 Staszyk C, Bienert A, Baumer W, *et al.* Stimulation of local anaesthetic nerve block of the infraorbital nerve within the pterygopalatine fossa; anatomical landmarks defined by computed tomography. *Res Vet Sci* 2008; **85**: 399–406.

3 Roberts VLH, Perkins JD, Skarlina E, *et al.* Caudal anaesthesia of the infraorbital nerve for diagnosis of idiopathic headshaking and caudal compression of the infraorbital nerve for its treatment, in 58 horses. *Equine Vet J* 2013; **45**: 107–110.

4 Newton SA, Knottenbelt DC, Eldridge PR. Headshaking in horses: possible aetiopathogenesis suggested by the results of diagnostic tests and several treatment regimes used in 20 cases. *Equine Vet J* 2000; **32**: 208–216.

5 Schumacher J. Anesthesia of the head and penis. In: Doherty T, Valverde A, eds. *Manual of Equine Anesthesia and Analgesia*. Oxford: Blackwell, 2006; 282–286.

6 Bardell D, Iff I, Mosing M. A cadaver study comparing two approaches to perform a maxillary nerve block in the horse. *Equine Vet J* 2010; **42**: 721–725.

7 Harding PG, Smith RL, Barakzai SZ. Comparison of two approaches to performing an inferior alveolar nerve block in the horse. *Aust Vet J* 2012; **90**: 146–150.

8 Lindsay WA, Hedberg EB. Performing facial nerve blocks, nasolacrimal catheterization and paranasal sinus centesis in horses. *Vet Med* 1991; **86**: 72–83.

9 Ward DS. Anesthesia of the eye. In: Doherty T, Valverde A, eds. *Manual of Equine Anesthesia and Analgesia*. Oxford: Blackwell, 2006; 287–292.

10 Monclin SJ, Farnir F, Grauwels M. Duration of corneal anaesthesia following multiple doses and two concentrations of tetracaine hydrochloride eyedrops on the normal equine cornea. *Equine Vet J* 2011; **43**: 69–73.

11 Pucket JD, Allbaugh RA, Rankin AJ, *et al.* Comparison of efficacy and duration of effect on corneal sensitivity among anesthetic agents following ocular administration in clinically normal horses. *Am J Vet Res* 2013; **74**: 459–464.

12 Merideth RE, Wolf ED. Ophthalmic examination and therapeutic techniques in the horse. *Compend Contin Educ* 1981; **3**: S426-S433.

13 Van Der Woerdt A, Gilger BC, Wilkie DA, Strauch SM. Effect of auriculopalpebral nerve block and intravenous administration of xylazine on intraocular pressure and corneal thickness. *Am J Vet Res* 1995; **56**: 155–158.

14 Manning JP, St Clair LE. Palpebral frontal and zygomatic nerve blocks for examination of the equine eye. *Vet Med* 1976; **71**: 187–189.

15 Pollock PJ, Russell T, Hughes TK, *et al.* Transpalpebral eye enucleation in 40 standing horses. *Vet Surg* 2008; **37**: 306–309.

16 Hewes CA, Keoughan GC, Gutierrez-Nibeyro S. Standing enucleation in the horse: a report of 5 cases. *Can Vet J* 2007; **48**: 512–514.

17 Hague BA, Honnas CM, Simpson RB, *et al.* Evaluation of skin bacterial flora before and after aseptic preparation of clipped and nonclipped arthrocentesis sites in horses. *Vet Surg* 1997; **26**: 121–125.

18 Wahl K, Adams SB, Moore GE. Contamination of joints with tissue debris and hair after arthrocentesis: the effect of needle insertion angle, spinal needle gauge, and insertion of spinal needles with and without a stylet. *Vet Surg* 2012; **41**: 391–398.

19 Buchner HH, Kübber P, Zohmann E, *et al.* Sedation and antisedation as tools in equine lameness examination. *Equine Vet J* 1999; (Suppl 30): 227–230.

20 Park J, Sutradhar BC, Hong G, *et al.* Comparison of the cytotoxic effects of bupivacaine, lidocaine, and mepivacaine in equine articular chondrocytes. *Vet Anesth Analg* 2011; **38**: 127–133.

21 Kearney CM, van Weeren PR, Cornelissen BP, *et al.* Which anatomical region determines a positive flexion test of the distal aspect of a forelimb in a nonlame horse? *Equine Vet J* 2010; **42**: 547–551.

22 Schumacher J, Livesey L, DeGraves FJ, *et al.* Effect of anaesthesia of the palmar digital nerves on proximal interphalangeal joint pain in the horse. *Equine Vet J* 2004; **36**: 409–414.

23 Schumacher J, Steiger R, Schumacher J, *et al.* Effects of analgesia of the distal interphalangeal joint or palmar digital nerves on lameness caused by solar pain in horses. *Vet Surg* 2000; **29**: 54–58.

24 Easter JL, Watkins JP, Stephens SL, *et al.* Effects of regional anesthesia on experimentally induced coffin joint synovitis. *Proc Annu Conv Am Assoc Equine Pract* 2000; **46**: 214–216.

25 Bidwell LA, Brown KE, Cordier A, *et al.* Mepivacaine local anaesthetic duration in equine palmar digital nerve blocks. *Equine Vet J* 2004; **36**: 723–726.

26 Keegan KG, Wilson DJ, Wilson DA, *et al.* Effects of anesthesia of the palmar digital nerves on kinematic gait analysis in horses with and without navicular disease. *Am J Vet Res* 1997; **58**: 218–223.

27 Nagy A, Bodo G, Dyson SJ, *et al.* Diffusion of contrast medium after perineural injection of the palmar nerves: an *in vivo* and *in vitro* study. *Equine Vet J* 2009; **41**: 379–383.

28 Seabaugh KA, Selberg KT, Valdes-Martinez A, *et al.* Assessment of the tissue diffusion of anesthetic agent following administration of a low palmar nerve block in horses. *J Am Vet Med Assoc* 2011; **239**: 1334–1340.

29 Nagy A, Bodo G, Dyson SJ, *et al.* Distribution of radiodense contrast medium after perineural injection of the palmar and palmar metacarpal nerves (low 4-point nerve block): an *in vivo* and *ex vivo* study in horses. *Equine Vet J* 2010; **42**: 512–518.

30 Nagy A, Bodo G, Dyson SJ. Diffusion of contrast medium after four different techniques for analgesia of the proximal metacarpal region: an *in vivo* and *in vitro* study. *Equine Vet J* 2012; **44**: 668–673.

31 Zekas LJ, Forrest LJ. Effect of perineural anesthesia on the ultrasonographic appearance of equine palmar metacarpal structures. *Vet Radiol Ultrasound* 2003; **44**: 59–64.

32 Castro FA, Schumacher JS, Pauwels F, Blackford JT. A new approach for perineural injection of the lateral palmar nerve in the horse. *Vet Surg* 2005; **34**: 539–542.

33 Hughes TK, Eliashar E, Smith RK. *In vitro* evaluation of a single injection technique for diagnostic analgesia of the proximal suspensory ligament of the equine pelvic limb. *Vet Surg* 2007; **36**: 760–764.

34 Gayle GM, Redding WR. Comparison of diagnostic anaesthetic techniques of the proximal plantar metatarsus in the horse. *Equine Vet Educ* 2007; **19**: 222–224.

35 Schramme MC, Boswell JC, Hamhougias K, *et al.* An *in vitro* study to compare 5 different techniques for injection of the navicular bursa in the horse. *Equine Vet J* 2000; **32**: 263–267.

36 Piccot-Crézollet C, Cauvin ER, Lepage OM. Comparison of two techniques for injection of the podotrochlear bursa in horses. *J Am Vet Med Assoc* 2005; **226**: 1524–1528.

37 Dyson SJ, Kidd L. A comparison of responses to analgesia of the navicular bursa and intra-articular analgesia of the distal interphalangeal joint in 59 horses. *Equine Vet J* 1992; **25**: 93–98.

38 Schumacher J, Schumacher J, Gillette R, *et al.* The effects of local anaesthetic solution in the navicular bursa of horses with lameness caused by distal interphalangeal joint pain. *Equine Vet J* 2003; **35**: 502–505.

39 Gough MR, Mayhew G, Munroe GA. Diffusion of mepivacaine between adjacent synovial structures in the horse. Part 1: forelimb foot and carpus. *Equine Vet J* 2002; **34**: 80–84.

40 Schumacher J, Schumacher J, DeGraves F. A comparison of the effects of local analgesic solution in the navicular bursa of horses with lameness caused by solar toe or solar heel pain. *Equine Vet J* 2001; **33**: 386–389.

41 Schumacher J, Schumacher J, DeGraves F, *et al.* A comparison of the effects of two volumes of local analgesic solution in the distal interphalangeal joint of horses with lameness caused by solar toe or solar heel pain. *Equine Vet J* 2001; **33**: 265–268.

42 Hassel DM, Stover SM, Yarbrough TB, *et al.* Palmar-plantar axial sesamoidean approach to the digital flexor tendon sheath in horses. *J Am Vet Med Assoc* 2000; **217**: 1343–1347.

43 Harper J, Schumacher J, DeGraves F, *et al.* Effects of analgesia of the digital flexor tendon sheath on pain originating in the sole, distal interphalangeal joint, or navicular bursa of horses. *Equine Vet J* 2007; **39**: 535–539.

44 Lewis RD. Techniques for arthrocentesis of the equine shoulder, elbow, stifle and hip joints. *Proc Annu Conv Am Assoc Equine Pract* 1996; **42**: 55–63.

45 Schumacher J, Livesey L, Brawner W, *et al.* Comparison of 2 methods of centesis of the bursa of the biceps brachii tendon of horses. *Equine Vet J* 2007; **39**: 356–359.

46 Schneeweiss W, Puggioni A, David F. Comparison of ultrasound-guided vs. 'blind' techniques for intra-synovial injections of the shoulder area in horses: scapulohumeral joint, bicipital and infraspinatus bursae. *Equine Vet J* 2012; **44**: 674–678.

47 Bell BT, Baker GJ, Foreman JH, Abbott LC. In vivo investigation of communication between the distal intertarsal and tarsometatarsal joints in horses and ponies. *Vet Surg* 1993; **22**: 289–292.

48 Dyson SJ, Romero JM. An investigation of techniques for local analgesia of the equine distal tarsus and proximal metatarsus. *Equine Vet J* 1993; **25**: 30–35.

49 Kraus-Hansen AE, Jann HW, Kerr DV, *et al.* Arthrographic analysis of communication between the tarsometatarsal and distal intertarsal joints of the horse. *Vet Surg* 1992; **21**: 139–144.

50 Sack WO, Orsini PG. Distal intertarsal and tarsometatarsal joints in the horse: communication and injection sites. *J Am Vet Med Assoc* 1981; **179**: 355–359.

51 Post EM, Singer ER, Clegg PD. An anatomic study of the calcaneal bursae in the horse. *Vet Surg* 2007; **36**: 3–9.

52 Vacek JR, Ford TS, Honnas CM. Communication between the femoropatellar and medial and lateral femorotibial joints in horses. *Am J Vet Res* 1992; **53**: 1431–1434.

53 Reeves MJ, Trotter GW, Kainer RA. Anatomical and functional communications between the synovial sacs of the equine stifle joint. *Equine Vet J* 1991; **23**: 215–218.

54 Gough MR, Munroe GA, Mayhew G. Diffusion of mepivacaine between adjacent synovial structures in the horse. Part 2: tarsus and stifle. *Equine Vet J* 2002; **34**: 85–90.

55 Hendrickson DA, Nixon AJ. A lateral approach for synovial fluid aspiration and joint injection of the femoropatellar joint of the horse. *Equine Vet J* 1992; **24**: 397–398.

56 Hendrickson DA, Nixon AJ. Comparison of the cranial and a new lateral approach to the femoropatellar joint for aspiration and injection in horses. *J Am Vet Med Assoc* 1994; **205**: 1177–1179.

57 Swiderski CE, Cooke E, Linford R. How to inject the medial femorotibial joint: an alternate approach. *Proc Annu Conv Am Assoc Equine Pract* 2005; **51**: 476–480.

58 Schumacher J, Schumacher J, Wilhite R. Comparison of four techniques of arthrocentesis of the lateral compartment of the femorotibial joint of the horse. *Equine Vet J* 2012; **44**: 664–667.

59 David F, Rougier M, Alexander K, *et al.* Ultrasound-guided coxofemoral arthrocentesis in horses. *Equine Vet J* 2007; **39**: 79–83.

60 Toth F, Schumacher J, Scramme M, Hecht S. Evaluation of four techniques for injecting the trochanteric bursa of horses. *Vet Surg* 2011; **40**: 489–493.

61 Skarda RT, Tranquilli WJ. Local and regional anesthetic and analgesic techniques: horses. In: Tranquilli WJ, Thurmon JC, Grimm KA, eds. *Lumb and Jones' Veterinary Anesthesia and Analgesia*, 4th edn. Ames, IA: Blackwell Publishing, 2007; 605–642.

62 Heavner JE. Local anesthetics. *Vet Clin North Am Large Anim Pract* 1991; **3**: 209–211.

63 Moon PF, Suter CM. Paravertebral thoracolumbar anaesthesia in 10 horses. *Equine Vet J* 1993; **25**: 304–308.

64 Haga HA, Lykkjen S, Revold T, Ranheim B. Effect of intratesticular injection of lidocaine on cardiovascular responses to castration in isoflurane anesthetized stallions. *Am J Vet Res* 2006; **67**: 403–408.

65 Portier KG, Jaillardon L, Leece EA, Walsh CM. Castration of horses under total intravenous anaesthesia: analgesic effects of lidocaine. *Vet Anaesth Analg* 2009; **36**: 173–179.

66 Joyce J, Hendrickson DA. Comparison of intraoperative pain responses following intratesticular or mesorchial injection of lidocaine in standing horses undergoing laparoscopic cryptorchidectomy. *J Am Vet Med Assoc* 2006; **229**: 1779–1783.

67 Magda JJ. Local anesthesia in operations on the male perineum in horses. *Veterinariya* 1948; **25**: 34–36.

68 Erkert RS, MacAllister CG, Campbell G, *et al.* Comparison of topical lidocaine/prilocaine anesthetic cream and local infiltration of 2% lidocaine for episioplasty in mares. *J Vet Pharmacol Ther* 2005; **28**: 299–304.

69 Doherty TJ, Geiser DR, Rohrbach BW. Effect of high volume epidural morphine, ketamine and butorphanol on halothane minimum alveolar concentration in ponies. *Equine Vet J* 1997; **29**: 370–373.

70 Doherty TJ, Geiser DR, Rohrbach BW. The effect of epidural xylazine on halothane minimum alveolar concentration in ponies. *J Vet Pharmacol Ther* 1997; **20**: 246–248.

71 Skarda RT, Muir WW. Segemental thoracolumbar spinal (subarachnoid) analgesia in conscious horses. *Am J Vet Res* 1982; **43**: 2121–2128.

72 Greene SA, Thurmon JC. Epidural anesthesia and sedation for selected equine surgeries. *Equine Pract* 1985; **7**: 14–19.

73 Lechner TJ, van Wijk MG, Maas AJ, *et al.* Clinical results with the acoustic puncture assist device, a new acoustic device to identify the epidural space. *Anesthes Analg* 2004; **96**: 1183–1187.

74 Iff I, Mosing M, Lechner T, Moens Y. The use of an acoustic device to identify the extradural space in standing horses. *Vet Anesth Analg* 2010; **37**: 57–62.

75 Martin CA, Kerr CL, Pearce SG, *et al.* Outcome of epidural catheterization for delivery of analgesics in horses: 43 cases (1998–2001). *J Am Vet Med Assoc* 2003; **222**: 1394–1398.

76 Sysel AM, Pleasant RS, Jacobson JD, *et al.* Systemic and local effects associated with long-term epidural catheterization and morphine-detomidine administration in horses. *Vet Surg* 1997; **26**: 141–149.

77 Skarda RT, Muir WW. Segmental and subarachnoid analgesia in conscious horses: a comparative study. *Am J Vet Res* 1983; **44**: 1870–1876.

78 Grubb TL, Riebold TW, Huber MJ. Comparison of lidocaine xylazine, and xylazine/lidocaine for caudal epidural analgesia in horses. *J Am Vet Med Assoc* 1992; **201**: 1187–1190.

79 Skarda RT, Muir WW, Ibrahim AL. Plasma mepivacaine concentrations after caudal epidural and subarachnoid injection in the horse: comparative study. *Am J Vet Res* 1984; **45**: 1967–1971.

80 DeRossi R, Breno FB, Varela JV, Junquieria AL. Perineal analgesia and hemodynamic effects of the epidural administration of meperidine or hyperbaric bupivacaine in conscious horses. *Can Vet J* 2004; **45**: 42–47.

81 Ganidalgi S, Cetin H, Biricik HS, Cimtay I. Comparison of ropivacaine with a combination of ropivacaine and fentanyl for the caudal epidural anaesthesia of mares. *Vet Rec* 2004; **154**: 329–332.

82 Skarda RT, Muir WW. Analgesic, hemodynamic and respiratory effects of caudally epidurally administered ropivacaine hydrochloride in mares. *Vet Anesth Analg* 2001; **28**: 61–74.

83 van Loon JPAM, Menke ES, Doornebal A, *et al.* Antinociceptive effects of low dose lumbosacral epidural ropivacaine in healthy ponies. *Vet J* 2012; **193**: 240–245.

84 Skarda RT, Muir WW. Influence of atipamezole on effects of midsacral subarachnoidally administered detomidine in mares. *Am J Vet Res* 1998; **59**: 468–478.

85 Skarda RT, Muir WW. Effects of intravenously administered yohimbine on antinociceptive, cardiorespiratory, and postural changes changes induced by epidural adminstration of detomidine hydrochloride solution in healthy mares. *Am J Vet Res* 1999; **60**: 1262–1270.

86 LeBlanc PH, Caron JP, Patterson JS, *et al.* Epidural injection of xylazine for perineal analgesia in horses. *J Am Vet Med Assoc* 1988; **193**: 1405–1408.

87 Skarda RT, Muir WW. Analgesic, hemodynamic and respiratory effects of caudally epidurally administered xylazine hydrochloride solution in mares. *Am J Vet Res* 1996; **57**: 193–200.

88 Teixeria Neto FJ, McDonell W, Pearce S, *et al.* Evaluation of anesthesia maintained with halothane and epidural xylazine for hind limb surgery in horses. *Vet Anaesth Analg* 2001; **28**: 107.

89 Skarda RT, Muir WW. Comparison of antinociceptive, cardiovascular, and respiratory effects, head ptosis, and position of pelvic limbs in mares after caudal epidural administration of xylazine and detomidine hydrochloride solution. *Am J Vet Res* 1996; **57**: 1338–1345.

90 Skarda RT, Muir WW. Caudal analgesia induced by epidural or subarachnoid administration of detomidine hydrochloride solution in mares. *Am J Vet Res* 1994: **55**: 670–680.

91 Kariman A, Ghamsari SM, Mokhber-Dezfooli MR. Evaluation of analgesia induced by epidural administration of medetomdine in horses. *J Fac Vet Med Tehran Univ* 2001; **56**: 49–51.

92 Kariman A. Cardiorespiratory and analgesic effects of epidurally administered romifidine in the horse [Abstract]. In: *Proceedings of the Seventh World Congress on Veterinary Anaesthesiology*, University of Bern, Bern, Switzerland, 2000; **55**.

93 Valverde A, Little CB, Dyson DH, Motter CH. Use of epidural morphine to relieve pain in a horse. *Can Vet J* 1990: **31**: 211–212.

94 Natalini CC, Robinson EP. Evaluation of the effects of epidurally administered morphine, alfentanil, butorphanol, tramadol and U50488H in horses. *Am J Vet Res* 2000; **61**: 1579–1586.

95 Freitas GC, Carregaro AB, Gehrcke MI, *et al.* Epidural analgesia with morphine or buprenorphine in ponies with lipopolysaccharide (LPS)-induced carpal synovitis. *Can J Vet Res* 2011; **75**: 141–146.

96 van Loon JPAM, Menke ES, L'Ami J, *et al.* Analgesic and anti-hyperalgesic effects of epidural morphine in an equine LPS-induced acute synovitis model. *Vet J* 2012; **193**: 464–470.

97 Van Hoogmoed LM, Galuppo LD. Laparoscopic ovariectomy using the endo-GIA stapling device and endo-catch pouches and evaluation of analgesic efficacy of epidural morphine sulfate in 10 mares. *Vet Surg* 2005; **34**: 646–650.

98 Sano H, Martin-Flores M, Santos LCP, *et al.* Effects of epidural morphine on gastrointestinal transit in unmedicated horses. *Vet Anaesth Analg* 2011; **38**: 121–126.

99 Natalini CC, Linardi RL. Analgesic effecs of epidural administration of hydromorphone in horses. *Am J Vet Res* 2006; **67**: 11–15.

100 Olbrich VH, Mosing M. A comparison of the analgesic effects of caudal epidural methadone and lidocaine in the horse. *Vet Anaesth Analg* 2003; **30**: 156–164.

101 van Loon JPAM, van Oostrom H, Doornenbal A, Hellebrekers LJ. Lumbosacral spinal cord somatosensory evoked potentials for quantification of nociception in horses. *Equine Vet J.* 2010; **42**: 255–260.

102 Skarda RT, Muir WW. Analgesic, hemodynamic and respiratory effects induced by caudally epidurally administered meperidine hydrochloride in mares. *Am J Vet Res* 2001; **62**: 1001–1007.

103 DeRossi R, Medeiros U, de Almeida RG, *et al.* Meperidine prolongs lidocaine caudal epidural anaesthesia in the horse. *Vet J* 2008; **178**: 294–297.

104 Gomez de Segura IA, DeRossi R, Lopez San-Roman J, *et al.* Epidural injection of ketamine for perineal analgesia in the horse. *Vet Surg* 1998; **27**: 384–391.

105 Giorgi M, Saccomanni G, Andreoni V. Pharmacokinetics of tramadol after epidural administration in horses. *J Equine Vet Sci* 2010; **30**: 44–46.

106 Natalini CC, Alves SD, Guedes AG, *et al.* Epidural administration of tiletamine/zolazepam in horses. *Vet Anesth Analg* 2004; **31**: 79–85.

107 Chopin JB, Wright JD. Complication after the use of a combination of lignocaine and xylazine for epidural anesthesia in a mare. *Aust Vet J* 1995; **72**: 354–355.

108 Sysel AM, Pleasant RS, Jacobson JD, *et al.* Efficacy of an epidural combination of morphine and detomidine in alleviating experimentally induced hindlimb lameness in horses. *Vet Surg* 1996; **25**: 511–518.

109 Goodrich LR, Nixon AJ, Fubini SL, *et al.* Epidural morphine and detomidine decreases postoperative hindlimb lameness in horses after bilateral stifle arthroscopy. *Vet Surg* 2002; **31**: 232–239.

110 Fischer BL, Ludders JW, Asakawa M, *et al.* A comparison of epidural buprenorphine plus detomidine with morphine plus detomidine in horses undergoing bilateral stifle arthroscopy. *Vet Anesth Analg* 2009; **36**: 67–76.

111 Natalini CC, Alves SD, Polydoro AS, *et al.* Epidural administration of morphine combined with romifidine in horses [Abstract]. In: *Proceedings of the Eighth World Congress of Veterinary Anesthesiologists*, University of Tennessee, Knoxville, TN, 2003; 168.

112 DeRossi R, Modolo TJC, Maciel FB, Pagliosa RC. Efficacy of epidural lidocaine combined with tramadol or neostigmine on perineal analgesia in the horse. *Equine Vet J* 2013; **45**: 497–502.

113 DeRossi R, Maciel FB, Modolo TJC, Pagliosa RC. Efficacy of concurrent epidural administration of neostigmine and lidocaine for perineal analgesia in geldings. *Am J Vet Res* 2012; **73**: 1356–1362.

114 Kariman A, Nowrouzian I, Bakhtiari J. Caudal epidural injection of a combination of ketamine and xylazine for perineal analgesia in horses [Abstract]. *Vet Anaesth Analg* 2000; **27**: 115.

115 DeRossi R, Modolo TJC, Pagliosa RC, *et al.* Comparison of analgesic effects of caudal epidural 0.25% bupivacaine with bupivacaine plus morphine or bupivacaine plus ketamine for analgesia in conscious horses. *J Equine Vet Sci* 2012; **32**: 190–195.

116 Haitjema H, Gibson KT. Severe pruritis associated with epidural morphine and detomidine in a horse. *Aust Vet J* 2001; **79**: 248–250.

117 Kalchofner KS, Kummer M, Price J, Bettschart-Wolfensberger R. Pruritis in two horses following epidurally administered morphine. *Equine Vet Educ* 2001; **19**: 590–594.

118 Burford JH, Corley KT. Morphine-associated pruritis after single extradural administration in a horse. *Vet Anaesth Analg* 2001; **33**: 193–198.

119 Sheehy JG, Hellyer PW, Sammonds GE, *et al.* Evaluation of opioid receptors in synovial membranes of horses. *Am J Vet Res* 2001; **62**: 1408–1412.

120 van Loon JPAM, de Grauw JC, Brunott A, *et al.* Upregulation of articular synovial membrane μ-opioid-like receptors in an acute equine synovitis model. *Vet J* 2013; **196**: 40–46.

121 van Loon JPAM, de Grauw JC, van Dierendonck M, *et al.* Intra-articular opioid analgesia is effective in reducing pain and inflammation in an equine LPS induced synovitis model. *Equine Vet J* 2010; **42**: 412–419.

122 Santos LCP, de Moraes AN, Saito ME. Effects of intraarticular ropivacaine and morphine on lipopolysaccharide-induced synovitis in horses. *Vet Anaesth Analg* 2009; **36**: 280–286.

123 Lopez-Sanroman FJ, Cruz JM, Santos M, *et al.* Evaluation of the local analgesic effect of ketamine in the palmar digital nerve block at the base of the proximal sesamoid (abaxial sesamoid block) in horses. *Am J Vet Res* 2003; **64**: 475–478.

124 Lopez-Sanroman FJ, Cruz JM, Santos M, *et al.* Effect of alkalinization on the local analgesic efficacy of ketamine in the abaxial sesamoid nerve block in horses. *J Vet Pharmacol Ther* 2003; **26**: 265–269.

125 Andreoni V, Giorgi M, Chem D. Evaluation of plasma detectable concentrations of two lidocaine transdermal formulations and their analgesic effect in the horse. *J Equine Vet Sci* 2009; **29**: 681–686.

126 Bidwell LA, Wilson DV, Caron JP. Lack of systemic absorption of lidocaine from 5% patches placed on horses. *Vet Anaesth Analg* 2007; **34**: 443–446.

127 Frisbie DD, McIlwraith CW, Kawcak CE, *et al.* Evaluation of topically administered diclofenac liposomal cream for treatment of horses with experimentally induced osteoarthritis. *Am J Vet Res* 2009; **70**: 210–215.

128 Levine DG, Epstein KL, Neelis DA, Ross MW. Effect of topical application of 1% diclofenac sodium liposomal cream on inflammation in healthy horses undergoing intravenous regional limb perfusion with amikacin sulfate. *Am J Vet Res* 2009; **70**: 1323–1325.

129 Lynn RC, Hepler DI, Keich WJ, *et al.* Double-blinded placebo-controlled clinical field trial to evaluate the safety and efficacy of topically applied 1% diclofenac liposomal cream for the relief of lameness in the horse. *Vet Ther* 2004; **5**: 128–138.

130 Villarino NF, Vispo TJ, Marcos F, Landoni MF. Inefficacy of topical diclofenac in arthritic horses. *Am J Anim Vet Sci* 2006; **1**: 8–12.

131 Ferrante M, Andreeta A, Landoni MF. Effect of different penetration enhancers on diclofenac permeation across horse skin. *Vet J* 2010; **186**: 312–315.

132 Driessen B, Scandella M, Zarucco L. Development of a technique for continuous perineural blockade of the palmar nerves in the distal equine thoracic limb. *Vet Anaesth Analg* 2008; **35**: 432–448.

133 Watts AE, Nixon AJ, Reesink HL, *et al.* Continuous peripheral neural blockade to alleviate signs of experimentally induced severe forelimb pain in horses. *J Am Vet Med Assoc* 2011; **238**: 1032–1039.

49 Ruminants

Thomas W. Riebold
Veterinary Teaching Hospital, College of Veterinary Medicine, Oregon State University, Corvallis, Oregon, USA

Chapter contents

Introduction

As in other species, sedation and anesthesia are often required for surgical or diagnostic procedures in ruminants. The decision to induce general anesthesia may be influenced by a ruminant's temperament and its specific anatomic and physiologic characteristics. Ruminants usually accept physical restraint well and that, in conjunction with local or regional anesthesia, is often sufficient to enable completion of many procedures. Other diagnostic and surgical procedures that are more complex require general anesthesia.

In addition to discussing techniques for cattle, goats, and sheep, anesthetic techniques for South American camelids, primarily llamas and alpacas, are discussed. South American camelids do not accept restraint as well as domestic ruminants and often require sedation before local or regional anesthesia. Although they have some unique species characteristics regarding anesthesia, many of the principles and techniques used in food animal and equine anesthesia also apply to South American camelids. Except for differences in size and that alpacas can require approximately 10% greater doses of sedatives, anesthetic management of alpacas and llamas is similar.

Preanesthetic preparation

Considerations for preanesthetic preparation include fasting, assessment of hematologic and blood chemistry values, venous catheterization, and estimation of body weight. Domestic ruminants have a multicompartment stomach with a large rumen that does not empty completely. South American camelids have a stomach divided into three compartments [1]. Each species, therefore, is susceptible to complications associated with recumbency and anesthesia: tympany, regurgitation, and aspiration pneumonia. To reduce the risks associated with these potential complications, calves, sheep, goats, and camelids should be fasted for 12–18 h and deprived of water for 8–12 h prior to anesthesia. Adult cattle should be fasted for 18–24 h and deprived of water for 12–18 h. In non-elective cases, this is often not possible, and precautions should be taken to avoid aspiration of gastric fluid and ingesta. Fasting of neonates is not advisable because hypoglycemia may result. Fasting and water deprivation will decrease the likelihood of tympany and regurgitation by decreasing the volume of fermentable ingesta. Fasting is also associated with bradycardia in cattle [2]. Additionally, pulmonary functional residual capacity may be better preserved in fasted anesthetized ruminants [3]. Although gas does not appear to accumulate in the first compartment of anesthetized camelids, these precautions are recommended to decrease the incidence of regurgitation. Even with these precautions, some ruminants will become tympanitic, and others will regurgitate.

Hematologic and blood chemistry values may be determined before anesthesia and the results should be compared with reference values [4–7]. Venipuncture and catheterization of the jugular

Veterinary Anesthesia and Analgesia: The Fifth Edition of Lumb and Jones.
Edited by Kurt A. Grimm, Leigh A. Lamont, William J. Tranquilli, Stephen A. Greene and Sheilah A. Robertson.

vein are often performed prior to anesthesia. Adult cattle require 12–14-gauge (G) catheters, whereas 16 G catheters are appropriate for adult camelids, calves, and large goats and sheep, and 18 G catheters are appropriate for juvenile camelids, sheep, and goats. Physical restraint during venipuncture or catheterization varies and can consist of a handler holding the animal's halter or use of head gates and chutes for adult cattle and llamas. If a camelid is fractious, grasping its ear may be helpful. Turning the animal's head excessively to either side may hinder venipuncture and catheter placement in goats and camelids and may increase the likelihood of carotid arterial puncture in camelids. Infiltration of local anesthetic at the site of catheterization is recommended.

Camelids do not have a jugular groove. The jugular vein lies deep to the sternomandibularis and brachiocephalicus muscles, ventral to cervical vertebral transverse processes and superficial to the carotid artery and vagosympathetic trunk within the carotid sheath for most of its length [8–10]. Beginning at a point about 15 cm caudal to the ramus of the mandible, the rostral course of the jugular vein is separated from the carotid artery by the omohyoideus muscle. The bifurcation of the jugular vein is located at the intersection of a line drawn caudally along the ventral aspect of the body of the mandible and another line connecting the base of the ear and the lateral aspect of the cervical transverse processes. Venipuncture or catheterization can be performed at the bifurcation or at any point caudal to it. Because of the close proximity of the carotid artery to the jugular vein, one must confirm that the vein has been catheterized and not the artery. After occlusion of the vessel, one will be unable to see the jugular vein distend; however, the vein can be palpated particularly rostrally and more easily in females and castrated males because their skin is thinner. On occasion, one will be able to see the jugular vein distend on crias and juvenile camelids. Camelids can have four to five jugular venous valves that prevent flow of venous blood into the head when the head is lowered during grazing [8]. Contact with jugular venous valves may prevent catheterization; a site caudal to the point where the valve was contacted should be used.

For accurate drug administration, body weight must be estimated or determined by weighing the animal. It is easy to overestimate the body weight of camelids because they are fairly tall, and their long haircoat obscures their body condition. Adult male llamas usually weigh 140–175 kg, occasionally reaching or exceeding 200 kg. Adult female llamas usually weigh 100–150 kg but may occasionally exceed 200 kg. Adult male alpacas usually weigh 60–100 kg and adult female alpacas usually weigh 50–80 kg. The body weight of crias and small juveniles may be determined on a bathroom scale.

Anticholinergics are usually not administered to domestic ruminants prior to induction of anesthesia. They do not consistently decrease salivary secretions unless used in high doses and frequently repeated. Anticholinergics, while decreasing the volume of secretions, make them more viscous and more difficult to clear from the trachea. The usual doses of atropine to prevent bradycardia in domestic ruminants, 0.06–0.1 mg/kg intravenously (IV), do not prevent salivation during anesthesia. Camelids are prone to increased vagal discharge during intubation or painful stimuli during surgery. Administration of atropine, 0.02 mg/kg IV or 0.04 mg/kg intramuscularly (IM), is recommended to prevent bradyarrhythmia and will also decrease salivary secretions [11]. Glycopyrrolate, 0.005–0.01 mg/kg IM or 0.002–0.005 mg/kg IV, may be substituted for atropine [12,13].

Sedation/chemical restraint

Drugs used to tranquilize and/or sedate ruminants include acepromazine, α_2-adrenergic receptor agonists (xylazine, detomidine, medetomidine, dexmedetomidine, and romifidine), pentobarbital, chloral hydrate, diazepam, and midazolam.

Acepromazine is the most commonly used phenothiazine derivative tranquilizer in veterinary anesthesia. It is not commonly used in ruminants but can be used in a manner similar to its use in horses, although lower doses are required for cattle than for horses. The usual doses of acepromazine in sheep and goats are 0.03–0.05 mg/kg IV and 0.05–0.1 mg/kg IM, which may increase the risk of regurgitation during anesthesia [14]. Acepromazine should not be injected into the coccygeal vein. The close proximity of the coccygeal artery makes the risk of inadvertent intra-arterial injection possible, with the potential loss of the tail (J.C. Thurmon, personal communication, 1970). Acepromazine can also cause prolapse of the penis and is not recommended in mature bulls prior to general anesthesia. Prolapse of the penis during recovery increases the risk of injury to that organ as the animal stands. Finally, acepromazine is relatively contraindicated in cachexic and/or hypovolemic patients.

Xylazine, detomidine, romifidine, medetomidine, and dexmedetomidine cause sedation by stimulating central α_2-adrenergic receptors. Xylazine is often used to sedate or, in higher doses, restrain ruminants by producing recumbency and light planes of general anesthesia. There appears to be some variation in response between species and within a species. Xylazine is much more potent in ruminants than in horses [15]. Goats appear to be more sensitive to xylazine than are sheep [13,14,16], with cattle appearing to be of intermediate sensitivity when compared with sheep and goats. South American camelids appear to be intermediate between cattle and horses in sensitivity to xylazine, and alpacas appear to be less sensitive to xylazine than are llamas. Hereford cattle are more sensitive to xylazine than are Holstein cattle [17], and anecdotal evidence indicates that Brahmans are perhaps the most sensitive of all cattle breeds [18]. Extreme environmental conditions can cause cattle to have a pronounced and prolonged response to xylazine [19]. Variation in response to the analgesic effects of xylazine between breeds of sheep has been reported [20,21]. Although complete data are not available on the cardiovascular and respiratory effects of xylazine in camelids, bradycardia [22] typically occurs as it does in other species [17,23–25]. Poorly trained or agitated male camelids tend to be less responsive, and debilitated individuals are more responsive to sedative doses of xylazine.

Detomidine has been used to a lesser extent in ruminants and provides sedation and/or analgesia in domestic ruminants not unlike that obtained in horses. Romifidine, medetomidine, and dexmedetomidine have also been used to a lesser extent in ruminants. All of these drugs have similar effects in ruminants and are more potent than xylazine. They can be used when xylazine is unavailable.

Xylazine causes hyperglycemia and hypoinsulinemia in cattle and sheep [26–31]. Hypoxemia and hypercapnia are common side-effects in domestic ruminants [14,17,22,32], and sheep are at risk of developing pulmonary edema [33]. Xylazine has an oxytocin-like effect on the uterus of pregnant cattle [34] and sheep [35]. Interestingly, detomidine may not have the same effect on the gravid uterus as xylazine in cattle [36].

The degree of sedation or restraint produced by α_2-adrenergic receptor agonists depends on the dose and animal temperament. Low doses of xylazine, 0.015–0.025 mg/kg IV or IM, typically provide sedation without recumbency in domestic ruminants [12,13,37]. Higher doses, 0.1–0.2 mg/kg IV, provide sedation without recumbency in camelids [38]. Detomidine can be given at 2.5–10 µg/kg IV in cattle [13,36,37,39,40] and at 10–20 µg/kg in sheep [14] to provide standing sedation for approximately 30–60 min. Medetomidine has been given at a dose of 5 µg/kg IV to cattle [40] or at 10 µg/kg IM to llamas [41] for brief periods of standing sedation with minimal analgesia.

Higher doses of xylazine will induce recumbency, heavy sedation, or possibly light planes of general anesthesia in domestic ruminants and camelids. Xylazine in goats at 0.05 mg/kg IV or 0.1 mg/kg IM [13,14,42], in sheep at 0.1–0.2 mg/kg IV or 0.2–0.3 mg/kg IM [13,14,42], and in cattle at 0.1 mg/kg IV or 0.2 mg/kg IM [18] will induce recumbency for approximately 1 h. Xylazine at 0.3–0.4 mg/kg IV usually induces 20–30 min of recumbency in llamas [8–11,38]. Alpacas may require an increased dose, by approximately 10–20%, to achieve the same result [43]. A high dose of detomidine, 30 µg/kg IV, will produce recumbency in sheep. This dose is equivalent to xylazine at 0.15 mg/kg IV, medetomidine at 10 µg/kg IV, or romifidine at 50 µg/kg IV [44]. In llamas, detomidine in doses as high as 40 µg/kg IV provides mild sedation but not restraint [38]. Romifidine has been used at 40, 80, and 120 µg/kg IV in Old World camels. Profound sedation and bradycardia of 4 h duration occurred with the highest dose [45]. Initially doses of 50–60 µg/kg IV are appropriate for South American camelids. Medetomidine given at 10 µg/kg IV induces recumbency in cattle [40]. When medetomidine is given at 30 µg/kg IV it causes bradycardia, decreased arterial oxygen tension (PaO_2), recumbency of 4 h duration, and sedation of 7 h duration in calves [46]. When given at 20–30 µg/kg IM to llamas, medetomidine provides profound sedation and recumbency lasting up to 120 min [41]. Higher doses of all α_2-adrenergic receptor agonists can be expected to induce longer periods of recumbency in all species. Dexmedetomidine would be substituted for medetomidine at 50% of the medetomidine dose.

Sedation following administration of α_2-adrenergic receptor agonists can be reversed by α_2-adrenergic receptor antagonists. They include atipamezole and yohimbine (specific to α_2-adrenergic receptors) and tolazoline (both α_2- and α_1-adrenergic receptor antagonist action). The dose of antagonist is dependent on the amount of agonist given and the interval between agonist and antagonist administration. The longer the interval between administration of the agonist and antagonist, the lower is the dose of antagonist that is needed as more metabolism of the agonist should have occurred. Giving the full dose of antagonist after significant metabolism of the agonist has occurred increases the likelihood that excitement will result, particularly if the antagonist is given IV. One could also consider giving the antagonist IM to make reversal more gradual.

When yohimbine is given at 0.12 mg/kg IV, its efficacy varies in cattle [47,48]. Low doses of yohimbine are ineffective in sheep [49]. Higher doses of yohimbine, 1 mg/kg IV, will generally reverse xylazine sedation in sheep [50]. Atipamezole at doses varying from 20 to 60 µg/kg IV has been used to reverse medetomidine sedation in calves [13]. Tolazoline is usually given at 0.5–2 mg/kg IV [48], but at 2 mg/kg IV it can cause hyperesthesia in unsedated cattle [51,52] and at doses of 4 mg/kg can cause seizure-like activity and death in llamas [38,53]. Tolazoline can induce unwanted cardiovascular effects such as transient bradycardia, sinus arrest, and hypotension [54]. Idazoxan can be given at doses of 0.05 mg/kg IV to sheep [49] and calves to reverse xylazine sedation [55].

Yohimbine, 0.12 mg/kg IV, has been used in llamas in combination with 4-aminopyridine, 0.3 mg/kg IV, to produce complete recovery from xylazine sedation [22]. Its use singly in camelids is also effective, and it can be administered at 0.12 mg/kg IV [38]. If sufficient arousal does not occur, additional yohimbine can be given. Atipamezole given at 30 µg/kg IV will reverse xylazine sedation in camelids. Tolazoline is effective for reversing xylazine sedation in camelids but caution is advised. When given at the recommended equine dose to camelids, tolazoline can cause severe complications, including transitory apnea, cardiac arrest, seizure-like activity, depression, and vague signs of abdominal pain, followed by death within 24 h. One method of administering tolazoline to healthy camelids is to give 50% of the calculated dose, 1–2 mg/kg IV, initially and the remainder if reversal is inadequate [38]. In most instances, the initial dose, 0.5–1 mg/kg IV, of tolazoline is adequate to provide sufficient arousal. Following tolazoline administration at the full calculated dose of 2 mg/kg IV, opisthotonus can occur in some animals. After excitement subsides, recovery is usually uneventful.

Doxapram, an analeptic, can be used to enhance the response to yohimbine or tolazoline. Doxapram, 1 mg/kg IV, has been somewhat effective in cattle [56] but is ineffective in llamas at 2 mg/kg IV [22]. For more information about doxapram, the reader is referred to Chapter 13.

Pentobarbital, 2 mg/kg IV, has been used in cattle for standing sedation and tranquilization [57]. Caution must be exercised to avoid inducing excitement. Pentobarbital provides moderate sedation for 30 min and mild sedation for an additional 60 min. Chloral hydrate or chloral hydrate–magnesium sulfate solutions can also be used to sedate ruminants [18]. These drugs must be injected slowly IV to avoid tissue necrosis. Diazepam, 0.25–0.5 mg/kg IV, injected slowly will provide 30 min of sedation without analgesia in sheep and goats [14,42]. Midazolam, 0.4–0.6 mg IM [58,59] or 0.3 mg/kg IV [60], will provide sedation and recumbency in sheep and goats for 10–20 min. Midazolam given at 1 mg/kg IM [58] or 0.6 mg/kg IV [60] can induce recumbency and profound sedation in goats. Increasing the dose to 1.2 mg/kg IV lengthens recumbency, lasting up to 30 min [59]. Midazolam given at 0.5 mg/kg IM to alpacas provides sedation without recumbency of approximately 100 min duration [61]. When given at 0.5 mg/kg IV to alpacas, midazolam provides sedation with recumbency of approximately 100 min duration [61].

Butorphanol is an opioid agonist–antagonist that provides sedation and analgesia in camelids and domestic ruminants. It is often given at 0.05–0.5 mg/kg IM in sheep and goats [14,62,63] and at 0.1–0.2 mg/kg IM in camelids [64]. Ataxia and dysphoria have been reported following butorphanol administration, 0.1–0.2 mg/kg IV, in sheep [63]. Camelids remain standing following butorphanol administration but may experience mild dysphoria.

Combinations of xylazine and butorphanol have been used in camelids and domestic ruminants to provide neuroleptanalgesia. Doses are 0.01–0.02 mg/kg IV of each drug administered separately to domestic ruminants (J.C. Thurmon, personal communication, 1993) and 0.2 mg/kg IV of xylazine with 0.02–0.04 mg/kg IV of butorphanol to camelids (M.J. Huber, personal communication, 2013). Action lasts approximately 1 h. Combinations of midazolam, 0.1 mg IV, and butorphanol, 0.1 mg/kg IV, simultaneously provide restraint of short duration [65].

Combinations of butorphanol, ketamine, and xylazine have also been used to restrain camelids [65]. The combination is prepared by combining 10 mg (1 mL) of butorphanol, 1000 mg (10 mL) of ketamine, and 100 mg (1 mL) of xylazine. It is administered at 1 mL/18 kg IM to alpacas and at 1 mL/23 kg IM to llamas [65]. Recumbency occurs within 5 min and lasts approximately 25 min. Other combinations of xylazine, ketamine, and butorphanol ('Ketamine Stun') have also been used in ruminants [37] and camelids [65]. Ruminant doses for the IV route of administration are xylazine at 0.025–0.05 mg/kg, ketamine at 0.3–0.5 mg/kg, and butorphanol at 0.05–0.1 mg/kg [37]. Animals will become recumbent for 15–25 min and administration of an additional partial dose of ketamine (50% of the original dose) will lengthen the duration of analgesia. If IV access is not feasible, the upper end of the doses cited above can also be administered IM or subcutaneously (SC) to achieve a longer but less intense form of chemical restraint. Alternatively, a combination of xylazine at 0.05 mg/kg, butorphanol at 0.025 mg/kg, and ketamine at 0.1 mg/kg can also be given IM to render ruminant patients more cooperative [37]. Onset occurs within 10 min, and duration of action is approximately 45 min with an additional 30 min needed to resume standing. Given IV, the combination of xylazine at 0.22–0.33 mg/kg, ketamine at 0.22–0.33 mg/kg, and butorphanol at 0.08–0.11 mg/kg induces more predictable restraint in camelids [65]. Animals will become recumbent and analgesia lasts for 15–20 min. Administration of an additional partial dose of ketamine will lengthen the duration of analgesia. When given IM to camelids, the dose range is increased to xylazine at 0.22–0.55 mg/kg, ketamine at 0.22–0.55 mg/kg, and butorphanol at 0.08–0.11 mg/kg [65]. Onset occurs within 10 min and duration of action is extended to approximately 45 min.

Induction

Ruminants do not require sedation prior to induction of anesthesia as other species do. Atraumatic physical restraint can be used in lieu of sedatives in some circumstances. Because ruminants seldom experience emergence delirium, sedation during the recovery period is not required as it is in the horse. In some instances, however, sedation is required to make handling of these animals, primarily fractious adult cattle, safer during the induction period. Sedation will tend to lengthen the recovery period from general anesthesia [39], increase the likelihood of regurgitation [14], and decrease anesthetic agent requirements.

General anesthesia can be induced by either injectable or inhalation techniques. Widely available drugs include ketamine, guaifenesin, tiletamine–zolazepam, propofol, alfaxalone, pentobarbital, isoflurane, and sevoflurane. If available, the thiobarbiturates and halothane could also be used. Anesthesia can be induced in small ruminants, weighing less than 50–100 kg, either by mask with isoflurane or sevoflurane or with injectable techniques. Anesthesia can be induced in larger animals with either IV or, if the animal's temperament dictates it, IM techniques. Anesthesia can be induced with isoflurane, or sevoflurane by face mask in small or debilitated camelids or in camelids restrained with xylazine–ketamine, tiletamine–zolazepam, etc. Mask induction in healthy untranquilized adult camelids is usually not attempted because application of the mask may provoke spitting. Addition of nitrous oxide (50% of total flow) to the inspired gas mixture will speed induction. However, administration of nitrous oxide to ruminants and camelids may cause distension of gas-containing organs, resulting in tympany.

Barbiturates/thiobarbiturates

When available, the thiobarbiturates thiopental and thiamylal were used extensively in veterinary anesthesia, both alone and in combination with guaifenesin. Used alone, they quickly induce anesthesia. Muscle relaxation is relatively poor but still sufficient to accomplish intubation. The acid–base status and physical status of patients affect the actions of these drugs. Acidemia increases the non-ionized fraction (i.e., the active portion) of the drug, increasing its activity and thus decreasing the dose required [66]. In addition, the heart, brain, and other vital organs receive a larger portion of cardiac output when patients are in shock [67]. Because patients in shock are often acidemic, altered pharmacokinetics and hemodynamics may cause a relative overdose.

Recovery from induction doses of thiobarbiturates is based on redistribution of the drug from the brain to other tissues in the body. Metabolism of the agent continues for some time following recovery until final elimination occurs. Maintenance of anesthesia with thiobarbiturates is not recommended because saturation of tissues causes recovery to be dependent on metabolism and recovery will be prolonged. Concurrent use of non-steroidal anti-inflammatory drugs (NSAIDs) may delay recovery as thiobarbiturate is displaced from protein [68], but the clinical significance of this drug interaction appears to be minimal.

Thiopental can be given at 6–10 mg/kg IV to unsedated animals and will provide approximately 10–15 min of anesthesia. Camelids often require additional thiopental for tracheal intubation [11]. Thiamylal is administered in a similar fashion although in slightly lower doses, usually 25–30% less.

Pentobarbital has been used to anesthetize domestic ruminants but is no longer commonly used. If a situation arises in which it is used, the dose is 20–25 mg/kg IV, half given rapidly and the remainder to effect. When given at an anesthetic dose, pentobarbital causes profound respiratory depression and is not an effective analgesic. Sheep appear to metabolize pentobarbital more quickly than other species [14]. Recovery in domestic ruminants is usually prolonged, and other anesthetic techniques are more appropriate.

Ketamine

Ketamine is a very versatile drug that has been used in many species. It is an *N*-methyl-D-aspartate receptor antagonist. It causes dysphoria, hallucinations, and excitement, in addition to tonic–clonic muscle activity when used alone in horses. Those same traits characterize its use in ruminants, although perhaps not to the same extent as in horses. It also provides mild cardiovascular stimulation. Although ketamine does not eliminate the swallowing reflex, tracheal intubation can be accomplished in most ruminants.

Ketamine will induce immobilization and incomplete analgesia when given alone, but it is usually combined with a sedative or tranquilizer. Most commonly, xylazine or a benzodiazepine is recommended. Xylazine at 0.1–0.2 mg/kg IM can be given first, followed by ketamine at 10–15 mg/kg IM in small domestic ruminants [14,42,69]. In goats, it is preferable to use the lower dose of xylazine followed by ketamine [14,42]. Anesthesia usually lasts about 45 min and can be prolonged by injection of 3–5 mg/kg IM or 1–2 mg/kg IV of ketamine. The longer duration of action of xylazine obviates the need for its readministration in most cases. Alternatively, xylazine at 0.03–0.05 mg/kg IV followed by ketamine at 3–5 mg/kg IV, or xylazine at 0.1 mg/kg in goats or 0.2 mg/kg in sheep IM followed by ketamine at 3–5 mg/kg IV, can provide anesthesia lasting 15–20 min [14]. Adult cattle can by anesthetized with xylazine at 0.1–0.2 mg/kg IV followed by ketamine at 2 mg/kg IV [70]. The lower dose of xylazine is used when cattle weigh more than 600 kg [70]. Anesthesia lasts approximately 30 min but can be prolonged for 15 min with additional ketamine at 0.75–1.25 mg/kg IV [70]. When evaluated in sheep, xylazine at 0.1 mg/kg IV and ketamine at 7.5 mg/kg IV provided anesthesia lasting 25 min and caused a decrease in cardiac output, mean arterial pressure, and peripheral vascular resistance [71]. Medetomidine has been combined with ketamine to induce anesthesia in calves. Because medetomidine (20 μg/kg IV) is much more potent that xylazine, lower doses of ketamine (0.5 mg/kg IV) can be used [72]. However, a local anesthetic at the surgical site may be required when ketamine is used at this dose [72]. Anesthesia can be reversed completely with α_2-adrenergic receptor antagonists without excitement occurring during recovery.

Diazepam at 0.1 mg/kg IV or midazolam at 0.1 mg/kg IV followed immediately by ketamine at 4.5 mg/kg IV can be used in domestic ruminants. Muscle relaxation is usually adequate for tracheal intubation, although the swallowing reflex may not be completely obtunded. Anesthesia usually lasts 10–15 min following benzodiazepine–ketamine administration, with recumbency of up to 30 min. Higher doses of diazepam (0.25–0.5 mg/kg IV) with ketamine (4–7.5 mg/kg IV) have also been used in sheep and provide the same duration of anesthesia [14,42,71]. Investigations into the cardiopulmonary effects of diazepam (0.375 mg/kg IV) and ketamine (7.5 mg/kg IV) in sheep have shown a decrease in cardiac output and an increase in peripheral vascular resistance without affecting arterial pressure [71]. Midazolam substituted for diazepam in goats and given at 0.4 mg/kg IM is followed by ketamine at 4 mg/kg IV after recumbency occurs (approximately 15 min). Anesthesia lasts approximately 15 min [58].

Xylazine (0.25–0.35 mg/kg IM) and ketamine (6–10 mg/kg IM) 15 min later usually provide 30–60 min of recumbency in camelids [8,11]. Simultaneous administration of xylazine (0.44 mg/kg IM) and ketamine (4 mg/kg IM) usually provides restraint for 15–20 min [10,73]. Higher doses of xylazine (0.8 mg/kg IM) and ketamine (8 mg/kg IM) given simultaneously usually induce sedation/anesthesia within 5 min that lasts 30 min [73]. Depth of anesthesia varies with the amount given and the camelid's temperament but is usually sufficient for minor procedures such as suturing lacerations, draining abscesses, or applying casts. When any of these combinations provides insufficient anesthetic depth, supplemental local anesthesia may be required in order to complete the procedure. Tracheal intubation may not be possible. However, these combinations heavily sedate and immobilize the animals, facilitating venipuncture and administration of additional anesthetic agent or application of a face mask to increase the depth of anesthesia when necessary. If desired, xylazine (0.25 mg/kg IV) and ketamine (3–5 mg/kg IV) may be administered 5 min apart to obtain a more uniform response and sufficient depth of anesthesia for tracheal intubation [8]. Diazepam (0.1–0.2 mg/kg IV) and ketamine (4.5 mg/kg IV) as used for domestic ruminants produces recumbency that lasts approximately 20 min and should provide enough muscle relaxation for tracheal intubation in camelids.

Guaifenesin

Guaifenesin is a centrally acting skeletal muscle relaxant that exerts its effect at the internuncial neurons in the spinal cord and at polysynaptic nerve endings [74]. It can be used alone to induce recumbency in domestic ruminants and camelids but is not recommended because it imparts little, if any, analgesia [75]. Addition of ketamine, or historically a thiobarbiturate, to guaifenesin solution improves induction quality and decreases the volume required for anesthetic induction. Muscle relaxation is improved compared with induction with ketamine or thiobarbiturates given alone. Typically, 5% guaifenesin solutions are used. Hemolysis can occur with 10% guaifenesin solutions [76]. Commonly, these solutions are given rapidly to effect, either by gravity and large-gauge catheter or by pressurizing the bag or bottle, in either tranquilized or untranquilized patients. The calculated volume dose when using 5% guaifenesin solution is 2 mL/kg. The amount of ketamine added to guaifenesin varies but is commonly 1 g per 50 g of guaifenesin. The amount of thiobarbiturate added to guaifenesin varies but is commonly 2 g per 50 g of guaifenesin. For convenience, guaifenesin-based mixtures may be injected with large (60–140 mL) syringes rather than administered by infusion to camelids and small ruminants to allow greater control over administration. If desired, xylazine can also be added to ketamine–guaifenesin solutions for induction and maintenance of anesthesia in cattle [70,77,78] and sheep [79]. Final concentrations are guaifenesin 50 mg/mL, ketamine 1–2 mg/mL, and xylazine 0.1 mg/mL. This solution is infused at 0.5 to 1 mL/kg IV for induction. For more information about guaifenesin, the reader is referred to Chapter 13.

Tiletamine–zolazepam

Tiletamine–zolazepam is a proprietary combination of equal parts of tiletamine and zolazepam available for use as an anesthetic agent in cats and dogs as Telazol®. When used alone, tiletamine induces poor muscle relaxation and causes excitement during recovery. The addition of zolazepam to tiletamine modifies these effects. As with ketamine, the swallowing reflex remains but is obtunded. Like ketamine, this combination provides slight cardiovascular stimulation, causing the heart rate to increase [80]. Elimination of tiletamine and zolazepam is not uniform, with variation occurring in each drug's clearance between species. Differential clearance of the two drugs can affect recovery quality [80].

In many respects, tiletamine–zolazepam can be considered to be similar to ketamine premixed with diazepam or midazolam. When used alone in horses, it provides unsatisfactory anesthesia [81]. Muscle relaxation is poor and recovery is characterized by excitement. However, when combined with a sedative such as xylazine, it can be used successfully in horses. Because of differences in temperament between horses and domestic ruminants and camelids, tiletamine–zolazepam can be used successfully with or without xylazine in these species. However, addition of xylazine to tiletamine–zolazepam will lengthen the effect.

Tiletamine–zolazepam given at 4 mg/kg IV in untranquilized calves caused minimal cardiovascular effects and provided anesthesia that lasted 45–60 min [82]. Xylazine at 0.1 mg/kg IM followed immediately by tiletamine–zolazepam at 4 mg/kg IM produced onset of anesthesia within 3 min, and anesthesia that lasted approximately 1 h [83]. Calves were able to stand approximately 130 min after injection. Increasing xylazine to 0.2 mg/kg IM increased the duration of anesthesia and recumbency and the incidence of apnea, necessitating intubation and ventilatory support [83]. Xylazine can also be administered at 0.05 mg/kg IV followed by tiletamine–zolazepam at 1 mg/kg IV [70].

Tiletamine–zolazepam given at 12 mg/kg IV in sheep provides approximately 2.5 h of surgical anesthesia, with a total recumbency time of 3.2 h [84]. More recent investigations in sheep have shown that tiletamine–zolazepam, dosed at 12–24 mg/kg IV, causes cardiopulmonary depression with anesthesia of approximately 40 min [85]. Rather than using these relatively large doses, it is more appropriate to decrease the initial dose of tiletamine–zolazepam to 2–4 mg/kg IV and administer additional drug as required to prolong anesthesia. Butorphanol at 0.5 mg/kg IV combined with tiletamine–zolazepam at 12 mg/kg IV given either simultaneously or 10 min apart induces 25–50 min of anesthesia in sheep, with mild cardiopulmonary depression [86]. Tiletamine–zolazepam at 4 mg/kg IM can immobilize llamas for up to 2 h [87]. The length of recumbency is unaffected by administration of flumazenil, indicating that the duration of action is more likely influenced by tiletamine rather than zolazepam [87]. Cardiovascular function is preserved although hypercapnia and hypoxemia can occur in some animals. Airway reflexes are maintained. Local anesthesia may be required for some surgical procedures [87]. Tiletamine–zolazepam at 2 mg/kg IM can immobilize llamas for approximately 1 h [88]. Tiletamine–zolazepam at 2 mg/kg IM can also be combined with acepromazine, butorphanol, or xylazine and will lengthen the duration of immobilization [88,89]. In camelids, tiletamine–zolazepam at 2 mg/kg IV can provide 15–20 min of anesthesia and 25–35 min of recumbency [38]. Depth of anesthesia is adequate to intubate nasally, but muscle relaxation is poor and oral intubation is difficult.

Propofol

Propofol is a non-barbiturate, non-steroidal hypnotic agent used to provide brief periods of anesthesia (5–10 min). The dose is 4–6 mg/kg IV for induction in unsedated ruminants [14,90–92]. Induction is smooth, as is recovery. If injected too rapidly, apnea may occur. Slow administration will reduce this complication. Propofol can also be used at 4 mg/kg IV following acepromazine at 0.05 mg/kg IM and papaveretum at 0.4 mg/kg IM [93]. Anesthesia can be induced in unsedated camelids with 2 mg/kg IV [94]. However, tracheal intubation is often difficult or impossible at this dose and additional propofol is usually needed.

Propofol at 3 mg/kg IV can be used in combination with ketamine at 1 mg/kg IV following acepromazine at 0.05 mg/kg IM and papaveretum at 0.4 mg/kg IM to induce anesthesia [93]. Anesthesia can be maintained with propofol at 0.2–0.3 mg/kg/min IV and ketamine at 0.1–0.2 mg/kg/min [93]. Recovery to standing occurs within 15 min [93].

Alfaxalone

The use of an earlier preparation of alfaxalone (alfaxalone and alphadolone solubilized in saline and Cremaphor) was investigated in ruminants in the late 1970s and early 1980s before the product was discontinued [95]. Alfaxalone has been re-released in a different formulation (2-hydroxypropyl-β-cyclodextrin) recently and has been investigated in sheep and camelids. Alfaxalone given at 2 mg/kg to unsedated sheep provided brief periods of anesthesia with less effect on cardiopulmonary variables than thiopental and propofol [96]. Anesthesia has also been induced in unsedated sheep with medetomidine at 2 μg/kg administered simultaneously with alfaxalone at 2 mg/kg IV [97]. Muscle relaxation was sufficient to allow intubation and duration of recumbency was brief, lasting less than 10 min [97]. Alfaxalone has been evaluated as a sole anesthetic agent in unsedated alpacas [98]. It is given at 2 mg/kg IV and provides sufficient depth of anesthesia to allow intubation. Duration was brief, lasting 10–15 min. Recovery to standing was complete within 35 min and was characterized as poor [98]. Use of alfaxalone would be improved by sedating camelids before induction or by using it as an induction agent to be followed by inhalant anesthesia.

Intubation

Tracheal intubation is recommended in all ruminants and camelids because it provides a secure airway and prevents aspiration of salivary and ruminal contents if active or passive regurgitation occurs. In lightly anesthetized ruminants, active regurgitation can occur during intubation [11,70], whereas passive regurgitation can occur at any time during anesthesia due to relaxation of the cardia. Because the rumen contents contain more solid material than do the gastric contents of monogastric animals, there is greater potential for ingesta to obstruct the larynx while the more fluid portion will drain from the mouth. Patients that are not intubated are at high risk. Intubated animals that have regurgitated during anesthesia are at risk following extubation. Treatment involves removal of ingesta from the buccal cavity or buccal lavage prior to extubation. If active regurgitation has occurred, anesthetic depth should be rapidly increased and the airway quickly protected to prevent aspiration.

Table 49.1 Sizes of endotracheal tubes needed for ruminants and camelids of various body weights.

Body Weight (kg)	Endotracheal Tube Size (mm i.d.)	
	Oral	Nasal
<30	4–7	4–6
30–60	8–10	6–8
60–100	10–12	8–10
100–200	12–14	10–12
200–300	14–16	
300–400	16–22	
400–600	22–26	
>600	26	

Several techniques can be used for intubation. Adult cattle can be intubated blindly or with digital palpation. Following insertion of a mouth speculum or the use of gauze loops, the animal's head and neck are hyperextended to make the orotracheal axis approach 180°. An endotracheal tube of appropriate size is inserted and manipulated into the larynx (Table 49.1). When that technique is unsuccessful, the anesthetist's hand should be inserted into the mouth with the tube. After the epiglottis has been located and depressed, a finger can be placed between the arytenoid cartilages and the tube inserted into the trachea. If desired, an equine nasogastric tube can be inserted into the larynx and serve as a guide for the endotracheal tube. Depending on the size of the animal and the individual's arm, airway obstruction may occur, hence it is important that intubation is performed promptly. If the technique requires more than 1 min, the hand and arm should be withdrawn from the oral cavity to allow the animal to ventilate before continuing to attempt intubation.

When blind orotracheal intubation is unsuccessful in calves, a laryngoscope with a 250–350 mm blade is required for laryngoscopy. Herbivores' mouths do not open widely, and can be held open by an assistant using gauze loops. Visibility of the pharynx and larynx will be improved by using an equine mouth speculum. Some effort is needed to keep the upper bar of the speculum against the dental pad but use of the speculum will allow an assistant to open the mouth more widely than can be accomplished otherwise and allow much better visibility of the larynx. Visibility of the larynx is also improved by hyperextending the animal's head and neck to make the orotracheal axis approach 180°. Using suction or gauze on a sponge forceps to swab the pharynx will improve visibility if secretions are an impediment. Attempting intubation when the anesthetic plane is insufficient may provoke active regurgitation. With adequate depth of anesthesia, this reflex is eliminated. The epiglottis is depressed to visualize the larynx. The endotracheal tube should be placed in the oral pharynx and inserted into the larynx during inspiration. If desired, a stylet [e.g., a 1 m × 0.5 cm stylet [99], a large male dog urinary catheter, or an endotracheal tube exchanger (Cook Airway Exchange Catheters, Cook Medical, Bloomington, IN, USA)] can be inserted through the endotracheal tube to facilitate intubation. The length of the stylet should be about 1.5–2 times that of the endotracheal tube. The stylet is placed through the larynx, and the endotracheal tube is then passed into the trachea.

Blind oral intubation is more difficult in sheep and goats, and intubation is best performed with laryngoscopy. To perform blind oral intubation, the animal's head and neck are extended after placement of the endotracheal tube in the oral pharynx. The larynx can be palpated and the tube directed into the larynx [42]. Members of both of these species have active laryngeal reflexes that may be obtunded by topical application of 2% lidocaine. This can be performed with an adjustable pattern plant sprayer [100] or with a syringe. Use of Cetacaine® is not recommended because overdosage can easily occur and because benzocaine-based local anesthetics can cause methemoglobinemia [101]. After desensitization of the larynx, intubation can be performed with the same technique as used in calves. Oral intubation in camelids is similar to that in domestic ruminants. Blind oral intubation is usually unsuccessful, and laryngoscopy with a 250–350 mm laryngoscope is recommended. Desensitization of the larynx is usually not required.

Blind nasotracheal intubation has been described in awake or mildly sedated calves, although it requires an endotracheal tube one size smaller than that used orally [102]. The technique in calves is very similar to that described for foals and is useful for induction of inhalation anesthesia or to facilitate oral surgery. Particular attention is needed to ensure that the tube is directed into the ventral meatus. Following placement of the tube in the nasopharynx, the calf's head and neck are extended to facilitate passage into the larynx. The tube is secured in place and connected to the anesthesia machine.

Nasotracheal intubation is also possible in sheep [39] and camelids [103], although it requires an endotracheal tube one size smaller than that used orally. Camelids are prone to epistaxis and use of a lubricant that contains phenylephrine is recommended. Blind nasal intubation is technically easier than blind oral intubation, but nasal intubation under laryngoscopic control is technically more difficult than orotracheal intubation. Even though nasotracheal intubation can be more difficult, it offers the option of recovering the animal with the endotracheal tube in place as a method of preventing airway obstruction during recovery. The endotracheal tube is advanced with slow, gentle pressure through the external nares into the ventral meatus. An obstruction encountered at approximately 10 cm in adults is usually due to placement of the tube in the middle meatus. If an obstruction is encountered more caudally, approximately 25 cm in adult llamas, the tube is likely in the nasopharyngeal diverticulum [103]. In either case, the tube should be partially or completely withdrawn and redirected. If the endotracheal tube cannot be redirected past the nasopharyngeal diverticulum, placement of a pre-bent stylet into the tube to direct its tip ventrally is usually effective.

After the endotracheal tube has been advanced into the nasopharynx, the camelid's head and neck should be extended and the tube manipulated into the larynx. If the tube will not enter the larynx, placing a pre-bent stylet in the endotracheal tube to direct the tube tip ventrally into the larynx instead of the esophagus is helpful. Although visibility of the larynx is somewhat limited, oral laryngoscopy will aid intubation and confirm correct placement of the tube.

Endotracheal intubation can be confirmed with several techniques. Initially, they include visualization of the endotracheal tube passing into the larynx. When transparent endotracheal tubes are used, condensed water vapor will appear and then disappear during each breath. One can feel gas being expelled from the tube during exhalation and, when the endotracheal tube is connected to the anesthesia machine, observation of synchrony between movement of the breathing bag and the thorax will be noted. If a suction bulb is evacuated and connected to the endotracheal tube, it will re-expand if the tube is in the trachea and will remain collapsed if the tube is in the esophagus, providing immediate confirmation of correct or incorrect placement of the tube (Fig. 49.1). Finally, if a capnograph is available, carbon dioxide will be noted in exhaled gas.

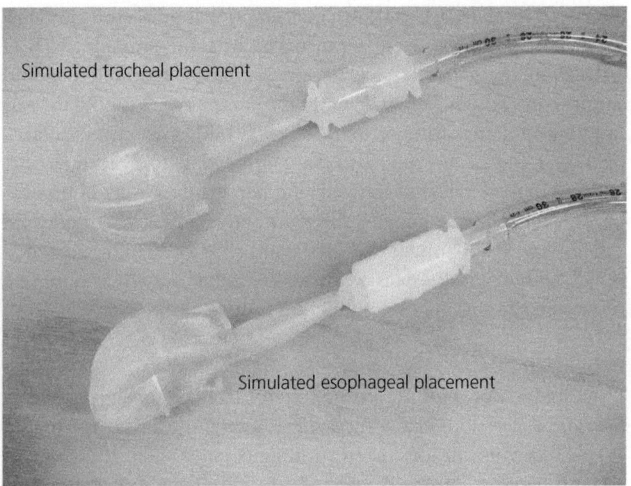

Figure 49.1 Evacuated bulbs attached to endotracheal tubes simulating esophageal (bottom) and tracheal (top) placement of the tube. The evacuated bulb will fill when attached to a correctly placed endotracheal tube.

Maintenance

Anesthesia in ruminants and camelids can be maintained with intravenous agents, commonly ketamine–guaifenesin–xylazine, and less commonly propofol or alfaxalone, or with the inhalant agents.

Injectable

Because ruminants may regurgitate during xylazine–ketamine–guaifenesin anesthesia, intubation is highly recommended. It is also often recommended that duration of anesthesia be limited to 60 min to limit recovery time and complications. The use of infusion pumps facilitates administration of the drugs and improves convenience and precision.

Following induction, xylazine–ketamine–guaifenesin solutions can be used for maintenance of anesthesia in cattle [71,77,78] and sheep [79]. Final concentrations are xylazine 0.1 mg/mL, ketamine 1–2 mg/mL, and guaifenesin 50 mg/mL. Anesthesia is maintained by infusion of the mixture at 1.5 mL/kg/h for calves [77,78], 2 mL/kg/h for adult cattle [70], and 2 mL/kg/h for sheep [79], although the final administration rate will vary with case requirements. If the procedure requires more than 2 mL/kg of the xylazine–ketamine–guaifenesin mixture in order to complete the procedure, the amount of xylazine added should be decreased by at least 50% because its duration of action is longer than that of the other two agents (J.C. Thurmon, personal communication, 1993). Alternatively, a solution with final concentrations of xylazine 0.05 mg/mL, ketamine 1 mg/mL, and guaifenesin 50 mg/mL can be formulated and infused at 2 mL/kg/h IV for maintenance to avoid the cumulative effects of xylazine. Following induction, xylazine–ketamine–guaifenesin solutions may be used for maintenance of anesthesia in llamas [104]. Final concentrations are xylazine 0.1–0.2 mg/mL, ketamine 2 mg/mL, and guaifenesin 50 mg/mL. Anesthesia is maintained by infusion of the mixture at 1.2–2.4 mL/kg/h, although the final administration rate will vary with case requirements.

Following induction in sedated sheep with propofol, anesthesia can be maintained with propofol at 0.3–0.5 mg/kg/min IV [93]. Recovery to standing occurs within 15 min [93]. A light plane of anesthesia can be maintained in unsedated llamas with a constant infusion of propofol at 0.4 mg/kg/min IV [94]. The approximate time from discontinuation of propofol infusion to sternal recumbency is 10–15 min [94]. Following induction of anesthesia in sedated sheep with propofol and ketamine, anesthesia can be maintained with propofol at 0.2–0.3 mg/kg/min and ketamine at 0.1–0.2 mg/kg/min IV [93]. Recovery to standing occurs within 15 min [93]. Anesthesia can also be maintained with alfaxalone at 10 mg/kg/h in unsedated sheep following induction with alfaxalone at 2 mg/kg [105]. Recovery following 70 min of anesthesia is within 25 min [105]. Alfaxalone can also be infused as an adjunct to inhalation anesthesia [106].

Inhalation

Inhalant agents that have been used historically in ruminants include methoxyflurane and halothane, but isoflurane and sevoflurane are the inhalant agents of choice in contemporary practice. Methoxyflurane has been utilized in small domestic ruminants and camelids, although induction and recovery were prolonged. Liver failure was reported in hyperimmunized goats subjected to halothane anesthesia [107], but another study performed in young, healthy goats showed that neither halothane nor isoflurane was likely to cause hepatic injury [108]. Reports of renal failure associated with flunixin meglumine administration immediately before or after methoxyflurane in dogs [109] caution against the use of this combination of drugs in ruminants.

Conventional small animal anesthesia machines can be used to anesthetize ruminants weighing less than 60 kg. Conventional human anesthesia machines or small animal machines with expanded carbon dioxide absorbent (e.g., soda lime) canisters are adequate for animals weighing up to 200 kg. Conventional large animal anesthesia machines can be used to anesthetize cattle weighing over 250 kg. Anesthesia is usually induced with 3–5% isoflurane or 4–6% sevoflurane and an oxygen flow rate of 20 mL/kg/min. Anesthesia is induced in animals of lower body weight by using agent concentrations at the lower end of the range. Anesthesia is usually maintained with 1.5–2.5% isoflurane or 2.5–3.5% sevoflurane with an oxygen flow rate of 12 mL/kg/min, with a minimum flow rate of 1 L/min being adequate. These vaporizer settings correspond to end-expired anesthetic concentrations of 1.25–1.5 minimum alveolar concentration (MAC) and should be adequate for ruminants that were not sedated prior to induction. Ruminants that have been sedated prior to induction can usually be maintained on end-expired anesthetic concentrations of 1–1.25 MAC, although final concentrations may vary depending on the sedative used. Because domestic ruminants have a respiratory pattern characterized by rapid respiratory rate and small tidal volume, higher vaporizer settings may be required to maintain anesthesia in spontaneously breathing patients.

Supportive therapy

Supportive therapy is an important part of anesthetic practice. As duration and difficulty increase, the likelihood of complications can also increase. Attention to supportive therapy in anesthetized ruminants and camelids can decrease the incidence of complications and improve outcome. Supportive therapy includes patient positioning, fluid administration, mechanical ventilation, cardiovascular support, and good monitoring techniques.

Patient positioning

Improper positioning and padding of anesthetized horses have been implicated as one cause of postanesthetic myopathy–neuropathy [110]. A similar situation may occur in adult cattle. Postanesthetic myopathy does not appear to occur in calves, goats, sheep, and South American camelids. Anesthetized ruminants should be positioned on a smooth, flat, padded surface. Adult cattle require water beds, dunnage bags, or 10–15 cm foam pads. Pads 5 cm thick are sufficient for sheep, goats, and South American camelids. Patients positioned in dorsal recumbency should be balanced squarely on their back with both gluteal areas bearing equal weight. The forelegs should be flexed and relaxed, and the hind legs relaxed and flexed. External support should be placed under the maxilla to prevent hyperextension of the neck.

Adult cattle in lateral recumbency should have an automobile inner tube (valve stem pointed down) placed under the shoulder of the dependent foreleg to help minimize pressure on the radial nerve as it traverses the musculospiral groove of the humerus. The point of the elbow should be positioned at five o'clock in the inner tube for cattle in right lateral recumbency or at seven o'clock for cattle in left lateral recumbency. In addition, the dependent foreleg is drawn anteriorly so that the weight of the thorax rests on the triceps rather than on the humerus. Non-elastic tape covering the portion of the inner tube not under the shoulder will prevent overexpansion of that section of inner tube and collapse of the inner tube under the shoulder and helps ensure that shoulder support remains (Fig. 49.2). The other three legs are positioned perpendicular to the body, with the uppermost legs elevated and parallel to the table surface. Support of these legs will improve venous drainage and prevent injury to the brachial plexus. The head and neck are maintained in a slightly extended position, with the head resting on a pad or towel (Fig. 49.3). If possible, the patient's head should be positioned so that salivary secretions and gastric contents, if regurgitation occurs, will drain from the mouth and not wick between the animal's head and the pad and contact the eye. The dependent eye should be closed prior to placing the head on the padding, and ophthalmic ointment should be instilled in the other eye. Camelids have

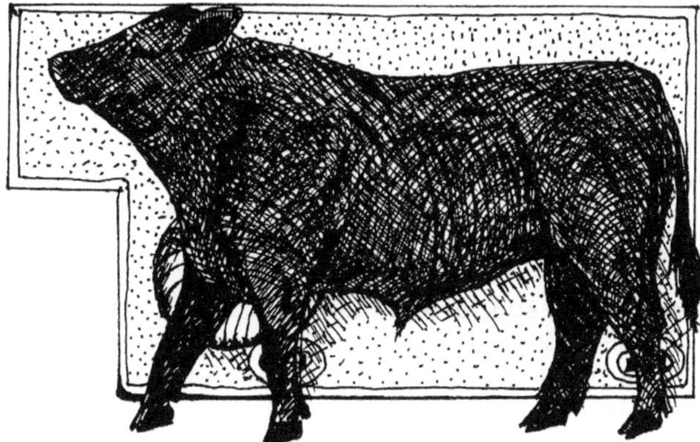

Figure 49.2 Cattle positioned in lateral recumbency should be placed on padding with an automobile inner tube placed under the dependent forelimb and that leg drawn cranially. Support should be placed under the non-dependent forelimb and hindlimb so that they are parallel to the table.

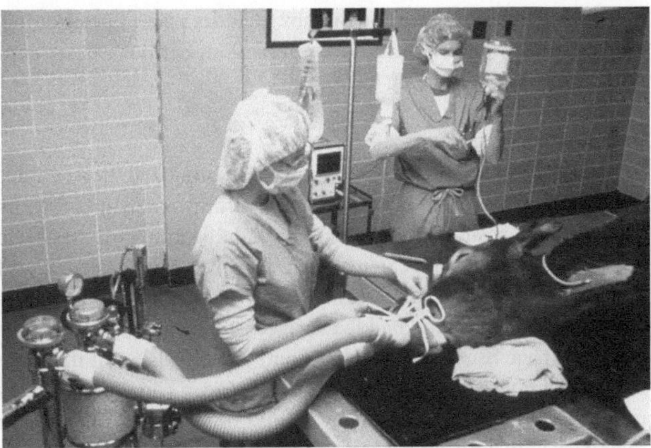

Figure 49.3 Position of the head and neck to enable fluid to drain from the oral cavity.

prominent eyes, and special attention should be given to the dependent eye to avoid injury. Use of circulating warm-water heating blankets or convective warm-air blowers should be considered to prevent hypothermia in juvenile cattle, sheep, camelids, and goats. Depending on size and duration of anesthesia, adults are less likely to become hypothermic, and use of active warming devices is not required.

Fluid administration

Fluid administration during anesthesia is important to correct pre-existing dehydration, if present, provide volume to offset anesthesia-related vasodilation, and provide maintenance needs. A balanced electrolyte solution is preferred. Lactated Ringer's solution, Normosol-R®, or the equivalent are most commonly used and are administered rapidly (10–25 mL/kg/h) in hypotensive patients. After hypotension is corrected, fluid administration may be slowed to 4–6 mL/kg/h. Although ruminants salivate copiously while anesthetized, replacement of bicarbonate is usually not required. Other fluids (e.g., saline) may be given when indicated. To increase the fluid delivery rate when needed, two administration sets can be connected to one catheter with a Y-connector, multiple catheters can be placed, a peristaltic pump can be used, or the fluid source may be pressurized. For convenience, fluids packaged in 3 or 5 L bags can be used for large-volume administration. When administering large volumes of fluid, serial determinations of hematocrit and plasma total solids should be performed to prevent hemodilution and pulmonary edema. Hematocrit should remain above 25% and plasma total solids above 4 g/dL. Use of synthetic colloids (e.g., hetastarch), plasma, or whole blood transfusion should be considered for hypoproteinemic or anemic individuals. Administration of sodium bicarbonate is indicated for correction of severe metabolic acidemia as determined by blood-gas analysis or total carbon dioxide measurement.

Respiratory supportive therapy

Although anesthetized South American camelids ventilate well, domestic ruminants tend to hypoventilate while anesthetized. Mechanical ventilation should be considered when the procedure will exceed 90 min and is indicated to prevent hypoventilation in individuals that will not maintain sufficient alveolar ventilation. To minimize the effects of mechanical ventilation on the cardiovascular system, the inspiratory time should be no more than 2–3 s, the inspiratory pressure should be 20–25 cmH_2O, the tidal volume should be between 13 and 18 mL/kg, and the respiratory rate should be 6–10 breaths/min. Hypocapnia can cause bradycardia in ruminants. In the absence of blood-gas analysis, the minute volume should be decreased if unexplained bradycardia occurs.

During intravenous anesthesia, ruminants also benefit from supplemental oxygen. If the animal is intubated, the endotracheal tube can be connected to a demand valve. This piece of equipment is connected to an oxygen source that enables the patient to breathe spontaneously [111]. Compression of a button on the demand valve enables the anesthetist to 'sigh' the patient. Because demand valves are designed for humans, there is an increase in the work of breathing associated with their use in large animals [112]. Intubated ruminants can also be insufflated with oxygen (5 L/min for small ruminants and 15 L/min for adult cattle). A flowmeter is connected to an oxygen source, and the tubing from the flowmeter is then inserted into the endotracheal tube [113].

Cardiovascular supportive therapy

Hypotension has been implicated as another cause of postanesthetic myopathy–neuropathy [110,114,115]. To help avoid this postanesthetic complication in ruminants, normotension should be maintained during anesthesia. Hypotension may often be corrected by adjusting the anesthetic depth. Although vasopressors can be used to correct hypotension, expansion of vascular volume with rapid fluid administration and/or augmentation of stroke volume and cardiac output with inotropic therapy are better alternatives. Calcium borogluconate (23% solution) may also increase myocardial contractility and can be given as a slow infusion (0.5–1 mL/kg/h IV) to effect. Calcium administration can cause bradycardia, however, necessitating the use of a chronotrope if hypotension due to bradycardia persists. Ephedrine, a mixed α- and β-sympathomimetic drug, can be used at 0.02–0.06 mg/kg IV to increase mean arterial pressure through an increase in cardiac contractility [116]. Lack of response at low doses can indicate excessive depth of anesthesia. Dobutamine, a synthetic β-adrenergic receptor agonist, can also be used to improve cardiac output. At low doses, it increases myocardial contractility and, at higher doses, also heart rate [117]. Dobutamine is preferred over dopamine because improvements in hemodynamic function are achieved with smaller increases in heart rate [118]. Dobutamine is infused at 1–2 μg/kg/min IV to effect [118]. Use of an infusion pump is recommended for convenience and consistency. After correction of hypotension, the infusion rate can often be decreased to maintain normotension.

Monitoring

As with any species, good anesthetic techniques require monitoring to ensure that drug administration meets the animal's requirements and to prevent excessive insult to the cardiovascular, respiratory, central nervous, and musculoskeletal systems, thereby decreasing the risk of complications. Monitoring includes techniques that require the tactile, visual, and auditory skills of the anesthetist, as well as more sophisticated techniques that require instrumentation. Attention is directed to three organ systems: the cardiovascular, the respiratory, and the central nervous systems. Ideally, one monitors variables that respond rapidly to changes in anesthetic depth, which gives the anesthetist sufficient time to alter anesthetic administration before the anesthetic plane becomes either excessive or insufficient. While monitoring is done constantly, most variables are recorded at 5 min intervals. In many instances, monitoring equipment is used to aid the evaluation of physiologic responses to anesthesia and therefore anesthetic depth. Use of these instruments can make evaluation more precise and the selection of ancillary drugs more rational.

Variables that can be used to monitor the cardiovascular system are heart rate, pulse pressure (pulse strength), mucous membrane color, and capillary refill time. In healthy anesthetized adult cattle, the heart rate is usually 60–90 beats/min. Animals that have received an anticholinergic will have an increased heart rate. The normal heart rate for calves, sheep, and goats varies with age. Juveniles will have a heart rate of 90–130 beats/min, which decreases as they mature. The normal heart rate for adult anesthetized camelids after administration of an anticholinergic is 80–100 beats/min, and for anesthetized juvenile camelids after the administration of an anticholinergic it is 100–125 beats/min. The heart rate may exceed the normal range at the beginning of anesthesia because of excitement associated with induction or hypotension but most often returns to the normal range within 10–20 min. In compromised patients, the heart rate begins to approach the normal range during anesthesia as oxygen, fluid, and analgesic support begin to stabilize the patient. The heart rate usually decreases as the depth of anesthesia increases, although that response is dependent on the agent used and can be masked by prior administration of anticholinergics.

Pulse pressure can be ascertained at several locations and should be full and bounding. The common digital, caudal auricular, radial, and saphenous arteries are commonly palpated. The facial artery can be palpated in young calves, but it becomes more difficult to do so as the animal ages. Pulse pressure should be strong and palpated at different locations for comparison. Noting the amount of turgor present in the vessel during diastole can give an indication of diastolic pressure. If the vessel is easily collapsed by digital pressure during diastole, then diastolic pressure and, therefore, systolic and mean pressure can be assumed to be low even though the pulse pressure may feel adequate. The availability of non-invasive blood pressure monitors suitable for patients the size of most ruminants and camelids should make blood pressure monitoring during anesthesia commonplace.

Mucous membranes should be pink, although those of some ruminants and camelids are pigmented, making assessment difficult. The presence of cyanosis must also be noted, although animals breathing oxygen and an inhalation agent may be apneic for several minutes before cyanosis occurs. Because at least 5 g/dL of reduced hemoglobin is required before cyanosis can be detected, severely anemic animals may not show this sign. Flushed mucous membranes are associated with vasodilation, which can be caused by hypercapnia, halothane, α_2-adrenergic receptor antagonists, or histamine release, or may be associated with postural hypostatic congestion [119]. Brick-red mucous membranes are associated with endotoxic shock. Following digital compression to blanch an area of the gum, capillary refill should occur in 1–2 s. Both of these variables give an imprecise indication of tissue perfusion. Excessive depth of anesthesia will cause the mucous membranes to become pale and the capillary refill time to increase.

The respiratory system is evaluated by monitoring respiratory rate and tidal volume. Spontaneous breathing rates are usually 20–30 breaths/min or higher in adult cattle; calves, sheep, and goats usually have respiratory rates of 20–40 breaths/min. Awake cattle have a decreased tidal volume compared with horses [120]. This relationship persists in anesthetized cattle and other domestic ruminants in that they have a decreased tidal volume compared with other species. Tidal volume is estimated by observing the decrease in size of the rebreathing bag during inspiration. Increasing depth of anesthesia can usually be expected to cause a decrease in tidal volume and eventually a decrease in respiratory rate. Normal values for respiratory rate in anesthetized camelids are 15–30 breaths/min for adults and 20–35 breaths/min for juveniles. Camelids tend to ventilate reasonably well when breathing spontaneously as judged by blood-gas and respiratory-gas analysis during sevoflurane and isoflurane anesthesia. End tidal CO_2 monitoring is available in many practices and is useful for monitoring ventilation in ruminants. Since CO_2 and other gases are produced during fermentation, the effect of these non-respiratory sources of gas should be assessed on each capnometer before use.

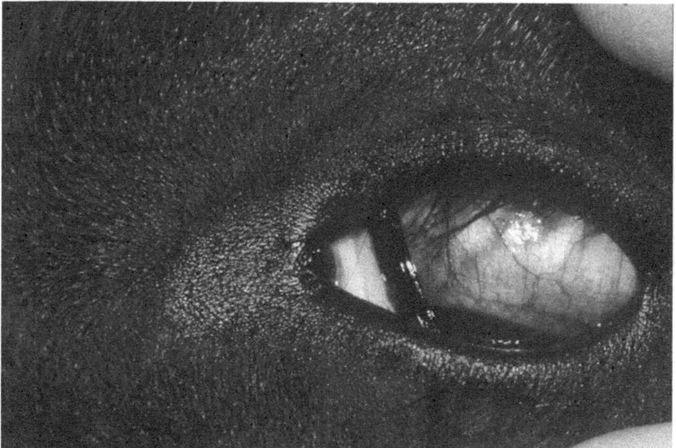

Figure 49.4 Ocular rotation in a ventral direction is indicative of a light plane of surgical anesthesia.

The central nervous system can be monitored by observation of ocular reflexes. The palpebral reflex disappears with minimal depth of anesthesia in cattle, sheep, and goats and is usually of no value during anesthesia. Rotation of the globe will occur as anesthetic depth changes in cattle (Fig. 49.4) [3,40,121]. The eyeball is normally centered between the palpebrae in awake cattle in lateral recumbency. As anesthesia is induced, the eyeball rotates ventrally, with the cornea being partially obscured by the lower eye lid. As depth of anesthesia increases, the pupil becomes completely hidden by the lower eyelid; this sign indicates the patient is at stage III, plane 2–3 anesthesia. A further increase in anesthetic depth is accompanied by dorsal rotation of the eyeball. Dorsal movement is complete when the cornea is centered between the palpebrae; this sign indicates deep surgical anesthesia with profound muscle relaxation. During recovery, the eyeball rotates in reverse order to that during induction [3,40,121]. Rotation of the globe does not occur in response to changes in depth of anesthesia in goats, sheep, or South American camelids. Usually, the palpebral reflex of the dorsal eyelid of camelids remains intact during surgical anesthesia. However, if the camelid can move its ventral eyelid without tactile stimulation, anesthetic depth is decreasing and eventually limb movement will occur [38]. Nystagmus usually does not occur during anesthesia of domestic ruminants or camelids. When it does occur, it cannot be correlated with changes in anesthetic depth. The corneal reflex should always be present.

Some ruminants will display involuntary swallowing motions under anesthesia without exhibiting other signs of insufficient anesthetic depth. This reflex may indicate that anesthetic depth is somewhat light but still appropriate. Response to pain from the surgical procedure can also be used to estimate depth of anesthesia. In some instances, camelids may respond by showing a more active palpebral reflex. Purposeful movement in all species indicates insufficient depth of anesthesia. A mild temporary increase in arterial pressure associated with surgical manipulation does not necessarily indicate inadequate anesthesia if purposeful movement does not occur.

Electrocardiography (ECG) is used with either standard limb leads (i.e., I, II, and III) or a dipole (augmented) lead for detection of cardiac rate and rhythm disturbances. The lead that has the largest amplitude should be selected. A recorder is optional and useful because it enables one to record an ECG at the beginning of the case for future reference. Most ECG units emit an audible tone when a QRS complex is detected. Anesthetists should learn to always listen to the audible rhythm in the background during the case, especially during distractions. Because an ECG gives no information regarding blood pressure or pulse strength, emphasis should be placed on monitoring pulse and arterial pressure instead of relying solely on the ECG.

Mean arterial pressure provides an accurate variable for assessing anesthetic depth. In most instances, changes in anesthetic depth become evident quickly through increases or decreases in blood pressure. Additionally, it is a more definitive variable than assessing pulse pressure alone. Monitoring pulse pressure determines the difference between systolic and diastolic pressure. An animal with systolic and diastolic pressures of 120/90 mmHg will have pulse pressure similar to that of another with pressures of 90/60 mmHg. However, a large difference exists in mean arterial pressure or perfusion pressure. The former case will have a mean pressure of about 100 mmHg whereas the latter will have a mean pressure of about 70 mmHg. Since animals with low mean pressure during anesthesia are more at risk of developing complications, identification of this situation is important [114,115]. Normal arterial pressure values in anesthetized cattle are systolic pressure 120–150, diastolic pressure 80–110, and mean pressure 90–120 mmHg, and are typically greater than in standing cattle [122]. Normal arterial pressure values in sheep, goats, and camelids are systolic pressure 90–120, diastolic pressure 60–80, and mean pressure 75–100 mmHg. However, if camelids are aroused by painful stimuli, mean arterial pressure may approach 150 mmHg. Arterial pressure can be monitored either indirectly or directly. Indirect methods of determining arterial pressure require the use of various infrasonic and ultrasonic devices to detect blood flow in peripheral arteries. A Doppler ultrasonic system or an oscillometric device (e.g., Cardell®) can be used with cuffs wrapped around the tail of cattle and the limbs of sheep and goats [18], or around the tail or the limbs of South American camelids [10]. The cuff diameter should be 40% of limb or tail circumference [123]. Unfortunately, there can be lack of agreement between pressures obtained with indirect and direct methods in domestic ruminants [124] and in camelids [125], and the use of direct techniques is recommended when feasible.

Direct methods require catheterization of an artery and use of a pressure transducer and amplifier or an aneroid manometer to determine pressure values. A transducer system determines systolic, diastolic, and mean arterial pressures. An aneroid manometer can be substituted for the pressure transducer and amplifier, but only mean pressure can be obtained [126]. However, changes in mean pressure occur rapidly in response to changes in anesthetic depth, and use of this system enables anesthetists to initiate appropriate responses.

Percutaneous arterial catheterization is easily performed in most ruminants and is relatively free of complications [126,127]. The caudal auricular, saphenous, and common digital arteries are the most commonly catheterized vessels. Over-the-needle catheters are preferred. Passage of this type of catheter through the unbroken skin will often damage the catheter, making arterial placement difficult. Therefore, incising the skin or piercing it with a slightly larger needle at the catheterization site prior to introducing the catheter is recommended [127]. A skin incision is usually unnecessary when the caudal auricular artery is catheterized, because the skin is relatively thin in that location and the artery is often inadvertently pierced because the skin is relatively immobile in that area. For adults 3–5 cm, 20 G catheters are used and for juveniles 2.5–3 cm, 20–22 G catheters are appropriate. An extension set with stopcock is used to connect the arterial catheter to a syringe containing heparinized (2 units/mL) saline and a piece of non-compliant tubing attached to the pressure transducer or aneroid manometer. After the arterial catheter has been removed, digital pressure is maintained at the site to prevent hematoma formation. If desired, a pressure bandage can be used.

Central venous pressure can be determined to assess venous return, myocardial function, and the need for fluid replacement. This is a good variable to use, along with serial determinations of hematocrit, plasma total solids, and urine production, in evaluating fluid replacement but often provides little information regarding changes in anesthetic depth. Normal values are 5–10 cmH_2O.

Normal values for arterial blood gas analysis are similar to those for other species [5,6]. Respiratory gas analysis can determine end-tidal carbon dioxide and anesthetic agent concentrations. Because domestic ruminants have a respiratory pattern characterized by small tidal volume, end-expired gas may not be sufficiently representative of alveolar gas and accurate results might not be obtained. End-tidal gas analysis is more accurate when assessing carbon dioxide during controlled ventilation. Anesthetic agent analyzers that use optical low-spectrum infrared measurement (i.e. measuring absorption in the lower region of the infrared spectrum) cannot distinguish between methane and halothane in the expired gas of herbivores and will report falsely increased concentrations of halothane, and to a lesser extent isoflurane, in the anesthetic circuit [128]. The presence of methane does not affect analyzers that use high-spectrum infrared measurement or piezoelectric measurement [128]. Analyzers that use low-spectrum infrared measurement can be used in herbivores by intermittently (i.e., every 15–30 min) placing a small container of activated charcoal in the sample path to adsorb the inhalant agent [129]. Methane will pass through the charcoal without adsorption and be measured. After removing the charcoal container from the sample path, one can subtract the concentration of background methane from the displayed value to determine the inhalant agent concentration.

Recovery

Ruminants and South American camelids recover well from general anesthesia and seldom experience emergence delirium, make premature attempts to stand, or sustain injuries. When an α_2-adrenergic receptor agonist is used as part of the anesthetic regimen, an α_2-adrenergic receptor antagonist can be used to hasten recovery [13,22,40,47,48,52,72,99,130].

Domestic ruminants should not be extubated until the laryngeal reflex has returned. If the patient has regurgitated, the buccal cavity and pharynx should be lavaged to prevent aspiration of the material. In these instances, the endotracheal tube should be withdrawn with the cuff inflated in an attempt to remove any material that may have entered the trachea. Since camelids are obligate nasal breathers [103], gas exchange must be confirmed after extubation. Airway obstruction can commonly occur in camelids during the transition from oral endotracheal intubation to nasal breathing and, in severe cases, can necessitate tracheotomy. Orally intubated camelids should not be extubated until the animal is swallowing, coughing, and actively trying to expel the endotracheal tube to decrease the incidence of this complication. Precautions should be taken to prevent the camelid from damaging or aspirating the endotracheal tube during 'awake' extubation. The endotracheal tube of nasally intubated camelids can be removed after they stand. Although ruminants recover well from general anesthesia with minimal assistance, an attendant should be available.

Intraoperative complications

Fortunately, major complications do not often occur during or following well-planned anesthesia in ruminants. However, one must be vigilant so that the unexpected occurrence of a complication can be recognized and effectively treated. As is the case in anesthesia of all species, potential complications are better prevented, and therefore emphasis should be placed on the formation and implementation of a rational anesthetic regimen. Airway obstruction, apnea, and hypothermia are diagnosed and treated in a manner similar to other domestic species as described elsewhere in this edition.

Although anesthetized camelids do not appear to become tympanitic, fermentation of ingesta and the animal's inability to eructate under anesthesia often cause ruminal tympany during anesthesia of domestic ruminants. As tympany develops, more pressure is placed on the diaphragm, decreasing functional residual capacity and impeding ventilation [131]. In addition, tympany increases the risk of regurgitation. Therapy involves passage of a stomach tube to decompress the rumen. On occasion, one will be unable to pass the stomach tube into the rumen. In these difficult cases, placing the animal in sternal recumbency will aid the procedure. When that is not possible, the rumen can be decompressed with a 12 G needle inserted through the abdominal wall. Fortunately, ruminal tympany is usually of the non-frothy type, and decompression is easily accomplished. External pressure placed on the rumen will help expel gas from the orogastric tube. Ruminal tympany can also occur during the use of nitrous oxide, which tends to accumulate in gas-filled viscid [132]. Discontinuation of nitrous oxide administration and decompression of the rumen are recommended.

Connective tissue is not as fibrous in the lungs of ruminants, and therefore excessive airway pressure can cause pneumothorax and emphysema more easily than in horses [133]. Signs include dyspnea and increased resistance to inspiration because of tension pneumothorax. Pneumothorax is treated by placement of a chest tube and aspiration of the gas. It is much easier to prevent than treat. Excessive airway pressure (i.e., pressures greater than 25 cmH_2O) should not be used when 'sighing' animals or when using controlled ventilation.

Cardiac arrhythmias usually do not occur in anesthetized ruminants. Atrial fibrillation can occur in cattle as a sequela to metabolic derangement secondary to another problem. Most often, it occurs secondary to gastrointestinal obstruction. Atrial fibrillation usually resolves when the primary problem is corrected. Because cattle are amenable to physical restraint and local anesthesia, corrective surgery can often be performed without general anesthesia. Diagnosis can be confirmed with ECG. The oculocardiac reflex is a well-recognized reflex in most animals and can be treated similarly in ruminants [134]. Cardiac arrest would be treated with similar techniques used in horses [135–137].

Postoperative complications

Because ruminants and camelids tend to recover well from general anesthesia, long-bone fractures, cervical fractures, or other catastrophic injuries seldom occur. Should they occur, therapy is based on severity of the fracture and the economic value of the animal. Postoperative myopathy–neuropathy can occur in larger cattle but is not a problem in calves, sheep, goats, or camelids. The problem is recognized when muscle weakness or motor nerve dysfunction are observed, with some animals being unable to stand. Therapy is symptomatic, with IV fluids administered to maintain hydration, acid–base status, and electrolyte balance, along with analgesics and NSAIDs as indicated. Depending on the type of sling used, slinging the animal may be helpful or could increase muscle injury. Myopathy may take several days to resolve and can be life threatening. Again, it is better to prevent muscle or nerve injury by positioning anesthetized animals properly and avoiding excessive depth of anesthesia.

Recovery from anesthesia can be delayed by hypothermia. Provision of thermal support to the patient with various warming devices including circulating warm-water pads and pumps, forced-air warmers, and resistive foam warming blankets will help maintain normothermia.

A less common cause of delayed recovery is muscle weakness caused by neuromuscular blockade. Because ruminants have very low levels of pseudocholinesterase, metabolism of succinylcholine is slow, causing prolonged effects of the drug [138]. Neuromuscular blockade may also be caused by interaction of anesthetics and aminoglycoside antibiotics [139], or by incomplete reversal of non-depolarizing muscle relaxants [140]. Muscle relaxants are rarely administered to ruminants.

Thrombophlebitis can occur after perivascular injection of irritating compounds, although usually not with the frequency or severity that occurs in horses, and is treated similarly [141]. Corneal ulcers can also occur following anesthesia and should be managed as in other species [142].

Aspiration pneumonia occurs after regurgitation of rumen or gastric contents and subsequent inhalation of the material. Active regurgitation may cause the material to be inhaled deeply into the pulmonary tree, initiating bronchospasm and physical obstruction of the airways. Signs include dyspnea and, depending on severity, cyanosis. If the patient survives the initial insult, pneumonia is certain. Broad-spectrum antibiotic and anti-inflammatory therapy is indicated [143]. Silent or passive regurgitation can occur with the same results, except that there usually is not as much particulate material in the regurgitant. Similar treatment is instituted. Because of the potential severity of this complication, prevention must be emphasized. Tracheal intubation is recommended and, if not possible, the occiput should be elevated to encourage fluids to drain from the mouth rather than into the trachea (Fig. 49.3) [39].

Analgesia

Providing postoperative analgesia is an important component of veterinary anesthesia. There are very few approved drugs for provision of analgesia in domestic ruminants and none approved for use in South American camelids. Drugs that have been used in other species include the NSAIDs carprofen, flunixin, phenylbutazone, meloxicam, and ketoprofen, the opioids butorphanol, buprenorphine, fentanyl, and morphine, the local anesthetic lidocaine, and ketamine. Although α_2-adrenergic receptor agonists can provide analgesia, their behavioral effects usually limit their use in ruminants.

When applicable, local anesthetic agents can be used to desensitize structures and tissue [144]. Epidural administration of local anesthetic agents and opioids may be appropriate for some procedures.

Flunixin can be given at 1.1–2.2 mg/kg IV daily. Carprofen can be given at 0.7 mg/kg IV daily [145]. When given at 4 mg/kg, therapeutic levels are maintained for at least 72 h [145]. Ketoprofen can be dosed at 3.3 mg/kg IV daily [145]. Phenylbutazone is recommended at a dose of 2.2 mg/kg orally every 48 h [145]. However, phenylbutazone is proscribed in some populations of food animals and should be avoided unless careful regulatory compliance is assured. Meloxicam is given at 0.5 mg/kg IV every 12 h to sheep or at 1 mg/kg orally every 24 h following a loading dose of 2 mg/kg orally [146]. Meloxicam is given at 0.5 mg/kg IV every 8 h to goats or at 0.5 mg/kg orally every 24 h following a loading dose of 2 mg/kg orally [146]. Except for flunixin, withdrawal times following the use of NSAIDs in ruminants are not well defined either for meat or for milk, and caution must be exercised to prevent residues from entering the food supply [145]. More latitude is available when administering NSAIDs to ruminants used in biomedical research.

The use of all the NSAIDs carries the risk of ulcer formation in the third gastric compartment of South American camelids. When extended use of these agents is anticipated, it is recommended that dose and frequency be decreased after the desired effect is obtained in an effort to determine the minimal dose needed to provide analgesic effect. Flunixin is commonly used for analgesia in South American camelids. The dose range is 0.5–1.1 mg/kg IV given once daily [147]. Flunixin has been given at 1.1 mg/kg twice daily in some instances. Meloxicam is given at 0.5 mg/kg IV or at 1 mg orally every 3 days to camelids [146]. Phenylbutazone is less commonly used in camelids. When used, it is administered in a manner similar to that in domestic ruminants (i.e., 2.2 mg/kg orally every 48 h) [148]. Ketoprofen has also been used in llamas at a dose of 1–2 mg/kg IV once daily [149].

Opioids have been used to provide analgesia to domestic ruminants and South American camelids. Most commonly, either butorphanol (0.05–0.2 mg/kg IM every 6 h) or morphine (0.05–0.1 mg/kg IM every 6 h) has been recommended [13]. Duration of effect for both drugs is 3–6 h. The use of other opioids, such as buprenorphine, fentanyl (both injectable and transdermal), hydromorphone, and oxymorphone, may be considered in dosages similar to those used in canine or equine patients [150–153]. Transdermal fentanyl patches have been used in llamas [154]. The dose of opioids may need to be adjusted if the behavioral effects cause problems (i.e., too much sedation, dysphoria, or excessive locomotor activity).

Epidural opioids have been used extensively to provide analgesia in companion animals [150,151,155,156] and in horses [157]. Morphine, which is the most commonly used agent, is typically administered at a dose of 0.1 mg/kg to treat postoperative abdominal and orthopedic pain and to prevent tenesmus in horses [157] and camelids [38]. Analgesia begins in 30–60 min with duration of action lasting 12–24 h. Injection is typically through the sacrocaudal space but can also be made at the lumbosacral space in anesthetized ruminants. A ruminant or camelid that becomes recumbent following sacrocaudal injection should be placed in sternal recumbency. As in other species, the lumbosacral space is caudal to a line connecting the anterior border of the wings of the ilium. In camelids, one can usually easily palpate the spinous process of the last lumbar vertebra and direct the needle caudal to it to enter the space. The spinous process of the first sacral vertebra is much smaller than that of the last lumbar vertebra and is difficult to palpate. Usually, a 7 cm, 18 G spinal needle is adequate. If the injection is made at the lumbosacral space, one must aspirate prior to injection to ensure that the intrathecal space has not been entered. Dose requirements of local anesthetics are 50–70% less when an agent is given intrathecally compared with epidural injection. If cerebrospinal fluid is obtained, the local anesthetic dose must be decreased or the needle must be withdrawn for epidural placement of the drug.

Infusions of ketamine and lidocaine have been used to provide analgesia in large and small animal patients. Ketamine is effective in small animal patients when administered at a loading dose of 0.5 mg/kg IV followed by an infusion at 10 μg/kg/min [158]. Ketamine has also been given alone at 6.6–13.3 μg/kg/min IV in horses [159] and at 25 μg/kg/min after a loading dose of 1 mg/kg [160]. Ketamine can be given at 40 μg/kg/min IV to awake camelids without untoward behavioral effects and will reduce anesthetic requirements by 35% when given to anesthetized camelids [161]. Systemic lidocaine administration has been effective in reducing overall anesthetic requirements in animals under inhalation anesthesia [162–164]. The reported lidocaine loading dose ranges from 2.5 to 5 mg/kg IV followed by an infusion of 50–100 μg/kg/min [162,164]. Starting at the lower end of the range for both loading and infusion doses is recommended. The infusion should be discontinued 30 min prior to recovery to avoid prolonged recoveries.

Provision of general anesthesia and analgesia to domestic ruminants and South American camelids for complex diagnostic and surgical procedures can be very rewarding. Although each species may exhibit unique characteristics, meeting the challenges of anesthetizing a wide variety of ruminants and camelids contributes greatly to the overall veterinary care of these species.

References

1 Vallenas A, Cummings JF, Munnell JF. A gross study of the compartmentalized stomach of two new-world camelids, the llama and guanaco. *J Morphol* 1971; **143**: 399–424.

2 McGuirk SM, Bednarski RM, Clayton MK. Bradycardia in cattle deprived of food. *J Am Vet Med Assoc* 1990; **196**: 894–896.

3 Tranquilli WJ. Techniques of inhalation anesthesia in ruminants and swine. *Vet Clin North Am Food Anim Pract* 1986; **2**: 593–619.

4 Lassen ED, Pearson EG, Long PO, *et al.* Serum biochemical values in llamas: reference values. *Am J Vet Res* 1986; **47**: 2278–2280.

5 Latimer KS, Mahaffey EA, Prasse KW, eds. *Duncan and Prasse's Veterinary Laboratory Medicine: Clinical Pathology*, 4th edn. Ames, IA: Iowa State University Press, 2003; 331–342.

6 Kaneko J, Harvey JW, Bruss ML. *Clinical Biochemistry of Domestic Animals*, 5th edn. San Diego, CA: Academic Press, 1997; 890–894.

7 Kramer JW. Normal hematology of cattle, sheep, and goats. In: Feldman BF, Zinkl JG, Jain NC, eds. *Schalm's Veterinary Hematology*, 5th edn. Philadelphia, PA: Lippincott Williams & Wilkins, 2000; 1075–1088.

8 Fowler ME. *Medicine and Surgery of the South American Camelid*, 3rd edn. Ames, IA: Iowa State University Press, 2010; 89–109.

9 Amsel SI, Kainer RA, Johnson LW. Choosing the best site to perform venipuncture in a llama. *Vet Med* 1987; **82**: 535–536.

10 Heath RB. Llama anesthetic programs. *Vet Clin North Am Food Anim Pract* 1989; **5**: 71–80.

11 Riebold TW, Kaneps AJ, Schmotzer WB. Anesthesia in the llama. *Vet Surg* 1989; **18**: 400–404.

12 Short CE. Preanesthetic medications in ruminants and swine. *Vet Clin North Am Food Anim Pract* 1986; **2**: 553–566.

13 Carroll GL, Hartsfield SM. General anesthetic techniques in ruminants. *Vet Clin North Am Food Anim Pract* 1996; **12**: 627–661.

14 Taylor PM. Anaesthesia in sheep and goats. *In Pract* 1991; **13**: 31–36.

15 Greene SA, Thurmon JC. Xylazine: a review of its pharmacology and use in veterinary medicine. *J Vet Pharmacol Ther* 1988; **11**: 295–313.

16 Gray PR, McDonell WN. Anesthesia in goats and sheep. Part I. Local analgesia. *Compend Contin Educ Pract Vet* 1986; **8**(Suppl): S33–S39.

17 Raptopoulos D, Weaver BMQ. Observations following intravenous xylazine administration in steers. *Vet Rec* 1984; **114**: 567–569.

18 Trim CM. Special anesthesia considerations in the ruminant. In: Short CE, ed. *Principles and Practice of Veterinary Anesthesia*. Baltimore, MD: Williams & Wilkins, 1987; 285–300.
19 Fayed AH, Abdalla EB, Anderson RR, *et al.* Effect of xylazine in heifers under thermoneutral or heat stress conditions. *Am J Vet Res* 1989; **50**: 151–153.
20 Ley S, Waterman A, Livingston A. Variation in the analgesic effects of xylazine in different breeds of sheep. *Vet Rec* 1990; **126**: 508.
21 O'Hair KC, McNeil JS, Phillips YY. Effects of xylazine in adult sheep. *Lab Anim Sci* 1986; **36**: 563.
22 Riebold TW, Kaneps AJ, Schmotzer WB. Reversal of xylazine-induced sedation in llamas using doxapram or 4-aminopyridine and yohimbine. *J Am Vet Med Assoc* 1986; **189**: 1059–1061.
23 Aouad JI, Wright EM, Shaner TW. Anesthesia evaluation on ketamine and xylazine in calves. *Bov Pract* 1981; **2**: 22–31.
24 Campbell KB, Klavano PA, Richardson P, Alexander JE. Hemodynamic effects of xylazine in the calf. *Am J Vet Res* 1979; **40**: 1777–1780.
25 Freire ACT, Gontijo RM, Pessoa JM, Souza R. Effect of xylazine on the electrocardiogram of the sheep. *Br Vet J* 1981; **137**: 590–595.
26 Symonds HW. The effect of xylazine upon hepatic glucose production and blood flow rate in the lactating dairy cow. *Vet Rec* 1976; **99**: 234–236.
27 Symonds HW, Mallison CB. The effect of xylazine and xylazine followed by insulin on blood glucose and insulin in the dairy cow. *Vet Rec* 1978; **102**: 27–29.
28 Eichner RD, Prior RL, Kvasnicka WG. Xylazine-induced hyperglycemia in beef cattle. *Am J Vet Res* 1979; **40**: 127–129.
29 Brockman RP. Effect of xylazine on plasma glucose, glucagon and insulin concentration in sheep. *Res Vet Sci* 1981; **30**: 383–384.
30 Muggaberg J, Brockman RP. Effect of adrenergic drugs on glucose and plasma glucagon and insulin response to xylazine in sheep. *Res Vet Sci* 1982; **33**: 118–120.
31 Thurmon JC, Nelson DR, Hartsfield SM, Rumore CA. Effects of xylazine hydrochloride on urine in cattle. *Aust Vet J* 1978; **54**: 178–180.
32 Hopkins TJ. The clinical pharmacology of xylazine in cattle. *Aust Vet J* 1972; **48**: 109–112.
33 Uggla A, Lindqvist A. Acute pulmonary oedema as an adverse reaction to the use of xylazine in sheep. *Vet Rec* 1983; **113**: 42.
34 LeBlanc MM, Hubbell JAE, Smith HC. The effect of xylazine hydrochloride on intrauterine pressure in the cow and the mare. In: *Proceedings of the Annual Meeting of the Society of Theriogenolgy*, 1984; 211–220.
35 Jansen CAM, Lowe KC, Nathanielsz PW. The effects of xylazine on uterine activity, fetal and maternal oxygenation, cardiovascular function, and fetal breathing. *Am J Obstet Gynecol* 1984; **148**: 386–390.
36 Jedruch J, Gajewski Z. The effect of detomidine hydrochloride (Domosedan) on the electrical activity of the uterus in cows. *Acta Vet Scand Suppl* 1986; **82**: 189–192.
37 Abrahamsen EJ. Chemical restraint and injectable anesthesia of ruminants. *Vet Clin North Am Food Anim Pract* 2013; **29**: 209–227.
38 Riebold TW. Anesthesia in South American camelids. In: *Proceedings of the American College of Veterinary Anesthesiologists/International Veterinary Academy of Pain Management /Academy of Veterinary Technician Anesthetists Meeting*, Phoenix, AZ, 2004; 155–169.
39 Hall LW, Clarke KW. *Veterinary Anaesthesia*, 9th edn. London: Baillière Tindall, 1991; 236–259.
40 Greene SA. Protocols for anesthesia of cattle. *Vet Clin North Am Food Anim Pract* 2003; **19**: 679–693.
41 Waldridge BM, Lin HC, DeGraves FJ, Pugh DG. Sedative effects of medetomidine and its reversal by atipamezole in llamas. *J Am Vet Med Assoc* 1997; **211**: 1562–1565.
42 Gray PR. Anesthesia in goats and sheep. Part II. General anesthesia. *Compend Contin Educ Pract Vet* 1986; **8**(**Suppl**): S127–S135.
43 Cebra CK, Tornquist SJ. Meta-analysis of glucose tolerance in llamas and alpacas [Abstract]. In: *Proceedings of the Fourth European Symposium on South American Camelids*, Göttingen, 2004; **27**.
44 Celly CS, McDonell WN, Young SS, Black WD. The comparative hypoxaemic effect of four α_2 adrenoceptor agonists (xylazine, romifidine, detomidine and medetomidine) in sheep. *J Vet Pharmacol Ther* 1997; **20**: 464–471.
45 Marzok M, El-Khodery S. Sedative and analgesic effects of romifidine in camels (*Camelus dromedarius*). *J Vet Anaesth Analg* 2009; **36**: 352–360.
46 Rioja E, Kerr CL, Enouri SS, McDonell WN. Sedative and cardiopulmonary effects of medetomidine hydrochloride and xylazine hydrochloride and their reversal with atipamezole hydrochloride in calves. *Am J Vet Res* 2008; **69**: 319–329.
47 Kitzman JV, Booth NH, Hatch RC, Wallner B. Antagonism of xylazine sedation by 4-aminopyridine and yohimbine in cattle. *Am J Vet Res* 1982; **43**: 2165–2169.
48 Thurmon JC, Lin HC, Tranquilli WJ, *et al.* A comparison of yohimbine and tolazoline as antagonists of xylazine sedation in calves [Abstract]. *Vet Surg* 1989; **18**: 170–171.
49 Hsu WH, Hanson CE, Hembrough FB, Schaffer DD. Effects of idazoxan, tolazoline, and yohimbine on xylazine-induced respiratory changes and central nervous system depression in ewes. *Am J Vet Res* 1989; **50**: 1570–1573.
50 Ko JCH, McGrath CJ. Effects of atipamezole and yohimbine on medetomidine-induced central nervous system depression and cardiorespiratory changes in lambs. *Am J Vet Res* 1995; **56**: 629–632.
51 Ruckenbusch Y, Toutain PL. Specific antagonism of xylazine effects on reticulo-rumen motor function in cattle. *Vet Med Rev* 1984; **5**: 3–12.
52 Young DB, Shawley RV, Barron SJ. Tolazoline reversal of xylazine–ketamine anesthesia in calves [Abstract]. *Vet Surg* 1988; **18**: 171.
53 Read MR, Duke T, Toews AR. Suspected tolazoline toxicosis in a llama. *J Am Vet Med Assoc* 2000; **216**: 227–229.
54 Lewis CA, Constable PD, Hun JC, Morin DE. Sedation with xylazine and lumbosacral epidural administration of lidocaine and xylazine for umbilical surgery in calves. *J Am Vet Med Assoc* 1999; **214**: 89–95.
55 Doherty TJ, Ballinger JA, McDonell WN, *et al.* Antagonism of xylazine-induced sedation by idazoxan in calves. *Can J Vet Res* 1987; **51**: 244–248.
56 Zahner JM, Hatch RC, Wilson RC, *et al.* Antagonism of xylazine sedation in steers by doxapram and 4-aminopyridine. *Am J Vet Res* 1984; **45**: 2546–2551.
57 Valverde A, Doherty TJ, Dyson D, Valliant AE. Evaluation of pentobarbital as a drug for standing sedation in cattle. *Vet Surg* 1989; **18**: 235–238.
58 Stegmann GF. Observations on the use of midazolam for sedation, and induction of anaesthesia with midazolam in combination with ketamine in the goat. *J S Afr Vet Assoc* 1998; **69**: 89–92.
59 Stegmann GF, Bester L. Sedative–hypnotic effects of midazolam in goats after intravenous and intramuscular administration. *J Vet Anaesth Analg* 2001; **28**: 49–55.
60 Kyles AE, Waterman AE, Livingston A. Antinociceptive activity of midazolam in sheep. *J Vet Pharmacol Ther* 1995; **18**: 54–60.
61 Aarnes TK, Fry PR, Hubbell JAE, *et al.* Pharmacokinetics and pharmacodynamics of midazolam after intravenous and intramuscular administration in alpacas. *Am J Vet Res* 2013; **74**: 294–299.
62 O'Hair KC, Dodd KT, Phillips YY, Beattie RJ. Cardiopulmonary effects of nalbuphine hydrochloride and butorphanol tartrate in sheep. *Lab Anim Sci* 1988; **38**: 58–61.
63 Waterman AE, Livingston A, Amin A. Analgesic activity and respiratory effects of butorphanol in sheep. *Res Vet Sci* 1991; **51**: 19–23.
64 Barrington GM, Meyer TF, Parish SM. Standing castration of the llama using butorphanol tartrate and local anesthesia. *Equine Pract* 1993; **15**: 35–39.
65 Abrahamsen EJ. Chemical restraint, anesthesia and analgesia for camelids. *Vet Clin North Am Food Anim Pract* 2009; **25**: 455–494.
66 Rouse S. Pharmacodynamics of thiobarbiturates. *Vet Anesth* 1978; **5**: 22–26.
67 Pascoe PJ. Emergency care medicine. In: Short CE, ed. *Principles and Practice of Veterinary Anesthesia*. Baltimore, MD: Williams & Wilkins, 1987; 558–598.
68 Chaplin MD, Roszkowski AP, Richards RK. Displacement of thiopental from plasma proteins by nonsteroidal anti-inflammatory agents. *Proc Soc Exp Biol Med* 1973; **143**: 667–671.
69 Blaze CA, Holland RE, Grant AL. Gas exchange during xylazine–ketamine anesthesia in neonatal calves. *Vet Surg* 1988; **17**: 155–159.
70 Thurmon JC, Benson GJ. Anesthesia in ruminants and swine. In: Howard JC, ed. *Current Veterinary Therapy 3: Food Animal Practice*, 3rd edn. Philadelphia, PA: WB Saunders, 1993; 58–76.
71 Coulson NM. The cardiorespiratory effects of diazepem/ketamine and xylazine/ketamine anesthetic combinations in sheep. *Lab Anim Sci* 1989; **39**: 591–597.
72 Raekallio M, Kivalo M, Jalanka H, Vainio O. Medetomidine/ketamine sedation in calves and its reversal with atipamezole. *J Vet Anaesth* 1991; **18**: 45–47.
73 DuBois WR, Prado TM, Ko JCH, *et al.* A comparison of two intramuscular doses of xylazine–ketamine combination and tolazoline reversal in llamas. *J Vet Anaesth Analg* 2004; **31**: 90–96.
74 Grandy JL, McDonell WN. Evaluation of concentrated solutions of guaifenesin for equine anesthesia. *J Am Vet Med Assoc* 1980; **176**: 619–622.
75 Thurmon JC. Injectable anesthetic agents and techniques in ruminants and swine. *Vet Clin North Am Food Anim Pract* 1986; **2**: 567–592.
76 Wall R, Muir WW. Hemolytic potential of guaifenesin in cattle. *Cornell Vet* 1990; **80**: 209–216.
77 Thurmon JC, Benson GJ, Tranquilli WJ, Olson WA. Cardiovascular effects of intravenous infusion of guaifenesin, ketamine, and xylazine in Holstein calves [Abstract]. *Vet Surg* 1986; **15**: 463.
78 Kerr CL, Windeyer C, Boure LP, *et al.* Cardiopulmonary effects of administration of a combination solution of xylazine, guaifenesin, and ketamine or inhaled isoflurane in mechanically ventilated calves. *Am J Vet Res* 2007; **68**: 1287–1293.
79 Lin HC, Tyler JW, Welles EG, *et al.* Effects of anesthesia induced and maintained by continuous intravenous administration of guaifenesin, ketamine, and xylazine in spontaneously breathing sheep. *Am J Vet Res* 1993; **54**: 1913–1916.
80 Tracy CH, Short CE, Clark BC. Comparing the effects of intravenous and intramuscular administration of Telazol®. *Vet Med* 1988; **83**: 104–111.
81 Hubbell JAE, Muir WW. Xylazine and tiletamine–zolazepam anesthesia in horses. *Am J Vet Res* 1989; **50**: 737–742.

82 Lin HC, Thurmon JC, Benson GJ, *et al*. The hemodynamic response of calves to tiletamine–zolazepam anesthesia. *Vet Surg* 1989; **18**: 328–334.

83 Thurmon JC, Lin HC, Benson GJ, *et al*. Combining Telazol® and xylazine for anesthesia in calves. *Vet Med* 1989; **84**: 824–830.

84 Conner GH, Coppock RW, Beck CC. Laboratory use of CI-744, a cataleptoid anesthetic, in sheep. *Vet Med Small Anim Clin* 1974; **69**: 479–482.

85 Lagutchik MS, Januszkiewicz AJ, Dodd KT, Martin DG. Cardiopulmonary effects of a tiletamine–zolazepam combination in sheep. *Am J Vet Res* 1991; **52**: 1441–1447.

86 Howard BW, Lagutchik MS, Januszkiewicz AJ, Martin DG. The cardiovascular response of sheep to tiletamine–zolazepam and butorphanol tartrate anesthesia. *Vet Surg* 1990; **19**: 461–467.

87 Klein LV, Tomasic M, Olsen K. Evaluation of Telazol® in llamas [Abstract]. *Vet Surg* 1990; **19**: 316–317.

88 Prado TM, Doherty TJ, Boggan EB, *et al*. Effects of acepromazine and butorphanol on tiletamine–zolazepam anesthesia in llamas. *Am J Vet Res* 2008; **69**: 182–188.

89 Seddighi R, Elliot SB, Whitlock BK, *et al*. Physiologic and antinociceptive effects following intramuscular administration of xylazine hydrochloride in combination with tiletamine–zolazepam in llamas. *Am J Vet Res* 2013; **74**: 530–534.

90 Waterman AE. Use of propofol in sheep. *Vet Rec* 1988; **122**: 260.

91 Nolan AM, Reid J, Welsh E. The use of propofol as an induction agent in goats [Abstract]. *J Vet Anaesth* 1991; **18**: 53–54.

92 Handel IG, Weaver BMQ, Staddon GE, Cruz Madorran JI. Observation on the pharmacokinetics of propofol in sheep. In: *Proceedings of the Fourth International Congress of Veterinary Anesthesia*, Utrecht, 1991; **143–154**.

93 Correia D, Nolan AM, Reid J. Pharmacokinetics of propofol infusions, either alone or with ketamine, in sheep premedicated with acepromazine and papaveretum. *Res Vet Sci* 1996; **60**: 213–217.

94 Duke T, Egger CM, Ferguson JG, Frketic MM. Cardiopulmonary effects of propofol infusion in llamas. *Am J Vet Res* 1997; **58**: 153–156.

95 Camburn MA. Use of alphazalone–alphadolone in ruminants. *Vet Rec* 1982; **111**: 166–167.

96 Andaluz A, Felez-Ocana N, Santos L, *et al*. The effects on cardio-respiratory and acid–base variables of the anaesthetic alfaxalone in a 2-hydroxypropyl-β-cyclodextrin (HPCD) formulation in sheep. *Vet J* 2012; **191**: 389–392.

97 Walsh VP, Gieseg M, Singh PM, *et al*. A comparison of two different ketamine and diazepam combinations with an alphaxalone and medetomidine combination for induction of anaesthesia in sheep. *N Z Vet J* 2012; **60**: 136–141.

98 del Alamo A, Mandsager R, Riebold T, Payton M. Anesthetic evaluation of administration of intravenous alfaxalone in comparison with propofol and ketamine/diazepam in alpacas [Abstract]. In: *Proceedings of the American College of Veterinary Anesthesiologists Meeting*, San Antonio, TX, 2012; **725**.

99 Hubbell JAE, Hull BL, Muir WW. Perianesthetic considerations in cattle. *Compend Contin Educ Pract Vet* 1986; **8**: F92–F102.

100 Kinyon GE. A new device for topical anesthesia. *Anesthesiology* 1982; **56**: 154–155.

101 Lagutchik MS, Mundie TG, Martin DG. Methemoglobinemia induced by a benzocaine-based topically administered anesthetic in eight sheep. *J Am Vet Med Assoc* 1992; **201**: 1407–1410.

102 Quandt JE, Robinson EP. Nasotracheal intubation in calves. *J Am Vet Med Assoc* 1996; **209**: 967–968.

103 Riebold TW, Engel HN, Grubb TL, *et al*. Anatomical considerations during intubation of the llama: the presence of a nasopharyngeal diverticulum. *J Am Vet Med Assoc* 1994; **204**: 779–783.

104 Wertz EA. A new parenteral anesthetic regime for llamas. In: *Proceedings of the Llama Medicine Workshop for Veterinarians*, Colorado State University, Fort Collins, CO, March 1993.

105 Moll X, Santos L, Garcia F, Andaluz A. The effects on cardio-respiratory and acid–base variable of a constant rate infusion of alfaxalone–HPCD in sheep. *Vet J* 2013; **196**: 209–212.

106 Granados MM, Dominguez JM, Fernandez-Sarmiento A, *et al*. Anaesthetic and cardiorespiratory effects of a constant-rate infusion of alfaxalone in desflurane-anaesthetised sheep. *Vet Rec* 2012; **171**: 125.

107 O'Brien TD, Raffe MR, Cox VS, *et al*. Hepatic necrosis following halothane anesthesia in goats. *J Am Vet Med Assoc* 1986; **189**: 1591–1595.

108 McEwan M-M, Gleed RD, Ludders JW, *et al*. Hepatic effects of halothane and isoflurane anesthesia in goats. *J Am Vet Med Assoc* 2000; **217**: 1697–1700.

109 Mathews K, Doherty T, Dyson D, *et al*. Nephrotoxicity in dogs associated with methoxyflurane anesthesia and flunixin meglumine analgesia. *Can Vet J* 1990; **31**: 766–771.

110 White NA. Postanesthetic recumbency myopathy in horses. *Compend Contin Educ Pract Vet* 1982; **4**(Suppl): S44–S52.

111 Riebold TW, Evans AT, Robinson NE. Evaluation of the demand valve for resuscitation of horses. *J Am Vet Med Assoc* 1980; **176**: 1736–1742.

112 Watney GCG, Watkins SB, Hall LW. Effects of a demand valve on pulmonary ventilation in spontaneously breathing, anaesthetized horses. *Vet Rec* 1985; **117**: 358–362.

113 Gabel AA, Heath RB, Ross JN, *et al*. Hypoxia: its prevention in inhalation anesthesia in horses. In: *Proceedings of the 12th Annual Meeting of the American Association of Equine Practitioners*, Los Angeles, CA, 1966; 179–196.

114 Cribb PH. The effects of prolonged hypotensive isoflurane anesthesia in horses: post-anesthetic myopathy [Abstract]. *Vet Surg* 1988; **17**: 164.

115 Grandy JL, Steffey EP, Hodgson DS, Woliner MJ. Arterial hypotension and the development of postanesthetic myopathy in halothane-anesthetized horses. *Am J Vet Res* 1987; **48**: 192–197.

116 Grandy JL, Hodgson DS, Dunlop CI, *et al*. Cardiopulmonary effects of ephedrine in halothane-anesthetized horses. *J Vet Pharmacol Ther* 1989; **12**: 389–396.

117 Daunt DA. Supportive therapy in the anesthetized horse. *Vet Clin North Am Equine Pract* 1990; **6**: 557–574.

118 Tranquilli WJ, Greene SA. Cardiovascular medications and the autonomic nervous system. In: Short CE, ed. *Principles and Practice of Veterinary Anesthesia*. Baltimore, MD: Williams & Wilkins, 1987; 426–454.

119 Manley SV. Monitoring the anesthetized horse. *Vet Clin North Am Large Anim Pract* 1981; **3**: 111–134.

120 Gallivan GJ, McDonell WN, Forrest JB. Comparative ventilation and gas exchange in the horse and cow. *Res Vet Sci* 1989; **46**: 331–336.

121 Thurmon JC, Romack FE, Garner HE. Excursion of the bovine eyeball during gaseous anesthesia. *Vet Med Small Anim Clin* 1968; **63**: 967–970.

122 Matthews NS, Gleed RD, Short CE. Cardiopulmonary effects of general anesthesia in adult cattle. *Mod Vet Pract* 1986; **67**: 618–620.

123 Grandy JL, Hodgson DS. Anesthetic considerations for emergency equine abdominal surgery. *Vet Clin North Am Equine Pract* 1988; **4**: 63–78.

124 Aarnes T, Hubbell JAE, Lerche P, Bednarski R. Comparison of invasive and oscillometric blood pressure measurement techniques in sheep, goats, and cattle anesthetized for surgery [Abstract]. In: *Proceedings of the American College of Veterinary Anesthesiologists Meeting*, San Antonio, TX, 2012.

125 Aarnes TK, Hubbell JAE, Lerche P, Bednarski RM. Comparison of invasive and oscillometric blood pressure measurement techniques in anesthetized camelids. *Can Vet J* 2012; **53**: 881–885.

126 Riebold TW, Evans AT. Comparison of simultaneous blood pressure determinations by four methods in the anesthetized horse. *Vet Surg* 1985; **14**: 332–337.

127 Riebold TW, Brunson DB, Lott RA, Evans AT. Percutaneous arterial catheterization in the horse. *Vet Med Small Anim Clin* 1980; **75**: 1736–1742.

128 Moens YP, Gootjes P, Lagerweij E. The influence of methane on the infrared measurement of halothane in the horse. *J Vet Anaesth* 1991; **18**: 4–7.

129 Gootjes P, Moens YP. A simple method to correct infrared measurement of anaesthetic vapour concentration in the presence of methane. *J Vet Anaesth* 1997; **24**: 24–25.

130 Kruse-Elliott KT, Riebold TW, Swanson CR. Reversal of xylazine–ketamine anesthesia in goats [Abstract]. *Vet Surg* 1987; **16**: 321.

131 Masewe VA, Gillespie JR, Berry JD. Influence of ruminal insufflation on pulmonary function and diaphragmatic electromyography in cattle. *Am J Vet Res* 1979; **40**: 26–31.

132 Lumb WV, Jones EW. *Veterinary Anesthesia*, 2nd edn. Philadelphia, PA: Lea & Febiger, 1984; 213–239.

133 Heath RB. General anesthesia in ruminants. In: Jennings PB, ed. *The Practice of Large Animal Surgery*. Philadelphia, PA: WB Saunders, 1984; 202–204.

134 Short CE, Rebhun WC. Complications caused by the oculocardiac reflex during anesthesia in the foal. *J Am Vet Med Assoc* 1980; **176**: 630–631.

135 Muir WW, Bednarski RM. Equine cardiopulmonary resuscitation. Part I. *Compend Contin Educ Pract Vet* 1983; **5**(Suppl): S228–S234.

136 Muir WW, Bednarski RM. Equine cardiopulmonary resuscitation. Part II. *Compend Contin Educ Pract Vet* 1983; **5**(Suppl):S287–S295.

137 Hubbell JAE, Muir WW, Gaynor JS. Cardiovascular effects of thoracic compression in horses subjected to euthanasia. *Equine Vet J* 1993; **25**: 282–284.

138 Tavernor WD. Muscle relaxants. In: Soma LR, ed. *Veterinary Anesthesia*. Baltimore, MD: Williams & Wilkins, 1971; 111–120.

139 Adams HR, Teske RH, Mercer HD. Anesthetic–antibiotic relationships. *J Am Vet Med Assoc* 1976; **169**: 409–412.

140 Hildebrand S. Neuromuscular blocking agents in equine anesthesia. *Vet Clin North Am Equine Pract* 1990; **6**: 587–606.

141 Courley KTT. Fluid therapy for horses with gastrointestinal disease. In: Smith BP, ed. *Large Animal Internal Medicine*, 3rd edn. St Louis, MO: Mosby, 2002; 682–694.

142 Whitley RD, Vygantas DR. Ocular trauma. In: Smith BP, ed. *Large Animal Internal Medicine*, 3rd edn. St Louis, MO: Mosby, 2002; 1159–1164.

143 Ames TR, Baker JC, Wikse SE. The bronchopneumonias (respiratory disease complex of cattle, sheep, and goats). In: Smith BP, ed. *Large Animal Internal Medicine*, 3rd edn. St Louis, MO: Mosby, 2002; 551–570.

144 Skarda RT. Local and regional anesthesia in ruminants and swine. *Vet Clin North Am Food Anim Pract* 1996; **12**: 579–626.

145 George LW. Pain control in food animals. In: Steffey EP, ed. *Recent Advances in Anesthetic Management of Large Domestic Animals.* Ithaca, NY: International Veterinary Information Service, 2003; A0615.1103.

146 Plummer PJ, Schleining JA. Assessment and management of pain in small ruminants and camelids. *Vet Clin North Am Food Anim Pract* 2013; **29**: 185–208.

147 Navarre CB, Ravis WR, Nagilla R, *et al.* Pharmacokinetics of flunixin meglumine in llamas following a single intravenous dose. *J Vet Pharmacol Ther* 2001; **24**: 361–364.

148 Navarre CB, Ravis WR, Nagilla R, *et al.* Pharmacokinetics of phenylbutazone in llamas following single intravenous and oral doses. *J Vet Pharmacol Ther* 2001; **24**: 227–231.

149 Navarre CB, Ravis WR, Campbell J, *et al.* Stereoselective pharmacokinetics of ketoprofen in llamas following intravenous administration. *J Vet Pharmacol Ther* 2001; **24**: 223–226.

150 Wagner AE. Opioids. In: Muir WW, Gaynor JS, eds. *Handbook of Veterinary Pain Management.* St Louis, MO: Mosby, 2002; 164–183.

151 Pascoe PJ. Opioid analgesics. *Vet Clin North Am Small Anim Pract* 2000; **30**: 757–772.

152 Bennett RC, Steffey EP. Use of opioids for pain and anesthetic management in horses. *Vet Clin North Am Equine Pract* 2002; **18**: 47–60.

153 Zimmel DN. How to manage pain and dehydration in horses with colic. In: *Proceedings of the 49th Annual Meeting of the American Association of Equine Practitioners*, New Orleans, LA, 2003; 127–131.

154 Grubb T, Gold J, Schlipf JW, *et al.* Assessment of serum concentrations and sedative effects of fentanyl after transdermal administration at three dosages in healthy llamas. *Am J Vet Res* 2005; **66**: 907–909.

155 Torske KE, Dyson DH. Epidural analgesia and anesthesia. *Vet Clin North Am Small Anim Pract* 2000; **30**: 859–874.

156 Gaynor JS, Mama KR. Local and regional anesthetic techniques for alleviation of perioperative pain. In: Muir WW, Gaynor JS, eds. *Handbook of Veterinary Pain Management.* St Louis, MO: Mosby, 2002; 261–280.

157 Robinson EP, Natalini CC. Epidural anesthesia and analgesia in horses. *Vet Clin North Am Equine Pract* 2002; **18**: 61–82.

158 Wagner AE, Walton JA, Hellyer PW, *et al.* Use of low doses of ketamine administered by constant rate infusion as an adjunct for postoperative analgesia in dogs. *J Am Vet Med Assoc* 2002; **221**: 72–75.

159 Matthews NS, Fielding CL, Swinebroad EL. How to use a ketamine constant rate infusion in horses for analgesia. In: *Proceedings of the 50th Annual Meeting of the American Association of Equine Practitioners*, Denver, CO, 2004; 227–228.

160 Queiroz-Castro P, Egger C, Redua MA, *et al.* Effects of ketamine and magnesium on the minimum alveolar concentration of isoflurane in goats. *Am J Vet Res* 2006; **67**: 1962–1966.

161 Schlipf JW Jr, Eaton K, Fulkerson P, *et al.* Constant rate infusion of ketamine reduces minimum alveolar concentration of isoflurane in alpacas [Abstract]. In: *Proceedings of the American College of Veterinary Anesthesiologists/International Veterinary Academy of Pain Management/Academy of Veterinary Technician Anesthetists Meeting*, Phoenix, AZ, 2004; 58.

162 Doherty TJ, Frazier D. Effect of intravenous lidocaine on halothane minimum alveolar concentration in ponies. *Equine Vet J* 1998; **30**: 300–303.

163 Valverde A, Doherty TJ, Hernandez J, Davies W. Effect of lidocaine on the minimum alveolar concentration of isoflurane in dogs. *J Vet Anaesth Analg* 2004; **31**: 264–271.

164 Doherty T, Redua MA, Queiroz-Castro P, *et al.* Effect of intravenous lidocaine and ketamine on isoflurane minimum alveolar concentration in goats. *Vet Anaesth Analg* 2007; **34**: 125–131.

50 Swine

Lais M. Malavasi
Department of Veterinary Clinical Sciences, College of Veterinary Medicine, Washington State University, Pullman, Washington, USA

Chapter contents

Preanesthetic considerations

Handling and restraint

Pigs are considered difficult animals to restrain because of their body shape and lack of appendages that can be readily grasped by handlers [1]. However, restraint can be facilitated by adapting the pig to human presence and manipulation, resulting in a less stressful environment. Since pigs can be very sensitive to stress, it is imperative for researchers to have their animals acclimatized at their institution 2–3 weeks prior to the experiment [2]. During this time, the pigs should be spoken to and handled in a calm manner. However, if time is limited and the animal is not trained, it can be isolated in a corner using a partition known as a 'hog board.' This partition may be constructed of wood or metal and should be the same height as the animal and two-thirds to the full length of the pig. The hog board is used to protect the handler during examination or intramuscular injection.

Pigs can be restrained using other methods as well. For piglets, the animal's hind legs can be lifted by one hand while the other is placed under the chest to provide support. However, pigs weighing more than 10 kg can be very strong and difficult to lift. These swine can be guided into a transport cart or coaxed out of the pen and into the cart with food. Another method of immobilization is the sling, where the pig is placed in a hammock with four holes for the limbs. This hammock is supported by a metal frame to which its limbs are loosely tied. One disadvantage is that the pig must be trained to use of the sling. Handlers can use a snout snare to temporarily restrain a pig for injections. However, the snare is not comfortable, as it acts like a tourniquet around the pig's snout and it is difficult to train a pig to accept. A snout snare should not be left on for more than a few minutes. In addition, only smooth rope or cable should be used, as a frayed cable can cut into the pig's nose.

Drug administration

Pigs have limited superficial veins that can be accessed easily to inject drugs. The marginal ear veins (i.e., auricular veins) are the only veins that are easily visible on pigs of any size (Fig. 50.1). In larger animals the lateral and medial veins on the outer surface of the ears are preferable because of their increased size. The central auricular vessels are usually arteries (as in the rabbit). Note that ear notching to identify pigs can damage some of these vessels.

Another option for venous access is the cephalic vein located, as in the dog, along the cranial surface of the leg before it crosses the ventral neck and enters the thoracic inlet. This vein usually cannot be visualized but may be entered using blind venepuncture after applying a tourniquet [3]. In small pigs it may be visualized across the ventral surface of the neck after applying digital pressure at the thoracic inlet. The saphenous vein, on the lateral surface of the rear leg, is usually not a reliable injection site. Larger vessels such as the external or internal jugular vein or anterior vena cava can be cannulated but are usually reserved for blood sample collection [4]. However, these latter options are most likely to be used for fluid therapy in pigs that are already under sedation or general anesthesia.

Under field conditions it is preferable to administer drugs for sedation and anesthesia either intraperitoneally or intramuscularly [5,6]. Intraperitoneal injection is considered cumbersome since it

Veterinary Anesthesia and Analgesia: The Fifth Edition of Lumb and Jones.
Edited by Kurt A. Grimm, Leigh A. Lamont, William J. Tranquilli, Stephen A. Greene and Sheilah A. Robertson.

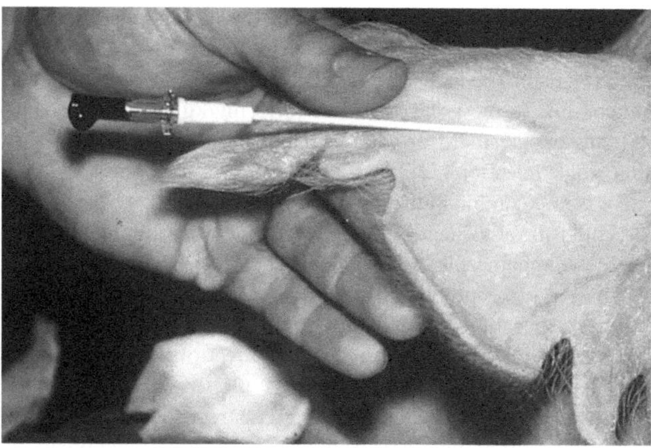

Figure 50.1 Cannulation of the auricular vein of a Landrace sow with a 16 gauge catheter. A tourniquet has been placed at the base of the ear to distend the veins.

requires specific training. Also, the consequences of improper administration can be severe if injection into the urinary bladder, intestines or other organs occurs [5]. For intramuscular injection in pigs, the muscles of the thigh are commonly used as the site of injection in piglets, but are not recommended in growers/finishers because of the possibility of causing an abscess or needle breakage in edible tissue. Appropriate intramuscular administration in adult pigs is behind the base of the ear where the layer of fat is thinner and the tissues have better perfusion [7]. Adequate needle size varies with the size of the animal, from a 20 G needle for a piglet up to a 14 G needle for a grower/finisher pig. This is important since shorter needles may result in injection of the drug into the fatty tissue, delaying the absorption, distribution and ultimately the action of the anesthetic agent [1].

Subcutaneous injection can be used in smaller or miniature pigs (e.g., Yorkshire and Yucatan). As pigs have very tight connective tissue, there are limited areas for subcutaneous injection such as the loose flap on the lateral cervical region [2,8]. It is advisable to slide the needle under the skin away from the site of skin puncture before depositing the compound to ensure proper injection.

Intranasal delivery can be used as a needleless route of drug administration in piglets. For example, Axiak described intranasal administration of a mixture of ketamine 15 mg/kg, climazolam 1.5 mg/kg and azaperone 1.0 mg/kg, 10 min prior to castration. Intranasal administration resulted in less effective anesthesia than intramuscular injection, but with the advantages of minor temperature loss and shorter recovery time [9]. Additionally, Lacoste and co-workers reported that optimal intranasal midazolam dose in piglets was 0.2 mg/kg, which produced rapid and reliable sedation [10].

Fasting

The presurgical fasting time for pigs should be at least 12 h. If the stomach is full, it may increase the risk of gastric dilation and regurgitation of food which may be aspirated, resulting in pneumonia. After 12 h of fasting, the stomach still contains food, due to the torus pyloricus which is well developed in pigs. An overloaded stomach can produce significant pressure on the diaphragm, decreasing the pulmonary functional residual capacity and alveolar ventilation [1]. When the surgical objective is to manipulate gastrointestinal or abdominal organs, the fasting time should be increased to 24–48 h to empty the large bowel. Neonates should be deprived of food for only 3 h in order to prevent hypoglycemia. All edible bedding must be removed from the cage in the fasting period, because pigs will readily consume it otherwise [11]. Water consumption is allowed until premedication is imminent although it will be restricted for 4–6 h if the pig is going to be submitted to stomach or upper small bowel surgery [4].

Premedication

The veterinary surgical procedures in pigs performed under field conditions are usually limited to minor operations such as hernia repair and castration [6]. In contrast, when used in biomedical research, the animal may be subjected to complicated and invasive surgical procedures that require more advanced analgesia and anesthesia techniques.

Parasympatholytic drugs

Atropine sulfate and glycopyrrolate are the two principal parasympatholytic drugs used in pigs. The use of these anticholinergic agents together with sedative/analgesic premedications may have a protective effect in domestic pigs and should be considered in Vietnamese pot-bellied pigs [12,13]. In some cases it may be helpful to decrease the possibility of bradycardia caused by such agents as morphine, thiopental, and xylazine [14,15]. Also, anticholinergic agents can avoid bronchoconstriction, diminish airway secretion volume and inhibit salivation that can create conditions for an easier orotracheal intubation. However, neither anticholinergic agent is routinely required.

During field anesthesia where orotracheal intubation will not occur, the use of these drugs will be limited to treating pre-existing bradycardia (heart rate less than 50 bpm) with atropine 0.02–0.05 mg/kg given IM or IV or glycopyrrolate 0.004–0.01 mg/kg given IM or IV. Anticholinergic agents increase heart rate and thus myocardial work and oxygen consumption. Since pigs have a normal heart rate between 60 to 120 bpm, higher rates can lead to other arrhythmias that, when not properly dealt with, may result in cardiac arrest. For pigs with pre-existing tachycardia caused by fever, extreme excitement or hyperthyroidism, anticholinergic agents should be avoided unless necessary for treatment of complications [1].

There is an alternative route of administering atropine in emergency situations to pigs that do not have an intravenous catheter. Hörnchen *et al.* concluded that 2 mg of atropine diluted in 5–10 mL of saline and instilled in the endotracheal tube was rapidly absorbed by the pulmonary circulation and increased heart rate within 1 min after administration [16]. The improvement in heart rate was found to occur between 9 and 30 min after endotracheal instillation compared to 12–15 min after IV injection.

Sedation

Anesthetic management of pigs can be complicated due to their behavior when physically restrained and the small number of vessels available for IV injections. Thus, IM administration of drugs is preferred for immobilization, and in some situations for induction of anesthesia in pigs. The major classes of drugs that are commonly used are the dissociative agents, tranquillizers (benzodiazepines, azaperone, acepromazine, droperidol) and the α_2-adrenergic receptor agonists [17]. The degree of sedation varies and hence the choice of agent is determined by the needs of the patient and anesthetist. As azaperone, acepromazine and the benzodiazepines offer little or no analgesia, these drugs should be given in combination with other agents to obtain adequate anesthesia and analgesia for various surgical procedures done in pigs.

Ketamine is the most used dissociative anesthetic in almost all the species, including human, non-human primates, cats, laboratory animals, and pigs. Ketamine is considered to have a wide safety margin and it generally causes minimal cardiovascular depression or it may stimulate cardiovascular function via its sympathomimetic effect [15,18]. The other advantage is that it can be given intramuscularly as well as intravenously, resulting in use when venous access is difficult to achieve. However, dissociative agents given alone can cause incomplete analgesia (somatic analgesia but no visceral analgesia) and muscle relaxation, often referred to as a cataleptoid state, and produce excessive salivation and hyperresponsiveness during recovery [1,3]. To minimize these negative effects, ketamine is combined with adjunctive agents to improve muscle relaxation and analgesia, which also decrease the ketamine dose required to achieve effective immobilization (Table 50.1).

α_2-Adrenergic receptor agonists, such as xylazine, romifidine, medetomidine, and dexmedetomidine, are agents that are used in pigs. Note that pigs are much more resistant to α_2-adrenergic receptor agonists than ruminants. Ketamine at a dose of 10–12 mg/kg IM with a dose of 1–2 mg/kg of xylazine will immobilize a pig in approximately 5 min [19]. However, this combination decreases the cardiac output significantly for 30 min after administration and the arterial partial pressure of oxygen (PaO_2) may decrease, whereas total vascular resistance increases [20]. Ketamine at a lower dose of 10 mg/kg IM, combined with medetomidine (0.1 mg/kg IM), gives better analgesia and fewer side-effects [6]. Sakaguchi *et al.* demonstrated that ketamine (10 mg/kg) and medetomidine (80 μg/kg) IM induced a chemical restraint of 49.4 min on average, which was 14.8 min longer than the xylazine (2 mg/kg) and ketamine (10 mg/kg) combination [21]. Another improvement provided by substituting medetomidine for xylazine is that the duration of muscle relaxation in pigs is twice as long as with the xylazine and ketamine mixture.

Table 50.1 Combination of drugs used as premedication in pigs and their dosages.

Drug	Dose (mg/kg)	Route	Primary references
Parasympatholytic agents			
Atropine	0.02–0.05	IM, IV	[1]
Glycopyrrolate	0.004–0.01	IM, IV	
Sedative and tranquilizer combinations			
Ketamine plus	10–12	IM	[19]
xylazine	1–2		
Ketamine plus	10	IM	[6]
medetomidine	0.08–0.1		
Ketamine plus	8	IM	[22]
romifidine plus	0.12		
butorphanol	0.1		
Ketamine plus	20	IM	[15]
xylazine plus	2		
midazolam	0.25		
Ketamine plus	10	IM	[25]
medetomidine plus	0.08		
butorphanol	0.2		
Ketamine plus	25	IM	[27]
xylazine plus	2.5		
tramadol	5		
Azaperone plus	4	IM	[11]
midazolam	1		
Azaperone plus	2	IM	[29]
xylazine	2		
Azaperone plus	2	IM	[30]
ketamine plus	15		
midazolam	0.3		
Acepromazine	0.03–0.1	IM	[3]

IM = intramuscular; IV = intravenous.

Sakaguchi *et al.* studied ketamine and medetomidine combined with 25 μg/kg of atropine and concluded that the cardiovascular effects were limited in healthy pigs [21]. Alternatively, a combination of ketamine (8 mg/kg), romifidine (0.12 mg/kg) and butorphanol (0.1 mg/kg) given IM provides reliable anesthesia for 20–30 min after single injection [22].

All of the combinations containing α_2-adrenergic receptor agonists offer the advantage of being reversible by yohimbine (0.1 mg/kg IM) or atipamezole (0.12 mg/kg IM) [23,24]. The reversal of the α_2-adrenergic receptor agonist is independent from the metabolism and clearance of ketamine. Therefore, when the α_2-adrenergic receptor agonist is reversed before the effect of the ketamine has waned, a undesirable recovery may result (e.g., hyperkinesia of limbs, severe and prolonged ataxia, and distress vocalization) [13].

Adding another muscle relaxant drug to anesthetic combinations should provide a better recovery following reversal of α_2-adrenergic agonists. Ajadi *et al.* reported using ketamine at 20 mg/kg IM with xylazine (2 mg/kg IM) and midazolam (0.25 mg/kg IM). This combination appeared to almost double the duration of the anesthesia period with adequate analgesia for at least 30 min compared to a lower dose of ketamine (10 mg/kg IM) added to this same combination of drugs [15]. However, recoveries after benzodiazepine-ketamine combinations are longer. The administration of one part flumazenil (benzodiazepine antagonist) to 13 parts of a benzodiazepine agonist should reduce the recovery time in pigs. However, if flumazenil is given before ketamine effects are diminishing, the recovery will be similar to that with ketamine alone [1,13]. Midazolam can also be given intranasally to produce sedation in pigs. At doses of 0.2–0.4 mg/kg, it will induce significant calming and sedation within 3–4 min in laboratory piglets [10].

Opioid receptor agonists can be used in anesthetic combinations in swine. Ketamine (10 mg/kg), medetomidine (80 μg/kg), and butorphanol (0.2 mg/kg) given intramuscularly prolonged the duration of the loss of protective reflexes in pigs and permitted surgical procedures to be performed for at least 30 min [25]. Another option is to use tramadol instead of butorphanol. Tramadol appears to cause less respiratory depression compared with morphine or other μ-opioid receptor agonists [26]. Pigs that received tramadol (5 mg/kg, IM) prior to sedation with ketamine (25 mg/kg), xylazine (2.5 mg/kg), and atropine (0.04 mg/kg) intramuscularly had better quality of sedation that facilitated endotracheal intubation. Also, this combination increased in about 26% the duration of analgesia compared to ketamine-xylazine sedation [27]. Unfortunately, at present, tramadol is not available in an injectable form in some countries such as the USA.

Yucatan and Yorkshire pigs usually need a higher dose of ketamine and midazolam to be fully sedated compared to other breeds. For 5–10 min of sedation in Yucatan pigs, a combination of ketamine (25 mg/kg) and midazolam (0.6 mg/kg) can be used. For Yorkshire pigs, a dose of ketamine 5 mg/kg and midazolam 0.5 mg/kg is usually sufficient [8]. It should be noted that in this study, the combination of drugs was given subcutaneously in the lateral cervical region which may have contributed to the relatively greater dosages needed. Note that the Göttingen miniature pig can also be sedated with ketamine (10 mg/kg) and midazolam (1 mg/kg) intramuscular injection behind the ear in the lateral cervical region. A disadvantage of IM injection is that it can be painful and stressful to the minipig compared with SC injection. As an alternative, a combination of azaperone (4 mg/kg) and midazolam (1 mg/kg) provides sedation in Göttingen minipigs [11].

Azaperone (Stresnil®) is one of the most widely used sedatives in pigs where it is available [3]. This drug is classified as a short acting butyrophenone neuroleptic and is relatively safe when given intramuscularly [13]. Intravenous injection of azaperone is contraindicated because it may cause excitation [12]. Azaperone may be used as a sedative in combination with local anesthetics for minor surgical procedures, as a premedicant with anxiolytic properties, as an anxiolytic in weanlings when they are mixed for the first time, and in maiden sows after their first litter to reduce the rejection of piglets [3]. The effects of azaperone are dose dependent, as suggested by Braun, where doses of 0.25 mg/kg produce mild sedation without ataxia in domestic pigs [28]. Doses of 0.5–2 mg/kg will produce greater sedation but with mild ataxia, and doses of 2–4 mg/kg produce significant sedation and possible recumbency in adult pigs [13]. In younger pigs it may be necessary to use a much higher dose of azaperone, such as 8 mg/kg, for appropriate sedation [1]. Also, pot-bellied Vietnamese pigs require a dose of 0.25–2 mg/kg for sedation and a higher dose of 2–8 mg/kg for induction of anesthesia. However, doses exceeding 2 mg/kg are also more likely to cause adverse effects such as hypotension, bradycardia, and decreased cardiac output and contractility [13]. Note that in large boars, it has been suggested that azaperone doses should not exceed 1 mg/kg in order to reduce the risk of priapism [12].

As mentioned for the Göttingen miniature pigs, azaperone can be combined with other drugs to improve sedation and reduce its dosage, avoiding its negative effects. Flores *et al.* suggested that azaperone (2 mg/kg) and xylazine (2 mg/kg) given intramuscularly produced good sedation and muscular relaxation [29]. Others have reported that animals pretreated with azaperone (2 mg/kg) and anesthetized with ketamine (15 mg/kg, IM) and midazolam (0.3 mg/kg, IM) demonstrated a good anesthetic induction and analgesia scores [30].

Acepromazine is a phenothiazine that can be used as part of a sedative combination in pigs, although by itself its sedative effects are considered inadequate. Acepromazine is usually contraindicated in debilitated animals due to its potential adverse effects such as hypotension, decrease in heart rate, hypothermia, and decrease of respiratory rate [12,13]. Acepromazine should be injected intramuscularly at the recommended dose of 0.03–0.1 mg/kg. In Göttingen minipigs it is recommended that higher doses of 0.1–0.45 mg/kg be used for sedation [11].

Induction of anesthesia

Depending on the surgical setting, the induction of anesthesia can be performed by inhalant or intravenous route, or a combination of both (Table 50.2). When anesthesia is being induced with an inhalant agent (ex. 3 to 5% isoflurane or 4 to 6% sevoflurane) in a mixture with oxygen (4 to 8 L/min) through a face mask there is a minimal amount of time to complete the intubation procedure once the face mask is removed. The moment that the face mask is applied against the nose of the pig the anesthetist should observe the breathing pattern (which should be regular) and determine the anesthetic stage the patient is in. Once relaxation is adequate, the face mask is removed and quickly the mouth of the pig is opened and the laryngeal opening is sprayed with lidocaine (if desired) prior to endotracheal intubation [1,2]. Although induction of anesthesia by administration of inhalant anesthetic agents through a mask is possible, it requires effective manual restraint. Pigs that are not trained will often resent handling and placement of the face mask [31]. Thus, to avoid stress it is appropriate to have a well sedated animal before the induction of anesthesia, either with inhalant or injectable agents [32].

Table 50.2 Doses of agents used for induction of anesthesia in pigs.

Drug	Dose (mg/kg)	Route	Primary references
Inhalant agents			
Isoflurane	To effect	Inhalation	
Sevoflurane	To effect	Inhalation	
Injectable agents and combinations			
Tiletamine/zolazepam plus	6	IM	[5,63]
xylazine[a]	2		
	or 1 mL/35–75 kg		
Tiletamine/zolazepam plus	5	IM	[32]
medetomidine	0.05		
Ketamine	4–6	IV	[1,3]
Thiopental	10–20	IV	[1]
Thiamylal	6–18	IV	[1,12]
Propofol	2–5	IV	[3,34]
Propofol plus	2	IV	[2]
fentanyl	0.005		
Propofol plus	2–4	IV	[1]
medetomidine or	0.02–0.04		
xylazine	1–2		
Etomidate plus	2–4	IV	[1]
xylazine or	1–2	IM, IV	
azaperone	2–4	IM	
Metomidate plus	4	IV	[37]
azaperone	2–4	IM	
Metomidate plus	10	IP	[5]
azaperone	2	IM	
Alfaxalone	5–6	IM	[1,3]
	6	IV	
α-Chloralose	40	IV	[46]
α-Chloralose plus	55–86	IV	[1]
morphine	0.3–0.9	IM	

IM = intramuscular; IV = intravenous; IP = intraperitoneal.
[a]In an unused vial of tiletamine/zolazepam, 2.5 mL of ketamine (100 mg/mL) and 2.5 mL of xylazine (100 mg/mL) are added to the powder, producing 100 mg of dissociative agents/mL (tiletamine and ketamine) and 50 mg/mL each of xylazine and zolazepam. This combination should be mixed just before use and should not be stored since the potency is diminished over time.

To speed induction of anesthesia with inhalants, nitrous oxide (N_2O) can be added to the mixture of oxygen (1:1 ratio) and the inhalant [33]. This is due to its high concentration gradient that results in a faster transport of this gas from the alveoli to the bloodstream. Thus, when given with a potent inhalant anesthetic, N_2O improves the uptake of the agent from the alveoli to the blood and increases the speed of induction. This rapid increase in anesthetic concentration gradient is known as the *second gas effect*. After intubation is complete, N_2O delivery is either decreased to less than 50% of the total fresh gas flow or discontinued altogether [1].

In most cases the anesthesia must be induced by IV injection of the anesthetic agent into an auricular vein. Placement of an indwelling intravenous catheter facilitates this process. Ketamine, thiopental, and propofol are the drugs most commonly used for inducing anesthesia in pigs, due to their fast-acting effects and short recovery time. In pigs that have been sedated with the IM combination of ketamine and xylazine, anesthesia can be induced using an additional 4–6 mg/kg of ketamine IV [1,3].

Thiopental and thiamylal are thiobarbiturates that have been extensively used for induction prior to inhalation maintenance. Like most injectable anesthetics, thiobarbiturates can cause apnea so a means of intubation and positive pressure ventilation should be available. A self-reinflating bag (i.e., Ambu-bag®) can be used for this purpose. To avoid tissue necrosis, the thiobarbiturates must be given IV, with induction doses for thiopental and thiamylal ranging from 10 to 20 mg/kg and 6 to 18 mg/kg, respectively. The higher dose is indicated for unpremedicated young pigs and the lower dose should be adequate for sedated animals. Prior to administration of a thiobarbiturate, adjunctive drugs such as xylazine (1–2 mg/kg IV), ketamine (2–4 mg/kg IV), or diazepam (2–4 mg/kg IV) may be given. Another use for thiopental is to abolish laryngeal reflexes with a small dose (4–6 mg/kg, IV) after administration of dissociative anesthetics (i.e., ketamine) [1]. Thiopental and thiamylal may produce prolonged recovery if an infusion or repeated doses are used to prolong anesthesia [13].

Propofol (2–5 mg/kg, IV) is an induction agent that can only be administered intravenously [3,34]. Unlike the thiobarbiturates, extravascular injection of propofol does not cause tissue injury (an advantage in unpremedicated swine) and can be given through the auricular vein without concern about phlebitis [13]. Propofol is often described as a hypnotic that has minimal analgesic effects, so it is frequently used for induction of anesthesia or combined with analgesic drugs (i.e., opioid or α_2-adrenergic receptor agonist). Induction of anesthesia in pigs with an IV bolus of fentanyl (5 μg/kg) followed by the administration of propofol (2 mg/kg, IV) allows tracheal intubation [2]. Alternatively, dexmedetomidine (20–40 μg/kg, IV) followed with propofol (2–4 mg/kg, IV) may be used for induction in 30–60 kg pigs. All these anesthetics are not given in fixed doses but are administered until the desired effects are observed, which include the absence of corneal reflexes and good muscular relaxation.

Other agents that can be used for anesthesia induction in pigs include etomidate, metomidate, alfaxalone and α-chloralose. Etomidate is rapidly hydrolyzed by plasma esterases, resulting in absence of accumulation after repeated injections. Available formulations of etomidate contain high concentrations of propylene glycol and are hypertonic, potentially causing hemolysis following high cumulative doses. Etomidate does not significantly affect the cardiovascular system, maintaining stability in critical patients, although it is reported to suppress the adrenocortical activity in humans and dogs for 24 h after administration [35,36]. In addition, etomidate may cause pain during IV administration, spontaneous involuntary muscle movement, tremor, and hypertonus when given alone [37]. Both metomidate and etomidate produce adequate sedation/hypnosis at doses of 2–4 mg/kg, but provide relatively poor analgesia and muscle relaxation. Therefore, it is recommended to administer other adjunctive drugs (e.g., α_2-adrenergic receptor agonists, benzodiazepines or opioids) concomitantly. Etomidate has been used in an experimental setting for induction of anesthesia at a dose of 0.6 mg/kg IV and then followed by a ketamine infusion rate of 10 mg/kg/h to maintain anesthesia [38]. Etomidate does not trigger malignant hyperthermia in susceptible pigs [39].

Metomidate (4 mg/kg, IV), similarly to etomidate, produces a hypnotic state with stable cardiovascular function, with poor muscle relaxation and little analgesia [37]. To improve the lack of analgesia, a local analgesic technique, an α_2-adrenergic receptor agonist, or an opioid is often included in the anesthetic protocol. Azaperone (2–4 mg/kg, IM) has been used as a premedicant for improving muscle relaxation associated with metomidate. Alternatively, anesthesia can be maintained with minimal analgesia by an intravenous infusion of azaperone (2 mg/kg/h) and metomidate (8 mg/kg/h) [1]. Due to the high incidence of peritonitis and intra-abdominal adhesions, intraperitoneal injection of metomidate is discouraged [1].

Alfaxalone is a neurosteroid anesthetic that has been previously combined with a weak anesthetic agent, alfadalone, to improve solubility. This combination then was used to induce or maintain anesthesia in various species. Most of the adverse effects with alfaxalone were related to the previous formulation which contained 20% of polyoxyethylated castor oil (Cremophor EL®). The vehicle caused histamine release when given rapidly IV, resulting in decreased blood pressure and edema of the pinnae and the paws in cats, and dose-dependent anaphylactoid reaction in dogs [40]. Alfaxalone is now available in solution with 2-hydroxypropyl-β-cyclodextrin (Alfaxan®CD-RTU) that is non-irritant, non-cumulative and has a high therapeutic index in most species. Alfaxalone at doses of 5–6 mg/kg IV provides anesthesia in pigs for 10–15 min. This dose can be decreased if xylazine (1–2 mg/kg, IM) or azaperone (4 mg/kg, IM) is given previously. The anesthesia produced by alfaxalone can be maintained by repeated IV injection of doses of 2–4 mg/kg [1]. Alfaxalone can also be given intramuscularly, but the maximum dose of 6 mg/kg should be observed. Anesthesia lasts for around 15 min and it may be rather unpredictable [3]. Also, intramuscular administration of alfaxalone requires a large volume to be injected, for example, a mean volume of 10.4 mL in gilts and 16.7 mL in mature sows [41].

α-Chloralose is an anesthetic compound which has mixed effects of dose-dependent central nervous system excitation and depression. It is exclusively used for non-survival experiments that require prolonged anesthesia with minimal surgical intervention since it provides poor analgesia when used alone. In particular, this agent may be selected when cardiovascular stability and lack of baroreceptor depression are desired [42]. However, its negative properties include poor solubility, slow onset (15–20 min), development of metabolic acidosis and hyper-reactivity to auditory stimulation, and when used in animals it has been reported to induce peritonitis and adynamic ileus [43]. To anesthetize pigs with α-chloralose, a loading dose of 40 mg/kg IV is required while surgical depth of anesthesia can be maintained with a constant infusion rate of 10 mg/kg/h [44]. Also, α-chloralose at a dose of 55–86 mg/kg IV can be combined with morphine (0.3–0.9 mg/kg, IM) or the combination of ketamine (5–10 mg/kg, IV or IM) and butorphanol (0.5 mg/kg, IV or IM) to improve analgesia and anesthesia. Artificial ventilation is recommended to prevent hypercapnia and respiratory acidosis [11].

Orotracheal intubation

Orotracheal intubation for maintenance of general anesthesia is important in pigs undergoing procedures longer than a few minutes or when unconscious animals are placed in dorsal recumbency which can otherwise result in hypoxia, hypercapnia or airway obstruction. Most sedatives, tranquilizers, and general anesthetic agents cause respiratory depression that can be severe in pigs due to the need for heavier sedation to decrease stress and also because of the high work of breathing imposed by the narrow upper airway of the pig. In addition, pigs are very prone to laryngospasm, and fluid tends to accumulate in the pharyngeal region under anesthesia. While intubation of swine may be challenging, after some training it can be successfully accomplished quickly.

The major difficulty during orotracheal intubation is visualization of the swine larynx due to the anatomy. Pigs have thick tongues and long, narrow oropharyngeal spaces. The elongated soft palate can hide the epiglottis. Swine also have a pharyngeal diverticulum that is long (3–4 cm in adults, 1 cm in piglets) which protrudes from the wall of the pharynx, above the esophagus. The angle between the floor of the lateral ventricles and the trachea, caudal to the opening of the larynx, is obtuse and can make the intubation difficult (Fig. 50.2) [45,46]. If an endotracheal tube is inserted too

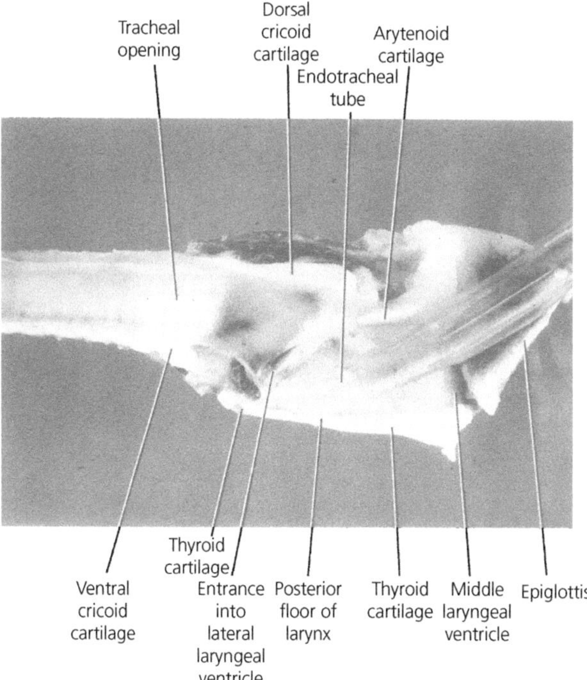

Figure 50.2 A sagittal view of a pig's larynx and trachea. Note the acute angle between the posterior portion of the larynx and the tracheal opening. Passage of the endotracheal tube is often difficult because of the entrapment of its tip in the floor of the larynx. Prior placement of a stylet through the tracheal opening will prevent entrapment of the endotracheal tube in the middle laryngeal ventricle just anterior to the thyroid cartilage and the posterior floor of the larynx anterior to the cricoid cartilage when the tube is passed into the trachea.

deeply, it may block the right cranial bronchus, thus compromising ventilation of that lung lobe and leading to poor gas exchange or difficulty in maintaining depth of inhaled anesthesia [13]. If an endotracheal tube is too wide for the tracheal, it can cause injuries to the delicate laryngeal mucosa, resulting in serious consequences. Formation of hematoma or generalized laryngeal edema may go unnoticed during anesthesia but after extubation the pig may present signs of respiratory distress [1,3].

When intubating a pig, the size of cuffed endotracheal tube should be selected according to the animal's weight. Tracheal tube sizes can range from 3–4 mm diameter for piglets up to 16–18 mm diameter in large boars or sows. Most pigs used in surgical research weigh 10–25 kg, and for these a 6–7 mm diameter endotracheal tube is appropriate [5]. The endotracheal tube should be measured and if necessary cut to a length equal to the distance from the tip of the animal's nostrils to the level of its shoulder [46]. Once selected, it is practical to have at hand three different sizes of endotracheal tube: the one thought to be correct, one size larger, and one size smaller [1].

Preoxygenation may be prudent in sick animals where orotracheal intubation may be challenging (e.g., mass-occupying space in the larynx) or when the anesthetist has little experience with swine intubation. It is recommended that the animal is preoxygenated with 100% oxygen through a face mask for 5–10 min unless the stress of restraint makes preoxygenation unreasonable [46].

Pigs can be intubated in dorsal or ventral recumbency, though ventral recumbency is easier and faster for less experienced personnel [45]. After placing the animal into a sling, gauze strips are placed behind the upper and lower canine teeth to assist in opening of the pig's mouth. Ideally the animal's head should not be extended which will make the arytenoid cartilages more difficult to identify and in some cases may even occlude the airway. To improve the visualization of the larynx, use of a laryngoscope with a long, straight (Miller) blade with a curved tip of at least 195 mm long for pigs up to 50 kg is helpful. For animals weighing more than 50 kg, a blade of 205 mm with an extension (4–8 cm) is more appropriate. Once the larynx is visualized, the arytenoids can be sprayed with 2% lidocaine to decrease laryngospasm and coughing when intubating a lightly anesthetized pig. Succinylcholine (1–2 mg/kg, IV) has been suggested for abolishing the laryngospasm; however, this drug causes transient muscle paralysis needing immediate ventilator support, and it is reported to trigger malignant hyperthermia in susceptible pigs. The laryngoscope should be inserted into the mouth of the pig and the tip gently pressed ventrally at the base of the tongue until the vocal cords can be visualized. If the larynx cannot be visualized, a plastic guide stylet to assist the intubation can be used. This stylet should be made of malleable atraumatic material and should be three times the length of the endotracheal tube chosen. The stylet can be first placed into the larynx and the endotracheal tube subsequently threaded over it. If the tube encounters resistance at the lateral laryngeal ventricle and cannot be inserted further, it should be gently rotated 180° so that it continues into the trachea. Note that when using a stiff guide stylet, it must be held in place while the endotracheal tube is being inserted in order to avoid deep advancement of the stylet, resulting in bronchial and peribronchial injuries. The guide stylet should then be carefully removed, leaving the endotracheal tube in place which can be secured with a gauze tie over the animal's snout or behind its ears. Correct placement of the endotracheal tube can be confirmed by noticing expired air moving through the tube, by visual confirmation via laryngoscopy, through bilateral chest auscultation, radiography, or capnography (i.e., end-tidal CO_2 waveform). Also, the tube cuff should be inflated to a pressure that prevents air escape around the tube when manual ventilation is applied to a pressure of 20–30 cmH_2O [1,13,46].

If orotracheal intubation is not possible or desired, alternatives for providing oxygen should be implemented. At a minimum, an oxygen mask can be employed and suction should be available in case of regurgitation or vomiting. The laryngeal mask airway and laryngeal tube airway have been evaluated for swine anesthesia. The researchers who first described the use of standard laryngeal mask, which was designed for humans, noted that airway management was greatly simplified compared to orotracheal intubation but it was also reported that gastric insufflation occurred in pigs during mechanical ventilation. The laryngeal mask airway may be used for induction of anesthesia with inhalation anesthetics [1,47].

Maintenance of anesthesia

Inhalation anesthesia

Both inhaled and injectable anesthetics can be used for maintaining anesthesia in pigs. Inhalation anesthesia is preferred for prolonged anesthesia, debilitated patients or for specific experimental studies because it provides smoother transitions, a more controlled plane of anesthesia, and a more rapid recovery than do many injectable combinations. All the current inhalant anesthetics have been used safely and effectively in pigs. Regardless of which anesthetic is chosen, the animal should be given oxygen from an appropriate anesthetic circuit. Anesthetic machines and delivery systems designed for humans or small animals can be used for most animals weighing up to 150 kg, provided that the carbon dioxide absorbent canister is of sufficient size. Adult pigs are normally maintained with an oxygen flow of 1–3 L/min [1,3].

For piglets, liquid volatile anesthetic is injected into a vaporization chamber which can be applied to the animal's snout. The apparatus is filled with a calculated amount of the volatile anesthetic agent and induction can be accomplished in less than 1 min. Recovery time is reported to be an average of 2 min after removal of the chamber from the animal. Hodgson compared the use of isoflurane and sevoflurane for short-term anesthesia in piglets and found that both agents can be used for castration without complications but isoflurane costs less [48].

Nitrous oxide (N_2O) is only used to supplement other anesthetics because it is not potent enough to provide anesthesia alone. To avoid hypoxia, the maximum concentration of N_2O for safe anesthesia in pigs is 75% N_2O with 25% O_2; however, 50–66% N_2O is more common in clinical practice. Nitrous oxide reduces the dose requirement of more potent anesthetics (i.e., MAC values are additive), thus minimizing the cardiopulmonary depression produced by the primary inhalant, and maintains a more physiologically stable state [11]. However, when a high concentration of N_2O is used to decrease that inhaled concentration it can accentuate hypoxic conditions. Rapid movement of N_2O from the blood to the alveoli at the end of anesthesia can result in diffusion hypoxia once oxygen supplementation ceases and the pig breathes ambient air. Therefore, it is indicated to provide 100% oxygen to the animal during the 5–10 min immediately after discontinuing N_2O delivery [1].

Other agents have been recently employed for maintenance of anesthesia in pigs, especially for research (i.e., xenon) or for field anesthesia (i.e., carbon dioxide). Xenon is an inert gas with many of the characteristics considered ideal for an anesthetic agent. One characteristic in particular is the fact that it is not harmful to the environment, since it is derived from a fractional distillation of the atmospheric air. Xenon has also been recently recognized for its systemic hemodynamic stability and analgesia. The MAC value of xenon has been established to be 119% in intubated pigs and has been reported to not trigger malignant hyperthermia [49,50]. Nevertheless, the production cost is prohibitive at this point and it requires low fresh gas flow rates with a xenon-recycling system [51].

Injectable anesthesia

Injectable maintenance of anesthesia is a suitable alternative to the use of inhalants in pigs. In field situations it is a useful method of anesthesia because it does not require specialized equipment (i.e., anesthetic machine with ventilator) or an oxygen delivery system, although intubation and oxygen delivery may be advisable in some situations. Drugs used for injectable anesthesia ideally should achieve the four elements of general anesthesia: amnesia, unconsciousness, analgesia, and muscle relaxation. Although total intravenous anesthesia (TIVA) requires an intravenous catheter (usually placed in an auricular vein), some injectable anesthetic combinations such as ketamine or tiletamine/zolazepam with xylazine can be given IM. There are disadvantages associated with injectable anesthesia: slower recovery, hypoventilation, and hypoxemia, especially in patients not given supplemental oxygen.

Common combinations of injectable anesthetics that have been used in pigs for field anesthesia are listed in Table 50.3. The tiletamine/zolazepam (TZ) mixture is effective and provides reliable immobilization in pigs (due to the tiletamine) and some muscle relaxation and sedation (due to the zolazepam). When given intramuscularly, TZ has the advantage over ketamine of requiring a smaller volume to be injected and provides 20 min of immobilization suitable for minor surgery [52]. However, TZ alone may not provide enough CNS depression and visceral analgesia for most surgical procedures and may require combination with an α_2-adrenergic receptor agonist (e.g., medetomidine) to provide effective anesthesia. Another reason to include a muscle relaxant with TZ or ketamine is its 'rough' and stressful recovery. Pigs may display excessive paddling, multiple failed attempts to return to sternal recumbency, hypersalivation, frequent vocalization, and hyperthermia [13]. Note that repeated doses of TZ result in prolonged recovery which appears to be caused in large part by the zolazepam's lingering effects. Zolazepam also is responsible for the posterior weakness observed in mature pigs during recovery. To decrease this effect, ketamine can be included in the TZ mixture (e.g., swine TXK). In an unused vial of TZ, 2.5 mL of ketamine (100 mg/mL) and 2.5 mL of xylazine (100 mg/mL) are added to the powder, thus producing 100 mg of dissociative agents/mL (tiletamine and ketamine) and 50 mg/mL each of xylazine and zolazepam. The recommended dose for commercial pigs is 1 mL per 35–75 kg, IM, depending on the depth of anesthesia required. It is suggested that the positive chronotropic effects of TZ and ketamine are partially counterbalanced by the enhanced vagal tone associated with xylazine [53].

Table 50.3 Doses of injectable agents used for maintenance of anesthesia in pigs.

Drug	Dose	Route	Primary references
Tiletamine/zolazepam plus xylazine plus tramadol	3.5 mg/kg 1.32 mg/kg 1.8 mg/kg	IM	[63]
Guaifenesine plus ketamine plus xylazine	0.67–1 mL/kg (induction) 2.2 mL/kg/h (maintenance)	IV	[5,19,66]
Medetomidine plus butorphanol plus ketamine	0.08 mg/kg 0.2 mg/kg 10 mg/kg	IM	[25]
Romifidine plus butorphanol plus ketamine	0.12 mg/kg 0.1 mg/kg 8 mg/kg 2 mL/kg/h (maintenance)	IV	[22]
Pentobarbital plus ketamine or fentanyl	8–10 mg/kg/h 5 mg/k/h 0.02 mg/kg/h	IV	[67]
Pentobarbital plus ketamine plus midazolam	6–8 mg/kg/h 3–5 mg/kg/h 0.1–0.2 mg/kg/h	IV IV IM	[68]
Propofol plus fentanyl	8 mg/kg/h 0.035 mg/kg/h	IV	[69]

IM = intramuscular; IV = intravenous.

For pot-bellied pigs the dose of TZ combination is one-half that of other pig types. Anesthetic drugs must be deposited into muscle tissue (not fat) and will require the use of a long needle (3.75 cm minimum length) since the pot-bellied pig's body is heavily covered with fatty tissue [1]. Also, the dose of TZ should be lower when given to miniature pigs compared to domestic pigs [53].

In a study by Ko *et al.* other drug combinations were evaluated in pigs: tiletamine/zolazepam (4.4 mg/kg), ketamine (2.2 mg/kg), and xylazine (2.2 mg/kg) were compared against TZ (4.4 mg/kg) with xylazine, TZ (4.4 mg/kg) and xylazine (4.4 mg/kg), and ketamine (2.2 mg/kg) with xylazine (2.2 mg/kg) [54]. After observing the quality of restraint and induction of surgical anesthesia, TZ with either dose of xylazine was preferred. All drug mixtures were mixed in a single syringe and given as a single intramuscular injection. All the combinations were considered safe and satisfactory for anesthesia induction in pigs aged 6–8 months [54]. For a greater depth and prolonged period of anesthesia in miniature pigs, TZ (3.5 mg/kg, IM) can be combined with xylazine (1.32 mg/kg, IM) and tramadol (1.8 mg/kg, IM). Animals became laterally recumbent within 3 min and were calmer during recovery compared with animals that received only TZ and xylazine. The time between administration of drugs and standing up was an average of 25 min. The inclusion of tramadol produced less pronounced cardiovascular depression, and did not cause additional respiratory depressant effects in miniature pigs [53]. Note that the combination of TZ, xylazine, and tramadol can be effectively antagonized when necessary with atipamezole (0.12 mg/kg, IM), flumazenil (0.1 mg/kg, IM), and naloxone (0.03 mg/kg, IM) [55].

Anesthesia can be maintained with a combination known as a *triple drip* which is a 5% solution of dextrose in water containing 50 mg/mL guaifenesin, 1–2 mg/mL ketamine, and 1 mg/mL xylazine (GKX) infused IV at a rate of 2.2 mL/kg/h. It is a satisfactory combination of drugs for induction and maintenance of surgical anesthesia in healthy swine for a period of up to 2 h [5,56]. Anesthesia can be induced using any drug combination or simply using GKX (0.67–1 mL/kg, IV) after adequate sedation and IV access are obtained. Sows that have been in prolonged labor usually require less drug for induction and maintenance, while young, healthy sows in labor for a short period of time may need a higher dose of GKX to provide adequate muscle relaxation and analgesia. Recovery occurs in 30–45 min after discontinuation of the IV infusion, and can be accelerated by administration of yohimbine (0.06–0.1 mg/kg, IV) or tolazoline (2–4 mg/kg, IV). Note that when the α_2-adrenergic receptor antagonist is used, postoperative analgesia will diminish, so pain management should rely on other analgesic techniques (e.g., epidural).

Medetomidine-butorphanol-ketamine (MBK) given IM also provides appropriate anesthesia and analgesia in pigs for 30–45 min. The dose of medetomidine is 80 μg/kg, butorphanol is 0.2 mg/kg, and ketamine at 10 mg/kg. Atropine (0.025 mg/kg) may also be given if desired. Anesthesia induction is rapid and the recovery is generally uneventful. Anesthesia can be quickly antagonized with atipamezole (0.24 mg/kg, IM) if necessary [25]. Alternatively, xylazine, butorphanol, and ketamine (XBK) can be mixed and given IM for anesthetizing Göttingen miniature pigs and pot-bellied pigs [1,11]. Yohimbine (0.05 mg/kg, IM) has been used to reverse XBK anesthesia in Göttingen minipigs [11]. Another group of researchers have reported that a combination of romifidine (0.12 mg/kg, IM), butorphanol (0.1 mg/kg, IM), and ketamine (8 mg/kg, IM) in pigs meets the requirements for anesthesia under field conditions. Immobilization was observed within 2–5 min after IM administration and reliable anesthesia was maintained for 20–30 min. All recoveries were smooth and smaller pigs were able to stand up 50–60 min after the injection, while larger animals needed more time (70–90 min).

Historically, the barbiturates have been extensively used for maintaining anesthesia in laboratory animals. Currently, due to lack of availability, use of barbiturates for general anesthesia has dramatically decreased. The recommendations for dosage must be considered as guidelines since barbiturates are administered IV to effect – pentobarbital 20–40 mg/kg and thiopental or thiamylal 6.6–30 mg/kg. This wide range of dosage is due to the animal's age and weight, and it is always reduced by one-half to two-thirds when barbiturates are combined with other agents [5,52]. Note that the use of a single injectable anesthetic is usually not enough to fulfill all the criteria of general anesthesia. Ketamine (5 mg/kg, IV) or fentanyl (20 μg/kg, IV) can be administered concomitantly with pentobarbital (20 mg/kg, IV) for induction of anesthesia after premedication with atropine (0.04 mg/kg, IM) and diazepam (0.5 mg/kg, IM). Maintenance of anesthesia using a constant infusion of ketamine (5 mg/kg/h) or fentanyl (20 μg/kg/h) in combination with a pentobarbital infusion of 8–10 mg/kg/h has been done. Both ketamine and fentanyl result in stable hemodynamics during induction and maintenance of anesthesia for pigs subjected to open heart surgery [57]. Miniature pigs may also be anesthetized with an infusion of low-dose ketamine combined with pentobarbital. After premedication with atropine (0.04 mg/kg, IM) and diazepam (0.4 mg/kg, IM), induction of anesthesia is achieved with IV ketamine (5 mg/kg) and pentobarbital (20 mg/kg). General anesthesia maintained with a constant intravenous infusion of ketamine (3–5 mg/kg/h) and pentobarbital (6–8 mg/kg/h) with intermittent midazolam injection hourly at 0.1–0.2 mg/kg demonstrated superior hemodynamic and respiratory indices in comparison with pentobarbital alone. Thus, this protocol resulted in both hypnosis and analgesia with stable circulatory parameters during a cardiopulmonary bypass procedure [58].

Propofol is rapidly cleared from plasma and therefore consciousness returns more quickly than with most other injectable anesthetic agents. Propofol is often combined with a potent analgesic drug, such as fentanyl, for maintenance of anesthesia in pigs. Schöffmann *et al.* reported that hemodynamic changes and stress responses in piglets subjected to superficial soft tissue surgery can be suppressed by total intravenous anesthesia with propofol and fentanyl [59]. After premedication with midazolam (0.5 mg/kg, IM), ketamine (10 mg/kg, IM) and butorphanol (0.5 mg/kg, IM), five piglets were induced with propofol at 1 mg/kg IV. Anesthesia was maintained with propofol (8 mg/kg/h) and fentanyl (35 μg/kg/h) during cannulation of blood vessels. There were no deaths or adverse events during anesthesia, and heart rate, mean arterial blood pressure, and lactate concentrations remained unaffected throughout the surgical procedure. Cortisol levels were suppressed by the combination, although fentanyl alone effectively suppresses the cortisol response of abdominal surgery in human patients [59,60].

Monitoring

Various parameters can be monitored during the anesthesia of pigs and it is possible to use the same monitors and equipment used during anesthesia of other domestic species. In general, the cardiovascular system, the respiratory system, and body temperature should be carefully monitored during anesthesia, and until the animal is stable and fully recovered from the effects of the anesthetic agents. Certainly the intensity of perioperative and postoperative monitoring depends on the type of surgical procedure and setting. Anesthesia ideally should be performed using continuous monitoring, with recording of vital signs at 5–10-min intervals. The intraoperative parameters must be recorded not only to provide useful physiologic trends, but are also required by regulatory agencies to assure that animals are properly anesthetized and monitored [2,61]. These parameters should include at least heart or pulse rate, mucous membrane color, respiratory rate, rectal or esophageal temperature, and absence of muscle reflexes in addition to the anesthetic levels. Advanced monitoring should include measurement of arterial blood pressure, capnography, and pulse oximetry.

Electrocardiography (ECG) can be easily performed in pigs, although alligator clips may not hold well due to the animal's thick skin and subcutaneous fat. Alternatives include 25 gauge needle electrodes inserted subcutaneously or patch electrodes held on the skin by adhesive. Esophageal ECG leads are also available for use in pigs [2,12]. ECG monitoring is recommended for detecting dysrhythmias, noting that normal pigs have a prolonged Q-T interval compared to other species [62].

Non-invasive blood pressure measurement is relatively easy in pigs, despite being less accurate than direct blood pressure measurements. Either oscillometric or Doppler flow monitors can be used. The cuff can be placed either immediately above or below the carpus or tarsus of the pig, and proper cuff width should be between 40% and 60% of the circumference of the limb. The values obtained through non-invasive blood pressure methods should be assessed depending on trends in these readings rather than absolute numbers. Also, blood pressures vary widely with anesthetic agents and the breed and size of the pig [12,61]. Arterial catheterization can be performed in pigs; it is easier in young or miniature animals where the auricular artery is preferred. The auricular artery runs down the center of the pinna and can be cannulated with a 24–22 gauge catheter and then connected to a direct blood pressure transducer and monitor. In larger pigs the medial saphenous, carotid or femoral arteries can be cannulated with a 5 cm (2 inch) or longer catheter, although a surgical cut-down may be required [12].

The pulse rate in pigs can be monitored at different sites that include the auricular arteries, the brachial artery on the medial aspect of the humeroradial joint, the saphenous artery over the medial aspect of the distal femur, or the sublingual artery on the ventral surface of the tongue. There are other locations which are considered less reliable, especially in larger animals with thick subcutaneous and muscular tissue, for example the femoral, carotid, or facial arteries [61]. Mucous membrane color can be observed in pigs by examination of the oral cavity, the snout or the ears, especially on unpigmented animals. Cyanotic mucous membranes can indicate hypoxemia from a number of etiologies, including inadequate lung ventilation or ventilation/perfusion mismatching while breathing unenriched air mixtures.

Rate, rhythm, and depth of respiration of the anesthetized animal can be assessed by observing thoracic cage movement, although capnography is a more sensitive and accurate measure of respiration. End-tidal carbon dioxide ($ETCO_2$) can be measured though a sampling line located between the end of the endotracheal tube and the anesthetic circuit. The normal physiologic range of $ETCO_2$ is 35–45 mmHg and higher values indicate that the animal may need to have ventilation assisted or controlled. A sudden rapid increase in $ETCO_2$ values might be related to the onset of malignant hyperthermia [12]. An increase in respiratory depth, regular rhythm, and decrease in respiratory rate signify surgical anesthesia. Opioids can cause severe respiratory depression, which can be reversed by the administration of an antagonist (i.e., naloxone).

The best method of assessing the lung's oxygen exchange is by performing blood gas analysis on an arterial blood sample or using a pulse oximeter [62]. Pulse oximetry is very practical to use in pigs and measures both pulse rate and the percentage of oxygenated hemoglobin that represents the relative ability of the lungs to deliver oxygen to the blood. The probe can be placed on the animal's tongue, eyelid, tip of its tail or interdigital space in unpigmented animals, or it can be placed intrarectally if a rectal probe is available and the rectum is cleared of feces [2,12].

A rectal or esophageal probe allows determination of the animal's temperature during the surgical procedure. Pigs are prone to hypothermia, because they are relatively hairless, and, depending on the sedation agent used, peripheral vasodilation of the cutaneous vessels [5]. Several techniques can be employed to slow or stop heat loss. Electrical heat pads or circulating hot water blankets under the animal, heat lamps over the animal, insulating material (e.g., rubber) in between the animal and the cold surgical tabletop, or wrapping the extremities in bubble sheeting minimize loss of heat [1,2,62]. Only electrical heating pads specifically designed for anesthetized patients (e.g., HotDog Patient Warmer) should be used to avoid skin burns. When hyperthermia is detected, it may be due to preanesthetic stress, capture, fever, or malignant hyperthermia [12].

The bispectral index (BIS) is a parameter derived from processing the electroencephalogram. It has been associated with the hypnotic component of the anesthetic state and has been used in humans and animals as a tool to assess anesthetic depth. BIS has been evaluated in the pig using various combinations of sevoflurane, isoflurane, propofol, fentanyl, and atracurium [63–65]. However, BIS values in pigs may have a poor correlation with anesthetic depth and may not predict changes in arterial blood pressure or heart rate during surgery [65].

A simple, yet reliable method for assessing anesthesia depth is by evaluation of muscle relaxation. Surgical depth of anesthesia is usually seen with laxity of the mandibular muscles (jaw tone) or absence of gross movement of the leg in response to a pinch or similar stimulus to the coronary band of the hoof. Also corneal and palpebral reflexes should be tested during anesthesia; their presence may indicate a lighter plane of anesthesia [2,11,61]. Ocular and pupillary reflexes are not reliable in pigs, particularly if atropine or ketamine is included in the anesthetic protocol.

Supportive therapies

When pigs are subjected to surgery or anesthesia that lasts longer than 1 h, a balanced electrolyte solution such as Ringer's lactate should be administered intravenously at a rate of 10–15 mL/kg/h, although allometric adjustments may be useful due to the range of body weights encountered [66]. Insufficient urine production, extensive blood loss, and hypotension are indications for a higher fluid infusion rate. Excessively high fluid rates may increase the likelihood of pulmonary edema [11]. In piglets, it is advisable to use warmed fluids (up to 37°C) to assist in the maintenance of body temperature [3,11,61]. In pigs that are hypovolemic or presenting with other signs of shock, fluid therapy should be initiated prior to anesthesia if reasonable. While fluids can be administered through various routes, generally the best during anesthesia is via an auricular vein. The intraosseous route for crystalloid and blood infusion in pigs can be used when necessary [67]. This route is a reasonable initial step for emergency fluid therapy until more conventional vascular access has been established. Note that intravenous access is a more efficient method of acute volume replacement than the intraosseous route [68]. Piglets and calves with mild dehydration will usually voluntarily drink oral rehydration solutions, resulting in a more cost-effective treatment [69].

For severe hypovolemia due to uncontrolled hemorrhage, hypotension can be minimized by adding colloid solution to the intravenous crystalloid fluid therapy. A slow (i.e., 5 min) administration of 1–2 mL/kg of 7.5% saline in 6% dextran 70 (HSD) decreased mortality by 30% in pigs with hemorrhagic hypovolemia. Colloid solutions (i.e., hydroxyethyl starch 130/0.4) markedly increase microcirculatory blood flow and tissue oxygen tension in the small intestinal mucosa, improve intestinal cellular substrate levels (e.g., lactate and glucose), and significantly enhance mixed venous saturation with less volume of fluid administration compared with crystalloid solutions [70]. In addition, a colloid/crystalloid solution ratio greater than 2 seems to promote coagulopathies [71,72].

Hypertonic saline can also be used to restore normovolemia in pigs [12]. The administration of 7.2% NaCl in 6% hydroxyethyl starch 200/0.5 at a dose of 5 mL/kg given IV demonstrated a positive inotropic effect with a significant increase in right ventricular contractility and cardiac output in pigs. Blood transfusions may be performed when necessary and blood donors are often littermates or close relatives. The risk of transfusion reaction from a non-cross-matched blood transfusion in pigs is relatively high since there are 16 recognized porcine blood groups that are not easily detectable [12,73].

During anesthesia, additional cardiovascular support using inotropes may be indicated. After studying the effects of hypothermia on hemodynamic responses to dopamine and dobutamine in pigs, Oung *et al.* found that profound hypothermia (30°C) causes significant depression of hemodynamic functions [74]. Infusion of either dopamine or dobutamine can be used safely and effectively for inotropic support during profound hypothermia. The optimal dosage for improving cardiac output in pigs is 10–20 μg/kg/min with minimal risk of inducing arrhythmias when IV infusion of either inotrope was given at the dosage of 30 μg/kg/min. Note that dopamine is the most effective inotropic agent in pigs. Dopamine administered at 15 μg/kg/min increased cardiac index by 18% and improved blood flow to the gastrointestinal tract by 33% in septic pigs [75]. In piglets, dopamine (15 μg/kg/min) better improved the blood flow to the heart and small intestine compared to dobutamine [76,77].

Mechanical ventilation is used to provide respiratory support in anesthetized pigs. The recommended peak inspiratory pressure is 20 cmH_2O and the respiratory rate should range between 8 and 18 breaths per minute depending on the age and size of the animal [78]. The arterial partial pressure of carbon dioxide is normally 40 ± 5 mmHg which would correspond to a $ETCO_2$ of 35–40 mmHg [79]. Pulmonary shunt fraction in pigs will depend on the inspired fraction of oxygen (FiO_2). Gianotti described that in pigs undergoing 2 h of general anesthesia with mechanical ventilation, there was a lower pulmonary shunt fraction when using an FiO_2 of 0.4 ($4.3 \pm 1.5\%$) compared to FiO_2 of 0.6 ($6.9 \pm 0.5\%$) and 0.8 ($9.5 \pm 2.5\%$) [80].

Recovery considerations

During recovery from anesthesia it is important to continue monitoring, to provide a smooth recovery, and to maintain homeostasis of the animal. The recovery should take place in a pen or cage lined with soft pads to preclude injury. The recovering animal should not be placed in a pen with other pigs, as they may attack and cannibalize the recovering animal. Room temperature should be 20–25°C to minimize hypothermia, or alternatively, a thermal blanket or lamp may be placed over the animal. Extubation should be performed when a strong laryngeal reflex is present. The endotracheal tube should be maintained until the pig is spontaneously moving its head or will no longer allow the presence of the tube. If extubation is performed too early, there is a high risk for hypoxia due to laryngospasm. If the intubation was known to be difficult, corticosteroids or diuretics (i.e., furosemide) can be given prophylactically prior to extubation. Some clinicians advocate spraying phenylephrine on the larynx to decrease vascular congestion and laryngeal edema. Severe upper airway obstruction is difficult to treat in pigs because it is difficult to restrain and reintubate the animal. If reintubation is required, it may be more effective in some instances to perform a tracheostomy. Pigs with surgical incisions should not be housed with other animals because of their tendency to cannibalize wounds [3,61]. If pre-emptive analgesics were not administered, postoperative analgesics should be given before the animal completely recovers from anesthesia. To assess postoperative pain in pigs, physiologic parameters (e.g., heart rate and respiratory rate), behavior parameters such as agitation, running, rooting, and evaluation of the animal's reaction during wound palpation can be used [81].

Malignant hyperthermia

Malignant hyperthermia is a genetic hypermetabolic syndrome in humans and pigs, and also has been diagnosed in other species, including dogs, horses, cats, birds, deer, and other wild animals (which then is known as *capture myopathy*). Pigs that are most affected by MH have a high ratio of muscle to total body mass and rapid growth. Therefore, the breeds that have high incidence of this syndrome are Pietran, Landrace, Spotted, Large White, Hampshire, and Poland-China. Some breeds are less susceptible such as Duroc and pot-bellied pigs [1,12,82]. In a susceptible animal MH can be trigged any type of stress, such as environmental (warm temperature) and pharmacologic (injectable and inhalant anesthetics). Even frequent procedures like restraint for blood sampling and castration can trigger MH in a highly susceptible pig. All commonly used volatile inhalation agents such as halothane, isoflurane, enflurane, desflurane and sevoflurane and depolarizing neuromuscular blockers (i.e., succinylcholine) will initiate MH in animals with the gene responsible for this syndrome. However, these volatile anesthetics do not have the same potential for triggering a MH episode.

Malignant hyperthermia is caused by an inherited autosomal recessive disorder that results in a single amino acid mutation in the ryanodine receptor type 1 (RYR1) associated with calcium channels in skeletal muscle. When MH is triggered, the muscle is not able to control calcium efflux from inside the sarcoplasmic reticulum, allowing calcium activation of myosin ATPase that causes muscle contracture and release of heat. Cell metabolism is increased significantly, requiring both aerobic and anaerobic respiration, leading to elevation in carbon dioxide, hydrogen ion and lactic acid, and decreased venous oxygen content [12,83]. Episodes of MH may present with increased core body temperature (up to 42°C), muscle rigidity, tachycardia, tachypnea, extreme hypercapnia ($ETCO_2$ as high as 70 mmHg), hypoxemia, metabolic acidosis, sympathetic activation with elevated catecholamine plasma concentration, and high values of serum magnesium, calcium, phosphorus, and potassium ion concentration. As this condition progresses, cell metabolism is unable to meet its demands and membrane integrity is compromised, resulting in increased permeability (i.e., edema). Also, the metabolic situation during a MH episode is known to cause ischemia of the heart, especially since the coronary perfusion is diminished while muscle metabolism is increased. Tachycardia may be followed by arrhythmias (e.g., ventricular tachycardia and fibrillation) that cause decreased cardiac output and, ultimately, cardiac failure with related hypotension. Myoglobinuria may also be observed if the patient lives long enough [1,12]. Since genetic testing has become available for determination of this RYR1 gene in pigs, the incidence of MH has been reduced drastically, although it is still present in some swine populations [1].

Once MH has been diagnosed, the volatile anesthetic should be discontinued and the pig should be ventilated with 100% oxygen, preferably using a different anesthetic machine or after changing the machine's rubber goods (i.e., hoses and rebreathing bag). Hypercapnia can be resolved by hyperventilating the animal. Body cooling can be achieved with alcohol baths, ice packs around large vessels (jugular and femoral veins), fans, and rectal lavage with ice water. When body temperature decreases to 38°C, the cooling methods should be terminated to avoid iatrogenic hypothermia. Dantrolene sodium is a skeletal muscle relaxant that inhibits excessive leak of calcium by RYR1 and can be employed both to prevent and to treat MH. This drug can be given orally (2–5 mg/kg) 6–10 h before induction of anesthesia, or it may be administered intravenously (1–5 mg/kg) immediately after MH symptoms are observed [1,3,12]. Despite the potency of dantrolene, this agent is highly lipophilic and poorly water soluble, making its preparation difficult for clinical use. A recently developed analogue, azumolene, has similar potency to dantrolene in relaxing skeletal muscle in MH-susceptible pigs. Azumolene (2 mg/kg, IV) is 30 times more soluble than dantrolene, and reverses the muscular contracture in pigs by reducing the opening rate of RYR1, without altering calcium uptake into the sarcoplasmic reticulum [83]. It has been reported in some patients that the increase of central temperature may be slow (i.e., several hours) until the fulminant episode develops which can be during the recovery time [84].

Analgesia

For any surgical procedure, it is good practice to administer an analgesic drug pre-emptively, i.e., prior to surgery. However, few drugs are currently approved for use in pigs that are destined for the human food chain. This scarcity is due to the lack of information about the minimal residual limit (MRL) and appropriate withdrawal time of these drugs [12]. Administration of analgesic drugs pre-emptively in pigs can reduce the degree of central hypersensitivity and therefore diminish the amount of drugs needed to control pain postoperatively.

Two major classes of drugs are used for analgesia in pigs: opioids and non-steroidal anti-inflammatory drugs (NSAIDs). In general, opioids have more pronounced analgesic and sedative effects than NSAIDs, but they have to be administered more frequently. Surgically induced pain may require the use of opioids for at least the first 2 days or even for a third day after major surgery, although effectiveness may diminish as inflammation becomes a major component of the discomfort. The most commonly used opioids in pigs are butorphanol and buprenorphine. Butorphanol (0.1–0.3 mg/kg, IM) has an analgesic effect of 4–6 h and produces fewer adverse effects in pigs [52]. Also, when given as part of the premedication, it will enhance depth of sedation and decrease the dose required for induction of anesthesia [59]. Buprenorphine (0.01–0.1 mg/kg, IM) can be given every 12 h and its onset of action is approximately 30–60 min after administration [85]. The analgesic effect of buprenorphine is reported to last 7–24 h when given in a high dose [32,86].

The short-acting opioids such as fentanyl can be used as a constant intravenous infusion at a rate varying from 10 to 100 μg/kg/h in pigs without major side-effects [1,11,52]. It has been shown that a fentanyl infusion rate of 35 μg/kg/h in piglets produces adequate analgesia for surgical procedures without affecting heart rate, mean arterial blood pressure and lactate concentrations during 5 h of anesthesia when maintained with a propofol infusion at 8 mg/kg/h [59]. This is most desirable for cardiovascular research where minimal effects on cardiovascular function are necessary. In addition, fentanyl can be administered to pigs through a transdermal patch that can be secured to the skin behind the ear. With this route, fentanyl is continuously administered for up to 72 h per patch application, and the discomfort and inconvenience of repeated parenteral injections are avoided [86–88]. Fentanyl patches come in different sizes: 12, 25, 50, 75, and 100 μg/h. For a 20 kg pig, the appropriate fentanyl patch will be a 50 μg/h patch applied at least 24 h prior to the surgery. Other opioids included in the short-acting category have been used in pigs: sufentanil (5–10 μg/h, IM every 2 h; 15–30 μg/h/h, IV), meperidine (2–10 mg/kg, IM every 4 h), and oxymorphone (0.15 mg/kg IM, every 4 h).

Note that morphine given systemically to non-painful pigs has been reported to cause excitement in a manner similar to that observed in cats and horses [52]. When administered intravenously to pigs, morphine produces not only analgesia but also respiratory depression [89]. Systemic morphine is also reported to produce other side-effects, such as decreased gastrointestinal motility, nausea and vomiting, pupillary constriction, bradycardia, euphoria, and histamine release in many species (e.g., dogs, cats, and horses) [87,90]. To avoid many of the systemic physiologic side-effects, morphine can be administered epidurally. It then acts locally on all opioid receptors located in the spinal cord, enhancing the analgesic effect [90,91]. In addition, because morphine has low lipid solubility, it remains for a longer period in the cerebrospinal fluid, prolonging the analgesic effect up to 33 h in pigs [92]. In many species, such as dogs, cats, horses, and cattle, this analgesic effect does not produce major motor impairment, in contrast to epidural administration of other drugs, such as lidocaine [87,90]. Epidural morphine can be given at a dosage of 0.1–0.12 mg/kg diluted in saline [93]. For maximal distribution of the drug into the spinal canal, morphine is diluted with saline to a final volume of 1 mL of solution for pigs with a vertebral length of up to 40 cm. Then, an additional 1.5 mL of saline is added for every additional 10 cm of vertebral length [93]. This final volume is delivered slowly over 1–2 min. Epidural morphine produced adequate analgesia without hemodynamic or respiratory effects on pigs during abdominal surgery [94].

Epidural anesthesia is helpful when performing obstetric and perineal surgery in pigs and in larger animals the landmarks can be difficult to locate. This technique, which is far easier in a heavily sedated animal, can be done with opioids, as mentioned before, or local anesthetics such as lidocaine where the dose should be 1 mL per 7.5 kg for pigs up to 50 kg, and then 1 mL per 10 kg above 50 kg [3]. This causes recumbency for 1–2 h. Also, there have been reports of bupivacaine (0.8 mg/kg) and ropivacaine (1.5 mg/kg) being administered epidurally in pigs [95,96]. Intratesticular analgesia is suitable for castration in young pigs up to 6 months old. For 1-week old piglets, a total of 0.5 mL of 2% lidocaine is injected into the stroma of each testicle, with a small amount being injected subcutaneously beneath the scrotal skin. At least 5 min should be allowed for the anesthetic to take effect and it will reduce pain responses during the surgical castration [97].

The NSAIDs are a group of analgesics that include organic acids, carboxylic acids (e.g., aspirin, flunixin, carprofen) and enolic acids such as phenylbutazone and meloxicam [90]. The analgesia produced by these drugs is related to the potent inhibitory effect on prostaglandin which is involved in the inflammatory process. In addition to the analgesia, the NSAIDs are reported to have anti-inflammatory and antipyretic properties [52,90,97]. Compared with opioids, NSAIDs are only effective against moderate pain but may be combined with opioids for treatment of more severe pain [11].

Although many NSAIDs must be dosed on a daily basis, they can be used in combination with opioids 1–1.5 days postoperatively and can be continued for another day and a half after the opioids are no longer administered to the animal [11]. Aspirin (10 mg/kg every 4–6 h) has been used orally in pigs; enteric-coated products are recommended due to the pig's predisposition for gastric ulcers [52]. Flunixin (2 mg/kg, IV; 1–4 mg/kg, SC or IM) has a prolonged effect of 12–24 h in pigs, but should not be administered for more than 3 days to minimize its adverse effects [98,99]. Carprofen (2 mg/kg, SC or IM) has a longer effect (12–24 h) in pigs and provides adequate analgesia for soft tissue and orthopedic pain. Ketoralac (1 mg/kg, IM or IV every 12 h), meloxicam (0.4 mg/kg, SC or IM every 24 h) and ketoprofen (1–3 mg/kg, IM, SC or PO every 12 h) have been reported to be effective as part of a balanced anesthetic regimen for postoperative and chronic pain. Phenylbutazone (10–20 mg/kg PO every 12 h) may be administered for treatment of musculoskeletal pain. Regulatory restrictions on the use of various NSAIDs in animals which could reach the human food chain should be strictly followed. Oral medications are readily accepted by pigs when hidden in canned dog food or in chocolate syrup [3,98].

References

1 Thurmon JC, Smith GW. Swine. In: Tranquili WJ, Thurmon JC, Grimm KA, eds. *Lumb and Jones' Veterinary Anesthesia and Analgesia*, 4th edn. Ames, IA: Blackwell Publishing, 2007; 747–764.

2 Kaiser GM, Heuer MM, Frühauf NR, *et al.* General handling and anesthesia for experimental surgery in pigs. *J Surg Res* 2006; **130**: 73–79.

3 Hodgkinson O. Practical sedation and anaesthesia in pigs. *Farm Anim Pract* 2007; **29**: 34–39.

4 Swindle MM. *Anesthesia and Analgesia in Swine: Technical Bulletin.* Sinclair Research Center, 2002. www.sinclairbioresources.com/Downloads/TechnicalBulletins/Anesthesia%20and%20Analgesia%20in%20Swine.pdf (accessed 3 October 2014).

5 Henrikson H, Jensen-Waern M, Nyman G. Anaesthetics for general anaesthesia in growing pigs. *Acta Vet Scand* 1995; **36**(3): 401–411.

6 Heinonen ML, Raekallio MR, Oliviero C, *et al.* Comparison azaperone-detomidine-butorphanol-ketamine and azaperone-tiletamine-zolazepam for anaesthesia in piglets. *Vet Anaesth Analg* 2009; **36**: 151–157.

7 Riviere JE, Papich MG. Potential and problems of developing transdermal patches for veterinary applications. *Adv Drug Deliv Rev* 2001; **50**: 175–203.

8 Linkenhoker JR, Burkholder TH, Linton CGG, *et al.* Effective and safe anesthesia for Yorkshire and Yucatan Swine with and without cardiovascular injury and intervention. *J Am Assoc Lab Anim Sci* 2010; **49**(3): 344–351.

9 Axiak SM, Jäggin N, Wenger S, *et al.* Anaesthesia for castration of piglets: comparison between intranasal and intramuscular application of ketamine, climazolam and azaperone. *Schweiz Arch Tierheilkd* 2007; **149**(9): 395–402.

10 Lacoste L, Bouquee S, Ingrand P, *et al.* Intranasal midazolam in piglets: pharmacodynamics (0.2 vs 0.4 mg/kg) and pharmacokinetics (0.4 mg/kg) with bioavailability determination. *Lab Anim* 2000; **34**; 29–35.

11 Alstrup AKO. *Anaesthesia and Analgesia in Ellegaard Göttingen Minipigs.* Arhus, Denmark: PET Centre, Aarhus University Hospital, 2010.

12 Moon PF, Smith LJ. General anesthetic techniques in swine. *Vet Clin North Am Food Anim Pract* 1996; **12**(3): 663–691.

13 Padilha LR, Ko JCH. Non-domestic suis. In: West G, Heard D, Caulkett N, eds. *Zoo Animal and Wild life Immobilization and Anesthesia.* Ames, IA: Blackwell Publishing, 2007; 567–578.

14 Gomez de Segura IA, Tendillo FJ, Mascias A, *et al.* Actions of xylazine in young swine. *Am J Vet Res* 1997; **58**(1): 99–102.

15 Ajadi RA, Smith OF, Makinde AFM, *et al.* Increasing ketamine dose enhances the anaesthetic properties of ketamine-xylazine-midazolam combination in growing pigs. *J S Afr Vet Assoc* 2008; **79**(4); 205–207.

16 Hörnchen U, Schüttler J, Stoeckel H, *et al.* Comparison of intravenous and endobronchial atropine: a pharmacokinetic and dynamic study in pigs. *Eur J Anaesthesiol* 1989; **6**: 95–102.

17 Lee JY, Jee HC, Jeong SM, *et al.* Comparison of anaesthetic and cardiorespiratory effects of xylazine or medetomidine in combination with tiletamine/zolazepam in pigs. *Vet Rec* 2010; **167**: 245–249.

18 Wagner AE, Helleyer PW. Survey of anesthetic techniques and concerns in private veterinary practice. *J Am Vet Med Assoc* 2000; **217**: 1652–1657.

19 Thurmon JC, Benson GJ. Anesthesia in ruminants and swine. In: Howard J, ed. *Current Veterinary Therapy*, 3rd edn. Philadelphia: WB Saunders, 1993; 58–76.

20 Trim CM, Gilroy BA. The cardiopulmonary effects of a xylazine and ketamine combination in pigs. *Res Vet Sci* 1985; **38**: 30–34.

21 Sakaguchi M, Nishimura R, Sasaki N, *et al.* Chemical restraint by medetomidine-ketamine and its cardiopulmonary effects in pigs. *J Vet Med* 1995; **42**: 293–299.

22 Nussbaumer I, Zimmermann W, Peterbauer C. Anaesthesia of pigs with a combination of romifidine, butorphanol and ketamine. *Vet Rec* 2008; **163**: 720–721.

23 Lu DZ, Fan HG, Kun M, *et al.* Antagonistic effect of atipamezole, flumazenil and naloxone following anaesthesia with xylazine, tramadol and tiletamine/zolazepam combinations in pigs. *Vet Anaesth Analg* 2011; **38**: 301–309.

24 Kim MJ, Park CS, Jun MH, *et al.* Antagonist effects of yohimbine in pigs anaesthetized with tiletamine/zolazepam and xylazine. *Vet Rec* 2007; **161**: 620–624.

25 Sakaguchi M, Nishimura R, Sasaki N, *et al.* Anesthesia induced in pigs by use of a combination of medetomidine, butorphanol, and ketamine and its reversal by administration of atipamezole. *Am J Vet Res* 1996; **57**: 529–534.

26 Natalini CC, Polydoro A, Crosignani N. Effects of morphine or tramadol on thiopental anaesthetic induction dosage and physiologic variables in halothane anaesthetized dogs. *Acta Sci Vet* 2007; **35**: 161–166.

27 Ajadi AR, Olusa TA, Smith OF, *et al.* Tramadol improved the efficacy of ketamine-xylazine anaesthesia in young pigs. *Vet Anaesth Analg* 2009; **36**: 562–566.

28 Braun W. Anesthetics and surgical techniques useful in the potbellied pig. *Vet Med* 1993; **88**: 441–447.

29 Flores FN, Tavares SG, Moraes AN, *et al.* Azaperone and its association with xylazine or dexmedetomidine in swine. *Ciência Rural* 2009; **39**(4): 1101–1107.

30 Rego Oliveira LC, Marques JA, Santos DAS, *et al.* Effects of ketamine and midazolam in pigs (*Sus scrofa*) pre-treated which acepromazine or azaperone. *Ars Vet* 2003; **19**(3): 235–240.

31 Ugarte CE, O'Flaherty KO. The use of a medetomidine, butorphanol and atropine combination to enable blood sampling in young pigs. *N Z Vet J* 2005; **53**(4): 249–252.

32 Malavasi LM, Jensen-Waern M, Augustsson H, *et al.* Changes in minimal alveolar concentration of isoflurane following treatment with medetomidine and tiletamine/zolazepam, epidural morphine or systemic buprenorphine in pigs. *Lab Anim* 2008; **42**: 62–70.

33 Brodbelt DC, Taylor PM. Comparison of two combinations of sedatives before anaesthetizing pigs with halothane and nitrous oxide. *Vet Rec* 1999; **145**: 283–287.

34 Mascoas A, Pera AM, Santos M, *et al.* Total intravenous anesthesia with propofol in pigs. *J Vet Anaesth* 1993; **20**: 53–54.

35 Archambault P, Dionne CE, Lortie G, *et al.* Adrenal inhibition following a single dose of etomidate in intubated traumatic brain injury victims. *Can Assoc Emerg Phys* 2012; **14**(5): 270–282.

36 Hirschman LJ. The cardiopulmonary and metabolic effects of hypoxia during acute adrenocortical suppression by etomidate in the dog. *AANA J* 1991; **59**(3): 281–287.

37 Clutton RE, Blissitt KJ, Bradley AA, *et al.* Comparison of three injectable anaesthetic techniques in pigs. *Vet Rec* 1997; **141**: 140–146.

38 Worek FS, Blumel G, Zaravik J, *et al.* Comparison of ketamine and pentobarbital anesthesia with the conscious state in a porcine model of *Pseudomonas aeruginosa* septicemia. *Acta Anaesth Scand* 1988; **32**: 509–515.

39 Suresh MS, Nelson TE. Malignant hyperthermia: is etomidate safe? *Anesth Analg* 1985; **64**: 420–424.

40 Hall LW, Clarke KW, Trim CM. Anaesthesia of the pig. In: Hall LW, Clarke KW, Trim CM, eds. *Veterinary Anesthesia*, 9th edn. London: WB Saunders, 1991.

41 Keates H. Induction of anaesthesia in pigs using a new alphaxalone formulation. *Vet Rec* 2003; **153**: 627–628.

42 Cunha DNQ, Buccellato M, Keene BW, *et al.* Electrocardiographic, hematologic, histopathologic, and recovery characteristics from repeated morphine-chloralose anesthesia in dogs. *Int J Appl Res Vet Med* 2008; **6**(3): 191–199.

43 Sommers MG, van Egmond J, Booji LHDJ, *et al.* Isoflurane anesthesia is a valuable alternative for α-chloralose anesthesia in the forepaw stimulation model in rats. *NMR Biomed* 2009; **22**: 414–418.

44 Seaberg DC, Menegazzi JJ, Check B, *et al.* Use of a cardiocerebral-protective drug cocktail prior to countershock in a porcine model of prolonged ventricular fibrillation. *Resuscitation* 2001; **51**: 301–308.

45 Theisen MM, Maas M, Grosse Hartlage MA, *et al.* Ventral recumbency is crucial for fast and safe orotracheal intubation in laboratory swine. *Lab Anim* 2009; **43**: 96–101.

46 Chum H, Pacharinsak C. Endotracheal intubation in swine. *Lab Anim* 2012; **41**: 309–311.

47 Patil VU, Fairbrother CR, Dunham BM. Use of laryngeal mask airway for emergency or elective airway management situations in pigs. *Contemp Top Lab Anim Sci* 1997; **36**: 47–49.

48 Hodgson DS. Comparison of isoflurane and sevoflurane for short-term anesthesia in piglets. *Vet Anaesth Analg* 2007; **34**: 117–124.

49 Hecker KE, Horn N, Baumert JH, *et al.* Minimum alveolar concentration (MAC) of xenon in intubated swine. *Br J Anaesth* 2004; **92**(3): 421–424.

50 Froeba G, Marx T, Pazhur J, *et al.* Xenon does not trigger malignant hyperthermia in susceptible swine. *Anesthesiology* 1999; **91**: 1047–1052.

51 Iber T, Hecker K, Vagts DA, *et al.* Xenon anesthesia inpairs hepatic oxygenation and perfusion in healthy pigs. *Minerva Anestesiol* 2008; **74**: 511–519.

52 Smith AC, Ehler WJ, Swindle MM. Anesthesia and analgesia in swine. In: Kohn DF, Winson SK, White WJ, Benson GJ, eds. *Anesthesia and Analgesia in Laboratory Animals*. San Diego, CA: Academic Press, 1997; 313–336.

53 Lu DZ, Fan HG, Wang HB, *et al.* Effect of the addition of tramadol to a combination of tiletamine-zolazepam and xylazine for anaesthesia of miniature pigs. *Vet Rec* 2010; **167**: 489–492.

54 Ko JC, Williams BL, Rogers ER, *et al.* Increased xylazine dose-enhanced anesthetic properties of telazol-xylazine combination in swine. *Lab Anim Sci* 1995; **45**: 290–294.

55 Lu DZ, Fan HG, Kun M, *et al.* Antagonistic effect of atipamezole, flumazenil and naloxone following anaesthesia with xylazine, tramadol and tiletamine/zolazepam combinations in pigs. *Vet Anaesth Analg* 2011; **4**: 301–309.

56 Thurmon JC, Tranquili WJ, Benson GJ. Cardiopulmonary responses of swine to intravenous infusion of guaifenesin, ketamine, and xylazine. *Am J Vet Res* 1986; **47**(10): 2138–2140.

57 Liu D, Shao YS, Luan X, *et al.* Comparison of ketamine-pentobarbital anesthesia and fentanyl-pentobarbital anesthesia for open-heart surgery in minipigs. *Lab Anim* 2009; **38**(7): 234–240.

58 Liu D, Hu J, Zhang M, *et al.* Low-dose ketamine combined with pentobarbital in a miniature porcine model for a cardiopulmonary bypass procedure: a randomized controlled study. *Eur J Anaesthesiol* 2009; **26**: 389–395.

59 Schöffmann G, Winter P, Palme R, *et al.* Haemodynamic changes and stress responses of piglets to surgery during total intravenous anaesthesia with propofol and fentanyl. *Lab Anim* 2009; **43**: 243–248.

60 Lacoumenta S, Yeo TH, Burrin JM, *et al.* Fentanyl and the beta-endorphin, ACTH and glycoregulatory hormonal response to surgery. *Br J Anaesth* 1987; **59**: 713–720.

61 Swindle MM. *Perioperative Care of Swine: Technical Bulletin*. Sinclair Research Center, 2002. www.sinclairresearch.com/PDF%20Files/perioperative%20care%20of%20swine.pdf (accessed 3 October 2014).

62 Smith AC, Swindle MM. Anesthesia and analgesia in swine. In: Fish RE, Brown MJ, Danneman PJ, Karas AZ, eds. *Anesthesia and Analgesia in Laboratory Animals*, 2nd edn. San Diego, CA: Academic Press, 2008; 413–440.

63 Greene SA, Benson GJ, Tranquili WJ, *et al.* Effect of isoflurane, atracurium, fentanyl, and noxious stimulation on bispectral index in pigs. *Compar Med* 2004; **54**(4): 397–403.

64 Martin-Cancho MF, Lima JR, Luis L, *et al.* Bispectral index, spectral edge frequency 95%, and median frequency recorded for various concentrations of isoflurane and sevoflurane in pigs. *Am J Vet Res* 2003; **64**(7): 866–873.

65 Martin-Cancho MF, Carrasco-Jimenez MS, Lima JR, *et al.* Assessment of the relationship of bispectral index values, hemodynamic changes, and recovery times associated with sevoflurane or propofol anesthesia in pigs. *Am J Vet Res* 2004; **65**(4): 409–416.

66 Hahn RG. Volume kinetics of infusion fluids (review). *Anesthesiology* 2010; **113**: 470–481.

67 Schoffstall JM, Spivey WH, Davidheiser S, *et al.* Intraosseous crystalloid and blood infusion in a swine model. *J Trauma* 1989; **29**(3): 384–387.

68 Warren DW, Kissoon N, Sommerauer JF, *et al.* Comparison of fluid rates among peripheral intravenous and humerus, femur, malleolus, and tibial intraosseous sites in normovolemic and hypovolemic piglets. *Ann Emerg Med* 1993; **22**(2): 183–186.

69 Rainger JE, Dart AJ. Enteral fluid therapy in large animals. *Aust Vet J* 2006; **84**(12): 447–451.

70 Hiltebrand LB, Kimberger O, Arnberger M, *et al.* Crystalloids versus colloids for goal-directed fluid therapy in major surgery. *Crit Care* 2009; **13**: 1–13.

71 Wafaisade A, Wutzler S, Lefering R, *et al.* Drivers of acute coagulopathy after severe trauma: a multivariate analysis of 1987 patients. *Emerg Med J* 2010; **22**: 934–939.

72 Hahn RG. Fluid therapy in uncontrolled hemorrhage – what experimental models have taught us. *Acta Anaesthesiol Scand* 2013; **57**: 16–28.

73 Smith DM, Newhouse M, Naziruddin B, *et al.* Blood group and transfusion in pigs. *Xenotransplantation* 2006; **13**: 186–194.

74 Oung CM, English M, Chiu RCJ, *et al.* Effects of hypothermia on hemodynamic responses to dopamine and dobutamine. *J Trauma* 1992; **33**(5): 671–678.

75 Hiltebrand LB, Krejci V, Sigurdsson GH. Effects of dopamine, dobutamine, and dopexamine on microcirculatory blood flow in the gastrointestinal tract during sepsis and anesthesia. *Anesthesiology* 2004; **100**: 1188–1197.

76 Ferrara JJ, Dyess DL, Peeples GL, *et al.* Effects of dopamine and dobutamine on regional blood flow distribution in the neonatal piglet. *Ann Surg* 1995; **221**(5): 531–542.

77 Priebe HJ, Nöldge GFE, Armbruster K, *et al.* Differential effects of dobutamine, dopamine, and noradrenaline on splanchnic haemodynamics and oxygenation I the pig. *Acta Anaesthesiol Scand* 1995; **39**: 1088–1096.

78 Massone, F. *Anestesiologia Veterinaria: Farmacologia e Tecnicas*, 5th edn. Rio de Janeiro, Brazil: Guanabara Koogan, 2008.

79 Haskins SC. Monitoring anesthetized patients. In: Short CE, ed. *Principles and Practice of Veterinary Anesthesia*. Baltimore, MD: Williams & Wilkins, 1987.

80 Gianotti GC, Beheregaray WK, Meyer FS, *et al.* Cardiorespiratory dynamics of sedated pigs submitted to different inspired oxygen fractions under controlled mechanical ventilation. *Acta Sci Vet* 2014; **42**: 1–8.

81 Dobromylsky P, Flecknell PA, Lascelles BD, *et al. Pain Management in Animals*. London: WB Saunders, 2001.

82 Claxton-Gill MS, Cornick-Seahorn JL, Gamboa JC, *et al.* Suspected malignant hyperthermia syndrome in a miniature pot-bellied pig anesthetized with isoflurane. *J Am Vet Med Assoc* 1993; **203**(10): 1434–1436.

83 Do Carmo PL, Zapata-Sudo MM, Trachez F, *et al.* Intravenous administration of azumolene to reverse malignant hyperthermia in swine. *J Vet Intern Med* 2010; **24**: 1224–1228.

84 Iaizzo PA, Kehler CH, Richard JC, *et al.* Prior hypothermia attenuates malignant hypothermia in susceptible swine. *Anesth Analg* 1996; **82**: 803–809.

85 Hermansen K, Pedersen LE, Olesen HO. The analgesic effect of buprenorphine, etorphine and pethidine in the pig: a randomized double blind cross-over study. *Acta Pharmacol Toxicol* 1986; **59**: 27–35.

86 Harvey-Clark CJ, Gillespie K, Riggs KW. Transdermal fentanyl compared with parenteral buprenorphine in post-surgical pain in swine: a case study. *Lab Anim* 2000; **34**: 386–398.

87 Branson KR, Gross ME. Opioid agonists and antagonists. In: *Veterinary Pharmacology and Therapeutics*, 8th edn. Ames, IA: Iowa State University Press, 2001.

88 Wilkinson AC, Thomas III ML, Morse BC. Evaluation of a transdermal fentanyl system in Yucatan miniature pigs. *Contemp Top Lab Anim Sci* 2001; **40**(3): 12–16.

89 Steffey EP, Baggot JD, Eisele JH, *et al.* Morphine-isoflurane interaction in dogs, swine and Rhesus monkeys. *J Vet Pharmacol Ther* 1994; **17**: 202–210.

90 Nolan AM. *Pain Management in Animals*. London: WB Saunders, 2001.

91 Rang HP, Dale MM, Ritter JM. *Pharmacology*, 3rd edn. London: Churchill Livingstone, 1996.

92 Ummenhofer WC, Arends R, Shen DD, *et al.* Comparative spinal distribution and clearance kinetics of intrathecally administered morphine, fentanyl, alfentanil, and sufentanil. *Anesthesiology* 2000; **92**: 739–753.

93 Strande A. Epidural anaesthesia in young pigs, dosage in relation to the length of the vertebral column. *Acta Vet Scand*; 1968: **9**(1): 41–49.

94 Malavasi LM, Nyman G, Augustsson H, *et al.* Effects of epidural morphine and transdermal fentanyl analgesia on physiology and behavior after abdominal surgery in pigs. *Lab Anim* 2006; **40**: 16–27.

95 Stegmann GF. Cardiovascular effects of epidural morphine or ropivacaine in isoflurane-anaesthetised pigs during surgical devascularisation of the liver. *J S Afr Vet Assoc* 2010; **81**(3): 143–147.

96 Mergner GW, Stolte AL, Frame WB, *et al.* Combined epidural analgesia and general anesthesia induce ischemia distal to a severe coronary artery stenosis in swine. *Anesth Analg* 1994; **78**: 37–45.

97 Boothe DM. Drugs affecting animal behavior. In: *Veterinary Pharmacology and Therapeutics*, 8th edn. Ames, IA: Iowa State University Press, 2001.

98 Swindle MM. *Swine in the Laboratory: Surgery, Anesthesia, Imaging, and Experimental Techniques*, 2nd edn. Boca Raton, FL: CRC Press, 2007.

99 Buur JL, Baynes RE, Smith G, *et al.* Pharmacokinetics of flunixin meglumine in swine after intravenous dosing. *J Vet Pharmacol Ther* 2006; **29**: 437–440.

51 Ruminant and Swine Local Anesthetic and Analgesic Techniques

Alexander Valverde and Melissa Sinclair
Department of Clinical Studies, Ontario Veterinary College, University of Guelph, Guelph, Ontario, Canada

Chapter contents

Introduction

In ruminant and swine practice, it is common to combine local anesthetics with restraint methods that may include physical and/or chemical means, to provide a cost-effective and humane alternative to general anesthesia. The choice of technique for a procedure and level of sedation required will depend on the species and breed of animal (dairy or beef cow, ovine or porcine), temperament, facilities available (farm or clinic location), and skills of the veterinarian. The economics of ruminant and swine practice does not allow for general anesthesia in most situations and local and regional anesthetic techniques are the basis of appropriate analgesia. Local anesthetic techniques do not require specialized equipment and avoid the potential complications of general anesthesia and recumbency. Most ruminants or swine are tolerant of humane restraint but appropriate sedation and facilities are necessary for successful application of these techniques. Most field surgeries are performed in standing adult cattle to minimize the risks associated with recumbency (e.g., bloat, regurgitation, hypoxemia, myopathy or neuropathy). Small ruminants or swine may be restrained in lateral or dorsal recumbency.

Local anesthetics can be infiltrated by perineural injection, infiltration at nerve endings in the skin or tissues, injection into the epidural or intrathecal space, and by injection into a peripheral vessel in combination with a tourniquet that prevents leakage into the systemic circulation. In cattle and small ruminants the most commonly used techniques are local anesthesia of the paralumbar fossa, caudal or lumbosacral epidural analgesia, horn blocks, and intravenous regional anesthesia of the foot. In swine, infiltrative local anesthesia, epidural anesthesia (caudal and lumbosacral) as well as intratesticular anesthesia are most common.

Local anesthetics

Local anesthetics block sodium channels and prevent depolarization of nerves. Lidocaine, bupivacaine, and mepivacaine are the most commonly used local anesthetics in ruminants and a specific drug is often chosen based on its onset and duration of action. Lidocaine and mepivacaine are shorter acting than bupivacaine due to their lower protein binding at the receptor, but faster in onset because their dissociation constant (pKA) is closer to plasma pH (7.4), which facilitates passage through cell membranes.

Toxicity of local anesthetics is related to their plasma concentration. Reported toxic doses are based on continuous intravenous (IV) infusion of the local anesthetic, which contrasts with clinical

Veterinary Anesthesia and Analgesia: The Fifth Edition of Lumb and Jones.
Edited by Kurt A. Grimm, Leigh A. Lamont, William J. Tranquilli, Stephen A. Greene and Sheilah A. Robertson.

Table 51.1 Approximate intravenous administration reported toxic doses (mg/kg) of local anesthetics in conscious sheep, lamb and pigs.

		Sheep	Lambs (1–5 days old)	Pig
Lidocaine	Seizure activity	5.8	18	30–60
	Hypotension and cardiovascular collapse	31–37	57–67	ND
Mepivacaine	Seizure activity	7.5–7.8	ND	ND
	Hypotension and cardiovascular collapse	49–69	ND	ND
Bupivacaine	Seizure activity	4.2–4.4	ND	ND
	Hypotension and cardiovascular collapse	8.3–9.2	ND	ND
Ropivacaine	Seizure activity	6.1–6.7	ND	ND
	Hypotension and cardiovascular collapse	11.3–11.9	ND	ND

ND = not determined.

situations where the local anesthetic drug is administered most commonly by extravascular infiltration; therefore a more gradual absorption from the injection site into the systemic circulation offsets the achievement of toxic doses.

Toxicity is dependent on multiple factors. In addition to dose, plasma concentrations are dependent on the site of injection, vascular supply and degree of absorption from the site, co-administration of other drugs (e.g., epinephrine), conscious versus anesthetized state, health status, and individual variation. In humans, peak plasma concentrations for routes other than IV are as follows: intercostal > epidural > brachial plexus > subcutaneous [1].

In ruminants, toxic doses of local anesthetics have only been determined for sheep which are often used as a model for humans (Table 51.1). The progressive manifestations of systemic toxicity in conscious sheep usually consist of mild cardiovascular depression, convulsions accompanied by cardiovascular stimulation, followed by hypotension, apnea, and finally circulatory collapse and death [2–4]. In sheep anesthetized with volatile anesthetic agents, no signs of central nervous system impairment (convulsions) are observed even when blood concentrations are two-fold higher than in conscious sheep exhibiting toxicity and although cardiovascular depression occurs, anesthesia has a protective role against arrhythmias and cardiovascular collapse [2].

Pregnancy may influence the toxic dose of local anesthetics. A slightly lower dose of bupivacaine (4.2 mg/kg versus 4.4 mg/kg) or ropivacaine (6.1 mg/kg versus 6.7 mg/kg) elicited the onset of convulsions in pregnant versus non-pregnant sheep after administration of 0.52 mg/kg/min of bupivacaine or 0.5 mg/kg/min of ropivacaine IV [3]. These differences are more statistically than clinically relevant. No differences between pregnant and non-pregnant sheep were detected for lidocaine or mepivacaine [5,6]. Signs of hypotension (a sudden 40% or greater drop in mean arterial blood pressure), apnea (>15 s), and circulatory collapse (loss of the peripheral pulse) occurred at approximately twice the convulsive dose: 8.3–9.2 mg/kg for bupivacaine and 11.3–11.9 mg/kg for ropivacaine [3].

Conscious non-pregnant adult sheep given intravenous lidocaine at 2 mg/kg/min showed convulsions after 5.8 mg/kg had been administered, whereas newborn lambs 1–5 days of age were more resistant and did not convulse until doses of 18 mg/kg were given [4]. Similarly, signs of hypotension (defined as a 20% drop in mean arterial blood pressure), apnea, and circulatory collapse occurred at 5–6 times (31–37 mg/kg) the convulsive dose for adult sheep and at 3.5 times (57–67 mg/kg) the convulsive dose for newborn lambs [4].

For mepivacaine, intravenous infusions of 2 mg/kg/min in conscious pregnant and non-pregnant sheep resulted in convulsions at doses of 7.5–7.8 mg/kg and signs of hypotension, apnea, and circulatory collapse at 6–9 times (49–69 mg/kg) the convulsive dose [6].

Pigs have been used as a model for the study of local anesthetic toxicity in human pediatric patients. Bupivacaine administered IV at 1 mg/kg/min in sevoflurane-anesthetized piglets aged 19–43 days of age (4.3–5.8 kg) induced hypotension (a 50% drop in mean arterial blood pressure) at a median doses of 4.6–5.2 mg/kg [7]. Older pigs (20–27 kg) administered 4 mg/kg of bupivacaine IV over 30 s under thiopental anesthesia showed an immediate drop in mean arterial blood pressure (24%), cardiac index (38%), and heart rate (14%) followed by a gradual recovery to baseline over 30 min [8].

In conscious piglets (12–60 hours old; 1–2.5 kg), lidocaine induced seizures at a total dose of 42 mg/kg IV administered as a 2 mg/kg bolus followed by an infusion at 2 mg/kg/min. Administration of 15 mg/kg within 30 s every 4 min resulted in seizures at cumulative doses of 30–60 mg [9]. In both groups, there were no detectable changes in heart rate or mean arterial blood pressure before the onset of seizures [9].

Lidocaine hydrochloride (2%) is approved in Canada and the United States for use in cattle as a local anesthetic, but not for small ruminants or swine. However, it is labeled in cattle without established withdrawal times for meat and milk. General recommendations are a 5-day withdrawal for meat and 3 days for milk after local infiltration techniques [10]. For caudal epidural anesthesia using volumes of less than 10 mL, recommended meat and milk withdrawal times of 24 h are listed [11,12]. Veterinarians should always check with the regulatory authorities of their region. Within the US, practitioners are referred to FARAD for withdrawal guidance and the Animal Medicinal Drug Use Clarification Act (AMDUCA) (www.farad.org/amduca) for regulatory considerations. Information on residue avoidance for Canada can be found at www.cgfarad.ca.

Blocks for regional anesthesia of the head

Horn blocks

There are similarities in desensitizing the nerve supply to the horn in cattle, goats, and sheep. In cattle, the main sensory nerve supply to the horn arises from the cornual branch and also the supraorbital and infratrochlear nerves, all of which originate from the ophthalmic branch of the trigeminal nerve (Fig. 51.1). The ophthalmic branch divides into three nerves while still within the foramen orbitorotundum: lacrimal, nasociliary, and frontal. The lacrimal nerve consists of two strands located along the lateral surface of the lateral rectus muscle that later join between them and with the communicating ramus of the zygomatic nerve to form the zygomaticotemporal branch, which is located at the level of the dorsal and caudal aspect of the orbit and exits along the ventral aspect of the zygomatic process (supraorbital) of the frontal bone. The zygomaticotemporal branch continues as the cornual branch as it travels caudally towards the base of the horn along the temporal ridge, between the supraorbital process and the lateral edge of the base of the horn [13].

In adult cattle, the site of injection for the cornual branch is 3–5 cm in front of the base of the horn, where the nerve veers from ventral to dorsal from the temporal fossa to the frontal bone and branches into endings along the base of the horn. A 2.5–3.8 cm, 20 gauge needle is inserted along the area of the temporal line and frontal bone and 10 mL of 2% lidocaine injected after negative

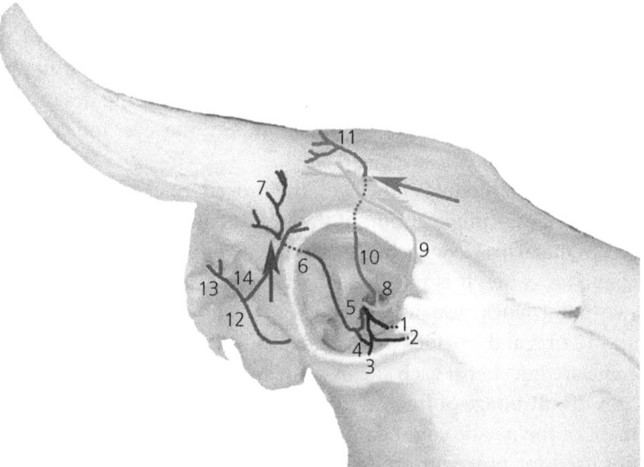

Figure 51.1 Innervation to the horn and surrounding tissue. Arrows indicate the sites for complete block to the horn, which includes the cornual branch (7), the infratrochlear nerve (9), the supraorbital nerve (11), and branches of the second cervical nerve (not shown, but injected at the caudal base of the horn). The branches of the ophthalmic nerve that give origin to these nerves (except second cervical nerve) are illustrated in color. (1) Maxillary nerve (black); (2) Zygomaticofacial branch; (3) Zygomatic nerve; (4) Communicating branch of zygomatic nerve to lacrimal nerve; (5) Lacrimal nerve (purple); (6) Zygomaticotemporal branch; (7) Cornual branch; (8) Nasociliary nerve (green); (9) Infratrochlear nerve; (10) Frontal nerve (red); (11) Supraorbital nerve. Also depicted are the auriculopalpebral nerve (12) and its branches the rostral auricular branch (13) and zygomatic branch (14).

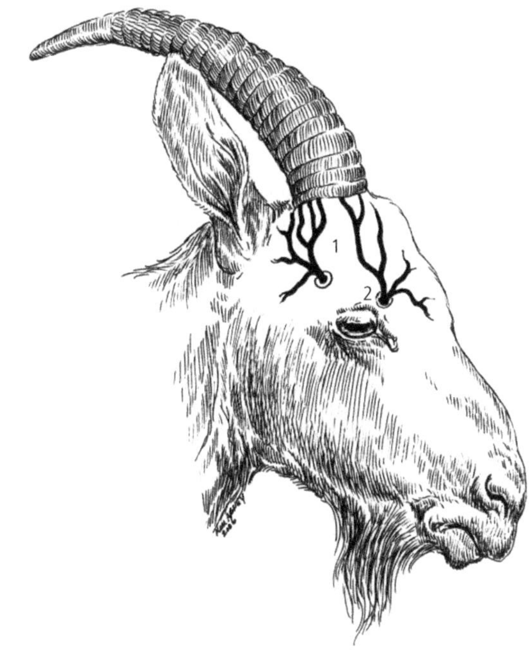

Figure 51.2 Locations for nerve block for dehorning an adult goat. The cornual branch of the lacrimal nerve (zygomaticotemporal) is blocked behind the root of the supraorbital process (1) and the cornual branch of the infratrochlear nerve is blocked at the dorsomedial margin of the orbit (2). From [15].

aspiration of blood has been verified to avoid injection into the cornual artery or vein in the surrounding area [14].

The nasociliary nerve branches into the infratrochlear nerve as it enters the orbit, which ascends to the dorsal margin of the orbit to the level of the lacrimal bone, dorsal to the medial canthus, where it curves around the frontal bony margin of the orbit to travel caudally and along the frontal bone; it may reach the base of the horn [13]. The site of injection for the infratrochlear nerve is 2–3 cm medial from the dorsal aspect of the rim of the orbit; a 2.5 cm, 20 gauge needle and 5 mL of 2% lidocaine are used. Alternatively, the branches that reach the horn can be blocked with the supraorbital nerve as described below.

The frontal nerve travels from the orbitorotundum foramen to the orbital opening of the supraorbital canal, on the caudal and dorsal aspect of the orbit, to emerge as the supraorbital nerve at the supraorbital foramen of the frontal bone. The supraorbital foramen can be located about 3–4 cm from the temporal ridge and halfway along the distance between the supraorbital process and the medial edge of the base of the horn [13]. The site of injection for the supraorbital nerve is at the level of the supraorbital foramen using a 2.5 cm, 20 gauge needle and 5 mL of 2% lidocaine and taking care to avoid the supraorbital vein. Because most of the cornual branches of the infratrochlear nerve travel to the horn at this same location, they can be blocked with this approach.

The proximity of the rostral auricular and zygomatic branches of the auriculopalpebral nerve to the sites of injection of the cornual, supraorbital, and nasociliary nerves [13] often results in their blockade, producing relaxation of the ear and inability to close the eyelids.

In addition to these three main nerves, the caudal aspect of the base of the horn may be supplied by cutaneous branches of the second cervical nerve and these can be blocked by injecting local anesthetic close to the dorsal midline of the neck at a point level with the base of the ear [14].

Following surgery on the horns, anesthesia and analgesia are provided for as long as the duration of action of the local anesthetic. Due to the invasive nature of dehorning surgery, a non-steroidal anti-inflammatory drug (e.g., flunixin meglumine 2 mg/kg, IV or IM) is suggested for postoperative analgesia after the anesthetic effect diminishes.

The cornual nerves of sheep and goats are very similar to those of cattle, although the cutaneous branches of the second cervical nerve are less likely to innervate the horn. The cornual branch of the lacrimal nerve (zygomaticotemporal) is blocked behind the root of the supraorbital process (Fig. 51.2). A 2.5 cm, 22 gauge needle is inserted to a depth of 1–1.5 cm and 2–3 mL of 2% lidocaine is injected, halfway between the lateral canthus and the lateral edge of the base of the horn. The cornual branches of the infratrochlear nerve are blocked close to the dorsal rim of the orbit, halfway between the medial canthus and the medial edge of the base of the horn, by inserting a 2.5 cm, 22 gauge needle to a depth of about 0.5 cm and injecting 1–2 mL of 2% lidocaine [14,15].

Eye and adnexa block

The orbit has a rich presence of nerves behind the globe that are not exclusive to the eye. These nerves emerge from the cranial cavity through various foramina (e.g., the foramen orbitorotundum and optic foramen) to supply the eye and adnexa in addition to other extraocular structures. Nerves present in this location include the optic nerve as it emerges from the optic foramen as well as the nerves emerging from the foramen orbitorotundum, including the ophthalmic branches of the trigeminal nerve or extensions of these branches that eventually give rise to the nerves to the horn (lacrimal nerve, infratrochlear nerve, frontal nerve), the oculomotor nerve, the trochlear nerve, the abducent nerve, and the zygomaticofacial branch of the maxillary nerve (part of the trigeminal nerve). Therefore, injection of local anesthetic in this area can result in sensory or motor blockade of those nerves and the structures they serve, and not just of the eye.

The structures potentially anesthetized or paralyzed by local anesthetic effects on the oculomotor nerve include the dorsal, ventral, and medial rectus muscles, the superior elevator palpebral muscle, the retractor globe muscle, and the ventral oblique muscle; by the trochlear nerve, the dorsal oblique muscle; by the ophthalmic branches of the trigeminal nerve, the upper eyelid, lacrimal gland, conjunctiva, third eyelid, skin of medial and lateral angle of the eye, iris, cornea, horn, sections of skin over the frontal bone; by the zygomaticofacial branch of the maxillary nerve, the lower eyelid; and by the abducent nerve the lateral rectus muscle and the lateral part of the retractor globe muscle [13].

Anesthesia of the eye is most commonly performed for enucleation surgery. It is possible to perform an enucleation in adult cattle with the animal standing, using either a four-point injection (retrobulbar block) to block the deep orbital nerves or a Peterson block to exclusively anesthetize the nerves as they exit the skull through the foramen orbitorotundum and optic foramen. Ocular surgery in small ruminants or young cattle is generally performed under general anesthesia but the use of an eye block is also recommended to decrease volatile anesthetic requirements, decrease the likelihood of eliciting the oculocardiac reflex (trigeminovagal), and provide postoperative analgesia.

Four-point block (retrobulbar)

In the awake, adult bovine, the animal can be restrained in a chute and the head is secured. A 9 cm, 18 or 20 gauge needle is bent into a curved shape and inserted into the orbit (i.e., the bony fossa surrounding the globe) at 12, 3, 6 and 9 o'clock positions to a depth of 7–9 cm (in the adult bovine). The injections can be made through the eyelids, if preferred. The operator uses an index finger to deflect the globe away from the needle as it is inserted. The orbital septum must be penetrated, otherwise the local anesthetic may be deposited subconjunctivally. The operator can generally perceive the point when the needle penetrates the septum. In adult cattle, 5–10 mL of 2% lidocaine are injected at each site and through the different tissue planes to provide good anesthetic spread [16] and desensitize all nerves present in the orbit that supply the eye and adnexa. Proptosis indicates a successful block.

In small ruminants and calves, the procedure can be performed to enhance antinociception of the eye during general anesthesia. A 3.8 cm, 20 or 22 gauge needle is curved and inserted as described above for cattle. It is possible to obtain good blockade by doing a two-point block, usually using two opposite locations (e.g., the 6 and 12 or 3 and 9 o'clock positions). Volumes of 2–3 mL of 2% lidocaine are injected at each site in adult small ruminants or calves.

A disadvantage of this technique is that the injection and placement of the needle could damage the optic nerve, so it is normally not used for procedures other than enucleation. There is also the possibility that the anesthetic could enter the cerebrospinal fluid, as the meninges extend around the optic nerve. This can result in acute CNS toxicity and potentially death. Other complications include penetration of the globe, retrobulbar hemorrhage, and initiation of the oculocardiac reflex from pressure generated during injection [14].

Peterson block

This is technically more difficult than the four-point block and requires careful needle positioning, making it less reliable. Its efficacy depends on accurate placement of the injected anesthetic at the site of emergence of the nerves from the foramen orbitorotundum since there is minimal distribution along tissue planes [16]. Due to the ventral location of the foramen orbitorotundum with respect to the optic foramen (about 1 cm ventral), direct blockade of the optic nerve may not result; however, increasing the volume of injection may facilitate reaching and therefore blocking the optic nerve (Fig. 51.3). In addition to the nerves emerging from the orbitorotundum foramen described for the retrobulbar block, the maxillary nerve (branch of the trigeminal nerve) is also involved and results in block of the zygomatic nerve and its zygomaticofacial branch (lower eyelid innervation) and the pterygopalatine and

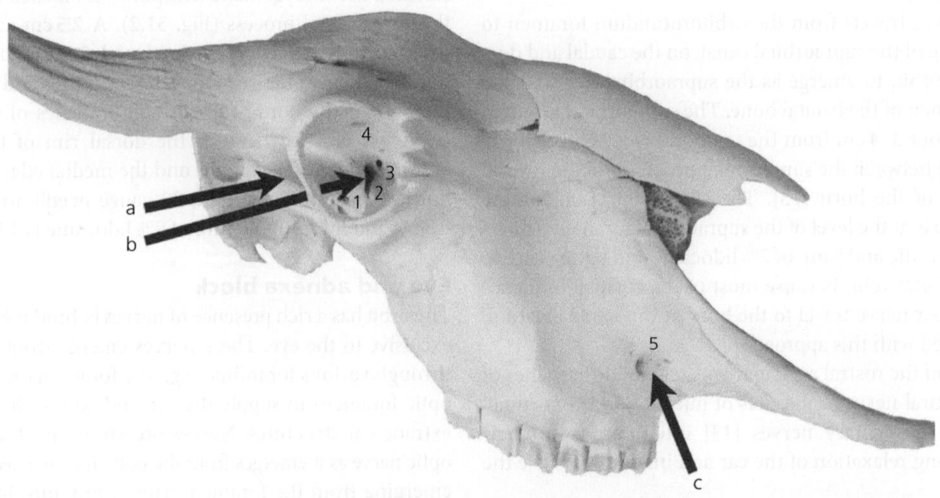

Figure 51.3 Location for needle placement for the auriculopalpebral block (a), the Peterson eye block (b), and the infraorbital block (c). (1) Oval foramen; (2) Foramen orbitorotundum; (3) Optic foramen; (4) Supraorbital foramen; (5) Infraorbital foramen.

infraorbital nerve for anesthesia of nasal passages and nose as described below [13]. The mandibular nerve (a branch of the trigeminal) is less likely to be affected because it exits the skull through the oval foramen, which is more ventrally located and separated from the orbitorotundum by the pterygoid crest (see Fig. 51.3) [13].

To perform this block, the animal is restrained with its nasal bones parallel to the ground. A 10 or 12 cm, 20 gauge needle is passed just in front of the rostral border of the coronoid process of the mandible, caudal to the notch formed by the zygomatic arch and supraorbital process, and directed slightly ventrally and posteriorly for the length of the needle or until it strikes bone. The local anesthetic (15–20 mL, 2% lidocaine) is injected once the needle strikes bone in the area where the nerves travel towards the orbit [14,15,17]. The same technique can be performed in small ruminants and calves using a 6.3 cm, 20 gauge needle and injecting 3–4 mL of 2% lidocaine.

Auriculopalpebral block

Eyelid akinesia (paralysis) can be produced by blocking the auriculopalpebral nerve (arising from the facial nerve) which provides innervation to the ear (rostral auricular branches) and to the eyelids (zygomatic branches). The zygomatic branches block the motor function of the orbicularis oculi muscle and elevator of the medial oculi angle muscle [13,14]. This type of anesthesia facilitates examination of the eye by preventing blinking but does not provide sensory blockade.

The auriculopapebral nerve is blocked by inserting a 2.5–3.8 cm, 22 gauge needle through the skin at the end of the zygomatic arch on the zygomatic process of the temporal bone and injecting 5–10 mL of 2% lidocaine, subcutaneously, at the dorsal border of the arch [14,15]. By injecting at this site, both the zygomatic and rostral auricular branches of the auriculopalpebral are blocked (see Fig. 51.3). Attempting to inject the zygomatic branch exclusively is more difficult due to the variable locations at which it branches from the auriculopapebral nerve once it has traveled dorsal from the zygomatic arch.

Nasal passages and nasal block

Anesthesia of nasal passages and nostrils can be achieved by blockade of the maxillary nerve at the foramen orbitorotundum as described for the Peterson eye block. This block will include the divisions of the maxillary nerve that enter the maxillary foramen, the pterygopalatine nerve, and infraorbital nerve. The pterygopalatine nerve supplies the soft palate (minor palatine nerve), hard palate (major palatine nerve), and ventral aspects of the nasal cavity and palate (caudal nasal nerve). The infraorbital nerve travels within the infraorbital canal from the maxillary foramen to the infraorbital foramen, where it emerges and continues to the nose and surrounding tissue, to supply the skin of the dorsal nasal area, nares, and upper lip [13]. To avoid including the innervation to the eye and adnexa, it is more common to only block the infraorbital nerve as it emerges from the infraorbital foramen, resulting in incomplete block of the nasal passages.

The infraorbital foramen can be readily localized by palpation, by extending a line from the nasoincisive notch to the first palpable cheek tooth (second premolar, since the first premolar is absent), approximately 5 cm above the tooth (see Fig. 51.3). A volume of 5–10 mL of 2% lidocaine can be injected into the infraorbital canal using a 3.8 cm, 20 gauge needle introduced through the infraorbital foramen.

Blocks for regional anesthesia of the flank or paralumbar fossa

Blocks to anesthetize the flank are commonly performed in ruminants to permit intra-abdominal surgery (e.g., cesarean section, abomasal, and rumenal procedures). They can be performed in the standing adult bovine and in the recumbent calf or small ruminant, using one of several described techniques, including line infiltration, inverted 'L' or '7,' proximal paravertebral, distal paravertebral, segmental dorsolumbar epidural, and segmental thoracolumbar subarachnoid anesthesia. Generally, for any of these techniques, the dermatomes intended to be blocked are those supplied by the thoracic nerve 13 (T13) and lumbar nerves 1 and 2 (L1, L2). The inclusion of lumbar nerve 3 (L3) provides superior anesthesia since it supplies the caudal third of the abdominal flank and may also supply branches that project to more cranial aspects of the flank. These techniques are not suitable for surgery of the ventral abdomen since not all spinal nerves involved in the sensory of this area are blocked.

Line infiltration block

Anesthesia of the body wall for abdominal surgery requires anesthesia of all layers including the peritoneum, which makes some of these techniques inadequate if the spread of the anesthetic does not reach all layers; this is especially likely with line infiltration techniques.

In adult cattle, this is the simplest block to perform since it involves the injection of small volumes (5–8 mL) of 2% lidocaine per site with a 3.8 cm, 18 gauge needle along the previously clipped and aseptically prepared predicted incision line; the anesthetic spreads in different directions and depths from the point of injection. Therefore, this block mostly affects the nerve endings proximal to the incision site. It is best to start from the most dorsal aspect of the flank and insert the needle in a dorsal to ventral direction and work towards the ventral end of the incision, as each injection provides progressive desensitization before the subsequent injection. A longer needle (8.9 cm) can be used instead of the shorter needle to reach the parietal peritoneum and improve the quality of the block [14]. This block is usually only effective for 60–90 min due to the rapid systemic uptake of anesthetic from the vascular abdominal wall.

Based on toxic doses for sheep, the total dose should not exceed 5–6 mg/kg since absorption from the muscle layers is probably rapid. This dose represents a volume of 83–100 mL of 2% lidocaine for a 500 kg cow.

In small ruminants or calves the technique is the same but a 2.5–3.8 cm, 20 gauge needle and volumes of 1–2 mL 2% lidocaine per site are used. In a 40 kg patient a volume of 10–12 mL of 2% lidocaine corresponds to the 5–6 mg/kg dose.

Inverted 'L' or '7' block

For correct nomenclature, the left flank is blocked with spread of local anesthetic in an inverted 'L' or reversed '7' shape, whereas the right flank is blocked with a '7' shape.

The injection of local anesthetic following the 'L' or '7' shape along the caudal aspect of the last rib and the ventral aspect of the lumbar vertebrae transverse processes blocks the transmission of pain from the periphery (flank area) to the spinal cord. The block is similar to the infiltration technique in that it requires similar volumes of 2% lidocaine and a 3.8 or 8.9 cm, 18 gauge needle for injection of anesthetic along the shape of the block. It is best to start from the angle of the 'L' or '7' and spread the anesthetic to the caudal aspect for the horizontal plane and to the ventral aspect for the vertical plane, to allow progressive desensitization before the subsequent injection. It is also important to remember that nerves will lie in different planes between muscle and facial layers so several different depths of injection may be required for complete block of deeper layers.

This block provides more spread of the local anesthetic than the line block; however, because it is done on two axes it is important to distribute the amount of local anesthetic evenly to avoid an incomplete block. Similar to the line block, the duration of action is approximately 60–90 min.

In small ruminants or calves the block follows the same technique using a 2.5–3.8 cm, 20 gauge needle and volumes of 1–2 mL 2% lidocaine per site.

Proximal paravertebral block

This block is also known as the Farquharson, Hall, or Cambridge technique [14] and the term *proximal* refers to the proximity to the spine. Generally, nerves T13, L1, and L2 are blocked. The inclusion of nerve L3 provides better anesthesia of the caudal third of the abdominal flank [15]. The latter nerve is sometimes considered one of the contributors to the femoral nerve and blocking it may potentially result in hindlimb weakness; however, the femoral nerve is mostly derived from L4, L5, and L6 [18], which makes ataxia very unlikely.

Dorsal and ventral branches from nerves T13 and L1 travel superimposed routes dorsoventrally for approximately 10 cm as the respective nerve emerges from the intervertebral foramen [19]. For nerves L2 and L3, the superimposition is less exact and a branch from the ventral branch of L2 joins the ventral branch from L3 at approximately 9–12 cm from the midline (Fig. 51.4). The ventral branch from L3 is the only one of the four nerves involved that travels rostral to the dorsal branch [19].

The proximal paravertebral technique involves the perineural injection of local anesthetic in proximity to the spinal nerves as they emerge from the vertebral canal. The dorsal and ventral branches of each nerve must be blocked if complete anesthesia of the flank is desired. To locate the site of injection, it is best to identify the lumbar transverse processes by counting them, starting at lumbar transverse process 5, which is the most proximal and cranial to the tuber coxae, then moving cranially, because lumbar transverse process 1 is not always palpable, depending on the degree of obesity of the animal, and may be confused with lumbar transverse process 2. Cattle have six lumbar vertebrae, but transverse process 6 is significantly smaller and hidden by the iliac wing. Each spinal nerve divides into a dorsal and ventral branch as it emerges and travels between lumbar transverse processes. Because the lumbar transverse processes are curved cranially, it is important to note that once a perpendicular line is traced from the middle of the width of the transverse process towards the spine, the nerve located in this area corresponds to the preceding process (e.g., for lumbar transverse process number 4, the nerve located using this method is L3 and so on). Therefore, to block nerves T13, L1, L2, and L3, it is necessary to locate lumbar transverse processes 1 through 4 (see Fig. 51.4).

The epaxial area from the last rib to lumbar transverse process 4 and from the tip of the transverse processes on the lateral aspect to 3–4 cm from the spinous processes on the midline is clipped and aseptically prepared for this block. In adult cattle, the distal end of lumbar transverse process 4 is identified by placing the thumb and index finger on either side of the process; a perpendicular line is traced from the midpoint of the process towards the spine and a 3.8 cm, 16 gauge needle is inserted its full length approximately 5–6 cm from the midline to act as a cannula for the subsequent insertion of a 8.9 cm, 20 gauge spinal needle and to prevent bending of the latter. Then, the spinal needle is directed towards the lumbar transverse process and once in contact with it, it is walked off towards the cranial edge until it advances through the intertransverse ligament and then situated ventrally for blockade of the ventral branch of nerve L3.

Avoid walking the needle off caudally because the blockade at this location is less effective due to the routing of the nerves from the vertebral foramen along the transverse process. Aspiration to confirm negative pressure is important to avoid placement of the needle in the abdominal cavity; then 20 mL of 2% lidocaine are injected. The needle is then retracted to the point of no friction, which indicates placement above the intertransverse ligament, and the dorsal branch is blocked with 5 mL of 2% lidocaine and the needles withdrawn. This method is repeated for nerves L2 and L1 by identifying the transverse processes of L3 and L2, respectively. If palpation of the transverse process of L1 is not feasible, the distances obtained between the previous injection sites should be symmetric and the distance between thoracic transverse processes 13 and lumbar transverse process 1 can be estimated and the

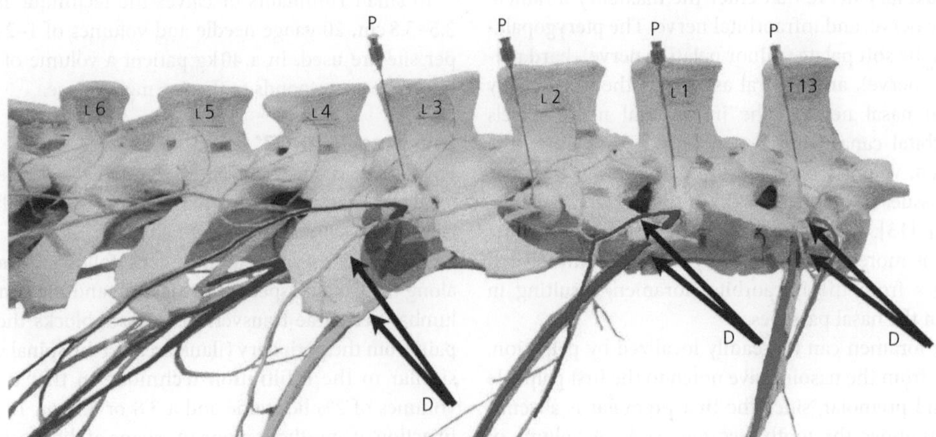

Figure 51.4 Proximal (P) and distal (D) paravertebral block at T13, L1, L2, L3 nerves. The colored thin lines depict the dorsal branch and the colored thick lines depict the ventral branch of each nerve. Note the communication between ventral branches of L2 and L3 nerves near the intertransverse space between L3 and L4 (*shaded circle*). The black arrows indicate the dorsal and ventral positioning of the needle for a distal paravertebral block.

method repeated to complete the block. Blockade of the four nerves as described requires approximately 100 mL of 2% lidocaine in a 500 kg cow, similar to the volume used for the infiltration block but it provides a more precise but extensive block of the flank; therefore, this technique is usually recommended. The duration of action tends to exceed that of the line infiltration and inverted 'L' or '7' blocks since the administration of anesthetic is more circumscribed to the main nerves; therefore blocks of 90–120 min are produced.

In addition to sensory blockade, motor and sympathetic fibers are also affected which results in relaxation of the epaxial lumbar muscles and vasodilation, respectively. Therefore, the spine curves (scoliosis) towards the blocked site and the skin temperature over the flank increases. From the surgeon's perspective, this means that tissues become tense due to the convexity that results on the surgical site which tends to spread the tissues when surgically approaching the abdominal cavity. This, combined with vasodilation of blood vessels, can result in increased bleeding if surgical hemostasis is poor.

In small ruminants or calves the block follows the same technique using a 2.5–3.8 cm, 20 gauge needle and the volumes of 2% lidocaine are 0.5–1 mL for the dorsal branch and 2–3 mL for the ventral branch, but not exceeding the 5–6 mg/kg that correspond to a toxic dose. Sheep have six (more common) or seven lumbar vertebrae, whereas goats have six but sometimes only five lumbar vertebrae, which can complicate the identification of vertebrae if counting backwards as described for cattle. However, it is simpler in these species to identify lumbar transverse process 1 and count from there to verify the proper sites for needle insertion.

Distal paravertebral block

This block is also known as the Magda, Cakala, or Cornell technique [14] and the term *distal* refers to the distance from the spine. This distal approach is used to block the dorsal and ventral branches of the same nerves as for the proximal paravertebral block (T13, L1–3) as they cross over and under, respectively, the transverse process.

For this block, a lateral approach with regard to the location of the lumbar transverse process is used and the area around the tips of the processes is clipped and aseptically prepared. The L2 and L3 nerves are blocked from the location of the lumbar transverse process 4, L1 from the location of the lumbar transverse process 2 and T13 from the location of the lumbar transverse process 1 (see Fig. 51.4) [14].

In adult cattle, approximately 5 mL of 2% lidocaine is injected above and 10–20 mL below the transverse process using a 6.4–8.9 cm, 18 gauge needle. The injection is started at the tip of the distal end of the transverse process and the local anesthetic is deposited along the process, as the needle is advanced towards the spine. It is important to keep the needle close to the process, otherwise the anesthetic is deposited in the surrounding soft tissue and the block may fail. The duration of action is similar to the proximal paravertebral block.

Segmental dorsolumbar epidural block

In cattle, the dermatomes innervated by nerves T13 and L1–3 can be blocked bilaterally or unilaterally by performing an epidural injection at the thoracolumbar (T13–L1) or first interlumbar (L1–2) space [14,20–23].

An epidural injection refers to depositing a drug in the space between the dura mater and the vertebral column. In reality, it is an intradural injection between two dural laminae because the dura mater only adheres closely as a fused double layer within the skull. In the vertebral column it is separated and only the internal lamina, made of fibrous tissue, surrounds the spinal cord and provides rigidity to help support the blood vessels that supply the spinal cord [24].

The injection of a reduced volume of local anesthetic or xylazine into the epidural space at T13–L1 or L1–2 allows these drugs to affect only those segments of the spinal cord that innervate the flank without interfering with motor function of the pelvic limbs; this allows the animal to remain standing and prevents ataxia. This technique can be used for surgery on or performed via the flank and needle tip placement in the epidural space can be directed towards one side of the spinal cord to emphasize the block on the corresponding ipsilateral flank or the needle kept on the median plane with respect to the spinal cord to block both sides. The block is more technically challenging than any of the other techniques previously described for flank anesthesia; however, it can be readily learned [25] and effectively used by practitioners [23].

Adequate restraint and sedation of the animal are necessary to facilitate the placement of the needle in the epidural space. The skin area caudal to the T13 or L1 spinous process and contralateral to the flank region to be desensitized is aseptically prepared and injected subcutaneously with 2–4 mL of 2% lidocaine adjacent to the interspinous ligaments between T13–L1 or L1–2 to facilitate the insertion of a short 2.5 cm, 14 gauge needle that serves as a cannula for the subsequent insertion of an 11.4 cm, 18 gauge spinal needle [14]. Alternatively, a 12 cm, 16 gauge Tuohy needle can be used by itself [26]. The mean distance from skin to the epidural space at this level is 8.1 cm in cows between 337 and 742 kg [27] but it is recommended to use needles that are slightly longer because if the needle does not reach the deeper planes of the epidural space, the injected anesthetic will remain between periosteum and epidural fat, when ideally it should distribute between epidural fat and dura mater [26]. The amount of fat in the thoracolumbar epidural space is greater in the dorsal than ventral aspect of the space and fat is considered a barrier because it is present in a semi-fluid state that impedes spread and also potentially prevents the actions of the anesthetic drug [26].

The L1–2 intervertebral space is localized on the path of an imaginary line drawn from side to side, 1–2 cm caudal to the tips of the two cranial edges of the second lumbar transverse process [14]. The operator can then decide to insert the needles at the depression between L1 and L2 or move to the next cranial depression between T13 and L1. The spinal needle is advanced gradually through the interspinous ligament until it reaches the ligamentum flavum which is pierced to enter the epidural space. Correct placement can be verified by use of the hanging drop technique in which the hub of the needle is filled with saline or local anesthetic after the stylet is removed and if the needle is correctly placed, the fluid is aspirated into the needle shaft and epidural space due to the subatmospheric epidural pressure. The stylet can also be removed before the needle penetrates the ligamentum flavum and the operator can detect the aspiration of the fluid once the needle enters the epidural space. The initial pressure of the epidural space is on average −21 mmHg (range of −17 to −23 mmHg), but within 1 min of needle insertion, it stabilizes at −14 mmHg (range of −9 to −17 mmHg) [27], and it is for this reason that it has been recommended to allow air to enter freely into the epidural space for approximately 1 min to decrease the effects of varying pressures on the distribution of anesthetic drug [22]. Additional verification of correct placement should include ease of injection into the epidural space and absence of cerebrospinal fluid (CSF) prior to injection, to ensure that the dura and arachnoid membrane have not been pierced and to avoid subarachnoid injection since epidural doses are significantly higher than subarachnoid doses. An alternative modified technique involves introducing the needle an additional 0.7–1.0 cm or until the cow shows signs of discomfort, such as sudden movement or dipping of the back, to bypass the epidural fat and enhance the spread of the anesthetic drug [22]. The needle should be removed immediately after injection to avoid damage to the spinal cord.

Studies using new methylene blue have shown that 5 mL injected at the L1–2 epidural space of adult Holstein cows spread to the T12–L3 spinal dermatomes, whereas 10 mL spread to the T11–L5 spinal dermatomes [26]. Volumes of 6–8 mL of 2% lidocaine (0.24–0.32 mg/kg) or 5% procaine (0.6–0.8 mg/kg) are recommended in a 500 kg cow to desensitize the dermatomes of T13–L3 [14]. Xylazine 2% (0.05 mg/kg) is also effective but the combination of xylazine (0.025 mg/kg) and lidocaine (0.1 mg/kg) diluted to a volume of 5 mL with 0.9% saline resulted in more consistent anesthesia than either drug alone diluted to the same volume [22]. Onset of anesthesia is approximately 10–15 min with a duration of 45–120 min [14,22,23].

Instead of injecting through a needle, an epidural catheter can be placed in the T13–L1 space to allow repeated injections of anesthetic drugs and prolonged duration of action. A 10.2 cm, 17 gauge Tuohy needle is placed in the epidural space as described above and the tip of the epidural catheter is advanced through the needle to the L1–2 space for injection of the anesthetic drugs [28]. Because of the probability of the catheter tip pointing to one side of the spinal cord, a unilateral block is more likely with this technique [14].

Segmental thoracolumbar subarachnoid block

For this block a catheter is advanced from the lumbosacral (L6–S1) subarachnoid space to the T13–L1 space for the injection of local anesthetic (lidocaine or procaine). The insertion of needles into the T13–L1 or L1–2 intervertebral spaces for subarachnoid injection of anesthetic is discouraged due to the high risk of trauma to the spinal cord when piercing of the dura mater and arachnoid membranes is attempted at these locations; hence the reason for advancing the catheter from the L6–S1 intervertebral subarachnoid space [28]. The distance from L6–S1 to T13–L1 is approximately 45 cm in adult cattle [14] and care must be taken while advancing the catheter rostrally within the subarachnoid space to avoid kinking or curling it, which results in patient discomfort and potential damage to the spinal cord. This technique is less likely to be performed under field conditions.

The L6–S1 intervertebral space is localized 1–4 cm caudal of an imaginary line traced between the cranial edges of the tuber coxae. A 15 cm, 17 gauge Tuohy needle is inserted at the L6–S1 intervertebral space after previous skin preparation, and the subcutaneous and deep interspinous ligaments are desensitized with 5 mL of 2% lidocaine using a 15 cm, 18 gauge needle. The Tuohy needle is advanced slowly with the bevel pointing cranially into the epidural space and continues to be advanced until it pierces the dura and arachnoid mater and enters the subarachnoid space. Correct placement is verified by aspiration of 2 mL of CSF. Then an 80–100 cm catheter (epidural catheters are used) with a spring guide is advanced into the subarachnoid space for the estimated distance required to reach the T13–L1 space, which is usually approximately 60 cm due to the length and angle of the needle. The Tuohy needle and spring guide are removed, the catheter distance adjusted to the correct location and secured in place. Doses of 1.5–2 mL of 2% lidocaine or 5% procaine have been injected at a rate of 0.5 mL/min to induce unilateral or bilateral anesthesia from T10 to L3 in 5–10 min and for a duration of 54 min [28].

One disadvantage of this technique is the uncertainty of whether the resulting block will be on the intended side of the animal. The variation in block has been suggested to result from trapping of the catheter ventral to the spinal cord, which may impede adequate distribution of the injected anesthetic around the circumference of the pia mater due to the presence of the dorsal and ventral longitudinal ligaments [14].

Blocks for regional anesthesia of the linea alba and paramedian

Line infiltration block

The abdomen, subcutaneous tissues, and skin of the abdomen can be desensitized by infiltration of local anesthetic to allow procedures such as correction of umbilical and abdominal wall hernias and a right paramedian abomasopexy to be performed. For these blocks, the technique and volumes described for the flank line infiltration block are used along the anatomic area selected for the surgery. Often a 'V' shape block can be used with the angle of the 'V' located at the cranial aspect of the incision and the wings along either side of the incision to create a shield that blocks sensory input towards the incision.

Lumbosacral, sacrococcygeal or intercoccygeal epidural (cranial epidural) block

This technique is often referred as a cranial (anterior) epidural and can be performed at any of the three sites (Fig. 51.5). Injections at the sacrococcygeal or first intercoccygeal epidural space require that the injectate volume of anesthetic drug is sufficient to facilitate its rostral spread from this site to the thoracolumbar area, so that it can affect structures cranial to the pelvis (navel region, flank). For lumbosacral epidurals less volume is required.

The same principles discussed for the segmental dorsolumbar epidural technique apply here. This technique is used commonly in small ruminants for abdominal or pelvic surgery, most often to supplement general anesthesia or sedation. Despite their popularity, epidural

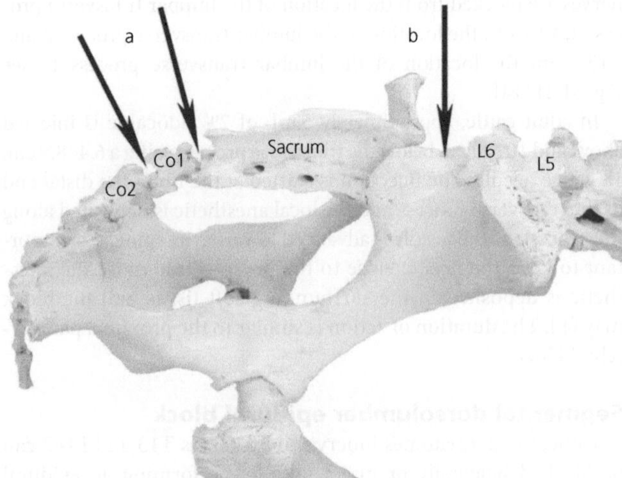

Figure 51.5 Locations for epidural injection in cattle. (a) Caudal epidural at the sacrococcygeal or intercoccygeal space. (b) Cranial epidural at the lumbosacral space. A caudal epidural approach can be used for a cranial epidural injection if sufficient volume is injected to spread the anesthetic rostrally.

Box 51.1 Reasons for failure of epidural injections.

Technique	Subcutaneous injection
	Intravascular injection
	Incomplete injection into epidural space
Drug	Inadequate drug for purpose of epidural
	Inadequate volume and fewer dermatomes blocked
	Inadequate dose
Timing	Insufficient time for onset of action
	Insufficient allowed duration of action
Anatomy	Malformations
	Trauma and distorted anatomy
	Fibrosis in epidural space from previous trauma/irritation
	Leakage from epidural space through intervertebral foramen into surrounding tissue
	Position of animal and asymmetric block due to deposition of anesthetic on one side or drainage into coccygeal epidural space
	Uptake into fat and/or vessels in epidural space

injections often fail in providing complete analgesia/anesthesia for multiple reasons, including those listed in Box 51.1.

In adult cattle, volumes of local anesthetic of up to 150 mL (0.2–0.3 mL/kg), injected in the sacrococcygeal or intercoccygeal epidural space, have been recommended to desensitize the flank and navel region but these volumes also result in motor block of the pelvic limbs and the animal is unable to remain standing. For this reason, cranial epidural blocks are not commonly practiced in adult cattle as they may injure themselves when motor control is lost or when attempting to stand. Another concern is that a high anterior epidural may result in hypotension secondary to blockade of sympathetic nerves, which results in vasodilation. Hypotension is more likely to develop in animals that are hypovolemic.

Calves and small ruminants require larger volumes on a mL per kg basis than adult cattle in order to achieve the same degree of rostral spread from the sacrococcygeal or intercoccygeal epidural space. Volumes of 0.4–0.6 mL/kg of local anesthetic are recommended to achieve analgesia of the navel region [29].

A lumbosacral epidural requires a smaller volume. In goats given 0.1, 0.2, or 0.3 mL/kg of new methylene blue at the lumbosacral space immediately after euthanasia, the average rostral spread was to L3–4, T13–L1, and T10–11, respectively [30]. To obtain sufficient anesthesia of the cranial abdomen and the corresponding abdominal wall, it is often necessary for the anesthetic to reach the T10 segment but due to the possible variation in further rostral spread, there is also an increased risk of impairing respiratory function. Doses of 0.2 mL/kg or 1 mL/5 kg of the local anesthetic of choice (lidocaine 2%, bupivacaine 0.5%, ropivacaine 0.75%) are commonly used, although lidocaine is the most common choice due to its rapid onset and adequate duration of action.

In goats and young calves, the lumbosacral space is easily palpable but may be less obvious in large, well-nourished sheep. A lumbosacral epidural injection can be made with the animal in sternal or lateral recumbency. More even spread of anesthetic which will produce a bilateral block occurs when the animal is placed in a sternal position. Otherwise the side to be approached should be the dependent side when performed in a lateral position; this facilitates contact of the local anesthetic with the desired nerve roots. The animal should be maintained in that position for at least 5–10 min to allow the block to take effect before moving it to the required position for surgery. Strict aseptic technique and use of sterile gloves are indicated for epidural injections at the lumbosacral space, due to the close proximity of the spinal cord within the spinal canal. For most small ruminants and calves, a 3.8 or 7.5 cm, 20 or 22 gauge spinal needle is suitable. The landmarks consist of the distinct dorsal spinous processes of the lumbar vertebrae which readily distinguish them from the sacral vertebrae. Calves and small ruminants have six lumbar vertebrae, but goats may only have five and sheep can have as many as seven lumbar vertebrae. Therefore it is advisable to palpate the anterior surfaces of both tuber coxae and draw an imaginary line between them; this borders the spinous process of the last lumbar vertebra. At this site, the index finger can palpate the space between the last lumbar vertebra and first sacral vertebra. At this point, the spinal needle enters the skin perpendicularly and is advanced into the epidural space, which can be determined by a popping sensation as it penetrates the ligamentum flavum and a loss of resistance upon injection. This distance is relatively short, especially in goats. An inadvertent 'spinal tap' (subarachnoid space) often occurs since the spinal cord is present at this location. In lateral recumbency the spinal fluid drips from the hub following removal of the stylet but in sternal recumbency this is less obvious. If CSF is encountered, the spinal needle can be withdrawn slightly to reposition it in the epidural space and avoid a subarachnoid injection.

In 1-month-old xylazine-sedated calves, one study compared epidural and subarachnoid injections of xylazine (0.025 mg/kg) combined with lidocaine (0.1 mg/kg; 0.05 mL/kg) diluted into 5 mL of sterile saline. Injections were made at the lumbosacral space with the calves in lateral recumbency for the subarachnoid injection and in sternal recumbency for the epidural injection. The subarachnoid injection was more effective and longer acting for providing complete antinociception to pinprick stimulation in the cranial abdomen, umbilicus, and caudal abdomen, than the epidural injection [31].

In pigs, lumbosacral epidural anesthesia can be used for cesarean section, repair of rectal, uterine, or vaginal prolapse, repair of umbilical, inguinal, or scrotal hernias, surgery of scirrhous cord and surgery of the prepuce, penis, or rear limbs [14]. Pigs have six or seven lumbar vertebrae and the location of the lumbosacral space can be located as described for ruminants. The imaginary line between the tuber coxae borders the spinous process of the last lumbar vertebra and the depression behind it, usually 0.5–2.5 cm caudal depending on the size of the pig, on the midline is the space between this vertebra and the sacrum. Alternatively, in the standing pig a line from the patella to the spine is usually 2–3 cm cranial to the lumbosacral space [14]. A 3.8 to 6.4 cm, 20 gauge spinal needle can be used in piglets less than 20 kg, and an 8.9 to 15.2 cm, 20 gauge spinal needle in larger pigs, especially boars and sows. Following aseptic preparation of the area and subcutaneous infiltration of 3–5 mL of lidocaine in larger pigs, a short 2.5 or 3.8 cm, 16 gauge needle can be introduced first in the depression of the lumbosacral space to act as a cannula and prevent bending of long spinal needles. The spinal needle is advanced between the vertebrae at a 0–20° angle perpendicular to the skin, until it perforates the ligamentum flavum, which can be felt as a pop. The spinal cord terminates with the conus medullaris between sacral vertebrae 2 and 3 [32]. The subarachnoid space is not easily penetrated due to its small size compared to the epidural space and the abundant adipose tissue causes anterior bulging of the dura mater with a consequent reduction in the subarachnoid space on the midline. The subarachnoid space and CSF is more readily accessed laterally [32]. It is possible to be in the subarachnoid space with the needle position exactly on the midline and not detect the presence of CSF;

therefore, proper verification of the epidural space is recommended before injection to avoid inadvertent subarachnoid injection of an epidural dose, since the latter can be 10 times that required for subarachnoid injection [24]. An epidural injection can also be performed at the first intersacral (S1–2) space in pigs, due to the presence of a significant dorsal foramen at this location, which is about 75% the size (diameter) of the lumbosacral space [33].

In 6–10-week-old pigs (18 kg) given new methylene blue at the lumbosacral space, immediately after euthanasia, the rostral spread was approximately eight spaces (range of L3–4 to T10–11) for a dose of 0.05 mL/kg; eight spaces (range of L2–3 to T8–9) for a dose of 0.1 mL/kg; 10 spaces (range of T13–L1 to T5–6) for a dose of 0.2 mL/kg; and 18 spaces (range of T8–9 to the brain) for a dose of 0.3 mL/kg [34]. Therefore, volumes of 0.05–0.1 mL/kg seem appropriate to desensitize structures caudal to the diaphragm and are less likely to result in adverse effects.

Clinically, doses of local anesthetics used in pigs at the lumbosacral space are similar to those of small ruminants, i.e., 0.13–0.22 mL/kg or 1 mL/4.5–7.5 kg, for pigs that are less than 50 kg, but reduced dose ranges (on a mg/kg basis) are suggested in larger pigs [14,35]. If the procedure involves the abdomen, such as in cesarean sections, maximum doses of 10 mL/100 kg, 15 mL/200 kg, and 20 mL/300 kg are used, whereas for standing castrations doses of 4 mL/100 kg, 6 mL/200 kg, and 8 mL/300 kg are recommended [14].

Xylazine has also been used for lumbosacral epidural injection in pigs; a dose of 2 mg/kg induced analgesia to electrical stimulation and skin-deep needle pricks to the perianal, flank and umbilical area [35] of similar duration (approximately 2 h) to lidocaine (0.13 mL/kg) [36].

Doses in pigs can also be calculated based on the length of the spinal canal. Pigs can show variations in the number of thoracic and lumbar vertebrae. In one study, 67% of pigs had a combined number of 22 thoracic and lumbar vertebrae, 14% had 21 vertebrae, and 19% had 23 vertebrae [33]. In addition, the combined number varies within each group, e.g., of those with 22 thoracic and lumbar vertebrae, 23% had 15 thoracic and seven lumbar vertebrae, whereas the remaining 77% had 16 thoracic and six lumbar vertebrae [33]. Therefore, measuring the distance from the external occipital protuberance to the first coccygeal vertebra may allow more precise dosing for epidural injections. For pigs weighing up to 65 kg, the distance from the external occipital protuberance to the first coccygeal vertebra varied between 40 and 99 cm. The estimated volumes required to spread contrast medium to the T10 vertebra was 0.8 mL/10 cm for pigs with distances between 40 and 69 cm, 0.9 mL/10 cm for pigs with distances between 70 and 79 cm, and 1.0 mL/10 cm for pigs with distances between 80 and 99 cm [33].

Blocks for regional anesthesia of the pelvic area and related tissues

Sacrococcygeal or intercoccygeal epidural (caudal epidural) block

The anatomic structures present in the pelvis and surrounding tissue can be blocked by injection of anesthetic drugs into the sacrococcygeal (S5–Co1 in cattle, S4–Co1 in small ruminants) or first intercoccygeal (Co1–Co2) spaces.

Maintaining motor control of the pelvic limbs and ensuring that the animal remains standing are possible by injecting lower volumes of anesthetic that selectively produce nociceptive blockade while sparing motor fibers (femoral and sciatic nerves) which are more cranially located. Thus, this technique, referred to as a caudal (posterior) epidural, is most commonly used to perform procedures on the perineum or tail in standing cattle, including obstetric procedures that involve the vulva and vagina, andrologic procedures of the prepuce and scrotum and procedures that involve the tail, perineum, anus, and rectum. This technique does not desensitize the udder. It is also less commonly used in small ruminants because injection at the lumbosacral space (cranial epidural) is easy to perform in these species and for ease of handling, recumbency is often desired in association with the sensory block.

The epidural space at the sacrococcygeal or intercoccygeal intervertebral spaces does not include the spinal cord since the caudal tip of the spinal cord (conus medullaris) extends only to sacral vertebrae 2–3 in young calves and to sacral vertebra 1 in the adult [37]. Only the last sacral nerve (S5) and caudal nerves are present at the level of S5–Co1 and only the caudal nerves at the level of Co1–Co2 in the form of the cauda equina. Therefore, compared to the L6–S1 epidural, all injections at the sacrococcygeal or first intercoccygeal space are strictly epidural and there is no risk of subarachnoid injection.

In cattle, the S5–Co1 or Co1–Co2 space is located by elevating and lowering the tail while palpating the area and identifying the space at which the tail hinges (see Fig. 51.5). In younger cattle, the movement of the tail ceases at the sacrococcygeal space but in older cattle the S5–Co1 space may be ossified and the preferred site of injection is the Co1–Co2 space.

A 3.8 cm, 20 or 18 gauge needle is passed, in the midline, between the vertebrae at a 0–15° angle to perpendicular. The needle is inserted to a depth of 1–2 cm, depending on the animal's size, and the hub of the needle is filled with saline or the local anesthetic, then the needle is advanced until the fluid is aspirated as it enters the epidural space, due to the subatmospheric epidural pressure. On occasion, blood will flow from the hub and, in this case, the needle should be withdrawn slightly. If the needle is correctly placed, there is minimal resistance to injection.

In neonatal calves, 0.05, 0.1, or 0.15 mL/kg of new methylene blue administered at the S5–Co1 epidural space immediately after euthanasia spread rostral for five spaces (range of L7–S1 to L5–6) for the low dose; for eight spaces (range of L7–S1 to L2–3) for the intermediate dose; and for eight spaces (range of L6–7 to L2–3) for the high dose [34]. The injection of 0.4 mL/kg of contrast medium in the same epidural space to calves weighing 50–60 kg resulted in rostral spread to the T12 vertebra [29]. In adult cattle (approximately 525 kg), epidural injection of new methylene blue at the Co1–Co2 space 20 min before euthanasia spread rostrally on average to L6–S1 with 5 mL (0.01 mL/kg), to L5–6 with 10 mL (0.02 mL/kg) and to L3–4 with 20 mL (0.04 mL/kg) [38]. This indicates that to avoid motor blockade and ataxia, significantly less volume (on a weight basis) is necessary for caudal epidural in adult cattle compared to younger animals. Clinically, in adult cattle 0.015 mL/kg of 0.75% ropivacaine at the S5–Co1 space resulted in analgesia of the dermatomes corresponding to the coccyx to S3 spinal cord segments without ataxia [39].

The usual volume of local anesthetic (lidocaine 2%, bupivacaine 0.5%, ropivacaine 0.75%) for a caudal epidural in adult cattle is recommended to be 5–6 mL (approximately 1 mL/100 kg) [14,15,39]. Volumes of greater than 10 mL may cause weakness of the pelvic limbs and recumbency due to involvement of the L4–6 nerves which are main contributors to the femoral nerve, and L5–S2, main contributors to the sciatic nerve [18]. Onset of anesthesia is usually 10–20 min, although tail flaccidity is obvious in less than 1–2 min with 2% lidocaine. The duration of anesthesia depends on the local anesthetic used, but usually is 0.5–1.5 h for lidocaine or mepivacaine and 1.5–3 h for bupivacaine or ropivacaine.

Anatomic structures blocked by a caudal epidural using the aforementioned doses include structures innervated by sacral and caudal segments, i.e., structures innervated by the pudendal nerve (S2–4) which include the skin of the perineum, skin over the semitendinosus and semimembranosus muscles, scrotum, labia, skin of the caudal surface of udder, perineal muscles, vagina, vulva, prepuce, penis, clitoris; the coccygeus and levator ani innervated by the corresponding nerves (S3, S4); structures innervated by the caudal rectal nerves (S4, S5) that include the caudal part of the rectum, coccygeus, levator ani, external anal sphincter, retractor penis (clotiris), constrictor vestibuli, labium, and skin of anal region; and the tail innervated by the caudal nerves from the cauda equina in the vertebral canal [18,40].

Analgesia or anesthesia appears more rapidly in the dermatomes proximal to the site of injection (tail) than at distant areas (perineal) and tends to disappear more quickly in distant compared to proximal areas. For adult cattle administered ropivacaine, time to onset of analgesia to needle pinprick and hemostat clamping was approximately 10 min on the tail (caudal nerve) and 15 min in the perineal area (pudendal nerve and its branches), whereas mean duration of analgesia was 368 min for the tail and 359 min for the perineal area, respectively [39].

Other drugs used for caudal epidural injection have included the α_2-adrenergic receptor agonists. Xylazine is the most effective for inducing analgesia and anesthesia, but the dose used is similar to systemic doses and absorption from the epidural space results in the known adverse effects of α_2-adrenergic receptor agonists, including sedation, ataxia, bradycardia, hypotension, respiratory acidosis, hypoxemia, increased uterine tone, and ruminal atony [14,41,42]. The increased uterine motility may interfere with fetotomy procedures [42]. Xylazine at 0.05–0.06 mg/kg diluted in 5 mL of saline induced more prolonged analgesia (four times) than 5 mL of lidocaine 2% (0.01 mL/kg; 0.2 mg/kg) in adult cows administered the drugs at the Co1–Co2 epidural space [41,42]. The co-administration of lidocaine and xylazine often results in more rapid onset and prolonged duration of analgesia than either drug alone. Other α_2-adrenergic receptor agonists, such as detomidine, dexmedetomidine, and medetomidine, are less reliable in their analgesic and anesthetic epidural effects or produce adverse effects that offer little advantage over xylazine [14].

The same technique can be used in small ruminants, calves, and South American camelids for castration and obstetric procedures, and for tail docking in lambs. A 2.5 or 3.8 cm, 20 gauge needle is introduced at the S4–Co1 or Co1–2 space for injection of 0.02–0.03 mL/kg of lidocaine 2% (1–1.5 mL/50 kg; 0.4–0.6 mg/kg) in small ruminants and calves [14,15,43]. In llamas, a dose of 0.01 mL/kg of lidocaine 2% (1 mL/100 kg; 0.22 mg/kg) or xylazine 0.17 mg/kg diluted with 2 mL of saline, or their combination with the same doses have been effective after S5–Co1 administration and as for other species the duration of analgesia was significantly longer for the combination (over 5.5 h) than for lidocaine (over 1 h) or xylazine (3 h) alone [44].

Sacral paravertebral block

This technique can produce effects similar to a caudal epidural, with the exception of the caudal nerves supplying the tail; therefore, tail tone is maintained. The block is specific to nerves S3, S4, and S5, so the animal does not become ataxic.

The blockade of S3–5 affects the nerves arising from these branches: the levatori ani nerve (S3, S4, and fibers from the pudendal nerve or caudal rectal nerve), the caudal rectal nerve (S4, S5), and the majority of fibers from the pudendal nerve (S2–4) [18].

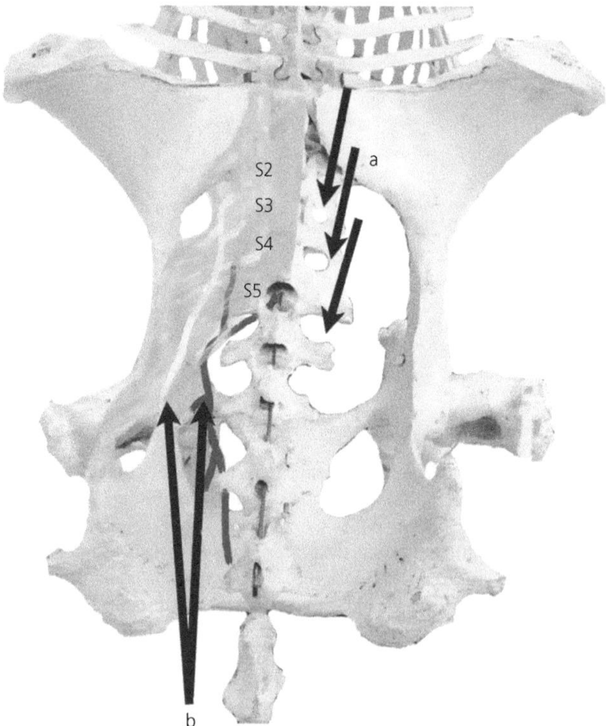

Figure 51.6 Dorsal view of the sacral paravertebral block (a) at S3, S4, and S5 foramina on the right side; this block should be performed bilaterally. Dorsal view of the pudendal (S2–4; orange) and caudal rectal nerve (S4, S5; blue) block (b) on the medial surface of the sacrosciatic ligament from a left ischiorectal fossa approach; this block is also performed bilaterally.

The block is performed with the animal standing and the area from the midsacrum to the base of the tail can be clipped and aseptically prepared at the specific points where the needle is inserted on both sides of midline (Figs 51.6, 51.7). The easiest site to locate is the S5–Co1 space. A 5 or 7.5 cm, 20 gauge spinal needle is inserted 1.0 cm lateral to the dorsal midline of the vertebral crest at the S5–Co1 space and advanced to the level of the transverse processes of those vertebrae; at the caudal border of S5, 5 mL of 2% lidocaine is injected to desensitize the dorsal and ventral branch and the procedure repeated on the contralateral side. Nerves S4 and S3 are approximately 3 and 6 cm cranial to the location of nerve S5, 1.0–1.5 cm lateral to the dorsal midline. At these two locations, the spinal needle penetrates the respective foramina and the volume of injection is also 5 mL of 2% lidocaine per nerve on each side of the dorsal midline [14].

Injection of alcohol for the alleviation of chronic rectal tenesmus for up to 5 weeks without affecting urination and defecation has been described; however, this treatment is not recommended in males because the pudendal nerve and caudal rectal nerve innervate the penis and preputial prolapse is likely to occur [45].

This block can also be performed in sheep and goats. The main differences are that sheep and goats only have four sacral vertebrae so the block is completed at S4–Co1 for nerve S4 and at the S3–4 space for nerve S3.

Pudendal block

The pudendal block involves injection around the pudendal and caudal rectal nerves through an ischiorectal fossa approach or a lateral

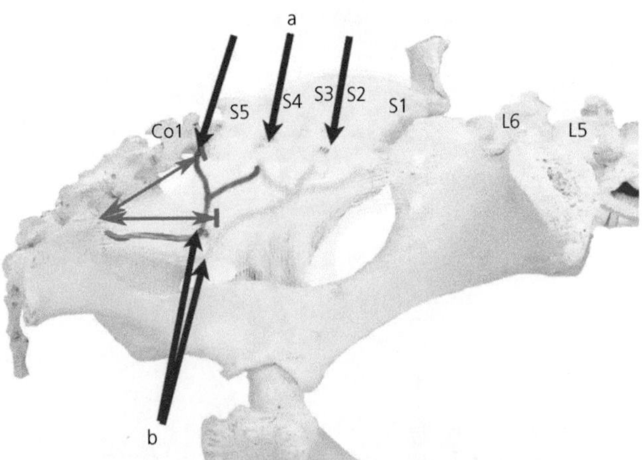

Figure 51.7 Lateral view of the sacral paravertebral block (a) at S3, S4, and S5 foramina on the right side; this block should be performed bilaterally. Lateral view of the pudendal (S2–4; orange) and caudal rectal nerve (S4, S5; blue) block (b) on the medial surface of the sacrosciatic ligament from a right lateral approach; this block is also performed bilaterally. The red arrows indicate the location of needle placement; the distance from the anterior and dorsal border of the ischial tuber to the caudal part of the sacrotuberous ligament corresponds to the point of needle insertion when this distance is applied to a line parallel to the midline and originating from the anterior border of the ischial tuber.

approach and has similar effects as a sacral paravertebral block. In standing males it is generally used for penile analgesia and to produce relaxation distal to the sigmoid flexure which allows examination of the prolapsed penis. In standing females this block relieves rectal and anal straining caused by uterine prolapse or chronic vaginal discharge and can be used for surgical ablation of masses in the rectum and anus and for manipulation of urethral calculi [14].

The pudendal nerve originates from sacral segments S2–4 and travels downward, partly embedded in the sacrosciatic ligament along the floor of the pelvis with the internal pudendal artery and vein and towards the ischial arch. It supplies several branches that innervate the whole perineal area. These branches include a proximal cutaneous branch to the skin of the semitendinosus area and a distal cutaneous branch to the skin of the semimembranosus area. This latter branch further extends to a superficial perineal branch that supplies the skin of the perineum and a dorsal scrotal (male) or dorsal labial (female) branch that supplies the scrotum or labia and skin of the caudal surface of the udder, respectively. Another major branch is the deep perineal nerve, which innervates the perineal muscles, vagina, vulva, major vestibular gland and skin of the perineum; this nerve also has a communication with the caudal rectal nerve (S4, S5). In the bull, the last segment of the pudendal nerve gives off the preputial and scrotal branch to supply the prepuce and scrotum and continues as the dorsal nerve of the penis to supply the penis. In the female, the pudendal nerve supplies a mammary branch to the udder and the dorsal nerve of the clitoris which supplies the clitoris [18,40].

The caudal rectal nerve (S4, S5) travels downward above the pudendal nerve and anastomoses with it. It supplies, as mentioned above, the caudal part of the rectum, external anal sphincter, and surrounding skin.

For the ischiorectal fossa approach, the block is performed with the animal standing, preferably under sedation. The skin over both ischiorectal fossae is clipped and aseptically prepared at the specific points where the needles are to be inserted and desensitized with 2–3 mL of 2% lidocaine (see Fig. 51.6). A hand is placed into the rectum to palpate the lesser sciatic notch of the ischium and the lesser sciatic foramen, the latter formed by the absence of attachment of the sacrosciatic ligament along the notch. The notch is located immediately after the hand enters the anus and descends from the ischial tuberosity. At the foramen, the caudal gluteal artery can be palpated as it leaves the pelvis towards the muscles in the thigh, and medial to it and within the pelvic area, the internal pudendal artery can be palpated which runs along with the pudendal nerve in a caudoventral direction on the internal surface of the sacrosciatic ligament [46]. A 2.5 cm, 16 gauge needle is inserted in the ischiorectal fossa to help direct an 8.9 cm, 20 gauge spinal needle, as the hand inside the rectum palpates the internal pudendal artery and helps direct the needle slightly dorsal towards the pudendal nerve. Up to 25 mL of 2% lidocaine is injected in the area and the needle redirected more dorsally (2–3 cm) to include the caudal rectal nerve, which is blocked with an additional 10 mL of anesthetic [14]. To block the nerves on the contralateral side of the pelvis, the hands are reversed and the procedure is repeated. Onset of the block may require from 5 to 30 min and will last 2–4 h [14].

In cattle and sheep this block can also be performed from the lateral side. In cattle the distance from the anterior and dorsal border of the ischial tuber to the lateral part of the sacrum, which corresponds to the location of the caudal (sacrotuberous) part of the sacrosciatic ligament, is measured and this same distance is used to establish the site of needle insertion on a line parallel to the midline and originating from the anterior border of the ischial tuber (see Fig. 51.7) [47]. A 3.8 cm, 20 gauge needle is used to inject 2–4 mL of 2% lidocaine subcutaneously at this site to facilitate the insertion of an 11.4 cm, 20 gauge spinal needle while the hand within the rectum locates the pudendal nerve as it passes medial and dorsal to the lesser sciatic foramen. The caudal rectal nerve is blocked by redirecting the needle 2–3 cm more dorsal, which requires penetrating the sacrosciatic ligament [47], and the procedure is then repeated on the other side. The volumes used can be the same as for the ischiorectal approach, although due to better accuracy less anesthetic may be required (10 mL for the pudendal nerve and 5 mL for the caudal rectal nerve) [47].

In sheep the lateral approach is performed by placing a finger into the rectum to locate the lesser sciatic foramen, usually at finger depth. The corresponding skin site is aseptically prepared and 3–7 mL of 2% lidocaine is injected using a 3.8 cm, 20 gauge needle directed towards the finger until it can be felt lying alongside the nerve. Immediately after injection the rectum is massaged to spread the anesthetic and the procedure repeated on the opposite side [47].

Dorsal nerve of the penis block

The dorsal nerve of the penis originates from the pudendal nerve, as the latter travels around the ischial arch [40]. This nerve is blocked to desensitize and relax the penis and areas of the prepuce and scrotum, without affecting other anatomic structures innervated by the pudendal nerve. The location of the block is approximately 10 cm ventral to the anus and 2.5 cm from the midline on both sides, where a 6.4 to 8.9 cm, 20 gauge spinal needle is directed along the border of the ischial arch to contact the pelvic floor, next to the penis at the 8 and 4 o'clock positions. The nerves are in a ventral position at the pelvic outlet as the penis has not veered around the ischial arch and are injected with 10–20 mL of 2% lidocaine on each side. Aspirate to verify absence of blood before injecting. The onset time of the block is 10–20 min with a duration of 1–2 h [14].

Blocks for regional anesthesia of the teats and udder

The skin and teats of the forequarters and the cranial part of the base of the udder are innervated by the iliohypogastric nerve (ventral branch of L1), the ilioinguinal nerve (ventral branches of L2 and L3), and the cranial branch of the genitofemoral nerve (ventral branches of L2–4). The skin and teats of the hindquarters are innervated by the caudal branch of the genitofemoral nerve and the mammary branch of the pudendal nerve (S2–4) (Fig. 51.8) [48]. Due to this innervation, a proximal or distal paravertebral block that includes T13–L3 nerves can provide significant anesthesia of the forequarters of the udder, but the block is incomplete because the genitofemoral nerve (L4 roots) is not included. A pudendal block (S2–4) can provide anesthesia of the caudal area of the hindquarters, but not their cranial area, which is innervated by the genitofemoral nerve. Therefore, a more simple and effective method is to desensitize the affected area locally using a ring block, inverted 'V' block, teat sinus infusion, or intravenous regional anesthesia of the teat, in combination with chemical and/or physical restraint (Fig. 51.9) [14]. The surgical procedure and block can be performed with the animal standing or recumbent, often dictated by the preference of the operator.

These blocks can be used for repair of lacerations and fistulae, release of cistern obstructions, wart removal, supernumerary teat removal, and teat removal.

Ring block

An elastic band or Doyen clamp is used as a tourniquet and applied to the base of the teat, to prolong the duration of action of the injected local anesthetic and to prevent blood and milk from entering the teat sinus and interfering with the surgical repair. Lidocaine 2%, 4–6 mL is injected subcutaneously with a 1.6 cm, 25 gauge needle, distal to the tourniquet, around the circumference of the teat and massaged to facilitate blockade of all layers, including the skin, subcutaneous, and muscularis (see Fig. 51.9).

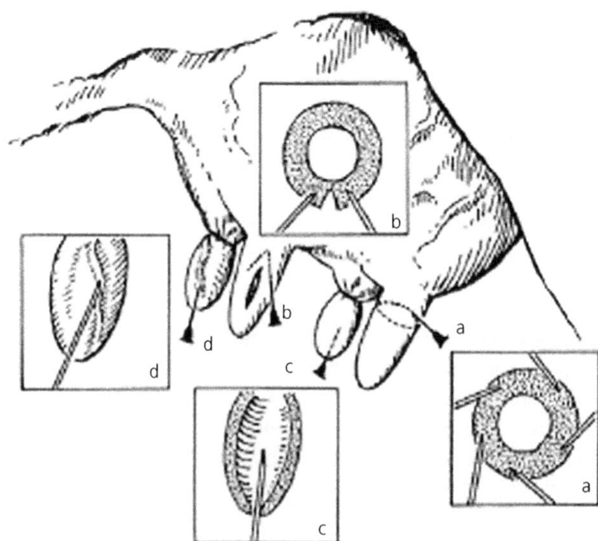

Figure 51.9 Needle placement for bovine ring block (a), inverted 'V' block (b), teat sinus infusion block (c), and intravenous regional teat block (d). From [14].

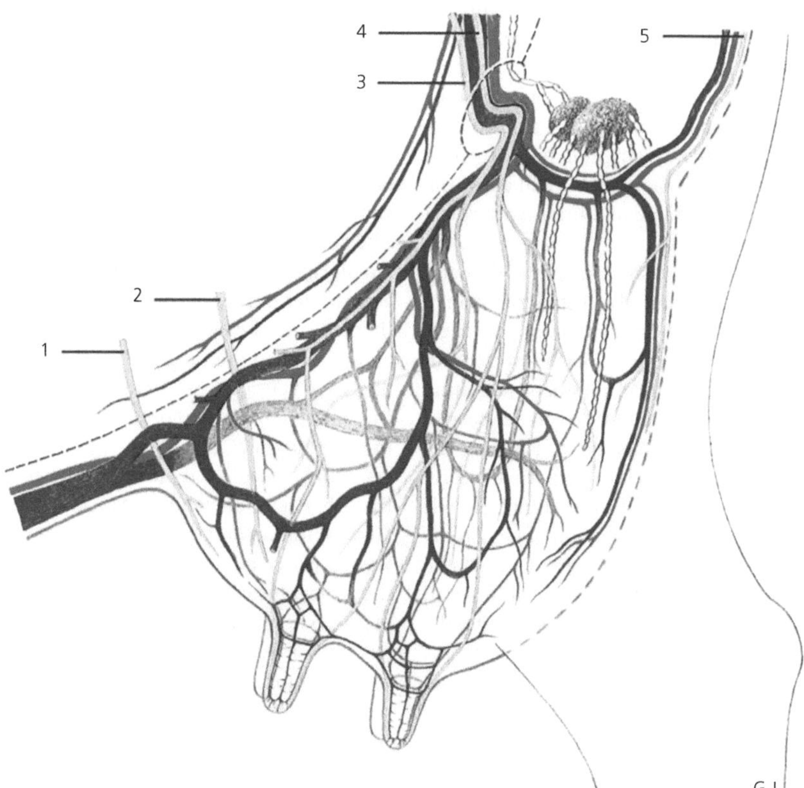

Figure 51.8 Innervation to skin and teats of the forequarters and hindquarters. (1) Iliohyhpogastric nerve; (2) Ilioinguinal nerve; (3) Cranial branch of the genitofemoral nerve; (4) Caudal branch of the genitofemoral nerve; and (5) Mammary branch of the pudendal nerve. Modified from [48].

Inverted 'V' block

Following placement of the tourniquet, 4–6 mL of 2% lidocaine is injected subcutaneously with a 1.6 cm, 25 gauge needle with the angle of the 'V' located at the cranial aspect of the incision and the wings along the incision to create a shield that blocks sensory input towards the incision (see Fig. 51.9).

Teat sinus infusion block

This block provides anesthesia of the mucous membranes lining the sinus of the teat without affecting the muscularis, subcutaneous layers, and skin. The block can be used to remove polyps within the mucosa, opening of contracted sphincters, and opening of spider teats. A tourniquet is placed as described above and a teat cannula is introduced into the sinus; 10 mL of lidocaine 2% is injected and held in place by blocking the cannula for 5–10 min to allow for absorption of the anesthetic by the mucosa; thereafter, the anesthetic is drained and the tourniquet removed (see Fig. 51.9).

Intravenous regional teat block

For this block, a superficial teat vein distal to a tourniquet is injected with 5–7 mL of lidocaine 2% using a 2.5 cm, 25 gauge needle (see Fig. 51.9). After injection, the needle is removed and pressure applied over the insertion site which should also be massaged to prevent hematoma formation. Analgesia occurs within 3–5 min and remains for as long as the tourniquet is left in place, which is usually for less than 2 h.

Blocks for castration

Castration of ruminants is routinely practiced and is usually performed in young animals. The procedure is usually performed under local anesthesia in cattle; however, smaller animals, especially young sheep and goats, could be anesthetized with xylazine (0.05 mg/kg, IM) and ketamine (10 mg/kg, IM) as described for disbudding. Castration of adult sheep and goats must be performed carefully to prevent postoperative hemorrhage. In such cases, sedation (e.g., xylazine 0.05–0.1 mg/kg, IM) will allow the animal to be restrained on a surgery table and improve surgical conditions.

For complete anesthesia of the surgical site, the scrotal skin and spermatic cord must be blocked or alternatively an epidural (cranial or caudal) as previously described can be performed. Local anesthetic can be injected directly into the center of each testicle until the testicle feels firm, which will result in local anesthetic migrating up to the spermatic cord. Alternatively the testicle can be grasped and pulled down and local anesthetic injected proximally into the surrounding subcutaneous tissues at the level of the spermatic cord. Complete desensitization occurs within 5–10 min. Using a small-bore needle (20–22 gauge) will reduce the likelihood of hematoma formation. When injected into the testicle, the local anesthetic passes out of the testicle along the lymph vessels and diffuses to block the nerve fibers in the spermatic cord. With either site, the bulk of the injected local anesthetic is systemically absorbed so it is important to be aware of the risk of toxicity. In small lambs and kids, 1 mL of lidocaine injected into each cord will be adequate. The scrotal skin is anesthetized by local infiltration of lidocaine along the proposed line of incision.

As in the case of dehorning or disbudding, a non-steroidal anti-inflammatory (e.g., flunixin meglumine 2 mg/kg, IV or IM) is suggested for postoperative analgesia.

Blocks for regional anesthesia of the limbs and feet

Most surgical procedures of the digit are performed in cattle using intravenous regional anesthesia (IVRA), a specific nerve block or simple infiltration of local anesthetic (ring block). Intravenous regional anesthesia is the method of choice for most surgical procedures of the foot or distal limb in ruminants and swine but digital nerve blocks can be a very useful diagnostic tool for localizing lameness in cattle. Additional regional anesthesia of the thoracic limb in cattle can be achieved with a brachial plexus nerve block or with digital nerve blocks distal to the carpus. Analgesia of the pelvic limb distal to the tarsus can be achieved by desensitizing the common peroneal and tibial nerves or by epidural techniques that include lumbosacral segments that include the femoral nerve (L4–6) and sciatic nerve (L5–S2). Intra-articular injections of local anesthetics or other medications can also be used as appropriate.

Thoracic limb blocks

Brachial plexus block

A brachial plexus block has been described in cattle [14] and sheep [49] to provide analgesia of the thoracic limb distal to and including the elbow. This block is likely to be most useful in calves, sheep, or goats in a clinical or research setting for procedures on the thoracic limb under general anesthesia. In swine, palpation of landmarks may be difficult, especially in pot-bellied pigs. The block can be performed blind or with nerve stimulation as is described in small animals (see also Chapter 45).

The brachial plexus block involves desensitization of the ventral roots of the sixth, seventh, and eighth cervical nerves (C6, C7, C8) as well as the first and second thoracic nerves (T1, T2) as they pass together over the lateral aspect of the middle third of the first rib [47]. The position and angle of the scapula can be used as a landmark by palpating the cranial and caudal angles and spine. The dorsal border of the scapula lies opposite the second to seventh thoracic vertebrae, but will only be palpable in thin animals. The shoulder joint is just lateral to the middle of the first and second thoracic vertebrae. The spine of the scapula is prominent in ruminants and juts out ventrally to form the acromion process. The point of needle insertion is 12–14 cm (adult cattle) or 6–10 cm (small ruminants) cranial to the palpable acromion of the scapula at the outer border of the scalenus ventralis muscle. The needle is then advanced caudally and slightly ventral, lateral to the thorax and parallel to the long axis of the animal's neck. In small ruminants and calves a 6.3–8.9 cm, 22–20 gauge spinal needle with stylet can be used to reach approximately 5 cm below the skin ventral to the scapula. In cattle an 8.9–16 cm, 18 gauge spinal needle is necessary. The needle is typically advanced until it hits the edge of the first rib. An initial volume of local anesthetic is injected at this site after aspiration and then the needle is redirected distally, dorsal to the rib where additional local anesthetic is injected. Lidocaine is the typical local anesthetic used in ruminants with total volumes of 20–25 mL described for adult cattle [14]; however, bupivacaine has been investigated in sheep [49]. The dosage of bupivacaine ranged from 0.5 to 4 mg/kg with a dose of 2 mg/kg resulting in the most effective brachial plexus block. No signs of toxicity were reported in sheep [49].

In ruminants the phrenic nerve is innervated by the C5–7 cervical nerves [18], so bilateral brachial plexus blockade should be avoided to minimize the risk of complete diaphragmatic motor block.

Digital nerve blocks for the thoracic limbs and feet

Cattle have four digits; the third and fourth digits correspond to the fully developed medial and lateral digits respectively whereas the second and fifth digits correspond to the medial and lateral dewclaws, respectively, which are positioned behind the fetlock and do not articulate with the limb.

Digital nerve blocks are more difficult to perform in cattle compared to horses, but may be useful for localizing lameness in cattle as they are in horses, or to desensitize the foot for surgery. Digital nerve blocks are more difficult because the skin below the tarsus and carpus is thick and the subcutaneous tissue is firm and fibrous, limiting palpation of the nerves and insertion of needles. The size of the needle used and total volume of local anesthetic injected are related to the size of the animal.

Innervation to the thoracic limb is supplied on the palmar aspect predominantly by the median nerve and also by the palmar branch of the ulnar nerve, and on the dorsal aspect by the radial nerve and also the dorsal branch of the ulnar nerve (Fig. 51.10) [50].

The median nerve passes through the carpal canal and divides halfway up the metacarpus into palmar common digital nerves II and III. Palmar common digital nerve II runs medially and divides at the level of the fetlock joint into the axial palmar digital nerve II, which ends near the dewclaw, and the abaxial palmar digital nerve III, which travels deep as far as the apex of the hoof. Palmar common digital nerve III is double and travels lateral to the interdigital space and gives rise to the axial palmar digital nerves III and IV (see Fig. 51.10) [50].

The ulnar nerve divides above the accessory carpal bone into dorsal and palmar branches. The palmar ulnar branch divides distal to the carpus into a deep branch that innervates the surrounding area of the third and fourth metacarpal bone, and a superficial branch that travels distally on the lateral aspect to become the palmar common digital nerve IV, which anastomoses at the midway point of the metacarpus with the median nerve via the communicating branch of the latter. Proximal to the fetlock joint of the fourth digit, the palmar common digital nerve IV divides into the axial palmar digital nerve V and abaxial palmar digital nerve IV (see Fig. 51.10) [50].

The dorsal branch of the ulnar nerve is located approximately 2 cm proximal to the accessory carpal bone and travels distally on the lateral surface between the third and fourth metacarpal bone as the dorsal common digital nerve, which divides on the dorsolateral aspect of the fetlock into the axial dorsal digital nerve V for the dewclaw and the abaxial dorsal digital nerve IV for the dorsolateral coronary region of the fourth digit (see Fig. 51.10) [50].

The dorsomedial aspect of the thoracic limb is supplied by the superficial branch of the radial nerve, which travels on the dorsomedial aspect of the forearm to cross to the dorsal aspect below the carpus and divides midway on the metacarpus into the dorsal common digital nerve III (dorsal aspect) and dorsal common digital nerve II (medial aspect). The latter divides at the level of the medial aspect of the fetlock into the axial dorsal digital nerve II to the dewclaw and the abaxial dorsal digital nerve III to the dorsomedial coronary region of the third digit. Dorsal common digital nerve III continues to travel dorsally and divides at the interdigital space into the axial dorsal digital nerves III and IV (see Fig. 51.10) [50].

The distribution of the nerve supply to the palmar surface of the digits of the forelimb is not always consistent, making digital nerve blocks of the forelimb less reliable for achieving complete digital analgesia and anesthesia which is necessary for surgery.

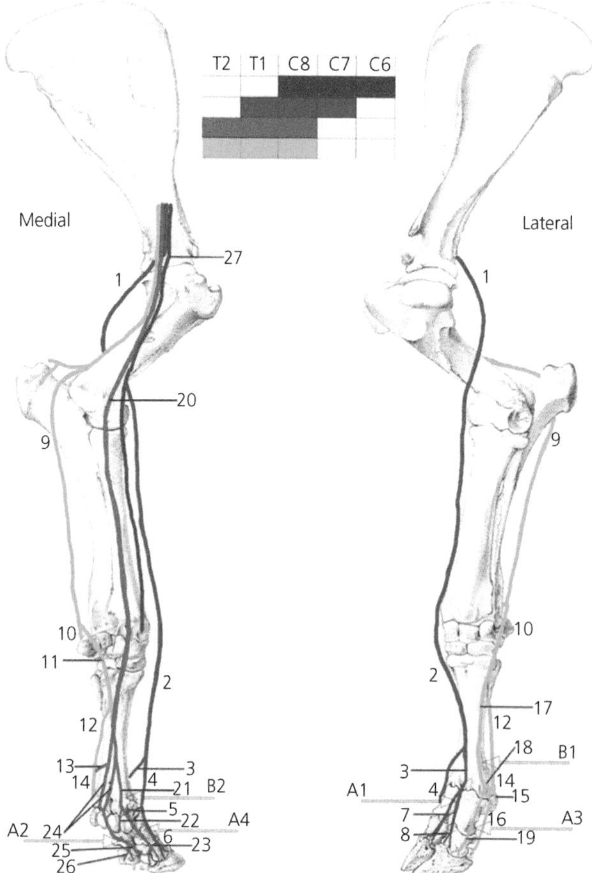

Figure 51.10 Innervation to the thoracic limb. (1) Radial nerve; (2) Superficial branch of the radial nerve; (3) Dorsal common digital nerve III; (4) Dorsal common digital nerve II; (5) Axial dorsal digital nerve II ; (6) Abaxial dorsal digital nerve III; (7) Axial dorsal digital nerve III; (8) Axial dorsal digital nerve IV; (9) Ulnar nerve; (10) Dorsal ulnar branch; (11) Palmar ulnar branch; (12) Superficial ulnar branch; (13) Communicating branch of the median nerve; (14) Palmar common digital nerve IV; (15) Axial palmar digital nerve V; (16) Abaxial palmar digital nerve IV; (17) Dorsal common digital nerve; (18) Axial dorsal digital nerve V; (19) Abaxial dorsal digital nerve IV; (20) Median nerve; (21) Palmar common digital nerve II; (22) Axial palmar digital nerve II; (23) Abaxial palmar digital nerve III; (24) Palmar common digital nerve III; (25) Axial palmar digital nerve III; (26) Axial palmar digital nerve IV; (27) Musculocutaneous nerve. (A) Block to the digit; (A1) Block to nerves numbered 7 and 8; (A2) Block to nerves numbered 25 and 26; (A3) Block to nerves numbered 16 and 19; (A4) Block to nerves numbered 6 and 23. (b) Block to dewclaws; (B1) Block to nerves numbered 15 and 18; (B2) Block to nerves numbered 5 and 22. Modified from [50].

To block the digits in the thoracic limb, it is necessary to block axial dorsal digital nerves III and IV which arise from the radial nerve. This block can be performed on the dorsal aspect proximal to the interdigital space, close to the metacarpal-phalangeal joint with a 3.8 cm, 20 or 18 gauge needle (see Fig. 51.10 A1). It is possible to encounter the axial dorsal digital artery and vein in this location so aspiration prior to injection is important. Ten mL of 2% lidocaine is required in adult cattle to desensitize the radial nerve at this location. The axial palmar digital nerves III and IV, originating from the median nerve, provide sensation to the medial aspect of the third and fourth digit and are blocked lower than on the dorsal site to avoid the cartilaginous palmar ligament. For these nerves, a

2.5 cm, 20 or 18 gauge needle is used to inject 5–10 mL of 2% lidocaine distal to the dewclaws on the palmar surface (see Fig. 51.10 A2). Desensitizing the lateral aspect of the fourth digit involves blocking the abaxial palmar digital nerve IV and the abaxial dorsal digital nerve IV, both originating from the ulnar nerve, using 3–5 mL of 2% lidocaine with a 3.8 cm, 20 or 18 gauge needle midway between the palmar lateral aspect of the dewclaw and the coronary band for the axial branch and at the same level but on the dorsolateral aspect for the abaxial branch (see Fig. 51.10 A3). A similar block to the one described for the fourth digit is used for the third digit and includes abaxial dorsal digital nerve III, originating from the radial nerve, and the abaxial palmar digital nerve III, originating from the median nerve (see Fig. 51.10 A4).

The dewclaws (second and fifth digits) can be blocked by injecting each with 5–10 mL of 2% lidocaine using a 3.8–5 cm, 20 or 18 gauge needle inserted in a horizontal direction above them. This blocks axial palmar and axial dorsal digital nerves V, originating from the ulnar nerve, which supply the lateral dewclaw (see Fig. 51.10 B1) and axial palmar digital nerve II, originating from the median nerve, and the axial dorsal digital nerve II, originating from the radial nerve, that supply the medial dewclaw (see Fig. 51.10 B2).

Pelvic limb blocks

The pelvic limb can be desensitized below the tarsus by blocking the peroneal and tibial nerves. These blocks are not commonly performed in clinical practice due to the ease and effectiveness of IVRA and caudal epidural anesthesia in ruminants.

The common peroneal nerve can be palpated at the caudal edge of the bony prominence of the lateral condyle of the tibia. At this level, the nerve is superficial and has not yet divided into the superficial and deep branches. A 2.5–3.8 cm, 18 or 20 gauge needle is inserted at the caudal edge of the lateral condyle of the tibia, over the fibula, until it touches the bony landmark. In adult cattle, 20 mL of lidocaine is required and 6–10 mL is sufficient in small ruminants with an onset time of approximately 15–20 min (Fig. 51.11).

Digital nerve blocks for the pelvic limbs and feet

Innervation to the pelvic limb is supplied on the plantar aspect by the tibial nerve and on the dorsal aspect by the superficial and deep peroneal nerves [51].

The tibial nerve divides into the medial and lateral plantar nerves at the distal third of the tibia, just above the calcaneus bone to innervate the plantar aspect of the pelvic limb. The medial plantar nerve runs in the groove between the interosseus and the deep flexor tendon and divides at the distal third of the metatarsus into plantar common digital nerves II and III (see Fig. 51.11) [51]. Both nerves travel down the fetlock where they divide into the axial and abaxial plantar digital nerves. From the plantar common digital nerve II, the axial plantar digital nerve II supplies the medial dewclaw and the abaxial plantar digital nerve III continues to the third digit on the medioplantar aspect. From the plantar common digital nerve III, the axial plantar digital nerve III and axial plantar digital nerve IV supply the axial bulb and hoof regions of the third and fourth digits (see Fig. 51.11) [51].

The lateral plantar nerve reaches below the tarsus and the lateral border of the deep flexor tendon and continues as plantar common digital nerve IV to divide at the level of the fetlock into the axial plantar digital nerve V, to supply the lateral dewclaw, and the abaxial plantar digital nerve IV, which continues to the fourth digit on the lateroplantar aspect (see Fig. 51.11) [51].

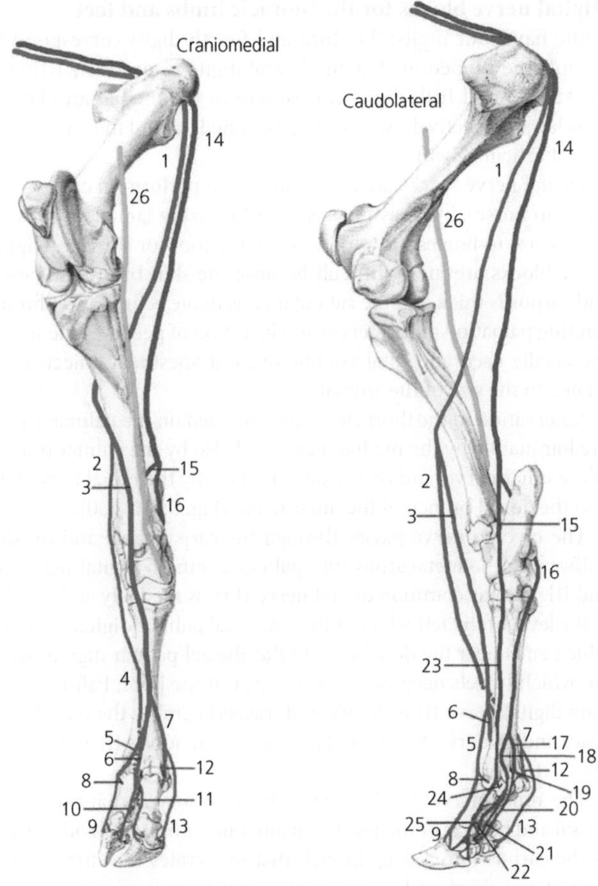

Figure 51.11 Innervation to the pelvic limb. (1) Peroneal nerve; (2) Deep peroneal nerve; (3) Superficial peroneal nerve; (4) Dorsal metatarsal III nerve; (5) Dorsal common digital nerve IV; (6) Dorsal common digital nerve III; (7) Dorsal common digital nerve II; (8) Axial dorsal digital nerve V; (9) Abaxial dorsal digital nerve IV; (10) Axial dorsal digital nerve IV; (11) Axial dorsal digital nerve III; (12) Axial dorsal digital nerve II; (13) Abaxial dorsal digital nerve III; (14) Tibial nerve; (15) Lateral plantar nerve; (16) Medial plantar nerve; (17) Plantar common digital nerve II; (18) Plantar common digital nerve III; (19) Axial plantar digital nerve II; (20) Abaxial plantar digital nerve III; (21) Axial plantar digital nerve III; (22) Axial plantar digital nerve IV; (23) Plantar common digital nerve IV; (24) Axial plantar digital nerve V; (25) Abaxial plantar digital nerve IV; (26) Saphenous nerve. Modified from [51].

The common peroneal nerve divides on the lateral aspect of the proximal third of the tibia into the superficial and deep peroneal nerves to innervate the dorsal aspect of the pelvic limb. The superficial peroneal nerve crosses to the dorsal aspect of the proximal metatarsus and divides in the proximal third into three branches: the dorsal common digital nerve II that travels medial, the dorsal common digital nerve III that continues on the dorsal aspect, and the dorsal common digital nerve IV that travels dorsolateral. Dorsal common digital nerve II travels dorsomedially along the metatarsus to the fetlock and divides into the axial dorsal digital nerve II, supplying the medial dewclaw, and the abaxial dorsal digital nerve III, which continues to the third digit on the medioplantar aspect. Dorsal common digital nerve III travels dorsally to the distal fetlock, where it divides into the axial dorsal digital nerves III and IV to supply the dorsal coronary aspect of the third and fourth digit. Dorsal common digital nerve IV reaches the fetlock on the dorsolateral aspect and divides into the axial dorsal digital nerve V, to supply the lateral dewclaw, and the abaxial dorsal digital nerve IV that continues to the dorsolateral coronary and bulbar regions of the fourth digit (see Fig. 51.11) [51].

The deep peroneal nerve runs from its lateral position at the tibia to a dorsal position at the metatarsus to become the dorsal metatarsal nerve III which runs lateral to the metatarsal bone, reaching the interdigital space and establishing communicating branches with the dorsal common digital nerve III, just before the latter divides into axial dorsal digital nerves III and IV. The new trunk then has communicating branches to the axial plantar digital nerves III and IV from the tibial nerve (see Fig. 51.11) [51].

To block the entire distal digit of the pelvic limb, the technique, equipment, and location of the nerves resemble the anatomy of the thoracic limb and can be completed in the same fashion as described above.

Ring block

Ring block of the foot or distal limb is the simplest method for producing anesthesia but is less precise than IVRA or digital nerve blocks. Advantages are its simplicity without the need for anatomic knowledge, and need for minimal equipment. However, it may not be fully efficacious and may allow for infection as a result of multiple injections, and can result in swelling.

It involves injection of local anesthetic superficially from the skin to the bone medial and lateral to the extensor tendons at the metatarsal or metacarpal level. It consists of multiple subcutaneous injections of local anesthetic solution into the tissue with aspiration after every movement to ensure the needle has not entered a blood vessel. The size of needle depends on the size of animal (2.5–3.8 cm, 25–20 gauge needle). The drug diffuses into the surrounding tissue from the sites of injection to anesthetize nerve fibers and endings. Large volumes of 2% lidocaine (1.5–2 mg/kg) are typically used in cattle, small ruminants, and swine. The amount of local anesthetic used will typically be dictated by the area to be infused. Epinephrine may be used in combination with infiltration of local anesthetic to reduce systemic absorption and prolong the anesthetic effect but the effects of vasoconstriction on regional blood flow should be considered.

Intravenous regional anesthesia (Bier block)

Intravenous regional anesthesia is a method suited to providing anesthesia of the distal limb for invasive hoof trimming of sole ulcers, draining of abscesses, claw amputation or other surgeries of the digits. The advantages of IVRA are that it is a relatively simple technique to perform compared to digital nerve blocks. Other advantages include rapid onset and recovery, the use of a single injection site, minimal blood at the surgical site, no need for specialized equipment, technical simplicity, and provision of effective analgesia and muscle relaxation during the surgical procedure and the ability of antibiotic administration. Disadvantages include the need to position and restrain the animal in lateral recumbency with the associated potential side-effects in adult ruminants, hematoma formation at the site of needle insertion, failure of the block, short duration of analgesia which is limited by the time the tourniquet can be applied, tourniquet discomfort, potential damage to nerves in the area under the tourniquet, and the possibility of local anesthetic toxicity when the tourniquet is released. The procedure is generally performed after manually casting the animal and restraining it in lateral recumbency or by using a tilting hoof-trimming table with the affected limb up. Attempts to perform IVRA in the standing bovine with the leg restrained tend to be unsuccessful as the animal typically becomes recumbent when the tourniquet is applied. Sedation is recommended for IVRA as discomfort from tourniquet application is common, especially when the procedure is prolonged. It is important to assess the degree of bloat in the laterally recumbent ruminant especially when abdominal bellybands are applied for restraint.

Intravenous regional anesthesia involves injection of local anesthetic into a superficial vein on the thoracic or pelvic limb after proximal application of a tourniquet to occlude arterial blood flow. The tourniquet is placed proximal to the region to be desensitized and interrupts arterial blood flow and removal of the local anesthetic from the surgical area. The local anesthetic is injected distal to the tourniquet and diffuses firstly into the superficial vascular space and then eventually into the deeper vasculature and venules. It passes out of the vasculature and into the small veins surrounding the nerves. From there it diffuses into the capillary plexi of the endoneurium and the vas nervorum capillary plexi that extend intraneurally, thereby blocking nerve conduction [52].

Minimal equipment is required consisting mainly of a tourniquet and regular sized needles (2.5–3.8 cm, 20 or 18 gauge), 4.8 cm, 20 to 16 gauge catheter, or simply a butterfly needle (20 to 16 gauge). Butterfly needles are ideal and can be fixed in place with adhesive tape to be used at the end of the procedure for antibiotic infusion. Tourniquet application can be manually applied using rubber tubing or a pneumatic cuff. The tourniquet used to occlude arterial flow manually can be round stout rubber tubing, a length of bicycle tire inner tube, or a wide flat rubber band. A length of 40–80 cm is usually necessary in adult cattle to allow the tourniquet to be wrapped around the limb and tied. The wide flat rubber band style tourniquet is generally preferable and minimizes discomfort to the animal. When the tourniquet is to be placed on the hindlimb above the hock, rolls of soft bandage should be applied on either side of the gastrocnemius tendon to minimize damage to this tendon and allow full occlusion of vasculature.

With either tourniquet method, the tourniquet needs to be inflated or secured sufficiently to occlude arterial blood flow. A cuff pressure of approximately 420 mmHg is used in equine patients [53]. Without a pneumatic cuff, the rubber style tourniquet is gradually wrapped around the animal's limb and tied or taped to maintain pressure. A more effective method is to exsanguinate the extremity using an Esmarch rubber bandage. The limb is tightly wrapped, from distal to proximal, before applying the tourniquet. A wide flat rubber band works best for this method. With use of an Esmarch technique, the vein may be initially difficult to visualize.

The common dorsal metacarpal vein, palmar metacarpal vein, or radial vein can be used in the thoracic limb [50]. In the pelvic limb, the cranial branch of the lateral saphenous vein or the lateral digital plantar digital vein is most easily accessed in the laterally recumbent animal (Fig. 51.12) [51]. Once isolated, the area over the vein can be clipped and disinfected prior to needle insertion. The direction of needle insertion into the now isolated vein is not crucial and depends on practitioner preference. However, it is important to inject the local anesthetic as close to the surgical site as possible. After injection of the local anesthetic, the needle can be removed and pressure and massage applied over the insertion site to prevent a hematoma forming.

The duration of analgesia is related to the time the tourniquet can safely be left in place. Complete desensitization of the area dissipates after tourniquet removal but some analgesia may persist for up to 30 min. The tourniquet can be left in place for 60–90 min but

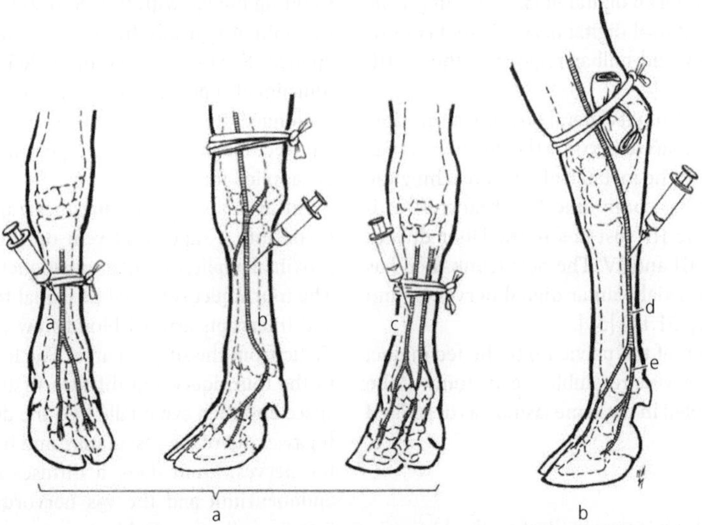

Figure 51.12 Tourniquet and needle placement for intravenous regional anesthesia of the bovine thoracic limb (a) and pelvic limb (b); a, dorsal metacarpal vein (dorsal view); b, radial vein (medial view); c, plantar metacarpal vein (palmar view); d, cranial branch of the lateral saphenous vein; and e, lateral plantar digital vein. From [14].

without sedation the animal will usually become restless and uncomfortable after 60 min of tourniquet application. The tourniquet should not be released earlier than 10 min after injection to minimize the chances of adverse effects from systemic local anesthetic. Other systemic analgesics, such as non-steroidal anti-inflammatory drugs, should be administered for long-term pain control whenever possible.

Lidocaine is the local anesthetic most commonly used for IVRA in ruminants and swine. It is important that solutions containing epinephrine are not used. Serious complications are uncommon with IVRA using lidocaine but seizures, convulsions, and cardiac arrest have been reported in humans undergoing IVRA with doses of lidocaine from 1.5 to 3 mg/kg [54]. Evidence of toxicity in cattle is rarely reported when the tourniquet is left in place for more than 20 min [55]. It may also help if the tourniquet is slowly released for 10–15 s and then reinflated for several minutes with this process being repeated several times prior to complete removal, so that the local anesthetic solution is released in stages, minimizing the potential for toxicity.

The volume of injectate will be influenced by the size of the limb and the location of the tourniquet. The presence of cellulitis in the limb will affect diffusion of anesthetic and a larger volume is required in such cases. A typical dose range for IVRA is 0.5–1.5 mg/kg. In adult cattle, this equates to 30–40 mL of 2% lidocaine. In sheep and goats, 3–10 mL of lidocaine will suffice. The local anesthetic is injected slowly and anesthesia develops in approximately 5 min. Pressure builds up in the venous system as the injection progresses, and to prevent leakage and hematoma formation around the site of venepuncture, gentle pressure should be applied over the site. Injection of saline (5–10 mL) after the local anesthetic to encourage spread of the local anesthetic through the limb has not been investigated for efficacy, although this technique is used by some bovine practitioners. Occasionally IVRA does not provide analgesia to the skin of the interdigital area. If necessary, this area can be desensitized by direct infiltration of local anesthetic (5–15 mL adult bovine; 2–5 mL small ruminants, calf, or swine).

Regional intravenous antibiotic perfusion may be useful in cases where the infected tissues or bone of the digital limb are unlikely to respond to topical or systemic antibiotic treatment. Antibiotics can be administered concurrently with regional intravenous anesthesia or on their own with similar techniques. The tourniquet should be left in place for a minimum of 20–30 min after antibiotic infusions.

References

1 Rosenberg PH, Veering BT, Urmey WF. Maximum recommended doses of local anesthetics: a multifactorial concept. *Reg Anesth Pain Med* 2004; **29**: 564–575.

2 Copeland SE, Ladd LA, Gu XO, *et al.* The effects of general anesthesia on the central nervous and cardiovascular system toxicity of local anesthetics. *Anesth Analg* 2008; **106**: 1429–1439.

3 Santos AC, DeArmas PI. Systemic toxicity of levobupivacaine, bupivacaine, and ropivacaine during continuous intravenous infusion to nonpregnant and pregnant ewes. *Anesthesiology* 2001; **95**: 1256–1264.

4 Morishima HO, Pederson H, Finster M, *et al.* Toxicity of lidocaine in adult, newborn, and fetal sheep. *Anesthesiology* 1981; **55**: 57–61.

5 Morishima HO, Finster M, Arthur GR, *et al.* Pregnancy does not alter lidocaine toxicity. *Am J Obstet Gynecol* 1990; **162**: 1320–1324.

6 Santos AC, Pedersen H, Harmon TW, *et al.* Does pregnancy alter the systemic toxicity of local anesthetics? *Anesthesiology* 1989; **70**: 991–995.

7 Mauch J, Martin Jurado O, Spielmann N, *et al.* Comparison of epinephrine vs lipid rescue to treat severe local anesthetic toxicity – an experimental study in piglets. *Pediatric Anesth* 2011; **21**: 1103–1108.

8 Udelsmann A, Lorena SE, Girioli SU, *et al.* Hemodynamic effects of local anesthetics intoxication. Experimental study in swine with levobupivacaine and bupivacaine *Acta Cir Bras* 2008; **23**: 55–64.

9 Satas S, Johannessen SI, Hoem NO, *et al.* Lidocaine pharmacokinetics and toxicity in newborn pigs. *Anesth Analg* 1997; **85**: 306–312.

10 Sellers G, Lin HC, Riddell MG, *et al.* Pharmacokinetics of lidocaine in serum and milk of mature Holstein cows. *J Vet Pharmacol Ther* 2009; **32**: 446–450.

11 Craigmill AL, Rangel-Lugo M, Damain P, *et al.* Extra-label use of tranquilizers and general anesthetics. *J Am Vet Med Assoc* 1997; **211**: 302–304.

12 Smith G. Extra-label drug use of anesthetics and analgesic compounds in cattle. *Vet Clin North Am Food Anim Pract* 2013; **29**: 29–45.

13 Habel R, Budras KD. Central nervous system and cranial nerves. In: Budras KD, Habel R, eds. *Bovine Anatomy*, 2nd edn. Hannover, Germany: Schlutersche, 2011; 30–49.

14 Skarda RT, Tranquilli WJ. Local and regional anesthetic and analgesic techniques: ruminants and swine. In: Tranquilli WJ, Thurmon JC, Grimm KA, eds. *Lumb and Jones' Veterinary Anesthesia and Analgesia*, 4th edn. Ames, IA: Blackwell Publishing, 2007; 643–681.

15 Valverde A, Doherty T. Anesthesia and analgesia of ruminants. In: Fish R, Danneman PJ, Brown M, Karas A, eds. *Anesthesia and Analgesia in Laboratory Animals*, 2nd edn. San Diego, CA: Academic Press, 2008; 385–412.

16 Pearce SG, Kerr CL, Boure LP, *et al.* Comparison of the retrobulbar and Peterson nerve block techniques via magnetic resonance imaging in bovine cadavers. *J Am Vet Med Assoc* 2003; **223**: 852–855.
17 Peterson DR. Nerve block of the eye and associated structures. *J Am Vet Med Assoc* 1951; **118**: 145–148.
18 Budras KD, Habel R. Special anatomy, tabular part. In: Budras KD, Habel R, eds. *Bovine Anatomy*, 2nd edn. Hannover, Germany: Schlutersche, 2011; 119, 123, 125.
19 Roe JM. Bovine paravertebral analgesia: radiographic analysis and suggested method for improvement. *Vet Rec* 1986; **119**: 236–238.
20 Arthur GH. Some notes on a preliminary trial of segmental epidural anesthesia of cattle. *Vet Rec* 1956; **68**: 254–256.
21 Skarda RT, Muir WW. Segmental lumbar epidural analgesia in cattle. *Am J Vet Res* 1979; **40**: 52–57.
22 Lee I, Yamagishi N, Oboshi K, *et al.* Comparison of xylazine, lidocaine and the two drugs combined for modified dorsolumbar epidural anaesthesia in cattle. *Vet Rec* 2004; **155**: 797–799.
23 Hiraoka M, Miyagawa T, Kobayashi H, *et al.* Successful introduction of modified dorsolumbar epidural anesthesia in a bovine referral center. *J Vet Sci* 2007; **8**: 181–184.
24 Valverde A. Epidural analgesia and anesthesia. *Vet Clin North Am Small Anim Pract* 2008; **38**: 1205–1230.
25 Lee I, Yamagishi N, Oboshi K, *et al.* Practical tips for the modified dorsolumbar epidural anesthesia in cattle. *J Vet Sci* 2006; **7**: 69–72.
26 Lee I, Soehartono RH, Yamagishi N, *et al.* Distribution of new methylene blue injected into the dorsolumbar epidural space in cows. *Vet Anaesth Analg* 2001; **28**: 140–145.
27 Lee I, Yamagishi N, Oboshi K, *et al.* Multivariate regression analysis of epidural pressure in cattle. *Am J Vet Res* 2002; **63**: 954–957.
28 Skarda RT, Muir WW, Hubbell JA. Comparative study of continuous lumbar segmental epidural and subarachnoid analgesia in Holstein cows. *Am J Vet Res* 1989; **50**: 39–44.
29 Meyer H, Starke A, Kehler W, *et al.* High caudal epidural anaesthesia with local anaesthetics or alpha(2)-agonists in calves. *J Vet Med A Physiol Pathol Clin Med* 2007; **54**: 384–389.
30 Johnson RA, Lopes MJ, Hendrickson DA, *et al.* Cephalad distribution of three different volumes of new methylene blue injected into the epidural space in adult goats. *Vet Surg* 1996; **25**: 448–451.
31 Condino MP, Suzuki K, Taguchi K. Antinociceptive, sedative and cardiopulmonary effects of subarachnoid and epidural xylazine-lidocaine in xylazine-sedated calves. *Vet Anaesth Analg* 2010; **37**: 70–78.
32 Pleticha J, Maus TP, Jeng-Singh C, *et al.* Pig lumbar spine anatomy and imaging-guided lateral lumbar puncture: a new large animal model for intrathecal drug delivery. *J Neurosci Methods* 2013; **216**: 10–15.
33 Strande A. Epidural anaesthesia in young pigs, dosage in relation to the length of the vertebral column. *Acta Vet Scand* 1968; **9**: 41–49.
34 Lopez MJ, Johnson R, Hendrickson DA, *et al.* Craniad migration of differing doses of new methylene blue injected into the epidural space after death of calves and juvenile pigs. *Am J Vet Res* 1997; **58**: 786–790.
35 Ko JCH, Thurmon JC, Benson GJ. Evaluation of analgesia induced by epidural injection of detomidine or xylazine in swine. *J Vet Anesth* 1992; **19**: 56–60.
36 Adetunji A, Ajao AO. Comparison of extradural injections of lignocaine and xylazine in azaperone-sedated pigs. *Vet J* 2001; **161**: 98–99.
37 Habel R, Budras KD. Head. In: Budras KD, Habel R, eds. *Bovine Anatomy*, 2nd edn. Hannover, Germany: Schlutersche, 2011; 50–57.
38 Lee I, Yamagishi N, Oboshi K, *et al.* Distribution of new methylene blue injected into the caudal epidural space in cattle. *Vet J* 2005; **169**: 257–261.
39 Araujo MA, Albuquerque VB, Deschk M, *et al.* Cardiopulmonary and analgesic effects of caudal epidurally administered ropivacaine in cattle. *Vet Anaesth Analg* 2012; **39**: 409–413.
40 Habel R, Budras KD. Perineum, pelvic diaphragm, ischiorectal fossa, and tail. In: Budras KD, Habel R, eds. *Bovine Anatomy*, 2nd edn. Hannover, Germany: Schlutersche, 2011; 94–95.
41 Caron JP, LeBlanc PH. Caudal epidural analgesia in cattle using xylazine. *Can J Vet Res* 1989; **53**: 486–489.
42 Ko JCH, Althouse GC, Hopkins SM, *et al.* Effects of epidural administration of xylazine or lidocaine on bovine uterine motility and perineal analgesia. *Theriogenology* 1989; **32**: 779–786.
43 Currah JM, Hendrick SH, Stookey JM. The behavioral assessment and alleviation of pain associated with castration in beef calves treated with flunixin meglumine and caudal lidocaine epidural anesthesia with epinephrine. *Can Vet J* 2009; **50**: 375–382.
44 Grubb TL, Riebold TW, Hubber MJ. Evaluation of lidocaine, xylazine, and a combination of lidocaine and xylazine for epidural analgesia in llamas. *J Am Vet Med Assoc* 1993; **203**: 1441–1444.
45 Noordsy JL. Sacral paravertebral alcohol nerve block as an aid in controlling chronic rectal tenesmus in cattle. *Vet Med Small Anim Clin* 1982; **77**: 797–801.
46 Wünsche A, Budras KD. Arteries, veins, and nerves of the pelvic cavity. In: Budras KD, Habel R, eds. *Bovine Anatomy*, 2nd edn. Hannover, Germany: Schlutersche, 2011; 84–85.
47 McFarlane IS. The lateral approach to the pudendal nerve block in the bovine and ovine. *J S Afr Vet Assoc* 1963; **34**: 73–76.
48 Bragulla H, König H, Budras KD. The udder with blood vessels, lymphatic system, nerves, and development. In: Budras KD, Habel R, eds. *Bovine Anatomy*, 2nd edn. Hannover, Germany: Schlutersche, 2011; 90–91.
49 Estebe JP, Le Corre P, du Plessis L, *et al.* The pharmacokinetics and pharmacodynamics of bupivacaine-loaded microspheres on a brachial plexus block model in sheep. *Anesth Analg* 2001; **93**: 447–455.
50 Wünsche A, Habel R, Budras KD. Thoracic limb. In: Budras KD, Habel R, eds. *Bovine Anatomy*, 2nd edn. Hannover, Germany: Schlutersche, 2011; 2–13.
51 Wünsche A, Habel R, Budras KD. Pelvic limb. In: Budras KD, Habel R, eds. *Bovine Anatomy*, 2nd edn. Hannover, Germany: Schlutersche, 2011; 14–29.
52 Ennevor SJ, Bobart V, Swamidoss CP. Intravenous regional anesthesia: a review. *Sem Anesth Perio M* 1998, **17**: 2–9.
53 Levine DG, Epstein KL, Ahern BJ, *et al.* Efficacy of three tourniquet types for intravenous antimicrobial regional limb perfusion in standing horses. *Vet Surg* 2010; **39**: 1021–1024.
54 Guay J. Adverse effects associated with intravenous regional anesthesia (Bier Block): a systematic review of complications. *J Clin Anesth* 2009; **21**: 585–594.
55 Elmore RG. Food animal regional anesthesia: bovine blocks-intravenous limb block. *Vet Med Small Anim Clin* 1980; **75**: 1835–1836.

SECTION 12

Anesthesia and Analgesia for Selected Patients or Procedures

52 Ophthalmic Patients

Marjorie E. Gross[1] **and Luisito S. Pablo**[2]

[1] Oklahoma State University, Center for Veterinary Health Sciences, Stillwater, Oklahoma, USA

[2] College of Veterinary Medicine, Auburn University, Auburn , Alabama, USA

Chapter contents

Introduction

Development of an anesthetic protocol for any ophthalmic patient involves not only appropriate anesthetic drug selection, but also a management plan to ensure an optimal postoperative outcome. This requires knowledge of the patient's physical status and the specific ophthalmic procedure to be performed. It also requires familiarity with ophthalmic physiology and the effects of current ophthalmic medications.

Physiologic considerations for the ophthalmic patient

Selection of an anesthetic protocol for ophthalmic surgery should include consideration of the effects on intraocular pressure (IOP), pupil size, globe position, tear production, and the potential for initiation of the oculocardiac reflex (OCR) during surgical manipulation of the globe.

Intraocular pressure (IOP)

Success of an ophthalmic procedure may depend on adequate control of IOP before, during, and after the procedure. The IOP is determined by aqueous humor dynamics, intraocular (choroidal) blood volume, central venous pressure, and extraocular muscle tone [1].

Normal IOP depends on the delicate balance between aqueous inflow (production) and outflow (filtration) [1,2]. Obstruction of outflow, which may dramatically increase IOP, may be induced by coughing, retching, vomiting, excessive restraint of the head and neck, or any maneuver or position that increases central venous pressure [3]. Indeed, coughing may increase IOP by as much as 40 mmHg.[1] Normal IOP has been reported for dogs (10–26 mmHg), cats (12–32 mmHg), and horses (23.5–28.6 mmHg) [4–6]. For intraocular surgery, a low-normal IOP is usually desirable [3]. Lens or vitreous prolapse, expulsive choroidal hemorrhage, and subsequent retinal detachment are possible sequelae to increased IOP during or after intraocular surgery, or in patients with penetrating eye wounds [3].

The effects of systemically administered anesthetic drugs on IOP should be taken into consideration when diagnostic tonometry is anticipated. The overall effect of most anesthetics is to decrease IOP [1]. This reduction may be attributable to a combination of factors, including depression of diencephalic centers regulating IOP, increased aqueous outflow, decreased venous and arterial blood pressures, and relaxation of extraocular musculature [1]. Many of the factors affecting IOP are listed in Table 52.1.

Aqueous humor is produced primarily by the ciliary body. It flows from the posterior chamber anteriorly through the pupil into the anterior chamber. Most of the aqueous humor exits the anterior chamber via the filtration angle of the eye, following a pattern of flow referred to as *conventional outflow* [2]. In conventional outflow, aqueous humor enters the venous vascular system via the scleral

Veterinary Anesthesia and Analgesia: The Fifth Edition of Lumb and Jones.
Edited by Kurt A. Grimm, Leigh A. Lamont, William J. Tranquilli, Stephen A. Greene and Sheilah A. Robertson.

Table 52.1 Factors altering intraocular pressure (IOP).

Altering factors	Change in IOP	Comments
Blockade of aqueous outflow	↑	Caused by any position/maneuver that increases CVP
Acute increase in arterial pressure	↑	Causes only a transient increase in IOP
Hypoventilation, airway obstruction, hypercapnia, choroidal vessel dilation	↑	
Hyperventilation, hypocapnia	↓	
Endotracheal intubation	↑	Topical or IV lidocaine may prevent coughing, gagging, straining
Eyeball pressure	↑	Caused by face mask, orbital tumors, surgical traction, eyeball position, retrobulbar injection
Anesthetic drugs		
Barbiturates	↓	May depress central control of IOP or promote aqueous outflow
Propofol	↓	May prevent intubation-associated increase in IOP; may suppress depolarizing NMB-induced increase in IOP
Etomidate	↑	May be predominantly due to etomidate-induced myoclonus
Ketamine	↑ or ↓	Contradictory; effect may depend on premedication
α_2-Agonists	↓	Induce bradycardia; may promote OCR; may induce vomiting; may suppress sympathetic input and aqueous production
Benzodiazepines	↓	May be in response to central relaxation of ocular muscles
Acepromazine	↓	Decreases arterial BP, suppresses vomiting/retching
Opioids	↓	IOP may increase with opioid-induced vomiting/retching
Neuromuscular blockers (NMBs)		
Depolarizing		
Succinylcholine	↑	Transient increase in IOP
Non-depolarizing	↓	Decrease or no effect
Pancuronium		
Vecuronium		
Atracurium		
Other drugs		
Osmotic (hyperosmotic) solutions	↓	Increase plasma osmotic pressure, decrease aqueous humor formation
Phenylephrine	↑ or ↓	Effect is dosage dependent
Epinephrine	↑ or ↓	Effect is dosage dependent

BP = blood pressure; CVP = central venous pressure; IV = intravenous; OCR-oculocardiac reflex.
Modified from Gross and Giuliano [161], p.945.

venous plexus (analogous to Schlemm's canal in humans), drains into the vortex veins, passes through the orbital vasculature, and ultimately enters the episcleral venous system. The small percentage of aqueous humor that exits the anterior chamber via diffusion through iris stroma and ciliary body musculature is referred to as uveoscleral or *unconventional outflow*. In unconventional outflow, aqueous humor flows caudally to enter the suprachoroidal and ultimately the scleral and choroidal vasculature [2].

Intraocular (choroidal) blood volume is determined by arterial inflow, venous outflow, and tone of the intraocular vasculature [7]. Autoregulation of choroidal blood flow minimizes the effects of systemic arterial blood pressure on choroidal blood volume and IOP. Sudden increases in systolic arterial blood pressure may cause a transient increase in choroidal blood volume and IOP, but a temporary increase in outflow will adjust IOP back to normal. Sudden increases in choroidal blood volume may also displace the vitreous forward into the anterior chamber during intraocular surgery or in patients with penetrating eye wounds. Marked IOP reductions may occur when systolic arterial blood pressure decreases below 90 mmHg and choroidal blood volume decreases [3].

A more direct, definitive relationship exists between central venous pressure and IOP [1,8]. Increases in central venous pressure can increase IOP and choroidal blood volume by diminishing aqueous humor outflow into the venous system [3]. To maintain normal central venous pressure and IOP in humans, a slightly head-up position is preferred for patients undergoing intraocular surgery [7]. The effect of head or body position on changes in IOP has also been reported in dogs, horses, and mice [9–11].

Choroidal blood volume, and consequently IOP, both increase in response to increases in the arterial partial pressure of carbon dioxide ($PaCO_2$) and decreases in the arterial partial pressure of oxygen (PaO_2) [12]. Hypercapnia and hypoxemia induce vasodilation which increases intraocular blood volume, leading to an increase in IOP. Conversely, respiratory alkalosis and hyperbaric oxygen conditions induce vasoconstriction and decrease aqueous humor formation through reduced carbonic anhydrase activity which decreases choroidal blood volume and IOP [12]. In anesthetized dogs, inspired concentrations of 5% carbon dioxide (CO_2) caused a mean increase in IOP of 35.2%. Concentrations of 10–15% of CO_2 increased IOP even higher [12]. It has been suggested, however, that hyperventilation may fail to decrease IOP because of the increases in intrathoracic and central venous pressure accompanying the use of mechanical ventilation [13]. There is no apparent correlation between increased $PaCO_2$ and IOP in anesthetized horses [14]. Unlike other species, horses have a greater dependence on unconventional outflow of aqueous humor which may result in a more constant IOP during hypercapnia [14].

Vitreous has been described as a hydrogel consisting of a loose fibrillar network of collagen that supports the lens anteriorly and the retina posteriorly [2]. Although the vitreous volume is fairly constant, it may be decreased by administration of osmotic (also called hyperosmotic) agents, such as mannitol or glycerin. As indicated previously, vitreous may be displaced by changes in intraocular blood volume, but also by extraocular and orbicularis oculi muscle contractions. Muscle contractions and vitreous displacement that occur during intraocular surgery, or with a penetrating eye wound, may cause expulsion of intraocular contents. Closure of the palpebrae may increase IOP anywhere from 10 to 50 mmHg depending on whether the closure is normal or forceful [7].

Pupil size

In mammals, iris musculature that controls pupil size is smooth muscle and is controlled primarily by the autonomic nervous system [15]. Parasympathetic stimulation of the iris constrictor muscle results in miosis (pupillary constriction) and sympathetic stimulation of the iris dilator muscle results in mydriasis (pupillary dilation). In contrast, avian species have striated pupillary muscles, which are unresponsive to topically applied parasympatholytic or sympathomimetic agents [16].

Pupil size as an indicator of anesthetic depth is not reliable [17]. In addition, pupils are typically inaccessible for anesthesia monitoring during ophthalmic surgery, although the ophthalmologist may be able to provide information about pupil size during the procedure.

Pupil size is of greatest concern in cataract removal surgery, which requires the pupil to be widely dilated and the eye immobilized.

Most anesthetic or sedative agents, with the exception of dissociative anesthetics (e.g., ketamine), will cause some degree of miosis [2]. Opioids have variable effects on pupil size among species [18] and may interfere with the mydriasis required for cataract surgery [19,20]. Administration of opioid antagonists (e.g., naloxone) may reverse miosis when it occurs, although direct mydriatics such as epinephrine have also been used during intraocular surgery [19,21]. Prostaglandins and other mediators of inflammation may cause miosis by a direct effect on the iris constrictor muscle [22]. Consequently, antiprostaglandins may be administered prior to intraocular surgery. Sympathomimetic, cholinergic, and anticholinergic drugs applied topically to the eye will affect pupil size. It has been suggested that mydriasis is more difficult to achieve after the onset of sedation or anesthesia [19] whereas mydriasis achieved prior to anesthetic induction or sedation is usually unaffected by the miotic properties of anesthetic and sedative drugs [2].

Globe position

Globe motion during general anesthesia is not unusual, and position of the globe may vary among species and stages of anesthesia. Motion is undesirable during corneal and intraocular surgery, but excessive manual traction to maintain a stable globe position may cause expulsion of intraocular contents or potentially initiate the OCR. Additionally, palpebral reflexes that may be maintained during anesthesia in some species may also interfere with procedures. Paralysis with neuromuscular blocking drugs or retrobulbar regional anesthesia with local anesthetics during general anesthesia should eliminate ocular reflexes and enable positioning of the globe without the need for manual traction, reducing the potential for expulsion of globe contents or initiation of the OCR.

Tear production

The precorneal tear film (PTF) has been described as three structurally and functionally unique layers consisting of lipid, aqueous, and mucin components. These three component layers appear to be intricately mingled, rather than having clear-cut barriers. The PTF is the primary oxygen source to the avascular cornea. It also provides lubrication between the lids and ocular surface, provides a protective antimicrobial protein source, and facilitates drainage of debris and exfoliated cells [23].

Reflex tears occur in response to light, cold, wind, or other irritants. Basal tears are continuously produced, and are necessary for normal functioning of the PTF. The Schirmer tear test (STT) is used to clinically evaluate aqueous tear production. The STT type I measures reflex tear production, while the STT type II measures basal tear production utilizing topical anesthesia and drying of the ventral conjunctival fornix [24,25]. Depression of both reflex and basal tear production has been demonstrated during anesthesia [26–30]. It has been suggested that depression of reflex tear formation during anesthesia may be due to depression of autonomic pathways responsible for production of reflex tears [28,31].

Tear production decreases during general anesthesia in people, dogs, horses, and possibly other species [26,28,32,33]. A study comparing the effects of sedative-tranquilizer and opioid combinations on tear production in dogs determined that acepromazine-oxymorphone, diazepam-butorphanol, and xylazine-butorphanol significantly decreased tear production (80%, 68%, and 33% of baseline, respectively) [34]. Based on retention studies in people and rabbits, it has been suggested that canine eyes be lubricated every 90 min during general anesthesia [28,35,36]. In horses undergoing general anesthesia with halothane, tear production decreased significantly but the volume of tear production remained higher than that of dogs or people [33]. Although this may seem to suggest that ocular lubrication may not be necessary to prevent corneal drying in horses, it is recommended that ocular lubrication be instilled in the eyes of all patients undergoing anesthesia unless otherwise directed by an ophthalmologist.

Oculocardiac reflex

The oculocardiac reflex (OCR) is a trigeminovagal (cranial nerves V and X) reflex that may be induced by pressure or traction on the eyeball, ocular trauma or pain, pressure from an orbital mass or hematoma, or retrobulbar blocks. Initiation of the OCR manifests as cardiac arrhythmias which may include bradycardia, nodal rhythms, ectopic beats, ventricular fibrillation, or asystole [1]. The afferent pathway of the reflex follows ciliary nerves to the ciliary ganglion and then along the ophthalmic division of the trigeminal nerve. The afferent pathway terminates in the main trigeminal sensory nucleus in the floor of the fourth ventricle. The efferent pathway starts in the fibers of the vagal cardiac depressor nerve, resulting in negative inotropic and conduction effects. Although the OCR may occur most commonly during ocular surgery, it may also occur during non-ocular surgery when excessive pressure is placed on the eyeball [1]. It has been suggested that the more acute the onset and the more sustained the pressure or traction, the more likely the OCR is to occur [1]. In people, OCR occurs most frequently during strabismus surgery in children and may be related to the degree of traction necessary to expose the medial rectus muscle during surgery [1]. Although it has been suggested that hypercapnia in these patients is an important adjuvant factor for the occurrence of OCR, it has not been clearly established that hypercapnia increases the risk of OCR [37].

Treatment of OCR should begin with discontinuing stimulation. The OCR ceases when stimulation ceases, so communication with the surgeon to discontinue procedural stimulation is vital if initiation of the OCR is suspected. Fortunately, it is possible for the OCR to fatigue with repeated, prolonged stimulation [1]. Atropine administration to prevent or treat the OCR is controversial in people [1]. Cardiac dysrhythmias may occur after atropine administration, especially in the presence of halothane, and may persist longer than the OCR response. In children, intravenous (IV) atropine or glycopyrrolate was more effective in preventing OCR than was intramuscular (IM) premedication with atropine, with glycopyrrolate producing less of a tachycardic effect than atropine [38].

Bradycardia is a common dysrhythmia associated with the OCR [39,40]. Treatment with atropine may be effective if the OCR persists, although the dosage and timing of atropine administration may greatly affect its ability to block the reflex [41]. Retrobulbar injection of lidocaine has been suggested if atropine is ineffective and the bradycardia is considered life-threatening [42] or as a prophylactic technique to prevent the OCR [43]. However, the possible complications associated with retrobulbar injection may pose a greater risk than those associated with occurrence of the OCR, and its use should be decided on a case-by-case basis [43]. Indeed, the prophylactic retrobulbar injection itself may elicit the OCR. The OCR was considered to be of minor clinical importance in dogs undergoing ophthalmic surgery when anesthesia provided adequate unconsciousness, good muscle relaxation, and mild hypocapnia [44].

Effects of ophthalmic medications on patient physiology

It is important to recognize that topical ophthalmic preparations are concentrated medications that may cause systemic side-effects, especially when administered to very small patients. Systemic effects may be minimized by diluting such medications and limiting their frequency of application prior to anesthesia; however, consultation with an ophthalmologist is recommended before changing or compounding any prescribed medications [1,45–47].

Cholinergic agonists and antagonists

Glaucoma may be treated with cholinergic agents that decrease IOP primarily by increasing aqueous outflow. Direct-acting cholinergic agonists are similar in structure and mimic the effects of acetylcholine. Indirect-acting cholinergic agonists are anticholinesterases, which facilitate the build-up of acetylcholine by slowing its enzymatic hydrolysis. Both types of agents may produce effects similar to acetylcholine when absorbed systemically, including bradycardia or atrioventricular blockade [2]. These dysrhythmias may be similar to, and difficult to distinguish from, those produced by the OCR [48]. If necessary, the systemic actions of acetylcholine may be blocked with the administration of an anticholinergic.

Topical administration of the direct-acting cholinergic agent pilocarpine is unlikely to produce systemic side-effects when given in solutions ranging in concentration from 0.5% to 8% or as a 4% gel formulation [49,50]. Systemic effects from indirect-acting anticholinesterases have the potential to interfere with metabolism of succinylcholine, and may result in prolongation of depolarizing neuromuscular blockade [48]. The anticholinesterase activity of organophosphates may also have an additive effect and should be avoided during administration of indirect-acting anticholinesterases [51]. Other systemic effects associated with indirect-acting anticholinesterases may include salivation, vomiting, diarrhea, and abdominal cramps [52].

Mydriatic agents are cholinergic antagonists (i.e., anticholinergics) that are generally administered topically and produce pupillary dilation by paralysis of the pupillary sphincter. Pupillary dilation facilitates visualization during ophthalmic examination and surgery of the lens and posterior segment. Salivation has been observed frequently and vomiting occasionally after topical administration of some anticholinergics, and are presumed to be due to their bitter taste [53–55]. In horses, systemic effects are of particular concern due to effects on intestinal motility and the potential for inducing colic. Abdominal pain and decreases in gastrointestinal myoelectric activity and borborygmi have been reported in horses following topical and subconjunctival administration of atropine [56,57].

Adrenergic agonists and antagonists

Adrenergic agonists may predispose patients to catecholamine-induced cardiac dysrhythmias, and topical application of adrenergic agonists has been associated with increased heart rate and blood pressure in people [58]. Phenylephrine is an adrenergic agonist that is used to produce mydriasis prior to cataract surgery or in patients with uveitis. Subconjunctival phenylephrine has been associated with hypertension and pulmonary edema in children and horses [47,49]. In dogs undergoing cataract surgery, topical treatment with phenylephrine has been associated with arterial hypertension [60]. Topical application of 10% phenylephrine increased arterial blood pressure and caused reflex bradycardia in normal dogs [61], and in a cat undergoing a conjunctival graft procedure [46]. Acepromazine may be useful in counteracting the hypertension produced by phenylephrine [60].

Both adrenergic agonists and antagonists are used to treat glaucoma. The mechanism by which the topical α_2-adrenergic receptor agonists decrease IOP is not fully understood. Decreases in aqueous humor formation appear to play a role [62,63] but a possible mechanism for a decrease in aqueous humor outflow remains unclear [64]. In the eyes of normal humans treated topically with 0.125% clonidine, there was a decrease in IOP, aqueous humor outflow, pupil size, and systolic blood pressure. This would suggest that topical 0.125% clonidine has both local and systemic effects [64]. Topical apraclonidine resulted in systemic effects in both dogs and cats, including decreases in heart rate that were greater in cats, and undesirable gastrointestinal effects that occurred in most of the cats [65,66]. In glaucomatous Beagle dogs, treatment with 0.2% brimonidine tartrate decreased heart rate by 12–22% [67]. Central nervous system depression, bradycardia, and hypotension were among the systemic effects that occurred in dogs after accidental ingestion of brimonidine ophthalmic solution [68].

Timolol, a non-selective β-adrenergic receptor antagonist that is commonly used to treat glaucoma, has been associated with more adverse systemic effects in people than have any other topically applied glaucoma medications [69]. Systemic effects in people may include bradycardia, hypotension, congestive heart failure, and exacerbation of asthma and myasthenia gravis [1]. Timolol is contraindicated in animals with atrioventricular block, cardiac failure, or obstructive pulmonary disease [70]. A significant decrease in heart rate was observed in normotensive and glaucomatous Beagle dogs administered topical timolol at concentrations ranging from 2% to 8% [71,72]. Significant decreases in heart rate and blood pressure have been observed in anesthetized dogs within 30 min of topical timolol administration [70]. Documented decreases in IOP of both treated and untreated eyes provide further evidence of systemic absorption of the drug in dogs and cats [73,74]. To help prevent undesirable systemic effects, it has been suggested that 0.25% timolol be used in cats and dogs weighing less than 10 kg, and 0.5% timolol in dogs above 12.5 kg [75].

Carbonic anhydrase inhibitors

Carbonic anhydrase inhibitors (CAIs) decrease IOP by decreasing aqueous humor production [76]. Carbonic anhydrase is also found in extraocular tissues, most notably red blood cells and kidneys [76,77]. Administration of systemic CAIs impacts ion exchange in the kidneys, resulting in retention of chloride and excretion of bicarbonate and potassium. Treated patients may develop metabolic acidosis and electrolyte imbalances, most notably hypokalemia and hyperchloremia. Some CAIs cause profound potassium excretion, resulting in hypokalemia even in the presence of metabolic acidosis, a condition that is typically accompanied by hyperkalemia [77]. Long-term administration of CAIs is more likely to result in adverse systemic effects [52].

Acidosis and electrolyte imbalances may disrupt cardiovascular and neurologic function. Hyperventilation would typically occur during metabolic acidosis as a compensatory mechanism, but hypoventilation during anesthesia may exacerbate the metabolic acidosis by inducing respiratory acidosis [78]. Acidosis may increase the potential for cardiac dysrhythmias during anesthesia. Ideally, metabolic acidosis and electrolyte imbalances would be corrected prior to anesthesia, and ventilatory support would be provided to prevent significant respiratory acidosis. No local or systemic side-effects were reported in short-term studies of topical CAIs in the dog, cat, and horse [79–82]. Recent focus has been on the development of topical CAIs with fewer adverse systemic effects [83].

Osmotic agents

Osmotic (also referred to as hyperosmotic) agents administered orally or intravenously result in a fluid shift that ultimately reduces the volume of the vitreous body, which allows for better drainage by opening the iridocorneal angle [52]. The resultant effect is a decrease in IOP. These agents are usually administered for emergency treatment of acute glaucoma and short-term control of IOP [84,85] rather than for prolonged treatment [86]. Water may be withheld for a period of time to enhance the effectiveness of the osmotic agent, unless otherwise contraindicated [52,87].

Examples of osmotic agents commonly used for treatment of glaucoma include glycerol and mannitol. Glycerol is administered orally, may have a slower onset, and is considered relatively nontoxic, although emesis has been reported [84,88,89]. Glycerol is metabolized into glucose, and should be used judiciously in diabetic patients [86]. Mannitol is administered intravenously, and is typically used for prompt, reliable reduction in IOP [87]. Mannitol is not metabolized to a significant degree. It is excreted in the urine, and increased urination should be anticipated during anesthesia and recovery [52]. Mannitol may be administered pre-, intra-, or postoperatively to decrease vitreous volume and IOP [86]. Both mannitol and glycerol have been used in combination for maintenance of normal IOP [85].

The major concern and potential toxicity associated with mannitol administration is rapid expansion of extracellular volume and overloading of the cardiovascular system [86–88]. Acute expansion of the extracellular fluid volume may precipitate the formation of pulmonary edema in patients with cardiovascular dysfunction, patients under general anesthesia, or those with renal dysfunction. Six dogs and one cat developed pulmonary edema prior to death after receiving 2.2 g/kg mannitol during methoxyflurane anesthesia [90]. Increased central venous pressure, increased serum osmolality, and pulmonary edema have been reported in dogs receiving 20% mannitol during methoxyflurane anesthesia [91]. The pulmonary edema was histologically but not clinically evident and reported changes were not as pronounced in dogs that were mechanically ventilated. This would suggest that positive pressure ventilation during and immediately after the administration of mannitol may prevent the development of pulmonary edema, compared with patients breathing spontaneously [91]. Dogs receiving a lower dose of mannitol (0.25 g/kg IV) during halothane anesthesia had no significant changes in cardiovascular variables, but also had no reduction in IOP either [92]. It has been suggested that decreased dose or rate of infusion, as well as thorough patient evaluation, may prevent complications associated with mannitol [87].

Other possible adverse effects associated with osmotic diuretic administration include nausea, vomiting, hypokalemia, dehydration (both systemic and cerebral), and central nervous system symptoms [87,88]. Osmotic agents are not routinely recommended in patients with pre-existing cardiac or pulmonary disease, renal dysfunction, or dehydration [2].

Corticosteroids

Topical or subconjunctival administration of corticosteroids has resulted in adverse effects in dogs, although these complications are much less likely than following systemic administration [93–97]. The occurrence of systemic effects appears to be both dose and duration dependent with signs of glucocorticoid-associated hepatopathy, marked reduction in corticosteroid production, and alopecia being reported [93–97]. In horses, repeated topical administration of dexamethasone ophthalmic ointment resulted in detectable corticosteroid concentrations in serum and urine [98]. It has also been proposed that topically applied glucocorticoids may be associated with abortion in llamas after administration of dexamethasone-containing ophthalmic ointment during late gestation [99]. It should be remembered that the co-administration of corticosteroids and non-steroidal anti-inflammatory drugs (NSAIDs) may exacerbate the toxicity of both classes of drugs.

Effects of anesthetic, analgesic, and adjunctive drugs on ophthalmic physiology

Inhalant anesthetics

Historically, methoxyflurane was the inhalation agent preferred by ophthalmologists. It was believed to provide greater extraocular muscle relaxation, as well as a hypotonic and centrally rotated eye [100,101]. Additionally, the slower recovery from anesthesia was preferred. Currently, isoflurane and sevoflurane are the inhalation agents most commonly used in veterinary patients. They provide rapid induction and recovery, although rapid recovery potentially increases the risk of iatrogenic trauma or intraocular bleeding if associated with emergence delirium. Appropriate perioperative medication should be used to facilitate calm recovery. In dogs, the dysrhythmogenic dose of epinephrine is higher for isoflurane [102] which made it preferable to halothane in patients receiving exogenously administered catecholamines or topical ophthalmic adrenergic agonist drugs. It has been suggested that extraocular muscle relaxation and position of the globe are superior with isoflurane, but this information is anecdotal [59].

Inhaled anesthetics reduce IOP in proportion to the depth of anesthesia in human patients during controlled ventilation and normocapnia. Reductions of 14–50% have been noted [1]. However, the effects of isoflurane on IOP have been described as being similar to those of halothane, which decreases IOP in a manner that is not dose dependent and has a ceiling effect in people [103]. In hypercapnic, halothane-anesthetized horses, there were no significant changes in IOP [14]. In a study comparing the effects of halothane and desflurane on IOP in dogs, it was concluded that desflurane decreases IOP similar to halothane. The decrease was attributed to a combination of decreased aqueous humor formation and increased outflow [104].

In a comparison of normocapnic dogs anesthetized with sevoflurane or desflurane, there were no significant differences in IOP between the two inhalants and IOP remained within normal limits [105]. In human patients undergoing elective non-ophthalmic surgery, desflurane significantly decreased IOP similar to isoflurane or propofol [106] and IOP was decreased equally in those patients receiving sevoflurane when compared with those receiving propofol [107]. In people undergoing elective ophthalmic surgery, IOP did not increase during sevoflurane and remifentanil anesthesia in response to endotracheal intubation or Laryngeal Mask Airway™ insertion [108]. In non-surgical human patients anesthetized with sevoflurane or desflurane, pupil size increased with increasing duration of constant levels of inhalant anesthesia [109].

In rabbits, sevoflurane anesthesia decreased IOP similar to halothane anesthesia; the addition of remifentanil to the sevoflurane protocol resulted in a greater decrease in IOP [110]. Both sevoflurane and sevoflurane-remifentanil decreased IOP compared with the average reported values in awake rabbits, with the magnitude of decrease being similar to previously reported values in rabbits anesthetized with ethyl urethane, pentobarbital, or halothane alone or in combination with propofol, cocaine, or lidocaine [110]. In pigs, isoflurane anesthesia caused a significant decrease in IOP, similar to that observed with propofol-ketamine administration [111]. In rats, isoflurane anesthesia decreased IOP in both normal eyes and eyes with experimental aqueous outflow obstruction [112].

Isoflurane and desflurane significantly decreased aqueous tear production in dogs during anesthesia durations of 1 and 4 h [30]. Tear production returned to normal immediately after recovery with no difference between the longer and shorter anesthesia durations. Tear production decreased in dogs during 30 min of sevoflurane anesthesia after acepromazine or morphine premedication but was not decreased before induction, at recovery from anesthesia, and at 2 and 10 h after recovery [27].

The addition of nitrous oxide (N_2O) to differing concentrations of desflurane during general anesthesia in dogs resulted in IOP measurements within normal limits [113]. This was in contrast to other reports of decreases in IOP with inhalant anesthetics [3,7]. In addition, no significant decrease in pupillary diameter was observed with the addition of N_2O. These results would suggest that the combination of desflurane and N_2O may be a suitable protocol for dogs undergoing ophthalmic surgery requiring mydriasis and normal IOP [113]. Nitrous oxide administration is contraindicated in ophthalmic surgeries when intraocular injection of a gas bubble is intended for a closed eye [48,114,115]. Examples of gases that have been used for intraocular injection include sulfur hexafluoride, perfluoropropane, and air [1]. Diffusion of N_2O into the intraocular gas bubble will cause it to expand and increase IOP and has been associated with loss of vision, presumably due to central retinal artery occlusion [115]. Prior to intraocular gas injection into a closed eye, N_2O should be discontinued for at least 15–20 min [114]. For repeat anesthetic episodes, it is recommended that N_2O not be administered for at least 5 days after intraocular air injection and for 10 days after sulfur hexafluoride injection [48,114].

Sedatives and injectable anesthetics

Barbiturates, propofol, and alfaxalone

Historically, pentobarbital and thiopental have been shown to decrease IOP [3,7]. The mechanism for reduction is believed to be depression of the areas of the central nervous system (diencephalon) influencing IOP, and facilitation of aqueous outflow [1]. Thiopental decreases IOP in both normal and glaucomatous eyes in people [116]. In cats with one normal eye and one glaucomatous eye administered two different doses of pentobarbital (25 mg/kg and 12.5 mg/kg intraperitoneal), the IOP decreased gradually and significantly by approximately 50% in the normal eye with the larger dose. The smaller dose also caused a significant but smaller decrease to approximately 30% of the preanesthetic IOP. In the glaucomatous eye, both doses caused a decrease of 20–30% of the preanesthetic IOP [117].

The effect of propofol on IOP during anesthesia induction in people is similar to thiopental [1]. In a study comparing the effects of propofol and thiopental in humans, both decreased IOP on induction, although the decrease was greater with propofol [118,119]. The administration of the depolarizing neuromuscular blocking agent succinylcholine increased IOP for both propofol and thiopental, although the increase was greater with thiopental and exceeded control values. Intubation resulted in significant increases in IOP for both propofol and thiopental, with an average increase of 25% above control values for both drugs, although individuals receiving additional boluses of propofol still maintained IOP below control values [118,119].

In contrast with humans, propofol does not appear to decrease IOP in dogs [120–122]. An evaluation of IOP and end-tidal carbon dioxide concentrations ($ETCO_2$) in dogs anesthetized with propofol failed to document a decrease in IOP after propofol administration and concluded that this was due to the opposing effect of increased $ETCO_2$ [120]. In dogs induced with propofol-atracurium, IV diazepam appears to blunt the increase in IOP associated with drug administration, but did not blunt the increase in IOP observed during intubation [121]. In a study comparing the peri-induction effects of propofol and thiopental on IOP in normal dogs, propofol caused a significant increase in IOP compared to baseline and to thiopental [122]. Thiopental caused an insignificant increase in IOP which decreased after intubation. It was suggested that propofol should be avoided for induction of anesthesia in dogs where a moderate increase in IOP could have harmful consequences [122].

An IV combination of propofol-ketamine caused a significant decrease in IOP in pigs, similar to the decrease observed with isoflurane anesthesia [111]. After IV administration of alfaxalone or propofol in sheep, IOP increased significantly at 15 min post injection for each drug, but IOP values remained within the normal range throughout the study period for all eyes. Miosis was observed for 8.89 ± 3.3 min after alfaxalone injection and 11.5 ± 3.38 min after propofol injection. Ventromedial positioning of the globe occurred for 10.5 ± 4.64 min after alfaxalone injection and 10.0 ± 2.35 min after propofol injection [123].

Dissociative anesthetics

Dissociative anesthetics are antagonists of the *N*-methyl-D-aspartate receptor (NMDAR), with ketamine and tiletamine (in combination with the benzodiazepine zolazepam in Telazol®) being commonly utilized in veterinary patients [124]. Ketamine induces extraocular muscle contraction, which may result in increased IOP, although the increase is not believed to be marked [100]. However, in patients with the potential for globe rupture any increase in IOP secondary to extraocular muscle contraction could be detrimental, suggesting that the use of ketamine should be avoided in patients when rupture of the globe is a concern. Muscular clonus was observed with tiletamine alone, but not with Telazol® [124].

The effect of ketamine on IOP can be variable. In people, ketamine does not affect IOP when administered after diazepam and meperidine in adults [125] and does not increase IOP when administered intramuscularly in children [126]. The IOP increased slightly in dogs administered a combination of ketamine-xylazine, but remained reasonably unchanged after ketamine-acepromazine administration [127]. In clinically normal dogs that did not receive premedication, ketamine at a dose of 5 mg/kg IV caused a significant and clinically relevant increase in IOP [128]. In cats with one normal eye and one glaucomatous eye administered two different doses of ketamine (25 mg/kg and 12.5 mg/kg IM), the IOP increased by approximately 10% in the normal eyes for both doses. In the glaucomatous eyes, the larger dose caused a 15% increase in IOP and the smaller dose caused a 5% increase [117]. In the same study, a low dose of Telazol® (2 mg/kg IM) had no significant effect on IOP in normal eyes. A higher dose of Telazol® (4 mg/kg IM) produced a small decrease in IOP in normal eyes that was significant only at 15 min after drug administration. In the glaucomatous eyes the smaller dose produced no change in IOP, while the larger dose caused a decrease of approximately 8%. When the Telazol® was administered as its separate components, tiletamine (1 mg/kg and 2 mg/kg IM) had no effect on IOP in normal or glaucomatous eyes, but both doses of zolazepam (1 mg/kg and 2 mg/kg IM) decreased

IOP approximately 10% in normal and glaucomatous eyes [117]. In horses, the administration of xylazine prior to ketamine attenuates the increase in IOP [129]. Both ketamine-diazepam and ketamine-acepromazine increased IOP after intramuscular administration in normal rabbits [130]. In rats, both intraperitoneal (IP) ketamine alone and an IP combination of ketamine-xylazine-acepromazine decreased IOP in both normal eyes and eyes with experimental aqueous outflow obstruction. After ketamine alone, IOP stabilized at approximately 50–60% of baseline values for both normal and affected eyes, whereas the ketamine combination continued to decrease IOP throughout the observation period [112].

Ketamine causes nystagmus, which may persist even when combined with xylazine, making ketamine unacceptable as the sole anesthetic agent for most ophthalmic procedures [100,129]. The palpebrae remain open, the pupils dilate, and the palpebrae and corneal reflexes persist after ketamine and Telazol® administration, [17,124] necessitating application of an ocular lubricant to prevent corneal drying, and decreasing the usefulness of eye position and ocular reflexes for evaluating anesthetic depth.

Ketamine combined with acepromazine did not decrease tear production in cats, but subcutaneous atropine administered prior to ketamine-acepromazine resulted in significant decreases in tear production [131]. Recoveries from ketamine administration can be very prolonged and unco-ordinated, predisposing patients to the potential for ocular trauma [100].

Etomidate

Etomidate significantly decreased IOP in human patients within 30 s of an IV injection. Mydriasis occurred within the first minute of injection which was then followed by miosis [132]. Also in human patients, etomidate anesthesia was compared with conventional inhalation anesthesia with halothane and N_2O. A greater significant decrease in mean IOP occurred with etomidate, with a maximum decrease of 61%, compared with a decrease of 45% in those patients receiving the conventional anesthesia protocol [133]. Although etomidate directly decreases IOP, etomidate-associated myoclonus may actually increase it [1,42]. Consequently, in patients with penetrating eye wounds and the potential for globe rupture, it is recommended that etomidate not be used alone for induction [42] but be administered in conjunction with a benzodiazepine such as diazepam or midazolam.

α_2-Adrenergic receptor agonists

In cats, rabbits, and monkeys, it has been reported that xylazine decreases IOP by depressing sympathetic function and decreasing aqueous production [134]. In horses, two studies determined that IOP could be decreased by 23% with the administration of 0.3 mg/kg xylazine IV, and by 27% with the administration of 1.0 mg/kg xylazine IV [135,136]. Xylazine produces mydriasis in some species, possibly by inhibiting central parasympathetic tone to the iris or through stimulation of α_2-adrenergic receptors located in the iris [137]. Systemically administered xylazine may cause acute reversible lens opacity in rats and mice [138]. Topical application of xylazine produces cataract formation in the treated eye, whereas the contralateral eye remains unaffected. The mechanism for this effect is unknown [138]. Xylazine alone does not significantly reduce tear production in dogs, but the combination of xylazine and butorphanol apparently works synergistically to decrease tear production significantly [34]. Premedication with xylazine prior to general anesthesia did not decrease tear production in horses [33].

The IV administration of detomidine in horses decreased IOP significantly from baseline, with the hypotensive effect remaining relatively static over time. Detomidine has a longer duration of sedation and analgesia when compared with xylazine and may be preferred for longer procedures [139].

Topical administration of medetomidine decreased IOP in cats and rabbits, while producing mydriasis, suggesting that there are α_2-adrenergic receptors in the eye that are involved in the regulation of IOP [140–142]. In contrast, IV administration of medetomidine resulted in miosis in normal dogs, without a decrease in IOP [143]. The IOP was not affected by systemically administered medetomidine in dogs that had received the anticholinergic and cyclopegic agent tropicamide, administered topically. The pupil size in these dogs increased after tropicamide administration and continued to increase slightly but significantly after medetomidine administration, although it was not determined whether the continued increase was exclusively caused by medetomidine; atipamezole did not affect pupil size [144]. Medetomidine alone, medetomidine-butorphanol, and medetomidine-buprenorphine have all caused significant decreases in tear production in dogs [145,146].

Dexmedetomidine (5 µg/kg), administered IV in clinically normal dogs, decreased IOP and produced significant miosis within the first 10 min after injection. It was concluded that mydriatics in combination with dexmedetomidine might be necessary to facilitate ophthalmic procedures requiring a dilated pupil [147]. In healthy dogs, both medetomidine-butorphanol and dexmedetomidine-butorphanol combinations induced a transient significant increase in IOP 10 min after IV administration, followed by a subsequent decrease. The increase in IOP at 10 min was significantly higher for dexmedetomidine-butorphanol when compared to medetomidine-butorphanol [148]. Unilateral topical administration of dexmedetomidine resulted in bilateral decreases in IOP in rabbits with normal or elevated IOP. In the rabbits with normal IOP, there was an initial increase followed by a decrease in IOP in the treated eye, but not in the untreated eye. No initial increase was observed in the rabbits with pre-existing elevations in IOP [149]. The potential systemic effects of dexmedetomidine when administered topically were studied in rabbits. A low dose of dexmedetomidine (12.5 µg) that was effective in decreasing IOP had no appreciable effects systemically, but when a higher dose (160 µg) was administered, there was a slow onset of hyperglycemia and a steady decrease in heart rate that resulted in bradycardia persisting for 2–3 h [150].

Benzodiazepines

Both diazepam and midazolam decrease IOP after IV administration in cats and dogs, respectively [7,151,152]. Topical (conjunctival) administration of diazepam in cats also decreased IOP [152]. One study suggests that diazepam may negate the increase in IOP that occurs after ketamine administration [3]. Although administration of diazepam alone caused no change in IOP, administration of diazepam along with ketamine did not prevent the increase in IOP caused by ketamine in clinically normal dogs [128]. Telazol® (2 mg/kg IM) had essentially no significant effect on IOP in normal eyes in cats, although a higher dose (4 mg/kg IM) produced a small decrease in IOP that was significant only at 15 min after drug administration [117]. In glaucomatous cat eyes, the smaller dose produced no change in IOP, while the higher dose caused an approximately 8% decrease. When the Telazol® was given as its separate components, tiletamine (1 mg/kg and 2 mg/kg IM) had no effect on IOP in normal or glaucomatous eyes, but both doses of zolazepam (1 mg/kg and 2 mg/kg IM) decreased IOP approximately

10% in normal and glaucomatous eyes [117]. Premedication with IV diazepam prevented an increase in IOP associated with induction of propofol-atracurium anesthesia in normal dogs, but did not prevent the increase in IOP associated with intubation [121]. No significant change in tear production occurred in rabbits after IM injection of diazepam [153].

Phenothiazines

Acepromazine is a tranquilizer with antiemetic properties that may prevent vomiting and gagging in ophthalmic patients who have undergone intraocular surgery, or have the potential for globe rupture. In horses, acepromazine IV has decreased IOP by as much as 20% [136]. In rhesus monkeys, acepromazine decreased IOP when injected IM; when administered topically, acepromazine was effective in decreasing elevated IOP but had no such effect in eyes with normal IOPs, and did not alter pupil size [154]. A significant decrease in tear production occurred in rabbits after IM injection with acepromazine.[153] The longer action of acepromazine may be useful in providing a slower, quieter anesthetic recovery, thereby reducing the potential for postoperative eye trauma.

Analgesics

Ocular and periocular structures are richly innervated and highly sensitive. Symptoms of ocular pain include blepharospasm, photophobia, ocular discharge, rubbing of the eyes, and avoidance behavior.

Opioids

Opioid selection for ophthalmic patients should include consideration of analgesic quality and duration of action. Opioids may be administered topically or systemically. Systemic administration may involve intermittent injections or IV continuous rate infusions (CRIs).

Topical administration of 1% morphine sulfate solution appears to provide local analgesia in dogs with corneal ulcers. The antinociceptive effect is possibly a result of interaction with μ-opioid receptors which have been identified in small numbers in normal canine corneas, and δ-opioid receptors which have been identified in the corneal epithelium and stroma of dogs [155]. In contrast with local anesthetics, this local analgesic effect is produced without delaying corneal wound healing or causing any discernible tissue damage [155–157]. In a pilot study comparing topical 1% nalbuphine and oral tramadol as analgesics for corneal pain in dogs, neither nalbuphine nor tramadol showed significant difference in pain relief from controls [158]. Considering the presence of μ- and δ-opioid receptors in the canine cornea, it was suggested that the weak κ-receptor agonist effects coupled with the μ- and δ-receptor antagonist effects of nalbuphine may account for the lack of corneal pain relief [158]. Another study reported that topical administration of 1% nalbuphine to normal dogs decreased corneal sensitivity significantly [159] but administration to normal horses had no effect [160].

High vagal efferent activity, which may predispose patients to the OCR, occurs with some opioids and may necessitate administration of an anticholinergic [161]. Emesis and the associated increase in IOP is a possible side-effect of systemic opioid administration [161]. This may suggest that opioid administration to patients at risk of globe rupture should be delayed until the patient is anesthetized and the risk of active vomiting has passed. Additionally, concurrent administration of antiemetics may be warranted. Morphine has been reported to decrease IOP in human patients [162] and other opioids are assumed to have the potential for a similar effect [7]. In an investigation of the effects of IV morphine, hydromorphone, buprenorphine, and butorphanol on IOP in normal dogs, mean IOP was statistically but not clinically significantly different from placebo for all drugs except buprenorphine, with changes varying from −1.6 to +1.1 mmHg [163]. The effects of acepromazine-butorphanol or acepromazine-meperidine premedication on IOP after midazolam-ketamine induction were compared in dogs [164]. The mean IOP 1 min after intubation showed an 8.4% decrease from baseline with acepromazine-butorphanol premedication, but a 14.1% increase with acepromazine-meperidine premedication. With both groups, there was an increase in IOP between 15 min after premedication and 1 min after induction. It has been suggested that this increase may be related to the sympathomimetic effects of ketamine counteracting the effects of the premedications [164].

The effects of opioids on pupil size are variable among species. Morphine has been reported to produce miosis in dogs, rabbits, and people, and mydriasis in cats, rats, mice, and monkeys [18]. The effects of IV morphine, hydromorphone, buprenorphine, and butorphanol on pupil size were investigated in normal dogs [163]. Pupil size was significantly decreased from placebo only after butorphanol injection, and only within the first 10 min after injection. No significant differences in pupil size occurred with morphine, hydromorphone, or buprenorphine, although morphine produced slight but insignificant mydriasis within 1.5 h of injection [163]. In contrast, an IM combination of hydromorphone-acepromazine caused significant miosis in dogs at 10 and 25 min after injection [20]. Opioid-induced miosis may prevent the mydriasis required for cataract surgery [19,20] although administration of an opioid antagonist such as naloxone may reverse miosis when it occurs [19,21].

Both meperidine and fentanyl cause a significant decrease in tear production in dogs, possibly as a result of central nervous system depression [165]. In a study comparing the effects of sedative and opioid combinations on tear production in dogs, it was determined that butorphanol alone significantly decreased tear production. Although xylazine alone had no significant effect, the combination of xylazine with butorphanol decreased tear production to a greater extent than that observed with butorphanol alone, suggesting a synergistic mechanism between xylazine and butorphanol for decreasing tear production in dogs [34]. Decreased tear production was also observed in dogs administered IV medetomidine-butorphanol [145] or medetomidine-buprenorphine [146]. In rats given subcutaneous fentanyl-fluanisone (Hypnorm®) tear production was not significantly decreased based on a fine-thread method of measurement [166].

Non-steroidal anti-inflammatory drugs

Both systemic and topical routes are routinely utilized for NSAID administration in ophthalmic patients. NSAIDs effectively prevent intraoperative miosis and control postoperative pain and inflammation after intraocular procedures, as well as controlling uveitis and alleviating pain from various other ophthalmic conditions or disease processes [167]. The responsiveness of the feline cornea to chemical stimuli of polymodal nociceptors was diminished by NSAIDs, suggesting that corneal pain may be alleviated by NSAIDs. This effect may be due not only to inhibition of cyclo-oxygenase activity but also to a direct effect of NSAIDs on the excitability of polymodal nerve endings [168].

Topical NSAID administration is associated with irritation of the conjunctiva and corneal cytotoxicity [169]. The use of NSAIDs in acutely inflamed canine eyes may increase IOP, possibly due to decreased aqueous outflow [170]. It has been suggested that corneal complications reported with topical use of NSAIDs in humans may be attributable to the solution's vehicle, solubilizer, or preservative, rather than the active drug itself [171].

Although rare, systemic effects may occur with topical ophthalmic NSAID administration due to absorption through nasal mucosa [171]. Systemic effects may include gastrointestinal irritation and ulceration, inhibition of platelet function, and renal disease [171]. Co-ordination of systemic and topical NSAID application is essential to prevent excessive administration and toxicity. The NSAIDs should be used cautiously in geriatric patients who often have pre-existing renal and gastrointestinal disease.

Intravenous lidocaine

In a preliminary study of dogs undergoing intraocular surgery, it was determined that lidocaine administered IV as a loading dose (1.0 mg/kg) followed by a CRI (0.025 mg/kg/min) may provide pre-emptive analgesia similar to morphine administered IV as a loading dose (0.15 mg/kg) followed by a CRI (0.1 mg/kg/h) [172]. The exact mechanism for the analgesic effects of IV lidocaine in these patients has not been established, although inhibition of A-δ fiber and C-fiber discharges from sensory neurons of the eye may be involved. It is also reasonable to speculate that the antinociceptive effects of systemic lidocaine may also prove to be effective for ophthalmic pain in equine patients [173].

Anticholinergics

Administration of atropine or glycopyrrolate to canine ophthalmic patients is controversial [44,100,174,175]. One potential benefit is preventing the OCR, but anticholinergic administration may increase the incidence of cardiac dysrhythmias and sinus tachycardia [175]. Conversely, anticholinergic administration may be appropriate in patients with pre-existing bradycardia or with concurrent administration of vagotonic injectable drugs (e.g., opioids and α_2-adrenergic receptor agonists). Cannulation of the parotid duct may be more difficult during parotid duct transposition surgery if secretions are dried up due to administration of preoperative anticholinergics [176]. In horses, topical administration of atropine has been associated with abdominal pain, decreases in gastrointestinal myoelectric activity, and borborygmi [56,57]. The potential for colic argues against the routine systemic administration of anticholinergics in horses [177].

Topically administered atropine produces cycloplegia which decreases aqueous filtration as well as mydriasis which predisposes patients to filtration angle closure [2]. Both of these effects will increase IOP in dogs and people with some forms of glaucoma, but the effects of systemically administered anticholinergics on pupil size and IOP are less clear [2]. In people, systemically administered atropine or glycopyrrolate had no effect on IOP in normal patients [174]. Glycopyrrolate administered parenterally had no effect on pupil size or IOP in normal dogs [178]. In a retrospective study of glaucomatous dogs, anticholinergic administration did not adversely affect IOP [178]. It has been suggested that glycopyrrolate may have a lesser effect on pupil size and IOP than atropine, possibly due to poor cellular penetration of end organs by quaternary ammonium compounds, such as glycopyrrolate, when compared with the tertiary amines, such as atropine [174]. Consequently, the use of glycopyrrolate may be preferred in glaucoma patients requiring anticholinergic treatment. Atropine administered with neostigmine to reverse non-depolarizing neuromuscular blockade does not seem to increase IOP [1].

Atropine has been shown to decrease tear production in the dog after topical or systemic administration [25,28,32,179]. In a short-term study in dogs, topical administration of atropine resulted in a significant decrease in tear production in both eyes within 30 min after unilateral instillation. The decrease reached a maximum at 120 min after instillation, and then returned to baseline values by 300 min. This would suggest that topically applied atropine may have a systemic effect on tear production in the short term [179]. In a related long-term study in dogs, tear production of the atropine-treated eye had decreased significantly by day 9, and continued to decrease until day 15 when atropine was discontinued. Tear production in the untreated eye also decreased significantly from baseline, but not from the treated eye, until day 9, but then seemed to plateau. On days 12 and 15, the tear production of the treated eye was significantly decreased when compared with the untreated eye. This would suggest that topically administered atropine may have local effects that become more pronounced over time [179]. Tear production in dogs decreased from baseline values within 10–15 min after subcutaneous administration of atropine and continued to decline after induction of general anesthesia with halothane or methoxyflurane [28,32]. Indeed, within 30–60 min of onset of general anesthesia, tear production in dogs can approach negligible amounts regardless of whether atropine was administered before surgery [32]. In a comparison of preanesthetic and postanesthetic Schirmer tear test values in dogs, significant decreases in tear production were evident for up to 24 h after the anesthetic procedure [29]. Anticholinergic administration before or during anesthesia further decreased the postanesthesia Schirmer tear test values [29].

Local and regional anesthesia

Local or regional anesthesia may be adequate for less invasive procedures or may be included as part of a balanced general anesthetic regimen. Topical anesthesia for diagnostic and therapeutic procedures in veterinary ophthalmic patients usually requires accompanying sedation to gain co-operation of the patient. Topical anesthesia and sedation may be the preferred technique in ruminants and horses in which a standing procedure is preferred, or in other patients in which general anesthesia would be accompanied by unacceptable risk. Tear production and the palpebral and corneal reflexes will be reduced after topical anesthetic administration, necessitating the application of ocular lubricant to protect the cornea after completion of the procedure [2].

Local anesthetics applied topically are readily absorbed through mucous membranes [2]. Systemic toxicosis is possible, though unlikely, but administration to small patients should be judicious [1,45]. Topical anesthetics can be irritating and cause transient conjunctival hyperemia as well as damage corneal epithelium, delay corneal wound healing, and mask signs of disease or discomfort [2]. Because of the toxic effects on the cornea, topical local anesthetics should be reserved for diagnostic use and never used as long-term therapeutic agents [180–193]. The use of topical proparacaine has been studied in dogs, cats, and horses [184–186]. In a study assessing the duration of effect of topical local anesthetic administration, it was determined that two applications of one drop of 0.5% proparacaine, with a 1 min interval between drops, resulted in 25 min of reduced corneal sensation in dogs [184]. Bupivacaine may be less toxic to the cornea than proparacaine but its duration of action is short [181]. Tetracaine and proparacaine have the same *in vivo* potency but tetracaine may be four times more toxic than proparacaine [183].

Splash blocks (i.e., administration of local anesthetic to the surface of an open wound) or local infiltration may be used for intraoperative and postoperative analgesia in ophthalmic patients [187]. Bupivacaine (0.5%) is commonly used for these techniques because of its longer action, but lidocaine has a quicker onset and may be combined with bupivacaine for that purpose [187]. The maximum dose of bupivacaine should not exceed 1.5 mg/kg to avoid potential toxicosis. Epinephrine may be added to the local anesthetic (1:100 000 or 1:200 000) to reduce bleeding and delay systemic absorption [187].

Regional anesthetic techniques commonly used for ophthalmic patients include auriculopalpebral nerve block, supraorbital nerve block, and retrobulbar injection. Techniques for these nerve blocks are described elsewhere in this text.

The auriculopalpebral nerve is a terminal branch of the facial nerve (cranial nerve VII) and provides motor innervation to the orbicularis oculi muscle. Blockade of the auriculopalpebral nerve eliminates forceful blepharospasms, thereby facilitating ocular examination or minor surgical or diagnostic procedures [2]. In horses, auriculopalpebral block has no adverse effects on tear production or IOP [135,188].

The supraorbital nerve is a termination of the ophthalmic branch of the trigeminal nerve (cranial nerve V) and provides sensory innervation to most of the superior palpebrae. Blockade of this nerve is commonly performed in sedated horses for placement of a subpalpebral lavage tube, repair of a palpebral laceration, or other similar minor procedures [2]. Other sensory nerves that are less commonly blocked include the infratrochlear, zygomatic, and lacrimal nerves.

Retrobulbar injection can be performed as an adjunct to sedation or general anesthesia. Retrobulbar injection of local anesthetic will block the optic (cranial nerve II), oculomotor (III), trochlear (IV), ophthalmic and maxillary divisions of the trigeminal (V), and the abducens (VI) nerves. Blockade of these nerves causes desensitization of the globe and palpebrae, akinesia of the globe, transient vision loss, pupil dilation, and decreased IOP [2]. During general anesthesia, retrobulbar injection has also been performed in horses to eliminate ocular movement without the accompanying disadvantages of deeper planes of anesthesia [59,189]. Retrobulbar injection has been associated with serious complications [190–197] and has prompted consideration of other techniques, including peribulbar, medial peribulbar, sub-Tenon's approaches, and topical anesthesia [198–202]. Retrobulbar injection has been advocated to prevent the OCR, but performance of the technique itself has the potential to elicit the OCR [1,2,41,48,189]. Large volumes of local anesthetic or orbital hemorrhage may cause either proptosis of the globe or displacement of the vitreous if the globe has been penetrated [2]. It has been suggested that increases in IOP that occur in dogs and cats during retrobulbar injection of saline to produce exophthalmos may be avoided by including lidocaine in the injectate and by injecting in small increments [203]. The Peterson eye block is a well-known alternative technique to retrobulbar injection for providing regional anesthesia of the eye in cattle, but carries some risk of accidental injection of drug into the cerebral spinal fluid and potentially death [204].

Neuromuscular blocking agents

Paralysis of extraocular muscles relaxes the eye, allowing the globe to roll centrally and proptose slightly. These effects greatly facilitate positioning of the globe for ophthalmic surgery, [205,206] thereby eliminating the need for significant surgical manipulation to obtain proper globe positioning and decreasing the potential for initiating the OCR [44].

An increase in IOP after administration of depolarizing neuromuscular blocking agents (NMBs), such as succinylcholine, has been observed in cats, rabbits, horses, and people [207–211] and has often been attributed to the contraction of extraocular muscles. However, other possible causes for succinylcholine-associated increases in IOP include distortion of the globe with axial shortening, choroidal vascular dilation secondary to increased arterial pressure, or contraction of orbital smooth muscle [209,212–214]. Endotracheal intubation, straining, or coughing may cause greater increases in IOP than those observed with succinylcholine [215].

In anesthetized cats, the increase in IOP after succinylcholine administration was not entirely due to increases in extraocular muscle tension. Increases in IOP in response to succinylcholine were also caused by contraction of orbital smooth muscle and increased arterial blood pressure, which may increase choroidal vascular dilation [209]. In anesthetized cats and rabbits, increases in IOP after IV succinylcholine injection appeared to be due to distortion of the globe in addition to the increased tension of the oculorotary muscles [212]. Axial shortening of the globe has also been demonstrated in anesthetized cats [213].

After anesthetic induction with thiopental in people, an increase in IOP occurs within 1 min of succinylcholine administration, with the peak significant increase occurring 2–4 min after administration and returning to baseline at 6 min [211]. The increase in IOP was exacerbated by simultaneous endotracheal intubation. Pretreatment with a subparalytic dose of succinylcholine, a subparalytic dose of d-tubocurarine, or IV diazepam did not prevent the increase in IOP associated with succinylcholine administration in human patients, although the increase in IOP was less with diazepam compared with the other pretreatments [208]. The potential effects of dosage and timing of succinylcholine administration on IOP have been investigated in human patients given a standard sleep dose of thiopental (3 mg/kg) followed by succinylcholine [216]. It was determined that thiopental alone decreases IOP; a low dose (0.5 mg/kg) of succinylcholine given immediately after thiopental returns IOP to normal; a high dose (1 mg/kg) of succinylcholine given immediately after thiopental maintains the decrease in IOP; a 2 min delay in administering a high dose of succinylcholine slightly increases IOP above preanesthetic levels; endotracheal intubation significantly increases IOP beyond any effect from succinylcholine alone; and succinylcholine infusion maintains a significant increase in IOP in some patients [216]. The increase in IOP associated with administration of succinylcholine would indicate that it should be avoided in patients with severely compromised eyes that are at risk for globe rupture. However, administration of succinylcholine in patients with intact globes would seem reasonable as long as enough time was allowed (8–10 min) for the increase in IOP to subside prior to incision [208,216].

As mentioned previously, indirect-acting cholinergic drugs are anticholinesterases that are used for treating glaucoma. Because anticholinesterases inhibit or inactivate the plasma pseudocholinesterases responsible for the metabolism of succinylcholine, they may prolong succinylcholine-induced paralysis [217]. It has been recommended that indirect-acting cholinergic drugs be discontinued 2–4 weeks prior to neuromuscular blockade with succinylcholine, although normal levels of plasma pseudocholinesterase activity may not be totally restored for 4–6 weeks [48]. Similarly, organophosphates also have anticholinesterase activity and succinylcholine should be avoided in patients that have been exposed [51]. There are no reversal agents for the effects of depolarizing NMBs [218].

Non-depolarizing NMBs do not appear to increase IOP [48]. Studies have indicated that vecuronium, pancuronium, and atracurium either decrease or have no effect on IOP in people and dogs [13,219–222]. In horses, rocuronium was used successfully to produce neuromuscular blockade and rotation of the globe to a central position [223]. The effects of the non-depolarizing NMBs are reversible with anticholinesterases, such as neostigmine or edrophonium [217]. In many species, an anticholinergic (e.g., atropine or glycopyrrolate) may be administered prior to the anticholinesterase to prevent profound bradycardia, [218] with horses as a possible exception. Although the use of systemic anticholinergics is usually avoided in horses, anticholinesterases may still be used for non-depolarizing NMB reversals, but should be administered very slowly while the heart rate is monitored. Alternatively, the use of non-depolarizing NMBs with a briefer action, such as atracurium, may be more desirable to avoid the need for reversal [42]. Isoflurane-anesthetized horses required larger doses of vecuronium than other domestic animals and humans to produce complete paralysis, which resulted in very long periods of neuromuscular blockade requiring reversal with edrophonium [224]. Neuromuscular paralysis reversal should be complete to prevent hypoventilation, struggling during recovery, self-trauma, and increases in IOP.

Birds have striated rather than smooth iris musculature and may require paralysis to produce mydriasis. Topically applied parasympatholytic or sympathomimetic agents are ineffective in birds [2]. Intracameral injection of d-tubocurarine has produced mydriasis in pigeons [225]. Apnea and salivation occurred in raptors after intracameral injection of muscle relaxants [16]. Topically applied vecuronium was found to produce the most consistent and greatest pupillary dilation in three species of psittacines with the fewest systemic side-effects when compared with d-tubocurarine and pancuronium [226]. However, the differences in systemic side-effects among the three psittacine species indicate that vecuronium should be used cautiously when applied bilaterally.

The use of sequential non-depolarizing and depolarizing NMBs is controversial [42]. In humans, a small amount of non-depolarizing NMB is administered first to block the initial muscle contractions of the depolarizing NMB. The depolarizing NMB is then administered to produce immobilization and allow intubation. Although this technique prevents coughing, gagging, and muscle fasciculations, IOP still increases during intubation [1].

Increases in IOP may occur with increases in $PaCO_2$, necessitating mechanical ventilation, which may be facilitated by the administration of NMBs. It has been suggested, however, that hyperventilation may fail to decrease IOP because of the increase in intrathoracic and central venous pressure accompanying the use of mechanical ventilation [13].

Anesthesia and the electroretinogram

The electroretinogram (ERG) is a widely used electrodiagnostic test in veterinary ophthalmology, [227] with the flash ERG (FERG) being most useful in detecting diffuse retinal disorders [228]. The a-wave, b-wave, and c-wave are the major components of the ERG waveform [229]. The a-wave is an initial negative deflection followed by the positive peak b-wave and a late slow positive c-wave. The a-wave and b-wave are the components most often measured [230]. The c-wave component is not usually included in animal protocols because of technical challenges associated with obtaining recordings in normal adult dogs [227,231]. The amplitude of the a-wave is measured from baseline to the negative trough; the larger b-wave is measured from the trough of the a-wave to the following peak of the b-wave [230]. The a-wave is generated by the cones and rods in the outer photoreceptor layer, whereas the b-wave is believed to be generated by the bipolar and Müller cells of the inner retina [232,233]. As a result, b/a-wave ratios can be used as an index of inner to outer retinal function [234]. The c-wave appears to be generated by the retinal pigment epithelium [232]. The time between stimulus onset and maximum amplitude is referred to as implicit time. Both amplitude and implicit time of each wave are used to measure the FERG response [228]. Decreases in response amplitudes and increases in implicit times for both rod- and cone-driven responses of the FERG are common effects of general anesthesia [235–237].

Sedation and a co-operative patient may prove adequate for a semi-quantitative ERG as is typically performed for preoperative screening of cataract patients, [2] although complete ocular akinesia is the gold standard and requires general anesthesia and possibly neuromuscular blockade. The ERG requires dark adaptation of the patient prior to performance of the ERG in the dark, which may make anesthetic monitoring a challenge during general anesthesia. The ERGs generated during sedation or general anesthesia are considered useful as long as the ERGs for the patient and the controls were generated under similar anesthetic conditions [227].

Several anesthetic protocols have been utilized for ERG evaluation in small animal patients. Medetomidine significantly affected all ERG responses examined in normal dogs but was considered to be a clinically viable choice for sedation during ERGs [238]. The combinations of xylazine-ketamine [239] and medetomidine-ketamine [240] were also considered acceptable for use during ERG evaluation in dogs. A significant decrease of the a-wave occurred in 11 dogs anesthetized with thiopental-halothane-nitrous oxide when compared to xylazine-ketamine anesthesia. Additional investigation of the selective actions of the different agents used in these protocols (excluding N_2O) determined that thiopental seemed to depress the a-wave selectively; halothane depressed both a- and b-wave amplitudes; ketamine (with vecuronium for intubation) showed responses almost identical to the xylazine-ketamine combination; and xylazine (with vecuronium for intubation) slightly depressed a- and b-waves in comparison to ketamine [237]. It was concluded that xylazine-ketamine was considered to be superior to the thiopental-halothane-nitrous oxide combination for ERG evaluation [240].

Propofol has been shown to produce a dose-related modulation of dark-adapted inner retinal signals during ERG evaluation in Beagle dogs [241] but appears to preserve the ERG photoreceptor response better in dogs than thiopental, and therefore may be more appropriate for ERG recordings [242]. Both halothane and sevoflurane significantly depressed components of the ERG in Beagles, suggesting that neither inhalation agent is appropriate for use during ERG evaluation in dogs [235]. The FERGs recorded in monocularly deprived cats anesthetized with a combination of xylazine-ketamine were similar to FERGs recorded from normal animals [243]. A combination of atropine-xylazine-pentobarbital has been used to anesthetize Abyssinian cats with progressive retinal atrophy for ERG evaluation [244]. Amplitudes were larger and implicit times longer for ERG responses recorded from infant and adult albino rats anesthetized with Telazol® (zolazepam and tiletamine) when compared with pentobarbital sodium [245]. ancuronium, vecuronium, and atracurium have been used to produce neuromuscular blockade with no apparent adverse effects on the performance of ERG evaluation in dogs [235,246–248].

In horses, FERGs have been recorded under halothane-nitrous oxide anesthesia [249,250] but significant complications may be associated with general anesthesia in large animals, making sedation a more desirable option. Detomidine has been used successfully for FERG recordings in standing horses [251,252]. Flash ERGs have also been recorded in awake, unsedated horses and cattle [227,253,254]. Dose-related changes in ERG recordings have been reported with thiopental in sheep [255–257].

Oxygenation and hypercapnia may affect FERG results, emphasizing the importance of verifying adequate patient oxygenation and ventilation. In cats, the a-wave amplitude decreased by a mean of 8.9% with mild hypoxemia (PaO_2 50–60 mmHg) but the b-wave amplitude was stable. During severe hypoxemia (PaO_2 20–30 mmHg), the a-wave was stable with no further decrease but the b-wave amplitude decreased by a mean of 35%. This implies that photoreceptor transduction performs almost normally during hypoxemia and that the decrease in b-wave amplitude may be a failure of inner retinal oxygen regulation [258,259]. In anesthetized dogs, hypoxemia (PaO_2 45 mmHg) resulted in a decrease in b-wave amplitude and an increase in latency (implicit time). In contrast, the a-wave was present long after the b-wave had decreased in amplitude or disappeared [260]. Hypercapnia depresses the amplitude of the ERG components, so anesthesia-related hypoventilation should be avoided during ERG evaluation [248]. In cats, it has been suggested that low arterial pH secondary to hypercapnia may interfere with inner retinal oxygen regulation. This may result in an observed decrease in b-wave amplitude, rather than the increase in amplitude typically associated with the dilatory effect of increased $PaCO_2$ [259]. In anesthetized dogs, the b-wave of the FERG was markedly increased by hyperventilation but no significant changes occurred in the a-wave. It was concluded that the mechanism of b-wave increases must be decreased $PaCO_2$ (hypocapnia) although the specific site of action and method of enhancement of the b-wave were not established [261].

General considerations for ophthalmic patients

Ophthalmic patients should receive thorough physical examinations and appropriate diagnostic tests to determine the presence of additional medical conditions beyond the ophthalmic problem. This is particularly important as ophthalmic patients are often either very young or geriatric, and may have additional medical problems that require special anesthetic considerations.

Ocular and periocular structures are often neglected during induction of anesthesia. Positioning of hands and equipment relative to the eyes should be noted during induction, especially when dealing with severely compromised globes with the potential to rupture. Mask induction may not be an option if the mask puts pressure on the eyes, and patient struggling during induction with a face mask may increase IOP or potentiate globe rupture. Providing analgesia is particularly important in ophthalmic patients with substantial discomfort from their primary ophthalmic disease. These patients may be more inclined to struggle when restrained which may result in increased IOP and additional damage to the globe during induction.

Positioning of the patient's head and application of any topical ophthalmic preparations should be co-ordinated between the anesthesiology personnel and ophthalmologist to ensure the best possible surgical outcome. Protection of the dependent, non-operated eye should be considered during positioning of patients for unilateral procedures. If intraocular surgery is planned or globe rupture has occurred, application of topical ophthalmic medications or lubrication should be restricted to aqueous-based formulations. Petroleum-based ointments that gain access to intraocular structures may cause severe uveitis and further compromise vision and ocular comfort. A flash fire involving ophthalmic ointment during anesthesia with nitrous oxide and oxygen has been reported [262] but a later study concluded that ophthalmic ointments do not pose a significant fire hazard [263]. Taping the palpebrae closed or performing a partial temporary tarsorrhaphy are additional techniques for protecting the globe and keeping it moist [2]. Resting the periocular region of the dependent eye on a soft padded eye ring or 'doughnut' may help protect the eye from corneal abrasion and external globe compression that may result in hypotony. Collapse of the anterior chamber of the dependent eye, possibly resulting from increased aqueous outflow caused by physical pressure on the globe, has been reported in birds positioned in lateral recumbency. The anterior chamber was re-established within a few minutes of repositioning [264]. A study in cats with postanesthetic cortical blindness suggests that spring-held mouth gags are a potential risk factor for cerebral ischemia due to compromise of the maxillary artery [265]. Of the 20 cats included in the study, 17 underwent either dentistry or endoscopy procedures, and in 16 of the 17 cats a spring-held mouth gag was used.

In people, the anesthesia-related practices most likely to increase IOP significantly (i.e., at least 10–20 mmHg) are laryngoscopy and endotracheal intubation (LETI) [1,3,7,45]. Although the mechanism is not clear, it has been suggested that it is related to sympathetic cardiovascular responses to laryngeal stimulation. The occurrence of increases in IOP during endotracheal intubation has not been clearly established in veterinary patients. No significant increase in IOP was demonstrated after intubation in dogs premedicated with acepromazine plus meperidine or butorphanol, and induced with ketamine and midazolam [164]. However, in dogs receiving IV diazepam prior to induction with propofol-atracurium, there was a non-significant increase in IOP after induction, but a significant increase in IOP after intubation when compared with preinduction [121]. Anesthetic induction with sevoflurane in dogs did not prevent sympathetic activation associated with endotracheal intubation, as indicated by an increase in the proprietary index [266]. It has been suggested that there may be a difference in the autonomic response to intubation in people compared to dogs. People may become both tachycardic and hypertensive with laryngoscopy and endotracheal intubation [267] whereas dogs appear to have more variability in the autonomic response to intubation [266]. Regardless, it is reasonable, and in the best interests of the patient, to attempt to minimize laryngeal stimulation and accomplish endotracheal intubation as smoothly as possible to avoid the potential for any increases in IOP [2]. Lidocaine applied topically to the larynx or administered intravenously (1.0 mg/kg) may be helpful in suppressing the cough reflex [42].

Positioning for the ophthalmic procedure may render ophthalmic patients less accessible for anesthetic monitoring and maintaining an appropriate level of anesthesia may become more difficult. Eye reflexes, jaw tone, and oral mucous membranes may not be accessible, although the ophthalmologist may be able to provide information about eye position and movement. Once the head has been surgically draped, the airway also becomes less accessible. A guarded (i.e., wire reinforced) endotracheal tube may be used to prevent unobserved kinking and occlusion of the airway during surgical positioning. Capnography is also useful for detection of an obstructed airway and pulse oximetry may help detect desaturation should the endotracheal tube become obstructed or the delivery system disconnected. However, the pulse oximeter may have to be placed somewhere other than on the tongue, lip, or other head structure to avoid interference with its function by the ophthalmologist's movements. Body position may also affect IOP. Intraocular pressure decreased significantly in dorsally recumbent or sitting dogs, but did not change significantly in dogs that were sternally recumbent. However, differences in IOP resulting from changes in head position disappeared after the position was maintained for 5 min [10]. The IOP increased significantly in horses when the head was below heart level, compared with IOP in the head-up position [11]. In mice, IOP increased when body position was changed from horizontal to head-down [9].

Monitoring heart rate and arterial blood pressure becomes essential in ophthalmic patients when other types of monitoring are limited and is particularly important when NMBs are included in the anesthetic protocol. Preventing movement during ophthalmic procedures and facilitation of eye positioning may be accomplished by using NMBs to paralyze patients, but the inability of patients to indicate inadequate anesthesia with movement makes monitoring all the more crucial. Increased heart rate or blood pressure may indicate an inadequate plane of anesthesia or the need for additional analgesics. Conversely, precipitous decreases in these parameters may indicate excessive anesthetic depth or initiation of the OCR. Increased respiration rate may also be indicative of inadequate anesthetic depth, but such a response may not be evident in mechanically ventilated or paralyzed patients.

Transient lens opacification may occur in rodents, such as mice, rats, and hamsters, during prolonged sedation or anesthesia. The opacification is believed to be caused by lack of blinking and subsequent evaporation of fluids from the shallow anterior chamber which then resolves upon awakening [268]. The instillation of ophthalmic ointment may help prevent this occurrence.

A smooth anesthetic recovery including appropriate analgesia and prevention of self-trauma is the primary postoperative management goal. For patients who have undergone intraocular surgery, periods of excitement, incoordination, coughing, gagging, or retching are particularly undesirable. Ideally, recovery should be in a quiet, dimly lit enclosure where external stimuli will be kept to a minimum. Patients may be kept comfortable and quiet by appropriate analgesia and sedation, but minimal physical restraint or words of reassurance while being held may be more effective for some small patients. Elizabethan collars for small patients may help protect the eyes, but may not be readily tolerated by some. Recovery cages and stalls should have extraneous structures such as feed-bowl rings or feeding bins removed to prevent ocular trauma during recovery. For small patients, small pads or rolled-up towels may provide a soft barrier to prevent the patient from bumping into and rubbing its eyes on the bars of the cage door.

Special considerations for equine ophthalmic patients

In equine ophthalmic patients, delicate ocular procedures are preferably performed under general anesthesia. However, certain ocular surgical procedures, such as enucleation, can also be performed under sedation with local anesthetic techniques. The decision to proceed with general anesthesia versus sedation and local anesthesia largely depends on the ophthalmologist's preference, cost, disposition of the horse, and available facilities. Some surgeons prefer a standing sedation technique to reduce the risk associated with general anesthesia [269,270]. Detomidine and butorphanol are commonly used for standing sedation in horses. Detomidine can be given in intermittent IV boluses as needed or as a CRI. For detomidine infusion, an IV loading dose of 7.5 μg/kg is administered, followed by a CRI of 1.87 μg/kg/min [271]. Local anesthetic nerve blocks assist in preventing sudden head movement in response to intense stimulation during standing surgical procedures. Local anesthetic techniques are described elsewhere in this text.

Equine patients with ocular problems that need surgical correction require a thorough physical examination before undergoing sedation or general anesthesia. If general anesthesia is required, hematologic and blood chemistry values should be determined to identify problems that cannot be detected by physical examination and also determine the severity of any additional medical problems.

Horses with a non-visual eye should be approached from the visual side. If approach from the non-visual side is necessary, it should be accompanied by words of reassurance and gentle hand contact. If an increase in IOP will jeopardize the primary ocular problem of the horse, steps should be taken to minimize factors that can potentially increase IOP during the physical examination. Horses that are excited or stressed are more difficult to handle and tend to have more fluctuations in IOP, [6] which may be deleterious to an eye with pre-existing intraocular hypertension. It is better to sedate these horses with xylazine or detomidine during the ophthalmic examination to prevent sudden changes in IOP. Both xylazine and detomidine have been shown to reduce IOP [129,135,139]. When examining a sedated horse, an effort should be made to raise the head above heart level as lowering of the head results in an increase in IOP [11]. When flushing the mouth of a horse before anesthesia, it is advisable to perform it after sedation has been administered to prevent excitement and increases in IOP.

Effective premedication is paramount to having a smooth anesthetic induction in horses. An IV α_2-adrenergic receptor agonist will provide profound sedation as well as analgesia and muscle relaxation. Recommended IV doses for the α_2-adrenergic receptor agonists are shown in Table 52.2. Administration of an opioid following an α_2-adrenergic receptor agonist will provide additional sedation and analgesia. To reduce the possibility of excitement, it is a good practice to give the opioid after signs of sedation from the α_2-adrenergic receptor agonist are observed, which generally occur about 2–3 min after administration. Butorphanol is the most commonly used opioid in equine practice. The IV dose for butorphanol ranges from 0.02 to 0.05 mg/kg. Morphine is an opioid that can be used as an alternative to butorphanol and is given IV at 0.2–0.6 mg/kg. Acepromazine is a tranquilizer that can be incorporated into the premedication. Acepromazine use is associated with lower mortality in equine anesthesia when used as part of the anesthetic regimen although the mechanism and relevance to ophthalmologic patients have not been determined [272]. It is given IV at 0.02 mg/kg 30 min prior to or simultaneously with the α_2-adrenergic receptor agonist. Acepromazine can also be administered IM before or during anesthesia. Since acepromazine has a long duration of action, its effect

Table 52.2 Recommended intravenous (IV) dosages of α_2-adrenergic receptor agonists for premedication in equine ophthalmic patients.

Agent	Dosage
Xylazine	0.5–1.0 mg/kg
Detomidine	5.0–20.0 μg/kg
Medetomidine	2.5–5.0 μg/kg
Dexmedetomidine	1.25–2.5 μg/kg
Romifidine	0.05–0.1 mg/kg

will persist into the recovery period which may contribute to a better recovery.

The choice of anesthetic induction agents for equine patients depends largely on the quality of induction associated with the injectable agents and the effect of the induction agents on IOP. Historically, thiopental was the agent of choice for inducing anesthesia in equine ophthalmic patients. It has been shown to reduce IOP in humans [2] but its effect on IOP has not been studied specifically in horses. It is associated with a smooth induction when administered after or concurrently with guaifenesin [273]. Unfortunately, neither of these drugs is currently available commercially. Presently, induction of anesthesia in equine patients typically involves a combination of diazepam or midazolam with ketamine, a combination of tiletamine with zolazepam (Telazol®), or propofol. Ketamine is associated with increases in IOP [117,128]. However, IV administra ion to horses after an α_2-adrenergic receptor agonist (xylazine) did not result in increased IOP [129]. The effects on IOP of a benzodiazepine (diazepam or midazolam) combined with ketamine for induction remain unclear [3,128]. The effects of propofol on IOP have not been studied in horses. It is known to increase IOP in dogs [122] but not in humans [274]. When an α_2-adrenergic receptor agonist is used as premedication, propofol may be an acceptable induction agent in foals. Telazol® can also be used for induction similar to a benzodiazepine and ketamine combination. It is imperative that profound sedation from an α_2-adrenergic receptor agonist be observed before inducing anesthesia with Telazol® to ensure a smooth induction and minimize the effect on IOP.

When a foal needs general anesthesia and is still nursing, the mare should be present during the induction of anesthesia to minimize the stress on the foal. Conversely, if the mare will undergo general anesthesia, it is important that the foal be near the induction stall to facilitate sedation of the mare and ensure a smooth induction. Mask induction may not be an option if the mask puts pressure on the eyes, and patient struggling during induction with a face mask may increase IOP or potentiate globe rupture. Nasotracheal intubation in a conscious foal requires heavy restraint and may be accompanied by coughing and gagging, which may increase IOP and further compromise the globe. Appropriate sedation may help calm the foal and decrease the amount of physical restraint that is needed as well as decrease the potential for additional ocular trauma or increases in IOP.

Endotracheal intubation should be accomplished quickly once the horse is in lateral recumbency. Adult horses rarely gag or cough during endotracheal intubation, making a sudden increase in IOP less likely to occur. Movement of equine patients to lateral recumbency after induction should include careful control of the head to prevent additional trauma to the eyes. In addition, lower positioning of the head relative to the body during hoist transport could result in increased IOP [11] and may be responsible for intraocular hemorrhage observed shortly after induction in horses with traumatized eyes [2]. Supporting the head to keep it level with the heart during transport is recommended to avoid such an occurrence.

Delicate ophthalmic procedures in horses may require extended anesthesia time. Partial IV anesthesia (PIVA) is a technique that may be implemented to reduce the amount of inhalation agent needed to maintain anesthesia, and minimize the cardiopulmonary depressant effects of the inhalation agents. This technique utilizes injectable agents that are administered as single-drug or multi-drug CRIs, thereby permitting reduction of the vaporizer setting over time while still maintaining an adequate plane of anesthesia. Injectable agents commonly utilized for this technique include ketamine, lidocaine, butorphanol, and α_2-adrenergic receptor agonists. Administration of CRIs requires close attention to detail especially if multiple drugs are being utilized. The PIVA technique has been associated with better recoveries and fewer attempts to stand in horses [275–277].

Analgesics administered during general anesthesia may reduce the inhalant anesthetic requirement, and may also improve recovery as the horse regains consciousness without the stimulus of postoperative pain. Non-steroidal anti-inflammatory drugs, opioids, lidocaine, ketamine, and appropriate nerve blocks have been recommended for pain control in equine ophthalmic patients [278]. One commonly administered NSAID for horses with ocular inflammation related to the primary disease or as a result of surgery is flunixin meglumine. It is administered at 1.1 mg/kg IV preoperatively. It is repeated postoperatively using the same dose every 12–24 h, with frequency of administration dependent on the ocular problem [279]. Butorphanol and morphine are opioids commonly used in horses. They can be administered as part of the premedication and may be re-dosed postoperatively. The intravenous doses for morphine and butorphanol are 0.2–0.6 mg/kg and 0.02–0.05 mg/kg, respectively. Lidocaine has been shown to provide analgesia in horses [280,281] and has been proven to provide analgesia in canine ophthalmic patients in particular [172]. In horses, a loading dose of 2.0 mg/kg is administered over 15 min followed by a CRI of 3.0 mg/kg/h. The CRI should be discontinued 30 min before recovery to minimize inco-ordination associated with lidocaine [282]. Administration of an α_2-adrenergic receptor agonist or ketamine as a CRI during anesthesia as part of a partial IV anesthetic technique will also provide additional analgesia. The analgesic effect may extend into the postoperative period. Nerve blockade from local anesthetic injection may provide analgesia both during surgery and postoperatively. Nerve blockade techniques commonly used for ophthalmic patients include auriculopalpebral nerve block, supraorbital nerve block, and retrobulbar injection.

Similar to other equine cases, the main goal of recovering anesthetized horses that have undergone an ophthalmic procedure is to have smooth and injury-free recoveries. This goal becomes more important in horses that have undergone intraocular procedures or corneal transplants. Recovery efforts should include preventing trauma to the eyes as the horse attempts to stand. The possibility of rough recoveries is higher in horses with ocular problems [283]. Many suggestions have been made to achieve quiet, predictable, smooth recoveries in horses but there is not any one single recommendation that will ensure this outcome. Administration of sedatives in recovery has been advocated to improve recovery [284]. α_2-Adrenergic receptor agonists like xylazine, romifidine, detomidine, medetomidine, and dexmedetomidine may be administered before the horse is moved to the recovery stall or when the horse reaches the recovery area. The dosages for α_2-adrenergic receptor agonists used during recovery are listed in Table 52.3. Note that these dosages are lower than those used for premedication. Acepromazine

Table 52.3 Recommended intravenous (IV) dosages of α_2-adrenergic receptor agonists for recovery of equine ophthalmic patients.

Agent	Dosage
Xylazine	0.2 mg/kg
Detomidine	2.0 μg/kg
Medetomidine	2.0 μg/kg
Dexmedetomidine	1.0 μg/kg
Romifidine	0.01–0.02 mg/kg

has also been given with or without the α_2-adrenergic receptor agonist. It should be given intravenously at 0.02 mg/kg at least 30 min before recovery because of its delayed onset of action compared with the α_2-adrenergic receptor agonists.

As discussed previously, effective analgesia will help improve the quality of recovery and ideally should be administered before the horse regains full consciousness. Horses that received a NMB during general anesthesia should be evaluated closely for muscle strength. Return of neuromuscular function as determined by the nerve stimulator does not rule out muscle weakness due to persistent low-level neuromuscular blockade. Horses with muscle weakness that attempt to stand are more prone to injuries. Muscle strength can be judged by determining the negative pressure that the horse can generate during inspiration when the connection to the rebreathing bag is occluded. A negative pressure of at least 15 cmH_2O indicates acceptable muscle strength. Conversely, signs of muscle weakness may include muscle fasciculations when the horse attempts to stand, inability to keep its head up, and failure to close its eyelids tightly [285]. When signs of muscle weakness are evident, and the reversal agent was not administered because the nerve stimulator indicated return to normal neuromuscular function, neostigmine or edrophonium should be given.

To protect the eye during recovery, a padded hood may be placed on the head, with a halter secured over the hood to keep it in place. However, a hood may not be tolerated by some horses, and may lead to premature attempts to rise. Weak attempts to rise may be controlled by kneeling on the horse's neck and lifting its muzzle toward the ceiling. Additional sedation may prevent horses with active nystagmus from attempting to rise. A head-and-tail rope technique is a practical way to assist horses that are making strong attempts to rise and remain standing in recovery. Ideally, there should be three individuals to execute this recovery technique. Ropes are tied to the tail and to a strong, reliable halter, and then passed through metal rings on the walls of the recovery stall. When the horse makes a strong attempt to rise, the person on the tail will forcefully pull the rope to assist the horse to rise. The person on the head rope will simply guide the head of the horse, rather than pulling forcefully on the rope and disorienting the horse. Once the horse stands, the third person will push the horse against the wall of the recovery stall for support. If this technique is to be used, recovery stalls should be constructed so that there are readily accessible exit routes, and the personnel handling the ropes will be outside the stall to avoid the hazards of an unco-ordinated horse attempting to stand. Quiet surroundings and a darkened recovery stall should be provided to minimize any stimulus that may excite a horse recovering from anesthesia, although it has been suggested that a darkened stall does not provide any benefit during recovery [286]. When the horse is standing and steady on its feet, a hard cup hood may be placed over the affected eye for additional ocular protection. A higher incidence of colic has been reported in horses with ocular disease[287] and such patients should be observed very closely postoperatively for signs of abdominal pain.

References

1 Donlon JV Jr. Anesthesia for eye, ear, nose, and throat surgery. In: Miller RD, ed. *Anesthesia*, 5th edn. Philadelphia: Churchill Livingstone, 2000; 2173–2198.

2 Collins BK, Gross ME, Moore CP, *et al.* Physiologic, pharmacologic, and practical considerations for anesthesia of domestic animals with eye disease. *J Am Vet Med Assoc* 1995; **207**: 220–230.

3 Cunningham AJ, Barry P. Intraocular pressure: physiology and implications for anaesthetic management. *Can Anaesth Soc J* 1986; **33**: 195–208.

4 Miller PE, Pickett JP. Comparison of the human and canine Schiotz tonometry conversion tables in clinically normal dogs. *J Am Vet Med Assoc* 1992; **201**: 1021–1025.

5 Miller PE, Pickett JP. Comparison of the human and canine Schiotz tonometry conversion tables in clinically normal cats. *J Am Vet Med Assoc* 1992; **201**: 1017–1020.

6 Miller PE, Pickett JP, Majors LJ. Evaluation of two applanation tonometers in horses. *Am J Vet Res* 1990; **51**: 935–937.

7 Murphy DF. Anesthesia and intraocular pressure. *Anesth Analg* 1985; **64**: 520–530.

8 Macri FJ. Interdependence of venous and eye pressure. *Arch Ophthalmol* 1961; **65**: 442–449.

9 Aihara M, Lindsey JD, Weinreb RN. Episcleral venous pressure of mouse eye and effect of body position. *Curr Eye Res* 2003; **27**: 355–362.

10 Broadwater JJ, Schorling JJ, Herring IP, *et al.* Effect of body position on intraocular pressure in dogs without glaucoma. *Am J Vet Res* 2008; **69**: 527–530.

11 Komaromy AM, Garg CD, Ying GS, *et al.* Effect of head position on intraocular pressure in horses. *Am J Vet Res* 2006; **67**: 1232–1235.

12 Duncalf D, Weitzner SW. The influence of ventilation and hypercapnia on intraocular pressure during anesthesia. *Anesth Analg* 1963; **42**: 232–246.

13 McMurphy RM, Davidson HJ, Hodgson DS. Effects of atracurium on intraocular pressure, eye position, and blood pressure in eucapnic and hypocapnic isoflurane-anesthetized dogs. *Am J Vet Res* 2004; **65**: 179–182.

14 Cullen LK, Steffey EP, Bailey CS, *et al.* Effect of high $PaCO_2$ and time on cerebrospinal fluid and intraocular pressure in halothane-anesthetized horses. *Am J Vet Res* 1990; **51**: 300–304.

15 Collins BK, O'Brien D. Autonomic dynfunction of the eye. *Semin Vet Med Surg (Small Anim)* 1990; **5**: 24–36.

16 Murphy CJ. Raptor ophthalmology. *Compend Contin Educ Vet* 1987; **9**: 241–260.

17 Haskins SC. General guidelines for judging anesthetic depth. *Vet Clin North Am Small Anim Pract* 1977; **1**: 432–434.

18 Murray RB, Adler MW, Korczyn AD. The pupillary effects of opioids. *Life Sci* 1983; **33**: 495–509.

19 Kaswan RL, Quandt JE, Moore PA. Narcotics, miosis, and cataract surgery [letter]. *J Am Vet Med Assoc* 1992; **201**: 1819–1820.

20 Stephen DD, Vestre WA, Stiles J, *et al.* Changes in intraocular pressure and pupil size following intramuscular administration of hydromorphone hydrochloride and acepromazine in clinically normal dogs. *Vet Ophthalmol* 2003; **6**: 73–76.

21 Sharpe LG, Pickworth WB. Opposite pupillary size effects in the cat and dog after microinjections of morphine, normorphine and clonidine in the Edinger–Westphal nucleus. *Brain Res Bull* 1985; **15**: 329–333.

22 Yoshitomi T, Ito Y. Effects of indomethacin and prostaglandins on the dog iris sphincter and dilator muscles. *Invest Ophthalmol Vis Sci* 1988; **29**: 127–132.

23 Giuliano EA, Moore CP. Diseases and surgery of the lacrimal secretory system. In: Gelatt KN, ed. *Veterinary Ophthalmology*, 4th edn. Ames, IA: Blackwell Publishing, 2007; 633–661.

24 Gum GG, Gelatt KN, Esson DW. Physiology of the eye. In: Gelatt KN, ed. *Veterinary Ophthalmology*, 4th edn. Ames, IA: Blackwell Publishing, 2007; 149–182.

25 Gelatt KN, Peiffer RL, Erickson JL, *et al.* Evaluation of tear formation in the dog, using a modification of the Schirmer tear test. *J Am Vet Med Assoc* 1975; **166**: 368–370.

26 Krupin T, Cross DA, Becker B. Decreased basal tear production associated with general anesthesia. *Arch Ophthalmol* 1977; **95**: 107–108.

27 Mouney MC, Accola PJ, Cremer J, *et al.* Effects of acepromazine maleate or morphine on tear production before, during, and after sevoflurane anesthesia in dogs. *Am J Vet Res* 2011; **72**: 1427–1430.

28 Vestre WA, Brightman AH, Helper LC, *et al.* Decreased tear production associated with general anesthesia in the dog. *J Am Vet Med Assoc* 1979; **174**: 1006–1007.

29 Herring IP, Pickett JP, Champagne ES, *et al.* Evaluation of aqueous tear production in dogs following general anesthesia. *J Am Anim Hosp Assoc* 2000; **36**: 427–430.

30 Shepard MK, Accola PJ, Lopez LA, *et al.* Effect of duration and type of anesthetic on tear production in dogs. *Am J Vet Res* 2011; **72**: 608–612.

31 Cross DA, Krupin T. Implications of the effects of general anesthesia on basal tear production. *Anesth Analg* 1977; **56**: 35–37.

32 Ludders JW, Heavner JE. Effect of atropine on tear formation in anesthetized dogs. *J Am Vet Med Assoc* 1979; **175**: 585–586.

33 Brightman AH, Manning JP, Benson GJ, *et al.* Decreased tear production associated with general anesthesia in the horse. *J Am Vet Med Assoc* 1983; **182**: 243–244.

34 Dodam JR, Branson KR, Martin DD. Effects of intramuscular sedative and opioid combinations on tear production in dogs. *Vet Ophthalmol* 1998; **1**: 57–59.

35 Hardberger R, Hanna C, Boyd CM. Effects of drug vehicles on ocular contact time. *Arch Ophthalmol* 1975; **93**: 42–45.

36 Holly FJ, Lemp MA. Tear physiology and dry eyes. *Surv Ophthalmol* 1977; **22**: 69–87.

37 Kil HK. Hypercapnea is an important adjuvant factor of oculocardiac reflex during strabismus surgery. *Anesth Analg* 2000; **91**: 1044–1045.

38 Mirakhur RK, Jones CJ, Dundee JW, *et al.* IM or IV atropine or glycopyrrolate for the prevention of oculocardiac reflex in children undergoing squint surgery. *Br J Anaesth* 1982; **54**: 1059–1063.

39 Steinmetz A, Ellenberger K, Marz I, *et al.* Oculocardiac reflex in a dog caused by a choroidal melanoma with orbital extension. *J Am Anim Hosp Assoc* 2012; **48**: 66–70.

40 Ghaffari MS, Marjani M, Masoudifard M. Oculocardiac reflex induced by zygomatic arch fracture in a crossbreed dog. *J Vet Cardiol* 2009; **11**: 67–69.

41 Short CE, Rebhun WC. Complications caused by the oculocardiac reflex during anesthesia in a foal. *J Am Vet Med Assoc* 1980; **176**: 630–631.

42 Thurmon JC, Tranquilli WJ, Benson GJ. Anesthesia for special patients: Ocular patients. In: Thurmon JC, Tranquilli WJ, Benson GJ, eds. *Lumb and Jones' Veterinary Anesthesia*, 3rd edn. Philadelphia: Williams and Wilkins, 1996; 812–818.

43 Berler DK. The oculocardiac reflex. *Am J Ophthalmol* 1963; **56**: 954–959.

44 Clutton RE, Boyd C, Richards DLS, *et al.* Significance of the oculocardiac reflex during ophthalmic surgery in the dog. *J Small Anim Pract* 1988; **29**: 573–579.

45 Donlon JV Jr. Anesthesia for ophthalmic surgery. In: Barash P, ed. *ASA Refresher Course Lectures*, vol **16**. Philadelphia: JB Lippincott, 1988; 81–92.

46 Franci P, Leece EA, McConnell JF. Arrhythmias and transient changes in cardiac function after topical administration of one drop of phenylephrine 10% in an adult cat undergoing conjunctival graft. *Vet Anaesth Analg* 2011; **38**: 208–212.

47 Venkatakrishnan J, Jagadeesh V, Kannan R. Pulmonary edema following instillation of topical phenylephrine eyedrops in a child under general anesthesia. *Eur J Opthalmol* 2011; **21**: 115–117.

48 Wolf GL, Goldfarb H. Complications of ophthalmologic anesthesia. *Semin Anesth* 1990; **9**: 108–118.

49 Whitley RD, Gelatt KN, Gum GG. Dose–response of topical pilocarpine in the normotensive and glaucomatous Beagle. *Am J Vet Res* 1980; **41**: 417–424.

50 Carrier M, Gum GG. Effects of 4% pilocarpine gel on normotensive and glaucomatous canine eyes. *Am J Vet Res* 1989; **50**: 239–244.

51 Gum GG, Gelatt KN, Gelatt JK, *et al.* Effect of topically applied demecarium bromide and echothiophate iodide on intraocular pressure and pupil size in Beagles with normotensive eyes and Beagles with inherited glaucoma. *Am J Vet Res* 1993; **54**: 287–293.

52 Regnier A. Clinical pharmacology and therapeutics: Part 2: Antimicrobials, anti-inflammatory agents, and antiglaucoma drugs. In: Gelatt KN, ed. *Veterinary Ophthalmology*, 4th edn. Ames, IA: Blackwell Publishing, 2007; 297–331.

53 Lynch R, Rubin LF. Salivation induced in dogs by conjunctival instillation of atropine. *J Am Vet Med Assoc* 1965; **147**: 511–513.

54 Rubin LF, Wolfes RL. Mydriatics for canine ophthalmoscopy. *J Am Vet Med Assoc* 1962; **140**: 137–141.

55 Gelatt KN, Boggess TS, Cure TH. Evaluation of mydriatics in the cat. *J Am Anim Hosp Assoc* 1973; **9**: 283–287.

56 Zekas LJ, Lester G, Brooks DE. The effect of ophthalmic atropine on intestinal transit and myoelectric activity in normal adult horses [abstract]. Proceedings of the 29th Annual Meeting of the American College of Veterinary Ophthalmologists, October 1998, Seattle, WA.

57 Williams MM, Spiess BM, Pascoe PJ, *et al.* Systemic effects of topical and subconjunctival ophthalmic atropine in the horse. *Vet Ophthalmol* 2000; **3**: 193–199.

58 Farrell TA. Minimizing the systemic effects of glaucoma medications. *Geriatrics* 1991; **46**: 61–73.

59 Hodgson DS, Dunlop CI. General anesthesia for horses with specific problems. *Vet Clin North Am Equine Pract* 1990; **6**: 625–650.

60 Pascoe PJ, Ilkiw JE, Stiles J, *et al.* Arterial hypertension associated with topical ocular use of phenylephrine in dogs. *J Am Vet Med Assoc* 1994; **205**: 1562–1564.

61 Herring IP, Jacobson JD, Pickett JP. Cardiovascular effects of topical ophthalmic 10% phenylephrine in dogs. *Vet Ophthalmol* 2004; **7**: 41–46.

62 Kaufman PL, Gabelt B'Ann. α_2-Adrenergic agonist effects on aqueous humor dynamics. *J Glaucoma* 1995; **4**: S8–S14.

63 Reitsamer HA, Posey M, Kiel JW. Effects of a topical α_2 adrenergic agonist on ciliary blood flow and aqueous production in rabbits. *Exper Eye Res* 2006; **82**: 405–415.

64 Lee DA, Topper JE, Brubaker RF. Effect of clonidine on aqueous humor flow in normal human eyes. *Exp Eye Res* 1984; **38**: 239–246.

65 Miller PE, Rhaesa SL. Effects of topical administration of 0.5% apraclonidine on intraocular pressure, pupil size, and heart rate in clinically normal cats. *Am J Vet Res* 1996; **57**: 83–86.

66 Miller PE, Nelson MJ, Rhaesa SL. Effects of topical administration of 0.5% apraclonidine on intraocular pressure, pupil size, and heart rate in clinically normal dogs. *Am J Vet Res* 1996; **57**: 79–82.

67 Gelatt KN, MacKay EO. Effect of single and multiple doses of 0.2% brimonidine tartrate in the glaucomatous Beagle. *Vet Ophthalmol* 2002; **5**: 253–262.

68 Welch SL, Richardson JA. Clinical effects of brimonidine ophthalmic drops ingestion in 52 dogs. *Vet Human Toxicol* 2002; **44**: 34–35.

69 Van Buskirk EM, Fraunfelder FT. Ocular beta blockers and systemic effects. *Am J Ophthalmol* 1984; **98**: 623–624.

70 Svec AL, Strosberg AM. Therapeutic and systemic side-effects of ocular β-adrenergic antagonists in anesthetized dogs. *Invest Ophthalmol Vis Sci* 1986; **27**: 401–405.

71 Gum GG, Larocca RD, Gelatt KN, *et al.* The effect of topical timolol maleate on intraocular pressure in normal Beagles and Beagles with inherited glaucoma. *Prog Vet Comp Ophthalmol* 1991; **1**: 141–149.

72 Gelatt KN, Larocca RD, Gelatt JK, *et al.* Evaluation of multiple doses of 4 and 6% timolol, and timolol combined with 2% pilocarpine in clinically normal Beagles and Beagles with glaucoma. *Am J Vet Res* 1995; **56**: 1325–1331.

73 Wilkie DA, Latimer CA. Effects of topical administration of timolol maleate on intraocular pressure and pupil size in dogs. *Am J Vet Res* 1991; **52**: 432–435.

74 Wilkie DA, Latimer CA. Effects of topical administration of timolol maleate on intraocular pressure and pupil size in cats. *Am J Vet Res* 1991; **52**: 436–440.

75 Willis AM. Ocular hypotensive drugs. *Vet Clin North Am Small Anim Pract* 2004; **34**: 755–776.

76 Maren TH. Carbonic anhydrase: chemistry, physiology, and inhibition. *Physiol Rev* 1967; **47**: 595–781.

77 Rose RJ, Carter J. Some physiological and biochemical effects of acetazolamide in the dog. *J Vet Pharmacol Ther* 1979; **2**: 215–221.

78 Ludders JW. Anesthesia for the patient with central nervous system or ophthalmic disease: anesthesia for the ophthalmic surgical patient. In: Slatter D, ed. *Textbook of Small Animal Surgery*, 3rd edn. Philadelphia: Saunders Elsevier, 2003; 2560–2564.

79 Cawrse MA, Ward DA, Hendrix DVH. Effects of topical application of a 2% solution of dorzolamide on intraocular pressure and aqueous humor flow rate in clinically normal dogs. *Am J Vet Res* 2001; **62**: 859–863.

80 Rainbow ME, Dziezyc J. Effects of twice daily application of 2% dorzolamide on intraocular pressure in normal cats. *Vet Ophthalmol* 2003; **6**: 147–150.

81 Willis AM, Robbin TE, Hoshaw-Woodard S, *et al.* Effect of topical administration of 2% dorzlamide hydrochloride or 2% dorzlamide hydrochloride – 0.5% timolol maleate on intraocular pressure in clinically normal horses. *Am J Vet Res* 2001; **62**: 709–713.

82 Rankin AJ, Crumley WR, Allbaugh RA. Effects of ocular administration of ophthalmic 2% dorzolamide hydrochloride solution on aqueous humor flow rate and intraocular pressure in clinically normal cats. *Am J Vet Res* 2012; **73**: 1074–1078.

83 Kass MA. Topical carbonic anhydrase inhibitors. *Am J Ophthalmol* 1989; **107**: 280–282.

84 Gwin RM. Current concepts in small animal glaucoma: recognition and treatment. *Vet Clin North Am Small Anim Pract* 1980; **10**: 357–376.

85 Brooks DE. Glaucoma in the dog and cat. *Vet Clin North Am Small Anim Pract* 1990; **20**: 775–797.

86 Singh K, Krupin T. Hyperosmotic agents. In: Zimmerman TJ, Kooner KS, Sharir M, eds. *Textbook of Ocular Pharmacology*, 3rd edn. Philadelphia: Lippincott William & Wilkins, 1997; 291–296.

87 Dugan SJ, Roberts SM, Severin GA. Systemic osmotherapy for ophthalmic disease in dogs and cats. *J Am Vet Med Assoc* 1989; **194**: 115–118.

88 Craig EL. Glaucoma therapy: Osmotic agents. In: Mauger TF, Craig EL, eds. *Havener's Ocular Pharmacology*, 6th edn. St Louis, MO: Mosby, 1994; 180–189.

89 Lorimer DW, Hakanson NE, Pion PD, *et al.* The effect of intravenous mannitol or oral glycerol on intraocular pressure in dogs. *Cornell Vet* 1989; **79**: 249–258.

90 Brock KA, Thurmon JC. Pulmonary edema associated with mannitol administration. *Can Pract* 1979; **6**: 31–34.

91 Brock KA, Thurmon JC, Benson GJ, *et al.* Selected hemodynamic and renal effects of intravenous infusions of hypertonic mannitol in dogs anesthetized with methoxyflurane in oxygen. *J Am Anim Hosp Assoc* 1985; **21**: 207–214.

92 Gilroy BA. Intraocular and cardiopulmonary effects of low-dose mannitol in the dog. *Vet Surg* 1986; **15**: 342–344.

93 Glaze MB, Crawford MA, Nachreiner RF, *et al.* Ophthalmic corticosteroid therapy: systemic effects in the dog. *J Am Vet Med Assoc* 1988; **192**: 73–75.

94 Roberts SM, Lavach JD, Macy DW, *et al.* Effect of ophthalmic prednisolone acetate on the canine adrenal gland and hepatic function. *Am J Vet Res* 1984; **45**: 1711–1714.

95 Regnier A, Toutain PL, Alvinerie M, *et al.* Adrenocortical function and plasma biochemical values in dogs after subconjunctival treatment with methylprednisolone acetate. *Res Vet Sci* 1982; **32**: 306–310.

96 Eichenbaum JD, Macy DW, Severin GA, *et al.* Effect in large dogs of ophthalmic prednisolone acetate on adrenal gland and hepatic function. *J Am Anim Hosp Assoc* 1988; **24**: 705–709.

97 Murphy CJ, Feldman E, Bellhorn R. Iatrogenic Cushing's syndrome in a dog caused by topical ophthalmic medications. *J Am Anim Hosp Assoc* 1990; **26**: 640–642.

98 Spiess BM, Nyikos S, Stummer E, *et al.* Systemic dexamethasone concentration in horses after continued topical treatment with an ophthalmic preparation of dexamethasone. *Am J Vet Res* 1999; **60**: 571–576.

99 Graham BP, Powell CC, Gionfriddo JR, *et al.* Evaluation of neomycin, polymixin B, dexamethasone ophthalmic ointment as a cause of abortion in llamas [abstract]. Proceedings of the 33rd Annual Meeting of the American College of Veterinary Ophthalmologists, October 2002, Denver, CO.

100 Brunson DB. Anesthesia in ophthalmic surgery. *Vet Clin North Am Small Anim Pract* 1980; **10**: 481–495.

101 Whitley RD, McLaughlin SA, Whitley EM, *et al.* Cataract removal in dogs: the surgical techniques. *Vet Med* 1993; **88**: 859–866.

102 Joas TA, Stevens WC. Comparison of the arrhythmic doses of epinephrine during Forane, halothane, and fluroxene anesthesia in dogs. *Anesthesiology* 1971; **35**: 48–53.

103 Mirakhur RK, Elliott P, Shepherd WFI, *et al.* Comparison of the effects of isoflurane and halothane on intraocular pressure. *Acta Anaesthesiol Scand* 1990; **34**: 282–285.

104 Artru AA. Rate of anterior chamber aqueous formation, trabecular outflow facility, and intraocular compliance during desflurane or halothane anesthesia in dogs. *Anesth Analg* 1995; **81**: 585–590.

105 Almeida DE, Rezende ML, Nunes N, *et al.* Evaluation of intraocular pressure in association with cardiovascular parameters in normocapnic dogs anesthetized with sevoflurane and desflurane. *Vet Ophthalmol* 2004; **7**: 265–269.

106 Sator S, Wildling E, Schabernig C, *et al.* Desflurane maintains intraocular pressure at an equivalent level to isoflurane and propofol during unstressed non-ophthalmic surgery. *Br J Anaesth* 1998; **80**: 243–244.

107 Sator-Katzenschlager S, Deusch E, Dolezal S, *et al.* Sevoflurane and propofol decrease intraocular pressure equally during non-ophthalmic surgery and recovery. *Br J Anaesth* 2002; **89**: 764–766.

108 Eltzschig HK, Darsow R, Schroeder TH, *et al.* Effect of tracheal intubation or Laryngeal Mask Airway™ insertion on intraocular pressure using balanced anesthesia with sevoflurane and remifentanil. *J Clin Anesth* 2001; **13**: 264–267.

109 Tayefeh F, Larson MD, Sessler DI, *et al.* Time-dependent changes in heart rate and pupil size during desflurane or sevoflurane anesthesia. *Anesth Analg* 1997; **85**: 1362–1366.

110 Artru AA, Momota Y. Trabecular outflow facility and formation rate of aqueous humor during anesthesia with sevoflurane-nitrous oxide or sevoflurane-remifentanil in rabbits. *Anesth Analg* 1999; **88**: 781–786.

111 Buehner E, Pietsch UC, Bringmann A, *et al.* Effects of propofol and isoflurane anesthesia on the intraocular pressure and hemodynamics of pigs. *Ophthalmic Res* 2011; **45**: 42–46.

112 Jia L, Cepurna WO, Johnson EC, *et al.* Effect of general anesthetics on IOP in rats with experimental aqueous outflow obstruction. *Invest Ophthalmol Vis Sci* 2000; **41**: 3415–3419.

113 Almeida DE, Nishimori CT, Oria AP, *et al.* Effects of nitrous oxide on IOP and pupillary diameter in dogs anesthetized with varying concentrations of desflurane. *Vet Ophthalmol* 2008; **11**: 170–176.

114 Wolf GL, Capuano C, Hartung J. Effect of nitrous oxide on gas bubble volume in the anterior chamber. *Arch Ophthalmol* 1985; **103**: 418–419.

115 Hart RH, Vote BJ, Borthwick JH, *et al.* Loss of vision caused by expansion of intraocular perfluoropropane (C_3F_8) gas during nitrous oxide anesthesia. *Am J Ophthalmol* 2002; **134**: 761–763.

116 de Roetth A, Schwartz H. Effect of ganglionic blocking agents and thiopental sodium (Pentothal) anesthesia on aqueous humor dynamics. *AMA Arch Ophthalmol* 1956; **55**: 755–764.

117 Hahnenberger RW. Influence of various anesthetic drugs on the intraocular pressure of cats. *Albrecht v Graefes Arch klin exp Ophthal* 1976; **199**: 179–186.

118 Langley MS, Heel RC. Propofol: a review of its pharmacodynamic and pharmacokinetic properties and use as an intravenous anaesthetic. *Drugs* 1988; **35**: 334–372.

119 Mirakhur RK, Shepherd WFI, Darrah WC. Propofol or thiopentone: effects on intraocular pressure associated with induction of anaesthesia and tracheal intubation (facilitated with suxamethonium). *Br J Anaesth* 1987; **59**: 431–436.

120 Batista CM, Laus JL, Nunes N, *et al.* Evaluation of intraocular and partial CO_2 pressure in dogs anesthetized with propofol. *Vet Ophthalmol* 2000; **3**: 17–19.

121 Hofmeister EH, Williams CO, Braun C, *et al.* Influence of lidocaine and diazepam on peri-induction intraocular pressures in dogs anesthetized with propofol-atracurium. *Can J Vet Res* 2006; **70**: 251–256.

122 Hofmeister EH, Williams CO, Braun C, *et al.* Propofol versus thiopental: effects on peri-induction intraocular pressures in normal dogs. *Vet Anaesth Analg* 2008; **35**: 275–281.

123 Torres MD, Andaluz A, Garcia F, *et al.* Effects of an intravenous bolus of alfaxalone versus propofol on intraocular pressure in sheep. *Vet Rec* 2012; **170**: 226–228.

124 Lin HC, Thurmon JC, Benson GJ, *et al.* Telazol – a review of its pharmacology and use in veterinary medicine. *J Vet Pharmacol Ther* 1993; **16**: 383–418.

125 Peuler M, Glass DD, Arens JF. Ketamine and intraocular pressure. *Anesthesiology* 1975; **43**: 575–578.

126 Ausinsch B, Rayburn RL, Munson ES, *et al.* Ketamine and intraocular pressure in children. *Anesth Analg* 1976; **55**: 773–775.

127 Gelatt KN, Gwin RM, Peiffer RL, *et al.* Tonography in the normal and glaucomatous Beagle. *Am J Vet Res* 1977; **38**: 515–520.

128 Hofmeister EH, Mosunic CB, Torres BT, *et al.* Effects of ketamine, diazepam, and their combination on intraocular pressures in clinically normal dogs. *Am J Vet Res* 2006; **67**: 1136–1139.

129 Trim CM, Colbern GT, Martin CL. Effect of xylazine and ketamine on intraocular pressure in horses. *Vet Rec* 1985; **117**: 442–443.

130 Ghaffari MS, Moghaddassi AP. Effects of ketamine-diazepam and ketamine-acepromazine combinations on intraocular pressure in rabbits. *Vet Anaesth Analg* 2010; **37**: 269–272.

131 Arnett BD, Brightman AH, Musselman EE. Effect of atropine sulfate on tear production in the cat when used with ketamine hydrochloride and acetylpromazine maleate. *J Am Vet Med Assoc* 1984; **185**: 214–215.

132 Oji EO, Holdcroft A. The ocular effects of etomidate. *Anaesthesia* 1979; **34**: 245–249.

133 Thomson MF, Brock-Utne JG, Bean P, *et al.* Anaesthesia and intra-ocular pressure: a comparison of total intravenous anaesthesia using etomidate with conventional inhalation anaesthesia. *Anaesthesia* 1982; **37**: 758–761.

134 Burke JA, Potter DE. The ocular effects of xylazine in rabbits, cats, and monkeys. *J Ocul Pharmacol* 1986; **2**: 9–21.

135 van der Woerdt A, Gilger BC, Wilkie DA, *et al.* Effect of auriculopalpebral nerve block and intravenous administration of xylazine on intraocular pressure and corneal thickness in horses. *Am J Vet Res* 1995; **56**: 155–158.

136 McClure JR, Gelatt KN, Gum GG, *et al.* The effect of parenteral acepromazine and xylazine on intraocular pressure in the horse. *Vet Med Small Anim Clin* 1976; **71**: 1727–1730.

137 Hsu WH, Lee P, Betts DM. Xylazine-induced mydriasis in rats and its antagonism by α-adrenergic blocking agents. *J Vet Pharmacol Ther* 1981; **4**: 97–101.

138 Calderone L, Grimes P, Shalev M. Acute reversible cataract induced by xylazine and by ketamine-xylazine anesthesia in rats and mice. *Exp Eye Res* 1986; **42**: 331–337.

139 Holve DL. Effect of sedation with detomidine on intraocular pressure with and without topical anesthesia in clinically normal horses. *J Am Vet Med Assoc* 2012; **240**: 308–311.

140 Jin Y, Wilson S, Elko EE, *et al.* Ocular hypotensive effects of medetomidine and its analogs. *J Ocul Pharmacol* 1991; **7**: 285–296.

141 Ogidigben MJ, Potter DE. Comparative effects of alpha-2 and DA_2 agonists on intraocular pressure in pigmented and nonpigmented rabbits. *J Ocul Pharmacol* 1993; **9**: 187–199.

142 Potter DE, Ogidigben MJ. Medetomidine-induced alterations of intraocular pressure and contraction of the nictitating membrane. *Invest Ophthalmol Vis Sci* 1991; **32**: 2799–2805.

143 Verbruggen AMJ, Akkerdaas LC, Hellebrekers LJ, *et al.* The effect of intravenous medetomidine on pupil size and intraocular pressure in normotensive dogs. *Vet Quart* 2000; **22**: 179–180.

144 Wallin-Hakanson N, Wallin-Hakanson B. The effects of topical tropicamide and systemic medetomidine, followed by atipamezole reversal, on pupil size and intraocular pressure in normal dogs. *Vet Ophthalmol* 2001; **4**: 3–6.

145 Sanchez RF, Mellor D, Mould J. Effects of medetomidine and medetomidine-butorphanol combination on Schirmer tear test 1 readings in dogs. *Vet Ophthalmol* 2006; **9**: 33–37.

146 Soontornvipart K, Rauser P, Kecova H, *et al.* Effect of intravenous medetomidine-buprenorphine on canine tear flow. *Online J Vet Res* 2003; **1**: 10–16.

147 Artigas C, Redondo JI, Lopez-Murcia MM. Effects of intravenous administration of dexmedetomidine on intraocular pressure and pupil size in clinically normal dogs. *Vet Ophthalmol* 2012; **15**: 79–82.

148 Rauser P, Pfeifr J, Proks P, *et al.* Effect of medetomidine-butorphanol and dexmedetomidine-butorphanol combinations on intraocular pressure in healthy dogs. *Vet Anaesth Analg* 2012; **39**: 301–305.

149 Vartiainen J, MacDonald E, Urtti A, *et al.* Dexmedetomidine-induced ocular hypotension in rabbits with normal or elevated intraocular pressures. *Invest Ophthalmol Vis Sci* 1992; **33**: 2019–2023.

150 MacDonald E, Vartiainen J, Jasberg K, *et al.* Systemic absorption and systemic effects of ocularly administered dexmedetomidine in rabbits. *Curr Eye Res* 1993; **12**: 451–460.

151 Artru AA. Intraocular pressure in anaesthetized dogs given flumazenil with and without prior administration of midazolam. *Can J Anaesth* 1991; **38**: 408–414.

152 Pino Capote JA. Decrease in intraocular pressure produced by I.V. or conjunctival diazepam. *Br J Anaesth* 1978; **50**: 865.

153 Ghaffari MS, Moghaddassi AP, Bokaie S. Effects of intramuscular acepromazine and diazepam on tear production in rabbits. *Vet Rec* 2009; **164**: 147–148.

154 Hayreh SS, Kardon RH, McAllister DL, *et al.* Acepromazine: effects on intraocular pressure. *Arch Ophthalmol* 1991; **109**: 119–124.

155 Stiles J, Honda CN, Krohne SG, *et al.* Effect of topical administration of 1% morphine sulfate solution on signs of pain and corneal wound healing in dogs. *Am J Vet Res* 2003; **64**: 813–818.
156 Peyman GA, Rahimy MH, Fernandes ML. Effects of morphine on corneal sensitivity and epithelial wound healing: implications for topical ophthalmic analgesia. *Br J Ophthalmol* 1994; **78**: 138–141.
157 Wenk HN, Nannenga MN, Honda CN. Effect of morphine sulphate eye drops on hyperalgesia in the rat cornea. *Pain* 2003; **105**: 455–465.
158 Clark JS, Bentley E, Smith LJ. Evaluation of topical nalbuphine or oral tramadol as analgesics for corneal pain in dogs: a pilot study. *Vet Ophthalmol* 2011; **14**: 358–364.
159 Aquino S, van der Woerdt A, Eaton JS. The effect of topical nalbuphine on corneal sensitivity in normal canine eyes [abstract]. Proceedings of the 36th Annual Meeting of the American College of Veterinary Ophthalmologists, October 2005, Nashville, TN.
160 Wotman KL, Utter ME. Effect of treatment with a topical ophthalmic preparation of 1% nalbuphine solution on corneal sensitivity in clinically normal horses. *Am J Vet Res* 2010; **71**: 223–228.
161 Gross ME, Giuliano EA. Anesthesia and analgesia for selected patients and procedures: ocular patients. In: Tranquilli WJ, Thurmon JC, Grimm KA, eds. *Lumb and Jones' Veterinary Anesthesia and Analgesia*, 4th edn. Ames, IA: Blackwell Publishing, 2007; 943–954.
162 Leopold IH, Comroe JH. Effect of intramuscular administration of morphine, atropine, scopolamine, and neostigmine on the human eye. *Arch Ophthalmol* 1948; **40**: 285–290.
163 Blaze C, Pirie CG, Casey E, *et al.* The effect of intravenous hydromorphone, butorphanol, morphine, and buprenorphine on pupil size and intraocular pressure in normal dogs [abstract]. Proceedings of the 10th World Congress of Veterinary Anesthesia, 2009, Glasgow, UK.
164 Tamura E, Barros P, Cortopassi S, *et al.* Effects of two preanesthetic regimens for ophthalmic surgery on intraocular pressure and cardiovascular measurements in dogs. *Vet Ther* 2002; **3**: 81–87.
165 Biricik HS, Ceylan C, Sakar M. Effects of pethidine and fentanyl on tear production in dogs. *Vet Rec* 2004; **155**: 564–565.
166 Thorig L, Halperin M, van Haeringen NJ. The fine-thread method: lacrimation test for measuring ocular side-effects of drugs in the rat. *Documenta Ophthalmol* 1983; **56**: 35–39.
167 Giuliano EA. Nonsteroidal anti-inflammatory drugs in veterinary ophthalmology. *Vet Clin North Am Small Anim Pract* 2004; **34**: 707–723.
168 Chen X, Gallar J, Belmonte C. Reduction by antiinflammatory drugs of the response of corneal sensory nerve fibers to chemical irritation. *Invest Ophthalmol Vis Sci* 1997; **38**: 1944–1953.
169 Schalnus R. Topical nonsteroidal anti-inflammatory therapy in ophthalmology. *Ophthalmologica* 2003; **217**: 89–98.
170 Millichamp NJ, Dziezyc J, Olsen JW. Effect of flurbiprofen on facility of aqueous outflow in the eyes of dogs. *Am J Vet Res* 1991; **52**: 1448–1451.
171 Gaynes BI, Fiscella R. Topical nonsteroidal anti-inflammatory drugs for ophthalmic use: a safety review. *Drug Saf* 2002; **25**: 233–250.
172 Smith LJ, Bentley E, Shih A, *et al.* Systemic lidocaine infusion as an analgesic for intraocular surgery in dogs: a pilot study. *Vet Anaesth Analg* 2004; **31**: 53–63.
173 Doherty TJ, Seddighi MR. Local anesthetics as pain therapy in horses. *Vet Clin Equine* 2010; **26**: 533–549.
174 Cozanitis DA, Dundee JW, Buchanan TAS, *et al.* Atropine versus glycopyrrolate: a study of intraocular pressure and pupil size in man. *Anaesthesia* 1979; **34**: 236–238.
175 Muir WW. Effects of atropine on cardiac rate and rhythm in dogs. *J Am Vet Med Assoc* 1978; **172**: 917–921.
176 Jensen HE. Keratitis sicca and parotid duct transposition. *Compend Contin Educ Pract Vet* 1979; **1**: 721–726.
177 Ducharme NG, Fubini SL. Gastrointestinal complications associated with the use of atropine in horses. *J Am Vet Med Assoc* 1983; **182**: 229–231.
178 Frischmeyer KJ, Miller PE, Bellay Y, *et al.* Parenteral anticholinergics in dogs with normal and elevated intraocular pressure. *Vet Surg* 1993; **22**: 230–234.
179 Hollingsworth SR, Canton DD, Buyukmihci NC, *et al.* Effect of topically administered atropine on tear production in dogs. *J Am Vet Med Assoc* 1992; **200**: 1481–1484.
180 Behrendt T. Experimental study of corneal lesions produced by topical anesthesia. *Am J Ophthalmol* 1956; **41**: 99–105.
181 Liu JC, Steinemann TL, McDonald MB, *et al.* Topical bupivacaine and proparacaine: a comparison of toxicity, onset of action, and duration of action. *Cornea* 1993; **12**: 228–232.
182 Marr WG, Wood R, Senterfit L, *et al.* Effect of topical anesthetics on regeneration of corneal epithelium. *Am J Ophthalmol* 1957; **43**: 606–610.
183 Grant RL, Acosta D. Comparative toxicity of tetracaine, proparacaine, and cocaine evaluated with primary cultures of rabbit corneal epithelial cells. *Exp Eye Res* 1994; **58**: 469–478.
184 Herring IP, Bobofchak MA, Landry MP, *et al.* Duration of effect and effect of multiple doses of topical ophthalmic 0.5% proparacaine hydrochloride in clinically normal dogs. *Am J Vet Res* 2005; **66**: 77–80.
185 Binder DR, Herring IP. Duration of corneal anesthesia following topical administration of 0.5% proparacaine hydrochloride solution in clinically normal cats. *Am J Vet Res* 2006; **67**: 1780–1782.
186 Kalf KL, Utter ME, Wotman KL. Evaluation of duration of corneal anesthesia induced with ophthalmic 0.5% proparacaine hydrochloride by use of a Cochet-Bonnet aesthesiometer in clinically normal horses. *Am J Vet Res* 2008; **69**: 1655–1658.
187 Giuliano EA. Regional anesthesia as an adjunct for eyelid surgery in dogs. *Top Compan Anim Med* 2008; **23**: 51–56.
188 Marts BS, Bryan GM, Prieur DJ. Schirmer tear test measurement and lysozyme concentration of equine tears. *J Equine Med Surg* 1977; **1**: 427–430.
189 Raffe MR, Bistner SI, Crimi AJ, *et al.* Retrobulbar block in combination with general anesthesia for equine ophthalmic surgery. *Vet Surg* 1986; **15**: 139–141.
190 Meyers EF, Ramirez RC, Boniuk I. Grand mal seizures after retrobulbar block. *Arch Ophthalmol* 1978; **96**: 847.
191 Klein ML, Jampol LM, Condon PI, *et al.* Central retinal artery occlusion without retrobulbar hemorrhage after retrobulbar anesthesia. *Am J Ophthalmol* 1982; **93**: 573–577.
192 Sullivan KL, Brown GC, Forman AR, *et al.* Retrobulbar anesthesia and retinal vascular obstruction. *Ophthalmology* 1983; **90**: 373–377.
193 Pautler SE, Grizzard WS, Thompson LN, *et al.* Blindness from retrobulbar injection into the optic nerve. *Ophthal Surg* 1986; **17**: 334–337.
194 Ramsay RC, Knobloch WH. Ocular perforation following retrobulbar anesthesia for retinal detachment surgery. *Am J Ophthalmol* 1978; **86**: 61–64.
195 Brookshire GL, Gleitsmann KY, Schenk EC. Life-threatening complication of retrobulbar block: a hypothesis. *Ophthalmology* 1986; **93**: 1476–1478.
196 Javitt JC, Addiego R, Friedberg HL, *et al.* Brain stem anesthesia after retrobulbar block. *Ophthalmology* 1987; **94**: 718–724.
197 Wittpenn JR, Rapoza P, Sternberg P, *et al.* Respiratory arrest following retrobulbar anesthesia. *Ophthalmology* 1986; **93**: 867–870.
198 Davis DB, Mandel MR. Posterior peribulbar anesthesia: an alternative to retrobulbar anesthesia. *Indian J Ophthalmol* 1989; **37**: 59–61.
199 Watkins R, Beigi B, Yates M, *et al.* Intraocular pressure and pulsatile ocular blood flow after retrobulbar and peribulbar anaesthesia. *Br J Ophthalmol* 2001; **85**: 796–798.
200 Evans TF, da Costa PD. Medial peribulbar (MPB) nerve block for corneal and intraocular surgery in the dog [abstract]. Proceedings of the 37th Annual Meeting of the American College of Veterinary Ophthalmologists, November 2006, San Antonio, TX.
201 Mein CE, Woodcock MG. Local anesthesia for vitreoretinal surgery. *Retina* 1990; **10**: 47–49.
202 Patel BCK, Clinch TE, Burns TA, *et al.* Prospective evaluation of topical versus retrobulbar anesthesia: a converting surgeon's experience. *J Cataract Refract Surg* 1998; **24**: 853–860.
203 Lampard DG, Morgan DL. Intra-ocular pressure during retrobulbar injection. *Aust Vet J* 1977; **53**: 490–491.
204 Peterson DR. Nerve block of the eye and associated structures. *J Am Vet Med Assoc* 1951; **118**: 145–148.
205 Young SS, Barnett KC, Taylor PM. Anaesthetic regimes for cataract removal in the dog. *J Sm Anim Pract* 1991; **32**: 236–240.
206 Donaldson LL, Holland M, Koch SA. Atracurium as an adjunct to halothane-oxygen anesthesia in a llama undergoing intraocular surgery: a case report. *Vet Surg* 1992; **21**: 76–79.
207 Benson GJ, Manning JP, Hartsfield SM, *et al.* Intraocular tension of the horse: effects of succinylcholine and halothane anesthesia. *Am J Vet Res* 1981; **42**: 1831–1832.
208 Varghese C, Chopra SK, Daniel R, *et al.* Intraocular pressure profile during general anesthesia. *Ophthal Surg* 1990; **21**: 856–859.
209 Katz RL, Eakins KE. Mode of action of succinylcholine on intraocular pressure. *J Pharmacol Exp Ther* 1968; **162**: 1–9.
210 Collins CC, Bach-y-Rita P. Succinylcholine, ocular pressure, and extraocular muscle tension in cats and rabbits. *J Appl Physiol* 1972; **33**: 788–791.
211 Pandey K, Badola RP, Kumar S. Time course of intraocular hypertension produced by suxamethonium. *Br J Anaesth* 1972; **44**: 191–196.
212 Collins CC, Bach-y-Rita P, Loeb DR. Intraocular pressure variation with oculorotary muscle tension. *Am J Physiol* 1967; **213**: 1039–1043.
213 Bach-y-Rita P, Collins C, Tengroth B. Effect of succinylcholine on length and refraction of eyes. *Proc West Pharmacol Soc* 1968; **11**: 21–22.
214 Bjork A, Halldin M, Wahlin A. Enophthalmos elicited by succinylcholine: some observations on the effect of succinylcholine and noradrenaline on the intraorbital muscles studied on man and experimental animals. *Acta Anaesth Scand* 1957; **1**: 41–53.

215 Thomas ET, Dobkin AB. Untoward effects of muscle relaxant drugs. *Int Anesthesiol Clin* 1972; **10**: 207–225.

216 Joshi C, Bruce DL. Thiopental and succinylcholine: action on intraocular pressure. *Anesth Analg* 1975; **54**: 471–475.

217 Adams HR. Cholinergic pharmacology: autonomic drugs. In: Adams HR, ed. *Veterinary Pharmacology and Therapeutics*, 8th edn. Ames, IA: Iowa State University Press,; 2001; 117–136.

218 Adams HR. Neuromuscular blocking agents. In: Adams HR, ed. *Veterinary Pharmacology and Therapeutics*, 8th edn. Ames, IA: Iowa State University Press,; 2001; 137–152.

219 Mirakhur RK, Shepherd WFI, Lavery GG, *et al.* The effects of vecuronium on intra-ocular pressure. *Anaesthesia* 1987; **42**: 944–949.

220 George R, Nursingh A, Downing JW, *et al.* Non-depolarizing neuromuscular blockers and the eye: a study of intraocular pressure: pancuronium versus alcuronium. *Br J Anaesth* 1979; **51**: 789–792.

221 Maharaj RJ, Humphrey D, Kaplan N, *et al.* Effects of atracurium on intraocular pressure. *Br J Anaesth* 1984; **56**: 459–463.

222 Jantzen JPAH, Earnshaw G, Hackett GH, *et al.* A study of the effects of neuromuscular blocking drugs on intraocular pressure. *Anaesthetist* 1987; **36**: 223–227.

223 Auer U, Moens Y. Neuromuscular blockade with rocuronium bromide for ophthalmic surgery in horses. *Vet Ophthalmol* 2011; **14**: 244–247.

224 Martin-Flores M, Pare MD, Adams W, *et al.* Observations of the potency and duration of vecuronium in isoflurane-anesthetized horses. *Vet Anaesth Analg* 2012; **39**: 385–389.

225 Verschueren CP, Lumeij JT. Mydriasis in pigeons (Columbia livia domestica) with d-tubocurarine: topical instillation versus intracameral injection. *J Vet Pharmacol Ther* 1991; **14**: 206–208.

226 Ramer JC, Paul-Murphy J, Brunson D, *et al.* Effects of mydriatic agents in cockatoos, African gray parrots, and Blue-fronted Amazon parrots. *J Am Vet Med Assoc* 1996; **208**: 227–230.

227 Ekesten B. Ophthalmic examination and diagnostics: electrodiagnostic evaluation of vision. In: Gelatt KN, ed. *Veterinary Ophthalmology*, 4th edn. Ames, IA: Blackwell Publishing, 2007; 520–535.

228 Young B, Eggenberger E, Kaufman D. Current electrophysiology in ophthalmology: a review. *Curr Opin Ophthalmol* 2012; **23**: 497–505.

229 Wachtmeister L. Oscillatory potentials in the retina: what do they reveal? *Prog Ret Eye Res* 1998; **17**: 485–521.

230 Creel DJ. The electroretinogram and electro-oculogram: clinical applications. http://webvision.med.utah.edu/book/electrophysiology/the-electroretinogram-clinical-applications/ (accessed 5 October 2014).

231 Dawson WW, Kommonen B. The late positive retinal potential in dogs. *Exp Eye Res* 1995; **60**: 173–179.

232 Miller RF, Dowling JE. Intracellular responses of the Muller (glial) cells of mudpuppy retina: their relation to b-wave of the electoretinogram. *J Neurophysiol* 1970; **33**: 323–341.

233 Stockton RA, Slaughter MM. B-wave of the electroretinogram: areflection of ON bipolar cell activity. *J Gen Physiol* 1989; **93**: 101–122.

234 Perlman I. Relationship between the amplitudes of the b wave and the a wave as a useful index for evaluating the electroretinogram. *Br J Ophthalmol* 1983; **67**: 443–448.

235 Yanase J, Ogawa H. Effects of halothane and sevoflurane on the electroretinogram of dogs. *Am J Vet Res* 1997; **58**: 904–909.

236 Acland GM, Forte S, Aguirre GD. Halothane effects on the canine electroretinogram. Proceedings of the 12th Annual Meeting of the College of Veterinary Ophthalmologists, November 1981, Atlanta, GA.

237 Kommonen B, Karhunen U, Raitta C. Effects of thiopentone-halothane-nitrous oxide anaesthesia compared to ketamine-xylazine anaesthesia on the DC recorded dog electroretinogram. *Acta Vet Scand* 1988; **29**: 23–33.

238 Norman JC, Narfstrom K, Barrett PM. The effects of medetomidine hydrochloride on the electroretinogram of normal dogs. *Vet Ophthalmol* 2008; **11**: 299–305.

239 Kommonen B, Raitta C. Electroretinography in Labrador Retrievers given ketamine-xylazine anesthesia. *Am J Vet Res* 1987; **48**: 1325–1331.

240 Kommonen B. The DC-recorded dog electroretinogram in ketamine-medetomidine anaesthesia. *Acta Vet Scand* 1988; **29**: 35–41.

241 Kommonen B, Hyvatti E, Dawson WW. Propofol modulates inner retina function in Beagles. *Vet Ophthalmol* 2007; **10**: 76–80.

242 Tanskanen P, Kylma T, Kommonen B, Karhunen U. Propofol influences the electroretinogram to a lesser degree than thiopentone. *Acta Anaesth Scand* 1996; **40**: 480–485.

243 Baro JA, Lehmkuhle S, Kratz KE. Electroretinograms and visual evoked potentials in long-term monocularly deprived cats. *Invest Ophthalmol Vis Sci* 1990; **31**: 1405–1409.

244 Narfstrom KL, Nilsson SE, Andersson BE. Progressive retinal atrophy in the Abyssinian cat: studies of the DC-recorded electroretinogram and the standing potential of the eye. *Br J Ophthalmol* 1985; **69**: 618–623.

245 Chaudhary V, Hansen R, Lindgren H, *et al.* Effects of Telazol and Nembutal on retinal responses. *Doc Ophthalmol* 2003; **107**: 45–51.

246 Ropstad EO, Bjerkas E, Narfstrom K. Electroretinographic findings in the standard wire haired Dachshund with inherited early onset cone-rod dystrophy. *Doc Ophthalmol* 2007; **114**: 27–36.

247 Yanase J, Ogawa H, Ohtsuka H. Rod and cone components in the dog electroretinogram during and after dark adaptation. *J Vet Med Sci* 1995; **57**: 877–881.

248 Lopez OV, Vazquez JCA, Cantalapiedra AG, *et al.* Effects of hypercapnia on the electroretinogram in sevoflurane and isoflurane anaesthetized dogs. *Doc Ophthalmol* 2010; **121**: 9–20.

249 Francois J, Wouters L, Victoria-Troncoso V, *et al.* Morphometric and electrophysiologic study of the photoreceptors in the horse. *Ophthalmologica* 1980; **181**: 340–349.

250 Wouters L, de Moor A, Moens Y. Rod and cone components in the electroretinogram of the horse. *Zbl Vet Med A* 1980; **27**: 330–338.

251 Komaromy AM, Andrew SE, Sapp HL, *et al.* Flash electroretinography in standing horses using the DTL™ microfiber electrode. *Vet Ophthalmol* 2003; **6**: 27–33.

252 Church ML, Norman JC. Electroretinogram responses of the normal thoroughbred horse sedated with detomidine hydrochloride. *Vet Ophthalmol* 2012; **15**: 77–83.

253 Kotani T, Kurosawa T, Numata Y, *et al.* The normal electroretinogram in cattle and its clinical application in calves with visual defects. *Prog Vet Comp Ophthalmol* 1993; **3**: 37–44.

254 Strain GM, Olcott BM, Hokett LD. Electroretinogram and visual-evoked potential measurements in Holstein cows. *Am J Vet Res* 1986; **47**: 1079–1081.

255 Knave B, Persson HE. The effect of barbiturate on retinal functions: I. Effects on the conventional electroretinogram of the sheep eye. *Acta Physiol Scand* 1974; **91**: 53–60.

256 Knave B, Persson HE, Nilsson SEG. The effect of barbiturate on retinal functions: II. Effects on the c-wave of the electroretinogram and the standing potential of the sheep eye. *Acta Physiol Scand* 1974; **91**: 180–186.

257 Knave B, Persson HE. The effect of barbiturate on retinal functions: III. Effects on the isolated receptor responses and the inner nuclear layer components in the low-intensity electroretinogram of the sheep eye. *Acta Physiol Scand* 1974; **91**: 187–195.

258 Derwent JK, Linsenmeier RA. Effects of hypoxemia on the a- and b-waves of the electroretinogram in the cat retina. *Invest Ophthalmol Vis Sci* 2000; **41**: 3634–3642.

259 Niemeyer G, Nagahara K, Demant E. Effects of changes in arterial PO_2 and PCO_2 on the electroretinogram in the cat. *Invest Ophthalmol Vis Sci* 1982; **23**: 678–683.

260 Howard DR, Sawyer DC. Electroretinography of acute hyoxic and increased intraocular pressure status in the dog. *Am J Vet Res* 1975; **36**: 81–84.

261 Murray MJ, Borda RP. Physiologic correlates of the ERG hyperventilatory response in dogs. *Acta Ophthalmol* 1984; **62**: 808–818.

262 Datta TD. Flash fire hazard with eye ointment. *Anesth Analg* 1984; **63**: 700–701.

263 Carpel EF, Rice SW, Lang M, *et al.* Fire risks with ophthalmic ointments. *Am J Ophthalmol* 1985; **100**: 477–478.

264 Karpinski LG, Clubb SL. Clinical aspects of ophthalmology in caged birds. In: Kirk RW, ed. *Current Veterinary Therapy IX: Small Animal Practice*. Philadelphia: WB Saunders, 1986; 616–621.

265 Stiles J, Weil AB, Packer RA, *et al.* Post-anesthetic cortical blindness in cats: twenty cases. *Vet J* 2012; **193**: 367–373.

266 Carrasco-Jimenez M, Cancho MFM, Lima JR, *et al.* Relationships between a proprietary index, bispectral index, and hemodynamic variables as a means for evaluating depth of anesthesia in dogs anesthetized with sevoflurane. *Am J Vet Res* 2004; **65**: 1128–1135.

267 Kovac AL. Controlling the hemodynamic response to laryngoscopy and endotracheal intubation. *J Clin Anesth* 1996; **8**: 63–79.

268 Bellhorn RW. Ophthalmologic disorders of exotic and laboratory animals. *Vet Clin North Am Small Anim Pract* 1973; **3**: 345–356.

269 Hewes CA, Keoughan GC, Gutierrez-Nibeyro S. Standing enucleation in the horse: a report of 5 cases. *Can Vet J* 2007; **48**: 512–514.

270 Pollock PJ, Russell T, Hughes TK, *et al.* Transpalpebral eye enucleation in 40 standing horses. *Vet Surg* 2008; **37**: 306–309.

271 Wilson DV, Bohart GV, Evans AT, *et al.* Retrospective analysis of detomidine infusion for standing chemical restraint in 51 horses. *Vet Anaesth Analg* 2002; **29**: 54–59.

272 Johnston GM, Eastment JK, Wood JLN, *et al.* The confidential enquiry into perioperative equine fatalities (CEPEF): mortality results of Phases 1 and 2. *Vet Anaesth Analg* 2002; **29**: 159–170.

273 Yamashita K, Muir WW. Intravenous anesthetic and analgesic adjuncts to inhalation anesthesia. In: Muir WW, Hubbell JAE, eds. *Equine Anesthesia*, 2nd edn. St Louis, MO: Saunders Elsevier, 2009; 260–276.

274 Neel S, Deitch R, Moorthy SS, *et al.* Changes in intraocular pressure during low dose intravenous sedation with propofol before cataract surgery. *Br J Ophthalmol* 1995; **79**; 1093–1097.

275 Yamashita K, Muir WW, Tsubakishita S, *et al.* Infusion of guaifenesin, ketamine, and medetomidine in combination with inhalation of sevoflurane versus inhalation of sevoflurane alone for anesthesia of horses. *J Am Vet Med Assoc* 2002; **221**: 1150–1155.

276 Bettschart-Wolfensberger R, Jaggin-Schmucker N, Lendl C, *et al.* Minimal alveolar concentration of desflurane in combination with an infusion of medetomidine for the anaesthesia of ponies. *Vet Rec* 2001; **148**: 264–267.

277 Ringer SK, Kalchofner K, Boller J, *et al.* A clinical comparison of two anaesthetic protocols using lidocaine or medetomidine in horses. *Vet Anaesth Analg* 2007; **34**: 257–268.

278 Robertson SA. Standing sedation and pain management for ophthalmic patients. *Vet Clin Equine* 2004; **20**: 485–497.

279 Cutler TJ. Diseases and surgery of the globe and orbit. In: Gilger BC, ed. *Equine Ophthalmology*. St Louis, MO: Saunders Elsevier, 2005; 63–106.

280 Robertson SA, Sanchez LC, Merritt AM, *et al.* Effect of systemic lidocaine on visceral and somatic nociception in conscious horses. *Equine Vet J* 2005; **37**: 122–127.

281 Murrell JC, White KL, Johnson CB, *et al.* Investigation of the EEG effects of intravenous lidocaine during halothane anaesthesia in ponies. *Vet Anaesth Analg* 2005; **32**: 212–221.

282 282.Valverde A, Gunkel C, Doherty TJ, *et al.* Effect of a constant rate infusion of lidocaine on the quality of recovery from sevoflurane or isoflurane general anesthesia in horses. *Equine Vet J* 2005; **37**: 559–564.

283 Parviainen AKJ, Trim CM. Complications associated with anaesthesia for ocular surgery: a retrospective study 1989–1996. *Equine Vet J* 2000; **32**: 555–559.

284 Santos M, Fuente M, Garcia-Iturralde G, *et al.* Effects of alpha-2 adrenoceptor agonists during recovery from isoflurane anaesthesia in horses. *Equine Vet J* 2003; **35**: 170–175.

285 Hubbell JAE, Muir WW. Peripheral muscle relaxants. In: Muir WW, Hubbell JAE, eds. *Equine Anesthesia*, 2nd edn. St Louis, MO: Saunders Elsevier, 2009; 358–368.

286 Clark-Price SC, Posner LP, Gleed RD. Recovery of horses from general anesthesia in a darkened or illuminated recovery stall. *Vet Anaesth Analg* 2008; **35**: 473–479.

287 Patipa LA, Sherlock CE, Witte SH, *et al.* Risk factors for colic in equids hospitalized for ocular disease. *J Am Vet Med Assoc* 2012; **240**: 1488–1493.

53 Neonatal and Pediatric Patients

Tamara L. Grubb[1], Tania E. Perez Jimenez[2] and Glenn R. Pettifer[3]

[1]Veterinary Clinical Sciences, Washington State University, Pullman, Washington, USA
[2]College of Veterinary Medicine, Washington State University, Pullman, Washington, USA
[3]College of Veterinarians of Ontario, Guelph, Ontario, Canada

Chapter contents

Introduction

With constantly advancing surgical techniques that promote correction of congenital defects in neonatal/pediatric patients and with the drive for 'early' spay/neuter programs (patients <6 weeks of age), extremely young patients have become a larger portion of our anesthetic caseload. In these patients, physiologic and pathologic immaturity or dysmaturity can impact the ability of the patient to tolerate anesthesia and increase the risk of anesthetic complications. Foals less than 1 month of age have been shown to be at increased risk for anesthetic death [1]. Puppies and kittens are also likely to be at increased risk. Although the neonatal/pediatric age group was not addressed in a recent study or factors contributing to anesthetic death in small animals, small body size did contribute to anesthetic risk for death and certainly neonatal/pediatric patients would fit into the small body category [2]. Attention to the unique physiology and particular requirements of individuals within neonatal/pediatric age group will improve our ability to provide safe, effective anesthesia and analgesia.

Physiology of neonatal and pediatric animals

Much of our knowledge of the delivery of anesthesia to pediatric/neonatal animals is based on our experience with young to middle-aged animals, or is extrapolated from information obtained from human neonates. Although the process of maturation and aging varies greatly between individual animals, species, and breeds, the neonatal and pediatric phases of life can be roughly defined. In dogs and cats, the neonatal period extends for the first 6 weeks of life and the pediatric period for the first 12 weeks [3–5]. Foals and calves are generally considered to be physiologically mature by 4–6 weeks of age [6].

Compared with young and middle-aged adults, neonatal and pediatric patients have a limited organ reserve, a decreased ability to respond to a physiologic challenge or change, and decreased dose requirements for some anesthetic and analgesic drugs. This results in an increased risk of perianesthetic complications in neonates, necessitating judicious administration of anesthetics and vigilant monitoring.

The physiology of neonates results in differences in pharmacokinetics and pharmacodynamics that contribute to altered response to drugs. These differences include the following.

- Hypoalbuminemia, which results in a greater free, active portion of protein-bound drugs. This may increase the response to highly protein-bound drugs like barbiturates, ketamine, etomidate, and the non-steroidal anti-inflammatory drugs (NSAIDs), although the clinical relevance of altered protein binding has been questioned (see Chapter 7).
- Increased permeability of the neonatal blood–brain barrier, which enables a larger percentage of a drug dose to reach the brain.
- An increased percentage of body water content, which alters the volume of distribution of some drugs. In foals, extracellular fluid volume is 43% of body weight, compared with 22% of body weight in adult horses [7]. The larger extracellular fluid volume results in a greater apparent volume of distribution of drugs that are highly ionized in plasma or relatively polar (e.g., NSAIDs).
- A circulating fluid volume that is fixed and relatively centralized, making the neonatal patient more susceptible to hypovolemia. The centralized circulation also causes greater delivery of anesthetic drugs to the highly perfused tissues, including the brain.
- Low body fat percentage, resulting in a smaller adipose tissue compartment for drug redistribution [8]. In foals, for example, total body fat is 2–3%, compared with 5% in adult horses [9].
- Lower hepatic enzymatic activity for the first 3–4 weeks (perhaps up to 12 weeks, particularly in small animals) of life [10–12] which can lead to prolongation of effects with drugs (or lower concentrations of active metabolites) that depend on hepatic metabolism for biotransformation.

Veterinary Anesthesia and Analgesia: The Fifth Edition of Lumb and Jones.
Edited by Kurt A. Grimm, Leigh A. Lamont, William J. Tranquilli, Stephen A. Greene and Sheilah A. Robertson.

- Lower glomerular filtration rate (GFR) in small animals for the first 2–3 weeks of life and slower tubular secretion for the first 4–8 weeks of life [10,13,14] which can lead to prolonged effects of drugs (or active metabolites of drugs) dependent on renal excretion. For example, the half-life of diazepam is increased in neonates due to decreased renal excretion [11]. Although the kidneys mature more rapidly in foals and calves (the GFR is at levels seen in mature animals by 2–4 days of life and tubular secretion by 2 weeks of life) [6,10] development of renal function may be prolonged in unhealthy or dysmature animals.
- A high metabolic rate with a concomitant higher rate of oxygen consumption. This necessitates the need for minute ventilation that is much greater than that of adults. Because of the increase in ventilation, anesthetic induction with inhalant anesthetics can occur more rapidly.

In addition to physiologic differences that result in altered clinical pharmacology of anesthetics, neonatal physiology alone can contribute to increased anesthetic risk (Table 53.1). These physiologic differences include the following.

- Compared with the adult heart, the neonatal heart has less contractile tissue per gram of myocardial tissue, and ventricular compliance is limited [15]. Stroke volume and cardiac reserve are limited in pediatric patients, and cardiac output is more dependent on heart rate. Furthermore, the resting cardiac index is much higher in neonates than adults and is very close to maximal cardiac index, making the cardiac reserve minimal. An adult can increase cardiac output by 300%, whereas the neonate can only increase output by 30% [16].
- The sympathetic nervous system is not fully functional in neonates, and sympathetic stimulation results in only minimal increases in heart rate and contractility, further impairing the ability to increase cardiac output [14]. Immaturity also manifests in poor vasomotor control and an incomplete or inadequate hypotension-induced baroresponse.

Table 53.1 Unique physiologic characteristics of neonatal and pediatric patients that may affect anesthesia (NOTE: the changes listed below are general changes associated with age but may not be present in all neonatal/pediatric patients).

Physiologic characteristic	Effect on anesthesia
General characteristics Hypoalbuminemia Increased permeability of blood–brain barrier Low percentage of body fat Circulating fluid volume is centralized Immature thermoregulatory system	Exaggerated effect from standard drug dosage for young adult patients, decreased dosage required; decreased tolerance to fluid load, don't overhydrate; hypothermia contributes to delayed recovery, keep warm
Renal/urinary system Immature renal function	Prolonged duration of action of renally cleared drugs, may prolong recovery time; decreased tolerance to fluid load, don't overhydrate
Hepatic system Immature hepatic function	Prolonged duration of hepatically cleared drugs, may prolong recovery time
Respiratory system High metabolic rate with high oxygen consumption High minute volume Limited pulmonary reserve Pliable rib cage	Decreased respiratory reserve, both oxygen and ventilatory support are required for most patients; mask induction occurs extremely quickly, induction must be closely supervised
Cardiovascular system Limited myocardial contractile tissue; low ventricular compliance; limited cardiac reserve; cardiac output heart rate dependent; poor vasomotor control	Decreased cardiac reserve, cardiovascular system must be supported with IV fluids and some patients may need chronotropic support

- Fetal circulation may persist for variable lengths of time. For example, normal healthy foals have a right-to-left intracardiac shunt for the first 3 days of life, and the duration of the shunt is often extended in unhealthy or dysmature foals [17].
- In the first 1–3 days (foals and calves) or 1–2 weeks of life (puppies and kittens), the kidneys may be less efficient than adult kidneys at eliminating fluid load and regulating electrolytes, so goal-directed use of appropriate intravenous fluids is necessary [8,10]. Rapid or excessive fluid administration may result in edema.
- Pulmonary functional reserve is minimal, increasing the risk of hypoxia during apnea or airway obstruction. The neonatal rib cage is very compliant, resulting in less efficient ventilation and greater work of breathing. This predisposes young patients to hypoxia and ventilatory fatigue, especially in the event of airway obstruction (e.g., endotracheal tube plugged with mucus) or respiratory disease.
- Alveolar minute ventilation is relatively high in neonates, raising the alveolar ventilation:functional residual capacity ratio above that of adults. Closing volume is higher in the neonate and overlaps within the lower range of the tidal volume. These factors make the neonate more susceptible to hypoxemia and increase the rapidity with which anesthesia is induced with inhalant drugs.
- Following birth, the production of erythropoietin is decreased because of the increased *extra-utero* oxygenation compared to *intra-utero*. This decrease leads to decreased production of erythrocytes. In small animals, the hematocrit (and with it, the hemoglobin) decreases by more than a third in the first 28 days of life [18,19]. Thus, even minor hemorrhage can greatly affect oxygen delivery to tissues.
- Neonates are more susceptible to hypothermia because of their immature thermoregulatory system, high body surface to mass ratio, and limited ability to vasoconstrict to conserve heat.

Anesthesia

Preparation for anesthesia

A thorough physical examination, including careful auscultation of the heart, is an essential component of preanesthetic assessment. Hydration status and fluid requirements should be evaluated. Fluid deficits should be corrected prior to anesthesia when possible. Preanesthetic blood analysis often includes a minimum of hematocrit, total and fractionated protein, and blood glucose. Other blood or serum chemistry analysis and diagnostic procedures should be performed as indicated from the history and physical exam. Neonates that are still suckling should not be held off food prior to anesthesia. Pediatric animals that are eating solid food should be denied food for only 3–4 h prior to anesthesia and should not be denied water at any time. The risk of hypoglycemia should be weighed against the risk of regurgitation and aspiration in each individual patient and fasting recommendations altered accordingly.

Anesthetic drugs

As with patients of any age, anesthetic drugs should be titrated 'to effect' and patients closely monitored. This is especially prudent in neonatal/pediatric patients because of physiologic changes that may result in unanticipated drug effects. The potential for adverse anesthetic effects is not solely dictated by drug dosing and may be more complicated than previously realized. General anesthesia has been implicated in cellular apoptosis with resultant neuronal degeneration in rodent, non-human primate, and human neonates [20]. Although the clinical impact of this degeneration is unknown, long-term behavioral and cognitive deficits have been identified in some rodents and non-human primates [20]. Of the drugs tested, ketamine and isoflurane appear to be the most likely to cause neuronal degeneration [21]. However, higher dosages than are clinically common were used in some studies, [21] decreasing the likelihood of an adverse impact when the drugs are used in clinical settings.

Premedication and pain management

Because of the immaturity of the neonatal nervous system, it has been a commonly held theory that mammalian neonates are incapable of experiencing pain. However, neonatal and pediatric humans experience pain [22] and pain experienced at an extremely young age may lead to changes in nociceptive processes, which could result in chronic pain conditions later in life [23]. These changes can also occur in neonatal and pediatric veterinary species. Using an EEG model to detect the response to pain of castration, Johnson *et al.* demonstrated that neonatal lambs progressed from almost no response at 3 h after birth to an 'adult-like' response at 1 week of age [24]. This might indicate that the often accepted practice of tail docking or dewclaw removal in extremely young patients without analgesia is acceptable. However, in a subsequent study, lambs castrated without analgesia at 1 day of age had increased expression of pain-related behaviors when their tails were docked at 1 month of age when compared to lambs that had been castrated without analgesia at 10 days of age followed by tail docking at 1 month of age [25]. This indicates that procedures performed in the early neonatal period can have increased pain-associated behavior later in life, perhaps because of alteration in inhibitory responses to pain. In addition to potentially limiting long-term effects on the nociceptive pathway, appropriate analgesia reduces the dose of drugs needed to maintain general anesthesia. This should improve anesthetic risk by decreasing dose-dependent adverse events.

Neonatal and pediatric patients often require lower dosages for most drugs. However, analgesic drug doses in some phases of human pediatric development are higher than those of adults [26,27]. The implication of this in veterinary medicine is that similar age-related dose adjustments may occur and emphasizes that analgesic drugs should be dosed 'to effect' rather than on a adult dose [28].

Opioid effects are reversible, making them an excellent choice for analgesia in neonates and pediatrics with limited metabolism. Adverse effects from opioids are usually manageable when used appropriately in adult animals but may be more problematic in neonatal patients. However, as the patient ages, adverse effects caused by opioids (specifically morphine and fentanyl) have been shown to decrease over the first month of life in dogs [29]. The specific opioid selected may influence the risk of adverse events. In puppies less than 1 month of age, morphine has been shown to cause more respiratory depression than equivalent doses of fentanyl [30]. Partial opioid recptor agonists (buprenorphine) and agonist-antagonists (butorphanol) appear to cause minimal cardiovascular and respiratory effects. Selection of an appropriate opioid should be based on the particular analgesic requirements of the intended procedure and the health status of the patient.

Local or regional blockade with local anesthetic drugs can provide anesthesia/analgesia. The reduction of general anesthetic requirements is of benefit in neonatal and pediatric patients. NSAIDs may be another option in older pediatric patients, but routine use of this class of drugs should be reserved for patients which are more developed with mature, competent renal and cardiovascular function.

Sedation may not be necessary in quiet or debilitated patients but sedatives can alleviate stress in anxious patients and decrease requirements of drugs needed for induction and maintenance of anesthesia. The adverse effects of longer acting sedatives should be weighed against the adverse effects of the shorter acting and titratable anesthetic drugs needed to induce and maintain anesthesia. The opioids often provide adequate sedation when used alone in neonatal and pediatric patients and have the added advantages of providing analgesia and producing effects that are reversible. Although benzodiazepines do not provide analgesia, they are reversible and produce little to no cardiovascular and respiratory depression. Benzodiazepines can produce adequate sedation in young patients, but may not produce consistent or deep sedation, and combination with other drugs (most commonly the opioids) may increase the likelihood that they provide sedation when used in healthy pediatric patients. The judicious use of low doses of α_2-adrenergic receptor agonists may be considered in selected pediatric patients with a healthy cardiovascular system. However, drugs in this class produce cardiovascular effects (increased peripheral vascular resistance, bradycardia, and decreased cardiac output) that may be detrimental to very young animals. Low dosages of xylazine have been shown to be safe and effective in foals as young as 10 days of age [31]. Acepromazine may be used for sedation of healthy pediatric animals, but the cardiovascular effects, including hypotension, may be poorly tolerated in neonatal and/or diseased animals. The vasodilation caused by acepromazine can also contribute to the development of hypothermia. Acepromazine is not reversible and does not provide analgesia.

The routine use of anticholinergics in adult veterinary patients is not often advocated. However, neonates depend on heart rate for maintenance of cardiac output so anticholinergics may be useful to treat or prevent bradycardia-associated hypotension.

Induction

Anesthesia can be induced by using a variety of anesthetic drugs. Mask delivery of inhaled anesthetics has been reported but use of inhalants alone (i.e., without concurrent administration of sedative or other anesthetic drugs) has been shown to increase the risk of anesthesia-related mortality in both small animals [2] and foals [1]. Thus, inhalant induction is no longer recommended as a routine induction technique and should be reserved for cases where animal behavior or medical conditions require inhalant induction.

Propofol, alfaxalone, and etomidate administration can be titrated. These drugs are rapidly redistributed and biotransformed by several routes so that termination of activity does not depend on the function of a single organ system [32]. Propofol has been studied for induction and maintenance of anesthesia in dogs <12 weeks of age following premedication with oxymorphone and atropine [33]. This protocol provided the 'best quality' and was deemed 'most effective' when compared to protocols that included other premedicants or other induction drugs such as tiletamine/zolazepam. Propofol has also been effectively and safely used to induce and maintain anesthesia in neontatal foals [34]. Alfaxalone has been studied for induction in dogs <12 weeks old following premedication of acepromazine, atropine and morphine [35] and in foals [36]. Alfaxalone can cause cardiovascular and respiratory depression similar to propofol [37,38]. Etomidate use has not been specifically reported in neonatal or pediatric animals but the drug is commonly used in neonatal and pediatric humans. As with adults, etomidate can cause adrenal insufficiency in septic neonates [39] but does not appear to cause long-term changes in adrenocortical function in healthy neonates [40]. Ketamine, in combination with a benzodiazepine, causes only mild respiratory depression and may actually improve cardiovascular function through stimulation of the sympathetic nervous system [41]. However, the latter response may be reduced in neonates because of their immature sympathetic nervous system. Ketamine requires either hepatic metabolism or renal clearance for termination of activity; thus, the effects of ketamine may be prolonged in patients with immature hepatic and renal systems [41]. Ketamine has been widely used in human neonates but use may become more controversial if the fears of ketamine-induced neuronal degeneration are valid [20,21].

Maintenance

Inhaled anesthetic drugs are minimally metabolized and primarily eliminated by the lungs, and are thus ideal for maintenance of anesthesia in animals with immature hepatic or renal function. However, inhaled anesthetic drugs do cause hypotension (secondary to both vasodilation and decreased cardiac contractility), hypoventilation, and hypothermia. Because of these adverse effects, inhaled anesthetic drug administration should be titrated and the patient must be carefully monitored to avoid serious complications. The concurrent administration of analgesic and sedative drugs will reduce the inhaled anesthetic dose required for maintenance of anesthesia.

Support

Along with a carefully chosen anesthetic protocol and appropriate drug dosing, physiologic support and vigilant monitoring are important during anesthesia to minimize patient risk. Compared with adults, fluid requirements are greater in neonates (60–180 mL/kg/day) [42] because of their greater body surface area, immature renal function (decreased ability to concentrate urine), higher percentage of body water, and higher respiratory rates leading to greater fluid losses [11]. However, overhydration should be avoided, because renal clearance may be limited and excessive dilution of serum protein can occur more readily in animals with pre-existing hypoalbuminemia. Using monitored endpoints (e.g., arterial blood pressure, lactate, heart rate) as a guide will facilitate making fluid administration decisions.

Neonates have minimal stores of hepatic glycogen and are prone to hypoglycemia, so periodic measurement of blood glucose is helpful. Hypoglycemia can be corrected or prevented with administration of dextrose-containing fluids.

Neonatal and pediatric animals are highly susceptible to hypothermia because of their high body surface area to body mass ratio. Every reasonable effort should be made to maintain body temperature. Hypothermia decreases anesthetic requirements, increases the incidence of adverse myocardial outcomes in high-risk patients, increases the incidence of surgical wound infection, adversely affects antibody- and cell-mediated immune defenses, changes the kinetics and action of various anesthetic and paralyzing agents, increases thermal discomfort, is associated with delayed postanesthetic recovery, [43] and may be a contributing factor in anesthesia-related death [2]. Shivering causes an increase in oxygen consumption (up to 200–300%), and this increased oxygen demand may not be met by an increase in oxygen delivery, particularly if anesthetic-induced hypoventilation occurs.

Monitoring is critical for the early detection of potential problems during the entire anesthetic period and well into recovery. In the perioperative mortality study by Brodbelt, [2] many factors significantly contributed to patient mortality but patient monitoring significantly decreased risk of death. Clinically acceptable ranges and/or normal values of commonly monitored indices can be different in neonates than in adults; therefore the anesthetist should be familiar with the acceptable ranges for each species and age group of individuals that are being anesthetized. Generally, neonatal and pediatric animals have a higher heart rate but lower blood pressure than adults. The normal heart rate in conscious neonatal dogs and cats is approximately 200–220 beats per minute, and the respiratory rate is approximately 15–40 breaths per minute [44]. Mean arterial blood pressure measured in 1-month-old puppies is only 49 mmHg [45]. The average heart rate in foals 1–2 days of age ranges from 70 to 90 beats per minute, and the normal respiratory rate is 30–40 breaths per minute [46,47].

Summary

Appropriate anesthetic management of neonatal and pediatric animals is often different than for adults. Patient evaluation and assessment, preoperative correction of identified abnormalities, vigilant perianesthetic monitoring, careful titration of anesthetic drugs, provision of analgesia, and appropriate perianesthetic support will all influence patient risk.

References

1 Johnston GM, Taylor PM, Holmes MA, *et al.* Confidential enquiry of perioperative equine fatalities (CEPEF-1): preliminary results. *Equine Vet J* 1995; **27**: 193–200.

2 Brodbelt DC. Perioperative mortality in small animal anaesthesia. *Vet J* 2009; **182**: 152–161.

3 Robinson EP. Anaesthesia of pediatric patients. *Compend Contin Educ Pract Vet* 1983; **5**: 1004–1011.

4 Breazile JE. Neurologic and behavioral development in the puppy. *Vet Clin North Am Small Anim Pract* 1978; **8**: 31–45.

5 Fox MW. *Canine Pediatrics*. Springfield, IL: Charles C Thomas, 1966.

6 Tranquilli WJ, Thurmon JC. Management of anesthesia in the foal. *Vet Clin North Am Equine Pract* 1990; **6**: 651–663.

7 Kami G, Merritt AM, Duelly P. Preliminary studies of plasma and extracellular fluid volume in neonatal ponies. *Equine Vet J* 1984; **16**: 356–358.

8 Baggot JD. Drug therapy in the neonatal animal. In: Baggot JD, ed. *Principles of Drug Disposition in Domestic Animals: The Basis of Veterinary Clinical Pharmacology*. Philadelphia: WB Saunders, 1992; 21–26.

9 Webb AI, Weaver BMQ. Body composition of the horse. *Equine Vet J* 1979; **11**: 39–47.

10 Baggot JD, Short CR. Drug disposition in the neonatal animal, with particular reference to the foal. *Equine Vet J* 1987; **19**: 169–171.

11 Boothe DM, Tannert K. Special considerations for drug and fluid therapy in the pediatric patient. *Compend Contin Educ Pract Vet* 1992; **14**: 313–329.

12 Short CR. Drug disposition in neonatal animals. *J Am Vet Med Assoc* 1984; **184**: 1161–1163.

13 Thurmon JC, Tranquilli WJ, Benson GJ, *et al.* Anesthesia for special patients: neonatal and geriatric patients. In: Thurmon JC, Tranquilli WJ, Benson GJ, eds. *Lumb and Jones' Veterinary Anesthesia*, 3rd edn. Baltimore, MD: Williams and Wilkins, 1996; 844–848.

14 Meyer RE. Anesthesia for neonatal and geriatric patients. In: Short CE, ed. *Principles and Practices of Veterinary Anesthesia*. Baltimore, MD: Williams and Wilkins, 1987; 330–337.

15 Friedman WF. The intrinsic physiologic properties of the developing heart. *Prog Cardiovasc Dis* 1972; **15**: 87–111.

16 Friedman WF, George BL. Treatment of congestive heart failure by altering loading conditions of the heart. *J Pediatr* 1985; **106**: 697–706.

17 Thomas WP, Madigan JE, Backus KQ, *et al.* Systemic and pulmonary haemodynamics in normal neonatal foals. *J Reprod Fertil* 1987; **35**: 623–628.

18 Earl FL, Melveger BE, Wilson RL. The hemogram and bone marrow profile of normal neonatal and weanling beagle dogs. *Lab Anim Sci* 1973; **23**: 690–695.

19 Meyers-Wallen VN, Haskins ME, Patterson DF. Hematologic values in healthy neonatal, weanling and juvenile kittens. *Am J Vet Res* 1984; **45**: 1322–1327.

20 Loftis GK, Collins S, McDowell M. Anesthesia-induced neuronal apoptosis during synaptogenesis: a review of the literature. *AANA J* 2012; **80**: 291–298.

21 Mellon RD, Simone AF, Rappaport BA. Use of anesthetic agents in neonates and young children. *Anesth Analg* 2007; **104**: 509–520.

22 Buskila D, Neumann L, Zmora E, *et al.* Pain sensitivity in prematurely born adolescents. *Arch Pediatr Adolesc Med* 2003; **157**: 1079–1082.

23 Grunnau RE. Long-term consequences of pain in neonates. In: Anand KJS, Stevens BJ, McGrath PJ, eds. *Pain in Neonates*. Amsterdam, Netherlands: Elsevier, 2000; 55–76.

24 Johnson CB, Sylvester SP, Stafford KJ, *et al.* Effects of age on the electroencephalographic response to castration in lambs anaesthetized with halothane in oxygen from birth to 6 weeks old. *Vet Anaesth Analg* 2009; **36**: 273–279.

25 McCracken L, Waran N, Mitchinson S, *et al.* Effect of age at castration on the behavioral response to tail docking (abstract). Proceedings of the New Zealand Biomedical and Medical Societies, 2006.

26 Collins JJ. Palliative care and the child with cancer. *Hematol Oncol Clin North Am* 2002; **16**: 657–670.

27 Berde CB, Sethna NF. Analgesics for the treatment of pain in children. *N Engl J Med* 2002; **347**: 1094–1103.

28 Mathews KA. Pain management for the pregnant, lactating, and neonatal to pediatric cat and dog. *Vet Clin North Am Small Anim Pract* 2008; **38**: 1291–1308.

29 Luks AM, Zwass MS, Brown RC, *et al.* Opioid-induced analgesia in neonatal dogs: pharmacodynamic differences between morphine and fentanyl. *J Pharmacol Exp Ther* 1998; **284**: 136–141.

30 Bragg P, Zwass MS, Lau M *et al.* Opioid pharmacodynamics in neonatal dogs: differences between morphine and fentanyl. *J Appl Physiol* 1995; **79**: 1519–1524.

31 Carter SW, Robertson SA, Steel CA, *et al.* Cardiopulmonary effects of xylazine sedation in the foal. *Equine Vet J* 1990; **22**: 384–388.

32 Simons PJ, Cockshott ID, Glen JB, *et al.* Disposition and pharmacology of propofol glucuronide administered intravenously to animals. *Xenobiotica* 1992; **22**: 1267–1273.

33 Fagella AM, Aronsohn MG. Evaluation of anesthetic protocols for neutering 6- to 14-week-old pups. *J Am Vet Med Assoc* 1993; **205**: 308–314.

34 Chaffin MK, Walker MA, McArthur NH, *et al.* Magnetic resonance imaging of the brain of normal neonatal foals. *Vet Radiol Ultrasound* 1997; **38**: 102–111.

35 O'Hagan B, Pasloske K, McKinnon C, *et al.* Clinical evaluation of alfaxalone as an anaesthetic induction agent in dogs less than 12 weeks of age. *Aust Vet J* 2012; **90**: 346–350.

36 Goodwin W, Keates H, Pasloske K, *et al.* Plasma pharmacokinetics and pharmacodynamics of alfaxalone in neonatal foals after an intravenous bolus of alfaxalone following premedication with butorphanol tartrate. *Vet Anaesth Analg* 2012; **39**: 503–510

37 Amengual M, Flaherty D, Auckburally A, *et al.* An evaluation of anaesthetic induction in healthy dogs using rapid intravenous injection of propofol or alfaxalone. *Vet Anaesth Analg* 2013; **40**: 115–123.

38 Maney JK, Shepard MK, Braun C, *et al.* A comparison of cardiopulmonary and anesthetic effects of an induction dose of alfaxalone or propofol in dogs. *Vet Anaesth Analg* 2013; **40**: 237–244.

39 Den Brinker M, Joosten KF, Liem O, *et al.* Adrenal insufficiency in meningococcal sepsis: bioavailable cortisol levels and impact of interleukin-6 levels and intubation with etomidate on adrenal function and mortality. *J Clin Endocrinol Metab* 2005; **90**: 5110–5117.

40 Sokolove PE, Price DD, Okada P. The safety of etomidate for emergency rapid sequence intubation of pediatric patients. *Pediatr Emerg Care* 2000; **16**: 18–21.

41 Wright M. Pharmacologic effects of ketamine and its use in veterinary medicine. *J Am Vet Med Assoc* 1982; **180**: 1462–1471.

42 Mosier JE. Canine pediatrics: the neonate. *AAHA Sci Present* 1981; **48**: 339–347.

43 Doufas AG. Consequences of inadvertent perioperative hypothermia. *Best Pract Res Clin Anaesthesiol* 2003; **17**: 535–549.

44 England GCW. Care of the neonate and fading pups. In: Ettinger SJ, Feldman EC, eds. *Veterinary Internal Medicine*, 7th edn. St Louis, MO: Elsevier, 2010; 1949–1954.

45 McMicheal M, Dhupa N. Pediatric critical care medicine: physiologic considerations. *Compend Contin Educ Pract Vet* 2000; **22**: 206–214.

46 Rossdale PD. Clinical studies in the newborn thoroughbred foal. II. Heart rate, auscultation and electrocardiogram. *Br Vet J* 1967; **123**: 521–532.

47 Rossdale PD. Some parameters of respiratory function in normal and abnormal newborn foals with specific reference to levels of PaO_2 during air and oxygen inhalation. *Res Vet Sci* 1970; **11**: 270–276.

54 Senior and Geriatric Patients

Tamara L. Grubb[1], Tania E. Perez Jimenez[2] and Glenn R. Pettifer[3]

[1] Veterinary Clinical Sciences, Washington State University, Pullman, Washington, USA
[2] College of Veterinary Medicine, Washington State University, Pullman, Washington, USA
[3] College of Veterinarians of Ontario, Guelph, Ontario, Canada

Chapter contents

Introduction

Companion animals are living increasingly longer lives and roughly 30% of the animal population is now considered to be geriatric [1–3]. Aging causes physiologic and pathologic changes, in addition to the presence of concurrent disease, that can impact the ability of the patient to tolerate anesthesia and surgery. These factors combine to increase anesthetic risk of mortality by as much as a factor of 7 in dogs and cats over 12 years of age [4]. Increasing age also increases the anesthetic risk in horses [5,6]. Attention to the unique physiology, presence of concurrent disease and particular requirements of individuals within the 'senior' age group will contribute to the provision of safe, effective anesthesia and analgesia.

Physiology of geriatric animals

The effect of age *per se* on perioperative morbidity and mortality appears to be related to the decreased physiologic reserve of the various organ systems that occur with aging. Aging is a progressive process that results in unavoidable alterations in organ system function. Within organ systems, reductions in functional reserve manifest as a decreased capacity for adaptation, a predisposition to the failure of homeostasis, and a reduced ability to respond to external stress. The effects of disease, stress, lack of exercise, genetics, malnutrition, and environment may hasten changes associated with aging. The time course of the aging process varies between organ systems within the same individual and between individuals. Assessment of the influence of aging on anatomic and physiologic function in animals is further complicated by the marked variations in life span and life expectancy within and between species. The campaign for 'senior at 7' is reasonable to aid in educating small animal owners about geriatric health issues. However, there is little correlation between chronologic and physiologic age.

For the purposes of this discussion, geriatric animals are considered to be those that have attained 75% of their expected life span [7]. With this definition, some giant breed dogs may be at the end of their expected life span at 7 years of age while toy breeds and cats may only be in early to mid-adulthood. For large animals, few definitions are available, but horses greater than 20 years of age could be considered geriatric [8,9].

Much of our knowledge of the impact of the aging process in animals is extrapolated from data obtained in aging humans. However, the impact of aging on physiologic systems should be similar across mammalian species and we can conclude that age-associated pathophysiologic changes in organ systems (Table 54.1) can potentially influence anesthetic management in veterinary patients. Cardiovascular changes are multifactorial, reflecting not only age-related degeneration but also age-related disease. In the absence of a particular cardiovascular disease, the major anatomic changes in aging hearts include an increase in the severity of myocardial fibrosis, valvular fibrocalcification, and ventricular wall thickening. Variable degrees of myocardial fiber atrophy result in decreased pump function and cardiac output. The heart rate may be affected if the pacemaker cells are involved. Fibrosis of the endocardium and valves leads to decreased compliance. Valvular incompetence may accompany valvular fibrocalcification. The vascular tree gradually loses elasticity, resulting in a decrease in distensibility, increased resistance to left ventricular output, and progressive hypertrophy of the ventricle. As ventricular hypertrophy and decreased chamber elasticity progress, the aging heart is more dependent on atrial contraction for diastolic ventricular filling. Thus, the atrial kick and normal sinus rhythm become more important in the maintenance of appropriate cardiac output [10,11]. It is difficult to make an all-encompassing statement about cardiovascular status since cardiac output in geriatric dogs can be

Veterinary Anesthesia and Analgesia: The Fifth Edition of Lumb and Jones.
Edited by Kurt A. Grimm, Leigh A. Lamont, William J. Tranquilli, Stephen A. Greene and Sheilah A. Robertson.

Table 54.1 Unique physiologic characteristics of geriatric patients that may affect anesthesia (NOTE: the changes listed below are general changes associated with age but may not be present in all geriatric patients).

Physiologic characteristic	Effect on anesthesia
General characteristics Hypoalbuminemia Neuronal degeneration Decrease in neurons and neurotransmitters Decrease in skeletal muscle Increase in body fat Impaired thermoregulatory system	Exaggerated effect from standard drug dosage for young adult patients, decreased dosage required; decreased tolerance to fluid load, don't overhydrate; fat may act as drug reservoir and contribute to delayed recovery; hypothermia contributes to delayed recovery, keep warm
Renal/urinary system Decreased RBF, GFR and tubular function Decreased filtration rate and excretory capacity	Prolonged duration of action of renally cleared drugs, may prolong recovery time; decreased tolerance to fluid load, don't overhydrate
Hepatic system Decreased hepatic mass and hepatic blood flow	Prolonged duration of action of hepatically cleared drugs, may prolong recovery time
Respiratory system Loss of strength of muscles of ventilation Thorax becomes rigid, lungs lose elasticity Increased closing volume Reduction in arterial oxygen	Decreased respiratory reserve, both oxygen and ventilatory support are required for most patients
Cardiovascular system Myocardial atrophy; fibrosis of the endocardium; decreased myocardial contractility; loss of vascular distensibility; maximum heart rate decreases, cardiac output is SV dependent; SNS less responsive to stress; decreased vasoconstrictor and baroreceptor responses	Decreased cardiac reserve, cardiovascular system must be supported with IV fluids and some patients may need chronotropic or inotropic support; anticipate need for dopamine or dobutamine

GFR = glomerular filtration rate; RBF = renal blood flow; SV = stroke volume; SNS = sympathetic nervous system.

decreased, [12] not different, [13] or even increased [14] relative to young adult dogs.

In geriatric individuals, the maximal chronotropic response during physiologic stress decreases. In addition, despite higher endogenous levels of norepinephrine, the response to stress is decreased. This appears to be due to receptor attrition and reduced affinity for agonist molecules. Whereas young adults increase cardiac output primarily through increased heart rate, geriatrics increase cardiac output by increasing stroke volume in association with an increase in end-diastolic volume. Thus, geriatric individuals rely more on preload than do younger animals and are not as tolerant of volume depletion in the perianesthetic period. This said, fit individuals maintain high levels of cardiac output and oxygen consumption, and reductions in cardiac index occur in direct proportion to reductions in skeletal muscle mass and metabolic rate associated with reductions in lean tissue mass [10,11,15].

Pulmonary changes associated with aging include a decrease in ventilatory volumes and a reduction in the efficiency of gas exchange. Vital capacity, total lung capacity, and maximum breathing capacity decrease as the intercostal and diaphragmatic muscle mass is reduced and the thorax becomes more rigid and less compliant. Functional alveoli and elasticity progressively decrease. As pulmonary elasticity decreases as a result of decreases in lung elastin, the ratio of residual volume and of functional residual capacity to total lung capacity increases. Closing volume is increased, resulting in air trapping and an increase in ventilation-perfusion mismatch. As a result, PaO_2 decreases with age [16].

In the central nervous system, aging is associated with a reduction in brain size that occurs with the loss of neurons. Cerebrospinal fluid volume increases to maintain normal intracranial pressure. Despite this loss in brain tissue, functional and anatomic redundancy within the nervous system provides for the maintenance of functioning at levels that approximate those observed at somatic maturity. With the loss of brain tissue, cerebral blood flow decreases, but cerebral autoregulation of blood flow is well maintained. In addition to the loss of functional neurons in aging individuals, generalized depletions of dopamine, norepinephrine, tyrosine, and serotonin occur. Receptor affinity for neurotransmitters may be reduced. Compared with the neuronal plasticity observed in the young, this process is slower and less complete in geriatric individuals. As a result of these functional and anatomic changes in the central nervous system, geriatric individuals generally have a decreased requirement for anesthetic agents. The minimum alveolar concentration for inhalant anesthetics decreases linearly with age, and the requirement for local anesthetics, opioids, barbiturates, benzodiazepines, and other intravenous drugs is likely similarly reduced [10,17,18].

With aging, there is a primary loss of cortical kidney mass and functional nephron units. Total renal blood flow decreases with age, with the majority of the loss occurring in the renal cortex. In humans, one-half of the glomeruli present in the young adult atrophy or are non-functional by the age of 80. Glomerular filtration rate decreases, partly in response to a reduction in renal plasma flow. Geriatric individuals are less responsive to antidiuretic hormone and have an impaired ability to conserve sodium or concentrate urine. A reduction in renal blood flow makes the geriatric animal more susceptible to renal failure in the face of renal ischemia. Since geriatric patients cannot maximally retain sodium or water under conditions of volume depletion, the ability to correct fluid, electrolyte, and acid–base disturbances or to tolerate hemodynamic insults is reduced. Because geriatric patients have difficulty excreting a salt and water load, vigorous fluid and electrolyte therapy may result in excessive intravascular and extravascular volume, with the possible sequelae of congestive heart failure and peripheral edema. Those anesthetic drugs eliminated primarily by renal excretion have a greater elimination half-time in geriatric individuals, necessitating a reduction in doses when these drugs are administered [19,20]. Glomerular filtration rate (GFR) is the same [21] or slightly decreased [22] in healthy geriatric dogs when compared to the GFR of middle-aged dogs but the presence of diseases that decrease renal blood flow could have a profound effect on GFR.

Hepatic clearance of drugs decreases with age as the mass of the liver decreases. In geriatric people, the liver mass, and consequently hepatic blood flow, may be decreased by 40–50%. Microsomal and non-microsomal enzyme function appears to be well maintained, although the reduction in hepatic mass significantly impairs overall hepatic function. Consequently, the metabolism of lipid-soluble drugs, particularly anesthetics, is decreased. Combined with decreased glomerular filtration and renal excretory capacity, the reduction in hepatic clearance of drugs results in an increase in the half-life and duration of effect of drugs that depend on these routes of elimination [10,19,20,23].

Aging results in changes in body composition that include a decrease in skeletal muscle, an increase in body fat as a percentage of total body weight, and a loss of intracellular water. A loss in total body water occurs as a result of decreased intracellular water and a reduction in plasma volume, although fit geriatric individuals maintain plasma volume well. Intravenous injection of anesthetic drugs into a contracted volume of distribution results in an increased initial plasma concentration that may be responsible for the observation that geriatric animals often require lower doses of injectable induction anesthetic drugs. Increased adipose tissue is associated with an increase in the fraction of a single dose of a lipid-soluble drug redistributed to adipose tissue, further delaying elimination from the body.

Reductions in serum albumin concentrations in association with aging can lead to reduced protein binding of some drugs. In addition, structural changes in the serum protein that occur with aging may decrease binding to the available protein. Theoretically, the administration of highly protein-bound drugs to animals with reduced serum proteins may lead to an exaggerated clinical effect [24].

A decrease in basal resting metabolic rate with age results in a reduction in the production of body heat. Consequently, geriatric individuals are less able to maintain core body temperature. This is particularly important in anesthetized animals placed in cold environments during anesthesia or recovery. Because shivering during recovery increases oxygen consumption by 200–300%, perianesthetic hypothermia alone may place severe demands on the cardiopulmonary system. If these demands are not met, tissue hypoxia may ensue [10].

Anesthesia

Preparation for anesthesia

A thorough physical examination, including careful auscultation of the heart, is an essential component of preanesthetic assessment. In geriatric people, exercise tolerance is one of the most important predictors of perioperative outcome, and this is likely an important predictor of outcome in the anesthesia of geriatric veterinary patients. Significant, pre-existing abnormalities should be medically managed or corrected prior to the induction of anesthesia when possible. Conditions of concern include chronic kidney disease, hepatobiliary disease, endocrine metabolic disorders (e.g., hyperadrenocorticism, diabetes mellitus, canine hypothyroidism, and feline hyperthyroidism) [25]. Left untreated, there is a risk that these abnormalities are likely to be decompensated by anesthesia. The preanesthetic assessment for a geriatric patient may include a complete blood count, serum chemistry profile with electrolytes, and urinalysis. In addition, analysis of serum T4 is recommended for geriatric cats [25]. Although the routine use of preanesthesia diagnostic tests is occasionally criticized, routine testing in geriatric human and veterinary patients is recommended. Previously undiagnosed subclinical disease was identified during preanesthesia screening in 30% of a geriatric pet population, almost half of which did not undergo anesthesia because of the new diagnosis [26]. In a separate study, new diagnoses were made in 80% of dogs over the age of 9 during routine geriatric screening [27]. Serum chemistry and urine analyses detected abnormalities in 55% and abdominal ultrasound detected abnormalities in 64% of geriatric golden retrievers [28].

Anesthetic drugs

As with patients of any age, anesthetic drugs should be titrated to effect and patients monitored closely during anesthesia. This is especially critical in geriatric patients because of the physiologic changes that result in decreased drug dosages required for clinical effect.

Premedication and pain management

Regardless of age, every patient anesthetized for a procedure that is anticipated to cause pain should receive appropriate analgesic therapy. Additionally, pre-existing painful conditions, like osteoarthritis and cancer, are common in geriatric dogs and cats and manipulation of the joints and tissues of these patients may result in increased pain and discomfort [29,30]. Although the full impact of pain in geriatric veterinary patients is unknown, when compared to untreated pain in young adult humans, untreated pain in geriatric humans contributes to a more rapid decline in physical abilities, cognitive function, and quality of life measures [31]. As with other drugs, dosages of the analgesic drugs may need to be decreased in geriatric animals and patients should be closely monitored for signs of adverse effects, but pain management should not be withheld because of age.

Opioid analgesics are reversible, making them a reasonable choice for analgesia in geriatrics with reduced hepatic or renal function. μ-Agonist opioids such as morphine, fentanyl, hydromorphone, and oxymorphone provide useful analgesia but may be more likely to cause respiratory depression and decreased GI motility, although both effects are generally clinically insignificant and are reversible. Partial agonists (buprenorphine) and agonist-antagonists (butorphanol) provide mild to moderate analgesia but also usually cause minimal impact on organ function. Selection of an appropriate opioid is best made based on the particular analgesic requirements, the health status of the patient, and the intended procedure.

The addition of local anesthetic techniques to anesthetic protocols is often appropriate. The inclusion of such techniques provides additional anesthesia/analgesia and an associated reduction in the requirement for general anesthetics. NSAIDs are appropriate in patients with competent hepatic and renal function and are commonly administered to geriatric patients with inflammatory disease, such as osteoarthritis or cancer.

Sedation may not appear necessary in quiet or debilitated patients. However, sedatives alleviate stress in anxious patients and decrease the dosage of drugs needed for induction and maintenance of anesthesia. The adverse effects of sedatives should be weighed against the adverse effects of having to use a larger dose of anesthetic drug (e.g., hypotension, hypoventilation). The older age of a patient is not a contraindication for the use of an α_2-adrenergic receptor agonist and administration to aged dogs with a healthy cardiovascular system usually does not cause adverse effects [32].

Induction

Anesthesia can be induced by using a variety of injectable anesthetic drugs. Mask induction with inhaled anesthetics, without sedative or induction drugs, increases the risk of anesthesia-related mortality [4] and is no longer recommended as a routine induction technique. Injectable drugs (e.g., alfaxalone, propofol, ketamine, etomidate, thiobarbiturates) can be easily titrated to effect [33]. The dose of propofol required to induce anesthesia in dogs >8.5 years of age has been shown to be lower than the dose reported for young adult dogs, and was eliminated more slowly than reported for young adult dogs [34]. Etomidate and alfaxalone depend on hepatic metabolism but redistribution and clearance are rapid following etomidate [35] or alfaxalone [36] administration to young adult cats and alfaxalone administration to young adult dogs [37]. No information on the effects of aging in animals is available for either drug but clinical experience suggests their use is acceptable. Etomidate causes minimal to no cardiovascular changes when compared to alfaxalone [38] or propofol [39] administered to young healthy dogs. There are no reports of the effects of etomidate in geriatric dogs but the cardiovascular effects were similar to those produced by propofol in geriatric humans [40]. Whether etomidate-induced adrenal suppression would have an impact in geriatric patients is unknown but adrenal disease is more common in geriatric animals and this should be considered when choosing an induction protocol.

Induction of anesthesia with ketamine, in combination with a benzodiazepine, causes only mild respiratory depression and may actually improve cardiovascular function through stimulation of the sympathetic nervous system [41]. Ketamine requires either hepatic metabolism or renal clearance for termination of activity; thus, the effects of ketamine may be prolonged in patients with failing hepatic and renal systems [41].

Inhalant anesthetics should not be used routinely for induction but could, if titrated very carefully, be used in patients that have received sedative/analgesic drugs. The prolonged excitement phase that occurs during induction in unsedated animals can be more physiologically detrimental than a judicious dose of an injectable anesthetic. Also, induction with inhalants can occur quickly, especially in geriatric or compromised patients, and excessive anesthetic depth may be reached very rapidly. Thus, constant assessment of response to the drugs is imperative. Environmental pollution and personnel exposure are also concerns during mask inductions with inhaled anesthetics.

Maintenance

Inhaled anesthetics allow rapid titration of anesthetic depth. This is very useful for geriatric patients where the response to a given dose can vary with age, pre-existing disease, and physiologic state of the patient. However, inhalant anesthetics can cause significant hypotension secondary to vasodilation so careful monitoring of cardiovascular function should be performed. The concurrent administration of analgesic and sedative drugs will reduce the inhaled anesthetic requirement while potentially decreasing the magnitude of their unwanted side-effects.

Support

Geriatric animals are highly susceptible to hypothermia, so every effort should be made to maintain body temperature. Hypothermia increases the incidence of adverse myocardial outcomes in high-risk patients, increases the incidence of surgical wound infection, adversely affects antibody- and cell-mediated immune defenses, changes the kinetics and action of various anesthetic and paralyzing agents, increases thermal discomfort, is associated with delayed postanesthetic recovery [42] and may contribute to increased anesthesia-related mortality [4]. Therefore vigilant monitoring is crucial during the entire anesthetic period and well into recovery.

Summary

No one ideal anesthetic protocol exists for all geriatric patients. An understanding of the pathophysiologic changes and the alterations in pharmacodynamics and pharmacokinetics that arise in conjunction with aging is necessary when choosing an anesthetic protocol for any geriatric animal. Particular attention to decreased dosage requirements and the titration of anesthetics to achieve the central nervous system depression necessary for a specific surgical procedure is advocated (see Table 54.1). Whenever possible, local and regional anesthetic techniques should be employed to reduce the dosage of concomitantly administered inhaled or injectable anesthetics. Appropriate anesthetic management of geriatric animals includes thorough evaluation and assessment; preoperative correction of identified abnormalities; vigilant, aggressive perianesthetic monitoring; careful titration of anesthetic drugs; provision of analgesia; and appropriate perianesthetic support. Other recent reviews of anesthesia and analgesia in geriatric patients are available [2,8,9,42–44].

References

1 Perrin T. Urban Animals Survey: the facts and statistics on companion animals in Canada. *Can Vet J* 2009; **50**: 48–52.
2 Carpenter R, Pettifer G, Tranquilli W. Anesthesia for geriatric patients. *Vet Clin North Am Small Anim Pract* 2005; **35**: 571–580.
3 Egenvall A, Nødtvedt A, Häggström J, *et al.* Mortality of life-insured Swedish cats during 1999–2006: age, breed, sex, and diagnosis. *J Vet Intern Med* 2009; **23**: 1175–1183.
4 Brodbelt DC, Blissitt, KJ, Hammond RA, *et al.* The risk of death: the confidential enquiry into perioperative small animal fatalities. *Vet Anaesth Analg* 2008; **35**: 365–373.
5 Proudman CJ, Dugdale AH, Senior JM, *et al.* Pre-operative and anaesthesia-related risk factors for mortality in equine colic cases. *Vet J* 2006; **171**: 89–97.
6 Johnston GM, Eastment JK, Wood JLN, *et al.* The confidential enquiry into perioperative equine fatalities (CEPEF): mortality results of Phases 1 and 2. *Vet Anaesth Analg* 2002; **29**: 159–170.
7 Hoskins J. *Geriatrics and Gerontology of the Dog and Cat*, 2nd edn. St Louis, MO: WB Saunders, 2004; 71–84.
8 Matthews NS. Anesthetic considerations of the older equine. *Vet Clin North Am Equine Pract* 2002; **18**: 403–409.
9 Seddighi R, Doherty TJ. Anesthesia of the geriatric equine. *Vet Med Res Rep* 2012; **3**: 53–64.
10 Muravchick S. Anesthesia for the elderly. In: Miller RD, ed. *Anesthesia*, 5th edn. Philadelphia: Churchill Livingstone, 2000; 2140–2156.
11 Wei JY. Age and the cardiovascular system. *N Engl J Med* 1992; **327**: 1735–1739.
12 Haidet GC, Parsons D. Reduced exercise capacity in senescent beagles: an evaluation of the periphery. *Am J Physiol* 1991; **260**: 173–182.
13 Mercier E, Mathieu M, Sandersen CF, *et al.* Evaluation of the influence of age on pulmonary arterial pressure by use of right ventricular catheterization, pulsed-wave Doppler echocardiography, and pulsed-wave tissue Doppler imaging in healthy Beagles. *Am J Vet Res* 2010; **71**: 891–897.
14 Haidet GC. Effects of age on beta-adrenergic-mediated reflex responses to induced muscular contraction in beagles. *Mech Ageing Dev* 1993; **68**: 89–104.
15 Lakatta EG. Diminished beta-adrenergic modulation of cardiovascular function in advanced age. *Cardiol Clin* 1986; **4**: 185–200.
16 Wahba WM. Influence of aging on lung function: clinical significance of changes from age twenty. *Anesth Analg* 1983; **62**: 764–776.
17 Stevens WD, Dolan WM, Gibbons RT, *et al.* Minimum alveolar concentrations (MAC) of isoflurane with and without nitrous oxide in patients of various ages. *Anesthesiology* 1975; **42**: 197–200.
18 Gregory GA, Eger EI, Munson ES. The relationship between age and halothane requirement in man. *Anesthesiology* 1969; **30**: 488–491.
19 Beck LH. The aging kidney: defending a delicate balance of fluid and electrolytes. *Geriatrics* 2000; **55**: 26–32.
20 Evers BM, Townsend CM, Thompson JC. Organ physiology of aging. *Surg Clin North Am* 1994; **74**: 23–39.
21 Bexfield NH, Heiene R, Gerritsen RJ, *et al.* Glomerular filtration rate estimated by 3-sample plasma clearance of iohexol in 118 healthy dogs. *J Vet Intern Med* 2008; **22**: 66–73.
22 Miyagawa Y, Takemura N, Hirose H. Assessments of factors that affect glomerular filtration rate and indirect markers of renal function in dogs and cats. *J Vet Med Sci* 2010; **72**: 1129–1136.
23 Geokas MC, Haverback BJ. The aging gastrointestinal tract. *Am J Surg* 1969; **117**: 881–892.
24 Homer TD, Stanski DR. The effect of increasing age on thiopental disposition and anesthetic requirement. *Anesthesiology* 1985; **62**: 714–724.
25 Metzger FL. Senior and geriatric care programs for veterinarians. *Vet Clin North Am Small Anim Pract* 2005; **35**: 743–753.
26 Joubert KE. Pre-anaesthetic screening of geriatric dogs. *J S Afr Vet Assoc* 2007; **78**: 31–35.
27 Davies M. Geriatric screening in first opinion practice – results from 45 dogs. *J Small Anim Pract* 2012; **53**: 507–513.
28 Webb JA, Kirby GM, Nykamp SG, Gauthier MJ. Ultrasonographic and laboratory screening in clinically normal mature golden retriever dogs. *Can Vet J* 2012; **53**: 626–630.
29 Vaughan LC. Orthopaedic problems in old dogs. *Vet Rec* 1990; **126**: 379–388.
30 Hardie EM, Roe SC, Martin FR. Radiographic evidence of degenerative joint disease in geriatric cats: 100 cases (1994–1997). *J Am Vet Med Assoc* 2002; **220**: 628–632.

31 Caltagirone C, Spoletini I, Gianni W, *et al*. Inadequate pain relief and consequences in oncological elderly patients. *Surg Oncol* 2010; **19**: 178–183.
32 Muir WW, Ford JL, Karpa GE, *et al*. Effects of intramuscular administration of low doses of medetomidine and medetomidine-butorphanol in middle-aged and old dogs. *J Am Vet Med Assoc* 1999; **215**: 1116–1120.
33 Simons PJ, Cockshott ID, Glen JB, *et al*. Disposition and pharmacology of propofol glucuronide administered intravenously to animals. *Xenobiotica* 1992; **22**: 1267–1273.
34 Reid J, Nolan AM. Pharmacokinetics of propofol as an induction agent in geriatric dogs. *Res Vet Sci* 1996; **61**: 169–171.
35 Wertz EM, Benson GJ, Thurmon JC, *et al*. Pharmacokinetics of etomidate in cats. *Am J Vet Res* 1990; **51**: 281–285.
36 Whittem T, Pasloske KS, Heit MC, *et al*. The pharmacokinetics and pharmacodynamics of alfaxalone in cats after single and multiple intravenous administration of Alfaxan at clinical and supraclinical doses. *J Vet Pharmacol Ther* 2008; **31**: 571–579.
37 Ferré PJ, Pasloske K, Whittem T, *et al*. Plasma pharmacokinetics of alfaxalone in dogs after an intravenous bolus of Alfaxan-CD RTU. *Vet Anaesth Analg* 2006; **33**: 229–236.
38 Rodríguez JM, Muñoz-Rascón P, Navarrete-Calvo R, *et al*. Comparison of the cardiopulmonary parameters after induction of anaesthesia with alphaxalone or etomidate in dogs. *Vet Anaesth Analg* 2012; **39**: 357–365.
39 Sams L, Braun C, Allman D, *et al*. A comparison of the effects of propofol and etomidate on the induction of anesthesia and on cardiopulmonary parameters in dogs. *Vet Anaesth Analg* 2008; **35**: 488–494.
40 Larsen R, Rathgeber J, Bagdahn A, *et al*. Effects of propofol on cardiovascular dynamics and coronary blood flow in geriatric patients: a comparison with etomidate. *Anaesthesia* 1988; **43**(Suppl): 25–31.
41 Wright M. Pharmacologic effects of ketamine and its use in veterinary medicine. *J Am Vet Med Assoc* 1982; **180**: 1462–1471.
42 Doufas AG. Consequences of inadvertent perioperative hypothermia. *Best Pract Res Clin Anaesthesiol* 2003; **17**: 535–549.
43 Baetge CL, Matthews NS. Anesthesia and analgesia for geriatric veterinary patients. *Vet Clin North Am Small Anim Pract* 2012; **42**: 643–653.
44 Hughes J. Anaesthesia for the geriatric dog and cat. *Ir Vet J* 2008; **61**: 380–387.

55 Cancer Patients

Timothy M. Fan

Department of Veterinary Clinical Medicine, College of Veterinary Medicine, University of Illinois at Urbana-Champaign, Urbana, Illinois, USA

Chapter contents

Commonality of cancer pain

The true prevalence of cancer pain in dogs and cats is unknown; however, given the conserved biology of cancer between companion animals and people [1–3], it is plausible that the incidence of cancer pain is comparable in these two populations. Pain is a common ailment in human cancer patients. Based upon epidemiologic studies, the incidence of cancer-related pain at initial diagnosis approaches 30%, and upon disease progression up to 65–85% of human cancer patients will experience pain at some point [4–8]. Correlating with its high reported incidence, pain is the most common physical symptom in people diagnosed with terminal cancer [9,10].

Cancer pain negatively affects quality of life as well as many important physiologic functions, and its alleviation in patients should be an utmost clinical and humane priority. No cures exist for many patients suffering from advanced cancer; however, effective analgesic strategies can diminish the discomfort and suffering associated with terminal disease progression. Estimates indicate that more than 70% of human cancer patients suffering from pain can be relieved with opioid-based regimens [4,11–13] and it is justifiable to believe that equally effective cancer pain management is achievable for companion animals too. However, for cancer pain to be adequately managed, it must be recognized early and frequently reassessed by veterinary caregivers and pet owners. Despite the treatability of cancer pain, many barriers obstruct its optimal management in animals, including poor recognition associated with many cancers, difficulty in response assessment, limited knowledge regarding the use of analgesics, and suboptimal communication between veterinary caregivers and pet owners [14,15].

Recognition and assessment of cancer pain

A major impediment to effectively managing cancer pain in companion animals is its accurate and timely recognition by veterinarians. By training, medical caregivers focus primarily on disease processes, and often lose sight of the global well-being of their animal patients. Because pets cannot directly communicate the sensation of pain through traditional verbal cues, alternative and reliable methods to identify pain are necessary.

One essential component of pain recognition is adequate communication with the pet owner [14,15]. Observant pet owners know their pet's personality well, and can recognize subtle changes in behavior that might represent pain or discomfort [16–19]. As such, it is imperative that veterinary caregivers make conscious efforts to believe the perceptions of pet owners who think their pet is experiencing pain. Mutual respect and dialogue between the veterinary caregiver and pet owner is an important step towards the early recognition of cancer pain, and the continued solicitation of pet owners' opinions during periodical reassessment of pain control is essential. Common behaviors noted by pet owners which might represent pain include changes in movement, posture, grooming, appetite and thirst, focal licking, drooling or dysphagia, vocalization, respiratory rate, and defecation and urination patterns.

Veterinary Anesthesia and Analgesia: The Fifth Edition of Lumb and Jones.
Edited by Kurt A. Grimm, Leigh A. Lamont, William J. Tranquilli, Stephen A. Greene and Sheilah A. Robertson.

To facilitate the recognition of pain and its assessment through behavioral observations, several validated observer pain scales have been used to estimate pain in animals [20–24]. However, the majority of conventional pain scales have been validated in the context of acute, postoperative pain or chronic osteoarthritic pain, and hence their suitability for cancer pain assessment might be limited. Two common standardized pain scales which are conceptually simplistic, and hence user friendly, include the visual analog scale (VAS) and the numerical rating scale (NRS). Both are unidimensional scales. The VAS is represented by a horizontal line, generally measuring 100 millimeters in length; the evaluator can make a vertical mark anywhere between 0 (no pain) and 100 (worst possible pain). With a NRS the evaluator chooses a number often between 0 and 5, but other numbers both higher and lower are used; again, 0 would represent no pain and the highest number in the scale the worst possible pain imaginable. There are many weaknesses with both assessment systems, but more crucial than the type of scale used is the importance of using a system that all observers understand and can use easily and in a repeatable manner.

Despite the simplicity of the NRS and VAS assessment methods, their utilization by pet owners and veterinary caregivers might not be completely applicable for the assessment of tumor-bearing animals, given the distinct pathophysiology of cancer pain. To address these limitations, alternative assessment schemes have been validated for pets that include either behavioral scales or health-related quality of life questionnaires specific to cancer pain [25–29]. Through the use of cancer pain-specific behavior scales or questionnaires, the objective assessment of pain and its alleviation can be more uniformly standardized in tumor-bearing pets.

In addition to cancer pain-specific scales, it would be ideal to have complementary and orthogonal methodologies for objectively characterizing cancer pain. Unfortunately, there are few reliable objective methods for measuring cancer pain which are confirmatory of pet owner-observed behavioral changes. Quantifiable physiologic parameters, such as heart and respiratory rates, temperature, pupil size, and blood pressure, have been evaluated as surrogate measures of pain, but lack specificity due to influence from other psychologic factors such as stress or fear [30]. Fortunately, some methodologies for quantifying cancer pain that directly affects bodily movement or ambulation can be objectively quantified by activity monitors or computerized force plate and gait analysis systems, respectively [31–35].

Types of cancer associated with pain

Cancer pain arises from the direct invasion of tumor cells into nerves, bones, soft tissue, ligaments, and fascia. Pain also can be elicited through the distension and obstruction of internal organs secondary to tumor infiltration. Erosive or inflammatory processes elicited by cancer cells within the microenvironment can generate pain too. Mechanistically, cancer pain can be categorized as nociceptive (somatic and visceral) or neuropathic in origin.

- Nociceptive pain is associated with direct tissue injury from tumor infiltration and peritumoral inflammation. Perception of pain is caused by the stimulation of peripheral pain receptors residing in the cutaneous and deeper musculoskeletal structures. Somatic and visceral pain syndromes can be characterized as nociceptive in nature.
- Somatic pain arises from direct injury due to cancer cell invasion into the skeleton, soft tissues, or tendons/ligaments, often manifesting as focal and stabbing in nature as described by human cancer patients.
- Visceral pain arises from cancer cell infiltration, compression, or distortion of internal organs within the abdominal, thoracic, or pelvic cavities, often manifesting as diffuse and squeezing in character as described by human cancer patients.
- Neuropathic pain is directly related to cancer cell infiltration of peripheral nerves, nerve plexi and roots, or spinal cord, often manifesting as burning, shooting, pins/needles, or numbness in nature as described by human cancer patients.

Although cancers associated with pain can be discretely categorized into either nociceptive or neuropathic, a singular tumor type can elicit pain which has blended characteristics of both nociceptive and neuropathic origin. A non-exhaustive list of common cancers arising in companion animals and the type of pain which they might elicit is summarized in Table 55.1.

Table 55.1 Common painful cancers in companion animals.

Type of cancer pain	Example
Nociceptive	
Somatic	Primary bone sarcomas (osteosarcoma, fibrosarcoma, chondrosarcoma)
	Joint sarcomas (histiocytic and synovial cell)
	Skeletal metastases (carcinoma of mammary, prostate, anal sac apocrine gland, lung, and transitional cell)
	Multiple myeloma or solitary osseous plasmacytoma
	Oral cavity tumors (melanoma, fibrosarcoma, squamous cell carcinoma)
	Nasal cavity tumors (adenocarcinoma, chondrosarcoma, squamous cell carcinoma)
	Skull and orbital tumors (multilobular osteochondrosarcoma)
	Ear tumors (ceruminous gland carcinoma)
	Cutaneous and subcutaneous tumors (mast cell tumor, basal cell carcinoma, apocrine gland carcinoma, injection site sarcoma)
	Mammary tumors (inflammatory mammary carcinoma)
Visceral	Urogenital tumors (transitional cell carcinoma, prostate carcinoma, renal carcinoma)
	Reproductive tumors (uterine leiomyosarcoma)
	Carcinomatosis (serosal surface-involving malignancy)
	Liver and splenic tumors (hepatocellular carcinoma, hemangiosarcoma)
	Pancreatic carcinoma
Neuropathic	Central nervous system (meningioma, astrocytoma)
	Brachial plexus tumor
	Vertebral body tumor with compression of spinal cord (osteosarcoma or other axillary bone sarcoma)

Specific underlying causes of cancer pain

Bone cancer pain

Bone is a living organ, rich in blood supply and nerves. Painful sensations arising from the skeleton can decrease quality-of-life scores in pets. Given its principal anatomic function for bearing weight and withstanding cyclic compressive forces, compromise in the structural integrity of bone (quantity and quality) poses risk for pain and pathologic fracture. Neoplasms involving the skeleton can arise primarily from the bone, or secondarily invade or metastasize to involve the skeleton. In dogs, osteosarcoma (OS) is the most common cancer that causes focal skeletal pain. However, other frequently diagnosed tumor types can involve bone too, including metastatic carcinoma and hematopoietic neoplasms such as multiple myeloma. In cats, primary bone tumors occur less frequently than in dogs; however, involvement of bone from secondary invasion is common for oral squamous cell carcinoma. Despite the diverse tumor histologies that can affect bone, the mechanisms for how tumor cells invade and cause skeletal pain are likely conserved among mammalian species.

Neurochemistry and bone cancer pain

Through the use of preclinical murine tumor models where tumor cells are directly implanted within the intramedullary cavity of bone [36–39], the pathophysiology and neurochemistry of bone cancer pain have been well characterized. Based upon these fundamental studies, it has been demonstrated that skeletal bone contains a mosaic of afferent nociceptors which are most densely concentrated within the periosteum and intramedullary cavity, and to a lesser extent within mineralized bone matrix [36,40]. Upon progressive intramedullary tumor cell growth and consequent chronic afferent nociceptor stimulation, neurochemical characteristics of chronic bone pain can be detected in both peripheral (afferent nociceptor and dorsal root ganglion) and central (dorsal horn) compartments [41,42]. Specific neuropathologic aberrations include enhanced release of substance P from primary afferent sensory neurons, marked reactive astrocytosis, and increased expression of glial fibrillary acidic protein within the dorsal horn of the spinal cord [42]. Importantly, the peripheral and central neurochemical signatures associated with bone cancer pain are distinct from the changes observed with either neuropathic or inflammatory pain [41]. Based upon these findings, it appears that unique pathophysiologic processes are required for the development of bone cancer pain.

Mechanisms of bone cancer pain

Bone cancer pain is attributed to specific host responses occurring within the bone microenvironment. First, the presence of cancer cells results in the release of chemical mediators by neoplastic and non-neoplastic stromal cells, which in turn stimulate sensory afferent nociceptors and cause painful sensations [43,44]. Specific ligands secreted by both cancer and stromal cells capable of nociceptor activation include endothelin-1, nerve growth factor, and prostaglandin E_2 [45]. Additionally, trafficking immune cells within the tumor microenvironment secrete proinflammatory cytokines including IL-1β, TNF-α, and bradykinin that also stimulate nociceptors [45]. Second, derived from preclinical studies, the generation and maintenance of bone cancer pain are directly attributed to pathologic osteoclastic bone resorption [46–48]. Mechanistically, osteoclastic bone resorption is mediated by the co-ordinated secretion of protons and cathepsin K, a cysteine protease [49,50]. Evidence suggests that the localized acidic environment created by osteoclasts stimulates afferent nociceptors through transient receptor potential vanilloid receptor-1 (TRPV-1) and acid sensing ion channels 2/3 (ASIC 2/3) [45,51]. Third, bone cancer pain can be generated as a consequence of bone erosion and subsequent mechanical instability, which allows for distortion of putative mechanotransducers belonging to the TRPV receptor family which innervate bone [52,53].

Based upon these unifying pathologic mechanisms, effective management of bone cancer pain requires a multi-pronged therapeutic approach which addresses the fundamental drivers that contribute to pain generation.

General therapeutic strategies for bone cancer pain

Several pathologic processes have been identified as the drivers of bone cancer pain, and allow for the rational institution of treatment modalities expected to be effective in diminishing pain associated with skeletal malignancies. Effective therapies should focus on the eradication of viable tumor cells; reduction of cancer-induced bone resorption; surgical stabilization of mechanically compromised bone; and administration of potent pharmacologic agents.

Viable cancer cells directly promote the generation of bone pain through the secretion of nociceptor-activating ligands, attraction of trafficking immune cells, and subversion of osteoclastic activities. As such, eradication of cancer cells remains a cornerstone for successful bone pain control. Reducing bone cancer burden is effectively achieved by cytotoxic therapies, including systemic chemotherapy and radiotherapy. Systemic chemotherapy can be effective in reducing tumor cell burdens within the bone microenvironment, but is contingent on the tumor histology (i.e., chemosensitive hematopoietic neoplasms) and favorable biodistribution kinetics. Ionizing radiation is the most effective treatment for alleviating bone cancer pain; the exact mechanisms of radiation-induced pain relief are incompletely understood, but likely depend upon radiation's cytotoxic effects on tumor cells and osteoclasts [47,54].

Osteoclasts, cells of the monocyte-macrophage cell lineage, are characterized by their high expressions of tartrate-resistant acid phosphatase and cathepsin K [49,50,55]. Under homeostatic conditions, osteoclasts resorb bone in balance with new bone formation by osteoblasts [56]. However, bone cancers of either primary (sarcomas) or metastatic (carcinomas) origin dysregulate osteoclastic activities in part through subversion of the receptor activator of nuclear factor κ-B/receptor activator of nuclear factor κ-B ligand/osteoprotegerin (RANK/RANKL/OPG) axis [57–59].

Given the role of osteoclasts in the generation of bone cancer pain through the secretion of protons and distortion of mechanotransducers, therapies that reduce osteoclast viability are useful in reducing the severity of bone cancer pain. Aminobisphosphonates induce osteoclast apoptosis through inhibition of the mevalonate pathway, and are first-line agents for the management of malignant skeletal events in human cancer patients [60–62]. Although aminobisphosphonates exert antiresorptive effects, based upon preclinical studies, the alleviation of focal bone cancer pain might be augmented by co-administering site-specific ionizing radiation therapy, which further augments osteoclast apoptosis [63–66].

When anatomically feasible, surgical stabilization of compromised bone integrity secondary to cancer infiltration can reduce excessive compression of mechanotransducers that stimulate afferent nociceptors. Diligence must be exercised in patient selection for surgical stabilization procedures, as successful outcomes require solid anchorage of stabilizing hardware into neighboring healthy bone [67]. As such, large or expansive areas of cancer-infiltrated bone will be prone to surgical failure, and alternative non-surgical treatment options should be considered first-line therapies for such patients.

For the majority of cancer patients experiencing pain, pharmacologic agents remain the cornerstone of successful pain management. Patients with bone cancer are likely to experience debilitating episodes of incident or breakthrough pain, and the medical armamentarium necessary to adequately manage bone cancer pain requires potent opioid-based regimens with adjuvant analgesic agents, corresponding with the highest level of the World Health Organization (WHO) three-step analgesic ladder (Fig. 55.1).

Radiotherapy-induced pain

Ionizing radiation is effective for managing localized forms of cancer. Mechanistically, ionizing radiation exerts cytotoxic effects by damaging DNA, either directly or indirectly. Following irreparable DNA damage, cancer cells undergo apoptosis. When applied therapeutically, ionizing radiation can be focally conformed to the shape of tumor masses through the use of linear accelerators equipped with three-dimensional planning software and sophisticated, multi-leaf collimators [68–71]. Even with advanced equipment, small volumes of normal tissue might be irradiated, potentially resulting in painful radiation-induced toxicity. Although the majority of caregivers who pursue radiation therapy for their pets consider the side-effects acceptable [72], some animals might experience considerable morbidity secondary to acute radiation burns. Depending upon the radiation field, acute moist dermatitis, mucositis, and colitis can be early radiation side-effects encountered with curative protocols (Fig. 55.2) [73–75].

Early radiation side-effects typically develop in the later stages of the treatment period, and may persist for several weeks upon completion of therapy. Common anatomic sites for the development of painful radiation-induced mucositis are the mouth, when oral or nasal tumors are irradiated, and the large colon/rectum (colitis, proctitis), when pelvic irradiation is performed [76,77]. Infrequently, late radiation side-effects might result in painful and unacceptable toxicity, including the development of osteoradionecrosis (Fig. 55.3) and peripheral neuropathies[78].

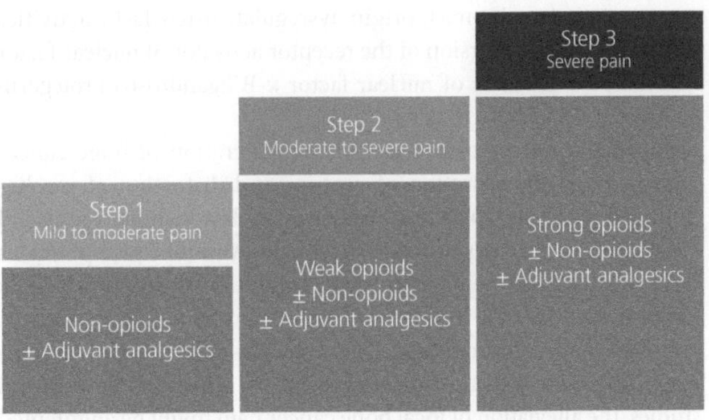

Figure 55.1 World Health Organization (WHO) analgesic ladder with indicated three-step approach to pain management. Companion animals diagnosed with bone cancer pain should be pre-emptively categorized into the highest tier and treated aggressively with potent opioid-based regimens.

Chemotherapy-induced pain

The administration of systemic chemotherapy is not typically uncomfortable; however, it can infrequently result in painful local and systemic side-effects. First, perivenous extravasation of certain chemotherapeutics, including vincristine, doxorubicin, vinblastine, mechlorethamine, and dactinomycin, might result in painful tissue irritation (Fig. 55.4), at times severe enough to necessitate surgical debridement [79,80].

Second, some chemotherapeutic agents have greater tendencies to perturb intestinal transit times and resident microflora, resulting in colitis (e.g., doxorubicin) or constipation (e.g., vinca alkaloids), which have the potential to generate visceral pain [81]. Third, bioconversion of some chemotherapeutic agents, like cyclophosphamide, can lead to the production of irritating metabolites which predisposes to the development of painful syndromes including sterile hemorrhagic cystitis [82,83]. Fourth, particular chemotherapeutic agents like dacarbazine which have a low pH (~3) can elicit

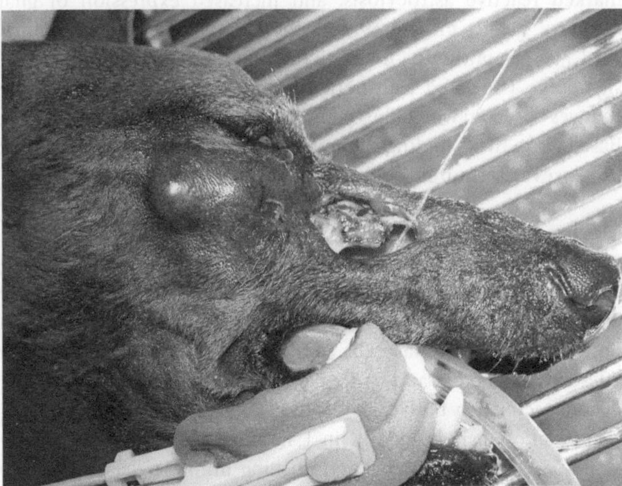

Figure 55.3 Irreparable late radiation toxicity in the form of osteoradionecrosis in a dog with nasal squamous cell carcinoma treated with high cumulative doses of radiation therapy.

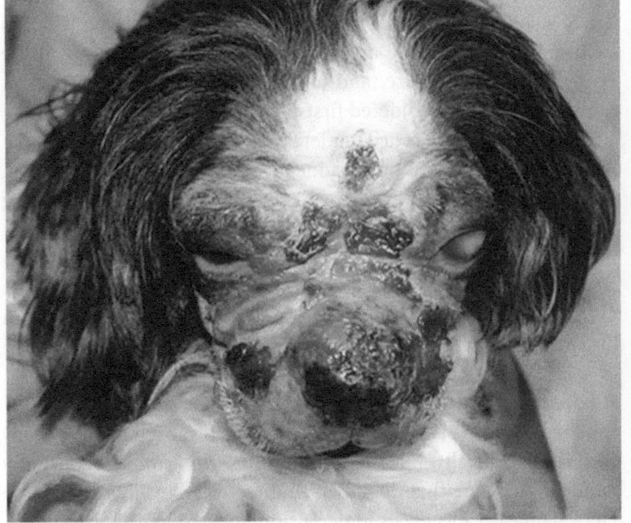

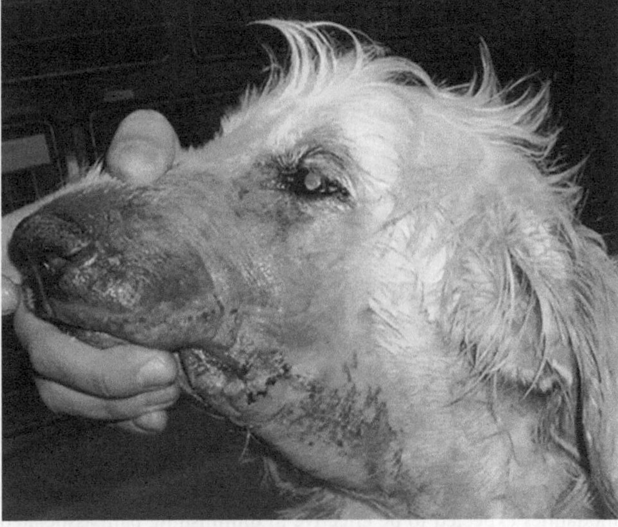

Figure 55.2 Resolving painful acute moist dermatitis in two different canine patients undergoing curative-intent radiation therapy for the treatment of cancer involving the nasal and perioral regions.

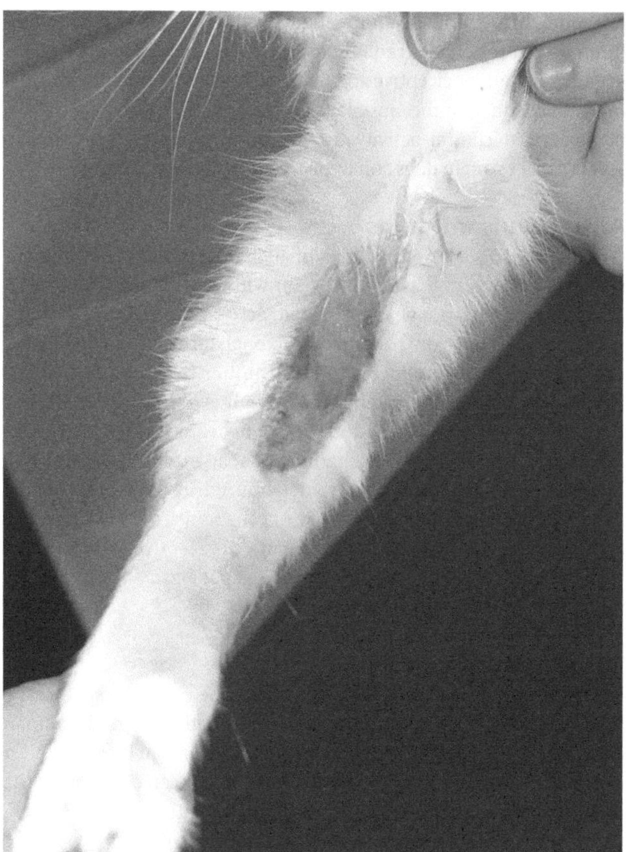

Figure 55.4 Painful soft tissue inflammation and dermal ulceration secondary to vinblastine extravasation in a cat.

burning sensations at the catheter site during intravenous infusion. Other chemotherapeutic agents like paclitaxel and docetaxel require Cremophor EL and polysorbate 80, respectively, for solubilization, and these solvents can directly activate complement and elicit systemic inflammatory cytokine release, resulting in diffuse pain sensations and systemic hypersensitivity reactions [84–87]. Fifth, certain chemotherapeutic formulations like liposome encapsulated doxorubicin (Doxil®) can induce palmar-plantar erythrodysesthesias, an unusual and painful cutaneous side-effect [88,89]. Lastly, painful peripheral neuropathies can be associated with the administration of certain drugs such as vincristine, cisplatin, and the taxanes in people [90], and similar side-effects have been documented in companion animals [91].

Surgery-induced pain

Invasive diagnostic or therapeutic procedures can cause acute nociceptive pain in veterinary cancer patients. Staging procedures such as tissue biopsies, bone marrow aspiration, and bone biopsies should be expected to cause mild to moderate pain that can be pre-emptively treated with analgesics. More aggressive surgeries such as amputation, hemipelvectomy, thoracotomy, radical mastectomy, large *en bloc* tumor resection including orbitectomy, mandibulectomy, or maxillectomy will generate severe postoperative pain and should be treated with aggressive pre-emptive analgesia, regional blocks, epidural or interpleural analgesia. The use of postoperative opioids should be a standard analgesic regimen for companion animals undergoing removal of painful invasive tumors through radical surgeries.

Pharmacologic treatment strategies

For the majority of pets diagnosed with cancer, pain becomes established early in the course of disease and rapidly intensifies during cancer progression. As such, pharmacologic strategies are often used in the setting of chronic pain management, where the primary intent of intervention is to minimize the clinical consequences of peripheral and central sensitization, as well as maintain quality of life. Tables 55.2 and 55.3 provide general guidelines for common analgesics that are easily administered by pet owners for the management of cancer pain in companion animals. General classes of analgesics are briefly summarized. For more detailed pharmacology and dosing regimens please refer to Section 2, Chapters 11–13.

Non-steroidal anti-inflammatory drugs (NSAIDs)

Non-steroidal anti-inflammatory drugs are used to control nociceptive pain in companion animals. The mechanism of action of NSAIDs is the inhibition of cyclo-oxygenases (COXs). For cancer

Table 55.2 Analgesic drug and oral dosages for dogs.

Class	Drug	Dosage
NSAIDs	Robenacoxib	1–2 mg/kg PO q 24 h
	Deracoxib	1–2 mg/kg PO q 24 h
	Carprofen	2.0 mg/kg PO q 12 h or 4.0 mg/kg PO q 24 h
	Etodolac	5–15 mg/kg PO q 24 h
	Meloxicam	0.1 mg/kg PO q 24 h
	Tepoxalin	10.0 mg/kg PO q 24 h
	Piroxicam	0.3 mg/kg PO q 24 h
	Ketoprofen	1.0 mg/kg PO q 24 h
	Aspirin	10.0 mg/kg PO q 12 h
Opioid	Morphine	
	Liquid	0.2–0.5 mg/kg PO q 6–8 h
	Slow release	0.5–3.0 mg/kg PO q 8–12 h
	Butorphanol	0.2–0.5 mg/kg PO q 8 h
	Codeine	1–2 mg/kg PO q 8–24 h
NMDA antagonist	Amantadine	3–5 mg/kg PO q 24 h
Combination analgesic	Tramadol	4–5 mg/kg PO q 6–12 h
Anticonvulsant	Gabapentin	2–10 mg/kg PO q 12–24 h
Tricyclic antidepressant	Amitriptyline	1–2 mg/kg PO q 12–24 h
	Clomipramine	1–2 mg/kg PO q 12 h
Corticosteroids	Prednisone	0.25–1.0 mg/kg PO q 24 h
	Dexamethasone	0.1–0.2 mg/kg PO q 24 h

Table 55.3 Analgesic drug and oral dosages for cats.

Class	Drug	Dosage
NSAIDs	Robenacoxib	1.0 mg/kg PO q 24 h; maximum 6 days
	Ketoprofen	1.0 mg/kg PO q 24 h; maximum 5 days
	Meloxicam	0.1 mg/kg PO day 1; 0.05 mg/kg PO days 2–5; then 0.05 mg/kg PO q 48 h
	Tolfenamic acid	4.0 mg/kg PO q 24 h; maximum 3 days
	Piroxicam	0.3 mg/kg PO q 48 h
Opioid	Buprenorphine	0.02 mg/kg oral transmucosal q 6–8 h
	Morphine liquid	0.2–0.5 mg/kg PO q 6–8 h
	Butorphanol	0.2–1.0 mg/kg PO q 6 h
NMDA antagonist	Amantadine	3.0 mg/kg PO q 24 h
Combination analgesic	Tramadol	1–2 mg/kg PO q 12–24 h
Anticonvulsant	Gabapentin	2–10 mg/kg PO q 12–24 h
Tricyclic antidepressant	Amitriptyline	1–2 mg/kg PO q 24 h
	Clomipramine	0.5–1.0 mg/kg PO q 24 h
Corticosteroids	Prednisone	0.5–1.5 mg/kg PO q 24 h
	Dexamethasone	0.1–0.2 mg/kg PO q 24 h

pain, COX-2 is the selective target of inhibition given its role in inflammatory pain, which is generated as a consequence of prostaglandin E_2 production. Prostaglandins play an important role in peripheral sensitization leading to a state of hyperalgesia or allodynia. Specifically, prostaglandins regulate the sensitivity of polymodal receptors, which typically cannot be easily activated by physiologic stimuli. However, following tissue injury and inflammation, the release of prostaglandins facilitates responsiveness of 'silent' polymodal receptors [92]. Prostaglandins can also activate certain sodium channels in the dorsal horn of the spinal cord, resulting in central sensitization and the establishment of chronic cancer pain [93]. The use of NSAIDs for managing cancer pain might be particularly relevant in companion animals given the multiple tumor histologies which overexpress COX-2 [94,95], and therefore have the potential for nociceptive sensitization through tumor-derived prostaglandin generation. In addition to alleviating cancer pain, another added benefit of NSAIDs for the treatment of patients with tumors expressing COX-2 is the theoretical exertion of antitumor activities, including reductions in cancer cell survival, proliferation, and angiogenesis.

Opioids

Three conventional opioid receptor subtypes have been cloned and isolated: μ, κ, and δ receptors. Opioid receptors are localized within the central nervous system, primarily in the superficial dorsal horn within laminae I–II. Within the dorsal horn, the majority of opioid receptors are located on the presynaptic terminal of afferent fibers; however, lower densities of opioid receptors are also found on postsynaptic sites and interneurons. The mechanism of analgesia is through reduced transmitter release from nociceptive C-fibers and postsynaptic inhibition of neurons conveying information from the spinal cord to higher centers of the brain. Binding of opioids to their presynaptic inhibitory receptor blocks the release of glutamate, substance P, and other transmitters, while binding to the postsynaptic receptor further inhibits neuronal depolarization. Opioids are readily available, can be titrated easily to desired effect, and demonstrate predictable toxicities that can be minimized preventatively. Side-effects in companion animals include diarrhea, vomiting, constipation, and excessive sedation. For further information on opioids and their use in dogs and cats, see Chapter 11.

N-methyl-D-aspartate (NMDA) antagonists

N-methyl-D-aspartate receptors play a key role in central sensitization within the dorsal horn of the spinal cord following the release of transmitters from nociceptor terminals. Sustained transmitter release leads to perturbations in synaptic receptor density, threshold, kinetics, and activation, with subsequent increases in pain transmissions. During central sensitization, glutamate-activated NDMA receptors undergo post-translational phosphorylation which increases their synaptic distribution and responsiveness to glutamate, with resultant hyperexcitability to normally subthreshold noxious stimuli. As such, NMDA antagonists such as amantadine, which has demonstrated adjuvant analgesia in dogs with osteoarthritis [96], might also have a role in the management of chronic cancer pain when central sensitization has been established.

Combination analgesics

Tramadol is a centrally acting analgesic and classified as an opioidergic/monoaminergic drug based upon its shared properties with both opioids and tricyclic antidepressants. Tramadol weakly binds to the μ opioid receptor, inhibits the reuptake of serotonin and norepinephrine, and promotes neuronal serotonin release. Based upon these properties, tramadol is a suitable analgesic for the management of both nociceptive and neuropathic pain. Recently, tramadol in combination with metamizole (dipyrone), with or without NSAIDs, demonstrated clinical activity for the management of moderate to severe cancer pain in dogs and improved quality of life scores [26].

Anticonvulsant drugs

Anticonvulsants are useful adjuvant analgesics in patients with neuropathic pain, as well as chronic pain with central sensitization. In companion animals, gabapentin, a structural analogue of γ-aminobutyric acid, acts on presynaptic axonal terminal voltage-gated calcium channels to reduce neurotransmitter release. Additionally, it induces postsynaptic inhibition through evoking hyperpolarization inhibitory potentials in dorsal horn neurons through the opening of potassium or chloride channels. Gabapentin is well tolerated, highly bioavailable, and rapidly metabolized in dogs [97]. Recent studies suggest that the adjuvant use of gabapentin does not improve analgesia for the management of acute nociceptive pain in dogs [98,99]; however, other studies suggest gabapentin's activity in the management of neuropathic pain [100].

Tricyclic antidepressants

Tricyclic antidepressants are used as first-line co-analgesic therapy for chronic cancer pain, especially of neuropathic origin in human cancer patients [101]. Chronic neuropathic pain can be the sequela of local nerve compression by expanding cancer cells, neuroma formation following surgical transection, radiation-induced fibrosis or neuritis, and systemic peripheral nerve damage from specific chemotherapeutic agents (vinca alkaloids). Mechanistically, the analgesia produced by tricyclic antidepressants such as amitriptyline, clomipramine, fluoxetine, and imipramine is attributable to their actions on endogenous monoaminergic pain modulating systems. Tricyclic antidepressants inhibit the reuptake of various monoamines such as serotonin and noradrenaline, allowing these biomolecules to remain present and act centrally on descending inhibitory serotonergic and noradrenergic pathways that modulate pain transmission at the level of the spinal cord.

Corticosteroids

Corticosteroid co-analgesic therapy can be helpful in nociceptive and neuropathic pain caused by inflammatory edema, which can exacerbate pain associated with acute nerve compression, visceral distension, increased intracranial pressure, and soft tissue infiltration.

Cancer-specific pain treatment options

Osteosarcoma

The most common and striking presenting sign of dogs with osteosarcoma (OS) is lameness associated with severe pain of the affected bone. The mechanisms of bone cancer pain have been characterized through the use of murine preclinical models. Given the evolutionary importance of adaptive pain, it is plausible that the same mechanisms responsible for pain generation in mouse models are also operative in spontaneously arising bone tumors in companion animals, such as canine OS. Since tumor cells and osteoclasts appear to play preponderant roles in the genesis of bone pain associated with malignant osteolysis, therapies that reduce the viability of resident cancer cells and inhibit pathologic osteoclastic activities are expected to be effective in decreasing bone pain in canine OS patients.

Aminobisphosphonates

Bisphosphonates are synthetic analogs of inorganic pyrophosphate (PP_i), initially utilized in the detergent industry as demineralizing agents and then for diagnostic purposes in bone scanning, based on their ability to adsorb to bone mineral. The pharmaceutical use of bisphosphonates has now gained wide acceptance for the management of human non-neoplastic bone disorders such as osteoporosis and Paget's disease [102–105], and currently several bisphosphonates have demonstrated activity for treating neoplastic bone pathologies including tumor-induced hypercalcemia, multiple myeloma, and skeletal metastases [106–108].

The effective treatment of bone disorders with bisphosphonates is attributed to their differential effects on bone resorption and bone mineralization. At biologically relevant concentrations, bisphosphonates inhibit bone resorption without inhibiting the process of bone mineralization. Bisphosphonates directly inhibit bone resorption by binding to hydroxyapatite crystals, which prevent further calcium and phosphorus mineral dissolution. Importantly, bisphosphonates impede osteoclast activity and induce osteoclast apoptosis, selectively reducing the cell population responsible for bone resorption [60,109–111]. Although several bisphosphonates prevent bone loss, nitrogen-containing bisphosphonates, also known as aminobisphosphonates (NBPs), possess the greatest relative antiresorptive potency. Pamidronate and zoledronate are the two intravenous NBPs formulations most commonly utilized in human oncology for their ability to decrease bone pain, improve quality of life, delay progression of the bone lesions, and decrease the frequency of malignant skeletal events.

Because OS is characterized by focal malignant osteolysis, the investigation of NBPs has been of clinical interest for reducing bone cancer pain by virtue of their antiresorptive properties. In two studies, intravenous pamidronate (1.0–2.0 mg/kg) administered as a 2-h constant rate infusion (CRI) every 28 days was well tolerated and exerted bone biologic and clinically relevant analgesic effects in dogs diagnosed with appendicular OS as supported by reductions in urine N-telopeptide (NTx) concentrations, increases in relative primary tumor bone mineral density (rBMD), and subjective pain alleviation [112,113]. In a third study, when used in combination with ionizing radiation, intravenous pamidronate did not appear to improve pain as determined by caregivers beyond the use of radiation alone; however, dogs receiving adjuvant pamidronate did demonstrate improved quality-of-life scores, and superior bone biologic effects represented by decreased malignant bone resorption at the level of the primary tumor [34].

Zoledronate possesses 100-fold greater antiresorptive potency than pamidronate, and has the advantage of being safely administered over a shorter period of time than other NBPs. In one case report, the use of intravenous zoledronate administered every 28 days was effective for the long-term pain management of a dog diagnosed with OS [114]. In a larger study, the bone biologic effects of intravenous zoledronate were evaluated in dogs diagnosed with primary and secondary skeletal tumors [115]. In 10 dogs with appendicular OS, zoledronate (0.25 mg/kg) was administered as a 15-min CRI every 28 days. Clinically relevant analgesia from bone cancer pain was achieved in 50% of dogs for greater than 4 months, and the primary tumor of responding dogs demonstrated significant increases in rBMD.

Radiotherapy

Conventional megavoltage

Radiation therapy is considered the most effective treatment modality in human cancer patients for the management of osteolytic bone pain, and mechanistically, the analgesic effects of ionizing radiation can be attributed to the induction of apoptosis in both cancer cells and resorbing osteoclasts [47]. In dogs with OS, there is histopathologic evidence to support the proapoptotic effects of ionizing radiation on malignant osteoblasts residing within the local bone microenvironment through percent necrosis quantification [116–118]. Collectively, the analgesic benefit afforded by ionizing radiation appears to be through the reduction of overall tumor burden and attenuation of osteoclastic resorption within the focal OS microenvironment. Mulitple palliative radiation protocols have been reported in the veterinary literature, with the majority of dosing schemes utilizing 2–4 individual treatments of 6–10 Gy fractions. Although variable and subjectively reported, the alleviation of bone cancer pain was achieved in the majority of OS dogs treated, with 74–93% of patients experiencing some degree of pain relief and improved limb function. Despite symptomatic improvement following palliative radiation therapy, the median time interval of subjective pain alleviation was not durable, and ranged from 53 to 130 days [119–123]. Some investigators have suggested that the concurrent administration of intravenous systemic chemotherapy along with palliative radiation might enhance analgesic response rates and durations [120,124].

Bone-seeking radionuclide

$^{[153]}$Samarium-EDTMP is commercially available for the treatment of skeletal metastases in human cancer patients, and is effective for alleviating bone pain associated with diffuse or multifocal skeletal lesions; it therefore has the advantage over palliative radiation therapy which is limited to treating only a few lesions [125,126]. The use of $^{[153]}$Samarium-EDTMP has been reported to alleviate bone cancer pain in dogs with appendicular and axial OS. Following intravenous $^{[153]}$Samarium-EDTMP administration, the majority (63–83%) of dogs with OS demonstrate improved lameness scores and activity levels, suggesting the achievement of pain palliation [127–130]. Despite clinical improvement in most treated dogs, the duration of pain alleviation has not been extensively documented, but appears to approximate similar durations of pain control achieved with megavoltage telotherapy. Overall, $^{[153]}$Samarium-EDTMP is well tolerated but side-effects associated with treatment include transient decreases in platelet and white blood cell counts as a consequence of β energy deposition within the proximity of pluripotent marrow stem cells [129].

Stereotactic radiosurgery (SRS)

Stereotactic radiosurgery involves the precise delivery of a single large dose of radiation to a designated tumor target, which is achieved by multiple arrays of overlapping radiation beams. Similar to its utility for treating brain tumors in people, stereotactic radiosurgery has also been evaluated for alleviating bone pain associated with appendicular OS in dogs. A non-surgical limb salvage technique using stereotactic radiosurgery was developed at the University of Florida (United States) and initial results were reported in 11 dogs [131]. Limb use in the dogs that received stereotactic radiosurgery was excellent, and the reported overall median survival was 363 days in this series. Advantages of this technique include limb preservation for anatomic sites not amenable to reliable surgical limb salvage, the sparing of normal tissue compared to conventional radiation therapy, no surgical procedures, clinically relevant pain alleviation, and good to excellent limb function.

Experimental therapeutics – intrathecal resiniferatoxin

Vanilloids belong to a family of small organic compounds that stimulate afferent sensory neurons through the binding of transient receptor potential vanilloid-1 (TRPV-1), a non-selective cation ionophore [132]. Upon binding by natural agonists like capsaicin, a chili pepper extract, TRPV-1 activation leads to noxious-mediated and inflammatory hyperalgesic responses [133,134]. Interestingly, prolonged exposure to TRPV-1 agonists has been shown to deplete vanilloid receptors in peripheral tissues and sensory ganglia, allowing for the potential of long-term desensitization of nociceptors [135].

Resiniferatoxin (RTX) is an ultrapotent analogue of capsaicin derived from the latex of a cactus-like plant (*Euphorbia resinifera*). Upon binding to TRPV-1, resiniferatoxin causes a large and prolonged increase in the free intracellular calcium concentration, resulting in lethal calcium cytotoxicity with subsequent apoptosis and depletion of only TRPV-1 expressing neurons, and hence reducing the sensitivity to nociceptive inputs [136]. Importantly, resiniferatoxin appears selective for only TRPV-1 expressing neurons which are typically unmyelinated C-fibers, while leaving large myelinated neurons responsible for proprioception and mechanosensation intact.

Depletion of TRPV-1 expression neurons by resiniferatoxin can be reversible or irreversible, and is dependent upon its spatial application within the nervous system. When administered peripherally, distantly located perikarya are spared from calcium-induced cytotoxicity, yet resiniferatoxin causes local, transient, and reversible loss of peripheral C-fiber endings. However, when resiniferatoxin is administered systemically, it potentially can exert wide-scale spatial depletion of both peripheral and central perikarya permanently, theoretically resulting in irreversible loss of nociception.

Intrathecal resiniferatoxin has been evaluated in pet dogs as an experimental therapeutic for the management of pain associated with osteoarthritis and bone cancer [137,138]. In the setting of bone cancer pain, dogs ($n=18$) receiving intrathecal resiniferatoxin achieved dramatic analgesia based upon caregiver-based visual analogue scores within 14 days of therapy. Although intrathecal resiniferatoxin provided substantive clinical analgesia in all dogs treated, significant physiologic perturbations including hypertension, tachycardia, and hypothermia were consistently observed during and following intrathecal administration, drawing some questions regarding the potential induction of pain while under general anesthesia or undesirable off-target effects. Nonetheless, these physiologic disturbances appeared to be self-limiting and transient in nature, and dogs returning for scheduled follow-up examinations continued to demonstrate clinically meaningful analgesia for up to 14 weeks post resiniferatoxin administration [137].

Radiation burns – acute side-effects

Ionizing radiation exerts its therapeutic effects by damaging cellular DNA through the generation of free radicals. Given that radiation therapy induces apoptosis preferentially in mitotically active cells, acute adverse effects tend to occur more commonly in normal cells with rapid division rates, which include those of mucosal surfaces, intestine, and skin, resulting in mucositis, colitis, and dermatitis, respectively.

The morbidity associated with mucositis, colitis, and dermatitis can be significant in companion animals given their inflammatory and ulcerative pathology. In particular, oral mucositis pain can negatively affect oral intake of fluids, food, and medications, with subsequent reduced quality of life (Fig. 55.5). The level of evidence-based medicine for the effective management of radiation-induced mucositis, colitis, and dermatitis is limited even for human cancer patients [139,140] and primarily anecdotal in companion animals [73,74].

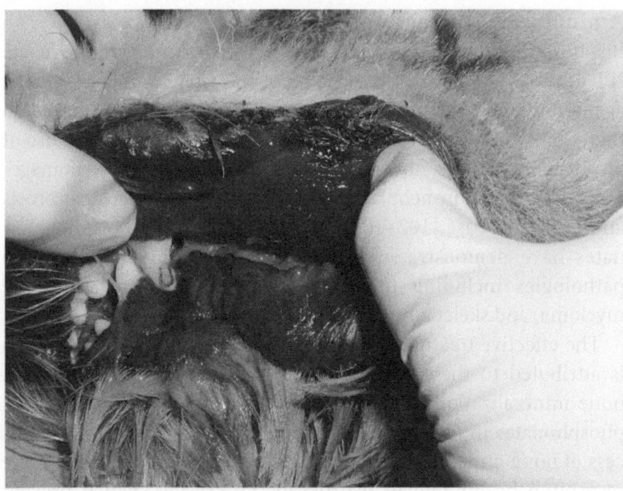

Figure 55.5 Severe and painful oral mucositis manifesting as erythema and coalescing mucosal blisters in a dog treated with curative-intent radiation therapy for perioral hamartoma.

Despite the absence of definitive clinical studies evaluating the effectiveness of various pain alleviating strategies, oral mucositis can be symptomatically treated with oral rinse solutions (weak tea solution, chlorhexidine rinse, or mixture of viscous lidocaine, liquid diphenhydramine, and magnesium hydroxide), and the systemic use of NSAIDs or corticosteroids with transmucosal buprenorphine as needed. Symptoms of colitis might be effectively relieved with the use of a corticosteroid enema and systemic medications consistent with step 2 of the WHO analgesic ladder. Acute moist dermatitis may benefit from topical application of colloidal oatmeal, wheat extracts, or aloe gel extract. As needed, the administration of broad-spectrum antibiotics or antifungal agents might prevent the establishment of opportunistic bacterial or fungal infections. Fortunately, the morbidity associated with acute radiation side-effects is temporary and limited to the first 4–6 weeks of therapy, and most clinical symptoms are self-resolving following supportive management.

Quality of life in cancer patients

Quality of life (QoL) is multidimensional and for its optimization, caregivers must consider various contextual parameters including physical, social, emotional, and cognitive well-being. Although the alleviation of cancer pain is paramount for improving many physiologic functions, additional supportive and alternative measures should be considered to lessen the suffering of companion animals diagnosed with cancer pain.

Supportive and complementary care

An emphasis on nutrition, emotional enrichment, and complementary therapies are accepted practices for the management of human cancer patients, and similar advancements are being made for companion animals too. Complementary therapies for improving quality of life in pets include acupuncture, massage, stretch and manipulation, hydrotherapy, play therapy, superficial heat and cold application, percutaneous electrical stimulation, laser therapy, and pulsed magnetic field therapy. While few studies have addressed the physiologic benefit derived from complementary therapies for improving quality-of-life scores, the excellent tolerability of these adjuvant therapies makes them an attractive addition to more conventional treatment regimens.

Promising innovative treatments

Advancements have been made in clarifying the fundamental underpinnings which drive different forms of pain, especially bone cancer pain through the use of murine preclinical models [43,44]. With a greater understanding of which tumor microenvironmental ligands are responsible for peripheral afferent nociceptor stimulation, it has become possible to rationally identify and design molecularly targeted therapeutics expected to provide analgesia in companion animals.

Although not exhaustive, at least three rational molecular targets warrant additional investigation for improving the alleviation of bone cancer pain in dogs and cats. First, small molecule inhibitors of cathepsin K, such as odanacatib (Merck & Co., Whitehouse Station, New Jersey), have demonstrated potent antiresorptive activities in women diagnosed with breast carcinoma skeletal metastases [141]. The pharmacology and metabolism of odanacatib have been characterized in multiple species, including dogs, allowing for its translational application to this species [142]. Recently, it was demonstrated that canine appendicular OS cells have the capacity to secrete cathepsin K, and theoretically could actively participate in malignant osteolysis and exacerbate bone pain [143]. As such, the evaluation of cathepsin K inhibitors, like odanacatib, for the alleviation of malignant osteolysis and pain in companion animals appears clinically justified.

Second, endothelin-1 is involved in peripheral nociceptor stimulation [144,145] and small molecule inhibitors, including atrasentan (ABT-627; Abbott Laboratories, Abbott Park, Illinois), have been developed to block endothelin-1 signaling through endothelin-A receptor antagonism. In preclinical models, atrasentan attenuates bone cancer pain associated with metastatic prostatic carcinoma [146,147]. Pharmacokinetic and preclinical toxicity studies for atrasentan have been conducted in normal dogs [148], which provides the opportunity to evaluate safe and biologically active dosing regimens for the treatment of canine bone cancer pain. Third, nerve growth factor (NGF) plays an important role for initiating nerve sprouting and bone cancer pain via binding to its cognate receptor, tropomyosin-related kinase A (Trk-A). In murine preclinical models, blockade of nerve growth factor signaling dramatically reduces bone cancer pain [149–151]. Additionally, Trk-A signaling appears to be involved in canine OS cell survival, and thereby incriminates NGF as a putative ligand that drives OS local tumor progression [152]. Potent and highly selective small molecule inhibitors of Trk-A signaling have been chemically designed [153,154]. Given the global role of NGF in nociception, therapeutic strategies that block Trk-A signaling are expected to provide analgesia in the setting of cancer pain in companion animals.

References

1 Breen M, Modiano JF. Evolutionarily conserved cytogenetic changes in hematological malignancies of dogs and humans – man and his best friend share more than companionship. *Chromosome Res* 2008; **16**(1): 145–154.

2 Paoloni M, *et al.* Canine tumor cross-species genomics uncovers targets linked to osteosarcoma progression. *BMC Genomics* 2009; **10**: 625.

3 Paoloni M, Khanna C. Translation of new cancer treatments from pet dogs to humans. *Nat Rev Cancer* 2008; **8**(2): 147–156.

4 Cleary J, Carbone PP. Pharmacologic management of cancer pain. *Hosp Pract* 1995; **30**(11): 41–49.

5 Cleeland CS, *et al.* Pain and its treatment in outpatients with metastatic cancer. *N Engl J Med* 1994; **330**(9): 592–596.

6 Foley KM. Improving palliative care for cancer: a national and international perspective. *Gynecol Oncol* 2005; **99**(3 Suppl 1): S213–214.

7 Jacox A, Carr DB, Payne R. New clinical-practice guidelines for the management of pain in patients with cancer. *N Engl J Med* 1994; **330**(9): 651–655.

8 Sykes NP. Pain control in terminal cancer. *Int Disabil Stud* 1987; **9**(1): 33–37.

9 Coyle N, *et al.* Character of terminal illness in the advanced cancer patient: pain and other symptoms during the last four weeks of life. *J Pain Symptom Manage* 1990; **5**(2): 83–93.

10 Grond S, *et al.* Prevalence and pattern of symptoms in patients with cancer pain: a prospective evaluation of 1635 cancer patients referred to a pain clinic. *J Pain Symptom Manage* 1994; **9**(6): 372–382.

11 Lussier D, Huskey AG, Portenoy RK. Adjuvant analgesics in cancer pain management. *Oncologist* 2004; **9**(5): 571–591.

12 Slavin KV, Tesoro EP, Mucksavage JJ. The treatment of cancer pain. *Drugs Today (Barc)* 2004; **40**(3): 235–245.

13 Yennurajalingam S, Peuckmann V, Bruera E. Recent developments in cancer pain assessment and management. *Support Cancer Ther* 2004; **1**(2): 97–110.

14 Kyles AE, Ruslander D. Chronic pain: osteoarthritis and cancer. *Semin Vet Med Surg (Small Anim)* 1997; **12**(2): 122–132.

15 Lester P, Gaynor JS. Management of cancer pain. *Vet Clin North Am Small Anim Pract* 2000; **30**(4): 951–966, ix.

16 Bennett D, Morton C. A study of owner observed behavioural and lifestyle changes in cats with musculoskeletal disease before and after analgesic therapy. *J Feline Med Surg* 2009; **11**(12): 997–1004.

17 Hielm-Bjorkman AK, *et al.* Evaluation of methods for assessment of pain associated with chronic osteoarthritis in dogs. *J Am Vet Med Assoc* 2003; **222**(11): 1552–1558.

18 Lascelles BD, *et al.* Evaluation of client-specific outcome measures and activity monitoring to measure pain relief in cats with osteoarthritis. *J Vet Intern Med* 2007; **21**(3): 410–416.

19 Brown DC, *et al.* Ability of the canine brief pain inventory to detect response to treatment in dogs with osteoarthritis. *J Am Vet Med Assoc* 2008; **233**(8): 1278–1283.

20 Hudson JT, *et al.* Assessing repeatability and validity of a visual analogue scale questionnaire for use in assessing pain and lameness in dogs. *Am J Vet Res* 2004; **65**(12): 1634–1643.

21 Holton LL, *et al.* Comparison of three methods used for assessment of pain in dogs. *J Am Vet Med Assoc* 1998; **212**(1): 61–66.

22 Morton CM, *et al.* Application of a scaling model to establish and validate an interval level pain scale for assessment of acute pain in dogs. *Am J Vet Res* 2005; **66**(12): 2154–2166.

23 Firth AM, Haldane SL. Development of a scale to evaluate postoperative pain in dogs. *J Am Vet Med Assoc* 1999; **214**(5): 651–659.

24 Holton LL, *et al.* Relationship between physiological factors and clinical pain in dogs scored using a numerical rating scale. *J Small Anim Pract* 1998; **39**(10): 469–474.

25 Carsten RE, *et al.* Correlations between acute radiation scores and pain scores in canine radiation patients with cancer of the forelimb. *Vet Anaesth Analg* 2008; **35**(4): 355–362.

26 Flor PB, *et al.* Tramadol plus metamizole combined or not with anti-inflammatory drugs is clinically effective for moderate to severe chronic pain treatment in cancer patients. *Vet Anaesth Analg* 2013; **40**(3): 316–327.

27 Yazbek KV, Fantoni DT. Validity of a health-related quality-of-life scale for dogs with signs of pain secondary to cancer. *J Am Vet Med Assoc* 2005; **226**(8): 1354–1358.

28 Lynch S, *et al.* Development of a questionnaire assessing health-related quality-of-life in dogs and cats with cancer. *Vet Comp Oncol* 2011; **9**(3): 172–182.

29 Tzannes S, *et al.* Owners' perception of their cats' quality of life during COP chemotherapy for lymphoma. *J Feline Med Surg* 2008; **10**(1): 73–81.

30 Conzemius MG, *et al.* Correlation between subjective and objective measures used to determine severity of postoperative pain in dogs. *J Am Vet Med Assoc* 1997; **210**(11): 1619–1622.

31 Brown DC, Boston RC, Farrar JT. Comparison of force plate gait analysis and owner assessment of pain using the Canine Brief Pain Inventory in dogs with osteoarthritis. *J Vet Intern Med* 2013; **27**(1): 22–30.

32 Feldsein JD, *et al.* Serum cortisol concentration and force plate analysis in the assessment of pain associated with sodium urate-induced acute synovitis in dogs. *Am J Vet Res* 2010; **71**(8): 940–945.

33 Jeunesse EC, *et al.* Paw inflammation model in dogs for preclinical pharmacokinetic/pharmacodynamic investigations of nonsteroidal anti-inflammatory drugs. *J Pharmacol Exp Ther* 2011; **338**(2): 548–558.

34 Fan TM, *et al.* Double-blind placebo-controlled trial of adjuvant pamidronate with palliative radiotherapy and intravenous doxorubicin for canine appendicular osteosarcoma bone pain. *J Vet Intern Med* 2009; **23**(1): 152–160.

35 Weinstein JI, *et al.* Use of force plate analysis to evaluate the efficacy of external beam radiation to alleviate osteosarcoma pain. *Vet Radiol Ultrasound* 2009; **50**(6): 673–678.

36 Mach DB, *et al.* Origins of skeletal pain: sensory and sympathetic innervation of the mouse femur. *Neuroscience* 2002; **113**(1): 155–166.

37 Medhurst SJ, *et al.* A rat model of bone cancer pain. *Pain* 2002; **96**(1–2): 129–140.

38 Sabino MA, *et al.* Simultaneous reduction in cancer pain, bone destruction, and tumor growth by selective inhibition of cyclooxygenase-2. *Cancer Res* 2002; **62**(24): 7343–7349.

39 Seong J, *et al.* Radiation-induced alteration of pain-related signals in an animal model with bone invasion from cancer. *Ann N Y Acad Sci* 2004; **1030**: 179–186.

40 Hukkanen M, *et al.* Innervation of bone from healthy and arthritic rats by substance P and calcitonin gene related peptide containing sensory fibers. *J Rheumatol* 1992; **19**(8): 1252–1259.

41 Honore P, *et al.* Murine models of inflammatory, neuropathic and cancer pain each generates a unique set of neurochemical changes in the spinal cord and sensory neurons. *Neuroscience* 2000; **98**(3): 585–598.

42 Schwei MJ, *et al.* Neurochemical and cellular reorganization of the spinal cord in a murine model of bone cancer pain. *J Neurosci* 1999; **19**(24): 10886–10897.

43 Clohisy DR, Mantyh PW. Bone cancer pain. *Cancer* 2003; **97**(3 Suppl): 866–873.

44 Mantyh PW, *et al.* Molecular mechanisms of cancer pain. *Nat Rev Cancer* 2002; **2**(3): 201–209.

45 Jimenez-Andrade JM, *et al.* Bone cancer pain. *Ann N Y Acad Sci* 2010; **1198**: 173–181.

46 Clohisy DR, Mantyh PW. Bone cancer pain and the role of RANKL/OPG. *J Musculoskelet Neuronal Interact* 2004; **4**(3): 293–300.

47 Goblirsch M, *et al.* Radiation treatment decreases bone cancer pain, osteolysis and tumor size. *Radiat Res* 2004; **161**(2): 228–234.

48 Luger NM, *et al.* Osteoprotegerin diminishes advanced bone cancer pain. *Cancer Res* 2001; **61**(10): 4038–4047.

49 Drake FH, *et al.* Cathepsin K, but not cathepsins B, L, or S, is abundantly expressed in human osteoclasts. *J Biol Chem* 1996; **271**(21): 12511–12516.

50 Inaoka T, *et al.* Molecular cloning of human cDNA for cathepsin K: novel cysteine proteinase predominantly expressed in bone. *Biochem Biophys Res Commun* 1995; **206**(1): 89–96.

51 Yoneda T, *et al.* Involvement of acidic microenvironment in the pathophysiology of cancer-associated bone pain. *Bone* 2011; **48**(1): 100–105.

52 Mizoguchi F, *et al.* Transient receptor potential vanilloid 4 deficiency suppresses unloading-induced bone loss. *J Cell Physiol* 2008; **216**(1): 47–53.

53 Guilak F, Leddy HA, Liedtke W. Transient receptor potential vanilloid 4: the sixth sense of the musculoskeletal system? *Ann N Y Acad Sci* 2010; **1192**: 404–409.

54 Hoskin PJ, *et al.* Effect of local radiotherapy for bone pain on urinary markers of osteoclast activity. *Lancet* 2000; **355**(9213): 1428–1429.

55 Lam KW, *et al.* Comparison of prostatic and nonprostatic acid phosphatase. *Ann N Y Acad Sci* 1982; **390**: 1–15.

56 Jilka RL. Biology of the basic multicellular unit and the pathophysiology of osteoporosis. *Med Pediatr Oncol* 2003; **41**(3): 182–185.

57 Lacey DL, *et al.* Osteoprotegerin ligand is a cytokine that regulates osteoclast differentiation and activation. *Cell* 1998; **93**(2): 165–176.

58 Brown JM, *et al.* Osteoprotegerin and rank ligand expression in prostate cancer. *Urology* 2001; **57**(4): 611–616.

59 Thomas RJ, *et al.* Breast cancer cells interact with osteoblasts to support osteoclast formation. *Endocrinology* 1999; **140**(10): 4451–4458.

60 Keller RK, Fliesler SJ. Mechanism of aminobisphosphonate action: characterization of alendronate inhibition of the isoprenoid pathway. *Biochem Biophys Res Commun* 1999; **266**(2): 560–563.

61 Aapro M, Saad F, Costa L. Optimizing clinical benefits of bisphosphonates in cancer patients with bone metastases. *Oncologist* 2010; **15**(11): 1147–1158.

62 Body JJ. Bisphosphonates for malignancy-related bone disease: current status, future developments. *Support Care Cancer* 2006; **14**(5): 408–418.

63 Krempien R, *et al.* Combination of early bisphosphonate administration and irradiation leads to improved remineralization and restabilization of osteolytic bone metastases in an animal tumor model. *Cancer* 2003; **98**(6): 1318–1324.

64 Vassiliou V, *et al.* Combination ibandronate and radiotherapy for the treatment of bone metastases: clinical evaluation and radiologic assessment. *Int J Radiat Oncol Biol Phys* 2007: **67**(1): 264–272.

65 Atahan L, *et al.* Zoledronic acid concurrent with either high- or reduced-dose palliative radiotherapy in the management of the breast cancer patients with bone metastases: a phase IV randomized clinical study. *Support Care Cancer* 2010; **18**(6): 691–698.

66 Arrington SA, *et al.* Concurrent administration of zoledronic acid and irradiation leads to improved bone density, biomechanical strength, and microarchitecture in a mouse model of tumor-induced osteolysis. *J Surg Oncol* 2008; **97**(3): 284–290.

67 Boston SE, *et al.* Outcome after repair of a sarcoma-related pathologic fracture in dogs: a Veterinary Society of Surgical Oncology Retrospective Study. *Vet Surg* 2011; **40**(4): 431–437.

68 Kippenes H, *et al.* Spatial accuracy of fractionated IMRT delivery studies in canine paraspinal irradiation. *Vet Radiol Ultrasound* 2003; **44**(3): 360–366.

69 Vaudaux C, Schneider U, Kaser-Hotz B. Potential for intensity-modulated radiation therapy to permit dose escalation for canine nasal cancer. *Vet Radiol Ultrasound* 2007; **48**(5): 475–481.

70 Lawrence JA, *et al.* Proof of principle of ocular sparing in dogs with sinonasal tumors treated with intensity-modulated radiation therapy. *Vet Radiol Ultrasound* 2010; **51**(5): 561–570.

71 Nolan MW, *et al.* Intensity-modulated and image-guided radiation therapy for treatment of genitourinary carcinomas in dogs. *J Vet Intern Med* 2012; **26**(4): 987–995.

72 Denneberg NA, Egenvall A. Evaluation of dog owners' perceptions concerning radiation therapy. *Acta Vet Scand* 2009; **51**: 19.

73 Flynn AK, Lurie DM. Canine acute radiation dermatitis, a survey of current management practices in North America. *Vet Comp Oncol* 2007; **5**(4): 197–207.

74 Flynn AK, *et al.* The clinical and histopathological effects of prednisone on acute radiation-induced dermatitis in dogs: a placebo-controlled, randomized, double-blind, prospective clinical trial. *Vet Dermatol* 2007; **18**(4): 217–226.

75 Collen EB, Mayer MN. Acute effects of radiation treatment: skin reactions. *Can Vet J* 2006; **47**(9): 931–932, 934–935.

76 Anderson CR, *et al.* Late complications of pelvic irradiation in 16 dogs. *Vet Radiol Ultrasound* 2002; **43**(2): 187–192.

77 Stryker JA, *et al.* The effect of prednisone and irradiation on the rectum in dogs. *Radiology* 1976; **121**(1): 183–187.

78 Harris D, King GK, Bergman PJ. Radiation therapy toxicities. *Vet Clin North Am Small Anim Pract* 1997; **27**(1): 37–46.

79 Venable RO, *et al.* Dexrazoxane treatment of doxorubicin extravasation injury in four dogs. *J Am Vet Med Assoc* 2012; **240**(3): 304–307.

80 Villalobos A. Dealing with chemotherapy extravasations: a new technique. *J Am Anim Hosp Assoc* 2006; **42**(4): 321–325.

81 Ogilvie GK, *et al.* Acute and short-term toxicoses associated with the administration of doxorubicin to dogs with malignant tumors. *J Am Vet Med Assoc* 1989; **195**(11): 1584–1587.

82 Charney SC, *et al.* Risk factors for sterile hemorrhagic cystitis in dogs with lymphoma receiving cyclophosphamide with or without concurrent administration of furosemide: 216 cases (1990–1996). *J Am Vet Med Assoc* 2003; **222**(10): 1388–1393.

83 Gaeta R, *et al.* Risk factors for development of sterile haemorrhagic cystitis in canine lymphoma patients receiving oral cyclophosphamide: a case–control study. *Vet Comp Oncol* 2012; DOI: 10.1111/vco.12009 (epub ahead of print).

84 Poirier VJ, *et al.* Efficacy and toxicity of paclitaxel (Taxol) for the treatment of canine malignant tumors. *J Vet Intern Med* 2004; **18**(2): 219–222.

85 McEntee MC, *et al.* Phase I and pharmacokinetic evaluation of the combination of orally administered docetaxel and cyclosporin A in tumor-bearing cats. *J Vet Intern Med* 2006; **20**(6): 1370–1375.

86 McEntee MC, *et al.* Phase I and pharmacokinetic evaluation of the combination of orally administered docetaxel and cyclosporin A in tumor-bearing dogs. *Am J Vet Res* 2006; **67**(6): 1057–1062.

87 Waite A, *et al.* Phase II study of oral docetaxel and cyclosporine in canine epithelial cancer. *Vet Comp Oncol* 2014; **12**(2): 160–168.

88 Vail DM, *et al.* Efficacy of pyridoxine to ameliorate the cutaneous toxicity associated with doxorubicin containing pegylated (Stealth) liposomes: a randomized, double-blind clinical trial using a canine model. *Clin Cancer Res* 1998; **4**(6): 1567–1571.

89 Vail DM, *et al.* Preclinical trial of doxorubicin entrapped in sterically stabilized liposomes in dogs with spontaneously arising malignant tumors. *Cancer Chemother Pharmacol* 1997; **39**(5): 410–416.

90 Carlson K, Ocean AJ. Peripheral neuropathy with microtubule-targeting agents: occurrence and management approach. *Clin Breast Cancer* 2011; **11**(2): 73–81.

91 Hamilton TA, *et al.* Vincristine-induced peripheral neuropathy in a dog. *J Am Vet Med Assoc* 1991; **198**(4): 635–638.

92 Neugebauer V, *et al.* Antinociceptive effects of R(−)- and S(+)-flurbiprofen on rat spinal dorsal horn neurons rendered hyperexcitable by an acute knee joint inflammation. *J Pharmacol Exp Ther* 1995; **275**(2): 618–628.

93 Gold MS, *et al.* Hyperalgesic agents increase a tetrodotoxin-resistant Na + current in nociceptors. *Proc Natl Acad Sci U S A* 1996; **93**(3): 1108–1112.

94 Dore, M. Cyclooxygenase-2 expression in animal cancers. *Vet Pathol* 2011; **48**(1): 254–265.

95 Spugnini EP, *et al.* COX-2 overexpression in canine tumors: potential therapeutic targets in oncology. *Histol Histopathol* 2005; **20**(4): 1309–1312.

96 Lascelles BD, *et al.* Amantadine in a multimodal analgesic regimen for alleviation of refractory osteoarthritis pain in dogs. *J Vet Intern Med* 2008; **22**(1): 53–59.

97 Radulovic LL, *et al.* Disposition of gabapentin (neurontin) in mice, rats, dogs, and monkeys. *Drug Metab Dispos* 1995; **23**(4): 441–448.

98 Aghighi SA, *et al.* Assessment of the effects of adjunctive gabapentin on postoperative pain after intervertebral disc surgery in dogs. *Vet Anaesth Analg* 2012; **39**(6): 636–646.

99 Wagner AE, *et al.* Clinical evaluation of perioperative administration of gabapentin as an adjunct for postoperative analgesia in dogs undergoing amputation of a forelimb. *J Am Vet Med Assoc* 2010; **236**(7): 751–756.

100 Cashmore RG, *et al.* Clinical diagnosis and treatment of suspected neuropathic pain in three dogs. *Aust Vet J* 2009; **87**(1): 45–50.

101 Berger A, *et al.* Use of antiepileptics and tricyclic antidepressants in cancer patients with neuropathic pain. *Eur J Cancer Care* 2006; **15**(2): 138–145.

102 Jeal W, Barradell LB, McTavish D. Alendronate. *A review of its pharmacological properties and therapeutic efficacy in postmenopausal osteoporosis. Drugs* 1997; **53**(3): 415–434.

103 Bone HG, Schurr W. Intravenous bisphosphonate therapy for osteoporosis: where do we stand? *Curr Osteoporos Rep* 2004; **2**(1): 24–30.

104 Gennari L, *et al.* The use of intravenous aminobisphosphonates for the treatment of Paget's disease of bone. *Mini Rev Med Chem* 2009; **9**(9): 1052–1063.

105 Maricic M. Zoledronic acid for Paget's disease of bone. *Drugs Today* 2007: **43**(12): 879–885.

106 Lipton A. Toward new horizons: the future of bisphosphonate therapy. *Oncologist* 2004; **9**(Suppl 4): 38–47.

107 Lipton A. Emerging role of bisphosphonates in the clinic – antitumor activity and prevention of metastasis to bone. *Cancer Treat Rev* 2008; **34**(Suppl 1): S25–30.

108 Morgan G, Lipton A. Antitumor effects and anticancer applications of bisphosphonates. *Semin Oncol* 2010; **37**(Suppl 2): S30–40.

109 Luckman SP, *et al.* Heterocycle-containing bisphosphonates cause apoptosis and inhibit bone resorption by preventing protein prenylation: evidence from structure–activity relationships in J774 macrophages. *J Bone Miner Res* 1998; **13**(11): 1668–1678.

110 Luckman SP, *et al.* Nitrogen-containing bisphosphonates inhibit the mevalonate pathway and prevent post-translational prenylation of GTP-binding proteins, including Ras. *J Bone Miner Res* 1998; **13**(4): 581–589.

111 Van Beek E, *et al.* Farnesyl pyrophosphate synthase is the molecular target of nitrogen-containing bisphosphonates. *Biochem Biophys Res Commun* 1999; **264**(1): 108–111.

112 Fan TM, *et al.* Evaluation of intravenous pamidronate administration in 33 cancer-bearing dogs with primary or secondary bone involvement. *J Vet Intern Med* 2005; **19**(1): 74–80.

113 Fan TM, *et al.* Single-agent pamidronate for palliative therapy of canine appendicular osteosarcoma bone pain. *J Vet Intern Med* 2007; **21**(3): 431–439.

114 Spugnini EP, *et al.* Zoledronic acid for the treatment of appendicular osteosarcoma in a dog. *J Small Anim Pract* 2009; **50**(1): 44–46.

115 Fan TM, *et al.* The bone biologic effects of zoledronate in healthy dogs and dogs with malignant osteolysis. *J Vet Intern Med* 2008; **22**(2): 380–387.

116 Powers BE, *et al.* Percent tumor necrosis as a predictor of treatment response in canine osteosarcoma. *Cancer* 1991; **67**(1): 126–134.

117 Withrow SJ, *et al.* Tumor necrosis following radiation therapy and/or chemotherapy for canine osteosarcoma. *Chir Organi Mov* 1990; **75**(1 Suppl): 29–31.

118 Withrow SJ, *et al.* Intra-arterial cisplatin with or without radiation in limb-sparing for canine osteosarcoma. *Cancer* 1993; **71**(8): 2484–2490.

119 Bateman KE, *et al.* 0-7-21 radiation therapy for the palliation of advanced cancer in dogs. *J Vet Intern Med* 1994; **8**(6): 394–399.

120 Green EM, Adams WM, Forrest LJ. Four fraction palliative radiotherapy for osteosarcoma in 24 dogs. *J Am Anim Hosp Assoc* 2002; **38**(5): 445–451.

121 Mueller F, *et al.* Palliative radiotherapy with electrons of appendicular osteosarcoma in 54 dogs. *In Vivo* 2005; **19**(4): 713–716.

122 Ramirez O III, *et al.* Palliative radiotherapy of appendicular osteosarcoma in 95 dogs. *Vet Radiol Ultrasound* 1999; **40**(5): 517–522.

123 Knapp-Hoch HM, *et al.* An expedited palliative radiation protocol for lytic or proliferative lesions of appendicular bone in dogs. *J Am Anim Hosp Assoc* 2009; **45**(1): 24–32.

124 Oblak ML, *et al.* The impact of pamidronate and chemotherapy on survival times in dogs with appendicular primary bone tumors treated with palliative radiation therapy. *Vet Surg* 2012; **41**(3): 430–435.

125 Holmes RA. [153Sm]EDTMP: a potential therapy for bone cancer pain. *Semin Nucl Med* 1992; **22**(1): 41–45.

126 Serafini AN. Systemic metabolic radiotherapy with samarium-153 EDTMP for the treatment of painful bone metastasis. *Q J Nucl Med* 2001; **45**(1): 91–99.

127 Aas M, *et al.* Internal radionuclide therapy of primary osteosarcoma in dogs, using 153Sm-ethylene-diamino-tetramethylene-phosphonate (EDTMP). *Clin Cancer Res* 1999; **5**(10 Suppl): 3148s–3152s.

128 Barnard SM, Zuber RM, Moore AS. Samarium Sm 153 lexidronam for the palliative treatment of dogs with primary bone tumors: 35 cases (1999–2005). *J Am Vet Med Assoc* 2007; **230**(12): 1877–1881.

129 Lattimer JC, *et al.* Clinical and clinicopathologic response of canine bone tumor patients to treatment with samarium-153-EDTMP. *J Nucl Med* 1990; **31**(8): 1316–1325.

130 Milner RJ, *et al.* Targeted radiotherapy with Sm-153-EDTMP in nine cases of canine primary bone tumours. *J S Afr Vet Assoc* 1998; **69**(1): 12–17.

131 Farese JP, *et al.* Stereotactic radiosurgery for treatment of osteosarcomas involving the distal portions of the limbs in dogs. *J Am Vet Med Assoc* 2004; **225**(10): 1548, 1567–1572.

132 Caterina MJ, *et al.* The capsaicin receptor: a heat-activated ion channel in the pain pathway. *Nature* 1997; **389**(6653): 816–824.

133 Caterina MJ, *et al.* Impaired nociception and pain sensation in mice lacking the capsaicin receptor. *Science* 2000; **288**(5464): 306–313.

134 Davis JB, *et al.* Vanilloid receptor-1 is essential for inflammatory thermal hyperalgesia. *Nature* 2000; **405**(6783): 183–187.

135 Szallasi A, Blumberg PM. Vanilloid receptor loss in rat sensory ganglia associated with long term desensitization to resiniferatoxin. *Neurosci Lett* 1992; **140**(1): 51–54.

136 Olah Z, *et al.* Ligand-induced dynamic membrane changes and cell deletion conferred by vanilloid receptor 1. *J Biol Chem* 2001; **276**(14): 11021–11030.

137 Brown DC, *et al.* Physiologic and antinociceptive effects of intrathecal resiniferatoxin in a canine bone cancer model. *Anesthesiology* 2005; **103**(5): 1052–1059.

138 Karai L, *et al.* Deletion of vanilloid receptor 1-expressing primary afferent neurons for pain control. *J Clin Invest* 2004; **113**(9): 1344–1352.

139 Saunders DP, *et al.* Systematic review of antimicrobials, mucosal coating agents, anesthetics, and analgesics for the management of oral mucositis in cancer patients. *Support Care Cancer* 2013; **21**(11): 3191–3207.

140 Yazbeck VY, *et al.* Management of normal tissue toxicity associated with chemoradiation (primary skin, esophagus, and lung). *Cancer J* 2013; **19**(3): 231–237.

141 Jensen AB, *et al.* The cathepsin K inhibitor odanacatib suppresses bone resorption in women with breast cancer and established bone metastases: results of a 4-week, double-blind, randomized, controlled trial. *Clin Breast Cancer* 2010; **10**(6): 452–458.

142 Kassahun K, *et al.* Pharmacokinetics and metabolism in rats, dogs, and monkeys of the cathepsin k inhibitor odanacatib: demethylation of a methylsulfonyl moiety as a major metabolic pathway. *Drug Metab Dispos* 2011; **39**(6): 1079–1087.

143 Schmit JM, *et al.* Cathepsin K expression and activity in canine osteosarcoma. *J Vet Intern Med* 2012; **26**(1): 126–134.

144 Hans G, Deseure K, Adriaensen H. Endothelin-1-induced pain and hyperalgesia: a review of pathophysiology, clinical manifestations and future therapeutic options. *Neuropeptides* 2008; **42**(2): 119–132.

145 Hans G, Schmidt BL, Strichartz G. Nociceptive sensitization by endothelin-1. *Brain Res Rev* 2009; **60**(1): 36–42.

146 Nelson JB, *et al.* Suppression of prostate cancer induced bone remodeling by the endothelin receptor A antagonist atrasentan. *J Urol* 2003; **169**(3): 1143–1149.

147 Carducci MA, *et al.* Effect of endothelin-A receptor blockade with atrasentan on tumor progression in men with hormone-refractory prostate cancer: a randomized, phase II, placebo-controlled trial. *J Clin Oncol* 2003; **21**(4): 679–689.

148 Wessale JL, *et al.* Pharmacology of endothelin receptor antagonists ABT-627, ABT-546, A-182086 and A-192621: ex vivo and in vivo studies. *Clin Sci (Lond)* 2002; **103**(Suppl 48): 112S–117S.

149 Jimenez-Andrade JM, *et al.* Preventive or late administration of anti-NGF therapy attenuates tumor-induced nerve sprouting, neuroma formation, and cancer pain. *Pain* 2011; **152**(11): 2564–2574.

150 Halvorson KG, *et al.* A blocking antibody to nerve growth factor attenuates skeletal pain induced by prostate tumor cells growing in bone. *Cancer Res* 2005; **65**(20): 9426–9435.

151 Sevcik MA, *et al.* Anti-NGF therapy profoundly reduces bone cancer pain and the accompanying increase in markers of peripheral and central sensitization. *Pain* 2005; **115**(1–2): 128–141.

152 Fan TM, *et al.* Investigating TrkA expression in canine appendicular osteosarcoma. *J Vet Intern Med* 2008; **22**(5): 1181–1188.

153 Thress K, *et al.* Identification and preclinical characterization of AZ-23, a novel, selective, and orally bioavailable inhibitor of the Trk kinase pathway. *Mol Cancer Ther* 2009; **8**(7): 1818–1827.

154 Wang T, *et al.* Identification of 4-aminopyrazolylpyrimidines as potent inhibitors of Trk kinases. *J Med Chem* 2008; **51**(15): 4672–4684.

56 Orthopedic Patients

Steven C. Budsberg
College of Veterinary Medicine, University of Georgia, Athens, Georgia, USA

Chapter contents

Introduction

As small animal clinicians attempt to treat chronic pain and the associated dysfunction in their patients with osteoarthritis (OA), they face several challenges. First, it must be understood that pain is a complex experience involving not only the transduction of noxious stimuli from the periphery to the central nervous system (CNS) but also processing of the stimuli by the higher centers in the brain [1,2]. Pain is perhaps the most profound but least well-studied component of OA [3,4]. Articular cartilage degeneration, inflammation, synovitis, and subchondral bone and periarticular tissue changes are believed to be a source of pain associated with OA in our companion animal patients [5–9]. Osteoarthritis is the most common joint disorder leading to significant disability and dysfunction seen by small animal clinicians. While considered a very common problem in small animal medicine, OA is likely the most underdiagnosed and misunderstood rheumatic disease of dogs and cats. OA is a slow, progressive, and often insidious problem and due to the wide range of clinical signs associated with the disease, it is frequently misdiagnosed or overlooked.

In the dog, primary OA is uncommon, with the development of OA mainly occurring secondary to another joint pathology. OA is estimated to affect 20% of the United States (US) canine population [10]. This widely referenced estimate, in practical terms, translates to over 14 million affected dogs based on an estimated US canine population of 70 million. Estimates of the number of cats in the US and United Kingdom (UK) range from 70 and 10 million to 80 and 12 million respectively [11–13]. The number of cats affected by joint disease is unknown but recent studies suggest it is far more common in this species than previously thought, with an incidence ranging from 24% to perhaps as high as 90% depending on the population studied [14–18]. Because of the large number of animals affected, recognition and management of this disease are of the utmost importance.

While OA and degenerative joint disease (DJD) are often considered as being almost synonymous in dogs, this may not be the case in cats. In cats, joint pathology may have a different etiology, with onset, clinical signs, and pathophysiology differing from dogs [19–21]. For the purposes of this chapter, when discussing the cat, the term DJD/OA will be used to highlight this potential difference [22].

The best current definition of OA has been proposed by the American Academy of Orthopedic Surgeons. The consensus definition states that: ‘Osteoarthritic diseases are a result of both mechanical and biologic events that destabilize the normal coupling of degradation and synthesis of articular cartilage chondrocytes, extracellular matrix (primarily collagen and aggrecan), and subchondral bone. Although they may be initiated by multiple factors, including genetic, developmental, metabolic, and traumatic factors, osteoarthritic diseases involve all of the tissues of the diarthrodial joint’[23]. Ultimately, osteoarthritic diseases are manifested by morphologic, biochemical, molecular, and biomechanical changes of both cells and matrix which lead to softening, fibrillation, ulceration, articular cartilage loss, sclerosis and subchondral bone eburnation, and osteophyte production [4–7,9]. When clinically evident, osteoarthritic diseases are characterized by joint pain, tenderness, limitation of mobility, crepitus, occasional effusion, and variable degrees of inflammation without systemic effects.

From a pathophysiologic viewpoint, OA is characterized by articular cartilage degeneration and changes in the periarticular soft tissues (synovium and joint capsule) and subchondral bone.

Veterinary Anesthesia and Analgesia: The Fifth Edition of Lumb and Jones.
Edited by Kurt A. Grimm, Leigh A. Lamont, William J. Tranquilli, Stephen A. Greene and Sheilah A. Robertson.

In essence, if a joint is considered as an organ, OA can be likened to the end-stage of organ failure [9,24]. Specifically, the pathologic changes of osteoarthritis encompass articular cartilage degeneration, which includes matrix fibrillation, fissure appearance, gross ulceration, and full-thickness loss of the cartilage matrix. This pathology is accompanied by hypertrophic bone changes with osteophyte formation and subchondral bone plate thickening. Failure to repair the damage affecting the surface cartilage and the inability of chondrocytes in injured articular cartilage to restore a functional matrix despite high metabolic activity remains a complex and challenging problem [4–7,9,24].

Clinical signs of OA occur with varying degrees of severity, ranging from a mild, intermittent condition that causes mild discomfort and minimal disability to a disease state characterized by constant pain along with severe functional disability. Painful mechanical stimuli are detected by nociceptor (type III or A-δ and IV or C-fibers) afferent nerve fibers located in the joint capsule, associated ligaments, periosteum, and subchondral bone. Joint movement induces mechano-gated ion channels to open, resulting in nerve firing [1–3,8]. When joint movement exceeds normal limits, nerve firing dramatically increases and the higher centers in the central nervous system interpret these signals as pain. Data from experimental models of OA suggest that mechanosensory fibers become sensitized, resulting in increased afferent firing even in response to normal physiologic joint motion [25]. Furthermore, as stated previously, trying to alter or reverse the structural changes in the joint is problematic. Currently, there are no proven methodologies to reverse the changes in an osteoarthritic joint.

Diagnosis

As stated earlier, clinical signs of OA can vary from mild to severe and from vague to obvious, with pain as a trademark component. However, accurate assessment of pain and dysfunction can be very difficult in dogs and cats. Typically, the diagnosis of OA is based upon history, clinical signs, physical examination, and radiographs of the affected joint(s). The clinician's goal when assessing a dog or cat with suspected OA is to identify the site of pain and discomfort as well as attempting to diagnose any initiating causes. While diagnosis of the inciting cause may be more important in the younger patient, it is never too late to address such things as stifle instability. When dealing with the chronic end-stage OA joint, initiating factors may be less relevant and management of the OA becomes the sole focus of therapy.

In the clinical situation owner input is paramount. To increase client awareness and involvement and to hopefully begin to quantify the clinical signs, the use of client questionnaires or clinical metrology instruments is becoming more common. Several questionnaires have been designed and validated in the dog including the Canine Brief Pain Inventory (CBPI), the Liverpool Osteoarthritis in Dogs (LOAD), and the Helsinki Chronic Pain Index (HCPI) [26–31]. Use of these questionnaires in practice may lead to improved outcomes as less biased and more accurate assessments will be available to the owner and clinician. In cats, we have fewer data and clinical manifestations are very different from the dog; however, our knowledge is increasing all the time and the Feline Musculoskeletal Pain Index (FMPI) has recently been developed [32–34].

Owner assessment of pain severity is an interesting paradox. While owners are most aware of a patient's daily routine, they are not always aware of how pain is manifested. In one study owners needed to see their dog after effective pain management before they knew what pain and dysfunction were like in their pet [30]. This is the rationale for using owner assessments in addition to veterinary examinations. Owner assessments should be initiated at the start of treatment to define the degree of disability, and thus help decide the level of treatment required. Their use should be continued to monitor treatment efficacy. It is safe to assume that because the owner sees the patient on a daily basis, they are able to assess the multidimensionality of the pain and the associated functional disability. Metrics like assessment protocols are mandatory as it is well known that owners and veterinarians are biased when subjectively evaluating the patient. In a recent study, placebo effect was common in the evaluation of response to treatment by both the owner (57% improvement noted on placebo) and veterinarian (between 40% and 45%) [35]. Additional data suggest lower placebo effects but they are still significant and can easily alter our assessment of success or failure of a product or procedure [36].

Current therapy focuses on palliative care, aiming to reduce pain and inflammation and maintain or improve joint function without altering the pathologic process in the tissues. Most osteoarthritis in the dog and perhaps the cat is secondary to some other pathologic state, and thus the underlying cause must be identified in an attempt to minimize the long-term effects. Certainly efforts are being made to provide treatments which may alter the course of the disease but these therapies are still largely unproven.

Treatment strategies for managing chronic OA pain

Management of OA should be thought of as a multi-step approach with 4–5 important components (multimodal approach) for both dogs and cats [19–21,37–42]. In the busy practice setting, some clinicians tend to reach for pharmacologic management alone (i.e., give drugs singularly or in a multimodal fashion), and this approach usually has limited success. Managing OA should be based on a well-thought-out comprehensive plan which can be presented as WEDDS: **W**eight reduction and control; an **E**xercise and physical therapy program; a plan for types of **D**iets and supplements that can be used; a **D**rug (pharmacologic plan); and a discussion of potential **S**urgical interventions (Box 56.1). Thus, starting a treatment plan for a patient with OA requires a lengthy discussion of all aspects of management with the client.

First and foremost in the initiation of a management plan for chronic OA pain, there are often some false assumptions made by clinicians and owners that must be addressed. Three of the most common are listed below and are used here to emphasize the need for a realistic and scientifically sound approach to pain management.

- Treatment of pain is an 'all or none' phenomenon – **False.**
- One drug, at one dose (i.e., approved label dose), will work for all patients – **False.**
- If treatment seems to work in people, it must work in small animal patients – **False.**

> Box 56.1 Components of the WEDDS strategy for managing osteoarthritis.
>
> - Weight management
> - Exercise and physical therapy plan
> - Diet modification
> - Drugs
> - Surgery

Box 56.2 Strength of evidence ranking for clinical studies where data were evaluated to provide recommendations of the confidence in the data and subsequent findings of each study.

High level of comfort

Advises that qualified scientists agree that a specific claim is scientifically valid. This highest level of ranking possesses a very low level of probability that new scientific data will overturn the conclusion that the relationship in question is valid or significant. This rank is based on relevant, high-quality studies of study design types I and II with sufficient numbers of individuals resulting in a high degree of confidence that the results are relevant to the target population.

Moderate level of comfort

Describes a relationship as promising but not definitive. The claim is based on relevant, high to moderate-quality studies of study design type III and higher and sufficient numbers resulting in a moderate degree of confidence that the results could be extrapolated to the target population.

Low level of comfort

Possesses a low consistency. The relationship is based on moderate to low-quality studies of study design type III and has insufficient numbers of individuals tested resulting in a low degree of confidence that the results could be extrapolated. Uncertainties would also exist as to whether the proposed benefit(s) would be physiologically meaningful and achievable.

Extremely low level of comfort

Very low consistency and is based on moderate to low-quality studies of design type III and insufficient numbers resulting in a very low degree of confidence that the results could be extrapolated.

Remember, one must examine each case individually, assessing the age, normal activity levels, and, most importantly, the owner's expectations for performance of their animal. Success largely depends on the accurate assessment of the client's expectations. During the following discussion of each potential treatment modality, the justification and recommendation for a given therapy will be evidence based Box 56.2.

Management components

Weight reduction

Weight control is essential when dealing with OA. The majority of patients seen with clinical manifestations of OA are overweight or obese. While clinicians often recommend weight loss programs, success is not common. Several articles are available which discuss how to increase the success of weight loss recommendations [43–47]. The available data support weight loss in canine OA patients but few data are available to guide management of cats; however, it is very reasonable to use the same logic in feline as for canine patients. Owner education and proper dietary management must be considered in every case. Several studies provide data to support improved quality of life and lameness in the dog related to weight loss [48–54]. On reviewing the strength of the evidence, one can conclude that weight loss has a positive effect resulting in a moderate level of comfort in affected patients.

Exercise modification/physical therapy

There is extensive interest in the use of exercise modification and physical therapy in dogs and cats suffering from OA/DJD. There are several programs providing extensive education (including various certifications) in this area although the description of them is beyond the scope of this chapter. There are also textbooks available on these topics to help guide the clinician [55]. While most clinicians who work extensively with OA patients will agree that controlled exercise and rehabilitation medicine are helpful, there are unfortunately limited peer-reviewed data to support specific programs for canine and feline patients. It is certainly beyond the scope of this chapter to discuss the many recommendations about the use of exercise and rehabilitation medicine, but it is important to be practical and pragmatic. One example that is commonly recommended is to protect the osteoarthritic joint from excessive mechanical stress (forced exercise, excessive vertical movements, etc.), as it is felt that limiting these activities will potentially limit the clinical signs. One study certainly shows that persistent trotting of OA dogs does exacerbate the lameness and lends credence to this concept [56]. Most patients with OA are comfortable with light to moderate exercise regimens that do not vary significantly. Rest and exercise modification are different for each animal, but exercise extremes tend to exacerbate clinical signs. A second example of a commonly recommended activity is water-based activities (swimming or underwater treadmill exercise) [57].

While data to support some therapy modalities are sparse, they are starting to emerge. One study showed improvements in subjective outcome measures in dogs with OA treated with pulsed signal therapy (PST) [58]. PST is the application of pulsed electromagnetic fields on the joint and surrounding tissues. The strength of these data is limited by the fact that while the study was randomized and prospective, it was not blinded. Furthermore, while subjective improvements were found, objective gait outcome measures were not significantly different between controls and treated animals, resulting in a low level of confidence in these data. A second prospective study found that a combination of caloric restriction and intense physiotherapy improved weight loss and force plate kinetic data in overweight dogs with OA [47]. The data for all published studies range from low to moderate quality and when rated overall, the strength of the evidence leads us to conclude that one can have a low to moderate level of comfort with the results of the aforementioned studies. It is up to veterinarians and rehabilitation medicine practitioners promoting, practicing and financially benefiting from rehabilitation services to perform clinical trials to support their methodologies and justify their recommendations to clients and colleagues.

Nutritional support

The introduction of diets formulated with high omega-3 polyunsaturated fatty acids (PUFA), specifically eicosopentanoic acid (EPA) and docosahexaenoic acid (DHA), is adding a whole new dimension to the management of OA [59–61]. The current concept on how they work in OA is two-fold. The omega-3 family of PUFAs includes α-linolenic acid (ALA), EPA, and DHA while the n-6 family includes linolenic acid (LA) and arachidonic acid (AA) [62]. EPA and DHA are precursors for anti-inflammatory lipid mediators while AA is a precursor for proinflammatory lipid mediators. The first effect is indirect; increased consumption of omega-3 PUFA lowers the AA concentration in the body and concurrently increases the concentrations of EPA and DHA. The functional significance is that these eicosanoids are less potent mediators of inflammation. Increased consumption of EPA and DHA results in increased proportions of these fatty acids in inflammatory cells and occurs in a dose–response fashion and at the expense of AA [63–65]. In addition to forming fewer inflammatory eicosanoids, less substrate is available for the formation of AA-derived eicosanoids. The second action is a direct effect on cartilage. Cartilage cell cultures treated with omega-3 PUFAS inhibit the transcription of major enzymes and cytokines tied to matrix degradation [66].

Several clinical trials have looked at the effects of diets high in omega-3 fatty acids on pain and dysfunction associated with OA in dogs [67–72]. All studies were prospective and randomized, and examination of the quality of the studies showed they had adequately addressed issues of scientific quality relating to data collection, analysis, bias, and generalizability. The studies were consistent in finding positive effects of the diets on the clinical signs associated with OA. Outcome measures varied between studies, creating some challenges in assessing their overall strength; however, these studies uniformly identified positive effects on clinical signs associated with OA in dogs. Based on the data from these studies, the overall rating of the strength of the evidence (Box 56.2) concludes that one can have a high level of comfort with the results. Given the data available, it is strongly recommended to switch canine patients to one of these diets. The data are less clear regarding supplementing an existing diet with n-3 fatty acid products (fish oil capsules as an example). In cats, one study evaluated the effects of an elevated n-3 fatty acid diet and the results were relatively inconclusive. Thus there are very few data to support or reject the use of these types of diets in the cat [73].

Pharmacologic management

Analgesic and anti-inflammatory agents are the most common final component in the management of OA. The efficacy of non-steroidal anti-inflammatory drugs (NSAIDs) in treating chronic pain associated with OA has been well documented in several systematic reviews in small animal medicine [42,74,75]. There is high confidence in the data supporting the use of NSAIDs in the management of OA in dogs. There are fewer data available in the cat but we still have moderate comfort in the data supporting the use of NSAIDs in management of DJD/OA in cats [76].

It is not surprising that as a class of drugs, NSAIDs are among the most prescribed in small animal medicine. There are more data on NSAID use and potential complications than for any other aspect of a multimodal OA plan. In addition to analgesic and anti-inflammatory effects of NSAIDs, other agents are being tested, including products which act at the level of cytokines and other mediators. We will not discuss these further as they are still in the testing phase and speculation does not benefit patients.

The concept of disease modification is beginning to enter the picture of OA management. Compounds now known as disease-modifying osteoarthritis drugs (DMOAD) or structure-modifying osteoarthritis drugs (STMOAD) are being developed. Agents that have been previously called chondroprotective are now considered DMOADs or STMOADs. These drugs can have effects on the inflammatory cascade and release of mediators and also direct effects on target tissues (e.g., cartilage, bone, synovium) [77].

NSAIDs

As stated previously, NSAIDs are one of the classes of drugs most commonly used for managing chronic pain in small animals. There are several reasons for the dramatic increase in NSAID use in companion animals, including the availability of NSAIDs with improved safety and efficacy targeted specifically for small animal use (primarily the dog) [75,78,79]. For the most part, currently prescribed NSAIDs are very safe drugs, with only a small percentage of patients experiencing serious complications [78].

The effectiveness of NSAIDs is comparable to opioids in many musculoskeletal and visceral pain states. However, for severe pain associated with some fractures, data are not available to substantiate the same claim [80]. NSAIDs can be used to alleviate acute pain, either traumatic or surgically induced, and for chronic pain such as OA. Efficacy and toxicity are often individualistic and monitoring of each animal is mandatory in all cases [78]. Choosing and monitoring NSAID usage is important but there are no definitive guidelines as to how this should be done. First, it is wise to use products with a history of extensive clinical use, use only one NSAID at a time, and ensure correct dosing. Observe for potential toxicity as soon as administration is begun, with increased vigilance and monitoring of high-risk patients. If indicated, establish the renal and hepatic status of the patient prior to NSAID administration. Review the treatment plan frequently, and change to an alternative NSAID if there is a poor response to therapy or patient intolerance.

Contraindications

One must adapt therapy to suit the patient's needs. In patients with chronic disease, begin with the recommended dose and if efficacious, attempt to reduce the dose at regular intervals (e.g., weekly) until the lowest dose that provides the desired benefit is reached; this is termed the lowest effective dose (LED). Determining this lowest effective dose can be difficult at best and one study suggested that it is difficult to decrease by more than 50% of the recommended (label) dose for most dogs [81]. Avoid NSAIDs in patients with known contraindications to their use. Contraindications for NSAID use range from fairly obvious to quite subtle reasons. The following is a list of general guidelines on *potential* contraindications for NSAID usage. These recommendations may change as more clinical data are generated [82].

- Patients receiving any type of systemic corticosteroids.
- Patients already receiving an NSAID.
- Patients with documented renal or hepatic insufficiency or dysfunction.
- Patients with any clinical syndrome that creates a decrease in the circulating blood volume (e.g., shock, dehydration, hypotension, or ascites).
- Patients with active gastrointestinal (GI) disease.
- Trauma patients with known or suspected significant active hemorrhage or blood loss.
- Pregnant patients or females intended for breeding
- Patients with significant pulmonary disease (this may be less important with COX-2-specific drugs).
- Patients with any type of confirmed or suspected coagulopathy (this may be less important with COX-2-specific drugs).

Adverse events

The most common problems associated with NSAID administration to dogs and cats involve the gastrointestinal (GI) tract [78]. Signs may range from vomiting and diarrhea, including hematemesis and melena, to a silent ulcer which results in perforation. The true overall incidence of GI toxicity in dogs or cats treated with NSAIDS is unknown. Concurrent administration of other medications (especially other NSAIDs or corticosteroids), previous GI bleeding, or the presence of other systemic diseases may contribute to adverse reactions. The effect that aging or disease has on an individual patient's ability to metabolize NSAIDs is likely to be quite variable. Hepatotoxicosis caused by NSAIDs is generally considered to be idiosyncratic [78,83]. Most dogs recover with cessation of treatment and supportive care. Renal dysfunction may occur with NSAID administration as a consequence of prostaglandin inhibition. Renal prostaglandin synthesis is low under normovolemic conditions but in the face of hypovolemia, prostaglandin synthesis is increased and is important for maintaining renal perfusion [84–86]. NSAID use must be considered very carefully in hypovolemic or hypotensive animals. Animals that are currently receiving NSAIDs may undergo anesthesia with or without surgery where hypotension and blood loss may occur, so this must be addressed so that renal function is not compromised.

Specific NSAIDs

The approved NSAIDs available to clinicians vary considerably around the world. It is very important for practitioners to remember that the clinical response of an individual to a particular drug is quite variable. Individuals may respond favorably to one product and not another, so if a NSAID is indicated in a case and the first product used does not achieve a positive clinical response, NSAIDs should not be abandoned but a different product tried. The following overview of data about these compounds is taken from a more complete description published elsewhere [82].

Carprofen

Carprofen is a member of the arylpropionic acid class of NSAIDs. Carprofen is approved, in both oral and injectable formulations, to treat pain and inflammation associated with OA. Carprofen improved limb function in clinical trials of dogs with naturally occurring OA [87–94]. Three long-term studies (84–120 days) found that carprofen was well tolerated and based on subjective assessment, dogs appeared to improve over the treatment period. In certain countries, a single injectable dose in cats is approved for the treatment of pain. While there are ample data to support single dose use for perioperative pain, repetitive dosing in cats is not recommended [95–99]. Given the data available, there is high comfort in data supporting the use of carprofen in the dog to treat OA pain.

Cimicoxib

Cimicoxib is a member of the coxib class of NSAIDs and is approved as an oral formulation in the European Union for the treatment of pain and inflammation associated with OA and postoperative pain in dogs [100,101]. Limited data are available on cimicoxib, with one study documenting non-inferiority compared to carprofen in managing postoperative pain for dogs undergoing either orthopedic or soft tissue surgery. There are some data available as part of cimicoxib's approval process in Europe to support its use for chronic pain [101,102]. Given the lack of peer-reviewed published data, comfort in the data supporting the effectiveness of cimicoxib to manage the pain of OA in dogs is low to moderate.

Deracoxib

Deracoxib is a member of the coxib class of NSAIDs. It is approved for use in dogs as an oral formulation for the treatment of pain and inflammation associated with OA and postoperative pain associated with orthopedic surgery. In a study which has not been published in a peer-reviewed journal but has been presented in abstract form, it was demonstrated to provide effective pain relief in clinical trials involving dogs with OA [103]. As with OA, there are only abstracts of its efficacy for relieving pain related to orthopedic surgery [104]. Due to lack of information, it is not possible to rate the comfort level for the use of deracoxib in the dog to treat OA pain.

Etodolac

Etodolac is a member of the pyranocarboxylic acid class of NSAIDs. It is approved as an oral formulation for use in managing pain and inflammation associated with canine OA. In a multicenter clinical study, it improved rear limb function in dogs with chronic OA [105]. There is moderate comfort in the data supporting use of etodolac in the dog to treat OA pain.

Firocoxib

Firocoxib is a member of the coxib class of NSAIDs. It is approved as an oral formulation for the management of pain and inflammation associated with OA in dogs. Clinically it has been shown to improve limb function in dogs with OA [106–111]. Clinical trials suggest that firocoxib may have some superiority based on subjective evaluations by owners and veterinarians with regard to lameness resolution when compared to carprofen and etodolac in dogs with OA [106,107]. Long-term dosing of firocoxib resulted in continued improvements in resolution of signs over the year of treatment. Therefore, there is high comfort in the data on the use of firocoxib to treat OA pain in dogs.

Ketoprofen

Ketoprofen is a member of the arylpropionic acid class of NSAIDs. The only data available to the practitioner regarding clinical use of this product are based on an acute pain model and its perioperative use in both dogs and cats [112–116]. One small study included cats with OA/DJD treated for 5 days but the study was very limited [116]. No evidence-based judgment on the effect of ketoprofen for treating chronic pain and dysfunction in OA/DJD in dogs and cats can be made.

Mavacoxib

Mavacoxib is a member of the coxib class of NSAIDs. It is approved in the European Union as an oral formulation for the treatment of pain and inflammation associated with OA in dogs. There are published pharmacologic data on mavacoxib but no clinical data beyond what is available in the application for approval in Europe and one abstract from a meeting in 2009 [117]. Mavacoxib is a long-acting agent with an approved dosing regimen consisting of a loading dose repeated at 14 days and thereafter at dosing intervals of 1 month. Given the lack of published data, it is difficult to provide any evaluation of the efficacy of mavacoxib.

Meloxicam

Meloxicam is a member of the oxicam family of NSAIDs. It is approved for use in dogs for the control of pain and inflammation associated with OA and is available in oral, transmucosal oral mist, and parenteral formulations. Based on the amount and quality of the published data available for its use in the management of acute postsurgical as well as chronic OA pain in dogs, confidence in this data is high [118–122].

Meloxicam is also approved for use in cats, but in the US that approval is limited to a single (injectable) dose to control pain and inflammation associated with orthopedic surgery, ovariohysterectomy, and castration. Long-term use of meloxicam for the treatment of musculoskeletal pain in cats has been approved in several countries outside the US. Use in cats from 5 days to indefinite dosing to provide analgesia for locomotor disorders including OA has been described at several different dosing levels (0.01–0.05 mg/kg PO) daily [123–126]. While these data exist, clinical efficacy is primarily supported by data generated from studies using the 0.05 mg/kg dose PO every 24 h. At lower dosing regimens (0.01–0.03 mg/kg PO q 24 h), meloxicam is well tolerated and seemingly safe in cats, including those with chronic renal dysfunction [124–126]. With the amount and quality of the published data on the use of meloxicam to manage chronic OA/DJD pain in cats, comfort in these data is moderate to high.

Robenacoxib

Robenacoxib is a member of the coxib class of NSAIDs. It is approved for use in dogs and cats but the specific species approval varies between countries; it is available in an oral and injectable formulation but this also varies between countries. Indications in the dog are for treatment of pain and inflammation associated with orthopedic or soft tissue surgery as well as the treatment of pain and inflammation associated with chronic osteoarthritis (depending on the country) [127–129]. Based on the published reports, there is high comfort in the data on the the use of robenacoxib to treat OA pain in the dog.

In the cat, approved indications (depending on the country) may include treatment of postoperative pain and inflammation associated with orthopedic and soft tissue surgeries as well as the acute pain and inflammation associated with musculoskeletal disorders [115,130–134]. Length of approved treatment time for robenacoxib in the cat varies from 3 to 11 days, depending on regulatory jurisdiction. Given the limited data available, there is low to moderate comfort in the data on the use of robenacoxib to treat chronic OA/DJD pain in the cat.

Tepoxalin

Tepoxalin is a dual cyclo-oxygenase/lipoxygenase (COX/LOX) inhibitor, inhibiting both COX isoenzymes and 5-lipoxygenase. This drug offers an alternative method of blocking the pathways responsible for pain and inflammation. Tepoxalin has been approved for use in dogs to control pain and inflammation associated with OA, and was available in an oral formulation. Unfortunately, there are no published reports available to support clinical efficacy and safety beyond data submitted as part of the approval process for use in dogs. There is one report of successful off-label use of tepoxalin in the cat [123]. Currently, there is limited to no availability of this drug. Given the limited data, there is a low degree of comfort to support the use of tepoxalin in the dog or cat to treat OA/DJD pain.

Tolfenamic acid

Tolfenamic acid is an anthranilic acid derivative and a member of the fenamates class of NSAIDs. It is approved in Canada and Europe in both an oral and parenteral formulation for dogs and cats. Some clinical data are available to support the use of tolfenamic acid in the dog and cat but all data reported are for short-term use (3–7 days) [135,136]. Given the lack of long-term data, we have low confidence in the data on the use of tolfenamic acid to treat OA/DJD pain in the dog or cat.

Washout period when switching between NSAIDs

A question that is commonly asked by clinicians is whether or not a washout period is needed when switching from one NSAID to another. Several sources, including crowd sourcing websites, conference proceedings, pharmaceutical company promotional materials and journal articles, have advocated washout periods of varying lengths (1–7 days) when changing NSAIDs [83,137–139]. These recommendations are not based on clinical data but rather are derived from extrapolations of pharmacokinetic data and conservative speculation.

There are several different situations that need to be addressed when discussing how to switch NSAIDs in our clinical patients. The first situation is a change in the route of administration; for example, administering a single dose of a perioperative parenteral NSAID (e.g., carprofen or meloxicam) followed by a different oral NSAID the next day. The only data to use in this situation come from a study of normal healthy dogs that were given parenteral (subcutaneous) carprofen followed by deracoxib orally 24 h later and repeated for 4 days. This was one arm of the study and when compared to continuous carprofen (subcutaneous and oral) or placebo, there were no differences in clinical findings or gastric lesions. Thus from these limited data it appears that it may be safe to switch from a single injection of one drug to an oral formulation of another NSAID the next day in healthy dogs [137]. However, without testing all the possible combinations of injectable and oral NSAIDs, one cannot be definitive about these treatment recommendations.

The second situation is switching NSAIDs for perceived lack of a response by the patient. This is a difficult question that a clinician often faces and where there is significant variation in recommendations. Many authors suggest waiting five half-lives of the first drug before initiating the second drug to reduce the plasma concentrations of the first drug to near zero. The only clinical data which may shed light on this situation come from a report of switching to firocoxib from another NSAID; this study showed no increase in documented side-effects whether firocoxib was started the next day or up to day 7 after stopping the original drug [149]. These data would again suggest that a washout period is not necessary, but most clinicians follow the recommendation of discontinuing a NSAID for 1–7 days before initiating another drug.

The final situation is transitioning to or from aspirin. If aspirin is the initial drug, it has been recommended that a minimum of a 7-day washout period be followed before starting another NSAID. The basis of this recommendation is to provide time for platelet regeneration due to aspirin's irreversible effects on platelets [83,141]. However, there are few clinical data to support this recommendation.

If for some reason a dog is on a product that is COX-1 sparing (a primary COX-2 inhibitor) and is then changed to aspirin, a 7-day washout is recommended due to the gastric adaptation and production of aspirin-triggered lipoxins (ATLs) [83,141]. The concern is that when a patient is on aspirin, ATLs are produced and have been shown to exert protective effects in the stomach by diminishing gastric injury, most likely via release of nitric oxide from the vascular endothelium. However, concurrent administration of COX-1 sparing drugs with aspirin results in the complete inhibition of ATLs and can potentially cause significant exacerbation of gastric mucosal injuries. It is important to remember that the formation of ATLs has yet to be proven in the dog.

NMDA receptor antagonists

A significant breakthrough in the understanding of nociceptive processing came when it was realized that the nervous system was plastic; which is to say, inputs from the periphery could, via activation of a variety of receptors (principally the NMDA receptor), produce changes in the way nociceptive signals were processed in the spinal cord. The characteristics of the NMDA receptor are such that with repeated stimulation, it can produce a state of prolonged depolarization in dorsal horn neurons. This cellular 'wind-up' is thought to produce the state of 'central sensitization' via the activation of a variety of second messenger systems, and the production of nitric oxide (NO), eicosanoids and induction of immediate early genes. Central sensitization is thought to contribute to injury- or disease-induced pain by amplification of afferent signals, and by altering processing of sensory information such that previously non-noxious signals are now encoded as noxious. The NMDA receptor appears to be central to the induction and maintenance of central sensitization, and the use of NMDA receptor antagonists would appear to offer benefit in the treatment of pain where central sensitization has become established (especially chronic pain). Ketamine, tiletamine, dextromethorphan, and amantadine all possess some degree of NMDA antagonist properties, among other actions [142–144].

Amantadine

One publication involving dogs with OA has documented that amantadine used in addition to an NSAID resulted in improvements over the use of the NSAID alone [145]. This study was a randomized, blinded, placebo-controlled trial. The study had positive efficacy data from objective and subjective outcome measures. Based on this single study, there is a moderate level of comfort to support the use of amantadine in combination with NSAIDs.

Opioids

Opioid receptors are involved in pain states, and the descending serotonergic system is known to be one of the body's endogenous 'analgesic' mechanisms [80]. For both pharmacologic and regulatory reasons, long-term classic oral opioid therapy has not been a viable treatment option in veterinary patients. However, the use of tramadol (classified as an opioidergic/monoaminergic drug), a synthetic derivative of codeine, which has actions at the μ opioid receptor and also facilitates the descending serotonergic system, has been commonplace in small animal practice. Tramadol usage has grown without any clinical data to support its use and in spite of unfavorable pharmacokinetic data. Tramadol and two of its major metabolites, O-desmethytramadol (ODM) and N,O-didesmethyltramadol (DDM), are credited with the pharmacologic effects of this drug [146]. Studies show that opioid analgesia (central analgesia due to μ opioid receptor agonist effects) is primarily caused by ODM, yet most dogs produce very little ODM through biotransformation of tramadol. However, DDM, which is readily produced by dogs, may provide some opioid effects [147]. Additionally, ODM and tramadol provide the serotonin and norepinephrine effects in the dog and the antimuscarinic effects are produced by ODM. The elimination half-life of tramadol in the dog is approximately 1 h. The elimination half-life of DDM is about 3.5 h and these short half-lives may account for some of the limited (or perceived) positive effects of tramadol administration. Finally, data on repetitive dosing with tramadol reveal a decrease in plasma concentrations of 60–70% in just one week [147]. Yet, because of crowd sourcing data sites and continuing education lectures purporting its safety despite limited pharmacokinetic data, veterinary medicine has embraced its use. One randomized, prospective clinical trial provides data showing limited improvements in both objective and subjective outcome measures in canine OA patients receiving tramadol [36]. A second study looking at tramadol used postoperatively after tibial plateau leveling (TPLO) found that used alone, tramadol may not provide sufficient analgesic efficacy [148]. From an evidence-based approach, the level of comfort in data supporting the use of tramadol is low in dogs.

Interestingly, cats produce significant amounts of ODM in the breakdown of tramadol which also has an elimination half-life of 4.5 h [149]. These data provide a basis for the investigation of tramadol in cats for the treatment of chronic pain [150]. However, because of the high ODM concentrations in cats, opioid-mediated adverse effects are more likely, including sedation, dysphoria, mydriasis, vomiting, and constipation. Given the lack of any data, no level of comfort can be measured for tramadol use in cats with chronic pain.

A variety of other drugs have been suggested for the relief of chronic pain in dogs and cats with minimal or no pharmacologic information or clinical trials. As examples, there have been no clinical trials assessing gabapentin, pregabalin, venlafaxine, duloxetine or amitriptyline for the relief of painful symptoms associated with any type of chronic pain (such as OA) in dogs or cats. Thus confidence in the use of these products is not measurable.

Alternative, complementary, and homeopathic compounds

Compounds based upon chondroitin sulfate and glucosamine hydrochloride

Two trials were identified describing the use of compounds with chondroitin sulfate and glucosamine hydrochloride as major components for improving clinical signs associated with OA in dogs. These studies were prospective, randomized, and receive a type I classification. One study subjectively showed a positive effect via a previously published veterinarian-based scoring system [151], while the other showed no positive objective effects measured by force plate analysis [89]. Examination of the quality of the studies showed that they had adequately addressed issues of scientific quality relating to data collection, analysis, bias, and generalizability. An overall rating of the strength of the evidence concludes that one can have a moderate level of comfort with the results of the aforementioned studies yet the inconsistencies of the findings are problematic.

Green-lipped mussel preparation

Four trials were identified using a compound whose main ingredient was green-lipped mussel (*Perna canaliculus*) for the treatment of OA in dogs. The studies were prospective, and randomized in design [152–155]. While all showed positive effects (subjectively and objectively), they all had small sample sizes. Additionally, there are some uncertainties relating to the scientific quality of two of the studies. There was a moderate level of consistency between the studies. The studies do provide information to conclude that the reported effect may be physiologically meaningful and achievable. Based on review of these studies, there is a moderate level of comfort with their results and the positive effects seen with these compounds.

Zeel® homeopathic preparation

Two trials were identified using Zeel® for the treatment of OA in dogs. While both were prospective, only one was randomized and blinded [156,157]. Both studies showed subjective positive effects of the product but in one study, the effects were less than those produced by carprofen. Given the small sample sizes and the study limitations, there are uncertainties relating to scientific quality. There was a moderate level of consistency between the studies. An overall rating of the strength of the evidence concludes that there is a low to moderate level of comfort in the results of these studies and the positive effects seen with these compounds.

Elk velvet preparation

Velvet from elk antlers was tested as a food additive for dogs with OA. One randomized, blinded, placebo-controlled, parallel group clinical trial was evaluated [158]. This is classified as a type I study. It had positive efficacy data from objective and subjective outcome measures. Examination of the quality of the study showed that it had adequately addressed issues of scientific quality relating to data collection, analysis, bias, and generalizability. The study does provide sufficient information to conclude that the effect may be physiologically meaningful and achievable. An overall rating of the strength of the evidence concludes that there is a moderate level of comfort with the results of this study.

Type II collagen

Four studies including a randomized, blinded, placebo-controlled clinical trial using type II collagen as a treatment for OA in dogs have been performed [159–162]. Subjective and objective data supported the use of this product but given the small sample sizes and study design limitations of two reports, there are uncertainties relating to the scientific quality. An overall rating of the strength of the evidence concludes that one can have a moderate level of comfort with the results of these studies and the positive effects seen with this compound.

Brachystemma calycinum D. don

Brachystemma calycinum D. don was tested in one randomized, blinded, placebo-controlled, parallel group clinical trial as a treatment for OA [163]. The study had positive efficacy data from objective and subjective outcome measures. Examination of the quality of the study showed that it had adequately addressed issues of scientific quality relating to data collection, analysis, bias, and generalizability. The study provides sufficient information to suggest that the effect will be physiologically meaningful and achievable. An overall rating of the strength of the evidence concludes that there is a moderate level of comfort with the results of this study.

Other products

There are several other single clinical trials for a variety of products with limited to no positive effects in the treatment of the pain and dysfunction of OA. These include a single study of S-adenosyl l-methionine which showed no effect [164] and two studies which found limited improvements with subjective scoring systems for P54FP (an extract of *Curcuma domestica* and *Curcum xanthorrhiza*) and resin extract of *Boswellia serrata* [165,166]. An overall rating of the strength of the evidence concludes there is a low level of comfort with the results of these studies. Additionally, there are several other products or procedures that result in negative or no improvement in patients with chronic pain. Again, these studies are difficult to evaluate due to either inadequate study design or the small numbers of patients enrolled in them.

Dealing with non-responders to treatment

There is a continued desire to find additional drugs and compounds to help in the alleviation of chronic pain in small animal patients. This is based on the fact that current products are not always effective and some result in more adverse reactions than some clinicians and clients are willing to accept. Given this set of circumstances, a discussion about non-responders to current treatments is appropriate.

After initiation of treatment, the veterinarian and client need to decide whether or not the animal is responding to the prescribed pain management plan. Clinicians need to ask this question every time a product or therapy is prescribed. Without verbal patient communication, veterinarians are hampered in all phases of treating pain, including diagnosis, accurate characterization and localization, and evaluation of efficacy of therapy. While veterinary patients possess many of the same nociceptive pathways (including neurotransmitter receptors) and perhaps even similar perceptions of painful stimuli as other species, including humans, one cannot assume the evaluation of responses should be similar for all patients. One needs to go no further than comparing cats, dogs, and pet birds to find striking examples of this conundrum. In recent years, strides have been made in evaluating the effects of different pain therapies in veterinary patients, but remember current limitations and proceed with caution when making claims about new treatments or therapeutic agents. In most cases, clinician additional time is not spent on cases that respond as expected to treatment plans.

Responders are defined not just by the level of response but also by the outcome measure used to define a response. The Initiative on Methods, Measurement, and Pain Assessment in Clinical Trials (IMMPACT) consortium statement defines the following outcome responses in clinical trials for human pain associated with chronic pain [167,168].

- 10–20% decrease in pain intensity – considered minimally important
- 30% decrease in pain intensity – considered moderately important
- 50% decrease in pain intensity – considered substantially important
- 70% decrease in pain intensity – considered extremely important

Given these guidelines, in many human studies a 30% improvement in a patient makes that case a positive responder. Veterinary clinical trials to demonstrate efficacy for pain control are usually performed for regulatory purposes, with outcomes typically reported as statistical comparisons between treatment group population means. Thus results represent the 'average' patient. These data are difficult to apply clinically because individual patients are being treated. In human medicine, managing the pain and dysfunction of OA has been often described as the 80/20 rule [169]. That is, 80% of patients experience 20% pain relief, while only 20% of patents experience 80% pain relief. About 50% have their pain halved. If one does an extensive review of the data available in human medicine, some interesting and sobering results emerge. Data clearly show that different NSAIDs produce a range of responses for pain relief. This is compounded by the fact that the same NSAID, at different doses, shows the same gradation of responses. Generally, only about 15–30% of patients actually show extensive improvement, while over 60–70% have minimal improvement (i.e., a benefit) [170,171]. In veterinary medicine outcome testing instruments cannot give such a differentiation of varying clinical responses and so there are no data supporting different doses of a given NSAID even though it has been observed that NSAID effects are dose dependent. Despite the limitations of being able to detect clinical improvements, many (including the Food and Drug Administration Center for Veterinary Medicine) suggest that clinicians titrate the dose of NSAIDs to the lowest effective dose.

Conclusion

Despite the strides which have been made in evaluating the effects of different pain therapies in veterinary patients, there are limitations and veterinary care providers should proceed with caution when making claims about new treatments or therapeutic agents. Treatment should be evidence based.

References

1 Malfait AM, Schnitzer TJ. Towards a mechanism-based approach to pain management in osteoarthritis. *Nat Rev Rheumatol* 2013; **9**: 654–664.
2 Dray A, Read SJ. Arthritis and pain. Future targets to control osteoarthritis pain. *Arthritis Res Ther* 2007; **9**: 212–215.

3 Schaible HG. Mechanisms of chronic pain in osteoarthritis. *Curr Rheumatol Rep* 2012; **14**: 549–556.

4 Lee AS, Ellman MB, Yan D, *et al.* A current review of molecular mechanisms regarding osteoarthritis and pain. *Gene* 2013; **527**: 440–447.

5 Krasnokutsky S, Attur M, Palmer G, *et al.* Current concepts in the pathogenesis of osteoarthritis. *Osteoarthritis Cartilage* 2008; **16**(Suppl 3): S1–3.

6 Pelletier JP, Martel-Pelletier J, Abramson SB. Osteoarthritis, an inflammatory disease: potential implication for the selection of new therapeutic targets. *Arthritis Rheum* 2001; **44**: 1237–1247.

7 Goldring MB, Goldring SR. Osteoarthritis. *J Cell Physiol* 2007; **213**: 626–634.

8 Zhang RX, Ren K, Dubner R. Osteoarthritis pain mechanisms: basic studies in animal models. *Osteoarthritis Cartilage* 2013; **21**: 1308–1315.

9 Loeser RF, Goldring SR, Scanzello CR, *et al.* Osteoarthritis: a disease of the joint as an organ. *Arthritis Rheum* 2012; **64**: 1697–1707.

10 Johnston SA. Osteoarthritis. Joint anatomy, physiology, and pathobiology. *Vet Clin North Am Small Anim Pract* 1997; **27**: 699–723.

11 Shepherd AJ. Results of the 2006 AVMA survey of companion animal ownership in US pet-owning households. *J Am Vet Med Assoc* 2008; **232**: 695–696.

12 US Pet Ownership & Demographics Sourcebook. 2012. www.avma.org/KB/Resources/Statistics/Pages/Market-research-statistics-US-pet-ownership.aspx (accessed 8 October 2014).

13 Murray JK, Browne WJ, Roberts MA, *et al.* Number and ownership profiles of cats and dogs in the UK. *Vet Rec* 2010; **166**: 163–168.

14 Lascelles BDX, Court MH, Hardie EM, *et al.* Nonsteroidal anti-inflammatory drugs in cats: a review. *Vet Anaesth Analg* 2007; **34**: 228–250.

15 Lascelles BD, Henry JB, Brown J, *et al.* Cross-sectional study of the prevalence of radiographic degenerative joint disease in domesticated cats. *Vet Surg* 2010; **39**: 535–544.

16 Clarke SP, Mellor D, Clements DN, *et al.* Prevalence of radiographic signs of degenerative joint disease in a hospital population of cats. *Vet Rec* 2005; **157**: 793–799.

17 Clarke SP, Bennett D. Feline osteoarthritis: a prospective study of 28 cases. *J Small Anim Pract* 2006; **47**: 439–445.

18 Bennett D, Zainal Ariffin SM, Johnston P. Osteoarthritis in the cat: 1. how common is it and how easy to recognise? *J Feline Med Surg* 2012; **14**: 65–75.

19 Lascelles BD, Robertson SA. DJD-associated pain in cats: what can we do to promote patient comfort? *J Feline Med Surg* 2010; **12**: 200–212.

20 Bennett D, Zainal Ariffin SM, Johnston P. Osteoarthritis in the cat: 2. how should it be managed and treated? *J Feline Med Surg* 2012; **14**: 76–84.

21 Taylor PM, Robertson SA. Pain management in cats – past, present and future. Part 1. The cat is unique. *J Feline Med Surg* 2004; **6**: 313–320.

22 Lascelles BD. Feline degenerative joint disease. *Vet Surg* 2010; **39**: 2–13.

23 Kuettner K, Goldberg VM. *Osteoarthritis Disorders.* Rosemont, IL: American Academy of Orthopedic Surgeons, 1995.

24 Heinegård D, Saxne T. The role of the cartilage matrix in osteoarthritis. *Nat Rev Rheumatol* 2011; **7**: 50–56.

25 Schuelert N, McDougall JJ. Electrophysiological evidence that the vasoactive intestinal peptide receptor antagonist VIP6-28 reduces nociception in an animal model of osteoarthritis. *Osteoarthritis Cartilage* 2006; **14**: 1155–1162.

26 Walton MB, Cowderoy E, Lascelles D. Evaluation of construct and criterion validity for the 'Liverpool Osteoarthritis in Dogs' (LOAD) clinical metrology instrument and comparison to two other instruments. *PLoS One* 2013; **8**: e58125.

27 Brown DC, Boston RC, Coyne JC, *et al.* Ability of the canine brief pain inventory to detect response to treatment in dogs with osteoarthritis. *J Am Vet Med Assoc* 2008; **233**: 1278–1283.

28 Brown DC, Boston RC, Farrar JT. Comparison of force plate gait analysis and owner assessment of pain using the Canine Brief Pain Inventory in dogs with osteoarthritis. *J Vet Intern Med* 2013; **27**: 22–30.

29 Hercock CA, Pinchbeck G, Giejda A, *et al.* Validation of a client-based clinical metrology instrument for the evaluation of canine elbow osteoarthritis. *J Small Anim Pract* 2009; **50**: 266–271.

30 Hielm-Björkman AK, Rita H, Tulamo RM. Psychometric testing of the Helsinki chronic pain index by completion of a questionnaire in Finnish by owners of dogs with chronic signs of pain caused by osteoarthritis. *Am J Vet Res* 2009; **70**: 727–734.

31 Hielm-Björkman AK, Kuusela E, Liman A, *et al.* Evaluation of methods for assessment of pain associated with chronic osteoarthritis in dogs. *J Am Vet Med Assoc* 2003; **222**: 1552–1558.

32 Lascelles BD, Hansen BD, Roe S, *et al.* Evaluation of client-specific outcome measures and activity monitoring to measure pain relief in cats with osteoarthritis. *J Vet Intern Med* 2007; **21**: 410–416.

33 Benito J, Hansen B, Depuy V, *et al.* Feline musculoskeletal pain index: responsiveness and testing of criterion validity. *J Vet Intern Med* 2013; **27**: 474–482.

34 Benito J, Depuy V, Hardie E, *et al.* Reliability and discriminatory testing of a client-based metrology instrument, feline musculoskeletal pain index (FMPI) for the evaluation of degenerative joint disease-associated pain in cats. *Vet J* 2013; **196**: 368–373.

35 Conzemius MG, Evans RB. Caregiver placebo effect for dogs with lameness from osteoarthritis. *J Am Vet Med Assoc* 2012; **241**: 1314–1319.

36 Malek S, Sample SJ, Schwartz Z, *et al.* Effect of analgesic therapy on clinical outcome measures in a randomized controlled trial using client-owned dogs with hip osteoarthritis. *BMC Vet Res* 2012; **8**: 185.

37 Johnston SA, McLaughlin RM, Budsberg SC. Nonsurgical management of osteoarthritis in dogs. *Vet Clin North Am Small Anim Pract* 2008; **38**: 1449–1470.

38 Innes JF, Walton MB. Update on the diagnosis and management of canine osteoarthritis. *CVL Compan Anim* 2013; **2**(4): 113–122.

39 Fox SM. Multimodal management of canine osteoarthritis. In: Fox SM, ed. *Chronic Pain in Small Animals.* London: Manson Publishing, 2010; 189–201.

40 Rychel JK. Diagnosis and treatment of osteoarthritis. *Top Compan Anim Med* 2010; **25**: 20–25.

41 Fox SM. Painful decisions for senior pets. *Vet Clin North Am Small Anim Pract* 2012; **42**: 727–748.

42 Sanderson RO, Beata C, Flipo JP, *et al.* Systematic review of the management of canine osteoarthritis. *Vet Rec* 2009; **164**: 418–424.

43 Laflamme DP. Understanding and managing obesity in dogs and cats. *Vet Clin North Am Small Anim Pract* 2006; **36**: 1283–1295.

44 Laflamme DP. Nutritional care for aging cats and dogs. *Vet Clin North Am Small Anim Pract* 2012; **42**: 769–791.

45 Churchill J. Increase the success of weight loss programs by creating an environment for change. *Compend Contin Educ Vet* 2010; **32**: E1.

46 Michel K, Scherk M. From problems to success: feline weight loss programs that work. *J Feline Med Surg* 2012; **14**: 327–336.

47 Brooks D, Churchill J, Fein K, *et al.* 2014 AAHA weight management guidelines for dogs and cats. *J Am Anim Hosp Assoc* 2014; **50**: 1–11.

48 Impellizeri JA, Tetrick MA, Muir P. Effect of weight reduction on clinical signs of lameness in dogs with hip osteoarthritis. *J Am Vet Med Assoc* 2000; **216**: 1089–1091.

49 Mlacnik E, Bockstahler BA, Müller M, *et al.* Effects of caloric restriction and a moderate or intense physiotherapy program for treatment of lameness in overweight dogs with osteoarthritis. *J Am Vet Med Assoc* 2006; **229**: 1756–1760.

50 Farrell M, Clements DN, Mellor D, *et al.* Retrospective evaluation of the long-term outcome of non-surgical management of 74 dogs with clinical hip dysplasia. *Vet Rec* 2007; **160**: 506–511.

51 Kealy RD, Lawler DF, Ballam JM, *et al.* Evaluation of the effect of limited food consumption on radiographic evidence of osteoarthritis in dogs. *J Am Vet Med Assoc* 2000; **217**: 1678–1680.

52 Smith GK, Paster ER, Powers MY, *et al.* Lifelong diet restriction and radiographic evidence of osteoarthritis of the hip joint in dogs. *J Am Vet Med Assoc* 2006; **229**: 690–693.

53 Kirkby KA, Lewis DD. Canine hip dysplasia: reviewing the evidence for nonsurgical management. *Vet Surg* 2012; **41**: 2–9.

54 Marshall W, Bockstahler B, Hulse D, *et al.* A review of osteoarthritis and obesity: current understanding of the relationship and benefit of obesity treatment and prevention in the dog. *Vet Comp Orthop Traumatol* 2009; **22**(5): 339–345.

55 Millis DL, Levine D, Taylor RA. *Canine Rehabilitation and Physical Therapy.* Philadelphia: WB Saunders, 2004.

56 Beraud R, Moreau M, Lussier B. Effect of exercise on kinetic gait analysis of dogs afflicted by osteoarthritis. *Vet Comp Orthop Traumatol* 2010; **23**: 87–92

57 Chauvet A, Laclair J, Elliott DA, *et al.* Incorporationof exercise, using an underwater treadmill, and active client education into a weight management program for obese dogs. *Can Vet J* 2011; **52**: 491–496.

58 Sullivan MO, Gordon-Evans WJ, Knap KE, *et al.* Randomized, controlled clinical trial evaluating the efficacy of pulsed signal therapy in dogs with osteoarthritis. *Vet Surg* 2013; **42**: 250–254.

59 Lenox CE, Bauer JE. Potential adverse effects of omega-3 fatty acids in dogs and cats. *J Vet Intern Med* 2013; **27**: 217–226.

60 Budsberg SC, Bartges JW. Nutrition and osteoarthritis in dogs: does it help? *Vet Clin North Am Small Anim Pract* 2006; **36**: 1307–1323.

61 Perea S. Nutritional management of osteoarthritis. *Compend Contin Educ Vet* 2012; **34**: E4.

62 Schuchardt JP, Hahn A. Bioavailability of long-chain omega-3 fatty acids. *Prostaglandins Leukot Essent Fatty Acids* 2013; **89**: 1–8.

63 Healy DA, Wallace FA, Miles EA, *et al.* Effect of low-to-moderate amounts of dietary fish oil on neutrophil lipid composition and function. *Lipids* 2000; **35**: 763–768.

64 Yaqoob P, Pala HS, Cortina-Borja M, *et al.* Encapsulated fish oil enriched in alpha-tocopherol alters plasma phospholipid and mononuclear cell fatty acid compositions but not mononuclear cell functions. *Eur J Clin Invest* 2000; **30**: 260–274.

65 Baker KR, Matthan NR, Lichtenstein A, *et al.* Association of Plasma n-6 and n-3 polyunsaturated fatty acids with synovitis in the knee: the MOST Study. *Osteoarthritis Cartilage* 2012; **20**: 382–387.

66 Zainal Z, Longman AJ, Hurst S, *et al.* Relative efficacies of omega-3 polyunsaturated fatty acids in reducing expression of key proteins in a model system for studying osteoarthritis. *Osteoarthritis Cartilage* 2009; **17**: 896–905.

67 Fritsch D, Allen TA, Dodd CE, *et al.* Dose-titration effects of fish oil in osteoarthritis dogs. *J Vet Intern Med* 2010; **24**: 1020–1026.

68 Fritsch DA, Allen TA, Dodd CE, *et al.* A multicenter study of the effects of dietary supplementation with fish oil omega-3 fatty acids on carprofen dosage in dogs with osteoarthritis. *J Am Vet Med Assoc* 2010; **236**: 535–539.

69 Roush JK, Dodd CE, Fritsch DA, *et al.* Multicenter veterinary practice assessment of the effects of omega-3 fatty acids on osteoarthritis in dogs. *J Am Vet Med Assoc* 2010; **236**: 59–66.

70 Roush JK, Cross AR, Renberg WC, *et al.* Evaluation of the effects of dietary supplementation with fish oil omega-3 fatty acids on weight bearing in dogs with osteoarthritis. *J Am Vet Med Assoc* 2010; **236**: 67–73.

71 Moreau M, Troncy E, del Castillo JR, *et al.* Effects of feeding a high omega-3 fatty acids diet in dogs with naturally occurring osteoarthritis. *J Anim Physiol Anim Nutr* 2013; **97**(5): 830–837.

72 Hielm-Björkman A, Roine J, Elo K, *et al.* An uncommissioned randomized, placebo-controlled double-blind study to test the effect of deep sea fish oil as a pain reliever for dogs suffering from canine OA. *BMC Vet Res* 2012; **8**: 157.

73 Lascelles BD, DePuy V, Thomson A, *et al.* Evaluation of a therapeutic diet for feline degenerative joint disease. *J Vet Intern Med* 2010; **24**: 487–495.

74 Aragon CL, Hofmeister EH, Budsberg SC. Systematic review of clinical trials of treatments for osteoarthritis in dogs. *J Am Vet Med Assoc* 2007; **230**: 514–521.

75 Innes JF, Clayton J, Lascelles BDX. Review of the safety and efficacy of long-term NSAID use in the treatment of canine osteoarthritis. *Vet Rec* 2010; **166**: 226–230.

76 ISFM and AAFP Consensus Guidelines. Long-term use of NSAIDs in cats. *J Feline Med Surg* 2012; **12**: 521–538.

77 Vandeweerd JM, Coisnon C, Clegg P, *et al.* Systematic review of efficacy of nutraceuticals to alleviate clinical signs of osteoarthritis. *J Vet Intern Med* 2012; **26**: 448–456.

78 Monteiro-Steagall BP, Steagall PVM, Lascelles BDX. Systematic review of nonsteroidal anti-inflammatory drug induced adverse effects in dogs. *J Vet Intern Med* 2013; **27**: 1011–1019.

79 Carmicheal S. Clinical use of non-steroidal anti-inflammatory agents (NSAIDs): the current position. *Eur J Compan Anim Prac* 2011; **21**: 171–177.

80 Freye E. *Opioids in Medicine – A Comprehensive Review on the Mode of Action and the Use of Analgesics in Different Clinical Pain States.* Dordrecht, Netherlands: Springer, 2008; 256–266.

81 Wernham BG, Trumpatori B, Hash J, *et al.* Dose reduction of meloxicam in dogs with osteoarthritis-associated pain and impaired mobility. *J Vet Intern Med* 2011; **25**: 1298–1305.

82 Budsberg SC. Nonsteroidal anti-inflammatory drugs. In: Gaynor JS, Muir WW, eds. *Handbook of Veterinary Pain Management*, 2nd edn. St Louis, MO: Mosby Elsevier, 2009; 183–209.

83 KuKanich B, Bidgood T, Knesl O. Clinical pharmacology of nonsteroidal anti-inflammatory drugs in dogs. *Vet Anaesth Analg* 2012; **39**: 69–90.

84 Surdyk KK, Brown CA, Brown SA. Evaluation of glomerular filtration rate in cats with reduced renal mass and administered meloxicam and acetylsalicylic acid. *Am J Vet Res* 2013; **74**: 648–651.

85 Surdyk KK, Sloan DL, Brown SA. Renal effects of carprofen and etodolac in euvolemic and volume-depleted dogs. *Am J Vet Res* 2012; **73**: 1485–1489.

86 Surdyk KK, Sloan DL, Brown SA. Evaluation of the renal effects of iburprofen and carprofen in euvolemic and volume-depleted dogs. *Intern J Appl Res Vet Med* 2011; **9**: 129–136.

87 Vasseur PB, Johnson AL, Budsberg SC, *et al.* Randomized, controlled trial of the efficacy of carprofen, a nonsteroidal antiinflammatory drug, in the treatment of osteoarthritis in dogs. *J Am Vet Med Assoc* 1995; **206**: 807–811.

88 Holtsinger RH, Parker RB, Beale BS, *et al.* The therapeutic efficacy of carprofen in 209 clinical cases of canine degenerative joint disease. *Vet Comp Orthop Traumat* 1992; **5**: 140–144.

89 Moreau M, Dubuis J, Bonneau NH, *et al.* Clinical evaluation of a nutraceutical, carprofen and meloxicam for the treatment of dogs with osteoarthritis. *Vet Rec* 2003; **152**: 323–329.

90 Pollmeier M, Toulemonde C, Fleishman C, *et al.* Clinical evaluation of firocoxib and carprofen for the treatment of dogs with osteoarthritis. *Vet Rec* 2006; **159**: 547–555.

91 Autefage A, Gossellin J. Efficacy and safety of the long-term oral administration of carprofen in the treatment of osteoarthritis in dogs. *Rev Med Vet* 2007; **158**: 119–127.

92 Mansa S, Palmér E, Grøndahl C, *et al.* Long-term treatment with carprofen of 805 dogs with osteoarthritis. *Vet Rec* 2007; **160**: 427–430.

93 Reymond N, Speranza C, Gruet P, *et al.* Robenacoxib vs. carprofen for the treatment of canine osteoarthritis: a randomized, noninferiority clinical trial. *J Vet Pharmacol Ther* 2012; **35**: 175–183.

94 Lascelles BDX, Cripps P, Mirchandani S, *et al.* Carprofen as an analgesic for postoperative pain in cats: dose titration and assessment of efficacy in comparison to pethidine hydrochloride. *J Small Anim Pract* 1995; **36**: 535–554.

95 Balmer TV, Irvine D, Jones RS, *et al.* Comparison of carprofen and pethidine as postoperative analgesics in the cat. *J Small Anim Pract* 1998; **39**: 158–164.

96 Slingsby LS, Waterman-Pearson AE. Postoperative analgesia in the cat after ovariohysterectomy by use of carprofen, ketoprofen, meloxicam or tolfenamic acid. *J Small Anim Pract* 2000; **41**: 447–450.

97 Slingsby LS, Waterman-Pearson AE. Comparison between meloxicam and carprofen for postoperative analgesia after feline ovariohysterectomy. *J Small Anim Pract* 2002; **43**: 286–289.

98 Al-Gizawiy MM, Rude PE. Comparison of preoperative carprofen and postoperative butorphanol as postsurgical analgesics in cats undergoing ovariohysterectomy. *Vet Anaesth Analg* 2004; **31**: 164–174.

99 Polson S, Taylor PM, Yates D. Analgesia after feline ovariohysterectomy under midazolam-medetomidine-ketamine anaesthesia with buprenorphine or butorphanol, and carprofen or meloxicam: a prospective, randomised clinical trial. *J Feline Med Surg* 2012; **14**: 553–559.

100 Grandemange E, Fournel S, Woehrlé F. Efficacy and safety of cimicoxib in the control of perioperative pain in dogs. *J Small Anim Pract* 2013; **54**: 304–312.

101 EMA. Cimalgex: summary to the public. EMA/532732/2010. www.ema.europa.eu/docs/en_GB/document_library/EPAR_-_Summary_for_the_public/veterinary/000162/WC500109401.pdf (accessed 8 October 2014).

102 EMA. Cimalgex: scientific discussion. EMA/CVMP/513842/2011. www.ema.europa.eu/docs/en_GB/document_library/EPAR_-_Public_assessment_report/veterinary/000162/WC500109399.pdf (accessed 8 october 2014).

103 Johnston SA, Conzemius MG, Cross AR, *et al.* A multi-center clinical study of the effects of Deracoxib, a COX-2 selective drug on chronic pain in dogs with osteoarthritis. *Vet Surg* 2001; **30**: 497.

104 Millis DL, Conzemius MG, Wells KL, *et al.* A multi-center clinical study on the effects of Dearcoxicb, a COX-2 selective drug on post-operative analgesia associated with cranial cruciate ligament stabilization in dogs. *Vet Surg* 2001; **30**: 502.

105 Budsberg SC, Johnston SA, Schwarz PD, *et al.* Evaluation of etodolac for the treatment of osteoarthritis of the hips in dogs: a prospective multicenter study. *J Am Vet Med Assoc* 1999; **214**: 1–5.

106 Pollmeier M, Toulemonde C, Fleishman C, *et al.* Clinical evaluation of firocoxib and carprofen for the treatment of dogs with osteoarthritis. *Vet Rec* 2006; **159**: 547–551.

107 Gordon WJ, Conzemius MG, Drag M, *et al.* Assessment of the efficacy of firocoxib and etodolac for the treatment of osteoarthritis in dogs. *Vet Surg* 2004; **33**: E9.

108 Hanson PD, Brooks KC, Case J, *et al.* Efficacy and safety of firocoxib in the management of canine osteoarthritis under field conditions. *Vet Ther* 2006; **7**: 127–140.

109 Autefage A, Palissier FM, Asimus E, *et al.* Long-term efficacy and safety of firocoxib in the treatment of dogs with osteoarthritis. *Vet Rec* 2011; **168**: 617–623.

110 Hanson PD, Brooks KC, Case J, *et al.* Efficacy and safety of firocoxib in the management of canine osteoarthritis under field conditions. *Vet Ther* 2006; **7**: 127–140.

111 Ryan WG, Moldave K, Carithers D. Clinical effectiveness and safety of a new NSAID, firocoxib: a 1000 dog study. *Vet Ther* 2006; **7**: 119–126.

112 Grisneaux E, Pibarot P, Dupuis J, *et al.* Comparison of ketoprofen and carprofen administered prior to orthopedic surgery for control of postoperative pain in dogs. *J Am Vet Med Assoc* 1999; **215**: 1105–1110.

113 Hazewinkel HA, van den Brom WE, Pollmeier M, *et al.* Reduced dosage of ketoprofen for the short-term and long-term treatment of joint pain in dogs. *Vet Rec* 2003; **152**: 11–14.

114 Morton CM, Grant D, Johnston L, *et al.* Clinical evaluation of meloxicam versus ketoprofen in cats suffering from painful acute locomotor disorders. *J Feline Med Surg* 2011; **13**: 237–243.

115 Sano T, King JN, Seewald W, *et al.* Comparison of oral robenacoxib and ketoprofen for the treatment of acute pain and inflammation associated with musculoskeletal disorders in cats: a randomised clinical trial. *Vet J* 2012; **93**: 397–403.

116 Lascelles BD, Henderson AJ, Hackett IJ. Evaluation of the clinical efficacy of meloxicam in cats with painful locomotor disorders. *J Small Anim Pract* 2001; **42**: 587–593.

117 Payne-Johnson M, Boucher JF, Stegemann MR. Efficacy and safety of mavacoxib in the treatment of pain and inflammation associated with degenerative joint disease in dogs presented as veterinary patients. 11th International Congress of European Association of Veterinary Pharmacology and Toxicology. *J Vet Pharmacol Ther* 2009; **32**: 106–107.

118 Doig PA, Purbrick KA, Hare JE, *et al.* Clinical efficacy and tolerance of meloxicam in dogs with chronic osteoarthritis. *Can Vet J* 2000; **41**: 296–300.

119 Nell T, Bergman J, Hoeijmakers M, *et al.* Comparison of vedaprofen and meloxicam in dogs with musculoskeletal pain and inflammation. *J Small Anim Pract* 2002; **43**: 208–212.

120 Peterson KD, Keefe TJ. Effects of meloxicam on severity of lameness and other clinical signs of osteoarthritis in dogs. *J Am Vet Med Assoc* 2004; **225**: 1056–1060.

121 Gruet P, Seewald W, King JN. Evaluation of subcutaneous and oral administration of robenacoxib and meloxicam for the treatment of acute pain and inflammation associated with orthopedic surgery in dogs. *Am J Vet Res* 2011; **72**: 184–193.

122 Laredo FG, Belda E, Murciano J, *et al.* Comparison of the analgesic effects of meloxicam and carprofen administered preoperatively to dogs undergoing orthopaedic surgery. *Vet Rec* 2004; **155**: 667–671.

123 Charlton AN, Benito J, Simpson W, *et al.* Evaluation of the clinical use of tepoxalin and meloxicam in cats. *J Feline Med Surg* 2013; **15**: 678–690.

124 Gunew MN, Menrath VH, Marshall RD. Long-term safety, efficacy and palatability of oral meloxicam at 0.01–0.03 mg/kg for treatment of osteoarthritic pain in cats. *J Feline Med Surg* 2008; **10**: 235–241.

125 Guillot M, Moreau M, Heit M, *et al.* Characterization of osteoarthritis in cats and meloxicam efficacy using objective chronic pain evaluation tools. *Vet J* 2013; **196**: 360–367.

126 Gowan RA, Lingard AE, Johnston L, *et al.* Retrospective case–control study of the effects of long-term dosing with meloxicam on renal function in aged cats with degenerative joint disease. *J Feline Med Surg* 2012; **13**: 752–761.

127 Reymond N, Speranza C, Gruet P, *et al.* Robenacoxib vs.carprofen for the treatment of canine osteoarthritis: a randomized, noninferiority clinical trial. *J Vet Pharmacol Ther* 2012; **35**: 175–183.

128 Gruet P, Seewald W, King JN. Evaluation of subcutaneous and oral administration of robenacoxib and meloxicam for the treatment of acute pain and inflammation associated with orthopedic surgery in dogs. *Am J Vet Res* 2011; **72**: 184–193.

129 Edamura K, King JN, Seewald W, *et al.* Comparison of oral robenacoxib and carprofen for the treatment of osteoarthritis in dogs: a randomized clinical trial. *J Vet Med Sci* 2012; **74**: 1121–1131.

130 Staffieri F, Centonze P, Gigante G, *et al.* Comparison of the analgesic effects of robenacoxib, buprenorphine and their combination in cats after ovariohysterectomy. *Vet J* 2013; **197**: 363–367.

131 Kamata M, King JN, Seewald W, *et al.* Comparison of injectable robenacoxib versus meloxicam for peri-operative use in cats: results of a randomised clinical trial. *Vet J* 2012; **193**: 114–118.

132 Giraudel JM, Gruet P, Alexander DG, *et al.* Evaluation of orally administered robenacoxib versus ketoprofen for treatment of acute pain and inflammation associated with musculoskeletal disorders in cats. *Am J Vet Res* 2010; **71**: 710–719.

133 King S, Roberts ES, Roycroft LM, *et al.* Evaluation of oral robenacoxib for the treatment of postoperative pain and inflammation in cats: results of a randomized clinical trial. *ISRN Vet Sci* 2012; **79**: 41–48.

134 King JN, Hotz R, Reagan EL, *et al.* Safety of oral robenacoxib in the cat. *J Vet Pharmacol Ther* 2011; **35**: 290–300.

135 Charette B, Dupuis J, Moreau M, *et al.* Assessing the efficacy of long-term administration of tolfenamic acid in dogs undergoing femoral head and neck excision. *Vet Comp Orthop Traumatol* 2003; **16**: 232–237.

136 Murison PJ, Tacke S, Wondratschek C, *et al.* Postoperative analgesic efficacy of meloxicam compared to tolfenamic acid in cats undergoing orthopaedic surgery. *J Small Anim Pract* 2010; **51**: 526–532.

137 Dowers KL, Uhrig SR, Mama KR, *et al.* Effect of short-term sequential administration of nonsteriodal anti-inflammatory drugs on the stomach and proximal portion of the duodenum in healthy dogs. *Am J Vet Res* 2006; **67**: 1794–1801.

138 Lascelles BD, McFarland JM, Swann H. Guidelines for safe and effective use of NSAIDs in dogs. *Vet Ther* 2005; **6**: 237–251.

139 Sharkey M, Brown M, Wilmot L. What veterinarians should tell clients about pain control and their pets. FDA Veterinarian Newsletter 2006, Volume XXI, No I. www.valheart.com/blog/what-veterinarians-should-tell-clients-about-pain-control-and-their-pets/ (accessed 8 October 2014).

140 Ryan WG, Moldave K, Carithers D. Switching NSAIDs in practice: insights from the Previcox (firocoxib) experience trial. *Vet Ther* 2007; **8**: 263–271.

141 Papich MG. An update on nonsteroidal anti-inflammatory drugs (NSAIDs) in small animals. *Vet Clin Small Anim* 2008; **38**: 1243–1266.

142 Gonda X. Basic pharmacology of NMDA receptors. *Curr Pharm Des* 2012; **18**: 1558–1567.

143 Pozzi A, Muir WW, Traverso F. Prevention of central sensitization and pain by N-methyl-D-aspartate receptor antagonists. *J Am Vet Med Assoc* 2006; **228**: 53–60.

144 Zhou HY, Chen SR, Pan HL. Targeting N-methyl-D-aspartate receptors for treatment of neuropathic pain. *Expert Rev Clin Pharmacol* 2011; **4**: 379–388.

145 Lascelles BD, Gaynor JS, Smith ES, *et al.* Amantadine in a multimodal analgesic regimen for alleviation of refractory osteoarthritis pain in dogs. *J Vet Intern Med* 2008; **22**: 53–59.

146 KuKanich B. Outpatient oral analgesics in dogs and cats beyond nonsteroidal anti-inflammatory drugs: an evidence-based approach. *Vet Clin Small Anim* 2013; **43**: 1109–1125.

147 KuKanich B, Papich MG. Pharmacokinetics and antinociceptive effects of oral tramadol hydrochloride administration in greyhounds. *Am J Vet Res* 2011; **72**: 256–262.

148 Davila D, Keeshen TP, Evans RB, *et al.* Comparison of the analgesic efficacy of perioperative firocoxib and tramadol administration in dogs undergoing tibial plateau leveling osteotomy. *J Am Vet Med Assoc* 2013; **243**: 225–231.

149 Pypendop BH, Ilkiw JE. Pharmacokinetics of tramadol and its metabolite O-desmethyl-tramadol, in cats. *J Vet Pharmacol Ther* 2008; **10**: 24–31.

150 Pypendop BH, Siao KT, Ilkiw JE. Effects of tramadol hydrochloride on the thermal threshold in cats. *Am J Vet Res* 2009; **70**: 1465–1470.

151 McCarthy G, O'Donovan J, Jones B, *et al.* Randomised double-blind, positive-controlled trial to assess the efficacy of glucosamine/chondroitin sulfate for the treatment of dogs with osteoarthritis. *Vet J* 2007; **174**: 54–61.

152 Bui LM, Bierer TL. Influence of green lipped mussels (perna canaliculus) in alleviating signs of arthritis in dogs. *Vet Therap* 2001; **2**: 101–111.

153 Bierer TL, Bui LM. Improvement of arthritic signs in dogs fed green-lipped mussel (perna canaliculus). *Am Soc Nutr Sci* 2002; **132**: 1634S–1636S.

154 Pollard B, Guilford WG, Ankenbauer-Perkins KL, *et al.* Clinical efficacy and tolerance of an extract of green-lipped mussel (Perna canaliculus) in dogs presumptively diagnosed with degenerative joint disease. *N Z Vet J* 2006; **54**: 114–118.

155 Rialland P, Bichot S, Lussier B, *et al.* Effect of a diet enriched with green-lipped mussel on pain behavior and functioning in dogs with clinical osteoarthritis. *Can J Vet Res* 2013; **77**: 66–74.

156 Hielm-Björkman A, Tulamo RM, Salonen H, *et al.* Evaluating complementary therapies for canine osteoarthritis – Part II: a homeopathic combination preparation (Zeel). *Evid Based Complement Alternat Med* 2009; **6**: 465–471.

157 Neumann S, Stolt P, Braun G, *et al.* Effectiveness of the homeopathic preparation Zeel compared with carprofen in dogs with osteoarthritis. *J Am Anim Hosp Assoc* 2011; **47**: 12–20.

158 Moreau M, Dupuis J, Bonneau NH, *et al.* Clinical evaluation of a powder of quality elk velvet antler for the treatment of osteoarthrosis in dogs. *Can Vet J* 2004; **45**: 133–139.

159 Deparle LA, Gupta RC, Canerdy TD, *et al.* Efficacy and safety of glycosylated undenatured type-II collagen (UC-II) in therapy of arthritic dogs. *J Vet Pharmacol Ther* 2005; **28**: 385–390.

160 Peal A, d'Altilio M, Simms C, *et al.* Therapeutic efficacy and safety of undenatured type-II collagen (UC-II) alone or in combination with (-)-hydroxycitric acid and chromemate in arthritic dogs. *J Vet Pharmacol Ther* 2007; **30**: 275–278.

161 D'Altilio M, Peal A, Alvey M, *et al.* Therapeutic efficacy and safety of undenatured type II collagen singly or in combination with glucosamine and chondroitin in arthritic dogs. *Toxicol Mech Methods* 2007; **17**: 189–196.

162 Gupta RC, Canerdy TD, Lindley J, *et al.* Comparative therapeutic efficacy and safety of type-II collagen (UC-II), glucosamine and chondroitin in arthritic dogs: pain evaluation by ground force plate. *J Anim Physiol Anim Nutr* 2012; **96**: 770–777.

163 Moreau M, Lussier B, Pelletier JP, *et al.* Brachystemma calycinum D. don effectively reduces the locomotor disability in dogs with naturally occurring osteoarthritis: a randomized placebo-controlled trial. *Evid Based Complement Alternat Med* 2012; doi:10.1155/2012/646191.

164 Imhoff DJ, Gordon-Evans WJ, Evans RB, *et al.* Evaluation of S-adenosyl l-methionine in a double-blinded, randomized, placebo-controlled, clinical trial for treatment of presumptive osteoarthritis in the dog. *Vet Surg* 2011; **40**: 228–232.

165 Innes JF, Fuller CJ, Grover ER, *et al.* Randomised, double-blind, placebo-controlled parallel group study of P54FP for the treatment of dogs with osteoarthritis. *Vet Rec* 2003; **152**: 457–460.

166 Reichling J, Schmokel H, Fitzi J, *et al.* Dietary support with Boswellia resin in canine inflammatory joint and spinal disease. *Schweiz Arch Tierheilkd* 2004; **146**: 71–79.

167 Dworkin RH, Turk DC, Peirce-Sandner S, *et al.* Considerations for improving assay sensitivity in chronic pain clinical trials: IMMPACT recommendations. *Pain* 2012; **153**: 1148–1158.

168 Dworkin RH, Turk DC, Peirce-Sandner S, *et al.* Research design considerations for confirmatory chronic pain clinical trials: IMMPACT recommendations. *Pain* 2010; **149**: 177–193.

169 Moore RA, Moore OA, Derry S, *et al.* Numbers needed to treat calculated from responder rates give a better indication of efficacy in osteoarthritis trials than mean pain scores. *Arthritis Res Ther* 2008; **10**: R39.

170 Moore RA, Moore OA, Derry S, *et al.* Responder analysis for pain relief and numbers needed to treat in a meta-analysis of etoricoxib osteoarthritis trials: bridging a gap between clinical trials and clinical practice. *Ann Rheum Dis* 2010; **69**: 374–379.

171 Moore RA, Derry S, McQuay HJ, *et al.* Clinical effectiveness: an approach to clinical trial design more relevant to clinical practice, acknowledging the importance of individual differences. *Pain* 2010; **149**: 173–176.

57 Patient and Anesthetist Safety Considerations for Laser and Radiographic Procedures and Magnetic Resonance Imaging

Julie A. Smith
MedVet Medical and Cancer Centers for Pets, Worthington, Ohio, USA

Chapter contents

Introduction

Anesthesia is often required for patients undergoing diagnostic or therapeutic procedures utilizing dangerous devices. Since the anesthetic requirements of patients can vary considerably, it is impractical to discuss specific protocols for each procedure; instead, the reader is directed to individual chapters on specific conditions (e.g., Chapter 28 for anesthetic considerations for neuroimaging of brain disease patients) for information about anesthetic drug selection and patient management considerations. Ensuring a safe environment for both the anesthetist and the patient during the use of lasers and diagnostic imaging procedures or high-strength magnetic fields is extremely important. Therefore, the subjects of this chapter are the patient and personnel safety considerations for diagnostic imaging and laser procedures.

Laser

The word laser is an acronym for Light Amplification by Stimulated Emission of Radiation. Surgical lasers produce an intense beam of pulsed or continuous invisible infrared light (radiation) that can be hazardous if proper precautions are not taken [1–3]. Laser devices are classified and labeled by the manufacturer according to their potential to cause biologic damage. The classifications range from Class 1, the safest, to Class 4, the most hazardous. Wavelength, output power, and tissue exposure time are parameters used to categorize lasers and determine which precautions are necessary [4]. The most common lasers utilized in veterinary procedures (Table 57.1) have high laser emission levels and are listed in Class 3b or Class 4. The American National Standards Institute's Z136.3 standards provide guidance for the safe operation of lasers in healthcare facilities including veterinary hospitals [5,6]. The primary hazard associated with Class 3b and Class 4 lasers is related to accidental exposure to laser emissions.

Laser beam hazard and safety

Exposure may occur directly from the laser beam or when the beam is reflected from a polished surface, metal instruments or other objects. Reflected laser beams are unaltered and contain the same energy as the direct beam. Backscattering can also occur as the energy partially reflects on impact with tissue. The energy reflected in backscatter is less than the direct or reflected beam, but may still have a damaging effect on staff and equipment if adequate safety precautions are not taken. The Nd:YAG and argon lasers are known to produce significant backscatter. The parts of the body at greatest risk are the eyes and skin.

The eye is extremely sensitive to laser radiation and can be permanently damaged from direct, diffuse or reflected beams. Even brief or partial exposures can instantaneously damage the cornea, lens or retina [1,3]. The extent of ocular damage is determined by the laser irradiance, exposure duration, and beam size. Infrared radiation is invisible, so it is possible for eye damage to occur without awareness that an exposure has occurred. Since the eye cannot detect the

Veterinary Anesthesia and Analgesia: The Fifth Edition of Lumb and Jones.
Edited by Kurt A. Grimm, Leigh A. Lamont, William J. Tranquilli, Stephen A. Greene and Sheilah A. Robertson.

Table 57.1 Most common surgical lasers used in veterinary medicine [1]. Common types of lasers used in veterinary procedures are listed along with their wavelengths and optical density number necessary for proper eye protection.

Laser type	Wavelength (nanometers)	Optical density number
Carbon dioxide	10 600	6+
Nd:YAG	1064	6
Ho:YAG	2100	4+
Diode laser	810, 980	5+
KTP	532	6+
Argon	488, 514	6+

Box 57.1 Guidelines for eye protection during laser use [1,3].

- ALWAYS wear appropriate protective eyewear (glasses or goggles) whenever lasers are in use.
- Prescription eyewear, sunglasses or contact lenses DO NOT protect eyes from laser beam.
- Wavelength number on protective eyewear should match laser being used.
- Optical density (OD) number on protective eyewear should match, or be greater than, manufacturer recommendations for laser in use.
- Eye protection should fit snugly around the nose and have side and top guards.
- NEVER look directly at the laser or into laser output port even when wearing eye protection.
- Protect glasses/goggles by returning them to their case or cover when not in use. Scratched, cracked, discolored, or loose lenses may allow injury to the eye.

invisible beam, it does not respond with a blink reflex or by averting the eye from the beam. Laser-induced eye injury can occur in one or both eyes, and may be temporary or permanent [3].

All persons within the operating area are at risk of eye injury so it is critical for the anesthesia provider to take precautions, and to be provided with protective eyewear (Box 57.1). Most regulatory jurisdictions, including the United States Occupational Safety and Health Administration (OSHA), require the use of eye protection for personnel in the presence of lasers that may result in eye injury [1]. Protective eyewear styles look similar but are not all the same. Selection is based on the particular type of laser in use and rated for the specified wavelength range. Eyewear is also rated for its optical density, which is its ability to reduce the beam power. The optical density protection level is unique to each laser (see Table 57.1) and will be recommended by the manufacturer in the laser operation manual. The wavelength and optical density for which the protective eyewear is rated can be found imprinted directly on the glasses (Fig. 57.1).

Eye protection is also important for the patient. Protect eyes from direct or scattered laser beam by making sure the eyelids are closed or protected by drapes. Pet eye protection goggles are available in a variety of sizes suitable for use with lasers classified OD 6+ and wavelength 800–1100 nm. Observe warning signs in areas where lasers are in use and do not enter without eye protection to prevent inadvertent exposure.

Skin damage from exposure to the direct laser beam is possible for personnel who are very close to the procedure site. The severity of skin damage depends on the total energy deposited and penetration depth of the laser beam. Injuries range from a mild erythematous reaction to a severe burn. Drapes are effective protection for patients and skin protection is usually not necessary for personnel

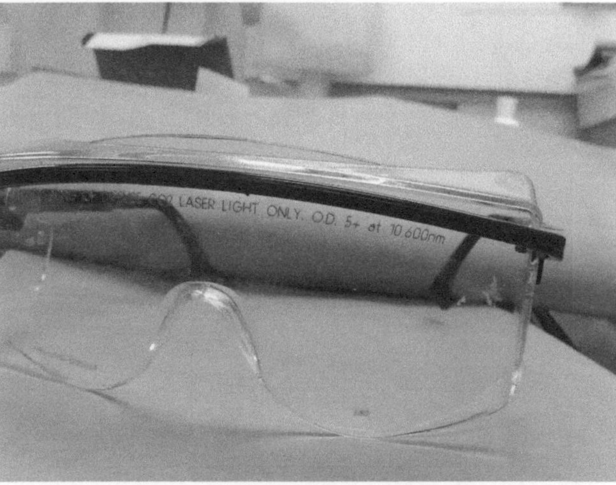

Figure 57.1 Protective eyewear performance characteristics will be recommended by the manufacturer in the laser operation manual. The wavelength and optical density for which the protective eyewear is rated can be found imprinted directly on the glasses. Image courtesy of Kendall Taney, with permission.

in the laser use area because the energy density decreases rapidly beyond the focal point [2,3].

Laser fire hazard and safety

The direct or reflected beam of a high-emission Class 3b or Class 4 laser can ignite combustible materials and is a fire risk. Devastating operating room fires and combustion of the endotracheal (ET) tube leading to fire in the trachea and lower airways have been reported in human medicine [7,8]. There is a single published report of a fire occurring during laser surgery in veterinary patients. It describes the ignition of the area around the face mask during inhalation anesthesia in two pet rodents, a mouse and a hamster, during cutaneous mass removal with diode laser. The fire resulted in life-threatening burns on the face, head, and upper body of both rodents; only one survived [9].

Anesthetic considerations for laser surgery

General anesthesia with inhalant anesthetics (e.g., isoflurane and sevoflurane) and high concentrations of oxygen are commonly used during laser procedures. Anesthesia may be delivered through an ET tube or by face mask, depending on the species and situation. Lasers are frequently utilized for procedures in the oral cavity and close to the airway in large and small veterinary patients where intubation is necessary to insure proper ventilatory support [10,11]. ET tubes made of polyvinyl chloride (PVC), red rubber, and silicone are combustible [7,12,13]. The intense heat of the laser can burn through the ET tube in seconds and cause a fire when the beam encounters the oxygen-enriched gas inside the tube [13]. Metal, copper-shielded and insulated ET tubes designed for use with laser procedures are commercially available. These tubes are expensive, bulky, and not universally safe for all types of lasers. Nor are they available in sizes suitable for horses or very small patients [7,14].

A standard red rubber ET tube, tightly wrapped with spirally overlapping loops of self-adhesive non-reflective aluminum or copper tape, has been evaluated and reported to be as safe or safer than the commercially available stainless steel or insulated ET tubes for use with CO_2 and Nd:YAG lasers [7,14–18]. the ET tube increases the external diameter and potentially makes the surface irritating to delicate tracheal tissue. Tape can also come loose from the wrapped tube during use. Carefully examine the ET tube following extubation to ensure that the tube and protective covering are completely intact [2,7,11,14,16].

A simple and effective method for protecting the ET tube from combustion is to cover it with a thick layer of saline-soaked sponges [7,19]. The sponges must remain moist throughout the procedure to dissipate the heat from any inadvertent exposure from the laser beam. A count of sponges before and after placement will ensure all sponges have been removed from the area of the airway.

The ET tube cuff and pilot tubing are also susceptible to damage by the laser [2,7]. Inadvertent deflation of the ET cuff will allow leakage of high oxygen concentration and anesthetic gases into the oral cavity and around the head of the patient. Fire may result if the enriched oxygen gas comes into contact with the laser beam and a flammable surface. Protecting the pilot tube with saline-soaked gauze sponges and using saline instead of air to fill the cuff can help dissipate heat and maintain patency of the cuff [2,7,19].

When using a face mask to deliver inhalant anesthesia in high concentrations of oxygen cannot be avoided, efforts should be made to fit the mask tightly around the face or head of the patient. Additionally, use of the lowest flow rates possible and a physical barrier to prevent oxygen-enriched gases from coming into contact with the laser beam can help reduce risk. The risk of fire hazard can also be minimized by choosing injectable anesthetic techniques, reducing oxygen concentrations or, in the case of laryngeal surgery, placing the ET tube nasotracheally or through a tracheostomy [2,10,11]. It may be necessary to remove the ET tube and oxygen source temporarily during a procedure to facilitate safe access to the laryngeal area.

To further reduce risk, the use of flammable prep solutions, drying agents, oil-based lubricants or ointments, or flammable plastics should be avoided whenever lasers are being used [2,7,20]. Box 57.2 lists the procedures to use if an airway or operating room fire occurs during laser surgery. Emergency procedures should be determined in advance and practiced by all potential participants.

Non-beam hazards and safety

Laser–tissue interactions produce a plume of smoke that may contain bacterial and viral particles as small as 0.1–0.3 microns and potentially toxic gases, some of which may be carcinogens. Bronchospasm from bronchial irritation, alveolar edema, interstitial pneumonia, and diffuse pulmonary atelectasis are potential consequences of inhaled laser smoke [2,3]. Air evacuation systems are used to remove laser-generated smoke and reduce pollution of the workspace. Laser-rated filtration surgical face masks are available for added protection. Standard surgical masks alone do not provide adequate protection during laser procedures [3]. Patients who are intubated and connected to an anesthesia machine are not at risk for inhaling the laser smoke. However, precautions should be taken for non-intubated patients to prevent inhalation exposure of smoke and potential pulmonary injury.

Box 57.2 Emergency procedures in the event of an airway or operating room fire during laser surgery [10,20].

1 ALERT the surgeon and other personnel of the fire. DISCONNECT the patient from the anesthesia circuit. TURN OFF the oxygen flow.
2 If the fire is in the airway/endotracheal (ET) tube:
 a remove the damaged ET tube
 b flush airway with saline or water
 c suction the airway to remove any debris
 d reintubate with a clean ET tube or maintain with a mask if feasible.
3 Support ventilation and treat symptomatically with oxygen, fluid support, anti-inflammatory administration, antibiotics and analgesics.
4 Determine extent of injury using bronchoscopy and/or radiographs.
5 If the fire does not involve the airway:
 a extinguish and remove all burning and flammable materials from the patient
 b provide adequate anesthesia and analgesia support while the burned area is irrigated and the condition of the patient and the full extent of the injury are evaluated.

Radiography

Plain radiography, contrast studies, fluoroscopy, computed tomography (CT), and radiation therapy (RT) all incorporate the use of ionizing radiation.

Ionizing radiation hazards and safety

Ionizing radiation exposure is potentially hazardous and causes injury at the cellular level by transferring high levels of energy into atoms and molecules such as DNA, RNA, and other cellular proteins. Energy transfer results in damage to chemical bonds and can create free radicals or ions [21–24]. If cellular damage is widespread and exceeds the body's ability to repair the cells, the resulting changes in structure and behavior of the damaged cells may result in adverse effects. Sensitivity to ionizing radiation is highest in the most actively replicating cells of the skin, bone marrow, small intestine, and reproductive cells. Developing embryos are particularly sensitive to the effects of ionizing radiation while slow-growing nerve and muscle cells are the most resistant to radiation damage [21–24].

Effects from the exposure to ionizing radiation may appear promptly or be delayed, depending on the type and duration of exposure. Effects resulting from chronic exposure to low levels of radiation are most relevant to veterinary anesthesia care providers. Chronic radiation exposure is associated with an increased incidence of cataracts, squamous cell carcinoma, leukemia, and premature aging [21–25].

Regulations require that personnel limit the level of radiation exposure to 'as low as reasonably achievable' or ALARA, an acronym coined by the Food and Drug Administration (FDA). ALARA can be achieved by increasing distance from the source, using shielding, and minimizing number of images and length of time of procedure.

The primary source of personnel occupational exposure is the x-rays that bounce off or scatter from objects in the path of the primary beam. The patient is the major source of scatter radiation. The amount of potential exposure from scatter radiation is directly related to the proximity of personnel to the source of the ionizing radiation and decreases rapidly with increased distance from the source. The best way to reduce exposure is to temporarily leave the radiology suite and view the sedated or anesthetized patient from the doorway or through leaded glass when the machine is in use. When leaving the room is not possible, standing at least 3 feet away from the patient during x-ray use and wearing a protective lead apron are advised [22,25].

An anesthesia provider may not be able to move away from the patient when involved with positioning patients for radiographs or during fluoroscopy and other special procedures. When this is the case, avoid direct beam exposure and avoid leaning over the patient during imaging. When in close proximity to the source of radiation, protective attire should include a lead apron, thyroid shield, and gloves. Consider wearing protective goggles if a lot of time is spent in the radiology suite. It is important to note that lead-lined protective apparel is not designed to provide protection from direct beam exposure [22].

The risk of potential radiation exposure is increased with CT and RT due to higher levels of radiation involved in the procedures. During these procedures, it is safest for the anesthetist to leave the patient and stand behind a portable barrier, move into the control room or leave the room altogether. Radiation exposure is cumulative so it is important to monitor radiation exposure by wearing a radiation exposure badge or dosimeter [22,23,25].

Anesthetic considerations for radiography

Radiology suites are rarely designed with anesthesia delivery in mind. Therefore, in order to provide optimal anesthesia support for every patient during radiology procedures, communication with the radiologist and other involved personnel is critical. It is important to understand the procedure being done, the contrast agents to be administered, and the estimated duration of the procedure.

Standard radiographs may be obtained easily with positioning devices without chemical restraint when the patient is co-operative. However, not all patients are co-operative and sedation allows good positioning and avoids the necessity of repeat x-ray exposure for patient and personnel. Procedures that take longer and may be invasive or painful, such as certain contrast studies and fluoroscopy, are best done using sedation or general anesthesia.

Computed tomography (CT) uses higher levels of radiation to obtain cross-sectional images and requires a motionless subject for best results. The imaging time varies depending on the type of CT being used (i.e., 1 slice/s versus 64 slice/s). While actual imaging time may be short, the time to position the patient and evaluate the study can be much longer. Patients experiencing pain may not want to lie still or allow positioning with just sedation. Even slight movement during the scan can result in motion artifacts that interfere with the quality of the images and diagnostic value. When this happens, the scan will have to be repeated, increasing overall anesthesia time and the amount of radiation exposure for the patient.

Radiation therapy (RT) uses a high dose of ionizing radiation delivered precisely by a direct beam into tumor tissue. The total treatment dose is divided into multiple sessions that are spread out over days or weeks. Patients must be motionless and positioned exactly the same for each treatment to limit damage to surrounding healthy tissue. A variety of devices are used to aid in positioning patients, depending on the location of the area being targeted. Certain positioning devices may interfere with anesthetic and monitoring equipment or influence placement of the IV catheter. Effective and safe anesthetic patient management depends on familiarity with the procedure and specific device being used. All personnel must leave the room during treatment for several minutes. Patients can be observed from outside the room using video camera(s), preferable with sound, positioned to provide a clear view of the monitor, the anesthesia machine, and the patient (Fig. 57.2). The treatment session can be paused if patient movement or problems are detected.

General anesthesia is recommended for horses and other large animals during selected radiographic studies and CT scanning to provide the necessary immobility to obtain diagnostic images quickly and safely by reducing scanning and anesthesia time. Inadequately immobilized large animals may cause damage to equipment or injury to themselves. Monitoring may consist of direct observation of respiratory rate and effort, evaluation of mucous membrane color, palpation of pulse quality and rate, and include the use of pulse oximetry and non-invasive blood pressure. Multiparameter monitors with easy-to-read screens, large numbers and visual alarms that can be easily seen in a dimly lit radiology suite from behind a screen or through an observation window may be helpful. There should be a source of oxygen available at all times. The anesthetist should be prepared to supplement sedation, intubate and support ventilation, induce general anesthesia, or perform rescue procedures when necessary.

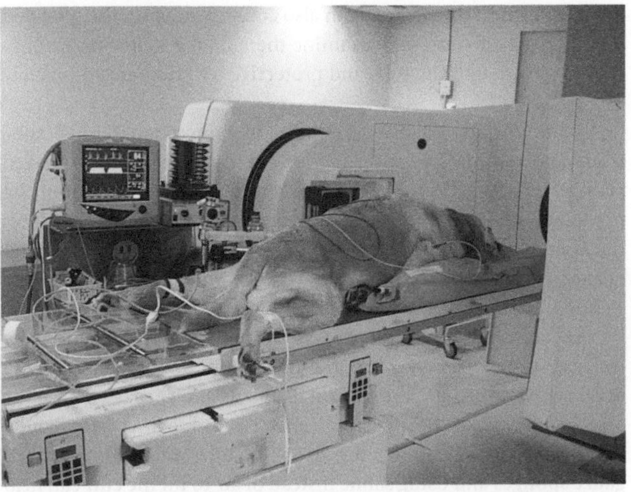

Figure 57.2 A dog undergoing radiation treatment for cancer. Note monitoring (ECG, SpO_2, $ETCO_2$, and body temperature) and supportive care (mechanical ventilation, emergency drugs, and fluids) are the same as for other anesthetic procedures. Image courtesy of Rebecca Acuña, VCA SouthPaws, Fairfax, VA 22031, with permission.

The radio-opaque stripe in most commonly used endotracheal tubes that allows visibility on radiographs causes an artifact on CT images, which may interfere with the diagnostic value of images of the neck and head (Fig. 57.3). ET tubes without the radio-opaque stripe are available and should be considered when the ET tube is in the area imaged.

During CT imaging, the presence of metal objects, such as electrocardiogram (ECG) clips and lead wires, in the scan field can lead to artifacts that can obscure or simulate pathology (see Fig. 57.3). If ECG leads need to be relocated, they can still provide rate and rhythm information when placed in non-standard sites such as paws, ears, and neck. It may be necessary to disconnect one of the ECG leads temporarily in order to avoid creating artifacts on the images.

During CT examination, the patient table will move in and out of the bore of the scanner. The anesthetist must make sure anesthesia delivery hoses are long enough to move with the patient during imaging without becoming kinked or disconnected. Monitoring cables and fluid administration lines are often positioned so that they will not get caught under the moving table or disconnected from the patient. Controlled ventilation is advisable for ensuring adequate ventilation and consistent anesthetic gas delivery during fluoroscopy, CT, and radiation therapy when the anesthetist leaves the room. Thoracic CT imaging, particularly the lungs, is best done immediately following induction. The patient is often kept in sternal recumbency to reduce positional atelectasis (personal correspondence, I Robertson, College of Veterinary Medicine, North Carolina State University).

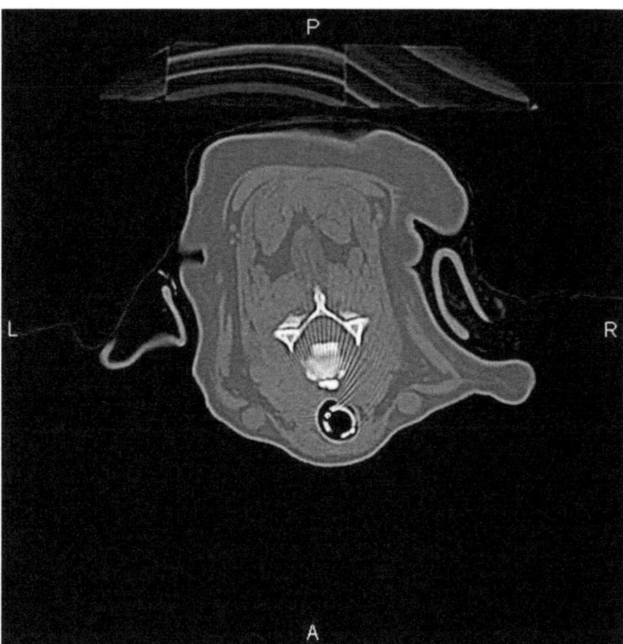

Figure 57.3 Computed tomography artifact created by the radio-opaque markers embedded in the wall of many common endotracheal tube models. The artifacts are the white lines radiating outward from the two markers embedded in the tube wall. Artifacts associated with anesthetic equipment may cause difficulty with obtaining optimal diagnostic images. ET tubes without the radio-opaque stripe are available and should be considered when the ET tube is located in the area being imaged.

Radiocontrast agents

Radiocontrast agents are used to improve the visibility of tissues during radiography and CT. The most common contrast agents used for radiographic procedures are compounds containing iodine or barium [26]. Barium compounds are used for gastrointestinal studies and are given orally. Barium studies do not usually require general anesthesia in companion animals, but it may be necessary for uncooperative, untamed or exotic species. Aspiration of barium can cause serious health effects ranging from pneumonia to acute death [26]. Prevention of barium aspiration is a critical part of anesthesia management during and after GI studies. An appropriately sized ET tube with inflated cuff and thorough inspection of the back of the mouth prior to extubation are important. When aspiration of barium is suspected, a chest radiograph will be able to verify barium in the lower airways and parenchyma.

Iodine-based solutions can be administered via oral, intravenous, intraluminal, or subarachnoid routes. Adverse effects are infrequent and depend on the site of administration and the type of contrast media used. Reactions are often related to the osmolality, molecular size, and complexity of the agent used. Effects range from minor physiologic alterations (e.g., mild hypertension) to bronchospasm, renal insufficiency, and life-threatening anaphylaxis [26].

Contrast-induced nephropathy (CIN) is a poorly understood pathology that is increasingly reported in diabetic people with pre-existing renal insufficiency given contrast agents [26,27]. Studies in dehydrated dogs have shown reduction in renal blood flow and glomerular filtration rate following parenteral administration of hypertonic contrast media. Prior to administration of contrast agents, it is prudent to evaluate renal and hydration status and correct hypotension if it exists (personal correspondence, I Robertson, College of Veterinary Medicine, North Carolina State University). Reduction in renal function due to contrast agents can usually be reversed with correction of hypotension and rapid rehydration [27].

Myelography is a contrast study of the subarachnoid space using radiography or CT scanning. It consists of injection of a water-soluble, non-ionic contrast medium in either the lumbar area or cerebello-medullary cistern. This is an invasive and noxious procedure so the patient must be adequately anesthetized prior to insertion of the needle and contrast injection. Patient movement can result in spinal cord damage or a non-diagnostic study. Adverse effects following subarachnoid injection depend on the agent selected, the site of administration, and needle placement and include tachycardia, bradycardia, vomiting, seizures, and cardiac arrest [28,29]. Postmyelographic adverse effects have become less frequent with the use of newer contrast agents.

Extravasation of contrast agents may lead to local tissue damage. The severity of the effects caused by perivascular injection depends on the osmolality of the contrast agent and the volume injected. They can range from mild swelling and erythema to ulceration and tissue necrosis [26,30–33]. Some radiographic studies require the rapid injection of the contrast agent by hand injection or via a rapid injector pump at flow rates of 0.5–5 ml/s. Large volumes of contrast can be injected perivascularly if the catheter is not properly placed. Box 57.3 lists steps to reduce the risk of extravasation and methods of treating accidental perivascular delivery.

> Box 57.3 Prevention and treatment of perivascular injection of radiocontrast agents [26,31–33].
>
> **Prevention**
>
> - Always inject contrast agents through an intravenous catheter.
> - Use largest bore catheter possible (>20 G is best).
> - Check catheter patency prior to injection.
> - Warm contrast media to decrease viscosity and resistance.
>
> **Treatment**
>
> - Early recognition of catheter failure is the best way to prevent serious side-effects.
> - Apply a cold compress to areas of perivascular injection.
> - Infiltrate area with saline to dilute radiocontrast agent and aid with absorption.
> - When large volume, hyaluronidase may be added to further increase absorption.
> - Provide symptomatic therapy.

Remote facilities

Advance planning for transportation to and from the imaging facility as well as consideration of monitoring and anesthesia maintenance during transfer are critical for patient safety. Emergency drugs and equipment should be available during transport and imaging.

Magnetic resonance imaging (MRI)

Magnetic resonance imaging (MRI) utilizes a powerful static magnetic field as well as several weaker, rapidly changing, gradient magnetic fields and high-frequency electromagnetic radiofrequency (RF) waves. Hazards include ferrometallic projectiles, high-level acoustic noise, and systemic and localized heating.

Strong static magnetic field

The main component of an MRI system is the magnet. MRI systems are classified by the basic shape (e.g., open or closed) and the way

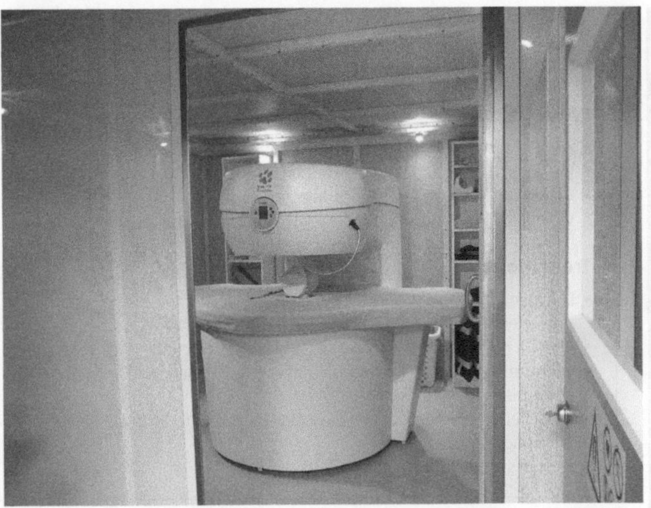

(a)

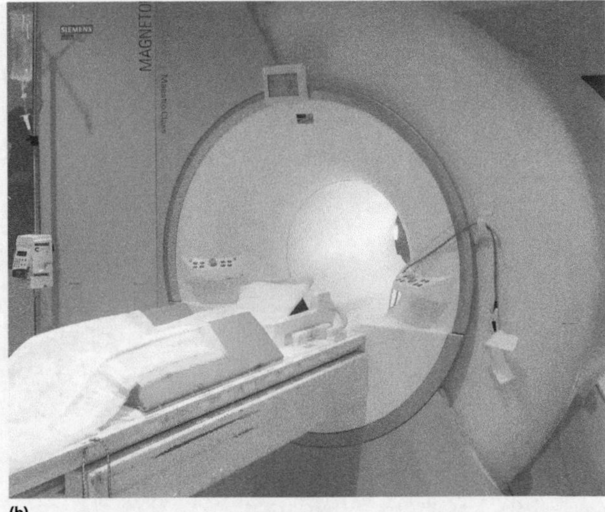

(b)

Figure 57.4 (a) An open magnetic resonance imaging machine. (b) A closed magnetic resonance imaging machine. Note the fiberoptic pulse oximeter cable/probe and the oscillometric blood pressure cuff and tubing located near the bore.

the magnetic field is generated (e.g., permanent magnet material or by currents in superconducting coils) [34]. The magnetic field strength is measured in tesla (T) units. Permanent magnets have low field strengths (less than 1.0 T) and an open configuration. Superconducting magnets have high field strengths and a closed cylindrical shape (Fig. 57.4). The clinically functional strengths are 1.0, 1.5, and 3.0 T. Stronger systems, 4.0, 7.0, and 9.4 T, are being evaluated for clinical and research use and their safety and health implications [34–42].

The magnetic field is always present (e.g., always on), extends outside the bore of the magnet in all directions and is one of the major hazards of the MR scanner. The extent of this 'fringe' or stray field depends on the strength and shielding of the magnet. The magnet vendor provides each facility with a map of the magnetic fields for onsite safety planning (Fig. 57.5). This magnetic field is weakest at the outside edge of the room and increases in strength as it approaches the scanner. It is critical to be familiar with the location of the 5 gauss line as the strength rises rapidly beyond this point, increasing the risk of projectile accidents and medical device malfunction. The 5 gauss line designates the perimeter of the MRI safety zone, inside which access is restricted to MRI safety-trained personnel, MRI safety-screened patients and MR designated safe or conditional devices (Box 57.4).

The closer a ferromagnetic object is to the magnet, the stronger the attraction, potentially causing it to become a projectile which can result in serious injury to anyone in the path. The 'missile' or projectile' effect is the most significant hazard to personnel and patients in a magnetic field environment. Large objects will be propelled faster and be more difficult to remove should they become attached to the scanner. Removal may require interruption of the magnetic field and lead to expensive restoration of the field, costly equipment damage, and loss of revenue [42–44]. In the bore of the magnet, where the magnetic field is the strongest, implanted, non-spherical, metallic objects, such as aneurysm clips, will torque or rotate as they attempt to align with the magnetic field. The induced rotation may cause the object to move in such a way as to tear vital structures [42–45]. Other implanted materials such as microchips, intravascular coils and stents, and vascular clamps can be safely imaged 6 weeks following placement once adequate scarring has occurred [42].

An individual is often exposed to static magnetic fields repeatedly for prolonged times. No substantial or harmful biologic effects have been reported in patients or MRI technologists following short-term exposures to static magnetic fields up to 9.4 T [42]. However, there are no current studies regarding prolonged, chronic exposure. The use of MRI during interventional procedures and surgery in humans is becoming more common, leading to increased exposure for the patient, anesthetist, surgeon, and other hospital personnel [46]. Until more evidence is available regarding long-term magnetic field exposure, it would seem prudent that all personnel try to limit their exposure.

Medical devices are tested and labeled safe, conditional or unsafe for use in a strong magnetic field using the American Society for Testing and Materials (ASTM) international classifications and icons [42]. Some common definitions include the following.

- *MRI safe.* Items made from materials considered safe in an MRI environment, such as glass, plastic, silicone, etc. and devices that have been tested and are considered safe for the patient,or the individuals working in specific MR environments.
- *MRI conditional.* Depending on the specific MR environment, objects may or may not be safe for the patient or personnel working with them. There are eight subcategories in this classification. MRI safety of a particular device or implant can be found at the manufacturer's website or from a list at www.mrisafety.com.
- *MRI unsafe.* Magnetic or metallic items known to pose human hazards in all MRI environments. There are two subcategories in this classification, depending on the type and degree of risk. It should be noted that the default magnetic field used to categorize devices is 1.5 T.

Gradient magnetic fields

Gradients (i.e., time varying magnetic fields) are created by weaker magnets located within the primary magnet. Gradients are switched on and off many times per second, producing variations in the magnetic field that allow image slices to be formed. Gradient switching induces electrical currents and conscious human patients have reported nerve stimulation or tingling during sequences using gradients. Safety standards have been installed in MR systems to protect patients from potential hazard

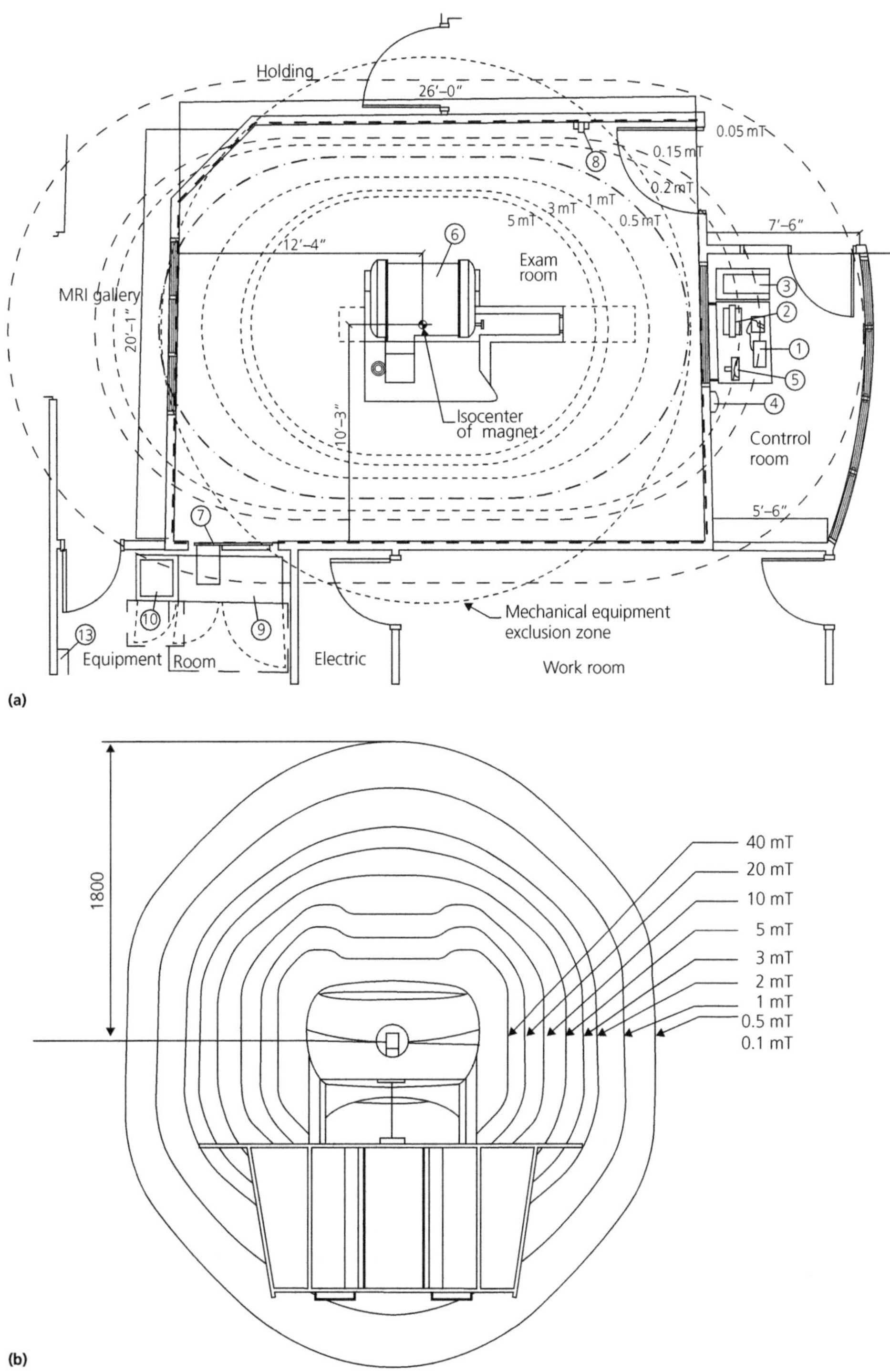

Figure 57.5 The magnetic field extends outside the bore of the magnet in all directions and is always present. The extent of this 'fringe' or stray field depends on the strength and shielding of the magnet. (a) A detailed map of the horizontal magnetic field strength diagrams the decrease in strength with increasing distance. Note the inclusion of a 'mechanical equipment exclusion zone.' (b) A diagram of varying magnetic field strength of an open magnetic resonance scanner.

or injury [42]. Gradient switching is also the source of the 'clanging' noise heard during MRI. The level of acoustic noise depends on the scan sequence and magnet strength. Noise levels range from 103–115 decibels (dB) for a 1.5 T magnet to 126–131 dB for a 3.0 T system [42,46]. The FDA and the International Electrotechnical Commission (IEC) limit permissible sound levels to 99 dB with hearing protection in place. The OSHA and the UK Department of Health recommend a maximum noise exposure of 85 dB over an 8 h period [42,47]. To prevent temporary or permanent hearing damage from exposure to high noise levels, always wear hearing protection in the MRI room during scanning. The best protection is provided by disposable or reusable ear plugs with a noise reduction rating (NRR) of 30–33 dB, or close-fitting headphones with NRR ratings of 20–30 dB. Optimal protection depends on how the

Box 57.4 Personnel, equipment, and patient screening guidelines for access to the MRI safety zone.

Personnel

- Inform ALL personnel that the **MAGNET IS ALWAYS ON.**
- Provide an MRI safety course for all anesthesia personnel. Make it mandatory and verify compliance.
- Restrict access to the MRI safety zone to individuals who have completed the MRI safety course.
- Be prepared for an anesthetic emergency and establish an emergency action plan – and practice it.
- Routinely update and review safety information and emergency procedures.
- Screen any personnel who will be providing patient care in the MRI suite for insulin pump, pacemaker, aneurysm clip, ocular metal, hearing aid, cochlear implant, metal piercings, recent surgery, etc.
- Pregnant personnel are not at risk in the MRI safety zone, but should not remain in the MRI room during imaging.
- Be vigilant to prevent any ferromagnetic objects from being inadvertently brought into the MRI safety zone (stethoscope, laryngoscope, medical instruments, clippers, oxygen tank, etc.).

Equipment

- Only equipment labeled conditional for the strength magnet in use should be taken into the MRI safety zone. Any other equipment must be tested and labeled as safe by the designated Safety Officer, MR technologist, and/or magnet engineer prior to entering the area.
- MRI-unsafe equipment located in close proximity to the MRI safety zone must be conspicuously labeled 'unsafe for MRI' to prevent inadvertent transfer into the scan room.
- Screen any equipment that leaves the MRI area when it returns, as ferromagnetic items may have been placed on it.
- Ferromagnetic devices used inside the MRI safety zone must be positioned outside the 5 gauss line and physically secured with plastic or rope ties, non-magnetic bolts, or a weighted base system. Conspicuously label the device 'unsafe for MRI' and mark the position of the 5 gauss line on the floor.

Patient

- Prior to entering the MRI safety zone, obtain a complete history and carefully screen patients for the presence of metal implants. Pacemakers, microchips, orthopedic implants, bullets or shrapnel, gold beads, ingested gravel or other metallic/magnetic substances in the gastrointestinal tract may pose a hazard for the patient or interfere with image acquisition.
- Remove collars, harnesses, halters, nose rings, hair clips, and any other items containing metal.
- Determine if the patient is ambulatory. Have a plan for getting large non-ambulatory patients into the facility/induction area.
- Transdermal patches (fentanyl and others) may contain aluminum that can heat up and cause skin irritation or burns. If the patch is located in the region being scanned, remove it prior to imaging.
- Have available a non-ferromagnetic gurney, stretcher, or table to transport heavy patients into the MRI safety zone.
- Carefully inspect any attached medical devices for metal parts or needles (urine collection systems, triple lumen catheters, infusion pumps, etc.).
- Remove towels, blankets and other items from around the patient before entering the MRI Safety zone. Ferromagnetic items may be hidden under blankets and become missiles when they get close to the magnet.

Equine checklist

- Remove shoes and clean all feet. Cover or wrap feet not being imaged.
- Verify region to be imaged. When imaging feet, radiograph before taking into the MRI safety zone to ensure that there are no metal pieces in the hoof.
- Review table orientation and pad configuration prior to anesthesia.
- Co-ordinate MRI safety trained personnel to assist with moving the patient into the MRI safety zone, to assist with positioning and later moving patient into recovery.
- Scan time should be as short as possible (i.e., not exceed 90 min).

ear plugs fit. Combining the ear plugs and the headphones will improve protection by 5–10 dB [42].

Hearing protection has not routinely been used for veterinary patients during MR imaging. The increased noise levels in the stronger magnets and extended scan times in clinical and research settings are reasons to consider using methods to reduce veterinary patient noise exposure [48]. Noise reduction may also allow lighter planes of anesthesia [49]. Interestingly, isoflurane anesthesia has a protective effect on noise-induced hearing loss in mice [50,51]. Testing the hearing of veterinary patients during and after MR imaging, and the effectiveness of protection devices during imaging, is problematic and there are currently no published studies on this subject. Hearing protection is commercially available for dogs and cats and has been tested to be safe during MRI [52].

Radiofrequency fields

Radiofrequency (RF) radiation is pulsed into tissue, eliciting the release of energy or a resonance signal which allows image construction. The majority of the RF energy is transformed into heat within the patient's tissues and can elevate body temperature [42,47], especially in large dogs and when scan times are long. The stronger the magnet, the more RF energy is required (3.0 T > 1.5 T). The specific absorption rate (SAR) of the RF radiation is measured throughout the scan to prevent systemic thermal overload. The SAR is strictly limited based on guidelines established by the FDA and limited by the MR scanner software. The SAR is calculated based on the weight of the patient. When potential overheating is detected, imaging will be interrupted by the system to allow more time between sequences and limit SAR [42,47].

The majority of MRI-related imaging injury reports in humans are related to RF burns resulting from the electrical currents induced in conductive materials (e.g., ECG cables) used during imaging. Cables placed against a patient's bare skin or looped to remove slack can create a voltage strong enough to cause tissue burning [42,53]. To reduce the risk of burns, all cables and wires should be straight and not looped. Cables should be run parallel to the bore of the magnet and insulated from areas of non-haired skin. Only MRI-conditional devices tested for the strength of magnet should be used.

The RF transmitter/receiver used to transfer energy into the tissue and capture the energy released from the tissue is called the RF coil. The most common types are body and local or surface coils. The body coil is part of the scanner and the surface soils are placed over or wrapped around the body part being scanned (Fig. 57.6). The resonance energy emitted from the patient is very weak and extraneous sources of RF noise cause artifacts and interfere with the acquisition of images. MRI suites are shielded from external sources of RF by copper sheeting in the walls or building a metal Faraday cage around the scanner (Fig. 57.7). Electrical devices produce RF signals and must be kept outside the 5 gauss line and the MRI room unless they are internally shielded and tested MRI safe or conditional. Waveguides that filter stray RF can be built into the shielding to allow the passage of plastic anesthetic delivery hoses and sampling tubing, fiberoptic pulse oximetry cables and non-conducting materials into the MRI room (see Fig. 57.7) [42–44].

Transdermal patches (e.g., fentanyl and some other agents) can contain aluminum or other metallic substances that could cause skin burns if exposed to an RF field. Second-degree burns have been reported in humans due to transdermal patches [42]. A warning about this hazard was issued by the FDA. Removal of the transdermal patch prior to imaging is recommended [54,55].

Cryogens

Superconducting high field strength magnets generate a large amount of energy and heat and must be encased in supercooled liquefied gas, usually liquid helium. If the system malfunctions and the temperature of the helium rises, enormous pressures can build up and cause an explosion called a boiling liquid expanding vapor explosion (BLEVE) or 'quench'. When this happens, the magnetic field is lost. MRI rooms are equipped with large vent pipes for the evacuation of the helium vapor if a quench occurs. A quench rarely happens spontaneously, but can be manually triggered in the event of a fire in the magnet room or other life-threatening situation requiring emergency termination of the magnetic field, such as a patient being crushed against the MRI scanner by a large ferromagnetic object [56].

If the vent pipe fails to contain the helium vapor, a cloud of vapor will enter the MRI room. This vapor is still very cold and can cause frostbite and asphyxiation due to displacement of oxygen in the room. In the event of a quench, the room should be evacuated immediately. The magnet could have a high voltage electrical charge and should not be touched. The patient should not be moved until the air in the room has returned to normal. Emergency and rescue personnel should not rush into the room as the magnetic field takes time to dissipate. Anesthesia providers should become familiar with and adhere to the quench protocol in place for the facility where they are working.

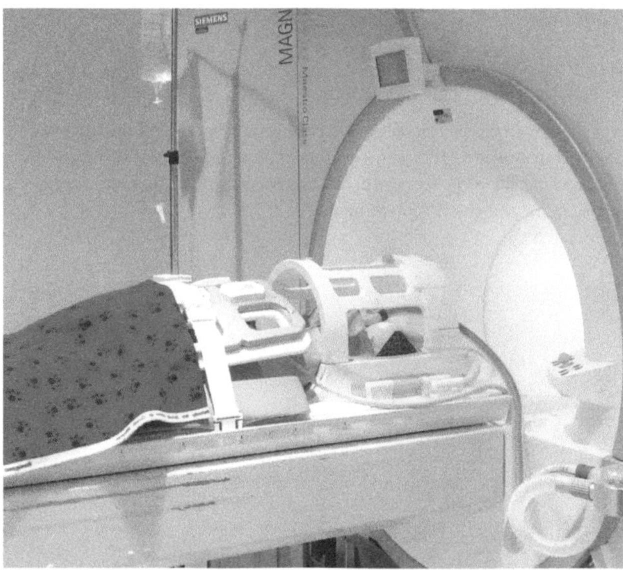

Figure 57.6 The radiofrequency coils placed near the body parts to be imaged create a 'cage' around the patient. Careful planning of the routes for breathing circuits, fluid lines, and monitoring leads can reduce artifacts and disruptions to the imaging sequences.

Anesthetic management considerations

For MR imaging, patients are placed on a long table, placed in devices to prevent motion, covered with RF coils and insulating blankets, and positioned in the center of the bore of the MRI scanner (see Fig. 57.6). Patients are difficult to visualize and access is limited, especially in smaller patients. The region being evaluated is imaged in different planes. Patients must remain in the exact same position for every sequence, otherwise the reconstruction of images will be suboptimal. Positioning devices, such as sandbags or foam cushions, are used to support the patient. These devices may interfere with monitoring or IV access so it is critical to be familiar with the scan being done and the equipment that will be used so that plans can be made for intravenous catheters and monitoring leads. Addition of extension lines and injection ports may be required for easy administration of fluids, contrast agents, and any other medications during scanning.

A light plane of anesthesia is usually adequate to prevent movement during the scan. Even small amounts of body motion due to

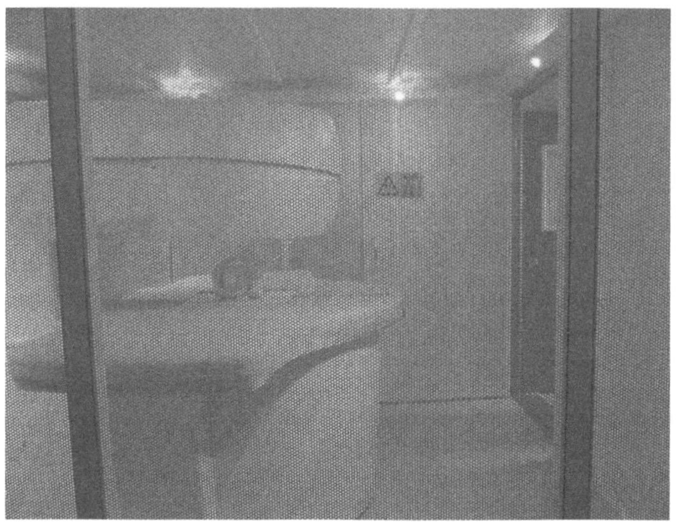

(a)

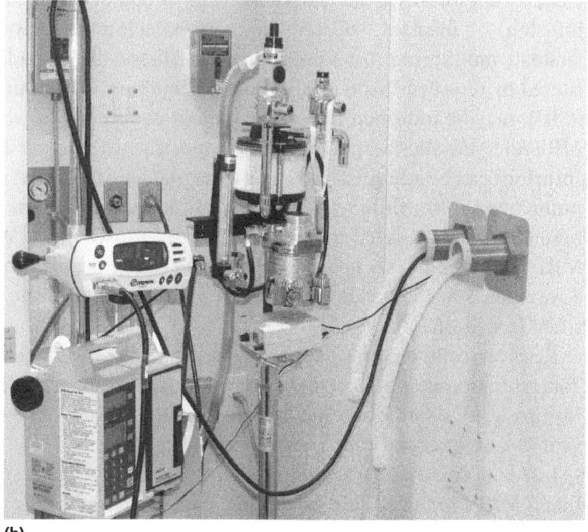

(b)

Figure 57.7 (a) A Faraday cage around the magnetic resonance imaging machine can reduce extraneous radiofrequency waves which may affect the image acquisition. (b) Waveguides that filter stray RF can be built into the shielding and walls to allow the passage of plastic anesthetic delivery hoses, monitoring leads, and other non-conducting materials into the MRI room. Note the magnetic resonance imaging machine is on the opposite side of the wall from the anesthetic equipment.

respiratory effort can interfere with some sequences. Controlled ventilation (manual or mechanical) can minimize motion.

A routine MRI scan can take 20–60 min depending on the strength of the magnet, the region being imaged, and the pathology discovered. Additional sedatives, anesthetic agents, support fluids, oxygen tanks, and other medications should be available. This is particularly critical when the MRI room is located outside the main anesthesia area. Large animal patients are often transported some distance from the induction area, and later back to the recovery area, so additional sedatives or injectable anesthetics may be required during transport.

Many patients needing an MRI are non-ambulatory and require transport to and from the MRI suite. The safest option is a magnet-safe gurney or stretcher. The MRI-safe gurneys designed for people may work well, especially for large breed dogs or other patients up to 150 kg in weight. Heavy patients can be transferred directly onto the MRI table, which aids in keeping them supported during repositioning and requires fewer personnel. Some magnets are equipped with a detachable table for transporting patients into and out of the room. Moving heavy, non-ambulatory patients into small MRI facilities, such as those located in trailers, requires additional personnel and an MRI-safe stretcher or other method.

Sedation versus general anesthesia

Monitoring is essential during scanning. Basic items to have available include additional endotracheal tubes, a self-inflating resuscitation bag, and an oxygen source. The oxygen source can be from piped-in oxygen and an MRI-safe anesthesia machine or a portable, magnetic field-compatible aluminum oxygen tank equipped with MRI-safe regulator and flowmeter assembly. Since many oxygen tanks look alike, conspicuously label all MRI-safe tanks to prevent a projectile accident. Mentally obtunded patients may require light (or no) sedation for short scans. Monitoring can be more challenging when the patient is not intubated or not anesthetized and the vibration and loud noises may cause unexpected arousal. It is recommended that someone stay in the room to visually monitor sedated patients during scanning in order to observe respirations and palpate pulses as electronic monitors may be unreliable. General anesthesia, either injectable (e.g., propofol or alfaxalone infusion) or inhalant, will provide more reliable immobility and facilitate monitoring. Total intravenous anesthesia (TIVA), administered by repeated IV bolus injections or continuous rate infusion (CRI), may be indicated for certain patient conditions or when a MRI-safe anesthesia machine and vaporizer is not available. Infusions can be administered using a magnet-safe fluid or syringe pump or an inline fluid regulator. Close monitoring of inline flow regulators is necessary to prevent fatal overdoses [57]. When MRI-safe equipment is not available, tubing can be passed through a waveguide to the patient from a pump located outside the MRI room (see Fig. 57.7).

Receiver coils plug into connections located in the MRI table. Take precautions to protect these connections from any organic fluids (urine, blood or feces) and leakage from the IV catheter to prevent short circuit and costly replacement (Fig. 57.8).

Inhalant anesthesia requires equipment and an oxygen source that is MRI conditional for the specific magnet strength being used. Oxygen can be piped into the room or MRI-safe aluminum tanks can be used. Incompatible anesthesia machines can be used outside the room with long hoses passed through waveguides (see Fig. 57.7) or, if used inside the MR room, positioned outside the 5 gauss line and secured to the wall or floor to prevent movement towards the magnet. Delivery hoses need to be long enough to reach the patient when they are moved inside the bore of the magnet and to accommodate any additional movement of the table. Coaxial delivery systems are commercially available up to 108 inches in length, or corrugated tubing can be cut to the desired length and attached to a Y-piece. Extra-long delivery hoses should be kept out of high traffic areas to prevent disconnection, kinking or obstruction of the tubing [57]. It should be remembered that the pilot tube of the ET tube contains a small amount of metal that will cause an artifact on the images if it is in the scan field (Fig. 57.9).

Ventilators can improve patient management and image quality by providing ventilatory support, a consistent plane of anesthesia, and control of respiratory motion. The ability to control ventilation

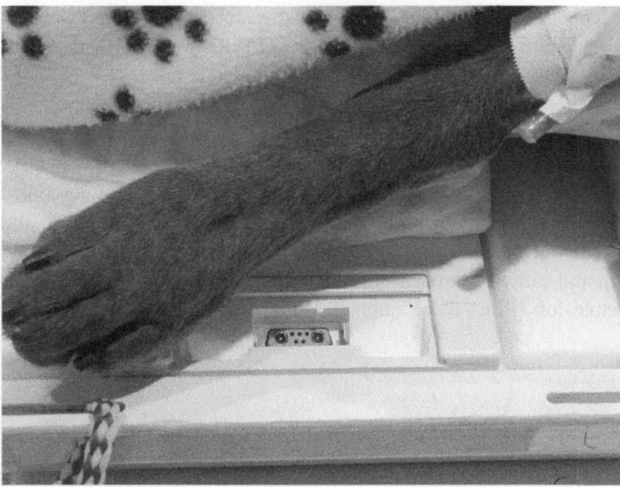

Figure 57.8 Receiver coils plug into connections located in the MRI table. Take precautions to protect these connections from any fluids (intravenous fluids, urine, blood or feces) and leakage from the IV catheter to prevent short circuit and costly replacement.

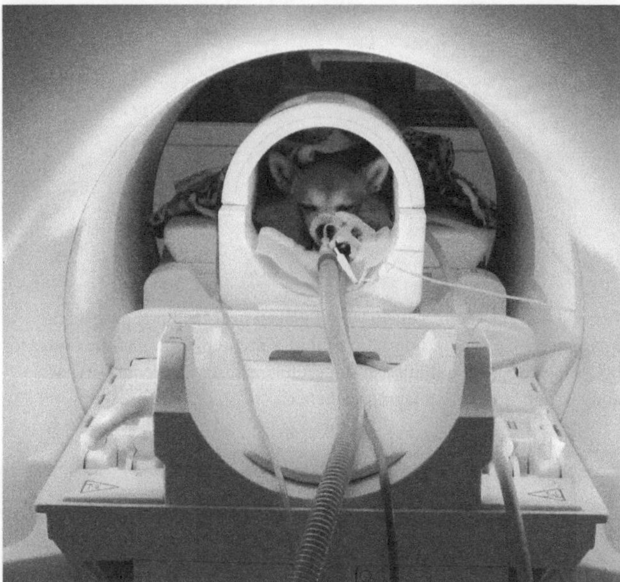

Figure 57.9 The pilot tube valve of the endotracheal tube often contains a small amount of metal that will cause an artifact on the images if it is near the body part being imaged.

is especially important for patients with pre-existing respiratory depression and those with suspected elevated intracranial pressure who require careful control of arterial carbon dioxide partial pressure.

Ideally, to prevent potential hazards, a MRI-compatible anesthesia machine should be dedicated for use in the MRI room and remain in the MRI safety zone at all times. Metallic objects or other MRI-unsafe items may be placed on anesthetic machines when out of the area and accidently be brought into the room when returned. An additional anesthesia machine, conspicuously labeled MRI unsafe, can be kept outside the MRI safety zone for induction, recovery, transport, and/or rescue procedures.

Patient monitoring

The patient monitoring in an MRI facility should be comparable to the surgical suite or any other area where general anesthesia is performed. However, most monitoring equipment and accessories are not designed for use in the MRI environment and the RF fields created can adversely affect their function. The dangers associated with using monitors and/or monitoring probes and cables not tested for use inside the 5 gauss line of the strength magnet being utilized include possible projectile hazard, patient burns, and degradation of MR images. Available MRI-safe monitors are designed for use with human patients, but are easily adaptable for use with most veterinary patients. Compared to standard monitoring systems, they are expensive. Increasing numbers of affordable, refurbished MRI-safe monitors are now available for purchase due to constant upgrading of such equipment in human facilities. It should not be assumed that a monitor safe for use with a 1.5 T magnet will be safe with a 3.0 T magnet. The anesthetist should check with the manufacturer before taking equipment into a new magnetic environment and be familiar with the location of the 5 gauss line.

Some MRI-safe monitoring systems are composed of a main monitor station with one or more wireless remote units so that anesthesia providers can monitor the patient when in the room as well as when outside the MRI room. If there is only one main monitor, the anesthetist may have to stay in the room for the entire procedure or the monitor can be positioned to be easily visualized through a window or door.

Gradient magnetic fields and radiofrequencies can interfere with the ECG, making it unreadable during many sequences. Newer MRI-safe monitoring systems have filters to help eliminate the interference. The appearance of the T wave or ST segment of the ECG complex may occur due to superimposed voltages generated by aortic flood flow in a magnetic field [56]. Newer monitors designed for MRI use have short wireless ECG cables to eliminate the hazard from looped or uninsulated wires and cables. Carbon graphite ECG electrodes and patches work best with direct skin contact so shaving is required in most patients. When a dysrhythmia is suspected, the scan can be stopped so that the rhythm can be evaluated.

Fiberoptic pulse oximetry is MRI safe and available in a variety of probe styles. The use of hard-wired pulse oximeters in the magnetic environment will result in unreliable readings, image degradation, and possibly patient burn injuries [47]. Capnography with side-stream sampling technology and extra-long sampling lines connected to a monitor inside or outside the magnet room is utilized during MR imaging. Direct and indirect arterial blood pressure monitoring can be used during MR imaging. Indirect oscillometric blood pressure is available on MRI-safe monitoring systems and the air-filled hoses are not hazardous. When monitoring arterial blood pressure directly using an arterial catheter and transducer, keep the transducer outside the bore of the magnet to reduce vibration interference.

Hypothermia is a concern as MRI rooms can be very cold. However, hyperthermia may also occur, especially in large, heavily coated dogs. There are no commercially available electrical warming systems specifically designed for use in an MRI room. Circulating hot water blankets have been used safely, but must be approved by the safety officer before they can be taken into the room. The water in the blanket will be visible on the scan if it is in the region being imaged. If this is a concern, the blanket can be removed for certain sequences. Body temperature fluctuations can be assessed during MRI using a digital thermometer, a fiberoptic temperature probe, or a modified standard esophageal temperature probe. Skin surface temperature technology is unreliable in both human and veterinary patients [42,58].

Gadolinium-based contrast agents (GBCA)

Gadolinium-based contrast agents (GBCA) are used to enhance the visibility of tissues for MRI studies. Gadolinium is a paramagnetic metal that is highly toxic in its natural state as it blocks physiologic pathways that rely on calcium. When gadolinium is chelated with a large organic molecule to form a stable complex, it is considered safe. The chelated compound has improved water solubility and is excreted predominantly unchanged by the kidneys [59]. The most common adverse effects observed in dogs and cats receiving a gadolinium chelate are bradycardia, tachycardia, hypotension, and hypertension [60–62]. Mild to severe anaphylactoid reactions have been reported in dogs. Dogs with a history of atopy may be more likely to have an adverse reaction [63]. An anaphylactoid reaction may be difficult to detect during MR imaging due to limited patient access and the effects of anesthesia.

After administration of a GBCA, closely monitor for any sudden changes in hemodynamic status or other signs of anaphylaxis. GBCA have been linked to a life-threatening skin disorder called nephrogenic systemic fibrosis (NSF) or nephrogenic fibrosing dermatopathy in humans. This condition has only been observed in individuals with severe renal failure or insufficiency with a GFR <15 mL/min [42]. It has not been reported in animals. GBCA are administered intravenously (IV), but have been given intramuscularly (IM) if IV access is unavailable.

Emergency procedures

Patients in the bore of the magnet are difficult to access during an emergency. An emergency plan specific to the facility being used should be determined in advance. Support staff and emergency personnel should not run into the MRI room in the case of an emergency. Designate an area outside the MRI safety zone where patient assessment and rescue procedures can be conducted. The designated area ideally should have an anesthesia machine, patient monitor, emergency drugs, additional IV catheters and fluids, ET tubes, laryngoscope, suction, and other relevant supplies.

Personnel considerations

Powerful, invisible hazards make working in an MRI environment extremely dangerous. Prior to entering the MRI area, personnel must be carefully screened and made familiar with the safety guidelines associated with working in an MRI environment, to prevent serious and life-threatening accidents.

References

1 OSHA Technical Manual (OTM), Section III, Chapter 6. www.osha.gov/dts/osta/otm/otm_iii/otm_iii_6.html (accessed 10 October 2014).

2 Hermens JM, Bennett MJ, Hirshman CA. Anesthesia for laser surgery. *Anesth Analg* 1983; **62**: 218–229.

3 *Lasers in Veterinary Practice: Safe Use Guidelines.* Version 2. Vancouver, BC: BC Centre for Disease Control, 2011.

4 *Laser Standards and Classifications.* Rockwell Laser Industries. www.rli.com/resources/articles/classification.aspx (accessed 10 October 2014).

5 American National Standards Institute (ANSI). *Safe Use of Lasers in Health Care.* ANSI Z136.3. Orlando, FL: Laser Institute of America, 2011.

6 Burns K. Laser guidelines encompass veterinarians. *JAVMA* 2012; **240**(7): 779.

7 Dorsch JA, Dorsch SE. Operating room fires and personnel injuries related to sources of ignition. In: Dorsch JA, Dorsch SE, eds. *Understanding Anesthesia Equipment*, 5th edn. Baltimore, MD: Lippincott, Williams and Wilkins, 2008; 907–928.

8 Stouffer DJ. Fires during surgery: two fatal incidents in Los Angeles. *J Burn Care Rehabil* 1992; **13**: 456–457.

9 Collarile T, DiGirolamo N, Nardini G, *et al.* Fire ignition during laser surgery in pet rodents. *BMC Vet Res* 2012; **8**: 177.

10 Driessen B, Zarucco L, Nann LE, *et al.* Hazards associated with laser surgery in the airway of the horse: implications for the anesthetic management. In: Steffey EP, ed. *Recent Advances in Anesthetic Management of Large Domestic Animals.* Ithaca, NY: International Veterinary Information Service, 2003. www.ivis.org.

11 Quandt JE. Airway management. In: Greene SA, ed. *Veterinary Anesthesia and Pain Management Secrets.* Philadelphia: Hanley and Belfus, 2002; 1–13.

12 Lai HC, Juang SE, Liu TJ, *et al.* Fires of endotracheal tubes of three different materials during carbon dioxide laser surgery. *Acta Anaesthesiol Sin* 2002; **40**(1): 47–51.

13 Steinberg TA. Combustion testing of non-metallic materials in ambient and oxygen-enriched atmospheres. In: Royals WT, Chou TC, Steinberg TA, eds. *Flammability and Sensitivity of Materials in Oxygen-Enriched Atmospheres*, vol. **8**. West Conshohocken, PA: American Society for Testing and Materials, 1997.

14 Dorsch JA, Dorsch SE. Tracheal tubes and associated equipment. In: Dorsch JA, Dorsch SE, eds. *Understanding Anesthesia Equipment*, 5th edn. Baltimore, MD: Lippincott, Williams and Wilkins, 2008; 561–628.

15 Mitchel B, Sosis MB. What is the safest endotracheal tube for Nd:YAG laser surgery? A comparative study. *Anesth Analg* 1989; **69**: 8024.

16 Sosis MB, Braverman B. Evaluation of foil coverings for protecting plastic endotracheal tubes from the potassium-titanyl-phosphate laser. *Anesth Analg* 1993; **77**(3): 589–591.

17 Mitchel B, Sosis MB, Braverman B, *et al.* Evaluation of a new laser-resistant fabric and copper foil-wrapped endotracheal tube. *Laryngoscope* 1996; **106**(7): 842–844.

18 Fried MP, Mallampati SR, Liu FC, *et al.* Laser resistant stainless steel endotracheal tube: experimental and clinical evaluation. *Lasers Surg Med* 1991; **11**(3): 301–306.

19 Sosis MB. Saline soaked pledgets prevent carbon dioxide laser-induced endotracheal tube cuff ignition. *J Clin Anesth* 1995; **7**(5): 395–397.

20 American Society of Anesthesiologists Task Force on Operating Room Fires. Practice advisory for the prevention and management of operating room fires. An updated report. *Anesthesiology* 2013; **118**(2): 271–290.

21 Committee to Assess Health Risks from Exposure to Low Levels of Ionizing Radiation. National Research Council. *Health Risks from Exposure to Low Levels of Ionizing Radiation.* Washington DC: National Academies Press, 2006.

22 California Veterinary Medical Board. *Radiation Safety Relating to Veterinary Medicine and Animal Health Technology in California.* Sacramento, CA: California Veterinary Medical Board, 2012.

23 *Radiation Protection Guidance for Hospital Staff.* Stanford, CA: Environmental Health and Safety, Stanford University, 2012.

24 Australian Radiation Protection and Nuclear Safety Agency. *Radiation Protection in Veterinary Medicine. Code of Practice and Safety Guide.* Radiation Protection Series No. 17. Yallambie, Australia: Australian Radiation Protection and Nuclear Safety Agency, 2009.

25 Marcus A. Glowing risk: anesthesiologists' exposure to radiation on the job. *Anesthesiol News* 2009; **35**(10): 1–5.

26 ACR Committee on Drugs and Contrast Media. *ACR Manual on Contrast Media*, Version 9. Reston, VA: American College of Radiology, 2013.

27 Katzberg RW. Contrast medium-induced nephrotoxicity: which pathway? *Radiology* 2005; **235**: 752–755.

28 Paithanpagare YM, Tank PH, Mankad MY, *et al.* Myelography in dogs. *Vet World* 2008; **1**(5): 152–154.

29 Roux FA, Deschamps JY. Inadvertent intrathecal administraton of ionic contrast medium to a dog. *Vet Radiol Ultrasound* 2007; **48**(5): 414–417.

30 Carroll GL, Keene BW, Forrest LJ. Asystole associated with iohexol myelography in a dog. *Vet Radiol Ultrasound* 1997; **38**(4): 284–287.

31 Belzunegui T, Louis CJ, Torrededia L, Oteiza J. Extravasation of radiographic contrast material and compartment syndrome in the hand: a case report. *Scand J Trauma Resus Emerg Med* 2011; **19**: 9.

32 Wang CL, Cohan RH, Ellis JH, *et al.* Frequency, management and outcome of extravasation of nonionic iodinated contrast medium in 69,657 intravenous injections. *Radiology* 2007; **243**(1): 80–87.

33 Miles SG, Rasmussen JF, Litwiller T, *et al.* Safe use of an intravenous power injector for CT: experience and protocol. *Radiology* 1990; **176**(1): 69–70.

34 Overweg J. *MRI Main Field Magnets.* Hamburg: Philips Research. http://afni.nimh.nih.gov/sscc/staff/rwcox/ISMRM_2006/ISMRM%20M-F%202006/files/TuA_08.pdf (accessed 10 October 2014).

35 Schenck JF, Dumoulin CL, Redington RW, *et al.* Human exposure to 4.0-Tesla magnetic fields in a whole-body scanner. *Med Phys* 1992; **19**(4): 1089–1098.

36 Theysohn JM, Maderwald S, Kraff O, *et al.* Subjective acceptance of 7 Tesla MRI for human imaging. *MAGMA* 2008; **21**(1-2): 63–72.

37 Van Nierop LE, Slottje P, Kingma H, *et al.* MRI-related static magnetic stray fields and postural body sway: a double-blind randomized crossover study. *Magn Reson Med* 2013; **70**(1): 232–240.

38 Van Nierop LE, Slottje P, van Zandvoort MJ, *et al.* Effects of magnetic stray fields from a 7 tesla MRI scanner on neurocognition: a double-blind randomised crossover study. *Occup Environ Med* 2012; **69**(10): 759–766.

39 Elbel GK, Kalisch R, Czisch M, *et al.* Design and importance of continuous physiologic monitoring for fMRI in rats at 7 T and first results with the novel anesthetic Sevoflurane. In: *Proceedings of the 8th International Society for Magnetic Resonance in Medicine* 2000; **2**: 928.

40 Elbel GL, Kalisch R, Schadrack J, *et al. Anesthesia and Monitoring for fMRI Experiments at 7T in Rats.* www.iars.org (accessed 10 October 2014).

41 Schmierer K, Parkes HG, So PW, *et al.* High field (9.4 Tesla) magnetic resonance imaging of cortical grey matter lesions in multiple sclerosis. *Brain* 2010; **133**: 858–867.

42 Shellock FG. *Reference Manual for Magnetic Resonance Safety, Implants, and Devices.* Los Angeles, CA: Biomedical Research Publishing Group, 2013.

43 Kanal E, Barkovich AJ, Bell C, *et al.* ACR guidance document on MR safe practices. *J Magn Reson Imag* 2013; **37**: 501–530.

44 Capizzani R. *Magnetic Resonance Imaging Hazards and Safety Guidelines.* Technical Advisory Bulletin, Strategic Outcomes Practice, 2009. www.koppdevelopment.com/articels/Willis%20MRI_Safety.pdf (accessed 10 October 2014).

45 Klucznik RP. Placement of a ferromagnetic intracerebral aneurysm clip in a magnetic field with a fatal outcome. *Radiology* 1993; **187**: 855–856.

46 Hattori Y, Fukatsu H, Ishigaki T. Measurement and evaluation of the acoustic noise of a 3 Tesla MR scanner. *Nagoya J Med Sci* 2007; **69**: 23–28.

47 Jerrolds J, Keene S. MRI-safety at 3T versus 1.5T. *Internet J Radiol* 2009; **11**(1). http://ispub.com/IJRA/11/1/10637 (accessed 10 October 2014).

48 Lauer AM, El-Sharkawy AM, Kraitchman DL, *et al.* MRI acoustic noise can harm experimental and companion animals. *J Magn Reson Imag* 2012; **36**(3): 743–747.

49 Oguriu M, Orhan ME, Cinar S, *et al.* Effect of headphones on sevoflurane requirement for MRI. *Pediatr Radiol* 2012; **42**: 1432–1436.

50 Chung JW, Ahn JH, Kim JY, *et al.* The effect of isoflurane, halothane and pentobarbital on noise-induced hearing loss in mice. *Anesth Analg* 2007; **6**: 1404–1408.

51 Kim JU, Lee HJ, Kang HH, *et al.* Protective effect of isoflurane anaesthesia on noise-induced hearing loss in mice. *Laryngoscope* 2005; **115**: 1996–1999.

52 Baker M. Evaluation of MR safety of a set of canine ear defenders (MuttMuffs®) at 1 T. *Radiography* 2013; **19**(4): 339–342.

53 Medical Device Safety Reports. Hazard, thermal injuries and patient monitoring during MRI studies. *Health Devices* 1991; **20**(9): 362–363.

54 Kuehn BM. FDA Warning: remove drug patches before mri to prevent burns to skin. *JAMA* 2009; **301**(13): 1328.

55 JAVMA News. Some metal-backed drug patches lack warning about MRI burn risk. *JAVMA* 2009; **235**: 16.

56 Menon DK, Peden CJ, Hall AS, *et al.* Magnetic resonance for the anaesthetist. Part I: physical principles, applications, safety aspects. *Anaesthesia* 1992; **47**: 240–255.

57 Kempen PM. Stand near by in the MRI. *ASPF Newsletter* 2005; **20**(2): 32–36.

58 Nasr VG, Schumann R, Bonney I, *et al.* Performance validation of a modified magnetic resonance imaging-compatible temperature probe in children. *Anesth Analg* 2012; **114**(6): 1230–1234.

59 Singer RM. *A Review of Gadolinium-Based Contrast Agents in Magnetic Resonance Imaging.* www.cewebsource.com/coursePDFs/ReviewGBCAsMRI.pdf (accessed 15 July 2013).

60 Pollard RE, Puchalski SM, Pascoe PJ. Hemodynamic and serum biochemical alterations associated with intravenous administration of three types of contrast media in anesthetized dogs. *AJVR* 2008; **69**(10): 1268–1273.

61 Pollard RE, Puchalski SM, Pascoe PJ. Hemodynamic and serum biochemical alterations associated with intravenous administration of three types of contrast medis in anesthetized cats. *AJVR* 2008; **69**(10): 1274–1278.

62 Mair AR, Woolley J, Martinez M. Cardiovascular effects of intravenous gadolinium administration to anaesthetized dogs undergoing magnetic resonance imaging. *Vet Anaesth Analg* 2010; **37**(4): 337–341.

63 Girard NM, Leece EA. Suspected anaphylactoid reaction following intravenous administration of a gadolinium-based contrast agent in three dogs undergoing magnetic resonance imaging. *Vet Anaesth Analg* 2010; **37**(4): 352–356.

Index

Page numbers in *italics* denote figures, those in **bold** denote tables.

Veterinary Anesthesia and Analgesia: The Fifth Edition of Lumb and Jones.
Edited by Kurt A. Grimm, Leigh A. Lamont, William J. Tranquilli, Stephen A. Greene and Sheilah A. Robertson.

Printed in the USA/Agawam, MA
January 5, 2021

767497.020

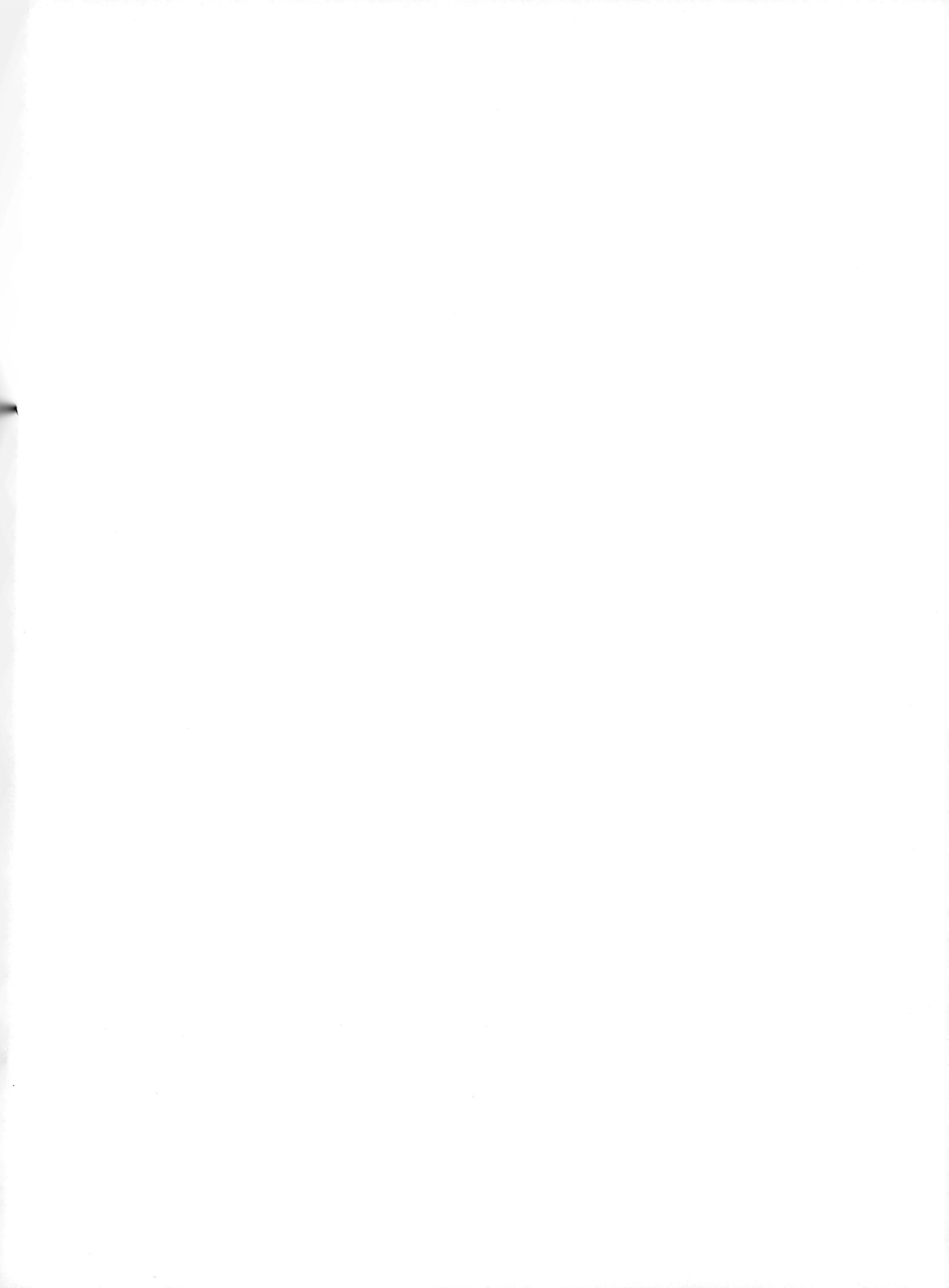